ICD·10·CM

International Classification of Diseases
10th Revision

Clinical Modification
Diagnosis Coding System

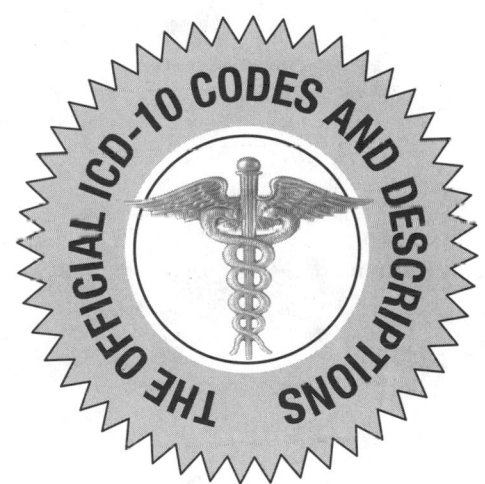

THE OFFICIAL ICD-10 CODES AND DESCRIPTIONS

2014

Transition & Training Edition

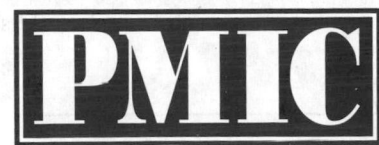

Volumes 1 & 2: Office, Hospital and Payer Edition

ISBN 978-1-939852-02-1 (Perfect bound)
ISBN 978-1-939852-05-2 (e-Book)

Volumes 1 & 2: Home Health Edition

ISBN 978-1-939852-34-2 (Perfect bound)
ISBN 978-1-939852-35-9 (e-Book)

Practice Management Information Corporation (PMIC)
4727 Wilshire Boulevard
Los Angeles, California 90010
http://www.pmiconline.com

Preface

On October 1, 2014 (subject to further delay by CMS) a key element of the data foundation of the United States' health care system will undergo a major transformation. We will transition from the decades-old Ninth Edition of the International Classification of Diseases (ICD-9) set of diagnosis and inpatient procedure codes to the far more contemporary, vastly larger, and much more detailed Tenth Edition of those code sets—or ICD-10—used by most developed countries throughout the world. This transition will have a major impact on anyone who uses health care information that contains a diagnosis and/or inpatient procedure code, including:

- Hospitals
- Health care practitioners and institutions
- Health insurers and other third-party payers
- Electronic-transaction clearinghouses
- Hardware and software manufacturers and vendors
- Billing and practice-management service providers
- Health care administrative and oversight agencies
- Public and private health care research institutions

All "covered entities"—as defined by the Health Insurance Portability and Accountability Act of 1996 (HIPAA)—are required to adopt ICD-10 codes for use in all HIPAA transactions with dates of service on or after the October 1, 2013 compliance date. for HIPAA inpatient claims, ICD-10 diagnosis and procedure codes are required for all inpatient stays with discharge dates on or after October 1, 2014 (or subsequently revised implementation date). Please note that the transition to ICD-10 does not directly affect provider use of the Current Procedural Terminology (CPT) and Healthcare Common Procedure Coding System (HCPCS) codes.

This edition of ICD-10-CM includes all official codes, descriptions and guidelines. A new edition is available approximately mid-September of each year. New editions may be purchased from:

Practice Management Information Corporation
4727 Wilshire Boulevard, Suite 300
Los Angeles, CA 90010
1-800-MED-SHOP
http://pmiconline.com

Disclaimer

This publication includes all official ICD-10-CM codes, descriptions, annotations and guidelines. This publication is revised annually so that we may present the most current information possible. Though all of the information is carefully researched and checked for accuracy and completeness, the publisher accepts no responsibility with regard to errors, omissions, misuse or misinterpretation.

Table of Contents

Introduction to ICD-10-CM

On October 1, 2014 (subject to further delay), the most significant change in medical coding requirements since the 1992 replacement of CPT visit codes with E & M codes will take place. On that date ICD-10 replaces ICD-9 as the mandated diagnosis coding system in the United States. All health insurance claims processed on or after October 1, 2014 must include ICD-10 codes. This change will have a tremendous impact on the health care industry.

- All health care providers must use ICD-10 instead of ICD-9 for new claims. All computer software that provides for storage of diagnosis codes must be revised to accommodate the additional digits of ICD-10 and maintain ICD-9 codes for previously filed claims.

- The conversion and implementation costs will be in the billions of dollars.

HISTORY OF THE INTERNATIONAL CLASSIFICATION OF DISEASES

For students of medical nomenclature and coding systems, the following history of the International Classification of Diseases excerpted from Wikipedia may be interesting.

HISTORICAL SYNOPSIS

In 1893, a French physician, Jacques Bertillon, introduced the *Bertillon Classification of Causes of Death* at a congress of the International Statistical Institute in Chicago. a number of countries and cities adopted Dr. Bertillon's system, which was based on the principle of distinguishing between general diseases and those localized to a particular organ or anatomical site, as used by the City of Paris for classifying deaths. Subsequent revisions represented a synthesis of English, German and Swiss classifications, expanding from the original 44 titles to 161 titles. in 1898, the American Public Health Association (APHA) recommended that the registrars of Canada, Mexico, and the United States also adopt it. The APHA also recommended revising the system every ten years to ensure the system remained current with medical practice advances. As a result, the first international conference to revise the International Classification of Causes of Death convened in 1900; with revisions occurring every ten years thereafter. At that time the classification system was contained in one book, which included an Alphabetic Index as well as a Tabular List. The book was small compared with current coding texts.

The revisions that followed contained minor changes, until the sixth revision of the classification system. with the sixth revision, the classification system expanded to two volumes. The sixth revision included morbidity and mortality conditions, and its title was modified to reflect the changes: *International Statistical Classification of Diseases, Injuries and Causes of Death (ICD)*. Prior to the sixth revision, responsibility for ICD revisions fell to the Mixed Commission, a group composed of representatives from the International Statistical Institute and the Health Organization of the League of Nations. in 1948, the World Health Organization (WHO) assumed responsibility for preparing and publishing the revisions to the ICD every ten years. WHO sponsored the seventh and eighth revisions in 1957 and 1968, respectively. It later become clear that the established ten-year interval between revisions was too short.

The ICD is currently the most widely used statistical classification system for diseases in the world. International health statistics using this system are available at the WHO Statistical Information System (WHOSIS). in addition, some countries—including Australia, Canada and the United States—have developed their own adaptations of ICD, with more procedure for classification of operative or diagnostic procedures.

HISTORY AND USAGE IN THE UNITED STATES

In the United States, the U.S. Public Health Service published the *International Classification of Diseases, Adapted for Indexing of Hospital Records and Operation Classification (ICDA)*, completed in 1962 and expanding the ICD-7 in a number of areas to more completely meet the indexing needs of hospitals. The U.S. Public Health Service later published the *Eighth Revision, International Classification of Diseases, Adapted for Use in the United States*, commonly referred to as ICDA-8, for official national morbidity and mortality statistics. This was followed by the *ICD, 9th Revision, Clinical Modification*, known as ICD-9-CM, published by the U.S. Department of Health and Human Services and used by hospitals and other healthcare facilities to better describe the clinical picture of the patient. The diagnosis component of ICD-9-CM is completely consistent with ICD-9 codes, and remains the data standard for reporting morbidity. National adaptations of the ICD-10 progressed to incorporate both clinical code (ICD-10-CM) and procedure code (ICD-10-PCS) with the revisions completed in 2003. in 2009, the U.S. Centers for Medicare and Medicaid Services announced that it would begin using ICD-10 on April 1, 2010, with full compliance by all involved parties by 2013.

BRIEF HISTORY OF ICD-10

ICD-10 was first published by the World Health Organization (WHO) in 1992. The National Center for Health Statistics (NCHS), the Federal agency responsible for use of the International Statistical Classification of Diseases and Related Health Problems, 10th revision (ICD-10) in the United States, has developed a clinical modification of the classification for morbidity purposes. The ICD-10 is used to code and classify mortality data from death certificates, having replaced ICD-9 for this purpose as of January 1, 1999. ICD-10-CM is planned as the replacement for ICD-9-CM, volumes 1 and 2. ICD-10-PCS is the replacement for ICD-9-CM volume 3, Procedures.

ICD-10-CM was developed following a thorough evaluation by a Technical Advisory Panel and extensive additional consultation with physician groups, clinical coders, and others to assure clinical accuracy and utility. Notable improvements in the content and format include: the addition of information relevant to ambulatory and managed care encounters; expanded injury codes; the creation of combination diagnosis/symptom codes to reduce the number of codes needed to fully describe a condition; the addition of a sixth character; incorporation of common 4th and 5th digit subclassifications; laterality; and greater specificity in code assignment. The new structure will allow further expansion than was possible with ICD-9-CM.

ICD-10 IS THE CHRONOLOGICAL SUCCESSOR TO ICD-9

The new classification system provides significant improvements through greater detailed information and the ability to expand in order to capture additional advancements in clinical medicine. ICD-10 consists of two different code sets:

- **ICD-10-CM** – the diagnosis classification system developed by the Centers for Disease Control and Prevention for use in all U.S. health care treatment settings. Diagnosis coding under this system uses 3–7 alpha and numeric digits and full code titles, but the format is very much the same as ICD-9-CM; and

- **ICD-10-PCS** – the procedure classification system developed by the Centers for Medicare & Medicaid Services (CMS) for use in the U.S. for inpatient hospital settings only. The new procedure coding system uses 7 alpha or numeric digits while the ICD-9-CM coding system uses 3 or 4 numeric digits.

The current system, International Classification of Diseases, 9th Edition, Clinical Modification (ICD-9-CM), does not provide the necessary detail for patients' medical conditions or the procedures and services performed on hospitalized patients. ICD-9-CM is 30 years old, has outdated and obsolete terminology, uses outdated codes that produce inaccurate and limited data, and is inconsistent with current medical practice. It cannot accurately describe the diagnoses and inpatient procedures of care delivered in the 21st century.

TERMINOLOGY

acute conditions	The medical conditions characterized by sudden onset, severe change, and/or short duration.
additional diagnosis	The secondary diagnosis code used, if available, to provide a more complete picture of the primary diagnosis.
alteration	Modifying the anatomic structure of a body part without affecting the function of the body part
applied mapping	Distillation of a reference mapping to conform to the needs of a particular application (e.g., data quality, research).
approach (5th character)	Defines the technique used to reach the site of the procedure.
backward mapping	mapping that proceeds from a newer code set to an older code set, for example from ICD-10-CM to ICD-9-CM.
bilateral	For bilateral sites, the final character of the codes in the ICD-10-CM indicates laterality. an unspecified side code is also provided should the side not be identified in the medical record. If no bilateral code is provided and the condition is bilateral, assign separate codes for both the left and right side.

body part or region (4th character)	Defines the specific anatomical site where the procedure is performed.
body system (2nd character)	Defines the general physiological system on which the procedure is performed or anatomical region where the procedure is performed.
bypass	Altering the route of passage of the contents of a tubular body part.
category	The three-digit diagnosis code classifications that broadly define each condition (e.g., 250 for diabetes mellitus).
Centers for Disease Control and Prevention (CDC)	A federal health data organization that helps maintain several code sets included in the HIPAA standards, including the ICD-9-CM codes. a division of the Department of Health and Human Services responsible for monitoring, researching and developing public health policies for the prevention of disease, injury and disability and the promotion of healthy behaviors. The National Center for Health Statistics is the part of the CDC that maintains health related statistics including the coordination with World Health Organization (WHO) on use of International Classification of Diseases (ICD) in North America.
Centers for Medicare & Medicaid Services (CMS)	The federal agency that runs the Medicare program. in addition, CMS works with the States to run the Medicaid program. CMS works to make sure that the beneficiaries in these programs are able to get high quality healthcare.
change	Taking out or off a device from a body part and putting back an identical or similar device in or on the same body part without cutting or puncturing the skin or a mucous membrane
character	One of the seven components that comprise an ICD-10-PCS procedure code.
chronic conditions	Medical conditions characterized by long duration, frequent recurrence over a long period of time, and/or slow progression over time.
cluster	in a combination entry, one instance where a code is chosen from each of the choice lists in the target system entry, that when combined satisfies the equivalent meaning of the corresponding code in the source system
combination codes	A single code used to classify any of the following: two diagnoses; a diagnosis with an associated secondary process (manifestation); or a diagnosis with an associated complication.
control	Stopping, or attempting to stop, postprocedural bleeding.
Conventions of ICD-10	The general rules for use of the classification independent of guidelines. These conventions are incorporated within the Index and Tabular of the ICD-10-CM as instructional notes.
creation	Making a new genital structure that does not take over the function of a body part.
crosswalk/mapping	A new test is determined to be similar to an existing test, multiple existing test codes, or a portion of an existing test code. The new test code is then assigned to the related existing local fee schedule amounts and resulting national limitation amount. in some instances, a test may only equate to a portion of a test, and, in those instances, payment at an appropriate percentage of the payment for the existing test is assigned.
Current Procedural Terminology (CPT) Codes	This is the procedural coding system that is currently used in America primarily to report physician professional services. Frequently called "CPT", the Current Procedural Terminology, is a code set, developed in 1966 and maintained by the American Medical Association (AMA), used to describe what healthcare professional services were provided or utilized by healthcare professionals. CPT codes are also known as "Level I" codes. Additional codes to describe use of healthcare facilities and services provided by healthcare professionals are known as "Level II" or "Healthcare Common Procedure Coding System" (HCPCS). Level II codes were developed are maintained by CMS.
destruction	Physical eradication of all or a portion of a body part by the direct use of energy, force or a destructive agent.
detachment	Cutting off all or a portion of the upper or lower extremities.

dilation	Expanding an orifice or the lumen of a tubular body part.
division	Cutting into a body part without draining fluids and/or gases from the body part in order to separate or transect a body part.
drainage	Taking or letting out fluids and/or gases from a body part.
excision	Cutting out or off, without replacement, a portion of a body part.
external (approach)	Procedures performed directly on the skin or mucous membrane and procedures performed indirectly by the application of external force through the skin or mucous membrane.
extirpation	Taking or cutting out solid matter from a body part.
extraction	Pulling or stripping out or off all or a portion of a body part by the use of force.
Federal Register	The "Federal Register" is the official daily publication for rules, proposed rules and notices of federal agencies and organizations, as well as Executive Orders and other Presidential documents.
forward mapping	mapping that proceeds from an older code set to a newer code set, for example from ICD-9-CM Volume 3 to ICD-10-PCS.
fragmentation	Breaking solid matter in a body part into pieces.
GEMs	This reference mapping attempts to include all valid relationships between the codes in the ICD-9-CM diagnosis classification and the ICD-10-CM diagnosis classification.
General Equivalence Map (GEM)	reference mapping that attempts to include all valid relationships between the codes in the ICD-9- CM diagnosis classification and the ICD-10-CM diagnosis classification
Health Insurance Portability & Accountability Act (HIPAA)	A law passed in 1996 which is also sometimes called the "Kassebaum-Kennedy" law. This law expands healthcare coverage for patients who have lost or changed jobs, or have pre-existing conditions. HIPAA does not replace the states' roles as primary regulators of insurance. The HIPAA legislation has the following broad goals, to provide: 1) a way to uniquely identify providers, employers and health plans, 2) a uniform level of protection of health information, known as the "Security Rule," 3) a uniform level of protection of the privacy of health data associated with patients, known as the "Privacy Rule" and 4) a simpler healthcare electronic transaction process by describing standards by which all healthcare administrative entities would use, which is known as the "Transactions and Code Sets Rule".
Healthcare Common Procedure Coding System (HCPCS)	A medical code set that identifies healthcare procedures, equipment, and supplies for claim submission purposes. It has been selected for use in the HIPAA transactions. HCPCS Level I contains numeric CPT codes which are maintained by the AMA. HCPCS Level II contains alphanumeric codes used to identify various items and services that are not included in the CPT medical code set. These are maintained by Health Care Financing Administration (HCFA), Blue Cross and Blue Shield Association (BCBSA), and the Health Insurance Association of America (HIAA). HCPCS Level III contains alphanumeric codes that are assigned by Medicaid state agencies to identify additional items and services not included in levels I or II. These are usually called "local codes", and must have "W", "X", "Y", or "Z" in the first position. HCPCS Procedure Modifier Codes can be used with all three levels, with the WA - ZY range used for locally assigned procedure modifiers.
HIPAA 4010	The original healthcare transactions version of HIPAA (officially known as Version 004010 of the ASC X12 transaction implementation guides) named as part of HIPAA's Electronic Transaction Standards regulation. Version 4010 was required to be used by HIPAA covered healthcare entities by Oct. 16, 2003.
HIPAA 5010	Required by Jan. 1, 2012 to be the new version of the HIPAA healthcare transactions. Officially known as Version 005010 of the ASC X12 transaction Technical Report Type 3. This new version was required as a result of Department of Health and Human Services (HHS) final rules published on Jan. 6, 2009.

ICD-10	The mortality and morbidity classification coding system implemented by WHO in 1993 to replace ICD-9.
ICD-10-CM	The updated version of the clinical modification coding set defined by the National Center for Health Statistics that will replace ICD-9-CM on Oct. 1, 2013.
ICD-10-PCS	The updated procedural coding system defined by CMS that will replace Volume 3 of ICD-9-CM for hospital inpatient services.
ICD-9	The mortality and morbidity classification coding system that is currently used throughout most of the world, including the United States. The ICD-9 classification of death and disease is based a series of classifications systems first adopted in 1893.
ICD-9-CM	The "clinical modification" to the ICD-9 code set that is currently used in America to report medical diagnoses. The "Clinical Modification" refers to the base WHO defined ICD-9 code set that has been defined for use in United State by the National Center for Health Statistics (NCHS) division of the Centers for Disease Control (CDC).
index (to diseases)	The ICD-10-CM is divided into the Alphabetic Index, an alphabetical list of terms and their corresponding code, and the Tabular List, a chronological list of codes divided into chapters based on body system or condition. The Alphabetic Index consists of the following parts: the Index of Diseases and Injury, the Index of External Causes of Injury, the Table of Neoplasms and the Table of Drugs and Chemicals.
insertion	Putting in a nonbiological device that monitors, assists, performs or prevents a physiological function but does not physically take the place of a body part.
inspection	Visually and/or manually exploring a body part.
International Classification of Diseases (ICD)	A medical code set maintained by the World Health Organization (WHO). The primary purpose of this code set is to classify both causes of death or mortality and diseases or morbidity. a U.S. extension, known as ICD-CM, "Clinical Modification," is maintained by the NCHS within the CDC to more precisely define ICD use in the U.S.
manifestation codes	Certain conditions have both an underlying etiology and multiple body system manifestations due to the underlying etiology. for such conditions, the ICD-10-CM has a coding convention that requires the underlying condition be sequenced first followed by the manifestation. Wherever such a combination exists, there is a "use additional code" note at the etiology code, and a "code first" note at the manifestation code. These instructional notes indicate the proper sequencing order of the codes, etiology followed by manifestation.
map	Locating the route of passage of electrical impulses and/or locating functional areas in a body part.
medical necessity	Services or supplies that: are proper and needed for the diagnosis or treatment of a medical condition; are provided for the diagnosis, direct care, and treatment of a medical condition; meet the standards of good medical practice in the local area; and are not mainly for the convenience of the patient or doctor.
morbidity	Term refers to the disease rate or number of cases of a particular disease in a given age range, gender, occupation, or other relevant population based grouping.
mortality	Term refers to the death rate reflected by the population in a given region, age range, or other relevant statistical grouping
National Center for Health Statistics (NCHS)	A federal organization within the CDC that collects, analyzes, and distributes healthcare statistics. The NCHS helps maintain the ICD-CM codes.
No Map Flag	attribute in a GEM that when turned on indicates that a code in the source system is not linked to any code in the target system .
occlusion	Completely closing an orifice or the lumen of a tubular body part.

open (approach)	Cutting through the skin or mucous membrane and any other body layers necessary to expose the site of the procedure.
percutaneous (approach)	Entry, by puncture or minor incision, of instrumentation through the skin or mucous membrane and any other body layers necessary to reach the site of the procedure.
percutaneous endoscopic (approach)	Entry, by puncture or minor incision, of instrumentation through the skin or mucous membrane and any other body layers necessary to reach and visualize the site of the procedure.
principle diagnosis	First-listed/primary diagnosis code. The code sequenced first on a medical record defines the primary reason for the encounter as determined at the end of the encounter.
procedure	The complete specification of the ICD-10-PCS seven characters.
reattachment	Putting back in or on all or a portion of a separated body part to its normal location or other suitable location.
release	Freeing a body part from an abnormal physical constraint by cutting or by use of force.
removal	Taking out or off a device from a body part.
repair	Restoring, to the extent possible, a body part to its normal anatomic structure and function.
replacement	Putting in or on biological or synthetic material that physically takes the place and/or function of all or a portion of a body part.
reposition	Moving to its normal location, or other suitable location, all or a portion of a body part.
resection	Cutting out or off, without replacement, all of a body part.
restriction	Partially closing an orifice or the lumen of a tubular body part.
reverse lookup	using a GEM by looking up a target system code to see all the codes in the source system that translate to it.
revision	Correcting, to the extent possible, a portion of a malfunctioning device or the position of a displaced device.
root operation/type (3rd character)	Defines the objective of the procedure.
section (1st character)	Defines the general type of procedure.
sequelae	A late effect is the residual effect (condition produced) after the acute phase of an illness or injury has terminated. There is no time limit on when a late effect code can be used. The residual may be apparent early, such as in cerebral infarction, or it may occur months or years later, such as that due to a previous injury.
signs/symptoms	Codes that describe symptoms and signs, as opposed to diagnoses, are acceptable for reporting purposes when a related definitive diagnosis has not been established (confirmed) by the provider.
source system	code set of origin in the mapping; the set being mapped 'from'
supplement	Putting in or on biological or synthetic material that physically reinforces and/or augments the function of a portion of a body part
Tabular List	It is essential to use both the Alphabetic Index and Tabular List when locating and assigning a code. The Alphabetic Index does not always provide the full code. Selection of the full code, including laterality and any applicable 7th character can only be done in the Tabular List. a dash (-) at the end of an Alphabetic Index entry indicates that additional characters are required. Even if a dash is not included at the Alphabetic Index entry, it is necessary to refer to the Tabular List to verify that no 7th character is required.
target system	destination code set in the mapping; the set being mapped 'to'.

transfer	Moving, without taking out, all or a portion of a body part to another location to take over the function of all or a portion of a body part.
transplantation	Putting in or on all or a portion of a living body part taken from another individual or animal to physically take the place and/or function of all or a portion of a similar body part.
Uniform Hospital Discharge Data Set (UHDDS)	The UHDDS definitions are used by hospitals to report inpatient data elements in a standardized manner. These data elements and their definitions can be found in the July 31, 1985, Federal Register (Vol. 50, No, 147), pp. 31038-40.
value	Individual units defined for each character of ICD-10-PCS and represented by a number or letter.
via natural or artificial opening (approach)	Entry of instrumentation through a natural or artificial external opening to reach the site of the procedure.
via natural or artificial opening endoscopic (approach)	Entry of instrumentation through a natural or artificial external opening to reach and visualize the site of the procedure.
via natural or artificial opening with percutaneous endoscopic assistance (approach)	Entry of instrumentation through a natural or artificial external opening and entry, by puncture or minor incision, of instrumentation through the skin or mucous membrane and any other body layers necessary to aid in the performance of the procedure.
Volume I	The detailed, tabular list of diagnosis codes in the ICD-9-CM manual.
Volume II	The alphabetical index to diseases in the ICD-9-CM diagnosis coding manual.
Volume III	The ICD-9/ICD-10 list of procedure codes, used in inpatient settings.
World Health Organization (WHO)	An organization that maintains the International Classification of Diseases (ICD) medical code set.

ICD-10-CM OVERVIEW

WHAT IS ICD-10-CM?

ICD-10-CM is an acronym for _**International Classification of Diseases, 10th Revision, Clinical Modification**_, published under different names since 1900. ICD-10-CM is a statistical classification system that arranges diseases and injuries into groups according to established criteria. Most ICD-9-CM codes are numeric and consist of three seven digits and a description. The codes are revised approximately every 10 years by the World Health Organization and annual updates are published by Center for Medicare and Medicaid Services (CMS).

KEY POINTS REGARDING ICD-10-CM

1. ICD-10-CM codes are three (3) to seven (7) digit alphanumeric codes.

2. ICD-10-CM codes describe illnesses, injuries, signs and symptoms, and procedures.

3. ICD-10-CM codes must be used on all health insurance claims as of October 1, 2014 (subject to extension by CMS).

4. Most ICD-10-CM codes have a specific definition; however, some ICD-10-CM codes have more than one definition.

5. Correct ICD-10-CM coding can make a significant difference in your reimbursement.

6. Accurate ICD-10-CM coding puts you in control of the reimbursement process.

STRUCTURE OF ICD-10-CM COMPARED TO ICD-9-CM

The easiest way to understand the structural difference between ICD-9-CM and ICD-10-CM is with a comparative visual representation of the two coding systems. The illustrations below clearly show the differences in structure and length.

STRUCTURE OF AN ICD-9-CM CODE

414.00   **Coronary atherosclerosis of unspecified type of vessel, native or graft**

Number or Letter (V/E)	Numbers Only			
1st Digit	2nd Digit	3rd Digit	4th Digit	5th Digit
4	**1**	**4 .**	**0**	**0**
Category			Etiology, anatomic site, manifestation	

Length: 3-5 digits

First character: Number or Letter (E or V)

Characters 2-5:   Numbers only

Minimum length: 3 characters

Decimal: After 3rd character

STRUCTURE OF AN ICD-10-CM CODE

S32.010A   **Wedge compression fracture of first lumbar vertebra, initial encounter for closed fracture**

Letter	Number or Letter					
1ST Digit	2nd Digit	3rd Digit	4th Digit	5th Digit	6th Digit	7th Digit
S	**3**	**2 .**	**0**	**1**	**0**	**A**
Category			Etiology, anatomic site, severity			Added code extensions for obstetrics, injuries and external causes of injury

Length: 3-7 digits

First character: Letter only (all letters except U are used)

Character 2:   Number only

Characters 3-7:   Numbers or letter

Decimal: After 3rd character

Placeholder: Use of "x" as a dummy placeholder

Letter format: Letters are case-sensitive

SIMILARITY OF ICD-10-CM TO ICD-9-CM

While there are more codes in the ICD-10-CM coding system than the ICD-9-CM coding system and the coding is a bit more complex, there are many similarities between the two systems. Experienced coders should be able to use the ICD-10-CM system relatively quickly due in part to these similarities.

1. Format – Both ICD-10-CM and ICD-9-CM have a Tabular List and Index.

2. Chapters in the ICD-10-CM Tabular list are structured similarly to ICD-9-CM, with minor exceptions.

    *   A few chapters have been restructured
    *   Sense organs (eye and ear) separated from Nervous System chapter and moved to their own Chapters

3. Index of ICD-10-CM is structured the same as ICD-9-CM.

    *   Alphabetic Index of Diseases and Injuries
    *   Alphabetic Index of External Causes
    *   Table of Neoplasms
    *   Table of Drugs and Chemicals

4. Divided into Alphabetic Index and Tabular List.

    *   Structure and format are the same
    *   Index is alphabetical list of terms and their corresponding codes

5. Alphabetic Index lists main terms in alphabetical order with indented subterms under main terms.

6. The Alphabetic Index is divided into 2 parts: Index to Diseases and Injuries and Index to External Causes.

7. The Tabular List is a chronological list of codes divided into chapters based on body system or condition.

8. The Tabular List is presented in code number order.

9. ICD-10-CM and ICD-9-CM have the same hierarchical structure.

10. Codes are invalid in both ICD-10-CM and ICD-9-CM if they are missing an applicable character.

11. ICD-10-CM and ICD-9-CM codes are looked up the same way.

    *   Look up diagnostic terms in Alphabetic Index
    *   Then verify code number in Tabular List

12. Many conventions have same meaning in ICD-10-CM and ICD-9-CM.

    *   Abbreviations, punctuation, symbols, notes such as "code first" and "use additional code"

13. Nonspecific codes ("unspecified" or "not otherwise specified") are available to use when detailed documentation to support more specific code is not available.

14. ICD-10-CM Official Guidelines for Coding and Reporting accompany and complement ICD-10-CM conventions and instructions.

15. Adherence to the official coding guidelines in all healthcare settings is required under the Health Insurance Portability and Accountability Act.

DIFFERENCES BETWEEN ICD-10-CM AND ICD-9-CM

While there are more similarities than differences between the ICD-10-CM and ICD-9-CM, the differences are significant. Understanding the differences will be the key to a successful transition to the new coding system.

1. All ICD-10-CM codes are alphanumeric (letter and numbers).

   - 1st character is always alpha and alpha characters may appear elsewhere in the code as well

2. ICD-10-CM codes can be up to 7 characters in length.

3. ICD-10-CM codes are more specific than ICD-9-CM codes.

4. ICD-10-CM code titles are more complete (no need to refer back to a category, subcategory, or subclassification level to determine complete meaning of code).

5. Laterality (side of the body affected) has been added to relevant ICD-10-CM codes.

6. ICD-10-CM features an expanded use of combination codes.

   - Certain conditions and associated common symptoms or manifestations
   - Poisonings and associated external cause

7. Injuries grouped by anatomical site rather than type of injury.

8. Codes reflect modern medicine and updated medical terminology.

9. Addition of 7th character

   - Used in certain chapters to provide information about the characteristic of the encounter
   - Must always be used in the 7th character position
   - If a code has an applicable 7th character, the code must be reported with an appropriate 7th character value in order to be valid

   Valid 7th Digit Character for Injuries and External Causes

   A Initial encounter
   D Subsequent encounter S Sequela

   Note: for aftercare of an injury, assign acute injury code with 7th character "D"

   Valid 7th Digit Character for Fractures

   A Initial encounter for closed fracture B Initial encounter for open fracture
   D Subsequent encounter for fracture with routine healing G Subsequent encounter for fracture with delayed healing
   K Subsequent encounter for fracture with nonunion
   P Subsequent encounter for fracture with malunion S Sequela

10. Addition of dummy placeholder "X" is used in certain codes to:

    - Allow for future expansion
    - Fill out empty characters when a code contains fewer than 6 characters and a 7th character applies

    When placeholder character applies, it must be used in order for the code to be considered valid.

11. ICD-10-CM includes two types of Excludes Notes.

- **Excludes 1 Note**

Indicates that code identified in the note and code where the note appears cannot be reported together because the 2 conditions cannot occur together.

Examples:

E10   Type 1 Diabetes mellitus

   Excludes 1: diabetes mellitus due to underlying condition (E08.-)
                    drug or chemical induced diabetes mellitus (E09.-)
                    gestational diabetes (O24.4-)
                    hyperglycemia NOS (R73.9)
                    neonatal diabetes mellitus (P70.2)
                    type 2 diabetes mellitus (E11.-)

M21   Other acquired deformities of limbs

   Excludes 1: acquired absence of limb (Z89.-)
                    congenital absence of limbs (Q71-Q73)

- **Excludes 2 Note**

Indicates that condition identified in the note is not part of the condition represented by the code where the note appears, so both codes may be reported together if the patient has both conditions.

Examples:

L89   Pressure ulcer

   Excludes 2: diabetic ulcers (E08.621, E08.622, E09.621, E09.622, E10.621, E10.622, E11.621, E11.622, E13.621, E13.622)
                    non-pressure chronic ulcer of skin (L97.-)
                    skin infections (L00-L08)
                    varicose ulcer (I83.0, I83.2)

I70.2   Atherosclerosis of native arteries of the extremities

   Excludes 2: atherosclerosis of bypass graft of extremities (I70.30-I70.79)

12. ICD-10-CM provides for increased specificity in comparison to ICD-9-CM.

   Examples

   S72.044G   Nondisplaced fracture of base of neck of right femur, subsequent encounter for closed fracture with delayed healing

   I69.351   Sequelae of cerebral infarction, Hemiplegia and hemiparesis following cerebral infarction affecting right dominant side

   Z47.81   Encounter for orthopedic aftercare following surgical amputation

   Z48.21   Encounter for aftercare following heart transplant

13. ICD-10-CM provides specific codes to identify laterality, i.e. left, right, unspecified. This applies to extremities as well as many organ systems; i.e. eyes, ears, shoulders, arms, hands, hips, legs, feet, lungs, kidneys, ovaries, testicles, etc.

Examples

C50.511   Malignant neoplasm of lower-outer quadrant of <u>right</u> female breast

C50.512   Malignant neoplasm of lower-outer quadrant of <u>left</u> female breast

C50.519   Malignant neoplasm of lower-outer quadrant of <u>unspecified</u> female breast

FORMAT OF ICD-10-CM

The Tabular List (Volume 1)

The ICD-10-CM Tabular List contains categories, subcategories and codes. Characters for categories, subcategories and codes may be either a letter or a number. All categories are 3 characters. a three-character category that has no further subdivision is equivalent to a code. Subcategories are either 4 or 5 characters. Codes may be 3, 4, 5, 6 or 7 characters. That is, each level of subdivision after a category is a subcategory. The final level of subdivision is a code. Codes that have applicable 7th characters are still referred to as codes, not subcategories. a code that has an applicable 7th character is considered invalid without the 7th character.

The Alphabetic Index (Volume 2)

The Alphabetic Index consists of the following parts: the Index of Diseases and Injury, the Index of External Causes of Injury, the Table of Neoplasms and the Table of Drugs and Chemicals.

CONVENTIONS USED IN THE TABULAR LIST

The ICD-10-CM Tabular List (Volume 1) makes use of certain abbreviations, punctuation, symbols, and other conventions that must be clearly understood. The purpose of these conventions is to provide special coding instructions and conserve space. Most of the conventions are defined in the ICD-10-CM Official Guidelines to Coding and Reporting following this chapter. There are sym

SYMBOLS AND COLOR CODING

All PMIC versions of ICD-10-CM include color-coding to alert the user to special coding situations or conditions that require additional attention. The use of color-coding is found in the Tabular List (Volume 1). The color is applied as solid rectangular bars over the codes only so that the descriptions remain clear and legible. The color codes and definitions are printed at the bottom of all right-sided pages of the Tabular List (Volume 1)

Color Coding

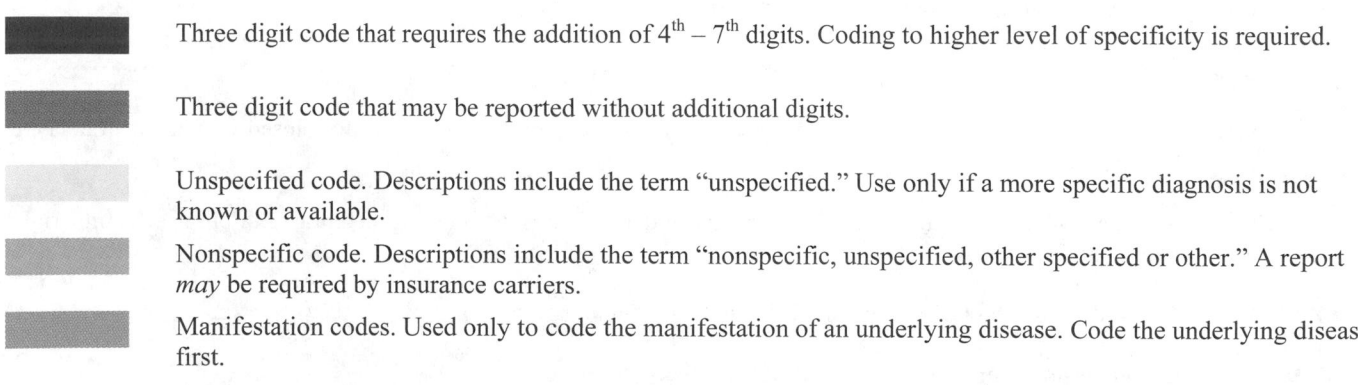

Three digit code that requires the addition of $4^{th} - 7^{th}$ digits. Coding to higher level of specificity is required.

Three digit code that may be reported without additional digits.

Unspecified code. Descriptions include the term "unspecified." Use only if a more specific diagnosis is not known or available.

Nonspecific code. Descriptions include the term "nonspecific, unspecified, other specified or other." A report *may* be required by insurance carriers.

Manifestation codes. Used only to code the manifestation of an underlying disease. Code the underlying disease first.

Symbols

- A filled BLACK CIRCLE preceding a code indicates that the code is new to this revision of ICD-9-CM. A symbol key appears on all left-hand pages of the Tabular List, Volume 1.

- ▲ A filled BLACK TRIANGLE preceding a code indicates that there is a revision to the text of an existing code. A symbol key appears on all left-hand pages of the Tabular List, Volume 1.

- ⑦ A red circle containing the number 7 preceding a code indicates that a seventh digit is required for coding to the highest level of specificity. The appropriate 7th character is to be added to each code from category. Definitions of valid seventh digits are found under the major category. If a code that requires a 7th character is not 6 characters, a placeholder X must be used to fill in the empty characters.

- ⊗ A red circle containing the letter P preceding a code indicates that a placeholder character "X" is required for the code to be complete. An example of this is at the poisoning, adverse effect and underdosing codes, categories T36-T50. Where a place holder exists, the X must be used in order for the code to be considered a valid code.

ICD-10-CM OFFICIAL GUIDELINES
FOR CODING AND REPORTING

The Centers for Medicare and Medicaid Services (CMS) and the National Center for Health Statistics (NCHS), two departments within the U.S. Federal Government's Department of Health and Human Services (DHHS) provide the following guidelines for coding and reporting using the International Classification of Diseases, 10th Revision, Clinical Modification (ICD-10-CM). These guidelines should be used as a companion document to the official version of the ICD-10-CM as published on the NCHS website. The ICD-10-CM is a morbidity classification published by the United States for classifying diagnoses and reason for visits in all health care settings. The ICD-10-CM is based on the ICD-10, the statistical classification of disease published by the World Health Organization (WHO).

These guidelines have been approved by the four organizations that make up the Cooperating Parties for the ICD-10-CM: the American Hospital Association (AHA), the American Health Information Management Association (AHIMA), CMS, and NCHS.

These guidelines are a set of rules that have been developed to accompany and complement the official conventions and instructions provided within the ICD-10-CM itself. The instructions and conventions of the classification take precedence over guidelines. These guidelines are based on the coding and sequencing instructions in the Tabular List and Alphabetic Index of ICD-10-CM, but provide additional instruction. Adherence to these guidelines when assigning ICD-10-CM diagnosis codes is required under the Health Insurance Portability and Accountability Act (HIPAA). The diagnosis codes (Tabular List and Alphabetic Index) have been adopted under HIPAA for all healthcare settings. A joint effort between the healthcare provider and the coder is essential to achieve complete and accurate documentation, code assignment, and reporting of diagnoses and procedures. These guidelines have been developed to assist both the healthcare provider and the coder in identifying those diagnoses that are to be reported. The importance of consistent, complete documentation in the medical record cannot be overemphasized. Without such documentation accurate coding cannot be achieved. The entire record should be reviewed to determine the specific reason for the encounter and the conditions treated.

The term encounter is used for all settings, including hospital admissions. In the context of these guidelines, the term provider is used throughout the guidelines to mean physician or any qualified health care practitioner who is legally accountable for establishing the patient's diagnosis. Only this set of guidelines, approved by the Cooperating Parties, is official.

The guidelines are organized into sections. Section I includes the structure and conventions of the classification and general guidelines that apply to the entire classification, and chapter-specific guidelines that correspond to the chapters as they are arranged in the classification. Section II includes guidelines for selection of principal diagnosis for non-outpatient settings. Section III includes guidelines for reporting additional diagnoses in non-outpatient settings. Section IV is for outpatient coding and reporting. It is necessary to review all sections of the guidelines to fully understand all of the rules and instructions needed to code properly.

SECTION I. CONVENTIONS, GENERAL CODING GUIDELINES AND CHAPTER SPECIFIC GUIDELINES

The conventions, general guidelines and chapter-specific guidelines are applicable to all health care settings unless otherwise indicated. The conventions and instructions of the classification take precedence over guidelines.

A. Conventions for the ICD-10-CM

The conventions for the ICD-10-CM are the general rules for use of the classification independent of the guidelines. These conventions are incorporated within the Alphabetic Index and Tabular List of the ICD-10-CM as instructional notes.

1. The Alphabetic Index and Tabular List

The ICD-10-CM is divided into the Alphabetic Index, an alphabetical list of terms and their corresponding code, and the Tabular List, a structured list of codes divided into chapters based on body system or condition. The Alphabetic Index consists of the following parts: the Index of Diseases and Injury, the Index of External Causes of Injury, the Table of Neoplasms and the Table of Drugs and Chemicals.

See Section I.C2. General guidelines
See Section I.C.19. Adverse effects, poisoning, underdosing and toxic effects

2. **Format and Structure:**

The ICD-10-CM Tabular List contains categories, subcategories and codes. Characters for categories, subcategories and codes may be either a letter or a number. All categories are 3 characters. A three-character category that has no further subdivision is equivalent to a code. Subcategories are either 4 or 5 characters. Codes may be 3, 4, 5, 6 or 7 characters. That is, each level of subdivision after a category is a subcategory. The final level of subdivision is a code. Codes that have applicable 7th characters are still referred to as codes, not subcategories. A code that has an applicable 7th character is considered invalid without the 7th character.

The ICD-10-CM uses an indented format for ease in reference.

3. **Use of codes for reporting purposes**

For reporting purposes only codes are permissible, not categories or subcategories, and any applicable 7th character is required.

4. **Placeholder character**

The ICD-10-CM utilizes a placeholder character "X". The "X" is used as a placeholder at certain codes to allow for future expansion. An example of this is at the poisoning, adverse effect and underdosing codes, categories T36-T50.

Where a placeholder exists, the X must be used in order for the code to be considered a valid code.

5. **7th Characters**

Certain ICD-10-CM categories have applicable 7th characters. The applicable 7th character is required for all codes within the category, or as the notes in the Tabular List instruct. The 7th character must always be the 7th character in the data field. If a code that requires a 7th character is not 6 characters, a placeholder X must be used to fill in the empty characters.

6. **Abbreviations**

   a. **Alphabetic Index abbreviations**

   NEC "Not elsewhere classifiable"

   This abbreviation in the Alphabetic Index represents "other specified". When a specific code is not available for a condition, the Alphabetic Index directs the coder to the "other specified" code in the Tabular List.

   NOS "Not otherwise specified"

   This abbreviation is the equivalent of unspecified.

   b. **Tabular List abbreviations**

   NEC   "Not elsewhere classifiable"

   This abbreviation in the Tabular List represents "other specified". When a specific code is not available for a condition the Tabular List includes an NEC entry under a code to identify the code as the "other specified" code.

   NOS "Not otherwise specified"

   This abbreviation is the equivalent of unspecified.

7. **Punctuation**

   [ ]   Brackets are used in the Tabular List to enclose synonyms, alternative wording or explanatory phrases. Brackets are used in the Alphabetic Index to identify manifestation codes.

( )   Parentheses are used in both the Alphabetic Index and Tabular List to enclose supplementary words that may be present or absent in the statement of a disease or procedure without affecting the code number to which it is assigned. The terms within the parentheses are referred to as nonessential modifiers. The nonessential modifiers in the Alphabetic Index to Diseases apply to subterms following a main term except when a nonessential modifier and a subentry are mutually exclusive, the subentry takes precedence. For example, in the ICD-10-CM Alphabetic Index under the main term Enteritis, "acute" is a nonessential modifier and "chronic" is a subentry. In this case, the nonessential modifier "acute" does not apply to the subentry "chronic".

:   Colons are used in the Tabular List after an incomplete term which needs one or more of the modifiers following the colon to make it assignable to a given category.

8. **Use of "and".**

   See Section I.A.14. Use of the term "And"

9. **Other and Unspecified codes**

   a. **"Other" codes**

   Codes titled "other" or "other specified" are for use when the information in the medical record provides detail for which a specific code does not exist. Alphabetic Index entries with NEC in the line designate "other" codes in the Tabular List. These Alphabetic Index entries represent specific disease entities for which no specific code exists so the term is included within an "other" code.

   b. **"Unspecified" codes**

   Codes titled "unspecified" are for use when the information in the medical record is insufficient to assign a more specific code. For those categories for which an unspecified code is not provided, the "other specified" code may represent both other and unspecified.

   See Section I.B.18 Use of Signs/Symptom/Unspecified Codes

10. **Includes Notes**

    This note appears immediately under a three character code title to further define, or give examples of, the content of the category.

11. **Inclusion terms**

    List of terms is included under some codes. These terms are the conditions for which that code is to be used. The terms may be synonyms of the code title, or, in the case of "other specified" codes, the terms are a list of the various conditions assigned to that code. The inclusion terms are not necessarily exhaustive. Additional terms found only in the Alphabetic Index may also be assigned to a code.

12. **Excludes Notes**

    The ICD-10-CM has two types of excludes notes. Each type of note has a different definition for use but they are all similar in that they indicate that codes excluded from each other are independent of each other.

    a. **Excludes 1**

    A type 1 Excludes note is a pure excludes note. It means "NOT CODED HERE!" An Excludes1 note indicates that the code excluded should never be used at the same time as the code above the Excludes1 note. An Excludes1 is used when two conditions cannot occur together, such as a congenital form versus an acquired form of the same condition.

    b. **Excludes 2**

    A type 2 Excludes note represents "Not included here". An excludes2 note indicates that the condition excluded is not part of the condition represented by the code, but a patient may have both conditions at the same time.

When an Excludes2 note appears under a code, it is acceptable to use both the code and the excluded code together, when appropriate.

13. Etiology/manifestation convention ("code first", "use additional code" and "in diseases classified elsewhere" notes)

Certain conditions have both an underlying etiology and multiple body system manifestations due to the underlying etiology. For such conditions, the ICD-10-CM has a coding convention that requires the underlying condition be sequenced first followed by the manifestation. Wherever such a combination exists, there is a "use additional code" note at the etiology code, and a "code first" note at the manifestation code. These instructional notes indicate the proper sequencing order of the codes, etiology followed by manifestation.

In most cases the manifestation codes will have in the code title, "in diseases classified elsewhere." Codes with this title are a component of the etiology/ manifestation convention. The code title indicates that it is a manifestation code. "In diseases classified elsewhere" codes are never permitted to be used as first-listed or principal diagnosis codes. They must be used in conjunction with an underlying condition code and they must be listed following the underlying condition. See category F02, Dementia in other diseases classified elsewhere, for an example of this convention.

There are manifestation codes that do not have "in diseases classified elsewhere" in the title. For such codes, there is a "use additional code" note at the etiology code and a "code first" note at the manifestation code and the rules for sequencing apply.

In addition to the notes in the Tabular List, these conditions also have a specific Alphabetic Index entry structure. In the Alphabetic Index both conditions are listed together with the etiology code first followed by the manifestation codes in brackets. The code in brackets is always to be sequenced second.

An example of the etiology/manifestation convention is dementia in Parkinson's disease. In the Alphabetic Index, code G20 is listed first, followed by code F02.80 or F02.81 in brackets. Code G20 represents the underlying etiology, Parkinson's disease, and must be sequenced first, whereas codes F02.80 and F02.81 represent the manifestation of dementia in diseases classified elsewhere, with or without behavioral disturbance.

"Code first" and "Use additional code" notes are also used as sequencing rules in the classification for certain codes that are not part of an etiology/ manifestation combination.

See Section I.B.7. Multiple coding for a single condition.

14. "And"

The word "and" should be interpreted to mean either "and" or "or" when it appears in a title.

For example, cases of "tuberculosis of bones", "tuberculosis of joints" and "tuberculosis of bones and joints" are classified to subcategory A18.0, Tuberculosis of bones and joints.

15. "With"

The word "with" should be interpreted to mean "associated with" or "due to" when it appears in a code title, the Alphabetic Index, or an instructional note in the Tabular List.

The word "with" in the Alphabetic Index is sequenced immediately following the main term, not in alphabetical order.

16. "See" and "See Also"

The "see" instruction following a main term in the Alphabetic Index indicates that another term should be referenced. It is necessary to go to the main term referenced with the "see" note to locate the correct code.

A "see also" instruction following a main term in the Alphabetic Index instructs that there is another main term that may also be referenced that may provide additional Alphabetic Index entries that may be useful. It is not necessary to follow the "see also" note when the original main term provides the necessary code.

17. "Code also note"

A "code also" note instructs that two codes may be required to fully describe a condition, but this note does not provide sequencing direction.

18. Default codes

A code listed next to a main term in the ICD-10-CM Alphabetic Index is referred to as a default code. The default code represents that condition that is most commonly associated with the main term, or is the unspecified code for the condition. If a condition is documented in a medical record (for example, appendicitis) without any additional information, such as acute or chronic, the default code should be assigned.

B. General Coding Guidelines

1. Locating a code in the ICD-10-CM

To select a code in the classification that corresponds to a diagnosis or reason for visit documented in a medical record, first locate the term in the Alphabetic Index, and then verify the code in the Tabular List. Read and be guided by instructional notations that appear in both the Alphabetic Index and the Tabular List.

It is essential to use both the Alphabetic Index and Tabular List when locating and assigning a code. The Alphabetic Index does not always provide the full code. Selection of the full code, including laterality and any applicable 7th character can only be done in the Tabular List. A dash (-) at the end of an Alphabetic Index entry indicates that additional characters are required. Even if a dash is not included at the Alphabetic Index entry, it is necessary to refer to the Tabular List to verify that no 7th character is required.

2. Level of Detail in Coding

Diagnosis codes are to be used and reported at their highest number of characters available.

ICD-10-CM diagnosis codes are composed of codes with 3, 4, 5, 6 or 7 characters. Codes with three characters are included in ICD-10-CM as the heading of a category of codes that may be further subdivided by the use of fourth and/or fifth characters and/or sixth characters, which provide greater detail.

A three-character code is to be used only if it is not further subdivided. A code is invalid if it has not been coded to the full number of characters required for that code, including the 7th character, if applicable.

3. Code or codes from A00.0 through T88.9, Z00-Z99.8

The appropriate code or codes from A00.0 through T88.9, Z00-Z99.8 must be used to identify diagnoses, symptoms, conditions, problems, complaints or other reason(s) for the encounter/visit.

4. Signs and symptoms

Codes that describe symptoms and signs, as opposed to diagnoses, are acceptable for reporting purposes when a related definitive diagnosis has not been established (confirmed) by the provider. Chapter 18 of ICD-10-CM, Symptoms, Signs, and Abnormal Clinical and Laboratory Findings, Not Elsewhere Classified (codes R00.0 - R99) contains many, but not all codes for symptoms.

See Section I.B.18 Use of Signs/Symptom/Unspecified Codes

5. Conditions that are an integral part of a disease process

Signs and symptoms that are associated routinely with a disease process should not be assigned as additional codes, unless otherwise instructed by the classification.

6. Conditions that are not an integral part of a disease process

Additional signs and symptoms that may not be associated routinely with a disease process should be coded when present.

7. **Multiple coding for a single condition**

In addition to the etiology/manifestation convention that requires two codes to fully describe a single condition that affects multiple body systems, there are other single conditions that also require more than one code. "Use additional code" notes are found in the Tabular List at codes that are not part of an etiology/manifestation pair where a secondary code is useful to fully describe a condition. The sequencing rule is the same as the etiology/manifestation pair, "use additional code" indicates that a secondary code should be added.

For example, for bacterial infections that are not included in chapter 1, a secondary code from category B95, Streptococcus, Staphylococcus, and Enterococcus, as the cause of diseases classified elsewhere, or B96, Other bacterial agents as the cause of diseases classified elsewhere, may be required to identify the bacterial organism causing the infection. A "use additional code" note will normally be found at the infectious disease code, indicating a need for the organism code to be added as a secondary code.

"Code first" notes are also under certain codes that are not specifically manifestation codes but may be due to an underlying cause. When there is a "code first" note and an underlying condition is present, the underlying condition should be sequenced first.

"Code, if applicable, any causal condition first", notes indicate that this code may be assigned as a principal diagnosis when the causal condition is unknown or not applicable. If a causal condition is known, then the code for that condition should be sequenced as the principal or first-listed diagnosis.

Multiple codes may be needed for sequela, complication codes and obstetric codes to more fully describe a condition. See the specific guidelines for these conditions for further instruction.

8. **Acute and Chronic Conditions**

If the same condition is described as both acute (subacute) and chronic, and separate subentries exist in the Alphabetic Index at the same indentation level, code both and sequence the acute (subacute) code first.

9. **Combination Code**

A combination code is a single code used to classify: Two diagnoses, or
A diagnosis with an associated secondary process (manifestation) A diagnosis with an associated complication

Combination codes are identified by referring to subterm entries in the Alphabetic Index and by reading the inclusion and exclusion notes in the Tabular List.

Assign only the combination code when that code fully identifies the diagnostic conditions involved or when the Alphabetic Index so directs. Multiple coding should not be used when the classification provides a combination code that clearly identifies all of the elements documented in the diagnosis. When the combination code lacks necessary specificity in describing the manifestation or complication, an additional code should be used as a secondary code.

10. **Sequela (Late Effects)**

A sequela is the residual effect (condition produced) after the acute phase of an illness or injury has terminated. There is no time limit on when a sequela code can be used. The residual may be apparent early, such as in cerebral infarction, or it may occur months or years later, such as that due to a previous injury. Coding of sequela generally requires two codes sequenced in the following order: The condition or nature of the sequela is sequenced first.

The sequela code is sequenced second.

An exception to the above guidelines are those instances where the code for the sequela is followed by a manifestation code identified in the Tabular List and title, or the sequela code has been expanded (at the fourth, fifth or sixth character levels) to include the manifestation(s). The code for the acute phase of an illness or injury that led to the sequela is never used with a code for the late effect.

See Section I.C.9. Sequelae of cerebrovascular disease
See Section I.C.15. Sequelae of complication of pregnancy, childbirth and the puerperium
See Section I.C.19. Application of 7th characters for Chapter 19

ICD-10-CM OFFICIAL GUIDELINES FOR CODING AND REPORTING

11. Impending or Threatened Condition

Code any condition described at the time of discharge as "impending" or "threatened" as follows:
If it did occur, code as confirmed diagnosis.
If it did not occur, reference the Alphabetic Index to determine if the condition has a subentry term for "impending" or "threatened" and also reference main term entries for "Impending" and for "Threatened."
If the subterms are listed, assign the given code.
If the subterms are not listed, code the existing underlying condition(s) and not the condition described as impending or threatened.

12. Reporting Same Diagnosis Code More than Once

Each unique ICD-10-CM diagnosis code may be reported only once for an encounter. This applies to bilateral conditions when there are no distinct codes identifying laterality or two different conditions classified to the same ICD-10-CM diagnosis code.

13. Laterality

Some ICD-10-CM codes indicate laterality, specifying whether the condition occurs on the left, right or is bilateral. If no bilateral code is provided and the condition is bilateral, assign separate codes for both the left and right side. If the side is not identified in the medical record, assign the code for the unspecified side.

14. Documentation for BMI, Non-pressure ulcers and Pressure Ulcer Stages

For the Body Mass Index (BMI), depth of non-pressure chronic ulcers and pressure ulcer stage codes, code assignment may be based on medical record documentation from clinicians who are not the patient's provider (i.e., physician or other qualified healthcare practitioner legally accountable for establishing the patient's diagnosis), since this information is typically documented by other clinicians involved in the care of the patient (e.g., a dietitian often documents the BMI and nurses often documents the pressure ulcer stages). However, the associated diagnosis (such as overweight, obesity, or pressure ulcer) must be documented by the patient's provider. If there is conflicting medical record documentation, either from the same clinician or different clinicians, the patient's attending provider should be queried for clarification.

The BMI codes should only be reported as secondary diagnoses. As with all other secondary diagnosis codes, the BMI codes should only be assigned when they meet the definition of a reportable additional diagnosis (see Section III, Reporting Additional Diagnoses).

15. Syndromes

Follow the Alphabetic Index guidance when coding syndromes. In the absence of Alphabetic Index guidance, assign codes for the documented manifestations of the syndrome. Additional codes for manifestations that are not an integral part of the disease process may also be assigned when the condition does not have a unique code.

16. Documentation of Complications of Care

Code assignment is based on the provider's documentation of the relationship between the condition and the care or procedure. The guideline extends to any complications of care, regardless of the chapter the code is located in. It is important to note that not all conditions that occur during or following medical care or surgery are classified as complications. There must be a cause-and-effect relationship between the care provided and the condition, and an indication in the documentation that it is a complication. Query the provider for clarification, if the complication is not clearly documented.

17. Borderline Diagnosis

If the provider documents a "borderline" diagnosis at the time of discharge, the diagnosis is coded as confirmed, unless the classification provides a specific entry (e.g., borderline diabetes). If a borderline condition has a specific index entry in ICD-10-CM, it should be coded as such. Since borderline conditions are not uncertain diagnoses, no distinction is made between the care setting (inpatient versus outpatient). Whenever the documentation is unclear regarding a borderline condition, coders are encouraged to query for clarification.

18. Use of Sign/Symptom/Unspecified Codes

Sign/symptom and "unspecified" codes have acceptable, even necessary, uses. While specific diagnosis codes should be reported when they are supported by the available medical record documentation and clinical knowledge of the patient's health condition, there are instances when signs/symptoms or unspecified codes are the best choices for accurately reflecting the healthcare encounter. Each healthcare encounter should be coded to the level of certainty known for that encounter.

If a definitive diagnosis has not been established by the end of the encounter, it is appropriate to report codes for sign(s) and/or symptom(s) in lieu of a definitive diagnosis. When sufficient clinical information isn't known or available about a particular health condition to assign a more specific code, it is acceptable to report the appropriate "unspecified" code (e.g., a diagnosis of pneumonia has been determined, but not the specific type). Unspecified codes should be reported when they are the codes that most accurately reflects what is known about the patient's condition at the time of that particular encounter. It would be inappropriate to select a specific code that is not supported by the medical record documentation or conduct medically unnecessary diagnostic testing in order to determine a more specific code.

C. Chapter-Specific Coding Guidelines

In addition to general coding guidelines, there are guidelines for specific diagnoses and/or conditions in the classification. Unless otherwise indicated, these guidelines apply to all health care settings. Please refer to Section II for guidelines on the selection of principal diagnosis.

1. Chapter 1: Certain Infectious and Parasitic Diseases (A00-B99)

a. Human Immunodeficiency Virus (HIV) Infections

1) Code only confirmed cases

Code only confirmed cases of HIV infection/illness. This is an exception to the hospital inpatient guideline Section II, H.

In this context, "confirmation" does not require documentation of positive serology or culture for HIV; the provider's diagnostic statement that the patient is HIV positive, or has an HIV-related illness is sufficient.

2) Selection and sequencing of HIV codes

(a) Patient admitted for HIV-related condition

If a patient is admitted for an HIV-related condition, the principal diagnosis should be B20, Human immunodeficiency virus [HIV] disease followed by additional diagnosis codes for all reported HIV-related conditions.

(b) Patient with HIV disease admitted for unrelated condition

If a patient with HIV disease is admitted for an unrelated condition (such as a traumatic injury), the code for the unrelated condition (e.g., the nature of injury code) should be the principal diagnosis. Other diagnoses would be B20 followed by additional diagnosis codes for all reported HIV-related conditions.

(c) Whether the patient is newly diagnosed

Whether the patient is newly diagnosed or has had previous admissions/encounters for HIV conditions is irrelevant to the sequencing decision.

(d) Asymptomatic human immunodeficiency virus

Z21, Asymptomatic human immunodeficiency virus [HIV] infection status, is to be applied when the patient without any documentation of symptoms is listed as being "HIV positive," "known HIV," "HIV test positive," or similar terminology. Do not use this code if the term "AIDS" is used or if the patient is treated for any HIV-related illness or is described as having any condition(s) resulting from his/her HIV positive status; use B20 in these cases.

(e) **Patients with inconclusive HIV serology**

Patients with inconclusive HIV serology, but no definitive diagnosis or manifestations of the illness, may be assigned code R75, Inconclusive laboratory evidence of human immunodeficiency virus [HIV].

(f) **Previously diagnosed HIV-related illness**

Patients with any known prior diagnosis of an HIV-related illness should be coded to B20. Once a patient has developed an HIV-related illness, the patient should always be assigned code B20 on every subsequent admission/encounter. Patients previously diagnosed with any HIV illness (B20) should never be assigned to R75 or Z21, Asymptomatic human immunodeficiency virus [HIV] infection status.

(g) **IIIV Infection in Pregnancy, Childbirth and the Puerperium**

During pregnancy, childbirth or the puerperium, a patient admitted (or presenting for a health care encounter) because of an HIV-related illness should receive a principal diagnosis code of O98.7-, Human immunodeficiency [HIV] disease complicating pregnancy, childbirth and the puerperium, followed by B20 and the code(s) for the HIV-related illness(es).

Codes from Chapter 15 always take sequencing priority.

Patients with asymptomatic HIV infection status admitted (or presenting for a health care encounter) during pregnancy, childbirth, or the puerperium should receive codes of O98.7- and Z21.

(h) **Encounters for testing for HIV**

If a patient is being seen to determine his/her HIV status, use code Z11.4, Encounter for screening for human immunodeficiency virus [HIV]. Use additional codes for any associated high risk behavior.

If a patient with signs or symptoms is being seen for HIV testing, code the signs and symptoms. An additional counseling code Z71.7, Human immunodeficiency virus [HIV] counseling, may be used if counseling is provided during the encounter for the test.

When a patient returns to be informed of his/her HIV test results and the test result is negative, use code Z71.7, Human immunodeficiency virus [HIV] counseling.

If the results are positive, see previous guidelines and assign codes as appropriate.

b. **Infectious agents as the cause of diseases classified to other chapters**

Certain infections are classified in chapters other than Chapter 1 and no organism is identified as part of the infection code. In these instances, it is necessary to use an additional code from Chapter 1 to identify the organism. A code from category B95, Streptococcus, Staphylococcus, and Enterococcus as the cause of diseases classified to other chapters, B96, Other bacterial agents as the cause of diseases classified to other chapters, or B97, Viral agents as the cause of diseases classified to other chapters, is to be used as an additional code to identify the organism. An instructional note will be found at the infection code advising that an additional organism code is required.

c. **Infections resistant to antibiotics**

Many bacterial infections are resistant to current antibiotics. It is necessary to identify all infections documented as antibiotic resistant. Assign a code from category Z16, Resistance to antimicrobial drugs, following the infection code only if the infection code does not identify drug resistance.

d. **Sepsis, Severe Sepsis, and Septic Shock**

1) **Coding of Sepsis and Severe Sepsis**

(a) **Sepsis**

For a diagnosis of sepsis, assign the appropriate code for the underlying systemic infection. If the type of infection or causal organism is not further specified, assign code A41.9, Sepsis, unspecified organism.

A code from subcategory R65.2, Severe sepsis, should not be assigned unless severe sepsis or an associated acute organ dysfunction is documented.

(i) Negative or inconclusive blood cultures and sepsis

Negative or inconclusive blood cultures do not preclude a diagnosis of sepsis in patients with clinical evidence of the condition, however, the provider should be queried.

(ii) Urosepsis

The term urosepsis is a nonspecific term. It is not to be considered synonymous with sepsis. It has no default code in the Alphabetic Index. Should a provider use this term, he/she must be queried for clarification.

(iii) Sepsis with organ dysfunction

If a patient has sepsis and associated acute organ dysfunction or multiple organ dysfunction (MOD), follow the instructions for coding severe sepsis.

(iv) Acute organ dysfunction that is not clearly associated with the sepsis

If a patient has sepsis and an acute organ dysfunction, but the medical record documentation indicates that the acute organ dysfunction is related to a medical condition other than the sepsis, do not assign a code from subcategory R65.2, Severe sepsis. An acute organ dysfunction must be associated with the sepsis in order to assign the severe sepsis code. If the documentation is not clear as to whether an acute organ dysfunction is related to the sepsis or another medical condition, query the provider.

(b) **Severe sepsis**

The coding of severe sepsis requires a minimum of 2 codes: first a code for the underlying systemic infection, followed by a code from subcategory R65.2, Severe sepsis. If the causal organism is not documented, assign code A41.9, Sepsis, unspecified organism, for the infection. Additional code(s) for the associated acute organ dysfunction are also required.

Due to the complex nature of severe sepsis, some cases may require querying the provider prior to assignment of the codes.

2) **Septic shock**

(a) Septic shock generally refers to circulatory failure associated with severe sepsis, and therefore, it represents a type of acute organ dysfunction.

For cases of septic shock, the code for the systemic infection should be sequenced first, followed by code R65.21, Severe sepsis with septic shock or code T81.12, Postprocedural septic shock. Any additional codes for the other acute organ dysfunctions should also be assigned. As noted in the sequencing instructions in the Tabular List, the code for septic shock cannot be assigned as a principal diagnosis.

3) **Sequencing of severe sepsis**

If severe sepsis is present on admission, and meets the definition of principal diagnosis, the underlying systemic infection should be assigned as principal diagnosis followed by the appropriate code from subcategory R65.2 as required by the sequencing rules in the Tabular List. A code from subcategory R65.2 can never be assigned as a principal diagnosis.

When severe sepsis develops during an encounter (it was not present on admission) the underlying systemic infection and the appropriate code from subcategory R65.2 should be assigned as secondary diagnoses.

Severe sepsis may be present on admission but the diagnosis may not be confirmed until sometime after admission. If the documentation is not clear whether severe sepsis was present on admission, the provider should be queried.

4) **Sepsis and severe sepsis with a localized infection**

If the reason for admission is both sepsis or severe sepsis and a localized infection, such as pneumonia or cellulitis, a code(s) for the underlying systemic infection should be assigned first and the code for the localized infection should be assigned as a secondary diagnosis. If the patient has severe sepsis, a code from subcategory R65.2 should also be assigned as a secondary diagnosis. If the patient is admitted with a localized infection, such as pneumonia, and sepsis/severe sepsis doesn't develop until after admission, the localized infection should be assigned first, followed by the appropriate sepsis/severe sepsis codes.

5) **Sepsis due to a postprocedural infection**

(a) **Documentation of causal relationship**

As with all postprocedural complications, code assignment is based on the provider's documentation of the relationship between the infection and the procedure.

(b) **Sepsis due to a postprocedural infection**

For such cases, the postprocedural infection code, such as, T80.2, Infections following infusion, transfusion, and therapeutic injection, T81.4, Infection following a procedure, T88.0, Infection following immunization, or O86.0, Infection of obstetric surgical wound, should be coded first, followed by the code for the specific infection. If the patient has severe sepsis the appropriate code from subcategory R65.2 should also be assigned with the additional code(s) for any acute organ dysfunction.

(c) **Postprocedural infection and postprocedural septic shock**

In cases where a postprocedural infection has occurred and has resulted in severe sepsis and postprocedural septic shock, the code for the precipitating complication such as code T81.4, Infection following a procedure, or O86.0, Infection of obstetrical surgical wound should be coded first followed by code R65.21, Severe sepsis with septic shock and a code for the systemic infection.

6) **Sepsis and severe sepsis associated with a noninfectious process (condition)**

In some cases a noninfectious process (condition), such as trauma, may lead to an infection which can result in sepsis or severe sepsis. If sepsis or severe sepsis is documented as associated with a noninfectious condition, such as a burn or serious injury, and this condition meets the definition for principal diagnosis, the code for the noninfectious condition should be sequenced first, followed by the code for the resulting infection. If severe sepsis, is present a code from subcategory R65.2 should also be assigned with any associated organ dysfunction(s) codes. It is not necessary to assign a code from subcategory R65.1, Systemic inflammatory response syndrome (SIRS) of non-infectious origin, for these cases.

If the infection meets the definition of principal diagnosis it should be sequenced before the non-infectious condition. When both the associated non-infectious condition and the infection meet the definition of principal diagnosis either may be assigned as principal diagnosis.

Only one code from category R65, Symptoms and signs specifically associated with systemic inflammation and infection, should be assigned. Therefore, when a non-infectious condition leads to an infection resulting in severe sepsis, assign the appropriate code from subcategory R65.2, Severe sepsis. Do not additionally assign a code from subcategory R65.1, Systemic inflammatory response syndrome (SIRS) of non-infectious origin.

See Section I.C.18. SIRS due to non-infectious process

7) **Sepsis and septic shock complicating abortion, pregnancy, childbirth, and the puerperium**

See Section I.C.15. Sepsis and septic shock complicating abortion, pregnancy, childbirth and the puerperium

8) **Newborn sepsis**

See Section I.C.16. f. Bacterial sepsis of Newborn

e. **Methicillin Resistant *Staphylococcus aureus* (MRSA) Conditions**

1) **Selection and sequencing of MRSA codes**

   (a) **Combination codes for MRSA infection**

When a patient is diagnosed with an infection that is due to methicillin resistant *Staphylococcus aureus* (MRSA), and that infection has a combination code that includes the causal organism (e.g., sepsis, pneumonia) assign the appropriate combination code for the condition (e.g., code A41.02, Sepsis due to Methicillin resistant Staphylococcus aureus or code J15.212, Pneumonia due to Methicillin resistant Staphylococcus aureus). Do not assign code B95.62, Methicillin resistant Staphylococcus aureus infection as the cause of diseases classified elsewhere, as an additional code because the combination code includes the type of infection and the MRSA organism. Do not assign a code from subcategory Z16.11, Resistance to penicillins, as an additional diagnosis.

See Section C.1. for instructions on coding and sequencing of sepsis and severe sepsis.

   (b) **Other codes for MRSA infection**

When there is documentation of a current infection (e.g., wound infection, stitch abscess, urinary tract infection) due to MRSA, and that infection does not have a combination code that includes the causal organism, assign the appropriate code to identify the condition along with code B95.62, Methicillin resistant Staphylococcus aureus infection as the cause of diseases classified elsewhere for the MRSA infection. Do not assign a code from subcategory Z16.11, Resistance to penicillins.

   (c) **Methicillin susceptible Staphylococcus aureus (MSSA) and MRSA colonization**

The condition or state of being colonized or carrying MSSA or MRSA is called colonization or carriage, while an individual person is described as being colonized or being a carrier. Colonization means that MSSA or MSRA is present on or in the body without necessarily causing illness. A positive MRSA colonization test might be documented by the provider as "MRSA screen positive" or "MRSA nasal swab positive".

Assign code Z22.322, Carrier or suspected carrier of Methicillin resistant Staphylococcus aureus, for patients documented as having MRSA colonization. Assign code Z22.321, Carrier or suspected carrier of Methicillin susceptible Staphylococcus aureus, for patient documented as having MSSA colonization. Colonization is not necessarily indicative of a disease process or as the cause of a specific condition the patient may have unless documented as such by the provider.

   (d) **MRSA colonization and infection**

If a patient is documented as having both MRSA colonization and infection during a hospital admission, code Z22.322, Carrier or suspected carrier of Methicillin resistant Staphylococcus aureus, and a code for the MRSA infection may both be assigned.

2. **Chapter 2: Neoplasms (C00-D49)**

General guidelines

Chapter 2 of the ICD-10-CM contains the codes for most benign and all malignant neoplasms. Certain benign neoplasms, such as prostatic adenomas, may be found in the specific body system chapters. To properly code a neoplasm it is necessary to determine from the record if the neoplasm is benign, in-situ, malignant, or of uncertain histologic behavior. If malignant, any secondary (metastatic) sites should also be determined.

Primary malignant neoplasms overlapping site boundaries

A primary malignant neoplasm that overlaps two or more contiguous (next to each other) sites should be classified to the subcategory/code .8 ('overlapping lesion'), unless the combination is specifically indexed elsewhere. For multiple neoplasms of the same site that are not contiguous such as tumors in different quadrants of the same breast, codes for each site should be assigned.

Malignant neoplasm of ectopic tissue

Malignant neoplasms of ectopic tissue are to be coded to the site of origin mentioned, e.g., ectopic pancreatic malignant neoplasms involving the stomach are coded to pancreas, unspecified (C25.9).

The neoplasm table in the Alphabetic Index should be referenced first. However, if the histological term is documented, that term should be referenced first, rather than going immediately to the Neoplasm Table, in order to determine which column in the Neoplasm Table is appropriate. For example, if the documentation indicates "adenoma," refer to the term in the Alphabetic Index to review the entries under this term and the instructional note to "see also neoplasm, by site, benign." The table provides the proper code based on the type of neoplasm and the site. It is important to select the proper column in the table that corresponds to the type of neoplasm. The Tabular List should then be referenced to verify that the correct code has been selected from the table and that a more specific site code does not exist.

See Section I.C.21. Factors influencing health status and contact with health services, Status, for information regarding Z15.0, codes for genetic susceptibility to cancer.

a. **Treatment directed at the malignancy**

If the treatment is directed at the malignancy, designate the malignancy as the principal diagnosis.

The only exception to this guideline is if a patient admission/encounter is solely for the administration of chemotherapy, immunotherapy or radiation therapy, assign the appropriate Z51.-- code as the first-listed or principal diagnosis, and the diagnosis or problem for which the service is being performed as a secondary diagnosis.

b. **Treatment of secondary site**

When a patient is admitted because of a primary neoplasm with metastasis and treatment is directed toward the secondary site only, the secondary neoplasm is designated as the principal diagnosis even though the primary malignancy is still present.

c. **Coding and sequencing of complications**

Coding and sequencing of complications associated with the malignancies or with the therapy thereof are subject to the following guidelines:

1) **Anemia associated with malignancy**

When admission/encounter is for management of an anemia associated with the malignancy, and the treatment is only for anemia, the appropriate code for the malignancy is sequenced as the principal or first-listed diagnosis followed by the appropriate code for the anemia (such as code D63.0, Anemia in neoplastic disease**).**

2) **Anemia associated with chemotherapy, immunotherapy and radiation therapy**

When the admission/encounter is for management of an anemia associated with an adverse effect of the administration of chemotherapy or immunotherapy and the only treatment is for the anemia, the anemia code is sequenced first followed by the appropriate codes for the neoplasm and the adverse effect (T45.1X5, Adverse effect of antineoplastic and immunosuppressive drugs).

When the admission/encounter is for management of an anemia associated with an adverse effect of radiotherapy, the anemia code should be sequenced first, followed by the appropriate neoplasm code and code Y84.2, Radiological procedure and radiotherapy as the cause of abnormal reaction of the patient, or of later complication, without mention of misadventure at the time of the procedure.

3) **Management of dehydration due to the malignancy**
When the admission/encounter is for management of dehydration due to the malignancy and only the dehydration is being treated (intravenous rehydration), the dehydration is sequenced first, followed by the code(s) for the malignancy.

4) **Treatment of a complication resulting from a surgical procedure**

When the admission/encounter is for treatment of a complication resulting from a surgical procedure, designate the complication as the principal or first-listed diagnosis if treatment is directed at resolving the complication.

d. **Primary malignancy previously excised**

When a primary malignancy has been previously excised or eradicated from its site and there is no further treatment directed to that site and there is no evidence of any existing primary malignancy, a code from category Z85, Personal history of malignant neoplasm, should be used to indicate the former site of the malignancy. Any mention of extension, invasion, or metastasis to another site is coded as a secondary malignant neoplasm to that site. The secondary site may be the principal or first-listed with the Z85 code used as a secondary code.

e. **Admissions/Encounters involving chemotherapy, immunotherapy and radiation therapy**

1) **Episode of care involves surgical removal of neoplasm**

When an episode of care involves the surgical removal of a neoplasm, primary or secondary site, followed by adjunct chemotherapy or radiation treatment during the same episode of care, the code for the neoplasm should be assigned as principal or first-listed diagnosis.

2) **Patient admission/encounter solely for administration of chemotherapy, immunotherapy and radiation therapy**

If a patient admission/encounter is solely for the administration of chemotherapy, immunotherapy or radiation therapy assign code Z51.0, Encounter for antineoplastic radiation therapy, or Z51.11, Encounter for antineoplastic chemotherapy, or Z51.12, Encounter for antineoplastic immunotherapy as the first-listed or principal diagnosis. If a patient receives more than one of these therapies during the same admission more than one of these codes may be assigned, in any sequence.

The malignancy for which the therapy is being administered should be assigned as a secondary diagnosis.

3) **Patient admitted for radiation therapy, chemotherapy or immunotherapy and develops complications**

When a patient is admitted for the purpose of radiotherapy, immunotherapy or chemotherapy and develops complications such as uncontrolled nausea and vomiting or dehydration, the principal or first-listed diagnosis is Z51.0, Encounter for antineoplastic radiation therapy, or Z51.11, Encounter for antineoplastic chemotherapy, or Z51.12, Encounter for antineoplastic immunotherapy followed by any codes for the complications.

f. **Admission/encounter to determine extent of malignancy**

When the reason for admission/encounter is to determine the extent of the malignancy, or for a procedure such as paracentesis or thoracentesis, the primary malignancy or appropriate metastatic site is designated as the principal or first-listed diagnosis, even though chemotherapy or radiotherapy is administered.

g. **Symptoms, signs, and abnormal findings listed in Chapter 18 associated with neoplasms**

Symptoms, signs, and ill-defined conditions listed in Chapter 18 characteristic of, or associated with, an existing primary or secondary site malignancy cannot be used to replace the malignancy as principal or first-listed diagnosis, regardless of the number of admissions or encounters for treatment and care of the neoplasm.

See section I.C.21. Factors influencing health status and contact with health services, Encounter for prophylactic organ removal.

h. Admission/encounter for pain control/management

See Section I.C.6. for information on coding admission/encounter for pain control/management.

i. Malignancy in two or more noncontiguous sites

A patient may have more than one malignant tumor in the same organ. These tumors may represent different primaries or metastatic disease, depending on the site. Should the documentation be unclear, the provider should be queried as to the status of each tumor so that the correct codes can be assigned.

j. Disseminated malignant neoplasm, unspecified

Code C80.0, Disseminated malignant neoplasm, unspecified, is for use only in those cases where the patient has advanced metastatic disease and no known primary or secondary sites are specified. It should not be used in place of assigning codes for the primary site and all known secondary sites.

k. Malignant neoplasm without specification of site

Code C80.1, Malignant (primary) neoplasm, unspecified, equates to Cancer, unspecified. This code should only be used when no determination can be made as to the primary site of a malignancy. This code should rarely be used in the inpatient setting.

l. Sequencing of neoplasm codes

1) Encounter for treatment of primary malignancy

If the reason for the encounter is for treatment of a primary malignancy, assign the malignancy as the principal/first-listed diagnosis. The primary site is to be sequenced first, followed by any metastatic sites.

2) Encounter for treatment of secondary malignancy

When an encounter is for a primary malignancy with metastasis and treatment is directed toward the metastatic (secondary) site(s) only, the metastatic site(s) is designated as the principal/first-listed diagnosis. The primary malignancy is coded as an additional code.

3) Malignant neoplasm in a pregnant patient

When a pregnant woman has a malignant neoplasm, a code from subcategory O9A.1-, Malignant neoplasm complicating pregnancy, childbirth, and the puerperium, should be sequenced first, followed by the appropriate code from Chapter 2 to indicate the type of neoplasm.

4) Encounter for complication associated with a neoplasm

When an encounter is for management of a complication associated with a neoplasm, such as dehydration, and the treatment is only for the complication, the complication is coded first, followed by the appropriate code(s) for the neoplasm.

The exception to this guideline is anemia. When the admission/encounter is for management of an anemia associated with the malignancy, and the treatment is only for anemia, the appropriate code for the malignancy is sequenced as the principal or first-listed diagnosis followed by code D63.0, Anemia in neoplastic disease.

5) Complication from surgical procedure for treatment of a neoplasm

When an encounter is for treatment of a complication resulting from a surgical procedure performed for the treatment of the neoplasm, designate the complication as the principal/first-listed diagnosis. See guideline regarding the coding of a current malignancy versus personal history to determine if the code for the neoplasm should also be assigned.

6) Pathologic fracture due to a neoplasm

When an encounter is for a pathological fracture due to a neoplasm, and the focus of treatment is the fracture, a code from subcategory M84.5, Pathological fracture in neoplastic disease, should be sequenced first, followed by the code for the neoplasm.

If the focus of treatment is the neoplasm with an associated pathological fracture, the neoplasm code should be sequenced first, followed by a code from M84.5 for the pathological fracture.

m. Current malignancy versus personal history of malignancy

When a primary malignancy has been excised but further treatment, such as an additional surgery for the malignancy, radiation therapy or chemotherapy is directed to that site, the primary malignancy code should be used until treatment is completed.

When a primary malignancy has been previously excised or eradicated from its site, there is no further treatment (of the malignancy) directed to that site, and there is no evidence of any existing primary malignancy, a code from category Z85, Personal history of malignant neoplasm, should be used to indicate the former site of the malignancy.

See Section I.C.21. Factors influencing health status and contact with health services, History (of)

n. Leukemia, Multiple Myeloma, and Malignant Plasma Cell Neoplasms in remission versus personal history

The categories for leukemia, and category C90, Multiple myeloma and malignant plasma cell neoplasms, have codes indicating whether or not the leukemia has achieved remission. There are also codes Z85.6, Personal history of leukemia, and Z85.79, Personal history of other malignant neoplasms of lymphoid, hematopoietic and related tissues. If the documentation is unclear, as to whether the leukemia has achieved remission, the provider should be queried.

See Section I.C.21. Factors influencing health status and contact with health services, History (of)

o. Aftercare following surgery for neoplasm

See Section I.C.21. Factors influencing health status and contact with health services, Aftercare

p. Follow-up care for completed treatment of a malignancy

See Section I.C.21. Factors influencing health status and contact with health services, Follow-up

q. Prophylactic organ removal for prevention of malignancy

See Section I.C.21, Factors influencing health status and contact with health services, Prophylactic organ removal

r. Malignant neoplasm associated with transplanted organ

A malignant neoplasm of a transplanted organ should be coded as a transplant complication. Assign first the appropriate code from category T86.-, Complications of transplanted organs and tissue, followed by code C80.2, Malignant neoplasm associated with transplanted organ. Use an additional code for the specific malignancy.

3. Chapter 3: Disease of the blood and blood-forming organs and certain disorders involving the immune mechanism (D50-D89)

Reserved for future guideline expansion

4. **Chapter 4: Endocrine, Nutritional, and Metabolic Diseases (E00-E89)**

   a. **Diabetes mellitus**

   The diabetes mellitus codes are combination codes that include the type of diabetes mellitus, the body system affected, and the complications affecting that body system. As many codes within a particular category as are necessary to describe all of the complications of the disease may be used. They should be sequenced based on the reason for a particular encounter. Assign as many codes from categories E08 – E13 as needed to identify all of the associated conditions that the patient has.

   1) **Type of diabetes**

   The age of a patient is not the sole determining factor, though most type 1 diabetics develop the condition before reaching puberty. For this reason type 1 diabetes mellitus is also referred to as juvenile diabetes.

   2) **Type of diabetes mellitus not documented**

   If the type of diabetes mellitus is not documented in the medical record the default is E11.-, Type 2 diabetes mellitus.

   3) **Diabetes mellitus and the use of insulin**

   If the documentation in a medical record does not indicate the type of diabetes but does indicate that the patient uses insulin, code E11, Type 2 diabetes mellitus, should be assigned. Code Z79.4, Long-term (current) use of insulin, should also be assigned to indicate that the patient uses insulin. Code Z79.4 should not be assigned if insulin is given temporarily to bring a type 2 patient's blood sugar under control during an encounter.

   4) **Diabetes mellitus in pregnancy and gestational diabetes**

   See Section I.C.15. Diabetes mellitus in pregnancy.
   See Section I.C.15. Gestational (pregnancy induced) diabetes

   5) **Complications due to insulin pump malfunction**

   (a) **Underdose of insulin due to insulin pump failure**

   An underdose of insulin due to an insulin pump failure should be assigned to a code from subcategory T85.6, Mechanical complication of other specified internal and external prosthetic devices, implants and grafts, that specifies the type of pump malfunction, as the principal or first-listed code, followed by code T38.3x6-, Underdosing of insulin and oral hypoglycemic [antidiabetic] drugs. Additional codes for the type of diabetes mellitus and any associated complications due to the underdosing should also be assigned.

   (b) **Overdose of insulin due to insulin pump failure**

   The principal or first-listed code for an encounter due to an insulin pump malfunction resulting in an overdose of insulin, should also be T85.6-, Mechanical complication of other specified internal and external prosthetic devices, implants and grafts, followed by code T38.3x1-, Poisoning by insulin and oral hypoglycemic [antidiabetic] drugs, accidental (unintentional).

   6) **Secondary diabetes mellitus**

   Codes under categories E08, Diabetes mellitus due to underlying condition, E09, Drug or chemical induced diabetes mellitus, and E13, Other specified diabetes mellitus, identify complications/manifestations associated with secondary diabetes mellitus. Secondary diabetes is always caused by another condition or event (e.g., cystic fibrosis, malignant neoplasm of pancreas, pancreatectomy, adverse effect of drug, or poisoning).

   (a) **Secondary diabetes mellitus and the use of insulin**

For patients who routinely use insulin, code Z79.4, Long-term (current) use of insulin, should also be assigned. Code Z79.4 should not be assigned if insulin is given temporarily to bring a patient's blood sugar under control during an encounter.

(b) **Assigning and sequencing secondary diabetes codes and its causes**

The sequencing of the secondary diabetes codes in relationship to codes for the cause of the diabetes is based on the Tabular List instructions for categories E08, E09 and E13.

(i) **Secondary diabetes mellitus due to pancreatectomy**

For postpancreatectomy diabetes mellitus (lack of insulin due to the surgical removal of all or part of the pancreas), assign code E89.1, Postprocedural hypoinsulinemia. Assign a code from category E13 and a code from subcategory Z90.41-, Acquired absence of pancreas, as additional codes.

(ii) **Secondary diabetes due to drugs**

Secondary diabetes may be caused by an adverse effect of correctly administered medications, poisoning or sequela of poisoning. *See section I.C.19.e for coding of adverse effects and poisoning, and section I.C.20 for external cause code reporting.*

5.   **Chapter 5: Mental, Behavioral and Neurodevelopmental disorders (F01 – F99)**

   a.   **Pain disorders related to psychological factors**

Assign code F45.41, for pain that is exclusively related to psychological disorders. As indicated by the Excludes 1 note under category G89, a code from category G89 should not be assigned with code F45.41

Code F45.42, Pain disorders with related psychological factors, should be used with a code from category G89, Pain, not elsewhere classified, if there is documentation of a psychological component for a patient with acute or chronic pain.

See Section I.C.6. Pain

   c.   **Mental and behavioral disorders due to psychoactive substance use**

   1)   **In Remission**

Selection of codes for "in remission" for categories F10-F19, Mental and behavioral disorders due to psychoactive substance use (categories F10-F19 with -.21) requires the provider's clinical judgment. The appropriate codes for "in remission" are assigned only on the basis of provider documentation (as defined in the Official Guidelines for Coding and Reporting).

   2)   **Psychoactive Substance Use, Abuse And Dependence**

When the provider documentation refers to use, abuse and dependence of the same substance (e.g. alcohol, opioid, cannabis, etc.), only one code should be assigned to identify the pattern of use based on the following hierarchy:

   •   If both use and abuse are documented, assign only the code for abuse
   •   If both abuse and dependence are documented, assign only the code for dependence
   •   If use, abuse and dependence are all documented, assign only the code for dependence
   •   If both use and dependence are documented, assign only the code for dependence.

   3)   **Psychoactive Substance Use**

As with all other diagnoses, the codes for psychoactive substance use (F10.9-, F11.9-, F12.9-, F13.9-, F14.9-, F15.9-, F16.9-) should only be assigned based on provider documentation and when they meet the definition of a reportable diagnosis (see Section III, Reporting Additional Diagnoses). The codes are to be used only when the psychoactive substance use is associated with a mental or behavioral disorder, and such a relationship is documented by the provider.

6. **Chapter 6: Diseases of the Nervous System (G00-G99)**

    a. **Dominant/nondominant side**

    Codes from category G81, Hemiplegia and hemiparesis, and subcategories, G83.1, Monoplegia of lower limb, G83.2, Monoplegia of upper limb, and G83.3, Monoplegia, unspecified, identify whether the dominant or nondominant side is affected. Should the affected side be documented, but not specified as dominant or nondominant, and the classification system does not indicate a default, code selection is as follows:

    - For ambidextrous patients, the default should be dominant.
    - If the left side is affected, the default is non-dominant.
    - If the right side is affected, the default is dominant.

    b. **Pain - Category G89**

    1) **General coding information**

        Codes in category G89, Pain, not elsewhere classified, may be used in conjunction with codes from other categories and chapters to provide more detail about acute or chronic pain and neoplasm-related pain, unless otherwise indicated below.

        If the pain is not specified as acute or chronic, post-thoracotomy, postprocedural, or neoplasm-related, do not assign codes from category G89.

        A code from category G89 should not be assigned if the underlying (definitive) diagnosis is known, unless the reason for the encounter is pain control/ management and not management of the underlying condition.

        When an admission or encounter is for a procedure aimed at treating the underlying condition (e.g., spinal fusion, kyphoplasty), a code for the underlying condition (e.g., vertebral fracture, spinal stenosis) should be assigned as the principal diagnosis. No code from category G89 should be assigned.

        (a) **Category G89 Codes as Principal or First-Listed Diagnosis**

             Category G89 codes are acceptable as principal diagnosis or the first-listed code:

             - When pain control or pain management is the reason for the admission/encounter (e.g., a patient with displaced intervertebral disc, nerve impingement and severe back pain presents for injection of steroid into the spinal canal). The underlying cause of the pain should be reported as an additional diagnosis, if known.

             - When a patient is admitted for the insertion of a neurostimulator for pain control, assign the appropriate pain code as the principal or first-listed diagnosis. When an admission or encounter is for a procedure aimed at treating the underlying condition and a neurostimulator is inserted for pain control during the same admission/encounter, a code for the underlying condition should be assigned as the principal diagnosis and the appropriate pain code should be assigned as a secondary diagnosis.

        (b) **Use of Category G89 Codes in Conjunction with Site Specific Pain Codes**

             (i) **Assigning Category G89 and Site-Specific Pain Codes**

                  Codes from category G89 may be used in conjunction with codes that identify the site of pain (including codes from chapter 18) if the category G89 code provides additional information. For example, if the code describes the site of the pain, but does not fully describe whether the pain is acute or chronic, then both codes should be assigned.

             (ii) **Sequencing of Category G89 Codes with Site-Specific Pain Codes**

                  The sequencing of category G89 codes with site-specific pain codes (including chapter 18 codes), is dependent on the circumstances of the encounter/admission as follows:

- If the encounter is for pain control or pain management, assign the code from category G89 followed by the code identifying the specific site of pain (e.g., encounter for pain management for acute neck pain from trauma is assigned code G89.11, Acute pain due to trauma, followed by code M54.2, Cervicalgia, to identify the site of pain).

- If the encounter is for any other reason except pain control or pain management, and a related definitive diagnosis has not been established (confirmed) by the provider, assign the code for the specific site of pain first, followed by the appropriate code from category G89.

2) Pain due to devices, implants and grafts

See Section I.C.19. Pain due to medical devices

3) Postoperative Pain

The provider's documentation should be used to guide the coding of postoperative pain, as well as *Section III. Reporting Additional Diagnoses* and *Section IV. Diagnostic Coding and Reporting in the Outpatient Setting.*

The default for post-thoracotomy and other postoperative pain not specified as acute or chronic is the code for the acute form.

Routine or expected postoperative pain immediately after surgery should not be coded.

(a) **Postoperative pain not associated with specific postoperative complication**

Postoperative pain not associated with a specific postoperative complication is assigned to the appropriate postoperative pain code in category G89.

(b) **Postoperative pain associated with specific postoperative complication**

Postoperative pain associated with a specific postoperative complication (such as painful wire sutures) is assigned to the appropriate code(s) found in Chapter 19, Injury, poisoning, and certain other consequences of external causes. If appropriate, use additional code(s) from category G89 to identify acute or chronic pain (G89.18 or G89.28).

4) Chronic pain

Chronic pain is classified to subcategory G89.2. There is no time frame defining when pain becomes chronic pain. The provider's documentation should be used to guide use of these codes.

5) Neoplasm Related Pain

Code G89.3 is assigned to pain documented as being related, associated or due to cancer, primary or secondary malignancy, or tumor. This code is assigned regardless of whether the pain is acute or chronic.

This code may be assigned as the principal or first-listed code when the stated reason for the admission/encounter is documented as pain control/pain management. The underlying neoplasm should be reported as an additional diagnosis.

When the reason for the admission/encounter is management of the neoplasm and the pain associated with the neoplasm is also documented, code G89.3 may be assigned as an additional diagnosis. It is not necessary to assign an additional code for the site of the pain.

See Section I.C.2 for instructions on the sequencing of neoplasms for all other stated reasons for the admission/encounter (except for pain control/pain management).

6) Chronic pain syndrome

Central pain syndrome (G89.0) and chronic pain syndrome (G89.4) are different than the term "chronic pain," and therefore codes should only be used when the provider has specifically documented this condition.

See Section I.C.5. Pain disorders related to psychological factors

7. **Chapter 7: Diseases of the Eye and Adnexa (H00-H59)**

   a. **Glaucoma**

      1) **Assigning Glaucoma Codes**

      Assign as many codes from category H40, Glaucoma, as needed to identify the type of glaucoma, the affected eye, and the glaucoma stage.

      2) **Bilateral glaucoma with same type and stage**

      When a patient has bilateral glaucoma and both eyes are documented as being the same type and stage, and there is a code for bilateral glaucoma, report only the code for the type of glaucoma, bilateral, with the seventh character for the stage.

      When a patient has bilateral glaucoma and both eyes are documented as being the same type and stage, and the classification does not provide a code for bilateral glaucoma (i.e. subcategories H40.10, H40.11 and H40.20) report only one code for the type of glaucoma with the appropriate seventh character for the stage.

      3) **Bilateral glaucoma stage with different types or stages**

      When a patient has bilateral glaucoma and each eye is documented as having a different type or stage, and the classification distinguishes laterality, assign the appropriate code for each eye rather than the code for bilateral glaucoma.

      When a patient has bilateral glaucoma and each eye is documented as having a different type, and the classification does not distinguish laterality (i.e. subcategories H40.10, H40.11 and H40.20), assign one code for each type of glaucoma with the appropriate seventh character for the stage.

      When a patient has bilateral glaucoma and each eye is documented as having the same type, but different stage, and the classification does not distinguish laterality (i.e. subcategories H40.10, H40.11 and H40.20), assign a code for the type of glaucoma for each eye with the seventh character for the specific glaucoma stage documented for each eye.

      4) **Patient admitted with glaucoma and stage evolves during the admission**

      If a patient is admitted with glaucoma and the stage progresses during the admission, assign the code for highest stage documented.

      5) **Indeterminate stage glaucoma**

      Assignment of the seventh character "4" for "indeterminate stage" should be based on the clinical documentation. The seventh character "4" is used for glaucomas whose stage cannot be clinically determined. This seventh character should not be confused with the seventh character "0", unspecified, which should be assigned when there is no documentation regarding the stage of the glaucoma.

8. **Chapter 8: Diseases of the Ear and Mastoid Process (H60-H95)**

   Reserved for future guideline expansion

9. **Chapter 9: Diseases of the Circulatory System (I00-I99)**

   a. **Hypertension**

      1) **Hypertension with Heart Disease**

Heart conditions classified to I50.- or I51.4-I51.9, are assigned to, a code from category I11, Hypertensive heart disease, when a causal relationship is stated (due to hypertension) or implied (hypertensive). Use an additional code from category I50, Heart failure, to identify the type of heart failure in those patients with heart failure.

The same heart conditions (I50.-, I51.4-I51.9) with hypertension, but without a stated causal relationship, are coded separately. Sequence according to the circumstances of the admission/encounter.

2) **Hypertensive Chronic Kidney Disease**

Assign codes from category I12, Hypertensive chronic kidney disease, when both hypertension and a condition classifiable to category N18, Chronic kidney disease (CKD), are present. Unlike hypertension with heart disease, ICD-10-CM presumes a cause-and-effect relationship and classifies chronic kidney disease with hypertension as hypertensive chronic kidney disease.

The appropriate code from category N18 should be used as a secondary code with a code from category I12 to identify the stage of chronic kidney disease.

See Section I.C.14. Chronic kidney disease.

If a patient has hypertensive chronic kidney disease and acute renal failure, an additional code for the acute renal failure is required.

3) **Hypertensive Heart and Chronic Kidney Disease**

Assign codes from combination category I13, Hypertensive heart and chronic kidney disease, when both hypertensive kidney disease and hypertensive heart disease are stated in the diagnosis. Assume a relationship between the hypertension and the chronic kidney disease, whether or not the condition is so designated. If heart failure is present, assign an additional code from category I50 to identify the type of heart failure.

The appropriate code from category N18, Chronic kidney disease, should be used as a secondary code with a code from category I13 to identify the stage of chronic kidney disease.

See Section I.C.14. Chronic kidney disease.

The codes in category I13, Hypertensive heart and chronic kidney disease, are combination codes that include hypertension, heart disease and chronic kidney disease. The Includes note at I13 specifies that the conditions included at I11 and I12 are included together in I13. If a patient has hypertension, heart disease and chronic kidney disease then a code from I13 should be used, not individual codes for hypertension, heart disease and chronic kidney disease, or codes from I11 or I12.

For patients with both acute renal failure and chronic kidney disease an additional code for acute renal failure is required.

4) **Hypertensive Cerebrovascular Disease**

For hypertensive cerebrovascular disease, first assign the appropriate code from categories I60-I69, followed by the appropriate hypertension code.

5) **Hypertensive Retinopathy**

Subcategory H35.0, Background retinopathy and retinal vascular changes, should be used with a code from category I10 – I15, Hypertensive disease to include the systemic hypertension. The sequencing is based on the reason for the encounter.

6) **Hypertension, Secondary**

Secondary hypertension is due to an underlying condition. Two codes are required: one to identify the underlying etiology and one from category I15 to identify the hypertension. Sequencing of codes is determined by the reason for admission/encounter.

7) **Hypertension, Transient**

Assign code R03.0, Elevated blood pressure reading without diagnosis of hypertension, unless patient has an established diagnosis of hypertension. Assign code O13.-, Gestational [pregnancy-induced] hypertension without significant proteinuria, or O14.-, Pre-eclampsia, for transient hypertension of pregnancy.

8) **Hypertension, Controlled**

This diagnostic statement usually refers to an existing state of hypertension under control by therapy. Assign the appropriate code from categories I10-I15, Hypertensive diseases.

9) **Hypertension, Uncontrolled**

Uncontrolled hypertension may refer to untreated hypertension or hypertension not responding to current therapeutic regimen. In either case, assign the appropriate code from categories I10-I15, Hypertensive diseases.

b. **Atherosclerotic Coronary Artery Disease and Angina**

ICD-10-CM has combination codes for atherosclerotic heart disease with angina pectoris. The subcategories for these codes are I25.11, Atherosclerotic heart disease of native coronary artery with angina pectoris and I25.7, Atherosclerosis of coronary artery bypass graft(s) and coronary artery of transplanted heart with angina pectoris.

When using one of these combination codes it is not necessary to use an additional code for angina pectoris. A causal relationship can be assumed in a patient with both atherosclerosis and angina pectoris, unless the documentation indicates the angina is due to something other than the atherosclerosis.

If a patient with coronary artery disease is admitted due to an acute myocardial infarction (AMI), the AMI should be sequenced before the coronary artery disease.

See Section I.C.9. Acute myocardial infarction (AMI)

c. **Intraoperative and Postprocedural Cerebrovascular Accident**

Medical record documentation should clearly specify the cause- and-effect relationship between the medical intervention and the cerebrovascular accident in order to assign a code for intraoperative or postprocedural cerebrovascular accident.

Proper code assignment depends on whether it was an infarction or hemorrhage and whether it occurred intraoperatively or postoperatively. If it was a cerebral hemorrhage, code assignment depends on the type of procedure performed.

d. **Sequelae of Cerebrovascular Disease**

1) **Category I69, Sequelae of Cerebrovascular disease**

Category I69 is used to indicate conditions classifiable to categories I60-I67 as the causes of sequela (neurologic deficits), themselves classified elsewhere. These "late effects" include neurologic deficits that persist after initial onset of conditions classifiable to categories I60-I67. The neurologic deficits caused by cerebrovascular disease may be present from the onset or may arise at any time after the onset of the condition classifiable to categories I60-I67.

Codes from category I69, Sequelae of cerebrovascular disease, that specify hemiplegia, hemiparesis and monoplegia identify whether the dominant or nondominant side is affected. Should the affected side be documented, but not specified as dominant or nondominant, and the classification system does not indicate a default, code selection is as follows:

- For ambidextrous patients, the default should be dominant.
- If the left side is affected, the default is non-dominant.
- If the right side is affected, the default is dominant.

2) **Codes from category I69 with codes from I60-I67**

Codes from category I69 may be assigned on a health care record with codes from I60-I67, if the patient has a current cerebrovascular disease and deficits from an old cerebrovascular disease.

3) **Codes from category I69 and Personal history of transient ischemic attack (TIA) and cerebral infarction (Z86.73)**

Codes from category I69 should not be assigned if the patient does not have neurologic deficits.

See Section I.C.21. 4. History (of) for use of personal history codes

e. **Acute myocardial infarction (AMI)**

1) **ST elevation myocardial infarction (STEMI) and non ST elevation myocardial infarction (NSTEMI)**

The ICD-10-CM codes for acute myocardial infarction (AMI) identify the site, such as anterolateral wall or true posterior wall. Subcategories I21.0-I21.2 and code I21.3 are used for ST elevation myocardial infarction (STEMI). Code I21.4, Non-ST elevation (NSTEMI) myocardial infarction, is used for non ST elevation myocardial infarction (NSTEMI) and nontransmural MIs.

If NSTEMI evolves to STEMI, assign the STEMI code. If STEMI converts to NSTEMI due to thrombolytic therapy, it is still coded as STEMI.

For encounters occurring while the myocardial infarction is equal to, or less than, four weeks old, including transfers to another acute setting or a postacute setting, and the patient requires continued care for the myocardial infarction, codes from category I21 may continue to be reported. For encounters after the 4 week time frame and the patient is still receiving care related to the myocardial infarction, the appropriate aftercare code should be assigned, rather than a code from category I21. For old or healed myocardial infarctions not requiring further care, code I25.2, Old myocardial infarction, may be assigned.

2) **Acute myocardial infarction, unspecified**

Code I21.3, ST elevation (STEMI) myocardial infarction of unspecified site, is the default for unspecified acute myocardial infarction. If only STEMI or transmural MI without the site is documented, assign code I21.3.

3) **AMI documented as nontransmural or subendocardial but site provided**

If an AMI is documented as nontransmural or subendocardial, but the site is provided, it is still coded as a subendocardial AMI.

See Section I.C.21.3 for information on coding status post administration of tPA in a different facility within the last 24 hours.

4) **Subsequent acute myocardial infarction**

A code from category I22, Subsequent ST elevation (STEMI) and non ST elevation (NSTEMI) myocardial infarction, is to be used when a patient who has suffered an AMI has a new AMI within the 4 week time frame of the initial AMI. A code from category I22 must be used in conjunction with a code from category I21. The sequencing of the I22 and I21 codes depends on the circumstances of the encounter.

10. **Chapter 10: Diseases of the Respiratory System (J00-J99)**

a. **Chronic Obstructive Pulmonary Disease [COPD] and Asthma**

1) **Acute exacerbation of chronic obstructive bronchitis and asthma**

The codes in categories J44 and J45 distinguish between uncomplicated cases and those in acute exacerbation. An acute exacerbation is a worsening or a decompensation of a chronic condition. An acute exacerbation is not equivalent to an infection superimposed on a chronic condition, though an exacerbation may be triggered by an infection.

b. Acute Respiratory Failure

1) Acute respiratory failure as principal diagnosis

A code from subcategory J96.0, Acute respiratory failure, or subcategory J96.2, Acute and chronic respiratory failure, may be assigned as a principal diagnosis when it is the condition established after study to be chiefly responsible for occasioning the admission to the hospital, and the selection is supported by the Alphabetic Index and Tabular List. However, chapter-specific coding guidelines (such as obstetrics, poisoning, HIV, newborn) that provide sequencing direction take precedence.

2) Acute respiratory failure as secondary diagnosis

Respiratory failure may be listed as a secondary diagnosis if it occurs after admission, or if it is present on admission, but does not meet the definition of principal diagnosis.

3) Sequencing of acute respiratory failure and another acute condition

When a patient is admitted with respiratory failure and another acute condition, (e.g., myocardial infarction, cerebrovascular accident, aspiration pneumonia), the principal diagnosis will not be the same in every situation. This applies whether the other acute condition is a respiratory or nonrespiratory condition. Selection of the principal diagnosis will be dependent on the circumstances of admission. If both the respiratory failure and the other acute condition are equally responsible for occasioning the admission to the hospital, and there are no chapter-specific sequencing rules, the guideline regarding two or more diagnoses that equally meet the definition for principal diagnosis *(Section II, C.)* may be applied in these situations.

If the documentation is not clear as to whether acute respiratory failure and another condition are equally responsible for occasioning the admission, query the provider for clarification.

c. Influenza due to certain identified influenza viruses

Code only confirmed cases of influenza due to certain identified influenza viruses (category J09), and due to other identified influenza virus (category J10). This is an exception to the hospital inpatient guideline Section II, H. (Uncertain Diagnosis).

In this context, "confirmation" does not require documentation of positive laboratory testing specific for avian or other novel influenza A or other identified influenza virus. However, coding should be based on the provider's diagnostic statement that the patient has avian influenza, or other novel influenza A, for category J09, or has another particular identified strain of influenza, such as H1N1 or H3N2, but not identified as novel or variant, for category J10.

If the provider records "suspected" or "possible" or "probable" avian influenza, or novel influenza, or other identified influenza, then the appropriate influenza code from category J11, Influenza due to unidentified influenza virus, should be assigned. A code from category J09, Influenza due to certain identified influenza viruses, should not be assigned nor should a code from category J10, Influenza due to other identified influenza virus.

d. Ventilator associated Pneumonia

1) Documentation of Ventilator associated Pneumonia

As with all procedural or postprocedural complications, code assignment is based on the provider's documentation of the relationship between the condition and the procedure.

Code J95.851, Ventilator associated pneumonia, should be assigned only when the provider has documented ventilator associated pneumonia (VAP). An additional code to identify the organism (e.g., Pseudomonas aeruginosa, code B96.5) should also be assigned. Do not assign an additional code from categories J12-J18 to identify the type of pneumonia.

Code J95.851 should not be assigned for cases where the patient has pneumonia and is on a mechanical ventilator and the provider has not specifically stated that the pneumonia is ventilator-associated pneumonia. If the documentation is unclear as to whether the patient has a pneumonia that is a complication attributable to the mechanical ventilator, query the provider.

2) Ventilator associated Pneumonia Develops after Admission

A patient may be admitted with one type of pneumonia (e.g., code J13, Pneumonia due to Streptococcus pneumonia) and subsequently develop VAP. In this instance, the principal diagnosis would be the appropriate code from categories J12-J18 for the pneumonia diagnosed at the time of admission. Code J95.851, Ventilator associated pneumonia, would be assigned as an additional diagnosis when the provider has also documented the presence of ventilator associated pneumonia.

11. Chapter 11: Diseases of the Digestive System (K00-K95)

Reserved for future guideline expansion

12. Chapter 12: Diseases of the Skin and Subcutaneous Tissue (L00-L99)

a. Pressure ulcer stage codes

1) Pressure ulcer stages

Codes from category L89, Pressure ulcer, are combination codes that identify the site of the pressure ulcer as well as the stage of the ulcer.

The ICD-10-CM classifies pressure ulcer stages based on severity, which is designated by stages 1-4, unspecified stage and unstageable.

Assign as many codes from category L89 as needed to identify all the pressure ulcers the patient has, if applicable.

2) Unstageable pressure ulcers

Assignment of the code for unstageable pressure ulcer (L89.--0) should be based on the clinical documentation. These codes are used for pressure ulcers whose stage cannot be clinically determined (e.g., the ulcer is covered by eschar or has been treated with a skin or muscle graft) and pressure ulcers that are documented as deep tissue injury but not documented as due to trauma. This code should not be confused with the codes for unspecified stage (L89.--9). When there is no documentation regarding the stage of the pressure ulcer, assign the appropriate code for unspecified stage (L89.--9).

3) Documented pressure ulcer stage

Assignment of the pressure ulcer stage code should be guided by clinical documentation of the stage or documentation of the terms found in the Alphabetic Index. For clinical terms describing the stage that are not found in the Alphabetic Index, and there is no documentation of the stage, the provider should be queried.

4) Patients admitted with pressure ulcers documented as healed

No code is assigned if the documentation states that the pressure ulcer is completely healed.

5) Patients admitted with pressure ulcers documented as healing

Pressure ulcers described as healing should be assigned the appropriate pressure ulcer stage code based on the documentation in the medical record. If the documentation does not provide information about the stage of the healing pressure ulcer, assign the appropriate code for unspecified stage.

If the documentation is unclear as to whether the patient has a current (new) pressure ulcer or if the patient is being treated for a healing pressure ulcer, query the provider.

6) **Patient admitted with pressure ulcer evolving into another stage during the admission**

If a patient is admitted with a pressure ulcer at one stage and it progresses to a higher stage, assign the code for the highest stage reported for that site.

13. **Chapter 13: Diseases of the Musculoskeletal System and Connective Tissue (M00-M99)**

a. **Site and laterality**

Most of the codes within Chapter 13 have site and laterality designations. The site represents the bone, joint or the muscle involved. For some conditions where more than one bone, joint or muscle is usually involved, such as osteoarthritis, there is a "multiple sites" code available. For categories where no multiple site code is provided and more than one bone, joint or muscle is involved, multiple codes should be used to indicate the different sites involved.

1) **Bone versus joint**

For certain conditions, the bone may be affected at the upper or lower end, (e.g., avascular necrosis of bone, M87, Osteoporosis, M80, M81). Though the portion of the bone affected may be at the joint, the site designation will be the bone, not the joint.

b. **Acute traumatic versus chronic or recurrent musculoskeletal conditions**

Many musculoskeletal conditions are a result of previous injury or trauma to a site, or are recurrent conditions. Bone, joint or muscle conditions that are the result of a healed injury are usually found in chapter 13. Recurrent bone, joint or muscle conditions are also usually found in chapter 13. Any current, acute injury should be coded to the appropriate injury code from chapter 19. Chronic or recurrent conditions should generally be coded with a code from chapter 13. If it is difficult to determine from the documentation in the record which code is best to describe a condition, query the provider.

c. **Coding of Pathologic Fractures**

7th character A is for use as long as the patient is receiving active treatment for the fracture. Examples of active treatment are: surgical treatment, emergency department encounter, evaluation and treatment by a new physician. 7th character, D is to be used for encounters after the patient has completed active treatment. The other 7th characters, listed under each subcategory in the Tabular List, are to be used for subsequent encounters for treatment of problems associated with the healing, such as malunions, nonunions, and sequelae.

Care for complications of surgical treatment for fracture repairs during the healing or recovery phase should be coded with the appropriate complication codes.

See Section I.C.19. Coding of traumatic fractures.

d. **Osteoporosis**

Osteoporosis is a systemic condition, meaning that all bones of the musculoskeletal system are affected. Therefore, site is not a component of the codes under category M81, Osteoporosis without current pathological fracture. The site codes under category M80, Osteoporosis with current pathological fracture, identify the site of the fracture, not the osteoporosis.

1) **Osteoporosis without pathological fracture**

Category M81, Osteoporosis without current pathological fracture, is for use for patients with osteoporosis who do not currently have a pathologic fracture due to the osteoporosis, even if they have had a fracture in the past. For patients with a history of osteoporosis fractures, status code Z87.310, Personal history of (healed) osteoporosis fracture, should follow the code from M81.

2) **Osteoporosis with current pathological fracture**

Category M80, Osteoporosis with current pathological fracture, is for patients who have a current pathologic fracture at the time of an encounter. The codes under M80 identify the site of the fracture. A code from category M80, not a traumatic fracture code, should be used for any patient with known osteoporosis who suffers a fracture, even if the patient had a minor fall or trauma, if that fall or trauma would not usually break a normal, healthy bone.

14. **Chapter 14: Diseases of Genitourinary System (N00-N99)**

    a. **Chronic kidney disease**

       1) **Stages of chronic kidney disease (CKD)**

          The ICD-10-CM classifies CKD based on severity. The severity of CKD is designated by stages 1-5. Stage 2, code N18.2, equates to mild CKD; stage 3, code N18.3, equates to moderate CKD; and stage 4, code N18.4, equates to severe CKD. Code N18.6, End stage renal disease (ESRD), is assigned when the provider has documented end-stage-renal disease (ESRD).

          If both a stage of CKD and ESRD are documented, assign code N18.6 only.

       2) **Chronic kidney disease and kidney transplant status**

          Patients who have undergone kidney transplant may still have some form of chronic kidney disease (CKD) because the kidney transplant may not fully restore kidney function. Therefore, the presence of CKD alone does not constitute a transplant complication. Assign the appropriate N18 code for the patient's stage of CKD and code Z94.0, Kidney transplant status. If a transplant complication such as failure or rejection or other transplant complication is documented, see section I.C.19.g for information on coding complications of a kidney transplant. If the documentation is unclear as to whether the patient has a complication of the transplant, query the provider.

       3) **Chronic kidney disease with other conditions**

          Patients with CKD may also suffer from other serious conditions, most commonly diabetes mellitus and hypertension. The sequencing of the CKD code in relationship to codes for other contributing conditions is based on the conventions in the Tabular List.

          See I.C.9. Hypertensive chronic kidney disease.
          See I.C.19. Chronic kidney disease and kidney transplant complications.

15. **Chapter 15: Pregnancy, Childbirth, and the Puerperium (O00-*O*9A)**

    a. **General Rules for Obstetric Cases**

       1) **Codes from chapter 15 and sequencing priority**

          Obstetric cases require codes from chapter 15, codes in the range O00-O9A, Pregnancy, Childbirth, and the Puerperium. Chapter 15 codes have sequencing priority over codes from other chapters. Additional codes from other chapters may be used in conjunction with chapter 15 codes to further specify conditions. Should the provider document that the pregnancy is incidental to the encounter, then code Z33.1, Pregnant state, incidental, should be used in place of any chapter 15 codes. It is the provider's responsibility to state that the condition being treated is not affecting the pregnancy.

       2) **Chapter 15 codes used only on the maternal record**

          Chapter 15 codes are to be used only on the maternal record, never on the record of the newborn.

       3) **Final character for trimester**

          The majority of codes in Chapter 15 have a final character indicating the trimester of pregnancy. The timeframes for the trimesters are indicated at the beginning of the chapter. If trimester is not a component of a code it is because the condition always occurs in a specific trimester, or the concept of trimester of pregnancy is not applicable. Certain codes have characters for only certain trimesters because the condition does not occur in all trimesters, but it may occur in more than just one.

Assignment of the final character for trimester should be based on the provider's documentation of the trimester (or number of weeks) for the current admission/encounter. This applies to the assignment of trimester for pre-existing conditions as well as those that develop during or are due to the pregnancy. The provider's documentation of the number of weeks may be used to assign the appropriate code identifying the trimester.

Whenever delivery occurs during the current admission, and there is an "in childbirth" option for the obstetric complication being coded, the "in childbirth" code should be assigned.

4) **Selection of trimester for inpatient admissions that encompass more than one trimester**

In instances when a patient is admitted to a hospital for complications of pregnancy during one trimester and remains in the hospital into a subsequent trimester, the trimester character for the antepartum complication code should be assigned on the basis of the trimester when the complication developed, not the trimester of the discharge. If the condition developed prior to the current admission/encounter or represents a pre-existing condition, the trimester character for the trimester at the time of the admission/encounter should be assigned.

5) **Unspecified trimester**

Each category that includes codes for trimester has a code for "unspecified trimester." The "unspecified trimester" code should rarely be used, such as when the documentation in the record is insufficient to determine the trimester and it is not possible to obtain clarification.

6) **7th character for Fetus Identification**

Where applicable, a 7th character is to be assigned for certain categories (O31, O32, O33.3 - O33.6, O35, O36, O40, O41, O60.1, O60.2, O64, and O69) to identify the fetus for which the complication code applies.

Assign 7th character "0":

- For single gestations
- When the documentation in the record is insufficient to determine the fetus affected and it is not possible to obtain clarification.
- When it is not possible to clinically determine which fetus is affected.

b. **Selection of OB Principal or First-listed Diagnosis**

1) **Routine outpatient prenatal visits**

For routine outpatient prenatal visits when no complications are present, a code from category Z34, Encounter for supervision of normal pregnancy, should be used as the first-listed diagnosis. These codes should not be used in conjunction with chapter 15 codes.

2) **Prenatal outpatient visits for high-risk patients**

For routine prenatal outpatient visits for patients with high-risk pregnancies, a code from category O09, Supervision of high-risk pregnancy, should be used as the first-listed diagnosis. Secondary chapter 15 codes may be used in conjunction with these codes if appropriate.

3) **Episodes when no delivery occurs**

In episodes when no delivery occurs, the principal diagnosis should correspond to the principal complication of the pregnancy which necessitated the encounter. Should more than one complication exist, all of which are treated or monitored, any of the complications codes may be sequenced first.

4) **When a delivery occurs**
When a delivery occurs, the principal diagnosis should correspond to the main circumstances or complication of the delivery. In cases of cesarean delivery, the selection of the principal diagnosis should be the condition established after study that was responsible for the patient's admission. If the patient was admitted with a condition that resulted in the performance of a cesarean procedure, that condition should be

selected as the principal diagnosis. If the reason for the admission/encounter was unrelated to the condition resulting in the cesarean delivery, the condition related to the reason for the admission/encounter should be selected as the principal diagnosis.

5) **Outcome of delivery**

A code from category Z37, Outcome of delivery, should be included on every maternal record when a delivery has occurred. These codes are not to be used on subsequent records or on the newborn record.

c. **Pre-existing conditions versus conditions due to the pregnancy**

Certain categories in Chapter 15 distinguish between conditions of the mother that existed prior to pregnancy (pre-existing) and those that are a direct result of pregnancy. When assigning codes from Chapter 15, it is important to assess if a condition was pre-existing prior to pregnancy or developed during or due to the pregnancy in order to assign the correct code.

Categories that do not distinguish between pre-existing and pregnancy-related conditions may be used for either. It is acceptable to use codes specifically for the puerperium with codes complicating pregnancy and childbirth if a condition arises postpartum during the delivery encounter.

d. **Pre-existing hypertension in pregnancy**

Category O10, Pre-existing hypertension complicating pregnancy, childbirth and the puerperium, includes codes for hypertensive heart and hypertensive chronic kidney disease. When assigning one of the O10 codes that includes hypertensive heart disease or hypertensive chronic kidney disease, it is necessary to add a secondary code from the appropriate hypertension category to specify the type of heart failure or chronic kidney disease.

See Section I.C.9. Hypertension.

e. **Fetal Conditions Affecting the Management of the Mother**

1) **Codes from categories O35 and O36**

Codes from categories O35, Maternal care for known or suspected fetal abnormality and damage, and O36, Maternal care for other fetal problems, are assigned only when the fetal condition is actually responsible for modifying the management of the mother, i.e., by requiring diagnostic studies, additional observation, special care, or termination of pregnancy. The fact that the fetal condition exists does not justify assigning a code from this series to the mother's record.

2) **In utero surgery**

In cases when surgery is performed on the fetus, a diagnosis code from category O35, Maternal care for known or suspected fetal abnormality and damage, should be assigned identifying the fetal condition. Assign the appropriate procedure code for the procedure performed.

No code from Chapter 16, the perinatal codes, should be used on the mother's record to identify fetal conditions. Surgery performed in utero on a fetus is still to be coded as an obstetric encounter.

f. **HIV Infection in Pregnancy, Childbirth and the Puerperium**

During pregnancy, childbirth or the puerperium, a patient admitted because of an HIV-related illness should receive a principal diagnosis from subcategory O98.7-, Human immunodeficiency [HIV] disease complicating pregnancy, childbirth and the puerperium, followed by the code(s) for the HIV-related illness(es).
Patients with asymptomatic HIV infection status admitted during pregnancy, childbirth, or the puerperium should receive codes of O98.7- and Z21, Asymptomatic human immunodeficiency virus [HIV] infection status.

g. **Diabetes mellitus in pregnancy**

Diabetes mellitus is a significant complicating factor in pregnancy. Pregnant women who are diabetic should be assigned a code from category O24, Diabetes mellitus in pregnancy, childbirth, and the puerperium, first, followed by the appropriate diabetes code(s) (E08-E13) from Chapter 4.

h.   Long term use of insulin

Code Z79.4, Long-term (current) use of insulin, should also be assigned if the diabetes mellitus is being treated with insulin.

i.   Gestational (pregnancy induced) diabetes

Gestational (pregnancy induced) diabetes can occur during the second and third trimester of pregnancy in women who were not diabetic prior to pregnancy. Gestational diabetes can cause complications in the pregnancy similar to those of pre-existing diabetes mellitus. It also puts the woman at greater risk of developing diabetes after the pregnancy. Codes for gestational diabetes are in subcategory O24.4, Gestational diabetes mellitus. No other code from category O24,

Diabetes mellitus in pregnancy, childbirth, and the puerperium, should be used with a code from O24.4

The codes under subcategory O24.4 include diet controlled and insulin controlled. If a patient with gestational diabetes is treated with both diet and insulin, only the code for insulin-controlled is required.

Code Z79.4, Long-term (current) use of insulin, should not be assigned with codes from subcategory O24.4.

An abnormal glucose tolerance in pregnancy is assigned a code from subcategory O99.81, Abnormal glucose complicating pregnancy, childbirth, and the puerperium.

j.   Sepsis and septic shock complicating abortion, pregnancy, childbirth and the puerperium

When assigning a chapter 15 code for sepsis complicating abortion, pregnancy, childbirth, and the puerperium, a code for the specific type of infection should be assigned as an additional diagnosis. If severe sepsis is present, a code from subcategory R65.2, Severe sepsis, and code(s) for associated organ dysfunction(s) should also be assigned as additional diagnoses.

k.   Puerperal sepsis

Code O85, Puerperal sepsis, should be assigned with a secondary code to identify the causal organism (e.g., for a bacterial infection, assign a code from category B95-B96, Bacterial infections in conditions classified elsewhere). A code from category A40, Streptococcal sepsis, or A41, Other sepsis, should not be used for puerperal sepsis. If applicable, use additional codes to identify severe sepsis (R65.2-) and any associated acute organ dysfunction.

l.   Alcohol and tobacco use during pregnancy, childbirth and the puerperium

1)   Alcohol use during pregnancy, childbirth and the puerperium

Codes under subcategory O99.31, Alcohol use complicating pregnancy, childbirth, and the puerperium, should be assigned for any pregnancy case when a mother uses alcohol during the pregnancy or postpartum. A secondary code from category F10, Alcohol related disorders, should also be assigned to identify manifestations of the alcohol use.

2)   Tobacco use during pregnancy, childbirth and the puerperium
Codes under subcategory O99.33, Smoking (tobacco) complicating pregnancy, childbirth, and the puerperium, should be assigned for any pregnancy case when a mother uses any type of tobacco product during the pregnancy or postpartum.

A secondary code from category F17, Nicotine dependence, should also be assigned to identify the type of nicotine dependence.

m.   Poisoning, toxic effects, adverse effects and underdosing in a pregnant patient

A code from subcategory O9A.2, Injury, poisoning and certain other consequences of external causes complicating pregnancy, childbirth, and the puerperium, should be sequenced first, followed by the appropriate injury, poisoning, toxic effect, adverse effect or underdosing code, and then the additional code(s) that specifies the condition caused by the poisoning, toxic effect, adverse effect or underdosing.

See Section I.C.19. Adverse effects, poisoning, underdosing and toxic effects.

n. **Normal Delivery, Code O80**

1) **Encounter for full term uncomplicated delivery**

Code O80 should be assigned when a woman is admitted for a full-term normal delivery and delivers a single, healthy infant without any complications antepartum, during the delivery, or postpartum during the delivery episode. Code O80 is always a principal diagnosis. It is not to be used if any other code from chapter 15 is needed to describe a current complication of the antenatal, delivery, or perinatal period. Additional codes from other chapters may be used with code O80 if they are not related to or are in any way complicating the pregnancy.

2) **Uncomplicated delivery with resolved antepartum complication**

Code O80 may be used if the patient had a complication at some point during the pregnancy, but the complication is not present at the time of the admission for delivery.

3) **Outcome of delivery for O80**

Z37.0, Single live birth, is the only outcome of delivery code appropriate for use with O80.

o. **The Peripartum and Postpartum Periods**

1) **Peripartum and Postpartum periods**

The postpartum period begins immediately after delivery and continues for six weeks following delivery. The peripartum period is defined as the last month of pregnancy to five months postpartum.

2) **Peripartum and postpartum complication**

A postpartum complication is any complication occurring within the six-week period.

3) **Pregnancy-related complications after 6 week period**

Chapter 15 codes may also be used to describe pregnancy-related complications after the peripartum or postpartum period if the provider documents that a condition is pregnancy related.

4) **Admission for routine postpartum care following delivery outside hospital**

When the mother delivers outside the hospital prior to admission and is admitted for routine postpartum care and no complications are noted, code Z39.0, Encounter for care and examination of mother immediately after delivery, should be assigned as the principal diagnosis.

5) **Pregnancy associated cardiomyopathy**

Pregnancy associated cardiomyopathy, code O90.3, is unique in that it may be diagnosed in the third trimester of pregnancy but may continue to progress months after delivery. For this reason, it is referred to as peripartum cardiomyopathy. Code O90.3 is only for use when the cardiomyopathy develops as a result of pregnancy in a woman who did not have pre-existing heart disease.

p. **Code O94, Sequelae of complication of pregnancy, childbirth, and the puerperium**

1) **Code O94**

Code O94, Sequelae of complication of pregnancy, childbirth, and the puerperium, is for use in those cases when an initial complication of a pregnancy develops a sequelae requiring care or treatment at a future date.

2) After the initial postpartum period

This code may be used at any time after the initial postpartum period.

3) Sequencing of Code O94

This code, like all sequela codes, is to be sequenced following the code describing the sequelae of the complication.

q. *Termination of Pregnancy and Spontaneous abortions*

1) Abortion with Liveborn Fetus

When an attempted termination of pregnancy results in a liveborn fetus, assign code Z33.2, Encounter for elective termination of pregnancy and a code from category Z37, Outcome of Delivery.

2) Retained Products of Conception following an abortion

Subsequent encounters for retained products of conception following a spontaneous abortion or elective termination of pregnancy are assigned the appropriate code from category O03, Spontaneous abortion, or codes O07.4, Failed attempted termination of pregnancy without complication and Z33.2, Encounter for elective termination of pregnancy. This advice is appropriate even when the patient was discharged previously with a discharge diagnosis of complete abortion.

3) Complications leading to abortion

Codes from Chapter 15 may be used as additional codes to identify any documented complications of the pregnancy in conjunction with codes in categories in O07 and O08.

r. Abuse in a pregnant patient

For suspected or confirmed cases of abuse of a pregnant patient, a code(s) from subcategories O9A.3, Physical abuse complicating pregnancy, childbirth, and the puerperium, O9A.4, Sexual abuse complicating pregnancy, childbirth, and the puerperium, and O9A.5, Psychological abuse complicating pregnancy, childbirth, and the puerperium, should be sequenced first, followed by the appropriate codes (if applicable) to identify any associated current injury due to physical abuse, sexual abuse, and the perpetrator of abuse.

See Section I.C.19. Adult and child abuse, neglect and other maltreatment.

16. Chapter 16: Certain Conditions Originating in the Perinatal Period (P00-P96)

For coding and reporting purposes the perinatal period is defined as before birth through the 28th day following birth. The following guidelines are provided for reporting purposes

a. General Perinatal Rules

1) Use of Chapter 16 Codes

Codes in this chapter are never for use on the maternal record. Codes from Chapter 15, the obstetric chapter, are never permitted on the newborn record. Chapter 16 codes may be used throughout the life of the patient if the condition is still present.

2) Principal Diagnosis for Birth Record

When coding the birth episode in a newborn record, assign a code from category Z38, Liveborn infants according to place of birth and type of delivery, as the principal diagnosis. A code from category Z38 is assigned only once, to a newborn at the time of birth. If a newborn is transferred to another institution, a code from category Z38 should not be used at the receiving hospital.

A code from category Z38 is used only on the newborn record, not on the mother's record.

3) Use of Codes from other Chapters with Codes from Chapter 16

Codes from other chapters may be used with codes from chapter 16 if the codes from the other chapters provide more specific detail. Codes for signs and symptoms may be assigned when a definitive diagnosis has not been established. If the reason for the encounter is a perinatal condition, the code from chapter 16 should be sequenced first.

4) Use of Chapter 16 Codes after the Perinatal Period

Should a condition originate in the perinatal period, and continue throughout the life of the patient, the perinatal code should continue to be used regardless of the patient's age.

5) Birth process or community acquired conditions

If a newborn has a condition that may be either due to the birth process or community acquired and the documentation does not indicate which it is, the default is due to the birth process and the code from Chapter 16 should be used. If the condition is community-acquired, a code from Chapter 16 should not be assigned.

6) Code all clinically significant conditions

All clinically significant conditions noted on routine newborn examination should be coded. A condition is clinically significant if it requires:

- clinical evaluation; or
- therapeutic treatment; or
- diagnostic procedures; or
- extended length of hospital stay; or
- increased nursing care and/or monitoring; or
- has implications for future health care needs

Note: The perinatal guidelines listed above are the same as the general coding guidelines for "additional diagnoses", except for the final point regarding implications for future health care needs. Codes should be assigned for conditions that have been specified by the provider as having implications for future health care needs.

b. Observation and Evaluation of Newborns for Suspected Conditions not Found

Reserved for future expansion

c. Coding Additional Perinatal Diagnoses

1) Assigning codes for conditions that require treatment

Assign codes for conditions that require treatment or further investigation, prolong the length of stay, or require resource utilization.

2) Codes for conditions specified as having implications for future health care needs

Assign codes for conditions that have been specified by the provider as having implications for future health care needs.

Note: This guideline should not be used for adult patients.

d. Prematurity and Fetal Growth Retardation

Providers utilize different criteria in determining prematurity. A code for prematurity should not be assigned unless it is documented. Assignment of codes in categories P05, Disorders of newborn related to slow fetal growth and fetal malnutrition, and P07, Disorders of newborn related to short gestation and low birth weight, not elsewhere classified, should be based on the recorded birth weight and estimated gestational age. Codes from category P05 should not be assigned with codes from category P07.

When both birth weight and gestational age are available, two codes from category P07 should be assigned, with the code for birth weight sequenced before the code for gestational age.

e. **Low birth weight and immaturity status**

Codes from category P07, Disorders of newborn related to short gestation and low birth weight, not elsewhere classified, are for use for a child or adult who was premature or had a low birth weight as a newborn and this is affecting the patient's current health status.

See Section I.C.21. Factors influencing health status and contact with health services, Status.

f. **Bacterial Sepsis of Newborn**

Category P36, Bacterial sepsis of newborn, includes congenital sepsis. If a perinate is documented as having sepsis without documentation of congenital or community acquired, the default is congenital and a code from category P36 should be assigned. If the P36 code includes the causal organism, an additional code from category B95, Streptococcus, Staphylococcus, and Enterococcus as the cause of diseases classified elsewhere, or B96, Other bacterial agents as the cause of diseases classified elsewhere, should not be assigned. If the P36 code does not include the causal organism, assign an additional code from category B96. If applicable, use additional codes to identify severe sepsis (R65.2-) and any associated acute organ dysfunction.

g. **Stillbirth**

Code P95, Stillbirth, is only for use in institutions that maintain separate records for stillbirths. No other code should be used with P95. Code P95 should not be used on the mother's record.

17. **Chapter 17: Congenital malformations, deformations, and chromosomal abnormalities (Q00-Q99)**

Assign an appropriate code(s) from categories Q00-Q99, Congenital malformations, deformations, and chromosomal abnormalities when a malformation/deformation or chromosomal abnormality is documented. A malformation/deformation/or chromosomal abnormality may be the principal/first-listed diagnosis on a record or a secondary diagnosis.

When a malformation/deformation/or chromosomal abnormality does not have a unique code assignment, assign additional code(s) for any manifestations that may be present.

When the code assignment specifically identifies the malformation/deformation/or chromosomal abnormality, manifestations that are an inherent component of the anomaly should not be coded separately. Additional codes should be assigned for manifestations that are not an inherent component.

Codes from Chapter 17 may be used throughout the life of the patient. If a congenital malformation or deformity has been corrected, a personal history code should be used to identify the history of the malformation or deformity. Although present at birth, malformation/deformation/or chromosomal abnormality may not be identified until later in life. Whenever the condition is diagnosed by the physician, it is appropriate to assign a code from codes Q00-Q99.For the birth admission, the appropriate code from category Z38, Liveborn infants, according to place of birth and type of delivery, should be sequenced as the principal diagnosis, followed by any congenital anomaly codes, Q00- Q99.

18. **Chapter 18: Symptoms, signs, and abnormal clinical and laboratory findings, not elsewhere classified (R00-R99)**

Chapter 18 includes symptoms, signs, abnormal results of clinical or other investigative procedures, and ill-defined conditions regarding which no diagnosis classifiable elsewhere is recorded. Signs and symptoms that point to a specific diagnosis have been assigned to a category in other chapters of the classification.

a. **Use of symptom codes**

Codes that describe symptoms and signs are acceptable for reporting purposes when a related definitive diagnosis has not been established (confirmed) by the provider.

b. **Use of a symptom code with a definitive diagnosis code**

Codes for signs and symptoms may be reported in addition to a related definitive diagnosis when the sign or symptom is not routinely associated with that diagnosis, such as the various signs and symptoms associated with complex syndromes. The definitive diagnosis code should be sequenced before the symptom code.

Signs or symptoms that are associated routinely with a disease process should not be assigned as additional codes, unless otherwise instructed by the classification.

c. **Combination codes that include symptoms**

ICD-10-CM contains a number of combination codes that identify both the definitive diagnosis and common symptoms of that diagnosis. When using one of these combination codes, an additional code should not be assigned for the symptom.

d. **Repeated falls**

Code R29.6, Repeated falls, is for use for encounters when a patient has recently fallen and the reason for the fall is being investigated.

Code Z91.81, History of falling, is for use when a patient has fallen in the past and is at risk for future falls. When appropriate, both codes R29.6 and Z91.81 may be assigned together.

e. **Coma scale**

The coma scale codes (R40.2-) can be used in conjunction with traumatic brain injury codes, acute cerebrovascular disease or sequelae of cerebrovascular disease codes. These codes are primarily for use by trauma registries, but they may be used in any setting where this information is collected. The coma scale codes should be sequenced after the diagnosis code(s).

These codes, one from each subcategory, are needed to complete the scale. The 7th character indicates when the scale was recorded. The 7th character should match for all three codes.

At a minimum, report the initial score documented on presentation at your facility. This may be a score from the emergency medicine technician (EMT) or in the emergency department. If desired, a facility may choose to capture multiple coma scale scores.

Assign code R40.24, Glasgow coma scale, total score, when only the total score is documented in the medical record and not the individual score(s).

f. **Functional quadriplegia**

Functional quadriplegia (code R53.2) is the lack of ability to use one's limbs or to ambulate due to extreme debility. It is not associated with neurologic deficit or injury, and code R53.2 should not be used for cases of neurologic quadriplegia. It should only be assigned if functional quadriplegia is specifically documented in the medical record.

g. **SIRS due to Non-Infectious Process**

The systemic inflammatory response syndrome (SIRS) can develop as a result of certain non-infectious disease processes, such as trauma, malignant neoplasm, or pancreatitis. When SIRS is documented with a noninfectious condition, and no subsequent infection is documented, the code for the underlying condition, such as an injury, should be assigned, followed by code R65.10, Systemic inflammatory response syndrome (SIRS) of non-infectious origin without acute organ dysfunction, or code R65.11, Systemic inflammatory response syndrome (SIRS) of non-infectious origin with acute organ dysfunction. If an associated acute organ dysfunction is documented, the appropriate code(s) for the specific type of organ dysfunction(s) should be assigned in addition to code R65.11. If acute organ dysfunction is documented, but it cannot be determined if the acute organ dysfunction is associated with SIRS or due to another condition (e.g., directly due to the trauma), the provider should be queried.

h. Death NOS

Code R99, Ill-defined and unknown cause of mortality, is only for use in the very limited circumstance when a patient who has already died is brought into an emergency department or other healthcare facility and is pronounced dead upon arrival. It does not represent the discharge disposition of death.

19. Chapter 19: Injury, poisoning, and certain other consequences of external causes (S00-T88)

a. Application of 7th Characters in Chapter 19

Most categories in chapter 19 have a 7th character requirement for each applicable code. Most categories in this chapter have three 7th character values (with the exception of fractures): A, initial encounter, D, subsequent encounter and S, sequela. Categories for traumatic fractures have additional 7th character values.

7th character "A", initial encounter is used while the patient is receiving active treatment for the condition. Examples of active treatment are: surgical treatment, emergency department encounter, and evaluation and treatment by a new physician.

7th character "D" subsequent encounter is used for encounters after the patient has received active treatment of the condition and is receiving routine care for the condition during the healing or recovery phase. Examples of subsequent care are: cast change or removal, removal of external or internal fixation device, medication adjustment, other aftercare and follow up visits following treatment of the injury or condition.

The aftercare Z codes should not be used for aftercare for conditions such as injuries or poisonings, where 7th characters are provided to identify subsequent care. For example, for aftercare of an injury, assign the acute injury code with the 7th character "D" (subsequent encounter).

7th character "S", sequela, is for use for complications or conditions that arise as a direct result of a condition, such as scar formation after a burn. The scars are sequelae of the burn. When using 7th character "S", it is necessary to use both the injury code that precipitated the sequela and the code for the sequela itself. The "S" is added only to the injury code, not the sequela code. The 7th character "S" identifies the injury responsible for the sequela. The specific type of sequela (e.g. scar) is sequenced first, followed by the injury code.

b. Coding of Injuries

When coding injuries, assign separate codes for each injury unless a combination code is provided, in which case the combination code is assigned. Code T07, Unspecified multiple injuries should not be assigned in the inpatient setting unless information for a more specific code is not available. Traumatic injury codes (S00-T14.9) are not to be used for normal, healing surgical wounds or to identify complications of surgical wounds.

The code for the most serious injury, as determined by the provider and the focus of treatment, is sequenced first.

1) Superficial injuries

Superficial injuries such as abrasions or contusions are not coded when associated with more severe injuries of the same site.

2) Primary injury with damage to nerves/blood vessels

When a primary injury results in minor damage to peripheral nerves or blood vessels, the primary injury is sequenced first with additional code(s) for injuries to nerves and spinal cord (such as category S04), and/or injury to blood vessels (such as category S15). When the primary injury is to the blood vessels or nerves, that injury should be sequenced first.

c. Coding of Traumatic Fractures

The principles of multiple coding of injuries should be followed in coding fractures. Fractures of specified sites are coded individually by site in accordance with both the provisions within categories S02, S12, S22, S32, S42, S49, S52, S59, S62, S72, S79, S82, S89, S92 and the level of detail furnished by medical record content.

A fracture not indicated as open or closed should be coded to closed. A fracture not indicated whether displaced or not displaced should be coded to displaced.

More specific guidelines are as follows:

1) **Initial vs. Subsequent Encounter for Fractures**

Traumatic fractures are coded using the appropriate 7th character for initial encounter (A, B, C) while the patient is receiving active treatment for the fracture. Examples of active treatment are: surgical treatment, emergency department encounter, and evaluation and treatment by a new physician. The appropriate 7th character for initial encounter should also be assigned for a patient who delayed seeking treatment for the fracture or nonunion.

Fractures are coded using the appropriate 7th character for subsequent care for encounters after the patient has completed active treatment of the fracture and is receiving routine care for the fracture during the healing or recovery phase. Examples of fracture aftercare are: cast change or removal, removal of external or internal fixation device, medication adjustment, and follow-up visits following fracture treatment.

Care for complications of surgical treatment for fracture repairs during the healing or recovery phase should be coded with the appropriate complication codes.

Care of complications of fractures, such as malunion and nonunion, should be reported with the appropriate 7th character for subsequent care with nonunion (K, M, N,) or subsequent care with malunion (P, Q, R).

A code from category M80, not a traumatic fracture code, should be used for any patient with known osteoporosis who suffers a fracture, even if the patient had a minor fall or trauma, if that fall or trauma would not usually break a normal, healthy bone.

See Section I.C.13. Osteoporosis.

The aftercare Z codes should not be used for aftercare for traumatic fractures. For aftercare of a traumatic fracture, assign the acute fracture code with the appropriate 7th character.

2) **Multiple fractures sequencing**

Multiple fractures are sequenced in accordance with the severity of the fracture.

d. **Coding of Burns and Corrosions**

The ICD-10-CM makes a distinction between burns and corrosions. The burn codes are for thermal burns, except sunburns, that come from a heat source, such as a fire or hot appliance. The burn codes are also for burns resulting from electricity and radiation. Corrosions are burns due to chemicals. The guidelines are the same for burns and corrosions.

Current burns (T20-T25) are classified by depth, extent and by agent (X code). Burns are classified by depth as first degree (erythema), second degree (blistering), and third degree (full-thickness involvement). Burns of the eye and internal organs (T26-T28) are classified by site, but not by degree.

1) **Sequencing of burn and related condition codes**

Sequence first the code that reflects the highest degree of burn when more than one burn is present.

a. When the reason for the admission or encounter is for treatment of external multiple burns, sequence first the code that reflects the burn of the highest degree.

b. When a patient has both internal and external burns, the circumstances of admission govern the selection of the principal diagnosis or first-listed diagnosis.

c. When a patient is admitted for burn injuries and other related conditions such as smoke inhalation and/or respiratory failure, the circumstances of admission govern the selection of the principal or first-listed diagnosis.

2) Burns of the same local site

Classify burns of the same local site (three-character category level, T20-T28) but of different degrees to the subcategory identifying the highest degree recorded in the diagnosis.

3) Non-healing burns

Non-healing burns are coded as acute burns.
Necrosis of burned skin should be coded as a non-healed burn.

4) Infected Burn

For any documented infected burn site, use an additional code for the infection.

5) Assign separate codes for each burn site

When coding burns, assign separate codes for each burn site. Category T30, Burn and corrosion, body region unspecified is extremely vague and should rarely be used.

6) Burns and Corrosions Classified According to Extent of Body Surface Involved

Assign codes from category T31, Burns classified according to extent of body surface involved, or T32, Corrosions classified according to extent of body surface involved, when the site of the burn is not specified or when there is a need for additional data. It is advisable to use category T31 as additional coding when needed to provide data for evaluating burn mortality, such as that needed by burn units. It is also advisable to use category T31 as an additional code for reporting purposes when there is mention of a third-degree burn involving 20 percent or more of the body surface.

Categories T31 and T32 are based on the classic "rule of nines" in estimating body surface involved: head and neck are assigned nine percent, each arm nine percent, each leg 18 percent, the anterior trunk 18 percent, posterior trunk 18 percent, and genitalia one percent. Providers may change these percentage assignments where necessary to accommodate infants and children who have proportionately larger heads than adults, and patients who have large buttocks, thighs, or abdomen that involve burns.

7) Encounters for treatment of sequela of burns

Encounters for the treatment of the late effects of burns or corrosions (i.e., scars or joint contractures) should be coded with a burn or corrosion code with the 7th character "S" for sequela.

8) Sequelae with a late effect code and current burn

When appropriate, both a code for a current burn or corrosion with 7th character "A" or "D" and a burn or corrosion code with 7th character "S" may be assigned on the same record (when both a current burn and sequelae of an old burn exist). Burns and corrosions do not heal at the same rate and a current healing wound may still exist with sequela of a healed burn or corrosion.

9) Use of an external cause code with burns and corrosions

An external cause code should be used with burns and corrosions to identify the source and intent of the burn, as well as the place where it occurred.

e. Adverse Effects, Poisoning, Underdosing and Toxic Effects

Codes in categories T36-T65 are combination codes that include the substance that was taken as well as the intent. No additional external cause code is required for poisonings, toxic effects, adverse effects and underdosing codes.

1) **Do not code directly from the Table of Drugs**

   Do not code directly from the Table of Drugs and Chemicals. Always refer back to the Tabular List.

2) **Use as many codes as necessary to describe**

   Use as many codes as necessary to describe completely all drugs, medicinal or biological substances.

3) **If the same code would describe the causative agent**

   If the same code would describe the causative agent for more than one adverse reaction, poisoning, toxic effect or underdosing, assign the code only once.

4) **If two or more drugs, medicinal or biological substances**

   If two or more drugs, medicinal or biological substances are reported, code each individually unless **a** combination code is listed in the Table of Drugs and Chemicals.

5) **The occurrence of drug toxicity is classified in ICD-10-CM as follows:**

   (a) **Adverse Effect**

   When coding an adverse effect of a drug that has been correctly prescribed and properly administered, assign the appropriate code for the nature of the adverse effect followed by the appropriate code for the adverse effect of the drug (T36-T50). The code for the drug should have a 5th or 6th character "5" (for example T36.0X5-) Examples of the nature of an adverse effect are tachycardia, delirium, gastrointestinal hemorrhaging, vomiting, hypokalemia, hepatitis, renal failure, or respiratory failure.

   (b) **Poisoning**

   When coding a poisoning or reaction to the improper use of a medication (e.g., overdose, wrong substance given or taken in error, wrong route of administration), first assign the appropriate code from categories T36-T50. The poisoning codes have an associated intent as their 5th or 6th character (accidental, intentional self-harm, assault and undetermined. Use additional code(s) for all manifestations of poisonings.

   If there is also a diagnosis of abuse or dependence of the substance, the abuse or dependence is assigned as an additional code.

   Examples of poisoning include:

   (i) Error was made in drug prescription

   Errors made in drug prescription or in the administration of the drug by provider, nurse, patient, or other person.

   (ii) Overdose of a drug intentionally taken

   If an overdose of a drug was intentionally taken or administered and resulted in drug toxicity, it would be coded as a poisoning.

   (iii) Nonprescribed drug taken with correctly prescribed and properly administered drug

   If a nonprescribed drug or medicinal agent was taken in combination with a correctly prescribed and properly administered drug, any drug toxicity or other reaction resulting from the interaction of the two drugs would be classified as a poisoning.

   (iv) Interaction of drug(s) and alcohol

   When a reaction results from the interaction of a drug(s) and alcohol, this would be classified as poisoning.

See Section I.C.4. if poisoning is the result of insulin pump malfunctions.

(c) Underdosing

Underdosing refers to taking less of a medication than is prescribed by a provider or a manufacturer's instruction. For underdosing, assign the code from categories T36-T50 (fifth or sixth character "6").

Codes for underdosing should never be assigned as principal or first-listed codes. If a patient has a relapse or exacerbation of the medical condition for which the drug is prescribed because of the reduction in dose, then the medical condition itself should be coded.

Noncompliance (Z91.12-, Z91.13-) or complication of care (Y63.6-Y63.9) codes are to be used with an underdosing code to indicate intent, if known.

(d) Toxic Effects

When a harmful substance is ingested or comes in contact with a person, this is classified as a toxic effect. The toxic effect codes are in categories T51-T65.

Toxic effect codes have an associated intent: accidental, intentional self-harm, assault and undetermined.

f. Adult and child abuse, neglect and other maltreatment

Sequence first the appropriate code from categories T74.- (Adult and child abuse, neglect and other maltreatment, confirmed) or T76.-(Adult and child abuse, neglect and other maltreatment, suspected) for abuse, neglect and other maltreatment, followed by any accompanying mental health or injury code(s).

If the documentation in the medical record states abuse or neglect it is coded as confirmed (T74.-). It is coded as suspected if it is documented as suspected (T76.-).

For cases of confirmed abuse or neglect an external cause code from the assault section (X92-Y08) should be added to identify the cause of any physical injuries. A perpetrator code (Y07) should be added when the perpetrator of the abuse is known. For suspected cases of abuse or neglect, do not report external cause or perpetrator code.

If a suspected case of abuse, neglect or mistreatment is ruled out during an encounter code Z04.71, Encounter for examination and observation following alleged physical adult abuse, ruled out, or code Z04.72, Encounter for examination and observation following alleged child physical abuse, ruled out, should be used, not a code from T76.

If a suspected case of alleged rape or sexual abuse is ruled out during an encounter code Z04.41, Encounter for examination and observation following alleged physical adult abuse, ruled out, or code Z04.42, Encounter for examination and observation following alleged rape or sexual abuse, ruled out, should be used, not a code from T76.

See Section I.C.15. Abuse in a pregnant patient.

g. Complications of care

1) General guidelines for complications of care

(a) Documentation of complications of care

See Section I.B.16. for information on documentation of complications of care.

2) Pain due to medical devices

Pain associated with devices, implants or grafts left in a surgical site (for example painful hip prosthesis) is assigned to the appropriate code(s) found in Chapter 19, Injury, poisoning, and certain other consequences of external causes. Specific codes for pain due to medical devices are found in the T code section of the

ICD-10-CM. Use additional code(s) from category G89 to identify acute or chronic pain due to presence of the device, implant or graft (G89.18 or G89.28).

3) Transplant complications

(a) Transplant complications other than kidney

Codes under category T86, Complications of transplanted organs and tissues, are for use for both complications and rejection of transplanted organs. A transplant complication code is only assigned if the complication affects the function of the transplanted organ. Two codes are required to fully describe a transplant complication: the appropriate code from category T86 and a secondary code that identifies the complication.

Pre-existing conditions or conditions that develop after the transplant are not coded as complications unless they affect the function of the transplanted organs.

See I.C.21. for transplant organ removal status See I.C.2. for malignant neoplasm associated with transplanted organ.

(b) Kidney transplant complications

Patients who have undergone kidney transplant may still have some form of chronic kidney disease (CKD) because the kidney transplant may not fully restore kidney function. Code T86.1- should be assigned for documented complications of a kidney transplant, such as transplant failure or rejection or other transplant complication. Code T86.1- should not be assigned for post kidney transplant patients who have chronic kidney (CKD) unless a transplant complication such as transplant failure or rejection is documented. If the documentation is unclear as to whether the patient has a complication of the transplant, query the provider.

Conditions that affect the function of the transplanted kidney, other than CKD, should be assigned a code from subcategory T86.1, Complications of transplanted organ, Kidney, and a secondary code that identifies the complication.

For patients with CKD following a kidney transplant, but who do not have a complication such as failure or rejection, *see section I.C.14. Chronic kidney disease and kidney transplant status*.

4) Complication codes that include the external cause

As with certain other T codes, some of the complications of care codes have the external cause included in the code. The code includes the nature of the complication as well as the type of procedure that caused the complication. No external cause code indicating the type of procedure is necessary for these codes.

5) Complications of care codes within the body system chapters

Intraoperative and postprocedural complication codes are found within the body system chapters with codes specific to the organs and structures of that body system. These codes should be sequenced first, followed by a code(s) for the specific complication, if applicable.

20. Chapter 20: External Causes of Morbidity (V00-Y99)

The external causes of morbidity codes should never be sequenced as the first-listed or principal diagnosis.

External cause codes are intended to provide data for injury research and evaluation of injury prevention strategies. These codes capture how the injury or health condition happened (cause), the intent (unintentional or accidental; or intentional, such as suicide or assault), the place where the event occurred the activity of the patient at the time of the event, and the person's status (e.g., civilian, military).

There is no national requirement for mandatory ICD-10-CM external cause code reporting. Unless a provider is subject to a state-based external cause code reporting mandate or these codes are required by a particular payer, reporting of ICD-10-CM codes in Chapter 20, External Causes of Morbidity, is not required. In the absence of a mandatory reporting requirement, providers are encouraged to voluntarily report external cause codes, as they provide valuable data for injury research and evaluation of injury prevention strategies.

a. General External Cause Coding Guidelines

1) Used with any code in the range of A00.0-T88.9, Z00-Z99

An external cause code may be used with any code in the range of A00.0-T88.9, Z00-Z99, classification that is a health condition due to an external cause. Though they are most applicable to injuries, they are also valid for use with such things as infections or diseases due to an external source, and other health conditions, such as a heart attack that occurs during strenuous physical activity.

2) External cause code used for length of treatment

Assign the external cause code, with the appropriate 7th character (initial encounter, subsequent encounter or sequela) for each encounter for which the injury or condition is being treated.

3) Use the full range of external cause codes

Use the full range of external cause codes to completely describe the cause, the intent, the place of occurrence, and if applicable, the activity of the patient at the time of the event, and the patient's status, for all injuries, and other health conditions due to an external cause.

4) Assign as many external cause codes as necessary

Assign as many external cause codes as necessary to fully explain each cause. If only one external code can be recorded, assign the code most related to the principal diagnosis.

5) The selection of the appropriate external cause code

The selection of the appropriate external cause code is guided by the Alphabetic Index of External Causes and by Inclusion and Exclusion notes in the Tabular List.

6) External cause code can never be a principal diagnosis

An external cause code can never be a principal (first-listed) diagnosis.

7) Combination external cause codes

Certain of the external cause codes are combination codes that identify sequential events that result in an injury, such as a fall which results in striking against an object. The injury may be due to either event or both. The combination external cause code used should correspond to the sequence of events regardless of which caused the most serious injury.

8) No external cause code needed in certain circumstances

No external cause code from Chapter 20 is needed if the external cause and intent are included in a code from another chapter (e.g. T36.0X1- Poisoning by penicillins, accidental (unintentional)).

b. Place of Occurrence Guideline

Codes from category Y92, Place of occurrence of the external cause, are secondary codes for use after other external cause codes to identify the location of the patient at the time of injury or other condition.

A place of occurrence code is used only once, at the initial encounter for treatment. No 7th characters are used for Y92. Only one code from Y92 should be recorded on a medical record.

Do not use place of occurrence code Y92.9 if the place is not stated or is not applicable.

c. Activity Code

Assign a code from category Y93, Activity code, to describe the activity of the patient at the time the injury or other health condition occurred.

An activity code is used only once, at the initial encounter for treatment. Only one code from Y93 should be recorded on a medical record.

The activity codes are not applicable to poisonings, adverse effects, misadventures or sequela .

Do not assign Y93.9, Unspecified activity, if the activity is not stated.

A code from category Y93 is appropriate for use with external cause and intent codes if identifying the activity provides additional information about the event.

d. Place of Occurrence, Activity, and Status Codes Used with other External Cause Code

When applicable, place of occurrence, activity, and external cause status codes are sequenced after the main external cause code(s). Regardless of the number of external cause codes assigned, there should be only one place of occurrence code, one activity code, and one external cause status code assigned to an encounter.

e. If the Reporting Format Limits the Number of External Cause Codes

If the reporting format limits the number of external cause codes that can be used in reporting clinical data, report the code for the cause/intent most related to the principal diagnosis. If the format permits capture of additional external cause codes, the cause/intent, including medical misadventures, of the additional events should be reported rather than the codes for place, activity, or external status.

f. Multiple External Cause Coding Guidelines

More than one external cause code is required to fully describe the external cause of an illness or injury. The assignment of external cause codes should be sequenced in the following priority:

If two or more events cause separate injuries, an external cause code should be assigned for each cause. The first-listed external cause code will be selected in the following order:

External codes for child and adult abuse take priority over all other external cause codes.

See Section I.C.19., Child and Adult abuse guidelines.

External cause codes for terrorism events take priority over all other external cause codes except child and adult abuse.

External cause codes for cataclysmic events take priority over all other external cause codes except child and adult abuse and terrorism.

External cause codes for transport accidents take priority over all other external cause codes except cataclysmic events, child and adult abuse and terrorism.

Activity and external cause status codes are assigned following all causal (intent) external cause codes.

The first-listed external cause code should correspond to the cause of the most serious diagnosis due to an assault, accident, or self-harm, following the order of hierarchy listed above.

g. Child and Adult Abuse Guideline

Adult and child abuse, neglect and maltreatment are classified as assault. Any of the assault codes may be used to indicate the external cause of any injury resulting from the confirmed abuse.

For confirmed cases of abuse, neglect and maltreatment, when the perpetrator is known, a code from Y07, Perpetrator of maltreatment and neglect, should accompany any other assault codes.

See Section I.C.19. Adult and child abuse, neglect and other maltreatment

h. Unknown or Undetermined Intent Guideline

If the intent (accident, self-harm, assault) of the cause of an injury or other condition is unknown or unspecified, code the intent as accidental intent. All transport accident categories assume accidental intent.

1) Use of undetermined intent

External cause codes for events of undetermined intent are only for use if the documentation in the record specifies that the intent cannot be determined.

i. Sequelae (Late Effects) of External Cause Guidelines

1) Sequelae external cause codes

Sequela are reported using the external cause code with the 7th character "S" for sequela. These codes should be used with any report of a late effect or sequela resulting from a previous injury.

2) Sequela external cause code with a related current injury

A sequela external cause code should never be used with a related current nature of injury code.

3) Use of sequela external cause codes for subsequent visits

Use a late effect external cause code for subsequent visits when a late effect of the initial injury is being treated. Do not use a late effect external cause code for subsequent visits for follow-up care (e.g., to assess healing, to receive rehabilitative therapy) of the injury when no late effect of the injury has been documented.

j. Terrorism Guidelines

1) Cause of injury identified by the Federal Government (FBI) as terrorism

When the cause of an injury is identified by the Federal Government (FBI) as terrorism, the first-listed external cause code should be a code from category Y38, Terrorism. The definition of terrorism employed by the FBI is found at the inclusion note at the beginning of category Y38. Use additional code for place of occurrence (Y92.-). More than one Y38 code may be assigned if the injury is the result of more than one mechanism of terrorism.

2) Cause of an injury is suspected to be the result of terrorism

When the cause of an injury is suspected to be the result of terrorism a code from category Y38 should not be assigned. Suspected cases should be classified as assault.

3) Code Y38.9, Terrorism, secondary effects

Assign code Y38.9, Terrorism, secondary effects, for conditions occurring subsequent to the terrorist event. This code should not be assigned for conditions that are due to the initial terrorist act.

It is acceptable to assign code Y38.9 with another code from Y38 if there is an injury due to the initial terrorist event and an injury that is a subsequent result of the terrorist event.

k. External cause status

A code from category Y99, External cause status, should be assigned whenever any other external cause code is assigned for an encounter, including an Activity code, except for the events noted below. Assign a code from category Y99, External cause status, to indicate the work status of the person at the time the event occurred. The status code indicates whether the event occurred during military activity, whether a non-military person was at work, whether an individual including a student or volunteer was involved in a non-work activity at the time of the causal event.

A code from Y99, External cause status, should be assigned, when applicable, with other external cause codes, such as transport accidents and falls. The external cause status codes are not applicable to poisonings, adverse effects, misadventures or late effects.

Do not assign a code from category Y99 if no other external cause codes (cause, activity) are applicable for the encounter.

An external cause status code is used only once, at the initial encounter for treatment. Only one code from Y99 should be recorded on a medical record.

Do not assign code Y99.9, Unspecified external cause status, if the status is not stated.

21. **Chapter 21: Factors influencing health status and contact with health services (Z00-Z99)**

    Note: The chapter specific guidelines provide additional information about the use of Z codes for specified encounters.

    a. **Use of Z codes in any healthcare setting**

    Z codes are for use in any healthcare setting. Z codes may be used as either a first-listed (principal diagnosis code in the inpatient setting) or secondary code, depending on the circumstances of the encounter. Certain Z codes may only be used as first-listed or principal diagnosis.

    b. **Z Codes indicate a reason for an encounter**

    Z codes are not procedure codes. A corresponding procedure code must accompany a Z code to describe any procedure performed.

    c. **Categories of Z Codes**

    1) **Contact/Exposure**

    Category Z20 indicates contact with, and suspected exposure to, communicable diseases. These codes are for patients who do not show any sign or symptom of a disease but are suspected to have been exposed to it by close personal contact with an infected individual or are in an area where a disease is epidemic.

    Category Z77, indicates contact with and suspected exposures hazardous to health.

    Contact/exposure codes may be used as a first-listed code to explain an encounter for testing, or, more commonly, as a secondary code to identify a potential risk.

    2) **Inoculations and vaccinations**

    Code Z23 is for encounters for inoculations and vaccinations. It indicates that a patient is being seen to receive a prophylactic inoculation against a disease. Procedure codes are required to identify the actual administration of the injection and the type(s) of immunizations given. Code Z23 may be used as a secondary code if the inoculation is given as a routine part of preventive health care, such as a well-baby visit.

    3) **Status**

    Status codes indicate that a patient is either a carrier of a disease or has the sequelae or residual of a past disease or condition. This includes such things as the presence of prosthetic or mechanical devices resulting from past treatment. A status code is informative, because the status may affect the course of treatment and its outcome. A status code is distinct from a history code. The history code indicates that the patient no longer has the condition.

    A status code should not be used with a diagnosis code from one of the body system chapters, if the diagnosis code includes the information provided by the status code. For example, code Z94.1, Heart transplant status, should not be used with a code from subcategory T86.2, Complications of heart transplant. The status code does not provide additional information. The complication code indicates that the patient is a heart transplant patient.

For encounters for weaning from a mechanical ventilator, assign a code from subcategory J96.1, Chronic respiratory failure, followed by code Z99.11, Dependence on respirator [ventilator] status.

The status Z codes/categories are:

Z14   Genetic carrier

Genetic carrier status indicates that a person carries a gene, associated with a particular disease, which may be passed to offspring who may develop that disease. The person does not have the disease and is not at risk of developing the disease.

Z15   Genetic susceptibility to disease

Genetic susceptibility indicates that a person has a gene that increases the risk of that person developing the disease.

Codes from category Z15 should not be used as principal or first-listed codes. If the patient has the condition to which he/she is susceptible, and that condition is the reason for the encounter, the code for the current condition should be sequenced first. If the patient is being seen for follow-up after completed treatment for this condition, and the condition no longer exists, a follow-up code should be sequenced first, followed by the appropriate personal history and genetic susceptibility codes. If the purpose of the encounter is genetic counseling associated with procreative management, code Z31.5, Encounter for genetic counseling, should be assigned as the first-listed code, followed by a code from category Z15. Additional codes should be assigned for any applicable family or personal history.

Z16   Resistance to antimicrobial drugs

This code indicates that a patient has a condition that is resistant to antimicrobial drug treatment. Sequence the infection code first.

Z17   Estrogen receptor status
Z18   Retained foreign body fragments
Z21   Asymptomatic HIV infection status

This code indicates that a patient has tested positive for HIV but has manifested no signs or symptoms of the disease.

Z22   Carrier of infectious disease

Carrier status indicates that a person harbors the specific organisms of a disease without manifest symptoms and is capable of transmitting the infection.

Z28.3   Underimmunization status Z33.1 Pregnant state, incidental

This code is a secondary code only for use when the pregnancy is in no way complicating the reason for visit. Otherwise, a code from the obstetric chapter is required.

Z66   Do not resuscitate

This code may be used when it is documented by the provider that a patient is on do not resuscitate status at any time during the stay.

Z67   Blood type
Z68   Body mass index (BMI)
Z74.01   Bed confinement status
Z76.82   Awaiting organ transplant status
Z78   Other specified health status

Code Z78.1, Physical restraint status, may be used when it is documented by the provider that a patient has been put in restraints during the current encounter. Please note that this code should not be reported when it is documented by the provider that a patient is temporarily restrained during a procedure.

Z79   Long-term (current) drug therapy

Codes from this category indicate a patient's continuous use of a prescribed drug (including such things as aspirin therapy) for the long-term treatment of a condition or for prophylactic use. It is not for use for patients who have addictions to drugs. This subcategory is not for use of medications for detoxification or maintenance programs to prevent withdrawal symptoms in patients with drug dependence (e.g., methadone maintenance for opiate dependence). Assign the appropriate code for the drug dependence instead.

Assign a code from Z79 if the patient is receiving a medication for an extended period as a prophylactic measure (such as for the prevention of deep vein thrombosis) or as treatment of a chronic condition (such as arthritis) or a disease requiring a lengthy course of treatment (such as cancer). Do not assign a code from category Z79 for medication being administered for a brief period of time to treat an acute illness or injury (such as a course of antibiotics to treat acute bronchitis).

Z88   Allergy status to drugs, medicaments and biological substances

Except: Z88.9, Allergy status to unspecified drugs, medicaments and biological substances status

Z89   Acquired absence of limb
Z90   Acquired absence of organs, not elsewhere classified
Z91.0 Allergy status, other than to drugs and biological substances
Z92.82 Status post administration of tPA (rtPA) in a different facility within the last 24 hours prior to admission to a current facility

Assign code Z92.82, Status post administration of tPA (rtPA) in a different facility within the last 24 hours prior to admission to current facility, as a secondary diagnosis when a patient is received by transfer into a facility and documentation indicates they were administered tissue plasminogen activator (tPA) within the last 24 hours prior to admission to the current facility.

This guideline applies even if the patient is still receiving the tPA at the time they are received into the current facility.

The appropriate code for the condition for which the tPA was administered (such as cerebrovascular disease or myocardial infarction) should be assigned first.

Code Z92.82 is only applicable to the receiving facility record and not to the transferring facility record.

Z93   Artificial opening status
Z94   Transplanted organ and tissue status
Z95   Presence of cardiac and vascular implants and grafts
Z96   Presence of other functional implants
Z97   Presence of other devices
Z98   Other postprocedural states

Assign code Z98.85, Transplanted organ removal status, to indicate that a transplanted organ has been previously removed. This code should not be assigned for the encounter in which the transplanted organ is removed. The complication necessitating removal of the transplant organ should be assigned for that encounter.

See section I.C19. for information on the coding of organ transplant complications.

Z99   Dependence on enabling machines and devices, not elsewhere classified

Note: Categories Z89-Z90 and Z93-Z99 are for use only if there are no complications or malfunctions of the organ or tissue replaced, the amputation site or the equipment on which the patient is dependent.

4)   **History (of)**

There are two types of history Z codes, personal and family. Personal history codes explain a patient's past medical condition that no longer exists and is not receiving any treatment, but that has the potential for recurrence, and therefore may require continued monitoring.

Family history codes are for use when a patient has a family member(s) who has had a particular disease that causes the patient to be at higher risk of also contracting the disease.

Personal history codes may be used in conjunction with follow-up codes and family history codes may be used in conjunction with screening codes to explain the need for a test or procedure. History codes are also acceptable on any medical record regardless of the reason for visit. A history of an illness, even if no longer present, is important information that may alter the type of treatment ordered.

The history Z code categories are:

Z80   Family history of primary malignant neoplasm
Z81   Family history of mental and behavioral disorders
Z82   Family history of certain disabilities and chronic diseases (leading to disablement)
Z83   Family history of other specific disorders
Z84   Family history of other conditions
Z85   Personal history of malignant neoplasm
Z86   Personal history of certain other diseases
Z87   Personal history of other diseases and conditions
Z91.4   Personal history of psychological trauma, not elsewhere classified
Z91.5   Personal history of self-harm
Z91.8   Other specified personal risk factors, not elsewhere classified Exception:
Z91.83 Wandering in diseases classified elsewhere
Z92   Personal history of medical treatment
        Except: Z92.0, Personal history of contraception
        Except: Z92.82, Status post administration of tPA (rtPA) in a different facility within the last 24
        hours prior to admission to a current facility

5) Screening

Screening is the testing for disease or disease precursors in seemingly well individuals so that early detection and treatment can be provided for those who test positive for the disease (e.g., screening mammogram).

The testing of a person to rule out or confirm a suspected diagnosis because the patient has some sign or symptom is a diagnostic examination, not a screening. In these cases, the sign or symptom is used to explain the reason for the test.

A screening code may be a first-listed code if the reason for the visit is specifically the screening exam. It may also be used as an additional code if the screening is done during an office visit for other health problems. A screening code is not necessary if the screening is inherent to a routine examination, such as a pap smear done during a routine pelvic examination.

Should a condition be discovered during the screening then the code for the condition may be assigned as an additional diagnosis.

The Z code indicates that a screening exam is planned. A procedure code is required to confirm that the screening was performed.

The screening Z codes/categories:

Z11   Encounter for screening for infectious and parasitic diseases
Z12   Encounter for screening for malignant neoplasms
Z13   Encounter for screening for other diseases and disorders
        Except: Z13.9, Encounter for screening, unspecified Z36 Encounter for antenatal screening for
        mother

6) Observation

There are two observation Z code categories. They are for use in very limited circumstances when a person is being observed for a suspected condition that is ruled out. The observation codes are not for use if an injury or illness or any signs or symptoms related to the suspected condition are present. In such cases the diagnosis/symptom code is used with the corresponding external cause code.

The observation codes are to be used as principal diagnosis only. Additional codes may be used in addition to the observation code but only if they are unrelated to the suspected condition being observed.

Codes from subcategory Z03.7, Encounter for suspected maternal and fetal conditions ruled out, may either be used as a first-listed or as an additional code assignment depending on the case. They are for use in very limited circumstances on a maternal record when an encounter is for a suspected maternal or fetal condition that is ruled out during that encounter (for example, a maternal or fetal condition may be suspected due to an abnormal test result). These codes should not be used when the condition is confirmed. In those cases, the confirmed condition should be coded. In addition, these codes are not for use if an illness or any signs or symptoms related to the suspected condition or problem are present. In such cases the diagnosis/symptom code is used.

Additional codes may be used in addition to the code from subcategory Z03.7, but only if they are unrelated to the suspected condition being evaluated.

Codes from subcategory Z03.7 may not be used for encounters for antenatal screening of mother. *See Section I.C.21. Screening.*

For encounters for suspected fetal condition that are inconclusive following testing and evaluation, assign the appropriate code from category O35, O36, O40 or O41. The observation Z code categories:

Z03   Encounter for medical observation for suspected diseases and conditions ruled out
Z04   Encounter for examination and observation for other reasons
        Except: Z04.9, Encounter for examination and observation for unspecified reason

7) Aftercare

Aftercare visit codes cover situations when the initial treatment of a disease has been performed and the patient requires continued care during the healing or recovery phase, or for the long-term consequences of the disease. The aftercare Z code should not be used if treatment is directed at a current, acute disease. The diagnosis code is to be used in these cases. Exceptions to this rule are codes Z51.0, Encounter for antineoplastic radiation therapy, and codes from subcategory Z51.1, Encounter for antineoplastic chemotherapy and immunotherapy. These codes are to be first-listed, followed by the diagnosis code when a patient's encounter is solely to receive radiation therapy, chemotherapy, or immunotherapy for the treatment of a neoplasm. If the reason for the encounter is more than one type of antineoplastic therapy, code Z51.0 and a code from subcategory Z51.1 may be assigned together, in which case one of these codes would be reported as a secondary diagnosis.

The aftercare Z codes should also not be used for aftercare for injuries. For aftercare of an injury, assign the acute injury code with the appropriate 7th character (for subsequent encounter).

The aftercare codes are generally first-listed to explain the specific reason for the encounter. An aftercare code may be used as an additional code when some type of aftercare is provided in addition to the reason for admission and no diagnosis code is applicable. An example of this would be the closure of a colostomy during an encounter for treatment of another condition.

Aftercare codes should be used in conjunction with other aftercare codes or diagnosis codes to provide better detail on the specifics of an aftercare encounter visit, unless otherwise directed by the classification. Should a patient receive multiple types of antineoplastic therapy during the same encounter, code Z51.0, Encounter for antineoplastic radiation therapy, and codes from subcategory Z51.1, Encounter for antineoplastic chemotherapy and immunotherapy, may be used together on a record. The sequencing of multiple aftercare codes depends on the circumstances of the encounter.

Certain aftercare Z code categories need a secondary diagnosis code to describe the resolving condition or sequelae. For others, the condition is included in the code title.

Additional Z code aftercare category terms include fitting and adjustment, and attention to artificial openings.

Status Z codes may be used with aftercare Z codes to indicate the nature of the aftercare. For example code Z95.1, Presence of aortocoronary bypass graft, may be used with code Z48.812,

Encounter for surgical aftercare following surgery on the circulatory system, to indicate the surgery for which the aftercare is being performed. A status code should not be used when the aftercare code indicates the type of status, such as using Z43.0, Encounter for attention to tracheostomy, with Z93.0, Tracheostomy status.

The aftercare Z category/codes:

Z42	Encounter for plastic and reconstructive surgery following medical procedure or healed injury
Z43	Encounter for attention to artificial openings
Z44	Encounter for fitting and adjustment of external prosthetic device
Z45	Encounter for adjustment and management of implanted device
Z46	Encounter for fitting and adjustment of other devices
Z47	Orthopedic aftercare
Z48	Encounter for other postprocedural aftercare
Z49	Encounter for care involving renal dialysis
Z51	Encounter for other aftercare

8) Follow-up

The follow-up codes are used to explain continuing surveillance following completed treatment of a disease, condition, or injury. They imply that the condition has been fully treated and no longer exists. They should not be confused with aftercare codes, or injury codes with a 7th character for subsequent encounter, that explain ongoing care of a healing condition or its sequelae. Follow-up codes may be used in conjunction with history codes to provide the full picture of the healed condition and its treatment. The follow-up code is sequenced first, followed by the history code.

A follow-up code may be used to explain multiple visits. Should a condition be found to have recurred on the follow-up visit, then the diagnosis code for the condition should be assigned in place of the follow-up code.

The follow-up Z code categories:

Z08	Encounter for follow-up examination after completed treatment for malignant neoplasm
Z09	Encounter for follow-up examination after completed treatment for conditions other than malignant neoplasm
Z39	Encounter for maternal postpartum care and examination

9) Donor

Codes in category Z52, Donors of organs and tissues, are used for living individuals who are donating blood or other body tissue. These codes are only for individuals donating for others, not for self-donations. They are not used to identify cadaveric donations.

10) Counseling

Counseling Z codes are used when a patient or family member receives assistance in the aftermath of an illness or injury, or when support is required in coping with family or social problems. They are not used in conjunction with a diagnosis code when the counseling component of care is considered integral to standard treatment.

The counseling Z codes/categories:

Z30.0	Encounter for general counseling and advice on contraception
Z31.5	Encounter for genetic counseling
Z31.6	Encounter for general counseling and advice on procreation

Z32.2   Encounter for childbirth instruction
Z32.3   Encounter for childcare instruction
Z69   Encounter for mental health services for victim and perpetrator of abuse
Z70   Counseling related to sexual attitude, behavior and orientation
Z71   Persons encountering health services for other counseling and medical advice, not elsewhere
        classified
Z76.81 Expectant mother prebirth pediatrician visit

11) Encounters for Obstetrical and Reproductive Services

See Section I.C.15. Pregnancy, Childbirth, and the Puerperium, for further instruction on the use of these codes.

Z codes for pregnancy are for use in those circumstances when none of the problems or complications included in the codes from the Obstetrics chapter exist (a routine prenatal visit or postpartum care). Codes in category Z34, Encounter for supervision of normal pregnancy, are always first-listed and are not to be used with any other code from the OB chapter.

Codes in category Z3A, Weeks of gestation, may be assigned to provide additional information about the pregnancy. The date of the admission should be used to determine weeks of gestation for inpatient admissions that encompass more than one gestational week.

The outcome of delivery, category Z37, should be included on all maternal delivery records. It is always a secondary code. Codes in category Z37 should not be used on the newborn record.

Z codes for family planning (contraceptive) or procreative management and counseling should be included on an obstetric record either during the pregnancy or the postpartum stage, if applicable.

Z codes/categories for obstetrical and reproductive services:

Z30   Encounter for contraceptive management
Z31   Encounter for procreative management
Z32.2   Encounter for childbirth instruction
Z32.3   Encounter for childcare instruction
Z33   Pregnant state
Z34   Encounter for supervision of normal pregnancy
Z36   Encounter for antenatal screening of mother
Z3A   Weeks of gestation
Z37   Outcome of delivery
Z39   Encounter for maternal postpartum care and examination
Z76.81 Expectant mother prebirth pediatrician visit

12) Newborns and Infants

See Section I.C.16. Newborn (Perinatal) Guidelines, for further instruction on the use of these codes.

Newborn Z codes/categories:

Z76.1   Encounter for health supervision and care of foundling
Z00.1   Encounter for routine child health examination
Z38   Liveborn infants according to place of birth and type of delivery

13) Routine and administrative examinations

The Z codes allow for the description of encounters for routine examinations, such as, a general check-up, or, examinations for administrative purposes, such as, a pre-employment physical. The codes are not to be used if the examination is for diagnosis of a suspected condition or for treatment purposes. In such cases the diagnosis code is used. During a routine exam, should a diagnosis or condition be discovered, it should be coded as an additional code. Pre-existing and chronic conditions and history codes may also be included as additional codes as long as the examination is for administrative purposes and not focused on any particular condition.

Some of the codes for routine health examinations distinguish between "with" and "without" abnormal findings. Code assignment depends on the information that is known at the time the encounter is being coded. For example, if no abnormal findings were found during the examination, but the encounter is being coded before test results are back, it is acceptable to assign the code for "without abnormal findings." When assigning a code for "with abnormal findings," additional code(s) should be assigned to identify the specific abnormal finding(s).

Pre-operative examination and pre-procedural laboratory examination Z codes are for use only in those situations when a patient is being cleared for a procedure or surgery and no treatment is given.

The Z codes/categories for routine and administrative examinations:

Z00	Encounter for general examination without complaint, suspected or reported diagnosis
Z01	Encounter for other special examination without complaint, suspected or reported diagnosis
Z02	Encounter for administrative examination
	Except: Z02.9, Encounter for administrative examinations, unspecified
Z32.0	Encounter for pregnancy test

14) Miscellaneous Z codes

The miscellaneous Z codes capture a number of other health care encounters that do not fall into one of the other categories. Certain of these codes identify the reason for the encounter; others are for use as additional codes that provide useful information on circumstances that may affect a patient's care and treatment.

Prophylactic Organ Removal

For encounters specifically for prophylactic removal of an organ (such as prophylactic removal of breasts due to a genetic susceptibility to cancer or a family history of cancer), the principal or first-listed code should be a code from category Z40, Encounter for prophylactic surgery, followed by the appropriate codes to identify the associated risk factor (such as genetic susceptibility or family history).

If the patient has a malignancy of one site and is having prophylactic removal at another site to prevent either a new primary malignancy or metastatic disease, a code for the malignancy should also be assigned in addition to a code from subcategory Z40.0, Encounter for prophylactic surgery for risk factors related to malignant neoplasms. A Z40.0 code should not be assigned if the patient is having organ removal for treatment of a malignancy, such as the removal of the testes for the treatment of prostate cancer.

Miscellaneous Z codes/categories:

Z28	Immunization not carried out
	Except: Z28.3, Underimmunization status
Z40	Encounter for prophylactic surgery
Z41	Encounter for procedures for purposes other than remedying health state
	Except: Z41.9, Encounter for procedure for purposes other than remedying health state, unspecified
Z53	Persons encountering health services for specific procedures and treatment, not carried out
Z55	Problems related to education and literacy
Z56	Problems related to employment and unemployment
Z57	Occupational exposure to risk factors
Z58	Problems related to physical environment
Z59	Problems related to housing and economic circumstances
Z60	Problems related to social environment
Z62	Problems related to upbringing
Z63	Other problems related to primary support group, including family circumstances
Z64	Problems related to certain psychosocial circumstances
Z65	Problems related to other psychosocial circumstances
Z72	Problems related to lifestyle
Z73	Problems related to life management difficulty
Z74	Problems related to care provider dependency
	Except: Z74.01, Bed confinement status

Z75	Problems related to medical facilities and other health care
Z76.0	Encounter for issue of repeat prescription
Z76.3	Healthy person accompanying sick person
Z76.4	Other boarder to healthcare facility
Z76.5	Malingerer [conscious simulation]
Z91.1	Patient's noncompliance with medical treatment and regimen
Z91.83	Wandering in diseases classified elsewhere
Z91.89	Other specified personal risk factors, not elsewhere classified

15) Nonspecific Z codes

Certain Z codes are so non-specific, or potentially redundant with other codes in the classification, that there can be little justification for their use in the inpatient setting. Their use in the outpatient setting should be limited to those instances when there is no further documentation to permit more precise coding. Otherwise, any sign or symptom or any other reason for visit that is captured in another code should be used.

Nonspecific Z codes/categories:

Z02.9	Encounter for administrative examinations, unspecified
Z04.9	Encounter for examination and observation for unspecified reason
Z13.9	Encounter for screening, unspecified
Z41.9	Encounter for procedure for purposes other than remedying health state, unspecified
Z52.9	Donor of unspecified organ or tissue
Z86.59	Personal history of other mental and behavioral disorders
Z88.9	Allergy status to unspecified drugs, medicaments and biological substances status
Z92.0	Personal history of contraception

16) Z Codes That May Only be Principal/First-Listed Diagnosis

The following Z codes/categories may only be reported as the principal/first-listed diagnosis, except when there are multiple encounters on the same day and the medical records for the encounters are combined:

Z00	Encounter for general examination without complaint, suspected or reported diagnosis
Z01	Encounter for other special examination without complaint, suspected or reported diagnosis
Z02	Encounter for administrative examination
Z03	Encounter for medical observation for suspected diseases and conditions ruled out
Z04	Encounter for examination and observation for other reasons
Z33.2	Encounter for elective termination of pregnancy
Z31.81	Encounter for male factor infertility in female patient
Z31.82	Encounter for Rh incompatibility status
Z31.83	Encounter for assisted reproductive fertility procedure cycle
Z31.84	Encounter for fertility preservation procedure
Z34	Encounter for supervision of normal pregnancy
Z39	Encounter for maternal postpartum care and examination
Z38	Liveborn infants according to place of birth and type of delivery
Z42	Encounter for plastic and reconstructive surgery following medical procedure or healed injury
Z51.0	Encounter for antineoplastic radiation therapy
Z51.1	Encounter for antineoplastic chemotherapy and immunotherapy
Z52	Donors of organs and tissues Except: Z52.9, Donor of unspecified organ or tissue
Z76.1	Encounter for health supervision and care of foundling
Z76.2	Encounter for health supervision and care of other healthy infant and child
Z99.12	Encounter for respirator [ventilator] dependence during power failure

SECTION II: SELECTION OF PRINCIPAL DIAGNOSIS

The circumstances of inpatient admission always govern the selection of principal diagnosis.

The principal diagnosis is defined in the Uniform Hospital Discharge Data Set (UHDDS) as "that condition established after study to be chiefly responsible for occasioning the admission of the patient to the hospital for care."

The UHDDS definitions are used by hospitals to report inpatient data elements in a standardized manner. These data elements and their definitions can be found in the July 31, 1985, Federal Register (Vol. 50, No, 147), pp. 31038-40.

Since that time the application of the UHDDS definitions has been expanded to include all non-outpatient settings (acute care, short term, long term care and psychiatric hospitals; home health agencies; rehab facilities; nursing homes, etc).

In determining principal diagnosis, coding conventions in the ICD-10-CM, the Tabular List and Alphabetic Index take precedence over these official coding guidelines.
(See Section I.A., Conventions for the ICD-10-CM)

The importance of consistent, complete documentation in the medical record cannot be overemphasized. Without such documentation the application of all coding guidelines is a difficult, if not impossible, task.

A. Codes for symptoms, signs, and ill-defined conditions

Codes for symptoms, signs, and ill-defined conditions from Chapter 18 are not to be used as principal diagnosis when a related definitive diagnosis has been established.

B. Two or more interrelated conditions, each potentially meeting the definition for principal diagnosis.

When there are two or more interrelated conditions (such as diseases in the same ICD-10-CM chapter or manifestations characteristically associated with a certain disease) potentially meeting the definition of principal diagnosis, either condition may be sequenced first, unless the circumstances of the admission, the therapy provided, the Tabular List, or the Alphabetic Index indicate otherwise.

C. Two or more diagnoses that equally meet the definition for principal diagnosis

In the unusual instance when two or more diagnoses equally meet the criteria for principal diagnosis as determined by the circumstances of admission, diagnostic workup and/or therapy provided, and the Alphabetic Index, Tabular List, or another coding guidelines does not provide sequencing direction, any one of the diagnoses may be sequenced first.

D. Two or more comparative or contrasting conditions

In those rare instances when two or more contrasting or comparative diagnoses are documented as "either/or" (or similar terminology), they are coded as if the diagnoses were confirmed and the diagnoses are sequenced according to the circumstances of the admission. If no further determination can be made as to which diagnosis should be principal, either diagnosis may be sequenced first.

E. A symptom(s) followed by contrasting/comparative diagnoses

When a symptom(s) is followed by contrasting/comparative diagnoses, the symptom code is sequenced first. **However, if the symptom code is integral to the conditions listed, no code for the symptom is reported.** All the contrasting/comparative diagnoses should be coded as additional diagnoses.

F. Original treatment plan not carried out

Sequence as the principal diagnosis the condition, which after study occasioned the admission to the hospital, even though treatment may not have been carried out due to unforeseen circumstances.

G. Complications of surgery and other medical care

When the admission is for treatment of a complication resulting from surgery or other medical care, the complication code is sequenced as the principal diagnosis. If the complication is classified to the T80-T88 series and the code lacks the necessary specificity in describing the complication, an additional code for the specific complication should be assigned.

H. Uncertain Diagnosis

If the diagnosis documented at the time of discharge is qualified as "probable", "suspected", "likely", "questionable", "possible", or "still to be ruled out", or other similar terms indicating uncertainty, code the condition as if it existed or was established. The bases for these guidelines are the diagnostic workup, arrangements for further workup or observation, and initial therapeutic approach that correspond most closely with the established diagnosis.

Note: This guideline is applicable only to inpatient admissions to short-term, acute, long-term care and psychiatric hospitals.

I. Admission from Observation Unit

1. Admission Following Medical Observation

When a patient is admitted to an observation unit for a medical condition, which either worsens or does not improve, and is subsequently admitted as an inpatient of the same hospital for this same medical condition, the principal diagnosis would be the medical condition which led to the hospital admission.

2. Admission Following Post-Operative Observation

When a patient is admitted to an observation unit to monitor a condition (or complication) that develops following outpatient surgery, and then is subsequently admitted as an inpatient of the same hospital, hospitals should apply the Uniform Hospital Discharge Data Set (UHDDS) definition of principal diagnosis as "that condition established after study to be chiefly responsible for occasioning the admission of the patient to the hospital for care."

J. Admission from Outpatient Surgery

When a patient receives surgery in the hospital's outpatient surgery department and is subsequently admitted for continuing inpatient care at the same hospital, the following guidelines should be followed in selecting the principal diagnosis for the inpatient admission:

- If the reason for the inpatient admission is a complication, assign the complication as the principal diagnosis.

- If no complication, or other condition, is documented as the reason for the inpatient admission, assign the reason for the outpatient surgery as the principal diagnosis.

- If the reason for the inpatient admission is another condition unrelated to the surgery, assign the unrelated condition as the principal diagnosis.

K. Admissions/Encounters for Rehabilitation

When the purpose for the admission/encounter is rehabilitation, sequence first the code for the condition for which the service is being performed. For example, for an admission/encounter for rehabilitation for right-sided dominant hemiplegia following a cerebrovascular infarction, report code I69.351, Hemiplegia and hemiparesis following cerebral infarction affecting right dominant side, as the first-listed or principal diagnosis.

If the condition for which the rehabilitation service is no longer present, report the appropriate aftercare code as the first-listed or principal diagnosis. For example, if a patient with severe degenerative osteoarthritis of the hip, underwent hip replacement and the current encounter/admission is for rehabilitation, report code Z47.1, Aftercare following joint replacement surgery, as the first-listed or principal diagnosis.

See Section I.C.21.c.7, Factors influencing health states and contact with health services, Aftercare.

SECTION III: REPORTING ADDITIONAL DIAGNOSES

GENERAL RULES FOR OTHER (ADDITIONAL) DIAGNOSES

For reporting purposes the definition for "other diagnoses" is interpreted as additional conditions that affect patient care in terms of requiring:

clinical evaluation;
or therapeutic treatment;
or diagnostic procedures;
or extended length of hospital stay;
or increased nursing care and/or monitoring.

The UHDDS item #11-b defines Other Diagnoses as "all conditions that coexist at the time of admission, that develop subsequently, or that affect the treatment received and/or the length of stay. Diagnoses that relate to an earlier episode which have no bearing on the current hospital stay are to be excluded." UHDDS definitions apply to inpatients in acute care, short-term, long term care and psychiatric hospital setting. The UHDDS definitions are used by acute care short-term hospitals to report inpatient data elements in a standardized manner. These data elements and their definitions can be found in the July 31, 1985, Federal Register (Vol. 50, No, 147), pp. 31038-40.

Since that time the application of the UHDDS definitions has been expanded to include all non-outpatient settings (acute care, short term, long term care and psychiatric hospitals; home health agencies; rehab facilities; nursing homes, etc).

The following guidelines are to be applied in designating "other diagnoses" when neither the Alphabetic Index nor the Tabular List in ICD-10-CM provide direction. The listing of the diagnoses in the patient record is the responsibility of the attending provider.

A. Previous conditions

If the provider has included a diagnosis in the final diagnostic statement, such as the discharge summary or the face sheet, it should ordinarily be coded. Some providers include in the diagnostic statement resolved conditions or diagnoses and status-post procedures from previous admission that have no bearing on the current stay. Such conditions are not to be reported and are coded only if required by hospital policy.

However, history codes (categories Z80-Z87) may be used as secondary codes if the historical condition or family history has an impact on current care or influences treatment.

B. Abnormal findings

Abnormal findings (laboratory, x-ray, pathologic, and other diagnostic results) are not coded and reported unless the provider indicates their clinical significance. If the findings are outside the normal range and the attending provider has ordered other tests to evaluate the condition or prescribed treatment, it is appropriate to ask the provider whether the abnormal finding should be added.

Please note: This differs from the coding practices in the outpatient setting for coding encounters for diagnostic tests that have been interpreted by a provider.

C. Uncertain Diagnosis

If the diagnosis documented at the time of discharge is qualified as "probable", "suspected", "likely", "questionable", "possible", or "still to be ruled out" or other similar terms indicating uncertainty, code the condition as if it existed or was established. The bases for these guidelines are the diagnostic workup, arrangements for further workup or observation, and initial therapeutic approach that correspond most closely with the established diagnosis.

Note: This guideline is applicable only to inpatient admissions to short-term, acute, long-term care and psychiatric hospitals.

SECTION IV: DIAGNOSTIC CODING AND REPORTING GUIDELINES FOR OUTPATIENT SERVICES

These coding guidelines for outpatient diagnoses have been approved for use by hospitals/ providers in coding and reporting hospital-based outpatient services and provider-based office visits.

Information about the use of certain abbreviations, punctuation, symbols, and other conventions used in the ICD-10-CM Tabular List (code numbers and titles), can be found in Section IA of these guidelines, under "Conventions Used in the Tabular List." Section I.B. contains general guidelines that apply to the entire classification. Section I.C. contains chapter-specific guidelines that correspond to the chapters as they are arranged in the classification. Information about the correct sequence to use in finding a code is also described in Section I.

The terms encounter and visit are often used interchangeably in describing outpatient service contacts and, therefore, appear together in these guidelines without distinguishing one from the other.

Though the conventions and general guidelines apply to all settings, coding guidelines for outpatient and provider reporting of diagnoses will vary in a number of instances from those for inpatient diagnoses, recognizing that:

The Uniform Hospital Discharge Data Set (UHDDS) definition of principal diagnosis applies only to inpatients in acute, short-term, long-term care and psychiatric hospitals.

Coding guidelines for inconclusive diagnoses (probable, suspected, rule out, etc.) were developed for inpatient reporting and do not apply to outpatients.

A. Selection of first-listed condition

In the outpatient setting, the term first-listed diagnosis is used in lieu of principal diagnosis.

In determining the first-listed diagnosis the coding conventions of ICD-10-CM, as well as the general and disease specific guidelines take precedence over the outpatient guidelines.

Diagnoses often are not established at the time of the initial encounter/visit. It may take two or more visits before the diagnosis is confirmed.

The most critical rule involves beginning the search for the correct code assignment through the Alphabetic Index. Never begin searching initially in the Tabular List as this will lead to coding errors.

1. Outpatient Surgery

When a patient presents for outpatient surgery (same day surgery), code the reason for the surgery as the first-listed diagnosis (reason for the encounter), even if the surgery is not performed due to a contraindication.

2. Observation Stay

When a patient is admitted for observation for a medical condition, assign a code for the medical condition as the first-listed diagnosis.

When a patient presents for outpatient surgery and develops complications requiring admission to observation, code the reason for the surgery as the first reported diagnosis (reason for the encounter), followed by codes for the complications as secondary diagnoses.

B. Codes from A00.0 through T88.9, Z00-Z99

The appropriate code(s) from A00.0 through T88.9, Z00-Z99 must be used to identify diagnoses, symptoms, conditions, problems, complaints, or other reason(s) for the encounter/visit.

C. Accurate reporting of ICD-10-CM diagnosis codes

For accurate reporting of ICD-10-CM diagnosis codes, the documentation should describe the patient's condition, using terminology which includes specific diagnoses as well as symptoms, problems, or reasons for the encounter. There are ICD-10-CM codes to describe all of these.

D. Codes that describe symptoms and signs

Codes that describe symptoms and signs, as opposed to diagnoses, are acceptable for reporting purposes when a diagnosis has not been established (confirmed) by the provider. Chapter 18 of ICD-10-CM, Symptoms, Signs, and Abnormal Clinical and Laboratory Findings Not Elsewhere Classified (codes R00-R99) contain many, but not all codes for symptoms.

E. Encounters for circumstances other than a disease or injury

ICD-10-CM provides codes to deal with encounters for circumstances other than a disease or injury. The Factors Influencing Health Status and Contact with Health Services codes (Z00-Z99) are provided to deal with occasions when circumstances other than a disease or injury are recorded as diagnosis or problems.
See Section I.C.21. Factors influencing health status and contact with health services.

F. **Level of Detail in Coding**

1. **ICD-10-CM codes with 3, 4, 5, 6 or 7 characters**

   ICD-10-CM is composed of codes with 3, 4, 5, 6 or 7 characters. Codes with three characters are included in ICD-10-CM as the heading of a category of codes that may be further subdivided by the use of fourth, fifth, sixth or seventh characters to provide greater specificity.

2. **Use of full number of *characters* required for a code**

   A three-character code is to be used only if it is not further subdivided. A code is invalid if it has not been coded to the full number of characters required for that code, including the 7th character, if applicable.

G. **ICD-10-CM code for the diagnosis, condition, problem, or other reason for encounter/visit**

List first the ICD-10-CM code for the diagnosis, condition, problem, or other reason for encounter/visit shown in the medical record to be chiefly responsible for the services provided. List additional codes that describe any coexisting conditions. In some cases the first-listed diagnosis may be a symptom when a diagnosis has not been established (confirmed) by the physician.

H. **Uncertain diagnosis**

Do not code diagnoses documented as "probable", "suspected," "questionable," "rule out," or "working diagnosis" or other similar terms indicating uncertainty. Rather, code the condition(s) to the highest degree of certainty for that encounter/visit, such as symptoms, signs, abnormal test results, or other reason for the visit.

Please note: This differs from the coding practices used by short-term, acute care, long-term care and psychiatric hospitals.

I. **Chronic diseases**

Chronic diseases treated on an ongoing basis may be coded and reported as many times as the patient receives treatment and care for the condition(s)

J. **Code all documented conditions that coexist**

Code all documented conditions that coexist at the time of the encounter/visit, and require or affect patient care treatment or management. Do not code conditions that were previously treated and no longer exist. However, history codes (categories Z80-Z87) may be used as secondary codes if the historical condition or family history has an impact on current care or influences treatment.

K. **Patients receiving diagnostic services only**

For patients receiving diagnostic services only during an encounter/visit, sequence first the diagnosis, condition, problem, or other reason for encounter/visit shown in the medical record to be chiefly responsible for the outpatient services provided during the encounter/visit. Codes for other diagnoses (e.g., chronic conditions) may be sequenced as additional diagnoses.

For encounters for routine laboratory/radiology testing in the absence of any signs, symptoms, or associated diagnosis, assign Z01.89, Encounter for other specified special examinations. If routine testing is performed during the same encounter as a test to evaluate a sign, symptom, or diagnosis, it is appropriate to assign both the **Z** code and the code describing the reason for the non-routine test.

For outpatient encounters for diagnostic tests that have been interpreted by a physician, and the final report is available at the time of coding, code any confirmed or definitive diagnosis(es) documented in the interpretation. Do not code related signs and symptoms as additional diagnoses.

Please note: This differs from the coding practice in the hospital inpatient setting regarding abnormal findings on test results.

L. **Patients receiving therapeutic services only**

For patients receiving therapeutic services only during an encounter/visit, sequence first the diagnosis, condition, problem, or other reason for encounter/visit shown in the medical record to be chiefly responsible for the outpatient services provided during the encounter/visit. Codes for other diagnoses (e.g., chronic conditions) may be sequenced as additional diagnoses.

The only exception to this rule is that when the primary reason for the admission/encounter is chemotherapy or radiation therapy, the appropriate Z code for the service is listed first, and the diagnosis or problem for which the service is being performed listed second.

M. Patients receiving preoperative evaluations only

For patients receiving preoperative evaluations only, sequence first a code from subcategory Z01.81, Encounter for pre-procedural examinations, to describe the pre-op consultations. Assign a code for the condition to describe the reason for the surgery as an additional diagnosis. Code also any findings related to the pre-op evaluation.

N. Ambulatory surgery

For ambulatory surgery, code the diagnosis for which the surgery was performed. If the postoperative diagnosis is known to be different from the preoperative diagnosis at the time the diagnosis is confirmed, select the postoperative diagnosis for coding, since it is the most definitive.

O. Routine outpatient prenatal visits

See Section I.C.15. Routine outpatient prenatal visits.

P. Encounters for general medical examinations with abnormal findings

The subcategories for encounters for general medical examinations, Z00.0-, provide codes for with and without abnormal findings. Should a general medical examination result in an abnormal finding, the code for general medical examination with abnormal finding should be assigned as the first-listed diagnosis. A secondary code for the abnormal finding should also be coded.

Q. Encounters for routine health screenings

See Section I.C.21. Factors influencing health status and contact with health services, Screening

APPENDIX I

PRESENT ON ADMISSION REPORTING GUIDELINES
Introduction

These guidelines are to be used as a supplement to the *ICD-10-CM Official Guidelines for Coding and Reporting* to facilitate the assignment of the Present on Admission (POA) indicator for each diagnosis and external cause of injury code reported on claim forms (UB-04 and 837 Institutional).

These guidelines are not intended to replace any guidelines in the main body of the *ICD-10-CM Official Guidelines for Coding and Reporting*. The POA guidelines are not intended to provide guidance on when a condition should be coded, but rather, how to apply the POA indicator to the final set of diagnosis codes that have been assigned in accordance with Sections I, II, and III of the official coding guidelines. Subsequent to the assignment of the ICD-10-CM codes, the POA indicator should then be assigned to those conditions that have been coded.

As stated in the Introduction to the ICD-10-CM Official Guidelines for Coding and Reporting, a joint effort between the healthcare provider and the coder is essential to achieve complete and accurate documentation, code assignment, and reporting of diagnoses and procedures. The importance of consistent, complete documentation in the medical record cannot be overemphasized. Medical record documentation from any provider involved in the care and treatment of the patient may be used to support the determination of whether a condition was present on admission or not. In the context of the official coding guidelines, the term "provider" means a physician or any qualified healthcare practitioner who is legally accountable for establishing the patient's diagnosis.

These guidelines are not a substitute for the provider's clinical judgment as to the determination of whether a condition was/was not present on admission. The provider should be queried regarding issues related to the linking of signs/symptoms, timing of test results, and the timing of findings.

General Reporting Requirements

All claims involving inpatient admissions to general acute care hospitals or other facilities that are subject to a law or regulation mandating collection of present on admission information.

Present on admission is defined as present at the time the order for inpatient admission occurs -- conditions that develop during an outpatient encounter, including emergency department, observation, or outpatient surgery, are considered as present on admission.

POA indicator is assigned to principal and secondary diagnoses (as defined in Section II of the Official Guidelines for Coding and Reporting) and the external cause of injury codes.

Issues related to inconsistent, missing, conflicting or unclear documentation must still be resolved by the provider.

If a condition would not be coded and reported based on UHDDS definitions and current official coding guidelines, then the POA indicator would not be reported.

Reporting Options

Y - Yes
N - No
U - Unknown
W – Clinically undetermined
Unreported/Not used – (Exempt from POA reporting)

Reporting Definitions

Y = present at the time of inpatient admission
N = not present at the time of inpatient admission
U = documentation is insufficient to determine if condition is present on admission
W = provider is unable to clinically determine whether condition was present on admission or not

Timeframe for POA Identification and Documentation

There is no required timeframe as to when a provider (per the definition of "provider" used in these guidelines) must identify or document a condition to be present on admission. In some clinical situations, it may not be possible for a provider to make a definitive diagnosis (or a condition may not be recognized or reported by the patient) for a period of time after admission. In some cases it may be several days before the provider arrives at a definitive diagnosis. This does not mean that the condition was not present on admission. Determination of whether the condition was present on admission or not will be based on the applicable POA guideline as identified in this document, or on the provider's best clinical judgment.

If at the time of code assignment the documentation is unclear as to whether a condition was present on admission or not, it is appropriate to query the provider for clarification.

Assigning the POA Indicator

Condition is on the "Exempt from Reporting" list
Leave the "present on admission" field blank if the condition is on the list of ICD-10-CM codes for which this field is not applicable. This is the only circumstance in which the field may be left blank.

POA Explicitly Documented

Assign Y for any condition the provider explicitly documents as being present on admission.

Assign N for any condition the provider explicitly documents as not present at the time of admission.

Conditions diagnosed prior to inpatient admission

Assign "Y" for conditions that were diagnosed prior to admission (example: hypertension, diabetes mellitus, asthma)

Conditions diagnosed during the admission but clearly present before admission

Assign "Y" for conditions diagnosed during the admission that were clearly present but not diagnosed until after admission occurred.

Diagnoses subsequently confirmed after admission are considered present on admission if at the time of admission they are documented as suspected, possible, rule out, differential diagnosis, or constitute an underlying cause of a symptom that is present at the time of admission.

Condition develops during outpatient encounter prior to inpatient admission

Assign Y for any condition that develops during an outpatient encounter prior to a written order for inpatient admission.

Documentation does not indicate whether condition was present on admission

Assign "U" when the medical record documentation is unclear as to whether the condition was present on admission. "U" should not be routinely assigned and used only in very limited circumstances. Coders are encouraged to query the providers when the documentation is unclear.

Documentation states that it cannot be determined whether the condition was or was not present on admission

Assign "W" when the medical record documentation indicates that it cannot be clinically determined whether or not the condition was present on admission.

Chronic condition with acute exacerbation during the admission

If a single code identifies both the chronic condition and the acute exacerbation, see POA guidelines pertaining to combination codes.

If a single code only identifies the chronic condition and not the acute exacerbation (e.g., acute exacerbation of chronic leukemia), assign "Y."

Conditions documented as possible, probable, suspected, or rule out at the time of discharge

If the final diagnosis contains a possible, probable, suspected, or rule out diagnosis, and this diagnosis was based on signs, symptoms or clinical findings suspected at the time of inpatient admission, assign "Y."

If the final diagnosis contains a possible, probable, suspected, or rule out diagnosis, and this diagnosis was based on signs, symptoms or clinical findings that were not present on admission, assign "N".

Conditions documented as impending or threatened at the time of discharge

If the final diagnosis contains an impending or threatened diagnosis, and this diagnosis is based on symptoms or clinical findings that were present on admission, assign "Y".

If the final diagnosis contains an impending or threatened diagnosis, and this diagnosis is based on symptoms or clinical findings that were not present on admission, assign "N".

Acute and Chronic Conditions

Assign "Y" for acute conditions that are present at time of admission and N for acute conditions that are not present at time of admission.

Assign "Y" for chronic conditions, even though the condition may not be diagnosed until after admission.

If a single code identifies both an acute and chronic condition, see the POA guidelines for combination codes.

Combination Codes

Assign "N" if any part of the combination code was not present on admission (e.g., COPD with acute exacerbation and the exacerbation was not present on admission; gastric ulcer that does not start bleeding until after admission; asthma patient develops status asthmaticus after admission)

Assign "Y" if all parts of the combination code were present on admission (e.g., patient with acute prostatitis admitted with hematuria)

If the final diagnosis includes comparative or contrasting diagnoses, and both were present, or suspected, at the time of admission, assign "Y".

For infection codes that include the causal organism, assign "Y" if the infection (or signs of the infection) was present on admission, even though the culture results may not be known until after admission (e.g., patient is admitted with pneumonia and the provider documents pseudomonas as the causal organism a few days later).

Same Diagnosis Code for Two or More Conditions

When the same ICD-10-CM diagnosis code applies to two or more conditions during the same encounter (e.g. two separate conditions classified to the same ICD-10-CM diagnosis code):

Assign "Y" if all conditions represented by the single ICD-10-CM code were present on admission (e.g. bilateral unspecified age-related cataracts).

Assign "N" if any of the conditions represented by the single ICD-10-CM code was not present on admission (e.g. traumatic secondary and recurrent hemorrhage and seroma is assigned to a single code T79.2, but only one of the conditions was present on admission).

Obstetrical conditions

Whether or not the patient delivers during the current hospitalization does not affect assignment of the POA indicator. The determining factor for POA assignment is whether the pregnancy complication or obstetrical condition described by the code was present at the time of admission or not.

If the pregnancy complication or obstetrical condition was present on admission (e.g., patient admitted in preterm labor), assign "Y".

If the pregnancy complication or obstetrical condition was not present on admission (e.g., 2nd degree laceration during delivery, postpartum hemorrhage that occurred during current hospitalization, fetal distress develops after admission), assign "N".

If the obstetrical code includes more than one diagnosis and any of the diagnoses identified by the code were not present on admission assign "N". (e.g., Category O11, Pre-existing hypertension with pre-eclampsia)

Perinatal conditions

Newborns are not considered to be admitted until after birth. Therefore, any condition present at birth or that developed in utero is considered present at admission and should be assigned "Y". This includes conditions that occur during delivery (e.g., injury during delivery, meconium aspiration, exposure to streptococcus B in the vaginal canal).

Congenital conditions and anomalies

Assign "Y" for congenital conditions and anomalies except for categories Q00-Q99, Congenital anomalies, which are on the exempt list. Congenital conditions are always considered present on admission.

External cause of injury codes

Assign "Y" for any external cause code representing an external cause of morbidity that occurred prior to inpatient admission (e.g., patient fell out of bed at home, patient fell out of bed in emergency room prior to admission)

Assign "N" for any external cause code representing an external cause of morbidity that occurred during inpatient hospitalization (e.g., patient fell out of hospital bed during hospital stay, patient experienced an adverse reaction to a medication administered after inpatient admission)

Categories and Codes Exempt from Diagnosis Present on Admission Requirement

Note: "Diagnosis present on admission" for these code categories are exempt because they represent circumstances regarding the healthcare encounter or factors influencing health status that do not represent a current disease or injury or are always present on admission

B90–B94	Sequelae of infectious and parasitic diseases
E64	Sequelae of malnutrition and other nutritional deficiencies
I25.2	Old myocardial infarction
I69	Sequelae of cerebrovascular disease
O09	Supervision of high risk pregnancy
O66.5	Attempted application of vacuum extractor and forceps
O80	Encounter for full-term uncomplicated delivery
O94	Sequelae of complication of pregnancy, childbirth, and the puerperium
P00	Newborn (suspected to be) affected by maternal conditions that may be unrelated to present pregnancy
Q00 – Q99	Congenital malformations, deformations and chromosomal abnormalities
S00-T88.9	Injury, poisoning and certain other consequences of external causes with 7th character representing subsequent encounter or sequela
V00- V09	Pedestrian injured in transport accident
	Except V00.81- Accident with wheelchair (powered)
V00.83-	Accident with motorized mobility scooter
V10-V19	Pedal cycle rider injured in transport accident
V20-V29	Motorcycle rider injured in transport accident
V30-V39	Occupant of three-wheeled motor vehicle injured in transport accident
V40-V49	Car occupant injured in transport accident
V50-V59	Occupant of pick-up truck or van injured in transport accident
V60-V69	Occupant of heavy transport vehicle injured in transport accident
V70-V79	Bus occupant injured in transport accident
V80-V89	Other land transport accidents
V90-V94	Water transport accidents
V95-V97	Air and space transport accidents
V98-V99	Other and unspecified transport accidents
W09	Fall on and from playground equipment
W14	Fall from tree
W15	Fall from cliff
W17.0	Fall into well
W17.1	Fall into storm drain or manhole
W18.01	Striking against sports equipment with subsequent fall
W21	Striking against or struck by sports equipment
W30	Contact with agricultural machinery
W31	Contact with other and unspecified machinery
W32-W34	Accidental handgun discharge and malfunction
W35- W40	Exposure to inanimate mechanical forces
W52	Crushed pushed or stepped on by crowd or human stampede
W56	Contact with nonvenomous marine animal
W58	Contact with crocodile or alligator
W61	Contact with birds (domestic) (wild)
W62	Contact with nonvenomous amphibians
W89	Exposure to man-made visible and ultraviolet light
X02	Exposure to controlled fire in building or structure
X03	Exposure to controlled fire, not in building or structure
X04	Exposure to ignition of highly flammable material
X52	Prolonged stay in weightless environment
X71	Intentional self-harm by drowning and submersion
	Except X71.0- Intentional self-harm by drowning and submersion while in bath tub
X72	Intentional self-harm by handgun discharge
X73	Intentional self-harm by rifle, shotgun and larger firearm discharge
X74	Intentional self-harm by other and unspecified firearm and gun discharge
X75	Intentional self-harm by explosive material
X76	Intentional self-harm by smoke, fire and flames
X77	Intentional self-harm by steam hot vapors and hot objects

X81	Intentional self-harm by jumping or lying in front of moving object
X82	Intentional self-harm by crashing of motor vehicle
X83	Intentional self-harm by other specified means
Y03	Assault by crashing of motor vehicle
Y07	Perpetrator of assault, maltreatment and neglect
Y08.8	Assault by strike by sports equipment
Y21	Drowning and submersion, undetermined intent
Y22	Handgun discharge, undetermined intent
Y23	Rifle, shotgun and larger firearm discharge, undetermined intent
Y24	Other and unspecified firearm discharge, undetermined intent
Y30	Falling, jumping or pushed from a high place, undetermined intent
Y32	Assault by crashing of motor vehicle, undetermined intent
Y37	Military operations
Y36	Operations of war
Y92	Place of occurrence of the external cause
Y93	Activity code
Y99	External cause status
Z00	Encounter for general examination without complaint, suspected or reported diagnosis
Z01	Encounter for other special examination without complaint, suspected or reported diagnosis
Z02	Encounter for administrative examination
Z03	Encounter for medical observation for suspected diseases and conditions ruled out
Z08	Encounter for follow-up examination following completed treatment for malignant neoplasm
Z09	Encounter for follow-up examination after completed treatment for conditions other than malignant neoplasm
Z11	Encounter for screening for infectious and parasitic diseases
Z11.8	Encounter for screening for other infectious and parasitic diseases
Z12	Encounter for screening for malignant neoplasms
Z13	Encounter for screening for other diseases and disorders
Z13.4	Encounter for screening for certain developmental disorders in childhood
Z13.5	Encounter for screening for eye and ear disorders
Z13.6	Encounter for screening for cardiovascular disorders
Z13.83	Encounter for screening for respiratory disorder NEC
Z13.89	Encounter for screening for other disorder
Z13.89	Encounter for screening for other disorder
Z14	Genetic carrier
Z15	Genetic susceptibility to disease
Z17	Estrogen receptor status
Z18	Retained foreign body fragments
Z22	Carrier of infectious disease
Z23	Encounter for immunization
Z28	Immunization not carried out and underimmunization status
Z28.3	Underimmunization status
Z30	Encounter for contraceptive management
Z31	Encounter for procreative management
Z34	Encounter for supervision of normal pregnancy
Z36	Encounter for antenatal screening of mother
Z37	Outcome of delivery
Z38	Liveborn infants according to place of birth and type of delivery
Z39	Encounter for maternal postpartum care and examination
Z41	Encounter for procedures for purposes other than remedying health state
Z42	Encounter for plastic and reconstructive surgery following medical procedure or healed injury
Z43	Encounter for attention to artificial openings
Z44	Encounter for fitting and adjustment of external prosthetic device
Z45	Encounter for adjustment and management of implanted device
Z46	Encounter for fitting and adjustment of other devices
Z47.8	Encounter for other orthopedic aftercare
Z49	Encounter for care involving renal dialysis
Z51	Encounter for other aftercare
Z51.5	Encounter for palliative care
Z51.8	Encounter for other specified aftercare
Z52	Donors of organs and tissues
Z59	Problems related to housing and economic circumstances

Z63	Other problems related to primary support group including family circumstances
Z65	Problems related to other psychosocial circumstances
Z65.8	Other specified problems related to psychosocial circumstances
Z67.1 –	
Z67.9	Blood type
Z68	Body mass index (BMI)
Z72	Problems related to lifestyle
Z74.01	Bed confinement status
Z76	Persons encountering health services in other circumstances
Z77.110-	
Z77.128	Environmental pollution and hazards in the physical environment
Z78	Other specified health status
Z79	Long term (current) drug therapy
Z80	Family history of primary malignant neoplasm
Z81	Family history of mental and behavioral disorders
Z82	Family history of certain disabilities and chronic diseases (leading to disablement)
Z83	Family history of other specific disorders
Z84	Family history of other conditions
Z85	Personal history of primary malignant neoplasm
Z86	Personal history of certain other diseases
Z87	Personal history of other diseases and conditions
Z87.828	Personal history of other (healed) physical injury and trauma
Z87.891	Personal history of nicotine dependence
Z88	Allergy status to drugs, medicaments and biological substances
Z89	Acquired absence of limb
Z90.710	Acquired absence of both cervix and uterus
Z91.0	Allergy status, other than to drugs and biological substances
Z91.4	Personal history of psychological trauma, not elsewhere classified
Z91.5	Personal history of self-harm
Z91.8	Other specified risk factors, not elsewhere classified
Z92	Personal history of medical treatment
Z93	Artificial opening status
Z94	Transplanted organ and tissue status
Z95	Presence of cardiac and vascular implants and grafts
Z97	Presence of other devices
Z98	Other postprocedural states
Z99	Dependence on enabling machines and devices, not elsewhere classified

Chapter 1: Certain Infectious And Parasitic Diseases (A00-B99)

Includes: diseases generally recognized as communicable or transmissible

Use additional code to identify resistance to antimicrobial drugs (Z16-)

Excludes 1: certain localized infections - see body system-related chapter

infectious and parasitic diseases complicating pregnancy, childbirth and the puerperium (O98.-)

influenza and other acute respiratory infections (J00-J22)

Excludes 2: carrier or suspected carrier of infectious disease (Z22.-)

infectious and parasitic diseases specific to the perinatal period (P35-P39)

This chapter contains the following blocks:

A00-A09	Intestinal infectious diseases
A15-A19	Tuberculosis
A20-A28	Certain zoonotic bacterial diseases
A30-A49	Other bacterial diseases
A50-A64	Infections with a predominantly sexual mode of transmission
A65-A69	Other spirochetal diseases
A70-A74	Other diseases caused by chlamydiae
A75-A79	Rickettsioses
A80-A89	Viral and prion infections of the central nervous system
A90-A99	Arthropod-borne viral fevers and viral hemorrhagic fevers
B00-B09	Viral infections characterized by skin and mucous membrane lesions
B10	Other human herpesviruses
B15-B19	Viral hepatitis
B20	Human immunodeficiency virus [HIV] disease
B25-B34	Other viral diseases
B35-B49	Mycoses
B50-B64	Protozoal diseases
B65-B83	Helminthiases
B85-B89	Pediculosis, acariasis and other infestations
B90-B94	Sequelae of infectious and parasitic diseases
B95-B97	Bacterial and viral infectious agents
B99	Other infectious diseases

INTESTINAL INFECTIOUS DISEASES (A00-A09)

A00 Cholera
- **A00.0** Cholera due to Vibrio cholerae 01, biovar cholerae
  - Classical cholera
- **A00.1** Cholera due to Vibrio cholerae 01, biovar eltor
  - Cholera eltor
- **A00.9** Cholera, unspecified

A01 Typhoid and paratyphoid fevers
- **A01.0** Typhoid fever
  - Infection due to Salmonella typhi
  - **A01.00** Typhoid fever, unspecified
  - **A01.01** Typhoid meningitis
  - **A01.02** Typhoid fever with heart involvement
    - Typhoid endocarditis
    - Typhoid myocarditis
  - **A01.03** Typhoid pneumonia
  - **A01.04** Typhoid arthritis
  - **A01.05** Typhoid osteomyelitis
  - **A01.09** Typhoid fever with other complications
- **A01.1** Paratyphoid fever A

- **A01.2** Paratyphoid fever B
- **A01.3** Paratyphoid fever C
- **A01.4** Paratyphoid fever, unspecified
  - Infection due to Salmonella paratyphi NOS

A02 Other salmonella infections
Includes: infection or foodborne intoxication due to any Salmonella species other than S. typhi and S. paratyphi
- **A02.0** Salmonella enteritis
  - Salmonellosis
- **A02.1** Salmonella sepsis
- **A02.2** Localized salmonella infections
  - **A02.20** Localized salmonella infection, unspecified
  - **A02.21** Salmonella meningitis
  - **A02.22** Salmonella pneumonia
  - **A02.23** Salmonella arthritis
  - **A02.24** Salmonella osteomyelitis
  - **A02.25** Salmonella pyelonephritis
    - Salmonella tubulo-interstitial nephropathy
  - **A02.29** Salmonella with other localized infection
- **A02.8** Other specified salmonella infections
- **A02.9** Salmonella infection, unspecified

A03 Shigellosis
- **A03.0** Shigellosis due to Shigella dysenteriae
  - Group A shigellosis [Shiga-Kruse dysentery]
- **A03.1** Shigellosis due to Shigella flexneri
  - Group B shigellosis
- **A03.2** Shigellosis due to Shigella boydii
  - Group C shigellosis
- **A03.3** Shigellosis due to Shigella sonnei
  - Group D shigellosis
- **A03.8** Other shigellosis
- **A03.9** Shigellosis, unspecified
  - Bacillary dysentery NOS

A04 Other bacterial intestinal infections
Excludes 1: bacterial foodborne intoxications, NEC (A05.-)
  tuberculous enteritis (A18.32)
- **A04.0** Enteropathogenic Escherichia coli infection
- **A04.1** Enterotoxigenic Escherichia coli infection
- **A04.2** Enteroinvasive Escherichia coli infection
- **A04.3** Enterohemorrhagic Escherichia coli infection
- **A04.4** Other intestinal Escherichia coli infections
  - Escherichia coli enteritis NOS
- **A04.5** Campylobacter enteritis
- **A04.6** Enteritis due to Yersinia enterocolitica
  Excludes 1: extraintestinal yersiniosis (A28.2)
- **A04.7** Enterocolitis due to Clostridium difficile
  - Foodborne intoxication by Clostridium difficile
  - Pseudomembraneous colitis
- **A04.8** Other specified bacterial intestinal infections
- **A04.9** Bacterial intestinal infection, unspecified
  - Bacterial enteritis NOS

A05 Other bacterial foodborne intoxications, not elsewhere classified
Excludes 1: Clostridium difficile foodborne intoxication and infection (A04.7)
  Escherichia coli infection (A04.0-A04.4)
  listeriosis (A32.-)
  salmonella foodborne intoxication and infection (A02.-)
  toxic effect of noxious foodstuffs (T61-T62)
- **A05.0** Foodborne staphylococcal intoxication
- **A05.1** Botulism food poisoning
  - Botulism NOS
  - Classical foodborne intoxication due to Clostridium

botulinum

    Excludes 1: infant botulism (A48.51)

                wound botulism (A48.52)

A05.2 Foodborne Clostridium perfringens [Clostridium welchii] intoxication

    Enteritis necroticans

    Pig-bel

A05.3 Foodborne Vibrio parahaemolyticus intoxication

A05.4 Foodborne Bacillus cereus intoxication

A05.5 Foodborne Vibrio vulnificus intoxication

A05.8 Other specified bacterial foodborne intoxications

A05.9 Bacterial foodborne intoxication, unspecified

A06 Amebiasis

    Includes: infection due to Entamoeba histolytica

    Excludes 1: other protozoal intestinal diseases (A07.-)

    Excludes 2: acanthamebiasis (B60.1-)

                Naegleriasis (B60.2)

A06.0 Acute amebic dysentery

    Acute amebiasis

    Intestinal amebiasis NOS

A06.1 Chronic intestinal amebiasis

A06.2 Amebic nondysenteric colitis

A06.3 Ameboma of intestine

    Ameboma NOS

A06.4 Amebic liver abscess

    Hepatic amebiasis

A06.5 Amebic lung abscess

    Amebic abscess of lung (and liver)

A06.6 Amebic brain abscess

    Amebic abscess of brain (and liver) (and lung)

A06.7 Cutaneous amebiasis

A06.8 Amebic infection of other sites

    A06.81 Amebic cystitis

    A06.82 Other amebic genitourinary infections

             Amebic balanitis

             Amebic vesiculitis

             Amebic vulvovaginitis

    A06.89 Other amebic infections

             Amebic appendicitis

             Amebic splenic abscess

A06.9 Amebiasis, unspecified

A07 Other protozoal intestinal diseases

A07.0 Balantidiasis

    Balantidial dysentery

A07.1 Giardiasis [lambliasis]

A07.2 Cryptosporidiosis

A07.3 Isosporiasis

    Infection due to Isospora belli and Isospora hominis

    Intestinal coccidiosis

    Isosporosis

A07.4 Cyclosporiasis

A07.8 Other specified protozoal intestinal diseases

    Intestinal microsporidiosis

    Intestinal trichomoniasis

    Sarcocystosis

    Sarcosporidiosis

A07.9 Protozoal intestinal disease, unspecified

    Flagellate diarrhea

    Protozoal colitis

    Protozoal diarrhea

    Protozoal dysentery

A08 Viral and other specified intestinal infections

    Excludes 1: influenza with involvement of gastrointestinal tract (J09.X3, J10.2, J11.2)

A08.0 Rotaviral enteritis

A08.1 Acute gastroenteropathy due to Norwalk agent and other small round viruses

    A08.11 Acute gastroenteropathy due to Norwalk agent

             Acute gastroenteropathy due to Norovirus

             Acute gastroenteropathy due to Norwalk-like agent

    A08.19 Acute gastroenteropathy due to other small round viruses

             Acute gastroenteropathy due to small round virus [SRV] NOS

A08.2 Adenoviral enteritis

A08.3 Other viral enteritis

    A08.31 Calicivirus enteritis

    A08.32 Astrovirus enteritis

    A08.39 Other viral enteritis

             Coxsackie virus enteritis

             Echovirus enteritis

             Enterovirus enteritis NEC

             Torovirus enteritis

A08.4 Viral intestinal infection, unspecified

    Viral enteritis NOS

    Viral gastroenteritis NOS

    Viral gastroenteropathy NOS

A08.8 Other specified intestinal infections

A09 Infectious gastroenteritis and colitis, unspecified

    Infectious colitis NOS

    Infectious enteritis NOS

    Infectious gastroenteritis NOS

    Excludes 1: colitis NOS (K52.9)

             diarrhea NOS (R19.7)

             enteritis NOS (K52.9)

             gastroenteritis NOS (K52.9)

             noninfective gastroenteritis and colitis, unspecified (K52.9)

TUBERCULOSIS (A15-A19)

Includes: infections due to Mycobacterium tuberculosis and Mycobacterium bovis

Excludes 1: congenital tuberculosis (P37.0)

    nonspecific reaction to test for tuberculosis without active tuberculosis (R76.1-)

    pneumoconiosis associated with tuberculosis, any type in A15 (J65)

    positive PPD (R76.11)

    positive tuberculin skin test without active tuberculosis (R76.11)

    sequelae of tuberculosis (B90.-)

    silicotuberculosis (J65)

A15 Respiratory tuberculosis

A15.0 Tuberculosis of lung

    Tuberculous bronchiectasis

    Tuberculous fibrosis of lung

    Tuberculous pneumonia

    Tuberculous pneumothorax

A15.4 Tuberculosis of intrathoracic lymph nodes

    Tuberculosis of hilar lymph nodes

    Tuberculosis of mediastinal lymph nodes

    Tuberculosis of tracheobronchial lymph nodes

    Excludes 1: tuberculosis specified as primary (A15.7)

A15.5 Tuberculosis of larynx, trachea and bronchus

    Tuberculosis of bronchus

    Tuberculosis of glottis

    Tuberculosis of larynx

Tuberculosis of trachea

A15.6 Tuberculous pleurisy

Tuberculosis of pleura Tuberculous empyema

Excludes 1: primary respiratory tuberculosis (A15.7)

A15.7 Primary respiratory tuberculosis

A15.8 Other respiratory tuberculosis

Mediastinal tuberculosis

Nasopharyngeal tuberculosis

Tuberculosis of nose

Tuberculosis of sinus [any nasal]

A15.9 Respiratory tuberculosis unspecified

A17 Tuberculosis of nervous system

A17.0 Tuberculous meningitis

Tuberculosis of meninges (cerebral)(spinal)

Tuberculous leptomeningitis

Excludes 1: tuberculous meningoencephalitis (A17.82)

A17.1 Meningeal tuberculoma

Tuberculoma of meninges (cerebral) (spinal)

Excludes 2: tuberculoma of brain and spinal cord (A17.81)

A17.8 Other tuberculosis of nervous system

A17.81 Tuberculoma of brain and spinal cord

Tuberculous abscess of brain and spinal cord

A17.82 Tuberculous meningoencephalitis

Tuberculous myelitis

A17.83 Tuberculous neuritis

Tuberculous mononeuropathy

A17.89 Other tuberculosis of nervous system

Tuberculous polyneuropathy

A17.9 Tuberculosis of nervous system, unspecified

A18 Tuberculosis of other organs

A18.0 Tuberculosis of bones and joints

A18.01 Tuberculosis of spine

Pott's disease or curvature of spine

Tuberculous arthritis

Tuberculous osteomyelitis of spine

Tuberculous spondylitis

A18.02 Tuberculous arthritis of other joints

Tuberculosis of hip (joint)

Tuberculosis of knee (joint)

A18.03 Tuberculosis of other bones

Tuberculous mastoiditis

Tuberculous osteomyelitis

A18.09 Other musculoskeletal tuberculosis

Tuberculous myositis

Tuberculous synovitis

Tuberculous tenosynovitis

A18.1 Tuberculosis of genitourinary system

A18.10 Tuberculosis of genitourinary system, unspecified

A18.11 Tuberculosis of kidney and ureter

A18.12 Tuberculosis of bladder

A18.13 Tuberculosis of other urinary organs

Tuberculous urethritis

A18.14 Tuberculosis of prostate

A18.15 Tuberculosis of other male genital organs

A18.16 Tuberculosis of cervix

A18.17 Tuberculous female pelvic inflammatory disease

Tuberculous endometritis

Tuberculous oophoritis and salpingitis

A18.18 Tuberculosis of other female genital organs

Tuberculous ulceration of vulva

A18.2 Tuberculous peripheral lymphadenopathy

Tuberculous adenitis

Excludes 2: tuberculosis of bronchial and mediastinal lymph nodes (A15.4)

tuberculosis of mesenteric and retroperitoneal lymph nodes (A18.39)

tuberculous tracheobronchial adenopathy (A15.4)

A18.3 Tuberculosis of intestines, peritoneum and mesenteric glands

A18.31 Tuberculous peritonitis

Tuberculous ascites

A18.32 Tuberculous enteritis

Tuberculosis of anus and rectum

Tuberculosis of intestine (large) (small)

A18.39 Retroperitoneal tuberculosis

Tuberculosis of mesenteric glands

Tuberculosis of retroperitoneal (lymph glands)

A18.4 Tuberculosis of skin and subcutaneous tissue

Erythema induratum, tuberculous

Lupus excedens

Lupus vulgaris NOS

Lupus vulgaris of eyelid

Scrofuloderma

Tuberculosis of external ear

Excludes 2: lupus erythematosus (L93.-)

lupus NOS (M32.9)

systemic (M32.-)

A18.5 Tuberculosis of eye

Excludes 2: lupus vulgaris of eyelid (A18.4)

A18.50 Tuberculosis of eye, unspecified

A18.51 Tuberculous episcleritis

A18.52 Tuberculous keratitis

Tuberculous interstitial keratitis

Tuberculous keratoconjunctivitis (interstitial) (phlyctenular)

A18.53 Tuberculous chorioretinitis

A18.54 Tuberculous iridocyclitis

A18.59 Other tuberculosis of eye

Tuberculous conjunctivitis

A18.6 Tuberculosis of (inner) (middle) ear

Tuberculous otitis media

Excludes 2: tuberculosis of external ear (A18.4)

tuberculous mastoiditis (A18.03)

A18.7 Tuberculosis of adrenal glands

Tuberculous Addison's disease

A18.8 Tuberculosis of other specified organs

A18.81 Tuberculosis of thyroid gland

A18.82 Tuberculosis of other endocrine glands

Tuberculosis of pituitary gland

Tuberculosis of thymus gland

A18.83 Tuberculosis of digestive tract organs, not elsewhere classified

Excludes 1: tuberculosis of intestine (A18.32)

A18.84 Tuberculosis of heart

Tuberculous cardiomyopathy

Tuberculous endocarditis

Tuberculous myocarditis

Tuberculous pericarditis

A18.85 Tuberculosis of spleen

A18.89 Tuberculosis of other sites

Tuberculosis of muscle

Tuberculous cerebral arteritis

A19 Miliary tuberculosis

Includes: disseminated tuberculosis
  generalized tuberculosis
  tuberculous polyserositis

A19.0 Acute miliary tuberculosis of a single specified site
A19.1 Acute miliary tuberculosis of multiple sites
A19.2 Acute miliary tuberculosis, unspecified
A19.8 Other miliary tuberculosis
A19.9 Miliary tuberculosis, unspecified

CERTAIN ZOONOTIC BACTERIAL DISEASES (A20-A28)

A20 Plague
  Includes: infection due to Yersinia pestis
A20.0 Bubonic plague
A20.1 Cellulocutaneous plague
A20.2 Pneumonic plague
A20.3 Plague meningitis
A20.7 Septicemic plague
A20.8 Other forms of plague
  Abortive plague
  Asymptomatic plague
  Pestis minor
A20.9 Plague, unspecified

A21 Tularemia
  Includes: deer-fly fever
  infection due to Francisella tularensis
  rabbit fever
A21.0 Ulceroglandular tularemia
A21.1 Oculoglandular tularemia
  Ophthalmic tularemia
A21.2 Pulmonary tularemia
A21.3 Gastrointestinal tularemia
  Abdominal tularemia
A21.7 Generalized tularemia
A21.8 Other forms of tularemia
A21.9 Tularemia, unspecified

A22 Anthrax
  Includes: infection due to Bacillus anthracis
A22.0 Cutaneous anthrax
  Malignant carbuncle
  Malignant pustule
A22.1 Pulmonary anthrax
  Inhalation anthrax
  Ragpicker's disease
  Woolsorter's disease
A22.2 Gastrointestinal anthrax
A22.7 Anthrax sepsis
A22.8 Other forms of anthrax
  Anthrax meningitis
A22.9 Anthrax, unspecified

A23 Brucellosis
  Includes: Malta fever
  Mediterranean fever
  undulant fever
A23.0 Brucellosis due to Brucella melitensis
A23.1 Brucellosis due to Brucella abortus
A23.2 Brucellosis due to Brucella suis
A23.3 Brucellosis due to Brucella canis
A23.8 Other brucellosis
A23.9 Brucellosis, unspecified

A24 Glanders and melioidosis
A24.0 Glanders

Infection due to Pseudomonas mallei
  Malleus
A24.1 Acute and fulminating melioidosis
  Melioidosis pneumonia
  Melioidosis sepsis
A24.2 Subacute and chronic melioidosis
A24.3 Other melioidosis
A24.9 Melioidosis, unspecified
  Infection due to Pseudomonas pseudomallei NOS
  Whitmore's disease

A25 Rat-bite fevers
A25.0 Spirillosis
  Sodoku
A25.1 Streptobacillosis
  Epidemic arthritic erythema
  Haverhill fever
  Streptobacillary rat-bite fever
A25.9 Rat-bite fever, unspecified

A26 Erysipeloid
A26.0 Cutaneous erysipeloid
  Erythema migrans
A26.7 Erysipelothrix sepsis
A26.8 Other forms of erysipeloid
A26.9 Erysipeloid, unspecified

A27 Leptospirosis
A27.0 Leptospirosis icterohemorrhagica
  Leptospiral or spirochetal jaundice (hemorrhagic)
  Weil's disease
A27.8 Other forms of leptospirosis
  A27.81 Aseptic meningitis in leptospirosis
  A27.89 Other forms of leptospirosis
A27.9 Leptospirosis, unspecified

A28 Other zoonotic bacterial diseases, not elsewhere classified
A28.0 Pasteurellosis
A28.1 Cat-scratch disease
  Cat-scratch fever
A28.2 Extraintestinal yersiniosis
  Excludes 1: enteritis due to Yersinia enterocolitica (A04.6)
  plague (A20.-)
A28.8 Other specified zoonotic bacterial diseases, not elsewhere classified
A28.9 Zoonotic bacterial disease, unspecified

OTHER BACTERIAL DISEASES (A30-A49)

A30 Leprosy [Hansen's disease]
  Includes: infection due to Mycobacterium leprae
  Excludes 1: sequelae of leprosy (B92)
A30.0 Indeterminate leprosy
  I leprosy
A30.1 Tuberculoid leprosy
  TT leprosy
A30.2 Borderline tuberculoid leprosy
  BT leprosy
A30.3 Borderline leprosy
  BB leprosy
A30.4 Borderline lepromatous leprosy
  BL leprosy
A30.5 Lepromatous leprosy
  LL leprosy
A30.8 Other forms of leprosy
A30.9 Leprosy, unspecified

A31 Infection due to other mycobacteria

> **Excludes 2:** leprosy (A30.-)
> tuberculosis (A15-A19)

A31.0 Pulmonary mycobacterial infection
Infection due to Mycobacterium avium
Infection due to Mycobacterium intracellulare [Battey bacillus]
Infection due to Mycobacterium kansasii

A31.1 Cutaneous mycobacterial infection
Buruli ulcer
Infection due to Mycobacterium marinum
Infection due to Mycobacterium ulcerans

A31.2 Disseminated mycobacterium avium-intracellulare complex (DMAC)
MAC sepsis

A31.8 Other mycobacterial infections

A31.9 Mycobacterial infection, unspecified
Atypical mycobacterial infection NOS
Mycobacteriosis NOS

A32 Listeriosis

> **Includes:** listerial foodborne infection
> **Excludes 1:** neonatal (disseminated) listeriosis (P37.2)

A32.0 Cutaneous listeriosis

A32.1 Listerial meningitis and meningoencephalitis

   A32.11 Listerial meningitis

   A32.12 Listerial meningoencephalitis

A32.7 Listerial sepsis

A32.8 Other forms of listeriosis

   A32.81 Oculoglandular listeriosis

   A32.82 Listerial endocarditis

   A32.89 Other forms of listeriosis
   Listerial cerebral arteritis

A32.9 Listeriosis, unspecified

A33 Tetanus neonatorum

A34 Obstetrical tetanus

A35 Other tetanus
Tetanus NOS

> **Excludes 1:** obstetrical tetanus (A34)
> tetanus neonatorum (A33)

A36 Diphtheria

A36.0 Pharyngeal diphtheria
Diphtheritic membranous angina
Tonsillar diphtheria

A36.1 Nasopharyngeal diphtheria

A36.2 Laryngeal diphtheria
Diphtheritic laryngotracheitis

A36.3 Cutaneous diphtheria

> **Excludes 2:** erythrasma (L08.1)

A36.8 Other diphtheria

   A36.81 Diphtheritic cardiomyopathy
   Diphtheritic myocarditis

   A36.82 Diphtheritic radiculomyelitis

   A36.83 Diphtheritic polyneuritis

   A36.84 Diphtheritic tubulo-interstitial nephropathy

   A36.85 Diphtheritic cystitis

   A36.86 Diphtheritic conjunctivitis

   A36.89 Other diphtheritic complications
   Diphtheritic peritonitis

A36.9 Diphtheria, unspecified

A37 Whooping cough

A37.0 Whooping cough due to Bordetella pertussis

   A37.00 Whooping cough due to Bordetella pertussis without pneumonia

   A37.01 Whooping cough due to Bordetella pertussis with pneumonia

A37.1 Whooping cough due to Bordetella parapertussis

   A37.10 Whooping cough due to Bordetella parapertussis without pneumonia

   A37.11 Whooping cough due to Bordetella parapertussis with pneumonia

A37.8 Whooping cough due to other Bordetella species

   A37.80 Whooping cough due to other Bordetella species without pneumonia

   A37.81 Whooping cough due to other Bordetella species with pneumonia

A37.9 Whooping cough, unspecified species

   A37.90 Whooping cough, unspecified species without pneumonia

   A37.91 Whooping cough, unspecified species with pneumonia

A38 Scarlet fever

> **Includes:** scarlatina
> **Excludes 2:** streptococcal sore throat (J02.0)

A38.0 Scarlet fever with otitis media

A38.1 Scarlet fever with myocarditis

A38.8 Scarlet fever with other complications

A38.9 Scarlet fever, uncomplicated
Scarlet fever, NOS

A39 Meningococcal infection

A39.0 Meningococcal meningitis

A39.1 Waterhouse-Friderichsen syndrome
Meningococcal hemorrhagic adrenalitis
Meningococcic adrenal syndrome

A39.2 Acute meningococcemia

A39.3 Chronic meningococcemia

A39.4 Meningococcemia, unspecified

A39.5 Meningococcal heart disease

   A39.50 Meningococcal carditis, unspecified

   A39.51 Meningococcal endocarditis

   A39.52 Meningococcal myocarditis

   A39.53 Meningococcal pericarditis

A39.8 Other meningococcal infections

   A39.81 Meningococcal encephalitis

   A39.82 Meningococcal retrobulbar neuritis

   A39.83 Meningococcal arthritis

   A39.84 Postmeningococcal arthritis

   A39.89 Other meningococcal infections
   Meningococcal conjunctivitis

A39.9 Meningococcal infection, unspecified
Meningococcal disease NOS

A40 Streptococcal sepsis

> **Code first** postprocedural streptococcal sepsis (T81.4)
> streptococcal sepsis during labor (O75.3)
> streptococcal sepsis following abortion or ectopic or molar pregnancy (O03-O07, O08.0)
> streptococcal sepsis following immunization (T88.0)
> streptococcal sepsis following infusion, transfusion or therapeutic injection (T80.2-)
> **Excludes 1:** neonatal (P36.0-P36.1)
> puerperal sepsis (O85)
> sepsis due to Streptococcus, group D (A41.81)

A40.0 Sepsis due to streptococcus, group A

A40.1 Sepsis due to streptococcus, group B

A40.3 Sepsis due to Streptococcus pneumoniae
Pneumococcal sepsis

A40.8 Other streptococcal sepsis

A40.9 Streptococcal sepsis, unspecified

A41 Other sepsis

<u>Code first</u> postprocedural sepsis (T81.4)

sepsis during labor (O75.3)

sepsis following abortion, ectopic or molar pregnancy (O03-O07, O08.0)

sepsis following immunization (T88.0)

sepsis following infusion, transfusion or therapeutic injection (T80.2-)

Excludes 1: bacteremia NOS (R78.81)

neonatal (P36.-)

puerperal sepsis (O85)

sepsis NOS (A41.9)

streptococcal sepsis (A40.-)

Excludes 2: sepsis (due to) (in) actinomycotic (A42.7)

sepsis (due to) (in) anthrax (A22.7)

sepsis (due to) (in) candidal (B37.7)

sepsis (due to) (in) Erysipelothrix (A26.7)

sepsis (due to) (in) extraintestinal yersiniosis (A28.2)

sepsis (due to) (in) gonococcal (A54.86)

sepsis (due to) (in) herpesviral (B00.7)

sepsis (due to) (in) listerial (A32.7)

sepsis (due to) (in) melioidosis (A24.1)

sepsis (due to) (in) meningococcal (A39.2-A39.4)

sepsis (due to) (in) plague (A20.7)

sepsis (due to) (in) tularemia (A21.7)

toxic shock syndrome (A48.3)

A41.0 Sepsis due to Staphylococcus aureus

A41.01 Sepsis due to Methicillin susceptible Staphylococcus aureus

MSSA sepsis

Staphylococcus aureus sepsis NOS

A41.02 Sepsis due to Methicillin resistant Staphylococcus aureus

A41.1 Sepsis due to other specified staphylococcus

Coagulase negative staphylococcus sepsis

A41.2 Sepsis due to unspecified staphylococcus

A41.3 Sepsis due to Hemophilus influenzae

A41.4 Sepsis due to anaerobes

Excludes 1: gas gangrene (A48.0)

A41.5 Sepsis due to other Gram-negative organisms

A41.50 Gram-negative sepsis, unspecified

Gram-negative sepsis NOS

A41.51 Sepsis due to Escherichia coli [E. coli]

A41.52 Sepsis due to Pseudomonas

Pseudomonas aeroginosa

A41.53 Sepsis due to Serratia

A41.59 Other Gram-negative sepsis

A41.8 Other specified sepsis

A41.81 Sepsis due to Enterococcus

A41.89 Other specified sepsis

A41.9 Sepsis, unspecified organism

Septicemia NOS

A42 Actinomycosis

Excludes 1: actinomycetoma (B47.1)

A42.0 Pulmonary actinomycosis

A42.1 Abdominal actinomycosis

A42.2 Cervicofacial actinomycosis

A42.7 Actinomycotic sepsis

A42.8 Other forms of actinomycosis

A42.81 Actinomycotic meningitis

A42.82 Actinomycotic encephalitis

A42.89 Other forms of actinomycosis

A42.9 Actinomycosis, unspecified

A43 Nocardiosis

A43.0 Pulmonary nocardiosis

A43.1 Cutaneous nocardiosis

A43.8 Other forms of nocardiosis

A43.9 Nocardiosis, unspecified

A44 Bartonellosis

A44.0 Systemic bartonellosis

Oroya fever

A44.1 Cutaneous and mucocutaneous bartonellosis

Verruga peruana

A44.8 Other forms of bartonellosis

A44.9 Bartonellosis, unspecified

A46 Erysipelas

Excludes 1: postpartum or puerperal erysipelas (O86.89)

A48 Other bacterial diseases, not elsewhere classified

Excludes 1: actinomycetoma (B47.1)

A48.0 Gas gangrene

Clostridial cellulitis

Clostridial myonecrosis

A48.1 Legionnaires' disease

A48.2 Nonpneumonic Legionnaires' disease [Pontiac fever]

A48.3 Toxic shock syndrome

Use additional code to identify the organism (B95, B96)

Excludes 1: endotoxic shock NOS (R57.8)

sepsis NOS (A41.9)

A48.4 Brazilian purpuric fever

Systemic Hemophilus aegyptius infection

A48.5 Other specified botulism

Non-foodborne intoxication due to toxins of Clostridium botulinum [C. botulinum]

Excludes 1: food poisoning due to toxins of Clostridium botulinum (A05.1)

A48.51 Infant botulism

A48.52 Wound botulism

Non-foodborne botulism NOS

Use additional code for associated wound

A48.8 Other specified bacterial diseases

A49 Bacterial infection of unspecified site

Excludes 1: bacterial agents as the cause of diseases classified elsewhere (B95-B96)

chlamydial infection NOS (A74.9)

meningococcal infection NOS (A39.9)

rickettsial infection NOS (A79.9)

spirochetal infection NOS (A69.9)

A49.0 Staphylococcal infection, unspecified site

A49.01 Methicillin susceptible Staphylococcus aureus infection, unspecified site

Methicillin susceptible Staphylococcus aureus (MSSA) infection

Staphylococcus aureus infection NOS

A49.02 Methicillin resistant Staphylococcus aureus infection, unspecified site

Methicillin resistant Staphylococcus aureus (MRSA) infection

A49.1 Streptococcal infection, unspecified site

A49.2 Hemophilus influenzae infection, unspecified site

A49.3 Mycoplasma infection, unspecified site

A49.8 Other bacterial infections of unspecified site

A49.9 Bacterial infection, unspecified

Excludes 1: bacteremia NOS (R78.81)

INFECTIONS WITH A PREDOMINANTLY SEXUAL MODE OF TRANSMISSION (A50-A64)

Excludes 1: human immunodeficiency virus [HIV] disease (B20)

nonspecific and nongonococcal urethritis (N34.1)

Reiter's disease (M02.3-)

A50 Congenital syphilis

A50.0 Early congenital syphilis, symptomatic

Any congenital syphilitic condition specified as early or manifest less than two years after birth.

A50.01 Early congenital syphilitic oculopathy

A50.02 Early congenital syphilitic osteochondropathy

A50.03 Early congenital syphilitic pharyngitis

Early congenital syphilitic laryngitis

A50.04 Early congenital syphilitic pneumonia

A50.05 Early congenital syphilitic rhinitis

A50.06 Early cutaneous congenital syphilis

A50.07 Early mucocutaneous congenital syphilis

A50.08 Early visceral congenital syphilis

A50.09 Other early congenital syphilis, symptomatic

A50.1 Early congenital syphilis, latent

Congenital syphilis without clinical manifestations, with positive serological reaction and negative spinal fluid test, less than two years after birth.

A50.2 Early congenital syphilis, unspecified

Congenital syphilis NOS less than two years after birth.

A50.3 Late congenital syphilitic oculopathy

Excludes 1: Hutchinson's triad (A50.53)

A50.30 Late congenital syphilitic oculopathy, unspecified

A50.31 Late congenital syphilitic interstitial keratitis

A50.32 Late congenital syphilitic chorioretinitis

A50.39 Other late congenital syphilitic oculopathy

A50.4 Late congenital neurosyphilis [juvenile neurosyphilis]

Use additional code to identify any associated mental disorder

Excludes 1: Hutchinson's triad (A50.53)

A50.40 Late congenital neurosyphilis, unspecified

Juvenile neurosyphilis NOS

A50.41 Late congenital syphilitic meningitis

A50.42 Late congenital syphilitic encephalitis

A50.43 Late congenital syphilitic polyneuropathy

A50.44 Late congenital syphilitic optic nerve atrophy

A50.45 Juvenile general paresis

Dementia paralytica juvenilis

Juvenile tabetoparetic neurosyphilis

A50.49 Other late congenital neurosyphilis

Juvenile tabes dorsalis

A50.5 Other late congenital syphilis, symptomatic

Any congenital syphilitic condition specified as late or manifest two years or more after birth.

A50.51 Clutton's joints

A50.52 Hutchinson's teeth

A50.53 Hutchinson's triad

A50.54 Late congenital cardiovascular syphilis

A50.55 Late congenital syphilitic arthropathy

A50.56 Late congenital syphilitic osteochondropathy

A50.57 Syphilitic saddle nose

A50.59 Other late congenital syphilis, symptomatic

A50.6 Late congenital syphilis, latent

Congenital syphilis without clinical manifestations, with positive serological reaction and negative spinal fluid test,

two years or more after birth.

A50.7 Late congenital syphilis, unspecified

Congenital syphilis NOS two years or more after birth.

A50.9 Congenital syphilis, unspecified

A51 Early syphilis

A51.0 Primary genital syphilis

Syphilitic chancre NOS

A51.1 Primary anal syphilis

A51.2 Primary syphilis of other sites

A51.3 Secondary syphilis of skin and mucous membranes

A51.31 Condyloma latum

A51.32 Syphilitic alopecia

A51.39 Other secondary syphilis of skin

Syphilitic leukoderma

Syphilitic mucous patch

Excludes 1: late syphilitic leukoderma (A52.79)

A51.4 Other secondary syphilis

A51.41 Secondary syphilitic meningitis

A51.42 Secondary syphilitic female pelvic disease

A51.43 Secondary syphilitic oculopathy

Secondary syphilitic chorioretinitis

Secondary syphilitic iridocyclitis, iritis

Secondary syphilitic uveitis

A51.44 Secondary syphilitic nephritis

A51.45 Secondary syphilitic hepatitis

A51.46 Secondary syphilitic osteopathy

A51.49 Other secondary syphilitic conditions

Secondary syphilitic lymphadenopathy

Secondary syphilitic myositis

A51.5 Early syphilis, latent

Syphilis (acquired) without clinical manifestations, with positive serological reaction and negative spinal fluid test, less than two years after infection.

A51.9 Early syphilis, unspecified

A52 Late syphilis

A52.0 Cardiovascular and cerebrovascular syphilis

A52.00 Cardiovascular syphilis, unspecified

A52.01 Syphilitic aneurysm of aorta

A52.02 Syphilitic aortitis

A52.03 Syphilitic endocarditis

Syphilitic aortic valve incompetence or stenosis

Syphilitic mitral valve stenosis

Syphilitic pulmonary valve regurgitation

A52.04 Syphilitic cerebral arteritis

A52.05 Other cerebrovascular syphilis

Syphilitic cerebral aneurysm (ruptured) (non-ruptured)

Syphilitic cerebral thrombosis

A52.06 Other syphilitic heart involvement

Syphilitic coronary artery disease

Syphilitic myocarditis

Syphilitic pericarditis

A52.09 Other cardiovascular syphilis

A52.1 Symptomatic neurosyphilis

A52.10 Symptomatic neurosyphilis, unspecified

A52.11 Tabes dorsalis

Locomotor ataxia (progressive)

Tabetic neurosyphilis

A52.12 Other cerebrospinal syphilis

A52.13 Late syphilitic meningitis

A52.14 Late syphilitic encephalitis

A52.15 Late syphilitic neuropathy

Late syphilitic acoustic neuritis

Late syphilitic optic (nerve) atrophy

Late syphilitic polyneuropathy

Late syphilitic retrobulbar neuritis

A52.16 Charcʃt's arthropathy (tabetic)

A52.17 General paresis

Dementia paralytica

A52.19 Other symptomatic neurosyphilis

Syphilitic parkinsonism

A52.2 Asymptomatic neurosyphilis

A52.3 Neurosyphilis, unspecified

Gumma (syphilitic)

Syphilis (late)

Syphiloma

A52.7 Other symptomatic late syphilis

A52.71 Late syphilitic oculopathy

Late syphilitic chorioretinitis

Late syphilitic episcleritis

A52.72 Syphilis of lung and bronchus

A52.73 Symptomatic late syphilis of other respiratory organs

A52.74 Syphilis of liver and other viscera

Late syphilitic peritonitis

A52.75 Syphilis of kidney and ureter

Syphilitic glomerular disease

A52.76 Other genitourinary symptomatic late syphilis

Late syphilitic female pelvic inflammatory disease

A52.77 Syphilis of bone and joint

A52.78 Syphilis of other musculoskeletal tissue

Late syphilitic bursitis

Syphilis [stage unspecified] of bursa

Syphilis [stage unspecified] of muscle

Syphilis [stage unspecified] of synovium

Syphilis [stage unspecified] of tendon

A52.79 Other symptomatic late syphilis

Late syphilitic leukoderma

Syphilis of adrenal gland

Syphilis of pituitary gland

Syphilis of thyroid gland

Syphilitic splenomegaly

Excludes 1: syphilitic leukoderma (secondary) (A51.39)

A52.8 Late syphilis, latent

Syphilis (acquired) without clinical manifestations, with positive serological reaction and negative spinal fluid test, two years or more after infection

A52.9 Late syphilis, unspecified

A53 Other and unspecified syphilis

A53.0 Latent syphilis, unspecified as early or late

Latent syphilis NOS

Positive serological reaction for syphilis

A53.9 Syphilis, unspecified

Infection due to Treponema pallidum NOS

Syphilis (acquired) NOS

Excludes 1: syphilis NOS under two years of age (A50.2)

A54 Gonococcal infection

A54.0 Gonococcal infection of lower genitourinary tract without periurethral or accessory gland abscess

Excludes 1: gonococcal infection with genitourinary gland abscess (A54.1)

gonococcal infection with periurethral abscess (A54.1)

A54.00 Gonococcal infection of lower genitourinary tract, unspecified

A54.01 Gonococcal cystitis and urethritis, unspecified

A54.02 Gonococcal vulvovaginitis, unspecified

A54.03 Gonococcal cervicitis, unspecified

A54.09 Other gonococcal infection of lower genitourinary tract

A54.1 Gonococcal infection of lower genitourinary tract with periurethral and accessory gland abscess

Gonococcal Bartholin's gland abscess

A54.2 Gonococcal pelviperitonitis and other gonococcal genitourinary infection

A54.21 Gonococcal infection of kidney and ureter

A54.22 Gonococcal prostatitis

A54.23 Gonococcal infection of other male genital organs

Gonococcal epididymitis

Gonococcal orchitis

A54.24 Gonococcal female pelvic inflammatory disease

Gonococcal pelviperitonitis

Excludes 1: gonococcal peritonitis (A54.85)

A54.29 Other gonococcal genitourinary infections

A54.3 Gonococcal infection of eye

A54.30 Gonococcal infection of eye, unspecified

A54.31 Gonococcal conjunctivitis

Ophthalmia neonatorum due to gonococcus

A54.32 Gonococcal iridocyclitis

A54.33 Gonococcal keratitis

A54.39 Other gonococcal eye infection

Gonococcal endophthalmia

A54.4 Gonococcal infection of musculoskeletal system

A54.40 Gonococcal infection of musculoskeletal system, unspecified

A54.41 Gonococcal spondylopathy

A54.42 Gonococcal arthritis

Excludes 2: gonococcal infection of spine (A54.41)

A54.43 Gonococcal osteomyelitis

Excludes 2: gonococcal infection of spine (A54.41)

A54.49 Gonococcal infection of other musculoskeletal tissue

Gonococcal bursitis

Gonococcal myositis

Gonococcal synovitis

Gonococcal tenosynovitis

A54.5 Gonococcal pharyngitis

A54.6 Gonococcal infection of anus and rectum

A54.8 Other gonococcal infections

A54.81 Gonococcal meningitis

A54.82 Gonococcal brain abscess

A54.83 Gonococcal heart infection

Gonococcal endocarditis

Gonococcal myocarditis

Gonococcal pericarditis

A54.84 Gonococcal pneumonia

A54.85 Gonococcal peritonitis

Excludes 1: gonococcal pelviperitonitis (A54.24)

A54.86 Gonococcal sepsis

A54.89 Other gonococcal infections

Gonococcal keratoderma

Gonococcal lymphadenitis

● New code   ▲ Revised code   ⑦ 7ᵗʰ digit required   ⊗ Placeholder required

A54.9 Gonococcal infection, unspecified

A55 Chlamydial lymphogranuloma (venereum)

Climatic or tropical bubo

Durand-Nicolas-Favre disease

Esthiomene

Lymphogranuloma inguinale

A56 Other sexually transmitted chlamydial diseases

Includes: sexually transmitted diseases due to Chlamydia trachomatis

Excludes 1: neonatal chlamydial conjunctivitis (P39.1)

neonatal chlamydial pneumonia (P23.1)

Excludes 2: chlamydial lymphogranuloma (A55)

conditions classified to A74.-

A56.0 Chlamydial infection of lower genitourinary tract

    A56.00 Chlamydial infection of lower genitourinary tract, unspecified

    A56.01 Chlamydial cystitis and urethritis

    A56.02 Chlamydial vulvovaginitis

    A56.09 Other chlamydial infection of lower genitourinary tract

        Chlamydial cervicitis

A56.1 Chlamydial infection of pelviperitoneum and other genitourinary organs

    A56.11 Chlamydial female pelvic inflammatory disease

    A56.19 Other chlamydial genitourinary infection

        Chlamydial epididymitis

        Chlamydial orchitis

A56.2 Chlamydial infection of genitourinary tract, unspecified

A56.3 Chlamydial infection of anus and rectum

A56.4 Chlamydial infection of pharynx

A56.8 Sexually transmitted chlamydial infection of other sites

A57 Chancroid

Ulcus molle

A58 Granuloma inguinale

Donovanosis

A59 Trichomoniasis

Excludes 2: intestinal trichomoniasis (A07.8)

A59.0 Urogenital trichomoniasis

    A59.00 Urogenital trichomoniasis, unspecified

        Fluor (vaginalis) due to Trichomonas

        Leukorrhea (vaginalis) due to Trichomonas

    A59.01 Trichomonal vulvovaginitis

    A59.02 Trichomonal prostatitis

    A59.03 Trichomonal cystitis and urethritis

    A59.09 Other urogenital trichomoniasis

        Trichomonas cervicitis

A59.8 Trichomoniasis of other sites

A59.9 Trichomoniasis, unspecified

A60 Anogenital herpesviral [herpes simplex] infections

A60.0 Herpesviral infection of genitalia and urogenital tract

    A60.00 Herpesviral infection of urogenital system, unspecified

    A60.01 Herpesviral infection of penis

    A60.02 Herpesviral infection of other male genital organs

    A60.03 Herpesviral cervicitis

    A60.04 Herpesviral vulvovaginitis

        Herpesviral [herpes simplex] ulceration

        Herpesviral [herpes simplex] vaginitis

        Herpesviral [herpes simplex] vulvitis

    A60.09 Herpesviral infection of other urogenital tract

A60.1 Herpesviral infection of perianal skin and rectum

A60.9 Anogenital herpesviral infection, unspecified

A63 Other predominantly sexually transmitted diseases, not elsewhere classified

Excludes 2: molluscum contagiosum (B08.1)

papilloma of cervix (D26.0)

A63.0 Anogenital (venereal) warts

Anogenital warts due to (human) papillomavirus [HPV]

Condyloma acuminatum

A63.8 Other specified predominantly sexually transmitted diseases

A64 Unspecified sexually transmitted disease

OTHER SPIROCHETAL DISEASES (A65-A69)

Excludes 2: leptospirosis (A27.-)

syphilis (A50-A53)

A65 Nonvenereal syphilis

Bejel

Endemic syphilis

Njovera

A66 Yaws

Includes: bouba

frambesia (tropica)

pian

A66.0 Initial lesions of yaws

Chancre of yaws

Frambesia, initial or primary

Initial frambesial ulcer

Mother yaw

A66.1 Multiple papillomata and wet crab yaws

Frambesioma

Pianoma

Plantar or palmar papilloma of yaws

A66.2 Other early skin lesions of yaws

Cutaneous yaws, less than five years after infection

Early yaws (cutaneous)(macular)(maculopapular)(micropapular)(papular)

Frambeside of early yaws

A66.3 Hyperkeratosis of yaws

Ghoul hand

Hyperkeratosis, palmar or plantar (early) (late) due to yaws

Worm-eaten soles

A66.4 Gummata and ulcers of yaws

Gummatous frambeside

Nodular late yaws (ulcerated)

A66.5 Gangosa

Rhinopharyngitis mutilans

A66.6 Bone and joint lesions of yaws

Yaws ganglion

Yaws goundou

Yaws gumma, bone

Yaws gummatous osteitis or periostitis

Yaws hydrarthrosis

Yaws osteitis

Yaws periostitis (hypertrophic)

A66.7 Other manifestations of yaws

Juxta-articular nodules of yaws

Mucosal yaws

A66.8 Latent yaws

Yaws without clinical manifestations, with positive serology

A66.9 Yaws, unspecified

A67 Pinta [carate]

A67.0 Primary lesions of pinta
  Chancre (primary) of pinta
  Papule (primary) of pinta
A67.1 Intermediate lesions of pinta
  Erythematous plaques of pinta
  Hyperchromic lesions of pinta
  Hyperkeratosis of pinta
  Pintids
A67.2 Late lesions of pinta
  Achromic skin lesions of pinta
  Cicatricial skin lesions of pinta
  Dyschromic skin lesions of pinta
A67.3 Mixed lesions of pinta
  Achromic with hyperchromic skin lesions of pinta [carate]
A67.9 Pinta, unspecified
A68 Relapsing fevers
  Includes: recurrent fever
  Excludes 2: Lyme disease (A69.2-)
A68.0 Louse-borne relapsing fever
  Relapsing fever due to Borrelia recurrentis
A68.1 Tick-borne relapsing fever
  Relapsing fever due to any Borrelia species other than Borrelia recurrentis
A68.9 Relapsing fever, unspecified
A69 Other spirochetal infections
A69.0 Necrotizing ulcerative stomatitis
  Cancrum oris
  Fusospirochetal gangrene
  Noma
  Stomatitis gangrenosa
A69.1 Other Vincent's infections
  Fusospirochetal pharyngitis
  Necrotizing ulcerative (acute) gingivitis
  Necrotizing ulcerative (acute) gingivostomatitis
  Spirochetal stomatitis
  Trench mouth
  Vincent's angina
  Vincent's gingivitis
A69.2 Lyme disease
  Erythema chronicum migrans due to Borrelia burgdorferi
  A69.20 Lyme disease, unspecified
  A69.21 Meningitis due to Lyme disease
  A69.22 Other neurologic disorders in Lyme disease
    Cranial neuritis
    Meningoencephalitis
    Polyneuropathy
  A69.23 Arthritis due to Lyme disease
  A69.29 Other conditions associated with Lyme disease
    Myopericarditis due to Lyme disease
A69.8 Other specified spirochetal infections
A69.9 Spirochetal infection, unspecified

OTHER DISEASES CAUSED BY CHLAMYDIAE (A70-A74)
Excludes 1: sexually transmitted chlamydial diseases (A55-A56)
A70 Chlamydia psittaci infections
  Ornithosis
  Parrot fever
  Psittacosis
A71 Trachoma
  Excludes 1: sequelae of trachoma (B94.0)
A71.0 Initial stage of trachoma
  Trachoma dubium

A71.1 Active stage of trachoma
  Granular conjunctivitis (trachomatous)
  Trachomatous follicular conjunctivitis
  Trachomatous pannus
A71.9 Trachoma, unspecified
A74 Other diseases caused by chlamydiae
  Excludes 1: neonatal chlamydial conjunctivitis (P39.1)
  neonatal chlamydial pneumonia (P23.1)
  Reiter's disease (M02.3-)
  sexually transmitted chlamydial diseases (A55-A56)
  Excludes 2: chlamydial pneumonia (J16.0)
A74.0 Chlamydial conjunctivitis
  Paratrachoma
A74.8 Other chlamydial diseases
  A74.81 Chlamydial peritonitis
  A74.89 Other chlamydial diseases
A74.9 Chlamydial infection, unspecified
  Chlamydiosis NOS

RICKETTSIOSES (A75-A79)
A75 Typhus fever
  Excludes 1: rickettsiosis due to Ehrlichia sennetsu (A79.2)
A75.0 Epidemic louse-borne typhus fever due to Rickettsia prowazekii
  Classical typhus (fever)
  Epidemic (louse-borne) typhus
A75.1 Recrudescent typhus [Brill's disease]
  Brill-Zinsser disease
A75.2 Typhus fever due to Rickettsia typhi
  Murine (flea-borne) typhus
A75.3 Typhus fever due to Rickettsia tsutsugamushi
  Scrub (mite-borne) typhus
  Tsutsugamushi fever
A75.9 Typhus fever, unspecified
  Typhus (fever) NOS
A77 Spotted fever [tick-borne rickettsioses]
A77.0 Spotted fever due to Rickettsia rickettsii
  Rocky Mountain spotted fever
  Sao Paulo fever
A77.1 Spotted fever due to Rickettsia conorii
  African tick typhus
  Boutonneuse fever
  India tick typhus
  Kenya tick typhus
  Marseilles fever
  Mediterranean tick fever
A77.2 Spotted fever due to Rickettsia siberica
  North Asian tick fever
  Siberian tick typhus
A77.3 Spotted fever due to Rickettsia australis
  Queensland tick typhus
A77.4 Ehrlichiosis
  Excludes 1: Rickettsiosis due to Ehrlichia sennetsu (A79.81)
  A77.40 Ehrlichiosis, unspecified
  A77.41 Ehrlichiosis chafeensis [E. chafeensis]
  A77.49 Other ehrlichiosis
A77.8 Other spotted fevers
A77.9 Spotted fever, unspecified
  Tick-borne typhus NOS
A78 Q fever
  Infection due to Coxiella burnetii

Nine Mile fever

Quadrilateral fever

A79 Other rickettsioses

A79.0 Trench fever

Quintan fever

Wolhynian fever

A79.1 Rickettsialpox due to Rickettsia akari

Kew Garden fever

Vesicular rickettsiosis

A79.8 Other specified rickettsioses

A79.81 Rickettsiosis due to Ehrlichia sennetsu

A79.89 Other specified rickettsioses

A79.9 Rickettsiosis, unspecified

Rickettsial infection NOS

VIRAL AND PRION INFECTIONS OF THE CENTRAL NERVOUS SYSTEM (A80-A89)

Excludes 1: postpolio syndrome (G14)

sequelae of poliomyelitis (B91)

sequelae of viral encephalitis (B94.1)

A80 Acute poliomyelitis

A80.0 Acute paralytic poliomyelitis, vaccine-associated

A80.1 Acute paralytic poliomyelitis, wild virus, imported

A80.2 Acute paralytic poliomyelitis, wild virus, indigenous

A80.3 Acute paralytic poliomyelitis, other and unspecified

A80.30 Acute paralytic poliomyelitis, unspecified

A80.39 Other acute paralytic poliomyelitis

A80.4 Acute nonparalytic poliomyelitis

A80.9 Acute poliomyelitis, unspecified

A81 Atypical virus infections of central nervous system

Includes: diseases of the central nervous system caused by prions

Use additional code to identify:

dementia with behavioral disturbance (F02.81)

dementia without behavioral disturbance (F02.80)

A81.0 Creutzfeldt-Jakob disease

A81.00 Creutzfeldt-Jakob disease, unspecified

Jakob-Creutzfeldt disease, unspecified

A81.01 Variant Creutzfeldt-Jakob disease

vCJD

A81.09 Other Creutzfeldt-Jakob disease

CJD

Familial Creutzfeldt-Jakob disease

Iatrogenic Creutzfeldt-Jakob disease

Sporadic Creutzfeldt-Jakob disease

Subacute spongiform encephalopathy (with dementia)

A81.1 Subacute sclerosing panencephalitis

Dawson's inclusion body encephalitis

Van Bogaert's sclerosing leukoencephalopathy

A81.2 Progressive multifocal leukoencephalopathy

Multifocal leukoencephalopathy NOS

A81.8 Other atypical virus infections of central nervous system

A81.81 Kuru

A81.82 Gerstmann-StrΣussler-Scheinker syndrome

GSS syndrome

A81.83 Fatal familial insomnia

FFI

A81.89 Other atypical virus infections of central nervous system

A81.9 Atypical virus infection of central nervous system, unspecified

Prion diseases of the central nervous system NOS

A82 Rabies

A82.0 Sylvatic rabies

A82.1 Urban rabies

A82.9 Rabies, unspecified

A83 Mosquito-borne viral encephalitis

Includes: mosquito-borne viral meningoencephalitis

Excludes 2: Venezuelan equine encephalitis (A92.2)

West Nile fever (A92.3-)

West Nile virus (A92.3-)

A83.0 Japanese encephalitis

A83.1 Western equine encephalitis

A83.2 Eastern equine encephalitis

A83.3 St Louis encephalitis

A83.4 Australian encephalitis

Kunjin virus disease

A83.5 California encephalitis

California meningoencephalitis

La Crosse encephalitis

A83.6 Rocio virus disease

A83.8 Other mosquito-borne viral encephalitis

A83.9 Mosquito-borne viral encephalitis, unspecified

A84 Tick-borne viral encephalitis

Includes: tick-borne viral meningoencephalitis

A84.0 Far Eastern tick-borne encephalitis [Russian spring-summer encephalitis]

A84.1 Central European tick-borne encephalitis

A84.8 Other tick-borne viral encephalitis

Louping ill

Powassan virus disease

A84.9 Tick-borne viral encephalitis, unspecified

A85 Other viral encephalitis, not elsewhere classified

Includes: specified viral encephalomyelitis NEC

specified viral meningoencephalitis NEC

Excludes 1: benign myalgic encephalomyelitis (G93.3)

encephalitis due to:

cytomegalovirus (B25.8)

herpesvirus NEC (B10.0-)

herpesvirus [herpes simplex] (B00.4)

measles virus (B05.0)

mumps virus (B26.2)

poliomyelitis virus (A80.)

zoster (B02.0)

lymphocytic choriomeningitis (A87.2)

A85.0 Enteroviral encephalitis

Enteroviral encephalomyelitis

A85.1 Adenoviral encephalitis

Adenoviral meningoencephalitis

A85.2 Arthropod-borne viral encephalitis, unspecified

Excludes 1: West nile virus with encephalitis (A92.31)

A85.8 Other specified viral encephalitis

Encephalitis lethargica

Von Economo-Cruchet disease

A86 Unspecified viral encephalitis

Viral encephalomyelitis NOS

Viral meningoencephalitis NOS

A87 Viral meningitis

Excludes 1: meningitis due to herpesvirus [herpes simplex] (B00.3)

meningitis due to herpesvirus [herpes simplex] (B00.3)

meningitis due to measles virus (B05.1)

meningitis due to mumps virus (B26.1)

meningitis due to poliomyelitis virus (A80.-)

meningitis due to zoster (B02.1)

A87.0 Enteroviral meningitis
Coxsackievirus meningitis
Echovirus meningitis
A87.1 Adenoviral meningitis
A87.2 Lymphocytic choriomeningitis
Lymphocytic meningoencephalitis
A87.8 Other viral meningitis
A87.9 Viral meningitis, unspecified
A88 Other viral infections of central nervous system, not elsewhere classified
Excludes 1: viral encephalitis NOS (A86)
viral meningitis NOS (A87.9)
A88.0 Enteroviral exanthematous fever [Boston exanthem]
A88.1 Epidemic vertigo
A88.8 Other specified viral infections of central nervous system
A89 Unspecified viral infection of central nervous system

ARTHROPOD-BORNE VIRAL FEVERS AND VIRAL HEMORRHAGIC FEVERS (A90-A99)

A90 Dengue fever [classical dengue]
Excludes 1: dengue hemorrhagic fever (A91)
A91 Dengue hemorrhagic fever
A92 Other mosquito-borne viral fevers
Excludes 1: Ross River disease (B33.1)
A92.0 Chikungunya virus disease
Chikungunya (hemorrhagic) fever
A92.1 O'nyong-nyong fever
A92.2 Venezuelan equine fever
Venezuelan equine encephalitis
Venezuelan equine encephalomyelitis virus disease
A92.3 West Nile virus infection
West Nile fever
   A92.30 West Nile virus infection, unspecified
West Nile fever NOS
West Nile fever without complications
West Nile virus NOS
   A92.31 West Nile virus infection with encephalitis
West Nile encephalitis
West Nile encephalomyelitis
   A92.32 West Nile virus infection with other neurologic manifestation
Use additional code to specify the neurologic manifestation
   A92.39 West Nile virus infection with other complications
Use additional code to specify the other conditions
A92.4 Rift Valley fever
A92.8 Other specified mosquito-borne viral fevers
A92.9 Mosquito-borne viral fever, unspecified
A93 Other arthropod-borne viral fevers, not elsewhere classified
A93.0 Oropouche virus disease
Oropouche fever
A93.1 Sandfly fever
Pappataci fever
Phlebotomus fever
A93.2 Colorado tick fever
A93.8 Other specified arthropod-borne viral fevers
Piry virus disease
Vesicular stomatitis virus disease [Indiana fever]
A94 Unspecified arthropod-borne viral fever
Arboviral fever NOS
Arbovirus infection NOS
A95 Yellow fever
A95.0 Sylvatic yellow fever
Jungle yellow fever
A95.1 Urban yellow fever
A95.9 Yellow fever, unspecified
A96 Arenaviral hemorrhagic fever
A96.0 Junin hemorrhagic fever
Argentinian hemorrhagic fever
A96.1 Machupo hemorrhagic fever
Bolivian hemorrhagic fever
A96.2 Lassa fever
A96.8 Other arenaviral hemorrhagic fevers
A96.9 Arenaviral hemorrhagic fever, unspecified
A98 Other viral hemorrhagic fevers, not elsewhere classified
Excludes 1: chikungunya hemorrhagic fever (A92.0)
dengue hemorrhagic fever (A91)
A98.0 Crimean-Congo hemorrhagic fever
Central Asian hemorrhagic fever
A98.1 Omsk hemorrhagic fever
A98.2 Kyasanur Forest disease
A98.3 Marburg virus disease
A98.4 Ebola virus disease
A98.5 Hemorrhagic fever with renal syndrome
Epidemic hemorrhagic fever
Korean hemorrhagic fever
Russian hemorrhagic fever
Hantaan virus disease
Hantavirus disease with renal manifestations
Nephropathia epidemica
Songo fever
Excludes 1: hantavirus (cardio)-pulmonary syndrome (B33.4)
A98.8 Other specified viral hemorrhagic fevers
A99 Unspecified viral hemorrhagic fever

VIRAL INFECTIONS CHARACTERIZED BY SKIN AND MUCOUS MEMBRANE LESIONS (B00-B09)

B00 Herpesviral [herpes simplex] infections
Excludes 1: congenital herpesviral infections (P35.2)
Excludes 2: anogenital herpesviral infection (A60.-)
gammaherpesviral mononucleosis (B27.0-)
herpangina (B08.5)
B00.0 Eczema herpeticum
Kaposi's varicelliform eruption
B00.1 Herpesviral vesicular dermatitis
Herpes simplex facialis
Herpes simplex labialis
Herpes simplex otitis externa
Vesicular dermatitis of ear
Vesicular dermatitis of lip
B00.2 Herpesviral gingivostomatitis and pharyngotonsillitis
Herpesviral pharyngitis
B00.3 Herpesviral meningitis
B00.4 Herpesviral encephalitis
Herpesviral meningoencephalitis
Simian B disease
Excludes 1: herpesviral encephalitis due to herpesvirus 6 and 7 (B10.01, B10.09)
non-simplex herpesviral encephalitis (B10.0-)
B00.5 Herpesviral ocular disease
   B00.50 Herpesviral ocular disease, unspecified
   B00.51 Herpesviral iridocyclitis

Herpesviral iritis

Herpesviral uveitis, anterior

B00.52 Herpesviral keratitis

Herpesviral keratoconjunctivitis

B00.53 Herpesviral conjunctivitis

B00.59 Other herpesviral disease of eye

Herpesviral dermatitis of eyelid

B00.7 Disseminated herpesviral disease

Herpesviral sepsis

B00.8 Other forms of herpesviral infections

B00.81 Herpesviral hepatitis

B00.82 Herpes simplex myelitis

B00.89 Other herpesviral infection

Herpesviral whitlow

B00.9 Herpesviral infection, unspecified

Herpes simplex infection NOS

B01 Varicella [chickenpox]

B01.0 Varicella meningitis

B01.1 Varicella encephalitis, myelitis and encephalomyelitis

Postchickenpox encephalitis, myelitis and encephalomyelitis

B01.11 Varicella encephalitis and encephalomyelitis

Postchickenpox encephalitis and encephalomyelitis

B01.12 Varicella myelitis

Postchickenpox myelitis

B01.2 Varicella pneumonia

B01.8 Varicella with other complications

B01.81 Varicella keratitis

B01.89 Other varicella complications

B01.9 Varicella without complication

Varicella NOS

B02 Zoster [herpes zoster]

Includes: shingles

zona

B02.0 Zoster encephalitis

Zoster meningoencephalitis

B02.1 Zoster meningitis

B02.2 Zoster with other nervous system involvement

B02.21 Postherpetic geniculate ganglionitis

B02.22 Postherpetic trigeminal neuralgia

B02.23 Postherpetic polyneuropathy

B02.24 Postherpetic myelitis

Herpes zoster myelitis

B02.29 Other postherpetic nervous system involvement

Postherpetic radiculopathy

B02.3 Zoster ocular disease

B02.30 Zoster ocular disease, unspecified

B02.31 Zoster conjunctivitis

B02.32 Zoster iridocyclitis

B02.33 Zoster keratitis

Herpes zoster keratoconjunctivitis

B02.34 Zoster scleritis

B02.39 Other herpes zoster eye disease

Zoster blepharitis

B02.7 Disseminated zoster

B02.8 Zoster with other complications

Herpes zoster otitis externa

B02.9 Zoster without complications

Zoster NOS

B03 Smallpox

Note: In 1980 the 33rd World Health Assembly declared that

smallpox had been eradicated. The classification is maintained for surveillance purposes.

B04 Monkeypox

B05 Measles

Includes: morbilli

Excludes 1: subacute sclerosing panencephalitis (A81.1)

B05.0 Measles complicated by encephalitis

Postmeasles encephalitis

B05.1 Measles complicated by meningitis

Postmeasles meningitis

B05.2 Measles complicated by pneumonia

Postmeasles pneumonia

B05.3 Measles complicated by otitis media

Postmeasles otitis media

B05.4 Measles with intestinal complications

B05.8 Measles with other complications

B05.81 Measles keratitis and keratoconjunctivitis

B05.89 Other measles complications

B05.9 Measles without complication

Measles NOS

B06 Rubella [German measles]

Excludes 1: congenital rubella (P35.0)

B06.0 Rubella with neurological complications

B06.00 Rubella with neurological complication, unspecified

B06.01 Rubella encephalitis

Rubella meningoencephalitis

B06.02 Rubella meningitis

B06.09 Other neurological complications of rubella

B06.8 Rubella with other complications

B06.81 Rubella pneumonia

B06.82 Rubella arthritis

B06.89 Other rubella complications

B06.9 Rubella without complication

Rubella NOS

B07 Viral warts

Includes: verruca simplex

verruca vulgaris

viral warts due to human papillomavirus

Excludes 2: anogenital (venereal) warts (A63.0)

papilloma of bladder (D41.4)

papilloma of cervix (D26.0)

papilloma larynx (D14.1)

B07.0 Plantar wart

Verruca plantaris

B07.8 Other viral warts

Common wart

Flat wart

Verruca plana

B07.9 Viral wart, unspecified

B08 Other viral infections characterized by skin and mucous membrane lesions, not elsewhere classified

Excludes 1: vesicular stomatitis virus disease (A93.8)

B08.0 Other orthopoxvirus infections

Excludes 2: monkeypox (B04)

B08.01 Cowpox and vaccinia not from vaccine

B08.010 Cowpox

B08.011 Vaccinia not from vaccine

Excludes 1: vaccinia (from vaccination) (generalized) (T88.1)

B08.02 Orf virus disease

Contagious pustular dermatitis

Ecthyma contagiosum

B08.03 Pseudocowpox [milker's node]

B08.04 Paravaccinia, unspecified

B08.09 Other orthopoxvirus infections

Orthopoxvirus infection NOS

B08.1 Molluscum contagiosum

B08.2 Exanthema subitum [sixth disease]

Roseola infantum

B08.20 Exanthema subitum [sixth disease], unspecified

Roseola infantum, unspecified

B08.21 Exanthema subitum [sixth disease] due to human herpesvirus 6

Roseola infantum due to human herpesvirus 6

B08.22 Exanthema subitum [sixth disease] due to human herpesvirus 7

Roseola infantum due to human herpesvirus 7

B08.3 Erythema infectiosum [fifth disease]

B08.4 Enteroviral vesicular stomatitis with exanthem

Hand, foot and mouth disease

B08.5 Enteroviral vesicular pharyngitis

Herpangina

B08.6 Parapoxvirus infections

B08.60 Parapoxvirus infection, unspecified

B08.61 Bovine stomatitis

B08.62 Sealpox

B08.69 Other parapoxvirus infections

B08.7 Yatapoxvirus infections

B08.70 Yatapoxvirus infection, unspecified

B08.71 Tanapox virus disease

B08.72 Yaba pox virus disease

Yaba monkey tumor disease

B08.79 Other yatapoxvirus infections

B08.8 Other specified viral infections characterized by skin and mucous membrane lesions

Enteroviral lymphonodular pharyngitis

Foot-and-mouth disease

Poxvirus NEC

B09 Unspecified viral infection characterized by skin and mucous membrane lesions

Viral enanthema NOS

Viral exanthema NOS

OTHER HUMAN HERPESVIRUSES (B10)

B10 Other human herpesviruses

Excludes 2: cytomegalovirus (B25.9)

Epstein-Barr virus (B27.0-)

herpes NOS (B00.9)

herpes simplex (B00.-)

herpes zoster (B02.-)

human herpesvirus NOS (B00.-)

human herpesvirus 1and 2 (B00.-)

human herpesvirus 3(B01.-, B02-)

human herpesvirus 4(B27.0-)

human herpesvirus 5(B25.-)

varicella (B01.-)

zoster (B02.-)

B10.0 Other human herpesvirus encephalitis

Excludes 2: herpes encephalitis NOS (B00.4)

herpes simplex encephalitis (B00.4)

human herpesvirus encephalitis (B00.4)

simian B herpes virus encephalitis (B00.4)

B10.01 Human herpesvirus 6encephalitis

B10.09 Other human herpesvirus encephalitis

Human herpesvirus 7encephalitis

B10.8 Other human herpesvirus infection

B10.81 Human herpesvirus 6infection

B10.82 Human herpesvirus 7infection

B10.89 Other human herpesvirus infection

Human herpesvirus 8infection

Kaposi's sarcoma-associated herpesvirus infection

VIRAL HEPATITIS (B15-B19)

Excludes 1: sequelae of viral hepatitis (B94.2)

Excludes 2: cytomegaloviral hepatitis (B25.1)

herpesviral [herpes simplex] hepatitis (B00.81)

B15 Acute hepatitis A

B15.0 Hepatitis A with hepatic coma

B15.9 Hepatitis A without hepatic coma

Hepatitis A (acute)(viral) NOS

B16 Acute hepatitis B

B16.0 Acute hepatitis B with delta-agent with hepatic coma

B16.1 Acute hepatitis B with delta-agent without hepatic coma

B16.2 Acute hepatitis B without delta-agent with hepatic coma

B16.9 Acute hepatitis B without delta-agent and without hepatic coma

Hepatitis B (acute) (viral) NOS

B17 Other acute viral hepatitis

B17.0 Acute delta-(super) infection of hepatitis B carrier

B17.1 Acute hepatitis C

B17.10 Acute hepatitis C without hepatic coma

Acute hepatitis C NOS

B17.11 Acute hepatitis C with hepatic coma

B17.2 Acute hepatitis E

B17.8 Other specified acute viral hepatitis

Hepatitis non-A non-B (acute) (viral) NEC

B17.9 Acute viral hepatitis, unspecified

Acute hepatitis NOS

B18 Chronic viral hepatitis

B18.0 Chronic viral hepatitis B with delta-agent

B18.1 Chronic viral hepatitis B without delta-agent

Chronic (viral) hepatitis B

B18.2 Chronic viral hepatitis C

B18.8 Other chronic viral hepatitis

B18.9 Chronic viral hepatitis, unspecified

B19 Unspecified viral hepatitis

B19.0 Unspecified viral hepatitis with hepatic coma

B19.1 Unspecified viral hepatitis B

B19.10 Unspecified viral hepatitis B without hepatic coma

Unspecified viral hepatitis B NOS

B19.11 Unspecified viral hepatitis B with hepatic coma

B19.2 Unspecified viral hepatitis C

B19.20 Unspecified viral hepatitis C without hepatic coma

Viral hepatitis C NOS

B19.21 Unspecified viral hepatitis C with hepatic coma

B19.9 Unspecified viral hepatitis without hepatic coma

Viral hepatitis NOS

HUMAN IMMUNODEFICIENCY VIRUS [HIV] DISEASE (B20)

B20 Human immunodeficiency virus [HIV] disease

Includes: acquired immune deficiency syndrome [AIDS]

AIDS-related complex [ARC]

HIV infection, symptomatic

Code first Human immunodeficiency virus [HIV] disease complicating pregnancy, childbirth and the puerperium, if applicable (O98.7-)

Use additional code(s) to identify all manifestations of HIV infection

Excludes 1: asymptomatic human immunodeficiency virus [HIV] infection status (Z21)

exposure to HIV virus (Z20.6)

inconclusive serologic evidence of HIV (R75)

OTHER VIRAL DISEASES (B25-B34)

B25 Cytomegaloviral disease

Excludes 1: congenital cytomegalovirus infection (P35.1)

cytomegaloviral mononucleosis (B27.1-)

B25.0 Cytomegaloviral pneumonitis

B25.1 Cytomegaloviral hepatitis

B25.2 Cytomegaloviral pancreatitis

B25.8 Other cytomegaloviral diseases

Cytomegaloviral encephalitis

B25.9 Cytomegaloviral disease, unspecified

B26 Mumps

Includes: epidemic parotitis

infectious parotitis

B26.0 Mumps orchitis

B26.1 Mumps meningitis

B26.2 Mumps encephalitis

B26.3 Mumps pancreatitis

B26.8 Mumps with other complications

B26.81 Mumps hepatitis

B26.82 Mumps myocarditis

B26.83 Mumps nephritis

B26.84 Mumps polyneuropathy

B26.85 Mumps arthritis

B26.89 Other mumps complications

B26.9 Mumps without complication

Mumps NOS

Mumps parotitis NOS

B27 Infectious mononucleosis

Includes: glandular fever

monocytic angina

Pfeiffer's disease

B27.0 Gammaherpesviral mononucleosis

Mononucleosis due to Epstein-Barr virus

B27.00 Gammaherpesviral mononucleosis without complication

B27.01 Gammaherpesviral mononucleosis with polyneuropathy

B27.02 Gammaherpesviral mononucleosis with meningitis

B27.09 Gammaherpesviral mononucleosis with other complications

Hepatomegaly in gammaherpesviral mononucleosis

B27.1 Cytomegaloviral mononucleosis

B27.10 Cytomegaloviral mononucleosis without complications

B27.11 Cytomegaloviral mononucleosis with polyneuropathy

B27.12 Cytomegaloviral mononucleosis with meningitis

B27.19 Cytomegaloviral mononucleosis with other complication

Hepatomegaly in cytomegaloviral mononucleosis

B27.8 Other infectious mononucleosis

B27.80 Other infectious mononucleosis without complication

B27.81 Other infectious mononucleosis with polyneuropathy

B27.82 Other infectious mononucleosis with meningitis

B27.89 Other infectious mononucleosis with other complication

Hepatomegaly in other infectious mononucleosis

B27.9 Infectious mononucleosis, unspecified

B27.90 Infectious mononucleosis, unspecified without complication

B27.91 Infectious mononucleosis, unspecified with polyneuropathy

B27.92 Infectious mononucleosis, unspecified with meningitis

B27.99 Infectious mononucleosis, unspecified with other complication

Hepatomegaly in unspecified infectious mononucleosis

B30 Viral conjunctivitis

Excludes 1: herpesviral [herpes simplex] ocular disease (B00.5)

ocular zoster (B02.3)

B30.0 Keratoconjunctivitis due to adenovirus

Epidemic keratoconjunctivitis

Shipyard eye

B30.1 Conjunctivitis due to adenovirus

Acute adenoviral follicular conjunctivitis

Swimming-pool conjunctivitis

B30.2 Viral pharyngoconjunctivitis

B30.3 Acute epidemic hemorrhagic conjunctivitis (enteroviral)

Conjunctivitis due to coxsackievirus 24

Conjunctivitis due to enterovirus 70

Hemorrhagic conjunctivitis (acute)(epidemic)

B30.8 Other viral conjunctivitis

Newcastle conjunctivitis

B30.9 Viral conjunctivitis, unspecified

B33 Other viral diseases, not elsewhere classified

B33.0 Epidemic myalgia

Bornholm disease

B33.1 Ross River disease

Epidemic polyarthritis and exanthema

Ross River fever

B33.2 Viral carditis

Coxsackie (virus) carditis

B33.20 Viral carditis, unspecified

B33.21 Viral endocarditis

B33.22 Viral myocarditis

B33.23 Viral pericarditis

B33.24 Viral cardiomyopathy

B33.3 Retrovirus infections, not elsewhere classified

Retrovirus infection NOS

B33.4 Hantavirus (cardio)-pulmonary syndrome [HPS] [HCPS]

Hantavirus disease with pulmonary manifestations

Sin nombre virus disease

Use additional code to identify any associated acute kidney failure (N17.9)

Excludes 1: hantavirus disease with renal manifestations (A98.5)

hemorrhagic fever with renal manifestations (A98.5)

B33.8 Other specified viral diseases

Excludes 1: anogenital human papillomavirus infection (A63.0)

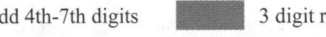 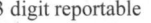

viral warts due to human papillomavirus infection (B07)

B34 Viral infection of unspecified site

Excludes 1: anogenital human papillomavirus infection (A63.0)

cytomegaloviral disease NOS (B25.9)

herpesvirus [herpes simplex] infection NOS (B00.9)

retrovirus infection NOS (B33.3)

viral agents as the cause of diseases classified elsewhere (B97.-)

viral warts due to human papillomavirus infection (B07)

B34.0 Adenovirus infection, unspecified

B34.1 Enterovirus infection, unspecified

Coxsackievirus infection NOS

Echovirus infection NOS

B34.2 Coronavirus infection, unspecified

Excludes 1: pneumonia due to SARS-associated coronavirus (J12.81)

B34.3 Parvovirus infection, unspecified

B34.4 Papovavirus infection, unspecified

B34.8 Other viral infections of unspecified site

B34.9 Viral infection, unspecified

Viremia NOS

MYCOSES (B35-B49)

Excludes 2: hypersensitivity pneumonitis due to organic dust (J67.-)

mycosis fungoides (C84.0-)

B35 Dermatophytosis

Includes: favus

infections due to species of Epidermophyton, Micro-sporum and Trichophyton

tinea, any type except those in B36.-

B35.0 Tinea barbae and tinea capitis

Beard ringworm

Kerion

Scalp ringworm

Sycosis, mycotic

B35.1 Tinea unguium

Dermatophytic onychia

Dermatophytosis of nail

Onychomycosis

Ringworm of nails

B35.2 Tinea manuum

Dermatophytosis of hand

Hand ringworm

B35.3 Tinea pedis

Athlete's foot

Dermatophytosis of foot

Foot ringworm

B35.4 Tinea corporis

Ringworm of the body

B35.5 Tinea imbricata

Tokelau

B35.6 Tinea cruris

Dhobi itch

Groin ringworm

Jock itch

B35.8 Other dermatophytoses

Disseminated dermatophytosis

Granulomatous dermatophytosis

B35.9 Dermatophytosis, unspecified

Ringworm NOS

B36 Other superficial mycoses

B36.0 Pityriasis versicolor

Tinea flava

Tinea versicolor

B36.1 Tinea nigra

Keratomycosis nigricans palmaris

Microsporosis nigra

Pityriasis nigra

B36.2 White piedra

Tinea blanca

B36.3 Black piedra

B36.8 Other specified superficial mycoses

B36.9 Superficial mycosis, unspecified

B37 Candidiasis

Includes: candidosis

moniliasis

Excludes 1: neonatal candidiasis (P37.5)

B37.0 Candidal stomatitis

Oral thrush

B37.1 Pulmonary candidiasis

Candidal bronchitis

Candidal pneumonia

B37.2 Candidiasis of skin and nail

Candidal onychia

Candidal paronychia

Excludes 2: diaper dermatitis (L22)

B37.3 Candidiasis of vulva and vagina

Candidal vulvovaginitis

Monilial vulvovaginitis

Vaginal thrush

B37.4 Candidiasis of other urogenital sites

B37.41 Candidal cystitis and urethritis

B37.42 Candidal balanitis

B37.49 Other urogenital candidiasis

Candidal pyelonephritis

B37.5 Candidal meningitis

B37.6 Candidal endocarditis

B37.7 Candidal sepsis

Disseminated candidiasis

Systemic candidiasis

B37.8 Candidiasis of other sites

B37.81 Candidal esophagitis

B37.82 Candidal enteritis

Candidal proctitis

B37.83 Candidal cheilitis

B37.84 Candidal otitis externa

B37.89 Other sites of candidiasis

Candidal osteomyelitis

B37.9 Candidiasis, unspecified

Thrush NOS

B38 Coccidioidomycosis

B38.0 Acute pulmonary coccidioidomycosis

B38.1 Chronic pulmonary coccidioidomycosis

B38.2 Pulmonary coccidioidomycosis, unspecified

B38.3 Cutaneous coccidioidomycosis

B38.4 Coccidioidomycosis meningitis

B38.7 Disseminated coccidioidomycosis

Generalized coccidioidomycosis

B38.8 Other forms of coccidioidomycosis

B38.81 Prostatic coccidioidomycosis

B38.89 Other forms of coccidioidomycosis

B38.9 Coccidioidomycosis, unspecified

B39 Histoplasmosis

Code first associated AIDS (B20)

● New code   ▲ Revised code   ⑦ 7th digit required   ⊗ Placeholder required

Use additional code for any associated manifestations, such as:

endocarditis (I39)

meningitis (G02)

pericarditis (I32)

retinitits (H32)

B39.0 Acute pulmonary histoplasmosis capsulati

B39.1 Chronic pulmonary histoplasmosis capsulati

B39.2 Pulmonary histoplasmosis capsulati, unspecified

B39.3 Disseminated histoplasmosis capsulati

Generalized histoplasmosis capsulati

B39.4 Histoplasmosis capsulati, unspecified

American histoplasmosis

B39.5 Histoplasmosis duboisii

African histoplasmosis

B39.9 Histoplasmosis, unspecified

B40 Blastomycosis

Excludes 1: Brazilian blastomycosis (B41.-)

keloidal blastomycosis (B48.0)

B40.0 Acute pulmonary blastomycosis

B40.1 Chronic pulmonary blastomycosis

B40.2 Pulmonary blastomycosis, unspecified

B40.3 Cutaneous blastomycosis

B40.7 Disseminated blastomycosis

Generalized blastomycosis

B40.8 Other forms of blastomycosis

B40.81 Blastomycotic meningoencephalitis

Meningomyelitis due to blastomycosis

B40.89 Other forms of blastomycosis

B40.9 Blastomycosis, unspecified

B41 Paracoccidioidomycosis

Includes: Brazilian blastomycosis

Lutz' disease

B41.0 Pulmonary paracoccidioidomycosis

B41.7 Disseminated paracoccidioidomycosis

Generalized paracoccidioidomycosis

B41.8 Other forms of paracoccidioidomycosis

B41.9 Paracoccidioidomycosis, unspecified

B42 Sporotrichosis

B42.0 Pulmonary sporotrichosis

B42.1 Lymphocutaneous sporotrichosis

B42.7 Disseminated sporotrichosis

Generalized sporotrichosis

B42.8 Other forms of sporotrichosis

B42.81 Cerebral sporotrichosis

Meningitis due to sporotrichosis

B42.82 Sporotrichosis arthritis

B42.89 Other forms of sporotrichosis

B42.9 Sporotrichosis, unspecified

B43 Chromomycosis and pheomycotic abscess

B43.0 Cutaneous chromomycosis

Dermatitis verrucosa

B43.1 Pheomycotic brain abscess

Cerebral chromomycosis

B43.2 Subcutaneous pheomycotic abscess and cyst

B43.8 Other forms of chromomycosis

B43.9 Chromomycosis, unspecified

B44 Aspergillosis

Includes: aspergilloma

B44.0 Invasive pulmonary aspergillosis

B44.1 Other pulmonary aspergillosis

B44.2 Tonsillar aspergillosis

B44.7 Disseminated aspergillosis

Generalized aspergillosis

B44.8 Other forms of aspergillosis

B44.81 Allergic bronchopulmonary aspergillosis

B44.89 Other forms of aspergillosis

B44.9 Aspergillosis, unspecified

B45 Cryptococcosis

B45.0 Pulmonary cryptococcosis

B45.1 Cerebral cryptococcosis

Cryptococcal meningitis

Cryptococcosis meningocerebralis

B45.2 Cutaneous cryptococcosis

B45.3 Osseous cryptococcosis

B45.7 Disseminated cryptococcosis

Generalized cryptococcosis

B45.8 Other forms of cryptococcosis

B45.9 Cryptococcosis, unspecified

B46 Zygomycosis

B46.0 Pulmonary mucormycosis

B46.1 Rhinocerebral mucormycosis

B46.2 Gastrointestinal mucormycosis

B46.3 Cutaneous mucormycosis

Subcutaneous mucormycosis

B46.4 Disseminated mucormycosis

Generalized mucormycosis

B46.5 Mucormycosis, unspecified

B46.8 Other zygomycoses

Entomophthoromycosis

B46.9 Zygomycosis, unspecified

Phycomycosis NOS

B47 Mycetoma

B47.0 Eumycetoma

Madura foot, mycotic

Maduromycosis

B47.1 Actinomycetoma

B47.9 Mycetoma, unspecified

Madura foot NOS

B48 Other mycoses, not elsewhere classified

B48.0 Lobomycosis

Keloidal blastomycosis

Lobo's disease

B48.1 Rhinosporidiosis

B48.2 Allescheriasis

Infection due to Pseudallescheria boydii

Excludes 1: eumycetoma (B47.0)

B48.3 Geotrichosis

Geotrichum stomatitis

B48.4 Penicillosis

B48.8 Other specified mycoses

Adiaspiromycosis

Infection of tissue and organs by Alternaria

Infection of tissue and organs by Drechslera

Infection of tissue and organs by Fusarium

Infection of tissue and organs by saprophytic fungi NEC

B49 Unspecified mycosis

Fungemia NOS

PROTOZOAL DISEASES (B50-B64)

Excludes 1: amebiasis (A06.-)

other protozoal intestinal diseases (A07.-)

B50 Plasmodium falciparum malaria

Includes: mixed infections of Plasmodium falciparum with any other Plasmodium species

B50.0 Plasmodium falciparum malaria with cerebral complications

Cerebral malaria NOS

B50.8 Other severe and complicated Plasmodium falciparum malaria

Severe or complicated Plasmodium falciparum malaria NOS

B50.9 Plasmodium falciparum malaria, unspecified

B51 Plasmodium vivax malaria

Includes: mixed infections of Plasmodium vivax with other Plasmodium species, except Plasmodium falciparum

Excludes 1: plasmodium vivav with Plasmodium falciparum (B50.-)

B51.0 Plasmodium vivax malaria with rupture of spleen

B51.8 Plasmodium vivax malaria with other complications

B51.9 Plasmodium vivax malaria without complication

Plasmodium vivax malaria NOS

B52 Plasmodium malariae malaria

Includes: mixed infections of Plasmodium malariae with other Plasmodium species, except Plasmodium falciparum and Plasmodium vivax

Excludes 1: Plasmodium falciparum (B50.-)

Plasmodium vivax (B51.-)

B52.0 Plasmodium malariae malaria with nephropathy

B52.8 Plasmodium malariae malaria with other complications

B52.9 Plasmodium malariae malaria without complication

Plasmodium malariae malaria NOS

B53 Other specified malaria

B53.0 Plasmodium ovale malaria

Excludes 1: Plasmodium ovale with Plasmodium falciparum (B50.-)

Plasmodium ovale with Plasmodium malariae (B52.-)

Plasmodium ovale with Plasmodium vivax (B51.-)

B53.1 Malaria due to simian plasmodia

Excludes 1: Malaria due to simian plasmodia with Plasmodium falciparum (B50.-)

Malaria due to simian plasmodia with Plasmodium malariae (B52.-)

Malaria due to simian plasmodia with Plasmodium ovale (B53.0)

Malaria due to simian plasmodia with Plasmodium vivax (B51.-)

B53.8 Other malaria, not elsewhere classified

B54 Unspecified malaria

B55 Leishmaniasis

B55.0 Visceral leishmaniasis

Kala-azar

Post-kala-azar dermal leishmaniasis

B55.1 Cutaneous leishmaniasis

B55.2 Mucocutaneous leishmaniasis

B55.9 Leishmaniasis, unspecified

B56 African trypanosomiasis

B56.0 Gambiense trypanosomiasis

Infection due to Trypanosoma brucei gambiense

West African sleeping sickness

B56.1 Rhodesiense trypanosomiasis

East African sleeping sickness

Infection due to Trypanosoma brucei rhodesiense

B56.9 African trypanosomiasis, unspecified

Sleeping sickness NOS

B57 Chagas' disease

Includes: American trypanosomiasis

infection due to Trypanosoma cruzi

B57.0 Acute Chagas' disease with heart involvement

Acute Chagas' disease with myocarditis

B57.1 Acute Chagas' disease without heart involvement

Acute Chagas' disease NOS

B57.2 Chagas' disease (chronic) with heart involvement

American trypanosomiasis NOS

Chagas' disease (chronic) NOS

Chagas' disease (chronic) with myocarditis

Trypanosomiasis NOS

B57.30 Chagas' disease with digestive system involvement, unspecified

B57.31 Megaesophagus in Chagas' disease

B57.32 Megacolon in Chagas' disease

B57.39 Other digestive system involvement in Chagas' disease

B57.4 Chagas' disease (chronic) with nervous system involvement

B57.40 Chagas' disease with nervous system involvement, unspecified

B57.41 Meningitis in Chagas' disease

B57.42 Meningoencephalitis in Chagas' disease

B57.49 Other nervous system involvement in Chagas' disease

B57.5 Chagas' disease (chronic) with other organ involvement

B58 Toxoplasmosis

Includes: infection due to Toxoplasma gondii

Excludes 1: congenital toxoplasmosis (P37.1)

B58.0 Toxoplasma oculopathy

B58.00 Toxoplasma oculopathy, unspecified

B58.01 Toxoplasma chorioretinitis

B58.09 Other toxoplasma oculopathy

Toxoplasma uveitis

B58.1 Toxoplasma hepatitis

B58.2 Toxoplasma meningoencephalitis

B58.3 Pulmonary toxoplasmosis

B58.8 Toxoplasmosis with other organ involvement

B58.81 Toxoplasma myocarditis

B58.82 Toxoplasma myositis

B58.83 Toxoplasma tubulo-interstitial nephropathy

Toxoplasma pyelonephritis

B58.89 Toxoplasmosis with other organ involvement

B58.9 Toxoplasmosis, unspecified

B59 Pneumocystosis

Pneumonia due to Pneumocystis carinii

Pneumonia due to Pneumocystis jiroveci

B60 Other protozoal diseases, not elsewhere classified

Excludes 1: cryptosporidiosis (A07.2)

intestinal microsporidiosis (A07.8)

isosporiasis (A07.3)

B60.0 Babesiosis

Piroplasmosis

B60.1 Acanthamebiasis

B60.10 Acanthamebiasis, unspecified

B60.11 Meningoencephalitis due to Acanthamoeba (culbertsoni)

B60.12 Conjunctivitis due to Acanthamoeba

B60.13 Keratoconjunctivitis due to Acanthamoeba

B60.19 Other acanthamebic disease

B60.2 Naegleriasis

Primary amebic meningoencephalitis

B60.8 Other specified protozoal diseases

Microsporidiosis

B64 Unspecified protozoal disease

● New code   ▲ Revised code   ⑦ 7th digit required   ⊗ Placeholder required

HELMINTHIASES (B65-B83)

B65 Schistosomiasis [bilharziasis]

Includes: snail fever

B65.0 Schistosomiasis due to Schistosoma haematobium [urinary schistosomiasis]

B65.1 Schistosomiasis due to Schistosoma mansoni [intestinal schistosomiasis]

B65.2 Schistosomiasis due to Schistosoma japonicum

Asiatic schistosomiasis

B65.3 Cercarial dermatitis

Swimmer's itch

B65.8 Other schistosomiasis

Infection due to Schistosoma intercalatum

Infection due to Schistosoma mattheei

Infection due to Schistosoma mekongi

B65.9 Schistosomiasis, unspecified

B66 Other fluke infections

B66.0 Opisthorchiasis

Infection due to cat liver fluke

Infection due to Opisthorchis (felineus)(viverrini)

B66.1 Clonorchiasis

Chinese liver fluke disease

Infection due to Clonorchis sinensis

Oriental liver fluke disease

B66.2 Dicroceliasis

Infection due to Dicrocoelium dendriticum

Lancet fluke infection

B66.3 Fascioliasis

Infection due to Fasciola gigantica

Infection due to Fasciola hepatica

Infection due to Fasciola indica

Sheep liver fluke disease

B66.4 Paragonimiasis

Infection due to Paragonimus species

Lung fluke disease

Pulmonary distomiasis

B66.5 Fasciolopsiasis

Infection due to Fasciolopsis buski

Intestinal distomiasis

B66.8 Other specified fluke infections

Echinostomiasis

Heterophyiasis

Metagonimiasis

Nanophyetiasis

Watsoniasis

B66.9 Fluke infection, unspecified

B67 Echinococcosis

Includes: hydatidosis

B67.0 Echinococcus granulosus infection of liver

B67.1 Echinococcus granulosus infection of lung

B67.2 Echinococcus granulosus infection of bone

B67.3 Echinococcus granulosus infection, other and multiple sites

B67.31 Echinococcus granulosus infection, thyroid gland

B67.32 Echinococcus granulosus infection, multiple sites

B67.39 Echinococcus granulosus infection, other sites

B67.4 Echinococcus granulosus infection, unspecified

Dog tapeworm (infection)

B67.5 Echinococcus multilocularis infection of liver

B67.6 Echinococcus multilocularis infection, other and multiple sites

B67.61 Echinococcus multilocularis infection, multiple sites

B67.69 Echinococcus multilocularis infection, other sites

B67.7 Echinococcus multilocularis infection, unspecified

B67.8 Echinococcosis, unspecified, of liver

B67.9 Echinococcosis, other and unspecified

B67.90 Echinococcosis, unspecified

Echinococcosis NOS

B67.99 Other echinococcosis

B68 Taeniasis

Excludes 1: cysticercosis (B69.-)

B68.0 Taenia solium taeniasis

Pork tapeworm (infection)

B68.1 Taenia saginata taeniasis

Beef tapeworm (infection)

Infection due to adult tapeworm Taenia saginata

B68.9 Taeniasis, unspecified

B69 Cysticercosis

Includes: cysticerciasis infection due to larval form of Taenia solium

B69.0 Cysticercosis of central nervous system

B69.1 Cysticercosis of eye

B69.8 Cysticercosis of other sites

B69.81 Myositis in cysticercosis

B69.89 Cysticercosis of other sites

B69.9 Cysticercosis, unspecified

B70 Diphyllobothriasis and sparganosis

B70.0 Diphyllobothriasis

Diphyllobothrium (adult) (latum) (pacificum) infection

Fish tapeworm (infection)

Excludes 2: larval diphyllobothriasis (B70.1)

B70.1 Sparganosis

Infection due to Sparganum (mansoni) (proliferum)

Infection due to Spirometra larva

Larval diphyllobothriasis

Spirometrosis

B71 Other cestode infections

B71.0 Hymenolepiasis

Dwarf tapeworm infection

Rat tapeworm (infection)

B71.1 Dipylidiasis

B71.8 Other specified cestode infections

Coenurosis

B71.9 Cestode infection, unspecified

Tapeworm (infection) NOS

B72 Dracunculiasis

Includes: guinea worm infection

infection due to Dracunculus medinensis

B73 Onchocerciasis

Includes: onchocerca volvulus infection

onchocercosis

river blindness

B73.0 Onchocerciasis with eye disease

B73.00 Onchocerciasis with eye involvement, unspecified

B73.01 Onchocerciasis with endophthalmitis

B73.02 Onchocerciasis with glaucoma

B73.09 Onchocerciasis with other eye involvement

Infestation of eyelid due to onchocerciasis

B73.1 Onchocerciasis without eye disease

B74 Filariasis

Excludes 2: onchocerciasis (B73)

tropical (pulmonary) eosinophilia NOS (J82)

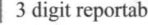

B74.0   Filariasis due to Wuchereria bancrofti
Bancroftian elephantiasis
Bancroftian filariasis

B74.1   Filariasis due to Brugia malayi

B74.2   Filariasis due to Brugia timori

B74.3   Loiasis
Calabar swelling
Eyeworm disease of Africa
Loa loa infection

B74.4   Mansonelliasis
Infection due to Mansonella ozzardi
Infection due to Mansonella perstans
Infection due to Mansonella streptocerca

B74.8   Other filariases
Dirofilariasis

B74.9   Filariasis, unspecified

B75   Trichinellosis
Includes: infection due to Trichinella species
trichiniasis

B76   Hookworm diseases
Includes: uncinariasis

B76.0   Ancylostomiasis
Infection due to Ancylostoma species

B76.1   Necatoriasis
Infection due to Necator americanus

B76.8   Other hookworm diseases

B76.9   Hookworm disease, unspecified
Cutaneous larva migrans NOS

B77   Ascariasis
Includes: ascaridiasis
roundworm infection

B77.0   Ascariasis with intestinal complications

B77.8   Ascariasis with other complications

B77.81   Ascariasis pneumonia

B77.89   Ascariasis with other complications

B77.9   Ascariasis, unspecified

B78   Strongyloidiasis
Excludes 1: trichostrongyliasis (B81.2)

B78.0   Intestinal strongyloidiasis

B78.1   Cutaneous strongyloidiasis

B78.7   Disseminated strongyloidiasis

B78.9   Strongyloidiasis, unspecified

B79   Trichuriasis
Includes: trichocephaliasis
whipworm (disease)(infection)

B80   Enterobiasis
Includes: oxyuriasis
pinworm infection
threadworm infection

B81   Other intestinal helminthiases, not elsewhere classified
Excludes 1: angiostrongyliasis due to Parastrongylus cantonensis (B83.2)

B81.0   Anisakiasis
Infection due to Anisakis larva

B81.1   Intestinal capillariasis
Capillariasis NOS
Infection due to Capillaria philippinensis
Excludes 2: hepatic capillariasis (B83.8)

B81.2   Trichostrongyliasis

B81.3   Intestinal angiostrongyliasis
Angiostrongyliasis due to Parastrongylus costaricensis

B81.4   Mixed intestinal helminthiases
Infection due to intestinal helminths classified to more than one of the categories B65.0-B81.3and B81.8
Mixed helminthiasis NOS

B81.8   Other specified intestinal helminthiases
Infection due to Oesophagostomum species [esophagostomiasis]
Infection due to Ternidens diminutus [ternidensiasis]

B82   Unspecified intestinal parasitism

B82.0   Intestinal helminthiasis, unspecified

B82.9   Intestinal parasitism, unspecified

B83   Other helminthiases
Excludes 1: capillariasis NOS (B81.1)
Excludes 2: intestinal capillariasis (B81.1)

B83.0   Visceral larva migrans
Toxocariasis

B83.1   Gnathostomiasis
Wandering swelling

B83.2   Angiostrongyliasis due to Parastrongylus cantonensis
Eosinophilic meningoencephalitis due to Parastrongylus cantonensis
Excludes 2: intestinal angiostrongyliasis (B81.3)

B83.3   Syngamiasis
Syngamosis

B83.4   Internal hirudiniasis
Excludes 2: external hirudiniasis (B88.3)

B83.8   Other specified helminthiases
Acanthocephaliasis
Gongylonemiasis
Hepatic capillariasis
Metastrongyliasis
Thelaziasis

B83.9   Helminthiasis, unspecified
Worms NOS
Excludes 1: intestinal helminthiasis NOS (B82.0)

PEDICULOSIS, ACARIASIS AND OTHER INFESTATIONS (B85-B89)

B85   Pediculosis and phthiriasis

B85.0   Pediculosis due to Pediculus humanus capitis
Head-louse infestation

B85.1   Pediculosis due to Pediculus humanus corporis
Body-louse infestation

B85.2   Pediculosis, unspecified

B85.3   Phthiriasis
Infestation by crab-louse
Infestation by Phthirus pubis

B85.4   Mixed pediculosis and phthiriasis
Infestation classifiable to more than one of the categories B85.0- B85.3

B86   Scabies
Sarcoptic itch

B87   Myiasis
Includes: infestation by larva of flies

B87.0   Cutaneous myiasis
Creeping myiasis

B87.1   Wound myiasis
Traumatic myiasis

B87.2   Ocular myiasis

B87.3   Nasopharyngeal myiasis
Laryngeal myiasis

B87.4   Aural myiasis

B87.8 Myiasis of other sites

    B87.81 Genitourinary myiasis

    B87.82 Intestinal myiasis

    B87.89 Myiasis of other sites

B87.9 Myiasis, unspecified

B88 Other infestations

B88.0 Other acariasis

    Acarine dermatitis

    Dermatitis due to Demodex species

    Dermatitis due to Dermanyssus gallinae

    Dermatitis due to Liponyssoides sanguineus

    Trombiculosis

    Excludes 2: scabies (B86)

B88.1 Tungiasis [sandflea infestation]

B88.2 Other arthropod infestations

    Scarabiasis

B88.3 External hirudiniasis

    Leech infestation NOS

    Excludes 2: internal hirudiniasis (B83.4)

B88.8 Other specified infestations

    Ichthyoparasitism due to Vandellia cirrhosa

    Linguatulosis

    Porocephaliasis

B88.9 Infestation, unspecified

    Infestation (skin) NOS

    Infestation by mites NOS

    Skin parasites NOS

B89 Unspecified parasitic disease

SEQUELAE OF INFECTIOUS AND PARASITIC DISEASES (B90-B94)

Note: Categories B90-B94 are to be used to indicate conditions in categories A00-B89 as the cause of sequelae, which are themselves classified elsewhere.

The 'sequelae' include conditions specified as such; they also include residuals of diseases classifiable to the above categories if there is evidence that the disease itself is no longer present. Codes from these categories are not to be used for chronic infections. Code chronic current infections to active infectious disease as appropriate. **Code first** condition resulting from (sequela) the infectious or parasitic disease

B90 Sequelae of tuberculosis

B90.0 Sequelae of central nervous system tuberculosis

B90.1 Sequelae of genitourinary tuberculosis

B90.2 Sequelae of tuberculosis of bones and joints

B90.8 Sequelae of tuberculosis of other organs

    Excludes 2: sequelae of respiratory tuberculosis (B90.9)

B90.9 Sequelae of respiratory and unspecified tuberculosis

    Sequelae of tuberculosis NOS

B91 Sequelae of poliomyelitis

    Excludes 1: postpolio syndrome (G14)

B92 Sequelae of leprosy

B94 Sequelae of other and unspecified infectious and parasitic diseases

B94.0 Sequelae of trachoma

B94.1 Sequelae of viral encephalitis

B94.2 Sequelae of viral hepatitis

B94.8 Sequelae of other specified infectious and parasitic diseases

B94.9 Sequelae of unspecified infectious and parasitic disease

    Bacterial and viral infectious agents (B95-B97)

Note: These categories are provided for use as supplementary or additional codes to identify the infectious agent(s) in diseases classified elsewhere.

B95 Streptococcus, Staphylococcus, and Enterococcus as the cause of diseases classified elsewhere

B95.0 Streptococcus, group A, as the cause of diseases classified elsewhere

B95.1 Streptococcus, group B, as the cause of diseases classified elsewhere

B95.2 Enterococcus as the cause of diseases classified elsewhere

B95.3 Streptococcus pneumoniae as the cause of diseases classified elsewhere

B95.4 Other streptococcus as the cause of diseases classified elsewhere

B95.5 Unspecified streptococcus as the cause of diseases classified elsewhere

B95.6 Staphylococcus aureus as the cause of diseases classified elsewhere

    B95.61 Methicillin susceptible Staphylococcus aureus infection as the cause of diseases classified elsewhere

        Methicillin susceptible Staphylococcus aureus (MSSA) infection as the cause of diseases classified elsewhere

        Staphylococcus aureus infection NOS as the cause of diseases classified elsewhere

    B95.62 Methicillin resistant Staphylococcus aureus infection as the cause of diseases classified elsewhere

        Methicillin resistant staphylococcus aureus (MRSA) infection as the cause of diseases classified elsewhere

B95.7 Other staphylococcus as the cause of diseases classified elsewhere

B95.8 Unspecified staphylococcus as the cause of diseases classified elsewhere

B96 Other bacterial agents as the cause of diseases classified elsewhere

B96.0 Mycoplasma pneumoniae [M. pneumoniae] as the cause of diseases classified elsewhere

    Pleuro-pneumonia-like-organism [PPLO]

B96.1 Klebsiella pneumoniae [K. pneumoniae] as the cause of diseases classified elsewhere

B96.2 Escherichia coli [E. coli] as the cause of diseases classified elsewhere

    B96.20 Unspecified Escherichia coli [E. coli] as the cause of diseases classified elsewhere

        Escherichia coli [E. coli] NOS

    B96.21 Shiga toxin-producing Escherichia coli [E. coli] (STEC) O157as the cause of diseases classified elsewhere

        E. coli O157:H- (nonmotile) with confirmation of Shiga toxin

        E. coli O157 with confirmation of Shiga toxin when H antigen is unknown, or is not H7

        O157:H7 Escherichia coli [E.coli] with or without confirmation of Shiga toxin-production

        Shiga toxin-producing Escherichia coli [E.coli] O157:H7 with or without confirmation of Shiga toxin-production

        STEC O157:H7with or without confirmation of Shiga toxin-production

    B96.22 Other specified Shiga toxin-producing Escherichia coli [E. coli] (STEC) as the cause of diseases classified elsewhere

        Non-O157 Shiga toxin-producing Escherichia coli [E.coli]

        Non-O157 Shiga toxin-producing Escherichia coli [E.coli] with known O group

    B96.23 Unspecified Shiga toxin-producing Escherichia

coli [E. coli] (STEC) as the cause of diseases classified elsewhere

Shiga toxin-producing Escherichia coli [E. coli] with unspecified O group

STEC NOS

B96.29 Other Escherichia coli [E. coli] as the cause of diseases classified elsewhere

Non-Shiga toxin-producing E. coli

B96.3 Hemophilus influenzae [H. influenzae] as the cause of diseases classified elsewhere

B96.4 Proteus (mirabilis) (morganii) as the cause of diseases classified elsewhere

B96.5 Pseudomonas (aeruginosa) (mallei) (pseudomallei) as the cause of diseases classified elsewhere

B96.6 Bacteroides fragilis [B. fragilis] as the cause of diseases classified elsewhere

B96.7 Clostridium perfringens [C. perfringens] as the cause of diseases classified elsewhere

B96.8 Other specified bacterial agents as the cause of diseases classified elsewhere

B96.81 Helicobacter pylori [H. pylori] as the cause of diseases classified elsewhere

B96.82 Vibrio vulnificus as the cause of diseases classified elsewhere

B96.89 Other specified bacterial agents as the cause of diseases classified elsewhere

B97 Viral agents as the cause of diseases classified elsewhere

B97.0 Adenovirus as the cause of diseases classified elsewhere

B97.1 Enterovirus as the cause of diseases classified elsewhere

B97.10 Unspecified enterovirus as the cause of diseases classified elsewhere

B97.11 Coxsackievirus as the cause of diseases classified elsewhere

B97.12 Echovirus as the cause of diseases classified elsewhere

B97.19 Other enterovirus as the cause of diseases classified elsewhere

B97.2 Coronavirus as the cause of diseases classified elsewhere

B97.21 SARS-associated coronavirus as the cause of diseases classified elsewhere

Excludes 1: pneumonia due to SARS-associated coronavirus (J12.81)

B97.29 Other coronavirus as the cause of diseases classified elsewhere

B97.3 Retrovirus as the cause of diseases classified elsewhere

Excludes 1: Human immunodeficiency virus [HIV] disease (B20)

B97.30 Unspecified retrovirus as the cause of diseases classified elsewhere

B97.31 Lentivirus as the cause of diseases classified elsewhere

B97.32 Oncovirus as the cause of diseases classified elsewhere

B97.33 Human T-cell lymphotrophic virus, type I [HTLV-I] as the cause of diseases classified elsewhere

B97.34 Human T-cell lymphotrophic virus, type II [HTLV-II] as the cause of diseases classified elsewhere

B97.35 Human immunodeficiency virus, type 2 [HIV 2] as the cause of diseases classified elsewhere

B97.39 Other retrovirus as the cause of diseases classified elsewhere

B97.4 Respiratory syncytial virus as the cause of diseases classified elsewhere

B97.5 Reovirus as the cause of diseases classified elsewhere

B97.6 Parvovirus as the cause of diseases classified elsewhere

B97.7 Papillomavirus as the cause of diseases classified elsewhere

B97.8 Other viral agents as the cause of diseases classified elsewhere

B97.81 Human metapneumovirus as the cause of diseases classified elsewhere

B97.89 Other viral agents as the cause of diseases classified elsewhere

OTHER INFECTIOUS DISEASES (B99)

B99 Other and unspecified infectious diseases

B99.8 Other infectious disease

B99.9 Unspecified infectious disease

● New code   ▲ Revised code   ⑦ 7th digit required   ⊗ Placeholder required

Chapter 2: Neoplasms (C00-D49)

Note: Functional activity

All neoplasms are classified in this chapter, whether they are functionally active or not. An additional code from Chapter 4 may be used, to identify functional activity associated with any neoplasm.

Morphology [Histology]

Chapter 2 classifies neoplasms primarily by site (topography), with broad groupings for behavior, malignant, in situ, benign, etc. The Table of Neoplasms should be used to identify the correct topography code. In a few cases, such as for malignant melanoma and certain neuroendocrine tumors, the morphology (histologic type) is included in the category and codes.

Primary malignant neoplasms overlapping site boundaries

A primary malignant neoplasm that overlaps two or more contiguous (next to each other) sites should be classified to the subcategory/code .8 ('overlapping lesion'), unless the combination is specifically indexed elsewhere. For multiple neoplasms of the same site that are not contiguous, such as tumors in different quadrants of the same breast, codes for each site should be assigned.

Malignant neoplasm of ectopic tissue

Malignant neoplasms of ectopic tissue are to be coded to the site mentioned, e.g., ectopic pancreatic malignant neoplasms are coded to pancreas, unspecified (C25.9).

This chapter contains the following blocks:

C00-C14	Malignant neoplasms of lip, oral cavity and pharynx
C15-C26	Malignant neoplasms of digestive organs
C30-C39	Malignant neoplasms of respiratory and intrathoracic organs
C40-C41	Malignant neoplasms of bone and articular cartilage
C43-C44	Melanoma and other malignant neoplasms of skin
C45-C49	Malignant neoplasms of mesothelial and soft tissue
C50	Malignant neoplasms of breast
C51-C58	Malignant neoplasms of female genital organs
C60-C63	Malignant neoplasms of male genital organs
C64-C68	Malignant neoplasms of urinary tract
C69-C72	Malignant neoplasms of eye, brain and other parts of central nervous system
C73-C75	Malignant neoplasms of thyroid and other endocrine glands
C7A	Malignant neuroendocrine tumors
C7B	Secondary neuroendocrine tumors
C76-C80	Malignant neoplasms of ill-defined, other secondary and unspecified sites
C81-C96	Malignant neoplasms of lymphoid, hematopoietic and related tissue
D00-D09	In situ neoplasms
D10-D36	Benign neoplasms, except benign neuroendocrine tumors
D3A	Benign neuroendocrine tumors
D37-D48	Neoplasms of uncertain behavior, polycythemia vera and myelodysplastic syndromes
D49	Neoplasms of unspecified behavior

MALIGNANT NEOPLASMS (C00-C96)

Malignant neoplasms, stated or presumed to be primary (of specified sites), and certain specified histologies, except neuroendocrine, and of lymphoid, hematopoietic and related tissue (C00-C75)
malignant neoplasms of lip, oral cavity and pharynx (C00-c14)

C00 Malignant neoplasm of lip
Use additional code to identify:
    alcohol abuse and dependence (F10.-)
    history of tobacco use (Z87.891)
    tobacco dependence (F17.-)
    tobacco use (Z72.0)
Excludes 1: malignant melanoma of lip (C43.0)
    Merkel cell carcinoma of lip (C4A.0)
    other and unspecified malignant neoplasm of skin of lip (C44.0-)

C00.0 Malignant neoplasm of external upper lip
Malignant neoplasm of lipstick area of upper lip
Malignant neoplasm of upper lip NOS
Malignant neoplasm of vermilion border of upper lip

C00.1 Malignant neoplasm of external lower lip
Malignant neoplasm of lower lip NOS
Malignant neoplasm of lipstick area of lower lip
Malignant neoplasm of vermilion border of lower lip

C00.2 Malignant neoplasm of external lip, unspecified
Malignant neoplasm of vermilion border of lip NOS

C00.3 Malignant neoplasm of upper lip, inner aspect
Malignant neoplasm of buccal aspect of upper lip
Malignant neoplasm of frenulum of upper lip
Malignant neoplasm of mucosa of upper lip
Malignant neoplasm of oral aspect of upper lip

C00.4 Malignant neoplasm of lower lip, inner aspect
Malignant neoplasm of buccal aspect of lower lip
Malignant neoplasm of frenulum of lower lip
Malignant neoplasm of mucosa of lower lip
Malignant neoplasm of oral aspect of lower lip

C00.5 Malignant neoplasm of lip, unspecified, inner aspect
Malignant neoplasm of buccal aspect of lip, unspecified
Malignant neoplasm of frenulum of lip, unspecified
Malignant neoplasm of mucosa of lip, unspecified
Malignant neoplasm of oral aspect of lip, unspecified

C00.6 Malignant neoplasm of commissure of lip, unspecified

C00.8 Malignant neoplasm of overlapping sites of lip

C00.9 Malignant neoplasm of lip, unspecified

C01 Malignant neoplasm of base of tongue
Malignant neoplasm of dorsal surface of base of tongue
Malignant neoplasm of fixed part of tongue NOS
Malignant neoplasm of posterior third of tongue
Use additional code to identify:
    alcohol abuse and dependence (F10.-)
    history of tobacco use (Z87.891)
    tobacco dependence (F17.-)
    tobacco use (Z72.0)

C02 Malignant neoplasm of other and unspecified parts of tongue
Use additional code to identify:
    alcohol abuse and dependence (F10.-)
    history of tobacco use (Z87.891)
    tobacco dependence (F17.-)
    tobacco use (Z72.0)

C02.0 Malignant neoplasm of dorsal surface of tongue
Malignant neoplasm of anterior two-thirds of tongue, dorsal surface
Excludes 2: malignant neoplasm of dorsal surface of base of tongue (C01)

C02.1 Malignant neoplasm of border of tongue
Malignant neoplasm of tip of tongue

C02.2 Malignant neoplasm of ventral surface of tongue
Malignant neoplasm of anterior two-thirds of tongue, ventral surface

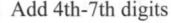 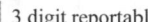

Malignant neoplasm of frenulum linguae

C02.3 Malignant neoplasm of anterior two-thirds of tongue, part unspecified

Malignant neoplasm of middle third of tongue NOS

Malignant neoplasm of mobile part of tongue NOS

C02.4 Malignant neoplasm of lingual tonsil

Excludes 2: malignant neoplasm of tonsil NOS (C09.9)

C02.8 Malignant neoplasm of overlapping sites of tongue

Malignant neoplasm of two or more contiguous sites of tongue

C02.9 Malignant neoplasm of tongue, unspecified

C03 Malignant neoplasm of gum

Includes: malignant neoplasm of alveolar (ridge) mucosa

malignant neoplasm of gingiva

Use additional code to identify:

alcohol abuse and dependence (F10.-)

history of tobacco use (Z87.891)

tobacco dependence (F17.-)

tobacco use (Z72.0)

Excludes 2: malignant odontogenic neoplasms (C41.0-C41.1)

C03.0 Malignant neoplasm of upper gum

C03.1 Malignant neoplasm of lower gum

C03.9 Malignant neoplasm of gum, unspecified

C04 Malignant neoplasm of floor of mouth

Use additional code to identify:

alcohol abuse and dependence (F10.-)

history of tobacco use (Z87.891)

tobacco dependence (F17.-)

tobacco use (Z72.0)

C04.0 Malignant neoplasm of anterior floor of mouth

Malignant neoplasm of anterior to the premolar-canine junction

C04.1 Malignant neoplasm of lateral floor of mouth

C04.8 Malignant neoplasm of overlapping sites of floor of mouth

C04.9 Malignant neoplasm of floor of mouth, unspecified

C05 Malignant neoplasm of palate

Use additional code to identify:

alcohol abuse and dependence (F10.-)

history of tobacco use (Z87.891)

tobacco dependence (F17.-)

tobacco use (Z72.0)

Excludes 1: Kaposi's sarcoma of palate (C46.2)

C05.0 Malignant neoplasm of hard palate

C05.1 Malignant neoplasm of soft palate

Excludes 2: malignant neoplasm of nasopharyngeal surface of soft palate (C11.3)

C05.2 Malignant neoplasm of uvula

C05.8 Malignant neoplasm of overlapping sites of palate

C05.9 Malignant neoplasm of palate, unspecified

Malignant neoplasm of roof of mouth

C06 Malignant neoplasm of other and unspecified parts of mouth

Use additional code to identify:

alcohol abuse and dependence (F10.-)

history of tobacco use (Z87.891)

tobacco dependence (F17.-)

tobacco use (Z72.0)

C06.0 Malignant neoplasm of cheek mucosa

Malignant neoplasm of buccal mucosa NOS

Malignant neoplasm of internal cheek

C06.1 Malignant neoplasm of vestibule of mouth

Malignant neoplasm of buccal sulcus (upper) (lower)

Malignant neoplasm of labial sulcus (upper) (lower)

C06.2 Malignant neoplasm of retromolar area

C06.8 Malignant neoplasm of overlapping sites of other and unspecified parts of mouth

C06.80 Malignant neoplasm of overlapping sites of unspecified parts of mouth

C06.89 Malignant neoplasm of overlapping sites of other parts of mouth

'book leaf' neoplasm [ventral surface of tongue and floor of mouth]

C06.9 Malignant neoplasm of mouth, unspecified

Malignant neoplasm of minor salivary gland, unspecified site

Malignant neoplasm of oral cavity NOS

C07 Malignant neoplasm of parotid gland

Use additional code to identify:

alcohol abuse and dependence (F10.-)

exposure to environmental tobacco smoke (Z77.22)

exposure to tobacco smoke in the perinatal period (P96.81)

history of tobacco use (Z87.891)

occupational exposure to environmental tobacco smoke (Z57.31)

tobacco dependence (F17.-)

tobacco use (Z72.0)

C08 Malignant neoplasm of other and unspecified major salivary glands

Includes: malignant neoplasm of salivary ducts

Use additional code to identify:

alcohol abuse and dependence (F10.-)

exposure to environmental tobacco smoke (Z77.22)

exposure to tobacco smoke in the perinatal period (P96.81)

history of tobacco use (Z87.891)

occupational exposure to environmental tobacco smoke (Z57.31)

tobacco dependence (F17.-)

tobacco use (Z72.0)

Excludes 1: malignant neoplasms of specified minor salivary glands which are classified according to their anatomical location

Excludes 2: malignant neoplasms of minor salivary glands NOS (C06.9)

malignant neoplasm of parotid gland (C07)

C08.0 Malignant neoplasm of submandibular gland

Malignant neoplasm of submaxillary gland

C08.1 Malignant neoplasm of sublingual gland

C08.9 Malignant neoplasm of major salivary gland, unspecified

Malignant neoplasm of salivary gland (major) NOS

C09 Malignant neoplasm of tonsil

Use additional code to identify:

alcohol abuse and dependence (F10.-)

exposure to environmental tobacco smoke (Z77.22)

exposure to tobacco smoke in the perinatal period (P96.81)

history of tobacco use (Z87.891)

occupational exposure to environmental tobacco smoke (Z57.31)

tobacco dependence (F17.-)

tobacco use (Z72.0)

Excludes 2: malignant neoplasm of lingual tonsil (C02.4)

malignant neoplasm of pharyngeal tonsil (C11.1)

C09.0 Malignant neoplasm of tonsillar fossa

C09.1 Malignant neoplasm of tonsillar pillar (anterior) (posterior)

C09.8 Malignant neoplasm of overlapping sites of tonsil

C09.9 Malignant neoplasm of tonsil, unspecified

Malignant neoplasm of tonsil NOS

Malignant neoplasm of faucial tonsils

Malignant neoplasm of palatine tonsils

C10 Malignant neoplasm of oropharynx

Use additional code to identify:

    alcohol abuse and dependence (F10.-)

    exposure to environmental tobacco smoke (Z77.22)

    exposure to tobacco smoke in the perinatal period (P96.81)

    history of tobacco use (Z87.891)

    occupational exposure to environmental tobacco smoke (Z57.31)

    tobacco dependence (F17.-)

    tobacco use (Z72.0)

    Excludes 2: malignant neoplasm of tonsil (C09.-)

C10.0 Malignant neoplasm of vallecula

C10.1 Malignant neoplasm of anterior surface of epiglottis

    Malignant neoplasm of epiglottis, free border [margin]

    Malignant neoplasm of glossoepiglottic fold(s)

    Excludes 2: malignant neoplasm of epiglottis (suprahyoid portion) NOS (C32.1)

C10.2 Malignant neoplasm of lateral wall of oropharynx

C10.3 Malignant neoplasm of posterior wall of oropharynx

C10.4 Malignant neoplasm of branchial cleft

    Malignant neoplasm of branchial cyst [site of neoplasm]

C10.8 Malignant neoplasm of overlapping sites of oropharynx

    Malignant neoplasm of junctional region of oropharynx

C10.9 Malignant neoplasm of oropharynx, unspecified

C11 Malignant neoplasm of nasopharynx

Use additional code to identify:

    exposure to environmental tobacco smoke (Z77.22)

    exposure to tobacco smoke in the perinatal period (P96.81)

    history of tobacco use (Z87.891)

    occupational exposure to environmental tobacco smoke (Z57.31)

    tobacco dependence (F17.-)

    tobacco use (Z72.0)

C11.0 Malignant neoplasm of superior wall of nasopharynx

    Malignant neoplasm of roof of nasopharynx

C11.1 Malignant neoplasm of posterior wall of nasopharynx

    Malignant neoplasm of adenoid

    Malignant neoplasm of pharyngeal tonsil

C11.2 Malignant neoplasm of lateral wall of nasopharynx

    Malignant neoplasm of fossa of Rosenmüller

    Malignant neoplasm of opening of auditory tube

    Malignant neoplasm of pharyngeal recess

C11.3 Malignant neoplasm of anterior wall of nasopharynx

    Malignant neoplasm of floor of nasopharynx

    Malignant neoplasm of nasopharyngeal (anterior) (posterior) surface of soft palate

    Malignant neoplasm of posterior margin of nasal choana

    Malignant neoplasm of posterior margin of nasal septum

C11.8 Malignant neoplasm of overlapping sites of nasopharynx

C11.9 Malignant neoplasm of nasopharynx, unspecified

    Malignant neoplasm of nasopharyngeal wall NOS

C12 Malignant neoplasm of pyriform sinus

    Malignant neoplasm of pyriform fossa

Use additional code to identify:

    exposure to environmental tobacco smoke (Z77.22)

    exposure to tobacco smoke in the perinatal period (P96.81)

    history of tobacco use (Z87.891)

    occupational exposure to environmental tobacco smoke (Z57.31)

    tobacco dependence (F17.-)

    tobacco use (Z72.0)

C13 Malignant neoplasm of hypopharynx

Use additional code to identify:

    exposure to environmental tobacco smoke (Z77.22)

    exposure to tobacco smoke in the perinatal period (P96.81)

    history of tobacco use (Z87.891)

    occupational exposure to environmental tobacco smoke (Z57.31)

    tobacco dependence (F17.-)

    tobacco use (Z72.0)

    Excludes 2: malignant neoplasm of pyriform sinus (C12)

C13.0 Malignant neoplasm of postcricoid region

C13.1 Malignant neoplasm of aryepiglottic fold, hypopharyngeal aspect

    Malignant neoplasm of aryepiglottic fold NOS

    Malignant neoplasm of interarytenoid fold NOS

    Malignant neoplasm of aryepiglottic fold marginal zone

    Malignant neoplasm of interarytenoid fold marginal zone

    Excludes 2: malignant neoplasm of aryepiglottic fold or interarytenoid fold, laryngeal aspect (C32.1)

C13.2 Malignant neoplasm of posterior wall of hypopharynx

C13.8 Malignant neoplasm of overlapping sites of hypopharynx

C13.9 Malignant neoplasm of hypopharynx, unspecified

    Malignant neoplasm of hypopharyngeal wall NOS

C14 Malignant neoplasm of other and ill-defined sites in the lip, oral cavity and pharynx

Use additional code to identify:

    alcohol abuse and dependence (F10.-)

    exposure to environmental tobacco smoke (Z77.22)

    exposure to tobacco smoke in the perinatal period (P96.81)

    history of tobacco use (Z87.891)

    occupational exposure to environmental tobacco smoke (Z57.31)

    tobacco dependence (F17.-)

    tobacco use (Z72.0)

    Excludes 1: malignant neoplasm of oral cavity NOS (C06.9)

C14.0 Malignant neoplasm of pharynx, unspecified

C14.2 Malignant neoplasm of Waldeyer's ring

C14.8 Malignant neoplasm of overlapping sites of lip, oral cavity and pharynx

    Primary malignant neoplasm of two or more contiguous sites of lip, oral cavity and pharynx

    Excludes 1: 'book leaf' neoplasm [ventral surface of tongue and floor of mouth] (C06.89)

MALIGNANT NEOPLASMS OF DIGESTIVE ORGANS (C15-C26)

Excludes 1: Kaposi's sarcoma of gastrointestinal sites (C46.4)

C15 Malignant neoplasm of esophagus

Use additional code to identify:

    alcohol abuse and dependence (F10.)

C15.3 Malignant neoplasm of upper third of esophagus

C15.4 Malignant neoplasm of middle third of esophagus

C15.5 Malignant neoplasm of lower third of esophagus

    Excludes 1: malignant neoplasm of cardio-esophageal junction (C16.0)

C15.8 Malignant neoplasm of overlapping sites of esophagus

C15.9 Malignant neoplasm of esophagus, unspecified

C16 Malignant neoplasm of stomach

Use additional code to identify:

alcohol abuse and dependence (F10.-)

Excludes 2: malignant carcinoid tumor of the stomach (C7A.092)

C16.0 Malignant neoplasm of cardia

    Malignant neoplasm of cardiac orifice

Malignant neoplasm of cardio-esophageal junction

Malignant neoplasm of esophagus and stomach

Malignant neoplasm of gastro-esophageal junction

C16.1 Malignant neoplasm of fundus of stomach

C16.2 Malignant neoplasm of body of stomach

C16.3 Malignant neoplasm of pyloric antrum

Malignant neoplasm of gastric antrum

C16.4 Malignant neoplasm of pylorus

Malignant neoplasm of prepylorus

Malignant neoplasm of pyloric canal

C16.5 Malignant neoplasm of lesser curvature of stomach, unspecified

Malignant neoplasm of lesser curvature of stomach, not classifiable to C16.1-C16.4

C16.6 Malignant neoplasm of greater curvature of stomach, unspecified

Malignant neoplasm of greater curvature of stomach, not classifiable to C16.0-C16.4

C16.8 Malignant neoplasm of overlapping sites of stomach

C16.9 Malignant neoplasm of stomach, unspecified

Gastric cancer NOS

C17 Malignant neoplasm of small intestine

Excludes 1: malignant carcinoid tumors of the small intestine (C7A.01)

C17.0 Malignant neoplasm of duodenum

C17.1 Malignant neoplasm of jejunum

C17.2 Malignant neoplasm of ileum

Excludes 1: malignant neoplasm of ileocecal valve (C18.0)

C17.3 Meckel's diverticulum, malignant

Excludes 1: Meckel's diverticulum, congenital (Q43.0)

C17.8 Malignant neoplasm of overlapping sites of small intestine

C17.9 Malignant neoplasm of small intestine, unspecified

C18 Malignant neoplasm of colon

Excludes 1: malignant carcinoid tumors of the colon (C7A.02-)

C18.0 Malignant neoplasm of cecum

Malignant neoplasm of ileocecal valve

C18.1 Malignant neoplasm of appendix

C18.2 Malignant neoplasm of ascending colon

C18.3 Malignant neoplasm of hepatic flexure

C18.4 Malignant neoplasm of transverse colon

C18.5 Malignant neoplasm of splenic flexure

C18.6 Malignant neoplasm of descending colon

C18.7 Malignant neoplasm of sigmoid colon

Malignant neoplasm of sigmoid (flexure)

Excludes 1: malignant neoplasm of rectosigmoid junction (C19)

C18.8 Malignant neoplasm of overlapping sites of colon

C18.9 Malignant neoplasm of colon, unspecified

Malignant neoplasm of large intestine NOS

C19 Malignant neoplasm of rectosigmoid junction

Malignant neoplasm of colon with rectum

Malignant neoplasm of rectosigmoid (colon)

Excludes 1: malignant carcinoid tumors of the colon (C7A.02-)

C20 Malignant neoplasm of rectum

Malignant neoplasm of rectal ampulla

Excludes 1: malignant carcinoid tumor of the rectum (C7A.026)

C21 Malignant neoplasm of anus and anal canal

Excludes 2: malignant carcinoid tumors of the colon (C7A.02-)

malignant melanoma of anal margin (C43.51)

malignant melanoma of anal skin (C43.51)

malignant melanoma of perianal skin (C43.51)

other and unspecified malignant neoplasm of anal margin (C44.500, C44.510, C44.520, C44.590)

other and unspecified malignant neoplasm of anal skin (C44.500, C44.510, C44.520, C44.590)

other and unspecified malignant neoplasm of perianal skin (C44.500, C44.510, C44.520, C44.590)

C21.0 Malignant neoplasm of anus, unspecified

C21.1 Malignant neoplasm of anal canal

Malignant neoplasm of anal sphincter

C21.2 Malignant neoplasm of cloacogenic zone

C21.8 Malignant neoplasm of overlapping sites of rectum, anus and anal canal

Malignant neoplasm of anorectal junction

Malignant neoplasm of anorectum

Primary malignant neoplasm of two or more contiguous sites of rectum, anus and anal canal

C22 Malignant neoplasm of liver and intrahepatic bile ducts

Excludes 1: malignant neoplasm of biliary tract NOS (C24.9)

secondary malignant neoplasm of liver and intrahepatic bile duct (C78.7)

Use additional code to identify:

alcohol abuse and dependence (F10.-)

hepatitis B (B16.-, B18.0-B18.1)

hepatitis C (B17.1-, B18.2)

C22.0 Liver cell carcinoma

Hepatocellular carcinoma

Hepatoma

C22.1 Intrahepatic bile duct carcinoma

Cholangiocarcinoma

Excludes 1: malignant neoplasm of hepatic duct (C24.0)

C22.2 Hepatoblastoma

C22.3 Angiosarcoma of liver

Kupffer cell sarcoma

C22.4 Other sarcomas of liver

C22.7 Other specified carcinomas of liver

C22.8 Malignant neoplasm of liver, primary, unspecified as to type

C22.9 Malignant neoplasm of liver, not specified as primary or secondary

C23 Malignant neoplasm of gallbladder

C24 Malignant neoplasm of other and unspecified parts of biliary tract

Excludes 1: malignant neoplasm of intrahepatic bile duct (C22.1)

C24.0 Malignant neoplasm of extrahepatic bile duct

Malignant neoplasm of biliary duct or passage NOS

Malignant neoplasm of common bile duct

Malignant neoplasm of cystic duct

Malignant neoplasm of hepatic duct

C24.1 Malignant neoplasm of ampulla of Vater

C24.8 Malignant neoplasm of overlapping sites of biliary tract

Malignant neoplasm involving both intrahepatic and extrahepatic bile ducts

Primary malignant neoplasm of two or more contiguous sites of biliary tract

C24.9 Malignant neoplasm of biliary tract, unspecified

C25 Malignant neoplasm of pancreas

Use additional code to identify:

alcohol abuse and dependence (F10.-)

C25.0 Malignant neoplasm of head of pancreas

C25.1 Malignant neoplasm of body of pancreas

C25.2 Malignant neoplasm of tail of pancreas

C25.3 Malignant neoplasm of pancreatic duct

C25.4 Malignant neoplasm of endocrine pancreas

Malignant neoplasm of islets of Langerhans
Use additional code to identify any functional activity.

C25.7 Malignant neoplasm of other parts of pancreas
Malignant neoplasm of neck of pancreas

C25.8 Malignant neoplasm of overlapping sites of pancreas

C25.9 Malignant neoplasm of pancreas, unspecified

C26 Malignant neoplasm of other and ill-defined digestive organs

Excludes 1: malignant neoplasm of peritoneum and retroperitoneum (C48.-)

C26.0 Malignant neoplasm of intestinal tract, part unspecified
Malignant neoplasm of intestine NOS

C26.1 Malignant neoplasm of spleen

Excludes 1: Hodgkin lymphoma (C81.-)
non-Hodgkin lymphoma (C82-C85)

C26.9 Malignant neoplasm of ill-defined sites within the digestive system
Malignant neoplasm of alimentary canal or tract NOS
Malignant neoplasm of gastrointestinal tract NOS

Excludes 1: malignant neoplasm of abdominal NOS (C76.2)
malignant neoplasm of intra-abdominal NOS (C76.2)

MALIGNANT NEOPLASMS OF RESPIRATORY AND INTRATHORACIC ORGANS (C30-C39)

Includes: malignant neoplasm of middle ear

Excludes 1: mesothelioma (C45.-)

C30 Malignant neoplasm of nasal cavity and middle ear

C30.0 Malignant neoplasm of nasal cavity
Malignant neoplasm of cartilage of nose
Malignant neoplasm of nasal concha
Malignant neoplasm of internal nose
Malignant neoplasm of septum of nose
Malignant neoplasm of vestibule of nose

Excludes 1: malignant neoplasm of nasal bone (C41.0)
malignant neoplasm of nose NOS (C76.0)
malignant neoplasm of olfactory bulb (C72.2-)
malignant neoplasm of posterior margin of nasal septum and choana (C11.3)
malignant melanoma of skin of nose (C43.31)
malignant neoplasm of turbinates (C41.0)
other and unspecified malignant neoplasm of skin of nose C44.301, C44.311, C44.321, C44.391)

C30.1 Malignant neoplasm of middle ear
Malignant neoplasm of antrum tympanicum
Malignant neoplasm of auditory tube
Malignant neoplasm of eustachian tube
Malignant neoplasm of inner ear
Malignant neoplasm of mastoid air cells
Malignant neoplasm of tympanic cavity

Excludes 1: malignant neoplasm of auricular canal (external) (C43.2-,C44.2-)
malignant neoplasm of bone of ear (meatus) (C41.0)
malignant neoplasm of cartilage of ear (C49.0)
malignant melanoma of skin of (external) ear (C43.2-)
other and unspecified malignant neoplasm of skin of (external) ear (C44.2-)

C31 Malignant neoplasm of accessory sinuses

C31.0 Malignant neoplasm of maxillary sinus

Malignant neoplasm of antrum (Highmore) (maxillary)

C31.1 Malignant neoplasm of ethmoidal sinus

C31.2 Malignant neoplasm of frontal sinus

C31.3 Malignant neoplasm of sphenoid sinus

C31.8 Malignant neoplasm of overlapping sites of accessory sinuses

C31.9 Malignant neoplasm of accessory sinus, unspecified

C32 Malignant neoplasm of larynx

Use additional code to identify:
alcohol abuse and dependence (F10.-)
exposure to environmental tobacco smoke (Z77.22)
exposure to tobacco smoke in the perinatal period (P96.81)
history of tobacco use (Z87.891)
occupational exposure to environmental tobacco smoke (Z57.31)
tobacco dependence (F17.-)
tobacco use (Z72.0)

C32.0 Malignant neoplasm of glottis
Malignant neoplasm of intrinsic larynx
Malignant neoplasm of laryngeal commissure (anterior)(posterior)
Malignant neoplasm of vocal cord (true) NOS

C32.1 Malignant neoplasm of supraglottis
Malignant neoplasm of aryepiglottic fold or interarytenoid fold, laryngeal aspect
Malignant neoplasm of epiglottis (suprahyoid portion) NOS
Malignant neoplasm of extrinsic larynx
Malignant neoplasm of false vocal cord
Malignant neoplasm of posterior (laryngeal) surface of epiglottis
Malignant neoplasm of ventricular bands

Excludes 2: malignant neoplasm of anterior surface of epiglottis (C10.1)
malignant neoplasm of aryepiglottic fold or interarytenoid fold:
NOS (C13.1)
hypopharyngeal aspect (C13.1)
marginal zone (C13.1)

C32.2 Malignant neoplasm of subglottis

C32.3 Malignant neoplasm of laryngeal cartilage

C32.8 Malignant neoplasm of overlapping sites of larynx

C32.9 Malignant neoplasm of larynx, unspecified

C33 Malignant neoplasm of trachea

Use additional code to identify:
exposure to environmental tobacco smoke (Z77.22)
exposure to tobacco smoke in the perinatal period (P96.81)
history of tobacco use (Z87.891)
occupational exposure to environmental tobacco smoke (Z57.31)
tobacco dependence (F17.-)
tobacco use (Z72.0)

C34 Malignant neoplasm of bronchus and lung

Use additional code to identify:
exposure to environmental tobacco smoke (Z77.22)
exposure to tobacco smoke in the perinatal period (P96.81)
history of tobacco use (Z87.891)
occupational exposure to environmental tobacco smoke (Z57.31)
tobacco dependence (F17.-)
tobacco use (Z72.0)

Excludes 1: Kaposi's sarcoma of lung (C46.5-)

---

malignant carcinoid tumor of the bronchus and lung (C7A.090)

C34.0 Malignant neoplasm of main bronchus

Malignant neoplasm of carina

Malignant neoplasm of hilus (of lung)

    C34.00 Malignant neoplasm of unspecified main bronchus

    C34.01 Malignant neoplasm of right main bronchus

    C34.02 Malignant neoplasm of left main bronchus

C34.1 Malignant neoplasm of upper lobe, bronchus or lung

    C34.10 Malignant neoplasm of upper lobe, unspecified bronchus or lung

    C34.11 Malignant neoplasm of upper lobe, right bronchus or lung

    C34.12 Malignant neoplasm of upper lobe, left bronchus or lung

C34.2 Malignant neoplasm of middle lobe, bronchus or lung

C34.3 Malignant neoplasm of lower lobe, bronchus or lung

    C34.30 Malignant neoplasm of lower lobe, unspecified bronchus or lung

    C34.31 Malignant neoplasm of lower lobe, right bronchus or lung

    C34.32 Malignant neoplasm of lower lobe, left bronchus or lung

C34.8 Malignant neoplasm of overlapping sites of bronchus and lung

    C34.80 Malignant neoplasm of overlapping sites of unspecified bronchus and lung

    C34.81 Malignant neoplasm of overlapping sites of right bronchus and lung

    C34.82 Malignant neoplasm of overlapping sites of left bronchus and lung

C34.9 Malignant neoplasm of unspecified part of bronchus or lung

    C34.90 Malignant neoplasm of unspecified part of unspecified bronchus or lung

        Lung cancer NOS

    C34.91 Malignant neoplasm of unspecified part of right bronchus or lung

    C34.92 Malignant neoplasm of unspecified part of left bronchus or lung

C37 Malignant neoplasm of thymus

  Excludes 1: malignant carcinoid tumor of the thymus (C7A.091)

C38 Malignant neoplasm of heart, mediastinum and pleura

  Excludes 1: mesothelioma (C45.-)

C38.0 Malignant neoplasm of heart

Malignant neoplasm of pericardium

  Excludes 1: malignant neoplasm of great vessels (C49.3)

C38.1 Malignant neoplasm of anterior mediastinum

C38.2 Malignant neoplasm of posterior mediastinum

C38.3 Malignant neoplasm of mediastinum, part unspecified

C38.4 Malignant neoplasm of pleura

C38.8 Malignant neoplasm of overlapping sites of heart, mediastinum and pleura

C39 Malignant neoplasm of other and ill-defined sites in the respiratory system and intrathoracic organs

Use additional code to identify:

exposure to environmental tobacco smoke (Z77.22)

exposure to tobacco smoke in the perinatal period (P96.81)

history of tobacco use (Z87.891)

occupational exposure to environmental tobacco smoke (Z57.31)

tobacco dependence (F17.-)

tobacco use (Z72.0)

  Excludes 1: intrathoracic malignant neoplasm NOS (C76.1)

thoracic malignant neoplasm NOS (C76.1)

C39.0 Malignant neoplasm of upper respiratory tract, part unspecified

C39.9 Malignant neoplasm of lower respiratory tract, part unspecified

Malignant neoplasm of respiratory tract NOS

MALIGNANT NEOPLASMS OF BONE AND ARTICULAR CARTILAGE (C40-C41)

Includes: malignant neoplasm of cartilage (articular) (joint)

malignant neoplasm of periosteum

Excludes 1: malignant neoplasm of bone marrow NOS (C96.9)

malignant neoplasm of synovia (C49.-)

C40 Malignant neoplasm of bone and articular cartilage of limbs

Use additional code to identify major osseous defect, if applicable (M89.7-)

C40.0 Malignant neoplasm of scapula and long bones of upper limb

    C40.00 Malignant neoplasm of scapula and long bones of unspecified upper limb

    C40.01 Malignant neoplasm of scapula and long bones of right upper limb

    C40.02 Malignant neoplasm of scapula and long bones of left upper limb

C40.1 Malignant neoplasm of short bones of upper limb

    C40.10 Malignant neoplasm of short bones of unspecified upper limb

    C40.11 Malignant neoplasm of short bones of right upper limb

    C40.12 Malignant neoplasm of short bones of left upper limb

C40.2 Malignant neoplasm of long bones of lower limb

    C40.20 Malignant neoplasm of long bones of unspecified lower limb

    C40.21 Malignant neoplasm of long bones of right lower limb

    C40.22 Malignant neoplasm of long bones of left lower limb

C40.3 Malignant neoplasm of short bones of lower limb

    C40.30 Malignant neoplasm of short bones of unspecified lower limb

    C40.31 Malignant neoplasm of short bones of right lower limb

    C40.32 Malignant neoplasm of short bones of left lower limb

C40.8 Malignant neoplasm of overlapping sites of bone and articular cartilage of limb

    C40.80 Malignant neoplasm of overlapping sites of bone and articular cartilage of unspecified limb

    C40.81 Malignant neoplasm of overlapping sites of bone and articular cartilage of right limb

    C40.82 Malignant neoplasm of overlapping sites of bone and articular cartilage of left limb

C40.9 Malignant neoplasm of unspecified bones and articular cartilage of limb

    C40.90 Malignant neoplasm of unspecified bones and articular cartilage of unspecified limb

    C40.91 Malignant neoplasm of unspecified bones and articular cartilage of right limb

    C40.92 Malignant neoplasm of unspecified bones and articular cartilage of left limb

C41 Malignant neoplasm of bone and articular cartilage of other and unspecified sites

Excludes 1: malignant neoplasm of bones of limbs (C40.-)
> malignant neoplasm of cartilage of:
>> ear (C49.0)
>> eyelid (C49.0)
>> larynx (C32.3)
>> limbs (C40.-)
>> nose (C30.0)

C41.0 Malignant neoplasm of bones of skull and face
Malignant neoplasm of maxilla (superior)
Malignant neoplasm of orbital bone
> Excludes 2: carcinoma, any type except intraosseous or odontogenic of:
>> maxillary sinus (C31.0)
>> upper jaw (C03.0)
>> malignant neoplasm of jaw bone (lower) (C41.1)

C41.1 Malignant neoplasm of mandible
Malignant neoplasm of inferior maxilla
Malignant neoplasm of lower jaw bone
> Excludes 2: carcinoma, any type except intraosseous or odontogenic of:
>> jaw NOS (C03.9)
>> lower (C03.1)
>> malignant neoplasm of upper jaw bone (C41.0)

C41.2 Malignant neoplasm of vertebral column
> Excludes 1: malignant neoplasm of sacrum and coccyx (C41.4)

C41.3 Malignant neoplasm of ribs, sternum and clavicle

C41.4 Malignant neoplasm of pelvic bones, sacrum and coccyx

C41.9 Malignant neoplasm of bone and articular cartilage, unspecified

MELANOMA AND OTHER MALIGNANT NEOPLASMS OF SKIN (C43-C44)

C43 Malignant melanoma of skin
Excludes 1: melanoma in situ (D03.-)
Excludes 2: malignant melanoma of skin of genital organs (C51-C52, C60.-, C63.-)
> Merkel cell carcinoma (C4A.-)
> sites other than skin-code to malignant neoplasm of the site

C43.0 Malignant melanoma of lip
> Excludes 1: malignant neoplasm of vermilion border of lip (C00.0-C00.2)

C43.1 Malignant melanoma of eyelid, including canthus
> **C43.10** Malignant melanoma of unspecified eyelid, including canthus
> **C43.11** Malignant melanoma of right eyelid, including canthus
> **C43.12** Malignant melanoma of left eyelid, including canthus

C43.2 Malignant melanoma of ear and external auricular canal
> **C43.20** Malignant melanoma of unspecified ear and external auricular canal
> **C43.21** Malignant melanoma of right ear and external auricular canal
> **C43.22** Malignant melanoma of left ear and external auricular canal

C43.3 Malignant melanoma of other and unspecified parts of face
> **C43.30** Malignant melanoma of unspecified part of face
> **C43.31** Malignant melanoma of nose
> **C43.39** Malignant melanoma of other parts of face

C43.4 Malignant melanoma of scalp and neck

C43.5 Malignant melanoma of trunk
> Excludes 2: malignant neoplasm of anus NOS (C21.0)
> malignant neoplasm of scrotum (C63.2)
> **C43.51** Malignant melanoma of anal skin
> Malignant melanoma of anal margin
> Malignant melanoma of perianal skin
> **C43.52** Malignant melanoma of skin of breast
> **C43.59** Malignant melanoma of other part of trunk

C43.6 Malignant melanoma of upper limb, including shoulder
> **C43.60** Malignant melanoma of unspecified upper limb, including shoulder
> **C43.61** Malignant melanoma of right upper limb, including shoulder
> **C43.62** Malignant melanoma of left upper limb, including shoulder

C43.7 Malignant melanoma of lower limb, including hip
> **C43.70** Malignant melanoma of unspecified lower limb, including hip
> **C43.71** Malignant melanoma of right lower limb, including hip
> **C43.72** Malignant melanoma of left lower limb, including hip

C43.8 Malignant melanoma of overlapping sites of skin

C43.9 Malignant melanoma of skin, unspecified
Malignant melanoma of unspecified site of skin
Melanoma (malignant) NOS

C4A Merkel cell carcinoma

C4A.0 Merkel cell carcinoma of lip
> Excludes 1: malignant neoplasm of vermilion border of lip (C00.0-C00.2)

C4A.1 Merkel cell carcinoma of eyelid, including canthus
> **C4A.10** Merkel cell carcinoma of unspecified eyelid, including canthus
> **C4A.11** Merkel cell carcinoma of right eyelid, including canthus
> **C4A.12** Merkel cell carcinoma of left eyelid, including canthus

C4A.2 Merkel cell carcinoma of ear and external auricular canal
> **C4A.20** Merkel cell carcinoma of unspecified ear and external auricular canal
> **C4A.21** Merkel cell carcinoma of right ear and external auricular canal
> **C4A.22** Merkel cell carcinoma of left ear and external auricular canal

C4A.3 Merkel cell carcinoma of other and unspecified parts of face
> **C4A.30** Merkel cell carcinoma of unspecified part of face
> **C4A.31** Merkel cell carcinoma of nose
> **C4A.39** Merkel cell carcinoma of other parts of face

C4A.4 Merkel cell carcinoma of scalp and neck

C4A.5 Merkel cell carcinoma of trunk
> Excludes 2: malignant neoplasm of anus NOS (C21.0)
> malignant neoplasm of scrotum (C63.2)
> **C4A.51** Merkel cell carcinoma of anal skin
> Merkel cell carcinoma of anal margin
> Merkel cell carcinoma of perianal skin
> **C4A.52** Merkel cell carcinoma of skin of breast
> **C4A.59** Merkel cell carcinoma of other part of trunk

C4A.6 Merkel cell carcinoma of upper limb, including shoulder
> **C4A.60** Merkel cell carcinoma of unspecified upper limb, including shoulder

---

C4A.61 Merkel cell carcinoma of right upper limb, including shoulder

C4A.62 Merkel cell carcinoma of left upper limb, including shoulder

C4A.7 Merkel cell carcinoma of lower limb, including hip

C4A.70 Merkel cell carcinoma of unspecified lower limb, including hip

C4A.71 Merkel cell carcinoma of right lower limb, including hip

C4A.72 Merkel cell carcinoma of left lower limb, including hip

C4A.8 Merkel cell carcinoma of overlapping sites

C4A.9 Merkel cell carcinoma, unspecified
Merkel cell carcinoma of unspecified site
Merkel cell carcinoma NOS

C44 Other and unspecified malignant neoplasm of skin
Includes: malignant neoplasm of sebaceous glands
malignant neoplasm of sweat glands
Excludes 1: Kaposi's sarcoma of skin (C46.0)
malignant melanoma of skin (C43.-)
malignant neoplasm of skin of genital organs (C51-C52, C60.-, C63.2)
Merkel cell carcinoma (C4A.-)

C44.0 Other and unspecified malignant neoplasm of skin of lip
Excludes 1: malignant neoplasm of lip (C00.-)

C44.00 Unspecified malignant neoplasm of skin of lip

C44.01 Basal cell carcinoma of skin of lip

C44.02 Squamous cell carcinoma of skin of lip

C44.09 Other specified malignant neoplasm of skin of lip

C44.1 Other and unspecified malignant neoplasm of skin of eyelid, including canthus
Excludes 1: connective tissue of eyelid (C49.0)

C44.10 Unspecified malignant neoplasm of skin of eyelid, including canthus

C44.101 Unspecified malignant neoplasm of skin of unspecified eyelid, including canthus

C44.102 Unspecified malignant neoplasm of skin of right eyelid, including canthus

C44.109 Unspecified malignant neoplasm of skin of left eyelid, including canthus

C44.11 Basal cell carcinoma of skin of eyelid, including canthus

C44.111 Basal cell carcinoma of skin of unspecified eyelid, including canthus

C44.112 Basal cell carcinoma of skin of right eyelid, including canthus

C44.119 Basal cell carcinoma of skin of left eyelid, including canthus

C44.12 Squamous cell carcinoma of skin of eyelid, including canthus

C44.121 Squamous cell carcinoma of skin of unspecified eyelid, including canthus

C44.122 Squamous cell carcinoma of skin of right eyelid, including canthus

C44.129 Squamous cell carcinoma of skin of left eyelid, including canthus

C44.19 Other specified malignant neoplasm of skin of eyelid, including canthus

C44.191 Other specified malignant neoplasm of skin of unspecified eyelid, including canthus

C44.192 Other specified malignant neoplasm of skin of right eyelid, including canthus

C44.199 Other specified malignant neoplasm of skin of left eyelid, including canthus

C44.2 Other and unspecified malignant neoplasm of skin of ear and external auricular canal
Excludes 1: connective tissue of ear (C49.0)

C44.20 Unspecified malignant neoplasm of skin of ear and external auricular canal

C44.201 Unspecified malignant neoplasm of skin of unspecified ear and external auricular canal

C44.202 Unspecified malignant neoplasm of skin of right ear and external auricular canal

C44.209 Unspecified malignant neoplasm of skin of left ear and external auricular canal

C44.21 Basal cell carcinoma of skin of ear and external auricular canal

C44.211 Basal cell carcinoma of skin of unspecified ear and external auricular canal

C44.212 Basal cell carcinoma of skin of right ear and external auricular canal

C44.219 Basal cell carcinoma of skin of left ear and external auricular canal

C44.22 Squamous cell carcinoma of skin of ear and external auricular canal

C44.221 Squamous cell carcinoma of skin of unspecified ear and external auricular canal

C44.222 Squamous cell carcinoma of skin of right ear and external auricular canal

C44.229 Squamous cell carcinoma of skin of left ear and external auricular canal

C44.29 Other specified malignant neoplasm of skin of ear and external auricular canal

C44.291 Other specified malignant neoplasm of skin of unspecified ear and external auricular canal

C44.292 Other specified malignant neoplasm of skin of right ear and external auricular canal

C44.299 Other specified malignant neoplasm of skin of left ear and external auricular canal

C44.3 Other and unspecified malignant neoplasm of skin of other and unspecified parts of face

C44.30 Unspecified malignant neoplasm of skin of other and unspecified parts of face

C44.300 Unspecified malignant neoplasm of skin of unspecified part of face

C44.301 Unspecified malignant neoplasm of skin of nose

C44.309 Unspecified malignant neoplasm of skin of other parts of face

C44.31 Basal cell carcinoma of skin of other and unspecified parts of face

C44.310 Basal cell carcinoma of skin of unspecified parts of face

C44.311 Basal cell carcinoma of skin of nose

● New code   ▲ Revised code   ⑦ 7th digit required   ⊗ Placeholder required

C44.319 Basal cell carcinoma of skin of other parts of face

C44.32 Squamous cell carcinoma of skin of other and unspecified parts of face

C44.320 Squamous cell carcinoma of skin of unspecified parts of face

C44.321 Squamous cell carcinoma of skin of nose

C44.329 Squamous cell carcinoma of skin of other parts of face

C44.39 Other specified malignant neoplasm of skin of other and unspecified parts of face

C44.390 Other specified malignant neoplasm of skin of unspecified parts of face

C44.391 Other specified malignant neoplasm of skin of nose

C44.399 Other specified malignant neoplasm of skin of other parts of face

C44.4 Other and unspecified malignant neoplasm of skin of scalp and neck

C44.40 Unspecified malignant neoplasm of skin of scalp and neck

C44.41 Basal cell carcinoma of skin of scalp and neck

C44.42 Squamous cell carcinoma of skin of scalp and neck

C44.49 Other specified malignant neoplasm of skin of scalp and neck

C44.5 Other and unspecified malignant neoplasm of skin of trunk

Excludes 1: anus NOS (C21.0)
scrotum (C63.2)

C44.50 Unspecified malignant neoplasm of skin of trunk

C44.500 Unspecified malignant neoplasm of anal skin
Unspecified malignant neoplasm of anal margin
Unspecified malignant neoplasm of perianal skin

C44.501 Unspecified malignant neoplasm of skin of breast

C44.509 Unspecified malignant neoplasm of skin of other part of trunk

C44.51 Basal cell carcinoma of skin of trunk

C44.510 Basal cell carcinoma of anal skin
Basal cell carcinoma of anal margin
Basal cell carcinoma of perianal skin

C44.511 Basal cell carcinoma of skin of breast

C44.519 Basal cell carcinoma of skin of other part of trunk

C44.52 Squamous cell carcinoma of skin of trunk

C44.520 Squamous cell carcinoma of anal skin
Squamous cell carcinoma of anal margin
Squamous cell carcinoma of perianal skin

C44.521 Squamous cell carcinoma of skin of breast

C44.529 Squamous cell carcinoma of skin of other part of trunk

C44.59 Other specified malignant neoplasm of skin of trunk

C44.590 Other specified malignant neoplasm of anal skin
Other specified malignant neoplasm of anal margin

Other specified malignant neoplasm of perianal skin

C44.591 Other specified malignant neoplasm of skin of breast

C44.599 Other specified malignant neoplasm of skin of other part of trunk

C44.6 Other and unspecified malignant neoplasm of skin of upper limb, including shoulder

C44.60 Unspecified malignant neoplasm of skin of upper limb, including shoulder

C44.601 Unspecified malignant neoplasm of skin of unspecified upper limb, including shoulder

C44.602 Unspecified malignant neoplasm of skin of right upper limb, including shoulder

C44.609 Unspecified malignant neoplasm of skin of left upper limb, including shoulder

C44.61 Basal cell carcinoma of skin of upper limb, including shoulder

C44.611 Basal cell carcinoma of skin of unspecified upper limb, including shoulder

C44.612 Basal cell carcinoma of skin of right upper limb, including shoulder

C44.619 Basal cell carcinoma of skin of left upper limb, including shoulder

C44.62 Squamous cell carcinoma of skin of upper limb, including shoulder

C44.621 Squamous cell carcinoma of skin of unspecified upper limb, including shoulder

C44.622 Squamous cell carcinoma of skin of right upper limb, including shoulder

C44.629 Squamous cell carcinoma of skin of left upper limb, including shoulder

C44.69 Other specified malignant neoplasm of skin of upper limb, including shoulder

C44.691 Other specified malignant neoplasm of skin of unspecified upper limb, including shoulder

C44.692 Other specified malignant neoplasm of skin of right upper limb, including shoulder

C44.699 Other specified malignant neoplasm of skin of left upper limb, including shoulder

C44.7 Other and unspecified malignant neoplasm of skin of lower limb, including hip

C44.70 Unspecified malignant neoplasm of skin of lower limb, including hip

C44.701 Unspecified malignant neoplasm of skin of unspecified lower limb, including hip

C44.702 Unspecified malignant neoplasm of skin of right lower limb, including hip

C44.709 Unspecified malignant neoplasm of skin of left lower limb, including hip

C44.71 Basal cell carcinoma of skin of lower limb, including hip

C44.711 Basal cell carcinoma of skin of unspecified lower limb, including hip

C44.712   Basal cell carcinoma of skin of right lower limb, including hip

C44.719   Basal cell carcinoma of skin of left lower limb, including hip

C44.72   Squamous cell carcinoma of skin of lower limb, including hip

C44.721   Squamous cell carcinoma of skin of unspecified lower limb, including hip

C44.722   Squamous cell carcinoma of skin of right lower limb, including hip

C44.729   Squamous cell carcinoma of skin of left lower limb, including hip

C44.79   Other specified malignant neoplasm of skin of lower limb, including hip

C44.791   Other specified malignant neoplasm of skin of unspecified lower limb, including hip

C44.792   Other specified malignant neoplasm of skin of right lower limb, including hip

C44.799   Other specified malignant neoplasm of skin of left lower limb, including hip

C44.8   Other and unspecified malignant neoplasm of overlapping sites of skin

C44.80   Unspecified malignant neoplasm of overlapping sites of skin

C44.81   Basal cell carcinoma of overlapping sites of skin

C44.82   Squamous cell carcinoma of overlapping sites of skin

C44.89   Other specified malignant neoplasm of overlapping sites of skin

C44.9   Other and unspecified malignant neoplasm of skin, unspecified

C44.90   Unspecified malignant neoplasm of skin, unspecified

Malignant neoplasm of unspecified site of skin

C44.91   Basal cell carcinoma of skin, unspecified

C44.92   Squamous cell carcinoma of skin, unspecified

C44.99   Other specified malignant neoplasm of skin, unspecified

MALIGNANT NEOPLASMS OF MESOTHELIAL AND SOFT TISSUE (C45-C49)

C45   Mesothelioma

C45.0   Mesothelioma of pleura

Excludes 1: other malignant neoplasm of pleura (C38.4)

C45.1   Mesothelioma of peritoneum

Mesothelioma of cul-de-sac

Mesothelioma of mesentery

Mesothelioma of mesocolon

Mesothelioma of omentum

Mesothelioma of peritoneum (parietal) (pelvic)

Excludes 1: other malignant neoplasm of soft tissue of peritoneum (C48.-)

C45.2   Mesothelioma of pericardium

Excludes 1: other malignant neoplasm of pericardium (C38.0)

C45.7   Mesothelioma of other sites

C45.9   Mesothelioma, unspecified

C46   Kaposi's sarcoma

Code first any human immunodeficiency virus [HIV] disease (B20)

C46.0   Kaposi's sarcoma of skin

C46.1   Kaposi's sarcoma of soft tissue

Kaposi's sarcoma of blood vessel

Kaposi's sarcoma of connective tissue

Kaposi's sarcoma of fascia

Kaposi's sarcoma of ligament

Kaposi's sarcoma of lymphatic(s) NEC

Kaposi's sarcoma of muscle

Excludes 2: Kaposi's sarcoma of lymph glands and nodes (C46.3)

C46.2   Kaposi's sarcoma of palate

C46.3   Kaposi's sarcoma of lymph nodes

C46.4   Kaposi's sarcoma of gastrointestinal sites

C46.5   Kaposi's sarcoma of lung

C46.50   Kaposi's sarcoma of unspecified lung

C46.51   Kaposi's sarcoma of right lung

C46.52   Kaposi's sarcoma of left lung

C46.7   Kaposi's sarcoma of other sites

C46.9   Kaposi's sarcoma, unspecified

Kaposi's sarcoma of unspecified site

C47   Malignant neoplasm of peripheral nerves and autonomic nervous system

Includes: malignant neoplasm of sympathetic and parasympathetic nerves and ganglia

Excludes 1: Kaposi's sarcoma of soft tissue (C46.1)

C47.0   Malignant neoplasm of peripheral nerves of head, face and neck

Excludes 1: malignant neoplasm of peripheral nerves of orbit (C69.6-)

C47.1   Malignant neoplasm of peripheral nerves of upper limb, including shoulder

C47.10   Malignant neoplasm of peripheral nerves of unspecified upper limb, including shoulder

C47.11   Malignant neoplasm of peripheral nerves of right upper limb, including shoulder

C47.12   Malignant neoplasm of peripheral nerves of left upper limb, including shoulder

C47.2   Malignant neoplasm of peripheral nerves of lower limb, including hip

C47.20   Malignant neoplasm of peripheral nerves of unspecified lower limb, including hip

C47.21   Malignant neoplasm of peripheral nerves of right lower limb, including hip

C47.22   Malignant neoplasm of peripheral nerves of left lower limb, including hip

C47.3   Malignant neoplasm of peripheral nerves of thorax

C47.4   Malignant neoplasm of peripheral nerves of abdomen

C47.5   Malignant neoplasm of peripheral nerves of pelvis

C47.6   Malignant neoplasm of peripheral nerves of trunk, unspecified

Malignant neoplasm of peripheral nerves of unspecified part of trunk

C47.8   Malignant neoplasm of overlapping sites of peripheral nerves and autonomic nervous system

C47.9   Malignant neoplasm of peripheral nerves and autonomic nervous system, unspecified

Malignant neoplasm of unspecified site of peripheral nerves and autonomic nervous system

C48   Malignant neoplasm of retroperitoneum and peritoneum

Excludes 1: Kaposi's sarcoma of connective tissue (C46.1)
mesothelioma (C45.-)

C48.0   Malignant neoplasm of retroperitoneum

C48.1   Malignant neoplasm of specified parts of peritoneum

Malignant neoplasm of cul-de-sac
Malignant neoplasm of mesentery
Malignant neoplasm of mesocolon
Malignant neoplasm of omentum
Malignant neoplasm of parietal peritoneum
Malignant neoplasm of pelvic peritoneum

C48.2 Malignant neoplasm of peritoneum, unspecified

C48.8 Malignant neoplasm of overlapping sites of retroperitoneum and peritoneum

C49 Malignant neoplasm of other connective and soft tissue

Includes: malignant neoplasm of blood vessel
malignant neoplasm of bursa
malignant neoplasm of cartilage
malignant neoplasm of fascia
malignant neoplasm of fat
malignant neoplasm of ligament, except uterine
malignant neoplasm of lymphatic vessel
malignant neoplasm of muscle
malignant neoplasm of synovia
malignant neoplasm of tendon (sheath)

Excludes 1: malignant neoplasm of cartilage (of):
articular (C40-C41)
larynx (C32.3)
nose (C30.0)
malignant neoplasm of connective tissue of breast (C50-)

Excludes 2: Kaposi's sarcoma of soft tissue (C46.1)
malignant neoplasm of heart (C38.0)
malignant neoplasm of peripheral nerves and autonomic nervous system (C47.-)
malignant neoplasm of peritoneum (C48.2)
malignant neoplasm of retroperitoneum (C48.0)
malignant neoplasm of uterine ligament (C57.3)
mesothelioma (C45.-)

C49.0 Malignant neoplasm of connective and soft tissue of head, face and neck
Malignant neoplasm of connective tissue of ear
Malignant neoplasm of connective tissue of eyelid
Excludes 1: connective tissue of orbit (C69.6-)

C49.1 Malignant neoplasm of connective and soft tissue of upper limb, including shoulder

C49.10 Malignant neoplasm of connective and soft tissue of unspecified upper limb, including shoulder

C49.11 Malignant neoplasm of connective and soft tissue of right upper limb, including shoulder

C49.12 Malignant neoplasm of connective and soft tissue of left upper limb, including shoulder

C49.2 Malignant neoplasm of connective and soft tissue of lower limb, including hip

C49.20 Malignant neoplasm of connective and soft tissue of unspecified lower limb, including hip

C49.21 Malignant neoplasm of connective and soft tissue of right lower limb, including hip

C49.22 Malignant neoplasm of connective and soft tissue of left lower limb, including hip

C49.3 Malignant neoplasm of connective and soft tissue of thorax
Malignant neoplasm of axilla
Malignant neoplasm of diaphragm
Malignant neoplasm of great vessels
Excludes 1: malignant neoplasm of breast (C50.-)
malignant neoplasm of heart (C38.0)

malignant neoplasm of mediastinum (C38.1-C38.3)
malignant neoplasm of thymus (C37)

C49.4 Malignant neoplasm of connective and soft tissue of abdomen
Malignant neoplasm of abdominal wall
Malignant neoplasm of hypochondrium

C49.5 Malignant neoplasm of connective and soft tissue of pelvis
Malignant neoplasm of buttock
Malignant neoplasm of groin
Malignant neoplasm of perineum

C49.6 Malignant neoplasm of connective and soft tissue of trunk, unspecified
Malignant neoplasm of back NOS

C49.8 Malignant neoplasm of overlapping sites of connective and soft tissue
Primary malignant neoplasm of two or more contiguous sites of connective and soft tissue

C49.9 Malignant neoplasm of connective and soft tissue, unspecified

MALIGNANT NEOPLASMS OF BREAST (C50)

C50 Malignant neoplasm of breast
Includes: connective tissue of breast
Paget's disease of breast
Paget's disease of nipple
Use additional code to identify estrogen receptor status (Z17.0, Z17.1)
Excludes 1: skin of breast (C44.501, C44.511, C44.521, C44.591)

C50.0 Malignant neoplasm of nipple and areola

C50.01 Malignant neoplasm of nipple and areola, female

C50.011 Malignant neoplasm of nipple and areola, right female breast

C50.012 Malignant neoplasm of nipple and areola, left female breast

C50.019 Malignant neoplasm of nipple and areola, unspecified female breast

C50.02 Malignant neoplasm of nipple and areola, male

C50.021 Malignant neoplasm of nipple and areola, right male breast

C50.022 Malignant neoplasm of nipple and areola, left male breast

C50.029 Malignant neoplasm of nipple and areola, unspecified male breast

C50.1 Malignant neoplasm of central portion of breast

C50.11 Malignant neoplasm of central portion of breast, female

C50.111 Malignant neoplasm of central portion of right female breast

C50.112 Malignant neoplasm of central portion of left female breast

C50.119 Malignant neoplasm of central portion of unspecified female breast

C50.12 Malignant neoplasm of central portion of breast, male

C50.121 Malignant neoplasm of central portion of right male breast

C50.122 Malignant neoplasm of central portion of left male breast

C50.129 Malignant neoplasm of central portion of unspecified male breast

C50.2 Malignant neoplasm of upper-inner quadrant of breast

C50.21 Malignant neoplasm of upper-inner quadrant of breast, female

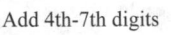 

C50.211 Malignant neoplasm of upper-inner quadrant of right female breast

C50.212 Malignant neoplasm of upper-inner quadrant of left female breast

C50.219 Malignant neoplasm of upper-inner quadrant of unspecified female breast

C50.22 Malignant neoplasm of upper-inner quadrant of breast, male

C50.221 Malignant neoplasm of upper-inner quadrant of right male breast

C50.222 Malignant neoplasm of upper-inner quadrant of left male breast

C50.229 Malignant neoplasm of upper-inner quadrant of unspecified male breast

C50.3 Malignant neoplasm of lower-inner quadrant of breast

C50.31 Malignant neoplasm of lower-inner quadrant of breast, female

C50.311 Malignant neoplasm of lower-inner quadrant of right female breast

C50.312 Malignant neoplasm of lower-inner quadrant of left female breast

C50.319 Malignant neoplasm of lower-inner quadrant of unspecified female breast

C50.32 Malignant neoplasm of lower-inner quadrant of breast, male

C50.321 Malignant neoplasm of lower-inner quadrant of right male breast

C50.322 Malignant neoplasm of lower-inner quadrant of left male breast

C50.329 Malignant neoplasm of lower-inner quadrant of unspecified male breast

C50.4 Malignant neoplasm of upper-outer quadrant of breast

C50.41 Malignant neoplasm of upper-outer quadrant of breast, female

C50.411 Malignant neoplasm of upper-outer quadrant of right female breast

C50.412 Malignant neoplasm of upper-outer quadrant of left female breast

C50.419 Malignant neoplasm of upper-outer quadrant of unspecified female breast

C50.42 Malignant neoplasm of upper-outer quadrant of breast, male

C50.421 Malignant neoplasm of upper-outer quadrant of right male breast

C50.422 Malignant neoplasm of upper-outer quadrant of left male breast

C50.429 Malignant neoplasm of upper-outer quadrant of unspecified male breast

C50.5 Malignant neoplasm of lower-outer quadrant of breast

C50.51 Malignant neoplasm of lower-outer quadrant of breast, female

C50.511 Malignant neoplasm of lower-outer quadrant of right female breast

C50.512 Malignant neoplasm of lower-outer quadrant of left female breast

C50.519 Malignant neoplasm of lower-outer quadrant of unspecified female breast

C50.52 Malignant neoplasm of lower-outer quadrant of breast, male

C50.521 Malignant neoplasm of lower-outer quadrant of right male breast

C50.522 Malignant neoplasm of lower-outer quadrant of left male breast

C50.529 Malignant neoplasm of lower-outer quadrant of unspecified male breast

C50.6 Malignant neoplasm of axillary tail of breast

C50.61 Malignant neoplasm of axillary tail of breast, female

C50.611 Malignant neoplasm of axillary tail of right female breast

C50.612 Malignant neoplasm of axillary tail of left female breast

C50.619 Malignant neoplasm of axillary tail of unspecified female breast

C50.62 Malignant neoplasm of axillary tail of breast, male

C50.621 Malignant neoplasm of axillary tail of right male breast

C50.622 Malignant neoplasm of axillary tail of left male breast

C50.629 Malignant neoplasm of axillary tail of unspecified male breast

C50.8 Malignant neoplasm of overlapping sites of breast

C50.81 Malignant neoplasm of overlapping sites of breast, female

C50.811 Malignant neoplasm of overlapping sites of right female breast

C50.812 Malignant neoplasm of overlapping sites of left female breast

C50.819 Malignant neoplasm of overlapping sites of unspecified female breast

C50.82 Malignant neoplasm of overlapping sites of breast, male

C50.821 Malignant neoplasm of overlapping sites of right male breast

C50.822 Malignant neoplasm of overlapping sites of left male breast

C50.829 Malignant neoplasm of overlapping sites of unspecified male breast

C50.9 Malignant neoplasm of breast of unspecified site

C50.91 Malignant neoplasm of breast of unspecified site, female

C50.911 Malignant neoplasm of unspecified site of right female breast

C50.912 Malignant neoplasm of unspecified site of left female breast

C50.919 Malignant neoplasm of unspecified site of unspecified female breast

C50.92 Malignant neoplasm of breast of unspecified site, male

C50.921 Malignant neoplasm of unspecified site of right male breast

C50.922 Malignant neoplasm of unspecified site of left male breast

C50.929 Malignant neoplasm of unspecified site of unspecified male breast

MALIGNANT NEOPLASMS OF FEMALE GENITAL ORGANS (C51-C58)

Includes: malignant neoplasm of skin of female genital organs

C51 Malignant neoplasm of vulva

Excludes 1: carcinoma in situ of vulva (D07.1)

C51.0 Malignant neoplasm of labium majus

Malignant neoplasm of Bartholin's [greater vestibular] gland

C51.1 Malignant neoplasm of labium minus

C51.2 Malignant neoplasm of clitoris

C51.8 Malignant neoplasm of overlapping sites of vulva

C51.9 Malignant neoplasm of vulva, unspecified

Malignant neoplasm of external female genitalia NOS

Malignant neoplasm of pudendum

C52 Malignant neoplasm of vagina

Excludes 1: carcinoma in situ of vagina (D07.2)

C53 Malignant neoplasm of cervix uteri

Excludes 1: carcinoma in situ of cervix uteri (D06.-)

C53.0 Malignant neoplasm of endocervix

C53.1 Malignant neoplasm of exocervix

C53.8 Malignant neoplasm of overlapping sites of cervix uteri

C53.9 Malignant neoplasm of cervix uteri, unspecified

C54 Malignant neoplasm of corpus uteri

C54.0 Malignant neoplasm of isthmus uteri

Malignant neoplasm of lower uterine segment

C54.1 Malignant neoplasm of endometrium

C54.2 Malignant neoplasm of myometrium

C54.3 Malignant neoplasm of fundus uteri

C54.8 Malignant neoplasm of overlapping sites of corpus uteri

C54.9 Malignant neoplasm of corpus uteri, unspecified

C55 Malignant neoplasm of uterus, part unspecified

C56 Malignant neoplasm of ovary

Use additional code to identify any functional activity

C56.1 Malignant neoplasm of right ovary

C56.2 Malignant neoplasm of left ovary

C56.9 Malignant neoplasm of unspecified ovary

C57 Malignant neoplasm of other and unspecified female genital organs

C57.0 Malignant neoplasm of fallopian tube

Malignant neoplasm of oviduct

Malignant neoplasm of uterine tube

C57.00 Malignant neoplasm of unspecified fallopian tube

C57.01 Malignant neoplasm of right fallopian tube

C57.02 Malignant neoplasm of left fallopian tube

C57.1 Malignant neoplasm of broad ligament

C57.10 Malignant neoplasm of unspecified broad ligament

C57.11 Malignant neoplasm of right broad ligament

C57.12 Malignant neoplasm of left broad ligament

C57.2 Malignant neoplasm of round ligament

C57.20 Malignant neoplasm of unspecified round ligament

C57.21 Malignant neoplasm of right round ligament

C57.22 Malignant neoplasm of left round ligament

C57.3 Malignant neoplasm of parametrium

Malignant neoplasm of uterine ligament NOS

C57.4 Malignant neoplasm of uterine adnexa, unspecified

C57.7 Malignant neoplasm of other specified female genital organs

Malignant neoplasm of wolffian body or duct

C57.8 Malignant neoplasm of overlapping sites of female genital organs

Primary malignant neoplasm of two or more contiguous sites of the female genital organs whose point of origin cannot be determined

Primary tubo-ovarian malignant neoplasm whose point of origin cannot be determined

Primary utero-ovarian malignant neoplasm whose point of origin cannot be determined

C57.9 Malignant neoplasm of female genital organ, unspecified

Malignant neoplasm of female genitourinary tract NOS

C58 Malignant neoplasm of placenta

Includes: choriocarcinoma NOS

chorionepithelioma NOS

Excludes 1: chorioadenoma (destruens) (D39.2)

hydatidiform mole NOS (O01.9)

invasive hydatidiform mole (D39.2)

male choriocarcinoma NOS (C62.9-)

malignant hydatidiform mole (D39.2)

MALIGNANT NEOPLASMS OF MALE GENITAL ORGANS (C60-C63)

Includes: malignant neoplasm of skin of male genital organs

C60 Malignant neoplasm of penis

C60.0 Malignant neoplasm of prepuce

Malignant neoplasm of foreskin

C60.1 Malignant neoplasm of glans penis

C60.2 Malignant neoplasm of body of penis

Malignant neoplasm of corpus cavernosum

C60.8 Malignant neoplasm of overlapping sites of penis

C60.9 Malignant neoplasm of penis, unspecified

Malignant neoplasm of skin of penis NOS

C61 Malignant neoplasm of prostate

Excludes 1: malignant neoplasm of seminal vesicle (C63.7)

C62 Malignant neoplasm of testis

Use additional code to identify any functional activity

C62.0 Malignant neoplasm of undescended testis

Malignant neoplasm of ectopic testis

Malignant neoplasm of retained testis

C62.00 Malignant neoplasm of unspecified undescended testis

C62.01 Malignant neoplasm of undescended right testis

C62.02 Malignant neoplasm of undescended left testis

C62.1 Malignant neoplasm of descended testis

Malignant neoplasm of scrotal testis

C62.10 Malignant neoplasm of unspecified descended testis

C62.11 Malignant neoplasm of descended right testis

C62.12 Malignant neoplasm of descended left testis

C62.9 Malignant neoplasm of testis, unspecified whether descended or undescended

C62.90 Malignant neoplasm of unspecified testis, unspecified whether descended or undescended

Malignant neoplasm of testis NOS

C62.91 Malignant neoplasm of right testis, unspecified whether descended or undescended

C62.92 Malignant neoplasm of left testis, unspecified whether descended or undescended

C63 Malignant neoplasm of other and unspecified male genital organs

C63.0 Malignant neoplasm of epididymis

C63.00 Malignant neoplasm of unspecified epididymis

C63.01 Malignant neoplasm of right epididymis

C63.02 Malignant neoplasm of left epididymis

C63.1 Malignant neoplasm of spermatic cord

C63.10 Malignant neoplasm of unspecified spermatic cord

C63.11 Malignant neoplasm of right spermatic cord

C63.12 Malignant neoplasm of left spermatic cord

C63.2 Malignant neoplasm of scrotum

Malignant neoplasm of skin of scrotum

C63.7 Malignant neoplasm of other specified male genital organs

Malignant neoplasm of seminal vesicle

Malignant neoplasm of tunica vaginalis

C63.8 Malignant neoplasm of overlapping sites of male genital organs

Primary malignant neoplasm of two or more contiguous
sites of male genital organs whose point of origin
cannot be determined

C63.9 Malignant neoplasm of male genital organ, unspecified
Malignant neoplasm of male genitourinary tract NOS

MALIGNANT NEOPLASMS OF URINARY TRACT (C64-C68)

C64 Malignant neoplasm of kidney, except renal pelvis
Excludes 1: malignant carcinoid tumor of the kidney (C7A.093)
malignant neoplasm of renal calyces (C65.-)
malignant neoplasm of renal pelvis (C65.-)
C64.1 Malignant neoplasm of right kidney, except renal pelvis
C64.2 Malignant neoplasm of left kidney, except renal pelvis
C64.9 Malignant neoplasm of unspecified kidney, except renal
pelvis
C65 Malignant neoplasm of renal pelvis
Includes: malignant neoplasm of pelviureteric junction
malignant neoplasm of renal calyces
C65.1 Malignant neoplasm of right renal pelvis
C65.2 Malignant neoplasm of left renal pelvis
C65.9 Malignant neoplasm of unspecified renal pelvis
C66 Malignant neoplasm of ureter
Excludes 1: malignant neoplasm of ureteric orifice of bladder
(C67.6)
C66.1 Malignant neoplasm of right ureter
C66.2 Malignant neoplasm of left ureter
C66.9 Malignant neoplasm of unspecified ureter
C67 Malignant neoplasm of bladder
C67.0 Malignant neoplasm of trigone of bladder
C67.1 Malignant neoplasm of dome of bladder
C67.2 Malignant neoplasm of lateral wall of bladder
C67.3 Malignant neoplasm of anterior wall of bladder
C67.4 Malignant neoplasm of posterior wall of bladder
C67.5 Malignant neoplasm of bladder neck
Malignant neoplasm of internal urethral orifice
C67.6 Malignant neoplasm of ureteric orifice
C67.7 Malignant neoplasm of urachus
C67.8 Malignant neoplasm of overlapping sites of bladder
C67.9 Malignant neoplasm of bladder, unspecified
C68 Malignant neoplasm of other and unspecified urinary organs
Excludes 1: malignant neoplasm of female genitourinary tract
NOS (C57.9)
malignant neoplasm of male genitourinary tract NOS
(C63.9)
C68.0 Malignant neoplasm of urethra
Excludes 1: malignant neoplasm of urethral orifice of
bladder (C67.5)
C68.1 Malignant neoplasm of paraurethral glands
C68.8 Malignant neoplasm of overlapping sites of urinary organs
Primary malignant neoplasm of two or more contiguous
sites of urinary organs whose point of origin cannot be
determined
C68.9 Malignant neoplasm of urinary organ, unspecified
Malignant neoplasm of urinary system NOS

MALIGNANT NEOPLASMS OF EYE, BRAIN AND OTHER PARTS OF CENTRAL NERVOUS SYSTEM (C69-C72)

C69 Malignant neoplasm of eye and adnexa
Excludes 1: malignant neoplasm of connective tissue of eyelid
(C49.0)
malignant neoplasm of eyelid (skin) (C43.1-, C44.1-)
malignant neoplasm of optic nerve (C72.3-)

C69.0 Malignant neoplasm of conjunctiva
C69.00 Malignant neoplasm of unspecified conjunctiva
C69.01 Malignant neoplasm of right conjunctiva
C69.02 Malignant neoplasm of left conjunctiva
C69.1 Malignant neoplasm of cornea
C69.10 Malignant neoplasm of unspecified cornea
C69.11 Malignant neoplasm of right cornea
C69.12 Malignant neoplasm of left cornea
C69.2 Malignant neoplasm of retina
Excludes 1: dark area on retina (D49.81)
neoplasm of unspecified behavior of retina
and choroid (D49.81)
retinal freckle (D49.81)
C69.20 Malignant neoplasm of unspecified retina
C69.21 Malignant neoplasm of right retina
C69.22 Malignant neoplasm of left retina
C69.3 Malignant neoplasm of choroid
C69.30 Malignant neoplasm of unspecified choroid
C69.31 Malignant neoplasm of right choroid
C69.32 Malignant neoplasm of left choroid
C69.4 Malignant neoplasm of ciliary body
C69.40 Malignant neoplasm of unspecified ciliary body
C69.41 Malignant neoplasm of right ciliary body
C69.42 Malignant neoplasm of left ciliary body
C69.5 Malignant neoplasm of lacrimal gland and duct
Malignant neoplasm of lacrimal sac
Malignant neoplasm of nasolacrimal duct
C69.50 Malignant neoplasm of unspecified lacrimal
gland and duct
C69.51 Malignant neoplasm of right lacrimal gland and
duct
C69.52 Malignant neoplasm of left lacrimal gland and
duct
C69.6 Malignant neoplasm of orbit
Malignant neoplasm of connective tissue of orbit
Malignant neoplasm of extraocular muscle
Malignant neoplasm of peripheral nerves of orbit
Malignant neoplasm of retrobulbar tissue
Malignant neoplasm of retro-ocular tissue
Excludes 1: malignant neoplasm of orbital bone (C41.0)
C69.60 Malignant neoplasm of unspecified orbit
C69.61 Malignant neoplasm of right orbit
C69.62 Malignant neoplasm of left orbit
C69.8 Malignant neoplasm of overlapping sites of eye and
adnexa
C69.80 Malignant neoplasm of overlapping sites of
unspecified eye and adnexa
C69.81 Malignant neoplasm of overlapping sites of right
eye and adnexa
C69.82 Malignant neoplasm of overlapping sites of left
eye and adnexa
C69.9 Malignant neoplasm of unspecified site of eye
Malignant neoplasm of eyeball
C69.90 Malignant neoplasm of unspecified site of
unspecified eye
C69.91 Malignant neoplasm of unspecified site of right
eye
C69.92 Malignant neoplasm of unspecified site of left
eye
C70 Malignant neoplasm of meninges
C70.0 Malignant neoplasm of cerebral meninges
C70.1 Malignant neoplasm of spinal meninges

● New code   ▲ Revised code   ⑦ 7th digit required   ⊗ Placeholder required

C70.9 Malignant neoplasm of meninges, unspecified

C71 Malignant neoplasm of brain

Excludes 1: malignant neoplasm of cranial nerves (C72.2-C72.5)

retrobulbar malignant neoplasm (C69.6-)

C71.0 Malignant neoplasm of cerebrum, except lobes and ventricles

Malignant neoplasm of supratentorial NOS

C71.1 Malignant neoplasm of frontal lobe

C71.2 Malignant neoplasm of temporal lobe

C71.3 Malignant neoplasm of parietal lobe

C71.4 Malignant neoplasm of occipital lobe

C71.5 Malignant neoplasm of cerebral ventricle

Excludes 1: malignant neoplasm of fourth cerebral ventricle (C71.7)

C71.6 Malignant neoplasm of cerebellum

C71.7 Malignant neoplasm of brain stem

Malignant neoplasm of fourth cerebral ventricle

Infratentorial malignant neoplasm NOS

C71.8 Malignant neoplasm of overlapping sites of brain

C71.9 Malignant neoplasm of brain, unspecified

C72 Malignant neoplasm of spinal cord, cranial nerves and other parts of central nervous system

Excludes 1: malignant neoplasm of meninges (C70.-)

malignant neoplasm of peripheral nerves and autonomic nervous system (C47.-)

C72.0 Malignant neoplasm of spinal cord

C72.1 Malignant neoplasm of cauda equina

C72.2 Malignant neoplasm of olfactory nerve

Malignant neoplasm of olfactory bulb

C72.20 Malignant neoplasm of unspecified olfactory nerve

C72.21 Malignant neoplasm of right olfactory nerve

C72.22 Malignant neoplasm of left olfactory nerve

C72.3 Malignant neoplasm of optic nerve

C72.30 Malignant neoplasm of unspecified optic nerve

C72.31 Malignant neoplasm of right optic nerve

C72.32 Malignant neoplasm of left optic nerve

C72.4 Malignant neoplasm of acoustic nerve

C72.40 Malignant neoplasm of unspecified acoustic nerve

C72.41 Malignant neoplasm of right acoustic nerve

C72.42 Malignant neoplasm of left acoustic nerve

C72.5 Malignant neoplasm of other and unspecified cranial nerves

C72.50 Malignant neoplasm of unspecified cranial nerve

Malignant neoplasm of cranial nerve NOS

C72.59 Malignant neoplasm of other cranial nerves

C72.9 Malignant neoplasm of central nervous system, unspecified

Malignant neoplasm of unspecified site of central nervous system

Malignant neoplasm of nervous system NOS

MALIGNANT NEOPLASMS OF THYROID AND OTHER ENDOCRINE GLANDS (C73-C75)

C73 Malignant neoplasm of thyroid gland

Use additional code to identify any functional activity

C74 Malignant neoplasm of adrenal gland

C74.0 Malignant neoplasm of cortex of adrenal gland

C74.00 Malignant neoplasm of cortex of unspecified adrenal gland

C74.01 Malignant neoplasm of cortex of right adrenal gland

C74.02 Malignant neoplasm of cortex of left adrenal gland

C74.1 Malignant neoplasm of medulla of adrenal gland

C74.10 Malignant neoplasm of medulla of unspecified adrenal gland

C74.11 Malignant neoplasm of medulla of right adrenal gland

C74.12 Malignant neoplasm of medulla of left adrenal gland

C74.9 Malignant neoplasm of unspecified part of adrenal gland

C74.90 Malignant neoplasm of unspecified part of unspecified adrenal gland

C74.91 Malignant neoplasm of unspecified part of right adrenal gland

C74.92 Malignant neoplasm of unspecified part of left adrenal gland

C75 Malignant neoplasm of other endocrine glands and related structures

Excludes 1: malignant carcinoid tumors (C7A.0-)

malignant neoplasm of adrenal gland (C74.-)

malignant neoplasm of endocrine pancreas (C25.4)

malignant neoplasm of islets of Langerhans (C25.4)

malignant neoplasm of ovary (C56-)

malignant neoplasm of testis (C62.-)

malignant neoplasm of thymus (C37)

malignant neoplasm of thyroid gland (C73)

malignant neuroendocrine tumors (C7A.-)

C75.0 Malignant neoplasm of parathyroid gland

C75.1 Malignant neoplasm of pituitary gland

C75.2 Malignant neoplasm of craniopharyngeal duct

C75.3 Malignant neoplasm of pineal gland

C75.4 Malignant neoplasm of carotid body

C75.5 Malignant neoplasm of aortic body and other paraganglia

C75.8 Malignant neoplasm with pluriglandular involvement, unspecified

C75.9 Malignant neoplasm of endocrine gland, unspecified

MALIGNANT NEUROENDOCRINE TUMORS (C7A)

C7A Malignant neuroendocrine tumors

Code also any associated multiple endocrine neoplasia [MEN] syndromes (E31.2-)

Use additional code to identify any associated endocrine syndrome, such as:

carcinoid syndrome (E34.0)

Excludes 2: malignant pancreatic islet cell tumors (C25.4)

Merkel cell carcinoma (C4A.-)

C7A.0 Malignant carcinoid tumors

C7A.00 Malignant carcinoid tumor of unspecified site

C7A.01 Malignant carcinoid tumors of the small intestine

C7A.010 Malignant carcinoid tumor of the duodenum

C7A.011 Malignant carcinoid tumor of the jejunum

C7A.012 Malignant carcinoid tumor of the ileum

C7A.019 Malignant carcinoid tumor of the small intestine, unspecified portion

C7A.02 Malignant carcinoid tumors of the appendix, large intestine, and rectum

C7A.020 Malignant carcinoid tumor of the appendix

C7A.021 Malignant carcinoid tumor of the cecum

C7A.022 Malignant carcinoid tumor of the ascending colon

C7A.023 Malignant carcinoid tumor of the transverse colon

C7A.024 Malignant carcinoid tumor of the descending colon

C7A.025 Malignant carcinoid tumor of the sigmoid colon

C7A.026 Malignant carcinoid tumor of the rectum

C7A.029 Malignant carcinoid tumor of the large intestine, unspecified portion

Malignant carcinoid tumor of the colon NOS

C7A.09 Malignant carcinoid tumors of other sites

C7A.090 Malignant carcinoid tumor of the bronchus and lung

C7A.091 Malignant carcinoid tumor of the thymus

C7A.092 Malignant carcinoid tumor of the stomach

C7A.093 Malignant carcinoid tumor of the kidney

C7A.094 Malignant carcinoid tumor of the foregut NOS

C7A.095 Malignant carcinoid tumor of the midgut NOS

C7A.096 Malignant carcinoid tumor of the hindgut NOS

C7A.098 Malignant carcinoid tumors of other sites

C7A.1 Malignant poorly differentiated neuroendocrine tumors

Malignant poorly differentiated neuroendocrine tumor NOS

Malignant poorly differentiated neuroendocrine carcinoma, any site

High grade neuroendocrine carcinoma, any site

C7A.8 Other malignant neuroendocrine tumors

SECONDARY NEUROENDOCRINE TUMORS (C7B)

C7B **Secondary neuroendocrine tumors**

Use additional code to identify any functional activity

C7B.0 Secondary carcinoid tumors

C7B.00 Secondary carcinoid tumors, unspecified site

C7B.01 Secondary carcinoid tumors of distant lymph nodes

C7B.02 Secondary carcinoid tumors of liver

C7B.03 Secondary carcinoid tumors of bone

C7B.04 Secondary carcinoid tumors of peritoneum

Mesentary metastasis of carcinoid tumor

C7B.09 Secondary carcinoid tumors of other sites

C7B.1 Secondary Merkel cell carcinoma

Merkel cell carcinoma nodal presentation

Merkel cell carcinoma visceral metastatic presentation

C7B.8 Other secondary neuroendocrine tumors

MALIGNANT NEOPLASMS OF ILL-DEFINED, OTHER SECONDARY AND UNSPECIFIED SITES (C76-C80)

C76 Malignant neoplasm of other and ill-defined sites

Excludes 1: malignant neoplasm of female genitourinary tract NOS (C57.9)

malignant neoplasm of male genitourinary tract NOS (C63.9)

malignant neoplasm of lymphoid, hematopoietic and related tissue (C81-C96)

malignant neoplasm of skin (C44.-)

malignant neoplasm of unspecified site NOS (C80.1)

C76.0 Malignant neoplasm of head, face and neck

Malignant neoplasm of cheek NOS

Malignant neoplasm of nose NOS

C76.1 Malignant neoplasm of thorax

Intrathoracic malignant neoplasm NOS

Malignant neoplasm of axilla NOS

Thoracic malignant neoplasm NOS

C76.2 Malignant neoplasm of abdomen

C76.3 Malignant neoplasm of pelvis

Malignant neoplasm of groin NOS

Malignant neoplasm of sites overlapping systems within the pelvis

Rectovaginal (septum) malignant neoplasm

Rectovesical (septum) malignant neoplasm

C76.4 Malignant neoplasm of upper limb

C76.40 Malignant neoplasm of unspecified upper limb

C76.41 Malignant neoplasm of right upper limb

C76.42 Malignant neoplasm of left upper limb

C76.5 Malignant neoplasm of lower limb

C76.50 Malignant neoplasm of unspecified lower limb

C76.51 Malignant neoplasm of right lower limb

C76.52 Malignant neoplasm of left lower limb

C76.8 Malignant neoplasm of other specified ill-defined sites

Malignant neoplasm of overlapping ill-defined sites

C77 Secondary and unspecified malignant neoplasm of lymph nodes

Excludes 1: malignant neoplasm of lymph nodes, specified as primary (C81-C86, C88, C96.-)

mesentary metastasis of carcinoid tumor (C7B.04)

secondary carcinoid tumors of distant lymph nodes (C7B.01)

C77.0 Secondary and unspecified malignant neoplasm of lymph nodes of head, face and neck

Secondary and unspecified malignant neoplasm of supraclavicular lymph nodes

C77.1 Secondary and unspecified malignant neoplasm of intrathoracic lymph nodes

C77.2 Secondary and unspecified malignant neoplasm of intra-abdominal lymph nodes

C77.3 Secondary and unspecified malignant neoplasm of axilla and upper limb lymph nodes

Secondary and unspecified malignant neoplasm of pectoral lymph nodes

C77.4 Secondary and unspecified malignant neoplasm of inguinal and lower limb lymph nodes

C77.5 Secondary and unspecified malignant neoplasm of intrapelvic lymph nodes

C77.8 Secondary and unspecified malignant neoplasm of lymph nodes of multiple regions

C77.9 Secondary and unspecified malignant neoplasm of lymph node, unspecified

C78 Secondary malignant neoplasm of respiratory and digestive organs

Excludes 1: lymph node metastases (C77.0)

secondary carcinoid tumors of liver (C7B.02)

secondary carcinoid tumors of peritoneum (C7B.04)

C78.0 Secondary malignant neoplasm of lung

C78.00 Secondary malignant neoplasm of unspecified lung

C78.01 Secondary malignant neoplasm of right lung

C78.02 Secondary malignant neoplasm of left lung

● New code   ▲ Revised code   ⑦ 7th digit required   ⊗ Placeholder required

C78.1   Secondary malignant neoplasm of mediastinum

C78.2   Secondary malignant neoplasm of pleura

C78.3   Secondary malignant neoplasm of other and unspecified respiratory organs

     C78.30   Secondary malignant neoplasm of unspecified respiratory organ

     C78.39   Secondary malignant neoplasm of other respiratory organs

C78.4   Secondary malignant neoplasm of small intestine

C78.5   Secondary malignant neoplasm of large intestine and rectum

C78.6   Secondary malignant neoplasm of retroperitoneum and peritoneum

C78.7   Secondary malignant neoplasm of liver and intrahepatic bile duct

C78.8   Secondary malignant neoplasm of other and unspecified digestive organs

     C78.80   Secondary malignant neoplasm of unspecified digestive organ

     C78.89   Secondary malignant neoplasm of other digestive organs

C79   Secondary malignant neoplasm of other and unspecified sites

     Excludes 1: lymph node metastases (C77.0)

         secondary carcinoid tumors (C7B.-)

         secondary neuroendocrine tumors (C7B.-)

C79.0   Secondary malignant neoplasm of kidney and renal pelvis

     C79.00   Secondary malignant neoplasm of unspecified kidney and renal pelvis

     C79.01   Secondary malignant neoplasm of right kidney and renal pelvis

     C79.02   Secondary malignant neoplasm of left kidney and renal pelvis

C79.1   Secondary malignant neoplasm of bladder and other and unspecified urinary organs

     C79.10   Secondary malignant neoplasm of unspecified urinary organs

     C79.11   Secondary malignant neoplasm of bladder

     C79.19   Secondary malignant neoplasm of other urinary organs

C79.2   Secondary malignant neoplasm of skin

     Excludes 1: secondary Merkel cell carcinoma (C7B.1)

C79.3   Secondary malignant neoplasm of brain and cerebral meninges

     C79.31   Secondary malignant neoplasm of brain

     C79.32   Secondary malignant neoplasm of cerebral meninges

C79.4   Secondary malignant neoplasm of other and unspecified parts of nervous system

     C79.40   Secondary malignant neoplasm of unspecified part of nervous system

     C79.49   Secondary malignant neoplasm of other parts of nervous system

C79.5   Secondary malignant neoplasm of bone and bone marrow

     Excludes 1: secondary carcinoid tumors of bone (C7B.03)

     C79.51   Secondary malignant neoplasm of bone

     C79.52   Secondary malignant neoplasm of bone marrow

C79.6   Secondary malignant neoplasm of ovary

     C79.60   Secondary malignant neoplasm of unspecified ovary

     C79.61   Secondary malignant neoplasm of right ovary

     C79.62   Secondary malignant neoplasm of left ovary

C79.7   Secondary malignant neoplasm of adrenal gland

C79.70   Secondary malignant neoplasm of unspecified adrenal gland

C79.71   Secondary malignant neoplasm of right adrenal gland

C79.72   Secondary malignant neoplasm of left adrenal gland

C79.8   Secondary malignant neoplasm of other specified sites

     C79.81   Secondary malignant neoplasm of breast

     C79.82   Secondary malignant neoplasm of genital organs

     C79.89   Secondary malignant neoplasm of other specified sites

C79.9   Secondary malignant neoplasm of unspecified site

     Metastatic cancer NOS

     Metastatic disease NOS

     Excludes 1: carcinomatosis NOS (C80.0)

         generalized cancer NOS (C80.0)

         malignant (primary) neoplasm of unspecified site (C80.1)

C80   Malignant neoplasm without specification of site

     Excludes 1: malignant carcinoid tumor of unspecified site (C7A.00)

         malignant neoplasm of specified multiple sites- code to each site

C80.0   Disseminated malignant neoplasm, unspecified

     Carcinomatosis NOS

     Generalized cancer, unspecified site (primary) (secondary)

     Generalized malignancy, unspecified site (primary) (secondary)

C80.1   Malignant (primary) neoplasm, unspecified

     Cancer NOS

     Cancer unspecified site (primary)

     Carcinoma unspecified site (primary)

     Malignancy unspecified site (primary)

     Excludes 1: secondary malignant neoplasm of unspecified site (C79.9)

C80.2   Malignant neoplasm associated with transplanted organ

     Code first complication of transplanted organ (T86.-)

     Use additional code to identify the specific malignancy

MALIGNANT NEOPLASMS OF LYMPHOID, HEMATOPOIETIC AND RELATED TISSUE (C81-C96)

Excludes 2: Kaposi's sarcoma of lymph nodes (C46.3)

     secondary and unspecified neoplasm of lymph nodes (C77.-)

     secondary neoplasm of bone marrow (C79.52)

     secondary neoplasm of spleen (C78.89)

C81   Hodgkin lymphoma

     Excludes 1: personal history of Hodgkin lymphoma (Z85.71)

C81.0   Nodular lymphocyte predominant Hodgkin lymphoma

     C81.00   Nodular lymphocyte predominant Hodgkin lymphoma, unspecified site

     C81.01   Nodular lymphocyte predominant Hodgkin lymphoma, lymph nodes of head, face, and neck

     C81.02   Nodular lymphocyte predominant Hodgkin lymphoma, intrathoracic lymph nodes

     C81.03   Nodular lymphocyte predominant Hodgkin lymphoma, intra-abdominal lymph nodes

     C81.04   Nodular lymphocyte predominant Hodgkin lymphoma, lymph nodes of axilla and upper limb

     C81.05   Nodular lymphocyte predominant Hodgkin lymphoma, lymph nodes of inguinal region and lower limb

     C81.06   Nodular lymphocyte predominant Hodgkin lymphoma, intrapelvic lymph nodes

C81.07   Nodular lymphocyte predominant Hodgkin lymphoma, spleen

C81.08   Nodular lymphocyte predominant Hodgkin lymphoma, lymph nodes of multiple sites

C81.09   Nodular lymphocyte predominant Hodgkin lymphoma, extranodal and solid organ sites

C81.1   Nodular sclerosis classical Hodgkin lymphoma

C81.10   Nodular sclerosis classical Hodgkin lymphoma, unspecified site

C81.11   Nodular sclerosis classical Hodgkin lymphoma, lymph nodes of head, face, and neck

C81.12   Nodular sclerosis classical Hodgkin lymphoma, intrathoracic lymph nodes

C81.13   Nodular sclerosis classical Hodgkin lymphoma, intra-abdominal lymph nodes

C81.14   Nodular sclerosis classical Hodgkin lymphoma, lymph nodes of axilla and upper limb

C81.15   Nodular sclerosis classical Hodgkin lymphoma, lymph nodes of inguinal region and lower limb

C81.16   Nodular sclerosis classical Hodgkin lymphoma, intrapelvic lymph nodes

C81.17   Nodular sclerosis classical Hodgkin lymphoma, spleen

C81.18   Nodular sclerosis classical Hodgkin lymphoma, lymph nodes of multiple sites

C81.19   Nodular sclerosis classical Hodgkin lymphoma, extranodal and solid organ sites

C81.2   Mixed cellularity classical Hodgkin lymphoma

C81.20   Mixed cellularity classical Hodgkin lymphoma, unspecified site

C81.21   Mixed cellularity classical Hodgkin lymphoma, lymph nodes of head, face, and neck

C81.22   Mixed cellularity classical Hodgkin lymphoma, intrathoracic lymph nodes

C81.23   Mixed cellularity classical Hodgkin lymphoma, intra-abdominal lymph nodes

C81.24   Mixed cellularity classical Hodgkin lymphoma, lymph nodes of axilla and upper limb

C81.25   Mixed cellularity classical Hodgkin lymphoma, lymph nodes of inguinal region and lower limb

C81.26   Mixed cellularity classical Hodgkin lymphoma, intrapelvic lymph nodes

C81.27   Mixed cellularity classical Hodgkin lymphoma, spleen

C81.28   Mixed cellularity classical Hodgkin lymphoma, lymph nodes of multiple sites

C81.29   Mixed cellularity classical Hodgkin lymphoma, extranodal and solid organ sites

C81.3   Lymphocyte depleted classical Hodgkin lymphoma

C81.30   Lymphocyte depleted classical Hodgkin lymphoma, unspecified site

C81.31   Lymphocyte depleted classical Hodgkin lymphoma, lymph nodes of head, face, and neck

C81.32   Lymphocyte depleted classical Hodgkin lymphoma, intrathoracic lymph nodes

C81.33   Lymphocyte depleted classical Hodgkin lymphoma, intra-abdominal lymph nodes

C81.34   Lymphocyte depleted classical Hodgkin lymphoma, lymph nodes of axilla and upper limb

C81.35   Lymphocyte depleted classical Hodgkin lymphoma, lymph nodes of inguinal region and lower limb

C81.36   Lymphocyte depleted classical Hodgkin lymphoma, intrapelvic lymph nodes

C81.37   Lymphocyte depleted classical Hodgkin lymphoma, spleen

C81.38   Lymphocyte depleted classical Hodgkin lymphoma, lymph nodes of multiple sites

C81.39   Lymphocyte depleted classical Hodgkin lymphoma, extranodal and solid organ sites

C81.4   Lymphocyte-rich classical Hodgkin lymphoma

Excludes 1: nodular lymphocyte predominant Hodgkin lymphoma (C81.0-)

C81.40   Lymphocyte-rich classical Hodgkin lymphoma, unspecified site

C81.41   Lymphocyte-rich classical Hodgkin lymphoma, lymph nodes of head, face, and neck

C81.42   Lymphocyte-rich classical Hodgkin lymphoma, intrathoracic lymph nodes

C81.43   Lymphocyte-rich classical Hodgkin lymphoma, intra-abdominal lymph nodes

C81.44   Lymphocyte-rich classical Hodgkin lymphoma, lymph nodes of axilla and upper limb

C81.45   Lymphocyte-rich classical Hodgkin lymphoma, lymph nodes of inguinal region and lower limb

C81.46   Lymphocyte-rich classical Hodgkin lymphoma, intrapelvic lymph nodes

C81.47   Lymphocyte-rich classical Hodgkin lymphoma, spleen

C81.48   Lymphocyte-rich classical Hodgkin lymphoma, lymph nodes of multiple sites

C81.49   Lymphocyte-rich classical Hodgkin lymphoma, extranodal and solid organ sites

C81.7   Other classical Hodgkin lymphoma

Classical Hodgkin lymphoma NOS

C81.70   Other classical Hodgkin lymphoma, unspecified site

C81.71   Other classical Hodgkin lymphoma, lymph nodes of head, face, and neck

C81.72   Other classical Hodgkin lymphoma, intrathoracic lymph nodes

C81.73   Other classical Hodgkin lymphoma, intra-abdominal lymph nodes

C81.74   Other classical Hodgkin lymphoma, lymph nodes of axilla and upper limb

C81.75   Other classical Hodgkin lymphoma, lymph nodes of inguinal region and lower limb

C81.76   Other classical Hodgkin lymphoma, intrapelvic lymph nodes

C81.77   Other classical Hodgkin lymphoma, spleen

C81.78   Other classical Hodgkin lymphoma, lymph nodes of multiple sites

C81.79   Other classical Hodgkin lymphoma, extranodal and solid organ sites

C81.9   Hodgkin lymphoma, unspecified

C81.90   Hodgkin lymphoma, unspecified, unspecified site

C81.91   Hodgkin lymphoma, unspecified, lymph nodes of head, face, and neck

C81.92   Hodgkin lymphoma, unspecified, intrathoracic lymph nodes

C81.93   Hodgkin lymphoma, unspecified, intra-abdominal lymph nodes

C81.94   Hodgkin lymphoma, unspecified, lymph nodes of axilla and upper limb

C81.95 Hodgkin lymphoma, unspecified, lymph nodes of inguinal region and lower limb

C81.96 Hodgkin lymphoma, unspecified, intrapelvic lymph nodes

C81.97 Hodgkin lymphoma, unspecified, spleen

C81.98 Hodgkin lymphoma, unspecified, lymph nodes of multiple sites

C81.99 Hodgkin lymphoma, unspecified, extranodal and solid organ sites

C82 Follicular lymphoma

Includes: follicular lymphoma with or without diffuse areas

Excludes 1: mature T/NK-cell lymphomas (C84.-)

personal history of non-Hodgkin lymphoma (Z85.72)

C82.0 Follicular lymphoma grade I

C82.00 Follicular lymphoma grade I, unspecified site

C82.01 Follicular lymphoma grade I, lymph nodes of head, face, and neck

C82.02 Follicular lymphoma grade I, intrathoracic lymph nodes

C82.03 Follicular lymphoma grade I, intra-abdominal lymph nodes

C82.04 Follicular lymphoma grade I, lymph nodes of axilla and upper limb

C82.05 Follicular lymphoma grade I, lymph nodes of inguinal region and lower limb

C82.06 Follicular lymphoma grade I, intrapelvic lymph nodes

C82.07 Follicular lymphoma grade I, spleen

C82.08 Follicular lymphoma grade I, lymph nodes of multiple sites

C82.09 Follicular lymphoma grade I, extranodal and solid organ sites

C82.1 Follicular lymphoma grade II

C82.10 Follicular lymphoma grade II, unspecified site

C82.11 Follicular lymphoma grade II, lymph nodes of head, face, and neck

C82.12 Follicular lymphoma grade II, intrathoracic lymph nodes

C82.13 Follicular lymphoma grade II, intra-abdominal lymph nodes

C82.14 Follicular lymphoma grade II, lymph nodes of axilla and upper limb

C82.15 Follicular lymphoma grade II, lymph nodes of inguinal region and lower limb

C82.16 Follicular lymphoma grade II, intrapelvic lymph nodes

C82.17 Follicular lymphoma grade II, spleen

C82.18 Follicular lymphoma grade II, lymph nodes of multiple sites

C82.19 Follicular lymphoma grade II, extranodal and solid organ sites

C82.2 Follicular lymphoma grade III, unspecified

C82.20 Follicular lymphoma grade III, unspecified, unspecified site

C82.21 Follicular lymphoma grade III, unspecified, lymph nodes of head, face, and neck

C82.22 Follicular lymphoma grade III, unspecified, intrathoracic lymph nodes

C82.23 Follicular lymphoma grade III, unspecified, intra-abdominal lymph nodes

C82.24 Follicular lymphoma grade III, unspecified, lymph nodes of axilla and upper limb

C82.25 Follicular lymphoma grade III, unspecified, lymph nodes of inguinal region and lower limb

C82.26 Follicular lymphoma grade III, unspecified, intrapelvic lymph nodes

C82.27 Follicular lymphoma grade III, unspecified, spleen

C82.28 Follicular lymphoma grade III, unspecified, lymph nodes of multiple sites

C82.29 Follicular lymphoma grade III, unspecified, extranodal and solid organ sites

C82.3 Follicular lymphoma grade IIIa

C82.30 Follicular lymphoma grade IIIa, unspecified site

C82.31 Follicular lymphoma grade IIIa, lymph nodes of head, face, and neck

C82.32 Follicular lymphoma grade IIIa, intrathoracic lymph nodes

C82.33 Follicular lymphoma grade IIIa, intra-abdominal lymph nodes

C82.34 Follicular lymphoma grade IIIa, lymph nodes of axilla and upper limb

C82.35 Follicular lymphoma grade IIIa, lymph nodes of inguinal region and lower limb

C82.36 Follicular lymphoma grade IIIa, intrapelvic lymph nodes

C82.37 Follicular lymphoma grade IIIa, spleen

C82.38 Follicular lymphoma grade IIIa, lymph nodes of multiple sites

C82.39 Follicular lymphoma grade IIIa, extranodal and solid organ sites

C82.4 Follicular lymphoma grade IIIb

C82.40 Follicular lymphoma grade IIIb, unspecified site

C82.41 Follicular lymphoma grade IIIb, lymph nodes of head, face, and neck

C82.42 Follicular lymphoma grade IIIb, intrathoracic lymph nodes

C82.43 Follicular lymphoma grade IIIb, intra-abdominal lymph nodes

C82.44 Follicular lymphoma grade IIIb, lymph nodes of axilla and upper limb

C82.45 Follicular lymphoma grade IIIb, lymph nodes of inguinal region and lower limb

C82.46 Follicular lymphoma grade IIIb, intrapelvic lymph nodes

C82.47 Follicular lymphoma grade IIIb, spleen

C82.48 Follicular lymphoma grade IIIb, lymph nodes of multiple sites

C82.49 Follicular lymphoma grade IIIb, extranodal and solid organ sites

C82.5 Diffuse follicle center lymphoma

C82.50 Diffuse follicle center lymphoma, unspecified site

C82.51 Diffuse follicle center lymphoma, lymph nodes of head, face, and neck

C82.52 Diffuse follicle center lymphoma, intrathoracic lymph nodes

C82.53 Diffuse follicle center lymphoma, intra-abdominal lymph nodes

C82.54 Diffuse follicle center lymphoma, lymph nodes of axilla and upper limb

C82.55 Diffuse follicle center lymphoma, lymph nodes of inguinal region and lower limb

C82.56 Diffuse follicle center lymphoma, intrapelvic lymph nodes

C82.57 Diffuse follicle center lymphoma, spleen

C82.58 Diffuse follicle center lymphoma, lymph nodes of multiple sites

C82.59 Diffuse follicle center lymphoma, extranodal and solid organ sites

C82.6 Cutaneous follicle center lymphoma

C82.60 Cutaneous follicle center lymphoma, unspecified site

C82.61 Cutaneous follicle center lymphoma, lymph nodes of head, face, and neck

C82.62 Cutaneous follicle center lymphoma, intrathoracic lymph nodes

C82.63 Cutaneous follicle center lymphoma, intra-abdominal lymph nodes

C82.64 Cutaneous follicle center lymphoma, lymph nodes of axilla and upper limb

C82.65 Cutaneous follicle center lymphoma, lymph nodes of inguinal region and lower limb

C82.66 Cutaneous follicle center lymphoma, intrapelvic lymph nodes

C82.67 Cutaneous follicle center lymphoma, spleen

C82.68 Cutaneous follicle center lymphoma, lymph nodes of multiple sites

C82.69 Cutaneous follicle center lymphoma, extranodal and solid organ sites

C82.8 Other types of follicular lymphoma

C82.80 Other types of follicular lymphoma, unspecified site

C82.81 Other types of follicular lymphoma, lymph nodes of head, face, and neck

C82.82 Other types of follicular lymphoma, intrathoracic lymph nodes

C82.83 Other types of follicular lymphoma, intra-abdominal lymph nodes

C82.84 Other types of follicular lymphoma, lymph nodes of axilla and upper limb

C82.85 Other types of follicular lymphoma, lymph nodes of inguinal region and lower limb

C82.86 Other types of follicular lymphoma, intrapelvic lymph nodes

C82.87 Other types of follicular lymphoma, spleen

C82.88 Other types of follicular lymphoma, lymph nodes of multiple sites

C82.89 Other types of follicular lymphoma, extranodal and solid organ sites

C82.9 Follicular lymphoma, unspecified

C82.90 Follicular lymphoma, unspecified, unspecified site

C82.91 Follicular lymphoma, unspecified, lymph nodes of head, face, and neck

C82.92 Follicular lymphoma, unspecified, intrathoracic lymph nodes

C82.93 Follicular lymphoma, unspecified, intra-abdominal lymph nodes

C82.94 Follicular lymphoma, unspecified, lymph nodes of axilla and upper limb

C82.95 Follicular lymphoma, unspecified, lymph nodes of inguinal region and lower limb

C82.96 Follicular lymphoma, unspecified, intrapelvic lymph nodes

C82.97 Follicular lymphoma, unspecified, spleen

C82.98 Follicular lymphoma, unspecified, lymph nodes of multiple sites

C82.99 Follicular lymphoma, unspecified, extranodal and solid organ sites

C83 Non-follicular lymphoma

Excludes 1: personal history of non-Hodgkin lymphoma (Z85.72)

C83.0 Small cell B-cell lymphoma

Lymphoplasmacytic lymphoma

Nodal marginal zone lymphoma

Non-leukemic variant of B-CLL

Splenic marginal zone lymphoma

Excludes 1: chronic lymphocytic leukemia (C91.1)
mature T/NK-cell lymphomas (C84.-)
Waldenstr÷m macroglobulinemia (C88.0)

C83.00 Small cell B-cell lymphoma, unspecified site

C83.01 Small cell B-cell lymphoma, lymph nodes of head, face, and neck

C83.02 Small cell B-cell lymphoma, intrathoracic lymph nodes

C83.03 Small cell B-cell lymphoma, intra-abdominal lymph nodes

C83.04 Small cell B-cell lymphoma, lymph nodes of axilla and upper limb

C83.05 Small cell B-cell lymphoma, lymph nodes of inguinal region and lower limb

C83.06 Small cell B-cell lymphoma, intrapelvic lymph nodes

C83.07 Small cell B-cell lymphoma, spleen

C83.08 Small cell B-cell lymphoma, lymph nodes of multiple sites

C83.09 Small cell B-cell lymphoma, extranodal and solid organ sites

C83.1 Mantle cell lymphoma

Centrocytic lymphoma

Malignant lymphomatous polyposis

C83.10 Mantle cell lymphoma, unspecified site

C83.11 Mantle cell lymphoma, lymph nodes of head, face, and neck

C83.12 Mantle cell lymphoma, intrathoracic lymph nodes

C83.13 Mantle cell lymphoma, intra-abdominal lymph nodes

C83.14 Mantle cell lymphoma, lymph nodes of axilla and upper limb

C83.15 Mantle cell lymphoma, lymph nodes of inguinal region and lower limb

C83.16 Mantle cell lymphoma, intrapelvic lymph nodes

C83.17 Mantle cell lymphoma, spleen

C83.18 Mantle cell lymphoma, lymph nodes of multiple sites

C83.19 Mantle cell lymphoma, extranodal and solid organ sites

C83.3 Diffuse large B-cell lymphoma

Anaplastic diffuse large B-cell lymphoma

CD30-positive diffuse large B-cell lymphoma

Centroblastic diffuse large B-cell lymphoma

Diffuse large B-cell lymphoma, subtype not specified

Immunoblastic diffuse large B-cell lymphoma

Plasmablastic diffuse large B-cell lymphoma

Diffuse large B-cell lymphoma, subtype not specified

T-cell rich diffuse large B-cell lymphoma

Excludes 1: mediastinal (thymic) large B-cell lymphoma (C85.2-)
mature T/NK-cell lymphomas (C84.-)

C83.30 Diffuse large B-cell lymphoma, unspecified site

C83.31 Diffuse large B-cell lymphoma, lymph nodes of head, face, and neck

C83.32 Diffuse large B-cell lymphoma, intrathoracic lymph nodes

C83.33 Diffuse large B-cell lymphoma, intra-abdominal lymph nodes

C83.34 Diffuse large B-cell lymphoma, lymph nodes of axilla and upper limb

C83.35 Diffuse large B-cell lymphoma, lymph nodes of inguinal region and lower limb

C83.36 Diffuse large B-cell lymphoma, intrapelvic lymph nodes

C83.37 Diffuse large B-cell lymphoma, spleen

C83.38 Diffuse large B-cell lymphoma, lymph nodes of multiple sites

C83.39 Diffuse large B-cell lymphoma, extranodal and solid organ sites

C83.5 Lymphoblastic (diffuse) lymphoma

B-precursor lymphoma

Lymphoblastic B-cell lymphoma

Lymphoblastic lymphoma NOS

Lymphoblastic T-cell lymphoma

T-precursor lymphoma

C83.50 Lymphoblastic (diffuse) lymphoma, unspecified site

C83.51 Lymphoblastic (diffuse) lymphoma, lymph nodes of head, face, and neck

C83.52 Lymphoblastic (diffuse) lymphoma, intrathoracic lymph nodes

C83.53 Lymphoblastic (diffuse) lymphoma, intra-abdominal lymph nodes

C83.54 Lymphoblastic (diffuse) lymphoma, lymph nodes of axilla and upper limb

C83.55 Lymphoblastic (diffuse) lymphoma, lymph nodes of inguinal region and lower limb

C83.56 Lymphoblastic (diffuse) lymphoma, intrapelvic lymph nodes

C83.57 Lymphoblastic (diffuse) lymphoma, spleen

C83.58 Lymphoblastic (diffuse) lymphoma, lymph nodes of multiple sites

C83.59 Lymphoblastic (diffuse) lymphoma, extranodal and solid organ sites

C83.7 Burkitt lymphoma

Atypical Burkitt lymphoma

Burkitt-like lymphoma

Excludes 1: mature B-cell leukemia Burkitt type (C91.A-)

C83.70 Burkitt lymphoma, unspecified site

C83.71 Burkitt lymphoma, lymph nodes of head, face, and neck

C83.72 Burkitt lymphoma, intrathoracic lymph nodes

C83.73 Burkitt lymphoma, intra-abdominal lymph nodes

C83.74 Burkitt lymphoma, lymph nodes of axilla and upper limb

C83.75 Burkitt lymphoma, lymph nodes of inguinal region and lower limb

C83.76 Burkitt lymphoma, intrapelvic lymph nodes

C83.77 Burkitt lymphoma, spleen

C83.78 Burkitt lymphoma, lymph nodes of multiple sites

C83.79 Burkitt lymphoma, extranodal and solid organ sites

C83.8 Other non-follicular lymphoma

Intravascular large B-cell lymphoma

Lymphoid granulomatosis

Primary effusion B-cell lymphoma

Excludes 1: mediastinal (thymic) large B-cell lymphoma (C85.2-)

T-cell rich B-cell lymphoma (C83.3-)

C83.80 Other non-follicular lymphoma, unspecified site

C83.81 Other non-follicular lymphoma, lymph nodes of head, face, and neck

C83.82 Other non-follicular lymphoma, intrathoracic lymph nodes

C83.83 Other non-follicular lymphoma, intra-abdominal lymph nodes

C83.84 Other non-follicular lymphoma, lymph nodes of axilla and upper limb

C83.85 Other non-follicular lymphoma, lymph nodes of inguinal region and lower limb

C83.86 Other non-follicular lymphoma, intrapelvic lymph nodes

C83.87 Other non-follicular lymphoma, spleen

C83.88 Other non-follicular lymphoma, lymph nodes of multiple sites

C83.89 Other non-follicular lymphoma, extranodal and solid organ sites

C83.9 Non-follicular (diffuse) lymphoma, unspecified

C83.90 Non-follicular (diffuse) lymphoma, unspecified, unspecified site

C83.91 Non-follicular (diffuse) lymphoma, unspecified, lymph nodes of head, face, and neck

C83.92 Non-follicular (diffuse) lymphoma, unspecified, intrathoracic lymph nodes

C83.93 Non-follicular (diffuse) lymphoma, unspecified, intra-abdominal lymph nodes

C83.94 Non-follicular (diffuse) lymphoma, unspecified, lymph nodes of axilla and upper limb

C83.95 Non-follicular (diffuse) lymphoma, unspecified, lymph nodes of inguinal region and lower limb

C83.96 Non-follicular (diffuse) lymphoma, unspecified, intrapelvic lymph nodes

C83.97 Non-follicular (diffuse) lymphoma, unspecified, spleen

C83.98 Non-follicular (diffuse) lymphoma, unspecified, lymph nodes of multiple sites

C83.99 Non-follicular (diffuse) lymphoma, unspecified, extranodal and solid organ sites

C84 Mature T/NK-cell lymphomas

Excludes 1: personal history of non-Hodgkin lymphoma (Z85.72)

C84.0 Mycosis fungoides

Excludes 1: peripheral T-cell lymphoma, not classified (C84.4-)

C84.00 Mycosis fungoides, unspecified site

C84.01 Mycosis fungoides, lymph nodes of head, face, and neck

C84.02 Mycosis fungoides, intrathoracic lymph nodes

C84.03 Mycosis fungoides, intra-abdominal lymph nodes

C84.04 Mycosis fungoides, lymph nodes of axilla and upper limb

C84.05 Mycosis fungoides, lymph nodes of inguinal region and lower limb

C84.06 Mycosis fungoides, intrapelvic lymph nodes

C84.07 Mycosis fungoides, spleen

C84.08 Mycosis fungoides, lymph nodes of multiple sites

C84.09 Mycosis fungoides, extranodal and solid organ sites

C84.1 Sezary disease

    C84.10 Sezary disease, unspecified site

    C84.11 Sezary disease, lymph nodes of head, face, and neck

    C84.12 Sezary disease, intrathoracic lymph nodes

    C84.13 Sezary disease, intra-abdominal lymph nodes

    C84.14 Sezary disease, lymph nodes of axilla and upper limb

    C84.15 Sezary disease, lymph nodes of inguinal region and lower limb

    C84.16 Sezary disease, intrapelvic lymph nodes

    C84.17 Sezary disease, spleen

    C84.18 Sezary disease, lymph nodes of multiple sites

    C84.19 Sezary disease, extranodal and solid organ sites

C84.4 Peripheral T-cell lymphoma, not classified

Lennert's lymphoma

Lymphoepithelioid lymphoma

Mature T-cell lymphoma, not elsewhere classified

    C84.40 Peripheral T-cell lymphoma, not classified, unspecified site

    C84.41 Peripheral T-cell lymphoma, not classified, lymph nodes of head, face, and neck

    C84.42 Peripheral T-cell lymphoma, not classified, intrathoracic lymph nodes

    C84.43 Peripheral T-cell lymphoma, not classified, intra-abdominal lymph nodes

    C84.44 Peripheral T-cell lymphoma, not classified, lymph nodes of axilla and upper limb

    C84.45 Peripheral T-cell lymphoma, not classified, lymph nodes of inguinal region and lower limb

    C84.46 Peripheral T-cell lymphoma, not classified, intrapelvic lymph nodes

    C84.47 Peripheral T-cell lymphoma, not classified, spleen

    C84.48 Peripheral T-cell lymphoma, not classified, lymph nodes of multiple sites

    C84.49 Peripheral T-cell lymphoma, not classified, extranodal and solid organ sites

C84.6 Anaplastic large cell lymphoma, ALK-positive

Anaplastic large cell lymphoma, CD30-positive

    C84.60 Anaplastic large cell lymphoma, ALK-positive, unspecified site

    C84.61 Anaplastic large cell lymphoma, ALK-positive, lymph nodes of head, face, and neck

    C84.62 Anaplastic large cell lymphoma, ALK-positive, intrathoracic lymph nodes

    C84.63 Anaplastic large cell lymphoma, ALK-positive, intra-abdominal lymph nodes

    C84.64 Anaplastic large cell lymphoma, ALK-positive, lymph nodes of axilla and upper limb

    C84.65 Anaplastic large cell lymphoma, ALK-positive, lymph nodes of inguinal region and lower limb

    C84.66 Anaplastic large cell lymphoma, ALK-positive, intrapelvic lymph nodes

    C84.67 Anaplastic large cell lymphoma, ALK-positive, spleen

    C84.68 Anaplastic large cell lymphoma, ALK-positive, lymph nodes of multiple sites

    C84.69 Anaplastic large cell lymphoma, ALK-positive, extranodal and solid organ sites

C84.7 Anaplastic large cell lymphoma, ALK-negative

Excludes 1: primary cutaneous CD30-positive T-cell proliferations (C86.6-)

    C84.70 Anaplastic large cell lymphoma, ALK-negative, unspecified site

    C84.71 Anaplastic large cell lymphoma, ALK-negative, lymph nodes of head, face, and neck

    C84.72 Anaplastic large cell lymphoma, ALK-negative, intrathoracic lymph nodes

    C84.73 Anaplastic large cell lymphoma, ALK-negative, intra-abdominal lymph nodes

    C84.74 Anaplastic large cell lymphoma, ALK-negative, lymph nodes of axilla and upper limb

    C84.75 Anaplastic large cell lymphoma, ALK-negative, lymph nodes of inguinal region and lower limb

    C84.76 Anaplastic large cell lymphoma, ALK-negative, intrapelvic lymph nodes

    C84.77 Anaplastic large cell lymphoma, ALK-negative, spleen

    C84.78 Anaplastic large cell lymphoma, ALK-negative, lymph nodes of multiple sites

    C84.79 Anaplastic large cell lymphoma, ALK-negative, extranodal and solid organ sites

C84.A Cutaneous T-cell lymphoma, unspecified

    C84.A0 Cutaneous T-cell lymphoma, unspecified, unspecified site

    C84.A1 Cutaneous T-cell lymphoma, unspecified lymph nodes of head, face, and neck

    C84.A2 Cutaneous T-cell lymphoma, unspecified, intrathoracic lymph nodes

    C84.A3 Cutaneous T-cell lymphoma, unspecified, intra-abdominal lymph nodes

    C84.A4 Cutaneous T-cell lymphoma, unspecified, lymph nodes of axilla and upper limb

    C84.A5 Cutaneous T-cell lymphoma, unspecified, lymph nodes of inguinal region and lower limb

    C84.A6 Cutaneous T-cell lymphoma, unspecified, intrapelvic lymph nodes

    C84.A7 Cutaneous T-cell lymphoma, unspecified, spleen

    C84.A8 Cutaneous T-cell lymphoma, unspecified, lymph nodes of multiple sites

    C84.A9 Cutaneous T-cell lymphoma, unspecified, extranodal and solid organ sites

C84.Z Other mature T/NK-cell lymphomas

Note: If T-cell lineage or involvement is mentioned in conjunction with a specific lymphoma, code to the more specific description.

Excludes 1: angioimmunoblastic T-cell lymphoma (C86.5)

    blastic NK-cell lymphoma (C86.4)

    enteropathy-type T-cell lymphoma (C86.2)

    extranodal NK-cell lymphoma, nasal type (C86.0)

    hepatosplenic T-cell lymphoma (C86.1)

    primary cutaneous CD30-positive T-cell proliferations (C86.6)

    subcutaneous panniculitis-like T-cell lymphoma (C86.3)

    T-cell leukemia (C91.1-)

    C84.Z0 Other mature T/NK-cell lymphomas, unspecified site

    C84.Z1 Other mature T/NK-cell lymphomas, lymph nodes of head, face, and neck

    C84.Z2 Other mature T/NK-cell lymphomas, intrathoracic lymph nodes

C84.Z3 Other mature T/NK-cell lymphomas, intra-abdominal lymph nodes

C84.Z4 Other mature T/NK-cell lymphomas, lymph nodes of axilla and upper limb

C84.Z5 Other mature T/NK-cell lymphomas, lymph nodes of inguinal region and lower limb

C84.Z6 Other mature T/NK-cell lymphomas, intrapelvic lymph nodes

C84.Z7 Other mature T/NK-cell lymphomas, spleen

C84.Z8 Other mature T/NK-cell lymphomas, lymph nodes of multiple sites

C84.Z9 Other mature T/NK-cell lymphomas, extranodal and solid organ sites

C84.9 Mature T/NK-cell lymphomas, unspecified

NK/T cell lymphoma NOS

Excludes 1: mature T-cell lymphoma, not elsewhere classified (C84.4-)

C84.90 Mature T/NK-cell lymphomas, unspecified, unspecified site

C84.91 Mature T/NK-cell lymphomas, unspecified, lymph nodes of head, face, and neck

C84.92 Mature T/NK-cell lymphomas, unspecified, intrathoracic lymph nodes

C84.93 Mature T/NK-cell lymphomas, unspecified, intra-abdominal lymph nodes

C84.94 Mature T/NK-cell lymphomas, unspecified, lymph nodes of axilla and upper limb

C84.95 Mature T/NK-cell lymphomas, unspecified, lymph nodes of inguinal region and lower limb

C84.96 Mature T/NK-cell lymphomas, unspecified, intrapelvic lymph nodes

C84.97 Mature T/NK-cell lymphomas, unspecified, spleen

C84.98 Mature T/NK-cell lymphomas, unspecified, lymph nodes of multiple sites

C84.99 Mature T/NK-cell lymphomas, unspecified, extranodal and solid organ sites

C85 Other specified and unspecified types of non-Hodgkin lymphoma

Excludes 1: other specified types of T/NK-cell lymphoma (C86.-)

personal history of non-Hodgkin lymphoma (Z85.72)

C85.1 Unspecified B-cell lymphoma

Note: If B-cell lineage or involvement is mentioned in conjunction with a specific lymphoma, code to the more specific description.

C85.10 Unspecified B-cell lymphoma, unspecified site

C85.11 Unspecified B-cell lymphoma, lymph nodes of head, face, and neck

C85.12 Unspecified B-cell lymphoma, intrathoracic lymph nodes

C85.13 Unspecified B-cell lymphoma, intra-abdominal lymph nodes

C85.14 Unspecified B-cell lymphoma, lymph nodes of axilla and upper limb

C85.15 Unspecified B-cell lymphoma, lymph nodes of inguinal region and lower limb

C85.16 Unspecified B-cell lymphoma, intrapelvic lymph nodes

C85.17 Unspecified B-cell lymphoma, spleen

C85.18 Unspecified B-cell lymphoma, lymph nodes of multiple sites

C85.19 Unspecified B-cell lymphoma, extranodal and solid organ sites

C85.2 Mediastinal (thymic) large B-cell lymphoma

C85.20 Mediastinal (thymic) large B-cell lymphoma, unspecified site

C85.21 Mediastinal (thymic) large B-cell lymphoma, lymph nodes of head, face, and neck

C85.22 Mediastinal (thymic) large B-cell lymphoma, intrathoracic lymph nodes

C85.23 Mediastinal (thymic) large B-cell lymphoma, intra-abdominal lymph nodes

C85.24 Mediastinal (thymic) large B-cell lymphoma, lymph nodes of axilla and upper limb

C85.25 Mediastinal (thymic) large B-cell lymphoma, lymph nodes of inguinal region and lower limb

C85.26 Mediastinal (thymic) large B-cell lymphoma, intrapelvic lymph nodes

C85.27 Mediastinal (thymic) large B-cell lymphoma, spleen

C85.28 Mediastinal (thymic) large B-cell lymphoma, lymph nodes of multiple sites

C85.29 Mediastinal (thymic) large B-cell lymphoma, extranodal and solid organ sites

C85.8 Other specified types of non-Hodgkin lymphoma

C85.80 Other specified types of non-Hodgkin lymphoma, unspecified site

C85.81 Other specified types of non-Hodgkin lymphoma, lymph nodes of head, face, and neck

C85.82 Other specified types of non-Hodgkin lymphoma, intrathoracic lymph nodes

C85.83 Other specified types of non-Hodgkin lymphoma, intra-abdominal lymph nodes

C85.84 Other specified types of non-Hodgkin lymphoma, lymph nodes of axilla and upper limb

C85.85 Other specified types of non-Hodgkin lymphoma, lymph nodes of inguinal region and lower limb

C85.86 Other specified types of non-Hodgkin lymphoma, intrapelvic lymph nodes

C85.87 Other specified types of non-Hodgkin lymphoma, spleen

C85.88 Other specified types of non-Hodgkin lymphoma, lymph nodes of multiple sites

C85.89 Other specified types of non-Hodgkin lymphoma, extranodal and solid organ sites

C85.9 Non-Hodgkin lymphoma, unspecified

Lymphoma NOS

Malignant lymphoma NOS

Non-Hodgkin lymphoma NOS

C85.90 Non-Hodgkin lymphoma, unspecified, unspecified site

C85.91 Non-Hodgkin lymphoma, unspecified, lymph nodes of head, face, and neck

C85.92 Non-Hodgkin lymphoma, unspecified, intrathoracic lymph nodes

C85.93 Non-Hodgkin lymphoma, unspecified, intra-abdominal lymph nodes

C85.94 Non-Hodgkin lymphoma, unspecified, lymph nodes of axilla and upper limb

C85.95 Non-Hodgkin lymphoma, unspecified, lymph nodes of inguinal region and lower limb

C85.96 Non-Hodgkin lymphoma, unspecified, intrapelvic lymph nodes

C85.97 Non-Hodgkin lymphoma, unspecified, spleen

C85.98 Non-Hodgkin lymphoma, unspecified, lymph nodes of multiple sites

C85.99 Non-Hodgkin lymphoma, unspecified, extranodal and solid organ sites

C86 Other specified types of T/NK-cell lymphoma
> **Excludes 1:** anaplastic large cell lymphoma, ALK negative
> (C84.7-)
> anaplastic large cell lymphoma, ALK positive
> (C84.6-)
> mature T/NK-cell lymphomas (C84.-)
> other specified types of non-Hodgkin lymphoma
> (C85.8-)

C86.0 Extranodal NK/T-cell lymphoma, nasal type

C86.1 Hepatosplenic T-cell lymphoma
Alpha-beta and gamma delta types

C86.2 Enteropathy-type (intestinal) T-cell lymphoma
Enteropathy associated T-cell lymphoma

C86.3 Subcutaneous panniculitis-like T-cell lymphoma

C86.4 Blastic NK-cell lymphoma

C86.5 Angioimmunoblastic T-cell lymphoma
Angioimmunoblastic lymphadenopathy with
dysproteinemia (AILD)

C86.6 Primary cutaneous CD30-positive T-cell proliferations
Lymphomatoid papulosis
Primary cutaneous anaplastic large cell lymphoma
Primary cutaneous CD30-positive large T-cell lymphoma

C88 Malignant immunoproliferative diseases and certain other B-cell
lymphomas
> **Excludes 1:** B-cell lymphoma, unspecified C85.1-
> personal history of other malignant neoplasms of
> lymphoid, hematopoietic and related tissues
> (Z85.79)

C88.0 Waldenstr÷m macroglobulinemia
Lymphoplasmacytic lymphoma with IgM-production
Macroglobulinemia (idiopathic) (primary)
> **Excludes 1:** small cell B-cell lymphoma (C83.0)

C88.2 Heavy chain disease
Franklin disease
Gamma heavy chain disease
Mu heavy chain disease

C88.3 Immunoproliferative small intestinal disease
Alpha heavy chain disease
Mediterranean lymphoma

C88.4 Extranodal marginal zone B-cell lymphoma of mucosa-
associated lymphoid tissue [MALT-lymphoma]
Lymphoma of skin-associated lymphoid tissue
[SALT-lymphoma]
Lymphoma of bronchial-associated lymphoid tissue
[BALT-lymphoma]
> **Excludes 1:** high malignant (diffuse large B-cell)
> lymphoma (C83.3-)

C88.8 Other malignant immunoproliferative diseases

C88.9 Malignant immunoproliferative disease, unspecified
Immunoproliferative disease NOS

C90 Multiple myeloma and malignant plasma cell neoplasms
> **Excludes 1:** personal history of other malignant neoplasms of
> lymphoid, hematopoietic and related tissues
> (Z85.79)

C90.0 Multiple myeloma
Kahler's disease
Medullary plasmacytoma
Myelomatosis
Plasma cell myeloma
> **Excludes 1:** solitary myeloma (C90.3-)
> solitary plasmactyoma (C90.3-)

C90.00 Multiple myeloma not having achieved
remission

Multiple myeloma with failed remission
Multiple myeloma NOS

C90.01 Multiple myeloma in remission

C90.02 Multiple myeloma in relapse

C90.1 Plasma cell leukemia
Plasmacytic leukemia

C90.10 Plasma cell leukemia not having achieved
remission
Plasma cell leukemia with failed remission
Plasma cell leukemia NOS

C90.11 Plasma cell leukemia in remission

C90.12 Plasma cell leukemia in relapse

C90.2 Extramedullary plasmacytoma

C90.20 Extramedullary plasmacytoma not having
achieved remission
Extramedullary plasmacytoma with failed
remission
Extramedullary plasmacytoma NOS

C90.21 Extramedullary plasmacytoma in remission

C90.22 Extramedullary plasmacytoma in relapse

C90.3 Solitary plasmacytoma
Localized malignant plasma cell tumor NOS
Plasmacytoma NOS
Solitary myeloma

C90.30 Solitary plasmacytoma not having achieved
remission
Solitary plasmacytoma with failed remission
Solitary plasmacytoma NOS

C90.31 Solitary plasmacytoma in remission

C90.32 Solitary plasmacytoma in relapse

C91 Lymphoid leukemia
> **Excludes 1:** personal history of leukemia (Z85.6)

C91.0 Acute lymphoblastic leukemia [ALL]
Note: Code C91.0 should only be used for T-cell and
B-cell precursor leukemia

C91.00 Acute lymphoblastic leukemia not having
achieved remission
Acute lymphoblastic leukemia with failed
remission
Acute lymphoblastic leukemia NOS

C91.01 Acute lymphoblastic leukemia, in remission

C91.02 Acute lymphoblastic leukemia, in relapse

C91.1 Chronic lymphocytic leukemia of B-cell type
Lymphoplasmacytic leukemia
Richter syndrome
> **Excludes 1:** lymphoplasmacytic lymphoma (C83.0-)

C91.10 Chronic lymphocytic leukemia of B-cell type not
having achieved remission
Chronic lymphocytic leukemia of B-cell type
with failed remission
Chronic lymphocytic leukemia of B-cell type
NOS

C91.11 Chronic lymphocytic leukemia of B-cell type in
remission

C91.12 Chronic lymphocytic leukemia of B-cell type in
relapse

C91.3 Prolymphocytic leukemia of B-cell type

C91.30 Prolymphocytic leukemia of B-cell type not
having achieved remission
Prolymphocytic leukemia of B-cell type with
failed remission
Prolymphocytic leukemia of B-cell type NOS

● New code   ▲ Revised code   ⑦ 7ᵗʰ digit required   ⊗ Placeholder required

C91.31　Prolymphocytic leukemia of B-cell type, in remission

C91.32　Prolymphocytic leukemia of B-cell type, in relapse

C91.4　Hairy cell leukemia

Leukemic reticuloendotheliosis

C91.40　Hairy cell leukemia not having achieved remission

Hairy cell leukemia with failed remission

Hairy cell leukemia NOS

C91.41　Hairy cell leukemia, in remission

C91.42　Hairy cell leukemia, in relapse

C91.5　Adult T-cell lymphoma/leukemia (HTLV-1-associated)

Acute variant of adult T-cell lymphoma/leukemia (HTLV-1-associated)

Chronic variant of adult T-cell lymphoma/leukemia (HTLV-1-associated)

Lymphomatoid variant of adult T-cell lymphoma/leukemia (HTLV-1-associated)

Smouldering variant of adult T-cell lymphoma/leukemia (HTLV-1-associated)

C91.50　Adult T-cell lymphoma/leukemia (HTLV-1-associated) not having achieved remission

Adult T-cell lymphoma/leukemia (HTLV-1-associated) with failed remission

Adult T-cell lymphoma/leukemia (HTLV-1-associated) NOS

C91.51　Adult T-cell lymphoma/leukemia (HTLV-1-associated), in remission

C91.52　Adult T-cell lymphoma/leukemia (HTLV-1-associated), in relapse

C91.6　Prolymphocytic leukemia of T-cell type

C91.60　Prolymphocytic leukemia of T-cell type not having achieved remission

Prolymphocytic leukemia of T-cell type with failed remission

Prolymphocytic leukemia of T-cell type NOS

C91.61　Prolymphocytic leukemia of T-cell type, in remission

C91.62　Prolymphocytic leukemia of T-cell type, in relapse

C91.A Mature B-cell leukemia Burkitt-type

Excludes 1: Burkitt lymphoma (C83.7-)

C91.A0　Mature B-cell leukemia Burkitt-type not having achieved remission

Mature B-cell leukemia Burkitt-type with failed remission

Mature B-cell leukemia Burkitt-type NOS

C91.A1　Mature B-cell leukemia Burkitt-type, in remission

C91.A2　Mature B-cell leukemia Burkitt-type, in relapse

C91.Z Other lymphoid leukemia

T-cell large granular lymphocytic leukemia (associated with rheumatoid arthritis)

C91.Z0　Other lymphoid leukemia not having achieved remission

Other lymphoid leukemia with failed remission

Other lymphoid leukemia NOS

C91.Z1　Other lymphoid leukemia, in remission

C91.Z2　Other lymphoid leukemia, in relapse

C91.9　Lymphoid leukemia, unspecified

C91.90　Lymphoid leukemia, unspecified not having achieved remission

Lymphoid leukemia with failed remission

Lymphoid leukemia NOS

C91.91　Lymphoid leukemia, unspecified, in remission

C91.92　Lymphoid leukemia, unspecified, in relapse

C92 Myeloid leukemia

Includes: granulocytic leukemia

myelogenous leukemia

Excludes 1: personal history of leukemia (Z85.6)

C92.0　Acute myeloblastic leukemia

Acute myeloblastic leukemia, minimal differentiation

Acute myeloblastic leukemia (with maturation)

Acute myeloblastic leukemia 1/ETO

Acute myeloblastic leukemia M0

Acute myeloblastic leukemia M1

Acute myeloblastic leukemia M2

Acute myeloblastic leukemia with t(8;21)

Acute myeloblastic leukemia (without a FAB classification) NOS

Refractory anemia with excess blasts in transformation [RAEB T]

Excludes 1: acute exacerbation of chronic myeloid leukemia (C92.10)

refractory anemia with excess of blasts not in transformation (D46.2-)

C92.00　Acute myeloblastic leukemia, not having achieved remission

Acute myeloblastic leukemia with failed remission

Acute myeloblastic leukemia NOS

C92.01　Acute myeloblastic leukemia, in remission

C92.02　Acute myeloblastic leukemia, in relapse

C92.1　Chronic myeloid leukemia, BCR/ABL-positive

Chronic myelogenous leukemia, Philadelphia chromosome (Ph1) positive

Chronic myelogenous leukemia, t(9;22) (q34;q11)

Chronic myelogenous leukemia with crisis of blast cells

Excludes 1: atypical chronic myeloid leukemia BCR/ABL-negative (C92.2-)

chronic myelomonocytic leukemia (C93.1-)

chronic myeloproliferative disease (D47.1)

C92.10　Chronic myeloid leukemia, BCR/ABL positive, not having achieved remission

Chronic myeloid leukemia, BCR/ABL-positive with failed remission

Chronic myeloid leukemia, BCR/ABL-positive NOS

C92.11　Chronic myeloid leukemia, BCR/ABL-positive, in remission

C92.12　Chronic myeloid leukemia, BCR/ABL-positive, in relapse

C92.2　Atypical chronic myeloid leukemia, BCR/ABL negative

C92.20　Atypical chronic myeloid leukemia, BCR/ABL-negative, not having achieved remission

Atypical chronic myeloid leukemia, BCR/ABL-negative with failed remission

Atypical chronic myeloid leukemia, BCR/ABL-negative NOS

C92.21　Atypical chronic myeloid leukemia, BCR/ABL-negative, in remission

C92.22　Atypical chronic myeloid leukemia, BCR/ABL-negative, in relapse

C92.3　Myeloid sarcoma

A malignant tumor of immature myeloid cells

Chloroma

Granulocytic sarcoma

C92.30 Myeloid sarcoma, not having achieved remission

Myeloid sarcoma with failed remission

Myeloid sarcoma NOS

C92.31 Myeloid sarcoma, in remission

C92.32 Myeloid sarcoma, in relapse

C92.4 Acute promyelocytic leukemia

AML M3

AML Me with t(15;17) and variants

C92.40 Acute promyelocytic leukemia, not having achieved remission

Acute promyelocytic leukemia with failed remission

Acute promyelocytic leukemia NOS

C92.41 Acute promyelocytic leukemia, in remission

C92.42 Acute promyelocytic leukemia, in relapse

C92.5 Acute myelomonocytic leukemia

AML M4

AML M4 Eo with inv(16) or t(16;16)

C92.50 Acute myelomonocytic leukemia, not having achieved remission

Acute myelomonocytic leukemia with failed remission

Acute myelomonocytic leukemia NOS

C92.51 Acute myelomonocytic leukemia, in remission

C92.52 Acute myelomonocytic leukemia, in relapse

C92.6 Acute myeloid leukemia with 11q23-abnormality

Acute myeloid leukemia with variation of MLL-gene

C92.60 Acute myeloid leukemia with 11q23-abnormality not having achieved remission

Acute myeloid leukemia with 11q23-abnormality with failed remission

Acute myeloid leukemia with 11q23-abnormality NOS

C92.61 Acute myeloid leukemia with 11q23-abnormality in remission

C92.62 Acute myeloid leukemia with 11q23-abnormality in relapse

C92.A Acute myeloid leukemia with multilineage dysplasia

Acute myeloid leukemia with dysplasia of remaining hematopoesis and/or myelodysplastic disease in its history

C92.A0 Acute myeloid leukemia with multilineage dysplasia, not having achieved remission

Acute myeloid leukemia with multilineage dysplasia with failed remission

Acute myeloid leukemia with multilineage dysplasia NOS

C92.A1 Acute myeloid leukemia with multilineage dysplasia, in remission

C92.A2 Acute myeloid leukemia with multilineage dysplasia, in relapse

C92.Z Other myeloid leukemia

C92.Z0 Other myeloid leukemia not having achieved remission

Myeloid leukemia NEC with failed remission

Myeloid leukemia NEC

C92.Z1 Other myeloid leukemia, in remission

C92.Z2 Other myeloid leukemia, in relapse

C92.9 Myeloid leukemia, unspecified

C92.90 Myeloid leukemia, unspecified, not having achieved remission

Myeloid leukemia, unspecified with failed remission

Myeloid leukemia, unspecified NOS

C92.91 Myeloid leukemia, unspecified in remission

C92.92 Myeloid leukemia, unspecified in relapse

C93 Monocytic leukemia

Includes: monocytoid leukemia

Excludes 1: personal history of leukemia (Z85.6)

C93.0 Acute monoblastic/monocytic leukemia

AML M5

AML M5a

AML M5b

C93.00 Acute monoblastic/monocytic leukemia, not having achieved remission

Acute monoblastic/monocytic leukemia with failed remission

Acute monoblastic/monocytic leukemia NOS

C93.01 Acute monoblastic/monocytic leukemia, in remission

C93.02 Acute monoblastic/monocytic leukemia, in relapse

C93.1 Chronic myelomonocytic leukemia

Chronic monocytic leukemia

cmML-1

cmML-2

cmML with eosinophilia

C93.10 Chronic myelomonocytic leukemia not having achieved remission

Chronic myelomonocytic leukemia with failed remission

Chronic myelomonocytic leukemia NOS

C93.11 Chronic myelomonocytic leukemia, in remission

C93.12 Chronic myelomonocytic leukemia, in relapse

C93.3 Juvenile myelomonocytic leukemia

C93.30 Juvenile myelomonocytic leukemia, not having achieved remission

Juvenile myelomonocytic leukemia with failed remission

Juvenile myelomonocytic leukemia NOS

C93.31 Juvenile myelomonocytic leukemia, in remission

C93.32 Juvenile myelomonocytic leukemia, in relapse

C93.Z Other monocytic leukemia

C93.Z0 Other monocytic leukemia, not having achieved remission

Other monocytic leukemia NOS

C93.Z1 Other monocytic leukemia, in remission

C93.Z2 Other monocytic leukemia, in relapse

C93.9 Monocytic leukemia, unspecified

C93.90 Monocytic leukemia, unspecified, not having achieved remission

Monocytic leukemia, unspecified with failed remission

Monocytic leukemia, unspecified NOS

C93.91 Monocytic leukemia, unspecified in remission

C93.92 Monocytic leukemia, unspecified in relapse

C94 Other leukemias of specified cell type

Excludes 1: leukemic reticuloendotheliosis (C91.4-)

myelodysplastic syndromes (D46.-)

personal history of leukemia (Z85.6)

plasma cell leukemia (C90.1-)

C94.0 Acute erythroid leukemia

Acute myeloid leukemia M6(a)(b)

Erythroleukemia

C94.00   Acute erythroid leukemia, not having achieved remission

Acute erythroid leukemia with failed remission

Acute erythroid leukemia NOS

C94.01   Acute erythroid leukemia, in remission

C94.02   Acute erythroid leukemia, in relapse

C94.2   Acute megakaryoblastic leukemia

Acute myeloid leukemia M7

Acute megakaryocytic leukemia

C94.20   Acute megakaryoblastic leukemia not having achieved remission

Acute megakaryoblastic leukemia with failed remission

Acute megakaryoblastic leukemia NOS

C94.21   Acute megakaryoblastic leukemia, in remission

C94.22   Acute megakaryoblastic leukemia, in relapse

C94.3   Mast cell leukemia

C94.30   Mast cell leukemia not having achieved remission

Mast cell leukemia with failed remission

Mast cell leukemia NOS

C94.31   Mast cell leukemia, in remission

C94.32   Mast cell leukemia, in relapse

C94.4   Acute panmyelosis with myelofibrosis

Acute myelofibrosis

Excludes 1: myelofibrosis NOS (D75.81)

secondary myelofibrosis NOS (D75.81)

C94.40   Acute panmyelosis with myelofibrosis not having achieved remission

Acute myelofibrosis NOS

Acute panmyelosis with myelofibrosis with failed remission

Acute panmyelosis NOS

C94.41   Acute panmyelosis with myelofibrosis, in remission

C94.42   Acute panmyelosis with myelofibrosis, in relapse

C94.6   Myelodysplastic disease, not classified

Myeloproliferative disease, not classified

C94.8   Other specified leukemias

Aggressive NK-cell leukemia

Acute basophilic leukemia

C94.80   Other specified leukemias not having achieved remission

Other specified leukemia with failed remission

Other specified leukemias NOS

C94.81   Other specified leukemias, in remission

C94.82   Other specified leukemias, in relapse

C95   Leukemia of unspecified cell type

Excludes 1: personal history of leukemia (Z85.6)

C95.0   Acute leukemia of unspecified cell type

Acute bilineal leukemia

Acute mixed lineage leukemia

Biphenotypic acute leukemia

Stem cell leukemia of unclear lineage

Excludes 1: acute exacerbation of unspecified chronic leukemia (C95.10)

C95.00   Acute leukemia of unspecified cell type not having achieved remission

Acute leukemia of unspecified cell type with failed remission

Acute leukemia NOS

C95.01   Acute leukemia of unspecified cell type, in remission

C95.02   Acute leukemia of unspecified cell type, in relapse

C95.1   Chronic leukemia of unspecified cell type

C95.10   Chronic leukemia of unspecified cell type not having achieved remission

Chronic leukemia of unspecified cell type with failed remission

Chronic leukemia NOS

C95.11   Chronic leukemia of unspecified cell type, in remission

C95.12   Chronic leukemia of unspecified cell type, in relapse

C95.9   Leukemia, unspecified

C95.90   Leukemia, unspecified not having achieved remission

Leukemia, unspecified with failed remission

Leukemia NOS

C95.91   Leukemia, unspecified, in remission

C95.92   Leukemia, unspecified, in relapse

C96   Other and unspecified malignant neoplasms of lymphoid, hematopoietic and related tissue

Excludes 1: personal history of other malignant neoplasms of lymphoid, hematopoietic and related tissues (Z85.79)

C96.0   Multifocal and multisystemic (disseminated) Langerhans-cell histiocytosis

Histiocytosis X, multisystemic

Letterer-Siwe disease

Excludes 1: adult pulmonary Langerhans cell histiocytosis (J84.82)

multifocal and unisystemic Langerhans-cell histiocytosis (C96.5)

unifocal Langerhans-cell histiocytosis (C96.6)

C96.2   Malignant mast cell tumor

Aggressive systemic mastocytosis

Mast cell sarcoma

Excludes 1: indolent mastocytosis (D47.0)

mast cell leukemia (C94.30)

mastocytosis (congenital) (cutaneous) (Q82.2)

C96.4   Sarcoma of dendritic cells (accessory cells)

Follicular dendritic cell sarcoma

Interdigitating dendritic cell sarcoma

Langerhans cell sarcoma

C96.5   Multifocal and unisystemic Langerhans-cell histiocytosis

Hand-Sch_ller-Christian disease

Histiocytosis X, multifocal

Excludes 1: multifocal and multisystemic (disseminated) Langerhans-cell histiocytosis (C96.0)

unifocal Langerhans-cell histiocytosis (C96.6)

C96.6   Unifocal Langerhans-cell histiocytosis

Eosinophilic granuloma

Histiocytosis X, unifocal

Histiocytosis X NOS

Langerhans-cell histiocytosis NOS

Excludes 1: multifocal and multisysemic (disseminated) Langerhans-cell histiocytosis (C96.0)

multifocal and unisystemic Langerhans-cell histiocytosis (C96.5)

C96.A   Histiocytic sarcoma

Malignant histiocytosis

C96.Z   Other specified malignant neoplasms of lymphoid, hematopoietic and related tissue

C96.9 Malignant neoplasm of lymphoid, hematopoietic and related tissue, unspecified

IN SITU NEOPLASMS (D00-D09)

Includes: Bowen's disease

erythroplasia

grade III intraepithelial neoplasia

Queyrat's erythroplasia

D00 Carcinoma in situ of oral cavity, esophagus and stomach

Excludes 1: melanoma in situ (D03.-)

D00.0 Carcinoma in situ of lip, oral cavity and pharynx

Use additional code to identify:

exposure to environmental tobacco smoke (Z77.22)

exposure to tobacco smoke in the perinatal period (P96.81)

history of tobacco use (Z87.891)

occupational exposure to environmental tobacco smoke (Z57.31)

tobacco dependence (F17.-)

tobacco use (Z72.0)

Excludes 1: carcinoma in situ of aryepiglottic fold or interarytenoid fold, laryngeal aspect (D02.0)

carcinoma in situ of epiglottis NOS (D02.0)

carcinoma in situ of epiglottis suprahyoid portion (D02.0)

carcinoma in situ of skin of lip (D03.0, D04.0)

D00.00 Carcinoma in situ of oral cavity, unspecified site

D00.01 Carcinoma in situ of labial mucosa and vermilion border

D00.02 Carcinoma in situ of buccal mucosa

D00.03 Carcinoma in situ of gingiva and edentulous alveolar ridge

D00.04 Carcinoma in situ of soft palate

D00.05 Carcinoma in situ of hard palate

D00.06 Carcinoma in situ of floor of mouth

D00.07 Carcinoma in situ of tongue

D00.08 Carcinoma in situ of pharynx

Carcinoma in situ of aryepiglottic fold NOS

Carcinoma in situ of hypopharyngeal aspect of aryepiglottic fold

Carcinoma in situ of marginal zone of aryepiglottic fold

D00.1 Carcinoma in situ of esophagus

D00.2 Carcinoma in situ of stomach

D01 Carcinoma in situ of other and unspecified digestive organs

Excludes 1: melanoma in situ (D03.-)

D01.0 Carcinoma in situ of colon

Excludes 1: carcinoma in situ of rectosigmoid junction (D01.1)

D01.1 Carcinoma in situ of rectosigmoid junction

D01.2 Carcinoma in situ of rectum

D01.3 Carcinoma in situ of anus and anal canal

Excludes 1: carcinoma in situ of anal margin (D04.5)

carcinoma in situ of anal skin (D04.5)

carcinoma in situ of perianal skin (D04.5)

D01.4 Carcinoma in situ of other and unspecified parts of intestine

Excludes 1: carcinoma in situ of ampulla of Vater (D01.5)

D01.40 Carcinoma in situ of unspecified part of intestine

D01.49 Carcinoma in situ of other parts of intestine

D01.5 Carcinoma in situ of liver, gallbladder and bile ducts

Carcinoma in situ of ampulla of Vater

D01.7 Carcinoma in situ of other specified digestive organs

Carcinoma in situ of pancreas

D01.9 Carcinoma in situ of digestive organ, unspecified

D02 Carcinoma in situ of middle ear and respiratory system

Use additional code to identify:

exposure to environmental tobacco smoke (Z77.22)

exposure to tobacco smoke in the perinatal period (P96.81)

history of tobacco use (Z87.891)

occupational exposure to environmental tobacco smoke (Z57.31)

tobacco dependence (F17.-)

tobacco use (Z72.0)

Excludes 1: melanoma in situ (D03.-)

D02.0 Carcinoma in situ of larynx

Carcinoma in situ of aryepiglottic fold or interarytenoid fold, laryngeal aspect

Carcinoma in situ of epiglottis (suprahyoid portion)

Excludes 1: carcinoma in situ of aryepiglottic fold or interarytenoid fold NOS (D00.08)

carcinoma in situ of hypopharyngeal aspect (D00.08)

carcinoma in situ of marginal zone (D00.08)

D02.1 Carcinoma in situ of trachea

D02.2 Carcinoma in situ of bronchus and lung

D02.20 Carcinoma in situ of unspecified bronchus and lung

D02.21 Carcinoma in situ of right bronchus and lung

D02.22 Carcinoma in situ of left bronchus and lung

D02.3 Carcinoma in situ of other parts of respiratory system

Carcinoma in situ of accessory sinuses

Carcinoma in situ of middle ear

Carcinoma in situ of nasal cavities

Excludes 1: carcinoma in situ of ear (external) (skin) (D04.2-)

carcinoma in situ of nose NOS D09.8

carcinoma in situ of skin of nose (D04.3)

D02.4 Carcinoma in situ of respiratory system, unspecified

D03 Melanoma in situ

D03.0 Melanoma in situ of lip

D03.1 Melanoma in situ of eyelid, including canthus

D03.10 Melanoma in situ of unspecified eyelid, including canthus

D03.11 Melanoma in situ of right eyelid, including canthus

D03.12 Melanoma in situ of left eyelid, including canthus

D03.2 Melanoma in situ of ear and external auricular canal

D03.20 Melanoma in situ of unspecified ear and external auricular canal

D03.21 Melanoma in situ of right ear and external auricular canal

D03.22 Melanoma in situ of left ear and external auricular canal

D03.3 Melanoma in situ of other and unspecified parts of face

D03.30 Melanoma in situ of unspecified part of face

D03.39 Melanoma in situ of other parts of face

D03.4 Melanoma in situ of scalp and neck

D03.5 Melanoma in situ of trunk

D03.51 Melanoma in situ of anal skin

Melanoma in situ of anal margin

Melanoma in situ of perianal skin

D03.52 Melanoma in situ of breast (skin) (soft tissue)

D03.59 Melanoma in situ of other part of trunk

D03.6 Melanoma in situ of upper limb, including shoulder
    D03.60 Melanoma in situ of unspecified upper limb, including shoulder
    D03.61 Melanoma in situ of right upper limb, including shoulder
    D03.62 Melanoma in situ of left upper limb, including shoulder

D03.7 Melanoma in situ of lower limb, including hip
    D03.70 Melanoma in situ of unspecified lower limb, including hip
    D03.71 Melanoma in situ of right lower limb, including hip
    D03.72 Melanoma in situ of left lower limb, including hip

D03.8 Melanoma in situ of other sites
    Melanoma in situ of scrotum
    Excludes 1: carcinoma in situ of scrotum (D07.61)

D03.9 Melanoma in situ, unspecified

D04 Carcinoma in situ of skin
    Excludes 1: erythroplasia of Queyrat (penis) NOS (D07.4)
    melanoma in situ (D03.-)

D04.0 Carcinoma in situ of skin of lip
    Excludes 1: carcinoma in situ of vermilion border of lip (D00.01)

D04.1 Carcinoma in situ of skin of eyelid, including canthus
    D04.10 Carcinoma in situ of skin of unspecified eyelid, including canthus
    D04.11 Carcinoma in situ of skin of right eyelid, including canthus
    D04.12 Carcinoma in situ of skin of left eyelid, including canthus

D04.2 Carcinoma in situ of skin of ear and external auricular canal
    D04.20 Carcinoma in situ of skin of unspecified ear and external auricular canal
    D04.21 Carcinoma in situ of skin of right ear and external auricular canal
    D04.22 Carcinoma in situ of skin of left ear and external auricular canal

D04.3 Carcinoma in situ of skin of other and unspecified parts of face
    D04.30 Carcinoma in situ of skin of unspecified part of face
    D04.39 Carcinoma in situ of skin of other parts of face

D04.4 Carcinoma in situ of skin of scalp and neck

D04.5 Carcinoma in situ of skin of trunk
    Carcinoma in situ of anal margin
    Carcinoma in situ of anal skin
    Carcinoma in situ of perianal skin
    Carcinoma in situ of skin of breast
    Excludes 1: carcinoma in situ of anus NOS (D01.3)
    carcinoma in situ of scrotum (D07.61)
    carcinoma in situ of skin of genital organs (D07.-)

D04.6 Carcinoma in situ of skin of upper limb, including shoulder
    D04.60 Carcinoma in situ of skin of unspecified upper limb, including shoulder
    D04.61 Carcinoma in situ of skin of right upper limb, including shoulder
    D04.62 Carcinoma in situ of skin of left upper limb, including shoulder

D04.7 Carcinoma in situ of skin of lower limb, including hip

D04.70 Carcinoma in situ of skin of unspecified lower limb, including hip
D04.71 Carcinoma in situ of skin of right lower limb, including hip
D04.72 Carcinoma in situ of skin of left lower limb, including hip
D04.8 Carcinoma in situ of skin of other sites
D04.9 Carcinoma in situ of skin, unspecified

D05 Carcinoma in situ of breast
    Excludes 1: carcinoma in situ of skin of breast (D04.5)
    melanoma in situ of breast (skin) (D03.5)
    Paget's disease of breast or nipple (C50.-)

D05.0 Lobular carcinoma in situ of breast
    D05.00 Lobular carcinoma in situ of unspecified breast
    D05.01 Lobular carcinoma in situ of right breast
    D05.02 Lobular carcinoma in situ of left breast

D05.1 Intraductal carcinoma in situ of breast
    D05.10 Intraductal carcinoma in situ of unspecified breast
    D05.11 Intraductal carcinoma in situ of right breast
    D05.12 Intraductal carcinoma in situ of left breast

D05.8 Other specified type of carcinoma in situ of breast
    D05.80 Other specified type of carcinoma in situ of unspecified breast
    D05.81 Other specified type of carcinoma in situ of right breast
    D05.82 Other specified type of carcinoma in situ of left breast

D05.9 Unspecified type of carcinoma in situ of breast
    D05.90 Unspecified type of carcinoma in situ of unspecified breast
    D05.91 Unspecified type of carcinoma in situ of right breast
    D05.92 Unspecified type of carcinoma in situ of left breast

D06 Carcinoma in situ of cervix uteri
    Includes: cervical adenocarcinoma in situ
    cervical intraepithelial glandular neoplasia
    cervical intraepithelial neoplasia III [CIN III]
    severe dysplasia of cervix uteri
    Excludes 1: cervical intraepithelial neoplasia II [CIN II] (N87.1)
    cytologic evidence of malignancy of cervix without histologic confirmation (R87.614)
    high grade squamous intraepithelial lesion (HGSIL) of cervix (R87.613)
    melanoma in situ of cervix (D03.5)
    moderate cervical dysplasia (N87.1)

D06.0 Carcinoma in situ of endocervix
D06.1 Carcinoma in situ of exocervix
D06.7 Carcinoma in situ of other parts of cervix
D06.9 Carcinoma in situ of cervix, unspecified

D07 Carcinoma in situ of other and unspecified genital organs
    Excludes 1: melanoma in situ of trunk (D03.5)
D07.0 Carcinoma in situ of endometrium
D07.1 Carcinoma in situ of vulva
    Severe dysplasia of vulva
    Vulvar intraepithelial neoplasia III [VIN III]
    Excludes 1: moderate dysplasia of vulva (N90.1)
    vulvar intraepithelial neoplasia II [VIN II] (N90.1)
D07.2 Carcinoma in situ of vagina
    Severe dysplasia of vagina
    Vaginal intraepithelial neoplasia III [VAIN III]

Excludes 1: moderate dysplasia of vagina (N89.1)
vaginal intraepithelial neoplasia II [VIN II] (N89.1)

D07.3 Carcinoma in situ of other and unspecified female genital organs

    D07.30 Carcinoma in situ of unspecified female genital organs

    D07.39 Carcinoma in situ of other female genital organs

D07.4 Carcinoma in situ of penis
Erythroplasia of Queyrat NOS

D07.5 Carcinoma in situ of prostate
Prostatic intraepithelial neoplasia III (PIN III)
Severe dysplasia of prostate
Excludes 1: dysplasia (mild) (moderate) of prostate (N42.3)

D07.6 Carcinoma in situ of other and unspecified male genital organs

    D07.60 Carcinoma in situ of unspecified male genital organs

    D07.61 Carcinoma in situ of scrotum

    D07.69 Carcinoma in situ of other male genital organs

D09 Carcinoma in situ of other and unspecified sites
Excludes 1: melanoma in situ (D03.-)

D09.0 Carcinoma in situ of bladder

D09.1 Carcinoma in situ of other and unspecified urinary organs

    D09.10 Carcinoma in situ of unspecified urinary organ

    D09.19 Carcinoma in situ of other urinary organs

D09.2 Carcinoma in situ of eye
Excludes 1: carcinoma in situ of skin of eyelid (D04.1-)

    D09.20 Carcinoma in situ of unspecified eye

    D09.21 Carcinoma in situ of right eye

    D09.22 Carcinoma in situ of left eye

D09.3 Carcinoma in situ of thyroid and other endocrine glands
Excludes 1: carcinoma in situ of endocrine pancreas (D01.7)
carcinoma in situ of ovary (D07.39)
carcinoma in situ of testis (D07.69)

D09.8 Carcinoma in situ of other specified sites

D09.9 Carcinoma in situ, unspecified

BENIGN NEOPLASMS, EXCEPT BENIGN NEUROENDOCRINE TUMORS (D10-D36)

D10 Benign neoplasm of mouth and pharynx

D10.0 Benign neoplasm of lip
Benign neoplasm of lip (frenulum) (inner aspect) (mucosa) (vermilion border)
Excludes 1: benign neoplasm of skin of lip (D22.0, D23.0)

D10.1 Benign neoplasm of tongue
Benign neoplasm of lingual tonsil

D10.2 Benign neoplasm of floor of mouth

D10.3 Other and unspecified parts of mouth

    D10.30 Benign neoplasm of unspecified part of mouth

    D10.39 Benign neoplasm of other parts of mouth
Benign neoplasm of minor salivary gland NOS
Excludes 1: benign odontogenic neoplasms (D16.4-D16.5)
benign neoplasm of mucosa of lip (D10.0)
benign neoplasm of nasopharyngeal surface of soft palate (D10.6)

D10.4 Benign neoplasm of tonsil

Benign neoplasm of tonsil (faucial) (palatine)
Excludes 1: benign neoplasm of lingual tonsil (D10.1)
benign neoplasm of pharyngeal tonsil (D10.6)
benign neoplasm of tonsillar fossa (D10.5)
benign neoplasm of tonsillar pillars (D10.5)

D10.5 Benign neoplasm of other parts of oropharynx
Benign neoplasm of epiglottis, anterior aspect
Benign neoplasm of tonsillar fossa
Benign neoplasm of tonsillar pillars
Benign neoplasm of vallecula
Excludes 1: benign neoplasm of epiglottis NOS (D14.1)
benign neoplasm of epiglottis, suprahyoid portion (D14.1)

D10.6 Benign neoplasm of nasopharynx
Benign neoplasm of pharyngeal tonsil
Benign neoplasm of posterior margin of septum and choanae

D10.7 Benign neoplasm of hypopharynx

D10.9 Benign neoplasm of pharynx, unspecified

D11 Benign neoplasm of major salivary glands
Excludes 1: benign neoplasms of specified minor salivary glands which are classified according to their anatomical location
benign neoplasms of minor salivary glands NOS (D10.39)

D11.0 Benign neoplasm of parotid gland

D11.7 Benign neoplasm of other major salivary glands
Benign neoplasm of sublingual salivary gland
Benign neoplasm of submandibular salivary gland

D11.9 Benign neoplasm of major salivary gland, unspecified

D12 Benign neoplasm of colon, rectum, anus and anal canal
Excludes 1: benign carcinoid tumors of the large intestine, and rectum (D3A.02-)

D12.0 Benign neoplasm of cecum
Benign neoplasm of ileocecal valve

D12.1 Benign neoplasm of appendix
Excludes 1: benign carcinoid tumor of the appendix (D3A.020)

D12.2 Benign neoplasm of ascending colon

D12.3 Benign neoplasm of transverse colon
Benign neoplasm of hepatic flexure
Benign neoplasm of splenic flexure

D12.4 Benign neoplasm of descending colon

D12.5 Benign neoplasm of sigmoid colon

D12.6 Benign neoplasm of colon, unspecified
Adenomatosis of colon
Benign neoplasm of large intestine NOS
Polyposis (hereditary) of colon
Excludes 1: inflammatory polyp of colon (K51.4-)
polyp of colon NOS (K63.5)

D12.7 Benign neoplasm of rectosigmoid junction

D12.8 Benign neoplasm of rectum
Excludes 1: benign carcinoid tumor of the rectum (D3A.026)

D12.9 Benign neoplasm of anus and anal canal
Benign neoplasm of anus NOS
Excludes 1: benign neoplasm of anal margin (D22.5, D23.5)
benign neoplasm of anal skin (D22.5, D23.5)
benign neoplasm of perianal skin (D22.5, D23.5)

D13 Benign neoplasm of other and ill-defined parts of digestive system

Excludes 1: benign stromal tumors of digestive system (D21.4)

D13.0 Benign neoplasm of esophagus

D13.1 Benign neoplasm of stomach

> **Excludes 1:** benign carcinoid tumor of the stomach (D3A.092)

D13.2 Benign neoplasm of duodenum

> **Excludes 1:** benign carcinoid tumor of the duodenum (D3A.010)

D13.3 Benign neoplasm of other and unspecified parts of small intestine

> **Excludes 1:** benign carcinoid tumors of the small intestine(D3A.01-)
>
> benign neoplasm of ileocecal valve (D12.0)

    D13.30 Benign neoplasm of unspecified part of small intestine

    D13.39 Benign neoplasm of other parts of small intestine

D13.4 Benign neoplasm of liver

Benign neoplasm of intrahepatic bile ducts

D13.5 Benign neoplasm of extrahepatic bile ducts

D13.6 Benign neoplasm of pancreas

> **Excludes 1:** benign neoplasm of endocrine pancreas (D13.7)

D13.7 Benign neoplasm of endocrine pancreas

Islet cell tumor

Benign neoplasm of islets of Langerhans

Use additional code to identify any functional activity.

D13.9 Benign neoplasm of ill-defined sites within the digestive system

Benign neoplasm of digestive system NOS

Benign neoplasm of intestine NOS

Benign neoplasm of spleen

D14 Benign neoplasm of middle ear and respiratory system

D14.0 Benign neoplasm of middle ear, nasal cavity and accessory sinuses

Benign neoplasm of cartilage of nose

> **Excludes 1:** benign neoplasm of auricular canal (external) (D22.2-, D23.2-)
>
> benign neoplasm of bone of ear (D16.4)
>
> benign neoplasm of bone of nose (D16.4)
>
> benign neoplasm of cartilage of ear (D21.0)
>
> benign neoplasm of ear (external)(skin) (D22.2-, D23.2-)
>
> benign neoplasm of nose NOS (D36.7)
>
> benign neoplasm of skin of nose (D22.39, D23.39)
>
> benign neoplasm of olfactory bulb (D33.3)
>
> benign neoplasm of posterior margin of septum and choanae (D10.6)
>
> polyp of accessory sinus (J33.8)
>
> polyp of ear (middle) (H74.4)
>
> polyp of nasal (cavity) (J33.-)

D14.1 Benign neoplasm of larynx

Adenomatous polyp of larynx

Benign neoplasm of epiglottis (suprahyoid portion)

> **Excludes 1:** benign neoplasm of epiglottis, anterior aspect (D10.5)
>
> polyp (nonadenomatous) of vocal cord or larynx (J38.1)

D14.2 Benign neoplasm of trachea

D14.3 Benign neoplasm of bronchus and lung

> **Excludes 1:** benign carcinoid tumor of the bronchus and lung (D3A.090)

    D14.30 Benign neoplasm of unspecified bronchus and lung

    D14.31 Benign neoplasm of right bronchus and lung

    D14.32 Benign neoplasm of left bronchus and lung

D14.4 Benign neoplasm of respiratory system, unspecified

D15 Benign neoplasm of other and unspecified intrathoracic organs

> **Excludes 1:** benign neoplasm of mesothelial tissue (D19.-)

D15.0 Benign neoplasm of thymus

> **Excludes 1:** benign carcinoid tumor of the thymus (D3A.091)

D15.1 Benign neoplasm of heart

> **Excludes 1:** benign neoplasm of great vessels (D21.3)

D15.2 Benign neoplasm of mediastinum

D15.7 Benign neoplasm of other specified intrathoracic organs

D15.9 Benign neoplasm of intrathoracic organ, unspecified

D16 Benign neoplasm of bone and articular cartilage

> **Excludes 1:** benign neoplasm of connective tissue of ear (D21.0)
>
> benign neoplasm of connective tissue of eyelid (D21.0)
>
> benign neoplasm of connective tissue of larynx (D14.1)
>
> benign neoplasm of connective tissue of nose (D14.0)
>
> benign neoplasm of synovia (D21.-)

D16.0 Benign neoplasm of scapula and long bones of upper limb

    D16.00 Benign neoplasm of scapula and long bones of unspecified upper limb

    D16.01 Benign neoplasm of scapula and long bones of right upper limb

    D16.02 Benign neoplasm of scapula and long bones of left upper limb

D16.1 Benign neoplasm of short bones of upper limb

    D16.10 Benign neoplasm of short bones of unspecified upper limb

    D16.11 Benign neoplasm of short bones of right upper limb

    D16.12 Benign neoplasm of short bones of left upper limb

D16.2 Benign neoplasm of long bones of lower limb

    D16.20 Benign neoplasm of long bones of unspecified lower limb

    D16.21 Benign neoplasm of long bones of right lower limb

    D16.22 Benign neoplasm of long bones of left lower limb

D16.3 Benign neoplasm of short bones of lower limb

    D16.30 Benign neoplasm of short bones of unspecified lower limb

    D16.31 Benign neoplasm of short bones of right lower limb

    D16.32 Benign neoplasm of short bones of left lower limb

D16.4 Benign neoplasm of bones of skull and face

Benign neoplasm of maxilla (superior)

Benign neoplasm of orbital bone

Keratocyst of maxilla

Keratocystic odontogenic tumor of maxilla

> **Excludes 1:** benign neoplasm of lower jaw bone (D16.5)

D16.5 Benign neoplasm of lower jaw bone

Keratocyst of mandible

Keratocystic odontogenic tumor of mandible

D16.6 Benign neoplasm of vertebral column

> **Excludes 1:** benign neoplasm of sacrum and coccyx (D16.8)

D16.7 Benign neoplasm of ribs, sternum and clavicle

D16.8 Benign neoplasm of pelvic bones, sacrum and coccyx

D16.9 Benign neoplasm of bone and articular cartilage, unspecified

D17 Benign lipomatous neoplasm

D17.0 Benign lipomatous neoplasm of skin and subcutaneous tissue of head, face and neck

D17.1 Benign lipomatous neoplasm of skin and subcutaneous tissue of trunk

D17.2 Benign lipomatous neoplasm of skin and subcutaneous tissue of limb

    D17.20 Benign lipomatous neoplasm of skin and subcutaneous tissue of unspecified limb

    D17.21 Benign lipomatous neoplasm of skin and subcutaneous tissue of right arm

    D17.22 Benign lipomatous neoplasm of skin and subcutaneous tissue of left arm

    D17.23 Benign lipomatous neoplasm of skin and subcutaneous tissue of right leg

    D17.24 Benign lipomatous neoplasm of skin and subcutaneous tissue of left leg

D17.3 Benign lipomatous neoplasm of skin and subcutaneous tissue of other and unspecified sites

    D17.30 Benign lipomatous neoplasm of skin and subcutaneous tissue of unspecified sites

    D17.39 Benign lipomatous neoplasm of skin and subcutaneous tissue of other sites

D17.4 Benign lipomatous neoplasm of intrathoracic organs

D17.5 Benign lipomatous neoplasm of intra-abdominal organs

    Excludes 1: benign lipomatous neoplasm of peritoneum and retroperitoneum (D17.79)

D17.6 Benign lipomatous neoplasm of spermatic cord

D17.7 Benign lipomatous neoplasm of other sites

    D17.71 Benign lipomatous neoplasm of kidney

    D17.72 Benign lipomatous neoplasm of other genitourinary organ

    D17.79 Benign lipomatous neoplasm of other sites

        Benign lipomatous neoplasm of peritoneum

        Benign lipomatous neoplasm of retroperitoneum

D17.9 Benign lipomatous neoplasm, unspecified

    Lipoma NOS

D18 Hemangioma and lymphangioma, any site

Excludes 1: benign neoplasm of glomus jugulare (D35.6)

        blue or pigmented nevus (D22.-)

        nevus NOS (D22.-)

        vascular nevus (Q82.5)

D18.0 Hemangioma

    Angioma NOS

    Cavernous nevus

    D18.00 Hemangioma unspecified site

    D18.01 Hemangioma of skin and subcutaneous tissue

    D18.02 Hemangioma of intracranial structures

    D18.03 Hemangioma of intra-abdominal structures

    D18.09 Hemangioma of other sites

D18.1 Lymphangioma, any site

D19 Benign neoplasm of mesothelial tissue

D19.0 Benign neoplasm of mesothelial tissue of pleura

D19.1 Benign neoplasm of mesothelial tissue of peritoneum

D19.7 Benign neoplasm of mesothelial tissue of other sites

D19.9 Benign neoplasm of mesothelial tissue, unspecified

    Benign mesothelioma NOS

D20 Benign neoplasm of soft tissue of retroperitoneum and peritoneum

    Excludes 1: benign lipomatous neoplasm of peritoneum and retroperitoneum (D17.79)

        benign neoplasm of mesothelial tissue (D19.-)

D20.0 Benign neoplasm of soft tissue of retroperitoneum

D20.1 Benign neoplasm of soft tissue of peritoneum

D21 Other benign neoplasms of connective and other soft tissue

Includes: benign neoplasm of blood vessel

    benign neoplasm of bursa

    benign neoplasm of cartilage

    benign neoplasm of fascia

    benign neoplasm of fat

    benign neoplasm of ligament, except uterine

    benign neoplasm of lymphatic channel

    benign neoplasm of muscle

    benign neoplasm of synovia

    benign neoplasm of tendon (sheath)

    benign stromal tumors

Excludes 1: benign neoplasm of articular cartilage (D16.-)

    benign neoplasm of cartilage of larynx (D14.1)

    benign neoplasm of cartilage of nose (D14.0)

    benign neoplasm of connective tissue of breast (D24.-)

    benign neoplasm of peripheral nerves and autonomic nervous system (D36.1-)

    benign neoplasm of peritoneum (D20.1)

    benign neoplasm of retroperitoneum (D20.0)

    benign neoplasm of uterine ligament, any (D28.2)

    benign neoplasm of vascular tissue (D18.-)

    hemangioma (D18.0-)

    lipomatous neoplasm (D17.-)

    lymphangioma (D18.1)

    uterine leiomyoma (D25.-)

D21.0 Benign neoplasm of connective and other soft tissue of head, face and neck

    Benign neoplasm of connective tissue of ear

    Benign neoplasm of connective tissue of eyelid

    Excludes 1: benign neoplasm of connective tissue of orbit (D31.6-)

D21.1 Benign neoplasm of connective and other soft tissue of upper limb, including shoulder

    D21.10 Benign neoplasm of connective and other soft tissue of unspecified upper limb, including shoulder

    D21.11 Benign neoplasm of connective and other soft tissue of right upper limb, including shoulder

    D21.12 Benign neoplasm of connective and other soft tissue of left upper limb, including shoulder

D21.2 Benign neoplasm of connective and other soft tissue of lower limb, including hip

    D21.20 Benign neoplasm of connective and other soft tissue of unspecified lower limb, including hip

    D21.21 Benign neoplasm of connective and other soft tissue of right lower limb, including hip

    D21.22 Benign neoplasm of connective and other soft tissue of left lower limb, including hip

D21.3 Benign neoplasm of connective and other soft tissue of thorax

    Benign neoplasm of axilla

    Benign neoplasm of diaphragm

    Benign neoplasm of great vessels

    Excludes 1: benign neoplasm of heart (D15.1)

        benign neoplasm of mediastinum (D15.2)

        benign neoplasm of thymus (D15.0)

D21.4 Benign neoplasm of connective and other soft tissue of abdomen

● New code   ▲ Revised code   ⑦ 7th digit required   ⊗ Placeholder required

Benign stromal tumors of abdomen

D21.5 Benign neoplasm of connective and other soft tissue of pelvis

Excludes 1: benign neoplasm of any uterine ligament (D28.2)

uterine leiomyoma (D25.-)

D21.6 Benign neoplasm of connective and other soft tissue of trunk, unspecified

Benign neoplasm of back NOS

D21.9 Benign neoplasm of connective and other soft tissue, unspecified

D22 Melanocytic nevi

Includes: atypical nevus

blue hairy pigmented nevus

nevus NOS

D22.0 Melanocytic nevi of lip

D22.1 Melanocytic nevi of eyelid, including canthus

D22.10 Melanocytic nevi of unspecified eyelid, including canthus

D22.11 Melanocytic nevi of right eyelid, including canthus

D22.12 Melanocytic nevi of left eyelid, including canthus

D22.2 Melanocytic nevi of ear and external auricular canal

D22.20 Melanocytic nevi of unspecified ear and external auricular canal

D22.21 Melanocytic nevi of right ear and external auricular canal

D22.22 Melanocytic nevi of left ear and external auricular canal

D22.3 Melanocytic nevi of other and unspecified parts of face

D22.30 Melanocytic nevi of unspecified part of face

D22.39 Melanocytic nevi of other parts of face

D22.4 Melanocytic nevi of scalp and neck

D22.5 Melanocytic nevi of trunk

Melanocytic nevi of anal margin

Melanocytic nevi of anal skin

Melanocytic nevi of perianal skin

Melanocytic nevi of skin of breast

D22.6 Melanocytic nevi of upper limb, including shoulder

D22.60 Melanocytic nevi of unspecified upper limb, including shoulder

D22.61 Melanocytic nevi of right upper limb, including shoulder

D22.62 Melanocytic nevi of left upper limb, including shoulder

D22.7 Melanocytic nevi of lower limb, including hip

D22.70 Melanocytic nevi of unspecified lower limb, including hip

D22.71 Melanocytic nevi of right lower limb, including hip

D22.72 Melanocytic nevi of left lower limb, including hip

D22.9 Melanocytic nevi, unspecified

D23 Other benign neoplasms of skin

Includes: benign neoplasm of hair follicles

benign neoplasm of sebaceous glands

benign neoplasm of sweat glands

Excludes 1: benign lipomatous neoplasms of skin (D17.0-D17.3)

melanocytic nevi (D22.-)

D23.0 Other benign neoplasm of skin of lip

Excludes 1: benign neoplasm of vermilion border of lip (D10.0)

D23.1 Other benign neoplasm of skin of eyelid, including canthus

D23.10 Other benign neoplasm of skin of unspecified eyelid, including canthus

D23.11 Other benign neoplasm of skin of right eyelid, including canthus

D23.12 Other benign neoplasm of skin of left eyelid, including canthus

D23.2 Other benign neoplasm of skin of ear and external auricular canal

D23.20 Other benign neoplasm of skin of unspecified ear and external auricular canal

D23.21 Other benign neoplasm of skin of right ear and external auricular canal

D23.22 Other benign neoplasm of skin of left ear and external auricular canal

D23.3 Other benign neoplasm of skin of other and unspecified parts of face

D23.30 Other benign neoplasm of skin of unspecified part of face

D23.39 Other benign neoplasm of skin of other parts of face

D23.4 Other benign neoplasm of skin of scalp and neck

D23.5 Other benign neoplasm of skin of trunk

Other benign neoplasm of anal margin

Other benign neoplasm of anal skin

Other benign neoplasm of perianal skin

Other benign neoplasm of skin of breast

Excludes 1: benign neoplasm of anus NOS (D12.9)

D23.6 Other benign neoplasm of skin of upper limb, including shoulder

D23.60 Other benign neoplasm of skin of unspecified upper limb, including shoulder

D23.61 Other benign neoplasm of skin of right upper limb, including shoulder

D23.62 Other benign neoplasm of skin of left upper limb, including shoulder

D23.7 Other benign neoplasm of skin of lower limb, including hip

D23.70 Other benign neoplasm of skin of unspecified lower limb, including hip

D23.71 Other benign neoplasm of skin of right lower limb, including hip

D23.72 Other benign neoplasm of skin of left lower limb, including hip

D23.9 Other benign neoplasm of skin, unspecified

D24 Benign neoplasm of breast

Includes: benign neoplasm of connective tissue of breast

benign neoplasm of soft parts of breast

fibroadenoma of breast

Excludes 2: adenofibrosis of breast (N60.2)

benign cyst of breast (N60.-)

benign mammary dysplasia (N60.-)

benign neoplasm of skin of breast (D22.5, D23.5)

fibrocystic disease of breast (N60.-)

D24.1 Benign neoplasm of right breast

D24.2 Benign neoplasm of left breast

D24.9 Benign neoplasm of unspecified breast

D25 Leiomyoma of uterus

Includes: uterine fibroid

uterine fibromyoma

uterine myoma

D25.0 Submucous leiomyoma of uterus

D25.1 Intramural leiomyoma of uterus

Interstitial leiomyoma of uterus

D25.2 Subserosal leiomyoma of uterus
Subperitoneal leiomyoma of uterus
D25.9 Leiomyoma of uterus, unspecified
D26 Other benign neoplasms of uterus
D26.0 Other benign neoplasm of cervix uteri
D26.1 Other benign neoplasm of corpus uteri
D26.7 Other benign neoplasm of other parts of uterus
D26.9 Other benign neoplasm of uterus, unspecified
D27 Benign neoplasm of ovary
Use additional code to identify any functional activity.
Excludes 2: corpus albicans cyst (N83.2)
corpus luteum cyst (N83.1)
endometrial cyst (N80.1)
follicular (atretic) cyst (N83.0)
graafian follicle cyst (N83.0)
ovarian cyst NEC (N83.2)
ovarian retention cyst (N83.2)
D27.0 Benign neoplasm of right ovary
D27.1 Benign neoplasm of left ovary
D27.9 Benign neoplasm of unspecified ovary
D28 Benign neoplasm of other and unspecified female genital organs
Includes: adenomatous polyp
benign neoplasm of skin of female genital organs
benign teratoma
Excludes 1: epoophoron cyst (Q50.5)
fimbrial cyst (Q50.4)
Gartner's duct cyst (Q52.4)
parovarian cyst (Q50.5)
D28.0 Benign neoplasm of vulva
D28.1 Benign neoplasm of vagina
D28.2 Benign neoplasm of uterine tubes and ligaments
Benign neoplasm of fallopian tube
Benign neoplasm of uterine ligament (broad) (round)
D28.7 Benign neoplasm of other specified female genital organs
D28.9 Benign neoplasm of female genital organ, unspecified
D29 Benign neoplasm of male genital organs
Includes: benign neoplasm of skin of male genital organs
D29.0 Benign neoplasm of penis
D29.1 Benign neoplasm of prostate
Excludes 1: enlarged prostate (N40.-)
D29.2 Benign neoplasm of testis
Use additional code to identify any functional activity.
D29.20 Benign neoplasm of unspecified testis
D29.21 Benign neoplasm of right testis
D29.22 Benign neoplasm of left testis
D29.3 Benign neoplasm of epididymis
D29.30 Benign neoplasm of unspecified epididymis
D29.31 Benign neoplasm of right epididymis
D29.32 Benign neoplasm of left epididymis
D29.4 Benign neoplasm of scrotum
Benign neoplasm of skin of scrotum
D29.8 Benign neoplasm of other specified male genital organs
Benign neoplasm of seminal vesicle
Benign neoplasm of spermatic cord
Benign neoplasm of tunica vaginalis
D29.9 Benign neoplasm of male genital organ, unspecified
D30 Benign neoplasm of urinary organs
D30.0 Benign neoplasm of kidney
Excludes 1: benign carcinoid tumor of the kidney (D3A.093)
benign neoplasm of renal calyces (D30.1-)

benign neoplasm of renal pelvis (D30.1-)
D30.00 Benign neoplasm of unspecified kidney
D30.01 Benign neoplasm of right kidney
D30.02 Benign neoplasm of left kidney
D30.1 Benign neoplasm of renal pelvis
D30.10 Benign neoplasm of unspecified renal pelvis
D30.11 Benign neoplasm of right renal pelvis
D30.12 Benign neoplasm of left renal pelvis
D30.2 Benign neoplasm of ureter
Excludes 1: benign neoplasm of ureteric orifice of bladder (D30.3)
D30.20 Benign neoplasm of unspecified ureter
D30.21 Benign neoplasm of right ureter
D30.22 Benign neoplasm of left ureter
D30.3 Benign neoplasm of bladder
Benign neoplasm of ureteric orifice of bladder
Benign neoplasm of urethral orifice of bladder
D30.4 Benign neoplasm of urethra
Excludes 1: benign neoplasm of urethral orifice of bladder (D30.3)
D30.8 Benign neoplasm of other specified urinary organs
Benign neoplasm of paraurethral glands
D30.9 Benign neoplasm of urinary organ, unspecified
Benign neoplasm of urinary system NOS
D31 Benign neoplasm of eye and adnexa
Excludes 1: benign neoplasm of connective tissue of eyelid (D21.0)
benign neoplasm of optic nerve (D33.3)
benign neoplasm of skin of eyelid (D22.1-, D23.1-)
D31.0 Benign neoplasm of conjunctiva
D31.00 Benign neoplasm of unspecified conjunctiva
D31.01 Benign neoplasm of right conjunctiva
D31.02 Benign neoplasm of left conjunctiva
D31.1 Benign neoplasm of cornea
D31.10 Benign neoplasm of unspecified cornea
D31.11 Benign neoplasm of right cornea
D31.12 Benign neoplasm of left cornea
D31.2 Benign neoplasm of retina
Excludes 1: dark area on retina (D49.81)
hemangioma of retina (D49.81)
neoplasm of unspecified behavior of retina and choroid (D49.81)
retinal freckle (D49.81)
D31.20 Benign neoplasm of unspecified retina
D31.21 Benign neoplasm of right retina
D31.22 Benign neoplasm of left retina
D31.3 Benign neoplasm of choroid
D31.30 Benign neoplasm of unspecified choroid
D31.31 Benign neoplasm of right choroid
D31.32 Benign neoplasm of left choroid
D31.4 Benign neoplasm of ciliary body
D31.40 Benign neoplasm of unspecified ciliary body
D31.41 Benign neoplasm of right ciliary body
D31.42 Benign neoplasm of left ciliary body
D31.5 Benign neoplasm of lacrimal gland and duct
Benign neoplasm of lacrimal sac
Benign neoplasm of nasolacrimal duct
D31.50 Benign neoplasm of unspecified lacrimal gland and duct
D31.51 Benign neoplasm of right lacrimal gland and duct
D31.52 Benign neoplasm of left lacrimal gland and duct

● New code ▲ Revised code ⑦ 7ᵗʰ digit required ⊗ Placeholder required

D31.6 Benign neoplasm of unspecified site of orbit
Benign neoplasm of connective tissue of orbit
Benign neoplasm of extraocular muscle
Benign neoplasm of peripheral nerves of orbit
Benign neoplasm of retrobulbar tissue
Benign neoplasm of retro-ocular tissue
Excludes 1: benign neoplasm of orbital bone (D16.4)

    D31.60 Benign neoplasm of unspecified site of unspecified orbit

    D31.61 Benign neoplasm of unspecified site of right orbit

    D31.62 Benign neoplasm of unspecified site of left orbit

D31.9 Benign neoplasm of unspecified part of eye
Benign neoplasm of eyeball

    D31.90 Benign neoplasm of unspecified part of unspecified eye

    D31.91 Benign neoplasm of unspecified part of right eye

    D31.92 Benign neoplasm of unspecified part of left eye

D32 Benign neoplasm of meninges

D32.0 Benign neoplasm of cerebral meninges

D32.1 Benign neoplasm of spinal meninges

D32.9 Benign neoplasm of meninges, unspecified
Meningioma NOS

D33 Benign neoplasm of brain and other parts of central nervous system
Excludes 1: angioma (D18.0-)
    benign neoplasm of meninges (D32.-)
    benign neoplasm of peripheral nerves and autonomic nervous system (D36.1-)
    hemangioma (D18.0-)
    neurofibromatosis (Q85.0-)
    retro-ocular benign neoplasm (D31.6-)

D33.0 Benign neoplasm of brain, supratentorial
Benign neoplasm of cerebral ventricle
Benign neoplasm of cerebrum
Benign neoplasm of frontal lobe
Benign neoplasm of occipital lobe
Benign neoplasm of parietal lobe
Benign neoplasm of temporal lobe
Excludes 1: benign neoplasm of fourth ventricle (D33.1)

D33.1 Benign neoplasm of brain, infratentorial
Benign neoplasm of brain stem
Benign neoplasm of cerebellum
Benign neoplasm of fourth ventricle

D33.2 Benign neoplasm of brain, unspecified

D33.3 Benign neoplasm of cranial nerves
Benign neoplasm of olfactory bulb

D33.4 Benign neoplasm of spinal cord

D33.7 Benign neoplasm of other specified parts of central nervous system

D33.9 Benign neoplasm of central nervous system, unspecified
Benign neoplasm of nervous system (central) NOS

D34 Benign neoplasm of thyroid gland
Use additional code to identify any functional activity

D35 Benign neoplasm of other and unspecified endocrine glands
Use additional code to identify any functional activity
Excludes 1: benign neoplasm of endocrine pancreas (D13.7)
    benign neoplasm of ovary (D27.-)
    benign neoplasm of testis (D29.2.-)
    benign neoplasm of thymus (D15.0)

D35.0 Benign neoplasm of adrenal gland

    D35.00 Benign neoplasm of unspecified adrenal gland

    D35.01 Benign neoplasm of right adrenal gland

    D35.02 Benign neoplasm of left adrenal gland

D35.1 Benign neoplasm of parathyroid gland

D35.2 Benign neoplasm of pituitary gland

D35.3 Benign neoplasm of craniopharyngeal duct

D35.4 Benign neoplasm of pineal gland

D35.5 Benign neoplasm of carotid body

D35.6 Benign neoplasm of aortic body and other paraganglia
Benign tumor of glomus jugulare

D35.7 Benign neoplasm of other specified endocrine glands

D35.9 Benign neoplasm of endocrine gland, unspecified
Benign neoplasm of unspecified endocrine gland

D36 Benign neoplasm of other and unspecified sites

D36.0 Benign neoplasm of lymph nodes
Excludes 1: lymphangioma (D18.1)

D36.1 Benign neoplasm of peripheral nerves and autonomic nervous system
Excludes 1: benign neoplasm of peripheral nerves of orbit (D31.6-)
    neurofibromatosis (Q85.0-)

    D36.10 Benign neoplasm of peripheral nerves and autonomic nervous system, unspecified

    D36.11 Benign neoplasm of peripheral nerves and autonomic nervous system of face, head, and neck

    D36.12 Benign neoplasm of peripheral nerves and autonomic nervous system, upper limb, including shoulder

    D36.13 Benign neoplasm of peripheral nerves and autonomic nervous system of lower limb, including hip

    D36.14 Benign neoplasm of peripheral nerves and autonomic nervous system of thorax

    D36.15 Benign neoplasm of peripheral nerves and autonomic nervous system of abdomen

    D36.16 Benign neoplasm of peripheral nerves and autonomic nervous system of pelvis

    D36.17 Benign neoplasm of peripheral nerves and autonomic nervous system of trunk, unspecified

D36.7 Benign neoplasm of other specified sites
Benign neoplasm of nose NOS

D36.9 Benign neoplasm, unspecified site

BENIGN NEUROENDOCRINE TUMORS (D3A)

D3A Benign neuroendocrine tumors
Code also any associated multiple endocrine neoplasia [MEN] syndromes (E31.2-)
Use additional code to identify any associated endocrine syndrome, such as:
carcinoid syndrome (E34.0)
Excludes 2: benign pancreatic islet cell tumors (D13.7)

D3A.0 Benign carcinoid tumors

    D3A.00 Benign carcinoid tumor of unspecified site
Carcinoid tumor NOS

    D3A.01 Benign carcinoid tumors of the small intestine

        D3A.010 Benign carcinoid tumor of the duodenum

        D3A.011 Benign carcinoid tumor of the jejunum

        D3A.012 Benign carcinoid tumor of the ileum

        D3A.019 Benign carcinoid tumor of the small intestine, unspecified portion

    D3A.02 Benign carcinoid tumors of the appendix, large intestine, and rectum

D3A.020   Benign carcinoid tumor of the appendix
D3A.021   Benign carcinoid tumor of the cecum
D3A.022   Benign carcinoid tumor of the ascending colon
D3A.023   Benign carcinoid tumor of the transverse colon
D3A.024   Benign carcinoid tumor of the descending colon
D3A.025   Benign carcinoid tumor of the sigmoid colon
D3A.026   Benign carcinoid tumor of the rectum
D3A.029   Benign carcinoid tumor of the large intestine, unspecified portion
           Benign carcinoid tumor of the colon NOS

D3A.09   Benign carcinoid tumors of other sites
D3A.090   Benign carcinoid tumor of the bronchus and lung
D3A.091   Benign carcinoid tumor of the thymus
D3A.092   Benign carcinoid tumor of the stomach
D3A.093   Benign carcinoid tumor of the kidney
D3A.094   Benign carcinoid tumor of the foregut NOS
D3A.095   Benign carcinoid tumor of the midgut NOS
D3A.096   Benign carcinoid tumor of the hindgut NOS
D3A.098   Benign carcinoid tumors of other sites

D3A.8   Other benign neuroendocrine tumors
         Neuroendocrine tumor NOS

NEOPLASMS OF UNCERTAIN BEHAVIOR, POLYCYTHEMIA VERA AND MYELODYSPLASTIC SYNDROMES (D37-D48)

Note: Categories D37-D44, and D48 classify by site neoplasms of uncertain behavior, i.e., histologic confirmation whether the neoplasm is malignant or benign cannot be made.

Excludes 1: neoplasms of unspecified behavior (D49-)

D37   Neoplasm of uncertain behavior of oral cavity and digestive organs
       Excludes 1: stromal tumors of uncertain behavior of digestive system (D48.1)

D37.0   Neoplasm of uncertain behavior of lip, oral cavity and pharynx
         Excludes 1: neoplasm of uncertain behavior of aryepiglottic fold or interarytenoid fold, laryngeal aspect (D38.0)
                     neoplasm of uncertain behavior of epiglottis NOS (D38.0)
                     neoplasm of uncertain behavior of skin of lip (D48.5)
                     neoplasm of uncertain behavior of suprahyoid portion of epiglottis (D38.0)
D37.01   Neoplasm of uncertain behavior of lip
          Neoplasm of uncertain behavior of vermilion border of lip
D37.02   Neoplasm of uncertain behavior of tongue
D37.03   Neoplasm of uncertain behavior of the major salivary glands
D37.030   Neoplasm of uncertain behavior of the parotid salivary glands
D37.031   Neoplasm of uncertain behavior of the sublingual salivary glands

D37.032   Neoplasm of uncertain behavior of the submandibular salivary glands
D37.039   Neoplasm of uncertain behavior of the major salivary glands, unspecified
D37.04   Neoplasm of uncertain behavior of the minor salivary glands
          Neoplasm of uncertain behavior of submucosal salivary glands of lip
          Neoplasm of uncertain behavior of submucosal salivary glands of cheek
          Neoplasm of uncertain behavior of submucosal salivary glands of hard palate
          Neoplasm of uncertain behavior of submucosal salivary glands of soft palate
D37.05   Neoplasm of uncertain behavior of pharynx
          Neoplasm of uncertain behavior of aryepiglottic fold of pharynx NOS
          Neoplasm of uncertain behavior of hypopharyngeal aspect of aryepiglottic fold of pharynx
          Neoplasm of uncertain behavior of marginal zone of aryepiglottic fold of pharynx
D37.09   Neoplasm of uncertain behavior of other specified sites of the oral cavity

D37.1   Neoplasm of uncertain behavior of stomach
D37.2   Neoplasm of uncertain behavior of small intestine
D37.3   Neoplasm of uncertain behavior of appendix
D37.4   Neoplasm of uncertain behavior of colon
D37.5   Neoplasm of uncertain behavior of rectum
         Neoplasm of uncertain behavior of rectosigmoid junction
D37.6   Neoplasm of uncertain behavior of liver, gallbladder and bile ducts
         Neoplasm of uncertain behavior of ampulla of Vater
D37.8   Neoplasm of uncertain behavior of other specified digestive organs
         Neoplasm of uncertain behavior of anal canal
         Neoplasm of uncertain behavior of anal sphincter
         Neoplasm of uncertain behavior of anus NOS
         Neoplasm of uncertain behavior of esophagus
         Neoplasm of uncertain behavior of intestine NOS
         Neoplasm of uncertain behavior of pancreas
         Excludes 1: neoplasm of uncertain behavior of anal margin (D48.5)
                     neoplasm of uncertain behavior of anal skin (D48.5)
                     neoplasm of uncertain behavior of perianal skin (D48.5)
D37.9   Neoplasm of uncertain behavior of digestive organ, unspecified

D38   Neoplasm of uncertain behavior of middle ear and respiratory and intrathoracic organs
       Excludes 1: neoplasm of uncertain behavior of heart (D48.7)
D38.0   Neoplasm of uncertain behavior of larynx
         Neoplasm of uncertain behavior of aryepiglottic fold or interarytenoid fold, laryngeal aspect
         Neoplasm of uncertain behavior of epiglottis (suprahyoid portion)
         Excludes 1: neoplasm of uncertain behavior of aryepiglottic fold or interarytenoid fold NOS (D37.05)
                     neoplasm of uncertain behavior of hypopharyngeal aspect of aryepiglottic fold (D37.05)

neoplasm of uncertain behavior of marginal zone of aryepiglottic fold (D37.05)

D38.1 Neoplasm of uncertain behavior of trachea, bronchus and lung

D38.2 Neoplasm of uncertain behavior of pleura

D38.3 Neoplasm of uncertain behavior of mediastinum

D38.4 Neoplasm of uncertain behavior of thymus

D38.5 Neoplasm of uncertain behavior of other respiratory organs

Neoplasm of uncertain behavior of accessory sinuses

Neoplasm of uncertain behavior of cartilage of nose

Neoplasm of uncertain behavior of middle ear

Neoplasm of uncertain behavior of nasal cavities

Excludes 1: neoplasm of uncertain behavior of ear (external) (skin) (D48.5)

neoplasm of uncertain behavior of nose NOS (D48.7)

neoplasm of uncertain behavior of skin of nose (D48.5)

D38.6 Neoplasm of uncertain behavior of respiratory organ, unspecified

D39 Neoplasm of uncertain behavior of female genital organs

D39.0 Neoplasm of uncertain behavior of uterus

D39.1 Neoplasm of uncertain behavior of ovary

Use additional code to identify any functional activity.

D39.10 Neoplasm of uncertain behavior of unspecified ovary

D39.11 Neoplasm of uncertain behavior of right ovary

D39.12 Neoplasm of uncertain behavior of left ovary

D39.2 Neoplasm of uncertain behavior of placenta

Chorioadenoma destruens

Invasive hydatidiform mole

Malignant hydatidiform mole

Excludes 1: hydatidiform mole NOS (O01.9)

D39.8 Neoplasm of uncertain behavior of other specified female genital organs

Neoplasm of uncertain behavior of skin of female genital organs

D39.9 Neoplasm of uncertain behavior of female genital organ, unspecified

D40 Neoplasm of uncertain behavior of male genital organs

D40.0 Neoplasm of uncertain behavior of prostate

D40.1 Neoplasm of uncertain behavior of testis

D40.10 Neoplasm of uncertain behavior of unspecified testis

D40.11 Neoplasm of uncertain behavior of right testis

D40.12 Neoplasm of uncertain behavior of left testis

D40.8 Neoplasm of uncertain behavior of other specified male genital organs

Neoplasm of uncertain behavior of skin of male genital organs

D40.9 Neoplasm of uncertain behavior of male genital organ, unspecified

D41 Neoplasm of uncertain behavior of urinary organs

D41.0 Neoplasm of uncertain behavior of kidney

Excludes 1: neoplasm of uncertain behavior of renal pelvis (D41.1-)

D41.00 Neoplasm of uncertain behavior of unspecified kidney

D41.01 Neoplasm of uncertain behavior of right kidney

D41.02 Neoplasm of uncertain behavior of left kidney

D41.1 Neoplasm of uncertain behavior of renal pelvis

D41.10 Neoplasm of uncertain behavior of unspecified renal pelvis

D41.11 Neoplasm of uncertain behavior of right renal pelvis

D41.12 Neoplasm of uncertain behavior of left renal pelvis

D41.2 Neoplasm of uncertain behavior of ureter

D41.20 Neoplasm of uncertain behavior of unspecified ureter

D41.21 Neoplasm of uncertain behavior of right ureter

D41.22 Neoplasm of uncertain behavior of left ureter

D41.3 Neoplasm of uncertain behavior of urethra

D41.4 Neoplasm of uncertain behavior of bladder

D41.8 Neoplasm of uncertain behavior of other specified urinary organs

D41.9 Neoplasm of uncertain behavior of unspecified urinary organ

D42 Neoplasm of uncertain behavior of meninges

D42.0 Neoplasm of uncertain behavior of cerebral meninges

D42.1 Neoplasm of uncertain behavior of spinal meninges

D42.9 Neoplasm of uncertain behavior of meninges, unspecified

D43 Neoplasm of uncertain behavior of brain and central nervous system

Excludes 1: neoplasm of uncertain behavior of peripheral nerves and autonomic nervous system (D48.2)

D43.0 Neoplasm of uncertain behavior of brain, supratentorial

Neoplasm of uncertain behavior of cerebral ventricle

Neoplasm of uncertain behavior of cerebrum

Neoplasm of uncertain behavior of frontal lobe

Neoplasm of uncertain behavior of occipital lobe

Neoplasm of uncertain behavior of parietal lobe

Neoplasm of uncertain behavior of temporal lobe

Excludes 1: neoplasm of uncertain behavior of fourth ventricle (D43.1)

D43.1 Neoplasm of uncertain behavior of brain, infratentorial

Neoplasm of uncertain behavior of brain stem

Neoplasm of uncertain behavior of cerebellum

Neoplasm of uncertain behavior of fourth ventricle

D43.2 Neoplasm of uncertain behavior of brain, unspecified

D43.4 Neoplasm of uncertain behavior of spinal cord

D43.8 Neoplasm of uncertain behavior of other specified parts of central nervous system

D43.9 Neoplasm of uncertain behavior of central nervous system, unspecified

Neoplasm of uncertain behavior of nervous system (central) NOS

D44 Neoplasm of uncertain behavior of endocrine glands

Excludes 1: multiple endocrine adenomatosis (E31.2-)

multiple endocrine neoplasia (E31.2-)

neoplasm of uncertain behavior of endocrine pancreas (D37.8)

neoplasm of uncertain behavior of ovary (D39.1-)

neoplasm of uncertain behavior of testis (D40.1-)

neoplasm of uncertain behavior of thymus (D38.4)

D44.0 Neoplasm of uncertain behavior of thyroid gland

D44.1 Neoplasm of uncertain behavior of adrenal gland

Use additional code to identify any functional activity.

D44.10 Neoplasm of uncertain behavior of unspecified adrenal gland

D44.11 Neoplasm of uncertain behavior of right adrenal gland

D44.12 Neoplasm of uncertain behavior of left adrenal gland

D44.2 Neoplasm of uncertain behavior of parathyroid gland

D44.3 Neoplasm of uncertain behavior of pituitary gland

Use additional code to identify any functional activity.

D44.4 Neoplasm of uncertain behavior of craniopharyngeal duct

D44.5 Neoplasm of uncertain behavior of pineal gland

D44.6 Neoplasm of uncertain behavior of carotid body

D44.7 Neoplasm of uncertain behavior of aortic body and other paraganglia

D44.9 Neoplasm of uncertain behavior of unspecified endocrine gland

D45 Polycythemia vera

Excludes 1: familial polycythemia (D75.0)
secondary polycythemia (D75.1)

D46 Myelodysplastic syndromes

Use additional code for adverse effect, if applicable, to identify drug (T36-T50 with fifth or sixth character 5)

Excludes 2: drug-induced aplastic anemia (D61.1)

D46.0 Refractory anemia without ring sideroblasts, so stated
Refractory anemia without sideroblasts, without excess of blasts

D46.1 Refractory anemia with ring sideroblasts
RARS

D46.2 Refractory anemia with excess of blasts

    D46.20 Refractory anemia with excess of blasts, unspecified
RAEB NOS

    D46.21 Refractory anemia with excess of blasts 1
RAEB 1

    D46.22 Refractory anemia with excess of blasts 2
RAEB 2

D46.A Refractory cytopenia with multilineage dysplasia

D46.B Refractory cytopenia with multilineage dysplasia and ring sideroblasts
RCMD RS

D46.C Myelodysplastic syndrome with isolated del(5q) chromosomal abnormality
Myelodysplastic syndrome with 5q deletion
5q minus syndrome NOS

D46.4 Refractory anemia, unspecified

D46.Z Other myelodysplastic syndromes

Excludes 1: chronic myelomonocytic leukemia (C93.1-)

D46.9 Myelodysplastic syndrome, unspecified
Myelodysplasia NOS

D47 Other neoplasms of uncertain behavior of lymphoid, hematopoietic and related tissue

D47.0 Histiocytic and mast cell tumors of uncertain behavior
Indolent systemic mastocytosis
Mast cell tumor NOS
Mastocytoma NOS

Excludes 1: malignant mast cell tumor (C96.2)
mastocytosis (congenital) (cutaneous) (Q82.2)

D47.1 Chronic myeloproliferative disease
Chronic neutrophilic leukemia
Myeloproliferative disease, unspecified

Excludes 1: atypical chronic myeloid leukemia BCR/ABL-negative (C92.2-)
chronic myeloid leukemia BCR/ABL-positive (C92.1-)
myelofibrosis NOS (D75.81)
myelophthisic anemia (D61.82)
myelophthisis (D61.82)
secondary myelofibrosis NOS (D75.81)

D47.2 Monoclonal gammopathy

Monoclonal gammopathy of undetermined significance [MGUS]

D47.3 Essential (hemorrhagic) thrombocythemia
Essential thrombocytosis
Idiopathic hemorrhagic thrombocythemia

D47.4 Osteomyelofibrosis
Chronic idiopathic myelofibrosis
Myelofibrosis (idiopathic) (with myeloid metaplasia)
Myelosclerosis (megakaryocytic) with myeloid metaplasia
Secondary myelofibrosis in myeloproliferative disease

Excludes 1: acute myelofibrosis (C94.4-)

D47.Z Other specified neoplasms of uncertain behavior of lymphoid, hematopoietic and related tissue

    D47.Z1 Post-transplant lymphoproliferative disorder (PTLD)

    Code first complications of transplanted organs and tissue (T86.-)

    D47.Z9 Other specified neoplasms of uncertain behavior of lymphoid, hematopoietic and related tissue
Histiocytic tumors of uncertain behavior

D47.9 Neoplasm of uncertain behavior of lymphoid, hematopoietic and related tissue, unspecified
Lymphoproliferative disease NOS

D48 Neoplasm of uncertain behavior of other and unspecified sites

Excludes 1: neurofibromatosis (nonmalignant) (Q85.0-)

D48.0 Neoplasm of uncertain behavior of bone and articular cartilage

Excludes 1: neoplasm of uncertain behavior of cartilage of ear (D48.1)
neoplasm of uncertain behavior of cartilage of larynx (D38.0)
neoplasm of uncertain behavior of cartilage of nose (D38.5)
neoplasm of uncertain behavior of connective tissue of eyelid (D48.1)
neoplasm of uncertain behavior of synovia (D48.1)

D48.1 Neoplasm of uncertain behavior of connective and other soft tissue
Neoplasm of uncertain behavior of connective tissue of ear
Neoplasm of uncertain behavior of connective tissue of eyelid
Stromal tumors of uncertain behavior of digestive system

Excludes 1: neoplasm of uncertain behavior of articular cartilage (D48.0)
neoplasm of uncertain behavior of cartilage of larynx (D38.0)
neoplasm of uncertain behavior of cartilage of nose (D38.5)
neoplasm of uncertain behavior of connective tissue of breast (D48.6-)

D48.2 Neoplasm of uncertain behavior of peripheral nerves and autonomic nervous system

Excludes 1: neoplasm of uncertain behavior of peripheral nerves of orbit (D48.7)

D48.3 Neoplasm of uncertain behavior of retroperitoneum

D48.4 Neoplasm of uncertain behavior of peritoneum

D48.5 Neoplasm of uncertain behavior of skin
Neoplasm of uncertain behavior of anal margin
Neoplasm of uncertain behavior of anal skin
Neoplasm of uncertain behavior of perianal skin
Neoplasm of uncertain behavior of skin of breast

Excludes 1: neoplasm of uncertain behavior of anus NOS (D37.8)

    ● New code   ▲ Revised code   ⑦ 7th digit required   ⊗ Placeholder required

neoplasm of uncertain behavior of skin of genital organs (D39.8, D40.7)

neoplasm of uncertain behavior of vermilion border of lip (D37.0)

D48.6 Neoplasm of uncertain behavior of breast

Neoplasm of uncertain behavior of connective tissue of breast

Cystosarcoma phyllodes

Excludes 1: neoplasm of uncertain behavior of skin of breast (D48.5)

D48.60 Neoplasm of uncertain behavior of unspecified breast

D48.61 Neoplasm of uncertain behavior of right breast

D48.62 Neoplasm of uncertain behavior of left breast

D48.7 Neoplasm of uncertain behavior of other specified sites

Neoplasm of uncertain behavior of eye

Neoplasm of uncertain behavior of heart

Neoplasm of uncertain behavior of peripheral nerves of orbit

Excludes 1: neoplasm of uncertain behavior of connective tissue (D48.1)

neoplasm of uncertain behavior of skin of eyelid (D48.5)

D48.9 Neoplasm of uncertain behavior, unspecified

NEOPLASMS OF UNSPECIFIED BEHAVIOR (D49)

D49 Neoplasms of unspecified behavior

Note: Category D49 classifies by site neoplasms of unspecified morphology and behavior. The term 'mass', unless otherwise stated, is not to be regarded as a neoplastic growth.

Includes: 'growth' NOS

neoplasm NOS

new growth NOS

tumor NOS

Excludes 1: neoplasms of uncertain behavior (D37-D44, D48)

D49.0 Neoplasm of unspecified behavior of digestive system

Excludes 1: neoplasm of unspecified behavior of margin of anus (D49.2)

neoplasm of unspecified behavior of perianal skin (D49.2)

neoplasm of unspecified behavior of skin of anus (D49.2)

D49.1 Neoplasm of unspecified behavior of respiratory system

D49.2 Neoplasm of unspecified behavior of bone, soft tissue, and skin

Excludes 1: neoplasm of unspecified behavior of anal canal (D49.0)

neoplasm of unspecified behavior of anus NOS (D49.0)

neoplasm of unspecified behavior of bone marrow (D49.9)

neoplasm of unspecified behavior of cartilage of larynx (D49.1)

neoplasm of unspecified behavior of cartilage of nose (D49.1)

neoplasm of unspecified behavior of connective tissue of breast (D49.3)

neoplasm of unspecified behavior of skin of genital organs (D49.5)

neoplasm of unspecified behavior of vermilion border of lip (D49.0)

D49.3 Neoplasm of unspecified behavior of breast

Excludes 1: neoplasm of unspecified behavior of skin of breast (D49.2)

D49.4 Neoplasm of unspecified behavior of bladder

D49.5 Neoplasm of unspecified behavior of other genitourinary organs

D49.6 Neoplasm of unspecified behavior of brain

Excludes 1: neoplasm of unspecified behavior of cerebral meninges (D49.7)

neoplasm of unspecified behavior of cranial nerves (D49.7)

D49.7 Neoplasm of unspecified behavior of endocrine glands and other parts of nervous system

Excludes 1: neoplasm of unspecified behavior of peripheral, sympathetic, and parasympathetic nerves and ganglia (D49.2)

D49.8 Neoplasm of unspecified behavior of other specified sites

Excludes 1: neoplasm of unspecified behavior of eyelid (skin) (D49.2)

neoplasm of unspecified behavior of eyelid cartilage (D49.2)

neoplasm of unspecified behavior of great vessels (D49.2)

neoplasm of unspecified behavior of optic nerve (D49.7)

D49.81 Neoplasm of unspecified behavior of retina and choroid

Dark area on retina

Retinal freckle

D49.89 Neoplasm of unspecified behavior of other specified sites

D49.9 Neoplasm of unspecified behavior of unspecified site

● New code   ▲ Revised code   ⑦ 7th digit required   ⊗ Placeholder required

Chapter 3: Diseases Of The Blood And Blood-Forming Organs and Certain Disorders Involving The Immune Mechanism (D50-D89)

Excludes 2: autoimmune disease (systemic) NOS (M35.9)

certain conditions originating in the perinatal period (P00-P96)

complications of pregnancy, childbirth and the puerperium (O00-O9A)

congenital malformations, deformations and chromosomal abnormalities (Q00-Q99)

endocrine, nutritional and metabolic diseases (E00-E88)

human immunodeficiency virus [HIV] disease (B20)

injury, poisoning and certain other consequences of external causes (S00-T88)

neoplasms (C00-D49)

symptoms, signs and abnormal clinical and laboratory findings, not elsewhere classified (R00-R94)

This chapter contains the following blocks:

D50-D53	Nutritional anemias
D55-D59	Hemolytic anemias
D60-D64	Aplastic and other anemias and other bone marrow failure syndromes
D65-D69	Coagulation defects, purpura and other hemorrhagic conditions
D70-D77	Other disorders of blood and blood-forming organs
D78	Intraoperative and postprocedural complications of the spleen
D80-D89	Certain disorders involving the immune mechanism

NUTRITIONAL ANEMIAS (D50-D53)

 Iron deficiency anemia

Includes: asiderotic anemia

hypochromic anemia

D50.0 Iron deficiency anemia secondary to blood loss (chronic)

Posthemorrhagic anemia (chronic)

Excludes 1: acute posthemorrhagic anemia (D62)

congenital anemia from fetal blood loss (P61.3)

D50.1 Sideropenic dysphagia

Kelly-Paterson syndrome

Plummer-Vinson syndrome

D50.8 Other iron deficiency anemias

Iron deficiency anemia due to inadequate dietary iron intake

D50.9 Iron deficiency anemia, unspecified

D51 Vitamin B12 deficiency anemia

Excludes 1: vitamin B12 deficiency (E53.8)

D51.0 Vitamin B12 deficiency anemia due to intrinsic factor deficiency

Addison anemia

Biermer anemia

Pernicious (congenital) anemia

Congenital intrinsic factor deficiency

D51.1 Vitamin B12 deficiency anemia due to selective vitamin B12 malabsorption with proteinuria

Imerslund (GrΣsbeck) syndrome

Megaloblastic hereditary anemia

D51.2 Transcobalamin II deficiency

D51.3 Other dietary vitamin B12 deficiency anemia

Vegan anemia

D51.8 Other vitamin B12 deficiency anemias

D51.9 Vitamin B12 deficiency anemia, unspecified

D52 Folate deficiency anemia

Excludes 1: folate deficiency without anemia (E53.8)

D52.0 Dietary folate deficiency anemia

Nutritional megaloblastic anemia

D52.1 Drug-induced folate deficiency anemia

Use additional code for adverse effect, if applicable, to identify drug (T36-T50 with fifth or sixth character 5)

D52.8 Other folate deficiency anemias

D52.9 Folate deficiency anemia, unspecified

Folic acid deficiency anemia NOS

D53 Other nutritional anemias

Includes: megaloblastic anemia unresponsive to vitamin B12 or folate therapy

D53.0 Protein deficiency anemia

Amino-acid deficiency anemia

Orotaciduric anemia

Excludes 1: Lesch-Nyhan syndrome (E79.1)

D53.1 Other megaloblastic anemias, not elsewhere classified

Megaloblastic anemia NOS

Excludes 1: Di Guglielmo's disease (C94.0)

D53.2 Scorbutic anemia

Excludes 1: scurvy (E54)

D53.8 Other specified nutritional anemias

Anemia associated with deficiency of copper

Anemia associated with deficiency of molybdenum

Anemia associated with deficiency of zinc

Excludes 1: nutritional deficiencies without anemia, such as:

copper deficiency NOS (E61.0)

molybdenum deficiency NOS (E61.5)

zinc deficiency NOS (E60)

D53.9 Nutritional anemia, unspecified

Simple chronic anemia

Excludes 1: anemia NOS (D64.9)

HEMOLYTIC ANEMIAS (D55-D59)

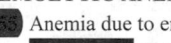 Anemia due to enzyme disorders

Excludes 1: drug-induced enzyme deficiency anemia (D59.2)

D55.0 Anemia due to glucose-6-phosphate dehydrogenase [G6PD] deficiency

Favism

G6PD deficiency anemia

D55.1 Anemia due to other disorders of glutathione metabolism

Anemia (due to) enzyme deficiencies, except G6PD, related to the hexose monophosphate [HMP] shunt pathway

Anemia (due to) hemolytic nonspherocytic (hereditary), type I

D55.2 Anemia due to disorders of glycolytic enzymes

Hemolytic nonspherocytic (hereditary) anemia, type II

Hexokinase deficiency anemia

Pyruvate kinase [PK] deficiency anemia

Triose-phosphate isomerase deficiency anemia

Excludes 1: disorders of glycolysis not associated with anemia (E74.8)

D55.3 Anemia due to disorders of nucleotide metabolism

D55.8 Other anemias due to enzyme disorders

D55.9 Anemia due to enzyme disorder, unspecified

D56 Thalassemia

Excludes 1: sickle-cell thalassemia (D57.4-)

D56.0 Alpha thalassemia

Alpha thalassemia major

Hemoglobin H Constant Spring

Hemoglobin H disease

Hydrops fetalis due to alpha thalassemia

Severe alpha thalassemia

Triple gene defect alpha thalassemia

Use additional code, if applicable, for hydrops fetalis due to alpha thalassemia (P56.99)

> **Excludes 1:** alpha thalassemia trait or minor (D56.3)
>
> asymptomatic alpha thalassemia (D56.3)
>
> hydrops fetalis due to isoimmunization (P56.0)
>
> hydrops fetalis not due to immune hemolysis (P83.2)

D56.1 Beta thalassemia

Beta thalassemia major

Cooley's anemia

Homozygous beta thalassemia

Severe beta thalassemia

Thalassemia intermedia

Thalassemia major

> **Excludes 1:** beta thalassemia minor (D56.3)
>
> beta thalassemia trait (D56.3)
>
> delta-beta thalassemia (D56.2)
>
> hemoglobin E-beta thalassemia (D56.5)
>
> sickle-cell beta thalassemia (D57.4-)

D56.2 Delta-beta thalassemia

Homozygous delta-beta thalassemia

> **Excludes 1:** delta-beta thalassemia minor (D56.3)
>
> delta-beta thalassemia trait (D56.3)

D56.3 Thalassemia minor

Alpha thalassemia minor

Alpha thalassemia silent carrier

Alpha thalassemia trait

Beta thalassemia minor

Beta thalassemia trait

Delta-beta thalassemia minor

Delta-beta thalassemia trait

Thalassemia trait NOS

> **Excludes 1:** alpha thalassemia (D56.0)
>
> beta thalassemia (D56.1)
>
> delta-beta thalassemia (D56.2)
>
> hemoglobin E-beta thalassemia (D56.5)
>
> sickle-cell trait (D57.3)

D56.4 Hereditary persistence of fetal hemoglobin [HPFH]

D56.5 Hemoglobin E-beta thalassemia

> **Excludes 1:** beta thalassemia (D56.1)
>
> beta thalassemia minor (D56.3)
>
> beta thalassemia trait (D56.3)
>
> delta-beta thalassemia (D56.2)
>
> delta-beta thalassemia trait (D56.3)
>
> hemoglobin E disease (D58.2)
>
> other hemoglobinopathies (D58.2)
>
> sickle-cell beta thalassemia (D57.4-)

D56.8 Other thalassemias

Dominant thalassemia

Hemoglobin C thalassemia

Mixed thalassemia

Thalassemia with other hemoglobinopathy

> **Excludes 1:** hemoglobin C disease (D58.2)
>
> hemoglobin E disease (D58.2)
>
> other hemoglobinopathies (D58.2)

sickle-cell anemia (D57.-)

sickle-cell thalassemia (D57.4)

D56.9 Thalassemia, unspecified

Mediterranean anemia (with other hemoglobinopathy)

D57 Sickle-cell disorders

Use additional code for any associated fever (R50.81)

> **Excludes 1:** other hemoglobinopathies (D58.-)

D57.0 Hb-SS disease with crisis

Sickle-cell disease NOS with crisis

Hb-SS disease with vasoocclusive pain

D57.00 Hb-SS disease with crisis, unspecified

D57.01 Hb-SS disease with acute chest syndrome

D57.02 Hb-SS disease with splenic sequestration

D57.1 Sickle-cell disease without crisis

Hb-SS disease without crisis

Sickle-cell anemia NOS

Sickle-cell disease NOS

Sickle-cell disorder NOS

D57.2 Sickle-cell/Hb-C disease

Hb-SC disease

Hb-S/Hb-C disease

D57.20 Sickle-cell/Hb-C disease without crisis

D57.21 Sickle-cell/Hb-C disease with crisis

D57.211 Sickle-cell/Hb-C disease with acute chest syndrome

D57.212 Sickle-cell/Hb-C disease with splenic sequestration

D57.219 Sickle-cell/Hb-C disease with crisis, unspecified

Sickle-cell/Hb-C disease with crisis NOS

D57.3 Sickle-cell trait

Hb-S trait

Heterozygous hemoglobin S

D57.4 Sickle-cell thalassemia

Sickle-cell beta thalassemia

Thalassemia Hb-S disease

D57.40 Sickle-cell thalassemia without crisis

Microdrepanocytosis

Sickle-cell thalassemia NOS

D57.41 Sickle-cell thalassemia with crisis

Sickle-cell thalassemia with vasoocclusive pain

D57.411 Sickle-cell thalassemia with acute chest syndrome

D57.412 Sickle-cell thalassemia with splenic sequestration

D57.419 Sickle-cell thalassemia with crisis, unspecified

Sickle-cell thalassemia with crisis NOS

D57.8 Other sickle-cell disorders

Hb-SD disease

Hb-SE disease

D57.80 Other sickle-cell disorders without crisis

D57.81 Other sickle-cell disorders with crisis

D57.811 Other sickle-cell disorders with acute chest syndrome

D57.812 Other sickle-cell disorders with splenic sequestration

D57.819 Other sickle-cell disorders with crisis, unspecified

Other sickle-cell disorders with crisis NOS

D58 Other hereditary hemolytic anemias

Excludes 1: hemolytic anemia of the newborn (P55.-)

D58.0 Hereditary spherocytosis

Acholuric (familial) jaundice

Congenital (spherocytic) hemolytic icterus

Minkowski-Chauffard syndrome

D58.1 Hereditary elliptocytosis

Elliptocytosis (congenital)

Ovalocytosis (congenital) (hereditary)

D58.2 Other hemoglobinopathies

Abnormal hemoglobin NOS

Congenital Heinz body anemia

Hb-C disease

Hb-D disease

Hb-E disease

Hemoglobinopathy NOS

Unstable hemoglobin hemolytic disease

Excludes 1: familial polycythemia (D75.0)

Hb-M disease (D74.0)

hemoglobin E-beta thalassemia (D56.5)

hereditary persistence of fetal hemoglobin [HPFH] (D56.4)

high-altitude polycythemia (D75.1)

methemoglobinemia (D74.-)

other hemoglobinopathies with thalassemia (D56.8)

D58.8 Other specified hereditary hemolytic anemias

Stomatocytosis

D58.9 Hereditary hemolytic anemia, unspecified

D59 Acquired hemolytic anemia

D59.0 Drug-induced autoimmune hemolytic anemia

Use additional code for adverse effect, if applicable, to identify drug (T36-T50 with fifth or sixth character 5)

D59.1 Other autoimmune hemolytic anemias

Autoimmune hemolytic disease (cold type) (warm type)

Chronic cold hemagglutinin disease

Cold agglutinin disease

Cold agglutinin hemoglobinuria

Cold type (secondary) (symptomatic) hemolytic anemia

Warm type (secondary) (symptomatic) hemolytic anemia

Excludes 1: Evans syndrome (D69.41)

hemolytic disease of newborn (P55.-)

paroxysmal cold hemoglobinuria (D59.6)

D59.2 Drug-induced nonautoimmune hemolytic anemia

Drug-induced enzyme deficiency anemia

Use additional code for adverse effect, if applicable, to identify drug (T36-T50 with fifth or sixth character 5)

D59.3 Hemolytic-uremic syndrome

Use additional code to identify associated:

E. coli infection (B96.2-)

Pneumococcal pneumonia (J13)

Shigella dysenteriae (A03.9)

D59.4 Other nonautoimmune hemolytic anemias

Mechanical hemolytic anemia

Microangiopathic hemolytic anemia

Toxic hemolytic anemia

D59.5 Paroxysmal nocturnal hemoglobinuria [Marchiafava-Micheli]

Excludes 1: hemoglobinuria NOS (R82.3)

D59.6 Hemoglobinuria due to hemolysis from other external causes

Hemoglobinuria from exertion

March hemoglobinuria

Paroxysmal cold hemoglobinuria

Use additional code (Chapter 20) to identify external cause

Excludes 1: hemoglobinuria NOS (R82.3)

D59.8 Other acquired hemolytic anemias

D59.9 Acquired hemolytic anemia, unspecified

Idiopathic hemolytic anemia, chronic

APLASTIC AND OTHER ANEMIAS AND OTHER BONE MARROW FAILURE SYNDROMES (D60-D64)

D60 Acquired pure red cell aplasia [erythroblastopenia]

Includes: red cell aplasia (acquired) (adult) (with thymoma)

Excludes 1: congenital red cell aplasia (D61.01)

D60.0 Chronic acquired pure red cell aplasia

D60.1 Transient acquired pure red cell aplasia

D60.8 Other acquired pure red cell aplasias

D60.9 Acquired pure red cell aplasia, unspecified

D61 Other aplastic anemias and other bone marrow failure syndromes

Excludes 1: neutropenia (D70.-)

D61.0 Constitutional aplastic anemia

D61.01 Constitutional (pure) red blood cell aplasia

Blackfan-Diamond syndrome

Congenital (pure) red cell aplasia

Familial hypoplastic anemia

Primary (pure) red cell aplasia

Red cell (pure) aplasia of infants

Excludes 1: acquired red cell aplasia (D60.9)

D61.09 Other constitutional aplastic anemia

Fanconi's anemia

Pancytopenia with malformations

D61.1 Drug-induced aplastic anemia

Use additional code for adverse effect, if applicable, to identify drug (T36-T50 with fifth or sixth character 5)

D61.2 Aplastic anemia due to other external agents

Code first, if applicable, toxic effects of substances chiefly nonmedicinal as to source (T51-T65)

D61.3 Idiopathic aplastic anemia

D61.8 Other specified aplastic anemias and other bone marrow failure syndromes

D61.81 Pancytopenia

Excludes 1: pancytopenia (due to) (with) aplastic anemia (D61.9)

pancytopenia (due to) (with) bone marrow infiltration (D61.82)

pancytopenia (due to) (with) congenital (pure) red cell aplasia (D61.01)

pancytopenia (due to) (with) hairy cell leukemia (C91.4-)

pancytopenia (due to) (with) human immunodeficiency virus disease (B20.-)

pancytopenia (due to) (with) leukoerythroblastic anemia (D61.82)

pancytopenia (due to) (with) myelodysplastic syndromes (D46.-)

pancytopenia (due to) (with) myeloproliferative disease (D47.1)

D61.810 Antineoplastic chemotherapy induced pancytopenia

Excludes 2: aplastic anemia due to antineoplastic chemotherapy (D61.1)

D61.811 Other drug-induced pancytopenia

Excludes 2: aplastic anemia due to drugs (D61.1)

D61.818 Other pancytopenia

D61.82 Myelophthisis

Leukoerythroblastic anemia

Myelophthisic anemia

Panmyelophthisis

Code also the underlying disorder, such as:

malignant neoplasm of breast (C50.-)

tuberculosis (A15.-)

Excludes 1: idiopathic myelofibrosis (D47.1)

myelofibrosis NOS (D75.81)

myelofibrosis with myeloid metaplasia (D47.4)

primary myelofibrosis (D47.1)

secondary myelofibrosis (D75.81)

D61.89 Other specified aplastic anemias and other bone marrow failure syndromes

D61.9 Aplastic anemia, unspecified

Hypoplastic anemia NOS

Medullary hypoplasia

D62 Acute posthemorrhagic anemia

Excludes 1: anemia due to chronic blood loss (D50.0)

blood loss anemia NOS (D50.0)

congenital anemia from fetal blood loss (P61.3)

D63 Anemia in chronic diseases classified elsewhere

D63.0 Anemia in neoplastic disease

Code first neoplasm (C00-D49)

Excludes 1: anemia due to antineoplastic chemotherapy (D64.81)

aplastic anemia due to antineoplastic chemotherapy (D61.1)

D63.1 Anemia in chronic kidney disease

Erythropoietin resistant anemia (EPO resistant anemia)

Code first underlying chronic kidney disease (CKD) (N18.-)

D63.8 Anemia in other chronic diseases classified elsewhere

Code first underlying disease, such as:

diphyllobothriasis (B70.0)

hookworm disease (B76.0-B76.9)

hypothyroidism (E00.0-E03.9)

malaria (B50.0-B54)

symptomatic late syphilis (A52.79)

tuberculosis (A18.89)

D64 Other anemias

Excludes 1: refractory anemia (D46.-)

refractory anemia with excess blasts in transformation [RAEB T] (C92.0-)

D64.0 Hereditary sideroblastic anemia

Sex-linked hypochromic sideroblastic anemia

D64.1 Secondary sideroblastic anemia due to disease

Code first underlying disease

D64.2 Secondary sideroblastic anemia due to drugs and toxins

Code first poisoning due to drug or toxin, if applicable (T36-T65 with fifth or sixth character 1-4 or 6)

Use additional code for adverse effect, if applicable, to identify drug (T36-T50 with fifth or sixth character 5)

D64.3 Other sideroblastic anemias

Sideroblastic anemia NOS

Pyridoxine-responsive sideroblastic anemia NEC

D64.4 Congenital dyserythropoietic anemia

Dyshematopoietic anemia (congenital)

Excludes 1: Blackfan-Diamond syndrome (D61.01)

Di Guglielmo's disease (C94.0)

D64.8 Other specified anemias

D64.81 Anemia due to antineoplastic chemotherapy

Antineoplastic chemotherapy induced anemia

Excludes 1: anemia in neoplastic disease (D63.0)

aplastic anemia due to antineoplastic chemotherapy (D61.1)

D64.89 Other specified anemias

Infantile pseudoleukemia

D64.9 Anemia, unspecified

COAGULATION DEFECTS, PURPURA AND OTHER HEMORRHAGIC CONDITIONS (D65-D69)

D65 Disseminated intravascular coagulation [defibrination syndrome]

Afibrinogenemia, acquired

Consumption coagulopathy

Diffuse or disseminated intravascular coagulation [DIC]

Fibrinolytic hemorrhage, acquired

Fibrinolytic purpura

Purpura fulminans

Excludes 1: disseminated intravascular coagulation(complicating):

abortion or ectopic or molar pregnancy (O00-O07, O08.1)

in newborn (P60)

pregnancy, childbirth and the puerperium (O45.0, O46.0, O67.0, O72.3)

D66 Hereditary factor VIII deficiency

Classical hemophilia

Deficiency factor VIII (with functional defect)

Hemophilia NOS

Hemophilia A

Excludes 1: factor VIII deficiency with vascular defect (D68.0)

D67 Hereditary factor IX deficiency

Christmas disease

Factor IX deficiency (with functional defect)

Hemophilia B

Plasma thromboplastin component [PTC] deficiency

D68 Other coagulation defects

Excludes 1: abnormal coagulation profile (R79.1)

coagulation defects complicating:

abortion or ectopic or molar pregnancy (O00-O07, O08.1)

pregnancy, childbirth and the puerperium (O45.0, O46.0, O67.0, O72.3)

D68.0 Von Willebrand's disease

Angiohemophilia

Factor VIII deficiency with vascular defect

Vascular hemophilia

Excludes 1: capillary fragility (hereditary) (D69.8)

factor VIII deficiency NOS (D66)

factor VIII deficiency with functional defect (D66)

D68.1 Hereditary factor XI deficiency

Hemophilia C

Plasma thromboplastin antecedent [PTA] deficiency

Rosenthal's disease

D68.2 Hereditary deficiency of other clotting factors

AC globulin deficiency

Congenital afibrinogenemia
deficiency of factor I [fibrinogen]
deficiency of factor II [prothrombin]
deficiency of factor V [labile]
deficiency of factor VII [stable]
deficiency of factor X [Stuart-Prower]
deficiency of factor XII [Hageman]
deficiency of factor XIII [fibrin stabilizing]
Dysfibrinogenemia (congenital)
Hypoproconvertinemia
Owren's disease
Proaccelerin deficiency

D68.3 Hemorrhagic disorder due to circulating anticoagulants

  D68.31 Hemorrhagic disorder due to intrinsic circulating anticoagulants, antibodies, or inhibitors

    D68.311 Acquired hemophilia
    Autoimmune hemophilia
    Autoimmune inhibitors to clotting factors
    Secondary hemophilia

    D68.312 Antiphospholipid antibody with hemorrhagic disorder
    Lupus anticoagulant (LAC) with hemorrhagic disorder
    Systemic lupus erythematosus [SLE] inhibitor with hemorrhagic disorder

    Excludes 1: antiphospholipid antibody, finding without diagnosis (R76.0)
    antiphospholipid antibody syndrome (D68.61)
    antiphospholipid antibody with hypercoagulable state (D68.61)
    lupus anticoagulant (LAC) finding without diagnosis (R76.0)
    lupus anticoagulant (LAC) with hypercoagulable state (D68.62)
    systemic lupus erythematosus [SLE] inhibitor finding without diagnosis (R76.0)
    systemic lupus erythematosus [SLE] inhibitor with hypercoagulable state (D68.62)

    D68.318 Other hemorrhagic disorder due to intrinsic circulating anticoagulants, antibodies, or inhibitors
    Antithromboplastinemia
    Antithromboplastinogenemia
    Hemorrhagic disorder due to intrinsic increase in antithrombin
    Hemorrhagic disorder due to intrinsic increase in anti-VIIIa
    Hemorrhagic disorder due to intrinsic increase in anti-IXa
    Hemorrhagic disorder due to intrinsic increase in anti-XIa

  D68.32 Hemorrhagic disorder due to extrinsic circulating anticoagulants
  Drug-induced hemorrhagic disorder
  Hemorrhagic disorder due to increase in anti-IIa
  Hemorrhagic disorder due to increase in anti-Xa
  Hyperheparinemia
  Use additional code for adverse effect, if applicable, to identify drug (T45.515, T45.525)

D68.4 Acquired coagulation factor deficiency
deficiency of coagulation factor due to liver disease
deficiency of coagulation factor due to vitamin K deficiency
Excludes 1: vitamin K deficiency of newborn (P53)

D68.5 Primary thrombophilia
Primary hypercoagulable states
Excludes 1: antiphospholipid syndrome (D68.61)
lupus anticoagulant (D68.62)
secondary activated protein C resistance (D68.69)
secondary antiphospholipid antibody syndrome (D68.69)
secondary lupus anticoagulant with hypercoagulable state (D68.69)
secondary systemic lupus erythematosus [SLE] inhibitor with hypercoagulable state (D68.69)
systemic lupus erythematosus [SLE] inhibitor finding without diagnosis (R76.0)
systemic lupus erythematosus [SLE] inhibitor with hemorrhagic disorder (D68.312)
thrombotic thrombocytopenic purpura (M31.1)

  D68.51 Activated protein C resistance
  Factor V Leiden mutation

  D68.52 Prothrombin gene mutation

  D68.59 Other primary thrombophilia
  Antithrombin III deficiency
  Hypercoagulable state NOS
  Primary hypercoagulable state NEC
  Primary thrombophilia NEC
  Protein C deficiency
  Protein S deficiency
  Thrombophilia NOS

D68.6 Other thrombophilia
Other hypercoagulable states
Excludes 1: diffuse or disseminated intravascular coagulation [DIC] (D65)
heparin induced thrombocytopenia (HIT) (D75.82)
hyperhomocysteinemia (E72.11)

  D68.61 Antiphospholipid syndrome
  Anticardiolipin syndrome
  Antiphospholipid antibody syndrome
  Excludes 1: anti-phospholipid antibody, finding without diagnosis (R76.0)
  anti-phospholipid antibody with hemorrhagic disorder (D68.312)
  lupus anticoagulant syndrome

(D68.62)

D68.62 Lupus anticoagulant syndrome
Lupus anticoagulant

Presence of systemic lupus erythematosus [SLE] inhibitor
Excludes 1: anticardiolipin syndrome (D68.61)
antiphospholipid syndrome (D68.61)
lupus anticoagulant (LAC) finding without diagnosis (R79.0)
lupus anticoagulant (LAC) with hemorrhagic disorder (D68.312)

D68.69 Other thrombophilia
Hypercoagulable states NEC
Secondary hypercoagulable state NOS

D68.8 Other specified coagulation defects
Excludes 1: hemorrhagic disease of newborn (P53)

D68.9 Coagulation defect, unspecified

D69 Purpura and other hemorrhagic conditions
Excludes 1: benign hypergammaglobulinemic purpura (D89.0)
cryoglobulinemic purpura (D89.1)
essential (hemorrhagic) thrombocythemia (D47.3)
hemorrhagic thrombocythemia (D47.3)
purpura fulminans (D65)
thrombotic thrombocytopenic purpura (M31.1)
Waldenstr÷m hypergammaglobulinemic purpura (D89.0)

D69.0 Allergic purpura
Allergic vasculitis
Nonthrombocytopenic hemorrhagic purpura
Nonthrombocytopenic idiopathic purpura
Purpura anaphylactoid
Purpura Henoch(-Sch÷nlein)
Purpura rheumatica
Vascular purpura
Excludes 1: thrombocytopenic hemorrhagic purpura (D69.3)

D69.1 Qualitative platelet defects
Bernard-Soulier [giant platelet] syndrome
Glanzmann's disease
Grey platelet syndrome
Thromboasthenia (hemorrhagic) (hereditary)
Thrombocytopathy
Excludes 1: von Willebrand's disease (D68.0)

D69.2 Other nonthrombocytopenic purpura
Purpura NOS
Purpura simplex
Senile purpura

D69.3 Immune thrombocytopenic purpura
Hemorrhagic (thrombocytopenic) purpura
Idiopathic thrombocytopenic purpura
Tidal platelet dysgenesis

D69.4 Other primary thrombocytopenia
Excludes 1: transient neonatal thrombocytopenia (P61.0)
Wiskott-Aldrich syndrome (D82.0)

D69.41 Evans syndrome

D69.42 Congenital and hereditary thrombocytopenia purpura
Congenital thrombocytopenia
Hereditary thrombocytopenia
Code first congenital or hereditary disorder,

such as:
thrombocytopenia with absent radius (TAR syndrome) (Q87.2)

D69.49 Other primary thrombocytopenia
Megakaryocytic hypoplasia
Primary thrombocytopenia NOS

D69.5 Secondary thrombocytopenia
Excludes 1: heparin induced thrombocytopenia (HIT) (D75.82)
transient thrombocytopenia of newborn (P61.0)

D69.51 Posttransfusion purpura
Posttransfusion purpura from whole blood (fresh) or blood products
PTP

D69.59 Other secondary thrombocytopenia

D69.6 Thrombocytopenia, unspecified

D69.8 Other specified hemorrhagic conditions
Capillary fragility (hereditary)
Vascular pseudohemophilia

D69.9 Hemorrhagic condition, unspecified

OTHER DISORDERS OF BLOOD AND BLOOD-FORMING ORGANS (D70-D77)

D70 Neutropenia
Includes: agranulocytosis
decreased absolute neurophile count (ANC)
Use additional code for any associated:
fever (R50.81)
mucositis (J34.81, K12.3-, K92.81, N76.81)
Excludes 1: neutropenic splenomegaly (D73.81)
transient neonatal neutropenia (P61.5)

D70.0 Congenital agranulocytosis
Congenital neutropenia
Infantile genetic agranulocytosis
Kostmann's disease

D70.1 Agranulocytosis secondary to cancer chemotherapy
Use additional code for adverse effect, if applicable, to identify drug (T45.1X5)
Code also underlying neoplasm

D70.2 Other drug-induced agranulocytosis
Use additional code for adverse effect, if applicable, to identify drug (T36-T50 with fifth or sixth character 5)

D70.3 Neutropenia due to infection

D70.4 Cyclic neutropenia
Cyclic hematopoiesis
Periodic neutropenia

D70.8 Other neutropenia

D70.9 Neutropenia, unspecified

D71 Functional disorders of polymorphonuclear neutrophils
Cell membrane receptor complex [CR3] defect
Chronic (childhood) granulomatous disease
Congenital dysphagocytosis
Progressive septic granulomatosis

D72 Other disorders of white blood cells
Excludes 1: basophilia (D72.824)
immunity disorders (D80-D89)
neutropenia (D70)
preleukemia (syndrome) (D46.9)

D72.0 Genetic anomalies of leukocytes
Alder (granulation) (granulocyte) anomaly
Alder syndrome
Hereditary leukocytic hypersegmentation

Hereditary leukocytic hyposegmentation
Hereditary leukomelanopathy
May-Hegglin (granulation) (granulocyte) anomaly
May-Hegglin syndrome
Pelger-Huðt (granulation) (granulocyte) anomaly
Pelger-Huðt syndrome
Excludes 1: ChΘdiak (-Steinbrinck)-Higashi syndrome
(E70.330)

D72.1 Eosinophilia
Allergic eosinophilia
Hereditary eosinophilia
Excludes 1: L÷ffler's syndrome (J82)
pulmonary eosinophilia (J82)

D72.8 Other specified disorders of white blood cells
Excludes 1: leukemia (C91-C95)

   D72.81 Decreased white blood cell count
     Excludes 1: neutropenia (D70.-)

     D72.810 Lymphocytopenia
Decreased lymphocytes

     D72.818 Other decreased white blood cell count
Basophilic leukopenia
Eosinophilic leukopenia
Monocytopenia
Other decreased leukocytes
Plasmacytopenia

     D72.819 Decreased white blood cell count, unspecified
Decreased leukocytes, unspecified
Leukocytopenia, unspecified
Leukopenia
Excludes 1: malignant leukopenia (D70.9)

   D72.82 Elevated white blood cell count
     Excludes 1: eosinophilia (D72.1)

     D72.820 Lymphocytosis (symptomatic)
Elevated lymphocytes

     D72.821 Monocytosis (symptomatic)
Excludes 1: infectious mononucleosis (B27.-)

     D72.822 Plasmacytosis

     D72.823 Leukemoid reaction
Basophilic leukemoid reaction
Leukemoid reaction NOS
Lymphocytic leukemoid reaction
Monocytic leukemoid reaction
Myelocytic leukemoid reaction
Neutrophilic leukemoid reaction

     D72.824 Basophilia

     D72.825 Bandemia
Bandemia without diagnosis of specific infection
Excludes 1: confirmed infection - code to infection
leukemia (C91.-, C92.-, C93.-, C94.-, C95.-)

     D72.828 Other elevated white blood cell count

     D72.829 Elevated white blood cell count, unspecified
Elevated leukocytes, unspecified
Leukocytosis, unspecified

   D72.89 Other specified disorders of white blood cells
Abnormality of white blood cells NEC

D72.9 Disorder of white blood cells, unspecified
Abnormal leukocyte differential NOS

D73 Diseases of spleen

D73.0 Hyposplenism
Atrophy of spleen
Excludes 1: asplenia (congenital) (Q89.01)
postsurgical absence of spleen (Z90.81)

D73.1 Hypersplenism
Excludes 1: neutropenic splenomegaly (D73.81)
primary splenic neutropenia (D73.81)
splenitis, splenomegaly in late syphilis (A52.79)
splenitis, splenomegaly in tuberculosis (A18.85)
splenomegaly NOS (R16.1)
splenomegaly congenital (Q89.0)

D73.2 Chronic congestive splenomegaly

D73.3 Abscess of spleen

D73.4 Cyst of spleen

D73.5 Infarction of spleen
Splenic rupture, nontraumatic
Torsion of spleen
Excludes 1: rupture of spleen due to Plasmodium vivax malaria (B51.0)
traumatic rupture of spleen (S36.03-)

D73.8 Other diseases of spleen

   D73.81 Neutropenic splenomegaly
Werner-Schultz disease

   D73.89 Other diseases of spleen
Fibrosis of spleen NOS
Perisplenitis
Splenitis NOS

D73.9 Disease of spleen, unspecified

D74 Methemoglobinemia

D74.0 Congenital methemoglobinemia
Congenital NADH-methemoglobin reductase deficiency
Hemoglobin-M [Hb-M] disease
Methemoglobinemia, hereditary

D74.8 Other methemoglobinemias
Acquired methemoglobinemia (with sulfhemoglobinemia)
Toxic methemoglobinemia

D74.9 Methemoglobinemia, unspecified

D75 Other and unspecified diseases of blood and blood-forming organs
Excludes 2: acute lymphadenitis (L04.-)
chronic lymphadenitis (I88.1)
enlarged lymph nodes (R59.-)
hypergammaglobulinemia NOS (D89.2)
lymphadenitis NOS (I88.9)
mesenteric lymphadenitis (acute) (chronic) (I88.0)

D75.0 Familial erythrocytosis
Benign polycythemia
Familial polycythemia
Excludes 1: hereditary ovalocytosis (D58.1)

D75.1 Secondary polycythemia
Acquired polycythemia
Emotional polycythemia
Erythrocytosis NOS
Hypoxemic polycythemia
Nephrogenous polycythemia
Polycythemia due to erythropoietin
Polycythemia due to fall in plasma volume
Polycythemia due to high altitude

Polycythemia due to stress

Polycythemia NOS

Relative polycythemia

Excludes 1: polycythemia neonatorum (P61.1)

polycythemia vera (D45)

D75.8 Other specified diseases of blood and blood-forming organs

D75.81 Myelofibrosis

Myelofibrosis NOS

Secondary myelofibrosis NOS

Code first the underlying disorder, such as:

malignant neoplasm of breast (C50.-)

Use additional code, if applicable, for associated therapy-related myelodysplastic syndrome (D46.-)

Use additional code for adverse effect, if applicable, to identify drug (T45.1X5)

Excludes 1: acute myelofibrosis (C94.4-)

idiopathic myelofibrosis (D47.1)

leukoerythroblastic anemia (D61.82)

myelofibrosis with myeloid metaplasia (D47.4)

myelophthisic anemia (D61.82)

myelophthisis (D61.82)

primary myelofibrosis (D47.1)

D75.82 Heparin induced thrombocytopenia (HIT)

D75.89 Other specified diseases of blood and blood-forming organs

D75.9 Disease of blood and blood-forming organs, unspecified

D76 Other specified diseases with participation of lymphoreticular and reticulohistiocytic tissue

Excludes 1: (Abt-) Letterer-Siwe disease (C96.0)

eosinophilic granuloma (C96.6)

Hand-Sch_ller-Christian disease (C96.5)

histiocytic sarcoma (C96.A)

histiocytosis X, multifocal (C96.5)

histiocytosis X, unifocal (C96.6)

malignant histiocytosis (C96.A)

Langerhans-cell histiocytosis, multifocal (C96.5)

Langerhans-cell histiocytosis NOS (C96.6)

Langerhans-cell histiocytosis, unifocal (C96.6)

leukemic reticuloendotheliosis or reticulosis (C91.4-)

lipomelanotic reticuloendotheliosis or reticulosis (I89.8)

D76.1 Hemophagocytic lymphohistiocytosis

Familial hemophagocytic reticulosis

Histiocytoses of mononuclear phagocytes

D76.2 Hemophagocytic syndrome, infection-associated

Use additional code to identify infectious agent or disease.

D76.3 Other histiocytosis syndromes

Reticulohistiocytoma (giant-cell)

Sinus histiocytosis with massive lymphadenopathy

Xanthogranuloma

D77 Other disorders of blood and blood-forming organs in diseases classified elsewhere

Code first underlying disease, such as:

amyloidosis (E85-)

congenital early syphilis (A50.0)

echinococcosis (B67.0-B67.9)

malaria (B50.0-B54)

schistosomiasis [bilharziasis] (B65.0-B65.9)

vitamin C deficiency (E54)

Excludes 1: rupture of spleen due to Plasmodium vivax malaria (B51.0)

splenitis, splenomegaly in:

late syphilis (A52.79)

tuberculosis (A18.85)

INTRAOPERATIVE AND POSTPROCEDURAL COMPLICATIONS OF THE SPLEEN (D78)

D78 Intraoperative and postprocedural complications of the spleen

D78.0 Intraoperative hemorrhage and hematoma of the spleen complicating a procedure

Excludes 1: intraoperative hemorrhage and hematoma of the spleen due to accidental puncture or laceration during a procedure (D78.1-)

D78.01 Intraoperative hemorrhage and hematoma of the spleen complicating a procedure on the spleen

D78.02 Intraoperative hemorrhage and hematoma of the spleen complicating other procedure

D78.1 Accidental puncture and laceration of the spleen during a procedure

D78.11 Accidental puncture and laceration of the spleen during a procedure on the spleen

D78.12 Accidental puncture and laceration of the spleen during other procedure

D78.2 Postprocedural hemorrhage and hematoma of the spleen following a procedure

D78.21 Postprocedural hemorrhage and hematoma of the spleen following a procedure on the spleen

D78.22 Postprocedural hemorrhage and hematoma of the spleen following other procedure

D78.8 Other intraoperative and postprocedural complications of the spleen

Use additional code, if applicable, to further specify disorder

D78.81 Other intraoperative complications of the spleen

D78.89 Other postprocedural complications of the spleen

CERTAIN DISORDERS INVOLVING THE IMMUNE MECHANISM (D80-D89)

Includes: defects in the complement system

immunodeficiency disorders, except human immunodeficiency virus [HIV] disease

sarcoidosis

Excludes 1: autoimmune disease (systemic) NOS (M35.9)

functional disorders of polymorphonuclear neutrophils (D71)

human immunodeficiency virus [HIV] disease (B20)

D80 Immunodeficiency with predominantly antibody defects

D80.0 Hereditary hypogammaglobulinemia

Autosomal recessive agammaglobulinemia (Swiss type)

X-linked agammaglobulinemia [Bruton] (with growth hormone deficiency)

D80.1 Nonfamilial hypogammaglobulinemia

Agammaglobulinemia with immunoglobulin-bearing B-lymphocytes

Common variable agammaglobulinemia [CVAgamma]

Hypogammaglobulinemia NOS

D80.2 Selective deficiency of immunoglobulin A [IgA]

D80.3 Selective deficiency of immunoglobulin G [IgG] subclasses

D80.4 Selective deficiency of immunoglobulin M [IgM]

D80.5 Immunodeficiency with increased immunoglobulin M [IgM]

D80.6   Antibody deficiency with near-normal immunoglobulins or with hyperimmunoglobulinemia

D80.7   Transient hypogammaglobulinemia of infancy

D80.8   Other immunodeficiencies with predominantly antibody defects

      Kappa light chain deficiency

D80.9   Immunodeficiency with predominantly antibody defects, unspecified

D81   Combined immunodeficiencies

     Excludes 1: autosomal recessive agammaglobulinemia (Swiss type) (D80.0)

D81.0   Severe combined immunodeficiency [SCID] with reticular dysgenesis

D81.1   Severe combined immunodeficiency [SCID] with low T- and B-cell numbers

D81.2   Severe combined immunodeficiency [SCID] with low or normal B-cell numbers

D81.3   Adenosine deaminase [ADA] deficiency

D81.4   Nezelof's syndrome

D81.5   Purine nucleoside phosphorylase [PNP] deficiency

D81.6   Major histocompatibility complex class I deficiency

      Bare lymphocyte syndrome

D81.7   Major histocompatibility complex class II deficiency

D81.8   Other combined immunodeficiencies

     D81.81   Biotin-dependent carboxylase deficiency

          Multiple carboxylase deficiency

          Excludes 1: biotin-dependent carboxylase deficiency due to dietary deficiency of biotin (E53.8)

         D81.810   Biotinidase deficiency

         D81.818   Other biotin-dependent carboxylase deficiency

               Holocarboxylase synthetase deficiency

               Other multiple carboxylase deficiency

         D81.819   Biotin-dependent carboxylase deficiency, unspecified

               Multiple carboxylase deficiency, unspecified

     D81.89   Other combined immunodeficiencies

D81.9   Combined immunodeficiency, unspecified

      Severe combined immunodeficiency disorder [SCID] NOS

D82   Immunodeficiency associated with other major defects

     Excludes 1: ataxia telangiectasia [Louis-Bar] (G11.3)

D82.0   Wiskott-Aldrich syndrome

      Immunodeficiency with thrombocytopenia and eczema

D82.1   Di George's syndrome

      Pharyngeal pouch syndrome

      Thymic alymphoplasia

      Thymic aplasia or hypoplasia with immunodeficiency

D82.2   Immunodeficiency with short-limbed stature

D82.3   Immunodeficiency following hereditary defective response to Epstein-Barr virus

      X-linked lymphoproliferative disease

D82.4   Hyperimmunoglobulin E [IgE] syndrome

D82.8   Immunodeficiency associated with other specified major defects

D82.9   Immunodeficiency associated with major defect, unspecified

D83   Common variable immunodeficiency

D83.0   Common variable immunodeficiency with predominant abnormalities of B-cell numbers and function

D83.1   Common variable immunodeficiency with predominant immunoregulatory T-cell disorders

D83.2   Common variable immunodeficiency with autoantibodies to B- or T-cells

D83.8   Other common variable immunodeficiencies

D83.9   Common variable immunodeficiency, unspecified

D84   Other immunodeficiencies

D84.0   Lymphocyte function antigen-1[LFA-1] defect

D84.1   Defects in the complement system

      C1esterase inhibitor [C1-INH] deficiency

D84.8   Other specified immunodeficiencies

D84.9   Immunodeficiency, unspecified

D86   Sarcoidosis

D86.0   Sarcoidosis of lung

D86.1   Sarcoidosis of lymph nodes

D86.2   Sarcoidosis of lung with sarcoidosis of lymph nodes

D86.3   Sarcoidosis of skin

D86.8   Sarcoidosis of other sites

     D86.81   Sarcoid meningitis

     D86.82   Multiple cranial nerve palsies in sarcoidosis

     D86.83   Sarcoid iridocyclitis

     D86.84   Sarcoid pyelonephritis

          Tubulo-interstitial nephropathy in sarcoidosis

     D86.85   Sarcoid myocarditis

     D86.86   Sarcoid arthropathy

          Polyarthritis in sarcoidosis

     D86.87   Sarcoid myositis

     D86.89   Sarcoidosis of other sites

          Hepatic granuloma

          Uveoparotid fever [Heerfordt]

D86.9   Sarcoidosis, unspecified

D89   Other disorders involving the immune mechanism, not elsewhere classified

     Excludes 1: hyperglobulinemia NOS (R77.1)

          monoclonal gammopathy (of undetermined significance) (D47.2)

     Excludes 2: transplant failure and rejection (T86.-)

D89.0   Polyclonal hypergammaglobulinemia

      Benign hypergammaglobulinemic purpura

      Polyclonal gammopathy NOS

D89.1   Cryoglobulinemia

      Cryoglobulinemic purpura

      Cryoglobulinemic vasculitis

      Essential cryoglobulinemia

      Idiopathic cryoglobulinemia

      Mixed cryoglobulinemia

      Primary cryoglobulinemia

      Secondary cryoglobulinemia

D89.2   Hypergammaglobulinemia, unspecified

D89.3   Immune reconstitution syndrome

      Immune reconstitution inflammatory syndrome [IRIS]

      Use additional code for adverse effect, if applicable, to identify drug (T36-T50 with fifth or sixth character 5)

D89.8   Other specified disorders involving the immune mechanism, not elsewhere classified

     D89.81   Graft-versus-host disease

          Code first underlying cause, such as:

               complications of transplanted organs and tissue (T86.-)

               complications of blood transfusion (T80.89)

          Use additional code to identify associated manifestations, such as:

               desquamative dermatitis (L30.8)

diarrhea (R19.7)

elevated bilirubin (R17)

hair loss (L65.9)

D89.810   Acute graft-versus-host disease

D89.811   Chronic graft-versus-host disease

D89.812   Acute on chronic graft-versus-host disease

D89.813   Graft-versus-host disease, unspecified

D89.82   Autoimmune lymphoproliferative syndrome [ALPS]

D89.89   Other specified disorders involving the immune mechanism, not elsewhere classified

Excludes 1:   human immunodeficiency virus disease (B20)

D89.9   Disorder involving the immune mechanism, unspecified

Immune disease NOS

Chapter 4: Endocrine, Nutritional And Metabolic Diseases (E00-E89)

Note: All neoplasms, whether functionally active or not, are classified in Chapter 2. Appropriate codes in this chapter (i.e. E05.8, E07.0, E16-E31, E34.-) may be used as additional codes to indicate either functional activity by neoplasms and ectopic endocrine tissue or hyperfunction and hypofunction of endocrine glands associated with neoplasms and other conditions classified elsewhere.

Excludes 1: transitory endocrine and metabolic disorders specific to newborn (P70-P74)

This chapter contains the following blocks:

E00-E07	Disorders of thyroid gland
E08-E13	Diabetes mellitus
E15-E16	Other disorders of glucose regulation and pancreatic internal secretion
E20-E35	Disorders of other endocrine glands
E36	Intraoperative complications of endocrine system
E40-E46	Malnutrition
E50-E64	Other nutritional deficiencies
E65-E68	Overweight, obesity and other hyperalimentation
E70-E88	Metabolic disorders
E89	Postprocedural endocrine and metabolic complications and disorders, not elsewhere classified

DISORDERS OF THYROID GLAND (E00-E07)

E00 Congenital iodine-deficiency syndrome

Use additional code (F70-F79) to identify associated intellectual disabilities.

Excludes 1: subclinical iodine-deficiency hypothyroidism (E02)

E00.0 Congenital iodine-deficiency syndrome, neurological type
Endemic cretinism, neurological type

E00.1 Congenital iodine-deficiency syndrome, myxedematous type
Endemic hypothyroid cretinism
Endemic cretinism, myxedematous type

E00.2 Congenital iodine-deficiency syndrome, mixed type
Endemic cretinism, mixed type

E00.9 Congenital iodine-deficiency syndrome, unspecified
Congenital iodine-deficiency hypothyroidism NOS
Endemic cretinism NOS

E01 Iodine-deficiency related thyroid disorders and allied conditions

Excludes 1: congenital iodine-deficiency syndrome (E00.-)
subclinical iodine-deficiency hypothyroidism (E02)

E01.0 Iodine-deficiency related diffuse (endemic) goiter

E01.1 Iodine-deficiency related multinodular (endemic) goiter
Iodine-deficiency related nodular goiter

E01.2 Iodine-deficiency related (endemic) goiter, unspecified
Endemic goiter NOS

E01.8 Other iodine-deficiency related thyroid disorders and allied conditions
Acquired iodine-deficiency hypothyroidism NOS

E02 Subclinical iodine-deficiency hypothyroidism

E03 Other hypothyroidism

Excludes 1: iodine-deficiency related hypothyroidism (E00-E02)
postprocedural hypothyroidism (E89.0)

E03.0 Congenital hypothyroidism with diffuse goiter
Congenital parenchymatous goiter (nontoxic)
Congenital goiter (nontoxic) NOS
Excludes 1: transitory congenital goiter with normal function (P72.0)

E03.1 Congenital hypothyroidism without goiter
Aplasia of thyroid (with myxedema)
Congenital atrophy of thyroid
Congenital hypothyroidism NOS

E03.2 Hypothyroidism due to medicaments and other exogenous substances
Code first poisoning due to drug or toxin, if applicable (T36-T65 with fifth or sixth character 1-4 or 6)
Use additional code for adverse effect, if applicable, to identify drug (T36-T50 with fifth or sixth character 5)

E03.3 Postinfectious hypothyroidism

E03.4 Atrophy of thyroid (acquired)
Excludes 1: congenital atrophy of thyroid (E03.1)

E03.5 Myxedema coma

E03.8 Other specified hypothyroidism

E03.9 Hypothyroidism, unspecified
Myxedema NOS

E04 Other nontoxic goiter

Excludes 1: congenital goiter (NOS) (diffuse) (parenchymatous) (E03.0)
iodine-deficiency related goiter (E00-E02)

E04.0 Nontoxic diffuse goiter
Diffuse (colloid) nontoxic goiter
Simple nontoxic goiter

E04.1 Nontoxic single thyroid nodule
Colloid nodule (cystic) (thyroid)
Nontoxic uninodular goiter
Thyroid (cystic) nodule NOS

E04.2 Nontoxic multinodular goiter
Cystic goiter NOS
Multinodular (cystic) goiter NOS

E04.8 Other specified nontoxic goiter

E04.9 Nontoxic goiter, unspecified
Goiter NOS
Nodular goiter (nontoxic) NOS

E05 Thyrotoxicosis [hyperthyroidism]

Excludes 1: chronic thyroiditis with transient thyrotoxicosis (E06.2)
neonatal thyrotoxicosis (P72.1)

E05.0 Thyrotoxicosis with diffuse goiter
Exophthalmic or toxic goiter NOS
Graves' disease
Toxic diffuse goiter
E05.00 Thyrotoxicosis with diffuse goiter without thyrotoxic crisis or storm
E05.01 Thyrotoxicosis with diffuse goiter with thyrotoxic crisis or storm

E05.1 Thyrotoxicosis with toxic single thyroid nodule
Thyrotoxicosis with toxic uninodular goiter
E05.10 Thyrotoxicosis with toxic single thyroid nodule without thyrotoxic crisis or storm
E05.11 Thyrotoxicosis with toxic single thyroid nodule with thyrotoxic crisis or storm

E05.2 Thyrotoxicosis with toxic multinodular goiter
Toxic nodular goiter NOS
E05.20 Thyrotoxicosis with toxic multinodular goiter without thyrotoxic crisis or storm
E05.21 Thyrotoxicosis with toxic multinodular goiter with thyrotoxic crisis or storm

E05.3 Thyrotoxicosis from ectopic thyroid tissue
E05.30 Thyrotoxicosis from ectopic thyroid tissue without thyrotoxic crisis or storm

E05.31   Thyrotoxicosis from ectopic thyroid tissue with thyrotoxic crisis or storm
E05.4   Thyrotoxicosis factitia
   E05.40   Thyrotoxicosis factitia without thyrotoxic crisis or storm
   E05.41   Thyrotoxicosis factitia with thyrotoxic crisis or storm
E05.8   Other thyrotoxicosis
   Overproduction of thyroid-stimulating hormone
   E05.80   Other thyrotoxicosis without thyrotoxic crisis or storm
   E05.81   Other thyrotoxicosis with thyrotoxic crisis or storm
E05.9   Thyrotoxicosis, unspecified
   Hyperthyroidism NOS
   E05.90   Thyrotoxicosis, unspecified without thyrotoxic crisis or storm
   E05.91   Thyrotoxicosis, unspecified with thyrotoxic crisis or storm

E06   Thyroiditis
   Excludes 1: postpartum thyroiditis (O90.5)
E06.0   Acute thyroiditis
   Abscess of thyroid
   Pyogenic thyroiditis
   Suppurative thyroiditis
   Use additional code (B95-B97) to identify infectious agent.
E06.1   Subacute thyroiditis
   de Quervain thyroiditis
   Giant-cell thyroiditis
   Granulomatous thyroiditis
   Nonsuppurative thyroiditis
   Viral thyroiditis
   Excludes 1: autoimmune thyroiditis (E06.3)
E06.2   Chronic thyroiditis with transient thyrotoxicosis
   Excludes 1: autoimmune thyroiditis (E06.3)
E06.3   Autoimmune thyroiditis
   Hashimoto's thyroiditis
   Hashitoxicosis (transient)
   Lymphadenoid goiter
   Lymphocytic thyroiditis
   Struma lymphomatosa
E06.4   Drug-induced thyroiditis
   Use additional code for adverse effect, if applicable, to identify drug (T36-T50 with fifth or sixth character 5)
E06.5   Other chronic thyroiditis
   Chronic fibrous thyroiditis
   Chronic thyroiditis NOS
   Ligneous thyroiditis
   Riedel thyroiditis
E06.9   Thyroiditis, unspecified

E07   Other disorders of thyroid
E07.0   Hypersecretion of calcitonin
   C-cell hyperplasia of thyroid
   Hypersecretion of thyrocalcitonin
E07.1   Dyshormogenetic goiter
   Familial dyshormogenetic goiter
   Pendred's syndrome
   Excludes 1: transitory congenital goiter with normal function (P72.0)
E07.8   Other specified disorders of thyroid
   E07.81   Sick-euthyroid syndrome

   Euthyroid sick-syndrome
   E07.89   Other specified disorders of thyroid
   Abnormality of thyroid-binding globulin
   Hemorrhage of thyroid
   Infarction of thyroid
E07.9   Disorder of thyroid, unspecified

DIABETES MELLITUS (E08-E13)

E08   Diabetes mellitus due to underlying condition
   Code first the underlying condition, such as:
   congenital rubella (P35.0)
   Cushing's syndrome (E24.-)
   cystic fibrosis (E84.-)
   malignant neoplasm (C00-C96)
   malnutrition (E40-E46)
   pancreatitis and other diseases of the pancreas (K85-K86.-)
   Use additional code to identify any insulin use (Z79.4)
   Excludes 1: drug or chemical induced diabetes mellitus (E09.-)
   gestational diabetes (O24.4-)
   neonatal diabetes mellitus (P70.2)
   postpancreatectomy diabetes mellitus (E13.-)
   postprocedural diabetes mellitus (E13.-)
   secondary diabetes mellitus NEC (E13.-)
   type 1 diabetes mellitus (E10.-)
   type 2 diabetes mellitus (E11.-)
E08.0   Diabetes mellitus due to underlying condition with hyperosmolarity
   E08.00   Diabetes mellitus due to underlying condition with hyperosmolarity without nonketotic hyperglycemic-hyperosmolar coma (NKHHC)
   E08.01   Diabetes mellitus due to underlying condition with hyperosmolarity with coma
E08.1   Diabetes mellitus due to underlying condition with ketoacidosis
   E08.10   Diabetes mellitus due to underlying condition with ketoacidosis without coma
   E08.11   Diabetes mellitus due to underlying condition with ketoacidosis with coma
E08.2   Diabetes mellitus due to underlying condition with kidney complications
   E08.21   Diabetes mellitus due to underlying condition with diabetic nephropathy
   Diabetes mellitus due to underlying condition with intercapillary glomerulosclerosis
   Diabetes mellitus due to underlying condition with intracapillary glomerulonephrosis
   Diabetes mellitus due to underlying condition with Kimmelstiel-Wilson disease
   E08.22   Diabetes mellitus due to underlying condition with diabetic chronic kidney disease
   Diabetes mellitus due to underlying condition with chronic kidney disease due to conditions classified to .21 and .22
   Use additional code to identify stage of chronic kidney disease (N18.1-N18.6)
   E08.29   Diabetes mellitus due to underlying condition with other diabetic kidney complication
   Renal tubular degeneration in diabetes mellitus due to underlying condition
E08.3   Diabetes mellitus due to underlying condition with ophthalmic complications

E08.31 Diabetes mellitus due to underlying condition with unspecified diabetic retinopathy

    E08.311 Diabetes mellitus due to underlying condition with unspecified diabetic retinopathy with macular edema

    E08.319 Diabetes mellitus due to underlying condition with unspecified diabetic retinopathy without macular edema

E08.32 Diabetes mellitus due to underlying condition with mild nonproliferative diabetic retinopathy

Diabetes mellitus due to underlying condition with nonproliferative diabetic retinopathy NOS

    E08.321 Diabetes mellitus due to underlying condition with mild nonproliferative diabetic retinopathy with macular edema

    E08.329 Diabetes mellitus due to underlying condition with mild nonproliferative diabetic retinopathy without macular edema

E08.33 Diabetes mellitus due to underlying condition with moderate nonproliferative diabetic retinopathy

    E08.331 Diabetes mellitus due to underlying condition with moderate nonproliferative diabetic retinopathy with macular edema

    E08.339 Diabetes mellitus due to underlying condition with moderate nonproliferative diabetic retinopathy without macular edema

E08.34 Diabetes mellitus due to underlying condition with severe nonproliferative diabetic retinopathy

    E08.341 Diabetes mellitus due to underlying condition with severe nonproliferative diabetic retinopathy with macular edema

    E08.349 Diabetes mellitus due to underlying condition with severe nonproliferative diabetic retinopathy without macular edema

E08.35 Diabetes mellitus due to underlying condition with proliferative diabetic retinopathy

    E08.351 Diabetes mellitus due to underlying condition with proliferative diabetic retinopathy with macular edema

    E08.359 Diabetes mellitus due to underlying condition with proliferative diabetic retinopathy without macular edema

E08.36 Diabetes mellitus due to underlying condition with diabetic cataract

E08.39 Diabetes mellitus due to underlying condition with other diabetic ophthalmic complication

E08.4 Diabetes mellitus due to underlying condition with neurological complications

E08.40 Diabetes mellitus due to underlying condition with diabetic neuropathy, unspecified

E08.41 Diabetes mellitus due to underlying condition with diabetic mononeuropathy

E08.42 Diabetes mellitus due to underlying condition with diabetic polyneuropathy

Diabetes mellitus due to underlying condition with diabetic neuralgia

E08.43 Diabetes mellitus due to underlying condition with diabetic autonomic (poly)neuropathy

Diabetes mellitus due to underlying condition with diabetic gastroparesis

E08.44 Diabetes mellitus due to underlying condition with diabetic amyotrophy

E08.49 Diabetes mellitus due to underlying condition with other diabetic neurological complication

E08.5 Diabetes mellitus due to underlying condition with circulatory complications

E08.51 Diabetes mellitus due to underlying condition with diabetic peripheral angiopathy without gangrene

E08.52 Diabetes mellitus due to underlying condition with diabetic peripheral angiopathy with gangrene

Diabetes mellitus due to underlying condition with diabetic gangrene

E08.59 Diabetes mellitus due to underlying condition with other circulatory complications

E08.6 Diabetes mellitus due to underlying condition with other specified complications

E08.61 Diabetes mellitus due to underlying condition with diabetic arthropathy

    E08.610 Diabetes mellitus due to underlying condition with diabetic neuropathic arthropathy

Diabetes mellitus due to underlying condition with Charcot's joints

    E08.618 Diabetes mellitus due to underlying condition with other diabetic arthropathy

E08.62 Diabetes mellitus due to underlying condition with skin complications

    E08.620 Diabetes mellitus due to underlying condition with diabetic dermatitis

Diabetes mellitus due to underlying condition with diabetic necrobiosis lipoidica

    E08.621 Diabetes mellitus due to underlying condition with foot ulcer

Use additional code to identify site of ulcer (L97.4-, L97.5-)

    E08.622 Diabetes mellitus due to underlying condition with other skin ulcer

Use additional code to identify site of ulcer (L97.1-L97.9, L98.41-L98.49)

    E08.628 Diabetes mellitus due to underlying condition with other skin complications

E08.63 Diabetes mellitus due to underlying condition with oral complications

    E08.630 Diabetes mellitus due to underlying condition with periodontal disease

    E08.638 Diabetes mellitus due to underlying condition with other oral complications

E08.64 Diabetes mellitus due to underlying condition with hypoglycemia

    E08.641 Diabetes mellitus due to underlying condition with hypoglycemia with coma

    E08.649 Diabetes mellitus due to underlying condition with hypoglycemia without coma

E08.65 Diabetes mellitus due to underlying condition with hyperglycemia

E08.69   Diabetes mellitus due to underlying condition with other specified complication
Use additional code to identify complication

E08.8   Diabetes mellitus due to underlying condition with unspecified complications

E08.9   Diabetes mellitus due to underlying condition without complications

E09   Drug or chemical induced diabetes mellitus

Code first poisoning due to drug or toxin, if applicable (T36-T65 with fifth or sixth character 1-4 or 6)

Use additional code for adverse effect, if applicable, to identify drug (T36-T50 with fifth or sixth character 5)

Use additional code to identify any insulin use (Z79.4)

Excludes 1: diabetes mellitus due to underlying condition (E08.-)
gestational diabetes (O24.4-)
neonatal diabetes mellitus (P70.2)
postpancreatectomy diabetes mellitus (E13.-)
postprocedural diabetes mellitus (E13.-)
secondary diabetes mellitus NEC (E13.-)
type 1 diabetes mellitus (E10.-)
type 2 diabetes mellitus (E11.-)

E09.0   Drug or chemical induced diabetes mellitus with hyperosmolarity

E09.00   Drug or chemical induced diabetes mellitus with hyperosmolarity without nonketotic hyperglycemic-hyperosmolar coma (NKHHC)

E09.01   Drug or chemical induced diabetes mellitus with hyperosmolarity with coma

E09.1   Drug or chemical induced diabetes mellitus with ketoacidosis

E09.10   Drug or chemical induced diabetes mellitus with ketoacidosis without coma

E09.11   Drug or chemical induced diabetes mellitus with ketoacidosis with coma

E09.2   Drug or chemical induced diabetes mellitus with kidney complications

E09.21   Drug or chemical induced diabetes mellitus with diabetic nephropathy
Drug or chemical induced diabetes mellitus with intercapillary glomerulosclerosis
Drug or chemical induced diabetes mellitus with intracapillary glomerulonephrosis
Drug or chemical induced diabetes mellitus with Kimmelstiel-Wilson disease

E09.22   Drug or chemical induced diabetes mellitus with diabetic chronic kidney disease
Drug or chemical induced diabetes mellitus with chronic kidney disease due to conditions classified to .21and .22
Use additional code to identify stage of chronic kidney disease (N18.1-N18.6)

E09.29   Drug or chemical induced diabetes mellitus with other diabetic kidney complication
Drug or chemical induced diabetes mellitus with renal tubular degeneration

E09.3   Drug or chemical induced diabetes mellitus with ophthalmic complications

E09.31   Drug or chemical induced diabetes mellitus with unspecified diabetic retinopathy

E09.311   Drug or chemical induced diabetes mellitus with unspecified diabetic retinopathy with macular edema

E09.319   Drug or chemical induced diabetes mellitus with unspecified diabetic retinopathy without macular edema

E09.32   Drug or chemical induced diabetes mellitus with mild nonproliferative diabetic retinopathy

Drug or chemical induced diabetes mellitus with nonproliferative diabetic retinopathy NOS

E09.321   Drug or chemical induced diabetes mellitus with mild nonproliferative diabetic retinopathy with macular edema

E09.329   Drug or chemical induced diabetes mellitus with mild nonproliferative diabetic retinopathy without macular edema

E09.33   Drug or chemical induced diabetes mellitus with moderate nonproliferative diabetic retinopathy

E09.331   Drug or chemical induced diabetes mellitus with moderate nonproliferative diabetic retinopathy with macular edema

E09.339   Drug or chemical induced diabetes mellitus with moderate nonproliferative diabetic retinopathy without macular edema

E09.34   Drug or chemical induced diabetes mellitus with severe nonproliferative diabetic retinopathy

E09.341   Drug or chemical induced diabetes mellitus with severe nonproliferative diabetic retinopathy with macular edema

E09.349   Drug or chemical induced diabetes mellitus with severe nonproliferative diabetic retinopathy without macular Edema

E09.35   Drug or chemical induced diabetes mellitus with proliferative diabetic retinopathy

E09.351   Drug or chemical induced diabetes mellitus with proliferative diabetic retinopathy with macular edema

E09.359   Drug or chemical induced diabetes mellitus with proliferative diabetic retinopathy without macular edema

E09.36   Drug or chemical induced diabetes mellitus with diabetic cataract

E09.39   Drug or chemical induced diabetes mellitus with other diabetic ophthalmic complication

E09.4   Drug or chemical induced diabetes mellitus with neurological complications

E09.40   Drug or chemical induced diabetes mellitus with neurological complications with diabetic neuropathy, unspecified

E09.41   Drug or chemical induced diabetes mellitus with neurological complications with diabetic mononeuropathy

E09.42   Drug or chemical induced diabetes mellitus with neurological complications with diabetic polyneuropathy
Drug or chemical induced diabetes mellitus with diabetic neuralgia

E09.43   Drug or chemical induced diabetes mellitus with neurological complications with diabetic autonomic (poly)neuropathy
Drug or chemical induced diabetes mellitus with diabetic gastroparesis

E09.44 Drug or chemical induced diabetes mellitus with neurological complications with diabetic amyotrophy

E09.49 Drug or chemical induced diabetes mellitus with neurological complications with other diabetic neurological complication

E09.5 Drug or chemical induced diabetes mellitus with circulatory complications

E09.51 Drug or chemical induced diabetes mellitus with diabetic peripheral angiopathy without gangrene

E09.52 Drug or chemical induced diabetes mellitus with diabetic peripheral angiopathy with gangrene

Drug or chemical induced diabetes mellitus with diabetic gangrene

E09.59 Drug or chemical induced diabetes mellitus with other circulatory complications

E09.6 Drug or chemical induced diabetes mellitus with other specified complications

E09.61 Drug or chemical induced diabetes mellitus with diabetic arthropathy

E09.610 Drug or chemical induced diabetes mellitus with diabetic neuropathic arthropathy

Drug or chemical induced diabetes mellitus with Charcot's joints

E09.618 Drug or chemical induced diabetes mellitus with other diabetic arthropathy

E09.62 Drug or chemical induced diabetes mellitus with skin complications

E09.620 Drug or chemical induced diabetes mellitus with diabetic dermatitis

Drug or chemical induced diabetes mellitus with diabetic necrobiosis lipoidica

E09.621 Drug or chemical induced diabetes mellitus with foot ulcer

Use additional code to identify site of ulcer (L97.4-, L97.5-)

E09.622 Drug or chemical induced diabetes mellitus with other skin ulcer

Use additional code to identify site of ulcer (L97.1-L97.9, L98.41-L98.49)

E09.628 Drug or chemical induced diabetes mellitus with other skin complications

E09.63 Drug or chemical induced diabetes mellitus with oral complications

E09.630 Drug or chemical induced diabetes mellitus with periodontal disease

E09.638 Drug or chemical induced diabetes mellitus with other oral complications

E09.64 Drug or chemical induced diabetes mellitus with hypoglycemia

E09.641 Drug or chemical induced diabetes mellitus with hypoglycemia with coma

E09.649 Drug or chemical induced diabetes mellitus with hypoglycemia without coma

E09.65 Drug or chemical induced diabetes mellitus with hyperglycemia

E09.69 Drug or chemical induced diabetes mellitus with other specified complication

Use additional code to identify complication

E09.8 Drug or chemical induced diabetes mellitus with unspecified complications

E09.9 Drug or chemical induced diabetes mellitus without complications

E10 Type 1 diabetes mellitus

Includes: brittle diabetes (mellitus)

diabetes (mellitus) due to autoimmune process

diabetes (mellitus) due to immune mediated pancreatic islet beta-cell destruction

idiopathic diabetes (mellitus)

juvenile onset diabetes (mellitus)

ketosis-prone diabetes (mellitus)

Excludes 1: diabetes mellitus due to underlying condition (E08.-)

drug or chemical induced diabetes mellitus (E09.-)

gestational diabetes (O24.4-)

hyperglycemia NOS (R73.9)

neonatal diabetes mellitus (P70.2)

postpancreatectomy diabetes mellitus (E13.-)

postprocedural diabetes mellitus (E13.-)

secondary diabetes mellitus NEC (E13.-)

type 2 diabetes mellitus (E11.-)

E10.1 Type 1 diabetes mellitus with ketoacidosis

E10.10 Type 1 diabetes mellitus with ketoacidosis without coma

E10.11 Type 1 diabetes mellitus with ketoacidosis with coma

E10.2 Type 1 diabetes mellitus with kidney complications

E10.21 Type 1 diabetes mellitus with diabetic nephropathy

Type 1 diabetes mellitus with intercapillary glomerulosclerosis

Type 1 diabetes mellitus with intracapillary glomerulonephrosis

Type 1 diabetes mellitus with Kimmelstiel-Wilson disease

E10.22 Type 1 diabetes mellitus with diabetic chronic kidney disease

Type 1 diabetes mellitus with chronic kidney disease due to conditions classified to .21 and .22

Use additional code to identify stage of chronic kidney disease (N18.1-N18.6)

E10.29 Type 1 diabetes mellitus with other diabetic kidney complication

Type 1 diabetes mellitus with renal tubular degeneration

E10.3 Type 1 diabetes mellitus with ophthalmic complications

E10.31 Type 1 diabetes mellitus with unspecified diabetic retinopathy

E10.311 Type 1 diabetes mellitus with unspecified diabetic retinopathy with macular edema

E10.319 Type 1 diabetes mellitus with unspecified diabetic retinopathy without macular edema

E10.32 Type 1 diabetes mellitus with mild nonproliferative diabetic retinopathy

Type 1 diabetes mellitus with nonproliferative diabetic retinopathy NOS

E10.321 Type 1 diabetes mellitus with mild nonproliferative diabetic retinopathy with macular edema

E10.329 Type 1 diabetes mellitus with mild nonproliferative diabetic retinopathy without macular edema

E10.33 Type 1 diabetes mellitus with moderate nonproliferative diabetic retinopathy

- **E10.331** Type 1 diabetes mellitus with moderate nonproliferative diabetic retinopathy with macular edema
- **E10.339** Type 1 diabetes mellitus with moderate nonproliferative diabetic retinopathy without macular edema

E10.34 Type 1 diabetes mellitus with severe nonproliferative diabetic retinopathy

- **E10.341** Type 1 diabetes mellitus with severe nonproliferative diabetic retinopathy with macular edema
- **E10.349** Type 1 diabetes mellitus with severe nonproliferative diabetic retinopathy without macular edema

E10.35 Type 1 diabetes mellitus with proliferative diabetic retinopathy

- **E10.351** Type 1 diabetes mellitus with proliferative diabetic retinopathy with macular edema
- **E10.359** Type 1 diabetes mellitus with proliferative diabetic retinopathy without macular edema

E10.36 Type 1 diabetes mellitus with diabetic cataract

E10.39 Type 1 diabetes mellitus with other diabetic ophthalmic complication

E10.4 Type 1 diabetes mellitus with neurological complications

E10.40 Type 1 diabetes mellitus with diabetic neuropathy, unspecified

E10.41 Type 1 diabetes mellitus with diabetic mononeuropathy

E10.42 Type 1 diabetes mellitus with diabetic polyneuropathy

Type 1 diabetes mellitus with diabetic neuralgia

E10.43 Type 1 diabetes mellitus with diabetic autonomic (poly)neuropathy

Type 1 diabetes mellitus with diabetic gastroparesis

E10.44 Type 1 diabetes mellitus with diabetic amyotrophy

E10.49 Type 1 diabetes mellitus with other diabetic neurological complication

E10.5 Type 1 diabetes mellitus with circulatory complications

E10.51 Type 1 diabetes mellitus with diabetic peripheral angiopathy without gangrene

E10.52 Type 1 diabetes mellitus with diabetic peripheral angiopathy with gangrene

Type 1 diabetes mellitus with diabetic gangrene

E10.59 Type 1 diabetes mellitus with other circulatory complications

E10.6 Type 1 diabetes mellitus with other specified complications

E10.61 Type 1 diabetes mellitus with diabetic arthropathy

- **E10.610** Type 1 diabetes mellitus with diabetic neuropathic arthropathy

  Type 1 diabetes mellitus with Charc ſt's joints
- **E10.618** Type 1 diabetes mellitus with other diabetic arthropathy

E10.62 Type 1 diabetes mellitus with skin complications

- **E10.620** Type 1 diabetes mellitus with diabetic dermatitis

  Type 1 diabetes mellitus with diabetic necrobiosis lipoidica
- **E10.621** Type 1 diabetes mellitus with foot ulcer

  Use additional code to identify site of ulcer (L97.4-, L97.5-)
- **E10.622** Type 1 diabetes mellitus with other skin ulcer

  Use additional code to identify site of ulcer (L97.1-L97.9, L98.41-L98.49)
- **E10.628** Type 1 diabetes mellitus with other skin complications

E10.63 Type 1 diabetes mellitus with oral complications

- **E10.630** Type 1 diabetes mellitus with periodontal disease
- **E10.638** Type 1 diabetes mellitus with other oral complications

E10.64 Type 1 diabetes mellitus with hypoglycemia

- **E10.641** Type 1 diabetes mellitus with hypoglycemia with coma
- **E10.649** Type 1 diabetes mellitus with hypoglycemia without coma

E10.65 Type 1 diabetes mellitus with hyperglycemia

E10.69 Type 1 diabetes mellitus with other specified complication

Use additional code to identify complication

E10.8 Type 1 diabetes mellitus with unspecified complications

E10.9 Type 1 diabetes mellitus without complications

E11 Type 2 diabetes mellitus

Includes: diabetes (mellitus) due to insulin secretory defect
diabetes NOS
insulin resistant diabetes (mellitus)

Use additional code to identify any insulin use (Z79.4)

Excludes 1: diabetes mellitus due to underlying condition (E08.-)
drug or chemical induced diabetes mellitus (E09.-)
gestational diabetes (O24.4-)
neonatal diabetes mellitus (P70.2)
postpancreatectomy diabetes mellitus (E13.-)
postprocedural diabetes mellitus (E13.-)
secondary diabetes mellitus NEC (E13.-)
type 1 diabetes mellitus (E10.-)

E11.0 Type 2 diabetes mellitus with hyperosmolarity

E11.00 Type 2 diabetes mellitus with hyperosmolarity without nonketotic hyperglycemic-hyperosmolar coma (NKHHC)

E11.01 Type 2 diabetes mellitus with hyperosmolarity with coma

E11.2 Type 2 diabetes mellitus with kidney complications

E11.21 Type 2 diabetes mellitus with diabetic nephropathy

Type 2 diabetes mellitus with intercapillary glomerulosclerosis

Type 2 diabetes mellitus with intracapillary glomerulonephrosis

Type 2 diabetes mellitus with Kimmelstiel-Wilson disease

E11.22 Type 2 diabetes mellitus with diabetic chronic kidney disease

Type 2 diabetes mellitus with chronic kidney disease due to conditions classified to .21 and .22

Use additional code to identify stage of chronic kidney disease (N18.1-N18.6)

E11.29 Type 2 diabetes mellitus with other diabetic kidney complication

Type 2 diabetes mellitus with renal tubular degeneration

E11.3 Type 2 diabetes mellitus with ophthalmic complications

E11.31 Type 2 diabetes mellitus with unspecified diabetic retinopathy

E11.311 Type 2 diabetes mellitus with unspecified diabetic retinopathy with macular edema

E11.319 Type 2 diabetes mellitus with unspecified diabetic retinopathy without macular edema

E11.32 Type 2 diabetes mellitus with mild nonproliferative diabetic retinopathy

Type 2 diabetes mellitus with nonproliferative diabetic retinopathy NOS

E11.321 Type 2 diabetes mellitus with mild nonproliferative diabetic retinopathy with macular edema

E11.329 Type 2 diabetes mellitus with mild nonproliferative diabetic retinopathy without macular edema

E11.33 Type 2 diabetes mellitus with moderate nonproliferative diabetic retinopathy

E11.331 Type 2 diabetes mellitus with moderate nonproliferative diabetic retinopathy with macular edema

E11.339 Type 2 diabetes mellitus with moderate nonproliferative diabetic retinopathy without macular edema

E11.34 Type 2 diabetes mellitus with severe nonproliferative diabetic retinopathy

E11.341 Type 2 diabetes mellitus with severe nonproliferative diabetic retinopathy with macular edema

E11.349 Type 2 diabetes mellitus with severe nonproliferative diabetic retinopathy without macular edema

E11.35 Type 2 diabetes mellitus with proliferative diabetic retinopathy

E11.351 Type 2 diabetes mellitus with proliferative diabetic retinopathy with macular edema

E11.359 Type 2 diabetes mellitus with proliferative diabetic retinopathy without macular edema

E11.36 Type 2 diabetes mellitus with diabetic cataract

E11.39 Type 2 diabetes mellitus with other diabetic ophthalmic complication

E11.4 Type 2 diabetes mellitus with neurological complications

E11.40 Type 2 diabetes mellitus with diabetic neuropathy, unspecified

E11.41 Type 2 diabetes mellitus with diabetic mononeuropathy

E11.42 Type 2 diabetes mellitus with diabetic polyneuropathy

Type 2 diabetes mellitus with diabetic neuralgia

E11.43 Type 2 diabetes mellitus with diabetic autonomic (poly)neuropathy

Type 2 diabetes mellitus with diabetic gastroparesis

E11.44 Type 2 diabetes mellitus with diabetic amyotrophy

E11.49 Type 2 diabetes mellitus with other diabetic neurological complication

E11.5 Type 2 diabetes mellitus with circulatory complications

E11.51 Type 2 diabetes mellitus with diabetic peripheral angiopathy without gangrene

E11.52 Type 2 diabetes mellitus with diabetic peripheral angiopathy with gangrene

Type 2 diabetes mellitus with diabetic gangrene

E11.59 Type 2 diabetes mellitus with other circulatory complications

E11.6 Type 2 diabetes mellitus with other specified complications

E11.61 Type 2 diabetes mellitus with diabetic arthropathy

E11.610 Type 2 diabetes mellitus with diabetic neuropathic arthropathy

Type 2 diabetes mellitus with Charcot's joints

E11.618 Type 2 diabetes mellitus with other diabetic arthropathy

E11.62 Type 2 diabetes mellitus with skin complications

E11.620 Type 2 diabetes mellitus with diabetic dermatitis

Type 2 diabetes mellitus with diabetic necrobiosis lipoidica

E11.621 Type 2 diabetes mellitus with foot ulcer

Use additional code to identify site of ulcer (L97.4-, L97.5-)

E11.622 Type 2 diabetes mellitus with other skin ulcer

Use additional code to identify site of ulcer (L97.1-L97.9, L98.41-L98.49)

E11.628 Type 2 diabetes mellitus with other skin complications

E11.63 Type 2 diabetes mellitus with oral complications

E11.630 Type 2 diabetes mellitus with periodontal disease

E11.638 Type 2 diabetes mellitus with other oral complications

E11.64 Type 2 diabetes mellitus with hypoglycemia

E11.641 Type 2 diabetes mellitus with hypoglycemia with coma

E11.649 Type 2 diabetes mellitus with hypoglycemia without coma

E11.65 Type 2 diabetes mellitus with hyperglycemia

E11.69 Type 2 diabetes mellitus with other specified complication

Use additional code to identify complication

E11.8 Type 2 diabetes mellitus with unspecified complications

E11.9 Type 2 diabetes mellitus without complications

E13 Other specified diabetes mellitus

Includes: diabetes mellitus due to genetic defects of beta-cell function

diabetes mellitus due to genetic defects in insulin action

postpancreatectomy diabetes mellitus

postprocedural diabetes mellitus

secondary diabetes mellitus NEC

Use additional code to identify any insulin use (Z79.4)

Excludes 1: diabetes (mellitus) due to autoimmune process (E10.-)

diabetes (mellitus) due to immune mediated pancreatic islet beta-cell destruction (E10.-)

diabetes mellitus due to underlying condition (E08.-)

drug or chemical induced diabetes mellitus (E09.-)
gestational diabetes (O24.4-)
neonatal diabetes mellitus (P70.2)
type 2 diabetes mellitus (E11.-)

E13.0 Other specified diabetes mellitus with hyperosmolarity

E13.00 Other specified diabetes mellitus with hyperosmolarity without nonketotic hyperglycemic-hyperosmolar coma (NKHHC)

E13.01 Other specified diabetes mellitus with hyperosmolarity with coma

E13.1 Other specified diabetes mellitus with ketoacidosis

E13.10 Other specified diabetes mellitus with ketoacidosis without coma

E13.11 Other specified diabetes mellitus with ketoacidosis with coma

E13.2 Other specified diabetes mellitus with kidney complications

E13.21 Other specified diabetes mellitus with diabetic nephropathy

Other specified diabetes mellitus with intercapillary glomerulosclerosis

Other specified diabetes mellitus with intracapillary glomerulonephrosis

Other specified diabetes mellitus with Kimmelstiel-Wilson disease

E13.22 Other specified diabetes mellitus with diabetic chronic kidney disease

Other specified diabetes mellitus with chronic kidney disease due to conditions classified to 21 and 22

Use additional code to identify stage of chronic kidney disease (N18.1-N18.6)

E13.29 Other specified diabetes mellitus with other diabetic kidney complication

Other specified diabetes mellitus with renal tubular degeneration

E13.3 Other specified diabetes mellitus with ophthalmic complications

E13.31 Other specified diabetes mellitus with unspecified diabetic retinopathy

E13.311 Other specified diabetes mellitus with unspecified diabetic retinopathy with macular edema

E13.319 Other specified diabetes mellitus with unspecified diabetic retinopathy without macular edema

E13.32 Other specified diabetes mellitus with mild nonproliferative diabetic retinopathy

Other specified diabetes mellitus with nonproliferative diabetic retinopathy NOS

E13.321 Other specified diabetes mellitus with mild nonproliferative diabetic retinopathy with macular edema

E13.329 Other specified diabetes mellitus with mild nonproliferative diabetic retinopathy without macular edema

E13.33 Other specified diabetes mellitus with moderate nonproliferative diabetic retinopathy

E13.331 Other specified diabetes mellitus with moderate nonproliferative diabetic retinopathy with macular edema

E13.339 Other specified diabetes mellitus with moderate nonproliferative diabetic retinopathy without macular edema

E13.34 Other specified diabetes mellitus with severe nonproliferative diabetic retinopathy

E13.341 Other specified diabetes mellitus with severe nonproliferative diabetic retinopathy with macular edema

E13.349 Other specified diabetes mellitus with severe nonproliferative diabetic retinopathy without macular edema

E13.35 Other specified diabetes mellitus with proliferative diabetic retinopathy

E13.351 Other specified diabetes mellitus with proliferative diabetic retinopathy with macular edema

E13.359 Other specified diabetes mellitus with proliferative diabetic retinopathy without macular edema

E13.36 Other specified diabetes mellitus with diabetic cataract

E13.39 Other specified diabetes mellitus with other diabetic ophthalmic complication

E13.4 Other specified diabetes mellitus with neurological complications

E13.40 Other specified diabetes mellitus with diabetic neuropathy, unspecified

E13.41 Other specified diabetes mellitus with diabetic mononeuropathy

E13.42 Other specified diabetes mellitus with diabetic polyneuropathy

Other specified diabetes mellitus with diabetic neuralgia

E13.43 Other specified diabetes mellitus with diabetic " autonomic (poly)neuropathy

Other specified diabetes mellitus with diabetic gastroparesis

E13.44 Other specified diabetes mellitus with diabetic amyotrophy

E13.49 Other specified diabetes mellitus with other diabetic neurological complication

E13.5 Other specified diabetes mellitus with circulatory complications

E13.51 Other specified diabetes mellitus with diabetic peripheral angiopathy without gangrene

E13.52 Other specified diabetes mellitus with diabetic peripheral angiopathy with gangrene

Other specified diabetes mellitus with diabetic gangrene

E13.59 Other specified diabetes mellitus with other circulatory complications

E13.6 Other specified diabetes mellitus with other specified complications

E13.61 Other specified diabetes mellitus with diabetic arthropathy

E13.610 Other specified diabetes mellitus with diabetic neuropathic arthropathy

Other specified diabetes mellitus with Charc∫t's joints

E13.618 Other specified diabetes mellitus with other diabetic arthropathy

E13.62 Other specified diabetes mellitus with skin complications

E13.620 Other specified diabetes mellitus with diabetic dermatitis

Other specified diabetes mellitus with diabetic necrobiosis lipoidica

● New code　　　　▲ Revised code　　　　⑦ 7th digit required　　　　⊗ Placeholder required

E13.621   Other specified diabetes mellitus with foot ulcer

Use additional code to identify site of ulcer (L97.4-, L97.5-)

E13.622   Other specified diabetes mellitus with other skin ulcer

Use additional code to identify site of ulcer (L97.1-L97.9, L98.41-L98.49)

E13.628   Other specified diabetes mellitus with other skin complications

E13.63   Other specified diabetes mellitus with oral complications

E13.630   Other specified diabetes mellitus with periodontal disease

E13.638   Other specified diabetes mellitus with other oral complications

E13.64   Other specified diabetes mellitus with hypoglycemia

E13.641   Other specified diabetes mellitus with hypoglycemia with coma

E13.649   Other specified diabetes mellitus with hypoglycemia without coma

E13.65   Other specified diabetes mellitus with hyperglycemia

E13.69   Other specified diabetes mellitus with other specified complication

Use additional code to identify complication

E13.8   Other specified diabetes mellitus with unspecified complications

E13.9   Other specified diabetes mellitus without complications

OTHER DISORDERS OF GLUCOSE REGULATION AND PANCREATIC INTERNAL SECRETION (E15-E16)

E15   Nondiabetic hypoglycemic coma

Includes: drug-induced insulin coma in nondiabetic

hyperinsulinism with hypoglycemic coma

hypoglycemic coma NOS

E16   Other disorders of pancreatic internal secretion

E16.0   Drug-induced hypoglycemia without coma

Use additional code for adverse effect, if applicable, to identify drug (T36-T50 with fifth or sixth character 5)

E16.1   Other hypoglycemia

Functional hyperinsulinism

Functional nonhyperinsulinemic hypoglycemia

Hyperinsulinism NOS

Hyperplasia of pancreatic islet beta cells NOS

Excludes 1: hypoglycemia in infant of diabetic mother (P70.1)

neonatal hypoglycemia (P70.4)

E16.2   Hypoglycemia, unspecified

E16.3   Increased secretion of glucagon

Hyperplasia of pancreatic endocrine cells with glucagon excess

E16.4   Increased secretion of gastrin

Hypergastrinemia

Hyperplasia of pancreatic endocrine cells with gastrin excess

Zollinger-Ellison syndrome

E16.8   Other specified disorders of pancreatic internal secretion

Increased secretion from endocrine pancreas of growth hormone-releasing hormone

Increased secretion from endocrine pancreas of pancreatic polypeptide

Increased secretion from endocrine pancreas of somatostatin

Increased secretion from endocrine pancreas of vasoactive-intestinal polypeptide

E16.9   Disorder of pancreatic internal secretion, unspecified

Islet-cell hyperplasia NOS

Pancreatic endocrine cell hyperplasia NOS

DISORDERS OF OTHER ENDOCRINE GLANDS (E20-E35)

Excludes 1: galactorrhea (N64.3)

gynecomastia (N62)

E20   Hypoparathyroidism

Excludes 1: Di George's syndrome (D82.1)

postprocedural hypoparathyroidism (E89.2)

tetany NOS (R29.0)

transitory neonatal hypoparathyroidism (P71.4)

E20.0   Idiopathic hypoparathyroidism

E20.1   Pseudohypoparathyroidism

E20.8   Other hypoparathyroidism

E20.9   Hypoparathyroidism, unspecified

Parathyroid tetany

E21   Hyperparathyroidism and other disorders of parathyroid gland

Excludes 1: adult osteomalacia (M83.-)

ectopic hyperparathyroidism (E34.2)

familial hypocalciuric hypercalcemia (E83.52)

hungry bone syndrome (E83.81)

infantile and juvenile osteomalacia (E55.0)

E21.0   Primary hyperparathyroidism

Hyperplasia of parathyroid

Osteitis fibrosa cystica generalisata [von Recklinghausen's disease of bone]

E21.1   Secondary hyperparathyroidism, not elsewhere classified

Excludes 1: secondary hyperparathyroidism of renal origin (N25.81)

E21.2   Other hyperparathyroidism

Tertiary hyperparathyroidism

Excludes 1: familial hypocalciuric hypercalcemia (E83.52)

E21.3   Hyperparathyroidism, unspecified

E21.4   Other specified disorders of parathyroid gland

E21.5   Disorder of parathyroid gland, unspecified

E22   Hyperfunction of pituitary gland

Excludes 1: Cushing's syndrome (E24.-)

Nelson's syndrome (E24.1)

overproduction of ACTH not associated with Cushing's disease (E27.0)

overproduction of pituitary ACTH (E24.0)

overproduction of thyroid-stimulating hormone (E05.8-)

E22.0   Acromegaly and pituitary gigantism

Overproduction of growth hormone

Excludes 1: constitutional gigantism (E34.4)

constitutional tall stature (E34.4)

increased secretion from endocrine pancreas of growth hormone-releasing hormone (E16.8)

E22.1   Hyperprolactinemia

Use additional code for adverse effect, if applicable, to identify drug (T36-T50 with fifth or sixth character 5)

E22.2   Syndrome of inappropriate secretion of antidiuretic hormone

E22.8   Other hyperfunction of pituitary gland

Central precocious puberty

E22.9   Hyperfunction of pituitary gland, unspecified

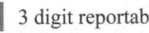

E23 Hypofunction and other disorders of the pituitary gland

Includes: the listed conditions whether the disorder is in the pituitary or the hypothalamus

Excludes 1: postprocedural hypopituitarism (E89.3)

E23.0 Hypopituitarism
Fertile eunuch syndrome
Hypogonadotropic hypogonadism
Idiopathic growth hormone deficiency
Isolated deficiency of gonadotropin
Isolated deficiency of growth hormone
Isolated deficiency of pituitary hormone
Kallmann's syndrome
Lorain-Levi short stature
Necrosis of pituitary gland (postpartum)
Panhypopituitarism
Pituitary cachexia
Pituitary insufficiency NOS
Pituitary short stature
Sheehan's syndrome
Simmonds' disease

E23.1 Drug-induced hypopituitarism
Use additional code for adverse effect, if applicable, to identify drug (T36-T50 with fifth or sixth character 5)

E23.2 diabetes insipidus
Excludes 1: nephrogenic diabetes insipidus (N25.1)

E23.3 Hypothalamic dysfunction, not elsewhere classified
Excludes 1: Prader-Willi syndrome (Q87.1)
Russell-Silver syndrome (Q87.1)

E23.6 Other disorders of pituitary gland
Abscess of pituitary
Adiposogenital dystrophy

E23.7 Disorder of pituitary gland, unspecified

E24 Cushing's syndrome

Excludes 1: congenital adrenal hyperplasia (E25.0)

E24.0 Pituitary-dependent Cushing's disease
Overproduction of pituitary ACTH
Pituitary-dependent hypercorticalism

E24.1 Nelson's syndrome

E24.2 Drug-induced Cushing's syndrome
Use additional code for adverse effect, if applicable, to identify drug (T36-T50 with fifth or sixth character 5)

E24.3 Ectopic ACTH syndrome

E24.4 Alcohol-induced pseudo-Cushing's syndrome

E24.8 Other Cushing's syndrome

E24.9 Cushing's syndrome, unspecified

E25 Adrenogenital disorders

Includes: adrenogenital syndromes, virilizing or feminizing, whether acquired or due to adrenal hyperplasia consequent on inborn enzyme defects in hormone synthesis
Female adrenal pseudohermaphroditism
Female heterosexual precocious pseudopuberty
Male isosexual precocious pseudopuberty
Male macrogenitosomia praecox
Male sexual precocity with adrenal hyperplasia
Male virilization (female)

Excludes 1: indeterminate sex and pseudohermaphroditism (Q56)
chromosomal abnormalities (Q90-Q99)

E25.0 Congenital adrenogenital disorders associated with enzyme deficiency
Congenital adrenal hyperplasia
21-Hydroxylase deficiency

Salt-losing congenital adrenal hyperplasia

E25.8 Other adrenogenital disorders
Idiopathic adrenogenital disorder
Use additional code for adverse effect, if applicable, to identify drug (T36-T50 with fifth or sixth character 5)

E25.9 Adrenogenital disorder, unspecified
Adrenogenital syndrome NOS

E26 Hyperaldosteronism

E26.0 Primary hyperaldosteronism

E26.01 Conn's syndrome
Code also adrenal adenoma (D35.0-)

E26.02 Glucocorticoid-remediable aldosteronism
Familial aldosteronism type I

E26.09 Other primary hyperaldosteronism
Primary aldosteronism due to adrenal hyperplasia (bilateral)

E26.1 Secondary hyperaldosteronism

E26.8 Other hyperaldosteronism

E26.81 Bartter's syndrome

E26.89 Other hyperaldosteronism

E26.9 Hyperaldosteronism, unspecified
Aldosteronism NOS
Hyperaldosteronism NOS

E27 Other disorders of adrenal gland

E27.0 Other adrenocortical overactivity
Overproduction of ACTH, not associated with Cushing's disease
Premature adrenarche
Excludes 1: Cushing's syndrome (E24.-)

E27.1 Primary adrenocortical insufficiency
Addison's disease
Autoimmune adrenalitis
Excludes 1: Addison only phenotype adrenoleukodystrophy (E71.528)
amyloidosis (E85-)
tuberculous Addison's disease (A18.7)
Waterhouse-Friderichsen syndrome (A39.1)

E27.2 Addisonian crisis
Adrenal crisis
Adrenocortical crisis

E27.3 Drug-induced adrenocortical insufficiency
Use additional code for adverse effect, if applicable, to identify drug (T36-T50 with fifth or sixth character 5)

E27.4 Other and unspecified adrenocortical insufficiency
Excludes 1: adrenoleukodystrophy [Addison-Schilder] (E71.528)
Waterhouse-Friderichsen syndrome (A39.1)

E27.40 Unspecified adrenocortical insufficiency
Adrenocortical insufficiency NOS
Hypoaldosteronism

E27.49 Other adrenocortical insufficiency
Adrenal hemorrhage
Adrenal infarction

E27.5 Adrenomedullary hyperfunction
Adrenomedullary hyperplasia
Catecholamine hypersecretion

E27.8 Other specified disorders of adrenal gland
Abnormality of cortisol-binding globulin

E27.9 Disorder of adrenal gland, unspecified

E28 Ovarian dysfunction

Excludes 1: isolated gonadotropin deficiency (E23.0)
postprocedural ovarian failure (E89.4-)

● New code   ▲ Revised code   ⑦ 7ᵗʰ digit required   ⊗ Placeholder required

E28.0 Estrogen excess
Use additional code for adverse effect, if applicable, to identify drug (T36-T50 with fifth or sixth character 5)

E28.1 Androgen excess
Hypersecretion of ovarian androgens
Use additional code for adverse effect, if applicable, to identify drug (T36-T50 with fifth or sixth character 5)

E28.2 Polycystic ovarian syndrome
Sclerocystic ovary syndrome
Stein-Leventhal syndrome

E28.3 Primary ovarian failure
Excludes 1: pure gonadal dysgenesis (Q99.1)
Turner's syndrome (Q96.-)

    E28.31 Premature menopause
        E28.310 Symptomatic premature menopause
Symptoms such as flushing, sleeplessness, headache, lack of concentration, associated with premature menopause
        E28.319 Asymptomatic premature menopause
Premature menopause NOS

    E28.39 Other primary ovarian failure
Decreased estrogen
Resistant ovary syndrome

E28.8 Other ovarian dysfunction
Ovarian hyperfunction NOS
Excludes 1: postprocedural ovarian failure (E89.4-)

E28.9 Ovarian dysfunction, unspecified

E29 Testicular dysfunction
Excludes 1: androgen insensitivity syndrome (E34.5-)
azoospermia or oligospermia NOS (N46.0-N46.1)
isolated gonadotropin deficiency (E23.0)
Klinefelter's syndrome (Q98.0-Q98.2, Q98.4)

E29.0 Testicular hyperfunction
Hypersecretion of testicular hormones

E29.1 Testicular hypofunction
Defective biosynthesis of testicular androgen NOS
5-delta-Reductase deficiency (with male pseudohermaphroditism)
Testicular hypogonadism NOS
Use additional code for adverse effect, if applicable, to identify drug (T36-T50 with fifth or sixth character 5)
Excludes 1: postprocedural testicular hypofunction (E89.5)

E29.8 Other testicular dysfunction

E29.9 Testicular dysfunction, unspecified

E30 Disorders of puberty, not elsewhere classified

E30.0 Delayed puberty
Constitutional delay of puberty
Delayed sexual development

E30.1 Precocious puberty
Precocious menstruation
Excludes 1: Albright (-McCune) (-Sternberg) syndrome (Q78.1)
central precocious puberty (E22.8)
congenital adrenal hyperplasia (E25.0)
female heterosexual precocious pseudopuberty (E25.-)
male isosexual precocious pseudopuberty (E25.-)

E30.8 Other disorders of puberty
Premature thelarche

E30.9 Disorder of puberty, unspecified

E31 Polyglandular dysfunction
Excludes 1: ataxia telangiectasia [Louis-Bar] (G11.3)
dystrophia myotonica [Steinert] (G71.11)
pseudohypoparathyroidism (E20.1)

E31.0 Autoimmune polyglandular failure
Schmidt's syndrome

E31.1 Polyglandular hyperfunction
Excludes 1: multiple endocrine adenomatosis (E31.2-)
multiple endocrine neoplasia (E31.2-)

E31.2 Multiple endocrine neoplasia [MEN] syndromes
Multiple endocrine adenomatosis
Code also any associated malignancies and other conditions associated with the syndromes

    E31.20 Multiple endocrine neoplasia [MEN] syndrome, unspecified
Multiple endocrine adenomatosis NOS
Multiple endocrine neoplasia [MEN] syndrome NOS
    E31.21 Multiple endocrine neoplasia [MEN] type I
Wermer's syndrome
    E31.22 Multiple endocrine neoplasia [MEN] type IIA
Sipple's syndrome
    E31.23 Multiple endocrine neoplasia [MEN] type IIB

E31.8 Other polyglandular dysfunction

E31.9 Polyglandular dysfunction, unspecified

E32 Diseases of thymus
Excludes 1: aplasia or hypoplasia of thymus with immunodeficiency (D82.1)
myasthenia gravis (G70.0)

E32.0 Persistent hyperplasia of thymus
Hypertrophy of thymus

E32.1 Abscess of thymus

E32.8 Other diseases of thymus
Excludes 1: aplasia or hypoplasia with immunodeficiency (D82.1)
thymoma (D15.0)

E32.9 Disease of thymus, unspecified

E34 Other endocrine disorders
Excludes 1: pseudohypoparathyroidism (E20.1)

E34.0 Carcinoid syndrome
Note: May be used as an additional code to identify functional activity associated with a carcinoid tumor.

E34.1 Other hypersecretion of intestinal hormones

E34.2 Ectopic hormone secretion, not elsewhere classified
Excludes 1: ectopic ACTH syndrome (E24.3)

E34.3 Short stature due to endocrine disorder
Constitutional short stature
Laron-type short stature
Excludes 1: achondroplastic short stature (Q77.4)
hypochondroplastic short stature (Q77.4)
nutritional short stature (E45)
pituitary short stature (E23.0)
progeria (E34.8)
renal short stature (N25.0)
Russell-Silver syndrome (Q87.1)
short-limbed stature with immunodeficiency (D82.2)
short stature in specific dysmorphic syndromes - code to syndrome - see Alphabetical Index
short stature NOS (R62.52)

E34.4 Constitutional tall stature
Constitutional gigantism

E34.5 Androgen insensitivity syndrome

    E34.50 Androgen insensitivity syndrome, unspecified
           Androgen insensitivity NOS

    E34.51 Complete androgen insensitivity syndrome
           Complete androgen insensitivity
           de Quervain syndrome
           Goldberg-Maxwell syndrome

    E34.52 Partial androgen insensitivity syndrome
           Partial androgen insensitivity
           Reifenstein syndrome

E34.8 Other specified endocrine disorders
    Pineal gland dysfunction
    Progeria
    Excludes 2: pseudohypoparathyroidism (E20.1)

E34.9 Endocrine disorder, unspecified
    Endocrine disturbance NOS
    Hormone disturbance NOS

E35 Disorders of endocrine glands in diseases classified elsewhere
    Code first underlying disease, such as:
        late congenital syphilis of thymus gland [Dubois disease] (A50.5)
        tuberculous calcification of adrenal gland (B90.8)
    Excludes 1: Echinococcus granulosus infection of thyroid gland (B67.3)
        meningococcal hemorrhagic adrenalitis (A39.1)
        syphilis of endocrine gland (A52.79)
        tuberculosis of adrenal gland, except calcification (A18.7)
        tuberculosis of endocrine gland NEC (A18.82)
        tuberculosis of thyroid gland (A18.81)
        Waterhouse-Friderichsen syndrome (A39.1)

INTRAOPERATIVE COMPLICATIONS OF ENDOCRINE SYSTEM (E36)

E36 Intraoperative complications of endocrine system
    Excludes 2: postprocedural endocrine and metabolic complications and disorders, not elsewhere classified (E89.-)

E36.0 Intraoperative hemorrhage and hematoma of an endocrine system organ or structure complicating a procedure
    Excludes 1: intraoperative hemorrhage and hematoma of an endocrine system organ or structure due to accidental puncture or laceration during a procedure (E36.1-)

    E36.01 Intraoperative hemorrhage and hematoma of an endocrine system organ or structure complicating an endocrine system procedure

    E36.02 Intraoperative hemorrhage and hematoma of an endocrine system organ or structure complicating other procedure

E36.1 Accidental puncture and laceration of an endocrine system organ or structure during a procedure
    E36.11 Accidental puncture and laceration of an endocrine system organ or structure during an endocrine system procedure
    E36.12 Accidental puncture and laceration of an endocrine system organ or structure during other procedure

E36.8 Other intraoperative complications of endocrine system
    Use additional code, if applicable, to further specify disorder

MALNUTRITION (E40-E46)
Excludes 1: intestinal malabsorption (K90.-)

        sequelae of protein-calorie malnutrition (E64.0)
Excludes 2: nutritional anemias (D50-D53)
        starvation (T73.0)

E40 Kwashiorkor
    Severe malnutrition with nutritional edema with dyspigmentation of skin and hair
    Excludes 1: marasmic kwashiorkor (E42)

E41 Nutritional marasmus
    Severe malnutrition with marasmus
    Excludes 1: marasmic kwashiorkor (E42)

E42 Marasmic kwashiorkor
    Intermediate form severe protein-calorie malnutrition
    Severe protein-calorie malnutrition with signs of both kwashiorkor and marasmus

E43 Unspecified severe protein-calorie malnutrition
    Starvation edema

E44 Protein-calorie malnutrition of moderate and mild degree
    E44.0 Moderate protein-calorie malnutrition
    E44.1 Mild protein-calorie malnutrition

E45 Retarded development following protein-calorie malnutrition
    Nutritional short stature
    Nutritional stunting
    Physical retardation due to malnutrition

E46 Unspecified protein-calorie malnutrition
    Malnutrition NOS
    Protein-calorie imbalance NOS
    Excludes 1: nutritional deficiency NOS (E63.9)

OTHER NUTRITIONAL DEFICIENCIES (E50-E64)
Excludes 2: nutritional anemias (D50-D53)

E50 Vitamin A deficiency
    Excludes 1: sequelae of vitamin A deficiency (E64.1)
    E50.0 Vitamin A deficiency with conjunctival xerosis
    E50.1 Vitamin A deficiency with Bitot's spot and conjunctival xerosis
        Bitot's spot in the young child
    E50.2 Vitamin A deficiency with corneal xerosis
    E50.3 Vitamin A deficiency with corneal ulceration and xerosis
    E50.4 Vitamin A deficiency with keratomalacia
    E50.5 Vitamin A deficiency with night blindness
    E50.6 Vitamin A deficiency with xerophthalmic scars of cornea
    E50.7 Other ocular manifestations of vitamin A deficiency
        Xerophthalmia NOS
    E50.8 Other manifestations of vitamin A deficiency
        Follicular keratosis
        Xeroderma
    E50.9 Vitamin A deficiency, unspecified
        Hypovitaminosis A NOS

E51 Thiamine deficiency
    Excludes 1: sequelae of thiamine deficiency (E64.8)
    E51.1 Beriberi
        E51.11 Dry beriberi
            Beriberi NOS
            Beriberi with polyneuropathy
        E51.12 Wet beriberi
            Beriberi with cardiovascular manifestations
            Cardiovascular beriberi
            Shoshin disease
    E51.2 Wernicke's encephalopathy
    E51.8 Other manifestations of thiamine deficiency
    E51.9 Thiamine deficiency, unspecified

E52 Niacin deficiency [pellagra]

Niacin (-tryptophan) deficiency
Nicotinamide deficiency
Pellagra (alcoholic)
Excludes 1: sequelae of niacin deficiency (E64.8)

E53 Deficiency of other B group vitamins
Excludes 1: sequelae of vitamin B deficiency (E64.8)

E53.0 Riboflavin deficiency
Ariboflavinosis
Vitamin B2 deficiency

E53.1 Pyridoxine deficiency
Vitamin B6 deficiency
Excludes 1: pyridoxine-responsive sideroblastic anemia (D64.3)

E53.8 Deficiency of other specified B group vitamins
Biotin deficiency
Cyanocobalamin deficiency
Folate deficiency
Folic acid deficiency
Pantothenic acid deficiency
Vitamin B12 deficiency
Excludes 1: folate deficiency anemia (D52.-)
vitamin B12 deficiency anemia (D51.-)

E53.9 Vitamin B deficiency, unspecified

E54 Ascorbic acid deficiency
Deficiency of vitamin C
Scurvy
Excludes 1: scorbutic anemia (D53.2)
sequelae of vitamin C deficiency (E64.2)

E55 Vitamin D deficiency
Excludes 1: adult osteomalacia (M83.-)
osteoporosis (M80-)
sequelae of rickets (E64.3)

E55.0 Rickets, active
Infantile Osteomalacia
Juvenile Osteomalacia
Excludes 1: celiac rickets (K90.0)
Crohn's rickets (K50.-)
hereditary vitamin D-dependent rickets (E83.32)
inactive rickets (E64.3)
renal rickets (N25.0)
sequelae of rickets (E64.3)
vitamin D-resistant rickets (E83.31)

E55.9 Vitamin D deficiency, unspecified
Avitaminosis D

E56 Other vitamin deficiencies
Excludes 1: sequelae of other vitamin deficiencies (E64.8)

E56.0 Deficiency of vitamin E

E56.1 Deficiency of vitamin K
Excludes 1: deficiency of coagulation factor due to vitamin K deficiency (D68.4)
vitamin K deficiency of newborn (P53)

E56.8 Deficiency of other vitamins

E56.9 Vitamin deficiency, unspecified

E58 Dietary calcium deficiency
Excludes 1: disorders of calcium metabolism (E83.5-)
sequelae of calcium deficiency (E64.8)

E59 Dietary selenium deficiency
Keshan disease
Excludes 1: sequelae of selenium deficiency (E64.8)

E60 Dietary zinc deficiency

E61 Deficiency of other nutrient elements

Use additional code for adverse effect, if applicable, to identify drug (T36-T50 with fifth or sixth character 5)
Excludes 1: disorders of mineral metabolism (E83.-)
iodine deficiency related thyroid disorders (E00-E02)
sequelae of malnutrition and other nutritional deficiencies (E64.-)

E61.0 Copper deficiency

E61.1 Iron deficiency
Excludes 1: iron deficiency anemia (D50.-)

E61.2 Magnesium deficiency

E61.3 Manganese deficiency

E61.4 Chromium deficiency

E61.5 Molybdenum deficiency

E61.6 Vanadium deficiency

E61.7 Deficiency of multiple nutrient elements

E61.8 Deficiency of other specified nutrient elements

E61.9 Deficiency of nutrient element, unspecified

E63 Other nutritional deficiencies
Excludes 1: dehydration (E86.0)
failure to thrive, adult (R62.7)
failure to thrive, child (R62.51)
feeding problems in newborn (P92.-)
sequelae of malnutrition and other nutritional deficiencies (E64.-)

E63.0 Essential fatty acid [EFA] deficiency

E63.1 Imbalance of constituents of food intake

E63.8 Other specified nutritional deficiencies

E63.9 Nutritional deficiency, unspecified

E64 Sequelae of malnutrition and other nutritional deficiencies
Note: This category is to be used to indicate conditions in categories E43, E44, E46, E50-E63 as the cause of sequelae, which are themselves classified elsewhere. The 'sequelae' include conditions specified as such; they also include the late effects of diseases classifiable to the above categories if the disease itself is no longer present.
Code first condition resulting from (sequela) of malnutrition and other nutritional deficiencies

E64.0 Sequelae of protein-calorie malnutrition
Excludes 2: retarded development following protein-calorie malnutrition (E45)

E64.1 Sequelae of vitamin A deficiency

E64.2 Sequelae of vitamin C deficiency

E64.3 Sequelae of rickets

E64.8 Sequelae of other nutritional deficiencies

E64.9 Sequelae of unspecified nutritional deficiency

OVERWEIGHT, OBESITY AND OTHER HYPERALIMENTATION (E65-E68)

E65 Localized adiposity
Fat pad

E66 Overweight and obesity
Code first obesity complicating pregnancy, childbirth and the puerperium, if applicable (O99.21-)
Use additional code to identify body mass index (BMI), if known (Z68.-)
Excludes 1: adiposogenital dystrophy (E23.6)
lipomatosis NOS (E88.2)
lipomatosis dolorosa [Dercum] (E88.2)
Prader-Willi syndrome (Q87.1)

E66.0 Obesity due to excess calories
E66.01 Morbid (severe) obesity due to excess calories
Excludes 1: morbid (severe) obesity with alveolar hypoventilation (E66.2)

E66.09   Other obesity due to excess calories

E66.1   Drug-induced obesity

Use additional code for adverse effect, if applicable, to identify drug (T36-T50 with fifth or sixth character 5)

E66.2   Morbid (severe) obesity with alveolar hypoventilation
Pickwickian syndrome

E66.3   Overweight

E66.8   Other obesity

E66.9   Obesity, unspecified
Obesity NOS

E67   Other hyperalimentation

Excludes 1: hyperalimentation NOS (R63.2)
sequelae of hyperalimentation (E68)

E67.0   Hypervitaminosis A

E67.1   Hypercarotinemia

E67.2   Megavitamin-B6 syndrome

E67.3   Hypervitaminosis D

E67.8   Other specified hyperalimentation

E68   Sequelae of hyperalimentation

Code first condition resulting from (sequela) of hyperalimentation

METABOLIC DISORDERS (E70-E88)

Excludes 1: androgen insensitivity syndrome (E34.5-)
congenital adrenal hyperplasia (E25.0)
Ehlers-Danlos syndrome (Q79.6)
hemolytic anemias attributable to enzyme disorders (D55.-)
Marfan's syndrome (Q87.4)
5-alpha-reductase deficiency (E29.1)

E70   Disorders of aromatic amino-acid metabolism

E70.0   Classical phenylketonuria

E70.1   Other hyperphenylalaninemias

E70.2   Disorders of tyrosine metabolism

Excludes 1: transitory tyrosinemia of newborn (P74.5)

E70.20   Disorder of tyrosine metabolism, unspecified

E70.21   Tyrosinemia
Hypertyrosinemia

E70.29   Other disorders of tyrosine metabolism
Alkaptonuria
Ochronosis

E70.3   Albinism

E70.30   Albinism, unspecified

E70.31   Ocular albinism

E70.310   X-linked ocular albinism

E70.311   Autosomal recessive ocular albinism

E70.318   Other ocular albinism

E70.319   Ocular albinism, unspecified

E70.32   Oculocutaneous albinism

Excludes 1: Chediak-Higashi syndrome (E70.330)
Hermansky-Pudlak syndrome (E70.331)

E70.320   Tyrosinase negative oculocutaneous albinism
Albinism I
Oculocutaneous albinism ty-neg

E70.321   Tyrosinase positive oculocutaneous albinism
Albinism II
Oculocutaneous albinism ty-pos

E70.328   Other oculocutaneous albinism
Cross syndrome

E70.329   Oculocutaneous albinism, unspecified

E70.33   Albinism with hematologic abnormality

E70.330   Chediak-Higashi syndrome

E70.331   Hermansky-Pudlak syndrome

E70.338   Other albinism with hematologic abnormality

E70.339   Albinism with hematologic abnormality, unspecified

E70.39   Other specified albinism
Piebaldism

E70.4   Disorders of histidine metabolism

E70.40   Disorders of histidine metabolism, unspecified

E70.41   Histidinemia

E70.49   Other disorders of histidine metabolism

E70.5   Disorders of tryptophan metabolism

E70.8   Other disorders of aromatic amino-acid metabolism

E70.9   Disorder of aromatic amino-acid metabolism, unspecified

E71   Disorders of branched-chain amino-acid metabolism and fatty-acid metabolism

E71.0   Maple-syrup-urine disease

E71.1   Other disorders of branched-chain amino-acid metabolism

E71.11   Branched-chain organic acidurias

E71.110   Isovaleric acidemia

E71.111   3-methylglutaconic aciduria

E71.118   Other branched-chain organic acidurias

E71.12   Disorders of propionate metabolism

E71.120   Methylmalonic acidemia

E71.121   Propionic acidemia

E71.128   Other disorders of propionate metabolism

E71.19   Other disorders of branched-chain amino-acid metabolism
Hyperleucine-isoleucinemia
Hypervalinemia

E71.2   Disorder of branched-chain amino-acid metabolism, unspecified

E71.3   Disorders of fatty-acid metabolism

Excludes 1: peroxisomal disorders (E71.5)
Refsum's disease (G60.1)
Schilder's disease (G37.0)

Excludes 2: carnitine deficiency due to inborn error of metabolism (E71.42)

E71.30   Disorder of fatty-acid metabolism, unspecified

E71.31   Disorders of fatty-acid oxidation

E71.310   Long chain/very long chain acyl CoA dehydrogenase deficiency
LCAD
VLCAD

E71.311   Medium chain acyl CoA dehydrogenase deficiency
MCAD

E71.312   Short chain acyl CoA dehydrogenase deficiency
SCAD

E71.313   Glutaric aciduria type II
Glutaric aciduria type II A
Glutaric aciduria type II B
Glutaric aciduria type II C

Excludes 1: glutaric aciduria (type 1) NOS (E72.3)

E71.314   Muscle carnitine palmitoyltransferase deficiency

E71.318 Other disorders of fatty-acid oxidation

E71.32 Disorders of ketone metabolism

E71.39 Other disorders of fatty-acid metabolism

E71.4 Disorders of carnitine metabolism

Excludes 1: Muscle carnitine palmitoyltransferase deficiency (E71.314)

E71.40 Disorder of carnitine metabolism, unspecified

E71.41 Primary carnitine deficiency

E71.42 Carnitine deficiency due to inborn errors of metabolism

Code also associated inborn error or metabolism

E71.43 Iatrogenic carnitine deficiency

Carnitine deficiency due to:

hemodialysis

Valproic acid therapy

E71.44 Other secondary carnitine deficiency

E71.440 Ruvalcaba-Myhre-Smith syndrome

E71.448 Other secondary carnitine deficiency

E71.5 Peroxisomal disorders

Excludes 1: Schilder's disease (G37.0)

E71.50 Peroxisomal disorder, unspecified

E71.51 Disorders of peroxisome biogenesis

Group 1 peroxisomal disorders

Excludes 1: Refsum's disease (G60.1)

E71.510 Zellweger syndrome

E71.511 Neonatal adrenoleukodystrophy

Excludes 1: X-linked adrenoleukodystrophy (E71.42-)

E71.518 Other disorders of peroxisome biogenesis

E71.52 X-linked adrenoleukodystrophy

E71.520 Childhood cerebral X-linked adrenoleukodystrophy

E71.521 Adolescent X-linked adrenoleukodystrophy

E71.522 Adrenomyeloneuropathy

E71.528 Other X-linked adrenoleukodystrophy

Addison only phenotype adrenoleukodystrophy

Addison-Schilder adrenoleukodystrophy

E71.529 X-linked adrenoleukodystrophy, unspecified type

E71.53 Other group 2 peroxisomal disorders

E71.54 Other peroxisomal disorders

E71.540 Rhizomelic chondrodysplasia punctata

Excludes 1: chondrodysplasia punctata NOS (Q77.3)

E71.541 Zellweger-like syndrome

E71.542 Other group 3 peroxisomal disorders

E71.548 Other peroxisomal disorders

E72 Other disorders of amino-acid metabolism

Excludes 1: disorders of:

aromatic amino-acid metabolism (E70.-)

branched-chain amino-acid metabolism (E71.0-E71.2)

fatty-acid metabolism (E71.3)

purine and pyrimidine metabolism (E79.-)

gout (M1A-, M10.-)

E72.0 Disorders of amino-acid transport

Excludes 1: disorders of tryptophan metabolism (E70.5)

E72.00 Disorders of amino-acid transport, unspecified

E72.01 Cystinuria

E72.02 Hartnup's disease

E72.03 Lowe's syndrome

Use additional code for associated glaucoma (H42)

E72.04 Cystinosis

Fanconi (-de Toni) (-DebrΘ) syndrome with cystinosis

Excludes 1: Fanconi (-de Toni) (-DebrΘ) syndrome without cystinosis (E72.09)

E72.09 Other disorders of amino-acid transport

Fanconi (-de Toni) (-DebrΘ) syndrome, unspecified

E72.1 Disorders of sulfur-bearing amino-acid metabolism

Excludes 1: cystinosis (E72.04)

cystinuria (E72.01)

transcobalamin II deficiency (D51.2)

E72.10 Disorders of sulfur-bearing amino-acid metabolism, unspecified

E72.11 Homocystinuria

Cystathionine synthase deficiency

E72.12 Methylenetetrahydrofolate reductase deficiency

E72.19 Other disorders of sulfur-bearing amino-acid metabolism

Cystathioninuria

Methioninemia

Sulfite oxidase deficiency

E72.2 Disorders of urea cycle metabolism

Excludes 1: disorders of ornithine metabolism (E72.4)

E72.20 Disorder of urea cycle metabolism, unspecified

Hyperammonemia

Excludes 1: hyperammonemia hyperornithinemia-homocitrullinemia syndrome E72.4

transient hyperammonemia of newborn (P74.6)

E72.21 Argininemia

E72.22 Arginosuccinic aciduria

E72.23 Citrullinemia

E72.29 Other disorders of urea cycle metabolism

E72.3 Disorders of lysine and hydroxylysine metabolism

Glutaric aciduria NOS

Glutaric aciduria (type I)

Hydroxylysinemia

Hyperlysinemia

Excludes 1: glutaric aciduria type II (E71.313)

Refsum's disease (G60.1)

Zellweger syndrome (E71.510)

E72.4 Disorders of ornithine metabolism

Hyperammonemia-Hyperornithinemia-Homocitrullinemia syndrome

Ornithinemia (types I, II)

Ornithine transcarbamylase deficiency

Excludes 1: hereditary choroidal dystrophy (H31.2-)

E72.5 Disorders of glycine metabolism

E72.50 Disorder of glycine metabolism, unspecified

E72.51 Non-ketotic hyperglycinemia

E72.52 Trimethylaminuria

E72.53 Hyperoxaluria

Oxalosis

Oxaluria

E72.59 Other disorders of glycine metabolism

Add 4th-7th digits	3 digit reportable	Nonspecific code	Unspecified code	Manifestation code

D-glycericacidemia

Hyperhydroxyprolinemia

Hyperprolinemia (types I, II)

Sarcosinemia

E72.8 Other specified disorders of amino-acid metabolism

Disorders of beta-amino-acid metabolism

Disorders of gamma-glutamyl cycle

E72.9 Disorder of amino-acid metabolism, unspecified

E73 Lactose intolerance

E73.0 Congenital lactase deficiency

E73.1 Secondary lactase deficiency

E73.8 Other lactose intolerance

E73.9 Lactose intolerance, unspecified

E74 Other disorders of carbohydrate metabolism

Excludes 1: diabetes mellitus (E08-E13)

hypoglycemia NOS (E16.2)

increased secretion of glucagon (E16.3)

mucopolysaccharidosis (E76.0-E76.3)

E74.0 Glycogen storage disease

E74.00 Glycogen storage disease, unspecified

E74.01 von Gierke disease

Type I glycogen storage disease

E74.02 Pompe disease

Cardiac glycogenosis

Type II glycogen storage disease

E74.03 Cori disease

Forbes disease

Type III glycogen storage disease

E74.04 McArdle disease

Type V glycogen storage disease

E74.09 Other glycogen storage disease

Andersen disease

Hers disease

Tauri disease

Glycogen storage disease, types 0, IV, VI-XI

Liver phosphorylase deficiency

Muscle phosphofructokinase deficiency

E74.1 Disorders of fructose metabolism

Excludes 1: muscle phosphofructokinase deficiency
(E74.09)

E74.10 Disorder of fructose metabolism, unspecified

E74.11 Essential fructosuria

Fructokinase deficiency

E74.12 Hereditary fructose intolerance

Fructosemia

E74.19 Other disorders of fructose metabolism

Fructose-1, 6-diphosphatase deficiency

E74.2 Disorders of galactose metabolism

E74.20 Disorders of galactose metabolism, unspecified

E74.21 Galactosemia

E74.29 Other disorders of galactose metabolism

Galactokinase deficiency

E74.3 Other disorders of intestinal carbohydrate absorption

Excludes 2: lactose intolerance (E73.-)

E74.31 Sucrase-isomaltase deficiency

E74.39 Other disorders of intestinal carbohydrate
absorption

Disorder of intestinal carbohydrate absorption
NOS

Glucose-galactose malabsorption

Sucrase deficiency

E74.4 Disorders of pyruvate metabolism and gluconeogenesis

Deficiency of phosphoenolpyruvate carboxykinase

Deficiency of pyruvate carboxylase

Deficiency of pyruvate dehydrogenase

Excludes 1: disorders of pyruvate metabolism and
gluconeogenesis with anemia (D55.-)

Leigh's syndrome (G31.82)

E74.8 Other specified disorders of carbohydrate metabolism

Essential pentosuria

Renal glycosuria

E74.9 Disorder of carbohydrate metabolism, unspecified

E75 Disorders of sphingolipid metabolism and other lipid storage
disorders

Excludes 1: mucolipidosis, types I-III (E77.0-E77.1)

Refsum's disease (G60.1)

E75.0 GM2 gangliosidosis

E75.00 GM2 gangliosidosis, unspecified

E75.01 Sandhoff disease

E75.02 Tay-Sachs disease

E75.09 Other GM2 gangliosidosis

Adult GM2 gangliosidosis

Juvenile GM2 gangliosidosis

E75.1 Other and unspecified gangliosidosis

E75.10 Unspecified gangliosidosis

Gangliosidosis NOS

E75.11 Mucolipidosis IV

E75.19 Other gangliosidosis

GM1 gangliosidosis

GM3 gangliosidosis

E75.2 Other sphingolipidosis

Excludes 1: adrenoleukodystrophy [Addison-Schilder]
(E71.528)

E75.21 Fabry (-Anderson) disease

E75.22 Gaucher disease

E75.23 Krabbe disease

E75.24 Niemann-Pick disease

E75.240 Niemann-Pick disease type A

E75.241 Niemann-Pick disease type B

E75.242 Niemann-Pick disease type C

E75.243 Niemann-Pick disease type D

E75.248 Other Niemann-Pick disease

E75.249 Niemann-Pick disease, unspecified

E75.25 Metachromatic leukodystrophy

E75.29 Other sphingolipidosis

Farber's syndrome

Sulfatase deficiency

Sulfatide lipidosis

E75.3 Sphingolipidosis, unspecified

E75.4 Neuronal ceroid lipofuscinosis

Batten disease

Bielschowsky-Jansky disease

Kufs disease

Spielmeyer-Vogt disease

E75.5 Other lipid storage disorders

Cerebrotendinous cholesterosis [van
Bogaert-Scherer-Epstein]

Wolman's disease

E75.6 Lipid storage disorder, unspecified

E76 Disorders of glycosaminoglycan metabolism

E76.0 Mucopolysaccharidosis, type I

E76.01 Hurler's syndrome

E76.02 Hurler-Scheie syndrome

E76.03 Scheie's syndrome

● New code ▲ Revised code ⑦ 7th digit required ⊗ Placeholder required

E76.1 Mucopolysaccharidosis, type II
Hunter's syndrome

E76.2 Other mucopolysaccharidoses

    E76.21 Morquio mucopolysaccharidoses

        E76.210 Morquio A mucopolysaccharidoses
Classic Morquio syndrome
Morquio syndrome A
Mucopolysaccharidosis, type IVA

        E76.211 Morquio B mucopolysaccharidoses
Morquio-like mucopolysaccharidoses
Morquio-like syndrome
Morquio syndrome B
Mucopolysaccharidosis, type IVB

        E76.219 Morquio mucopolysaccharidoses, unspecified
Morquio syndrome
Mucopolysaccharidosis, type IV

    E76.22 Sanfilippo mucopolysaccharidoses
Mucopolysaccharidosis, type III (A) (B) (C) (D)
Sanfilippo A syndrome
Sanfilippo B syndrome
Sanfilippo C syndrome
Sanfilippo D syndrome

    E76.29 Other mucopolysaccharidoses
beta-Glucuronidase deficiency
Maroteaux-Lamy (mild) (severe) syndrome
Mucopolysaccharidosis, types VI, VII

E76.3 Mucopolysaccharidosis, unspecified

E76.8 Other disorders of glucosaminoglycan metabolism

E76.9 Glucosaminoglycan metabolism disorder, unspecified

E77 Disorders of glycoprotein metabolism

E77.0 Defects in post-translational modification of lysosomal enzymes
Mucolipidosis II [I-cell disease]
Mucolipidosis III [pseudo-Hurler polydystrophy]

E77.1 Defects in glycoprotein degradation
Aspartylglucosaminuria
Fucosidosis
Mannosidosis
Sialidosis [mucolipidosis I]

E77.8 Other disorders of glycoprotein metabolism

E77.9 Disorder of glycoprotein metabolism, unspecified

E78 Disorders of lipoprotein metabolism and other lipidemias

    Excludes 1: sphingolipidosis (E75.0-E75.3)

E78.0 Pure hypercholesterolemia
Familial hypercholesterolemia
Fredrickson's hyperlipoproteinemia, type IIa
Hyperbetalipoproteinemia
Hyperlipidemia, Group A
Low-density-lipoprotein-type [LDL] hyperlipoproteinemia

E78.1 Pure hyperglyceridemia
Elevated fasting triglycerides
Endogenous hyperglyceridemia
Fredrickson's hyperlipoproteinemia, type IV
Hyperlipidemia, group B
Hyperprebetalipoproteinemia
Very-low-density-lipoprotein-type [VLDL] hyperlipoproteinemia

E78.2 Mixed hyperlipidemia
Broad- or floating-betalipoproteinemia
Combined hyperlipidemia NOS
Elevated cholesterol with elevated triglycerides NEC

Fredrickson's hyperlipoproteinemia, type IIb or III
Hyperbetalipoproteinemia with prebetalipoproteinemia
Hypercholesteremia with endogenous hyperglyceridemia
Hyperlipidemia, group C
Tubo-eruptive xanthoma
Xanthoma tuberosum

    Excludes 1: cerebrotendinous cholesterosis [van Bogaert-Scherer- Epstein] (E75.5)
familial combined hyperlipidemia (E78.4)

E78.3 Hyperchylomicronemia
Chylomicron retention disease
Fredrickson's hyperlipoproteinemia, type I or V
Hyperlipidemia, group D
Mixed hyperglyceridemia

E78.4 Other hyperlipidemia
Familial combined hyperlipidemia

E78.5 Hyperlipidemia, unspecified

E78.6 Lipoprotein deficiency
Abetalipoproteinemia
Depressed HDL cholesterol
High-density lipoprotein deficiency
Hypoalphalipoproteinemia
Hypobetalipoproteinemia (familial)
Lecithin cholesterol acyltransferase deficiency
Tangier disease

E78.7 Disorders of bile acid and cholesterol metabolism

    Excludes 1: Niemann-Pick disease type C (E75.242)

    E78.70 Disorder of bile acid and cholesterol metabolism, unspecified

    E78.71 Barth syndrome

    E78.72 Smith-Lemli-Opitz syndrome

    E78.79 Other disorders of bile acid and cholesterol metabolism

E78.8 Other disorders of lipoprotein metabolism

    E78.81 Lipoid dermatoarthritis

    E78.89 Other lipoprotein metabolism disorders

E78.9 Disorder of lipoprotein metabolism, unspecified

E79 Disorders of purine and pyrimidine metabolism

    Excludes 1: Ataxia-telangiectasia (Q87.1)
Bloom's syndrome (Q82.8)
Cockayne's syndrome (Q87.1)
calculus of kidney (N20.0)
combined immunodeficiency disorders (D81.-)
Fanconi's anemia (D61.09)
gout (M1A-, M10.-)
orotaciduric anemia (D53.0)
progeria (E34.8)
Werner's syndrome (E34.8)
xeroderma pigmentosum (Q82.1)

E79.0 Hyperuricemia without signs of inflammatory arthritis and tophaceous disease
Asymptomatic hyperuricemia

E79.1 Lesch-Nyhan syndrome
HGPRT deficiency

E79.2 Myoadenylate deaminase deficiency

E79.8 Other disorders of purine and pyrimidine metabolism
Hereditary xanthinuria

E79.9 Disorder of purine and pyrimidine metabolism, unspecified

E80 Disorders of porphyrin and bilirubin metabolism

    Includes: defects of catalase and peroxidase

E80.0 Hereditary erythropoietic porphyria

Congenital erythropoietic porphyria

Erythropoietic protoporphyria

E80.1 Porphyria cutanea tarda

E80.2 Other and unspecified porphyria

    E80.20 Unspecified porphyria

        Porphyria NOS

    E80.21 Acute intermittent (hepatic) porphyria

    E80.29 Other porphyria

        Hereditary coproporphyria

E80.3 Defects of catalase and peroxidase

    Acatalasia [Takahara]

E80.4 Gilbert syndrome

E80.5 Crigler-Najjar syndrome

E80.6 Other disorders of bilirubin metabolism

    Dubin-Johnson syndrome

    Rotor's syndrome

E80.7 Disorder of bilirubin metabolism, unspecified

E83 Disorders of mineral metabolism

Excludes 1: dietary mineral deficiency (E58-E61)

        parathyroid disorders (E20-E21)

        vitamin D deficiency (E55.-)

E83.0 Disorders of copper metabolism

    E83.00 Disorder of copper metabolism, unspecified

    E83.01 Wilson's disease

        Code also associated Kayser Fleischer ring (H18.04-)

    E83.09 Other disorders of copper metabolism

        Menkes' (kinky hair) (steely hair) disease

E83.1 Disorders of iron metabolism

Excludes 1: iron deficiency anemia (D50.-)

        sideroblastic anemia (D64.0-D64.3)

    E83.10 Disorder of iron metabolism, unspecified

    E83.11 Hemochromatosis

        E83.110 Hereditary hemochromatosis

            Bronzed diabetes

            Pigmentary cirrhosis (of liver)

            Primary (hereditary) hemochromatosis

        E83.111 Hemochromatosis due to repeated red blood cell transfusions

            Iron overload due to repeated red blood cell transfusions

            Transfusion (red blood cell) associated hemochromatosis

        E83.118 Other hemochromatosis

        E83.119 Hemochromatosis, unspecified

    E83.19 Other disorders of iron metabolism

        Use additional code, if applicable, for idiopathic pulmonary hemosiderosis (J84.03)

E83.2 Disorders of zinc metabolism

    Acrodermatitis enteropathica

E83.3 Disorders of phosphorus metabolism and phosphatases

Excludes 1: adult osteomalacia (M83.-)

        osteoporosis (M80-)

    E83.30 Disorder of phosphorus metabolism, unspecified

    E83.31 Familial hypophosphatemia

        Vitamin D-resistant osteomalacia

        Vitamin D-resistant rickets

        Excludes 1: vitamin D-deficiency rickets (E55.0)

    E83.32 Hereditary vitamin D-dependent rickets (type 1) (type 2)

25-hydroxyvitamin D 1-alpha-hydroxylase deficiency

Pseudovitamin D deficiency

Vitamin D receptor defect

    E83.39 Other disorders of phosphorus metabolism

        Acid phosphatase deficiency

        Hypophosphatasia

E83.4 Disorders of magnesium metabolism

    E83.40 Disorders of magnesium metabolism, unspecified

    E83.41 Hypermagnesemia

    E83.42 Hypomagnesemia

    E83.49 Other disorders of magnesium metabolism

E83.5 Disorders of calcium metabolism

Excludes 1: chondrocalcinosis (M11.1-M11.2)

        hungry bone syndrome (E83.81)

        hyperparathyroidism (E21.0-E21.3)

    E83.50 Unspecified disorder of calcium metabolism

    E83.51 Hypocalcemia

    E83.52 Hypercalcemia

        Familial hypocalciuric hypercalcemia

    E83.59 Other disorders of calcium metabolism

        Idiopathic hypercalciuria

E83.8 Other disorders of mineral metabolism

    E83.81 Hungry bone syndrome

    E83.89 Other disorders of mineral metabolism

E83.9 Disorder of mineral metabolism, unspecified

E84 Cystic fibrosis

Includes: mucoviscidosis

E84.0 Cystic fibrosis with pulmonary manifestations

    Use additional code to identify any infectious organism present, such as:

    Pseudomonas (B96.5)

E84.1 Cystic fibrosis with intestinal manifestations

    E84.11 Meconium ileus in cystic fibrosis

        Excludes 1: meconium ileus not due to cystic fibrosis (P76.0)

    E84.19 Cystic fibrosis with other intestinal manifestations

        Distal intestinal obstruction syndrome

E84.8 Cystic fibrosis with other manifestations

E84.9 Cystic fibrosis, unspecified

E85 Amyloidosis

Excludes 1: Alzheimer's disease (G30.0-)

E85.0 Non-neuropathic heredofamilial amyloidosis

    Familial Mediterranean fever

    Hereditary amyloid nephropathy

E85.1 Neuropathic heredofamilial amyloidosis

    Amyloid polyneuropathy (Portuguese)

E85.2 Heredofamilial amyloidosis, unspecified

E85.3 Secondary systemic amyloidosis

    Hemodialysis-associated amyloidosis

E85.4 Organ-limited amyloidosis

    Localized amyloidosis

E85.8 Other amyloidosis

E85.9 Amyloidosis, unspecified

E86 Volume depletion

Excludes 1: dehydration of newborn (P74.1)

        hypovolemic shock NOS (R57.1)

        postprocedural hypovolemic shock (T81.11)

        traumatic hypovolemic shock (T79.4)

E86.0 Dehydration

E86.1 Hypovolemia

Depletion of volume of plasma

E86.9 Volume depletion, unspecified

E87 Other disorders of fluid, electrolyte and acid-base balance

Excludes 1: diabetes insipidus (E23.2)

electrolyte imbalance associated with hyperemesis gravidarum (O21.1)

electrolyte imbalance following ectopic or molar pregnancy (O08.5)

familial periodic paralysis (G72.3)

E87.0 Hyperosmolality and hypernatremia

Sodium [Na] excess

Sodium [Na] overload

E87.1 Hypo-osmolality and hyponatremia

Sodium [Na] deficiency

Excludes 1: syndrome of inappropriate secretion of antidiuretic hormone (E22.2)

E87.2 Acidosis

Acidosis NOS

Lactic acidosis

Metabolic acidosis

Respiratory acidosis

Excludes 1: diabetic acidosis - see categories E08-E13 with ketoacidosis

E87.3 Alkalosis

Alkalosis NOS

Metabolic alkalosis

Respiratory alkalosis

E87.4 Mixed disorder of acid-base balance

E87.5 Hyperkalemia

Potassium [K] excess

Potassium [K] overload

E87.6 Hypokalemia

Potassium [K] deficiency

E87.7 Fluid overload

Excludes 1: edema NOS (R60.9)

fluid retention (R60.9)

E87.70 Fluid overload, unspecified

E87.71 Transfusion associated circulatory overload

Fluid overload due to transfusion (blood) (blood components)

TACO

E87.79 Other fluid overload

E87.8 Other disorders of electrolyte and fluid balance, not elsewhere classified

Electrolyte imbalance NOS

Hyperchloremia

Hypochloremia

E88 Other and unspecified metabolic disorders

Use additional codes for associated conditions

Excludes 1: histiocytosis X (chronic) (C96.6)

E88.0 Disorders of plasma-protein metabolism, not elsewhere classified

Excludes 1: disorder of lipoprotein metabolism (E78.-)

monoclonal gammopathy (of undetermined significance) (D47.2)

polyclonal hypergammaglobulinemia (D89.0)

Waldenstr÷m macroglobulinemia (C88.0)

E88.01 Alpha-1-antitrypsin deficiency

AAT deficiency

E88.09 Other disorders of plasma-protein metabolism, not elsewhere classified

Bisalbuminemia

E88.1 Lipodystrophy, not elsewhere classified

Lipodystrophy NOS

Excludes 1: Whipple's disease (K90.81)

E88.2 Lipomatosis, not elsewhere classified

Lipomatosis NOS

Lipomatosis (Check) dolorosa [Dercum]

E88.3 Tumor lysis syndrome

Tumor lysis syndrome (spontaneous)

Tumor lysis syndrome following antineoplastic drug chemotherapy

Use additional code for adverse effect, if applicable, to identify drug (T45.1X5)

E88.4 Mitochondrial metabolism disorders

Excludes 1: disorders of pyruvate metabolism (E74.4)

Kearns-Sayre syndrome (H49.81)

Leber's disease (H47.22)

Leigh's encephalopathy (G31.82)

Mitochondrial myopathy, NEC (G71.3)

Reye's syndrome (G93.7)

E88.40 Mitochondrial metabolism disorder, unspecified

E88.41 MELAS syndrome

Mitochondrial myopathy, encephalopathy, lactic acidosis and stroke-like episodes

E88.42 MERRF syndrome

Myoclonic epilepsy associated with ragged-red fibers

Code also myoclonic epilepsy (G40.3-)

E88.49 Other mitochondrial metabolism disorders

E88.8 Other specified metabolic disorders

E88.81 Metabolic syndrome

Dysmetabolic syndrome X

Use additional codes for associated manifestations, such as:

obesity (E66.-)

E88.89 Other specified metabolic disorders

Launois-Bensaude adenolipomatosis

Excludes 1: adult pulmonary Langerhans cell histiocytosis (J84.82)

E88.9 Metabolic disorder, unspecified

POSTPROCEDURAL ENDOCRINE AND METABOLIC COMPLICATIONS AND DISORDERS, NOT ELSEWHERE CLASSIFIED (E89)

E89 Postprocedural endocrine and metabolic complications and disorders, not elsewhere classified

Excludes 2: intraoperative complications of endocrine system organ or structure (E36.0-, E36.1-, E36.8)

E89.0 Postprocedural hypothyroidism

Postirradiation hypothyroidism

Postsurgical hypothyroidism

E89.1 Postprocedural hypoinsulinemia

Postpancreatectomy hyperglycemia

Postsurgical hypoinsulinemia

Use additional code, if applicable, to identify:

acquired absence of pancreas (Z90.41-)

diabetes mellitus (postpancreatectomy) (postprocedural) (E13.-)

insulin use (Z79.4)

Excludes 1: transient postprocedural hyperglycemia (R73.9)

transient postprocedural hypoglycemia (E16.2)

 Add 4th-7th digits   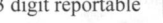 3 digit reportable   Nonspecific code   Unspecified code   Manifestation code

E89.2 Postprocedural hypoparathyroidism
  Parathyroprival tetany
E89.3 Postprocedural hypopituitarism
  Postirradiation hypopituitarism
E89.4 Postprocedural ovarian failure
  E89.40 Asymptomatic postprocedural ovarian failure
    Postprocedural ovarian failure NOS
  E89.41 Symptomatic postprocedural ovarian failure
    Symptoms such as flushing, sleeplessness, headache, lack of concentration, associated with postprocedural menopause
E89.5 Postprocedural testicular hypofunction
E89.6 Postprocedural adrenocortical (-medullary) hypofunction
E89.8 Other postprocedural endocrine and metabolic complications and disorders

  E89.81 Postprocedural hemorrhage and hematoma of an endocrine system organ or structure following a procedure
    E89.810 Postprocedural hemorrhage and hematoma of an endocrine system organ or structure following an endocrine system procedure
    E89.811 Postprocedural hemorrhage and hematoma of an endocrine system organ or structure following other procedure
  E89.89 Other postprocedural endocrine and metabolic complications and disorders
    Use additional code, if applicable, to further specify disorder

● New code   ▲ Revised code   ⑦ 7th digit required   ⊗ Placeholder required

Chapter 5: Mental, Behavioral And Neurodevelopmental Disorders (F01-F99)

Includes: disorders of psychological development

Excludes 2: symptoms, signs and abnormal clinical laboratory findings, not elsewhere classified (R00-R99)

This chapter contains the following blocks:

F01-F09	Mental disorders due to known physiological conditions
F10-F19	Mental and behavioral disorders due to psychoactive substance use
F20-F29	Schizophrenia, schizotypal, delusional, and other non-mood psychotic disorders
F30-F39	Mood [affective] disorders
F40-F48	Anxiety, dissociative, stress-related, somatoform and other nonpsychotic mental disorders
F50-F59	Behavioral syndromes associated with physiological disturbances and physical factors
F60-F69	Disorders of adult personality and behavior
F70-F79	Intellectual disabilities
F80-F89	Pervasive and specific developmental disorders
F90-F98	Behavioral and emotional disorders with onset usually occurring in childhood and adolescence
F99	Unspecified mental disorder

MENTAL DISORDERS DUE TO KNOWN PHYSIOLOGICAL CONDITIONS (F01-F09)

Note: This block comprises a range of mental disorders grouped together on the basis of their having in common a demonstrable etiology in cerebral disease, brain injury, or other insult leading to cerebral dysfunction. The dysfunction may be primary, as in diseases, injuries, and insults that affect the brain directly and selectively; or secondary, as in systemic diseases and disorders that attack the brain only as one of the multiple organs or systems of the body that are involved.

F01 Vascular dementia

Vascular dementia as a result of infarction of the brain due to vascular disease, including hypertensive cerebrovascular disease.

Includes: arteriosclerotic dementia

Code first the underlying physiological condition or sequelae of cerebrovascular disease.

F01.5 Vascular dementia

F01.50 Vascular dementia without behavioral disturbance

F01.51 Vascular dementia with behavioral disturbance

Vascular dementia with aggressive behavior

Vascular dementia with combative behavior

Vascular dementia with violent behavior

Use additional code, if applicable, to identify wandering in vascular dementia (Z91.83)

F02 Dementia in other diseases classified elsewhere

Code first the underlying physiological condition, such as:

Alzheimer's (G30.-)

cerebral lipidosis (E75.4)

Creutzfeldt-Jakob disease (A81.0-)

dementia with Lewy bodies (G31.83)

epilepsy and recurrent seizures (G40.-)

frontotemporal dementia (G31.09)

hepatolenticular degeneration (E83.0)

human immunodeficiency virus [HIV] disease (B20)

hypercalcemia (E83.52)

hypothyroidism, acquired (E00-E03.-)

intoxications (T36-T65)

Jakob-Creutzfeldt disease (A81.0-)

multiple sclerosis (G35)

neurosyphilis (A52.17)

niacin deficiency [pellagra] (E52)

Parkinson's disease (G20)

Pick's disease (G31.01)

polyarteritis nodosa (M30.0)

systemic lupus erythematosus (M32.-)

trypanosomiasis (B56.-, B57.-)

vitamin B deficiency (E53.8)

Excludes 1: dementia with Parkinsonism (G31.83)

Excludes 2: dementia in alcohol and psychoactive substance disorders (F10-F19, with .17, .27, .97)

vascular dementia (F01.5-)

F02.8 Dementia in other diseases classified elsewhere

F02.80 Dementia in other diseases classified elsewhere without behavioral disturbance

Dementia in other diseases classified elsewhere NOS

F02.81 Dementia in other diseases classified elsewhere with behavioral disturbance

Dementia in other diseases classified elsewhere with aggressive behavior

Dementia in other diseases classified elsewhere with combative behavior

Dementia in other diseases classified elsewhere with violent behavior

Use additional code, if applicable, to identify wandering in dementia in conditions classified elsewhere (Z91.83)

F03 Unspecified dementia

Presenile dementia NOS

Presenile psychosis NOS

Primary degenerative dementia NOS

Senile dementia NOS

Senile dementia depressed or paranoid type

Senile psychosis NOS

Excludes 1: senility NOS (R41.81)

Excludes 2: mild memory disturbance due to known physiological condition (F06.8)

senile dementia with delirium or acute confusional state (F05)

F03.9 Unspecified dementia

F03.90 Unspecified dementia without behavioral disturbance

Dementia NOS

F03.91 Unspecified dementia with behavioral disturbance

Unspecified dementia with aggressive behavior

Unspecified dementia with combative behavior

Unspecified dementia with violent behavior

Use additional code, if applicable, to identify wandering in unspecified dementia (Z91.83)

F04 Amnestic disorder due to known physiological condition

Korsakov's psychosis or syndrome, nonalcoholic

Code first the underlying physiological condition

Excludes 1: amnesia NOS (R41.3)

anterograde amnesia (R41.1)

dissociative amnesia (F44.0)

retrograde amnesia (R41.2)

Excludes 2: alcohol-induced or unspecified Korsakov's syndrome (F10.26, F10.96)

Korsakov's syndrome induced by other psychoactive substances (F13.26, F13.96, F19.16, F19.26, F19.96)

F05 Delirium due to known physiological condition

Acute or subacute brain syndrome
Acute or subacute confusional state (nonalcoholic)
Acute or subacute infective psychosis
Acute or subacute organic reaction
Acute or subacute psycho-organic syndrome
Delirium of mixed etiology
Delirium superimposed on dementia
Sundowning
Code first the underlying physiological condition
Excludes 1: delirium NOS (R41.0)
Excludes 2: delirium tremens alcohol-induced or unspecified
(F10.231, F10.921)

F06 Other mental disorders due to known physiological condition
Includes: mental disorders due to endocrine disorder
mental disorders due to exogenous hormone
mental disorders due to exogenous toxic substance
mental disorders due to primary cerebral disease
mental disorders due to somatic illness
mental disorders due to systemic disease affecting the brain
Code first the underlying physiological condition
Excludes 1: unspecified dementia (F03)
Excludes 2: delirium due to known physiological condition (F05)
dementia as classified in F01-F02
other mental disorders associated with alcohol and other
psychoactive substances (F10-F19)

F06.0 Psychotic disorder with hallucinations due to known
physiological condition
Organic hallucinatory state (nonalcoholic)
Excludes 2: hallucinations and perceptual disturbance
induced by alcohol and other psychoactive substances
(F10-F19 with .151, .251, .951)
schizophrenia (F20.-)

F06.1 Catatonic disorder due to known physiological condition
Excludes 1: catatonic stupor (R40.1)
stupor NOS (R40.1)
Excludes 2: catatonic schizophrenia (F20.2)
dissociative stupor (F44.2)

F06.2 Psychotic disorder with delusions due to known
physiological condition
Paranoid and paranoid-hallucinatory organic states
Schizophrenia-like psychosis in epilepsy
Excludes 2: alcohol and drug-induced psychotic disorder
(F10-F19 with .150, .250, .950)
brief psychotic disorder (F23)
delusional disorder (F22)
schizophrenia (F20.-)

F06.3 Mood disorder due to known physiological condition
Excludes 2: mood disorders due to alcohol and
other psychoactive substances (F10-F19 with .14,
.24, .94)
mood disorders, not due to known physiological
condition or unspecified (F30-F39)

F06.30 Mood disorder due to known physiological
condition, unspecified
F06.31 Mood disorder due to known physiological
condition with depressive features
F06.32 Mood disorder due to known physiological
condition with major depressive-like episode
F06.33 Mood disorder due to known physiological
condition with manic features
F06.34 Mood disorder due to known physiological
condition with mixed features

F06.4 Anxiety disorder due to known physiological condition

Excludes 2: anxiety disorders due to alcohol and other
psychoactive substances (F10-F19
with .180, .280, .980)
anxiety disorders, not due to known
physiological condition or unspecified (F40.-,
F41.-)

F06.8 Other specified mental disorders due to known
physiological condition
Epileptic psychosis NOS
Organic dissociative disorder
Organic emotionally labile [asthenic] disorder

F07 Personality and behavioral disorders due to known physiological
condition
Code first the underlying physiological condition

F07.0 Personality change due to known physiological condition
Frontal lobe syndrome
Limbic epilepsy personality syndrome
Lobotomy syndrome
Organic personality disorder
Organic pseudopsychopathic personality
Organic pseudoretarded personality
Postleucotomy syndrome
Code first underlying physiological condition
Excludes 1: mild cognitive impairment (G31.84)
postconcussional syndrome (F07.81)
postencephalitic syndrome (F07.89)
signs and symptoms involving emotional state
(R45.-)
Excludes 2: specific personality disorder (F60.-)

F07.8 Other personality and behavioral disorders due to known
physiological condition
F07.81 Postconcussional syndrome
Postcontusional syndrome (encephalopathy)
Post-traumatic brain syndrome, nonpsychotic
Use additional code to identify associated
post-traumatic headache, if applicable (G44.3-)
Excludes 1: current concussion (brain) (S06.0-)
postencephalitic syndrome (F07.89)

F07.89 Other personality and behavioral disorders due to
known physiological condition
Postencephalitic syndrome
Right hemispheric organic affective disorder

F07.9 Unspecified personality and behavioral disorder due to
known physiological condition
Organic psychosyndrome

F09 Unspecified mental disorder due to known physiological condition
Mental disorder NOS due to known physiological condition
Organic brain syndrome NOS
Organic mental disorder NOS
Organic psychosis NOS
Symptomatic psychosis NOS
Code first the underlying physiological condition
Excludes 1: psychosis NOS (F29)

MENTAL AND BEHAVIORAL DISORDERS DUE TO PSYCHOACTIVE SUBSTANCE USE (F10-F19)

F10 Alcohol related disorders
Use additional code for blood alcohol level, if applicable (Y90.-)
F10.1 Alcohol abuse
Excludes 1: alcohol dependence (F10.2-)
alcohol use, unspecified (F10.9-)
F10.10 Alcohol abuse, uncomplicated
F10.12 Alcohol abuse with intoxication

F10.120 Alcohol abuse with intoxication, uncomplicated

F10.121 Alcohol abuse with intoxication delirium

F10.129 Alcohol abuse with intoxication, unspecified

F10.14 Alcohol abuse with alcohol-induced mood disorder

F10.15 Alcohol abuse with alcohol-induced psychotic disorder

    F10.150 Alcohol abuse with alcohol-induced psychotic disorder with delusions

    F10.151 Alcohol abuse with alcohol-induced psychotic disorder with hallucinations

    F10.159 Alcohol abuse with alcohol-induced psychotic disorder, unspecified

F10.18 Alcohol abuse with other alcohol-induced disorders

    F10.180 Alcohol abuse with alcohol-induced anxiety disorder

    F10.181 Alcohol abuse with alcohol-induced sexual dysfunction

    F10.182 Alcohol abuse with alcohol-induced sleep disorder

    F10.188 Alcohol abuse with other alcohol-induced disorder

F10.19 Alcohol abuse with unspecified alcohol-induced disorder

F10.2 Alcohol dependence

Excludes 1: alcohol abuse (F10.1-)
alcohol use, unspecified (F10.9-)

Excludes 2: toxic effect of alcohol (T51.0-)

F10.20 Alcohol dependence, uncomplicated

F10.21 Alcohol dependence, in remission

F10.22 Alcohol dependence with intoxication
Acute drunkenness (in alcoholism)

Excludes 1: alcohol dependence with withdrawal (F10.23-)

    F10.220 Alcohol dependence with intoxication, uncomplicated

    F10.221 Alcohol dependence with intoxication delirium

    F10.229 Alcohol dependence with intoxication, unspecified

F10.23 Alcohol dependence with withdrawal

Excludes 1: Alcohol dependence with intoxication (F10.22-)

    F10.230 Alcohol dependence with withdrawal, uncomplicated

    F10.231 Alcohol dependence with withdrawal delirium

    F10.232 Alcohol dependence with withdrawal with perceptual disturbance

    F10.239 Alcohol dependence with withdrawal, unspecified

F10.24 Alcohol dependence with alcohol-induced mood disorder

F10.25 Alcohol dependence with alcohol-induced psychotic disorder

    F10.250 Alcohol dependence with alcohol-induced psychotic disorder with delusions

    F10.251 Alcohol dependence with alcohol-induced psychotic disorder with hallucinations

    F10.259 Alcohol dependence with alcohol-induced psychotic disorder, unspecified

F10.26 Alcohol dependence with alcohol-induced persisting amnestic disorder

F10.27 Alcohol dependence with alcohol-induced persisting dementia

F10.28 Alcohol dependence with other alcohol-induced disorders

    F10.280 Alcohol dependence with alcohol-induced anxiety disorder

    F10.281 Alcohol dependence with alcohol-induced sexual dysfunction

    F10.282 Alcohol dependence with alcohol-induced sleep disorder

    F10.288 Alcohol dependence with other alcohol-induced disorder

F10.29 Alcohol dependence with unspecified alcohol-induced disorder

F10.9 Alcohol use, unspecified

Excludes 1: alcohol abuse (F10.1-)
alcohol dependence (F10.2-)

F10.92 Alcohol use, unspecified with intoxication

    F10.920 Alcohol use, unspecified with intoxication, uncomplicated

    F10.921 Alcohol use, unspecified with intoxication delirium

    F10.929 Alcohol use, unspecified with intoxication, unspecified

F10.94 Alcohol use, unspecified with alcohol-induced mood disorder

F10.95 Alcohol use, unspecified with alcohol-induced psychotic disorder

    F10.950 Alcohol use, unspecified with alcohol-induced psychotic disorder with delusions

    F10.951 Alcohol use, unspecified with alcohol-induced psychotic disorder with hallucinations

    F10.959 Alcohol use, unspecified with alcohol-induced psychotic disorder, unspecified

F10.96 Alcohol use, unspecified with alcohol-induced persisting amnestic disorder

F10.97 Alcohol use, unspecified with alcohol-induced persisting dementia

F10.98 Alcohol use, unspecified with other alcohol-induced disorders

    F10.980 Alcohol use, unspecified with alcohol-induced anxiety disorder

    F10.981 Alcohol use, unspecified with alcohol-induced sexual dysfunction

    F10.982 Alcohol use, unspecified with alcohol-induced sleep disorder

    F10.988 Alcohol use, unspecified with other alcohol-induced disorder

F10.99 Alcohol use, unspecified with unspecified alcohol-induced disorder

F11 Opioid related disorders

F11.1 Opioid abuse

Excludes 1: opioid dependence (F11.2-)
opioid use, unspecified (F11.9-)

F11.10 Opioid abuse, uncomplicated

F11.12 Opioid abuse with intoxication

F11.120   Opioid abuse with intoxication, uncomplicated

F11.121   Opioid abuse with intoxication delirium

F11.122   Opioid abuse with intoxication with perceptual disturbance

F11.129   Opioid abuse with intoxication, unspecified

F11.14   Opioid abuse with opioid-induced mood disorder

F11.15   Opioid abuse with opioid-induced psychotic disorder

F11.150   Opioid abuse with opioid-induced psychotic disorder with delusions

F11.151   Opioid abuse with opioid-induced psychotic disorder with hallucinations

F11.159   Opioid abuse with opioid-induced psychotic disorder, unspecified

F11.18   Opioid abuse with other opioid-induced disorder

F11.181   Opioid abuse with opioid-induced sexual dysfunction

F11.182   Opioid abuse with opioid-induced sleep disorder

F11.188   Opioid abuse with other opioid-induced disorder

F11.19   Opioid abuse with unspecified opioid-induced disorder

F11.2   Opioid dependence

Excludes 1: opioid abuse (F11.1-)

opioid use, unspecified (F11.9-)

Excludes 2: opioid poisoning (T40.0-T40.2-)

F11.20   Opioid dependence, uncomplicated

F11.21   Opioid dependence, in remission

F11.22   Opioid dependence with intoxication

Excludes 1: opioid dependence with withdrawal (F11.23)

F11.220   Opioid dependence with intoxication, uncomplicated

F11.221   Opioid dependence with intoxication delirium

F11.222   Opioid dependence with intoxication with perceptual disturbance

F11.229   Opioid dependence with intoxication, unspecified

F11.23   Opioid dependence with withdrawal

Excludes 1: opioid dependence with intoxication (F11.22-)

F11.24   Opioid dependence with opioid-induced mood disorder

F11.25   Opioid dependence with opioid-induced psychotic disorder

F11.250   Opioid dependence with opioid-induced psychotic disorder with delusions

F11.251   Opioid dependence with opioid-induced psychotic disorder with hallucinations

F11.259   Opioid dependence with opioid-induced psychotic disorder, unspecified

F11.28   Opioid dependence with other opioid-induced disorder

F11.281   Opioid dependence with opioid-induced sexual dysfunction

F11.282   Opioid dependence with opioid-induced sleep disorder

F11.288   Opioid dependence with other opioid-induced disorder

F11.29   Opioid dependence with unspecified opioid-induced disorder

F11.9   Opioid use, unspecified

Excludes 1: opioid abuse (F11.1-)

opioid dependence (F11.2-)

F11.90   Opioid use, unspecified, uncomplicated

F11.92   Opioid use, unspecified with intoxication

Excludes 1: opioid use, unspecified with withdrawal (F11.93)

F11.920   Opioid use, unspecified with intoxication, uncomplicated

F11.921   Opioid use, unspecified with intoxication delirium

F11.922   Opioid use, unspecified with intoxication with perceptual disturbance

F11.929   Opioid use, unspecified with intoxication, unspecified

F11.93   Opioid use, unspecified with withdrawal

Excludes 1: opioid use, unspecified with intoxication (F11.92-)

F11.94   Opioid use, unspecified with opioid-induced mood disorder

F11.95   Opioid use, unspecified with opioid-induced psychotic disorder

F11.950   Opioid use, unspecified with opioid-induced psychotic disorder with delusions

F11.951   Opioid use, unspecified with opioid-induced psychotic disorder with hallucinations

F11.959   Opioid use, unspecified with opioid-induced psychotic disorder, unspecified

F11.98   Opioid use, unspecified with other specified opioid-induced disorder

F11.981   Opioid use, unspecified with opioid-induced sexual dysfunction

F11.982   Opioid use, unspecified with opioid-induced sleep disorder

F11.988   Opioid use, unspecified with other opioid-induced disorder

F11.99   Opioid use, unspecified with unspecified opioid-induced disorder

F12   Cannabis related disorders

Includes: marijuana

F12.1   Cannabis abuse

Excludes 1: cannabis dependence (F12.2-)

cannabis use, unspecified (F12.9-)

F12.10   Cannabis abuse, uncomplicated

F12.12   Cannabis abuse with intoxication

F12.120   Cannabis abuse with intoxication, uncomplicated

F12.121   Cannabis abuse with intoxication delirium

F12.122   Cannabis abuse with intoxication with perceptual disturbance

F12.129   Cannabis abuse with intoxication, unspecified

F12.15   Cannabis abuse with psychotic disorder

F12.150 Cannabis abuse with psychotic disorder with delusions
F12.151 Cannabis abuse with psychotic disorder with hallucinations
F12.159 Cannabis abuse with psychotic disorder, unspecified
F12.18 Cannabis abuse with other cannabis-induced disorder
F12.180 Cannabis abuse with cannabis-induced anxiety disorder
F12.188 Cannabis abuse with other cannabis-induced disorder
F12.19 Cannabis abuse with unspecified cannabis-induced disorder
F12.2 Cannabis dependence
Excludes 1: cannabis abuse (F12.1-)
cannabis use, unspecified (F12.9-)
Excludes 2: cannabis poisoning (T40.7-)
F12.20 Cannabis dependence, uncomplicated
F12.21 Cannabis dependence, in remission
F12.22 Cannabis dependence with intoxication
F12.220 Cannabis dependence with intoxication, uncomplicated
F12.221 Cannabis dependence with intoxication delirium
F12.222 Cannabis dependence with intoxication with perceptual disturbance
F12.229 Cannabis dependence with intoxication, unspecified
F12.25 Cannabis dependence with psychotic disorder
F12.250 Cannabis dependence with psychotic disorder with delusions
F12.251 Cannabis dependence with psychotic disorder with hallucinations
F12.259 Cannabis dependence with psychotic disorder, unspecified
F12.28 Cannabis dependence with other cannabis-induced disorder
F12.280 Cannabis dependence with cannabis-induced anxiety disorder
F12.288 Cannabis dependence with other cannabis-induced disorder
F12.29 Cannabis dependence with unspecified cannabis-induced disorder
F12.9 Cannabis use, unspecified
Excludes 1: cannabis abuse (F12.1-)
cannabis dependence (F12.2-)
F12.90 Cannabis use, unspecified, uncomplicated
F12.92 Cannabis use, unspecified with intoxication
F12.920 Cannabis use, unspecified with intoxication, uncomplicated
F12.921 Cannabis use, unspecified with intoxication delirium
F12.922 Cannabis use, unspecified with intoxication with perceptual disturbance
F12.929 Cannabis use, unspecified with intoxication, unspecified
F12.95 Cannabis use, unspecified with psychotic disorder
F12.950 Cannabis use, unspecified with psychotic disorder with delusions

F12.951 Cannabis use, unspecified with psychotic disorder with hallucinations
F12.959 Cannabis use, unspecified with psychotic disorder, unspecified
F12.98 Cannabis use, unspecified with other cannabis-induced disorder
F12.980 Cannabis use, unspecified with anxiety disorder
F12.988 Cannabis use, unspecified with other cannabis-induced disorder
F12.99 Cannabis use, unspecified with unspecified cannabis-induced disorder
F13 Sedative, hypnotic, or anxiolytic related disorders
F13.1 Sedative, hypnotic or anxiolytic-related abuse
Excludes 1: sedative, hypnotic or anxiolytic-related dependence (F13.2-)
sedative, hypnotic, or anxiolytic use, unspecified (F13.9-)
F13.10 Sedative, hypnotic or anxiolytic abuse, uncomplicated
F13.12 Sedative, hypnotic or anxiolytic abuse with intoxication
F13.120 Sedative, hypnotic or anxiolytic abuse with intoxication, uncomplicated
F13.121 Sedative, hypnotic or anxiolytic abuse with intoxication delirium
F13.129 Sedative, hypnotic or anxiolytic abuse with intoxication, unspecified
F13.14 Sedative, hypnotic or anxiolytic abuse with sedative, hypnotic or anxiolytic-induced mood disorder
F13.15 Sedative, hypnotic or anxiolytic abuse with sedative, hypnotic or anxiolytic-induced psychotic disorder
F13.150 Sedative, hypnotic or anxiolytic abuse with sedative, hypnotic or anxiolytic-induced psychotic disorder with delusions
F13.151 Sedative, hypnotic or anxiolytic abuse with sedative, hypnotic or anxiolytic-induced psychotic disorder with hallucinations
F13.159 Sedative, hypnotic or anxiolytic abuse with sedative, hypnotic or anxiolytic-induced psychotic disorder, unspecified
F13.18 Sedative, hypnotic or anxiolytic abuse with other sedative, hypnotic or anxiolytic-induced disorders
F13.180 Sedative, hypnotic or anxiolytic abuse with sedative, hypnotic or anxiolytic-induced anxiety disorder
F13.181 Sedative, hypnotic or anxiolytic abuse with sedative, hypnotic or anxiolytic-induced sexual dysfunction
F13.182 Sedative, hypnotic or anxiolytic abuse with sedative, hypnotic or anxiolytic-induced sleep disorder
F13.188 Sedative, hypnotic or anxiolytic abuse with other sedative, hypnotic or anxiolytic-induced disorder
F13.19 Sedative, hypnotic or anxiolytic abuse with unspecified sedative, hypnotic or anxiolytic-induced disorder
F13.2 Sedative, hypnotic or anxiolytic-related dependence

Excludes 1: sedative, hypnotic or anxiolytic-related abuse (F13.1-)

sedative, hypnotic, or anxiolytic use, unspecified (F13.9-)

Excludes 2: sedative, hypnotic, or anxiolytic poisoning (T42.-)

F13.20 Sedative, hypnotic or anxiolytic dependence, uncomplicated

F13.21 Sedative, hypnotic or anxiolytic dependence, in remission

F13.22 Sedative, hypnotic or anxiolytic dependence with intoxication

    Excludes 1: sedative, hypnotic or anxiolytic dependence with withdrawal (F13.23-)

F13.220 Sedative, hypnotic or anxiolytic dependence with intoxication, uncomplicated

F13.221 Sedative, hypnotic or anxiolytic dependence with intoxication delirium

F13.229 Sedative, hypnotic or anxiolytic dependence with intoxication, unspecified

F13.23 Sedative, hypnotic or anxiolytic dependence with withdrawal

    Excludes 1: sedative, hypnotic or anxiolytic dependence with intoxication (F13.22-)

F13.230 Sedative, hypnotic or anxiolytic dependence with withdrawal, uncomplicated

F13.231 Sedative, hypnotic or anxiolytic dependence with withdrawal delirium

F13.232 Sedative, hypnotic or anxiolytic dependence with withdrawal with perceptual disturbance

F13.239 Sedative, hypnotic or anxiolytic dependence with withdrawal, unspecified

F13.24 Sedative, hypnotic or anxiolytic dependence with sedative, hypnotic or anxiolytic-induced mood disorder

F13.25 Sedative, hypnotic or anxiolytic dependence with sedative, hypnotic or anxiolytic-induced psychotic disorder

F13.250 Sedative, hypnotic or anxiolytic dependence with sedative, hypnotic or anxiolytic-induced psychotic disorder with delusions

F13.251 Sedative, hypnotic or anxiolytic dependence with sedative, hypnotic or anxiolytic-induced psychotic disorder with hallucinations

F13.259 Sedative, hypnotic or anxiolytic dependence with sedative, hypnotic or anxiolytic-induced psychotic disorder, unspecified

F13.26 Sedative, hypnotic or anxiolytic dependence with sedative, hypnotic or anxiolytic-induced persisting amnestic disorder

F13.27 Sedative, hypnotic or anxiolytic dependence with sedative, hypnotic or anxiolytic-induced persisting dementia

F13.28 Sedative, hypnotic or anxiolytic dependence with other sedative, hypnotic or anxiolytic-induced disorders

F13.280 Sedative, hypnotic or anxiolytic dependence with sedative, hypnotic or anxiolytic-induced anxiety disorder

F13.281 Sedative, hypnotic or anxiolytic dependence with sedative, hypnotic or anxiolytic-induced sexual dysfunction

F13.282 Sedative, hypnotic or anxiolytic dependence with sedative, hypnotic or anxiolytic-induced sleep disorder

F13.288 Sedative, hypnotic or anxiolytic dependence with other sedative, hypnotic or anxiolytic-induced disorder

F13.29 Sedative, hypnotic or anxiolytic dependence with unspecified sedative, hypnotic or anxiolytic-induced disorder

F13.9 Sedative, hypnotic or anxiolytic-related use, unspecified

    Excludes 1: sedative, hypnotic or anxiolytic-related abuse (F13.1-)

sedative, hypnotic or anxiolytic-related dependence (F13.2-)

F13.90 Sedative, hypnotic, or anxiolytic use, unspecified, uncomplicated

F13.92 Sedative, hypnotic or anxiolytic use, unspecified with intoxication

    Excludes 1: sedative, hypnotic or anxiolytic use, unspecified with withdrawal (F13.93-)

F13.920 Sedative, hypnotic or anxiolytic use, unspecified with intoxication, uncomplicated

F13.921 Sedative, hypnotic or anxiolytic use, unspecified with intoxication delirium

F13.929 Sedative, hypnotic or anxiolytic use, unspecified with intoxication, unspecified

F13.93 Sedative, hypnotic or anxiolytic use, unspecified with withdrawal

    Excludes 1: sedative, hypnotic or anxiolytic use, unspecified with intoxication (F13.92-)

F13.930 Sedative, hypnotic or anxiolytic use, unspecified with withdrawal, uncomplicated

F13.931 Sedative, hypnotic or anxiolytic use, unspecified with withdrawal delirium

F13.932 Sedative, hypnotic or anxiolytic use, unspecified with withdrawal with perceptual disturbances

F13.939 Sedative, hypnotic or anxiolytic use, unspecified with withdrawal, unspecified

F13.94 Sedative, hypnotic or anxiolytic use, unspecified with sedative, hypnotic or anxiolytic-induced mood disorder

F13.95 Sedative, hypnotic or anxiolytic use, unspecified with sedative, hypnotic or anxiolytic-induced psychotic disorder

F13.950 Sedative, hypnotic or anxiolytic use, unspecified with sedative, hypnotic or anxiolytic-induced psychotic disorder with delusions

F13.951 Sedative, hypnotic or anxiolytic use, unspecified with sedative, hypnotic or anxiolytic-induced psychotic disorder with hallucinations

F13.959 Sedative, hypnotic or anxiolytic use, unspecified with sedative, hypnotic or anxiolytic-induced psychotic disorder, unspecified

F13.96 Sedative, hypnotic or anxiolytic use, unspecified with sedative, hypnotic or anxiolytic-induced persisting amnestic disorder

F13.97 Sedative, hypnotic or anxiolytic use, unspecified with sedative, hypnotic or anxiolytic-induced persisting dementia

F13.98 Sedative, hypnotic or anxiolytic use, unspecified with other sedative, hypnotic or anxiolytic-induced disorders

F13.980 Sedative, hypnotic or anxiolytic use, unspecified with sedative, hypnotic or anxiolytic-induced anxiety disorder

F13.981 Sedative, hypnotic or anxiolytic use, unspecified with sedative, hypnotic or anxiolytic-induced sexual dysfunction

F13.982 Sedative, hypnotic or anxiolytic use, unspecified with sedative, hypnotic or anxiolytic-induced sleep disorder

F13.988 Sedative, hypnotic or anxiolytic use, unspecified with other sedative, hypnotic or anxiolytic-induced disorder

F13.99 Sedative, hypnotic or anxiolytic use, unspecified with unspecified sedative, hypnotic or anxiolytic-induced disorder

F14 Cocaine related disorders
Excludes 2: other stimulant-related disorders (F15.-)

F14.1 Cocaine abuse
Excludes 1: cocaine dependence (F14.2-)
cocaine use, unspecified (F14.9-)

F14.10 Cocaine abuse, uncomplicated

F14.12 Cocaine abuse with intoxication

F14.120 Cocaine abuse with intoxication, uncomplicated

F14.121 Cocaine abuse with intoxication with delirium

F14.122 Cocaine abuse with intoxication with perceptual disturbance

F14.129 Cocaine abuse with intoxication, unspecified

F14.14 Cocaine abuse with cocaine-induced mood disorder

F14.15 Cocaine abuse with cocaine-induced psychotic disorder

F14.150 Cocaine abuse with cocaine-induced psychotic disorder with delusions

F14.151 Cocaine abuse with cocaine-induced psychotic disorder with hallucinations

F14.159 Cocaine abuse with cocaine-induced psychotic disorder, unspecified

F14.18 Cocaine abuse with other cocaine-induced disorder

F14.180 Cocaine abuse with cocaine-induced anxiety disorder

F14.181 Cocaine abuse with cocaine-induced sexual dysfunction

F14.182 Cocaine abuse with cocaine-induced sleep disorder

F14.188 Cocaine abuse with other cocaine-induced disorder

F14.19 Cocaine abuse with unspecified cocaine-induced disorder

F14.2 Cocaine dependence
Excludes 1: cocaine abuse (F14.1-)
cocaine use, unspecified (F14.9-)
Excludes 2: cocaine poisoning (T40.5-)

F14.20 Cocaine dependence, uncomplicated

F14.21 Cocaine dependence, in remission

F14.22 Cocaine dependence with intoxication
Excludes 1: cocaine dependence with withdrawal (F14.23)

F14.220 Cocaine dependence with intoxication, uncomplicated

F14.221 Cocaine dependence with intoxication delirium

F14.222 Cocaine dependence with intoxication with perceptual disturbance

F14.229 Cocaine dependence with intoxication, unspecified

F14.23 Cocaine dependence with withdrawal
Excludes 1: cocaine dependence with intoxication (F14.22-)

F14.24 Cocaine dependence with cocaine-induced mood disorder

F14.25 Cocaine dependence with cocaine-induced psychotic disorder

F14.250 Cocaine dependence with cocaine-induced psychotic disorder with delusions

F14.251 Cocaine dependence with cocaine-induced psychotic disorder with hallucinations

F14.259 Cocaine dependence with cocaine-induced psychotic disorder, unspecified

F14.28 Cocaine dependence with other cocaine-induced disorder

F14.280 Cocaine dependence with cocaine-induced anxiety disorder

F14.281 Cocaine dependence with cocaine-induced sexual dysfunction

F14.282 Cocaine dependence with cocaine-induced sleep disorder

F14.288 Cocaine dependence with other cocaine-induced disorder

F14.29 Cocaine dependence with unspecified cocaine-induced disorder

F14.9 Cocaine use, unspecified
Excludes 1: cocaine abuse (F14.1-)
cocaine dependence (F14.2-)

F14.90 Cocaine use, unspecified, uncomplicated

F14.92 Cocaine use, unspecified with intoxication

F14.920 Cocaine use, unspecified with intoxication, uncomplicated

F14.921 Cocaine use, unspecified with intoxication delirium

F14.922 Cocaine use, unspecified with intoxication with perceptual disturbance

F14.929 Cocaine use, unspecified with intoxication, unspecified

F14.94 Cocaine use, unspecified with cocaine-induced mood disorder

F14.95 Cocaine use, unspecified with cocaine-induced psychotic disorder

    F14.950 Cocaine use, unspecified with cocaine-induced psychotic disorder with delusions

    F14.951 Cocaine use, unspecified with cocaine-induced psychotic disorder with hallucinations

    F14.959 Cocaine use, unspecified with cocaine-induced psychotic disorder, unspecified

F14.98 Cocaine use, unspecified with other specified cocaine-induced disorder

    F14.980 Cocaine use, unspecified with cocaine-induced anxiety disorder

    F14.981 Cocaine use, unspecified with cocaine-induced sexual dysfunction

    F14.982 Cocaine use, unspecified with cocaine-induced sleep disorder

    F14.988 Cocaine use, unspecified with other cocaine-induced disorder

F14.99 Cocaine use, unspecified with unspecified cocaine-induced disorder

F15 Other stimulant related disorders

Includes: amphetamine-related disorders

    Caffeine

Excludes 2: cocaine-related disorders (F14.-)

F15.1 Other stimulant abuse

Excludes 1: other stimulant dependence (F15.2-)

    other stimulant use, unspecified (F15.9-)

    F15.10 Other stimulant abuse, uncomplicated

F15.12 Other stimulant abuse with intoxication

    F15.120 Other stimulant abuse with intoxication, uncomplicated

    F15.121 Other stimulant abuse with intoxication delirium

    F15.122 Other stimulant abuse with intoxication with perceptual disturbance

    F15.129 Other stimulant abuse with intoxication, unspecified

    F15.14 Other stimulant abuse with stimulant-induced mood disorder

F15.15 Other stimulant abuse with stimulant-induced psychotic disorder

    F15.150 Other stimulant abuse with stimulant-induced psychotic disorder with delusions

    F15.151 Other stimulant abuse with stimulant-induced psychotic disorder with hallucinations

    F15.159 Other stimulant abuse with stimulant-induced psychotic disorder, unspecified

F15.18 Other stimulant abuse with other stimulant-induced disorder

    F15.180 Other stimulant abuse with stimulant-induced anxiety disorder

    F15.181 Other stimulant abuse with stimulant-induced sexual dysfunction

    F15.182 Other stimulant abuse with stimulant-induced sleep disorder

    F15.188 Other stimulant abuse with other stimulant-induced disorder

    F15.19 Other stimulant abuse with unspecified stimulant-induced disorder

F15.2 Other stimulant dependence

Excludes 1: other stimulant abuse (F15.1-)

    other stimulant use, unspecified (F15.9-)

    F15.20 Other stimulant dependence, uncomplicated

    F15.21 Other stimulant dependence, in remission

F15.22 Other stimulant dependence with intoxication

Excludes 1: other stimulant dependence with withdrawal (F15.23)

    F15.220 Other stimulant dependence with intoxication, uncomplicated

    F15.221 Other stimulant dependence with intoxication delirium

    F15.222 Other stimulant dependence with intoxication with perceptual disturbance

    F15.229 Other stimulant dependence with intoxication, unspecified

    F15.23 Other stimulant dependence with withdrawal

Excludes 1: other stimulant dependence with intoxication (F15.22-)

    F15.24 Other stimulant dependence with stimulant-induced mood disorder

F15.25 Other stimulant dependence with stimulant-induced psychotic disorder

    F15.250 Other stimulant dependence with stimulant-induced psychotic disorder with delusions

    F15.251 Other stimulant dependence with stimulant-induced psychotic disorder with hallucinations

    F15.259 Other stimulant dependence with stimulant-induced psychotic disorder, unspecified

F15.28 Other stimulant dependence with other stimulant-induced disorder

    F15.280 Other stimulant dependence with stimulant-induced anxiety disorder

    F15.281 Other stimulant dependence with stimulant-induced sexual dysfunction

    F15.282 Other stimulant dependence with stimulant-induced sleep disorder

    F15.288 Other stimulant dependence with other stimulant-induced disorder

    F15.29 Other stimulant dependence with unspecified stimulant-induced disorder

F15.9 Other stimulant use, unspecified

Excludes 1: other stimulant abuse (F15.1-)

    other stimulant dependence (F15.2-)

    F15.90 Other stimulant use, unspecified, uncomplicated

F15.92 Other stimulant use, unspecified with intoxication

Excludes 1: other stimulant use, unspecified with withdrawal (F15.93)

    F15.920 Other stimulant use, unspecified with intoxication, uncomplicated

    F15.921 Other stimulant use, unspecified with intoxication delirium

    F15.922 Other stimulant use, unspecified with intoxication with perceptual disturbance

    F15.929 Other stimulant use, unspecified with intoxication, unspecified

F15.93   Other stimulant use, unspecified with withdrawal
          Excludes 1: other stimulant use, unspecified with intoxication (F15.92-)
F15.94   Other stimulant use, unspecified with stimulant-induced mood disorder
F15.95   Other stimulant use, unspecified with stimulant-induced psychotic disorder
          F15.950   Other stimulant use, unspecified with stimulant-induced psychotic disorder with delusions
          F15.951   Other stimulant use, unspecified with stimulant-induced psychotic disorder with hallucinations
          F15.959   Other stimulant use, unspecified with stimulant-induced psychotic disorder, unspecified
F15.98   Other stimulant use, unspecified with other stimulant-induced disorder
          F15.980   Other stimulant use, unspecified with stimulant-induced anxiety disorder
          F15.981   Other stimulant use, unspecified with stimulant-induced sexual dysfunction
          F15.982   Other stimulant use, unspecified with stimulant-induced sleep disorder
          F15.988   Other stimulant use, unspecified with other stimulant-induced disorder
F15.99   Other stimulant use, unspecified with unspecified stimulant-induced disorder

F16 Hallucinogen related disorders
         Includes: ecstasy
                       PCP
                       phencyclidine
F16.1   Hallucinogen abuse
         Excludes 1: hallucinogen dependence (F16.2-)
                         hallucinogen use, unspecified (F16.9-)
F16.10   Hallucinogen abuse, uncomplicated
F16.12   Hallucinogen abuse with intoxication
          F16.120   Hallucinogen abuse with intoxication, uncomplicated
          F16.121   Hallucinogen abuse with intoxication with delirium
          F16.122   Hallucinogen abuse with intoxication with perceptual disturbance
          F16.129   Hallucinogen abuse with intoxication, unspecified
F16.14   Hallucinogen abuse with hallucinogen-induced mood disorder
F16.15   Hallucinogen abuse with hallucinogen-induced psychotic disorder
          F16.150   Hallucinogen abuse with hallucinogen-induced psychotic disorder with delusions
          F16.151   Hallucinogen abuse with hallucinogen-induced psychotic disorder with hallucinations
          F16.159   Hallucinogen abuse with hallucinogen-induced psychotic disorder, unspecified
F16.18   Hallucinogen abuse with other hallucinogen-induced disorder
          F16.180   Hallucinogen abuse with hallucinogen-induced anxiety disorder
          F16.183   Hallucinogen abuse with hallucinogen persisting perception disorder (flashbacks)

          F16.188   Hallucinogen abuse with other hallucinogen-induced disorder
F16.19   Hallucinogen abuse with unspecified hallucinogen-induced disorder
F16.2   Hallucinogen dependence
         Excludes 1: hallucinogen abuse (F16.1-)
                         hallucinogen use, unspecified (F16.9-)
F16.20   Hallucinogen dependence, uncomplicated
F16.21   Hallucinogen dependence, in remission
F16.22   Hallucinogen dependence with intoxication
          F16.220   Hallucinogen dependence with intoxication, uncomplicated
          F16.221   Hallucinogen dependence with intoxication with delirium
          F16.229   Hallucinogen dependence with intoxication, unspecified
F16.24   Hallucinogen dependence with hallucinogen-induced mood disorder
F16.25   Hallucinogen dependence with hallucinogen-induced psychotic disorder
          F16.250   Hallucinogen dependence with hallucinogen-induced psychotic disorder with delusions
          F16.251   Hallucinogen dependence with hallucinogen-induced psychotic disorder with hallucinations
          F16.259   Hallucinogen dependence with hallucinogen-induced psychotic disorder, unspecified
F16.28   Hallucinogen dependence with other hallucinogen-induced disorder
          F16.280   Hallucinogen dependence with hallucinogen-induced anxiety disorder
          F16.283   Hallucinogen dependence with hallucinogen persisting perception disorder (flashbacks)
          F16.288   Hallucinogen dependence with other hallucinogen-induced disorder
F16.29   Hallucinogen dependence with unspecified hallucinogen-induced disorder
F16.9   Hallucinogen use, unspecified
         Excludes 1: hallucinogen abuse (F16.1-)
                         hallucinogen dependence (F16.2-)
F16.90   Hallucinogen use, unspecified, uncomplicated
F16.92   Hallucinogen use, unspecified with intoxication
          F16.920   Hallucinogen use, unspecified with intoxication, uncomplicated
          F16.921   Hallucinogen use, unspecified with intoxication with delirium
          F16.929   Hallucinogen use, unspecified with intoxication, unspecified
F16.94   Hallucinogen use, unspecified with hallucinogen-induced mood disorder
F16.95   Hallucinogen use, unspecified with hallucinogen-induced psychotic disorder
          F16.950   Hallucinogen use, unspecified with hallucinogen-induced psychotic disorder with delusions
          F16.951   Hallucinogen use, unspecified with hallucinogen-induced psychotic disorder with hallucinations
          F16.959   Hallucinogen use, unspecified with hallucinogen-induced psychotic disorder, unspecified

F16.98 Hallucinogen use, unspecified with other specified hallucinogen-induced disorder

    F16.980 Hallucinogen use, unspecified with hallucinogen-induced anxiety disorder

    F16.983 Hallucinogen use, unspecified with hallucinogen persisting perception disorder (flashbacks)

    F16.988 Hallucinogen use, unspecified with other hallucinogen-induced disorder

F16.99 Hallucinogen use, unspecified with unspecified hallucinogen-induced disorder

F17 Nicotine dependence

Excludes 1: history of tobacco dependence (Z87.891)
tobacco use NOS (Z72.0)

Excludes 2: tobacco use (smoking) during pregnancy, childbirth and the puerperium (O99.33-)
toxic effect of nicotine (T65.2-)

F17.2 Nicotine dependence

  F17.20 Nicotine dependence, unspecified

    F17.200 Nicotine dependence, unspecified, uncomplicated

    F17.201 Nicotine dependence, unspecified, in remission

    F17.203 Nicotine dependence unspecified, with withdrawal

    F17.208 Nicotine dependence, unspecified, with other nicotine-induced disorders

    F17.209 Nicotine dependence, unspecified, with unspecified nicotine-induced disorders

  F17.21 Nicotine dependence, cigarettes

    F17.210 Nicotine dependence, cigarettes, uncomplicated

    F17.211 Nicotine dependence, cigarettes, in remission

    F17.213 Nicotine dependence, cigarettes, with withdrawal

    F17.218 Nicotine dependence, cigarettes, with other nicotine-induced disorders

    F17.219 Nicotine dependence, cigarettes, with unspecified nicotine-induced disorders

  F17.22 Nicotine dependence, chewing tobacco

    F17.220 Nicotine dependence, chewing tobacco, uncomplicated

    F17.221 Nicotine dependence, chewing tobacco, in remission

    F17.223 Nicotine dependence, chewing tobacco, with withdrawal

    F17.228 Nicotine dependence, chewing tobacco, with other nicotine-induced disorders

    F17.229 Nicotine dependence, chewing tobacco, with unspecified nicotine-induced disorders

  F17.29 Nicotine dependence, other tobacco product

    F17.290 Nicotine dependence, other tobacco product, uncomplicated

    F17.291 Nicotine dependence, other tobacco product, in remission

    F17.293 Nicotine dependence, other tobacco product, with withdrawal

    F17.298 Nicotine dependence, other tobacco product, with other nicotine-induced disorders

    F17.299 Nicotine dependence, other tobacco product, with unspecified nicotine-induced disorders

F18 Inhalant related disorders

Includes: volatile solvents

F18.1 Inhalant abuse

Excludes 1: inhalant dependence (F18.2-)
inhalant use, unspecified (F18.9-)

  F18.10 Inhalant abuse, uncomplicated

  F18.12 Inhalant abuse with intoxication

    F18.120 Inhalant abuse with intoxication, uncomplicated

    F18.121 Inhalant abuse with intoxication delirium

    F18.129 Inhalant abuse with intoxication, unspecified

  F18.14 Inhalant abuse with inhalant-induced mood disorder

  F18.15 Inhalant abuse with inhalant-induced psychotic disorder

    F18.150 Inhalant abuse with inhalant-induced psychotic disorder with delusions

    F18.151 Inhalant abuse with inhalant-induced psychotic disorder with hallucinations

    F18.159 Inhalant abuse with inhalant-induced psychotic disorder, unspecified

  F18.17 Inhalant abuse with inhalant-induced dementia

  F18.18 Inhalant abuse with other inhalant-induced disorders

    F18.180 Inhalant abuse with inhalant-induced anxiety disorder

    F18.188 Inhalant abuse with other inhalant-induced disorder

  F18.19 Inhalant abuse with unspecified inhalant-induced disorder

F18.2 Inhalant dependence

Excludes 1: inhalant abuse (F18.1-)
inhalant use, unspecified (F18.9-)

  F18.20 Inhalant dependence, uncomplicated

  F18.21 Inhalant dependence, in remission

  F18.22 Inhalant dependence with intoxication

    F18.220 Inhalant dependence with intoxication, uncomplicated

    F18.221 Inhalant dependence with intoxication delirium

    F18.229 Inhalant dependence with intoxication, unspecified

  F18.24 Inhalant dependence with inhalant-induced mood disorder

  F18.25 Inhalant dependence with inhalant-induced psychotic disorder

    F18.250 Inhalant dependence with inhalant-induced psychotic disorder with delusions

    F18.251 Inhalant dependence with inhalant-induced psychotic disorder with hallucinations

    F18.259 Inhalant dependence with inhalant-induced psychotic disorder, unspecified

F18.27   Inhalant dependence with inhalant-induced dementia

F18.28   Inhalant dependence with other inhalant-induced disorders

 F18.280   Inhalant dependence with inhalant-induced anxiety disorder

 F18.288   Inhalant dependence with other inhalant-induced disorder

F18.29   Inhalant dependence with unspecified inhalant-induced disorder

F18.9   Inhalant use, unspecified

Excludes 1: inhalant abuse (F18.1-)
inhalant dependence (F18.2-)

F18.90   Inhalant use, unspecified, uncomplicated

F18.92   Inhalant use, unspecified with intoxication

 F18.920   Inhalant use, unspecified with intoxication, uncomplicated

 F18.921   Inhalant use, unspecified with intoxication with delirium

 F18.929   Inhalant use, unspecified with intoxication, unspecified

F18.94   Inhalant use, unspecified with inhalant-induced mood disorder

F18.95   Inhalant use, unspecified with inhalant-induced psychotic disorder

 F18.950   Inhalant use, unspecified with inhalant-induced psychotic disorder with delusions

 F18.951   Inhalant use, unspecified with inhalant-induced psychotic disorder with hallucinations

 F18.959   Inhalant use, unspecified with inhalant-induced psychotic disorder, unspecified

F18.97   Inhalant use, unspecified with inhalant-induced persisting dementia

F18.98   Inhalant use, unspecified with other inhalant-induced disorders

 F18.980   Inhalant use, unspecified with inhalant-induced anxiety disorder

 F18.988   Inhalant use, unspecified with other inhalant-induced disorder

F18.99   Inhalant use, unspecified with unspecified inhalant-induced disorder

F19   Other psychoactive substance related disorders

Includes: polysubstance drug use (indiscriminate drug use)

F19.1   Other psychoactive substance abuse

Excludes 1: other psychoactive substance dependence (F19.2-)
other psychoactive substance use, unspecified (F19.9-)

F19.10   Other psychoactive substance abuse, uncomplicated

F19.12   Other psychoactive substance abuse with intoxication

 F19.120   Other psychoactive substance abuse with intoxication, uncomplicated

 F19.121   Other psychoactive substance abuse with intoxication delirium

 F19.122   Other psychoactive substance abuse with intoxication with perceptual disturbances

 F19.129   Other psychoactive substance abuse with intoxication, unspecified

F19.14   Other psychoactive substance abuse with psychoactive substance-induced mood disorder

F19.15   Other psychoactive substance abuse with psychoactive substance-induced psychotic disorder

 F19.150   Other psychoactive substance abuse with psychoactive substance-induced psychotic disorder with delusions

 F19.151   Other psychoactive substance abuse with psychoactive substance-induced psychotic disorder with hallucinations

 F19.159   Other psychoactive substance abuse with psychoactive substance-induced psychotic disorder, unspecified

F19.16   Other psychoactive substance abuse with psychoactive substance-induced persisting amnestic disorder

F19.17   Other psychoactive substance abuse with psychoactive substance-induced persisting dementia

F19.18   Other psychoactive substance abuse with other psychoactive substance-induced disorders

 F19.180   Other psychoactive substance abuse with psychoactive substance-induced anxiety disorder

 F19.181   Other psychoactive substance abuse with psychoactive substance-induced sexual dysfunction

 F19.182   Other psychoactive substance abuse with psychoactive substance-induced sleep disorder

 F19.188   Other psychoactive substance abuse with other psychoactive substance-induced disorder

F19.19   Other psychoactive substance abuse with unspecified psychoactive substance-induced disorder

F19.2   Other psychoactive substance dependence

Excludes 1: other psychoactive substance abuse (F19.1-)
other psychoactive substance use, unspecified (F19.9-)

F19.20   Other psychoactive substance dependence, uncomplicated

F19.21   Other psychoactive substance dependence, in remission

F19.22   Other psychoactive substance dependence with intoxication

Excludes 1: other psychoactive substance dependence with withdrawal (F19.23-)

 F19.220   Other psychoactive substance dependence with intoxication, uncomplicated

 F19.221   Other psychoactive substance dependence with intoxication delirium

 F19.222   Other psychoactive substance dependence with intoxication with perceptual disturbance

 F19.229   Other psychoactive substance dependence with intoxication, unspecified

F19.23   Other psychoactive substance dependence with withdrawal

Excludes 1: other psychoactive substance dependence with intoxication (F19.22-)

F19.230 Other psychoactive substance dependence with withdrawal, uncomplicated

F19.231 Other psychoactive substance dependence with withdrawal delirium

F19.232 Other psychoactive substance dependence with withdrawal with perceptual disturbance

F19.239 Other psychoactive substance dependence with withdrawal, unspecified

F19.24 Other psychoactive substance dependence with psychoactive substance-induced mood disorder

F19.25 Other psychoactive substance dependence with psychoactive substance-induced psychotic disorder

F19.250 Other psychoactive substance dependence with psychoactive substance-induced psychotic disorder with delusions

F19.251 Other psychoactive substance dependence with psychoactive substance-induced psychotic disorder with hallucinations

F19.259 Other psychoactive substance dependence with psychoactive substance-induced psychotic disorder, unspecified

F19.26 Other psychoactive substance dependence with psychoactive substance-induced persisting amnestic disorder

F19.27 Other psychoactive substance dependence with psychoactive substance-induced persisting dementia

F19.28 Other psychoactive substance dependence with other psychoactive substance-induced disorders

F19.280 Other psychoactive substance dependence with psychoactive substance-induced anxiety disorder

F19.281 Other psychoactive substance dependence with psychoactive substance-induced sexual dysfunction

F19.282 Other psychoactive substance dependence with psychoactive substance-induced sleep disorder

F19.288 Other psychoactive substance dependence with other psychoactive substance-induced disorder

F19.29 Other psychoactive substance dependence with unspecified psychoactive substance-induced disorder

F19.9 Other psychoactive substance use, unspecified

Excludes 1: other psychoactive substance abuse (F19.1-)
other psychoactive substance dependence (F19.2-)

F19.90 Other psychoactive substance use, unspecified, uncomplicated

F19.92 Other psychoactive substance use, unspecified with intoxication

Excludes 1: other psychoactive substance use, unspecified with withdrawal (F19.93)

F19.920 Other psychoactive substance use, unspecified with intoxication, uncomplicated

F19.921 Other psychoactive substance use, unspecified with intoxication with delirium

F19.922 Other psychoactive substance use, unspecified with intoxication with perceptual disturbance

F19.929 Other psychoactive substance use, unspecified with intoxication, unspecified

F19.93 Other psychoactive substance use, unspecified with withdrawal

Excludes 1: other psychoactive substance use, unspecified with intoxication (F19.92-)

F19.930 Other psychoactive substance use, unspecified with withdrawal, uncomplicated

F19.931 Other psychoactive substance use, unspecified with withdrawal delirium

F19.932 Other psychoactive substance use, unspecified with withdrawal with perceptual disturbance

F19.939 Other psychoactive substance use, unspecified with withdrawal, unspecified

F19.94 Other psychoactive substance use, unspecified with psychoactive substance-induced mood disorder

F19.95 Other psychoactive substance use, unspecified with psychoactive substance-induced psychotic disorder

F19.950 Other psychoactive substance use, unspecified with psychoactive substance-induced psychotic disorder with delusions

F19.951 Other psychoactive substance use, unspecified with psychoactive substance-induced psychotic disorder with hallucinations

F19.959 Other psychoactive substance use, unspecified with psychoactive substance-induced psychotic disorder, unspecified

F19.96 Other psychoactive substance use, unspecified with psychoactive substance-induced persisting amnestic disorder

F19.97 Other psychoactive substance use, unspecified with psychoactive substance-induced persisting dementia

F19.98 Other psychoactive substance use, unspecified with other psychoactive substance-induced disorders

F19.980 Other psychoactive substance use, unspecified with psychoactive substance-induced anxiety disorder

F19.981 Other psychoactive substance use, unspecified with psychoactive substance-induced sexual dysfunction

F19.982 Other psychoactive substance use, unspecified with psychoactive substance-induced sleep disorder

F19.988 Other psychoactive substance use, unspecified with other psychoactivesubstance-induced disorder

F19.99 Other psychoactive substance use, unspecified with unspecified psychoactive substance-induced disorder

SCHIZOPHRENIA, SCHIZOTYPAL, DELUSIONAL, AND OTHER NON-MOOD PSYCHOTIC DISORDERS (F20-F29)

F20 Schizophrenia

Excludes 1: brief psychotic disorder (F23)
cyclic schizophrenia (F25.0)
mood [affective] disorders with psychotic symptoms (F30.2, F31.2, F31.5, F31.64, F32.3, F33.3)
schizoaffective disorder (F25.-)
schizophrenic reaction NOS (F23)

Excludes 2: schizophrenic reaction in:
alcoholism (F10.15-, F10.25-, F10.95-)
brain disease (F06.2)
epilepsy (F06.2)
psychoactive drug use (F11-F19 with .15, .25, .95)
schizotypal disorder (F21)

F20.0 Paranoid schizophrenia
Paraphrenic schizophrenia
Excludes 1: involutional paranoid state (F22)
paranoia (F22)

F20.1 Disorganized schizophrenia
Hebephrenic schizophrenia
Hebephrenia

F20.2 Catatonic schizophrenia
Schizophrenic catalepsy
Schizophrenic catatonia
Schizophrenic flexibilitas cerea
Excludes 1: catatonic stupor (R40.1)

F20.3 Undifferentiated schizophrenia
Atypical schizophrenia
Excludes 1: acute schizophrenia-like psychotic disorder (F23)
Excludes 2: post-schizophrenic depression (F32.8)

F20.5 Residual schizophrenia
Restzustand (schizophrenic)
Schizophrenic residual state

F20.8 Other schizophrenia
F20.81 Schizophreniform disorder
Schizophreniform psychosis NOS
F20.89 Other schizophrenia
Cenesthopathic schizophrenia
Simple schizophrenia

F20.9 Schizophrenia, unspecified

F21 Schizotypal disorder
Borderline schizophrenia
Latent schizophrenia
Latent schizophrenic reaction
Prepsychotic schizophrenia
Prodromal schizophrenia
Pseudoneurotic schizophrenia
Pseudopsychopathic schizophrenia
Schizotypal personality disorder
Excludes 2: Asperger's syndrome (F84.5)
schizoid personality disorder (F60.1)

F22 Delusional disorders
Delusional dysmorphophobia
Involutional paranoid state
Paranoia
Paranoia querulans

Paranoid psychosis
Paranoid state
Paraphrenia (late)
Sensitiver Beziehungswahn
Excludes 1: mood [affective] disorders with psychotic symptoms (F30.2, F31.2, F31.5, F31.64, F32.3, F33.3)
paranoid schizophrenia (F20.0)
Excludes 2: paranoid personality disorder (F60.0)
paranoid psychosis, psychogenic (F23)
paranoid reaction (F23)

F23 Brief psychotic disorder
Paranoid reaction
Psychogenic paranoid psychosis
Excludes 2: mood [affective] disorders with psychotic symptoms (F30.2, F31.2, F31.5, F31.64, F32.3, F33.3)

F24 Shared psychotic disorder
Folie α deux
Induced paranoid disorder
Induced psychotic disorder

F25 Schizoaffective disorders
Excludes 1: mood [affective] disorders with psychotic symptoms (F30.2, F31.2, F31.5, F31.64, F32.3, F33.3)
schizophrenia (F20.-)

F25.0 Schizoaffective disorder, bipolar type
Cyclic schizophrenia
Schizoaffective disorder, manic type
Schizoaffective disorder, mixed type
Schizoaffective psychosis, bipolar type
Schizophreniform psychosis, manic type

F25.1 Schizoaffective disorder, depressive type
Schizoaffective psychosis, depressive type
Schizophreniform psychosis, depressive type

F25.8 Other schizoaffective disorders

F25.9 Schizoaffective disorder, unspecified
Schizoaffective psychosis NOS

F28 Other psychotic disorder not due to a substance or known physiological condition
Chronic hallucinatory psychosis

F29 Unspecified psychosis not due to a substance or known physiological condition
Psychosis NOS
Excludes 1: mental disorder NOS (F99)
unspecified mental disorder due to known physiological condition (F09)

MOOD [AFFECTIVE] DISORDERS (F30-F39)

F30 Manic episode
Includes: bipolar disorder, single manic episode
mixed affective episode
Excludes 1: bipolar disorder (F31.-)
major depressive disorder, single episode (F32.-)
major depressive disorder, recurrent (F33.-)

F30.1 Manic episode without psychotic symptoms
F30.10 Manic episode without psychotic symptoms, unspecified
F30.11 Manic episode without psychotic symptoms, mild
F30.12 Manic episode without psychotic symptoms, moderate
F30.13 Manic episode, severe, without psychotic symptoms

F30.2 Manic episode, severe with psychotic symptoms
Manic stupor
Mania with mood-congruent psychotic symptoms

Mania with mood-incongruent psychotic symptoms

F30.3 Manic episode in partial remission

F30.4 Manic episode in full remission

F30.8 Other manic episodes

Hypomania

F30.9 Manic episode, unspecified

Mania NOS

F31 Bipolar disorder

Includes: manic-depressive illness

manic-depressive psychosis

manic-depressive reaction

Excludes 1: bipolar disorder, single manic episode (F30.-)

major depressive disorder, single episode (F32.-)

major depressive disorder, recurrent (F33.-)

Excludes 2: cyclothymia (F34.0)

F31.0 Bipolar disorder, current episode hypomanic

F31.1 Bipolar disorder, current episode manic without psychotic features

    F31.10 Bipolar disorder, current episode manic without psychotic features, unspecified

    F31.11 Bipolar disorder, current episode manic without psychotic features, mild

    F31.12 Bipolar disorder, current episode manic without psychotic features, moderate

    F31.13 Bipolar disorder, current episode manic without psychotic features, severe

F31.2 Bipolar disorder, current episode manic severe with psychotic features

Bipolar disorder, current episode manic with mood-congruent psychotic symptoms

Bipolar disorder, current episode manic with mood-incongruent psychotic symptoms

F31.3 Bipolar disorder, current episode depressed, mild or moderate severity

    F31.30 Bipolar disorder, current episode depressed, mild or moderate severity, unspecified

    F31.31 Bipolar disorder, current episode depressed, mild

    F31.32 Bipolar disorder, current episode depressed, moderate

F31.4 Bipolar disorder, current episode depressed, severe, without psychotic features

F31.5 Bipolar disorder, current episode depressed, severe, with psychotic features

Bipolar disorder, current episode depressed with mood-incongruent psychotic symptoms

Bipolar disorder, current episode depressed with mood-congruent psychotic symptoms

F31.6 Bipolar disorder, current episode mixed

    F31.60 Bipolar disorder, current episode mixed, unspecified

    F31.61 Bipolar disorder, current episode mixed, mild

    F31.62 Bipolar disorder, current episode mixed, moderate

    F31.63 Bipolar disorder, current episode mixed, severe, without psychotic features

    F31.64 Bipolar disorder, current episode mixed, severe, with psychotic features

Bipolar disorder, current episode mixed with mood-congruent psychotic symptoms

Bipolar disorder, current episode mixed with mood-incongruent psychotic symptoms

F31.7 Bipolar disorder, currently in remission

    F31.70 Bipolar disorder, currently in remission, most recent episode unspecified

    F31.71 Bipolar disorder, in partial remission, most recent episode hypomanic

    F31.72 Bipolar disorder, in full remission, most recent episode hypomanic

    F31.73 Bipolar disorder, in partial remission, most recent episode manic

    F31.74 Bipolar disorder, in full remission, most recent episode manic

    F31.75 Bipolar disorder, in partial remission, most recent episode depressed

    F31.76 Bipolar disorder, in full remission, most recent episode depressed

    F31.77 Bipolar disorder, in partial remission, most recent episode mixed

    F31.78 Bipolar disorder, in full remission, most recent episode mixed

F31.8 Other bipolar disorders

    F31.81 Bipolar II disorder

    F31.89 Other bipolar disorder

Recurrent manic episodes NOS

F31.9 Bipolar disorder, unspecified

F32 Major depressive disorder, single episode

Includes: single episode of agitated depression

single episode of depressive reaction

single episode of major depression

single episode of psychogenic depression

single episode of reactive depression

single episode of vital depression

Excludes 1: bipolar disorder (F31-)

manic episode (F30-)

recurrent depressive disorder (F33.-)

Excludes 2: adjustment disorder (F43.2)

F32.0 Major depressive disorder, single episode, mild

F32.1 Major depressive disorder, single episode, moderate

F32.2 Major depressive disorder, single episode, severe without psychotic features

F32.3 Major depressive disorder, single episode, severe with psychotic features

Single episode of major depression with mood-congruent psychotic symptoms

Single episode of major depression with mood-incongruent psychotic symptoms

Single episode of major depression with psychotic symptoms

Single episode of psychogenic depressive psychosis

Single episode of psychotic depression

Single episode of reactive depressive psychosis

F32.4 Major depressive disorder, single episode, in partial remission

F32.5 Major depressive disorder, single episode, in full remission

F32.8 Other depressive episodes

Atypical depression

Post-schizophrenic depression

Single episode of 'masked' depression NOS

F32.9 Major depressive disorder, single episode, unspecified

Depression NOS

Depressive disorder NOS

Major depression NOS

F33 Major depressive disorder, recurrent

Includes: recurrent episodes of depressive reaction

recurrent episodes of endogenous depression

recurrent episodes of major depression

recurrent episodes of psychogenic depression

   ● New code   ▲ Revised code   ⑦ 7th digit required   ⊗ Placeholder required

recurrent episodes of reactive depression

recurrent episodes of seasonal depressive disorder

recurrent episodes of vital depression

Excludes 1: bipolar disorder (F31.-)

manic episode (F30.-)

F33.0   Major depressive disorder, recurrent, mild

F33.1   Major depressive disorder, recurrent, moderate

F33.2   Major depressive disorder, recurrent severe without psychotic features

F33.3   Major depressive disorder, recurrent, severe with psychotic symptoms

Endogenous depression with psychotic symptoms

Recurrent severe episodes of major depression with mood-congruent psychotic symptoms

Recurrent severe episodes of major depression with mood-incongruent psychotic symptoms

Recurrent severe episodes of major depression with psychotic symptoms

Recurrent severe episodes of psychogenic depressive psychosis

Recurrent severe episodes of psychotic depression

Recurrent severe episodes of reactive depressive psychosis

F33.4   Major depressive disorder, recurrent, in remission

   F33.40   Major depressive disorder, recurrent, in remission, unspecified

   F33.41   Major depressive disorder, recurrent, in partial remission

   F33.42   Major depressive disorder, recurrent, in full remission

F33.8   Other recurrent depressive disorders

Recurrent brief depressive episodes

F33.9   Major depressive disorder, recurrent, unspecified

Monopolar depression NOS

F34   Persistent mood [affective] disorders

F34.0   Cyclothymic disorder

Affective personality disorder

Cycloid personality

Cyclothymia

Cyclothymic personality

F34.1   Dysthymic disorder

Depressive neurosis

Depressive personality disorder

Dysthymia

Neurotic depression

Persistent anxiety depression

Excludes 2: anxiety depression (mild or not persistent) (F41.8)

F34.8   Other persistent mood [affective] disorders

F34.9   Persistent mood [affective] disorder, unspecified

F39   Unspecified mood [affective] disorder

Affective psychosis NOS

ANXIETY, DISSOCIATIVE, STRESS-RELATED, SOMATOFORM AND OTHER NONPSYCHOTIC MENTAL DISORDERS (F40-F48)

F40   Phobic anxiety disorders

F40.0   Agoraphobia

   F40.00   Agoraphobia, unspecified

   F40.01   Agoraphobia with panic disorder

Panic disorder with agoraphobia

Excludes 1: panic disorder without agoraphobia (F41.0)

   F40.02   Agoraphobia without panic disorder

F40.1   Social phobias

Anthropophobia

Social anxiety disorder of childhood

Social neurosis

   F40.10   Social phobia, unspecified

   F40.11   Social phobia, generalized

F40.2   Specific (isolated) phobias

Excludes 2: dysmorphophobia (nondelusional) (F45.22)

nosophobia (F45.22)

   F40.21   Animal type phobia

      F40.210   Arachnophobia

Fear of spiders

      F40.218   Other animal type phobia

   F40.22   Natural environment type phobia

      F40.220   Fear of thunderstorms

      F40.228   Other natural environment type phobia

   F40.23   Blood, injection, injury type phobia

      F40.230   Fear of blood

      F40.231   Fear of injections and transfusions

      F40.232   Fear of other medical care

      F40.233   Fear of injury

   F40.24   Situational type phobia

      F40.240   Claustrophobia

      F40.241   Acrophobia

      F40.242   Fear of bridges

      F40.243   Fear of flying

      F40.248   Other situational type phobia

   F40.29   Other specified phobia

      F40.290   Androphobia

Fear of men

      F40.291   Gynephobia

Fear of women

      F40.298   Other specified phobia

F40.8   Other phobic anxiety disorders

Phobic anxiety disorder of childhood

F40.9   Phobic anxiety disorder, unspecified

Phobia NOS

Phobic state NOS

F41   Other anxiety disorders

Excludes 2: anxiety in:

acute stress reaction (F43.0)

transient adjustment reaction (F43.2)

neurasthenia (F48.8)

psychophysiologic disorders (F45.-)

separation anxiety (F93.0)

F41.0   Panic disorder [episodic paroxysmal anxiety] without agoraphobia

Panic attack

Panic state

Excludes 1: panic disorder with agoraphobia (F40.01)

F41.1   Generalized anxiety disorder

Anxiety neurosis

Anxiety reaction

Anxiety state

Overanxious disorder

Excludes 2: neurasthenia (F48.8)

F41.3   Other mixed anxiety disorders

F41.8   Other specified anxiety disorders

Anxiety depression (mild or not persistent)

Anxiety hysteria

Mixed anxiety and depressive disorder

F41.9 Anxiety disorder, unspecified

Anxiety NOS

F42 Obsessive-compulsive disorder

Anancastic neurosis

Obsessive-compulsive neurosis

Excludes 2: obsessive-compulsive personality (disorder) (F60.5)

obsessive-compulsive symptoms occurring in:

depression (F32-F33)

schizophrenia (F20.-)

F43 Reaction to severe stress, and adjustment disorders

F43.0 Acute stress reaction

Acute crisis reaction

Acute reaction to stress

Combat and operational stress reaction

Combat fatigue

Crisis state

Psychic shock

F43.1 Post-traumatic stress disorder (PTSD)

Traumatic neurosis

F43.10 Post-traumatic stress disorder, unspecified

F43.11 Post-traumatic stress disorder, acute

F43.12 Post-traumatic stress disorder, chronic

F43.2 Adjustment disorders

Culture shock

Grief reaction

Hospitalism in children

Excludes 2: separation anxiety disorder of childhood (F93.0)

F43.20 Adjustment disorder, unspecified

F43.21 Adjustment disorder with depressed mood

F43.22 Adjustment disorder with anxiety

F43.23 Adjustment disorder with mixed anxiety and depressed mood

F43.24 Adjustment disorder with disturbance of conduct

F43.25 Adjustment disorder with mixed disturbance of emotions and conduct

F43.29 Adjustment disorder with other symptoms

F43.8 Other reactions to severe stress

F43.9 Reaction to severe stress, unspecified

F44 Dissociative and conversion disorders

Includes: conversion hysteria

conversion reaction

hysteria

hysterical psychosis

Excludes 2: malingering [conscious simulation] (Z76.5)

F44.0 Dissociative amnesia

Excludes 1: amnesia NOS (R41.3)

anterograde amnesia (R41.1)

retrograde amnesia (R41.2)

Excludes 2: alcohol-or other psychoactive substance-induced amnestic disorder (F10, F13, F19with .26, .96)

amnestic disorder due to known physiological condition (F04)

postictal amnesia in epilepsy (G40.-)

F44.1 Dissociative fugue

Excludes 2: postictal fugue in epilepsy (G40.-)

F44.2 Dissociative stupor

Excludes 1: catatonic stupor (R40.1)

stupor NOS (R40.1)

Excludes 2: catatonic disorder due to known physiological condition (F06.1)

depressive stupor (F32, F33)

manic stupor (F30, F31)

F44.4 Conversion disorder with motor symptom or deficit

Dissociative motor disorders

Psychogenic aphonia

Psychogenic dysphonia

F44.5 Conversion disorder with seizures or convulsions

Dissociative convulsions

F44.6 Conversion disorder with sensory symptom or deficit

Dissociative anesthesia and sensory loss

Psychogenic deafness

F44.7 Conversion disorder with mixed symptom presentation

F44.8 Other dissociative and conversion disorders

F44.81 Dissociative identity disorder

Multiple personality disorder

F44.89 Other dissociative and conversion disorders

Ganser's syndrome

Psychogenic confusion

Psychogenic twilight state

Trance and possession disorders

F44.9 Dissociative and conversion disorder, unspecified

Dissociative disorder NOS

F45 Somatoform disorders

Excludes 2: dissociative and conversion disorders (F44.-)

factitious disorders (F68.1-)

hair-plucking (F63.3)

lalling (F80.0)

lisping (F80.0)

malingering [conscious simulation] (Z76.5)

nail-biting (F98.8)

psychological or behavioral factors associated with disorders or diseases classified elsewhere (F54)

sexual dysfunction, not due to a substance or known physiological condition (F52.-)

thumb-sucking (F98.8)

tic disorders (in childhood and adolescence) (F95.-)

Tourette's syndrome (F95.2)

trichotillomania (F63.3)

F45.0 Somatization disorder

Briquet's disorder

Multiple psychosomatic disorder

F45.1 Undifferentiated somatoform disorder

Undifferentiated psychosomatic disorder

F45.2 Hypochondriacal disorders

Excludes 2: delusional dysmorphophobia (F22)

fixed delusions about bodily functions or shape (F22)

F45.20 Hypochondriacal disorder, unspecified

F45.21 Hypochondriasis

Hypochondriacal neurosis

F45.22 Body dysmorphic disorder

Dysmorphophobia (nondelusional)

Nosophobia

F45.29 Other hypochondriacal disorders

F45.4 Pain disorders related to psychological factors

Excludes 1: pain NOS (R52)

F45.41 Pain disorder exclusively related to psychological factors

Somatoform pain disorder (persistent)

F45.42 Pain disorder with related psychological factors

Code also associated acute or chronic pain (G89.-)

F45.8 Other somatoform disorders

Psychogenic dysmenorrhea

Psychogenic dysphagia, including 'globus hystericus'

Psychogenic pruritus

Psychogenic torticollis

Somatoform autonomic dysfunction

Teeth grinding

> Excludes 1: sleep related teeth grinding (G47.63)

F45.9 Somatoform disorder, unspecified

Psychosomatic disorder NOS

F48 Other nonpsychotic mental disorders

F48.1 Depersonalization-derealization syndrome

F48.2 Pseudobulbar affect

Involuntary emotional expression disorder

Code first underlying cause, if known, such as:

amyotrophic lateral sclerosis (G12.21)

multiple sclerosis (G35)

sequelae of cerebrovascular disease (I69.-)

sequelae of traumatic intracranial injury (S06.-)

F48.8 Other specified nonpsychotic mental disorders

Dhat syndrome

Neurasthenia

Occupational neurosis, including writer's cramp

Psychasthenia

Psychasthenic neurosis

Psychogenic syncope

F48.9 Nonpsychotic mental disorder, unspecified

Neurosis NOS

BEHAVIORAL SYNDROMES ASSOCIATED WITH PHYSIOLOGICAL DISTURBANCES AND PHYSICAL FACTORS (F50-F59)

F50 Eating disorders

> Excludes 1: anorexia NOS (R63.0)
>
> feeding difficulties (R63.3)
>
> polyphagia (R63.2)
>
> Excludes 2: feeding disorder in infancy or childhood (F98.2-)

F50.0 Anorexia nervosa

> Excludes 1: loss of appetite (R63.0)
>
> psychogenic loss of appetite (F50.8)

F50.00 Anorexia nervosa, unspecified

F50.01 Anorexia nervosa, restricting type

F50.02 Anorexia nervosa, binge eating/purging type

> Excludes 1: bulimia nervosa (F50.2)

F50.2 Bulimia nervosa

Bulimia NOS

Hyperorexia nervosa

> Excludes 1: anorexia nervosa, binge eating/purging type (F50.02)

F50.8 Other eating disorders

Pica in adults

Psychogenic loss of appetite

> Excludes 2: pica of infancy and childhood (F98.3)

F50.9 Eating disorder, unspecified

Atypical anorexia nervosa

Atypical bulimia nervosa

F51 Sleep disorders not due to a substance or known physiological condition

> Excludes 2: organic sleep disorders (G47.-)

F51.0 Insomnia not due to a substance or known physiological condition

> Excludes 2: alcohol related insomnia (F10.182, F10.282, F10.982)

drug related insomnia (F11.182, F11.282, F11.982, F13.182, F13.282, F13.982, F14.182, F14.282, F14.982, F15.182, F15.282, F15.982, F19.182, F19.282, F19.982)

insomnia NOS (G47.0-)

insomnia due to known physiological condition (G47.0-)

organic insomnia (G47.0-)

sleep deprivation (Z72.820)

F51.01 Primary insomnia

Idiopathic insomnia

F51.02 Adjustment insomnia

F51.03 Paradoxical insomnia

F51.04 Psychophysiologic insomnia

F51.05 Insomnia due to other mental disorder

Code also associated mental disorder

F51.09 Other insomnia not due to a substance or known physiological condition

F51.1 Hypersomnia not due to a substance or known physiological condition

> Excludes 2: alcohol related hypersomnia (F10.182, F10.282, F10.982)
>
> drug related hypersomnia (F11.182, F11.282, F11.982, F13.182, F13.282, F13.982, F14.182, F14.282, F14.982, F15.182, F15.282, F15.982, F19.182, F19.282, F19.982)
>
> hypersomnia NOS (G47.10)
>
> hypersomnia due to known physiological condition (G47.10)
>
> idiopathic hypersomnia (G47.11, G47.12)
>
> narcolepsy (G47.4-)

F51.11 Primary hypersomnia

F51.12 Insufficient sleep syndrome

> Excludes 1: sleep deprivation (Z72.820)

F51.13 Hypersomnia due to other mental disorder

Code also associated mental disorder

F51.19 Other hypersomnia not due to a substance or known physiological condition

F51.3 Sleepwalking [somnambulism]

F51.4 Sleep terrors [night terrors]

F51.5 Nightmare disorder

Dream anxiety disorder

F51.8 Other sleep disorders not due to a substance or known physiological condition

F51.9 Sleep disorder not due to a substance or known physiological condition, unspecified

Emotional sleep disorder NOS

F52 Sexual dysfunction not due to a substance or known physiological condition

> Excludes 2: Dhat syndrome (F48.8)

F52.0 Hypoactive sexual desire disorder

Anhedonia (sexual)

Lack or loss of sexual desire

> Excludes 1: decreased libido (R68.82)

F52.1 Sexual aversion disorder

Sexual aversion and lack of sexual enjoyment

F52.2 Sexual arousal disorders

Failure of genital response

F52.21 Male erectile disorder

Psychogenic impotence

> Excludes 1: impotence of organic origin (N52.-)
>
> impotence NOS (N52.-)

F52.22 Female sexual arousal disorder

Frigidity

F52.3 Orgasmic disorder

Inhibited orgasm

Psychogenic anorgasmy

F52.31 Female orgasmic disorder

F52.32 Male orgasmic disorder

F52.4 Premature ejaculation

F52.5 Vaginismus not due to a substance or known physiological condition

Psychogenic vaginismus

Excludes 2: vaginismus (due to a known physiological condition) (N94.2)

F52.6 Dyspareunia not due to a substance or known physiological condition

Psychogenic dyspareunia

Excludes 2: dyspareunia (due to a known physiological condition) (N94.1)

F52.8 Other sexual dysfunction not due to a substance or known physiological condition

Excessive sexual drive

Nymphomania

Satyriasis

F52.9 Unspecified sexual dysfunction not due to a substance or known physiological condition

Sexual dysfunction NOS

F53 Puerperal psychosis

Postpartum depression

Excludes 1: mood disorders with psychotic features (F30.2, F31.2, F31.5, F31.64, F32.3, F33.3)

postpartum dysphoria (O90.6)

psychosis in schizophrenia, schizotypal, delusional, and other psychotic disorders (F20-F29)

F54 Psychological and behavioral factors associated with disorders or diseases classified elsewhere

Psychological factors affecting physical conditions

Code first the associated physical disorder, such as:

asthma (J45.-)

dermatitis (L23-L25)

gastric ulcer (K25.-)

mucous colitis (K58.-)

ulcerative colitis (K51.-)

urticaria (L50.-)

Excludes 2: tension-type headache (G44.2)

F55 Abuse of non-psychoactive substances

Excludes 2: abuse of psychoactive substances (F10-F19)

F55.0 Abuse of antacids

F55.1 Abuse of herbal or folk remedies

F55.2 Abuse of laxatives

F55.3 Abuse of steroids or hormones

F55.4 Abuse of vitamins

F55.8 Abuse of other non-psychoactive substances

F59 Unspecified behavioral syndromes associated with physiological disturbances and physical factors

Psychogenic physiological dysfunction NOS

DISORDERS OF ADULT PERSONALITY AND BEHAVIOR (F60-F69)

F60 Specific personality disorders

F60.0 Paranoid personality disorder

Expansive paranoid personality (disorder)

Fanatic personality (disorder)

Querulant personality (disorder)

Paranoid personality (disorder)

Sensitive paranoid personality (disorder)

Excludes 2: paranoia (F22)

paranoia querulans (F22)

paranoid psychosis (F22)

paranoid schizophrenia (F20.0)

paranoid state (F22)

F60.1 Schizoid personality disorder

Excludes 2: Asperger's syndrome (F84.5)

delusional disorder (F22)

schizoid disorder of childhood (F84.5)

schizophrenia (F20.-)

schizotypal disorder (F21)

F60.2 Antisocial personality disorder

Amoral personality (disorder)

Asocial personality (disorder)

Dissocial personality disorder

Psychopathic personality (disorder)

Sociopathic personality (disorder)

Excludes 1: conduct disorders (F91.-)

Excludes 2: borderline personality disorder (F60.3)

F60.3 Borderline personality disorder

Aggressive personality (disorder)

Emotionally unstable personality disorder

Explosive personality (disorder)

Excludes 2: antisocial personality disorder (F60.2)

F60.4 Histrionic personality disorder

Hysterical personality (disorder)

Psychoinfantile personality (disorder)

F60.5 Obsessive-compulsive personality disorder

Anankastic personality (disorder)

Compulsive personality (disorder)

Obsessional personality (disorder)

Excludes 2: obsessive-compulsive disorder (F42)

F60.6 Avoidant personality disorder

Anxious personality disorder

F60.7 Dependent personality disorder

Asthenic personality (disorder)

Inadequate personality (disorder)

Passive personality (disorder)

F60.8 Other specific personality disorders

F60.81 Narcissistic personality disorder

F60.89 Other specific personality disorders

Eccentric personality disorder

'Haltlose' type personality disorder

Immature personality disorder

Passive-aggressive personality disorder

Psychoneurotic personality disorder

Self-defeating personality disorder

F60.9 Personality disorder, unspecified

Character disorder NOS

Character neurosis NOS

Pathological personality NOS

F63 Impulse disorders

Excludes 2: habitual excessive use of alcohol or psychoactive substances (F10-F19)

impulse disorders involving sexual behavior (F65.-)

F63.0 Pathological gambling

Compulsive gambling

Excludes 1: gambling and betting NOS (Z72.6)

Excludes 2: excessive gambling by manic patients (F30, F31)

gambling in antisocial personality disorder (F60.2)

F63.1 Pyromania

Pathological fire-setting

Excludes 2: fire-setting (by) (in):

adult with antisocial personality disorder (F60.2)

alcohol or psychoactive substance intoxication (F10-F19)

conduct disorders (F91.-)

mental disorders due to known physiological condition (F01-F09)

schizophrenia (F20.-)

F63.2 Kleptomania

Pathological stealing

Excludes 1: shoplifting as the reason for observation for suspected mental disorder (Z03.8)

Excludes 2: depressive disorder with stealing (F31-F33)

stealing due to underlying mental condition-code to mental condition

stealing in mental disorders due to known physiological condition (F01-F09)

F63.3 Trichotillomania

Hair plucking

Excludes 2: other stereotyped movement disorder (F98.4)

F63.8 Other impulse disorders

F63.81 Intermittent explosive disorder

F63.89 Other impulse disorders

F63.9 Impulse disorder, unspecified

Impulse control disorder NOS

F64 Gender identity disorders

F64.1 Gender identity disorder in adolescence and adulthood

Dual role transvestism

Transsexualism

Use additional code to identify sex reassignment status (Z87.890)

Excludes 1: gender identity disorder in childhood (F64.2)

Excludes 2: fetishistic transvestism (F65.1)

F64.2 Gender identity disorder of childhood

Excludes 1: gender identity disorder in adolescence and adulthood (F64.1)

Excludes 2: sexual maturation disorder (F66)

F64.8 Other gender identity disorders

F64.9 Gender identity disorder, unspecified

Gender-role disorder NOS

F65 Paraphilias

F65.0 Fetishism

F65.1 Transvestic fetishism

Fetishistic transvestism

F65.2 Exhibitionism

F65.3 Voyeurism

F65.4 Pedophilia

F65.5 Sadomasochism

F65.50 Sadomasochism, unspecified

F65.51 Sexual masochism

F65.52 Sexual sadism

F65.8 Other paraphilias

F65.81 Frotteurism

F65.89 Other paraphilias

Necrophilia

F65.9 Paraphilia, unspecified

Sexual deviation NOS

F66 Other sexual disorders

Sexual maturation disorder

Sexual relationship disorder

F68 Other disorders of adult personality and behavior

F68.1 Factitious disorder

Compensation neurosis

Elaboration of physical symptoms for psychological reasons

Hospital hopper syndrome

M_nchausen's syndrome

Peregrinating patient

Excludes 2: factitial dermatitis (L98.1)

person feigning illness (with obvious motivation) (Z76.5)

F68.10 Factitious disorder, unspecified

F68.11 Factitious disorder with predominantly psychological signs and symptoms

F68.12 Factitious disorder with predominantly physical signs and symptoms

F68.13 Factitious disorder with combined psychological and physical signs and symptoms

F68.8 Other specified disorders of adult personality and behavior

F69 Unspecified disorder of adult personality and behavior

INTELLECTUAL DISABILITIES (F70-F79)

Code first any associated physical or developmental disorders

Excludes 1: borderline intellectual functioning, IQ above 70 to 84(R41.83)

F70 Mild intellectual disabilities

IQ level 50-55 to approximately 70

Mild mental subnormality

F71 Moderate intellectual disabilities

IQ level 35-40 to 50-55

Moderate mental subnormality

F72 Severe intellectual disabilities

IQ 20-25 to 35-40

Severe mental subnormality

F73 Profound intellectual disabilities

IQ level below 20-25

Profound mental subnormality

F78 Other intellectual disabilities

F79 Unspecified intellectual disabilities

Mental deficiency NOS

Mental subnormality NOS

PERVASIVE AND SPECIFIC DEVELOPMENTAL DISORDERS (F80-F89)

F80 Specific developmental disorders of speech and language

F80.0 Phonological disorder

Dyslalia

Functional speech articulation disorder

Lalling

Lisping

Phonological developmental disorder

Speech articulation developmental disorder

Excludes 1: speech articulation impairment due to aphasia NOS (R47.01)

speech articulation impairment due to apraxia (R48.2)

Excludes 2: speech articulation impairment due to hearing loss (F80.4)

speech articulation impairment due to intellectual disabilities (F70-F79)

speech articulation impairment with expressive language developmental disorder (F80.1)

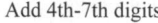 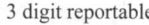

speech articulation impairment with mixed receptive expressive language developmental disorder (F80.2)

F80.1 Expressive language disorder

Developmental dysphasia or aphasia, expressive type

Excludes 1: mixed receptive-expressive language disorder (F80.2)

dysphasia and aphasia NOS (R47.-)

Excludes 2: acquired aphasia with epilepsy [Landau-Kleffner] (G40.80-)

selective mutism (F94.0)

intellectual disabilities (F70-F79)

pervasive developmental disorders (F84.-)

F80.2 Mixed receptive-expressive language disorder

Developmental dysphasia or aphasia, receptive type

Developmental Wernicke's aphasia

Excludes 1: central auditory processing disorder (H93.25)

dysphasia or aphasia NOS (R47.-)

expressive language disorder (F80.1)

expressive type dysphasia or aphasia (F80.1)

word deafness (H93.25)

Excludes 2: acquired aphasia with epilepsy [Landau-Kleffner] (G40.80-)

pervasive developmental disorders (F84.-)

selective mutism (F94.0)

intellectual disabilities (F70-F79)

F80.4 Speech and language development delay due to hearing loss

Code also type of hearing loss (H90.-, H91.-)

F80.8 Other developmental disorders of speech and language

F80.81 Childhood onset fluency disorder

Cluttering NOS

Stuttering NOS

Excludes 1: adult onset fluency disorder (F98.5)

fluency disorder in conditions classified elsewhere (R47.82)

fluency disorder (stuttering) following cerebrovascular disease (I69. with final characters -23)

F80.89 Other developmental disorders of speech and language

F80.9 Developmental disorder of speech and language, unspecified

Communication disorder NOS

Language disorder NOS

F81 Specific developmental disorders of scholastic skills

F81.0 Specific reading disorder

'Backward reading'

Developmental dyslexia

Specific reading retardation

Excludes 1: alexia NOS (R48.0)

dyslexia NOS (R48.0)

F81.2 Mathematics disorder

Developmental acalculia

Developmental arithmetical disorder

Developmental Gerstmann's syndrome

Excludes 1: acalculia NOS (R48.8)

Excludes 2: arithmetical difficulties associated with a reading disorder (F81.0)

arithmetical difficulties associated with a spelling disorder (F81.81)

arithmetical difficulties due to inadequate teaching (Z55.8)

F81.8 Other developmental disorders of scholastic skills

F81.81 Disorder of written expression

Specific spelling disorder

F81.89 Other developmental disorders of scholastic skills

F81.9 Developmental disorder of scholastic skills, unspecified

Knowledge acquisition disability NOS

Learning disability NOS

Learning disorder NOS

F82 Specific developmental disorder of motor function

Clumsy child syndrome

Developmental coordination disorder

Developmental dyspraxia

Excludes 1: abnormalities of gait and mobility (R26.-)

lack of coordination (R27.-)

Excludes 2: lack of coordination secondary to intellectual disabilities (F70-F79)

F84 Pervasive developmental disorders

Use additional code to identify any associated medical condition and intellectual disabilities.

F84.0 Autistic disorder

Infantile autism

Infantile psychosis

Kanner's syndrome

Excludes 1: Asperger's syndrome (F84.5)

F84.2 Rett's syndrome

Excludes 1: Asperger's syndrome (F84.5)

Autistic disorder (F84.0)

Other childhood disintegrative disorder (F84.3)

F84.3 Other childhood disintegrative disorder

Dementia infantilis

Disintegrative psychosis

Heller's syndrome

Symbiotic psychosis

Use additional code to identify any associated neurological condition.

Excludes 1: Asperger's syndrome (F84.5)

Autistic disorder (F84.0)

Rett's syndrome (F84.2)

F84.5 Asperger's syndrome

Asperger's disorder

Autistic psychopathy

Schizoid disorder of childhood

F84.8 Other pervasive developmental disorders

Overactive disorder associated with intellectual disabilities and stereotyped movements

F84.9 Pervasive developmental disorder, unspecified

Atypical autism

F88 Other disorders of psychological development

Developmental agnosia

F89 Unspecified disorder of psychological development

Developmental disorder NOS

BEHAVIORAL AND EMOTIONAL DISORDERS WITH ONSET USUALLY OCCURRING IN CHILDHOOD AND ADOLESCENCE (F90-F98)

Note: Codes within categories F90-F98 may be used regardless of the age of a patient. These disorders generally have onset within the childhood or adolescent years, but may continue throughout life or not be diagnosed until adulthood

F90 Attention-deficit hyperactivity disorders

Includes: attention deficit disorder with hyperactivity

attention deficit syndrome with hyperactivity

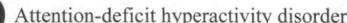

Excludes 2: anxiety disorders (F40.-, F41.-)

mood [affective] disorders (F30-F39)

pervasive developmental disorders (F84.-)

schizophrenia (F20.-)

F90.0 Attention-deficit hyperactivity disorder, predominantly inattentive type

F90.1 Attention-deficit hyperactivity disorder, predominantly hyperactive type

F90.2 Attention-deficit hyperactivity disorder, combined type

F90.8 Attention-deficit hyperactivity disorder, other type

F90.9 Attention-deficit hyperactivity disorder, unspecified type

Attention-deficit hyperactivity disorder of childhood or adolescence NOS

Attention-deficit hyperactivity disorder NOS

F91 Conduct disorders

Excludes 1: antisocial behavior (Z72.81-)

antisocial personality disorder (F60.2)

Excludes 2: conduct problems associated with attention-deficit hyperactivity disorder (F90.-)

mood [affective] disorders (F30-F39)

pervasive developmental disorders (F84.-)

schizophrenia (F20.-)

F91.0 Conduct disorder confined to family context

F91.1 Conduct disorder, childhood-onset type

Unsocialized conduct disorder

Conduct disorder, solitary aggressive type

Unsocialized aggressive disorder

F91.2 Conduct disorder, adolescent-onset type

Socialized conduct disorder

Conduct disorder, group type

F91.3 Oppositional defiant disorder

F91.8 Other conduct disorders

F91.9 Conduct disorder, unspecified

Behavioral disorder NOS

Conduct disorder NOS

Disruptive behavior disorder NOS

F93 Emotional disorders with onset specific to childhood

F93.0 Separation anxiety disorder of childhood

Excludes 2: mood [affective] disorders (F30-F39)

nonpsychotic mental disorders (F40-F48)

phobic anxiety disorder of childhood (F40.8)

social phobia (F40.1)

F93.8 Other childhood emotional disorders

Identity disorder

Excludes 2: gender identity disorder of childhood (F64.2)

F93.9 Childhood emotional disorder, unspecified

F94 Disorders of social functioning with onset specific to childhood and adolescence

F94.0 Selective mutism

Elective mutism

Excludes 2: pervasive developmental disorders (F84.-)

schizophrenia (F20.-)

specific developmental disorders of speech and language (F80.-)

transient mutism as part of separation anxiety in young children (F93.0)

F94.1 Reactive attachment disorder of childhood

Use additional code to identify any associated failure to thrive or growth retardation

Excludes 1: disinhibited attachment disorder of childhood (F94.2)

normal variation in pattern of selective attachment

Excludes 2: Asperger's syndrome (F84.5)

maltreatment syndromes (T74.-)

sexual or physical abuse in childhood, resulting in psychosocial problems (Z62.81-)

F94.2 Disinhibited attachment disorder of childhood

Affectionless psychopathy

Institutional syndrome

Excludes 1: reactive attachment disorder of childhood (F94.l)

Excludes 2: Asperger's syndrome (F84.5)

attention-deficit hyperactivity disorders (F90.-)

hospitalism in children (F43.2-)

F94.8 Other childhood disorders of social functioning

F94.9 Childhood disorder of social functioning, unspecified

F95 Tic disorder

F95.0 Transient tic disorder

F95.1 Chronic motor or vocal tic disorder

F95.2 Tourette's disorder

Combined vocal and multiple motor tic disorder [de la Tourette]

Tourette's syndrome

F95.8 Other tic disorders

F95.9 Tic disorder, unspecified

Tic NOS

F98 Other behavioral and emotional disorders with onset usually occurring in childhood and adolescence

Excludes 2: breath-holding spells (R06.89)

gender identity disorder of childhood (F64.2)

Kleine-Levin syndrome (G47.13)

obsessive-compulsive disorder (F42)

sleep disorders not due to a substance or known physiological condition (F51.-)

F98.0 Enuresis not due to a substance or known physiological condition

Enuresis (primary) (secondary) of nonorganic origin

Functional enuresis

Psychogenic enuresis

Urinary incontinence of nonorganic origin

Excludes 1: enuresis NOS (R32)

F98.1 Encopresis not due to a substance or known physiological condition

Functional encopresis

Incontinence of feces of nonorganic origin

Psychogenic encopresis

Use additional code to identify the cause of any coexisting constipation.

Excludes 1: encopresis NOS (R15-)

F98.2 Other feeding disorders of infancy and childhood

Excludes 1: feeding difficulties (R63.3)

Excludes 2: anorexia nervosa and other eating disorders (F50.-)

feeding problems of newborn (P92.-)

pica of infancy or childhood (F98.3)

F98.21 Rumination disorder of infancy

F98.29 Other feeding disorders of infancy and early childhood

F98.3 Pica of infancy and childhood

F98.4 Stereotyped movement disorders

Stereotype/habit disorder

Excludes 1: abnormal involuntary movements (R25.-)

Excludes 2: compulsions in obsessive-compulsive disorder (F42)

hair plucking (F63.3)

movement disorders of organic origin (G20-G25)

                  nail-biting (F98.8)

                  nose-picking (F98.8)

                  stereotypies that are part of a broader psychiatric condition (F01-F95)

                  thumb-sucking (F98.8)

                  tic disorders (F95.-)

                  trichotillomania (F63.3)

F98.5   Adult onset fluency disorder

         Excludes 1: childhood onset fluency disorder (F80.81)

                  dysphasia (R47.02)

                  fluency disorder in conditions classified elsewhere (R47.82)

                  fluency disorder (stuttering) following cerebrovascular disease (I69. with final characters -23)

                  tic disorders (F95.-)

F98.8   Other specified behavioral and emotional disorders with onset usually occurring in childhood and adolescence

         Excessive masturbation

         Nail-biting

         Nose-picking

         Thumb-sucking

F98.9   Unspecified behavioral and emotional disorders with onset usually occurring in childhood and adolescence

UNSPECIFIED MENTAL DISORDER (F99)

F99   Mental disorder, not otherwise specified

         Mental illness NOS

         Excludes 1: unspecified mental disorder due to known physiological condition (F09)

Chapter 6: Diseases Of The Nervous System (G00-G99)

Excludes 2: certain conditions originating in the perinatal period (P04-P96)

certain infectious and parasitic diseases (A00-B99)

complications of pregnancy, childbirth and the puerperium (O00-O9A)

congenital malformations, deformations, and chromosomal abnormalities (Q00-Q99)

endocrine, nutritional and metabolic diseases (E00-E88)

injury, poisoning and certain other consequences of external causes (S00-T88)

neoplasms (C00-D49)

symptoms, signs and abnormal clinical and laboratory findings, not elsewhere classified (R00-R94)

This chapter contains the following blocks:

G00-G09	Inflammatory diseases of the central nervous system
G10-G14	Systemic atrophies primarily affecting the central nervous system
G20-G26	Extrapyramidal and movement disorders
G30-G32	Other degenerative diseases of the nervous system
G35-G37	Demyelinating diseases of the central nervous system
G40-G47	Episodic and paroxysmal disorders
G50-G59	Nerve, nerve root and plexus disorders
G60-G65	Polyneuropathies and other disorders of the peripheral nervous system
G70-G73	Diseases of myoneural junction and muscle
G80-G83	Cerebral palsy and other paralytic syndromes
G89-G99	Other disorders of the nervous system

INFLAMMATORY DISEASES OF THE CENTRAL NERVOUS SYSTEM (G00-G09)

G00 Bacterial meningitis, not elsewhere classified

Includes: bacterial arachnoiditis

bacterial leptomeningitis

bacterial meningitis

bacterial pachymeningitis

Excludes 1: bacterial:

meningoencephalitis (G04.2)

meningomyelitis (G04.2)

G00.0 Hemophilus meningitis

Meningitis due to Hemophilus influenzae

G00.1 Pneumococcal meningitis

G00.2 Streptococcal meningitis

Use additional code to further identify organism (B95.0-B95.5)

G00.3 Staphylococcal meningitis

Use additional code to further identify organism (B95.61-B95.8)

G00.8 Other bacterial meningitis

Meningitis due to Escherichia coli

Meningitis due to Friedländer's bacillus

Meningitis due to Klebsiella

Use additional code to further identify organism (B96.-)

G00.9 Bacterial meningitis, unspecified

Meningitis due to gram-negative bacteria, unspecified

Purulent meningitis NOS

Pyogenic meningitis NOS

Suppurative meningitis NOS

G01 Meningitis in bacterial diseases classified elsewhere

Code first underlying disease

Excludes 1: meningitis (in):

gonococcal (A54.81)

leptospirosis (A27.81)

listeriosis (A32.11)

Lyme disease (A69.21)

meningococcal (A39.0)

neurosyphilis (A52.13)

tuberculosis (A17.0)

meningoencephalitis and meningomyelitis in bacterial diseases classified elsewhere (G05)

G02 Meningitis in other infectious and parasitic diseases classified elsewhere

Code first underlying disease, such as:

African trypanosomiasis (B56.-)

poliovirus infection (A80.-)

Excludes 1: candidal meningitis (B37.5)

coccidioidomycosis meningitis (B38.4)

cryptococcal meningitis (B45.1)

herpesviral [herpes simplex] meningitis (B00.3)

infectious mononucleosis complicated by meningitis (B27.- with fourth character 2)

measles complicated by meningitis (B05.1)

meningoencephalitis and meningomyelitis in other infectious and parasitic diseases classified elsewhere (G05)

mumps meningitis (B26.1)

rubella meningitis (B06.02)

varicella [chickenpox] meningitis (B01.0)

zoster meningitis (B02.1)

G03 Meningitis due to other and unspecified causes

Includes: arachnoiditis NOS

leptomeningitis NOS

meningitis NOS

pachymeningitis NOS

Excludes 1: meningoencephalitis (G04.-)

meningomyelitis (G04.-)

G03.0 Nonpyogenic meningitis

Aseptic meningitis

Nonbacterial meningitis

G03.1 Chronic meningitis

G03.2 Benign recurrent meningitis [Mollaret]

G03.8 Meningitis due to other specified causes

G03.9 Meningitis, unspecified

Arachnoiditis (spinal) NOS

G04 Encephalitis, myelitis and encephalomyelitis

Includes: acute ascending myelitis

meningoencephalitis

meningomyelitis

Excludes 1: encephalopathy NOS (G93.40)

Excludes 2: acute transverse myelitis (G37.3)

alcoholic encephalopathy (G31.2)

benign myalgic encephalomyelitis (G93.3)

multiple sclerosis (G35)

subacute necrotizing myelitis (G37.4)

toxic encephalitis (G92)

toxic encephalopathy (G92)

G04.0 Acute disseminated encephalitis and encephalomyelitis (ADEM)

Excludes 1: acute necrotizing hemorrhagic encephalopathy (G04.3-)

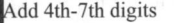

other noninfectious acute disseminated encephalomyelitis (noninfectious ADEM) (G04.81)

G04.00 Acute disseminated encephalitis and encephalomyelitis, unspecified

G04.01 Postinfectious acute disseminated encephalitis and encephalomyelitis (postinfectious ADEM)

Excludes 1: post chickenpox encephalitis (B01.1)

post measles encephalitis (B05.0)

post measles myelitis (B05.1)

G04.02 Postimmunization acute disseminated encephalitis, myelitis and encephalomyelitis

Encephalitis, post immunization

Encephalomyelitis, post immunization

Use additional code to identify the vaccine (T50.A-, T50.B-, T50.Z-)

G04.1 Tropical spastic paraplegia

G04.2 Bacterial meningoencephalitis and meningomyelitis, not elsewhere classified

G04.3 Acute necrotizing hemorrhagic encephalopathy

Excludes 1: acute disseminated encephalitis and encephalomyelitis (G04.0-)

G04.30 Acute necrotizing hemorrhagic encephalopathy, unspecified

G04.31 Postinfectious acute necrotizing hemorrhagic encephalopathy

G04.32 Postimmunization acute necrotizing hemorrhagic encephalopathy

Use additional code to identify the vaccine (T50.A-, T50.B-, T50.Z-)

G04.39 Other acute necrotizing hemorrhagic encephalopathy

Code also underlying etiology, if applicable

G04.8 Other encephalitis, myelitis and encephalomyelitis

Code also any associated seizure (G40.-, R56.9)

G04.81 Other encephalitis and encephalomyelitis

Noninfectious acute disseminated encephalomyelitis (noninfectious ADEM)

G04.89 Other myelitis

G04.9 Encephalitis, myelitis and encephalomyelitis, unspecified

G04.90 Encephalitis and encephalomyelitis, unspecified

Ventriculitis (cerebral) NOS

G04.91 Myelitis, unspecified

G05 Encephalitis, myelitis and encephalomyelitis in diseases classified elsewhere

Code first underlying disease, such as:

human immunodeficiency virus [HIV] disease (B20)

poliovirus (A80.-)

suppurative otitis media (H66.01-H66.4)

trichinellosis (B75)

Excludes 1: adenoviral encephalitis, myelitis and encephalomyelitis (A85.1)

congenital toxoplasmosis encephalitis, myelitis and encephalomyelitis (P37.1)

cytomegaloviral encephalitis, myelitis and encephalomyelitis (B25.8)

encephalitis, myelitis and encephalomyelitis (in) measles (B05.0)

encephalitis, myelitis and encephalomyelitis (in) systemic lupus erythematosus (M32.19)

enteroviral encephalitis, myelitis and encephalomyelitis (A85.0)

eosinophilic meningoencephalitis (B83.2)

herpesviral [herpes simplex] encephalitis, myelitis and encephalomyelitis (B00.4)

listerial encephalitis, myelitis and encephalomyelitis (A32.12)

meningococcal encephalitis, myelitis and encephalomyelitis (A39.81)

mumps encephalitis, myelitis and encephalomyelitis (B26.2)

postchickenpox encephalitis, myelitis and encephalomyelitis (B01.1-)

rubella encephalitis, myelitis and encephalomyelitis (B06.01)

toxoplasmosis encephalitis, myelitis and encephalomyelitis (B58.2)

zoster encephalitis, myelitis and encephalomyelitis (B02.0)

G05.3 Encephalitis and encephalomyelitis in diseases classified elsewhere

Meningoencephalitis in diseases classified elsewhere

G05.4 Myelitis in diseases classified elsewhere

Meningomyelitis in diseases classified elsewhere

G06 Intracranial and intraspinal abscess and granuloma

Use additional code (B95-B97) to identify infectious agent.

G06.0 Intracranial abscess and granuloma

Brain [any part] abscess (embolic)

Cerebellar abscess (embolic)

Cerebral abscess (embolic)

Intracranial epidural abscess or granuloma

Intracranial extradural abscess or granuloma

Intracranial subdural abscess or granuloma

Otogenic abscess (embolic)

Excludes 1: tuberculous intracranial abscess and granuloma (A17.81)

G06.1 Intraspinal abscess and granuloma

Abscess (embolic) of spinal cord [any part]

Intraspinal epidural abscess or granuloma

Intraspinal extradural abscess or granuloma

Intraspinal subdural abscess or granuloma

Excludes 1: tuberculous intraspinal abscess and granuloma (A17.81)

G06.2 Extradural and subdural abscess, unspecified

G07 Intracranial and intraspinal abscess and granuloma in diseases classified elsewhere

Code first , underlying disease, such as:

schistosomiasis granuloma of brain (B65.-)

Excludes 1: abscess of brain:

amebic (A06.6)

chromomycotic (B43.1)

gonococcal (A54.82)

tuberculous (A17.81)

tuberculoma of meninges (A17.1)

G08 Intracranial and intraspinal phlebitis and thrombophlebitis

Septic embolism of intracranial or intraspinal venous sinuses and veins

Septic endophlebitis of intracranial or intraspinal venous sinuses and veins

Septic phlebitis of intracranial or intraspinal venous sinuses and veins

Septic thrombophlebitis of intracranial or intraspinal venous sinuses and veins

Septic thrombosis of intracranial or intraspinal venous sinuses and veins

Excludes 1: intracranial phlebitis and thrombophlebitis complicating:

 abortion, ectopic or molar pregnancy (O00-O07, O08.7)

 pregnancy, childbirth and the puerperium (O22.5, O87.3)

 nonpyogenic intracranial phlebitis and thrombophlebitis (I67.6)

 nonpyogenic intraspinal phlebitis and thrombophlebitis (G95.1)

G09 Sequelae of inflammatory diseases of central nervous system

Note: Category G09 is to be used to indicate conditions whose primary classification is to G00-G08 as the cause of sequelae, themselves classifiable elsewhere. The 'sequelae' include conditions specified as residuals.

Code first condition resulting from (sequela) of inflammatory diseases of central nervous system

SYSTEMIC ATROPHIES PRIMARILY AFFECTING THE CENTRAL NERVOUS SYSTEM (G10-G14)

G10 Huntington's disease

Huntington's chorea

Huntington's dementia

G11 Hereditary ataxia

 Excludes 2: cerebral palsy (G80.-)

  hereditary and idiopathic neuropathy (G60.-)

  metabolic disorders (E70-E88)

G11.0 Congenital nonprogressive ataxia

G11.1 Early-onset cerebellar ataxia

Early-onset cerebellar ataxia with essential tremor

Early-onset cerebellar ataxia with myoclonus [Hunt's ataxia]

Early-onset cerebellar ataxia with retained tendon reflexes

Friedreich's ataxia (autosomal recessive)

X-linked recessive spinocerebellar ataxia

G11.2 Late-onset cerebellar ataxia

G11.3 Cerebellar ataxia with defective DNA repair

Ataxia telangiectasia [Louis-Bar]

 Excludes 2: Cockayne's syndrome (Q87.1)

  other disorders of purine and pyrimidine metabolism (E79.-)

  xeroderma pigmentosum (Q82.1)

G11.4 Hereditary spastic paraplegia

G11.8 Other hereditary ataxias

G11.9 Hereditary ataxia, unspecified

Hereditary cerebellar ataxia NOS

Hereditary cerebellar degeneration

Hereditary cerebellar disease

Hereditary cerebellar syndrome

G12 Spinal muscular atrophy and related syndromes

G12.0 Infantile spinal muscular atrophy, type I [Werdnig-Hoffman]

G12.1 Other inherited spinal muscular atrophy

Adult form spinal muscular atrophy

Childhood form, type II spinal muscular atrophy

Distal spinal muscular atrophy

Juvenile form, type III spinal muscular atrophy [Kugelberg-Welander]

Progressive bulbar palsy of childhood [Fazio-Londe]

Scapuloperoneal form spinal muscular atrophy

G12.2 Motor neuron disease

 G12.20 Motor neuron disease, unspecified

 G12.21 Amyotrophic lateral sclerosis

 Progressive spinal muscle atrophy

 G12.22 Progressive bulbar palsy

 G12.29 Other motor neuron disease

 Familial motor neuron disease

 Primary lateral sclerosis

G12.8 Other spinal muscular atrophies and related syndromes

G12.9 Spinal muscular atrophy, unspecified

G13 Systemic atrophies primarily affecting central nervous system in diseases classified elsewhere

G13.0 Paraneoplastic neuromyopathy and neuropathy

Carcinomatous neuromyopathy

Sensorial paraneoplastic neuropathy [Denny Brown]

Code first underlying neoplasm (C00-D49)

G13.1 Other systemic atrophy primarily affecting central nervous system in neoplastic disease

Paraneoplastic limbic encephalopathy

Code first underlying neoplasm (C00-D49)

G13.2 Systemic atrophy primarily affecting the central nervous system in myxedema

Code first underlying disease, such as:

 hypothyroidism (E03.-)

 myxedematous congenital iodine deficiency (E00.1)

G13.8 Systemic atrophy primarily affecting central nervous system in other diseases classified elsewhere

Code first underlying disease

G14 Postpolio syndrome

 Includes: postpolio myelitic syndrome

 Excludes 1: sequelae of poliomyelitis (B91)

EXTRAPYRAMIDAL AND MOVEMENT DISORDERS (G20-G26)

G20 Parkinson's disease

Hemiparkinsonism

Idiopathic Parkinsonism or Parkinson's disease

Paralysis agitans

Parkinsonism or Parkinson's disease NOS

Primary Parkinsonism or Parkinson's disease

 Excludes 1: dementia with Parkinsonism (G31.83)

G21 Secondary parkinsonism

 Excludes 1: dementia with Parkinsonism (G31.83)

  Huntington's disease (G10)

  Shy-Drager syndrome (G90.3)

  syphilitic Parkinsonism (A52.19)

G21.0 Malignant neuroleptic syndrome

Use additional code for adverse effect, if applicable, to identify drug (T43.3X5, T43.4X5, T43.505, T43.595)

 Excludes 1: neuroleptic induced parkinsonism (G21.11)

G21.1 Other drug-induced secondary parkinsonism

 G21.11 Neuroleptic induced parkinsonism

Use additional code for adverse effect, if applicable, to identify drug (T43.3X5, T43.4X5, T43.505, T43.595)

  Excludes 1: malignant neuroleptic syndrome (G21.0)

 G21.19 Other drug induced secondary parkinsonism

Use additional code for adverse effect, if applicable, to identify drug (T36-T50 ith fifth or sixth character 5)

G21.2 Secondary parkinsonism due to other external agents

Code first (T51-T65) to identify external agent

G21.3 Postencephalitic parkinsonism

G21.4 Vascular parkinsonism

G21.8 Other secondary parkinsonism

G21.9 Secondary parkinsonism, unspecified

G23 Other degenerative diseases of basal ganglia

Excludes 2: multi-system degeneration of the autonomic nervous system (G90.3)

G23.0 Hallervorden-Spatz disease

Pigmentary pallidal degeneration

G23.1 Progressive supranuclear ophthalmoplegia [Steele-Richardson-Olszewski]

Progressive supranuclear palsy

G23.2 Striatonigral degeneration

G23.8 Other specified degenerative diseases of basal ganglia

Calcification of basal ganglia

G23.9 Degenerative disease of basal ganglia, unspecified

G24 Dystonia

Includes: dyskinesia

Excludes 2: athetoid cerebral palsy (G80.3)

G24.0 Drug induced dystonia

Use additional code code for adverse effect, if applicable, to identify drug (T36-T50 with fifth or sixth character 5)

G24.01 Drug induced subacute dyskinesia

Drug induced blepharospasm

Drug induced orofacial dyskinesia

Neuroleptic induced tardive dyskinesia

Tardive dyskinesia

G24.02 Drug induced acute dystonia

Acute dystonic reaction to drugs

Neuroleptic induced acute dystonia

G24.09 Other drug induced dystonia

G24.1 Genetic torsion dystonia

Dystonia deformans progressiva

Dystonia musculorum deformans

Familial torsion dystonia

Idiopathic familial dystonia

Idiopathic (torsion) dystonia NOS

(Schwalbe-) Ziehen-Oppenheim disease

G24.2 Idiopathic nonfamilial dystonia

G24.3 Spasmodic torticollis

Excludes 1: congenital torticollis (Q68.0)

hysterical torticollis (F44.4)

ocular torticollis (R29.891)

psychogenic torticollis (F45.8)

torticollis NOS (M43.6)

traumatic recurrent torticollis (S13.4)

G24.4 Idiopathic orofacial dystonia

Orofacial dyskinesia

Excludes 1: drug induced orofacial dyskinesia (G24.01)

G24.5 Blepharospasm

Excludes 1: drug induced blepharospasm (G24.01)

G24.8 Other dystonia

Acquired torsion dystonia NOS

G24.9 Dystonia, unspecified

Dyskinesia NOS

G25 Other extrapyramidal and movement disorders

Excludes 2: sleep related movement disorders (G47.6-)

G25.0 Essential tremor

Familial tremor

Excludes 1: tremor NOS (R25.1)

G25.1 Drug-induced tremor

Use additional code for adverse effect, if applicable, to identify drug (T36-T50 with fifth or sixth character 5)

G25.2 Other specified forms of tremor

Intention tremor

G25.3 Myoclonus

Drug-induced myoclonus

Palatal myoclonus

Use additional code for adverse effect, if applicable, to identify drug (T36-T50 with fifth or sixth character 5)

Excludes 1: facial myokymia (G51.4)

myoclonic epilepsy (G40.-)

G25.4 Drug-induced chorea

Use additional code for adverse effect, if applicable, to identify drug (T36-T50 with fifth or sixth character 5)

G25.5 Other chorea

Chorea NOS

Excludes 1: chorea NOS with heart involvement (I02.0)

Huntington's chorea (G10)

rheumatic chorea (I02.-)

Sydenham's chorea (I02.-)

G25.6 Drug induced tics and other tics of organic origin

G25.61 Drug induced tics

Use additional code for adverse effect, if applicable, to identify drug (T36-T50 with fifth or sixth character 5)

G25.69 Other tics of organic origin

Excludes 1: habit spasm (F95.9)

tic NOS (F95.9)

Tourette's syndrome (F95.2)

G25.7 Other and unspecified drug induced movement disorders

Use additional code for adverse effect, if applicable, to identify drug (T36-T50 with fifth or sixth character 5)

G25.70 Drug induced movement disorder, unspecified

G25.71 Drug induced akathisia

Drug induced acathisia

Neuroleptic induced acute akathisia

G25.79 Other drug induced movement disorders

G25.8 Other specified extrapyramidal and movement disorders

G25.81 Restless legs syndrome

G25.82 Stiff-man syndrome

G25.83 Benign shuddering attacks

G25.89 Other specified extrapyramidal and movement disorders

G25.9 Extrapyramidal and movement disorder, unspecified

G26 Extrapyramidal and movement disorders in diseases classified elsewhere

Code first underlying disease

OTHER DEGENERATIVE DISEASES OF THE NERVOUS SYSTEM (G30-G32)

G30 Alzheimer's disease

Includes: Alzheimer's dementia senile and presenile forms

Use additional code to identify:

delirium, if applicable (F05)

dementia with behavioral disturbance (F02.81)

dementia without behavioral disturbance (F02.80)

Excludes 1: senile degeneration of brain NEC (G31.1)

senile dementia NOS (F03)

senility NOS (R41.81)

G30.0 Alzheimer's disease with early onset

G30.1 Alzheimer's disease with late onset

G30.8 Other Alzheimer's disease

G30.9 Alzheimer's disease, unspecified

G31 Other degenerative diseases of nervous system, not elsewhere classified

Use additional code to identify:

dementia with behavioral disturbance (F02.81)

  ● New code   ▲ Revised code   ⑦ 7th digit required   ⊗ Placeholder required

dementia without behavioral disturbance (F02.80)

Excludes 2: Reye's syndrome (G93.7)

G31.0 Frontotemporal dementia

    G31.01 Pick's disease

        Primary progressive aphasia

        Progressive isolated aphasia

    G31.09 Other frontotemporal dementia

        Frontal dementia

G31.1 Senile degeneration of brain, not elsewhere classified

    Excludes 1: Alzheimer's disease (G30.-)

        senility NOS (R41.81)

G31.2 Degeneration of nervous system due to alcohol

    Alcoholic cerebellar ataxia

    Alcoholic cerebellar degeneration

    Alcoholic cerebral degeneration

    Alcoholic encephalopathy

    Dysfunction of the autonomic nervous system due to alcohol

    Code also associated alcoholism (F10.-)

G31.8 Other specified degenerative diseases of nervous system

    G31.81 Alpers disease

        Grey-matter degeneration

    G31.82 Leigh's disease

        Subacute necrotizing encephalopathy

    G31.83 Dementia with Lewy bodies

        Dementia with Parkinsonism

        Lewy body dementia

        Lewy body disease

    G31.84 Mild cognitive impairment, so stated

        Excludes 1: age related cognitive decline (R41.81)

            altered mental status (R41.82)

            cerebral degeneration (G31.9)

            change in mental status (R41.82)

            cognitive deficits following (sequelae of) cerebral hemorrhage or infarction (I69.01, I69.11, I69.21, I69.31, I69.81, I69.91)

            cognitive impairment due to intracranial or head injury (S06.-)

            dementia (F01.-, F02.-, F03)

            mild memory disturbance (F06.8)

            neurologic neglect syndrome (R41.4)

            personality change, nonpsychotic (F68.8)

    G31.85 Corticobasal degeneration

    G31.89 Other specified degenerative diseases of nervous system

G31.9 Degenerative disease of nervous system, unspecified

G32 Other degenerative disorders of nervous system in diseases classified elsewhere

    G32.0 Subacute combined degeneration of spinal cord in diseases classified elsewhere

        Dana-Putnam syndrome

        Sclerosis of spinal cord (combined) (dorsolateral) (posterolateral)

        Code first underlying disease, such as:

            vitamin B12 deficiency (E53.8)

            anemia (D51.9)

            dietary (D51.3)

            pernicious (D51.0)

Excludes 1: syphilitic combined degeneration of spinal cord (A52.11)

G32.8 Other specified degenerative disorders of nervous system in diseases classified elsewhere

    Code first underlying disease, such as:

        amyloidosis cerebral degeneration (E85-)

        cerebral degeneration (due to) hypothyroidism (E00.0-E03.9)

        cerebral degeneration (due to) neoplasm (C00-D49)

        cerebral degeneration (due to) vitamin B deficiency, except thiamine (E52-E53.-)

    Excludes 1: superior hemorrhagic polioencephalitis [Wernicke's encephalopathy] (E51.2)

    G32.81 Cerebellar ataxia in diseases classified elsewhere

        Code first underlying disease, such as:

            cerebellar ataxia (in) neoplastic disease (paraneoplastic cerebellar degeneration) (C00-D49)

        Excludes 1: systemic atrophy primarily affecting the central nervous system in alcoholic cerebellar ataxia (G31.2)

            systemic atrophy primarily affecting the central nervous system in myxedema (G13.2)

    G32.89 Other specified degenerative disorders of nervous system in diseases classified elsewhere

        Degenerative encephalopathy in diseases classified elsewhere

DEMYELINATING DISEASES OF THE CENTRAL NERVOUS SYSTEM (G35-G37)

G35 Multiple sclerosis

    Disseminated multiple sclerosis

    Generalized multiple sclerosis

    Multiple sclerosis NOS

    Multiple sclerosis of brain stem

    Multiple sclerosis of cord

G36 Other acute disseminated demyelination

    Excludes 1: postinfectious encephalitis and encephalomyelitis NOS (G04.01)

    G36.0 Neuromyelitis optica [Devic]

        Demyelination in optic neuritis

        Excludes 1: optic neuritis NOS (H46)

    G36.1 Acute and subacute hemorrhagic leukoencephalitis [Hurst]

    G36.8 Other specified acute disseminated demyelination

    G36.9 Acute disseminated demyelination, unspecified

G37 Other demyelinating diseases of central nervous system

    G37.0 Diffuse sclerosis of central nervous system

        Periaxial encephalitis

        Schilder's disease

        Excludes 1: X linked adrenoleukodystrophy (E71.52-)

    G37.1 Central demyelination of corpus callosum

    G37.2 Central pontine myelinolysis

    G37.3 Acute transverse myelitis in demyelinating disease of central nervous system

        Acute transverse myelitis NOS

        Acute transverse myelopathy

        Excludes 1: multiple sclerosis (G35)

            neuromyelitis optica [Devic] (G36.0)

    G37.4 Subacute necrotizing myelitis of central nervous system

    G37.5 Concentric sclerosis [Balo] of central nervous system

G37.8 Other specified demyelinating diseases of central nervous system

G37.9 Demyelinating disease of central nervous system, unspecified

EPISODIC AND PAROXYSMAL DISORDERS (G40-G47)

G40 Epilepsy and recurrent seizures

Note: the following terms are to be considered equivalent to intractable: pharmacoresistant (pharmacologically resistant), treatment resistant, refractory (medically) and poorly controlled

Excludes 1: conversion disorder with seizures (F44.5)
    convulsions NOS (R56.9)
    hippocampal sclerosis (G93.81)
    mesial temporal sclerosis (G93.81)
    post traumatic seizures (R56.1)
    seizure (convulsive) NOS (R56.9)
    seizure of newborn (P90)
    temporal sclerosis (G93.81)
    Todd's paralysis (G83.8)

G40.0 Localization-related (focal) (partial) idiopathic epilepsy and epileptic syndromes with seizures of localized onset

Benign childhood epilepsy with centrotemporal EEGspikes

Childhood epilepsy with occipital EEG paroxysms

Excludes 1: adult onset localization-related epilepsy (G40.1-, G40.2-)

G40.00 Localization-related (focal) (partial) idiopathic epilepsy and epileptic syndromes with seizures of localized onset, not intractable

Localization-related (focal) (partial) idiopathic epilepsy and epileptic syndromes with seizures of localized onset without intractability

G40.001 Localization-related (focal) (partial) idiopathic epilepsy and epileptic syndromes with seizures of localized onset, not intractable, with status epilepticus

G40.009 Localization-related (focal) (partial) idiopathic epilepsy and epileptic syndromes with seizures of localized onset, not intractable, without status epilepticus

Localization-related (focal) (partial) idiopathic epilepsy and epileptic syndromes with seizures of localized onset NOS

G40.01 Localization-related (focal) (partial) idiopathic epilepsy and epileptic syndromes with seizures of localized onset, intractable

G40.011 Localization-related (focal) (partial) idiopathic epilepsy and epileptic syndromes with seizures of localized onset, intractable, with status epilepticus

G40.019 Localization-related (focal) (partial) idiopathic epilepsy and epileptic syndromes with seizures of localized onset, intractable, without status epilepticus

G40.1 Localization-related (focal) (partial) symptomatic epilepsy and epileptic syndromes with simple partial seizures

Attacks without alteration of consciousness

Epilepsia partialis continua [Kozhevnikof]

Simple partial seizures developing into secondarily generalized seizures

G40.10 Localization-related (focal) (partial) symptomatic epilepsy and epileptic syndromes with simple partial seizures, not intractable

Localization-related (focal) (partial) symptomatic epilepsy and epileptic syndromes with simple partial seizures without intractability

G40.101 Localization-related (focal) (partial) symptomatic epilepsy and epileptic syndromes with simple partial seizures, not intractable, with status epilepticus

G40.109 Localization-related (focal) (partial) symptomatic epilepsy and epileptic syndromes with simple partial seizures, not intractable, without status epilepticus

Localization-related (focal) (partial) symptomatic epilepsy and epileptic syndromes with simple partial seizures NOS

G40.11 Localization-related (focal) (partial) symptomatic epilepsy and epileptic syndromes with simple partial seizures, intractable

G40.111 Localization-related (focal) (partial) symptomatic epilepsy and epileptic syndromes with simple partial seizures, intractable, with status epilepticus

G40.119 Localization-related (focal) (partial) symptomatic epilepsy and epileptic syndromes with simple partial seizures, intractable, without status epilepticus

G40.2 Localization-related (focal) (partial) symptomatic epilepsy and epileptic syndromes with complex partial seizures

Attacks with alteration of consciousness, often with automatisms

Complex partial seizures developing into secondarily generalized seizures

G40.20 Localization-related (focal) (partial) symptomatic epilepsy and epileptic syndromes with complex partial seizures, not intractable

Localization-related (focal) (partial) symptomatic epilepsy and epileptic syndromes with complex partial seizures without intractability

G40.201 Localization-related (focal) (partial) symptomatic epilepsy and epileptic syndromes with complex partial seizures, not intractable, with status epilepticus

G40.209 Localization-related (focal) (partial) symptomatic epilepsy and epileptic syndromes with complex partial seizures, not intractable, without status epilepticus

Localization-related (focal) (partial) symptomatic epilepsy and epileptic syndromes with complex partial seizures NOS

G40.21 Localization-related (focal) (partial) symptomatic epilepsy and epileptic syndromes with complex partial seizures, intractable

G40.211 Localization-related (focal) (partial) symptomatic epilepsy and epileptic syndromes with complex partial seizures, intractable, with status epilepticus

G40.219 Localization-related (focal) (partial) symptomatic epilepsy and epileptic syndromes with complex partial seizures, intractable, without status epilepticus

G40.3 Generalized idiopathic epilepsy and epileptic syndromes
Code also MERRF syndrome, if applicable (E88.42)

G40.30 Generalized idiopathic epilepsy and epileptic syndromes, not intractable
Generalized idiopathic epilepsy and epileptic syndromes without intractability

G40.301 Generalized idiopathic epilepsy and epileptic syndromes, not intractable, with status epilepticus

G40.309 Generalized idiopathic epilepsy and epileptic syndromes, not intractable, without status epilepticus
Generalized idiopathic epilepsy and epileptic syndromes NOS

G40.31 Generalized idiopathic epilepsy and epileptic syndromes, intractable

G40.311 Generalized idiopathic epilepsy and epileptic syndromes, intractable, with status epilepticus

G40.319 Generalized idiopathic epilepsy and epileptic syndromes, intractable, without status epilepticus

G40.A Absence epileptic syndrome
Childhood absence epilepsy [pyknolepsy]
Juvenile absence epilepsy
Absence epileptic syndrome, NOS

G40.A0 Absence epileptic syndrome, not intractable

G40.A01 Absence epileptic syndrome, not intractable, with status epilepticus

G40.A09 Absence epileptic syndrome, not intractable, without status epilepticus

G40.A1 Absence epileptic syndrome, intractable

G40.A11 Absence epileptic syndrome, intractable, with status epilepticus

G40.A19 Absence epileptic syndrome, intractable, without status epilepticus

G40.B Juvenile myoclonic epilepsy [impulsive petit mal]

G40.B0 Juvenile myoclonic epilepsy, not intractable

G40.B01 Juvenile myoclonic epilepsy, not intractable, with status epilepticus

G40.B09 Juvenile myoclonic epilepsy, not intractable, without status epilepticus

G40.B1 Juvenile myoclonic epilepsy, intractable

G40.B11 Juvenile myoclonic epilepsy, intractable, with status epilepticus

G40.B19 Juvenile myoclonic epilepsy, intractable, without status epilepticus

G40.4 Other generalized epilepsy and epileptic syndromes
Epilepsy with grand mal seizures on awakening
Epilepsy with myoclonic absences
Epilepsy with myoclonic-astatic seizures
Grand mal seizure NOS
Nonspecific atonic epileptic seizures
Nonspecific clonic epileptic seizures
Nonspecific myoclonic epileptic seizures
Nonspecific tonic epileptic seizures
Nonspecific tonic-clonic epileptic seizures

Symptomatic early myoclonic encephalopathy

G40.40 Other generalized epilepsy and epileptic syndromes, not intractable
Other generalized epilepsy and epileptic syndromes without intractability
Other generalized epilepsy and epileptic syndromes NOS

G40.401 Other generalized epilepsy and epileptic syndromes, not intractable, with status epilepticus

G40.409 Other generalized epilepsy and epileptic syndromes, not intractable, without status epilepticus

G40.41 Other generalized epilepsy and epileptic syndromes, intractable

G40.411 Other generalized epilepsy and epileptic syndromes, intractable, with status epilepticus

G40.419 Other generalized epilepsy and epileptic syndromes, intractable, without status epilepticus

G40.5 Epileptic seizures related to external causes
Epileptic seizures related to alcohol
Epileptic seizures related to drugs
Epileptic seizures related to hormonal changes
Epileptic seizures related to sleep deprivation
Epileptic seizures related to stress
Use additional code for adverse effect, if applicable, to identify drug (T36-T50 with fifth or sixth character 5)
Code also , if applicable, associated epilepsy and recurrent seizures (G40.-)

G40.50 Epileptic seizures related to external causes, not intractable

G40.501 Epileptic seizures related to external causes, not intractable, with status epilepticus

G40.509 Epileptic seizures related to external causes, not intractable, without status epilepticus
Epileptic seizures related to external causes, NOS

G40.8 Other epilepsy and recurrent seizures
Epilepsies and epileptic syndromes undetermined as to whether they are focal or generalized
Landau-Kleffner syndrome

G40.80 Other epilepsy

G40.801 Other epilepsy, not intractable, with status epilepticus
Other epilepsy without intractability with status epilepticus

G40.802 Other epilepsy, not intractable, without status epilepticus
Other epilepsy NOS
Other epilepsy without intractability without status epilepticus

G40.803 Other epilepsy, intractable, with status epilepticus

G40.804 Other epilepsy, intractable, without status epilepticus

G40.81 Lennox-Gastaut syndrome

G40.811 Lennox-Gastaut syndrome, not intractable, with status epilepticus

G40.812 Lennox-Gastaut syndrome, not intractable, without status epilepticus

G40.813   Lennox-Gastaut syndrome, intractable, with status epilepticus

G40.814   Lennox-Gastaut syndrome, intractable, without status epilepticus

G40.82   Epileptic spasms
Infantile spasms
Salaam attacks
West's syndrome

G40.821   Epileptic spasms, not intractable, with status epilepticus

G40.822   Epileptic spasms, not intractable, without status epilepticus

G40.823   Epileptic spasms, intractable, with status epilepticus

G40.824   Epileptic spasms, intractable, without status epilepticus

G40.89   Other seizures
Excludes 1: post traumatic seizures (R56.1)
recurrent seizures NOS (G40.909)
seizure NOS (R56.9)

G40.9   Epilepsy, unspecified

G40.90   Epilepsy, unspecified, not intractable
Epilepsy, unspecified, without intractability

G40.901   Epilepsy, unspecified, not intractable, with status epilepticus

G40.909   Epilepsy, unspecified, not intractable, without status epilepticus
Epilepsy NOS
Epileptic convulsions NOS
Epileptic fits NOS
Epileptic seizures NOS
Recurrent seizures NOS
Seizure disorder NOS

G40.91   Epilepsy, unspecified, intractable
Intractable seizure disorder NOS

G40.911   Epilepsy, unspecified, intractable, with status epilepticus

G40.919   Epilepsy, unspecified, intractable, without status epilepticus

G43   Migraine
Note: the following terms are to be considered equivalent to intractable: pharmacoresistant (pharmacologically resistant), treatment resistant, refractory (medically) and poorly controlled
Use additional code for adverse effect, if applicable, to identify drug (T36-T50 with fifth or sixth character 5)
Excludes 1: headache NOS (R51)
headache syndromes (G44.-)
lower half migraine (G44.00)

G43.0   Migraine without aura
Common migraine
Excludes 1: chronic migraine without aura (G43.7-)

G43.00   Migraine without aura, not intractable
Migraine without aura without mention of refractory migraine

G43.001   Migraine without aura, not intractable, with status migrainosus

G43.009   Migraine without aura, not intractable, without status migrainosus
Migraine without aura NOS

G43.01   Migraine without aura, intractable
Migraine without aura with refractory migraine

G43.011   Migraine without aura, intractable, with status migrainosus

G43.019   Migraine without aura, intractable, without status migrainosus

G43.1   Migraine with aura
Basilar migraine
Classical migraine
Migraine equivalents
Migraine preceded or accompanied by transient focal neurological phenomena
Migraine triggered seizures
Migraine with acute-onset aura
Migraine with aura without headache (migraine equivalents)
Migraine with prolonged aura
Migraine with typical aura
Retinal migraine
Code also any associated seizure (G40.-, R56.9)
Excludes 1: persistent migraine aura (G43.5-, G43.6-)

G43.10   Migraine with aura, not intractable
Migraine with aura without mention of refractory migraine

G43.101   Migraine with aura, not intractable, with status migrainosus

G43.109   Migraine with aura, not intractable, without status migrainosus
Migraine with aura NOS

G43.11   Migraine with aura, intractable
Migraine with aura with refractory migraine

G43.111   Migraine with aura, intractable, with status migrainosus

G43.119   Migraine with aura, intractable, without status migrainosus

G43.4   Hemiplegic migraine
Familial migraine
Sporadic migraine

G43.40   Hemiplegic migraine, not intractable
Hemiplegic migraine without refractory migraine

G43.401   Hemiplegic migraine, not intractable, with status migrainosus

G43.409   Hemiplegic migraine, not intractable, without status migrainosus
Hemiplegic migraine NOS

G43.41   Hemiplegic migraine, intractable
Hemiplegic migraine with refractory migraine

G43.411   Hemiplegic migraine, intractable, with status migrainosus

G43.419   Hemiplegic migraine, intractable, without status migrainosus

G43.5   Persistent migraine aura without cerebral infarction

G43.50   Persistent migraine aura without cerebral infarction, not intractable
Persistent migraine aura without cerebral infarction, without refractory migraine

G43.501   Persistent migraine aura without cerebral infarction, not intractable, with status migrainosus

G43.509   Persistent migraine aura without cerebral infarction, not intractable, without status migrainosus
Persistent migraine aura NOS

G43.51   Persistent migraine aura without cerebral infarction, intractable

Persistent migraine aura without cerebral infarction, with refractory migraine

G43.511   Persistent migraine aura without cerebral infarction, intractable, with status migrainosus

G43.519   Persistent migraine aura without cerebral infarction, intractable, without status migrainosus

G43.6 Persistent migraine aura with cerebral infarction

Code also the type of cerebral infarction (I63.-)

G43.60 Persistent migraine aura with cerebral infarction, not intractable

Persistent migraine aura with cerebral infarction, without refractory migraine

G43.601   Persistent migraine aura with cerebral infarction, not intractable, with status migrainosus

G43.609   Persistent migraine aura with cerebral infarction, not intractable, without status migrainosus

G43.61 Persistent migraine aura with cerebral infarction, intractable

Persistent migraine aura with cerebral infarction, with refractory migraine

G43.611   Persistent migraine aura with cerebral infarction, intractable, with status migrainosus

G43.619   Persistent migraine aura with cerebral infarction, intractable, without status migrainosus

G43.7 Chronic migraine without aura

Transformed migraine

Excludes 1: migraine without aura (G43.0-)

G43.70 Chronic migraine without aura, not intractable

Chronic migraine without aura, without refractory migraine

G43.701   Chronic migraine without aura, not intractable, with status migrainosus

G43.709   Chronic migraine without aura, not intractable, without status migrainosus

Chronic migraine without aura NOS

G43.71 Chronic migraine without aura, intractable

Chronic migraine without aura, with refractory migraine

G43.711   Chronic migraine without aura, intractable, with status migrainosus

G43.719   Chronic migraine without aura, intractable, without status migrainosus

G43.A Cyclical vomiting

G43.A0 Cyclical vomiting, not intractable

Cyclical vomiting, without refractory migraine

G43.A1 Cyclical vomiting, intractable

Cyclical vomiting, with refractory migraine

G43.B Ophthalmoplegic migraine

G43.B0 Ophthalmoplegic migraine, not intractable

Ophthalmoplegic migraine, without refractory migraine

G43.B1 Ophthalmoplegic migraine, intractable

Ophthalmoplegic migraine, with refractory migraine

G43.C Periodic headache syndromes in child or adult

G43.C0 Periodic headache syndromes in child or adult, not intractable

Periodic headache syndromes in child or adult, without refractory migraine

G43.C1 Periodic headache syndromes in child or adult, intractable

Periodic headache syndromes in child or adult, with refractory migraine

G43.D Abdominal migraine

G43.D0 Abdominal migraine, not intractable

Abdominal migraine, without refractory migraine

G43.D1 Abdominal migraine, intractable

Abdominal migraine, with refractory migraine

G43.8 Other migraine

G43.80 Other migraine, not intractable

Other migraine, without refractory migraine

G43.801   Other migraine, not intractable, with status migrainosus

G43.809   Other migraine, not intractable, without status migrainosus

G43.81 Other migraine, intractable

Other migraine, with refractory migraine

G43.811   Other migraine, intractable, with status migrainosus

G43.819   Other migraine, intractable, without status migrainosus

G43.82 Menstrual migraine, not intractable

Menstrual headache, not intractable

Menstrual migraine, without refractory migraine

Menstrually related migraine, not intractable

Pre-menstrual headache, not intractable

Pre-menstrual migraine, not intractable

Pure menstrual migraine, not intractable

Code also associated premenstrual tension syndrome (N94.3)

G43.821   Menstrual migraine, not intractable, with status migrainosus

G43.829   Menstrual migraine, not intractable, without status migrainosus

Menstrual migraine NOS

G43.83 Menstrual migraine, intractable

Menstrual headache, intractable

Menstrual migraine, with refractory migraine

Menstrually related migraine, intractable

Pre-menstrual headache, intractable

Pre-menstrual migraine, intractable

Pure menstrual migraine, intractable

Code also associated premenstrual tension syndrome (N94.3)

G43.831   Menstrual migraine, intractable, with status migrainosus

G43.839   Menstrual migraine, intractable, without status migrainosus

G43.9 Migraine, unspecified

G43.90 Migraine, unspecified, not intractable

Migraine, unspecified, without refractory migraine

G43.901   Migraine, unspecified, not intractable, with status migrainosus

Status migrainosus NOS

G43.909   Migraine, unspecified, not intractable, without status migrainosus

Migraine NOS

G43.91 Migraine, unspecified, intractable

Migraine, unspecified, with refractory migraine

G43.911 Migraine, unspecified, intractable, with status migrainosus

G43.919 Migraine, unspecified, intractable, without status migrainosus

G44 Other headache syndromes

Excludes 1: headache NOS (R51)

Excludes 2: atypical facial pain (G50.1)

headache due to lumbar puncture (G97.1)

migraines (G43.-)

trigeminal neuralgia (G50.0)

G44.0 Cluster headaches and other trigeminal autonomic cephalgias (TAC)

G44.00 Cluster headache syndrome, unspecified

Ciliary neuralgia

Cluster headache NOS

Histamine cephalgia

Lower half migraine

Migrainous neuralgia

G44.001 Cluster headache syndrome, unspecified, intractable

G44.009 Cluster headache syndrome, unspecified, not intractable

Cluster headache syndrome NOS

G44.01 Episodic cluster headache

G44.011 Episodic cluster headache, intractable

G44.019 Episodic cluster headache, not intractable

Episodic cluster headache NOS

G44.02 Chronic cluster headache

G44.021 Chronic cluster headache, intractable

G44.029 Chronic cluster headache, not intractable

Chronic cluster headache NOS

G44.03 Episodic paroxysmal hemicrania

Paroxysmal hemicrania NOS

G44.031 Episodic paroxysmal hemicrania, intractable

G44.039 Episodic paroxysmal hemicrania, not intractable

Episodic paroxysmal hemicrania NOS

G44.04 Chronic paroxysmal hemicrania

G44.041 Chronic paroxysmal hemicrania, intractable

G44.049 Chronic paroxysmal hemicrania, not intractable

Chronic paroxysmal hemicrania NOS

G44.05 Short lasting unilateral neuralgiform headache with conjunctival injection and tearing (SUNCT)

G44.051 Short lasting unilateral neuralgiform headache with conjunctival injection and tearing (SUNCT), intractable

G44.059 Short lasting unilateral neuralgiform headache with conjunctival injection and tearing (SUNCT), not intractable

Short lasting unilateral neuralgiform headache with conjunctival injection and tearing (SUNCT) NOS

G44.09 Other trigeminal autonomic cephalgias (TAC)

G44.091 Other trigeminal autonomic cephalgias (TAC), intractable

G44.099 Other trigeminal autonomic cephalgias (TAC), not intractable

G44.1 Vascular headache, not elsewhere classified

Excludes 2: cluster headache (G44.0)

complicated headache syndromes (G44.5-)

drug-induced headache (G44.4-)

migraine (G43.-)

other specified headache syndromes (G44.8-)

post-traumatic headache (G44.3-)

tension-type headache (G44.2-)

G44.2 Tension-type headache

G44.20 Tension-type headache, unspecified

G44.201 Tension-type headache, unspecified, intractable

G44.209 Tension-type headache, unspecified, not intractable

Tension headache NOS

G44.21 Episodic tension-type headache

G44.211 Episodic tension-type headache, intractable

G44.219 Episodic tension-type headache, not intractable

Episodic tension-type headache NOS

G44.22 Chronic tension-type headache

G44.221 Chronic tension-type headache, intractable

G44.229 Chronic tension-type headache, not intractable

Chronic tension-type headache NOS

G44.3 Post-traumatic headache

G44.30 Post-traumatic headache, unspecified

G44.301 Post-traumatic headache, unspecified, intractable

G44.309 Post-traumatic headache, unspecified, not intractable

Post-traumatic headache NOS

G44.31 Acute post-traumatic headache

G44.311 Acute post-traumatic headache, intractable

G44.319 Acute post-traumatic headache, not intractable

Acute post-traumatic headache NOS

G44.32 Chronic post-traumatic headache

G44.321 Chronic post-traumatic headache, intractable

G44.329 Chronic post-traumatic headache, not intractable

Chronic post-traumatic headache NOS

G44.4 Drug-induced headache, not elsewhere classified

Medication overuse headache

Use additional code for adverse effect, if applicable, to identify drug (T36-T50 with fifth or sixth character 5)

G44.40 Drug-induced headache, not elsewhere classified, not intractable

G44.41 Drug-induced headache, not elsewhere classified, intractable

G44.5 Complicated headache syndromes

G44.51 Hemicrania continua

G44.52 New daily persistent headache (NDPH)

G44.53 Primary thunderclap headache

● New code   ▲ Revised code   ⑦ 7ᵗʰ digit required   ⊗ Placeholder required

G44.59 Other complicated headache syndrome

G44.8 Other specified headache syndromes

    G44.81 Hypnic headache

    G44.82 Headache associated with sexual activity

        Orgasmic headache

        Preorgasmic headache

    G44.83 Primary cough headache

    G44.84 Primary exertional headache

    G44.85 Primary stabbing headache

    G44.89 Other headache syndrome

G45 Transient cerebral ischemic attacks and related syndromes

  Excludes 1: neonatal cerebral ischemia (P91.0)

        transient retinal artery occlusion (H34.0-)

G45.0 Vertebro-basilar artery syndrome

G45.1 Carotid artery syndrome (hemispheric)

G45.2 Multiple and bilateral precerebral artery syndromes

G45.3 Amaurosis fugax

G45.4 Transient global amnesia

  Excludes 1: amnesia NOS (R41.3)

G45.8 Other transient cerebral ischemic attacks and related syndromes

G45.9 Transient cerebral ischemic attack, unspecified

    Spasm of cerebral artery

    TIA

    Transient cerebral ischemia NOS

G46 Vascular syndromes of brain in cerebrovascular diseases

  Code first underlying cerebrovascular disease (I60-I69)

G46.0 Middle cerebral artery syndrome

G46.1 Anterior cerebral artery syndrome

G46.2 Posterior cerebral artery syndrome

G46.3 Brain stem stroke syndrome

    Benedikt syndrome

    Claude syndrome

    Foville syndrome

    Millard-Gubler syndrome

    Wallenberg syndrome

    Weber syndrome

G46.4 Cerebellar stroke syndrome

G46.5 Pure motor lacunar syndrome

G46.6 Pure sensory lacunar syndrome

G46.7 Other lacunar syndromes

G46.8 Other vascular syndromes of brain in cerebrovascular diseases

G47 Sleep disorders

  Excludes 2: nightmares (F51.5)

        nonorganic sleep disorders (F51.-)

        sleep terrors (F51.4)

        sleepwalking (F51.3)

G47.0 Insomnia

  Excludes 2: alcohol related insomnia (F10.182, F10.282, F10.982)

        drug related insomnia (F11.182, F11.282, F11.982, F13.182, F13.282, F13.982, F14.182, F14.282, F14.982, F15.182, F15.282, F15.982, F19.182, F19.282, F19.982)

        idiopathic insomnia (F51.01)

        insomnia due to a mental disorder (F51.05)

        insomnia not due to a substance or known physiological condition (F51.0-)

        nonorganic insomnia (F51.0-)

        primary insomnia (F51.01)

        sleep apnea (G47.3-)

G47.00 Insomnia, unspecified

    Insomnia NOS

G47.01 Insomnia due to medical condition

    Code also associated medical condition

G47.09 Other insomnia

G47.1 Hypersomnia

  Excludes 2: alcohol-related hypersomnia (F10.182, F10.282, F10.982)

        drug-related hypersomnia (F11.182, F11.282, F11.982, F13.182, F13.282, F13.982, F14.182, F14.282, F14.982, F15.182, F15.282, F15.982, F19.182, F19.282, F19.982)

        hypersomnia due to a mental disorder (F51.13)

        hypersomnia not due to a substance or known physiological condition (F51.1-)

        primary hypersomnia (F51.11)

        sleep apnea (G47.3-)

G47.10 Hypersomnia, unspecified

    Hypersomnia NOS

G47.11 Idiopathic hypersomnia with long sleep time

    Idiopathic hypersomnia NOS

G47.12 Idiopathic hypersomnia without long sleep time

G47.13 Recurrent hypersomnia

    Kleine-Levin syndrome

    Menstrual related hypersomnia

G47.14 Hypersomnia due to medical condition

    Code also associated medical condition

G47.19 Other hypersomnia

G47.2 Circadian rhythm sleep disorders

  Disorders of the sleep wake schedule

  Inversion of nyctohemeral rhythm

  Inversion of sleep rhythm

G47.20 Circadian rhythm sleep disorder, unspecified type

    Sleep wake schedule disorder NOS

G47.21 Circadian rhythm sleep disorder, delayed sleep phase type

    Delayed sleep phase syndrome

G47.22 Circadian rhythm sleep disorder, advanced sleep phase type

G47.23 Circadian rhythm sleep disorder, irregular sleep wake type

    Irregular sleep-wake pattern

G47.24 Circadian rhythm sleep disorder, free running type

G47.25 Circadian rhythm sleep disorder, jet lag type

G47.26 Circadian rhythm sleep disorder, shift work type

G47.27 Circadian rhythm sleep disorder in conditions classified elsewhere

    Code first underlying condition

G47.29 Other circadian rhythm sleep disorder

G47.3 Sleep apnea

  Code also any associated underlying condition

  Excludes 1: apnea NOS R06.81

        Cheyne-Stokes breathing (R06.3)

        pickwickian syndrome (E66.2)

        sleep apnea of newborn (P28.3)

G47.30 Sleep apnea, unspecified

    Sleep apnea NOS

G47.31 Primary central sleep apnea

G47.32 High altitude periodic breathing

G47.33 Obstructive sleep apnea (adult) (pediatric)

  Add 4th-7th digits   3 digit reportable   Nonspecific code   Unspecified code   Manifestation code

Excludes 1: obstructive sleep apnea of newborn (P28.3)

G47.34   Idiopathic sleep related nonobstructive alveolar hypoventilation
Sleep related hypoxia

G47.35   Congenital central alveolar hypoventilation syndrome

G47.36   Sleep related hypoventilation in conditions classified elsewhere
Sleep related hypoxemia in conditions classified elsewhere
Code first underlying condition

G47.37   Central sleep apnea in conditions classified elsewhere
Code first underlying condition

G47.39   Other sleep apnea

G47.4   Narcolepsy and cataplexy

   G47.41   Narcolepsy

     G47.411   Narcolepsy with cataplexy

     G47.419   Narcolepsy without cataplexy
Narcolepsy NOS

   G47.42   Narcolepsy in conditions classified elsewhere

     G47.421   Narcolepsy in conditions classified elsewhere with cataplexy

     G47.429   Narcolepsy in conditions classified elsewhere without cataplexy

G47.5   Parasomnia

Excludes 1: alcohol induced parasomnia (F10.182, F10.282, F10.982)
drug induced parasomnia (F11.182, F11.282, F11.982, F13.182, F13.282, F13.982, F14.182, F14.282, F14.982, F15.182, F15.282, F15.982, F19.182, F19.282, F19.982)
parasomnia not due to a substance or known physiological condition (F51.8)

   G47.50   Parasomnia, unspecified
Parasomnia NOS

   G47.51   Confusional arousals

   G47.52   REM sleep behavior disorder

   G47.53   Recurrent isolated sleep paralysis

   G47.54   Parasomnia in conditions classified elsewhere
Code first underlying condition

   G47.59   Other parasomnia

G47.6   Sleep related movement disorders

Excludes 2: restless legs syndrome (G25.81)

   G47.61   Periodic limb movement disorder
Periodic limb movement disorder

   G47.62   Sleep related leg cramps

   G47.63   Sleep related bruxism
Excludes 1: psychogenic bruxism (F45.8)

   G47.69   Other sleep related movement disorders

G47.8   Other sleep disorders

G47.9   Sleep disorder, unspecified
Sleep disorder NOS

NERVE, NERVE ROOT AND PLEXUS DISORDERS (G50-G59)

Excludes 1: current traumatic nerve, nerve root and plexus disorders - see Injury, nerve by body region
neuralgia NOS (M79.2)
neuritis NOS (M79.2)
peripheral neuritis in pregnancy (O26.82-)
radiculitis NOS (M54.1-)

G50   Disorders of trigeminal nerve

Includes: disorders of 5th cranial nerve

   G50.0   Trigeminal neuralgia
Syndrome of paroxysmal facial pain
Tic douloureux

   G50.1   Atypical facial pain

   G50.8   Other disorders of trigeminal nerve

   G50.9   Disorder of trigeminal nerve, unspecified

G51   Facial nerve disorders

Includes: disorders of 7th cranial nerve

   G51.0   Bell's palsy
Facial palsy

   G51.1   Geniculate ganglionitis
Excludes 1: postherpetic geniculate ganglionitis (B02.21)

   G51.2   Melkersson's syndrome
Melkersson-Rosenthal syndrome

   G51.3   Clonic hemifacial spasm

   G51.4   Facial myokymia

   G51.8   Other disorders of facial nerve

   G51.9   Disorder of facial nerve, unspecified

G52   Disorders of other cranial nerves

Excludes 2: disorders of acoustic [8th] nerve (H93.3)
disorders of optic [2nd] nerve (H46, H47.0)
paralytic strabismus due to nerve palsy (H49.0-H49.2)

   G52.0   Disorders of olfactory nerve
Disorders of 1st cranial nerve

   G52.1   Disorders of glossopharyngeal nerve
Disorder of 9th cranial nerve
Glossopharyngeal neuralgia

   G52.2   Disorders of vagus nerve
Disorders of pneumogastric [10th] nerve

   G52.3   Disorders of hypoglossal nerve
Disorders of 12th cranial nerve

   G52.7   Disorders of multiple cranial nerves
Polyneuritis cranialis

   G52.8   Disorders of other specified cranial nerves

   G52.9   Cranial nerve disorder, unspecified

G53   Cranial nerve disorders in diseases classified elsewhere

Code first underlying disease, such as:
neoplasm (C00-D49)

Excludes 1: multiple cranial nerve palsy in sarcoidosis (D86.82)
multiple cranial nerve palsy in syphilis (A52.15)
postherpetic geniculate ganglionitis (B02.21)
postherpetic trigeminal neuralgia (B02.22)

G54   Nerve root and plexus disorders

Excludes 1: current traumatic nerve root and plexus disorders - see nerve injury by body region
intervertebral disc disorders (M50-M51)
neuralgia or neuritis NOS (M79.2)
neuritis or radiculitis:
brachial NOS (M54.13)
lumbar NOS (M54.16)
lumbosacral NOS (M54.17)
thoracic NOS (M54.14)
radiculitis NOS (M54.10)
radiculopathy NOS (M54.10)
spondylosis (M47.-)

   G54.0   Brachial plexus disorders
Thoracic outlet syndrome

   G54.1   Lumbosacral plexus disorders

   G54.2   Cervical root disorders, not elsewhere classified

G54.3 Thoracic root disorders, not elsewhere classified

G54.4 Lumbosacral root disorders, not elsewhere classified

G54.5 Neuralgic amyotrophy

Parsonage-Aldren-Turner syndrome

Shoulder-girdle neuritis

Excludes 1: neuralgic amyotrophy in diabetes mellitus (E08-E13 with .44)

G54.6 Phantom limb syndrome with pain

G54.7 Phantom limb syndrome without pain

Phantom limb syndrome NOS

G54.8 Other nerve root and plexus disorders

G54.9 Nerve root and plexus disorder, unspecified

G55 Nerve root and plexus compressions in diseases classified elsewhere

Code first underlying disease, such as:

neoplasm (C00-D49)

Excludes 1: nerve root compression (due to) (in) ankylosing spondylitis (M45.-)

nerve root compression (due to) (in) ankylosing spondylitis (M45.-)

nerve root compression (due to) (in) dorsopathies (M53.-, M54.-)

nerve root compression (due to) (in) intervertebral disc disorders (M50.1.-, M51.1.-)

nerve root compression (due to) (in) spondylopathies (M46.-, M48.-)

nerve root compression (due to) (in) spondylosis (M47.0-M47.2.-)

G56 Mononeuropathies of upper limb

Excludes 1: current traumatic nerve disorder - see nerve injury by body region

G56.0 Carpal tunnel syndrome

G56.00 Carpal tunnel syndrome, unspecified upper limb

G56.01 Carpal tunnel syndrome, right upper limb

G56.02 Carpal tunnel syndrome, left upper limb

G56.1 Other lesions of median nerve

G56.10 Other lesions of median nerve, unspecified upper limb

G56.11 Other lesions of median nerve, right upper limb

G56.12 Other lesions of median nerve, left upper limb

G56.2 Lesion of ulnar nerve

Tardy ulnar nerve palsy

G56.20 Lesion of ulnar nerve, unspecified upper limb

G56.21 Lesion of ulnar nerve, right upper limb

G56.22 Lesion of ulnar nerve, left upper limb

G56.3 Lesion of radial nerve

G56.30 Lesion of radial nerve, unspecified upper limb

G56.31 Lesion of radial nerve, right upper limb

G56.32 Lesion of radial nerve, left upper limb

G56.4 Causalgia of upper limb

Complex regional pain syndrome II of upper limb

Excludes 1: complex regional pain syndrome I of lower limb (G90.52-)

complex regional pain syndrome I of upper limb (G90.51-)

complex regional pain syndrome II of lower limb (G57.7-)

reflex sympathetic dystrophy of lower limb (G90.52-)

reflex sympathetic dystrophy of upper limb (G90.51-)

G56.40 Causalgia of unspecified upper limb

G56.41 Causalgia of right upper limb

G56.42 Causalgia of left upper limb

G56.8 Other specified mononeuropathies of upper limb

Interdigital neuroma of upper limb

G56.80 Other specified mononeuropathies of unspecified upper limb

G56.81 Other specified mononeuropathies of right upper limb

G56.82 Other specified mononeuropathies of left upper limb

G56.9 Unspecified mononeuropathy of upper limb

G56.90 Unspecified mononeuropathy of unspecified upper limb

G56.91 Unspecified mononeuropathy of right upper limb

G56.92 Unspecified mononeuropathy of left upper limb

G57 Mononeuropathies of lower limb

Excludes 1: current traumatic nerve disorder - see nerve injury by body region

G57.0 Lesion of sciatic nerve

Excludes 1: sciatica NOS (M54.3-)

Excludes 2: sciatica attributed to intervertebral disc disorder (M51.1.-)

G57.00 Lesion of sciatic nerve, unspecified lower limb

G57.01 Lesion of sciatic nerve, right lower limb

G57.02 Lesion of sciatic nerve, left lower limb

G57.1 Meralgia paresthetica

Lateral cutaneous nerve of thigh syndrome

G57.10 Meralgia paresthetica, unspecified lower limb

G57.11 Meralgia paresthetica, right lower limb

G57.12 Meralgia paresthetica, left lower limb

G57.2 Lesion of femoral nerve

G57.20 Lesion of femoral nerve, unspecified lower limb

G57.21 Lesion of femoral nerve, right lower limb

G57.22 Lesion of femoral nerve, left lower limb

G57.3 Lesion of lateral popliteal nerve

Peroneal nerve palsy

G57.30 Lesion of lateral popliteal nerve, unspecified lower limb

G57.31 Lesion of lateral popliteal nerve, right lower limb

G57.32 Lesion of lateral popliteal nerve, left lower limb

G57.4 Lesion of medial popliteal nerve

G57.40 Lesion of medial popliteal nerve, unspecified lower limb

G57.41 Lesion of medial popliteal nerve, right lower limb

G57.42 Lesion of medial popliteal nerve, left lower limb

G57.5 Tarsal tunnel syndrome

G57.50 Tarsal tunnel syndrome, unspecified lower limb

G57.51 Tarsal tunnel syndrome, right lower limb

G57.52 Tarsal tunnel syndrome, left lower limb

G57.6 Lesion of plantar nerve

Morton's metatarsalgia

G57.60 Lesion of plantar nerve, unspecified lower limb

G57.61 Lesion of plantar nerve, right lower limb

G57.62 Lesion of plantar nerve, left lower limb

G57.7 Causalgia of lower limb

Complex regional pain syndrome II of lower limb

Excludes 1: complex regional pain syndrome I of lower limb (G90.52-)

complex regional pain syndrome I of upper limb (G90.51-)

complex regional pain syndrome II of upper limb (G56.4-)

reflex sympathetic dystrophy of lower limb
(G90.52-)

reflex sympathetic dystrophy of upper limb
(G90.51-)

G57.70   Causalgia of unspecified lower limb
G57.71   Causalgia of right lower limb
G57.72   Causalgia of left lower limb
G57.8   Other specified mononeuropathies of lower limb
Interdigital neuroma of lower limb
G57.80   Other specified mononeuropathies of unspecified lower limb
G57.81   Other specified mononeuropathies of right lower limb
G57.82   Other specified mononeuropathies of left lower limb
G57.9   Unspecified mononeuropathy of lower limb
G57.90   Unspecified mononeuropathy of unspecified lower limb
G57.91   Unspecified mononeuropathy of right lower limb
G57.92   Unspecified mononeuropathy of left lower limb
G58   Other mononeuropathies
G58.0   Intercostal neuropathy
G58.7   Mononeuritis multiplex
G58.8   Other specified mononeuropathies
G58.9   Mononeuropathy, unspecified
G59   Mononeuropathy in diseases classified elsewhere
Code first underlying disease
Excludes 1: diabetic mononeuropathy (E09-E14 with .41)
syphilitic nerve paralysis (A52.19)
syphilitic neuritis (A52.15)
tuberculous mononeuropathy (A17.83)

POLYNEUROPATHIES AND OTHER DISORDERS OF THE PERIPHERAL NERVOUS SYSTEM (G60-G65)

Excludes 1: neuralgia NOS (M79.2)
neuritis NOS (M79.2)
peripheral neuritis in pregnancy (O26.82-)
radiculitis NOS (M54.10)
G60   Hereditary and idiopathic neuropathy
G60.0   Hereditary motor and sensory neuropathy
Charcot-Marie-Tooth disease
DⓈjⒺrine-Sottas disease
Hereditary motor and sensory neuropathy, types I-IV
Hypertrophic neuropathy of infancy
Peroneal muscular atrophy (axonal type) (hypertrophic type)
Roussy-Levy syndrome
G60.1   Refsum's disease
Infantile Refsum disease
G60.2   Neuropathy in association with hereditary ataxia
G60.3   Idiopathic progressive neuropathy
G60.8   Other hereditary and idiopathic neuropathies
Dominantly inherited sensory neuropathy
Morvan's disease
Nelaton's syndrome
Recessively inherited sensory neuropathy
G60.9   Hereditary and idiopathic neuropathy, unspecified
G61   Inflammatory polyneuropathy
G61.0   Guillain-Barre syndrome
Acute (post-)infective polyneuritis
Miller Fisher Syndrome
G61.1   Serum neuropathy

Use additional code for adverse effect, if applicable, to identify serum (T50.-)
G61.8   Other inflammatory polyneuropathies
G61.81   Chronic inflammatory demyelinating polyneuritis
G61.89   Other inflammatory polyneuropathies
G61.9   Inflammatory polyneuropathy, unspecified
G62   Other and unspecified polyneuropathies
G62.0   Drug-induced polyneuropathy
Use additional code for adverse effect, if applicable, to identify drug (T36-T50 with fifth or sixth character 5)
G62.1   Alcoholic polyneuropathy
G62.2   Polyneuropathy due to other toxic agents
Code first (T51-T65) to identify toxic agent
G62.8   Other specified polyneuropathies
G62.81   Critical illness polyneuropathy
Acute motor neuropathy
G62.82   Radiation-induced polyneuropathy
Use additional external cause code (W88-W90, X39.0-) to identify cause
G62.89   Other specified polyneuropathies
G62.9   Polyneuropathy, unspecified
Neuropathy NOS
G63   Polyneuropathy in diseases classified elsewhere
Code first underlying disease, such as:
amyloidosis (E85-)
endocrine disease, except diabetes (E00-E07, E15-E16, E20-E34)
metabolic diseases (E70-E88)
neoplasm (C00-D49)
nutritional deficiency (E40-E64)
Excludes 1: polyneuropathy (in):
diabetes mellitus (E08-E13 with .42)
diphtheria (A36.83)
infectious mononucleosis (B27.0-B27.9 with 1)
Lyme disease (A69.22)
mumps (B26.84)
postherpetic (B02.23)
rheumatoid arthritis (M05.33)
scleroderma (M34.83)
systemic lupus erythematosus (M32.19)
G64   Other disorders of peripheral nervous system
Disorder of peripheral nervous system NOS
G65   Sequelae of inflammatory and toxic polyneuropathies
Code first condition resulting from (sequela) of inflammatory and toxic polyneuropathies
G65.0   Sequelae of Guillain-Barr syndrome
G65.1   Sequelae of other inflammatory polyneuropathy
G65.2   Sequelae of toxic polyneuropathy

DISEASES OF MYONEURAL JUNCTION AND MUSCLE (G70-G73)

G70   Myasthenia gravis and other myoneural disorders
Excludes 1: botulism (A05.1, A48.51-A48.52)
transient neonatal myasthenia gravis (P94.0)
G70.0   Myasthenia gravis
G70.00   Myasthenia gravis without (acute) exacerbation
Myasthenia gravis NOS
G70.01   Myasthenia gravis with (acute) exacerbation
Myasthenia gravis in crisis
G70.1   Toxic myoneural disorders
Code first (T51-T65) to identify toxic agent

G70.2 Congenital and developmental myasthenia

G70.8 Other specified myoneural disorders

    G70.80 Lambert-Eaton syndrome, unspecified
          Lambert-Eaton syndrome NOS

    G70.81 Lambert-Eaton syndrome in disease classified elsewhere
          Code first underlying disease
          Excludes 1: Lambert-Eaton syndrome in neoplastic disease (G73.1)

    G70.89 Other specified myoneural disorders

G70.9 Myoneural disorder, unspecified

G71 Primary disorders of muscles

  Excludes 2: arthrogryposis multiplex congenita (Q74.3)
      metabolic disorders (E70-E88)
      myositis (M60.-)

G71.0 Muscular dystrophy
  Autosomal recessive, childhood type, muscular dystrophy resembling Duchenne or Becker muscular dystrophy
  Benign [Becker] muscular dystrophy
  Benign scapuloperoneal muscular dystrophy with early contractures [Emery-Dreifuss]
  Congenital muscular dystrophy NOS
  Congenital muscular dystrophy with specific morphological abnormalities of the muscle fiber
  Distal muscular dystrophy
  Facioscapulohumeral muscular dystrophy
  Limb-girdle muscular dystrophy
  Ocular muscular dystrophy
  Oculopharyngeal muscular dystrophy
  Scapuloperoneal muscular dystrophy
  Severe [Duchenne] muscular dystrophy

G71.1 Myotonic disorders

    G71.11 Myotonic muscular dystrophy
      Dystrophia myotonica [Steinert]
      Myotonia atrophica
      Myotonic dystrophy
      Proximal myotonic myopathy (PROMM)
      Steinert disease

    G71.12 Myotonia congenita
      Acetazolamide responsive myotonia congenita
      Dominant myotonia congenita [Thomsen disease]
      Myotonia levior
      Recessive myotonia congenita [Becker disease]

    G71.13 Myotonic chondrodystrophy
      Chondrodystrophic myotonia
      Congenital myotonic chondrodystrophy
      Schwartz-Jampel disease

    G71.14 Drug induced myotonia
      Use additional code for adverse effect, if applicable, to identify drug (T36-T50 with fifth or sixth character 5)

    G71.19 Other specified myotonic disorders
      Myotonia fluctuans
      Myotonia permanens
      Neuromyotonia [Isaacs]
      Paramyotonia congenita (of von Eulenburg)
      Pseudomyotonia
      Symptomatic myotonia

G71.2 Congenital myopathies
  Central core disease
  Fiber-type disproportion

  Minicore disease
  Multicore disease
  Myotubular (centronuclear) myopathy
  Nemaline myopathy
  Excludes 1: arthrogryposis multiplex congenita (Q74.3)

G71.3 Mitochondrial myopathy, not elsewhere classified
  Excludes 1: Kearns-Sayre syndrome (H49.81)
      Leber's disease (H47.21)
      Leigh's encephalopathy (G31.82)
      mitochondrial metabolism disorders (E88.4.-)
      Reye's syndrome (G93.7)

G71.8 Other primary disorders of muscles

G71.9 Primary disorder of muscle, unspecified
  Hereditary myopathy NOS

G72 Other and unspecified myopathies
  Excludes 1: arthrogryposis multiplex congenita (Q74.3)
      dermatopolymyositis (M33.-)
      ischemic infarction of muscle (M62.2-)
      myositis (M60.-)
      polymyositis (M33.2.-)

G72.0 Drug-induced myopathy
  Use additional code for adverse effect, if applicable, to identify drug (T36-T50 with fifth or sixth character 5)

G72.1 Alcoholic myopathy
  Use additional code to identify alcoholism (F10.-)

G72.2 Myopathy due to other toxic agents
  Code first (T51-T65) to identify toxic agent

G72.3 Periodic paralysis
  Familial periodic paralysis
  Hyperkalemic periodic paralysis (familial)
  Hypokalemic periodic paralysis (familial)
  Myotonic periodic paralysis (familial)
  Normokalemic paralysis (familial)
  Potassium sensitive periodic paralysis
  Excludes 1: paramyotonia congenita (of von Eulenburg) (G71.19)

G72.4 Inflammatory and immune myopathies, not elsewhere classified
    G72.41 Inclusion body myositis [IBM]
    G72.49 Other inflammatory and immune myopathies, not elsewhere classified
      Inflammatory myopathy NOS

G72.8 Other specified myopathies
    G72.81 Critical illness myopathy
      Acute necrotizing myopathy
      Acute quadriplegic myopathy
      Intensive care (ICU) myopathy
      Myopathy of critical illness
    G72.89 Other specified myopathies

G72.9 Myopathy, unspecified

G73 Disorders of myoneural junction and muscle in diseases classified elsewhere

G73.1 Lambert-Eaton syndrome in neoplastic disease
  Code first underlying neoplasm (C00-D49)
  Excludes 1: Lambert-Eaton syndrome not associated with neoplasm (G70.80-G70.81)

G73.3 Myasthenic syndromes in other diseases classified elsewhere
  Code first underlying disease, such as:
      neoplasm (C00-D49)
      thyrotoxicosis (E05.-)

G73.7 Myopathy in diseases classified elsewhere

Code first underlying disease, such as:

    hyperparathyroidism (E21.0, E21.3)

    hypoparathyroidism (E20.-)

    glycogen storage disease (E74.0)

    lipid storage disorders (E75.-)

Excludes 1: myopathy in:

    rheumatoid arthritis (M05.32)

    sarcoidosis (D86.87)

    scleroderma (M34.82)

    sicca syndrome [Sj÷gren] (M35.03)

    systemic lupus erythematosus (M32.19)

CEREBRAL PALSY AND OTHER PARALYTIC SYNDROMES (G80-G83)

G80 Cerebral palsy

Excludes 1: hereditary spastic paraplegia (G11.4)

G80.0 Spastic quadriplegic cerebral palsy

Congenital spastic paralysis (cerebral)

G80.1 Spastic diplegic cerebral palsy

Spastic cerebral palsy NOS

G80.2 Spastic hemiplegic cerebral palsy

G80.3 Athetoid cerebral palsy

Double athetosis (syndrome)

Dyskinetic cerebral palsy

Dystonic cerebral palsy

Vogt disease

G80.4 Ataxic cerebral palsy

G80.8 Other cerebral palsy

Mixed cerebral palsy syndromes

G80.9 Cerebral palsy, unspecified

Cerebral palsy NOS

G81 Hemiplegia and hemiparesis

Note: This category is to be used only when hemiplegia (complete)(incomplete) is reported without further specification, or is stated to be old or longstanding but of unspecified cause. The category is also for use in multiple coding to identify these types of hemiplegia resulting from any cause.

Excludes 1: congenital cerebral palsy (G80.-)

    hemiplegia and hemiparesis due to sequela of cerebrovascular disease (I69.05-, I69.15-, I69.25-, I69.35-, I69.85-, I69.95-)

G81.0 Flaccid hemiplegia

  G81.00 Flaccid hemiplegia affecting unspecified side

  G81.01 Flaccid hemiplegia affecting right dominant side

  G81.02 Flaccid hemiplegia affecting left dominant side

  G81.03 Flaccid hemiplegia affecting right nondominant side

  G81.04 Flaccid hemiplegia affecting left nondominant side

G81.1 Spastic hemiplegia

  G81.10 Spastic hemiplegia affecting unspecified side

  G81.11 Spastic hemiplegia affecting right dominant side

  G81.12 Spastic hemiplegia affecting left dominant side

  G81.13 Spastic hemiplegia affecting right nondominant side

  G81.14 Spastic hemiplegia affecting left nondominant side

G81.9 Hemiplegia, unspecified

  G81.90 Hemiplegia, unspecified affecting unspecified side

  G81.91 Hemiplegia, unspecified affecting right dominant side

  G81.92 Hemiplegia, unspecified affecting left dominant side

  G81.93 Hemiplegia, unspecified affecting right nondominant side

  G81.94 Hemiplegia, unspecified affecting left nondominant side

G82 Paraplegia (paraparesis) and quadriplegia (quadriparesis)

Note: This category is to be used only when the listed conditions are reported without further specification, or are stated to be old or longstanding but of unspecified cause. The category is also for use in multiple coding to identify these conditions resulting from any cause

Excludes 1: congenital cerebral palsy (G80.-)

    functional quadriplegia (R53.2)

    hysterical paralysis (F44.4)

G82.2 Paraplegia

Paralysis of both lower limbs NOS

Paraparesis (lower) NOS

Paraplegia (lower) NOS

  G82.20 Paraplegia, unspecified

  G82.21 Paraplegia, complete

  G82.22 Paraplegia, incomplete

G82.5 Quadriplegia

  G82.50 Quadriplegia, unspecified

  G82.51 Quadriplegia, C1-C4 complete

  G82.52 Quadriplegia, C1-C4 incomplete

  G82.53 Quadriplegia, C5-C7 complete

  G82.54 Quadriplegia, C5-C7 incomplete

G83 Other paralytic syndromes

Note: This category is to be used only when the listed conditions are reported without further specification, or are stated to be old or longstanding but of unspecified cause. The category is also for use in multiple coding to identify these conditions resulting from any cause.

Includes: paralysis (complete) (incomplete), except as in G80-G82

G83.0 Diplegia of upper limbs

Diplegia (upper)

Paralysis of both upper limbs

G83.1 Monoplegia of lower limb

Paralysis of lower limb

Excludes 1: monoplegia of lower limbs due to sequela of cerebrovascular disease (I69.04-, I69.14-, I69.24-, I69.34-, I69.84-, I69.94-)

  G83.10 Monoplegia of lower limb affecting unspecified side

  G83.11 Monoplegia of lower limb affecting right dominant side

  G83.12 Monoplegia of lower limb affecting left dominant side

  G83.13 Monoplegia of lower limb affecting right nondominant side

  G83.14 Monoplegia of lower limb affecting left nondominant side

G83.2 Monoplegia of upper limb

Paralysis of upper limb

Excludes 1: monoplegia of upper limbs due to sequela of cerebrovascular disease (I69.03-, I69.13-, I69.23-, I69.33-, I69.83-, I69.93-)

  G83.20 Monoplegia of upper limb affecting unspecified side

  G83.21 Monoplegia of upper limb affecting right dominant side

  G83.22 Monoplegia of upper limb affecting left dominant side

  ● New code   ▲ Revised code   ⑦ 7th digit required   ⊗ Placeholder required

G83.23 Monoplegia of upper limb affecting right nondominant side

G83.24 Monoplegia of upper limb affecting left nondominant side

G83.3 Monoplegia, unspecified

G83.30 Monoplegia, unspecified affecting unspecified side

G83.31 Monoplegia, unspecified affecting right dominant side

G83.32 Monoplegia, unspecified affecting left dominant side

G83.33 Monoplegia, unspecified affecting right nondominant side

G83.34 Monoplegia, unspecified affecting left nondominant side

G83.4 Cauda equina syndrome

Neurogenic bladder due to cauda equina syndrome

Excludes 1: cord bladder NOS (G95.89)

neurogenic bladder NOS (N31.9)

G83.5 Locked-in state

G83.8 Other specified paralytic syndromes

Excludes 1: paralytic syndromes due to current spinal cord injury-code to spinal cord injury (S14, S24, S34)

G83.81 Brown-Sequard syndrome

G83.82 Anterior cord syndrome

G83.83 Posterior cord syndrome

G83.84 Todd's paralysis (postepileptic)

G83.89 Other specified paralytic syndromes

G83.9 Paralytic syndrome, unspecified

OTHER DISORDERS OF THE NERVOUS SYSTEM (G89-G99)

G89 Pain, not elsewhere classified

Code also related psychological factors associated with pain (F45.42)

Excludes 1: generalized pain NOS (R52)

pain disorders exclusively related to psychological factors (F45.41)

pain NOS (R52)

Excludes 2: atypical face pain (G50.1)

headache syndromes (G44.-)

localized pain, unspecified type - code to pain by site, such as:

abdomen pain (R10.-)

back pain (M54.9)

breast pain (N64.4)

chest pain (R07.1-R07.9)

ear pain (H92.0-)

eye pain (H57.1)

headache (R51)

joint pain (M25.5-)

limb pain (M79.6-)

lumbar region pain (M54.5)

painful urination (R30.9)

pelvic and perineal pain (R10.2)

shoulder pain (M25.51-)

spine pain (M54.-)

throat pain (R07.0)

tongue pain (K14.6)

tooth pain (K08.8)

renal colic (N23)

migraines (G43.-)

myalgia (M79.1)

pain from prosthetic devices, implants, and grafts (T82.84, T83.84, T84.84, T85.84)

phantom limb syndrome with pain (G54.6)

vulvar vestibulitis (N94.810)

vulvodynia (N94.81-)

G89.0 Central pain syndrome

Dejerine-Roussy syndrome

Myelopathic pain syndrome

Thalamic pain syndrome (hyperesthetic)

G89.1 Acute pain, not elsewhere classified

G89.11 Acute pain due to trauma

G89.12 Acute post-thoracotomy pain

Post-thoracotomy pain NOS

G89.18 Other acute postprocedural pain

Postoperative pain NOS

Postprocedural pain NOS

G89.2 Chronic pain, not elsewhere classified

Excludes 1: causalgia, lower limb (G57.7-)

causalgia, upper limb (G56.4-)

central pain syndrome (G89.0)

chronic pain syndrome (G89.4)

complex regional pain syndrome II, lower limb (G57.7-)

complex regional pain syndrome II, upper limb (G56.4-)

neoplasm related chronic pain (G89.3)

reflex sympathetic dystrophy (G90.5-)

G89.21 Chronic pain due to trauma

G89.22 Chronic post-thoracotomy pain

G89.28 Other chronic postprocedural pain

Other chronic postoperative pain

G89.29 Other chronic pain

G89.3 Neoplasm related pain (acute) (chronic)

Cancer associated pain

Pain due to malignancy (primary) (secondary)

Tumor associated pain

G89.4 Chronic pain syndrome

Chronic pain associated with significant psychosocial dysfunction

G90 Disorders of autonomic nervous system

Excludes 1: dysfunction of the autonomic nervous system due to alcohol (G31.2)

G90.0 Idiopathic peripheral autonomic neuropathy

G90.01 Carotid sinus syncope

Carotid sinus syndrome

G90.09 Other idiopathic peripheral autonomic neuropathy

Idiopathic peripheral autonomic neuropathy NOS

G90.1 Familial dysautonomia [Riley-Day]

G90.2 Horner's syndrome

Bernard(-Horner) syndrome

Cervical sympathetic dystrophy or paralysis

G90.3 Multi-system degeneration of the autonomic nervous system

Neurogenic orthostatic hypotension [Shy-Drager]

Excludes 1: orthostatic hypotension NOS (I95.1)

G90.4 Autonomic dysreflexia

Use additional code to identify the cause, such as:

fecal impaction (K56.41)

pressure ulcer (pressure area) (L89.-)

urinary tract infection (N39.0)

G90.5 Complex regional pain syndrome I (CRPS I)
Reflex sympathetic dystrophy
Excludes 1: causalgia of lower limb (G57.7-)
causalgia of upper limb (G56.4-)
complex regional pain syndrome II of lower limb (G57.7-)
complex regional pain syndrome II of upper limb (G56.4-)
G90.50 Complex regional pain syndrome I, unspecified
G90.51 Complex regional pain syndrome I of upper limb
G90.511 Complex regional pain syndrome I of right upper limb
G90.512 Complex regional pain syndrome I of left upper limb
G90.513 Complex regional pain syndrome I of upper limb, bilateral
G90.519 Complex regional pain syndrome I of unspecified upper limb
G90.52 Complex regional pain syndrome I of lower limb
G90.521 Complex regional pain syndrome I of right lower limb
G90.522 Complex regional pain syndrome I of left lower limb
G90.523 Complex regional pain syndrome I of lower limb, bilateral
G90.529 Complex regional pain syndrome I of unspecified lower limb
G90.59 Complex regional pain syndrome I of other specified site
G90.8 Other disorders of autonomic nervous system
G90.9 Disorder of the autonomic nervous system, unspecified
G91 Hydrocephalus
Includes: acquired hydrocephalus
Excludes 1: Arnold-Chiari syndrome with hydrocephalus (Q07.-)
congenital hydrocephalus (Q03.-)
spina bifida with hydrocephalus (Q05.-)
G91.0 Communicating hydrocephalus
Secondary normal pressure hydrocephalus
G91.1 Obstructive hydrocephalus
G91.2 (Idiopathic) normal pressure hydrocephalus
Normal pressure hydrocephalus NOS
G91.3 Post-traumatic hydrocephalus, unspecified
G91.4 Hydrocephalus in diseases classified elsewhere
Code first underlying condition, such as:
congenital syphilis (A50.4-)
neoplasm (C00-D49)
Excludes 1: hydrocephalus due to congenital toxoplasmosis (P37.1)
G91.8 Other hydrocephalus
G91.9 Hydrocephalus, unspecified
G92 Toxic encephalopathy
Toxic encephalitis
Toxic metabolic encephalopathy
Code first (T51-T65) to identify toxic agent
G93 Other disorders of brain
G93.0 Cerebral cysts
Arachnoid cyst
Porencephalic cyst, acquired
Excludes 1: acquired periventricular cysts of newborn (P91.1)
congenital cerebral cysts (Q04.6)
G93.1 Anoxic brain damage, not elsewhere classified

Excludes 1: cerebral anoxia due to anesthesia during labor and delivery (O74.3)
cerebral anoxia due to anesthesia during the puerperium (O89.2)
neonatal anoxia (P84)
G93.2 Benign intracranial hypertension
Excludes 1: hypertensive encephalopathy (I67.4)
G93.3 Postviral fatigue syndrome
Benign myalgic encephalomyelitis
Excludes 1: chronic fatigue syndrome NOS (R53.82)
G93.4 Other and unspecified encephalopathy
Excludes 1: alcoholic encephalopathy (G31.2)
encephalopathy in diseases classified elsewhere (G94)
hypertensive encephalopathy (I67.4)
toxic (metabolic) encephalopathy (G92)
G93.40 Encephalopathy, unspecified
G93.41 Metabolic encephalopathy
Septic encephalopathy
G93.49 Other encephalopathy
Encephalopathy NEC
G93.5 Compression of brain
Arnold-Chiari type 1 compression of brain
Compression of brain (stem)
Herniation of brain (stem)
Excludes 1: diffuse traumatic compression of brain (S06.2-)
focal traumatic compression of brain (S06.3-)
G93.6 Cerebral edema
Excludes 1: cerebral edema due to birth injury (P11.0)
traumatic cerebral edema (S06.1-)
G93.7 Reye's syndrome
Code first (T39.0-), if salicylates-induced
G93.8 Other specified disorders of brain
G93.81 Temporal sclerosis
Hippocampal sclerosis
Mesial temporal sclerosis
G93.82 Brain death
G93.89 Other specified disorders of brain
Postradiation encephalopathy
G93.9 Disorder of brain, unspecified
G94 Other disorders of brain in diseases classified elsewhere
Code first underlying disease
Excludes 1: encephalopathy in congenital syphilis (A50.49)
encephalopathy in influenza (J09.X9, J10.81, J11.81)
encephalopathy in syphilis (A52.19)
hydrocephalus in diseases classified elsewhere (G91.4)
G95 Other and unspecified diseases of spinal cord
Excludes 2: myelitis (G04.-)
G95.0 Syringomyelia and syringobulbia
G95.1 Vascular myelopathies
Excludes 2: intraspinal phlebitis and thrombophlebitis, except non-pyogenic (G08)
G95.11 Acute infarction of spinal cord (embolic) (nonembolic)
Anoxia of spinal cord
Arterial thrombosis of spinal cord
G95.19 Other vascular myelopathies
Edema of spinal cord
Hematomyelia

Nonpyogenic intraspinal phlebitis and thrombophlebitis

Subacute necrotic myelopathy

G95.2 Other and unspecified cord compression

    G95.20 Unspecified cord compression

    G95.29 Other cord compression

G95.8 Other specified diseases of spinal cord

    Excludes 1: neurogenic bladder NOS (N31.9)

          neurogenic bladder due to cauda equina syndrome (G83.4)

          neuromuscular dysfunction of bladder without spinal cord lesion (N31.-)

    G95.81 Conus medullaris syndrome

    G95.89 Other specified diseases of spinal cord

    Cord bladder NOS

    Drug-induced myelopathy

    Radiation-induced myelopathy

    Excludes 1: myelopathy NOS (G95.9)

G95.9 Disease of spinal cord, unspecified

Myelopathy NOS

G96 Other disorders of central nervous system

G96.0 Cerebrospinal fluid leak

    Excludes 1: cerebrospinal fluid leak from spinal puncture (G97.0)

G96.1 Disorders of meninges, not elsewhere classified

    G96.11 Dural tear

        Excludes 1: accidental puncture or laceration of dura during a procedure (G97.41)

    G96.12 Meningeal adhesions (cerebral) (spinal)

    G96.19 Other disorders of meninges, not elsewhere classified

G96.8 Other specified disorders of central nervous system

G96.9 Disorder of central nervous system, unspecified

G97 Intraoperative and postprocedural complications and disorders of nervous system, not elsewhere classified

    Excludes 2: intraoperative and postprocedural cerebrovascular infarction (I97.81-, I97.82-)

G97.0 Cerebrospinal fluid leak from spinal puncture

G97.1 Other reaction to spinal and lumbar puncture

Headache due to lumbar puncture

G97.2 Intracranial hypotension following ventricular shunting

G97.3 Intraoperative hemorrhage and hematoma of a nervous system organ or structure complicating a procedure

    Excludes 1: intraoperative hemorrhage and hematoma of a nervous system organ or structure due to accidental puncture and laceration during a procedure (G97.4-)

    G97.31 Intraoperative hemorrhage and hematoma of a nervous system organ or structure complicating a nervous system procedure

    G97.32 Intraoperative hemorrhage and hematoma of a nervous system organ or structure complicating other procedure

G97.4 Accidental puncture and laceration of a nervous system organ or structure during a procedure

    G97.41 Accidental puncture or laceration of dura during a procedure

    Incidental (inadvertent) durotomy

    G97.48 Accidental puncture and laceration of other nervous system organ or structure during a nervous system procedure

    G97.49 Accidental puncture and laceration of other nervous system organ or structure during other procedure

G97.5 Postprocedural hemorrhage and hematoma of a nervous system organ or structure following a procedure

    G97.51 Postprocedural hemorrhage and hematoma of a nervous system organ or structure following a nervous system procedure

    G97.52 Postprocedural hemorrhage and hematoma of a nervous system organ or structure following other procedure

G97.8 Other intraoperative and postprocedural complications and disorders of nervous system

Use additional code to further specify disorder

    G97.81 Other intraoperative complications of nervous system

    G97.82 Other postprocedural complications and disorders of nervous system

G98 Other disorders of nervous system not elsewhere classified

Includes: nervous system disorder NOS

G98.0 Neurogenic arthritis, not elsewhere classified

Nonsyphilitic neurogenic arthropathy NEC

Nonsyphilitic neurogenic spondylopathy NEC

    Excludes 1: spondylopathy (in):

        syringomyelia and syringobulbia (G95.0)

        tabes dorsalis (A52.11)

G98.8 Other disorders of nervous system

Nervous system disorder NOS

G99 Other disorders of nervous system in diseases classified elsewhere

G99.0 Autonomic neuropathy in diseases classified elsewhere

    Code first underlying disease, such as:

        amyloidosis (E85-)

        gout (M1A-, M10.-)

        hyperthyroidism (E05.-)

    Excludes 1: diabetic autonomic neuropathy (E09-14 with .43)

G99.2 Myelopathy in diseases classified elsewhere

    Code first underlying disease, such as:

        neoplasm (C00-D49)

    Excludes 1: myelopathy in:

        intervertebral disease (M50.0-, M51.0-)

        spondylosis (M47.0-, M47.1-)

G99.8 Other specified disorders of nervous system in diseases classified elsewhere

    Code first underlying disorder, such as:

        amyloidosis (E85-)

        avitaminosis (E56.9)

    Excludes 1: nervous system involvement in:

        cysticercosis (B69.0)

        rubella (B06.0-)

        syphilis (A52.1-)

● New code   ▲ Revised code   ⑦ 7th digit required   ⊗ Placeholder required

Chapter 7: Diseases Of The Eye And Adnexa (H00-H59)

Note: Use an external cause code following the code for the eye condition, if applicable, to identify the cause of the eye condition

Excludes 2: certain conditions originating in the perinatal period (P04-P96)

certain infectious and parasitic diseases (A00-B99)

complications of pregnancy, childbirth and the puerperium (O00-O9A)

congenital malformations, deformations, and chromosomal abnormalities (Q00-Q99)

diabetes mellitus related eye conditions (E09.3-, E10.3-, E11.3-, E13.3-)

endocrine, nutritional and metabolic diseases (E00-E88)

injury (trauma) of eye and orbit (S05.-)

injury, poisoning and certain other consequences of external causes (S00-T88)

neoplasms (C00-D49)

symptoms, signs and abnormal clinical and laboratory findings, not elsewhere classified (R00-R94)

syphilis related eye disorders (A50.01, A50.3-, A51.43, A52.71)

This chapter contains the following blocks:

H00-H05	Disorders of eyelid, lacrimal system and orbit
H10-H11	Disorders of conjunctiva
H15-H22	Disorders of sclera, cornea, iris and ciliary body
H25-H28	Disorders of lens
H30-H36	Disorders of choroid and retina
H40-H42	Glaucoma
H43-H44	Disorders of vitreous body and globe
H46-H47	Disorders of optic nerve and visual pathways
H49-H52	Disorders of ocular muscles, binocular movement, accommodation and refraction
H53-H54	Visual disturbances and blindness
H55-H57	Other disorders of eye and adnexa
H59	Intraoperative and postprocedural complications and disorders of eye and adnexa, not elsewhere classified

DISORDERS OF EYELID, LACRIMAL SYSTEM AND ORBIT (H00-H05)

Excludes 2: open wound of eyelid (S01.1-)

superficial injury of eyelid (S00.1-, S00.2-)

H00 Hordeolum and chalazion

H00.0 Hordeolum (externum) (internum) of eyelid

    H00.01 Hordeolum externum

    Hordeolum NOS

    Stye

        H00.011 Hordeolum externum right upper eyelid

        H00.012 Hordeolum externum right lower eyelid

        H00.013 Hordeolum externum right eye, unspecified eyelid

        H00.014 Hordeolum externum left upper eyelid

        H00.015 Hordeolum externum left lower eyelid

        H00.016 Hordeolum externum left eye, unspecified eyelid

        H00.019 Hordeolum externum unspecified eye, unspecified eyelid

    H00.02 Hordeolum internum

    Infection of meibomian gland

        H00.021 Hordeolum internum right upper eyelid

        H00.022 Hordeolum internum right lower eyelid

        H00.023 Hordeolum internum right eye, unspecified eyelid

        H00.024 Hordeolum internum left upper eyelid

        H00.025 Hordeolum internum left lower eyelid

        H00.026 Hordeolum internum left eye, unspecified eyelid

        H00.029 Hordeolum internum unspecified eye, unspecified eyelid

    H00.03 Abscess of eyelid

    Furuncle of eyelid

        H00.031 Abscess of right upper eyelid

        H00.032 Abscess of right lower eyelid

        H00.033 Abscess of eyelid right eye, unspecified eyelid

        H00.034 Abscess of left upper eyelid

        H00.035 Abscess of left lower eyelid

        H00.036 Abscess of eyelid left eye, unspecified eyelid

        H00.039 Abscess of eyelid unspecified eye, unspecified eyelid

H00.1 Chalazion

Meibomian (gland) cyst

Excludes 2: infected meibomian gland (H00.02-)

    H00.11 Chalazion right upper eyelid

    H00.12 Chalazion right lower eyelid

    H00.13 Chalazion right eye, unspecified eyelid

    H00.14 Chalazion left upper eyelid

    H00.15 Chalazion left lower eyelid

    H00.16 Chalazion left eye, unspecified eyelid

    H00.19 Chalazion unspecified eye, unspecified eyelid

H01 Other inflammation of eyelid

H01.0 Blepharitis

Excludes 1: blepharoconjunctivitis (H10.5-)

    H01.00 Unspecified blepharitis

        H01.001 Unspecified blepharitis right upper eyelid

        H01.002 Unspecified blepharitis right lower eyelid

        H01.003 Unspecified blepharitis right eye, unspecified eyelid

        H01.004 Unspecified blepharitis left upper eyelid

        H01.005 Unspecified blepharitis left lower eyelid

        H01.006 Unspecified blepharitis left eye, unspecified eyelid

        H01.009 Unspecified blepharitis unspecified eye, unspecified eyelid

    H01.01 Ulcerative blepharitis

        H01.011 Ulcerative blepharitis right upper eyelid

        H01.012 Ulcerative blepharitis right lower eyelid

        H01.013 Ulcerative blepharitis right eye, unspecified eyelid

        H01.014 Ulcerative blepharitis left upper eyelid

        H01.015 Ulcerative blepharitis left lower eyelid

        H01.016 Ulcerative blepharitis left eye, unspecified eyelid

H01.019   Ulcerative blepharitis unspecified eye, unspecified eyelid

H01.02   Squamous blepharitis

H01.021   Squamous blepharitis right upper eyelid

H01.022   Squamous blepharitis right lower eyelid

H01.023   Squamous blepharitis right eye, unspecified eyelid

H01.024   Squamous blepharitis left upper eyelid

H01.025   Squamous blepharitis left lower eyelid

H01.026   Squamous blepharitis left eye, unspecified eyelid

H01.029   Squamous blepharitis unspecified eye, unspecified eyelid

H01.1   Noninfectious dermatoses of eyelid

H01.11   Allergic dermatitis of eyelid
Contact dermatitis of eyelid

H01.111   Allergic dermatitis of right upper eyelid

H01.112   Allergic dermatitis of right lower eyelid

H01.113   Allergic dermatitis of right eye, unspecified eyelid

H01.114   Allergic dermatitis of left upper eyelid

H01.115   Allergic dermatitis of left lower eyelid

H01.116   Allergic dermatitis of left eye, unspecified eyelid

H01.119   Allergic dermatitis of unspecified eye, unspecified eyelid

H01.12   Discoid lupus erythematosus of eyelid

H01.121   Discoid lupus erythematosus of right upper eyelid

H01.122   Discoid lupus erythematosus of right lower eyelid

H01.123   Discoid lupus erythematosus of right eye, unspecified eyelid

H01.124   Discoid lupus erythematosus of left upper eyelid

H01.125   Discoid lupus erythematosus of left lower eyelid

H01.126   Discoid lupus erythematosus of left eye, unspecified eyelid

H01.129   Discoid lupus erythematosus of unspecified eye, unspecified eyelid

H01.13   Eczematous dermatitis of eyelid

H01.131   Eczematous dermatitis of right upper eyelid

H01.132   Eczematous dermatitis of right lower eyelid

H01.133   Eczematous dermatitis of right eye, unspecified eyelid

H01.134   Eczematous dermatitis of left upper eyelid

H01.135   Eczematous dermatitis of left lower eyelid

H01.136   Eczematous dermatitis of left eye, unspecified eyelid

H01.139   Eczematous dermatitis of unspecified eye, unspecified eyelid

H01.14   Xeroderma of eyelid

H01.141   Xeroderma of right upper eyelid

H01.142   Xeroderma of right lower eyelid

H01.143   Xeroderma of right eye, unspecified eyelid

H01.144   Xeroderma of left upper eyelid

H01.145   Xeroderma of left lower eyelid

H01.146   Xeroderma of left eye, unspecified eyelid

H01.149   Xeroderma of unspecified eye, unspecified eyelid

H01.8   Other specified inflammations of eyelid

H01.9   Unspecified inflammation of eyelid
Inflammation of eyelid NOS

H02   Other disorders of eyelid

Excludes 1: congenital malformations of eyelid (Q10.0-Q10.3)

H02.0   Entropion and trichiasis of eyelid

H02.00   Unspecified entropion of eyelid

H02.001   Unspecified entropion of right upper eyelid

H02.002   Unspecified entropion of right lower eyelid

H02.003   Unspecified entropion of right eye, unspecified eyelid

H02.004   Unspecified entropion of left upper eyelid

H02.005   Unspecified entropion of left lower eyelid

H02.006   Unspecified entropion of left eye, unspecified eyelid

H02.009   Unspecified entropion of unspecified eye, unspecified eyelid

H02.01   Cicatricial entropion of eyelid

H02.011   Cicatricial entropion of right upper eyelid

H02.012   Cicatricial entropion of right lower eyelid

H02.013   Cicatricial entropion of right eye, unspecified eyelid

H02.014   Cicatricial entropion of left upper eyelid

H02.015   Cicatricial entropion of left lower eyelid

H02.016   Cicatricial entropion of left eye, unspecified eyelid

H02.019   Cicatricial entropion of unspecified eye, unspecified eyelid

H02.02   Mechanical entropion of eyelid

H02.021   Mechanical entropion of right upper eyelid

H02.022   Mechanical entropion of right lower eyelid

H02.023   Mechanical entropion of right eye, unspecified eyelid

H02.024   Mechanical entropion of left upper eyelid

H02.025   Mechanical entropion of left lower eyelid

H02.026   Mechanical entropion of left eye, unspecified eyelid

H02.029   Mechanical entropion of unspecified eye, unspecified eyelid

H02.03   Senile entropion of eyelid

H02.031   Senile entropion of right upper eyelid

H02.032   Senile entropion of right lower eyelid

H02.033 Senile entropion of right eye, unspecified eyelid

H02.034 Senile entropion of left upper eyelid

H02.035 Senile entropion of left lower eyelid

H02.036 Senile entropion of left eye, unspecified eyelid

H02.039 Senile entropion of unspecified eye, unspecified eyelid

H02.04 Spastic entropion of eyelid

H02.041 Spastic entropion of right upper eyelid

H02.042 Spastic entropion of right lower eyelid

H02.043 Spastic entropion of right eye, unspecified eyelid

H02.044 Spastic entropion of left upper eyelid

H02.045 Spastic entropion of left lower eyelid

H02.046 Spastic entropion of left eye, unspecified eyelid

H02.049 Spastic entropion of unspecified eye, unspecified eyelid

H02.05 Trichiasis without entropian

H02.051 Trichiasis without entropian right upper eyelid

H02.052 Trichiasis without entropian right lower eyelid

H02.053 Trichiasis without entropian right eye, unspecified eyelid

H02.054 Trichiasis without entropian left upper eyelid

H02.055 Trichiasis without entropian left lower eyelid

H02.056 Trichiasis without entropian left eye, unspecified eyelid

H02.059 Trichiasis without entropian unspecified eye, unspecified eyelid

H02.1 Ectropion of eyelid

H02.10 Unspecified ectropion of eyelid

H02.101 Unspecified ectropion of right upper eyelid

H02.102 Unspecified ectropion of right lower eyelid

H02.103 Unspecified ectropion of right eye, unspecified eyelid

H02.104 Unspecified ectropion of left upper eyelid

H02.105 Unspecified ectropion of left lower eyelid

H02.106 Unspecified ectropion of left eye, unspecified eyelid

H02.109 Unspecified ectropion of unspecified eye, unspecified eyelid

H02.11 Cicatricial ectropion of eyelid

H02.111 Cicatricial ectropion of right upper eyelid

H02.112 Cicatricial ectropion of right lower eyelid

H02.113 Cicatricial ectropion of right eye, unspecified eyelid

H02.114 Cicatricial ectropion of left upper eyelid

H02.115 Cicatricial ectropion of left lower eyelid

H02.116 Cicatricial ectropion of left eye, unspecified eyelid

H02.119 Cicatricial ectropion of unspecified eye, unspecified eyelid

H02.12 Mechanical ectropion of eyelid

H02.121 Mechanical ectropion of right upper eyelid

H02.122 Mechanical ectropion of right lower eyelid

H02.123 Mechanical ectropion of right eye, unspecified eyelid

H02.124 Mechanical ectropion of left upper eyelid

H02.125 Mechanical ectropion of left lower eyelid

H02.126 Mechanical ectropion of left eye, unspecified eyelid

H02.129 Mechanical ectropion of unspecified eye, unspecified eyelid

H02.13 Senile ectropion of eyelid

H02.131 Senile ectropion of right upper eyelid

H02.132 Senile ectropion of right lower eyelid

H02.133 Senile ectropion of right eye, unspecified eyelid

H02.134 Senile ectropion of left upper eyelid

H02.135 Senile ectropion of left lower eyelid

H02.136 Senile ectropion of left eye, unspecified eyelid

H02.139 Senile ectropion of unspecified eye, unspecified eyelid

H02.14 Spastic ectropion of eyelid

H02.141 Spastic ectropion of right upper eyelid

H02.142 Spastic ectropion of right lower eyelid

H02.143 Spastic ectropion of right eye, unspecified eyelid

H02.144 Spastic ectropion of left upper eyelid

H02.145 Spastic ectropion of left lower eyelid

H02.146 Spastic ectropion of left eye, unspecified eyelid

H02.149 Spastic ectropion of unspecified eye, unspecified eyelid

H02.2 Lagophthalmos

H02.20 Unspecified lagophthalmos

H02.201 Unspecified lagophthalmos right upper eyelid

H02.202 Unspecified lagophthalmos right lower eyelid

H02.203 Unspecified lagophthalmos right eye, unspecified eyelid

H02.204 Unspecified lagophthalmos left upper eyelid

H02.205 Unspecified lagophthalmos left lower eyelid

H02.206 Unspecified lagophthalmos left eye, unspecified eyelid

H02.209 Unspecified lagophthalmos unspecified eye, unspecified eyelid

H02.21 Cicatricial lagophthalmos

H02.211 Cicatricial lagophthalmos right upper eyelid

H02.212 Cicatricial lagophthalmos right lower eyelid

H02.213 Cicatricial lagophthalmos right eye, unspecified eyelid

H02.214 Cicatricial lagophthalmos left upper eyelid

H02.215 Cicatricial lagophthalmos left lower eyelid

H02.216 Cicatricial lagophthalmos left eye, unspecified eyelid

H02.219 Cicatricial lagophthalmos unspecified eye, unspecified eyelid

H02.22 Mechanical lagophthalmos

H02.221 Mechanical lagophthalmos right upper eyelid

H02.222 Mechanical lagophthalmos right lower eyelid

H02.223 Mechanical lagophthalmos right eye, unspecified eyelid

H02.224 Mechanical lagophthalmos left upper eyelid

H02.225 Mechanical lagophthalmos left lower eyelid

H02.226 Mechanical lagophthalmos left eye, unspecified eyelid

H02.229 Mechanical lagophthalmos unspecified eye, unspecified eyelid

H02.23 Paralytic lagophthalmos

H02.231 Paralytic lagophthalmos right upper eyelid

H02.232 Paralytic lagophthalmos right lower eyelid

H02.233 Paralytic lagophthalmos right eye, unspecified eyelid

H02.234 Paralytic lagophthalmos left upper eyelid

H02.235 Paralytic lagophthalmos left lower eyelid

H02.236 Paralytic lagophthalmos left eye, unspecified eyelid

H02.239 Paralytic lagophthalmos unspecified eye, unspecified eyelid

H02.3 Blepharochalasis

Pseudoptosis

H02.30 Blepharochalasis unspecified eye, unspecified eyelid

H02.31 Blepharochalasis right upper eyelid

H02.32 Blepharochalasis right lower eyelid

H02.33 Blepharochalasis right eye, unspecified eyelid

H02.34 Blepharochalasis left upper eyelid

H02.35 Blepharochalasis left lower eyelid

H02.36 Blepharochalasis left eye, unspecified eyelid

H02.4 Ptosis of eyelid

H02.40 Unspecified ptosis of eyelid

H02.401 Unspecified ptosis of right eyelid

H02.402 Unspecified ptosis of left eyelid

H02.403 Unspecified ptosis of bilateral eyelids

H02.409 Unspecified ptosis of unspecified eyelid

H02.41 Mechanical ptosis of eyelid

H02.411 Mechanical ptosis of right eyelid

H02.412 Mechanical ptosis of left eyelid

H02.413 Mechanical ptosis of bilateral eyelids

H02.419 Mechanical ptosis of unspecified eyelid

H02.42 Myogenic ptosis of eyelid

H02.421 Myogenic ptosis of right eyelid

H02.422 Myogenic ptosis of left eyelid

H02.423 Myogenic ptosis of bilateral eyelids

H02.429 Myogenic ptosis of unspecified eyelid

H02.43 Paralytic ptosis of eyelid

Neurogenic ptosis of eyelid

H02.431 Paralytic ptosis of right eyelid

H02.432 Paralytic ptosis of left eyelid

H02.433 Paralytic ptosis of bilateral eyelids

H02.439 Paralytic ptosis unspecified eyelid

H02.5 Other disorders affecting eyelid function

Excludes 2: blepharospasm (G24.5)

organic tic (G25.69)

psychogenic tic (F95.-)

H02.51 Abnormal innervation syndrome

H02.511 Abnormal innervation syndrome right upper eyelid

H02.512 Abnormal innervation syndrome right lower eyelid

H02.513 Abnormal innervation syndrome right eye, unspecified eyelid

H02.514 Abnormal innervation syndrome left upper eyelid

H02.515 Abnormal innervation syndrome left lower eyelid

H02.516 Abnormal innervation syndrome left eye, unspecified eyelid

H02.519 Abnormal innervation syndrome unspecified eye, unspecified eyelid

H02.52 Blepharophimosis

Ankyloblepharon

H02.521 Blepharophimosis right upper eyelid

H02.522 Blepharophimosis right lower eyelid

H02.523 Blepharophimosis right eye, unspecified eyelid

H02.524 Blepharophimosis left upper eyelid

H02.525 Blepharophimosis left lower eyelid

H02.526 Blepharophimosis left eye, unspecified eyelid

H02.529 Blepharophimosis unspecified eye, unspecified lid

H02.53 Eyelid retraction

Eyelid lag

H02.531 Eyelid retraction right upper eyelid

H02.532 Eyelid retraction right lower eyelid

H02.533 Eyelid retraction right eye, unspecified eyelid

H02.534 Eyelid retraction left upper eyelid

H02.535 Eyelid retraction left lower eyelid

H02.536 Eyelid retraction left eye, unspecified eyelid

H02.539 Eyelid retraction unspecified eye, unspecified lid

H02.59 Other disorders affecting eyelid function

Deficient blink reflex

Sensory disorders

H02.6 Xanthelasma of eyelid

H02.60 Xanthelasma of unspecified eye, unspecified eyelid

H02.61 Xanthelasma of right upper eyelid

H02.62 Xanthelasma of right lower eyelid

H02.63 Xanthelasma of right eye, unspecified eyelid

H02.64 Xanthelasma of left upper eyelid

H02.65 Xanthelasma of left lower eyelid

H02.66 Xanthelasma of left eye, unspecified eyelid

H02.7 Other and unspecified degenerative disorders of eyelid and periocular area

H02.70 Unspecified degenerative disorders of eyelid and periocular area

H02.71 Chloasma of eyelid and periocular area

Dyspigmentation of eyelid

Hyperpigmentation of eyelid

H02.711 Chloasma of right upper eyelid and periocular area

H02.712 Chloasma of right lower eyelid and periocular area

H02.713 Chloasma of right eye, unspecified eyelid and periocular area

H02.714 Chloasma of left upper eyelid and periocular area

H02.715 Chloasma of left lower eyelid and periocular area

H02.716 Chloasma of left eye, unspecified eyelid and periocular area

H02.719 Chloasma of unspecified eye, unspecified eyelid and periocular area

H02.72 Madarosis of eyelid and periocular area

Hypotrichosis of eyelid

H02.721 Madarosis of right upper eyelid and periocular area

H02.722 Madarosis of right lower eyelid and periocular area

H02.723 Madarosis of right eye, unspecified eyelid and periocular area

H02.724 Madarosis of left upper eyelid and periocular area

H02.725 Madarosis of left lower eyelid and periocular area

H02.726 Madarosis of left eye, unspecified eyelid and periocular area

H02.729 Madarosis of unspecified eye, unspecified eyelid and periocular area

H02.73 Vitiligo of eyelid and periocular area

Hypopigmentation of eyelid

H02.731 Vitiligo of right upper eyelid and periocular area

H02.732 Vitiligo of right lower eyelid and periocular area

H02.733 Vitiligo of right eye, unspecified eyelid and periocular area

H02.734 Vitiligo of left upper eyelid and periocular area

H02.735 Vitiligo of left lower eyelid and periocular area

H02.736 Vitiligo of left eye, unspecified eyelid and periocular area

H02.739 Vitiligo of unspecified eye, unspecified eyelid and periocular area

H02.79 Other degenerative disorders of eyelid and periocular area

H02.8 Other specified disorders of eyelid

H02.81 Retained foreign body in eyelid

Use additional code to identify the type of retained foreign body (Z18.-)

Excludes 1: laceration of eyelid with foreign body (S01.12-)

retained intraocular foreign body (H44.6-, H44.7-)

superficial foreign body of eyelid and periocular area (S00.25-)

H02.811 Retained foreign body in right upper eyelid

H02.812 Retained foreign body in right lower eyelid

H02.813 Retained foreign body in right eye, unspecified eyelid

H02.814 Retained foreign body in left upper eyelid

H02.815 Retained foreign body in left lower eyelid

H02.816 Retained foreign body in left eye, unspecified eyelid

H02.819 Retained foreign body in unspecified eye, unspecified eyelid

H02.82 Cysts of eyelid

Sebaceous cyst of eyelid

H02.821 Cysts of right upper eyelid

H02.822 Cysts of right lower eyelid

H02.823 Cysts of right eye, unspecified eyelid

H02.824 Cysts of left upper eyelid

H02.825 Cysts of left lower eyelid

H02.826 Cysts of left eye, unspecified eyelid

H02.829 Cysts of unspecified eye, unspecified eyelid

H02.83 Dermatochalasis of eyelid

H02.831 Dermatochalasis of right upper eyelid

H02.832 Dermatochalasis of right lower eyelid

H02.833 Dermatochalasis of right eye, unspecified eyelid

H02.834 Dermatochalasis of left upper eyelid

H02.835 Dermatochalasis of left lower eyelid

H02.836 Dermatochalasis of left eye, unspecified eyelid

H02.839 Dermatochalasis of unspecified eye, unspecified eyelid

H02.84 Edema of eyelid

Hyperemia of eyelid

H02.841 Edema of right upper eyelid

H02.842 Edema of right lower eyelid

H02.843 Edema of right eye, unspecified eyelid

H02.844 Edema of left upper eyelid

H02.845 Edema of left lower eyelid

H02.846 Edema of left eye, unspecified eyelid

H02.849 Edema of unspecified eye, unspecified eyelid

H02.85 Elephantiasis of eyelid

H02.851 Elephantiasis of right upper eyelid

H02.852 Elephantiasis of right lower eyelid

H02.853 Elephantiasis of right eye, unspecified eyelid

H02.854 Elephantiasis of left upper eyelid

H02.855 Elephantiasis of left lower eyelid

H02.856 Elephantiasis of left eye, unspecified eyelid

H02.859 Elephantiasis of unspecified eye, unspecified eyelid

H02.86 Hypertrichosis of eyelid

H02.861 Hypertrichosis of right upper eyelid

H02.862 Hypertrichosis of right lower eyelid
H02.863 Hypertrichosis of right eye, unspecified eyelid
H02.864 Hypertrichosis of left upper eyelid
H02.865 Hypertrichosis of left lower eyelid
H02.866 Hypertrichosis of left eye, unspecified eyelid
H02.869 Hypertrichosis of unspecified eye, unspecified eyelid

H02.87 Vascular anomalies of eyelid
H02.871 Vascular anomalies of right upper eyelid
H02.872 Vascular anomalies of right lower eyelid
H02.873 Vascular anomalies of right eye, unspecified eyelid
H02.874 Vascular anomalies of left upper eyelid
H02.875 Vascular anomalies of left lower eyelid
H02.876 Vascular anomalies of left eye, unspecified eyelid
H02.879 Vascular anomalies of unspecified eye, unspecified eyelid

H02.89 Other specified disorders of eyelid
Hemorrhage of eyelid

H02.9 Unspecified disorder of eyelid
Disorder of eyelid NOS

H04 Disorders of lacrimal system
Excludes 1: congenital malformations of lacrimal system (Q10.4-Q10.6)

H04.0 Dacryoadenitis
H04.00 Unspecified dacryoadenitis
H04.001 Unspecified dacryoadenitis, right lacrimal gland
H04.002 Unspecified dacryoadenitis, left lacrimal gland
H04.003 Unspecified dacryoadenitis, bilateral lacrimal glands
H04.009 Unspecified dacryoadenitis, unspecified lacrimal gland

H04.01 Acute dacryoadenitis
H04.011 Acute dacryoadenitis, right lacrimal gland
H04.012 Acute dacryoadenitis, left lacrimal gland
H04.013 Acute dacryoadenitis, bilateral lacrimal glands
H04.019 Acute dacryoadenitis, unspecified lacrimal gland

H04.02 Chronic dacryoadenitis
H04.021 Chronic dacryoadenitis, right lacrimal gland
H04.022 Chronic dacryoadenitis, left lacrimal gland
H04.023 Chronic dacryoadenitis, bilateral lacrimal gland
H04.029 Chronic dacryoadenitis, unspecified lacrimal gland

H04.03 Chronic enlargement of lacrimal gland
H04.031 Chronic enlargement of right lacrimal gland
H04.032 Chronic enlargement of left lacrimal gland

H04.033 Chronic enlargement of bilateral lacrimal glands
H04.039 Chronic enlargement of unspecified lacrimal gland

H04.1 Other disorders of lacrimal gland
H04.11 Dacryops
H04.111 Dacryops of right lacrimal gland
H04.112 Dacryops of left lacrimal gland
H04.113 Dacryops of bilateral lacrimal glands
H04.119 Dacryops of unspecified lacrimal gland

H04.12 Dry eye syndrome
Tear film insufficiency, NOS
H04.121 Dry eye syndrome of right lacrimal gland
H04.122 Dry eye syndrome of left lacrimal gland
H04.123 Dry eye syndrome of bilateral lacrimal glands
H04.129 Dry eye syndrome of unspecified lacrimal gland

H04.13 Lacrimal cyst
Lacrimal cystic degeneration
H04.131 Lacrimal cyst, right lacrimal gland
H04.132 Lacrimal cyst, left lacrimal gland
H04.133 Lacrimal cyst, bilateral lacrimal glands
H04.139 Lacrimal cyst, unspecified lacrimal gland

H04.14 Primary lacrimal gland atrophy
H04.141 Primary lacrimal gland atrophy, right lacrimal gland
H04.142 Primary lacrimal gland atrophy, left lacrimal gland
H04.143 Primary lacrimal gland atrophy, bilateral lacrimal glands
H04.149 Primary lacrimal gland atrophy, unspecified lacrimal gland

H04.15 Secondary lacrimal gland atrophy
H04.151 Secondary lacrimal gland atrophy, right lacrimal gland
H04.152 Secondary lacrimal gland atrophy, left lacrimal gland
H04.153 Secondary lacrimal gland atrophy, bilateral lacrimal glands
H04.159 Secondary lacrimal gland atrophy, unspecified lacrimal gland

H04.16 Lacrimal gland dislocation
H04.161 Lacrimal gland dislocation, right lacrimal gland
H04.162 Lacrimal gland dislocation, left lacrimal gland
H04.163 Lacrimal gland dislocation, bilateral lacrimal glands
H04.169 Lacrimal gland dislocation, unspecified lacrimal gland

H04.19 Other specified disorders of lacrimal gland
H04.2 Epiphora
H04.20 Unspecified epiphora
H04.201 Unspecified epiphora, right lacrimal gland
H04.202 Unspecified epiphora, left lacrimal gland

H04.203 Unspecified epiphora, bilateral lacrimal glands
H04.209 Unspecified epiphora, unspecified lacrimal gland
H04.21 Epiphora due to excess lacrimation
H04.211 Epiphora due to excess lacrimation, right lacrimal gland
H04.212 Epiphora due to excess lacrimation, left lacrimal gland
H04.213 Epiphora due to excess lacrimation, bilateral lacrimal glands
H04.219 Epiphora due to excess lacrimation, unspecified lacrimal gland
H04.22 Epiphora due to insufficient drainage
H04.221 Epiphora due to insufficient drainage, right lacrimal gland
H04.222 Epiphora due to insufficient drainage, left lacrimal gland
H04.223 Epiphora due to insufficient drainage, bilateral lacrimal glands
H04.229 Epiphora due to insufficient drainage, unspecified lacrimal gland
H04.3 Acute and unspecified inflammation of lacrimal passages
Excludes 1: neonatal dacryocystitis (P39.1)
H04.30 Unspecified dacryocystitis
H04.301 Unspecified dacryocystitis of right lacrimal passage
H04.302 Unspecified dacryocystitis of left lacrimal passage
H04.303 Unspecified dacryocystitis of bilateral lacrimal passages
H04.309 Unspecified dacryocystitis of unspecified lacrimal passage
H04.31 Phlegmonous dacryocystitis
H04.311 Phlegmonous dacryocystitis of right lacrimal passage
H04.312 Phlegmonous dacryocystitis of left lacrimal passage
H04.313 Phlegmonous dacryocystitis of bilateral lacrimal passages
H04.319 Phlegmonous dacryocystitis of unspecified lacrimal passage
H04.32 Acute dacryocystitis
Acute dacryopericystitis
H04.321 Acute dacryocystitis of right lacrimal passage
H04.322 Acute dacryocystitis of left lacrimal passage
H04.323 Acute dacryocystitis of bilateral lacrimal passages
H04.329 Acute dacryocystitis of unspecified lacrimal passage
H04.33 Acute lacrimal canaliculitis
H04.331 Acute lacrimal canaliculitis of right lacrimal passage
H04.332 Acute lacrimal canaliculitis of left lacrimal passage
H04.333 Acute lacrimal canaliculitis of bilateral lacrimal passages
H04.339 Acute lacrimal canaliculitis of unspecified lacrimal passage
H04.4 Chronic inflammation of lacrimal passages
H04.41 Chronic dacryocystitis

H04.411 Chronic dacryocystitis of right lacrimal passage
H04.412 Chronic dacryocystitis of left lacrimal passage
H04.413 Chronic dacryocystitis of bilateral lacrimal passages
H04.419 Chronic dacryocystitis of unspecified lacrimal passage
H04.42 Chronic lacrimal canaliculitis
H04.421 Chronic lacrimal canaliculitis of right lacrimal passage
H04.422 Chronic lacrimal canaliculitis of left lacrimal passage
H04.423 Chronic lacrimal canaliculitis of bilateral lacrimal passages
H04.429 Chronic lacrimal canaliculitis of unspecified lacrimal passage
H04.43 Chronic lacrimal mucocele
H04.431 Chronic lacrimal mucocele of right lacrimal passage
H04.432 Chronic lacrimal mucocele of left lacrimal passage
H04.433 Chronic lacrimal mucocele of bilateral lacrimal passages
H04.439 Chronic lacrimal mucocele of unspecified lacrimal passage
H04.5 Stenosis and insufficiency of lacrimal passages
H04.51 Dacryolith
H04.511 Dacryolith of right lacrimal passage
H04.512 Dacryolith of left lacrimal passage
H04.513 Dacryolith of bilateral lacrimal passages
H04.519 Dacryolith of unspecified lacrimal passage
H04.52 Eversion of lacrimal punctum
H04.521 Eversion of right lacrimal punctum
H04.522 Eversion of left lacrimal punctum
H04.523 Eversion of bilateral lacrimal punctum
H04.529 Eversion of unspecified lacrimal punctum
H04.53 Neonatal obstruction of nasolacrimal duct
Excludes 1: congenital stenosis and stricture of lacrimal duct (Q10.5)
H04.531 Neonatal obstruction of right nasolacrimal duct
H04.532 Neonatal obstruction of left nasolacrimal duct
H04.533 Neonatal obstruction of bilateral nasolacrimal duct
H04.539 Neonatal obstruction of unspecified nasolacrimal duct
H04.54 Stenosis of lacrimal canaliculi
H04.541 Stenosis of right lacrimal canaliculi
H04.542 Stenosis of left lacrimal canaliculi
H04.543 Stenosis of bilateral lacrimal canaliculi
H04.549 Stenosis of unspecified lacrimal canaliculi
H04.55 Acquired stenosis of nasolacrimal duct
H04.551 Acquired stenosis of right nasolacrimal duct
H04.552 Acquired stenosis of left nasolacrimal duct

H04.553　Acquired stenosis of bilateral nasolacrimal duct

H04.559　Acquired stenosis of unspecified nasolacrimal duct

H04.56　Stenosis of lacrimal punctum

H04.561　Stenosis of right lacrimal punctum

H04.562　Stenosis of left lacrimal punctum

H04.563　Stenosis of bilateral lacrimal punctum

H04.569　Stenosis of unspecified lacrimal punctum

H04.57　Stenosis of lacrimal sac

H04.571　Stenosis of right lacrimal sac

H04.572　Stenosis of left lacrimal sac

H04.573　Stenosis of bilateral lacrimal sac

H04.579　Stenosis of unspecified lacrimal sac

H04.6　Other changes of lacrimal passages

H04.61　Lacrimal fistula

H04.611　Lacrimal fistula right lacrimal passage

H04.612　Lacrimal fistula left lacrimal passage

H04.613　Lacrimal fistula bilateral lacrimal passages

H04.619　Lacrimal fistula unspecified lacrimal passage

H04.69　Other changes of lacrimal passages

H04.8　Other disorders of lacrimal system

H04.81　Granuloma of lacrimal passages

H04.811　Granuloma of right lacrimal passage

H04.812　Granuloma of left lacrimal passage

H04.813　Granuloma of bilateral lacrimal passages

H04.819　Granuloma of unspecified lacrimal passage

H04.89　Other disorders of lacrimal system

H04.9　Disorder of lacrimal system, unspecified

H05　Disorders of orbit

Excludes 1: congenital malformation of orbit (Q10.7)

H05.0　Acute inflammation of orbit

H05.00　Unspecified acute inflammation of orbit

H05.01　Cellulitis of orbit

Abscess of orbit

H05.011　Cellulitis of right orbit

H05.012　Cellulitis of left orbit

H05.013　Cellulitis of bilateral orbits

H05.019　Cellulitis of unspecified orbit

H05.02　Osteomyelitis of orbit

H05.021　Osteomyelitis of right orbit

H05.022　Osteomyelitis of left orbit

H05.023　Osteomyelitis of bilateral orbits

H05.029　Osteomyelitis of unspecified orbit

H05.03　Periostitis of orbit

H05.031　Periostitis of right orbit

H05.032　Periostitis of left orbit

H05.033　Periostitis of bilateral orbits

H05.039　Periostitis of unspecified orbit

H05.04　Tenonitis of orbit

H05.041　Tenonitis of right orbit

H05.042　Tenonitis of left orbit

H05.043　Tenonitis of bilateral orbits

H05.049　Tenonitis of unspecified orbit

H05.1　Chronic inflammatory disorders of orbit

H05.10　Unspecified chronic inflammatory disorders of orbit

H05.11　Granuloma of orbit

Pseudotumor (inflammatory) of orbit

H05.111　Granuloma of right orbit

H05.112　Granuloma of left orbit

H05.113　Granuloma of bilateral orbits

H05.119　Granuloma of unspecified orbit

H05.12　Orbital myositis

H05.121　Orbital myositis, right orbit

H05.122　Orbital myositis, left orbit

H05.123　Orbital myositis, bilateral

H05.129　Orbital myositis, unspecified orbit

H05.2　Exophthalmic conditions

H05.20　Unspecified exophthalmos

H05.21　Displacement (lateral) of globe

H05.211　Displacement (lateral) of globe, right eye

H05.212　Displacement (lateral) of globe, left eye

H05.213　Displacement (lateral) of globe, bilateral

H05.219　Displacement (lateral) of globe, unspecified eye

H05.22　Edema of orbit

Orbital congestion

H05.221　Edema of right orbit

H05.222　Edema of left orbit

H05.223　Edema of bilateral orbit

H05.229　Edema of unspecified orbit

H05.23　Hemorrhage of orbit

H05.231　Hemorrhage of right orbit

H05.232　Hemorrhage of left orbit

H05.233　Hemorrhage of bilateral orbit

H05.239　Hemorrhage of unspecified orbit

H05.24　Constant exophthalmos

H05.241　Constant exophthalmos, right eye

H05.242　Constant exophthalmos, left eye

H05.243　Constant exophthalmos, bilateral

H05.249　Constant exophthalmos, unspecified eye

H05.25　Intermittent exophthalmos

H05.251　Intermittent exophthalmos, right eye

H05.252　Intermittent exophthalmos, left eye

H05.253　Intermittent exophthalmos, bilateral

H05.259　Intermittent exophthalmos, unspecified eye

H05.26　Pulsating exophthalmos

H05.261　Pulsating exophthalmos, right eye

H05.262　Pulsating exophthalmos, left eye

H05.263　Pulsating exophthalmos, bilateral

H05.269　Pulsating exophthalmos, unspecified eye

H05.3　Deformity of orbit

Excludes 1: congenital deformity of orbit (Q10.7)
hypertelorism (Q75.2)

H05.30　Unspecified deformity of orbit

H05.31　Atrophy of orbit

H05.311　Atrophy of right orbit

H05.312　Atrophy of left orbit

H05.313　Atrophy of bilateral orbit

H05.319　Atrophy of unspecified orbit

H05.32 Deformity of orbit due to bone disease
Code also associated bone disease
- H05.321 Deformity of right orbit due to bone disease
- H05.322 Deformity of left orbit due to bone disease
- H05.323 Deformity of bilateral orbits due to bone disease
- H05.329 Deformity of unspecified orbit due to bone disease

H05.33 Deformity of orbit due to trauma or surgery
- H05.331 Deformity of right orbit due to trauma or surgery
- H05.332 Deformity of left orbit due to trauma or surgery
- H05.333 Deformity of bilateral orbits due to trauma or surgery
- H05.339 Deformity of unspecified orbit due to trauma or surgery

H05.34 Enlargement of orbit
- H05.341 Enlargement of right orbit
- H05.342 Enlargement of left orbit
- H05.343 Enlargement of bilateral orbits
- H05.349 Enlargement of unspecified orbit

H05.35 Exostosis of orbit
- H05.351 Exostosis of right orbit
- H05.352 Exostosis of left orbit
- H05.353 Exostosis of bilateral orbits
- H05.359 Exostosis of unspecified orbit

H05.4 Enophthalmos
- H05.40 Unspecified enophthalmos
  - H05.401 Unspecified enophthalmos, right eye
  - H05.402 Unspecified enophthalmos, left eye
  - H05.403 Unspecified enophthalmos, bilateral
  - H05.409 Unspecified enophthalmos, unspecified eye
- H05.41 Enophthalmos due to atrophy of orbital tissue
  - H05.411 Enophthalmos due to atrophy of orbital tissue, right eye
  - H05.412 Enophthalmos due to atrophy of orbital tissue, left eye
  - H05.413 Enophthalmos due to atrophy of orbital tissue, bilateral
  - H05.419 Enophthalmos due to atrophy of orbital tissue, unspecified eye
- H05.42 Enophthalmos due to trauma or surgery
  - H05.421 Enophthalmos due to trauma or surgery, right eye
  - H05.422 Enophthalmos due to trauma or surgery, left eye
  - H05.423 Enophthalmos due to trauma or surgery, bilateral
  - H05.429 Enophthalmos due to trauma or surgery, unspecified eye

H05.5 Retained (old) foreign body following penetrating wound of orbit
Retrobulbar foreign body
Use additional code to identify the type of retained foreign body (Z18.-)
Excludes 1: current penetrating wound of orbit (S05.4-)
Excludes 2: retained foreign body of eyelid (H02.81-)
retained intraocular foreign body (H44.6-, H44.7-)

H05.50 Retained (old) foreign body following penetrating wound of unspecified orbit
- H05.51 Retained (old) foreign body following penetrating wound of right orbit
- H05.52 Retained (old) foreign body following penetrating wound of left orbit
- H05.53 Retained (old) foreign body following penetrating wound of bilateral orbits

H05.8 Other disorders of orbit
- H05.81 Cyst of orbit
  Encephalocele of orbit
  - H05.811 Cyst of right orbit
  - H05.812 Cyst of left orbit
  - H05.813 Cyst of bilateral orbits
  - H05.819 Cyst of unspecified orbit
- H05.82 Myopathy of extraocular muscles
  - H05.821 Myopathy of extraocular muscles, right orbit
  - H05.822 Myopathy of extraocular muscles, left orbit
  - H05.823 Myopathy of extraocular muscles, bilateral
  - H05.829 Myopathy of extraocular muscles, unspecified orbit
- H05.89 Other disorders of orbit

H05.9 Unspecified disorder of orbit

DISORDERS OF CONJUNCTIVA (H10-H11)

H10 Conjunctivitis
Excludes 1: keratoconjunctivitis (H16.2-)

H10.0 Mucopurulent conjunctivitis
- H10.01 Acute follicular conjunctivitis
  - H10.011 Acute follicular conjunctivitis, right eye
  - H10.012 Acute follicular conjunctivitis, left eye
  - H10.013 Acute follicular conjunctivitis, bilateral
  - H10.019 Acute follicular conjunctivitis, unspecified eye
- H10.02 Other mucopurulent conjunctivitis
  - H10.021 Other mucopurulent conjunctivitis, right eye
  - H10.022 Other mucopurulent conjunctivitis, left eye
  - H10.023 Other mucopurulent conjunctivitis, bilateral
  - H10.029 Other mucopurulent conjunctivitis, unspecified eye

H10.1 Acute atopic conjunctivitis
Acute papillary conjunctivitis
- H10.10 Acute atopic conjunctivitis, unspecified eye
- H10.11 Acute atopic conjunctivitis, right eye
- H10.12 Acute atopic conjunctivitis, left eye
- H10.13 Acute atopic conjunctivitis, bilateral

H10.2 Other acute conjunctivitis
- H10.21 Acute toxic conjunctivitis
  Acute chemical conjunctivitis
  Code first (T51-T65) to identify chemical and intent
  Excludes 1: burn and corrosion of eye and adnexa (T26.-)
  - H10.211 Acute toxic conjunctivitis, right eye

H10.212   Acute toxic conjunctivitis, left eye
H10.213   Acute toxic conjunctivitis, bilateral
H10.219   Acute toxic conjunctivitis, unspecified eye
H10.22   Pseudomembranous conjunctivitis
    H10.221   Pseudomembranous conjunctivitis, right eye
    H10.222   Pseudomembranous conjunctivitis, left eye
    H10.223   Pseudomembranous conjunctivitis, bilateral
    H10.229   Pseudomembranous conjunctivitis, unspecified eye
H10.23   Serous conjunctivitis, except viral
    Excludes 1: viral conjunctivitis (B30.-)
    H10.231   Serous conjunctivitis, except viral, right eye
    H10.232   Serous conjunctivitis, except viral, left eye
    H10.233   Serous conjunctivitis, except viral, bilateral
    H10.239   Serous conjunctivitis, except viral, unspecified eye
H10.3   Unspecified acute conjunctivitis
    Excludes 1: ophthalmia neonatorum NOS (P39.1)
    H10.30   Unspecified acute conjunctivitis, unspecified eye
    H10.31   Unspecified acute conjunctivitis, right eye
    H10.32   Unspecified acute conjunctivitis, left eye
    H10.33   Unspecified acute conjunctivitis, bilateral
H10.4   Chronic conjunctivitis
    H10.40   Unspecified chronic conjunctivitis
        H10.401   Unspecified chronic conjunctivitis, right eye
        H10.402   Unspecified chronic conjunctivitis, left eye
        H10.403   Unspecified chronic conjunctivitis, bilateral
        H10.409   Unspecified chronic conjunctivitis, unspecified eye
    H10.41   Chronic giant papillary conjunctivitis
        H10.411   Chronic giant papillary conjunctivitis, right eye
        H10.412   Chronic giant papillary conjunctivitis, left eye
        H10.413   Chronic giant papillary conjunctivitis, bilateral
        H10.419   Chronic giant papillary conjunctivitis, unspecified eye
    H10.42   Simple chronic conjunctivitis
        H10.421   Simple chronic conjunctivitis, right eye
        H10.422   Simple chronic conjunctivitis, left eye
        H10.423   Simple chronic conjunctivitis, bilateral
        H10.429   Simple chronic conjunctivitis, unspecified eye
    H10.43   Chronic follicular conjunctivitis
        H10.431   Chronic follicular conjunctivitis, right eye
        H10.432   Chronic follicular conjunctivitis, left eye
        H10.433   Chronic follicular conjunctivitis, bilateral

H10.439   Chronic follicular conjunctivitis, unspecified eye
H10.44   Vernal conjunctivitis
    Excludes 1: vernal keratoconjunctivitis with limbar and corneal involvement (H16.26-)
H10.45   Other chronic allergic conjunctivitis
H10.5   Blepharoconjunctivitis
    H10.50   Unspecified blepharoconjunctivitis
        H10.501   Unspecified blepharoconjunctivitis, right eye
        H10.502   Unspecified blepharoconjunctivitis, left eye
        H10.503   Unspecified blepharoconjunctivitis, bilateral
        H10.509   Unspecified blepharoconjunctivitis, unspecified eye
    H10.51   Ligneous conjunctivitis
        H10.511   Ligneous conjunctivitis, right eye
        H10.512   Ligneous conjunctivitis, left eye
        H10.513   Ligneous conjunctivitis, bilateral
        H10.519   Ligneous conjunctivitis, unspecified eye
    H10.52   Angular blepharoconjunctivitis
        H10.521   Angular blepharoconjunctivitis, right eye
        H10.522   Angular blepharoconjunctivitis, left eye
        H10.523   Angular blepharoconjunctivitis, bilateral
        H10.529   Angular blepharoconjunctivitis, unspecified eye
    H10.53   Contact blepharoconjunctivitis
        H10.531   Contact blepharoconjunctivitis, right eye
        H10.532   Contact blepharoconjunctivitis, left eye
        H10.533   Contact blepharoconjunctivitis, bilateral
        H10.539   Contact blepharoconjunctivitis, unspecified eye
H10.8   Other conjunctivitis
    H10.81   Pingueculitis
        Excludes 1: pinguecula (H11.15-)
        H10.811   Pingueculitis, right eye
        H10.812   Pingueculitis, left eye
        H10.813   Pingueculitis, bilateral
        H10.819   Pingueculitis, unspecified eye
    H10.89   Other conjunctivitis
H10.9   Unspecified conjunctivitis
H11   Other disorders of conjunctiva
Excludes 1: keratoconjunctivitis (H16.2-)
H11.0   Pterygium of eye
    Excludes 1: pseudopterygium (H11.81-)
    H11.00   Unspecified pterygium of eye
        H11.001   Unspecified pterygium of right eye
        H11.002   Unspecified pterygium of left eye
        H11.003   Unspecified pterygium of eye, bilateral
        H11.009   Unspecified pterygium of unspecified eye
    H11.01   Amyloid pterygium

H11.011 Amyloid pterygium of right eye

H11.012 Amyloid pterygium of left eye

H11.013 Amyloid pterygium of eye, bilateral

H11.019 Amyloid pterygium of unspecified eye

H11.02 Central pterygium of eye

H11.021 Central pterygium of right eye

H11.022 Central pterygium of left eye

H11.023 Central pterygium of eye, bilateral

H11.029 Central pterygium of unspecified eye

H11.03 Double pterygium of eye

H11.031 Double pterygium of right eye

H11.032 Double pterygium of left eye

H11.033 Double pterygium of eye, bilateral

H11.039 Double pterygium of unspecified eye

H11.04 Peripheral pterygium of eye, stationary

H11.041 Peripheral pterygium, stationary, right eye

H11.042 Peripheral pterygium, stationary, left eye

H11.043 Peripheral pterygium, stationary, bilateral

H11.049 Peripheral pterygium, stationary, unspecified eye

H11.05 Peripheral pterygium of eye, progressive

H11.051 Peripheral pterygium, progressive, right eye

H11.052 Peripheral pterygium, progressive, left eye

H11.053 Peripheral pterygium, progressive, bilateral

H11.059 Peripheral pterygium, progressive, unspecified eye

H11.06 Recurrent pterygium of eye

H11.061 Recurrent pterygium of right eye

H11.062 Recurrent pterygium of left eye

H11.063 Recurrent pterygium of eye, bilateral

H11.069 Recurrent pterygium of unspecified eye

H11.1 Conjunctival degenerations and deposits

Excludes 2: pseudopterygium (H11.81)

H11.10 Unspecified conjunctival degenerations

H11.11 Conjunctival deposits

H11.111 Conjunctival deposits, right eye

H11.112 Conjunctival deposits, left eye

H11.113 Conjunctival deposits, bilateral

H11.119 Conjunctival deposits, unspecified eye

H11.12 Conjunctival concretions

H11.121 Conjunctival concretions, right eye

H11.122 Conjunctival concretions, left eye

H11.123 Conjunctival concretions, bilateral

H11.129 Conjunctival concretions, unspecified eye

H11.13 Conjunctival pigmentations

Conjunctival argyrosis [argyria]

H11.131 Conjunctival pigmentations, right eye

H11.132 Conjunctival pigmentations, left eye

H11.133 Conjunctival pigmentations, bilateral

H11.139 Conjunctival pigmentations, unspecified eye

H11.14 Conjunctival xerosis, unspecified

Excludes 1: xerosis of conjunctiva due to vitamin A deficiency (E50.0, E50.1)

H11.141 Conjunctival xerosis, unspecified, right eye

H11.142 Conjunctival xerosis, unspecified, left eye

H11.143 Conjunctival xerosis, unspecified, bilateral

H11.149 Conjunctival xerosis, unspecified, unspecified eye

H11.15 Pinguecula

Excludes 1: pingueculitis (H10.81-)

H11.151 Pinguecula, right eye

H11.152 Pinguecula, left eye

H11.153 Pinguecula, bilateral

H11.159 Pinguecula, unspecified eye

H11.2 Conjunctival scars

H11.21 Conjunctival adhesions and strands (localized)

H11.211 Conjunctival adhesions and strands (localized), right eye

H11.212 Conjunctival adhesions and strands (localized), left eye

H11.213 Conjunctival adhesions and strands (localized), bilateral

H11.219 Conjunctival adhesions and strands (localized), unspecified eye

H11.22 Conjunctival granuloma

H11.221 Conjunctival granuloma, right eye

H11.222 Conjunctival granuloma, left eye

H11.223 Conjunctival granuloma, bilateral

H11.229 Conjunctival granuloma, unspecified

H11.23 Symblepharon

H11.231 Symblepharon, right eye

H11.232 Symblepharon, left eye

H11.233 Symblepharon, bilateral

H11.239 Symblepharon, unspecified eye

H11.24 Scarring of conjunctiva

H11.241 Scarring of conjunctiva, right eye

H11.242 Scarring of conjunctiva, left eye

H11.243 Scarring of conjunctiva, bilateral

H11.249 Scarring of conjunctiva, unspecified eye

H11.3 Conjunctival hemorrhage

Subconjunctival hemorrhage

H11.30 Conjunctival hemorrhage, unspecified eye

H11.31 Conjunctival hemorrhage, right eye

H11.32 Conjunctival hemorrhage, left eye

H11.33 Conjunctival hemorrhage, bilateral

H11.4 Other conjunctival vascular disorders and cysts

H11.41 Vascular abnormalities of conjunctiva

Conjunctival aneurysm

H11.411 Vascular abnormalities of conjunctiva, right eye

H11.412 Vascular abnormalities of conjunctiva, left eye

H11.413 Vascular abnormalities of conjunctiva, bilateral

H11.419 Vascular abnormalities of conjunctiva, unspecified eye

H11.42 Conjunctival edema

H11.421 Conjunctival edema, right eye

H11.422 Conjunctival edema, left eye

H11.423   Conjunctival edema, bilateral
H11.429   Conjunctival edema, unspecified eye
H11.43   Conjunctival hyperemia
H11.431   Conjunctival hyperemia, right eye
H11.432   Conjunctival hyperemia, left eye
H11.433   Conjunctival hyperemia, bilateral
H11.439   Conjunctival hyperemia, unspecified eye
H11.44   Conjunctival cysts
H11.441   Conjunctival cysts, right eye
H11.442   Conjunctival cysts, left eye
H11.443   Conjunctival cysts, bilateral
H11.449   Conjunctival cysts, unspecified eye
H11.8   Other specified disorders of conjunctiva
H11.81   Pseudopterygium of conjunctiva
H11.811   Pseudopterygium of conjunctiva, right eye
H11.812   Pseudopterygium of conjunctiva, left eye
H11.813   Pseudopterygium of conjunctiva, bilateral
H11.819   Pseudopterygium of conjunctiva, unspecified eye
H11.82   Conjunctivochalasis
H11.821   Conjunctivochalasis, right eye
H11.822   Conjunctivochalasis, left eye
H11.823   Conjunctivochalasis, bilateral
H11.829   Conjunctivochalasis, unspecified eye
H11.89   Other specified disorders of conjunctiva
H11.9   Unspecified disorder of conjunctiva

DISORDERS OF SCLERA, CORNEA, IRIS AND CILIARY BODY (H15-H22)

H15   Disorders of sclera
H15.0   Scleritis
H15.00   Unspecified scleritis
H15.001   Unspecified scleritis, right eye
H15.002   Unspecified scleritis, left eye
H15.003   Unspecified scleritis, bilateral
H15.009   Unspecified scleritis, unspecified eye
H15.01   Anterior scleritis
H15.011   Anterior scleritis, right eye
H15.012   Anterior scleritis, left eye
H15.013   Anterior scleritis, bilateral
H15.019   Anterior scleritis, unspecified eye
H15.02   Brawny scleritis
H15.021   Brawny scleritis, right eye
H15.022   Brawny scleritis, left eye
H15.023   Brawny scleritis, bilateral
H15.029   Brawny scleritis, unspecified eye
H15.03   Posterior scleritis
Sclerotenonitis
H15.031   Posterior scleritis, right eye
H15.032   Posterior scleritis, left eye
H15.033   Posterior scleritis, bilateral
H15.039   Posterior scleritis, unspecified eye
H15.04   Scleritis with corneal involvement
H15.041   Scleritis with corneal involvement, right eye
H15.042   Scleritis with corneal involvement, left eye

H15.043   Scleritis with corneal involvement, bilateral
H15.049   Scleritis with corneal involvement, unspecified eye
H15.05   Scleromalacia perforans
H15.051   Scleromalacia perforans, right eye
H15.052   Scleromalacia perforans, left eye
H15.053   Scleromalacia perforans, bilateral
H15.059   Scleromalacia perforans, unspecified eye
H15.09   Other scleritis
Scleral abscess
H15.091   Other scleritis, right eye
H15.092   Other scleritis, left eye
H15.093   Other scleritis, bilateral
H15.099   Other scleritis, unspecified eye
H15.1   Episcleritis
H15.10   Unspecified episcleritis
H15.101   Unspecified episcleritis, right eye
H15.102   Unspecified episcleritis, left eye
H15.103   Unspecified episcleritis, bilateral
H15.109   Unspecified episcleritis, unspecified eye
H15.11   Episcleritis periodica fugax
H15.111   Episcleritis periodica fugax, right eye
H15.112   Episcleritis periodica fugax, left eye
H15.113   Episcleritis periodica fugax, bilateral
H15.119   Episcleritis periodica fugax, unspecified eye
H15.12   Nodular episcleritis
H15.121   Nodular episcleritis, right eye
H15.122   Nodular episcleritis, left eye
H15.123   Nodular episcleritis, bilateral
H15.129   Nodular episcleritis, unspecified eye
H15.8   Other disorders of sclera
Excludes 2: blue sclera (Q13.5)
degenerative myopia (H44.2-)
H15.81   Equatorial staphyloma
H15.811   Equatorial staphyloma, right eye
H15.812   Equatorial staphyloma, left eye
H15.813   Equatorial staphyloma, bilateral
H15.819   Equatorial staphyloma, unspecified eye
H15.82   Localized anterior staphyloma
H15.821   Localized anterior staphyloma, right eye
H15.822   Localized anterior staphyloma, left eye
H15.823   Localized anterior staphyloma, bilateral
H15.829   Localized anterior staphyloma, unspecified eye
H15.83   Staphyloma posticum
H15.831   Staphyloma posticum, right eye
H15.832   Staphyloma posticum, left eye
H15.833   Staphyloma posticum, bilateral
H15.839   Staphyloma posticum, unspecified eye
H15.84   Scleral ectasia
H15.841   Scleral ectasia, right eye
H15.842   Scleral ectasia, left eye
H15.843   Scleral ectasia, bilateral

H15.849 Scleral ectasia, unspecified eye

H15.85 Ring staphyloma

    H15.851 Ring staphyloma, right eye

    H15.852 Ring staphyloma, left eye

    H15.853 Ring staphyloma, bilateral

    H15.859 Ring staphyloma, unspecified eye

H15.89 Other disorders of sclera

H15.9 Unspecified disorder of sclera

H16 Keratitis

H16.0 Corneal ulcer

  H16.00 Unspecified corneal ulcer

    H16.001 Unspecified corneal ulcer, right eye

    H16.002 Unspecified corneal ulcer, left eye

    H16.003 Unspecified corneal ulcer, bilateral

    H16.009 Unspecified corneal ulcer, unspecified eye

  H16.01 Central corneal ulcer

    H16.011 Central corneal ulcer, right eye

    H16.012 Central corneal ulcer, left eye

    H16.013 Central corneal ulcer, bilateral

    H16.019 Central corneal ulcer, unspecified eye

  H16.02 Ring corneal ulcer

    H16.021 Ring corneal ulcer, right eye

    H16.022 Ring corneal ulcer, left eye

    H16.023 Ring corneal ulcer, bilateral

    H16.029 Ring corneal ulcer, unspecified eye

  H16.03 Corneal ulcer with hypopyon

    H16.031 Corneal ulcer with hypopyon, right eye

    H16.032 Corneal ulcer with hypopyon, left eye

    H16.033 Corneal ulcer with hypopyon, bilateral

    H16.039 Corneal ulcer with hypopyon, unspecified eye

  H16.04 Marginal corneal ulcer

    H16.041 Marginal corneal ulcer, right eye

    H16.042 Marginal corneal ulcer, left eye

    H16.043 Marginal corneal ulcer, bilateral

    H16.049 Marginal corneal ulcer, unspecified eye

  H16.05 Mooren's corneal ulcer

    H16.051 Mooren's corneal ulcer, right eye

    H16.052 Mooren's corneal ulcer, left eye

    H16.053 Mooren's corneal ulcer, bilateral

    H16.059 Mooren's corneal ulcer, unspecified eye

  H16.06 Mycotic corneal ulcer

    H16.061 Mycotic corneal ulcer, right eye

    H16.062 Mycotic corneal ulcer, left eye

    H16.063 Mycotic corneal ulcer, bilateral

    H16.069 Mycotic corneal ulcer, unspecified eye

  H16.07 Perforated corneal ulcer

    H16.071 Perforated corneal ulcer, right eye

    H16.072 Perforated corneal ulcer, left eye

    H16.073 Perforated corneal ulcer, bilateral

    H16.079 Perforated corneal ulcer, unspecified eye

H16.1 Other and unspecified superficial keratitis without conjunctivitis

  H16.10 Unspecified superficial keratitis

    H16.101 Unspecified superficial keratitis, right eye

    H16.102 Unspecified superficial keratitis, left eye

    H16.103 Unspecified superficial keratitis, bilateral

    H16.109 Unspecified superficial keratitis, unspecified eye

  H16.11 Macular keratitis

    Areolar keratitis

    Nummular keratitis

    Stellate keratitis

    Striate keratitis

    H16.111 Macular keratitis, right eye

    H16.112 Macular keratitis, left eye

    H16.113 Macular keratitis, bilateral

    H16.119 Macular keratitis, unspecified eye

  H16.12 Filamentary keratitis

    H16.121 Filamentary keratitis, right eye

    H16.122 Filamentary keratitis, left eye

    H16.123 Filamentary keratitis, bilateral

    H16.129 Filamentary keratitis, unspecified eye

  H16.13 Photokeratitis

    Snow blindness

    Welders keratitis

    H16.131 Photokeratitis, right eye

    H16.132 Photokeratitis, left eye

    H16.133 Photokeratitis, bilateral

    H16.139 Photokeratitis, unspecified eye

  H16.14 Punctate keratitis

    H16.141 Punctate keratitis, right eye

    H16.142 Punctate keratitis, left eye

    H16.143 Punctate keratitis, bilateral

    H16.149 Punctate keratitis, unspecified eye

H16.2 Keratoconjunctivitis

  H16.20 Unspecified keratoconjunctivitis

    Superficial keratitis with conjunctivitis NOS

    H16.201 Unspecified keratoconjunctivitis, right eye

    H16.202 Unspecified keratoconjunctivitis, left eye

    H16.203 Unspecified keratoconjunctivitis, bilateral

    H16.209 Unspecified keratoconjunctivitis, unspecified eye

  H16.21 Exposure keratoconjunctivitis

    H16.211 Exposure keratoconjunctivitis, right eye

    H16.212 Exposure keratoconjunctivitis, left eye

    H16.213 Exposure keratoconjunctivitis, bilateral

    H16.219 Exposure keratoconjunctivitis, unspecified eye

  H16.22 Keratoconjunctivitis sicca, not specified as Sjogren's

    Excludes 1: Sjogren's syndrome (M35.01)

    H16.221 Keratoconjunctivitis sicca, not specified as Sjogren's, right eye

    H16.222 Keratoconjunctivitis sicca, not specified as Sjogren's, left eye

    H16.223 Keratoconjunctivitis sicca, not specified as Sjogren's, bilateral

H16.229   Keratoconjunctivitis sicca, not specified as Sjogren's, unspecified eye

H16.23   Neurotrophic keratoconjunctivitis

H16.231   Neurotrophic keratoconjunctivitis, right eye

H16.232   Neurotrophic keratoconjunctivitis, left eye

H16.233   Neurotrophic keratoconjunctivitis, bilateral

H16.239   Neurotrophic keratoconjunctivitis, unspecified eye

H16.24   Ophthalmia nodosa

H16.241   Ophthalmia nodosa, right eye

H16.242   Ophthalmia nodosa, left eye

H16.243   Ophthalmia nodosa, bilateral

H16.249   Ophthalmia nodosa, unspecified eye

H16.25   Phlyctenular keratoconjunctivitis

H16.251   Phlyctenular keratoconjunctivitis, right eye

H16.252   Phlyctenular keratoconjunctivitis, left eye

H16.253   Phlyctenular keratoconjunctivitis, bilateral

H16.259   Phlyctenular keratoconjunctivitis, unspecified eye

H16.26   Vernal keratoconjunctivitis, with limbar and corneal involvement

Excludes 1: vernal conjunctivitis without limbar and corneal involvement (H10.44)

H16.261   Vernal keratoconjunctivitis, with limbar and corneal involvement, right eye

H16.262   Vernal keratoconjunctivitis, with limbar and corneal involvement, left eye

H16.263   Vernal keratoconjunctivitis, with limbar and corneal involvement, bilateral

H16.269   Vernal keratoconjunctivitis, with limbar and corneal involvement, unspecified eye

H16.29   Other keratoconjunctivitis

H16.291   Other keratoconjunctivitis, right eye

H16.292   Other keratoconjunctivitis, left eye

H16.293   Other keratoconjunctivitis, bilateral

H16.299   Other keratoconjunctivitis, unspecified eye

H16.3   Interstitial and deep keratitis

H16.30   Unspecified interstitial keratitis

H16.301   Unspecified interstitial keratitis, right eye

H16.302   Unspecified interstitial keratitis, left eye

H16.303   Unspecified interstitial keratitis, bilateral

H16.309   Unspecified interstitial keratitis, unspecified eye

H16.31   Corneal abscess

H16.311   Corneal abscess, right eye

H16.312   Corneal abscess, left eye

H16.313   Corneal abscess, bilateral

H16.319   Corneal abscess, unspecified eye

H16.32   Diffuse interstitial keratitis

Cogan's syndrome

H16.321   Diffuse interstitial keratitis, right eye

H16.322   Diffuse interstitial keratitis, left eye

H16.323   Diffuse interstitial keratitis, bilateral

H16.329   Diffuse interstitial keratitis, unspecified eye

H16.33   Sclerosing keratitis

H16.331   Sclerosing keratitis, right eye

H16.332   Sclerosing keratitis, left eye

H16.333   Sclerosing keratitis, bilateral

H16.339   Sclerosing keratitis, unspecified eye

H16.39   Other interstitial and deep keratitis

H16.391   Other interstitial and deep keratitis, right eye

H16.392   Other interstitial and deep keratitis, left eye

H16.393   Other interstitial and deep keratitis, bilateral

H16.399   Other interstitial and deep keratitis, unspecified eye

H16.4   Corneal neovascularization

H16.40   Unspecified corneal neovascularization

H16.401   Unspecified corneal neovascularization, right eye

H16.402   Unspecified corneal neovascularization, left eye

H16.403   Unspecified corneal neovascularization, bilateral

H16.409   Unspecified corneal neovascularization, unspecified eye

H16.41   Ghost vessels (corneal)

H16.411   Ghost vessels (corneal), right eye

H16.412   Ghost vessels (corneal), left eye

H16.413   Ghost vessels (corneal), bilateral

H16.419   Ghost vessels (corneal), unspecified eye

H16.42   Pannus (corneal)

H16.421   Pannus (corneal), right eye

H16.422   Pannus (corneal), left eye

H16.423   Pannus (corneal), bilateral

H16.429   Pannus (corneal), unspecified eye

H16.43   Localized vascularization of cornea

H16.431   Localized vascularization of cornea, right eye

H16.432   Localized vascularization of cornea, left eye

H16.433   Localized vascularization of cornea, bilateral

H16.439   Localized vascularization of cornea, unspecified eye

H16.44   Deep vascularization of cornea

H16.441   Deep vascularization of cornea, right eye

H16.442   Deep vascularization of cornea, left eye

H16.443   Deep vascularization of cornea, bilateral

H16.449   Deep vascularization of cornea, unspecified eye

H16.8   Other keratitis

H16.9   Unspecified keratitis

H17   Corneal scars and opacities

H17.0   Adherent leukoma

H17.00   Adherent leukoma, unspecified eye

● New code   ▲ Revised code   ⑦ 7th digit required   ⊗ Placeholder required

H17.01   Adherent leukoma, right eye
H17.02   Adherent leukoma, left eye
H17.03   Adherent leukoma, bilateral
H17.1   Central corneal opacity
    H17.10   Central corneal opacity, unspecified eye
    H17.11   Central corneal opacity, right eye
    H17.12   Central corneal opacity, left eye
    H17.13   Central corneal opacity, bilateral
H17.8   Other corneal scars and opacities
    H17.81   Minor opacity of cornea
       Corneal nebula
       H17.811   Minor opacity of cornea, right eye
       H17.812   Minor opacity of cornea, left eye
       H17.813   Minor opacity of cornea, bilateral
       H17.819   Minor opacity of cornea, unspecified eye
    H17.82   Peripheral opacity of cornea
       H17.821   Peripheral opacity of cornea, right eye
       H17.822   Peripheral opacity of cornea, left eye
       H17.823   Peripheral opacity of cornea, bilateral
       H17.829   Peripheral opacity of cornea, unspecified eye
    H17.89   Other corneal scars and opacities
H17.9   Unspecified corneal scar and opacity
H18   Other disorders of cornea
H18.0   Corneal pigmentations and deposits
    H18.00   Unspecified corneal deposit
       H18.001   Unspecified corneal deposit, right eye
       H18.002   Unspecified corneal deposit, left eye
       H18.003   Unspecified corneal deposit, bilateral
       H18.009   Unspecified corneal deposit, unspecified eye
    H18.01   Anterior corneal pigmentations
       Staehli's line
       H18.011   Anterior corneal pigmentations, right eye
       H18.012   Anterior corneal pigmentations, left eye
       H18.013   Anterior corneal pigmentations, bilateral
       H18.019   Anterior corneal pigmentations, unspecified eye
    H18.02   Argentous corneal deposits
       H18.021   Argentous corneal deposits, right eye
       H18.022   Argentous corneal deposits, left eye
       H18.023   Argentous corneal deposits, bilateral
       H18.029   Argentous corneal deposits, unspecified eye
    H18.03   Corneal deposits in metabolic disorders
       Code also associated metabolic disorder
       H18.031   Corneal deposits in metabolic disorders, right eye
       H18.032   Corneal deposits in metabolic disorders, left eye
       H18.033   Corneal deposits in metabolic disorders, bilateral
       H18.039   Corneal deposits in metabolic disorders, unspecified eye
    H18.04   Kayser-Fleischer ring
       Code also associated Wilson's disease (E83.01)
       H18.041   Kayser-Fleischer ring, right eye
       H18.042   Kayser-Fleischer ring, left eye
       H18.043   Kayser-Fleischer ring, bilateral

       H18.049   Kayser-Fleischer ring, unspecified eye
    H18.05   Posterior corneal pigmentations
       Krukenberg's spindle
       H18.051   Posterior corneal pigmentations, right eye
       H18.052   Posterior corneal pigmentations, left eye
       H18.053   Posterior corneal pigmentations, bilateral
       H18.059   Posterior corneal pigmentations, unspecified eye
    H18.06   Stromal corneal pigmentations
       Hematocornea
       H18.061   Stromal corneal pigmentations, right eye
       H18.062   Stromal corneal pigmentations, left eye
       H18.063   Stromal corneal pigmentations, bilateral
       H18.069   Stromal corneal pigmentations, unspecified eye
H18.1   Bullous keratopathy
    H18.10   Bullous keratopathy, unspecified eye
    H18.11   Bullous keratopathy, right eye
    H18.12   Bullous keratopathy, left eye
    H18.13   Bullous keratopathy, bilateral
H18.2   Other and unspecified corneal edema
    H18.20   Unspecified corneal edema
    H18.21   Corneal edema secondary to contact lens
       Excludes 2: other corneal disorders due to contact lens (H18.82-)
       H18.211   Corneal edema secondary to contact lens, right eye
       H18.212   Corneal edema secondary to contact lens, left eye
       H18.213   Corneal edema secondary to contact lens, bilateral
       H18.219   Corneal edema secondary to contact lens, unspecified eye
    H18.22   Idiopathic corneal edema
       H18.221   Idiopathic corneal edema, right eye
       H18.222   Idiopathic corneal edema, left eye
       H18.223   Idiopathic corneal edema, bilateral
       H18.229   Idiopathic corneal edema, unspecified eye
    H18.23   Secondary corneal edema
       H18.231   Secondary corneal edema, right eye
       H18.232   Secondary corneal edema, left eye
       H18.233   Secondary corneal edema, bilateral
       H18.239   Secondary corneal edema, unspecified eye
H18.3   Changes of corneal membranes
    H18.30   Unspecified corneal membrane change
    H18.31   Folds and rupture in Bowman's membrane
       H18.311   Folds and rupture in Bowman's membrane, right eye
       H18.312   Folds and rupture in Bowman's membrane, left eye
       H18.313   Folds and rupture in Bowman's membrane, bilateral
       H18.319   Folds and rupture in Bowman's membrane, unspecified eye
    H18.32   Folds in Descemet's membrane

H18.321 Folds in Descemet's membrane, right eye

H18.322 Folds in Descemet's membrane, left eye

H18.323 Folds in Descemet's membrane, bilateral

H18.329 Folds in Descemet's membrane, unspecified eye

H18.33 Rupture in Descemet's membrane

H18.331 Rupture in Descemet's membrane, right eye

H18.332 Rupture in Descemet's membrane, left eye

H18.333 Rupture in Descemet's membrane, bilateral

H18.339 Rupture in Descemet's membrane, unspecified eye

H18.4 Corneal degeneration

Excludes 1: Mooren's ulcer (H16.0-)
  recurrent erosion of cornea (H18.83-)

H18.40 Unspecified corneal degeneration

H18.41 Arcus senilis
  Senile corneal changes

H18.411 Arcus senilis, right eye

H18.412 Arcus senilis, left eye

H18.413 Arcus senilis, bilateral

H18.419 Arcus senilis, unspecified eye

H18.42 Band keratopathy

H18.421 Band keratopathy, right eye

H18.422 Band keratopathy, left eye

H18.423 Band keratopathy, bilateral

H18.429 Band keratopathy, unspecified eye

H18.43 Other calcerous corneal degeneration

H18.44 Keratomalacia

Excludes 1: keratomalacia due to vitamin A deficiency (E50.4)

H18.441 Keratomalacia, right eye

H18.442 Keratomalacia, left eye

H18.443 Keratomalacia, bilateral

H18.449 Keratomalacia, unspecified eye

H18.45 Nodular corneal degeneration

H18.451 Nodular corneal degeneration, right eye

H18.452 Nodular corneal degeneration, left eye

H18.453 Nodular corneal degeneration, bilateral

H18.459 Nodular corneal degeneration, unspecified eye

H18.46 Peripheral corneal degeneration

H18.461 Peripheral corneal degeneration, right eye

H18.462 Peripheral corneal degeneration, left eye

H18.463 Peripheral corneal degeneration, bilateral

H18.469 Peripheral corneal degeneration, unspecified eye

H18.49 Other corneal degeneration

H18.5 Hereditary corneal dystrophies

H18.50 Unspecified hereditary corneal dystrophies

H18.51 Endothelial corneal dystrophy
  Fuchs' dystrophy

H18.52 Epithelial (juvenile) corneal dystrophy

H18.53 Granular corneal dystrophy

H18.54 Lattice corneal dystrophy

H18.55 Macular corneal dystrophy

H18.59 Other hereditary corneal dystrophies

H18.6 Keratoconus

H18.60 Keratoconus, unspecified

H18.601 Keratoconus, unspecified, right eye

H18.602 Keratoconus, unspecified, left eye

H18.603 Keratoconus, unspecified, bilateral

H18.609 Keratoconus, unspecified, unspecified eye

H18.61 Keratoconus, stable

H18.611 Keratoconus, stable, right eye

H18.612 Keratoconus, stable, left eye

H18.613 Keratoconus, stable, bilateral

H18.619 Keratoconus, stable, unspecified eye

H18.62 Keratoconus, unstable
  Acute hydrops

H18.621 Keratoconus, unstable, right eye

H18.622 Keratoconus, unstable, left eye

H18.623 Keratoconus, unstable, bilateral

H18.629 Keratoconus, unstable, unspecified eye

H18.7 Other and unspecified corneal deformities

Excludes 1: congenital malformations of cornea (Q13.3-Q13.4)

H18.70 Unspecified corneal deformity

H18.71 Corneal ectasia

H18.711 Corneal ectasia, right eye

H18.712 Corneal ectasia, left eye

H18.713 Corneal ectasia, bilateral

H18.719 Corneal ectasia, unspecified eye

H18.72 Corneal staphyloma

H18.721 Corneal staphyloma, right eye

H18.722 Corneal staphyloma, left eye

H18.723 Corneal staphyloma, bilateral

H18.729 Corneal staphyloma, unspecified eye

H18.73 Descemetocele

H18.731 Descemetocele, right eye

H18.732 Descemetocele, left eye

H18.733 Descemetocele, bilateral

H18.739 Descemetocele, unspecified eye

H18.79 Other corneal deformities

H18.791 Other corneal deformities, right eye

H18.792 Other corneal deformities, left eye

H18.793 Other corneal deformities, bilateral

H18.799 Other corneal deformities, unspecified eye

H18.8 Other specified disorders of cornea

H18.81 Anesthesia and hypoesthesia of cornea

H18.811 Anesthesia and hypoesthesia of cornea, right eye

H18.812 Anesthesia and hypoesthesia of cornea, left eye

H18.813 Anesthesia and hypoesthesia of cornea, bilateral

H18.819 Anesthesia and hypoesthesia of cornea, unspecified eye

H18.82 Corneal disorder due to contact lens

Excludes 2: corneal edema due to contact lens (H18.21-)

● New code   ▲ Revised code   ⑦ 7th digit required   ⊗ Placeholder required

H18.821 Corneal disorder due to contact lens, right eye

H18.822 Corneal disorder due to contact lens, left eye

H18.823 Corneal disorder due to contact lens, bilateral

H18.829 Corneal disorder due to contact lens, unspecified eye

H18.83 Recurrent erosion of cornea

H18.831 Recurrent erosion of cornea, right eye

H18.832 Recurrent erosion of cornea, left eye

H18.833 Recurrent erosion of cornea, bilateral

H18.839 Recurrent erosion of cornea, unspecified eye

H18.89 Other specified disorders of cornea

H18.891 Other specified disorders of cornea, right eye

H18.892 Other specified disorders of cornea, left eye

H18.893 Other specified disorders of cornea, bilateral

H18.899 Other specified disorders of cornea, unspecified eye

H18.9 Unspecified disorder of cornea

H20 Iridocyclitis

H20.0 Acute and subacute iridocyclitis

Acute anterior uveitis

Acute cyclitis

Acute iritis

Subacute anterior uveitis

Subacute cyclitis

Subacute iritis

Excludes 1: iridocyclitis, iritis, uveitis (due to) (in) diabetes mellitus (E08-E13 with .39)

iridocyclitis, iritis, uveitis (due to) (in) diphtheria (A36.89)

iridocyclitis, iritis, uveitis (due to) (in) gonococcal (A54.32)

iridocyclitis, iritis, uveitis (due to) (in) herpes (simplex) (B00.51)

iridocyclitis, iritis, uveitis (due to) (in) herpes zoster (B02.32)

iridocyclitis, iritis, uveitis (due to) (in) late congenital syphilis (A50.39)

iridocyclitis, iritis, uveitis (due to) (in) late syphilis (A52.71)

iridocyclitis, iritis, uveitis (due to) (in) sarcoidosis (D86.83)

iridocyclitis, iritis, uveitis (due to) (in) syphilis (A51.43)

iridocyclitis, iritis, uveitis (due to) (in) toxoplasmosis (B58.09)

iridocyclitis, iritis, uveitis (due to) (in) tuberculosis (A18.54)

H20.00 Unspecified acute and subacute iridocyclitis

H20.01 Primary iridocyclitis

H20.011 Primary iridocyclitis, right eye

H20.012 Primary iridocyclitis, left eye

H20.013 Primary iridocyclitis, bilateral

H20.019 Primary iridocyclitis, unspecified eye

H20.02 Recurrent acute iridocyclitis

H20.021 Recurrent acute iridocyclitis, right eye

H20.022 Recurrent acute iridocyclitis, left eye

H20.023 Recurrent acute iridocyclitis, bilateral

H20.029 Recurrent acute iridocyclitis, unspecified eye

H20.03 Secondary infectious iridocyclitis

H20.031 Secondary infectious iridocyclitis, right eye

H20.032 Secondary infectious iridocyclitis, left eye

H20.033 Secondary infectious iridocyclitis, bilateral

H20.039 Secondary infectious iridocyclitis, unspecified eye

H20.04 Secondary noninfectious iridocyclitis

H20.041 Secondary noninfectious iridocyclitis, right eye

H20.042 Secondary noninfectious iridocyclitis, left eye

H20.043 Secondary noninfectious iridocyclitis, bilateral

H20.049 Secondary noninfectious iridocyclitis, unspecified eye

H20.05 Hypopyon

H20.051 Hypopyon, right eye

H20.052 Hypopyon, left eye

H20.053 Hypopyon, bilateral

H20.059 Hypopyon, unspecified eye

H20.1 Chronic iridocyclitis

Use additional code for any associated cataract (H26.21-)

Excludes 2: posterior cyclitis (H30.2-)

H20.10 Chronic iridocyclitis, unspecified eye

H20.11 Chronic iridocyclitis, right eye

H20.12 Chronic iridocyclitis, left eye

H20.13 Chronic iridocyclitis, bilateral

H20.2 Lens-induced iridocyclitis

H20.20 Lens-induced iridocyclitis, unspecified eye

H20.21 Lens-induced iridocyclitis, right eye

H20.22 Lens-induced iridocyclitis, left eye

H20.23 Lens-induced iridocyclitis, bilateral

H20.8 Other iridocyclitis

Excludes 2: glaucomatocyclitis crises (H40.4-)

posterior cyclitis (H30.2-)

sympathetic uveitis (H44.13-)

H20.81 Fuchs' heterochromic cyclitis

H20.811 Fuchs' heterochromic cyclitis, right eye

H20.812 Fuchs' heterochromic cyclitis, left eye

H20.813 Fuchs' heterochromic cyclitis, bilateral

H20.819 Fuchs' heterochromic cyclitis, unspecified eye

H20.82 Vogt-Koyanagi syndrome

H20.821 Vogt-Koyanagi syndrome, right eye

H20.822 Vogt-Koyanagi syndrome, left eye

H20.823 Vogt-Koyanagi syndrome, bilateral

H20.829 Vogt-Koyanagi syndrome, unspecified eye

H20.9 Unspecified iridocyclitis

Uveitis NOS

H21 Other disorders of iris and ciliary body

Excludes 2: sympathetic uveitis (H44.1-)

H21.0 Hyphema

Excludes 1: traumatic hyphema (S05.1-)

H21.00   Hyphema, unspecified eye
H21.01   Hyphema, right eye
H21.02   Hyphema, left eye
H21.03   Hyphema, bilateral
H21.1   Other vascular disorders of iris and ciliary body
Neovascularization of iris or ciliary body
Rubeosis iridis
Rubeosis of iris
H21.1X   Other vascular disorders of iris and ciliary body
H21.1X1   Other vascular disorders of iris and ciliary body, right eye
H21.1X2   Other vascular disorders of iris and ciliary body, left eye
H21.1X3   Other vascular disorders of iris and ciliary body, bilateral
H21.1X9   Other vascular disorders of iris and ciliary body, unspecified eye
H21.2   Degeneration of iris and ciliary body
H21.21   Degeneration of chamber angle
H21.211   Degeneration of chamber angle, right eye
H21.212   Degeneration of chamber angle, left eye
H21.213   Degeneration of chamber angle, bilateral
H21.219   Degeneration of chamber angle, unspecified eye
H21.22   Degeneration of ciliary body
H21.221   Degeneration of ciliary body, right eye
H21.222   Degeneration of ciliary body, left eye
H21.223   Degeneration of ciliary body, bilateral
H21.229   Degeneration of ciliary body, unspecified eye
H21.23   Degeneration of iris (pigmentary)
Translucency of iris
H21.231   Degeneration of iris (pigmentary), right eye
H21.232   Degeneration of iris (pigmentary), left eye
H21.233   Degeneration of iris (pigmentary), bilateral
H21.239   Degeneration of iris (pigmentary), unspecified eye
H21.24   Degeneration of pupillary margin
H21.241   Degeneration of pupillary margin, right eye
H21.242   Degeneration of pupillary margin, left eye
H21.243   Degeneration of pupillary margin, bilateral
H21.249   Degeneration of pupillary margin, unspecified eye
H21.25   Iridoschisis
H21.251   Iridoschisis, right eye
H21.252   Iridoschisis, left eye
H21.253   Iridoschisis, bilateral
H21.259   Iridoschisis, unspecified eye
H21.26   Iris atrophy (essential) (progressive)
H21.261   Iris atrophy (essential) (progressive), right eye

H21.262   Iris atrophy (essential) (progressive), left eye
H21.263   Iris atrophy (essential) (progressive), bilateral
H21.269   Iris atrophy (essential) (progressive), unspecified eye
H21.27   Miotic pupillary cyst
H21.271   Miotic pupillary cyst, right eye
H21.272   Miotic pupillary cyst, left eye
H21.273   Miotic pupillary cyst, bilateral
H21.279   Miotic pupillary cyst, unspecified eye
H21.29   Other iris atrophy
H21.3   Cyst of iris, ciliary body and anterior chamber
Excludes 2: miotic pupillary cyst (H21.27-)
H21.30   Idiopathic cysts of iris, ciliary body or anterior chamber
Cyst of iris, ciliary body or anterior chamber NOS
H21.301   Idiopathic cysts of iris, ciliary body or anterior chamber, right eye
H21.302   Idiopathic cysts of iris, ciliary body or anterior chamber, left eye
H21.303   Idiopathic cysts of iris, ciliary body or anterior chamber, bilateral
H21.309   Idiopathic cysts of iris, ciliary body or anterior chamber, unspecified eye
H21.31   Exudative cysts of iris or anterior chamber
H21.311   Exudative cysts of iris or anterior chamber, right eye
H21.312   Exudative cysts of iris or anterior chamber, left eye
H21.313   Exudative cysts of iris or anterior chamber, bilateral
H21.319   Exudative cysts of iris or anterior chamber, unspecified eye
H21.32   Implantation cysts of iris, ciliary body or anterior chamber
H21.321   Implantation cysts of iris, ciliary body or anterior chamber, right eye
H21.322   Implantation cysts of iris, ciliary body or anterior chamber, left eye
H21.323   Implantation cysts of iris, ciliary body or anterior chamber, bilateral
H21.329   Implantation cysts of iris, ciliary body or anterior chamber, unspecified eye
H21.33   Parasitic cyst of iris, ciliary body or anterior chamber
H21.331   Parasitic cyst of iris, ciliary body or anterior chamber, right eye
H21.332   Parasitic cyst of iris, ciliary body or anterior chamber, left eye
H21.333   Parasitic cyst of iris, ciliary body or anterior chamber, bilateral
H21.339   Parasitic cyst of iris, ciliary body or anterior chamber, unspecified eye
H21.34   Primary cyst of pars plana
H21.341   Primary cyst of pars plana, right eye
H21.342   Primary cyst of pars plana, left eye
H21.343   Primary cyst of pars plana, bilateral
H21.349   Primary cyst of pars plana, unspecified eye
H21.35   Exudative cyst of pars plana
H21.351   Exudative cyst of pars plana, right eye

H21.352 Exudative cyst of pars plana, left eye

H21.353 Exudative cyst of pars plana, bilateral

H21.359 Exudative cyst of pars plana, unspecified eye

H21.4 Pupillary membranes

Iris bombΘ

Pupillary occlusion

Pupillary seclusion

Excludes 1: congenital pupillary membranes (Q13.8)

H21.40 Pupillary membranes, unspecified eye

H21.41 Pupillary membranes, right eye

H21.42 Pupillary membranes, left eye

H21.43 Pupillary membranes, bilateral

H21.5 Other and unspecified adhesions and disruptions of iris and ciliary body

Excludes 1: corectopia (Q13.2)

H21.50 Unspecified adhesions of iris

Synechia (iris) NOS

H21.501 Unspecified adhesions of iris, right eye

H21.502 Unspecified adhesions of iris, left eye

H21.503 Unspecified adhesions of iris, bilateral

H21.509 Unspecified adhesions of iris and ciliary body, unspecified eye

H21.51 Anterior synechiae (iris)

H21.511 Anterior synechiae (iris), right eye

H21.512 Anterior synechiae (iris), left eye

H21.513 Anterior synechiae (iris), bilateral

H21.519 Anterior synechiae (iris), unspecified eye

H21.52 Goniosynechiae

H21.521 Goniosynechiae, right eye

H21.522 Goniosynechiae, left eye

H21.523 Goniosynechiae, bilateral

H21.529 Goniosynechiae, unspecified eye

H21.53 Iridodialysis

H21.531 Iridodialysis, right eye

H21.532 Iridodialysis, left eye

H21.533 Iridodialysis, bilateral

H21.539 Iridodialysis, unspecified eye

H21.54 Posterior synechiae (iris)

H21.541 Posterior synechiae (iris), right eye

H21.542 Posterior synechiae (iris), left eye

H21.543 Posterior synechiae (iris), bilateral

H21.549 Posterior synechiae (iris), unspecified eye

H21.55 Recession of chamber angle

H21.551 Recession of chamber angle, right eye

H21.552 Recession of chamber angle, left eye

H21.553 Recession of chamber angle, bilateral

H21.559 Recession of chamber angle, unspecified eye

H21.56 Pupillary abnormalities

Deformed pupil

Ectopic pupil

Rupture of sphincter, pupil

Excludes 1: congenital deformity of pupil (Q13.2-)

H21.561 Pupillary abnormality, right eye

H21.562 Pupillary abnormality, left eye

H21.563 Pupillary abnormality, bilateral

H21.569 Pupillary abnormality, unspecified eye

H21.8 Other specified disorders of iris and ciliary body

H21.81 Floppy iris syndrome

Intraoperative floppy iris syndrome (IFIS)

Use additional code for adverse effect, if applicable, to identify drug (T36-T50 with fifth or sixth character 5)

H21.82 Plateau iris syndrome (post-iridectomy) (postprocedural)

H21.89 Other specified disorders of iris and ciliary body

H21.9 Unspecified disorder of iris and ciliary body

H22 Disorders of iris and ciliary body in diseases classified elsewhere

Code first underlying disease, such as:

gout (M1A-, M10.-)

DISORDERS OF LENS (H25-H28)

H25 Age-related cataract

Senile cataract

Excludes 2: capsular glaucoma with pseudoexfoliation of lens (H40.1-)

H25.0 Age-related incipient cataract

H25.01 Cortical age-related cataract

H25.011 Cortical age-related cataract, right eye

H25.012 Cortical age-related cataract, left eye

H25.013 Cortical age-related cataract, bilateral

H25.019 Cortical age-related cataract, unspecified eye

H25.03 Anterior subcapsular polar age-related cataract

H25.031 Anterior subcapsular polar age-related cataract, right eye

H25.032 Anterior subcapsular polar age-related cataract, left eye

H25.033 Anterior subcapsular polar age-related cataract, bilateral

H25.039 Anterior subcapsular polar age-related cataract, unspecified eye

H25.04 Posterior subcapsular polar age-related cataract

H25.041 Posterior subcapsular polar age-related cataract, right eye

H25.042 Posterior subcapsular polar age-related cataract, left eye

H25.043 Posterior subcapsular polar age-related cataract, bilateral

H25.049 Posterior subcapsular polar age-related cataract, unspecified eye

H25.09 Other age-related incipient cataract

Coronary age-related cataract

Punctate age-related cataract

Water clefts

H25.091 Other age-related incipient cataract, right eye

H25.092 Other age-related incipient cataract, left eye

H25.093 Other age-related incipient cataract, bilateral

H25.099 Other age-related incipient cataract, unspecified eye

H25.1 Age-related nuclear cataract

Cataracta brunescens

Nuclear sclerosis cataract

H25.10 Age-related nuclear cataract, unspecified eye

H25.11 Age-related nuclear cataract, right eye

H25.12 Age-related nuclear cataract, left eye

H25.13　Age-related nuclear cataract, bilateral

H25.2　Age-related cataract, morgagnian type

Age-related hypermature cataract

H25.20　Age-related cataract, morgagnian type, unspecified eye

H25.21　Age-related cataract, morgagnian type, right eye

H25.22　Age-related cataract, morgagnian type, left eye

H25.23　Age-related cataract, morgagnian type, bilateral

H25.8　Other age-related cataract

H25.81　Combined forms of age-related cataract

H25.811　Combined forms of age-related cataract, right eye

H25.812　Combined forms of age-related cataract, left eye

H25.813　Combined forms of age-related cataract, bilateral

H25.819　Combined forms of age-related cataract, unspecified eye

H25.89　Other age-related cataract

H25.9　Unspecified age-related cataract

H26　Other cataract

Excludes 1: congenital cataract (Q12.0)

H26.0　Infantile and juvenile cataract

H26.00　Unspecified infantile and juvenile cataract

H26.001　Unspecified infantile and juvenile cataract, right eye

H26.002　Unspecified infantile and juvenile cataract, left eye

H26.003　Unspecified infantile and juvenile cataract, bilateral

H26.009　Unspecified infantile and juvenile cataract, unspecified eye

H26.01　Infantile and juvenile cortical, lamellar, or zonular cataract

H26.011　Infantile and juvenile cortical, lamellar, or zonular cataract, right eye

H26.012　Infantile and juvenile cortical, lamellar, or zonular cataract, left eye

H26.013　Infantile and juvenile cortical, lamellar, or zonular cataract, bilateral

H26.019　Infantile and juvenile cortical, lamellar, or zonular cataract, unspecified eye

H26.03　Infantile and juvenile nuclear cataract

H26.031　Infantile and juvenile nuclear cataract, right eye

H26.032　Infantile and juvenile nuclear cataract, left eye

H26.033　Infantile and juvenile nuclear cataract, bilateral

H26.039　Infantile and juvenile nuclear cataract, unspecified eye

H26.04　Anterior subcapsular polar infantile and juvenile cataract

H26.041　Anterior subcapsular polar infantile and juvenile cataract, right eye

H26.042　Anterior subcapsular polar infantile and juvenile cataract, left eye

H26.043　Anterior subcapsular polar infantile and juvenile cataract, bilateral

H26.049　Anterior subcapsular polar infantile and juvenile cataract, unspecified eye

H26.05　Posterior subcapsular polar infantile and juvenile cataract

H26.051　Posterior subcapsular polar infantile and juvenile cataract, right eye

H26.052　Posterior subcapsular polar infantile and juvenile cataract, left eye

H26.053　Posterior subcapsular polar infantile and juvenile cataract, bilateral

H26.059　Posterior subcapsular polar infantile and juvenile cataract, unspecified eye

H26.06　Combined forms of infantile and juvenile cataract

H26.061　Combined forms of infantile and juvenile cataract, right eye

H26.062　Combined forms of infantile and juvenile cataract, left eye

H26.063　Combined forms of infantile and juvenile cataract, bilateral

H26.069　Combined forms of infantile and juvenile cataract, unspecified eye

H26.09　Other infantile and juvenile cataract

H26.1　Traumatic cataract

Use additional code (Chapter 20) to identify external cause

H26.10　Unspecified traumatic cataract

H26.101　Unspecified traumatic cataract, right eye

H26.102　Unspecified traumatic cataract, left eye

H26.103　Unspecified traumatic cataract, bilateral

H26.109　Unspecified traumatic cataract, unspecified eye

H26.11　Localized traumatic opacities

H26.111　Localized traumatic opacities, right eye

H26.112　Localized traumatic opacities, left eye

H26.113　Localized traumatic opacities, bilateral

H26.119　Localized traumatic opacities, unspecified eye

H26.12　Partially resolved traumatic cataract

H26.121　Partially resolved traumatic cataract, right eye

H26.122　Partially resolved traumatic cataract, left eye

H26.123　Partially resolved traumatic cataract, bilateral

H26.129　Partially resolved traumatic cataract, unspecified eye

H26.13　Total traumatic cataract

H26.131　Total traumatic cataract, right eye

H26.132　Total traumatic cataract, left eye

H26.133　Total traumatic cataract, bilateral

H26.139　Total traumatic cataract, unspecified eye

H26.2　Complicated cataract

H26.20　Unspecified complicated cataract

Cataracta complicata NOS

H26.21　Cataract with neovascularization

Code also associated condition, such as:

chronic iridocyclitis (H20.1-)

H26.211　Cataract with neovascularization, right eye

H26.212　Cataract with neovascularization, left eye

H26.213 Cataract with neovascularization, bilateral

H26.219 Cataract with neovascularization, unspecified eye

H26.22 Cataract secondary to ocular disorders (degenerative) (inflammatory)

Code also associated ocular disorder

H26.221 Cataract secondary to ocular disorders (degenerative) (inflammatory), right eye

H26.222 Cataract secondary to ocular disorders degenerative) (inflammatory), left eye

H26.223 Cataract secondary to ocular disorders (degenerative) (inflammatory), bilateral

H26.229 Cataract secondary to ocular disorders (degenerative) (inflammatory), unspecified eye

H26.23 Glaucomatous flecks (subcapsular)

Code first underlying glaucoma (H40-H42)

H26.231 Glaucomatous flecks (subcapsular), right eye

H26.232 Glaucomatous flecks (subcapsular), left eye

H26.233 Glaucomatous flecks (subcapsular), bilateral

H26.239 Glaucomatous flecks (subcapsular), unspecified eye

H26.3 Drug-induced cataract

Toxic cataract

Use additional code for adverse effect, if applicable, to identify drug (T36-T50 with fifth or sixth character 5)

H26.30 Drug-induced cataract, unspecified eye

H26.31 Drug-induced cataract, right eye

H26.32 Drug-induced cataract, left eye

H26.33 Drug-induced cataract, bilateral

H26.4 Secondary cataract

H26.40 Unspecified secondary cataract

H26.41 Soemmering's ring

H26.411 Soemmering's ring, right eye

H26.412 Soemmering's ring, left eye

H26.413 Soemmering's ring, bilateral

H26.419 Soemmering's ring, unspecified eye

H26.49 Other secondary cataract

H26.491 Other secondary cataract, right eye

H26.492 Other secondary cataract, left eye

H26.493 Other secondary cataract, bilateral

H26.499 Other secondary cataract, unspecified eye

H26.8 Other specified cataract

H26.9 Unspecified cataract

H27 Other disorders of lens

Excludes 1: congenital lens malformations (Q12.-)

mechanical complications of intraocular lens implant (T85.2)

pseudophakia (Z96.1)

H27.0 Aphakia

Acquired absence of lens

Acquired aphakia

Aphakia due to trauma

Excludes 1: cataract extraction status (Z98.4-)

congenital absence of lens (Q12.3)

congenital aphakia (Q12.3)

H27.00 Aphakia, unspecified eye

H27.01 Aphakia, right eye

H27.02 Aphakia, left eye

H27.03 Aphakia, bilateral

H27.1 Dislocation of lens

H27.10 Unspecified dislocation of lens

H27.11 Subluxation of lens

H27.111 Subluxation of lens, right eye

H27.112 Subluxation of lens, left eye

H27.113 Subluxation of lens, bilateral

H27.119 Subluxation of lens, unspecified eye

H27.12 Anterior dislocation of lens

H27.121 Anterior dislocation of lens, right eye

H27.122 Anterior dislocation of lens, left eye

H27.123 Anterior dislocation of lens, bilateral

H27.129 Anterior dislocation of lens, unspecified eye

H27.13 Posterior dislocation of lens

H27.131 Posterior dislocation of lens, right eye

H27.132 Posterior dislocation of lens, left eye

H27.133 Posterior dislocation of lens, bilateral

H27.139 Posterior dislocation of lens, unspecified eye

H27.8 Other specified disorders of lens

H27.9 Unspecified disorder of lens

H28 Cataract in diseases classified elsewhere

Code first underlying disease, such as:

hypoparathyroidism (E20.-)

myotonia (G71.1-)

myxedema (E03.-)

protein-calorie malnutrition (E40-E46)

Excludes 1: cataract in diabetes mellitus (E08.33, E09.33, E10.33, E11.33, E13.33)

DISORDERS OF CHOROID AND RETINA (H30-H36)

H30 Chorioretinal inflammation

H30.0 Focal chorioretinal inflammation

Focal chorioretinitis

Focal choroiditis

Focal retinitis

Focal retinochoroiditis

H30.00 Unspecified focal chorioretinal inflammation

Focal chorioretinitis NOS

Focal choroiditis NOS

Focal retinitis NOS

Focal retinochoroiditis NOS

H30.001 Unspecified focal chorioretinal inflammation, right eye

H30.002 Unspecified focal chorioretinal inflammation, left eye

H30.003 Unspecified focal chorioretinal inflammation, bilateral

H30.009 Unspecified focal chorioretinal inflammation, unspecified eye

H30.01 Focal chorioretinal inflammation, juxtapapillary

H30.011 Focal chorioretinal inflammation, juxtapapillary, right eye

H30.012 Focal chorioretinal inflammation, juxtapapillary, left eye

H30.013 Focal chorioretinal inflammation, juxtapapillary, bilateral

H30.019 Focal chorioretinal inflammation, juxtapapillary, unspecified eye

H30.02 Focal chorioretinal inflammation of posterior pole

    H30.021 Focal chorioretinal inflammation of posterior pole, right eye

    H30.022 Focal chorioretinal inflammation of posterior pole, left eye

    H30.023 Focal chorioretinal inflammation of posterior pole, bilateral

    H30.029 Focal chorioretinal inflammation of posterior pole, unspecified eye

H30.03 Focal chorioretinal inflammation, peripheral

    H30.031 Focal chorioretinal inflammation, peripheral, right eye

    H30.032 Focal chorioretinal inflammation, peripheral, left eye

    H30.033 Focal chorioretinal inflammation, peripheral, bilateral

    H30.039 Focal chorioretinal inflammation, peripheral, unspecified eye

H30.04 Focal chorioretinal inflammation, macular or paramacular

    H30.041 Focal chorioretinal inflammation, macular or paramacular, right eye

    H30.042 Focal chorioretinal inflammation, macular or paramacular, left eye

    H30.043 Focal chorioretinal inflammation, macular or paramacular, bilateral

    H30.049 Focal chorioretinal inflammation, macular or paramacular, unspecified eye

H30.1 Disseminated chorioretinal inflammation

Disseminated chorioretinitis

Disseminated choroiditis

Disseminated retinitis

Disseminated retinochoroiditis'

Excludes 2: exudative retinopathy (H35.02-)

H30.10 Unspecified disseminated chorioretinal inflammation

Disseminated chorioretinitis NOS

Disseminated choroiditis NOS

Disseminated retinitis NOS

Disseminated retinochoroiditis NOS

    H30.101 Unspecified disseminated chorioretinal inflammation, right eye

    H30.102 Unspecified disseminated chorioretinal inflammation, left eye

    H30.103 Unspecified disseminated chorioretinal inflammation, bilateral

    H30.109 Unspecified disseminated chorioretinal inflammation, unspecified eye

H30.11 Disseminated chorioretinal inflammation of posterior pole

    H30.111 Disseminated chorioretinal inflammation of posterior pole, right eye

    H30.112 Disseminated chorioretinal inflammation of posterior pole, left eye

    H30.113 Disseminated chorioretinal inflammation of posterior pole, bilateral

    H30.119 Disseminated chorioretinal inflammation of posterior pole, unspecified eye

H30.12 Disseminated chorioretinal inflammation, peripheral

    H30.121 Disseminated chorioretinal inflammation, peripheral right eye

    H30.122 Disseminated chorioretinal inflammation, peripheral, left eye

    H30.123 Disseminated chorioretinal inflammation, peripheral, bilateral

    H30.129 Disseminated chorioretinal inflammation, peripheral, unspecified eye

H30.13 Disseminated chorioretinal inflammation, generalized

    H30.131 Disseminated chorioretinal inflammation, generalized, right eye

    H30.132 Disseminated chorioretinal inflammation, generalized, left eye

    H30.133 Disseminated chorioretinal inflammation, generalized, bilateral

    H30.139 Disseminated chorioretinal inflammation, generalized, unspecified eye

H30.14 Acute posterior multifocal placoid pigment epitheliopathy

    H30.141 Acute posterior multifocal placoid pigment epitheliopathy, right eye

    H30.142 Acute posterior multifocal placoid pigment epitheliopathy, left eye

    H30.143 Acute posterior multifocal placoid pigment epitheliopathy, bilateral

    H30.149 Acute posterior multifocal placoid pigment epitheliopathy, unspecified eye

H30.2 Posterior cyclitis

Pars planitis

  H30.20 Posterior cyclitis, unspecified eye

  H30.21 Posterior cyclitis, right eye

  H30.22 Posterior cyclitis, left eye

  H30.23 Posterior cyclitis, bilateral

H30.8 Other chorioretinal inflammations

  H30.81 Harada's disease

    H30.811 Harada's disease, right eye

    H30.812 Harada's disease, left eye

    H30.813 Harada's disease, bilateral

    H30.819 Harada's disease, unspecified eye

  H30.89 Other chorioretinal inflammations

    H30.891 Other chorioretinal inflammations, right eye

    H30.892 Other chorioretinal inflammations, left eye

    H30.893 Other chorioretinal inflammations, bilateral

    H30.899 Other chorioretinal inflammations, unspecified eye

H30.9 Unspecified chorioretinal inflammation

Chorioretinitis NOS

Choroiditis NOS

Neuroretinitis NOS

Retinitis NOS

Retinochoroiditis NOS

H30.90 Unspecified chorioretinal inflammation, unspecified eye

H30.91 Unspecified chorioretinal inflammation, right eye

H30.92 Unspecified chorioretinal inflammation, left eye

H30.93 Unspecified chorioretinal inflammation, bilateral

H31 Other disorders of choroid

H31.0 Chorioretinal scars

Excludes 2: postsurgical chorioretinal scars (H59.81-)

H31.00 Unspecified chorioretinal scars

H31.001 Unspecified chorioretinal scars, right eye

H31.002 Unspecified chorioretinal scars, left eye

H31.003 Unspecified chorioretinal scars, bilateral

H31.009 Unspecified chorioretinal scars, unspecified eye

H31.01 Macula scars of posterior pole (postinflammatory) (post-traumatic)

Excludes 1: postprocedural choriorentinal scar (H59.81-)

H31.011 Macula scars of posterior pole (postinflammatory) (post-traumatic), right eye

H31.012 Macula scars of posterior pole (postinflammatory) (post-traumatic), left eye

H31.013 Macula scars of posterior pole (postinflammatory) (post-traumatic), bilateral

H31.019 Macula scars of posterior pole (postinflammatory) (post-traumatic), unspecified eye

H31.02 Solar retinopathy

H31.021 Solar retinopathy, right eye

H31.022 Solar retinopathy, left eye

H31.023 Solar retinopathy, bilateral

H31.029 Solar retinopathy, unspecified eye

H31.09 Other chorioretinal scars

H31.091 Other chorioretinal scars, right eye

H31.092 Other chorioretinal scars, left eye

H31.093 Other chorioretinal scars, bilateral

H31.099 Other chorioretinal scars, unspecified eye

H31.1 Choroidal degeneration

Excludes 2: angioid streaks of macula (H35.33)

H31.10 Unspecified choroidal degeneration

Choroidal sclerosis NOS

H31.101 Choroidal degeneration, unspecified, right eye

H31.102 Choroidal degeneration, unspecified, left eye

H31.103 Choroidal degeneration, unspecified, bilateral

H31.109 Choroidal degeneration, unspecified, unspecified eye

H31.11 Age-related choroidal atrophy

H31.111 Age-related choroidal atrophy, right eye

H31.112 Age-related choroidal atrophy, left eye

H31.113 Age-related choroidal atrophy, bilateral

H31.119 Age-related choroidal atrophy, unspecified eye

H31.12 Diffuse secondary atrophy of choroid

H31.121 Diffuse secondary atrophy of choroid, right eye

H31.122 Diffuse secondary atrophy of choroid, left eye

H31.123 Diffuse secondary atrophy of choroid, bilateral

H31.129 Diffuse secondary atrophy of choroid, unspecified eye

H31.2 Hereditary choroidal dystrophy

Excludes 2: hyperornithinemia (E72.4)

ornithinemia (E72.4)

H31.20 Hereditary choroidal dystrophy, unspecified

H31.21 Choroideremia

H31.22 Choroidal dystrophy (central areolar) (generalized) (peripapillary)

H31.23 Gyrate atrophy, choroid

H31.29 Other hereditary choroidal dystrophy

H31.3 Choroidal hemorrhage and rupture

H31.30 Unspecified choroidal hemorrhage

H31.301 Unspecified choroidal hemorrhage, right eye

H31.302 Unspecified choroidal hemorrhage, left eye

H31.303 Unspecified choroidal hemorrhage, bilateral

H31.309 Unspecified choroidal hemorrhage, unspecified eye

H31.31 Expulsive choroidal hemorrhage

H31.311 Expulsive choroidal hemorrhage, right eye

H31.312 Expulsive choroidal hemorrhage, left eye

H31.313 Expulsive choroidal hemorrhage, bilateral

H31.319 Expulsive choroidal hemorrhage, unspecified eye

H31.32 Choroidal rupture

H31.321 Choroidal rupture, right eye

H31.322 Choroidal rupture, left eye

H31.323 Choroidal rupture, bilateral

H31.329 Choroidal rupture, unspecified eye

H31.4 Choroidal detachment

H31.40 Unspecified choroidal detachment

H31.401 Unspecified choroidal detachment, right eye

H31.402 Unspecified choroidal detachment, left eye

H31.403 Unspecified choroidal detachment, bilateral

H31.409 Unspecified choroidal detachment, unspecified eye

H31.41 Hemorrhagic choroidal detachment

H31.411 Hemorrhagic choroidal detachment, right eye

H31.412 Hemorrhagic choroidal detachment, left eye

H31.413 Hemorrhagic choroidal detachment, bilateral

H31.419 Hemorrhagic choroidal detachment, unspecified eye

H31.42 Serous choroidal detachment

H31.421 Serous choroidal detachment, right eye

H31.422 Serous choroidal detachment, left eye

H31.423 Serous choroidal detachment, bilateral

H31.429 Serous choroidal detachment, unspecified eye

H31.8 Other specified disorders of choroid

H31.9 Unspecified disorder of choroid

H32 Chorioretinal disorders in diseases classified elsewhere

Code first underlying disease, such as:

congenital toxoplasmosis (P37.1)

histoplasmosis (B39.-)

leprosy (A30.-)

Excludes 1: chorioretinitis (in):

toxoplasmosis (acquired) (B58.01)

tuberculosis (A18.53)

H33 Retinal detachments and breaks

Excludes 1: detachment of retinal pigment epithelium (H35.72-, H35.73-)

H33.0 Retinal detachment with retinal break

Rhegmatogenous retinal detachment

Excludes 1: serous retinal detachment (without retinal break) (H33.2-)

H33.00 Unspecified retinal detachment with retinal break

H33.001 Unspecified retinal detachment with retinal break, right eye

H33.002 Unspecified retinal detachment with retinal break, left eye

H33.003 Unspecified retinal detachment with retinal break, bilateral

H33.009 Unspecified retinal detachment with retinal break, unspecified eye

H33.01 Retinal detachment with single break

H33.011 Retinal detachment with single break, right eye

H33.012 Retinal detachment with single break, left eye

H33.013 Retinal detachment with single break, bilateral

H33.019 Retinal detachment with single break, unspecified eye

H33.02 Retinal detachment with multiple breaks

H33.021 Retinal detachment with multiple breaks, right eye

H33.022 Retinal detachment with multiple breaks, left eye

H33.023 Retinal detachment with multiple breaks, bilateral

H33.029 Retinal detachment with multiple breaks, unspecified eye

H33.03 Retinal detachment with giant retinal tear

H33.031 Retinal detachment with giant retinal tear, right eye

H33.032 Retinal detachment with giant retinal tear, left eye

H33.033 Retinal detachment with giant retinal tear, bilateral

H33.039 Retinal detachment with giant retinal tear, unspecified eye

H33.04 Retinal detachment with retinal dialysis

H33.041 Retinal detachment with retinal dialysis, right eye

H33.042 Retinal detachment with retinal dialysis, left eye

H33.043 Retinal detachment with retinal dialysis, bilateral

H33.049 Retinal detachment with retinal dialysis, unspecified eye

H33.05 Total retinal detachment

H33.051 Total retinal detachment, right eye

H33.052 Total retinal detachment, left eye

H33.053 Total retinal detachment, bilateral

H33.059 Total retinal detachment, unspecified eye

H33.1 Retinoschisis and retinal cysts

Excludes 1: congenital retinoschisis (Q14.1)

microcystoid degeneration of retina (H35.42-)

H33.10 Unspecified retinoschisis

H33.101 Unspecified retinoschisis, right eye

H33.102 Unspecified retinoschisis, left eye

H33.103 Unspecified retinoschisis, bilateral

H33.109 Unspecified retinoschisis, unspecified eye

H33.11 Cyst of ora serrata

H33.111 Cyst of ora serrata, right eye

H33.112 Cyst of ora serrata, left eye

H33.113 Cyst of ora serrata, bilateral

H33.119 Cyst of ora serrata, unspecified eye

H33.12 Parasitic cyst of retina

H33.121 Parasitic cyst of retina, right eye

H33.122 Parasitic cyst of retina, left eye

H33.123 Parasitic cyst of retina, bilateral

H33.129 Parasitic cyst of retina, unspecified eye

H33.19 Other retinoschisis and retinal cysts

Pseudocyst of retina

H33.191 Other retinoschisis and retinal cysts, right eye

H33.192 Other retinoschisis and retinal cysts, left eye

H33.193 Other retinoschisis and retinal cysts, bilateral

H33.199 Other retinoschisis and retinal cysts, unspecified eye

H33.2 Serous retinal detachment

Retinal detachment NOS

Retinal detachment without retinal break

Excludes 1: central serous chorioretinopathy (H35.71-)

H33.20 Serous retinal detachment, unspecified eye

H33.21 Serous retinal detachment, right eye

H33.22 Serous retinal detachment, left eye

H33.23 Serous retinal detachment, bilateral

H33.3 Retinal breaks without detachment

Excludes 1: chorioretinal scars after surgery for detachment (H59.81-)

peripheral retinal degeneration without break (H35.4-)

H33.30 Unspecified retinal break

H33.301 Unspecified retinal break, right eye

H33.302 Unspecified retinal break, left eye

H33.303 Unspecified retinal break, bilateral

H33.309 Unspecified retinal break, unspecified eye

H33.31 Horseshoe tear of retina without detachment

Operculum of retina without detachment

H33.311   Horseshoe tear of retina without detachment, right eye

H33.312   Horseshoe tear of retina without detachment, left eye

H33.313   Horseshoe tear of retina without detachment, bilateral

H33.319   Horseshoe tear of retina without detachment, unspecified eye

H33.32   Round hole of retina without detachment

H33.321   Round hole, right eye

H33.322   Round hole, left eye

H33.323   Round hole, bilateral

H33.329   Round hole, unspecified eye

H33.33   Multiple defects of retina without detachment

H33.331   Multiple defects of retina without detachment, right eye

H33.332   Multiple defects of retina without detachment, left eye

H33.333   Multiple defects of retina without detachment, bilateral

H33.339   Multiple defects of retina without detachment, unspecified eye

H33.4   Traction detachment of retina

Proliferative vitreo-retinopathy with retinal detachment

H33.40   Traction detachment of retina, unspecified eye

H33.41   Traction detachment of retina, right eye

H33.42   Traction detachment of retina, left eye

H33.43   Traction detachment of retina, bilateral

H33.8   Other retinal detachments

H34   Retinal vascular occlusions

Excludes 1: amaurosis fugax (G45.3)

H34.0   Transient retinal artery occlusion

H34.00   Transient retinal artery occlusion, unspecified eye

H34.01   Transient retinal artery occlusion, right eye

H34.02   Transient retinal artery occlusion, left eye

H34.03   Transient retinal artery occlusion, bilateral

H34.1   Central retinal artery occlusion

H34.10   Central retinal artery occlusion, unspecified eye

H34.11   Central retinal artery occlusion, right eye

H34.12   Central retinal artery occlusion, left eye

H34.13   Central retinal artery occlusion, bilateral

H34.2   Other retinal artery occlusions

H34.21   Partial retinal artery occlusion

Hollenhorst's plaque

Retinal microembolism

H34.211   Partial retinal artery occlusion, right eye

H34.212   Partial retinal artery occlusion, left eye

H34.213   Partial retinal artery occlusion, bilateral

H34.219   Partial retinal artery occlusion, unspecified eye

H34.23   Retinal artery branch occlusion

H34.231   Retinal artery branch occlusion, right eye

H34.232   Retinal artery branch occlusion, left eye

H34.233   Retinal artery branch occlusion, bilateral

H34.239   Retinal artery branch occlusion, unspecified eye

H34.8   Other retinal vascular occlusions

H34.81   Central retinal vein occlusion

H34.811   Central retinal vein occlusion, right eye

H34.812   Central retinal vein occlusion, left eye

H34.813   Central retinal vein occlusion, bilateral

H34.819   Central retinal vein occlusion, unspecified eye

H34.82   Venous engorgement

Incipient retinal vein occlusion

Partial retinal vein occlusion

H34.821   Venous engorgement, right eye

H34.822   Venous engorgement, left eye

H34.823   Venous engorgement, bilateral

H34.829   Venous engorgement, unspecified eye

H34.83   Tributary (branch) retinal vein occlusion

H34.831   Tributary (branch) retinal vein occlusion, right eye

H34.832   Tributary (branch) retinal vein occlusion, left eye

H34.833   Tributary (branch) retinal vein occlusion, bilateral

H34.839   Tributary (branch) retinal vein occlusion, unspecified eye

H34.9   Unspecified retinal vascular occlusion

H35   Other retinal disorders

Excludes 2: diabetic retinal disorders (E08.311- E08.359, E09.311- E09.359, E10.311- E10.359, E11.311- E11.359, E13.311- E13.359)

H35.0   Background retinopathy and retinal vascular changes

Code also any associated hypertension (I10-)

H35.00   Unspecified background retinopathy

H35.01   Changes in retinal vascular appearance

Retinal vascular sheathing

H35.011   Changes in retinal vascular appearance, right eye

H35.012   Changes in retinal vascular appearance, left eye

H35.013   Changes in retinal vascular appearance, bilateral

H35.019   Changes in retinal vascular appearance, unspecified eye

H35.02   Exudative retinopathy

Coats retinopathy

H35.021   Exudative retinopathy, right eye

H35.022   Exudative retinopathy, left eye

H35.023   Exudative retinopathy, bilateral

H35.029   Exudative retinopathy, unspecified eye

H35.03   Hypertensive retinopathy

H35.031   Hypertensive retinopathy, right eye

H35.032   Hypertensive retinopathy, left eye

H35.033   Hypertensive retinopathy, bilateral

H35.039   Hypertensive retinopathy, unspecified eye

H35.04   Retinal micro-aneurysms, unspecified

H35.041   Retinal micro-aneurysms, unspecified, right eye

H35.042   Retinal micro-aneurysms, unspecified, left eye

H35.043 Retinal micro-aneurysms, unspecified, bilateral

H35.049 Retinal micro-aneurysms, unspecified, unspecified eye

H35.05 Retinal neovascularization, unspecified

H35.051 Retinal neovascularization, unspecified, right eye

H35.052 Retinal neovascularization, unspecified, left eye

H35.053 Retinal neovascularization, unspecified, bilateral

H35.059 Retinal neovascularization, unspecified, unspecified eye

H35.06 Retinal vasculitis

Eales disease

Retinal perivasculitis

H35.061 Retinal vasculitis, right eye

H35.062 Retinal vasculitis, left eye

H35.063 Retinal vasculitis, bilateral

H35.069 Retinal vasculitis, unspecified eye

H35.07 Retinal telangiectasis

H35.071 Retinal telangiectasis, right eye

H35.072 Retinal telangiectasis, left eye

H35.073 Retinal telangiectasis, bilateral

H35.079 Retinal telangiectasis, unspecified eye

H35.09 Other intraretinal microvascular abnormalities

Retinal varices

H35.1 Retinopathy of prematurity

H35.10 Retinopathy of prematurity, unspecified

Retinopathy of prematurity NOS

H35.101 Retinopathy of prematurity, unspecified, right eye

H35.102 Retinopathy of prematurity, unspecified, left eye

H35.103 Retinopathy of prematurity, unspecified, bilateral

H35.109 Retinopathy of prematurity, unspecified, unspecified eye

H35.11 Retinopathy of prematurity, stage 0

H35.111 Retinopathy of prematurity, stage 0, right eye

H35.112 Retinopathy of prematurity, stage 0, left eye

H35.113 Retinopathy of prematurity, stage 0, bilateral

H35.119 Retinopathy of prematurity, stage 0, unspecified eye

H35.12 Retinopathy of prematurity, stage 1

H35.121 Retinopathy of prematurity, stage 1, right eye

H35.122 Retinopathy of prematurity, stage 1, left eye

H35.123 Retinopathy of prematurity, stage 1, bilateral

H35.129 Retinopathy of prematurity, stage 1, unspecified eye

H35.13 Retinopathy of prematurity, stage 2

H35.131 Retinopathy of prematurity, stage 2, right eye

H35.132 Retinopathy of prematurity, stage 2, left eye

H35.133 Retinopathy of prematurity, stage 2, bilateral

H35.139 Retinopathy of prematurity, stage 2, unspecified eye

H35.14 Retinopathy of prematurity, stage 3

H35.141 Retinopathy of prematurity, stage 3, right eye

H35.142 Retinopathy of prematurity, stage 3, left eye

H35.143 Retinopathy of prematurity, stage 3, bilateral

H35.149 Retinopathy of prematurity, stage 3, unspecified eye

H35.15 Retinopathy of prematurity, stage 4

H35.151 Retinopathy of prematurity, stage 4, right eye

H35.152 Retinopathy of prematurity, stage 4, left eye

H35.153 Retinopathy of prematurity, stage 4, bilateral

H35.159 Retinopathy of prematurity, stage 4, unspecified eye

H35.16 Retinopathy of prematurity, stage 5

H35.161 Retinopathy of prematurity, stage 5, right eye

H35.162 Retinopathy of prematurity, stage 5, left eye

H35.163 Retinopathy of prematurity, stage 5, bilateral

H35.169 Retinopathy of prematurity, stage 5, unspecified eye

H35.17 Retrolental fibroplasia

H35.171 Retrolental fibroplasia, right eye

H35.172 Retrolental fibroplasia, left eye

H35.173 Retrolental fibroplasia, bilateral

H35.179 Retrolental fibroplasia, unspecified eye

H35.2 Other non-diabetic proliferative retinopathy

Proliferative vitreo-retinopathy

Excludes 1: proliferative vitreo-retinopathy with retinal detachment (H33.4-)

H35.20 Other non-diabetic proliferative retinopathy, unspecified eye

H35.21 Other non-diabetic proliferative retinopathy, right eye

H35.22 Other non-diabetic proliferative retinopathy, left eye

H35.23 Other non-diabetic proliferative retinopathy, bilateral

H35.3 Degeneration of macula and posterior pole

H35.30 Unspecified macular degeneration

Age-related macular degeneration

H35.31 Nonexudative age-related macular degeneration

Atrophic age-related macular degeneration

H35.32 Exudative age-related macular degeneration

H35.33 Angioid streaks of macula

H35.34 Macular cyst, hole, or pseudohole

H35.341 Macular cyst, hole, or pseudohole, right eye

H35.342 Macular cyst, hole, or pseudohole, left eye

H35.343 Macular cyst, hole, or pseudohole, bilateral

H35.349 Macular cyst, hole, or pseudohole, unspecified eye

H35.35 Cystoid macular degeneration

Excludes 1: cystoid macular edema following cataract surgery (H59.03-)

H35.351 Cystoid macular degeneration, right eye

H35.352 Cystoid macular degeneration, left eye

H35.353 Cystoid macular degeneration, bilateral

H35.359 Cystoid macular degeneration, unspecified eye

H35.36 Drusen (degenerative) of macula

H35.361 Drusen (degenerative) of macula, right eye

H35.362 Drusen (degenerative) of macula, left eye

H35.363 Drusen (degenerative) of macula, bilateral

H35.369 Drusen (degenerative) of macula, unspecified eye

H35.37 Puckering of macula

H35.371 Puckering of macula, right eye

H35.372 Puckering of macula, left eye

H35.373 Puckering of macula, bilateral

H35.379 Puckering of macula, unspecified eye

H35.38 Toxic maculopathy

Code first poisoning due to drug or toxin, if applicable (T36-T65 with fifth or sixth character 1-4 or 6)

Use additional code for adverse effect, if applicable, to identify drug (T36-T50 with fifth or sixth character 5)

H35.381 Toxic maculopathy, right eye

H35.382 Toxic maculopathy, left eye

H35.383 Toxic maculopathy, bilateral

H35.389 Toxic maculopathy, unspecified eye

H35.4 Peripheral retinal degeneration

Excludes 1: hereditary retinal degeneration (dystrophy) (H35.5-)

peripheral retinal degeneration with retinal break (H33.3-)

H35.40 Unspecified peripheral retinal degeneration

H35.41 Lattice degeneration of retina

Palisade degeneration of retina

H35.411 Lattice degeneration of retina, right eye

H35.412 Lattice degeneration of retina, left eye

H35.413 Lattice degeneration of retina, bilateral

H35.419 Lattice degeneration of retina, unspecified eye

H35.42 Microcystoid degeneration of retina

H35.421 Microcystoid degeneration of retina, right eye

H35.422 Microcystoid degeneration of retina, left eye

H35.423 Microcystoid degeneration of retina, bilateral

H35.429 Microcystoid degeneration of retina, unspecified eye

H35.43 Paving stone degeneration of retina

H35.431 Paving stone degeneration of retina, right eye

H35.432 Paving stone degeneration of retina, left eye

H35.433 Paving stone degeneration of retina, bilateral

H35.439 Paving stone degeneration of retina, unspecified eye

H35.44 Age-related reticular degeneration of retina

H35.441 Age-related reticular degeneration of retina, right eye

H35.442 Age-related reticular degeneration of retina, left eye

H35.443 Age-related reticular degeneration of retina, bilateral

H35.449 Age-related reticular degeneration of retina, unspecified eye

H35.45 Secondary pigmentary degeneration

H35.451 Secondary pigmentary degeneration, right eye

H35.452 Secondary pigmentary degeneration, left eye

H35.453 Secondary pigmentary degeneration, bilateral

H35.459 Secondary pigmentary degeneration, unspecified eye

H35.46 Secondary vitreoretinal degeneration

H35.461 Secondary vitreoretinal degeneration, right eye

H35.462 Secondary vitreoretinal degeneration, left eye

H35.463 Secondary vitreoretinal degeneration, bilateral

H35.469 Secondary vitreoretinal degeneration, unspecified eye

H35.5 Hereditary retinal dystrophy

Excludes 1: dystrophies primarily involving Bruch's membrane (H31.1-)

H35.50 Unspecified hereditary retinal dystrophy

H35.51 Vitreoretinal dystrophy

H35.52 Pigmentary retinal dystrophy

Albipunctate retinal dystrophy

Retinitis pigmentosa

Tapetoretinal dystrophy

H35.53 Other dystrophies primarily involving the sensory retina

Stargardt's disease

H35.54 Dystrophies primarily involving the retinal pigment epithelium

Vitelliform retinal dystrophy

H35.6 Retinal hemorrhage

H35.60 Retinal hemorrhage, unspecified eye

H35.61 Retinal hemorrhage, right eye

H35.62 Retinal hemorrhage, left eye

H35.63 Retinal hemorrhage, bilateral

H35.7 Separation of retinal layers

Excludes 1: retinal detachment (serous) (H33.2-)

rhegmatogenous retinal detachment (H33.0-)

H35.70 Unspecified separation of retinal layers

H35.71 Central serous chorioretinopathy

H35.711 Central serous chorioretinopathy, right eye

H35.712 Central serous chorioretinopathy, left eye

H35.713 Central serous chorioretinopathy, bilateral

H35.719 Central serous chorioretinopathy, unspecified eye

H35.72 Serous detachment of retinal pigment epithelium

H35.721 Serous detachment of retinal pigment epithelium, right eye

H35.722 Serous detachment of retinal pigment epithelium, left eye

H35.723 Serous detachment of retinal pigment epithelium, bilateral

H35.729 Serous detachment of retinal pigment epithelium, unspecified eye

H35.73 Hemorrhagic detachment of retinal pigment epithelium

H35.731 Hemorrhagic detachment of retinal pigment epithelium, right eye

H35.732 Hemorrhagic detachment of retinal pigment epithelium, left eye

H35.733 Hemorrhagic detachment of retinal pigment epithelium, bilateral

H35.739 Hemorrhagic detachment of retinal pigment epithelium, unspecified eye

H35.8 Other specified retinal disorders

Excludes 2: retinal hemorrhage (H35.6-)

H35.81 Retinal edema

Retinal cotton wool spots

H35.82 Retinal ischemia

H35.89 Other specified retinal disorders

H35.9 Unspecified retinal disorder

H36 Retinal disorders in diseases classified elsewhere

Code first underlying disease, such as:

lipid storage disorders (E75.-)

sickle-cell disorders (D57.-)

Excludes 1: arteriosclerotic retinopathy (H35.0-)

diabetic retinopathy (E08.3-, E09.3-, E10.3-, E11.3-, E13.3-)

GLAUCOMA (H40-H42)

H40 Glaucoma

Excludes 1: absolute glaucoma (H44.51-)

congenital glaucoma (Q15.0)

traumatic glaucoma due to birth injury (P15.3)

H40.0 Glaucoma suspect

H40.00 Preglaucoma, unspecified

H40.001 Preglaucoma, unspecified, right eye

H40.002 Preglaucoma, unspecified, left eye

H40.003 Preglaucoma, unspecified, bilateral

H40.009 Preglaucoma, unspecified, unspecified eye

H40.01 Open angle with borderline findings, low risk

Open angle, low risk

H40.011 Open angle with borderline findings, low risk, right eye

H40.012 Open angle with borderline findings, low risk, left eye

H40.013 Open angle with borderline findings, low risk, bilateral

H40.019 Open angle with borderline findings, low risk, unspecified eye

H40.02 Open angle with borderline findings, high risk

Open angle, high risk

H40.021 Open angle with borderline findings, high risk, right eye

H40.022 Open angle with borderline findings, high risk, left eye

H40.023 Open angle with borderline findings, high risk, bilateral

H40.029 Open angle with borderline findings, high risk, unspecified eye

H40.03 Anatomical narrow angle

Primary angle closure suspect

H40.031 Anatomical narrow angle, right eye

H40.032 Anatomical narrow angle, left eye

H40.033 Anatomical narrow angle, bilateral

H40.039 Anatomical narrow angle, unspecified eye

H40.04 Steroid responder

H40.041 Steroid responder, right eye

H40.042 Steroid responder, left eye

H40.043 Steroid responder, bilateral

H40.049 Steroid responder, unspecified eye

H40.05 Ocular hypertension

H40.051 Ocular hypertension, right eye

H40.052 Ocular hypertension, left eye

H40.053 Ocular hypertension, bilateral

H40.059 Ocular hypertension, unspecified eye

H40.06 Primary angle closure without glaucoma damage

H40.061 Primary angle closure without glaucoma damage, right eye

H40.062 Primary angle closure without glaucoma damage, left eye

H40.063 Primary angle closure without glaucoma damage, bilateral

H40.069 Primary angle closure without glaucoma damage, unspecified eye

H40.1 Open-angle glaucoma

⊗⑦**H40.10** Unspecified open-angle glaucoma

One of the following 7th characters is to be assigned to code H40.10 to designate the stage of glaucoma

0 - stage unspecified

1 - mild stage

2 - moderate stage

3 - severe stage

4 - indeterminate stage

⊗⑦**H40.11** Primary open-angle glaucoma

Chronic simple glaucoma

One of the following 7th characters is to be assigned to code H40.11 to designate the stage of glaucoma

0 - stage unspecified

1 - mild stage

2 - moderate stage

3 - severe stage

4 - indeterminate stage

H40.12 Low-tension glaucoma

One of the following 7th characters is to be assigned to each code in subcategory H40.12 to designate the stage of glaucoma

0 - stage unspecified

1 - mild stage

2 - moderate stage

3 - severe stage

4 - indeterminate stage

⑦**H40.121** Low-tension glaucoma, right eye

⑦**H40.122** Low-tension glaucoma, left eye

⑦**H40.123** Low-tension glaucoma, bilateral

⑦**H40.129** Low-tension glaucoma, unspecified eye

H40.13 Pigmentary glaucoma

One of the following 7th characters is to be assigned to each code in subcategory H40.13 to designate the stage of glaucoma

0 - stage unspecified

1 - mild stage

2 - moderate stage

3 - severe stage

4 - indeterminate stage

⑦**H40.131** Pigmentary glaucoma, right eye

⑦**H40.132** Pigmentary glaucoma, left eye

⑦**H40.133** Pigmentary glaucoma, bilateral

⑦**H40.139** Pigmentary glaucoma, unspecified eye

H40.14 Capsular glaucoma with pseudoexfoliation of lens

One of the following 7th characters is to be assigned to each code in subcategory H40.14 to designate the stage of glaucoma

0 - stage unspecified

1 - mild stage

2 - moderate stage

3 - severe stage

4 - indeterminate stage

⑦**H40.141** Capsular glaucoma with pseudoexfoliation of lens, right eye

⑦**H40.142** Capsular glaucoma with pseudoexfoliation of lens, left eye

⑦**H40.143** Capsular glaucoma with pseudoexfoliation of lens, bilateral

⑦**H40.149** Capsular glaucoma with pseudoexfoliation of lens, unspecified eye

H40.15 Residual stage of open-angle glaucoma

H40.151 Residual stage of open-angle glaucoma, right eye

H40.152 Residual stage of open-angle glaucoma, left eye

H40.153 Residual stage of open-angle glaucoma, bilateral

H40.159 Residual stage of open-angle glaucoma, unspecified eye

H40.2 Primary angle-closure glaucoma

Excludes 1: aqueous misdirection (H40.83-)

malignant glaucoma (H40.83-)

⊗⑦**H40.20** Unspecified primary angle-closure glaucoma

One of the following 7th characters is to be assigned to code H40.20 to designate the stage of glaucoma

0 - stage unspecified

1 - mild stage

2 - moderate stage

3 - severe stage

4 - indeterminate stage

H40.21 Acute angle-closure glaucoma

Acute angle-closure glaucoma attack

Acute angle-closure glaucoma crisis

H40.211 Acute angle-closure glaucoma, right eye

H40.212 Acute angle-closure glaucoma, left eye

H40.213 Acute angle-closure glaucoma, bilateral

H40.219 Acute angle-closure glaucoma, unspecified eye

H40.22 Chronic angle-closure glaucoma

Chronic primary angle closure glaucoma

One of the following 7th characters is to be assigned to each code in subcategory H40.22 to designate the stage of glaucoma

0 - stage unspecified

1 - mild stage

2 - moderate stage

3 - severe stage

4 - indeterminate stage

⑦**H40.221** Chronic angle-closure glaucoma, right eye

⑦**H40.222** Chronic angle-closure glaucoma, left eye

⑦**H40.223** Chronic angle-closure glaucoma, bilateral

⑦**H40.229** Chronic angle-closure glaucoma, unspecified eye

H40.23 Intermittent angle-closure glaucoma

H40.231 Intermittent angle-closure glaucoma, right eye

H40.232 Intermittent angle-closure glaucoma, left eye

H40.233 Intermittent angle-closure glaucoma, bilateral

H40.239 Intermittent angle-closure glaucoma, unspecified eye

H40.24 Residual stage of angle-closure glaucoma

H40.241 Residual stage of angle-closure glaucoma, right eye

H40.242 Residual stage of angle-closure glaucoma, left eye

H40.243 Residual stage of angle-closure glaucoma, bilateral

H40.249 Residual stage of angle-closure glaucoma, unspecified eye

H40.3 Glaucoma secondary to eye trauma

Code also underlying condition

One of the following 7th characters is to be assigned to each code in subcategory H40.3 to designate the stage of glaucoma

0 - stage unspecified

1 - mild stage

2 - moderate stage

3 - severe stage

4 - indeterminate stage

⊗⑦**H40.30** Glaucoma secondary to eye trauma, unspecified eye

⊗⑦**H40.31** Glaucoma secondary to eye trauma, right eye

⊗⑦**H40.32** Glaucoma secondary to eye trauma, left eye

⊗⑦**H40.33** Glaucoma secondary to eye trauma, bilateral

H40.4 Glaucoma secondary to eye inflammation

Code also underlying condition

One of the following 7th characters is to be assigned to each code in subcategory H40.4 to designate the stage of glaucoma

0 - stage unspecified
1 - mild stage
2 - moderate stage
3 - severe stage
4 - indeterminate stage

⊗ ⑦ **H40.40** Glaucoma secondary to eye inflammation, unspecified eye

⊗ ⑦ **H40.41** Glaucoma secondary to eye inflammation, right eye

⊗ ⑦ **H40.42** Glaucoma secondary to eye inflammation, left eye

⊗ ⑦ **H40.43** Glaucoma secondary to eye inflammation, bilateral

H40.5 Glaucoma secondary to other eye disorders
Code also underlying eye disorder
One of the following 7th characters is to be assigned to each code in subcategory H40.5 to designate the stage of glaucoma
0 - stage unspecified
1 - mild stage
2 - moderate stage
3 - severe stage
4 - indeterminate stage

⊗ ⑦ **H40.50** Glaucoma secondary to other eye disorders, unspecified eye

⊗ ⑦ **H40.51** Glaucoma secondary to other eye disorders, right eye

⊗ ⑦ **H40.52** Glaucoma secondary to other eye disorders, left eye

⊗ ⑦ **H40.53** Glaucoma secondary to other eye disorders, bilateral

H40.6 Glaucoma secondary to drugs
Use additional code for adverse effect, if applicable, to identify drug (T36-T50 with fifth or sixth character 5)
One of the following 7th characters is to be assigned to each code in subcategory H40.6 to designate the stage of glaucoma
0 - stage unspecified
1 - mild stage
2 - moderate stage
3 - severe stage
4 - indeterminate stage

⊗ ⑦ **H40.60** Glaucoma secondary to drugs, unspecified eye

⊗ ⑦ **H40.61** Glaucoma secondary to drugs, right eye

⊗ ⑦ **H40.62** Glaucoma secondary to drugs, left eye

⊗ ⑦ **H40.63** Glaucoma secondary to drugs, bilateral

H40.8 Other glaucoma

H40.81 Glaucoma with increased episcleral venous pressure

H40.811 Glaucoma with increased episcleral venous pressure, right eye

H40.812 Glaucoma with increased episcleral venous pressure, left eye

H40.813 Glaucoma with increased episcleral venous pressure, bilateral

H40.819 Glaucoma with increased episcleral venous pressure, unspecified eye

H40.82 Hypersecretion glaucoma

H40.821 Hypersecretion glaucoma, right eye

H40.822 Hypersecretion glaucoma, left eye

H40.823 Hypersecretion glaucoma, bilateral

H40.829 Hypersecretion glaucoma, unspecified eye

H40.83 Aqueous misdirection
Malignant glaucoma

H40.831 Aqueous misdirection, right eye

H40.832 Aqueous misdirection, left eye

H40.833 Aqueous misdirection, bilateral

H40.839 Aqueous misdirection, unspecified eye

H40.89 Other specified glaucoma

H40.9 Unspecified glaucoma

H42 Glaucoma in diseases classified elsewhere
Code first underlying condition, such as:
amyloidosis (E85-)
aniridia (Q13.1)
Lowe's syndrome (E72.03)
Reiger's anomaly (Q13.81)
specified metabolic disorder (E70-E88)
Excludes 1: glaucoma (in):
    diabetes mellitus (E08.39, E09.39, E10.39, E11.39, E13.39)
    onchocerciasis (B73.02)
    syphilis (A52.71)
    tuberculous (A18.59)

DISORDERS OF VITREOUS BODY AND GLOBE (H43-H44)

H43 Disorders of vitreous body

H43.0 Vitreous prolapse
Excludes 1: vitreous syndrome following cataract surgery (H59.0-)
    traumatic vitreous prolapse (S05.2-)

H43.00 Vitreous prolapse, unspecified eye

H43.01 Vitreous prolapse, right eye

H43.02 Vitreous prolapse, left eye

H43.03 Vitreous prolapse, bilateral

H43.1 Vitreous hemorrhage

H43.10 Vitreous hemorrhage, unspecified eye

H43.11 Vitreous hemorrhage, right eye

H43.12 Vitreous hemorrhage, left eye

H43.13 Vitreous hemorrhage, bilateral

H43.2 Crystalline deposits in vitreous body

H43.20 Crystalline deposits in vitreous body, unspecified eye

H43.21 Crystalline deposits in vitreous body, right eye

H43.22 Crystalline deposits in vitreous body, left eye

H43.23 Crystalline deposits in vitreous body, bilateral

H43.3 Other vitreous opacities

H43.31 Vitreous membranes and strands

H43.311 Vitreous membranes and strands, right eye

H43.312 Vitreous membranes and strands, left eye

H43.313 Vitreous membranes and strands, bilateral

H43.319 Vitreous membranes and strands, unspecified eye

H43.39 Other vitreous opacities
Vitreous floaters

H43.391 Other vitreous opacities, right eye

H43.392 Other vitreous opacities, left eye

H43.393 Other vitreous opacities, bilateral

H43.399 Other vitreous opacities, unspecified eye

H43.8 Other disorders of vitreous body

Excludes 1: proliferative vitreo-retinopathy with retinal detachment (H33.4-)

Excludes 2: vitreous abscess (H44.02-)

H43.81 Vitreous degeneration
Vitreous detachment
- H43.811 Vitreous degeneration, right eye
- H43.812 Vitreous degeneration, left eye
- H43.813 Vitreous degeneration, bilateral
- H43.819 Vitreous degeneration, unspecified eye

H43.82 Vitreomacular adhesion
Vitreomacular traction
- H43.821 Vitreomacular adhesion, right eye
- H43.822 Vitreomacular adhesion, left eye
- H43.823 Vitreomacular adhesion, bilateral
- H43.829 Vitreomacular adhesion, unspecified eye

H43.89 Other disorders of vitreous body

H43.9 Unspecified disorder of vitreous body

H44 Disorders of globe

Includes: disorders affecting multiple structures of eye

H44.0 Purulent endophthalmitis
Use additional code to identify organism

Excludes 1: bleb associated endophthalmitis (H59.4-)

H44.00 Unspecified purulent endophthalmitis
- H44.001 Unspecified purulent endophthalmitis, right eye
- H44.002 Unspecified purulent endophthalmitis, left eye
- H44.003 Unspecified purulent endophthalmitis, bilateral
- H44.009 Unspecified purulent endophthalmitis, unspecified eye

H44.01 Panophthalmitis (acute)
- H44.011 Panophthalmitis (acute), right eye
- H44.012 Panophthalmitis (acute), left eye
- H44.013 Panophthalmitis (acute), bilateral
- H44.019 Panophthalmitis (acute), unspecified eye

H44.02 Vitreous abscess (chronic)
- H44.021 Vitreous abscess (chronic), right eye
- H44.022 Vitreous abscess (chronic), left eye
- H44.023 Vitreous abscess (chronic), bilateral
- H44.029 Vitreous abscess (chronic), unspecified eye

H44.1 Other endophthalmitis

Excludes 1: bleb associated endophthalmitis (H59.4-)

Excludes 2: ophthalmia nodosa (H16.2-)

H44.11 Panuveitis
- H44.111 Panuveitis, right eye
- H44.112 Panuveitis, left eye
- H44.113 Panuveitis, bilateral
- H44.119 Panuveitis, unspecified eye

H44.12 Parasitic endophthalmitis, unspecified
- H44.121 Parasitic endophthalmitis, unspecified, right eye
- H44.122 Parasitic endophthalmitis, unspecified, left eye
- H44.123 Parasitic endophthalmitis, unspecified, bilateral

H44.129 Parasitic endophthalmitis, unspecified, unspecified eye

H44.13 Sympathetic uveitis
- H44.131 Sympathetic uveitis, right eye
- H44.132 Sympathetic uveitis, left eye
- H44.133 Sympathetic uveitis, bilateral
- H44.139 Sympathetic uveitis, unspecified eye

H44.19 Other endophthalmitis

H44.2 Degenerative myopia
Malignant myopia
- H44.20 Degenerative myopia, unspecified eye
- H44.21 Degenerative myopia, right eye
- H44.22 Degenerative myopia, left eye
- H44.23 Degenerative myopia, bilateral

H44.3 Other and unspecified degenerative disorders of globe
- H44.30 Unspecified degenerative disorder of globe

H44.31 Chalcosis
- H44.311 Chalcosis, right eye
- H44.312 Chalcosis, left eye
- H44.313 Chalcosis, bilateral
- H44.319 Chalcosis, unspecified eye

H44.32 Siderosis of eye
- H44.321 Siderosis of eye, right eye
- H44.322 Siderosis of eye, left eye
- H44.323 Siderosis of eye, bilateral
- H44.329 Siderosis of eye, unspecified eye

H44.39 Other degenerative disorders of globe
- H44.391 Other degenerative disorders of globe, right eye
- H44.392 Other degenerative disorders of globe, left eye
- H44.393 Other degenerative disorders of globe, bilateral
- H44.399 Other degenerative disorders of globe, unspecified eye

H44.4 Hypotony of eye
- H44.40 Unspecified hypotony of eye

H44.41 Flat anterior chamber hypotony of eye
- H44.411 Flat anterior chamber hypotony of right eye
- H44.412 Flat anterior chamber hypotony of left eye
- H44.413 Flat anterior chamber hypotony of eye, bilateral
- H44.419 Flat anterior chamber hypotony of unspecified eye

H44.42 Hypotony of eye due to ocular fistula
- H44.421 Hypotony of right eye due to ocular fistula
- H44.422 Hypotony of left eye due to ocular fistula
- H44.423 Hypotony of eye due to ocular fistula, bilateral
- H44.429 Hypotony of unspecified eye due to ocular fistula

H44.43 Hypotony of eye due to other ocular disorders
- H44.431 Hypotony of eye due to other ocular disorders, right eye
- H44.432 Hypotony of eye due to other ocular disorders, left eye
- H44.433 Hypotony of eye due to other ocular disorders, bilateral

H44.439 Hypotony of eye due to other ocular disorders, unspecified eye

H44.44 Primary hypotony of eye

    H44.441 Primary hypotony of right eye

    H44.442 Primary hypotony of left eye

    H44.443 Primary hypotony of eye, bilateral

    H44.449 Primary hypotony of unspecified eye

H44.5 Degenerated conditions of globe

  H44.50 Unspecified degenerated conditions of globe

  H44.51 Absolute glaucoma

    H44.511 Absolute glaucoma, right eye

    H44.512 Absolute glaucoma, left eye

    H44.513 Absolute glaucoma, bilateral

    H44.519 Absolute glaucoma, unspecified eye

  H44.52 Atrophy of globe

    Phthisis bulbi

    H44.521 Atrophy of globe, right eye

    H44.522 Atrophy of globe, left eye

    H44.523 Atrophy of globe, bilateral

    H44.529 Atrophy of globe, unspecified eye

  H44.53 Leucocoria

    H44.531 Leucocoria, right eye

    H44.532 Leucocoria, left eye

    H44.533 Leucocoria, bilateral

    H44.539 Leucocoria, unspecified eye

H44.6 Retained (old) intraocular foreign body, magnetic

Use additional code to identify magnetic foreign body (Z18.11)

Excludes 1: current intraocular foreign body (S05.-)

Excludes 2: retained foreign body in eyelid (H02.81-)

    retained (old) foreign body following penetrating wound of orbit (H05.5-)

    retained (old) intraocular foreign body, nonmagnetic (H44.7-)

  H44.60 Unspecified retained (old) intraocular foreign body, magnetic

    H44.601 Unspecified retained (old) intraocular foreign body, magnetic, right eye

    H44.602 Unspecified retained (old) intraocular foreign body, magnetic, left eye

    H44.603 Unspecified retained (old) intraocular foreign body, magnetic, bilateral

    H44.609 Unspecified retained (old) intraocular foreign body, magnetic, unspecified eye

  H44.61 Retained (old) magnetic foreign body in anterior chamber

    H44.611 Retained (old) magnetic foreign body in anterior chamber, right eye

    H44.612 Retained (old) magnetic foreign body in anterior chamber, left eye

    H44.613 Retained (old) magnetic foreign body in anterior chamber, bilateral

    H44.619 Retained (old) magnetic foreign body in anterior chamber, unspecified eye

  H44.62 Retained (old) magnetic foreign body in iris or ciliary body

    H44.621 Retained (old) magnetic foreign body in iris or ciliary body, right eye

    H44.622 Retained (old) magnetic foreign body in iris or ciliary body, left eye

    H44.623 Retained (old) magnetic foreign body in iris or ciliary body, bilateral

    H44.629 Retained (old) magnetic foreign body in iris or ciliary body, unspecified eye

  H44.63 Retained (old) magnetic foreign body in lens

    H44.631 Retained (old) magnetic foreign body in lens, right eye

    H44.632 Retained (old) magnetic foreign body in lens, left eye

    H44.633 Retained (old) magnetic foreign body in lens, bilateral

    H44.639 Retained (old) magnetic foreign body in lens, unspecified eye

  H44.64 Retained (old) magnetic foreign body in posterior wall of globe

    H44.641 Retained (old) magnetic foreign body in posterior wall of globe, right eye

    H44.642 Retained (old) magnetic foreign body in posterior wall of globe, left eye

    H44.643 Retained (old) magnetic foreign body in posterior wall of globe, bilateral

    H44.649 Retained (old) magnetic foreign body in posterior wall of globe, unspecified eye

  H44.65 Retained (old) magnetic foreign body in vitreous body

    H44.651 Retained (old) magnetic foreign body in vitreous body, right eye

    H44.652 Retained (old) magnetic foreign body in vitreous body, left eye

    H44.653 Retained (old) magnetic foreign body in vitreous body, bilateral

    H44.659 Retained (old) magnetic foreign body in vitreous body, unspecified eye

  H44.69 Retained (old) intraocular foreign body, magnetic, in other or multiple sites

    H44.691 Retained (old) intraocular foreign body, magnetic, in other or multiple sites, right eye

    H44.692 Retained (old) intraocular foreign body, magnetic, in other or multiple sites, left eye

    H44.693 Retained (old) intraocular foreign body, magnetic, in other or multiple sites, bilateral

    H44.699 Retained (old) intraocular foreign body, magnetic, in other or multiple sites, unspecified eye

H44.7 Retained (old) intraocular foreign body, nonmagnetic

Use additional code to identify nonmagnetic foreign body (Z18.01-Z18.10, Z18.12, Z18.2-Z18.9)

Excludes 1: current intraocular foreign body (S05.-)

Excludes 2: retained foreign body in eyelid (H02.81-)

    retained (old) foreign body following penetrating wound of orbit (H05.5-)

    retained (old) intraocular foreign body, magnetic (H44.6-)

  H44.70 Unspecified retained (old) intraocular foreign body, nonmagnetic

    H44.701 Unspecified retained (old) intraocular foreign body, nonmagnetic, right eye

    H44.702 Unspecified retained (old) intraocular foreign body, nonmagnetic, left eye

    H44.703 Unspecified retained (old) intraocular foreign body, nonmagnetic, bilateral

● New code   ▲ Revised code   ⑦ 7th digit required   ⊗ Placeholder required

H44.709 Unspecified retained (old) intraocular foreign body, nonmagnetic, unspecified eye

Retained (old) intraocular foreign body NOS

H44.71 Retained (nonmagnetic) (old) foreign body in anterior chamber

H44.711 Retained (nonmagnetic) (old) foreign body in anterior chamber, right eye

H44.712 Retained (nonmagnetic) (old) foreign body in anterior chamber, left eye

H44.713 Retained (nonmagnetic) (old) foreign body in anterior chamber, bilateral

H44.719 Retained (nonmagnetic) (old) foreign body in anterior chamber, unspecified eye

H44.72 Retained (nonmagnetic) (old) foreign body in iris or ciliary body

H44.721 Retained (nonmagnetic) (old) foreign body in iris or ciliary body, right eye

H44.722 Retained (nonmagnetic) (old) foreign body in iris or ciliary body, left eye

H44.723 Retained (nonmagnetic) (old) foreign body in iris or ciliary body, bilateral

H44.729 Retained (nonmagnetic) (old) foreign body in iris or ciliary body, unspecified eye

H44.73 Retained (nonmagnetic) (old) foreign body in lens

H44.731 Retained (nonmagnetic) (old) foreign body in lens, right eye

H44.732 Retained (nonmagnetic) (old) foreign body in lens, left eye

H44.733 Retained (nonmagnetic) (old) foreign body in lens, bilateral

H44.739 Retained (nonmagnetic) (old) foreign body in lens, unspecified eye

H44.74 Retained (nonmagnetic) (old) foreign body in posterior wall of globe

H44.741 Retained (nonmagnetic) (old) foreign body in posterior wall of globe, right eye

H44.742 Retained (nonmagnetic) (old) foreign body in posterior wall of globe, left eye

H44.743 Retained (nonmagnetic) (old) foreign body in posterior wall of globe, bilateral

H44.749 Retained (nonmagnetic) (old) foreign body in posterior wall of globe, unspecified eye

H44.75 Retained (nonmagnetic) (old) foreign body in vitreous body

H44.751 Retained (nonmagnetic) (old) foreign body in vitreous body, right eye

H44.752 Retained (nonmagnetic) (old) foreign body in vitreous body, left eye

H44.753 Retained (nonmagnetic) (old) foreign body in vitreous body, bilateral

H44.759 Retained (nonmagnetic) (old) foreign body in vitreous body, unspecified eye

H44.79 Retained (old) intraocular foreign body, nonmagnetic, in other or multiple sites

H44.791 Retained (old) intraocular foreign body, nonmagnetic, in other or multiple sites, right eye

H44.792 Retained (old) intraocular foreign body, nonmagnetic, in other or multiple sites, left eye

H44.793 Retained (old) intraocular foreign body, nonmagnetic, in other or multiple sites, bilateral

H44.799 Retained (old) intraocular foreign body, nonmagnetic, in other or multiple sites, unspecified eye

H44.8 Other disorders of globe

H44.81 Hemophthalmos

H44.811 Hemophthalmos, right eye

H44.812 Hemophthalmos, left eye

H44.813 Hemophthalmos, bilateral

H44.819 Hemophthalmos, unspecified eye

H44.82 Luxation of globe

H44.821 Luxation of globe, right eye

H44.822 Luxation of globe, left eye

H44.823 Luxation of globe, bilateral

H44.829 Luxation of globe, unspecified eye

H44.89 Other disorders of globe

H44.9 Unspecified disorder of globe

DISORDERS OF OPTIC NERVE AND VISUAL PATHWAYS (H46-H47)

H46 Optic neuritis

Excludes 2: ischemic optic neuropathy (H47.01-)
neuromyelitis optica [Devic] (G36.0)

H46.0 Optic papillitis

H46.00 Optic papillitis, unspecified eye

H46.01 Optic papillitis, right eye

H46.02 Optic papillitis, left eye

H46.03 Optic papillitis, bilateral

H46.1 Retrobulbar neuritis

Retrobulbar neuritis NOS

Excludes 1: syphilitic retrobulbar neuritis (A52.15)

H46.10 Retrobulbar neuritis, unspecified eye

H46.11 Retrobulbar neuritis, right eye

H46.12 Retrobulbar neuritis, left eye

H46.13 Retrobulbar neuritis, bilateral

H46.2 Nutritional optic neuropathy

H46.3 Toxic optic neuropathy

Code first (T51-T65) to identify cause

H46.8 Other optic neuritis

H46.9 Unspecified optic neuritis

H47 Other disorders of optic [2nd] nerve and visual pathways

H47.0 Disorders of optic nerve, not elsewhere classified

H47.01 Ischemic optic neuropathy

H47.011 Ischemic optic neuropathy, right eye

H47.012 Ischemic optic neuropathy, left eye

H47.013 Ischemic optic neuropathy, bilateral

H47.019 Ischemic optic neuropathy, unspecified eye

H47.02 Hemorrhage in optic nerve sheath

H47.021 Hemorrhage in optic nerve sheath, right eye

H47.022 Hemorrhage in optic nerve sheath, left eye

H47.023 Hemorrhage in optic nerve sheath, bilateral

H47.029   Hemorrhage in optic nerve sheath, unspecified eye

H47.03   Optic nerve hypoplasia
H47.031   Optic nerve hypoplasia, right eye
H47.032   Optic nerve hypoplasia, left eye
H47.033   Optic nerve hypoplasia, bilateral
H47.039   Optic nerve hypoplasia, unspecified eye

H47.09   Other disorders of optic nerve, not elsewhere classified
Compression of optic nerve
H47.091   Other disorders of optic nerve, not elsewhere classified, right eye
H47.092   Other disorders of optic nerve, not elsewhere classified, left eye
H47.093   Other disorders of optic nerve, not elsewhere classified, bilateral
H47.099   Other disorders of optic nerve, not elsewhere classified, unspecified eye

H47.1   Papilledema
H47.10   Unspecified papilledema
H47.11   Papilledema associated with increased intracranial pressure
H47.12   Papilledema associated with decreased ocular pressure
H47.13   Papilledema associated with retinal disorder
H47.14   Foster-Kennedy syndrome
H47.141   Foster-Kennedy syndrome, right eye
H47.142   Foster-Kennedy syndrome, left eye
H47.143   Foster-Kennedy syndrome, bilateral
H47.149   Foster-Kennedy syndrome, unspecified eye

H47.2   Optic atrophy
H47.20   Unspecified optic atrophy
H47.21   Primary optic atrophy
H47.211   Primary optic atrophy, right eye
H47.212   Primary optic atrophy, left eye
H47.213   Primary optic atrophy, bilateral
H47.219   Primary optic atrophy, unspecified eye
H47.22   Hereditary optic atrophy
Leber's optic atrophy
H47.23   Glaucomatous optic atrophy
H47.231   Glaucomatous optic atrophy, right eye
H47.232   Glaucomatous optic atrophy, left eye
H47.233   Glaucomatous optic atrophy, bilateral
H47.239   Glaucomatous optic atrophy, unspecified eye
H47.29   Other optic atrophy
Temporal pallor of optic disc
H47.291   Other optic atrophy, right eye
H47.292   Other optic atrophy, left eye
H47.293   Other optic atrophy, bilateral
H47.299   Other optic atrophy, unspecified eye

H47.3   Other disorders of optic disc
H47.31   Coloboma of optic disc
H47.311   Coloboma of optic disc, right eye
H47.312   Coloboma of optic disc, left eye
H47.313   Coloboma of optic disc, bilateral
H47.319   Coloboma of optic disc, unspecified eye
H47.32   Drusen of optic disc

H47.321   Drusen of optic disc, right eye
H47.322   Drusen of optic disc, left eye
H47.323   Drusen of optic disc, bilateral
H47.329   Drusen of optic disc, unspecified eye
H47.33   Pseudopapilledema of optic disc
H47.331   Pseudopapilledema of optic disc, right eye
H47.332   Pseudopapilledema of optic disc, left eye
H47.333   Pseudopapilledema of optic disc, bilateral
H47.339   Pseudopapilledema of optic disc, unspecified eye
H47.39   Other disorders of optic disc
H47.391   Other disorders of optic disc, right eye
H47.392   Other disorders of optic disc, left eye
H47.393   Other disorders of optic disc, bilateral
H47.399   Other disorders of optic disc, unspecified eye

H47.4   Disorders of optic chiasm
Code also underlying condition
H47.41   Disorders of optic chiasm in (due to) inflammatory disorders
H47.42   Disorders of optic chiasm in (due to) neoplasm
H47.43   Disorders of optic chiasm in (due to) vascular disorders
H47.49   Disorders of optic chiasm in (due to) other disorders

H47.5   Disorders of other visual pathways
Disorders of optic tracts, geniculate nuclei and optic radiations
Code also underlying condition
H47.51   Disorders of visual pathways in (due to) inflammatory disorders
H47.511   Disorders of visual pathways in (due to) inflammatory disorders, right side
H47.512   Disorders of visual pathways in (due to) inflammatory disorders, left side
H47.519   Disorders of visual pathways in (due to) inflammatory disorders, unspecified side
H47.52   Disorders of visual pathways in (due to) neoplasm
H47.521   Disorders of visual pathways in (due to) neoplasm, right side
H47.522   Disorders of visual pathways in (due to) neoplasm, left side
H47.529   Disorders of visual pathways in (due to) neoplasm, unspecified side
H47.53   Disorders of visual pathways in (due to) vascular disorders
H47.531   Disorders of visual pathways in (due to) vascular disorders, right side
H47.532   Disorders of visual pathways in (due to) vascular disorders, left side
H47.539   Disorders of visual pathways in (due to) vascular disorders, unspecified side

H47.6   Disorders of visual cortex
Code also underlying condition
Excludes 1: injury to visual cortex S04.04
H47.61   Cortical blindness
H47.611   Cortical blindness, right side of brain

● New code   ▲ Revised code   ⑦ 7th digit required   ⊗ Placeholder required

H47.612 Cortical blindness, left side of brain
H47.619 Cortical blindness, unspecified side of brain
H47.62 Disorders of visual cortex in (due to) inflammatory disorders
H47.621 Disorders of visual cortex in (due to) inflammatory disorders, right side of brain
H47.622 Disorders of visual cortex in (due to) inflammatory disorders, left side of brain
H47.629 Disorders of visual cortex in (due to) inflammatory disorders, unspecified side of brain
H47.63 Disorders of visual cortex in (due to) neoplasm
H47.631 Disorders of visual cortex in (due to) neoplasm, right side of brain
H47.632 Disorders of visual cortex in (due to) neoplasm, left side of brain
H47.639 Disorders of visual cortex in (due to) neoplasm, unspecified side of brain
H47.64 Disorders of visual cortex in (due to) vascular disorders
H47.641 Disorders of visual cortex in (due to) vascular disorders, right side of brain
H47.642 Disorders of visual cortex in (due to) vascular disorders, left side of brain
H47.649 Disorders of visual cortex in (due to) vascular disorders, unspecified side of brain
H47.9 Unspecified disorder of visual pathways

DISORDERS OF OCULAR MUSCLES, BINOCULAR MOVEMENT, ACCOMMODATION AND REFRACTION (H49-H52)

Excludes 2: nystagmus and other irregular eye movements (H55)

H49 Paralytic strabismus
Excludes 2: internal ophthalmoplegia (H52.51-)
internuclear ophthalmoplegia (H51.2-)
progressive supranuclear ophthalmoplegia (G23.1)
H49.0 Third [oculomotor] nerve palsy
H49.00 Third [oculomotor] nerve palsy, unspecified eye
H49.01 Third [oculomotor] nerve palsy, right eye
H49.02 Third [oculomotor] nerve palsy, left eye
H49.03 Third [oculomotor] nerve palsy, bilateral
H49.1 Fourth [trochlear] nerve palsy
H49.10 Fourth [trochlear] nerve palsy, unspecified eye
H49.11 Fourth [trochlear] nerve palsy, right eye
H49.12 Fourth [trochlear] nerve palsy, left eye
H49.13 Fourth [trochlear] nerve palsy, bilateral
H49.2 Sixth [abducent] nerve palsy
H49.20 Sixth [abducent] nerve palsy, unspecified eye
H49.21 Sixth [abducent] nerve palsy, right eye
H49.22 Sixth [abducent] nerve palsy, left eye
H49.23 Sixth [abducent] nerve palsy, bilateral
H49.3 Total (external) ophthalmoplegia
H49.30 Total (external) ophthalmoplegia, unspecified eye
H49.31 Total (external) ophthalmoplegia, right eye
H49.32 Total (external) ophthalmoplegia, left eye
H49.33 Total (external) ophthalmoplegia, bilateral
H49.4 Progressive external ophthalmoplegia
Excludes 1: Kearns-Sayre syndrome (H49.81-)
H49.40 Progressive external ophthalmoplegia, unspecified eye

H49.41 Progressive external ophthalmoplegia, right eye
H49.42 Progressive external ophthalmoplegia, left eye
H49.43 Progressive external ophthalmoplegia, bilateral
H49.8 Other paralytic strabismus
H49.81 Kearns-Sayre syndrome
Progressive external ophthalmoplegia with pigmentary retinopathy
Use additional code for other manifestation, such as:
heart block (I45.9)
H49.811 Kearns-Sayre syndrome, right eye
H49.812 Kearns-Sayre syndrome, left eye
H49.813 Kearns-Sayre syndrome, bilateral
H49.819 Kearns-Sayre syndrome, unspecified eye
H49.88 Other paralytic strabismus
External ophthalmoplegia NOS
H49.881 Other paralytic strabismus, right eye
H49.882 Other paralytic strabismus, left eye
H49.883 Other paralytic strabismus, bilateral
H49.889 Other paralytic strabismus, unspecified eye
H49.9 Unspecified paralytic strabismus
H50 Other strabismus
H50.0 Esotropia
Convergent concomitant strabismus
Excludes 1: intermittent esotropia (H50.31-, H50.32)
H50.00 Unspecified esotropia
H50.01 Monocular esotropia
H50.011 Monocular esotropia, right eye
H50.012 Monocular esotropia, left eye
H50.02 Monocular esotropia with A pattern
H50.021 Monocular esotropia with A pattern, right eye
H50.022 Monocular esotropia with A pattern, left eye
H50.03 Monocular esotropia with V pattern
H50.031 Monocular esotropia with V pattern, right eye
H50.032 Monocular esotropia with V pattern, left eye
H50.04 Monocular esotropia with other noncomitancies
H50.041 Monocular esotropia with other noncomitancies, right eye
H50.042 Monocular esotropia with other noncomitancies, left eye
H50.05 Alternating esotropia
H50.06 Alternating esotropia with A pattern
H50.07 Alternating esotropia with V pattern
H50.08 Alternating esotropia with other noncomitancies
H50.1 Exotropia
Divergent concomitant strabismus
Excludes 1: intermittent exotropia (H50.33-, H50.34)
H50.10 Unspecified exotropia
H50.11 Monocular exotropia
H50.111 Monocular exotropia, right eye
H50.112 Monocular exotropia, left eye
H50.12 Monocular exotropia with A pattern
H50.121 Monocular exotropia with A pattern, right eye
H50.122 Monocular exotropia with A pattern, left eye
H50.13 Monocular exotropia with V pattern

H50.131 Monocular exotropia with V pattern, right eye

H50.132 Monocular exotropia with V pattern, left eye

H50.14 Monocular exotropia with other noncomitancies

H50.141 Monocular exotropia with other noncomitancies, right eye

H50.142 Monocular exotropia with other noncomitancies, left eye

H50.15 Alternating exotropia

H50.16 Alternating exotropia with A pattern

H50.17 Alternating exotropia with V pattern

H50.18 Alternating exotropia with other noncomitancies

H50.2 Vertical strabismus
Hypertropia

H50.21 Vertical strabismus, right eye

H50.22 Vertical strabismus, left eye

H50.3 Intermittent heterotropia

H50.30 Unspecified intermittent heterotropia

H50.31 Intermittent monocular esotropia

H50.311 Intermittent monocular esotropia, right eye

H50.312 Intermittent monocular esotropia, left eye

H50.32 Intermittent alternating esotropia

H50.33 Intermittent monocular exotropia

H50.331 Intermittent monocular exotropia, right eye

H50.332 Intermittent monocular exotropia, left eye

H50.34 Intermittent alternating exotropia

H50.4 Other and unspecified heterotropia

H50.40 Unspecified heterotropia

H50.41 Cyclotropia

H50.411 Cyclotropia, right eye

H50.412 Cyclotropia, left eye

H50.42 Monofixation syndrome

H50.43 Accommodative component in esotropia

H50.5 Heterophoria

H50.50 Unspecified heterophoria

H50.51 Esophoria

H50.52 Exophoria

H50.53 Vertical heterophoria

H50.54 Cyclophoria

H50.55 Alternating heterophoria

H50.6 Mechanical strabismus

H50.60 Mechanical strabismus, unspecified

H50.61 Brown's sheath syndrome

H50.611 Brown's sheath syndrome, right eye

H50.612 Brown's sheath syndrome, left eye

H50.69 Other mechanical strabismus
Strabismus due to adhesions
Traumatic limitation of duction of eye muscle

H50.8 Other specified strabismus

H50.81 Duane's syndrome

H50.811 Duane's syndrome, right eye

H50.812 Duane's syndrome, left eye

H50.89 Other specified strabismus

H50.9 Unspecified strabismus

H51 Other disorders of binocular movement

H51.0 Palsy (spasm) of conjugate gaze

H51.1 Convergence insufficiency and excess

H51.11 Convergence insufficiency

H51.12 Convergence excess

H51.2 Internuclear ophthalmoplegia

H51.20 Internuclear ophthalmoplegia, unspecified eye

H51.21 Internuclear ophthalmoplegia, right eye

H51.22 Internuclear ophthalmoplegia, left eye

H51.23 Internuclear ophthalmoplegia, bilateral

H51.8 Other specified disorders of binocular movement

H51.9 Unspecified disorder of binocular movement

H52 Disorders of refraction and accommodation

H52.0 Hypermetropia

H52.00 Hypermetropia, unspecified eye

H52.01 Hypermetropia, right eye

H52.02 Hypermetropia, left eye

H52.03 Hypermetropia, bilateral

H52.1 Myopia

Excludes 1: degenerative myopia (H44.2-)

H52.10 Myopia, unspecified eye

H52.11 Myopia, right eye

H52.12 Myopia, left eye

H52.13 Myopia, bilateral

H52.2 Astigmatism

H52.20 Unspecified astigmatism

H52.201 Unspecified astigmatism, right eye

H52.202 Unspecified astigmatism, left eye

H52.203 Unspecified astigmatism, bilateral

H52.209 Unspecified astigmatism, unspecified eye

H52.21 Irregular astigmatism

H52.211 Irregular astigmatism, right eye

H52.212 Irregular astigmatism, left eye

H52.213 Irregular astigmatism, bilateral

H52.219 Irregular astigmatism, unspecified eye

H52.22 Regular astigmatism

H52.221 Regular astigmatism, right eye

H52.222 Regular astigmatism, left eye

H52.223 Regular astigmatism, bilateral

H52.229 Regular astigmatism, unspecified eye

H52.3 Anisometropia and aniseikonia

H52.31 Anisometropia

H52.32 Aniseikonia

H52.4 Presbyopia

H52.5 Disorders of accommodation

H52.51 Internal ophthalmoplegia (complete) (total)

H52.511 Internal ophthalmoplegia (complete) (total), right eye

H52.512 Internal ophthalmoplegia (complete) (total), left eye

H52.513 Internal ophthalmoplegia (complete) (total), bilateral

H52.519 Internal ophthalmoplegia (complete) (total), unspecified eye

H52.52 Paresis of accommodation

H52.521 Paresis of accommodation, right eye

H52.522 Paresis of accommodation, left eye

H52.523 Paresis of accommodation, bilateral

H52.529 Paresis of accommodation, unspecified eye

H52.53 Spasm of accommodation

H52.531 Spasm of accommodation, right eye

H52.532 Spasm of accommodation, left eye

H52.533 Spasm of accommodation, bilateral

● New code ▲ Revised code ⑦ 7th digit required ⊗ Placeholder required

H52.539 Spasm of accommodation, unspecified eye

H52.6 Other disorders of refraction

H52.7 Unspecified disorder of refraction

VISUAL DISTURBANCES AND BLINDNESS (H53-H54)

H53 Visual disturbances

H53.0 Amblyopia ex anopsia

Excludes 1: amblyopia due to vitamin A deficiency (E50.5)

    H53.00 Unspecified amblyopia

        H53.001 Unspecified amblyopia, right eye

        H53.002 Unspecified amblyopia, left eye

        H53.003 Unspecified amblyopia, bilateral

        H53.009 Unspecified amblyopia, unspecified eye

    H53.01 Deprivation amblyopia

        H53.011 Deprivation amblyopia, right eye

        H53.012 Deprivation amblyopia, left eye

        H53.013 Deprivation amblyopia, bilateral

        H53.019 Deprivation amblyopia, unspecified eye

    H53.02 Refractive amblyopia

        H53.021 Refractive amblyopia, right eye

        H53.022 Refractive amblyopia, left eye

        H53.023 Refractive amblyopia, bilateral

        H53.029 Refractive amblyopia, unspecified eye

    H53.03 Strabismic amblyopia

    Excludes 1: strabismus (H50.-)

        H53.031 Strabismic amblyopia, right eye

        H53.032 Strabismic amblyopia, left eye

        H53.033 Strabismic amblyopia, bilateral

        H53.039 Strabismic amblyopia, unspecified eye

H53.1 Subjective visual disturbances

Excludes 1: subjective visual disturbances due to vitamin A deficiency (E50.5)

visual hallucinations (R44.1)

    H53.10 Unspecified subjective visual disturbances

    H53.11 Day blindness

Hemeralopia

    H53.12 Transient visual loss

Scintillating scotoma

    Excludes 1: amaurosis fugax (G45.3-)

transient retinal artery occlusion (H34.0-)

        H53.121 Transient visual loss, right eye

        H53.122 Transient visual loss, left eye

        H53.123 Transient visual loss, bilateral

        H53.129 Transient visual loss, unspecified eye

    H53.13 Sudden visual loss

        H53.131 Sudden visual loss, right eye

        H53.132 Sudden visual loss, left eye

        H53.133 Sudden visual loss, bilateral

        H53.139 Sudden visual loss, unspecified eye

    H53.14 Visual discomfort

Asthenopia

Photophobia

        H53.141 Visual discomfort, right eye

        H53.142 Visual discomfort, left eye

        H53.143 Visual discomfort, bilateral

        H53.149 Visual discomfort, unspecified

    H53.15 Visual distortions of shape and size

Metamorphopsia

    H53.16 Psychophysical visual disturbances

    H53.19 Other subjective visual disturbances

Visual halos

H53.2 Diplopia

Double vision

H53.3 Other and unspecified disorders of binocular vision

    H53.30 Unspecified disorder of binocular vision

    H53.31 Abnormal retinal correspondence

    H53.32 Fusion with defective stereopsis

    H53.33 Simultaneous visual perception without fusion

    H53.34 Suppression of binocular vision

H53.4 Visual field defects

    H53.40 Unspecified visual field defects

    H53.41 Scotoma involving central area

Central scotoma

        H53.411 Scotoma involving central area, right eye

        H53.412 Scotoma involving central area, left eye

        H53.413 Scotoma involving central area, bilateral

        H53.419 Scotoma involving central area, unspecified eye

    H53.42 Scotoma of blind spot area

Enlarged blind spot

        H53.421 Scotoma of blind spot area, right eye

        H53.422 Scotoma of blind spot area, left eye

        H53.423 Scotoma of blind spot area, bilateral

        H53.429 Scotoma of blind spot area, unspecified eye

    H53.43 Sector or arcuate defects

Arcuate scotoma

Bjerrum scotoma

        H53.431 Sector or arcuate defects, right eye

        H53.432 Sector or arcuate defects, left eye

        H53.433 Sector or arcuate defects, bilateral

        H53.439 Sector or arcuate defects, unspecified eye

    H53.45 Other localized visual field defect

Peripheral visual field defect

Ring scotoma NOS

Scotoma NOS

        H53.451 Other localized visual field defect, right eye

        H53.452 Other localized visual field defect, left eye

        H53.453 Other localized visual field defect, bilateral

        H53.459 Other localized visual field defect, unspecified eye

    H53.46 Homonymous bilateral field defects

Homonymous hemianop(s)ia

Quadrant anop(s)ia

        H53.461 Homonymous bilateral field defects, right side

        H53.462 Homonymous bilateral field defects, left side

        H53.469 Homonymous bilateral field defects, unspecified side

Homonymous bilateral field defects NOS

H53.47 Heteronymous bilateral field defects
Heteronymous hemianop(s)ia

H53.48 Generalized contraction of visual field

    H53.481 Generalized contraction of visual field, right eye

    H53.482 Generalized contraction of visual field, left eye

    H53.483 Generalized contraction of visual field, bilateral

    H53.489 Generalized contraction of visual field, unspecified eye

H53.5 Color vision deficiencies
Color blindness
Excludes 2: day blindness (H53.11)

    H53.50 Unspecified color vision deficiencies
Color blindness NOS

    H53.51 Achromatopsia

    H53.52 Acquired color vision deficiency

    H53.53 Deuteranomaly
Deuteranopia

    H53.54 Protanomaly
Protanopia

    H53.55 Tritanomaly
Tritanopia

    H53.59 Other color vision deficiencies

H53.6 Night blindness
Excludes 1: night blindness due to vitamin A deficiency (E50.5)

    H53.60 Unspecified night blindness

    H53.61 Abnormal dark adaptation curve

    H53.62 Acquired night blindness

    H53.63 Congenital night blindness

    H53.69 Other night blindness

H53.7 Vision sensitivity deficiencies

    H53.71 Glare sensitivity

    H53.72 Impaired contrast sensitivity

H53.8 Other visual disturbances

H53.9 Unspecified visual disturbance

H54 Blindness and low vision
Note: For definition of visual impairment categories see table below
Code first any associated underlying cause of the blindness
Excludes 1: amaurosis fugax (G45.3)

H54.0 Blindness, both eyes
Visual impairment categories 3, 4, 5 in both eyes.

H54.1 Blindness, one eye, low vision other eye
Visual impairment categories 3, 4, 5 in one eye, with categories 1or 2 in the other eye.

    H54.10 Blindness, one eye, low vision other eye, unspecified eyes

    H54.11 Blindness, right eye, low vision left eye

    H54.12 Blindness, left eye, low vision right eye

H54.2 Low vision, both eyes
Visual impairment categories 1 or 2 in both eyes.

H54.3 Unqualified visual loss, both eyes
Visual impairment category 9 in both eyes.

H54.4 Blindness, one eye
Visual impairment categories 3, 4, 5 in one eye [normal vision in other eye]

    H54.40 Blindness, one eye, unspecified eye

    H54.41 Blindness, right eye, normal vision left eye

    H54.42 Blindness, left eye, normal vision right eye

H54.5 Low vision, one eye
Visual impairment categories 1or 2 in one eye [normal vision in other eye].

    H54.50 Low vision, one eye, unspecified eye

    H54.51 Low vision, right eye, normal vision left eye

    H54.52 Low vision, left eye, normal vision right eye

H54.6 Unqualified visual loss, one eye
Visual impairment category 9 in one eye [normal vision in other eye].

    H54.60 Unqualified visual loss, one eye, unspecified

    H54.61 Unqualified visual loss, right eye, normal vision left eye

    H54.62 Unqualified visual loss, left eye, normal vision right eye

H54.7 Unspecified visual loss
Visual impairment category 9 NOS

H54.8 Legal blindness, as defined in USA
Blindness NOS according to USA definition
Excludes 1: legal blindness with specification of impairment level (H54.0-H54.7)

Note: The table below gives a classification of severity of visual impairment recommended by a WHO Study Group on the Prevention of Blindness, Geneva, 6-10 November 1972. The term 'low vision' in category H54 comprises categories 1 and 2 of the table, the term 'blindness' categories 3, 4 and 5, and the term 'unqualified visual loss' category 9. If the extent of the visual field is taken into account, patients with a field no greater than 10 but greater than 5 around central fixation should be placed in category 3 and patients with a field no greater than 5 around central fixation should be placed in category 4, even if the central acuity is not impaired.

Category of visual impairment	Visual acuity with best possible correction	
	Maximum less than:	Minimum equal to or better than:
	6/18	6/60
33/10 (0.3)	1/10 (0.1)	
220/70	20/200	
	6/60	3/60
1/10 (0.1)	1/20 (0.05)	
20/200	20/400	
	3/60	1/60 (finger counting at one meter)
1/20 (0.05)	1/50 (0.02)	
20/400	5/300 (20/1200)	
	1/60 (finger counting at one meter)	Light perception
1/50 (0.02)		
5/300		
	No light perception	
	Undetermined or unspecified	

OTHER DISORDERS OF EYE AND ADNEXA (H55-H57)

H55 Nystagmus and other irregular eye movements

H55.0 Nystagmus
- **H55.00** Unspecified nystagmus
- **H55.01** Congenital nystagmus
- **H55.02** Latent nystagmus
- **H55.03** Visual deprivation nystagmus
- **H55.04** Dissociated nystagmus
- **H55.09** Other forms of nystagmus

H55.8 Other irregular eye movements
- **H55.81** Saccadic eye movements
- **H55.89** Other irregular eye movements

H57 Other disorders of eye and adnexa

H57.0 Anomalies of pupillary function
- **H57.00** Unspecified anomaly of pupillary function
- **H57.01** Argyll Robertson pupil, atypical
  - **Excludes 1:** syphilitic Argyll Robertson pupil (A52.19)
- **H57.02** Anisocoria
- **H57.03** Miosis
- **H57.04** Mydriasis
- **H57.05** Tonic pupil
  - **H57.051** Tonic pupil, right eye
  - **H57.052** Tonic pupil, left eye
  - **H57.053** Tonic pupil, bilateral
  - **H57.059** Tonic pupil, unspecified eye
- **H57.09** Other anomalies of pupillary function

H57.1 Ocular pain
- **H57.10** Ocular pain, unspecified eye
- **H57.11** Ocular pain, right eye
- **H57.12** Ocular pain, left eye
- **H57.13** Ocular pain, bilateral

H57.8 Other specified disorders of eye and adnexa

H57.9 Unspecified disorder of eye and adnexa

INTRAOPERATIVE AND POSTPROCEDURAL COMPLICATIONS AND DISORDERS OF EYE AND ADNEXA, NOT ELSEWHERE CLASSIFIED (H59)

H59 Intraoperative and postprocedural complications and disorders of eye and adnexa, not elsewhere classified
- **Excludes 1:** mechanical complication of intraocular lens (T85.2)
  - mechanical complication of other ocular prosthetic devices, implants and grafts (T85.3)
  - pseudophakia (Z96.1)
  - secondary cataracts (H26.4-)

H59.0 Disorders of the eye following cataract surgery
- **H59.01** Keratopathy (bullous aphakic) following cataract surgery
  - Vitreal corneal syndrome
  - Vitreous (touch) syndrome
  - **H59.011** Keratopathy (bullous aphakic) following cataract surgery, right eye
  - **H59.012** Keratopathy (bullous aphakic) following cataract surgery, left eye
  - **H59.013** Keratopathy (bullous aphakic) following cataract surgery, bilateral
  - **H59.019** Keratopathy (bullous aphakic) following cataract surgery, unspecified eye
- **H59.02** Cataract (lens) fragments in eye following cataract surgery
  - **H59.021** Cataract (lens) fragments in eye following cataract surgery, right eye
  - **H59.022** Cataract (lens) fragments in eye following cataract surgery, left eye
  - **H59.023** Cataract (lens) fragments in eye following cataract surgery, bilateral
  - **H59.029** Cataract (lens) fragments in eye following cataract surgery, unspecified eye
- **H59.03** Cystoid macular edema following cataract surgery
  - **H59.031** Cystoid macular edema following cataract surgery, right eye
  - **H59.032** Cystoid macular edema following cataract surgery, left eye
  - **H59.033** Cystoid macular edema following cataract surgery, bilateral
  - **H59.039** Cystoid macular edema following cataract surgery, unspecified eye
- **H59.09** Other disorders of the eye following cataract surgery
  - **H59.091** Other disorders of the right eye following cataract surgery
  - **H59.092** Other disorders of the left eye following cataract surgery
  - **H59.093** Other disorders of the eye following cataract surgery, bilateral
  - **H59.099** Other disorders of unspecified eye following cataract surgery

H59.1 Intraoperative hemorrhage and hematoma of eye and adnexa complicating a procedure
- **Excludes 1:** intraoperative hemorrhage and hematoma of eye and adnexa due to accidental puncture
  - or
  - laceration during a procedure (H59.2-)
- **H59.11** Intraoperative hemorrhage and hematoma of eye and adnexa complicating an ophthalmic procedure
  - **H59.111** Intraoperative hemorrhage and hematoma of right eye and adnexa complicating an ophthalmic procedure
  - **H59.112** Intraoperative hemorrhage and hematoma of left eye and adnexa complicating an ophthalmic procedure
  - **H59.113** Intraoperative hemorrhage and hematoma of eye and adnexa complicating an ophthalmic procedure, bilateral
  - **H59.119** Intraoperative hemorrhage and hematoma of unspecified eye and adnexa complicating an ophthalmic procedure
- **H59.12** Intraoperative hemorrhage and hematoma of eye and adnexa complicating other procedure
  - **H59.121** Intraoperative hemorrhage and hematoma of right eye and adnexa complicating other procedure
  - **H59.122** Intraoperative hemorrhage and hematoma of left eye and adnexa complicating other procedure
  - **H59.123** Intraoperative hemorrhage and hematoma of eye and adnexa complicating other procedure, bilateral
  - **H59.129** Intraoperative hemorrhage and hematoma of unspecified eye and adnexa complicating other procedure

H59.2 Accidental puncture and laceration of eye and adnexa during a procedure

H59.21 Accidental puncture and laceration of eye and adnexa during an ophthalmic procedure

    H59.211 Accidental puncture and laceration of right eye and adnexa during an ophthalmic procedure

    H59.212 Accidental puncture and laceration of left eye and adnexa during an ophthalmic procedure

    H59.213 Accidental puncture and laceration of eye and adnexa during an ophthalmic procedure, bilateral

    H59.219 Accidental puncture and laceration of unspecified eye and adnexa during an ophthalmic procedure

H59.22 Accidental puncture and laceration of eye and adnexa during other procedure

    H59.221 Accidental puncture and laceration of right eye and adnexa during other procedure

    H59.222 Accidental puncture and laceration of left eye and adnexa during other procedure

    H59.223 Accidental puncture and laceration of eye and adnexa during other procedure, bilateral

    H59.229 Accidental puncture and laceration of unspecified eye and adnexa during other procedure

H59.3 Postprocedural hemorrhage and hematoma of eye and adnexa following a procedure

  H59.31 Postprocedural hemorrhage and hematoma of eye and adnexa following an ophthalmic procedure

    H59.311 Postprocedural hemorrhage and hematoma of right eye and adnexa following an ophthalmic procedure

    H59.312 Postprocedural hemorrhage and hematoma of left eye and adnexa following an ophthalmic procedure

    H59.313 Postprocedural hemorrhage and hematoma of eye and adnexa following an ophthalmic procedure, bilateral

    H59.319 Postprocedural hemorrhage and hematoma of unspecified eye and adnexa following an ophthalmic procedure

  H59.32 Postprocedural hemorrhage and hematoma of eye and adnexa following other procedure

    H59.321 Postprocedural hemorrhage and hematoma of right eye and adnexa following other procedure

    H59.322 Postprocedural hemorrhage and hematoma of left eye and adnexa following other procedure

    H59.323 Postprocedural hemorrhage and hematoma of eye and adnexa following other procedure, bilateral

    H59.329 Postprocedural hemorrhage and hematoma of unspecified eye and adnexa following other procedure

H59.4 Inflammation (infection) of postprocedural bleb

Postprocedural blebitis

Excludes 1: filtering (vitreous) bleb after glaucoma surgery status (Z98.83)

H59.40 Inflammation (infection) of postprocedural bleb, unspecified

H59.41 Inflammation (infection) of postprocedural bleb, stage 1

H59.42 Inflammation (infection) of postprocedural bleb, stage 2

H59.43 Inflammation (infection) of postprocedural bleb, stage 3

Bleb endophthalmitis

H59.8 Other intraoperative and postprocedural complications and disorders of eye and adnexa, not elsewhere classified

  H59.81 Chorioretinal scars after surgery for detachment

    H59.811 Chorioretinal scars after surgery for detachment, right eye

    H59.812 Chorioretinal scars after surgery for detachment, left eye

    H59.813 Chorioretinal scars after surgery for detachment, bilateral

    H59.819 Chorioretinal scars after surgery for detachment, unspecified eye

  H59.88 Other intraoperative complications of eye and adnexa, not elsewhere classified

  H59.89 Other postprocedural complications and disorders of eye and adnexa, not elsewhere classified

CHAPTER 8: DISEASES OF THE EAR AND MASTOID PROCESS (H60-H95)

Note: Use an external cause code following the code for the ear condition, if applicable, to identify the cause of the ear condition

Excludes 2: certain conditions originating in the perinatal period (P04-P96)

certain infectious and parasitic diseases (A00-B99)

complications of pregnancy, childbirth and the puerperium (O00-O9A)

congenital malformations, deformations and chromosomal abnormalities (Q00-Q99)

endocrine, nutritional and metabolic diseases (E00-E88)

injury, poisoning and certain other consequences of external causes (S00-T88)

neoplasms (C00-D49)

symptoms, signs and abnormal clinical and laboratory findings, not elsewhere classified (R00-R94)

This chapter contains the following blocks:

H60-H62	Diseases of external ear
H65-H75	Diseases of middle ear and mastoid
H80-H83	Diseases of inner ear
H90-H94	Other disorders of ear
H95	Intraoperative and postprocedural complications and disorders of ear and mastoid process, not elsewhere classified

DISEASES OF EXTERNAL EAR (H60-H62)

H60 Otitis externa

H60.0 Abscess of external ear
Boil of external ear
Carbuncle of auricle or external auditory canal
Furuncle of external ear
- **H60.00** Abscess of external ear, unspecified ear
- **H60.01** Abscess of right external ear
- **H60.02** Abscess of left external ear
- **H60.03** Abscess of external ear, bilateral

H60.1 Cellulitis of external ear
Cellulitis of auricle
Cellulitis of external auditory canal
- **H60.10** Cellulitis of external ear, unspecified ear
- **H60.11** Cellulitis of right external ear
- **H60.12** Cellulitis of left external ear
- **H60.13** Cellulitis of external ear, bilateral

H60.2 Malignant otitis externa
- **H60.20** Malignant otitis externa, unspecified ear
- **H60.21** Malignant otitis externa, right ear
- **H60.22** Malignant otitis externa, left ear
- **H60.23** Malignant otitis externa, bilateral

H60.3 Other infective otitis externa
- **H60.31** Diffuse otitis externa
  - **H60.311** Diffuse otitis externa, right ear
  - **H60.312** Diffuse otitis externa, left ear
  - **H60.313** Diffuse otitis externa, bilateral
  - **H60.319** Diffuse otitis externa, unspecified ear
- **H60.32** Hemorrhagic otitis externa
  - **H60.321** Hemorrhagic otitis externa, right ear
  - **H60.322** Hemorrhagic otitis externa, left ear
  - **H60.323** Hemorrhagic otitis externa, bilateral
  - **H60.329** Hemorrhagic otitis externa, unspecified ear

- **H60.33** Swimmer's ear
  - **H60.331** Swimmer's ear, right ear
  - **H60.332** Swimmer's ear, left ear
  - **H60.333** Swimmer's ear, bilateral
  - **H60.339** Swimmer's ear, unspecified ear
- **H60.39** Other infective otitis externa
  - **H60.391** Other infective otitis externa, right ear
  - **H60.392** Other infective otitis externa, left ear
  - **H60.393** Other infective otitis externa, bilateral
  - **H60.399** Other infective otitis externa, unspecified ear

H60.4 Cholesteatoma of external ear
Keratosis obturans of external ear (canal)
Excludes 2: cholesteatoma of middle ear (H71.-)
recurrent cholesteatoma of postmastoidectomy cavity (H95.0-)
- **H60.40** Cholesteatoma of external ear, unspecified ear
- **H60.41** Cholesteatoma of right external ear
- **H60.42** Cholesteatoma of left external ear
- **H60.43** Cholesteatoma of external ear, bilateral

H60.5 Acute noninfective otitis externa
- **H60.50** Unspecified acute noninfective otitis externa
  Acute otitis externa NOS
  - **H60.501** Unspecified acute noninfective otitis externa, right ear
  - **H60.502** Unspecified acute noninfective otitis externa, left ear
  - **H60.503** Unspecified acute noninfective otitis externa, bilateral
  - **H60.509** Unspecified acute noninfective otitis externa, unspecified ear
- **H60.51** Acute actinic otitis externa
  - **H60.511** Acute actinic otitis externa, right ear
  - **H60.512** Acute actinic otitis externa, left ear
  - **H60.513** Acute actinic otitis externa, bilateral
  - **H60.519** Acute actinic otitis externa, unspecified ear
- **H60.52** Acute chemical otitis externa
  - **H60.521** Acute chemical otitis externa, right ear
  - **H60.522** Acute chemical otitis externa, left ear
  - **H60.523** Acute chemical otitis externa, bilateral
  - **H60.529** Acute chemical otitis externa, unspecified ear
- **H60.53** Acute contact otitis externa
  - **H60.531** Acute contact otitis externa, right ear
  - **H60.532** Acute contact otitis externa, left ear
  - **H60.533** Acute contact otitis externa, bilateral
  - **H60.539** Acute contact otitis externa, unspecified ear
- **H60.54** Acute eczematoid otitis externa
  - **H60.541** Acute eczematoid otitis externa, right ear
  - **H60.542** Acute eczematoid otitis externa, left ear
  - **H60.543** Acute eczematoid otitis externa, bilateral
  - **H60.549** Acute eczematoid otitis externa, unspecified ear
- **H60.55** Acute reactive otitis externa
  - **H60.551** Acute reactive otitis externa, right ear
  - **H60.552** Acute reactive otitis externa, left ear

H60.553 Acute reactive otitis externa, bilateral

H60.559 Acute reactive otitis externa, unspecified ear

H60.59 Other noninfective acute otitis externa

H60.591 Other noninfective acute otitis externa, right ear

H60.592 Other noninfective acute otitis externa, left ear

H60.593 Other noninfective acute otitis externa, bilateral

H60.599 Other noninfective acute otitis externa, unspecified ear

H60.6 Unspecified chronic otitis externa

H60.60 Unspecified chronic otitis externa, unspecified ear

H60.61 Unspecified chronic otitis externa, right ear

H60.62 Unspecified chronic otitis externa, left ear

H60.63 Unspecified chronic otitis externa, bilateral

H60.8 Other otitis externa

H60.8X Other otitis externa

H60.8X1 Other otitis externa, right ear

H60.8X2 Other otitis externa, left ear

H60.8X3 Other otitis externa, bilateral

H60.8X9 Other otitis externa, unspecified ear

H60.9 Unspecified otitis externa

H60.90 Unspecified otitis externa, unspecified ear

H60.91 Unspecified otitis externa, right ear

H60.92 Unspecified otitis externa, left ear

H60.93 Unspecified otitis externa, bilateral

H61 Other disorders of external ear

H61.0 Chondritis and perichondritis of external ear

Chondrodermatitis nodularis chronica helicis

Perichondritis of auricle

Perichondritis of pinna

H61.00 Unspecified perichondritis of external ear

H61.001 Unspecified perichondritis of right external ear

H61.002 Unspecified perichondritis of left external ear

H61.003 Unspecified perichondritis of external ear, bilateral

H61.009 Unspecified perichondritis of external ear, unspecified ear

H61.01 Acute perichondritis of external ear

H61.011 Acute perichondritis of right external ear

H61.012 Acute perichondritis of left external ear

H61.013 Acute perichondritis of external ear, bilateral

H61.019 Acute perichondritis of external ear, unspecified ear

H61.02 Chronic perichondritis of external ear

H61.021 Chronic perichondritis of right external ear

H61.022 Chronic perichondritis of left external ear

H61.023 Chronic perichondritis of external ear, bilateral

H61.029 Chronic perichondritis of external ear, unspecified ear

H61.03 Chondritis of external ear

Chondritis of auricle

Chondritis of pinna

H61.031 Chondritis of right external ear

H61.032 Chondritis of left external ear

H61.033 Chondritis of external ear, bilateral

H61.039 Chondritis of external ear, unspecified ear

H61.1 Noninfective disorders of pinna

Excludes 2: cauliflower ear (M95.1-)

gouty tophi of ear (M1A-, M10.-)

H61.10 Unspecified noninfective disorders of pinna

Disorder of pinna NOS

H61.101 Unspecified noninfective disorders of pinna, right ear

H61.102 Unspecified noninfective disorders of pinna, left ear

H61.103 Unspecified noninfective disorders of pinna, bilateral

H61.109 Unspecified noninfective disorders of pinna, unspecified ear

H61.11 Acquired deformity of pinna

Acquired deformity of auricle

Excludes 2: cauliflower ear (M95.1-)

H61.111 Acquired deformity of pinna, right ear

H61.112 Acquired deformity of pinna, left ear

H61.113 Acquired deformity of pinna, bilateral

H61.119 Acquired deformity of pinna, unspecified ear

H61.12 Hematoma of pinna

Hematoma of auricle

H61.121 Hematoma of pinna, right ear

H61.122 Hematoma of pinna, left ear

H61.123 Hematoma of pinna, bilateral

H61.129 Hematoma of pinna, unspecified ear

H61.19 Other noninfective disorders of pinna

H61.191 Noninfective disorders of pinna, right ear

H61.192 Noninfective disorders of pinna, left ear

H61.193 Noninfective disorders of pinna, bilateral

H61.199 Noninfective disorders of pinna, unspecified ear

H61.2 Impacted cerumen

Wax in ear

H61.20 Impacted cerumen, unspecified ear

H61.21 Impacted cerumen, right ear

H61.22 Impacted cerumen, left ear

H61.23 Impacted cerumen, bilateral

H61.3 Acquired stenosis of external ear canal

Collapse of external ear canal

Excludes 1: postprocedural stenosis of external ear canal (H95.81-)

H61.30 Acquired stenosis of external ear canal, unspecified

H61.301 Acquired stenosis of right external ear canal, unspecified

H61.302 Acquired stenosis of left external ear canal, unspecified

H61.303 Acquired stenosis of external ear canal, unspecified, bilateral

H61.309 Acquired stenosis of external ear canal, unspecified, unspecified ear

● New code   ▲ Revised code   ⑦ 7th digit required   ⊗ Placeholder required

H61.31 Acquired stenosis of external ear canal secondary to trauma

   H61.311 Acquired stenosis of right external ear canal secondary to trauma

   H61.312 Acquired stenosis of left external ear canal secondary to trauma

   H61.313 Acquired stenosis of external ear canal secondary to trauma, bilateral

   H61.319 Acquired stenosis of external ear canal secondary to trauma, unspecified ear

H61.32 Acquired stenosis of external ear canal secondary to inflammation and infection

   H61.321 Acquired stenosis of right external ear canal secondary to inflammation and infection

   H61.322 Acquired stenosis of left external ear canal secondary to inflammation and infection

   H61.323 Acquired stenosis of external ear canal secondary to inflammation and infection, bilateral

   H61.329 Acquired stenosis of external ear canal secondary to inflammation and infection, unspecified ear

H61.39 Other acquired stenosis of external ear canal

   H61.391 Other acquired stenosis of right external ear canal

   H61.392 Other acquired stenosis of left external ear canal

   H61.393 Other acquired stenosis of external ear canal, bilateral

   H61.399 Other acquired stenosis of external ear canal, unspecified ear

H61.8 Other specified disorders of external ear

H61.81 Exostosis of external canal

   H61.811 Exostosis of right external canal

   H61.812 Exostosis of left external canal

   H61.813 Exostosis of external canal, bilateral

   H61.819 Exostosis of external canal, unspecified ear

H61.89 Other specified disorders of external ear

   H61.891 Other specified disorders of right external ear

   H61.892 Other specified disorders of left external ear

   H61.893 Other specified disorders of external ear, bilateral

   H61.899 Other specified disorders of external ear, unspecified ear

H61.9 Disorder of external ear, unspecified

H61.90 Disorder of external ear, unspecified, unspecified ear

H61.91 Disorder of right external ear, unspecified

H61.92 Disorder of left external ear, unspecified

H61.93 Disorder of external ear, unspecified, bilateral

H62 Disorders of external ear in diseases classified elsewhere

H62.4 Otitis externa in other diseases classified elsewhere

Code first underlying disease, such as:
erysipelas (A46)
impetigo (L01.0)

Excludes 1: otitis externa (in):
candidiasis (B37.84)
herpes viral [herpes simplex] (B00.1)
herpes zoster (B02.8)

H62.40 Otitis externa in other diseases classified elsewhere, unspecified ear

H62.41 Otitis externa in other diseases classified elsewhere, right ear

H62.42 Otitis externa in other diseases classified elsewhere, left ear

H62.43 Otitis externa in other diseases classified elsewhere, bilateral

H62.8 Other disorders of external ear in diseases classified elsewhere

Code first underlying disease, such as:
gout (M1A-, M10.-)

H62.8X Other disorders of external ear in diseases classified elsewhere

   H62.8X1 Other disorders of right external ear in diseases classified elsewhere

   H62.8X2 Other disorders of left external ear in diseases classified elsewhere

   H62.8X3 Other disorders of external ear in diseases classified elsewhere, bilateral

   H62.8X9 Other disorders of external ear in diseases classified elsewhere, unspecified ear

DISEASES OF MIDDLE EAR AND MASTOID (H65-H75)

H65 Nonsuppurative otitis media

Includes: nonsuppurative otitis media with myringitis

Use additional code for any associated perforated tympanic membrane (H72.-)

Use additional code to identify:
exposure to environmental tobacco smoke (Z77.22)
exposure to tobacco smoke in the perinatal period (P96.81)
history of tobacco use (Z87.891)
occupational exposure to environmental tobacco smoke (Z57.31)
tobacco dependence (F17.-)
tobacco use (Z72.0)

H65.0 Acute serous otitis media
Acute and subacute secretory otitis

H65.00 Acute serous otitis media, unspecified ear

H65.01 Acute serous otitis media, right ear

H65.02 Acute serous otitis media, left ear

H65.03 Acute serous otitis media, bilateral

H65.04 Acute serous otitis media, recurrent, right ear

H65.05 Acute serous otitis media, recurrent, left ear

H65.06 Acute serous otitis media, recurrent, bilateral

H65.07 Acute serous otitis media, recurrent, unspecified ear

H65.1 Other acute nonsuppurative otitis media

Excludes 1: otitic barotrauma (T70.0)
otitis media (acute) NOS (H66.9)

H65.11 Acute and subacute allergic otitis media (mucoid) (sanguinous) (serous)

   H65.111 Acute and subacute allergic otitis media (mucoid) (sanguinous) (serous), right ear

   H65.112 Acute and subacute allergic otitis media (mucoid) (sanguinous) (serous), left ear

   H65.113 Acute and subacute allergic otitis media (mucoid) (sanguinous) (serous), bilateral

H65.114   Acute and subacute allergic otitis media (mucoid) (sanguinous) (serous), recurrent, right ear

H65.115   Acute and subacute allergic otitis media (mucoid) (sanguinous) (serous), recurrent, left ear

H65.116   Acute and subacute allergic otitis media (mucoid) (sanguinous) (serous), recurrent, bilateral

H65.117   Acute and subacute allergic otitis media (mucoid) (sanguinous) (serous), recurrent, unspecified ear

H65.119   Acute and subacute allergic otitis media (mucoid) (sanguinous) (serous), unspecified ear

H65.19   Other acute nonsuppurative otitis media

Acute and subacute mucoid otitis media

Acute and subacute nonsuppurative otitis media NOS

Acute and subacute sanguinous otitis media

Acute and subacute seromucinous otitis media

H65.191   Other acute nonsuppurative otitis media, right ear

H65.192   Other acute nonsuppurative otitis media, left ear

H65.193   Other acute nonsuppurative otitis media, bilateral

H65.194   Other acute nonsuppurative otitis media, recurrent, right ear

H65.195   Other acute nonsuppurative otitis media, recurrent, left ear

H65.196   Other acute nonsuppurative otitis media, recurrent, bilateral

H65.197   Other acute nonsuppurative otitis media recurrent, unspecified ear

H65.199   Other acute nonsuppurative otitis media, unspecified ear

H65.2   Chronic serous otitis media

Chronic tubotympanal catarrh

H65.20   Chronic serous otitis media, unspecified ear

H65.21   Chronic serous otitis media, right ear

H65.22   Chronic serous otitis media, left ear

H65.23   Chronic serous otitis media, bilateral

H65.3   Chronic mucoid otitis media

Chronic mucinous otitis media

Chronic secretory otitis media

Chronic transudative otitis media

Glue ear

Excludes 1: adhesive middle ear disease (H74.1)

H65.30   Chronic mucoid otitis media, unspecified ear

H65.31   Chronic mucoid otitis media, right ear

H65.32   Chronic mucoid otitis media, left ear

H65.33   Chronic mucoid otitis media, bilateral

H65.4   Other chronic nonsuppurative otitis media

H65.41   Chronic allergic otitis media

H65.411   Chronic allergic otitis media, right ear

H65.412   Chronic allergic otitis media, left ear

H65.413   Chronic allergic otitis media, bilateral

H65.419   Chronic allergic otitis media, unspecified ear

H65.49   Other chronic nonsuppurative otitis media

Chronic exudative otitis media

Chronic nonsuppurative otitis media NOS

Chronic otitis media with effusion (nonpurulent)

Chronic seromucinous otitis media

H65.491   Other chronic nonsuppurative otitis media, right ear

H65.492   Other chronic nonsuppurative otitis media, left ear

H65.493   Other chronic nonsuppurative otitis media, bilateral

H65.499   Other chronic nonsuppurative otitis media, unspecified ear

H65.9   Unspecified nonsuppurative otitis media

Allergic otitis media NOS

Catarrhal otitis media NOS

Exudative otitis media NOS

Mucoid otitis media NOS

Otitis media with effusion (nonpurulent) NOS

Secretory otitis media NOS

Seromucinous otitis media NOS

Serous otitis media NOS

Transudative otitis media NOS

H65.90   Unspecified nonsuppurative otitis media, unspecified ear

H65.91   Unspecified nonsuppurative otitis media, right ear

H65.92   Unspecified nonsuppurative otitis media, left ear

H65.93   Unspecified nonsuppurative otitis media, bilateral

H66   Suppurative and unspecified otitis media

Includes: suppurative and unspecified otitis media with myringitis

Use additional code for any associated perforated tympanic membrane (H72.-)

Use additional code to identify:

exposure to environmental tobacco smoke (Z77.22)

exposure to tobacco smoke in the perinatal period (P96.81)

history of tobacco use (Z87.891)

occupational exposure to environmental tobacco smoke (Z57.31)

tobacco dependence (F17.-)

tobacco use (Z72.0)

H66.0   Acute suppurative otitis media

H66.00   Acute suppurative otitis media without spontaneous rupture of ear drum

H66.001   Acute suppurative otitis media without spontaneous rupture of ear drum, right ear

H66.002   Acute suppurative otitis media without spontaneous rupture of ear drum, left ear

H66.003   Acute suppurative otitis media without spontaneous rupture of ear drum, bilateral

H66.004   Acute suppurative otitis media without spontaneous rupture of ear drum, recurrent, right ear

H66.005   Acute suppurative otitis media without spontaneous rupture of ear drum, recurrent, left ear

H66.006   Acute suppurative otitis media without spontaneous rupture of ear drum, recurrent, bilateral

H66.007   Acute suppurative otitis media without spontaneous rupture of ear drum, recurrent, unspecified ear

● New code   ▲ Revised code   ⑦ 7th digit required   ⊗ Placeholder required

H66.009   Acute suppurative otitis media without spontaneous rupture of ear drum, unspecified ear

H66.01   Acute suppurative otitis media with spontaneous rupture of ear drum

     H66.011   Acute suppurative otitis media with spontaneous rupture of ear drum, right ear

     H66.012   Acute suppurative otitis media with spontaneous rupture of ear drum, left ear

     H66.013   Acute suppurative otitis media with spontaneous rupture of ear drum, bilateral

     H66.014   Acute suppurative otitis media with spontaneous rupture of ear drum, recurrent, right ear

     H66.015   Acute suppurative otitis media with spontaneous rupture of ear drum, recurrent, left ear

     H66.016   Acute suppurative otitis media with spontaneous rupture of ear drum, recurrent, bilateral

     H66.017   Acute suppurative otitis media with spontaneous rupture of ear drum, recurrent, unspecified ear

     H66.019   Acute suppurative otitis media with spontaneous rupture of ear drum, unspecified ear

H66.1   Chronic tubotympanic suppurative otitis media

Benign chronic suppurative otitis media

Chronic tubotympanic disease

     H66.10   Chronic tubotympanic suppurative otitis media, unspecified

     H66.11   Chronic tubotympanic suppurative otitis media, right ear

     H66.12   Chronic tubotympanic suppurative otitis media, left ear

     H66.13   Chronic tubotympanic suppurative otitis media, bilateral

H66.2   Chronic atticoantral suppurative otitis media

Chronic atticoantral disease

     H66.20   Chronic atticoantral suppurative otitis media, unspecified ear

     H66.21   Chronic atticoantral suppurative otitis media, right ear

     H66.22   Chronic atticoantral suppurative otitis media, left ear

     H66.23   Chronic atticoantral suppurative otitis media, bilateral

H66.3   Other chronic suppurative otitis media

Chronic suppurative otitis media NOS

Excludes 1: tuberculous otitis media (A18.6)

     H66.3X   Other chronic suppurative otitis media

         H66.3X1   Other chronic suppurative otitis media, right ear

         H66.3X2   Other chronic suppurative otitis media, left ear

         H66.3X3   Other chronic suppurative otitis media, bilateral

         H66.3X9   Other chronic suppurative otitis media, unspecified ear

H66.4   Suppurative otitis media, unspecified

Purulent otitis media NOS

H66.40   Suppurative otitis media, unspecified, unspecified ear

H66.41   Suppurative otitis media, unspecified, right ear

H66.42   Suppurative otitis media, unspecified, left ear

H66.43   Suppurative otitis media, unspecified, bilateral

H66.9   Otitis media, unspecified

Otitis media NOS

Acute otitis media NOS

Chronic otitis media NOS

     H66.90   Otitis media, unspecified, unspecified ear

     H66.91   Otitis media, unspecified, right ear

     H66.92   Otitis media, unspecified, left ear

     H66.93   Otitis media, unspecified, bilateral

H67   Otitis media in diseases classified elsewhere

Code first underlying disease, such as:

     viral disease NEC (B00-B34)

Use additional code for any associated perforated tympanic membrane (H72.-)

Excludes 1: otitis media in:

     influenza (J09.X9, J10.83, J11.83)

     measles (B05.3)

     scarlet fever (A38.0)

     tuberculosis (A18.6)

H67.1   Otitis media in diseases classified elsewhere, right ear

H67.2   Otitis media in diseases classified elsewhere, left ear

H67.3   Otitis media in diseases classified elsewhere, bilateral

H67.9   Otitis media in diseases classified elsewhere, unspecified ear

H68   Eustachian salpingitis and obstruction

H68.0   Eustachian salpingitis

     H68.00   Unspecified Eustachian salpingitis

         H68.001   Unspecified Eustachian salpingitis, right ear

         H68.002   Unspecified Eustachian salpingitis, left ear

         H68.003   Unspecified Eustachian salpingitis, bilateral

         H68.009   Unspecified Eustachian salpingitis, unspecified ear

     H68.01   Acute Eustachian salpingitis

         H68.011   Acute Eustachian salpingitis, right ear

         H68.012   Acute Eustachian salpingitis, left ear

         H68.013   Acute Eustachian salpingitis, bilateral

         H68.019   Acute Eustachian salpingitis, unspecified ear

     H68.02   Chronic Eustachian salpingitis

         H68.021   Chronic Eustachian salpingitis, right ear

         H68.022   Chronic Eustachian salpingitis, left ear

         H68.023   Chronic Eustachian salpingitis, bilateral

         H68.029   Chronic Eustachian salpingitis, unspecified ear

H68.1   Obstruction of Eustachian tube

Stenosis of Eustachian tube

Stricture of Eustachian tube

     H68.10   Unspecified obstruction of Eustachian tube

         H68.101   Unspecified obstruction of Eustachian tube, right ear

         H68.102   Unspecified obstruction of Eustachian tube, left ear

H68.103 Unspecified obstruction of Eustachian tube, bilateral

H68.109 Unspecified obstruction of Eustachian tube, unspecified ear

H68.11 Osseous obstruction of Eustachian tube

H68.111 Osseous obstruction of Eustachian tube, right ear

H68.112 Osseous obstruction of Eustachian tube, left ear

H68.113 Osseous obstruction of Eustachian tube, bilateral

H68.119 Osseous obstruction of Eustachian tube, unspecified ear

H68.12 Intrinsic cartilagenous obstruction of Eustachian tube

H68.121 Intrinsic cartilagenous obstruction of Eustachian tube, right ear

H68.122 Intrinsic cartilagenous obstruction of Eustachian tube, left ear

H68.123 Intrinsic cartilagenous obstruction of Eustachian tube, bilateral

H68.129 Intrinsic cartilagenous obstruction of Eustachian tube, unspecified ear

H68.13 Extrinsic cartilagenous obstruction of Eustachian tube

Compression of Eustachian tube

H68.131 Extrinsic cartilagenous obstruction of Eustachian tube, right ear

H68.132 Extrinsic cartilagenous obstruction of Eustachian tube, left ear

H68.133 Extrinsic cartilagenous obstruction of Eustachian tube, bilateral

H68.139 Extrinsic cartilagenous obstruction of Eustachian tube, unspecified ear

H69 Other and unspecified disorders of Eustachian tube

H69.0 Patulous Eustachian tube

H69.00 Patulous Eustachian tube, unspecified ear

H69.01 Patulous Eustachian tube, right ear

H69.02 Patulous Eustachian tube, left ear

H69.03 Patulous Eustachian tube, bilateral

H69.8 Other specified disorders of Eustachian tube

H69.80 Other specified disorders of Eustachian tube, unspecified ear

H69.81 Other specified disorders of Eustachian tube, right ear

H69.82 Other specified disorders of Eustachian tube, left ear

H69.83 Other specified disorders of Eustachian tube, bilateral

H69.9 Unspecified Eustachian tube disorder

H69.90 Unspecified Eustachian tube disorder, unspecified ear

H69.91 Unspecified Eustachian tube disorder, right ear

H69.92 Unspecified Eustachian tube disorder, left ear

H69.93 Unspecified Eustachian tube disorder, bilateral

H70 Mastoiditis and related conditions

H70.0 Acute mastoiditis

Abscess of mastoid

Empyema of mastoid

H70.00 Acute mastoiditis without complications

H70.001 Acute mastoiditis without complications, right ear

H70.002 Acute mastoiditis without complications, left ear

H70.003 Acute mastoiditis without complications, bilateral

H70.009 Acute mastoiditis without complications, unspecified ear

H70.01 Subperiosteal abscess of mastoid

H70.011 Subperiosteal abscess of mastoid, right ear

H70.012 Subperiosteal abscess of mastoid, left ear

H70.013 Subperiosteal abscess of mastoid, bilateral

H70.019 Subperiosteal abscess of mastoid, unspecified ear

H70.09 Acute mastoiditis with other complications

H70.091 Acute mastoiditis with other complications, right ear

H70.092 Acute mastoiditis with other complications, left ear

H70.093 Acute mastoiditis with other complications, bilateral

H70.099 Acute mastoiditis with other complications, unspecified ear

H70.1 Chronic mastoiditis

Caries of mastoid

Fistula of mastoid

Excludes 1: tuberculous mastoiditis (A18.03)

H70.10 Chronic mastoiditis, unspecified ear

H70.11 Chronic mastoiditis, right ear

H70.12 Chronic mastoiditis, left ear

H70.13 Chronic mastoiditis, bilateral

H70.2 Petrositis

Inflammation of petrous bone

H70.20 Unspecified petrositis

H70.201 Unspecified petrositis, right ear

H70.202 Unspecified petrositis, left ear

H70.203 Unspecified petrositis, bilateral

H70.209 Unspecified petrositis, unspecified ear

H70.21 Acute petrositis

H70.211 Acute petrositis, right ear

H70.212 Acute petrositis, left ear

H70.213 Acute petrositis, bilateral

H70.219 Acute petrositis, unspecified ear

H70.22 Chronic petrositis

H70.221 Chronic petrositis, right ear

H70.222 Chronic petrositis, left ear

H70.223 Chronic petrositis, bilateral

H70.229 Chronic petrositis, unspecified ear

H70.8 Other mastoiditis and related conditions

Excludes 1: preauricular sinus and cyst (Q18.1)

sinus, fistula, and cyst of branchial cleft (Q18.0)

H70.81 Postauricular fistula

H70.811 Postauricular fistula, right ear

H70.812 Postauricular fistula, left ear

H70.813 Postauricular fistula, bilateral

H70.819 Postauricular fistula, unspecified ear

H70.89 Other mastoiditis and related conditions

H70.891 Other mastoiditis and related conditions, right ear

H70.892 Other mastoiditis and related conditions, left ear

H70.893 Other mastoiditis and related conditions, bilateral

● New code   ▲ Revised code   ⑦ 7th digit required   ⊗ Placeholder required

H70.899 Other mastoiditis and related conditions, unspecified ear

H70.9 Unspecified mastoiditis

H70.90 Unspecified mastoiditis, unspecified ear

H70.91 Unspecified mastoiditis, right ear

H70.92 Unspecified mastoiditis, left ear

H70.93 Unspecified mastoiditis, bilateral

H71 Cholesteatoma of middle ear

Excludes 2: cholesteatoma of external ear (H60.4-)

recurrent cholesteatoma of postmastoidectomy cavity (H95.0-)

H71.0 Cholesteatoma of attic

H71.00 Cholesteatoma of attic, unspecified ear

H71.01 Cholesteatoma of attic, right ear

H71.02 Cholesteatoma of attic, left ear

H71.03 Cholesteatoma of attic, bilateral

H71.1 Cholesteatoma of tympanum

H71.10 Cholesteatoma of tympanum, unspecified ear

H71.11 Cholesteatoma of tympanum, right ear

H71.12 Cholesteatoma of tympanum, left ear

H71.13 Cholesteatoma of tympanum, bilateral

H71.2 Cholesteatoma of mastoid

H71.20 Cholesteatoma of mastoid, unspecified ear

H71.21 Cholesteatoma of mastoid, right ear

H71.22 Cholesteatoma of mastoid, left ear

H71.23 Cholesteatoma of mastoid, bilateral

H71.3 Diffuse cholesteatosis

H71.30 Diffuse cholesteatosis, unspecified ear

H71.31 Diffuse cholesteatosis, right ear

H71.32 Diffuse cholesteatosis, left ear

H71.33 Diffuse cholesteatosis, bilateral

H71.9 Unspecified cholesteatoma

H71.90 Unspecified cholesteatoma, unspecified ear

H71.91 Unspecified cholesteatoma, right ear

H71.92 Unspecified cholesteatoma, left ear

H71.93 Unspecified cholesteatoma, bilateral

H72 Perforation of tympanic membrane

Includes: persistent post-traumatic perforation of ear drum

postinflammatory perforation of ear drum

Code first any associated otitis media (H65.-, H66.1-, H66.2-, H66.3-, H66.4-, H66.9-, H67.-)

Excludes 1: acute suppurative otitis media with rupture of the tympanic membrane (H66.01-)

traumatic rupture of ear drum (S09.2-)

H72.0 Central perforation of tympanic membrane

H72.00 Central perforation of tympanic membrane, unspecified ear

H72.01 Central perforation of tympanic membrane, right ear

H72.02 Central perforation of tympanic membrane, left ear

H72.03 Central perforation of tympanic membrane, bilateral

H72.1 Attic perforation of tympanic membrane

Perforation of pars flaccida

H72.10 Attic perforation of tympanic membrane, unspecified ear

H72.11 Attic perforation of tympanic membrane, right ear

H72.12 Attic perforation of tympanic membrane, left ear

H72.13 Attic perforation of tympanic membrane, bilateral

H72.2 Other marginal perforations of tympanic membrane

H72.2X Other marginal perforations of tympanic membrane

H72.2X1 Other marginal perforations of tympanic membrane, right ear

H72.2X2 Other marginal perforations of tympanic membrane, left ear

H72.2X3 Other marginal perforations of tympanic membrane, bilateral

H72.2X9 Other marginal perforations of tympanic membrane, unspecified ear

H72.8 Other perforations of tympanic membrane

H72.81 Multiple perforations of tympanic membrane

H72.811 Multiple perforations of tympanic membrane, right ear

H72.812 Multiple perforations of tympanic membrane, left ear

H72.813 Multiple perforations of tympanic membrane, bilateral

H72.819 Multiple perforations of tympanic membrane, unspecified ear

H72.82 Total perforations of tympanic membrane

H72.821 Total perforations of tympanic membrane, right ear

H72.822 Total perforations of tympanic membrane, left ear

H72.823 Total perforations of tympanic membrane, bilateral

H72.829 Total perforations of tympanic membrane, unspecified ear

H72.9 Unspecified perforation of tympanic membrane

H72.90 Unspecified perforation of tympanic membrane, unspecified ear

H72.91 Unspecified perforation of tympanic membrane, right ear

H72.92 Unspecified perforation of tympanic membrane, left ear

H72.93 Unspecified perforation of tympanic membrane, bilateral

H73 Other disorders of tympanic membrane

H73.0 Acute myringitis

Excludes 1: acute myringitis with otitis media (H65, H66)

H73.00 Unspecified acute myringitis

Acute tympanitis NOS

H73.001 Acute myringitis, right ear

H73.002 Acute myringitis, left ear

H73.003 Acute myringitis, bilateral

H73.009 Acute myringitis, unspecified ear

H73.01 Bullous myringitis

H73.011 Bullous myringitis, right ear

H73.012 Bullous myringitis, left ear

H73.013 Bullous myringitis, bilateral

H73.019 Bullous myringitis, unspecified ear

H73.09 Other acute myringitis

H73.091 Other acute myringitis, right ear

H73.092 Other acute myringitis, left ear

H73.093 Other acute myringitis, bilateral

H73.099 Other acute myringitis, unspecified ear

H73.1 Chronic myringitis

Chronic tympanitis

Excludes 1: chronic myringitis with otitis media (H65, H66)

H73.10 Chronic myringitis, unspecified ear

H73.11   Chronic myringitis, right ear
H73.12   Chronic myringitis, left ear
H73.13   Chronic myringitis, bilateral
H73.2   Unspecified myringitis
   H73.20   Unspecified myringitis, unspecified ear
   H73.21   Unspecified myringitis, right ear
   H73.22   Unspecified myringitis, left ear
   H73.23   Unspecified myringitis, bilateral
H73.8   Other specified disorders of tympanic membrane
   H73.81   Atrophic flaccid tympanic membrane
      H73.811   Atrophic flaccid tympanic membrane, right ear
      H73.812   Atrophic flaccid tympanic membrane, left ear
      H73.813   Atrophic flaccid tympanic membrane, bilateral
      H73.819   Atrophic flaccid tympanic membrane, unspecified ear
   H73.82   Atrophic nonflaccid tympanic membrane
      H73.821   Atrophic nonflaccid tympanic membrane, right ear
      H73.822   Atrophic nonflaccid tympanic membrane, left ear
      H73.823   Atrophic nonflaccid tympanic membrane, bilateral
      H73.829   Atrophic nonflaccid tympanic membrane, unspecified ear
   H73.89   Other specified disorders of tympanic membrane
      H73.891   Other specified disorders of tympanic membrane, right ear
      H73.892   Other specified disorders of tympanic membrane, left ear
      H73.893   Other specified disorders of tympanic membrane, bilateral
      H73.899   Other specified disorders of tympanic membrane, unspecified ear
H73.9   Unspecified disorder of tympanic membrane
   H73.90   Unspecified disorder of tympanic membrane, unspecified ear
   H73.91   Unspecified disorder of tympanic membrane, right ear
   H73.92   Unspecified disorder of tympanic membrane, left ear
   H73.93   Unspecified disorder of tympanic membrane, bilateral

H74   Other disorders of middle ear mastoid
Excludes 2: mastoiditis (H70.-)
H74.0   Tympanosclerosis
   H74.01   Tympanosclerosis, right ear
   H74.02   Tympanosclerosis, left ear
   H74.03   Tympanosclerosis, bilateral
   H74.09   Tympanosclerosis, unspecified ear
H74.1   Adhesive middle ear disease
   Adhesive otitis
   Excludes 1: glue ear (H65.3-)
   H74.11   Adhesive right middle ear disease
   H74.12   Adhesive left middle ear disease
   H74.13   Adhesive middle ear disease, bilateral
   H74.19   Adhesive middle ear disease, unspecified ear
H74.2   Discontinuity and dislocation of ear ossicles
   H74.20   Discontinuity and dislocation of ear ossicles, unspecified ear
   H74.21   Discontinuity and dislocation of right ear ossicles

H74.22   Discontinuity and dislocation of left ear ossicles
H74.23   Discontinuity and dislocation of ear ossicles, bilateral
H74.3   Other acquired abnormalities of ear ossicles
   H74.31   Ankylosis of ear ossicles
      H74.311   Ankylosis of ear ossicles, right ear
      H74.312   Ankylosis of ear ossicles, left ear
      H74.313   Ankylosis of ear ossicles, bilateral
      H74.319   Ankylosis of ear ossicles, unspecified ear
   H74.32   Partial loss of ear ossicles
      H74.321   Partial loss of ear ossicles, right ear
      H74.322   Partial loss of ear ossicles, left ear
      H74.323   Partial loss of ear ossicles, bilateral
      H74.329   Partial loss of ear ossicles, unspecified ear
   H74.39   Other acquired abnormalities of ear ossicles
      H74.391   Other acquired abnormalities of right ear ossicles
      H74.392   Other acquired abnormalities of left ear ossicles
      H74.393   Other acquired abnormalities of ear ossicles, bilateral
      H74.399   Other acquired abnormalities of ear ossicles, unspecified ear
H74.4   Polyp of middle ear
   H74.40   Polyp of middle ear, unspecified ear
   H74.41   Polyp of right middle ear
   H74.42   Polyp of left middle ear
   H74.43   Polyp of middle ear, bilateral
H74.8   Other specified disorders of middle ear and mastoid
   H74.8X   Other specified disorders of middle ear and mastoid
      H74.8X1   Other specified disorders of right middle ear and mastoid
      H74.8X2   Other specified disorders of left middle ear and mastoid
      H74.8X3   Other specified disorders of middle ear and mastoid, bilateral
      H74.8X9   Other specified disorders of middle ear and mastoid, unspecified ear
H74.9   Unspecified disorder of middle ear and mastoid
   H74.90   Unspecified disorder of middle ear and mastoid, unspecified ear
   H74.91   Unspecified disorder of right middle ear and mastoid
   H74.92   Unspecified disorder of left middle ear and mastoid
   H74.93   Unspecified disorder of middle ear and mastoid, bilateral

H75   Other disorders of middle ear and mastoid in diseases classified elsewhere
Code first underlying disease
H75.0   Mastoiditis in infectious and parasitic diseases classified elsewhere
   Excludes 1: mastoiditis (in):
      syphilis (A52.77)
      tuberculosis (A18.03)
   H75.00   Mastoiditis in infectious and parasitic diseases classified elsewhere, unspecified ear
   H75.01   Mastoiditis in infectious and parasitic diseases classified elsewhere, right ear

● New code   ▲ Revised code   ⑦ 7th digit required   ⊗ Placeholder required

H75.02 Mastoiditis in infectious and parasitic diseases classified elsewhere, left ear

H75.03 Mastoiditis in infectious and parasitic diseases classified elsewhere, bilateral

H75.8 Other specified disorders of middle ear and mastoid in diseases classified elsewhere

H75.80 Other specified disorders of middle ear and mastoid in diseases classified elsewhere, unspecified ear

H75.81 Other specified disorders of right middle ear and mastoid in diseases classified elsewhere

H75.82 Other specified disorders of left middle ear and mastoid in diseases classified elsewhere

H75.83 Other specified disorders of middle ear and mastoid in diseases classified elsewhere, bilateral

DISEASES OF INNER EAR (H80-H83)

H80 Otosclerosis

Includes: Otospongiosis

H80.0 Otosclerosis involving oval window, nonobliterative

H80.00 Otosclerosis involving oval window, nonobliterative, unspecified ear

H80.01 Otosclerosis involving oval window, nonobliterative, right ear

H80.02 Otosclerosis involving oval window, nonobliterative, left ear

H80.03 Otosclerosis involving oval window, nonobliterative, bilateral

H80.1 Otosclerosis involving oval window, obliterative

H80.10 Otosclerosis involving oval window, obliterative, unspecified ear

H80.11 Otosclerosis involving oval window, obliterative, right ear

H80.12 Otosclerosis involving oval window, obliterative, left ear

H80.13 Otosclerosis involving oval window, obliterative, bilateral

H80.2 Cochlear otosclerosis

Otosclerosis involving otic capsule

Otosclerosis involving round window

H80.20 Cochlear otosclerosis, unspecified ear

H80.21 Cochlear otosclerosis, right ear

H80.22 Cochlear otosclerosis, left ear

H80.23 Cochlear otosclerosis, bilateral

H80.8 Other otosclerosis

H80.80 Other otosclerosis, unspecified ear

H80.81 Other otosclerosis, right ear

H80.82 Other otosclerosis, left ear

H80.83 Other otosclerosis, bilateral

H80.9 Unspecified otosclerosis

H80.90 Unspecified otosclerosis, unspecified ear

H80.91 Unspecified otosclerosis, right ear

H80.92 Unspecified otosclerosis, left ear

H80.93 Unspecified otosclerosis, bilateral

H81 Disorders of vestibular function

Excludes 1: epidemic vertigo (A88.1)

vertigo NOS (R42)

H81.0 Meniere's disease

Labyrinthine hydrops

Meniere's syndrome or vertigo

H81.01 Meniere's disease, right ear

H81.02 Meniere's disease, left ear

H81.03 Meniere's disease, bilateral

H81.09 Meniere's disease, unspecified ear

H81.1 Benign paroxysmal vertigo

H81.10 Benign paroxysmal vertigo, unspecified ear

H81.11 Benign paroxysmal vertigo, right ear

H81.12 Benign paroxysmal vertigo, left ear

H81.13 Benign paroxysmal vertigo, bilateral

H81.2 Vestibular neuronitis

H81.20 Vestibular neuronitis, unspecified ear

H81.21 Vestibular neuronitis, right ear

H81.22 Vestibular neuronitis, left ear

H81.23 Vestibular neuronitis, bilateral

H81.3 Other peripheral vertigo

H81.31 Aural vertigo

H81.311 Aural vertigo, right ear

H81.312 Aural vertigo, left ear

H81.313 Aural vertigo, bilateral

H81.319 Aural vertigo, unspecified ear

H81.39 Other peripheral vertigo

Lermoyez' syndrome

Otogenic vertigo

Peripheral vertigo NOS

H81.391 Other peripheral vertigo, right ear

H81.392 Other peripheral vertigo, left ear

H81.393 Other peripheral vertigo, bilateral

H81.399 Other peripheral vertigo, unspecified ear

H81.4 Vertigo of central origin

Central positional nystagmus

H81.41 Vertigo of central origin, right ear

H81.42 Vertigo of central origin, left ear

H81.43 Vertigo of central origin, bilateral

H81.49 Vertigo of central origin, unspecified ear

H81.8 Other disorders of vestibular function

H81.8X Other disorders of vestibular function

H81.8X1 Other disorders of vestibular function, right ear

H81.8X2 Other disorders of vestibular function, left ear

H81.8X3 Other disorders of vestibular function, bilateral

H81.8X9 Other disorders of vestibular function, unspecified ear

H81.9 Unspecified disorder of vestibular function

Vertiginous syndrome NOS

H81.90 Unspecified disorder of vestibular function, unspecified ear

H81.91 Unspecified disorder of vestibular function, right ear

H81.92 Unspecified disorder of vestibular function, left ear

H81.93 Unspecified disorder of vestibular function, bilateral

H82 Vertiginous syndromes in diseases classified elsewhere

Code first underlying disease

Excludes 1: epidemic vertigo (A88.1)

H82.1 Vertiginous syndromes in diseases classified elsewhere, right ear

H82.2 Vertiginous syndromes in diseases classified elsewhere, left ear

H82.3 Vertiginous syndromes in diseases classified elsewhere, bilateral

H82.9 Vertiginous syndromes in diseases classified elsewhere, unspecified ear

---

H83 Other diseases of inner ear

H83.0 Labyrinthitis

H83.01 Labyrinthitis, right ear

H83.02 Labyrinthitis, left ear

H83.03 Labyrinthitis, bilateral

H83.09 Labyrinthitis, unspecified ear

H83.1 Labyrinthine fistula

H83.11 Labyrinthine fistula, right ear

H83.12 Labyrinthine fistula, left ear

H83.13 Labyrinthine fistula, bilateral

H83.19 Labyrinthine fistula, unspecified ear

H83.2 Labyrinthine dysfunction

Labyrinthine hypersensitivity

Labyrinthine hypofunction

Labyrinthine loss of function

H83.2X Labyrinthine dysfunction

H83.2X1 Labyrinthine dysfunction, right ear

H83.2X2 Labyrinthine dysfunction, left ear

H83.2X3 Labyrinthine dysfunction, bilateral

H83.2X9 Labyrinthine dysfunction, unspecified ear

H83.3 Noise effects on inner ear

Acoustic trauma of inner ear

Noise-induced hearing loss of inner ear

H83.3X Noise effects on inner ear

H83.3X1 Noise effects on right inner ear

H83.3X2 Noise effects on left inner ear

H83.3X3 Noise effects on inner ear, bilateral

H83.3X9 Noise effects on inner ear, unspecified ear

H83.8 Other specified diseases of inner ear

H83.8X Other specified diseases of inner ear

H83.8X1 Other specified diseases of right inner ear

H83.8X2 Other specified diseases of left inner ear

H83.8X3 Other specified diseases of inner ear, bilateral

H83.8X9 Other specified diseases of inner ear, unspecified ear

H83.9 Unspecified disease of inner ear

H83.90 Unspecified disease of inner ear, unspecified ear

H83.91 Unspecified disease of right inner ear

H83.92 Unspecified disease of left inner ear

H83.93 Unspecified disease of inner ear, bilateral

OTHER DISORDERS OF EAR (H90-H94)

H90 Conductive and sensorineural hearing loss

Excludes 1: deaf nonspeaking NEC (H91.3)

deafness NOS (H91.9-)

hearing loss NOS (H91.9-)

noise-induced hearing loss (H83.3-)

ototoxic hearing loss (H91.0-)

sudden (idiopathic) hearing loss (H91.2-)

H90.0 Conductive hearing loss, bilateral

H90.1 Conductive hearing loss, unilateral with unrestricted hearing on the contralateral side

H90.11 Conductive hearing loss, unilateral, right ear, with unrestricted hearing on the contralateral side

H90.12 Conductive hearing loss, unilateral, left ear, with unrestricted hearing on the contralateral side

H90.2 Conductive hearing loss, unspecified

Conductive deafness NOS

H90.3 Sensorineural hearing loss, bilateral

H90.4 Sensorineural hearing loss, unilateral with unrestricted hearing on the contralateral side

H90.41 Sensorineural hearing loss, unilateral, right ear, with unrestricted hearing on the contralateral side

H90.42 Sensorineural hearing loss, unilateral, left ear, with unrestricted hearing on the contralateral side

H90.5 Unspecified sensorineural hearing loss

Central hearing loss NOS

Congenital deafness NOS

Neural hearing loss NOS

Perceptive hearing loss NOS

Sensorineural deafness NOS

Sensory hearing loss NOS

Excludes 1: abnormal auditory perception (H93.2-)

psychogenic deafness (F44.6)

H90.6 Mixed conductive and sensorineural hearing loss, bilateral

H90.7 Mixed conductive and sensorineural hearing loss, unilateral with unrestricted hearing on the contralateral side

H90.71 Mixed conductive and sensorineural hearing loss, unilateral, right ear, with unrestricted hearing on the contralateral side

H90.72 Mixed conductive and sensorineural hearing loss, unilateral, left ear, with unrestricted hearing on the contralateral side

H90.8 Mixed conductive and sensorineural hearing loss, unspecified

H91 Other and unspecified hearing loss

Excludes 1: abnormal auditory perception (H93.2-)

hearing loss as classified in H90.-

impacted cerumen (H61.2-)

noise-induced hearing loss (H83.3-)

psychogenic deafness (F44.6)

transient ischemic deafness (H93.01-)

H91.0 Ototoxic hearing loss

Code first poisoning due to drug or toxin, if applicable (T36-T65 with fifth or sixth character 1-4 or 6)

Use additional code for adverse effect, if applicable, to identify drug (T36-T50 with fifth or sixth character 5)

H91.01 Ototoxic hearing loss, right ear

H91.02 Ototoxic hearing loss, left ear

H91.03 Ototoxic hearing loss, bilateral

H91.09 Ototoxic hearing loss, unspecified ear

H91.1 Presbycusis

Presbyacusia

H91.10 Presbycusis, unspecified ear

H91.11 Presbycusis, right ear

H91.12 Presbycusis, left ear

H91.13 Presbycusis, bilateral

H91.2 Sudden idiopathic hearing loss

Sudden hearing loss NOS

H91.20 Sudden idiopathic hearing loss, unspecified ear

H91.21 Sudden idiopathic hearing loss, right ear

H91.22 Sudden idiopathic hearing loss, left ear

H91.23 Sudden idiopathic hearing loss, bilateral

H91.3 Deaf nonspeaking, not elsewhere classified

H91.8 Other specified hearing loss

H91.8X Other specified hearing loss

H91.8X1 Other specified hearing loss, right ear

H91.8X2 Other specified hearing loss, left ear

H91.8X3 Other specified hearing loss, bilateral

H91.8X9 Other specified hearing loss, unspecified ear

H91.9 Unspecified hearing loss
Deafness NOS
High frequency deafness
Low frequency deafness

H91.90 Unspecified hearing loss, unspecified ear

H91.91 Unspecified hearing loss, right ear

H91.92 Unspecified hearing loss, left ear

H91.93 Unspecified hearing loss, bilateral

H92 Otalgia and effusion of ear

H92.0 Otalgia

H92.01 Otalgia, right ear

H92.02 Otalgia, left ear

H92.03 Otalgia, bilateral

H92.09 Otalgia, unspecified ear

H92.1 Otorrhea

Excludes 1: leakage of cerebrospinal fluid through ear (G96.0)

H92.10 Otorrhea, unspecified ear

H92.11 Otorrhea, right ear

H92.12 Otorrhea, left ear

H92.13 Otorrhea, bilateral

H92.2 Otorrhagia

Excludes 1: traumatic otorrhagia - code to injury

H92.20 Otorrhagia, unspecified ear

H92.21 Otorrhagia, right ear

H92.22 Otorrhagia, left ear

H92.23 Otorrhagia, bilateral

H93 Other disorders of ear, not elsewhere classified

H93.0 Degenerative and vascular disorders of ear

Excludes 1: presbycusis (H91.1)

H93.01 Transient ischemic deafness

H93.011 Transient ischemic deafness, right ear

H93.012 Transient ischemic deafness, left ear

H93.013 Transient ischemic deafness, bilateral

H93.019 Transient ischemic deafness, unspecified ear

H93.09 Unspecified degenerative and vascular disorders of ear

H93.091 Unspecified degenerative and vascular disorders of right ear

H93.092 Unspecified degenerative and vascular disorders of left ear

H93.093 Unspecified degenerative and vascular disorders of ear, bilateral

H93.099 Unspecified degenerative and vascular disorders of unspecified ear

H93.1 Tinnitus

H93.11 Tinnitus, right ear

H93.12 Tinnitus, left ear

H93.13 Tinnitus, bilateral

H93.19 Tinnitus, unspecified ear

H93.2 Other abnormal auditory perceptions

Excludes 2: auditory hallucinations (R44.0)

H93.21 Auditory recruitment

H93.211 Auditory recruitment, right ear

H93.212 Auditory recruitment, left ear

H93.213 Auditory recruitment, bilateral

H93.219 Auditory recruitment, unspecified ear

H93.22 Diplacusis

H93.221 Diplacusis, right ear

H93.222 Diplacusis, left ear

H93.223 Diplacusis, bilateral

H93.229 Diplacusis, unspecified ear

H93.23 Hyperacusis

H93.231 Hyperacusis, right ear

H93.232 Hyperacusis, left ear

H93.233 Hyperacusis, bilateral

H93.239 Hyperacusis, unspecified ear

H93.24 Temporary auditory threshold shift

H93.241 Temporary auditory threshold shift, right ear

H93.242 Temporary auditory threshold shift, left ear

H93.243 Temporary auditory threshold shift, bilateral

H93.249 Temporary auditory threshold shift, unspecified ear

H93.25 Central auditory processing disorder
Congenital auditory imperception
Word deafness

Excludes 1: mixed receptive-expressive language disorder (F80.2)

H93.29 Other abnormal auditory perceptions

H93.291 Other abnormal auditory perceptions, right ear

H93.292 Other abnormal auditory perceptions, left ear

H93.293 Other abnormal auditory perceptions, bilateral

H93.299 Other abnormal auditory perceptions, unspecified ear

H93.3 Disorders of acoustic nerve
Disorder of 8th cranial nerve

Excludes 1: acoustic neuroma (D33.3)
syphilitic acoustic neuritis (A52.15)

H93.3X Disorders of acoustic nerve

H93.3X1 Disorders of right acoustic nerve

H93.3X2 Disorders of left acoustic nerve

H93.3X3 Disorders of bilateral acoustic nerves

H93.3X9 Disorders of unspecified acoustic nerve

H93.8 Other specified disorders of ear

H93.8X Other specified disorders of ear

H93.8X1 Other specified disorders of right ear

H93.8X2 Other specified disorders of left ear

H93.8X3 Other specified disorders of ear, bilateral

H93.8X9 Other specified disorders of ear, unspecified ear

H93.9 Unspecified disorder of ear

H93.90 Unspecified disorder of ear, unspecified ear

H93.91 Unspecified disorder of right ear

H93.92 Unspecified disorder of left ear

H93.93 Unspecified disorder of ear, bilateral

H94 Other disorders of ear in diseases classified elsewhere

H94.0 Acoustic neuritis in infectious and parasitic diseases classified elsewhere

Code first underlying disease, such as:
parasitic disease (B65-B89)

Excludes 1: acoustic neuritis (in):
herpes zoster (B02.29)
syphilis (A52.15)

H94.00   Acoustic neuritis in infectious and parasitic diseases classified elsewhere, unspecified ear

H94.01   Acoustic neuritis in infectious and parasitic diseases classified elsewhere, right ear

H94.02   Acoustic neuritis in infectious and parasitic diseases classified elsewhere, left ear

H94.03   Acoustic neuritis in infectious and parasitic diseases classified elsewhere, bilateral

H94.8   Other specified disorders of ear in diseases classified elsewhere

Code first underlying disease, such as:

congenital syphilis (A50.0)

Excludes 1: aural myiasis (B87.4)

syphilitic labyrinthitis (A52.79)

H94.80   Other specified disorders of ear in diseases classified elsewhere, unspecified ear

H94.81   Other specified disorders of right ear in diseases classified elsewhere

H94.82   Other specified disorders of left ear in diseases classified elsewhere

H94.83   Other specified disorders of ear in diseases classified elsewhere, bilateral

INTRAOPERATIVE AND POSTPROCEDURAL COMPLICATIONS AND DISORDERS OF EAR AND MASTOID PROCESS, NOT ELSEWHERE CLASSIFIED (H95)

H95   Intraoperative and postprocedural complications and disorders of ear and mastoid process, not elsewhere classified

H95.0   Recurrent cholesteatoma of postmastoidectomy cavity

H95.00   Recurrent cholesteatoma of postmastoidectomy cavity, unspecified ear

H95.01   Recurrent cholesteatoma of postmastoidectomy cavity, right ear

H95.02   Recurrent cholesteatoma of postmastoidectomy cavity, left ear

H95.03   Recurrent cholesteatoma of postmastoidectomy cavity, bilateral ears

H95.1   Other disorders of ear and mastoid process following mastoidectomy

H95.11   Chronic inflammation of postmastoidectomy cavity

H95.111   Chronic inflammation of postmastoidectomy cavity, right ear

H95.112   Chronic inflammation of postmastoidectomy cavity, left ear

H95.113   Chronic inflammation of postmastoidectomy cavity, bilateral ears

H95.12   Granulation of postmastoidectomy cavity

H95.121   Granulation of postmastoidectomy cavity, right ear

H95.122   Granulation of postmastoidectomy cavity, left ear

H95.123   Granulation of postmastoidectomy cavity, bilateral ears

H95.129   Granulation of postmastoidectomy cavity, unspecified ear

H95.13   Mucosal cyst of postmastoidectomy cavity

H95.131   Mucosal cyst of postmastoidectomy cavity, right ear

H95.132   Mucosal cyst of postmastoidectomy cavity, left ear

H95.133   Mucosal cyst of postmastoidectomy cavity, bilateral ears

H95.139   Mucosal cyst of postmastoidectomy cavity, unspecified ear

H95.19   Other disorders following mastoidectomy

H95.191   Other disorders following mastoidectomy, right ear

H95.192   Other disorders following mastoidectomy, left ear

H95.193   Other disorders following mastoidectomy, bilateral ears

H95.199   Other disorders following mastoidectomy, unspecified ear

H95.2   Intraoperative hemorrhage and hematoma of ear and mastoid process complicating a procedure

Excludes 1: intraoperative hemorrhage and hematoma of ear and mastoid process due to accidental puncture or laceration during a procedure (H95.3-)

H95.21   Intraoperative hemorrhage and hematoma of ear and mastoid process complicating a procedure on the ear and mastoid process

H95.22   Intraoperative hemorrhage and hematoma of ear and mastoid process complicating other procedure

H95.3   Accidental puncture and laceration of ear and mastoid process during a procedure

H95.31   Accidental puncture and laceration of the ear and mastoid process during a procedure on the ear and mastoid process

H95.32   Accidental puncture and laceration of the ear and mastoid process during other procedure

H95.4   Postprocedural hemorrhage and hematoma of ear and mastoid process following a procedure

H95.41   Postprocedural hemorrhage and hematoma of ear and mastoid process following a procedure on the ear and mastoid process

H95.42   Postprocedural hemorrhage and hematoma of ear and mastoid process following other procedure

H95.8   Other intraoperative and postprocedural complications and disorders of the ear and mastoid process, not elsewhere classified

Excludes 2: postprocedural complications and disorders following mastoidectomy (H95.0-, H95.1-)

H95.81   Postprocedural stenosis of external ear canal

H95.811   Postprocedural stenosis of right external ear canal

H95.812   Postprocedural stenosis of left external ear canal

H95.813   Postprocedural stenosis of external ear canal, bilateral

H95.819   Postprocedural stenosis of unspecified external ear canal

H95.88   Other intraoperative complications and disorders of the ear and mastoid process, not elsewhere classified

Use additional code, if applicable, to further specify disorder

elsewhere classified

Use additional code, if applicable, to further specify disorder

Chapter 9: Diseases Of The Circulatory System (I00-I99)

Excludes 2: certain conditions originating in the perinatal period (P04-P96)

certain infectious and parasitic diseases (A00-B99)

complications of pregnancy, childbirth and the puerperium (O00-O9A)

congenital malformations, deformations, and chromosomal abnormalities (Q00-Q99)

endocrine, nutritional and metabolic diseases (E00-E88)

injury, poisoning and certain other consequences of external causes (S00-T88)

neoplasms (C00-D49)

symptoms, signs and abnormal clinical and laboratory findings, not elsewhere classified (R00-R94)

systemic connective tissue disorders (M30-M36)

transient cerebral ischemic attacks and related syndromes (G45.-)

This chapter contains the following blocks:

I00-I02	Acute rheumatic fever
I05-I09	Chronic rheumatic heart diseases
I10-I15	Hypertensive diseases
I20-I25	Ischemic heart diseases
I26-I28	Pulmonary heart disease and diseases of pulmonary circulation
I30-I52	Other forms of heart disease
I60-I69	Cerebrovascular diseases
I70-I79	Diseases of arteries, arterioles and capillaries
I80-I89	Diseases of veins, lymphatic vessels and lymph nodes, not elsewhere classified
I95-I99	Other and unspecified disorders of the circulatory system

ACUTE RHEUMATIC FEVER (I00-I02)

I00 Rheumatic fever without heart involvement

Includes: arthritis, rheumatic, acute or subacute

Excludes 1: rheumatic fever with heart involvement (I01.0 - I01.9)

I01 Rheumatic fever with heart involvement

Excludes 1: chronic diseases of rheumatic origin (I05-I09) unless rheumatic fever is also present or there is evidence of reactivation or activity of the rheumatic process.

I01.0 Acute rheumatic pericarditis

Any condition in I00 with pericarditis

Rheumatic pericarditis (acute)

Excludes 1: acute pericarditis not specified as rheumatic (I30.-)

I01.1 Acute rheumatic endocarditis

Any condition in I00 with endocarditis or valvulitis

Acute rheumatic valvulitis

I01.2 Acute rheumatic myocarditis

Any condition in I00 with myocarditis

I01.8 Other acute rheumatic heart disease

Any condition in I00 with other or multiple types of heart involvement

Acute rheumatic pancarditis

I01.9 Acute rheumatic heart disease, unspecified

Any condition in I00 with unspecified type of heart involvement

Rheumatic carditis, acute

Rheumatic heart disease, active or acute

I02 Rheumatic chorea

Includes: Sydenham's chorea

Excludes 1: chorea NOS (G25.5)

Huntington's chorea (G10)

I02.0 Rheumatic chorea with heart involvement

Chorea NOS with heart involvement

Rheumatic chorea with heart involvement of any type classifiable under I01.-

I02.9 Rheumatic chorea without heart involvement

Rheumatic chorea NOS

CHRONIC RHEUMATIC HEART DISEASES (I05-I09)

I05 Rheumatic mitral valve diseases

Includes: conditions classifiable to both I05.0 and I05.2-I05.9, whether specified as rheumatic or not

Excludes 1: mitral valve disease specified as nonrheumatic (I34.-)

mitral valve disease with aortic and/or tricuspid valve involvement (I08.-)

I05.0 Rheumatic mitral stenosis

Mitral (valve) obstruction (rheumatic)

I05.1 Rheumatic mitral insufficiency

Rheumatic mitral incompetence

Rheumatic mitral regurgitation

Excludes 1: mitral insufficiency not specified as rheumatic (I34.0)

I05.2 Rheumatic mitral stenosis with insufficiency

Rheumatic mitral stenosis with incompetence or regurgitation

I05.8 Other rheumatic mitral valve diseases

Rheumatic mitral (valve) failure

I05.9 Rheumatic mitral valve disease, unspecified

Rheumatic mitral (valve) disorder (chronic) NOS

I06 Rheumatic aortic valve diseases

Excludes 1: aortic valve disease not specified as rheumatic (I35.-)

aortic valve disease with mitral and/or tricuspid valve involvement (I08.-)

I06.0 Rheumatic aortic stenosis

Rheumatic aortic (valve) obstruction

I06.1 Rheumatic aortic insufficiency

Rheumatic aortic incompetence

Rheumatic aortic regurgitation

I06.2 Rheumatic aortic stenosis with insufficiency

Rheumatic aortic stenosis with incompetence or regurgitation

I06.8 Other rheumatic aortic valve diseases

I06.9 Rheumatic aortic valve disease, unspecified

Rheumatic aortic (valve) disease NOS

I07 Rheumatic tricuspid valve diseases

Includes: rheumatic tricuspid valve diseases specified as rheumatic or unspecified

Excludes 1: tricuspid valve disease specified as nonrheumatic (I36.-)

tricuspid valve disease with aortic and/or mitral valve involvement (I08.-)

I07.0 Rheumatic tricuspid stenosis

Tricuspid (valve) stenosis (rheumatic)

I07.1 Rheumatic tricuspid insufficiency

Tricuspid (valve) insufficiency (rheumatic)

I07.2 Rheumatic tricuspid stenosis and insufficiency

I07.8 Other rheumatic tricuspid valve diseases

I07.9 Rheumatic tricuspid valve disease, unspecified

Rheumatic tricuspid valve disorder NOS

I08 Multiple valve diseases

Includes: multiple valve diseases specified as rheumatic or unspecified

---

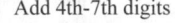 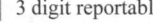

Excludes 1: endocarditis, valve unspecified (I38)

multiple valve disease specified a nonrheumatic (I34.-, I35.-, I36.-, I37.-, I38.-, Q22.-, Q23.-, Q24.8-)

rheumatic valve disease NOS (I09.1)

I08.0 Rheumatic disorders of both mitral and aortic valves

Involvement of both mitral and aortic valves specified as rheumatic or unspecified

I08.1 Rheumatic disorders of both mitral and tricuspid valves

I08.2 Rheumatic disorders of both aortic and tricuspid valves

I08.3 Combined rheumatic disorders of mitral, aortic and tricuspid valves

I08.8 Other rheumatic multiple valve diseases

I08.9 Rheumatic multiple valve disease, unspecified

I09 Other rheumatic heart diseases

I09.0 Rheumatic myocarditis

Excludes 1: myocarditis not specified as rheumatic (I51.4)

I09.1 Rheumatic diseases of endocardium, valve unspecified

Rheumatic endocarditis (chronic)

Rheumatic valvulitis (chronic)

Excludes 1: endocarditis, valve unspecified (I38)

I09.2 Chronic rheumatic pericarditis

Adherent pericardium, rheumatic

Chronic rheumatic mediastinopericarditis

Chronic rheumatic myopericarditis

Excludes 1: chronic pericarditis not specified as rheumatic (I31.-)

I09.8 Other specified rheumatic heart diseases

I09.81 Rheumatic heart failure

Use additional code to identify type of heart failure (I50.-)

I09.89 Other specified rheumatic heart diseases

Rheumatic disease of pulmonary valve

I09.9 Rheumatic heart disease, unspecified

Rheumatic carditis

Excludes 1: rheumatoid carditis (M05.31)

HYPERTENSIVE DISEASES (I10-I15)

Use additional code to identify:

exposure to environmental tobacco smoke (Z77.22)

history of tobacco use (Z87.891)

occupational exposure to environmental tobacco smoke (Z57.31)

tobacco dependence (F17.-)

tobacco use (Z72.0)

Excludes 1: hypertensive disease complicating pregnancy, childbirth and the puerperium (O10-O11, O13-O16)

neonatal hypertension (P29.2)

primary pulmonary hypertension (I27.0)

I10 Essential (primary) hypertension

Includes: high blood pressure

hypertension (arterial) (benign) (essential) (malignant) (primary) (systemic)

Excludes 1: hypertensive disease complicating pregnancy, childbirth and the puerperium (O10-O11, O13-O16)

Excludes 2: essential (primary) hypertension involving vessels of brain (I60-I69)

essential (primary) hypertension involving vessels of eye (H35.0-)

I11 Hypertensive heart disease

Includes: any condition in I51.4-I51.9 due to hypertension

I11.0 Hypertensive heart disease with heart failure

Hypertensive heart failure

Use additional code to identify type of heart failure (I50.-)

I11.9 Hypertensive heart disease without heart failure

Hypertensive heart disease NOS

I12 Hypertensive chronic kidney disease

Includes: any condition in N18 and N26 - due to hypertension

arteriosclerosis of kidney

arteriosclerotic nephritis (chronic) (interstitial)

hypertensive nephropathy

nephrosclerosis

Excludes 1: hypertension due to kidney disease (I15.0, I15.1)

renovascular hypertension (I15.0)

secondary hypertension (I15.-)

Excludes 2: acute kidney failure (N17.-)

I12.0 Hypertensive chronic kidney disease with stage 5 chronic kidney disease or end stage renal disease

Use additional code to identify the stage of chronic kidney disease (N18.5, N18.6)

I12.9 Hypertensive chronic kidney disease with stage 1 through stage 4 chronic kidney disease, or unspecified chronic kidney disease

Hypertensive chronic kidney disease NOS

Hypertensive renal disease NOS

Use additional code to identify the stage of chronic kidney disease (N18.1-N18.4, N18.9)

I13 Hypertensive heart and chronic kidney disease

Includes: any condition in I11.- with any condition in I12.-

cardiorenal disease

cardiovascular renal disease

I13.0 Hypertensive heart and chronic kidney disease with heart failure and stage 1 through stage 4 chronic kidney disease, or unspecified chronic kidney disease

Use additional code to identify type of heart failure (I50.-)

Use additional code to identify stage of chronic kidney disease (N18.1-N18.4, N18.9)

I13.1 Hypertensive heart and chronic kidney disease without heart failure

I13.10 Hypertensive heart and chronic kidney disease without heart failure, with stage 1throughstage 4 chronic kidney disease, or unspecified chronic kidney disease

Hypertensive heart disease and hypertensive chronic kidney disease NOS

Use additional code to identify the stage of chronic kidney disease (N18.1-N18.4, N18.9)

I13.11 Hypertensive heart and chronic kidney disease without heart failure, with stage 5chronic kidney disease, or end stage renal disease

Use additional code to identify the stage of chronic kidney disease (N18.5, N18.6)

I13.2 Hypertensive heart and chronic kidney disease with heart failure and with stage 5 chronic kidney disease, or end stage renal disease

Use additional code to identify type of heart failure (I50.-)

Use additional code to identify the stage of chronic kidney disease (N18.5, N18.6)

I15 Secondary hypertension

Code also underlying condition

Excludes 1: postprocedural hypertension (I97.3)

Excludes 2: secondary hypertension involving vessels of brain (I60-I69)

secondary hypertension involving vessels of eye (H35.0-)

I15.0 Renovascular hypertension

● New code ▲ Revised code ⑦ 7th digit required ⊗ Placeholder required

I15.1   Hypertension secondary to other renal disorders
I15.2   Hypertension secondary to endocrine disorders
I15.8   Other secondary hypertension
I15.9   Secondary hypertension, unspecified

ISCHEMIC HEART DISEASES (I20-I25)

Use additional code to identify presence of hypertension (I10-I15)

I20   Angina pectoris

Use additional code to identify:

exposure to environmental tobacco smoke (Z77.22)

history of tobacco use (Z87.891)

occupational exposure to environmental tobacco smoke (Z57.31)

tobacco dependence (F17.-)

tobacco use (Z72.0)

Excludes 1: angina pectoris with atherosclerotic heart disease of native coronary arteries (I25.1-)

atherosclerosis of coronary artery bypass graft(s) and coronary artery of transplanted heart with angina pectoris (I25.7-)

postinfarction angina (I23.7)

I20.0   Unstable angina
Accelerated angina
Crescendo angina
De novo effort angina
Intermediate coronary syndrome
Preinfarction syndrome
Worsening effort angina

I20.1   Angina pectoris with documented spasm
Angiospastic angina
Prinzmetal angina
Spasm-induced angina
Variant angina

I20.8   Other forms of angina pectoris
Angina equivalent
Angina of effort
Coronary slow flow syndrome
Stenocardia
Use additional code(s) for symptoms associated with angina equivalent

I20.9   Angina pectoris, unspecified
Angina NOS
Anginal syndrome
Cardiac angina
Ischemic chest pain

I21   ST elevation (STEMI) and non-ST elevation (NSTEMI) myocardial infarction

Includes: cardiac infarction

coronary (artery) embolism

coronary (artery) occlusion

coronary (artery) rupture

coronary (artery) thrombosis

infarction of heart, myocardium, or ventricle

myocardial infarction specified as acute or with a stated duration of 4 weeks (28 days) or less from onset

Use additional code, if applicable, to identify:

exposure to environmental tobacco smoke (Z77.22)

history of tobacco use (Z87.891)

occupational exposure to environmental tobacco smoke(Z57.31)

status post administration of tPA (rtPA) in a different facility within the last 24 hours prior to admission to current facility (Z92.82)

tobacco dependence (F17.-)

tobacco use (Z72.0)

Excludes 2: old myocardial infarction (I25.2)

postmyocardial infarction syndrome (I24.1)

subsequent myocardial infarction (I22.-)

I21.0   ST elevation (STEMI) myocardial infarction of anterior wall

I21.01   ST elevation (STEMI) myocardial infarction involving left main coronary artery

I21.02   ST elevation (STEMI) myocardial infarction involving left anterior descending coronary artery
ST elevation (STEMI) myocardial infarction involving diagonal coronary artery

I21.09   ST elevation (STEMI) myocardial infarction involving other coronary artery of anterior wall
Acute transmural myocardial infarction of anterior wall
Anteroapical transmural (Q wave) infarction (acute)
Anterolateral transmural (Q wave) infarction (acute)
Anteroseptal transmural (Q wave) infarction (acute)
Transmural (Q wave) infarction (acute) (of) anterior (wall) NOS

I21.1   ST elevation (STEMI) myocardial infarction of inferior wall

I21.11   ST elevation (STEMI) myocardial infarction involving right coronary artery
Inferoposterior transmural (Q wave) infarction (acute)

I21.19   ST elevation (STEMI) myocardial infarction involving other coronary artery of inferior wall
Acute transmural myocardial infarction of inferior wall
Inferolateral transmural (Q wave) infarction (acute)
Transmural (Q wave) infarction (acute) (of) diaphragmatic wall
Transmural (Q wave) infarction (acute) (of) inferior (wall) NOS
Excludes 2: ST elevation (STEMI) myocardial infarction involving left circumflex coronary artery (I21.21)

I21.2   ST elevation (STEMI) myocardial infarction of other sites

I21.21   ST elevation (STEMI) myocardial infarction involving left circumflex coronary artery
ST elevation (STEMI) myocardial infarction involving oblique marginal coronary artery

I21.29   ST elevation (STEMI) myocardial infarction involving other sites
Acute transmural myocardial infarction of other sites
Apical-lateral transmural (Q wave) infarction (acute)
Basal-lateral transmural (Q wave) infarction (acute)
High lateral transmural (Q wave) infarction (acute)
Lateral (wall) NOS transmural (Q wave) infarction (acute)
Posterior (true) transmural (Q wave) infarction (acute)

Posterobasal transmural (Q wave) infarction (acute)

Posterolateral transmural (Q wave) infarction (acute)

Posteroseptal transmural (Q wave) infarction (acute)

Septal transmural (Q wave) infarction (acute) NOS

I21.3 ST elevation (STEMI) myocardial infarction of unspecified site

Acute transmural myocardial infarction of unspecified site

Myocardial infarction (acute) NOS

Transmural (Q wave) myocardial infarction NOS

I21.4 Non-ST elevation (NSTEMI) myocardial infarction

Acute subendocardial myocardial infarction

Non-Q wave myocardial infarction NOS

Nontransmural myocardial infarction NOS

I22 Subsequent ST elevation (STEMI) and non-ST elevation (NSTEMI) myocardial infarction

Includes: acute myocardial infarction occurring within four weeks (28 days) of a previous acute myocardial infarction, regardless of site

cardiac infarction

coronary (artery) embolism

coronary (artery) occlusion

coronary (artery) rupture

coronary (artery) thrombosis

infarction of heart, myocardium, or ventricle

recurrent myocardial infarction

reinfarction of myocardium

rupture of heart, myocardium, or ventricle

Use additional code, if applicable, to identify:

exposure to environmental tobacco smoke (Z77.22)

history of tobacco use (Z87.891)

occupational exposure to environmental tobacco smoke (Z57.31)

status post administration of tPA (rtPA) in a different facility within the last 24 hours prior to admission to current
facility (Z92.82)

tobacco dependence (F17.-)

tobacco use (Z72.0)

I22.0 Subsequent ST elevation (STEMI) myocardial infarction of anterior wall

Subsequent acute transmural myocardial infarction of anterior wall

Subsequent transmural (Q wave) infarction (acute)(of) anterior (wall) NOS

Subsequent anteroapical transmural (Q wave) infarction (acute)

Subsequent anterolateral transmural (Q wave) infarction (acute)

Subsequent anteroseptal transmural (Q wave) infarction (acute)

I22.1 Subsequent ST elevation (STEMI) myocardial infarction of inferior wall

Subsequent acute transmural myocardial infarction of inferior wall

Subsequent transmural (Q wave) infarction (acute)(of) diaphragmatic wall

Subsequent transmural (Q wave) infarction (acute)(of) inferior (wall) NOS

Subsequent inferolateral transmural (Q wave) infarction (acute)

Subsequent inferoposterior transmural (Q wave) infarction (acute)

I22.2 Subsequent non-ST elevation (NSTEMI) myocardial infarction

Subsequent acute subendocardial myocardial infarction

Subsequent non-Q wave myocardial infarction NOS

Subsequent nontransmural myocardial infarction NOS

I22.8 Subsequent ST elevation (STEMI) myocardial infarction of other sites

Subsequent acute transmural myocardial infarction of other sites

Subsequent apical-lateral transmural (Q wave) myocardial infarction (acute)

Subsequent basal-lateral transmural (Q wave) myocardial infarction (acute)

Subsequent high lateral transmural (Q wave) myocardial infarction (acute)

Subsequent transmural (Q wave) myocardial infarction (acute)(of) lateral (wall) NOS

Subsequent posterior (true)transmural (Q wave) myocardial infarction (acute)

Subsequent posterobasal transmural (Q wave) myocardial infarction (acute)

Subsequent posterolateral transmural (Q wave) myocardial infarction (acute)

Subsequent posteroseptal transmural (Q wave) myocardial infarction (acute)

Subsequent septal NOS transmural (Q wave) myocardial infarction (acute)

I22.9 Subsequent ST elevation (STEMI) myocardial infarction of unspecified site

Subsequent acute myocardial infarction of unspecified site

Subsequent myocardial infarction (acute) NOS

I23 Certain current complications following ST elevation (STEMI) and non-ST elevation (NSTEMI) myocardial infarction (within the 28 day period)

Note: A code from category I23 must be used in conjunction with a code from category I21 or category I22. The I23 code should be sequenced first, if it is the reason for encounter, or, it should be sequenced after the I21 or I22 code if the complication of the MI occurs during the encounter for the MI.

I23.0 Hemopericardium as current complication following acute myocardial infarction

Excludes 1: hemopericardium not specified as current complication following acute myocardial infarction (I31.2)

I23.1 Atrial septal defect as current complication following acute myocardial infarction

Excludes 1: acquired atrial septal defect not specified as current complication following acute myocardial infarction (I51.0)

I23.2 Ventricular septal defect as current complication following acute myocardial infarction

Excludes 1: acquired ventricular septal defect not specified as current complication following acute myocardial infarction (I51.0)

I23.3 Rupture of cardiac wall without hemopericardium as current complication following acute myocardial infarction

I23.4 Rupture of chordae tendineae as current complication following acute myocardial infarction

Excludes 1: rupture of chordae tendineae not specified as current complication following acute myocardial infarction (I51.1)

I23.5 Rupture of papillary muscle as current complication following acute myocardial infarction

● New code   ▲ Revised code   ⑦ 7th digit required   ⊗ Placeholder required

Excludes 1: rupture of papillary muscle not specified as current complication following acute myocardial infarction (I51.2)

I23.6 Thrombosis of atrium, auricular appendage, and ventricle as current complications following acute myocardial infarction

Excludes 1: thrombosis of atrium, auricular appendage, and ventricle not specified as current complication following acute myocardial infarction (I51.3)

I23.7 Postinfarction angina

I23.8 Other current complications following acute myocardial infarction

I24 Other acute ischemic heart diseases

Excludes 1: angina pectoris (I20.-)
　　　　　　transient myocardial ischemia in newborn (P29.4)

I24.0 Acute coronary thrombosis not resulting in myocardial infarction
Acute coronary (artery) (vein) embolism not resulting in myocardial infarction
Acute coronary (artery) (vein) occlusion not resulting in myocardial infarction
Acute coronary (artery) (vein) thromboembolism not resulting in myocardial infarction

Excludes 1: atherosclerotic heart disease (I25.1-)

I24.1 Dressler's syndrome
Postmyocardial infarction syndrome

Excludes 1: postinfarction angina (I23.7)

I24.8 Other forms of acute ischemic heart disease

I24.9 Acute ischemic heart disease, unspecified

Excludes 1: ischemic heart disease (chronic) NOS (I25.9)

I25 Chronic ischemic heart disease

Use additional code to identify:
chronic total occlusion of coronary artery (I25.82)
exposure to environmental tobacco smoke (Z77.22)
history of tobacco use (Z87.891)
occupational exposure to environmental tobacco smoke (Z57.31)
tobacco dependence (F17.-)
tobacco use (Z72.0)

I25.1 Atherosclerotic heart disease of native coronary artery
Atherosclerotic cardiovascular disease
Coronary (artery) atheroma
Coronary (artery) atherosclerosis
Coronary (artery) disease
Coronary (artery) sclerosis
Use additional code, if applicable, to identify:
coronary atherosclerosis due to calcified coronary lesion (I25.84)
coronary atherosclerosis due to lipid rich plaque (I25.83)

Excludes 2: atheroembolism (I75.-)
　　　　　　atherosclerosis of coronary artery bypass graft(s) and transplanted heart (I25.7-)

I25.10 Atherosclerotic heart disease of native coronary artery without angina pectoris
Atherosclerotic heart disease NOS

I25.11 Atherosclerotic heart disease of native coronary artery with angina pectoris

I25.110 Atherosclerotic heart disease of native coronary artery with unstable angina pectoris

Excludes 1: unstable angina without atherosclerotic heart disease (I20.0)

I25.111 Atherosclerotic heart disease of native coronary artery with angina pectoris with documented spasm

Excludes 1: angina pectoris with documented spasm without atherosclerotic heart disease (I20.1)

I25.118 Atherosclerotic heart disease of native coronary artery with other forms of angina pectoris

Excludes 1: other forms of angina pectoris without atherosclerotic heart disease (I20.8)

I25.119 Atherosclerotic heart disease of native coronary artery with unspecified angina pectoris
Atherosclerotic heart disease with angina NOS
Atherosclerotic heart disease with ischemic chest pain

Excludes 1: unspecified angina pectoris without atherosclerotic heart disease (I20.9)

I25.2 Old myocardial infarction
Healed myocardial infarction
Past myocardial infarction diagnosed by ECG or other investigation, but currently presenting no symptoms

I25.3 Aneurysm of heart
Mural aneurysm
Ventricular aneurysm

I25.4 Coronary artery aneurysm and dissection

I25.41 Coronary artery aneurysm
Coronary arteriovenous fistula, acquired

Excludes 1: congenital coronary (artery) aneurysm (Q24.5)

I25.42 Coronary artery dissection

I25.5 Ischemic cardiomyopathy

Excludes 2: coronary atherosclerosis (I25.1-, I25.7-)

I25.6 Silent myocardial ischemia

I25.7 Atherosclerosis of coronary artery bypass graft(s) and coronary artery of transplanted heart with angina pectoris
Use additional code, if applicable, to identify:
coronary atherosclerosis due to calcified coronary lesion (I25.84)
coronary atherosclerosis due to lipid rich plaque (I25.83)

Excludes 1: atherosclerosis of bypass graft(s) of transplanted heart without angina pectoris (I25.812)
　　　　　　atherosclerosis of coronary artery bypass graft(s) without angina pectoris (I25.810)
　　　　　　atherosclerosis of native coronary artery of transplanted heart without angina pectoris (I25.811)
　　　　　　embolism or thrombus of coronary artery bypass graft(s) (T82.8-)

I25.70 Atherosclerosis of coronary artery bypass graft(s), unspecified, with angina pectoris

I25.700 Atherosclerosis of coronary artery bypass graft(s), unspecified, with unstable angina pectoris

Excludes 1: unstable angina pectoris without atherosclerosis of coronary artery bypass graft (I20.0)

I25.701 Atherosclerosis of coronary artery bypass graft(s), unspecified, with angina pectoris with documented spasm

Excludes 1: angina pectoris with documented spasm without atherosclerosis of coronary artery bypass graft (I20.1)

I25.708 Atherosclerosis of coronary artery bypass graft(s), unspecified, with other forms of angina pectoris

Excludes 1: other forms of angina pectoris without atherosclerosis of coronary artery bypass graft (I20.8)

I25.709 Atherosclerosis of coronary artery bypass graft(s), unspecified, with unspecified angina pectoris

Excludes 1: unspecified angina pectoris without atherosclerosis of coronary artery bypass graft (I20.9)

I25.71 Atherosclerosis of autologous vein coronary artery bypass graft(s) with angina pectoris

I25.710 Atherosclerosis of autologous vein coronary artery bypass graft(s) with unstable angina pectoris

Excludes 1: unstable angina without atherosclerosis of autologous vein coronary artery bypass graft(s) (I20.0)

I25.711 Atherosclerosis of autologous vein coronary artery bypass graft(s) with angina pectoris with documented spasm

Excludes 1: angina pectoris with documented spasm without atherosclerosis of autologous vein coronary artery bypass graft(s) I20.1)

I25.718 Atherosclerosis of autologous vein coronary artery bypass graft(s) with other forms of angina pectoris

Excludes 1: other forms of angina pectoris without atherosclerosis of autologous vein coronary artery bypass graft(s)(I20.8)

I25.719 Atherosclerosis of autologous vein coronary artery bypass graft(s) with unspecified angina pectoris

Excludes 1: unspecified angina pectoris without atherosclerosis of autologous vein coronary

artery bypass graft(s) (I20.9)

I25.72 Atherosclerosis of autologous artery coronary artery bypass graft(s) with angina pectoris

Atherosclerosis of internal mammary artery graft with angina pectoris

I25.720 Atherosclerosis of autologous artery coronary artery bypass graft(s) with unstable angina pectoris

Excludes 1: unstable angina without atherosclerosis of autologous artery coronary artery bypass graft(s) (I20.0)

I25.721 Atherosclerosis of autologous artery coronary artery bypass graft(s) with angina pectoris with documented spasm

Excludes 1: angina pectoris with documented spasm without atherosclerosis of autologous artery coronary artery bypass graft(s) (I20.1

I25.728 Atherosclerosis of autologous artery coronary artery bypass graft(s) with other forms of angina pectoris

Excludes 1: other forms of angina pectoris without atherosclerosis of autologous artery coronary artery bypass graft(s) I20.8)

I25.729 Atherosclerosis of autologous artery coronary artery bypass graft(s) with unspecified angina pectoris

Excludes 1: unspecified angina pectoris without atherosclerosis of autologous artery coronary artery bypass graft(s) (I20.9)

I25.73 Atherosclerosis of nonautologous biological coronary artery bypass graft(s) with angina pectoris

I25.730 Atherosclerosis of nonautologous biological coronary artery bypass graft(s) with unstable angina pectoris

Excludes 1: unstable angina without atherosclerosis of nonautologous biological coronary artery bypass graft(s) (I20.0)

I25.731 Atherosclerosis of nonautologous biological coronary artery bypass graft(s) with angina pectoris with documented spasm

Excludes 1: angina pectoris with documented spasm without atherosclerosis of nonautologous biological coronary artery bypass graft(s) (I20.1)

● New code   ▲ Revised code   ⑦ 7th digit required   ⊗ Placeholder required

I25.738   Atherosclerosis of nonautologous biological coronary artery bypass graft(s) with other forms of angina pectoris
Excludes 1: other forms of angina pectoris without atherosclerosis of nonautologous biological coronary artery bypass graft(s) (I20.8)

I25.739   Atherosclerosis of nonautologous biological coronary artery bypass graft(s) with unspecified angina pectoris
Excludes 1: unspecified angina pectoris without atherosclerosis of nonautologous biological coronary artery bypass graft(s) (I20.9)

I25.75   Atherosclerosis of native coronary artery of transplanted heart with angina pectoris
Excludes 1: atherosclerosis of native coronary artery of transplanted heart without angina pectoris (I25.811)

I25.750   Atherosclerosis of native coronary artery of transplanted heart with unstable angina

I25.751   Atherosclerosis of native coronary artery of transplanted heart with angina pectoris with documented spasm

I25.758   Atherosclerosis of native coronary artery of transplanted heart with other forms of angina pectoris

I25.759   Atherosclerosis of native coronary artery of transplanted heart with unspecified angina pectoris

I25.76   Atherosclerosis of bypass graft of coronary artery of transplanted heart with angina pectoris
Excludes 1: atherosclerosis of bypass graft of coronary artery of transplanted heart without angina pectoris (I25.812)

I25.760   Atherosclerosis of bypass graft of coronary artery of transplanted heart with unstable angina

I25.761   Atherosclerosis of bypass graft of coronary artery of transplanted heart with angina pectoris with documented spasm

I25.768   Atherosclerosis of bypass graft of coronary artery of transplanted heart with other forms of angina pectoris

I25.769   Atherosclerosis of bypass graft of coronary artery of transplanted heart with unspecified angina pectoris

I25.79   Atherosclerosis of other coronary artery bypass graft(s) with angina pectoris

I25.790   Atherosclerosis of other coronary artery bypass graft(s) with unstable angina pectoris
Excludes 1: unstable angina without atherosclerosis of other coronary artery bypass graft(s) (I20.0)

I25.791   Atherosclerosis of other coronary artery bypass graft(s) with angina pectoris with documented spasm
Excludes 1: angina pectoris with documented spasm without atherosclerosis of other coronary artery bypass graft(s) (I20.1)

I25.798   Atherosclerosis of other coronary artery bypass graft(s) with other forms of angina pectoris
Excludes 1: other forms of angina pectoris without atherosclerosis of other coronary artery bypass graft(s)(I20.8)

I25.799   Atherosclerosis of other coronary artery bypass graft(s) with unspecified angina pectoris
Excludes 1: unspecified angina pectoris without atherosclerosis of other coronary artery bypass graft(s) (I20.9)

I25.8   Other forms of chronic ischemic heart disease

I25.81   Atherosclerosis of other coronary vessels without angina pectoris
Use additional code, if applicable, to identify:
coronary atherosclerosis due to calcified coronary lesion (I25.84)
coronary atherosclerosis due to lipid rich plaque (I25.83)
Excludes 1: atherosclerotic heart disease of native coronary artery without angina pectoris (I25.10)

I25.810   Atherosclerosis of coronary artery bypass graft(s) without angina pectoris
Atherosclerosis of coronary artery bypass graft NOS
Excludes 1: atherosclerosis of coronary bypass graft(s) with angina pectoris (I25.70-I25.73-, I25.79-)

I25.811   Atherosclerosis of native coronary artery of transplanted heart without angina pectoris
Atherosclerosis of native coronary artery of transplanted heart NOS
Excludes 1: atherosclerosis of native coronary artery of transplanted heart with angina pectoris (I25.75-)

I25.812   Atherosclerosis of bypass graft of coronary artery of transplanted heart without angina pectoris
Atherosclerosis of bypass graft of transplanted heart NOS
Excludes 1: atherosclerosis of bypass graft of transplanted heart with angina pectoris (I25.76)

I25.82 Chronic total occlusion of coronary artery
Complete occlusion of coronary artery
Total occlusion of coronary artery
Code first coronary atherosclerosis (I25.1-, I25.7-, I25.81-)
Excludes 1: acute coronary occlusion with myocardial infarction (I21.-, I22.-)
acute coronary occlusion without myocardial infarction (I24.0)

I25.83 Coronary atherosclerosis due to lipid rich plaque
Code first coronary atherosclerosis (I25.1-, I25.7-, I25.81-)

I25.84 Coronary atherosclerosis due to calcified coronary lesion
Coronary atherosclerosis due to severely calcified coronary lesion
Code first coronary atherosclerosis (I25.1-, I25.7-, I25.81-)

I25.89 Other forms of chronic ischemic heart disease

I25.9 Chronic ischemic heart disease, unspecified
Ischemic heart disease (chronic) NOS

PULMONARY HEART DISEASE AND DISEASES OF PULMONARY CIRCULATION (I26-I28)

I26 Pulmonary embolism
Includes: pulmonary (acute) (artery)(vein) infarction
pulmonary (acute) (artery)(vein) thromboembolism
pulmonary (acute) (artery)(vein) thrombosis
Excludes 2: chronic pulmonary embolism (I27.82)
personal history of pulmonary embolism (Z86.711)
pulmonary embolism due to trauma (T79.0, T79.1)
pulmonary embolism due to complications of surgical and medical care (T80.0, T81.7-, T82.8-)
pulmonary embolism complicating: abortion, ectopic or molar pregnancy (O00-O07, O08.2)
pregnancy, childbirth and the puerperium (O88.-)
septic (non-pulmonary) arterial embolism (I76)

I26.0 Pulmonary embolism with acute cor pulmonale
I26.01 Septic pulmonary embolism with acute cor pulmonale
Code first underlying infection

I26.02 Saddle embolus of pulmonary artery with acute cor pulmonale

I26.09 Other pulmonary embolism with acute cor pulmonale
Acute cor pulmonale NOS

I26.9 Pulmonary embolism without acute cor pulmonale
I26.90 Septic pulmonary embolism without acute cor pulmonale
Code first underlying infection

I26.92 Saddle embolus of pulmonary artery without acute cor pulmonale

I26.99 Other pulmonary embolism without acute cor pulmonale
Acute pulmonary embolism NOS
Pulmonary embolism NOS

I27 Other pulmonary heart diseases
I27.0 Primary pulmonary hypertension
Excludes 1: pulmonary hypertension NOS (I27.2)
secondary pulmonary hypertension (I27.2)

I27.1 Kyphoscoliotic heart disease

I27.2 Other secondary pulmonary hypertension
Pulmonary hypertension NOS

Code also associated underlying condition
I27.8 Other specified pulmonary heart diseases
I27.81 Cor pulmonale (chronic)
Cor pulmonale NOS
Excludes 1: acute cor pulmonale (I26.0-)

I27.82 Chronic pulmonary embolism
Use additional code, if applicable, for associated long-term (current) use of anticoagulants (Z79.01)
Excludes 1: personal history of pulmonary embolism (Z86.711)

I27.89 Other specified pulmonary heart diseases
Eisenmenger's complex
Eisenmenger's syndrome
Excludes 1: Eisenmenger's defect (Q21.8)

I27.9 Pulmonary heart disease, unspecified
Chronic cardiopulmonary disease

I28 Other diseases of pulmonary vessels
I28.0 Arteriovenous fistula of pulmonary vessels
Excludes 1: congenital arteriovenous fistula (Q25.72)

I28.1 Aneurysm of pulmonary artery
Excludes 1: congenital aneurysm (Q25.79)
congenital arteriovenous aneurysm (Q25.72)

I28.8 Other diseases of pulmonary vessels
Pulmonary arteritis
Pulmonary endarteritis
Rupture of pulmonary vessels
Stenosis of pulmonary vessels
Stricture of pulmonary vessels

I28.9 Disease of pulmonary vessels, unspecified

OTHER FORMS OF HEART DISEASE (I30-I52)

I30 Acute pericarditis
Includes: acute mediastinopericarditis
acute myopericarditis
acute pericardial effusion
acute pleuropericarditis
acute pneumopericarditis
Excludes 1: Dressler's syndrome (I24.1)
rheumatic pericarditis (acute) (I01.0)

I30.0 Acute nonspecific idiopathic pericarditis

I30.1 Infective pericarditis
Pneumococcal pericarditis
Pneumopyopericardium
Purulent pericarditis
Pyopericarditis
Pyopericardium
Pyopneumopericardium
Staphylococcal pericarditis
Streptococcal pericarditis
Suppurative pericarditis
Viral pericarditis
Use additional code (B95-B97) to identify infectious agent

I30.8 Other forms of acute pericarditis

I30.9 Acute pericarditis, unspecified

I31 Other diseases of pericardium
Excludes 1: diseases of pericardium specified as rheumatic (I09.2)
postcardiotomy syndrome (I97.0)
traumatic injury to pericardium (S26.-)

I31.0 Chronic adhesive pericarditis
Accretio cordis
Adherent pericardium
Adhesive mediastinopericarditis

I31.1 Chronic constrictive pericarditis
Concretio cordis
Pericardial calcification

I31.2 Hemopericardium, not elsewhere classified
Excludes 1: hemopericardium as current complication following acute myocardial infarction (I23.0)

I31.3 Pericardial effusion (noninflammatory)
Chylopericardium
Excludes 1: acute pericardial effusion (I30.9)

I31.4 Cardiac tamponade
Code first underlying cause

I31.8 Other specified diseases of pericardium
Epicardial plaques
Focal pericardial adhesions

I31.9 Disease of pericardium, unspecified
Pericarditis (chronic) NOS

I32 Pericarditis in diseases classified elsewhere
Code first underlying disease
Excludes 1: pericarditis (in):
coxsackie (virus) (B33.23)
gonococcal (A54.83)
meningococcal (A39.53)
rheumatoid (arthritis) (M05.31)
syphilitic (A52.06)
systemic lupus crythematosus (M32.12)
tuberculosis (A18.84)

I33 Acute and subacute endocarditis
Excludes 1: acute rheumatic endocarditis (I01.1)
endocarditis NOS (I38)

I33.0 Acute and subacute infective endocarditis
Bacterial endocarditis (acute) (subacute)
Infective endocarditis (acute) (subacute) NOS
Endocarditis lenta (acute) (subacute)
Malignant endocarditis (acute) (subacute)
Purulent endocarditis (acute) (subacute)
Septic endocarditis (acute) (subacute)
Ulcerative endocarditis (acute) (subacute)
Vegetative endocarditis (acute) (subacute)
Use additional code (B95-B97) to identify infectious agent

I33.9 Acute and subacute endocarditis, unspecified
Acute endocarditis NOS
Acute myoendocarditis NOS
Acute periendocarditis NOS
Subacute endocarditis NOS
Subacute myoendocarditis NOS
Subacute periendocarditis NOS

I34 Nonrheumatic mitral valve disorders
Excludes 1: mitral valve disease (I05.9)
mitral valve failure (I05.8)
mitral valve stenosis (I05.0)
mitral valve disorder of unspecified cause with diseases of aortic and/or tricuspid valve(s) (I08.-)
mitral valve disorder of unspecified cause with mitral stenosis or obstruction (I05.0)
mitral valve disorder specified as congenital (Q23.2, Q23.3)
mitral valve disorder specified as rheumatic (I05.-)

I34.0 Nonrheumatic mitral (valve) insufficiency
Nonrheumatic mitral (valve) incompetence NOS
Nonrheumatic mitral (valve) regurgitation NOS

I34.1 Nonrheumatic mitral (valve) prolapse
Floppy nonrheumatic mitral valve syndrome

Excludes 1: Marfan's syndrome (Q87.4-)

I34.2 Nonrheumatic mitral (valve) stenosis

I34.8 Other nonrheumatic mitral valve disorders

I34.9 Nonrheumatic mitral valve disorder, unspecified

I35 Nonrheumatic aortic valve disorders
Excludes 1: aortic valve disorder of unspecified cause but with diseases of mitral and/or tricuspid valve(s) (I08.-)
aortic valve disorder specified as congenital (Q23.0, Q23.1)
aortic valve disorder specified as rheumatic (I06.-)
hypertrophic subaortic stenosis (I42.1)

I35.0 Nonrheumatic aortic (valve) stenosis

I35.1 Nonrheumatic aortic (valve) insufficiency
Nonrheumatic aortic (valve) incompetence NOS
Nonrheumatic aortic (valve) regurgitation NOS

I35.2 Nonrheumatic aortic (valve) stenosis with insufficiency

I35.8 Other nonrheumatic aortic valve disorders

I35.9 Nonrheumatic aortic valve disorder, unspecified

I36 Nonrheumatic tricuspid valve disorders
Excludes 1: tricuspid valve disorders of unspecified cause (I07.-)
tricuspid valve disorders specified as congenital (Q22.4, Q22.8, Q22.9)
tricuspid valve disorders specified as rheumatic (I07.-)
tricuspid valve disorders with aortic and/or mitral valve involvement (I08.-)

I36.0 Nonrheumatic tricuspid (valve) stenosis

I36.1 Nonrheumatic tricuspid (valve) insufficiency
Nonrheumatic tricuspid (valve) incompetence
Nonrheumatic tricuspid (valve) regurgitation

I36.2 Nonrheumatic tricuspid (valve) stenosis with insufficiency

I36.8 Other nonrheumatic tricuspid valve disorders

I36.9 Nonrheumatic tricuspid valve disorder, unspecified

I37 Nonrheumatic pulmonary valve disorders
Excludes 1: pulmonary valve disorder specified as congenital (Q22.1, Q22.2, Q22.3)
pulmonary valve disorder specified as rheumatic (I09.89)

I37.0 Nonrheumatic pulmonary valve stenosis

I37.1 Nonrheumatic pulmonary valve insufficiency
Nonrheumatic pulmonary valve incompetence
Nonrheumatic pulmonary valve regurgitation

I37.2 Nonrheumatic pulmonary valve stenosis with insufficiency

I37.8 Other nonrheumatic pulmonary valve disorders

I37.9 Nonrheumatic pulmonary valve disorder, unspecified

I38 Endocarditis, valve unspecified
Includes: endocarditis (chronic) NOS
valvular incompetence NOS
valvular insufficiency NOS
valvular regurgitation NOS
valvular stenosis NOS
valvulitis (chronic) NOS
Excludes 1: congenital insufficiency of cardiac valve NOS (Q24.8)
congenital stenosis of cardiac valve NOS (Q24.8)
endocardial fibroelastosis (I42.4)
endocarditis specified as rheumatic (I09.1)

I39 Endocarditis and heart valve disorders in diseases classified elsewhere
Code first underlying disease, such as:
Q fever (A78)
Excludes 1: endocardial involvement in:
candidiasis (B37.6)
gonococcal infection (A54.83)
Libman-Sacks disease (M32.11)

listerosis (A32.82)
meningococcal infection (A39.51)
rheumatoid arthritis (M05.31)
syphilis (A52.03)
tuberculosis (A18.84)
typhoid fever (A01.02)

I40 Acute myocarditis
Includes: subacute myocarditis
Excludes 1: acute rheumatic myocarditis (I01.2)
I40.0 Infective myocarditis
Septic myocarditis
Use additional code (B95-B97) to identify infectious agent
I40.1 Isolated myocarditis
Fiedler's myocarditis
Giant cell myocarditis
Idiopathic myocarditis
I40.8 Other acute myocarditis
I40.9 Acute myocarditis, unspecified

I41 Myocarditis in diseases classified elsewhere
Code first underlying disease, such as:
typhus (A75.0-A75.9)
Excludes 1: myocarditis (in):
Chagas' disease (chronic) (B57.2)
acute (B57.0)
coxsackie (virus) infection (B33.22)
diphtheritic (A36.81)
gonococcal (A54.83)
influenzal (J09.X9, J10.82, J11.82)
meningococcal (A39.52)
mumps (B26.82)
rheumatoid arthritis (M05.31)
sarcoid (D86.85)
syphilis (A52.06)
toxoplasmosis (B58.81)
tuberculous (A18.84)

I42 Cardiomyopathy
Includes: myocardiopathy
Code first cardiomyopathy complicating pregnancy and
puerperium (O99.4)
Excludes 1: ischemic cardiomyopathy (I25.5)
peripartum cardiomyopathy (O90.3)
Excludes 2: ventricular hypertrophy (I51.7)

I42.0 Dilated cardiomyopathy
Congestive cardiomyopathy
I42.1 Obstructive hypertrophic cardiomyopathy
Hypertrophic subaortic stenosis (idiopathic)
I42.2 Other hypertrophic cardiomyopathy
Nonobstructive hypertrophic cardiomyopathy
I42.3 Endomyocardial (eosinophilic) disease
Endomyocardial (tropical) fibrosis
Loeffler's endocarditis
I42.4 Endocardial fibroelastosis
Congenital cardiomyopathy
Elastomyofibrosis
I42.5 Other restrictive cardiomyopathy
Constrictive cardiomyopathy NOS
I42.6 Alcoholic cardiomyopathy
Code also presence of alcoholism (F10.-)
I42.7 Cardiomyopathy due to drug and external agent
Code first poisoning due to drug or toxin, if applicable
(T36-T65with fifth or sixth character 1-4or 6)

Use additional code for adverse effect, if applicable, to
identify drug (T36-T50with fifth or sixth character 5)
I42.8 Other cardiomyopathies
I42.9 Cardiomyopathy, unspecified
Cardiomyopathy (primary) (secondary) NOS
I43 Cardiomyopathy in diseases classified elsewhere
Code first underlying disease, such as:
amyloidosis (E85-)
glycogen storage disease (E74.0)
gout (M10.0-)
thyrotoxicosis (E05.0-E05.9-)
Excludes 1: cardiomyopathy (in):
coxsackie (virus) (B33.24)
diphtheria (A36.81)
sarcoidosis (D86.85)
tuberculosis (A18.84)
I44 Atrioventricular and left bundle-branch block
I44.0 Atrioventricular block, first degree
I44.1 Atrioventricular block, second degree
Atrioventricular block, type I and II
Mobitz block, type I and II
Second degree block, type I and II
Wenckebach's block
I44.2 Atrioventricular block, complete
Complete heart block NOS
Third degree block
I44.3 Other and unspecified atrioventricular block
Atrioventricular block NOS
I44.30 Unspecified atrioventricular block
I44.39 Other atrioventricular block
I44.4 Left anterior fascicular block
I44.5 Left posterior fascicular block
I44.6 Other and unspecified fascicular block
I44.60 Unspecified fascicular block
Left bundle-branch hemiblock NOS
I44.69 Other fascicular block
I44.7 Left bundle-branch block, unspecified
I45 Other conduction disorders
I45.0 Right fascicular block
I45.1 Other and unspecified right bundle-branch block
I45.10 Unspecified right bundle-branch block
Right bundle-branch block NOS
I45.19 Other right bundle-branch block
I45.2 Bifascicular block
I45.3 Trifascicular block
I45.4 Nonspecific intraventricular block
Bundle-branch block NOS
I45.5 Other specified heart block
Sinoatrial block
Sinoauricular block
Excludes 1: heart block NOS (I45.9)
I45.6 Pre-excitation syndrome
Accelerated atrioventricular conduction
Accessory atrioventricular conduction
Anomalous atrioventricular excitation
Lown-Ganong-Levine syndrome
Pre-excitation atrioventricular conduction
Wolff-Parkinson-White syndrome
I45.8 Other specified conduction disorders
I45.81 Long QT syndrome
I45.89 Other specified conduction disorders
Atrioventricular [AV] dissociation

Interference dissociation

Isorhythmic dissociation

Nonparoxysmal AV nodal tachycardia

I45.9 Conduction disorder, unspecified

Heart block NOS

Stokes-Adams syndrome

I46 Cardiac arrest

Excludes 1: cardiogenic shock (R57.0)

I46.2 Cardiac arrest due to underlying cardiac condition

Code first underlying cardiac condition

I46.8 Cardiac arrest due to other underlying condition

Code first underlying condition

I46.9 Cardiac arrest, cause unspecified

I47 Paroxysmal tachycardia

Code first tachycardia complicating:

abortion or ectopic or molar pregnancy (O00-O07, O08.8)

obstetric surgery and procedures (O75.4)

Excludes 1: tachycardia: NOS (R00.0)

sinoauricular NOS (R00.0)

sinus [sinusal] NOS (R00.0)

I47.0 Re-entry ventricular arrhythmia

I47.1 Supraventricular tachycardia

Atrial (paroxysmal) tachycardia

Atrioventricular [AV] (paroxysmal) tachycardia

Atrioventricular re-entrant (nodal) tachycardia [AVNRT] [AVRT]

Junctional (paroxysmal) tachycardia

Nodal (paroxysmal) tachycardia

I47.2 Ventricular tachycardia

I47.9 Paroxysmal tachycardia, unspecified

Bouveret (-Hoffman) syndrome

I48 Atrial fibrillation and flutter

I48.0 Paroxysmal atrial fibrillation

I48.1 Persistent atrial fibrillation

I48.2 Chronic atrial fibrillation

Permanent atrial fibrillation

I48.3 Typical atrial flutter

Type I atrial flutter

I48.4 Atypical atrial flutter

Type II atrial flutter

I48.9 Unspecified atrial fibrillation and atrial flutter

I48.91 Unspecified atrial fibrillation

I48.92 Unspecified atrial flutter

I49 Other cardiac arrhythmias

Code first cardiac arrhythmia complicating:

abortion or ectopic or molar pregnancy (O00-O07, O08.8)

obstetric surgery and procedures (O75.4)

Excludes 1: bradycardia:

NOS (R00.1)

sinoatrial (R00.1)

sinus (R00.1)

vagal (R00.1)

neonatal dysrhythmia (P29.1-)

I49.0 Ventricular fibrillation and flutter

I49.01 Ventricular fibrillation

I49.02 Ventricular flutter

I49.1 Atrial premature depolarization

Atrial premature beats

I49.2 Junctional premature depolarization

I49.3 Ventricular premature depolarization

I49.4 Other and unspecified premature depolarization

I49.40 Unspecified premature depolarization

Premature beats NOS

I49.49 Other premature depolarization

Ectopic beats

Extrasystoles

Extrasystolic arrhythmias

Premature contractions

I49.5 Sick sinus syndrome

Tachycardia-bradycardia syndrome

I49.8 Other specified cardiac arrhythmias

Coronary sinus rhythm disorder

Ectopic rhythm disorder

Nodal rhythm disorder

I49.9 Cardiac arrhythmia, unspecified

Arrhythmia (cardiac) NOS

I50 Heart failure

Code first heart failure complicating abortion or ectopic or molar pregnancy (O00-O07, O08.8)

heart failure following surgery (I97.13-)

heart failure due to hypertension (I11.0)

heart failure due to hypertension with chronic kidney disease (I13.-)

obstetric surgery and procedures (O75.4)

rheumatic heart failure (I09.81)

Excludes 1: cardiac arrest (I46.-)

neonatal cardiac failure (P29.0)

I50.1 Left ventricular failure

Cardiac asthma

Edema of lung with heart disease NOS

Edema of lung with heart failure

Left heart failure

Pulmonary edema with heart disease NOS

Pulmonary edema with heart failure

Excludes 1: edema of lung without heart disease or heart failure (J81.-)

pulmonary edema without heart disease or failure (J81.-)

I50.2 Systolic (congestive) heart failure

Excludes 1: combined systolic (congestive) and diastolic (congestive) heart failure (I50.4-)

I50.20 Unspecified systolic (congestive) heart failure

I50.21 Acute systolic (congestive) heart failure

I50.22 Chronic systolic (congestive) heart failure

I50.23 Acute on chronic systolic (congestive) heart failure

I50.3 Diastolic (congestive) heart failure

Excludes 1: combined systolic (congestive) and diastolic (congestive) heart failure (I50.4-)

I50.30 Unspecified diastolic (congestive) heart failure

I50.31 Acute diastolic (congestive) heart failure

I50.32 Chronic diastolic (congestive) heart failure

I50.33 Acute on chronic diastolic (congestive) heart failure

I50.4 Combined systolic (congestive) and diastolic (congestive) heart failure

I50.40 Unspecified combined systolic (congestive) and diastolic (congestive) heart failure

I50.41 Acute combined systolic (congestive) and diastolic (congestive) heart failure

I50.42 Chronic combined systolic (congestive) and diastolic (congestive) heart failure

I50.43 Acute on chronic combined systolic (congestive) and diastolic (congestive) heart failure

I50.9 Heart failure, unspecified

Biventricular (heart) failure NOS

Cardiac, heart or myocardial failure NOS

Congestive heart disease

Congestive heart failure NOS

Right ventricular failure (secondary to left heart failure)

Excludes 1: fluid overload (E87.70)

I51 Complications and ill-defined descriptions of heart disease

Excludes 1: any condition in I51.4-I51.9 due to hypertension (I11.-)

any condition in I51.4-I51.9 due to hypertension and chronic kidney disease (I13.-)

heart disease specified as rheumatic (I00-I09)

I51.0 Cardiac septal defect, acquired

Acquired septal atrial defect (old)

Acquired septal auricular defect (old)

Acquired septal ventricular defect (old)

Excludes 1: cardiac septal defect as current complication following acute myocardial infarction (I23.1, I23.2)

I51.1 Rupture of chordae tendineae, not elsewhere classified

Excludes 1: rupture of chordae tendineae as current complication following acute myocardial infarction (I23.4)

I51.2 Rupture of papillary muscle, not elsewhere classified

Excludes 1: rupture of papillary muscle as current complication following acute myocardial infarction (I23.5)

I51.3 Intracardiac thrombosis, not elsewhere classified

Apical thrombosis (old)

Atrial thrombosis (old)

Auricular thrombosis (old)

Mural thrombosis (old)

Ventricular thrombosis (old)

Excludes 1: intracardiac thrombosis as current complication following acute myocardial infarction (I23.6)

I51.4 Myocarditis, unspecified

Chronic (interstitial) myocarditis

Myocardial fibrosis

Myocarditis NOS

Excludes 1: acute or subacute myocarditis (I40.-)

I51.5 Myocardial degeneration

Fatty degeneration of heart or myocardium

Myocardial disease

Senile degeneration of heart or myocardium

I51.7 Cardiomegaly

Cardiac dilatation

Cardiac hypertrophy

Ventricular dilatation

I51.8 Other ill-defined heart diseases

I51.81 Takotsubo syndrome

Reversible left ventricular dysfunction following sudden emotional stress

Stress induced cardiomyopathy

Takotsubo cardiomyopathy

Transient left ventricular apical ballooning syndrome

I51.89 Other ill-defined heart diseases

Carditis (acute)(chronic)

Pancarditis (acute)(chronic)

I51.9 Heart disease, unspecified

I52 Other heart disorders in diseases classified elsewhere

Code first underlying disease, such as:

congenital syphilis (A50.5)

mucopolysaccharidosis (E76.3)

schistosomiasis (B65.0-B65.9)

Excludes 1: heart disease (in):

gonococcal infection (A54.83)

meningococcal infection (A39.50)

rheumatoid arthritis (M05.31)

syphilis (A52.06)

CEREBROVASCULAR DISEASES (I60-I69)

Use additional code to identify presence of:

alcohol abuse and dependence (F10.-)

exposure to environmental tobacco smoke (Z77.22)

history of tobacco use (Z87.891)

hypertension (I10-I15)

occupational exposure to environmental tobacco smoke (Z57.31)

tobacco dependence (F17.-)

tobacco use (Z72.0)

Excludes 1: transient cerebral ischemic attacks and related syndromes (G45.-)

traumatic intracranial hemorrhage (S06.-)

I60 Nontraumatic subarachnoid hemorrhage

Includes: ruptured cerebral aneurysm

Excludes 1: sequelae of subarachnoid hemorrhage (I69.0-)

syphilitic ruptured cerebral aneurysm (A52.05)

I60.0 Nontraumatic subarachnoid hemorrhage from carotid siphon and bifurcation

I60.00 Nontraumatic subarachnoid hemorrhage from unspecified carotid siphon and bifurcation

I60.01 Nontraumatic subarachnoid hemorrhage from right carotid siphon and bifurcation

I60.02 Nontraumatic subarachnoid hemorrhage from left carotid siphon and bifurcation

I60.1 Nontraumatic subarachnoid hemorrhage from middle cerebral artery

I60.10 Nontraumatic subarachnoid hemorrhage from unspecified middle cerebral artery

I60.11 Nontraumatic subarachnoid hemorrhage from right middle cerebral artery

I60.12 Nontraumatic subarachnoid hemorrhage from left middle cerebral artery

I60.2 Nontraumatic subarachnoid hemorrhage from anterior communicating artery

I60.20 Nontraumatic subarachnoid hemorrhage from unspecified anterior communicating artery

I60.21 Nontraumatic subarachnoid hemorrhage from right anterior communicating artery

I60.22 Nontraumatic subarachnoid hemorrhage from left anterior communicating artery

I60.3 Nontraumatic subarachnoid hemorrhage from posterior communicating artery

I60.30 Nontraumatic subarachnoid hemorrhage from unspecified posterior communicating artery

I60.31 Nontraumatic subarachnoid hemorrhage from right posterior communicating artery

I60.32 Nontraumatic subarachnoid hemorrhage from left posterior communicating artery

I60.4 Nontraumatic subarachnoid hemorrhage from basilar artery

I60.5 Nontraumatic subarachnoid hemorrhage from vertebral artery

I60.50 Nontraumatic subarachnoid hemorrhage from unspecified vertebral artery

I60.51   Nontraumatic subarachnoid hemorrhage from right vertebral artery

I60.52   Nontraumatic subarachnoid hemorrhage from left vertebral artery

I60.6   Nontraumatic subarachnoid hemorrhage from other intracranial arteries

I60.7   Nontraumatic subarachnoid hemorrhage from unspecified intracranial artery

Ruptured (congenital) berry aneurysm

Ruptured (congenital) cerebral aneurysm

Subarachnoid hemorrhage (nontraumatic) from cerebral artery NOS

Subarachnoid hemorrhage (nontraumatic) from communicating artery NOS

Excludes 1: berry aneurysm, nonruptured (I67.1)

I60.8   Other nontraumatic subarachnoid hemorrhage

Meningeal hemorrhage

Rupture of cerebral arteriovenous malformation

I60.9   Nontraumatic subarachnoid hemorrhage, unspecified

I61   Nontraumatic intracerebral hemorrhage

Excludes 1: sequelae of intracerebral hemorrhage (I69.1-)

I61.0   Nontraumatic intracerebral hemorrhage in hemisphere, subcortical

Deep intracerebral hemorrhage (nontraumatic)

I61.1   Nontraumatic intracerebral hemorrhage in hemisphere, cortical

Cerebral lobe hemorrhage (nontraumatic)

Superficial intracerebral hemorrhage (nontraumatic)

I61.2   Nontraumatic intracerebral hemorrhage in hemisphere, unspecified

I61.3   Nontraumatic intracerebral hemorrhage in brain stem

I61.4   Nontraumatic intracerebral hemorrhage in cerebellum

I61.5   Nontraumatic intracerebral hemorrhage, intraventricular

I61.6   Nontraumatic intracerebral hemorrhage, multiple localized

I61.8   Other nontraumatic intracerebral hemorrhage

I61.9   Nontraumatic intracerebral hemorrhage, unspecified

I62   Other and unspecified nontraumatic intracranial hemorrhage

Excludes 1: sequelae of intracranial hemorrhage (I69.2)

I62.0   Nontraumatic subdural hemorrhage

    I62.00   Nontraumatic subdural hemorrhage, unspecified

    I62.01   Nontraumatic acute subdural hemorrhage

    I62.02   Nontraumatic subacute subdural hemorrhage

    I62.03   Nontraumatic chronic subdural hemorrhage

I62.1   Nontraumatic extradural hemorrhage

Nontraumatic epidural hemorrhage

I62.9   Nontraumatic intracranial hemorrhage, unspecified

I63   Cerebral infarction

Includes: occlusion and stenosis of cerebral and precerebral arteries, resulting in cerebral infarction

Use additional code, if applicable, to identify status post administration of tPA (rtPA) in a different facility within the last 24 hours prior to admission to current facility (Z92.82)

Excludes 1: sequelae of cerebral infarction (I69.3-)

I63.0   Cerebral infarction due to thrombosis of precerebral arteries

    I63.00   Cerebral infarction due to thrombosis of unspecified precerebral artery

    I63.01   Cerebral infarction due to thrombosis of vertebral artery

        I63.011   Cerebral infarction due to thrombosis of right vertebral artery

        I63.012   Cerebral infarction due to thrombosis of left vertebral artery

        I63.019   Cerebral infarction due to thrombosis of unspecified vertebral artery

    I63.02   Cerebral infarction due to thrombosis of basilar artery

    I63.03   Cerebral infarction due to thrombosis of carotid artery

        I63.031   Cerebral infarction due to thrombosis of right carotid artery

        I63.032   Cerebral infarction due to thrombosis of left carotid artery

        I63.039   Cerebral infarction due to thrombosis of unspecified carotid artery

    I63.09   Cerebral infarction due to thrombosis of other precerebral artery

I63.1   Cerebral infarction due to embolism of precerebral arteries

    I63.10   Cerebral infarction due to embolism of unspecified precerebral artery

    I63.11   Cerebral infarction due to embolism of vertebral artery

        I63.111   Cerebral infarction due to embolism of right vertebral artery

        I63.112   Cerebral infarction due to embolism of left vertebral artery

        I63.119   Cerebral infarction due to embolism of unspecified vertebral artery

    I63.12   Cerebral infarction due to embolism of basilar artery

    I63.13   Cerebral infarction due to embolism of carotid artery

        I63.131   Cerebral infarction due to embolism of right carotid artery

        I63.132   Cerebral infarction due to embolism of left carotid artery

        I63.139   Cerebral infarction due to embolism of unspecified carotid artery

    I63.19   Cerebral infarction due to embolism of other precerebral artery

I63.2   Cerebral infarction due to unspecified occlusion or stenosis of precerebral arteries

    I63.20   Cerebral infarction due to unspecified occlusion or stenosis of unspecified precerebral arteries

    I63.21   Cerebral infarction due to unspecified occlusion or stenosis of vertebral arteries

        I63.211   Cerebral infarction due to unspecified occlusion or stenosis of right vertebral arteries

        I63.212   Cerebral infarction due to unspecified occlusion or stenosis of left vertebral arteries

        I63.219   Cerebral infarction due to unspecified occlusion or stenosis of unspecified vertebral arteries

    I63.22   Cerebral infarction due to unspecified occlusion or stenosis of basilar arteries

    I63.23   Cerebral infarction due to unspecified occlusion or stenosis of carotid arteries

        I63.231   Cerebral infarction due to unspecified occlusion or stenosis of right carotid arteries

        I63.232   Cerebral infarction due to unspecified occlusion or stenosis of left carotid arteries

        I63.239   Cerebral infarction due to unspecified occlusion or stenosis of unspecified carotid arteries

I63.29 Cerebral infarction due to unspecified occlusion or stenosis of other precerebral arteries

I63.3 Cerebral infarction due to thrombosis of cerebral arteries

I63.30 Cerebral infarction due to thrombosis of unspecified cerebral artery

I63.31 Cerebral infarction due to thrombosis of middle cerebral artery

I63.311 Cerebral infarction due to thrombosis of right middle cerebral artery

I63.312 Cerebral infarction due to thrombosis of left middle cerebral artery

I63.319 Cerebral infarction due to thrombosis of unspecified middle cerebral artery

I63.32 Cerebral infarction due to thrombosis of anterior cerebral artery

I63.321 Cerebral infarction due to thrombosis of right anterior cerebral artery

I63.322 Cerebral infarction due to thrombosis of left anterior cerebral artery

I63.329 Cerebral infarction due to thrombosis of unspecified anterior cerebral artery

I63.33 Cerebral infarction due to thrombosis of posterior cerebral artery

I63.331 Cerebral infarction due to thrombosis of right posterior cerebral artery

I63.332 Cerebral infarction due to thrombosis of left posterior cerebral artery

I63.339 Cerebral infarction due to thrombosis of unspecified posterior cerebral artery

I63.34 Cerebral infarction due to thrombosis of cerebellar artery

I63.341 Cerebral infarction due to thrombosis of right cerebellar artery

I63.342 Cerebral infarction due to thrombosis of left cerebellar artery

I63.349 Cerebral infarction due to thrombosis of unspecified cerebellar artery

I63.39 Cerebral infarction due to thrombosis of other cerebral artery

I63.4 Cerebral infarction due to embolism of cerebral arteries

I63.40 Cerebral infarction due to embolism of unspecified cerebral artery

I63.41 Cerebral infarction due to embolism of middle cerebral artery

I63.411 Cerebral infarction due to embolism of right middle cerebral artery

I63.412 Cerebral infarction due to embolism of left middle cerebral artery

I63.419 Cerebral infarction due to embolism of unspecified middle cerebral artery

I63.42 Cerebral infarction due to embolism of anterior cerebral artery

I63.421 Cerebral infarction due to embolism of right anterior cerebral artery

I63.422 Cerebral infarction due to embolism of left anterior cerebral artery

I63.429 Cerebral infarction due to embolism of unspecified anterior cerebral artery

I63.43 Cerebral infarction due to embolism of posterior cerebral artery

I63.431 Cerebral infarction due to embolism of right posterior cerebral artery

I63.432 Cerebral infarction due to embolism of left posterior cerebral artery

I63.439 Cerebral infarction due to embolism of unspecified posterior cerebral artery

I63.44 Cerebral infarction due to embolism of cerebellar artery

I63.441 Cerebral infarction due to embolism of right cerebellar artery

I63.442 Cerebral infarction due to embolism of left cerebellar artery

I63.449 Cerebral infarction due to embolism of unspecified cerebellar artery

I63.49 Cerebral infarction due to embolism of other cerebral artery

I63.5 Cerebral infarction due to unspecified occlusion or stenosis of cerebral arteries

I63.50 Cerebral infarction due to unspecified occlusion or stenosis of unspecified cerebral artery

I63.51 Cerebral infarction due to unspecified occlusion or stenosis of middle cerebral artery

I63.511 Cerebral infarction due to unspecified occlusion or stenosis of right middle cerebral artery

I63.512 Cerebral infarction due to unspecified occlusion or stenosis of left middle cerebral artery

I63.519 Cerebral infarction due to unspecified occlusion or stenosis of unspecified middle cerebral artery

I63.52 Cerebral infarction due to unspecified occlusion or stenosis of anterior cerebral artery

I63.521 Cerebral infarction due to unspecified occlusion or stenosis of right anterior cerebral artery

I63.522 Cerebral infarction due to unspecified occlusion or stenosis of left anterior cerebral artery

I63.529 Cerebral infarction due to unspecified occlusion or stenosis of unspecified anterior cerebral artery

I63.53 Cerebral infarction due to unspecified occlusion or stenosis of posterior cerebral artery

I63.531 Cerebral infarction due to unspecified occlusion or stenosis of right posterior cerebral artery

I63.532 Cerebral infarction due to unspecified occlusion or stenosis of left posterior cerebral artery

I63.539 Cerebral infarction due to unspecified occlusion or stenosis of unspecified posterior cerebral artery

I63.54 Cerebral infarction due to unspecified occlusion or stenosis of cerebellar artery

I63.541 Cerebral infarction due to unspecified occlusion or stenosis of right cerebellar artery

I63.542 Cerebral infarction due to unspecified occlusion or stenosis of left cerebellar artery

I63.549 Cerebral infarction due to unspecified occlusion or stenosis of unspecified cerebellar artery

I63.59 Cerebral infarction due to unspecified occlusion or stenosis of other cerebral artery

● New code   ▲ Revised code   ⑦ 7ᵗʰ digit required   ⊗ Placeholder required

I63.6 Cerebral infarction due to cerebral venous thrombosis, nonpyogenic

I63.8 Other cerebral infarction

I63.9 Cerebral infarction, unspecified
Stroke NOS

I65 Occlusion and stenosis of precerebral arteries, not resulting in cerebral infarction

Includes: embolism of precerebral artery
narrowing of precerebral artery
obstruction (complete) (partial) of precerebral artery
thrombosis of precerebral artery

Excludes 1: insufficiency, NOS, of precerebral artery (G45.-)
insufficiency of precerebral arteries causing cerebral infarction (I63.0-I63.2)

I65.0 Occlusion and stenosis of vertebral artery

  I65.01 Occlusion and stenosis of right vertebral artery

  I65.02 Occlusion and stenosis of left vertebral artery

  I65.03 Occlusion and stenosis of bilateral vertebral arteries

  I65.09 Occlusion and stenosis of unspecified vertebral artery

I65.1 Occlusion and stenosis of basilar artery

I65.2 Occlusion and stenosis of carotid artery

  I65.21 Occlusion and stenosis of right carotid artery

  I65.22 Occlusion and stenosis of left carotid artery

  I65.23 Occlusion and stenosis of bilateral carotid arteries

  I65.29 Occlusion and stenosis of unspecified carotid artery

I65.8 Occlusion and stenosis of other precerebral arteries

I65.9 Occlusion and stenosis of unspecified precerebral artery
Occlusion and stenosis of precerebral artery NOS

I66 Occlusion and stenosis of cerebral arteries, not resulting in cerebral infarction

Includes: embolism of cerebral artery
narrowing of cerebral artery
obstruction (complete) (partial) of cerebral artery
thrombosis of cerebral artery

Excludes 1: Occlusion and stenosis of cerebral artery causing cerebral infarction (I63.3-I63.5)

I66.0 Occlusion and stenosis of middle cerebral artery

  I66.01 Occlusion and stenosis of right middle cerebral artery

  I66.02 Occlusion and stenosis of left middle cerebral artery

  I66.03 Occlusion and stenosis of bilateral middle cerebral arteries

  I66.09 Occlusion and stenosis of unspecified middle cerebral artery

I66.1 Occlusion and stenosis of anterior cerebral artery

  I66.11 Occlusion and stenosis of right anterior cerebral artery

  I66.12 Occlusion and stenosis of left anterior cerebral artery

  I66.13 Occlusion and stenosis of bilateral anterior cerebral arteries

  I66.19 Occlusion and stenosis of unspecified anterior cerebral artery

I66.2 Occlusion and stenosis of posterior cerebral artery

  I66.21 Occlusion and stenosis of right posterior cerebral artery

  I66.22 Occlusion and stenosis of left posterior cerebral artery

  I66.23 Occlusion and stenosis of bilateral posterior cerebral arteries

  I66.29 Occlusion and stenosis of unspecified posterior cerebral artery

I66.3 Occlusion and stenosis of cerebellar arteries

I66.8 Occlusion and stenosis of other cerebral arteries
Occlusion and stenosis of perforating arteries

I66.9 Occlusion and stenosis of unspecified cerebral artery

I67 Other cerebrovascular diseases

Excludes 1: sequelae of the listed conditions (I69.8)

I67.0 Dissection of cerebral arteries, nonruptured

Excludes 1: ruptured cerebral arteries (I60.7)

I67.1 Cerebral aneurysm, nonruptured
Cerebral aneurysm NOS
Cerebral arteriovenous fistula, acquired
Internal carotid artery aneurysm, intracranial portion
Internal carotid artery aneurysm, NOS

Excludes 1: congenital cerebral aneurysm, nonruptured (Q28.-)
ruptured cerebral aneurysm (I60.7)

I67.2 Cerebral atherosclerosis
Atheroma of cerebral and precerebral arteries

I67.3 Progressive vascular leukoencephalopathy
Binswanger's disease

I67.4 Hypertensive encephalopathy

I67.5 Moyamoya disease

I67.6 Nonpyogenic thrombosis of intracranial venous system
Nonpyogenic thrombosis of cerebral vein
Nonpyogenic thrombosis of intracranial venous sinus

Excludes 1: nonpyogenic thrombosis of intracranial venous system causing infarction (I63.6)

I67.7 Cerebral arteritis, not elsewhere classified
Granulomatous angiitis of the nervous system

Excludes 1: allergic granulomatous angiitis (M30.1)

I67.8 Other specified cerebrovascular diseases

  I67.81 Acute cerebrovascular insufficiency
Acute cerebrovascular insufficiency unspecified as to location or reversibility

  I67.82 Cerebral ischemia
Chronic cerebral ischemia

  I67.83 Posterior reversible encephalopathy syndrome
PRES

  I67.84 Cerebral vasospasm and vasoconstriction

    I67.841 Reversible cerebrovascular vasoconstriction syndrome
Call-Fleming syndrome
Code first underlying condition, if applicable, such as eclampsia (O15.00-O15.9)

    I67.848 Other cerebrovascular vasospasm and vasoconstriction

  I67.89 Other cerebrovascular disease

I67.9 Cerebrovascular disease, unspecified

I68 Cerebrovascular disorders in diseases classified elsewhere

I68.0 Cerebral amyloid angiopathy
Code first underlying amyloidosis (E85-)

I68.2 Cerebral arteritis in other diseases classified elsewhere
Code first underlying disease

Excludes 1: cerebral arteritis (in):
listerosis (A32.89)
systemic lupus erythematosus (M32.19)
syphilis (A52.04)
tuberculosis (A18.89)

I68.8 Other cerebrovascular disorders in diseases classified elsewhere

Code first underlying disease

Excludes 1: syphilitic cerebral aneurysm (A52.05)

I69 Sequelae of cerebrovascular disease

Note: Category I69 is to be used to indicate conditions in I60-I67 as the cause of sequelae. The 'sequelae' include conditions specified as such or as residuals which may occur at any time after the onset of the causal condition

Excludes 1: personal history of cerebral infarction without residual deficit (Z86.73)

personal history of prolonged reversible ischemic neurologic deficit (PRIND) (Z86.73)

personal history of reversible ischemic neurological deficit (RIND) (Z86.73)

sequelae of traumatic intracranial injury (S06.-)

transient ischemic attack (TIA) (G45.9)

I69.0 Sequelae of nontraumatic subarachnoid hemorrhage

I69.00 Unspecified sequelae of nontraumatic subarachnoid hemorrhage

I69.01 Cognitive deficits following nontraumatic subarachnoid hemorrhage

I69.02 Speech and language deficits following nontraumatic subarachnoid hemorrhage

I69.020 Aphasia following nontraumatic subarachnoid hemorrhage

I69.021 Dysphasia following nontraumatic subarachnoid hemorrhage

I69.022 Dysarthria following nontraumatic subarachnoid hemorrhage

I69.023 Fluency disorder following nontraumatic subarachnoid hemorrhage

Stuttering following nontraumatic subarachnoid hemorrhage

I69.028 Other speech and language deficits following nontraumatic subarachnoid hemorrhage

I69.03 Monoplegia of upper limb following nontraumatic subarachnoid hemorrhage

I69.031 Monoplegia of upper limb following nontraumatic subarachnoid hemorrhage affecting right dominant side

I69.032 Monoplegia of upper limb following nontraumatic subarachnoid hemorrhage affecting left dominant side

I69.033 Monoplegia of upper limb following nontraumatic subarachnoid hemorrhage affecting right non-dominant side

I69.034 Monoplegia of upper limb following nontraumatic subarachnoid hemorrhage affecting left non-dominant side

I69.039 Monoplegia of upper limb following nontraumatic subarachnoid hemorrhage affecting unspecified side

I69.04 Monoplegia of lower limb following nontraumatic subarachnoid hemorrhage

I69.041 Monoplegia of lower limb following nontraumatic subarachnoid hemorrhage affecting right dominant side

I69.042 Monoplegia of lower limb following nontraumatic subarachnoid hemorrhage affecting left dominant side

I69.043 Monoplegia of lower limb following nontraumatic subarachnoid hemorrhage affecting right non-dominant side

I69.044 Monoplegia of lower limb following nontraumatic subarachnoid hemorrhage affecting left non-dominant side

I69.049 Monoplegia of lower limb following nontraumatic subarachnoid hemorrhage affecting unspecified side

I69.05 Hemiplegia and hemiparesis following nontraumatic subarachnoid hemorrhage

I69.051 Hemiplegia and hemiparesis following nontraumatic subarachnoid hemorrhage affecting right dominant side

I69.052 Hemiplegia and hemiparesis following nontraumatic subarachnoid hemorrhage affecting left dominant side

I69.053 Hemiplegia and hemiparesis following nontraumatic subarachnoid hemorrhage affecting right non-dominant side

I69.054 Hemiplegia and hemiparesis following nontraumatic subarachnoid hemorrhage affecting left non-dominant side

I69.059 Hemiplegia and hemiparesis following nontraumatic subarachnoid hemorrhage affecting unspecified side

I69.06 Other paralytic syndrome following nontraumatic subarachnoid hemorrhage

Use additional code to identify type of paralytic syndrome, such as:

locked-in state (G83.5)

quadriplegia (G82.5-)

Excludes 1: hemiplegia/hemiparesis following nontraumatic subarachnoid hemorrhage (I69.05-)

monoplegia of lower limb following nontraumatic subarachnoid hemorrhage (I69.04-)

monoplegia of upper limb following nontraumatic subarachnoid hemorrhage (I69.03-)

I69.061 Other paralytic syndrome following nontraumatic subarachnoid hemorrhage affecting right dominant side

I69.062 Other paralytic syndrome following nontraumatic subarachnoid hemorrhage affecting left dominant side

I69.063 Other paralytic syndrome following nontraumatic subarachnoid hemorrhage affecting right non-dominant side

I69.064 Other paralytic syndrome following nontraumatic subarachnoid hemorrhage affecting left non-dominant side

● New code   ▲ Revised code   ⑦ 7th digit required   ⊗ Placeholder required

I69.065 Other paralytic syndrome following nontraumatic subarachnoid hemorrhage, bilateral

I69.069 Other paralytic syndrome following nontraumatic subarachnoid hemorrhage affecting unspecified side

I69.09 Other sequelae of nontraumatic subarachnoid hemorrhage

I69.090 Apraxia following nontraumatic subarachnoid hemorrhage

I69.091 Dysphagia following nontraumatic subarachnoid hemorrhage

Use additional code to identify the type of dysphagia, if known (R13.1-)

I69.092 Facial weakness following nontraumatic subarachnoid hemorrhage

Facial droop following nontraumatic subarachnoid hemorrhage

I69.093 Ataxia following nontraumatic subarachnoid hemorrhage

I69.098 Other sequelae following nontraumatic subarachnoid hemorrhage

Alterations of sensation following nontraumatic subarachnoid hemorrhage

Disturbance of vision following nontraumatic subarachnoid hemorrhage

Use additional code to identify the sequelae

I69.1 Sequelae of nontraumatic intracerebral hemorrhage

I69.10 Unspecified sequelae of nontraumatic intracerebral hemorrhage

I69.11 Cognitive deficits following nontraumatic intracerebral hemorrhage

I69.12 Speech and language deficits following nontraumatic intracerebral hemorrhage

I69.120 Aphasia following nontraumatic intracerebral hemorrhage

I69.121 Dysphasia following nontraumatic intracerebral hemorrhage

I69.122 Dysarthria following nontraumatic intracerebral hemorrhage

I69.123 Fluency disorder following nontraumatic intracerebral hemorrhage

Stuttering following nontraumatic subarachnoid hemorrhage

I69.128 Other speech and language deficits following nontraumatic intracerebral hemorrhage

I69.13 Monoplegia of upper limb following nontraumatic intracerebral hemorrhage

I69.131 Monoplegia of upper limb following nontraumatic intracerebral hemorrhage affecting right dominant side

I69.132 Monoplegia of upper limb following nontraumatic intracerebral hemorrhage affecting left dominant side

I69.133 Monoplegia of upper limb following nontraumatic intracerebral

hemorrhage affecting right non-dominant side

I69.134 Monoplegia of upper limb following nontraumatic intracerebral hemorrhage affecting left non-dominant side

I69.139 Monoplegia of upper limb following nontraumatic intracerebral hemorrhage affecting unspecified side

I69.14 Monoplegia of lower limb following nontraumatic intracerebral hemorrhage

I69.141 Monoplegia of lower limb following nontraumatic intracerebral hemorrhage affecting right dominant side

I69.142 Monoplegia of lower limb following nontraumatic intracerebral hemorrhage affecting left dominant side

I69.143 Monoplegia of lower limb following nontraumatic intracerebral hemorrhage affecting right non-dominant side

I69.144 Monoplegia of lower limb following nontraumatic intracerebral hemorrhage affecting left non-dominant side

I69.149 Monoplegia of lower limb following nontraumatic intracerebral hemorrhage affecting unspecified side

I69.15 Hemiplegia and hemiparesis following nontraumatic intracerebral hemorrhage

I69.151 Hemiplegia and hemiparesis following nontraumatic intracerebral hemorrhage affecting right dominant side

I69.152 Hemiplegia and hemiparesis following nontraumatic intracerebral hemorrhage affecting left dominant side

I69.153 Hemiplegia and hemiparesis following nontraumatic intracerebral hemorrhage affecting right non-dominant side

I69.154 Hemiplegia and hemiparesis following nontraumatic intracerebral hemorrhage affecting left non-dominant side

I69.159 Hemiplegia and hemiparesis following nontraumatic intracerebral hemorrhage affecting unspecified side

I69.16 Other paralytic syndrome following nontraumatic intracerebral hemorrhage

Use additional code to identify type of paralytic syndrome, such as:

locked-in state (G83.5)

quadriplegia (G82.5-)

Excludes 1: hemiplegia/hemiparesis following nontraumatic intracerebral hemorrhage (I69.15-)

monoplegia of lower limb following nontraumatic intracerebral hemorrhage (I69.14-)

monoplegia of upper limb following nontraumatic intracerebral hemorrhage (I69.13-)

I69.161   Other paralytic syndrome following nontraumatic intracerebral hemorrhage affecting right dominant side

I69.162   Other paralytic syndrome following nontraumatic intracerebral hemorrhage affecting left dominant side

I69.163   Other paralytic syndrome following nontraumatic intracerebral hemorrhage affecting right non-dominant side

I69.164   Other paralytic syndrome following nontraumatic intracerebral hemorrhage affecting left non-dominant side

I69.165   Other paralytic syndrome following nontraumatic intracerebral hemorrhage, bilateral

I69.169   Other paralytic syndrome following nontraumatic intracerebral hemorrhage affecting unspecified side

I69.19   Other sequelae of nontraumatic intracerebral hemorrhage

     I69.190   Apraxia following nontraumatic intracerebral hemorrhage

     I69.191   Dysphagia following nontraumatic intracerebral hemorrhage

       Use additional code to identify the type of dysphagia, if known (R13.1-)

     I69.192   Facial weakness following nontraumatic intracerebral hemorrhage

       Facial droop following nontraumatic intracerebral hemorrhage

     I69.193   Ataxia following nontraumatic intracerebral hemorrhage

     I69.198   Other sequelae of nontraumatic intracerebral hemorrhage

       Alteration of sensations following nontraumatic intracerebral hemorrhage

       Disturbance of vision following nontraumatic intracerebral hemorrhage

       Use additional code to identify the sequelae

I69.2   Sequelae of other nontraumatic intracranial hemorrhage

   I69.20   Unspecified sequelae of other nontraumatic intracranial hemorrhage

   I69.21   Cognitive deficits following other nontraumatic intracranial hemorrhage

   I69.22   Speech and language deficits following other nontraumatic intracranial hemorrhage

     I69.220   Aphasia following other nontraumatic intracranial hemorrhage

     I69.221   Dysphasia following other nontraumatic intracranial hemorrhage

     I69.222   Dysarthria following other nontraumatic intracranial hemorrhage

     I69.223   Fluency disorder following other nontraumatic intracranial hemorrhage

       Stuttering following nontraumatic subarachnoid hemorrhage

     I69.228   Other speech and language deficits following other nontraumatic intracranial hemorrhage

   I69.23   Monoplegia of upper limb following other nontraumatic intracranial hemorrhage

     I69.231   Monoplegia of upper limb following other nontraumatic intracranial hemorrhage affecting right dominant side

     I69.232   Monoplegia of upper limb following other nontraumatic intracranial hemorrhage affecting left dominant side

     I69.233   Monoplegia of upper limb following other nontraumatic intracranial hemorrhage affecting right non-dominant side

     I69.234   Monoplegia of upper limb following other nontraumatic intracranial hemorrhage affecting left non-dominant side

     I69.239   Monoplegia of upper limb following other nontraumatic intracranial hemorrhage affecting unspecified side

   I69.24   Monoplegia of lower limb following other nontraumatic intracranial hemorrhage

     I69.241   Monoplegia of lower limb following other nontraumatic intracranial hemorrhage affecting right dominant side

     I69.242   Monoplegia of lower limb following other nontraumatic intracranial hemorrhage affecting left dominant side

     I69.243   Monoplegia of lower limb following other nontraumatic intracranial hemorrhage affecting right non-dominant side

     I69.244   Monoplegia of lower limb following other nontraumatic intracranial hemorrhage affecting left non-dominant side

     I69.249   Monoplegia of lower limb following other nontraumatic intracranial hemorrhage affecting unspecified side

   I69.25   Hemiplegia and hemiparesis following other nontraumatic intracranial hemorrhage

     I69.251   Hemiplegia and hemiparesis following other nontraumatic intracranial hemorrhage affecting right dominant side

     I69.252   Hemiplegia and hemiparesis following other nontraumatic intracranial hemorrhage affecting left dominant side

     I69.253   Hemiplegia and hemiparesis following other nontraumatic intracranial hemorrhage affecting right non-dominant side

     I69.254   Hemiplegia and hemiparesis following other nontraumatic intracranial hemorrhage affecting left non-dominant side

I69.259　Hemiplegia and hemiparesis following other nontraumatic intracranial hemorrhage affecting unspecified side

I69.26　Other paralytic syndrome following other nontraumatic intracranial hemorrhage

Use additional code to identify type of paralytic syndrome, such as:

locked-in state (G83.5)

quadriplegia (G82.5-)

Excludes 1: hemiplegia/hemiparesis following other nontraumatic intracranial hemorrhage (I69.25-)

monoplegia of lower limb following other nontraumatic intracranial hemorrhage (I69.24-)

monoplegia of upper limb following other nontraumatic intracranial hemorrhage (I69.23-)

I69.261　Other paralytic syndrome following other nontraumatic intracranial hemorrhage affecting right dominant side

I69.262　Other paralytic syndrome following other nontraumatic intracranial hemorrhage affecting left dominant side

I69.263　Other paralytic syndrome following other nontraumatic intracranial hemorrhage affecting right non-dominant side

I69.264　Other paralytic syndrome following other nontraumatic intracranial hemorrhage affecting left non-dominant side

I69.265　Other paralytic syndrome following other nontraumatic intracranial hemorrhage, bilateral

I69.269　Other paralytic syndrome following other nontraumatic intracranial hemorrhage affecting unspecified side

I69.29　Other sequelae of other nontraumatic intracranial hemorrhage

I69.290　Apraxia following other nontraumatic intracranial hemorrhage

I69.291　Dysphagia following other nontraumatic intracranial hemorrhage

Use additional code to identify the type of dysphagia, if known (R13.1-)

I69.292　Facial weakness following other nontraumatic intracranial hemorrhage

Facial droop following other nontraumatic intracranial hemorrhage

I69.293　Ataxia following other nontraumatic intracranial hemorrhage

I69.298　Other sequelae of other nontraumatic intracranial hemorrhage

Alteration of sensation following other nontraumatic intracranial hemorrhage

Disturbance of vision following other nontraumatic intracranial hemorrhage

Use additional code to identify the sequelae

I69.3　Sequelae of cerebral infarction

Sequelae of stroke NOS

I69.30　Unspecified sequelae of cerebral infarction

I69.31　Cognitive deficits following cerebral infarction

I69.32　Speech and language deficits following cerebral infarction

I69.320　Aphasia following cerebral infarction

I69.321　Dysphasia following cerebral infarction

I69.322　Dysarthria following cerebral infarction

I69.323　Fluency disorder following cerebral infarction

Stuttering following nontraumatic subarachnoid hemorrhage

I69.328　Other speech and language deficits following cerebral infarction

I69.33　Monoplegia of upper limb following cerebral infarction

I69.331　Monoplegia of upper limb following cerebral infarction affecting right dominant side

I69.332　Monoplegia of upper limb following cerebral infarction affecting left dominant side

I69.333　Monoplegia of upper limb following cerebral infarction affecting right non-dominant side

I69.334　Monoplegia of upper limb following cerebral infarction affecting left non-dominant side

I69.339　Monoplegia of upper limb following cerebral infarction affecting unspecified side

I69.34　Monoplegia of lower limb following cerebral infarction

I69.341　Monoplegia of lower limb following cerebral infarction affecting right dominant side

I69.342　Monoplegia of lower limb following cerebral infarction affecting left dominant side

I69.343　Monoplegia of lower limb following cerebral infarction affecting right non-dominant side

I69.344　Monoplegia of lower limb following cerebral infarction affecting left non-dominant side

I69.349　Monoplegia of lower limb following cerebral infarction affecting unspecified side

I69.35　Hemiplegia and hemiparesis following cerebral infarction

I69.351　Hemiplegia and hemiparesis following cerebral infarction affecting right dominant side

I69.352　Hemiplegia and hemiparesis following cerebral infarction affecting left dominant side

I69.353　Hemiplegia and hemiparesis following cerebral infarction affecting right non-dominant side

I69.354 Hemiplegia and hemiparesis following cerebral infarction affecting left non-dominant side

I69.359 Hemiplegia and hemiparesis following cerebral infarction affecting unspecified side

I69.36 Other paralytic syndrome following cerebral infarction

Use additional code to identify type of paralytic syndrome, such as:

locked-in state (G83.5)

quadriplegia (G82.5-)

Excludes 1: hemiplegia/hemiparesis following cerebral infarction (I69.35-)

monoplegia of lower limb following cerebral infarction (I69.34-)

monoplegia of upper limb following cerebral infarction (I69.33-)

I69.361 Other paralytic syndrome following cerebral infarction affecting right dominant side

I69.362 Other paralytic syndrome following cerebral infarction affecting left dominant side

I69.363 Other paralytic syndrome following cerebral infarction affecting right non-dominant side

I69.364 Other paralytic syndrome following cerebral infarction affecting left non-dominant side

I69.365 Other paralytic syndrome following cerebral infarction, bilateral

I69.369 Other paralytic syndrome following cerebral infarction affecting unspecified side

I69.39 Other sequelae of cerebral infarction

I69.390 Apraxia following cerebral infarction

I69.391 Dysphagia following cerebral infarction

Use additional code to identify the type of dysphagia, if known (R13.1-)

I69.392 Facial weakness following cerebral infarction

Facial droop following cerebral infarction

I69.393 Ataxia following cerebral infarction

I69.398 Other sequelae of cerebral infarction

Alteration of sensation following cerebral infarction

Disturbance of vision following cerebral infarction

Use additional code to identify the sequelae

I69.8 Sequelae of other cerebrovascular diseases

Excludes 1: sequelae of traumatic intracranial injury (S06.-)

I69.80 Unspecified sequelae of other cerebrovascular disease

I69.81 Cognitive deficits following other cerebrovascular disease

I69.82 Speech and language deficits following other cerebrovascular disease

I69.820 Aphasia following other cerebrovascular disease

I69.821 Dysphasia following other cerebrovascular disease

I69.822 Dysarthria following other cerebrovascular disease

I69.823 Fluency disorder following other cerebrovascular disease

Stuttering following nontraumatic subarachnoid hemorrhage

I69.828 Other speech and language deficits following other cerebrovascular disease

I69.83 Monoplegia of upper limb following other cerebrovascular disease

I69.831 Monoplegia of upper limb following other cerebrovascular disease affecting right dominant side

I69.832 Monoplegia of upper limb following other cerebrovascular disease affecting left dominant side

I69.833 Monoplegia of upper limb following other cerebrovascular disease affecting right non-dominant side

I69.834 Monoplegia of upper limb following other cerebrovascular disease affecting left non-dominant side

I69.839 Monoplegia of upper limb following other cerebrovascular disease affecting unspecified side

I69.84 Monoplegia of lower limb following other cerebrovascular disease

I69.841 Monoplegia of lower limb following other cerebrovascular disease affecting right dominant side

I69.842 Monoplegia of lower limb following other cerebrovascular disease affecting left dominant side

I69.843 Monoplegia of lower limb following other cerebrovascular disease affecting right non-dominant side

I69.844 Monoplegia of lower limb following other cerebrovascular disease affecting left non-dominant side

I69.849 Monoplegia of lower limb following other cerebrovascular disease affecting unspecified side

I69.85 Hemiplegia and hemiparesis following other cerebrovascular disease

I69.851 Hemiplegia and hemiparesis following other cerebrovascular disease affecting right dominant side

I69.852 Hemiplegia and hemiparesis following other cerebrovascular disease affecting left dominant side

I69.853 Hemiplegia and hemiparesis following other cerebrovascular disease affecting right non-dominant side

I69.854 Hemiplegia and hemiparesis following other cerebrovascular disease affecting left non-dominant side

I69.859 Hemiplegia and hemiparesis following other cerebrovascular disease affecting unspecified side

I69.86 Other paralytic syndrome following other cerebrovascular disease

Use additional code to identify type of paralytic syndrome, such as:

locked-in state (G83.5)

quadriplegia (G82.5-)

Excludes 1: hemiplegia/hemiparesis following other cerebrovascular disease (I69.85-)

monoplegia of lower limb following other cerebrovascular disease (I69.84-)

monoplegia of upper limb following other cerebrovascular disease (I69.83-)

I69.861   Other paralytic syndrome following other cerebrovascular disease affecting right dominant side

I69.862   Other paralytic syndrome following other cerebrovascular disease affecting left dominant side

I69.863   Other paralytic syndrome following other cerebrovascular disease affecting right non-dominant side

I69.864   Other paralytic syndrome following other cerebrovascular disease affecting left non-dominant side

I69.865   Other paralytic syndrome following other cerebrovascular disease, bilateral

I69.869   Other paralytic syndrome following other cerebrovascular disease affecting unspecified side

I69.89   Other sequelae of other cerebrovascular disease

I69.890   Apraxia following other cerebrovascular disease

I69.891   Dysphagia following other cerebrovascular disease

Use additional code to identify the type of dysphagia, if known (R13.1-)

I69.892   Facial weakness following other cerebrovascular disease

Facial droop following other cerebrovascular disease

I69.893   Ataxia following other cerebrovascular disease

I69.898   Other sequelae of other cerebrovascular disease

Alteration of sensation following other cerebrovascular disease

Disturbance of vision following other cerebrovascular disease

Use additional code to identify the sequelae

I69.9   Sequelae of unspecified cerebrovascular diseases

Excludes 1: sequelae of stroke (I69.3)

sequelae of traumatic intracranial injury (S06.-)

I69.90   Unspecified sequelae of unspecified cerebrovascular disease

I69.91   Cognitive deficits following unspecified cerebrovascular disease

I69.92   Speech and language deficits following unspecified cerebrovascular disease

I69.920   Aphasia following unspecified cerebrovascular disease

I69.921   Dysphasia following unspecified cerebrovascular disease

I69.922   Dysarthria following unspecified cerebrovascular disease

I69.923   Fluency disorder following unspecified cerebrovascular disease

Stuttering following nontraumatic subarachnoid hemorrhage

I69.928   Other speech and language deficits following unspecified cerebrovascular disease

I69.93   Monoplegia of upper limb following unspecified cerebrovascular disease

I69.931   Monoplegia of upper limb following unspecified cerebrovascular disease affecting right dominant side

I69.932   Monoplegia of upper limb following unspecified cerebrovascular disease affecting left dominant side

I69.933   Monoplegia of upper limb following unspecified cerebrovascular disease affecting right non-dominant side

I69.934   Monoplegia of upper limb following unspecified cerebrovascular disease affecting left non-dominant side

I69.939   Monoplegia of upper limb following unspecified cerebrovascular disease affecting unspecified side

I69.94   Monoplegia of lower limb following unspecified cerebrovascular disease

I69.941   Monoplegia of lower limb following unspecified cerebrovascular disease affecting right dominant side

I69.942   Monoplegia of lower limb following unspecified cerebrovascular disease affecting left dominant side

I69.943   Monoplegia of lower limb following unspecified cerebrovascular disease affecting right non-dominant side

I69.944   Monoplegia of lower limb following unspecified cerebrovascular disease affecting left non-dominant side

I69.949   Monoplegia of lower limb following unspecified cerebrovascular disease affecting unspecified side

I69.95   Hemiplegia and hemiparesis following unspecified cerebrovascular disease

I69.951   Hemiplegia and hemiparesis following unspecified cerebrovascular disease affecting right dominant side

I69.952   Hemiplegia and hemiparesis following unspecified cerebrovascular disease affecting left dominant side

I69.953   Hemiplegia and hemiparesis following unspecified cerebrovascular disease affecting right non-dominant side

I69.954   Hemiplegia and hemiparesis following unspecified cerebrovascular disease affecting left non-dominant side

I69.959   Hemiplegia and hemiparesis following unspecified cerebrovascular disease affecting unspecified side

I69.96   Other paralytic syndrome following unspecified cerebrovascular disease

Use additional code to identify type of paralytic syndrome, such as:

locked-in state (G83.5)

quadriplegia (G82.5-)

Excludes 1: hemiplegia/hemiparesis following unspecified cerebrovascular disease (I69.95-)

monoplegia of lower limb following unspecified cerebrovascular disease (I69.94-)

monoplegia of upper limb following unspecified cerebrovascular disease (I69.93-)

I69.961   Other paralytic syndrome following unspecified cerebrovascular disease affecting right dominant side

I69.962   Other paralytic syndrome following unspecified cerebrovascular disease affecting left dominant side

I69.963   Other paralytic syndrome following unspecified cerebrovascular disease affecting right non-dominant side

I69.964   Other paralytic syndrome following unspecified cerebrovascular disease affecting left non-dominant side

I69.965   Other paralytic syndrome following unspecified cerebrovascular disease, bilateral

I69.969   Other paralytic syndrome following unspecified cerebrovascular disease affecting unspecified side

I69.99   Other sequelae of unspecified cerebrovascular disease

I69.990   Apraxia following unspecified cerebrovascular disease

I69.991   Dysphagia following unspecified cerebrovascular disease

Use additional code to identify the type of dysphagia, if known (R13.1-)

I69.992   Facial weakness following unspecified cerebrovascular disease

Facial droop following unspecified cerebrovascular disease

I69.993   Ataxia following unspecified cerebrovascular disease

I69.998   Other sequelae following unspecified cerebrovascular disease

Alteration in sensation following unspecified cerebrovascular disease

Disturbance of vision following unspecified cerebrovascular disease

Use additional code to identify the sequelae

DISEASES OF ARTERIES, ARTERIOLES AND CAPILLARIES (I70-I79)

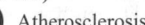 Atherosclerosis

Includes: arteriolosclerosis

arterial degeneration

arteriosclerosis

arteriosclerotic vascular disease

arteriovascular degeneration

atheroma

endarteritis deformans or obliterans

senile arteritis

senile endarteritis

vascular degeneration

Use additional code to identify:

exposure to environmental tobacco smoke (Z77.22)

history of tobacco use (Z87.891)

occupational exposure to environmental tobacco smoke (Z57.31)

tobacco dependence (F17.-)

tobacco use (Z72.0)

Excludes 2: arteriosclerotic cardiovascular disease (I25.1-)

arteriosclerotic heart disease (I25.1-)

atheroembolism (I75.-)

cerebral atherosclerosis (I67.2)

coronary atherosclerosis (I25.1-)

mesenteric atherosclerosis (K55.1)

precerebral atherosclerosis (I67.2)

primary pulmonary atherosclerosis (I27.0)

I70.0   Atherosclerosis of aorta

I70.1   Atherosclerosis of renal artery

Goldblatt's kidney

Excludes 2: atherosclerosis of renal arterioles (I12.-)

I70.2   Atherosclerosis of native arteries of the extremities

Mönckeberg's (medial) sclerosis

Use additional code, if applicable, to identify chronic total occlusion of artery of extremity (I70.92)

Excludes 2: atherosclerosis of bypass graft of extremities (I70.30-I70.79)

I70.20   Unspecified atherosclerosis of native arteries of extremities

I70.201   Unspecified atherosclerosis of native arteries of extremities, right leg

I70.202   Unspecified atherosclerosis of native arteries of extremities, left leg

I70.203   Unspecified atherosclerosis of native arteries of extremities, bilateral legs

I70.208   Unspecified atherosclerosis of native arteries of extremities, other extremity

I70.209   Unspecified atherosclerosis of native arteries of extremities, unspecified extremity

I70.21   Atherosclerosis of native arteries of extremities with intermittent claudication

I70.211   Atherosclerosis of native arteries of extremities with intermittent claudication, right leg

I70.212   Atherosclerosis of native arteries of extremities with intermittent claudication, left leg

I70.213   Atherosclerosis of native arteries of extremities with intermittent claudication, bilateral legs

I70.218   Atherosclerosis of native arteries of extremities with intermittent claudication, other extremity

I70.219   Atherosclerosis of native arteries of extremities with intermittent claudication, unspecified extremity

I70.22   Atherosclerosis of native arteries of extremities with rest pain

Includes: any condition classifiable to I70.21-

I70.221   Atherosclerosis of native arteries of extremities with rest pain, right leg

I70.222 Atherosclerosis of native arteries of extremities with rest pain, left leg

I70.223 Atherosclerosis of native arteries of extremities with rest pain, bilateral legs

I70.228 Atherosclerosis of native arteries of extremities with rest pain, other extremity

I70.229 Atherosclerosis of native arteries of extremities with rest pain, unspecified extremity

I70.23 Atherosclerosis of native arteries of right leg with ulceration

Includes: any condition classifiable to I70.211 and I70.221

Use additional code to identify severity of ulcer (L97.- with fifth character 1)

I70.231 Atherosclerosis of native arteries of right leg with ulceration of thigh

I70.232 Atherosclerosis of native arteries of right leg with ulceration of calf

I70.233 Atherosclerosis of native arteries of right leg with ulceration of ankle

I70.234 Atherosclerosis of native arteries of right leg with ulceration of heel and midfoot

Atherosclerosis of native arteries of right leg with ulceration of plantar surface of midfoot

I70.235 Atherosclerosis of native arteries of right leg with ulceration of other part of foot

Atherosclerosis of native arteries of right leg extremities with ulceration of toe

I70.238 Atherosclerosis of native arteries of right leg with ulceration of other part of lower right leg

I70.239 Atherosclerosis of native arteries of right leg with ulceration of unspecified site

I70.24 Atherosclerosis of native arteries of left leg with ulceration

Includes: any condition classifiable to I70.212 and I70.222

Use additional code to identify severity of ulcer (L97.- with fifth character 2)

I70.241 Atherosclerosis of native arteries of left leg with ulceration of thigh

I70.242 Atherosclerosis of native arteries of left leg with ulceration of calf

I70.243 Atherosclerosis of native arteries of left leg with ulceration of ankle

I70.244 Atherosclerosis of native arteries of left leg with ulceration of heel and midfoot

Atherosclerosis of native arteries of left leg with ulceration of plantar surface of midfoot

I70.245 Atherosclerosis of native arteries of left leg with ulceration of other part of foot

Atherosclerosis of native arteries of left leg extremities with ulceration of toe

I70.248 Atherosclerosis of native arteries of left leg with ulceration of other part of lower left leg

I70.249 Atherosclerosis of native arteries of left leg with ulceration of unspecified site

I70.25 Atherosclerosis of native arteries of other extremities with ulceration

Includes: any condition classifiable to I70.218 and I70.228

Use additional code to identify the severity of the ulcer (L98.49-)

I70.26 Atherosclerosis of native arteries of extremities with gangrene

Includes: any condition classifiable to I70.21-, I70.22-, I70.23-, I70.24-, and I70.25-

Use additional code to identify the severity of any ulcer (L98.49-), if applicable

I70.261 Atherosclerosis of native arteries of extremities with gangrene, right leg

I70.262 Atherosclerosis of native arteries of extremities with gangrene, left leg

I70.263 Atherosclerosis of native arteries of extremities with gangrene, bilateral legs

I70.268 Atherosclerosis of native arteries of extremities with gangrene, other extremity

I70.269 Atherosclerosis of native arteries of extremities with gangrene, unspecified extremity

I70.29 Other atherosclerosis of native arteries of extremities

I70.291 Other atherosclerosis of native arteries of extremities, right leg

I70.292 Other atherosclerosis of native arteries of extremities, left leg

I70.293 Other atherosclerosis of native arteries of extremities, bilateral legs

I70.298 Other atherosclerosis of native arteries of extremities, other extremity

I70.299 Other atherosclerosis of native arteries of extremities, unspecified extremity

I70.3 Atherosclerosis of unspecified type of bypass graft(s) of the extremities

Use additional code, if applicable, to identify chronic total occlusion of artery of extremity (I70.92)

Excludes 1: embolism or thrombus of bypass graft(s) of extremities (T82.8-)

I70.30 Unspecified atherosclerosis of unspecified type of bypass graft(s) of the extremities

I70.301 Unspecified atherosclerosis of unspecified type of bypass graft(s) of the extremities, right leg

I70.302 Unspecified atherosclerosis of unspecified type of bypass graft(s) of the extremities, left leg

I70.303 Unspecified atherosclerosis of unspecified type of bypass graft(s) of the extremities, bilateral legs

I70.308 Unspecified atherosclerosis of unspecified type of bypass graft(s) of the extremities, other extremity

I70.309 Unspecified atherosclerosis of unspecified type of bypass graft(s) of the extremities, unspecified extremity

I70.31 Atherosclerosis of unspecified type of bypass graft(s) of the extremities with intermittent claudication

I70.311 Atherosclerosis of unspecified type of bypass graft(s) of the extremities with intermittent claudication, right leg

I70.312 Atherosclerosis of unspecified type of bypass graft(s) of the extremities with intermittent claudication, left leg

I70.313 Atherosclerosis of unspecified type of bypass graft(s) of the extremities with intermittent claudication, bilateral legs

I70.318 Atherosclerosis of unspecified type of bypass graft(s) of the extremities with intermittent claudication, other extremity

I70.319 Atherosclerosis of unspecified type of bypass graft(s) of the extremities with intermittent claudication, unspecified extremity

I70.32 Atherosclerosis of unspecified type of bypass graft(s) of the extremities with rest pain
Includes: any condition classifiable to I70.31-

I70.321 Atherosclerosis of unspecified type of bypass graft(s) of the extremities with rest pain, right leg

I70.322 Atherosclerosis of unspecified type of bypass graft(s) of the extremities with rest pain, left leg

I70.323 Atherosclerosis of unspecified type of bypass graft(s) of the extremities with rest pain, bilateral legs

I70.328 Atherosclerosis of unspecified type of bypass graft(s) of the extremities with rest pain, other extremity

I70.329 Atherosclerosis of unspecified type of bypass graft(s) of the extremities with rest pain, unspecified extremity

I70.33 Atherosclerosis of unspecified type of bypass graft(s) of the right leg with ulceration
Includes: any condition classifiable to I70.311 and I70.321
Use additional code to identify severity of ulcer (L97.- with fifth character 1)

I70.331 Atherosclerosis of unspecified type of bypass graft(s) of the right leg with ulceration of thigh

I70.332 Atherosclerosis of unspecified type of bypass graft(s) of the right leg with ulceration of calf

I70.333 Atherosclerosis of unspecified type of bypass graft(s) of the right leg with ulceration of ankle

I70.334 Atherosclerosis of unspecified type of bypass graft(s) of the right leg with ulceration of heel and midfoot
Atherosclerosis of unspecified type of bypass graft(s) of right leg with ulceration of plantar surface of midfoot

I70.335 Atherosclerosis of unspecified type of bypass graft(s) of the right leg with ulceration of other part of foot

Atherosclerosis of unspecified type of bypass graft(s) of the right leg with ulceration of toe

I70.338 Atherosclerosis of unspecified type of bypass graft(s) of the right leg with ulceration of other part of lower leg

I70.339 Atherosclerosis of unspecified type of bypass graft(s) of the right leg with ulceration of unspecified site

I70.34 Atherosclerosis of unspecified type of bypass graft(s) of the left leg with ulceration
Includes: any condition classifiable to I70.312 and I70.322
Use additional code to identify severity of ulcer (L97.- with fifth character 2)

I70.341 Atherosclerosis of unspecified type of bypass graft(s) of the left leg with ulceration of thigh

I70.342 Atherosclerosis of unspecified type of bypass graft(s) of the left leg with ulceration of calf

I70.343 Atherosclerosis of unspecified type of bypass graft(s) of the left leg with ulceration of ankle

I70.344 Atherosclerosis of unspecified type of bypass graft(s) of the left leg with ulceration of heel and midfoot
Atherosclerosis of unspecified type of bypass graft(s) of left leg with ulceration of plantar surface of midfoot

I70.345 Atherosclerosis of unspecified type of bypass graft(s) of the left leg with ulceration of other part of foot
Atherosclerosis of unspecified type of bypass graft(s) of the left leg with ulceration of toe

I70.348 Atherosclerosis of unspecified type of bypass graft(s) of the left leg with ulceration of other part of lower leg

I70.349 Atherosclerosis of unspecified type of bypass graft(s) of the left leg with ulceration of unspecified site

I70.35 Atherosclerosis of unspecified type of bypass graft(s) of other extremity with ulceration
Includes: any condition classifiable to I70.318 and I70.328
Use additional code to identify severity of ulcer (L98.49-)

I70.36 Atherosclerosis of unspecified type of bypass graft(s) of the extremities with gangrene
Includes: any condition classifiable to I70.31-, I70.32-, I70.33-, I70.34-, I70.35
Use additional code to identify the severity of any ulcer (L98.49-), if applicable

I70.361 Atherosclerosis of unspecified type of bypass graft(s) of the extremities with gangrene, right leg

I70.362 Atherosclerosis of unspecified type of bypass graft(s) of the extremities with gangrene, left leg

I70.363 Atherosclerosis of unspecified type of bypass graft(s) of the extremities with gangrene, bilateral legs

● New code   ▲ Revised code   ⑦ 7th digit required   ⊗ Placeholder required

I70.368 Atherosclerosis of unspecified type of bypass graft(s) of the extremities with gangrene, other extremity

I70.369 Atherosclerosis of unspecified type of bypass graft(s) of the extremities with gangrene, unspecified extremity

I70.39 Other atherosclerosis of unspecified type of bypass graft(s) of the extremities

I70.391 Other atherosclerosis of unspecified type of bypass graft(s) of the extremities, right leg

I70.392 Other atherosclerosis of unspecified type of bypass graft(s) of the extremities, left leg

I70.393 Other atherosclerosis of unspecified type of bypass graft(s) of the extremities, bilateral legs

I70.398 Other atherosclerosis of unspecified type of bypass graft(s) of the extremities, other extremity

I70.399 Other atherosclerosis of unspecified type of bypass graft(s) of the extremities, unspecified extremity

I70.4 Atherosclerosis of autologous vein bypass graft(s) of the extremities

Use additional code, if applicable, to identify chronic total occlusion of artery of extremity (I70.92)

I70.40 Unspecified atherosclerosis of autologous vein bypass graft(s) of the extremities

I70.401 Unspecified atherosclerosis of autologous vein bypass graft(s) of the extremities, right leg

I70.402 Unspecified atherosclerosis of autologous vein bypass graft(s) of the extremities, left leg

I70.403 Unspecified atherosclerosis of autologous vein bypass graft(s) of the extremities, bilateral legs

I70.408 Unspecified atherosclerosis of autologous vein bypass graft(s) of the extremities, other extremity

I70.409 Unspecified atherosclerosis of autologous vein bypass graft(s) of the extremities, unspecified extremity

I70.41 Atherosclerosis of autologous vein bypass graft(s) of the extremities with intermittent claudication

I70.411 Atherosclerosis of autologous vein bypass graft(s) of the extremities with intermittent claudication, right leg

I70.412 Atherosclerosis of autologous vein bypass graft(s) of the extremities with intermittent claudication, left leg

I70.413 Atherosclerosis of autologous vein bypass graft(s) of the extremities with intermittent claudication, bilateral legs

I70.418 Atherosclerosis of autologous vein bypass graft(s) of the extremities with intermittent claudication, other extremity

I70.419 Atherosclerosis of autologous vein bypass graft(s) of the extremities with intermittent claudication, unspecified extremity

I70.42 Atherosclerosis of autologous vein bypass graft(s) of the extremities with rest pain
Includes: any condition classifiable to I70.41-

I70.421 Atherosclerosis of autologous vein bypass graft(s) of the extremities with rest pain, right leg

I70.422 Atherosclerosis of autologous vein bypass graft(s) of the extremities with rest pain, left leg

I70.423 Atherosclerosis of autologous vein bypass graft(s) of the extremities with rest pain, bilateral legs

I70.428 Atherosclerosis of autologous vein bypass graft(s) of the extremities with rest pain, other extremity

I70.429 Atherosclerosis of autologous vein bypass graft(s) of the extremities with rest pain, unspecified extremity

I70.43 Atherosclerosis of autologous vein bypass graft(s) of the right leg with ulceration
Includes: any condition classifiable to I70.411 and I70.421
Use additional code to identify severity of ulcer (L97.- with fifth character 1)

I70.431 Atherosclerosis of autologous vein bypass graft(s) of the right leg with ulceration of thigh

I70.432 Atherosclerosis of autologous vein bypass graft(s) of the right leg with ulceration of calf

I70.433 Atherosclerosis of autologous vein bypass graft(s) of the right leg with ulceration of ankle

I70.434 Atherosclerosis of autologous vein bypass graft(s) of the right leg with ulceration of heel and midfoot
Atherosclerosis of autologous vein bypass graft(s) of right leg with ulceration of plantar surface of midfoot

I70.435 Atherosclerosis of autologous vein bypass graft(s) of the right leg with ulceration of other part of foot
Atherosclerosis of autologous vein bypass graft(s) of right leg with ulceration of toe

I70.438 Atherosclerosis of autologous vein bypass graft(s) of the right leg with ulceration of other part of lower leg

I70.439 Atherosclerosis of autologous vein bypass graft(s) of the right leg with ulceration of unspecified site

I70.44 Atherosclerosis of autologous vein bypass graft(s) of the left leg with ulceration
Includes: any condition classifiable to I70.412 and I70.422
Use additional code to identify severity of ulcer (L97.- with fifth character 2)

I70.441 Atherosclerosis of autologous vein bypass graft(s) of the left leg with ulceration of thigh

I70.442 Atherosclerosis of autologous vein bypass graft(s) of the left leg with ulceration of calf

I70.443 Atherosclerosis of autologous vein bypass graft(s) of the left leg with ulceration of ankle

I70.444 Atherosclerosis of autologous vein bypass graft(s) of the left leg with ulceration of heel and midfoot

Atherosclerosis of autologous vein bypass graft(s) of left leg with ulceration of plantar surface of midfoot

I70.445 Atherosclerosis of autologous vein bypass graft(s) of the left leg with ulceration of other part of foot

Atherosclerosis of autologous vein bypass graft(s) of left leg with ulceration of toe

I70.448 Atherosclerosis of autologous vein bypass graft(s) of the left leg with ulceration of other part of lower leg

I70.449 Atherosclerosis of autologous vein bypass graft(s) of the left leg with ulceration of unspecified site

I70.45 Atherosclerosis of autologous vein bypass graft(s) of other extremity with ulceration

Includes: any condition classifiable to I70.418, I70.428, and I70.438

Use additional code to identify severity of ulcer (L98.49)

I70.46 Atherosclerosis of autologous vein bypass graft(s) of the extremities with gangrene

Includes: any condition classifiable to I70.41-, I70.42-, and I70.43-, I70.44-, I70.45

Use additional code to identify the severity of any ulcer (L98.49-), if applicable

I70.461 Atherosclerosis of autologous vein bypass graft(s) of the extremities with gangrene, right leg

I70.462 Atherosclerosis of autologous vein bypass graft(s) of the extremities with gangrene, left leg

I70.463 Atherosclerosis of autologous vein bypass graft(s) of the extremities with gangrene, bilateral legs

I70.468 Atherosclerosis of autologous vein bypass graft(s) of the extremities with gangrene, other extremity

I70.469 Atherosclerosis of autologous vein bypass graft(s) of the extremities with gangrene, unspecified extremity

I70.49 Other atherosclerosis of autologous vein bypass graft(s) of the extremities

I70.491 Other atherosclerosis of autologous vein bypass graft(s) of the extremities, right leg

I70.492 Other atherosclerosis of autologous vein bypass graft(s) of the extremities, left leg

I70.493 Other atherosclerosis of autologous vein bypass graft(s) of the extremities, bilateral legs

I70.498 Other atherosclerosis of autologous vein bypass graft(s) of the extremities, other extremity

I70.499 Other atherosclerosis of autologous vein bypass graft(s) of the extremities, unspecified extremity

I70.5 Atherosclerosis of nonautologous biological bypass graft(s) of the extremities

Use additional code, if applicable, to identify chronic total occlusion of artery of extremity (I70.92)

I70.50 Unspecified atherosclerosis of nonautologous biological bypass graft(s) of the extremities

I70.501 Unspecified atherosclerosis of nonautologous biological bypass graft(s) of the extremities, right leg

I70.502 Unspecified atherosclerosis of nonautologous biological bypass graft(s) of the extremities, left leg

I70.503 Unspecified atherosclerosis of nonautologous biological bypass graft(s) of the extremities, bilateral legs

I70.508 Unspecified atherosclerosis of nonautologous biological bypass graft(s) of the extremities, other extremity

I70.509 Unspecified atherosclerosis of nonautologous biological bypass graft(s) of the extremities, unspecified extremity

I70.51 Atherosclerosis of nonautologous biological bypass graft(s) of the extremities intermittent claudication

I70.511 Atherosclerosis of nonautologous biological bypass graft(s) of the extremities with intermittent claudication, right leg

I70.512 Atherosclerosis of nonautologous biological bypass graft(s) of the extremities with intermittent claudication, left leg

I70.513 Atherosclerosis of nonautologous biological bypass graft(s) of the extremities with intermittent claudication, bilateral legs

I70.518 Atherosclerosis of nonautologous biological bypass graft(s) of the extremities with intermittent claudication, other extremity

I70.519 Atherosclerosis of nonautologous biological bypass graft(s) of the extremities with intermittent claudication, unspecified extremity

I70.52 Atherosclerosis of nonautologous biological bypass graft(s) of the extremities with rest pain

Includes: any condition classifiable to I70.51-

I70.521 Atherosclerosis of nonautologous biological bypass graft(s) of the extremities with rest pain, right leg

I70.522 Atherosclerosis of nonautologous biological bypass graft(s) of the extremities with rest pain, left leg

I70.523 Atherosclerosis of nonautologous biological bypass graft(s) of the extremities with rest pain, bilateral legs

I70.528 Atherosclerosis of nonautologous biological bypass graft(s) of the extremities with rest pain, other extremity

I70.529 Atherosclerosis of nonautologous biological bypass graft(s) of the extremities with rest pain, unspecified extremity

I70.53 Atherosclerosis of nonautologous biological bypass graft(s) of the right leg with ulceration

Includes: any condition classifiable to I70.511 and I70.521

Use additional code to identify severity of ulcer (L97.- with fifth character 1)

I70.531 Atherosclerosis of nonautologous biological bypass graft(s) of the right leg with ulceration of thigh

I70.532 Atherosclerosis of nonautologous biological bypass graft(s) of the right leg with ulceration of calf

I70.533 Atherosclerosis of nonautologous biological bypass graft(s) of the right leg with ulceration of ankle

I70.534 Atherosclerosis of nonautologous biological bypass graft(s) of the right leg with ulceration of heel and midfoot

Atherosclerosis of nonautologous biological bypass graft(s) of right leg with ulceration of plantar surface of midfoot

I70.535 Atherosclerosis of nonautologous biological bypass graft(s) of the right leg with ulceration of other part of foot

Atherosclerosis of nonautologous biological bypass graft(s) of the right leg with ulceration of toe

I70.538 Atherosclerosis of nonautologous biological bypass graft(s) of the right leg with ulceration of other part of lower leg

I70.539 Atherosclerosis of nonautologous biological bypass graft(s) of the right leg with ulceration of unspecified site

I70.54 Atherosclerosis of nonautologous biological bypass graft(s) of the left leg with ulceration

Includes: any condition classifiable to I70.512 and I70.522

Use additional code to identify severity of ulcer (L97.- with fifth character 2)

I70.541 Atherosclerosis of nonautologous biological bypass graft(s) of the left leg with ulceration of thigh

I70.542 Atherosclerosis of nonautologous biological bypass graft(s) of the left leg with ulceration of calf

I70.543 Atherosclerosis of nonautologous biological bypass graft(s) of the left leg with ulceration of ankle

I70.544 Atherosclerosis of nonautologous biological bypass graft(s) of the left leg with ulceration of heel and midfoot

Atherosclerosis of nonautologous biological bypass graft(s) of left leg with ulceration of plantar surface of midfoot

I70.545 Atherosclerosis of nonautologous biological bypass graft(s) of the left leg with ulceration of other part of foot

Atherosclerosis of nonautologous biological bypass graft(s) of the left leg with ulceration of toe

I70.548 Atherosclerosis of nonautologous biological bypass graft(s) of the left leg with ulceration of other part of lower leg

I70.549 Atherosclerosis of nonautologous biological bypass graft(s) of the left leg with ulceration of unspecified site

I70.55 Atherosclerosis of nonautologous biological bypass graft(s) of other extremity with ulceration

Includes: any condition classifiable to I70.518, I70.528, and I70.538

Use additional code to identify severity of ulcer (L98.49)

I70.56 Atherosclerosis of nonautologous biological bypass graft(s) of the extremities with gangrene

Includes: any condition classifiable to I70.51-, I70.52-, and I70.53-, I70.54-, I70.55

Use additional code to identify the severity of any ulcer (L98.49-), if applicable

I70.561 Atherosclerosis of nonautologous biological bypass graft(s) of the extremities with gangrene, right leg

I70.562 Atherosclerosis of nonautologous biological bypass graft(s) of the extremities with gangrene, left leg

I70.563 Atherosclerosis of nonautologous biological bypass graft(s) of the extremities with gangrene, bilateral legs

I70.568 Atherosclerosis of nonautologous biological bypass graft(s) of the extremities with gangrene, other extremity

I70.569 Atherosclerosis of nonautologous biological bypass graft(s) of the extremities with gangrene, unspecified extremity

I70.59 Other atherosclerosis of nonautologous biological bypass graft(s) of the extremities

I70.591 Other atherosclerosis of nonautologous biological bypass graft(s) of the extremities, right leg

I70.592 Other atherosclerosis of nonautologous biological bypass graft(s) of the extremities, left leg

I70.593 Other atherosclerosis of nonautologous biological bypass graft(s) of the extremities, bilateral legs

I70.598 Other atherosclerosis of nonautologous biological bypass graft(s) of the extremities, other extremity

I70.599 Other atherosclerosis of nonautologous biological bypass graft(s) of the extremities, unspecified extremity

I70.6 Atherosclerosis of nonbiological bypass graft(s) of the extremities

Use additional code, if applicable, to identify chronic total occlusion of artery of extremity (I70.92)

I70.60 Unspecified atherosclerosis of nonbiological bypass graft(s) of the extremities

I70.601 Unspecified atherosclerosis of nonbiological bypass graft(s) of the extremities, right leg

I70.602 Unspecified atherosclerosis of nonbiological bypass graft(s) of the extremities, left leg

I70.603 Unspecified atherosclerosis of nonbiological bypass graft(s) of the extremities, bilateral legs

I70.608 Unspecified atherosclerosis of nonbiological bypass graft(s) of the extremities, other extremity

I70.609 Unspecified atherosclerosis of nonbiological bypass graft(s) of the extremities, unspecified extremity

I70.61 Atherosclerosis of nonbiological bypass graft(s) of the extremities with intermittent claudication

I70.611 Atherosclerosis of nonbiological bypass graft(s) of the extremities with intermittent claudication, right leg

I70.612 Atherosclerosis of nonbiological bypass graft(s) of the extremities with intermittent claudication, left leg

I70.613 Atherosclerosis of nonbiological bypass graft(s) of the extremities with intermittent claudication, bilateral legs

I70.618 Atherosclerosis of nonbiological bypass graft(s) of the extremities with intermittent claudication, other extremity

I70.619 Atherosclerosis of nonbiological bypass graft(s) of the extremities with intermittent claudication, unspecified extremity

I70.62 Atherosclerosis of nonbiological bypass graft(s) of the extremities with rest pain
Includes: any condition classifiable to I70.61-

I70.621 Atherosclerosis of nonbiological bypass graft(s) of the extremities with rest pain, right leg

I70.622 Atherosclerosis of nonbiological bypass graft(s) of the extremities with rest pain, left leg

I70.623 Atherosclerosis of nonbiological bypass graft(s) of the extremities with rest pain, bilateral legs

I70.628 Atherosclerosis of nonbiological bypass graft(s) of the extremities with rest pain, other extremity

I70.629 Atherosclerosis of nonbiological bypass graft(s) of the extremities with rest pain, unspecified extremity

I70.63 Atherosclerosis of nonbiological bypass graft(s) of the right leg with ulceration
Includes: any condition classifiable to I70.611 and I70.621
Use additional code to identify severity of ulcer (L97.- with fifth character 1)

I70.631 Atherosclerosis of nonbiological bypass graft(s) of the right leg with ulceration of thigh

I70.632 Atherosclerosis of nonbiological bypass graft(s) of the right leg with ulceration of calf

I70.633 Atherosclerosis of nonbiological bypass graft(s) of the right leg with ulceration of ankle

I70.634 Atherosclerosis of nonbiological bypass graft(s) of the right leg with ulceration of heel and midfoot
Atherosclerosis of nonbiological bypass graft(s) of right leg with ulceration of plantar surface of midfoot

I70.635 Atherosclerosis of nonbiological bypass graft(s) of the right leg with ulceration of other part of foot
Atherosclerosis of nonbiological bypass graft(s) of the right leg with ulceration of toe

I70.638 Atherosclerosis of nonbiological bypass graft(s) of the right leg with ulceration of other part of lower leg

I70.639 Atherosclerosis of nonbiological bypass graft(s) of the right leg with ulceration of unspecified site

I70.64 Atherosclerosis of nonbiological bypass graft(s) of the left leg with ulceration
Includes: any condition classifiable to I70.612 and I70.622
Use additional code to identify severity of ulcer (L97.- with fifth character 2)

I70.641 Atherosclerosis of nonbiological bypass graft(s) of the left leg with ulceration of thigh

I70.642 Atherosclerosis of nonbiological bypass graft(s) of the left leg with ulceration of calf

I70.643 Atherosclerosis of nonbiological bypass graft(s) of the left leg with ulceration of ankle

I70.644 Atherosclerosis of nonbiological bypass graft(s) of the left leg with ulceration of heel and midfoot
Atherosclerosis of nonbiological bypass graft(s) of left leg with ulceration of plantar surface of midfoot

I70.645 Atherosclerosis of nonbiological bypass graft(s) of the left leg with ulceration of other part of foot
Atherosclerosis of nonbiological bypass graft(s) of the left leg with ulceration of toe

I70.648 Atherosclerosis of nonbiological bypass graft(s) of the left leg with ulceration of other part of lower leg

I70.649 Atherosclerosis of nonbiological bypass graft(s) of the left leg with ulceration of unspecified site

I70.65 Atherosclerosis of nonbiological bypass graft(s) of other extremity with ulceration
Includes: any condition classifiable to I70.618 and I70.628
Use additional code to identify severity of ulcer (L98.49)

I70.66 Atherosclerosis of nonbiological bypass graft(s) of the extremities with gangrene
Includes: any condition classifiable to I70.61-, I70.62-, I70.63-, I70.64-, I70.65

● New code   ▲ Revised code   ⑦ 7th digit required   ⊗ Placeholder required

Use additional code to identify the severity of any ulcer (L98.49-), if applicable

I70.661 Atherosclerosis of nonbiological bypass graft(s) of the extremities with gangrene, right leg

I70.662 Atherosclerosis of nonbiological bypass graft(s) of the extremities with gangrene, left leg

I70.663 Atherosclerosis of nonbiological bypass graft(s) of the extremities with gangrene, bilateral legs

I70.668 Atherosclerosis of nonbiological bypass graft(s) of the extremities with gangrene, other extremity

I70.669 Atherosclerosis of nonbiological bypass graft(s) of the extremities with gangrene, unspecified extremity

I70.69 Other atherosclerosis of nonbiological bypass graft(s) of the extremities

I70.691 Other atherosclerosis of nonbiological bypass graft(s) of the extremities, right leg

I70.692 Other atherosclerosis of nonbiological bypass graft(s) of the extremities, left leg

I70.693 Other atherosclerosis of nonbiological bypass graft(s) of the extremities, bilateral legs

I70.698 Other atherosclerosis of nonbiological bypass graft(s) of the extremities, other extremity

I70.699 Other atherosclerosis of nonbiological bypass graft(s) of the extremities, unspecified extremity

I70.7 Atherosclerosis of other type of bypass graft(s) of the extremities

Use additional code, if applicable, to identify chronic total occlusion of artery of extremity (I70.92)

I70.70 Unspecified atherosclerosis of other type of bypass graft(s) of the extremities

I70.701 Unspecified atherosclerosis of other type of bypass graft(s) of the extremities, right leg

I70.702 Unspecified atherosclerosis of other type of bypass graft(s) of the extremities, left leg

I70.703 Unspecified atherosclerosis of other type of bypass graft(s) of the extremities, bilateral legs

I70.708 Unspecified atherosclerosis of other type of bypass graft(s) of the extremities, other extremity

I70.709 Unspecified atherosclerosis of other type of bypass graft(s) of the extremities, unspecified extremity

I70.71 Atherosclerosis of other type of bypass graft(s) of the extremities with intermittent claudication

I70.711 Atherosclerosis of other type of bypass graft(s) of the extremities with intermittent claudication, right leg

I70.712 Atherosclerosis of other type of bypass graft(s) of the extremities with intermittent claudication, left leg

I70.713 Atherosclerosis of other type of bypass graft(s) of the extremities with intermittent claudication, bilateral legs

I70.718 Atherosclerosis of other type of bypass graft(s) of the extremities with intermittent claudication, other extremity

I70.719 Atherosclerosis of other type of bypass graft(s) of the extremities with intermittent claudication, unspecified extremity

I70.72 Atherosclerosis of other type of bypass graft(s) of the extremities with rest pain
Includes: any condition classifiable to I70.71-

I70.721 Atherosclerosis of other type of bypass graft(s) of the extremities with rest pain, right leg

I70.722 Atherosclerosis of other type of bypass graft(s) of the extremities with rest pain, left leg

I70.723 Atherosclerosis of other type of bypass graft(s) of the extremities with rest pain, bilateral legs

I70.728 Atherosclerosis of other type of bypass graft(s) of the extremities with rest pain, other extremity

I70.729 Atherosclerosis of other type of bypass graft(s) of the extremities with rest pain, unspecified extremity

I70.73 Atherosclerosis of other type of bypass graft(s) of the right leg with ulceration
Includes: any condition classifiable to I70.711 and I70.721
Use additional code to identify severity of ulcer (L97.- with fifth character 1)

I70.731 Atherosclerosis of other type of bypass graft(s) of the right leg with ulceration of thigh

I70.732 Atherosclerosis of other type of bypass graft(s) of the right leg with ulceration of calf

I70.733 Atherosclerosis of other type of bypass graft(s) of the right leg with ulceration of ankle

I70.734 Atherosclerosis of other type of bypass graft(s) of the right leg with ulceration of heel and midfoot
Atherosclerosis of other type of bypass graft(s) of right leg with ulceration of plantar surface of midfoot

I70.735 Atherosclerosis of other type of bypass graft(s) of the right leg with ulceration of other part of foot
Atherosclerosis of other type of bypass graft(s) of right leg with ulceration of toe

I70.738 Atherosclerosis of other type of bypass graft(s) of the right leg with ulceration of other part of lower leg

I70.739 Atherosclerosis of other type of bypass graft(s) of the right leg with ulceration of unspecified site

I70.74 Atherosclerosis of other type of bypass graft(s) of the left leg with ulceration
Includes: any condition classifiable to I70.712 and I70.722
Use additional code to identify severity of ulcer (L97.- with fifth character 2)

I70.741 Atherosclerosis of other type of bypass graft(s) of the left leg with ulceration of thigh

I70.742 Atherosclerosis of other type of bypass graft(s) of the left leg with ulceration of calf

I70.743 Atherosclerosis of other type of bypass graft(s) of the left leg with ulceration of ankle

I70.744 Atherosclerosis of other type of bypass graft(s) of the left leg with ulceration of heel and midfoot

Atherosclerosis of other type of bypass graft(s) of left leg with ulceration of plantar surface of midfoot

I70.745 Atherosclerosis of other type of bypass graft(s) of the left leg with ulceration of other part of foot

Atherosclerosis of other type of bypass graft(s) of left leg with ulceration of toe

I70.748 Atherosclerosis of other type of bypass graft(s) of the left leg with ulceration of other part of lower leg

I70.749 Atherosclerosis of other type of bypass graft(s) of the left leg with ulceration of unspecified site

I70.75 Atherosclerosis of other type of bypass graft(s) of other extremity with ulceration

Includes: any condition classifiable to I70.718 and I70.728

Use additional code to identify severity of ulcer (L98.49)

I70.76 Atherosclerosis of other type of bypass graft(s) of the extremities with gangrene

Includes: any condition classifiable to I70.71-, I70.72-, I70.73-, I70.74-, I70.75

Use additional code to identify the severity of any ulcer (L98.49-), if applicable

I70.761 Atherosclerosis of other type of bypass graft(s) of the extremities with gangrene, right leg

I70.762 Atherosclerosis of other type of bypass graft(s) of the extremities with gangrene, left leg

I70.763 Atherosclerosis of other type of bypass graft(s) of the extremities with gangrene, bilateral legs

I70.768 Atherosclerosis of other type of bypass graft(s) of the extremities with gangrene, other extremity

I70.769 Atherosclerosis of other type of bypass graft(s) of the extremities with gangrene, unspecified extremity

I70.79 Other atherosclerosis of other type of bypass graft(s) of the extremities

I70.791 Other atherosclerosis of other type of bypass graft(s) of the extremities, right leg

I70.792 Other atherosclerosis of other type of bypass graft(s) of the extremities, left leg

I70.793 Other atherosclerosis of other type of bypass graft(s) of the extremities, bilateral legs

I70.798 Other atherosclerosis of other type of bypass graft(s) of the extremities, other extremity

I70.799 Other atherosclerosis of other type of bypass graft(s) of the extremities, unspecified extremity

I70.8 Atherosclerosis of other arteries

I70.9 Other and unspecified atherosclerosis

I70.90 Unspecified atherosclerosis

I70.91 Generalized atherosclerosis

I70.92 Chronic total occlusion of artery of the extremities

Complete occlusion of artery of the extremities

Total occlusion of artery of the extremities

Code first atherosclerosis of arteries of the extremities (I70.2-, I70.3-, I70.4-, I70.5-, I70.6-, I70.7-)

Excludes 1: acute occlusion of artery of the extremity (I70.2-, I70.3-, I70.4-)

I71 Aortic aneurysm and dissection

Excludes 1: aortic ectasia (I77.81-)

syphilitic aortic aneurysm (A52.01)

traumatic aortic aneurysm (S25.09, S35.09)

I71.0 Dissection of aorta

I71.00 Dissection of unspecified site of aorta

I71.01 Dissection of thoracic aorta

I71.02 Dissection of abdominal aorta

I71.03 Dissection of thoracoabdominal aorta

I71.1 Thoracic aortic aneurysm, ruptured

I71.2 Thoracic aortic aneurysm, without rupture

I71.3 Abdominal aortic aneurysm, ruptured

I71.4 Abdominal aortic aneurysm, without rupture

I71.5 Thoracoabdominal aortic aneurysm, ruptured

I71.6 Thoracoabdominal aortic aneurysm, without rupture

I71.8 Aortic aneurysm of unspecified site, ruptured

Rupture of aorta NOS

I71.9 Aortic aneurysm of unspecified site, without rupture

Aneurysm of aorta

Dilatation of aorta

Hyaline necrosis of aorta

I72 Other aneurysm

Includes: aneurysm (cirsoid) (false) (ruptured)

Excludes 2: acquired aneurysm (I77.0)

aneurysm (of) aorta (I71.-)

aneurysm (of) arteriovenous NOS (Q27.3-)

carotid artery dissection (I77.71)

cerebral (nonruptured) aneurysm (I67.1)

coronary aneurysm (I25.4)

coronary artery dissection (I25.42)

dissection of artery NEC (I77.79)

heart aneurysm (I25.3)

iliac artery dissection (I77.72)

pulmonary artery aneurysm (I28.1)

renal artery dissection (I77.73)

retinal aneurysm (H35.0)

ruptured cerebral aneurysm (I60.7)

varicose aneurysm (I77.0)

vertebral artery dissection (I77.74)

I72.0 Aneurysm of carotid artery

Aneurysm of common carotid artery

Aneurysm of external carotid artery

Aneurysm of internal carotid artery, extracranial portion

Excludes 1: aneurysm of internal carotid artery, intracranial portion (I67.1)

aneurysm of internal carotid artery NOS (I67.1)

I72.1 Aneurysm of artery of upper extremity

I72.2 Aneurysm of renal artery

I72.3 Aneurysm of iliac artery

I72.4 Aneurysm of artery of lower extremity

I72.8 Aneurysm of other specified arteries

I72.9 Aneurysm of unspecified site

I73 Other peripheral vascular diseases

Excludes 2: chilblains (T69.1)

frostbite (T33- T34)

immersion hand or foot (T69.0-)

spasm of cerebral artery (G45.9)

I73.0 Raynaud's syndrome

Raynaud's disease

Raynaud's phenomenon (secondary)

I73.00 Raynaud's syndrome without gangrene

I73.01 Raynaud's syndrome with gangrene

I73.1 Thromboangiitis obliterans [Buerger's disease]

I73.8 Other specified peripheral vascular diseases

Excludes 1: diabetic (peripheral) angiopathy (E08-E13 with .51-.52)

I73.81 Erythromelalgia

I73.89 Other specified peripheral vascular diseases

Acrocyanosis

Erythrocyanosis

Simple acroparesthesia [Schultze's type]

Vasomotor acroparesthesia [Nothnagel's type]

I73.9 Peripheral vascular disease, unspecified

Intermittent claudication

Peripheral angiopathy NOS

Spasm of artery

Excludes 1: atherosclerosis of the extremities (I70.2--I70.7-)

I74 Arterial embolism and thrombosis

Includes: embolic infarction

embolic occlusion

thrombotic infarction

thrombotic occlusion

Code first embolism and thrombosis complicating abortion or ectopic or molar pregnancy (O00-O07, O08.2)

embolism and thrombosis complicating pregnancy, childbirth and the puerperium (O88.-)

Excludes 2: atheroembolism (I75.-)

basilar embolism and thrombosis (I63.0-I63.2, I65.1)

carotid embolism and thrombosis (I63.0-I63.2, I65.2)

cerebral embolism and thrombosis (I63.3-I63.5, I66.-)

coronary embolism and thrombosis (I21-I25)

mesenteric embolism and thrombosis (K55.0)

ophthalmic embolism and thrombosis (H34.-)

precerebral embolism and thrombosis NOS (I63.0-I63.2, I65.9)

pulmonary embolism and thrombosis (I26.-)

renal embolism and thrombosis (N28.0)

retinal embolism and thrombosis (H34.-)

septic embolism and thrombosis (I76)

vertebral embolism and thrombosis (I63.0-I63.2, I65.0)

I74.0 Embolism and thrombosis of abdominal aorta

I74.01 Saddle embolus of abdominal aorta

I74.09 Other arterial embolism and thrombosis of abdominal aorta

Aortic bifurcation syndrome

Aortoiliac obstruction

Leriche's syndrome

I74.1 Embolism and thrombosis of other and unspecified parts of aorta

I74.10 Embolism and thrombosis of unspecified parts of aorta

I74.11 Embolism and thrombosis of thoracic aorta

I74.19 Embolism and thrombosis of other parts of aorta

I74.2 Embolism and thrombosis of arteries of the upper extremities

I74.3 Embolism and thrombosis of arteries of the lower extremities

I74.4 Embolism and thrombosis of arteries of extremities, unspecified

Peripheral arterial embolism NOS

I74.5 Embolism and thrombosis of iliac artery

I74.8 Embolism and thrombosis of other arteries

I74.9 Embolism and thrombosis of unspecified artery

I75 Atheroembolism

Includes: atherothrombotic microembolism

cholesterol embolism

I75.0 Atheroembolism of extremities

I75.01 Atheroembolism of upper extremity

I75.011 Atheroembolism of right upper extremity

I75.012 Atheroembolism of left upper extremity

I75.013 Atheroembolism of bilateral upper extremities

I75.019 Atheroembolism of unspecified upper extremity

I75.02 Atheroembolism of lower extremity

I75.021 Atheroembolism of right lower extremity

I75.022 Atheroembolism of left lower extremity

I75.023 Atheroembolism of bilateral lower extremities

I75.029 Atheroembolism of unspecified lower extremity

I75.8 Atheroembolism of other sites

I75.81 Atheroembolism of kidney

Use additional code for any associated acute kidney failure and chronic kidney disease (N17.-, N18.-)

I75.89 Atheroembolism of other site

I76 Septic arterial embolism

Code first underlying infection, such as:

infective endocarditis (I33.0)

lung abscess (J85.-)

Use additional code to identify the site of the embolism (I74.-)

Excludes 2: septic pulmonary embolism (I26.01, I26.90)

I77 Other disorders of arteries and arterioles

Excludes 2: collagen (vascular) diseases (M30-M36)

hypersensitivity angiitis (M31.0)

pulmonary artery (I28.-)

I77.0 Arteriovenous fistula, acquired

Aneurysmal varix

Arteriovenous aneurysm, acquired

Excludes 1: arteriovenous aneurysm NOS (Q27.3-)

presence of arteriovenous shunt (fistula) for dialysis (Z99.2) traumatic - see injury of blood vessel by body region

Excludes 2: cerebral (I67.1)

coronary (I25.4)

I77.1 Stricture of artery

Narrowing of artery

I77.2 Rupture of artery

Erosion of artery

Fistula of artery

Ulcer of artery

Excludes 1: traumatic rupture of artery - see injury of blood vessel by body region

I77.3 Arterial fibromuscular dysplasia

Fibromuscular hyperplasia (of) carotid artery

Fibromuscular hyperplasia (of) renal artery

I77.4 Celiac artery compression syndrome

I77.5 Necrosis of artery

I77.6 Arteritis, unspecified

Aortitis NOS

Endarteritis NOS

Excludes 1: arteritis or endarteritis:

aortic arch (M31.4)

cerebral NEC (I67.7)

coronary (I25.89)

deformans (I70.-)

giant cell (M31.5., M31.6)

obliterans (I70.-)

senile (I70.-)

I77.7 Other arterial dissection

Excludes 2: dissection of aorta (I71.0-)

dissection of coronary artery (I25.42)

I77.71 Dissection of carotid artery

I77.72 Dissection of iliac artery

I77.73 Dissection of renal artery

I77.74 Dissection of vertebral artery

I77.79 Dissection of other artery

I77.8 Other specified disorders of arteries and arterioles

I77.81 Aortic ectasia

Ectasis aorta

Excludes 1: aortic aneurysm and dissection (I71.0-)

I77.810 Thoracic aortic ectasia

I77.811 Abdominal aortic ectasia

I77.812 Thoracoabdominal aortic ectasia

I77.819 Aortic ectasia, unspecified site

I77.89 Other specified disorders of arteries and arterioles

I77.9 Disorder of arteries and arterioles, unspecified

I78 Diseases of capillaries

I78.0 Hereditary hemorrhagic telangiectasia

Rendu-Osler-Weber disease

I78.1 Nevus, non-neoplastic

Araneus nevus

Senile nevus

Spider nevus

Stellar nevus

Excludes 1: nevus NOS (D22.-)

vascular NOS (Q82.5)

Excludes 2: blue nevus (D22.-)

flammeus nevus (Q82.5)

hairy nevus (D22.-)

melanocytic nevus (D22.-)

pigmented nevus (D22.-)

port wine nevus (Q82.5)

sanguineous nevus (Q82.5)

strawberry nevus (Q82.5)

verrucous nevus (Q82.5)

I78.8 Other diseases of capillaries

I78.9 Disease of capillaries, unspecified

I79 Disorders of arteries, arterioles and capillaries in diseases classified elsewhere

I79.0 Aneurysm of aorta in diseases classified elsewhere

Code first underlying disease

Excludes 1: syphilitic aneurysm (A52.01)

I79.1 Aortitis in diseases classified elsewhere

Code first underlying disease

Excludes 1: syphilitic aortitis (A52.02)

I79.8 Other disorders of arteries, arterioles and capillaries in diseases classified elsewhere

Code first underlying disease, such as:

amyloidosis (E85-)

Excludes 1: diabetic (peripheral) angiopathy (E08-E13 with .51-.52)

endarteritis:

syphilitic (A52.09)

tuberculous (A18.89)

DISEASES OF VEINS, LYMPHATIC VESSELS AND LYMPH NODES, NOT ELSEWHERE CLASSIFIED (I80-I89)

I80 Phlebitis and thrombophlebitis

Includes: endophlebitis

inflammation, vein

periphlebitis

suppurative phlebitis

Code first phlebitis and thrombophlebitis complicating abortion, ectopic or molar pregnancy (O00-O07, O08.7)

phlebitis and thrombophlebitis complicating pregnancy, childbirth and the puerperium (O22.-, O87.-)

Excludes 1: venous embolism and thrombosis of lower extremities (I82.4-, I82.5-, I82.81-)

I80.0 Phlebitis and thrombophlebitis of superficial vessels of lower extremities

Phlebitis and thrombophlebitis of femoropopliteal vein

I80.00 Phlebitis and thrombophlebitis of superficial vessels of unspecified lower extremity

I80.01 Phlebitis and thrombophlebitis of superficial vessels of right lower extremity

I80.02 Phlebitis and thrombophlebitis of superficial vessels of left lower extremity

I80.03 Phlebitis and thrombophlebitis of superficial vessels of lower extremities, bilateral

I80.1 Phlebitis and thrombophlebitis of femoral vein

I80.10 Phlebitis and thrombophlebitis of unspecified femoral vein

I80.11 Phlebitis and thrombophlebitis of right femoral vein

I80.12 Phlebitis and thrombophlebitis of left femoral vein

I80.13 Phlebitis and thrombophlebitis of femoral vein, bilateral

I80.2 Phlebitis and thrombophlebitis of other and unspecified deep vessels of lower extremities

I80.20 Phlebitis and thrombophlebitis of unspecified deep vessels of lower extremities

I80.201 Phlebitis and thrombophlebitis of unspecified deep vessels of right lower extremity

I80.202 Phlebitis and thrombophlebitis of unspecified deep vessels of left lower extremity

I80.203 Phlebitis and thrombophlebitis of unspecified deep vessels of lower extremities, bilateral

I80.209 Phlebitis and thrombophlebitis of unspecified deep vessels of unspecified lower extremity

I80.21 Phlebitis and thrombophlebitis of iliac vein

I80.211 Phlebitis and thrombophlebitis of right iliac vein

I80.212 Phlebitis and thrombophlebitis of left iliac vein

I80.213 Phlebitis and thrombophlebitis of iliac vein, bilateral

I80.219 Phlebitis and thrombophlebitis of unspecified iliac vein

I80.22 Phlebitis and thrombophlebitis of popliteal vein

I80.221 Phlebitis and thrombophlebitis of right popliteal vein

I80.222 Phlebitis and thrombophlebitis of left popliteal vein

I80.223 Phlebitis and thrombophlebitis of popliteal vein, bilateral

I80.229 Phlebitis and thrombophlebitis of unspecified popliteal vein

I80.23 Phlebitis and thrombophlebitis of tibial vein

I80.231 Phlebitis and thrombophlebitis of right tibial vein

I80.232 Phlebitis and thrombophlebitis of left tibial vein

I80.233 Phlebitis and thrombophlebitis of tibial vein, bilateral

I80.239 Phlebitis and thrombophlebitis of unspecified tibial vein

I80.29 Phlebitis and thrombophlebitis of other deep vessels of lower extremities

I80.291 Phlebitis and thrombophlebitis of other deep vessels of right lower extremity

I80.292 Phlebitis and thrombophlebitis of other deep vessels of left lower extremity

I80.293 Phlebitis and thrombophlebitis of other deep vessels of lower extremity, bilateral

I80.299 Phlebitis and thrombophlebitis of other deep vessels of unspecified lower extremity

I80.3 Phlebitis and thrombophlebitis of lower extremities, unspecified

I80.8 Phlebitis and thrombophlebitis of other sites

I80.9 Phlebitis and thrombophlebitis of unspecified site

I81 Portal vein thrombosis

Portal (vein) obstruction

Excludes 2: hepatic vein thrombosis (I82.0)

phlebitis of portal vein (K75.1)

I82 Other venous embolism and thrombosis

Code first venous embolism and thrombosis complicating:

abortion, ectopic or molar pregnancy (O00-O07, O08.7)

pregnancy, childbirth and the puerperium (O22.-, O87.-)

Excludes 2: venous embolism and thrombosis (of):

cerebral (I63.6, I67.6)

coronary (I21-I25)

intracranial and intraspinal, septic or NOS (G08)

intracranial, nonpyogenic (I67.6)

intraspinal, nonpyogenic (G95.1)

mesenteric (K55.0)

portal (I81)

pulmonary (I26.-)

I82.0 Budd-Chiari syndrome

Hepatic vein thrombosis

I82.1 Thrombophlebitis migrans

I82.2 Embolism and thrombosis of vena cava and other thoracic veins

I82.21 Embolism and thrombosis of superior vena cava

I82.210 Acute embolism and thrombosis of superior vena cava

Embolism and thrombosis of superior vena cava NOS

I82.211 Chronic embolism and thrombosis of superior vena cava

I82.22 Embolism and thrombosis of inferior vena cava

I82.220 Acute embolism and thrombosis of inferior vena cava

Embolism and thrombosis of inferior vena cava NOS

I82.221 Chronic embolism and thrombosis of inferior vena cava

I82.29 Embolism and thrombosis of other thoracic veins

Embolism and thrombosis of brachiocephalic (innominate) vein

I8.290 Acute embolism and thrombosis of other thoracic veins

I82.291 Chronic embolism and thrombosis of other thoracic veins

I82.3 Embolism and thrombosis of renal vein

I82.4 Acute embolism and thrombosis of deep veins of lower extremity

I82.40 Acute embolism and thrombosis of unspecified deep veins of lower extremity

Deep vein thrombosis NOS

DVT NOS

Excludes 1: acute embolism and thrombosis of unspecified deep veins of distal lower extremity (I82.4b-)

acute embolism and thrombosis of unspecified deep veins of proximal lower extremity (I82.4a-)

I82.401 Acute embolism and thrombosis of unspecified deep veins of right lower extremity

I82.402 Acute embolism and thrombosis of unspecified deep veins of left lower extremity

I82.403 Acute embolism and thrombosis of unspecified deep veins of lower extremity, bilateral

I82.409 Acute embolism and thrombosis of unspecified deep veins of unspecified lower extremity

I82.41 Acute embolism and thrombosis of femoral vein

I82.411 Acute embolism and thrombosis of right femoral vein

I82.412 Acute embolism and thrombosis of left femoral vein

I82.413 Acute embolism and thrombosis of femoral vein, bilateral

I82.419 Acute embolism and thrombosis of unspecified femoral vein

I82.42 Acute embolism and thrombosis of iliac vein

I82.421 Acute embolism and thrombosis of right iliac vein

I82.422 Acute embolism and thrombosis of left iliac vein

I82.423 Acute embolism and thrombosis of iliac vein, bilateral

I82.429 Acute embolism and thrombosis of unspecified iliac vein

I82.43 Acute embolism and thrombosis of popliteal vein

I82.431 Acute embolism and thrombosis of right popliteal vein

I82.432 Acute embolism and thrombosis of left popliteal vein

I82.433 Acute embolism and thrombosis of popliteal vein, bilateral

I82.439 Acute embolism and thrombosis of unspecified popliteal vein

I82.44 Acute embolism and thrombosis of tibial vein

I82.441 Acute embolism and thrombosis of right tibial vein

I82.442 Acute embolism and thrombosis of left tibial vein

I82.443 Acute embolism and thrombosis of tibial vein, bilateral

I82.449 Acute embolism and thrombosis of unspecified tibial vein

I82.49 Acute embolism and thrombosis of other specified deep vein of lower extremity

I82.491 Acute embolism and thrombosis of other specified deep vein of right lower extremity

I82.492 Acute embolism and thrombosis of other specified deep vein of left lower extremity

I82.493 Acute embolism and thrombosis of other specified deep vein of lower extremity, bilateral

I82.499 Acute embolism and thrombosis of other specified deep vein of unspecified lower extremity

I82.4Y Acute embolism and thrombosis of unspecified deep veins of proximal lower extremity

Acute embolism and thrombosis of deep vein of thigh NOS

Acute embolism and thrombosis of deep vein of upper leg NOS

I82.4Y1 Acute embolism and thrombosis of unspecified deep veins of right proximal lower extremity

I82.4Y2 Acute embolism and thrombosis of unspecified deep veins of left proximal lower extremity

I82.4Y3 Acute embolism and thrombosis of unspecified deep veins of proximal lower extremity, bilateral

I82.4Y9 Acute embolism and thrombosis of unspecified deep veins of unspecified proximal lower extremity

I82.4Z Acute embolism and thrombosis of unspecified deep veins of distal lower extremity

Acute embolism and thrombosis of deep vein of calf NOS

Acute embolism and thrombosis of deep vein of lower leg NOS

I82.4Z1 Acute embolism and thrombosis of unspecified deep veins of right distal lower extremity

I82.4Z2 Acute embolism and thrombosis of unspecified deep veins of left distal lower extremity

I82.4Z3 Acute embolism and thrombosis of unspecified deep veins of distal lower extremity, bilateral

I82.4Z9 Acute embolism and thrombosis of unspecified deep veins of unspecified distal lower extremity

I82.5 Chronic embolism and thrombosis of deep veins of lower extremity

Use additional code, if applicable, for associated long-term (current) use of anticoagulants (Z79.01)

Excludes 1: personal history of venous embolism and thrombosis (Z86.718)

I82.50 Chronic embolism and thrombosis of unspecified deep veins of lower extremity

Excludes 1: chronic embolism and thrombosis of unspecified deep veins of distal lower extremity (I82.5b-)

chronic embolism and thrombosis of unspecified deep veins of proximal lower extremity (I82.5a-)

I82.501 Chronic embolism and thrombosis of unspecified deep veins of right lower extremity

I82.502 Chronic embolism and thrombosis of unspecified deep veins of left lower extremity

I82.503 Chronic embolism and thrombosis of unspecified deep veins of lower extremity, bilateral

I82.509 Chronic embolism and thrombosis of unspecified deep veins of unspecified lower extremity

I82.51 Chronic embolism and thrombosis of femoral vein

I82.511 Chronic embolism and thrombosis of right femoral vein

I82.512 Chronic embolism and thrombosis of left femoral vein

I82.513 Chronic embolism and thrombosis of femoral vein, bilateral

I82.519 Chronic embolism and thrombosis of unspecified femoral vein

I82.52 Chronic embolism and thrombosis of iliac vein

I82.521 Chronic embolism and thrombosis of right iliac vein

I82.522 Chronic embolism and thrombosis of left iliac vein

I82.523 Chronic embolism and thrombosis of iliac vein, bilateral

I82.529 Chronic embolism and thrombosis of unspecified iliac vein

I82.53 Chronic embolism and thrombosis of popliteal vein

I82.531   Chronic embolism and thrombosis of right popliteal vein

I82.532   Chronic embolism and thrombosis of left popliteal vein

I82.533   Chronic embolism and thrombosis of popliteal vein, bilateral

I82.539   Chronic embolism and thrombosis of unspecified popliteal vein

I82.54   Chronic embolism and thrombosis of tibial vein

I82.541   Chronic embolism and thrombosis of right tibial vein

I82.542   Chronic embolism and thrombosis of left tibial vein

I82.543   Chronic embolism and thrombosis of tibial vein, bilateral

I82.549   Chronic embolism and thrombosis of unspecified tibial vein

I82.59   Chronic embolism and thrombosis of other specified deep vein of lower extremity

I82.591   Chronic embolism and thrombosis of other specified deep vein of right lower extremity

I82.592   Chronic embolism and thrombosis of other specified deep vein of left lower extremity

I82.593   Chronic embolism and thrombosis of other specified deep vein of lower extremity, bilateral

I82.599   Chronic embolism and thrombosis of other specified deep vein of unspecified lower extremity

I82.5Y   Chronic embolism and thrombosis of unspecified deep veins of proximal lower extremity

Chronic embolism and thrombosis of deep veins of thigh NOS

Chronic embolism and thrombosis of deep veins of upper leg NOS

I82.5Y1   Chronic embolism and thrombosis of unspecified deep veins of right proximal lower extremity

I82.5Y2   Chronic embolism and thrombosis of unspecified deep veins of left proximal lower extremity

I82.5Y3   Chronic embolism and thrombosis of unspecified deep veins of proximal lower extremity, bilateral

I82.5Y9   Chronic embolism and thrombosis of unspecified deep veins of unspecified proximal lower extremity

I82.5Z   Chronic embolism and thrombosis of unspecified deep veins of distal lower extremity

Chronic embolism and thrombosis of deep veins of calf NOS

Chronic embolism and thrombosis of deep veins of lower leg NOS

I82.5Z1   Chronic embolism and thrombosis of unspecified deep veins of right distal lower extremity

I82.5Z2   Chronic embolism and thrombosis of unspecified deep veins of left distal lower extremity

I82.5Z3   Chronic embolism and thrombosis of unspecified deep veins of distal lower extremity, bilateral

I82.5Z9   Chronic embolism and thrombosis of unspecified deep veins of unspecified distal lower extremity

I82.6   Acute embolism and thrombosis of veins of upper extremity

I82.60   Acute embolism and thrombosis of unspecified veins of upper extremity

I82.601   Acute embolism and thrombosis of unspecified veins of right upper extremity

I82.602   Acute embolism and thrombosis of unspecified veins of left upper extremity

I82.603   Acute embolism and thrombosis of unspecified veins of upper extremity, bilateral

I82.609   Acute embolism and thrombosis of unspecified veins of unspecified upper extremity

I82.61   Acute embolism and thrombosis of superficial veins of upper extremity

Acute embolism and thrombosis of antecubital vein

Acute embolism and thrombosis of basilic vein

Acute embolism and thrombosis of cephalic vein

I82.611   Acute embolism and thrombosis of superficial veins of right upper extremity

I82.612   Acute embolism and thrombosis of superficial veins of left upper extremity

I82.613   Acute embolism and thrombosis of superficial veins of upper extremity, bilateral

I82.619   Acute embolism and thrombosis of superficial veins of unspecified upper extremity

I82.62   Acute embolism and thrombosis of deep veins of upper extremity

Acute embolism and thrombosis of brachial vein

Acute embolism and thrombosis of radial vein

Acute embolism and thrombosis of ulnar vein

I82.621   Acute embolism and thrombosis of deep veins of right upper extremity

I82.622   Acute embolism and thrombosis of deep veins of left upper extremity

I82.623   Acute embolism and thrombosis of deep veins of upper extremity, bilateral

I82.629   Acute embolism and thrombosis of deep veins of unspecified upper extremity

I82.7   Chronic embolism and thrombosis of veins of upper extremity

Use additional code, if applicable, for associated long-term (current) use of anticoagulants (Z79.01)

Excludes 1: personal history of venous embolism and thrombosis (Z86.718)

I82.70   Chronic embolism and thrombosis of unspecified veins of upper extremity

I82.701   Chronic embolism and thrombosis of unspecified veins of right upper extremity

I82.702   Chronic embolism and thrombosis of unspecified veins of left upper extremity

I82.703 Chronic embolism and thrombosis of unspecified veins of upper extremity, bilateral

I82.709 Chronic embolism and thrombosis of unspecified veins of unspecified upper extremity

I82.71 Chronic embolism and thrombosis of superficial veins of upper extremity

Chronic embolism and thrombosis of antecubital vein

Chronic embolism and thrombosis of basilic vein

Chronic embolism and thrombosis of cephalic vein

I82.711 Chronic embolism and thrombosis of superficial veins of right upper extremity

I82.712 Chronic embolism and thrombosis of superficial veins of left upper extremity

I82.713 Chronic embolism and thrombosis of superficial veins of upper extremity, bilateral

I82.719 Chronic embolism and thrombosis of superficial veins of unspecified upper extremity

I82.72 Chronic embolism and thrombosis of deep veins of upper extremity

Chronic embolism and thrombosis of brachial vein

Chronic embolism and thrombosis of radial vein

Chronic embolism and thrombosis of ulnar vein

I82.721 Chronic embolism and thrombosis of deep veins of right upper extremity

I82.722 Chronic embolism and thrombosis of deep veins of left upper extremity

I82.723 Chronic embolism and thrombosis of deep veins of upper extremity, bilateral

I82.729 Chronic embolism and thrombosis of deep veins of unspecified upper extremity

I82.A Embolism and thrombosis of axillary vein

I82.A1 Acute embolism and thrombosis of axillary vein

I82.A11 Acute embolism and thrombosis of right axillary vein

I82.A12 Acute embolism and thrombosis of left axillary vein

I82.A13 Acute embolism and thrombosis of axillary vein, bilateral

I82.A19 Acute embolism and thrombosis of unspecified axillary vein

I82.A2 Chronic embolism and thrombosis of axillary vein

I82.A21 Chronic embolism and thrombosis of right axillary vein

I82.A22 Chronic embolism and thrombosis of left axillary vein

I82.A23 Chronic embolism and thrombosis of axillary vein, bilateral

I82.A29 Chronic embolism and thrombosis of unspecified axillary vein

I82.B Embolism and thrombosis of subclavian vein

I82.B1 Acute embolism and thrombosis of subclavian vein

I82.B11 Acute embolism and thrombosis of right subclavian vein

I82.B12 Acute embolism and thrombosis of left subclavian vein

I82.B13 Acute embolism and thrombosis of subclavian vein, bilateral

I82.B19 Acute embolism and thrombosis of unspecified subclavian vein

I82.B2 Chronic embolism and thrombosis of subclavian vein

I82.B21 Chronic embolism and thrombosis of right subclavian vein

I82.B22 Chronic embolism and thrombosis of left subclavian vein

I82.B23 Chronic embolism and thrombosis of subclavian vein, bilateral

I82.B29 Chronic embolism and thrombosis of unspecified subclavian vein

I82.C Embolism and thrombosis of internal jugular vein

I82.C1 Acute embolism and thrombosis of internal jugular vein

I82.C11 Acute embolism and thrombosis of right internal jugular vein

I82.C12 Acute embolism and thrombosis of left internal jugular vein

I82.C13 Acute embolism and thrombosis of internal jugular vein, bilateral

I82.C19 Acute embolism and thrombosis of unspecified internal jugular vein

I82.C2 Chronic embolism and thrombosis of internal jugular vein

I82.C21 Chronic embolism and thrombosis of right internal jugular vein

I82.C22 Chronic embolism and thrombosis of left internal jugular vein

I82.C23 Chronic embolism and thrombosis of internal jugular vein, bilateral

I82.C29 Chronic embolism and thrombosis of unspecified internal jugular vein

I82.8 Embolism and thrombosis of other specified veins

Use additional code, if applicable, for associated long-term (current) use of anticoagulants (Z79.01)

I82.81 Embolism and thrombosis of superficial veins of lower extremities

Embolism and thrombosis of saphenous vein (greater) (lesser)

I82.811 Embolism and thrombosis of superficial veins of right lower extremities

I82.812 Embolism and thrombosis of superficial veins of left lower extremities

I82.813 Embolism and thrombosis of superficial veins of lower extremities, bilateral

I82.819 Embolism and thrombosis of superficial veins of unspecified lower extremities

I82.89 Embolism and thrombosis of other specified veins

I82.890 Acute embolism and thrombosis of other specified veins

I82.891 Chronic embolism and thrombosis of other specified veins

I82.9 Embolism and thrombosis of unspecified vein

● New code   ▲ Revised code   ⑦ 7th digit required   ⊗ Placeholder required

I82.90 Acute embolism and thrombosis of unspecified vein

Embolism of vein NOS

Thrombosis (vein) NOS

I82.91 Chronic embolism and thrombosis of unspecified vein

I83 Varicose veins of lower extremities

Excludes 1: varicose veins complicating pregnancy (O22.0-)

varicose veins complicating the puerperium (O87.4)

I83.0 Varicose veins of lower extremities with ulcer

Use additional code to identify severity of ulcer (L97.-)

I83.00 Varicose veins of unspecified lower extremity with ulcer

I83.001 Varicose veins of unspecified lower extremity with ulcer of thigh

I83.002 Varicose veins of unspecified lower extremity with ulcer of calf

I83.003 Varicose veins of unspecified lower extremity with ulcer of ankle

I83.004 Varicose veins of unspecified lower extremity with ulcer of heel and midfoot

Varicose veins of unspecified lower extremity with ulcer of plantar surface of midfoot

I83.005 Varicose veins of unspecified lower extremity with ulcer other part of foot

Varicose veins of unspecified lower extremity with ulcer of toe

I83.008 Varicose veins of unspecified lower extremity with ulcer other part of lower leg

I83.009 Varicose veins of unspecified lower extremity with ulcer of unspecified site

I83.01 Varicose veins of right lower extremity with ulcer

I83.011 Varicose veins of right lower extremity with ulcer of thigh

I83.012 Varicose veins of right lower extremity with ulcer of calf

I83.013 Varicose veins of right lower extremity with ulcer of ankle

I83.014 Varicose veins of right lower extremity with ulcer of heel and midfoot

Varicose veins of right lower extremity with ulcer of plantar surface of midfoot

I83.015 Varicose veins of right lower extremity with ulcer other part of foot

Varicose veins of right lower extremity with ulcer of toe

I83.018 Varicose veins of right lower extremity with ulcer other part of lower leg

I83.019 Varicose veins of right lower extremity with ulcer of unspecified site

I83.02 Varicose veins of left lower extremity with ulcer

I83.021 Varicose veins of left lower extremity with ulcer of thigh

I83.022 Varicose veins of left lower extremity with ulcer of calf

I83.023 Varicose veins of left lower extremity with ulcer of ankle

I83.024 Varicose veins of left lower extremity with ulcer of heel and midfoot

Varicose veins of left lower extremity with ulcer of plantar surface of midfoot

I83.025 Varicose veins of left lower extremity with ulcer other part of foot

Varicose veins of left lower extremity with ulcer of toe

I83.028 Varicose veins of left lower extremity with ulcer other part of lower leg

I83.029 Varicose veins of left lower extremity with ulcer of unspecified site

I83.1 Varicose veins of lower extremities with inflammation

Stasis dermatitis

I83.10 Varicose veins of unspecified lower extremity with inflammation

I83.11 Varicose veins of right lower extremity with inflammation

I83.12 Varicose veins of left lower extremity with inflammation

I83.2 Varicose veins of lower extremities with both ulcer and inflammation

Use additional code to identify severity of ulcer (L97.-)

I83.20 Varicose veins of unspecified lower extremity with both ulcer and inflammation

I83.201 Varicose veins of unspecified lower extremity with both ulcer of thigh and inflammation

I83.202 Varicose veins of unspecified lower extremity with both ulcer of calf and inflammation

I83.203 Varicose veins of unspecified lower extremity with both ulcer of ankle and inflammation

I83.204 Varicose veins of unspecified lower extremity with both ulcer of heel and midfoot and inflammation

Varicose veins of unspecified lower extremity with both ulcer of plantar surface of midfoot and inflammation

I83.205 Varicose veins of unspecified lower extremity with both ulcer other part of foot and inflammation

Varicose veins of unspecified lower extremity with both ulcer of toe and inflammation

I83.208 Varicose veins of unspecified lower extremity with both ulcer of other part of lower extremity and inflammation

I83.209 Varicose veins of unspecified lower extremity with both ulcer of unspecified site and inflammation

I83.21 Varicose veins of right lower extremity with both ulcer and inflammation

I83.211 Varicose veins of right lower extremity with both ulcer of thigh and inflammation

I83.212 Varicose veins of right lower extremity with both ulcer of calf and inflammation

I83.213 Varicose veins of right lower extremity with both ulcer of ankle and inflammation

I83.214   Varicose veins of right lower extremity with both ulcer of heel and midfoot and inflammation

Varicose veins of right lower extremity with both ulcer of plantar surface of midfoot and inflammation

I83.215   Varicose veins of right lower extremity with both ulcer other part of foot and inflammation

Varicose veins of right lower extremity with both ulcer of toe and inflammation

I83.218   Varicose veins of right lower extremity with both ulcer of other part of lower extremity and inflammation

I83.219   Varicose veins of right lower extremity with both ulcer of unspecified site and inflammation

I83.22   Varicose veins of left lower extremity with both ulcer and inflammation

I83.221   Varicose veins of left lower extremity with both ulcer of thigh and inflammation

I83.222   Varicose veins of left lower extremity with both ulcer of calf and inflammation

I83.223   Varicose veins of left lower extremity with both ulcer of ankle and inflammation

I83.224   Varicose veins of left lower extremity with both ulcer of heel and midfoot and inflammation

Varicose veins of left lower extremity with both ulcer of plantar surface of midfoot and inflammation

I83.225   Varicose veins of left lower extremity with both ulcer other part of foot and inflammation

Varicose veins of left lower extremity with both ulcer of toe and inflammation

I83.228   Varicose veins of left lower extremity with both ulcer of other part of lower extremity and inflammation

I83.229   Varicose veins of left lower extremity with both ulcer of unspecified site and inflammation

I83.8   Varicose veins of lower extremities with other complications

I83.81   Varicose veins of lower extremities with pain

I83.811   Varicose veins of right lower extremities with pain

I83.812   Varicose veins of left lower extremities with pain

I83.813   Varicose veins of bilateral lower extremities with pain

I83.819   Varicose veins of unspecified lower extremities with pain

I83.89   Varicose veins of lower extremities with other complications

Varicose veins of lower extremities with edema

Varicose veins of lower extremities with swelling

I83.891   Varicose veins of right lower extremities with other complications

I83.892   Varicose veins of left lower extremities with other complications

I83.893   Varicose veins of bilateral lower extremities with other complications

I83.899   Varicose veins of unspecified lower extremities with other complications

I83.9   Asymptomatic varicose veins of lower extremities

Phlebectasia of lower extremities

Varicose veins of lower extremities

Varix of lower extremities

I83.90   Asymptomatic varicose veins of unspecified lower extremity

Varicose veins NOS

I83.91   Asymptomatic varicose veins of right lower extremity

I83.92   Asymptomatic varicose veins of left lower extremity

I83.93   Asymptomatic varicose veins of bilateral lower extremities

I85   Esophageal varices

Use additional code to identify:

alcohol abuse and dependence (F10.-)

I85.0   Esophageal varices

Idiopathic esophageal varices

Primary esophageal varices

I85.00   Esophageal varices without bleeding

Esophageal varices NOS

I85.01   Esophageal varices with bleeding

I85.1   Secondary esophageal varices

Esophageal varices secondary to alcoholic liver disease

Esophageal varices secondary to cirrhosis of liver

Esophageal varices secondary to schistosomiasis

Esophageal varices secondary to toxic liver disease

Code first underlying disease

I85.10   Secondary esophageal varices without bleeding

I85.11   Secondary esophageal varices with bleeding

I86   Varicose veins of other sites

Excludes 1: varicose veins of unspecified site (I83.9-)

Excludes 2: retinal varices (H35.0-)

I86.0   Sublingual varices

I86.1   Scrotal varices

Varicocele

I86.2   Pelvic varices

I86.3   Vulval varices

Excludes 1: vulval varices complicating childbirth and the puerperium (O87.8)

vulval varices complicating pregnancy (O22.1-)

I86.4   Gastric varices

I86.8   Varicose veins of other specified sites

Varicose ulcer of nasal septum

I87   Other disorders of veins

I87.0   Postthrombotic syndrome

Chronic venous hypertension due to deep vein thrombosis

Postphlebitic syndrome

Excludes 1: chronic venous hypertension without deep vein thrombosis (I87.3-)

I87.00   Postthrombotic syndrome without complications

Asymptomatic Postthrombotic syndrome

I87.001   Postthrombotic syndrome without complications of right lower extremity

I87.002   Postthrombotic syndrome without complications of left lower extremity

I87.003   Postthrombotic syndrome without complications of bilateral lower extremity

I87.009   Postthrombotic syndrome without complications of unspecified extremity
Postthrombotic syndrome NOS

I87.01   Postthrombotic syndrome with ulcer
Use additional code to specify site and severity of ulcer (L97.-)

I87.011   Postthrombotic syndrome with ulcer of right lower extremity

I87.012   Postthrombotic syndrome with ulcer of left lower extremity

I87.013   Postthrombotic syndrome with ulcer of bilateral lower extremity

I87.019   Postthrombotic syndrome with ulcer of unspecified lower extremity

I87.02   Postthrombotic syndrome with inflammation

I87.021   Postthrombotic syndrome with inflammation of right lower extremity

I87.022   Postthrombotic syndrome with inflammation of left lower extremity

I87.023   Postthrombotic syndrome with inflammation of bilateral lower extremity

I87.029   Postthrombotic syndrome with inflammation of unspecified lower extremity

I87.03   Postthrombotic syndrome with ulcer and inflammation
Use additional code to specify site and severity of ulcer (L97.-)

I87.031   Postthrombotic syndrome with ulcer and inflammation of right lower extremity

I87.032   Postthrombotic syndrome with ulcer and inflammation of left lower extremity

I87.033   Postthrombotic syndrome with ulcer and inflammation of bilateral lower extremity

I87.039   Postthrombotic syndrome with ulcer and inflammation of unspecified lower extremity

I87.09   Postthrombotic syndrome with other complications

I87.091   Postthrombotic syndrome with other complications of right lower extremity

I87.092   Postthrombotic syndrome with other complications of left lower extremity

I87.093   Postthrombotic syndrome with other complications of bilateral lower extremity

I87.099   Postthrombotic syndrome with other complications of unspecified lower extremity

I87.1   Compression of vein
Stricture of vein
Vena cava syndrome (inferior) (superior)
Excludes 2: compression of pulmonary vein (I28.8)

I87.2   Venous insufficiency (chronic) (peripheral)

I87.3   Chronic venous hypertension (idiopathic)
Stasis edema

Excludes 1: chronic venous hypertension due to deep vein thrombosis (I87.0-)
varicose veins of lower extremities (I83.-)

I87.30   Chronic venous hypertension (idiopathic) without complications
Asymptomatic chronic venous hypertension (idiopathic)

I87.301   Chronic venous hypertension (idiopathic) without complications of right lower extremity

I87.302   Chronic venous hypertension (idiopathic) without complications of left lower extremity

I87.303   Chronic venous hypertension (idiopathic) without complications of bilateral lower extremity

I87.309   Chronic venous hypertension (idiopathic) without complications of unspecified lower extremity
Chronic venous hypertension NOS

I87.31   Chronic venous hypertension (idiopathic) with ulcer
Use additional code to specify site and severity of ulcer (L97.-)

I87.311   Chronic venous hypertension (idiopathic) with ulcer of right lower extremity

I87.312   Chronic venous hypertension (idiopathic) with ulcer of left lower extremity

I87.313   Chronic venous hypertension (idiopathic) with ulcer of bilateral lower extremity

I87.319   Chronic venous hypertension (idiopathic) with ulcer of unspecified lower extremity

I87.32   Chronic venous hypertension (idiopathic) with inflammation

I87.321   Chronic venous hypertension (idiopathic) with inflammation of right lower extremity

I87.322   Chronic venous hypertension (idiopathic) with inflammation of left lower extremity

I87.323   Chronic venous hypertension (idiopathic) with inflammation of bilateral lower extremity

I87.329   Chronic venous hypertension (idiopathic) with inflammation of unspecified lower extremity

I87.33   Chronic venous hypertension (idiopathic) with ulcer and inflammation
Use additional code to specify site and severity of ulcer (L97.-)

I87.331   Chronic venous hypertension (idiopathic) with ulcer and inflammation of right lower extremity

I87.332   Chronic venous hypertension (idiopathic) with ulcer and inflammation of left lower extremity

I87.333   Chronic venous hypertension (idiopathic) with ulcer and inflammation of bilateral lower extremity

I87.339   Chronic venous hypertension (idiopathic) with ulcer and inflammation of unspecified lower extremity

I87.39　Chronic venous hypertension (idiopathic) with other complications

　　I87.391　Chronic venous hypertension (idiopathic) with other complications of right lower extremity

　　I87.392　Chronic venous hypertension (idiopathic) with other complications of left lower extremity

　　I87.393　Chronic venous hypertension (idiopathic) with other complications of bilateral lower extremity

　　I87.399　Chronic venous hypertension (idiopathic) with other complications of unspecified lower extremity

I87.8　Other specified disorders of veins

Phlebosclerosis

Venofibrosis

I87.9　Disorder of vein, unspecified

I88　Nonspecific lymphadenitis

Excludes 1: acute lymphadenitis, except mesenteric (L04.-)

enlarged lymph nodes NOS (R59.-)

human immunodeficiency virus [HIV] disease resulting in generalized lymphadenopathy (B20)

I88.0　Nonspecific mesenteric lymphadenitis

Mesenteric lymphadenitis (acute)(chronic)

I88.1　Chronic lymphadenitis, except mesenteric

Adenitis

Lymphadenitis

I88.8　Other nonspecific lymphadenitis

I88.9　Nonspecific lymphadenitis, unspecified

Lymphadenitis NOS

I89　Other noninfective disorders of lymphatic vessels and lymph nodes

Excludes 1: chylocele, tunica vaginalis (nonfilarial) NOS (N50.8)

enlarged lymph nodes NOS (R59.-)

filarial chylocele (B74.-)

hereditary lymphedema (Q82.0)

I89.0　Lymphedema, not elsewhere classified

Elephantiasis (nonfilarial) NOS

Lymphangiectasis

Obliteration, lymphatic vessel

Praecox lymphedema

Secondary lymphedema

Excludes 1: postmastectomy lymphedema (I97.2)

I89.1　Lymphangitis

Chronic lymphangitis

Lymphangitis NOS

Subacute lymphangitis

Excludes 1: acute lymphangitis (L03.-)

I89.8　Other specified noninfective disorders of lymphatic vessels and lymph nodes

Chylocele (nonfilarial)

Chylous ascites

Chylous cyst

Lipomelanotic reticulosis

Lymph node or vessel fistula

Lymph node or vessel infarction

Lymph node or vessel rupture

I89.9　Noninfective disorder of lymphatic vessels and lymph nodes, unspecified

Disease of lymphatic vessels NOS

OTHER AND UNSPECIFIED DISORDERS OF THE CIRCULATORY SYSTEM (I95-I99)

I95　Hypotension

Excludes 1: cardiovascular collapse (R57.9)

maternal hypotension syndrome (O26.5-)

nonspecific low blood pressure reading NOS (R03.1)

I95.0　Idiopathic hypotension

I95.1　Orthostatic hypotension

Hypotension, postural

Excludes 1: neurogenic orthostatic hypotension [Shy-Drager] (G90.3)

orthostatic hypotension due to drugs (I95.2)

I95.2　Hypotension due to drugs

Orthostatic hypotension due to drugs

Use additional code for adverse effect, if applicable, to identify drug (T36-T50 with fifth or sixth character 5)

I95.3　Hypotension of hemodialysis

Intra-dialytic hypotension

I95.8　Other hypotension

　　I95.81　Postprocedural hypotension

　　I95.89　Other hypotension

Chronic hypotension

I95.9　Hypotension, unspecified

I96　Gangrene, not elsewhere classified

Gangrenous cellulitis

Excludes 1: gangrene in atherosclerosis of native arteries of the extremities (I70.26)

gangrene in diabetes mellitus (E08-E13)

gangrene in hernia (K40.1, K40.4, K41.1, K41.4, K42.1, K43.1-, K44.1, K45.1, K46.1)

gangrene in other peripheral vascular diseases (I73.-)

gangrene of certain specified sites - see Alphabetical Index

gas gangrene (A48.0)

pyoderma gangrenosum (L88)

I97　Intraoperative and postprocedural complications and disorders of circulatory system, not elsewhere classified

Excludes 2: postprocedural shock (T81.1-)

I97.0　Postcardiotomy syndrome

I97.1　Other postprocedural cardiac functional disturbances

Excludes 2: acute pulmonary insufficiency following thoracic surgery (J95.1)

intraoperative cardiac functional disturbances (I97.7-)

　　I97.11　Postprocedural cardiac insufficiency

　　　I97.110　Postprocedural cardiac insufficiency following cardiac surgery

　　　I97.111　Postprocedural cardiac insufficiency following other surgery

　　I97.12　Postprocedural cardiac arrest

　　　I97.120　Postprocedural cardiac arrest following cardiac surgery

　　　I97.121　Postprocedural cardiac arrest following other surgery

　　I97.13　Postprocedural heart failure

Use additional code to identify the heart failure (I50.-)

　　　I97.130　Postprocedural heart failure following cardiac surgery

　　　I97.131　Postprocedural heart failure following other surgery

　　I97.19　Other postprocedural cardiac functional disturbances

Use additional code, if applicable, to further specify disorder

I97.190   Other postprocedural cardiac functional disturbances following cardiac surgery

I97.191   Other postprocedural cardiac functional disturbances following other surgery

I97.2   Postmastectomy lymphedema syndrome

Elephantiasis due to mastectomy

Obliteration of lymphatic vessels

I97.3   Postprocedural hypertension

I97.4   Intraoperative hemorrhage and hematoma of a circulatory system organ or structure complicating a procedure

Excludes 1: intraoperative hemorrhage and hematoma of a circulatory system organ or structure due to accidental puncture and laceration during a procedure (I97.5-)

Excludes 2: intraoperative cerebrovascular hemorrhage complicating a procedure (G97.3-)

I97.41   Intraoperative hemorrhage and hematoma of a circulatory system organ or structure complicating a circulatory system procedure

I97.410   Intraoperative hemorrhage and hematoma of a circulatory system organ or structure complicating a cardiac catheterization

I97.411   Intraoperative hemorrhage and hematoma of a circulatory system organ or structure complicating a cardiac bypass

I97.418   Intraoperative hemorrhage and hematoma of a circulatory system organ or structure complicating other circulatory system procedure

I97.42   Intraoperative hemorrhage and hematoma of a circulatory system organ or structure complicating other procedure

I97.5   Accidental puncture and laceration of a circulatory system organ or structure during a procedure

Excludes 2: accidental puncture and laceration of brain during a procedure (G97.4-)

I97.51   Accidental puncture and laceration of a circulatory system organ or structure during a circulatory system procedure

I97.52   Accidental puncture and laceration of a circulatory system organ or structure during other procedure

I97.6   Postprocedural hemorrhage and hematoma of a circulatory system organ or structure following a procedure

Excludes 2: postprocedural cerebrovascular hemorrhage complicating a procedure (G97.5-)

I97.61   Postprocedural hemorrhage and hematoma of a circulatory system organ or structure following a circulatory system procedure

I97.610   Postprocedural hemorrhage and hematoma of a circulatory system organ or structure following a cardiac catheterization

I97.611   Postprocedural hemorrhage and hematoma of a circulatory system organ or structure following cardiac bypass

I97.618   Postprocedural hemorrhage and hematoma of a circulatory system

organ or structure following other circulatory system procedure

I97.62   Postprocedural hemorrhage and hematoma of a circulatory system organ or structure following other procedure

I97.7   Intraoperative cardiac functional disturbances

Excludes 2: acute pulmonary insufficiency following thoracic surgery (J95.1)

postprocedural cardiac functional disturbances (I97.1-)

I97.71   Intraoperative cardiac arrest

I97.710   Intraoperative cardiac arrest during cardiac surgery

I97.711   Intraoperative cardiac arrest during other surgery

I97.79   Other intraoperative cardiac functional disturbances

Use additional code, if applicable, to further specify disorder

I97.790   Other intraoperative cardiac functional disturbances during cardiac surgery

I97.791   Other intraoperative cardiac functional disturbances during other surgery

197.8   Other intraoperative and postprocedural complications and disorders of the circulatory system, not elsewhere classified

Use additional code, if applicable, to further specify disorder

I97.81   Intraoperative cerebrovascular infarction

I97.810   Intraoperative cerebrovascular infarction during cardiac surgery

I97.811   Intraoperative cerebrovascular infarction during other surgery

I97.82   Postprocedural cerebrovascular infarction

I97.820   Postprocedural cerebrovascular infarction during cardiac surgery

I97.821   Postprocedural cerebrovascular infarction during other surgery

I97.88   Other intraoperative complications of the circulatory system, not elsewhere classified

I97.89   Other postprocedural complications and disorders of the circulatory system, not elsewhere classified

I99   Other and unspecified disorders of circulatory system

I99.8   Other disorder of circulatory system

I99.9   Unspecified disorder of circulatory system

● New code ▲ Revised code ⑦ 7th digit required ⊗ Placeholder required

Chapter 10: Diseases Of The Respiratory System (J00-J99)

Note: When a respiratory condition is described as occurring in more than one site and is not specifically indexed, it should be classified to the lower anatomic site (e.g. tracheobronchitis to bronchitis in J40).

Use additional code, where applicable, to identify:
exposure to environmental tobacco smoke (Z77.22)
exposure to tobacco smoke in the perinatal period (P96.81)
history of tobacco use (Z87.891)
occupational exposure to environmental tobacco smoke (Z57.31)
tobacco dependence (F17.-)
tobacco use (Z72.0)

Excludes 2: certain conditions originating in the perinatal period (P04-P96)
certain infectious and parasitic diseases (A00-B99)
complications of pregnancy, childbirth and the puerperium (O00-O9A)
congenital malformations, deformations and chromosomal abnormalities (Q00-Q99)
endocrine, nutritional and metabolic diseases (E00-E88)
injury, poisoning and certain other consequences of external causes (S00-T88)
neoplasms (C00-D49)
smoke inhalation (T59.81-)
symptoms, signs and abnormal clinical and laboratory findings, not elsewhere classified (R00-R94)

This chapter contains the following blocks:

J00-J06	Acute upper respiratory infections
J09-J18	Influenza and pneumonia
J20-J22	Other acute lower respiratory infections
J30-J39	Other diseases of upper respiratory tract
J40-J47	Chronic lower respiratory diseases
J60-J70	Lung diseases due to external agents
J80-J84	Other respiratory diseases principally affecting the interstitium
J85-J86	Suppurative and necrotic conditions of the lower respiratory tract
J90-J94	Other diseases of the pleura
J95	Intraoperative and postprocedural complications and disorders of respiratory system, not elsewhere classified
J96-J99	Other diseases of the respiratory system

ACUTE UPPER RESPIRATORY INFECTIONS (J00-J06)

Excludes 1: chronic obstructive pulmonary disease with acute lower respiratory infection (J44.0)
influenza virus with other respiratory manifestations (J09.X2, J10.1, J11.1)

J00 Acute nasopharyngitis [common cold]
Acute rhinitis
Coryza (acute)
Infective nasopharyngitis NOS
Infective rhinitis
Nasal catarrh, acute
Nasopharyngitis NOS
Excludes 1: acute pharyngitis (J02.-)
acute sore throat NOS (J02.9)
pharyngitis NOS (J02.9)
rhinitis NOS (J31.0)

sore throat NOS (J02.9)
Excludes 2: allergic rhinitis (J30.1-J30.9)
chronic pharyngitis (J31.2)
chronic rhinitis (J31.0)
chronic sore throat (J31.2)
nasopharyngitis, chronic (J31.1)
vasomotor rhinitis (J30.0)

J01 Acute sinusitis
Includes: acute abscess of sinus
acute empyema of sinus
acute infection of sinus
acute inflammation of sinus
acute suppuration of sinus
Use additional code (B95-B97) to identify infectious agent.
Excludes 1: sinusitis NOS (J32.9)
Excludes 2: chronic sinusitis (J32.0-J32.8)
J01.0   Acute maxillary sinusitis
Acute antritis
    J01.00   Acute maxillary sinusitis, unspecified
    J01.01   Acute recurrent maxillary sinusitis
J01.1   Acute frontal sinusitis
    J01.10   Acute frontal sinusitis, unspecified
    J01.11   Acute recurrent frontal sinusitis
J01.2   Acute ethmoidal sinusitis
    J01.20   Acute ethmoidal sinusitis, unspecified
    J01.21   Acute recurrent ethmoidal sinusitis
J01.3   Acute sphenoidal sinusitis
    J01.30   Acute sphenoidal sinusitis, unspecified
    J01.31   Acute recurrent sphenoidal sinusitis
J01.4   Acute pansinusitis
    J01.40   Acute pansinusitis, unspecified
    J01.41   Acute recurrent pansinusitis
J01.8   Other acute sinusitis
    J01.80   Other acute sinusitis
        Acute sinusitis involving more than one sinus but not pansinusitis
    J01.81   Other acute recurrent sinusitis
        Acute recurrent sinusitis involving more than one sinus but not pansinusitis
J01.9   Acute sinusitis, unspecified
    J01.90   Acute sinusitis, unspecified
    J01.91   Acute recurrent sinusitis, unspecified

J02 Acute pharyngitis
Includes: acute sore throat
Excludes 1: acute laryngopharyngitis (J06.0)
peritonsillar abscess (J36)
pharyngeal abscess (J39.1)
retropharyngeal abscess (J39.0)
Excludes 2: chronic pharyngitis (J31.2)
J02.0   Streptococcal pharyngitis
Septic pharyngitis
Streptococcal sore throat
    Excludes 2: scarlet fever (A38.-)
J02.8   Acute pharyngitis due to other specified organisms
Use additional code (B95-B97) to identify infectious agent
    Excludes 1: acute pharyngitis due to coxsackie virus (B08.5)
    acute pharyngitis due to gonococcus (A54.5)
    acute pharyngitis due to herpes [simplex] virus (B00.2)
    acute pharyngitis due to infectious mononucleosis (B27.-)

enteroviral vesicular pharyngitis (B08.5)

J02.9 Acute pharyngitis, unspecified

Gangrenous pharyngitis (acute)

Infective pharyngitis (acute) NOS

Pharyngitis (acute) NOS

Sore throat (acute) NOS

Suppurative pharyngitis (acute)

Ulcerative pharyngitis (acute)

J03 Acute tonsillitis

Excludes 1: acute sore throat (J02.-)

hypertrophy of tonsils (J35.1)

peritonsillar abscess (J36)

sore throat NOS (J02.9)

streptococcal sore throat (J02.0)

Excludes 2: chronic tonsillitis (J35.0)

J03.0 Streptococcal tonsillitis

J03.00 Acute streptococcal tonsillitis, unspecified

J03.01 Acute recurrent streptococcal tonsillitis

J03.8 Acute tonsillitis due to other specified organisms

Use additional code (B95-B97) to identify infectious agent.

Excludes 1: diphtheritic tonsillitis (A36.0)

herpesviral pharyngotonsillitis (B00.2)

streptococcal tonsillitis (J03.0)

tuberculous tonsillitis (A15.8)

Vincent's tonsillitis (A69.1)

J03.80 Acute tonsillitis due to other specified organisms

J03.81 Acute recurrent tonsillitis due to other specified organisms

J03.9 Acute tonsillitis, unspecified

Follicular tonsillitis (acute)

Gangrenous tonsillitis (acute)

Infective tonsillitis (acute)

Tonsillitis (acute) NOS

Ulcerative tonsillitis (acute)

J03.90 Acute tonsillitis, unspecified

J03.91 Acute recurrent tonsillitis, unspecified

J04 Acute laryngitis and tracheitis

Use additional code (B95-B97) to identify infectious agent.

Excludes 1: acute obstructive laryngitis [croup] and epiglottitis (J05.-)

Excludes 2: laryngismus (stridulus) (J38.5)

J04.0 Acute laryngitis

Edematous laryngitis (acute)

Laryngitis (acute) NOS

Subglottic laryngitis (acute)

Suppurative laryngitis (acute)

Ulcerative laryngitis (acute)

Excludes 1: acute obstructive laryngitis (J05.0)

Excludes 2: chronic laryngitis (J37.0)

J04.1 Acute tracheitis

Acute viral tracheitis

Catarrhal tracheitis (acute)

Tracheitis (acute) NOS

Excludes 2: chronic tracheitis (J42)

J04.10 Acute tracheitis without obstruction

J04.11 Acute tracheitis with obstruction

J04.2 Acute laryngotracheitis

Laryngotracheitis NOS

Tracheitis (acute) with laryngitis (acute)

Excludes 1: acute obstructive laryngotracheitis (J05.0)

Excludes 2: chronic laryngotracheitis (J37.1)

J04.3 Supraglottitis, unspecified

J04.30 Supraglottitis, unspecified, without obstruction

J04.31 Supraglottitis, unspecified, with obstruction

J05 Acute obstructive laryngitis [croup] and epiglottitis

Use additional code (B95-B97) to identify infectious agent.

J05.0 Acute obstructive laryngitis [croup]

Obstructive laryngitis (acute) NOS

Obstructive laryngotracheitis NOS

J05.1 Acute epiglottitis

Excludes 2: epiglottitis, chronic (J37.0)

J05.10 Acute epiglottitis without obstruction

Epiglottitis NOS

J05.11 Acute epiglottitis with obstruction

J06 Acute upper respiratory infections of multiple and unspecified sites

Excludes 1: acute respiratory infection NOS (J22)

streptococcal pharyngitis (J02.0)

J06.0 Acute laryngopharyngitis

J06.9 Acute upper respiratory infection, unspecified

Upper respiratory disease, acute

Upper respiratory infection NOS

INFLUENZA AND PNEUMONIA (J09-J18)

Excludes 2: allergic or eosinophilic pneumonia (J82)

aspiration pneumonia NOS (J69.0)

meconium pneumonia (P24.01)

neonatal aspiration pneumonia (P24.-)

pneumonia due to solids and liquids (J69-)

congenital pneumonia (P23.9)

lipid pneumonia (J69.1)

rheumatic pneumonia (I00)

ventilator associated pneumonia (J95.851)

J09 Influenza due to certain identified influenza viruses

Excludes 1: influenza due to other identified influenza virus (J10.-)

influenza due to unidentified influenza virus (J11.-)

seasonal influenza due to other identified influenza virus (J10.-)

seasonal influenza due to unidentified influenza virus (J11.-)

J09.X Influenza due to identified novel influenza A virus

Avian influenza

Bird influenza

Influenza A/H5N1

Influenza of other animal origin, not bird or swine

Swine influenza virus (viruses that normally cause infections in pigs)

J09.X1 Influenza due to identified novel influenza A virus with pneumonia

Code also , if applicable, associated:

lung abscess (J85.1)

other specified type of pneumonia

J09.X2 Influenza due to identified novel influenza A virus with other respiratory manifestations

Influenza due to identified novel influenza A virus NOS

Influenza due to identified novel influenza A virus with laryngitis

Influenza due to identified novel influenza A virus with pharyngitis

Influenza due to identified novel influenza A virus with upper respiratory symptoms

Use additional code, if applicable, for associated:

pleural effusion (J91.8)

sinusitis (J01.-)

● New code ▲ Revised code ⑦ 7ᵗʰ digit required ⊗ Placeholder required

J09.X3 Influenza due to identified novel influenza A virus with gastrointestinal manifestations

Influenza due to identified novel influenza A virus gastroenteritis

Excludes 1: 'intestinal flu' [viral gastroenteritis] (A08.-)

J09.X9 Influenza due to identified novel influenza A virus with other manifestations

Influenza due to identified novel influenza A virus with encephalopathy

Influenza due to identified novel influenza A virus with myocarditis

Influenza due to identified novel influenza A virus with otitis media

Use additional code to identify manifestation

J10 Influenza due to other identified influenza virus

Use additional code to identify the virus (B97.-)

Excludes 1: influenza due to avian influenza virus (J09.X-)

influenza due to swine flu (J09.X-)

influenza due to unidentified influenza virus (J11.-)

J10.0 Influenza due to other identified influenza virus with pneumonia

Code also associated lung abscess, if applicable (J85.1)

J10.00 Influenza due to other identified influenza virus with unspecified type of pneumonia

J10.01 Influenza due to other identified influenza virus with the same other identified influenza virus pneumonia

J10.08 Influenza due to other identified influenza virus with other specified pneumonia

Code also other specified type of pneumonia

J10.1 Influenza due to other identified influenza virus with other respiratory manifestations

Influenza due to other identified influenza virus NOS

Influenza due to other identified influenza virus with laryngitis

Influenza due to other identified influenza virus with pharyngitis

Influenza due to other identified influenza virus with upper respiratory symptoms

Use additional code for associated pleural effusion, if applicable (J91.8)

Use additional code for associated sinusitis, if applicable (J01.-)

J10.2 Influenza due to other identified influenza virus with gastrointestinal manifestations

Influenza due to other identified influenza virus gastroenteritis

Excludes 1: 'intestinal flu' [viral gastroenteritis] (A08.-)

J10.8 Influenza due to other identified influenza virus with other manifestations

J10.81 Influenza due to other identified influenza virus with encephalopathy

J10.82 Influenza due to other identified influenza virus with myocarditis

J10.83 Influenza due to other identified influenza virus with otitis media

Use additional code for any associated perforated tympanic membrane (H72.-)

J10.89 Influenza due to other identified influenza virus with other manifestations

Use additional codes to identify the manifestations

J11 Influenza due to unidentified influenza virus

J11.0 Influenza due to unidentified influenza virus with pneumonia

Code also associated lung abscess, if applicable (J85.1)

J11.00 Influenza due to unidentified influenza virus with unspecified type of pneumonia

Influenza with pneumonia NOS

J11.08 Influenza due to unidentified influenza virus with specified pneumonia

Code also other specified type of pneumonia

J11.1 Influenza due to unidentified influenza virus with other respiratory manifestations

Influenza NOS

Influenzal laryngitis NOS

Influenzal pharyngitis NOS

Influenza with upper respiratory symptoms NOS

Use additional code for associated pleural effusion, if applicable (J91.8)

Use additional code for associated sinusitis, if applicable (J01.-)

J11.2 Influenza due to unidentified influenza virus with gastrointestinal manifestations

Influenza gastroenteritis NOS

Excludes 1: 'intestinal flu' [viral gastroenteritis] (A08.-)

J11.8 Influenza due to unidentified influenza virus with other manifestations

J11.81 Influenza due to unidentified influenza virus with encephalopathy

Influenzal encephalopathy NOS

J11.82 Influenza due to unidentified influenza virus with myocarditis

Influenzal myocarditis NOS

J11.83 Influenza due to unidentified influenza virus with otitis media

Influenzal otitis media NOS

Use additional code for any associated perforated tympanic membrane (H72.-)

J11.89 Influenza due to unidentified influenza virus with other manifestations

Use additional codes to identify the manifestations

J12 Viral pneumonia, not elsewhere classified

Includes: bronchopneumonia due to viruses other than influenza viruses

Code first associated influenza, if applicable (J09.X1, J10.0-, J11.0-)

Code also associated abscess, if applicable (J85.1)

Excludes 1: aspiration pneumonia due to anesthesia during labor and delivery (O74.0)

aspiration pneumonia due to anesthesia during pregnancy (O29)

aspiration pneumonia due to anesthesia during puerperium (O89.0)

aspiration pneumonia due to solids and liquids (J69.-)

aspiration pneumonia NOS (J69.0)

congenital pneumonia (P23.0)

congenital rubella pneumonitis (P35.0)

interstitial pneumonia NOS (J84.9)

lipid pneumonia (J69.1)

neonatal aspiration pneumonia (P24.-)

J12.0 Adenoviral pneumonia

J12.1 Respiratory syncytial virus pneumonia

J12.2 Parainfluenza virus pneumonia

J12.3 Human metapneumovirus pneumonia

J12.8 Other viral pneumonia

	Add 4th-7th digits		3 digit reportable		Nonspecific code		Unspecified code		Manifestation code	

J12.81 Pneumonia due to SARS-associated coronavirus

Severe acute respiratory syndrome NOS

J12.89 Other viral pneumonia

J12.9 Viral pneumonia, unspecified

J13 Pneumonia due to Streptococcus pneumoniae

Bronchopneumonia due to S. pneumoniae

Code first associated influenza, if applicable (J09.X1, J10.0-, -J11.0-)

Code also associated abscess, if applicable (J85.1)

Excludes 1: congenital pneumonia due to S. pneumoniae (P23.6)

lobar pneumonia, unspecified organism (J18.1)

pneumonia due to other streptococci (J15.3-J15.4)

J14 Pneumonia due to Hemophilus influenzae

Bronchopneumonia due to H. influenzae

Code first associated influenza, if applicable (J09.X1, J10.0-, -J11.0-)

Code also associated abscess, if applicable (J85.1)

Excludes 1: congenital pneumonia due to H. influenzae (P23.6)

J15 Bacterial pneumonia, not elsewhere classified

Includes: bronchopneumonia due to bacteria other than S. pneumoniae and H. influenzae

Code first associated influenza, if applicable (J09.X1, J10.0-, -J11.0-)

Code also associated abscess, if applicable (J85.1)

Excludes 1: chlamydial pneumonia (J16.0)

congenital pneumonia (P23.-)

Legionnaires' disease (A48.1)

spirochetal pneumonia (A69.8)

J15.0 Pneumonia due to Klebsiella pneumoniae

J15.1 Pneumonia due to Pseudomonas

J15.2 Pneumonia due to staphylococcus

J15.20 Pneumonia due to staphylococcus, unspecified

J15.21 Pneumonia due to staphylococcus aureus

J15.211 Pneumonia due to Methicillin susceptible Staphylococcus aureus

MSSA pneumonia

Pneumonia due to Staphylococcus aureus NOS

J15.212 Pneumonia due to Methicillin resistant Staphylococcus aureus

J15.29 Pneumonia due to other staphylococcus

J15.3 Pneumonia due to streptococcus, group B

J15.4 Pneumonia due to other streptococci

Excludes 1: pneumonia due to streptococcus, group B (J15.3)

pneumonia due to Streptococcus pneumoniae (J13)

J15.5 Pneumonia due to Escherichia coli

J15.6 Pneumonia due to other aerobic Gram-negative bacteria

Pneumonia due to Serratia marcescens

J15.7 Pneumonia due to Mycoplasma pneumoniae

J15.8 Pneumonia due to other specified bacteria

J15.9 Unspecified bacterial pneumonia

Pneumonia due to gram-positive bacteria

J16 Pneumonia due to other infectious organisms, not elsewhere classified

Code first associated influenza, if applicable (J09.X1, J10.0-, -J11.0-)

Code also associated abscess, if applicable (J85.1)

Excludes 1: congenital pneumonia (P23.-)

ornithosis (A70)

pneumocystosis (B59)

pneumonia NOS (J18.9)

J16.0 Chlamydial pneumonia

J16.8 Pneumonia due to other specified infectious organisms

J17 Pneumonia in diseases classified elsewhere

Code first underlying disease, such as:

Q fever (A78)

rheumatic fever (I00)

schistosomiasis (B65.0-B65.9)

Excludes 1: candidal pneumonia (B37.1)

chlamydial pneumonia (J16.0)

gonorrheal pneumonia (A54.84)

histoplasmosis pneumonia (B39.0-B39.2)

measles pneumonia (B05.2)

nocardiosis pneumonia (A43.0)

pneumocystosis (B59)

pneumonia due to Pneumocystis carinii (B59)

pneumonia due to Pneumocystis jiroveci (B59)

pneumonia in actinomycosis (A42.0)

pneumonia in anthrax (A22.1)

pneumonia in ascariasis (B77.81)

pneumonia in aspergillosis (B44.0-B44.1)

pneumonia in coccidioidomycosis (B38.0-B38.2)

pneumonia in cytomegalovirus disease (B25.0)

pneumonia in toxoplasmosis (B58.3)

rubella pneumonia (B06.81)

salmonella pneumonia (A02.22)

spirochetal infection NEC with pneumonia (A69.8)

tularemia pneumonia (A21.2)

typhoid fever with pneumonia (A01.03)

varicella pneumonia (B01.2)

whooping cough with pneumonia (A37 with fifth-character 1)

J18 Pneumonia, unspecified organism

Code first associated influenza, if applicable (J09.X1, J10.0-, -J11.0-)

Excludes 1: abscess of lung with pneumonia (J85.1)

aspiration pneumonia due to anesthesia during labor and delivery (O74.0)

aspiration pneumonia due to anesthesia during pregnancy (O29)

aspiration pneumonia due to anesthesia during puerperium (O89.0)

aspiration pneumonia due to solids and liquids (J69.-)

aspiration pneumonia NOS (J69.0)

congenital pneumonia (P23.0)

drug-induced interstitial lung disorder (J70.2-J70.4)

interstitial pneumonia NOS (J84.9)

lipid pneumonia (J69.1)

neonatal aspiration pneumonia (P24.-)

pneumonitis due to external agents (J67-J70)

pneumonitis due to fumes and vapors (J68.0)

usual interstitial pneumonia (J84.17)

J18.0 Bronchopneumonia, unspecified organism

Excludes 1: hypostatic bronchopneumonia (J18.2)

lipid pneumonia (J69.1)

Excludes 2: acute bronchiolitis (J21.-)

chronic bronchiolitis (J44.9)

J18.1 Lobar pneumonia, unspecified organism

J18.2 Hypostatic pneumonia, unspecified organism

Hypostatic bronchopneumonia

Passive pneumonia

J18.8 Other pneumonia, unspecified organism

J18.9 Pneumonia, unspecified organism

● New code ▲ Revised code ⑦ 7th digit required ⊗ Placeholder required

OTHER ACUTE LOWER RESPIRATORY INFECTIONS (J20-J22)

Excludes 2: chronic obstructive pulmonary disease with acute lower respiratory infection (J44.0)

J20 Acute bronchitis

Includes: acute and subacute bronchitis (with) bronchospasm
acute and subacute bronchitis (with) tracheitis
acute and subacute bronchitis (with) tracheobronchitis, acute
acute and subacute fibrinous bronchitis
acute and subacute membranous bronchitis
acute and subacute purulent bronchitis
acute and subacute septic bronchitis

Excludes 2: acute bronchitis with bronchiectasis (J47.0)
acute bronchitis with chronic obstructive asthma (J44.0)
acute bronchitis with chronic obstructive pulmonary disease (J44.0)
allergic bronchitis NOS (J45.909-)
bronchitis due to chemicals, fumes and vapors (J68.0)
bronchitis NOS (J40)
chronic bronchitis NOS (J42)
chronic mucopurulent bronchitis (J41.1)
chronic obstructive bronchitis (J44.-)
chronic obstructive tracheobronchitis (J44.-)
chronic simple bronchitis (J41.0)
chronic tracheobronchitis (J42)
tracheobronchitis NOS (J40)

J20.0 Acute bronchitis due to Mycoplasma pneumoniae
J20.1 Acute bronchitis due to Hemophilus influenzae
J20.2 Acute bronchitis due to streptococcus
J20.3 Acute bronchitis due to coxsackievirus
J20.4 Acute bronchitis due to parainfluenza virus
J20.5 Acute bronchitis due to respiratory syncytial virus
J20.6 Acute bronchitis due to rhinovirus
J20.7 Acute bronchitis due to echovirus
J20.8 Acute bronchitis due to other specified organisms
J20.9 Acute bronchitis, unspecified

J21 Acute bronchiolitis

Includes: acute bronchiolitis with bronchospasm

Excludes 2: respiratory bronchiolitis interstitial lung disease (J84.115)

J21.0 Acute bronchiolitis due to respiratory syncytial virus
J21.1 Acute bronchiolitis due to human metapneumovirus
J21.8 Acute bronchiolitis due to other specified organisms
J21.9 Acute bronchiolitis, unspecified
Bronchiolitis (acute)
Excludes 1: chronic bronchiolitis (J44.-)

J22 Unspecified acute lower respiratory infection
Acute (lower) respiratory (tract) infection NOS
Excludes 1: upper respiratory infection (acute) (J06.9)

OTHER DISEASES OF UPPER RESPIRATORY TRACT (J30-J39)

J30 Vasomotor and allergic rhinitis
Includes: spasmodic rhinorrhea
Excludes 1: allergic rhinitis with asthma (bronchial) (J45.909)
rhinitis NOS (J31.0)
J30.0 Vasomotor rhinitis
J30.1 Allergic rhinitis due to pollen
Allergy NOS due to pollen
Hay fever
Pollinosis
J30.2 Other seasonal allergic rhinitis

J30.5 Allergic rhinitis due to food
J30.8 Other allergic rhinitis
J30.81 Allergic rhinitis due to animal (cat) (dog) hair and dander
J30.89 Other allergic rhinitis
Perennial allergic rhinitis
J30.9 Allergic rhinitis, unspecified

J31 Chronic rhinitis, nasopharyngitis and pharyngitis
Use additional code to identify:
exposure to environmental tobacco smoke (Z77.22)
exposure to tobacco smoke in the perinatal period (P96.81)
history of tobacco use (Z87.891)
occupational exposure to environmental tobacco smoke (Z57.31)
tobacco dependence (F17.-)
tobacco use (Z72.0)

J31.0 Chronic rhinitis
Atrophic rhinitis (chronic)
Granulomatous rhinitis (chronic)
Hypertrophic rhinitis (chronic)
Obstructive rhinitis (chronic)
Ozena
Purulent rhinitis (chronic)
Rhinitis (chronic) NOS
Ulcerative rhinitis (chronic)
Excludes 1: allergic rhinitis (J30.1-J30.9)
vasomotor rhinitis (J30.0)
J31.1 Chronic nasopharyngitis
Excludes 2: acute nasopharyngitis (J00)
J31.2 Chronic pharyngitis
Chronic sore throat
Atrophic pharyngitis (chronic)
Granular pharyngitis (chronic)
Hypertrophic pharyngitis (chronic)
Excludes 2: acute pharyngitis (J02.9)

J32 Chronic sinusitis
Includes: sinus abscess
sinus empyema
sinus infection
sinus suppuration
Use additional code to identify:
exposure to environmental tobacco smoke (Z77.22)
exposure to tobacco smoke in the perinatal period (P96.81)
history of tobacco use (Z87.891)
infectious agent (B95-B97)
occupational exposure to environmental tobacco smoke (Z57.31)
tobacco dependence (F17.-)
tobacco use (Z72.0)
Excludes 2: acute sinusitis (J01.-)
J32.0 Chronic maxillary sinusitis
Antritis (chronic)
Maxillary sinusitis NOS
J32.1 Chronic frontal sinusitis
Frontal sinusitis NOS
J32.2 Chronic ethmoidal sinusitis
Ethmoidal sinusitis NOS
Excludes 1: Woakes' ethmoiditis (J33.1)
J32.3 Chronic sphenoidal sinusitis
Sphenoidal sinusitis NOS
J32.4 Chronic pansinusitis
Pansinusitis NOS

J32.8 Other chronic sinusitis
Sinusitis (chronic) involving more than one sinus but not pansinusitis

J32.9 Chronic sinusitis, unspecified
Sinusitis (chronic) NOS

J33 Nasal polyp
Use additional code to identify:
exposure to environmental tobacco smoke (Z77.22)
exposure to tobacco smoke in the perinatal period (P96.81)
history of tobacco use (Z87.891)
occupational exposure to environmental tobacco smoke (Z57.31)
tobacco dependence (F17.-)
tobacco use (Z72.0)
Excludes 1: adenomatous polyps (D14.0)

J33.0 Polyp of nasal cavity
Choanal polyp
Nasopharyngeal polyp

J33.1 Polypoid sinus degeneration
Woakes' syndrome or ethmoiditis

J33.8 Other polyp of sinus
Accessory polyp of sinus
Ethmoidal polyp of sinus
Maxillary polyp of sinus
Sphenoidal polyp of sinus

J33.9 Nasal polyp, unspecified

J34 Other and unspecified disorders of nose and nasal sinuses
Excludes 2: varicose ulcer of nasal septum (I86.8)

J34.0 Abscess, furuncle and carbuncle of nose
Cellulitis of nose
Necrosis of nose
Ulceration of nose

J34.1 Cyst and mucocele of nose and nasal sinus

J34.2 Deviated nasal septum
Deflection or deviation of septum (nasal) (acquired)
Excludes 1: congenital deviated nasal septum (Q67.4)

J34.3 Hypertrophy of nasal turbinates

J34.8 Other specified disorders of nose and nasal sinuses

J34.81 Nasal mucositis (ulcerative)
Code also type of associated therapy, such as:
antineoplastic and immunosuppressive drugs (T45.1x-)
radiological procedure and radiotherapy (Y84.2)
Excludes 2: gastrointestinal mucositis (ulcerative) (K92.81)
mucositis (ulcerative) of vagina and vulva (N76.81)
oral mucositis (ulcerative) (K12.3-)

J34.89 Other specified disorders of nose and nasal sinuses
Perforation of nasal septum NOS
Rhinolith

J34.9 Unspecified disorder of nose and nasal sinuses

J35 Chronic diseases of tonsils and adenoids
Use additional code to identify:
exposure to environmental tobacco smoke (Z77.22)
exposure to tobacco smoke in the perinatal period (P96.81)
history of tobacco use (Z87.891)
occupational exposure to environmental tobacco smoke (Z57.31)
tobacco dependence (F17.-)
tobacco use (Z72.0)

J35.0 Chronic tonsillitis and adenoiditis
Excludes 2: acute tonsillitis (J03.-)

J35.01 Chronic tonsillitis

J35.02 Chronic adenoiditis

J35.03 Chronic tonsillitis and adenoiditis

J35.1 Hypertrophy of tonsils
Enlargement of tonsils
Excludes 1: hypertrophy of tonsils with tonsillitis (J35.0-)

J35.2 Hypertrophy of adenoids
Enlargement of adenoids
Excludes 1: hypertrophy of adenoids with adenoiditis (J35.0-)

J35.3 Hypertrophy of tonsils with hypertrophy of adenoids
Excludes 1: hypertrophy of tonsils and adenoids with tonsillitis and adenoiditis (J35.03)

J35.8 Other chronic diseases of tonsils and adenoids
Adenoid vegetations
Amygdalolith
Calculus, tonsil
Cicatrix of tonsil (and adenoid)
Tonsillar tag
Ulcer of tonsil

J35.9 Chronic disease of tonsils and adenoids, unspecified
Disease (chronic) of tonsils and adenoids NOS

J36 Peritonsillar abscess
Includes: abscess of tonsil
peritonsillar cellulitis
quinsy
Use additional code (B95-B97) to identify infectious agent.
Excludes 1: acute tonsillitis (J03.-)
chronic tonsillitis (J35.0)
retropharyngeal abscess (J39.0)
tonsillitis NOS (J03.9-)

J37 Chronic laryngitis and laryngotracheitis
Use additional code to identify:
exposure to environmental tobacco smoke (Z77.22)
exposure to tobacco smoke in the perinatal period (P96.81)
history of tobacco use (Z87.891)
infectious agent (B95-B97)
occupational exposure to environmental tobacco smoke (Z57.31)
tobacco dependence (F17.-)
tobacco use (Z72.0)

J37.0 Chronic laryngitis
Catarrhal laryngitis
Hypertrophic laryngitis
Sicca laryngitis
Excludes 2: acute laryngitis (J04.0)
obstructive (acute) laryngitis (J05.0)

J37.1 Chronic laryngotracheitis
Laryngitis, chronic, with tracheitis (chronic)
Tracheitis, chronic, with laryngitis
Excludes 1: chronic tracheitis (J42)
Excludes 2: acute laryngotracheitis (J04.2)
acute tracheitis (J04.1)

J38 Diseases of vocal cords and larynx, not elsewhere classified
Use additional code to identify:
exposure to environmental tobacco smoke (Z77.22)
exposure to tobacco smoke in the perinatal period (P96.81)
history of tobacco use (Z87.891)
occupational exposure to environmental tobacco smoke (Z57.31)

● New code ▲ Revised code ⑦ 7th digit required ⊗ Placeholder required

tobacco dependence (F17.-)

tobacco use (Z72.0)

Excludes 1: congenital laryngeal stridor (P28.89)

obstructive laryngitis (acute) (J05.0)

postprocedural subglottic stenosis (J95.5)

stridor (R06.1)

ulcerative laryngitis (J04.0)

J38.0 Paralysis of vocal cords and larynx

Laryngoplegia

Paralysis of glottis

J38.00 Paralysis of vocal cords and larynx, unspecified

J38.01 Paralysis of vocal cords and larynx, unilateral

J38.02 Paralysis of vocal cords and larynx, bilateral

J38.1 Polyp of vocal cord and larynx

Excludes 1: adenomatous polyps (D14.1)

J38.2 Nodules of vocal cords

Chorditis (fibrinous)(nodosa)(tuberosa)

Singer's nodes

Teacher's nodes

J38.3 Other diseases of vocal cords

Abscess of vocal cords

Cellulitis of vocal cords

Granuloma of vocal cords

Leukokeratosis of vocal cords

Leukoplakia of vocal cords

J38.4 Edema of larynx

Edema (of) glottis

Subglottic edema

Supraglottic edema

Excludes 1: acute obstructive laryngitis [croup] (J05.0)

edematous laryngitis (J04.0)

J38.5 Laryngeal spasm

Laryngismus (stridulus)

J38.6 Stenosis of larynx

J38.7 Other diseases of larynx

Abscess of larynx

Cellulitis of larynx

Disease of larynx NOS

Necrosis of larynx

Pachyderma of larynx

Perichondritis of larynx

Ulcer of larynx

J39 Other diseases of upper respiratory tract

Excludes 1: acute respiratory infection NOS (J22)

acute upper respiratory infection (J06.9)

upper respiratory inflammation due to chemicals, gases, fumes or vapors (J68.2)

J39.0 Retropharyngeal and parapharyngeal abscess

Peripharyngeal abscess

Excludes 1: peritonsillar abscess (J36)

J39.1 Other abscess of pharynx

Cellulitis of pharynx

Nasopharyngeal abscess

J39.2 Other diseases of pharynx

Cyst of pharynx

Edema of pharynx

Excludes 2: chronic pharyngitis (J31.2)

ulcerative pharyngitis (J02.9)

J39.3 Upper respiratory tract hypersensitivity reaction, site unspecified

Excludes 1: hypersensitivity reaction of upper respiratory tract, such as:

extrinsic allergic alveolitis (J67.9)

pneumoconiosis (J60-J67.9)

J39.8 Other specified diseases of upper respiratory tract

J39.9 Disease of upper respiratory tract, unspecified

CHRONIC LOWER RESPIRATORY DISEASES (J40-J47)

Excludes 1: bronchitis due to chemicals, gases, fumes and vapors (J68.0)

Excludes 2: cystic fibrosis (E84.-)

J40 Bronchitis, not specified as acute or chronic

Bronchitis NOS

Bronchitis with tracheitis NOS

Catarrhal bronchitis

Tracheobronchitis NOS

Use additional code to identify:

exposure to environmental tobacco smoke (Z77.22)

exposure to tobacco smoke in the perinatal period (P96.81)

history of tobacco use (Z87.891)

occupational exposure to environmental tobacco smoke (Z57.31)

tobacco dependence (F17.-)

tobacco use (Z72.0)

Excludes 1: allergic bronchitis NOS (J45.909-)

asthmatic bronchitis NOS (J45.9-)

bronchitis due to chemicals, gases, fumes and vapors (J68.0)

J41 Simple and mucopurulent chronic bronchitis

Use additional code to identify:

exposure to environmental tobacco smoke (Z77.22)

exposure to tobacco smoke in the perinatal period (P96.81)

history of tobacco use (Z87.891)

occupational exposure to environmental tobacco smoke (Z57.31)

tobacco dependence (F17.-)

tobacco use (Z72.0)

Excludes 1: chronic bronchitis NOS (J42)

chronic obstructive bronchitis (J44.-)

J41.0 Simple chronic bronchitis

J41.1 Mucopurulent chronic bronchitis

J41.8 Mixed simple and mucopurulent chronic bronchitis

J42 Unspecified chronic bronchitis

Chronic bronchitis NOS

Chronic tracheitis

Chronic tracheobronchitis

Use additional code to identify:

exposure to environmental tobacco smoke (Z77.22)

exposure to tobacco smoke in the perinatal period (P96.81)

history of tobacco use (Z87.891)

occupational exposure to environmental tobacco smoke (Z57.31)

tobacco dependence (F17.-)

tobacco use (Z72.0)

Excludes 1: chronic asthmatic bronchitis (J44.-)

chronic bronchitis with airways obstruction (J44.-)

chronic emphysematous bronchitis (J44.-)

chronic obstructive pulmonary disease NOS (J44.9)

simple and mucopurulent chronic bronchitis (J41.-)

J43 Emphysema

Use additional code to identify:

exposure to environmental tobacco smoke (Z77.22)

history of tobacco use (Z87.891)

occupational exposure to environmental tobacco smoke (Z57.31)

tobacco dependence (F17.-)

     tobacco use (Z72.0)

Excludes 1: compensatory emphysema (J98.3)

     emphysema due to inhalation of chemicals, gases, fumes or vapors (J68.4)

     emphysema with chronic (obstructive) bronchitis (J44.-)

     emphysematous (obstructive) bronchitis (J44.-)

     interstitial emphysema (J98.2)

     mediastinal emphysema (J98.2)

     neonatal interstitial emphysema (P25.0)

     surgical (subcutaneous) emphysema (T81.82)

     traumatic subcutaneous emphysema (T79.7)

J43.0 Unilateral pulmonary emphysema [MacLeod's syndrome]

     Swyer-James syndrome

     Unilateral emphysema

     Unilateral hyperlucent lung

     Unilateral pulmonary artery functional hypoplasia

     Unilateral transparency of lung

J43.1 Panlobular emphysema

     Panacinar emphysema

J43.2 Centrilobular emphysema

J43.8 Other emphysema

J43.9 Emphysema, unspecified

     Bullous emphysema (lung)(pulmonary)

     Emphysema (lung)(pulmonary) NOS

     Emphysematous bleb

     Vesicular emphysema (lung)(pulmonary)

J44 Other chronic obstructive pulmonary disease

Includes: asthma with chronic obstructive pulmonary disease

     chronic asthmatic (obstructive) bronchitis

     chronic bronchitis with airways obstruction

     chronic bronchitis with emphysema

     chronic emphysematous bronchitis

     chronic obstructive asthma

     chronic obstructive bronchitis

     chronic obstructive tracheobronchitis

Code also type of asthma, if applicable (J45.-):

Use additional code to identify:

     exposure to environmental tobacco smoke (Z77.22)

     history of tobacco use (Z87.891)

     occupational exposure to environmental tobacco smoke (Z57.31)

     tobacco dependence (F17.-)

     tobacco use (Z72.0)

Excludes 1: bronchiectasis (J47.-)

     chronic bronchitis NOS (J42)

     chronic simple and mucopurulent bronchitis (J41.-)

     chronic tracheitis (J42)

     chronic tracheobronchitis (J42)

     emphysema without chronic bronchitis (J43.-)

     lung diseases due to external agents (J60-J70)

J44.0 Chronic obstructive pulmonary disease with acute lower respiratory infection

     Use additional code to identify the infection

J44.1 Chronic obstructive pulmonary disease with (acute) exacerbation

     Decompensated COPD

     Decompensated COPD with (acute) exacerbation

     Excludes 2: chronic obstructive pulmonary disease [COPD] with acute bronchitis (J44.0)

J44.9 Chronic obstructive pulmonary disease, unspecified

     Chronic obstructive airway disease NOS

     Chronic obstructive lung disease NOS

J45 Asthma

Includes: allergic (predominantly) asthma

     allergic bronchitis NOS

     allergic rhinitis with asthma

     atopic asthma

     extrinsic allergic asthma

     hay fever with asthma

     idiosyncratic asthma

     intrinsic nonallergic asthma

     nonallergic asthma

Use additional code to identify:

     exposure to environmental tobacco smoke (Z77.22)

     exposure to tobacco smoke in the perinatal period (P96.81)

     history of tobacco use (Z87.891)

     occupational exposure to environmental tobacco smoke (Z57.31)

     tobacco dependence (F17.-)

     tobacco use (Z72.0)

Excludes 1: detergent asthma (J69.8)

     eosinophilic asthma (J82)

     lung diseases due to external agents (J60-J70)

     miner's asthma (J60)

     wheezing NOS (R06.2)

     wood asthma (J67.8)

Excludes 2: asthma with chronic obstructive pulmonary disease (J44.9)

     chronic asthmatic (obstructive) bronchitis (J44.9)

     chronic obstructive asthma (J44.9)

J45.2 Mild intermittent asthma

     J45.20 Mild intermittent asthma, uncomplicated

          Mild intermittent asthma NOS

     J45.21 Mild intermittent asthma with (acute) exacerbation

     J45.22 Mild intermittent asthma with status asthmaticus

J45.3 Mild persistent asthma

     J45.30 Mild persistent asthma, uncomplicated

          Mild persistent asthma NOS

     J45.31 Mild persistent asthma with (acute) exacerbation

     J45.32 Mild persistent asthma with status asthmaticus

J45.4 Moderate persistent asthma

     J45.40 Moderate persistent asthma, uncomplicated

          Moderate persistent asthma NOS

     J45.41 Moderate persistent asthma with (acute) exacerbation

     J45.42 Moderate persistent asthma with status asthmaticus

J45.5 Severe persistent asthma

     J45.50 Severe persistent asthma, uncomplicated

          Severe persistent asthma NOS

     J45.51 Severe persistent asthma with (acute) exacerbation

     J45.52 Severe persistent asthma with status asthmaticus

J45.9 Other and unspecified asthma

     J45.90 Unspecified asthma

          Asthmatic bronchitis NOS

          Childhood asthma NOS

          Late onset asthma

          J45.901 Unspecified asthma with (acute) exacerbation

          J45.902 Unspecified asthma with status asthmaticus

          J45.909 Unspecified asthma, uncomplicated

Asthma NOS

J45.99 Other asthma

    J45.990 Exercise induced bronchospasm

    J45.991 Cough variant asthma

    J45.998 Other asthma

J47 Bronchiectasis

Includes: bronchiolectasis

Use additional code to identify:

exposure to environmental tobacco smoke (Z77.22)

exposure to tobacco smoke in the perinatal period (P96.81)

history of tobacco use (Z87.891)

occupational exposure to environmental tobacco smoke (Z57.31)

tobacco dependence (F17.-)

tobacco use (Z72.0)

Excludes 1: congenital bronchiectasis (Q33.4)

tuberculous bronchiectasis (current disease) (A15.0)

J47.0 Bronchiectasis with acute lower respiratory infection

Bronchiectasis with acute bronchitis

J47.1 Bronchiectasis with (acute) exacerbation

J47.9 Bronchiectasis, uncomplicated

Bronchiectasis NOS

LUNG DISEASES DUE TO EXTERNAL AGENTS (J60-J70)

Excludes 2: asthma (J45.-)

malignant neoplasm of bronchus and lung (C34.-)

J60 Coalworker's pneumoconiosis

Anthracosilicosis

Anthracosis

Black lung disease

Coalworker's lung

Excludes 1: coal worker pneumoconiosis with tuberculosis, any type in A15(J65)

J61 Pneumoconiosis due to asbestos and other mineral fibers

Asbestosis

Excludes 1: pleural plaque with asbestosis (J92.0)

pneumoconiosis with tuberculosis, any type in A15(J65)

J62 Pneumoconiosis due to dust containing silica

Includes: silicotic fibrosis (massive) of lung

Excludes 1: pneumoconiosis with tuberculosis, any type in A15 (J65)

J62.0 Pneumoconiosis due to talc dust

J62.8 Pneumoconiosis due to other dust containing silica

Silicosis NOS

J63 Pneumoconiosis due to other inorganic dusts

Excludes 1: pneumoconiosis with tuberculosis, any type in A15(J65)

J63.0 Aluminosis (of lung)

J63.1 Bauxite fibrosis (of lung)

J63.2 Berylliosis

J63.3 Graphite fibrosis (of lung)

J63.4 Siderosis

J63.5 Stannosis

J63.6 Pneumoconiosis due to other specified inorganic dusts

J64 Unspecified pneumoconiosis

Excludes 1: pneumonoconiosis with tuberculosis, any type in A15 (J65)

J65 Pneumoconiosis associated with tuberculosis

Any condition in J60-J64 with tuberculosis, any type in A15

Silicotuberculosis

J66 Airway disease due to specific organic dust

Excludes 2: allergic alveolitis (J67.-)

asbestosis (J61)

bagassosis (J67.1)

farmer's lung (J67.0)

hypersensitivity pneumonitis due to organic dust (J67.-)

reactive airways dysfunction syndrome (J68.3)

J66.0 Byssinosis

Airway disease due to cotton dust

J66.1 Flax-dressers' disease

J66.2 Cannabinosis

J66.8 Airway disease due to other specific organic dusts

J67 Hypersensitivity pneumonitis due to organic dust

Includes: allergic alveolitis and pneumonitis due to inhaled organic dust and particles of fungal, actinomycetic or other origin

Excludes 1: pneumonitis due to inhalation of chemicals, gases, fumes or vapors (J68.0)

J67.0 Farmer's lung

Harvester's lung

Haymaker's lung

Moldy hay disease

J67.1 Bagassosis

Bagasse disease

Bagasse pneumonitis

J67.2 Bird fancier's lung

Budgerigar fancier's disease or lung

Pigeon fancier's disease or lung

J67.3 Suberosis

Cork handler's disease or lung

Cork worker's disease or lung

J67.4 Maltworker's lung

Alveolitis due to Aspergillus clavatus

J67.5 Mushroom-worker's lung

J67.6 Maple-bark-stripper's lung

Alveolitis due to Cryptostroma corticale

Cryptostromosis

J67.7 Air conditioner and humidifier lung

Allergic alveolitis due to fungal, thermophilic actinomycetes and other organisms growing in ventilation [air conditioning] systems

J67.8 Hypersensitivity pneumonitis due to other organic dusts

Cheese-washer's lung

Coffee-worker's lung

Fish-meal worker's lung

Furrier's lung

Sequoiosis

J67.9 Hypersensitivity pneumonitis due to unspecified organic dust

Allergic alveolitis (extrinsic) NOS

Hypersensitivity pneumonitis NOS

J68 Respiratory conditions due to inhalation of chemicals, gases, fumes and vapors

Code first (T51-T65) to identify cause

Use additional code to identify associated respiratory conditions, such as:

acute respiratory failure (J96.0-)

J68.0 Bronchitis and pneumonitis due to chemicals, gases, fumes and vapors

Chemical bronchitis (acute)

J68.1 Pulmonary edema due to chemicals, gases, fumes and vapors

Chemical pulmonary edema (acute) (chronic)

Excludes 1: pulmonary edema (acute) (chronic) NOS (J81.-)

J68.2 Upper respiratory inflammation due to chemicals, gases, fumes and vapors, not elsewhere classified

J68.3 Other acute and subacute respiratory conditions due to chemicals, gases, fumes and vapors

Reactive airways dysfunction syndrome

J68.4 Chronic respiratory conditions due to chemicals, gases, fumes and vapors

Emphysema (diffuse) (chronic) due to inhalation of chemicals, gases, fumes and vapors

Obliterative bronchiolitis (chronic) (subacute) due to inhalation of chemicals, gases, fumes and vapors

Pulmonary fibrosis (chronic) due to inhalation of chemicals, gases, fumes and vapors

Excludes 1: chronic pulmonary edema due to chemicals, gases, fumes and vapors (J68.1)

J68.8 Other respiratory conditions due to chemicals, gases, fumes and vapors

J68.9 Unspecified respiratory condition due to chemicals, gases, fumes and vapors

J69 Pneumonitis due to solids and liquids

Excludes 1: neonatal aspiration syndromes (P24.-)

postprocedural pneumonitis (J95.4)

J69.0 Pneumonitis due to inhalation of food and vomit

Aspiration pneumonia NOS

Aspiration pneumonia (due to) food (regurgitated)

Aspiration pneumonia (due to) gastric secretions

Aspiration pneumonia (due to) milk

Aspiration pneumonia (due to) vomit

Code also any associated foreign body in respiratory tract (T17.-)

Excludes 1: chemical pneumonitis due to anesthesia (J95.4)

obstetric aspiration pneumonitis (O74.0)

J69.1 Pneumonitis due to inhalation of oils and essences

Exogenous lipoid pneumonia

Lipid pneumonia NOS

Code first (T51-T65) to identify substance

Excludes 1: endogenous lipoid pneumonia (J84.89)

J69.8 Pneumonitis due to inhalation of other solids and liquids

Pneumonitis due to aspiration of blood

Pneumonitis due to aspiration of detergent

Code first (T51-T65) to identify substance

J70 Respiratory conditions due to other external agents

J70.0 Acute pulmonary manifestations due to radiation

Radiation pneumonitis

Use additional code (W88-W90, X39.0-) to identify the external cause

J70.1 Chronic and other pulmonary manifestations due to radiation

Fibrosis of lung following radiation

Use additional code (W88-W90, X39.0-) to identify the external cause

J70.2 Acute drug-induced interstitial lung disorders

Use additional code for adverse effect, if applicable, to identify drug (T36-T50 with fifth or sixth character 5)

Excludes 1: interstitial pneumonia NOS (J84.9)

lymphoid interstitial pneumonia (J84.2)

J70.3 Chronic drug-induced interstitial lung disorders

Use additional code for adverse effect, if applicable, to identify drug (T36-T50 with fifth or sixth character 5)

Excludes 1: interstitial pneumonia NOS (J84.9)

lymphoid interstitial pneumonia (J84.2)

J70.4 Drug-induced interstitial lung disorders, unspecified

Use additional code for adverse effect, if applicable, to identify drug (T36-T50 with fifth or sixth character 5)

Excludes 1: interstitial pneumonia NOS (J84.9)

lymphoid interstitial pneumonia (J84.2)

J70.5 Respiratory conditions due to smoke inhalation

Smoke inhalation NOS

Excludes 1: smoke inhalation due to chemicals, gases, fumes and vapors (J68.9)

J70.8 Respiratory conditions due to other specified external agents

J70.9 Respiratory conditions due to unspecified external agent

Code first (T51-T65) to identify the external agent

OTHER RESPIRATORY DISEASES PRINCIPALLY AFFECTING THE INTERSTITIUM (J80-J84)

J80 Acute respiratory distress syndrome

Acute respiratory distress syndrome in adult or child

Adult hyaline membrane disease

Excludes 1: respiratory distress syndrome in newborn (perinatal) (P22.0)

J81 Pulmonary edema

Use additional code to identify:

exposure to environmental tobacco smoke (Z77.22)

history of tobacco use (Z87.891)

occupational exposure to environmental tobacco smoke (Z57.31)

tobacco dependence (F17.-)

tobacco use (Z72.0)

Excludes 1: chemical (acute) pulmonary edema (J68.1)

hypostatic pneumonia (J18.2)

passive pneumonia (J18.2)

pulmonary edema due to external agents (J60-J70)

pulmonary edema with heart disease NOS (I50.1)

pulmonary edema with heart failure (I50.1)

J81.0 Acute pulmonary edema

Acute edema of lung

J81.1 Chronic pulmonary edema

Pulmonary congestion (chronic) (passive)

Pulmonary edema NOS

J82 Pulmonary eosinophilia, not elsewhere classified

Allergic pneumonia

Eosinophilic asthma

Eosinophilic pneumonia

Loeffler's pneumonia

Tropical (pulmonary) eosinophilia NOS

Excludes 1: pulmonary eosinophilia due to aspergillosis (B44.-)

pulmonary eosinophilia due to drugs (J70.2-J70.4)

pulmonary eosinophilia due to specified parasitic infection (B50-B83)

pulmonary eosinophilia due to systemic connective tissue disorders (M30-M36)

pulmonary infiltrate NOS (R91.8)

J84 Other interstitial pulmonary diseases

Excludes 1: drug-induced interstitial lung disorders (J70.2-J70.4)

interstitial emphysema (J98.2)

lung diseases due to external agents (J60-J70)

J84.0 Alveolar and parieto-alveolar conditions

J84.01 Alveolar proteinosis

J84.02 Pulmonary alveolar microlithiasis

J84.03 Idiopathic pulmonary hemosiderosis

Essential brown induration of lung

Code first underlying disease, such as:

● New code   ▲ Revised code   ⑦ 7th digit required   ⊗ Placeholder required

disorders of iron metabolism (E83.1-)

Excludes 1: acute idiopathic pulmonary hemorrhage in infants [AIPHI] (R04.81)

J84.09 Other alveolar and parieto-alveolar conditions

J84.1 Other interstitial pulmonary diseases with fibrosis

Excludes 1: pulmonary fibrosis (chronic) due to inhalation of chemicals, gases, fumes or vapors (J68.4)
pulmonary fibrosis (chronic) following radiation (J70.1)

J84.10 Pulmonary fibrosis, unspecified
Capillary fibrosis of lung
Cirrhosis of lung (chronic) NOS
Fibrosis of lung (atrophic) (chronic) (confluent) (massive) (perialveolar) (peribronchial) NOS
Induration of lung (chronic) NOS
Postinflammatory pulmonary fibrosis

J84.11 Idiopathic interstitial pneumonia

Excludes 1: lymphoid interstitial pneumonia (J84.2)
pneumocystis pneumonia (B59)

J84.111 Idiopathic interstitial pneumonia, not otherwise specified

J84.112 Idiopathic pulmonary fibrosis
Cryptogenic fibrosing alveolitis
Idiopathic fibrosing alveolitis

J84.113 Idiopathic non-specific interstitial pneumonitis

Excludes 1: non-specific interstitial pneumonia NOS, or due to known underlying cause (J84.89)

J84.114 Acute interstitial pneumonitis
Hamman-Rich syndrome

Excludes 1: pneumocystis pneumonia (B59)

J84.115 Respiratory bronchiolitis interstitial lung disease

J84.116 Cryptogenic organizing pneumonia

Excludes 1: organizing pneumonia NOS, or due to known underlying cause (J84.89)

J84.117 Desquamative interstitial pneumonia

J84.17 Other interstitial pulmonary diseases with fibrosis in diseases classified elsewhere
Interstitial pneumonia (nonspecific) (usual) due to collagen vascular disease
Interstitial pneumonia (nonspecific) (usual) in diseases classified elsewhere
Organizing pneumonia due to collagen vascular disease
Organizing pneumonia in diseases classified elsewhere

Code first underlying disease, such as:
progressive systemic sclerosis (M34.0)
rheumatoid arthritis (M05.00-M06.9)
systemic lupus erythematosus (M32.0-M32.9)

J84.2 Lymphoid interstitial pneumonia
Lymphoid interstitial pneumonitis

J84.8 Other specified interstitial pulmonary diseases

Excludes 1: exogenous lipoid pneumonia (J69.1)

unspecified lipoid pneumonia (J69.1)

J84.81 Lymphangioleiomyomatosis
Lymphangiomyomatosis

J84.82 Adult pulmonary Langerhans cell histiocytosis
Adult PLCH

J84.83 Surfactant mutations of the lung

J84.84 Other interstitial lung diseases of childhood

J84.841 Neuroendocrine cell hyperplasia of infancy

J84.842 Pulmonary interstitial glycogenosis

J84.843 Alveolar capillary dysplasia with vein misalignment

J84.848 Other interstitial lung diseases of childhood

J84.89 Other specified interstitial pulmonary diseases
Endogenous lipoid pneumonia
Interstitial pneumonitis
Non-specific interstitial pneumonitis NOS
Organizing pneumonia due to known underlying cause
Organizing pneumonia NOS

Code first , if applicable:
poisoning due to drug or toxin (T51-T65 with fifth or sixth character to indicate intent), for toxic pneumonopathy
underlying cause of pneumonopathy, if known

Use additional code, for adverse effect, to identify drug (T36-T50 with fifth or sixth character 5), if drug-induced

Excludes 1: cryptogenic organizing pneumonia (J84.116)
idiopathic non-specific interstitial pneumonitis (J84.843)
lipoid pneumonia, exogenous or unspecified (J69.1)
lymphoid interstitial pneumonia (J84.2)

J84.9 Interstitial pulmonary disease, unspecified
Interstitial pneumonia NOS

SUPPURATIVE AND NECROTIC CONDITIONS OF THE LOWER RESPIRATORY TRACT (J85-J86)

J85 Abscess of lung and mediastinum
Use additional code (B95-B97) to identify infectious agent.

J85.0 Gangrene and necrosis of lung

J85.1 Abscess of lung with pneumonia
Code also the type of pneumonia

J85.2 Abscess of lung without pneumonia
Abscess of lung NOS

J85.3 Abscess of mediastinum

J86 Pyothorax
Use additional code (B95-B97) to identify infectious agent.

Excludes 1: abscess of lung (J85.-)
pyothorax due to tuberculosis (A15.6)

J86.0 Pyothorax with fistula
Bronchocutaneous fistula
Bronchopleural fistula
Hepatopleural fistula
Mediastinal fistula
Pleural fistula
Thoracic fistula

Any condition classifiable to J86.9 with fistula

J86.9 Pyothorax without fistula

Abscess of pleura

Abscess of thorax

Empyema (chest) (lung) (pleura)

Fibrinopurulent pleurisy

Purulent pleurisy

Pyopneumothorax

Septic pleurisy

Seropurulent pleurisy

Suppurative pleurisy

OTHER DISEASES OF THE PLEURA (J90-J94)

J90 Pleural effusion, not elsewhere classified

Encysted pleurisy

Pleural effusion NOS

Pleurisy with effusion (exudative) (serous)

Excludes 1: chylous (pleural) effusion (J94.0)

malignant pleural effusion (J91.0))

pleurisy NOS (R09.1)

tuberculous pleural effusion (A15.6)

J91 Pleural effusion in conditions classified elsewhere

Excludes 2: pleural effusion in heart failure (I50.-)

pleural effusion in systemic lupus erythematosus (M32.13)

J91.0 Malignant pleural effusion

Code first underlying neoplasm

J91.8 Pleural effusion in other conditions classified elsewhere

Code first underlying disease, such as:

filariasis (B74.0-B74.9)

influenza (J09.X2, J10.1, J11.1)

J92 Pleural plaque

Includes: pleural thickening

J92.0 Pleural plaque with presence of asbestos

J92.9 Pleural plaque without asbestos

Pleural plaque NOS

J93 Pneumothorax and air leak

Excludes 1: congenital or perinatal pneumothorax (P25.1)

postprocedural air leak (J95.812)

postprocedural pneumothorax (J95.811)

traumatic pneumothorax (S27.0)

tuberculous (current disease) pneumothorax (A15.-)

pyopneumothorax (J86.-)

J93.0 Spontaneous tension pneumothorax

J93.1 Other spontaneous pneumothorax

J93.11 Primary spontaneous pneumothorax

J93.12 Secondary spontaneous pneumothorax

Code first underlying condition, such as:

catamenial pneumothorax due to endometriosis (N80.8)

cystic fibrosis (E84.-)

eosinophilic pneumonia (J82)

lymphangioleiomyomatosis (J84.81)

malignant neoplasm of bronchus and lung (C34.-)

Marfan's syndrome (Q87.4)

pneumonia due to Pneumocystis carinii (B59)

secondary malignant neoplasm of lung (C78.0-)

spontaneous rupture of the esophagus (K22.3)

J93.8 Other pneumothorax and air leak

J93.81 Chronic pneumothorax

J93.82 Other air leak

Persistent air leak

J93.83 Other pneumothorax

Acute pneumothorax

Spontaneous pneumothorax NOS

J93.9 Pneumothorax, unspecified

Pneumothorax NOS

J94 Other pleural conditions

Excludes 1: pleurisy NOS (R09.1)

traumatic hemopneumothorax (S27.2)

traumatic hemothorax (S27.1)

tuberculous pleural conditions (current disease) A15.-)

J94.0 Chylous effusion

Chyliform effusion

J94.1 Fibrothorax

J94.2 Hemothorax

Hemopneumothorax

J94.8 Other specified pleural conditions

Hydropneumothorax

Hydrothorax

J94.9 Pleural condition, unspecified

INTRAOPERATIVE AND POSTPROCEDURAL COMPLICATIONS AND DISORDERS OF RESPIRATORY SYSTEM, NOT ELSEWHERE CLASSIFIED (J95)

J95 Intraoperative and postprocedural complications and disorders of respiratory system, not elsewhere classified

Excludes 2: aspiration pneumonia (J69.-)

emphysema (subcutaneous) resulting from a procedure (T81.82)

hypostatic pneumonia (J18.2)

pulmonary manifestations due to radiation (J70.0- J70.1)

J95.0 Tracheostomy complications

J95.00 Unspecified tracheostomy complication

J95.01 Hemorrhage from tracheostomy stoma

J95.02 Infection of tracheostomy stoma

Use additional code to identify type of infection, such as:

cellulitis of neck (L03.8)

sepsis (A40, A41.-)

J95.03 Malfunction of tracheostomy stoma

Mechanical complication of tracheostomy stoma

Obstruction of tracheostomy airway

Tracheal stenosis due to tracheostomy

J95.04 Tracheo-esophageal fistula following tracheostomy

J95.09 Other tracheostomy complication

J95.1 Acute pulmonary insufficiency following thoracic surgery

Excludes 2: Functional disturbances following cardiac surgery (I97.0, I97.1-)

J95.2 Acute pulmonary insufficiency following nonthoracic surgery

Excludes 2: Functional disturbances following cardiac surgery (I97.0, I97.1-)

J95.3 Chronic pulmonary insufficiency following surgery

Excludes 2: Functional disturbances following cardiac surgery (I97.0, I97.1-)

J95.4 Chemical pneumonitis due to anesthesia

Mendelson's syndrome

Postprocedural aspiration pneumonia

Use additional code for adverse effect, if applicable, to identify drug (T41.- with fifth or sixth character 5)

Excludes 1: aspiration pneumonitis due to anesthesia complicating labor and delivery (O74.0)

aspiration pneumonitis due to anesthesia complicating pregnancy (O29)

aspiration pneumonitis due to anesthesia complicating the puerperium (O89.01)

J95.5 Postprocedural subglottic stenosis

J95.6 Intraoperative hemorrhage and hematoma of a respiratory system organ or structure complicating a procedure

Excludes 1: intraoperative hemorrhage and hematoma of a respiratory system organ or structure due to accidental puncture and laceration during procedure (J95.7-)

J95.61 Intraoperative hemorrhage and hematoma of a respiratory system organ or structure complicating a respiratory system procedure

J95.62 Intraoperative hemorrhage and hematoma of a respiratory system organ or structure complicating other procedure

J95.7 Accidental puncture and laceration of a respiratory system organ or structure during a procedure

Excludes 2: postprocedural pneumothorax (J95.8)

J95.71 Accidental puncture and laceration of a respiratory system organ or structure during a respiratory system procedure

J95.72 Accidental puncture and laceration of a respiratory system organ or structure during other procedure

J95.8 Other intraoperative and postprocedural complications and disorders of respiratory system, not elsewhere classified

J95.81 Postprocedural pneumothorax and air leak

J95.811 Postprocedural pneumothorax

J95.812 Postprocedural air leak

J95.82 Postprocedural respiratory failure

Excludes 1: Respiratory failure in other conditions (J96.-)

J95.821 Acute postprocedural respiratory failure

Postprocedural respiratory failure NOS

J95.822 Acute and chronic postprocedural respiratory failure

J95.83 Postprocedural hemorrhage and hematoma of a respiratory system organ or structure following a procedure

J95.830 Postprocedural hemorrhage and hematoma of a respiratory system organ or structure following a respiratory system procedure

J95.831 Postprocedural hemorrhage and hematoma of a respiratory system organ or structure following other procedure

J95.84 Transfusion related acute lung injury (TRALI)

J95.85 Complication of respirator [ventilator]

J95.850 Mechanical complication of respirator

Excludes 1: encounter for respirator [ventilator] dependence during power failure (Z99.12)

J95.851 Ventilator associated pneumonia

Ventilator associated pneumonitis

Use additional code to identify the organism, if known (B95.-, B96.-, B97.-)

Excludes 1: ventilator lung in newborn (P27.8)

J95.859 Other complication of respirator [ventilator]

J95.88 Other intraoperative complications of respiratory system, not elsewhere classified

J95.89 Other postprocedural complications and disorders of respiratory system, not elsewhere classified

Use additional code to identify disorder, such as:

aspiration pneumonia (J69.-)

bacterial or viral pneumonia (J12-J18)

Excludes 2: acute pulmonary insufficiency following thoracic surgery (J95.1)

postprocedural subglottic stenosis (J95.5)

OTHER DISEASES OF THE RESPIRATORY SYSTEM (J96-J99)

J96 Respiratory failure, not elsewhere classified

Excludes 1: acute respiratory distress syndrome (J80)

cardiorespiratory failure (R09.2)

newborn respiratory distress syndrome (P22.0)

postprocedural respiratory failure (J95.82-)

respiratory arrest (R09.2)

respiratory arrest of newborn (P28.81)

respiratory failure of newborn (P28.5)

J96.0 Acute respiratory failure

J96.00 Acute respiratory failure, unspecified whether with hypoxia or hypercapnia

J96.01 Acute respiratory failure with hypoxia

J96.02 Acute respiratory failure with hypercapnia

J96.1 Chronic respiratory failure

J96.10 Chronic respiratory failure, unspecified whether with hypoxia or hypercapnia

J96.11 Chronic respiratory failure with hypoxia

J96.12 Chronic respiratory failure with hypercapnia

J96.2 Acute and chronic respiratory failure

Acute on chronic respiratory failure

J96.20 Acute and chronic respiratory failure, unspecified whether with hypoxia or hypercapnia

J96.21 Acute and chronic respiratory failure with hypoxia

J96.22 Acute and chronic respiratory failure with hypercapnia

J96.9 Respiratory failure, unspecified

J96.90 Respiratory failure, unspecified, unspecified whether with hypoxia or hypercapnia

J96.91 Respiratory failure, unspecified with hypoxia

J96.92 Respiratory failure, unspecified with hypercapnia

J98 Other respiratory disorders

Use additional code to identify:

exposure to environmental tobacco smoke (Z77.22)

exposure to tobacco smoke in the perinatal period (P96.81)

history of tobacco use (Z87.891)

occupational exposure to environmental tobacco smoke (Z57.31)

tobacco dependence (F17.-)

tobacco use (Z72.0)

Excludes 1: newborn apnea (P28.4)

newborn sleep apnea (P28.3)

Excludes 2: apnea NOS (R06.81)

sleep apnea (G47.3-)

J98.0 Diseases of bronchus, not elsewhere classified

J98.01 Acute bronchospasm

Excludes 1: acute bronchiolitis with bronchospasm (J21.-)
acute bronchitis with bronchospasm (J20.-)
asthma (J45.-)
exercise induced bronchospasm (J45.990)

J98.09 Other diseases of bronchus, not elsewhere classified
Broncholithiasis
Calcification of bronchus
Stenosis of bronchus
Tracheobronchial collapse
Tracheobronchial dyskinesia
Ulcer of bronchus

J98.1 Pulmonary collapse
Excludes 1: therapeutic collapse of lung status (Z98.3)

J98.11 Atelectasis
Excludes 1: newborn atelectasis
tuberculous atelectasis (current disease) (A15)

J98.19 Other pulmonary collapse

J98.2 Interstitial emphysema
Mediastinal emphysema
Excludes 1: emphysema NOS (J43.9)
emphysema in newborn (P25.0)
surgical emphysema (subcutaneous) (T81.82)
traumatic subcutaneous emphysema (T79.7)

J98.3 Compensatory emphysema

J98.4 Other disorders of lung
Calcification of lung
Cystic lung disease (acquired)
Lung disease NOS
Pulmolithiasis
Excludes 1: acute interstitial pneumonitis (J84.114)
pulmonary insufficiency following surgery (J95.1-J95.2)

J98.5 Diseases of mediastinum, not elsewhere classified
Fibrosis of mediastinum
Hernia of mediastinum
Retraction of mediastinum
Mediastinitis
Excludes 2: abscess of mediastinum (J85.3)

J98.6 Disorders of diaphragm
Diaphragmatitis
Paralysis of diaphragm
Relaxation of diaphragm
Excludes 1: congenital malformation of diaphragm NEC (Q79.1)
congenital diaphragmatic hernia (Q79.0)
Excludes 2: diaphragmatic hernia (K44.-)

J98.8 Other specified respiratory disorders

J98.9 Respiratory disorder, unspecified
Respiratory disease (chronic) NOS

J99 Respiratory disorders in diseases classified elsewhere
Code first underlying disease, such as:
amyloidosis (E85-)
ankylosing spondylitis (M45)
congenital syphilis (A50.5)
cryoglobulinemia (D89.1)
early congenital syphilis (A50.0)
schistosomiasis (B65.0-B65.9)
Excludes 1: respiratory disorders in:
amebiasis (A06.5)

blastomycosis (B40.0-B40.2)
candidiasis (B37.1)
coccidioidomycosis (B38.0-B38.2)
cystic fibrosis with pulmonary manifestations (E84.0)
dermatomyositis (M33.01, M33.11)
histoplasmosis (B39.0-B39.2)
late syphilis (A52.72, A52.73)
polymyositis (M33.21)
sicca syndrome (M35.02)
systemic lupus erythematosus (M32.13)
systemic sclerosis (M34.81)
Wegener's granulomatosis (M31.30-M31.31)

Chapter 11: Diseases Of The Digestive System (K00-K95)

Excludes 2: certain conditions originating in the perinatal period (P04-P96)

certain infectious and parasitic diseases (A00-B99)

complications of pregnancy, childbirth and the puerperium (O00-O9A)

congenital malformations, deformations and chromosomal abnormalities (Q00-Q99)

endocrine, nutritional and metabolic diseases (E00-E88)

injury, poisoning and certain other consequences of external causes (S00-T88)

neoplasms (C00-D49)

symptoms, signs and abnormal clinical and laboratory findings, not elsewhere classified (R00-R94)

This chapter contains the following blocks:

K00-K14   Diseases of oral cavity and salivary glands
K20-K31   Diseases of esophagus, stomach and duodenum
K35-K38   Diseases of appendix
K40-K46   Hernia
K50-K52   Noninfective enteritis and colitis
K55-K64   Other diseases of intestines
K65-K68   Diseases of peritoneum and retroperitoneum
K70-K77   Diseases of liver
K80-K87   Disorders of gallbladder, biliary tract and pancreas
K90-K95   Other diseases of the digestive system

DISEASES OF ORAL CAVITY AND SALIVARY GLANDS (K00-K14)

K00 Disorders of tooth development and eruption

Excludes 2: embedded and impacted teeth (K01.-)

K00.0   Anodontia
Hypodontia
Oligodontia
Excludes 1: acquired absence of teeth (K08.1-)

K00.1   Supernumerary teeth
Distomolar
Fourth molar
Mesiodens
Paramolar
Supplementary teeth
Excludes 2: supernumerary roots (K00.2)

K00.2   Abnormalities of size and form of teeth
Concrescence of teeth
Fusion of teeth
Gemination of teeth
Dens evaginatus
Dens in dente
Dens invaginatus
Enamel pearls
Macrodontia
Microdontia
Peg-shaped [conical] teeth
Supernumerary roots
Taurodontism
Tuberculum paramolare
Excludes 1: abnormalities of teeth due to congenital syphilis (A50.5)
tuberculum Carabelli, which is regarded as a normal variation and should not be coded

K00.3   Mottled teeth
Dental fluorosis
Mottling of enamel
Nonfluoride enamel opacities
Excludes 2: deposits [accretions] on teeth (K03.6)

K00.4   Disturbances in tooth formation
Aplasia and hypoplasia of cementum
Dilaceration of tooth
Enamel hypoplasia (neonatal) (postnatal) (prenatal)
Regional odontodysplasia
Turner's tooth
Excludes 1: Hutchinson's teeth and mulberry molars in congenital syphilis (A50.5)
Excludes 2: mottled teeth (K00.3)

K00.5   Hereditary disturbances in tooth structure, not elsewhere classified
Amelogenesis imperfecta
Dentinogenesis imperfecta
Odontogenesis imperfecta
Dentinal dysplasia
Shell teeth

K00.6   Disturbances in tooth eruption
Dentia praecox
Natal tooth
Neonatal tooth
Premature eruption of tooth
Premature shedding of primary [deciduous] tooth
Prenatal teeth
Retained [persistent] primary tooth
Excludes 2: embedded and impacted teeth (K01.-)

K00.7   Teething syndrome

K00.8   Other disorders of tooth development
Color changes during tooth formation
Intrinsic staining of teeth NOS
Excludes 2: posteruptive color changes (K03.7)

K00.9   Disorder of tooth development, unspecified
Disorder of odontogenesis NOS

K01 Embedded and impacted teeth

Excludes 1: abnormal position of fully erupted teeth (M26.3-)

K01.0   Embedded teeth
K01.1   Impacted teeth

K02 Dental caries

dental cavities

tooth decay

K02.3   Arrested dental caries
Arrested coronal and root caries

K02.5   Dental caries on pit and fissure surface
Dental caries on chewing surface of tooth

     K02.51   Dental caries on pit and fissure surface limited to enamel
White spot lesions [initial caries] on pit and fissure surface of tooth

     K02.52   Dental caries on pit and fissure surface penetrating into dentin

     K02.53   Dental caries on pit and fissure surface penetrating into pulp

K02.6   Dental caries on smooth surface

     K02.61   Dental caries on smooth surface limited to enamel
White spot lesions [initial caries] on smooth surface of tooth

     K02.62   Dental caries on smooth surface penetrating into dentin

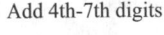 

K02.63 Dental caries on smooth surface penetrating into pulp

K02.7 Dental root caries

K02.9 Dental caries, unspecified

K03 Other diseases of hard tissues of teeth

Excludes 2: bruxism (F45.8)
dental caries (K02.-)
teeth-grinding NOS (F45.8)

K03.0 Excessive attrition of teeth
Approximal wear of teeth
Occlusal wear of teeth

K03.1 Abrasion of teeth
Dentifrice abrasion of teeth
Habitual abrasion of teeth
Occupational abrasion of teeth
Ritual abrasion of teeth
Traditional abrasion of teeth
Wedge defect NOS

K03.2 Erosion of teeth
Erosion of teeth due to diet
Erosion of teeth due to drugs and medicaments
Erosion of teeth due to persistent vomiting
Erosion of teeth NOS
Idiopathic erosion of teeth
Occupational erosion of teeth

K03.3 Pathological resorption of teeth
Internal granuloma of pulp
Resorption of teeth (external)

K03.4 Hypercementosis
Cementation hyperplasia

K03.5 Ankylosis of teeth

K03.6 Deposits [accretions] on teeth
Betel deposits [accretions] on teeth
Black deposits [accretions] on teeth
Extrinsic staining of teeth NOS
Green deposits [accretions] on teeth
Materia alba deposits [accretions] on teeth
Orange deposits [accretions] on teeth
Staining of teeth NOS
Subgingival dental calculus
Supragingival dental calculus
Tobacco deposits [accretions] on teeth

K03.7 Posteruptive color changes of dental hard tissues
Excludes 2: deposits [accretions] on teeth (K03.6)

K03.8 Other specified diseases of hard tissues of teeth

K03.81 Cracked tooth
Excludes 1: asymptomatic craze lines in enamel - omit code
broken or fractured tooth due to trauma (S02.5)

K03.89 Other specified diseases of hard tissues of teeth

K03.9 Disease of hard tissues of teeth, unspecified

K04 Diseases of pulp and periapical tissues

K04.0 Pulpitis
Acute pulpitis
Chronic (hyperplastic) (ulcerative) pulpitis
Irreversible pulpitis
Reversible pulpitis

K04.1 Necrosis of pulp
Pulpal gangrene

K04.2 Pulp degeneration
Denticles
Pulpal calcifications

Pulpal stones

K04.3 Abnormal hard tissue formation in pulp
Secondary or irregular dentine

K04.4 Acute apical periodontitis of pulpal origin
Acute apical periodontitis NOS
Excludes 1: acute periodontitis (K05.2-)

K04.5 Chronic apical periodontitis
Apical or periapical granuloma
Apical periodontitis NOS
Excludes 1: chronic periodontitis (K05.3-)

K04.6 Periapical abscess with sinus
Dental abscess with sinus
Dentoalveolar abscess with sinus

K04.7 Periapical abscess without sinus
Dental abscess without sinus
Dentoalveolar abscess without sinus
Periapical abscess without sinus

K04.8 Radicular cyst
Apical (periodontal) cyst
Periapical cyst
Residual radicular cyst
Excludes 2: lateral periodontal cyst (K09.0)

K04.9 Other and unspecified diseases of pulp and periapical tissues

K04.90 Unspecified diseases of pulp and periapical tissues

K04.99 Other diseases of pulp and periapical tissues

K05 Gingivitis and periodontal diseases

Use additional code to identify:
alcohol abuse and dependence (F10.-)
exposure to environmental tobacco smoke (Z77.22)
exposure to tobacco smoke in the perinatal period (P96.81)
history of tobacco use (Z87.891)
occupational exposure to environmental tobacco smoke (Z57.31)
tobacco dependence (F17.-)
tobacco use (Z72.0)

K05.0 Acute gingivitis
Excludes 1: acute necrotizing ulcerative gingivitis (A69.1)
herpesviral [herpes simplex] gingivostomatitis (B00.2)

K05.00 Acute gingivitis, plaque induced
Acute gingivitis NOS

K05.01 Acute gingivitis, non-plaque induced

K05.1 Chronic gingivitis
Desquamative gingivitis (chronic)
Gingivitis (chronic) NOS
Hyperplastic gingivitis (chronic)
Simple marginal gingivitis (chronic)
Ulcerative gingivitis (chronic)

K05.10 Chronic gingivitis, plaque induced
Chronic gingivitis NOS
Gingivitis NOS

K05.11 Chronic gingivitis, non-plaque induced

K05.2 Aggressive periodontitis
Acute pericoronitis
Excludes 1: acute apical periodontitis (K04.4)
periapical abscess (K04.7)
periapical abscess with sinus (K04.6)

K05.20 Aggressive periodontitis, unspecified

K05.21 Aggressive periodontitis, localized
Periodontal abscess

K05.22 Aggressive periodontitis, generalized

K05.3 Chronic periodontitis
Chronic pericoronitis
Complex periodontitis
Periodontitis NOS
Simplex periodontitis
Excludes 1: chronic apical periodontitis (K04.5)

K05.30 Chronic periodontitis, unspecified
K05.31 Chronic periodontitis, localized
K05.32 Chronic periodontitis, generalized

K05.4 Periodontosis
Juvenile periodontosis

K05.5 Other periodontal diseases
Excludes 2: leukoplakia of gingiva (K13.21)

K05.6 Periodontal disease, unspecified

K06 Other disorders of gingiva and edentulous alveolar ridge
Excludes 2: acute gingivitis (K05.0)
atrophy of edentulous alveolar ridge (K08.2)
chronic gingivitis (K05.1)
gingivitis NOS (K05.1)

K06.0 Gingival recession
Gingival recession (generalized) (localized) (postinfective) (postprocedural)

K06.1 Gingival enlargement
Gingival fibromatosis

K06.2 Gingival and edentulous alveolar ridge lesions associated with trauma
Irritative hyperplasia of edentulous ridge [denture hyperplasia]
Use additional code (Chapter 20) to identify external cause or denture status (Z97.2)

K06.8 Other specified disorders of gingiva and edentulous alveolar ridge
Fibrous epulis
Flabby alveolar ridge
Giant cell epulis
Peripheral giant cell granuloma of gingiva
Pyogenic granuloma of gingiva
Excludes 2: gingival cyst (K09.0)

K06.9 Disorder of gingiva and edentulous alveolar ridge, unspecified

K08 Other disorders of teeth and supporting structures
Excludes 2: dentofacial anomalies [including malocclusion] (M26.-)
disorders of jaw (M27.-)

K08.0 Exfoliation of teeth due to systemic causes
Code also underlying systemic condition

K08.1 Complete loss of teeth
Acquired loss of teeth, complete
Excludes 1: congenital absence of teeth (K00.0)
exfoliation of teeth due to systemic causes (K08.0)
partial loss of teeth (K08.4-)

K08.10 Complete loss of teeth, unspecified cause
K08.101 Complete loss of teeth, unspecified cause, class I
K08.102 Complete loss of teeth, unspecified cause, class II
K08.103 Complete loss of teeth, unspecified cause, class III
K08.104 Complete loss of teeth, unspecified cause, class IV

K08.109 Complete loss of teeth, unspecified cause, unspecified class
Edentulism NOS

K08.11 Complete loss of teeth due to trauma
K08.111 Complete loss of teeth due to trauma, class I
K08.112 Complete loss of teeth due to trauma, class II
K08.113 Complete loss of teeth due to trauma, class III
K08.114 Complete loss of teeth due to trauma, class IV
K08.119 Complete loss of teeth due to trauma, unspecified class

K08.12 Complete loss of teeth due to periodontal diseases
K08.121 Complete loss of teeth due to periodontal diseases, class I
K08.122 Complete loss of teeth due to periodontal diseases, class II
K08.123 Complete loss of teeth due to periodontal diseases, class III
K08.124 Complete loss of teeth due to periodontal diseases, class IV
K08.129 Complete loss of teeth due to periodontal diseases, unspecified class

K08.13 Complete loss of teeth due to caries
K08.131 Complete loss of teeth due to caries, class I
K08.132 Complete loss of teeth due to caries, class II
K08.133 Complete loss of teeth due to caries, class III
K08.134 Complete loss of teeth due to caries, class IV
K08.139 Complete loss of teeth due to caries, unspecified class

K08.19 Complete loss of teeth due to other specified cause
K08.191 Complete loss of teeth due to other specified cause, class I
K08.192 Complete loss of teeth due to other specified cause, class II
K08.193 Complete loss of teeth due to other specified cause, class III
K08.194 Complete loss of teeth due to other specified cause, class IV
K08.199 Complete loss of teeth due to other specified cause, unspecified class

K08.2 Atrophy of edentulous alveolar ridge
K08.20 Unspecified atrophy of edentulous alveolar ridge
Atrophy of the mandible NOS
Atrophy of the maxilla NOS
K08.21 Minimal atrophy of the mandible
Minimal atrophy of the edentulous mandible
K08.22 Moderate atrophy of the mandible
Moderate atrophy of the edentulous mandible
K08.23 Severe atrophy of the mandible
Severe atrophy of the edentulous mandible
K08.24 Minimal atrophy of maxilla
Minimal atrophy of the edentulous maxilla
K08.25 Moderate atrophy of the maxilla
Moderate atrophy of the edentulous maxilla

K08.26   Severe atrophy of the maxilla
          Severe atrophy of the edentulous maxilla
K08.3   Retained dental root
K08.4   Partial loss of teeth
        Acquired loss of teeth, partial
        Excludes 1: complete loss of teeth (K08.1-)
                  congenital absence of teeth (K00.0)
        Excludes 2: exfoliation of teeth due to systemic causes
                  (K08.0)
  K08.40   Partial loss of teeth, unspecified cause
      K08.401   Partial loss of teeth, unspecified
                 cause, class I
      K08.402   Partial loss of teeth, unspecified
                 cause, class II
      K08.403   Partial loss of teeth, unspecified
                 cause, class III
      K08.404   Partial loss of teeth, unspecified
                 cause, class IV
      K08.409   Partial loss of teeth, unspecified
                 cause, unspecified class
                 Tooth extraction status NOS
  K08.41   Partial loss of teeth due to trauma
      K08.411   Partial loss of teeth due to trauma,
                 class I
      K08.412   Partial loss of teeth due to trauma,
                 class II
      K08.413   Partial loss of teeth due to trauma,
                 class III
      K08.414   Partial loss of teeth due to trauma,
                 class IV
      K08.419   Partial loss of teeth due to trauma,
                 unspecified class
  K08.42   Partial loss of teeth due to periodontal diseases
      K08.421   Partial loss of teeth due to
                 periodontal diseases, class I
      K08.422   Partial loss of teeth due to
                 periodontal diseases, class II
      K08.423   Partial loss of teeth due to
                 periodontal diseases, class III
      K08.424   Partial loss of teeth due to
                 periodontal diseases, class IV
      K08.429   Partial loss of teeth due to
                 periodontal diseases, unspecified
                 class
  K08.43   Partial loss of teeth due to caries
      K08.431   Partial loss of teeth due to caries,
                 class I
      K08.432   Partial loss of teeth due to caries,
                 class II
      K08.433   Partial loss of teeth due to caries,
                 class III
      K08.434   Partial loss of teeth due to caries,
                 class IV
      K08.439   Partial loss of teeth due to caries,
                 unspecified class
  K08.49   Partial loss of teeth due to other specified cause
      K08.491   Partial loss of teeth due to other
                 specified cause, class I
      K08.492   Partial loss of teeth due to other
                 specified cause, class II
      K08.493   Partial loss of teeth due to other
                 specified cause, class III
      K08.494   Partial loss of teeth due to other
                 specified cause, class IV

      K08.499   Partial loss of teeth due to other
                 specified cause, unspecified class
K08.5   Unsatisfactory restoration of tooth
        Defective bridge, crown, filling
        Defective dental restoration
        Excludes 1: dental restoration status (Z98.811)
        Excludes 2: endosseous dental implant failure (M27.6-)
                  unsatisfactory endodontic treatment (M27.5-)
  K08.50   Unsatisfactory restoration of tooth, unspecified
            Defective dental restoration NOS
  K08.51   Open restoration margins of tooth
            Dental restoration failure of marginal integrity
            Open margin on tooth restoration
            Poor gingival margin to tooth restoration
  K08.52   Unrepairable overhanging of dental restorative
            materials
            Overhanging of tooth restoration
  K08.53   Fractured dental restorative material
        Excludes 1: cracked tooth (K03.81)
                      traumatic fracture of tooth (S02.5)
      K08.530   Fractured dental restorative material
                 without loss of material
      K08.531   Fractured dental restorative material
                 with loss of material
      K08.539   Fractured dental restorative material,
                 unspecified
  K08.54   Contour of existing restoration of tooth
            biologically incompatible with oral health
            Dental restoration failure of periodontal
            anatomical integrity
            Unacceptable contours of existing restoration of
            tooth
            Unacceptable morphology of existing restoration
            of tooth
  K08.55   Allergy to existing dental restorative material
            Use additional code to identify the specific type
            of allergy
  K08.56   Poor aesthetic of existing restoration of tooth
            Dental restoration aesthetically inadequate or
            displeasing
  K08.59   Other unsatisfactory restoration of tooth
            Other defective dental restoration
K08.8   Other specified disorders of teeth and supporting structures
        Enlargement of alveolar ridge NOS
        Irregular alveolar process
        Toothache NOS
K08.9   Disorder of teeth and supporting structures, unspecified
K09   Cysts of oral region, not elsewhere classified
      Includes: lesions showing histological features both of aneurysmal
               cyst and of another fibro-osseous lesion
      Excludes 2: cysts of jaw (M27.0-, M27.4-)
               radicular cyst (K04.8)
K09.0   Developmental odontogenic cysts
        Dentigerous cyst
        Eruption cyst
        Follicular cyst
        Gingival cyst
        Lateral periodontal cyst
        Primordial cyst
        Excludes 2: keratocysts D16.4, D16.5
                  odontogenic keratocystic tumors D16.4, D16.5
K09.1   Developmental (nonodontogenic) cysts of oral region
        Cyst (of) incisive canal

● New code   ▲ Revised code   ⑦ 7th digit required   ⊗ Placeholder required

Cyst (of) palatine of papilla
Globulomaxillary cyst
Median palatal cyst
Nasoalveolar cyst
Nasolabial cyst
Nasopalatine duct cyst

K09.8 Other cysts of oral region, not elsewhere classified
Dermoid cyst
Epidermoid cyst
Lymphoepithelial cyst
Epstein's pearl

K09.9 Cyst of oral region, unspecified

K11 Diseases of salivary glands

Use additional code to identify:
alcohol abuse and dependence (F10.-)
exposure to environmental tobacco smoke (Z77.22)
exposure to tobacco smoke in the perinatal period (P96.81)
history of tobacco use (Z87.891)
occupational exposure to environmental tobacco smoke (Z57.31)
tobacco dependence (F17.-)
tobacco use (Z72.0)

K11.0 Atrophy of salivary gland

K11.1 Hypertrophy of salivary gland

K11.2 Sialoadenitis
Parotitis
Excludes 1: epidemic parotitis (B26.-)
mumps (B26.-)
uveoparotid fever [Heerfordt] (D86.89)

K11.20 Sialoadenitis, unspecified

K11.21 Acute sialoadenitis
Excludes 1: acute recurrent sialoadenitis (K11.22)

K11.22 Acute recurrent sialoadenitis

K11.23 Chronic sialoadenitis

K11.3 Abscess of salivary gland

K11.4 Fistula of salivary gland
Excludes 1: congenital fistula of salivary gland (Q38.4)

K11.5 Sialolithiasis
Calculus of salivary gland or duct
Stone of salivary gland or duct

K11.6 Mucocele of salivary gland
Mucous extravasation cyst of salivary gland
Mucous retention cyst of salivary gland
Ranula

K11.7 Disturbances of salivary secretion
Hypoptyalism
Ptyalism
Xerostomia
Excludes 2: dry mouth NOS (R68.2)

K11.8 Other diseases of salivary glands
Benign lymphoepithelial lesion of salivary gland
Mikulicz' disease
Necrotizing sialometaplasia
Sialectasia
Stenosis of salivary duct
Stricture of salivary duct
Excludes 1: sicca syndrome [Sjogren] (M35.0-)

K11.9 Disease of salivary gland, unspecified
Sialadenopathy NOS

K12 Stomatitis and related lesions

Use additional code to identify:

alcohol abuse and dependence (F10.-)
exposure to environmental tobacco smoke (Z77.22)
exposure to tobacco smoke in the perinatal period (P96.81)
history of tobacco use (Z87.891)
occupational exposure to environmental tobacco smoke (Z57.31)
tobacco dependence (F17.-)
tobacco use (Z72.0)
Excludes 1: cancrum oris (A69.0)
cheilitis (K13.0)
gangrenous stomatitis (A69.0)
herpesviral [herpes simplex] gingivostomatitis (B00.2)
noma (A69.0)

K12.0 Recurrent oral aphthae
Aphthous stomatitis (major) (minor)
Bednar's aphthae
Periadenitis mucosa necrotica recurrens
Recurrent aphthous ulcer
Stomatitis herpetiformis

K12.1 Other forms of stomatitis
Stomatitis NOS
Denture stomatitis
Ulcerative stomatitis
Vesicular stomatitis
Excludes 1: acute necrotizing ulcerative stomatitis (A69.1)
Vincent's stomatitis (A69.1)

K12.2 Cellulitis and abscess of mouth
Cellulitis of mouth (floor)
Submandibular abscess
Excludes 2: abscess of salivary gland (K11.3)
abscess of tongue (K14.0)
periapical abscess (K04.6-K04.7)
periodontal abscess (K05.21)
peritonsillar abscess (J36)

K12.3 Oral mucositis (ulcerative)
Mucositis (oral) (oropharyngeal)
Excludes 2: gastrointestinal mucositis (ulcerative) (K92.81)
mucositis (ulcerative) of vagina and vulva (N76.81)
nasal mucositis (ulcerative) (J34.81)

K12.30 Oral mucositis (ulcerative), unspecified

K12.31 Oral mucositis (ulcerative) due to antineoplastic therapy
Use additional code for adverse effect, if applicable, to identify antineoplastic and immunosuppressive drugs (T45.1x5)
Use additional code for other antineoplastic therapy, such as:
radiological procedure and radiotherapy (Y84.2)

K12.32 Oral mucositis (ulcerative) due to other drugs
Use additional code for adverse effect, if applicable, to identify drug (T36-T50with fifth or sixth character 5)

K12.33 Oral mucositis (ulcerative) due to radiation
Use additional external cause code (W88-W90, X39.0-) to identify cause

K12.39 Other oral mucositis (ulcerative)
Viral oral mucositis (ulcerative)

K13 Other diseases of lip and oral mucosa
Includes: epithelial disturbances of tongue

Use additional code to identify:
alcohol abuse and dependence (F10.-)

---

exposure to environmental tobacco smoke (Z77.22)

exposure to tobacco smoke in the perinatal period (P96.81)

history of tobacco use (Z87.891)

occupational exposure to environmental tobacco smoke (Z57.31)

tobacco dependence (F17.-)

tobacco use (Z72.0)

Excludes 2: certain disorders of gingiva and edentulous alveolar ridge (K05-K06)

cysts of oral region (K09.-)

diseases of tongue (K14.-)

stomatitis and related lesions (K12.-)

K13.0 Diseases of lips

Abscess of lips

Angular cheilitis

Cellulitis of lips

Cheilitis NOS

Cheilodynia

Cheilosis

Exfoliative cheilitis

Fistula of lips

Glandular cheilitis

Hypertrophy of lips

Perlèche NEC

Excludes 1: ariboflavinosis (E53.0)

cheilitis due to radiation-related disorders (L55-L59)

congenital fistula of lips (Q38.0)

congenital hypertrophy of lips (Q18.6)

Perlèche due to candidiasis (B37.83)

Perlèche due to riboflavin deficiency (E53.0)

K13.1 Cheek and lip biting

K13.2 Leukoplakia and other disturbances of oral epithelium, including tongue

Excludes 1: carcinoma in situ of oral epithelium (D00.0-)

hairy leukoplakia (K13.3)

K13.21 Leukoplakia of oral mucosa, including tongue

Leukokeratosis of oral mucosa

Leukoplakia of gingiva, lips, tongue

Excludes 1: hairy leukoplakia (K13.3)

leukokeratosis nicotina palati (K13.24)

K13.22 Minimal keratinized residual ridge mucosa

Minimal keratinization of alveolar ridge mucosa

K13.23 Excessive keratinized residual ridge mucosa

Excessive keratinization of alveolar ridge mucosa

K13.24 Leukokeratosis nicotina palati

Smoker's palate

K13.29 Other disturbances of oral epithelium, including tongue

Erythroplakia of mouth or tongue

Focal epithelial hyperplasia of mouth or tongue

Leukoedema of mouth or tongue

Other oral epithelium disturbances

K13.3 Hairy leukoplakia

K13.4 Granuloma and granuloma-like lesions of oral mucosa

Eosinophilic granuloma

Granuloma pyogenicum

Verrucous xanthoma

K13.5 Oral submucous fibrosis

Submucous fibrosis of tongue

K13.6 Irritative hyperplasia of oral mucosa

Excludes 2: irritative hyperplasia of edentulous ridge [denture hyperplasia] (K06.2)

K13.7 Other and unspecified lesions of oral mucosa

K13.70 Unspecified lesions of oral mucosa

K13.79 Other lesions of oral mucosa

Focal oral mucinosis

K14 Diseases of tongue

Use additional code to identify:

alcohol abuse and dependence (F10.-)

exposure to environmental tobacco smoke (Z77.22)

history of tobacco use (Z87.891)

occupational exposure to environmental tobacco smoke (Z57.31)

tobacco dependence (F17.-)

tobacco use (Z72.0)

Excludes 2: erythroplakia (K13.29)

focal epithelial hyperplasia (K13.29)

leukoedema of tongue (K13.29)

leukoplakia of tongue (K13.21)

hairy leukoplakia (K13.3)

macroglossia (congenital) (Q38.2)

submucous fibrosis of tongue (K13.5)

K14.0 Glossitis

Abscess of tongue

Ulceration (traumatic) of tongue

Excludes 1: atrophic glossitis (K14.4)

K14.1 Geographic tongue

Benign migratory glossitis

Glossitis areata exfoliativa

K14.2 Median rhomboid glossitis

K14.3 Hypertrophy of tongue papillae

Black hairy tongue

Coated tongue

Hypertrophy of foliate papillae

Lingua villosa nigra

K14.4 Atrophy of tongue papillae

Atrophic glossitis

K14.5 Plicated tongue

Fissured tongue

Furrowed tongue

Scrotal tongue

Excludes 1: fissured tongue, congenital (Q38.3)

K14.6 Glossodynia

Glossopyrosis

Painful tongue

K14.8 Other diseases of tongue

Atrophy of tongue

Crenated tongue

Enlargement of tongue

Glossocele

Glossoptosis

Hypertrophy of tongue

K14.9 Disease of tongue, unspecified

Glossopathy NOS

DISEASES OF ESOPHAGUS, STOMACH AND DUODENUM (K20-K31)

Excludes 2: hiatus hernia (K44.-)

K20 Esophagitis

Use additional code to identify:

alcohol abuse and dependence (F10.-)

Excludes 1: erosion of esophagus (K22.1-)

esophagitis with gastro-esophageal reflux disease (K21.0)

reflux esophagitis (K21.0)

ulcerative esophagitis (K22.1-)

Excludes 2: eosinophilic gastritis or gastroenteritis (K52.81)

K20.0 Eosinophilic esophagitis

K20.8 Other esophagitis

Abscess of esophagus

K20.9 Esophagitis, unspecified

Esophagitis NOS

K21 Gastro-esophageal reflux disease

Excludes 1: newborn esophageal reflux (P78.83)

K21.0 Gastro-esophageal reflux disease with esophagitis

Reflux esophagitis

K21.9 Gastro-esophageal reflux disease without esophagitis

Esophageal reflux NOS

K22 Other diseases of esophagus

Excludes 2: esophageal varices (I85.-)

K22.0 Achalasia of cardia

Achalasia NOS

Cardiospasm

Excludes 1: congenital cardiospasm (Q39.5)

K22.1 Ulcer of esophagus

Barrett's ulcer

Erosion of esophagus

Fungal ulcer of esophagus

Peptic ulcer of esophagus

Ulcer of esophagus due to ingestion of chemicals

Ulcer of esophagus due to ingestion of drugs and medicaments

Ulcerative esophagitis

Code first poisoning due to drug or toxin, if applicable (T36-T65 with fifth or sixth character 1-4 or 6)

Use additional code for adverse effect, if applicable, to identify drug (T36-T50 with fifth or sixth character 5)

Excludes 1: Barrett's esophagus (K22.7-)

K22.10 Ulcer of esophagus without bleeding

Ulcer of esophagus NOS

K22.11 Ulcer of esophagus with bleeding

Excludes 2: bleeding esophageal varices (I85.01, I85.11)

K22.2 Esophageal obstruction

Compression of esophagus

Constriction of esophagus

Stenosis of esophagus

Stricture of esophagus

Excludes 1: congenital stenosis or stricture of esophagus (Q39.3)

K22.3 Perforation of esophagus

Rupture of esophagus

Excludes 1: traumatic perforation of (thoracic) esophagus (S27.8-)

K22.4 Dyskinesia of esophagus

Corkscrew esophagus

Diffuse esophageal spasm

Spasm of esophagus

Excludes 1: cardiospasm (K22.0)

K22.5 Diverticulum of esophagus, acquired

Esophageal pouch, acquired

Excludes 1: diverticulum of esophagus (congenital) (Q39.6)

K22.6 Gastro-esophageal laceration-hemorrhage syndrome

Mallory-Weiss syndrome

K22.7 Barrett's esophagus

Barrett's disease

Barrett's syndrome

Excludes 1: Barrett's ulcer (K22.1)

malignant neoplasm of esophagus (C15.-)

K22.70 Barrett's esophagus without dysplasia

Barrett's esophagus NOS

K22.71 Barrett's esophagus with dysplasia

K22.710 Barrett's esophagus with low grade dysplasia

K22.711 Barrett's esophagus with high grade dysplasia

K22.719 Barrett's esophagus with dysplasia, unspecified

K22.8 Other specified diseases of esophagus

Hemorrhage of esophagus NOS

Excludes 2: esophageal varices (I85.-)

Paterson-Kelly syndrome (D50.1)

K22.9 Disease of esophagus, unspecified

K23 Disorders of esophagus in diseases classified elsewhere

Code first underlying disease, such as:

congenital syphilis (A50.5)

Excludes 1: late syphilis (A52.79)

megaesophagus due to Chagas' disease (B57.31)

tuberculosis (A18.83)

K25 Gastric ulcer

Includes: erosion (acute) of stomach

pylorus ulcer (peptic)

stomach ulcer (peptic)

Use additional code to identify:

alcohol abuse and dependence (F10.-)

Excludes 1: acute gastritis (K29.0-)

peptic ulcer NOS (K27.-)

K25.0 Acute gastric ulcer with hemorrhage

K25.1 Acute gastric ulcer with perforation

K25.2 Acute gastric ulcer with both hemorrhage and perforation

K25.3 Acute gastric ulcer without hemorrhage or perforation

K25.4 Chronic or unspecified gastric ulcer with hemorrhage

K25.5 Chronic or unspecified gastric ulcer with perforation

K25.6 Chronic or unspecified gastric ulcer with both hemorrhage and perforation

K25.7 Chronic gastric ulcer without hemorrhage or perforation

K25.9 Gastric ulcer, unspecified as acute or chronic, without hemorrhage or perforation

K26 Duodenal ulcer

Includes: erosion (acute) of duodenum

duodenum ulcer (peptic)

postpyloric ulcer (peptic)

Use additional code to identify:

alcohol abuse and dependence (F10.-)

Excludes 1: peptic ulcer NOS (K27.-)

K26.0 Acute duodenal ulcer with hemorrhage

K26.1 Acute duodenal ulcer with perforation

K26.2 Acute duodenal ulcer with both hemorrhage and perforation

K26.3 Acute duodenal ulcer without hemorrhage or perforation

K26.4 Chronic or unspecified duodenal ulcer with hemorrhage

K26.5 Chronic or unspecified duodenal ulcer with perforation

K26.6 Chronic or unspecified duodenal ulcer with both hemorrhage and perforation

K26.7 Chronic duodenal ulcer without hemorrhage or perforation

K26.9 Duodenal ulcer, unspecified as acute or chronic, without hemorrhage or perforation

K27 Peptic ulcer, site unspecified

Add 4th-7th digits   3 digit reportable   Nonspecific code   Unspecified code   Manifestation code

Includes: gastroduodenal ulcer NOS
peptic ulcer NOS

Use additional code to identify:
alcohol abuse and dependence (F10.-)

Excludes 1: peptic ulcer of newborn (P78.82)

K27.0 Acute peptic ulcer, site unspecified, with hemorrhage

K27.1 Acute peptic ulcer, site unspecified, with perforation

K27.2 Acute peptic ulcer, site unspecified, with both hemorrhage and perforation

K27.3 Acute peptic ulcer, site unspecified, without hemorrhage or perforation

K27.4 Chronic or unspecified peptic ulcer, site unspecified, with hemorrhage

K27.5 Chronic or unspecified peptic ulcer, site unspecified, with perforation

K27.6 Chronic or unspecified peptic ulcer, site unspecified, with both hemorrhage and perforation

K27.7 Chronic peptic ulcer, site unspecified, without hemorrhage or perforation

K27.9 Peptic ulcer, site unspecified, unspecified as acute or chronic, without hemorrhage or perforation

K28 Gastrojejunal ulcer

Includes: anastomotic ulcer (peptic) or erosion
gastrocolic ulcer (peptic) or erosion
gastrointestinal ulcer (peptic) or erosion
gastrojejunal ulcer (peptic) or erosion
jejunal ulcer (peptic) or erosion
marginal ulcer (peptic) or erosion
stomal ulcer (peptic) or erosion

Use additional code to identify:
alcohol abuse and dependence (F10.-)

Excludes 1: primary ulcer of small intestine (K63.3)

K28.0 Acute gastrojejunal ulcer with hemorrhage

K28.1 Acute gastrojejunal ulcer with perforation

K28.2 Acute gastrojejunal ulcer with both hemorrhage and perforation

K28.3 Acute gastrojejunal ulcer without hemorrhage or perforation

K28.4 Chronic or unspecified gastrojejunal ulcer with hemorrhage

K28.5 Chronic or unspecified gastrojejunal ulcer with perforation

K28.6 Chronic or unspecified gastrojejunal ulcer with both hemorrhage and perforation

K28.7 Chronic gastrojejunal ulcer without hemorrhage or perforation

K28.9 Gastrojejunal ulcer, unspecified as acute or chronic, without hemorrhage or perforation

K29 Gastritis and duodenitis

Excludes 1: eosinophilic gastritis or gastroenteritis (K52.81)
Zollinger-Ellison syndrome (E16.4)

K29.0 Acute gastritis

Use additional code to identify:
alcohol abuse and dependence (F10.-)

Excludes 1: erosion (acute) of stomach (K25.-)

K29.00 Acute gastritis without bleeding

K29.01 Acute gastritis with bleeding

K29.2 Alcoholic gastritis

Use additional code to identify:
alcohol abuse and dependence (F10.-)

K29.20 Alcoholic gastritis without bleeding

K29.21 Alcoholic gastritis with bleeding

K29.3 Chronic superficial gastritis

K29.30 Chronic superficial gastritis without bleeding

K29.31 Chronic superficial gastritis with bleeding

K29.4 Chronic atrophic gastritis
Gastric atrophy

K29.40 Chronic atrophic gastritis without bleeding

K29.41 Chronic atrophic gastritis with bleeding

K29.5 Unspecified chronic gastritis
Chronic antral gastritis
Chronic fundal gastritis

K29.50 Unspecified chronic gastritis without bleeding

K29.51 Unspecified chronic gastritis with bleeding

K29.6 Other gastritis
Giant hypertrophic gastritis
Granulomatous gastritis
Ménétrier's disease

K29.60 Other gastritis without bleeding

K29.61 Other gastritis with bleeding

K29.7 Gastritis, unspecified

K29.70 Gastritis, unspecified, without bleeding

K29.71 Gastritis, unspecified, with bleeding

K29.8 Duodenitis

K29.80 Duodenitis without bleeding

K29.81 Duodenitis with bleeding

K29.9 Gastroduodenitis, unspecified

K29.90 Gastroduodenitis, unspecified, without bleeding

K29.91 Gastroduodenitis, unspecified, with bleeding

K30 Functional dyspepsia
Indigestion

Excludes 1: dyspepsia NOS (R10.13)
heartburn (R12)
nervous dyspepsia (F45.8)
neurotic dyspepsia (F45.8)
psychogenic dyspepsia (F45.8)

K31 Other diseases of stomach and duodenum

Includes: functional disorders of stomach

Excludes 2: diabetic gastroparesis (E08.43, E09.43, E10.43, E11.43, E13.43)
diverticulum of duodenum (K57.00-K57.13)

K31.0 Acute dilatation of stomach
Acute distention of stomach

K31.1 Adult hypertrophic pyloric stenosis
Pyloric stenosis NOS

Excludes 1: congenital or infantile pyloric stenosis (Q40.0)

K31.2 Hourglass stricture and stenosis of stomach

Excludes 1: congenital hourglass stomach (Q40.2)
hourglass contraction of stomach (K31.89)

K31.3 Pylorospasm, not elsewhere classified

Excludes 1: congenital or infantile pylorospasm (Q40.0)
neurotic pylorospasm (F45.8)
psychogenic pylorospasm (F45.8)

K31.4 Gastric diverticulum

Excludes 1: congenital diverticulum of stomach (Q40.2)

K31.5 Obstruction of duodenum
Constriction of duodenum
Duodenal ileus (chronic)
Stenosis of duodenum
Stricture of duodenum
Volvulus of duodenum

Excludes 1: congenital stenosis of duodenum (Q41.0)

K31.6 Fistula of stomach and duodenum
Gastrocolic fistula
Gastrojejunocolic fistula

● New code   ▲ Revised code   ⑦ 7ᵗʰ digit required   ⊗ Placeholder required

K31.7 Polyp of stomach and duodenum

    Excludes 1: adenomatous polyp of stomach (D13.1)

K31.8 Other specified diseases of stomach and duodenum

    K31.81 Angiodysplasia of stomach and duodenum

        K31.811 Angiodysplasia of stomach and duodenum with bleeding

        K31.819 Angiodysplasia of stomach and duodenum without bleeding

        Angiodysplasia of stomach and duodenum NOS

    K31.82 Dieulafoy lesion (hemorrhagic) of stomach and duodenum

        Excludes 2: Dieulafoy lesion of intestine (K63.81)

    K31.83 Achlorhydria

    K31.84 Gastroparesis

    Gastroparalysis

    Code first underlying disease, if known, such as:

    anorexia nervosa (F50.0-)

    diabetes mellitus (E08.43, E09.43, E10.43, E11.43, E13.43)

    scleroderma (M34.-)

    K31.89 Other diseases of stomach and duodenum

K31.9 Disease of stomach and duodenum, unspecified

DISEASES OF APPENDIX (K35-K38)

K35 Acute appendicitis

    K35.2 Acute appendicitis with generalized peritonitis

    Appendicitis (acute) with generalized (diffuse) peritonitis following rupture or perforation of appendix

    Appendicitis with peritonitis NOS

    Perforated appendix NOS

    Ruptured appendix NOS

    K35.3 Acute appendicitis with localized peritonitis

    Acute appendicitis with localized peritonitis with or without rupture or perforation of appendix

    Acute appendicitis with peritoneal abscess

    K35.8 Other and unspecified acute appendicitis

        K35.80 Unspecified acute appendicitis

        Acute appendicitis NOS

        Acute appendicitis without (localized) (generalized) peritonitis

        K35.89 Other acute appendicitis

K36 Other appendicitis

Chronic appendicitis

Recurrent appendicitis

K37 Unspecified appendicitis

    Excludes 1: -unspecified appendicitis with peritonitis (K35.2-K35.3)

K38 Other diseases of appendix

    K38.0 Hyperplasia of appendix

    K38.1 Appendicular concretions

    Fecalith of appendix

    Stercolith of appendix

    K38.2 Diverticulum of appendix

    K38.3 Fistula of appendix

    K38.8 Other specified diseases of appendix

    Intussusception of appendix

    K38.9 Disease of appendix, unspecified

HERNIA (K40-K46)

Note: Hernia with both gangrene and obstruction is classified to hernia with gangrene.

Includes: acquired hernia

congenital [except diaphragmatic or hiatus] hernia

recurrent hernia

K40 Inguinal hernia

Includes: bubonocele

    direct inguinal hernia

    double inguinal hernia

    indirect inguinal hernia

    inguinal hernia NOS

    oblique inguinal hernia

    scrotal hernia

    K40.0 Bilateral inguinal hernia, with obstruction, without gangrene

    Inguinal hernia (bilateral) causing obstruction without gangrene

    Incarcerated inguinal hernia (bilateral) without gangrene

    Irreducible inguinal hernia (bilateral) without gangrene

    Strangulated inguinal hernia (bilateral) without gangrene

        K40.00 Bilateral inguinal hernia, with obstruction, without gangrene, not specified as recurrent

        Bilateral inguinal hernia, with obstruction, without gangrene NOS

        K40.01 Bilateral inguinal hernia, with obstruction, without gangrene, recurrent

    K40.1 Bilateral inguinal hernia, with gangrene

        K40.10 Bilateral inguinal hernia, with gangrene, not specified as recurrent

        Bilateral inguinal hernia, with gangrene NOS

        K40.11 Bilateral inguinal hernia, with gangrene, recurrent

    K40.2 Bilateral inguinal hernia, without obstruction or gangrene

        K40.20 Bilateral inguinal hernia, without obstruction or gangrene, not specified as recurrent

        Bilateral inguinal hernia NOS

        K40.21 Bilateral inguinal hernia, without obstruction or gangrene, recurrent

    K40.3 Unilateral inguinal hernia, with obstruction, without gangrene

    Inguinal hernia (unilateral) causing obstruction without gangrene

    Incarcerated inguinal hernia (unilateral) without gangrene

    Irreducible inguinal hernia (unilateral) without gangrene

    Strangulated inguinal hernia (unilateral) without gangrene

        K40.30 Unilateral inguinal hernia, with obstruction, without gangrene, not specified as recurrent

        Inguinal hernia, with obstruction NOS

        Unilateral inguinal hernia, with obstruction, without gangrene NOS

        K40.31 Unilateral inguinal hernia, with obstruction, without gangrene, recurrent

    K40.4 Unilateral inguinal hernia, with gangrene

        K40.40 Unilateral inguinal hernia, with gangrene, not specified as recurrent

        Inguinal hernia with gangrene NOS

        Unilateral inguinal hernia with gangrene NOS

        K40.41 Unilateral inguinal hernia, with gangrene, recurrent

    K40.9 Unilateral inguinal hernia, without obstruction or gangrene

        K40.90 Unilateral inguinal hernia, without obstruction or gangrene, not specified as recurrent

        Inguinal hernia NOS

        Unilateral inguinal hernia NOS

        K40.91 Unilateral inguinal hernia, without obstruction or gangrene, recurrent

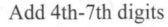 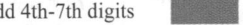

K41 Femoral hernia

K41.0 Bilateral femoral hernia, with obstruction, without gangrene
Femoral hernia (bilateral) causing obstruction, without gangrene
Incarcerated femoral hernia (bilateral), without gangrene
Irreducible femoral hernia (bilateral), without gangrene
Strangulated femoral hernia (bilateral), without gangrene

K41.00 Bilateral femoral hernia, with obstruction, without gangrene, not specified as recurrent
Bilateral femoral hernia, with obstruction, without gangrene NOS

K41.01 Bilateral femoral hernia, with obstruction, without gangrene, recurrent

K41.1 Bilateral femoral hernia, with gangrene

K41.10 Bilateral femoral hernia, with gangrene, not specified as recurrent
Bilateral femoral hernia, with gangrene NOS

K41.11 Bilateral femoral hernia, with gangrene, recurrent

K41.2 Bilateral femoral hernia, without obstruction or gangrene

K41.20 Bilateral femoral hernia, without obstruction or gangrene, not specified as recurrent
Bilateral femoral hernia NOS

K41.21 Bilateral femoral hernia, without obstruction or gangrene, recurrent

K41.3 Unilateral femoral hernia, with obstruction, without gangrene
Femoral hernia (unilateral) causing obstruction, without gangrene
Incarcerated femoral hernia (unilateral), without gangrene
Irreducible femoral hernia (unilateral), without gangrene
Strangulated femoral hernia (unilateral), without gangrene

K41.30 Unilateral femoral hernia, with obstruction, without gangrene, not specified as recurrent
Femoral hernia, with obstruction NOS
Unilateral femoral hernia, with obstruction NOS

K41.31 Unilateral femoral hernia, with obstruction, without gangrene, recurrent

K41.4 Unilateral femoral hernia, with gangrene

K41.40 Unilateral femoral hernia, with gangrene, not specified as recurrent
Femoral hernia, with gangrene NOS
Unilateral femoral hernia, with gangrene NOS

K41.41 Unilateral femoral hernia, with gangrene, recurrent

K41.9 Unilateral femoral hernia, without obstruction or gangrene

K41.90 Unilateral femoral hernia, without obstruction or gangrene, not specified as recurrent
Femoral hernia NOS
Unilateral femoral hernia NOS

K41.91 Unilateral femoral hernia, without obstruction or gangrene, recurrent

K42 Umbilical hernia
Includes: paraumbilical hernia
Excludes 1: omphalocele (Q79.2)

K42.0 Umbilical hernia with obstruction, without gangrene
Umbilical hernia causing obstruction, without gangrene
Incarcerated umbilical hernia, without gangrene
Irreducible umbilical hernia, without gangrene
Strangulated umbilical hernia, without gangrene

K42.1 Umbilical hernia with gangrene
Gangrenous umbilical hernia

K42.9 Umbilical hernia without obstruction or gangrene

Umbilical hernia NOS

K43 Ventral hernia

K43.0 Incisional hernia with obstruction, without gangrene
Incisional hernia causing obstruction, without gangrene
Incarcerated incisional hernia, without gangrene
Irreducible incisional hernia, without gangrene
Strangulated incisional hernia, without gangrene

K43.1 Incisional hernia with gangrene
Gangrenous incisional hernia

K43.2 Incisional hernia without obstruction or gangrene
Incisional hernia NOS

K43.3 Parastomal hernia with obstruction, without gangrene
Incarcerated parastomal hernia, without gangrene
Irreducible parastomal hernia, without gangrene
Parastomal hernia causing obstruction, without gangrene
Strangulated parastomal hernia, without gangrene

K43.4 Parastomal hernia with gangrene
Gangrenous parastomal hernia

K43.5 Parastomal hernia without obstruction or gangrene
Parastomal hernia NOS

K43.6 Other and unspecified ventral hernia with obstruction, without gangrene
Epigastric hernia causing obstruction, without gangrene
Hypogastric hernia causing obstruction, without gangrene
Incarcerated epigastric hernia without gangrene
Incarcerated hypogastric hernia without gangrene
Incarcerated midline hernia without gangrene
Incarcerated spigelian hernia without gangrene
Incarcerated subxiphoid hernia without gangrene
Irreducible epigastric hernia without gangrene
Irreducible hypogastric hernia without gangrene
Irreducible midline hernia without gangrene
Irreducible spigelian hernia without gangrene
Irreducible subxiphoid hernia without gangrene
Midline hernia causing obstruction, without gangrene
Spigelian hernia causing obstruction, without gangrene
Strangulated epigastric hernia without gangrene
Strangulated hypogastric hernia without gangrene
Strangulated midline hernia without gangrene
Strangulated spigelian hernia without gangrene
Strangulated subxiphoid hernia without gangrene
Subxiphoid hernia causing obstruction, without gangrene

K43.7 Other and unspecified ventral hernia with gangrene
Any condition listed under K43.6 specified as gangrenous

K43.9 Ventral hernia without obstruction or gangrene
Epigastric hernia
Ventral hernia NOS

K44 Diaphragmatic hernia
Includes: hiatus hernia (esophageal) (sliding)
paraesophageal hernia
Excludes 1: congenital diaphragmatic hernia (Q79.0)
congenital hiatus hernia (Q40.1)

K44.0 Diaphragmatic hernia with obstruction, without gangrene
Diaphragmatic hernia causing obstruction
Incarcerated diaphragmatic hernia
Irreducible diaphragmatic hernia
Strangulated diaphragmatic hernia

K44.1 Diaphragmatic hernia with gangrene
Gangrenous diaphragmatic hernia

K44.9 Diaphragmatic hernia without obstruction or gangrene
Diaphragmatic hernia NOS

K45 Other abdominal hernia

　● New code　　▲ Revised code　　⑦ 7th digit required　　⊗ Placeholder required

Includes: abdominal hernia, specified site NEC
　lumbar hernia
　　　obturator hernia
　　　pudendal hernia
　　　retroperitoneal hernia
　　　sciatic hernia

K45.0 Other specified abdominal hernia with obstruction, without gangrene
　　　Other specified abdominal hernia causing obstruction
　　　Other specified incarcerated abdominal hernia
　　　Other specified irreducible abdominal hernia
　　　Other specified strangulated abdominal hernia

K45.1 Other specified abdominal hernia with gangrene
　　　Any condition listed under K45specified as gangrenous

K45.8 Other specified abdominal hernia without obstruction or gangrene

K46 Unspecified abdominal hernia
　Includes: enterocele
　　　epiplocele
　　　hernia NOS
　　　interstitial hernia
　　　intestinal hernia
　　　intra-abdominal hernia
　Excludes 1: vaginal enterocele (N81.5)

K46.0 Unspecified abdominal hernia with obstruction, without gangrene
　　　Unspecified abdominal hernia causing obstruction
　　　Unspecified incarcerated abdominal hernia
　　　Unspecified irreducible abdominal hernia
　　　Unspecified strangulated abdominal hernia

K46.1 Unspecified abdominal hernia with gangrene
　　　Any condition listed under K46specified as gangrenous

K46.9 Unspecified abdominal hernia without obstruction or gangrene
　　　Abdominal hernia NOS

NONINFECTIVE ENTERITIS AND COLITIS (K50-K52)

Includes: noninfective inflammatory bowel disease
Excludes 1: irritable bowel syndrome (K58.-)
　megacolon (K59.3)

K50 Crohn's disease [regional enteritis]
　Includes: granulomatous enteritis
　Use additional code to identify manifestations, such as:
　pyoderma gangrenosum (L88)
　Excludes 1: ulcerative colitis (K51.-)

K50.0 Crohn's disease of small intestine
　　　Crohn's disease [regional enteritis] of duodenum
　　　Crohn's disease [regional enteritis] of ileum
　　　Crohn's disease [regional enteritis] of jejunum
　　　Regional ileitis
　　　Terminal ileitis
　　Excludes 1: Crohn's disease of both small and large intestine (K50.8-)

K50.00 Crohn's disease of small intestine without complications

K50.01 Crohn's disease of small intestine with complications
　　　K50.011 Crohn's disease of small intestine with rectal bleeding
　　　K50.012 Crohn's disease of small intestine with intestinal obstruction
　　　K50.013 Crohn's disease of small intestine with fistula

K50.014 Crohn's disease of small intestine with abscess
K50.018 Crohn's disease of small intestine with other complication
K50.019 Crohn's disease of small intestine with unspecified complications

K50.1 Crohn's disease of large intestine
　　Crohn's disease [regional enteritis] of colon
　　Crohn's disease [regional enteritis] of large bowel
　　Crohn's disease [regional enteritis] of rectum
　　Granulomatous colitis
　　Regional colitis
　Excludes 1: Crohn's disease of both small and large intestine (K50.8)

K50.10 Crohn's disease of large intestine without complications

K50.11 Crohn's disease of large intestine with complications
　　　K50.111 Crohn's disease of large intestine with rectal bleeding
　　　K50.112 Crohn's disease of large intestine with intestinal obstruction
　　　K50.113 Crohn's disease of large intestine with fistula
　　　K50.114 Crohn's disease of large intestine with abscess
　　　K50.118 Crohn's disease of large intestine with other complication
　　　K50.119 Crohn's disease of large intestine with unspecified complications

K50.8 Crohn's disease of both small and large intestine
　K50.80 Crohn's disease of both small and large intestine without complications
　K50.81 Crohn's disease of both small and large intestine with complications
　　　K50.811 Crohn's disease of both small and large intestine with rectal bleeding
　　　K50.812 Crohn's disease of both small and large intestine with intestinal obstruction
　　　K50.813 Crohn's disease of both small and large intestine with fistula
　　　K50.814 Crohn's disease of both small and large intestine with abscess
　　　K50.818 Crohn's disease of both small and large intestine with other complication
　　　K50.819 Crohn's disease of both small and large intestine with unspecified complications

K50.9 Crohn's disease, unspecified
　K50.90 Crohn's disease, unspecified, without complications
　　　Crohn's disease NOS
　　　Regional enteritis NOS
　K50.91 Crohn's disease, unspecified, with complications
　　　K50.911 Crohn's disease, unspecified, with rectal bleeding
　　　K50.912 Crohn's disease, unspecified, with intestinal obstruction
　　　K50.913 Crohn's disease, unspecified, with fistula
　　　K50.914 Crohn's disease, unspecified, with abscess

K50.918   Crohn's disease, unspecified, with other complication

K50.919   Crohn's disease, unspecified, with unspecified complications

K51   Ulcerative colitis

Use additional code to identify manifestations, such as:
     pyoderma gangrenosum (L88)

Excludes 1: Crohn's disease [regional enteritis] (K50.-)

K51.0   Ulcerative (chronic) pancolitis
     Backwash ileitis

   K51.00   Ulcerative (chronic) pancolitis without complications
       Ulcerative (chronic) pancolitis NOS

   K51.01   Ulcerative (chronic) pancolitis with complications

     K51.011   Ulcerative (chronic) pancolitis with rectal bleeding

     K51.012   Ulcerative (chronic) pancolitis with intestinal obstruction

     K51.013   Ulcerative (chronic) pancolitis with fistula

     K51.014   Ulcerative (chronic) pancolitis with abscess

     K51.018   Ulcerative (chronic) pancolitis with other complication

     K51.019   Ulcerative (chronic) pancolitis with unspecified complications

K51.2   Ulcerative (chronic) proctitis

   K51.20   Ulcerative (chronic) proctitis without complications
       Ulcerative (chronic) proctitis NOS

   K51.21   Ulcerative (chronic) proctitis with complications

     K51.211   Ulcerative (chronic) proctitis with rectal bleeding

     K51.212   Ulcerative (chronic) proctitis with intestinal obstruction

     K51.213   Ulcerative (chronic) proctitis with fistula

     K51.214   Ulcerative (chronic) proctitis with abscess

     K51.218   Ulcerative (chronic) proctitis with other complication

     K51.219   Ulcerative (chronic) proctitis with unspecified complications

K51.3   Ulcerative (chronic) rectosigmoiditis

   K51.30   Ulcerative (chronic) rectosigmoiditis without complications
       Ulcerative (chronic) rectosigmoiditis NOS

   K51.31   Ulcerative (chronic) rectosigmoiditis with complications

     K51.311   Ulcerative (chronic) rectosigmoiditis with rectal bleeding

     K51.312   Ulcerative (chronic) rectosigmoiditis with intestinal obstruction

     K51.313   Ulcerative (chronic) rectosigmoiditis with fistula

     K51.314   Ulcerative (chronic) rectosigmoiditis with abscess

     K51.318   Ulcerative (chronic) rectosigmoiditis with other complication

     K51.319   Ulcerative (chronic) rectosigmoiditis with unspecified complications

K51.4   Inflammatory polyps of colon

   Excludes 1: adenomatous polyp of colon (D12.6)

       polyposis of colon (D12.6)
       polyps of colon NOS (K63.5)

K51.40   Inflammatory polyps of colon without complications
     Inflammatory polyps of colon NOS

K51.41   Inflammatory polyps of colon with complications

   K51.411   Inflammatory polyps of colon with rectal bleeding

   K51.412   Inflammatory polyps of colon with intestinal obstruction

   K51.413   Inflammatory polyps of colon with fistula

   K51.414   Inflammatory polyps of colon with abscess

   K51.418   Inflammatory polyps of colon with other complication

   K51.419   Inflammatory polyps of colon with unspecified complications

K51.5   Left sided colitis
     Left hemicolitis

   K51.50   Left sided colitis without complications
       Left sided colitis NOS

   K51.51   Left sided colitis with complications

     K51.511   Left sided colitis with rectal bleeding

     K51.512   Left sided colitis with intestinal obstruction

     K51.513   Left sided colitis with fistula

     K51.514   Left sided colitis with abscess

     K51.518   Left sided colitis with other complication

     K51.519   Left sided colitis with unspecified complications

K51.8   Other ulcerative colitis

   K51.80   Other ulcerative colitis without complications

   K51.81   Other ulcerative colitis with complications

     K51.811   Other ulcerative colitis with rectal bleeding

     K51.812   Other ulcerative colitis with intestinal obstruction

     K51.813   Other ulcerative colitis with fistula

     K51.814   Other ulcerative colitis with abscess

     K51.818   Other ulcerative colitis with other complication

     K51.819   Other ulcerative colitis with unspecified complications

K51.9   Ulcerative colitis, unspecified

   K51.90   Ulcerative colitis, unspecified, without complications

   K51.91   Ulcerative colitis, unspecified, with complications

     K51.911   Ulcerative colitis, unspecified with rectal bleeding

     K51.912   Ulcerative colitis, unspecified with intestinal obstruction

     K51.913   Ulcerative colitis, unspecified with fistula

     K51.914   Ulcerative colitis, unspecified with abscess

     K51.918   Ulcerative colitis, unspecified with other complication

     K51.919   Ulcerative colitis, unspecified with unspecified complications

K52   Other and unspecified noninfective gastroenteritis and colitis

K52.0 Gastroenteritis and colitis due to radiation

K52.1 Toxic gastroenteritis and colitis

Drug-induced gastroenteritis and colitis

Code first (T51-T65) to identify toxic agent

Use additional code for adverse effect, if applicable, to identify drug (T36-T50 with fifth or sixth character 5)

K52.2 Allergic and dietetic gastroenteritis and colitis

Food hypersensitivity gastroenteritis or colitis

Use additional code to identify type of food allergy (Z91.01-, Z91.02-)

K52.8 Other specified noninfective gastroenteritis and colitis

K52.81 Eosinophilic gastritis or gastroenteritis

Eosinophilic enteritis

Excludes 1: eosinophilic esophagitis (K20.0)

K52.82 Eosinophilic colitis

K52.89 Other specified noninfective gastroenteritis and colitis

Collagenous colitis

Lymphocytic colitis

Microscopic colitis (collagenous or lymphocytic)

K52.9 Noninfective gastroenteritis and colitis, unspecified

Colitis NOS

Enteritis NOS

Gastroenteritis NOS

Ileitis NOS

Jejunitis NOS

Sigmoiditis NOS

Excludes 1: diarrhea NOS (R19.7)

functional diarrhea (K59.1)

infectious gastroenteritis and colitis NOS (A09)

neonatal diarrhea (noninfective) (P78.3)

psychogenic diarrhea (F45.8)

OTHER DISEASES OF INTESTINES (K55-K64)

K55 Vascular disorders of intestine

Excludes 1: necrotizing enterocolitis of newborn (P77.-)

K55.0 Acute vascular disorders of intestine

Acute fulminant ischemic colitis

Acute intestinal infarction

Acute small intestine ischemia

Infarction of appendices epiploicae

Mesenteric (artery) (vein) embolism

Mesenteric (artery) (vein) infarction

Mesenteric (artery) (vein) thrombosis

Necrosis of intestine

Subacute ischemic colitis

K55.1 Chronic vascular disorders of intestine

Chronic ischemic colitis

Chronic ischemic enteritis

Chronic ischemic enterocolitis

Ischemic stricture of intestine

Mesenteric atherosclerosis

Mesenteric vascular insufficiency

K55.2 Angiodysplasia of colon

K55.20 Angiodysplasia of colon without hemorrhage

K55.21 Angiodysplasia of colon with hemorrhage

K55.8 Other vascular disorders of intestine

K55.9 Vascular disorder of intestine, unspecified

Ischemic colitis

Ischemic enteritis

Ischemic enterocolitis

K56 Paralytic ileus and intestinal obstruction without hernia

Excludes 1: congenital stricture or stenosis of intestine (Q41-Q42)

cystic fibrosis with meconium ileus (E84.11)

ischemic stricture of intestine (K55.1)

meconium ileus NOS (P76.0)

neonatal intestinal obstructions classifiable to P76.-

obstruction of duodenum (K31.5)

postprocedural intestinal obstruction (K91.3)

stenosis of anus or rectum (K62.4)

intestinal obstruction with hernia (K40-K46)

K56.0 Paralytic ileus

Paralysis of bowel

Paralysis of colon

Paralysis of intestine

Excludes 1: gallstone ileus (K56.3)

ileus NOS (K56.7)

obstructive ileus NOS (K56.69)

K56.1 Intussusception

Intussusception or invagination of bowel

Intussusception or invagination of colon

Intussusception or invagination of intestine

Intussusception or invagination of rectum

Excludes 2: intussusception of appendix (K38.8)

K56.2 Volvulus

Strangulation of colon or intestine

Torsion of colon or intestine

Twist of colon or intestine

Excludes 2: volvulus of duodenum (K31.5)

K56.3 Gallstone ileus

Obstruction of intestine by gallstone

K56.4 Other impaction of intestine

K56.41 Fecal impaction

Excludes 1: constipation (K59.0-)

incomplete defecation (R15.0)

K56.49 Other impaction of intestine

K56.5 Intestinal adhesions [bands] with obstruction (postprocedural) (postinfection)

Abdominal hernia due to adhesions with obstruction

Peritoneal adhesions [bands] with intestinal obstruction (postprocedural) (postinfection)

K56.6 Other and unspecified intestinal obstruction

K56.60 Unspecified intestinal obstruction

Intestinal obstruction NOS

Excludes 1: intestinal obstruction due to specified condition-code to condition

K56.69 Other intestinal obstruction

Enterostenosis NOS

Obstructive ileus NOS

Occlusion of colon or intestine NOS

Stenosis of colon or intestine NOS

Stricture of colon or intestine NOS

Excludes 1: intestinal obstruction due to specified condition-code to condition

K56.7 Ileus, unspecified

Excludes 1: obstructive ileus (K56.69)

K57 Diverticular disease of intestine

Excludes 1: congenital diverticulum of intestine (Q43.8)

Meckel's diverticulum (Q43.0)

Excludes 2: diverticulum of appendix (K38.2)

K57.0 Diverticulitis of small intestine with perforation and abscess

Diverticulitis of small intestine with peritonitis

| | Add 4th-7th digits | | 3 digit reportable | | Nonspecific code | | Unspecified code | | Manifestation code | 335 |

Excludes 1: diverticulitis of both small and large intestine with perforation and abscess (K57.4-)

K57.00 Diverticulitis of small intestine with perforation and abscess without bleeding

K57.01 Diverticulitis of small intestine with perforation and abscess with bleeding

K57.1 Diverticular disease of small intestine without perforation or abscess

Excludes 1: diverticular disease of both small and large intestine without perforation or abscess (K57.5-)

K57.10 Diverticulosis of small intestine without perforation or abscess without bleeding
Diverticular disease of small intestine NOS

K57.11 Diverticulosis of small intestine without perforation or abscess with bleeding

K57.12 Diverticulitis of small intestine without perforation or abscess without bleeding

K57.13 Diverticulitis of small intestine without perforation or abscess with bleeding

K57.2 Diverticulitis of large intestine with perforation and abscess
Diverticulitis of colon with peritonitis

Excludes 1: diverticulitis of both small and large intestine with perforation and abscess (K57.4-)

K57.20 Diverticulitis of large intestine with perforation and abscess without bleeding

K57.21 Diverticulitis of large intestine with perforation and abscess with bleeding

K57.3 Diverticular disease of large intestine without perforation or abscess

Excludes 1: diverticular disease of both small and large intestine without perforation or abscess (K57.5-)

K57.30 Diverticulosis of large intestine without perforation or abscess without bleeding
Diverticular disease of colon NOS

K57.31 Diverticulosis of large intestine without perforation or abscess with bleeding

K57.32 Diverticulitis of large intestine without perforation or abscess without bleeding

K57.33 Diverticulitis of large intestine without perforation or abscess with bleeding

K57.4 Diverticulitis of both small and large intestine with perforation and abscess
Diverticulitis of both small and large intestine with peritonitis

K57.40 Diverticulitis of both small and large intestine with perforation and abscess without bleeding

K57.41 Diverticulitis of both small and large intestine with perforation and abscess with bleeding

K57.5 Diverticular disease of both small and large intestine without perforation or abscess

K57.50 Diverticulosis of both small and large intestine without perforation or abscess without bleeding
Diverticular disease of both small and large intestine NOS

K57.51 Diverticulosis of both small and large intestine without perforation or abscess with bleeding

K57.52 Diverticulitis of both small and large intestine without perforation or abscess without bleeding

K57.53 Diverticulitis of both small and large intestine without perforation or abscess with bleeding

K57.8 Diverticulitis of intestine, part unspecified, with perforation and abscess
Diverticulitis of intestine NOS with peritonitis

K57.80 Diverticulitis of intestine, part unspecified, with perforation and abscess without bleeding

K57.81 Diverticulitis of intestine, part unspecified, with perforation and abscess with bleeding

K57.9 Diverticular disease of intestine, part unspecified, without perforation or abscess

K57.90 Diverticulosis of intestine, part unspecified, without perforation or abscess without bleeding
Diverticular disease of intestine NOS

K57.91 Diverticulosis of intestine, part unspecified, without perforation or abscess with bleeding

K57.92 Diverticulitis of intestine, part unspecified, without perforation or abscess without bleeding

K57.93 Diverticulitis of intestine, part unspecified, without perforation or abscess with bleeding

K58 Irritable bowel syndrome
Includes: irritable colon
spastic colon

K58.0 Irritable bowel syndrome with diarrhea

K58.9 Irritable bowel syndrome without diarrhea
Irritable bowel syndrome NOS

K59 Other functional intestinal disorders
Excludes 1: change in bowel habit NOS (R19.4)
intestinal malabsorption (K90.-)
psychogenic intestinal disorders (F45.8)
Excludes 2: functional disorders of stomach (K31.-)

K59.0 Constipation
Excludes 1: fecal impaction (K56.41)
incomplete defecation (R15.0)

K59.00 Constipation, unspecified

K59.01 Slow transit constipation

K59.02 Outlet dysfunction constipation

K59.09 Other constipation

K59.1 Functional diarrhea
Excludes 1: diarrhea NOS (R19.7)
irritable bowel syndrome with diarrhea (K58.0)

K59.2 Neurogenic bowel, not elsewhere classified

K59.3 Megacolon, not elsewhere classified
Dilatation of colon
Toxic megacolon
Code first (T51-T65) to identify toxic agent
Excludes 1: congenital megacolon (aganglionic) (Q43.1)
megacolon (due to) (in) Chagas' disease (B57.32)
megacolon (due to) (in) Clostridium difficile (A04.7)
megacolon (due to) (in) Hirschsprung's disease (Q43.1)

K59.4 Anal spasm
Proctalgia fugax

K59.8 Other specified functional intestinal disorders
Atony of colon
Pseudo-obstruction (acute) (chronic) of intestine

K59.9 Functional intestinal disorder, unspecified

K60 Fissure and fistula of anal and rectal regions
Excludes 1: fissure and fistula of anal and rectal regions with abscess or cellulitis (K61.-)
Excludes 2: anal sphincter tear (healed) (nontraumatic) (old) (K62.81)

K60.0 Acute anal fissure

K60.1 Chronic anal fissure

K60.2 Anal fissure, unspecified

K60.3 Anal fistula

K60.4 Rectal fistula
Fistula of rectum to skin
Excludes 1: rectovaginal fistula (N82.3)
vesicorectal fistula (N32.1)

K60.5 Anorectal fistula

K61 Abscess of anal and rectal regions
Includes: abscess of anal and rectal regions
cellulitis of anal and rectal regions

K61.0 Anal abscess
Perianal abscess
Excludes 1: intrasphincteric abscess (K61.4)

K61.1 Rectal abscess
Perirectal abscess
Excludes 1: ischiorectal abscess (K61.3)

K61.2 Anorectal abscess

K61.3 Ischiorectal abscess
Abscess of ischiorectal fossa

K61.4 Intrasphincteric abscess

K62 Other diseases of anus and rectum
Includes: anal canal
Excludes 2: colostomy and enterostomy malfunction (K94.0-, K94.1-)
fecal incontinence (R15-)
hemorrhoids (K64.-)

K62.0 Anal polyp

K62.1 Rectal polyp
Excludes 1: adenomatous polyp (D12.8)

K62.2 Anal prolapse
Prolapse of anal canal

K62.3 Rectal prolapse
Prolapse of rectal mucosa

K62.4 Stenosis of anus and rectum
Stricture of anus (sphincter)

K62.5 Hemorrhage of anus and rectum
Excludes 1: gastrointestinal bleeding NOS (K92.2)
melena (K92.1)
neonatal rectal hemorrhage (P54.2)

K62.6 Ulcer of anus and rectum
Solitary ulcer of anus and rectum
Stercoral ulcer of anus and rectum
Excludes 1: fissure and fistula of anus and rectum (K60.-)
ulcerative colitis (K51.-)

K62.7 Radiation proctitis
Use additional code to identify the type of radiation (W90.-)

K62.8 Other specified diseases of anus and rectum
Excludes 2: ulcerative proctitis (K51.2)

  K62.81 Anal sphincter tear (healed) (nontraumatic) (old)
  Tear of anus, nontraumatic
  Use additional code for any associated fecal incontinence (R15-)
  Excludes 2: anal fissure (K60.-)
  anal sphincter tear (healed) (old) complicating delivery (O34.7-)
  traumatic tear of anal sphincter (S31.831)

  K62.82 Dysplasia of anus
  Anal intraepithelial neoplasia I and II (AIN I and II) (histologically confirmed)
  Dysplasia of anus NOS
  Mild and moderate dysplasia of anus (histologically confirmed)

Excludes 1: abnormal results from anal cytologic examination without histologic confirmation (R85.61-)
anal intraepithelial neoplasia III (D01.3)
carcinoma in situ of anus (D01.3)
HGSIL of anus (R85.613)
severe dysplasia of anus (D01.3)

  K62.89 Other specified diseases of anus and rectum
  Proctitis NOS
  Use additional code for any associated fecal incontinence (R15-)

K62.9 Disease of anus and rectum, unspecified

K63 Other diseases of intestine

K63.0 Abscess of intestine
Excludes 1: abscess of intestine with Crohn's disease (K50.014, K50.114, K50.814, K50.914,)
abscess of intestine with diverticular disease (K57.0, K57.2, K57.4, K57.8)
abscess of intestine with ulcerative colitis (K51.014, K51.114, K51.214, K51.314, K51.414, K51.514, K51.814, K51.914)
Excludes 2: abscess of anal and rectal regions (K61.-)
abscess of appendix (K35.3)

K63.1 Perforation of intestine (nontraumatic)
Perforation (nontraumatic) of rectum
Excludes 1: perforation (nontraumatic) of duodenum (K26.-)
perforation (nontraumatic) of intestine with diverticular disease (K57.0, K57.2, K57.4, K57.8)
Excludes 2: perforation (nontraumatic) of appendix (K35.2, K35.3)

K63.2 Fistula of intestine
Excludes 1: fistula of duodenum (K31.6)
fistula of intestine with Crohn's disease (K50.013, K50.113, K50.813, K50.913,)
fistula of intestine with ulcerative colitis (K51.013, K51.113, K51.213, K51.313, K51.413, K51.513, K51.813, K51.913)
Excludes 2: fistula of anal and rectal regions (K60.-)
fistula of appendix (K38.3)
intestinal-genital fistula, female (N82.2-N82.4)
vesicointestinal fistula (N32.1)

K63.3 Ulcer of intestine
Primary ulcer of small intestine
Excludes 1: duodenal ulcer (K26.-)
gastrointestinal ulcer (K28.-)
gastrojejunal ulcer (K28.-)
jejunal ulcer (K28.-)
peptic ulcer, site unspecified (K27.-)
ulcer of intestine with perforation (K63.1)
ulcer of anus or rectum (K62.6)
ulcerative colitis (K51.-)

K63.4 Enteroptosis

K63.5 Polyp of colon
Excludes 1: adenomatous polyp of colon (D12.6)
inflammatory polyp of colon (K51.4-)
polyposis of colon (D12.6)

K63.8 Other specified diseases of intestine

  K63.81 Dieulafoy lesion of intestine
  Excludes 2: Dieulafoy lesion of stomach and duodenum (K31.82)

  K63.89 Other specified diseases of intestine

K63.9 Disease of intestine, unspecified

K64 Hemorrhoids and perianal venous thrombosis
Includes: piles
Excludes 1: hemorrhoids complicating childbirth and the
puerperium (O87.2)
hemorrhoids complicating pregnancy (O22.4)

K64.0 First degree hemorrhoids
Grade/stage I hemorrhoids
Hemorrhoids (bleeding) without prolapse outside of anal
canal

K64.1 Second degree hemorrhoids
Grade/stage II hemorrhoids
Hemorrhoids (bleeding) that prolapse with straining, but
retract spontaneously

K64.2 Third degree hemorrhoids
Grade/stage III hemorrhoids
Hemorrhoids (bleeding) that prolapse with straining and
require manual replacement back inside anal canal

K64.3 Fourth degree hemorrhoids
Grade/stage IV hemorrhoids
Hemorrhoids (bleeding) with prolapsed tissue that cannot
be manually replaced

K64.4 Residual hemorrhoidal skin tags
External hemorrhoids, NOS
Skin tags of anus

K64.5 Perianal venous thrombosis
External hemorrhoids with thrombosis
Perianal hematoma
Thrombosed hemorrhoids NOS

K64.8 Other hemorrhoids
Internal hemorrhoids, without mention of degree
Prolapsed hemorrhoids, degree not specified

K64.9 Unspecified hemorrhoids
Hemorrhoids (bleeding) NOS
Hemorrhoids (bleeding) without mention of degree

DISEASES OF PERITONEUM AND RETROPERITONEUM (K65-K68)

K65 Peritonitis
Use additional code (B95-B97), to identify infectious agent
Excludes 1: acute appendicitis with generalized peritonitis (K35.2)
aseptic peritonitis (T81.6)
benign paroxysmal peritonitis (E85.0)
chemical peritonitis (T81.6)
diverticulitis of both small and large intestine with
peritonitis (K57.4-)
diverticulitis of colon with peritonitis (K57.2-)
diverticulitis of intestine, NOS, with peritonitis (K57.8-)
diverticulitis of small intestine with peritonitis (K57.0-)
gonococcal peritonitis (A54.85)
neonatal peritonitis (P78.0-P78.1)
pelvic peritonitis, female (N73.3-N73.5)
periodic familial peritonitis (E85.0)
peritonitis due to talc or other foreign substance (T81.6)
peritonitis in chlamydia (A74.81)
peritonitis in diphtheria (A36.89)
peritonitis in syphilis (late) (A52.74)
peritonitis in tuberculosis (A18.31)
peritonitis with or following abortion or ectopic or molar
pregnancy (O00-O07, O08.0)
peritonitis with or following appendicitis (K35.-)
peritonitis with or following diverticular disease of
intestine (K57.-)

puerperal peritonitis (O85)
retroperitoneal infections (K68.-)

K65.0 Generalized (acute) peritonitis
Pelvic peritonitis (acute), male
Subphrenic peritonitis (acute)
Suppurative peritonitis (acute)

K65.1 Peritoneal abscess
Abdominopelvic abscess
Abscess (of) omentum
Abscess (of) peritoneum
Mesenteric abscess
Retrocecal abscess
Subdiaphragmatic abscess
Subhepatic abscess
Subphrenic abscess

K65.2 Spontaneous bacterial peritonitis
Excludes 1: bacterial peritonitis NOS K65.9

K65.3 Choleperitonitis
Peritonitis due to bile

K65.4 Sclerosing mesenteritis
Fat necrosis of peritoneum
(Idiopathic) sclerosing mesenteric fibrosis
Mesenteric lipodystrophy
Mesenteric panniculitis
Retractile mesenteritis

K65.8 Other peritonitis
Chronic proliferative peritonitis
Peritonitis due to urine

K65.9 Peritonitis, unspecified
Bacterial peritonitis NOS

K66 Other disorders of peritoneum
Excludes 2: ascites (R18.-)
peritoneal effusion (chronic) (R18.8)

K66.0 Peritoneal adhesions (postprocedural) (postinfection)
Adhesions (of) abdominal (wall)
Adhesions (of) diaphragm
Adhesions (of) intestine
Adhesions (of) male pelvis
Adhesions (of) omentum
Adhesions (of) stomach
Adhesive bands
Mesenteric adhesions
Excludes 1: female pelvic adhesions [bands] (N73.6)
peritoneal adhesions with intestinal obstruction
(K56.5)

K66.1 Hemoperitoneum
Excludes 1: traumatic hemoperitoneum (S36.8-)

K66.8 Other specified disorders of peritoneum

K66.9 Disorder of peritoneum, unspecified

K67 Disorders of peritoneum in infectious diseases classified elsewhere
Code first underlying disease, such as :
congenital syphilis (A50.0)
helminthiasis (B65.0 - B83.9)
Excludes 1: peritonitis in chlamydia (A74.81)
peritonitis in diphtheria (A36.89)
peritonitis in gonococcal (A54.85)
peritonitis in syphilis (late) (A52.74)
peritonitis in tuberculosis (A18.31)

K68 Disorders of retroperitoneum

K68.1 Retroperitoneal abscess

K68.11 Postprocedural retroperitoneal abscess

K68.12 Psoas muscle abscess

K68.19   Other retroperitoneal abscess

K68.9   Other disorders of retroperitoneum

DISEASES OF LIVER (K70-K77)

Excludes 1: jaundice NOS (R17)

Excludes 2: hemochromatosis (E83.11-)

Reye's syndrome (G93.7)

viral hepatitis (B15-B19)

Wilson's disease (E83.0)

K70   Alcoholic liver disease

Use additional code to identify:

alcohol abuse and dependence (F10.-)

K70.0   Alcoholic fatty liver

K70.1   Alcoholic hepatitis

K70.10   Alcoholic hepatitis without ascites

K70.11   Alcoholic hepatitis with ascites

K70.2   Alcoholic fibrosis and sclerosis of liver

K70.3   Alcoholic cirrhosis of liver

Alcoholic cirrhosis NOS

K70.30   Alcoholic cirrhosis of liver without ascites

K70.31   Alcoholic cirrhosis of liver with ascites

K70.4   Alcoholic hepatic failure

Acute alcoholic hepatic failure

Alcoholic hepatic failure NOS

Chronic alcoholic hepatic failure

Subacute alcoholic hepatic failure

K70.40   Alcoholic hepatic failure without coma

K70.41   Alcoholic hepatic failure with coma

K70.9   Alcoholic liver disease, unspecified

K71   Toxic liver disease

Includes: drug-induced idiosyncratic (unpredictable) liver disease

drug-induced toxic (predictable) liver disease

Code first poisoning due to drug or toxin, if applicable (T36-T65 with fifth or sixth character 1-4 or 6)

Use additional code for adverse effect, if applicable, to identify drug (T36-T50 with fifth or sixth character 5)

Excludes 2: alcoholic liver disease (K70.-)

Budd-Chiari syndrome (I82.0)

K71.0   Toxic liver disease with cholestasis

Cholestasis with hepatocyte injury

'Pure' cholestasis

K71.1   Toxic liver disease with hepatic necrosis

Hepatic failure (acute) (chronic) due to drugs

K71.10   Toxic liver disease with hepatic necrosis, without coma

K71.11   Toxic liver disease with hepatic necrosis, with coma

K71.2   Toxic liver disease with acute hepatitis

K71.3   Toxic liver disease with chronic persistent hepatitis

K71.4   Toxic liver disease with chronic lobular hepatitis

K71.5   Toxic liver disease with chronic active hepatitis

Toxic liver disease with lupoid hepatitis

K71.50   Toxic liver disease with chronic active hepatitis without ascites

K71.51   Toxic liver disease with chronic active hepatitis with ascites

K71.6   Toxic liver disease with hepatitis, not elsewhere classified

K71.7   Toxic liver disease with fibrosis and cirrhosis of liver

K71.8   Toxic liver disease with other disorders of liver

Toxic liver disease with focal nodular hyperplasia

Toxic liver disease with hepatic granulomas

Toxic liver disease with peliosis hepatis

Toxic liver disease with veno-occlusive disease of liver

K71.9   Toxic liver disease, unspecified

K72   Hepatic failure, not elsewhere classified

Includes: acute hepatitis NEC, with hepatic failure

fulminant hepatitis NEC, with hepatic failure

hepatic encephalopathy NOS

liver (cell) necrosis with hepatic failure

malignant hepatitis NEC, with hepatic failure

yellow liver atrophy or dystrophy

Excludes 1: alcoholic hepatic failure (K70.4)

hepatic failure complicating abortion or ectopic or molar pregnancy (O00-O07, O08.8)

hepatic failure complicating pregnancy, childbirth and the puerperium (O26.6-)

hepatic failure with toxic liver disease (K71.1-)

icterus of newborn (P55-P59)

postprocedural hepatic failure (K91.82)

viral hepatitis with hepatic coma (B15-B19)

K72.0   Acute and subacute hepatic failure

K72.00   Acute and subacute hepatic failure without coma

K72.01   Acute and subacute hepatic failure with coma

K72.1   Chronic hepatic failure

K72.10   Chronic hepatic failure without coma

K72.11   Chronic hepatic failure with coma

K72.9   Hepatic failure, unspecified

K72.90   Hepatic failure, unspecified without coma

K72.91   Hepatic failure, unspecified with coma

Hepatic coma NOS

K73   Chronic hepatitis, not elsewhere classified

Excludes 1: alcoholic hepatitis (chronic) (K70.1-)

drug-induced hepatitis (chronic) (K71.-)

granulomatous hepatitis (chronic) NEC (K75.3)

reactive, nonspecific hepatitis (chronic) (K75.2)

viral hepatitis (chronic) (B15-B19)

K73.0   Chronic persistent hepatitis, not elsewhere classified

K73.1   Chronic lobular hepatitis, not elsewhere classified

K73.2   Chronic active hepatitis, not elsewhere classified

K73.8   Other chronic hepatitis, not elsewhere classified

K73.9   Chronic hepatitis, unspecified

K74   Fibrosis and cirrhosis of liver

Code also , if applicable, viral hepatitis (acute) (chronic) (B15-B19)

Excludes 1: alcoholic cirrhosis (of liver) (K70.3)

alcoholic fibrosis of liver (K70.2)

cardiac sclerosis of liver (K76.1)

cirrhosis (of liver) with toxic liver disease (K71.7)

congenital cirrhosis (of liver) (P78.81)

pigmentary cirrhosis (of liver) (E83.110)

K74.0   Hepatic fibrosis

K74.1   Hepatic sclerosis

K74.2   Hepatic fibrosis with hepatic sclerosis

K74.3   Primary biliary cirrhosis

Chronic nonsuppurative destructive cholangitis

K74.4   Secondary biliary cirrhosis

K74.5   Biliary cirrhosis, unspecified

K74.6   Other and unspecified cirrhosis of liver

K74.60   Unspecified cirrhosis of liver

Cirrhosis (of liver) NOS

K74.69   Other cirrhosis of liver

Cryptogenic cirrhosis (of liver)

Macronodular cirrhosis (of liver)

Micronodular cirrhosis (of liver)

Mixed type cirrhosis (of liver)

Portal cirrhosis (of liver)

Postnecrotic cirrhosis (of liver)

K75 Other inflammatory liver diseases

Excludes 2: toxic liver disease (K71.-)

K75.0 Abscess of liver

Cholangitic hepatic abscess

Hematogenic hepatic abscess

Hepatic abscess NOS

Lymphogenic hepatic abscess

Pylephlebitic hepatic abscess

Excludes 1: amebic liver abscess (A06.4)

cholangitis without liver abscess (K83.0)

pylephlebitis without liver abscess (K75.1)

K75.1 Phlebitis of portal vein

Pylephlebitis

Excludes 1: pylephlebitic liver abscess (K75.0)

K75.2 Nonspecific reactive hepatitis

Excludes 1: acute or subacute hepatitis (K72.0-)

chronic hepatitis NEC (K73.-)

viral hepatitis (B15-B19)

K75.3 Granulomatous hepatitis, not elsewhere classified

Excludes 1: acute or subacute hepatitis (K72.0-)

chronic hepatitis NEC (K73.-)

viral hepatitis (B15-B19)

K75.4 Autoimmune hepatitis

Lupoid hepatitis NEC

K75.8 Other specified inflammatory liver diseases

K75.81 Nonalcoholic steatohepatitis (NASH)

K75.89 Other specified inflammatory liver diseases

K75.9 Inflammatory liver disease, unspecified

Hepatitis NOS

Excludes 1: acute or subacute hepatitis (K72.0-)

chronic hepatitis NEC (K73.-)

viral hepatitis (B15-B19)

K76 Other diseases of liver

Excludes 2: alcoholic liver disease (K70.-)

amyloid degeneration of liver (E85-)

cystic disease of liver (congenital) (Q44.6)

hepatic vein thrombosis (I82.0)

hepatomegaly NOS (R16.0)

pigmentary cirrhosis (of liver) (E83.110)

portal vein thrombosis (I81)

toxic liver disease (K71.-)

K76.0 Fatty (change of) liver, not elsewhere classified

Nonalcoholic fatty liver disease (NAFLD)

Excludes 1: nonalcoholic steatohepatitis (NASH) (K75.81)

K76.1 Chronic passive congestion of liver

Cardiac cirrhosis

Cardiac sclerosis

K76.2 Central hemorrhagic necrosis of liver

Excludes 1: liver necrosis with hepatic failure (K72.-)

K76.3 Infarction of liver

K76.4 Peliosis hepatis

Hepatic angiomatosis

K76.5 Hepatic veno-occlusive disease

Excludes 1: Budd-Chiari syndrome (I82.0)

K76.6 Portal hypertension

Use additional code for any associated complications, such as:

portal hypertensive gastropathy (K31.89)

K76.7 Hepatorenal syndrome

Excludes 1: hepatorenal syndrome following labor and delivery (O90.4)

postprocedural hepatorenal syndrome (K91.82)

K76.8 Other specified diseases of liver

K76.81 Hepatopulmonary syndrome

Code first underlying liver disease, such as:

alcoholic cirrhosis of liver (K70.3-)

cirrhosis of liver without mention of alcohol (K74.6-)

K76.89 Other specified diseases of liver

Cyst (simple) of liver

Focal nodular hyperplasia of liver

Hepatoptosis

K76.9 Liver disease, unspecified

K77 Liver disorders in diseases classified elsewhere

Code first underlying disease, such as:

amyloidosis (E85-)

congenital syphilis (A50.0, A50.5)

congenital toxoplasmosis (P37.1)

schistosomiasis (B65.0-B65.9)

Excludes 1: alcoholic hepatitis (K70.1-)

alcoholic liver disease (K70.-)

cytomegaloviral hepatitis (B25.1)

herpesviral [herpes simplex] hepatitis (B00.81)

infectious mononucleosis with liver disease (B27.0-B27.9 with .9)

mumps hepatitis (B26.81)

sarcoidosis with liver disease (D86.89)

secondary syphilis with liver disease (A51.45)

syphilis (late) with liver disease (A52.74)

toxoplasmosis (acquired) hepatitis (B58.1)

tuberculosis with liver disease (A18.83)

DISORDERS OF GALLBLADDER, BILIARY TRACT AND PANCREAS (K80-K87)

K80 Cholelithiasis

Excludes 1: retained cholelithiasis following cholecystectomy (K91.86)

K80.0 Calculus of gallbladder with acute cholecystitis

Any condition listed in K80.2 with acute cholecystitis

K80.00 Calculus of gallbladder with acute cholecystitis without obstruction

K80.01 Calculus of gallbladder with acute cholecystitis with obstruction

K80.1 Calculus of gallbladder with other cholecystitis

K80.10 Calculus of gallbladder with chronic cholecystitis without obstruction

Cholelithiasis with cholecystitis NOS

K80.11 Calculus of gallbladder with chronic cholecystitis with obstruction

K80.12 Calculus of gallbladder with acute and chronic cholecystitis without obstruction

K80.13 Calculus of gallbladder with acute and chronic cholecystitis with obstruction

K80.18 Calculus of gallbladder with other cholecystitis without obstruction

K80.19 Calculus of gallbladder with other cholecystitis with obstruction

K80.2 Calculus of gallbladder without cholecystitis

Cholecystolithiasis without cholecystitis

Cholelithiasis (without cholecystitis)

Colic (recurrent) of gallbladder (without cholecystitis)

Gallstone (impacted) of cystic duct (without cholecystitis)

Gallstone (impacted) of gallbladder (without cholecystitis)

K80.20 Calculus of gallbladder without cholecystitis without obstruction

K80.21 Calculus of gallbladder without cholecystitis with obstruction

K80.3 Calculus of bile duct with cholangitis

Any condition listed in K80.5 with cholangitis

K80.30 Calculus of bile duct with cholangitis, unspecified, without obstruction

K80.31 Calculus of bile duct with cholangitis, unspecified, with obstruction

K80.32 Calculus of bile duct with acute cholangitis without obstruction

K80.33 Calculus of bile duct with acute cholangitis with obstruction

K80.34 Calculus of bile duct with chronic cholangitis without obstruction

K80.35 Calculus of bile duct with chronic cholangitis with obstruction

K80.36 Calculus of bile duct with acute and chronic cholangitis without obstruction

K80.37 Calculus of bile duct with acute and chronic cholangitis with obstruction

K80.4 Calculus of bile duct with cholecystitis

Any condition listed in K80.5 with cholecystitis (with cholangitis)

K80.40 Calculus of bile duct with cholecystitis, unspecified, without obstruction

K80.41 Calculus of bile duct with cholecystitis, unspecified, with obstruction

K80.42 Calculus of bile duct with acute cholecystitis without obstruction

K80.43 Calculus of bile duct with acute cholecystitis with obstruction

K80.44 Calculus of bile duct with chronic cholecystitis without obstruction

K80.45 Calculus of bile duct with chronic cholecystitis with obstruction

K80.46 Calculus of bile duct with acute and chronic cholecystitis without obstruction

K80.47 Calculus of bile duct with acute and chronic cholecystitis with obstruction

K80.5 Calculus of bile duct without cholangitis or cholecystitis

Choledocholithiasis (without cholangitis or cholecystitis)

Gallstone (impacted) of bile duct NOS (without cholangitis or cholecystitis)

Gallstone (impacted) of common duct (without cholangitis or cholecystitis)

Gallstone (impacted) of hepatic duct (without cholangitis or cholecystitis)

Hepatic cholelithiasis (without cholangitis or cholecystitis)

Hepatic colic (recurrent) (without cholangitis or cholecystitis)

K80.50 Calculus of bile duct without cholangitis or cholecystitis without obstruction

K80.51 Calculus of bile duct without cholangitis or cholecystitis with obstruction

K80.6 Calculus of gallbladder and bile duct with cholecystitis

K80.60 Calculus of gallbladder and bile duct with cholecystitis, unspecified, without obstruction

K80.61 Calculus of gallbladder and bile duct with cholecystitis, unspecified, with obstruction

K80.62 Calculus of gallbladder and bile duct with acute cholecystitis without obstruction

K80.63 Calculus of gallbladder and bile duct with acute cholecystitis with obstruction

K80.64 Calculus of gallbladder and bile duct with chronic cholecystitis without obstruction

K80.65 Calculus of gallbladder and bile duct with chronic cholecystitis with obstruction

K80.66 Calculus of gallbladder and bile duct with acute and chronic cholecystitis without obstruction

K80.67 Calculus of gallbladder and bile duct with acute and chronic cholecystitis with obstruction

K80.7 Calculus of gallbladder and bile duct without cholecystitis

K80.70 Calculus of gallbladder and bile duct without cholecystitis without obstruction

K80.71 Calculus of gallbladder and bile duct without cholecystitis with obstruction

K80.8 Other cholelithiasis

K80.80 Other cholelithiasis without obstruction

K80.81 Other cholelithiasis with obstruction

K81 Cholecystitis

Excludes 1: cholecystitis with cholelithiasis (K80.-)

K81.0 Acute cholecystitis

Abscess of gallbladder

Angiocholecystitis

Emphysematous (acute) cholecystitis

Empyema of gallbladder

Gangrene of gallbladder

Gangrenous cholecystitis

Suppurative cholecystitis

K81.1 Chronic cholecystitis

K81.2 Acute cholecystitis with chronic cholecystitis

K81.9 Cholecystitis, unspecified

K82 Other diseases of gallbladder

Excludes 1: nonvisualization of gallbladder (R93.2)

postcholecystectomy syndrome (K91.5)

K82.0 Obstruction of gallbladder

Occlusion of cystic duct or gallbladder without cholelithiasis

Stenosis of cystic duct or gallbladder without cholelithiasis

Stricture of cystic duct or gallbladder without cholelithiasis

Excludes 1: obstruction of gallbladder with cholelithiasis (K80.-)

K82.1 Hydrops of gallbladder

Mucocele of gallbladder

K82.2 Perforation of gallbladder

Rupture of cystic duct or gallbladder

K82.3 Fistula of gallbladder

Cholecystocolic fistula

Cholecystoduodenal fistula

K82.4 Cholesterolosis of gallbladder

Strawberry gallbladder

Excludes 1: cholesterolosis of gallbladder with cholecystitis (K81.-)

cholesterolosis of gallbladder with cholelithiasis (K80.-)

K82.8 Other specified diseases of gallbladder

Adhesions of cystic duct or gallbladder

Atrophy of cystic duct or gallbladder

Cyst of cystic duct or gallbladder

Dyskinesia of cystic duct or gallbladder

Hypertrophy of cystic duct or gallbladder

Nonfunctioning of cystic duct or gallbladder

Ulcer of cystic duct or gallbladder

K82.9 Disease of gallbladder, unspecified

K83 Other diseases of biliary tract

Excludes 1: postcholecystectomy syndrome (K91.5)

Excludes 2: conditions involving the gallbladder (K81-K82)

conditions involving the cystic duct (K81-K82)

K83.0 Cholangitis

Ascending cholangitis

Cholangitis NOS

Primary cholangitis

Recurrent cholangitis

Sclerosing cholangitis

Secondary cholangitis

Stenosing cholangitis

Suppurative cholangitis

Excludes 1: cholangitic liver abscess (K75.0)

cholangitis with choledocholithiasis (K80.3-, K80.4-)

chronic nonsuppurative destructive cholangitis (K74.3)

K83.1 Obstruction of bile duct

Occlusion of bile duct without cholelithiasis

Stenosis of bile duct without cholelithiasis

Stricture of bile duct without cholelithiasis

Excludes 1: congenital obstruction of bile duct (Q44.3)

obstruction of bile duct with cholelithiasis (K80.-)

K83.2 Perforation of bile duct

Rupture of bile duct

K83.3 Fistula of bile duct

Choledochoduodenal fistula

K83.4 Spasm of sphincter of Oddi

K83.5 Biliary cyst

K83.8 Other specified diseases of biliary tract

Adhesions of biliary tract

Atrophy of biliary tract

Hypertrophy of biliary tract

Ulcer of biliary tract

K83.9 Disease of biliary tract, unspecified

K85 Acute pancreatitis

Includes: abscess of pancreas

acute necrosis of pancreas

acute (recurrent) pancreatitis

gangrene of (gangrenous) pancreas

hemorrhagic pancreatitis

infective necrosis of pancreas

subacute pancreatitis

suppurative pancreatitis

K85.0 Idiopathic acute pancreatitis

K85.1 Biliary acute pancreatitis

Gallstone pancreatitis

K85.2 Alcohol induced acute pancreatitis

Excludes 2: alcohol induced chronic pancreatitis (K86.0)

K85.3 Drug induced acute pancreatitis

Use additional code for adverse effect, if applicable, to identify drug (T36-T50 with fifth or sixth character 5)

Use additional code to identify drug abuse and dependence (F11.- F17.-)

K85.8 Other acute pancreatitis

K85.9 Acute pancreatitis, unspecified

Pancreatitis NOS

K86 Other diseases of pancreas

Excludes 2: fibrocystic disease of pancreas (E84.-)

islet cell tumor (of pancreas) (D13.7)

pancreatic steatorrhea (K90.3)

K86.0 Alcohol-induced chronic pancreatitis

Use additional code to identify:

alcohol abuse and dependence (F10.-)

Excludes 2: alcohol induced acute pancreatitis (K85.2)

K86.1 Other chronic pancreatitis

Chronic pancreatitis NOS

Infectious chronic pancreatitis

Recurrent chronic pancreatitis

Relapsing chronic pancreatitis

K86.2 Cyst of pancreas

K86.3 Pseudocyst of pancreas

K86.8 Other specified diseases of pancreas

Aseptic pancreatic necrosis

Atrophy of pancreas

Calculus of pancreas

Cirrhosis of pancreas

Fibrosis of pancreas

Pancreatic fat necrosis

Pancreatic infantilism

Pancreatic necrosis NOS

K86.9 Disease of pancreas, unspecified

K87 Disorders of gallbladder, biliary tract and pancreas in diseases classified elsewhere

Code first underlying disease

Excludes 1: cytomegaloviral pancreatitis (B25.2)

mumps pancreatitis (B26.3)

syphilitic gallbladder (A52.74)

syphilitic pancreas (A52.74)

tuberculosis of gallbladder (A18.83)

tuberculosis of pancreas (A18.83)

OTHER DISEASES OF THE DIGESTIVE SYSTEM (K90-K95)

K90 Intestinal malabsorption

Excludes 1: intestinal malabsorption following gastrointestinal surgery (K91.2)

K90.0 Celiac disease

Gluten-sensitive enteropathy

Idiopathic steatorrhea

Nontropical sprue

K90.1 Tropical sprue

Sprue NOS

Tropical steatorrhea

K90.2 Blind loop syndrome, not elsewhere classified

Blind loop syndrome NOS

Excludes 1: congenital blind loop syndrome (Q43.8)

postsurgical blind loop syndrome (K91.2)

K90.3 Pancreatic steatorrhea

K90.4 Malabsorption due to intolerance, not elsewhere classified

Malabsorption due to intolerance to carbohydrate

Malabsorption due to intolerance to fat

Malabsorption due to intolerance to protein

Malabsorption due to intolerance to starch

Excludes 2: gluten-sensitive enteropathy (K90.0)

lactose intolerance (E73.-)

K90.8 Other intestinal malabsorption

K90.81 Whipple's disease

K90.89 Other intestinal malabsorption

K90.9 Intestinal malabsorption, unspecified

K91 Intraoperative and postprocedural complications and disorders of digestive system, not elsewhere classified

● New code ▲ Revised code ⑦ 7th digit required ⊗ Placeholder required

Excludes 2: complications of artificial opening of digestive system (K94.-)

complications of bariatric procedures (K95.-)

gastrojejunal ulcer (K28.-)

postprocedural (radiation) retroperitoneal abscess (K68.11)

radiation colitis (K52.0)

radiation gastroenteritis (K52.0)

radiation proctitis (K62.7)

K91.0 Vomiting following gastrointestinal surgery

K91.1 Postgastric surgery syndromes

Dumping syndrome

Postgastrectomy syndrome

Postvagotomy syndrome

K91.2 Postsurgical malabsorption, not elsewhere classified

Postsurgical blind loop syndrome

Excludes 1: malabsorption osteomalacia in adults (M83.2)

malabsorption osteoporosis, postsurgical (M80.8-, M81.8)

K91.3 Postprocedural intestinal obstruction

K91.5 Postcholecystectomy syndrome

K91.6 Intraoperative hemorrhage and hematoma of a digestive system organ or structure complicating a procedure

Excludes 1: intraoperative hemorrhage and hematoma of a digestive system organ or structure due to accidental puncture and laceration during a procedure (K91.7-)

K91.61 Intraoperative hemorrhage and hematoma of a digestive system organ or structure complicating a digestive system procedure

K91.62 Intraoperative hemorrhage and hematoma of a digestive system organ or structure complicating other procedure

K91.7 Accidental puncture and laceration of a digestive system organ or structure during a procedure

K91.71 Accidental puncture and laceration of a digestive system organ or structure during a digestive system procedure

K91.72 Accidental puncture and laceration of a digestive system organ or structure during other procedure

K91.8 Other intraoperative and postprocedural complications and disorders of digestive system

K91.81 Other intraoperative complications of digestive system

K91.82 Postprocedural hepatic failure

K91.83 Postprocedural hepatorenal syndrome

K91.84 Postprocedural hemorrhage and hematoma of a digestive system organ or structure following a procedure

K91.840 Postprocedural hemorrhage and hematoma of a digestive system organ or structure following a digestive system procedure

K91.841 Postprocedural hemorrhage and hematoma of a digestive system organ or structure following other procedure

K91.85 Complications of intestinal pouch

K91.850 Pouchitis

Inflammation of internal ileoanal pouch

K91.858 Other complications of intestinal pouch

K91.86 Retained cholelithiasis following cholecystectomy

K91.89 Other postprocedural complications and disorders of digestive system

Use additional code, if applicable, to further specify disorder

Excludes 2: postprocedural retroperitoneal abscess (K68.11)

K92 Other diseases of digestive system

Excludes 1: neonatal gastrointestinal hemorrhage (P54.0-P54.3)

K92.0 Hematemesis

K92.1 Melena

Excludes 1: occult blood in feces (R19.5)

K92.2 Gastrointestinal hemorrhage, unspecified

Gastric hemorrhage NOS

Intestinal hemorrhage NOS

Excludes 1: acute hemorrhagic gastritis (K29.01)

hemorrhage of anus and rectum (K62.5)

angiodysplasia of stomach with hemorrhage (K31.811)

diverticular disease with hemorrhage (K57.-)

gastritis and duodenitis with hemorrhage (K29.-)

peptic ulcer with hemorrhage (K25-K28)

K92.8 Other specified diseases of the digestive system

K92.81 Gastrointestinal mucositis (ulcerative)

Code also type of associated therapy, such as: antineoplastic and immunosuppressive drugs (T45.1x-)

radiological procedure and radiotherapy (Y84.2)

Excludes 2: mucositis (ulcerative) of vagina and vulva (N76.81)

nasal mucositis (ulcerative) (J34.81)

oral mucositis (ulcerative) (K12.3-)

K92.89 Other specified diseases of the digestive system

K92.9 Disease of digestive system, unspecified

K94 Complications of artificial openings of the digestive system

K94.0 Colostomy complications

K94.00 Colostomy complication, unspecified

K94.01 Colostomy hemorrhage

K94.02 Colostomy infection

Use additional code to specify type of infection, such as:

cellulitis of abdominal wall (L03.311)

sepsis (A40.-, A41.-)

K94.03 Colostomy malfunction

Mechanical complication of colostomy

K94.09 Other complications of colostomy

K94.1 Enterostomy complications

K94.10 Enterostomy complication, unspecified

K94.11 Enterostomy hemorrhage

K94.12 Enterostomy infection

Use additional code to specify type of infection, such as:

cellulitis of abdominal wall (L03.311)

sepsis (A40.-, A41.-)

K94.13 Enterostomy malfunction

Mechanical complication of enterostomy

K94.19 Other complications of enterostomy

K94.2 Gastrostomy complications

K94.20 Gastrostomy complication, unspecified

K94.21 Gastrostomy hemorrhage

K94.22 Gastrostomy infection

Use additional code to specify type of infection, such as:

cellulitis of abdominal wall (L03.311)

sepsis (A40.-, A41.-)

K94.23 Gastrostomy malfunction

Mechanical complication of gastrostomy

K94.29   Other complications of gastrostomy

K94.3   Esophagostomy complications

K94.30   Esophagostomy complications, unspecified

K94.31   Esophagostomy hemorrhage

K94.32   Esophagostomy infection

Use additional code to identify the infection

K94.33   Esophagostomy malfunction

Mechanical complication of esophagostomy

K94.39   Other complications of esophagostomy

K95   Complications of bariatric procedures

K95.0   Complications of gastric band procedure

K95.01   Infection due to gastric band procedure

Use additional code to specify type of infection or organism, such as:

bacterial and viral infectious agents(B95-, B96-)

cellulitis of abdominal wall (L03.311)

sepsis (A40.-, A41.-)

K95.09   Other complications of gastric band procedure

Use additional code, if applicable, to further specify complication

K95.8   Complications of other bariatric procedure

Excludes 1: complications of gastric band surgery (K95.0-)

K95.81   Infection due to other bariatric procedure

Use additional code to specify type of infection or organism, such as:

bacterial and viral infectious agents(B95-, B96-)

cellulitis of abdominal wall (L03.311)

sepsis (A40.-, A41.-)

K95.89   Other complications of other bariatric procedure

Use additional code, if applicable, to further specify complication

Chapter 12: Diseases Of The Skin And Subcutaneous Tissue (L00-L99)

Excludes 2: certain conditions originating in the perinatal period (P04-P96)

certain infectious and parasitic diseases (A00-B99)

complications of pregnancy, childbirth and the puerperium (O00-O9A)

congenital malformations, deformations, and chromosomal abnormalities (Q00-Q99)

endocrine, nutritional and metabolic diseases (E00-E88)

lipomelanotic reticulosis (I89.8)

neoplasms (C00-D49)

symptoms, signs and abnormal clinical and laboratory findings, not elsewhere classified (R00-R94)

systemic connective tissue disorders (M30-M36)

viral warts (B07.-)

This chapter contains the following blocks:

L00-L08	Infections of the skin and subcutaneous tissue
L10-L14	Bullous disorders
L20-L30	Dermatitis and eczema
L40-L45	Papulosquamous disorders
L49-L54	Urticaria and erythema
L55-L59	Radiation-related disorders of the skin and subcutaneous tissue
L60-L75	Disorders of skin appendages
L76	Intraoperative and postprocedural complications of skin and subcutaneous tissue
L80-L99	Other disorders of the skin and subcutaneous tissue

INFECTIONS OF THE SKIN AND SUBCUTANEOUS TISSUE (L00-L08)

Use additional code (B95-B97) to identify infectious agent.

Excludes 2: hordeolum (H00.0)

infective dermatitis (L30.3)

local infections of skin classified in Chapter 1

lupus panniculitis (L93.2)

panniculitis NOS (M79.3)

panniculitis of neck and back (M54.0-)

Perleche NOS (K13.0)

Perleche due to candidiasis (B37.0)

Perleche due to riboflavin deficiency (E53.0)

pyogenic granuloma (L98.0)

relapsing panniculitis [Weber-Christian] (M35.6)

viral warts (B07.-)

zoster (B02.-)

L00 Staphylococcal scalded skin syndrome

Ritter's disease

Use additional code to identify percentage of skin exfoliation (L49-)

Excludes 1: bullous impetigo (L01.03)

pemphigus neonatorum (L01.03)

toxic epidermal necrolysis [Lyell] (L51.2)

L01 Impetigo

Excludes 1: impetigo herpetiformis (L40.1)

L01.0 Impetigo

Impetigo contagiosa

Impetigo vulgaris

L01.00 Impetigo, unspecified

Impetigo NOS

L01.01 Non-bullous impetigo

L01.02 Bockhart's impetigo

Impetigo follicularis

Perifolliculitis NOS

Superficial pustular perifolliculitis

L01.03 Bullous impetigo

Impetigo neonatorum

Pemphigus neonatorum

L01.09 Other impetigo

Ulcerative impetigo

L01.1 Impetiginization of other dermatoses

L02 Cutaneous abscess, furuncle and carbuncle

Use additional code to identify organism (B95-B96)

Excludes 2: abscess of anus and rectal regions (K61.-)

abscess of female genital organs (external) (N76.4)

abscess of male genital organs (external) (N48.2, N49.-)

L02.0 Cutaneous abscess, furuncle and carbuncle of face

Excludes 2: abscess of ear, external (H60.0)

abscess of eyelid (H00.0)

abscess of head [any part, except face] (L02.8)

abscess of lacrimal gland (H04.0)

abscess of lacrimal passages (H04.3)

abscess of mouth (K12.2)

abscess of nose (J34.0)

abscess of orbit (H05.0)

submandibular abscess (K12.2)

L02.01 Cutaneous abscess of face

L02.02 Furuncle of face

Boil of face

Folliculitis of face

L02.03 Carbuncle of face

L02.1 Cutaneous abscess, furuncle and carbuncle of neck

L02.11 Cutaneous abscess of neck

L02.12 Furuncle of neck

Boil of neck

Folliculitis of neck

L02.13 Carbuncle of neck

L02.2 Cutaneous abscess, furuncle and carbuncle of trunk

Excludes 1: non-newborn omphalitis (L08.82)

omphalitis of newborn (P38.-)

Excludes 2: abscess of breast (N61)

abscess of buttocks (L02.3)

abscess of female external genital organs (N76.4)

abscess of male external genital organs (N48.2, N49.-)

abscess of hip (L02.4)

L02.21 Cutaneous abscess of trunk

L02.211 Cutaneous abscess of abdominal wall

L02.212 Cutaneous abscess of back [any part, except buttock]

L02.213 Cutaneous abscess of chest wall

L02.214 Cutaneous abscess of groin

L02.215 Cutaneous abscess of perineum

L02.216 Cutaneous abscess of umbilicus

L02.219 Cutaneous abscess of trunk, unspecified

L02.22 Furuncle of trunk

Boil of trunk

Folliculitis of trunk

L02.221 Furuncle of abdominal wall

	L02.222	Furuncle of back [any part, except buttock]
	L02.223	Furuncle of chest wall
	L02.224	Furuncle of groin
	L02.225	Furuncle of perineum
	L02.226	Furuncle of umbilicus
	L02.229	Furuncle of trunk, unspecified
L02.23	Carbuncle of trunk	
	L02.231	Carbuncle of abdominal wall
	L02.232	Carbuncle of back [any part, except buttock]
	L02.233	Carbuncle of chest wall
	L02.234	Carbuncle of groin
	L02.235	Carbuncle of perineum
	L02.236	Carbuncle of umbilicus
	L02.239	Carbuncle of trunk, unspecified

L02.3 Cutaneous abscess, furuncle and carbuncle of buttock

Excludes 1: pilonidal cyst with abscess (L05.01)

L02.31 Cutaneous abscess of buttock
Cutaneous abscess of gluteal region

L02.32 Furuncle of buttock
Boil of buttock
Folliculitis of buttock
Furuncle of gluteal region

L02.33 Carbuncle of buttock
Carbuncle of gluteal region

L02.4 Cutaneous abscess, furuncle and carbuncle of limb

Excludes 2: Cutaneous abscess, furuncle and carbuncle of groin (L02.214, L02.224, L02.234)
Cutaneous abscess, furuncle and carbuncle of hand (L02.5-)
Cutaneous abscess, furuncle and carbuncle of foot (L02.6-)

L02.41	Cutaneous abscess of limb	
	L02.411	Cutaneous abscess of right axilla
	L02.412	Cutaneous abscess of left axilla
	L02.413	Cutaneous abscess of right upper limb
	L02.414	Cutaneous abscess of left upper limb
	L02.415	Cutaneous abscess of right lower limb
	L02.416	Cutaneous abscess of left lower limb
	L02.419	Cutaneous abscess of limb, unspecified
L02.42	Furuncle of limb	
	Boil of limb	
	Folliculitis of limb	
	L02.421	Furuncle of right axilla
	L02.422	Furuncle of left axilla
	L02.423	Furuncle of right upper limb
	L02.424	Furuncle of left upper limb
	L02.425	Furuncle of right lower limb
	L02.426	Furuncle of left lower limb
	L02.429	Furuncle of limb, unspecified
L02.43	Carbuncle of limb	
	L02.431	Carbuncle of right axilla
	L02.432	Carbuncle of left axilla
	L02.433	Carbuncle of right upper limb
	L02.434	Carbuncle of left upper limb
	L02.435	Carbuncle of right lower limb
	L02.436	Carbuncle of left lower limb
	L02.439	Carbuncle of limb, unspecified

L02.5 Cutaneous abscess, furuncle and carbuncle of hand

L02.51	Cutaneous abscess of hand	
	L02.511	Cutaneous abscess of right hand
	L02.512	Cutaneous abscess of left hand
	L02.519	Cutaneous abscess of unspecified hand
L02.52	Furuncle hand	
	Boil of hand	
	Folliculitis of hand	
	L02.521	Furuncle right hand
	L02.522	Furuncle left hand
	L02.529	Furuncle unspecified hand
L02.53	Carbuncle of hand	
	L02.531	Carbuncle of right hand
	L02.532	Carbuncle of left hand
	L02.539	Carbuncle of unspecified hand

L02.6 Cutaneous abscess, furuncle and carbuncle of foot

L02.61	Cutaneous abscess of foot	
	L02.611	Cutaneous abscess of right foot
	L02.612	Cutaneous abscess of left foot
	L02.619	Cutaneous abscess of unspecified foot
L02.62	Furuncle of foot	
	Boil of foot	
	Folliculitis of foot	
	L02.621	Furuncle of right foot
	L02.622	Furuncle of left foot
	L02.629	Furuncle of unspecified foot
L02.63	Carbuncle of foot	
	L02.631	Carbuncle of right foot
	L02.632	Carbuncle of left foot
	L02.639	Carbuncle of unspecified foot

L02.8 Cutaneous abscess, furuncle and carbuncle of other sites

L02.81	Cutaneous abscess of other sites	
	L02.811	Cutaneous abscess of head [any part, except face]
	L02.818	Cutaneous abscess of other sites
L02.82	Furuncle of other sites	
	Boil of other sites	
	Folliculitis of other sites	
	L02.821	Furuncle of head [any part, except face]
	L02.828	Furuncle of other sites
L02.83	Carbuncle of other sites	
	L02.831	Carbuncle of head [any part, except face]
	L02.838	Carbuncle of other sites

L02.9 Cutaneous abscess, furuncle and carbuncle, unspecified

L02.91 Cutaneous abscess, unspecified

L02.92 Furuncle, unspecified
Boil NOS
Furunculosis NOS

L02.93 Carbuncle, unspecified

L03 Cellulitis and acute lymphangitis

Excludes 2: cellulitis of anal and rectal region (K61.-)
cellulitis of external auditory canal (H60.1)
cellulitis of eyelid (H00.0)
cellulitis of female external genital organs (N76.4)
cellulitis of lacrimal apparatus (H04.3)
cellulitis of male external genital organs (N48.2, N49.-)
cellulitis of mouth (K12.2)
cellulitis of nose (J34.0)

eosinophilic cellulitis [Wells] (L98.3)

febrile neutrophilic dermatosis [Sweet] (L98.2)

lymphangitis (chronic) (subacute) (I89.1)

L03.0 Cellulitis and acute lymphangitis of finger and toe

Infection of nail

Onychia

Paronychia

Perionychia

    L03.01 Cellulitis of finger

      Felon

      Whitlow

      Excludes 1: herpetic whitlow (B00.89)

      L03.011 Cellulitis of right finger

      L03.012 Cellulitis of left finger

      L03.019 Cellulitis of unspecified finger

    L03.02 Acute lymphangitis of finger

      Hangnail with lymphangitis of finger

      L03.021 Acute lymphangitis of right finger

      L03.022 Acute lymphangitis of left finger

      L03.029 Acute lymphangitis of unspecified finger

    L03.03 Cellulitis of toe

      L03.031 Cellulitis of right toe

      L03.032 Cellulitis of left toe

      L03.039 Cellulitis of unspecified toe

    L03.04 Acute lymphangitis of toe

      Hangnail with lymphangitis of toe

      L03.041 Acute lymphangitis of right toe

      L03.042 Acute lymphangitis of left toe

      L03.049 Acute lymphangitis of unspecified toe

L03.1 Cellulitis and acute lymphangitis of other parts of limb

    L03.11 Cellulitis of other parts of limb

      Excludes 2: cellulitis of fingers (L03.01-)

        cellulitis of toes (L03.03-)

        groin (L03.314)

      L03.111 Cellulitis of right axilla

      L03.112 Cellulitis of left axilla

      L03.113 Cellulitis of right upper limb

      L03.114 Cellulitis of left upper limb

      L03.115 Cellulitis of right lower limb

      L03.116 Cellulitis of left lower limb

      L03.119 Cellulitis of unspecified part of limb

    L03.12 Acute lymphangitis of other parts of limb

      Excludes 2: acute lymphangitis of fingers (L03.2-)

        acute lymphangitis of toes (L03.4-)

        acute lymphangitis of groin (L03.324)

      L03.121 Acute lymphangitis of right axilla

      L03.122 Acute lymphangitis of left axilla

      L03.123 Acute lymphangitis of right upper limb

      L03.124 Acute lymphangitis of left upper limb

      L03.125 Acute lymphangitis of right lower limb

      L03.126 Acute lymphangitis of left lower limb

      L03.129 Acute lymphangitis of unspecified part of limb

L03.2 Cellulitis and acute lymphangitis of face and neck

    L03.21 Cellulitis and acute lymphangitis of face

      L03.211 Cellulitis of face

        Excludes 2: cellulitis of ear (H60.1-)

          cellulitis of eyelid (H00.0-)

          cellulitis of head (L03.81)

          cellulitis of lacrimal apparatus (H04.3)

          cellulitis of lip (K13.0)

          cellulitis of mouth (K12.2)

          cellulitis of nose (internal) (J34.0)

          cellulitis of orbit (H05.0)

          cellulitis of scalp (L03.81)

      L03.212 Acute lymphangitis of face

    L03.22 Cellulitis and acute lymphangitis of neck

      L03.221 Cellulitis of neck

      L03.222 Acute lymphangitis of neck

L03.3 Cellulitis and acute lymphangitis of trunk

    L03.31 Cellulitis of trunk

      Excludes 2: cellulitis of anal and rectal regions (K61.-)

        cellulitis of breast NOS (N61)

        cellulitis of female external genital organs (N76.4)

        cellulitis of male external genital organs (N48.2, N49.-)

        omphalitis of newborn (P38.-)

        puerperal cellulitis of breast (O91.2)

      L03.311 Cellulitis of abdominal wall

        Excludes 2: cellulitis of umbilicus (L03.316)

          cellulitis of groin (L03.314)

      L03.312 Cellulitis of back [any part except buttock]

      L03.313 Cellulitis of chest wall

      L03.314 Cellulitis of groin

      L03.315 Cellulitis of perineum

      L03.316 Cellulitis of umbilicus

      L03.317 Cellulitis of buttock

      L03.319 Cellulitis of trunk, unspecified

    L03.32 Acute lymphangitis of trunk

      L03.321 Acute lymphangitis of abdominal wall

      L03.322 Acute lymphangitis of back [any part except buttock]

      L03.323 Acute lymphangitis of chest wall

      L03.324 Acute lymphangitis of groin

      L03.325 Acute lymphangitis of perineum

      L03.326 Acute lymphangitis of umbilicus

      L03.327 Acute lymphangitis of buttock

      L03.329 Acute lymphangitis of trunk, unspecified

L03.8 Cellulitis and acute lymphangitis of other sites

    L03.81 Cellulitis of other sites

      L03.811 Cellulitis of head [any part, except face]

        Cellulitis of scalp

        Excludes 2: cellulitis of face (L03.211)

      L03.818 Cellulitis of other sites

    L03.89 Acute lymphangitis of other sites

      L03.891 Acute lymphangitis of head [any part, except face]

L03.898　　Acute lymphangitis of other sites

L03.9　　Cellulitis and acute lymphangitis, unspecified

　　L03.90　　Cellulitis, unspecified

　　L03.91　　Acute lymphangitis, unspecified

　　　　Excludes 1: lymphangitis NOS (I89.1)

L04 Acute lymphadenitis

Includes: abscess (acute) of lymph nodes, except mesenteric

acute lymphadenitis, except mesenteric

Excludes 1: chronic or subacute lymphadenitis, except mesenteric (I88.1)

enlarged lymph nodes (R59.-)

human immunodeficiency virus [HIV] disease resulting in generalized lymphadenopathy (B20)

lymphadenitis NOS (I88.9)

nonspecific mesenteric lymphadenitis (I88.0)

L04.0　　Acute lymphadenitis of face, head and neck

L04.1　　Acute lymphadenitis of trunk

L04.2　　Acute lymphadenitis of upper limb

Acute lymphadenitis of axilla

Acute lymphadenitis of shoulder

L04.3　　Acute lymphadenitis of lower limb

Acute lymphadenitis of hip

　　Excludes 2: acute lymphadenitis of groin (L04.1)

L04.8　　Acute lymphadenitis of other sites

L04.9　　Acute lymphadenitis, unspecified

L05 Pilonidal cyst and sinus

L05.0　　Pilonidal cyst and sinus with abscess

　　L05.01　　Pilonidal cyst with abscess

Parasacral dimple with abscess

Pilonidal abscess

Pilonidal dimple with abscess

Postanal dimple with abscess

　　L05.02　　Pilonidal sinus with abscess

Coccygeal fistula with abscess

Coccygeal sinus with abscess

Pilonidal fistula with abscess

L05.9　　Pilonidal cyst and sinus without abscess

　　L05.91　　Pilonidal cyst without abscess

Parasacral dimple

Pilonidal dimple

Postanal dimple

Pilonidal cyst NOS

　　L05.92　　Pilonidal sinus without abscess

Coccygeal fistula

Coccygeal sinus without abscess

Pilonidal fistula

L08 Other local infections of skin and subcutaneous tissue

L08.0　　Pyoderma

Dermatitis gangrenosa

Purulent dermatitis

Septic dermatitis

Suppurative dermatitis

　　Excludes 1: pyoderma gangrenosum (L88)

　　　　　pyoderma vegetans (L08.81)

L08.1　　Erythrasma

L08.8　　Other specified local infections of the skin and subcutaneous tissue

　　L08.81　　Pyoderma vegetans

　　　　Excludes 1: pyoderma gangrenosum (L88)

　　　　　　pyoderma NOS (L08.0)

　　L08.82　　Omphalitis not of newborn

　　　　Excludes 1: omphalitis of newborn (P38.-)

L08.89　　Other specified local infections of the skin and subcutaneous tissue

L08.9　　Local infection of the skin and subcutaneous tissue, unspecified

BULLOUS DISORDERS (L10-L14)

Excludes 1: benign familial pemphigus [Hailey-Hailey] (Q82.8)

staphylococcal scalded skin syndrome (L00)

toxic epidermal necrolysis [Lyell] (L51.2)

L10 Pemphigus

Excludes 1: pemphigus neonatorum (L01.03)

L10.0　　Pemphigus vulgaris

L10.1　　Pemphigus vegetans

L10.2　　Pemphigus foliaceous

L10.3　　Brazilian pemphigus [fogo selvagem]

L10.4　　Pemphigus erythematosus

Senear-Usher syndrome

L10.5　　Drug-induced pemphigus

Use additional code for adverse effect, if applicable, to identify drug (T36-T50 with fifth or sixth character 5)

L10.8　　Other pemphigus

　　L10.81　　Paraneoplastic pemphigus

　　L10.89　　Other pemphigus

L10.9　　Pemphigus, unspecified

L11 Other acantholytic disorders

L11.0　　Acquired keratosis follicularis

　　Excludes 1: keratosis follicularis (congenital) [Darier-White] (Q82.8)

L11.1　　Transient acantholytic dermatosis [Grover]

L11.8　　Other specified acantholytic disorders

L11.9　　Acantholytic disorder, unspecified

L12 Pemphigoid

Excludes 1: herpes gestationis (O26.4-)

impetigo herpetiformis (L40.1)

L12.0　　Bullous pemphigoid

L12.1　　Cicatricial pemphigoid

Benign mucous membrane pemphigoid

L12.2　　Chronic bullous disease of childhood

Juvenile dermatitis herpetiformis

L12.3　　Acquired epidermolysis bullosa

　　Excludes 1: epidermolysis bullosa (congenital) (Q81.-)

　　L12.30　　Acquired epidermolysis bullosa, unspecified

　　L12.31　　Epidermolysis bullosa due to drug

Use additional code for adverse effect, if applicable, to identify drug (T36-T50 with fifth or sixth character 5)

　　L12.35　　Other acquired epidermolysis bullosa

L12.8　　Other pemphigoid

L12.9　　Pemphigoid, unspecified

L13 Other bullous disorders

L13.0　　Dermatitis herpetiformis

Duhring's disease

Hydroa herpetiformis

　　Excludes 1: juvenile dermatitis herpetiformis (L12.2)

　　　　senile dermatitis herpetiformis (L12.0)

L13.1　　Subcorneal pustular dermatitis

Sneddon-Wilkinson disease

L13.8　　Other specified bullous disorders

L13.9　　Bullous disorder, unspecified

L14 Bullous disorders in diseases classified elsewhere

Code first underlying disease

● New code　　　　▲ Revised code　　　　⑦ 7th digit required　　　　⊗ Placeholder required

DERMATITIS AND ECZEMA (L20-L30)

Note: In this block the terms dermatitis and eczema are used synonymously and interchangeably.

Excludes 2: chronic (childhood) granulomatous disease (D71)

dermatitis gangrenosa (L08.0)

dermatitis herpetiformis (L13.0)

dry skin dermatitis (L85.3)

factitial dermatitis (L98.1)

perioral dermatitis (L71.0)

radiation-related disorders of the skin and subcutaneous tissue (L55-L59)

stasis dermatitis (I83.1-I83.2)

L20 Atopic dermatitis

L20.0 Besnier's prurigo

L20.8 Other atopic dermatitis

Excludes 2: circumscribed neurodermatitis (L28.0)

L20.81 Atopic neurodermatitis

Diffuse neurodermatitis

L20.82 Flexural eczema

L20.83 Infantile (acute) (chronic) eczema

L20.84 Intrinsic (allergic) eczema

L20.89 Other atopic dermatitis

L20.9 Atopic dermatitis, unspecified

L21 Seborrheic dermatitis

Excludes 2: infective dermatitis (L30.3)

seborrheic keratosis (L82.-)

L21.0 Seborrhea capitis

Cradle cap

L21.1 Seborrheic infantile dermatitis

L21.8 Other seborrheic dermatitis

L21.9 Seborrheic dermatitis, unspecified

Seborrhea NOS

L22 Diaper dermatitis

Diaper erythema

Diaper rash

Psoriasiform diaper rash

L23 Allergic contact dermatitis

Excludes 1: allergy NOS (T78.40)

contact dermatitis NOS (L25.9)

dermatitis NOS (L30.9)

Excludes 2: dermatitis due to substances taken internally (L27.-)

dermatitis of eyelid (H01.1-)

diaper dermatitis (L22)

eczema of external ear (H60.5-)

irritant contact dermatitis (L24.-)

perioral dermatitis (L71.0)

radiation-related disorders of the skin and subcutaneous tissue (L55-L59)

L23.0 Allergic contact dermatitis due to metals

Allergic contact dermatitis due to chromium

Allergic contact dermatitis due to nickel

L23.1 Allergic contact dermatitis due to adhesives

L23.2 Allergic contact dermatitis due to cosmetics

L23.3 Allergic contact dermatitis due to drugs in contact with skin

Use additional code for adverse effect, if applicable, to identify drug (T36-T50 with fifth or sixth character 5)

Excludes 2: dermatitis due to ingested drugs and medicaments (L27.0-L27.1)

L23.4 Allergic contact dermatitis due to dyes

L23.5 Allergic contact dermatitis due to other chemical products

Allergic contact dermatitis due to cement

Allergic contact dermatitis due to insecticide

Allergic contact dermatitis due to plastic

Allergic contact dermatitis due to rubber

L23.6 Allergic contact dermatitis due to food in contact with the skin

Excludes 2: dermatitis due to ingested food (L27.2)

L23.7 Allergic contact dermatitis due to plants, except food

Excludes 2: allergy NOS due to pollen (J30.1)

L23.8 Allergic contact dermatitis due to other agents

L23.81 Allergic contact dermatitis due to animal (cat) (dog) dander

Allergic contact dermatitis due to animal (cat) (dog) hair

L23.89 Allergic contact dermatitis due to other agents

L23.9 Allergic contact dermatitis, unspecified cause

Allergic contact eczema NOS

L24 Irritant contact dermatitis

Excludes 1: allergy NOS (T78.40)

contact dermatitis NOS (L25.9)

dermatitis NOS (L30.9)

Excludes 2: allergic contact dermatitis (L23.-)

dermatitis due to substances taken internally (L27.-)

dermatitis of eyelid (H01.1-)

diaper dermatitis (L22)

eczema of external ear (H60.5-)

perioral dermatitis (L71.0)

radiation-related disorders of the skin and subcutaneous tissue (L55-L59)

L24.0 Irritant contact dermatitis due to detergents

L24.1 Irritant contact dermatitis due to oils and greases

L24.2 Irritant contact dermatitis due to solvents

Irritant contact dermatitis due to chlorocompound

Irritant contact dermatitis due to cyclohexane

Irritant contact dermatitis due to ester

Irritant contact dermatitis due to glycol

Irritant contact dermatitis due to hydrocarbon

Irritant contact dermatitis due to ketone

L24.3 Irritant contact dermatitis due to cosmetics

L24.4 Irritant contact dermatitis due to drugs in contact with skin

Use additional code for adverse effect, if applicable, to identify drug (T36-T50 with fifth or sixth character 5)

L24.5 Irritant contact dermatitis due to other chemical products

Irritant contact dermatitis due to cement

Irritant contact dermatitis due to insecticide

Irritant contact dermatitis due to plastic

Irritant contact dermatitis due to rubber

L24.6 Irritant contact dermatitis due to food in contact with skin

Excludes 2: dermatitis due to ingested food (L27.2)

L24.7 Irritant contact dermatitis due to plants, except food

Excludes 2: allergy NOS to pollen (J30.1)

L24.8 Irritant contact dermatitis due to other agents

L24.81 Irritant contact dermatitis due to metals

Irritant contact dermatitis due to chromium

Irritant contact dermatitis due to nickel

L24.89 Irritant contact dermatitis due to other agents

Irritant contact dermatitis due to dyes

L24.9 Irritant contact dermatitis, unspecified cause

Irritant contact eczema NOS

L25 Unspecified contact dermatitis

Excludes 1: allergic contact dermatitis (L23.-)

allergy NOS (T78.40)

dermatitis NOS (L30.9)

irritant contact dermatitis (L24.-)

Excludes 2: dermatitis due to ingested substances (L27.-)
dermatitis of eyelid (H01.1-)
eczema of external ear (H60.5-)
perioral dermatitis (L71.0)
radiation-related disorders of the skin and subcutaneous tissue (L55-L59)

L25.0 Unspecified contact dermatitis due to cosmetics

L25.1 Unspecified contact dermatitis due to drugs in contact with skin

Use additional code for adverse effect, if applicable, to identify drug (T36-T50 with fifth or sixth character 5)

Excludes 2: dermatitis due to ingested drugs and medicaments (L27.0-L27.1)

L25.2 Unspecified contact dermatitis due to dyes

L25.3 Unspecified contact dermatitis due to other chemical products

Unspecified contact dermatitis due to cement
Unspecified contact dermatitis due to insecticide

L25.4 Unspecified contact dermatitis due to food in contact with skin

Excludes 2: dermatitis due to ingested food (L27.2)

L25.5 Unspecified contact dermatitis due to plants, except food

Excludes 1: nettle rash (L50.9)

Excludes 2: allergy NOS due to pollen (J30.1)

L25.8 Unspecified contact dermatitis due to other agents

L25.9 Unspecified contact dermatitis, unspecified cause

Contact dermatitis (occupational) NOS
Contact eczema (occupational) NOS

L26 Exfoliative dermatitis

Hebra's pityriasis

Excludes 1: Ritter's disease (L00)

L27 Dermatitis due to substances taken internally

Excludes 1: allergy NOS (T78.40)

Excludes 2: adverse food reaction, except dermatitis (T78.0-T78.1)
contact dermatitis (L23-L25)
drug photoallergic response (L56.1)
drug phototoxic response (L56.0)
urticaria (L50.-)

L27.0 Generalized skin eruption due to drugs and medicaments taken internally

Use additional code for adverse effect, if applicable, to identify drug (T36-T50 with fifth or sixth character 5)

L27.1 Localized skin eruption due to drugs and medicaments taken internally

Use additional code for adverse effect, if applicable, to identify drug (T36-T50 with fifth or sixth character 5)

L27.2 Dermatitis due to ingested food

Excludes 2: dermatitis due to food in contact with skin (L23.6, L24.6, L25.4)

L27.8 Dermatitis due to other substances taken internally

L27.9 Dermatitis due to unspecified substance taken internally

L28 Lichen simplex chronicus and prurigo

L28.0 Lichen simplex chronicus

Circumscribed neurodermatitis
Lichen NOS

L28.1 Prurigo nodularis

L28.2 Other prurigo

Prurigo NOS
Prurigo Hebra
Prurigo mitis
Urticaria papulosa

L29 Pruritus

Excludes 1: neurotic excoriation (L98.1)

psychogenic pruritus (F45.8)

L29.0 Pruritus ani

L29.1 Pruritus scroti

L29.2 Pruritus vulvae

L29.3 Anogenital pruritus, unspecified

L29.8 Other pruritus

L29.9 Pruritus, unspecified

Itch NOS

L30 Other and unspecified dermatitis

Excludes 2: contact dermatitis (L23-L25)
dry skin dermatitis (L85.3)
small plaque parapsoriasis (L41.3)
stasis dermatitis (I83.1-.2)

L30.0 Nummular dermatitis

L30.1 Dyshidrosis [pompholyx]

L30.2 Cutaneous autosensitization

Candidid [levurid]
Dermatophytid
Eczematid

L30.3 Infective dermatitis

Infectious eczematoid dermatitis

L30.4 Erythema intertrigo

L30.5 Pityriasis alba

L30.8 Other specified dermatitis

L30.9 Dermatitis, unspecified

Eczema NOS

PAPULOSQUAMOUS DISORDERS (L40-L45)

L40 Psoriasis

L40.0 Psoriasis vulgaris

Nummular psoriasis
Plaque psoriasis

L40.1 Generalized pustular psoriasis

Impetigo herpetiformis
Von Zumbusch's disease

L40.2 Acrodermatitis continua

L40.3 Pustulosis palmaris et plantaris

L40.4 Guttate psoriasis

L40.5 Arthropathic psoriasis

L40.50 Arthropathic psoriasis, unspecified

L40.51 Distal interphalangeal psoriatic arthropathy

L40.52 Psoriatic arthritis mutilans

L40.53 Psoriatic spondylitis

L40.54 Psoriatic juvenile arthropathy

L40.59 Other psoriatic arthropathy

L40.8 Other psoriasis

Flexural psoriasis

L40.9 Psoriasis, unspecified

L41 Parapsoriasis

Excludes 1: poikiloderma vasculare atrophicans (L94.5)

L41.0 Pityriasis lichenoides et varioliformis acuta

Mucha-Habermann disease

L41.1 Pityriasis lichenoides chronica

L41.3 Small plaque parapsoriasis

L41.4 Large plaque parapsoriasis

L41.5 Retiform parapsoriasis

L41.8 Other parapsoriasis

L41.9 Parapsoriasis, unspecified

L42 Pityriasis rosea

L43 Lichen planus

Excludes 1: lichen planopilaris (L66.1)

● New code   ▲ Revised code   ⑦ 7th digit required   ⊗ Placeholder required

L43.0   Hypertrophic lichen planus

L43.1   Bullous lichen planus

L43.2   Lichenoid drug reaction

Use additional code for adverse effect, if applicable, to identify drug (T36-T50 with fifth or sixth character 5)

L43.3   Subacute (active) lichen planus

Lichen planus tropicus

L43.8   Other lichen planus

L43.9   Lichen planus, unspecified

L44   Other papulosquamous disorders

L44.0   Pityriasis rubra pilaris

L44.1   Lichen nitidus

L44.2   Lichen striatus

L44.3   Lichen ruber moniliformis

L44.4   Infantile papular acrodermatitis [Gianotti-Crosti]

L44.8   Other specified papulosquamous disorders

L44.9   Papulosquamous disorder, unspecified

L45   Papulosquamous disorders in diseases classified elsewhere

Code first underlying disease.

URTICARIA AND ERYTHEMA (L49-L54)

Excludes 1: Lyme disease (A69.2-)

rosacea (L71.-)

L49   Exfoliation due to erythematous conditions according to extent of body surface involved

Code first erythematous condition causing exfoliation, such as:

Ritter's disease (L00)

(Staphylococcal) scalded skin syndrom (L00)

Stevens-Johnson syndrome (L51.1)

Stevens-Johnson syndrome-toxic epidermal necrolysis overlap syndrome (L51.3)

Toxic epidermal necrolysis (L51.2)

L49.0   Exfoliation due to erythematous condition involving less than 10 percent of body surface

Exfoliation due to erythematous condition NOS

L49.1   Exfoliation due to erythematous condition involving 10-19 percent of body surface

L49.2   Exfoliation due to erythematous condition involving 20-29 percent of body surface

L49.3   Exfoliation due to erythematous condition involving 30-39 percent of body surface

L49.4   Exfoliation due to erythematous condition involving 40-49 percent of body surface

L49.5   Exfoliation due to erythematous condition involving 50-59 percent of body surface

L49.6   Exfoliation due to erythematous condition involving 60-69 percent of body surface

L49.7   Exfoliation due to erythematous condition involving 70-79 percent of body surface

L49.8   Exfoliation due to erythematous condition involving 80-89 percent of body surface

L49.9   Exfoliation due to erythematous condition involving 90 or more percent of body surface

L50   Urticaria

Excludes 1: allergic contact dermatitis (L23.-)

angioneurotic edema (T78.3)

giant urticaria (T78.3)

hereditary angio-edema (D84.1)

Quincke's edema (T78.3)

serum urticaria (T80.6-)

solar urticaria (L56.3)

urticaria neonatorum (P83.8)

urticaria papulosa (L28.2)

urticaria pigmentosa (Q82.2)

L50.0   Allergic urticaria

L50.1   Idiopathic urticaria

L50.2   Urticaria due to cold and heat

L50.3   Dermatographic urticaria

L50.4   Vibratory urticaria

L50.5   Cholinergic urticaria

L50.6   Contact urticaria

L50.8   Other urticaria

Chronic urticaria

Recurrent periodic urticaria

L50.9   Urticaria, unspecified

L51   Erythema multiforme

Use additional code for adverse effect, if applicable, to identify drug (T36-T50 with fifth or sixth character 5)

Use additional code to identify associated manifestations, such as:

arthropathy associated with dermatological disorders (M14.8-)

conjunctival edema (H11.42)

conjunctivitis (H10.22-)

corneal scars and opacities (H17.-)

corneal ulcer (H16.0-)

edema of eyelid (H02.84)

inflammation of eyelid (H01.8)

keratoconjunctivitis sicca (H16.22-)

mechanical lagophthalmos (H02.22-)

stomatitis (K12.-)

symblepharon (H11.23-)

Use additional code to identify percentage of skin exfoliation (L49-)

Excludes 1: staphylococcal scalded skin syndrome (L00)

Ritter's disease (L00)

L51.0   Nonbullous erythema multiforme

L51.1   Stevens-Johnson syndrome

L51.2   Toxic epidermal necrolysis [Lyell]

L51.3   Stevens-Johnson syndrome-toxic epidermal necrolysis overlap syndrome

SJS-TEN overlap syndrome

L51.8   Other erythema multiforme

L51.9   Erythema multiforme, unspecified

Erythema iris

Erythema multiforme major NOS

Erythema multiforme minor NOS

Herpes iris

L52   Erythema nodosum

Excludes 1: tuberculous erythema nodosum (A18.4)

L53   Other erythematous conditions

Excludes 1: erythema ab igne (L59.0)

erythema due to external agents in contact with skin (L23-L25)

erythema intertrigo (L30.4)

L53.0   Toxic erythema

Code first poisoning due to drug or toxin, if applicable (T36-T65 with fifth or sixth character 1-4 or 6)

Use additional code for adverse effect, if applicable, to identify drug (T36-T50 with fifth or sixth character 5)

Excludes 1: neonatal erythema toxicum (P83.1)

L53.1   Erythema annulare centrifugum

L53.2   Erythema marginatum

L53.3   Other chronic figurate erythema

L53.8   Other specified erythematous conditions

L53.9   Erythematous condition, unspecified

Erythema NOS

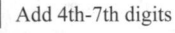 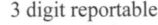

Erythroderma NOS

L54 Erythema in diseases classified elsewhere
Code first underlying disease.

RADIATION-RELATED DISORDERS OF THE SKIN AND SUBCUTANEOUS TISSUE (L55-L59)

L55 Sunburn

L55.0 Sunburn of first degree

L55.1 Sunburn of second degree

L55.2 Sunburn of third degree

L55.9 Sunburn, unspecified

L56 Other acute skin changes due to ultraviolet radiation
Use additional code to identify the source of the ultraviolet radiation (W89, X32)

L56.0 Drug phototoxic response
Use additional code for adverse effect, if applicable, to identify drug (T36-T50 with fifth or sixth character 5)

L56.1 Drug photoallergic response
Use additional code for adverse effect, if applicable, to identify drug (T36-T50 with fifth or sixth character 5)

L56.2 Photocontact dermatitis [berloque dermatitis]

L56.3 Solar urticaria

L56.4 Polymorphous light eruption

L56.5 Disseminated superficial actinic porokeratosis (DSAP)

L56.8 Other specified acute skin changes due to ultraviolet radiation

L56.9 Acute skin change due to ultraviolet radiation, unspecified

L57 Skin changes due to chronic exposure to nonionizing radiation
Use additional code to identify the source of the ultraviolet radiation (W89, X32)

L57.0 Actinic keratosis
Keratosis NOS
Senile keratosis
Solar keratosis

L57.1 Actinic reticuloid

L57.2 Cutis rhomboidalis nuchae

L57.3 Poikiloderma of Civatte

L57.4 Cutis laxa senilis
Elastosis senilis

L57.5 Actinic granuloma

L57.8 Other skin changes due to chronic exposure to nonionizing radiation
Farmer's skin
Sailor's skin
Solar dermatitis

L57.9 Skin changes due to chronic exposure to nonionizing radiation, unspecified

L58 Radiodermatitis
Use additional code to identify the source of the radiation (W88, W90)

L58.0 Acute radiodermatitis

L58.1 Chronic radiodermatitis

L58.9 Radiodermatitis, unspecified

L59 Other disorders of skin and subcutaneous tissue related to radiation

L59.0 Erythema ab igne [dermatitis ab igne]

L59.8 Other specified disorders of the skin and subcutaneous tissue related to radiation

L59.9 Disorder of the skin and subcutaneous tissue related to radiation, unspecified

DISORDERS OF SKIN APPENDAGES (L60-L75)

Excludes 1: congenital malformations of integument (Q84.-)

L60 Nail disorders
Excludes 2: clubbing of nails (R68.3)
onychia and paronychia (L03.0-)

L60.0 Ingrowing nail

L60.1 Onycholysis

L60.2 Onychogryphosis

L60.3 Nail dystrophy

L60.4 Beau's lines

L60.5 Yellow nail syndrome

L60.8 Other nail disorders

L60.9 Nail disorder, unspecified

L62 Nail disorders in diseases classified elsewhere
Code first underlying disease, such as:
pachydermoperiostosis (M89.4-)

L63 Alopecia areata

L63.0 Alopecia (capitis) totalis

L63.1 Alopecia universalis

L63.2 Ophiasis

L63.8 Other alopecia areata

L63.9 Alopecia areata, unspecified

L64 Androgenic alopecia
Includes: male-pattern baldness

L64.0 Drug-induced androgenic alopecia
Use additional code for adverse effect, if applicable, to identify drug (T36-T50 with fifth or sixth character 5)

L64.8 Other androgenic alopecia

L64.9 Androgenic alopecia, unspecified

L65 Other nonscarring hair loss
Use additional code for adverse effect, if applicable, to identify drug (T36-T50 with fifth or sixth character 5)
Excludes 1: trichotillomania (F63.3)

L65.0 Telogen effluvium

L65.1 Anagen effluvium

L65.2 Alopecia mucinosa

L65.8 Other specified nonscarring hair loss

L65.9 Nonscarring hair loss, unspecified
Alopecia NOS

L66 Cicatricial alopecia [scarring hair loss]

L66.0 Pseudopelade

L66.1 Lichen planopilaris
Follicular lichen planus

L66.2 Folliculitis decalvans

L66.3 Perifolliculitis capitis abscedens

L66.4 Folliculitis ulerythematosa reticulata

L66.8 Other cicatricial alopecia

L66.9 Cicatricial alopecia, unspecified

L67 Hair color and hair shaft abnormalities
Excludes 1: monilethrix (Q84.1)
pili annulati (Q84.1)
telogen effluvium (L65.0)

L67.0 Trichorrhexis nodosa

L67.1 Variations in hair color
Canities
Greyness, hair (premature)
Heterochromia of hair
Poliosis circumscripta, acquired
Poliosis NOS

L67.8 Other hair color and hair shaft abnormalities
Fragilitas crinium

L67.9 Hair color and hair shaft abnormality, unspecified

L68 Hypertrichosis

Includes: excess hair
Excludes 1: congenital hypertrichosis (Q84.2)
  persistent lanugo (Q84.2)
L68.0 Hirsutism
L68.1 Acquired hypertrichosis lanuginosa
L68.2 Localized hypertrichosis
L68.3 Polytrichia
L68.8 Other hypertrichosis
L68.9 Hypertrichosis, unspecified

L70 Acne
Excludes 2: acne keloid (L73.0)
L70.0 Acne vulgaris
L70.1 Acne conglobata
L70.2 Acne varioliformis
  Acne necrotica miliaris
L70.3 Acne tropica
L70.4 Infantile acne
▲ **L70.5** Acne excoriee des jeunes filles
  Picker's acne
L70.8 Other acne
L70.9 Acne, unspecified

L71 Rosacea
Use additional code for adverse effect, if applicable, to identify drug (T36-T50 with fifth or sixth character 5)
L71.0 Perioral dermatitis
L71.1 Rhinophyma
L71.8 Other rosacea
L71.9 Rosacea, unspecified

L72 Follicular cysts of skin and subcutaneous tissue
L72.0 Epidermal cyst
L72.1 Pilar and trichodermal cyst
  L72.11 Pilar cyst
  L72.12 Trichodermal cyst
    Trichilemmal (proliferating) cyst
L72.2 Steatocystoma multiplex
L72.3 Sebaceous cyst
  Excludes 2: pilar cyst (L72.11)
    trichilemmal (proliferating) cyst (L72.12)
L72.8 Other follicular cysts of the skin and subcutaneous tissue
L72.9 Follicular cyst of the skin and subcutaneous tissue, unspecified

L73 Other follicular disorders
L73.0 Acne keloid
L73.1 Pseudofolliculitis barbae
L73.2 Hidradenitis suppurativa
L73.8 Other specified follicular disorders
  Sycosis barbae
L73.9 Follicular disorder, unspecified

L74 Eccrine sweat disorders
Excludes 2: generalized hyperhidrosis (R61)
L74.0 Miliaria rubra
L74.1 Miliaria crystallina
L74.2 Miliaria profunda
  Miliaria tropicalis
L74.3 Miliaria, unspecified
L74.4 Anhidrosis
  Hypohidrosis
L74.5 Focal hyperhidrosis
  L74.51 Primary focal hyperhidrosis
    L74.510 Primary focal hyperhidrosis, axilla
    L74.511 Primary focal hyperhidrosis, face
    L74.512 Primary focal hyperhidrosis, palms
    L74.513 Primary focal hyperhidrosis, soles
    L74.519 Primary focal hyperhidrosis, unspecified
  L74.52 Secondary focal hyperhidrosis
    Frey's syndrome
L74.8 Other eccrine sweat disorders
L74.9 Eccrine sweat disorder, unspecified
  Sweat gland disorder NOS

L75 Apocrine sweat disorders
Excludes 1: dyshidrosis (L30.1)
  hidradenitis suppurativa (L73.2)
L75.0 Bromhidrosis
L75.1 Chromhidrosis
L75.2 Apocrine miliaria
  Fox-Fordyce disease
L75.8 Other apocrine sweat disorders
L75.9 Apocrine sweat disorder, unspecified

INTRAOPERATIVE AND POSTPROCEDURAL COMPLICATIONS OF SKIN AND SUBCUTANEOUS TISSUE (L76)

L76 Intraoperative and postprocedural complications of skin and subcutaneous tissue
L76.0 Intraoperative hemorrhage and hematoma of skin and subcutaneous tissue complicating a procedure
  Excludes 1: intraoperative hemorrhage and hematoma of skin and subcutaneous tissue due to accidental puncture and laceration during a procedure (L76.1-)
  L76.01 Intraoperative hemorrhage and hematoma of skin and subcutaneous tissue complicating a dermatologic procedure
  L76.02 Intraoperative hemorrhage and hematoma of skin and subcutaneous tissue complicating other procedure
L76.1 Accidental puncture and laceration of skin and subcutaneous tissue during a procedure
  L76.11 Accidental puncture and laceration of skin and subcutaneous tissue during a dermatologic procedure
  L76.12 Accidental puncture and laceration of skin and subcutaneous tissue during other procedure
L76.2 Postprocedural hemorrhage and hematoma of skin and subcutaneous tissue following a procedure
  L76.21 Postprocedural hemorrhage and hematoma of skin and subcutaneous tissue following a dermatologic procedure
  L76.22 Postprocedural hemorrhage and hematoma of skin and subcutaneous tissue following other procedure
L76.8 Other intraoperative and postprocedural complications of skin and subcutaneous tissue
  Use additional code, if applicable, to further specify disorder
  L76.81 Other intraoperative complications of skin and subcutaneous tissue
  L76.82 Other postprocedural complications of skin and subcutaneous tissue

OTHER DISORDERS OF THE SKIN AND SUBCUTANEOUS TISSUE (L80-L99)

L80 Vitiligo
Excludes 2: vitiligo of eyelids (H02.73-)
  vitiligo of vulva (N90.89)

L81 Other disorders of pigmentation
Excludes 1: birthmark NOS (Q82.5)
Peutz-Jeghers syndrome (Q85.8)
Excludes 2: nevus - see Alphabetical Index
L81.0 Postinflammatory hyperpigmentation
L81.1 Chloasma
L81.2 Freckles
L81.3 Cafe au lait spots
L81.4 Other melanin hyperpigmentation
Lentigo
L81.5 Leukoderma, not elsewhere classified
L81.6 Other disorders of diminished melanin formation
L81.7 Pigmented purpuric dermatosis
Angioma serpiginosum
L81.8 Other specified disorders of pigmentation
Iron pigmentation
Tattoo pigmentation
L81.9 Disorder of pigmentation, unspecified
L82 Seborrheic keratosis
Includes: dermatosis papulosa nigra
Leser-Trelat disease
Excludes 2: seborrheic dermatitis (L21.-)
L82.0 Inflamed seborrheic keratosis
L82.1 Other seborrheic keratosis
Seborrheic keratosis NOS
L83 Acanthosis nigricans
Confluent and reticulated papillomatosis
L84 Corns and callosities
Callus
Clavus
L85 Other epidermal thickening
Excludes 2: hypertrophic disorders of the skin (L91.-)
L85.0 Acquired ichthyosis
Excludes 1: congenital ichthyosis (Q80.-)
L85.1 Acquired keratosis [keratoderma] palmaris et plantaris
Excludes 1: inherited keratosis palmaris et plantaris (Q82.8)
L85.2 Keratosis punctata (palmaris et plantaris)
L85.3 Xerosis cutis
Dry skin dermatitis
L85.8 Other specified epidermal thickening
Cutaneous horn
L85.9 Epidermal thickening, unspecified
L86 Keratoderma in diseases classified elsewhere
Code first underlying disease, such as:
Reiter's disease (M02.3-)
Excludes 1: gonococcal keratoderma (A54.89)
gonococcal keratosis (A54.89)
keratoderma due to vitamin A deficiency (E50.8)
keratosis due to vitamin A deficiency (E50.8)
xeroderma due to vitamin A deficiency (E50.8)
L87 Transepidermal elimination disorders
Excludes 1: granuloma annulare (perforating) (L92.0)
L87.0 Keratosis follicularis et parafollicularis in cutem penetrans
Kyrle disease
Hyperkeratosis follicularis penetrans
L87.1 Reactive perforating collagenosis
L87.2 Elastosis perforans serpiginosa
L87.8 Other transepidermal elimination disorders
L87.9 Transepidermal elimination disorder, unspecified
L88 Pyoderma gangrenosum

Phagedenic pyoderma
Excludes 1: dermatitis gangrenosa (L08.0)
L89 Pressure ulcer
Includes: bed sore
decubitus ulcer
plaster ulcer
pressure area
pressure sore
Code first any associated gangrene (I96)
Excludes 2: decubitus (trophic) ulcer of cervix (uteri) (N86)
diabetic ulcers (E08.621, E08.622, E09.621, E09.622, E10.621, E10.622, E11.621, E11.622, E13.621, E13.622)
non-pressure chronic ulcer of skin (L97.-)
skin infections (L00-L08)
varicose ulcer (I83.0, I83.2)
L89.0 Pressure ulcer of elbow
L89.00 Pressure ulcer of unspecified elbow
L89.000 Pressure ulcer of unspecified elbow, unstageable
L89.001 Pressure ulcer of unspecified elbow, stage 1
Healing pressure ulcer of unspecified elbow, stage 1
Pressure pre-ulcer skin changes limited to persistent focal edema, unspecified elbow
L89.002 Pressure ulcer of unspecified elbow, stage 2
Healing pressure ulcer of unspecified elbow, stage 2
Pressure ulcer with abrasion, blister, partial thickness skin loss involving epidermis and/or dermis, unspecified elbow
L89.003 Pressure ulcer of unspecified elbow, stage 3
Healing pressure ulcer of unspecified elbow, stage 3
Pressure ulcer with full thickness skin loss involving damage or necrosis of subcutaneous tissue, unspecified elbow
L89.004 Pressure ulcer of unspecified elbow, stage 4
Healing pressure ulcer of unspecified elbow, stage 4
Pressure ulcer with necrosis of soft tissues through to underlying muscle, tendon, or bone, unspecified elbow
L89.009 Pressure ulcer of unspecified elbow, unspecified stage
Healing pressure ulcer of elbow NOS
Healing pressure ulcer of unspecified elbow, unspecified stage
L89.01 Pressure ulcer of right elbow
L89.010 Pressure ulcer of right elbow, unstageable
L89.011 Pressure ulcer of right elbow, stage 1
Healing pressure ulcer of right elbow, stage 1

Pressure pre-ulcer skin changes limited to persistent focal edema, right elbow

L89.012 Pressure ulcer of right elbow, stage 2

Healing pressure ulcer of right elbow, stage 2

Pressure ulcer with abrasion, blister, partial thickness skin loss involving epidermis and/or dermis, right elbow

L89.013 Pressure ulcer of right elbow, stage 3

Healing pressure ulcer of right elbow, stage 3

Pressure ulcer with full thickness skin loss involving damage or necrosis of subcutaneous tissue, right elbow

L89.014 Pressure ulcer of right elbow, stage 4

Healing pressure ulcer of right elbow, stage 4

Pressure ulcer with necrosis of soft tissues through to underlying muscle, tendon, or bone, right elbow

L89.019 Pressure ulcer of right elbow, unspecified stage

Healing pressure right of elbow NOS

Healing pressure ulcer of unspecified elbow, unspecified stage

L89.02 Pressure ulcer of left elbow

L89.020 Pressure ulcer of left elbow, unstageable

L89.021 Pressure ulcer of left elbow, stage 1

Healing pressure ulcer of left elbow, stage 1

Pressure pre-ulcer skin changes limited to persistent focal edema, left elbow

L89.022 Pressure ulcer of left elbow, stage 2

Healing pressure ulcer of left elbow, stage 2

Pressure ulcer with abrasion, blister, partial thickness skin loss involving epidermis and/or dermis, left elbow

L89.023 Pressure ulcer of left elbow, stage 3

Healing pressure ulcer of left elbow, stage 3

Pressure ulcer with full thickness skin loss involving damage or necrosis of subcutaneous tissue, left elbow

L89.024 Pressure ulcer of left elbow, stage 4

Healing pressure ulcer of left elbow, stage 4

Pressure ulcer with necrosis of soft tissues through to underlying muscle, tendon, or bone, left elbow

L89.029 Pressure ulcer of left elbow, unspecified stage

Healing pressure ulcer of left of elbow NOS

Healing pressure ulcer of unspecified elbow, unspecified stage

L89.1 Pressure ulcer of back

L89.10 Pressure ulcer of unspecified part of back

L89.100 Pressure ulcer of unspecified part of back, unstageable

L89.101 Pressure ulcer of unspecified part of back, stage 1

Healing pressure ulcer of unspecified part of back, stage 1

Pressure pre-ulcer skin changes limited to persistent focal edema, unspecified part of back

L89.102 Pressure ulcer of unspecified part of back, stage 2

Healing pressure ulcer of unspecified part of back, stage 2

Pressure ulcer with abrasion, blister, partial thickness skin loss involving epidermis and/or dermis, unspecified part of back

L89.103 Pressure ulcer of unspecified part of back, stage 3

Healing pressure ulcer of unspecified part of back, stage 3

Pressure ulcer with full thickness skin loss involving damage or necrosis of subcutaneous tissue, unspecified part of back

L89.104 Pressure ulcer of unspecified part of back, stage 4

Healing pressure ulcer of unspecified part of back, stage 4

Pressure ulcer with necrosis of soft tissues through to underlying muscle, tendon, or bone, unspecified part of back

L89.109 Pressure ulcer of unspecified part of back, unspecified stage

Healing pressure ulcer of unspecified part of back NOS

Healing pressure ulcer of unspecified part of back, unspecified stage

L89.11 Pressure ulcer of right upper back

Pressure ulcer of right shoulder blade

L89.110 Pressure ulcer of right upper back, unstageable

L89.111 Pressure ulcer of right upper back, stage 1

Healing pressure ulcer of right upper back, stage 1

Pressure pre-ulcer skin changes limited to persistent focal edema, right upper back

L89.112 Pressure ulcer of right upper back, stage 2

Healing pressure ulcer of right upper back, stage 2

Pressure ulcer with abrasion, blister, partial thickness skin loss involving epidermis and/or dermis, right upper back

L89.113 Pressure ulcer of right upper back, stage 3

Healing pressure ulcer of right upper back, stage 3

Pressure ulcer with full thickness skin loss involving damage or necrosis of subcutaneous tissue, right upper back

L89.114 Pressure ulcer of right upper back, stage 4

Healing pressure ulcer of right upper back, stage 4

Pressure ulcer with necrosis of soft tissues through to underlying muscle, tendon, or bone, right upper back

L89.119 Pressure ulcer of right upper back, unspecified stage

Healing pressure ulcer of right upper back NOS

Healing pressure ulcer of right upper back, unspecified stage

L89.12 Pressure ulcer of left upper back

Pressure ulcer of left shoulder blade

L89.120 Pressure ulcer of left upper back, unstageable

L89.121 Pressure ulcer of left upper back, stage 1

Healing pressure ulcer of left upper back, stage 1

Pressure pre-ulcer skin changes limited to persistent focal edema, left upper back

L89.122 Pressure ulcer of left upper back, stage 2

Healing pressure ulcer of left upper back, stage 2

Pressure ulcer with abrasion, blister, partial thickness skin loss involving epidermis and/or dermis, left upper back

L89.123 Pressure ulcer of left upper back, stage 3

Healing pressure ulcer of left upper back, stage 3

Pressure ulcer with full thickness skin loss involving damage or necrosis of subcutaneous tissue, left upper back

L89.124 Pressure ulcer of left upper back, stage 4

Healing pressure ulcer of left upper back, stage 4

Pressure ulcer with necrosis of soft tissues through to underlying muscle, tendon, or bone, left upper back

L89.129 Pressure ulcer of left upper back, unspecified stage

Healing pressure ulcer of left upper back NOS

Healing pressure ulcer of left upper back, unspecified stage

L89.13 Pressure ulcer of right lower back

L89.130 Pressure ulcer of right lower back, unstageable

L89.131 Pressure ulcer of right lower back, stage 1

Healing pressure ulcer of right lower back, stage 1

Pressure pre-ulcer skin changes limited to persistent focal edema, right lower back

L89.132 Pressure ulcer of right lower back, stage 2

Healing pressure ulcer of right lower back, stage 2

Pressure ulcer with abrasion, blister, partial thickness skin loss involving epidermis and/or dermis, right lower back

L89.133 Pressure ulcer of right lower back, stage 3

Healing pressure ulcer of right lower back, stage 3

Pressure ulcer with full thickness skin loss involving damage or necrosis of subcutaneous tissue, right lower back

L89.134 Pressure ulcer of right lower back, stage 4

Healing pressure ulcer of right lower back, stage 4

Pressure ulcer with necrosis of soft tissues through to underlying muscle, tendon, or bone, right lower back

L89.139 Pressure ulcer of right lower back, unspecified stage

Healing pressure ulcer of right lower back NOS

Healing pressure ulcer of right lower back, unspecified stage

L89.14 Pressure ulcer of left lower back

L89.140 Pressure ulcer of left lower back, unstageable

L89.141 Pressure ulcer of left lower back, stage 1

Healing pressure ulcer of left lower back, stage 1

Pressure pre-ulcer skin changes limited to persistent focal edema, left lower back

L89.142 Pressure ulcer of left lower back, stage 2

Healing pressure ulcer of left lower back, stage 2

Pressure ulcer with abrasion, blister, partial thickness skin loss involving epidermis and/or dermis, left lower back

L89.143 Pressure ulcer of left lower back, stage 3

Healing pressure ulcer of left lower back, stage 3

Pressure ulcer with full thickness skin loss involving damage or necrosis of subcutaneous tissue, left lower back

L89.144 Pressure ulcer of left lower back, stage 4

Healing pressure ulcer of left lower back, stage 4

Pressure ulcer with necrosis of soft tissues through to underlying muscle, tendon, or bone, left lower back

L89.149 Pressure ulcer of left lower back, unspecified stage

Healing pressure ulcer of left lower back NOS

Healing pressure ulcer of left lower back, unspecified stage

L89.15 Pressure ulcer of sacral region

Pressure ulcer of coccyx

Pressure ulcer of tailbone

L89.150 Pressure ulcer of sacral region, unstageable

L89.151 Pressure ulcer of sacral region, stage 1

Healing pressure ulcer of sacral region, stage 1

Pressure pre-ulcer skin changes limited to persistent focal edema, sacral region

L89.152 Pressure ulcer of sacral region, stage 2

Healing pressure ulcer of sacral region, stage 2

Pressure ulcer with abrasion, blister, partial thickness skin loss involving epidermis and/or dermis, sacral region

L89.153 Pressure ulcer of sacral region, stage 3

Healing pressure ulcer of sacral region, stage 3

Pressure ulcer with full thickness skin loss involving damage or necrosis of subcutaneous tissue, sacral region

L89.154 Pressure ulcer of sacral region, stage 4

Healing pressure ulcer of sacral region, stage 4

Pressure ulcer with necrosis of soft tissues through to underlying muscle, tendon, or bone, sacral region

L89.159 Pressure ulcer of sacral region, unspecified stage

Healing pressure ulcer of sacral region NOS

Healing pressure ulcer of sacral region, unspecified stage

L89.2 Pressure ulcer of hip

L89.20 Pressure ulcer of unspecified hip

L89.200 Pressure ulcer of unspecified hip, unstageable

L89.201 Pressure ulcer of unspecified hip, stage 1

Healing pressure ulcer of unspecified hip back, stage 1

Pressure pre-ulcer skin changes limited to persistent focal edema, unspecified hip

L89.202 Pressure ulcer of unspecified hip, stage 2

Healing pressure ulcer of unspecified hip, stage 2

Pressure ulcer with abrasion, blister, partial thickness skin loss involving epidermis and/or dermis, unspecified hip

L89.203 Pressure ulcer of unspecified hip, stage 3

Healing pressure ulcer of unspecified hip, stage 3

Pressure ulcer with full thickness skin loss involving damage or necrosis of subcutaneous tissue, unspecified hip

L89.204 Pressure ulcer of unspecified hip, stage 4

Healing pressure ulcer of unspecified hip, stage 4

Pressure ulcer with necrosis of soft tissues through to underlying muscle, tendon, or bone, unspecified hip

L89.209 Pressure ulcer of unspecified hip, unspecified stage

Healing pressure ulcer of unspecified hip NOS

Healing pressure ulcer of unspecified hip, unspecified stage

L89.21 Pressure ulcer of right hip

L89.210 Pressure ulcer of right hip, unstageable

L89.211 Pressure ulcer of right hip, stage 1

Healing pressure ulcer of right hip back, stage 1

Pressure pre-ulcer skin changes limited to persistent focal edema, right hip

L89.212 Pressure ulcer of right hip, stage 2

Healing pressure ulcer of right hip, stage 2

Pressure ulcer with abrasion, blister, partial thickness skin loss involving epidermis and/or dermis, right hip

L89.213 Pressure ulcer of right hip, stage 3

Healing pressure ulcer of right hip, stage 3

Pressure ulcer with full thickness skin loss involving damage or necrosis of subcutaneous tissue, right hip

L89.214 Pressure ulcer of right hip, stage 4

Healing pressure ulcer of right hip, stage 4

Pressure ulcer with necrosis of soft tissues through to underlying muscle, tendon, or bone, right hip

L89.219 Pressure ulcer of right hip, unspecified stage

Healing pressure ulcer of right hip NOS

Healing pressure ulcer of right hip, unspecified stage

L89.22 Pressure ulcer of left hip

L89.220 Pressure ulcer of left hip, unstageable

L89.221 Pressure ulcer of left hip, stage 1

Healing pressure ulcer of left hip back, stage 1

Pressure pre-ulcer skin changes limited to persistent focal edema, left hip

L89.222   Pressure ulcer of left hip, stage 2

Healing pressure ulcer of left hip, stage 2

Pressure ulcer with abrasion, blister, partial thickness skin loss involving epidermis and/or dermis, left hip

L89.223   Pressure ulcer of left hip, stage 3

Healing pressure ulcer of left hip, stage 3

Pressure ulcer with full thickness skin loss involving damage or necrosis of subcutaneous tissue, left hip

L89.224   Pressure ulcer of left hip, stage 4

Healing pressure ulcer of left hip, stage 4

Pressure ulcer with necrosis of soft tissues through to underlying muscle, tendon, or bone, left hip

L89.229   Pressure ulcer of left hip, unspecified stage

Healing pressure ulcer of left hip NOS

Healing pressure ulcer of left hip, unspecified stage

L89.3   Pressure ulcer of buttock

L89.30   Pressure ulcer of unspecified buttock

L89.300   Pressure ulcer of unspecified buttock, unstageable

L89.301   Pressure ulcer of unspecified buttock, stage 1

Healing pressure ulcer of unspecified buttock, stage 1

Pressure pre-ulcer skin changes limited to persistent focal edema, unspecified buttock

L89.302   Pressure ulcer of unspecified buttock, stage 2

Healing pressure ulcer of unspecified buttock, stage 2

Pressure ulcer with abrasion, blister, partial thickness skin loss involving epidermis and/or dermis, unspecified buttock

L89.303   Pressure ulcer of unspecified buttock, stage 3

Healing pressure ulcer of unspecified buttock, stage 3

Pressure ulcer with full thickness skin loss involving damage or necrosis of subcutaneous tissue, unspecified buttock

L89.304   Pressure ulcer of unspecified buttock, stage 4

Healing pressure ulcer of unspecified buttock, stage 4

Pressure ulcer with necrosis of soft tissues through to underlying muscle, tendon, or bone, unspecified buttock

L89.309   Pressure ulcer of unspecified buttock, unspecified stage

Healing pressure ulcer of unspecified buttock NOS

Healing pressure ulcer of unspecified buttock, unspecified stage

L89.31   Pressure ulcer of right buttock

L89.310   Pressure ulcer of right buttock, unstageable

L89.311   Pressure ulcer of right buttock, stage 1

Healing pressure ulcer of right buttock, stage 1

Pressure pre-ulcer skin changes limited to persistent focal edema, right buttock

L89.312   Pressure ulcer of right buttock, stage 2

Healing pressure ulcer of right buttock, stage 2

Pressure ulcer with abrasion, blister, partial thickness skin loss involving epidermis and/or dermis, right buttock

L89.313   Pressure ulcer of right buttock, stage 3

Healing pressure ulcer of right buttock, stage 3

Pressure ulcer with full thickness skin loss involving damage or necrosis of subcutaneous tissue, right buttock

L89.314   Pressure ulcer of right buttock, stage 4

Healing pressure ulcer of right buttock, stage 4

Pressure ulcer with necrosis of soft tissues through to underlying muscle, tendon, or bone, right buttock

L89.319   Pressure ulcer of right buttock, unspecified stage

Healing pressure ulcer of right buttock NOS

Healing pressure ulcer of right buttock, unspecified stage

L89.32   Pressure ulcer of left buttock

L89.320   Pressure ulcer of left buttock, unstageable

L89.321   Pressure ulcer of left buttock, stage 1

Healing pressure ulcer of left buttock, stage 1

Pressure pre-ulcer skin changes limited to persistent focal edema, left buttock

L89.322   Pressure ulcer of left buttock, stage 2

Healing pressure ulcer of left buttock, stage 2

Pressure ulcer with abrasion, blister, partial thickness skin loss involving epidermis and/or dermis, left buttock

L89.323   Pressure ulcer of left buttock, stage 3

Healing pressure ulcer of left buttock, stage 3

● New code   ▲ Revised code   ⑦ 7th digit required   ⊗ Placeholder required

Pressure ulcer with full thickness skin loss involving damage or necrosis of subcutaneous tissue, left buttock

L89.324 Pressure ulcer of left buttock, stage 4

Healing pressure ulcer of left buttock, stage 4

Pressure ulcer with necrosis of soft tissues through to underlying muscle, tendon, or bone, left buttock

L89.329 Pressure ulcer of left buttock, unspecified stage

Healing pressure ulcer of left buttock NOS

Healing pressure ulcer of left buttock, unspecified stage

L89.4 Pressure ulcer of contiguous site of back, buttock and hip

L89.40 Pressure ulcer of contiguous site of back, buttock and hip, unspecified stage

Healing pressure ulcer of contiguous site of back, buttock and hip NOS

Healing pressure ulcer of contiguous site of back, buttock and hip, unspecified stage

L89.41 Pressure ulcer of contiguous site of back, buttock and hip, stage 1

Healing pressure ulcer of contiguous site of back, buttock and hip, stage 1

Pressure pre-ulcer skin changes limited to persistent focal edema, contiguous site of back, buttock and hip

L89.42 Pressure ulcer of contiguous site of back, buttock and hip, stage 2

Healing pressure ulcer of contiguous site of back, buttock and hip, stage 2

Pressure ulcer with abrasion, blister, partial thickness skin loss involving epidermis and/or dermis, contiguous site of back, buttock and hip

L89.43 Pressure ulcer of contiguous site of back, buttock and hip, stage 3

Healing pressure ulcer of contiguous site of back, buttock and hip, stage 3

Pressure ulcer with full thickness skin loss involving damage or necrosis of subcutaneous tissue, contiguous site of back, buttock and hip

L89.44 Pressure ulcer of contiguous site of back, buttock and hip, stage 4

Healing pressure ulcer of contiguous site of back, buttock and hip, stage 4

Pressure ulcer with necrosis of soft tissues through to underlying muscle, tendon, or bone, contiguous site of back, buttock and hip

L89.45 Pressure ulcer of contiguous site of back, buttock and hip, unstageable

L89.5 Pressure ulcer of ankle

L89.50 Pressure ulcer of unspecified ankle

L89.500 Pressure ulcer of unspecified ankle, unstageable

L89.501 Pressure ulcer of unspecified ankle, stage 1

Healing pressure ulcer of unspecified ankle, stage 1

Pressure pre-ulcer skin changes limited to persistent focal edema, unspecified ankle

L89.502 Pressure ulcer of unspecified ankle, stage 2

Healing pressure ulcer of unspecified ankle, stage 2

Pressure ulcer with abrasion, blister, partial thickness skin loss involving epidermis and/or dermis, unspecified ankle

L89.503 Pressure ulcer of unspecified ankle, stage 3

Healing pressure ulcer of unspecified ankle, stage 3

Pressure ulcer with full thickness skin loss involving damage or necrosis of subcutaneous tissue, unspecified ankle

L89.504 Pressure ulcer of unspecified ankle, stage 4

Healing pressure ulcer of unspecified ankle, stage 4

Pressure ulcer with necrosis of soft tissues through to underlying muscle, tendon, or bone, unspecified ankle

L89.509 Pressure ulcer of unspecified ankle, unspecified stage

Healing pressure ulcer of unspecified ankle NOS

Healing pressure ulcer of unspecified ankle, unspecified stage

L89.51 Pressure ulcer of right ankle

L89.510 Pressure ulcer of right ankle, unstageable

L89.511 Pressure ulcer of right ankle, stage 1

Healing pressure ulcer of right ankle, stage 1

Pressure pre-ulcer skin changes limited to persistent focal edema, right ankle

L89.512 Pressure ulcer of right ankle, stage 2

Healing pressure ulcer of right ankle, stage 2

Pressure ulcer with abrasion, blister, partial thickness skin loss involving epidermis and/or dermis, right ankle

L89.513 Pressure ulcer of right ankle, stage 3

Healing pressure ulcer of right ankle, stage 3

Pressure ulcer with full thickness skin loss involving damage or necrosis of subcutaneous tissue, right ankle

L89.514 Pressure ulcer of right ankle, stage 4

Healing pressure ulcer of right ankle, stage 4

Pressure ulcer with necrosis of soft tissues through to underlying muscle, tendon, or bone, right ankle

L89.519 Pressure ulcer of right ankle, unspecified stage

Healing pressure ulcer of right ankle NOS

Healing pressure ulcer of right ankle, unspecified stage

L89.52 Pressure ulcer of left ankle

L89.520 Pressure ulcer of left ankle, unstageable

L89.521 Pressure ulcer of left ankle, stage 1

Healing pressure ulcer of left ankle, stage 1

Pressure pre-ulcer skin changes limited to persistnt focal edema, left ankle

L89.522 Pressure ulcer of left ankle, stage 2

Healing pressure ulcer of left ankle, stage 2

Pressure ulcer with abrasion, blister, partial thickness skin loss involving epidermis and/or dermis, left ankle

L89.523 Pressure ulcer of left ankle, stage 3

Healing pressure ulcer of left ankle, stage 3

Pressure ulcer with full thickness skin loss involving damage or necrosis of subcutaneous tissue, left ankle

L89.524 Pressure ulcer of left ankle, stage 4

Healing pressure ulcer of left ankle, stage 4

Pressure ulcer with necrosis of soft tissues through to underlying muscle, tendon, or bone, left ankle

L89.529 Pressure ulcer of left ankle, unspecified stage

Healing pressure ulcer of left ankle NOS

Healing pressure ulcer of left ankle, unspecified stage

L89.6 Pressure ulcer of heel

L89.60 Pressure ulcer of unspecified heel

L89.600 Pressure ulcer of unspecified heel, unstageable

L89.601 Pressure ulcer of unspecified heel, stage 1

Healing pressure ulcer of unspecified heel, stage 1

Pressure pre-ulcer skin changes limited to persistent focal edema, unspecified heel

L89.602 Pressure ulcer of unspecified heel, stage 2

Healing pressure ulcer of unspecified heel, stage 2

Pressure ulcer with abrasion, blister, partial thickness skin loss involving epidermis and/or dermis, unspecified heel

L89.603 Pressure ulcer of unspecified heel, stage 3

Healing pressure ulcer of unspecified heel, stage 3

Pressure ulcer with full thickness skin loss involving damage or necrosis of subcutaneous tissue, unspecified heel

L89.604 Pressure ulcer of unspecified heel, stage 4

Healing pressure ulcer of unspecified heel, stage 4

Pressure ulcer with necrosis of soft tissues through to underlying muscle, tendon, or bone, unspecified heel

L89.609 Pressure ulcer of unspecified heel, unspecified stage

Healing pressure ulcer of unspecified heel NOS

Healing pressure ulcer of unspecified heel, unspecified stage

L89.61 Pressure ulcer of right heel

L89.610 Pressure ulcer of right heel, unstageable

L89.611 Pressure ulcer of right heel, stage 1

Healing pressure ulcer of right heel, stage 1

Pressure pre-ulcer skin changes limited to persistent focal edema, right heel

L89.612 Pressure ulcer of right heel, stage 2

Healing pressure ulcer of right heel, stage 2

Pressure ulcer with abrasion, blister, partial thickness skin loss involving epidermis and/or dermis, right heel

L89.613 Pressure ulcer of right heel, stage 3

Healing pressure ulcer of right heel, stage 3

Pressure ulcer with full thickness skin loss involving damage or necrosis of subcutaneous tissue, right heel

L89.614 Pressure ulcer of right heel, stage 4

Healing pressure ulcer of right heel, stage 4

Pressure ulcer with necrosis of soft tissues through to underlying muscle, tendon, or bone, right heel

L89.619 Pressure ulcer of right heel, unspecified stage

Healing pressure ulcer of right heel NOS

Healing pressure ulcer of unspecified heel, right stage

L89.62 Pressure ulcer of left heel

L89.620 Pressure ulcer of left heel, unstageable

L89.621 Pressure ulcer of left heel, stage 1

Healing pressure ulcer of left heel, stage 1

Pressure pre-ulcer skin changes limited to persistent focal edema, left heel

L89.622 Pressure ulcer of left heel, stage 2

Healing pressure ulcer of left heel, stage 2

Pressure ulcer with abrasion, blister, partial thickness skin loss involving epidermis and/or dermis, left heel

L89.623 Pressure ulcer of left heel, stage 3

Healing pressure ulcer of left heel, stage 3

Pressure ulcer with full thickness skin loss involving damage or necrosis of subcutaneous tissue, left heel

L89.624 Pressure ulcer of left heel, stage 4

Healing pressure ulcer of left heel, stage 4

Pressure ulcer with necrosis of soft tissues through to underlying muscle, tendon, or bone, left heel

L89.629 Pressure ulcer of left heel, unspecified stage

Healing pressure ulcer of left heel NOS

Healing pressure ulcer of left heel, unspecified stage

L89.8 Pressure ulcer of other site

L89.81 Pressure ulcer of head

Pressure ulcer of face

L89.810 Pressure ulcer of head, unstageable

L89.811 Pressure ulcer of head, stage 1

Healing pressure ulcer of head, stage 1

Pressure pre-ulcer skin changes limited to persistent focal edema, head

L89.812 Pressure ulcer of head, stage 2

Healing pressure ulcer of head, stage 2

Pressure ulcer with abrasion, blister, partial thickness skin loss involving epidermis and/or dermis, head

L89.813 Pressure ulcer of head, stage 3

Healing pressure ulcer of head, stage 3

Pressure ulcer with full thickness skin loss involving damage or necrosis of subcutaneous tissue, head

L89.814 Pressure ulcer of head, stage 4

Healing pressure ulcer of head, stage 4

Pressure ulcer with necrosis of soft tissues through to underlying muscle, tendon, or bone, head

L89.819 Pressure ulcer of head, unspecified stage

Healing pressure ulcer of head NOS

Healing pressure ulcer of head, unspecified stage

L89.89 Pressure ulcer of other site

L89.890 Pressure ulcer of other site, unstageable

L89.891 Pressure ulcer of other site, stage 1

Healing pressure ulcer of other site, stage 1

Pressure pre-ulcer skin changes limited to persistent focal edema, other site

L89.892 Pressure ulcer of other site, stage 2

Healing pressure ulcer of other site, stage 2

Pressure ulcer with abrasion, blister, partial thickness skin loss involving epidermis and/or dermis, other site

L89.893 Pressure ulcer of other site, stage 3

Healing pressure ulcer of other site, stage 3

Pressure ulcer with full thickness skin loss involving damage or necrosis of subcutaneous tissue, other site

L89.894 Pressure ulcer of other site, stage 4

Healing pressure ulcer of other site, stage 4

Pressure ulcer with necrosis of soft tissues through to underlying muscle, tendon, or bone, other site

L89.899 Pressure ulcer of other site, unspecified stage

Healing pressure ulcer of other site NOS

Healing pressure ulcer of other site, unspecified stage

L89.9 Pressure ulcer of unspecified site

L89.90 Pressure ulcer of unspecified site, unspecified stage

Healing pressure ulcer of unspecified site NOS

Healing pressure ulcer of unspecified site, unspecified stage

L89.91 Pressure ulcer of unspecified site, stage 1

Healing pressure ulcer of unspecified site, stage 1

Pressure pre-ulcer skin changes limited to persistent focal edema, unspecified site

L89.92 Pressure ulcer of unspecified site, stage 2

Healing pressure ulcer of unspecified site, stage 2

Pressure ulcer with abrasion, blister, partial thickness skin loss involving epidermis and/or dermis, unspecified site

L89.93 Pressure ulcer of unspecified site, stage 3

Healing pressure ulcer of unspecified site, stage 3

Pressure ulcer with full thickness skin loss involving damage or necrosis of subcutaneous tissue, unspecified site

L89.94 Pressure ulcer of unspecified site, stage 4

Healing pressure ulcer of unspecified site, stage 4

Pressure ulcer with necrosis of soft tissues through to underlying muscle, tendon, or bone, unspecified site

L89.95 Pressure ulcer of unspecified site, unstageable

L90 Atrophic disorders of skin

L90.0 Lichen sclerosus et atrophicus

Excludes 2: lichen sclerosus of external female genital organs (N90.4)

lichen sclerosus of external male genital organs (N48.0)

L90.1 Anetoderma of Schweninger-Buzzi

L90.2 Anetoderma of Jadassohn-Pellizzari

L90.3 Atrophoderma of Pasini and Pierini

L90.4 Acrodermatitis chronica atrophicans

L90.5 Scar conditions and fibrosis of skin

Adherent scar (skin)

Cicatrix

Disfigurement of skin due to scar

Fibrosis of skin NOS

Scar NOS

Excludes 2: hypertrophic scar (L91.0)

keloid scar (L91.0)

L90.6 Striae atrophicae

L90.8 Other atrophic disorders of skin

L90.9 Atrophic disorder of skin, unspecified

L91 Hypertrophic disorders of skin

L91.0 Hypertrophic scar

Keloid

Keloid scar

> **Excludes 2:** acne keloid (L73.0)
>
> scar NOS (L90.5)

L91.8 Other hypertrophic disorders of the skin

L91.9 Hypertrophic disorder of the skin, unspecified

L92 Granulomatous disorders of skin and subcutaneous tissue

> **Excludes 2:** actinic granuloma (L57.5)

L92.0 Granuloma annulare

Perforating granuloma annulare

L92.1 Necrobiosis lipoidica, not elsewhere classified

> **Excludes 1:** necrobiosis lipoidica associated with diabetes mellitus (E08-E13 with .620)

L92.2 Granuloma faciale [eosinophilic granuloma of skin]

L92.3 Foreign body granuloma of the skin and subcutaneous tissue

Use additional code to identify the type of retained foreign body (Z18.-)

L92.8 Other granulomatous disorders of the skin and subcutaneous tissue

L92.9 Granulomatous disorder of the skin and subcutaneous tissue, unspecified

L93 Lupus erythematosus

Use additional code for adverse effect, if applicable, to identify drug (T36-T50 with fifth or sixth character 5)

> **Excludes 1:** lupus exedens (A18.4)
>
> lupus vulgaris (A18.4)
>
> scleroderma (M34.-)
>
> systemic lupus erythematosus (M32.-)

L93.0 Discoid lupus erythematosus

Lupus erythematosus NOS

L93.1 Subacute cutaneous lupus erythematosus

L93.2 Other local lupus erythematosus

Lupus erythematosus profundus

Lupus panniculitis

L94 Other localized connective tissue disorders

> **Excludes 1:** systemic connective tissue disorders (M30-M36)

L94.0 Localized scleroderma [morphea]

Circumscribed scleroderma

L94.1 Linear scleroderma

En coup de sabre lesion

L94.2 Calcinosis cutis

L94.3 Sclerodactyly

L94.4 Gottron's papules

L94.5 Poikiloderma vasculare atrophicans

L94.6 Ainhum

L94.8 Other specified localized connective tissue disorders

L94.9 Localized connective tissue disorder, unspecified

L95 Vasculitis limited to skin, not elsewhere classified

> **Excludes 1:** angioma serpiginosum (L81.7)
>
> Henoch (-Schonlein) purpura (D69.0)
>
> hypersensitivity angiitis (M31.0)
>
> lupus panniculitis (L93.2)
>
> panniculitis NOS (M79.3)
>
> panniculitis of neck and back (M54.0-)
>
> polyarteritis nodosa (M30.0)
>
> relapsing panniculitis (M35.6)
>
> rheumatoid vasculitis (M05.2)
>
> serum sickness (T80.6-)

> urticaria (L50.-)
>
> Wegener's granulomatosis (M31.3-)

L95.0 Livedoid vasculitis

Atrophie blanche (en plaque)

L95.1 Erythema elevatum diutinum

L95.8 Other vasculitis limited to the skin

L95.9 Vasculitis limited to the skin, unspecified

L97 Non-pressure chronic ulcer of lower limb, not elsewhere classified

> **Includes:** chronic ulcer of skin of lower limb NOS
>
> non-healing ulcer of skin
>
> non-infected sinus of skin
>
> trophic ulcer NOS
>
> tropical ulcer NOS
>
> ulcer of skin of lower limb NOS

Code first any associated underlying condition, such as:

any associated gangrene (I96)

atherosclerosis of the lower extremities (I70.23-, I70.24-, I70.33-, I70.34-, I70.43-, I70.44-, I70.53-, I70.54-, I70.63-, I70.64-, I70.73-, I70.74-)

chronic venous hypertension (I87.31-, I87.33-)

diabetic ulcers (E08.621, E08.622, E09.621, E09.622, E10.621, E10.622, E11.621, E11.622, E13.621, E13.622)

postphlebitic syndrome (I87.01-, I87.03-)

postthrombotic syndrome (I87.01-, I87.03-)

varicose ulcer (I83.0-, I83.2-)

> **Excludes 2:** pressure ulcer (pressure area) (L89.-)
>
> skin infections (L00-L08)
>
> specific infections classified to A00-B99

L97.1 Non-pressure chronic ulcer of thigh

    L97.10 Non-pressure chronic ulcer of unspecified thigh

        L97.101 Non-pressure chronic ulcer of unspecified thigh limited to breakdown of skin

        L97.102 Non-pressure chronic ulcer of unspecified thigh with fat layer exposed

        L97.103 Non-pressure chronic ulcer of unspecified thigh with necrosis of muscle

        L97.104 Non-pressure chronic ulcer of unspecified thigh with necrosis of bone

        L97.109 Non-pressure chronic ulcer of unspecified thigh with unspecified severity

    L97.11 Non-pressure chronic ulcer of right thigh

        L97.111 Non-pressure chronic ulcer of right thigh limited to breakdown of skin

        L97.112 Non-pressure chronic ulcer of right thigh with fat layer exposed

        L97.113 Non-pressure chronic ulcer of right thigh with necrosis of muscle

        L97.114 Non-pressure chronic ulcer of right thigh with necrosis of bone

        L97.119 Non-pressure chronic ulcer of right thigh with unspecified severity

    L97.12 Non-pressure chronic ulcer of left thigh

        L97.121 Non-pressure chronic ulcer of left thigh limited to breakdown of skin

        L97.122 Non-pressure chronic ulcer of left thigh with fat layer exposed

        L97.123 Non-pressure chronic ulcer of left thigh with necrosis of muscle

● New code   ▲ Revised code   ⑦ 7th digit required   ⊗ Placeholder required

L97.124 Non-pressure chronic ulcer of left thigh with necrosis of bone

L97.129 Non-pressure chronic ulcer of left thigh with unspecified severity

L97.2 Non-pressure chronic ulcer of calf

L97.20 Non-pressure chronic ulcer of unspecified calf

L97.201 Non-pressure chronic ulcer of unspecified calf limited to breakdown of skin

L97.202 Non-pressure chronic ulcer of unspecified calf with fat layer exposed

L97.203 Non-pressure chronic ulcer of unspecified calf with necrosis of muscle

L97.204 Non-pressure chronic ulcer of unspecified calf with necrosis of bone

L97.209 Non-pressure chronic ulcer of unspecified calf with unspecified severity

L97.21 Non-pressure chronic ulcer of right calf

L97.211 Non-pressure chronic ulcer of right calf limited to breakdown of skin

L97.212 Non-pressure chronic ulcer of right calf with fat layer exposed

L97.213 Non-pressure chronic ulcer of right calf with necrosis of muscle

L97.214 Non-pressure chronic ulcer of right calf with necrosis of bone

L97.219 Non-pressure chronic ulcer of right calf with unspecified severity

L97.22 Non-pressure chronic ulcer of left calf

L97.221 Non-pressure chronic ulcer of left calf limited to breakdown of skin

L97.222 Non-pressure chronic ulcer of left calf with fat layer exposed

L97.223 Non-pressure chronic ulcer of left calf with necrosis of muscle

L97.224 Non-pressure chronic ulcer of left calf with necrosis of bone

L97.229 Non-pressure chronic ulcer of left calf with unspecified severity

L97.3 Non-pressure chronic ulcer of ankle

L97.30 Non-pressure chronic ulcer of unspecified ankle

L97.301 Non-pressure chronic ulcer of unspecified ankle limited to breakdown of skin

L97.302 Non-pressure chronic ulcer of unspecified ankle with fat layer exposed

L97.303 Non-pressure chronic ulcer of unspecified ankle with necrosis of muscle

L97.304 Non-pressure chronic ulcer of unspecified ankle with necrosis of bone

L97.309 Non-pressure chronic ulcer of unspecified ankle with unspecified severity

L97.31 Non-pressure chronic ulcer of right ankle

L97.311 Non-pressure chronic ulcer of right ankle limited to breakdown of skin

L97.312 Non-pressure chronic ulcer of right ankle with fat layer exposed

L97.313 Non-pressure chronic ulcer of right ankle with necrosis of muscle

L97.314 Non-pressure chronic ulcer of right ankle with necrosis of bone

L97.319 Non-pressure chronic ulcer of right ankle with unspecified severity

L97.32 Non-pressure chronic ulcer of left ankle

L97.321 Non-pressure chronic ulcer of left ankle limited to breakdown of skin

L97.322 Non-pressure chronic ulcer of left ankle with fat layer exposed

L97.323 Non-pressure chronic ulcer of left ankle with necrosis of muscle

L97.324 Non-pressure chronic ulcer of left ankle with necrosis of bone

L97.329 Non-pressure chronic ulcer of left ankle with unspecified severity

L97.4 Non-pressure chronic ulcer of heel and midfoot
Non-pressure chronic ulcer of plantar surface of midfoot

L97.40 Non-pressure chronic ulcer of unspecified heel and midfoot

L97.401 Non-pressure chronic ulcer of unspecified heel and midfoot limited to breakdown of skin

L97.402 Non-pressure chronic ulcer of unspecified heel and midfoot with fat layer exposed

L97.403 Non-pressure chronic ulcer of unspecified heel and midfoot with necrosis of muscle

L97.404 Non-pressure chronic ulcer of unspecified heel and midfoot with necrosis of bone

L97.409 Non-pressure chronic ulcer of unspecified heel and midfoot with unspecified severity

L97.41 Non-pressure chronic ulcer of right heel and midfoot

L97.411 Non-pressure chronic ulcer of right heel and midfoot limited to breakdown of skin

L97.412 Non-pressure chronic ulcer of right heel and midfoot with fat layer exposed

L97.413 Non-pressure chronic ulcer of right heel and midfoot with necrosis of muscle

L97.414 Non-pressure chronic ulcer of right heel and midfoot with necrosis of bone

L97.419 Non-pressure chronic ulcer of right heel and midfoot with unspecified severity

L97.42 Non-pressure chronic ulcer of left heel and midfoot

L97.421 Non-pressure chronic ulcer of left heel and midfoot limited to breakdown of skin

L97.422 Non-pressure chronic ulcer of left heel and midfoot with fat layer exposed

L97.423 Non-pressure chronic ulcer of left heel and midfoot with necrosis of muscle

L97.424 Non-pressure chronic ulcer of left heel and midfoot with necrosis of bone

L97.429 Non-pressure chronic ulcer of left heel and midfoot with unspecified severity

L97.5 Non-pressure chronic ulcer of other part of foot
Non-pressure chronic ulcer of toe

    L97.50 Non-pressure chronic ulcer of other part of unspecified foot

L97.501 Non-pressure chronic ulcer of other part of unspecified foot limited to breakdown of skin

L97.502 Non-pressure chronic ulcer of other part of unspecified foot with fat layer exposed

L97.503 Non-pressure chronic ulcer of other part of unspecified foot with necrosis of muscle

L97.504 Non-pressure chronic ulcer of other part of unspecified foot with necrosis of bone

L97.509 Non-pressure chronic ulcer of other part of unspecified foot with unspecified severity

    L97.51 Non-pressure chronic ulcer of other part of right foot

L97.511 Non-pressure chronic ulcer of other part of right foot limited to breakdown of skin

L97.512 Non-pressure chronic ulcer of other part of right foot with fat layer exposed

L97.513 Non-pressure chronic ulcer of other part of right foot with necrosis of muscle

L97.514 Non-pressure chronic ulcer of other part of right foot with necrosis of bone

L97.519 Non-pressure chronic ulcer of other part of right foot with unspecified severity

    L97.52 Non-pressure chronic ulcer of other part of left foot

L97.521 Non-pressure chronic ulcer of other part of left foot limited to breakdown of skin

L97.522 Non-pressure chronic ulcer of other part of left foot with fat layer exposed

L97.523 Non-pressure chronic ulcer of other part of left foot with necrosis of muscle

L97.524 Non-pressure chronic ulcer of other part of left foot with necrosis of bone

L97.529 Non-pressure chronic ulcer of other part of left foot with unspecified severity

L97.8 Non-pressure chronic ulcer of other part of lower leg

    L97.80 Non-pressure chronic ulcer of other part of unspecified lower leg

L97.801 Non-pressure chronic ulcer of other part of unspecified lower leg limited to breakdown of skin

L97.802 Non-pressure chronic ulcer of other part of unspecified lower leg with fat layer exposed

L97.803 Non-pressure chronic ulcer of other part of unspecified lower leg with necrosis of muscle

L97.804 Non-pressure chronic ulcer of other part of unspecified lower leg with necrosis of bone

L97.809 Non-pressure chronic ulcer of other part of unspecified lower leg with unspecified severity

    L97.81 Non-pressure chronic ulcer of other part of right lower leg

L97.811 Non-pressure chronic ulcer of other part of right lower leg limited to breakdown of skin

L97.812 Non-pressure chronic ulcer of other part of right lower leg with fat layer exposed

L97.813 Non-pressure chronic ulcer of other part of right lower leg with necrosis of muscle

L97.814 Non-pressure chronic ulcer of other part of right lower leg with necrosis of bone

L97.819 Non-pressure chronic ulcer of other part of right lower leg with unspecified severity

    L97.82 Non-pressure chronic ulcer of other part of left lower leg

L97.821 Non-pressure chronic ulcer of other part of left lower leg limited to breakdown of skin

L97.822 Non-pressure chronic ulcer of other part of left lower leg with fat layer exposed

L97.823 Non-pressure chronic ulcer of other part of left lower leg with necrosis of muscle

L97.824 Non-pressure chronic ulcer of other part of left lower leg with necrosis of bone

L97.829 Non-pressure chronic ulcer of other part of left lower leg with unspecified severity

L97.9 Non-pressure chronic ulcer of unspecified part of lower leg

    L97.90 Non-pressure chronic ulcer of unspecified part of unspecified lower leg

L97.901 Non-pressure chronic ulcer of unspecified part of unspecified lower leg limited to breakdown of skin

L97.902 Non-pressure chronic ulcer of unspecified part of unspecified lower leg with fat layer exposed

L97.903 Non-pressure chronic ulcer of unspecified part of unspecified lower leg with necrosis of muscle

L97.904 Non-pressure chronic ulcer of unspecified part of unspecified lower leg with necrosis of bone

L97.909 Non-pressure chronic ulcer of unspecified part of unspecified lower leg with unspecified severity

    L97.91 Non-pressure chronic ulcer of unspecified part of right lower leg

● New code   ▲ Revised code   ⑦ 7th digit required   ⊗ Placeholder required

L97.911 Non-pressure chronic ulcer of unspecified part of right lower leg limited to breakdown of skin

L97.912 Non-pressure chronic ulcer of unspecified part of right lower leg with fat layer exposed

L97.913 Non-pressure chronic ulcer of unspecified part of right lower leg with necrosis of muscle

L97.914 Non-pressure chronic ulcer of unspecified part of right lower leg with necrosis of bone

L97.919 Non-pressure chronic ulcer of unspecified part of right lower leg with unspecified severity

L97.92 Non-pressure chronic ulcer of unspecified part of left lower leg

L97.921 Non-pressure chronic ulcer of unspecified part of left lower leg limited to breakdown of skin

L97.922 Non-pressure chronic ulcer of unspecified part of left lower leg with fat layer exposed

L97.923 Non-pressure chronic ulcer of unspecified part of left lower leg with necrosis of muscle

L97.924 Non-pressure chronic ulcer of unspecified part of left lower leg with necrosis of bone

L97.929 Non-pressure chronic ulcer of unspecified part of left lower leg with unspecified severity

L98 Other disorders of skin and subcutaneous tissue, not elsewhere classified

L98.0 Pyogenic granuloma

Excludes 2: pyogenic granuloma of gingiva (K06.8)

pyogenic granuloma of maxillary alveolar ridge (K04.5)

pyogenic granuloma of oral mucosa (K13.4)

L98.1 Factitial dermatitis

Neurotic excoriation

L98.2 Febrile neutrophilic dermatosis [Sweet]

L98.3 Eosinophilic cellulitis [Wells]

L98.4 Non-pressure chronic ulcer of skin, not elsewhere classified

Chronic ulcer of skin NOS

Tropical ulcer NOS

Ulcer of skin NOS

Excludes 2: pressure ulcer (pressure area) (L89.-)

gangrene (I96)

skin infections (L00-L08)

specific infections classified to A00-B99

ulcer of lower limb NEC (L97.-)

varicose ulcer (I83.0-I82.2)

L98.41 Non-pressure chronic ulcer of buttock

L98.411 Non-pressure chronic ulcer of buttock limited to breakdown of skin

L98.412 Non-pressure chronic ulcer of buttock with fat layer exposed

L98.413 Non-pressure chronic ulcer of buttock with necrosis of muscle

L98.414 Non-pressure chronic ulcer of buttock with necrosis of bone

L98.419 Non-pressure chronic ulcer of buttock with unspecified severity

L98.42 Non-pressure chronic ulcer of back

L98.421 Non-pressure chronic ulcer of back limited to breakdown of skin

L98.422 Non-pressure chronic ulcer of back with fat layer exposed

L98.423 Non-pressure chronic ulcer of back with necrosis of muscle

L98.424 Non-pressure chronic ulcer of back with necrosis of bone

L98.429 Non-pressure chronic ulcer of back with unspecified severity

L98.49 Non-pressure chronic ulcer of skin of other sites

Non-pressure chronic ulcer of skin NOS

L98.491 Non-pressure chronic ulcer of skin of other sites limited to breakdown of skin

L98.492 Non-pressure chronic ulcer of skin of other sites with fat layer exposed

L98.493 Non-pressure chronic ulcer of skin of other sites with necrosis of muscle

L98.494 Non-pressure chronic ulcer of skin of other sites with necrosis of bone

L98.499 Non-pressure chronic ulcer of skin of other sites with unspecified severity

L98.5 Mucinosis of the skin

Focal mucinosis

Lichen myxedematosus

Reticular erythematous mucinosis

Excludes 1: focal oral mucinosis (K13.79)

myxedema (E03.9)

L98.6 Other infiltrative disorders of the skin and subcutaneous tissue

Excludes 1: hyalinosis cutis et mucosae (E78.89)

L98.8 Other specified disorders of the skin and subcutaneous tissue

L98.9 Disorder of the skin and subcutaneous tissue, unspecified

L99 Other disorders of skin and subcutaneous tissue in diseases classified elsewhere

Code first underlying disease, such as:

amyloidosis (E85-)

Excludes 1: skin disorders in diabetes (E08-E13 with .62)

skin disorders in gonorrhea (A54.89)

skin disorders in syphilis (A51.31, A52.79)

Add 4th-7th digits   3 digit reportable   Nonspecific code   Unspecified code   Manifestation code

● New code ▲ Revised code ⑦ 7th digit required ⊗ Placeholder required

Chapter 13: Diseases Of The Musculoskeletal System And Connective Tissue (M00-M99)

Note: Use an external cause code following the code for the musculoskeletal condition, if applicable, to identify the cause of the musculoskeletal condition

Excludes 2: arthropathic psoriasis (L40.5-)

certain conditions originating in the perinatal period (P04-P96)

certain infectious and parasitic diseases (A00-B99)

compartment syndrome (traumatic) (T79.A-)

complications of pregnancy, childbirth and the puerperium (O00-O9A)

congenital malformations, deformations, and chromosomal abnormalities (Q00-Q99)

endocrine, nutritional and metabolic diseases (E00-E88)

injury, poisoning and certain other consequences of external causes (S00-T88)

neoplasms (C00-D49)

symptoms, signs and abnormal clinical and laboratory findings, not elsewhere classified (R00-R94)

This chapter contains the following blocks:

M00-M02	Infectious arthropathies
M05-M14	Inflammatory polyarthropathies
M15-M19	Osteoarthritis
M20-M25	Other joint disorders
M26-M27	Dentofacial anomalies [including malocclusion] and other disorders of jaw
M30-M36	Systemic connective tissue disorders
M40-M43	Deforming dorsopathies
M45-M49	Spondylopathies
M50-M54	Other dorsopathies
M60-M63	Disorders of muscles
M65-M67	Disorders of synovium and tendon
M70-M79	Other soft tissue disorders
M80-M85	Disorders of bone density and structure
M86-M90	Other osteopathies
M91-M94	Chondropathies
M95	Other disorders of the musculoskeletal system and connective tissue
M96	Intraoperative and postprocedural complications and disorders of musculoskeletal system, not elsewhere classified
M99	Biomechanical lesions, not elsewhere classified

ARTHROPATHIES (M00-M25)

Includes: Disorders affecting predominantly peripheral (limb) joints

Infectious arthropathies (M00-M02)

Note: This block comprises arthropathies due to microbiological agents. Distinction is made between the following types of etiological relationship:

a) direct infection of joint, where organisms invade synovial tissue and microbial antigen is present in the joint;

b) indirect infection, which may be of two types: a reactive arthropathy, where microbial infection of the body is established but neither organisms nor antigens can be identified in the joint, and a postinfective arthropathy, where microbial antigen is present but recovery of an organism is inconstant and evidence of local multiplication is lacking.

M00 Pyogenic arthritis

M00.0 Staphylococcal arthritis and polyarthritis

Use additional code (B95.61-B95.8) to identify bacterial agent

Excludes 2: infection and inflammatory reaction due to internal joint prosthesis (T84.5-)

M00.00 Staphylococcal arthritis, unspecified joint

M00.01 Staphylococcal arthritis, shoulder

    M00.011 Staphylococcal arthritis, right shoulder

    M00.012 Staphylococcal arthritis, left shoulder

    M00.019 Staphylococcal arthritis, unspecified shoulder

M00.02 Staphylococcal arthritis, elbow

    M00.021 Staphylococcal arthritis, right elbow

    M00.022 Staphylococcal arthritis, left elbow

    M00.029 Staphylococcal arthritis, unspecified elbow

M00.03 Staphylococcal arthritis, wrist

Staphylococcal arthritis of carpal bones

    M00.031 Staphylococcal arthritis, right wrist

    M00.032 Staphylococcal arthritis, left wrist

    M00.039 Staphylococcal arthritis, unspecified wrist

M00.04 Staphylococcal arthritis, hand

Staphylococcal arthritis of metacarpus and phalanges

    M00.041 Staphylococcal arthritis, right hand

    M00.042 Staphylococcal arthritis, left hand

    M00.049 Staphylococcal arthritis, unspecified hand

M00.05 Staphylococcal arthritis, hip

    M00.051 Staphylococcal arthritis, right hip

    M00.052 Staphylococcal arthritis, left hip

    M00.059 Staphylococcal arthritis, unspecified hip

M00.06 Staphylococcal arthritis, knee

    M00.061 Staphylococcal arthritis, right knee

    M00.062 Staphylococcal arthritis, left knee

    M00.069 Staphylococcal arthritis, unspecified knee

M00.07 Staphylococcal arthritis, ankle and foot

Staphylococcal arthritis, tarsus, metatarsus and phalanges

    M00.071 Staphylococcal arthritis, right ankle and foot

    M00.072 Staphylococcal arthritis, left ankle and foot

    M00.079 Staphylococcal arthritis, unspecified ankle and foot

M00.08 Staphylococcal arthritis, vertebrae

M00.09 Staphylococcal polyarthritis

M00.1 Pneumococcal arthritis and polyarthritis

M00.10 Pneumococcal arthritis, unspecified joint

M00.11 Pneumococcal arthritis, shoulder

    M00.111 Pneumococcal arthritis, right shoulder

    M00.112 Pneumococcal arthritis, left shoulder

M00.119 Pneumococcal arthritis, unspecified shoulder

M00.12 Pneumococcal arthritis, elbow

    M00.121 Pneumococcal arthritis, right elbow

    M00.122 Pneumococcal arthritis, left elbow

    M00.129 Pneumococcal arthritis, unspecified elbow

M00.13 Pneumococcal arthritis, wrist

    Pneumococcal arthritis of carpal bones

    M00.131 Pneumococcal arthritis, right wrist

    M00.132 Pneumococcal arthritis, left wrist

    M00.139 Pneumococcal arthritis, unspecified wrist

M00.14 Pneumococcal arthritis, hand

    Pneumococcal arthritis of metacarpus and phalanges

    M00.141 Pneumococcal arthritis, right hand

    M00.142 Pneumococcal arthritis, left hand

    M00.149 Pneumococcal arthritis, unspecified hand

M00.15 Pneumococcal arthritis, hip

    M00.151 Pneumococcal arthritis, right hip

    M00.152 Pneumococcal arthritis, left hip

    M00.159 Pneumococcal arthritis, unspecified hip

M00.16 Pneumococcal arthritis, knee

    M00.161 Pneumococcal arthritis, right knee

    M00.162 Pneumococcal arthritis, left knee

    M00.169 Pneumococcal arthritis, unspecified knee

M00.17 Pneumococcal arthritis, ankle and foot

    Pneumococcal arthritis, tarsus, metatarsus and phalanges

    M00.171 Pneumococcal arthritis, right ankle and foot

    M00.172 Pneumococcal arthritis, left ankle and foot

    M00.179 Pneumococcal arthritis, unspecified ankle and foot

M00.18 Pneumococcal arthritis, vertebrae

M00.19 Pneumococcal polyarthritis

M00.2 Other streptococcal arthritis and polyarthritis

Use additional code (B95.0-B95.2, B95.4-B95.5) to identify bacterial agent

M00.20 Other streptococcal arthritis, unspecified joint

M00.21 Other streptococcal arthritis, shoulder

    M00.211 Other streptococcal arthritis, right shoulder

    M00.212 Other streptococcal arthritis, left shoulder

    M00.219 Other streptococcal arthritis, unspecified shoulder

M00.22 Other streptococcal arthritis, elbow

    M00.221 Other streptococcal arthritis, right elbow

    M00.222 Other streptococcal arthritis, left elbow

    M00.229 Other streptococcal arthritis, unspecified elbow

M00.23 Other streptococcal arthritis, wrist

    Other streptococcal arthritis of carpal bones

    M00.231 Other streptococcal arthritis, right wrist

    M00.232 Other streptococcal arthritis, left wrist

    M00.239 Other streptococcal arthritis, unspecified wrist

M00.24 Other streptococcal arthritis, hand

    Other streptococcal arthritis metacarpus and phalanges

    M00.241 Other streptococcal arthritis, right hand

    M00.242 Other streptococcal arthritis, left hand

    M00.249 Other streptococcal arthritis, unspecified hand

M00.25 Other streptococcal arthritis, hip

    M00.251 Other streptococcal arthritis, right hip

    M00.252 Other streptococcal arthritis, left hip

    M00.259 Other streptococcal arthritis, unspecified hip

M00.26 Other streptococcal arthritis, knee

    M00.261 Other streptococcal arthritis, right knee

    M00.262 Other streptococcal arthritis, left knee

    M00.269 Other streptococcal arthritis, unspecified knee

M00.27 Other streptococcal arthritis, ankle and foot

    Other streptococcal arthritis, tarsus, metatarsus and phalanges

    M00.271 Other streptococcal arthritis, right ankle and foot

    M00.272 Other streptococcal arthritis, left ankle and foot

    M00.279 Other streptococcal arthritis, unspecified ankle and foot

M00.28 Other streptococcal arthritis, vertebrae

M00.29 Other streptococcal polyarthritis

M00.8 Arthritis and polyarthritis due to other bacteria

Use additional code (B96) to identify bacteria

M00.80 Arthritis due to other bacteria, unspecified joint

M00.81 Arthritis due to other bacteria, shoulder

    M00.811 Arthritis due to other bacteria, right shoulder

    M00.812 Arthritis due to other bacteria, left shoulder

    M00.819 Arthritis due to other bacteria, unspecified shoulder

M00.82 Arthritis due to other bacteria, elbow

    M00.821 Arthritis due to other bacteria, right elbow

    M00.822 Arthritis due to other bacteria, left elbow

    M00.829 Arthritis due to other bacteria, unspecified elbow

M00.83 Arthritis due to other bacteria, wrist

    Arthritis due to other bacteria, carpal bones

● New code   ▲ Revised code   ⑦ 7ᵗʰ digit required   ⊗ Placeholder required

M00.831   Arthritis due to other bacteria, right wrist

M00.832   Arthritis due to other bacteria, left wrist

M00.839   Arthritis due to other bacteria, unspecified wrist

M00.84   Arthritis due to other bacteria, hand

Arthritis due to other bacteria, metacarpus and phalanges

M00.841   Arthritis due to other bacteria, right hand

M00.842   Arthritis due to other bacteria, left hand

M00.849   Arthritis due to other bacteria, unspecified hand

M00.85   Arthritis due to other bacteria, hip

M00.851   Arthritis due to other bacteria, right hip

M00.852   Arthritis due to other bacteria, left hip

M00.859   Arthritis due to other bacteria, unspecified hip

M00.86   Arthritis due to other bacteria, knee

M00.861   Arthritis due to other bacteria, right knee

M00.862   Arthritis due to other bacteria, left knee

M00.869   Arthritis due to other bacteria, unspecified knee

M00.87   Arthritis due to other bacteria, ankle and foot

Arthritis due to other bacteria, tarsus, metatarsus, and phalanges

M00.871   Arthritis due to other bacteria, right ankle and foot

M00.872   Arthritis due to other bacteria, left ankle and foot

M00.879   Arthritis due to other bacteria, unspecified ankle and foot

M00.88   Arthritis due to other bacteria, vertebrae

M00.89   Polyarthritis due to other bacteria

M00.9   Pyogenic arthritis, unspecified

Infective arthritis NOS

M01   Direct infections of joint in infectious and parasitic diseases classified elsewhere

Code first underlying disease, such as:

leprosy [Hansen's disease] (A30.-)

mycoses (B35-B49)

O'nyong-nyong fever (A92.1)

paratyphoid fever (A01.1-A01.4)

Excludes 1: arthritis, arthropathy (in):

gonococcal (A54.42)

Lyme disease (A69.23)

meningococcal (A39.83)

postmeningococcal (A39.84)

mumps (B26.85)

postinfective (M02.-)

reactive (M04.0-)

rubella (B06.82)

sarcoidosis (D86.86)

typhoid fever (A01.04)

tuberculosis (A18.02)

spine (A18.01)

M01.X   Direct infection of joint in infectious and parasitic diseases classified elsewhere

M01.X0   Direct infection of unspecified joint in infectious and parasitic diseases classified elsewhere

M01.X1   Direct infection of shoulder joint in infectious and parasitic diseases classified elsewhere

M01.X11   Direct infection of right shoulder in infectious and parasitic diseases classified elsewhere

M01.X12   Direct infection of left shoulder in infectious and parasitic diseases classified elsewhere

M01.X19   Direct infection of unspecified shoulder in infectious and parasitic diseases classified elsewhere

M01.X2   Direct infection of elbow in infectious and parasitic diseases classified elsewhere

M01.X21   Direct infection of right elbow in infectious and parasitic diseases classified elsewhere

M01.X22   Direct infection of left elbow in infectious and parasitic diseases classified elsewhere

M01.X29   Direct infection of unspecified elbow in infectious and parasitic diseases classified elsewhere

M01.X3   Direct infection of wrist in infectious and parasitic diseases classified elsewhere

Direct infection of carpal bones in infectious and parasitic diseases classified elsewhere

M01.X31   Direct infection of right wrist in infectious and parasitic diseases classified elsewhere

M01.X32   Direct infection of left wrist in infectious and parasitic diseases classified elsewhere

M01.X39   Direct infection of unspecified wrist in infectious and parasitic diseases classified elsewhere

M01.X4   Direct infection of hand in infectious and parasitic diseases classified elsewhere

Direct infection of metacarpus and phalanges in infectious and parasitic diseases classified elsewhere

M01.X41   Direct infection of right hand in infectious and parasitic diseases classified elsewhere

M01.X42   Direct infection of left hand in infectious and parasitic diseases classified elsewhere

M01.X49   Direct infection of unspecified hand in infectious and parasitic diseases classified elsewhere

M01.X5   Direct infection of hip in infectious and parasitic diseases classified elsewhere

M01.X51   Direct infection of right hip in infectious and parasitic diseases classified elsewhere

M01.X52 Direct infection of left hip in infectious and parasitic diseases classified elsewhere

M01.X59 Direct infection of unspecified hip in infectious and parasitic diseases classified elsewhere

M01.X6 Direct infection of knee in infectious and parasitic diseases classified elsewhere

M01.X61 Direct infection of right knee in infectious and parasitic diseases classified elsewhere

M01.X62 Direct infection of left knee in infectious and parasitic diseases classified elsewhere

M01.X69 Direct infection of unspecified knee in infectious and parasitic diseases classified elsewhere

M01.X7 Direct infection of ankle and foot in infectious and parasitic diseases classified elsewhere

Direct infection of tarsus, metatarsus and phalanges in infectious and parasitic diseases classified elsewhere

M01.X71 Direct infection of right ankle and foot in infectious and parasitic diseases classified elsewhere

M01.X72 Direct infection of left ankle and foot in infectious and parasitic diseases classified elsewhere

M01.X79 Direct infection of unspecified ankle and foot in infectious and parasitic diseases classified elsewhere

M01.X8 Direct infection of vertebrae in infectious and parasitic diseases classified elsewhere

M01.X9 Direct infection of multiple joints in infectious and parasitic diseases classified elsewhere

M02 Postinfective and reactive arthropathies

Code first underlying disease, such as:

congenital syphilis [Clutton's joints] (A50.5)

enteritis due to Yersinia enterocolitica (A04.6)

infective endocarditis (I33.0)

viral hepatitis (B15-B19)

Excludes 1: Behcet's disease (M35.2)

direct infections of joint in infectious and parasitic diseases classified elsewhere (M01.-)

postinfectious arthritis (in):

meningococcal (A39.84)

mumps (B26.85)

rubella (B06.82)

syphilis (late) (A52.77)

rheumatic fever (I00)

tabetic arthropathy [Charcot's] (A52.16)

M02.0 Arthropathy following intestinal bypass

M02.00 Arthropathy following intestinal bypass, unspecified site

M02.01 Arthropathy following intestinal bypass, shoulder

M02.011 Arthropathy following intestinal bypass, right shoulder

M02.012 Arthropathy following intestinal bypass, left shoulder

M02.019 Arthropathy following intestinal bypass, unspecified shoulder

M02.02 Arthropathy following intestinal bypass, elbow

M02.021 Arthropathy following intestinal bypass, right elbow

M02.022 Arthropathy following intestinal bypass, left elbow

M02.029 Arthropathy following intestinal bypass, unspecified elbow

M02.03 Arthropathy following intestinal bypass, wrist

Arthropathy following intestinal bypass, carpal bones

M02.031 Arthropathy following intestinal bypass, right wrist

M02.032 Arthropathy following intestinal bypass, left wrist

M02.039 Arthropathy following intestinal bypass, unspecified wrist

M02.04 Arthropathy following intestinal bypass, hand

Arthropathy following intestinal bypass, metacarpals and phalanges

M02.041 Arthropathy following intestinal bypass, right hand

M02.042 Arthropathy following intestinal bypass, left hand

M02.049 Arthropathy following intestinal bypass, unspecified hand

M02.05 Arthropathy following intestinal bypass, hip

M02.051 Arthropathy following intestinal bypass, right hip

M02.052 Arthropathy following intestinal bypass, left hip

M02.059 Arthropathy following intestinal bypass, unspecified hip

M02.06 Arthropathy following intestinal bypass, knee

M02.061 Arthropathy following intestinal bypass, right knee

M02.062 Arthropathy following intestinal bypass, left knee

M02.069 Arthropathy following intestinal bypass, unspecified knee

M02.07 Arthropathy following intestinal bypass, ankle and foot

Arthropathy following intestinal bypass, tarsus, metatarsus and phalanges

M02.071 Arthropathy following intestinal bypass, right ankle and foot

M02.072 Arthropathy following intestinal bypass, left ankle and foot

M02.079 Arthropathy following intestinal bypass, unspecified ankle and foot

M02.08 Arthropathy following intestinal bypass, vertebrae

M02.09 Arthropathy following intestinal bypass, multiple sites

M02.1 Postdysenteric arthropathy

M02.10 Postdysenteric arthropathy, unspecified site

M02.11 Postdysenteric arthropathy, shoulder

M02.111 Postdysenteric arthropathy, right shoulder

M02.112 Postdysenteric arthropathy, left shoulder

● New code   ▲ Revised code   ⑦ 7th digit required   ⊗ Placeholder required

M02.119 Postdysenteric arthropathy, unspecified shoulder

M02.12 Postdysenteric arthropathy, elbow

  M02.121 Postdysenteric arthropathy, right elbow

  M02.122 Postdysenteric arthropathy, left elbow

  M02.129 Postdysenteric arthropathy, unspecified elbow

M02.13 Postdysenteric arthropathy, wrist

Postdysenteric arthropathy, carpal bones

  M02.131 Postdysenteric arthropathy, right wrist

  M02.132 Postdysenteric arthropathy, left wrist

  M02.139 Postdysenteric arthropathy, unspecified wrist

M02.14 Postdysenteric arthropathy, hand

Postdysenteric arthropathy, metacarpus and phalanges

  M02.141 Postdysenteric arthropathy, right hand

  M02.142 Postdysenteric arthropathy, left hand

  M02.149 Postdysenteric arthropathy, unspecified hand

M02.15 Postdysenteric arthropathy, hip

  M02.151 Postdysenteric arthropathy, right hip

  M02.152 Postdysenteric arthropathy, left hip

  M02.159 Postdysenteric arthropathy, unspecified hip

M02.16 Postdysenteric arthropathy, knee

  M02.161 Postdysenteric arthropathy, right knee

  M02.162 Postdysenteric arthropathy, left knee

  M02.169 Postdysenteric arthropathy, unspecified knee

M02.17 Postdysenteric arthropathy, ankle and foot

Postdysenteric arthropathy, tarsus, metatarsus and phalanges

  M02.171 Postdysenteric arthropathy, right ankle and foot

  M02.172 Postdysenteric arthropathy, left ankle and foot

  M02.179 Postdysenteric arthropathy, unspecified ankle and foot

M02.18 Postdysenteric arthropathy, vertebrae

M02.19 Postdysenteric arthropathy, multiple sites

M02.2 Postimmunization arthropathy

  M02.20 Postimmunization arthropathy, unspecified site

  M02.21 Postimmunization arthropathy, shoulder

    M02.211 Postimmunization arthropathy, right shoulder

    M02.212 Postimmunization arthropathy, left shoulder

    M02.219 Postimmunization arthropathy, unspecified shoulder

  M02.22 Postimmunization arthropathy, elbow

    M02.221 Postimmunization arthropathy, right elbow

    M02.222 Postimmunization arthropathy, left elbow

    M02.229 Postimmunization arthropathy, unspecified elbow

  M02.23 Postimmunization arthropathy, wrist

Postimmunization arthropathy, carpal bones

    M02.231 Postimmunization arthropathy, right wrist

    M02.232 Postimmunization arthropathy, left wrist

    M02.239 Postimmunization arthropathy, unspecified wrist

  M02.24 Postimmunization arthropathy, hand

Postimmunization arthropathy, metacarpus and phalanges

    M02.241 Postimmunization arthropathy, right hand

    M02.242 Postimmunization arthropathy, left hand

    M02.249 Postimmunization arthropathy, unspecified hand

  M02.25 Postimmunization arthropathy, hip

    M02.251 Postimmunization arthropathy, right hip

    M02.252 Postimmunization arthropathy, left hip

    M02.259 Postimmunization arthropathy, unspecified hip

  M02.26 Postimmunization arthropathy, knee

    M02.261 Postimmunization arthropathy, right knee

    M02.262 Postimmunization arthropathy, left knee

    M02.269 Postimmunization arthropathy, unspecified knee

  M02.27 Postimmunization arthropathy, ankle and foot

Postimmunization arthropathy, tarsus, metatarsus and phalanges

    M02.271 Postimmunization arthropathy, right ankle and foot

    M02.272 Postimmunization arthropathy, left ankle and foot

    M02.279 Postimmunization arthropathy, unspecified ankle and foot

  M02.28 Postimmunization arthropathy, vertebrae

  M02.29 Postimmunization arthropathy, multiple sites

M02.3 Reiter's disease

Reactive arthritis

  M02.30 Reiter's disease, unspecified site

  M02.31 Reiter's disease, shoulder

    M02.311 Reiter's disease, right shoulder

    M02.312 Reiter's disease, left shoulder

    M02.319 Reiter's disease, unspecified shoulder

  M02.32 Reiter's disease, elbow

    M02.321 Reiter's disease, right elbow

    M02.322 Reiter's disease, left elbow

    M02.329 Reiter's disease, unspecified elbow

  M02.33 Reiter's disease, wrist

Reiter's disease, carpal bones

    M02.331 Reiter's disease, right wrist

    M02.332 Reiter's disease, left wrist

M02.339   Reiter's disease, unspecified wrist

M02.34 Reiter's disease, hand
    Reiter's disease, metacarpus and phalanges
- M02.341   Reiter's disease, right hand
- M02.342   Reiter's disease, left hand
- M02.349   Reiter's disease, unspecified hand

M02.35 Reiter's disease, hip
- M02.351   Reiter's disease, right hip
- M02.352   Reiter's disease, left hip
- M02.359   Reiter's disease, unspecified hip

M02.36 Reiter's disease, knee
- M02.361   Reiter's disease, right knee
- M02.362   Reiter's disease, left knee
- M02.369   Reiter's disease, unspecified knee

M02.37 Reiter's disease, ankle and foot
    Reiter's disease, tarsus, metatarsus and phalanges
- M02.371   Reiter's disease, right ankle and foot
- M02.372   Reiter's disease, left ankle and foot
- M02.379   Reiter's disease, unspecified ankle and foot

M02.38 Reiter's disease, vertebrae

M02.39 Reiter's disease, multiple sites

M02.8 Other reactive arthropathies
- M02.80   Other reactive arthropathies, unspecified site

M02.81 Other reactive arthropathies, shoulder
- M02.811   Other reactive arthropathies, right shoulder
- M02.812   Other reactive arthropathies, left shoulder
- M02.819   Other reactive arthropathies, unspecified shoulder

M02.82 Other reactive arthropathies, elbow
- M02.821   Other reactive arthropathies, right elbow
- M02.822   Other reactive arthropathies, left elbow
- M02.829   Other reactive arthropathies, unspecified elbow

M02.83 Other reactive arthropathies, wrist
    Other reactive arthropathies, carpal bones
- M02.831   Other reactive arthropathies, right wrist
- M02.832   Other reactive arthropathies, left wrist
- M02.839   Other reactive arthropathies, unspecified wrist

M02.84 Other reactive arthropathies, hand
    Other reactive arthropathies, metacarpus and phalanges
- M02.841   Other reactive arthropathies, right hand
- M02.842   Other reactive arthropathies, left hand
- M02.849   Other reactive arthropathies, unspecified hand

M02.85 Other reactive arthropathies, hip
- M02.851   Other reactive arthropathies, right hip
- M02.852   Other reactive arthropathies, left hip

M02.859   Other reactive arthropathies, unspecified hip

M02.86 Other reactive arthropathies, knee
- M02.861   Other reactive arthropathies, right knee
- M02.862   Other reactive arthropathies, left knee
- M02.869   Other reactive arthropathies, unspecified knee

M02.87 Other reactive arthropathies, ankle and foot
    Other reactive arthropathies, tarsus, metatarsus and phalanges
- M02.871   Other reactive arthropathies, right ankle and foot
- M02.872   Other reactive arthropathies, left ankle and foot
- M02.879   Other reactive arthropathies, unspecified ankle and foot

M02.88 Other reactive arthropathies, vertebrae

M02.89 Other reactive arthropathies, multiple sites

M02.9 Reactive arthropathy, unspecified

INFLAMMATORY POLYARTHROPATHIES (M05-M14)

M05 Rheumatoid arthritis with rheumatoid factor
    Excludes 1: rheumatic fever (I00)
        juvenile rheumatoid arthritis (M08.-)
        rheumatoid arthritis of spine (M45.-)

M05.0 Felty's syndrome
    Rheumatoid arthritis with splenoadenomegaly and leukopenia
- M05.00   Felty's syndrome, unspecified site

M05.01 Felty's syndrome, shoulder
- M05.011   Felty's syndrome, right shoulder
- M05.012   Felty's syndrome, left shoulder
- M05.019   Felty's syndrome, unspecified shoulder

M05.02 Felty's syndrome, elbow
- M05.021   Felty's syndrome, right elbow
- M05.022   Felty's syndrome, left elbow
- M05.029   Felty's syndrome, unspecified elbow

M05.03 Felty's syndrome, wrist
    Felty's syndrome, carpal bones
- M05.031   Felty's syndrome, right wrist
- M05.032   Felty's syndrome, left wrist
- M05.039   Felty's syndrome, unspecified wrist

M05.04 Felty's syndrome, hand
    Felty's syndrome, metacarpus and phalanges
- M05.041   Felty's syndrome, right hand
- M05.042   Felty's syndrome, left hand
- M05.049   Felty's syndrome, unspecified hand

M05.05 Felty's syndrome, hip
- M05.051   Felty's syndrome, right hip
- M05.052   Felty's syndrome, left hip
- M05.059   Felty's syndrome, unspecified hip

M05.06 Felty's syndrome, knee
- M05.061   Felty's syndrome, right knee
- M05.062   Felty's syndrome, left knee
- M05.069   Felty's syndrome, unspecified knee

M05.07 Felty's syndrome, ankle and foot

Felty's syndrome, tarsus, metatarsus and phalanges

    M05.071 Felty's syndrome, right ankle and foot

    M05.072 Felty's syndrome, left ankle and foot

    M05.079 Felty's syndrome, unspecified ankle and foot

M05.09 Felty's syndrome, multiple sites

M05.1 Rheumatoid lung disease with rheumatoid arthritis

  M05.10 Rheumatoid lung disease with rheumatoid arthritis of unspecified site

  M05.11 Rheumatoid lung disease with rheumatoid arthritis of shoulder

    M05.111 Rheumatoid lung disease with rheumatoid arthritis of right shoulder

    M05.112 Rheumatoid lung disease with rheumatoid arthritis of left shoulder

    M05.119 Rheumatoid lung disease with rheumatoid arthritis of unspecified shoulder

  M05.12 Rheumatoid lung disease with rheumatoid arthritis of elbow

    M05.121 Rheumatoid lung disease with rheumatoid arthritis of right elbow

    M05.122 Rheumatoid lung disease with rheumatoid arthritis of left elbow

    M05.129 Rheumatoid lung disease with rheumatoid arthritis of unspecified elbow

  M05.13 Rheumatoid lung disease with rheumatoid arthritis of wrist

Rheumatoid lung disease with rheumatoid arthritis, carpal bones

    M05.131 Rheumatoid lung disease with rheumatoid arthritis of right wrist

    M05.132 Rheumatoid lung disease with rheumatoid arthritis of left wrist

    M05.139 Rheumatoid lung disease with rheumatoid arthritis of unspecified wrist

  M05.14 Rheumatoid lung disease with rheumatoid arthritis of hand

Rheumatoid lung disease with rheumatoid arthritis, metacarpus and phalanges

    M05.141 Rheumatoid lung disease with rheumatoid arthritis of right hand

    M05.142 Rheumatoid lung disease with rheumatoid arthritis of left hand

    M05.149 Rheumatoid lung disease with rheumatoid arthritis of unspecified hand

  M05.15 Rheumatoid lung disease with rheumatoid arthritis of hip

    M05.151 Rheumatoid lung disease with rheumatoid arthritis of right hip

    M05.152 Rheumatoid lung disease with rheumatoid arthritis of left hip

    M05.159 Rheumatoid lung disease with rheumatoid arthritis of unspecified hip

  M05.16 Rheumatoid lung disease with rheumatoid arthritis of knee

    M05.161 Rheumatoid lung disease with rheumatoid arthritis of right knee

    M05.162 Rheumatoid lung disease with rheumatoid arthritis of left knee

    M05.169 Rheumatoid lung disease with rheumatoid arthritis of unspecified knee

  M05.17 Rheumatoid lung disease with rheumatoid arthritis of ankle and foot

Rheumatoid lung disease with rheumatoid arthritis, tarsus, metatarsus and phalanges

    M05.171 Rheumatoid lung disease with rheumatoid arthritis of right ankle and foot

    M05.172 Rheumatoid lung disease with rheumatoid arthritis of left ankle and foot

    M05.179 Rheumatoid lung disease with rheumatoid arthritis of unspecified ankle and foot

  M05.19 Rheumatoid lung disease with rheumatoid arthritis of multiple sites

M05.2 Rheumatoid vasculitis with rheumatoid arthritis

  M05.20 Rheumatoid vasculitis with rheumatoid arthritis of unspecified site

  M05.21 Rheumatoid vasculitis with rheumatoid arthritis of shoulder

    M05.211 Rheumatoid vasculitis with rheumatoid arthritis of right shoulder

    M05.212 Rheumatoid vasculitis with rheumatoid arthritis of left shoulder

    M05.219 Rheumatoid vasculitis with rheumatoid arthritis of unspecified shoulder

  M05.22 Rheumatoid vasculitis with rheumatoid arthritis of elbow

    M05.221 Rheumatoid vasculitis with rheumatoid arthritis of right elbow

    M05.222 Rheumatoid vasculitis with rheumatoid arthritis of left elbow

    M05.229 Rheumatoid vasculitis with rheumatoid arthritis of unspecified elbow

  M05.23 Rheumatoid vasculitis with rheumatoid arthritis of wrist

Rheumatoid vasculitis with rheumatoid arthritis, carpal bones

    M05.231 Rheumatoid vasculitis with rheumatoid arthritis of right wrist

    M05.232 Rheumatoid vasculitis with rheumatoid arthritis of left wrist

    M05.239 Rheumatoid vasculitis with rheumatoid arthritis of unspecified wrist

  M05.24 Rheumatoid vasculitis with rheumatoid arthritis of hand

Rheumatoid vasculitis with rheumatoid arthritis, metacarpus and phalanges

    M05.241 Rheumatoid vasculitis with rheumatoid arthritis of right hand

    M05.242 Rheumatoid vasculitis with rheumatoid arthritis of left hand

M05.249 Rheumatoid vasculitis with rheumatoid arthritis of unspecified hand

M05.25 Rheumatoid vasculitis with rheumatoid arthritis of hip

M05.251 Rheumatoid vasculitis with rheumatoid arthritis of right hip

M05.252 Rheumatoid vasculitis with rheumatoid arthritis of left hip

M05.259 Rheumatoid vasculitis with rheumatoid arthritis of unspecified hip

M05.26 Rheumatoid vasculitis with rheumatoid arthritis of knee

M05.261 Rheumatoid vasculitis with rheumatoid arthritis of right knee

M05.262 Rheumatoid vasculitis with rheumatoid arthritis of left knee

M05.269 Rheumatoid vasculitis with rheumatoid arthritis of unspecified knee

M05.27 Rheumatoid vasculitis with rheumatoid arthritis of ankle and foot
Rheumatoid vasculitis with rheumatoid arthritis, tarsus, metatarsus and phalanges

M05.271 Rheumatoid vasculitis with rheumatoid arthritis of right ankle and foot

M05.272 Rheumatoid vasculitis with rheumatoid arthritis of left ankle and foot

M05.279 Rheumatoid vasculitis with rheumatoid arthritis of unspecified ankle and foot

M05.29 Rheumatoid vasculitis with rheumatoid arthritis of multiple sites

M05.3 Rheumatoid heart disease with rheumatoid arthritis
Rheumatoid carditis
Rheumatoid endocarditis
Rheumatoid myocarditis
Rheumatoid pericarditis

M05.30 Rheumatoid heart disease with rheumatoid arthritis of unspecified site

M05.31 Rheumatoid heart disease with rheumatoid arthritis of shoulder

M05.311 Rheumatoid heart disease with rheumatoid arthritis of right shoulder

M05.312 Rheumatoid heart disease with rheumatoid arthritis of left shoulder

M05.319 Rheumatoid heart disease with rheumatoid arthritis of unspecified shoulder

M05.32 Rheumatoid heart disease with rheumatoid arthritis of elbow

M05.321 Rheumatoid heart disease with rheumatoid arthritis of right elbow

M05.322 Rheumatoid heart disease with rheumatoid arthritis of left elbow

M05.329 Rheumatoid heart disease with rheumatoid arthritis of unspecified elbow

M05.33 Rheumatoid heart disease with rheumatoid arthritis of wrist
Rheumatoid heart disease with rheumatoid arthritis, carpal bones

M05.331 Rheumatoid heart disease with rheumatoid arthritis of right wrist

M05.332 Rheumatoid heart disease with rheumatoid arthritis of left wrist

M05.339 Rheumatoid heart disease with rheumatoid arthritis of unspecified wrist

M05.34 Rheumatoid heart disease with rheumatoid arthritis of hand
Rheumatoid heart disease with rheumatoid arthritis, metacarpus and phalanges

M05.341 Rheumatoid heart disease with rheumatoid arthritis of right hand

M05.342 Rheumatoid heart disease with rheumatoid arthritis of left hand

M05.349 Rheumatoid heart disease with rheumatoid arthritis of unspecified hand

M05.35 Rheumatoid heart disease with rheumatoid arthritis of hip

M05.351 Rheumatoid heart disease with rheumatoid arthritis of right hip

M05.352 Rheumatoid heart disease with rheumatoid arthritis of left hip

M05.359 Rheumatoid heart disease with rheumatoid arthritis of unspecified hip

M05.36 Rheumatoid heart disease with rheumatoid arthritis of knee

M05.361 Rheumatoid heart disease with rheumatoid arthritis of right knee

M05.362 Rheumatoid heart disease with rheumatoid arthritis of left knee

M05.369 Rheumatoid heart disease with rheumatoid arthritis of unspecified knee

M05.37 Rheumatoid heart disease with rheumatoid arthritis of ankle and foot
Rheumatoid heart disease with rheumatoid arthritis, tarsus, metatarsus and phalanges

M05.371 Rheumatoid heart disease with rheumatoid arthritis of right ankle and foot

M05.372 Rheumatoid heart disease with rheumatoid arthritis of left ankle and foot

M05.379 Rheumatoid heart disease with rheumatoid arthritis of unspecified ankle and foot

M05.39 Rheumatoid heart disease with rheumatoid arthritis of multiple sites

M05.4 Rheumatoid myopathy with rheumatoid arthritis

M05.40 Rheumatoid myopathy with rheumatoid arthritis of unspecified site

M05.41 Rheumatoid myopathy with rheumatoid arthritis of shoulder

● New code   ▲ Revised code   ⑦ 7th digit required   ⊗ Placeholder required

M05.411 Rheumatoid myopathy with rheumatoid arthritis of right shoulder

M05.412 Rheumatoid myopathy with rheumatoid arthritis of left shoulder

M05.419 Rheumatoid myopathy with rheumatoid arthritis of unspecified shoulder

M05.42 Rheumatoid myopathy with rheumatoid arthritis of elbow

M05.421 Rheumatoid myopathy with rheumatoid arthritis of right elbow

M05.422 Rheumatoid myopathy with rheumatoid arthritis of left elbow

M05.429 Rheumatoid myopathy with rheumatoid arthritis of unspecified elbow

M05.43 Rheumatoid myopathy with rheumatoid arthritis of wrist

Rheumatoid myopathy with rheumatoid arthritis, carpal bones

M05.431 Rheumatoid myopathy with rheumatoid arthritis of right wrist

M05.432 Rheumatoid myopathy with rheumatoid arthritis of left wrist

M05.439 Rheumatoid myopathy with rheumatoid arthritis of unspecified wrist

M05.44 Rheumatoid myopathy with rheumatoid arthritis of hand

Rheumatoid myopathy with rheumatoid arthritis, metacarpus and phalanges

M05.441 Rheumatoid myopathy with rheumatoid arthritis of right hand

M05.442 Rheumatoid myopathy with rheumatoid arthritis of left hand

M05.449 Rheumatoid myopathy with rheumatoid arthritis of unspecified hand

M05.45 Rheumatoid myopathy with rheumatoid arthritis of hip

M05.451 Rheumatoid myopathy with rheumatoid arthritis of right hip

M05.452 Rheumatoid myopathy with rheumatoid arthritis of left hip

M05.459 Rheumatoid myopathy with rheumatoid arthritis of unspecified hip

M05.46 Rheumatoid myopathy with rheumatoid arthritis of knee

M05.461 Rheumatoid myopathy with rheumatoid arthritis of right knee

M05.462 Rheumatoid myopathy with rheumatoid arthritis of left knee

M05.469 Rheumatoid myopathy with rheumatoid arthritis of unspecified knee

M05.47 Rheumatoid myopathy with rheumatoid arthritis of ankle and foot

Rheumatoid myopathy with rheumatoid arthritis, tarsus, metatarsus and phalanges

M05.471 Rheumatoid myopathy with rheumatoid arthritis of right ankle and foot

M05.472 Rheumatoid myopathy with rheumatoid arthritis of left ankle and foot

M05.479 Rheumatoid myopathy with rheumatoid arthritis of unspecified ankle and foot

M05.49 Rheumatoid myopathy with rheumatoid arthritis of multiple sites

M05.5 Rheumatoid polyneuropathy with rheumatoid arthritis

M05.50 Rheumatoid polyneuropathy with rheumatoid arthritis of unspecified site

M05.51 Rheumatoid polyneuropathy with rheumatoid arthritis of shoulder

M05.511 Rheumatoid polyneuropathy with rheumatoid arthritis of right shoulder

M05.512 Rheumatoid polyneuropathy with rheumatoid arthritis of left shoulder

M05.519 Rheumatoid polyneuropathy with rheumatoid arthritis of unspecified shoulder

M05.52 Rheumatoid polyneuropathy with rheumatoid arthritis of elbow

M05.521 Rheumatoid polyneuropathy with rheumatoid arthritis of right elbow

M05.522 Rheumatoid polyneuropathy with rheumatoid arthritis of left elbow

M05.529 Rheumatoid polyneuropathy with rheumatoid arthritis of unspecified elbow

M05.53 Rheumatoid polyneuropathy with rheumatoid arthritis of wrist

Rheumatoid polyneuropathy with rheumatoid arthritis, carpal bones

M05.531 Rheumatoid polyneuropathy with rheumatoid arthritis of right wrist

M05.532 Rheumatoid polyneuropathy with rheumatoid arthritis of left wrist

M05.539 Rheumatoid polyneuropathy with rheumatoid arthritis of unspecified wrist

M05.54 Rheumatoid polyneuropathy with rheumatoid arthritis of hand

Rheumatoid polyneuropathy with rheumatoid arthritis, metacarpus and phalanges

M05.541 Rheumatoid polyneuropathy with rheumatoid arthritis of right hand

M05.542 Rheumatoid polyneuropathy with rheumatoid arthritis of left hand

M05.549 Rheumatoid polyneuropathy with rheumatoid arthritis of unspecified hand

M05.55 Rheumatoid polyneuropathy with rheumatoid arthritis of hip

M05.551 Rheumatoid polyneuropathy with rheumatoid arthritis of right hip

M05.552 Rheumatoid polyneuropathy with rheumatoid arthritis of left hip

M05.559 Rheumatoid polyneuropathy with rheumatoid arthritis of unspecified hip

M05.56 Rheumatoid polyneuropathy with rheumatoid arthritis of knee

    M05.561 Rheumatoid polyneuropathy with rheumatoid arthritis of right knee

    M05.562 Rheumatoid polyneuropathy with rheumatoid arthritis of left knee

    M05.569 Rheumatoid polyneuropathy with rheumatoid arthritis of unspecified knee

M05.57 Rheumatoid polyneuropathy with rheumatoid arthritis of ankle and foot

Rheumatoid polyneuropathy with rheumatoid arthritis, tarsus, metatarsus and phalanges

    M05.571 Rheumatoid polyneuropathy with rheumatoid arthritis of right ankle and foot

    M05.572 Rheumatoid polyneuropathy with rheumatoid arthritis of left ankle and foot

    M05.579 Rheumatoid polyneuropathy with rheumatoid arthritis of unspecified ankle and foot

M05.59 Rheumatoid polyneuropathy with rheumatoid arthritis of multiple sites

M05.6 Rheumatoid arthritis with involvement of other organs and systems

  M05.60 Rheumatoid arthritis of unspecified site with involvement of other organs and systems

  M05.61 Rheumatoid arthritis of shoulder with involvement of other organs and systems

    M05.611 Rheumatoid arthritis of right shoulder with involvement of other organs and systems

    M05.612 Rheumatoid arthritis of left shoulder with involvement of other organs and systems

    M05.619 Rheumatoid arthritis of unspecified shoulder with involvement of other organs and systems

  M05.62 Rheumatoid arthritis of elbow with involvement of other organs and systems

    M05.621 Rheumatoid arthritis of right elbow with involvement of other organs and systems

    M05.622 Rheumatoid arthritis of left elbow with involvement of other organs and systems

    M05.629 Rheumatoid arthritis of unspecified elbow with involvement of other organs and systems

  M05.63 Rheumatoid arthritis of wrist with involvement of other organs and systems

Rheumatoid arthritis of carpal bones with involvement of other organs and systems

    M05.631 Rheumatoid arthritis of right wrist with involvement of other organs and systems

    M05.632 Rheumatoid arthritis of left wrist with involvement of other organs and systems

    M05.639 Rheumatoid arthritis of unspecified wrist with involvement of other organs and systems

  M05.64 Rheumatoid arthritis of hand with involvement of other organs and systems

Rheumatoid arthritis of metacarpus and phalanges with involvement of other organs and systems

    M05.641 Rheumatoid arthritis of right hand with involvement of other organs and systems

    M05.642 Rheumatoid arthritis of left hand with involvement of other organs and systems

    M05.649 Rheumatoid arthritis of unspecified hand with involvement of other organs and systems

  M05.65 Rheumatoid arthritis of hip with involvement of other organs and systems

    M05.651 Rheumatoid arthritis of right hip with involvement of other organs and systems

    M05.652 Rheumatoid arthritis of left hip with involvement of other organs and systems

    M05.659 Rheumatoid arthritis of unspecified hip with involvement of other organs and systems

  M05.66 Rheumatoid arthritis of knee with involvement of other organs and systems

    M05.661 Rheumatoid arthritis of right knee with involvement of other organs and systems

    M05.662 Rheumatoid arthritis of left knee with involvement of other organs and systems

    M05.669 Rheumatoid arthritis of unspecified knee with involvement of other organs and systems

  M05.67 Rheumatoid arthritis of ankle and foot with involvement of other organs and systems

Rheumatoid arthritis of tarsus, metatarsus and phalanges with involvement of other organs and systems

    M05.671 Rheumatoid arthritis of right ankle and foot with involvement of other organs and systems

    M05.672 Rheumatoid arthritis of left ankle and foot with involvement of other organs and systems

    M05.679 Rheumatoid arthritis of unspecified ankle and foot with involvement of other organs and systems

  M05.69 Rheumatoid arthritis of multiple sites with involvement of other organs and systems

M05.7 Rheumatoid arthritis with rheumatoid factor without organ or systems involvement

M05.70 Rheumatoid arthritis with rheumatoid factor of unspecified site without organ or systems involvement

M05.71 Rheumatoid arthritis with rheumatoid factor of shoulder without organ or systems involvement

M05.711 Rheumatoid arthritis with rheumatoid factor of right shoulder without organ or systems involvement

M05.712 Rheumatoid arthritis with rheumatoid factor of left shoulder without organ or systems involvement

M05.719 Rheumatoid arthritis with rheumatoid factor of unspecified shoulder without organ or systems involvement

M05.72 Rheumatoid arthritis with rheumatoid factor of elbow without organ or systems involvement

M05.721 Rheumatoid arthritis with rheumatoid factor of right elbow without organ or systems involvement

M05.722 Rheumatoid arthritis with rheumatoid factor of left elbow without organ or systems involvement

M05.729 Rheumatoid arthritis with rheumatoid factor of unspecified elbow without organ or systems involvement

M05.73 Rheumatoid arthritis with rheumatoid factor of wrist without organ or systems involvement

M05.731 Rheumatoid arthritis with rheumatoid factor of right wrist without organ or systems involvement

M05.732 Rheumatoid arthritis with rheumatoid factor of left wrist without organ or systems involvement

M05.739 Rheumatoid arthritis with rheumatoid factor of unspecified wrist without organ or systems involvement

M05.74 Rheumatoid arthritis with rheumatoid factor of hand without organ or systems involvement

M05.741 Rheumatoid arthritis with rheumatoid factor of right hand without organ or systems involvement

M05.742 Rheumatoid arthritis with rheumatoid factor of left hand without organ or systems involvement

M05.749 Rheumatoid arthritis with rheumatoid factor of unspecified hand without organ or systems involvement

M05.75 Rheumatoid arthritis with rheumatoid factor of hip without organ or systems involvement

M05.751 Rheumatoid arthritis with rheumatoid factor of right hip without organ or systems involvement

M05.752 Rheumatoid arthritis with rheumatoid factor of left hip without organ or systems involvement

M05.759 Rheumatoid arthritis with rheumatoid factor of unspecified hip without organ or systems involvement

M05.76 Rheumatoid arthritis with rheumatoid factor of knee without organ or systems involvement

M05.761 Rheumatoid arthritis with rheumatoid factor of right knee without organ or systems involvement

M05.762 Rheumatoid arthritis with rheumatoid factor of left knee without organ or systems involvement

M05.769 Rheumatoid arthritis with rheumatoid factor of unspecified knee without organ or systems involvement

M05.77 Rheumatoid arthritis with rheumatoid factor of ankle and foot without organ or systems involvement

M05.771 Rheumatoid arthritis with rheumatoid factor of right ankle and foot without organ or systems involvement

M05.772 Rheumatoid arthritis with rheumatoid factor of left ankle and foot without organ or systems involvement

M05.779 Rheumatoid arthritis with rheumatoid factor of unspecified ankle and foot without organ or systems involvement

M05.79 Rheumatoid arthritis with rheumatoid factor of multiple sites without organ or systems involvement

M05.8 Other rheumatoid arthritis with rheumatoid factor

M05.80 Other rheumatoid arthritis with rheumatoid factor of unspecified site

M05.81 Other rheumatoid arthritis with rheumatoid factor of shoulder

M05.811 Other rheumatoid arthritis with rheumatoid factor of right shoulder

M05.812 Other rheumatoid arthritis with rheumatoid factor of left shoulder

M05.819 Other rheumatoid arthritis with rheumatoid factor of unspecified shoulder

M05.82 Other rheumatoid arthritis with rheumatoid factor of elbow

M05.821 Other rheumatoid arthritis with rheumatoid factor of right elbow

M05.822 Other rheumatoid arthritis with rheumatoid factor of left elbow

M05.829 Other rheumatoid arthritis with rheumatoid factor of unspecified elbow

M05.83   Other rheumatoid arthritis with rheumatoid factor of wrist

    M05.831   Other rheumatoid arthritis with rheumatoid factor of right wrist

    M05.832   Other rheumatoid arthritis with rheumatoid factor of left wrist

    M05.839   Other rheumatoid arthritis with rheumatoid factor of unspecified wrist

M05.84   Other rheumatoid arthritis with rheumatoid factor of hand

    M05.841   Other rheumatoid arthritis with rheumatoid factor of right hand

    M05.842   Other rheumatoid arthritis with rheumatoid factor of left hand

    M05.849   Other rheumatoid arthritis with rheumatoid factor of unspecified hand

M05.85   Other rheumatoid arthritis with rheumatoid factor of hip

    M05.851   Other rheumatoid arthritis with rheumatoid factor of right hip

    M05.852   Other rheumatoid arthritis with rheumatoid factor of left hip

    M05.859   Other rheumatoid arthritis with rheumatoid factor of unspecified hip

M05.86   Other rheumatoid arthritis with rheumatoid factor of knee

    M05.861   Other rheumatoid arthritis with rheumatoid factor of right knee

    M05.862   Other rheumatoid arthritis with rheumatoid factor of left knee

    M05.869   Other rheumatoid arthritis with rheumatoid factor of unspecified knee

M05.87   Other rheumatoid arthritis with rheumatoid factor of ankle and foot

    M05.871   Other rheumatoid arthritis with rheumatoid factor of right ankle and foot

    M05.872   Other rheumatoid arthritis with rheumatoid factor of left ankle and foot

    M05.879   Other rheumatoid arthritis with rheumatoid factor of unspecified ankle and foot

M05.89   Other rheumatoid arthritis with rheumatoid factor of multiple sites

M05.9   Rheumatoid arthritis with rheumatoid factor, unspecified

M06   Other rheumatoid arthritis

M06.0   Rheumatoid arthritis without rheumatoid factor

    M06.00   Rheumatoid arthritis without rheumatoid factor, unspecified site

    M06.01   Rheumatoid arthritis without rheumatoid factor, shoulder

        M06.011   Rheumatoid arthritis without rheumatoid factor, right shoulder

        M06.012   Rheumatoid arthritis without rheumatoid factor, left shoulder

        M06.019   Rheumatoid arthritis without rheumatoid factor, unspecified shoulder

    M06.02   Rheumatoid arthritis without rheumatoid factor, elbow

        M06.021   Rheumatoid arthritis without rheumatoid factor, right elbow

        M06.022   Rheumatoid arthritis without rheumatoid factor, left elbow

        M06.029   Rheumatoid arthritis without rheumatoid factor, unspecified elbow

    M06.03   Rheumatoid arthritis without rheumatoid factor, wrist

        M06.031   Rheumatoid arthritis without rheumatoid factor, right wrist

        M06.032   Rheumatoid arthritis without rheumatoid factor, left wrist

        M06.039   Rheumatoid arthritis without rheumatoid factor, unspecified wrist

    M06.04   Rheumatoid arthritis without rheumatoid factor, hand

        M06.041   Rheumatoid arthritis without rheumatoid factor, right hand

        M06.042   Rheumatoid arthritis without rheumatoid factor, left hand

        M06.049   Rheumatoid arthritis without rheumatoid factor, unspecified hand

    M06.05   Rheumatoid arthritis without rheumatoid factor, hip

        M06.051   Rheumatoid arthritis without rheumatoid factor, right hip

        M06.052   Rheumatoid arthritis without rheumatoid factor, left hip

        M06.059   Rheumatoid arthritis without rheumatoid factor, unspecified hip

    M06.06   Rheumatoid arthritis without rheumatoid factor, knee

        M06.061   Rheumatoid arthritis without rheumatoid factor, right knee

        M06.062   Rheumatoid arthritis without rheumatoid factor, left knee

        M06.069   Rheumatoid arthritis without rheumatoid factor, unspecified knee

    M06.07   Rheumatoid arthritis without rheumatoid factor, ankle and foot

        M06.071   Rheumatoid arthritis without rheumatoid factor, right ankle and foot

        M06.072   Rheumatoid arthritis without rheumatoid factor, left ankle and foot

        M06.079   Rheumatoid arthritis without rheumatoid factor, unspecified ankle and foot

    M06.08   Rheumatoid arthritis without rheumatoid factor, vertebrae

    M06.09   Rheumatoid arthritis without rheumatoid factor, multiple sites

M06.1   Adult-onset Still's disease

    Excludes 1: Still's disease NOS (M08.2-)

M06.2 Rheumatoid bursitis
    M06.20 Rheumatoid bursitis, unspecified site
    M06.21 Rheumatoid bursitis, shoulder
        M06.211 Rheumatoid bursitis, right shoulder
        M06.212 Rheumatoid bursitis, left shoulder
        M06.219 Rheumatoid bursitis, unspecified shoulder
    M06.22 Rheumatoid bursitis, elbow
        M06.221 Rheumatoid bursitis, right elbow
        M06.222 Rheumatoid bursitis, left elbow
        M06.229 Rheumatoid bursitis, unspecified elbow
    M06.23 Rheumatoid bursitis, wrist
        M06.231 Rheumatoid bursitis, right wrist
        M06.232 Rheumatoid bursitis, left wrist
        M06.239 Rheumatoid bursitis, unspecified wrist
    M06.24 Rheumatoid bursitis, hand
        M06.241 Rheumatoid bursitis, right hand
        M06.242 Rheumatoid bursitis, left hand
        M06.249 Rheumatoid bursitis, unspecified hand
    M06.25 Rheumatoid bursitis, hip
        M06.251 Rheumatoid bursitis, right hip
        M06.252 Rheumatoid bursitis, left hip
        M06.259 Rheumatoid bursitis, unspecified hip
    M06.26 Rheumatoid bursitis, knee
        M06.261 Rheumatoid bursitis, right knee
        M06.262 Rheumatoid bursitis, left knee
        M06.269 Rheumatoid bursitis, unspecified knee
    M06.27 Rheumatoid bursitis, ankle and foot
        M06.271 Rheumatoid bursitis, right ankle and foot
        M06.272 Rheumatoid bursitis, left ankle and foot
        M06.279 Rheumatoid bursitis, unspecified ankle and foot
    M06.28 Rheumatoid bursitis, vertebrae
    M06.29 Rheumatoid bursitis, multiple sites
M06.3 Rheumatoid nodule
    M06.30 Rheumatoid nodule, unspecified site
    M06.31 Rheumatoid nodule, shoulder
        M06.311 Rheumatoid nodule, right shoulder
        M06.312 Rheumatoid nodule, left shoulder
        M06.319 Rheumatoid nodule, unspecified shoulder
    M06.32 Rheumatoid nodule, elbow
        M06.321 Rheumatoid nodule, right elbow
        M06.322 Rheumatoid nodule, left elbow
        M06.329 Rheumatoid nodule, unspecified elbow
    M06.33 Rheumatoid nodule, wrist
        M06.331 Rheumatoid nodule, right wrist
        M06.332 Rheumatoid nodule, left wrist
        M06.339 Rheumatoid nodule, unspecified wrist
    M06.34 Rheumatoid nodule, hand
        M06.341 Rheumatoid nodule, right hand

M06.342 Rheumatoid nodule, left hand
M06.349 Rheumatoid nodule, unspecified hand
    M06.35 Rheumatoid nodule, hip
        M06.351 Rheumatoid nodule, right hip
        M06.352 Rheumatoid nodule, left hip
        M06.359 Rheumatoid nodule, unspecified hip
    M06.36 Rheumatoid nodule, knee
        M06.361 Rheumatoid nodule, right knee
        M06.362 Rheumatoid nodule, left knee
        M06.369 Rheumatoid nodule, unspecified knee
    M06.37 Rheumatoid nodule, ankle and foot
        M06.371 Rheumatoid nodule, right ankle and foot
        M06.372 Rheumatoid nodule, left ankle and foot
        M06.379 Rheumatoid nodule, unspecified ankle and foot
    M06.38 Rheumatoid nodule, vertebrae
    M06.39 Rheumatoid nodule, multiple sites
M06.4 Inflammatory polyarthropathy
    Excludes 1: polyarthritis NOS (M13.0)
M06.8 Other specified rheumatoid arthritis
    M06.80 Other specified rheumatoid arthritis, unspecified site
    M06.81 Other specified rheumatoid arthritis, shoulder
        M06.811 Other specified rheumatoid arthritis, right shoulder
        M06.812 Other specified rheumatoid arthritis, left shoulder
        M06.819 Other specified rheumatoid arthritis, unspecified shoulder
    M06.82 Other specified rheumatoid arthritis, elbow
        M06.821 Other specified rheumatoid arthritis, right elbow
        M06.822 Other specified rheumatoid arthritis, left elbow
        M06.829 Other specified rheumatoid arthritis, unspecified elbow
    M06.83 Other specified rheumatoid arthritis, wrist
        M06.831 Other specified rheumatoid arthritis, right wrist
        M06.832 Other specified rheumatoid arthritis, left wrist
        M06.839 Other specified rheumatoid arthritis, unspecified wrist
    M06.84 Other specified rheumatoid arthritis, hand
        M06.841 Other specified rheumatoid arthritis, right hand
        M06.842 Other specified rheumatoid arthritis, left hand
        M06.849 Other specified rheumatoid arthritis, unspecified hand
    M06.85 Other specified rheumatoid arthritis, hip
        M06.851 Other specified rheumatoid arthritis, right hip
        M06.852 Other specified rheumatoid arthritis, left hip

M06.859 Other specified rheumatoid arthritis, unspecified hip

M06.86 Other specified rheumatoid arthritis, knee

M06.861 Other specified rheumatoid arthritis, right knee

M06.862 Other specified rheumatoid arthritis, left knee

M06.869 Other specified rheumatoid arthritis, unspecified knee

M06.87 Other specified rheumatoid arthritis, ankle and foot

M06.871 Other specified rheumatoid arthritis, right ankle and foot

M06.872 Other specified rheumatoid arthritis, left ankle and foot

M06.879 Other specified rheumatoid arthritis, unspecified ankle and foot

M06.88 Other specified rheumatoid arthritis, vertebrae

M06.89 Other specified rheumatoid arthritis, multiple sites

M06.9 Rheumatoid arthritis, unspecified

M07 Enteropathic arthropathies

Code also associated enteropathy, such as:
regional enteritis [Crohn's disease] (K50.-)
ulcerative colitis (K51.-)

Excludes 1: psoriatic arthropathies (L40.5-)

M07.6 Enteropathic arthropathies

M07.60 Enteropathic arthropathies, unspecified site

M07.61 Enteropathic arthropathies, shoulder

M07.611 Enteropathic arthropathies, right shoulder

M07.612 Enteropathic arthropathies, left shoulder

M07.619 Enteropathic arthropathies, unspecified shoulder

M07.62 Enteropathic arthropathies, elbow

M07.621 Enteropathic arthropathies, right elbow

M07.622 Enteropathic arthropathies, left elbow

M07.629 Enteropathic arthropathies, unspecified elbow

M07.63 Enteropathic arthropathies, wrist

M07.631 Enteropathic arthropathies, right wrist

M07.632 Enteropathic arthropathies, left wrist

M07.639 Enteropathic arthropathies, unspecified wrist

M07.64 Enteropathic arthropathies, hand

M07.641 Enteropathic arthropathies, right hand

M07.642 Enteropathic arthropathies, left hand

M07.649 Enteropathic arthropathies, unspecified hand

M07.65 Enteropathic arthropathies, hip

M07.651 Enteropathic arthropathies, right hip

M07.652 Enteropathic arthropathies, left hip

M07.659 Enteropathic arthropathies, unspecified hip

M07.66 Enteropathic arthropathies, knee

M07.661 Enteropathic arthropathies, right knee

M07.662 Enteropathic arthropathies, left knee

M07.669 Enteropathic arthropathies, unspecified knee

M07.67 Enteropathic arthropathies, ankle and foot

M07.671 Enteropathic arthropathies, right ankle and foot

M07.672 Enteropathic arthropathies, left ankle and foot

M07.679 Enteropathic arthropathies, unspecified ankle and foot

M07.68 Enteropathic arthropathies, vertebrae

M07.69 Enteropathic arthropathies, multiple sites

M08 Juvenile arthritis

Code also any associated underlying condition, such as:
regional enteritis [Crohn's disease] (K50.-)
ulcerative colitis (K51.-)

Excludes 1: arthropathy in Whipple's disease (M14.8)
Felty's syndrome (M05.0)
juvenile dermatomyositis (M33.0-)
psoriatic juvenile arthropathy (L40.54)

M08.0 Unspecified juvenile rheumatoid arthritis

Juvenile rheumatoid arthritis with or without rheumatoid factor

M08.00 Unspecified juvenile rheumatoid arthritis of unspecified site

M08.01 Unspecified juvenile rheumatoid arthritis, shoulder

M08.011 Unspecified juvenile rheumatoid arthritis, right shoulder

M08.012 Unspecified juvenile rheumatoid arthritis, left shoulder

M08.019 Unspecified juvenile rheumatoid arthritis, unspecified shoulder

M08.02 Unspecified juvenile rheumatoid arthritis of elbow

M08.021 Unspecified juvenile rheumatoid arthritis, right elbow

M08.022 Unspecified juvenile rheumatoid arthritis, left elbow

M08.029 Unspecified juvenile rheumatoid arthritis, unspecified elbow

M08.03 Unspecified juvenile rheumatoid arthritis, wrist

M08.031 Unspecified juvenile rheumatoid arthritis, right wrist

M08.032 Unspecified juvenile rheumatoid arthritis, left wrist

M08.039 Unspecified juvenile rheumatoid arthritis, unspecified wrist

M08.04 Unspecified juvenile rheumatoid arthritis, hand

M08.041 Unspecified juvenile rheumatoid arthritis, right hand

M08.042 Unspecified juvenile rheumatoid arthritis, left hand

M08.049 Unspecified juvenile rheumatoid arthritis, unspecified hand

M08.05 Unspecified juvenile rheumatoid arthritis, hip

M08.051 Unspecified juvenile rheumatoid arthritis, right hip

● New code   ▲ Revised code   ⑦ 7ᵗʰ digit required   ⊗ Placeholder required

M08.052 Unspecified juvenile rheumatoid arthritis, left hip

M08.059 Unspecified juvenile rheumatoid arthritis, unspecified hip

M08.06 Unspecified juvenile rheumatoid arthritis, knee

M08.061 Unspecified juvenile rheumatoid arthritis, right knee

M08.062 Unspecified juvenile rheumatoid arthritis, left knee

M08.069 Unspecified juvenile rheumatoid arthritis, unspecified knee

M08.07 Unspecified juvenile rheumatoid arthritis, ankle and foot

M08.071 Unspecified juvenile rheumatoid arthritis, right ankle and foot

M08.072 Unspecified juvenile rheumatoid arthritis, left ankle and foot

M08.079 Unspecified juvenile rheumatoid arthritis, unspecified ankle and foot

M08.08 Unspecified juvenile rheumatoid arthritis, vertebrae

M08.09 Unspecified juvenile rheumatoid arthritis, multiple sites

M08.1 Juvenile ankylosing spondylitis
Excludes 1: ankylosing spondylitis in adults (M45.0-)

M08.2 Juvenile rheumatoid arthritis with systemic onset
Still's disease NOS
Excludes 1: adult-onset Still's disease (M06.1-)

M08.20 Juvenile rheumatoid arthritis with systemic onset, unspecified site

M08.21 Juvenile rheumatoid arthritis with systemic onset, shoulder

M08.211 Juvenile rheumatoid arthritis with systemic onset, right shoulder

M08.212 Juvenile rheumatoid arthritis with systemic onset, left shoulder

M08.219 Juvenile rheumatoid arthritis with systemic onset, unspecified shoulder

M08.22 Juvenile rheumatoid arthritis with systemic onset, elbow

M08.221 Juvenile rheumatoid arthritis with systemic onset, right elbow

M08.222 Juvenile rheumatoid arthritis with systemic onset, left elbow

M08.229 Juvenile rheumatoid arthritis with systemic onset, unspecified elbow

M08.23 Juvenile rheumatoid arthritis with systemic onset, wrist

M08.231 Juvenile rheumatoid arthritis with systemic onset, right wrist

M08.232 Juvenile rheumatoid arthritis with systemic onset, left wrist

M08.239 Juvenile rheumatoid arthritis with systemic onset, unspecified wrist

M08.24 Juvenile rheumatoid arthritis with systemic onset, hand

M08.241 Juvenile rheumatoid arthritis with systemic onset, right hand

M08.242 Juvenile rheumatoid arthritis with systemic onset, left hand

M08.249 Juvenile rheumatoid arthritis with systemic onset, unspecified hand

M08.25 Juvenile rheumatoid arthritis with systemic onset, hip

M08.251 Juvenile rheumatoid arthritis with systemic onset, right hip

M08.252 Juvenile rheumatoid arthritis with systemic onset, left hip

M08.259 Juvenile rheumatoid arthritis with systemic onset, unspecified hip

M08.26 Juvenile rheumatoid arthritis with systemic onset, knee

M08.261 Juvenile rheumatoid arthritis with systemic onset, right knee

M08.262 Juvenile rheumatoid arthritis with systemic onset, left knee

M08.269 Juvenile rheumatoid arthritis with systemic onset, unspecified knee

M08.27 Juvenile rheumatoid arthritis with systemic onset, ankle and foot

M08.271 Juvenile rheumatoid arthritis with systemic onset, right ankle and foot

M08.272 Juvenile rheumatoid arthritis with systemic onset, left ankle and foot

M08.279 Juvenile rheumatoid arthritis with systemic onset, unspecified ankle and foot

M08.28 Juvenile rheumatoid arthritis with systemic onset, vertebrae

M08.29 Juvenile rheumatoid arthritis with systemic onset, multiple sites

M08.3 Juvenile rheumatoid polyarthritis (seronegative)

M08.4 Pauciarticular juvenile rheumatoid arthritis

M08.40 Pauciarticular juvenile rheumatoid arthritis, unspecified site

M08.41 Pauciarticular juvenile rheumatoid arthritis, shoulder

M08.411 Pauciarticular juvenile rheumatoid arthritis, right shoulder

M08.412 Pauciarticular juvenile rheumatoid arthritis, left shoulder

M08.419 Pauciarticular juvenile rheumatoid arthritis, unspecified shoulder

M08.42 Pauciarticular juvenile rheumatoid arthritis, elbow

M08.421 Pauciarticular juvenile rheumatoid arthritis, right elbow

M08.422 Pauciarticular juvenile rheumatoid arthritis, left elbow

M08.429 Pauciarticular juvenile rheumatoid arthritis, unspecified elbow

M08.43 Pauciarticular juvenile rheumatoid arthritis, wrist

M08.431 Pauciarticular juvenile rheumatoid arthritis, right wrist

M08.432 Pauciarticular juvenile rheumatoid arthritis, left wrist

M08.439 Pauciarticular juvenile rheumatoid arthritis, unspecified wrist

M08.44 Pauciarticular juvenile rheumatoid arthritis, hand

M08.441 Pauciarticular juvenile rheumatoid arthritis, right hand

M08.442   Pauciarticular juvenile rheumatoid arthritis, left hand

M08.449   Pauciarticular juvenile rheumatoid arthritis, unspecified hand

M08.45   Pauciarticular juvenile rheumatoid arthritis, hip

M08.451   Pauciarticular juvenile rheumatoid arthritis, right hip

M08.452   Pauciarticular juvenile rheumatoid arthritis, left hip

M08.459   Pauciarticular juvenile rheumatoid arthritis, unspecified hip

M08.46   Pauciarticular juvenile rheumatoid arthritis, knee

M08.461   Pauciarticular juvenile rheumatoid arthritis, right knee

M08.462   Pauciarticular juvenile rheumatoid arthritis, left knee

M08.469   Pauciarticular juvenile rheumatoid arthritis, unspecified knee

M08.47   Pauciarticular juvenile rheumatoid arthritis, ankle and foot

M08.471   Pauciarticular juvenile rheumatoid arthritis, right ankle and foot

M08.472   Pauciarticular juvenile rheumatoid arthritis, left ankle and foot

M08.479   Pauciarticular juvenile rheumatoid arthritis, unspecified ankle and foot

M08.48   Pauciarticular juvenile rheumatoid arthritis, vertebrae

M08.8   Other juvenile arthritis

M08.80   Other juvenile arthritis, unspecified site

M08.81   Other juvenile arthritis, shoulder

M08.811   Other juvenile arthritis, right shoulder

M08.812   Other juvenile arthritis, left shoulder

M08.819   Other juvenile arthritis, unspecified shoulder

M08.82   Other juvenile arthritis, elbow

M08.821   Other juvenile arthritis, right elbow

M08.822   Other juvenile arthritis, left elbow

M08.829   Other juvenile arthritis, unspecified elbow

M08.83   Other juvenile arthritis, wrist

M08.831   Other juvenile arthritis, right wrist

M08.832   Other juvenile arthritis, left wrist

M08.839   Other juvenile arthritis, unspecified wrist

M08.84   Other juvenile arthritis, hand

M08.841   Other juvenile arthritis, right hand

M08.842   Other juvenile arthritis, left hand

M08.849   Other juvenile arthritis, unspecified hand

M08.85   Other juvenile arthritis, hip

M08.851   Other juvenile arthritis, right hip

M08.852   Other juvenile arthritis, left hip

M08.859   Other juvenile arthritis, unspecified hip

M08.86   Other juvenile arthritis, knee

M08.861   Other juvenile arthritis, right knee

M08.862   Other juvenile arthritis, left knee

M08.869   Other juvenile arthritis, unspecified knee

M08.87   Other juvenile arthritis, ankle and foot

M08.871   Other juvenile arthritis, right ankle and foot

M08.872   Other juvenile arthritis, left ankle and foot

M08.879   Other juvenile arthritis, unspecified ankle and foot

▲ **M08.88**   Other juvenile arthritis, other specified site

M08.89   Other juvenile arthritis, multiple sites

M08.9   Juvenile arthritis, unspecified

Excludes 1: juvenile rheumatoid arthritis, unspecified (M08.0-)

M08.90   Juvenile arthritis, unspecified, unspecified site

M08.91   Juvenile arthritis, unspecified, shoulder

M08.911   Juvenile arthritis, unspecified, right shoulder

M08.912   Juvenile arthritis, unspecified, left shoulder

M08.919   Juvenile arthritis, unspecified, unspecified shoulder

M08.92   Juvenile arthritis, unspecified, elbow

M08.921   Juvenile arthritis, unspecified, right elbow

M08.922   Juvenile arthritis, unspecified, left elbow

M08.929   Juvenile arthritis, unspecified, unspecified elbow

M08.93   Juvenile arthritis, unspecified, wrist

M08.931   Juvenile arthritis, unspecified, right wrist

M08.932   Juvenile arthritis, unspecified, left wrist

M08.939   Juvenile arthritis, unspecified, unspecified wrist

M08.94   Juvenile arthritis, unspecified, hand

M08.941   Juvenile arthritis, unspecified, right hand

M08.942   Juvenile arthritis, unspecified, left hand

M08.949   Juvenile arthritis, unspecified, unspecified hand

M08.95   Juvenile arthritis, unspecified, hip

M08.951   Juvenile arthritis, unspecified, right hip

M08.952   Juvenile arthritis, unspecified, left hip

M08.959   Juvenile arthritis, unspecified, unspecified hip

M08.96   Juvenile arthritis, unspecified, knee

M08.961   Juvenile arthritis, unspecified, right knee

M08.962   Juvenile arthritis, unspecified, left knee

M08.969   Juvenile arthritis, unspecified, unspecified knee

M08.97   Juvenile arthritis, unspecified, ankle and foot

M08.971   Juvenile arthritis, unspecified, right ankle and foot

M08.972	Juvenile arthritis, unspecified, left ankle and foot	
M08.979	Juvenile arthritis, unspecified, unspecified ankle and foot	

M08.98 Juvenile arthritis, unspecified, vertebrae

M08.99 Juvenile arthritis, unspecified, multiple sites

M1A Chronic gout

Use additional code to identify:

Autonomic neuropathy in diseases classified elsewhere (G99.0)

Calculus of urinary tract in diseases classified elsewhere (N22)

Cardiomyopathy in diseases classified elsewhere (I43)

Disorders of external ear in diseases classified elsewhere (H61.1-, H62.8-)

Disorders of iris and ciliary body in diseases classified elsewhere (H22)

Glomerular disorders in diseases classified elsewhere (N08)

Excludes 1: acute gout (M10-)
gout NOS (M10.-)

The appropriate 7th character is to be added to each code from category M1A

0 - without tophus (tophi)

1 - with tophus (tophi)

M1A.0 Idiopathic chronic gout

Chronic gouty bursitis

Primary chronic gout

⊗⑦**M1A.00** Idiopathic chronic gout, unspecified site

M1A.01 Idiopathic chronic gout, shoulder

⑦**M1A.011** Idiopathic chronic gout, right shoulder

⑦**M1A.012** Idiopathic chronic gout, left shoulder

⑦**M1A.019** Idiopathic chronic gout, unspecified shoulder

M1A.02 Idiopathic chronic gout, elbow

⑦**M1A.021** Idiopathic chronic gout, right elbow

⑦**M1A.022** Idiopathic chronic gout, left elbow

⑦**M1A.029** Idiopathic chronic gout, unspecified elbow

M1A.03 Idiopathic chronic gout, wrist

⑦**M1A.031** Idiopathic chronic gout, right wrist

⑦**M1A.032** Idiopathic chronic gout, left wrist

⑦**M1A.039** Idiopathic chronic gout, unspecified wrist

M1A.04 Idiopathic chronic gout, hand

⑦**M1A.041** Idiopathic chronic gout, right hand

⑦**M1A.042** Idiopathic chronic gout, left hand

⑦**M1A.049** Idiopathic chronic gout, unspecified hand

M1A.05 Idiopathic chronic gout, hip

⑦**M1A.051** Idiopathic chronic gout, right hip

⑦**M1A.052** Idiopathic chronic gout, left hip

⑦**M1A.059** Idiopathic chronic gout, unspecified hip

M1A.06 Idiopathic chronic gout, knee

⑦**M1A.061** Idiopathic chronic gout, right knee

⑦**M1A.062** Idiopathic chronic gout, left knee

⑦**M1A.069** Idiopathic chronic gout, unspecified knee

M1A.07 Idiopathic chronic gout, ankle and foot

⑦**M1A.071** Idiopathic chronic gout, right ankle and foot

⑦**M1A.072** Idiopathic chronic gout, left ankle and foot

⑦**M1A.079** Idiopathic chronic gout, unspecified ankle and foot

⊗⑦**M1A.08** Idiopathic chronic gout, vertebrae

⊗⑦**M1A.09** Idiopathic chronic gout, multiple sites

M1A.1 Lead-induced chronic gout

Code first toxic effects of lead and its compounds (T56.0-)

M1A.10 Lead-induced chronic gout, unspecified site

M1A.11 Lead-induced chronic gout, shoulder

⑦**M1A.111** Lead-induced chronic gout, right shoulder

⑦**M1A.112** Lead-induced chronic gout, left shoulder

⑦**M1A.119** Lead-induced chronic gout, unspecified shoulder

M1A.12 Lead-induced chronic gout, elbow

⑦**M1A.121** Lead-induced chronic gout, right elbow

⑦**M1A.122** Lead-induced chronic gout, left elbow

⑦**M1A.129** Lead-induced chronic gout, unspecified elbow

M1A.13 Lead-induced chronic gout, wrist

⑦**M1A.131** Lead-induced chronic gout, right wrist

⑦**M1A.132** Lead-induced chronic gout, left wrist

⑦**M1A.139** Lead-induced chronic gout, unspecified wrist

M1A.14 Lead-induced chronic gout, hand

⑦**M1A.141** Lead-induced chronic gout, right hand

⑦**M1A.142** Lead-induced chronic gout, left hand

⑦**M1A.149** Lead-induced chronic gout, unspecified hand

M1A.15 Lead-induced chronic gout, hip

⑦**M1A.151** Lead-induced chronic gout, right hip

⑦**M1A.152** Lead-induced chronic gout, left hip

⑦**M1A.159** Lead-induced chronic gout, unspecified hip

M1A.16 Lead-induced chronic gout, knee

⑦**M1A.161** Lead-induced chronic gout, right knee

⑦**M1A.162** Lead-induced chronic gout, left knee

⑦**M1A.169** Lead-induced chronic gout, unspecified knee

M1A.17 Lead-induced chronic gout, ankle and foot

⑦**M1A.171** Lead-induced chronic gout, right ankle and foot

⑦**M1A.172** Lead-induced chronic gout, left ankle and foot

⑦**M1A.179** Lead-induced chronic gout, unspecified ankle and foot

⊗⑦**M1A.18** Lead-induced chronic gout, vertebrae

⊗⑦**M1A.19** Lead-induced chronic gout, multiple sites

M1A.2 Drug-induced chronic gout

Use additional code for adverse effect, if applicable, to identify drug (T36-T50 with fifth or sixth character 5)

⊗⑦**M1A.20** Drug-induced chronic gout, unspecified site

M1A.21 Drug-induced chronic gout, shoulder

⑦**M1A.211** Drug-induced chronic gout, right shoulder

⑦**M1A.212** Drug-induced chronic gout, left shoulder

⑦**M1A.219** Drug-induced chronic gout, unspecified shoulder

M1A.22 Drug-induced chronic gout, elbow

⑦**M1A.221** Drug-induced chronic gout, right elbow

⑦**M1A.222** Drug-induced chronic gout, left elbow

⑦**M1A.229** Drug-induced chronic gout, unspecified elbow

M1A.23 Drug-induced chronic gout, wrist

⑦**M1A.231** Drug-induced chronic gout, right wrist

⑦**M1A.232** Drug-induced chronic gout, left wrist

⑦**M1A.239** Drug-induced chronic gout, unspecified wrist

M1A.24 Drug-induced chronic gout, hand

⑦**M1A.241** Drug-induced chronic gout, right hand

⑦**M1A.242** Drug-induced chronic gout, left hand

⑦**M1A.249** Drug-induced chronic gout, unspecified hand

M1A.25 Drug-induced chronic gout, hip

⑦**M1A.251** Drug-induced chronic gout, right hip

⑦**M1A.252** Drug-induced chronic gout, left hip

⑦**M1A.259** Drug-induced chronic gout, unspecified hip

M1A.26 Drug-induced chronic gout, knee

⑦**M1A.261** Drug-induced chronic gout, right knee

⑦**M1A.262** Drug-induced chronic gout, left knee

⑦**M1A.269** Drug-induced chronic gout, unspecified knee

M1A.27 Drug-induced chronic gout, ankle and foot

⑦**M1A.271** Drug-induced chronic gout, right ankle and foot

⑦**M1A.272** Drug-induced chronic gout, left ankle and foot

⑦**M1A.279** Drug-induced chronic gout, unspecified ankle and foot

⊗⑦**M1A.28** Drug-induced chronic gout, vertebrae

⊗⑦**M1A.29** Drug-induced chronic gout, multiple sites

M1A.3 Chronic gout due to renal impairment

Code first associated renal disease

⊗⑦**M1A.30** Chronic gout due to renal impairment, unspecified site

M1A.31 Chronic gout due to renal impairment, shoulder

⑦**M1A.311** Chronic gout due to renal impairment, right shoulder

⑦**M1A.312** Chronic gout due to renal impairment, left shoulder

⑦**M1A.319** Chronic gout due to renal impairment, unspecified shoulder

M1A.32 Chronic gout due to renal impairment, elbow

⑦**M1A.321** Chronic gout due to renal impairment, right elbow

⑦**M1A.322** Chronic gout due to renal impairment, left elbow

⑦**M1A.329** Chronic gout due to renal impairment, unspecified elbow

M1A.33 Chronic gout due to renal impairment, wrist

⑦**M1A.331** Chronic gout due to renal impairment, right wrist

⑦**M1A.332** Chronic gout due to renal impairment, left wrist

⑦**M1A.339** Chronic gout due to renal impairment, unspecified wrist

M1A.34 Chronic gout due to renal impairment, hand

⑦**M1A.341** Chronic gout due to renal impairment, right hand

⑦**M1A.342** Chronic gout due to renal impairment, left hand

⑦**M1A.349** Chronic gout due to renal impairment, unspecified hand

M1A.35 Chronic gout due to renal impairment, hip

⑦**M1A.351** Chronic gout due to renal impairment, right hip

⑦**M1A.352** Chronic gout due to renal impairment, left hip

⑦**M1A.359** Chronic gout due to renal impairment, unspecified hip

M1A.36 Chronic gout due to renal impairment, knee

⑦**M1A.361** Chronic gout due to renal impairment, right knee

⑦**M1A.362** Chronic gout due to renal impairment, left knee

⑦**M1A.369** Chronic gout due to renal impairment, unspecified knee

M1A.37 Chronic gout due to renal impairment, ankle and foot

⑦**M1A.371** Chronic gout due to renal impairment, right ankle and foot

⑦**M1A.372** Chronic gout due to renal impairment, left ankle and foot

⑦**M1A.379** Chronic gout due to renal impairment, unspecified ankle and foot

⊗⑦**M1A.38** Chronic gout due to renal impairment, vertebrae

⊗⑦**M1A.39** Chronic gout due to renal impairment, multiple sites

M1A.4 Other secondary chronic gout

Code first associated condition

⊗⑦**M1A.40** Other secondary chronic gout, unspecified site

M1A.41 Other secondary chronic gout, shoulder

● New code   ▲ Revised code   ⑦ 7ᵗʰ digit required   ⊗ Placeholder required

⑦**M1A.411** Other secondary chronic gout, right shoulder

⑦**M1A.412** Other secondary chronic gout, left shoulder

⑦**M1A.419** Other secondary chronic gout, unspecified shoulder

M1A.42 Other secondary chronic gout, elbow

⑦**M1A.421** Other secondary chronic gout, right elbow

⑦**M1A.422** Other secondary chronic gout, left elbow

⑦**M1A.429** Other secondary chronic gout, unspecified elbow

M1A.43 Other secondary chronic gout, wrist

⑦**M1A.431** Other secondary chronic gout, right wrist

⑦**M1A.432** Other secondary chronic gout, left wrist

⑦**M1A.439** Other secondary chronic gout, unspecified wrist

M1A.44 Other secondary chronic gout, hand

⑦**M1A.441** Other secondary chronic gout, right hand

⑦**M1A.442** Other secondary chronic gout, left hand

⑦**M1A.449** Other secondary chronic gout, unspecified hand

M1A.45 Other secondary chronic gout, hip

⑦**M1A.451** Other secondary chronic gout, right hip

⑦**M1A.452** Other secondary chronic gout, left hip

⑦**M1A.459** Other secondary chronic gout, unspecified hip

M1A.46 Other secondary chronic gout, knee

⑦**M1A.461** Other secondary chronic gout, right knee

⑦**M1A.462** Other secondary chronic gout, left knee

⑦**M1A.469** Other secondary chronic gout, unspecified knee

M1A.47 Other secondary chronic gout, ankle and foot

⑦**M1A.471** Other secondary chronic gout, right ankle and foot

⑦**M1A.472** Other secondary chronic gout, left ankle and foot

⑦**M1A.479** Other secondary chronic gout, unspecified ankle and foot

⊗⑦**M1A.48** Other secondary chronic gout, vertebrae

⊗⑦**M1A.49** Other secondary chronic gout, multiple sites

M1A.9 Chronic gout, unspecified

M10 Gout

Acute gout

Gout attack

Gout flare

Gout NOS

Podagra

Use additional code to identify:

Autonomic neuropathy in diseases classified elsewhere (G99.0)

Calculus of urinary tract in diseases classified elsewhere (N22)

Cardiomyopathy in diseases classified elsewhere (I43)

Disorders of external ear in diseases classified elsewhere (H61.1-, H62.8-)

Disorders of iris and ciliary body in diseases classified elsewhere (H22)

Glomerular disorders in diseases classified elsewhere (N08)

Excludes 1: chronic gout (M1A-)

M10.0 Idiopathic gout

Gouty bursitis

Primary gout

M10.00 Idiopathic gout, unspecified site

M10.01 Idiopathic gout, shoulder

M10.011 Idiopathic gout, right shoulder

M10.012 Idiopathic gout, left shoulder

M10.019 Idiopathic gout, unspecified shoulder

M10.02 Idiopathic gout, elbow

M10.021 Idiopathic gout, right elbow

M10.022 Idiopathic gout, left elbow

M10.029 Idiopathic gout, unspecified elbow

M10.03 Idiopathic gout, wrist

M10.031 Idiopathic gout, right wrist

M10.032 Idiopathic gout, left wrist

M10.039 Idiopathic gout, unspecified wrist

M10.04 Idiopathic gout, hand

M10.041 Idiopathic gout, right hand

M10.042 Idiopathic gout, left hand

M10.049 Idiopathic gout, unspecified hand

M10.05 Idiopathic gout, hip

M10.051 Idiopathic gout, right hip

M10.052 Idiopathic gout, left hip

M10.059 Idiopathic gout, unspecified hip

M10.06 Idiopathic gout, knee

M10.061 Idiopathic gout, right knee

M10.062 Idiopathic gout, left knee

M10.069 Idiopathic gout, unspecified knee

M10.07 Idiopathic gout, ankle and foot

M10.071 Idiopathic gout, right ankle and foot

M10.072 Idiopathic gout, left ankle and foot

M10.079 Idiopathic gout, unspecified ankle and foot

M10.08 Idiopathic gout, vertebrae

M10.09 Idiopathic gout, multiple sites

M10.1 Lead-induced gout

Code first toxic effects of lead and its compounds (T56.0-)

M10.10 Lead-induced gout, unspecified site

M10.11 Lead-induced gout, shoulder

M10.111 Lead-induced gout, right shoulder

M10.112 Lead-induced gout, left shoulder

M10.119 Lead-induced gout, unspecified shoulder

M10.12 Lead-induced gout, elbow

M10.121 Lead-induced gout, right elbow

M10.122 Lead-induced gout, left elbow

M10.129 Lead-induced gout, unspecified elbow

M10.13 Lead-induced gout, wrist

M10.131 Lead-induced gout, right wrist

M10.132 Lead-induced gout, left wrist

M10.139 Lead-induced gout, unspecified wrist

M10.14 Lead-induced gout, hand

M10.141 Lead-induced gout, right hand

M10.142 Lead-induced gout, left hand

M10.149 Lead-induced gout, unspecified hand

M10.15 Lead-induced gout, hip

M10.151 Lead-induced gout, right hip

M10.152 Lead-induced gout, left hip

M10.159 Lead-induced gout, unspecified hip

M10.16 Lead-induced gout, knee

M10.161 Lead-induced gout, right knee

M10.162 Lead-induced gout, left knee

M10.169 Lead-induced gout, unspecified knee

M10.17 Lead-induced gout, ankle and foot

M10.171 Lead-induced gout, right ankle and foot

M10.172 Lead-induced gout, left ankle and foot

M10.179 Lead-induced gout, unspecified ankle and foot

M10.18 Lead-induced gout, vertebrae

M10.19 Lead-induced gout, multiple sites

M10.2 Drug-induced gout

Use additional code for adverse effect, if applicable, to identify drug (T36-T50 with fifth or sixth character 5)

M10.20 Drug-induced gout, unspecified site

M10.21 Drug-induced gout, shoulder

M10.211 Drug-induced gout, right shoulder

M10.212 Drug-induced gout, left shoulder

M10.219 Drug-induced gout, unspecified shoulder

M10.22 Drug-induced gout, elbow

M10.221 Drug-induced gout, right elbow

M10.222 Drug-induced gout, left elbow

M10.229 Drug-induced gout, unspecified elbow

M10.23 Drug-induced gout, wrist

M10.231 Drug-induced gout, right wrist

M10.232 Drug-induced gout, left wrist

M10.239 Drug-induced gout, unspecified wrist

M10.24 Drug-induced gout, hand

M10.241 Drug-induced gout, right hand

M10.242 Drug-induced gout, left hand

M10.249 Drug-induced gout, unspecified hand

M10.25 Drug-induced gout, hip

M10.251 Drug-induced gout, right hip

M10.252 Drug-induced gout, left hip

M10.259 Drug-induced gout, unspecified hip

M10.26 Drug-induced gout, knee

M10.261 Drug-induced gout, right knee

M10.262 Drug-induced gout, left knee

M10.269 Drug-induced gout, unspecified knee

M10.27 Drug-induced gout, ankle and foot

M10.271 Drug-induced gout, right ankle and foot

M10.272 Drug-induced gout, left ankle and foot

M10.279 Drug-induced gout, unspecified ankle and foot

M10.28 Drug-induced gout, vertebrae

M10.29 Drug-induced gout, multiple sites

M10.3 Gout due to renal impairment

Code first associated renal disease

M10.30 Gout due to renal impairment, unspecified site

M10.31 Gout due to renal impairment, shoulder

M10.311 Gout due to renal impairment, right shoulder

M10.312 Gout due to renal impairment, left shoulder

M10.319 Gout due to renal impairment, unspecified shoulder

M10.32 Gout due to renal impairment, elbow

M10.321 Gout due to renal impairment, right elbow

M10.322 Gout due to renal impairment, left elbow

M10.329 Gout due to renal impairment, unspecified elbow

M10.33 Gout due to renal impairment, wrist

M10.331 Gout due to renal impairment, right wrist

M10.332 Gout due to renal impairment, left wrist

M10.339 Gout due to renal impairment, unspecified wrist

M10.34 Gout due to renal impairment, hand

M10.341 Gout due to renal impairment, right hand

M10.342 Gout due to renal impairment, left hand

M10.349 Gout due to renal impairment, unspecified hand

M10.35 Gout due to renal impairment, hip

M10.351 Gout due to renal impairment, right hip

M10.352 Gout due to renal impairment, left hip

M10.359 Gout due to renal impairment, unspecified hip

M10.36 Gout due to renal impairment, knee

M10.361 Gout due to renal impairment, right knee

M10.362 Gout due to renal impairment, left knee

M10.369 Gout due to renal impairment, unspecified knee

M10.37 Gout due to renal impairment, ankle and foot

M10.371 Gout due to renal impairment, right ankle and foot

M10.372 Gout due to renal impairment, left ankle and foot

M10.379 Gout due to renal impairment, unspecified ankle and foot

M10.38 Gout due to renal impairment, vertebrae

M10.39 Gout due to renal impairment, multiple sites

● New code   ▲ Revised code   ⑦ 7th digit required   ⊗ Placeholder required

M10.4 Other secondary gout
Code first associated condition
M10.40 Other secondary gout, unspecified site
M10.41 Other secondary gout, shoulder
M10.411 Other secondary gout, right shoulder
M10.412 Other secondary gout, left shoulder
M10.419 Other secondary gout, unspecified shoulder
M10.42 Other secondary gout, elbow
M10.421 Other secondary gout, right elbow
M10.422 Other secondary gout, left elbow
M10.429 Other secondary gout, unspecified elbow
M10.43 Other secondary gout, wrist
M10.431 Other secondary gout, right wrist
M10.432 Other secondary gout, left wrist
M10.439 Other secondary gout, unspecified wrist
M10.44 Other secondary gout, hand
M10.441 Other secondary gout, right hand
M10.442 Other secondary gout, left hand
M10.449 Other secondary gout, unspecified hand
M10.45 Other secondary gout, hip
M10.451 Other secondary gout, right hip
M10.452 Other secondary gout, left hip
M10.459 Other secondary gout, unspecified hip
M10.46 Other secondary gout, knee
M10.461 Other secondary gout, right knee
M10.462 Other secondary gout, left knee
M10.469 Other secondary gout, unspecified knee
M10.47 Other secondary gout, ankle and foot
M10.471 Other secondary gout, right ankle and foot
M10.472 Other secondary gout, left ankle and foot
M10.479 Other secondary gout, unspecified ankle and foot
M10.48 Other secondary gout, vertebrae
M10.49 Other secondary gout, multiple sites
M10.9 Gout, unspecified
Gout NOS
M11 Other crystal arthropathies
M11.0 Hydroxyapatite deposition disease
M11.00 Hydroxyapatite deposition disease, unspecified site
M11.01 Hydroxyapatite deposition disease, shoulder
M11.011 Hydroxyapatite deposition disease, right shoulder
M11.012 Hydroxyapatite deposition disease, left shoulder
M11.019 Hydroxyapatite deposition disease, unspecified shoulder
M11.02 Hydroxyapatite deposition disease, elbow
M11.021 Hydroxyapatite deposition disease, right elbow
M11.022 Hydroxyapatite deposition disease, left elbow

M11.029 Hydroxyapatite deposition disease, unspecified elbow
M11.03 Hydroxyapatite deposition disease, wrist
M11.031 Hydroxyapatite deposition disease, right wrist
M11.032 Hydroxyapatite deposition disease, left wrist
M11.039 Hydroxyapatite deposition disease, unspecified wrist
M11.04 Hydroxyapatite deposition disease, hand
M11.041 Hydroxyapatite deposition disease, right hand
M11.042 Hydroxyapatite deposition disease, left hand
M11.049 Hydroxyapatite deposition disease, unspecified hand
M11.05 Hydroxyapatite deposition disease, hip
M11.051 Hydroxyapatite deposition disease, right hip
M11.052 Hydroxyapatite deposition disease, left hip
M11.059 Hydroxyapatite deposition disease, unspecified hip
M11.06 Hydroxyapatite deposition disease, knee
M11.061 Hydroxyapatite deposition disease, right knee
M11.062 Hydroxyapatite deposition disease, left knee
M11.069 Hydroxyapatite deposition disease, unspecified knee
M11.07 Hydroxyapatite deposition disease, ankle and foot
M11.071 Hydroxyapatite deposition disease, right ankle and foot
M11.072 Hydroxyapatite deposition disease, left ankle and foot
M11.079 Hydroxyapatite deposition disease, unspecified ankle and foot
M11.08 Hydroxyapatite deposition disease, vertebrae
M11.09 Hydroxyapatite deposition disease, multiple sites
M11.1 Familial chondrocalcinosis
M11.10 Familial chondrocalcinosis, unspecified site
M11.11 Familial chondrocalcinosis, shoulder
M11.111 Familial chondrocalcinosis, right shoulder
M11.112 Familial chondrocalcinosis, left shoulder
M11.119 Familial chondrocalcinosis, unspecified shoulder
M11.12 Familial chondrocalcinosis, elbow
M11.121 Familial chondrocalcinosis, right elbow
M11.122 Familial chondrocalcinosis, left elbow
M11.129 Familial chondrocalcinosis, unspecified elbow
M11.13 Familial chondrocalcinosis, wrist
M11.131 Familial chondrocalcinosis, right wrist
M11.132 Familial chondrocalcinosis, left wrist

M11.139 Familial chondrocalcinosis, unspecified wrist

M11.14 Familial chondrocalcinosis, hand

M11.141 Familial chondrocalcinosis, right hand

M11.142 Familial chondrocalcinosis, left hand

M11.149 Familial chondrocalcinosis, unspecified hand

M11.15 Familial chondrocalcinosis, hip

M11.151 Familial chondrocalcinosis, right hip

M11.152 Familial chondrocalcinosis, left hip

M11.159 Familial chondrocalcinosis, unspecified hip

M11.16 Familial chondrocalcinosis, knee

M11.161 Familial chondrocalcinosis, right knee

M11.162 Familial chondrocalcinosis, left knee

M11.169 Familial chondrocalcinosis, unspecified knee

M11.17 Familial chondrocalcinosis, ankle and foot

M11.171 Familial chondrocalcinosis, right ankle and foot

M11.172 Familial chondrocalcinosis, left ankle and foot

M11.179 Familial chondrocalcinosis, unspecified ankle and foot

M11.18 Familial chondrocalcinosis, vertebrae

M11.19 Familial chondrocalcinosis, multiple sites

M11.2 Other chondrocalcinosis

Chondrocalcinosis NOS

M11.20 Other chondrocalcinosis, unspecified site

M11.21 Other chondrocalcinosis, shoulder

M11.211 Other chondrocalcinosis, right shoulder

M11.212 Other chondrocalcinosis, left shoulder

M11.219 Other chondrocalcinosis, unspecified shoulder

M11.22 Other chondrocalcinosis, elbow

M11.221 Other chondrocalcinosis, right elbow

M11.222 Other chondrocalcinosis, left elbow

M11.229 Other chondrocalcinosis, unspecified elbow

M11.23 Other chondrocalcinosis, wrist

M11.231 Other chondrocalcinosis, right wrist

M11.232 Other chondrocalcinosis, left wrist

M11.239 Other chondrocalcinosis, unspecified wrist

M11.24 Other chondrocalcinosis, hand

M11.241 Other chondrocalcinosis, right hand

M11.242 Other chondrocalcinosis, left hand

M11.249 Other chondrocalcinosis, unspecified hand

M11.25 Other chondrocalcinosis, hip

M11.251 Other chondrocalcinosis, right hip

M11.252 Other chondrocalcinosis, left hip

M11.259 Other chondrocalcinosis, unspecified hip

M11.26 Other chondrocalcinosis, knee

M11.261 Other chondrocalcinosis, right knee

M11.262 Other chondrocalcinosis, left knee

M11.269 Other chondrocalcinosis, unspecified knee

M11.27 Other chondrocalcinosis, ankle and foot

M11.271 Other chondrocalcinosis, right ankle and foot

M11.272 Other chondrocalcinosis, left ankle and foot

M11.279 Other chondrocalcinosis, unspecified ankle and foot

M11.28 Other chondrocalcinosis, vertebrae

M11.29 Other chondrocalcinosis, multiple sites

M11.8 Other specified crystal arthropathies

M11.80 Other specified crystal arthropathies, unspecified site

M11.81 Other specified crystal arthropathies, shoulder

M11.811 Other specified crystal arthropathies, right shoulder

M11.812 Other specified crystal arthropathies, left shoulder

M11.819 Other specified crystal arthropathies, unspecified shoulder

M11.82 Other specified crystal arthropathies, elbow

M11.821 Other specified crystal arthropathies, right elbow

M11.822 Other specified crystal arthropathies, left elbow

M11.829 Other specified crystal arthropathies, unspecified elbow

M11.83 Other specified crystal arthropathies, wrist

M11.831 Other specified crystal arthropathies, right wrist

M11.832 Other specified crystal arthropathies, left wrist

M11.839 Other specified crystal arthropathies, unspecified wrist

M11.84 Other specified crystal arthropathies, hand

M11.841 Other specified crystal arthropathies, right hand

M11.842 Other specified crystal arthropathies, left hand

M11.849 Other specified crystal arthropathies, unspecified hand

M11.85 Other specified crystal arthropathies, hip

M11.851 Other specified crystal arthropathies, right hip

M11.852 Other specified crystal arthropathies, left hip

M11.859 Other specified crystal arthropathies, unspecified hip

M11.86 Other specified crystal arthropathies, knee

M11.861 Other specified crystal arthropathies, right knee

M11.862 Other specified crystal arthropathies, left knee

M11.869 Other specified crystal arthropathies, unspecified knee

M11.87 Other specified crystal arthropathies, ankle and foot

● New code   ▲ Revised code   ⑦ 7ᵗʰ digit required   ⊗ Placeholder required

M11.871 Other specified crystal arthropathies, right ankle and foot

M11.872 Other specified crystal arthropathies, left ankle and foot

M11.879 Other specified crystal arthropathies, unspecified ankle and foot

M11.88 Other specified crystal arthropathies, vertebrae

M11.89 Other specified crystal arthropathies, multiple sites

M11.9 Crystal arthropathy, unspecified

M12 Other and unspecified arthropathy

Excludes 1: arthrosis (M15-M19)

cricoarytenoid arthropathy (J38.7)

M12.0 Chronic postrheumatic arthropathy [Jaccoud]

M12.00 Chronic postrheumatic arthropathy [Jaccoud], unspecified site

M12.01 Chronic postrheumatic arthropathy [Jaccoud], shoulder

M12.011 Chronic postrheumatic arthropathy [Jaccoud], right shoulder

M12.012 Chronic postrheumatic arthropathy [Jaccoud], left shoulder

M12.019 Chronic postrheumatic arthropathy [Jaccoud], unspecified shoulder

M12.02 Chronic postrheumatic arthropathy [Jaccoud], elbow

M12.021 Chronic postrheumatic arthropathy [Jaccoud], right elbow

M12.022 Chronic postrheumatic arthropathy [Jaccoud], left elbow

M12.029 Chronic postrheumatic arthropathy [Jaccoud], unspecified elbow

M12.03 Chronic postrheumatic arthropathy [Jaccoud], wrist

M12.031 Chronic postrheumatic arthropathy [Jaccoud], right wrist

M12.032 Chronic postrheumatic arthropathy [Jaccoud], left wrist

M12.039 Chronic postrheumatic arthropathy [Jaccoud], unspecified wrist

M12.04 Chronic postrheumatic arthropathy [Jaccoud], hand

M12.041 Chronic postrheumatic arthropathy [Jaccoud], right hand

M12.042 Chronic postrheumatic arthropathy [Jaccoud], left hand

M12.049 Chronic postrheumatic arthropathy [Jaccoud], unspecified hand

M12.05 Chronic postrheumatic arthropathy [Jaccoud], hip

M12.051 Chronic postrheumatic arthropathy [Jaccoud], right hip

M12.052 Chronic postrheumatic arthropathy [Jaccoud], left hip

M12.059 Chronic postrheumatic arthropathy [Jaccoud], unspecified hip

M12.06 Chronic postrheumatic arthropathy [Jaccoud], knee

M12.061 Chronic postrheumatic arthropathy [Jaccoud], right knee

M12.062 Chronic postrheumatic arthropathy [Jaccoud], left knee

M12.069 Chronic postrheumatic arthropathy [Jaccoud], unspecified knee

M12.07 Chronic postrheumatic arthropathy [Jaccoud], ankle and foot

M12.071 Chronic postrheumatic arthropathy [Jaccoud], right ankle and foot

M12.072 Chronic postrheumatic arthropathy [Jaccoud], left ankle and foot

M12.079 Chronic postrheumatic arthropathy [Jaccoud], unspecified ankle and foot

▲ **M12.08** Chronic postrheumatic arthropathy [Jaccoud], other specified site

M12.09 Chronic postrheumatic arthropathy [Jaccoud], multiple sites

M12.1 Kaschin-Beck disease

Osteochondroarthrosis deformans endemica

M12.10 Kaschin-Beck disease, unspecified site

M12.11 Kaschin-Beck disease, shoulder

M12.111 Kaschin-Beck disease, right shoulder

M12.112 Kaschin-Beck disease, left shoulder

M12.119 Kaschin-Beck disease, unspecified shoulder

M12.12 Kaschin-Beck disease, elbow

M12.121 Kaschin-Beck disease, right elbow

M12.122 Kaschin-Beck disease, left elbow

M12.129 Kaschin-Beck disease, unspecified elbow

M12.13 Kaschin-Beck disease, wrist

M12.131 Kaschin-Beck disease, right wrist

M12.132 Kaschin-Beck disease, left wrist

M12.139 Kaschin-Beck disease, unspecified wrist

M12.14 Kaschin-Beck disease, hand

M12.141 Kaschin-Beck disease, right hand

M12.142 Kaschin-Beck disease, left hand

M12.149 Kaschin-Beck disease, unspecified hand

M12.15 Kaschin-Beck disease, hip

M12.151 Kaschin-Beck disease, right hip

M12.152 Kaschin-Beck disease, left hip

M12.159 Kaschin-Beck disease, unspecified hip

M12.16 Kaschin-Beck disease, knee

M12.161 Kaschin-Beck disease, right knee

M12.162 Kaschin-Beck disease, left knee

M12.169 Kaschin-Beck disease, unspecified knee

M12.17 Kaschin-Beck disease, ankle and foot

M12.171 Kaschin-Beck disease, right ankle and foot

M12.172 Kaschin-Beck disease, left ankle and foot

M12.179 Kaschin-Beck disease, unspecified ankle and foot

M12.18 Kaschin-Beck disease, vertebrae

M12.19 Kaschin-Beck disease, multiple sites

M12.2 Villonodular synovitis (pigmented)

M12.20 Villonodular synovitis (pigmented), unspecified site

M12.21 Villonodular synovitis (pigmented), shoulder

    M12.211 Villonodular synovitis (pigmented), right shoulder

    M12.212 Villonodular synovitis (pigmented), left shoulder

    M12.219 Villonodular synovitis (pigmented), unspecified shoulder

M12.22 Villonodular synovitis (pigmented), elbow

    M12.221 Villonodular synovitis (pigmented), right elbow

    M12.222 Villonodular synovitis (pigmented), left elbow

    M12.229 Villonodular synovitis (pigmented), unspecified elbow

M12.23 Villonodular synovitis (pigmented), wrist

    M12.231 Villonodular synovitis (pigmented), right wrist

    M12.232 Villonodular synovitis (pigmented), left wrist

    M12.239 Villonodular synovitis (pigmented), unspecified wrist

M12.24 Villonodular synovitis (pigmented), hand

    M12.241 Villonodular synovitis (pigmented), right hand

    M12.242 Villonodular synovitis (pigmented), left hand

    M12.249 Villonodular synovitis (pigmented), unspecified hand

M12.25 Villonodular synovitis (pigmented), hip

    M12.251 Villonodular synovitis (pigmented), right hip

    M12.252 Villonodular synovitis (pigmented), left hip

    M12.259 Villonodular synovitis (pigmented), unspecified hip

M12.26 Villonodular synovitis (pigmented), knee

    M12.261 Villonodular synovitis (pigmented), right knee

    M12.262 Villonodular synovitis (pigmented), left knee

    M12.269 Villonodular synovitis (pigmented), unspecified knee

M12.27 Villonodular synovitis (pigmented), ankle and foot

    M12.271 Villonodular synovitis (pigmented), right ankle and foot

    M12.272 Villonodular synovitis (pigmented), left ankle and foot

    M12.279 Villonodular synovitis (pigmented), unspecified ankle and foot

▲ M12.28 Villonodular synovitis (pigmented), other specified

M12.29 Villonodular synovitis (pigmented), multiple sites

M12.3 Palindromic rheumatism

M12.30 Palindromic rheumatism, unspecified site

M12.31 Palindromic rheumatism, shoulder

    M12.311 Palindromic rheumatism, right shoulder

    M12.312 Palindromic rheumatism, left shoulder

    M12.319 Palindromic rheumatism, unspecified shoulder

M12.32 Palindromic rheumatism, elbow

    M12.321 Palindromic rheumatism, right elbow

    M12.322 Palindromic rheumatism, left elbow

    M12.329 Palindromic rheumatism, unspecified elbow

M12.33 Palindromic rheumatism, wrist

    M12.331 Palindromic rheumatism, right wrist

    M12.332 Palindromic rheumatism, left wrist

    M12.339 Palindromic rheumatism, unspecified wrist

M12.34 Palindromic rheumatism, hand

    M12.341 Palindromic rheumatism, right hand

    M12.342 Palindromic rheumatism, left hand

    M12.349 Palindromic rheumatism, unspecified hand

M12.35 Palindromic rheumatism, hip

    M12.351 Palindromic rheumatism, right hip

    M12.352 Palindromic rheumatism, left hip

    M12.359 Palindromic rheumatism, unspecified hip

M12.36 Palindromic rheumatism, knee

    M12.361 Palindromic rheumatism, right knee

    M12.362 Palindromic rheumatism, left knee

    M12.369 Palindromic rheumatism, unspecified knee

M12.37 Palindromic rheumatism, ankle and foot

    M12.371 Palindromic rheumatism, right ankle and foot

    M12.372 Palindromic rheumatism, left ankle and foot

    M12.379 Palindromic rheumatism, unspecified ankle and foot

▲ M12.38 Palindromic rheumatism, other specified site

M12.39 Palindromic rheumatism, multiple sites

M12.4 Intermittent hydrarthrosis

M12.40 Intermittent hydrarthrosis, unspecified site

M12.41 Intermittent hydrarthrosis, shoulder

    M12.411 Intermittent hydrarthrosis, right shoulder

    M12.412 Intermittent hydrarthrosis, left shoulder

    M12.419 Intermittent hydrarthrosis, unspecified shoulder

M12.42 Intermittent hydrarthrosis, elbow

    M12.421 Intermittent hydrarthrosis, right elbow

    M12.422 Intermittent hydrarthrosis, left elbow

    M12.429 Intermittent hydrarthrosis, unspecified elbow

M12.43 Intermittent hydrarthrosis, wrist

    M12.431 Intermittent hydrarthrosis, right wrist

    M12.432 Intermittent hydrarthrosis, left wrist

    M12.439 Intermittent hydrarthrosis, unspecified wrist

M12.44 Intermittent hydrarthrosis, hand

M12.441	Intermittent hydrarthrosis, right hand	
M12.442	Intermittent hydrarthrosis, left hand	
M12.449	Intermittent hydrarthrosis, unspecified hand	

M12.45 Intermittent hydrarthrosis, hip
    M12.451 Intermittent hydrarthrosis, right hip
    M12.452 Intermittent hydrarthrosis, left hip
    M12.459 Intermittent hydrarthrosis, unspecified hip

M12.46 Intermittent hydrarthrosis, knee
    M12.461 Intermittent hydrarthrosis, right knee
    M12.462 Intermittent hydrarthrosis, left knee
    M12.469 Intermittent hydrarthrosis, unspecified knee

M12.47 Intermittent hydrarthrosis, ankle and foot
    M12.471 Intermittent hydrarthrosis, right ankle and foot
    M12.472 Intermittent hydrarthrosis, left ankle and foot
    M12.479 Intermittent hydrarthrosis, unspecified ankle and foot

M12.48 Intermittent hydrarthrosis, other site
M12.49 Intermittent hydrarthrosis, multiple sites

M12.5 Traumatic arthropathy
    Excludes 1: current injury-see Alphabetic Index
    post-traumatic osteoarthritis (of):
    NOS (M19.1-)
    first carpometacarpal joint (M18.2-M18.3)
    hip (M16.4-M16.5)
    knee (M17.2-M17.3)
    other single joints (M19.1-)

M12.50 Traumatic arthropathy, unspecified site
M12.51 Traumatic arthropathy, shoulder
    M12.511 Traumatic arthropathy, right shoulder
    M12.512 Traumatic arthropathy, left shoulder
    M12.519 Traumatic arthropathy, unspecified shoulder

M12.52 Traumatic arthropathy, elbow
    M12.521 Traumatic arthropathy, right elbow
    M12.522 Traumatic arthropathy, left elbow
    M12.529 Traumatic arthropathy, unspecified elbow

M12.53 Traumatic arthropathy, wrist
    M12.531 Traumatic arthropathy, right wrist
    M12.532 Traumatic arthropathy, left wrist
    M12.539 Traumatic arthropathy, unspecified wrist

M12.54 Traumatic arthropathy, hand
    M12.541 Traumatic arthropathy, right hand
    M12.542 Traumatic arthropathy, left hand
    M12.549 Traumatic arthropathy, unspecified hand

M12.55 Traumatic arthropathy, hip
    M12.551 Traumatic arthropathy, right hip
    M12.552 Traumatic arthropathy, left hip
    M12.559 Traumatic arthropathy, unspecified hip

M12.56 Traumatic arthropathy, knee
    M12.561 Traumatic arthropathy, right knee

    M12.562 Traumatic arthropathy, left knee
    M12.569 Traumatic arthropathy, unspecified knee

M12.57 Traumatic arthropathy, ankle and foot
    M12.571 Traumatic arthropathy, right ankle and foot
    M12.572 Traumatic arthropathy, left ankle and foot
    M12.579 Traumatic arthropathy, unspecified ankle and foot

▲ **M12.58** Traumatic arthropathy, other specified site
M12.59 Traumatic arthropathy, multiple sites

M12.8 Other specific arthropathies, not elsewhere classified
Transient arthropathy
    M12.80 Other specific arthropathies, not elsewhere classified, unspecified site

M12.81 Other specific arthropathies, not elsewhere classified, shoulder
    M12.811 Other specific arthropathies, not elsewhere classified, right shoulder
    M12.812 Other specific arthropathies, not elsewhere classified, left shoulder
    M12.819 Other specific arthropathies, not elsewhere classified, unspecified shoulder

M12.82 Other specific arthropathies, not elsewhere classified, elbow
    M12.821 Other specific arthropathies, not elsewhere classified, right elbow
    M12.822 Other specific arthropathies, not elsewhere classified, left elbow
    M12.829 Other specific arthropathies, not elsewhere classified, unspecified elbow

M12.83 Other specific arthropathies, not elsewhere classified, wrist
    M12.831 Other specific arthropathies, not elsewhere classified, right wrist
    M12.832 Other specific arthropathies, not elsewhere classified, left wrist
    M12.839 Other specific arthropathies, not elsewhere classified, unspecified wrist

M12.84 Other specific arthropathies, not elsewhere classified, hand
    M12.841 Other specific arthropathies, not elsewhere classified, right hand
    M12.842 Other specific arthropathies, not elsewhere classified, left hand
    M12.849 Other specific arthropathies, not elsewhere classified, unspecified hand

M12.85 Other specific arthropathies, not elsewhere classified, hip
    M12.851 Other specific arthropathies, not elsewhere classified, right hip
    M12.852 Other specific arthropathies, not elsewhere classified, left hip
    M12.859 Other specific arthropathies, not elsewhere classified, unspecified hip

M12.86 Other specific arthropathies, not elsewhere classified, knee

    M12.861 Other specific arthropathies, not elsewhere classified, right knee

    M12.862 Other specific arthropathies, not elsewhere classified, left knee

    M12.869 Other specific arthropathies, not elsewhere classified, unspecified knee

M12.87 Other specific arthropathies, not elsewhere classified, ankle and foot

    M12.871 Other specific arthropathies, not elsewhere classified, right ankle and foot

    M12.872 Other specific arthropathies, not elsewhere classified, left ankle and foot

    M12.879 Other specific arthropathies, not elsewhere classified, unspecified ankle and foot

▲ **M12.88** Other specific arthropathies, not elsewhere classified, other specified site

M12.89 Other specific arthropathies, not elsewhere classified, multiple sites

M12.9 Arthropathy, unspecified

M13 Other arthritis

Excludes 1: arthrosis (M15-M19)

    osteoarthritis (M15-M19)

M13.0 Polyarthritis, unspecified

M13.1 Monoarthritis, not elsewhere classified

  M13.10 Monoarthritis, not elsewhere classified, unspecified site

  M13.11 Monoarthritis, not elsewhere classified, shoulder

    M13.111 Monoarthritis, not elsewhere classified, right shoulder

    M13.112 Monoarthritis, not elsewhere classified, left shoulder

    M13.119 Monoarthritis, not elsewhere classified, unspecified shoulder

  M13.12 Monoarthritis, not elsewhere classified, elbow

    M13.121 Monoarthritis, not elsewhere classified, right elbow

    M13.122 Monoarthritis, not elsewhere classified, left elbow

    M13.129 Monoarthritis, not elsewhere classified, unspecified elbow

  M13.13 Monoarthritis, not elsewhere classified, wrist

    M13.131 Monoarthritis, not elsewhere classified, right wrist

    M13.132 Monoarthritis, not elsewhere classified, left wrist

    M13.139 Monoarthritis, not elsewhere classified, unspecified wrist

  M13.14 Monoarthritis, not elsewhere classified, hand

    M13.141 Monoarthritis, not elsewhere classified, right hand

    M13.142 Monoarthritis, not elsewhere classified, left hand

    M13.149 Monoarthritis, not elsewhere classified, unspecified hand

  M13.15 Monoarthritis, not elsewhere classified, hip

    M13.151 Monoarthritis, not elsewhere classified, right hip

    M13.152 Monoarthritis, not elsewhere classified, left hip

    M13.159 Monoarthritis, not elsewhere classified, unspecified hip

  M13.16 Monoarthritis, not elsewhere classified, knee

    M13.161 Monoarthritis, not elsewhere classified, right knee

    M13.162 Monoarthritis, not elsewhere classified, left knee

    M13.169 Monoarthritis, not elsewhere classified, unspecified knee

  M13.17 Monoarthritis, not elsewhere classified, ankle and foot

    M13.171 Monoarthritis, not elsewhere classified, right ankle and foot

    M13.172 Monoarthritis, not elsewhere classified, left ankle and foot

    M13.179 Monoarthritis, not elsewhere classified, unspecified ankle and foot

M13.8 Other specified arthritis

Allergic arthritis

Excludes 1: osteoarthritis (M15-M19)

  M13.80 Other specified arthritis, unspecified site

  M13.81 Other specified arthritis, shoulder

    M13.811 Other specified arthritis, right shoulder

    M13.812 Other specified arthritis, left shoulder

    M13.819 Other specified arthritis, unspecified shoulder

  M13.82 Other specified arthritis, elbow

    M13.821 Other specified arthritis, right elbow

    M13.822 Other specified arthritis, left elbow

    M13.829 Other specified arthritis, unspecified elbow

  M13.83 Other specified arthritis, wrist

    M13.831 Other specified arthritis, right wrist

    M13.832 Other specified arthritis, left wrist

    M13.839 Other specified arthritis, unspecified wrist

  M13.84 Other specified arthritis, hand

    M13.841 Other specified arthritis, right hand

    M13.842 Other specified arthritis, left hand

    M13.849 Other specified arthritis, unspecified hand

  M13.85 Other specified arthritis, hip

    M13.851 Other specified arthritis, right hip

    M13.852 Other specified arthritis, left hip

    M13.859 Other specified arthritis, unspecified hip

  M13.86 Other specified arthritis, knee

    M13.861 Other specified arthritis, right knee

    M13.862 Other specified arthritis, left knee

    M13.869 Other specified arthritis, unspecified knee

  M13.87 Other specified arthritis, ankle and foot

M13.871 Other specified arthritis, right ankle and foot

M13.872 Other specified arthritis, left ankle and foot

M13.879 Other specified arthritis, unspecified ankle and foot

M13.88 Other specified arthritis, other site

M13.89 Other specified arthritis, multiple sites

M14 Arthropathies in other diseases classified elsewhere

Excludes 1: arthropathy in:

diabetes mellitus (E08-E13 with 4th character 61)

hematological disorders (M36.2-M36.3)

hypersensitivity reactions (M36.4)

neoplastic disease (M36.1)

neurosyphillis (A52.16)

sarcoidosis (D86.86)

enteropathic arthropathies (M07.-)

juvenile psoriatic arthropathy (L40.54)

lipoid dermatoarthritis (E78.81)

M14.6 Charcot's joint

Neuropathic arthropathy

Excludes 1: Charcot's joint in diabetes mellitus (E08-E13 with final characters 610)

Charcot's joint in tabes dorsalis (A52.16)

M14.60 Charcot's joint, unspecified site

M14.61 Charcot's joint, shoulder

    M14.611 Charcot's joint, right shoulder

    M14.612 Charcot's joint, left shoulder

    M14.619 Charcot's joint, unspecified shoulder

M14.62 Charcot's joint, elbow

    M14.621 Charcot's joint, right elbow

    M14.622 Charcot's joint, left elbow

    M14.629 Charcot's joint, unspecified elbow

M14.63 Charcot's joint, wrist

    M14.631 Charcot's joint, right wrist

    M14.632 Charcot's joint, left wrist

    M14.639 Charcot's joint, unspecified wrist

M14.64 Charcot's joint, hand

    M14.641 Charcot's joint, right hand

    M14.642 Charcot's joint, left hand

    M14.649 Charcot's joint, unspecified hand

M14.65 Charcot's joint, hip

    M14.651 Charcot's joint, right hip

    M14.652 Charcot's joint, left hip

    M14.659 Charcot's joint, unspecified hip

M14.66 Charcot's joint, knee

    M14.661 Charcot's joint, right knee

    M14.662 Charcot's joint, left knee

    M14.669 Charcot's joint, unspecified knee

M14.67 Charcot's joint, ankle and foot

    M14.671 Charcot's joint, right ankle and foot

    M14.672 Charcot's joint, left ankle and foot

    M14.679 Charcot's joint, unspecified ankle and foot

M14.68 Charcot's joint, vertebrae

M14.69 Charcot's joint, multiple sites

M14.8 Arthropathies in other specified diseases classified elsewhere

Code first underlying disease, such as:

amyloidosis (E85-)

erythema multiforme (L51.-)

erythema nodosum (L52)

hemochromatosis (E83.11-)

hyperparathyroidism (E21.-)

hypothyroidism (E00-E03)

sickle-cell disorders (D57.-)

thyrotoxicosis [hyperthyroidism] (E05.-)

Whipple's disease (K90.81)

M14.80 Arthropathies in other specified diseases classified elsewhere, unspecified site

M14.81 Arthropathies in other specified diseases classified elsewhere, shoulder

    M14.811 Arthropathies in other specified diseases classified elsewhere, right shoulder

    M14.812 Arthropathies in other specified diseases classified elsewhere, left shoulder

    M14.819 Arthropathies in other specified diseases classified elsewhere, unspecified shoulder

M14.82 Arthropathies in other specified diseases classified elsewhere, elbow

    M14.821 Arthropathies in other specified diseases classified elsewhere, right elbow

    M14.822 Arthropathies in other specified diseases classified elsewhere, left elbow

    M14.829 Arthropathies in other specified diseases classified elsewhere, unspecified elbow

M14.83 Arthropathies in other specified diseases classified elsewhere, wrist

    M14.831 Arthropathies in other specified diseases classified elsewhere, right wrist

    M14.832 Arthropathies in other specified diseases classified elsewhere, left wrist

    M14.839 Arthropathies in other specified diseases classified elsewhere, unspecified wrist

M14.84 Arthropathies in other specified diseases classified elsewhere, hand

    M14.841 Arthropathies in other specified diseases classified elsewhere, right hand

    M14.842 Arthropathies in other specified diseases classified elsewhere, left hand

    M14.849 Arthropathies in other specified diseases classified elsewhere, unspecified hand

M14.85 Arthropathies in other specified diseases classified elsewhere, hip

    M14.851 Arthropathies in other specified diseases classified elsewhere, right hip

M14.852 Arthropathies in other specified diseases classified elsewhere, left hip

M14.859 Arthropathies in other specified diseases classified elsewhere, unspecified hip

M14.86 Arthropathies in other specified diseases classified elsewhere, knee

M14.861 Arthropathies in other specified diseases classified elsewhere, right knee

M14.862 Arthropathies in other specified diseases classified elsewhere, left knee

M14.869 Arthropathies in other specified diseases classified elsewhere, unspecified knee

M14.87 Arthropathies in other specified diseases classified elsewhere, ankle and foot

M14.871 Arthropathies in other specified diseases classified elsewhere, right ankle and foot

M14.872 Arthropathies in other specified diseases classified elsewhere, left ankle and foot

M14.879 Arthropathies in other specified diseases classified elsewhere, unspecified ankle and foot

M14.88 Arthropathies in other specified diseases classified elsewhere, vertebrae

M14.89 Arthropathies in other specified diseases classified elsewhere, multiple sites

OSTEOARTHRITIS (M15-M19)

Excludes 2: osteoarthritis of spine (M47.-)

M15 Polyosteoarthritis

Includes: arthritis of multiple sites

Excludes 1: bilateral involvement of single joint (M16-M19)

M15.0 Primary generalized (osteo) arthritis

M15.1 Heberden's nodes (with arthropathy)
Interphalangeal distal osteoarthritis

M15.2 Bouchard's nodes (with arthropathy)
Juxtaphalangeal distal osteoarthritis

M15.3 Secondary multiple arthritis
Post-traumatic polyosteoarthritis

M15.4 Erosive (osteo)arthritis

M15.8 Other polyosteoarthritis

M15.9 Polyosteoarthritis, unspecified
Generalized osteoarthritis NOS

M16 Osteoarthritis of hip

M16.0 Bilateral primary osteoarthritis of hip

M16.1 Unilateral primary osteoarthritis of hip
Primary osteoarthritis of hip NOS

M16.10 Unilateral primary osteoarthritis, unspecified hip

M16.11 Unilateral primary osteoarthritis, right hip

M16.12 Unilateral primary osteoarthritis, left hip

M16.2 Bilateral osteoarthritis resulting from hip dysplasia

M16.3 Unilateral osteoarthritis resulting from hip dysplasia
Dysplastic osteoarthritis of hip NOS

M16.30 Unilateral osteoarthritis resulting from hip dysplasia, unspecified hip

M16.31 Unilateral osteoarthritis resulting from hip dysplasia, right hip

M16.32 Unilateral osteoarthritis resulting from hip dysplasia, left hip

M16.4 Bilateral post-traumatic osteoarthritis of hip

M16.5 Unilateral post-traumatic osteoarthritis of hip
Post-traumatic osteoarthritis of hip NOS

M16.50 Unilateral post-traumatic osteoarthritis, unspecified hip

M16.51 Unilateral post-traumatic osteoarthritis, right hip

M16.52 Unilateral post-traumatic osteoarthritis, left hip

M16.6 Other bilateral secondary osteoarthritis of hip

M16.7 Other unilateral secondary osteoarthritis of hip
Secondary osteoarthritis of hip NOS

M16.9 Osteoarthritis of hip, unspecified

M17 Osteoarthritis of knee

M17.0 Bilateral primary osteoarthritis of knee

M17.1 Unilateral primary osteoarthritis of knee
Primary osteoarthritis of knee NOS

M17.10 Unilateral primary osteoarthritis, unspecified knee

M17.11 Unilateral primary osteoarthritis, right knee

M17.12 Unilateral primary osteoarthritis, left knee

M17.2 Bilateral post-traumatic osteoarthritis of knee

M17.3 Unilateral post-traumatic osteoarthritis of knee
Post-traumatic osteoarthritis of knee NOS

M17.30 Unilateral post-traumatic osteoarthritis, unspecified knee

M17.31 Unilateral post-traumatic osteoarthritis, right knee

M17.32 Unilateral post-traumatic osteoarthritis, left knee

M17.4 Other bilateral secondary osteoarthritis of knee

M17.5 Other unilateral secondary osteoarthritis of knee
Secondary osteoarthritis of knee NOS

M17.9 Osteoarthritis of knee, unspecified

M18 Osteoarthritis of first carpometacarpal joint

M18.0 Bilateral primary osteoarthritis of first carpometacarpal joints

M18.1 Unilateral primary osteoarthritis of first carpometacarpal joint
Primary osteoarthritis of first carpometacarpal joint NOS

M18.10 Unilateral primary osteoarthritis of first carpometacarpal joint, unspecified hand

M18.11 Unilateral primary osteoarthritis of first carpometacarpal joint, right hand

M18.12 Unilateral primary osteoarthritis of first carpometacarpal joint, left hand

M18.2 Bilateral post-traumatic osteoarthritis of first carpometacarpal joints

M18.3 Unilateral post-traumatic osteoarthritis of first carpometacarpal joint
Post-traumatic osteoarthritis of first carpometacarpal joint NOS

M18.30 Unilateral post-traumatic osteoarthritis of first carpometacarpal joint, unspecified hand

M18.31 Unilateral post-traumatic osteoarthritis of first carpometacarpal joint, right hand

M18.32 Unilateral post-traumatic osteoarthritis of first carpometacarpal joint, left hand

M18.4 Other bilateral secondary osteoarthritis of first carpometacarpal joints

M18.5 Other unilateral secondary osteoarthritis of first carpometacarpal joint

Secondary osteoarthritis of first carpometacarpal joint NOS

M18.50 Other unilateral secondary osteoarthritis of first carpometacarpal joint, unspecified hand

M18.51 Other unilateral secondary osteoarthritis of first carpometacarpal joint, right hand

M18.52 Other unilateral secondary osteoarthritis of first carpometacarpal joint, left hand

M18.9 Osteoarthritis of first carpometacarpal joint, unspecified

M19 Other and unspecified osteoarthritis

Excludes 1: polyarthritis (M15.-)

Excludes 2: arthrosis of spine (M47.-)

hallux rigidus (M20.2)

osteoarthritis of spine (M47.-)

M19.0 Primary osteoarthritis of other joints

M19.01 Primary osteoarthritis, shoulder

M19.011 Primary osteoarthritis, right shoulder

M19.012 Primary osteoarthritis, left shoulder

M19.019 Primary osteoarthritis, unspecified shoulder

M19.02 Primary osteoarthritis, elbow

M19.021 Primary osteoarthritis, right elbow

M19.022 Primary osteoarthritis, left elbow

M19.029 Primary osteoarthritis, unspecified elbow

M19.03 Primary osteoarthritis, wrist

M19.031 Primary osteoarthritis, right wrist

M19.032 Primary osteoarthritis, left wrist

M19.039 Primary osteoarthritis, unspecified wrist

M19.04 Primary osteoarthritis, hand

Excludes 2: primary osteoarthritis of first carpometacarpal joint (M18.0-, M18.1-)

M19.041 Primary osteoarthritis, right hand

M19.042 Primary osteoarthritis, left hand

M19.049 Primary osteoarthritis, unspecified hand

M19.07 Primary osteoarthritis ankle and foot

M19.071 Primary osteoarthritis, right ankle and foot

M19.072 Primary osteoarthritis, left ankle and foot

M19.079 Primary osteoarthritis, unspecified ankle and foot

M19.1 Post-traumatic osteoarthritis of other joints

M19.11 Post-traumatic osteoarthritis, shoulder

M19.111 Post-traumatic osteoarthritis, right shoulder

M19.112 Post-traumatic osteoarthritis, left shoulder

M19.119 Post-traumatic osteoarthritis, unspecified shoulder

M19.12 Post-traumatic osteoarthritis, elbow

M19.121 Post-traumatic osteoarthritis, right elbow

M19.122 Post-traumatic osteoarthritis, left elbow

M19.129 Post-traumatic osteoarthritis, unspecified elbow

M19.13 Post-traumatic osteoarthritis, wrist

M19.131 Post-traumatic osteoarthritis, right wrist

M19.132 Post-traumatic osteoarthritis, left wrist

M19.139 Post-traumatic osteoarthritis, unspecified wrist

M19.14 Post-traumatic osteoarthritis, hand

Excludes 2: post-traumatic osteoarthritis of first carpometacarpal joint (M18.2-, M18.3-)

M19.141 Post-traumatic osteoarthritis, right hand

M19.142 Post-traumatic osteoarthritis, left hand

M19.149 Post-traumatic osteoarthritis, unspecified hand

M19.17 Post-traumatic osteoarthritis, ankle and foot

M19.171 Post-traumatic osteoarthritis, right ankle and foot

M19.172 Post-traumatic osteoarthritis, left ankle and foot

M19.179 Post-traumatic osteoarthritis, unspecified ankle and foot

M19.2 Secondary osteoarthritis of other joints

M19.21 Secondary osteoarthritis, shoulder

M19.211 Secondary osteoarthritis, right shoulder

M19.212 Secondary osteoarthritis, left shoulder

M19.219 Secondary osteoarthritis, unspecified shoulder

M19.22 Secondary osteoarthritis, elbow

M19.221 Secondary osteoarthritis, right elbow

M19.222 Secondary osteoarthritis, left elbow

M19.229 Secondary osteoarthritis, unspecified elbow

M19.23 Secondary osteoarthritis, wrist

M19.231 Secondary osteoarthritis, right wrist

M19.232 Secondary osteoarthritis, left wrist

M19.239 Secondary osteoarthritis, unspecified wrist

M19.24 Secondary osteoarthritis, hand

M19.241 Secondary osteoarthritis, right hand

M19.242 Secondary osteoarthritis, left hand

M19.249 Secondary osteoarthritis, unspecified hand

M19.27 Secondary osteoarthritis, ankle and foot

M19.271 Secondary osteoarthritis, right ankle and foot

M19.272 Secondary osteoarthritis, left ankle and foot

M19.279 Secondary osteoarthritis, unspecified ankle and foot

M19.9 Osteoarthritis, unspecified site

M19.90 Unspecified osteoarthritis, unspecified site

Arthrosis NOS

Arthritis NOS
Osteoarthritis NOS

M19.91 Primary osteoarthritis, unspecified site
Primary osteoarthritis NOS

M19.92 Post-traumatic osteoarthritis, unspecified site
Post-traumatic osteoarthritis NOS

M19.93 Secondary osteoarthritis, unspecified site
Secondary osteoarthritis NOS

OTHER JOINT DISORDERS (M20-M25)

Excludes 2: joints of the spine (M40-M54)

M20 Acquired deformities of fingers and toes

Excludes 1: acquired absence of fingers and toes (Z89.-)
congenital absence of fingers and toes (Q71.3-, Q72.3-)
congenital deformities and malformations of fingers and toes (Q66.-, Q68-Q70, Q74.-)

M20.0 Deformity of finger(s)

Excludes 1: clubbing of fingers (R68.3)
palmar fascial fibromatosis [Dupuytren] (M72.0)
trigger finger (M65.3)

M20.00 Unspecified deformity of finger(s)

M20.001 Unspecified deformity of right finger(s)

M20.002 Unspecified deformity of left finger(s)

M20.009 Unspecified deformity of unspecified finger(s)

M20.01 Mallet finger

M20.011 Mallet finger of right finger(s)

M20.012 Mallet finger of left finger(s)

M20.019 Mallet finger of unspecified finger(s)

M20.02 Boutonniere deformity

M20.021 Boutonniere deformity of right finger(s)

M20.022 Boutonniere deformity of left finger(s)

M20.029 Boutonniere deformity of unspecified finger(s)

M20.03 Swan-neck deformity

M20.031 Swan-neck deformity of right finger(s)

M20.032 Swan-neck deformity of left finger(s)

M20.039 Swan-neck deformity of unspecified finger(s)

M20.09 Other deformity of finger(s)

M20.091 Other deformity of right finger(s)

M20.092 Other deformity of left finger(s)

M20.099 Other deformity of finger(s), unspecified finger(s)

M20.1 Hallux valgus (acquired)
Bunion

M20.10 Hallux valgus (acquired), unspecified foot

M20.11 Hallux valgus (acquired), right foot

M20.12 Hallux valgus (acquired), left foot

M20.2 Hallux rigidus

M20.20 Hallux rigidus, unspecified foot

M20.21 Hallux rigidus, right foot

M20.22 Hallux rigidus, left foot

M20.3 Hallux varus (acquired)

M20.30 Hallux varus (acquired), unspecified foot

M20.31 Hallux varus (acquired), right foot

M20.32 Hallux varus (acquired), left foot

M20.4 Other hammer toe(s) (acquired)

M20.40 Other hammer toe(s) (acquired), unspecified foot

M20.41 Other hammer toe(s) (acquired), right foot

M20.42 Other hammer toe(s) (acquired), left foot

M20.5 Other deformities of toe(s) (acquired)

M20.5X Other deformities of toe(s) (acquired)

M20.5X1 Other deformities of toe(s) (acquired), right foot

M20.5X2 Other deformities of toe(s) (acquired), left foot

M20.5X9 Other deformities of toe(s) (acquired), unspecified foot

M20.6 Acquired deformities of toe(s), unspecified

M20.60 Acquired deformities of toe(s), unspecified, unspecified foot

M20.61 Acquired deformities of toe(s), unspecified, right foot

M20.62 Acquired deformities of toe(s), unspecified, left foot

M21 Other acquired deformities of limbs

Excludes 1: acquired absence of limb (Z89.-)
congenital absence of limbs (Q71-Q73)
congenital deformities and malformations of limbs (Q65-Q66, Q68-Q74)

Excludes 2: acquired deformities of fingers or toes (M20.-)
coxa plana (M91.2)

M21.0 Valgus deformity, not elsewhere classified

Excludes 1: metatarsus valgus (Q66.6)
talipes calcaneovalgus (Q66.4)

M21.00 Valgus deformity, not elsewhere classified, unspecified site

M21.02 Valgus deformity, not elsewhere classified, elbow
Cubitus valgus

M21.021 Valgus deformity, not elsewhere classified, right elbow

M21.022 Valgus deformity, not elsewhere classified, left elbow

M21.029 Valgus deformity, not elsewhere classified, unspecified elbow

M21.05 Valgus deformity, not elsewhere classified, hip

M21.051 Valgus deformity, not elsewhere classified, right hip

M21.052 Valgus deformity, not elsewhere classified, left hip

M21.059 Valgus deformity, not elsewhere classified, unspecified hip

M21.06 Valgus deformity, not elsewhere classified, knee
Genu valgum
Knock knee

M21.061 Valgus deformity, not elsewhere classified, right knee

M21.062 Valgus deformity, not elsewhere classified, left knee

M21.069 Valgus deformity, not elsewhere classified, unspecified knee

M21.07 Valgus deformity, not elsewhere classified, ankle

M21.071 Valgus deformity, not elsewhere classified, right ankle

M21.072 Valgus deformity, not elsewhere classified, left ankle

M21.079 Valgus deformity, not elsewhere classified, unspecified ankle

M21.1 Varus deformity, not elsewhere classified

Excludes 1: metatarsus varus (Q66.2)
tibia vara (M92.5)

M21.10 Varus deformity, not elsewhere classified, unspecified site

M21.12 Varus deformity, not elsewhere classified, elbow
Cubitus varus, elbow

M21.121 Varus deformity, not elsewhere classified, right elbow

M21.122 Varus deformity, not elsewhere classified, left elbow

M21.129 Varus deformity, not elsewhere classified, unspecified elbow

M21.15 Varus deformity, not elsewhere classified, hip

M21.151 Varus deformity, not elsewhere classified, right hip

M21.152 Varus deformity, not elsewhere classified, left hip

M21.159 Varus deformity, not elsewhere classified, unspecified

M21.16 Varus deformity, not elsewhere classified, knee
Bow leg
Genu varum

M21.161 Varus deformity, not elsewhere classified, right knee

M21.162 Varus deformity, not elsewhere classified, left knee

M21.169 Varus deformity, not elsewhere classified, unspecified knee

M21.17 Varus deformity, not elsewhere classified, ankle

M21.171 Varus deformity, not elsewhere classified, right ankle

M21.172 Varus deformity, not elsewhere classified, left ankle

M21.179 Varus deformity, not elsewhere classified, unspecified ankle

M21.2 Flexion deformity

M21.20 Flexion deformity, unspecified site

M21.21 Flexion deformity, shoulder

M21.211 Flexion deformity, right shoulder

M21.212 Flexion deformity, left shoulder

M21.219 Flexion deformity, unspecified shoulder

M21.22 Flexion deformity, elbow

M21.221 Flexion deformity, right elbow

M21.222 Flexion deformity, left elbow

M21.229 Flexion deformity, unspecified elbow

M21.23 Flexion deformity, wrist

M21.231 Flexion deformity, right wrist

M21.232 Flexion deformity, left wrist

M21.239 Flexion deformity, unspecified wrist

M21.24 Flexion deformity, finger joints

M21.241 Flexion deformity, right finger joints

M21.242 Flexion deformity, left finger joints

M21.249 Flexion deformity, unspecified finger joints

M21.25 Flexion deformity, hip

M21.251 Flexion deformity, right hip

M21.252 Flexion deformity, left hip

M21.259 Flexion deformity, unspecified hip

M21.26 Flexion deformity, knee

M21.261 Flexion deformity, right knee

M21.262 Flexion deformity, left knee

M21.269 Flexion deformity, unspecified knee

M21.27 Flexion deformity, ankle and toes

M21.271 Flexion deformity, right ankle and toes

M21.272 Flexion deformity, left ankle and toes

M21.279 Flexion deformity, unspecified ankle and toes

M21.3 Wrist or foot drop (acquired)

M21.33 Wrist drop (acquired)

M21.331 Wrist drop, right wrist

M21.332 Wrist drop, left wrist

M21.339 Wrist drop, unspecified wrist

M21.37 Foot drop (acquired)

M21.371 Foot drop, right foot

M21.372 Foot drop, left foot

M21.379 Foot drop, unspecified foot

M21.4 Flat foot [pes planus] (acquired)

Excludes 1: congenital pes planus (Q66.5-)

M21.40 Flat foot [pes planus] (acquired), unspecified foot

M21.41 Flat foot [pes planus] (acquired), right foot

M21.42 Flat foot [pes planus] (acquired), left foot

M21.5 Acquired clawhand, clubhand, clawfoot and clubfoot

Excludes 1: clubfoot, not specified as acquired (Q66.89)

M21.51 Acquired clawhand

M21.511 Acquired clawhand, right hand

M21.512 Acquired clawhand, left hand

M21.519 Acquired clawhand, unspecified hand

M21.52 Acquired clubhand

M21.521 Acquired clubhand, right hand

M21.522 Acquired clubhand, left hand

M21.529 Acquired clubhand, unspecified hand

M21.53 Acquired clawfoot

M21.531 Acquired clawfoot, right foot

M21.532 Acquired clawfoot, left foot

M21.539 Acquired clawfoot, unspecified foot

M21.54 Acquired clubfoot

M21.541 Acquired clubfoot, right foot

M21.542 Acquired clubfoot, left foot

M21.549 Acquired clubfoot, unspecified foot

M21.6 Other acquired deformities of foot

Excludes 2: deformities of toe (acquired) (M20.1-(M20.6)

M21.6X Other acquired deformities of foot

M21.6X1 Other acquired deformities of right foot

M21.6X2 Other acquired deformities of left foot

M21.6X9 Other acquired deformities of unspecified foot

M21.7 Unequal limb length (acquired)

Note: The site used should correspond to the shorter limb

M21.70 Unequal limb length (acquired), unspecified site

M21.72 Unequal limb length (acquired), humerus

M21.721 Unequal limb length (acquired), right humerus

M21.722 Unequal limb length (acquired), left humerus

M21.729 Unequal limb length (acquired), unspecified humerus

M21.73 Unequal limb length (acquired), ulna and radius

M21.731 Unequal limb length (acquired), right ulna

M21.732 Unequal limb length (acquired), left ulna

M21.733 Unequal limb length (acquired), right radius

M21.734 Unequal limb length (acquired), left radius

M21.739 Unequal limb length (acquired), unspecified ulna and radius

M21.75 Unequal limb length (acquired), femur

M21.751 Unequal limb length (acquired), right femur

M21.752 Unequal limb length (acquired), left femur

M21.759 Unequal limb length (acquired), unspecified femur

M21.76 Unequal limb length (acquired), tibia and fibula

M21.761 Unequal limb length (acquired), right tibia

M21.762 Unequal limb length (acquired), left tibia

M21.763 Unequal limb length (acquired), right fibula

M21.764 Unequal limb length (acquired), left fibula

M21.769 Unequal limb length (acquired), unspecified tibia and fibula

M21.8 Other specified acquired deformities of limbs

Excludes 2: coxa plana (M91.2)

M21.80 Other specified acquired deformities of unspecified limb

M21.82 Other specified acquired deformities of upper arm

M21.821 Other specified acquired deformities of right upper arm

M21.822 Other specified acquired deformities of left upper arm

M21.829 Other specified acquired deformities of unspecified upper arm

M21.83 Other specified acquired deformities of forearm

M21.831 Other specified acquired deformities of right forearm

M21.832 Other specified acquired deformities of left forearm

M21.839 Other specified acquired deformities of unspecified forearm

M21.85 Other specified acquired deformities of thigh

M21.851 Other specified acquired deformities of right thigh

M21.852 Other specified acquired deformities of left thigh

M21.859 Other specified acquired deformities of unspecified thigh

M21.86 Other specified acquired deformities of lower leg

M21.861 Other specified acquired deformities of right lower leg

M21.862 Other specified acquired deformities of left lower leg

M21.869 Other specified acquired deformities of unspecified lower leg

M21.9 Unspecified acquired deformity of limb and hand

M21.90 Unspecified acquired deformity of unspecified limb

M21.92 Unspecified acquired deformity of upper arm

M21.921 Unspecified acquired deformity of right upper arm

M21.922 Unspecified acquired deformity of left upper arm

M21.929 Unspecified acquired deformity of unspecified upper arm

M21.93 Unspecified acquired deformity of forearm

M21.931 Unspecified acquired deformity of right forearm

M21.932 Unspecified acquired deformity of left forearm

M21.939 Unspecified acquired deformity of unspecified forearm

M21.94 Unspecified acquired deformity of hand

M21.941 Unspecified acquired deformity of hand, right hand

M21.942 Unspecified acquired deformity of hand, left hand

M21.949 Unspecified acquired deformity of hand, unspecified hand

M21.95 Unspecified acquired deformity of thigh

M21.951 Unspecified acquired deformity of right thigh

M21.952 Unspecified acquired deformity of left thigh

M21.959 Unspecified acquired deformity of unspecified thigh

M21.96 Unspecified acquired deformity of lower leg

M21.961 Unspecified acquired deformity of right lower leg

M21.962 Unspecified acquired deformity of left lower leg

M21.969 Unspecified acquired deformity of unspecified lower leg

M22 Disorder of patella

Excludes 1: traumatic dislocation of patella (S83.0-)

M22.0 Recurrent dislocation of patella

M22.00 Recurrent dislocation of patella, unspecified knee

● New code   ▲ Revised code   ⑦ 7th digit required   ⊗ Placeholder required

M22.01 Recurrent dislocation of patella, right knee
M22.02 Recurrent dislocation of patella, left knee
M22.1 Recurrent subluxation of patella
Incomplete dislocation of patella
M22.10 Recurrent subluxation of patella, unspecified knee
M22.11 Recurrent subluxation of patella, right knee
M22.12 Recurrent subluxation of patella, left knee
M22.2 Patellofemoral disorders
M22.2X Patellofemoral disorders
M22.2X1 Patellofemoral disorders, right knee
M22.2X2 Patellofemoral disorders, left knee
M22.2X9 Patellofemoral disorders, unspecified knee
M22.3 Other derangements of patella
M22.3X Other derangements of patella
M22.3X1 Other derangements of patella, right knee
M22.3X2 Other derangements of patella, left knee
M22.3X9 Other derangements of patella, unspecified knee
M22.4 Chondromalacia patellae
M22.40 Chondromalacia patellae, unspecified knee
M22.41 Chondromalacia patellae, right knee
M22.42 Chondromalacia patellae, left knee
M22.8 Other disorders of patella
M22.8X Other disorders of patella
M22.8X1 Other disorders of patella, right knee
M22.8X2 Other disorders of patella, left knee
M22.8X9 Other disorders of patella, unspecified knee
M22.9 Unspecified disorder of patella
M22.90 Unspecified disorder of patella, unspecified knee
M22.91 Unspecified disorder of patella, right knee
M22.92 Unspecified disorder of patella, left knee
M23 Internal derangement of knee
Excludes 1: ankylosis (M24.66)
current injury - see injury of knee and lower leg (S80-S89)
deformity of knee (M21.-)
osteochondritis dissecans (M93.2)
recurrent dislocation or subluxation of joints (M24.4)
recurrent dislocation or subluxation of patella (M22.0-M22.1)
M23.0 Cystic meniscus
M23.00 Cystic meniscus, unspecified meniscus
Cystic meniscus, unspecified lateral meniscus
Cystic meniscus, unspecified medial meniscus
M23.000 Cystic meniscus, unspecified lateral meniscus, right knee
M23.001 Cystic meniscus, unspecified lateral meniscus, left knee
M23.002 Cystic meniscus, unspecified lateral meniscus, unspecified knee
M23.003 Cystic meniscus, unspecified medial meniscus, right knee
M23.004 Cystic meniscus, unspecified medial meniscus, left knee
M23.005 Cystic meniscus, unspecified medial meniscus, unspecified knee

M23.006 Cystic meniscus, unspecified meniscus, right knee
M23.007 Cystic meniscus, unspecified meniscus, left knee
M23.009 Cystic meniscus, unspecified meniscus, unspecified knee
M23.01 Cystic meniscus, anterior horn of medial meniscus
M23.011 Cystic meniscus, anterior horn of medial meniscus, right knee
M23.012 Cystic meniscus, anterior horn of medial meniscus, left knee
M23.019 Cystic meniscus, anterior horn of medial meniscus, unspecified knee
M23.02 Cystic meniscus, posterior horn of medial meniscus
M23.021 Cystic meniscus, posterior horn of medial meniscus, right knee
M23.022 Cystic meniscus, posterior horn of medial meniscus, left knee
M23.029 Cystic meniscus, posterior horn of medial meniscus, unspecified knee
M23.03 Cystic meniscus, other medial meniscus
M23.031 Cystic meniscus, other medial meniscus, right knee
M23.032 Cystic meniscus, other medial meniscus, left knee
M23.039 Cystic meniscus, other medial meniscus, unspecified knee
M23.04 Cystic meniscus, anterior horn of lateral meniscus
M23.041 Cystic meniscus, anterior horn of lateral meniscus, right knee
M23.042 Cystic meniscus, anterior horn of lateral meniscus, left knee
M23.049 Cystic meniscus, anterior horn of lateral meniscus, unspecified knee
M23.05 Cystic meniscus, posterior horn of lateral meniscus
M23.051 Cystic meniscus, posterior horn of lateral meniscus, right knee
M23.052 Cystic meniscus, posterior horn of lateral meniscus, left knee
M23.059 Cystic meniscus, posterior horn of lateral meniscus, unspecified knee
M23.06 Cystic meniscus, other lateral meniscus
M23.061 Cystic meniscus, other lateral meniscus, right knee
M23.062 Cystic meniscus, other lateral meniscus, left knee
M23.069 Cystic meniscus, other lateral meniscus, unspecified knee
M23.2 Derangement of meniscus due to old tear or injury
Old bucket-handle tear
M23.20 Derangement of unspecified meniscus due to old tear or injury
Derangement of unspecified lateral meniscus due to old tear or injury
Derangement of unspecified medial meniscus due to old tear or injury

M23.200 Derangement of unspecified lateral meniscus due to old tear or injury, right knee

M23.201 Derangement of unspecified lateral meniscus due to old tear or injury, left knee

M23.202 Derangement of unspecified lateral meniscus due to old tear or injury, unspecified knee

M23.203 Derangement of unspecified medial meniscus due to old tear or injury, right knee

M23.204 Derangement of unspecified medial meniscus due to old tear or injury, left knee

M23.205 Derangement of unspecified medial meniscus due to old tear or injury, unspecified knee

M23.206 Derangement of unspecified meniscus due to old tear or injury, right knee

M23.207 Derangement of unspecified meniscus due to old tear or injury, left knee

M23.209 Derangement of unspecified meniscus due to old tear or injury, unspecified knee

M23.21 Derangement of anterior horn of medial meniscus due to old tear or injury

M23.211 Derangement of anterior horn of medial meniscus due to old tear or injury, right knee

M23.212 Derangement of anterior horn of medial meniscus due to old tear or injury, left knee

M23.219 Derangement of anterior horn of medial meniscus due to old tear or injury, unspecified knee

M23.22 Derangement of posterior horn of medial meniscus due to old tear or injury

M23.221 Derangement of posterior horn of medial meniscus due to old tear or injury, right knee

M23.222 Derangement of posterior horn of medial meniscus due to old tear or injury, left knee

M23.229 Derangement of posterior horn of medial meniscus due to old tear or injury, unspecified knee

M23.23 Derangement of other medial meniscus due to old tear or injury

M23.231 Derangement of other medial meniscus due to old tear or injury, right knee

M23.232 Derangement of other medial meniscus due to old tear or injury, left knee

M23.239 Derangement of other medial meniscus due to old tear or injury, unspecified knee

M23.24 Derangement of anterior horn of lateral meniscus due to old tear or injury

M23.241 Derangement of anterior horn of lateral meniscus due to old tear or injury, right knee

M23.242 Derangement of anterior horn of lateral meniscus due to old tear or injury, left knee

M23.249 Derangement of anterior horn of lateral meniscus due to old tear or injury, unspecified knee

M23.25 Derangement of posterior horn of lateral meniscus due to old tear or injury

M23.251 Derangement of posterior horn of lateral meniscus due to old tear or injury, right knee

M23.252 Derangement of posterior horn of lateral meniscus due to old tear or injury, left knee

M23.259 Derangement of posterior horn of lateral meniscus due to old tear or injury, unspecified knee

M23.26 Derangement of other lateral meniscus due to old tear or injury

M23.261 Derangement of other lateral meniscus due to old tear or injury, right knee

M23.262 Derangement of other lateral meniscus due to old tear or injury, left knee

M23.269 Derangement of other lateral meniscus due to old tear or injury, unspecified knee

M23.3 Other meniscus derangements

Degenerate meniscus

Detached meniscus

Retained meniscus

M23.30 Other meniscus derangements, unspecified meniscus

Other meniscus derangements, unspecified lateral meniscus

Other meniscus derangements, unspecified medial meniscus

M23.300 Other meniscus derangements, unspecified lateral meniscus, right knee

M23.301 Other meniscus derangements, unspecified lateral meniscus, left knee

M23.302 Other meniscus derangements, unspecified lateral meniscus, unspecified knee

M23.303 Other meniscus derangements, unspecified medial meniscus, right knee

M23.304 Other meniscus derangements, unspecified medial meniscus, left knee

M23.305 Other meniscus derangements, unspecified medial meniscus, unspecified knee

M23.306 Other meniscus derangements, unspecified meniscus, right knee

● New code   ▲ Revised code   ⑦ 7th digit required   ⊗ Placeholder required

M23.307   Other meniscus derangements, unspecified meniscus, left knee

M23.309   Other meniscus derangements, unspecified meniscus, unspecified knee

M23.31   Other meniscus derangements, anterior horn of medial meniscus

M23.311   Other meniscus derangements, anterior horn of medial meniscus, right knee

M23.312   Other meniscus derangements, anterior horn of medial meniscus, left knee

M23.319   Other meniscus derangements, anterior horn of medial meniscus, unspecified knee

M23.32   Other meniscus derangements, posterior horn of medial meniscus

M23.321   Other meniscus derangements, posterior horn of medial meniscus, right knee

M23.322   Other meniscus derangements, posterior horn of medial meniscus, left knee

M23.329   Other meniscus derangements, posterior horn of medial meniscus, unspecified knee

M23.33   Other meniscus derangements, other medial meniscus

M23.331   Other meniscus derangements, other medial meniscus, right knee

M23.332   Other meniscus derangements, other medial meniscus, left knee

M23.339   Other meniscus derangements, other medial meniscus, unspecified knee

M23.34   Other meniscus derangements, anterior horn of lateral meniscus

M23.341   Other meniscus derangements, anterior horn of lateral meniscus, right knee

M23.342   Other meniscus derangements, anterior horn of lateral meniscus, left knee

M23.349   Other meniscus derangements, anterior horn of lateral meniscus, unspecified knee

M23.35   Other meniscus derangements, posterior horn of lateral meniscus

M23.351   Other meniscus derangements, posterior horn of lateral meniscus, right knee

M23.352   Other meniscus derangements, posterior horn of lateral meniscus, left knee

M23.359   Other meniscus derangements, posterior horn of lateral meniscus, unspecified knee

M23.36   Other meniscus derangements, other lateral meniscus

M23.361   Other meniscus derangements, other lateral meniscus, right knee

M23.362   Other meniscus derangements, other lateral meniscus, left knee

M23.369   Other meniscus derangements, other lateral meniscus, unspecified knee

M23.4   Loose body in knee

M23.40   Loose body in knee, unspecified knee

M23.41   Loose body in knee, right knee

M23.42   Loose body in knee, left knee

M23.5   Chronic instability of knee

M23.50   Chronic instability of knee, unspecified knee

M23.51   Chronic instability of knee, right knee

M23.52   Chronic instability of knee, left knee

M23.6   Other spontaneous disruption of ligament(s) of knee

M23.60   Other spontaneous disruption of unspecified ligament of knee

M23.601   Other spontaneous disruption of unspecified ligament of right knee

M23.602   Other spontaneous disruption of unspecified ligament of left knee

M23.609   Other spontaneous disruption of unspecified ligament of unspecified knee

M23.61   Other spontaneous disruption of anterior cruciate ligament of knee

M23.611   Other spontaneous disruption of anterior cruciate ligament of right knee

M23.612   Other spontaneous disruption of anterior cruciate ligament of left knee

M23.619   Other spontaneous disruption of anterior cruciate ligament of unspecified knee

M23.62   Other spontaneous disruption of posterior cruciate ligament of knee

M23.621   Other spontaneous disruption of posterior cruciate ligament of right knee

M23.622   Other spontaneous disruption of posterior cruciate ligament of left knee

M23.629   Other spontaneous disruption of posterior cruciate ligament of unspecified knee

M23.63   Other spontaneous disruption of medial collateral ligament of knee

M23.631   Other spontaneous disruption of medial collateral ligament of right knee

M23.632   Other spontaneous disruption of medial collateral ligament of left knee

M23.639   Other spontaneous disruption of medial collateral ligament of unspecified knee

M23.64   Other spontaneous disruption of lateral collateral ligament of knee

M23.641   Other spontaneous disruption of lateral collateral ligament of right knee

M23.642 Other spontaneous disruption of lateral collateral ligament of left knee

M23.649 Other spontaneous disruption of lateral collateral ligament of unspecified knee

M23.67 Other spontaneous disruption of capsular ligament of knee

M23.671 Other spontaneous disruption of capsular ligament of right knee

M23.672 Other spontaneous disruption of capsular ligament of left knee

M23.679 Other spontaneous disruption of capsular ligament of unspecified knee

M23.8 Other internal derangements of knee

Laxity of ligament of knee

Snapping knee

M23.8X Other internal derangements of knee

M23.8X1 Other internal derangements of right knee

M23.8X2 Other internal derangements of left knee

M23.8X9 Other internal derangements of unspecified knee

M23.9 Unspecified internal derangement of knee

M23.90 Unspecified internal derangement of unspecified knee

M23.91 Unspecified internal derangement of right knee

M23.92 Unspecified internal derangement of left knee

M24 Other specific joint derangements

Excludes 1: current injury - see injury of joint by body region

Excludes 2: ganglion (M67.4)

snapping knee (M23.8-)

temporomandibular joint disorders (M26.6-)

M24.0 Loose body in joint

Excludes 2: loose body in knee (M23.4)

M24.00 Loose body in unspecified joint

M24.01 Loose body in shoulder

M24.011 Loose body in right shoulder

M24.012 Loose body in left shoulder

M24.019 Loose body in unspecified shoulder

M24.02 Loose body in elbow

M24.021 Loose body in right elbow

M24.022 Loose body in left elbow

M24.029 Loose body in unspecified elbow

M24.03 Loose body in wrist

M24.031 Loose body in right wrist

M24.032 Loose body in left wrist

M24.039 Loose body in unspecified wrist

M24.04 Loose body in finger joints

M24.041 Loose body in right finger joint(s)

M24.042 Loose body in left finger joint(s)

M24.049 Loose body in unspecified finger joint(s)

M24.05 Loose body in hip

M24.051 Loose body in right hip

M24.052 Loose body in left hip

M24.059 Loose body in unspecified hip

M24.07 Loose body in ankle and toe joints

M24.071 Loose body in right ankle

M24.072 Loose body in left ankle

M24.073 Loose body in unspecified ankle

M24.074 Loose body in right toe joint(s)

M24.075 Loose body in left toe joint(s)

M24.076 Loose body in unspecified toe joints

M24.08 Loose body, other site

M24.1 Other articular cartilage disorders

Excludes 2: chondrocalcinosis (M11.1, M11.2-)

internal derangement of knee (M23.-)

metastatic calcification (E83.5)

ochronosis (E70.2)

M24.10 Other articular cartilage disorders, unspecified site

M24.11 Other articular cartilage disorders, shoulder

M24.111 Other articular cartilage disorders, right shoulder

M24.112 Other articular cartilage disorders, left shoulder

M24.119 Other articular cartilage disorders, unspecified shoulder

M24.12 Other articular cartilage disorders, elbow

M24.121 Other articular cartilage disorders, right elbow

M24.122 Other articular cartilage disorders, left elbow

M24.129 Other articular cartilage disorders, unspecified elbow

M24.13 Other articular cartilage disorders, wrist

M24.131 Other articular cartilage disorders, right wrist

M24.132 Other articular cartilage disorders, left wrist

M24.139 Other articular cartilage disorders, unspecified wrist

M24.14 Other articular cartilage disorders, hand

M24.141 Other articular cartilage disorders, right hand

M24.142 Other articular cartilage disorders, left hand

M24.149 Other articular cartilage disorders, unspecified hand

M24.15 Other articular cartilage disorders, hip

M24.151 Other articular cartilage disorders, right hip

M24.152 Other articular cartilage disorders, left hip

M24.159 Other articular cartilage disorders, unspecified hip

M24.17 Other articular cartilage disorders, ankle and foot

M24.171 Other articular cartilage disorders, right ankle

M24.172 Other articular cartilage disorders, left ankle

M24.173 Other articular cartilage disorders, unspecified ankle

M24.174 Other articular cartilage disorders, right foot

M24.175 Other articular cartilage disorders, left foot

M24.176 Other articular cartilage disorders, unspecified foot

M24.2 Disorder of ligament
Instability secondary to old ligament injury
Ligamentous laxity NOS
Excludes 1: familial ligamentous laxity (M35.7)
Excludes 2: internal derangement of knee (M23.5-M23.89)

M24.20 Disorder of ligament, unspecified site

M24.21 Disorder of ligament, shoulder
    M24.211 Disorder of ligament, right shoulder
    M24.212 Disorder of ligament, left shoulder
    M24.219 Disorder of ligament, unspecified shoulder

M24.22 Disorder of ligament, elbow
    M24.221 Disorder of ligament, right elbow
    M24.222 Disorder of ligament, left elbow
    M24.229 Disorder of ligament, unspecified elbow

M24.23 Disorder of ligament, wrist
    M24.231 Disorder of ligament, right wrist
    M24.232 Disorder of ligament, left wrist
    M24.239 Disorder of ligament, unspecified wrist

M24.24 Disorder of ligament, hand
    M24.241 Disorder of ligament, right hand
    M24.242 Disorder of ligament, left hand
    M24.249 Disorder of ligament, unspecified hand

M24.25 Disorder of ligament, hip
    M24.251 Disorder of ligament, right hip
    M24.252 Disorder of ligament, left hip
    M24.259 Disorder of ligament, unspecified hip

M24.27 Disorder of ligament, ankle and foot
    M24.271 Disorder of ligament, right ankle
    M24.272 Disorder of ligament, left ankle
    M24.273 Disorder of ligament, unspecified ankle
    M24.274 Disorder of ligament, right foot
    M24.275 Disorder of ligament, left foot
    M24.276 Disorder of ligament, unspecified foot

M24.28 Disorder of ligament, vertebrae

M24.3 Pathological dislocation of joint, not elsewhere classified
Excludes 1: congenital dislocation or displacement of joint- see congenital malformations and deformations of the musculoskeletal system (Q65-Q79)
current injury - see injury of joints and ligaments by body region
recurrent dislocation of joint (M24.4-)

M24.30 Pathological dislocation of unspecified joint, not elsewhere classified

M24.31 Pathological dislocation of shoulder, not elsewhere classified
    M24.311 Pathological dislocation of right shoulder, not elsewhere classified

M24.312 Pathological dislocation of left shoulder, not elsewhere classified

M24.319 Pathological dislocation of unspecified shoulder, not elsewhere classified

M24.32 Pathological dislocation of elbow, not elsewhere classified
    M24.321 Pathological dislocation of right elbow, not elsewhere classified
    M24.322 Pathological dislocation of left elbow, not elsewhere classified
    M24.329 Pathological dislocation of unspecified elbow, not elsewhere classified

M24.33 Pathological dislocation of wrist, not elsewhere classified
    M24.331 Pathological dislocation of right wrist, not elsewhere classified
    M24.332 Pathological dislocation of left wrist, not elsewhere classified
    M24.339 Pathological dislocation of unspecified wrist, not elsewhere classified

M24.34 Pathological dislocation of hand, not elsewhere classified
    M24.341 Pathological dislocation of right hand, not elsewhere classified
    M24.342 Pathological dislocation of left hand, not elsewhere classified
    M24.349 Pathological dislocation of unspecified hand, not elsewhere classified

M24.35 Pathological dislocation of hip, not elsewhere classified
    M24.351 Pathological dislocation of right hip, not elsewhere classified
    M24.352 Pathological dislocation of left hip, not elsewhere classified
    M24.359 Pathological dislocation of unspecified hip, not elsewhere classified

M24.36 Pathological dislocation of knee, not elsewhere classified
    M24.361 Pathological dislocation of right knee, not elsewhere classified
    M24.362 Pathological dislocation of left knee, not elsewhere classified
    M24.369 Pathological dislocation of unspecified knee, not elsewhere classified

M24.37 Pathological dislocation of ankle and foot, not elsewhere classified
    M24.371 Pathological dislocation of right ankle, not elsewhere classified
    M24.372 Pathological dislocation of left ankle, not elsewhere classified
    M24.373 Pathological dislocation of unspecified ankle, not elsewhere classified
    M24.374 Pathological dislocation of right foot, not elsewhere classified

M24.375 Pathological dislocation of left foot, not elsewhere classified

M24.376 Pathological dislocation of unspecified foot, not elsewhere classified

M24.4 Recurrent dislocation of joint

Recurrent subluxation of joint

Excludes 2: recurrent dislocation of patella (M22.0-M22.1)

recurrent vertebral dislocation (M43.3-, M43.4, M43.5-)

M24.40 Recurrent dislocation, unspecified joint

M24.41 Recurrent dislocation, shoulder

M24.411 Recurrent dislocation, right shoulder

M24.412 Recurrent dislocation, left shoulder

M24.419 Recurrent dislocation, unspecified shoulder

M24.42 Recurrent dislocation, elbow

M24.421 Recurrent dislocation, right elbow

M24.422 Recurrent dislocation, left elbow

M24.429 Recurrent dislocation, unspecified elbow

M24.43 Recurrent dislocation, wrist

M24.431 Recurrent dislocation, right wrist

M24.432 Recurrent dislocation, left wrist

M24.439 Recurrent dislocation, unspecified wrist

M24.44 Recurrent dislocation, hand and finger(s)

M24.441 Recurrent dislocation, right hand

M24.442 Recurrent dislocation, left hand

M24.443 Recurrent dislocation, unspecified hand

M24.444 Recurrent dislocation, right finger

M24.445 Recurrent dislocation, left finger

M24.446 Recurrent dislocation, unspecified finger

M24.45 Recurrent dislocation, hip

M24.451 Recurrent dislocation, right hip

M24.452 Recurrent dislocation, left hip

M24.459 Recurrent dislocation, unspecified hip

M24.46 Recurrent dislocation, knee

M24.461 Recurrent dislocation, right knee

M24.462 Recurrent dislocation, left knee

M24.469 Recurrent dislocation, unspecified knee

M24.47 Recurrent dislocation, ankle, foot and toes

M24.471 Recurrent dislocation, right ankle

M24.472 Recurrent dislocation, left ankle

M24.473 Recurrent dislocation, unspecified ankle

M24.474 Recurrent dislocation, right foot

M24.475 Recurrent dislocation, left foot

M24.476 Recurrent dislocation, unspecified foot

M24.477 Recurrent dislocation, right toe(s)

M24.478 Recurrent dislocation, left toe(s)

M24.479 Recurrent dislocation, unspecified toe(s)

M24.5 Contracture of joint

Excludes 1: contracture of muscle without contracture of joint (M62.4-)

contracture of tendon (sheath) without contracture of joint (M62.4-)

Dupuytren's contracture (M72.0)

Excludes 2: acquired deformities of limbs (M20-M21)

M24.50 Contracture, unspecified joint

M24.51 Contracture, shoulder

M24.511 Contracture, right shoulder

M24.512 Contracture, left shoulder

M24.519 Contracture, unspecified shoulder

M24.52 Contracture, elbow

M24.521 Contracture, right elbow

M24.522 Contracture, left elbow

M24.529 Contracture, unspecified elbow

M24.53 Contracture, wrist

M24.531 Contracture, right wrist

M24.532 Contracture, left wrist

M24.539 Contracture, unspecified wrist

M24.54 Contracture, hand

M24.541 Contracture, right hand

M24.542 Contracture, left hand

M24.549 Contracture, unspecified hand

M24.55 Contracture, hip

M24.551 Contracture, right hip

M24.552 Contracture, left hip

M24.559 Contracture, unspecified hip

M24.56 Contracture, knee

M24.561 Contracture, right knee

M24.562 Contracture, left knee

M24.569 Contracture, unspecified knee

M24.57 Contracture, ankle and foot

M24.571 Contracture, right ankle

M24.572 Contracture, left ankle

M24.573 Contracture, unspecified ankle

M24.574 Contracture, right foot

M24.575 Contracture, left foot

M24.576 Contracture, unspecified foot

M24.6 Ankylosis of joint

Excludes 1: stiffness of joint without ankylosis (M25.6-)

Excludes 2: spine (M43.2-)

M24.60 Ankylosis, unspecified joint

M24.61 Ankylosis, shoulder

M24.611 Ankylosis, right shoulder

M24.612 Ankylosis, left shoulder

M24.619 Ankylosis, unspecified shoulder

M24.62 Ankylosis, elbow

M24.621 Ankylosis, right elbow

M24.622 Ankylosis, left elbow

M24.629 Ankylosis, unspecified elbow

M24.63 Ankylosis, wrist

M24.631 Ankylosis, right wrist

M24.632 Ankylosis, left wrist

M24.639 Ankylosis, unspecified wrist

M24.64 Ankylosis, hand

M24.641 Ankylosis, right hand

M24.642 Ankylosis, left hand

M24.649   Ankylosis, unspecified hand

M24.65   Ankylosis, hip

     M24.651   Ankylosis, right hip

     M24.652   Ankylosis, left hip

     M24.659   Ankylosis, unspecified hip

M24.66   Ankylosis, knee

     M24.661   Ankylosis, right knee

     M24.662   Ankylosis, left knee

     M24.669   Ankylosis, unspecified knee

M24.67   Ankylosis, ankle and foot

     M24.671   Ankylosis, right ankle

     M24.672   Ankylosis, left ankle

     M24.673   Ankylosis, unspecified ankle

     M24.674   Ankylosis, right foot

     M24.675   Ankylosis, left foot

     M24.676   Ankylosis, unspecified foot

M24.7   Protrusio acetabuli

M24.8   Other specific joint derangements, not elsewhere classified

   Excludes 2: iliotibial band syndrome (M76.3)

   M24.80   Other specific joint derangements of unspecified joint, not elsewhere classified

   M24.81   Other specific joint derangements of shoulder, not elsewhere classified

     M24.811   Other specific joint derangements of right shoulder, not elsewhere classified

     M24.812   Other specific joint derangements of left shoulder, not elsewhere classified

     M24.819   Other specific joint derangements of unspecified shoulder, not elsewhere classified

   M24.82   Other specific joint derangements of elbow, not elsewhere classified

     M24.821   Other specific joint derangements of right elbow, not elsewhere classified

     M24.822   Other specific joint derangements of left elbow, not elsewhere classified

     M24.829   Other specific joint derangements of unspecified elbow, not elsewhere classified

   M24.83   Other specific joint derangements of wrist, not elsewhere classified

     M24.831   Other specific joint derangements of right wrist, not elsewhere classified

     M24.832   Other specific joint derangements of left wrist, not elsewhere classified

     M24.839   Other specific joint derangements of unspecified wrist, not elsewhere classified

   M24.84   Other specific joint derangements of hand, not elsewhere classified

     M24.841   Other specific joint derangements of right hand, not elsewhere classified

     M24.842   Other specific joint derangements of left hand, not elsewhere classified

     M24.849   Other specific joint derangements of unspecified hand, not elsewhere classified

   M24.85   Other specific joint derangements of hip, not elsewhere classified

Irritable hip

     M24.851   Other specific joint derangements of right hip, not elsewhere classified

     M24.852   Other specific joint derangements of left hip, not elsewhere classified

     M24.859   Other specific joint derangements of unspecified hip, not elsewhere classified

M24.87   Other specific joint derangements of ankle and foot, not elsewhere classified

     M24.871   Other specific joint derangements of right ankle, not elsewhere classified

     M24.872   Other specific joint derangements of left ankle, not elsewhere classified

     M24.873   Other specific joint derangements of unspecified ankle, not elsewhere classified

     M24.874   Other specific joint derangements of right foot, not elsewhere classified

     M24.875   Other specific joint derangements left foot, not elsewhere classified

     M24.876   Other specific joint derangements of unspecified foot, not elsewhere classified

M24.9   Joint derangement, unspecified

M25   Other joint disorder, not elsewhere classified

   Excludes 2: abnormality of gait and mobility (R26.-)

     acquired deformities of limb (M20-M21)

     calcification of bursa (M71.4-)

     calcification of shoulder (joint) (M75.3)

     calcification of tendon (M65.2-)

     difficulty in walking (R26.2)

     temporomandibular joint disorder (M26.6-)

M25.0   Hemarthrosis

   Excludes 1: current injury - see injury of joint by body region

     hemophilic arthropathy (M36.2)

   M25.00   Hemarthrosis, unspecified joint

   M25.01   Hemarthrosis, shoulder

     M25.011   Hemarthrosis, right shoulder

     M25.012   Hemarthrosis, left shoulder

     M25.019   Hemarthrosis, unspecified shoulder

   M25.02   Hemarthrosis, elbow

     M25.021   Hemarthrosis, right elbow

     M25.022   Hemarthrosis, left elbow

     M25.029   Hemarthrosis, unspecified elbow

   M25.03   Hemarthrosis, wrist

     M25.031   Hemarthrosis, right wrist

     M25.032   Hemarthrosis, left wrist

     M25.039   Hemarthrosis, unspecified wrist

   M25.04   Hemarthrosis, hand

     M25.041   Hemarthrosis, right hand

     M25.042   Hemarthrosis, left hand

     M25.049   Hemarthrosis, unspecified hand

   M25.05   Hemarthrosis, hip

     M25.051   Hemarthrosis, right hip

     M25.052   Hemarthrosis, left hip

     M25.059   Hemarthrosis, unspecified hip

   M25.06   Hemarthrosis, knee

     M25.061   Hemarthrosis, right knee

M25.062   Hemarthrosis, left knee
M25.069   Hemarthrosis, unspecified knee
M25.07 Hemarthrosis, ankle and foot
M25.071   Hemarthrosis, right ankle
M25.072   Hemarthrosis, left ankle
M25.073   Hemarthrosis, unspecified ankle
M25.074   Hemarthrosis, right foot
M25.075   Hemarthrosis, left foot
M25.076   Hemarthrosis, unspecified foot
▲ M25.08 Hemarthrosis, other specified site
M25.1 Fistula of joint
M25.10 Fistula, unspecified joint
M25.11 Fistula, shoulder
M25.111   Fistula, right shoulder
M25.112   Fistula, left shoulder
M25.119   Fistula, unspecified shoulder
M25.12 Fistula, elbow
M25.121   Fistula, right elbow
M25.122   Fistula, left elbow
M25.129   Fistula, unspecified elbow
M25.13 Fistula, wrist
M25.131   Fistula, right wrist
M25.132   Fistula, left wrist
M25.139   Fistula, unspecified wrist
M25.14 Fistula, hand
M25.141   Fistula, right hand
M25.142   Fistula, left hand
M25.149   Fistula, unspecified hand
M25.15 Fistula, hip
M25.151   Fistula, right hip
M25.152   Fistula, left hip
M25.159   Fistula, unspecified hip
M25.16 Fistula, knee
M25.161   Fistula, right knee
M25.162   Fistula, left knee
M25.169   Fistula, unspecified knee
M25.17 Fistula, ankle and foot
M25.171   Fistula, right ankle
M25.172   Fistula, left ankle
M25.173   Fistula, unspecified ankle
M25.174   Fistula, right foot
M25.175   Fistula, left foot
M25.176   Fistula, unspecified foot
▲ M25.18 Fistula, other specified site
M25.2 Flail joint
M25.20 Flail joint, unspecified joint
M25.21 Flail joint, shoulder
M25.211   Flail joint, right shoulder
M25.212   Flail joint, left shoulder
M25.219   Flail joint, unspecified shoulder
M25.22 Flail joint, elbow
M25.221   Flail joint, right elbow
M25.222   Flail joint, left elbow
M25.229   Flail joint, unspecified elbow
M25.23 Flail joint, wrist
M25.231   Flail joint, right wrist
M25.232   Flail joint, left wrist
M25.239   Flail joint, unspecified wrist

M25.24 Flail joint, hand
M25.241   Flail joint, right hand
M25.242   Flail joint, left hand
M25.249   Flail joint, unspecified hand
M25.25 Flail joint, hip
M25.251   Flail joint, right hip
M25.252   Flail joint, left hip
M25.259   Flail joint, unspecified hip
M25.26 Flail joint, knee
M25.261   Flail joint, right knee
M25.262   Flail joint, left knee
M25.269   Flail joint, unspecified knee
M25.27 Flail joint, ankle and foot
M25.271   Flail joint, right ankle and foot
M25.272   Flail joint, left ankle and foot
M25.279   Flail joint, unspecified ankle and foot
M25.28 Flail joint, other site
M25.3 Other instability of joint
Excludes 1: instability of joint secondary to old ligament injury (M24.2-)
            instability of joint secondary to removal of joint prosthesis (M96.8-)
Excludes 2: spinal instabilities (M53.2-)
M25.30 Other instability, unspecified joint
M25.31 Other instability, shoulder
M25.311   Other instability, right shoulder
M25.312   Other instability, left shoulder
M25.319   Other instability, unspecified shoulder
M25.32 Other instability, elbow
M25.321   Other instability, right elbow
M25.322   Other instability, left elbow
M25.329   Other instability, unspecified elbow
M25.33 Other instability, wrist
M25.331   Other instability, right wrist
M25.332   Other instability, left wrist
M25.339   Other instability, unspecified wrist
M25.34 Other instability, hand
M25.341   Other instability, right hand
M25.342   Other instability, left hand
M25.349   Other instability, unspecified hand
M25.35 Other instability, hip
M25.351   Other instability, right hip
M25.352   Other instability, left hip
M25.359   Other instability, unspecified hip
M25.36 Other instability, knee
M25.361   Other instability, right knee
M25.362   Other instability, left knee
M25.369   Other instability, unspecified knee
M25.37 Other instability, ankle and foot
M25.371   Other instability, right ankle
M25.372   Other instability, left ankle
M25.373   Other instability, unspecified ankle
M25.374   Other instability, right foot
M25.375   Other instability, left foot
M25.376   Other instability, unspecified foot
M25.4 Effusion of joint

Excludes 1: hydrarthrosis in yaws (A66.6)
intermittent hydrarthrosis (M12.4-)
other infective (teno)synovitis (M65.1-)

M25.40 Effusion, unspecified joint
M25.41 Effusion, shoulder
    M25.411   Effusion, right shoulder
    M25.412   Effusion, left shoulder
    M25.419   Effusion, unspecified shoulder
M25.42 Effusion, elbow
    M25.421   Effusion, right elbow
    M25.422   Effusion, left elbow
    M25.429   Effusion, unspecified elbow
M25.43 Effusion, wrist
    M25.431   Effusion, right wrist
    M25.432   Effusion, left wrist
    M25.439   Effusion, unspecified wrist
M25.44 Effusion, hand
    M25.441   Effusion, right hand
    M25.442   Effusion, left hand
    M25.449   Effusion, unspecified hand
M25.45 Effusion, hip
    M25.451   Effusion, right hip
    M25.452   Effusion, left hip
    M25.459   Effusion, unspecified hip
M25.46 Effusion, knee
    M25.461   Effusion, right knee
    M25.462   Effusion, left knee
    M25.469   Effusion, unspecified knee
M25.47 Effusion, ankle and foot
    M25.471   Effusion, right ankle
    M25.472   Effusion, left ankle
    M25.473   Effusion, unspecified ankle
    M25.474   Effusion, right foot
    M25.475   Effusion, left foot
    M25.476   Effusion, unspecified foot
M25.48 Effusion, other site
M25.5 Pain in joint
Excludes 2: pain in hand (M79.64-)
pain in fingers (M79.64-)
pain in foot (M79.67-)
pain in limb (M79.6-)
pain in toes (M79.67-)
M25.50 Pain in unspecified joint
M25.51 Pain in shoulder
    M25.511   Pain in right shoulder
    M25.512   Pain in left shoulder
    M25.519   Pain in unspecified shoulder
M25.52 Pain in elbow
    M25.521   Pain in right elbow
    M25.522   Pain in left elbow
    M25.529   Pain in unspecified elbow
M25.53 Pain in wrist
    M25.531   Pain in right wrist
    M25.532   Pain in left wrist
    M25.539   Pain in unspecified wrist
M25.55 Pain in hip
    M25.551   Pain in right hip
    M25.552   Pain in left hip

    M25.559   Pain in unspecified hip
M25.56 Pain in knee
    M25.561   Pain in right knee
    M25.562   Pain in left knee
    M25.569   Pain in unspecified knee
M25.57 Pain in ankle and joints of foot
    M25.571   Pain in right ankle and joints of right foot
    M25.572   Pain in left ankle and joints of left foot
    M25.579   Pain in unspecified ankle and joints of unspecified foot
M25.6 Stiffness of joint, not elsewhere classified
Excludes 1: ankylosis of joint (M24.6-)
contracture of joint (M24.5-)
M25.60 Stiffness of unspecified joint, not elsewhere classified
M25.61 Stiffness of shoulder, not elsewhere classified
    M25.611   Stiffness of right shoulder, not elsewhere classified
    M25.612   Stiffness of left shoulder, not elsewhere classified
    M25.619   Stiffness of unspecified shoulder, not elsewhere classified
M25.62 Stiffness of elbow, not elsewhere classified
    M25.621   Stiffness of right elbow, not elsewhere classified
    M25.622   Stiffness of left elbow, not elsewhere classified
    M25.629   Stiffness of unspecified elbow, not elsewhere classified
M25.63 Stiffness of wrist, not elsewhere classified
    M25.631   Stiffness of right wrist, not elsewhere classified
    M25.632   Stiffness of left wrist, not elsewhere classified
    M25.639   Stiffness of unspecified wrist, not elsewhere classified
M25.64 Stiffness of hand, not elsewhere classified
    M25.641   Stiffness of right hand, not elsewhere classified
    M25.642   Stiffness of left hand, not elsewhere classified
    M25.649   Stiffness of unspecified hand, not elsewhere classified
M25.65 Stiffness of hip, not elsewhere classified
    M25.651   Stiffness of right hip, not elsewhere classified
    M25.652   Stiffness of left hip, not elsewhere classified
    M25.659   Stiffness of unspecified hip, not elsewhere classified
M25.66 Stiffness of knee, not elsewhere classified
    M25.661   Stiffness of right knee, not elsewhere classified
    M25.662   Stiffness of left knee, not elsewhere classified
    M25.669   Stiffness of unspecified knee, not elsewhere classified
M25.67 Stiffness of ankle and foot, not elsewhere classified

M25.671   Stiffness of right ankle, not elsewhere classified

M25.672   Stiffness of left ankle, not elsewhere classified

M25.673   Stiffness of unspecified ankle, not elsewhere classified

M25.674   Stiffness of right foot, not elsewhere classified

M25.675   Stiffness of left foot, not elsewhere classified

M25.676   Stiffness of unspecified foot, not elsewhere classified

M25.7   Osteophyte

   M25.70   Osteophyte, unspecified joint

   M25.71   Osteophyte, shoulder

     M25.711   Osteophyte, right shoulder

     M25.712   Osteophyte, left shoulder

     M25.719   Osteophyte, unspecified shoulder

   M25.72   Osteophyte, elbow

     M25.721   Osteophyte, right elbow

     M25.722   Osteophyte, left elbow

     M25.729   Osteophyte, unspecified elbow

   M25.73   Osteophyte, wrist

     M25.731   Osteophyte, right wrist

     M25.732   Osteophyte, left wrist

     M25.739   Osteophyte, unspecified wrist

   M25.74   Osteophyte, hand

     M25.741   Osteophyte, right hand

     M25.742   Osteophyte, left hand

     M25.749   Osteophyte, unspecified hand

   M25.75   Osteophyte, hip

     M25.751   Osteophyte, right hip

     M25.752   Osteophyte, left hip

     M25.759   Osteophyte, unspecified hip

   M25.76   Osteophyte, knee

     M25.761   Osteophyte, right knee

     M25.762   Osteophyte, left knee

     M25.769   Osteophyte, unspecified knee

   M25.77   Osteophyte, ankle and foot

     M25.771   Osteophyte, right ankle

     M25.772   Osteophyte, left ankle

     M25.773   Osteophyte, unspecified ankle

     M25.774   Osteophyte, right foot

     M25.775   Osteophyte, left foot

     M25.776   Osteophyte, unspecified foot

   M25.78   Osteophyte, vertebrae

M25.8   Other specified joint disorders

   M25.80   Other specified joint disorders, unspecified joint

   M25.81   Other specified joint disorders, shoulder

     M25.811   Other specified joint disorders, right shoulder

     M25.812   Other specified joint disorders, left shoulder

     M25.819   Other specified joint disorders, unspecified shoulder

   M25.82   Other specified joint disorders, elbow

     M25.821   Other specified joint disorders, right elbow

     M25.822   Other specified joint disorders, left elbow

     M25.829   Other specified joint disorders, unspecified elbow

   M25.83   Other specified joint disorders, wrist

     M25.831   Other specified joint disorders, right wrist

     M25.832   Other specified joint disorders, left wrist

     M25.839   Other specified joint disorders, unspecified wrist

   M25.84   Other specified joint disorders, hand

     M25.841   Other specified joint disorders, right hand

     M25.842   Other specified joint disorders, left hand

     M25.849   Other specified joint disorders, unspecified hand

   M25.85   Other specified joint disorders, hip

     M25.851   Other specified joint disorders, right hip

     M25.852   Other specified joint disorders, left hip

     M25.859   Other specified joint disorders, unspecified hip

   M25.86   Other specified joint disorders, knee

     M25.861   Other specified joint disorders, right knee

     M25.862   Other specified joint disorders, left knee

     M25.869   Other specified joint disorders, unspecified knee

   M25.87   Other specified joint disorders, ankle and foot

     M25.871   Other specified joint disorders, right ankle and foot

     M25.872   Other specified joint disorders, left ankle and foot

     M25.879   Other specified joint disorders, unspecified ankle and foot

M25.9   Joint disorder, unspecified

DENTOFACIAL ANOMALIES [INCLUDING MALOCCLUSION] AND OTHER DISORDERS OF JAW (M26-M27)

Excludes 1: hemifacial atrophy or hypertrophy (Q67.4)

unilateral condylar hyperplasia or hypoplasia (M27.8)

M26 Dentofacial anomalies [including malocclusion]

   M26.0   Major anomalies of jaw size

     Excludes 1: acromegaly (E22.0)

       Robin's syndrome (Q87.0)

     M26.00   Unspecified anomaly of jaw size

     M26.01   Maxillary hyperplasia

     M26.02   Maxillary hypoplasia

     M26.03   Mandibular hyperplasia

     M26.04   Mandibular hypoplasia

     M26.05   Macrogenia

     M26.06   Microgenia

     M26.07   Excessive tuberosity of jaw

       Entire maxillary tuberosity

     M26.09   Other specified anomalies of jaw size

   M26.1   Anomalies of jaw-cranial base relationship

M26.10 Unspecified anomaly of jaw-cranial base relationship

M26.11 Maxillary asymmetry

M26.12 Other jaw asymmetry

M26.19 Other specified anomalies of jaw-cranial base relationship

M26.2 Anomalies of dental arch relationship

M26.20 Unspecified anomaly of dental arch relationship

M26.21 Malocclusion, Angle's class

    M26.211 Malocclusion, Angle's class I
            Neutro-occlusion

    M26.212 Malocclusion, Angle's class II
            Disto-occlusion Division I
            Disto-occlusion Division II

    M26.213 Malocclusion, Angle's class III
            Mesio-occlusion

    M26.219 Malocclusion, Angle's class, unspecified

M26.22 Open occlusal relationship

    M26.220 Open anterior occlusal relationship
            Anterior openbite

    M26.221 Open posterior occlusal relationship
            Posterior openbite

M26.23 Excessive horizontal overlap
    Excessive horizontal overjet

M26.24 Reverse articulation
    Crossbite (anterior) (posterior)

M26.25 Anomalies of interarch distance

M26.29 Other anomalies of dental arch relationship
    Midline deviation of dental arch
    Overbite (excessive) deep
    Overbite (excessive) horizontal
    Overbite (excessive) vertical
    Posterior lingual occlusion of mandibular teeth

M26.3 Anomalies of tooth position of fully erupted tooth or teeth

Excludes 2: embedded and impacted teeth (K01.-)

M26.30 Unspecified anomaly of tooth position of fully erupted tooth or teeth
    Abnormal spacing of fully erupted tooth or teeth NOS
    Displacement of fully erupted tooth or teeth NOS
    Transposition of fully erupted tooth or teeth NOS

M26.31 Crowding of fully erupted teeth

M26.32 Excessive spacing of fully erupted teeth
    Diastema of fully erupted tooth or teeth NOS

M26.33 Horizontal displacement of fully erupted tooth or teeth
    Tipped tooth or teeth
    Tipping of fully erupted tooth

M26.34 Vertical displacement of fully erupted tooth or teeth
    Extruded tooth
    Infraeruption of tooth or teeth
    Supraeruption of tooth or teeth

M26.35 Rotation of fully erupted tooth or teeth

M26.36 Insufficient interocclusal distance of fully erupted teeth (ridge)
    Lack of adequate intermaxillary vertical dimension of fully erupted teeth

M26.37 Excessive interocclusal distance of fully erupted teeth
    Excessive intermaxillary vertical dimension of fully erupted teeth
    Loss of occlusal vertical dimension of fully erupted teeth

M26.39 Other anomalies of tooth position of fully erupted tooth or teeth

M26.4 Malocclusion, unspecified

M26.5 Dentofacial functional abnormalities

Excludes 1: bruxism (F45.8)
    teeth-grinding NOS (F45.8)

M26.50 Dentofacial functional abnormalities, unspecified

M26.51 Abnormal jaw closure

M26.52 Limited mandibular range of motion

M26.53 Deviation in opening and closing of the mandible

M26.54 Insufficient anterior guidance
    Insufficient anterior occlusal guidance

M26.55 Centric occlusion maximum intercuspation discrepancy

Excludes 1: centric occlusion NOS (M26.59)

M26.56 Non-working side interference
    Balancing side interference

M26.57 Lack of posterior occlusal support

M26.59 Other dentofacial functional abnormalities
    Centric occlusion (of teeth) NOS
    Malocclusion due to abnormal swallowing
    Malocclusion due to mouth breathing
    Malocclusion due to tongue, lip or finger habits

M26.6 Temporomandibular joint disorders

Excludes 2: current temporomandibular joint dislocation (S03.0)
    current temporomandibular joint sprain (S03.4)

M26.60 Temporomandibular joint disorder, unspecified

M26.61 Adhesions and ankylosis of temporomandibular joint

M26.62 Arthralgia of temporomandibular joint

M26.63 Articular disc disorder of temporomandibular joint

M26.69 Other specified disorders of temporomandibular joint

M26.7 Dental alveolar anomalies

M26.70 Unspecified alveolar anomaly

M26.71 Alveolar maxillary hyperplasia

M26.72 Alveolar mandibular hyperplasia

M26.73 Alveolar maxillary hypoplasia

M26.74 Alveolar mandibular hypoplasia

M26.79 Other specified alveolar anomalies

M26.8 Other dentofacial anomalies

M26.81 Anterior soft tissue impingement
    Anterior soft tissue impingement on teeth

M26.82 Posterior soft tissue impingement
    Posterior soft tissue impingement on teeth

M26.89 Other dentofacial anomalies

M26.9 Dentofacial anomaly, unspecified

M27 Other diseases of jaws

M27.0 Developmental disorders of jaws
    Latent bone cyst of jaw
    Stafne's cyst

Torus mandibularis

Torus palatinus

M27.1 Giant cell granuloma, central

Giant cell granuloma NOS

Excludes 1: peripheral giant cell granuloma (K06.8)

M27.2 Inflammatory conditions of jaws

Osteitis of jaw(s)

Osteomyelitis (neonatal) jaw(s)

Osteoradionecrosis jaw(s)

Periostitis jaw(s)

Sequestrum of jaw bone

Use additional code (W88-W90, X39.0) to identify radiation, if radiation-induced

Excludes 2: osteonecrosis of jaw due to drug (M87.180)

M27.3 Alveolitis of jaws

Alveolar osteitis

Dry socket

M27.4 Other and unspecified cysts of jaw

Excludes 1: cysts of oral region (K09.-)

latent bone cyst of jaw (M27.0)

Stafne's cyst (M27.0)

M27.40 Unspecified cyst of jaw

Cyst of jaw NOS

M27.49 Other cysts of jaw

Aneurysmal cyst of jaw

Hemorrhagic cyst of jaw

Traumatic cyst of jaw

M27.5 Periradicular pathology associated with previous endodontic treatment

M27.51 Perforation of root canal space due to endodontic treatment

M27.52 Endodontic overfill

M27.53 Endodontic underfill

M27.59 Other periradicular pathology associated with previous endodontic treatment

M27.6 Endosseous dental implant failure

M27.61 Osseointegration failure of dental implant

Hemorrhagic complications of dental implant placement

Iatrogenic osseointegration failure of dental implant

Osseointegration failure of dental implant due to complications of systemic disease

Osseointegration failure of dental implant due to poor bone quality

Pre-integration failure of dental implant NOS

Pre-osseointegration failure of dental implant

M27.62 Post-osseointegration biological failure of dental implant

Failure of dental implant due to lack of attached gingiva

Failure of dental implant due to occlusal trauma (caused by poor prosthetic design)

Failure of dental implant due to parafunctional habits

Failure of dental implant due to periodontal infection (peri-implantitis)

Failure of dental implant due to poor oral hygiene

Iatrogenic post-osseointegration failure of dental implant

Post-osseointegration failure of dental implant due to complications of systemic disease

M27.63 Post-osseointegration mechanical failure of dental implant

Failure of dental prosthesis causing loss of dental implant

Fracture of dental implant

Excludes 2: cracked tooth (K03.81)

fractured dental restorative material with loss of material (K08.531)

fractured dental restorative material without loss of material (K08.530)

fractured tooth (S02.5)

M27.69 Other endosseous dental implant failure

Dental implant failure NOS

M27.8 Other specified diseases of jaws

Cherubism

Exostosis

Fibrous dysplasia

Unilateral condylar hyperplasia

Unilateral condylar hypoplasia

Excludes 1: jaw pain (R68.84)

M27.9 Disease of jaws, unspecified

SYSTEMIC CONNECTIVE TISSUE DISORDERS (M30-M36)

Includes: autoimmune disease NOS

collagen (vascular) disease NOS

systemic autoimmune disease

systemic collagen (vascular) disease

Excludes 1: autoimmune disease, single organ or single cell-type -code to relevant condition category

M30 Polyarteritis nodosa and related conditions

Excludes 1: microscopic polyarteritis (M31.7)

M30.0 Polyarteritis nodosa

M30.1 Polyarteritis with lung involvement [Churg-Strauss]

Allergic granulomatous angiitis

M30.2 Juvenile polyarteritis

M30.3 Mucocutaneous lymph node syndrome [Kawasaki]

M30.8 Other conditions related to polyarteritis nodosa

Polyangiitis overlap syndrome

M31 Other necrotizing vasculopathies

M31.0 Hypersensitivity angiitis

Goodpasture's syndrome

M31.1 Thrombotic microangiopathy

Thrombotic thrombocytopenic purpura

M31.2 Lethal midline granuloma

M31.3 Wegener's granulomatosis

Necrotizing respiratory granulomatosis

M31.30 Wegener's granulomatosis without renal involvement

Wegener's granulomatosis NOS

M31.31 Wegener's granulomatosis with renal involvement

M31.4 Aortic arch syndrome [Takayasu]

M31.5 Giant cell arteritis with polymyalgia rheumatica

M31.6 Other giant cell arteritis

M31.7 Microscopic polyangiitis

Microscopic polyarteritis

Excludes 1: polyarteritis nodosa (M30.0)

● New code   ▲ Revised code   ⑦ 7th digit required   ⊗ Placeholder required

M31.8 Other specified necrotizing vasculopathies
Hypocomplementemic vasculitis
Septic vasculitis
M31.9 Necrotizing vasculopathy, unspecified
M32 Systemic lupus erythematosus (SLE)
Excludes 1: lupus erythematosus (discoid) (NOS) (L93.0)
M32.0 Drug-induced systemic lupus erythematosus
Use additional code for adverse effect, if applicable, to identify drug (T36-T50 with fifth or sixth character 5)
M32.1 Systemic lupus erythematosus with organ or system involvement
  M32.10 Systemic lupus erythematosus, organ or system involvement unspecified
  M32.11 Endocarditis in systemic lupus erythematosus
Libman-Sacks disease
  M32.12 Pericarditis in systemic lupus erythematosus
Lupus pericarditis
  M32.13 Lung involvement in systemic lupus erythematosus
Pleural effusion due to systemic lupus erythematosus
  M32.14 Glomerular disease in systemic lupus erythematosus
Lupus renal disease NOS
  M32.15 Tubulointerstitial nephropathy in systemic lupus erythematosus
  M32.19 Other organ or system involvement in systemic lupus erythematosus
M32.8 Other forms of systemic lupus erythematosus
M32.9 Systemic lupus erythematosus, unspecified
SLE NOS
Systemic lupus erythematosus NOS
Systemic lupus erythematosus without organ involvement
M33 Dermatopolymyositis
M33.0 Juvenile dermatopolymyositis
  M33.00 Juvenile dermatopolymyositis, organ involvement unspecified
  M33.01 Juvenile dermatopolymyositis with respiratory involvement
  M33.02 Juvenile dermatopolymyositis with myopathy
  M33.09 Juvenile dermatopolymyositis with other organ involvement
M33.1 Other dermatopolymyositis
  M33.10 Other dermatopolymyositis, organ involvement unspecified
  M33.11 Other dermatopolymyositis with respiratory involvement
  M33.12 Other dermatopolymyositis with myopathy
  M33.19 Other dermatopolymyositis with other organ involvement
M33.2 Polymyositis
  M33.20 Polymyositis, organ involvement unspecified
  M33.21 Polymyositis with respiratory involvement
  M33.22 Polymyositis with myopathy
  M33.29 Polymyositis with other organ involvement
M33.9 Dermatopolymyositis, unspecified
  M33.90 Dermatopolymyositis, unspecified, organ involvement unspecified
  M33.91 Dermatopolymyositis, unspecified with respiratory involvement

  M33.92 Dermatopolymyositis, unspecified with myopathy
  M33.99 Dermatopolymyositis, unspecified with other organ involvement
M34 Systemic sclerosis [scleroderma]
Excludes 1: circumscribed scleroderma (L94.0)
neonatal scleroderma (P83.8)
M34.0 Progressive systemic sclerosis
M34.1 CR(E)ST syndrome
Combination of calcinosis, Raynaud's phenomenon, esophageal dysfunction, sclerodactyly, telangiectasia
M34.2 Systemic sclerosis induced by drug and chemical
Code first poisoning due to drug or toxin, if applicable (T36-T65 with fifth or sixth character 1-4 or 6)
Use additional code for adverse effect, if applicable, to identify drug (T36-T50 with fifth or sixth character 5)
M34.8 Other forms of systemic sclerosis
  M34.81 Systemic sclerosis with lung involvement
  M34.82 Systemic sclerosis with myopathy
  M34.83 Systemic sclerosis with polyneuropathy
  M34.89 Other systemic sclerosis
M34.9 Systemic sclerosis, unspecified
M35 Other systemic involvement of connective tissue
Excludes 1: reactive perforating collagenosis (L87.1)
M35.0 Sicca syndrome [Sjogren]
  M35.00 Sicca syndrome, unspecified
  M35.01 Sicca syndrome with keratoconjunctivitis
  M35.02 Sicca syndrome with lung involvement
  M35.03 Sicca syndrome with myopathy
  M35.04 Sicca syndrome with tubulointerstitial nephropathy
Renal tubular acidosis in sicca syndrome
  M35.09 Sicca syndrome with other organ involvement
M35.1 Other overlap syndromes
Mixed connective tissue disease
Excludes 1: polyangiitis overlap syndrome (M30.8)
M35.2 Behcet's disease
M35.3 Polymyalgia rheumatica
Excludes 1: polymyalgia rheumatica with giant cell arteritis (M31.5)
M35.4 Diffuse (eosinophilic) fasciitis
M35.5 Multifocal fibrosclerosis
M35.6 Relapsing panniculitis [Weber-Christian]
Excludes 1: lupus panniculitis (L93.2)
panniculitis NOS (M79.3-)
M35.7 Hypermobility syndrome
Familial ligamentous laxity
Excludes 1: Ehlers-Danlos syndrome (Q79.6)
ligamentous laxity, NOS (M24.2-)
M35.8 Other specified systemic involvement of connective tissue
M35.9 Systemic involvement of connective tissue, unspecified
Autoimmune disease (systemic) NOS
Collagen (vascular) disease NOS
M36 Systemic disorders of connective tissue in diseases classified elsewhere
Excludes 2: arthropathies in diseases classified elsewhere (M14.-)
M36.0 Dermato(poly)myositis in neoplastic disease
Code first underlying neoplasm (C00-D49)
M36.1 Arthropathy in neoplastic disease

Code first underlying neoplasm, such as:

    leukemia (C91-C95)

    malignant histiocytosis (C96.A)

    multiple myeloma (C90.0)

M36.2 Hemophilic arthropathy

Hemarthrosis in hemophilic arthropathy

Code first underlying disease, such as:

    factor VIII deficiency (D66)

    with vascular defect (D68.0)

    factor IX deficiency (D67)

    hemophilia (classical) (D66)

    hemophilia B (D67)

    hemophilia C (D68.1)

M36.3 Arthropathy in other blood disorders

M36.4 Arthropathy in hypersensitivity reactions classified elsewhere

Code first underlying disease, such as:

    Henoch (-Schönlein) purpura (D69.0)

    serum sickness (T80.6-)

M36.8 Systemic disorders of connective tissue in other diseases classified elsewhere

Code first underlying disease, such as:

alkaptonuria (E70.2)

hypogammaglobulinemia (D80.-)

ochronosis (E70.2)

DORSOPATHIES (M40-M54)

DEFORMING DORSOPATHIES (M40-M43)

M40 Kyphosis and lordosis

Excludes 1: congenital kyphosis and lordosis (Q76.4)

kyphoscoliosis (M41.-)

postprocedural kyphosis and lordosis (M96.-)

M40.0 Postural kyphosis

    Excludes 1: osteochondrosis of spine (M42.-)

    M40.00 Postural kyphosis, site unspecified

    M40.03 Postural kyphosis, cervicothoracic region

    M40.04 Postural kyphosis, thoracic region

    M40.05 Postural kyphosis, thoracolumbar region

M40.1 Other secondary kyphosis

    M40.10 Other secondary kyphosis, site unspecified

    M40.12 Other secondary kyphosis, cervical region

    M40.13 Other secondary kyphosis, cervicothoracic region

    M40.14 Other secondary kyphosis, thoracic region

    M40.15 Other secondary kyphosis, thoracolumbar region

M40.2 Other and unspecified kyphosis

    M40.20 Unspecified kyphosis

        M40.202 Unspecified kyphosis, cervical region

        M40.203 Unspecified kyphosis, cervicothoracic region

        M40.204 Unspecified kyphosis, thoracic region

        M40.205 Unspecified kyphosis, thoracolumbar region

        M40.209 Unspecified kyphosis, site unspecified

    M40.29 Other kyphosis

        M40.292 Other kyphosis, cervical region

        M40.293 Other kyphosis, cervicothoracic region

        M40.294 Other kyphosis, thoracic region

        M40.295 Other kyphosis, thoracolumbar region

        M40.299 Other kyphosis, site unspecified

M40.3 Flatback syndrome

    M40.30 Flatback syndrome, site unspecified

    M40.35 Flatback syndrome, thoracolumbar region

    M40.36 Flatback syndrome, lumbar region

    M40.37 Flatback syndrome, lumbosacral region

M40.4 Postural lordosis

Acquired lordosis

    M40.40 Postural lordosis, site unspecified

    M40.45 Postural lordosis, thoracolumbar region

    M40.46 Postural lordosis, lumbar region

    M40.47 Postural lordosis, lumbosacral region

M40.5 Lordosis, unspecified

    M40.50 Lordosis, unspecified, site unspecified

    M40.55 Lordosis, unspecified, thoracolumbar region

    M40.56 Lordosis, unspecified, lumbar region

    M40.57 Lordosis, unspecified, lumbosacral region

M41 Scoliosis

Includes: kyphoscoliosis

Excludes 1: congenital scoliosis NOS (Q67.5)

congenital scoliosis due to bony malformation (Q76.3)

postural congenital scoliosis (Q67.5)

kyphoscoliotic heart disease (I27.1)

postprocedural scoliosis (M96.-)

M41.0 Infantile idiopathic scoliosis

    M41.00 Infantile idiopathic scoliosis, site unspecified

    M41.02 Infantile idiopathic scoliosis, cervical region

    M41.03 Infantile idiopathic scoliosis, cervicothoracic region

    M41.04 Infantile idiopathic scoliosis, thoracic region

    M41.05 Infantile idiopathic scoliosis, thoracolumbar region

    M41.06 Infantile idiopathic scoliosis, lumbar region

    M41.07 Infantile idiopathic scoliosis, lumbosacral region

    M41.08 Infantile idiopathic scoliosis, sacral and sacrococcygeal region

M41.1 Juvenile and adolescent idiopathic scoliosis

    M41.11 Juvenile idiopathic scoliosis

        M41.112 Juvenile idiopathic scoliosis, cervical region

        M41.113 Juvenile idiopathic scoliosis, cervicothoracic region

        M41.114 Juvenile idiopathic scoliosis, thoracic region

        M41.115 Juvenile idiopathic scoliosis, thoracolumbar region

        M41.116 Juvenile idiopathic scoliosis, lumbar region

        M41.117 Juvenile idiopathic scoliosis, lumbosacral region

        M41.119 Juvenile idiopathic scoliosis, site unspecified

    M41.12 Adolescent scoliosis

● New code   ▲ Revised code   ⑦ 7th digit required   ⊗ Placeholder required

M41.122 Adolescent idiopathic scoliosis, cervical region

M41.123 Adolescent idiopathic scoliosis, cervicothoracic region

M41.124 Adolescent idiopathic scoliosis, thoracic region

M41.125 Adolescent idiopathic scoliosis, thoracolumbar region

M41.126 Adolescent idiopathic scoliosis, lumbar region

M41.127 Adolescent idiopathic scoliosis, lumbosacral region

M41.129 Adolescent idiopathic scoliosis, site unspecified

M41.2 Other idiopathic scoliosis

M41.20 Other idiopathic scoliosis, site unspecified

M41.22 Other idiopathic scoliosis, cervical region

M41.23 Other idiopathic scoliosis, cervicothoracic region

M41.24 Other idiopathic scoliosis, thoracic region

M41.25 Other idiopathic scoliosis, thoracolumbar region

M41.26 Other idiopathic scoliosis, lumbar region

M41.27 Other idiopathic scoliosis, lumbosacral region

M41.3 Thoracogenic scoliosis

M41.30 Thoracogenic scoliosis, site unspecified

M41.34 Thoracogenic scoliosis, thoracic region

M41.35 Thoracogenic scoliosis, thoracolumbar region

M41.4 Neuromuscular scoliosis

Scoliosis secondary to cerebral palsy, Friedreich's ataxia, poliomyelitis and other neuromuscular disorders

Code also underlying condition

M41.40 Neuromuscular scoliosis, site unspecified

M41.41 Neuromuscular scoliosis, occipito-atlanto-axial region

M41.42 Neuromuscular scoliosis, cervical region

M41.43 Neuromuscular scoliosis, cervicothoracic region

M41.44 Neuromuscular scoliosis, thoracic region

M41.45 Neuromuscular scoliosis, thoracolumbar region

M41.46 Neuromuscular scoliosis, lumbar region

M41.47 Neuromuscular scoliosis, lumbosacral region

M41.5 Other secondary scoliosis

M41.50 Other secondary scoliosis, site unspecified

M41.52 Other secondary scoliosis, cervical region

M41.53 Other secondary scoliosis, cervicothoracic region

M41.54 Other secondary scoliosis, thoracic region

M41.55 Other secondary scoliosis, thoracolumbar region

M41.56 Other secondary scoliosis, lumbar region

M41.57 Other secondary scoliosis, lumbosacral region

M41.8 Other forms of scoliosis

M41.80 Other forms of scoliosis, site unspecified

M41.82 Other forms of scoliosis, cervical region

M41.83 Other forms of scoliosis, cervicothoracic region

M41.84 Other forms of scoliosis, thoracic region

M41.85 Other forms of scoliosis, thoracolumbar region

M41.86 Other forms of scoliosis, lumbar region

M41.87 Other forms of scoliosis, lumbosacral region

M41.9 Scoliosis, unspecified

M42 Spinal osteochondrosis

M42.0 Juvenile osteochondrosis of spine

Calvé's disease

Scheuermann's disease

Excludes 1: postural kyphosis (M40.0)

M42.00 Juvenile osteochondrosis of spine, site unspecified

M42.01 Juvenile osteochondrosis of spine, occipito-atlanto-axial region

M42.02 Juvenile osteochondrosis of spine, cervical region

M42.03 Juvenile osteochondrosis of spine, cervicothoracic region

M42.04 Juvenile osteochondrosis of spine, thoracic region

M42.05 Juvenile osteochondrosis of spine, thoracolumbar region

M42.06 Juvenile osteochondrosis of spine, lumbar region

M42.07 Juvenile osteochondrosis of spine, lumbosacral region

M42.08 Juvenile osteochondrosis of spine, sacral and sacrococcygeal region

M42.09 Juvenile osteochondrosis of spine, multiple sites in spine

M42.1 Adult osteochondrosis of spine

M42.10 Adult osteochondrosis of spine, site unspecified

M42.11 Adult osteochondrosis of spine, occipito-atlanto-axial region

M42.12 Adult osteochondrosis of spine, cervical region

M42.13 Adult osteochondrosis of spine, cervicothoracic region

M42.14 Adult osteochondrosis of spine, thoracic region

M42.15 Adult osteochondrosis of spine, thoracolumbar region

M42.16 Adult osteochondrosis of spine, lumbar region

M42.17 Adult osteochondrosis of spine, lumbosacral region

M42.18 Adult osteochondrosis of spine, sacral and sacrococcygeal region

M42.19 Adult osteochondrosis of spine, multiple sites in spine

M42.9 Spinal osteochondrosis, unspecified

M43 Other deforming dorsopathies

Excludes 1: congenital spondylolysis and spondylolisthesis (Q76.2)

hemivertebra (Q76.3-Q76.4)

Klippel-Feil syndrome (Q76.1)

lumbarization and sacralization (Q76.4)

platyspondylisis (Q76.4)

spina bifida occulta (Q76.0)

spinal curvature in osteoporosis (M80-)

spinal curvature in Paget's disease of bone [osteitis deformans] (M88.-)

M43.0 Spondylolysis

Excludes 1: congenital spondylolysis (Q76.2)

spondylolisthesis (M43.1)

M43.00 Spondylolysis, site unspecified

M43.01 Spondylolysis, occipito-atlanto-axial region

M43.02 Spondylolysis, cervical region

M43.03 Spondylolysis, cervicothoracic region

M43.04 Spondylolysis, thoracic region

M43.05 Spondylolysis, thoracolumbar region

M43.06 Spondylolysis, lumbar region

M43.07 Spondylolysis, lumbosacral region

M43.08 Spondylolysis, sacral and sacrococcygeal region

M43.09 Spondylolysis, multiple sites in spine

M43.1 Spondylolisthesis

Excludes 1: acute traumatic of lumbosacral region (S33.1)

acute traumatic of sites other than lumbosacral-code to Fracture, vertebra, by region

congenital spondylolisthesis (Q76.2)

M43.10 Spondylolisthesis, site unspecified

M43.11 Spondylolisthesis, occipito-atlanto-axial region

M43.12 Spondylolisthesis, cervical region

M43.13 Spondylolisthesis, cervicothoracic region

M43.14 Spondylolisthesis, thoracic region

M43.15 Spondylolisthesis, thoracolumbar region

M43.16 Spondylolisthesis, lumbar region

M43.17 Spondylolisthesis, lumbosacral region

M43.18 Spondylolisthesis, sacral and sacrococcygeal region

M43.19 Spondylolisthesis, multiple sites in spine

M43.2 Fusion of spine

Ankylosis of spinal joint

Excludes 1: ankylosing spondylitis (M45.0-)

congenital fusion of spine (Q76.4)

Excludes 2: arthrodesis status (Z98.1)

pseudoarthrosis after fusion or arthrodesis (M96.0)

M43.20 Fusion of spine, site unspecified

M43.21 Fusion of spine, occipito-atlanto-axial region

M43.22 Fusion of spine, cervical region

M43.23 Fusion of spine, cervicothoracic region

M43.24 Fusion of spine, thoracic region

M43.25 Fusion of spine, thoracolumbar region

M43.26 Fusion of spine, lumbar region

M43.27 Fusion of spine, lumbosacral region

M43.28 Fusion of spine, sacral and sacrococcygeal region

M43.3 Recurrent atlantoaxial dislocation with myelopathy

M43.4 Other recurrent atlantoaxial dislocation

M43.5 Other recurrent vertebral dislocation

Excludes 1: biomechanical lesions NEC (M99.-)

M43.5X Other recurrent vertebral dislocation

M43.5X2 Other recurrent vertebral dislocation, cervical region

M43.5X3 Other recurrent vertebral dislocation, cervicothoracic region

M43.5X4 Other recurrent vertebral dislocation, thoracic region

M43.5X5 Other recurrent vertebral dislocation, thoracolumbar region

M43.5X6 Other recurrent vertebral dislocation, lumbar region

M43.5X7 Other recurrent vertebral dislocation, lumbosacral region

M43.5X8 Other recurrent vertebral dislocation, sacral and sacrococcygeal region

M43.5X9 Other recurrent vertebral dislocation, site unspecified

M43.6 Torticollis

Excludes 1: congenital (sternomastoid) torticollis (Q68.0)

current injury - see Injury, of spine, by body region

ocular torticollis (R29.891)

psychogenic torticollis (F45.8)

spasmodic torticollis (G24.3)

torticollis due to birth injury (P15.2)

M43.8 Other specified deforming dorsopathies

Excludes 2: kyphosis and lordosis (M40.-)

scoliosis (M41.-)

M43.8X Other specified deforming dorsopathies

M43.8X1 Other specified deforming dorsopathies, occipito-atlanto-axial region

M43.8X2 Other specified deforming dorsopathies, cervical region

M43.8X3 Other specified deforming dorsopathies, cervicothoracic region

M43.8X4 Other specified deforming dorsopathies, thoracic region

M43.8X5 Other specified deforming dorsopathies, thoracolumbar region

M43.8X6 Other specified deforming dorsopathies, lumbar region

M43.8X7 Other specified deforming dorsopathies, lumbosacral region

M43.8X8 Other specified deforming dorsopathies, sacral and sacrococcygeal region

M43.8X9 Other specified deforming dorsopathies, site unspecified

M43.9 Deforming dorsopathy, unspecified

Curvature of spine NOS

SPONDYLOPATHIES (M45-M49)

M45 Ankylosing spondylitis

Rheumatoid arthritis of spine

Excludes 1: arthropathy in Reiter's disease (M02.3-)

juvenile (ankylosing) spondylitis (M08.1)

Excludes 2: Behcet's disease (M35.2)

M45.0 Ankylosing spondylitis of multiple sites in spine

M45.1 Ankylosing spondylitis of occipito-atlanto-axial region

M45.2 Ankylosing spondylitis of cervical region

M45.3 Ankylosing spondylitis of cervicothoracic region

M45.4 Ankylosing spondylitis of thoracic region

M45.5 Ankylosing spondylitis of thoracolumbar region

M45.6 Ankylosing spondylitis lumbar region

M45.7 Ankylosing spondylitis of lumbosacral region

M45.8 Ankylosing spondylitis sacral and sacrococcygeal region

M45.9 Ankylosing spondylitis of unspecified sites in spine

M46 Other inflammatory spondylopathies

M46.0 Spinal enthesopathy

Disorder of ligamentous or muscular attachments of spine

M46.00 Spinal enthesopathy, site unspecified

M46.01 Spinal enthesopathy, occipito-atlanto-axial region

M46.02 Spinal enthesopathy, cervical region

M46.03 Spinal enthesopathy, cervicothoracic region

M46.04 Spinal enthesopathy, thoracic region

M46.05 Spinal enthesopathy, thoracolumbar region

M46.06 Spinal enthesopathy, lumbar region

● New code   ▲ Revised code   ⑦ 7th digit required   ⊗ Placeholder required

M46.07　Spinal enthesopathy, lumbosacral region
M46.08　Spinal enthesopathy, sacral and sacrococcygeal region
M46.09　Spinal enthesopathy, multiple sites in spine
M46.1　Sacroiliitis, not elsewhere classified
M46.2　Osteomyelitis of vertebra
M46.20　Osteomyelitis of vertebra, site unspecified
M46.21　Osteomyelitis of vertebra, occipito-atlanto-axial region
M46.22　Osteomyelitis of vertebra, cervical region
M46.23　Osteomyelitis of vertebra, cervicothoracic region
M46.24　Osteomyelitis of vertebra, thoracic region
M46.25　Osteomyelitis of vertebra, thoracolumbar region
M46.26　Osteomyelitis of vertebra, lumbar region
M46.27　Osteomyelitis of vertebra, lumbosacral region
M46.28　Osteomyelitis of vertebra, sacral and sacrococcygeal region
M46.3　Infection of intervertebral disc (pyogenic)
Use additional code (B95-B97) to identify infectious agent.
M46.30　Infection of intervertebral disc (pyogenic), site unspecified
M46.31　Infection of intervertebral disc (pyogenic), occipito-atlanto-axial region
M46.32　Infection of intervertebral disc (pyogenic), cervical region
M46.33　Infection of intervertebral disc (pyogenic), cervicothoracic region
M46.34　Infection of intervertebral disc (pyogenic), thoracic region
M46.35　Infection of intervertebral disc (pyogenic), thoracolumbar region
M46.36　Infection of intervertebral disc (pyogenic), lumbar region
M46.37　Infection of intervertebral disc (pyogenic), lumbosacral region
M46.38　Infection of intervertebral disc (pyogenic), sacral and sacrococcygeal region
M46.39　Infection of intervertebral disc (pyogenic), multiple sites in spine
M46.4　Discitis, unspecified
M46.40　Discitis, unspecified, site unspecified
M46.41　Discitis, unspecified, occipito-atlanto-axial region
M46.42　Discitis, unspecified, cervical region
M46.43　Discitis, unspecified, cervicothoracic region
M46.44　Discitis, unspecified, thoracic region
M46.45　Discitis, unspecified, thoracolumbar region
M46.46　Discitis, unspecified, lumbar region
M46.47　Discitis, unspecified, lumbosacral region
M46.48　Discitis, unspecified, sacral and sacrococcygeal region
M46.49　Discitis, unspecified, multiple sites in spine
M46.5　Other infective spondylopathies
M46.50　Other infective spondylopathies, site unspecified
M46.51　Other infective spondylopathies, occipito-atlanto-axial region
M46.52　Other infective spondylopathies, cervical region
M46.53　Other infective spondylopathies, cervicothoracic region
M46.54　Other infective spondylopathies, thoracic region

M46.55　Other infective spondylopathies, thoracolumbar region
M46.56　Other infective spondylopathies, lumbar region
M46.57　Other infective spondylopathies, lumbosacral region
M46.58　Other infective spondylopathies, sacral and sacrococcygeal region
M46.59　Other infective spondylopathies, multiple sites in spine
M46.8　Other specified inflammatory spondylopathies
M46.80　Other specified inflammatory spondylopathies, site unspecified
M46.81　Other specified inflammatory spondylopathies, occipito-atlanto-axial region
M46.82　Other specified inflammatory spondylopathies, cervical region
M46.83　Other specified inflammatory spondylopathies, cervicothoracic region
M46.84　Other specified inflammatory spondylopathies, thoracic region
M46.85　Other specified inflammatory spondylopathies, thoracolumbar region
M46.86　Other specified inflammatory spondylopathies, lumbar region
M46.87　Other specified inflammatory spondylopathies, lumbosacral region
M46.88　Other specified inflammatory spondylopathies, sacral and sacrococcygeal region
M46.89　Other specified inflammatory spondylopathies, multiple sites in spine
M46.9　Unspecified inflammatory spondylopathy
M46.90　Unspecified inflammatory spondylopathy, site unspecified
M46.91　Unspecified inflammatory spondylopathy, occipito-atlanto-axial region
M46.92　Unspecified inflammatory spondylopathy, cervical region
M46.93　Unspecified inflammatory spondylopathy, cervicothoracic region
M46.94　Unspecified inflammatory spondylopathy, thoracic region
M46.95　Unspecified inflammatory spondylopathy, thoracolumbar region
M46.96　Unspecified inflammatory spondylopathy, lumbar region
M46.97　Unspecified inflammatory spondylopathy, lumbosacral region
M46.98　Unspecified inflammatory spondylopathy, sacral and sacrococcygeal region
M46.99　Unspecified inflammatory spondylopathy, multiple sites in spine
M47　Spondylosis
Includes: arthrosis or osteoarthritis of spine
degeneration of facet joints
M47.0　Anterior spinal and vertebral artery compression syndromes
M47.01　Anterior spinal artery compression syndromes
M47.011　Anterior spinal artery compression syndromes, occipito-atlanto-axial region

M47.012 Anterior spinal artery compression syndromes, cervical region

M47.013 Anterior spinal artery compression syndromes, cervicothoracic region

M47.014 Anterior spinal artery compression syndromes, thoracic region

M47.015 Anterior spinal artery compression syndromes, thoracolumbar region

M47.016 Anterior spinal artery compression syndromes, lumbar region

M47.019 Anterior spinal artery compression syndromes, site unspecified

M47.02 Vertebral artery compression syndromes

M47.021 Vertebral artery compression syndromes, occipito-atlanto-axial region

M47.022 Vertebral artery compression syndromes, cervical region

M47.029 Vertebral artery compression syndromes, site unspecified

M47.1 Other spondylosis with myelopathy
Spondylogenic compression of spinal cord
Excludes 1: vertebral subluxation (M43.3-M43.59)

M47.10 Other spondylosis with myelopathy, site unspecified

M47.11 Other spondylosis with myelopathy, occipito-atlanto-axial region

M47.12 Other spondylosis with myelopathy, cervical region

M47.13 Other spondylosis with myelopathy, cervicothoracic region

M47.14 Other spondylosis with myelopathy, thoracic region

M47.15 Other spondylosis with myelopathy, thoracolumbar region

M47.16 Other spondylosis with myelopathy, lumbar region

M47.17 Other spondylosis with myelopathy, lumbosacral region (deleted 2014)

M47.18 Other spondylosis with myelopathy, sacral and sacrococcygeal region (deleted 2014)

M47.2 Other spondylosis with radiculopathy

M47.20 Other spondylosis with radiculopathy, site unspecified

M47.21 Other spondylosis with radiculopathy, occipito-atlanto-axial region

M47.22 Other spondylosis with radiculopathy, cervical region

M47.23 Other spondylosis with radiculopathy, cervicothoracic region

M47.24 Other spondylosis with radiculopathy, thoracic region

M47.25 Other spondylosis with radiculopathy, thoracolumbar region

M47.26 Other spondylosis with radiculopathy, lumbar region

M47.27 Other spondylosis with radiculopathy, lumbosacral region

M47.28 Other spondylosis with radiculopathy, sacral and sacrococcygeal region

M47.8 Other spondylosis

M47.81 Spondylosis without myelopathy or radiculopathy

M47.811 Spondylosis without myelopathy or radiculopathy, occipito-atlanto-axial region

M47.812 Spondylosis without myelopathy or radiculopathy, cervical region

M47.813 Spondylosis without myelopathy or radiculopathy, cervicothoracic region

M47.814 Spondylosis without myelopathy or radiculopathy, thoracic region

M47.815 Spondylosis without myelopathy or radiculopathy, thoracolumbar region

M47.816 Spondylosis without myelopathy or radiculopathy, lumbar region

M47.817 Spondylosis without myelopathy or radiculopathy, lumbosacral region

M47.818 Spondylosis without myelopathy or radiculopathy, sacral and sacrococcygeal region

M47.819 Spondylosis without myelopathy or radiculopathy, site unspecified

M47.89 Other spondylosis

M47.891 Other spondylosis, occipito-atlanto-axial region

M47.892 Other spondylosis, cervical region

M47.893 Other spondylosis, cervicothoracic region

M47.894 Other spondylosis, thoracic region

M47.895 Other spondylosis, thoracolumbar region

M47.896 Other spondylosis, lumbar region

M47.897 Other spondylosis, lumbosacral region

M47.898 Other spondylosis, sacral and sacrococcygeal region

M47.899 Other spondylosis, site unspecified

M47.9 Spondylosis, unspecified

M48 Other spondylopathies

M48.0 Spinal stenosis
Caudal stenosis

M48.00 Spinal stenosis, site unspecified

M48.01 Spinal stenosis, occipito-atlanto-axial region

M48.02 Spinal stenosis, cervical region

M48.03 Spinal stenosis, cervicothoracic region

M48.04 Spinal stenosis, thoracic region

M48.05 Spinal stenosis, thoracolumbar region

M48.06 Spinal stenosis, lumbar region

M48.07 Spinal stenosis, lumbosacral region

M48.08 Spinal stenosis, sacral and sacrococcygeal region

M48.1 Ankylosing hyperostosis [Forestier]
Diffuse idiopathic skeletal hyperostosis [DISH]

M48.10 Ankylosing hyperostosis [Forestier], site unspecified

M48.11 Ankylosing hyperostosis [Forestier], occipito-atlanto-axial region

M48.12 Ankylosing hyperostosis [Forestier], cervical region

● New code   ▲ Revised code   ⑦ 7th digit required   ⊗ Placeholder required

M48.13 Ankylosing hyperostosis [Forestier], cervicothoracic region

M48.14 Ankylosing hyperostosis [Forestier], thoracic region

M48.15 Ankylosing hyperostosis [Forestier], thoracolumbar region

M48.16 Ankylosing hyperostosis [Forestier], lumbar region

M48.17 Ankylosing hyperostosis [Forestier], lumbosacral region

M48.18 Ankylosing hyperostosis [Forestier], sacral and sacrococcygeal region

M48.19 Ankylosing hyperostosis [Forestier], multiple sites in spine

M48.2 Kissing spine

M48.20 Kissing spine, site unspecified

M48.21 Kissing spine, occipito-atlanto-axial region

M48.22 Kissing spine, cervical region

M48.23 Kissing spine, cervicothoracic region

M48.24 Kissing spine, thoracic region

M48.25 Kissing spine, thoracolumbar region

M48.26 Kissing spine, lumbar region

M48.27 Kissing spine, lumbosacral region

M48.3 Traumatic spondylopathy

M48.30 Traumatic spondylopathy, site unspecified

M48.31 Traumatic spondylopathy, occipito-atlanto-axial region

M48.32 Traumatic spondylopathy, cervical region

M48.33 Traumatic spondylopathy, cervicothoracic region

M48.34 Traumatic spondylopathy, thoracic region

M48.35 Traumatic spondylopathy, thoracolumbar region

M48.36 Traumatic spondylopathy, lumbar region

M48.37 Traumatic spondylopathy, lumbosacral region

M48.38 Traumatic spondylopathy, sacral and sacrococcygeal region

M48.4 Fatigue fracture of vertebra
Stress fracture of vertebra
Excludes 1: pathological fracture NOS (M84.4-)
pathological fracture of vertebra due to neoplasm (M84.58)
pathological fracture of vertebra due to other diagnosis (M84.68)
pathological fracture of vertebra due to osteoporosis (M80.-)
traumatic fracture of vertebrae (S12.0-S12.3-, S22.0-, S32.0-)
The appropriate 7th character is to be added to each code from subcategory M48.4:
A - initial encounter for fracture
D - subsequent encounter for fracture with routine healing
G - subsequent encounter for fracture with delayed healing
S - sequela of fracture

⊗⑦**M48.40** Fatigue fracture of vertebra, site unspecified

⊗⑦**M48.41** Fatigue fracture of vertebra, occipito-atlanto-axial region

⊗⑦**M48.42** Fatigue fracture of vertebra, cervical region

⊗⑦**M48.43** Fatigue fracture of vertebra, cervicothoracic region

⊗⑦**M48.44** Fatigue fracture of vertebra, thoracic region

⊗⑦**M48.45** Fatigue fracture of vertebra, thoracolumbar region

⊗⑦**M48.46** Fatigue fracture of vertebra, lumbar region

⊗⑦**M48.47** Fatigue fracture of vertebra, lumbosacral region

⊗⑦**M48.48** Fatigue fracture of vertebra, sacral and sacrococcygeal region

M48.5 Collapsed vertebra, not elsewhere classified
Collapsed vertebra NOS
Wedging of vertebra NOS
Excludes 1: current injury - see Injury of spine, by body region
fatigue fracture of vertebra (M48.4)
pathological fracture of vertebra due to other diagnosis (M84.68)
pathological fracture of vertebra due to osteoporosis (M80.-)
pathological fracture NOS (M84.4-)
stress fracture of vertebra (M48.4-)
traumatic fracture of vertebra (S12.-, S22.-, S32.-)
The appropriate 7th character is to be added to each code from subcategory M48.5:
A - initial encounter for fracture
D - subsequent encounter for fracture with routine healing
G - subsequent encounter for fracture with delayed healing
S - sequela of fracture

⊗⑦**M48.50** Collapsed vertebra, not elsewhere classified, site unspecified

⊗⑦**M48.51** Collapsed vertebra, not elsewhere classified, occipito-atlanto-axial region

⊗⑦**M48.52** Collapsed vertebra, not elsewhere classified, cervical region

⊗⑦**M48.53** Collapsed vertebra, not elsewhere classified, cervicothoracic region

⊗⑦**M48.54** Collapsed vertebra, not elsewhere classified, thoracic region

⊗⑦**M48.55** Collapsed vertebra, not elsewhere classified, thoracolumbar region

⊗⑦**M48.56** Collapsed vertebra, not elsewhere classified, lumbar region

⊗⑦**M48.57** Collapsed vertebra, not elsewhere classified, lumbosacral region

⊗⑦**M48.58** Collapsed vertebra, not elsewhere classified, sacral and sacrococcygeal region

M48.8 Other specified spondylopathies
Ossification of posterior longitudinal ligament
M48.8X Other specified spondylopathies

⑦**M48.8X1** Other specified spondylopathies, occipito-atlanto-axial region

⑦**M48.8X2** Other specified spondylopathies, cervical region

⑦**M48.8X3** Other specified spondylopathies, cervicothoracic region

⑦**M48.8X4** Other specified spondylopathies, thoracic region

⑦**M48.8X5** Other specified spondylopathies, thoracolumbar region

⑦**M48.8X6** Other specified spondylopathies, lumbar region

⑦ **M48.8X7** Other specified spondylopathies, lumbosacral region

⑦ **M48.8X8** Other specified spondylopathies, sacral and sacrococcygeal region

⑦ **M48.8X9** Other specified spondylopathies, site unspecified

M48.9 Spondylopathy, unspecified

M49 Spondylopathies in diseases classified elsewhere

Includes: curvature of spine in diseases classified elsewhere
deformity of spine in diseases classified elsewhere
kyphosis in diseases classified elsewhere
scoliosis in diseases classified elsewhere
spondylopathy in diseases classified elsewhere

Excludes 1: curvature of spine in tuberculosis [Pott's] (A18.01)
enteropathic arthropathies (M07.-)
neuropathic spondylopathy (in):
nonsyphilitic NEC (G98.0)
syringomyelia (G95.0)
tabes dorsalis (A52.11)
spondylitis (in):
gonococcal (A54.41)
syphilis (acquired) (A52.77)
neuropathic [tabes dorsalis] (A52.11)
tuberculosis (A18.01)
typhoid fever (A01.05)

Code first underlying disease, such as:
brucellosis (A23.-)
Charcot-Marie-Tooth disease (G60.0)
enterobacterial infections (A01-A04)
osteitis fibrosa cystica (E21.0)

M49.8 Spondylopathy in diseases classified elsewhere

M49.80 Spondylopathy in diseases classified elsewhere, site unspecified

M49.81 Spondylopathy in diseases classified elsewhere, occipito-atlanto-axial region

M49.82 Spondylopathy in diseases classified elsewhere, cervical region

M49.83 Spondylopathy in diseases classified elsewhere, cervicothoracic region

M49.84 Spondylopathy in diseases classified elsewhere, thoracic region

M49.85 Spondylopathy in diseases classified elsewhere, thoracolumbar region

M49.86 Spondylopathy in diseases classified elsewhere, lumbar region

M49.87 Spondylopathy in diseases classified elsewhere, lumbosacral region

M49.88 Spondylopathy in diseases classified elsewhere, sacral and sacrococcygeal region

M49.89 Spondylopathy in diseases classified elsewhere, multiple sites in spine

OTHER DORSOPATHIES (M50-M54)

Excludes 1: current injury - see injury of spine by body region
discitis NOS (M46.4-)

M50 Cervical disc disorders

Note: code to the most superior level of disorder

Includes: cervicothoracic disc disorders with cervicalgia
cervicothoracic disc disorders

M50.0 Cervical disc disorder with myelopathy

M50.00 Cervical disc disorder with myelopathy, unspecified cervical region

▲ **M50.01** Cervical disc disorder with myelopathy, high cervical region

M50.02 Cervical disc disorder with myelopathy, mid-cervical region

M50.03 Cervical disc disorder with myelopathy, cervicothoracic region

M50.1 Cervical disc disorder with radiculopathy

Excludes 2: brachial radiculitis NOS (M54.13)

M50.10 Cervical disc disorder with radiculopathy, unspecified cervical region

▲ **M50.11** Cervical disc disorder with radiculopathy, high cervical region

M50.12 Cervical disc disorder with radiculopathy, mid-cervical region

M50.13 Cervical disc disorder with radiculopathy, cervicothoracic region

M50.2 Other cervical disc displacement

M50.20 Other cervical disc displacement, unspecified cervical region

▲ **M50.21** Other cervical disc displacement, high cervical region

M50.22 Other cervical disc displacement, mid-cervical region

M50.23 Other cervical disc displacement, cervicothoracic region

M50.3 Other cervical disc degeneration

M50.30 Other cervical disc degeneration, unspecified cervical region

▲ **M50.31** Other cervical disc degeneration, high cervical region

M50.32 Other cervical disc degeneration, region mid-cervical

M50.33 Other cervical disc degeneration, cervicothoracic region

M50.8 Other cervical disc disorders

M50.80 Other cervical disc disorders, unspecified cervical region

▲ **M50.81** Other cervical disc disorders, high cervical region

M50.82 Other cervical disc disorders, mid-cervical region

M50.83 Other cervical disc disorders, cervicothoracic region

M50.9 Cervical disc disorder, unspecified

M50.90 Cervical disc disorder, unspecified, unspecified cervical region

▲ **M50.91** Cervical disc disorder, unspecified, high cervical region

M50.92 Cervical disc disorder, unspecified, mid-cervical region

M50.93 Cervical disc disorder, unspecified, cervicothoracic region

M51 Thoracic, thoracolumbar, and lumbosacral intervertebral disc disorders

Excludes 2: cervical and cervicothoracic disc disorders (M50.-)
sacral and sacrococcygeal disorders (M53.3)

M51.0 Thoracic, thoracolumbar and lumbosacral intervertebral disc disorders with myelopathy

M51.04 Intervertebral disc disorders with myelopathy, thoracic region

M51.05 Intervertebral disc disorders with myelopathy, thoracolumbar region

M51.06 Intervertebral disc disorders with myelopathy, lumbar region

M51.07 ~~Intervertebral disc disorders with myelopathy, lumbosacral region~~ (deleted 2014)

M51.1 Thoracic, thoracolumbar and lumbosacral intervertebral disc disorders with radiculopathy
Sciatica due to intervertebral disc disorder
Excludes 1: lumbar radiculitis NOS (M54.16)
sciatica NOS (M54.3)

M51.14 Intervertebral disc disorders with radiculopathy, thoracic region

M51.15 Intervertebral disc disorders with radiculopathy, thoracolumbar region

M51.16 Intervertebral disc disorders with radiculopathy, lumbar region

M51.17 Intervertebral disc disorders with radiculopathy, lumbosacral region

M51.2 Other thoracic, thoracolumbar and lumbosacral intervertebral disc displacement
Lumbago due to displacement of intervertebral disc

M51.24 Other intervertebral disc displacement, thoracic region

M51.25 Other intervertebral disc displacement, thoracolumbar region

M51.26 Other intervertebral disc displacement, lumbar region

M51.27 Other intervertebral disc displacement, lumbosacral region

M51.3 Other thoracic, thoracolumbar and lumbosacral intervertebral disc degeneration

M51.34 Other intervertebral disc degeneration, thoracic region

M51.35 Other intervertebral disc degeneration, thoracolumbar region

M51.36 Other intervertebral disc degeneration, lumbar region

M51.37 Other intervertebral disc degeneration, lumbosacral region

M51.4 Schmorl's nodes

M51.44 Schmorl's nodes, thoracic region

M51.45 Schmorl's nodes, thoracolumbar region

M51.46 Schmorl's nodes, lumbar region

M51.47 Schmorl's nodes, lumbosacral region

M51.8 Other thoracic, thoracolumbar and lumbosacral intervertebral disc disorders

M51.84 Other intervertebral disc disorders, thoracic region

M51.85 Other intervertebral disc disorders, thoracolumbar region

M51.86 Other intervertebral disc disorders, lumbar region

M51.87 Other intervertebral disc disorders, lumbosacral region

M51.9 Unspecified thoracic, thoracolumbar and lumbosacral intervertebral disc disorder

M53 Other and unspecified dorsopathies, not elsewhere classified

M53.0 Cervicocranial syndrome
Posterior cervical sympathetic syndrome

M53.1 Cervicobrachial syndrome
Excludes 2: cervical disc disorder (M50.-)
thoracic outlet syndrome (G54.0)

M53.2 Spinal instabilities

M53.2X Spinal instabilities

M53.2X1 Spinal instabilities, occipito-atlanto-axial region

M53.2X2 Spinal instabilities, cervical region

M53.2X3 Spinal instabilities, cervicothoracic region

M53.2X4 Spinal instabilities, thoracic region

M53.2X5 Spinal instabilities, thoracolumbar region

M53.2X6 Spinal instabilities, lumbar region

M53.2X7 Spinal instabilities, lumbosacral region

M53.2X8 Spinal instabilities, sacral and sacrococcygeal region

M53.2X9 Spinal instabilities, site unspecified

M53.3 Sacrococcygeal disorders, not elsewhere classified
Coccygodynia

M53.8 Other specified dorsopathies

M53.80 Other specified dorsopathies, site unspecified

M53.81 Other specified dorsopathies, occipito-atlanto-axial region

M53.82 Other specified dorsopathies, cervical region

M53.83 Other specified dorsopathies, cervicothoracic region

M53.84 Other specified dorsopathies, thoracic region

M53.85 Other specified dorsopathies, thoracolumbar region

M53.86 Other specified dorsopathies, lumbar region

M53.87 Other specified dorsopathies, lumbosacral region

M53.88 Other specified dorsopathies, sacral and sacrococcygeal region

M53.9 Dorsopathy, unspecified

M54 Dorsalgia
Excludes 1: psychogenic dorsalgia (F45.41)

M54.0 Panniculitis affecting regions of neck and back
Excludes 1: lupus panniculitis (L93.2)
panniculitis NOS (M79.3)
relapsing [Weber-Christian] panniculitis (M35.6)

M54.00 Panniculitis affecting regions of neck and back, site unspecified

M54.01 Panniculitis affecting regions of neck and back, occipito-atlanto-axial region

M54.02 Panniculitis affecting regions of neck and back, cervical region

M54.03 Panniculitis affecting regions of neck and back, cervicothoracic region

M54.04 Panniculitis affecting regions of neck and back, thoracic region

M54.05 Panniculitis affecting regions of neck and back, thoracolumbar region

M54.06 Panniculitis affecting regions of neck and back, lumbar region

M54.07 Panniculitis affecting regions of neck and back, lumbosacral region

M54.08 Panniculitis affecting regions of neck and back, sacral and sacrococcygeal region

M54.09 Panniculitis affecting regions, neck and back, multiple sites in spine

M54.1 Radiculopathy

Brachial neuritis or radiculitis NOS

lumbar neuritis or radiculitis NOS

Lumbosacral neuritis or radiculitis NOS

thoracic neuritis or radiculitis NOS

Radiculitis NOS

Excludes 1: neuralgia and neuritis NOS (M79.2)

radiculopathy with cervical disc disorder (M50.1)

radiculopathy with lumbar and other intervertebral disc disorder (M51.1-)

radiculopathy with spondylosis (M47.2-)

M54.10 Radiculopathy, site unspecified

M54.11 Radiculopathy, occipito-atlanto-axial region

M54.12 Radiculopathy, cervical region

M54.13 Radiculopathy, cervicothoracic region

M54.14 Radiculopathy, thoracic region

M54.15 Radiculopathy, thoracolumbar region

M54.16 Radiculopathy, lumbar region

M54.17 Radiculopathy, lumbosacral region

M54.18 Radiculopathy, sacral and sacrococcygeal region

M54.2 Cervicalgia

Excludes 1: cervicalgia due to intervertebral cervical disc disorder (M50.-)

M54.3 Sciatica

Excludes 1: lesion of sciatic nerve (G57.0)

sciatica due to intervertebral disc disorder (M51.1-)

sciatica with lumbago (M54.4-)

M54.30 Sciatica, unspecified side

M54.31 Sciatica, right side

M54.32 Sciatica, left side

M54.4 Lumbago with sciatica

Excludes 1: lumbago with sciatica due to intervertebral disc disorder (M51.1-)

M54.40 Lumbago with sciatica, unspecified side

M54.41 Lumbago with sciatica, right side

M54.42 Lumbago with sciatica, left side

M54.5 Low back pain

Loin pain

Lumbago NOS

Excludes 1: low back strain S39.012

lumbago due to intervertebral disc displacement (M51.2-)

lumbago with sciatica (M54.4-)

M54.6 Pain in thoracic spine

Excludes 1: pain in thoracic spine due to intervertebral disc disorder (M51.-)

M54.8 Other dorsalgia

Excludes 1: dorsalgia in thoracic region (M54.6)

low back pain (M54.5)

M54.81 Occipital neuralgia

M54.89 Other dorsalgia

M54.9 Dorsalgia, unspecified

Backache NOS

Back pain NOS

SOFT TISSUE DISORDERS (M60-M79)

DISORDERS OF MUSCLES (M60-M63)

Excludes 1: dermatopolymyositis (M33.-)

muscular dystrophies and myopathies (G71-G72)

myopathy in:

amyloidosis (E85-)

polyarteritis nodosa (M30.0)

rheumatoid arthritis (M05.32)

scleroderma (M34.-)

Sjogren's syndrome (M35.03)

systemic lupus erythematosus (M32.-)

M60 Myositis

Excludes 2: inclusion body myositis [IBM] (G72.41)

M60.0 Infective myositis

Tropical pyomyositis

Use additional code (B95-B97) to identify infectious agent

M60.00 Infective myositis, unspecified site

M60.000 Infective myositis, unspecified right arm

Infective myositis, right upper limb NOS

M60.001 Infective myositis, unspecified left arm

Infective myositis, left upper limb NOS

M60.002 Infective myositis, unspecified arm

Infective myositis, upper limb NOS

M60.003 Infective myositis, unspecified right leg

Infective myositis, right lower limb NOS

M60.004 Infective myositis, unspecified left leg

Infective myositis, left lower limb NOS

M60.005 Infective myositis, unspecified leg

Infective myositis, lower limb NOS

M60.009 Infective myositis, unspecified site

M60.01 Infective myositis, shoulder

M60.011 Infective myositis, right shoulder

M60.012 Infective myositis, left shoulder

M60.019 Infective myositis, unspecified shoulder

M60.02 Infective myositis, upper arm

M60.021 Infective myositis, right upper arm

M60.022 Infective myositis, left upper arm

M60.029 Infective myositis, unspecified upper arm

M60.03 Infective myositis, forearm

M60.031 Infective myositis, right forearm

M60.032 Infective myositis, left forearm

M60.039 Infective myositis, unspecified forearm

M60.04 Infective myositis, hand and fingers

M60.041 Infective myositis, right hand

M60.042 Infective myositis, left hand

M60.043 Infective myositis, unspecified hand

M60.044 Infective myositis, right finger(s)

M60.045 Infective myositis, left finger(s)

M60.046 Infective myositis, unspecified finger(s)

M60.05 Infective myositis, thigh
- **M60.051** Infective myositis, right thigh
- **M60.052** Infective myositis, left thigh
- **M60.059** Infective myositis, unspecified thigh

M60.06 Infective myositis, lower leg
- **M60.061** Infective myositis, right lower leg
- **M60.062** Infective myositis, left lower leg
- **M60.069** Infective myositis, unspecified lower leg

M60.07 Infective myositis, ankle, foot and toes
- **M60.070** Infective myositis, right ankle
- **M60.071** Infective myositis, left ankle
- **M60.072** Infective myositis, unspecified ankle
- **M60.073** Infective myositis, right foot
- **M60.074** Infective myositis, left foot
- **M60.075** Infective myositis, unspecified foot
- **M60.076** Infective myositis, right toe(s)
- **M60.077** Infective myositis, left toe(s)
- **M60.078** Infective myositis, unspecified toe(s)

M60.08 Infective myositis, other site

M60.09 Infective myositis, multiple sites

M60.1 Interstitial myositis

M60.10 Interstitial myositis of unspecified site

M60.11 Interstitial myositis, shoulder
- **M60.111** Interstitial myositis, right shoulder
- **M60.112** Interstitial myositis, left shoulder
- **M60.119** Interstitial myositis, unspecified shoulder

M60.12 Interstitial myositis, upper arm
- **M60.121** Interstitial myositis, right upper arm
- **M60.122** Interstitial myositis, left upper arm
- **M60.129** Interstitial myositis, unspecified upper arm

M60.13 Interstitial myositis, forearm
- **M60.131** Interstitial myositis, right forearm
- **M60.132** Interstitial myositis, left forearm
- **M60.139** Interstitial myositis, unspecified forearm

M60.14 Interstitial myositis, hand
- **M60.141** Interstitial myositis, right hand
- **M60.142** Interstitial myositis, left hand
- **M60.149** Interstitial myositis, unspecified hand

M60.15 Interstitial myositis, thigh
- **M60.151** Interstitial myositis, right thigh
- **M60.152** Interstitial myositis, left thigh
- **M60.159** Interstitial myositis, unspecified thigh

M60.16 Interstitial myositis, lower leg
- **M60.161** Interstitial myositis, right lower leg
- **M60.162** Interstitial myositis, left lower leg
- **M60.169** Interstitial myositis, unspecified lower leg

M60.17 Interstitial myositis, ankle and foot
- **M60.171** Interstitial myositis, right ankle and foot

M60.172 Interstitial myositis, left ankle and foot

M60.179 Interstitial myositis, unspecified ankle and foot

M60.18 Interstitial myositis, other site

M60.19 Interstitial myositis, multiple sites

M60.2 Foreign body granuloma of soft tissue, not elsewhere classified

Use additional code to identify the type of retained foreign body (Z18.-)

Excludes 1: foreign body granuloma of skin and subcutaneous tissue (L92.3)

M60.20 Foreign body granuloma of soft tissue, not elsewhere classified, unspecified site

M60.21 Foreign body granuloma of soft tissue, not elsewhere classified, shoulder
- **M60.211** Foreign body granuloma of soft tissue, not elsewhere classified, right shoulder
- **M60.212** Foreign body granuloma of soft tissue, not elsewhere classified, left shoulder
- **M60.219** Foreign body granuloma of soft tissue, not elsewhere classified, unspecified shoulder

M60.22 Foreign body granuloma of soft tissue, not elsewhere classified, upper arm
- **M60.221** Foreign body granuloma of soft tissue, not elsewhere classified, right upper arm
- **M60.222** Foreign body granuloma of soft tissue, not elsewhere classified, left upper arm
- **M60.229** Foreign body granuloma of soft tissue, not elsewhere classified, unspecified upper arm

M60.23 Foreign body granuloma of soft tissue, not elsewhere classified, forearm
- **M60.231** Foreign body granuloma of soft tissue, not elsewhere classified, right forearm
- **M60.232** Foreign body granuloma of soft tissue, not elsewhere classified, left forearm
- **M60.239** Foreign body granuloma of soft tissue, not elsewhere classified, unspecified forearm

M60.24 Foreign body granuloma of soft tissue, not elsewhere classified, hand
- **M60.241** Foreign body granuloma of soft tissue, not elsewhere classified, right hand
- **M60.242** Foreign body granuloma of soft tissue, not elsewhere classified, left hand
- **M60.249** Foreign body granuloma of soft tissue, not elsewhere classified, unspecified hand

M60.25 Foreign body granuloma of soft tissue, not elsewhere classified, thigh

M60.251 Foreign body granuloma of soft tissue, not elsewhere classified, right thigh

M60.252 Foreign body granuloma of soft tissue, not elsewhere classified, left thigh

M60.259 Foreign body granuloma of soft tissue, not elsewhere classified, unspecified thigh

M60.26 Foreign body granuloma of soft tissue, not elsewhere classified, lower leg

M60.261 Foreign body granuloma of soft tissue, not elsewhere classified, right lower leg

M60.262 Foreign body granuloma of soft tissue, not elsewhere classified, left lower leg

M60.269 Foreign body granuloma of soft tissue, not elsewhere classified, unspecified lower leg

M60.27 Foreign body granuloma of soft tissue, not elsewhere classified, ankle and foot

M60.271 Foreign body granuloma of soft tissue, not elsewhere classified, right ankle and foot

M60.272 Foreign body granuloma of soft tissue, not elsewhere classified, left ankle and foot

M60.279 Foreign body granuloma of soft tissue, not elsewhere classified, unspecified ankle and foot

M60.28 Foreign body granuloma of soft tissue, not elsewhere classified, other site

M60.8 Other myositis

M60.80 Other myositis, unspecified site

M60.81 Other myositis shoulder

M60.811 Other myositis, right shoulder

M60.812 Other myositis, left shoulder

M60.819 Other myositis, unspecified shoulder

M60.82 Other myositis, upper arm

M60.821 Other myositis, right upper arm

M60.822 Other myositis, left upper arm

M60.829 Other myositis, unspecified upper arm

M60.83 Other myositis, forearm

M60.831 Other myositis, right forearm

M60.832 Other myositis, left forearm

M60.839 Other myositis, unspecified forearm

M60.84 Other myositis, hand

M60.841 Other myositis, right hand

M60.842 Other myositis, left hand

M60.849 Other myositis, unspecified hand

M60.85 Other myositis, thigh

M60.851 Other myositis, right thigh

M60.852 Other myositis, left thigh

M60.859 Other myositis, unspecified thigh

M60.86 Other myositis, lower leg

M60.861 Other myositis, right lower leg

M60.862 Other myositis, left lower leg

M60.869 Other myositis, unspecified lower leg

M60.87 Other myositis, ankle and foot

M60.871 Other myositis, right ankle and foot

M60.872 Other myositis, left ankle and foot

M60.879 Other myositis, unspecified ankle and foot

M60.88 Other myositis, other site

M60.89 Other myositis, multiple sites

M60.9 Myositis, unspecified

M61 Calcification and ossification of muscle

M61.0 Myositis ossificans traumatica

M61.00 Myositis ossificans traumatica, unspecified site

M61.01 Myositis ossificans traumatica, shoulder

M61.011 Myositis ossificans traumatica, right shoulder

M61.012 Myositis ossificans traumatica, left shoulder

M61.019 Myositis ossificans traumatica, unspecified shoulder

M61.02 Myositis ossificans traumatica, upper arm

M61.021 Myositis ossificans traumatica, right upper arm

M61.022 Myositis ossificans traumatica, left upper arm

M61.029 Myositis ossificans traumatica, unspecified upper arm

M61.03 Myositis ossificans traumatica, forearm

M61.031 Myositis ossificans traumatica, right forearm

M61.032 Myositis ossificans traumatica, left forearm

M61.039 Myositis ossificans traumatica, unspecified forearm

M61.04 Myositis ossificans traumatica, hand

M61.041 Myositis ossificans traumatica, right hand

M61.042 Myositis ossificans traumatica, left hand

M61.049 Myositis ossificans traumatica, unspecified hand

M61.05 Myositis ossificans traumatica, thigh

M61.051 Myositis ossificans traumatica, right thigh

M61.052 Myositis ossificans traumatica, left thigh

M61.059 Myositis ossificans traumatica, unspecified thigh

M61.06 Myositis ossificans traumatica, lower leg

M61.061 Myositis ossificans traumatica, right lower leg

M61.062 Myositis ossificans traumatica, left lower leg

M61.069 Myositis ossificans traumatica, unspecified lower leg

M61.07 Myositis ossificans traumatica, ankle and foot

M61.071 Myositis ossificans traumatica, right ankle and foot

M61.072 Myositis ossificans traumatica, left ankle and foot

● New code   ▲ Revised code   ⑦ 7ᵗʰ digit required   ⊗ Placeholder required

M61.079 Myositis ossificans traumatica, unspecified ankle and foot

M61.08 Myositis ossificans traumatica, other site

M61.09 Myositis ossificans traumatica, multiple sites

M61.1 Myositis ossificans progressiva

Fibrodysplasia ossificans progressiva

M61.10 Myositis ossificans progressiva, unspecified site

M61.11 Myositis ossificans progressiva, shoulder

M61.111 Myositis ossificans progressiva, right shoulder

M61.112 Myositis ossificans progressiva, left shoulder

M61.119 Myositis ossificans progressiva, unspecified shoulder

M61.12 Myositis ossificans progressiva, upper arm

M61.121 Myositis ossificans progressiva, right upper arm

M61.122 Myositis ossificans progressiva, left upper arm

M61.129 Myositis ossificans progressiva, unspecified arm

M61.13 Myositis ossificans progressiva, forearm

M61.131 Myositis ossificans progressiva, right forearm

M61.132 Myositis ossificans progressiva, left forearm

M61.139 Myositis ossificans progressiva, unspecified forearm

M61.14 Myositis ossificans progressiva, hand and finger(s)

M61.141 Myositis ossificans progressiva, right hand

M61.142 Myositis ossificans progressiva, left hand

M61.143 Myositis ossificans progressiva, unspecified hand

M61.144 Myositis ossificans progressiva, right finger(s)

M61.145 Myositis ossificans progressiva, left finger(s)

M61.146 Myositis ossificans progressiva, unspecified finger(s)

M61.15 Myositis ossificans progressiva, thigh

M61.151 Myositis ossificans progressiva, right thigh

M61.152 Myositis ossificans progressiva, left thigh

M61.159 Myositis ossificans progressiva, unspecified thigh

M61.16 Myositis ossificans progressiva, lower leg

M61.161 Myositis ossificans progressiva, right lower leg

M61.162 Myositis ossificans progressiva, left lower leg

M61.169 Myositis ossificans progressiva, unspecified lower leg

M61.17 Myositis ossificans progressiva, ankle, foot and toe(s)

M61.171 Myositis ossificans progressiva, right ankle

M61.172 Myositis ossificans progressiva, left ankle

M61.173 Myositis ossificans progressiva, unspecified ankle

M61.174 Myositis ossificans progressiva, right foot

M61.175 Myositis ossificans progressiva, left foot

M61.176 Myositis ossificans progressiva, unspecified foot

M61.177 Myositis ossificans progressiva, right toe(s)

M61.178 Myositis ossificans progressiva, left toe(s)

M61.179 Myositis ossificans progressiva, unspecified toe(s)

M61.18 Myositis ossificans progressiva, other site

M61.19 Myositis ossificans progressiva, multiple sites

M61.2 Paralytic calcification and ossification of muscle

Myositis ossificans associated with quadriplegia or paraplegia

M61.20 Paralytic calcification and ossification of muscle, unspecified site

M61.21 Paralytic calcification and ossification of muscle, shoulder

M61.211 Paralytic calcification and ossification of muscle, right shoulder

M61.212 Paralytic calcification and ossification of muscle, left shoulder

M61.219 Paralytic calcification and ossification of muscle, unspecified shoulder

M61.22 Paralytic calcification and ossification of muscle, upper arm

M61.221 Paralytic calcification and ossification of muscle, right upper arm

M61.222 Paralytic calcification and ossification of muscle, left upper arm

M61.229 Paralytic calcification and ossification of muscle, unspecified upper arm

M61.23 Paralytic calcification and ossification of muscle, forearm

M61.231 Paralytic calcification and ossification of muscle, right forearm

M61.232 Paralytic calcification and ossification of muscle, left forearm

M61.239 Paralytic calcification and ossification of muscle, unspecified forearm

M61.24 Paralytic calcification and ossification of muscle, hand

M61.241 Paralytic calcification and ossification of muscle, right hand

M61.242 Paralytic calcification and ossification of muscle, left hand

M61.249 Paralytic calcification and ossification of muscle, unspecified hand

M61.25 Paralytic calcification and ossification of muscle, thigh

    M61.251 Paralytic calcification and ossification of muscle, right thigh

    M61.252 Paralytic calcification and ossification of muscle, left thigh

    M61.259 Paralytic calcification and ossification of muscle, unspecified thigh

M61.26 Paralytic calcification and ossification of muscle, lower leg

    M61.261 Paralytic calcification and ossification of muscle, right lower leg

    M61.262 Paralytic calcification and ossification of muscle, left lower leg

    M61.269 Paralytic calcification and ossification of muscle, unspecified lower leg

M61.27 Paralytic calcification and ossification of muscle, ankle and foot

    M61.271 Paralytic calcification and ossification of muscle, right ankle and foot

    M61.272 Paralytic calcification and ossification of muscle, left ankle and foot

    M61.279 Paralytic calcification and ossification of muscle, unspecified ankle and foot

M61.28 Paralytic calcification and ossification of muscle, other site

M61.29 Paralytic calcification and ossification of muscle, multiple sites

M61.3 Calcification and ossification of muscles associated with burns

Myositis ossificans associated with burns

M61.30 Calcification and ossification of muscles associated with burns, unspecified site

M61.31 Calcification and ossification of muscles associated with burns, shoulder

    M61.311 Calcification and ossification of muscles associated with burns, right shoulder

    M61.312 Calcification and ossification of muscles associated with burns, left shoulder

    M61.319 Calcification and ossification of muscles associated with burns, unspecified shoulder

M61.32 Calcification and ossification of muscles associated with burns, upper arm

    M61.321 Calcification and ossification of muscles associated with burns, right upper arm

    M61.322 Calcification and ossification of muscles associated with burns, left upper arm

    M61.329 Calcification and ossification of muscles associated with burns, unspecified upper arm

M61.33 Calcification and ossification of muscles associated with burns, forearm

    M61.331 Calcification and ossification of muscles associated with burns, right forearm

    M61.332 Calcification and ossification of muscles associated with burns, left forearm

    M61.339 Calcification and ossification of muscles associated with burns, unspecified forearm

M61.34 Calcification and ossification of muscles associated with burns, hand

    M61.341 Calcification and ossification of muscles associated with burns, right hand

    M61.342 Calcification and ossification of muscles associated with burns, left hand

    M61.349 Calcification and ossification of muscles associated with burns, unspecified hand

M61.35 Calcification and ossification of muscles associated with burns, thigh

    M61.351 Calcification and ossification of muscles associated with burns, right thigh

    M61.352 Calcification and ossification of muscles associated with burns, left thigh

    M61.359 Calcification and ossification of muscles associated with burns, unspecified thigh

M61.36 Calcification and ossification of muscles associated with burns, lower leg

    M61.361 Calcification and ossification of muscles associated with burns, right lower leg

    M61.362 Calcification and ossification of muscles associated with burns, left lower leg

    M61.369 Calcification and ossification of muscles associated with burns, unspecified lower leg

M61.37 Calcification and ossification of muscles associated with burns, ankle and foot

    M61.371 Calcification and ossification of muscles associated with burns, right ankle and foot

    M61.372 Calcification and ossification of muscles associated with burns, left ankle and foot

    M61.379 Calcification and ossification of muscles associated with burns, unspecified ankle and foot

M61.38 Calcification and ossification of muscles associated with burns, other site

M61.39 Calcification and ossification of muscles associated with burns, multiple sites

M61.4 Other calcification of muscle

    Excludes 1: calcific tendinitis NOS (M65.2-)

                 calcific tendinitis of shoulder (M75.3)

M61.40 Other calcification of muscle, unspecified site

M61.41 Other calcification of muscle, shoulder

M61.411 Other calcification of muscle, right shoulder

M61.412 Other calcification of muscle, left shoulder

M61.419 Other calcification of muscle, unspecified shoulder

M61.42 Other calcification of muscle, upper arm

M61.421 Other calcification of muscle, right upper arm

M61.422 Other calcification of muscle, left upper arm

M61.429 Other calcification of muscle, unspecified upper arm

M61.43 Other calcification of muscle, forearm

M61.431 Other calcification of muscle, right forearm

M61.432 Other calcification of muscle, left forearm

M61.439 Other calcification of muscle, unspecified forearm

M61.44 Other calcification of muscle, hand

M61.441 Other calcification of muscle, right hand

M61.442 Other calcification of muscle, left hand

M61.449 Other calcification of muscle, unspecified hand

M61.45 Other calcification of muscle, thigh

M61.451 Other calcification of muscle, right thigh

M61.452 Other calcification of muscle, left thigh

M61.459 Other calcification of muscle, unspecified thigh

M61.46 Other calcification of muscle, lower leg

M61.461 Other calcification of muscle, right lower leg

M61.462 Other calcification of muscle, left lower leg

M61.469 Other calcification of muscle, unspecified lower leg

M61.47 Other calcification of muscle, ankle and foot

M61.471 Other calcification of muscle, right ankle and foot

M61.472 Other calcification of muscle, left ankle and foot

M61.479 Other calcification of muscle, unspecified ankle and foot

M61.48 Other calcification of muscle, other site

M61.49 Other calcification of muscle, multiple sites

M61.5 Other ossification of muscle

M61.50 Other ossification of muscle, unspecified site

M61.51 Other ossification of muscle, shoulder

M61.511 Other ossification of muscle, right shoulder

M61.512 Other ossification of muscle, left shoulder

M61.519 Other ossification of muscle, unspecified shoulder

M61.52 Other ossification of muscle, upper arm

M61.521 Other ossification of muscle, right upper arm

M61.522 Other ossification of muscle, left upper arm

M61.529 Other ossification of muscle, unspecified upper arm

M61.53 Other ossification of muscle, forearm

M61.531 Other ossification of muscle, right forearm

M61.532 Other ossification of muscle, left forearm

M61.539 Other ossification of muscle, unspecified forearm

M61.54 Other ossification of muscle, hand

M61.541 Other ossification of muscle, right hand

M61.542 Other ossification of muscle, left hand

M61.549 Other ossification of muscle, unspecified hand

M61.55 Other ossification of muscle, thigh

M61.551 Other ossification of muscle, right thigh

M61.552 Other ossification of muscle, left thigh

M61.559 Other ossification of muscle, unspecified thigh

M61.56 Other ossification of muscle, lower leg

M61.561 Other ossification of muscle, right lower leg

M61.562 Other ossification of muscle, left lower leg

M61.569 Other ossification of muscle, unspecified lower leg

M61.57 Other ossification of muscle, ankle and foot

M61.571 Other ossification of muscle, right ankle and foot

M61.572 Other ossification of muscle, left ankle and foot

M61.579 Other ossification of muscle, unspecified ankle and foot

M61.58 Other ossification of muscle, other site

M61.59 Other ossification of muscle, multiple sites

M61.9 Calcification and ossification of muscle, unspecified

M62 Other disorders of muscle

Excludes 1: alcoholic myopathy (G72.1)

cramp and spasm (R25.2)

drug-induced myopathy (G72.0)

myalgia (M79.1)

stiff-man syndrome (G25.82)

Excludes 2: nontraumatic hematoma of muscle (M79.81)

M62.0 Separation of muscle (nontraumatic)

Diastasis of muscle

Excludes 1: diastasis recti complicating pregnancy, labor and delivery (O71.8)

traumatic separation of muscle- see strain of muscle by body region

M62.00 Separation of muscle (nontraumatic), unspecified site

M62.01 Separation of muscle (nontraumatic), shoulder

M62.011 Separation of muscle (nontraumatic), right shoulder

M62.012 Separation of muscle (nontraumatic), left shoulder

M62.019 Separation of muscle (nontraumatic), unspecified shoulder

M62.02 Separation of muscle (nontraumatic), upper arm

M62.021 Separation of muscle (nontraumatic), right upper arm

M62.022 Separation of muscle (nontraumatic), left upper arm

M62.029 Separation of muscle (nontraumatic), unspecified upper arm

M62.03 Separation of muscle (nontraumatic), forearm

M62.031 Separation of muscle (nontraumatic), right forearm

M62.032 Separation of muscle (nontraumatic), left forearm

M62.039 Separation of muscle (nontraumatic), unspecified forearm

M62.04 Separation of muscle (nontraumatic), hand

M62.041 Separation of muscle (nontraumatic), right hand

M62.042 Separation of muscle (nontraumatic), left hand

M62.049 Separation of muscle (nontraumatic), unspecified hand

M62.05 Separation of muscle (nontraumatic), thigh

M62.051 Separation of muscle (nontraumatic), right thigh

M62.052 Separation of muscle (nontraumatic), left thigh

M62.059 Separation of muscle (nontraumatic), unspecified thigh

M62.06 Separation of muscle (nontraumatic), lower leg

M62.061 Separation of muscle (nontraumatic), right lower leg

M62.062 Separation of muscle (nontraumatic), left lower leg

M62.069 Separation of muscle (nontraumatic), unspecified lower leg

M62.07 Separation of muscle (nontraumatic), ankle and foot

M62.071 Separation of muscle (nontraumatic), right ankle and foot

M62.072 Separation of muscle (nontraumatic), left ankle and foot

M62.079 Separation of muscle (nontraumatic), unspecified ankle and foot

M62.08 Separation of muscle (nontraumatic), other site

M62.1 Other rupture of muscle (nontraumatic)

Excludes 1: traumatic rupture of muscle - see strain of muscle by body region

Excludes 2: rupture of tendon (M66.-)

M62.10 Other rupture of muscle (nontraumatic), unspecified site

M62.11 Other rupture of muscle (nontraumatic), shoulder

M62.111 Other rupture of muscle (nontraumatic), right shoulder

M62.112 Other rupture of muscle (nontraumatic), left shoulder

M62.119 Other rupture of muscle (nontraumatic), unspecified shoulder

M62.12 Other rupture of muscle (nontraumatic), upper arm

M62.121 Other rupture of muscle (nontraumatic), right upper arm

M62.122 Other rupture of muscle (nontraumatic), left upper arm

M62.129 Other rupture of muscle (nontraumatic), unspecified upper arm

M62.13 Other rupture of muscle (nontraumatic), forearm

M62.131 Other rupture of muscle (nontraumatic), right forearm

M62.132 Other rupture of muscle (nontraumatic), left forearm

M62.139 Other rupture of muscle (nontraumatic), unspecified forearm

M62.14 Other rupture of muscle (nontraumatic), hand

M62.141 Other rupture of muscle (nontraumatic), right hand

M62.142 Other rupture of muscle (nontraumatic), left hand

M62.149 Other rupture of muscle (nontraumatic), unspecified hand

M62.15 Other rupture of muscle (nontraumatic), thigh

M62.151 Other rupture of muscle (nontraumatic), right thigh

M62.152 Other rupture of muscle (nontraumatic), left thigh

M62.159 Other rupture of muscle (nontraumatic), unspecified thigh

M62.16 Other rupture of muscle (nontraumatic), lower leg

M62.161 Other rupture of muscle (nontraumatic), right lower leg

M62.162 Other rupture of muscle (nontraumatic), left lower leg

M62.169 Other rupture of muscle (nontraumatic), unspecified lower leg

M62.17 Other rupture of muscle (nontraumatic), ankle and foot

M62.171 Other rupture of muscle (nontraumatic), right ankle and foot

M62.172 Other rupture of muscle (nontraumatic), left ankle and foot

M62.179 Other rupture of muscle (nontraumatic), unspecified ankle and foot

M62.18 Other rupture of muscle (nontraumatic), other site

M62.2 Nontraumatic ischemic infarction of muscle

Excludes 1: compartment syndrome (traumatic) (T79.A-)
nontraumatic compartment syndrome (M79.A-)
traumatic ischemia of muscle (T79.6)
rhabdomyolysis (M62.82)
Volkmann's ischemic contracture (T79.6)

M62.20 Nontraumatic ischemic infarction of muscle, unspecified site

M62.21 Nontraumatic ischemic infarction of muscle, shoulder

M62.211 Nontraumatic ischemic infarction of muscle, right shoulder

M62.212 Nontraumatic ischemic infarction of muscle, left shoulder

M62.219 Nontraumatic ischemic infarction of muscle, unspecified shoulder

M62.22 Nontraumatic ischemic infarction of muscle, upper arm

M62.221 Nontraumatic ischemic infarction of muscle, right upper arm

M62.222 Nontraumatic ischemic infarction of muscle, left upper arm

M62.229 Nontraumatic ischemic infarction of muscle, unspecified upper arm

M62.23 Nontraumatic ischemic infarction of muscle, forearm

M62.231 Nontraumatic ischemic infarction of muscle, right forearm

M62.232 Nontraumatic ischemic infarction of muscle, left forearm

M62.239 Nontraumatic ischemic infarction of muscle, unspecified forearm

M62.24 Nontraumatic ischemic infarction of muscle, hand

M62.241 Nontraumatic ischemic infarction of muscle, right hand

M62.242 Nontraumatic ischemic infarction of muscle, left hand

M62.249 Nontraumatic ischemic infarction of muscle, unspecified hand

M62.25 Nontraumatic ischemic infarction of muscle, thigh

M62.251 Nontraumatic ischemic infarction of muscle, right thigh

M62.252 Nontraumatic ischemic infarction of muscle, left thigh

M62.259 Nontraumatic ischemic infarction of muscle, unspecified thigh

M62.26 Nontraumatic ischemic infarction of muscle, lower leg

M62.261 Nontraumatic ischemic infarction of muscle, right lower leg

M62.262 Nontraumatic ischemic infarction of muscle, left lower leg

M62.269 Nontraumatic ischemic infarction of muscle, unspecified lower leg

M62.27 Nontraumatic ischemic infarction of muscle, ankle and foot

M62.271 Nontraumatic ischemic infarction of muscle, right ankle and foot

M62.272 Nontraumatic ischemic infarction of muscle, left ankle and foot

M62.279 Nontraumatic ischemic infarction of muscle, unspecified ankle and foot

M62.28 Nontraumatic ischemic infarction of muscle, other site

M62.3 Immobility syndrome (paraplegic)

M62.4 Contracture of muscle
Contracture of tendon (sheath)
Excludes 1: contracture of joint (M24.5-)

M62.40 Contracture of muscle, unspecified site

M62.41 Contracture of muscle, shoulder

M62.411 Contracture of muscle, right shoulder

M62.412 Contracture of muscle, left shoulder

M62.419 Contracture of muscle, unspecified shoulder

M62.42 Contracture of muscle, upper arm

M62.421 Contracture of muscle, right upper arm

M62.422 Contracture of muscle, left upper arm

M62.429 Contracture of muscle, unspecified upper arm

M62.43 Contracture of muscle, forearm

M62.431 Contracture of muscle, right forearm

M62.432 Contracture of muscle, left forearm

M62.439 Contracture of muscle, unspecified forearm

M62.44 Contracture of muscle, hand

M62.441 Contracture of muscle, right hand

M62.442 Contracture of muscle, left hand

M62.449 Contracture of muscle, unspecified hand

M62.45 Contracture of muscle, thigh

M62.451 Contracture of muscle, right thigh

M62.452 Contracture of muscle, left thigh

M62.459 Contracture of muscle, unspecified thigh

M62.46 Contracture of muscle, lower leg

M62.461 Contracture of muscle, right lower leg

M62.462 Contracture of muscle, left lower leg

M62.469 Contracture of muscle, unspecified lower leg

M62.47 Contracture of muscle, ankle and foot

M62.471 Contracture of muscle, right ankle and foot

M62.472 Contracture of muscle, left ankle and foot

M62.479 Contracture of muscle, unspecified ankle and foot

M62.48 Contracture of muscle, other site

M62.49 Contracture of muscle, multiple sites

M62.5 Muscle wasting and atrophy, not elsewhere classified
Disuse atrophy NEC
Excludes 1: neuralgic amyotrophy (G54.5)
progressive muscular atrophy (G12.29)
Excludes 2: pelvic muscle wasting (N81.84)

M62.50 Muscle wasting and atrophy, not elsewhere classified, unspecified site

M62.51 Muscle wasting and atrophy, not elsewhere classified, shoulder

M62.511 Muscle wasting and atrophy, not elsewhere classified, right shoulder

M62.512 Muscle wasting and atrophy, not elsewhere classified, left shoulder

M62.519 Muscle wasting and atrophy, not elsewhere classified, unspecified shoulder

M62.52 Muscle wasting and atrophy, not elsewhere classified, upper arm
    M62.521 Muscle wasting and atrophy, not elsewhere classified, right upper arm
    M62.522 Muscle wasting and atrophy, not elsewhere classified, left upper arm
    M62.529 Muscle wasting and atrophy, not elsewhere classified, unspecified upper arm
M62.53 Muscle wasting and atrophy, not elsewhere classified, forearm
    M62.531 Muscle wasting and atrophy, not elsewhere classified, right forearm
    M62.532 Muscle wasting and atrophy, not elsewhere classified, left forearm
    M62.539 Muscle wasting and atrophy, not elsewhere classified, unspecified forearm
M62.54 Muscle wasting and atrophy, not elsewhere classified, hand
    M62.541 Muscle wasting and atrophy, not elsewhere classified, right hand
    M62.542 Muscle wasting and atrophy, not elsewhere classified, left hand
    M62.549 Muscle wasting and atrophy, not elsewhere classified, unspecified hand
M62.55 Muscle wasting and atrophy, not elsewhere classified, thigh
    M62.551 Muscle wasting and atrophy, not elsewhere classified, right thigh
    M62.552 Muscle wasting and atrophy, not elsewhere classified, left thigh
    M62.559 Muscle wasting and atrophy, not elsewhere classified, unspecified thigh
M62.56 Muscle wasting and atrophy, not elsewhere classified, lower leg
    M62.561 Muscle wasting and atrophy, not elsewhere classified, right lower leg
    M62.562 Muscle wasting and atrophy, not elsewhere classified, left lower leg
    M62.569 Muscle wasting and atrophy, not elsewhere classified, unspecified lower leg
M62.57 Muscle wasting and atrophy, not elsewhere classified, ankle and foot
    M62.571 Muscle wasting and atrophy, not elsewhere classified, right ankle and foot
    M62.572 Muscle wasting and atrophy, not elsewhere classified, left ankle and foot
    M62.579 Muscle wasting and atrophy, not elsewhere classified, unspecified ankle and foot
M62.58 Muscle wasting and atrophy, not elsewhere classified, other site
M62.59 Muscle wasting and atrophy, not elsewhere classified, multiple sites
M62.8 Other specified disorders of muscle

    Excludes 2: nontraumatic hematoma of muscle (M79.81)
M62.81 Muscle weakness (generalized)
M62.82 Rhabdomyolysis
    Excludes 1: traumatic rhabdomyolysis (T79.6)
M62.83 Muscle spasm
    M62.830 Muscle spasm of back
    M62.831 Muscle spasm of calf
        Charley-horse
    M62.838 Other muscle spasm
M62.89 Other specified disorders of muscle
    Muscle (sheath) hernia
M62.9 Disorder of muscle, unspecified
M63 Disorders of muscle in diseases classified elsewhere
Code first underlying disease, such as:
    leprosy (A30.-)
    neoplasm (C49.-, C79.89, D21.-, D48.1)
    schistosomiasis (B65.-)
    trichinellosis (B75)
Excludes 1: myopathy in cysticercosis (B69.81)
    myopathy in endocrine diseases (G73.7)
    myopathy in metabolic diseases (G73.7)
    myopathy in sarcoidosis (D86.87)
    myopathy in secondary syphilis (A51.49)
    myopathy in syphilis (late) (A52.78)
    myopathy in toxoplasmosis (B58.82)
    myopathy in tuberculosis (A18.09)
M63.8 Disorders of muscle in diseases classified elsewhere
  M63.80 Disorders of muscle in diseases classified elsewhere, unspecified site
  M63.81 Disorders of muscle in diseases classified elsewhere, shoulder
    M63.811 Disorders of muscle in diseases classified elsewhere, right shoulder
    M63.812 Disorders of muscle in diseases classified elsewhere, left shoulder
    M63.819 Disorders of muscle in diseases classified elsewhere, unspecified shoulder
  M63.82 Disorders of muscle in diseases classified elsewhere, upper arm
    M63.821 Disorders of muscle in diseases classified elsewhere, right upper arm
    M63.822 Disorders of muscle in diseases classified elsewhere, left upper arm
    M63.829 Disorders of muscle in diseases classified elsewhere, unspecified upper arm
  M63.83 Disorders of muscle in diseases classified elsewhere, forearm
    M63.831 Disorders of muscle in diseases classified elsewhere, right forearm
    M63.832 Disorders of muscle in diseases classified elsewhere, left forearm
    M63.839 Disorders of muscle in diseases classified elsewhere, unspecified forearm
  M63.84 Disorders of muscle in diseases classified elsewhere, hand
    M63.841 Disorders of muscle in diseases classified elsewhere, right hand

M63.842   Disorders of muscle in diseases classified elsewhere, left hand

M63.849   Disorders of muscle in diseases classified elsewhere, unspecified hand

M63.85   Disorders of muscle in diseases classified elsewhere, thigh

M63.851   Disorders of muscle in diseases classified elsewhere, right thigh

M63.852   Disorders of muscle in diseases classified elsewhere, left thigh

M63.859   Disorders of muscle in diseases classified elsewhere, unspecified thigh

M63.86   Disorders of muscle in diseases classified elsewhere, lower leg

M63.861   Disorders of muscle in diseases classified elsewhere, right lower leg

M63.862   Disorders of muscle in diseases classified elsewhere, left lower leg

M63.869   Disorders of muscle in diseases classified elsewhere, unspecified lower leg

M63.87   Disorders of muscle in diseases classified elsewhere, ankle and foot

M63.871   Disorders of muscle in diseases classified elsewhere, right ankle and foot

M63.872   Disorders of muscle in diseases classified elsewhere, left ankle and foot

M63.879   Disorders of muscle in diseases classified elsewhere, unspecified ankle and foot

M63.88   Disorders of muscle in diseases classified elsewhere, other site

M63.89   Disorders of muscle in diseases classified elsewhere, multiple sites

DISORDERS OF SYNOVIUM AND TENDON (M65-M67)

M65   Synovitis and tenosynovitis

Excludes 1: chronic crepitant synovitis of hand and wrist (M70.0-)
current injury - see injury of ligament or tendon by body region
soft tissue disorders related to use, overuse and pressure (M70.-)

M65.0   Abscess of tendon sheath
Use additional code (B95-B96) to identify bacterial agent.

M65.00   Abscess of tendon sheath, unspecified site

M65.01   Abscess of tendon sheath, shoulder

M65.011   Abscess of tendon sheath, right shoulder

M65.012   Abscess of tendon sheath, left shoulder

M65.019   Abscess of tendon sheath, unspecified shoulder

M65.02   Abscess of tendon sheath, upper arm

M65.021   Abscess of tendon sheath, right upper arm

M65.022   Abscess of tendon sheath, left upper arm

M65.029   Abscess of tendon sheath, unspecified upper arm

M65.03   Abscess of tendon sheath, forearm

M65.031   Abscess of tendon sheath, right forearm

M65.032   Abscess of tendon sheath, left forearm

M65.039   Abscess of tendon sheath, unspecified forearm

M65.04   Abscess of tendon sheath, hand

M65.041   Abscess of tendon sheath, right hand

M65.042   Abscess of tendon sheath, left hand

M65.049   Abscess of tendon sheath, unspecified hand

M65.05   Abscess of tendon sheath, thigh

M65.051   Abscess of tendon sheath, right thigh

M65.052   Abscess of tendon sheath, left thigh

M65.059   Abscess of tendon sheath, unspecified thigh

M65.06   Abscess of tendon sheath, lower leg

M65.061   Abscess of tendon sheath, right lower leg

M65.062   Abscess of tendon sheath, left lower leg

M65.069   Abscess of tendon sheath, unspecified lower leg

M65.07   Abscess of tendon sheath, ankle and foot

M65.071   Abscess of tendon sheath, right ankle and foot

M65.072   Abscess of tendon sheath, left ankle and foot

M65.079   Abscess of tendon sheath, unspecified ankle and foot

M65.08   Abscess of tendon sheath, other site

M65.1   Other infective (teno)synovitis

M65.10   Other infective (teno)synovitis, unspecified site

M65.11   Other infective (teno)synovitis, shoulder

M65.111   Other infective (teno)synovitis, right shoulder

M65.112   Other infective (teno)synovitis, left shoulder

M65.119   Other infective (teno)synovitis, unspecified shoulder

M65.12   Other infective (teno)synovitis, elbow

M65.121   Other infective (teno)synovitis, right elbow

M65.122   Other infective (teno)synovitis, left elbow

M65.129   Other infective (teno)synovitis, unspecified elbow

M65.13   Other infective (teno)synovitis, wrist

M65.131   Other infective (teno)synovitis, right wrist

M65.132   Other infective (teno)synovitis, left wrist

M65.139   Other infective (teno)synovitis, unspecified wrist

M65.14   Other infective (teno)synovitis, hand

M65.141   Other infective (teno)synovitis, right hand

M65.142 Other infective (teno)synovitis, left hand

M65.149 Other infective (teno)synovitis, unspecified hand

M65.15 Other infective (teno)synovitis, hip

M65.151 Other infective (teno)synovitis, right hip

M65.152 Other infective (teno)synovitis, left hip

M65.159 Other infective (teno)synovitis, unspecified hip

M65.16 Other infective (teno)synovitis, knee

M65.161 Other infective (teno)synovitis, right knee

M65.162 Other infective (teno)synovitis, left knee

M65.169 Other infective (teno)synovitis, unspecified knee

M65.17 Other infective (teno)synovitis, ankle and foot

M65.171 Other infective (teno)synovitis, right ankle and foot

M65.172 Other infective (teno)synovitis, left ankle and foot

M65.179 Other infective (teno)synovitis, unspecified ankle and foot

M65.18 Other infective (teno)synovitis, other site

M65.19 Other infective (teno)synovitis, multiple sites

M65.2 Calcific tendinitis

Excludes 1: tendinitis as classified in M75-M77

calcified tendinitis of shoulder (M75.3)

M65.20 Calcific tendinitis, unspecified site

M65.22 Calcific tendinitis, upper arm

M65.221 Calcific tendinitis, right upper arm

M65.222 Calcific tendinitis, left upper arm

M65.229 Calcific tendinitis, unspecified upper arm

M65.23 Calcific tendinitis, forearm

M65.231 Calcific tendinitis, right forearm

M65.232 Calcific tendinitis, left forearm

M65.239 Calcific tendinitis, unspecified forearm

M65.24 Calcific tendinitis, hand

M65.241 Calcific tendinitis, right hand

M65.242 Calcific tendinitis, left hand

M65.249 Calcific tendinitis, unspecified hand

M65.25 Calcific tendinitis, thigh

M65.251 Calcific tendinitis, right thigh

M65.252 Calcific tendinitis, left thigh

M65.259 Calcific tendinitis, unspecified thigh

M65.26 Calcific tendinitis, lower leg

M65.261 Calcific tendinitis, right lower leg

M65.262 Calcific tendinitis, left lower leg

M65.269 Calcific tendinitis, unspecified lower leg

M65.27 Calcific tendinitis, ankle and foot

M65.271 Calcific tendinitis, right ankle and foot

M65.272 Calcific tendinitis, left ankle and foot

M65.279 Calcific tendinitis, unspecified ankle and foot

M65.28 Calcific tendinitis, other site

M65.29 Calcific tendinitis, multiple sites

M65.3 Trigger finger

Nodular tendinous disease

M65.30 Trigger finger, unspecified finger

M65.31 Trigger thumb

M65.311 Trigger thumb, right thumb

M65.312 Trigger thumb, left thumb

M65.319 Trigger thumb, unspecified thumb

M65.32 Trigger finger, index finger

M65.321 Trigger finger, right index finger

M65.322 Trigger finger, left index finger

M65.329 Trigger finger, unspecified index finger

M65.33 Trigger finger, middle finger

M65.331 Trigger finger, right middle finger

M65.332 Trigger finger, left middle finger

M65.339 Trigger finger, unspecified middle finger

M65.34 Trigger finger, ring finger

M65.341 Trigger finger, right ring finger

M65.342 Trigger finger, left ring finger

M65.349 Trigger finger, unspecified ring finger

M65.35 Trigger finger, little finger

M65.351 Trigger finger, right little finger

M65.352 Trigger finger, left little finger

M65.359 Trigger finger, unspecified little finger

M65.4 Radial styloid tenosynovitis [de Quervain]

M65.8 Other synovitis and tenosynovitis

M65.80 Other synovitis and tenosynovitis, unspecified site

M65.81 Other synovitis and tenosynovitis, shoulder

M65.811 Other synovitis and tenosynovitis, right shoulder

M65.812 Other synovitis and tenosynovitis, left shoulder

M65.819 Other synovitis and tenosynovitis, unspecified shoulder

M65.82 Other synovitis and tenosynovitis, upper arm

M65.821 Other synovitis and tenosynovitis, right upper arm

M65.822 Other synovitis and tenosynovitis, left upper arm

M65.829 Other synovitis and tenosynovitis, unspecified upper arm

M65.83 Other synovitis and tenosynovitis, forearm

M65.831 Other synovitis and tenosynovitis, right forearm

M65.832 Other synovitis and tenosynovitis, left forearm

M65.839 Other synovitis and tenosynovitis, unspecified forearm

M65.84 Other synovitis and tenosynovitis, hand

M65.841 Other synovitis and tenosynovitis, right hand

M65.842 Other synovitis and tenosynovitis, left hand

M65.849 Other synovitis and tenosynovitis, unspecified hand

M65.85 Other synovitis and tenosynovitis, thigh

M65.851 Other synovitis and tenosynovitis, right thigh

M65.852 Other synovitis and tenosynovitis, left thigh

M65.859 Other synovitis and tenosynovitis, unspecified thigh

M65.86 Other synovitis and tenosynovitis, lower leg

M65.861 Other synovitis and tenosynovitis, right lower leg

M65.862 Other synovitis and tenosynovitis, left lower leg

M65.869 Other synovitis and tenosynovitis, unspecified lower leg

M65.87 Other synovitis and tenosynovitis, ankle and foot

M65.871 Other synovitis and tenosynovitis, right ankle and foot

M65.872 Other synovitis and tenosynovitis, left ankle and foot

M65.879 Other synovitis and tenosynovitis, unspecified ankle and foot

M65.88 Other synovitis and tenosynovitis, other site

M65.89 Other synovitis and tenosynovitis, multiple sites

M65.9 Synovitis and tenosynovitis, unspecified

M66 Spontaneous rupture of synovium and tendon

Includes: rupture that occurs when a normal force is applied to tissues that are inferred to have less than normal strength

Excludes 2: rotator cuff syndrome (M75.1-)

rupture where an abnormal force is applied to normal tissue - see injury of tendon by body region

M66.0 Rupture of popliteal cyst

M66.1 Rupture of synovium

Rupture of synovial cyst

Excludes 2: rupture of popliteal cyst (M66.0)

M66.10 Rupture of synovium, unspecified joint

M66.11 Rupture of synovium, shoulder

M66.111 Rupture of synovium, right shoulder

M66.112 Rupture of synovium, left shoulder

M66.119 Rupture of synovium, unspecified shoulder

M66.12 Rupture of synovium, elbow

M66.121 Rupture of synovium, right elbow

M66.122 Rupture of synovium, left elbow

M66.129 Rupture of synovium, unspecified elbow

M66.13 Rupture of synovium, wrist

M66.131 Rupture of synovium, right wrist

M66.132 Rupture of synovium, left wrist

M66.139 Rupture of synovium, unspecified wrist

M66.14 Rupture of synovium, hand and fingers

M66.141 Rupture of synovium, right hand

M66.142 Rupture of synovium, left hand

M66.143 Rupture of synovium, unspecified hand

M66.144 Rupture of synovium, right finger(s)

M66.145 Rupture of synovium, left finger(s)

M66.146 Rupture of synovium, unspecified finger(s)

M66.15 Rupture of synovium, hip

M66.151 Rupture of synovium, right hip

M66.152 Rupture of synovium, left hip

M66.159 Rupture of synovium, unspecified hip

M66.17 Rupture of synovium, ankle, foot and toes

M66.171 Rupture of synovium, right ankle

M66.172 Rupture of synovium, left ankle

M66.173 Rupture of synovium, unspecified ankle

M66.174 Rupture of synovium, right foot

M66.175 Rupture of synovium, left foot

M66.176 Rupture of synovium, unspecified foot

M66.177 Rupture of synovium, right toe(s)

M66.178 Rupture of synovium, left toe(s)

M66.179 Rupture of synovium, unspecified toe(s)

M66.18 Rupture of synovium, other site

M66.2 Spontaneous rupture of extensor tendons

M66.20 Spontaneous rupture of extensor tendons, unspecified site

M66.21 Spontaneous rupture of extensor tendons, shoulder

M66.211 Spontaneous rupture of extensor tendons, right shoulder

M66.212 Spontaneous rupture of extensor tendons, left shoulder

M66.219 Spontaneous rupture of extensor tendons, unspecified shoulder

M66.22 Spontaneous rupture of extensor tendons, upper arm

M66.221 Spontaneous rupture of extensor tendons, right upper arm

M66.222 Spontaneous rupture of extensor tendons, left upper arm

M66.229 Spontaneous rupture of extensor tendons, unspecified upper arm

M66.23 Spontaneous rupture of extensor tendons, forearm

M66.231 Spontaneous rupture of extensor tendons, right forearm

M66.232 Spontaneous rupture of extensor tendons, left forearm

M66.239 Spontaneous rupture of extensor tendons, unspecified forearm

M66.24 Spontaneous rupture of extensor tendons, hand

M66.241 Spontaneous rupture of extensor tendons, right hand

M66.242 Spontaneous rupture of extensor tendons, left hand

M66.249 Spontaneous rupture of extensor tendons, unspecified hand

M66.25 Spontaneous rupture of extensor tendons, thigh

M66.251 Spontaneous rupture of extensor tendons, right thigh

M66.252 Spontaneous rupture of extensor tendons, left thigh

M66.259 Spontaneous rupture of extensor tendons, unspecified thigh

M66.26 Spontaneous rupture of extensor tendons, lower leg

M66.261 Spontaneous rupture of extensor tendons, right lower leg

M66.262 Spontaneous rupture of extensor tendons, left lower leg

M66.269 Spontaneous rupture of extensor tendons, unspecified lower leg

M66.27 Spontaneous rupture of extensor tendons, ankle and foot

M66.271 Spontaneous rupture of extensor tendons, right ankle and foot

M66.272 Spontaneous rupture of extensor tendons, left ankle and foot

M66.279 Spontaneous rupture of extensor tendons, unspecified ankle and foot

M66.28 Spontaneous rupture of extensor tendons, other site

M66.29 Spontaneous rupture of extensor tendons, multiple sites

M66.3 Spontaneous rupture of flexor tendons

M66.30 Spontaneous rupture of flexor tendons, unspecified site

M66.31 Spontaneous rupture of flexor tendons, shoulder

M66.311 Spontaneous rupture of flexor tendons, right shoulder

M66.312 Spontaneous rupture of flexor tendons, left shoulder

M66.319 Spontaneous rupture of flexor tendons, unspecified shoulder

M66.32 Spontaneous rupture of flexor tendons, upper arm

M66.321 Spontaneous rupture of flexor tendons, right upper arm

M66.322 Spontaneous rupture of flexor tendons, left upper arm

M66.329 Spontaneous rupture of flexor tendons, unspecified upper arm

M66.33 Spontaneous rupture of flexor tendons, forearm

M66.331 Spontaneous rupture of flexor tendons, right forearm

M66.332 Spontaneous rupture of flexor tendons, left forearm

M66.339 Spontaneous rupture of flexor tendons, unspecified forearm

M66.34 Spontaneous rupture of flexor tendons, hand

M66.341 Spontaneous rupture of flexor tendons, right hand

M66.342 Spontaneous rupture of flexor tendons, left hand

M66.349 Spontaneous rupture of flexor tendons, unspecified hand

M66.35 Spontaneous rupture of flexor tendons, thigh

M66.351 Spontaneous rupture of flexor tendons, right thigh

M66.352 Spontaneous rupture of flexor tendons, left thigh

M66.359 Spontaneous rupture of flexor tendons, unspecified thigh

M66.36 Spontaneous rupture of flexor tendons, lower leg

M66.361 Spontaneous rupture of flexor tendons, right lower leg

M66.362 Spontaneous rupture of flexor tendons, left lower leg

M66.369 Spontaneous rupture of flexor tendons, unspecified lower leg

M66.37 Spontaneous rupture of flexor tendons, ankle and foot

M66.371 Spontaneous rupture of flexor tendons, right ankle and foot

M66.372 Spontaneous rupture of flexor tendons, left ankle and foot

M66.379 Spontaneous rupture of flexor tendons, unspecified ankle and foot

M66.38 Spontaneous rupture of flexor tendons, other site

M66.39 Spontaneous rupture of flexor tendons, multiple sites

M66.8 Spontaneous rupture of other tendons

M66.80 Spontaneous rupture of other tendons, unspecified site

M66.81 Spontaneous rupture of other tendons, shoulder

M66.811 Spontaneous rupture of other tendons, right shoulder

M66.812 Spontaneous rupture of other tendons, left shoulder

M66.819 Spontaneous rupture of other tendons, unspecified shoulder

M66.82 Spontaneous rupture of other tendons, upper arm

M66.821 Spontaneous rupture of other tendons, right upper arm

M66.822 Spontaneous rupture of other tendons, left upper arm

M66.829 Spontaneous rupture of other tendons, unspecified upper arm

M66.83 Spontaneous rupture of other tendons, forearm

M66.831 Spontaneous rupture of other tendons, right forearm

M66.832 Spontaneous rupture of other tendons, left forearm

M66.839 Spontaneous rupture of other tendons, unspecified forearm

M66.84 Spontaneous rupture of other tendons, hand

M66.841 Spontaneous rupture of other tendons, right hand

M66.842 Spontaneous rupture of other tendons, left hand

M66.849 Spontaneous rupture of other tendons, unspecified hand

M66.85 Spontaneous rupture of other tendons, thigh

M66.851 Spontaneous rupture of other tendons, right thigh

M66.852 Spontaneous rupture of other tendons, left thigh

M66.859 Spontaneous rupture of other tendons, unspecified thigh

M66.86 Spontaneous rupture of other tendons, lower leg

M66.861 Spontaneous rupture of other tendons, right lower leg

M66.862 Spontaneous rupture of other tendons, left lower leg

● New code　　　　▲ Revised code　　　　⑦ 7th digit required　　　　⊗ Placeholder required

M66.869 Spontaneous rupture of other tendons, unspecified lower leg

M66.87 Spontaneous rupture of other tendons, ankle and foot

M66.871 Spontaneous rupture of other tendons, right ankle and foot

M66.872 Spontaneous rupture of other tendons, left ankle and foot

M66.879 Spontaneous rupture of other tendons, unspecified ankle and foot

M66.88 Spontaneous rupture of other tendons, other

M66.89 Spontaneous rupture of other tendons, multiple sites

M66.9 Spontaneous rupture of unspecified tendon

Rupture at musculotendinous junction, nontraumatic

M67 Other disorders of synovium and tendon

Excludes 1: palmar fascial fibromatosis [Dupuytren] (M72.0)

tendinitis NOS (M77.9-)

xanthomatosis localized to tendons (E78.2)

M67.0 Short Achilles tendon (acquired)

M67.00 Short Achilles tendon (acquired), unspecified ankle

M67.01 Short Achilles tendon (acquired), right ankle

M67.02 Short Achilles tendon (acquired), left ankle

M67.2 Synovial hypertrophy, not elsewhere classified

Excludes 1: villonodular synovitis (pigmented) (M12.2-)

M67.20 Synovial hypertrophy, not elsewhere classified, unspecified site

M67.21 Synovial hypertrophy, not elsewhere classified, shoulder

M67.211 Synovial hypertrophy, not elsewhere classified, right shoulder

M67.212 Synovial hypertrophy, not elsewhere classified, left shoulder

M67.219 Synovial hypertrophy, not elsewhere classified, unspecified shoulder

M67.22 Synovial hypertrophy, not elsewhere classified, upper arm

M67.221 Synovial hypertrophy, not elsewhere classified, right upper arm

M67.222 Synovial hypertrophy, not elsewhere classified, left upper arm

M67.229 Synovial hypertrophy, not elsewhere classified, unspecified upper arm

M67.23 Synovial hypertrophy, not elsewhere classified, forearm

M67.231 Synovial hypertrophy, not elsewhere classified, right forearm

M67.232 Synovial hypertrophy, not elsewhere classified, left forearm

M67.239 Synovial hypertrophy, not elsewhere classified, unspecified forearm

M67.24 Synovial hypertrophy, not elsewhere classified, hand

M67.241 Synovial hypertrophy, not elsewhere classified, right hand

M67.242 Synovial hypertrophy, not elsewhere classified, left hand

M67.249 Synovial hypertrophy, not elsewhere classified, unspecified hand

M67.25 Synovial hypertrophy, not elsewhere classified, thigh

M67.251 Synovial hypertrophy, not elsewhere classified, right thigh

M67.252 Synovial hypertrophy, not elsewhere classified, left thigh

M67.259 Synovial hypertrophy, not elsewhere classified, unspecified thigh

M67.26 Synovial hypertrophy, not elsewhere classified, lower leg

M67.261 Synovial hypertrophy, not elsewhere classified, right lower leg

M67.262 Synovial hypertrophy, not elsewhere classified, left lower leg

M67.269 Synovial hypertrophy, not elsewhere classified, unspecified lower leg

M67.27 Synovial hypertrophy, not elsewhere classified, ankle and foot

M67.271 Synovial hypertrophy, not elsewhere classified, right ankle and foot

M67.272 Synovial hypertrophy, not elsewhere classified, left ankle and foot

M67.279 Synovial hypertrophy, not elsewhere classified, unspecified ankle and foot

M67.28 Synovial hypertrophy, not elsewhere classified, other site

M67.29 Synovial hypertrophy, not elsewhere classified, multiple sites

M67.3 Transient synovitis

Toxic synovitis

Excludes 1: palindromic rheumatism (M12.3-)

M67.30 Transient synovitis, unspecified site

M67.31 Transient synovitis, shoulder

M67.311 Transient synovitis, right shoulder

M67.312 Transient synovitis, left shoulder

M67.319 Transient synovitis, unspecified shoulder

M67.32 Transient synovitis, elbow

M67.321 Transient synovitis, right elbow

M67.322 Transient synovitis, left elbow

M67.329 Transient synovitis, unspecified elbow

M67.33 Transient synovitis, wrist

M67.331 Transient synovitis, right wrist

M67.332 Transient synovitis, left wrist

M67.339 Transient synovitis, unspecified wrist

M67.34 Transient synovitis, hand

M67.341 Transient synovitis, right hand

M67.342 Transient synovitis, left hand

M67.349 Transient synovitis, unspecified hand

M67.35 Transient synovitis, hip

M67.351 Transient synovitis, right hip

M67.352 Transient synovitis, left hip

M67.359 Transient synovitis, unspecified hip

M67.36 Transient synovitis, knee

M67.361 Transient synovitis, right knee

M67.362 Transient synovitis, left knee

M67.369 Transient synovitis, unspecified knee

M67.37 Transient synovitis, ankle and foot

M67.371 Transient synovitis, right ankle and foot

M67.372 Transient synovitis, left ankle and foot

M67.379 Transient synovitis, unspecified ankle and foot

M67.38 Transient synovitis, other site

M67.39 Transient synovitis, multiple sites

M67.4 Ganglion

Ganglion of joint or tendon (sheath)

Excludes 1: ganglion in yaws (A66.6)

Excludes 2: cyst of bursa (M71.2-M71.3)

cyst of synovium (M71.2-M71.3)

M67.40 Ganglion, unspecified site

M67.41 Ganglion, shoulder

M67.411 Ganglion, right shoulder

M67.412 Ganglion, left shoulder

M67.419 Ganglion, unspecified shoulder

M67.42 Ganglion, elbow

M67.421 Ganglion, right elbow

M67.422 Ganglion, left elbow

M67.429 Ganglion, unspecified elbow

M67.43 Ganglion, wrist

M67.431 Ganglion, right wrist

M67.432 Ganglion, left wrist

M67.439 Ganglion, unspecified wrist

M67.44 Ganglion, hand

M67.441 Ganglion, right hand

M67.442 Ganglion, left hand

M67.449 Ganglion, unspecified hand

M67.45 Ganglion, hip

M67.451 Ganglion, right hip

M67.452 Ganglion, left hip

M67.459 Ganglion, unspecified hip

M67.46 Ganglion, knee

M67.461 Ganglion, right knee

M67.462 Ganglion, left knee

M67.469 Ganglion, unspecified knee

M67.47 Ganglion, ankle and foot

M67.471 Ganglion, right ankle and foot

M67.472 Ganglion, left ankle and foot

M67.479 Ganglion, unspecified ankle and foot

M67.48 Ganglion, other site

M67.49 Ganglion, multiple sites

M67.5 Plica syndrome

Plica knee

M67.50 Plica syndrome, unspecified knee

M67.51 Plica syndrome, right knee

M67.52 Plica syndrome, left knee

M67.8 Other specified disorders of synovium and tendon

M67.80 Other specified disorders of synovium and tendon, unspecified site

M67.81 Other specified disorders of synovium and tendon, shoulder

M67.811 Other specified disorders of synovium, right shoulder

M67.812 Other specified disorders of synovium, left shoulder

M67.813 Other specified disorders of tendon, right shoulder

M67.814 Other specified disorders of tendon, left shoulder

M67.819 Other specified disorders of synovium and tendon, unspecified shoulder

M67.82 Other specified disorders of synovium and tendon, elbow

M67.821 Other specified disorders of synovium, right elbow

M67.822 Other specified disorders of synovium, left elbow

M67.823 Other specified disorders of tendon, right elbow

M67.824 Other specified disorders of tendon, left elbow

M67.829 Other specified disorders of synovium and tendon, unspecified elbow

M67.83 Other specified disorders of synovium and tendon, wrist

M67.831 Other specified disorders of synovium, right wrist

M67.832 Other specified disorders of synovium, left wrist

M67.833 Other specified disorders of tendon, right wrist

M67.834 Other specified disorders of tendon, left wrist

M67.839 Other specified disorders of synovium and tendon, unspecified forearm

M67.84 Other specified disorders of synovium and tendon, hand

M67.841 Other specified disorders of synovium, right hand

M67.842 Other specified disorders of synovium, left hand

M67.843 Other specified disorders of tendon, right hand

M67.844 Other specified disorders of tendon, left hand

M67.849 Other specified disorders of synovium and tendon, unspecified hand

M67.85 Other specified disorders of synovium and tendon, hip

M67.851 Other specified disorders of synovium, right hip

M67.852 Other specified disorders of synovium, left hip

M67.853 Other specified disorders of tendon, right hip

M67.854 Other specified disorders of tendon, left hip

M67.859 Other specified disorders of synovium and tendon, unspecified hip

● New code   ▲ Revised code   ⑦ 7th digit required   ⊗ Placeholder required

M67.86 Other specified disorders of synovium and tendon, knee

    M67.861 Other specified disorders of synovium, right knee

    M67.862 Other specified disorders of synovium, left knee

    M67.863 Other specified disorders of tendon, right knee

    M67.864 Other specified disorders of tendon, left knee

    M67.869 Other specified disorders of synovium and tendon, unspecified knee

M67.87 Other specified disorders of synovium and tendon, ankle and foot

    M67.871 Other specified disorders of synovium, right ankle and foot

    M67.872 Other specified disorders of synovium, left ankle and foot

    M67.873 Other specified disorders of tendon, right ankle and foot

    M67.874 Other specified disorders of tendon, left ankle and foot

    M67.879 Other specified disorders of synovium and tendon, unspecified ankle and foot

M67.88 Other specified disorders of synovium and tendon, other site

M67.89 Other specified disorders of synovium and tendon, multiple sites

M67.9 Unspecified disorder of synovium and tendon

  M67.90 Unspecified disorder of synovium and tendon, unspecified site

  M67.91 Unspecified disorder of synovium and tendon, shoulder

    M67.911 Unspecified disorder of synovium and tendon, right shoulder

    M67.912 Unspecified disorder of synovium and tendon, left shoulder

    M67.919 Unspecified disorder of synovium and tendon, unspecified shoulder

  M67.92 Unspecified disorder of synovium and tendon, upper arm

    M67.921 Unspecified disorder of synovium and tendon, right upper arm

    M67.922 Unspecified disorder of synovium and tendon, left upper arm

    M67.929 Unspecified disorder of synovium and tendon, unspecified upper arm

  M67.93 Unspecified disorder of synovium and tendon, forearm

    M67.931 Unspecified disorder of synovium and tendon, right forearm

    M67.932 Unspecified disorder of synovium and tendon, left forearm

    M67.939 Unspecified disorder of synovium and tendon, unspecified forearm

  M67.94 Unspecified disorder of synovium and tendon, hand

    M67.941 Unspecified disorder of synovium and tendon, right hand

    M67.942 Unspecified disorder of synovium and tendon, left hand

    M67.949 Unspecified disorder of synovium and tendon, unspecified hand

  M67.95 Unspecified disorder of synovium and tendon, thigh

    M67.951 Unspecified disorder of synovium and tendon, right thigh

    M67.952 Unspecified disorder of synovium and tendon, left thigh

    M67.959 Unspecified disorder of synovium and tendon, unspecified thigh

  M67.96 Unspecified disorder of synovium and tendon, lower leg

    M67.961 Unspecified disorder of synovium and tendon, right lower leg

    M67.962 Unspecified disorder of synovium and tendon, left lower leg

    M67.969 Unspecified disorder of synovium and tendon, unspecified lower leg

  M67.97 Unspecified disorder of synovium and tendon, ankle and foot

    M67.971 Unspecified disorder of synovium and tendon, right ankle and foot

    M67.972 Unspecified disorder of synovium and tendon, left ankle and foot

    M67.979 Unspecified disorder of synovium and tendon, unspecified ankle and foot

  M67.98 Unspecified disorder of synovium and tendon, other site

  M67.99 Unspecified disorder of synovium and tendon, multiple sites

OTHER SOFT TISSUE DISORDERS (M70-M79)

M70 Soft tissue disorders related to use, overuse and pressure

Includes: soft tissue disorders of occupational origin

Use additional external cause code to identify activity causing disorder (Y93.-)

Excludes 1: bursitis NOS (M71.9-)

Excludes 2: bursitis of shoulder (M75.5)

enthesopathies (M76-M77)

pressure ulcer (pressure area) (L89.-)

M70.0 Crepitant synovitis (acute) (chronic) of hand and wrist

  M70.03 Crepitant synovitis (acute) (chronic), wrist

    M70.031 Crepitant synovitis (acute) (chronic), right wrist

    M70.032 Crepitant synovitis (acute) (chronic), left wrist

    M70.039 Crepitant synovitis (acute) (chronic), unspecified wrist

  M70.04 Crepitant synovitis (acute) (chronic), hand

    M70.041 Crepitant synovitis (acute) (chronic), right hand

    M70.042 Crepitant synovitis (acute) (chronic), left hand

    M70.049 Crepitant synovitis (acute) (chronic), unspecified hand

M70.1 Bursitis of hand

  M70.10 Bursitis, unspecified hand

  M70.11 Bursitis, right hand

M70.12 Bursitis, left hand

M70.2 Olecranon bursitis

    M70.20 Olecranon bursitis, unspecified elbow

    M70.21 Olecranon bursitis, right elbow

    M70.22 Olecranon bursitis, left elbow

M70.3 Other bursitis of elbow

    M70.30 Other bursitis of elbow, unspecified elbow

    M70.31 Other bursitis of elbow, right elbow

    M70.32 Other bursitis of elbow, left elbow

M70.4 Prepatellar bursitis

    M70.40 Prepatellar bursitis, unspecified knee

    M70.41 Prepatellar bursitis, right knee

    M70.42 Prepatellar bursitis, left knee

M70.5 Other bursitis of knee

    M70.50 Other bursitis of knee, unspecified knee

    M70.51 Other bursitis of knee, right knee

    M70.52 Other bursitis of knee, left knee

M70.6 Trochanteric bursitis

Trochanteric tendinitis

    M70.60 Trochanteric bursitis, unspecified hip

    M70.61 Trochanteric bursitis, right hip

    M70.62 Trochanteric bursitis, left hip

M70.7 Other bursitis of hip

Ischial bursitis

    M70.70 Other bursitis of hip, unspecified hip

    M70.71 Other bursitis of hip, right hip

    M70.72 Other bursitis of hip, left hip

M70.8 Other soft tissue disorders related to use, overuse and pressure

    M70.80 Other soft tissue disorders related to use, overuse and pressure of unspecified site

    M70.81 Other soft tissue disorders related to use, overuse and pressure of shoulder

        M70.811 Other soft tissue disorders related to use, overuse and pressure, right shoulder

        M70.812 Other soft tissue disorders related to use, overuse and pressure, left shoulder

        M70.819 Other soft tissue disorders related to use, overuse and pressure, unspecified shoulder

    M70.82 Other soft tissue disorders related to use, overuse and pressure of upper arm

        M70.821 Other soft tissue disorders related to use, overuse and pressure, right upper arm

        M70.822 Other soft tissue disorders related to use, overuse and pressure, left upper arm

        M70.829 Other soft tissue disorders related to use, overuse and pressure, unspecified upper arms

    M70.83 Other soft tissue disorders related to use, overuse and pressure of forearm

        M70.831 Other soft tissue disorders related to use, overuse and pressure, right forearm

        M70.832 Other soft tissue disorders related to use, overuse and pressure, left forearm

        M70.839 Other soft tissue disorders related to use, overuse and pressure, unspecified forearm

M70.84 Other soft tissue disorders related to use, overuse and pressure of hand

    M70.841 Other soft tissue disorders related to use, overuse and pressure, right hand

    M70.842 Other soft tissue disorders related to use, overuse and pressure, left hand

    M70.849 Other soft tissue disorders related to use, overuse and pressure, unspecified hand

M70.85 Other soft tissue disorders related to use, overuse and pressure of thigh

    M70.851 Other soft tissue disorders related to use, overuse and pressure, right thigh

    M70.852 Other soft tissue disorders related to use, overuse and pressure, left thigh

    M70.859 Other soft tissue disorders related to use, overuse and pressure, unspecified thigh

M70.86 Other soft tissue disorders related to use, overuse and pressure lower leg

    M70.861 Other soft tissue disorders related to use, overuse and pressure, right lower leg

    M70.862 Other soft tissue disorders related to use, overuse and pressure, left lower leg

    M70.869 Other soft tissue disorders related to use, overuse and pressure, unspecified leg

M70.87 Other soft tissue disorders related to use, overuse and pressure of ankle and foot

    M70.871 Other soft tissue disorders related to use, overuse and pressure, right ankle and foot

    M70.872 Other soft tissue disorders related to use, overuse and pressure, left ankle and foot

    M70.879 Other soft tissue disorders related to use, overuse and pressure, unspecified ankle and foot

    M70.88 Other soft tissue disorders related to use, overuse and pressure other site

    M70.89 Other soft tissue disorders related to use, overuse and pressure multiple sites

M70.9 Unspecified soft tissue disorder related to use, overuse and pressure

    M70.90 Unspecified soft tissue disorder related to use, overuse and pressure of unspecified site

    M70.91 Unspecified soft tissue disorder related to use, overuse and pressure of shoulder

        M70.911 Unspecified soft tissue disorder related to use, overuse and pressure, right shoulder

● New code   ▲ Revised code   ⑦ 7th digit required   ⊗ Placeholder required

M70.912 Unspecified soft tissue disorder related to use, overuse and pressure, left shoulder

M70.919 Unspecified soft tissue disorder related to use, overuse and pressure, unspecified shoulder

M70.92 Unspecified soft tissue disorder related to use, overuse and pressure of upper arm

M70.921 Unspecified soft tissue disorder related to use, overuse and pressure, right upper arm

M70.922 Unspecified soft tissue disorder related to use, overuse and pressure, left upper arm

M70.929 Unspecified soft tissue disorder related to use, overuse and pressure, unspecified upper arm

M70.93 Unspecified soft tissue disorder related to use, overuse and pressure of forearm

M70.931 Unspecified soft tissue disorder related to use, overuse and pressure, right forearm

M70.932 Unspecified soft tissue disorder related to use, overuse and pressure, left forearm

M70.939 Unspecified soft tissue disorder related to use, overuse and pressure, unspecified forearm

M70.94 Unspecified soft tissue disorder related to use, overuse and pressure of hand

M70.941 Unspecified soft tissue disorder related to use, overuse and pressure, right hand

M70.942 Unspecified soft tissue disorder related to use, overuse and pressure, left hand

M70.949 Unspecified soft tissue disorder related to use, overuse and pressure, unspecified hand

M70.95 Unspecified soft tissue disorder related to use, overuse and pressure of thigh

M70.951 Unspecified soft tissue disorder related to use, overuse and pressure, right thigh

M70.952 Unspecified soft tissue disorder related to use, overuse and pressure, left thigh

M70.959 Unspecified soft tissue disorder related to use, overuse and pressure, unspecified thigh

M70.96 Unspecified soft tissue disorder related to use, overuse and pressure lower leg

M70.961 Unspecified soft tissue disorder related to use, overuse and pressure, right lower leg

M70.962 Unspecified soft tissue disorder related to use, overuse and pressure, left lower leg

M70.969 Unspecified soft tissue disorder related to use, overuse and pressure, unspecified lower leg

M70.97 Unspecified soft tissue disorder related to use, overuse and pressure of ankle and foot

M70.971 Unspecified soft tissue disorder related to use, overuse and pressure, right ankle and foot

M70.972 Unspecified soft tissue disorder related to use, overuse and pressure, left ankle and foot

M70.979 Unspecified soft tissue disorder related to use, overuse and pressure, unspecified ankle and foot

M70.98 Unspecified soft tissue disorder related to use, overuse and pressure other

M70.99 Unspecified soft tissue disorder related to use, overuse and pressure multiple sites

M71 Other bursopathies

Excludes 1: bunion (M20.1)

bursitis related to use, overuse or pressure (M70.-)

enthesopathies (M76-M77)

M71.0 Abscess of bursa

Use additional code (B95.-, B96.-) to identify causative organism

M71.00 Abscess of bursa, unspecified site

M71.01 Abscess of bursa, shoulder

M71.011 Abscess of bursa, right shoulder

M71.012 Abscess of bursa, left shoulder

M71.019 Abscess of bursa, unspecified shoulder

M71.02 Abscess of bursa, elbow

M71.021 Abscess of bursa, right elbow

M71.022 Abscess of bursa, left elbow

M71.029 Abscess of bursa, unspecified elbow

M71.03 Abscess of bursa, wrist

M71.031 Abscess of bursa, right wrist

M71.032 Abscess of bursa, left wrist

M71.039 Abscess of bursa, unspecified wrist

M71.04 Abscess of bursa, hand

M71.041 Abscess of bursa, right hand

M71.042 Abscess of bursa, left hand

M71.049 Abscess of bursa, unspecified hand

M71.05 Abscess of bursa, hip

M71.051 Abscess of bursa, right hip

M71.052 Abscess of bursa, left hip

M71.059 Abscess of bursa, unspecified hip

M71.06 Abscess of bursa, knee

M71.061 Abscess of bursa, right knee

M71.062 Abscess of bursa, left knee

M71.069 Abscess of bursa, unspecified knee

M71.07 Abscess of bursa, ankle and foot

M71.071 Abscess of bursa, right ankle and foot

M71.072 Abscess of bursa, left ankle and foot

M71.079 Abscess of bursa, unspecified ankle and foot

M71.08 Abscess of bursa, other site

M71.09 Abscess of bursa, multiple sites

M71.1 Other infective bursitis

Use additional code (B95.-, B96.-) to identify causative organism

M71.10 Other infective bursitis, unspecified site

M71.11 Other infective bursitis, shoulder
- M71.111 Other infective bursitis, right shoulder
- M71.112 Other infective bursitis, left shoulder
- M71.119 Other infective bursitis, unspecified shoulder

M71.12 Other infective bursitis, elbow
- M71.121 Other infective bursitis, right elbow
- M71.122 Other infective bursitis, left elbow
- M71.129 Other infective bursitis, unspecified elbow

M71.13 Other infective bursitis, wrist
- M71.131 Other infective bursitis, right wrist
- M71.132 Other infective bursitis, left wrist
- M71.139 Other infective bursitis, unspecified wrist

M71.14 Other infective bursitis, hand
- M71.141 Other infective bursitis, right hand
- M71.142 Other infective bursitis, left hand
- M71.149 Other infective bursitis, unspecified hand

M71.15 Other infective bursitis, hip
- M71.151 Other infective bursitis, right hip
- M71.152 Other infective bursitis, left hip
- M71.159 Other infective bursitis, unspecified hip

M71.16 Other infective bursitis, knee
- M71.161 Other infective bursitis, right knee
- M71.162 Other infective bursitis, left knee
- M71.169 Other infective bursitis, unspecified knee

M71.17 Other infective bursitis, ankle and foot
- M71.171 Other infective bursitis, right ankle and foot
- M71.172 Other infective bursitis, left ankle and foot
- M71.179 Other infective bursitis, unspecified ankle and foot

M71.18 Other infective bursitis, other site

M71.19 Other infective bursitis, multiple sites

M71.2 Synovial cyst of popliteal space [Baker]

Excludes 1: synovial cyst of popliteal space with rupture (M66.0)

M71.20 Synovial cyst of popliteal space [Baker], unspecified knee

M71.21 Synovial cyst of popliteal space [Baker], right knee

M71.22 Synovial cyst of popliteal space [Baker], left knee

M71.3 Other bursal cyst

Synovial cyst NOS

Excludes 1: synovial cyst with rupture (M66.1-)

M71.30 Other bursal cyst, unspecified site

M71.31 Other bursal cyst, shoulder
- M71.311 Other bursal cyst, right shoulder
- M71.312 Other bursal cyst, left shoulder
- M71.319 Other bursal cyst, unspecified shoulder

M71.32 Other bursal cyst, elbow
- M71.321 Other bursal cyst, right elbow
- M71.322 Other bursal cyst, left elbow
- M71.329 Other bursal cyst, unspecified elbow

M71.33 Other bursal cyst, wrist
- M71.331 Other bursal cyst, right wrist
- M71.332 Other bursal cyst, left wrist
- M71.339 Other bursal cyst, unspecified wrist

M71.34 Other bursal cyst, hand
- M71.341 Other bursal cyst, right hand
- M71.342 Other bursal cyst, left hand
- M71.349 Other bursal cyst, unspecified hand

M71.35 Other bursal cyst, hip
- M71.351 Other bursal cyst, right hip
- M71.352 Other bursal cyst, left hip
- M71.359 Other bursal cyst, unspecified hip

M71.37 Other bursal cyst, ankle and foot
- M71.371 Other bursal cyst, right ankle and foot
- M71.372 Other bursal cyst, left ankle and foot
- M71.379 Other bursal cyst, unspecified ankle and foot

M71.38 Other bursal cyst, other site

M71.39 Other bursal cyst, multiple sites

M71.4 Calcium deposit in bursa

Excludes 2: calcium deposit in bursa of shoulder (M75.3)

M71.40 Calcium deposit in bursa, unspecified site

M71.42 Calcium deposit in bursa, elbow
- M71.421 Calcium deposit in bursa, right elbow
- M71.422 Calcium deposit in bursa, left elbow
- M71.429 Calcium deposit in bursa, unspecified elbow

M71.43 Calcium deposit in bursa, wrist
- M71.431 Calcium deposit in bursa, right wrist
- M71.432 Calcium deposit in bursa, left wrist
- M71.439 Calcium deposit in bursa, unspecified wrist

M71.44 Calcium deposit in bursa, hand
- M71.441 Calcium deposit in bursa, right hand
- M71.442 Calcium deposit in bursa, left hand
- M71.449 Calcium deposit in bursa, unspecified hand

M71.45 Calcium deposit in bursa, hip
- M71.451 Calcium deposit in bursa, right hip
- M71.452 Calcium deposit in bursa, left hip
- M71.459 Calcium deposit in bursa, unspecified hip

M71.46 Calcium deposit in bursa, knee
- M71.461 Calcium deposit in bursa, right knee
- M71.462 Calcium deposit in bursa, left knee
- M71.469 Calcium deposit in bursa, unspecified knee

M71.47 Calcium deposit in bursa, ankle and foot
- M71.471 Calcium deposit in bursa, right ankle and foot
- M71.472 Calcium deposit in bursa, left ankle and foot
- M71.479 Calcium deposit in bursa, unspecified ankle and foot

M71.48 Calcium deposit in bursa, other site

M71.49 Calcium deposit in bursa, multiple sites

M71.5 Other bursitis, not elsewhere classified

Excludes 1: bursitis NOS (M71.9-)

Excludes 2: bursitis of shoulder (M75.5)

bursitis of tibial collateral [Pellegrini-Stieda] (M76.4)

M71.50 Other bursitis, not elsewhere classified, unspecified site

M71.52 Other bursitis, not elsewhere classified, elbow

M71.521 Other bursitis, not elsewhere classified, right elbow

M71.522 Other bursitis, not elsewhere classified, left elbow

M71.529 Other bursitis, not elsewhere classified, unspecified elbow

M71.53 Other bursitis, not elsewhere classified, wrist

M71.531 Other bursitis, not elsewhere classified, right wrist

M71.532 Other bursitis, not elsewhere classified, left wrist

M71.539 Other bursitis, not elsewhere classified, unspecified wrist

M71.54 Other bursitis, not elsewhere classified, hand

M71.541 Other bursitis, not elsewhere classified, right hand

M71.542 Other bursitis, not elsewhere classified, left hand

M71.549 Other bursitis, not elsewhere classified, unspecified hand

M71.55 Other bursitis, not elsewhere classified, hip

M71.551 Other bursitis, not elsewhere classified, right hip

M71.552 Other bursitis, not elsewhere classified, left hip

M71.559 Other bursitis, not elsewhere classified, unspecified hip

M71.56 Other bursitis, not elsewhere classified, knee

M71.561 Other bursitis, not elsewhere classified, right knee

M71.562 Other bursitis, not elsewhere classified, left knee

M71.569 Other bursitis, not elsewhere classified, unspecified knee

M71.57 Other bursitis, not elsewhere classified, ankle and foot

M71.571 Other bursitis, not elsewhere classified, right ankle and foot

M71.572 Other bursitis, not elsewhere classified, left ankle and foot

M71.579 Other bursitis, not elsewhere classified, unspecified ankle and foot

M71.58 Other bursitis, not elsewhere classified, other site

M71.8 Other specified bursopathies

M71.80 Other specified bursopathies, unspecified site

M71.81 Other specified bursopathies, shoulder

M71.811 Other specified bursopathies, right shoulder

M71.812 Other specified bursopathies, left shoulder

M71.819 Other specified bursopathies, unspecified shoulder

M71.82 Other specified bursopathies, elbow

M71.821 Other specified bursopathies, right elbow

M71.822 Other specified bursopathies, left elbow

M71.829 Other specified bursopathies, unspecified elbow

M71.83 Other specified bursopathies, wrist

M71.831 Other specified bursopathies, right wrist

M71.832 Other specified bursopathies, left wrist

M71.839 Other specified bursopathies, unspecified wrist

M71.84 Other specified bursopathies, hand

M71.841 Other specified bursopathies, right hand

M71.842 Other specified bursopathies, left hand

M71.849 Other specified bursopathies, unspecified hand

M71.85 Other specified bursopathies, hip

M71.851 Other specified bursopathies, right hip

M71.852 Other specified bursopathies, left hip

M71.859 Other specified bursopathies, unspecified hip

M71.86 Other specified bursopathies, knee

M71.861 Other specified bursopathies, right knee

M71.862 Other specified bursopathies, left knee

M71.869 Other specified bursopathies, unspecified knee

M71.87 Other specified bursopathies, ankle and foot

M71.871 Other specified bursopathies, right ankle and foot

M71.872 Other specified bursopathies, left ankle and foot

M71.879 Other specified bursopathies, unspecified ankle and foot

M71.88 Other specified bursopathies, other site

M71.89 Other specified bursopathies, multiple sites

M71.9 Bursopathy, unspecified

Bursitis NOS

M72 Fibroblastic disorders

Excludes 2: retroperitoneal fibromatosis (D48.3)

M72.0 Palmar fascial fibromatosis [Dupuytren]

M72.1 Knuckle pads

M72.2 Plantar fascial fibromatosis

Plantar fasciitis

M72.4 Pseudosarcomatous fibromatosis

Nodular fasciitis

M72.6 Necrotizing fasciitis

Use additional code (B95.-, B96.-) to identify causative organism

M72.8 Other fibroblastic disorders

Abscess of fascia

Fasciitis NEC

Other infective fasciitis

Use additional code to (B95.-, B96.-) identify causative organism

Excludes 1: diffuse (eosinophilic) fasciitis (M35.4)

necrotizing fasciitis (M72.6)

nodular fasciitis (M72.4)

perirenal fasciitis NOS (N13.5)

perirenal fasciitis with infection (N13.6)

plantar fasciitis (M72.2)

M72.9 Fibroblastic disorder, unspecified

Fasciitis NOS

Fibromatosis NOS

M75 Shoulder lesions

Excludes 2: shoulder-hand syndrome (M89.0-)

M75.0 Adhesive capsulitis of shoulder

Frozen shoulder

Periarthritis of shoulder

M75.00 Adhesive capsulitis of unspecified shoulder

M75.01 Adhesive capsulitis of right shoulder

M75.02 Adhesive capsulitis of left shoulder

M75.1 Rotator cuff tear or rupture, not specified as traumatic

Rotator cuff syndrome

Supraspinatus tear or rupture, not specified as traumatic

Supraspinatus syndrome

Excludes 1: tear of rotator cuff, traumatic (S46.01-)

M75.10 Unspecified rotator cuff tear or rupture, not specified as traumatic

M75.100 Unspecified rotator cuff tear or rupture of unspecified shoulder, not specified as traumatic

M75.101 Unspecified rotator cuff tear or rupture of right shoulder, not specified as traumatic

M75.102 Unspecified rotator cuff tear or rupture of left shoulder, not specified as traumatic

M75.11 Incomplete rotator cuff tear or rupture not specified as traumatic

M75.110 Incomplete rotator cuff tear or rupture of unspecified shoulder, not specified as traumatic

M75.111 Incomplete rotator cuff tear or rupture of right shoulder, not specified as traumatic

M75.112 Incomplete rotator cuff tear or rupture of left shoulder, not specified as traumatic

M75.12 Complete rotator cuff tear or rupture not specified as traumatic

M75.120 Complete rotator cuff tear or rupture of unspecified shoulder, not specified as traumatic

M75.121 Complete rotator cuff tear or rupture of right shoulder, not specified as traumatic

M75.122 Complete rotator cuff tear or rupture of left shoulder, not specified as traumatic

M75.2 Bicipital tendinitis

M75.20 Bicipital tendinitis, unspecified shoulder

M75.21 Bicipital tendinitis, right shoulder

M75.22 Bicipital tendinitis, left shoulder

M75.3 Calcific tendinitis of shoulder

Calcified bursa of shoulder

M75.30 Calcific tendinitis of unspecified shoulder

M75.31 Calcific tendinitis of right shoulder

M75.32 Calcific tendinitis of left shoulder

M75.4 Impingement syndrome of shoulder

M75.40 Impingement syndrome of unspecified shoulder

M75.41 Impingement syndrome of right shoulder

M75.42 Impingement syndrome of left shoulder

M75.5 Bursitis of shoulder

M75.50 Bursitis of unspecified shoulder

M75.51 Bursitis of right shoulder

M75.52 Bursitis of left shoulder

M75.8 Other shoulder lesions

M75.80 Other shoulder lesions, unspecified shoulder

M75.81 Other shoulder lesions, right shoulder

M75.82 Other shoulder lesions, left shoulder

M75.9 Shoulder lesion, unspecified

M75.90 Shoulder lesion, unspecified, unspecified shoulder

M75.91 Shoulder lesion, unspecified, right shoulder

M75.92 Shoulder lesion, unspecified, left shoulder

M76 Enthesopathies, lower limb, excluding foot

Excludes 2: bursitis due to use, overuse and pressure (M70.-)

enthesopathies of ankle and foot (M77.5-)

M76.0 Gluteal tendinitis

M76.00 Gluteal tendinitis, unspecified hip

M76.01 Gluteal tendinitis, right hip

M76.02 Gluteal tendinitis, left hip

M76.1 Psoas tendinitis

M76.10 Psoas tendinitis, unspecified hip

M76.11 Psoas tendinitis, right hip

M76.12 Psoas tendinitis, left hip

M76.2 Iliac crest spur

M76.20 Iliac crest spur, unspecified hip

M76.21 Iliac crest spur, right hip

M76.22 Iliac crest spur, left hip

M76.3 Iliotibial band syndrome

M76.30 Iliotibial band syndrome, unspecified leg

M76.31 Iliotibial band syndrome, right leg

M76.32 Iliotibial band syndrome, left leg

M76.4 Tibial collateral bursitis [Pellegrini-Stieda]

M76.40 Tibial collateral bursitis [Pellegrini-Stieda], unspecified leg

M76.41 Tibial collateral bursitis [Pellegrini-Stieda], right leg

M76.42 Tibial collateral bursitis [Pellegrini-Stieda], left leg

M76.5 Patellar tendinitis

M76.50 Patellar tendinitis, unspecified knee

M76.51 Patellar tendinitis, right knee

M76.52 Patellar tendinitis, left knee

M76.6 Achilles tendinitis

Achilles bursitis

M76.60 Achilles tendinitis, unspecified leg

M76.61 Achilles tendinitis, right leg
M76.62 Achilles tendinitis, left leg
M76.7 Peroneal tendinitis
  M76.70 Peroneal tendinitis, unspecified leg
  M76.71 Peroneal tendinitis, right leg
  M76.72 Peroneal tendinitis, left leg
M76.8 Other specified enthesopathies of lower limb, excluding foot
  M76.81 Anterior tibial syndrome
    M76.811 Anterior tibial syndrome, right leg
    M76.812 Anterior tibial syndrome, left leg
    M76.819 Anterior tibial syndrome, unspecified leg
  M76.82 Posterior tibial tendinitis
    M76.821 Posterior tibial tendinitis, right leg
    M76.822 Posterior tibial tendinitis, left leg
    M76.829 Posterior tibial tendinitis, unspecified leg
  M76.89 Other specified enthesopathies of lower limb, excluding foot
    M76.891 Other specified enthesopathies of right lower limb, excluding foot
    M76.892 Other specified enthesopathies of left lower limb, excluding foot
    M76.899 Other specified enthesopathies of unspecified lower limb, excluding foot
M76.9 Unspecified enthesopathy, lower limb, excluding foot
M77 Other enthesopathies
Excludes 1: bursitis NOS (M71.9-)
Excludes 2: bursitis due to use, overuse and pressure (M70.-)
  osteophyte (M25.7)
  spinal enthesopathy (M46.0-)
M77.0 Medial epicondylitis
  M77.00 Medial epicondylitis, unspecified elbow
  M77.01 Medial epicondylitis, right elbow
  M77.02 Medial epicondylitis, left elbow
M77.1 Lateral epicondylitis
Tennis elbow
  M77.10 Lateral epicondylitis, unspecified elbow
  M77.11 Lateral epicondylitis, right elbow
  M77.12 Lateral epicondylitis, left elbow
M77.2 Periarthritis of wrist
  M77.20 Periarthritis, unspecified wrist
  M77.21 Periarthritis, right wrist
  M77.22 Periarthritis, left wrist
M77.3 Calcaneal spur
  M77.30 Calcaneal spur, unspecified foot
  M77.31 Calcaneal spur, right foot
  M77.32 Calcaneal spur, left foot
M77.4 Metatarsalgia
Excludes 1: Morton's metatarsalgia (G57.6)
  M77.40 Metatarsalgia, unspecified foot
  M77.41 Metatarsalgia, right foot
  M77.42 Metatarsalgia, left foot
M77.5 Other enthesopathy of foot
  M77.50 Other enthesopathy of unspecified foot
  M77.51 Other enthesopathy of right foot
  M77.52 Other enthesopathy of left foot

M77.8 Other enthesopathies, not elsewhere classified
M77.9 Enthesopathy, unspecified
Bone spur NOS
Capsulitis NOS
Periarthritis NOS
Tendinitis NOS
M79 Other and unspecified soft tissue disorders, not elsewhere classified
Excludes 1: psychogenic rheumatism (F45.8)
  soft tissue pain, psychogenic (F45.41)
M79.0 Rheumatism, unspecified
Excludes 1: fibromyalgia (M79.7)
  palindromic rheumatism (M12.3-)
M79.1 Myalgia
Myofascial pain syndrome
Excludes 1: fibromyalgia (M79.7)
  myositis (M60.-)
M79.2 Neuralgia and neuritis, unspecified
Excludes 1: brachial radiculitis NOS (M54.1)
  lumbosacral radiculitis NOS (M54.1)
  mononeuropathies (G56-G58)
  radiculitis NOS (M54.1)
  sciatica (M54.3-M54.4)
M79.3 Panniculitis, unspecified
Excludes 1: lupus panniculitis (L93.2)
  neck and back panniculitis (M54.0-)
  relapsing [Weber-Christian] panniculitis (M35.6)
M79.4 Hypertrophy of (infrapatellar) fat pad
M79.5 Residual foreign body in soft tissue
Excludes 1: foreign body granuloma of skin and subcutaneous tissue (L92.3)
  foreign body granuloma of soft tissue (M60.2-)
M79.6 Pain in limb, hand, foot, fingers and toes
Excludes 2: pain in joint (M25.5-)
  M79.60 Pain in limb, unspecified
    M79.601 Pain in right arm
      Pain in right upper limb NOS
    M79.602 Pain in left arm
      Pain in left upper limb NOS
    M79.603 Pain in arm, unspecified
      Pain in upper limb NOS
    M79.604 Pain in right leg
      Pain in right lower limb NOS
    M79.605 Pain in left leg
      Pain in left lower limb NOS
    M79.606 Pain in leg, unspecified
      Pain in lower limb NOS
    M79.609 Pain in unspecified limb
      Pain in limb NOS
  M79.62 Pain in upper arm
  Pain in axillary region
    M79.621 Pain in right upper arm
    M79.622 Pain in left upper arm
    M79.629 Pain in unspecified upper arm
  M79.63 Pain in forearm
    M79.631 Pain in right forearm
    M79.632 Pain in left forearm
    M79.639 Pain in unspecified forearm
  M79.64 Pain in hand and fingers
    M79.641 Pain in right hand

M79.642 Pain in left hand

M79.643 Pain in unspecified hand

M79.644 Pain in right finger(s)

M79.645 Pain in left finger(s)

M79.646 Pain in unspecified finger(s)

M79.65 Pain in thigh

M79.651 Pain in right thigh

M79.652 Pain in left thigh

M79.659 Pain in unspecified thigh

M79.66 Pain in lower leg

M79.661 Pain in right lower leg

M79.662 Pain in left lower leg

M79.669 Pain in unspecified lower leg

M79.67 Pain in foot and toes

M79.671 Pain in right foot

M79.672 Pain in left foot

M79.673 Pain in unspecified foot

M79.674 Pain in right toe(s)

M79.675 Pain in left toe(s)

M79.676 Pain in unspecified toe(s)

M79.7 Fibromyalgia

Fibromyositis

Fibrositis

Myofibrositis

M79.A Nontraumatic compartment syndrome

Code first , if applicable, associated postprocedural complication

Excludes 1: compartment syndrome NOS (T79.A-)

fibromyalgia (M79.7)

nontraumatic ischemic infarction of muscle (M62.2-)

traumatic compartment syndrome (T79.A-)

M79.A1 Nontraumatic compartment syndrome of upper extremity

Nontraumatic compartment syndrome of shoulder, arm, forearm, wrist, hand, and fingers

M79.A11 Nontraumatic compartment syndrome of right upper extremity

M79.A12 Nontraumatic compartment syndrome of left upper extremity

M79.A19 Nontraumatic compartment syndrome of unspecified upper extremity

M79.A2 Nontraumatic compartment syndrome of lower extremity

Nontraumatic compartment syndrome of hip, buttock, thigh, leg, foot, and toes

M79.A21 Nontraumatic compartment syndrome of right lower extremity

M79.A22 Nontraumatic compartment syndrome of left lower extremity

M79.A29 Nontraumatic compartment syndrome of unspecified lower extremity

M79.A3 Nontraumatic compartment syndrome of abdomen

M79.A9 Nontraumatic compartment syndrome of other sites

M79.8 Other specified soft tissue disorders

M79.81 Nontraumatic hematoma of soft tissue

Nontraumatic hematoma of muscle

Nontraumatic seroma of muscle and soft tissue

M79.89 Other specified soft tissue disorders

Polyalgia

M79.9 Soft tissue disorder, unspecified

OSTEOPATHIES AND CHONDROPATHIES (M80-M94)
DISORDERS OF BONE DENSITY AND STRUCTURE (M80-M85)

M80 Osteoporosis with current pathological fracture

Includes: osteoporosis with current fragility fracture

Use additional code to identify major osseous defect, if applicable (M89.7-)

Excludes 1: collapsed vertebra NOS (M48.5)

pathological fracture NOS (M84.4)

wedging of vertebra NOS (M48.5)

Excludes 2: personal history of (healed) osteoporosis fracture (Z87.310)

The appropriate M5 character is to be added to each code from category M80:

A - initial encounter for fracture

D - subsequent encounter for fracture with routine healing

G - subsequent encounter for fracture with delayed healing

K - subsequent encounter for fracture with nonunion

P - subsequent encounter for fracture with malunion

S - sequela

M80.0 Age-related osteoporosis with current pathological fracture

Involutional osteoporosis with current pathological fracture

Osteoporosis NOS with current pathological fracture

Postmenopausal osteoporosis with current pathological fracture

Senile osteoporosis with current pathological fracture

M80.00 Age-related osteoporosis with current pathological fracture, unspecified site

M80.01 Age-related osteoporosis with current pathological fracture, shoulder

M80.011 Age-related osteoporosis with current pathological fracture, right shoulder

M80.012 Age-related osteoporosis with current pathological fracture, left shoulder

M80.019 Age-related osteoporosis with current pathological fracture, unspecified shoulder

M80.02 Age-related osteoporosis with current pathological fracture, humerus

M80.021 Age-related osteoporosis with current pathological fracture, right humerus

M80.022 Age-related osteoporosis with current pathological fracture, left humerus

M80.029 Age-related osteoporosis with current pathological fracture, unspecified humerus

M80.03 Age-related osteoporosis with current pathological fracture, forearm

Age-related osteoporosis with current pathological fracture of wrist

● New code   ▲ Revised code   ⑦ 7th digit required   ⊗ Placeholder required

M80.031 Age-related osteoporosis with current pathological fracture, right forearm

M80.032 Age-related osteoporosis with current pathological fracture, left forearm

M80.039 Age-related osteoporosis with current pathological fracture, unspecified forearm

M80.04 Age-related osteoporosis with current pathological fracture, hand

M80.041 Age-related osteoporosis with current pathological fracture, right hand

M80.042 Age-related osteoporosis with current pathological fracture, left hand

M80.049 Age-related osteoporosis with current pathological fracture, unspecified hand

M80.05 Age-related osteoporosis with current pathological fracture, femur

Age-related osteoporosis with current pathological fracture of hip

M80.051 Age-related osteoporosis with current pathological fracture, right femur

M80.052 Age-related osteoporosis with current pathological fracture, left femur

M80.059 Age-related osteoporosis with current pathological fracture, unspecified femur

M80.06 Age-related osteoporosis with current pathological fracture, lower leg

M80.061 Age-related osteoporosis with current pathological fracture, right lower leg

M80.062 Age-related osteoporosis with current pathological fracture, left lower leg

M80.069 Age-related osteoporosis with current pathological fracture, unspecified lower leg

M80.07 Age-related osteoporosis with current pathological fracture, ankle and foot

M80.071 Age-related osteoporosis with current pathological fracture, right ankle and foot

M80.072 Age-related osteoporosis with current pathological fracture, left ankle and foot

M80.079 Age-related osteoporosis with current pathological fracture, unspecified ankle and foot

M80.08 Age-related osteoporosis with current pathological fracture, vertebra(e)

M80.8 Other osteoporosis with current pathological fracture

Drug-induced osteoporosis with current pathological fracture

Idiopathic osteoporosis with current pathological fracture

Osteoporosis of disuse with current pathological fracture

Post oophorectomy osteoporosis with current pathological fracture

Postsurgical malabsorption osteoporosis with current pathological fracture

Post-traumatic osteoporosis with current pathological fracture

Use additional code for adverse effect, if applicable, to identify drug (T36-T50 with fifth or sixth character 5)

M80.80 Other osteoporosis with current pathological fracture, unspecified site

M80.81 Other osteoporosis with pathological fracture, shoulder

M80.811 Other osteoporosis with current pathological fracture, right shoulder

M80.812 Other osteoporosis with current pathological fracture, left shoulder

M80.819 Other osteoporosis with current pathological fracture, unspecified shoulder

M80.82 Other osteoporosis with current pathological fracture, humerus

M80.821 Other osteoporosis with current pathological fracture, right humerus

M80.822 Other osteoporosis with current pathological fracture, left humerus

M80.829 Other osteoporosis with current pathological fracture, unspecified humerus

M80.83 Other osteoporosis with current pathological fracture, forearm

Other osteoporosis with current pathological fracture of wrist

M80.831 Other osteoporosis with current pathological fracture, right forearm

M80.832 Other osteoporosis with current pathological fracture, left forearm

M80.839 Other osteoporosis with current pathological fracture, unspecified forearm

M80.84 Other osteoporosis with current pathological fracture, hand

M80.841 Other osteoporosis with current pathological fracture, right hand

M80.842 Other osteoporosis with current pathological fracture, left hand

M80.849 Other osteoporosis with current pathological fracture, unspecified hand

M80.85 Other osteoporosis with current pathological fracture, femur

Other osteoporosis with current pathological fracture of hip

M80.851 Other osteoporosis with current pathological fracture, right femur

M80.852 Other osteoporosis with current pathological fracture, left femur

M80.859 Other osteoporosis with current pathological fracture, unspecified femur

M80.86 Other osteoporosis with current pathological fracture, lower leg

M80.861 Other osteoporosis with current pathological fracture, right lower leg

M80.862 Other osteoporosis with current pathological fracture, left lower leg

M80.869 Other osteoporosis with current pathological fracture, unspecified lower leg

M80.87 Other osteoporosis with current pathological fracture, ankle and foot

M80.871 Other osteoporosis with current pathological fracture, right ankle and foot

M80.872 Other osteoporosis with current pathological fracture, left ankle and foot

M80.879 Other osteoporosis with current pathological fracture, unspecified ankle and foot

M80.88 Other osteoporosis with current pathological fracture, vertebra(e)

M81 Osteoporosis without current pathological fracture

Use additional code to identify:

major osseous defect, if applicable (M89.7-)

personal history of (healed) osteoporosis fracture, if applicable (Z87.310)

Excludes 1: osteoporosis with current pathological fracture (M80.-)

Sudeck's atrophy (M89.0)

M81.0 Age-related osteoporosis without current pathological fracture

Involutional osteoporosis without current pathological fracture

Osteoporosis NOS

Postmenopausal osteoporosis without current pathological fracture

Senile osteoporosis without current pathological fracture

M81.6 Localized osteoporosis [Lequesne]

Excludes 1: Sudeck's atrophy (M89.0)

M81.8 Other osteoporosis without current pathological fracture

Drug-induced osteoporosis without current pathological fracture

Idiopathic osteoporosis without current pathological fracture

Osteoporosis of disuse without current pathological fracture

Post oophorectomy osteoporosis without current pathological fracture

Postsurgical malabsorption osteoporosis without current pathological fracture

Post-traumatic osteoporosis without current pathological fracture

Use additional code for adverse effect, if applicable, to identify drug (T36-T50 with fifth or sixth character 5)

M83 Adult osteomalacia

Excludes 1: infantile and juvenile osteomalacia (E55.0)

renal osteodystrophy (N25.0)

rickets (active) (E55.0)

rickets (active) sequelae (E64.3)

vitamin D-resistant osteomalacia (E83.3)

vitamin D-resistant rickets (active) (E83.3)

M83.0 Puerperal osteomalacia

M83.1 Senile osteomalacia

M83.2 Adult osteomalacia due to malabsorption

Postsurgical malabsorption osteomalacia in adults

M83.3 Adult osteomalacia due to malnutrition

M83.4 Aluminum bone disease

M83.5 Other drug-induced osteomalacia in adults

Use additional code for adverse effect, if applicable, to identify drug (T36-T50 with fifth or sixth character 5)

M83.8 Other adult osteomalacia

M83.9 Adult osteomalacia, unspecified

M84 Disorder of continuity of bone

Excludes 2: traumatic fracture of bone-see fracture, by site

M84.3 Stress fracture

Fatigue fracture

March fracture

Stress fracture NOS

Stress reaction

Use additional external cause code(s) to identify the cause of the stress fracture

Excludes 1: pathological fracture NOS (M84.4.-)

pathological fracture due to osteoporosis (M80.-)

traumatic fracture (S12.-, S22.-, S32.-, S42.-, S52.-, S62.-, S72.-, S82.-, S92.-)

Excludes 2: personal history of (healed) stress (fatigue) fracture (Z87.312)

stress fracture of vertebra (M48.4-)

The appropriate 7th character is to be added to each code from subcategory M84.3:

A - initial encounter for fracture

D - subsequent encounter for fracture with routine healing

G - subsequent encounter for fracture with delayed healing

K - subsequent encounter for fracture with nonunion

P - subsequent encounter for fracture with malunion

S - sequela

⊗⑦**M84.30** Stress fracture, unspecified site

M84.31 Stress fracture, shoulder

⑦**M84.311** Stress fracture, right shoulder

⑦**M84.312** Stress fracture, left shoulder

⑦**M84.319** Stress fracture, unspecified shoulder

M84.32 Stress fracture, humerus

⑦**M84.321** Stress fracture, right humerus

⑦**M84.322** Stress fracture, left humerus

⑦**M84.329** Stress fracture, unspecified humerus

M84.33 Stress fracture, ulna and radius

⑦**M84.331** Stress fracture, right ulna

⑦**M84.332** Stress fracture, left ulna

⑦**M84.333** Stress fracture, right radius

⑦**M84.334** Stress fracture, left radius

⑦**M84.339** Stress fracture, unspecified ulna and radius

M84.34 Stress fracture, hand and fingers

⑦**M84.341** Stress fracture, right hand

⑦**M84.342** Stress fracture, left hand

⑦**M84.343** Stress fracture, unspecified hand

⑦**M84.344** Stress fracture, right finger(s)

⑦**M84.345** Stress fracture, left finger(s)

⑦**M84.346** Stress fracture, unspecified finger(s)

M84.35 Stress fracture, pelvis and femur

Stress fracture, hip

⑦**M84.350**   Stress fracture, pelvis

⑦**M84.351**   Stress fracture, right femur

⑦**M84.352**   Stress fracture, left femur

⑦**M84.353**   Stress fracture, unspecified femur

⑦**M84.359**   Stress fracture, hip, unspecified

M84.36   Stress fracture, tibia and fibula

⑦**M84.361**   Stress fracture, right tibia

⑦**M84.362**   Stress fracture, left tibia

⑦**M84.363**   Stress fracture, right fibula

⑦**M84.364**   Stress fracture, left fibula

⑦**M84.369**   Stress fracture, unspecified tibia and fibula

M84.37   Stress fracture, ankle, foot and toes

⑦**M84.371**   Stress fracture, right ankle

⑦**M84.372**   Stress fracture, left ankle

⑦**M84.373**   Stress fracture, unspecified ankle

⑦**M84.374**   Stress fracture, right foot

⑦**M84.375**   Stress fracture, left foot

⑦**M84.376**   Stress fracture, unspecified foot

⑦**M84.377**   Stress fracture, right toe(s)

⑦**M84.378**   Stress fracture, left toe(s)

⑦**M84.379**   Stress fracture, unspecified toe(s)

⊗⑦**M84.38**   Stress fracture, other site

Excludes 2: stress fracture of vertebra (M48.4-)

M84.4   Pathological fracture, not elsewhere classified

Chronic fracture

Pathological fracture NOS

Excludes 1: collapsed vertebra NEC (M48.5)

pathological fracture in neoplastic disease (M84.5-)

pathological fracture in osteoporosis (M80.-)

pathological fracture in other disease (M84.6-)

stress fracture (M84.3-)

traumatic fracture (S12.-, S22.-, S32.-, S42.-, S52.-, S62.-, S72.-, S82.-, S92.-)

Excludes 2: personal history of (healed) pathological fracture (Z87.311)

The appropriate 7th character is to be added to each code from subcategory M84.4:

A - initial encounter for fracture

D - subsequent encounter for fracture with routine healing

G - subsequent encounter for fracture with delayed healing

K - subsequent encounter for fracture with nonunion

P - subsequent encounter for fracture with malunion

S - sequela

⊗⑦**M84.40**   Pathological fracture, unspecified site

M84.41   Pathological fracture, shoulder

⑦**M84.411**   Pathological fracture, right shoulder

⑦**M84.412**   Pathological fracture, left shoulder

⑦**M84.419**   Pathological fracture, unspecified shoulder

M84.42   Pathological fracture, humerus

⑦**M84.421**   Pathological fracture, right humerus

⑦**M84.422**   Pathological fracture, left humerus

⑦**M84.429**   Pathological fracture, unspecified humerus

M84.43   Pathological fracture, ulna and radius

⑦**M84.431**   Pathological fracture, right ulna

⑦**M84.432**   Pathological fracture, left ulna

⑦**M84.433**   Pathological fracture, right radius

⑦**M84.434**   Pathological fracture, left radius

⑦**M84.439**   Pathological fracture, unspecified ulna and radius

M84.44   Pathological fracture, hand and fingers

⑦**M84.441**   Pathological fracture, right hand

⑦**M84.442**   Pathological fracture, left hand

⑦**M84.443**   Pathological fracture, unspecified hand

⑦**M84.444**   Pathological fracture, right finger(s)

⑦**M84.445**   Pathological fracture, left finger(s)

⑦**M84.446**   Pathological fracture, unspecified finger(s)

M84.45   Pathological fracture, femur and pelvis

⑦**M84.451**   Pathological fracture, right femur

⑦**M84.452**   Pathological fracture, left femur

⑦**M84.453**   Pathological fracture, unspecified femur

⑦**M84.454**   Pathological fracture, pelvis

⑦**M84.459**   Pathological fracture, hip, unspecified

M84.46   Pathological fracture, tibia and fibula

⑦**M84.461**   Pathological fracture, right tibia

⑦**M84.462**   Pathological fracture, left tibia

⑦**M84.463**   Pathological fracture, right fibula

⑦**M84.464**   Pathological fracture, left fibula

⑦**M84.469**   Pathological fracture, unspecified tibia and fibula

M84.47   Pathological fracture, ankle, foot and toes

⑦**M84.471**   Pathological fracture, right ankle

⑦**M84.472**   Pathological fracture, left ankle

⑦**M84.473**   Pathological fracture, unspecified ankle

⑦**M84.474**   Pathological fracture, right foot

⑦**M84.475**   Pathological fracture, left foot

⑦**M84.476**   Pathological fracture, unspecified foot

⑦**M84.477**   Pathological fracture, right toe(s)

⑦**M84.478**   Pathological fracture, left toe(s)

⑦**M84.479**   Pathological fracture, unspecified toe(s)

⊗⑦**M84.48**   Pathological fracture, other site

M84.5   Pathological fracture in neoplastic disease

Code also underlying neoplasm

The appropriate 7th character is to be added to each code from subcategory M84.5:

A - initial encounter for fracture

D - subsequent encounter for fracture with routine healing

G - subsequent encounter for fracture with delayed healing

K - subsequent encounter for fracture with nonunion

P - subsequent encounter for fracture with malunion

S - sequela

⊗⑦**M84.50**   Pathological fracture in neoplastic disease, unspecified site

M84.51 Pathological fracture in neoplastic disease, shoulder

⑦**M84.511** Pathological fracture in neoplastic disease, right shoulder

⑦**M84.512** Pathological fracture in neoplastic disease, left shoulder

⑦**M84.519** Pathological fracture in neoplastic disease, unspecified shoulder

M84.52 Pathological fracture in neoplastic disease, humerus

⑦**M84.521** Pathological fracture in neoplastic disease, right humerus

⑦**M84.522** Pathological fracture in neoplastic disease, left humerus

⑦**M84.529** Pathological fracture in neoplastic disease, unspecified humerus

M84.53 Pathological fracture in neoplastic disease, ulna and radius

⑦**M84.531** Pathological fracture in neoplastic disease, right ulna

⑦**M84.532** Pathological fracture in neoplastic disease, left ulna

⑦**M84.533** Pathological fracture in neoplastic disease, right radius

⑦**M84.534** Pathological fracture in neoplastic disease, left radius

⑦**M84.539** Pathological fracture in neoplastic disease, unspecified ulna and radius

M84.54 Pathological fracture in neoplastic disease, hand

⑦**M84.541** Pathological fracture in neoplastic disease, right hand

⑦**M84.542** Pathological fracture in neoplastic disease, left hand

⑦**M84.549** Pathological fracture in neoplastic disease, unspecified hand

M84.55 Pathological fracture in neoplastic disease, pelvis and femur

⑦**M84.550** Pathological fracture in neoplastic disease, pelvis

⑦**M84.551** Pathological fracture in neoplastic disease, right femur

⑦**M84.552** Pathological fracture in neoplastic disease, left femur

⑦**M84.553** Pathological fracture in neoplastic disease, unspecified femur

⑦**M84.559** Pathological fracture in neoplastic disease, hip, unspecified

M84.56 Pathological fracture in neoplastic disease, tibia and fibula

⑦**M84.561** Pathological fracture in neoplastic disease, right tibia

⑦**M84.562** Pathological fracture in neoplastic disease, left tibia

⑦**M84.563** Pathological fracture in neoplastic disease, right fibula

⑦**M84.564** Pathological fracture in neoplastic disease, left fibula

⑦**M84.569** Pathological fracture in neoplastic disease, unspecified tibia and fibula

M84.57 Pathological fracture in neoplastic disease, ankle and foot

⑦**M84.571** Pathological fracture in neoplastic disease, right ankle

⑦**M84.572** Pathological fracture in neoplastic disease, left ankle

⑦**M84.573** Pathological fracture in neoplastic disease, unspecified ankle

⑦**M84.574** Pathological fracture in neoplastic disease, right foot

⑦**M84.575** Pathological fracture in neoplastic disease, left foot

⑦**M84.576** Pathological fracture in neoplastic disease, unspecified foot

▲⊗⑦**M84.58** Pathological fracture in neoplastic disease, other specified site

M84.6 Pathological fracture in other disease

Code also underlying condition

Excludes 1: pathological fracture in osteoporosis (M80.-)

The appropriate 7th character is to be added to each code from subcategory M84.6:

A - initial encounter for fracture

D - subsequent encounter for fracture with routine healing

G - subsequent encounter for fracture with delayed healing

K - subsequent encounter for fracture with nonunion

P - subsequent encounter for fracture with malunion

S - sequela

⊗⑦**M84.60** Pathological fracture in other disease, unspecified site

M84.61 Pathological fracture in other disease, shoulder

⑦**M84.611** Pathological fracture in other disease, right shoulder

⑦**M84.612** Pathological fracture in other disease, left shoulder

⑦**M84.619** Pathological fracture in other disease, unspecified shoulder

M84.62 Pathological fracture in other disease, humerus

⑦**M84.621** Pathological fracture in other disease, right humerus

⑦**M84.622** Pathological fracture in other disease, left humerus

⑦**M84.629** Pathological fracture in other disease, unspecified humerus

M84.63 Pathological fracture in other disease, ulna and radius

⑦**M84.631** Pathological fracture in other disease, right ulna

⑦**M84.632** Pathological fracture in other disease, left ulna

⑦**M84.633** Pathological fracture in other disease, right radius

⑦**M84.634** Pathological fracture in other disease, left radius

⑦**M84.639** Pathological fracture in other disease, unspecified ulna and radius

M84.64 Pathological fracture in other disease, hand

⑦**M84.641** Pathological fracture in other disease, right hand

⑦M84.642 Pathological fracture in other disease, left hand

⑦M84.649 Pathological fracture in other disease, unspecified hand

M84.65 Pathological fracture in other disease, pelvis and femur

⑦M84.650 Pathological fracture in other disease, pelvis

⑦M84.651 Pathological fracture in other disease, right femur

⑦M84.652 Pathological fracture in other disease, left femur

⑦M84.653 Pathological fracture in other disease, unspecified femur

⑦M84.659 Pathological fracture in other disease, hip, unspecified

M84.66 Pathological fracture in other disease, tibia and fibula

⑦M84.661 Pathological fracture in other disease, right tibia

⑦M84.662 Pathological fracture in other disease, left tibia

⑦M84.663 Pathological fracture in other disease, right fibula

⑦M84.664 Pathological fracture in other disease, left fibula

⑦M84.669 Pathological fracture in other disease, unspecified tibia and fibula

M84.67 Pathological fracture in other disease, ankle and foot

⑦M84.671 Pathological fracture in other disease, right ankle

⑦M84.672 Pathological fracture in other disease, left ankle

⑦M84.673 Pathological fracture in other disease, unspecified ankle

⑦M84.674 Pathological fracture in other disease, right foot

⑦M84.675 Pathological fracture in other disease, left foot

⑦M84.676 Pathological fracture in other disease, unspecified foot

⊗⑦M84.68 Pathological fracture in other disease, other site

M84.8 Other disorders of continuity of bone

⊗⑦M84.80 Other disorders of continuity of bone, unspecified site

M84.81 Other disorders of continuity of bone, shoulder

⑦M84.811 Other disorders of continuity of bone, right shoulder

⑦M84.812 Other disorders of continuity of bone, left shoulder

⑦M84.819 Other disorders of continuity of bone, unspecified shoulder

M84.82 Other disorders of continuity of bone, humerus

⑦M84.821 Other disorders of continuity of bone, right humerus

⑦M84.822 Other disorders of continuity of bone, left humerus

⑦M84.829 Other disorders of continuity of bone, unspecified humerus

M84.83 Other disorders of continuity of bone, ulna and radius

⑦M84.831 Other disorders of continuity of bone, right ulna

⑦M84.832 Other disorders of continuity of bone, left ulna

⑦M84.833 Other disorders of continuity of bone, right radius

⑦M84.834 Other disorders of continuity of bone, left radius

⑦M84.839 Other disorders of continuity of bone, unspecified ulna and radius

M84.84 Other disorders of continuity of bone, hand

⑦M84.841 Other disorders of continuity of bone, right hand

⑦M84.842 Other disorders of continuity of bone, left hand

⑦M84.849 Other disorders of continuity of bone, unspecified hand

M84.85 Other disorders of continuity of bone, pelvic region and thigh

⑦M84.851 Other disorders of continuity of bone, right pelvic region and thigh

⑦M84.852 Other disorders of continuity of bone, left pelvic region and thigh

⑦M84.859 Other disorders of continuity of bone, unspecified pelvic region and thigh

M84.86 Other disorders of continuity of bone, tibia and fibula

⑦M84.861 Other disorders of continuity of bone, right tibia

⑦M84.862 Other disorders of continuity of bone, left tibia

⑦M84.863 Other disorders of continuity of bone, right fibula

⑦M84.864 Other disorders of continuity of bone, left fibula

⑦M84.869 Other disorders of continuity of bone, unspecified tibia and fibula

M84.87 Other disorders of continuity of bone, ankle and foot

⑦M84.871 Other disorders of continuity of bone, right ankle and foot

⑦M84.872 Other disorders of continuity of bone, left ankle and foot

⑦M84.879 Other disorders of continuity of bone, unspecified ankle and foot

⊗⑦M84.88 Other disorders of continuity of bone, other site

M84.9 Disorder of continuity of bone, unspecified

M85 Other disorders of bone density and structure

Excludes 1: osteogenesis imperfecta (Q78.0)
osteopetrosis (Q78.2)
osteopoikilosis (Q78.8)
polyostotic fibrous dysplasia (Q78.1)

M85.0 Fibrous dysplasia (monostotic)
Excludes 2: fibrous dysplasia of jaw (M27.8)

M85.00 Fibrous dysplasia (monostotic), unspecified site

M85.01 Fibrous dysplasia (monostotic), shoulder

    M85.011 Fibrous dysplasia (monostotic), right shoulder

    M85.012 Fibrous dysplasia (monostotic), left shoulder

    M85.019 Fibrous dysplasia (monostotic), unspecified shoulder

M85.02 Fibrous dysplasia (monostotic), upper arm

    M85.021 Fibrous dysplasia (monostotic), right upper arm

    M85.022 Fibrous dysplasia (monostotic), left upper arm

    M85.029 Fibrous dysplasia (monostotic), unspecified upper arm

M85.03 Fibrous dysplasia (monostotic), forearm

    M85.031 Fibrous dysplasia (monostotic), right forearm

    M85.032 Fibrous dysplasia (monostotic), left forearm

    M85.039 Fibrous dysplasia (monostotic), unspecified forearm

M85.04 Fibrous dysplasia (monostotic), hand

    M85.041 Fibrous dysplasia (monostotic), right hand

    M85.042 Fibrous dysplasia (monostotic), left hand

    M85.049 Fibrous dysplasia (monostotic), unspecified hand

M85.05 Fibrous dysplasia (monostotic), thigh

    M85.051 Fibrous dysplasia (monostotic), right thigh

    M85.052 Fibrous dysplasia (monostotic), left thigh

    M85.059 Fibrous dysplasia (monostotic), unspecified thigh

M85.06 Fibrous dysplasia (monostotic), lower leg

    M85.061 Fibrous dysplasia (monostotic), right lower leg

    M85.062 Fibrous dysplasia (monostotic), left lower leg

    M85.069 Fibrous dysplasia (monostotic), unspecified lower leg

M85.07 Fibrous dysplasia (monostotic), ankle and foot

    M85.071 Fibrous dysplasia (monostotic), right ankle and foot

    M85.072 Fibrous dysplasia (monostotic), left ankle and foot

    M85.079 Fibrous dysplasia (monostotic), unspecified ankle and foot

M85.08 Fibrous dysplasia (monostotic), other site

M85.09 Fibrous dysplasia (monostotic), multiple sites

M85.1 Skeletal fluorosis

M85.10 Skeletal fluorosis, unspecified site

M85.11 Skeletal fluorosis, shoulder

    M85.111 Skeletal fluorosis, right shoulder

    M85.112 Skeletal fluorosis, left shoulder

    M85.119 Skeletal fluorosis, unspecified shoulder

M85.12 Skeletal fluorosis, upper arm

    M85.121 Skeletal fluorosis, right upper arm

    M85.122 Skeletal fluorosis, left upper arm

    M85.129 Skeletal fluorosis, unspecified upper arm

M85.13 Skeletal fluorosis, forearm

    M85.131 Skeletal fluorosis, right forearm

    M85.132 Skeletal fluorosis, left forearm

    M85.139 Skeletal fluorosis, unspecified forearm

M85.14 Skeletal fluorosis, hand

    M85.141 Skeletal fluorosis, right hand

    M85.142 Skeletal fluorosis, left hand

    M85.149 Skeletal fluorosis, unspecified hand

M85.15 Skeletal fluorosis, thigh

    M85.151 Skeletal fluorosis, right thigh

    M85.152 Skeletal fluorosis, left thigh

    M85.159 Skeletal fluorosis, unspecified thigh

M85.16 Skeletal fluorosis, lower leg

    M85.161 Skeletal fluorosis, right lower leg

    M85.162 Skeletal fluorosis, left lower leg

    M85.169 Skeletal fluorosis, unspecified lower leg

M85.17 Skeletal fluorosis, ankle and foot

    M85.171 Skeletal fluorosis, right ankle and foot

    M85.172 Skeletal fluorosis, left ankle and foot

    M85.179 Skeletal fluorosis, unspecified ankle and foot

M85.18 Skeletal fluorosis, other site

M85.19 Skeletal fluorosis, multiple sites

M85.2 Hyperostosis of skull

M85.3 Osteitis condensans

M85.30 Osteitis condensans, unspecified site

M85.31 Osteitis condensans, shoulder

    M85.311 Osteitis condensans, right shoulder

    M85.312 Osteitis condensans, left shoulder

    M85.319 Osteitis condensans, unspecified shoulder

M85.32 Osteitis condensans, upper arm

    M85.321 Osteitis condensans, right upper arm

    M85.322 Osteitis condensans, left upper arm

    M85.329 Osteitis condensans, unspecified upper arm

M85.33 Osteitis condensans, forearm

    M85.331 Osteitis condensans, right forearm

    M85.332 Osteitis condensans, left forearm

    M85.339 Osteitis condensans, unspecified forearm

M85.34 Osteitis condensans, hand

    M85.341 Osteitis condensans, right hand

    M85.342 Osteitis condensans, left hand

    M85.349 Osteitis condensans, unspecified hand

M85.35 Osteitis condensans, thigh

    M85.351 Osteitis condensans, right thigh

    M85.352 Osteitis condensans, left thigh

    M85.359 Osteitis condensans, unspecified thigh

M85.36 Osteitis condensans, lower leg

● New code   ▲ Revised code   ⑦ 7th digit required   ⊗ Placeholder required

M85.361 Osteitis condensans, right lower leg
M85.362 Osteitis condensans, left lower leg
M85.369 Osteitis condensans, unspecified lower leg
M85.37 Osteitis condensans, ankle and foot
    M85.371 Osteitis condensans, right ankle and foot
    M85.372 Osteitis condensans, left ankle and foot
    M85.379 Osteitis condensans, unspecified ankle and foot
M85.38 Osteitis condensans, other site
M85.39 Osteitis condensans, multiple sites
M85.4 Solitary bone cyst
    Excludes 2: solitary cyst of jaw (M27.4)
M85.40 Solitary bone cyst, unspecified site
M85.41 Solitary bone cyst, shoulder
    M85.411 Solitary bone cyst, right shoulder
    M85.412 Solitary bone cyst, left shoulder
    M85.419 Solitary bone cyst, unspecified shoulder
M85.42 Solitary bone cyst, humerus
    M85.421 Solitary bone cyst, right humerus
    M85.422 Solitary bone cyst, left humerus
    M85.429 Solitary bone cyst, unspecified humerus
M85.43 Solitary bone cyst, ulna and radius
    M85.431 Solitary bone cyst, right ulna and radius
    M85.432 Solitary bone cyst, left ulna and radius
    M85.439 Solitary bone cyst, unspecified ulna and radius
M85.44 Solitary bone cyst, hand
    M85.441 Solitary bone cyst, right hand
    M85.442 Solitary bone cyst, left hand
    M85.449 Solitary bone cyst, unspecified hand
M85.45 Solitary bone cyst, pelvis
    M85.451 Solitary bone cyst, right pelvis
    M85.452 Solitary bone cyst, left pelvis
    M85.459 Solitary bone cyst, unspecified pelvis
M85.46 Solitary bone cyst, tibia and fibula
    M85.461 Solitary bone cyst, right tibia and fibula
    M85.462 Solitary bone cyst, left tibia and fibula
    M85.469 Solitary bone cyst, unspecified tibia and fibula
M85.47 Solitary bone cyst, ankle and foot
    M85.471 Solitary bone cyst, right ankle and foot
    M85.472 Solitary bone cyst, left ankle and foot
    M85.479 Solitary bone cyst, unspecified ankle and foot
M85.48 Solitary bone cyst, other site
M85.5 Aneurysmal bone cyst
    Excludes 2: aneurysmal cyst of jaw (M27.4)
M85.50 Aneurysmal bone cyst, unspecified site

M85.51 Aneurysmal bone cyst, shoulder
    M85.511 Aneurysmal bone cyst, right shoulder
    M85.512 Aneurysmal bone cyst, left shoulder
    M85.519 Aneurysmal bone cyst, unspecified shoulder
M85.52 Aneurysmal bone cyst, upper arm
    M85.521 Aneurysmal bone cyst, right upper arm
    M85.522 Aneurysmal bone cyst, left upper arm
    M85.529 Aneurysmal bone cyst, unspecified upper arm
M85.53 Aneurysmal bone cyst, forearm
    M85.531 Aneurysmal bone cyst, right forearm
    M85.532 Aneurysmal bone cyst, left forearm
    M85.539 Aneurysmal bone cyst, unspecified forearm
M85.54 Aneurysmal bone cyst, hand
    M85.541 Aneurysmal bone cyst, right hand
    M85.542 Aneurysmal bone cyst, left hand
    M85.549 Aneurysmal bone cyst, unspecified hand
M85.55 Aneurysmal bone cyst, thigh
    M85.551 Aneurysmal bone cyst, right thigh
    M85.552 Aneurysmal bone cyst, left thigh
    M85.559 Aneurysmal bone cyst, unspecified thigh
M85.56 Aneurysmal bone cyst, lower leg
    M85.561 Aneurysmal bone cyst, right lower leg
    M85.562 Aneurysmal bone cyst, left lower leg
    M85.569 Aneurysmal bone cyst, unspecified lower leg
M85.57 Aneurysmal bone cyst, ankle and foot
    M85.571 Aneurysmal bone cyst, right ankle and foot
    M85.572 Aneurysmal bone cyst, left ankle and foot
    M85.579 Aneurysmal bone cyst, unspecified ankle and foot
M85.58 Aneurysmal bone cyst, other site
M85.59 Aneurysmal bone cyst, multiple sites
M85.6 Other cyst of bone
    Excludes 1: cyst of jaw NEC (M27.4)
    osteitis fibrosa cystica generalisata [von Recklinghausen's disease of bone] (E21.0)
M85.60 Other cyst of bone, unspecified site
M85.61 Other cyst of bone, shoulder
    M85.611 Other cyst of bone, right shoulder
    M85.612 Other cyst of bone, left shoulder
    M85.619 Other cyst of bone, unspecified shoulder
M85.62 Other cyst of bone, upper arm
    M85.621 Other cyst of bone, right upper arm
    M85.622 Other cyst of bone, left upper arm
    M85.629 Other cyst of bone, unspecified upper arm
M85.63 Other cyst of bone, forearm
    M85.631 Other cyst of bone, right forearm

M85.632 Other cyst of bone, left forearm

M85.639 Other cyst of bone, unspecified forearm

M85.64 Other cyst of bone, hand

M85.641 Other cyst of bone, right hand

M85.642 Other cyst of bone, left hand

M85.649 Other cyst of bone, unspecified hand

M85.65 Other cyst of bone, thigh

M85.651 Other cyst of bone, right thigh

M85.652 Other cyst of bone, left thigh

M85.659 Other cyst of bone, unspecified thigh

M85.66 Other cyst of bone, lower leg

M85.661 Other cyst of bone, right lower leg

M85.662 Other cyst of bone, left lower leg

M85.669 Other cyst of bone, unspecified lower leg

M85.67 Other cyst of bone, ankle and foot

M85.671 Other cyst of bone, right ankle and foot

M85.672 Other cyst of bone, left ankle and foot

M85.679 Other cyst of bone, unspecified ankle and foot

M85.68 Other cyst of bone, other site

M85.69 Other cyst of bone, multiple sites

M85.8 Other specified disorders of bone density and structure

Hyperostosis of bones, except skull

Osteosclerosis, acquired

Excludes 1: diffuse idiopathic skeletal hyperostosis [DISH] (M48.1)

osteosclerosis congenita (Q77.4)

osteosclerosis fragilitas (generalisata) (Q78.2)

osteosclerosis myelofibrosis (D75.81)

M85.80 Other specified disorders of bone density and structure, unspecified site

M85.81 Other specified disorders of bone density and structure, shoulder

M85.811 Other specified disorders of bone density and structure, right shoulder

M85.812 Other specified disorders of bone density and structure, left shoulder

M85.819 Other specified disorders of bone density and structure, unspecified shoulder

M85.82 Other specified disorders of bone density and structure, upper arm

M85.821 Other specified disorders of bone density and structure, right upper arm

M85.822 Other specified disorders of bone density and structure, left upper arm

M85.829 Other specified disorders of bone density and structure, unspecified upper arm

M85.83 Other specified disorders of bone density and structure, forearm

M85.831 Other specified disorders of bone density and structure, right forearm

M85.832 Other specified disorders of bone density and structure, left forearm

M85.839 Other specified disorders of bone density and structure, unspecified forearm

M85.84 Other specified disorders of bone density and structure, hand

M85.841 Other specified disorders of bone density and structure, right hand

M85.842 Other specified disorders of bone density and structure, left hand

M85.849 Other specified disorders of bone density and structure, unspecified hand

M85.85 Other specified disorders of bone density and structure, thigh

M85.851 Other specified disorders of bone density and structure, right thigh

M85.852 Other specified disorders of bone density and structure, left thigh

M85.859 Other specified disorders of bone density and structure, unspecified thigh

M85.86 Other specified disorders of bone density and structure, lower leg

M85.861 Other specified disorders of bone density and structure, right lower leg

M85.862 Other specified disorders of bone density and structure, left lower leg

M85.869 Other specified disorders of bone density and structure, unspecified lower leg

M85.87 Other specified disorders of bone density and structure, ankle and foot

M85.871 Other specified disorders of bone density and structure, right ankle and foot

M85.872 Other specified disorders of bone density and structure, left ankle and foot

M85.879 Other specified disorders of bone density and structure, unspecified ankle and foot

M85.88 Other specified disorders of bone density and structure, other site

M85.89 Other specified disorders of bone density and structure, multiple sites

M85.9 Disorder of bone density and structure, unspecified

OTHER OSTEOPATHIES (M86-M90)

Excludes 1: postprocedural osteopathies (M96.-)

M86 Osteomyelitis

Use additional code (B95-B97) to identify infectious agent

Use additional code to identify major osseous defect, if applicable (M89.7-)

Excludes 1: osteomyelitis due to:

echinococcus (B67.2)

gonococcus (A54.43)

salmonella (A02.24)

Excludes 2: osteomyelitis of:

orbit (H05.0-)

petrous bone (H70.2-)

vertebra (M46.2-)

M86.0   Acute hematogenous osteomyelitis
    M86.00   Acute hematogenous osteomyelitis, unspecified site
    M86.01   Acute hematogenous osteomyelitis, shoulder
        M86.011   Acute hematogenous osteomyelitis, right shoulder
        M86.012   Acute hematogenous osteomyelitis, left shoulder
        M86.019   Acute hematogenous osteomyelitis, unspecified shoulder
    M86.02   Acute hematogenous osteomyelitis, humerus
        M86.021   Acute hematogenous osteomyelitis, right humerus
        M86.022   Acute hematogenous osteomyelitis, left humerus
        M86.029   Acute hematogenous osteomyelitis, unspecified humerus
    M86.03   Acute hematogenous osteomyelitis, radius and ulna
        M86.031   Acute hematogenous osteomyelitis, right radius and ulna
        M86.032   Acute hematogenous osteomyelitis, left radius and ulna
        M86.039   Acute hematogenous osteomyelitis, unspecified radius and ulna
    M86.04   Acute hematogenous osteomyelitis, hand
        M86.041   Acute hematogenous osteomyelitis, right hand
        M86.042   Acute hematogenous osteomyelitis, left hand
        M86.049   Acute hematogenous osteomyelitis, unspecified hand
    M86.05   Acute hematogenous osteomyelitis, femur
        M86.051   Acute hematogenous osteomyelitis, right femur
        M86.052   Acute hematogenous osteomyelitis, left femur
        M86.059   Acute hematogenous osteomyelitis, unspecified femur
    M86.06   Acute hematogenous osteomyelitis, tibia and fibula
        M86.061   Acute hematogenous osteomyelitis, right tibia and fibula
        M86.062   Acute hematogenous osteomyelitis, left tibia and fibula
        M86.069   Acute hematogenous osteomyelitis, unspecified tibia and fibula
    M86.07   Acute hematogenous osteomyelitis, ankle and foot
        M86.071   Acute hematogenous osteomyelitis, right ankle and foot
        M86.072   Acute hematogenous osteomyelitis, left ankle and foot
        M86.079   Acute hematogenous osteomyelitis, unspecified ankle and foot
    M86.08   Acute hematogenous osteomyelitis, other sites
    M86.09   Acute hematogenous osteomyelitis, multiple sites
M86.1   Other acute osteomyelitis
    M86.10   Other acute osteomyelitis, unspecified site
    M86.11   Other acute osteomyelitis, shoulder

        M86.111   Other acute osteomyelitis, right shoulder
        M86.112   Other acute osteomyelitis, left shoulder
        M86.119   Other acute osteomyelitis, unspecified shoulder
    M86.12   Other acute osteomyelitis, humerus
        M86.121   Other acute osteomyelitis, right humerus
        M86.122   Other acute osteomyelitis, left humerus
        M86.129   Other acute osteomyelitis, unspecified humerus
    M86.13   Other acute osteomyelitis, radius and ulna
        M86.131   Other acute osteomyelitis, right radius and ulna
        M86.132   Other acute osteomyelitis, left radius and ulna
        M86.139   Other acute osteomyelitis, unspecified radius and ulna
    M86.14   Other acute osteomyelitis, hand
        M86.141   Other acute osteomyelitis, right hand
        M86.142   Other acute osteomyelitis, left hand
        M86.149   Other acute osteomyelitis, unspecified hand
    M86.15   Other acute osteomyelitis, femur
        M86.151   Other acute osteomyelitis, right femur
        M86.152   Other acute osteomyelitis, left femur
        M86.159   Other acute osteomyelitis, unspecified femur
    M86.16   Other acute osteomyelitis, tibia and fibula
        M86.161   Other acute osteomyelitis, right tibia and fibula
        M86.162   Other acute osteomyelitis, left tibia and fibula
        M86.169   Other acute osteomyelitis, unspecified tibia and fibula
    M86.17   Other acute osteomyelitis, ankle and foot
        M86.171   Other acute osteomyelitis, right ankle and foot
        M86.172   Other acute osteomyelitis, left ankle and foot
        M86.179   Other acute osteomyelitis, unspecified ankle and foot
    M86.18   Other acute osteomyelitis, other site
    M86.19   Other acute osteomyelitis, multiple sites
M86.2   Subacute osteomyelitis
    M86.20   Subacute osteomyelitis, unspecified site
    M86.21   Subacute osteomyelitis, shoulder
        M86.211   Subacute osteomyelitis, right shoulder
        M86.212   Subacute osteomyelitis, left shoulder
        M86.219   Subacute osteomyelitis, unspecified shoulder
    M86.22   Subacute osteomyelitis, humerus
        M86.221   Subacute osteomyelitis, right humerus
        M86.222   Subacute osteomyelitis, left humerus
        M86.229   Subacute osteomyelitis, unspecified humerus

M86.23 Subacute osteomyelitis, radius and ulna
    M86.231 Subacute osteomyelitis, right radius and ulna
    M86.232 Subacute osteomyelitis, left radius and ulna
    M86.239 Subacute osteomyelitis, unspecified radius and ulna
M86.24 Subacute osteomyelitis, hand
    M86.241 Subacute osteomyelitis, right hand
    M86.242 Subacute osteomyelitis, left hand
    M86.249 Subacute osteomyelitis, unspecified hand
M86.25 Subacute osteomyelitis, femur
    M86.251 Subacute osteomyelitis, right femur
    M86.252 Subacute osteomyelitis, left femur
    M86.259 Subacute osteomyelitis, unspecified femur
M86.26 Subacute osteomyelitis, tibia and fibula
    M86.261 Subacute osteomyelitis, right tibia and fibula
    M86.262 Subacute osteomyelitis, left tibia and fibula
    M86.269 Subacute osteomyelitis, unspecified tibia and fibula
M86.27 Subacute osteomyelitis, ankle and foot
    M86.271 Subacute osteomyelitis, right ankle and foot
    M86.272 Subacute osteomyelitis, left ankle and foot
    M86.279 Subacute osteomyelitis, unspecified ankle and foot
M86.28 Subacute osteomyelitis, other site
M86.29 Subacute osteomyelitis, multiple sites
M86.3 Chronic multifocal osteomyelitis
M86.30 Chronic multifocal osteomyelitis, unspecified site
M86.31 Chronic multifocal osteomyelitis, shoulder
    M86.311 Chronic multifocal osteomyelitis, right shoulder
    M86.312 Chronic multifocal osteomyelitis, left shoulder
    M86.319 Chronic multifocal osteomyelitis, unspecified shoulder
M86.32 Chronic multifocal osteomyelitis, humerus
    M86.321 Chronic multifocal osteomyelitis, right humerus
    M86.322 Chronic multifocal osteomyelitis, left humerus
    M86.329 Chronic multifocal osteomyelitis, unspecified humerus
M86.33 Chronic multifocal osteomyelitis, radius and ulna
    M86.331 Chronic multifocal osteomyelitis, right radius and ulna
    M86.332 Chronic multifocal osteomyelitis, left radius and ulna
    M86.339 Chronic multifocal osteomyelitis, unspecified radius and ulna
M86.34 Chronic multifocal osteomyelitis, hand
    M86.341 Chronic multifocal osteomyelitis, right hand

    M86.342 Chronic multifocal osteomyelitis, left hand
    M86.349 Chronic multifocal osteomyelitis, unspecified hand
M86.35 Chronic multifocal osteomyelitis, femur
    M86.351 Chronic multifocal osteomyelitis, right femur
    M86.352 Chronic multifocal osteomyelitis, left femur
    M86.359 Chronic multifocal osteomyelitis, unspecified femur
M86.36 Chronic multifocal osteomyelitis, tibia and fibula
    M86.361 Chronic multifocal osteomyelitis, right tibia and fibula
    M86.362 Chronic multifocal osteomyelitis, left tibia and fibula
    M86.369 Chronic multifocal osteomyelitis, unspecified tibia and fibula
M86.37 Chronic multifocal osteomyelitis, ankle and foot
    M86.371 Chronic multifocal osteomyelitis, right ankle and foot
    M86.372 Chronic multifocal osteomyelitis, left ankle and foot
    M86.379 Chronic multifocal osteomyelitis, unspecified ankle and foot
M86.38 Chronic multifocal osteomyelitis, other site
M86.39 Chronic multifocal osteomyelitis, multiple sites
M86.4 Chronic osteomyelitis with draining sinus
M86.40 Chronic osteomyelitis with draining sinus, unspecified site
M86.41 Chronic osteomyelitis with draining sinus, shoulder
    M86.411 Chronic osteomyelitis with draining sinus, right shoulder
    M86.412 Chronic osteomyelitis with draining sinus, left shoulder
    M86.419 Chronic osteomyelitis with draining sinus, unspecified shoulder
M86.42 Chronic osteomyelitis with draining sinus, humerus
    M86.421 Chronic osteomyelitis with draining sinus, right humerus
    M86.422 Chronic osteomyelitis with draining sinus, left humerus
    M86.429 Chronic osteomyelitis with draining sinus, unspecified humerus
M86.43 Chronic osteomyelitis with draining sinus, radius and ulna
    M86.431 Chronic osteomyelitis with draining sinus, right radius and ulna
    M86.432 Chronic osteomyelitis with draining sinus, left radius and ulna
    M86.439 Chronic osteomyelitis with draining sinus, unspecified radius and ulna
M86.44 Chronic osteomyelitis with draining sinus, hand
    M86.441 Chronic osteomyelitis with draining sinus, right hand
    M86.442 Chronic osteomyelitis with draining sinus, left hand
    M86.449 Chronic osteomyelitis with draining sinus, unspecified hand

● New code   ▲ Revised code   ⑦ 7th digit required   ⊗ Placeholder required

M86.45 Chronic osteomyelitis with draining sinus, femur
    M86.451 Chronic osteomyelitis with draining sinus, right femur
    M86.452 Chronic osteomyelitis with draining sinus, left femur
    M86.459 Chronic osteomyelitis with draining sinus, unspecified femur

M86.46 Chronic osteomyelitis with draining sinus, tibia and fibula
    M86.461 Chronic osteomyelitis with draining sinus, right tibia and fibula
    M86.462 Chronic osteomyelitis with draining sinus, left tibia and fibula
    M86.469 Chronic osteomyelitis with draining sinus, unspecified tibia and fibula

M86.47 Chronic osteomyelitis with draining sinus, ankle and foot
    M86.471 Chronic osteomyelitis with draining sinus, right ankle and foot
    M86.472 Chronic osteomyelitis with draining sinus, left ankle and foot
    M86.479 Chronic osteomyelitis with draining sinus, unspecified ankle and foot

M86.48 Chronic osteomyelitis with draining sinus, other site

M86.49 Chronic osteomyelitis with draining sinus, multiple sites

M86.5 Other chronic hematogenous osteomyelitis
  M86.50 Other chronic hematogenous osteomyelitis, unspecified site

  M86.51 Other chronic hematogenous osteomyelitis, shoulder
    M86.511 Other chronic hematogenous osteomyelitis, right shoulder
    M86.512 Other chronic hematogenous osteomyelitis, left shoulder
    M86.519 Other chronic hematogenous osteomyelitis, unspecified shoulder

  M86.52 Other chronic hematogenous osteomyelitis, humerus
    M86.521 Other chronic hematogenous osteomyelitis, right humerus
    M86.522 Other chronic hematogenous osteomyelitis, left humerus
    M86.529 Other chronic hematogenous osteomyelitis, unspecified humerus

  M86.53 Other chronic hematogenous osteomyelitis, radius and ulna
    M86.531 Other chronic hematogenous osteomyelitis, right radius and ulna
    M86.532 Other chronic hematogenous osteomyelitis, left radius and ulna
    M86.539 Other chronic hematogenous osteomyelitis, unspecified radius and ulna

  M86.54 Other chronic hematogenous osteomyelitis, hand
    M86.541 Other chronic hematogenous osteomyelitis, right hand
    M86.542 Other chronic hematogenous osteomyelitis, left hand

    M86.549 Other chronic hematogenous osteomyelitis, unspecified hand

  M86.55 Other chronic hematogenous osteomyelitis, femur
    M86.551 Other chronic hematogenous osteomyelitis, right femur
    M86.552 Other chronic hematogenous osteomyelitis, left femur
    M86.559 Other chronic hematogenous osteomyelitis, unspecified femur

  M86.56 Other chronic hematogenous osteomyelitis, tibia and fibula
    M86.561 Other chronic hematogenous osteomyelitis, right tibia and fibula
    M86.562 Other chronic hematogenous osteomyelitis, left tibia and fibula
    M86.569 Other chronic hematogenous osteomyelitis, unspecified tibia and fibula

  M86.57 Other chronic hematogenous osteomyelitis, ankle and foot
    M86.571 Other chronic hematogenous osteomyelitis, right ankle and foot
    M86.572 Other chronic hematogenous osteomyelitis, left ankle and foot
    M86.579 Other chronic hematogenous osteomyelitis, unspecified ankle and foot

  M86.58 Other chronic hematogenous osteomyelitis, other site

  M86.59 Other chronic hematogenous osteomyelitis, multiple sites

M86.6 Other chronic osteomyelitis
  M86.60 Other chronic osteomyelitis, unspecified site

  M86.61 Other chronic osteomyelitis, shoulder
    M86.611 Other chronic osteomyelitis, right shoulder
    M86.612 Other chronic osteomyelitis, left shoulder
    M86.619 Other chronic osteomyelitis, unspecified shoulder

  M86.62 Other chronic osteomyelitis, humerus
    M86.621 Other chronic osteomyelitis, right humerus
    M86.622 Other chronic osteomyelitis, left humerus
    M86.629 Other chronic osteomyelitis, unspecified humerus

  M86.63 Other chronic osteomyelitis, radius and ulna
    M86.631 Other chronic osteomyelitis, right radius and ulna
    M86.632 Other chronic osteomyelitis, left radius and ulna
    M86.639 Other chronic osteomyelitis, unspecified radius and ulna

  M86.64 Other chronic osteomyelitis, hand
    M86.641 Other chronic osteomyelitis, right hand
    M86.642 Other chronic osteomyelitis, left hand

M86.649 Other chronic osteomyelitis, unspecified hand

M86.65 Other chronic osteomyelitis, thigh

M86.651 Other chronic osteomyelitis, right thigh

M86.652 Other chronic osteomyelitis, left thigh

M86.659 Other chronic osteomyelitis, unspecified thigh

M86.66 Other chronic osteomyelitis, tibia and fibula

M86.661 Other chronic osteomyelitis, right tibia and fibula

M86.662 Other chronic osteomyelitis, left tibia and fibula

M86.669 Other chronic osteomyelitis, unspecified tibia and fibula

M86.67 Other chronic osteomyelitis, ankle and foot

M86.671 Other chronic osteomyelitis, right ankle and foot

M86.672 Other chronic osteomyelitis, left ankle and foot

M86.679 Other chronic osteomyelitis, unspecified ankle and foot

M86.68 Other chronic osteomyelitis, other site

M86.69 Other chronic osteomyelitis, multiple sites

M86.8 Other osteomyelitis

Brodie's abscess

M86.8X Other osteomyelitis

M86.8X0 Other osteomyelitis, multiple sites

M86.8X1 Other osteomyelitis, shoulder

M86.8X2 Other osteomyelitis, upper arm

M86.8X3 Other osteomyelitis, forearm

M86.8X4 Other osteomyelitis, hand

M86.8X5 Other osteomyelitis, thigh

M86.8X6 Other osteomyelitis, lower leg

M86.8X7 Other osteomyelitis, ankle and foot

M86.8X8 Other osteomyelitis, other site

M86.8X9 Other osteomyelitis, unspecified sites

M86.9 Osteomyelitis, unspecified

Infection of bone NOS

Periostitis without osteomyelitis

M87 Osteonecrosis

Includes: avascular necrosis of bone

Use additional code to identify major osseous defect, if applicable (M89.7-)

Excludes 1: juvenile osteonecrosis (M91-M92)

osteochondropathies (M90-M93)

M87.0 Idiopathic aseptic necrosis of bone

M87.00 Idiopathic aseptic necrosis of unspecified bone

M87.01 Idiopathic aseptic necrosis of shoulder

Idiopathic aseptic necrosis of clavicle and scapula

M87.011 Idiopathic aseptic necrosis of right shoulder

M87.012 Idiopathic aseptic necrosis of left shoulder

M87.019 Idiopathic aseptic necrosis of unspecified shoulder

M87.02 Idiopathic aseptic necrosis of humerus

M87.021 Idiopathic aseptic necrosis of right humerus

M87.022 Idiopathic aseptic necrosis of left humerus

M87.029 Idiopathic aseptic necrosis of unspecified humerus

M87.03 Idiopathic aseptic necrosis of radius, ulna and carpus

M87.031 Idiopathic aseptic necrosis of right radius

M87.032 Idiopathic aseptic necrosis of left radius

M87.033 Idiopathic aseptic necrosis of unspecified radius

M87.034 Idiopathic aseptic necrosis of right ulna

M87.035 Idiopathic aseptic necrosis of left ulna

M87.036 Idiopathic aseptic necrosis of unspecified ulna

M87.037 Idiopathic aseptic necrosis of right carpus

M87.038 Idiopathic aseptic necrosis of left carpus

M87.039 Idiopathic aseptic necrosis of unspecified carpus

M87.04 Idiopathic aseptic necrosis of hand and fingers

Idiopathic aseptic necrosis of metacarpals and phalanges of hands

M87.041 Idiopathic aseptic necrosis of right hand

M87.042 Idiopathic aseptic necrosis of left hand

M87.043 Idiopathic aseptic necrosis of unspecified hand

M87.044 Idiopathic aseptic necrosis of right finger(s)

M87.045 Idiopathic aseptic necrosis of left finger(s)

M87.046 Idiopathic aseptic necrosis of unspecified finger(s)

M87.05 Idiopathic aseptic necrosis of pelvis and femur

M87.050 Idiopathic aseptic necrosis of pelvis

M87.051 Idiopathic aseptic necrosis of right femur

M87.052 Idiopathic aseptic necrosis of left femur

M87.059 Idiopathic aseptic necrosis of unspecified femur

Idiopathic aseptic necrosis of hip NOS

M87.06 Idiopathic aseptic necrosis of tibia and fibula

M87.061 Idiopathic aseptic necrosis of right tibia

M87.062 Idiopathic aseptic necrosis of left tibia

M87.063 Idiopathic aseptic necrosis of unspecified tibia

M87.064 Idiopathic aseptic necrosis of right fibula

M87.065   Idiopathic aseptic necrosis of left fibula

M87.066   Idiopathic aseptic necrosis of unspecified fibula

M87.07   Idiopathic aseptic necrosis of ankle, foot and toes

Idiopathic aseptic necrosis of metatarsus, tarsus, and phalanges of toes

M87.071   Idiopathic aseptic necrosis of right ankle

M87.072   Idiopathic aseptic necrosis of left ankle

M87.073   Idiopathic aseptic necrosis of unspecified ankle

M87.074   Idiopathic aseptic necrosis of right foot

M87.075   Idiopathic aseptic necrosis of left foot

M87.076   Idiopathic aseptic necrosis of unspecified foot

M87.077   Idiopathic aseptic necrosis of right toe(s)

M87.078   Idiopathic aseptic necrosis of left toe(s)

M87.079   Idiopathic aseptic necrosis of unspecified toe(s)

M87.08   Idiopathic aseptic necrosis of bone, other site

M87.09   Idiopathic aseptic necrosis of bone, multiple sites

M87.1   Osteonecrosis due to drugs

Use additional code for adverse effect, if applicable, to identify drug (T36-T50 with fifth or sixth character 5)

M87.10   Osteonecrosis due to drugs, unspecified bone

M87.11   Osteonecrosis due to drugs, shoulder

M87.111   Osteonecrosis due to drugs, right shoulder

M87.112   Osteonecrosis due to drugs, left shoulder

M87.119   Osteonecrosis due to drugs, unspecified shoulder

M87.12   Osteonecrosis due to drugs, humerus

M87.121   Osteonecrosis due to drugs, right humerus

M87.122   Osteonecrosis due to drugs, left humerus

M87.129   Osteonecrosis due to drugs, unspecified humerus

M87.13   Osteonecrosis due to drugs of radius, ulna and carpus

M87.131   Osteonecrosis due to drugs of right radius

M87.132   Osteonecrosis due to drugs of left radius

M87.133   Osteonecrosis due to drugs of unspecified radius

M87.134   Osteonecrosis due to drugs of right ulna

M87.135   Osteonecrosis due to drugs of left ulna

M87.136   Osteonecrosis due to drugs of unspecified ulna

M87.137   Osteonecrosis due to drugs of right carpus

M87.138   Osteonecrosis due to drugs of left carpus

M87.139   Osteonecrosis due to drugs of unspecified carpus

M87.14   Osteonecrosis due to drugs, hand and fingers

M87.141   Osteonecrosis due to drugs, right hand

M87.142   Osteonecrosis due to drugs, left hand

M87.143   Osteonecrosis due to drugs, unspecified hand

M87.144   Osteonecrosis due to drugs, right finger(s)

M87.145   Osteonecrosis due to drugs, left finger(s)

M87.146   Osteonecrosis due to drugs, unspecified finger(s)

M87.15   Osteonecrosis due to drugs, pelvis and femur

M87.150   Osteonecrosis due to drugs, pelvis

M87.151   Osteonecrosis due to drugs, right femur

M87.152   Osteonecrosis due to drugs, left femur

M87.159   Osteonecrosis due to drugs, unspecified femur

M87.16   Osteonecrosis due to drugs, tibia and fibula

M87.161   Osteonecrosis due to drugs, right tibia

M87.162   Osteonecrosis due to drugs, left tibia

M87.163   Osteonecrosis due to drugs, unspecified tibia

M87.164   Osteonecrosis due to drugs, right fibula

M87.165   Osteonecrosis due to drugs, left fibula

M87.166   Osteonecrosis due to drugs, unspecified fibula

M87.17   Osteonecrosis due to drugs, ankle, foot and toes

M87.171   Osteonecrosis due to drugs, right ankle

M87.172   Osteonecrosis due to drugs, left ankle

M87.173   Osteonecrosis due to drugs, unspecified ankle

M87.174   Osteonecrosis due to drugs, right foot

M87.175   Osteonecrosis due to drugs, left foot

M87.176   Osteonecrosis due to drugs, unspecified foot

M87.177   Osteonecrosis due to drugs, right toe(s)

M87.178   Osteonecrosis due to drugs, left toe(s)

M87.179   Osteonecrosis due to drugs, unspecified toe(s)

M87.18   Osteonecrosis due to drugs, other site

M87.180   Osteonecrosis due to drugs, jaw

M87.188   Osteonecrosis due to drugs, other site

M87.19   Osteonecrosis due to drugs, multiple sites

M87.2   Osteonecrosis due to previous trauma

M87.20 Osteonecrosis due to previous trauma, unspecified bone

M87.21 Osteonecrosis due to previous trauma, shoulder

 M87.211 Osteonecrosis due to previous trauma, right shoulder

 M87.212 Osteonecrosis due to previous trauma, left shoulder

 M87.219 Osteonecrosis due to previous trauma, unspecified shoulder

M87.22 Osteonecrosis due to previous trauma, humerus

 M87.221 Osteonecrosis due to previous trauma, right humerus

 M87.222 Osteonecrosis due to previous trauma, left humerus

 M87.229 Osteonecrosis due to previous trauma, unspecified humerus

M87.23 Osteonecrosis due to previous trauma of radius, ulna and carpus

 M87.231 Osteonecrosis due to previous trauma of right radius

 M87.232 Osteonecrosis due to previous trauma of left radius

 M87.233 Osteonecrosis due to previous trauma of unspecified radius

 M87.234 Osteonecrosis due to previous trauma of right ulna

 M87.235 Osteonecrosis due to previous trauma of left ulna

 M87.236 Osteonecrosis due to previous trauma of unspecified ulna

 M87.237 Osteonecrosis due to previous trauma of right carpus

 M87.238 Osteonecrosis due to previous trauma of left carpus

 M87.239 Osteonecrosis due to previous trauma of unspecified carpus

M87.24 Osteonecrosis due to previous trauma, hand and fingers

 M87.241 Osteonecrosis due to previous trauma, right hand

 M87.242 Osteonecrosis due to previous trauma, left hand

 M87.243 Osteonecrosis due to previous trauma, unspecified hand

 M87.244 Osteonecrosis due to previous trauma, right finger(s)

 M87.245 Osteonecrosis due to previous trauma, left finger(s)

 M87.246 Osteonecrosis due to previous trauma, unspecified finger(s)

M87.25 Osteonecrosis due to previous trauma, pelvis and femur

 M87.250 Osteonecrosis due to previous trauma, pelvis

 M87.251 Osteonecrosis due to previous trauma, right femur

 M87.252 Osteonecrosis due to previous trauma, left femur

 M87.256 Osteonecrosis due to previous trauma, unspecified femur

M87.26 Osteonecrosis due to previous trauma, tibia and fibula

 M87.261 Osteonecrosis due to previous trauma, right tibia

 M87.262 Osteonecrosis due to previous trauma, left tibia

 M87.263 Osteonecrosis due to previous trauma, unspecified tibia

 M87.264 Osteonecrosis due to previous trauma, right fibula

 M87.265 Osteonecrosis due to previous trauma, left fibula

 M87.266 Osteonecrosis due to previous trauma, unspecified fibula

M87.27 Osteonecrosis due to previous trauma, ankle, foot and toes

 M87.271 Osteonecrosis due to previous trauma, right ankle

 M87.272 Osteonecrosis due to previous trauma, left ankle

 M87.273 Osteonecrosis due to previous trauma, unspecified ankle

 M87.274 Osteonecrosis due to previous trauma, right foot

 M87.275 Osteonecrosis due to previous trauma, left foot

 M87.276 Osteonecrosis due to previous trauma, unspecified foot

 M87.277 Osteonecrosis due to previous trauma, right toe(s)

 M87.278 Osteonecrosis due to previous trauma, left toe(s)

 M87.279 Osteonecrosis due to previous trauma, unspecified toe(s)

M87.28 Osteonecrosis due to previous trauma, other site

M87.29 Osteonecrosis due to previous trauma, multiple sites

M87.3 Other secondary osteonecrosis

 M87.30 Other secondary osteonecrosis, unspecified bone

 M87.31 Other secondary osteonecrosis, shoulder

  M87.311 Other secondary osteonecrosis, right shoulder

  M87.312 Other secondary osteonecrosis, left shoulder

  M87.319 Other secondary osteonecrosis, unspecified shoulder

 M87.32 Other secondary osteonecrosis, humerus

  M87.321 Other secondary osteonecrosis, right humerus

  M87.322 Other secondary osteonecrosis, left humerus

  M87.329 Other secondary osteonecrosis, unspecified humerus

 M87.33 Other secondary osteonecrosis of radius, ulna and carpus

  M87.331 Other secondary osteonecrosis of right radius

  M87.332 Other secondary osteonecrosis of left radius

  M87.333 Other secondary osteonecrosis of unspecified radius

M87.334 Other secondary osteonecrosis of right ulna

M87.335 Other secondary osteonecrosis of left ulna

M87.336 Other secondary osteonecrosis of unspecified ulna

M87.337 Other secondary osteonecrosis of right carpus

M87.338 Other secondary osteonecrosis of left carpus

M87.339 Other secondary osteonecrosis of unspecified carpus

M87.34 Other secondary osteonecrosis, hand and fingers

M87.341 Other secondary osteonecrosis, right hand

M87.342 Other secondary osteonecrosis, left hand

M87.343 Other secondary osteonecrosis, unspecified hand

M87.344 Other secondary osteonecrosis, right finger(s)

M87.345 Other secondary osteonecrosis, left finger(s)

M87.346 Other secondary osteonecrosis, unspecified finger(s)

M87.35 Other secondary osteonecrosis, pelvis and femur

M87.350 Other secondary osteonecrosis, pelvis

M87.351 Other secondary osteonecrosis, right femur

M87.352 Other secondary osteonecrosis, left femur

M87.353 Other secondary osteonecrosis, unspecified femur

M87.36 Other secondary osteonecrosis, tibia and fibula

M87.361 Other secondary osteonecrosis, right tibia

M87.362 Other secondary osteonecrosis, left tibia

M87.363 Other secondary osteonecrosis, unspecified tibia

M87.364 Other secondary osteonecrosis, right fibula

M87.365 Other secondary osteonecrosis, left fibula

M87.366 Other secondary osteonecrosis, unspecified fibula

M87.37 Other secondary osteonecrosis, ankle and foot

M87.371 Other secondary osteonecrosis, right ankle

M87.372 Other secondary osteonecrosis, left ankle

M87.373 Other secondary osteonecrosis, unspecified ankle

M87.374 Other secondary osteonecrosis, right foot

M87.375 Other secondary osteonecrosis, left foot

M87.376 Other secondary osteonecrosis, unspecified foot

M87.377 Other secondary osteonecrosis, right toe(s)

M87.378 Other secondary osteonecrosis, left toe(s)

M87.379 Other secondary osteonecrosis, unspecified toe(s)

M87.38 Other secondary osteonecrosis, other site

M87.39 Other secondary osteonecrosis, multiple sites

M87.8 Other osteonecrosis

M87.80 Other osteonecrosis, unspecified bone

M87.81 Other osteonecrosis, shoulder

M87.811 Other osteonecrosis, right shoulder

M87.812 Other osteonecrosis, left shoulder

M87.819 Other osteonecrosis, unspecified shoulder

M87.82 Other osteonecrosis, humerus

M87.821 Other osteonecrosis, right humerus

M87.822 Other osteonecrosis, left humerus

M87.829 Other osteonecrosis, unspecified humerus

M87.83 Other osteonecrosis of radius, ulna and carpus

M87.831 Other osteonecrosis of right radius

M87.832 Other osteonecrosis of left radius

M87.833 Other osteonecrosis of unspecified radius

M87.834 Other osteonecrosis of right ulna

M87.835 Other osteonecrosis of left ulna

M87.836 Other osteonecrosis of unspecified ulna

M87.837 Other osteonecrosis of right carpus

M87.838 Other osteonecrosis of left carpus

M87.839 Other osteonecrosis of unspecified carpus

M87.84 Other osteonecrosis, hand and fingers

M87.841 Other osteonecrosis, right hand

M87.842 Other osteonecrosis, left hand

M87.843 Other osteonecrosis, unspecified hand

M87.844 Other osteonecrosis, right finger(s)

M87.845 Other osteonecrosis, left finger(s)

M87.849 Other osteonecrosis, unspecified finger(s)

M87.85 Other osteonecrosis, pelvis and femur

M87.850 Other osteonecrosis, pelvis

M87.851 Other osteonecrosis, right femur

M87.852 Other osteonecrosis, left femur

M87.859 Other osteonecrosis, unspecified femur

M87.86 Other osteonecrosis, tibia and fibula

M87.861 Other osteonecrosis, right tibia

M87.862 Other osteonecrosis, left tibia

M87.863 Other osteonecrosis, unspecified tibia

M87.864 Other osteonecrosis, right fibula

M87.865 Other osteonecrosis, left fibula

M87.869 Other osteonecrosis, unspecified fibula

M87.87 Other osteonecrosis, ankle, foot and toes

M87.871 Other osteonecrosis, right ankle

M87.872 Other osteonecrosis, left ankle

M87.873 Other osteonecrosis, unspecified ankle

M87.874 Other osteonecrosis, right foot

M87.875 Other osteonecrosis, left foot

M87.876 Other osteonecrosis, unspecified foot

M87.877 Other osteonecrosis, right toe(s)

M87.878 Other osteonecrosis, left toe(s)

M87.879 Other osteonecrosis, unspecified toe(s)

M87.88 Other osteonecrosis, other site

M87.89 Other osteonecrosis, multiple sites

M87.9 Osteonecrosis, unspecified

Necrosis of bone NOS

M88 Osteitis deformans [Paget's disease of bone]

Excludes 1: osteitis deformans in neoplastic disease (M90.6)

M88.0 Osteitis deformans of skull

M88.1 Osteitis deformans of vertebrae

M88.8 Osteitis deformans of other bones

M88.81 Osteitis deformans of shoulder

M88.811 Osteitis deformans of right shoulder

M88.812 Osteitis deformans of left shoulder

M88.819 Osteitis deformans of unspecified shoulder

M88.82 Osteitis deformans of upper arm

M88.821 Osteitis deformans of right upper arm

M88.822 Osteitis deformans of left upper arm

M88.829 Osteitis deformans of unspecified upper arm

M88.83 Osteitis deformans of forearm

M88.831 Osteitis deformans of right forearm

M88.832 Osteitis deformans of left forearm

M88.839 Osteitis deformans of unspecified forearm

M88.84 Osteitis deformans of hand

M88.841 Osteitis deformans of right hand

M88.842 Osteitis deformans of left hand

M88.849 Osteitis deformans of unspecified hand

M88.85 Osteitis deformans of thigh

M88.851 Osteitis deformans of right thigh

M88.852 Osteitis deformans of left thigh

M88.859 Osteitis deformans of unspecified thigh

M88.86 Osteitis deformans of lower leg

M88.861 Osteitis deformans of right lower leg

M88.862 Osteitis deformans of left lower leg

M88.869 Osteitis deformans of unspecified lower leg

M88.87 Osteitis deformans of ankle and foot

M88.871 Osteitis deformans of right ankle and foot

M88.872 Osteitis deformans of left ankle and foot

M88.879 Osteitis deformans of unspecified ankle and foot

M88.88 Osteitis deformans of other bones

Excludes 2: osteitis deformans of skull (M88.0)

osteitis deformans of vertebrae (M88.1)

M88.89 Osteitis deformans of multiple sites

M88.9 Osteitis deformans of unspecified bone

M89 Other disorders of bone

M89.0 Algoneurodystrophy

Shoulder-hand syndrome

Sudeck's atrophy

Excludes 1: causalgia, lower limb (G57.7-)

causalgia, upper limb (G56.4-)

complex regional pain syndrome II, lower limb (G57.7-)

complex regional pain syndrome II, upper limb (G56.4-)

reflex sympathetic dystrophy (G90.5-)

M89.00 Algoneurodystrophy, unspecified site

M89.01 Algoneurodystrophy, shoulder

M89.011 Algoneurodystrophy, right shoulder

M89.012 Algoneurodystrophy, left shoulder

M89.019 Algoneurodystrophy, unspecified shoulder

M89.02 Algoneurodystrophy, upper arm

M89.021 Algoneurodystrophy, right upper arm

M89.022 Algoneurodystrophy, left upper arm

M89.029 Algoneurodystrophy, unspecified upper arm

M89.03 Algoneurodystrophy, forearm

M89.031 Algoneurodystrophy, right forearm

M89.032 Algoneurodystrophy, left forearm

M89.039 Algoneurodystrophy, unspecified forearm

M89.04 Algoneurodystrophy, hand

M89.041 Algoneurodystrophy, right hand

M89.042 Algoneurodystrophy, left hand

M89.049 Algoneurodystrophy, unspecified hand

M89.05 Algoneurodystrophy, thigh

M89.051 Algoneurodystrophy, right thigh

M89.052 Algoneurodystrophy, left thigh

M89.059 Algoneurodystrophy, unspecified thigh

M89.06 Algoneurodystrophy, lower leg

M89.061 Algoneurodystrophy, right lower leg

M89.062 Algoneurodystrophy, left lower leg

M89.069 Algoneurodystrophy, unspecified lower leg

M89.07 Algoneurodystrophy, ankle and foot

M89.071 Algoneurodystrophy, right ankle and foot

M89.072 Algoneurodystrophy, left ankle and foot

M89.079 Algoneurodystrophy, unspecified ankle and foot

M89.08 Algoneurodystrophy, other site

M89.09 Algoneurodystrophy, multiple sites

M89.1 Physeal arrest

Arrest of growth plate

Epiphyseal arrest

● New code   ▲ Revised code   ⑦ 7th digit required   ⊗ Placeholder required

Growth plate arrest

M89.12 Physeal arrest, humerus

 M89.121 Complete physeal arrest, right proximal humerus

 M89.122 Complete physeal arrest, left proximal humerus

 M89.123 Partial physeal arrest, right proximal humerus

 M89.124 Partial physeal arrest, left proximal humerus

 M89.125 Complete physeal arrest, right distal humerus

 M89.126 Complete physeal arrest, left distal humerus

 M89.127 Partial physeal arrest, right distal humerus

 M89.128 Partial physeal arrest, left distal humerus

 M89.129 Physeal arrest, humerus, unspecified

M89.13 Physeal arrest, forearm

 M89.131 Complete physeal arrest, right distal radius

 M89.132 Complete physeal arrest, left distal radius

 M89.133 Partial physeal arrest, right distal radius

 M89.134 Partial physeal arrest, left distal radius

 M89.138 Other physeal arrest of forearm

 M89.139 Physeal arrest, forearm, unspecified

M89.15 Physeal arrest, femur

 M89.151 Complete physeal arrest, right proximal femur

 M89.152 Complete physeal arrest, left proximal femur

 M89.153 Partial physeal arrest, right proximal femur

 M89.154 Partial physeal arrest, left proximal femur

 M89.155 Complete physeal arrest, right distal femur

 M89.156 Complete physeal arrest, left distal femur

 M89.157 Partial physeal arrest, right distal femur

 M89.158 Partial physeal arrest, left distal femur

 M89.159 Physeal arrest, femur, unspecified

M89.16 Physeal arrest, lower leg

 M89.160 Complete physeal arrest, right proximal tibia

 M89.161 Complete physeal arrest, left proximal tibia

 M89.162 Partial physeal arrest, right proximal tibia

 M89.163 Partial physeal arrest, left proximal tibia

 M89.164 Complete physeal arrest, right distal tibia

 M89.165 Complete physeal arrest, left distal tibia

 M89.166 Partial physeal arrest, right distal tibia

 M89.167 Partial physeal arrest, left distal tibia

 M89.168 Other physeal arrest of lower leg

 M89.169 Physeal arrest, lower leg, unspecified

M89.18 Physeal arrest, other site

M89.2 Other disorders of bone development and growth

 M89.20 Other disorders of bone development and growth, unspecified site

M89.21 Other disorders of bone development and growth, shoulder

 M89.211 Other disorders of bone development and growth, right shoulder

 M89.212 Other disorders of bone development and growth, left shoulder

 M89.219 Other disorders of bone development and growth, unspecified shoulder

M89.22 Other disorders of bone development and growth, humerus

 M89.221 Other disorders of bone development and growth, right humerus

 M89.222 Other disorders of bone development and growth, left humerus

 M89.229 Other disorders of bone development and growth, unspecified humerus

M89.23 Other disorders of bone development and growth, ulna and radius

 M89.231 Other disorders of bone development and growth, right ulna

 M89.232 Other disorders of bone development and growth, left ulna

 M89.233 Other disorders of bone development and growth, right radius

 M89.234 Other disorders of bone development and growth, left radius

 M89.239 Other disorders of bone development and growth, unspecified ulna and radius

M89.24 Other disorders of bone development and growth, hand

 M89.241 Other disorders of bone development and growth, right hand

 M89.242 Other disorders of bone development and growth, left hand

 M89.249 Other disorders of bone development and growth, unspecified hand

M89.25 Other disorders of bone development and growth, femur

 M89.251 Other disorders of bone development and growth, right femur

 M89.252 Other disorders of bone development and growth, left femur

M89.259 Other disorders of bone development and growth, unspecified femur

M89.26 Other disorders of bone development and growth, tibia and fibula

M89.261 Other disorders of bone development and growth, right tibia

M89.262 Other disorders of bone development and growth, left tibia

M89.263 Other disorders of bone development and growth, right fibula

M89.264 Other disorders of bone development and growth, left fibula

M89.269 Other disorders of bone development and growth, unspecified lower leg

M89.27 Other disorders of bone development and growth, ankle and foot

M89.271 Other disorders of bone development and growth, right ankle and foot

M89.272 Other disorders of bone development and growth, left ankle and foot

M89.279 Other disorders of bone development and growth, unspecified ankle and foot

M89.28 Other disorders of bone development and growth, other site

M89.29 Other disorders of bone development and growth, multiple sites

M89.3 Hypertrophy of bone

M89.30 Hypertrophy of bone, unspecified site

M89.31 Hypertrophy of bone, shoulder

M89.311 Hypertrophy of bone, right shoulder

M89.312 Hypertrophy of bone, left shoulder

M89.319 Hypertrophy of bone, unspecified shoulder

M89.32 Hypertrophy of bone, humerus

M89.321 Hypertrophy of bone, right humerus

M89.322 Hypertrophy of bone, left humerus

M89.329 Hypertrophy of bone, unspecified humerus

M89.33 Hypertrophy of bone, ulna and radius

M89.331 Hypertrophy of bone, right ulna

M89.332 Hypertrophy of bone, left ulna

M89.333 Hypertrophy of bone, right radius

M89.334 Hypertrophy of bone, left radius

M89.339 Hypertrophy of bone, unspecified ulna and radius

M89.34 Hypertrophy of bone, hand

M89.341 Hypertrophy of bone, right hand

M89.342 Hypertrophy of bone, left hand

M89.349 Hypertrophy of bone, unspecified hand

M89.35 Hypertrophy of bone, femur

M89.351 Hypertrophy of bone, right femur

M89.352 Hypertrophy of bone, left femur

M89.359 Hypertrophy of bone, unspecified femur

M89.36 Hypertrophy of bone, tibia and fibula

M89.361 Hypertrophy of bone, right tibia

M89.362 Hypertrophy of bone, left tibia

M89.363 Hypertrophy of bone, right fibula

M89.364 Hypertrophy of bone, left fibula

M89.369 Hypertrophy of bone, unspecified tibia and fibula

M89.37 Hypertrophy of bone, ankle and foot

M89.371 Hypertrophy of bone, right ankle and foot

M89.372 Hypertrophy of bone, left ankle and foot

M89.379 Hypertrophy of bone, unspecified ankle and foot

M89.38 Hypertrophy of bone, other site

M89.39 Hypertrophy of bone, multiple sites

M89.4 Other hypertrophic osteoarthropathy
Marie-Bamberger disease

M89.40 Other hypertrophic osteoarthropathy, unspecified site

M89.41 Other hypertrophic osteoarthropathy, shoulder

M89.411 Other hypertrophic osteoarthropathy, right shoulder

M89.412 Other hypertrophic osteoarthropathy, left shoulder

M89.419 Other hypertrophic osteoarthropathy, unspecified shoulder

M89.42 Other hypertrophic osteoarthropathy, upper arm

M89.421 Other hypertrophic osteoarthropathy, right upper arm

M89.422 Other hypertrophic osteoarthropathy, left upper arm

M89.429 Other hypertrophic osteoarthropathy, unspecified upper arm

M89.43 Other hypertrophic osteoarthropathy, forearm

M89.431 Other hypertrophic osteoarthropathy, right forearm

M89.432 Other hypertrophic osteoarthropathy, left forearm

M89.439 Other hypertrophic osteoarthropathy, unspecified forearm

M89.44 Other hypertrophic osteoarthropathy, hand

M89.441 Other hypertrophic osteoarthropathy, right hand

M89.442 Other hypertrophic osteoarthropathy, left hand

M89.449 Other hypertrophic osteoarthropathy, unspecified hand

M89.45 Other hypertrophic osteoarthropathy, thigh

M89.451 Other hypertrophic osteoarthropathy, right thigh

M89.452 Other hypertrophic osteoarthropathy, left thigh

M89.459 Other hypertrophic osteoarthropathy, unspecified thigh

M89.46 Other hypertrophic osteoarthropathy, lower leg

M89.461 Other hypertrophic osteoarthropathy, right lower leg

M89.462 Other hypertrophic osteoarthropathy, left lower leg

M89.469 Other hypertrophic osteoarthropathy, unspecified lower leg

M89.47 Other hypertrophic osteoarthropathy, ankle and foot

    M89.471 Other hypertrophic osteoarthropathy, right ankle and foot

    M89.472 Other hypertrophic osteoarthropathy, left ankle and foot

    M89.479 Other hypertrophic osteoarthropathy, unspecified ankle and foot

M89.48 Other hypertrophic osteoarthropathy, other site

M89.49 Other hypertrophic osteoarthropathy, multiple sites

M89.5 Osteolysis

Use additional code to identify major osseous defect, if applicable (M89.7-)

Excludes 2: periprosthetic osteolysis of internal prosthetic joint (T84.05-)

M89.50 Osteolysis, unspecified site

M89.51 Osteolysis, shoulder

    M89.511 Osteolysis, right shoulder

    M89.512 Osteolysis, left shoulder

    M89.519 Osteolysis, unspecified shoulder

M89.52 Osteolysis, upper arm

    M89.521 Osteolysis, right upper arm

    M89.522 Osteolysis, left upper arm

    M89.529 Osteolysis, unspecified upper arm

M89.53 Osteolysis, forearm

    M89.531 Osteolysis, right forearm

    M89.532 Osteolysis, left forearm

    M89.539 Osteolysis, unspecified forearm

M89.54 Osteolysis, hand

    M89.541 Osteolysis, right hand

    M89.542 Osteolysis, left hand

    M89.549 Osteolysis, unspecified hand

M89.55 Osteolysis, thigh

    M89.551 Osteolysis, right thigh

    M89.552 Osteolysis, left thigh

    M89.559 Osteolysis, unspecified thigh

M89.56 Osteolysis, lower leg

    M89.561 Osteolysis, right lower leg

    M89.562 Osteolysis, left lower leg

    M89.569 Osteolysis, unspecified lower leg

M89.57 Osteolysis, ankle and foot

    M89.571 Osteolysis, right ankle and foot

    M89.572 Osteolysis, left ankle and foot

    M89.579 Osteolysis, unspecified ankle and foot

M89.58 Osteolysis, other site

M89.59 Osteolysis, multiple sites

M89.6 Osteopathy after poliomyelitis

Use additional code (B91) to identify previous poliomyelitis

Excludes 1: postpolio syndrome (G14)

M89.60 Osteopathy after poliomyelitis, unspecified site

M89.61 Osteopathy after poliomyelitis, shoulder

    M89.611 Osteopathy after poliomyelitis, right shoulder

    M89.612 Osteopathy after poliomyelitis, left shoulder

    M89.619 Osteopathy after poliomyelitis, unspecified shoulder

M89.62 Osteopathy after poliomyelitis, upper arm

    M89.621 Osteopathy after poliomyelitis, right upper arm

    M89.622 Osteopathy after poliomyelitis, left upper arm

    M89.629 Osteopathy after poliomyelitis, unspecified upper arm

M89.63 Osteopathy after poliomyelitis, forearm

    M89.631 Osteopathy after poliomyelitis, right forearm

    M89.632 Osteopathy after poliomyelitis, left forearm

    M89.639 Osteopathy after poliomyelitis, unspecified forearm

M89.64 Osteopathy after poliomyelitis, hand

    M89.641 Osteopathy after poliomyelitis, right hand

    M89.642 Osteopathy after poliomyelitis, left hand

    M89.649 Osteopathy after poliomyelitis, unspecified hand

M89.65 Osteopathy after poliomyelitis, thigh

    M89.651 Osteopathy after poliomyelitis, right thigh

    M89.652 Osteopathy after poliomyelitis, left thigh

    M89.659 Osteopathy after poliomyelitis, unspecified thigh

M89.66 Osteopathy after poliomyelitis, lower leg

    M89.661 Osteopathy after poliomyelitis, right lower leg

    M89.662 Osteopathy after poliomyelitis, left lower leg

    M89.669 Osteopathy after poliomyelitis, unspecified lower leg

M89.67 Osteopathy after poliomyelitis, ankle and foot

    M89.671 Osteopathy after poliomyelitis, right ankle and foot

    M89.672 Osteopathy after poliomyelitis, left ankle and foot

    M89.679 Osteopathy after poliomyelitis, unspecified ankle and foot

M89.68 Osteopathy after poliomyelitis, other site

M89.69 Osteopathy after poliomyelitis, multiple sites

M89.7 Major osseous defect

Code first underlying disease, if known, such as:

    aseptic necrosis of bone (M87.-)

    malignant neoplasm of bone (C40.-)

    osteolysis (M89.5)

    osteomyelitis (M86.-)

    osteonecrosis (M87.-)

    osteoporosis (M80.-, M81.-)

    periprosthetic osteolysis (T84.05-)

M89.70 Major osseous defect, unspecified site

M89.71 Major osseous defect, shoulder region

    Major osseous defect clavicle or scapula

M89.711 Major osseous defect, right shoulder region

M89.712 Major osseous defect, left shoulder region

M89.719 Major osseous defect, unspecified shoulder region

M89.72 Major osseous defect, humerus

M89.721 Major osseous defect, right humerus

M89.722 Major osseous defect, left humerus

M89.729 Major osseous defect, unspecified humerus

M89.73 Major osseous defect, forearm

Major osseous defect of radius and ulna

M89.731 Major osseous defect, right forearm

M89.732 Major osseous defect, left forearm

M89.739 Major osseous defect, unspecified forearm

M89.74 Major osseous defect, hand

Major osseous defect of carpus, fingers, metacarpus

M89.741 Major osseous defect, right hand

M89.742 Major osseous defect, left hand

M89.749 Major osseous defect, unspecified hand

M89.75 Major osseous defect, pelvic region and thigh

Major osseous defect of femur and pelvis

M89.751 Major osseous defect, right pelvic region and thigh

M89.752 Major osseous defect, left pelvic region and thigh

M89.759 Major osseous defect, unspecified pelvic region and thigh

M89.76 Major osseous defect, lower leg

Major osseous defect of fibula and tibia

M89.761 Major osseous defect, right lower leg

M89.762 Major osseous defect, left lower leg

M89.769 Major osseous defect, unspecified lower leg

M89.77 Major osseous defect, ankle and foot

Major osseous defect of metatarsus, tarsus, toes

M89.771 Major osseous defect, right ankle and foot

M89.772 Major osseous defect, left ankle and foot

M89.779 Major osseous defect, unspecified ankle and foot

M89.78 Major osseous defect, other site

M89.79 Major osseous defect, multiple sites

M89.8 Other specified disorders of bone

Infantile cortical hyperostoses

Post-traumatic subperiosteal ossification

M89.8X Other specified disorders of bone

M89.8X0 Other specified disorders of bone, multiple sites

M89.8X1 Other specified disorders of bone, shoulder

M89.8X2 Other specified disorders of bone, upper arm

M89.8X3 Other specified disorders of bone, forearm

M89.8X4 Other specified disorders of bone, hand

M89.8X5 Other specified disorders of bone, thigh

M89.8X6 Other specified disorders of bone, lower leg

M89.8X7 Other specified disorders of bone, ankle and foot

M89.8X8 Other specified disorders of bone, other site

M89.8X9 Other specified disorders of bone, unspecified site

M89.9 Disorder of bone, unspecified

M90 Osteopathies in diseases classified elsewhere

Excludes 1: osteochondritis, osteomyelitis, and osteopathy (in):

cryptococcosis (B45.3)

diabetes mellitus (E08-E13 with 4th character .61-)

gonococcal (A54.43)

neurogenic syphilis (A52.11)

renal osteodystrophy (N25.0)

salmonellosis (A02.24)

secondary syphilis (A51.46)

syphilis (late) (A52.77)

M90.5 Osteonecrosis in diseases classified elsewhere

Code first underlying disease, such as:

caisson disease (T70.3)

hemoglobinopathy (D50-D64)

M90.50 Osteonecrosis in diseases classified elsewhere, unspecified site

M90.51 Osteonecrosis in diseases classified elsewhere, shoulder

M90.511 Osteonecrosis in diseases classified elsewhere, right shoulder

M90.512 Osteonecrosis in diseases classified elsewhere, left shoulder

M90.519 Osteonecrosis in diseases classified elsewhere, unspecified shoulder

M90.52 Osteonecrosis in diseases classified elsewhere, upper arm

M90.521 Osteonecrosis in diseases classified elsewhere, right upper arm

M90.522 Osteonecrosis in diseases classified elsewhere, left upper arm

M90.529 Osteonecrosis in diseases classified elsewhere, unspecified upper arm

M90.53 Osteonecrosis in diseases classified elsewhere, forearm

M90.531 Osteonecrosis in diseases classified elsewhere, right forearm

M90.532 Osteonecrosis in diseases classified elsewhere, left forearm

M90.539 Osteonecrosis in diseases classified elsewhere, unspecified forearm

M90.54 Osteonecrosis in diseases classified elsewhere, hand

M90.541 Osteonecrosis in diseases classified elsewhere, right hand

M90.542 Osteonecrosis in diseases classified elsewhere, left hand

M90.549 Osteonecrosis in diseases classified elsewhere, unspecified hand

M90.55 Osteonecrosis in diseases classified elsewhere, thigh

M90.551 Osteonecrosis in diseases classified elsewhere, right thigh

M90.552 Osteonecrosis in diseases classified elsewhere, left thigh

M90.559 Osteonecrosis in diseases classified elsewhere, unspecified thigh

M90.56 Osteonecrosis in diseases classified elsewhere, lower leg

M90.561 Osteonecrosis in diseases classified elsewhere, right lower leg

M90.562 Osteonecrosis in diseases classified elsewhere, left lower leg

M90.569 Osteonecrosis in diseases classified elsewhere, unspecified lower leg

M90.57 Osteonecrosis in diseases classified elsewhere, ankle and foot

M90.571 Osteonecrosis in diseases classified elsewhere, right ankle and foot

M90.572 Osteonecrosis in diseases classified elsewhere, left ankle and foot

M90.579 Osteonecrosis in diseases classified elsewhere, unspecified ankle and foot

M90.58 Osteonecrosis in diseases classified elsewhere, other site

M90.59 Osteonecrosis in diseases classified elsewhere, multiple sites

M90.6 Osteitis deformans in neoplastic diseases

Osteitis deformans in malignant neoplasm of bone

Code first the neoplasm (C40.-, C41.-)

Excludes 1: osteitis deformans [Paget's disease of bone] (M88.-)

M90.60 Osteitis deformans in neoplastic diseases, unspecified site

M90.61 Osteitis deformans in neoplastic diseases, shoulder

M90.611 Osteitis deformans in neoplastic diseases, right shoulder

M90.612 Osteitis deformans in neoplastic diseases, left shoulder

M90.619 Osteitis deformans in neoplastic diseases, unspecified shoulder

M90.62 Osteitis deformans in neoplastic diseases, upper arm

M90.621 Osteitis deformans in neoplastic diseases, right upper arm

M90.622 Osteitis deformans in neoplastic diseases, left upper arm

M90.629 Osteitis deformans in neoplastic diseases, unspecified upper arm

M90.63 Osteitis deformans in neoplastic diseases, forearm

M90.631 Osteitis deformans in neoplastic diseases, right forearm

M90.632 Osteitis deformans in neoplastic diseases, left forearm

M90.639 Osteitis deformans in neoplastic diseases, unspecified forearm

M90.64 Osteitis deformans in neoplastic diseases, hand

M90.641 Osteitis deformans in neoplastic diseases, right hand

M90.642 Osteitis deformans in neoplastic diseases, left hand

M90.649 Osteitis deformans in neoplastic diseases, unspecified hand

M90.65 Osteitis deformans in neoplastic diseases, thigh

M90.651 Osteitis deformans in neoplastic diseases, right thigh

M90.652 Osteitis deformans in neoplastic diseases, left thigh

M90.659 Osteitis deformans in neoplastic diseases, unspecified thigh

M90.66 Osteitis deformans in neoplastic diseases, lower leg

M90.661 Osteitis deformans in neoplastic diseases, right lower leg

M90.662 Osteitis deformans in neoplastic diseases, left lower leg

M90.669 Osteitis deformans in neoplastic diseases, unspecified lower leg

M90.67 Osteitis deformans in neoplastic diseases, ankle and foot

M90.671 Osteitis deformans in neoplastic diseases, right ankle and foot

M90.672 Osteitis deformans in neoplastic diseases, left ankle and foot

M90.679 Osteitis deformans in neoplastic diseases, unspecified ankle and foot

M90.68 Osteitis deformans in neoplastic diseases, other site

M90.69 Osteitis deformans in neoplastic diseases, multiple sites

M90.8 Osteopathy in diseases classified elsewhere

Code first underlying disease, such as:

    rickets (E55.0)

    vitamin-D-resistant rickets (E83.3)

M90.80 Osteopathy in diseases classified elsewhere, unspecified site

M90.81 Osteopathy in diseases classified elsewhere, shoulder

M90.811 Osteopathy in diseases classified elsewhere, right shoulder

M90.812 Osteopathy in diseases classified elsewhere, left shoulder

M90.819 Osteopathy in diseases classified elsewhere, unspecified shoulder

M90.82 Osteopathy in diseases classified elsewhere, upper arm

M90.821 Osteopathy in diseases classified elsewhere, right upper arm

M90.822 Osteopathy in diseases classified elsewhere, left upper arm

M90.829 Osteopathy in diseases classified elsewhere, unspecified upper arm

M90.83 Osteopathy in diseases classified elsewhere, forearm

    M90.831 Osteopathy in diseases classified elsewhere, right forearm

    M90.832 Osteopathy in diseases classified elsewhere, left forearm

    M90.839 Osteopathy in diseases classified elsewhere, unspecified forearm

M90.84 Osteopathy in diseases classified elsewhere, hand

    M90.841 Osteopathy in diseases classified elsewhere, right hand

    M90.842 Osteopathy in diseases classified elsewhere, left hand

    M90.849 Osteopathy in diseases classified elsewhere, unspecified hand

M90.85 Osteopathy in diseases classified elsewhere, thigh

    M90.851 Osteopathy in diseases classified elsewhere, right thigh

    M90.852 Osteopathy in diseases classified elsewhere, left thigh

    M90.859 Osteopathy in diseases classified elsewhere, unspecified thigh

M90.86 Osteopathy in diseases classified elsewhere, lower leg

    M90.861 Osteopathy in diseases classified elsewhere, right lower leg

    M90.862 Osteopathy in diseases classified elsewhere, left lower leg

    M90.869 Osteopathy in diseases classified elsewhere, unspecified lower leg

M90.87 Osteopathy in diseases classified elsewhere, ankle and foot

    M90.871 Osteopathy in diseases classified elsewhere, right ankle and foot

    M90.872 Osteopathy in diseases classified elsewhere, left ankle and foot

    M90.879 Osteopathy in diseases classified elsewhere, unspecified ankle and foot

M90.88 Osteopathy in diseases classified elsewhere, other site

M90.89 Osteopathy in diseases classified elsewhere, multiple sites

CHONDROPATHIES (M91-M94)

Excludes 1: postprocedural chondropathies (M96.-)

M91 Juvenile osteochondrosis of hip and pelvis

Excludes 1: slipped upper femoral epiphysis (nontraumatic) (M93.0)

M91.0 Juvenile osteochondrosis of pelvis

Osteochondrosis (juvenile) of:

acetabulum

iliac crest [Buchanan]

ischiopubic synchondrosis [van Neck]

symphysis pubis [Pierson]

M91.1 Juvenile osteochondrosis of head of femur [Legg-Calvé-Perthes-Perthes]

    M91.10 Juvenile osteochondrosis of head of femur [Legg-Calvé-Perthes-Perthes], unspecified leg

    M91.11 Juvenile osteochondrosis of head of femur [Legg-Calve-Perthes], right leg

    M91.12 Juvenile osteochondrosis of head of femur [Legg-Calve-Perthes], left leg

M91.2 Coxa plana

Hip deformity due to previous juvenile osteochondrosis

    M91.20 Coxa plana, unspecified hip

    M91.21 Coxa plana, right hip

    M91.22 Coxa plana, left hip

M91.3 Pseudocoxalgia

    M91.30 Pseudocoxalgia, unspecified hip

    M91.31 Pseudocoxalgia, right hip

    M91.32 Pseudocoxalgia, left hip

M91.4 Coxa magna

    M91.40 Coxa magna, unspecified hip

    M91.41 Coxa magna, right hip

    M91.42 Coxa magna, left hip

M91.8 Other juvenile osteochondrosis of hip and pelvis

Juvenile osteochondrosis after reduction of congenital dislocation of hip

    M91.80 Other juvenile osteochondrosis of hip and pelvis, unspecified leg

    M91.81 Other juvenile osteochondrosis of hip and pelvis, right leg

    M91.82 Other juvenile osteochondrosis of hip and pelvis, left leg

M91.9 Juvenile osteochondrosis of hip and pelvis, unspecified

    M91.90 Juvenile osteochondrosis of hip and pelvis, unspecified, unspecified leg

    M91.91 Juvenile osteochondrosis of hip and pelvis, unspecified, right leg

    M91.92 Juvenile osteochondrosis of hip and pelvis, unspecified, left leg

M92 Other juvenile osteochondrosis

M92.0 Juvenile osteochondrosis of humerus

Osteochondrosis (juvenile) of capitulum of humerus [Panner]

Osteochondrosis (juvenile) of head of humerus [Haas]

    M92.00 Juvenile osteochondrosis of humerus, unspecified arm

    M92.01 Juvenile osteochondrosis of humerus, right arm

    M92.02 Juvenile osteochondrosis of humerus, left arm

M92.1 Juvenile osteochondrosis of radius and ulna

Osteochondrosis (juvenile) of lower ulna [Burns]

Osteochondrosis (juvenile) of radial head [Brailsford]

    M92.10 Juvenile osteochondrosis of radius and ulna, unspecified arm

    M92.11 Juvenile osteochondrosis of radius and ulna, right arm

    M92.12 Juvenile osteochondrosis of radius and ulna, left arm

M92.2 Juvenile osteochondrosis, hand

    M92.20 Unspecified juvenile osteochondrosis, hand

        M92.201 Unspecified juvenile osteochondrosis, right hand

        M92.202 Unspecified juvenile osteochondrosis, left hand

        M92.209 Unspecified juvenile osteochondrosis, unspecified hand

● New code   ▲ Revised code   ⑦ 7th digit required   ⊗ Placeholder required

M92.21 Osteochondrosis (juvenile) of carpal lunate [Kienbock]

    M92.211 Osteochondrosis (juvenile) of carpal lunate [Kienbock], right hand

    M92.212 Osteochondrosis (juvenile) of carpal lunate [Kienbock], left hand

    M92.219 Osteochondrosis (juvenile) of carpal lunate [Kienbock], unspecified hand

M92.22 Osteochondrosis (juvenile) of metacarpal heads [Mauclaire]

    M92.221 Osteochondrosis (juvenile) of metacarpal heads [Mauclaire], right hand

    M92.222 Osteochondrosis (juvenile) of metacarpal heads [Mauclaire], left hand

    M92.229 Osteochondrosis (juvenile) of metacarpal heads [Mauclaire], unspecified hand

M92.29 Other juvenile osteochondrosis, hand

    M92.291 Other juvenile osteochondrosis, right hand

    M92.292 Other juvenile osteochondrosis, left hand

    M92.299 Other juvenile osteochondrosis, unspecified hand

M92.3 Other juvenile osteochondrosis, upper limb

    M92.30 Other juvenile osteochondrosis, unspecified upper limb

    M92.31 Other juvenile osteochondrosis, right upper limb

    M92.32 Other juvenile osteochondrosis, left upper limb

M92.4 Juvenile osteochondrosis of patella

Osteochondrosis (juvenile) of primary patellar center [Kohler]

Osteochondrosis (juvenile) of secondary patellar centre [Sinding Larsen]

    M92.40 Juvenile osteochondrosis of patella, unspecified knee

    M92.41 Juvenile osteochondrosis of patella, right knee

    M92.42 Juvenile osteochondrosis of patella, left knee

M92.5 Juvenile osteochondrosis of tibia and fibula

Osteochondrosis (juvenile) of proximal tibia [Blount]

Osteochondrosis (juvenile) of tibial tubercle [Osgood-Schlatter]

Tibia vara

    M92.50 Juvenile osteochondrosis of tibia and fibula, unspecified leg

    M92.51 Juvenile osteochondrosis of tibia and fibula, right leg

    M92.52 Juvenile osteochondrosis of tibia and fibula, left leg

M92.6 Juvenile osteochondrosis of tarsus

Osteochondrosis (juvenile) of calcaneum [Sever]

Osteochondrosis (juvenile) of os tibiale externum [Haglund]

Osteochondrosis (juvenile) of talus [Diaz]

Osteochondrosis (juvenile) of tarsal navicular [Kohler]

    M92.60 Juvenile osteochondrosis of tarsus, unspecified ankle

    M92.61 Juvenile osteochondrosis of tarsus, right ankle

    M92.62 Juvenile osteochondrosis of tarsus, left ankle

M92.7 Juvenile osteochondrosis of metatarsus

Osteochondrosis (juvenile) of fifth metatarsus [Iselin]

Osteochondrosis (juvenile) of second metatarsus [Freiberg]

    M92.70 Juvenile osteochondrosis of metatarsus, unspecified foot

    M92.71 Juvenile osteochondrosis of metatarsus, right foot

    M92.72 Juvenile osteochondrosis of metatarsus, left foot

M92.8 Other specified juvenile osteochondrosis

Calcaneal apophysitis

M92.9 Juvenile osteochondrosis, unspecified

Juvenile apophysitis NOS

Juvenile epiphysitis NOS

Juvenile osteochondritis NOS

Juvenile osteochondrosis NOS

M93 Other osteochondropathies

    Excludes 2: osteochondrosis of spine (M42.-)

M93.0 Slipped upper femoral epiphysis (nontraumatic)

Use additional code for associated chondrolysis (M94.3)

    M93.00 Unspecified slipped upper femoral epiphysis (nontraumatic)

        M93.001 Unspecified slipped upper femoral epiphysis (nontraumatic), right hip

        M93.002 Unspecified slipped upper femoral epiphysis (nontraumatic), left hip

        M93.003 Unspecified slipped upper femoral epiphysis (nontraumatic), unspecified hip

    M93.01 Acute slipped upper femoral epiphysis (nontraumatic)

        M93.011 Acute slipped upper femoral epiphysis (nontraumatic), right hip

        M93.012 Acute slipped upper femoral epiphysis (nontraumatic), left hip

        M93.013 Acute slipped upper femoral epiphysis (nontraumatic), unspecified hip

    M93.02 Chronic slipped upper femoral epiphysis (nontraumatic)

        M93.021 Chronic slipped upper femoral epiphysis (nontraumatic), right hip

        M93.022 Chronic slipped upper femoral epiphysis (nontraumatic), left hip

        M93.023 Chronic slipped upper femoral epiphysis (nontraumatic), unspecified hip

    M93.03 Acute on chronic slipped upper femoral epiphysis (nontraumatic)

        M93.031 Acute on chronic slipped upper femoral epiphysis (nontraumatic), right hip

        M93.032 Acute on chronic slipped upper femoral epiphysis (nontraumatic), left hip

        M93.033 Acute on chronic slipped upper femoral epiphysis (nontraumatic), unspecified hip

M93.1 Kienbock's disease of adults

Adult osteochondrosis of carpal lunates

M93.2 Osteochondritis dissecans

    M93.20 Osteochondritis dissecans of unspecified site

    M93.21 Osteochondritis dissecans of shoulder

M93.211 Osteochondritis dissecans, right shoulder

M93.212 Osteochondritis dissecans, left shoulder

M93.219 Osteochondritis dissecans, unspecified shoulder

M93.22 Osteochondritis dissecans of elbow

M93.221 Osteochondritis dissecans, right elbow

M93.222 Osteochondritis dissecans, left elbow

M93.229 Osteochondritis dissecans, unspecified elbow

M93.23 Osteochondritis dissecans of wrist

M93.231 Osteochondritis dissecans, right wrist

M93.232 Osteochondritis dissecans, left wrist

M93.239 Osteochondritis dissecans, unspecified wrist

M93.24 Osteochondritis dissecans of joints of hand

M93.241 Osteochondritis dissecans, joints of right hand

M93.242 Osteochondritis dissecans, joints of left hand

M93.249 Osteochondritis dissecans, joints of unspecified hand

M93.25 Osteochondritis dissecans of hip

M93.251 Osteochondritis dissecans, right hip

M93.252 Osteochondritis dissecans, left hip

M93.259 Osteochondritis dissecans, unspecified hip

M93.26 Osteochondritis dissecans knee

M93.261 Osteochondritis dissecans, right knee

M93.262 Osteochondritis dissecans, left knee

M93.269 Osteochondritis dissecans, unspecified knee

M93.27 Osteochondritis dissecans of ankle and joints of foot

M93.271 Osteochondritis dissecans, right ankle and joints of right foot

M93.272 Osteochondritis dissecans, left ankle and joints of left foot

M93.279 Osteochondritis dissecans, unspecified ankle and joints of foot

M93.28 Osteochondritis dissecans other site

M93.29 Osteochondritis dissecans multiple sites

M93.8 Other specified osteochondropathies

M93.80 Other specified osteochondropathies of unspecified site

M93.81 Other specified osteochondropathies of shoulder

M93.811 Other specified osteochondropathies, right shoulder

M93.812 Other specified osteochondropathies, left shoulder

M93.819 Other specified osteochondropathies, unspecified shoulder

M93.82 Other specified osteochondropathies of upper arm

M93.821 Other specified osteochondropathies, right upper arm

M93.822 Other specified osteochondropathies, left upper arm

M93.829 Other specified osteochondropathies, unspecified upper arm

M93.83 Other specified osteochondropathies of forearm

M93.831 Other specified osteochondropathies, right forearm

M93.832 Other specified osteochondropathies, left forearm

M93.839 Other specified osteochondropathies, unspecified forearm

M93.84 Other specified osteochondropathies of hand

M93.841 Other specified osteochondropathies, right hand

M93.842 Other specified osteochondropathies, left hand

M93.849 Other specified osteochondropathies, unspecified hand

M93.85 Other specified osteochondropathies of thigh

M93.851 Other specified osteochondropathies, right thigh

M93.852 Other specified osteochondropathies, left thigh

M93.859 Other specified osteochondropathies, unspecified thigh

M93.86 Other specified osteochondropathies lower leg

M93.861 Other specified osteochondropathies, right lower leg

M93.862 Other specified osteochondropathies, left lower leg

M93.869 Other specified osteochondropathies, unspecified lower leg

M93.87 Other specified osteochondropathies of ankle and foot

M93.871 Other specified osteochondropathies, right ankle and foot

M93.872 Other specified osteochondropathies, left ankle and foot

M93.879 Other specified osteochondropathies, unspecified ankle and foot

M93.88 Other specified osteochondropathies other

M93.89 Other specified osteochondropathies multiple sites

M93.9 Osteochondropathy, unspecified

Apophysitis NOS

Epiphysitis NOS

Osteochondritis NOS

Osteochondrosis NOS

M93.90 Osteochondropathy, unspecified of unspecified site

M93.91 Osteochondropathy, unspecified of shoulder
    M93.911 Osteochondropathy, unspecified, right shoulder
    M93.912 Osteochondropathy, unspecified, left shoulder
    M93.919 Osteochondropathy, unspecified, unspecified shoulder
M93.92 Osteochondropathy, unspecified of upper arm
    M93.921 Osteochondropathy, unspecified, right upper arm
    M93.922 Osteochondropathy, unspecified, left upper arm
    M93.929 Osteochondropathy, unspecified, unspecified upper arm
M93.93 Osteochondropathy, unspecified of forearm
    M93.931 Osteochondropathy, unspecified, right forearm
    M93.932 Osteochondropathy, unspecified, left forearm
    M93.939 Osteochondropathy, unspecified, unspecified forearm
M93.94 Osteochondropathy, unspecified of hand
    M93.941 Osteochondropathy, unspecified, right hand
    M93.942 Osteochondropathy, unspecified, left hand
    M93.949 Osteochondropathy, unspecified, unspecified hand
M93.95 Osteochondropathy, unspecified of thigh
    M93.951 Osteochondropathy, unspecified, right thigh
    M93.952 Osteochondropathy, unspecified, left thigh
    M93.959 Osteochondropathy, unspecified, unspecified thigh
M93.96 Osteochondropathy, unspecified lower leg
    M93.961 Osteochondropathy, unspecified, right lower leg
    M93.962 Osteochondropathy, unspecified, left lower leg
    M93.969 Osteochondropathy, unspecified, unspecified lower leg
M93.97 Osteochondropathy, unspecified of ankle and foot
    M93.971 Osteochondropathy, unspecified, right ankle and foot
    M93.972 Osteochondropathy, unspecified, left ankle and foot
    M93.979 Osteochondropathy, unspecified, unspecified ankle and foot
M93.98 Osteochondropathy, unspecified other
M93.99 Osteochondropathy, unspecified multiple sites

M94 Other disorders of cartilage
M94.0 Chondrocostal junction syndrome [Tietze]
Costochondritis
M94.1 Relapsing polychondritis
M94.2 Chondromalacia
    Excludes 1: chondromalacia patellae (M22.4)
  M94.20 Chondromalacia, unspecified site
  M94.21 Chondromalacia, shoulder
    M94.211 Chondromalacia, right shoulder

    M94.212 Chondromalacia, left shoulder
    M94.219 Chondromalacia, unspecified shoulder
M94.22 Chondromalacia, elbow
    M94.221 Chondromalacia, right elbow
    M94.222 Chondromalacia, left elbow
    M94.229 Chondromalacia, unspecified elbow
M94.23 Chondromalacia, wrist
    M94.231 Chondromalacia, right wrist
    M94.232 Chondromalacia, left wrist
    M94.239 Chondromalacia, unspecified wrist
M94.24 Chondromalacia, joints of hand
    M94.241 Chondromalacia, joints of right hand
    M94.242 Chondromalacia, joints of left hand
    M94.249 Chondromalacia, joints of unspecified hand
M94.25 Chondromalacia, hip
    M94.251 Chondromalacia, right hip
    M94.252 Chondromalacia, left hip
    M94.259 Chondromalacia, unspecified hip
M94.26 Chondromalacia, knee
    M94.261 Chondromalacia, right knee
    M94.262 Chondromalacia, left knee
    M94.269 Chondromalacia, unspecified knee
M94.27 Chondromalacia, ankle and joints of foot
    M94.271 Chondromalacia, right ankle and joints of right foot
    M94.272 Chondromalacia, left ankle and joints of left foot
    M94.279 Chondromalacia, unspecified ankle and joints of foot
M94.28 Chondromalacia, other site
M94.29 Chondromalacia, multiple sites
M94.3 Chondrolysis
Code first any associated slipped upper femoral epiphysis (nontraumatic) (M93.0-)
  M94.35 Chondrolysis, hip
    M94.351 Chondrolysis, right hip
    M94.352 Chondrolysis, left hip
    M94.359 Chondrolysis, unspecified hip
M94.8 Other specified disorders of cartilage
  M94.8X Other specified disorders of cartilage
    M94.8X0 Other specified disorders of cartilage, multiple sites
    M94.8X1 Other specified disorders of cartilage, shoulder
    M94.8X2 Other specified disorders of cartilage, upper arm
    M94.8X3 Other specified disorders of cartilage, forearm
    M94.8X4 Other specified disorders of cartilage, hand
    M94.8X5 Other specified disorders of cartilage, thigh
    M94.8X6 Other specified disorders of cartilage, lower leg
    M94.8X7 Other specified disorders of cartilage, ankle and foot
    M94.8X8 Other specified disorders of cartilage, other site

M94.8X9 Other specified disorders of cartilage, unspecified sites

M94.9 Disorder of cartilage, unspecified

OTHER DISORDERS OF THE MUSCULOSKELETAL SYSTEM AND CONNECTIVE TISSUE (M95)

M95 Other acquired deformities of musculoskeletal system and connective tissue

Excludes 2: acquired absence of limbs and organs (Z89-Z90)

acquired deformities of limbs (M20-M21)

congenital malformations and deformations of the musculoskeletal system (Q65-Q79)

deforming dorsopathies (M40-M43)

dentofacial anomalies [including malocclusion] (M26.-)

postprocedural musculoskeletal disorders (M96.-)

M95.0 Acquired deformity of nose

Excludes 2: deviated nasal septum (J34.2)

M95.1 Cauliflower ear

Excludes 2: other acquired deformities of ear (H61.1)

M95.10 Cauliflower ear, unspecified ear

M95.11 Cauliflower ear, right ear

M95.12 Cauliflower ear, left ear

M95.2 Other acquired deformity of head

M95.3 Acquired deformity of neck

M95.4 Acquired deformity of chest and rib

M95.5 Acquired deformity of pelvis

Excludes 1: maternal care for known or suspected disproportion (O33.-)

M95.8 Other specified acquired deformities of musculoskeletal system

M95.9 Acquired deformity of musculoskeletal system, unspecified

INTRAOPERATIVE AND POSTPROCEDURAL COMPLICATIONS AND DISORDERS OF MUSCULOSKELETAL SYSTEM, NOT ELSEWHERE CLASSIFIED (M96)

M96 Intraoperative and postprocedural complications and disorders of musculoskeletal system, not elsewhere classified

Excludes 2: arthropathy following intestinal bypass (M02.0-)

complications of internal orthopedic prosthetic devices, implants and grafts (T84.-)

disorders associated with osteoporosis (M80)

presence of functional implants and other devices (Z96-Z97)

M96.0 Pseudarthrosis after fusion or arthrodesis

M96.1 Postlaminectomy syndrome, not elsewhere classified

M96.2 Postradiation kyphosis

M96.3 Postlaminectomy kyphosis

M96.4 Postsurgical lordosis

M96.5 Postradiation scoliosis

M96.6 Fracture of bone following insertion of orthopedic implant, joint prosthesis, or bone plate

Intraoperative fracture of bone during insertion of orthopedic implant, joint prosthesis, or bone plate

Excludes 2: complication of internal orthopedic devices, implants or grafts (T84.-)

M96.62 Fracture of humerus following insertion of orthopedic implant, joint prosthesis, or bone plate

M96.621 Fracture of humerus following insertion of orthopedic implant, joint prosthesis, or bone plate, right arm

M96.622 Fracture of humerus following insertion of orthopedic implant, joint prosthesis, or bone plate, left arm

M96.629 Fracture of humerus following insertion of orthopedic implant, joint prosthesis, or bone plate, unspecified arm

M96.63 Fracture of radius or ulna following insertion of orthopedic implant, joint prosthesis, or bone plate

M96.631 Fracture of radius or ulna following insertion of orthopedic implant, joint prosthesis, or bone plate, right arm

M96.632 Fracture of radius or ulna following insertion of orthopedic implant, joint prosthesis, or bone plate, left arm

M96.639 Fracture of radius or ulna following insertion of orthopedic implant, joint prosthesis, or bone plate, unspecified arm

M96.65 Fracture of pelvis following insertion of orthopedic implant, joint prosthesis, or bone plate

M96.66 Fracture of femur following insertion of orthopedic implant, joint prosthesis, or bone plate

M96.661 Fracture of femur following insertion of orthopedic implant, joint prosthesis, or bone plate, right leg

M96.662 Fracture of femur following insertion of orthopedic implant, joint prosthesis, or bone plate, left leg

M96.669 Fracture of femur following insertion of orthopedic implant, joint prosthesis, or bone plate, unspecified leg

M96.67 Fracture of tibia or fibula following insertion of orthopedic implant, joint prosthesis, or bone plate

M96.671 Fracture of tibia or fibula following insertion of orthopedic implant, joint prosthesis, or bone plate, right leg

M96.672 Fracture of tibia or fibula following insertion of orthopedic implant, joint prosthesis, or bone plate, left leg

M96.679 Fracture of tibia or fibula following insertion of orthopedic implant, joint prosthesis, or bone plate, unspecified leg

M96.69 Fracture of other bone following insertion of orthopedic implant, joint prosthesis, or bone plate

M96.8 Other intraoperative and postprocedural complications and disorders of musculoskeletal system, not elsewhere classified

M96.81 Intraoperative hemorrhage and hematoma of a musculoskeletal structure complicating a procedure

Excludes 1: intraoperative hemorrhage and hematoma of a musculoskeletal structure due to accidental puncture and laceration during a procedure (M98.82-)

● New code   ▲ Revised code   ⑦ 7th digit required   ⊗ Placeholder required

M96.810 Intraoperative hemorrhage and hematoma of a musculoskeletal structure complicating a musculoskeletal system procedure

M96.811 Intraoperative hemorrhage and hematoma of a musculoskeletal structure complicating other procedure

M96.82 Accidental puncture and laceration of a musculoskeletal structure during a procedure

M96.820 Accidental puncture and laceration of a musculoskeletal structure during a musculoskeletal system procedure

M96.821 Accidental puncture and laceration of a musculoskeletal structure during other procedure

M96.83 Postprocedural hemorrhage and hematoma of a musculoskeletal structure following a procedure

M96.830 Postprocedural hemorrhage and hematoma of a musculoskeletal structure following a musculoskeletal system procedure

M96.831 Postprocedural hemorrhage and hematoma of a musculoskeletal structure following other procedure

M96.89 Other intraoperative and postprocedural complications and disorders of the musculoskeletal system

Instability of joint secondary to removal of joint prosthesis

Use additional code, if applicable, to further specify disorder

BIOMECHANICAL LESIONS, NOT ELSEWHERE CLASSIFIED (M99)

M99 Biomechanical lesions, not elsewhere classified

Note: This category should not be used if the condition can be classified elsewhere.

M99.0 Segmental and somatic dysfunction

M99.00 Segmental and somatic dysfunction of head region

M99.01 Segmental and somatic dysfunction of cervical region

M99.02 Segmental and somatic dysfunction of thoracic region

M99.03 Segmental and somatic dysfunction of lumbar region

M99.04 Segmental and somatic dysfunction of sacral region

M99.05 Segmental and somatic dysfunction of pelvic region

M99.06 Segmental and somatic dysfunction of lower extremity

M99.07 Segmental and somatic dysfunction of upper extremity

M99.08 Segmental and somatic dysfunction of rib cage

M99.09 Segmental and somatic dysfunction of abdomen and other regions

M99.1 Subluxation complex (vertebral)

M99.10 Subluxation complex (vertebral) of head region

M99.11 Subluxation complex (vertebral) of cervical region

M99.12 Subluxation complex (vertebral) of thoracic region

M99.13 Subluxation complex (vertebral) of lumbar region

M99.14 Subluxation complex (vertebral) of sacral region

M99.15 Subluxation complex (vertebral) of pelvic region

M99.16 Subluxation complex (vertebral) of lower extremity

M99.17 Subluxation complex (vertebral) of upper extremity

M99.18 Subluxation complex (vertebral) of rib cage

M99.19 Subluxation complex (vertebral) of abdomen and other regions

M99.2 Subluxation stenosis of neural canal

M99.20 Subluxation stenosis of neural canal of head region

M99.21 Subluxation stenosis of neural canal of cervical region

M99.22 Subluxation stenosis of neural canal of thoracic region

M99.23 Subluxation stenosis of neural canal of lumbar region

M99.24 Subluxation stenosis of neural canal of sacral region

M99.25 Subluxation stenosis of neural canal of pelvic region

M99.26 Subluxation stenosis of neural canal of lower extremity

M99.27 Subluxation stenosis of neural canal of upper extremity

M99.28 Subluxation stenosis of neural canal of rib cage

M99.29 Subluxation stenosis of neural canal of abdomen and other regions

M99.3 Osseous stenosis of neural canal

M99.30 Osseous stenosis of neural canal of head region

M99.31 Osseous stenosis of neural canal of cervical region

M99.32 Osseous stenosis of neural canal of thoracic region

M99.33 Osseous stenosis of neural canal of lumbar region

M99.34 Osseous stenosis of neural canal of sacral region

M99.35 Osseous stenosis of neural canal of pelvic region

M99.36 Osseous stenosis of neural canal of lower extremity

M99.37 Osseous stenosis of neural canal of upper extremity

M99.38 Osseous stenosis of neural canal of rib cage

M99.39 Osseous stenosis of neural canal of abdomen and other regions

M99.4 Connective tissue stenosis of neural canal

M99.40 Connective tissue stenosis of neural canal of head region

M99.41 Connective tissue stenosis of neural canal of cervical region

M99.42 Connective tissue stenosis of neural canal of thoracic region

M99.43 Connective tissue stenosis of neural canal of lumbar region

M99.44 Connective tissue stenosis of neural canal of sacral region

M99.45 Connective tissue stenosis of neural canal of pelvic region

M99.46 Connective tissue stenosis of neural canal of lower extremity

M99.47 Connective tissue stenosis of neural canal of upper extremity

M99.48 Connective tissue stenosis of neural canal of rib cage

M99.49 Connective tissue stenosis of neural canal of abdomen and other regions

M99.5 Intervertebral disc stenosis of neural canal

M99.50 Intervertebral disc stenosis of neural canal of head region

M99.51 Intervertebral disc stenosis of neural canal of cervical region

M99.52 Intervertebral disc stenosis of neural canal of thoracic region

M99.53 Intervertebral disc stenosis of neural canal of lumbar region

M99.54 Intervertebral disc stenosis of neural canal of sacral region

M99.55 Intervertebral disc stenosis of neural canal of pelvic region

M99.56 Intervertebral disc stenosis of neural canal of lower extremity

M99.57 Intervertebral disc stenosis of neural canal of upper extremity

M99.58 Intervertebral disc stenosis of neural canal of rib cage

M99.59 Intervertebral disc stenosis of neural canal of abdomen and other regions

M99.6 Osseous and subluxation stenosis of intervertebral foramina

M99.60 Osseous and subluxation stenosis of intervertebral foramina of head region

M99.61 Osseous and subluxation stenosis of intervertebral foramina of cervical region

M99.62 Osseous and subluxation stenosis of intervertebral foramina of thoracic region

M99.63 Osseous and subluxation stenosis of intervertebral foramina of lumbar region

M99.64 Osseous and subluxation stenosis of intervertebral foramina of sacral region

M99.65 Osseous and subluxation stenosis of intervertebral foramina of pelvic region

M99.66 Osseous and subluxation stenosis of intervertebral foramina of lower extremity

M99.67 Osseous and subluxation stenosis of intervertebral foramina of upper extremity

M99.68 Osseous and subluxation stenosis of intervertebral foramina of rib cage

M99.69 Osseous and subluxation stenosis of intervertebral foramina of abdomen and other regions

M99.7 Connective tissue and disc stenosis of intervertebral foramina

M99.70 Connective tissue and disc stenosis of intervertebral foramina of head region

M99.71 Connective tissue and disc stenosis of intervertebral foramina of cervical region

M99.72 Connective tissue and disc stenosis of intervertebral foramina of thoracic region

M99.73 Connective tissue and disc stenosis of intervertebral foramina of lumbar region

M99.74 Connective tissue and disc stenosis of intervertebral foramina of sacral region

M99.75 Connective tissue and disc stenosis of intervertebral foramina of pelvic region

M99.76 Connective tissue and disc stenosis of intervertebral foramina of lower extremity

M99.77 Connective tissue and disc stenosis of intervertebral foramina of upper extremity

M99.78 Connective tissue and disc stenosis of intervertebral foramina of rib cage

M99.79 Connective tissue and disc stenosis of intervertebral foramina of abdomen and other regions

M99.8 Other biomechanical lesions

M99.80 Other biomechanical lesions of head region

M99.81 Other biomechanical lesions of cervical region

M99.82 Other biomechanical lesions of thoracic region

M99.83 Other biomechanical lesions of lumbar region

M99.84 Other biomechanical lesions of sacral region

M99.85 Other biomechanical lesions of pelvic region

M99.86 Other biomechanical lesions of lower extremity

M99.87 Other biomechanical lesions of upper extremity

M99.88 Other biomechanical lesions of rib cage

M99.89 Other biomechanical lesions of abdomen and other regions

M99.9 Biomechanical lesion, unspecified

● New code   ▲ Revised code   ⑦ 7th digit required   ⊗ Placeholder required

● New code ▲ Revised code ⑦ 7th digit required ⊗ Placeholder required

Chapter 14: Diseases Of The Genitourinary System (N00-N99)

Excludes 2: certain conditions originating in the perinatal period (P04-P96)

certain infectious and parasitic diseases (A00-B99)

complications of pregnancy, childbirth and the puerperium (O00-O9A)

congenital malformations, deformations and chromosomal abnormalities (Q00-Q99)

endocrine, nutritional and metabolic diseases (E00-E88)

injury, poisoning and certain other consequences of external causes (S00-T88)

neoplasms (C00-D49)

symptoms, signs and abnormal clinical and laboratory findings, not elsewhere classified (R00-R94)

This chapter contains the following blocks:

N00-N08	Glomerular diseases
N10-N16	Renal tubulointerstitial diseases
N17-N19	Acute kidney failure and chronic kidney disease
N20-N23	Urolithiasis
N25-N29	Other disorders of kidney and ureter
N30-N39	Other diseases of the urinary system
N40-N53	Diseases of male genital organs
N60-N65	Disorders of breast
N70-N77	Inflammatory diseases of female pelvic organs
N80-N98	Noninflammatory disorders of female genital tract
N99	Intraoperative and postprocedural complications and disorders of genitourinary system, not elsewhere classified

GLOMERULAR DISEASES (N00-N08)

Code also any associated kidney failure (N17-N19).

Excludes 1: hypertensive chronic kidney disease (I12.-)

N00 Acute nephritic syndrome

Includes: acute glomerular disease

acute glomerulonephritis

acute nephritis

Excludes 1: acute tubulointerstitial nephritis (N10)

nephritic syndrome NOS (N05.-)

N00.0 Acute nephritic syndrome with minor glomerular abnormality

Acute nephritic syndrome with minimal change lesion

N00.1 Acute nephritic syndrome with focal and segmental glomerular lesions

Acute nephritic syndrome with focal and segmental hyalinosis

Acute nephritic syndrome with focal and segmental sclerosis

Acute nephritic syndrome with focal glomerulonephritis

N00.2 Acute nephritic syndrome with diffuse membranous glomerulonephritis

N00.3 Acute nephritic syndrome with diffuse mesangial proliferative glomerulonephritis

N00.4 Acute nephritic syndrome with diffuse endocapillary proliferative glomerulonephritis

N00.5 Acute nephritic syndrome with diffuse mesangiocapillary glomerulonephritis

Acute nephritic syndrome with membranoproliferative glomerulonephritis, types 1and 3, or NOS

N00.6 Acute nephritic syndrome with dense deposit disease

Acute nephritic syndrome with membranoproliferative glomerulonephritis, type 2

N00.7 Acute nephritic syndrome with diffuse crescentic glomerulonephritis

Acute nephritic syndrome with extracapillary glomerulonephritis

N00.8 Acute nephritic syndrome with other morphologic changes

Acute nephritic syndrome with proliferative glomerulonephritis NOS

N00.9 Acute nephritic syndrome with unspecified morphologic changes

N01 Rapidly progressive nephritic syndrome

Includes: rapidly progressive glomerular disease

rapidly progressive glomerulonephritis

rapidly progressive nephritis

Excludes 1: nephritic syndrome NOS (N05.-)

N01.0 Rapidly progressive nephritic syndrome with minor glomerular abnormality

Rapidly progressive nephritic syndrome with minimal change lesion

N01.1 Rapidly progressive nephritic syndrome with focal and segmental glomerular lesions

Rapidly progressive nephritic syndrome with focal and segmental hyalinosis

Rapidly progressive nephritic syndrome with focal and segmental sclerosis

Rapidly progressive nephritic syndrome with focal glomerulonephritis

N01.2 Rapidly progressive nephritic syndrome with diffuse membranous glomerulonephritis

N01.3 Rapidly progressive nephritic syndrome with diffuse mesangial proliferative glomerulonephritis

N01.4 Rapidly progressive nephritic syndrome with diffuse endocapillary proliferative glomerulonephritis

N01.5 Rapidly progressive nephritic syndrome with diffuse mesangiocapillary glomerulonephritis

Rapidly progressive nephritic syndrome with membranoproliferative glomerulonephritis, types 1and 3, or NOS

N01.6 Rapidly progressive nephritic syndrome with dense deposit disease

Rapidly progressive nephritic syndrome with membranoproliferative glomerulonephritis, type 2

N01.7 Rapidly progressive nephritic syndrome with diffuse crescentic glomerulonephritis

Rapidly progressive nephritic syndrome with extracapillary glomerulonephritis

N01.8 Rapidly progressive nephritic syndrome with other morphologic changes

Rapidly progressive nephritic syndrome with proliferative glomerulonephritis NOS

N01.9 Rapidly progressive nephritic syndrome with unspecified morphologic changes

N02 Recurrent and persistent hematuria

Excludes 1: acute cystitis with hematuria (N30.01)

acute prostatitis with hematuria (N41.01)

chronic prostatitis with hematuria (N41.11)

hematuria NOS (R31.9)

hematuria not associated with specified morphologic lesions (R31.-)

N02.0 Recurrent and persistent hematuria with minor glomerular abnormality
Recurrent and persistent hematuria with minimal change lesion

N02.1 Recurrent and persistent hematuria with focal and segmental glomerular lesions
Recurrent and persistent hematuria with focal and segmental hyalinosis
Recurrent and persistent hematuria with focal and segmental sclerosis
Recurrent and persistent hematuria with focal glomerulonephritis

N02.2 Recurrent and persistent hematuria with diffuse membranous glomerulonephritis

N02.3 Recurrent and persistent hematuria with diffuse mesangial proliferative glomerulonephritis

N02.4 Recurrent and persistent hematuria with diffuse endocapillary proliferative glomerulonephritis

N02.5 Recurrent and persistent hematuria with diffuse mesangiocapillary glomerulonephritis
Recurrent and persistent hematuria with membranoproliferative glomerulonephritis, types 1 and 3, or NOS

N02.6 Recurrent and persistent hematuria with dense deposit disease
Recurrent and persistent hematuria with membranoproliferative glomerulonephritis, type 2

N02.7 Recurrent and persistent hematuria with diffuse crescentic glomerulonephritis
Recurrent and persistent hematuria with extracapillary glomerulonephritis

N02.8 Recurrent and persistent hematuria with other morphologic changes
Recurrent and persistent hematuria with proliferative glomerulonephritis NOS

N02.9 Recurrent and persistent hematuria with unspecified morphologic changes

N03 Chronic nephritic syndrome
Includes: chronic glomerular disease
chronic glomerulonephritis
chronic nephritis
Excludes 1: chronic tubulointerstitial nephritis (N11.-)
diffuse sclerosing glomerulonephritis (N05.8-)
nephritic syndrome NOS (N05.-)

N03.0 Chronic nephritic syndrome with minor glomerular abnormality
Chronic nephritic syndrome with minimal change lesion

N03.1 Chronic nephritic syndrome with focal and segmental glomerular lesions
Chronic nephritic syndrome with focal and segmental hyalinosis
Chronic nephritic syndrome with focal and segmental sclerosis
Chronic nephritic syndrome with focal glomerulonephritis

N03.2 Chronic nephritic syndrome with diffuse membranous glomerulonephritis

N03.3 Chronic nephritic syndrome with diffuse mesangial proliferative glomerulonephritis

N03.4 Chronic nephritic syndrome with diffuse endocapillary proliferative glomerulonephritis

N03.5 Chronic nephritic syndrome with diffuse mesangiocapillary glomerulonephritis
Chronic nephritic syndrome with membranoproliferative glomerulonephritis, types 1 and 3, or NOS

N03.6 Chronic nephritic syndrome with dense deposit disease
Chronic nephritic syndrome with membranoproliferative glomerulonephritis, type 2

N03.7 Chronic nephritic syndrome with diffuse crescentic glomerulonephritis
Chronic nephritic syndrome with extracapillary glomerulonephritis

N03.8 Chronic nephritic syndrome with other morphologic changes
Chronic nephritic syndrome with proliferative glomerulonephritis NOS

N03.9 Chronic nephritic syndrome with unspecified morphologic changes

N04 Nephrotic syndrome
Includes: congenital nephrotic syndrome
lipoid nephrosis

N04.0 Nephrotic syndrome with minor glomerular abnormality
Nephrotic syndrome with minimal change lesion

N04.1 Nephrotic syndrome with focal and segmental glomerular lesions
Nephrotic syndrome with focal and segmental hyalinosis
Nephrotic syndrome with focal and segmental sclerosis
Nephrotic syndrome with focal glomerulonephritis

N04.2 Nephrotic syndrome with diffuse membranous glomerulonephritis

N04.3 Nephrotic syndrome with diffuse mesangial proliferative glomerulonephritis

N04.4 Nephrotic syndrome with diffuse endocapillary proliferative glomerulonephritis

N04.5 Nephrotic syndrome with diffuse mesangiocapillary glomerulonephritis
Nephrotic syndrome with membranoproliferative glomerulonephritis, types 1 and 3, or NOS

N04.6 Nephrotic syndrome with dense deposit disease
Nephrotic syndrome with membranoproliferative glomerulonephritis, type 2

N04.7 Nephrotic syndrome with diffuse crescentic glomerulonephritis
Nephrotic syndrome with extracapillary glomerulonephritis

N04.8 Nephrotic syndrome with other morphologic changes
Nephrotic syndrome with proliferative glomerulonephritis NOS

N04.9 Nephrotic syndrome with unspecified morphologic changes

N05 Unspecified nephritic syndrome
Includes: glomerular disease NOS
glomerulonephritis NOS
nephritis NOS
nephropathy NOS and renal disease NOS with morphological lesion specified in .0-.8
Excludes 1: nephropathy NOS with no stated morphological lesion (N28.9)
renal disease NOS with no stated morphological lesion (N28.9)
tubulo-interstitial nephritis NOS (N12)

● New code ▲ Revised code ⑦ 7th digit required ⊗ Placeholder required

N05.0   Unspecified nephritic syndrome with minor glomerular abnormality

Unspecified nephritic syndrome with minimal change lesion

N05.1   Unspecified nephritic syndrome with focal and segmental glomerular lesions

Unspecified nephritic syndrome with focal and segmental hyalinosis

Unspecified nephritic syndrome with focal and segmental sclerosis

Unspecified nephritic syndrome with focal glomerulonephritis

N05.2   Unspecified nephritic syndrome with diffuse membranous glomerulonephritis

N05.3   Unspecified nephritic syndrome with diffuse mesangial proliferative glomerulonephritis

N05.4   Unspecified nephritic syndrome with diffuse endocapillary proliferative glomerulonephritis

N05.5   Unspecified nephritic syndrome with diffuse mesangiocapillary glomerulonephritis

Unspecified nephritic syndrome with membranoproliferative glomerulonephritis, types 1 and 3, or NOS

N05.6   Unspecified nephritic syndrome with dense deposit disease

Unspecified nephritic syndrome with membranoproliferative glomerulonephritis, type 2

N05.7   Unspecified nephritic syndrome with diffuse crescentic glomerulonephritis

Unspecified nephritic syndrome with extracapillary glomerulonephritis

N05.8   Unspecified nephritic syndrome with other morphologic changes

Unspecified nephritic syndrome with proliferative glomerulonephritis NOS

N05.9   Unspecified nephritic syndrome with unspecified morphologic changes

N06   Isolated proteinuria with specified morphological lesion

Excludes 1: Proteinuria not associated with specific morphologic lesions (R80.0)

N06.0   Isolated proteinuria with minor glomerular abnormality

Isolated proteinuria with minimal change lesion

N06.1   Isolated proteinuria with focal and segmental glomerular lesions

Isolated proteinuria with focal and segmental hyalinosis

Isolated proteinuria with focal and segmental sclerosis

Isolated proteinuria with focal glomerulonephritis

N06.2   Isolated proteinuria with diffuse membranous glomerulonephritis

N06.3   Isolated proteinuria with diffuse mesangial proliferative glomerulonephritis

N06.4   Isolated proteinuria with diffuse endocapillary proliferative glomerulonephritis

N06.5   Isolated proteinuria with diffuse mesangiocapillary glomerulonephritis

Isolated proteinuria with membranoproliferative glomerulonephritis, types 1 and 3, or NOS

N06.6   Isolated proteinuria with dense deposit disease

Isolated proteinuria with membranoproliferative glomerulonephritis, type 2

N06.7   Isolated proteinuria with diffuse crescentic glomerulonephritis

Isolated proteinuria with extracapillary glomerulonephritis

N06.8   Isolated proteinuria with other morphologic lesion

Isolated proteinuria with proliferative glomerulonephritis NOS

N06.9   Isolated proteinuria with unspecified morphologic lesion

N07   Hereditary nephropathy, not elsewhere classified

Excludes 2: Alport's syndrome (Q87.81-)

hereditary amyloid nephropathy (E85-)

nail patella syndrome (Q87.2)

non-neuropathic heredofamilial amyloidosis (E85-)

N07.0   Hereditary nephropathy, not elsewhere classified with minor glomerular abnormality

Hereditary nephropathy, not elsewhere classified with minimal change lesion

N07.1   Hereditary nephropathy, not elsewhere classified with focal and segmental glomerular lesions

Hereditary nephropathy, not elsewhere classified with focal and segmental hyalinosis

Hereditary nephropathy, not elsewhere classified with focal and segmental sclerosis

Hereditary nephropathy, not elsewhere classified with focal glomerulonephritis

N07.2   Hereditary nephropathy, not elsewhere classified with diffuse membranous glomerulonephritis

N07.3   Hereditary nephropathy, not elsewhere classified with diffuse mesangial proliferative glomerulonephritis

N07.4   Hereditary nephropathy, not elsewhere classified with diffuse endocapillary proliferative glomerulonephritis

N07.5   Hereditary nephropathy, not elsewhere classified with diffuse mesangiocapillary glomerulonephritis

Hereditary nephropathy, not elsewhere classified with membranoproliferative glomerulonephritis, types 1 and 3, or NOS

N07.6   Hereditary nephropathy, not elsewhere classified with dense deposit disease

Hereditary nephropathy, not elsewhere classified with membranoproliferative glomerulonephritis, type 2

N07.7   Hereditary nephropathy, not elsewhere classified with diffuse crescentic glomerulonephritis

Hereditary nephropathy, not elsewhere classified with extracapillary glomerulonephritis

N07.8   Hereditary nephropathy, not elsewhere classified with other morphologic lesions

Hereditary nephropathy, not elsewhere classified with proliferative glomerulonephritis NOS

N07.9   Hereditary nephropathy, not elsewhere classified with unspecified morphologic lesions

N08   Glomerular disorders in diseases classified elsewhere

Glomerulonephritis

Nephritis

Nephropathy

Code first underlying disease, such as:

amyloidosis (E85-)

congenital syphilis (A50.5)

cryoglobulinemia (D89.1)

disseminated intravascular coagulation (D65)

gout (M1A-, M10.-)

microscopic polyangiitis (M31.7)

multiple myeloma (C90.0-)

sepsis (A40.0-A41.9)

sickle-cell disease (D57.0-D57.8)

Excludes 1: glomerulonephritis, nephritis and nephropathy (in):

antiglomerular basement membrane disease (M31.0)

diabetes (E08-E13 with .21)

gonococcal (A54.21)

Goodpasture's syndrome (M31.0)

hemolytic-uremic syndrome (D59.3)

lupus (M32.14)

mumps (B26.83)

syphilis (A52.75)

systemic lupus erythematosus (M32.14)

Wegener's granulomatosis (M31.31)

pyelonephritis in diseases classified elsewhere (N16)

renal tubulo-interstitial disorders classified elsewhere (N16)

RENAL TUBULO-INTERSTITIAL DISEASES (N10-N16)

Includes: pyelonephritis

Excludes 1: pyeloureteritis cystica (N28.85)

N10 Acute tubulo-interstitial nephritis

Acute infectious interstitial nephritis

Acute pyelitis

Acute pyelonephritis

Hemoglobin nephrosis

Myoglobin nephrosis

Use additional code (B95-B97), to identify infectious agent.

N11 Chronic tubulo-interstitial nephritis

Includes: chronic infectious interstitial nephritis

chronic pyelitis

chronic pyelonephritis

Use additional code (B95-B97), to identify infectious agent.

N11.0 Nonobstructive reflux-associated chronic pyelonephritis

Pyelonephritis (chronic) associated with (vesicoureteral) reflux

Excludes 1: vesicoureteral reflux NOS (N13.70)

N11.1 Chronic obstructive pyelonephritis

Pyelonephritis (chronic) associated with anomaly of pelviureteric junction

Pyelonephritis (chronic) associated with anomaly of pyeloureteric junction

Pyelonephritis (chronic) associated with crossing of vessel

Pyelonephritis (chronic) associated with kinking of ureter

Pyelonephritis (chronic) associated with obstruction of ureter

Pyelonephritis (chronic) associated with stricture of pelviureteric junction

Pyelonephritis (chronic) associated with stricture of ureter

Excludes 1: calculous pyelonephritis (N20.9)

obstructive uropathy (N13.-)

N11.8 Other chronic tubulo-interstitial nephritis

Nonobstructive chronic pyelonephritis NOS

N11.9 Chronic tubulo-interstitial nephritis, unspecified

Chronic interstitial nephritis NOS

Chronic pyelitis NOS

Chronic pyelonephritis NOS

N12 Tubulo-interstitial nephritis, not specified as acute or chronic

Interstitial nephritis NOS

Pyelitis NOS

Pyelonephritis NOS

Excludes 1: calculous pyelonephritis (N20.9)

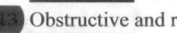 Obstructive and reflux uropathy

Excludes 2: calculus of kidney and ureter without hydronephrosis (N20.-)

congenital obstructive defects of renal pelvis and ureter (Q62.0-Q62.3)

hydronephrosis with ureteropelvic junction obstruction (Q62.1)

obstructive pyelonephritis (N11.1)

N13.1 Hydronephrosis with ureteral stricture, not elsewhere classified

Excludes 1: Hydronephrosis with ureteral stricture with infection (N13.6)

N13.2 Hydronephrosis with renal and ureteral calculous obstruction

Excludes 1: Hydronephrosis with renal and ureteral calculous obstruction with infection (N13.6)

N13.3 Other and unspecified hydronephrosis

Excludes 1: hydronephrosis with infection (N13.6)

N13.30 Unspecified hydronephrosis

N13.39 Other hydronephrosis

N13.4 Hydroureter

Excludes 1: congenital hydroureter (Q62.3-)

hydroureter with infection (N13.6)

vesicoureteral-reflux with hydroureter (N13.73-)

N13.5 Crossing vessel and stricture of ureter without hydronephrosis

Kinking and stricture of ureter without hydronephrosis

Excludes 1: Crossing vessel and stricture of ureter without hydronephrosis with infection (N13.6)

N13.6 Pyonephrosis

Conditions in N13.1-N13.5 with infection

Obstructive uropathy with infection

Use additional code (B95-B97), to identify infectious agent.

N13.7 Vesicoureteral-reflux

Excludes 1: reflux-associated pyelonephritis (N11.0)

N13.70 Vesicoureteral-reflux, unspecified

Vesicoureteral-reflux NOS

N13.71 Vesicoureteral-reflux without reflux nephropathy

N13.72 Vesicoureteral-reflux with reflux nephropathy without hydroureter

N13.721 Vesicoureteral-reflux with reflux nephropathy without hydroureter, unilateral

N13.722 Vesicoureteral-reflux with reflux nephropathy without hydroureter, bilateral

N13.729 Vesicoureteral-reflux with reflux nephropathy without hydroureter, unspecified

N13.73 Vesicoureteral-reflux with reflux nephropathy with hydroureter

N13.731 Vesicoureteral-reflux with reflux nephropathy with hydroureter, unilateral

N13.732 Vesicoureteral-reflux with reflux nephropathy with hydroureter, bilateral

● New code   ▲ Revised code   ⑦ 7th digit required   ⊗ Placeholder required

N13.739 Vesicoureteral-reflux with reflux nephropathy with hydroureter, unspecified

N13.8 Other obstructive and reflux uropathy

Urinary tract obstruction due to specified cause

Code first , if applicable, any causal condition, such as:

enlarged prostate (N40.1)

N13.9 Obstructive and reflux uropathy, unspecified

Urinary tract obstruction NOS

N14 Drug- and heavy-metal-induced tubulo-interstitial and tubular conditions

Code first poisoning due to drug or toxin, if applicable (T36-T65 with fifth or sixth character 1-4 or 6)

Use additional code for adverse effect, if applicable, to identify drug (T36-T50 with fifth or sixth character 5)

N14.0 Analgesic nephropathy

N14.1 Nephropathy induced by other drugs, medicaments and biological substances

N14.2 Nephropathy induced by unspecified drug, medicament or biological substance

N14.3 Nephropathy induced by heavy metals

N14.4 Toxic nephropathy, not elsewhere classified

N15 Other renal tubulo-interstitial diseases

N15.0 Balkan nephropathy

Balkan endemic nephropathy

N15.1 Renal and perinephric abscess

N15.8 Other specified renal tubulo-interstitial diseases

N15.9 Renal tubulo-interstitial disease, unspecified

Infection of kidney NOS

Excludes 1: urinary tract infection NOS (N39.0)

N16 Renal tubulo-interstitial disorders in diseases classified elsewhere

Pyelonephritis

Tubulo-interstitial nephritis

Code first underlying disease, such as:

brucellosis (A23.0-A23.9)

cryoglobulinemia (D89.1)

glycogen storage disease (E74.0)

leukemia (C91-C95)

lymphoma (C81.0-C85.9, C96.0-C96.9)

multiple myeloma (C90.0-)

sepsis (A40.0-A41.9)

Wilson's disease (E83.0)

Excludes 1: diphtheritic pyelonephritis and tubulo-interstitial nephritis (A36.84)

pyelonephritis and tubulo-interstitial nephritis in candidiasis (B37.49)

pyelonephritis and tubulo-interstitial nephritis in cystinosis (E72.04)

pyelonephritis and tubulo-interstitial nephritis in salmonella infection (A02.25)

pyelonephritis and tubulo-interstitial nephritis in sarcoidosis (D86.84)

pyelonephritis and tubulo-interstitial nephritis in sicca syndrome [Sjogren's] (M35.04)

pyelonephritis and tubulo-interstitial nephritis in systemic lupus erythematosus (M32.15)

pyelonephritis and tubulo-interstitial nephritis in toxoplasmosis (B58.83)

renal tubular degeneration in diabetes (E08-E13 with .29)

syphilitic pyelonephritis and tubulo-interstitial nephritis (A52.75)

ACUTE KIDNEY FAILURE AND CHRONIC KIDNEY DISEASE (N17-N19)

Excludes 2: congenital renal failure (P96.0)

drug- and heavy-metal-induced tubulo-interstitial and tubular conditions (N14.-)

extrarenal uremia (R39.2)

hemolytic-uremic syndrome (D59.3)

hepatorenal syndrome (K76.7)

postpartum hepatorenal syndrome (O90.4)

posttraumatic renal failure (T79.5)

prerenal uremia (R39.2)

renal failure:

complicating abortion or ectopic or molar pregnancy (O00-O07, O08.4)

following labor and delivery (O90.4)

postprocedural (N99.0)

N17 Acute kidney failure

Code also associated underlying condition

Excludes 1: posttraumatic renal failure (T79.5)

N17.0 Acute kidney failure with tubular necrosis

Acute tubular necrosis

Renal tubular necrosis

Tubular necrosis NOS

N17.1 Acute kidney failure with acute cortical necrosis

Acute cortical necrosis

Cortical necrosis NOS

Renal cortical necrosis

N17.2 Acute kidney failure with medullary necrosis

Medullary [papillary] necrosis NOS

Acute medullary [papillary] necrosis

Renal medullary [papillary] necrosis

N17.8 Other acute kidney failure

N17.9 Acute kidney failure, unspecified

Acute kidney injury (nontraumatic)

Excludes 2: traumatic kidney injury (S37.0-)

N18 Chronic kidney disease (CKD)

Code first any associated:

diabetic chronic kidney disease (E08.22, E09.22, E10.22, E11.22, E13.22)

hypertensive chronic kidney disease (I12.-, I13.-)

Use additional code to identify kidney transplant status, if applicable, (Z94.0)

N18.1 Chronic kidney disease, stage 1

N18.2 Chronic kidney disease, stage 2 (mild)

N18.3 Chronic kidney disease, stage 3(moderate)

N18.4 Chronic kidney disease, stage 4(severe)

N18.5 Chronic kidney disease, stage 5

Excludes 1: chronic kidney disease, stage 5requiring chronic dialysis (N18.6)

N18.6 End stage renal disease

Chronic kidney disease requiring chronic dialysis

Use additional code to identify dialysis status (Z99.2)

N18.9 Chronic kidney disease, unspecified

Chronic renal disease

Chronic renal failure NOS

Chronic renal insufficiency

Chronic uremia

Renal disease NOS

N19 Unspecified kidney failure

Uremia NOS

Excludes 1: acute kidney failure (N17.-)

chronic kidney disease (N18.-)

chronic uremia (N18.9)

extrarenal uremia (R39.2)

prerenal uremia (R39.2)

renal insufficiency (acute) (N28.9)

uremia of newborn (P96.0)

UROLITHIASIS (N20-N23)

N20 Calculus of kidney and ureter

Calculous pyelonephritis

Excludes 1: nephrocalcinosis (E83.5)

that with hydronephrosis (N13.2)

N20.0 Calculus of kidney

Nephrolithiasis NOS

Renal calculus

Renal stone

Staghorn calculus

Stone in kidney

N20.1 Calculus of ureter

Ureteric stone

N20.2 Calculus of kidney with calculus of ureter

N20.9 Urinary calculus, unspecified

N21 Calculus of lower urinary tract

Includes: calculus of lower urinary tract with cystitis and urethritis

N21.0 Calculus in bladder

Calculus in diverticulum of bladder

Urinary bladder stone

Excludes 2: staghorn calculus (N20.0)

N21.1 Calculus in urethra

Excludes 2: calculus of prostate (N42.0)

N21.8 Other lower urinary tract calculus

N21.9 Calculus of lower urinary tract, unspecified

Excludes 1: calculus of urinary tract NOS (N20.9)

N22 Calculus of urinary tract in diseases classified elsewhere

Code first underlying disease, such as:

gout (M1A-, M10.-)

schistosomiasis (B65.0-B65.9)

N23 Unspecified renal colic

OTHER DISORDERS OF KIDNEY AND URETER (N25-N29)

Excludes 2: disorders of kidney and ureter with urolithiasis (N20-N23)

N25 Disorders resulting from impaired renal tubular function

Excludes 1: metabolic disorders classifiable to E70-E88

N25.0 Renal osteodystrophy

Azotemic osteodystrophy

Phosphate-losing tubular disorders

Renal rickets

Renal short stature

N25.1 Nephrogenic diabetes insipidus

Excludes 1: diabetes insipidus NOS (E23.2)

N25.8 Other disorders resulting from impaired renal tubular function

N25.81 Secondary hyperparathyroidism of renal origin

Excludes 1: secondary hyperparathyroidism,

non-renal (E21.1)

N25.89 Other disorders resulting from impaired renal tubular function

Hypokalemic nephropathy

Lightwood-Albright syndrome

Renal tubular acidosis NOS

N25.9 Disorder resulting from impaired renal tubular function, unspecified

N26 Unspecified contracted kidney

Excludes 1: contracted kidney due to hypertension (I12.-)

diffuse sclerosing glomerulonephritis (N05.8.-)

hypertensive nephrosclerosis (arteriolar) (arteriosclerotic) (I12.-)

small kidney of unknown cause (N27.-)

N26.1 Atrophy of kidney (terminal)

N26.2 Page kidney

N26.9 Renal sclerosis, unspecified

N27 Small kidney of unknown cause

Includes: oligonephronia

N27.0 Small kidney, unilateral

N27.1 Small kidney, bilateral

N27.9 Small kidney, unspecified

N28 Other disorders of kidney and ureter, not elsewhere classified

N28.0 Ischemia and infarction of kidney

Renal artery embolism

Renal artery obstruction

Renal artery occlusion

Renal artery thrombosis

Renal infarct

Excludes 1: atherosclerosis of renal artery (extrarenal part) (I70.1)

congenital stenosis of renal artery (Q27.1)

Goldblatt's kidney (I70.1)

N28.1 Cyst of kidney, acquired

Cyst (multiple)(solitary) of kidney, acquired

Excludes 1: cystic kidney disease (congenital) (Q61.-)

N28.8 Other specified disorders of kidney and ureter

Excludes 1: hydroureter (N13.4)

ureteric stricture with hydronephrosis (N13.1)

ureteric stricture without hydronephrosis (N13.5)

N28.81 Hypertrophy of kidney

N28.82 Megaloureter

N28.83 Nephroptosis

N28.84 Pyelitis cystica

N28.85 Pyeloureteritis cystica

N28.86 Ureteritis cystica

N28.89 Other specified disorders of kidney and ureter

N28.9 Disorder of kidney and ureter, unspecified

Nephropathy NOS

Renal disease (acute) NOS

Renal insufficiency (acute)

Excludes 1: chronic renal insufficiency (N18.9)

unspecified nephritic syndrome (N05-)

N29 Other disorders of kidney and ureter in diseases classified elsewhere

Code first underlying disease, such as:

amyloidosis (E85-)

nephrocalcinosis (E83.5)

schistosomiasis (B65.0-B65.9)

Excludes 1: disorders of kidney and ureter in:
    cystinosis (E72.0)
    gonorrhea (A54.21)
    syphilis (A52.75)
    tuberculosis (A18.11)

OTHER DISEASES OF THE URINARY SYSTEM (N30-N39)

Excludes 1: urinary infection (complicating):
    abortion or ectopic or molar pregnancy (O00-O07, O08.8)
    pregnancy, childbirth and the puerperium (O23.-, O75.3, O86.2-)

N30 Cystitis
Use additional code to identify infectious agent (B95-B97)
Excludes 1: prostatocystitis (N41.3)
- **N30.0** Acute cystitis
  Excludes 1: irradiation cystitis (N30.4-)
      trigonitis (N30.3-)
  - **N30.00** Acute cystitis without hematuria
  - **N30.01** Acute cystitis with hematuria
- **N30.1** Interstitial cystitis (chronic)
  - **N30.10** Interstitial cystitis (chronic) without hematuria
  - **N30.11** Interstitial cystitis (chronic) with hematuria
- **N30.2** Other chronic cystitis
  - **N30.20** Other chronic cystitis without hematuria
  - **N30.21** Other chronic cystitis with hematuria
- **N30.3** Trigonitis
  Urethrotrigonitis
  - **N30.30** Trigonitis without hematuria
  - **N30.31** Trigonitis with hematuria
- **N30.4** Irradiation cystitis
  - **N30.40** Irradiation cystitis without hematuria
  - **N30.41** Irradiation cystitis with hematuria
- **N30.8** Other cystitis
  Abscess of bladder
  - **N30.80** Other cystitis without hematuria
  - **N30.81** Other cystitis with hematuria
- **N30.9** Cystitis, unspecified
  - **N30.90** Cystitis, unspecified without hematuria
  - **N30.91** Cystitis, unspecified with hematuria

N31 Neuromuscular dysfunction of bladder, not elsewhere classified
Use additional code to identify any associated urinary incontinence (N39.3-N39.4-)
Excludes 1: cord bladder NOS (G95.89)
    neurogenic bladder due to cauda equina syndrome (G83.4)
    neuromuscular dysfunction due to spinal cord lesion (G95.89)
- **N31.0** Uninhibited neuropathic bladder, not elsewhere classified
- **N31.1** Reflex neuropathic bladder, not elsewhere classified
- **N31.2** Flaccid neuropathic bladder, not elsewhere classified
  Atonic (motor) (sensory) neuropathic bladder
  Autonomous neuropathic bladder
  Nonreflux neuropathic bladder
- **N31.8** Other neuromuscular dysfunction of bladder
- **N31.9** Neuromuscular dysfunction of bladder, unspecified
  Neurogenic bladder dysfunction NOS

N32 Other disorders of bladder
Excludes 2: calculus of bladder (N21.0)
    cystocele (N81.1-)
    hernia or prolapse of bladder, female (N81.1-)
- **N32.0** Bladder-neck obstruction

Bladder-neck stenosis (acquired)
Excludes 1: congenital bladder-neck obstruction (Q64.3-)
- **N32.1** Vesicointestinal fistula
  Vesicorectal fistula
- **N32.2** Vesical fistula, not elsewhere classified
  Excludes 1: fistula between bladder and female genital tract (N82.0-N82.1)
- **N32.3** Diverticulum of bladder
  Excludes 1: congenital diverticulum of bladder (Q64.6)
      diverticulitis of bladder (N30.8-)
- **N32.8** Other specified disorders of bladder
  - **N32.81** Overactive bladder
    Detrusor muscle hyperactivity
    Excludes 1: frequent urination due to specified bladder condition- code to condition
  - **N32.89** Other specified disorders of bladder
    Bladder hemorrhage
    Bladder hypertrophy
    Calcified bladder
    Contracted bladder
- **N32.9** Bladder disorder, unspecified

N33 Bladder disorders in diseases classified elsewhere
Code first underlying disease, such as:
    schistosomiasis (B65.0-B65.9)
Excludes 1: bladder disorder in:
    syphilis (A52.76)
    tuberculosis (A18.12)
    cystitis (in):
    candidal infection (B37.41)
    chlamydial (A56.01)
    diphtheritic (A36.85)
    gonorrhea (A54.01)
    syphilitic (A52.76)
    trichomonal infection (A59.03)
    neurogenic bladder (N31.-)

N34 Urethritis and urethral syndrome
Use additional code (B95-B97), to identify infectious agent.
Excludes 2: Reiter's disease (M02.3-)
    urethritis in diseases with a predominantly sexual mode of transmission (A50-A64)
    urethrotrigonitis (N30.3-)
- **N34.0** Urethral abscess
  Abscess (of) Cowper's gland
  Abscess (of) Littre's gland
  Abscess (of) urethral (gland)
  Periurethral abscess
  Excludes 1: urethral caruncle (N36.2)
- **N34.1** Nonspecific urethritis
  Nongonococcal urethritis
  Nonvenereal urethritis
- **N34.2** Other urethritis
  Meatitis, urethral
  Postmenopausal urethritis
  Ulcer of urethra (meatus)
  Urethritis NOS
- **N34.3** Urethral syndrome, unspecified

N35 Urethral stricture
Excludes 1: congenital urethral stricture (Q64.3-)
    postprocedural urethral stricture (N99.1-)

N35.0   Post-traumatic urethral stricture
        Urethral stricture due to injury
        Excludes 1: postprocedural urethral stricture (N99.1-)
        N35.01   Post-traumatic urethral stricture, male
                 N35.010   Post-traumatic urethral stricture, male, meatal
                 N35.011   Post-traumatic bulbous urethral stricture
                 N35.012   Post-traumatic membranous urethral stricture
                 N35.013   Post-traumatic anterior urethral stricture
                 N35.014   Post-traumatic urethral stricture, male, unspecified
        N35.02   Post-traumatic urethral stricture, female
                 N35.021   Urethral stricture due to childbirth
                 N35.028   Other post-traumatic urethral stricture, female
N35.1   Postinfective urethral stricture, not elsewhere classified
        Excludes 1: urethral stricture associated with schistosomiasis (B65.-, N29)
                        gonococcal urethral stricture (A54.01)
                        syphilitic urethral stricture (A52.76)
        N35.11   Postinfective urethral stricture, not elsewhere classified, male
                 N35.111   Postinfective urethral stricture, not elsewhere classified, male, meatal
                 N35.112   Postinfective bulbous urethral stricture, not elsewhere classified
                 N35.113   Postinfective membranous urethral stricture, not elsewhere classified
                 N35.114   Postinfective anterior urethral stricture, not elsewhere classified
                 N35.119   Postinfective urethral stricture, not elsewhere classified, male, unspecified
        N35.12   Postinfective urethral stricture, not elsewhere classified, female
N35.8   Other urethral stricture
        Excludes 1: postprocedural urethral stricture (N99.1-)
N35.9   Urethral stricture, unspecified
N36   Other disorders of urethra
N36.0   Urethral fistula
        Urethroperineal fistula
        Urethrorectal fistula
        Urinary fistula NOS
        Excludes 1: urethroscrotal fistula (N50.8)
                        urethrovaginal fistula (N82.1)
                        urethrovesicovaginal fistula (N82.1)
N36.1   Urethral diverticulum
N36.2   Urethral caruncle
N36.4   Urethral functional and muscular disorders
        Use additional code to identify associated urinary stress incontinence (N39.3)
        N36.41   Hypermobility of urethra
        N36.42   Intrinsic sphincter deficiency (ISD)
        N36.43   Combined hypermobility of urethra and intrinsic sphincter deficiency
        N36.44   Muscular disorders of urethra

        Bladder sphincter dyssynergy
N36.5   Urethral false passage
N36.8   Other specified disorders of urethra
N36.9   Urethral disorder, unspecified
N37   Urethral disorders in diseases classified elsewhere
        Code first underlying disease
        Excludes 1: urethritis (in):
                        candidal infection (B37.41)
                        chlamydial (A56.01)
                        gonorrhea (A54.01)
                        syphilis (A52.76)
                        trichomonal infection (A59.03)
                        tuberculosis (A18.13)
N39   Other disorders of urinary system
        Excludes 2: hematuria NOS (R31-)
                        recurrent or persistent hematuria (N02.-)
                        recurrent or persistent hematuria with specified morphological lesion (N02.-)
                        proteinuria NOS (R80.-)
N39.0   Urinary tract infection, site not specified
        Use additional code (B95-B97), to identify infectious agent.
        Excludes 1: candidiasis of urinary tract (B37.4-)
                        neonatal urinary tract infection (P39.3)
                        urinary tract infection of specified site, such as:
                        cystitis (N30.-)
                        urethritis (N34.-)
N39.3   Stress incontinence (female) (male)
        Code also any associated overactive bladder (N32.81)
        Excludes 1: mixed incontinence (N39.46)
N39.4   Other specified urinary incontinence
        Code also any associated overactive bladder (N32.81)
        Excludes 1: enuresis NOS (R32)
                        functional urinary incontinence (R39.81)
                        urinary incontinence associated with cognitive impairment (R39.81)
                        urinary incontinence NOS (R32)
                        urinary incontinence of nonorganic origin (F98.0)
        N39.41   Urge incontinence
                 Excludes 1: mixed incontinence (N39.46)
        N39.42   Incontinence without sensory awareness
        N39.43   Post-void dribbling
        N39.44   Nocturnal enuresis
        N39.45   Continuous leakage
        N39.46   Mixed incontinence
                 Urge and stress incontinence
        N39.49   Other specified urinary incontinence
                 N39.490   Overflow incontinence
                 N39.498   Other specified urinary incontinence
                           Reflex incontinence
                           Total incontinence
N39.8   Other specified disorders of urinary system
N39.9   Disorder of urinary system, unspecified

DISEASES OF MALE GENITAL ORGANS (N40-N53)
N40   Enlarged prostate
        Includes: adenofibromatous hypertrophy of prostate

benign hypertrophy of the prostate
benign prostatic hyperplasia
benign prostatic hypertrophy
BPH
nodular prostate
polyp of prostate
Excludes 1: benign neoplasms of prostate (adenoma, benign) (fibroadenoma) (fibroma) (myoma) (D29.1)
Excludes 2: malignant neoplasm of prostate (C61)

N40.0 Enlarged prostate without lower urinary tract symptoms
Enlarged prostate without LUTS
Enlarged prostate NOS

N40.1 Enlarged prostate with lower urinary tract symptoms
Enlarged prostate with LUTS
Use additional code for associated symptoms, when specified:
incomplete bladder emptying (R39.14)
nocturia (R35.1)
straining on urination (R39.16)
urinary frequency (R35.0)
urinary hesitancy (R39.11)
urinary incontinence (N39.4-)
urinary obstruction (N13.8)
urinary retention (R33.8)
urinary urgency (R39.15)
weak urinary stream (R39.12)

N40.2 Nodular prostate without lower urinary tract symptoms
Nodular prostate without LUTS

N40.3 Nodular prostate with lower urinary tract symptoms
Use additional code for associated symptoms, when specified:
incomplete bladder emptying (R39.14)
nocturia (R35.1)
straining on urination (R39.16)
urinary frequency (R35.0)
urinary hesitancy (R39.11)
urinary incontinence (N39.4-)
urinary obstruction (N13.8)
urinary retention (R33.8)
urinary urgency (R39.15)
weak urinary stream (R39.12)

N41 Inflammatory diseases of prostate
Use additional code (B95-B97), to identify infectious agent.

N41.0 Acute prostatitis
N41.1 Chronic prostatitis
N41.2 Abscess of prostate
N41.3 Prostatocystitis
N41.4 Granulomatous prostatitis
N41.8 Other inflammatory diseases of prostate
N41.9 Inflammatory disease of prostate, unspecified
Prostatitis NOS

N42 Other and unspecified disorders of prostate
N42.0 Calculus of prostate
Prostatic stone
N42.1 Congestion and hemorrhage of prostate
Excludes 1: enlarged prostate (N40.-)
hematuria (R31.-)
hyperplasia of prostate (N40.-)
inflammatory diseases of prostate (N41.-)

N42.3 Dysplasia of prostate
Prostatic intraepithelial neoplasia I (PIN I)
Prostatic intraepithelial neoplasia II (PIN II)
Excludes 1: prostatic intraepithelial neoplasia III (PIN III) (D07.5)

N42.8 Other specified disorders of prostate
N42.81 Prostatodynia syndrome
Painful prostate syndrome
N42.82 Prostatosis syndrome
N42.83 Cyst of prostate
N42.89 Other specified disorders of prostate

N42.9 Disorder of prostate, unspecified

N43 Hydrocele and spermatocele
Includes: hydrocele of spermatic cord, testis or tunica vaginalis
Excludes 1: congenital hydrocele (P83.5)

N43.0 Encysted hydrocele
N43.1 Infected hydrocele
Use additional code (B95-B97), to identify infectious agent
N43.2 Other hydrocele
N43.3 Hydrocele, unspecified
N43.4 Spermatocele of epididymis
Spermatic cyst
N43.40 Spermatocele of epididymis, unspecified
N43.41 Spermatocele of epididymis, single
N43.42 Spermatocele of epididymis, multiple

N44 Noninflammatory disorders of testis
N44.0 Torsion of testis
N44.00 Torsion of testis, unspecified
N44.01 Extravaginal torsion of spermatic cord
N44.02 Intravaginal torsion of spermatic cord
Torsion of spermatic cord NOS
N44.03 Torsion of appendix testis
N44.04 Torsion of appendix epididymis
N44.1 Cyst of tunica albuginea testis
N44.2 Benign cyst of testis
N44.8 Other noninflammatory disorders of the testis

N45 Orchitis and epididymitis
Use additional code (B95-B97), to identify infectious agent.
N45.1 Epididymitis
N45.2 Orchitis
N45.3 Epididymo-orchitis
N45.4 Abscess of epididymis or testis

N46 Male infertility
Excludes 1: vasectomy status (Z98.52)
N46.0 Azoospermia
Absolute male infertility
Male infertility due to germinal (cell) aplasia
Male infertility due to spermatogenic arrest (complete)
N46.01 Organic azoospermia
Azoospermia NOS
N46.02 Azoospermia due to extratesticular causes
Code also associated cause
N46.021 Azoospermia due to drug therapy
N46.022 Azoospermia due to infection
N46.023 Azoospermia due to obstruction of efferent ducts
N46.024 Azoospermia due to radiation
N46.025 Azoospermia due to systemic disease

 N46.029 Azoospermia due to other extratesticular causes

N46.1 Oligospermia

Male infertility due to germinal cell desquamation

Male infertility due to hypospermatogenesis

Male infertility due to incomplete spermatogenic arrest

 N46.11 Organic oligospermia

 Oligospermia NOS

 N46.12 Oligospermia due to extratesticular causes

 Code also associated cause

 N46.121 Oligospermia due to drug therapy

 N46.122 Oligospermia due to infection

 N46.123 Oligospermia due to obstruction of efferent ducts

 N46.124 Oligospermia due to radiation

 N46.125 Oligospermia due to systemic disease

 N46.129 Oligospermia due to other extratesticular causes

N46.8 Other male infertility

N46.9 Male infertility, unspecified

N47 Disorders of prepuce

N47.0 Adherent prepuce, newborn

N47.1 Phimosis

N47.2 Paraphimosis

N47.3 Deficient foreskin

N47.4 Benign cyst of prepuce

N47.5 Adhesions of prepuce and glans penis

N47.6 Balanoposthitis

Use additional code (B95-B97), to identify infectious agent.

Excludes 1: balanitis (N48.1)

N47.7 Other inflammatory diseases of prepuce

Use additional code (B95-B97), to identify infectious agent.

N47.8 Other disorders of prepuce

N48 Other disorders of penis

N48.0 Leukoplakia of penis

Balanitis xerotica obliterans

Kraurosis of penis

Lichen sclerosus of external male genital organs

Excludes 1: carcinoma in situ of penis (D07.4)

N48.1 Balanitis

Use additional code (B95-B97), to identify infectious agent

Excludes 1: amebic balanitis (A06.8)

 balanitis xerotica obliterans (N48.0)

 candidal balanitis (B37.42)

 gonococcal balanitis (A54.23)

 herpesviral [herpes simplex] balanitis (A60.01)

N48.2 Other inflammatory disorders of penis

Use additional code (B95-B97), to identify infectious agent.

Excludes 1: balanitis (N48.1)

 balanitis xerotica obliterans (N48.0)

 balanoposthitis (N47.6)

N48.21 Abscess of corpus cavernosum and penis

N48.22 Cellulitis of corpus cavernosum and penis

N48.29 Other inflammatory disorders of penis

N48.3 Priapism

Painful erection

Code first underlying cause

 N48.30 Priapism, unspecified

 N48.31 Priapism due to trauma

 N48.32 Priapism due to disease classified elsewhere

 N48.33 Priapism, drug-induced

 N48.39 Other priapism

N48.5 Ulcer of penis

N48.6 Induration penis plastica

Peyronie's disease

Plastic induration of penis

N48.8 Other specified disorders of penis

 N48.81 Thrombosis of superficial vein of penis

 N48.82 Acquired torsion of penis

 Acquired torsion of penis NOS

 Excludes 1: congenital torsion of penis (Q55.63)

 N48.83 Acquired buried penis

 Excludes 1: congenital hidden penis (Q55.64)

 N48.89 Other specified disorders of penis

N48.9 Disorder of penis, unspecified

N49 Inflammatory disorders of male genital organs, not elsewhere classified

Use additional code (B95-B97), to identify infectious agent

Excludes 1: inflammation of penis (N48.1, N48.2-)

 orchitis and epididymitis (N45.-)

N49.0 Inflammatory disorders of seminal vesicle

Vesiculitis NOS

N49.1 Inflammatory disorders of spermatic cord, tunica vaginalis and vas deferens

Vasitis

N49.2 Inflammatory disorders of scrotum

N49.3 Fournier gangrene

N49.8 Inflammatory disorders of other specified male genital organs

Inflammation of multiple sites in male genital organs

N49.9 Inflammatory disorder of unspecified male genital organ

Abscess of unspecified male genital organ

Boil of unspecified male genital organ

Carbuncle of unspecified male genital organ

Cellulitis of unspecified male genital organ

N50 Other and unspecified disorders of male genital organs

Excludes 2: torsion of testis (N44.0-)

N50.0 Atrophy of testis

N50.1 Vascular disorders of male genital organs

Hematocele, NOS, of male genital organs

Hemorrhage of male genital organs

Thrombosis of male genital organs

N50.3 Cyst of epididymis

N50.8 Other specified disorders of male genital organs

Atrophy of scrotum, seminal vesicle, spermatic cord, tunica vaginalis and vas deferens

Edema of scrotum, seminal vesicle, spermatic cord, testis, tunica vaginalis and vas deferens

Hypertrophy of scrotum, seminal vesicle, spermatic cord, testis, tunica vaginalis and vas deferens

Ulcer of scrotum, seminal vesicle, spermatic cord, testis, tunica vaginalis and vas deferens

Chylocele, tunica vaginalis (nonfilarial) NOS

Urethroscrotal fistula

● New code   ▲ Revised code   ⑦ 7th digit required   ⊗ Placeholder required

Stricture of spermatic cord, tunica vaginalis, and vas deferens

N50.9 Disorder of male genital organs, unspecified

N51 Disorders of male genital organs in diseases classified elsewhere
Code first underlying disease, such as:
filariasis (B74.0-B74.9)
Excludes 1: amebic balanitis (A06.8)
candidal balanitis (B37.42)
gonococcal balanitis (A54.23)
gonococcal prostatitis (A54.22)
herpesviral [herpes simplex] balanitis (A60.01)
trichomonal prostatitis (A59.02)
tuberculous prostatitis (A18.14)

N52 Male erectile dysfunction
Excludes 1: psychogenic impotence (F52.21)

N52.0 Vasculogenic erectile dysfunction
N52.01 Erectile dysfunction due to arterial insufficiency
N52.02 Corporo-venous occlusive erectile dysfunction
N52.03 Combined arterial insufficiency and corporo-venous occlusive erectile dysfunction

N52.1 Erectile dysfunction due to diseases classified elsewhere
Code first underlying disease

N52.2 Drug-induced erectile dysfunction

N52.3 Post-surgical erectile dysfunction
N52.31 Erectile dysfunction following radical prostatectomy
N52.32 Erectile dysfunction following radical cystectomy
N52.33 Erectile dysfunction following urethral surgery
N52.34 Erectile dysfunction following simple prostatectomy
N52.39 Other post-surgical erectile dysfunction

N52.8 Other male erectile dysfunction

N52.9 Male erectile dysfunction, unspecified
Impotence NOS

N53 Other male sexual dysfunction
Excludes 1: psychogenic sexual dysfunction (F52.-)

N53.1 Ejaculatory dysfunction
Excludes 1: premature ejaculation (F52.4)
N53.11 Retarded ejaculation
N53.12 Painful ejaculation
N53.13 Anejaculatory orgasm
N53.14 Retrograde ejaculation
N53.19 Other ejaculatory dysfunction
Ejaculatory dysfunction NOS

N53.8 Other male sexual dysfunction

N53.9 Unspecified male sexual dysfunction

DISORDERS OF BREAST (N60-N65)

Excludes 1: disorders of breast associated with childbirth (O91-O92)

N60 Benign mammary dysplasia
Includes: fibrocystic mastopathy

N60.0 Solitary cyst of breast
Cyst of breast
N60.01 Solitary cyst of right breast
N60.02 Solitary cyst of left breast
N60.09 Solitary cyst of unspecified breast

N60.1 Diffuse cystic mastopathy
Cystic breast

Fibrocystic disease of breast
Excludes 1: diffuse cystic mastopathy with epithelial proliferation (N60.3-)
N60.11 Diffuse cystic mastopathy of right breast
N60.12 Diffuse cystic mastopathy of left breast
N60.19 Diffuse cystic mastopathy of unspecified breast

N60.2 Fibroadenosis of breast
Adenofibrosis of breast
Excludes 2: fibroadenoma of breast (D24.-)
N60.21 Fibroadenosis of right breast
N60.22 Fibroadenosis of left breast
N60.29 Fibroadenosis of unspecified breast

N60.3 Fibrosclerosis of breast
Cystic mastopathy with epithelial proliferation
N60.31 Fibrosclerosis of right breast
N60.32 Fibrosclerosis of left breast
N60.39 Fibrosclerosis of unspecified breast

N60.4 Mammary duct ectasia
N60.41 Mammary duct ectasia of right breast
N60.42 Mammary duct ectasia of left breast
N60.49 Mammary duct ectasia of unspecified breast

N60.8 Other benign mammary dysplasias
N60.81 Other benign mammary dysplasias of right breast
N60.82 Other benign mammary dysplasias of left breast
N60.89 Other benign mammary dysplasias of unspecified breast

N60.9 Unspecified benign mammary dysplasia
N60.91 Unspecified benign mammary dysplasia of right breast
N60.92 Unspecified benign mammary dysplasia of left breast
N60.99 Unspecified benign mammary dysplasia of unspecified breast

N61 Inflammatory disorders of breast
Abscess (acute) (chronic) (nonpuerperal) of areola
Abscess (acute) (chronic) (nonpuerperal) of breast
Carbuncle of breast
Infective mastitis (acute) (subacute) (nonpuerperal)
Mastitis (acute) (subacute) (nonpuerperal) NOS
Excludes 1: inflammatory carcinoma of breast (C50.9)
inflammatory disorder of breast associated with childbirth (O91.-)
neonatal infective mastitis (P39.0)
thrombophlebitis of breast [Mondor's disease] (I80.8)

N62 Hypertrophy of breast
Gynecomastia
Hypertrophy of breast NOS
Massive pubertal hypertrophy of breast
Excludes 1: breast engorgement of newborn (P83.4)
disproportion of reconstructed breast (N65.1)

N63 Unspecified lump in breast
Nodule(s) NOS in breast

N64 Other disorders of breast
Excludes 2: mechanical complication of breast prosthesis and implant (T85.4-)

N64.0 Fissure and fistula of nipple

N64.1 Fat necrosis of breast
Fat necrosis (segmental) of breast
Code first breast necrosis due to breast graft (T85.89)

■ Add 4th-7th digits	▨ 3 digit reportable	▨ Nonspecific code	▨ Unspecified code	▨ Manifestation code	483

N64.2 Atrophy of breast

N64.3 Galactorrhea not associated with childbirth

N64.4 Mastodynia

N64.5 Other signs and symptoms in breast

  Excludes 2: abnormal findings on diagnostic imaging of
    breast (R92.-)

   N64.51 Induration of breast

   N64.52 Nipple discharge

  Excludes 1: abnormal findings in nipple
    discharge (R89.-)

   N64.53 Retraction of nipple

   N64.59 Other signs and symptoms in breast

N64.8 Other specified disorders of breast

   N64.81 Ptosis of breast

  Excludes 1: ptosis of native breast in relation to
    reconstructed breast (N65.1)

   N64.82 Hypoplasia of breast
    Micromastia

  Excludes 1: congenital absence of breast
    (Q83.0)
    hypoplasia of native breast in
    relation to reconstructed breast
    (N65.1)

   N64.89 Other specified disorders of breast
    Galactocele
    Subinvolution of breast (post lactational)

N64.9 Disorder of breast, unspecified

N65 Deformity and disproportion of reconstructed breast

N65.0 Deformity of reconstructed breast
  Contour irregularity in reconstructed breast
  Excess tissue in reconstructed breast
  Misshapen reconstructed breast

N65.1 Disproportion of reconstructed breast
  Breast asymmetry between native breast and reconstructed
  breast
  Disproportion between native breast and reconstructed
  breast

INFLAMMATORY DISEASES OF FEMALE PELVIC ORGANS (N70-N77)

Excludes 1: inflammatory diseases of female pelvic organs complicating:
    abortion or ectopic or molar pregnancy (O00-O07, O08.0)
    pregnancy, childbirth and the puerperium (O23.-, O75.3,
    O85, O86.-)

N70 Salpingitis and oophoritis

  Includes: abscess (of) fallopian tube
    abscess (of) ovary
    pyosalpinx
    salpingo-oophoritis
    tubo-ovarian abscess
    tubo-ovarian inflammatory disease

  Use additional code (B95-B97), to identify infectious agent

  Excludes 1: gonococcal infection (A54.24)
    tuberculous infection (A18.17)

N70.0 Acute salpingitis and oophoritis

   N70.01 Acute salpingitis

   N70.02 Acute oophoritis

   N70.03 Acute salpingitis and oophoritis

N70.1 Chronic salpingitis and oophoritis

  Hydrosalpinx

   N70.11 Chronic salpingitis

   N70.12 Chronic oophoritis

   N70.13 Chronic salpingitis and oophoritis

N70.9 Salpingitis and oophoritis, unspecified

   N70.91 Salpingitis, unspecified

   N70.92 Oophoritis, unspecified

   N70.93 Salpingitis and oophoritis, unspecified

N71 Inflammatory disease of uterus, except cervix

  Includes: endo (myo) metritis
    metritis
    myometritis
    pyometra
    uterine abscess

  Use additional code (B95-B97), to identify infectious agent

  Excludes 1: hyperplastic endometritis (N85.0-)
    infection of uterus following delivery (O85, O86-)

N71.0 Acute inflammatory disease of uterus

N71.1 Chronic inflammatory disease of uterus

N71.9 Inflammatory disease of uterus, unspecified

N72 Inflammatory disease of cervix uteri

  Includes: cervicitis (with or without erosion or ectropion)
    endocervicitis (with or without erosion or ectropion)
    exocervicitis (with or without erosion or ectropion)

  Use additional code (B95-B97), to identify infectious agent

  Excludes 1: erosion and ectropion of cervix without cervicitis
    (N86)

N73 Other female pelvic inflammatory diseases

  Use additional code (B95-B97), to identify infectious agent.

N73.0 Acute parametritis and pelvic cellulitis
  Abscess of broad ligament
  Abscess of parametrium
  Pelvic cellulitis, female

N73.1 Chronic parametritis and pelvic cellulitis
  Any condition in N73.0 specified as chronic

  Excludes 1: tuberculous parametritis and pelvic cellulitis
    (A18.17)

N73.2 Unspecified parametritis and pelvic cellulitis
  Any condition in N73.0 unspecified whether acute or
  chronic

N73.3 Female acute pelvic peritonitis

N73.4 Female chronic pelvic peritonitis

  Excludes 1: tuberculous pelvic (female) peritonitis
    (A18.17)

N73.5 Female pelvic peritonitis, unspecified

N73.6 Female pelvic peritoneal adhesions (postinfective)

  Excludes 2: postprocedural pelvic peritoneal adhesions
    (N99.4)

N73.8 Other specified female pelvic inflammatory diseases

N73.9 Female pelvic inflammatory disease, unspecified
  Female pelvic infection or inflammation NOS

N74 Female pelvic inflammatory disorders in diseases classified
  elsewhere

  Code first underlying disease

  Excludes 1: cervicitis:
    chlamydial (A56.02)
    gonococcal (A54.03)
    herpesviral [herpes simplex] (A60.03)

syphilitic (A52.76)

trichomonal (A59.09)

tuberculous (A18.16)

pelvic inflammatory disease:

chlamydial (A56.11)

gonococcal (A54.24)

herpesviral [herpes simplex] (A60.09)

syphilitic (A52.76)

tuberculous (A18.17)

N75 Diseases of Bartholin's gland

N75.0 Cyst of Bartholin's gland

N75.1 Abscess of Bartholin's gland

N75.8 Other diseases of Bartholin's gland

Bartholinitis

N75.9 Disease of Bartholin's gland, unspecified

N76 Other inflammation of vagina and vulva

Use additional code (B95-B97), to identify infectious agent

Excludes 2: senile (atrophic) vaginitis (N95.2)

vulvar vestibulitis (N94.810)

N76.0 Acute vaginitis

Acute vulvovaginitis

Vaginitis NOS

Vulvovaginitis NOS

N76.1 Subacute and chronic vaginitis

Chronic vulvovaginitis

Subacute vulvovaginitis

N76.2 Acute vulvitis

Vulvitis NOS

N76.3 Subacute and chronic vulvitis

N76.4 Abscess of vulva

Furuncle of vulva

N76.5 Ulceration of vagina

N76.6 Ulceration of vulva

N76.8 Other specified inflammation of vagina and vulva

N76.81 Mucositis (ulcerative) of vagina and vulva

Code also type of associated therapy, such as:

antineoplastic and immunosuppressive drugs (T45.1x-)

radiological procedure and radiotherapy (Y84.2)

Excludes 2: gastrointestinal mucositis (ulcerative) (K92.81)

nasal mucositis (ulcerative) (J34.81)

oral mucositis (ulcerative) (K12.3-)

N76.89 Other specified inflammation of vagina and vulva

N77 Vulvovaginal ulceration and inflammation in diseases classified elsewhere

N77.0 Ulceration of vulva in diseases classified elsewhere

Code first underlying disease, such as:

Behcet's disease (M35.2)

Excludes 1: ulceration of vulva in gonococcal infection (A54.02)

ulceration of vulva in herpesviral [herpes simplex] infection (A60.04)

ulceration of vulva in syphilis (A51.0)

ulceration of vulva in tuberculosis (A18.18)

N77.1 Vaginitis, vulvitis and vulvovaginitis in diseases classified elsewhere

Code first underlying disease, such as:

pinworm (B80)

Excludes 1: vaginitis, vulvitis and vulvovaginitis (in):

candidiasis (B37.3)

chlamydial (A56.02)

gonococcal infection (A54.02)

herpesviral [herpes simplex] infection (A60.04)

syphilitic, early (A51.0)

syphilitic, late (A52.76)

trichomonal (A59.01)

tuberculous (A18.18)

NONINFLAMMATORY DISORDERS OF FEMALE GENITAL TRACT (N80-N98)

N80 Endometriosis

N80.0 Endometriosis of uterus

Adenomyosis

Excludes 1: stromal endometriosis (D39.0)

N80.1 Endometriosis of ovary

N80.2 Endometriosis of fallopian tube

N80.3 Endometriosis of pelvic peritoneum

N80.4 Endometriosis of rectovaginal septum and vagina

N80.5 Endometriosis of intestine

N80.6 Endometriosis in cutaneous scar

N80.8 Other endometriosis

N80.9 Endometriosis, unspecified

N81 Female genital prolapse

Excludes 1: genital prolapse complicating pregnancy, labor or delivery (O34.5-)

prolapse and hernia of ovary and fallopian tube (N83.4)

prolapse of vaginal vault after hysterectomy (N99.3)

N81.0 Urethrocele

Excludes 1: urethrocele with cystocele (N81.1-)

urethrocele with prolapse of uterus (N81.2-N81.4)

N81.1 Cystocele

Cystocele with urethrocele

Cystourethrocele

Excludes 1: cystocele with prolapse of uterus (N81.2-N81.4)

N81.10 Cystocele, unspecified

Prolapse of (anterior) vaginal wall NOS

N81.11 Cystocele, midline

N81.12 Cystocele, lateral

Paravaginal cystocele

N81.2 Incomplete uterovaginal prolapse

First degree uterine prolapse

Prolapse of cervix NOS

Second degree uterine prolapse

Excludes 1: cervical stump prolapse (N81.85)

N81.3 Complete uterovaginal prolapse

Procidentia (uteri) NOS

Third degree uterine prolapse

N81.4 Uterovaginal prolapse, unspecified

Prolapse of uterus NOS

N81.5 Vaginal enterocele

Excludes 1: enterocele with prolapse of uterus (N81.2-N81.4)

N81.6 Rectocele

Prolapse of posterior vaginal wall

Use additional code for any associated fecal incontinence, if applicable (R15-)

Excludes 2: perineocele N81.81

rectal prolapse (K62.3)

rectocele with prolapse of uterus (N81.2-N81.4)

N81.8 Other female genital prolapse

N81.81 Perineocele

N81.82 Incompetence or weakening of pubocervical tissue

N81.83 Incompetence or weakening of rectovaginal tissue

N81.84 Pelvic muscle wasting

Disuse atrophy of pelvic muscles and anal sphincter

N81.85 Cervical stump prolapse

N81.89 Other female genital prolapse

Deficient perineum

Old laceration of muscles of pelvic floor

N81.9 Female genital prolapse, unspecified

N82 Fistulae involving female genital tract

Excludes 1: vesicointestinal fistulae (N32.1)

N82.0 Vesicovaginal fistula

N82.1 Other female urinary-genital tract fistulae

Cervicovesical fistula

Ureterovaginal fistula

Urethrovaginal fistula

Uteroureteric fistula

Uterovesical fistula

N82.2 Fistula of vagina to small intestine

N82.3 Fistula of vagina to large intestine

Rectovaginal fistula

N82.4 Other female intestinal-genital tract fistulae

Intestinouterine fistula

N82.5 Female genital tract-skin fistulae

Uterus to abdominal wall fistula

Vaginoperineal fistula

N82.8 Other female genital tract fistulae

N82.9 Female genital tract fistula, unspecified

N83 Noninflammatory disorders of ovary, fallopian tube and broad ligament

Excludes 2: hydrosalpinx (N70.1-)

N83.0 Follicular cyst of ovary

Cyst of graafian follicle

Hemorrhagic follicular cyst (of ovary)

N83.1 Corpus luteum cyst

Hemorrhagic corpus luteum cyst

N83.2 Other and unspecified ovarian cysts

Excludes 1: developmental ovarian cyst (Q50.1)

neoplastic ovarian cyst (D27.-)

polycystic ovarian syndrome (E28.2)

Stein-Leventhal syndrome (E28.2)

N83.20 Unspecified ovarian cysts

N83.29 Other ovarian cysts

Retention cyst of ovary

Simple cyst of ovary

N83.3 Acquired atrophy of ovary and fallopian tube

N83.31 Acquired atrophy of ovary

N83.32 Acquired atrophy of fallopian tube

N83.33 Acquired atrophy of ovary and fallopian tube

N83.4 Prolapse and hernia of ovary and fallopian tube

N83.5 Torsion of ovary, ovarian pedicle and fallopian tube

Torsion of accessory tube

N83.51 Torsion of ovary and ovarian pedicle

N83.52 Torsion of fallopian tube

Torsion of hydatid of Morgagni

N83.53 Torsion of ovary, ovarian pedicle and fallopian tube

N83.6 Hematosalpinx

Excludes 1: hematosalpinx (with) (in):

hematocolpos (N89.7)

hematometra (N85.7)

tubal pregnancy (O00.1)

N83.7 Hematoma of broad ligament

N83.8 Other noninflammatory disorders of ovary, fallopian tube and broad ligament

Broad ligament laceration syndrome [Allen-Masters]

N83.9 Noninflammatory disorder of ovary, fallopian tube and broad ligament, unspecified

N84 Polyp of female genital tract

Excludes 1: adenomatous polyp (D28.-)

placental polyp (O90.89)

N84.0 Polyp of corpus uteri

Polyp of endometrium

Polyp of uterus NOS

Excludes 1: polypoid endometrial hyperplasia (N85.0-)

N84.1 Polyp of cervix uteri

Mucous polyp of cervix

N84.2 Polyp of vagina

N84.3 Polyp of vulva

Polyp of labia

N84.8 Polyp of other parts of female genital tract

N84.9 Polyp of female genital tract, unspecified

N85 Other noninflammatory disorders of uterus, except cervix

Excludes 1: endometriosis (N80.-)

inflammatory diseases of uterus (N71.-)

noninflammatory disorders of cervix, except malposition (N86-N88)

polyp of corpus uteri (N84.0)

uterine prolapse (N81.-)

N85.0 Endometrial hyperplasia

N85.00 Endometrial hyperplasia, unspecified

Hyperplasia (adenomatous) (cystic) (glandular) of endometrium

Hyperplastic endometritis

N85.01 Benign endometrial hyperplasia

Endometrial hyperplasia (complex) (simple) without atypia

N85.02 Endometrial intraepithelial neoplasia [EIN]

Endometrial hyperplasia with atypia

Excludes 1: malignant neoplasm of endometrium (with endometrial intraepithelial neoplasia [EIN]) (C54.1)

N85.2 Hypertrophy of uterus

Bulky or enlarged uterus

Excludes 1: puerperal hypertrophy of uterus (O90.89)

N85.3 Subinvolution of uterus

Excludes 1: puerperal subinvolution of uterus (O90.89)

N85.4 Malposition of uterus
Anteversion of uterus
Retroflexion of uterus
Retroversion of uterus
Excludes 1: malposition of uterus complicating
pregnancy, labor or delivery (O34.5-, O65.5)

N85.5 Inversion of uterus
Excludes 1: current obstetric trauma (O71.2)
postpartum inversion of uterus (O71.2)

N85.6 Intrauterine synechiae

N85.7 Hematometra
Hematosalpinx with hematometra
Excludes 1: hematometra with hematocolpos (N89.7)

N85.8 Other specified noninflammatory disorders of uterus
Atrophy of uterus, acquired
Fibrosis of uterus NOS

N85.9 Noninflammatory disorder of uterus, unspecified
Disorder of uterus NOS

N86 Erosion and ectropion of cervix uteri
Decubitus (trophic) ulcer of cervix
Eversion of cervix
Excludes 1: erosion and ectropion of cervix with cervicitis (N72)

N87 Dysplasia of cervix uteri
Excludes 1: abnormal results from cervical cytologic examination
without histologic confirmation (R87.61-)
carcinoma in situ of cervix uteri (D06.-)
cervical intraepithelial neoplasia III [CIN III] (D06.-)
HGSIL of cervix (R87.613)
severe dysplasia of cervix uteri (D06.-)

N87.0 Mild cervical dysplasia
Cervical intraepithelial neoplasia I [CIN I]

N87.1 Moderate cervical dysplasia
Cervical intraepithelial neoplasia II [CIN II]

N87.9 Dysplasia of cervix uteri, unspecified
Anaplasia of cervix
Cervical atypism
Cervical dysplasia NOS

N88 Other noninflammatory disorders of cervix uteri
Excludes 2: inflammatory disease of cervix (N72)
polyp of cervix (N84.1)

N88.0 Leukoplakia of cervix uteri

N88.1 Old laceration of cervix uteri
Adhesions of cervix
Excludes 1: current obstetric trauma (O71.3)

N88.2 Stricture and stenosis of cervix uteri
Excludes 1: stricture and stenosis of cervix uteri
complicating labor (O65.5)

N88.3 Incompetence of cervix uteri
Investigation and management of (suspected) cervical
incompetence in a nonpregnant woman
Excludes 1: cervical incompetence complicating
pregnancy (O34.3-)

N88.4 Hypertrophic elongation of cervix uteri

N88.8 Other specified noninflammatory disorders of cervix uteri
Excludes 1: current obstetric trauma (O71.3)

N88.9 Noninflammatory disorder of cervix uteri, unspecified

N89 Other noninflammatory disorders of vagina
Excludes 1: abnormal results from vaginal cytologic examination
without histologic confirmation (R87.62-)

carcinoma in situ of vagina (D07.2)
HGSIL of vagina (R87.623)
inflammation of vagina (N76.-)
senile (atrophic) vaginitis (N95.2)
severe dysplasia of vagina (D07.2)
trichomonal leukorrhea (A59.00)
vaginal intraepithelial neoplasia [VAIN], grade III (D07.2)

N89.0 Mild vaginal dysplasia
Vaginal intraepithelial neoplasia [VAIN], grade I

N89.1 Moderate vaginal dysplasia
Vaginal intraepithelial neoplasia [VAIN], grade II

N89.3 Dysplasia of vagina, unspecified

N89.4 Leukoplakia of vagina

N89.5 Stricture and atresia of vagina
Vaginal adhesions
Vaginal stenosis
Excludes 1: congenital atresia or stricture (Q52.4)
postprocedural adhesions of vagina (N99.2)

N89.6 Tight hymenal ring
Rigid hymen
Tight introitus
Excludes 1: imperforate hymen (Q52.3)

N89.7 Hematocolpos
Hematocolpos with hematometra or hematosalpinx

N89.8 Other specified noninflammatory disorders of vagina
Leukorrhea NOS
Old vaginal laceration
Pessary ulcer of vagina
Excludes 1: current obstetric trauma (O70.-, O71.4,
O71.7-O71.8)
old laceration involving muscles of pelvic floor
(N81.8)

N89.9 Noninflammatory disorder of vagina, unspecified

N90 Other noninflammatory disorders of vulva and perineum
Excludes 1: anogenital (venereal) warts (A63.0)
carcinoma in situ of vulva (D07.1)
condyloma acuminatum (A63.0)
current obstetric trauma (O70.-, O71.7-O71.8)
inflammation of vulva (N76.-)
severe dysplasia of vulva (D07.1)
vulvar intraepithelial neoplasm III [VIN III] (D07.1)

N90.0 Mild vulvar dysplasia
Vulvar intraepithelial neoplasia [VIN], grade I

N90.1 Moderate vulvar dysplasia
Vulvar intraepithelial neoplasia [VIN], grade II

N90.3 Dysplasia of vulva, unspecified

N90.4 Leukoplakia of vulva
Dystrophy of vulva
Kraurosis of vulva
Lichen sclerosus of external female genital organs

N90.5 Atrophy of vulva
Stenosis of vulva

N90.6 Hypertrophy of vulva
Hypertrophy of labia

N90.7 Vulvar cyst

N90.8 Other specified noninflammatory disorders of vulva and
perineum

N90.81 Female genital mutilation status
Female genital cutting status

N90.810 Female genital mutilation status, unspecified
Female genital cutting status, unspecified
Female genital mutilation status NOS

N90.811 Female genital mutilation Type I status
Clitorectomy status
Female genital cutting Type I status

N90.812 Female genital mutilation Type II status
Clitorectomy with excision of labia minora status
Female genital cutting Type II status

N90.813 Female genital mutilation Type III status
Female genital cutting Type III status
Infibulation status

N90.818 Other female genital mutilation status
Female genital cutting Type IV status
Female genital mutilation Type IV status
Other female genital cutting status

N90.89 Other specified noninflammatory disorders of vulva and perineum
Adhesions of vulva
Hypertrophy of clitoris

N90.9 Noninflammatory disorder of vulva and perineum, unspecified

N91 Absent, scanty and rare menstruation
Excludes 1: ovarian dysfunction (E28.-)

N91.0 Primary amenorrhea

N91.1 Secondary amenorrhea

N91.2 Amenorrhea, unspecified

N91.3 Primary oligomenorrhea

N91.4 Secondary oligomenorrhea

N91.5 Oligomenorrhea, unspecified
Hypomenorrhea NOS

N92 Excessive, frequent and irregular menstruation
Excludes 1: postmenopausal bleeding (N95.0)
precocious puberty (menstruation) (E30.1)

N92.0 Excessive and frequent menstruation with regular cycle
Heavy periods NOS
Menorrhagia NOS
Polymenorrhea

N92.1 Excessive and frequent menstruation with irregular cycle
Irregular intermenstrual bleeding
Irregular, shortened intervals between menstrual bleeding
Menometrorrhagia
Metrorrhagia

N92.2 Excessive menstruation at puberty
Excessive bleeding associated with onset of menstrual periods
Pubertal menorrhagia
Puberty bleeding

N92.3 Ovulation bleeding
Regular intermenstrual bleeding

N92.4 Excessive bleeding in the premenopausal period
Climacteric menorrhagia or metrorrhagia
Menopausal menorrhagia or metrorrhagia
Preclimacteric menorrhagia or metrorrhagia
Premenopausal menorrhagia or metrorrhagia

N92.5 Other specified irregular menstruation

N92.6 Irregular menstruation, unspecified
Irregular bleeding NOS
Irregular periods NOS
Excludes 1: irregular menstruation with:
lengthened intervals or scanty bleeding (N91.3-N91.5)
shortened intervals or excessive bleeding (N92.1)

N93 Other abnormal uterine and vaginal bleeding
Excludes 1: neonatal vaginal hemorrhage (P54.6)
precocious puberty (menstruation) (E30.1)
pseudomenses (P54.6)

N93.0 Postcoital and contact bleeding

N93.8 Other specified abnormal uterine and vaginal bleeding
Dysfunctional or functional uterine or vaginal bleeding NOS

N93.9 Abnormal uterine and vaginal bleeding, unspecified

N94 Pain and other conditions associated with female genital organs and menstrual cycle

N94.0 Mittelschmerz

N94.1 Dyspareunia
Excludes 1: psychogenic dyspareunia (F52.6)

N94.2 Vaginismus
Excludes 1: psychogenic vaginismus (F52.5)

N94.3 Premenstrual tension syndrome
Premenstrual dysphoric disorder
Code also associated menstrual migraine (G43.82-, G43.83-)

N94.4 Primary dysmenorrhea

N94.5 Secondary dysmenorrhea

N94.6 Dysmenorrhea, unspecified
Excludes 1: psychogenic dysmenorrhea (F45.8)

N94.8 Other specified conditions associated with female genital organs and menstrual cycle

N94.81 Vulvodynia

N94.810 Vulvar vestibulitis

N94.818 Other vulvodynia

N94.819 Vulvodynia, unspecified
Vulvodynia NOS

N94.89 Other specified conditions associated with female genital organs and menstrual cycle

N94.9 Unspecified condition associated with female genital organs and menstrual cycle

N95 Menopausal and other perimenopausal disorders
Menopausal and other perimenopausal disorders due to naturally occurring (age-related) menopause and perimenopause
Excludes 1: excessive bleeding in the premenopausal period (N92.4)
menopausal and perimenopausal disorders due to artificial or premature menopause (E89.4-, E28.31-)
premature menopause (E28.31-)

● New code   ▲ Revised code   ⑦ 7ᵗʰ digit required   ⊗ Placeholder required

postmenopausal osteoporosis (M81.0-)

postmenopausal osteoporosis with current pathological fracture (M80.0-)

postmenopausal urethritis (N34.2)

N95.0 Postmenopausal bleeding

N95.1 Menopausal and female climacteric states

Symptoms such as flushing, sleeplessness, headache, lack of concentration, associated with natural (age-related) menopause

Use additional code for associated symptoms

Excludes 1: asymptomatic menopausal state (Z78.0)

symptoms associated with artificial menopause (E89.41)

symptoms associated with premature menopause (E28.310)

N95.2 Postmenopausal atrophic vaginitis

Senile (atrophic) vaginitis

N95.8 Other specified menopausal and perimenopausal disorders

N95.9 Unspecified menopausal and perimenopausal disorder

N96 Recurrent pregnancy loss

Investigation or care in a nonpregnant woman with history of recurrent pregnancy loss

Excludes 1: recurrent pregnancy loss with current pregnancy (O26.2-)

N97 Female infertility

Includes: inability to achieve a pregnancy

sterility, female NOS

Excludes 1: female infertility associated with:

hypopituitarism (E23.0)

Stein-Leventhal syndrome (E28.2)

Excludes 2: incompetence of cervix uteri (N88.3)

N97.0 Female infertility associated with anovulation

N97.1 Female infertility of tubal origin

Female infertility associated with congenital anomaly of tube

Female infertility due to tubal block

Female infertility due to tubal occlusion

Female infertility due to tubal stenosis

N97.2 Female infertility of uterine origin

Female infertility associated with congenital anomaly of uterus

Female infertility due to nonimplantation of ovum

N97.8 Female infertility of other origin

N97.9 Female infertility, unspecified

N98 Complications associated with artificial fertilization

N98.0 Infection associated with artificial insemination

N98.1 Hyperstimulation of ovaries

Hyperstimulation of ovaries NOS

Hyperstimulation of ovaries associated with induced ovulation

N98.2 Complications of attempted introduction of fertilized ovum following in vitro fertilization

N98.3 Complications of attempted introduction of embryo in embryo transfer

N98.8 Other complications associated with artificial fertilization

N98.9 Complication associated with artificial fertilization, unspecified

INTRAOPERATIVE AND POSTPROCEDURAL COMPLICATIONS AND DISORDERS OF

GENITOURINARY SYSTEM, NOT ELSEWHERE CLASSIFIED (N99)

N99 Intraoperative and postprocedural complications and disorders of genitourinary system, not elsewhere classified

Excludes 2: irradiation cystitis (N30.4-)

post oophorectomy osteoporosis with current pathological fracture (M80.8-)

post oophorectomy osteoporosis without current pathological fracture (M81.8)

N99.0 Postprocedural (acute) (chronic) kidney failure

Use additional code to type of kidney disease

N99.1 Postprocedural urethral stricture

Postcatheterization urethral stricture

N99.11 Postprocedural urethral stricture, male

N99.110 Postprocedural urethral stricture, male, meatal

N99.111 Postprocedural bulbous urethral stricture

N99.112 Postprocedural membranous urethral stricture

N99.113 Postprocedural anterior urethral stricture

N99.114 Postprocedural urethral stricture, male, unspecified

N99.12 Postprocedural urethral stricture, female

N99.2 Postprocedural adhesions of vagina

N99.3 Prolapse of vaginal vault after hysterectomy

N99.4 Postprocedural pelvic peritoneal adhesions

Excludes 2: pelvic peritoneal adhesions NOS (N73.6)

postinfective pelvic peritoneal adhesions (N73.6)

N99.5 Complications of stoma of urinary tract

Excludes 2: mechanical complication of urinary (indwelling) catheter (T83.0-)

N99.51 Complication of cystostomy

N99.510 Cystostomy hemorrhage

N99.511 Cystostomy infection

N99.512 Cystostomy malfunction

N99.518 Other cystostomy complication

N99.52 Complication of other external stoma of urinary tract

N99.520 Hemorrhage of other external stoma of urinary tract

N99.521 Infection of other external stoma of urinary tract

N99.522 Malfunction of other external stoma of urinary tract

N99.528 Other complication of other external stoma of urinary tract

N99.53 Complication of other stoma of urinary tract

N99.530 Hemorrhage of other stoma of urinary tract

N99.531 Infection of other stoma of urinary tract

N99.532 Malfunction of other stoma of urinary tract

N99.538 Other complication of other stoma of urinary tract

N99.6 Intraoperative hemorrhage and hematoma of a genitourinary system organ or structure complicating a procedure

Excludes 1: intraoperative hemorrhage and hematoma of a genitourinary system organ or structure due to accidental puncture or laceration during a procedure (N99.7-)

N99.61 Intraoperative hemorrhage and hematoma of a genitourinary system organ or structure complicating a genitourinary system procedure

N99.62 Intraoperative hemorrhage and hematoma of a genitourinary system organ or structure complicating other procedure

N99.7 Accidental puncture and laceration of a genitourinary system organ or structure during a procedure

N99.71 Accidental puncture and laceration of a genitourinary system organ or structure during a genitourinary system procedure

N99.72 Accidental puncture and laceration of a genitourinary system organ or structure during other procedure

N99.8 Other intraoperative and postprocedural complications and disorders of genitourinary system

N99.81 Other intraoperative complications of genitourinary system

N99.82 Postprocedural hemorrhage and hematoma of a genitourinary system organ or structure following a procedure

N99.820 Postprocedural hemorrhage and hematoma of a genitourinary system organ or structure following a genitourinary system procedure

N99.821 Postprocedural hemorrhage and hematoma of a genitourinary system organ or structure following other procedure

N99.83 Residual ovary syndrome

N99.89 Other postprocedural complications and disorders of genitourinary system

● New code   ▲ Revised code   ⑦ 7th digit required   ⊗ Placeholder required

Chapter 15: Pregnancy, Childbirth And The Puerperium (O00-O9A)

Note: codes from this chapter are for use only on maternal records, never on newborn records.

Codes from this chapter are for use for conditions related to or aggravated by the pregnancy, childbirth, or by the puerperium (maternal causes or obstetric causes)

Trimesters are counted from the first day of the last menstrual period. They are defined as follows:

1st trimester- less than 14weeks 0days

2nd trimester- 14weeks 0days to less than 28weeks 0days

3rd trimester- 28weeks 0days until delivery

Use additional code from category Z3A, Weeks of gestation, to identify the specific week of the pregnancy

Excludes 1: supervision of normal pregnancy (Z34.-)

Excludes 2: mental and behavioral disorders associated with the puerperium (F53)

obstetrical tetanus (A34)

postpartum necrosis of pituitary gland (E23.0)

puerperal osteomalacia (M83.0)

This chapter contains the following blocks:

O00-O08	Pregnancy with abortive outcome
O09	Supervision of high risk pregnancy
O10-O16	Edema, proteinuria and hypertensive disorders in pregnancy, childbirth and the puerperium
O20-O29	Other maternal disorders predominantly related to pregnancy
O30-O48	Maternal care related to the fetus and amniotic cavity and possible delivery problems
O60-O77	Complications of labor and delivery
O80-O82	Encounter for delivery
O85-O92	Complications predominantly related to the puerperium
O94-O9A	Other obstetric conditions, not elsewhere classified

PREGNANCY WITH ABORTIVE OUTCOME (O00-O08)

Excludes 1: continuing pregnancy in multiple gestation after abortion of one fetus or more (O31.1-, O31.3-)

O00 Ectopic pregnancy

Includes: ruptured ectopic pregnancy

Use additional code from category O08 to identify any associated complication

O00.0 Abdominal pregnancy

Excludes 1: maternal care for viable fetus in abdominal pregnancy (O36.7-)

O00.1 Tubal pregnancy

Fallopian pregnancy

Rupture of (fallopian) tube due to pregnancy

Tubal abortion

O00.2 Ovarian pregnancy

O00.8 Other ectopic pregnancy

Cervical pregnancy

Cornual pregnancy

Intraligamentous pregnancy

Mural pregnancy

O00.9 Ectopic pregnancy, unspecified

O01 Hydatidiform mole

Use additional code from category O08 to identify any associated complication.

Excludes 1: chorioadenoma (destruens) (D39.2)

malignant hydatidiform mole (D39.2)

O01.0 Classical hydatidiform mole

Complete hydatidiform mole

O01.1 Incomplete and partial hydatidiform mole

O01.9 Hydatidiform mole, unspecified

Trophoblastic disease NOS

Vesicular mole NOS

O02 Other abnormal products of conception

Use additional code from category O08 to identify any associated complication.

Excludes 1: papyraceous fetus (O31.0-)

O02.0 Blighted ovum and nonhydatidiform mole

Carneous mole

Fleshy mole

Intrauterine mole NOS

Molar pregnancy NEC

Pathological ovum

O02.1 Missed abortion

Early fetal death, before completion of 20 weeks of gestation, with retention of dead fetus

Excludes 1: failed induced abortion (O07.-)

fetal death (intrauterine) (late) (O36.4)

missed abortion with blighted ovum (O02.0)

missed abortion with hydatidiform mole (O01.-)

missed abortion with nonhydatidiform (O02.0)

missed abortion with other abnormal products of conception (O02.8-)

missed delivery (O36.4)

stillbirth (P95)

O02.8 Other specified abnormal products of conception

Excludes 1: abnormal products of conception with blighted ovum (O02.0)

abnormal products of conception with hydatidiform mole (O01.-)

abnormal products of conception with nonhydatidiform mole (O02.0)

O02.81 Inappropriate change in quantitative human chorionic gonadotropin (hCG) in early pregnancy

Biochemical pregnancy

Chemical pregnancy

Inappropriate level of quantitative human chorionic gonadotropin (hCG) for gestational age in early pregnancy

O02.89 Other abnormal products of conception

O02.9 Abnormal product of conception, unspecified

O03 Spontaneous abortion

Note: Incomplete abortion includes retained products of conception following spontaneous abortion

Includes: miscarriage

O03.0 Genital tract and pelvic infection following incomplete spontaneous abortion

Endometritis following incomplete spontaneous abortion

Oophoritis following incomplete spontaneous abortion

Parametritis following incomplete spontaneous abortion

Pelvic peritonitis following incomplete spontaneous abortion

Salpingitis following incomplete spontaneous abortion

Salpingo-oophoritis following incomplete spontaneous abortion

Excludes 1: sepsis following incomplete spontaneous abortion (O03.37)

urinary tract infection following incomplete spontaneous abortion (O03.38)

O03.1 Delayed or excessive hemorrhage following incomplete spontaneous abortion

Afibrinogenemia following incomplete spontaneous abortion

Defibrination syndrome following incomplete spontaneous abortion

Hemolysis following incomplete spontaneous abortion

Intravascular coagulation following incomplete spontaneous abortion

O03.2 Embolism following incomplete spontaneous abortion

Air embolism following incomplete spontaneous abortion

Amniotic fluid embolism following incomplete spontaneous abortion

Blood-clot embolism following incomplete spontaneous abortion

Embolism NOS following incomplete spontaneous abortion

Fat embolism following incomplete spontaneous abortion

Pulmonary embolism following incomplete spontaneous abortion

Pyemic embolism following incomplete spontaneous abortion

Septic or septicopyemic embolism following incomplete spontaneous abortion

Soap embolism following incomplete spontaneous abortion

O03.3 Other and unspecified complications following incomplete spontaneous abortion

O03.30 Unspecified complication following incomplete spontaneous abortion

O03.31 Shock following incomplete spontaneous abortion

Circulatory collapse following incomplete spontaneous abortion

Shock (postprocedural) following incomplete spontaneous abortion

Excludes 1: shock due to infection following incomplete spontaneous abortion (O03.37)

O03.32 Renal failure following incomplete spontaneous abortion

Kidney failure (acute) following incomplete spontaneous abortion

Oliguria following incomplete spontaneous abortion

Renal shutdown following incomplete spontaneous abortion

Renal tubular necrosis following incomplete spontaneous abortion

Uremia following incomplete spontaneous abortion

O03.33 Metabolic disorder following incomplete spontaneous abortion

O03.34 Damage to pelvic organs following incomplete spontaneous abortion

Laceration, perforation, tear or chemical damage of bladder following incomplete spontaneous abortion

Laceration, perforation, tear or chemical damage of bowel following incomplete spontaneous abortion

Laceration, perforation, tear or chemical damage of broad ligament following incomplete spontaneous abortion

Laceration, perforation, tear or chemical damage of cervix following incomplete spontaneous abortion

Laceration, perforation, tear or chemical damage of periurethral tissue following incomplete spontaneous abortion

Laceration, perforation, tear or chemical damage of uterus following incomplete spontaneous abortion

Laceration, perforation, tear or chemical damage of vagina following incomplete spontaneous abortion

O03.35 Other venous complications following incomplete spontaneous abortion

O03.36 Cardiac arrest following incomplete spontaneous abortion

O03.37 Sepsis following incomplete spontaneous abortion

Use additional code to identify infectious agent (B95-B97)

Use additional code to identify severe sepsis, if applicable (R65.2-)

Excludes 1: septic or septicopyemic embolism following incomplete spontaneous abortion (O03.2)

O03.38 Urinary tract infection following incomplete spontaneous abortion

Cystitis following incomplete spontaneous abortion

O03.39 Incomplete spontaneous abortion with other complications

O03.4 Incomplete spontaneous abortion without complication

O03.5 Genital tract and pelvic infection following complete or unspecified spontaneous abortion

Endometritis following complete or unspecified spontaneous abortion

Oophoritis following complete or unspecified spontaneous abortion

Parametritis following complete or unspecified spontaneous abortion

Pelvic peritonitis following complete or unspecified spontaneous abortion

Salpingitis following complete or unspecified spontaneous abortion

Salpingo-oophoritis following complete or unspecified spontaneous abortion

Excludes 1: sepsis following complete or unspecified spontaneous abortion (O03.87)

urinary tract infection following complete or unspecified spontaneous abortion (O03.88)

O03.6 Delayed or excessive hemorrhage following complete or unspecified spontaneous abortion

Afibrinogenemia following complete or unspecified spontaneous abortion

Defibrination syndrome following complete or unspecified spontaneous abortion

Hemolysis following complete or unspecified spontaneous abortion

Intravascular coagulation following complete or unspecified spontaneous abortion

O03.7 Embolism following complete or unspecified spontaneous abortion

Air embolism following complete or unspecified spontaneous abortion

Amniotic fluid embolism following complete or unspecified spontaneous abortion

Blood-clot embolism following complete or unspecified spontaneous abortion

Embolism NOS following complete or unspecified spontaneous abortion

Fat embolism following complete or unspecified spontaneous abortion

Pulmonary embolism following complete or unspecified spontaneous abortion

Pyemic embolism following complete or unspecified spontaneous abortion

Septic or septicopyemic embolism following complete or unspecified spontaneous abortion

Soap embolism following complete or unspecified spontaneous abortion

O03.8 Other and unspecified complications following complete or unspecified spontaneous abortion

O03.80 Unspecified complication following complete or unspecified spontaneous abortion

O03.81 Shock following complete or unspecified spontaneous abortion

Circulatory collapse following complete or unspecified spontaneous abortion

Shock (postprocedural) following complete or unspecified spontaneous abortion

Excludes 1: shock due to infection following complete or unspecified spontaneous abortion (O03.87)

O03.82 Renal failure following complete or unspecified spontaneous abortion

Kidney failure (acute) following complete or unspecified spontaneous abortion

Oliguria following complete or unspecified spontaneous abortion

Renal shutdown following complete or unspecified spontaneous abortion

Renal tubular necrosis following complete or unspecified spontaneous abortion

Uremia following complete or unspecified spontaneous abortion

O03.83 Metabolic disorder following complete or unspecified spontaneous abortion

O03.84 Damage to pelvic organs following complete or unspecified spontaneous abortion

Laceration, perforation, tear or chemical damage of bladder following complete or unspecified spontaneous abortion

Laceration, perforation, tear or chemical damage of bowel following complete or unspecified spontaneous abortion

Laceration, perforation, tear or chemical damage of broad ligament following complete or unspecified spontaneous abortion

Laceration, perforation, tear or chemical damage of cervix following complete or unspecified spontaneous abortion

Laceration, perforation, tear or chemical damage of periurethral tissue following complete or unspecified spontaneous abortion

Laceration, perforation, tear or chemical damage of uterus following complete or unspecified spontaneous abortion

Laceration, perforation, tear or chemical damage of vagina following complete or unspecified spontaneous abortion

O03.85 Other venous complications following complete or unspecified spontaneous abortion

O03.86 Cardiac arrest following complete or unspecified spontaneous abortion

O03.87 Sepsis following complete or unspecified spontaneous abortion

Use additional code to identify infectious agent (B95-B97)

Use additional code to identify severe sepsis, if applicable (R65.2-)

Excludes 1: septic or septicopyemic embolism following complete or unspecified spontaneous abortion (O03.7)

O03.88 Urinary tract infection following complete or unspecified spontaneous abortion

Cystitis following complete or unspecified spontaneous abortion

O03.89 Complete or unspecified spontaneous abortion with other complications

O03.9 Complete or unspecified spontaneous abortion without complication

Miscarriage NOS

Spontaneous abortion NOS

O04 Complications following (induced) termination of pregnancy

Includes: complications following (induced) termination of pregnancy

Excludes 1: encounter for elective termination of pregnancy, uncomplicated (Z33.2)

failed attempted termination of pregnancy (O07.-)

O04.5 Genital tract and pelvic infection following (induced) termination of pregnancy

Endometritis following (induced) termination of pregnancy

Oophoritis following (induced) termination of pregnancy

Parametritis following (induced) termination of pregnancy

Pelvic peritonitis following (induced) termination of pregnancy

Salpingitis following (induced) termination of pregnancy

Salpingo-oophoritis following (induced) termination of pregnancy

Excludes 1: sepsis following (induced) termination of pregnancy (O04.87)

urinary tract infection following (induced) termination of pregnancy (O04.88)

O04.6 Delayed or excessive hemorrhage following (induced) termination of pregnancy

Afibrinogenemia following (induced) termination of pregnancy

Defibrination syndrome following (induced) termination of pregnancy

Hemolysis following (induced) termination of pregnancy

Intravascular coagulation following (induced) termination of pregnancy

O04.7 Embolism following (induced) termination of pregnancy

Air embolism following (induced) termination of pregnancy

Amniotic fluid embolism following (induced) termination of pregnancy

Blood-clot embolism following (induced) termination of pregnancy

Embolism NOS following (induced) termination of pregnancy

Fat embolism following (induced) termination of pregnancy

Pulmonary embolism following (induced) termination of pregnancy

Pyemic embolism following (induced) termination of pregnancy

Septic or septicopyemic embolism following (induced) termination of pregnancy

Soap embolism following (induced) termination of pregnancy

O04.8 (Induced) termination of pregnancy with other and unspecified complications

O04.80 (Induced) termination of pregnancy with unspecified complications

O04.81 Shock following (induced) termination of pregnancy

Circulatory collapse following (induced) termination of pregnancy

Shock (postprocedural) following (induced) termination of pregnancy

Excludes 1: shock due to infection following (induced) termination of pregnancy (O04.87)

O04.82 Renal failure following (induced) termination of pregnancy

Kidney failure (acute) following (induced) termination of pregnancy

Oliguria following (induced) termination of pregnancy

Renal shutdown following (induced) termination of pregnancy

Renal tubular necrosis following (induced) termination of pregnancy

Uremia following (induced) termination of pregnancy

O04.83 Metabolic disorder following (induced) termination of pregnancy

O04.84 Damage to pelvic organs following (induced) termination of pregnancy

Laceration, perforation, tear or chemical damage of bladder following (induced) termination of pregnancy

Laceration, perforation, tear or chemical damage of bowel following (induced) termination of pregnancy

Laceration, perforation, tear or chemical damage of broad ligament following (induced) termination of pregnancy

Laceration, perforation, tear or chemical damage of cervix following (induced) termination of Pregnancy

Laceration, perforation, tear or chemical damage of periurethral tissue following (induced) termination of pregnancy

Laceration, perforation, tear or chemical damage of uterus following (induced) termination of pregnancy

Laceration, perforation, tear or chemical damage of vagina following (induced) termination of pregnancy

O04.85 Other venous complications following (induced) termination of pregnancy

O04.86 Cardiac arrest following (induced) termination of pregnancy

O04.87 Sepsis following (induced) termination of pregnancy

Use additional code to identify infectious agent (B95-B97)

Use additional code to identify severe sepsis, if applicable (R65.2-)

Excludes 1: septic or septicopyemic embolism following (induced) termination of pregnancy (O04.7)

O04.88 Urinary tract infection following (induced) termination of pregnancy

Cystitis following (induced) termination of pregnancy

O04.89 (Induced) termination of pregnancy with other complications

O07 Failed attempted termination of pregnancy

Includes: failure of attempted induction of termination of pregnancy

incomplete elective abortion

Excludes 1: incomplete spontaneous abortion (O03.0-)

O07.0 Genital tract and pelvic infection following failed attempted termination of pregnancy

Endometritis following failed attempted termination of pregnancy

Oophoritis following failed attempted termination of pregnancy

Parametritis following failed attempted termination of pregnancy

Pelvic peritonitis following failed attempted termination of pregnancy

Salpingitis following failed attempted termination of pregnancy

Salpingo-oophoritis following failed attempted termination of pregnancy

Excludes 1: sepsis following failed attempted termination of pregnancy (O07.37)

urinary tract infection following failed attempted termination of pregnancy (O07.38)

O07.1 Delayed or excessive hemorrhage following failed attempted termination of pregnancy

Afibrinogenemia following failed attempted termination of pregnancy

Defibrination syndrome following failed attempted termination of pregnancy

Hemolysis following failed attempted termination of pregnancy

Intravascular coagulation following failed attempted termination of pregnancy

O07.2 Embolism following failed attempted termination of pregnancy

Air embolism following failed attempted termination of pregnancy

Amniotic fluid embolism following failed attempted termination of pregnancy

Blood-clot embolism following failed attempted termination of pregnancy

Embolism NOS following failed attempted termination of pregnancy

Fat embolism following failed attempted termination of pregnancy

Pulmonary embolism following failed attempted termination of pregnancy

Pyemic embolism following failed attempted termination of pregnancy

Septic or septicopyemic embolism following failed attempted termination of pregnancy

Soap embolism following failed attempted termination of pregnancy

O07.3 Failed attempted termination of pregnancy with other and unspecified complications

O07.30 Failed attempted termination of pregnancy with unspecified complications

O07.31 Shock following failed attempted termination of pregnancy

Circulatory collapse following failed attempted termination of pregnancy

Shock (postprocedural) following failed attempted termination of pregnancy

Excludes 1: shock due to infection following failed attempted termination of pregnancy (O07.37)

O07.32 Renal failure following failed attempted termination of pregnancy

Kidney failure (acute) following failed attempted termination of pregnancy

Oliguria following failed attempted termination of pregnancy

Renal shutdown following failed attempted termination of pregnancy

Renal tubular necrosis following failed attempted termination of pregnancy

Uremia following failed attempted termination of pregnancy

O07.33 Metabolic disorder following failed attempted termination of pregnancy

O07.34 Damage to pelvic organs following failed attempted termination of pregnancy

Laceration, perforation, tear or chemical damage of bladder following failed attempted termination of pregnancy

Laceration, perforation, tear or chemical damage of bowel following failed attempted termination of pregnancy

Laceration, perforation, tear or chemical damage of broad ligament following failed attempted termination of pregnancy

Laceration, perforation, tear or chemical damage of cervix following failed attempted termination of pregnancy

Laceration, perforation, tear or chemical damage of periurethral tissue following failed attempted termination of pregnancy

Laceration, perforation, tear or chemical damage of uterus following failed attempted termination of pregnancy

Laceration, perforation, tear or chemical damage of vagina following failed attempted termination of pregnancy

O07.35 Other venous complications following failed attempted termination of pregnancy

O07.36 Cardiac arrest following failed attempted termination of pregnancy

O07.37 Sepsis following failed attempted termination of pregnancy

Use additional code (B95-B97), to identify infectious agent

Use additional code (R65.2-) to identify severe sepsis, if applicable

Excludes 1: septic or septicopyemic embolism following failed attempted termination of pregnancy (O07.2)

O07.38 Urinary tract infection following failed attempted termination of pregnancy

Cystitis following failed attempted termination of pregnancy

O07.39 Failed attempted termination of pregnancy with other complications

O07.4 Failed attempted termination of pregnancy without complication

O08 Complications following ectopic and molar pregnancy

This category is for use with categories O00-O02 to identify any associated complications

O08.0 Genital tract and pelvic infection following ectopic and molar pregnancy

Endometritis following ectopic and molar pregnancy

Oophoritis following ectopic and molar pregnancy

Parametritis following ectopic and molar pregnancy

Pelvic peritonitis following ectopic and molar pregnancy

Salpingitis following ectopic and molar pregnancy

Salpingo-oophoritis following ectopic and molar pregnancy

Excludes 1: sepsis following ectopic and molar pregnancy (O08.82)

urinary tract infection (O08.83)

O08.1 Delayed or excessive hemorrhage following ectopic and molar pregnancy

Afibrinogenemia following ectopic and molar pregnancy

Defibrination syndrome following ectopic and molar pregnancy

Hemolysis following ectopic and molar pregnancy

Intravascular coagulation following ectopic and molar pregnancy

Excludes 1: delayed or excessive hemorrhage due to incomplete abortion (O03.1)

O08.2   Embolism following ectopic and molar pregnancy
Air embolism following ectopic and molar pregnancy
Amniotic fluid embolism following ectopic and molar pregnancy
Blood-clot embolism following ectopic and molar pregnancy
Embolism NOS following ectopic and molar pregnancy
Fat embolism following ectopic and molar pregnancy
Pulmonary embolism following ectopic and molar pregnancy
Pyemic embolism following ectopic and molar pregnancy
Septic or septicopyemic embolism following ectopic and molar pregnancy
Soap embolism following ectopic and molar pregnancy

O08.3   Shock following ectopic and molar pregnancy
Circulatory collapse following ectopic and molar pregnancy
Shock (postprocedural) following ectopic and molar pregnancy
Excludes 1: shock due to infection following ectopic and molar pregnancy (O08.82)

O08.4   Renal failure following ectopic and molar pregnancy
Kidney failure (acute) following ectopic and molar pregnancy
Oliguria following ectopic and molar pregnancy
Renal shutdown following ectopic and molar pregnancy
Renal tubular necrosis following ectopic and molar pregnancy
Uremia following ectopic and molar pregnancy

O08.5   Metabolic disorders following an ectopic and molar pregnancy

O08.6   Damage to pelvic organs and tissues following an ectopic and molar pregnancy
Laceration, perforation, tear or chemical damage of bladder following an ectopic and molar pregnancy
Laceration, perforation, tear or chemical damage of bowel following an ectopic and molar pregnancy
Laceration, perforation, tear or chemical damage of broad ligament following an ectopic and molar pregnancy
Laceration, perforation, tear or chemical damage of cervix following an ectopic and molar pregnancy
Laceration, perforation, tear or chemical damage of periurethral tissue following an ectopic and molar pregnancy
Laceration, perforation, tear or chemical damage of uterus following an ectopic and molar pregnancy
Laceration, perforation, tear or chemical damage of vagina following an ectopic and molar pregnancy

O08.7   Other venous complications following an ectopic and molar pregnancy

O08.8   Other complications following an ectopic and molar pregnancy
O08.81   Cardiac arrest following an ectopic and molar pregnancy
O08.82   Sepsis following ectopic and molar pregnancy
Use additional code (B95-B97), to identify infectious agent
Use additional code (R65.2-) to identify severe sepsis, if applicable

Excludes 1: septic or septicopyemic embolism following ectopic and molar pregnancy (O08.2)

O08.83   Urinary tract infection following an ectopic and molar pregnancy
Cystitis following an ectopic and molar pregnancy
O08.89   Other complications following an ectopic and molar pregnancy

O08.9   Unspecified complication following an ectopic and molar pregnancy

SUPERVISION OF HIGH RISK PREGNANCY (O09)

O09   Supervision of high risk pregnancy

O09.0   Supervision of pregnancy with history of infertility
O09.00   Supervision of pregnancy with history of infertility, unspecified trimester
O09.01   Supervision of pregnancy with history of infertility, first trimester
O09.02   Supervision of pregnancy with history of infertility, second trimester
O09.03   Supervision of pregnancy with history of infertility, third trimester

O09.1   Supervision of pregnancy with history of ectopic or molar pregnancy
O09.10   Supervision of pregnancy with history of ectopic or molar pregnancy, unspecified trimester
O09.11   Supervision of pregnancy with history of ectopic or molar pregnancy, first trimester
O09.12   Supervision of pregnancy with history of ectopic or molar pregnancy, second trimester
O09.13   Supervision of pregnancy with history of ectopic or molar pregnancy, third trimester

O09.2   Supervision of pregnancy with other poor reproductive or obstetric history
Excludes 2: pregnancy care for patient with history of recurrent pregnancy loss (O26.2-)

O09.21   Supervision of pregnancy with history of pre-term labor
O09.211   Supervision of pregnancy with history of pre-term labor, first trimester
O09.212   Supervision of pregnancy with history of pre-term labor, second trimester
O09.213   Supervision of pregnancy with history of pre-term labor, third trimester
O09.219   Supervision of pregnancy with history of pre-term labor, unspecified trimester

O09.29   Supervision of pregnancy with other poor reproductive or obstetric history
Supervision of pregnancy with history of neonatal death
Supervision of pregnancy with history of stillbirth
O09.291   Supervision of pregnancy with other poor reproductive or obstetric history, first trimester

O09.292 Supervision of pregnancy with other poor reproductive or obstetric history, second trimester

O09.293 Supervision of pregnancy with other poor reproductive or obstetric history, third trimester

O09.299 Supervision of pregnancy with other poor reproductive or obstetric history, unspecified trimester

O09.3 Supervision of pregnancy with insufficient antenatal care
Supervision of concealed pregnancy
Supervision of hidden pregnancy

O09.30 Supervision of pregnancy with insufficient antenatal care, unspecified trimester

O09.31 Supervision of pregnancy with insufficient antenatal care, first trimester

O09.32 Supervision of pregnancy with insufficient antenatal care, second trimester

O09.33 Supervision of pregnancy with insufficient antenatal care, third trimester

O09.4 Supervision of pregnancy with grand multiparity

O09.40 Supervision of pregnancy with grand multiparity, unspecified trimester

O09.41 Supervision of pregnancy with grand multiparity, first trimester

O09.42 Supervision of pregnancy with grand multiparity, second trimester

O09.43 Supervision of pregnancy with grand multiparity, third trimester

O09.5 Supervision of elderly primigravida and multigravida
Pregnancy for a female 35 years and older at expected date of delivery

O09.51 Supervision of elderly primigravida

O09.511 Supervision of elderly primigravida, first trimester

O09.512 Supervision of elderly primigravida, second trimester

O09.513 Supervision of elderly primigravida, third trimester

O09.519 Supervision of elderly primigravida, unspecified trimester

O09.52 Supervision of elderly multigravida

O09.521 Supervision of elderly multigravida, first trimester

O09.522 Supervision of elderly multigravida, second trimester

O09.523 Supervision of elderly multigravida, third trimester

O09.529 Supervision of elderly multigravida, unspecified trimester

O09.6 Supervision of young primigravida and multigravida
Supervision of pregnancy for a female less than 16 years old at expected date of delivery

O09.61 Supervision of young primigravida

O09.611 Supervision of young primigravida, first trimester

O09.612 Supervision of young primigravida, second trimester

O09.613 Supervision of young primigravida, third trimester

O09.619 Supervision of young primigravida, unspecified trimester

O09.62 Supervision of young multigravida

O09.621 Supervision of young multigravida, first trimester

O09.622 Supervision of young multigravida, second trimester

O09.623 Supervision of young multigravida, third trimester

O09.629 Supervision of young multigravida, unspecified trimester

O09.7 Supervision of high risk pregnancy due to social problems

O09.70 Supervision of high risk pregnancy due to social problems, unspecified trimester

O09.71 Supervision of high risk pregnancy due to social problems, first trimester

O09.72 Supervision of high risk pregnancy due to social problems, second trimester

O09.73 Supervision of high risk pregnancy due to social problems, third trimester

O09.8 Supervision of other high risk pregnancies

O09.81 Supervision of pregnancy resulting from assisted reproductive technology
Supervision of pregnancy resulting from in-vitro fertilization

O09.811 Supervision of pregnancy resulting from assisted reproductive technology, first trimester

O09.812 Supervision of pregnancy resulting from assisted reproductive technology, second trimester

O09.813 Supervision of pregnancy resulting from assisted reproductive technology, third trimester

O09.819 Supervision of pregnancy resulting from assisted reproductive technology, unspecified trimester

O09.82 Supervision of pregnancy with history of in utero procedure during previous pregnancy

O09.821 Supervision of pregnancy with history of in utero procedure during previous pregnancy, first trimester

O09.822 Supervision of pregnancy with history of in utero procedure during previous pregnancy, second trimester

O09.823 Supervision of pregnancy with history of in utero procedure during previous pregnancy, third trimester

O09.829 Supervision of pregnancy with history of in utero procedure during previous pregnancy, unspecified trimester

Excludes 1: supervision of pregnancy affected by in utero procedure during current pregnancy (O35.7)

O09.89 Supervision of other high risk pregnancies

O09.891 Supervision of other high risk pregnancies, first trimester

O09.892   Supervision of other high risk pregnancies, second trimester

O09.893   Supervision of other high risk pregnancies, third trimester

O09.899   Supervision of other high risk pregnancies, unspecified trimester

O09.9   Supervision of high risk pregnancy, unspecified

    O09.90   Supervision of high risk pregnancy, unspecified, unspecified trimester

    O09.91   Supervision of high risk pregnancy, unspecified, first trimester

    O09.92   Supervision of high risk pregnancy, unspecified, second trimester

    O09.93   Supervision of high risk pregnancy, unspecified, third trimester

EDEMA, PROTEINURIA AND HYPERTENSIVE DISORDERS IN PREGNANCY, CHILDBIRTH AND THE PUERPERIUM (O10-O16)

O10   Pre-existing hypertension complicating pregnancy, childbirth and the puerperium

Includes: pre-existing hypertension with pre-existing proteinuria complicating pregnancy, childbirth and the puerperium

Excludes 2: pre-existing hypertension with superimposed pre-eclampsia complicating pregnancy, childbirth and the puerperium (O11.-)

O10.0   Pre-existing essential hypertension complicating pregnancy, childbirth and the puerperium

Any condition in I10 specified as a reason for obstetric care during pregnancy, childbirth or the puerperium

    O10.01   Pre-existing essential hypertension complicating pregnancy,

       O10.011   Pre-existing essential hypertension complicating pregnancy, first trimester

       O10.012   Pre-existing essential hypertension complicating pregnancy, second trimester

       O10.013   Pre-existing essential hypertension complicating pregnancy, third trimester

       O10.019   Pre-existing essential hypertension complicating pregnancy, unspecified trimester

    O10.02   Pre-existing essential hypertension complicating childbirth

    O10.03   Pre-existing essential hypertension complicating the puerperium

O10.1   Pre-existing hypertensive heart disease complicating pregnancy, childbirth and the puerperium

Any condition in I11 specified as a reason for obstetric care during pregnancy, childbirth or the puerperium

Use additional code from I11 to identify the type of hypertensive heart disease

    O10.11   Pre-existing hypertensive heart disease complicating pregnancy

       O10.111   Pre-existing hypertensive heart disease complicating pregnancy, first trimester

       O10.112   Pre-existing hypertensive heart disease complicating pregnancy, second trimester

       O10.113   Pre-existing hypertensive heart disease complicating pregnancy, third trimester

       O10.119   Pre-existing hypertensive heart disease complicating pregnancy, unspecified trimester

    O10.12   Pre-existing hypertensive heart disease complicating childbirth

    O10.13   Pre-existing hypertensive heart disease complicating the puerperium

O10.2   Pre-existing hypertensive chronic kidney disease complicating pregnancy, childbirth and the puerperium

Any condition in I12 specified as a reason for obstetric care during pregnancy, childbirth or the puerperium

Use additional code from I12 to identify the type of hypertensive chronic kidney disease

    O10.21   Pre-existing hypertensive chronic kidney disease complicating pregnancy

       O10.211   Pre-existing hypertensive chronic kidney disease complicating pregnancy, first trimester

       O10.212   Pre-existing hypertensive chronic kidney disease complicating pregnancy, second trimester

       O10.213   Pre-existing hypertensive chronic kidney disease complicating pregnancy, third trimester

       O10.219   Pre-existing hypertensive chronic kidney disease complicating pregnancy, unspecified trimester

    O10.22   Pre-existing hypertensive chronic kidney disease complicating childbirth

    O10.23   Pre-existing hypertensive chronic kidney disease complicating the puerperium

O10.3   Pre-existing hypertensive heart and chronic kidney disease complicating pregnancy, childbirth and the puerperium

Any condition in I13 specified as a reason for obstetric care during pregnancy, childbirth or the puerperium

Use additional code from I13 to identify the type of hypertensive heart and chronic kidney disease

    O10.31   Pre-existing hypertensive heart and chronic kidney disease complicating pregnancy

       O10.311   Pre-existing hypertensive heart and chronic kidney disease complicating pregnancy, first trimester

       O10.312   Pre-existing hypertensive heart and chronic kidney disease complicating pregnancy, second trimester

       O10.313   Pre-existing hypertensive heart and chronic kidney disease complicating pregnancy, third trimester

       O10.319   Pre-existing hypertensive heart and chronic kidney disease complicating pregnancy, unspecified trimester

    O10.32   Pre-existing hypertensive heart and chronic kidney disease complicating childbirth

    O10.33   Pre-existing hypertensive heart and chronic kidney disease complicating the puerperium

O10.4   Pre-existing secondary hypertension complicating pregnancy, childbirth and the puerperium

Any condition in I15 specified as a reason for obstetric care during pregnancy, childbirth or the puerperium

Use additional code from I15 to identify the type of secondary hypertension

O10.41 Pre-existing secondary hypertension complicating pregnancy

O10.411 Pre-existing secondary hypertension complicating pregnancy, first trimester

O10.412 Pre-existing secondary hypertension complicating pregnancy, second trimester

O10.413 Pre-existing secondary hypertension complicating pregnancy, third trimester

O10.419 Pre-existing secondary hypertension complicating pregnancy, unspecified trimester

O10.42 Pre-existing secondary hypertension complicating childbirth

O10.43 Pre-existing secondary hypertension complicating the puerperium

O10.9 Unspecified pre-existing hypertension complicating pregnancy, childbirth and the puerperium

O10.91 Unspecified pre-existing hypertension complicating pregnancy

O10.911 Unspecified pre-existing hypertension complicating pregnancy, first trimester

O10.912 Unspecified pre-existing hypertension complicating pregnancy, second trimester

O10.913 Unspecified pre-existing hypertension complicating pregnancy, third trimester

O10.919 Unspecified pre-existing hypertension complicating pregnancy, unspecified trimester

O10.92 Unspecified pre-existing hypertension complicating childbirth

O10.93 Unspecified pre-existing hypertension complicating the puerperium

O11 Pre-existing hypertension with pre-eclampsia

Includes: conditions in O10 complicated by pre-eclampsia pre-eclampsia superimposed pre-existing hypertension

Use additional code from O10 to identify the type of hypertension

O11.1 Pre-existing hypertension with pre-eclampsia, first trimester

O11.2 Pre-existing hypertension with pre-eclampsia, second trimester

O11.3 Pre-existing hypertension with pre-eclampsia, third trimester

O11.9 Pre-existing hypertension with pre-eclampsia, unspecified trimester

O12 Gestational [pregnancy-induced] edema and proteinuria without hypertension

O12.0 Gestational edema

O12.00 Gestational edema, unspecified trimester

O12.01 Gestational edema, first trimester

O12.02 Gestational edema, second trimester

O12.03 Gestational edema, third trimester

O12.1 Gestational proteinuria

O12.10 Gestational proteinuria, unspecified trimester

O12.11 Gestational proteinuria, first trimester

O12.12 Gestational proteinuria, second trimester

O12.13 Gestational proteinuria, third trimester

O12.2 Gestational edema with proteinuria

O12.20 Gestational edema with proteinuria, unspecified trimester

O12.21 Gestational edema with proteinuria, first trimester

O12.22 Gestational edema with proteinuria, second trimester

O12.23 Gestational edema with proteinuria, third trimester

O13 Gestational [pregnancy-induced] hypertension without significant proteinuria

Includes: gestational hypertension NOS

O13.1 Gestational [pregnancy-induced] hypertension without significant proteinuria, first trimester

O13.2 Gestational [pregnancy-induced] hypertension without significant proteinuria, second trimester

O13.3 Gestational [pregnancy-induced] hypertension without significant proteinuria, third trimester

O13.9 Gestational [pregnancy-induced] hypertension without significant proteinuria, unspecified trimester

O14 Pre-eclampsia

Excludes 1: pre-existing hypertension with pre-eclampsia (O11)

O14.0 Mild to moderate pre-eclampsia

O14.00 Mild to moderate pre-eclampsia, unspecified trimester

O14.02 Mild to moderate pre-eclampsia, second trimester

O14.03 Mild to moderate pre-eclampsia, third trimester

O14.1 Severe pre-eclampsia

Excludes 1: HELLP syndrome (O14.2-)

O14.10 Severe pre-eclampsia, unspecified trimester

O14.12 Severe pre-eclampsia, second trimester

O14.13 Severe pre-eclampsia, third trimester

O14.2 HELLP syndrome

Severe pre-eclampsia with hemolysis, elevated liver enzymes and low platelet count (HELLP)

O14.20 HELLP syndrome (HELLP), unspecified trimester

O14.22 HELLP syndrome (HELLP), second trimester

O14.23 HELLP syndrome (HELLP), third trimester

O14.9 Unspecified pre-eclampsia

O14.90 Unspecified pre-eclampsia, unspecified trimester

O14.92 Unspecified pre-eclampsia, second trimester

O14.93 Unspecified pre-eclampsia, third trimester

O15 Eclampsia

Includes: convulsions following conditions in O10-O14 and O16

O15.0 Eclampsia in pregnancy

O15.00 Eclampsia in pregnancy, unspecified trimester

O15.02 Eclampsia in pregnancy, second trimester

O15.03 Eclampsia in pregnancy, third trimester

O15.1 Eclampsia in labor

O15.2 Eclampsia in the puerperium

O15.9 Eclampsia, unspecified as to time period

Eclampsia NOS

O16 Unspecified maternal hypertension

O16.1 Unspecified maternal hypertension, first trimester

O16.2 Unspecified maternal hypertension, second trimester

O16.3 Unspecified maternal hypertension, third trimester

O16.9 Unspecified maternal hypertension, unspecified trimester

OTHER MATERNAL DISORDERS PREDOMINANTLY RELATED TO PREGNANCY (O20-O29)

Excludes 2: maternal care related to the fetus and amniotic cavity and possible delivery problems (O30-O48)

maternal diseases classifiable elsewhere but complicating pregnancy, labor and delivery, and the puerperium (O98-O99)

O20 Hemorrhage in early pregnancy

Includes: hemorrhage before completion of 20 weeks gestation

Excludes 1: pregnancy with abortive outcome (O00-O08)

O20.0 Threatened abortion

Hemorrhage specified as due to threatened abortion

O20.8 Other hemorrhage in early pregnancy

O20.9 Hemorrhage in early pregnancy, unspecified

O21 Excessive vomiting in pregnancy

O21.0 Mild hyperemesis gravidarum

Hyperemesis gravidarum, mild or unspecified, starting before the end of the 20th week of gestation

O21.1 Hyperemesis gravidarum with metabolic disturbance

Hyperemesis gravidarum, starting before the end of the 20th week of gestation, with metabolic disturbance such as carbohydrate depletion

Hyperemesis gravidarum, starting before the end of the 20th week of gestation, with metabolic disturbance such as dehydration

Hyperemesis gravidarum, starting before the end of the 20th week of gestation, with metabolic disturbance such as electrolyte imbalance

O21.2 Late vomiting of pregnancy

Excessive vomiting starting after 20completed weeks of gestation

O21.8 Other vomiting complicating pregnancy

Vomiting due to diseases classified elsewhere, complicating pregnancy

Use additional code, to identify cause.

O21.9 Vomiting of pregnancy, unspecified

O22 Venous complications and hemorrhoids in pregnancy

Excludes 1: venous complications of:

abortion NOS (O03.9)

ectopic or molar pregnancy (O08.7)

failed attempted abortion (O07.35)

induced abortion (O04.85)

spontaneous abortion (O03.89)

Excludes 2: obstetric pulmonary embolism (O88.-)

venous complications and hemorrhoids of childbirth and the puerperium (O87.-)

O22.0 Varicose veins of lower extremity in pregnancy

Varicose veins NOS in pregnancy

O22.00 Varicose veins of lower extremity in pregnancy, unspecified trimester

O22.01 Varicose veins of lower extremity in pregnancy, first trimester

O22.02 Varicose veins of lower extremity in pregnancy, second trimester

O22.03 Varicose veins of lower extremity in pregnancy, third trimester

O22.1 Genital varices in pregnancy

Perineal varices in pregnancy

Vaginal varices in pregnancy

Vulval varices in pregnancy

O22.10 Genital varices in pregnancy, unspecified trimester

O22.11 Genital varices in pregnancy, first trimester

O22.12 Genital varices in pregnancy, second trimester

O22.13 Genital varices in pregnancy, third trimester

O22.2 Superficial thrombophlebitis in pregnancy

Phlebitis in pregnancy NOS

Thrombophlebitis of legs in pregnancy

Thrombosis in pregnancy NOS

Use additional code to identify the superficial thrombophlebitis (I80.0-)

O22.20 Superficial thrombophlebitis in pregnancy, unspecified trimester

O22.21 Superficial thrombophlebitis in pregnancy, first trimester

O22.22 Superficial thrombophlebitis in pregnancy, second trimester

O22.23 Superficial thrombophlebitis in pregnancy, third trimester

O22.3 Deep phlebothrombosis in pregnancy

Deep vein thrombosis, antepartum

Use additional code to identify the deep vein thrombosis (I82.4-, I82.5-, I82.62-. I82.72-)

Use additional code, if applicable, for associated long-term (current) use of anticoagulants (Z79.01)

O22.30 Deep phlebothrombosis in pregnancy, unspecified trimester

O22.31 Deep phlebothrombosis in pregnancy, first trimester

O22.32 Deep phlebothrombosis in pregnancy, second trimester

O22.33 Deep phlebothrombosis in pregnancy, third trimester

O22.4 Hemorrhoids in pregnancy

O22.40 Hemorrhoids in pregnancy, unspecified trimester

O22.41 Hemorrhoids in pregnancy, first trimester

O22.42 Hemorrhoids in pregnancy, second trimester

O22.43 Hemorrhoids in pregnancy, third trimester

O22.5 Cerebral venous thrombosis in pregnancy

Cerebrovenous sinus thrombosis in pregnancy

O22.50 Cerebral venous thrombosis in pregnancy, unspecified trimester

O22.51 Cerebral venous thrombosis in pregnancy, first trimester

O22.52 Cerebral venous thrombosis in pregnancy, second trimester

O22.53 Cerebral venous thrombosis in pregnancy, third trimester

O22.8 Other venous complications in pregnancy

O22.8X Other venous complications in pregnancy

O22.8X1 Other venous complications in pregnancy, first trimester

O22.8X2 Other venous complications in pregnancy, second trimester

O22.8X3 Other venous complications in pregnancy, third trimester

O22.8X9 Other venous complications in pregnancy, unspecified trimester

O22.9 Venous complication in pregnancy, unspecified

Gestational phlebitis NOS

Gestational phlebopathy NOS

Gestational thrombosis NOS

O22.90 Venous complication in pregnancy, unspecified, unspecified trimester

O22.91 Venous complication in pregnancy, unspecified, first trimester

O22.92 Venous complication in pregnancy, unspecified, second trimester

O22.93 Venous complication in pregnancy, unspecified, third trimester

O23 Infections of genitourinary tract in pregnancy

Use additional code to identify organism (B95.-, B96.-)

Excludes 2: gonococcal infections complicating pregnancy, childbirth and the puerperium (O98.2)

infections with a predominantly sexual mode of transmission NOS complicating pregnancy, childbirth and the puerperium (O98.3)

syphilis complicating pregnancy, childbirth and the puerperium (O98.1)

tuberculosis of genitourinary system complicating pregnancy, childbirth and the puerperium (O98.0)

venereal disease NOS complicating pregnancy, childbirth and the puerperium (O98.3)

O23.0 Infections of kidney in pregnancy

Pyelonephritis in pregnancy

O23.00 Infections of kidney in pregnancy, unspecified trimester

O23.01 Infections of kidney in pregnancy, first trimester

O23.02 Infections of kidney in pregnancy, second trimester

O23.03 Infections of kidney in pregnancy, third trimester

O23.1 Infections of bladder in pregnancy

O23.10 Infections of bladder in pregnancy, unspecified trimester

O23.11 Infections of bladder in pregnancy, first trimester

O23.12 Infections of bladder in pregnancy, second trimester

O23.13 Infections of bladder in pregnancy, third trimester

O23.2 Infections of urethra in pregnancy

O23.20 Infections of urethra in pregnancy, unspecified trimester

O23.21 Infections of urethra in pregnancy, first trimester

O23.22 Infections of urethra in pregnancy, second trimester

O23.23 Infections of urethra in pregnancy, third trimester

O23.3 Infections of other parts of urinary tract in pregnancy

O23.30 Infections of other parts of urinary tract in pregnancy, unspecified trimester

O23.31 Infections of other parts of urinary tract in pregnancy, first trimester

O23.32 Infections of other parts of urinary tract in pregnancy, second trimester

O23.33 Infections of other parts of urinary tract in pregnancy, third trimester

O23.4 Unspecified infection of urinary tract in pregnancy

O23.40 Unspecified infection of urinary tract in pregnancy, unspecified trimester

O23.41 Unspecified infection of urinary tract in pregnancy, first trimester

O23.42 Unspecified infection of urinary tract in pregnancy, second trimester

O23.43 Unspecified infection of urinary tract in pregnancy, third trimester

O23.5 Infections of the genital tract in pregnancy

O23.51 Infection of cervix in pregnancy

O23.511 Infections of cervix in pregnancy, first trimester

O23.512 Infections of cervix in pregnancy, second trimester

O23.513 Infections of cervix in pregnancy, third trimester

O23.519 Infections of cervix in pregnancy, unspecified trimester

O23.52 Salpingo-oophoritis in pregnancy

Oophoritis in pregnancy

Salpingitis in pregnancy

O23.521 Salpingo-oophoritis in pregnancy, first trimester

O23.522 Salpingo-oophoritis in pregnancy, second trimester

O23.523 Salpingo-oophoritis in pregnancy, third trimester

O23.529 Salpingo-oophoritis in pregnancy, unspecified trimester

O23.59 Infection of other part of genital tract in pregnancy

O23.591 Infection of other part of genital tract in pregnancy, first trimester

O23.592 Infection of other part of genital tract in pregnancy, second trimester

O23.593 Infection of other part of genital tract in pregnancy, third trimester

O23.599 Infection of other part of genital tract in pregnancy, unspecified trimester

O23.9 Unspecified genitourinary tract infection in pregnancy

Genitourinary tract infection in pregnancy NOS

O23.90 Unspecified genitourinary tract infection in pregnancy, unspecified trimester

O23.91 Unspecified genitourinary tract infection in pregnancy, first trimester

O23.92 Unspecified genitourinary tract infection in pregnancy, second trimester

O23.93 Unspecified genitourinary tract infection in pregnancy, third trimester

O24 diabetes mellitus in pregnancy, childbirth, and the puerperium

O24.0 Pre-existing diabetes mellitus, type 1, in pregnancy, childbirth and the puerperium

Juvenile onset diabetes mellitus, in pregnancy, childbirth and the puerperium

Ketosis-prone diabetes mellitus in pregnancy, childbirth and the puerperium

Use additional code from category E10 to further identify any manifestations

O24.01 Pre-existing diabetes mellitus, type 1, in pregnancy

O24.011 Pre-existing diabetes mellitus, type 1, in pregnancy, first trimester

O24.012 Pre-existing diabetes mellitus, type 1, in pregnancy, second trimester

O24.013 Pre-existing diabetes mellitus, type 1, in pregnancy, third trimester

O24.019 Pre-existing diabetes mellitus, type 1, in pregnancy, unspecified trimester

O24.02 Pre-existing diabetes mellitus, type 1, in childbirth

O24.03 Pre-existing diabetes mellitus, type 1, in the puerperium

O24.1 Pre-existing diabetes mellitus, type 2, in pregnancy, childbirth and the puerperium

Insulin-resistant diabetes mellitus in pregnancy, childbirth and the puerperium

Use additional code (for):

from category E11to further identify any manifestations

long-term (current) use of insulin (Z79.4)

O24.11 Pre-existing diabetes mellitus, type 2, in pregnancy

O24.111 Pre-existing diabetes mellitus, type 2, in pregnancy, first trimester

O24.112 Pre-existing diabetes mellitus, type 2, in pregnancy, second trimester

O24.113 Pre-existing diabetes mellitus, type 2, in pregnancy, third trimester

O24.119 Pre-existing diabetes mellitus, type 2, in pregnancy, unspecified trimester

O24.12 Pre-existing diabetes mellitus, type 2, in childbirth

O24.13 Pre-existing diabetes mellitus, type 2, in the puerperium

O24.3 Unspecified pre-existing diabetes mellitus in pregnancy, childbirth and the puerperium

Use additional code (for):

from category E11 to further identify any manifestation

long-term (current) use of insulin (Z79.4)

O24.31 Unspecified pre-existing diabetes mellitus in pregnancy

O24.311 Unspecified pre-existing diabetes mellitus in pregnancy, first trimester

O24.312 Unspecified pre-existing diabetes mellitus in pregnancy, second trimester

O24.313 Unspecified pre-existing diabetes mellitus in pregnancy, third trimester

O24.319 Unspecified pre-existing diabetes mellitus in pregnancy, unspecified trimester

O24.32 Unspecified pre-existing diabetes mellitus in childbirth

O24.33 Unspecified pre-existing diabetes mellitus in the puerperium

O24.4 Gestational diabetes mellitus

diabetes mellitus arising in pregnancy

Gestational diabetes mellitus NOS

O24.41 Gestational diabetes mellitus in pregnancy

O24.410 Gestational diabetes mellitus in pregnancy, diet controlled

O24.414 Gestational diabetes mellitus in pregnancy, insulin controlled

O24.419 Gestational diabetes mellitus in pregnancy, unspecified control

O24.42 Gestational diabetes mellitus in childbirth

O24.420 Gestational diabetes mellitus in childbirth, diet controlled

O24.424 Gestational diabetes mellitus in childbirth, insulin controlled

O24.429 Gestational diabetes mellitus in childbirth, unspecified control

O24.43 Gestational diabetes mellitus in the puerperium

O24.430 Gestational diabetes mellitus in the puerperium, diet controlled

O24.434 Gestational diabetes mellitus in the puerperium, insulin controlled

O24.439 Gestational diabetes mellitus in the puerperium, unspecified control

O24.8 Other pre-existing diabetes mellitus in pregnancy, childbirth, and the puerperium

Use additional code (for):

from categories E08, E09and E13 to further identify any manifestation

long-term (current) use of insulin (Z79.4)

O24.81 Other pre-existing diabetes mellitus in pregnancy

O24.811 Other pre-existing diabetes mellitus in pregnancy, first trimester

O24.812 Other pre-existing diabetes mellitus in pregnancy, second trimester

O24.813 Other pre-existing diabetes mellitus in pregnancy, third trimester

O24.819 Other pre-existing diabetes mellitus in pregnancy, unspecified trimester

O24.82 Other pre-existing diabetes mellitus in childbirth

O24.83 Other pre-existing diabetes mellitus in the puerperium

O24.9 Unspecified diabetes mellitus in pregnancy, childbirth and the puerperium

Use additional code for long-term (current) use of insulin (Z79.4)

O24.91 Unspecified diabetes mellitus in pregnancy

O24.911 Unspecified diabetes mellitus in pregnancy, first trimester

O24.912 Unspecified diabetes mellitus in pregnancy, second trimester

O24.913 Unspecified diabetes mellitus in pregnancy, third trimester

O24.919 Unspecified diabetes mellitus in pregnancy, unspecified trimester

O24.92 Unspecified diabetes mellitus in childbirth

O24.93 Unspecified diabetes mellitus in the puerperium

O25 Malnutrition in pregnancy, childbirth and the puerperium

O25.1 Malnutrition in pregnancy

O25.10 Malnutrition in pregnancy, unspecified trimester

O25.11 Malnutrition in pregnancy, first trimester

O25.12 Malnutrition in pregnancy, second trimester

O25.13 Malnutrition in pregnancy, third trimester

O25.2 Malnutrition in childbirth

O25.3 Malnutrition in the puerperium

O26 Maternal care for other conditions predominantly related to pregnancy

O26.0 Excessive weight gain in pregnancy

Excludes 2: gestational edema (O12.0, O12.2)

O26.00 Excessive weight gain in pregnancy, unspecified trimester

O26.01 Excessive weight gain in pregnancy, first trimester

O26.02 Excessive weight gain in pregnancy, second trimester

O26.03 Excessive weight gain in pregnancy, third trimester

O26.1 Low weight gain in pregnancy

    O26.10 Low weight gain in pregnancy, unspecified trimester

    O26.11 Low weight gain in pregnancy, first trimester

    O26.12 Low weight gain in pregnancy, second trimester

    O26.13 Low weight gain in pregnancy, third trimester

O26.2 Pregnancy care for patient with recurrent pregnancy loss

    O26.20 Pregnancy care for patient with recurrent pregnancy loss, unspecified trimester

    O26.21 Pregnancy care for patient with recurrent pregnancy loss, first trimester

    O26.22 Pregnancy care for patient with recurrent pregnancy loss, second trimester

    O26.23 Pregnancy care for patient with recurrent pregnancy loss, third trimester

O26.3 Retained intrauterine contraceptive device in pregnancy

    O26.30 Retained intrauterine contraceptive device in pregnancy, unspecified trimester

    O26.31 Retained intrauterine contraceptive device in pregnancy, first trimester

    O26.32 Retained intrauterine contraceptive device in pregnancy, second trimester

    O26.33 Retained intrauterine contraceptive device in pregnancy, third trimester

O26.4 Herpes gestationis

    O26.40 Herpes gestationis, unspecified trimester

    O26.41 Herpes gestationis, first trimester

    O26.42 Herpes gestationis, second trimester

    O26.43 Herpes gestationis, third trimester

O26.5 Maternal hypotension syndrome

Supine hypotensive syndrome

    O26.50 Maternal hypotension syndrome, unspecified trimester

    O26.51 Maternal hypotension syndrome, first trimester

    O26.52 Maternal hypotension syndrome, second trimester

    O26.53 Maternal hypotension syndrome, third trimester

O26.6 Liver and biliary tract disorders in pregnancy, childbirth and the puerperium

Use additional code to identify the specific disorder

Excludes 2: hepatorenal syndrome following labor and delivery (O90.4)

    O26.61 Liver and biliary tract disorders in pregnancy

        O26.611 Liver and biliary tract disorders in pregnancy, first trimester

        O26.612 Liver and biliary tract disorders in pregnancy, second trimester

        O26.613 Liver and biliary tract disorders in pregnancy, third trimester

        O26.619 Liver and biliary tract disorders in pregnancy, unspecified trimester

O26.62 Liver and biliary tract disorders in childbirth

O26.63 Liver and biliary tract disorders in the puerperium

O26.7 Subluxation of symphysis (pubis) in pregnancy, childbirth and the puerperium

Excludes 1: traumatic separation of symphysis (pubis) during childbirth (O71.6)

    O26.71 Subluxation of symphysis (pubis) in pregnancy

        O26.711 Subluxation of symphysis (pubis) in pregnancy, first trimester

        O26.712 Subluxation of symphysis (pubis) in pregnancy, second trimester

        O26.713 Subluxation of symphysis (pubis) in pregnancy, third trimester

        O26.719 Subluxation of symphysis (pubis) in pregnancy, unspecified trimester

    O26.72 Subluxation of symphysis (pubis) in childbirth

    O26.73 Subluxation of symphysis (pubis) in the puerperium

O26.8 Other specified pregnancy related conditions

    O26.81 Pregnancy related exhaustion and fatigue

        O26.811 Pregnancy related exhaustion and fatigue, first trimester

        O26.812 Pregnancy related exhaustion and fatigue, second trimester

        O26.813 Pregnancy related exhaustion and fatigue, third trimester

        O26.819 Pregnancy related exhaustion and fatigue, unspecified trimester

    O26.82 Pregnancy related peripheral neuritis

        O26.821 Pregnancy related peripheral neuritis, first trimester

        O26.822 Pregnancy related peripheral neuritis, second trimester

        O26.823 Pregnancy related peripheral neuritis, third trimester

        O26.829 Pregnancy related peripheral neuritis, unspecified trimester

    O26.83 Pregnancy related renal disease

Use additional code to identify the specific disorder

        O26.831 Pregnancy related renal disease, first trimester

        O26.832 Pregnancy related renal disease, second trimester

        O26.833 Pregnancy related renal disease, third trimester

        O26.839 Pregnancy related renal disease, unspecified trimester

    O26.84 Uterine size-date discrepancy complicating pregnancy

Excludes 1: encounter for suspected problem with fetal growth ruled out (Z03.74)

        O26.841 Uterine size-date discrepancy, first trimester

        O26.842 Uterine size-date discrepancy, second trimester

        O26.843 Uterine size-date discrepancy, third trimester

        O26.849 Uterine size-date discrepancy, unspecified trimester

O26.85 Spotting complicating pregnancy

    O26.851 Spotting complicating pregnancy, first trimester

    O26.852 Spotting complicating pregnancy, second trimester

    O26.853 Spotting complicating pregnancy, third trimester

    O26.859 Spotting complicating pregnancy, unspecified trimester

O26.86 Pruritic urticarial papules and plaques of pregnancy (PUPPP)

    Polymorphic eruption of pregnancy

O26.87 Cervical shortening

    Excludes 1: encounter for suspected cervical shortening ruled out (Z03.75)

    O26.872 Cervical shortening, second trimester

    O26.873 Cervical shortening, third trimester

    O26.879 Cervical shortening, unspecified trimester

O26.89 Other specified pregnancy related conditions

    O26.891 Other specified pregnancy related conditions, first trimester

    O26.892 Other specified pregnancy related conditions, second trimester

    O26.893 Other specified pregnancy related conditions, third trimester

    O26.899 Other specified pregnancy related conditions, unspecified trimester

O26.9 Pregnancy related conditions, unspecified

    O26.90 Pregnancy related conditions, unspecified, unspecified trimester

    O26.91 Pregnancy related conditions, unspecified, first trimester

    O26.92 Pregnancy related conditions, unspecified, second trimester

    O26.93 Pregnancy related conditions, unspecified, third trimester

O28 Abnormal findings on antenatal screening of mother

    Excludes 1: diagnostic findings classified elsewhere - see Alphabetical Index

O28.0 Abnormal hematological finding on antenatal screening of mother

O28.1 Abnormal biochemical finding on antenatal screening of mother

O28.2 Abnormal cytological finding on antenatal screening of mother

O28.3 Abnormal ultrasonic finding on antenatal screening of mother

O28.4 Abnormal radiological finding on antenatal screening of mother

O28.5 Abnormal chromosomal and genetic finding on antenatal screening of mother

O28.8 Other abnormal findings on antenatal screening of mother

O28.9 Unspecified abnormal findings on antenatal screening of mother

O29 Complications of anesthesia during pregnancy

    Includes: maternal complications arising from the administration of a general, regional or local anesthetic, analgesic or other sedation during pregnancy

    Use additional code, if necessary, to identify the complication

    Excludes 2: complications of anesthesia during labor and delivery (O74.-)

    complications of anesthesia during the puerperium (O89.-)

O29.0 Pulmonary complications of anesthesia during pregnancy

    O29.01 Aspiration pneumonitis due to anesthesia during pregnancy

        Inhalation of stomach contents or secretions NOS due to anesthesia during pregnancy

        Mendelson's syndrome due to anesthesia during pregnancy

        O29.011 Aspiration pneumonitis due to anesthesia during pregnancy, first trimester

        O29.012 Aspiration pneumonitis due to anesthesia during pregnancy, second trimester

        O29.013 Aspiration pneumonitis due to anesthesia during pregnancy, third trimester

        O29.019 Aspiration pneumonitis due to anesthesia during pregnancy, unspecified trimester

    O29.02 Pressure collapse of lung due to anesthesia during pregnancy

        O29.021 Pressure collapse of lung due to anesthesia during pregnancy, first trimester

        O29.022 Pressure collapse of lung due to anesthesia during pregnancy, second trimester

        O29.023 Pressure collapse of lung due to anesthesia during pregnancy, third trimester

        O29.029 Pressure collapse of lung due to anesthesia during pregnancy, unspecified trimester

    O29.09 Other pulmonary complications of anesthesia during pregnancy

        O29.091 Other pulmonary complications of anesthesia during pregnancy, first trimester

        O29.092 Other pulmonary complications of anesthesia during pregnancy, second trimester

        O29.093 Other pulmonary complications of anesthesia during pregnancy, third trimester

        O29.099 Other pulmonary complications of anesthesia during pregnancy, unspecified trimester

O29.1 Cardiac complications of anesthesia during pregnancy

    O29.11 Cardiac arrest due to anesthesia during pregnancy

        O29.111 Cardiac arrest due to anesthesia during pregnancy, first trimester

        O29.112 Cardiac arrest due to anesthesia during pregnancy, second trimester

        O29.113 Cardiac arrest due to anesthesia during pregnancy, third trimester

        O29.119 Cardiac arrest due to anesthesia during pregnancy, unspecified trimester

● New code   ▲ Revised code   ⑦ 7th digit required   ⊗ Placeholder required

O29.12 Cardiac failure due to anesthesia during pregnancy
- O29.121 Cardiac failure due to anesthesia during pregnancy, first trimester
- O29.122 Cardiac failure due to anesthesia during pregnancy, second trimester
- O29.123 Cardiac failure due to anesthesia during pregnancy, third trimester
- O29.129 Cardiac failure due to anesthesia during pregnancy, unspecified trimester

O29.19 Other cardiac complications of anesthesia during pregnancy
- O29.191 Other cardiac complications of anesthesia during pregnancy, first trimester
- O29.192 Other cardiac complications of anesthesia during pregnancy, second trimester
- O29.193 Other cardiac complications of anesthesia during pregnancy, third trimester
- O29.199 Other cardiac complications of anesthesia during pregnancy, unspecified trimester

O29.2 Central nervous system complications of anesthesia during pregnancy
- O29.21 Cerebral anoxia due to anesthesia during pregnancy
  - O29.211 Cerebral anoxia due to anesthesia during pregnancy, first trimester
  - O29.212 Cerebral anoxia due to anesthesia during pregnancy, second trimester
  - O29.213 Cerebral anoxia due to anesthesia during pregnancy, third trimester
  - O29.219 Cerebral anoxia due to anesthesia during pregnancy, unspecified trimester
- O29.29 Other central nervous system complications of anesthesia during pregnancy
  - O29.291 Other central nervous system complications of anesthesia during pregnancy, first trimester
  - O29.292 Other central nervous system complications of anesthesia during pregnancy, second trimester
  - O29.293 Other central nervous system complications of anesthesia during pregnancy, third trimester
  - O29.299 Other central nervous system complications of anesthesia during pregnancy, unspecified trimester

O29.3 Toxic reaction to local anesthesia during pregnancy
- O29.3X Toxic reaction to local anesthesia during pregnancy
  - O29.3X1 Toxic reaction to local anesthesia during pregnancy, first trimester
  - O29.3X2 Toxic reaction to local anesthesia during pregnancy, second trimester
  - O29.3X3 Toxic reaction to local anesthesia during pregnancy, third trimester

O29.3X9 Toxic reaction to local anesthesia during pregnancy, unspecified trimester

O29.4 Spinal and epidural anesthesia induced headache during pregnancy
- O29.40 Spinal and epidural anesthesia induced headache during pregnancy, unspecified trimester
- O29.41 Spinal and epidural anesthesia induced headache during pregnancy, first trimester
- O29.42 Spinal and epidural anesthesia induced headache during pregnancy, second trimester
- O29.43 Spinal and epidural anesthesia induced headache during pregnancy, third trimester

O29.5 Other complications of spinal and epidural anesthesia during pregnancy
- O29.5X Other complications of spinal and epidural anesthesia during pregnancy
  - O29.5X1 Other complications of spinal and epidural anesthesia during pregnancy, first trimester
  - O29.5X2 Other complications of spinal and epidural anesthesia during pregnancy, second trimester
  - O29.5X3 Other complications of spinal and epidural anesthesia during pregnancy, third trimester
  - O29.5X9 Other complications of spinal and epidural anesthesia during pregnancy, unspecified trimester

O29.6 Failed or difficult intubation for anesthesia during pregnancy
- O29.60 Failed or difficult intubation for anesthesia during pregnancy, unspecified trimester
- O29.61 Failed or difficult intubation for anesthesia during pregnancy, first trimester
- O29.62 Failed or difficult intubation for anesthesia during pregnancy, second trimester
- O29.63 Failed or difficult intubation for anesthesia during pregnancy, third trimester

O29.8 Other complications of anesthesia during pregnancy
- O29.8X Other complications of anesthesia during pregnancy
  - O29.8X1 Other complications of anesthesia during pregnancy, first trimester
  - O29.8X2 Other complications of anesthesia during pregnancy, second trimester
  - O29.8X3 Other complications of anesthesia during pregnancy, third trimester
  - O29.8X9 Other complications of anesthesia during pregnancy, unspecified trimester

O29.9 Unspecified complication of anesthesia during pregnancy
- O29.90 Unspecified complication of anesthesia during pregnancy, unspecified trimester
- O29.91 Unspecified complication of anesthesia during pregnancy, first trimester
- O29.92 Unspecified complication of anesthesia during pregnancy, second trimester
- O29.93 Unspecified complication of anesthesia during pregnancy, third trimester

MATERNAL CARE RELATED TO THE FETUS AND AMNIOTIC CAVITY AND POSSIBLE DELIVERY PROBLEMS (O30-O48)

O30 Multiple gestation

Code also any complications specific to multiple gestation

O30.0 Twin pregnancy

    O30.00 Twin pregnancy, unspecified number of placenta and unspecified number of amniotic sacs

        O30.001 Twin pregnancy, unspecified number of placenta and unspecified number of amniotic sacs, first trimester

        O30.002 Twin pregnancy, unspecified number of placenta and unspecified number of amniotic sacs, second trimester

        O30.003 Twin pregnancy, unspecified number of placenta and unspecified number of amniotic sacs, third trimester

        O30.009 Twin pregnancy, unspecified number of placenta and unspecified number of amniotic sacs, unspecified trimester

    O30.01 Twin pregnancy, monochorionic/monoamniotic

Twin pregnancy, one placenta, one amniotic sac

Excludes 1: conjoined twins (O30.02-)

        O30.011 Twin pregnancy, monochorionic/monoamniotic, first trimester

        O30.012 Twin pregnancy, monochorionic/monoamniotic, second trimester

        O30.013 Twin pregnancy, monochorionic/monoamniotic, third trimester

        O30.019 Twin pregnancy, monochorionic/monoamniotic, unspecified trimester

    O30.02 Conjoined twin pregnancy

        O30.021 Conjoined twin pregnancy, first trimester

        O30.022 Conjoined twin pregnancy, second trimester

        O30.023 Conjoined twin pregnancy, third trimester

        O30.029 Conjoined twin pregnancy, unspecified trimester

    O30.03 Twin pregnancy, monochorionic/diamniotic

Twin pregnancy, one placenta, two amniotic sacs

        O30.031 Twin pregnancy, monochorionic/diamniotic, first trimester

        O30.032 Twin pregnancy, monochorionic/diamniotic, second trimester

        O30.033 Twin pregnancy, monochorionic/diamniotic, third trimester

        O30.039 Twin pregnancy, monochorionic/diamniotic, unspecified trimester

    O30.04 Twin pregnancy, dichorionic/diamniotic

Twin pregnancy, two placentae, two amniotic sacs

        O30.041 Twin pregnancy, dichorionic/diamniotic, first trimester

        O30.042 Twin pregnancy, dichorionic/diamniotic, second trimester

        O30.043 Twin pregnancy, dichorionic/diamniotic, third trimester

        O30.049 Twin pregnancy, dichorionic/diamniotic, unspecified trimester

    O30.09 Twin pregnancy, unable to determine number of placenta and number of amniotic sacs

        O30.091 Twin pregnancy, unable to determine number of placenta and number of amniotic sacs, first trimester

        O30.092 Twin pregnancy, unable to determine number of placenta and number of amniotic sacs, second trimester

        O30.093 Twin pregnancy, unable to determine number of placenta and number of amniotic sacs, third trimester

        O30.099 Twin pregnancy, unable to determine number of placenta and number of amniotic sacs, unspecified trimester

O30.1 Triplet pregnancy

    O30.10 Triplet pregnancy, unspecified number of placenta and unspecified number of amniotic sacs

        O30.101 Triplet pregnancy, unspecified number of placenta and unspecified number of amniotic sacs, first trimester

        O30.102 Triplet pregnancy, unspecified number of placenta and unspecified number of amniotic sacs, second trimester

        O30.103 Triplet pregnancy, unspecified number of placenta and unspecified number of amniotic sacs, third trimester

        O30.109 Triplet pregnancy, unspecified number of placenta and unspecified number of amniotic sacs, unspecified trimester

    O30.11 Triplet pregnancy with two or more monochorionic fetuses

        O30.111 Triplet pregnancy with two or more monochorionic fetuses, first trimester

        O30.112 Triplet pregnancy with two or more monochorionic fetuses, second trimester

O30.113 Triplet pregnancy with two or more monochorionic fetuses, third trimester

O30.119 Triplet pregnancy with two or more monochorionic fetuses, unspecified trimester

O30.12 Triplet pregnancy with two or more monoamniotic fetuses

O30.121 Triplet pregnancy with two or more monoamniotic fetuses, first trimester

O30.122 Triplet pregnancy with two or more monoamniotic fetuses, second trimester

O30.123 Triplet pregnancy with two or more monoamniotic fetuses, third trimester

O30.129 Triplet pregnancy with two or more monoamniotic fetuses, unspecified trimester

O30.19 Triplet pregnancy, unable to determine number of placenta and number of amniotic sacs

O30.191 Triplet pregnancy, unable to determine number of placenta and number of amniotic sacs, first trimester

O30.192 Triplet pregnancy, unable to determine number of placenta and number of amniotic sacs, second trimester

O30.193 Triplet pregnancy, unable to determine number of placenta and number of amniotic sacs, third trimester

O30.199 Triplet pregnancy, unable to determine number of placenta and number of amniotic sacs, unspecified trimester

O30.2 Quadruplet pregnancy

O30.20 Quadruplet pregnancy, unspecified number of placenta and unspecified number of amniotic sacs

O30.201 Quadruplet pregnancy, unspecified number of placenta and unspecified number of amniotic sacs, first trimester

O30.202 Quadruplet pregnancy, unspecified number of placenta and unspecified number of amniotic sacs, second trimester

O30.203 Quadruplet pregnancy, unspecified number of placenta and unspecified number of amniotic sacs, third trimester

O30.209 Quadruplet pregnancy, unspecified number of placenta and unspecified number of amniotic sacs, unspecified trimester

O30.21 Quadruplet pregnancy with two or more monochorionic fetuses

O30.211 Quadruplet pregnancy with two or more monochorionic fetuses, first trimester

O30.212 Quadruplet pregnancy with two or more monochorionic fetuses, second trimester

O30.213 Quadruplet pregnancy with two or more monochorionic fetuses, third trimester

O30.219 Quadruplet pregnancy with two or more monochorionic fetuses, unspecified trimester

O30.22 Quadruplet pregnancy with two or more monoamniotic fetuses

O30.221 Quadruplet pregnancy with two or more monoamniotic fetuses, first trimester

O30.222 Quadruplet pregnancy with two or more monoamniotic fetuses, second trimester

O30.223 Quadruplet pregnancy with two or more monoamniotic fetuses, third trimester

O30.229 Quadruplet pregnancy with two or more monoamniotic fetuses, unspecified Trimester

O30.29 Quadruplet pregnancy, unable to determine number of placenta and number of amniotic sacs

O30.291 Quadruplet pregnancy, unable to determine number of placenta and number of amniotic sacs, first trimester

O30.292 Quadruplet pregnancy, unable to determine number of placenta and number of amniotic sacs, second trimester

O30.293 Quadruplet pregnancy, unable to determine number of placenta and number of amniotic sacs, third trimester

O30.299 Quadruplet pregnancy, unable to determine number of placenta and number of amniotic sacs, unspecified trimester

O30.8 Other specified multiple gestation

Multiple gestation pregnancy greater then quadruplets

O30.80 Other specified multiple gestation, unspecified number of placenta and unspecified number of amniotic sacs

O30.801 Other specified multiple gestation, unspecified number of placenta and unspecified number of amniotic sacs, first trimester

O30.802 Other specified multiple gestation, unspecified number of placenta and unspecified number of amniotic sacs, second trimester

O30.803 Other specified multiple gestation, unspecified number of placenta and unspecified number of amniotic sacs, third trimester

O30.809 Other specified multiple gestation, unspecified number of placenta and unspecified number of amniotic sacs, unspecified trimester

O30.81 Other specified multiple gestation with two or more monochorionic fetuses

    O30.811 Other specified multiple gestation with two or more monochorionic fetuses, first trimester

    O30.812 Other specified multiple gestation with two or more monochorionic fetuses, second trimester

    O30.813 Other specified multiple gestation with two or more monochorionic fetuses, third trimester

    O30.819 Other specified multiple gestation with two or more monochorionic fetuses, unspecified trimester

O30.82 Other specified multiple gestation with two or more monoamniotic fetuses

    O30.821 Other specified multiple gestation with two or more monoamniotic fetuses, first trimester

    O30.822 Other specified multiple gestation with two or more monoamniotic fetuses, second trimester

    O30.823 Other specified multiple gestation with two or more monoamniotic fetuses, third trimester

    O30.829 Other specified multiple gestation with two or more monoamniotic fetuses, unspecified trimester

O30.89 Other specified multiple gestation, unable to determine number of placenta and number of amniotic sacs

    O30.891 Other specified multiple gestation, unable to determine number of placenta and number of amniotic sacs, first trimester

    O30.892 Other specified multiple gestation, unable to determine number of placenta and number of amniotic sacs, second trimester

    O30.893 Other specified multiple gestation, unable to determine number of placenta and number of amniotic sacs, third trimester

    O30.899 Other specified multiple gestation, unable to determine number of placenta and number of amniotic sacs, unspecified trimester

O30.9 Multiple gestation, unspecified
Multiple pregnancy NOS

  ⊗⑦**O30.90** Multiple gestation, unspecified, unspecified trimester

  ⊗⑦**O30.91** Multiple gestation, unspecified, first trimester

  ⊗⑦**O30.92** Multiple gestation, unspecified, second trimester

  ⊗⑦**O30.93** Multiple gestation, unspecified, third trimester

O31 Complications specific to multiple gestation

Excludes 2: delayed delivery of second twin, triplet, etc. (O63.2)
malpresentation of one fetus or more (O32.5)
placental transfusion syndromes (O43.0-)

One of the following 7th characters is to be assigned to each code under category O31. 7th character 0 is for single gestations and multiple gestations where the fetus is unspecified. 7th characters 1 through 9 are for cases of multiple gestations to identify the fetus for which the code applies. The appropriate code from category O30, Multiple gestation, must also be assigned when assigning a code from category O31 that has a 7th character of 1 through 9.

0 - not applicable or unspecified
1 - fetus 1
2 - fetus 2
3 - fetus 3
4 - fetus 4
5 - fetus 5
9 - other fetus

O31.0 Papyraceous fetus
Fetus compressus

  ⊗⑦**O31.00** Papyraceous fetus, unspecified trimester

  ⊗⑦**O31.01** Papyraceous fetus, first trimester

  ⊗⑦**O31.02** Papyraceous fetus, second trimester

  ⊗⑦**O31.03** Papyraceous fetus, third trimester

O31.1 Continuing pregnancy after spontaneous abortion of one fetus or more

  ⊗⑦**O31.10** Continuing pregnancy after spontaneous abortion of one fetus or more, unspecified trimester

  ⊗⑦**O31.11** Continuing pregnancy after spontaneous abortion of one fetus or more, first trimester

  ⊗⑦**O31.12** Continuing pregnancy after spontaneous abortion of one fetus or more, second trimester

  ⊗⑦**O31.13** Continuing pregnancy after spontaneous abortion of one fetus or more, third trimester

O31.2 Continuing pregnancy after intrauterine death of one fetus or more

  ⊗⑦**O31.20** Continuing pregnancy after intrauterine death of one fetus or more, unspecified trimester

  ⊗⑦**O31.21** Continuing pregnancy after intrauterine death of one fetus or more, first trimester

  ⊗⑦**O31.22** Continuing pregnancy after intrauterine death of one fetus or more, second trimester

  ⊗⑦**O31.23** Continuing pregnancy after intrauterine death of one fetus or more, third trimester

O31.3 Continuing pregnancy after elective fetal reduction of one fetus or more
Continuing pregnancy after selective termination of one fetus or more

  ⊗⑦**O31.30** Continuing pregnancy after elective fetal reduction of one fetus or more, unspecified trimester

  ⊗⑦**O31.31** Continuing pregnancy after elective fetal reduction of one fetus or more, first trimester

  ⊗⑦**O31.32** Continuing pregnancy after elective fetal reduction of one fetus or more, second trimester

  ⊗⑦**O31.33** Continuing pregnancy after elective fetal reduction of one fetus or more, third trimester

O31.8 Other complications specific to multiple gestation

  O31.8X Other complications specific to multiple gestation

    ⑦**O31.8X1** Other complications specific to multiple gestation, first trimester

    ⑦**O31.8X2** Other complications specific to multiple gestation, second trimester

    ⑦**O31.8X3** Other complications specific to multiple gestation, third trimester

  ● New code   ▲ Revised code   ⑦ 7th digit required   ⊗ Placeholder required

⑦ O31.8X9　Other complications specific to multiple gestation, unspecified trimester

O32　Maternal care for malpresentation of fetus

Includes: the listed conditions as a reason for observation, hospitalization or other obstetric care of the mother, or for cesarean delivery before onset of labor

Excludes 1: malpresentation of fetus with obstructed labor (O64.-)

One of the following 7th characters is to be assigned to each code under category O32. 7th character 0 is for single gestations and multiple gestations

where the fetus is unspecified. 7th characters 1 through 9 are for cases of multiple gestations to identify the fetus for which the code applies. The appropriate code from category O30, Multiple gestation, must also be assigned when assigning a code from category O32 that has a 7th character of 1 through 9.

0 - not applicable or unspecified
1 - fetus 1
2 - fetus 2
3 - fetus 3
4 - fetus 4
5 - fetus 5
9 - other fetus

⊗⑦ O32.0　Maternal care for unstable lie

⊗⑦ O32.1　Maternal care for breech presentation
Maternal care for buttocks presentation
Maternal care for complete breech
Maternal care for frank breech
Excludes 1: footling presentation (O32.8)
　　　　　　incomplete breech (O32.8)

⊗⑦ O32.2　Maternal care for transverse and oblique lie
Maternal care for oblique presentation
Maternal care for transverse presentation

⊗⑦ O32.3　Maternal care for face, brow and chin presentation

⊗⑦ O32.4　Maternal care for high head at term
Maternal care for failure of head to enter pelvic brim

⊗⑦ O32.6　Maternal care for compound presentation

⊗⑦ O32.8　Maternal care for other malpresentation of fetus
Maternal care for footling presentation
Maternal care for incomplete breech

⊗⑦ O32.9　Maternal care for malpresentation of fetus, unspecified

O33　Maternal care for disproportion

Includes: the listed conditions as a reason for observation, hospitalization or other obstetric care of the mother, or for cesarean delivery before onset of labor

Excludes 1: disproportion with obstructed labor (O65- O66)

O33.0　Maternal care for disproportion due to deformity of maternal pelvic bones
Maternal care for disproportion due to pelvic deformity causing disproportion NOS

O33.1　Maternal care for disproportion due to generally contracted pelvis
Maternal care for disproportion due to contracted pelvis NOS causing disproportion

O33.2　Maternal care for disproportion due to inlet contraction of pelvis
Maternal care for disproportion due to inlet contraction (pelvis) causing disproportion

⊗⑦ O33.3　Maternal care for disproportion due to outlet contraction of pelvis

Maternal care for disproportion due to mid-cavity contraction (pelvis)
Maternal care for disproportion due to outlet contraction (pelvis)

One of the following 7th characters is to be assigned to code O33.3. 7th character 0 is for single gestations and multiple gestations where the fetus is unspecified. 7th characters 1 through 9 are for cases of multiple gestations to identify the fetus for which the code applies. The appropriate code from category O30, Multiple gestation, must also be assigned when assigning code O33.3 with a 7th character of 1 through 9.

0 - not applicable or unspecified
1 - fetus 1
2 - fetus 2
3 - fetus 3
4 - fetus 4
5 - fetus 5
9 - other fetus

⊗⑦ O33.4　Maternal care for disproportion of mixed maternal and fetal origin

One of the following 7th characters is to be assigned to code O33.4. 7th character 0 is for single gestations and multiple gestations where the fetus is unspecified. 7th characters 1 through 9 are for cases of multiple gestations to identify the fetus for which the code applies. The appropriate code from category O30, Multiple gestation, must also be assigned when assigning code O33.4 with a 7th character of 1 through 9.

0 - not applicable or unspecified
1 - fetus 1
2 - fetus 2
3 - fetus 3
4 - fetus 4
5 - fetus 5
9 - other fetus

⊗⑦ O33.5　Maternal care for disproportion due to unusually large fetus
Maternal care for disproportion due to disproportion of fetal origin with normally formed fetus
Maternal care for disproportion due to fetal disproportion NOS

One of the following 7th characters is to be assigned to code O33.5. 7th character 0 is for single gestations and multiple gestations where the fetus is unspecified. 7th characters 1 through 9 are for cases of multiple gestations to identify the fetus for which the code applies. The appropriate code from category O30, Multiple gestation, must also be assigned when assigning code O33.5 with a 7th character of 1 through 9.

0 - not applicable or unspecified
1 - fetus 1
2 - fetus 2
3 - fetus 3
4 - fetus 4
5 - fetus 5
9 - other fetus

⊗⑦ O33.6　Maternal care for disproportion due to hydrocephalic fetus
One of the following 7th characters is to be assigned to code O33.6. 7th character 0 is for single gestations and multiple gestations where the fetus is unspecified. 7th characters 1 through 9 are for cases of multiple gestations

to identify the fetus for which the code applies. The appropriate code from category O30, Multiple gestation, must also be assigned when assigning code O33.6 with a 7th character of 1 through 9.

0 - not applicable or unspecified
1 - fetus 1
2 - fetus 2
3 - fetus 3
4 - fetus 4
5 - fetus 5
9 - other fetus

O33.7 Maternal care for disproportion due to other fetal deformities

Maternal care for disproportion due to fetal ascites

Maternal care for disproportion due to fetal hydrops

Maternal care for disproportion due to fetal meningomyelocele

Maternal care for disproportion due to fetal sacral teratoma

Maternal care for disproportion due to fetal tumor

Excludes 1: obstructed labor due to other fetal deformities (O66.3)

O33.8 Maternal care for disproportion of other origin

O33.9 Maternal care for disproportion, unspecified

Maternal care for disproportion due to cephalopelvic disproportion NOS

Maternal care for disproportion due to fetopelvic disproportion NOS

O34 Maternal care for abnormality of pelvic organs

Includes: the listed conditions as a reason for hospitalization or other obstetric care of the mother, or for cesarean delivery before onset of labor

Code first any associated obstructed labor (O65.5)

Use additional code for specific condition

O34.0 Maternal care for congenital malformation of uterus

O34.00 Maternal care for unspecified congenital malformation of uterus, unspecified trimester

O34.01 Maternal care for unspecified congenital malformation of uterus, first trimester

O34.02 Maternal care for unspecified congenital malformation of uterus, second trimester

O34.03 Maternal care for unspecified congenital malformation of uterus, third trimester

O34.1 Maternal care for benign tumor of corpus uteri

Excludes 2: maternal care for benign tumor of cervix (O34.4-)

maternal care for malignant neoplasm of uterus (O9A.1-)

O34.10 Maternal care for benign tumor of corpus uteri, unspecified trimester

O34.11 Maternal care for benign tumor of corpus uteri, first trimester

O34.12 Maternal care for benign tumor of corpus uteri, second trimester

O34.13 Maternal care for benign tumor of corpus uteri, third trimester

O34.2 Maternal care due to uterine scar from previous surgery

O34.21 Maternal care for scar from previous cesarean delivery

O34.29 Maternal care due to uterine scar from other previous surgery

O34.3 Maternal care for cervical incompetence

Maternal care for cerclage with or without cervical incompetence

Maternal care for Shirodkar suture with or without cervical incompetence

O34.30 Maternal care for cervical incompetence, unspecified trimester

O34.31 Maternal care for cervical incompetence, first trimester

O34.32 Maternal care for cervical incompetence, second trimester

O34.33 Maternal care for cervical incompetence, third trimester

O34.4 Maternal care for other abnormalities of cervix

O34.40 Maternal care for other abnormalities of cervix, unspecified trimester

O34.41 Maternal care for other abnormalities of cervix, first trimester

O34.42 Maternal care for other abnormalities of cervix, second trimester

O34.43 Maternal care for other abnormalities of cervix, third trimester

O34.5 Maternal care for other abnormalities of gravid uterus

O34.51 Maternal care for incarceration of gravid uterus

O34.511 Maternal care for incarceration of gravid uterus, first trimester

O34.512 Maternal care for incarceration of gravid uterus, second trimester

O34.513 Maternal care for incarceration of gravid uterus, third trimester

O34.519 Maternal care for incarceration of gravid uterus, unspecified trimester

O34.52 Maternal care for prolapse of gravid uterus

O34.521 Maternal care for prolapse of gravid uterus, first trimester

O34.522 Maternal care for prolapse of gravid uterus, second trimester

O34.523 Maternal care for prolapse of gravid uterus, third trimester

O34.529 Maternal care for prolapse of gravid uterus, unspecified trimester

O34.53 Maternal care for retroversion of gravid uterus

O34.531 Maternal care for retroversion of gravid uterus, first trimester

O34.532 Maternal care for retroversion of gravid uterus, second trimester

O34.533 Maternal care for retroversion of gravid uterus, third trimester

O34.539 Maternal care for retroversion of gravid uterus, unspecified trimester

O34.59 Maternal care for other abnormalities of gravid uterus

O34.591 Maternal care for other abnormalities of gravid uterus, first trimester

O34.592 Maternal care for other abnormalities of gravid uterus, second trimester

O34.593 Maternal care for other abnormalities of gravid uterus, third trimester

O34.599 Maternal care for other abnormalities of gravid uterus, unspecified trimester

O34.6 Maternal care for abnormality of vagina

Excludes 2: maternal care for vaginal varices in pregnancy (O22.1-)

O34.60 Maternal care for abnormality of vagina, unspecified trimester

O34.61 Maternal care for abnormality of vagina, first trimester

O34.62 Maternal care for abnormality of vagina, second trimester

O34.63 Maternal care for abnormality of vagina, third trimester

O34.7 Maternal care for abnormality of vulva and perineum

Excludes 2: maternal care for perineal and vulval varices in pregnancy (O22.1-)

O34.70 Maternal care for abnormality of vulva and perineum, unspecified trimester

O34.71 Maternal care for abnormality of vulva and perineum, first trimester

O34.72 Maternal care for abnormality of vulva and perineum, second trimester

O34.73 Maternal care for abnormality of vulva and perineum, third trimester

O34.8 Maternal care for other abnormalities of pelvic organs

O34.80 Maternal care for other abnormalities of pelvic organs, unspecified trimester

O34.81 Maternal care for other abnormalities of pelvic organs, first trimester

O34.82 Maternal care for other abnormalities of pelvic organs, second trimester

O34.83 Maternal care for other abnormalities of pelvic organs, third trimester

O34.9 Maternal care for abnormality of pelvic organ, unspecified

O34.90 Maternal care for abnormality of pelvic organ, unspecified, unspecified trimester

O34.91 Maternal care for abnormality of pelvic organ, unspecified, first trimester

O34.92 Maternal care for abnormality of pelvic organ, unspecified, second trimester

O34.93 Maternal care for abnormality of pelvic organ, unspecified, third trimester

O35 Maternal care for known or suspected fetal abnormality and damage

Includes: the listed conditions in the fetus as a reason for hospitalization or other obstetric care to the mother, or for termination of pregnancy

Code also any associated maternal condition

Excludes 1: encounter for suspected maternal and fetal conditions ruled out (Z03.7-)

One of the following 7th characters is to be assigned to each code under category O35. 7th character 0 is for single gestations and multiple gestations where the fetus is unspecified. 7th characters 1 through 9 are for cases of multiple gestations to identify the fetus for which the code applies. The appropriate code from category O30, Multiple gestation, must also be assigned when assigning a code from category O35 that has a 7th character of 1 through 9.

0 - not applicable or unspecified

1 - fetus 1

2 - fetus 2

3 - fetus 3

4 - fetus 4

5 - fetus 5

9 - other fetus

⊗⑦**O35.0** Maternal care for (suspected) central nervous system malformation in fetus

Maternal care for fetal anencephaly

Maternal care for fetal hydrocephalus

Maternal care for fetal spina bifida

Excludes 2: chromosomal abnormality in fetus (O35.1)

⊗⑦**O35.1** Maternal care for (suspected) chromosomal abnormality in fetus

⊗⑦**O35.2** Maternal care for (suspected) hereditary disease in fetus

Excludes 2: chromosomal abnormality in fetus (O35.1)

⊗⑦**O35.3** Maternal care for (suspected) damage to fetus from viral disease in mother

Maternal care for damage to fetus from maternal cytomegalovirus infection

Maternal care for damage to fetus from maternal rubella

⊗⑦**O35.4** Maternal care for (suspected) damage to fetus from alcohol

⊗⑦**O35.5** Maternal care for (suspected) damage to fetus by drugs

Maternal care for damage to fetus from drug addiction

⊗⑦**O35.6** Maternal care for (suspected) damage to fetus by radiation

⊗⑦**O35.7** Maternal care for (suspected) damage to fetus by other medical procedures

Maternal care for damage to fetus by amniocentesis

Maternal care for damage to fetus by biopsy procedures

Maternal care for damage to fetus by hematological investigation

Maternal care for damage to fetus by intrauterine contraceptive device

Maternal care for damage to fetus by intrauterine surgery

⊗⑦**O35.8** Maternal care for other (suspected) fetal abnormality and damage

Maternal care for damage to fetus from maternal listeriosis

Maternal care for damage to fetus from maternal toxoplasmosis

⊗⑦**O35.9** Maternal care for (suspected) fetal abnormality and damage, unspecified

O36 Maternal care for other fetal problems

Includes: the listed conditions in the fetus as a reason for hospitalization or other obstetric care of the mother, or for termination of pregnancy

Excludes 1: encounter for suspected maternal and fetal conditions ruled out (Z03.7-)

placental transfusion syndromes (O43.0-)

Excludes 2: labor and delivery complicated by fetal stress (O77.-)

One of the following 7th characters is to be assigned to each code under category O36. 7th character 0 is for single gestations and multiple gestations where the fetus is unspecified. 7th characters 1 through 9 are for cases of multiple gestations to identify the fetus for which the code applies. The appropriate code from category O30, Multiple gestation, must also be assigned when assigning a code from category O36 that has a 7th character of 1 through 9.

0 - not applicable or unspecified

1 - fetus 1

2 - fetus 2

3 - fetus 3

4 - fetus 4

5 - fetus 5

9 - other fetus

O36.0 Maternal care for rhesus isoimmunization

Maternal care for Rh incompatibility (with hydrops fetalis)

O36.01 Maternal care for anti-D [Rh] antibodies

⑦**O36.011** Maternal care for anti-D [Rh] antibodies, first trimester

⑦**O36.012** Maternal care for anti-D [Rh] antibodies, second trimester

⑦**O36.013** Maternal care for anti-D [Rh] antibodies, third trimester

⑦**O36.019** Maternal care for anti-D [Rh] antibodies, unspecified trimester

O36.09 Maternal care for other rhesus isoimmunization

⑦**O36.091** Maternal care for other rhesus isoimmunization, first trimester

⑦**O36.092** Maternal care for other rhesus isoimmunization, second trimester

⑦**O36.093** Maternal care for other rhesus isoimmunization, third trimester

⑦**O36.099** Maternal care for other rhesus isoimmunization, unspecified trimester

O36.1 Maternal care for other isoimmunization

Maternal care for ABO isoimmunization

O36.11 Maternal care for Anti-A sensitization

Maternal care for isoimmunization NOS (with hydrops fetalis)

⑦**O36.111** Maternal care for Anti-A sensitization, first trimester

⑦**O36.112** Maternal care for Anti-A sensitization, second trimester

⑦**O36.113** Maternal care for Anti-A sensitization, third trimester

⑦**O36.119** Maternal care for Anti-A sensitization, unspecified trimester

O36.19 Maternal care for other isoimmunization

Maternal care for Anti-B sensitization

⑦**O36.191** Maternal care for other isoimmunization, first trimester

⑦**O36.192** Maternal care for other isoimmunization, second trimester

⑦**O36.193** Maternal care for other isoimmunization, third trimester

⑦**O36.199** Maternal care for other isoimmunization, unspecified trimester

O36.2 Maternal care for hydrops fetalis

Maternal care for hydrops fetalis NOS

Maternal care for hydrops fetalis not associated with isoimmunization

Excludes 1: hydrops fetalis associated with ABO isoimmunization (O36.1-)

hydrops fetalis associated with rhesus isoimmunization (O36.0-)

⊗⑦**O36.20** Maternal care for hydrops fetalis, unspecified trimester

⊗⑦**O36.21** Maternal care for hydrops fetalis, first trimester

⊗⑦**O36.22** Maternal care for hydrops fetalis, second trimester

⊗⑦**O36.23** Maternal care for hydrops fetalis, third trimester

O36.4 Maternal care for intrauterine death

Maternal care for intrauterine fetal death NOS

Maternal care for intrauterine fetal death after completion of 20 weeks of gestation

Maternal care for late fetal death

Maternal care for missed delivery

Excludes 1: missed abortion (O02.1)

stillbirth (P95)

O36.5 Maternal care for known or suspected poor fetal growth

O36.51 Maternal care for known or suspected placental insufficiency

⑦**O36.511** Maternal care for known or suspected placental insufficiency, first trimester

⑦**O36.512** Maternal care for known or suspected placental insufficiency, second trimester

⑦**O36.513** Maternal care for known or suspected placental insufficiency, third trimester

⑦**O36.519** Maternal care for known or suspected placental insufficiency, unspecified trimester

O36.59 Maternal care for other known or suspected poor fetal growth

Maternal care for known or suspected light-for-dates NOS

Maternal care for known or suspected small-for-dates NOS

⑦**O36.591** Maternal care for other known or suspected poor fetal growth, first trimester

⑦**O36.592** Maternal care for other known or suspected poor fetal growth, second trimester

⑦**O36.593** Maternal care for other known or suspected poor fetal growth, third trimester

⑦**O36.599** Maternal care for other known or suspected poor fetal growth, unspecified trimester

O36.6 Maternal care for excessive fetal growth

Maternal care for known or suspected large-for-dates

⊗⑦**O36.60** Maternal care for excessive fetal growth, unspecified trimester

⊗⑦**O36.61** Maternal care for excessive fetal growth, first trimester

⊗⑦**O36.62** Maternal care for excessive fetal growth, second trimester

⊗⑦**O36.63** Maternal care for excessive fetal growth, third trimester

O36.7 Maternal care for viable fetus in abdominal pregnancy

⊗⑦**O36.70** Maternal care for viable fetus in abdominal pregnancy, unspecified trimester

⊗⑦**O36.71** Maternal care for viable fetus in abdominal pregnancy, first trimester

⊗⑦**O36.72** Maternal care for viable fetus in abdominal pregnancy, second trimester

● New code   ▲ Revised code   ⑦ 7th digit required   ⊗ Placeholder required

⊗⑦O36.73 Maternal care for viable fetus in abdominal pregnancy, third trimester

O36.8 Maternal care for other specified fetal problems

⊗⑦O36.80 Pregnancy with inconclusive fetal viability
Encounter to determine fetal viability of pregnancy

O36.81 Decreased fetal movements

⑦O36.812 Decreased fetal movements, second trimester

⑦O36.813 Decreased fetal movements, third trimester

⑦O36.819 Decreased fetal movements, unspecified trimester

O36.82 Fetal anemia and thrombocytopenia

⑦O36.821 Fetal anemia and thrombocytopenia, first trimester

⑦O36.822 Fetal anemia and thrombocytopenia, second trimester

⑦O36.823 Fetal anemia and thrombocytopenia, third trimester

⑦O36.829 Fetal anemia and thrombocytopenia, unspecified trimester

O36.89 Maternal care for other specified fetal problems

⑦O36.891 Maternal care for other specified fetal problems, first trimester

⑦O36.892 Maternal care for other specified fetal problems, second trimester

⑦O36.893 Maternal care for other specified fetal problems, third trimester

⑦O36.899 Maternal care for other specified fetal problems, unspecified trimester

O36.9 Maternal care for fetal problem, unspecified

⊗⑦O36.90 Maternal care for fetal problem, unspecified, unspecified trimester

⊗⑦O36.91 Maternal care for fetal problem, unspecified, first trimester

⊗⑦O36.92 Maternal care for fetal problem, unspecified, second trimester

⊗⑦O36.93 Maternal care for fetal problem, unspecified, third trimester

O40 Polyhydramnios
Includes: hydramnios
Excludes 1: encounter for suspected maternal and fetal conditions ruled out (Z03.7-)

One of the following 7th characters is to be assigned to each code under category O40. 7th character 0 is for single gestations and multiple gestations where the fetus is unspecified. 7th characters 1 through 9 are for cases of multiple gestations to identify the fetus for which the code applies. The appropriate code from category O30, Multiple gestation, must also be assigned when assigning a code from category O40 that has a 7th character of 1 through 9.

0 - not applicable or unspecified
1 - fetus 1
2 - fetus 2
3 - fetus 3
4 - fetus 4
5 - fetus 5
9 - other fetus

⊗⑦O40.1 Polyhydramnios, first trimester

⊗⑦O40.2 Polyhydramnios, second trimester

⊗⑦O40.3 Polyhydramnios, third trimester

⊗⑦O40.9 Polyhydramnios, unspecified trimester

O41 Other disorders of amniotic fluid and membranes
Excludes 1: encounter for suspected maternal and fetal conditions ruled out (Z03.7-)

One of the following 7th characters is to be assigned to each code under category O41. 7th character 0 is for single gestations and multiple gestations where the fetus is unspecified. 7th characters 1 through 9 are for cases of multiple gestations to identify the fetus for which the code applies. The appropriate code from category O30, Multiple gestation, must also be assigned when assigning a code from category O41 that has a 7th character of 1 through 9.

0 - not applicable or unspecified
1 - fetus 1
2 - fetus 2
3 - fetus 3
4 - fetus 4
5 - fetus 5
9 - other fetus

O41.0 Oligohydramnios
Oligohydramnios without rupture of membranes

⊗⑦O41.00 Oligohydramnios, unspecified trimester

⊗⑦O41.01 Oligohydramnios, first trimester

⊗⑦O41.02 Oligohydramnios, second trimester

⊗⑦O41.03 Oligohydramnios, third trimester

O41.1 Infection of amniotic sac and membranes

O41.10 Infection of amniotic sac and membranes, unspecified

⑦O41.101 Infection of amniotic sac and membranes, unspecified, first trimester

⑦O41.102 Infection of amniotic sac and membranes, unspecified, second trimester

⑦O41.103 Infection of amniotic sac and membranes, unspecified, third trimester

⑦O41.109 Infection of amniotic sac and membranes, unspecified, unspecified trimester

O41.12 Chorioamnionitis

⑦O41.121 Chorioamnionitis, first trimester

⑦O41.122 Chorioamnionitis, second trimester

⑦O41.123 Chorioamnionitis, third trimester

⑦O41.129 Chorioamnionitis, unspecified trimester

O41.14 Placentitis

⑦O41.141 Placentitis, first trimester

⑦O41.142 Placentitis, second trimester

⑦O41.143 Placentitis, third trimester

⑦O41.149 Placentitis, unspecified trimester

O41.8 Other specified disorders of amniotic fluid and membranes

O41.8X Other specified disorders of amniotic fluid and membranes

⑦O41.8X1 Other specified disorders of amniotic fluid and membranes, first trimester

⑦ O41.8X2 Other specified disorders of amniotic fluid and membranes, second trimester

⑦ O41.8X3 Other specified disorders of amniotic fluid and membranes, third trimester

⑦ O41.8X9 Other specified disorders of amniotic fluid and membranes, unspecified trimester

O41.9 Disorder of amniotic fluid and membranes, unspecified

⊗⑦ O41.90 Disorder of amniotic fluid and membranes, unspecified, unspecified trimester

⊗⑦ O41.91 Disorder of amniotic fluid and membranes, unspecified, first trimester

⊗⑦ O41.92 Disorder of amniotic fluid and membranes, unspecified, second trimester

⊗⑦ O41.93 Disorder of amniotic fluid and membranes, unspecified, third trimester

O42 Premature rupture of membranes

O42.0 Premature rupture of membranes, onset of labor within 24 hours of rupture

O42.00 Premature rupture of membranes, onset of labor within 24 hours of rupture, unspecified weeks of gestation

O42.01 Preterm premature rupture of membranes, onset of labor within 24 hours of rupture
Premature rupture of membranes before 37 completed weeks of gestation

O42.011 Preterm premature rupture of membranes, onset of labor within 24 hours of rupture, first trimester

O42.012 Preterm premature rupture of membranes, onset of labor within 24 hours of rupture, second trimester

O42.013 Preterm premature rupture of membranes, onset of labor within 24 hours of rupture, third trimester

O42.019 Preterm premature rupture of membranes, onset of labor within 24 hours of rupture, unspecified trimester

O42.02 Full-term premature rupture of membranes, onset of labor within 24 hours of rupture
Premature rupture of membranes after 37 completed weeks of gestation

O42.1 Premature rupture of membranes, onset of labor more than 24 hours following rupture

O42.10 Premature rupture of membranes, onset of labor more than 24 hours following rupture, unspecified weeks of gestation

O42.11 Preterm premature rupture of membranes, onset of labor more than 24 hours following rupture
Premature rupture of membranes before 37 completed weeks of gestation

O42.111 Preterm premature rupture of membranes, onset of labor more than 24 hours following rupture, first trimester

O42.112 Preterm premature rupture of membranes, onset of labor more than

24 hours following rupture, second trimester

O42.113 Preterm premature rupture of membranes, onset of labor more than 24 hours following rupture, third trimester

O42.119 Preterm premature rupture of membranes, onset of labor more than 24 hours following rupture, unspecified trimester

O42.12 Full-term premature rupture of membranes, onset of labor more than 24 hours following rupture
Premature rupture of membranes after 37 completed weeks of gestation

O42.9 Premature rupture of membranes, unspecified as to length of time between rupture and onset of labor

O42.90 Premature rupture of membranes, unspecified as to length of time between rupture and onset of labor, unspecified weeks of gestation

O42.91 Preterm premature rupture of membranes, unspecified as to length of time between rupture and onset of labor
Premature rupture of membranes before 37 completed weeks of gestation

O42.911 Preterm premature rupture of membranes, unspecified as to length of time between rupture and onset of labor, first trimester

O42.912 Preterm premature rupture of membranes, unspecified as to length of time between rupture and onset of labor, second trimester

O42.913 Preterm premature rupture of membranes, unspecified as to length of time between rupture and onset of labor, third trimester

O42.919 Preterm premature rupture of membranes, unspecified as to length of time between rupture and onset of labor, unspecified trimester

O42.92 Full-term premature rupture of membranes, unspecified as to length of time between rupture and onset of labor
Premature rupture of membranes after 37 completed weeks of gestation

O43 Placental disorders

Excludes 2: maternal care for poor fetal growth due to placental insufficiency (O36.5-)
placenta previa (O44.-)
placental polyp (O90.89)
placentitis (O41.14-)
premature separation of placenta [abruptio placentae] (O45.-)

O43.0 Placental transfusion syndromes

O43.01 Fetomaternal placental transfusion syndrome
Maternofetal placental transfusion syndrome

O43.011 Fetomaternal placental transfusion syndrome, first trimester

O43.012 Fetomaternal placental transfusion syndrome, second trimester

O43.013 Fetomaternal placental transfusion syndrome, third trimester

● New code   ▲ Revised code   ⑦ 7th digit required   ⊗ Placeholder required

O43.019   Fetomaternal placental transfusion syndrome, unspecified trimester

O43.02   Fetus-to-fetus placental transfusion syndrome

     O43.021   Fetus-to-fetus placental transfusion syndrome, first trimester

     O43.022   Fetus-to-fetus placental transfusion syndrome, second trimester

     O43.023   Fetus-to-fetus placental transfusion syndrome, third trimester

     O43.029   Fetus-to-fetus placental transfusion syndrome, unspecified trimester

O43.1   Malformation of placenta

   O43.10   Malformation of placenta, unspecified
     Abnormal placenta NOS

     O43.101   Malformation of placenta, unspecified, first trimester

     O43.102   Malformation of placenta, unspecified, second trimester

     O43.103   Malformation of placenta, unspecified, third trimester

     O43.109   Malformation of placenta, unspecified, unspecified trimester

   O43.11   Circumvallate placenta

     O43.111   Circumvallate placenta, first trimester

     O43.112   Circumvallate placenta, second trimester

     O43.113   Circumvallate placenta, third trimester

     O43.119   Circumvallate placenta, unspecified trimester

   O43.12   Velamentous insertion of umbilical cord

     O43.121   Velamentous insertion of umbilical cord, first trimester

     O43.122   Velamentous insertion of umbilical cord, second trimester

     O43.123   Velamentous insertion of umbilical cord, third trimester

     O43.129   Velamentous insertion of umbilical cord, unspecified trimester

   O43.19   Other malformation of placenta

     O43.191   Other malformation of placenta, first trimester

     O43.192   Other malformation of placenta, second trimester

     O43.193   Other malformation of placenta, third trimester

     O43.199   Other malformation of placenta, unspecified trimester

O43.2   Morbidly adherent placenta

   Code also associated third stage postpartum hemorrhage, if applicable (O72.0)

   Excludes 1: retained placenta (O73.-)

   O43.21   Placenta accreta

     O43.211   Placenta accreta, first trimester

     O43.212   Placenta accreta, second trimester

     O43.213   Placenta accreta, third trimester

     O43.219   Placenta accreta, unspecified trimester

   O43.22   Placenta increta

     O43.221   Placenta increta, first trimester

     O43.222   Placenta increta, second trimester

     O43.223   Placenta increta, third trimester

     O43.229   Placenta increta, unspecified trimester

   O43.23   Placenta percreta

     O43.231   Placenta percreta, first trimester

     O43.232   Placenta percreta, second trimester

     O43.233   Placenta percreta, third trimester

     O43.239   Placenta percreta, unspecified trimester

O43.8   Other placental disorders

   O43.81   Placental infarction

     O43.811   Placental infarction, first trimester

     O43.812   Placental infarction, second trimester

     O43.813   Placental infarction, third trimester

     O43.819   Placental infarction, unspecified trimester

   O43.89   Other placental disorders
     Placental dysfunction

     O43.891   Other placental disorders, first trimester

     O43.892   Other placental disorders, second trimester

     O43.893   Other placental disorders, third trimester

     O43.899   Other placental disorders, unspecified trimester

O43.9   Unspecified placental disorder

   O43.90   Unspecified placental disorder, unspecified trimester

   O43.91   Unspecified placental disorder, first trimester

   O43.92   Unspecified placental disorder, second trimester

   O43.93   Unspecified placental disorder, third trimester

O44   Placenta previa

   O44.0   Placenta previa specified as without hemorrhage
     Low implantation of placenta specified as without hemorrhage

     O44.00   Placenta previa specified as without hemorrhage, unspecified trimester

     O44.01   Placenta previa specified as without hemorrhage, first trimester

     O44.02   Placenta previa specified as without hemorrhage, second trimester

     O44.03   Placenta previa specified as without hemorrhage, third trimester

   O44.1   Placenta previa with hemorrhage
     Low implantation of placenta, NOS or with hemorrhage
     Marginal placenta previa, NOS or with hemorrhage
     Partial placenta previa, NOS or with hemorrhage
     Total placenta previa, NOS or with hemorrhage

     Excludes 1: labor and delivery complicated by hemorrhage from vasa previa (O69.4)

     O44.10   Placenta previa with hemorrhage, unspecified trimester

     O44.11   Placenta previa with hemorrhage, first trimester

     O44.12   Placenta previa with hemorrhage, second trimester

     O44.13   Placenta previa with hemorrhage, third trimester

O45   Premature separation of placenta [abruptio placentae]

   O45.0   Premature separation of placenta with coagulation defect

---

| | Add 4th-7th digits | | 3 digit reportable | | Nonspecific code | | Unspecified code | | Manifestation code | 515 |

O45.00   Premature separation of placenta with coagulation defect, unspecified

   O45.001   Premature separation of placenta with coagulation defect, unspecified, first trimester

   O45.002   Premature separation of placenta with coagulation defect, unspecified, second trimester

   O45.003   Premature separation of placenta with coagulation defect, unspecified, third trimester

   O45.009   Premature separation of placenta with coagulation defect, unspecified, unspecified trimester

O45.01   Premature separation of placenta with afibrinogenemia

   Premature separation of placenta with hypofibrinogenemia

   O45.011   Premature separation of placenta with afibrinogenemia, first trimester

   O45.012   Premature separation of placenta with afibrinogenemia, second trimester

   O45.013   Premature separation of placenta with afibrinogenemia, third trimester

   O45.019   Premature separation of placenta with afibrinogenemia, unspecified trimester

O45.02   Premature separation of placenta with disseminated intravascular coagulation

   O45.021   Premature separation of placenta with disseminated intravascular coagulation, first trimester

   O45.022   Premature separation of placenta with disseminated intravascular coagulation, second trimester

   O45.023   Premature separation of placenta with disseminated intravascular coagulation, third trimester

   O45.029   Premature separation of placenta with disseminated intravascular coagulation, unspecified trimester

O45.09   Premature separation of placenta with other coagulation defect

   O45.091   Premature separation of placenta with other coagulation defect, first trimester

   O45.092   Premature separation of placenta with other coagulation defect, second trimester

   O45.093   Premature separation of placenta with other coagulation defect, third trimester

   O45.099   Premature separation of placenta with other coagulation defect, unspecified trimester

O45.8   Other premature separation of placenta

   O45.8X   Other premature separation of placenta

      O45.8X1   Other premature separation of placenta, first trimester

      O45.8X2   Other premature separation of placenta, second trimester

      O45.8X3   Other premature separation of placenta, third trimester

      O45.8X9   Other premature separation of placenta, unspecified trimester

O45.9   Premature separation of placenta, unspecified

   Abruptio placentae NOS

   O45.90   Premature separation of placenta, unspecified, unspecified trimester

   O45.91   Premature separation of placenta, unspecified, first trimester

   O45.92   Premature separation of placenta, unspecified, second trimester

   O45.93   Premature separation of placenta, unspecified, third trimester

O46   Antepartum hemorrhage, not elsewhere classified

   Excludes 1: hemorrhage in early pregnancy (O20.-)

   intrapartum hemorrhage NEC (O67.-)

   placenta previa (O44.-)

   premature separation of placenta [abruptio placentae] (O45.-)

   O46.0   Antepartum hemorrhage with coagulation defect

      O46.00   Antepartum hemorrhage with coagulation defect, unspecified

         O46.001   Antepartum hemorrhage with coagulation defect, unspecified, first trimester

         O46.002   Antepartum hemorrhage with coagulation defect, unspecified, second trimester

         O46.003   Antepartum hemorrhage with coagulation defect, unspecified, third trimester

         O46.009   Antepartum hemorrhage with coagulation defect, unspecified, unspecified trimester

      O46.01   Antepartum hemorrhage with afibrinogenemia

         Antepartum hemorrhage with hypofibrinogenemia

         O46.011   Antepartum hemorrhage with afibrinogenemia, first trimester

         O46.012   Antepartum hemorrhage with afibrinogenemia, second trimester

         O46.013   Antepartum hemorrhage with afibrinogenemia, third trimester

         O46.019   Antepartum hemorrhage with afibrinogenemia, unspecified trimester

      O46.02   Antepartum hemorrhage with disseminated intravascular coagulation

         O46.021   Antepartum hemorrhage with disseminated intravascular coagulation, first trimester

         O46.022   Antepartum hemorrhage with disseminated intravascular coagulation, second trimester

         O46.023   Antepartum hemorrhage with disseminated intravascular coagulation, third trimester

         O46.029   Antepartum hemorrhage with disseminated intravascular coagulation, unspecified trimester

● New code   ▲ Revised code   ⑦ 7th digit required   ⊗ Placeholder required

O46.09 Antepartum hemorrhage with other coagulation defect

    O46.091 Antepartum hemorrhage with other coagulation defect, first trimester

    O46.092 Antepartum hemorrhage with other coagulation defect, second trimester

    O46.093 Antepartum hemorrhage with other coagulation defect, third trimester

    O46.099 Antepartum hemorrhage with other coagulation defect, unspecified trimester

O46.8 Other antepartum hemorrhage

  O46.8X Other antepartum hemorrhage

    O46.8X1 Other antepartum hemorrhage, first trimester

    O46.8X2 Other antepartum hemorrhage, second trimester

    O46.8X3 Other antepartum hemorrhage, third trimester

    O46.8X9 Other antepartum hemorrhage, unspecified trimester

O46.9 Antepartum hemorrhage, unspecified

  O46.90 Antepartum hemorrhage, unspecified, unspecified trimester

  O46.91 Antepartum hemorrhage, unspecified, first trimester

  O46.92 Antepartum hemorrhage, unspecified, second trimester

  O46.93 Antepartum hemorrhage, unspecified, third trimester

O47 False labor

Includes: Braxton Hicks contractions
threatened labor

Excludes 1: preterm labor (O60.-)

O47.0 False labor before 37 completed weeks of gestation

  O47.00 False labor before 37 completed weeks of gestation, unspecified trimester

  O47.02 False labor before 37 completed weeks of gestation, second trimester

  O47.03 False labor before 37 completed weeks of gestation, third trimester

O47.1 False labor at or after 37completed weeks of gestation

O47.9 False labor, unspecified

O48 Late pregnancy

O48.0 Post-term pregnancy
Pregnancy over 40completed weeks to 42completed weeks gestation

O48.1 Prolonged pregnancy
Pregnancy which has advanced beyond 42completed weeks gestation

COMPLICATIONS OF LABOR AND DELIVERY (O60-O77)

O60 Preterm labor

Includes: onset (spontaneous) of labor before 37 completed weeks of gestation

Excludes 1: false labor (O47.0-)
threatened labor NOS (O47.0-)

O60.0 Preterm labor without delivery

  O60.00 Preterm labor without delivery, unspecified trimester

  O60.02 Preterm labor without delivery, second trimester

  O60.03 Preterm labor without delivery, third trimester

O60.1 Preterm labor with preterm delivery

One of the following 7th characters is to be assigned to each code under subcategory O60.1. 7th character 0 is for single gestations and multiple Gestations where the fetus is unspecified. 7th characters 1through 9are for cases of multiple gestations to identify the fetus for which the code applies. The appropriate code from category O30, Multiple gestation, must also be assigned when assigning a code from subcategory O60.1that has a 7th character of 1through 9.

0- not applicable or unspecified
1- fetus 1
2- fetus 2
3- fetus 3
4- fetus 4
5- fetus 5
9- other fetus

  ⊗⑦**O60.10** Preterm labor with preterm delivery, unspecified trimester
Preterm labor with delivery NOS

  ⊗⑦**O60.12** Preterm labor second trimester with preterm delivery second trimester

  ⊗⑦**O60.13** Preterm labor second trimester with preterm delivery third trimester

  ⊗⑦**O60.14** Preterm labor third trimester with preterm delivery third trimester

O60.2 Term delivery with preterm labor

One of the following 7th characters is to be assigned to each code under subcategory O60.2. 7th character 0 is for single gestations and multiple gestations where the fetus is unspecified. 7th characters 1through 9 are for cases of multiple gestations to identify the fetus for which the code applies. The appropriate code from category O30, Multiple gestation, must also be assigned when assigning a code from subcategory O60.2 that has a 7th character of 1 through 9.

0- not applicable or unspecified
1- fetus 1
2- fetus 2
3- fetus 3
4- fetus 4
5- fetus 5
9- other fetus

  ⊗⑦**O60.20** Term delivery with preterm labor, unspecified trimester

  ⊗⑦**O60.22** Term delivery with preterm labor, second trimester

  ⊗⑦**O60.23** Term delivery with preterm labor, third trimester

O61 Failed induction of labor

O61.0 Failed medical induction of labor
Failed induction (of labor) by oxytocin
Failed induction (of labor) by prostaglandins

O61.1 Failed instrumental induction of labor
Failed mechanical induction (of labor)
Failed surgical induction (of labor)

O61.8 Other failed induction of labor

O61.9 Failed induction of labor, unspecified

O62 Abnormalities of forces of labor

	Add 4th-7th digits		3 digit reportable		Nonspecific code		Unspecified code		Manifestation code	517

O62.0 Primary inadequate contractions
Failure of cervical dilatation
Primary hypotonic uterine dysfunction
Uterine inertia during latent phase of labor

O62.1 Secondary uterine inertia
Arrested active phase of labor
Secondary hypotonic uterine dysfunction

O62.2 Other uterine inertia
Atony of uterus without hemorrhage
Atony of uterus NOS
Desultory labor
Hypotonic uterine dysfunction NOS
Irregular labor
Poor contractions
Slow slope active phase of labor
Uterine inertia NOS
Excludes 1: atony of uterus with hemorrhage (postpartum) (O72.1)
postpartum atony of uterus without hemorrhage (O75.89)

O62.3 Precipitate labor

O62.4 Hypertonic, incoordinate, and prolonged uterine contractions
Cervical spasm
Contraction ring dystocia
Dyscoordinate labor
Hour-glass contraction of uterus
Hypertonic uterine dysfunction
Incoordinate uterine action
Tetanic contractions
Uterine dystocia NOS
Uterine spasm
Excludes 1: dystocia (fetal) (maternal) NOS (O66.9)

O62.8 Other abnormalities of forces of labor

O62.9 Abnormality of forces of labor, unspecified

O63 Long labor

O63.0 Prolonged first stage (of labor)

O63.1 Prolonged second stage (of labor)

O63.2 Delayed delivery of second twin, triplet, etc.

O63.9 Long labor, unspecified
Prolonged labor NOS

O64 Obstructed labor due to malposition and malpresentation of fetus
One of the following 7th characters is to be assigned to each code under category O64. 7th character 0is for single gestations and multiple gestations where the fetus is unspecified. 7th characters 1through 9are for cases of multiple gestations to identify the fetus for which the code applies. The appropriate code from category O30, Multiple gestation, must also be assigned when assigning a code from category O64that has a 7th character of 1 through 9.
0- not applicable or unspecified
1- fetus 1
2- fetus 2
3- fetus 3
4- fetus 4
5- fetus 5
9- other fetus

⊗⑦**O64.0** Obstructed labor due to incomplete rotation of fetal head
Deep transverse arrest
Obstructed labor due to persistent occipitoiliac (position)
Obstructed labor due to persistent occipitoposterior (position)
Obstructed labor due to persistent occipitosacral (position)
Obstructed labor due to persistent occipitotransverse (position)

⊗⑦**O64.1** Obstructed labor due to breech presentation
Obstructed labor due to buttocks presentation
Obstructed labor due to complete breech presentation
Obstructed labor due to frank breech presentation

⊗⑦**O64.2** Obstructed labor due to face presentation
Obstructed labor due to chin presentation

⊗⑦**O64.3** Obstructed labor due to brow presentation

⊗⑦**O64.4** Obstructed labor due to shoulder presentation
Prolapsed arm
Excludes 1: impacted shoulders (O66.0)
shoulder dystocia (O66.0)

⊗⑦**O64.5** Obstructed labor due to compound presentation

⊗⑦**O64.8** Obstructed labor due to other malposition and malpresentation
Obstructed labor due to footling presentation
Obstructed labor due to incomplete breech presentation

⊗⑦**O64.9** Obstructed labor due to malposition and malpresentation, unspecified

O65 Obstructed labor due to maternal pelvic abnormality

O65.0 Obstructed labor due to deformed pelvis

O65.1 Obstructed labor due to generally contracted pelvis

O65.2 Obstructed labor due to pelvic inlet contraction

O65.3 Obstructed labor due to pelvic outlet and mid-cavity contraction

O65.4 Obstructed labor due to fetopelvic disproportion, unspecified
Excludes 1: dystocia due to abnormality of fetus (O66.2-O66.3)

O65.5 Obstructed labor due to abnormality of maternal pelvic organs
Obstructed labor due to conditions listed in O34.-
Use additional code to identify abnormality of pelvic organs O34.-

O65.8 Obstructed labor due to other maternal pelvic abnormalities

O65.9 Obstructed labor due to maternal pelvic abnormality, unspecified

O66 Other obstructed labor

O66.0 Obstructed labor due to shoulder dystocia
Impacted shoulders

O66.1 Obstructed labor due to locked twins

O66.2 Obstructed labor due to unusually large fetus

O66.3 Obstructed labor due to other abnormalities of fetus
Dystocia due to fetal ascites
Dystocia due to fetal hydrops
Dystocia due to fetal meningomyelocele
Dystocia due to fetal sacral teratoma
Dystocia due to fetal tumor
Dystocia due to hydrocephalic fetus
Use additional code to identify cause of obstruction

O66.4 Failed trial of labor

O66.40 Failed trial of labor, unspecified

O66.41 Failed attempted vaginal birth after previous cesarean delivery

Code first rupture of uterus, if applicable (O71.0-, O71.1)

O66.5 Attempted application of vacuum extractor and forceps

Attempted application of vacuum or forceps, with subsequent delivery by forceps or cesarean delivery

O66.6 Obstructed labor due to other multiple fetuses

O66.8 Other specified obstructed labor

Use additional code to identify cause of obstruction

O66.9 Obstructed labor, unspecified

Dystocia NOS

Fetal dystocia NOS

Maternal dystocia NOS

O67 Labor and delivery complicated by intrapartum hemorrhage, not elsewhere classified

Excludes 1: antepartum hemorrhage NEC (O46.-)

placenta previa (O44.-)

premature separation of placenta [abruptio placentae] (O45.-)

Excludes 2: postpartum hemorrhage (O72.-)

O67.0 Intrapartum hemorrhage with coagulation defect

Intrapartum hemorrhage (excessive) associated with afibrinogenemia

Intrapartum hemorrhage (excessive) associated with disseminated intravascular coagulation

Intrapartum hemorrhage (excessive) associated with hyperfibrinolysis

Intrapartum hemorrhage (excessive) associated with hypofibrinogenemia

O67.8 Other intrapartum hemorrhage

Excessive intrapartum hemorrhage

O67.9 Intrapartum hemorrhage, unspecified

O68 Labor and delivery complicated by abnormality of fetal acid-base balance

Fetal acidemia complicating labor and delivery

Fetal acidosis complicating labor and delivery

Fetal alkalosis complicating labor and delivery

Fetal metabolic acidemia complicating labor and delivery

Excludes 1: fetal stress NOS (O77.9)

labor and delivery complicated by electrocardiographic evidence of fetal stress (O77.8)

labor and delivery complicated by ultrasonic evidence of fetal stress (O77.8)

Excludes 2: abnormality in fetal heart rate or rhythm (O76)

labor and delivery complicated by meconium in amniotic fluid (O77.0)

O69 Labor and delivery complicated by umbilical cord complications

One of the following 7th characters is to be assigned to each code under category O69. 7th character 0 is for single gestations and multiple gestations where the fetus is unspecified. 7th characters 1 through 9 are for cases of multiple gestations to identify the fetus for which the code applies. The appropriate code from category O30, Multiple gestation, must also be assigned when assigning a code from category O69 that has a 7th character of 1 through 9.

0- not applicable or unspecified

1- fetus 1

2- fetus 2

3- fetus 3

4- fetus 4

5- fetus 5

9- other fetus

⊗⑦**O69.0** Labor and delivery complicated by prolapse of cord

⊗⑦**O69.1** Labor and delivery complicated by cord around neck, with compression

Excludes 1: labor and delivery complicated by cord around neck, without compression (O69.81)

⊗⑦**O69.2** Labor and delivery complicated by other cord entanglement, with compression

Labor and delivery complicated by compression of cord NOS

Labor and delivery complicated by entanglement of cords of twins in monoamniotic sac

Labor and delivery complicated by knot in cord

Excludes 1: labor and delivery complicated by other cord entanglement, without compression (O69.82)

⊗⑦**O69.3** Labor and delivery complicated by short cord

⊗⑦**O69.4** Labor and delivery complicated by vasa previa

Labor and delivery complicated by hemorrhage from vasa previa

⊗⑦**O69.5** Labor and delivery complicated by vascular lesion of cord

Labor and delivery complicated by cord bruising

Labor and delivery complicated by cord hematoma

Labor and delivery complicated by thrombosis of umbilical vessels

O69.8 Labor and delivery complicated by other cord complications

⊗⑦**O69.81** Labor and delivery complicated by cord around neck, without compression

⊗⑦**O69.82** Labor and delivery complicated by other cord entanglement, without compression

⊗⑦**O69.89** Labor and delivery complicated by other cord complications

O69.9 Labor and delivery complicated by cord complication, unspecified

O70 Perineal laceration during delivery

Includes: episiotomy extended by laceration

Excludes 1: obstetric high vaginal laceration alone (O71.4)

O70.0 First degree perineal laceration during delivery

Perineal laceration, rupture or tear involving fourchette during delivery

Perineal laceration, rupture or tear involving labia during delivery

Perineal laceration, rupture or tear involving skin during delivery

Perineal laceration, rupture or tear involving vagina during delivery

Perineal laceration, rupture or tear involving vulva during delivery

Slight perineal laceration, rupture or tear during delivery

O70.1 Second degree perineal laceration during delivery

Perineal laceration, rupture or tear during delivery as in O70.0, also involving pelvic floor

Perineal laceration, rupture or tear during delivery as in O70.0, also involving perineal muscles

Perineal laceration, rupture or tear during delivery as in O70.0, also involving vaginal muscles

Excludes 1: perineal laceration involving anal sphincter (O70.2)

O70.2 Third degree perineal laceration during delivery

Perineal laceration, rupture or tear during delivery as in O70.1, also involving anal sphincter

Perineal laceration, rupture or tear during delivery as in O70.1, also involving rectovaginal septum

Perineal laceration, rupture or tear during delivery as in O70.1, also involving sphincter NOS

Excludes 1: anal sphincter tear during delivery without third degree perineal laceration (O70.4)

perineal laceration involving anal or rectal mucosa (O70.3)

O70.3 Fourth degree perineal laceration during delivery

Perineal laceration, rupture or tear during delivery as in O70.2, also involving anal mucosa

Perineal laceration, rupture or tear during delivery as in O70.2, also involving rectal mucosa

O70.4 Anal sphincter tear complicating delivery, not associated with third degree laceration

Excludes 1: anal sphincter tear with third degree perineal laceration (O70.2)

O70.9 Perineal laceration during delivery, unspecified

O71 Other obstetric trauma

Includes: obstetric damage from instruments

O71.0 Rupture of uterus (spontaneous) before onset of labor

Excludes 1: disruption of (current) cesarean delivery wound (O90.0)

laceration of uterus, NEC (O71.81)

O71.00 Rupture of uterus before onset of labor, unspecified trimester

O71.02 Rupture of uterus before onset of labor, second trimester

O71.03 Rupture of uterus before onset of labor, third trimester

O71.1 Rupture of uterus during labor

Rupture of uterus not stated as occurring before onset of labor

Excludes 1: disruption of cesarean delivery wound (O90.0)

laceration of uterus, NEC (O71.81)

O71.2 Postpartum inversion of uterus

O71.3 Obstetric laceration of cervix

Annular detachment of cervix

O71.4 Obstetric high vaginal laceration alone

Laceration of vaginal wall without perineal laceration

Excludes 1: obstetric high vaginal laceration with perineal laceration (O70.-)

O71.5 Other obstetric injury to pelvic organs

Obstetric injury to bladder

Obstetric injury to urethra

Excludes 2: obstetric periurethral trauma (O71.82)

O71.6 Obstetric damage to pelvic joints and ligaments

Obstetric avulsion of inner symphyseal cartilage

Obstetric damage to coccyx

Obstetric traumatic separation of symphysis (pubis)

O71.7 Obstetric hematoma of pelvis

Obstetric hematoma of perineum

Obstetric hematoma of vagina

Obstetric hematoma of vulva

O71.8 Other specified obstetric trauma

O71.81 Laceration of uterus, not elsewhere classified

O71.82 Other specified trauma to perineum and vulva

Obstetric periurethral trauma

O71.89 Other specified obstetric trauma

O71.9 Obstetric trauma, unspecified

O72 Postpartum hemorrhage

Includes: hemorrhage after delivery of fetus or infant

O72.0 Third-stage hemorrhage

Hemorrhage associated with retained, trapped or adherent placenta

Retained placenta NOS

Code also type of adherent placenta (O43.2-)

O72.1 Other immediate postpartum hemorrhage

Hemorrhage following delivery of placenta

Postpartum hemorrhage (atonic) NOS

Uterine atony with hemorrhage

Excludes 1: uterine atony NOS (O62.2)

uterine atony without hemorrhage (O62.2)

postpartum atony of uterus without hemorrhage (O75.89)

O72.2 Delayed and secondary postpartum hemorrhage

Hemorrhage associated with retained portions of placenta or membranes after the first 24 hours following delivery of placenta

Retained products of conception NOS, following delivery

O72.3 Postpartum coagulation defects

Postpartum afibrinogenemia

Postpartum fibrinolysis

O73 Retained placenta and membranes, without hemorrhage

Excludes 1: placenta accreta (O43.21-)

placenta increta (O43.22-)

placenta percreta (O43.23-)

O73.0 Retained placenta without hemorrhage

Adherent placenta, without hemorrhage

Trapped placenta without hemorrhage

O73.1 Retained portions of placenta and membranes, without hemorrhage

Retained products of conception following delivery, without hemorrhage

O74 Complications of anesthesia during labor and delivery

Includes: maternal complications arising from the administration of a general, regional or local anesthetic, analgesic or other sedation during labor and delivery

Use additional code, if applicable, to identify specific complication

O74.0 Aspiration pneumonitis due to anesthesia during labor and delivery

Inhalation of stomach contents or secretions NOS due to anesthesia during labor and delivery

Mendelson's syndrome due to anesthesia during labor and delivery

O74.1 Other pulmonary complications of anesthesia during labor and delivery

O74.2 Cardiac complications of anesthesia during labor and delivery

O74.3 Central nervous system complications of anesthesia during labor and delivery

O74.4 Toxic reaction to local anesthesia during labor and delivery

O74.5 Spinal and epidural anesthesia-induced headache during labor and delivery

O74.6 Other complications of spinal and epidural anesthesia during labor and delivery

O74.7 Failed or difficult intubation for anesthesia during labor and delivery

O74.8 Other complications of anesthesia during labor and delivery

O74.9 Complication of anesthesia during labor and delivery, unspecified

O75 Other complications of labor and delivery, not elsewhere classified

Excludes 2: puerperal (postpartum) infection (O86.-)
puerperal (postpartum) sepsis (O85)

O75.0 Maternal distress during labor and delivery

O75.1 Shock during or following labor and delivery
Obstetric shock following labor and delivery

O75.2 Pyrexia during labor, not elsewhere classified

O75.3 Other infection during labor
Sepsis during labor
Use additional code (B95-B97), to identify infectious agent

O75.4 Other complications of obstetric surgery and procedures
Cardiac arrest following obstetric surgery or procedures
Cardiac failure following obstetric surgery or procedures
Cerebral anoxia following obstetric surgery or procedures
Pulmonary edema following obstetric surgery or procedures
Use additional code to identify specific complication
Excludes 2: complications of anesthesia during labor and delivery (O74.-)
disruption of obstetrical (surgical) wound (O90.0-O90.1)
hematoma of obstetrical (surgical) wound (O90.2)
infection of obstetrical (surgical) wound (O86.0)

O75.5 Delayed delivery after artificial rupture of membranes

O75.8 Other specified complications of labor and delivery

O75.81 Maternal exhaustion complicating labor and delivery

O75.82 Onset (spontaneous) of labor after 37 completed weeks of gestation but before 39 completed weeks gestation, with delivery by (planned) cesarean section
Delivery by (planned) cesarean section occurring after 37 completed weeks of gestation but before 39 completed weeks gestation due to (spontaneous) onset of labor
Use additional code to specify reason for planned cesarean section such as:
cephalopelvic disproportion (normally formed fetus) (O33.9)
previous cesarean delivery (O34.21)

O75.89 Other specified complications of labor and delivery

O75.9 Complication of labor and delivery, unspecified

O76 Abnormality in fetal heart rate and rhythm complicating labor and delivery
Depressed fetal heart rate tones complicating labor and delivery
Fetal bradycardia complicating labor and delivery
Fetal heart rate decelerations complicating labor and delivery
Fetal heart rate irregularity complicating labor and delivery
Fetal heart rate abnormal variability complicating labor and delivery
Fetal tachycardia complicating labor and delivery
Non-reassuring fetal heart rate or rhythm complicating labor and delivery
Excludes 1: fetal stress NOS (O77.9)

labor and delivery complicated by electrocardiographic evidence of fetal stress (O77.8)
labor and delivery complicated by ultrasonic evidence of fetal stress (O77.8)
Excludes 2: fetal metabolic acidemia (O68)
other fetal stress (O77.0-O77.1)

O77 Other fetal stress complicating labor and delivery

O77.0 Labor and delivery complicated by meconium in amniotic fluid

O77.1 Fetal stress in labor or delivery due to drug administration

O77.8 Labor and delivery complicated by other evidence of fetal stress
Labor and delivery complicated by electrocardiographic evidence of fetal stress
Labor and delivery complicated by ultrasonic evidence of fetal stress
Excludes 1: abnormality of fetal acid-base balance (O68)
abnormality in fetal heart rate or rhythm (O76)
fetal metabolic acidemia (O68)

O77.9 Labor and delivery complicated by fetal stress, unspecified
Excludes 1: abnormality of fetal acid-base balance (O68)
abnormality in fetal heart rate or rhythm (O76)
fetal metabolic acidemia (O68)

ENCOUNTER FOR DELIVERY (O80-O82)

O80 Encounter for full-term uncomplicated delivery
Delivery requiring minimal or no assistance, with or without episiotomy, without fetal manipulation [e.g., rotation version] or instrumentation [forceps] of a spontaneous, cephalic, vaginal, full-term, single, live-born infant. This code is for use as a single diagnosis code and is not to be used with any other code from chapter 15. This code must be accompanied by a delivery code from the appropriate procedure classification.
Use additional code to indicate outcome of delivery (Z37.0)

O82 Encounter for cesarean delivery without indication
This code must be accompanied by a delivery code from the appropriate procedure classification.
Use additional code to indicate outcome of delivery (Z37.0)

COMPLICATIONS PREDOMINANTLY RELATED TO THE PUERPERIUM (O85-O92)

Excludes 2: mental and behavioral disorders associated with the puerperium (F53)
obstetrical tetanus (A34)
puerperal osteomalacia (M83.0)

O85 Puerperal sepsis
Postpartum sepsis
Puerperal peritonitis
Puerperal pyemia
Use additional code (B95-B97), to identify infectious agent
Use additional code (R65.2) to identify severe sepsis, if applicable
Excludes 1: fever of unknown origin following delivery (O86.4)
genital tract infection following delivery (O86.1-)
obstetric pyemic and septic embolism (O88.3-)
puerperal septic thrombophlebitis (O86.81)
urinary tract infection following delivery (O86.2-)
Excludes 2: sepsis during labor (O75.3)

O86 Other puerperal infections
Use additional code (B95-B97), to identify infectious agent
Excludes 2: infection during labor (O75.3)

obstetrical tetanus (A34)

O86.0 Infection of obstetric surgical wound

Infected cesarean delivery wound following delivery

Infected perineal repair following delivery

O86.1 Other infection of genital tract following delivery

O86.11 Cervicitis following delivery

O86.12 Endometritis following delivery

O86.13 Vaginitis following delivery

O86.19 Other infection of genital tract following delivery

O86.2 Urinary tract infection following delivery

O86.20 Urinary tract infection following delivery, unspecified

Puerperal urinary tract infection NOS

O86.21 Infection of kidney following delivery

O86.22 Infection of bladder following delivery

Infection of urethra following delivery

O86.29 Other urinary tract infection following delivery

O86.4 Pyrexia of unknown origin following delivery

Puerperal infection NOS following delivery

Puerperal pyrexia NOS following delivery

Excludes 2: pyrexia during labor (O75.2)

O86.8 Other specified puerperal infections

O86.81 Puerperal septic thrombophlebitis

O86.89 Other specified puerperal infections

O87 Venous complications and hemorrhoids in the puerperium

Includes: venous complications in labor, delivery and the puerperium

Excludes 2: obstetric embolism (O88.-)

puerperal septic thrombophlebitis (O86.81)

venous complications in pregnancy (O22.-)

O87.0 Superficial thrombophlebitis in the puerperium

Puerperal phlebitis NOS

Puerperal thrombosis NOS

O87.1 Deep phlebothrombosis in the puerperium

Deep vein thrombosis, postpartum

Pelvic thrombophlebitis, postpartum

Use additional code to identify the deep vein thrombosis (I82.4-, I82.5-, I82.62-. I82.72-)

Use additional code, if applicable, for associated long-term (current) use of anticoagulants (Z79.01)

O87.2 Hemorrhoids in the puerperium

O87.3 Cerebral venous thrombosis in the puerperium

Cerebrovenous sinus thrombosis in the puerperium

O87.4 Varicose veins of lower extremity in the puerperium

O87.8 Other venous complications in the puerperium

Genital varices in the puerperium

O87.9 Venous complication in the puerperium, unspecified

Puerperal phlebopathy NOS

O88 Obstetric embolism

Excludes 1: embolism complicating abortion NOS (O03.2)

embolism complicating ectopic or molar pregnancy (O08.2)

embolism complicating failed attempted abortion (O07.2, O07.7)

embolism complicating induced abortion (O04.7)

embolism complicating spontaneous abortion (O03.2, O03.7)

O88.0 Obstetric air embolism

O88.01 Obstetric air embolism in pregnancy

O88.011 Air embolism in pregnancy, first trimester

O88.012 Air embolism in pregnancy, second trimester

O88.013 Air embolism in pregnancy, third trimester

O88.019 Air embolism in pregnancy, unspecified trimester

O88.02 Air embolism in childbirth

O88.03 Air embolism in the puerperium

O88.1 Amniotic fluid embolism

Anaphylactoid syndrome in pregnancy

O88.11 Amniotic fluid embolism in pregnancy

O88.111 Amniotic fluid embolism in pregnancy, first trimester

O88.112 Amniotic fluid embolism in pregnancy, second trimester

O88.113 Amniotic fluid embolism in pregnancy, third trimester

O88.119 Amniotic fluid embolism in pregnancy, unspecified trimester

O88.12 Amniotic fluid embolism in childbirth

O88.13 Amniotic fluid embolism in the puerperium

O88.2 Obstetric thromboembolism

O88.21 Thromboembolism in pregnancy

Obstetric (pulmonary) embolism NOS

O88.211 Thromboembolism in pregnancy, first trimester

O88.212 Thromboembolism in pregnancy, second trimester

O88.213 Thromboembolism in pregnancy, third trimester

O88.219 Thromboembolism in pregnancy, unspecified trimester

O88.22 Thromboembolism in childbirth

O88.23 Thromboembolism in the puerperium

Puerperal (pulmonary) embolism NOS

O88.3 Obstetric pyemic and septic embolism

O88.31 Pyemic and septic embolism in pregnancy

O88.311 Pyemic and septic embolism in pregnancy, first trimester

O88.312 Pyemic and septic embolism in pregnancy, second trimester

O88.313 Pyemic and septic embolism in pregnancy, third trimester

O88.319 Pyemic and septic embolism in pregnancy, unspecified trimester

O88.32 Pyemic and septic embolism in childbirth

O88.33 Pyemic and septic embolism in the puerperium

O88.8 Other obstetric embolism

Obstetric fat embolism

O88.81 Other embolism in pregnancy

O88.811 Other embolism in pregnancy, first trimester

O88.812 Other embolism in pregnancy, second trimester

O88.813 Other embolism in pregnancy, third trimester

O88.819 Other embolism in pregnancy, unspecified trimester

O88.82 Other embolism in childbirth

O88.83 Other embolism in the puerperium

O89 Complications of anesthesia during the puerperium

Includes: maternal complications arising from the administration of a general, regional or local anesthetic, analgesic or other sedation during the puerperium

Use additional code, if applicable, to identify specific complication

O89.0 Pulmonary complications of anesthesia during the puerperium

O89.01 Aspiration pneumonitis due to anesthesia during the puerperium

Inhalation of stomach contents or secretions NOS due to anesthesia during the puerperium

Mendelson's syndrome due to anesthesia during the puerperium

O89.09 Other pulmonary complications of anesthesia during the puerperium

O89.1 Cardiac complications of anesthesia during the puerperium

O89.2 Central nervous system complications of anesthesia during the puerperium

O89.3 Toxic reaction to local anesthesia during the puerperium

O89.4 Spinal and epidural anesthesia-induced headache during the puerperium

O89.5 Other complications of spinal and epidural anesthesia during the puerperium

O89.6 Failed or difficult intubation for anesthesia during the puerperium

O89.8 Other complications of anesthesia during the puerperium

O89.9 Complication of anesthesia during the puerperium, unspecified

O90 Complications of the puerperium, not elsewhere classified

O90.0 Disruption of cesarean delivery wound

Dehiscence of cesarean delivery wound

Excludes 1: rupture of uterus (spontaneous) before onset of labor (O71.0-)

rupture of uterus during labor (O71.1)

O90.1 Disruption of perineal obstetric wound

Disruption of wound of episiotomy

Disruption of wound of perineal laceration

Secondary perineal tear

O90.2 Hematoma of obstetric wound

O90.3 Peripartum cardiomyopathy

Conditions in I42.- arising during pregnancy and the puerperium

Excludes 1: pre-existing heart disease complicating pregnancy and the puerperium (O99.4-)

O90.4 Postpartum acute kidney failure

Hepatorenal syndrome following labor and delivery

O90.5 Postpartum thyroiditis

O90.6 Postpartum mood disturbance

Postpartum blues

Postpartum dysphoria

Postpartum sadness

Excludes 1: postpartum depression (F53)

puerperal psychosis (F53)

O90.8 Other complications of the puerperium, not elsewhere classified

O90.81 Anemia of the puerperium

Postpartum anemia NOS

Excludes 1: pre-existing anemia complicating the puerperium (O99.03)

O90.89 Other complications of the puerperium, not elsewhere classified

Placental polyp

O90.9 Complication of the puerperium, unspecified

O91 Infections of breast associated with pregnancy, the puerperium and lactation

Use additional code to identify infection

O91.0 Infection of nipple associated with pregnancy, the puerperium and lactation

O91.01 Infection of nipple associated with pregnancy

Gestational abscess of nipple

O91.011 Infection of nipple associated with pregnancy, first trimester

O91.012 Infection of nipple associated with pregnancy, second trimester

O91.013 Infection of nipple associated with pregnancy, third trimester

O91.019 Infection of nipple associated with pregnancy, unspecified trimester

O91.02 Infection of nipple associated with the puerperium

Puerperal abscess of nipple

O91.03 Infection of nipple associated with lactation

Abscess of nipple associated with lactation

O91.1 Abscess of breast associated with pregnancy, the puerperium and lactation

O91.11 Abscess of breast associated with pregnancy

Gestational mammary abscess

Gestational purulent mastitis

Gestational subareolar abscess

O91.111 Abscess of breast associated with pregnancy, first trimester

O91.112 Abscess of breast associated with pregnancy, second trimester

O91.113 Abscess of breast associated with pregnancy, third trimester

O91.119 Abscess of breast associated with pregnancy, unspecified trimester

O91.12 Abscess of breast associated with the puerperium

Puerperal mammary abscess

Puerperal purulent mastitis

Puerperal subareolar abscess

O91.13 Abscess of breast associated with lactation

Mammary abscess associated with lactation

Purulent mastitis associated with lactation

Subareolar abscess associated with lactation

O91.2 Nonpurulent mastitis associated with pregnancy, the puerperium and lactation

O91.21 Nonpurulent mastitis associated with pregnancy

Gestational interstitial mastitis

Gestational lymphangitis of breast

Gestational mastitis NOS

Gestational parenchymatous mastitis

O91.211 Nonpurulent mastitis associated with pregnancy, first trimester

O91.212 Nonpurulent mastitis associated with pregnancy, second trimester

O91.213 Nonpurulent mastitis associated with pregnancy, third trimester

O91.219 Nonpurulent mastitis associated with pregnancy, unspecified trimester

O91.22 Nonpurulent mastitis associated with the puerperium
Puerperal interstitial mastitis
Puerperal lymphangitis of breast
Puerperal mastitis NOS
Puerperal parenchymatous mastitis

O91.23 Nonpurulent mastitis associated with lactation
Interstitial mastitis associated with lactation
Lymphangitis of breast associated with lactation
Mastitis NOS associated with lactation
Parenchymatous mastitis associated with lactation

O92 Other disorders of breast and disorders of lactation associated with pregnancy and the puerperium

O92.0 Retracted nipple associated with pregnancy, the puerperium, and lactation

O92.01 Retracted nipple associated with pregnancy

O92.011 Retracted nipple associated with pregnancy, first trimester

O92.012 Retracted nipple associated with pregnancy, second trimester

O92.013 Retracted nipple associated with pregnancy, third trimester

O92.019 Retracted nipple associated with pregnancy, unspecified trimester

O92.02 Retracted nipple associated with the puerperium

O92.03 Retracted nipple associated with lactation

O92.1 Cracked nipple associated with pregnancy, the puerperium, and lactation
Fissure of nipple, gestational or puerperal

O92.11 Cracked nipple associated with pregnancy

O92.111 Cracked nipple associated with pregnancy, first trimester

O92.112 Cracked nipple associated with pregnancy, second trimester

O92.113 Cracked nipple associated with pregnancy, third trimester

O92.119 Cracked nipple associated with pregnancy, unspecified trimester

O92.12 Cracked nipple associated with the puerperium

O92.13 Cracked nipple associated with lactation

O92.2 Other and unspecified disorders of breast associated with pregnancy and the puerperium

O92.20 Unspecified disorder of breast associated with pregnancy and the puerperium

O92.29 Other disorders of breast associated with pregnancy and the puerperium

O92.3 Agalactia
Primary agalactia
Excludes 1: Elective agalactia (O92.5)
Secondary agalactia (O92.5)
Therapeutic agalactia (O92.5)

O92.4 Hypogalactia

O92.5 Suppressed lactation
Elective agalactia
Secondary agalactia

Therapeutic agalactia
Excludes 1: primary agalactia (O92.3)

O92.6 Galactorrhea

O92.7 Other and unspecified disorders of lactation

O92.70 Unspecified disorders of lactation

O92.79 Other disorders of lactation
Puerperal galactocele

OTHER OBSTETRIC CONDITIONS, NOT ELSEWHERE CLASSIFIED (O94-O9A)

O94 Sequelae of complication of pregnancy, childbirth, and the puerperium
Note: This category is to be used to indicate conditions in O00-O77.-, O85-O94 and O98-O9A.- as the cause of late effects. The sequelae include conditions specified as such, or as late effects, which may occur at any time after the puerperium. Code first condition resulting from (sequela) of complication of pregnancy, childbirth, and the puerperium

O98 Maternal infectious and parasitic diseases classifiable elsewhere but complicating pregnancy, childbirth and the puerperium
Includes: the listed conditions when complicating the pregnant state, when aggravated by the pregnancy, or as a reason for obstetric care
Use additional code (Chapter 1), to identify specific infectious or parasitic disease
Excludes 2: herpes gestationis (O26.4-)
infectious carrier state (O99.82-, O99.83-)
obstetrical tetanus (A34)
puerperal infection (O86.-)
puerperal sepsis (O85)
when the reason for maternal care is that the disease is known or suspected to have affected the fetus (O35-O36)

O98.0 Tuberculosis complicating pregnancy, childbirth and the puerperium
Conditions in A15-A19

O98.01 Tuberculosis complicating pregnancy

O98.011 Tuberculosis complicating pregnancy, first trimester

O98.012 Tuberculosis complicating pregnancy, second trimester

O98.013 Tuberculosis complicating pregnancy, third trimester

O98.019 Tuberculosis complicating pregnancy, unspecified trimester

O98.02 Tuberculosis complicating childbirth

O98.03 Tuberculosis complicating the puerperium

O98.1 Syphilis complicating pregnancy, childbirth and the puerperium
Conditions in A50-A53

O98.11 Syphilis complicating pregnancy

O98.111 Syphilis complicating pregnancy, first trimester

O98.112 Syphilis complicating pregnancy, second trimester

O98.113 Syphilis complicating pregnancy, third trimester

O98.119 Syphilis complicating pregnancy, unspecified trimester

O98.12 Syphilis complicating childbirth

O98.13 Syphilis complicating the puerperium

O98.2 Gonorrhea complicating pregnancy, childbirth and the puerperium
Conditions in A54.-

    O98.21 Gonorrhea complicating pregnancy

        O98.211 Gonorrhea complicating pregnancy, first trimester

        O98.212 Gonorrhea complicating pregnancy, second trimester

        O98.213 Gonorrhea complicating pregnancy, third trimester

        O98.219 Gonorrhea complicating pregnancy, unspecified trimester

    O98.22 Gonorrhea complicating childbirth

    O98.23 Gonorrhea complicating the puerperium

O98.3 Other infections with a predominantly sexual mode of transmission complicating pregnancy, childbirth and the puerperium
Conditions in A55-A64

    O98.31 Other infections with a predominantly sexual mode of transmission complicating pregnancy

        O98.311 Other infections with a predominantly sexual mode of transmission complicating pregnancy, first trimester

        O98.312 Other infections with a predominantly sexual mode of transmission complicating pregnancy, second trimester

        O98.313 Other infections with a predominantly sexual mode of transmission complicating pregnancy, third trimester

        O98.319 Other infections with a predominantly sexual mode of transmission complicating pregnancy, unspecified trimester

    O98.32 Other infections with a predominantly sexual mode of transmission complicating childbirth

    O98.33 Other infections with a predominantly sexual mode of transmission complicating the puerperium

O98.4 Viral hepatitis complicating pregnancy, childbirth and the puerperium
Conditions in B15-B19

    O98.41 Viral hepatitis complicating pregnancy

        O98.411 Viral hepatitis complicating pregnancy, first trimester

        O98.412 Viral hepatitis complicating pregnancy, second trimester

        O98.413 Viral hepatitis complicating pregnancy, third trimester

        O98.419 Viral hepatitis complicating pregnancy, unspecified trimester

    O98.42 Viral hepatitis complicating childbirth

    O98.43 Viral hepatitis complicating the puerperium

O98.5 Other viral diseases complicating pregnancy, childbirth and the puerperium
Conditions in A80-B09, B25-B34, R87.81-, R87.82-

Excludes 1: human immunodeficiency virus [HIV] disease complicating pregnancy, childbirth and the puerperium (O98.7-)

    O98.51 Other viral diseases complicating pregnancy

        O98.511 Other viral diseases complicating pregnancy, first trimester

        O98.512 Other viral diseases complicating pregnancy, second trimester

        O98.513 Other viral diseases complicating pregnancy, third trimester

        O98.519 Other viral diseases complicating pregnancy, unspecified trimester

    O98.52 Other viral diseases complicating childbirth

    O98.53 Other viral diseases complicating the puerperium

O98.6 Protozoal diseases complicating pregnancy, childbirth and the puerperium
Conditions in B50-B64

    O98.61 Protozoal diseases complicating pregnancy

        O98.611 Protozoal diseases complicating pregnancy, first trimester

        O98.612 Protozoal diseases complicating pregnancy, second trimester

        O98.613 Protozoal diseases complicating pregnancy, third trimester

        O98.619 Protozoal diseases complicating pregnancy, unspecified trimester

    O98.62 Protozoal diseases complicating childbirth

    O98.63 Protozoal diseases complicating the puerperium

O98.7 Human immunodeficiency virus [HIV] disease complicating pregnancy, childbirth and the puerperium
Use additional code to identify the type of HIV disease:
Acquired immune deficiency syndrome (AIDS) (B20)
Asymptomatic HIV status (Z21)
HIV positive NOS (Z21)
Symptomatic HIV disease (B20)

    O98.71 Human immunodeficiency virus [HIV] disease complicating pregnancy

        O98.711 Human immunodeficiency virus [HIV] disease complicating pregnancy, first trimester

        O98.712 Human immunodeficiency virus [HIV] disease complicating pregnancy, second trimester

        O98.713 Human immunodeficiency virus [HIV] disease complicating pregnancy, third trimester

        O98.719 Human immunodeficiency virus [HIV] disease complicating pregnancy, unspecified trimester

    O98.72 Human immunodeficiency virus [HIV] disease complicating childbirth

    O98.73 Human immunodeficiency virus [HIV] disease complicating the puerperium

O98.8 Other maternal infectious and parasitic diseases complicating pregnancy, childbirth and the puerperium

    O98.81 Other maternal infectious and parasitic diseases complicating pregnancy

        O98.811 Other maternal infectious and parasitic diseases complicating pregnancy, first trimester

        O98.812 Other maternal infectious and parasitic diseases complicating pregnancy, second trimester

O98.813   Other maternal infectious and parasitic diseases complicating pregnancy, third trimester

O98.819   Other maternal infectious and parasitic diseases complicating pregnancy, unspecified trimester

O98.82   Other maternal infectious and parasitic diseases complicating childbirth

O98.83   Other maternal infectious and parasitic diseases complicating the puerperium

O98.9   Unspecified maternal infectious and parasitic disease complicating pregnancy, childbirth and the puerperium

O98.91   Unspecified maternal infectious and parasitic disease complicating pregnancy

O98.911   Unspecified maternal infectious and parasitic disease complicating pregnancy, first trimester

O98.912   Unspecified maternal infectious and parasitic disease complicating pregnancy, second trimester

O98.913   Unspecified maternal infectious and parasitic disease complicating pregnancy, third trimester

O98.919   Unspecified maternal infectious and parasitic disease complicating pregnancy, unspecified trimester

O98.92   Unspecified maternal infectious and parasitic disease complicating childbirth

O98.93   Unspecified maternal infectious and parasitic disease complicating the puerperium

O99   Other maternal diseases classifiable elsewhere but complicating pregnancy, childbirth and the puerperium

Includes: conditions which complicate the pregnant state, are aggravated by the pregnancy or are a main reason for obstetric care

Use additional code to identify specific condition

Excludes 2: when the reason for maternal care is that the condition is known or suspected to have affected the fetus (O35-O36)

O99.0   Anemia complicating pregnancy, childbirth and the puerperium

Conditions in D50-D64

Excludes 1: anemia arising in the puerperium (O90.81)

postpartum anemia NOS (O90.81)

O99.01   Anemia complicating pregnancy

O99.011   Anemia complicating pregnancy, first trimester

O99.012   Anemia complicating pregnancy, second trimester

O99.013   Anemia complicating pregnancy, third trimester

O99.019   Anemia complicating pregnancy, unspecified trimester

O99.02   Anemia complicating childbirth

O99.03   Anemia complicating the puerperium

Excludes 1: postpartum anemia not pre-existing prior to delivery (O90-.81)

O99.1   Other diseases of the blood and blood-forming organs and certain disorders involving the immune mechanism complicating pregnancy, childbirth and the puerperium

Conditions in D65-D89

Excludes 2: hemorrhage with coagulation defects (O45.-, O46.0-, O67.0, O72.3)

O99.11   Other diseases of the blood and blood-forming organs and certain disorders involving the immune mechanism complicating pregnancy

O99.111   Other diseases of the blood and blood-forming organs and certain disorders involving the immune mechanism complicating pregnancy, first trimester

O99.112   Other diseases of the blood and blood-forming organs and certain disorders involving the immune mechanism complicating pregnancy, second trimester

O99.113   Other diseases of the blood and blood-forming organs and certain disorders involving the immune mechanism complicating pregnancy, third trimester

O99.119   Other diseases of the blood and blood-forming organs and certain disorders involving the immune mechanism complicating pregnancy, unspecified trimester

O99.12   Other diseases of the blood and blood-forming organs and certain disorders involving the immune mechanism complicating childbirth

O99.13   Other diseases of the blood and blood-forming organs and certain disorders involving the immune mechanism complicating the puerperium

O99.2   Endocrine, nutritional and metabolic diseases complicating pregnancy, childbirth and the puerperium

Conditions in E00-E88

Excludes 2: diabetes mellitus (O24.-)

malnutrition (O25.-)

postpartum thyroiditis (O90.5)

O99.21   Obesity complicating pregnancy, childbirth, and the puerperium

Use additional code to identify the type of obesity (E66.-)

O99.210   Obesity complicating pregnancy, unspecified trimester

O99.211   Obesity complicating pregnancy, first trimester

O99.212   Obesity complicating pregnancy, second trimester

O99.213   Obesity complicating pregnancy, third trimester

O99.214   Obesity complicating childbirth

O99.215   Obesity complicating the puerperium

O99.28   Other endocrine, nutritional and metabolic diseases complicating pregnancy, childbirth and the puerperium

O99.280   Endocrine, nutritional and metabolic diseases complicating pregnancy, unspecified trimester

O99.281   Endocrine, nutritional and metabolic diseases complicating pregnancy, first trimester

O99.282   Endocrine, nutritional and metabolic diseases complicating pregnancy, second trimester

O99.283   Endocrine, nutritional and metabolic diseases complicating pregnancy, third trimester

O99.284   Endocrine, nutritional and metabolic diseases complicating childbirth

O99.285   Endocrine, nutritional and metabolic diseases complicating the puerperium

O99.3   Mental disorders and diseases of the nervous system complicating pregnancy, childbirth and the puerperium

O99.31   Alcohol use complicating pregnancy, childbirth, and the puerperium

Use additional code(s) from F10 to identify manifestations of the alcohol use

O99.310   Alcohol use complicating pregnancy, unspecified trimester

O99.311   Alcohol use complicating pregnancy, first trimester

O99.312   Alcohol use complicating pregnancy, second trimester

O99.313   Alcohol use complicating pregnancy, third trimester

O99.314   Alcohol use complicating childbirth

O99.315   Alcohol use complicating the puerperium

O99.32   Drug use complicating pregnancy, childbirth, and the puerperium

Use additional code(s) from F11-F16 and F18-F19 to identify manifestations of the drug use

O99.320   Drug use complicating pregnancy, unspecified trimester

O99.321   Drug use complicating pregnancy, first trimester

O99.322   Drug use complicating pregnancy, second trimester

O99.323   Drug use complicating pregnancy, third trimester

O99.324   Drug use complicating childbirth

O99.325   Drug use complicating the puerperium

O99.33   Smoking (tobacco) complicating pregnancy, childbirth, and the puerperium

Use additional code from F17 to identify type of tobacco

O99.330   Smoking (tobacco) complicating pregnancy, unspecified trimester

O99.331   Smoking (tobacco) complicating pregnancy, first trimester

O99.332   Smoking (tobacco) complicating pregnancy, second trimester

O99.333   Smoking (tobacco) complicating pregnancy, third trimester

O99.334   Smoking (tobacco) complicating childbirth

O99.335   Smoking (tobacco) complicating the puerperium

O99.34   Other mental disorders complicating pregnancy, childbirth, and the puerperium

Conditions in F01-F09 and F20-F99

Excludes 2: postpartum mood disturbance (O90.6)

postnatal psychosis (F53)

puerperal psychosis (F53)

O99.340   Other mental disorders complicating pregnancy, unspecified trimester

O99.341   Other mental disorders complicating pregnancy, first trimester

O99.342   Other mental disorders complicating pregnancy, second trimester

O99.343   Other mental disorders complicating pregnancy, third trimester

O99.344   Other mental disorders complicating childbirth

O99.345   Other mental disorders complicating the puerperium

O99.35   Diseases of the nervous system complicating pregnancy, childbirth, and the puerperium

Conditions in G00-G99

Excludes 2: pregnancy related peripheral neuritis (O26.8-)

O99.350   Diseases of the nervous system complicating pregnancy, unspecified trimester

O99.351   Diseases of the nervous system complicating pregnancy, first trimester

O99.352   Diseases of the nervous system complicating pregnancy, second trimester

O99.353   Diseases of the nervous system complicating pregnancy, third trimester

O99.354   Diseases of the nervous system complicating childbirth

O99.355   Diseases of the nervous system complicating the puerperium

O99.4   Diseases of the circulatory system complicating pregnancy, childbirth and the puerperium

Conditions in I00-I99

Excludes 1: peripartum cardiomyopathy (O90.3)

Excludes 2: hypertensive disorders (O10-O16)

obstetric embolism (O88.-)

venous complications and cerebrovenous sinus thrombosis in labor, childbirth and the puerperium (O87.-)

venous complications and cerebrovenous sinus thrombosis in pregnancy (O22.-)

O99.41   Diseases of the circulatory system complicating pregnancy

O99.411   Diseases of the circulatory system complicating pregnancy, first trimester

O99.412   Diseases of the circulatory system complicating pregnancy, second trimester

O99.413   Diseases of the circulatory system complicating pregnancy, third trimester

O99.419 Diseases of the circulatory system complicating pregnancy, unspecified trimester

O99.42 Diseases of the circulatory system complicating childbirth

O99.43 Diseases of the circulatory system complicating the puerperium

O99.5 Diseases of the respiratory system complicating pregnancy, childbirth and the puerperium
Conditions in J00-J99

O99.51 Diseases of the respiratory system complicating pregnancy

O99.511 Diseases of the respiratory system complicating pregnancy, first trimester

O99.512 Diseases of the respiratory system complicating pregnancy, second trimester

O99.513 Diseases of the respiratory system complicating pregnancy, third trimester

O99.519 Diseases of the respiratory system complicating pregnancy, unspecified trimester

O99.52 Diseases of the respiratory system complicating childbirth

O99.53 Diseases of the respiratory system complicating the puerperium

O99.6 Diseases of the digestive system complicating pregnancy, childbirth and the puerperium
Conditions in K00-K93
Excludes 2: liver and biliary tract disorders in pregnancy, childbirth and the puerperium (O26.6-)

O99.61 Diseases of the digestive system complicating pregnancy

O99.611 Diseases of the digestive system complicating pregnancy, first trimester

O99.612 Diseases of the digestive system complicating pregnancy, second trimester

O99.613 Diseases of the digestive system complicating pregnancy, third trimester

O99.619 Diseases of the digestive system complicating pregnancy, unspecified trimester

O99.62 Diseases of the digestive system complicating childbirth

O99.63 Diseases of the digestive system complicating the puerperium

O99.7 Diseases of the skin and subcutaneous tissue complicating pregnancy, childbirth and the puerperium
Conditions in L00-L99
Excludes 2: herpes gestationis (O26.4)
pruritic urticarial papules and plaques of pregnancy (PUPPP) (O26.86)

O99.71 Diseases of the skin and subcutaneous tissue complicating pregnancy

O99.711 Diseases of the skin and subcutaneous tissue complicating pregnancy, first trimester

O99.712 Diseases of the skin and subcutaneous tissue complicating pregnancy, second trimester

O99.713 Diseases of the skin and subcutaneous tissue complicating pregnancy, third trimester

O99.719 Diseases of the skin and subcutaneous tissue complicating pregnancy, unspecified trimester

O99.72 Diseases of the skin and subcutaneous tissue complicating childbirth

O99.73 Diseases of the skin and subcutaneous tissue complicating the puerperium

O99.8 Other specified diseases and conditions complicating pregnancy, childbirth and the puerperium
Conditions in D00-D48, H00-H95, M00-N99, and Q00-Q99
Use additional code to identify condition
Excludes 2: genitourinary infections in pregnancy (O23.-)
infection of genitourinary tract following delivery (O86.1-O86.3)
malignant neoplasm complicating pregnancy, childbirth and the puerperium (O9A.1-)
maternal care for known or suspected abnormality of maternal pelvic organs (O34.-)
postpartum acute kidney failure (O90.4)
traumatic injuries in pregnancy (O9A.2-)

O99.81 Abnormal glucose complicating pregnancy, childbirth and the puerperium
Excludes 1: gestational diabetes (O24.4-)

O99.810 Abnormal glucose complicating pregnancy

O99.814 Abnormal glucose complicating childbirth

O99.815 Abnormal glucose complicating the puerperium

O99.82 Streptococcus B carrier state complicating pregnancy, childbirth and the puerperium

O99.820 Streptococcus B carrier state complicating pregnancy

O99.824 Streptococcus B carrier state complicating childbirth

O99.825 Streptococcus B carrier state complicating the puerperium

O99.83 Other infection carrier state complicating pregnancy, childbirth and the puerperium
Use additional code to identify the carrier state (Z22.-)

O99.830 Other infection carrier state complicating pregnancy

O99.834 Other infection carrier state complicating childbirth

O99.835 Other infection carrier state complicating the puerperium

O99.84 Bariatric surgery status complicating pregnancy, childbirth and the puerperium
Gastric banding status complicating pregnancy, childbirth and the puerperium

Gastric bypass status for obesity complicating pregnancy, childbirth and the puerperium

Obesity surgery status complicating pregnancy, childbirth and the puerperium

O99.840 Bariatric surgery status complicating pregnancy, unspecified trimester

O99.841 Bariatric surgery status complicating pregnancy, first trimester

O99.842 Bariatric surgery status complicating pregnancy, second trimester

O99.843 Bariatric surgery status complicating pregnancy, third trimester

O99.844 Bariatric surgery status complicating childbirth

O99.845 Bariatric surgery status complicating the puerperium

O99.89 Other specified diseases and conditions complicating pregnancy, childbirth and the puerperium

O9A Maternal malignant neoplasms, traumatic injuries and abuse classifiable elsewhere but complicating pregnancy, childbirth and the puerperium

O9A.1 Malignant neoplasm complicating pregnancy, childbirth and the puerperium

Conditions in C00-C96

Use additional code to identify neoplasm

Excludes 2: maternal care for benign tumor of corpus uteri (O34.1-)

maternal care for benign tumor of cervix (O34.4-)

O9A.11 Malignant neoplasm complicating pregnancy

O9A.111 Malignant neoplasm complicating pregnancy, first trimester

O9A.112 Malignant neoplasm complicating pregnancy, second trimester

O9A.113 Malignant neoplasm complicating pregnancy, third trimester

O9A.119 Malignant neoplasm complicating pregnancy, unspecified trimester

O9A.12 Malignant neoplasm complicating childbirth

O9A.13 Malignant neoplasm complicating the puerperium

O9A.2 Injury, poisoning and certain other consequences of external causes complicating pregnancy, childbirth and the puerperium

Conditions in S00-T88, except T74 and T76

Use additional code(s) to identify the injury or poisoning

Excludes 2: physical, sexual and psychological abuse complicating pregnancy, childbirth and the puerperium (O9A.3-, O9A.4-, O9A.5-)

O9A.21 Injury, poisoning and certain other consequences of external causes complicating pregnancy

O9A.211 Injury, poisoning and certain other consequences of external causes complicating pregnancy, first trimester

O9A.212 Injury, poisoning and certain other consequences of external causes complicating pregnancy, second trimester

O9A.213 Injury, poisoning and certain other consequences of external causes

complicating pregnancy, third trimester

O9A.219 Injury, poisoning and certain other consequences of external causes complicating pregnancy, unspecified trimester

O9A.22 Injury, poisoning and certain other consequences of external causes complicating childbirth

O9A.23 Injury, poisoning and certain other consequences of external causes complicating the puerperium

O9A.3 Physical abuse complicating pregnancy, childbirth and the puerperium

Conditions in T74.11 or T76.11

Use additional code (if applicable):

to identify any associated current injury due to physical abuse

to identify the perpetrator of abuse (Y07.-)

Excludes 2: sexual abuse complicating pregnancy, childbirth and the puerperium (O9A.4)

O9A.31 Physical abuse complicating pregnancy

O9A.311 Physical abuse complicating pregnancy, first trimester

O9A.312 Physical abuse complicating pregnancy, second trimester

O9A.313 Physical abuse complicating pregnancy, third trimester

O9A.319 Physical abuse complicating pregnancy, unspecified trimester

O9A.32 Physical abuse complicating childbirth

O9A.33 Physical abuse complicating the puerperium

O9A.4 Sexual abuse complicating pregnancy, childbirth and the puerperium

Conditions in T74.21 or T76.21

Use additional code (if applicable):

to identify any associated current injury due to sexual abuse

to identify the perpetrator of abuse (Y07.-)

O9A.41 Sexual abuse complicating pregnancy

O9A.411 Sexual abuse complicating pregnancy, first trimester

O9A.412 Sexual abuse complicating pregnancy, second trimester

O9A.413 Sexual abuse complicating pregnancy, third trimester

O9A.419 Sexual abuse complicating pregnancy, unspecified trimester

O9A.42 Sexual abuse complicating childbirth

O9A.43 Sexual abuse complicating the puerperium

O9A.5 Psychological abuse complicating pregnancy, childbirth and the puerperium

Conditions in T74.31 or T76.31

Use additional code to identify the perpetrator of abuse (Y07.-)

O9A.51 Psychological abuse complicating pregnancy

O9A.511 Psychological abuse complicating pregnancy, first trimester

O9A.512 Psychological abuse complicating pregnancy, second trimester

O9A.513 Psychological abuse complicating pregnancy, third trimester

               O9A.519   Psychological abuse complicating
                                     pregnancy, unspecified trimester
O9A.52 Psychological abuse complicating childbirth
O9A.53 Psychological abuse complicating the puerperium

   ● New code   ▲ Revised code   ⑦ 7th digit required   ⊗ Placeholder required

Chapter 16: Certain Conditions Originating In The Perinatal Period (P00-P96)

Note: Codes from this chapter are for use on newborn records only, never on maternal records

Includes: conditions that have their origin in the fetal or perinatal period (before birth through the first 28 days after birth) even if morbidity occurs later

Excludes 2: congenital malformations, deformations and chromosomal abnormalities (Q00-Q99)

endocrine, nutritional and metabolic diseases (E00-E88)

injury, poisoning and certain other consequences of external causes (S00-T88)

neoplasms (C00-D49)

tetanus neonatorum (A33)

This chapter contains the following blocks:

P00-P04	Newborn affected by maternal factors and by complications of pregnancy, labor, and delivery
P05-P08	Disorders of newborn related to length of gestation and fetal growth
P09	Abnormal findings on neonatal screening
P10-P15	Birth trauma
P19-P29	Respiratory and cardiovascular disorders specific to the perinatal period
P35-P39	Infections specific to the perinatal period
P50-P61	Hemorrhagic and hematological disorders of newborn
P70-P74	Transitory endocrine and metabolic disorders specific to newborn
P76-P78	Digestive system disorders of newborn
P80-P83	Conditions involving the integument and temperature regulation of newborn
P84	Other problems with newborn
P90-P96	Other disorders originating in the perinatal period

NEWBORN AFFECTED BY MATERNAL FACTORS AND BY COMPLICATIONS OF PREGNANCY, LABOR, AND DELIVERY (P00-P04)

Note: These codes are for use when the listed maternal conditions are specified as the cause of confirmed morbidity or potential morbidity which have their origin in the perinatal period (before birth through the first 28 days after birth). Codes from these categories are also for use for newborns who are suspected of having an abnormal condition resulting from exposure from the mother or the birth process, but without signs or symptoms, and, which after examination and observation, is found not to exist. These codes may be used even if treatment is begun for a suspected condition that is ruled out.

 Newborn (suspected to be) affected by maternal conditions that may be unrelated to present pregnancy

Code first any current condition in newborn

Excludes 2: newborn (suspected to be) affected by maternal complications of pregnancy (P01.-)

newborn affected by maternal endocrine and metabolic disorders (P70-P74)

newborn affected by noxious substances transmitted via placenta or breast milk (P04.-)

P00.0 Newborn (suspected to be) affected by maternal hypertensive disorders

Newborn (suspected to be) affected by maternal conditions classifiable to O10-O11, O13-O16

P00.1 Newborn (suspected to be) affected by maternal renal and urinary tract diseases

Newborn (suspected to be) affected by maternal conditions classifiable to N00-N39

P00.2 Newborn (suspected to be) affected by maternal infectious and parasitic diseases

Newborn (suspected to be) affected by maternal infectious disease classifiable to A00-B99, J09and J10

Excludes 1: infections specific to the perinatal period (P35-P39)

maternal genital tract or other localized infections (P00.8)

P00.3 Newborn (suspected to be) affected by other maternal circulatory and respiratory diseases

Newborn (suspected to be) affected by maternal conditions classifiable to I00-I99, J00-J99, Q20-Q34 and not included in P00.0, P00.2

P00.4 Newborn (suspected to be) affected by maternal nutritional disorders

Newborn (suspected to be) affected by maternal disorders classifiable to E40-E64

Maternal malnutrition NOS

P00.5 Newborn (suspected to be) affected by maternal injury

Newborn (suspected to be) affected by maternal conditions classifiable to O9A.2-

P00.6 Newborn (suspected to be) affected by surgical procedure on mother

Newborn (suspected to be) affected by amniocentesis

Excludes 1: Cesarean delivery for present delivery (P03.4)

damage to placenta from amniocentesis, Cesarean delivery or surgical induction (P02.1)

previous surgery to uterus or pelvic organs (P03.89)

Excludes 2: newborn affected by complication of (fetal) intrauterine procedure (P96.5)

P00.7 Newborn (suspected to be) affected by other medical procedures on mother, not elsewhere classified

Newborn (suspected to be) affected by radiation to mother

Excludes 1: damage to placenta from amniocentesis, cesarean delivery or surgical induction (P02.1)

newborn affected by other complications of labor and delivery (P03.-)

P00.8 Newborn (suspected to be) affected by other maternal conditions

P00.81 Newborn (suspected to be) affected by periodontal disease in mother

P00.89 Newborn (suspected to be) affected by other maternal conditions

Newborn (suspected to be) affected by conditions classifiable to T80-T88

Newborn (suspected to be) affected by maternal genital tract or other localized infections

Newborn (suspected to be) affected by maternal systemic lupus erythematosus

P00.9 Newborn (suspected to be) affected by unspecified maternal condition

P01 Newborn (suspected to be) affected by maternal complications of pregnancy

Code first any current condition in newborn

P01.0 Newborn (suspected to be) affected by incompetent cervix

P01.1 Newborn (suspected to be) affected by premature rupture of membranes

P01.2 Newborn (suspected to be) affected by oligohydramnios
Excludes 1: oligohydramnios due to premature rupture of membranes (P01.1)

P01.3 Newborn (suspected to be) affected by polyhydramnios
Newborn (suspected to be) affected by hydramnios

P01.4 Newborn (suspected to be) affected by ectopic pregnancy
Newborn (suspected to be) affected by abdominal pregnancy

P01.5 Newborn (suspected to be) affected by multiple pregnancy
Newborn (suspected to be) affected by triplet (pregnancy)
Newborn (suspected to be) affected by twin (pregnancy)

P01.6 Newborn (suspected to be) affected by maternal death

P01.7 Newborn (suspected to be) affected by malpresentation before labor
Newborn (suspected to be) affected by breech presentation before labor
Newborn (suspected to be) affected by external version before labor
Newborn (suspected to be) affected by face presentation before labor
Newborn (suspected to be) affected by transverse lie before labor
Newborn (suspected to be) affected by unstable lie before labor

P01.8 Newborn (suspected to be) affected by other maternal complications of pregnancy

P01.9 Newborn (suspected to be) affected by maternal complication of pregnancy, unspecified

P02 Newborn (suspected to be) affected by complications of placenta, cord and membranes
Code first any current condition in newborn

P02.0 Newborn (suspected to be) affected by placenta previa

P02.1 Newborn (suspected to be) affected by other forms of placental separation and hemorrhage
Newborn (suspected to be) affected by abruptio placenta
Newborn (suspected to be) affected by accidental hemorrhage
Newborn (suspected to be) affected by antepartum hemorrhage
Newborn (suspected to be) affected by damage to placenta from amniocentesis, cesarean delivery or surgical induction
Newborn (suspected to be) affected by maternal blood loss
Newborn (suspected to be) affected by premature separation of placenta

P02.2 Newborn (suspected to be) affected by other and unspecified morphological and functional abnormalities of placenta
P02.20 Newborn (suspected to be) affected by unspecified morphological and functional abnormalities of placenta
P02.29 Newborn (suspected to be) affected by other morphological and functional abnormalities of placenta
Newborn (suspected to be) affected by placental dysfunction
Newborn (suspected to be) affected by placental infarction

Newborn (suspected to be) affected by placental insufficiency

P02.3 Newborn (suspected to be) affected by placental transfusion syndromes
Newborn (suspected to be) affected by placental and cord abnormalities resulting in twin-to-twin or other transplacental transfusion

P02.4 Newborn (suspected to be) affected by prolapsed cord

P02.5 Newborn (suspected to be) affected by other compression of umbilical cord
Newborn (suspected to be) affected by umbilical cord (tightly) around neck
Newborn (suspected to be) affected by entanglement of umbilical cord
Newborn (suspected to be) affected by knot in umbilical cord

P02.6 Newborn (suspected to be) affected by other and unspecified conditions of umbilical cord
P02.60 Newborn (suspected to be) affected by unspecified conditions of umbilical cord
P02.69 Newborn (suspected to be) affected by other conditions of umbilical cord
Newborn (suspected to be) affected by short umbilical cord
Newborn (suspected to be) affected by vasa previa
Excludes 1: newborn affected by single umbilical artery (Q27.0)

P02.7 Newborn (suspected to be) affected by chorioamnionitis
Newborn (suspected to be) affected by amnionitis
Newborn (suspected to be) affected by membranitis
Newborn (suspected to be) affected by placentitis

P02.8 Newborn (suspected to be) affected by other abnormalities of membranes

P02.9 Newborn (suspected to be) affected by abnormality of membranes, unspecified

P03 Newborn (suspected to be) affected by other complications of labor and delivery
Code first any current condition in newborn

P03.0 Newborn (suspected to be) affected by breech delivery and extraction

P03.1 Newborn (suspected to be) affected by other malpresentation, malposition and disproportion during labor and delivery
Newborn (suspected to be) affected by contracted pelvis
Newborn (suspected to be) affected by conditions classifiable to O64-O66
Newborn (suspected to be) affected by persistent occipitoposterior
Newborn (suspected to be) affected by transverse lie

P03.2 Newborn (suspected to be) affected by forceps delivery

P03.3 Newborn (suspected to be) affected by delivery by vacuum extractor [ventouse]

P03.4 Newborn (suspected to be) affected by Cesarean delivery

P03.5 Newborn (suspected to be) affected by precipitate delivery
Newborn (suspected to be) affected by rapid second stage

P03.6 Newborn (suspected to be) affected by abnormal uterine contractions
Newborn (suspected to be) affected by conditions classifiable to O62.-, except O62.3
Newborn (suspected to be) affected by hypertonic labor

● New code   ▲ Revised code   ⑦ 7th digit required   ⊗ Placeholder required

Newborn (suspected to be) affected by uterine inertia

P03.8 Newborn (suspected to be) affected by other specified complications of labor and delivery

    P03.81 Newborn (suspected to be) affected by abnormality in fetal (intrauterine) heart rate or rhythm

        Excludes 1: neonatal cardiac dysrhythmia (P29.1-)

        P03.810 Newborn (suspected to be) affected by abnormality in fetal (intrauterine) heart rate or rhythm before the onset of labor

        P03.811 Newborn (suspected to be) affected by abnormality in fetal (intrauterine) heart rate or rhythm during labor

        P03.819 Newborn (suspected to be) affected by abnormality in fetal (intrauterine) heart rate or rhythm, unspecified as to time of onset

    P03.82 Meconium passage during delivery

        Excludes 1: meconium aspiration (P24.00, P24.01)

        meconium staining (P96.83)

    P03.89 Newborn (suspected to be) affected by other specified complications of labor and delivery

        Newborn (suspected to be) affected by abnormality of maternal soft tissues

        Newborn (suspected to be) affected by conditions classifiable to O60-O75 and by procedures used in labor and delivery not included in P02.- and P03.0-P03.6

        Newborn (suspected to be) affected by induction of labor

P03.9 Newborn (suspected to be) affected by complication of labor and delivery, unspecified

P04 Newborn (suspected to be) affected by noxious substances transmitted via placenta or breast milk

Includes: nonteratogenic effects of substances transmitted via placenta

Excludes 2: congenital malformations (Q00-Q99)

    neonatal jaundice from excessive hemolysis due to drugs or toxins transmitted from mother (P58.4)

    newborn in contact with and (suspected) exposures hazardous to health not transmitted via placenta or breast milk (Z77.-)

P04.0 Newborn (suspected to be) affected by maternal anesthesia and analgesia in pregnancy, labor and delivery

    Newborn (suspected to be) affected by reactions and intoxications from maternal opiates and tranquilizer administered during labor and delivery

P04.1 Newborn (suspected to be) affected by other maternal medication

    Newborn (suspected to be) affected by cancer chemotherapy

    Newborn (suspected to be) affected by cytotoxic drugs

    Excludes 1: dysmorphism due to warfarin (Q86.2)

        fetal hydantoin syndrome (Q86.1)

        maternal use of drugs of addiction (P04.4-)

P04.2 Newborn (suspected to be) affected by maternal use of tobacco

    Newborn (suspected to be) affected by exposure in utero to tobacco smoke

    Excludes 2: newborn exposure to environmental tobacco smoke (P96.81)

P04.3 Newborn (suspected to be) affected by maternal use of alcohol

    Excludes 1: fetal alcohol syndrome (Q86.0)

P04.4 Newborn (suspected to be) affected by maternal use of drugs of addiction

    P04.41 Newborn (suspected to be) affected by maternal use of cocaine

        'Crack baby'

    P04.49 Newborn (suspected to be) affected by maternal use of other drugs of addiction

        Excludes 2: newborn (suspected to be) affected by maternal anesthesia and analgesia (P04.0)

        withdrawal symptoms from maternal use of drugs of addiction (P96.1)

P04.5 Newborn (suspected to be) affected by maternal use of nutritional chemical substances

P04.6 Newborn (suspected to be) affected by maternal exposure to environmental chemical substances

P04.8 Newborn (suspected to be) affected by other maternal noxious substances

P04.9 Newborn (suspected to be) affected by maternal noxious substance, unspecified

DISORDERS OF NEWBORN RELATED TO LENGTH OF GESTATION AND FETAL GROWTH (P05-P08)

P05 Disorders of newborn related to slow fetal growth and fetal malnutrition

P05.0 Newborn light for gestational age

Newborn light-for-dates

    P05.00 Newborn light for gestational age, unspecified weight

    P05.01 Newborn light for gestational age, less than 500 grams

    P05.02 Newborn light for gestational age, 500-749 grams

    P05.03 Newborn light for gestational age, 750-999 grams

    P05.04 Newborn light for gestational age, 1000-1249 grams

    P05.05 Newborn light for gestational age, 1250-1499 grams

    P05.06 Newborn light for gestational age, 1500-1749 grams

    P05.07 Newborn light for gestational age, 1750-1999 grams

    P05.08 Newborn light for gestational age, 2000-2499 grams

P05.1 Newborn small for gestational age

Newborn small-and-light-for-dates

Newborn small-for-dates

    P05.10 Newborn small for gestational age, unspecified weight

    P05.11 Newborn small for gestational age, less than 500 grams

    P05.12 Newborn small for gestational age, 500-749 grams

    P05.13 Newborn small for gestational age, 750-999 grams

P05.14 Newborn small for gestational age, 1000-1249 grams

P05.15 Newborn small for gestational age, 1250-1499 grams

P05.16 Newborn small for gestational age, 1500-1749 grams

P05.17 Newborn small for gestational age, 1750-1999 grams

P05.18 Newborn small for gestational age, 2000-2499 grams

P05.2 Newborn affected by fetal (intrauterine) malnutrition not light or small for gestational age

Infant, not light or small for gestational age, showing signs of fetal malnutrition, such as dry, peeling skin and loss of subcutaneous tissue

Excludes 1: newborn affected by fetal malnutrition with light for gestational age (P05.0-)

newborn affected by fetal malnutrition with small for gestational age (P05.1-)

P05.9 Newborn affected by slow intrauterine growth, unspecified

Newborn affected by fetal growth retardation NOS

P07 Disorders of newborn related to short gestation and low birth weight, not elsewhere classified

Note: When both birth weight and gestational age of the newborn are available, both should be coded with birth weight sequenced before gestational age

Includes: the listed conditions, without further specification, as the cause of morbidity or additional care, in newborn

Excludes 1: low birth weight due to slow fetal growth and fetal malnutrition (P05.-)

P07.0 Extremely low birth weight newborn

Newborn birth weight 999 g. or less

P07.00 Extremely low birth weight newborn, unspecified weight

P07.01 Extremely low birth weight newborn, less than 500 grams

P07.02 Extremely low birth weight newborn, 500-749 grams

P07.03 Extremely low birth weight newborn, 750-999 grams

P07.1 Other low birth weight newborn

Newborn birth weight 1000-2499 grams

P07.10 Other low birth weight newborn, unspecified weight

P07.14 Other low birth weight newborn, 1000-1249 grams

P07.15 Other low birth weight newborn, 1250-1499 grams

P07.16 Other low birth weight newborn, 1500-1749 grams

P07.17 Other low birth weight newborn, 1750-1999 grams

P07.18 Other low birth weight newborn, 2000-2499 grams

P07.2 Extreme immaturity of newborn

Less than 28 completed weeks (less than 196 completed days) of gestation.

P07.20 Extreme immaturity of newborn, unspecified weeks of gestation

Gestational age less than 28 completed weeks NOS

P07.21 Extreme immaturity of newborn, gestational age less than 23 completed weeks

Extreme immaturity of newborn, gestational age less than 23 weeks, 0 days

P07.22 Extreme immaturity of newborn, gestational age 23 completed weeks

Extreme immaturity of newborn, gestational age 23 weeks, 0 days through 23 weeks, 6 days

P07.23 Extreme immaturity of newborn, gestational age 24 completed weeks

Extreme immaturity of newborn, gestational age 24 weeks, 0 days through 24 weeks, 6 days

P07.24 Extreme immaturity of newborn, gestational age 25 completed weeks

Extreme immaturity of newborn, gestational age 25 weeks, 0 days through 25 weeks, 6 days

P07.25 Extreme immaturity of newborn, gestational age 26 completed weeks

Extreme immaturity of newborn, gestational age 26 weeks, 0 days through 26 weeks, 6 days

P07.26 Extreme immaturity of newborn, gestational age 27 completed weeks

Extreme immaturity of newborn, gestational age 27 weeks, 0 days through 27 weeks, 6 days

P07.3 Preterm [premature] newborn [other]

28 completed weeks or more but less than 37 completed weeks (196 completed days but less than 259 completed days) of gestation.

Prematurity NOS

P07.30 Preterm newborn, unspecified weeks of gestation

P07.31 Preterm newborn, gestational age 28 completed weeks

Preterm newborn, gestational age 28 weeks, 0 days through 28 weeks, 6 days

P07.32 Preterm newborn, gestational age 29 completed weeks

Preterm newborn, gestational age 29 weeks, 0 days through 29 weeks, 6 days

P07.33 Preterm newborn, gestational age 30 completed weeks

Preterm newborn, gestational age 30 weeks, 0 days through 30 weeks, 6 days

P07.34 Preterm newborn, gestational age 31 completed weeks

Preterm newborn, gestational age 31 weeks, 0 days through 31 weeks, 6 days

P07.35 Preterm newborn, gestational age 32 completed weeks

Preterm newborn, gestational age 32 weeks, 0 days through 32 weeks, 6 days

P07.36 Preterm newborn, gestational age 33 completed weeks

Preterm newborn, gestational age 33 weeks, 0 days through 33 weeks, 6 days

P07.37 Preterm newborn, gestational age 34 completed weeks

Preterm newborn, gestational age 34 weeks, 0 days through 34 weeks, 6 days

P07.38 Preterm newborn, gestational age 35 completed weeks

● New code   ▲ Revised code   ⑦ 7th digit required   ⊗ Placeholder required

Preterm newborn, gestational age 35 weeks, 0 days through 35 weeks, 6 days

P07.39   Preterm newborn, gestational age 36 completed weeks

Preterm newborn, gestational age 36 weeks, 0 days through 36 weeks, 6 days

P08   Disorders of newborn related to long gestation and high birth weight

Note: When both birth weight and gestational age of the newborn are available, priority of assignment should be given to birth weight

Includes: the listed conditions, without further specification, as causes of morbidity or additional care, in newborn

P08.0   Exceptionally large newborn baby

Usually implies a birth weight of 4500 g. or more

Excludes 1: syndrome of infant of diabetic mother (P70.1)

syndrome of infant of mother with gestational diabetes (P70.0)

P08.1   Other heavy for gestational age newborn

Other newborn heavy- or large-for-dates regardless of period of gestation

Usually implies a birth weight of 4000 g. to 4499 g.

Excludes 1: newborn with a birth weight of 4500 or more (P08.0)

syndrome of infant of diabetic mother (P70.1)

syndrome of infant of mother with gestational diabetes (P70.0).

P08.2   Late newborn, not heavy for gestational age

P08.21   Post-term newborn

Newborn with gestation period over 40 completed weeks to 42 completed weeks

P08.22   Prolonged gestation of newborn

Newborn with gestation period over 42 completed weeks (294 days or more), not heavy- or large-for-dates.

Postmaturity NOS

ABNORMAL FINDINGS ON NEONATAL SCREENING (P09)

P09   Abnormal findings on neonatal screening

Use additional code to identify signs, symptoms and conditions associated with the screening

Excludes 2: nonspecific serologic evidence of human immunodeficiency virus [HIV] (R75)

BIRTH TRAUMA (P10-P15)

P10   Intracranial laceration and hemorrhage due to birth injury

Excludes 1: intracranial hemorrhage of newborn NOS (P52.9)

intracranial hemorrhage of newborn due to anoxia or hypoxia (P52.-)

nontraumatic intracranial hemorrhage of newborn (P52.-)

P10.0   Subdural hemorrhage due to birth injury

Subdural hematoma (localized) due to birth injury

Excludes 1: subdural hemorrhage accompanying tentorial tear (P10.4)

P10.1   Cerebral hemorrhage due to birth injury

P10.2   Intraventricular hemorrhage due to birth injury

P10.3   Subarachnoid hemorrhage due to birth injury

P10.4   Tentorial tear due to birth injury

P10.8   Other intracranial lacerations and hemorrhages due to birth injury

P10.9   Unspecified intracranial laceration and hemorrhage due to birth injury

P11   Other birth injuries to central nervous system

P11.0   Cerebral edema due to birth injury

P11.1   Other specified brain damage due to birth injury

P11.2   Unspecified brain damage due to birth injury

P11.3   Birth injury to facial nerve

Facial palsy due to birth injury

P11.4   Birth injury to other cranial nerves

P11.5   Birth injury to spine and spinal cord

Fracture of spine due to birth injury

P11.9   Birth injury to central nervous system, unspecified

P12   Birth injury to scalp

P12.0   Cephalhematoma due to birth injury

P12.1   Chignon (from vacuum extraction) due to birth injury

P12.2   Epicranial subaponeurotic hemorrhage due to birth injury

Subgaleal hemorrhage

P12.3   Bruising of scalp due to birth injury

P12.4   Injury of scalp of newborn due to monitoring equipment

Sampling incision of scalp of newborn

Scalp clip (electrode) injury of newborn

P12.8   Other birth injuries to scalp

P12.81   Caput succedaneum

P12.89   Other birth injuries to scalp

P12.9   Birth injury to scalp, unspecified

P13   Birth injury to skeleton

Excludes 2: birth injury to spine (P11.5)

P13.0   Fracture of skull due to birth injury

P13.1   Other birth injuries to skull

Excludes 1: cephalhematoma (P12.0)

P13.2   Birth injury to femur

P13.3   Birth injury to other long bones

P13.4   Fracture of clavicle due to birth injury

P13.8   Birth injuries to other parts of skeleton

P13.9   Birth injury to skeleton, unspecified

P14   Birth injury to peripheral nervous system

P14.0   Erb's paralysis due to birth injury

P14.1   Klumpke's paralysis due to birth injury

P14.2   Phrenic nerve paralysis due to birth injury

P14.3   Other brachial plexus birth injuries

P14.8   Birth injuries to other parts of peripheral nervous system

P14.9   Birth injury to peripheral nervous system, unspecified

P15   Other birth injuries

P15.0   Birth injury to liver

Rupture of liver due to birth injury

P15.1   Birth injury to spleen

Rupture of spleen due to birth injury

P15.2   Sternomastoid injury due to birth injury

P15.3   Birth injury to eye

Subconjunctival hemorrhage due to birth injury

Traumatic glaucoma due to birth injury

P15.4   Birth injury to face

Facial congestion due to birth injury

P15.5   Birth injury to external genitalia

P15.6   Subcutaneous fat necrosis due to birth injury

P15.8   Other specified birth injuries

P15.9   Birth injury, unspecified

RESPIRATORY AND CARDIOVASCULAR DISORDERS SPECIFIC TO THE PERINATAL PERIOD (P19-P29)

P19 Metabolic acidemia in newborn

Includes: metabolic acidemia in newborn

P19.0 Metabolic acidemia in newborn first noted before onset of labor

P19.1 Metabolic acidemia in newborn first noted during labor

P19.2 Metabolic acidemia noted at birth

P19.9 Metabolic acidemia, unspecified

P22 Respiratory distress of newborn

Excludes 1: respiratory arrest of newborn (P28.81)

respiratory failure of newborn NOS (P28.5)

P22.0 Respiratory distress syndrome of newborn

Cardiorespiratory distress syndrome of newborn

Hyaline membrane disease

Idiopathic respiratory distress syndrome [IRDS or RDS] of newborn

Pulmonary hypoperfusion syndrome

Respiratory distress syndrome, type I

P22.1 Transient tachypnea of newborn

Idiopathic tachypnea of newborn

Respiratory distress syndrome, type II

Wet lung syndrome

P22.8 Other respiratory distress of newborn

P22.9 Respiratory distress of newborn, unspecified

P23 Congenital pneumonia

Includes: infective pneumonia acquired in utero or during birth

Excludes 1: neonatal pneumonia resulting from aspiration (P24.-)

P23.0 Congenital pneumonia due to viral agent

Use additional code (B97) to identify organism

Excludes 1: congenital rubella pneumonitis (P35.0)

P23.1 Congenital pneumonia due to Chlamydia

P23.2 Congenital pneumonia due to staphylococcus

P23.3 Congenital pneumonia due to streptococcus, group B

P23.4 Congenital pneumonia due to Escherichia coli

P23.5 Congenital pneumonia due to Pseudomonas

P23.6 Congenital pneumonia due to other bacterial agents

Congenital pneumonia due to Hemophilus influenzae

Congenital pneumonia due to Klebsiella pneumoniae

Congenital pneumonia due to Mycoplasma

Congenital pneumonia due to Streptococcus, except group B

Use additional code (B95-B96) to identify organism

P23.8 Congenital pneumonia due to other organisms

P23.9 Congenital pneumonia, unspecified

P24 Neonatal aspiration

Includes: aspiration in utero and during delivery

P24.0 Meconium aspiration

Excludes 1: meconium passage (without aspiration) during delivery (P03.82)

meconium staining (P96.83   )

P24.00 Meconium aspiration without respiratory symptoms

Meconium aspiration NOS

P24.01 Meconium aspiration with respiratory symptoms

Meconium aspiration pneumonia

Meconium aspiration pneumonitis

Meconium aspiration syndrome NOS

Use additional code to identify any secondary pulmonary hypertension, if applicable (I27.2)

P24.1 Neonatal aspiration of (clear) amniotic fluid and mucus

Neonatal aspiration of liquor (amnii)

P24.10 Neonatal aspiration of (clear) amniotic fluid and mucus without respiratory symptoms

Neonatal aspiration of amniotic fluid and mucus NOS

P24.11 Neonatal aspiration of (clear) amniotic fluid and mucus with respiratory symptoms

Neonatal aspiration of amniotic fluid and mucus with pneumonia

Neonatal aspiration of amniotic fluid and mucus with pneumonitis

Use additional code to identify any secondary pulmonary hypertension, if applicable (I27.2)

P24.2 Neonatal aspiration of blood

P24.20 Neonatal aspiration of blood without respiratory symptoms

Neonatal aspiration of blood NOS

P24.21 Neonatal aspiration of blood with respiratory symptoms

Neonatal aspiration of blood with pneumonia

Neonatal aspiration of blood with pneumonitis

Use additional code to identify any secondary pulmonary hypertension, if applicable (I27.2)

P24.3 Neonatal aspiration of milk and regurgitated food

Neonatal aspiration of stomach contents

P24.30 Neonatal aspiration of milk and regurgitated food without respiratory symptoms

Neonatal aspiration of milk and regurgitated food NOS

P24.31 Neonatal aspiration of milk and regurgitated food with respiratory symptoms

Neonatal aspiration of milk and regurgitated food with pneumonia

Neonatal aspiration of milk and regurgitated food with pneumonitis

Use additional code to identify any secondary pulmonary hypertension, if applicable (I27.2)

P24.8 Other neonatal aspiration

P24.80 Other neonatal aspiration without respiratory symptoms

Neonatal aspiration NEC

P24.81 Other neonatal aspiration with respiratory symptoms

Neonatal aspiration pneumonia NEC

Neonatal aspiration with pneumonitis NEC

Neonatal aspiration with pneumonia NOS

Neonatal aspiration with pneumonitis NOS

Use additional code to identify any secondary pulmonary hypertension, if applicable (I27.2)

P24.9 Neonatal aspiration, unspecified

P25 Interstitial emphysema and related conditions originating in the perinatal period

P25.0 Interstitial emphysema originating in the perinatal period

P25.1 Pneumothorax originating in the perinatal period

P25.2 Pneumomediastinum originating in the perinatal period

P25.3 Pneumopericardium originating in the perinatal period

● New code   ▲ Revised code   ⑦ 7th digit required   ⊗ Placeholder required

P25.8 Other conditions related to interstitial emphysema originating in the perinatal period

P26 Pulmonary hemorrhage originating in the perinatal period

Excludes 1: acute idiopathic hemorrhage in infants over 28 days old (R04.81)

P26.0 Tracheobronchial hemorrhage originating in the perinatal period

P26.1 Massive pulmonary hemorrhage originating in the perinatal period

P26.8 Other pulmonary hemorrhages originating in the perinatal period

P26.9 Unspecified pulmonary hemorrhage originating in the perinatal period

P27 Chronic respiratory disease originating in the perinatal period

Excludes 1: respiratory distress of newborn (P22.0-P22.9)

P27.0 Wilson-Mikity syndrome
Pulmonary dysmaturity

P27.1 Bronchopulmonary dysplasia originating in the perinatal period

P27.8 Other chronic respiratory diseases originating in the perinatal period
Congenital pulmonary fibrosis
Ventilator lung in newborn

P27.9 Unspecified chronic respiratory disease originating in the perinatal period

P28 Other respiratory conditions originating in the perinatal period

Excludes 1: congenital malformations of the respiratory system (Q30-Q34)

P28.0 Primary atelectasis of newborn
Primary failure to expand terminal respiratory units
Pulmonary hypoplasia associated with short gestation
Pulmonary immaturity NOS

P28.1 Other and unspecified atelectasis of newborn

P28.10 Unspecified atelectasis of newborn
Atelectasis of newborn NOS

P28.11 Resorption atelectasis without respiratory distress syndrome
Excludes 1: resorption atelectasis with respiratory distress syndrome (P22.0)

P28.19 Other atelectasis of newborn
Partial atelectasis of newborn
Secondary atelectasis of newborn

P28.2 Cyanotic attacks of newborn
Excludes 1: apnea of newborn (P28.3-P28.4)

P28.3 Primary sleep apnea of newborn
Central sleep apnea of newborn
Obstructive sleep apnea of newborn
Sleep apnea of newborn NOS

P28.4 Other apnea of newborn
Apnea of prematurity
Obstructive apnea of newborn
Excludes 1: obstructive sleep apnea of newborn (P28.3)

P28.5 Respiratory failure of newborn
Excludes 1: respiratory arrest of newborn (P28.81)
respiratory distress of newborn (P22.0-)

P28.8 Other specified respiratory conditions of newborn

P28.81 Respiratory arrest of newborn

P28.89 Other specified respiratory conditions of newborn

Congenital laryngeal stridor
Sniffles in newborn
Snuffles in newborn
Excludes 1: early congenital syphilitic rhinitis (A50.0)

P28.9 Respiratory condition of newborn, unspecified
Respiratory depression in newborn

P29 Cardiovascular disorders originating in the perinatal period

Excludes 1: congenital malformations of the circulatory system (Q20-Q28)

P29.0 Neonatal cardiac failure

P29.1 Neonatal cardiac dysrhythmia

P29.11 Neonatal tachycardia

P29.12 Neonatal bradycardia

P29.2 Neonatal hypertension

P29.3 Persistent fetal circulation
Delayed closure of ductus arteriosus
(Persistent) pulmonary hypertension of newborn

P29.4 Transient myocardial ischemia in newborn

P29.8 Other cardiovascular disorders originating in the perinatal period

P29.81 Cardiac arrest of newborn

P29.89 Other cardiovascular disorders originating in the perinatal period

P29.9 Cardiovascular disorder originating in the perinatal period, unspecified

INFECTIONS SPECIFIC TO THE PERINATAL PERIOD (P35-P39)

Infections acquired in utero, during birth via the umbilicus, or during the first 28 days after birth

Excludes 2: asymptomatic human immunodeficiency virus [HIV] infection status (Z21)
congenital gonococcal infection (A54.-)
congenital pneumonia (P23.-)
congenital syphilis (A50.-)
human immunodeficiency virus [HIV] disease (B20)
infant botulism (A48.51)
infectious diseases not specific to the perinatal period (A00-B99, J09, J10.-)
intestinal infectious disease (A00-A09)
laboratory evidence of human immunodeficiency virus [HIV] (R75)
tetanus neonatorum (A33)

P35 Congenital viral diseases

Includes: infections acquired in utero or during birth

P35.0 Congenital rubella syndrome
Congenital rubella pneumonitis

P35.1 Congenital cytomegalovirus infection

P35.2 Congenital herpesviral [herpes simplex] infection

P35.3 Congenital viral hepatitis

P35.8 Other congenital viral diseases
Congenital varicella [chickenpox]

P35.9 Congenital viral disease, unspecified

P36 Bacterial sepsis of newborn

Includes: congenital sepsis

Use additional code(s), if applicable, to identify severe sepsis (R65.2-) and associated acute organ dysfunction(s)

P36.0 Sepsis of newborn due to streptococcus, group B

P36.1 Sepsis of newborn due to other and unspecified streptococci

P36.10 Sepsis of newborn due to unspecified streptococci

P36.19 Sepsis of newborn due to other streptococci

P36.2 Sepsis of newborn due to Staphylococcus aureus

P36.3 Sepsis of newborn due to other and unspecified staphylococci

P36.30 Sepsis of newborn due to unspecified staphylococci

P36.39 Sepsis of newborn due to other staphylococci

P36.4 Sepsis of newborn due to Escherichia coli

P36.5 Sepsis of newborn due to anaerobes

P36.8 Other bacterial sepsis of newborn

Use additional code from category B96 to identify organism

P36.9 Bacterial sepsis of newborn, unspecified

P37 Other congenital infectious and parasitic diseases

Excludes 2: congenital syphilis (A50.-)

infectious neonatal diarrhea (A00-A09)

necrotizing enterocolitis in newborn (P77.-)

noninfectious neonatal diarrhea (P78.3)

ophthalmia neonatorum due to gonococcus (A54.31)

tetanus neonatorum (A33)

P37.0 Congenital tuberculosis

P37.1 Congenital toxoplasmosis

Hydrocephalus due to congenital toxoplasmosis

P37.2 Neonatal (disseminated) listeriosis

P37.3 Congenital falciparum malaria

P37.4 Other congenital malaria

P37.5 Neonatal candidiasis

P37.8 Other specified congenital infectious and parasitic diseases

P37.9 Congenital infectious or parasitic disease, unspecified

P38 Omphalitis of newborn

Excludes 1: omphalitis not of newborn (L08.82)

tetanus omphalitis (A33)

umbilical hemorrhage of newborn (P51.-)

P38.1 Omphalitis with mild hemorrhage

P38.9 Omphalitis without hemorrhage

Omphalitis of newborn NOS

P39 Other infections specific to the perinatal period

Use additional code to identify organism or specific infection

P39.0 Neonatal infective mastitis

Excludes 1: breast engorgement of newborn (P83.4)

noninfective mastitis of newborn (P83.4)

P39.1 Neonatal conjunctivitis and dacryocystitis

Neonatal chlamydial conjunctivitis

Ophthalmia neonatorum NOS

Excludes 1: gonococcal conjunctivitis (A54.31)

P39.2 Intra-amniotic infection affecting newborn, not elsewhere classified

P39.3 Neonatal urinary tract infection

P39.4 Neonatal skin infection

Neonatal pyoderma

Excludes 1: pemphigus neonatorum (L00)

staphylococcal scalded skin syndrome (L00)

P39.8 Other specified infections specific to the perinatal period

P39.9 Infection specific to the perinatal period, unspecified

HEMORRHAGIC AND HEMATOLOGICAL DISORDERS OF NEWBORN (P50-P61)

Excludes 1: congenital stenosis and stricture of bile ducts (Q44.3)

Crigler-Najjar syndrome (E80.5)

Dubin-Johnson syndrome (E80.6)

Gilbert syndrome (E80.4)

hereditary hemolytic anemias (D55-D58)

P50 Newborn affected by intrauterine (fetal) blood loss

Excludes 1: congenital anemia from intrauterine (fetal) blood loss (P61.3)

P50.0 Newborn affected by intrauterine (fetal) blood loss from vasa previa

P50.1 Newborn affected by intrauterine (fetal) blood loss from ruptured cord

P50.2 Newborn affected by intrauterine (fetal) blood loss from placenta

P50.3 Newborn affected by hemorrhage into co-twin

P50.4 Newborn affected by hemorrhage into maternal circulation

P50.5 Newborn affected by intrauterine (fetal) blood loss from cut end of co-twin's cord

P50.8 Newborn affected by other intrauterine (fetal) blood loss

P50.9 Newborn affected by intrauterine (fetal) blood loss, unspecified

Newborn affected by fetal hemorrhage NOS

P51 Umbilical hemorrhage of newborn

Excludes 1: omphalitis with mild hemorrhage (P38.1)

umbilical hemorrhage from cut end of co-twins cord (P50.5)

P51.0 Massive umbilical hemorrhage of newborn

P51.8 Other umbilical hemorrhages of newborn

Slipped umbilical ligature NOS

P51.9 Umbilical hemorrhage of newborn, unspecified

P52 Intracranial nontraumatic hemorrhage of newborn

Includes: intracranial hemorrhage due to anoxia or hypoxia

Excludes 1: intracranial hemorrhage due to birth injury (P10.-)

intracranial hemorrhage due to other injury (S06.-)

P52.0 Intraventricular (nontraumatic) hemorrhage, grade 1, of newborn

Subependymal hemorrhage (without intraventricular extension)

Bleeding into germinal matrix

P52.1 Intraventricular (nontraumatic) hemorrhage, grade 2, of newborn

Subependymal hemorrhage with intraventricular extension

Bleeding into ventricle

P52.2 Intraventricular (nontraumatic) hemorrhage, grade 3 and grade 4, of newborn

P52.21 Intraventricular (nontraumatic) hemorrhage, grade 3, of newborn

Subependymal hemorrhage with intraventricular extension with enlargement of ventricle

P52.22 Intraventricular (nontraumatic) hemorrhage, grade 4, of newborn

Bleeding into cerebral cortex

Subependymal hemorrhage with intracerebral extension

P52.3 Unspecified intraventricular (nontraumatic) hemorrhage of newborn

P52.4 Intracerebral (nontraumatic) hemorrhage of newborn

P52.5 Subarachnoid (nontraumatic) hemorrhage of newborn

P52.6 Cerebellar (nontraumatic) and posterior fossa hemorrhage of newborn

P52.8 Other intracranial (nontraumatic) hemorrhages of newborn

P52.9 Intracranial (nontraumatic) hemorrhage of newborn, unspecified

P53 Hemorrhagic disease of newborn
Vitamin K deficiency of newborn

P54 Other neonatal hemorrhages
Excludes 1: newborn affected by (intrauterine) blood loss (P50.-)
pulmonary hemorrhage originating in the perinatal period (P26.-)

P54.0 Neonatal hematemesis
Excludes 1: neonatal hematemesis due to swallowed maternal blood (P78.2)

P54.1 Neonatal melena
Excludes 1: neonatal melena due to swallowed maternal blood (P78.2)

P54.2 Neonatal rectal hemorrhage

P54.3 Other neonatal gastrointestinal hemorrhage

P54.4 Neonatal adrenal hemorrhage

P54.5 Neonatal cutaneous hemorrhage
Neonatal bruising
Neonatal ecchymoses
Neonatal petechiae
Neonatal superficial hematomata
Excludes 2: bruising of scalp due to birth injury (P12.3)
cephalhematoma due to birth injury (P12.0)

P54.6 Neonatal vaginal hemorrhage
Neonatal pseudomenses

P54.8 Other specified neonatal hemorrhages

P54.9 Neonatal hemorrhage, unspecified

P55 Hemolytic disease of newborn

P55.0 Rh isoimmunization of newborn

P55.1 ABO isoimmunization of newborn

P55.8 Other hemolytic diseases of newborn

P55.9 Hemolytic disease of newborn, unspecified

P56 Hydrops fetalis due to hemolytic disease
Excludes 1: hydrops fetalis NOS (P83.2)

P56.0 Hydrops fetalis due to isoimmunization

P56.9 Hydrops fetalis due to other and unspecified hemolytic disease

P56.90 Hydrops fetalis due to unspecified hemolytic disease

P56.99 Hydrops fetalis due to other hemolytic disease

P57 Kernicterus

P57.0 Kernicterus due to isoimmunization

P57.8 Other specified kernicterus
Excludes 1: Crigler-Najjar syndrome (E80.5)

P57.9 Kernicterus, unspecified

P58 Neonatal jaundice due to other excessive hemolysis
Excludes 1: jaundice due to isoimmunization (P55-P57)

P58.0 Neonatal jaundice due to bruising

P58.1 Neonatal jaundice due to bleeding

P58.2 Neonatal jaundice due to infection

P58.3 Neonatal jaundice due to polycythemia

P58.4 Neonatal jaundice due to drugs or toxins transmitted from mother or given to newborn
Code first poisoning due to drug or toxin, if applicable (T36-T65 with fifth or sixth character 1-4or 6)

Use additional code for adverse effect, if applicable, to identify drug (T36-T50 with fifth or sixth character 5)

P58.41 Neonatal jaundice due to drugs or toxins transmitted from mother

P58.42 Neonatal jaundice due to drugs or toxins given to newborn

P58.5 Neonatal jaundice due to swallowed maternal blood

P58.8 Neonatal jaundice due to other specified excessive hemolysis

P58.9 Neonatal jaundice due to excessive hemolysis, unspecified

P59 Neonatal jaundice from other and unspecified causes
Excludes 1: jaundice due to inborn errors of metabolism (E70-E88)
kernicterus (P57.-)

P59.0 Neonatal jaundice associated with preterm delivery
Hyperbilirubinemia of prematurity
Jaundice due to delayed conjugation associated with preterm delivery

P59.1 Inspissated bile syndrome

P59.2 Neonatal jaundice from other and unspecified hepatocellular damage
Excludes 1: congenital viral hepatitis (P35.3)

P59.20 Neonatal jaundice from unspecified hepatocellular damage

P59.29 Neonatal jaundice from other hepatocellular damage
Neonatal giant cell hepatitis
Neonatal (idiopathic) hepatitis

P59.3 Neonatal jaundice from breast milk inhibitor

P59.8 Neonatal jaundice from other specified causes

P59.9 Neonatal jaundice, unspecified
Neonatal physiological jaundice (intense)(prolonged) NOS

P60 Disseminated intravascular coagulation of newborn
Defibrination syndrome of newborn

P61 Other perinatal hematological disorders
Excludes 1: transient hypogammaglobulinemia of infancy (D80.7)

P61.0 Transient neonatal thrombocytopenia
Neonatal thrombocytopenia due to exchange transfusion
Neonatal thrombocytopenia due to idiopathic maternal thrombocytopenia
Neonatal thrombocytopenia due to isoimmunization

P61.1 Polycythemia neonatorum

P61.2 Anemia of prematurity

P61.3 Congenital anemia from fetal blood loss

P61.4 Other congenital anemias, not elsewhere classified
Congenital anemia NOS

P61.5 Transient neonatal neutropenia
Excludes 1: congenital neutropenia (nontransient) (D70.0)

P61.6 Other transient neonatal disorders of coagulation

P61.8 Other specified perinatal hematological disorders

P61.9 Perinatal hematological disorder, unspecified

TRANSITORY ENDOCRINE AND METABOLIC DISORDERS SPECIFIC TO NEWBORN (P70-P74)

Includes: transitory endocrine and metabolic disturbances caused by the infant's response to maternal endocrine and metabolic factors, or its adjustment to extrauterine environment

P70 Transitory disorders of carbohydrate metabolism specific to newborn

P70.0 Syndrome of infant of mother with gestational diabetes

Newborn (with hypoglycemia) affected by maternal gestational diabetes

Excludes 1: newborn (with hypoglycemia) affected by maternal (pre-existing) diabetes mellitus (P70.1)

syndrome of infant of a diabetic mother (P70.1)

P70.1 Syndrome of infant of a diabetic mother

Newborn (with hypoglycemia) affected by maternal (pre-existing) diabetes mellitus

Excludes 1: newborn (with hypoglycemia) affected by maternal gestational diabetes (P70.0)

syndrome of infant of mother with gestational diabetes (P70.0)

P70.2 Neonatal diabetes mellitus

P70.3 Iatrogenic neonatal hypoglycemia

P70.4 Other neonatal hypoglycemia

Transitory neonatal hypoglycemia

P70.8 Other transitory disorders of carbohydrate metabolism of newborn

P70.9 Transitory disorder of carbohydrate metabolism of newborn, unspecified

P71 Transitory neonatal disorders of calcium and magnesium metabolism

P71.0 Cow's milk hypocalcemia in newborn

P71.1 Other neonatal hypocalcemia

Excludes 1: neonatal hypoparathyroidism (P71.4)

P71.2 Neonatal hypomagnesemia

P71.3 Neonatal tetany without calcium or magnesium deficiency

Neonatal tetany NOS

P71.4 Transitory neonatal hypoparathyroidism

P71.8 Other transitory neonatal disorders of calcium and magnesium metabolism

P71.9 Transitory neonatal disorder of calcium and magnesium metabolism, unspecified

P72 Other transitory neonatal endocrine disorders

Excludes 1: congenital hypothyroidism with or without goiter (E03.0-E03.1)

dyshormogenetic goiter (E07.1)

Pendred's syndrome (E07.1)

P72.0 Neonatal goiter, not elsewhere classified

Transitory congenital goiter with normal functioning

P72.1 Transitory neonatal hyperthyroidism

Neonatal thyrotoxicosis

P72.2 Other transitory neonatal disorders of thyroid function, not elsewhere classified

Transitory neonatal hypothyroidism

P72.8 Other specified transitory neonatal endocrine disorders

P72.9 Transitory neonatal endocrine disorder, unspecified

P74 Other transitory neonatal electrolyte and metabolic disturbances

P74.0 Late metabolic acidosis of newborn

Excludes 1: (fetal) metabolic acidosis of newborn (P19)

P74.1 Dehydration of newborn

P74.2 Disturbances of sodium balance of newborn

P74.3 Disturbances of potassium balance of newborn

P74.4 Other transitory electrolyte disturbances of newborn

P74.5 Transitory tyrosinemia of newborn

P74.6 Transitory hyperammonemia of newborn

P74.8 Other transitory metabolic disturbances of newborn

Amino-acid metabolic disorders described as transitory

P74.9 Transitory metabolic disturbance of newborn, unspecified

DIGESTIVE SYSTEM DISORDERS OF NEWBORN (P76-P78)

P76 Other intestinal obstruction of newborn

P76.0 Meconium plug syndrome

Meconium ileus NOS

Excludes 1: meconium ileus in cystic fibrosis (E84.11)

P76.1 Transitory ileus of newborn

Excludes 1: Hirschsprung's disease (Q43.1)

P76.2 Intestinal obstruction due to inspissated milk

P76.8 Other specified intestinal obstruction of newborn

Excludes 1: intestinal obstruction classifiable to K56.-

P76.9 Intestinal obstruction of newborn, unspecified

P77 Necrotizing enterocolitis of newborn

P77.1 Stage 1 necrotizing enterocolitis in newborn

Necrotizing enterocolitis without pneumatosis, without perforation

P77.2 Stage 2 necrotizing enterocolitis in newborn

Necrotizing enterocolitis with pneumatosis, without perforation

P77.3 Stage 3 necrotizing enterocolitis in newborn

Necrotizing enterocolitis with perforation

Necrotizing enterocolitis with pneumatosis and perforation

P77.9 Necrotizing enterocolitis in newborn, unspecified

Necrotizing enterocolitis in newborn, NOS

P78 Other perinatal digestive system disorders

Excludes 1: cystic fibrosis (E84.0-E84.9)

neonatal gastrointestinal hemorrhages (P54.0-P54.3)

P78.0 Perinatal intestinal perforation

Meconium peritonitis

P78.1 Other neonatal peritonitis

Neonatal peritonitis NOS

P78.2 Neonatal hematemesis and melena due to swallowed maternal blood

P78.3 Noninfective neonatal diarrhea

Neonatal diarrhea NOS

P78.8 Other specified perinatal digestive system disorders

P78.81 Congenital cirrhosis (of liver)

P78.82 Peptic ulcer of newborn

P78.83 Newborn esophageal reflux

Neonatal esophageal reflux

P78.89 Other specified perinatal digestive system disorders

P78.9 Perinatal digestive system disorder, unspecified

CONDITIONS INVOLVING THE INTEGUMENT AND TEMPERATURE REGULATION OF NEWBORN (P80-P83)

P80 Hypothermia of newborn

P80.0 Cold injury syndrome

Severe and usually chronic hypothermia associated with a pink flushed appearance, edema and neurological and biochemical abnormalities.

Excludes 1: mild hypothermia of newborn (P80.8)

P80.8 Other hypothermia of newborn

Mild hypothermia of newborn

P80.9 Hypothermia of newborn, unspecified

P81 Other disturbances of temperature regulation of newborn

P81.0 Environmental hyperthermia of newborn

P81.8 Other specified disturbances of temperature regulation of newborn

P81.9 Disturbance of temperature regulation of newborn, unspecified

Fever of newborn NOS

P83 Other conditions of integument specific to newborn

Excludes 1: congenital malformations of skin and integument (Q80-Q84)

hydrops fetalis due to hemolytic disease (P56.-)

neonatal skin infection (P39.4)

staphylococcal scalded skin syndrome (L00)

Excludes 2: cradle cap (L21.0)

diaper [napkin] dermatitis (L22)

P83.0 Sclerema neonatorum

P83.1 Neonatal erythema toxicum

P83.2 Hydrops fetalis not due to hemolytic disease

Hydrops fetalis NOS

P83.3 Other and unspecified edema specific to newborn

P83.30 Unspecified edema specific to newborn

P83.39 Other edema specific to newborn

P83.4 Breast engorgement of newborn

Noninfective mastitis of newborn

P83.5 Congenital hydrocele

P83.6 Umbilical polyp of newborn

P83.8 Other specified conditions of integument specific to newborn

Bronze baby syndrome

Neonatal scleroderma

Urticaria neonatorum

P83.9 Condition of the integument specific to newborn, unspecified

OTHER PROBLEMS WITH NEWBORN (P84)

P84 Other problems with newborn

Acidemia of newborn

Acidosis of newborn

Anoxia of newborn NOS

Asphyxia of newborn NOS

Hypercapnia of newborn

Hypoxemia of newborn

Hypoxia of newborn NOS

Mixed metabolic and respiratory acidosis of newborn

Excludes 1: intracranial hemorrhage due to anoxia or hypoxia (P52.-)

hypoxic ischemic encephalopathy [HIE] (P91.6-)

late metabolic acidosis of newborn (P74.0)

Other disorders originating in the perinatal period (P90-P96)

P90 Convulsions of newborn

Excludes 1: benign myoclonic epilepsy in infancy (G40.3-)

benign neonatal convulsions (familial) (G40.3-)

P91 Other disturbances of cerebral status of newborn

P91.0 Neonatal cerebral ischemia

P91.1 Acquired periventricular cysts of newborn

P91.2 Neonatal cerebral leukomalacia

Periventricular leukomalacia

P91.3 Neonatal cerebral irritability

P91.4 Neonatal cerebral depression

P91.5 Neonatal coma

P91.6 Hypoxic ischemic encephalopathy [HIE]

P91.60 Hypoxic ischemic encephalopathy [HIE], unspecified

P91.61 Mild hypoxic ischemic encephalopathy [HIE]

P91.62 Moderate hypoxic ischemic encephalopathy [HIE]

P91.63 Severe hypoxic ischemic encephalopathy [HIE]

P91.8 Other specified disturbances of cerebral status of newborn

P91.9 Disturbance of cerebral status of newborn, unspecified

P92 Feeding problems of newborn

Excludes 1: feeding problems in child over 28 days old (R63.3)

P92.0 Vomiting of newborn

Excludes 1: vomiting of child over 28 days old (R11.-)

P92.01 Bilious vomiting of newborn

Excludes 1: bilious vomiting in child over 28 days old (R11.4)

P92.09 Other vomiting of newborn

Excludes 1: regurgitation of food in newborn (P92.1)

P92.1 Regurgitation and rumination of newborn

P92.2 Slow feeding of newborn

P92.3 Underfeeding of newborn

P92.4 Overfeeding of newborn

P92.5 Neonatal difficulty in feeding at breast

P92.6 Failure to thrive in newborn

Excludes 1: failure to thrive in child over 28 days old (R62.51)

P92.8 Other feeding problems of newborn

P92.9 Feeding problem of newborn, unspecified

P93 Reactions and intoxications due to drugs administered to newborn

Includes: reactions and intoxications due to drugs administered to fetus affecting newborn

Excludes 1: jaundice due to drugs or toxins transmitted from mother or given to newborn (P58.4-)

reactions and intoxications from maternal opiates, tranquilizers and other medication (P04.0-P04.1, P04.4)

withdrawal symptoms from maternal use of drugs of addiction (P96.1)

withdrawal symptoms from therapeutic use of drugs in newborn (P96.2)

P93.0 Grey baby syndrome

Grey syndrome from chloramphenicol administration in newborn

P93.8 Other reactions and intoxications due to drugs administered to newborn

Use additional code for adverse effect, if applicable, to identify drug (T36-T50 with fifth or sixth character 5)

P94 Disorders of muscle tone of newborn

P94.0 Transient neonatal myasthenia gravis

Excludes 1: myasthenia gravis (G70.0)

P94.1 Congenital hypertonia

P94.2 Congenital hypotonia

Floppy baby syndrome, unspecified

P94.8 Other disorders of muscle tone of newborn

P94.9 Disorder of muscle tone of newborn, unspecified

P95 Stillbirth

Dead born fetus NOS

Fetal death of unspecified cause

Stillbirth NOS

Excludes 1: maternal care for intrauterine death (O36.4)

missed abortion (O02.1)

outcome of delivery, stillbirth (Z37.1, Z37.3, Z37.4, Z37.7)

P96 Other conditions originating in the perinatal period

P96.0 Congenital renal failure
Uremia of newborn

P96.1 Neonatal withdrawal symptoms from maternal use of drugs of addiction
Drug withdrawal syndrome in infant of dependent mother
Neonatal abstinence syndrome
Excludes 1: reactions and intoxications from maternal opiates and tranquilizers administered during labor and delivery (P04.0)

P96.2 Withdrawal symptoms from therapeutic use of drugs in newborn

P96.3 Wide cranial sutures of newborn
Neonatal craniotabes

P96.5 Complication to newborn due to (fetal) intrauterine procedure
Excludes 2: newborn (suspected to be) affected by amniocentesis (P00.6)

P96.8 Other specified conditions originating in the perinatal period

    P96.81 Exposure to (parental) (environmental) tobacco smoke in the perinatal period
        Excludes 2: newborn affected by in utero exposure to tobacco (P04.2)
            exposure to environmental tobacco smoke after the perinatal period (Z77.22)

    P96.82 Delayed separation of umbilical cord

    P96.83 Meconium staining
        Excludes 1: meconium aspiration (P24.00, P24.01)
            meconium passage during delivery (P03.82)

    P96.89 Other specified conditions originating in the perinatal period
        Use additional code to specify condition

P96.9 Condition originating in the perinatal period, unspecified
Congenital debility NOS

● New code   ▲ Revised code   ⑦ 7ᵗʰ digit required   ⊗ Placeholder required

Chapter 17: Congenital Malformations, Deformations And Chromosomal Abnormalities (Q00-Q99)

Note: Codes from this chapter are not for use on maternal or fetal records

Excludes 2: inborn errors of metabolism (E70-E88)

This chapter contains the following blocks:

Q00-Q07	Congenital malformations of the nervous system
Q10-Q18	Congenital malformations of eye, ear, face and neck
Q20-Q28	Congenital malformations of the circulatory system
Q30-Q34	Congenital malformations of the respiratory system
Q35-Q37	Cleft lip and cleft palate
Q38-Q45	Other congenital malformations of the digestive system
Q50-Q56	Congenital malformations of genital organs
Q60-Q64	Congenital malformations of the urinary system
Q65-Q79	Congenital malformations and deformations of the musculoskeletal system
Q80-Q89	Other congenital malformations
Q90-Q99	Chromosomal abnormalities, not elsewhere classified

CONGENITAL MALFORMATIONS OF THE NERVOUS SYSTEM (Q00-Q07)

Q00 Anencephaly and similar malformations

- Q00.0   Anencephaly
  - Acephaly
  - Acrania
  - Amyelencephaly
  - Hemianencephaly
  - Hemicephaly
- Q00.1   Craniorachischisis
- Q00.2   Iniencephaly

Q01 Encephalocele

Includes: Arnold-Chiari syndrome, type III
- encephalocystocele
- encephalomyelocele
- hydroencephalocele
- hydromeningocele, cranial
- meningocele, cerebral
- meningoencephalocele

Excludes 1: Meckel-Gruber syndrome (Q61.9)
- Q01.0   Frontal encephalocele
- Q01.1   Nasofrontal encephalocele
- Q01.2   Occipital encephalocele
- Q01.8   Encephalocele of other sites
- Q01.9   Encephalocele, unspecified

Q02   Microcephaly

Includes: hydromicrocephaly
- micrencephalon

Excludes 1: Meckel-Gruber syndrome (Q61.9)

Q03 Congenital hydrocephalus

Includes: hydrocephalus in newborn

Excludes 1: Arnold-Chiari syndrome, type II (Q07.0-)
- acquired hydrocephalus (G91.-)
- hydrocephalus due to congenital toxoplasmosis (P37.1)
- hydrocephalus with spina bifida (Q05.0-Q05.4)

- Q03.0   Malformations of aqueduct of Sylvius
  - Anomaly of aqueduct of Sylvius
  - Obstruction of aqueduct of Sylvius, congenital
  - Stenosis of aqueduct of Sylvius
- Q03.1   Atresia of foramina of Magendie and Luschka
  - Dandy-Walker syndrome
- Q03.8   Other congenital hydrocephalus
- Q03.9   Congenital hydrocephalus, unspecified

Q04 Other congenital malformations of brain

Excludes 1: cyclopia (Q87.0)
- macrocephaly (Q75.3)

- Q04.0   Congenital malformations of corpus callosum
  - Agenesis of corpus callosum
- Q04.1   Arhinencephaly
- Q04.2   Holoprosencephaly
- Q04.3   Other reduction deformities of brain
  - Absence of part of brain
  - Agenesis of part of brain
  - Agyria
  - Aplasia of part of brain
  - Hydranencephaly
  - Hypoplasia of part of brain
  - Lissencephaly
  - Microgyria
  - Pachygyria

  Excludes 1: congenital malformations of corpus callosum (Q04.0)
- Q04.4   Septo-optic dysplasia of brain
- Q04.5   Megalencephaly
- Q04.6   Congenital cerebral cysts
  - Porencephaly
  - Schizencephaly

  Excludes 1: acquired porencephalic cyst (G93.0)
- Q04.8   Other specified congenital malformations of brain
  - Arnold-Chiari syndrome, type IV
  - Macrogyria
- Q04.9   Congenital malformation of brain, unspecified
  - Congenital anomaly NOS of brain
  - Congenital deformity NOS of brain
  - Congenital disease or lesion NOS of brain
  - Multiple anomalies NOS of brain, congenital

Q05 Spina bifida

Includes: hydromeningocele (spinal)
- meningocele (spinal)
- meningomyelocele
- myelocele
- myelomeningocele
- rachischisis
- spina bifida (aperta)(cystica)
- syringomyelocele

Use additional code for any associated paraplegia (paraparesis) (G82.2-)

Excludes 1: Arnold-Chiari syndrome, type II (Q07.0-)
- spina bifida occulta (Q76.0)

- Q05.0   Cervical spina bifida with hydrocephalus
- Q05.1   Thoracic spina bifida with hydrocephalus
  - Dorsal spina bifida with hydrocephalus
  - Thoracolumbar spina bifida with hydrocephalus
- Q05.2   Lumbar spina bifida with hydrocephalus
  - Lumbosacral spina bifida with hydrocephalus
- Q05.3   Sacral spina bifida with hydrocephalus
- Q05.4   Unspecified spina bifida with hydrocephalus

Q05.5 Cervical spina bifida without hydrocephalus

Q05.6 Thoracic spina bifida without hydrocephalus

Dorsal spina bifida NOS

Thoracolumbar spina bifida NOS

Q05.7 Lumbar spina bifida without hydrocephalus

Lumbosacral spina bifida NOS

Q05.8 Sacral spina bifida without hydrocephalus

Q05.9 Spina bifida, unspecified

Q06 Other congenital malformations of spinal cord

Q06.0 Amyelia

Q06.1 Hypoplasia and dysplasia of spinal cord

Atelomyelia

Myelatelia

Myelodysplasia of spinal cord

Q06.2 Diastematomyelia

Q06.3 Other congenital cauda equina malformations

Q06.4 Hydromyelia

Hydrorachis

Q06.8 Other specified congenital malformations of spinal cord

Q06.9 Congenital malformation of spinal cord, unspecified

Congenital anomaly NOS of spinal cord

Congenital deformity NOS of spinal cord

Congenital disease or lesion NOS of spinal cord

Q07 Other congenital malformations of nervous system

Excludes 2: congenital central alveolar hypoventilation syndrome (G47.35)

familial dysautonomia [Riley-Day] (G90.1)

neurofibromatosis (nonmalignant) (Q85.0-)

Q07.0 Arnold-Chiari syndrome

Arnold-Chiari syndrome, type II

Excludes 1: Arnold-Chiari syndrome, type III (Q01.-)

Arnold-Chiari syndrome, type IV (Q04.8)

Q07.00 Arnold-Chiari syndrome without spina bifida or hydrocephalus

Q07.01 Arnold-Chiari syndrome with spina bifida

Q07.02 Arnold-Chiari syndrome with hydrocephalus

Q07.03 Arnold-Chiari syndrome with spina bifida and hydrocephalus

Q07.8 Other specified congenital malformations of nervous system

Agenesis of nerve

Displacement of brachial plexus

Jaw-winking syndrome

Marcus Gunn's syndrome

Q07.9 Congenital malformation of nervous system, unspecified

Congenital anomaly NOS of nervous system

Congenital deformity NOS of nervous system

Congenital disease or lesion NOS of nervous system

CONGENITAL MALFORMATIONS OF EYE, EAR, FACE AND NECK (Q10-Q18)

Excludes 2: cleft lip and cleft palate (Q35-Q37)

congenital malformation of:

cervical spine (Q05.0, Q05.5, Q67.5, Q76.0-Q76.4)

larynx (Q31.-)

lip NEC (Q38.0)

nose (Q30.-)

parathyroid gland (Q89.2)

thyroid gland (Q89.2)

Q10 Congenital malformations of eyelid, lacrimal apparatus and orbit

Excludes 1: cryptophthalmos NOS (Q11.2)

cryptophthalmos syndrome (Q87.0)

Q10.0 Congenital ptosis

Q10.1 Congenital ectropion

Q10.2 Congenital entropion

Q10.3 Other congenital malformations of eyelid

Ablepharon

Blepharophimosis, congenital

Coloboma of eyelid

Congenital absence or agenesis of cilia

Congenital absence or agenesis of eyelid

Congenital accessory eyelid

Congenital accessory eye muscle

Congenital malformation of eyelid NOS

Q10.4 Absence and agenesis of lacrimal apparatus

Congenital absence of punctum lacrimale

Q10.5 Congenital stenosis and stricture of lacrimal duct

Q10.6 Other congenital malformations of lacrimal apparatus

Congenital malformation of lacrimal apparatus NOS

Q10.7 Congenital malformation of orbit

Q11 Anophthalmos, microphthalmos and macrophthalmos

Q11.0 Cystic eyeball

Q11.1 Other anophthalmos

Anophthalmos NOS

Agenesis of eye

Aplasia of eye

Q11.2 Microphthalmos

Cryptophthalmos NOS

Dysplasia of eye

Hypoplasia of eye

Rudimentary eye

Excludes 1: cryptophthalmos syndrome (Q87.0)

Q11.3 Macrophthalmos

Excludes 1: macrophthalmos in congenital glaucoma (Q15.0)

Q12 Congenital lens malformations

Q12.0 Congenital cataract

Q12.1 Congenital displaced lens

Q12.2 Coloboma of lens

Q12.3 Congenital aphakia

Q12.4 Spherophakia

Q12.8 Other congenital lens malformations

Microphakia

Q12.9 Congenital lens malformation, unspecified

Q13 Congenital malformations of anterior segment of eye

Q13.0 Coloboma of iris

Coloboma NOS

Q13.1 Absence of iris

Aniridia

Use additional code for associated glaucoma (H42)

Q13.2 Other congenital malformations of iris

Anisocoria, congenital

Atresia of pupil

Congenital malformation of iris NOS

Corectopia

Q13.3 Congenital corneal opacity

Q13.4 Other congenital corneal malformations

Congenital malformation of cornea NOS

● New code   ▲ Revised code   ⑦ 7th digit required   ⊗ Placeholder required

Microcornea

Peter's anomaly

Q13.5 Blue sclera

Q13.8 Other congenital malformations of anterior segment of eye

    Q13.81 Rieger's anomaly

        Use additional code for associated glaucoma (H42)

    Q13.89 Other congenital malformations of anterior segment of eye

Q13.9 Congenital malformation of anterior segment of eye, unspecified

Q14 Congenital malformations of posterior segment of eye

Excludes 2: optic nerve hypoplasia (H47.03-)

Q14.0 Congenital malformation of vitreous humor

Congenital vitreous opacity

Q14.1 Congenital malformation of retina

Congenital retinal aneurysm

Q14.2 Congenital malformation of optic disc

Coloboma of optic disc

Q14.3 Congenital malformation of choroid

Q14.8 Other congenital malformations of posterior segment of eye

Coloboma of the fundus

Q14.9 Congenital malformation of posterior segment of eye, unspecified

Q15 Other congenital malformations of eye

Excludes 1: congenital nystagmus (H55.01)

ocular albinism (E70.31-)

optic nerve hypoplasia (H47.03-)

retinitis pigmentosa (H35.52)

Q15.0 Congenital glaucoma

Axenfeld's anomaly

Buphthalmos

Glaucoma of childhood

Glaucoma of newborn

Hydrophthalmos

Keratoglobus, congenital, with glaucoma

Macrocornea with glaucoma

Macrophthalmos in congenital glaucoma

Megalocornea with glaucoma

Q15.8 Other specified congenital malformations of eye

Q15.9 Congenital malformation of eye, unspecified

Congenital anomaly of eye

Congenital deformity of eye

Q16 Congenital malformations of ear causing impairment of hearing

Excludes 1: congenital deafness (H90.-)

Q16.0 Congenital absence of (ear) auricle

Q16.1 Congenital absence, atresia and stricture of auditory canal (external)

Congenital atresia or stricture of osseous meatus

Q16.2 Absence of eustachian tube

Q16.3 Congenital malformation of ear ossicles

Congenital fusion of ear ossicles

Q16.4 Other congenital malformations of middle ear

Congenital malformation of middle ear NOS

Q16.5 Congenital malformation of inner ear

Congenital anomaly of membranous labyrinth

Congenital anomaly of organ of Corti

Q16.9 Congenital malformation of ear causing impairment of hearing, unspecified

Congenital absence of ear NOS

Q17 Other congenital malformations of ear

Excludes 1: congenital malformations of ear with impairment of hearing (Q16.0-Q16.9)

preauricular sinus (Q18.1)

Q17.0 Accessory auricle

Accessory tragus

Polyotia

Preauricular appendage or tag

Supernumerary ear

Supernumerary lobule

Q17.1 Macrotia

Q17.2 Microtia

Q17.3 Other misshapen ear

Pointed ear

Q17.4 Misplaced ear

Low-set ears

Excludes 1: cervical auricle (Q18.2)

Q17.5 Prominent ear

Bat ear

Q17.8 Other specified congenital malformations of ear

Congenital absence of lobe of ear

Q17.9 Congenital malformation of ear, unspecified

Congenital anomaly of ear NOS

Q18 Other congenital malformations of face and neck

Excludes 1: cleft lip and cleft palate (Q35-Q37)

conditions classified to Q67.0-Q67.4

congenital malformations of skull and face bones (Q75.-)

cyclopia (Q87.0)

dentofacial anomalies [including malocclusion] (M26.-)

malformation syndromes affecting facial appearance (Q87.0)

persistent thyroglossal duct (Q89.2)

Q18.0 Sinus, fistula and cyst of branchial cleft

Branchial vestige

Q18.1 Preauricular sinus and cyst

Fistula of auricle, congenital

Cervicoaural fistula

Q18.2 Other branchial cleft malformations

Branchial cleft malformation NOS

Cervical auricle

Otocephaly

Q18.3 Webbing of neck

Pterygium colli

Q18.4 Macrostomia

Q18.5 Microstomia

Q18.6 Macrocheilia

Hypertrophy of lip, congenital

Q18.7 Microcheilia

Q18.8 Other specified congenital malformations of face and neck

Medial cyst of face and neck

Medial fistula of face and neck

Medial sinus of face and neck

Q18.9 Congenital malformation of face and neck, unspecified

Congenital anomaly NOS of face and neck

CONGENITAL MALFORMATIONS OF THE CIRCULATORY SYSTEM (Q20-Q28)

Q20 Congenital malformations of cardiac chambers and connections

Excludes 1: dextrocardia with situs inversus (Q89.3)

mirror-image atrial arrangement with situs inversus (Q89.3)

Q20.0 Common arterial trunk

Persistent truncus arteriosus

Excludes 1: aortic septal defect (Q21.4)

Q20.1 Double outlet right ventricle

Taussig-Bing syndrome

Q20.2 Double outlet left ventricle

Q20.3 Discordant ventriculoarterial connection

Dextrotransposition of aorta

Transposition of great vessels (complete)

Q20.4 Double inlet ventricle

Common ventricle

Cor triloculare biatriatum

Single ventricle

Q20.5 Discordant atrioventricular connection

Corrected transposition

Levotransposition

Ventricular inversion

Q20.6 Isomerism of atrial appendages

Isomerism of atrial appendages with asplenia or polysplenia

Q20.8 Other congenital malformations of cardiac chambers and connections

Cor binoculare

Q20.9 Congenital malformation of cardiac chambers and connections, unspecified

Q21 Congenital malformations of cardiac septa

Excludes 1: acquired cardiac septal defect (I51.0)

Q21.0 Ventricular septal defect

Roger's disease

Q21.1 Atrial septal defect

Coronary sinus defect

Patent or persistent foramen ovale

Patent or persistent ostium secundum defect (type II)

Patent or persistent sinus venosus defect

Q21.2 Atrioventricular septal defect

Common atrioventricular canal

Endocardial cushion defect

Ostium primum atrial septal defect (type I)

Q21.3 Tetralogy of Fallot

Ventricular septal defect with pulmonary stenosis or atresia, dextroposition of aorta and hypertrophy of right ventricle.

Q21.4 Aortopulmonary septal defect

Aortic septal defect

Aortopulmonary window

Q21.8 Other congenital malformations of cardiac septa

Eisenmenger's defect

Pentalogy of Fallot

Excludes 1: Eisenmenger's complex (I27.8)

Eisenmenger's syndrome (I27.8)

Q21.9 Congenital malformation of cardiac septum, unspecified

Septal (heart) defect NOS

Q22 Congenital malformations of pulmonary and tricuspid valves

Q22.0 Pulmonary valve atresia

Q22.1 Congenital pulmonary valve stenosis

Q22.2 Congenital pulmonary valve insufficiency

Congenital pulmonary valve regurgitation

Q22.3 Other congenital malformations of pulmonary valve

Congenital malformation of pulmonary valve NOS

Supernumerary cusps of pulmonary valve

Q22.4 Congenital tricuspid stenosis

Congenital tricuspid atresia

Q22.5 Ebstein's anomaly

Q22.6 Hypoplastic right heart syndrome

Q22.8 Other congenital malformations of tricuspid valve

Q22.9 Congenital malformation of tricuspid valve, unspecified

Q23 Congenital malformations of aortic and mitral valves

Q23.0 Congenital stenosis of aortic valve

Congenital aortic atresia

Congenital aortic stenosis NOS

Excludes 1: congenital stenosis of aortic valve in hypoplastic left heart syndrome (Q23.4)

congenital subaortic stenosis (Q24.4)

supravalvular aortic stenosis (congenital) (Q25.3)

Q23.1 Congenital insufficiency of aortic valve

Bicuspid aortic valve

Congenital aortic insufficiency

Q23.2 Congenital mitral stenosis

Congenital mitral atresia

Q23.3 Congenital mitral insufficiency

Q23.4 Hypoplastic left heart syndrome

Q23.8 Other congenital malformations of aortic and mitral valves

Q23.9 Congenital malformation of aortic and mitral valves, unspecified

Q24 Other congenital malformations of heart

Excludes 1: endocardial fibroelastosis (I42.4)

Q24.0 Dextrocardia

Excludes 1: dextrocardia with situs inversus (Q89.3)

isomerism of atrial appendages (with asplenia or polysplenia) (Q20.6)

mirror-image atrial arrangement with situs inversus (Q89.3)

Q24.1 Levocardia

Q24.2 Cor triatriatum

Q24.3 Pulmonary infundibular stenosis

Subvalvular pulmonic stenosis

Q24.4 Congenital subaortic stenosis

Q24.5 Malformation of coronary vessels

Congenital coronary (artery) aneurysm

Q24.6 Congenital heart block

Q24.8 Other specified congenital malformations of heart

Congenital diverticulum of left ventricle

Congenital malformation of myocardium

Congenital malformation of pericardium

Malposition of heart

Uhl's disease

Q24.9 Congenital malformation of heart, unspecified

Congenital anomaly of heart

Congenital disease of heart

Q25 Congenital malformations of great arteries

Q25.0 Patent ductus arteriosus

Patent ductus Botallo

Persistent ductus arteriosus

Q25.1 Coarctation of aorta

● New code   ▲ Revised code   ⑦ 7th digit required   ⊗ Placeholder required

Coarctation of aorta (preductal) (postductal)

Q25.2 Atresia of aorta

Q25.3 Supravalvular aortic stenosis

> **Excludes 1:** congenital aortic stenosis NOS (Q23.0)
> congenital stenosis of aortic valve (Q23.0)

Q25.4 Other congenital malformations of aorta

Absence of aorta

Aneurysm of sinus of Valsalva (ruptured)

Aplasia of aorta

Congenital aneurysm of aorta

Congenital malformations of aorta

Congenital dilatation of aorta

Double aortic arch [vascular ring of aorta]

Hypoplasia of aorta

Persistent convolutions of aortic arch

Persistent right aortic arch

> **Excludes 1:** hypoplasia of aorta in hypoplastic left heart
> syndrome (Q23.4)

Q25.5 Atresia of pulmonary artery

Q25.6 Stenosis of pulmonary artery

Supravalvular pulmonary stenosis

Q25.7 Other congenital malformations of pulmonary artery

Q25.71 Coarctation of pulmonary artery

Q25.72 Congenital pulmonary arteriovenous
malformation

Congenital pulmonary arteriovenous aneurysm

Q25.79 Other congenital malformations of pulmonary
artery

Aberrant pulmonary artery

Agenesis of pulmonary artery

Congenital aneurysm of pulmonary artery

Congenital anomaly of pulmonary artery

Hypoplasia of pulmonary artery

Q25.8 Other congenital malformations of other great arteries

Q25.9 Congenital malformation of great arteries, unspecified

Q26 Congenital malformations of great veins

Q26.0 Congenital stenosis of vena cava

Congenital stenosis of vena cava (inferior)(superior)

Q26.1 Persistent left superior vena cava

Q26.2 Total anomalous pulmonary venous connection

Total anomalous pulmonary venous return [TAPVR],
subdiaphragmatic

Total anomalous pulmonary venous return [TAPVR],
supradiaphragmatic

Q26.3 Partial anomalous pulmonary venous connection

Partial anomalous pulmonary venous return

Q26.4 Anomalous pulmonary venous connection, unspecified

Q26.5 Anomalous portal venous connection

Q26.6 Portal vein-hepatic artery fistula

Q26.8 Other congenital malformations of great veins

Absence of vena cava (inferior) (superior)

Azygos continuation of inferior vena cava

Persistent left posterior cardinal vein

Scimitar syndrome

Q26.9 Congenital malformation of great vein, unspecified

Congenital anomaly of vena cava (inferior) (superior) NOS

Q27 Other congenital malformations of peripheral vascular system

> **Excludes 2:** anomalies of cerebral and precerebral vessels
> (Q28.0-Q28.3)

anomalies of coronary vessels (Q24.5)

anomalies of pulmonary artery (Q25.5-Q25.7)

congenital retinal aneurysm (Q14.1)

hemangioma and lymphangioma (D18.-)

Q27.0 Congenital absence and hypoplasia of umbilical artery

Single umbilical artery

Q27.1 Congenital renal artery stenosis

Q27.2 Other congenital malformations of renal artery

Congenital malformation of renal artery NOS

Multiple renal arteries

Q27.3 Arteriovenous malformation (peripheral)

Arteriovenous aneurysm

> **Excludes 1:** acquired arteriovenous aneurysm (I77.0)
> **Excludes 2:** arteriovenous malformation of cerebral
> vessels (Q28.2)

arteriovenous malformation of precerebral vessels (Q28.0)

Q27.30 Arteriovenous malformation, site unspecified

Q27.31 Arteriovenous malformation of vessel of upper
limb

Q27.32 Arteriovenous malformation of vessel of lower
limb

Q27.33 Arteriovenous malformation of digestive system
vessel

Q27.34 Arteriovenous malformation of renal vessel

Q27.39 Arteriovenous malformation, other site

Q27.4 Congenital phlebectasia

Q27.8 Other specified congenital malformations of peripheral
vascular system

Absence of peripheral vascular system

Atresia of peripheral vascular system

Congenital aneurysm (peripheral)

Congenital stricture, artery

Congenital varix

> **Excludes 1:** arteriovenous malformation (Q27.3-)

Q27.9 Congenital malformation of peripheral vascular system,
unspecified

Anomaly of artery or vein NOS

Q28 Other congenital malformations of circulatory system

> **Excludes 1:** congenital aneurysm NOS (Q27.8)
> congenital coronary aneurysm (Q24.5)
> ruptured cerebral arteriovenous malformation (I60.8)
> ruptured malformation of precerebral vessels (I72.0)
> **Excludes 2:** congenital peripheral aneurysm (Q27.8)
> congenital pulmonary aneurysm (Q25.79)
> congenital retinal aneurysm (Q14.1)

Q28.0 Arteriovenous malformation of precerebral vessels

Congenital arteriovenous precerebral aneurysm
(nonruptured)

Q28.1 Other malformations of precerebral vessels

Congenital malformation of precerebral vessels NOS

Congenital precerebral aneurysm (nonruptured)

Q28.2 Arteriovenous malformation of cerebral vessels

Arteriovenous malformation of brain NOS

Congenital arteriovenous cerebral aneurysm (nonruptured)

Q28.3 Other malformations of cerebral vessels

Congenital cerebral aneurysm (nonruptured)

Congenital malformation of cerebral vessels NOS

Developmental venous anomaly

Q28.8 Other specified congenital malformations of circulatory
system

Congenital aneurysm, specified site NEC

Spinal vessel anomaly

Q28.9 Congenital malformation of circulatory system, unspecified

CONGENITAL MALFORMATIONS OF THE RESPIRATORY SYSTEM (Q30-Q34)

Q30 Congenital malformations of nose

Excludes 1: congenital deviation of nasal septum (Q67.4)

Q30.0 Choanal atresia

Atresia of nares (anterior) (posterior)

Congenital stenosis of nares (anterior) (posterior)

Q30.1 Agenesis and underdevelopment of nose

Congenital absent of nose

Q30.2 Fissured, notched and cleft nose

Q30.3 Congenital perforated nasal septum

Q30.8 Other congenital malformations of nose

Accessory nose

Congenital anomaly of nasal sinus wall

Q30.9 Congenital malformation of nose, unspecified

Q31 Congenital malformations of larynx

Excludes 1: congenital laryngeal stridor NOS (P28.89)

Q31.0 Web of larynx

Glottic web of larynx

Subglottic web of larynx

Web of larynx NOS

Q31.1 Congenital subglottic stenosis

Q31.2 Laryngeal hypoplasia

Q31.3 Laryngocele

Q31.5 Congenital laryngomalacia

Q31.8 Other congenital malformations of larynx

Absence of larynx

Agenesis of larynx

Atresia of larynx

Congenital cleft thyroid cartilage

Congenital fissure of epiglottis

Congenital stenosis of larynx NEC

Posterior cleft of cricoid cartilage

Q31.9 Congenital malformation of larynx, unspecified

Q32 Congenital malformations of trachea and bronchus

Excludes 1: congenital bronchiectasis (Q33.4)

Q32.0 Congenital tracheomalacia

Q32.1 Other congenital malformations of trachea

Atresia of trachea

Congenital anomaly of tracheal cartilage

Congenital dilatation of trachea

Congenital malformation of trachea

Congenital stenosis of trachea

Congenital tracheocele

Q32.2 Congenital bronchomalacia

Q32.3 Congenital stenosis of bronchus

Q32.4 Other congenital malformations of bronchus

Absence of bronchus

Agenesis of bronchus

Atresia of bronchus

Congenital diverticulum of bronchus

Congenital malformation of bronchus NOS

Q33 Congenital malformations of lung

Q33.0 Congenital cystic lung

Congenital cystic lung disease

Congenital honeycomb lung

Congenital polycystic lung disease

Excludes 1: cystic fibrosis (E84.0)

cystic lung disease, acquired or unspecified (J98.4)

Q33.1 Accessory lobe of lung

Azygos lobe (fissured), lung

Q33.2 Sequestration of lung

Q33.3 Agenesis of lung

Congenital absence of lung (lobe)

Q33.4 Congenital bronchiectasis

Q33.5 Ectopic tissue in lung

Q33.6 Congenital hypoplasia and dysplasia of lung

Excludes 1: pulmonary hypoplasia associated with short gestation (P28.0)

Q33.8 Other congenital malformations of lung

Q33.9 Congenital malformation of lung, unspecified

Q34 Other congenital malformations of respiratory system

Excludes 2: congenital central alveolar hypoventilation syndrome (G47.35)

Q34.0 Anomaly of pleura

Q34.1 Congenital cyst of mediastinum

Q34.8 Other specified congenital malformations of respiratory system

Atresia of nasopharynx

Q34.9 Congenital malformation of respiratory system, unspecified

Congenital absence of respiratory system

Congenital anomaly of respiratory system NOS

CLEFT LIP AND CLEFT PALATE (Q35-Q37)

Use additional code to identify associated malformation of the nose (Q30.2)

Excludes 1: Robin's syndrome (Q87.0)

Q35 Cleft palate

Includes: fissure of palate

palatoschisis

Excludes 1: cleft palate with cleft lip (Q37.-)

Q35.1 Cleft hard palate

Q35.3 Cleft soft palate

Q35.5 Cleft hard palate with cleft soft palate

Q35.7 Cleft uvula

Q35.9 Cleft palate, unspecified

Cleft palate NOS

Q36 Cleft lip

Includes: cheiloschisis

congenital fissure of lip

harelip

labium leporinum

Excludes 1: cleft lip with cleft palate (Q37.-)

Q36.0 Cleft lip, bilateral

Q36.1 Cleft lip, median

Q36.9 Cleft lip, unilateral

Cleft lip NOS

Q37 Cleft palate with cleft lip

Includes: cheilopalatoschisis

Q37.0 Cleft hard palate with bilateral cleft lip

Q37.1 Cleft hard palate with unilateral cleft lip

Cleft hard palate with cleft lip NOS

Q37.2 Cleft soft palate with bilateral cleft lip

Q37.3 Cleft soft palate with unilateral cleft lip
Cleft soft palate with cleft lip NOS

Q37.4 Cleft hard and soft palate with bilateral cleft lip

Q37.5 Cleft hard and soft palate with unilateral cleft lip
Cleft hard and soft palate with cleft lip NOS

Q37.8 Unspecified cleft palate with bilateral cleft lip

Q37.9 Unspecified cleft palate with unilateral cleft lip
Cleft palate with cleft lip NOS

OTHER CONGENITAL MALFORMATIONS OF THE DIGESTIVE SYSTEM (Q38-Q45)

Q38 Other congenital malformations of tongue, mouth and pharynx
Excludes 1: dentofacial anomalies (M26.-)
macrostomia (Q18.4)
microstomia (Q18.5)

Q38.0 Congenital malformations of lips, not elsewhere classified
Congenital fistula of lip
Congenital malformation of lip NOS
Van der Woude's syndrome
Excludes 1: cleft lip (Q36.-)
cleft lip with cleft palate (Q37.-)
macrocheilia (Q18.6)
microcheilia (Q18.7)

Q38.1 Ankyloglossia
Tongue tie

Q38.2 Macroglossia
Congenital hypertrophy of tongue

Q38.3 Other congenital malformations of tongue
Aglossia
Bifid tongue
Congenital adhesion of tongue
Congenital fissure of tongue
Congenital malformation of tongue NOS
Double tongue
Hypoglossia
Hypoplasia of tongue
Microglossia

Q38.4 Congenital malformations of salivary glands and ducts
Atresia of salivary glands and ducts
Congenital absence of salivary glands and ducts
Congenital accessory salivary glands and ducts
Congenital fistula of salivary gland

Q38.5 Congenital malformations of palate, not elsewhere classified
Congenital absence of uvula
Congenital malformation of palate NOS
Congenital high arched palate
Excludes 1: cleft palate (Q35.-)
cleft palate with cleft lip (Q37.-)

Q38.6 Other congenital malformations of mouth
Congenital malformation of mouth NOS

Q38.7 Congenital pharyngeal pouch
Congenital diverticulum of pharynx
Excludes 1: pharyngeal pouch syndrome (D82.1)

Q38.8 Other congenital malformations of pharynx
Congenital malformation of pharynx NOS
Imperforate pharynx

Q39 Congenital malformations of esophagus

Q39.0 Atresia of esophagus without fistula

Atresia of esophagus NOS

Q39.1 Atresia of esophagus with tracheo-esophageal fistula
Atresia of esophagus with broncho-esophageal fistula

Q39.2 Congenital tracheo-esophageal fistula without atresia
Congenital tracheo-esophageal fistula NOS

Q39.3 Congenital stenosis and stricture of esophagus

Q39.4 Esophageal web

Q39.5 Congenital dilatation of esophagus
Congenital cardiospasm

Q39.6 Congenital diverticulum of esophagus
Congenital esophageal pouch

Q39.8 Other congenital malformations of esophagus
Congenital absence of esophagus
Congenital displacement of esophagus
Congenital duplication of esophagus

Q39.9 Congenital malformation of esophagus, unspecified

Q40 Other congenital malformations of upper alimentary tract

Q40.0 Congenital hypertrophic pyloric stenosis
Congenital or infantile constriction
Congenital or infantile hypertrophy
Congenital or infantile spasm
Congenital or infantile stenosis
Congenital or infantile stricture

Q40.1 Congenital hiatus hernia
Congenital displacement of cardia through esophageal hiatus
Excludes 1: congenital diaphragmatic hernia (Q79.0)

Q40.2 Other specified congenital malformations of stomach
Congenital displacement of stomach
Congenital diverticulum of stomach
Congenital hourglass stomach
Congenital duplication of stomach
Megalogastria
Microgastria

Q40.3 Congenital malformation of stomach, unspecified

Q40.8 Other specified congenital malformations of upper alimentary tract

Q40.9 Congenital malformation of upper alimentary tract, unspecified
Congenital anomaly of upper alimentary tract
Congenital deformity of upper alimentary tract

Q41 Congenital absence, atresia and stenosis of small intestine
Includes: congenital obstruction, occlusion or stricture of small intestine or intestine NOS
Excludes 1: cystic fibrosis with intestinal manifestation (E84.11)
meconium ileus NOS (without cystic fibrosis) (P76.0)

Q41.0 Congenital absence, atresia and stenosis of duodenum

Q41.1 Congenital absence, atresia and stenosis of jejunum
Apple peel syndrome
Imperforate jejunum

Q41.2 Congenital absence, atresia and stenosis of ileum

Q41.8 Congenital absence, atresia and stenosis of other specified parts of small intestine

Q41.9 Congenital absence, atresia and stenosis of small intestine, part unspecified
Congenital absence, atresia and stenosis of intestine NOS

Q42 Congenital absence, atresia and stenosis of large intestine
Includes: congenital obstruction, occlusion and stricture of large intestine

Q42.0 Congenital absence, atresia and stenosis of rectum with fistula

Q42.1 Congenital absence, atresia and stenosis of rectum without fistula

Imperforate rectum

Q42.2 Congenital absence, atresia and stenosis of anus with fistula

Q42.3 Congenital absence, atresia and stenosis of anus without fistula

Imperforate anus

Q42.8 Congenital absence, atresia and stenosis of other parts of large intestine

Q42.9 Congenital absence, atresia and stenosis of large intestine, part unspecified

Q43 Other congenital malformations of intestine

Q43.0 Meckel's diverticulum (displaced) (hypertrophic)

Persistent omphalomesenteric duct

Persistent vitelline duct

Q43.1 Hirschsprung's disease

Aganglionosis

Congenital (aganglionic) megacolon

Q43.2 Other congenital functional disorders of colon

Congenital dilatation of colon

Q43.3 Congenital malformations of intestinal fixation

Congenital omental, anomalous adhesions [bands]

Congenital peritoneal adhesions [bands]

Incomplete rotation of cecum and colon

Insufficient rotation of cecum and colon

Jackson's membrane

Malrotation of colon

Rotation failure of cecum and colon

Universal mesentery

Q43.4 Duplication of intestine

Q43.5 Ectopic anus

Q43.6 Congenital fistula of rectum and anus

Excludes 1: congenital fistula of anus with absence, atresia and stenosis (Q42.2)

congenital fistula of rectum with absence, atresia and stenosis (Q42.0)

congenital rectovaginal fistula (Q52.2)

congenital urethrorectal fistula (Q64.7)

pilonidal fistula or sinus (L05.-)

Q43.7 Persistent cloaca

Cloaca NOS

Q43.8 Other specified congenital malformations of intestine

Congenital blind loop syndrome

Congenital diverticulitis, colon

Congenital diverticulum, intestine

Dolichocolon

Megaloappendix

Megaloduodenum

Microcolon

Transposition of appendix

Transposition of colon

Transposition of intestine

Q43.9 Congenital malformation of intestine, unspecified

Q44 Congenital malformations of gallbladder, bile ducts and liver

Q44.0 Agenesis, aplasia and hypoplasia of gallbladder

Congenital absence of gallbladder

Q44.1 Other congenital malformations of gallbladder

Congenital malformation of gallbladder NOS

Intrahepatic gallbladder

Q44.2 Atresia of bile ducts

Q44.3 Congenital stenosis and stricture of bile ducts

Q44.4 Choledochal cyst

Q44.5 Other congenital malformations of bile ducts

Accessory hepatic duct

Biliary duct duplication

Congenital malformation of bile duct NOS

Cystic duct duplication

Q44.6 Cystic disease of liver

Fibrocystic disease of liver

Q44.7 Other congenital malformations of liver

Accessory liver

Alagille's syndrome

Congenital absence of liver

Congenital hepatomegaly

Congenital malformation of liver NOS

Q45 Other congenital malformations of digestive system

Excludes 2: congenital diaphragmatic hernia (Q79.0)

congenital hiatus hernia (Q40.1)

Q45.0 Agenesis, aplasia and hypoplasia of pancreas

Congenital absence of pancreas

Q45.1 Annular pancreas

Q45.2 Congenital pancreatic cyst

Q45.3 Other congenital malformations of pancreas and pancreatic duct

Accessory pancreas

Congenital malformation of pancreas or pancreatic duct NOS

Excludes 1: congenital diabetes mellitus (E10.-)

cystic fibrosis (E84.0-E84.9)

fibrocystic disease of pancreas (E84.-)

neonatal diabetes mellitus (P70.2)

Q45.8 Other specified congenital malformations of digestive system

Absence (complete) (partial) of alimentary tract NOS

Duplication of digestive system

Malposition, congenital of digestive system

Q45.9 Congenital malformation of digestive system, unspecified

Congenital anomaly of digestive system

Congenital deformity of digestive system

CONGENITAL MALFORMATIONS OF GENITAL ORGANS (Q50-Q56)

Excludes 1: androgen insensitivity syndrome (E34.5-)

syndromes associated with anomalies in the number and form of chromosomes (Q90-Q99)

Q50 Congenital malformations of ovaries, fallopian tubes and broad ligaments

Q50.0 Congenital absence of ovary

Excludes 1: Turner's syndrome (Q96.-)

Q50.01 Congenital absence of ovary, unilateral

Q50.02 Congenital absence of ovary, bilateral

Q50.1 Developmental ovarian cyst

Q50.2 Congenital torsion of ovary

Q50.3 Other congenital malformations of ovary

Q50.31 Accessory ovary

Q50.32 Ovarian streak

46, XX with streak gonads

Q50.39 Other congenital malformation of ovary

Congenital malformation of ovary NOS

Q50.4 Embryonic cyst of fallopian tube

Fimbrial cyst

Q50.5 Embryonic cyst of broad ligament

Epoophoron cyst

Parovarian cyst

Q50.6 Other congenital malformations of fallopian tube and broad ligament

Absence of fallopian tube and broad ligament

Accessory fallopian tube and broad ligament

Atresia of fallopian tube and broad ligament

Congenital malformation of fallopian tube or broad ligament NOS

Q51 Congenital malformations of uterus and cervix

Q51.0 Agenesis and aplasia of uterus

Congenital absence of uterus

Q51.1 Doubling of uterus with doubling of cervix and vagina

Q51.10 Doubling of uterus with doubling of cervix and vagina without obstruction

Doubling of uterus with doubling of cervix and vagina NOS

Q51.11 Doubling of uterus with doubling of cervix and vagina with obstruction

Q51.2 Other doubling of uterus

Doubling of uterus NOS

Septate uterus, complete or partial

Q51.3 Bicornate uterus

Bicornate uterus, complete or partial

Q51.4 Unicornate uterus

Unicornate uterus with or without a separate uterine horn

Uterus with only one functioning horn

Q51.5 Agenesis and aplasia of cervix

Congenital absence of cervix

Q51.6 Embryonic cyst of cervix

Q51.7 Congenital fistulae between uterus and digestive and urinary tracts

Q51.8 Other congenital malformations of uterus and cervix

Q51.81 Other congenital malformations of uterus

Q51.810 Arcuate uterus

Arcuatus uterus

Q51.811 Hypoplasia of uterus

Q51.818 Other congenital malformations of uterus

M_llerian anomaly of uterus NEC

Q51.82 Other congenital malformations of cervix

Q51.820 Cervical duplication

Q51.821 Hypoplasia of cervix

Q51.828 Other congenital malformations of cervix

Q51.9 Congenital malformation of uterus and cervix, unspecified

Q52 Other congenital malformations of female genitalia

Q52.0 Congenital absence of vagina

Vaginal agenesis, total or partial

Q52.1 Doubling of vagina

Excludes 1: doubling of vagina with doubling of uterus and cervix (Q51.1-)

Q52.10 Doubling of vagina, unspecified

Septate vagina NOS

Q52.11 Transverse vaginal septum

Q52.12 Longitudinal vaginal septum

Longitudinal vaginal septum with or without obstruction

Q52.2 Congenital rectovaginal fistula

Excludes 1: cloaca (Q43.7)

Q52.3 Imperforate hymen

Q52.4 Other congenital malformations of vagina

Canal of Nuck cyst, congenital

Congenital malformation of vagina NOS

Embryonic vaginal cyst

Gartner's duct cyst

Q52.5 Fusion of labia

Q52.6 Congenital malformation of clitoris

Q52.7 Other and unspecified congenital malformations of vulva

Q52.70 Unspecified congenital malformations of vulva

Congenital malformation of vulva NOS

Q52.71 Congenital absence of vulva

Q52.79 Other congenital malformations of vulva

Congenital cyst of vulva

Q52.8 Other specified congenital malformations of female genitalia

Q52.9 Congenital malformation of female genitalia, unspecified

Q53 Undescended and ectopic testicle

Q53.0 Ectopic testis

Q53.00 Ectopic testis, unspecified

Q53.01 Ectopic testis, unilateral

Q53.02 Ectopic testes, bilateral

Q53.1 Undescended testicle, unilateral

Q53.10 Unspecified undescended testicle, unilateral

Q53.11 Abdominal testis, unilateral

Q53.12 Ectopic perineal testis, unilateral

Q53.2 Undescended testicle, bilateral

Q53.20 Undescended testicle, unspecified, bilateral

Q53.21 Abdominal testis, bilateral

Q53.22 Ectopic perineal testis, bilateral

Q53.9 Undescended testicle, unspecified

Cryptorchism NOS

Q54 Hypospadias

Excludes 1: epispadias (Q64.0)

Q54.0 Hypospadias, balanic

Hypospadias, coronal

Hypospadias, glandular

Q54.1 Hypospadias, penile

Q54.2 Hypospadias, penoscrotal

Q54.3 Hypospadias, perineal

Q54.4 Congenital chordee

Chordee without hypospadias

Q54.8 Other hypospadias

Hypospadias with intersex state

Q54.9 Hypospadias, unspecified

Q55 Other congenital malformations of male genital organs

Excludes 1: congenital hydrocele (P83.5)

hypospadias (Q54.-)

Q55.0 Absence and aplasia of testis

Monorchism

Q55.1 Hypoplasia of testis and scrotum

Fusion of testes

Q55.2 Other and unspecified congenital malformations of testis and scrotum

    Q55.20 Unspecified congenital malformations of testis and scrotum

        Congenital malformation of testis or scrotum NOS

    Q55.21 Polyorchism

    Q55.22 Retractile testis

    Q55.23 Scrotal transposition

    Q55.29 Other congenital malformations of testis and scrotum

Q55.3 Atresia of vas deferens

    Code first any associated cystic fibrosis (E84.-)

Q55.4 Other congenital malformations of vas deferens, epididymis, seminal vesicles and prostate

    Absence or aplasia of prostate

    Absence or aplasia of spermatic cord

    Congenital malformation of vas deferens, epididymis, seminal vesicles or prostate NOS

Q55.5 Congenital absence and aplasia of penis

Q55.6 Other congenital malformations of penis

    Q55.61 Curvature of penis (lateral)

    Q55.62 Hypoplasia of penis

        Micropenis

    Q55.63 Congenital torsion of penis

        Excludes 1: acquired torsion of penis (N48.82)

    Q55.64 Hidden penis

        Buried penis

        Concealed penis

        Excludes 1: acquired buried penis (N48.83)

    Q55.69 Other congenital malformation of penis

        Congenital malformation of penis NOS

Q55.7 Congenital vasocutaneous fistula

Q55.8 Other specified congenital malformations of male genital organs

Q55.9 Congenital malformation of male genital organ, unspecified

    Congenital anomaly of male genital organ

    Congenital deformity of male genital organ

Q56 Indeterminate sex and pseudohermaphroditism

Excludes 1: 46,XX true hermaphrodite (Q99.1)

    androgen insensitivity syndrome (E34.5-)

    chimera 46,XX/46,XY true hermaphrodite (Q99.0)

    female pseudohermaphroditism with adrenocortical disorder (E25.-)

    pseudohermaphroditism with specified chromosomal anomaly (Q96-Q99)

    pure gonadal dysgenesis (Q99.1)

Q56.0 Hermaphroditism, not elsewhere classified

    Ovotestis

Q56.1 Male pseudohermaphroditism, not elsewhere classified

    46, XY with streak gonads

    Male pseudohermaphroditism NOS

Q56.2 Female pseudohermaphroditism, not elsewhere classified

    Female pseudohermaphroditism NOS

Q56.3 Pseudohermaphroditism, unspecified

Q56.4 Indeterminate sex, unspecified

    Ambiguous genitalia

CONGENITAL MALFORMATIONS OF THE URINARY SYSTEM (Q60-Q64)

Q60 Renal agenesis and other reduction defects of kidney

Includes: congenital absence of kidney

    congenital atrophy of kidney

    infantile atrophy of kidney

Q60.0 Renal agenesis, unilateral

Q60.1 Renal agenesis, bilateral

Q60.2 Renal agenesis, unspecified

Q60.3 Renal hypoplasia, unilateral

Q60.4 Renal hypoplasia, bilateral

Q60.5 Renal hypoplasia, unspecified

Q60.6 Potter's syndrome

Q61 Cystic kidney disease

Excludes 1: acquired cyst of kidney (N28.1)

    Potter's syndrome (Q60.6)

Q61.0 Congenital renal cyst

    Q61.00 Congenital renal cyst, unspecified

        Cyst of kidney NOS (congenital)

    Q61.01 Congenital single renal cyst

    Q61.02 Congenital multiple renal cysts

Q61.1 Polycystic kidney, infantile type

    Polycystic kidney, autosomal recessive

    Q61.11 Cystic dilatation of collecting ducts

    Q61.19 Other polycystic kidney, infantile type

Q61.2 Polycystic kidney, adult type

    Polycystic kidney, autosomal dominant

Q61.3 Polycystic kidney, unspecified

Q61.4 Renal dysplasia

    Multicystic dysplastic kidney

    Multicystic kidney (development)

    Multicystic kidney disease

    Multicystic renal dysplasia

    Excludes 1: polycystic kidney disease (Q61.11-Q61.3)

Q61.5 Medullary cystic kidney

    Nephronopthisis

    Sponge kidney NOS

Q61.8 Other cystic kidney diseases

    Fibrocystic kidney

    Fibrocystic renal degeneration or disease

Q61.9 Cystic kidney disease, unspecified

    Meckel-Gruber syndrome

Q62 Congenital obstructive defects of renal pelvis and congenital malformations of ureter

Q62.0 Congenital hydronephrosis

Q62.1 Congenital occlusion of ureter

    Atresia and stenosis of ureter

    Q62.10 Congenital occlusion of ureter, unspecified

    Q62.11 Congenital occlusion of ureteropelvic junction

    Q62.12 Congenital occlusion of ureterovesical orifice

Q62.2 Congenital megaureter

    Congenital dilatation of ureter

Q62.3 Other obstructive defects of renal pelvis and ureter

    Q62.31 Congenital ureterocele, orthotopic

    Q62.32 Cecoureterocele

        Ectopic ureterocele

● New code   ▲ Revised code   ⑦ 7th digit required   ⊗ Placeholder required

Q62.39 Other obstructive defects of renal pelvis and ureter

Ureteropelvic junction obstruction NOS

Q62.4 Agenesis of ureter

Congenital absence ureter

Q62.5 Duplication of ureter

Accessory ureter

Double ureter

Q62.6 Malposition of ureter

Q62.60 Malposition of ureter, unspecified

Q62.61 Deviation of ureter

Q62.62 Displacement of ureter

Q62.63 Anomalous implantation of ureter

Ectopia of ureter

Ectopic ureter

Q62.69 Other malposition of ureter

Q62.7 Congenital vesico-uretero-renal reflux

Q62.8 Other congenital malformations of ureter

Anomaly of ureter NOS

Q63 Other congenital malformations of kidney

Excludes 1: congenital nephrotic syndrome (N04.-)

Q63.0 Accessory kidney

Q63.1 Lobulated, fused and horseshoe kidney

Q63.2 Ectopic kidney

Congenital displaced kidney

Malrotation of kidney

Q63.3 Hyperplastic and giant kidney

Compensatory hypertrophy of kidney

Q63.8 Other specified congenital malformations of kidney

Congenital renal calculi

Q63.9 Congenital malformation of kidney, unspecified

Q64 Other congenital malformations of urinary system

Q64.0 Epispadias

Excludes 1: hypospadias (Q54.-)

Q64.1 Exstrophy of urinary bladder

Q64.10 Exstrophy of urinary bladder, unspecified

Ectopia vesicae

Q64.11 Supravesical fissure of urinary bladder

Q64.12 Cloacal exstrophy of urinary bladder

Q64.19 Other exstrophy of urinary bladder

Extroversion of bladder

Q64.2 Congenital posterior urethral valves

Q64.3 Other atresia and stenosis of urethra and bladder neck

Q64.31 Congenital bladder neck obstruction

Congenital obstruction of vesicourethral orifice

Q64.32 Congenital stricture of urethra

Q64.33 Congenital stricture of urinary meatus

Q64.39 Other atresia and stenosis of urethra and bladder neck

Atresia and stenosis of urethra and bladder neck NOS

Q64.4 Malformation of urachus

Cyst of urachus

Patent urachus

Prolapse of urachus

Q64.5 Congenital absence of bladder and urethra

Q64.6 Congenital diverticulum of bladder

Q64.7 Other and unspecified congenital malformations of bladder and urethra

Excludes 1: congenital prolapse of bladder (mucosa) (Q79.4)

Q64.70 Unspecified congenital malformation of bladder and urethra

Malformation of bladder or urethra NOS

Q64.71 Congenital prolapse of urethra

Q64.72 Congenital prolapse of urinary meatus

Q64.73 Congenital urethrorectal fistula

Q64.74 Double urethra

Q64.75 Double urinary meatus

Q64.79 Other congenital malformations of bladder and urethra

Q64.8 Other specified congenital malformations of urinary system

Q64.9 Congenital malformation of urinary system, unspecified

Congenital anomaly NOS of urinary system

Congenital deformity NOS of urinary system

CONGENITAL MALFORMATIONS AND DEFORMATIONS OF THE MUSCULOSKELETAL SYSTEM (Q65-Q79)

Q65 Congenital deformities of hip

Excludes 1: clicking hip (R29.4)

Q65.0 Congenital dislocation of hip, unilateral

Q65.00 Congenital dislocation of unspecified hip, unilateral

Q65.01 Congenital dislocation of right hip, unilateral

Q65.02 Congenital dislocation of left hip, unilateral

Q65.1 Congenital dislocation of hip, bilateral

Q65.2 Congenital dislocation of hip, unspecified

Q65.3 Congenital partial dislocation of hip, unilateral

Q65.30 Congenital partial dislocation of unspecified hip, unilateral

Q65.31 Congenital partial dislocation of right hip, unilateral

Q65.32 Congenital partial dislocation of left hip, unilateral

Q65.4 Congenital partial dislocation of hip, bilateral

Q65.5 Congenital partial dislocation of hip, unspecified

Q65.6 Congenital unstable hip

Congenital dislocatable hip

Q65.8 Other congenital deformities of hip

Q65.81 Congenital coxa valga

Q65.82 Congenital coxa vara

Q65.89 Other specified congenital deformities of hip

Anteversion of femoral neck

Congenital acetabular dysplasia

Q65.9 Congenital deformity of hip, unspecified

Q66 Congenital deformities of feet

Excludes 1: reduction defects of feet (Q72.-)

valgus deformities (acquired) (M21.0-)

varus deformities (acquired) (M21.1-)

Q66.0 Congenital talipes equinovarus

Q66.1 Congenital talipes calcaneovarus

Q66.2 Congenital metatarsus (primus) varus

Q66.3 Other congenital varus deformities of feet

Hallux varus, congenital

Q66.4 Congenital talipes calcaneovalgus

Q66.5 Congenital pes planus

Congenital flat foot

Congenital rigid flat foot

Congenital spastic (everted) flat foot
Excludes 1: pes planus, acquired (M21.4)
   Q66.50 Congenital pes planus, unspecified foot
   Q66.51 Congenital pes planus, right foot
   Q66.52 Congenital pes planus, left foot
Q66.6 Other congenital valgus deformities of feet
Congenital metatarsus valgus
Q66.7 Congenital pes cavus
Q66.8 Other congenital deformities of feet
   Q66.80 Congenital vertical talus deformity, unspecified foot
   Q66.81 Congenital vertical talus deformity, right foot
   Q66.82 Congenital vertical talus deformity, left foot
   Q66.89 Other specified congenital deformities of feet
     Congenital asymmetric talipes
     Congenital clubfoot NOS
     Congenital talipes NOS
     Congenital tarsal coalition
     Hammer toe, congenital
Q66.9 Congenital deformity of feet, unspecified

Q67 Congenital musculoskeletal deformities of head, face, spine and chest
Excludes 1: congenital malformation syndromes classified to Q87.-
     Potter's syndrome (Q60.6)
Q67.0 Congenital facial asymmetry
Q67.1 Congenital compression facies
Q67.2 Dolichocephaly
Q67.3 Plagiocephaly
Q67.4 Other congenital deformities of skull, face and jaw
Congenital depressions in skull
Congenital hemifacial atrophy or hypertrophy
Deviation of nasal septum, congenital
Squashed or bent nose, congenital
Excludes 1: dentofacial anomalies [including malocclusion] (M26-)
     syphilitic saddle nose (A50.5)
Q67.5 Congenital deformity of spine
Congenital postural scoliosis
Congenital scoliosis NOS
Excludes 1: infantile idiopathic scoliosis (M41.0)
     scoliosis due to congenital bony malformation (Q76.3)
Q67.6 Pectus excavatum
Congenital funnel chest
Q67.7 Pectus carinatum
Congenital pigeon chest
Q67.8 Other congenital deformities of chest
Congenital deformity of chest wall NOS
Q68 Other congenital musculoskeletal deformities
Excludes 1: reduction defects of limb(s) (Q71-Q73)
Excludes 2: congenital myotonic chondrodystrophy (G71.13)
Q68.0 Congenital deformity of sternocleidomastoid muscle
Congenital contracture of sternocleidomastoid (muscle)
Congenital (sternomastoid) torticollis
Sternomastoid tumor (congenital)
Q68.1 Congenital deformity of finger(s) and hand
Congenital clubfinger
Spade-like hand (congenital)
Q68.2 Congenital deformity of knee

Congenital dislocation of knee
Congenital genu recurvatum
Q68.3 Congenital bowing of femur
Excludes 1: anteversion of femur (neck) (Q65.89)
Q68.4 Congenital bowing of tibia and fibula
Q68.5 Congenital bowing of long bones of leg, unspecified
Q68.6 Discoid meniscus
Q68.8 Other specified congenital musculoskeletal deformities
Congenital deformity of clavicle
Congenital deformity of elbow
Congenital deformity of forearm
Congenital deformity of scapula
Congenital deformity of wrist
Congenital dislocation of elbow
Congenital dislocation of shoulder
Congenital dislocation of wrist
Q69 Polydactyly
Q69.0 Accessory finger(s)
Q69.1 Accessory thumb(s)
Q69.2 Accessory toe(s)
Accessory hallux
Q69.9 Polydactyly, unspecified
Supernumerary digit(s) NOS
Q70 Syndactyly
Q70.0 Fused fingers
Complex syndactyly of fingers with synostosis
   Q70.00 Fused fingers, unspecified hand
   Q70.01 Fused fingers, right hand
   Q70.02 Fused fingers, left hand
   Q70.03 Fused fingers, bilateral
Q70.1 Webbed fingers
Simple syndactyly of fingers without synostosis
   Q70.10 Webbed fingers, unspecified hand
   Q70.11 Webbed fingers, right hand
   Q70.12 Webbed fingers, left hand
   Q70.13 Webbed fingers, bilateral
Q70.2 Fused toes
Complex syndactyly of toes with synostosis
   Q70.20 Fused toes, unspecified foot
   Q70.21 Fused toes, right foot
   Q70.22 Fused toes, left foot
   Q70.23 Fused toes, bilateral
Q70.3 Webbed toes
Simple syndactyly of toes without synostosis
   Q70.30 Webbed toes, unspecified foot
   Q70.31 Webbed toes, right foot
   Q70.32 Webbed toes, left foot
   Q70.33 Webbed toes, bilateral
Q70.4 Polysyndactyly, unspecified
Excludes 1: specified syndactyly of hand and feet - code to specified conditions (Q70.0- - Q70.3-)
Q70.9 Syndactyly, unspecified
Symphalangy NOS
Q71 Reduction defects of upper limb
Q71.0 Congenital complete absence of upper limb
   Q71.00 Congenital complete absence of unspecified upper limb
   Q71.01 Congenital complete absence of right upper limb

CONGENITAL MALFORMATIONS, DEFORMATIONS AND CHROMOSOMAL ABNORMALITIES

Q71.02 Congenital complete absence of left upper limb

Q71.03 Congenital complete absence of upper limb, bilateral

Q71.1 Congenital absence of upper arm and forearm with hand present

Q71.10 Congenital absence of unspecified upper arm and forearm with hand present

Q71.11 Congenital absence of right upper arm and forearm with hand present

Q71.12 Congenital absence of left upper arm and forearm with hand present

Q71.13 Congenital absence of upper arm and forearm with hand present, bilateral

Q71.2 Congenital absence of both forearm and hand

Q71.20 Congenital absence of both forearm and hand, unspecified upper limb

Q71.21 Congenital absence of both forearm and hand, right upper limb

Q71.22 Congenital absence of both forearm and hand, left upper limb

Q71.23 Congenital absence of both forearm and hand, bilateral

Q71.3 Congenital absence of hand and finger

Q71.30 Congenital absence of unspecified hand and finger

Q71.31 Congenital absence of right hand and finger

Q71.32 Congenital absence of left hand and finger

Q71.33 Congenital absence of hand and finger, bilateral

Q71.4 Longitudinal reduction defect of radius

Clubhand (congenital)

Radial clubhand

Q71.40 Longitudinal reduction defect of unspecified radius

Q71.41 Longitudinal reduction defect of right radius

Q71.42 Longitudinal reduction defect of left radius

Q71.43 Longitudinal reduction defect of radius, bilateral

Q71.5 Longitudinal reduction defect of ulna

Q71.50 Longitudinal reduction defect of unspecified ulna

Q71.51 Longitudinal reduction defect of right ulna

Q71.52 Longitudinal reduction defect of left ulna

Q71.53 Longitudinal reduction defect of ulna, bilateral

Q71.6 Lobster-claw hand

Q71.60 Lobster-claw hand, unspecified hand

Q71.61 Lobster-claw right hand

Q71.62 Lobster-claw left hand

Q71.63 Lobster-claw hand, bilateral

Q71.8 Other reduction defects of upper limb

Q71.81 Congenital shortening of upper limb

Q71.811 Congenital shortening of right upper limb

Q71.812 Congenital shortening of left upper limb

Q71.813 Congenital shortening of upper limb, bilateral

Q71.819 Congenital shortening of unspecified upper limb

Q71.89 Other reduction defects of upper limb

Q71.891 Other reduction defects of right upper limb

Q71.892 Other reduction defects of left upper limb

Q71.893 Other reduction defects of upper limb, bilateral

Q71.899 Other reduction defects of unspecified upper limb

Q71.9 Unspecified reduction defect of upper limb

Q71.90 Unspecified reduction defect of unspecified upper limb

Q71.91 Unspecified reduction defect of right upper limb

Q71.92 Unspecified reduction defect of left upper limb

Q71.93 Unspecified reduction defect of upper limb, bilateral

Q72 Reduction defects of lower limb

Q72.0 Congenital complete absence of lower limb

Q72.00 Congenital complete absence of unspecified lower limb

Q72.01 Congenital complete absence of right lower limb

Q72.02 Congenital complete absence of left lower limb

Q72.03 Congenital complete absence of lower limb, bilateral

Q72.1 Congenital absence of thigh and lower leg with foot present

Q72.10 Congenital absence of unspecified thigh and lower leg with foot present

Q72.11 Congenital absence of right thigh and lower leg with foot present

Q72.12 Congenital absence of left thigh and lower leg with foot present

Q72.13 Congenital absence of thigh and lower leg with foot present, bilateral

Q72.2 Congenital absence of both lower leg and foot

Q72.20 Congenital absence of both lower leg and foot, unspecified lower limb

Q72.21 Congenital absence of both lower leg and foot, right lower limb

Q72.22 Congenital absence of both lower leg and foot, left lower limb

Q72.23 Congenital absence of both lower leg and foot, bilateral

Q72.3 Congenital absence of foot and toe(s)

Q72.30 Congenital absence of unspecified foot and toe(s)

Q72.31 Congenital absence of right foot and toe(s)

Q72.32 Congenital absence of left foot and toe(s)

Q72.33 Congenital absence of foot and toe(s), bilateral

Q72.4 Longitudinal reduction defect of femur

Proximal femoral focal deficiency

Q72.40 Longitudinal reduction defect of unspecified femur

Q72.41 Longitudinal reduction defect of right femur

Q72.42 Longitudinal reduction defect of left femur

Q72.43 Longitudinal reduction defect of femur, bilateral

Q72.5 Longitudinal reduction defect of tibia

Q72.50 Longitudinal reduction defect of unspecified tibia

Q72.51 Longitudinal reduction defect of right tibia

Q72.52 Longitudinal reduction defect of left tibia

Q72.53 Longitudinal reduction defect of tibia, bilateral

Q72.6 Longitudinal reduction defect of fibula

Q72.60 Longitudinal reduction defect of unspecified fibula

Add 4th-7th digits   3 digit reportable   Nonspecific code   Unspecified code   Manifestation code   555

Q72.61   Longitudinal reduction defect of right fibula

Q72.62   Longitudinal reduction defect of left fibula

Q72.63   Longitudinal reduction defect of fibula, bilateral

Q72.7   Split foot

   Q72.70   Split foot, unspecified lower limb

   Q72.71   Split foot, right lower limb

   Q72.72   Split foot, left lower limb

   Q72.73   Split foot, bilateral

Q72.8   Other reduction defects of lower limb

   Q72.81   Congenital shortening of lower limb

      Q72.811   Congenital shortening of right lower limb

      Q72.812   Congenital shortening of left lower limb

      Q72.813   Congenital shortening of lower limb, bilateral

      Q72.819   Congenital shortening of unspecified lower limb

   Q72.89   Other reduction defects of lower limb

      Q72.891   Other reduction defects of right lower limb

      Q72.892   Other reduction defects of left lower limb

      Q72.893   Other reduction defects of lower limb, bilateral

      Q72.899   Other reduction defects of unspecified lower limb

Q72.9   Unspecified reduction defect of lower limb

   Q72.90   Unspecified reduction defect of unspecified lower limb

   Q72.91   Unspecified reduction defect of right lower limb

   Q72.92   Unspecified reduction defect of left lower limb

   Q72.93   Unspecified reduction defect of lower limb, bilateral

Q73   Reduction defects of unspecified limb

Q73.0   Congenital absence of unspecified limb(s)

   Amelia NOS

Q73.1   Phocomelia, unspecified limb(s)

   Phocomelia NOS

Q73.8   Other reduction defects of unspecified limb(s)

   Longitudinal reduction deformity of unspecified limb(s)

   Ectromelia of limb NOS

   Hemimelia of limb NOS

   Reduction defect of limb NOS

Q74   Other congenital malformations of limb(s)

Excludes 1: polydactyly (Q69.-)

   reduction defect of limb (Q71-Q73)

   syndactyly (Q70.-)

Q74.0   Other congenital malformations of upper limb(s), including shoulder girdle

   Accessory carpal bones

   Cleidocranial dysostosis

   Congenital pseudarthrosis of clavicle

   Macrodactylia (fingers)

   Madelung's deformity

   Radioulnar synostosis

   Sprengel's deformity

   Triphalangeal thumb

Q74.1   Congenital malformation of knee

   Congenital absence of patella

   Congenital dislocation of patella

   Congenital genu valgum

   Congenital genu varum

   Rudimentary patella

   Excludes 1: congenital dislocation of knee (Q68.2)

      congenital genu recurvatum (Q68.2)

      nail patella syndrome (Q87.2)

Q74.2   Other congenital malformations of lower limb(s), including pelvic girdle

   Congenital fusion of sacroiliac joint

   Congenital malformation of ankle joint

   Congenital malformation of sacroiliac joint

   Excludes 1: anteversion of femur (neck) (Q65.89)

Q74.3   Arthrogryposis multiplex congenita

Q74.8   Other specified congenital malformations of limb(s)

Q74.9   Unspecified congenital malformation of limb(s)

   Congenital anomaly of limb(s) NOS

Q75   Other congenital malformations of skull and face bones

Excludes 1: congenital malformation of face NOS (Q18.-)

   congenital malformation syndromes classified to Q87.-

   dentofacial anomalies [including malocclusion] (M26.-)

   musculoskeletal deformities of head and face (Q67.0-Q67.4)

   skull defects associated with congenital anomalies of brain such as:

   anencephaly (Q00.0)

   encephalocele (Q01.-)

   hydrocephalus (Q03.-)

   microcephaly (Q02)

Q75.0   Craniosynostosis

   Acrocephaly

   Imperfect fusion of skull

   Oxycephaly

   Trigonocephaly

Q75.1   Craniofacial dysostosis

   Crouzon's disease

Q75.2   Hypertelorism

Q75.3   Macrocephaly

Q75.4   Mandibulofacial dysostosis

   Franceschetti syndrome

   Treacher Collins syndrome

Q75.5   Oculomandibular dysostosis

Q75.8   Other specified congenital malformations of skull and face bones

   Absence of skull bone, congenital

   Congenital deformity of forehead

   Platybasia

Q75.9   Congenital malformation of skull and face bones, unspecified

   Congenital anomaly of face bones NOS

   Congenital anomaly of skull NOS

Q76   Congenital malformations of spine and bony thorax

Excludes 1: congenital musculoskeletal deformities of spine and chest (Q67.5-Q67.8)

Q76.0   Spina bifida occulta

   Excludes 1: meningocele (spinal) (Q05.-)

      spina bifida (aperta) (cystica) (Q05.-)

Q76.1   Klippel-Feil syndrome

Cervical fusion syndrome

Q76.2 Congenital spondylolisthesis

Congenital spondylolysis

Excludes 1: spondylolisthesis (acquired) (M43.1-)

spondylolysis (acquired) (M43.0-)

Q76.3 Congenital scoliosis due to congenital bony malformation

Hemivertebra fusion or failure of segmentation with scoliosis

Q76.4 Other congenital malformations of spine, not associated with scoliosis

Q76.41 Congenital kyphosis

Q76.411 Congenital kyphosis, occipito-atlanto-axial region

Q76.412 Congenital kyphosis, cervical region

Q76.413 Congenital kyphosis, cervicothoracic region

Q76.414 Congenital kyphosis, thoracic region

Q76.415 Congenital kyphosis, thoracolumbar region

Q76.419 Congenital kyphosis, unspecified region

Q76.42 Congenital lordosis

Q76.425 Congenital lordosis, thoracolumbar region

Q76.426 Congenital lordosis, lumbar region

Q76.427 Congenital lordosis, lumbosacral region

Q76.428 Congenital lordosis, sacral and sacrococcygeal region

Q76.429 Congenital lordosis, unspecified region

Q76.49 Other congenital malformations of spine, not associated with scoliosis

Congenital absence of vertebra NOS

Congenital fusion of spine NOS

Congenital malformation of lumbosacral (joint) (region) NOS

Congenital malformation of spine NOS

Hemivertebra NOS

Malformation of spine NOS

Platyspondylisis NOS

Supernumerary vertebra NOS

Q76.5 Cervical rib

Supernumerary rib in cervical region

Q76.6 Other congenital malformations of ribs

Accessory rib

Congenital absence of rib

Congenital fusion of ribs

Congenital malformation of ribs NOS

Excludes 1: short rib syndrome (Q77.2)

Q76.7 Congenital malformation of sternum

Congenital absence of sternum

Sternum bifidum

Q76.8 Other congenital malformations of bony thorax

Q76.9 Congenital malformation of bony thorax, unspecified

Q77 Osteochondrodysplasia with defects of growth of tubular bones and spine

Excludes 1: mucopolysaccharidosis (E76.0-E76.3)

Excludes 2: congenital myotonic chondrodystrophy (G71.13)

Q77.0 Achondrogenesis

Hypochondrogenesis

Q77.1 Thanatophoric short stature

Q77.2 Short rib syndrome

Asphyxiating thoracic dysplasia [Jeune]

Q77.3 Chondrodysplasia punctata

Excludes 1: Rhizomelic chondrodysplasia punctata (E71.43)

Q77.4 Achondroplasia

Hypochondroplasia

Osteosclerosis congenita

Q77.5 Diastrophic dysplasia

Q77.6 Chondroectodermal dysplasia

Ellis-van Creveld syndrome

Q77.7 Spondyloepiphyseal dysplasia

Q77.8 Other osteochondrodysplasia with defects of growth of tubular bones and spine

Q77.9 Osteochondrodysplasia with defects of growth of tubular bones and spine, unspecified

Q78 Other osteochondrodysplasias

Excludes 2: congenital myotonic chondrodystrophy (G71.13)

Q78.0 Osteogenesis imperfecta

Fragilitas ossium

Osteopsathyrosis

Q78.1 Polyostotic fibrous dysplasia

Albright(-McCune)(-Sternberg) syndrome

Q78.2 Osteopetrosis

Albers-Sch÷nberg syndrome

Osteosclerosis NOS

Q78.3 Progressive diaphyseal dysplasia

Camurati-Engelmann syndrome

Q78.4 Enchondromatosis

Maffucci's syndrome

Ollier's disease

Q78.5 Metaphyseal dysplasia

Pyle's syndrome

Q78.6 Multiple congenital exostoses

Diaphyseal aclasis

Q78.8 Other specified osteochondrodysplasias

Osteopoikilosis

Q78.9 Osteochondrodysplasia, unspecified

Chondrodystrophy NOS

Osteodystrophy NOS

Q79 Congenital malformations of musculoskeletal system, not elsewhere classified

Excludes 2: congenital (sternomastoid) torticollis (Q68.0)

Q79.0 Congenital diaphragmatic hernia

Excludes 1: congenital hiatus hernia (Q40.1)

Q79.1 Other congenital malformations of diaphragm

Absence of diaphragm

Congenital malformation of diaphragm NOS

Eventration of diaphragm

Q79.2 Exomphalos

Omphalocele

Excludes 1: umbilical hernia (K42.-)

Q79.3 Gastroschisis

Q79.4 Prune belly syndrome

Congenital prolapse of bladder mucosa

Eagle-Barrett syndrome

Q79.5 Other congenital malformations of abdominal wall

Excludes 1: umbilical hernia (K42.-)

Q79.51 Congenital hernia of bladder

Q79.59 Other congenital malformations of abdominal wall

Q79.6 Ehlers-Danlos syndrome

Q79.8 Other congenital malformations of musculoskeletal system

Absence of muscle

Absence of tendon

Accessory muscle

Amyotrophia congenita

Congenital constricting bands

Congenital shortening of tendon

Poland syndrome

Q79.9 Congenital malformation of musculoskeletal system, unspecified

Congenital anomaly of musculoskeletal system NOS

Congenital deformity of musculoskeletal system NOS

OTHER CONGENITAL MALFORMATIONS (Q80-Q89)

Q80 Congenital ichthyosis

Excludes 1: Refsum's disease (G60.1)

Q80.0 Ichthyosis vulgaris

Q80.1 X-linked ichthyosis

Q80.2 Lamellar ichthyosis

Collodion baby

Q80.3 Congenital bullous ichthyosiform erythroderma

Q80.4 Harlequin fetus

Q80.8 Other congenital ichthyosis

Q80.9 Congenital ichthyosis, unspecified

Q81 Epidermolysis bullosa

Q81.0 Epidermolysis bullosa simplex

Excludes 1: Cockayne's syndrome (Q87.1)

Q81.1 Epidermolysis bullosa letalis

Herlitz' syndrome

Q81.2 Epidermolysis bullosa dystrophica

Q81.8 Other epidermolysis bullosa

Q81.9 Epidermolysis bullosa, unspecified

Q82 Other congenital malformations of skin

Excludes 1: acrodermatitis enteropathica (E83.2)

congenital erythropoietic porphyria (E80.0)

pilonidal cyst or sinus (L05.-)

Sturge-Weber (-Dimitri) syndrome (Q85.8)

Q82.0 Hereditary lymphedema

Q82.1 Xeroderma pigmentosum

Q82.2 Mastocytosis

Urticaria pigmentosa

Excludes 1: malignant mastocytosis (C96.2)

Q82.3 Incontinentia pigmenti

Q82.4 Ectodermal dysplasia (anhidrotic)

Excludes 1: Ellis-van Creveld syndrome (Q77.6)

Q82.5 Congenital non-neoplastic nevus

Birthmark NOS

Flammeus Nevus

Portwine Nevus

Sanguineous Nevus

Strawberry Nevus

Vascular Nevus NOS

Verrucous Nevus

Excludes 2: CafΘ au lait spots (L81.3)

lentigo (L81.4)

nevus NOS (D22.-)

araneus nevus (I78.1)

melanocytic nevus (D22.-)

pigmented nevus (D22.-)

spider nevus (I78.1)

stellar nevus (I78.1)

Q82.8 Other specified congenital malformations of skin

Abnormal palmar creases

Accessory skin tags

Benign familial pemphigus [Hailey-Hailey]

Congenital poikiloderma

Cutis laxa (hyperelastica)

Dermatoglyphic anomalies

Inherited keratosis palmaris et plantaris

Keratosis follicularis [Darier-White]

Excludes 1: Ehlers-Danlos syndrome (Q79.6)

Q82.9 Congenital malformation of skin, unspecified

Q83 Congenital malformations of breast

Excludes 2: absence of pectoral muscle (Q79.8)

hypoplasia of breast (N64.82)

micromastia (N64.82)

Q83.0 Congenital absence of breast with absent nipple

Q83.1 Accessory breast

Supernumerary breast

Q83.2 Absent nipple

Q83.3 Accessory nipple

Supernumerary nipple

Q83.8 Other congenital malformations of breast

Q83.9 Congenital malformation of breast, unspecified

Q84 Other congenital malformations of integument

Q84.0 Congenital alopecia

Congenital atrichosis

Q84.1 Congenital morphological disturbances of hair, not elsewhere classified

Beaded hair

Monilethrix

Pili annulati

Excludes 1: Menkes' kinky hair syndrome (E83.0)

Q84.2 Other congenital malformations of hair

Congenital hypertrichosis

Congenital malformation of hair NOS

Persistent lanugo

Q84.3 Anonychia

Excludes 1: nail patella syndrome (Q87.2)

Q84.4 Congenital leukonychia

Q84.5 Enlarged and hypertrophic nails

Congenital onychauxis

Pachyonychia

Q84.6 Other congenital malformations of nails

Congenital clubnail

Congenital koilonychia

Congenital malformation of nail NOS

Q84.8 Other specified congenital malformations of integument

Aplasia cutis congenita

Q84.9 Congenital malformation of integument, unspecified

Congenital anomaly of integument NOS

● New code   ▲ Revised code   ⑦ 7th digit required   ⊗ Placeholder required

Congenital deformity of integument NOS

Q85 Phakomatoses, not elsewhere classified

Excludes 1: ataxia telangiectasia [Louis-Bar] (G11.3)

familial dysautonomia [Riley-Day] (G90.1)

Q85.0 Neurofibromatosis (nonmalignant)

Q85.00 Neurofibromatosis, unspecified

Q85.01 Neurofibromatosis, type 1

Von Recklinghausen disease

Q85.02 Neurofibromatosis, type 2

Acoustic neurofibromatosis

Q85.03 Schwannomatosis

Q85.09 Other neurofibromatosis

Q85.1 Tuberous sclerosis

Bourneville's disease

Epiloia

Q85.8 Other phakomatoses, not elsewhere classified

Peutz-Jeghers Syndrome

Sturge-Weber(-Dimitri) syndrome

von Hippel-Lindau syndrome

Excludes 1: Meckel-Gruber syndrome (Q61.9)

Q85.9 Phakomatosis, unspecified

Hamartosis NOS

Q86 Congenital malformation syndromes due to known exogenous causes, not elsewhere classified

Excludes 2: iodine-deficiency-related hypothyroidism (E00-E02)

nonteratogenic effects of substances transmitted via placenta or breast milk (P04.-)

Q86.0 Fetal alcohol syndrome (dysmorphic)

Q86.1 Fetal hydantoin syndrome

Meadow's syndrome

Q86.2 Dysmorphism due to warfarin

Q86.8 Other congenital malformation syndromes due to known exogenous causes

Q87 Other specified congenital malformation syndromes affecting multiple systems

Use additional code(s) to identify all associated manifestations

Q87.0 Congenital malformation syndromes predominantly affecting facial appearance

Acrocephalopolysyndactyly

Acrocephalosyndactyly [Apert]

Cryptophthalmos syndrome

Cyclopia

Goldenhar syndrome

Moebius syndrome

Oro-facial-digital syndrome

Robin syndrome

Whistling face

Q87.1 Congenital malformation syndromes predominantly associated with short stature

Aarskog syndrome

Cockayne syndrome

De Lange syndrome

Dubowitz syndrome

Noonan syndrome

Prader-Willi syndrome

Robinow-Silverman-Smith syndrome

Russell-Silver syndrome

Seckel syndrome

Excludes 1: Ellis-van Creveld syndrome (Q77.6)

Smith-Lemli-Opitz syndrome (E78.72)

Q87.2 Congenital malformation syndromes predominantly involving limbs

Holt-Oram syndrome

Klippel-Trenaunay-Weber syndrome

Nail patella syndrome

Rubinstein-Taybi syndrome

Sirenomelia syndrome

Thrombocytopenia with absent radius [TAR] syndrome

VATER syndrome

Q87.3 Congenital malformation syndromes involving early overgrowth

Beckwith-Wiedemann syndrome

Sotos syndrome

Weaver syndrome

Q87.4 Marfan's syndrome

Q87.40 Marfan's syndrome, unspecified

Q87.41 Marfan's syndrome with cardiovascular manifestations

Q87.410 Marfan's syndrome with aortic dilation

Q87.418 Marfan's syndrome with other cardiovascular manifestations

Q87.42 Marfan's syndrome with ocular manifestations

Q87.43 Marfan's syndrome with skeletal manifestation

Q87.5 Other congenital malformation syndromes with other skeletal changes

Q87.8 Other specified congenital malformation syndromes, not elsewhere classified

Excludes 1: Zellweger syndrome (E71.510)

Q87.81 Alport syndrome

Use additional code to identify stage of chronic kidney disease (N18.1-N18.6)

Q87.89 Other specified congenital malformation syndromes, not elsewhere classified

Laurence-Moon (-Bardet)-Biedl syndrome

Q89 Other congenital malformations, not elsewhere classified

Q89.0 Congenital absence and malformations of spleen

Excludes 1: isomerism of atrial appendages (with asplenia or polysplenia) (Q20.6)

Q89.01 Asplenia (congenital)

Q89.09 Congenital malformations of spleen

Congenital splenomegaly

Q89.1 Congenital malformations of adrenal gland

Excludes 1: adrenogenital disorders (E25.-)

congenital adrenal hyperplasia (E25.0)

Q89.2 Congenital malformations of other endocrine glands

Congenital malformation of parathyroid or thyroid gland

Persistent thyroglossal duct

Thyroglossal cyst

Excludes 1: congenital goiter (E03.0)

congenital hypothyroidism (E03.1)

Q89.3 Situs inversus

Dextrocardia with situs inversus

Mirror-image atrial arrangement with situs inversus

Situs inversus or transversus abdominalis

Situs inversus or transversus thoracis

Transposition of abdominal viscera

Transposition of thoracic viscera

Excludes 1: dextrocardia NOS (Q24.0)

Q89.4   Conjoined twins
Craniopagus
Dicephaly
Pygopagus
Thoracopagus

Q89.7   Multiple congenital malformations, not elsewhere classified
Multiple congenital anomalies NOS
Multiple congenital deformities NOS
> **Excludes 1:** congenital malformation syndromes affecting multiple systems (Q87.-)

Q89.8   Other specified congenital malformations
Use additional code(s) to identify all associated manifestations

Q89.9   Congenital malformation, unspecified
Congenital anomaly NOS
Congenital deformity NOS

CHROMOSOMAL ABNORMALITIES, NOT ELSEWHERE CLASSIFIED (Q90-Q99)

Excludes 2: mitochondrial metabolic disorders (E88.4-)

Q90   Down syndrome
Use additional code(s) to identify any associated physical conditions and degree of intellectual disabilities (F70-F79)

Q90.0   Trisomy 21, nonmosaicism (meiotic nondisjunction)

Q90.1   Trisomy 21, mosaicism (mitotic nondisjunction)

Q90.2   Trisomy 21, translocation

Q90.9   Down syndrome, unspecified
Trisomy 21 NOS

Q91   Trisomy 18 and Trisomy 13

Q91.0   Trisomy 18, nonmosaicism (meiotic nondisjunction)

Q91.1   Trisomy 18, mosaicism (mitotic nondisjunction)

Q91.2   Trisomy 18, translocation

Q91.3   Trisomy 18, unspecified

Q91.4   Trisomy 13, nonmosaicism (meiotic nondisjunction)

Q91.5   Trisomy 13, mosaicism (mitotic nondisjunction)

Q91.6   Trisomy 13, translocation

Q91.7   Trisomy 13, unspecified

Q92   Other trisomies and partial trisomies of the autosomes, not elsewhere classified
Includes: unbalanced translocations and insertions
Excludes 1: trisomies of chromosomes 13, 18, 21 (Q90-Q91)

Q92.0   Whole chromosome trisomy, nonmosaicism (meiotic nondisjunction)

Q92.1   Whole chromosome trisomy, mosaicism (mitotic nondisjunction)

Q92.2   Partial trisomy
Less than whole arm duplicated
Whole arm or more duplicated
> **Excludes 1:** partial trisomy due to unbalanced translocation (Q92.5)

Q92.5   Duplications with other complex rearrangements
Partial trisomy due to unbalanced translocations
Code also any associated deletions due to unbalanced translocations, inversions and insertions (Q93.7)

Q92.6   Marker chromosomes
Trisomies due to dicentrics
Trisomies due to extra rings

Trisomies due to isochromosomes
Individual with marker heterochromatin

Q92.61   Marker chromosomes in normal individual

Q92.62   Marker chromosomes in abnormal individual

Q92.7   Triploidy and polyploidy

Q92.8   Other specified trisomies and partial trisomies of autosomes
Duplications identified by fluorescence in situ hybridization (FISH)
Duplications identified by in situ hybridization (ISH)
Duplications seen only at prometaphase

Q92.9   Trisomy and partial trisomy of autosomes, unspecified

Q93   Monosomies and deletions from the autosomes, not elsewhere classified

Q93.0   Whole chromosome monosomy, nonmosaicism (meiotic nondisjunction)

Q93.1   Whole chromosome monosomy, mosaicism (mitotic nondisjunction)

Q93.2   Chromosome replaced with ring, dicentric or isochromosome

Q93.3   Deletion of short arm of chromosome 4
Wolff-Hirschorn syndrome

Q93.4   Deletion of short arm of chromosome 5
Cri-du-chat syndrome

Q93.5   Other deletions of part of a chromosome
Angelman syndrome

Q93.7   Deletions with other complex rearrangements
Deletions due to unbalanced translocations, inversions and insertions
Code also any associated duplications due to unbalanced translocations, inversions and insertions (Q92.5)

Q93.8   Other deletions from the autosomes

Q93.81   Velo-cardio-facial syndrome
Deletion 22q11.2

Q93.88   Other microdeletions
Miller-Dieker syndrome
Smith-Magenis syndrome

Q93.89   Other deletions from the autosomes
Deletions identified by fluorescence in situ hybridization (FISH)
Deletions identified by in situ hybridization (ISH)
Deletions seen only at prometaphase

Q93.9   Deletion from autosomes, unspecified

Q95   Balanced rearrangements and structural markers, not elsewhere classified
Includes: Robertsonian and balanced reciprocal translocations and insertions

Q95.0   Balanced translocation and insertion in normal individual

Q95.1   Chromosome inversion in normal individual

Q95.2   Balanced autosomal rearrangement in abnormal individual

Q95.3   Balanced sex/autosomal rearrangement in abnormal individual

Q95.5   Individual with autosomal fragile site

Q95.8   Other balanced rearrangements and structural markers

Q95.9   Balanced rearrangement and structural marker, unspecified

Q96   Turner's syndrome
Excludes 1: Noonan syndrome (Q87.1)

Q96.0   Karyotype 45, X

● New code   ▲ Revised code   ⑦ 7th digit required   ⊗ Placeholder required

Q96.1 Karyotype 46, X iso (Xq)

Karyotype 46, isochromosome Xq

Q96.2 Karyotype 46, X with abnormal sex chromosome, except iso (Xq)

Karyotype 46, X with abnormal sex chromosome, except isochromosome Xq

Q96.3 Mosaicism, 45, X/46, XX or XY

Q96.4 Mosaicism, 45, X/other cell line(s) with abnormal sex chromosome

Q96.8 Other variants of Turner's syndrome

Q96.9 Turner's syndrome, unspecified

Q97 Other sex chromosome abnormalities, female phenotype, not elsewhere classified

Excludes 1: Turner's syndrome (Q96.-)

Q97.0 Karyotype 47, XXX

Q97.1 Female with more than three X chromosomes

Q97.2 Mosaicism, lines with various numbers of X chromosomes

Q97.3 Female with 46, XY karyotype

Q97.8 Other specified sex chromosome abnormalities, female phenotype

Q97.9 Sex chromosome abnormality, female phenotype, unspecified

Q98 Other sex chromosome abnormalities, male phenotype, not elsewhere classified

Q98.0 Klinefelter syndrome karyotype 47, XXY

Q98.1 Klinefelter syndrome, male with more than two X chromosomes

Q98.3 Other male with 46, XX karyotype

Q98.4 Klinefelter syndrome, unspecified

Q98.5 Karyotype 47, XYY

Q98.6 Male with structurally abnormal sex chromosome

Q98.7 Male with sex chromosome mosaicism

Q98.8 Other specified sex chromosome abnormalities, male phenotype

Q98.9 Sex chromosome abnormality, male phenotype, unspecified

Q99 Other chromosome abnormalities, not elsewhere classified

Q99.0 Chimera 46, XX/46, XY

Chimera 46, XX/46, XY true hermaphrodite

Q99.1 46, XX true hermaphrodite

46, XX with streak gonads

46, XY with streak gonads

Pure gonadal dysgenesis

Q99.2 Fragile X chromosome

Fragile X syndrome

Q99.8 Other specified chromosome abnormalities

Q99.9 Chromosomal abnormality, unspecified

● New code   ▲ Revised code   ⑦ 7th digit required   ⊗ Placeholder required

Chapter 18: Symptoms, Signs And Abnormal Clinical And Laboratory Findings, Not Elsewhere Classified (R00-R99)

Note: This chapter includes symptoms, signs, abnormal results of clinical or other investigative procedures, and ill-defined conditions regarding which no diagnosis classifiable elsewhere is recorded.

Signs and symptoms that point rather definitely to a given diagnosis have been assigned to a category in other chapters of the classification. In general, categories in this chapter include the less well-defined conditions and symptoms that, without the necessary study of the case to establish a final diagnosis, point perhaps equally to two or more diseases or to two or more systems of the body. Practically all categories in the chapter could be designated 'not otherwise specified', 'unknown etiology' or 'transient'. The Alphabetical Index should be consulted to determine which symptoms and signs are to be allocated here and which to other chapters. The residual subcategories, numbered .8, are generally provided for other relevant symptoms that cannot be allocated elsewhere in the classification.

The conditions and signs or symptoms included in categories R00-R94 consist of:

(a) cases for which no more specific diagnosis can be made even after all the facts bearing on the case have been investigated;

(b) signs or symptoms existing at the time of initial encounter that proved to be transient and whose causes could not be determined;

(c) provisional diagnosis in a patient who failed to return for further investigation or care;

(d) cases referred elsewhere for investigation or treatment before the diagnosis was made;

(e) cases in which a more precise diagnosis was not available for any other reason;

(f) certain symptoms, for which supplementary information is provided, that represent important problems in medical care in their own right.

Excludes 2: abnormal findings on antenatal screening of mother (O28.-)
certain conditions originating in the perinatal period (P04-P96)
signs and symptoms classified in the body system chapters
signs and symptoms of breast (N63, N64.5)

This chapter contains the following blocks:

R00-R09	Symptoms and signs involving the circulatory and respiratory systems
R10-R19	Symptoms and signs involving the digestive system and abdomen
R20-R23	Symptoms and signs involving the skin and subcutaneous tissue
R25-R29	Symptoms and signs involving the nervous and musculoskeletal systems
R30-R39	Symptoms and signs involving the genitourinary system
R40-R46	Symptoms and signs involving cognition, perception, emotional state and behavior
R47-R49	Symptoms and signs involving speech and voice
R50-R69	General symptoms and signs
R70-R79	Abnormal findings on examination of blood, without diagnosis
R80-R82	Abnormal findings on examination of urine, without diagnosis
R83-R89	Abnormal findings on examination of other body fluids, substances and tissues, without diagnosis
R90-R94	Abnormal findings on diagnostic imaging and in function studies, without diagnosis
R97	Abnormal tumor markers
R99	Ill-defined and unknown cause of mortality

SYMPTOMS AND SIGNS INVOLVING THE CIRCULATORY AND RESPIRATORY SYSTEMS (R00-R09)

R00 Abnormalities of heart beat

Excludes 1: abnormalities originating in the perinatal period (P29.1-)
specified arrhythmias (I47-I49)

R00.0 Tachycardia, unspecified
Rapid heart beat
Sinoauricular tachycardia NOS
Sinus [sinusal] tachycardia NOS
Excludes 1: neonatal tachycardia (P29.11)
paroxysmal tachycardia (I47.-)

R00.1 Bradycardia, unspecified
Sinoatrial bradycardia
Sinus bradycardia
Slow heart beat
Vagal bradycardia
Use additional code for adverse effect, if applicable, to identify drug (T36-T50 with fifth or sixth character 5)
Excludes 1: neonatal bradycardia (P29.12)

R00.2 Palpitations
Awareness of heart beat

R00.8 Other abnormalities of heart beat

R00.9 Unspecified abnormalities of heart beat

R01 Cardiac murmurs and other cardiac sounds

Excludes 1: cardiac murmurs and sounds originating in the perinatal period (P29.8)

R01.0 Benign and innocent cardiac murmurs
Functional cardiac murmur

R01.1 Cardiac murmur, unspecified
Cardiac bruit NOS
Heart murmur NOS

R01.2 Other cardiac sounds
Cardiac dullness, increased or decreased
Precordial friction

R03 Abnormal blood-pressure reading, without diagnosis

R03.0 Elevated blood-pressure reading, without diagnosis of hypertension
Note: This category is to be used to record an episode of elevated blood pressure in a patient in whom no formal diagnosis of hypertension has been made, or as an isolated incidental finding.

R03.1 Nonspecific low blood-pressure reading
Excludes 1: hypotension (I95.-)
maternal hypotension syndrome (O26.5-)
neurogenic orthostatic hypotension (G90.3)

R04 Hemorrhage from respiratory passages

R04.0 Epistaxis
Hemorrhage from nose
Nosebleed

R04.1 Hemorrhage from throat
Excludes 2: hemoptysis (R04.2)

R04.2 Hemoptysis
Blood-stained sputum
Cough with hemorrhage

R04.8 Hemorrhage from other sites in respiratory passages

    R04.81 Acute idiopathic pulmonary hemorrhage in infants
        AIPHI
        Acute idiopathic hemorrhage in infants over 28 days old
        Excludes 1: perinatal pulmonary hemorrhage (P26.-)
            von Willebrand's disease (D68.0)

    R04.89 Hemorrhage from other sites in respiratory passages
        Pulmonary hemorrhage NOS

R04.9 Hemorrhage from respiratory passages, unspecified

R05 Cough
Excludes 1: cough with hemorrhage (R04.2)
    smoker's cough (J41.0)

R06 Abnormalities of breathing
Excludes 1: acute respiratory distress syndrome (J80)
    respiratory arrest (R09.2)
    respiratory arrest of newborn (P28.81)
    respiratory distress syndrome of newborn (P22.-)
    respiratory failure (J96.-)
    respiratory failure of newborn (P28.5)

R06.0 Dyspnea
Excludes 1: tachypnea NOS (R06.82)
    transient tachypnea of newborn (P22.1)

    R06.00 Dyspnea, unspecified
    R06.01 Orthopnea
    R06.02 Shortness of breath
    R06.09 Other forms of dyspnea

R06.1 Stridor
Excludes 1: congenital laryngeal stridor (P28.89)
    laryngismus (stridulus) (J38.5)

R06.2 Wheezing
Excludes 1: Asthma (J45.-)

R06.3 Periodic breathing
Cheyne-Stokes breathing

R06.4 Hyperventilation
Excludes 1: psychogenic hyperventilation (F45.8)

R06.5 Mouth breathing
Excludes 2: dry mouth NOS (R68.2)

R06.6 Hiccough
Excludes 1: psychogenic hiccough (F45.8)

R06.7 Sneezing

R06.8 Other abnormalities of breathing

    R06.81 Apnea, not elsewhere classified
        Apnea NOS
        Excludes 1: apnea (of) newborn (P28.4)
            sleep apnea (G47.3-)
            sleep apnea of newborn (primary) (P28.3)

    R06.82 Tachypnea, not elsewhere classified
        Tachypnea NOS

        Excludes 1: transitory tachypnea of newborn (P22.1)

    R06.83 Snoring

    R06.89 Other abnormalities of breathing
        Breath-holding (spells)
        Sighing

R06.9 Unspecified abnormalities of breathing

R07 Pain in throat and chest
Excludes 1: epidemic myalgia (B33.0)
Excludes 2: jaw pain R68.84
    pain in breast (N64.4)

R07.0 Pain in throat
Excludes 1: chronic sore throat (J31.2)
    sore throat (acute) NOS (J02.9)
Excludes 2: dysphagia (R13.1-)
    pain in neck (M54.2)

R07.1 Chest pain on breathing
Painful respiration

R07.2 Precordial pain

R07.8 Other chest pain

    R07.81 Pleurodynia
        Pleurodynia NOS
        Excludes 1: epidemic pleurodynia (B33.0)

    R07.82 Intercostal pain

    R07.89 Other chest pain
        Anterior chest-wall pain NOS

R07.9 Chest pain, unspecified

R09 Other symptoms and signs involving the circulatory and respiratory system
Excludes 1: acute respiratory distress syndrome (J80)
    respiratory arrest of newborn (P28.81)
    respiratory distress syndrome of newborn (P22.0)
    respiratory failure (J96.-)
    respiratory failure of newborn (P28.5)

R09.0 Asphyxia and hypoxemia
Excludes 1: asphyxia due to carbon monoxide (T58.-)
asphyxia due to foreign body in respiratory tract (T17.-)
    birth (intrauterine) asphyxia (P84)
    hypercapnia (R06.4)
    hyperventilation (R06.4)
    traumatic asphyxia (T71-)

    R09.01 Asphyxia
    R09.02 Hypoxemia

R09.1 Pleurisy
Excludes 1: pleurisy with effusion (J90)

R09.2 Respiratory arrest
Cardiorespiratory failure
Excludes 1: cardiac arrest (I46.-)
    respiratory arrest of newborn (P28.81)
    respiratory distress of newborn (P22.0)
    respiratory failure (J96.-)
    respiratory failure of newborn (P28.5)
    respiratory insufficiency (R06.89)
    respiratory insufficiency of newborn (P28.5)

R09.3 Abnormal sputum
Abnormal amount of sputum
Abnormal color of sputum
Abnormal odor of sputum

Excessive sputum
Excludes 1: blood-stained sputum (R04.2)

R09.8   Other specified symptoms and signs involving the
circulatory and respiratory systems
    R09.81   Nasal congestion
    R09.82   Postnasal drip
    R09.89   Other specified symptoms and signs involving
the circulatory and respiratory systems
Bruit (arterial)
Abnormal chest percussion
Feeling of foreign body in throat
Friction sounds in chest
Chest tympany
Choking sensation
Rales
Weak pulse
Excludes 2: foreign body in throat (T17.2-)
wheezing (R06.2)

SYMPTOMS AND SIGNS INVOLVING THE DIGESTIVE SYSTEM AND ABDOMEN (R10-R19)

Excludes 1: congenital or infantile pylorospasm (Q40.0)
gastrointestinal hemorrhage (K92.0-K92.2)
intestinal obstruction (K56.)
newborn gastrointestinal hemorrhage (P54.0-P54.3)
newborn intestinal obstruction (P76.-)
pylorospasm (K31.3)
signs and symptoms involving the urinary system (R30-R39)
symptoms referable to female genital organs (N94.-)
symptoms referable to male genital organs male (N48-N50)

R10   Abdominal and pelvic pain
    Excludes 1: renal colic (N23)
    Excludes 2: dorsalgia (M54.-)
flatulence and related conditions (R14.-)
    R10.0   Acute abdomen
Severe abdominal pain (generalized) (with abdominal
rigidity)
Excludes 1: abdominal rigidity NOS (R19.3)
generalized abdominal pain NOS (R10.84)
localized abdominal pain (R10.1-R10.3-)
    R10.1   Pain localized to upper abdomen
        R10.10   Upper abdominal pain, unspecified
        R10.11   Right upper quadrant pain
        R10.12   Left upper quadrant pain
        R10.13   Epigastric pain
Dyspepsia
Excludes 1: functional dyspepsia (K30)
    R10.2   Pelvic and perineal pain
Excludes 1: vulvodynia (N94.81)
    R10.3   Pain localized to other parts of lower abdomen
        R10.30   Lower abdominal pain, unspecified
        R10.31   Right lower quadrant pain
        R10.32   Left lower quadrant pain
        R10.33   Periumbilical pain
    R10.8   Other abdominal pain
        R10.81   Abdominal tenderness
Abdominal tenderness NOS
            R10.811   Right upper quadrant abdominal
tenderness

            R10.812   Left upper quadrant abdominal
tenderness
            R10.813   Right lower quadrant abdominal
tenderness
            R10.814   Left lower quadrant abdominal
tenderness
            R10.815   Periumbilic abdominal tenderness
            R10.816   Epigastric abdominal tenderness
            R10.817   Generalized abdominal tenderness
            R10.819   Abdominal tenderness, unspecified
site
        R10.82   Rebound abdominal tenderness
            R10.821   Right upper quadrant rebound
abdominal tenderness
            R10.822   Left upper quadrant rebound
abdominal tenderness
            R10.823   Right lower quadrant rebound
abdominal tenderness
            R10.824   Left lower quadrant rebound
abdominal tenderness
            R10.825   Periumbilic rebound abdominal
tenderness
            R10.826   Epigastric rebound abdominal
tenderness
            R10.827   Generalized rebound abdominal
tenderness
            R10.829   Rebound abdominal tenderness,
unspecified site
        R10.83   Colic
Colic NOS
Infantile colic
Excludes 1: colic in adult and child over 12
months old (R10.84)
        R10.84   Generalized abdominal pain
Excludes 1: generalized abdominal pain
associated with acute abdomen
(R10.0)
    R10.9   Unspecified abdominal pain
R11   Nausea and vomiting
Excludes 1: cyclical vomiting associated with migraine (G43.A-)
excessive vomiting in pregnancy (O21.-)
hematemesis (K92.0)
neonatal hematemesis (P54.0)
newborn vomiting (P92.0-)
psychogenic vomiting (F50.8)
vomiting associated with bulimia nervosa (F50.2)
vomiting following gastrointestinal surgery (K91.0)
    R11.0   Nausea
Nausea NOS
Nausea without vomiting
    R11.1   Vomiting
        R11.10   Vomiting, unspecified
Vomiting NOS
        R11.11   Vomiting without nausea
        R11.12   Projectile vomiting
        R11.13   Vomiting of fecal matter
        R11.14   Bilious vomiting
Bilious emesis
    R11.2   Nausea with vomiting, unspecified
Persistent nausea with vomiting NOS

R12 Heartburn
Excludes 1: dyspepsia NOS (R10.13)
functional dyspepsia (K30)

R13 Aphagia and dysphagia

R13.0 Aphagia
Inability to swallow
Excludes 1: psychogenic aphagia (F50.9)

R13.1 Dysphagia
Code first , if applicable, dysphagia following cerebrovascular disease (I69. with final characters -91)
Excludes 1: psychogenic dysphagia (F45.8)

R13.10 Dysphagia, unspecified
Difficulty in swallowing NOS

R13.11 Dysphagia, oral phase

R13.12 Dysphagia, oropharyngeal phase

R13.13 Dysphagia, pharyngeal phase

R13.14 Dysphagia, pharyngoesophageal phase

R13.19 Other dysphagia
Cervical dysphagia
Neurogenic dysphagia

R14 Flatulence and related conditions
Excludes 1: psychogenic aerophagy (F45.8)

R14.0 Abdominal distension (gaseous)
Bloating
Tympanites (abdominal) (intestinal)

R14.1 Gas pain

R14.2 Eructation

R14.3 Flatulence

R15 Fecal incontinence
Includes: encopresis NOS
Excludes 1: fecal incontinence of nonorganic origin (F98.1)

R15.0 Incomplete defecation
Excludes 1: constipation (K59.0-)
fecal impaction (K56.41)

R15.1 Fecal smearing
Fecal soiling

R15.2 Fecal urgency

R15.9 Full incontinence of feces
Fecal incontinence NOS

R16 Hepatomegaly and splenomegaly, not elsewhere classified

R16.0 Hepatomegaly, not elsewhere classified
Hepatomegaly NOS

R16.1 Splenomegaly, not elsewhere classified
Splenomegaly NOS

R16.2 Hepatomegaly with splenomegaly, not elsewhere classified
Hepatosplenomegaly NOS

R17 Unspecified jaundice
Excludes 1: neonatal jaundice (P55, P57-P59)

R18 Ascites
Includes: fluid in peritoneal cavity
Excludes 1: ascites in alcoholic cirrhosis (K70.31)
ascites in alcoholic hepatitis (K70.11)
ascites in toxic liver disease with chronic active hepatitis (K71.51)

R18.0 Malignant ascites
Code first malignancy, such as:
malignant neoplasm of ovary (C56.-)
secondary malignant neoplasm of

retroperitoneum and peritoneum (C78.6)

R18.8 Other ascites
Ascites NOS
Peritoneal effusion (chronic)

R19 Other symptoms and signs involving the digestive system and abdomen
Excludes 1: acute abdomen (R10.0)

R19.0 Intra-abdominal and pelvic swelling, mass and lump
Excludes 1: abdominal distension (gaseous) (R14.-)
ascites (R18.-)

R19.00 Intra-abdominal and pelvic swelling, mass and lump, unspecified site

R19.01 Right upper quadrant abdominal swelling, mass and lump

R19.02 Left upper quadrant abdominal swelling, mass and lump

R19.03 Right lower quadrant abdominal swelling, mass and lump

R19.04 Left lower quadrant abdominal swelling, mass and lump

R19.05 Periumbilic swelling, mass or lump
Diffuse or generalized umbilical swelling or mass

R19.06 Epigastric swelling, mass or lump

R19.07 Generalized intra-abdominal and pelvic swelling, mass and lump
Diffuse or generalized intra-abdominal swelling or mass NOS
Diffuse or generalized pelvic swelling or mass NOS

R19.09 Other intra-abdominal and pelvic swelling, mass and lump

R19.1 Abnormal bowel sounds

R19.11 Absent bowel sounds

R19.12 Hyperactive bowel sounds

R19.15 Other abnormal bowel sounds
Abnormal bowel sounds NOS

R19.2 Visible peristalsis
Hyperperistalsis

R19.3 Abdominal rigidity
Excludes 1: abdominal rigidity with severe abdominal pain (R10.0)

R19.30 Abdominal rigidity, unspecified site

R19.31 Right upper quadrant abdominal rigidity

R19.32 Left upper quadrant abdominal rigidity

R19.33 Right lower quadrant abdominal rigidity

R19.34 Left lower quadrant abdominal rigidity

R19.35 Periumbilic abdominal rigidity

R19.36 Epigastric abdominal rigidity

R19.37 Generalized abdominal rigidity

R19.4 Change in bowel habit
Excludes 1: constipation (K59.0-)
functional diarrhea (K59.1)

R19.5 Other fecal abnormalities
Abnormal stool color
Bulky stools
Mucus in stools
Occult blood in feces
Occult blood in stools
Excludes 1: melena (K92.1)

● New code   ▲ Revised code   ⑦ 7th digit required   ⊗ Placeholder required

neonatal melena (P54.1)

R19.6 Halitosis

R19.7 Diarrhea, unspecified

Diarrhea NOS

Excludes 1: functional diarrhea (K59.1)

neonatal diarrhea (P78.3)

psychogenic diarrhea (F45.8)

R19.8 Other specified symptoms and signs involving the digestive system and abdomen

SYMPTOMS AND SIGNS INVOLVING THE SKIN AND SUBCUTANEOUS TISSUE (R20-R23)

Excludes 2: symptoms relating to breast (N64.4-N64.5)

R20 Disturbances of skin sensation

Excludes 1: dissociative anesthesia and sensory loss (F44.6)

psychogenic disturbances (F45.8)

R20.0 Anesthesia of skin

R20.1 Hypoesthesia of skin

R20.2 Paresthesia of skin

Formication

Pins and needles

Tingling skin

Excludes 1: acroparesthesia (I73.8)

R20.3 Hyperesthesia

R20.8 Other disturbances of skin sensation

R20.9 Unspecified disturbances of skin sensation

R21 Rash and other nonspecific skin eruption

Includes: rash NOS

Excludes 1: specified type of rash- code to condition

vesicular eruption (R23.8)

R22 Localized swelling, mass and lump of skin and subcutaneous tissue

Includes: subcutaneous nodules (localized)(superficial)

Excludes 1: abnormal findings on diagnostic imaging (R90-R93)

edema (R60.-)

enlarged lymph nodes (R59.-)

localized adiposity (E65)

swelling of joint (M25.4-)

R22.0 Localized swelling, mass and lump, head

R22.1 Localized swelling, mass and lump, neck

R22.2 Localized swelling, mass and lump, trunk

Excludes 1: intra-abdominal or pelvic mass and lump (R19.0-)

intra-abdominal or pelvic swelling (R19.0-)

Excludes 2: breast mass and lump (N63)

R22.3 Localized swelling, mass and lump, upper limb

R22.30 Localized swelling, mass and lump, unspecified upper limb

R22.31 Localized swelling, mass and lump, right upper limb

R22.32 Localized swelling, mass and lump, left upper limb

R22.33 Localized swelling, mass and lump, upper limb, bilateral

R22.4 Localized swelling, mass and lump, lower limb

R22.40 Localized swelling, mass and lump, unspecified lower limb

R22.41 Localized swelling, mass and lump, right lower limb

R22.42 Localized swelling, mass and lump, left lower limb

R22.43 Localized swelling, mass and lump, lower limb, bilateral

R22.9 Localized swelling, mass and lump, unspecified

R23 Other skin changes

R23.0 Cyanosis

Excludes 1: acrocyanosis (I73.8)

cyanotic attacks of newborn (P28.2)

R23.1 Pallor

Clammy skin

R23.2 Flushing

Excessive blushing

Code first , if applicable, menopausal and female climacteric states (N95.1)

R23.3 Spontaneous ecchymoses

Petechiae

Excludes 1: ecchymoses of newborn (P54.5)

purpura (D69.-)

R23.4 Changes in skin texture

Desquamation of skin

Induration of skin

Scaling of skin

Excludes 1: epidermal thickening NOS (L85.9)

R23.8 Other skin changes

R23.9 Unspecified skin changes

SYMPTOMS AND SIGNS INVOLVING THE NERVOUS AND MUSCULOSKELETAL SYSTEMS (R25-R29)

R25 Abnormal involuntary movements

Excludes 1: specific movement disorders (G20-G26)

stereotyped movement disorders (F98.4)

tic disorders (F95.-)

R25.0 Abnormal head movements

R25.1 Tremor, unspecified

Excludes 1: chorea NOS (G25.5)

essential tremor (G25.0)

hysterical tremor (F44.4)

intention tremor (G25.2)

R25.2 Cramp and spasm

Excludes 2: carpopedal spasm (R29.0)

charley-horse (M62.831)

infantile spasms (G40.4-)

muscle spasm of back (M62.830)

muscle spasm of calf (M62.831)

R25.3 Fasciculation

Twitching NOS

R25.8 Other abnormal involuntary movements

R25.9 Unspecified abnormal involuntary movements

R26 Abnormalities of gait and mobility

Excludes 1: ataxia NOS (R27.0)

hereditary ataxia (G11.-)

locomotor (syphilitic) ataxia (A52.11)

immobility syndrome (paraplegic) (M62.3)

R26.0 Ataxic gait

Staggering gait

R26.1 Paralytic gait

Spastic gait

R26.2 Difficulty in walking, not elsewhere classified

Excludes 1: falling (R29.6)

unsteadiness on feet (R26.81)

R26.8 Other abnormalities of gait and mobility

R26.81 Unsteadiness on feet

R26.89 Other abnormalities of gait and mobility

R26.9 Unspecified abnormalities of gait and mobility

R27 Other lack of coordination

Excludes 1: ataxic gait (R26.0)

hereditary ataxia (G11.-)

vertigo NOS (R42)

R27.0 Ataxia, unspecified

Excludes 1: ataxia following cerebrovascular disease (I69. with final characters -93)

R27.8 Other lack of coordination

R27.9 Unspecified lack of coordination

R29 Other symptoms and signs involving the nervous and musculoskeletal systems

R29.0 Tetany

Carpopedal spasm

Excludes 1: hysterical tetany (F44.5)

neonatal tetany (P71.3)

parathyroid tetany (E20.9)

post-thyroidectomy tetany (E89.2)

R29.1 Meningismus

R29.2 Abnormal reflex

Excludes 2: abnormal pupillary reflex (H57.0)

hyperactive gag reflex (J39.2)

vasovagal reaction or syncope (R55)

R29.3 Abnormal posture

R29.4 Clicking hip

Excludes 1: congenital deformities of hip (Q65.-)

R29.5 Transient paralysis

Code first any associated spinal cord injury (S14.0, S14.1-, S24.0, S24.1-, S34.0-, S34.1-)

Excludes 1: transient ischemic attack (G45.9)

R29.6 Repeated falls

Falling

Tendency to fall

Excludes 2: at risk for falling (Z91.81)

history of falling (Z91.81)

R29.8 Other symptoms and signs involving the nervous and musculoskeletal systems

R29.81 Other symptoms and signs involving the nervous system

R29.810 Facial weakness

Facial droop

Excludes 1: Bell's palsy (G51.0)

facial weakness following cerebrovascular disease (I69. with final characters -92)

R29.818 Other symptoms and signs involving the nervous system

R29.89 Other symptoms and signs involving the musculoskeletal system

Excludes 2: pain in limb (M79.6-)

R29.890 Loss of height

Excludes 1: osteoporosis (M80-M81)

R29.891 Ocular torticollis

Excludes 1: congenital (sternomastoid) torticollis Q68.0

psychogenic torticollis (F45.8)

spasmodic torticollis (G24.3)

torticollis due to birth injury (P15.8)

torticollis NOS M43.6

R29.898 Other symptoms and signs involving the musculoskeletal system

R29.9 Unspecified symptoms and signs involving the nervous and musculoskeletal systems

R29.90 Unspecified symptoms and signs involving the nervous system

R29.91 Unspecified symptoms and signs involving the musculoskeletal system

SYMPTOMS AND SIGNS INVOLVING THE GENITOURINARY SYSTEM (R30-R39)

R30 Pain associated with micturition

Excludes 1: psychogenic pain associated with micturition (F45.8)

R30.0 Dysuria

Strangury

R30.1 Vesical tenesmus

R30.9 Painful micturition, unspecified

Painful urination NOS

R31 Hematuria

Excludes 1: hematuria included with underlying conditions, such as:

acute cystitis with hematuria (N30.01)

acute prostatitis with hematuria (N41.01)

recurrent and persistent hematuria in glomerular diseases (N02.-)

R31.0 Gross hematuria

R31.1 Benign essential microscopic hematuria

R31.2 Other microscopic hematuria

R31.9 Hematuria, unspecified

R32 Unspecified urinary incontinence

Enuresis NOS

Excludes 1: functional urinary incontinence (R39.81)

nonorganic enuresis (F98.0)

stress incontinence and other specified urinary incontinence (N39.3-N39.4-)

urinary incontinence associated with cognitive impairment (R39.81)

R33 Retention of urine

Excludes 1: psychogenic retention of urine (F45.8)

R33.0 Drug induced retention of urine

Use additional code for adverse effect, if applicable, to identify drug (T36-T50 with fifth or sixth character 5)

R33.8 Other retention of urine

Code first , if applicable, any causal condition, such as: enlarged prostate (N40.1)

R33.9 Retention of urine, unspecified

R34 Anuria and oliguria

Excludes 1: anuria and oliguria complicating abortion or ectopic or molar pregnancy (O00-O07, O08.4)

anuria and oliguria complicating pregnancy (O26.83-)

anuria and oliguria complicating the puerperium (O90.4)

● New code   ▲ Revised code   ⑦ 7th digit required   ⊗ Placeholder required

R35 Polyuria

Code first , if applicable, any causal condition, such as:

enlarged prostate (N40.1)

Excludes 1: psychogenic polyuria (F45.8)

R35.0 Frequency of micturition

R35.1 Nocturia

R35.8 Other polyuria

Polyuria NOS

R36 Urethral discharge

R36.0 Urethral discharge without blood

R36.1 Hematospermia

R36.9 Urethral discharge, unspecified

Penile discharge NOS

Urethrorrhea

R37 Sexual dysfunction, unspecified

R39 Other and unspecified symptoms and signs involving the genitourinary system

R39.0 Extravasation of urine

R39.1 Other difficulties with micturition

Code first , if applicable, any causal condition, such as:

enlarged prostate (N40.1)

R39.11 Hesitancy of micturition

R39.12 Poor urinary stream

Weak urinary steam

R39.13 Splitting of urinary stream

R39.14 Feeling of incomplete bladder emptying

R39.15 Urgency of urination

Excludes 1: urge incontinence (N39.41, N39.46)

R39.16 Straining to void

R39.19 Other difficulties with micturition

R39.2 Extrarenal uremia

Prerenal uremia

Excludes 1: uremia NOS (N19)

R39.8 Other symptoms and signs involving the genitourinary system

R39.81 Functional urinary incontinence

Urinary incontinence due to cognitive impairment, or severe physical disability or immobility

Excludes 1: stress incontinence and other specified urinary incontinence (N39.3-N39.4-)

urinary incontinence NOS (R32)

R39.89 Other symptoms and signs involving the genitourinary system

R39.9 Unspecified symptoms and signs involving the genitourinary system

SYMPTOMS AND SIGNS INVOLVING COGNITION, PERCEPTION, EMOTIONAL STATE AND BEHAVIOR (R40-R46)

Excludes 1: symptoms and signs constituting part of a pattern of mental disorder (F01-F99)

R40 Somnolence, stupor and coma

Excludes 1: neonatal coma (P91.5)

somnolence, stupor and coma in diabetes (E08-E13)

somnolence, stupor and coma in hepatic failure (K72.-)

somnolence, stupor and coma in hypoglycemia (nondiabetic) (E15)

R40.0 Somnolence

Drowsiness

Excludes 1: coma (R40.2-)

R40.1 Stupor

Catatonic stupor

Semicoma

Excludes 1: catatonic schizophrenia (F20.2)

coma (R40.2-)

depressive stupor (F31-F33)

dissociative stupor (F44.2)

manic stupor (F30.2)

R40.2 Coma

Code first any associated:

coma in fracture of skull (S02.-)

coma in intracranial injury (S06.-)

The appropriate 7th character is to be added to each code from subcategory R40.21-, R40.22-, R40.23-:

0- unspecified time

1- in the field [EMT or ambulance]

2- at arrival to emergency department

3- at hospital admission

4- 24 hours or more after hospital admission

Note: A code from each subcategory is required to complete the coma scale

⊗⑦ **R40.20** Unspecified coma

Coma NOS

Unconsciousness NOS

R40.21 Coma scale, eyes open

⑦ **R40.211** Coma scale, eyes open, never

⑦ **R40.212** Coma scale, eyes open, to pain

⑦ **R40.213** Coma scale, eyes open, to sound

⑦ **R40.214** Coma scale, eyes open, spontaneous

R40.22 Coma scale, best verbal response

⑦ **R40.221** Coma scale, best verbal response, none

⑦ **R40.222** Coma scale, best verbal response, incomprehensible words

⑦ **R40.223** Coma scale, best verbal response, inappropriate words

⑦ **R40.224** Coma scale, best verbal response, confused conversation

⑦ **R40.225** Coma scale, best verbal response, oriented

R40.23 Coma scale, best motor response

⑦ **R40.231** Coma scale, best motor response, none

⑦ **R40.232** Coma scale, best motor response, extension

⑦ **R40.233** Coma scale, best motor response, abnormal

⑦ **R40.234** Coma scale, best motor response, flexion withdrawal

⑦ **R40.235** Coma scale, best motor response, localizes pain

⑦ **R40.236** Coma scale, best motor response, obeys commands

R40.24 Glasgow coma scale, total score

Use codes R40.21- through R40.23- only when the individual score(s) are documented

---

Add 4th-7th digits   3 digit reportable   Nonspecific code   Unspecified code   Manifestation code

R40.241	Glasgow coma scale score 13-15	
R40.242	Glasgow coma scale score 9-12	
R40.243	Glasgow coma scale score 3-8	
R40.244	Other coma, without documented Glasgow coma scale score, or with partial score reported	

R40.3 Persistent vegetative state

R40.4 Transient alteration of awareness

R41 Other symptoms and signs involving cognitive functions and awareness

Excludes 1: dissociative [conversion] disorders (F44.-)
mild cognitive impairment, so stated (G31.84)

R41.0 Disorientation, unspecified
Confusion NOS
Delirium NOS

R41.1 Anterograde amnesia

R41.2 Retrograde amnesia

R41.3 Other amnesia
Amnesia NOS
Memory loss NOS

Excludes 1: amnestic disorder due to known physiologic condition (F04)
amnestic syndrome due to psychoactive substance use (F10-F19 with 5th character .6)
mild memory disturbance due to known physiological condition (F06.8)
transient global amnesia (G45.4)

R41.4 Neurologic neglect syndrome
Asomatognosia
Hemi-akinesia
Hemi-inattention
Hemispatial neglect
Left-sided neglect
Sensory neglect
Visuospatial neglect

Excludes 1: visuospatial deficit (R41.842)

R41.8 Other symptoms and signs involving cognitive functions and awareness

R41.81 Age-related cognitive decline
Senility NOS

R41.82 Altered mental status, unspecified
Change in mental status NOS

Excludes 1: altered level of consciousness (R40.-)
altered mental status due to known condition - code to condition
delirium NOS (R41.0)

R41.83 Borderline intellectual functioning
IQ level 71 to 84

Excludes 1: intellectual disabilities (F70-F79)

R41.84 Other specified cognitive deficit

R41.840 Attention and concentration deficit

Excludes 1: attention-deficit hyperactivity disorders (F90.-)

R41.841 Cognitive communication deficit

R41.842 Visuospatial deficit

R41.843 Psychomotor deficit

R41.844 Frontal lobe and executive function deficit

R41.89 Other symptoms and signs involving cognitive functions and awareness
Anosognosia

R41.9 Unspecified symptoms and signs involving cognitive functions and awareness

R42 Dizziness and giddiness
Light-headedness
Vertigo NOS

Excludes 1: vertiginous syndromes (H81.-)
vertigo from infrasound (T75.23)

R43 Disturbances of smell and taste

R43.0 Anosmia

R43.1 Parosmia

R43.2 Parageusia

R43.8 Other disturbances of smell and taste
Mixed disturbance of smell and taste

R43.9 Unspecified disturbances of smell and taste

R44 Other symptoms and signs involving general sensations and perceptions

Excludes 1: alcoholic hallucinations (F1.5)
hallucinations in drug psychosis (F11-F19 with .5)
hallucinations in mood disorders with psychotic symptoms (F30.2, F31.5, F32.3, F33.3)
hallucinations in schizophrenia, schizotypal and delusional disorders (F20-F29)

Excludes 2: disturbances of skin sensation (R20.-)

R44.0 Auditory hallucinations

R44.1 Visual hallucinations

R44.2 Other hallucinations

R44.3 Hallucinations, unspecified

R44.8 Other symptoms and signs involving general sensations and perceptions

R44.9 Unspecified symptoms and signs involving general sensations and perceptions

R45 Symptoms and signs involving emotional state

R45.0 Nervousness
Nervous tension

R45.1 Restlessness and agitation

R45.2 Unhappiness

R45.3 Demoralization and apathy

Excludes 1: anhedonia (R45.84)

R45.4 Irritability and anger

R45.5 Hostility

R45.6 Violent behavior

R45.7 State of emotional shock and stress, unspecified

R45.8 Other symptoms and signs involving emotional state

R45.81 Low self-esteem

R45.82 Worries

R45.83 Excessive crying of child, adolescent or adult

Excludes 1: excessive crying of infant (baby) R68.11

R45.84 Anhedonia

R45.85 Homicidal and suicidal ideations

Excludes 1: suicide attempt (T14.91)

R45.850 Homicidal ideations

R45.851 Suicidal ideations

R45.86 Emotional lability

R45.87 Impulsiveness

R45.89 Other symptoms and signs involving emotional state

R46 Symptoms and signs involving appearance and behavior

> **Excludes 1:** appearance and behavior in schizophrenia, schizotypal and delusional disorders (F20-F29)
> mental and behavioral disorders (F01-F99)

R46.0 Very low level of personal hygiene

R46.1 Bizarre personal appearance

R46.2 Strange and inexplicable behavior

R46.3 Overactivity

R46.4 Slowness and poor responsiveness

> **Excludes 1:** stupor (R40.1)

R46.5 Suspiciousness and marked evasiveness

R46.6 Undue concern and preoccupation with stressful events

R46.7 Verbosity and circumstantial detail obscuring reason for contact

R46.8 Other symptoms and signs involving appearance and behavior

R46.81 Obsessive-compulsive behavior

> **Excludes 1:** obsessive-compulsive disorder (F42)

R46.89 Other symptoms and signs involving appearance and behavior

SYMPTOMS AND SIGNS INVOLVING SPEECH AND VOICE (R47-R49)

R47 Speech disturbances, not elsewhere classified

> **Excludes 1:** autism (F84.0)
> cluttering (F80.81)
> specific developmental disorders of speech and language (F80.-)
> stuttering (F80.81)

R47.0 Dysphasia and aphasia

R47.01 Aphasia

> **Excludes 1:** aphasia following cerebrovascular disease (I69. with final characters -20)
> progressive isolated aphasia (G31.01)

R47.02 Dysphasia

> **Excludes 1:** dysphasia following cerebrovascular disease (I69. with final characters -21)

R47.1 Dysarthria and anarthria

> **Excludes 1:** dysarthria following cerebrovascular disease (I69. with final characters -22)

R47.8 Other speech disturbances

> **Excludes 1:** dysarthria following cerebrovascular disease (I69. with final characters -28)

R47.81 Slurred speech

R47.82 Fluency disorder in conditions classified elsewhere
Stuttering in conditions classified elsewhere
Code first underlying disease or condition, such as:
Parkinson's disease (G20)

> **Excludes 1:** adult onset fluency disorder (F98.5)
> childhood onset fluency disorder (F80.81)

fluency disorder (stuttering) following cerebrovascular disease (I69. with final characters -23)

R47.89 Other speech disturbances

R47.9 Unspecified speech disturbances

R48 Dyslexia and other symbolic dysfunctions, not elsewhere classified

> **Excludes 1:** specific developmental disorders of scholastic skills (F81.-)

R48.0 Dyslexia and alexia

R48.1 Agnosia
Astereognosia (astereognosis)
Autotopagnosia

> **Excludes 1:** visual object agnosia (R48.3)

R48.2 Apraxia

> **Excludes 1:** apraxia following cerebrovascular disease (I69. with final characters -90)

R48.3 Visual agnosia
Prosopagnosia
Simultanagnosia (asimultagnosia)

R48.8 Other symbolic dysfunctions
Acalculia
Agraphia

R48.9 Unspecified symbolic dysfunctions

R49 Voice and resonance disorders

> **Excludes 1:** psychogenic voice and resonance disorders (F44.4)

R49.0 Dysphonia
Hoarseness

R49.1 Aphonia
Loss of voice

R49.2 Hypernasality and hyponasality

R49.21 Hypernasality

R49.22 Hyponasality

R49.8 Other voice and resonance disorders

R49.9 Unspecified voice and resonance disorder
Change in voice NOS
Resonance disorder NOS

GENERAL SYMPTOMS AND SIGNS (R50-R69)

R50 Fever of other and unknown origin

> **Excludes 1:** chills without fever (R68.83)
> febrile convulsions (R56.0-)
> fever of unknown origin during labor (O75.2)
> fever of unknown origin in newborn (P81.9)
> hypothermia due to illness (R68.0)
> malignant hyperthermia due to anesthesia (T88.3)
> puerperal pyrexia NOS (O86.4)

R50.2 Drug induced fever
Use additional code for adverse effect, if applicable, to identify drug (T36-T50 with fifth or sixth character 5)

> **Excludes 1:** postvaccination (postimmunization) fever (R50.83)

R50.8 Other specified fever

R50.81 Fever presenting with conditions classified elsewhere
Code first underlying condition when associated fever is present, such as with:
leukemia (C91-C95)
neutropenia (D70.-)
sickle-cell disease (D57.-)

R50.82 Postprocedural fever
    Excludes 1: postprocedural infection (T81.4)
        posttransfusion fever (R50.84)
        postvaccination (postimmunization)
        fever (R50.83)
R50.83 Postvaccination fever
    Postimmunization fever
R50.84 Febrile nonhemolytic transfusion reaction
    FNHTR
    Posttransfusion fever
R50.9 Fever, unspecified
    Fever NOS
    Fever of unknown origin [FUO]
    Fever with chills
    Fever with rigors
    Hyperpyrexia NOS
    Persistent fever
    Pyrexia NOS
R51 Headache
Facial pain NOS
Excludes 1: atypical face pain (G50.1)
    migraine and other headache syndromes (G43-G44)
    trigeminal neuralgia (G50.0)
R52 Pain, unspecified
Acute pain NOS
Generalized pain NOS
Pain NOS
Excludes 1: acute and chronic pain, not elsewhere classified
    (G89.-)
    localized pain, unspecified type - code to pain by site, such
    as:
    abdomen pain (R10.-)
    back pain (M54.9)
    breast pain (N64.4)
    chest pain (R07.1-R07.9)
    ear pain (H92.0-)
    eye pain (H57.1)
    headache (R51)
    joint pain (M25.5-)
    limb pain (M79.6-)
    lumbar region pain (M54.5)
    pelvic and perineal pain (R10.2)
    shoulder pain (M25.51-)
    spine pain (M54.-)
    throat pain (R07.0)
    tongue pain (K14.6)
    tooth pain (K08.8)
    renal colic (N23)
    pain disorders exclusively related to psychological factors
    (F45.41)
R53 Malaise and fatigue
R53.0 Neoplastic (malignant) related fatigue
    Code first associated neoplasm
R53.1 Weakness
    Asthenia NOS
    Excludes 1: age-related weakness (R54)
        muscle weakness (M62.8-)
        senile asthenia (R54)

R53.2 Functional quadriplegia
    Complete immobility due to severe physical disability or
    frailty
    Excludes 1: frailty NOS (R54)
        hysterical paralysis (F44.4)
        immobility syndrome (M62.3)
        neurologic quadriplegia (G82.5-)
        quadriplegia (G82.50)
R53.8 Other malaise and fatigue
    Excludes 1: combat exhaustion and fatigue (F43.0)
        congenital debility (P96.9)
        exhaustion and fatigue due to:
        depressive episode (F32.-)
        excessive exertion (T73.3)
        exposure (T73.2)
        heat (T67.-)
        pregnancy (O26.8-)
        recurrent depressive episode (F33)
        senile debility (R54)
R53.81 Other malaise
    Chronic debility
    Debility NOS
    General physical deterioration
    Malaise NOS
    Nervous debility
    Excludes 1: age-related physical debility (R54)
R53.82 Chronic fatigue, unspecified
    Chronic fatigue syndrome NOS
    Excludes 1: postviral fatigue syndrome (G93.3)
R53.83 Other fatigue
    Fatigue NOS
    Lack of energy
    Lethargy
    Tiredness
R54 Age-related physical debility
Frailty
Old age
Senescence
Senile asthenia
Senile debility
Excludes 1: age-related cognitive decline (R41.81)
    senile psychosis (F03)
    senility NOS (R41.81)
R55 Syncope and collapse
Blackout
Fainting
Vasovagal attack
Excludes 1: cardiogenic shock (R57.0)
    carotid sinus syncope (G90.01)
    heat syncope (T67.1)
    neurocirculatory asthenia (F45.8)
    neurogenic orthostatic hypotension (G90.3)
    orthostatic hypotension (I95.1)
    postprocedural shock (T81.1-)
    psychogenic syncope (F48.8)
    shock NOS (R57.9)
    shock complicating or following abortion or ectopic or
    molar pregnancy (O00-O07, O08.3)
    shock complicating or following labor and delivery

(O75.1)

Stokes-Adams attack (I45.9)

unconsciousness NOS (R40.2-)

R56 Convulsions, not elsewhere classified

Excludes 1: dissociative convulsions and seizures (F44.5)

epileptic convulsions and seizures (G40.-)

newborn convulsions and seizures (P90)

R56.0 Febrile convulsions

R56.00 Simple febrile convulsions

Febrile convulsion NOS

Febrile seizure NOS

R56.01 Complex febrile convulsions

Atypical febrile seizure

Complex febrile seizure

Complicated febrile seizure

Excludes 1: status epilepticus (G40.901)

R56.1 Post traumatic seizures

Excludes 1: post traumatic epilepsy (G40.-)

R56.9 Unspecified convulsions

Convulsion disorder

Fit NOS

Recurrent convulsions

Seizure(s) (convulsive) NOS

R57 Shock, not elsewhere classified

Excludes 1: anaphylactic shock NOS (T78.2)

anaphylactic reaction or shock due to adverse food reaction (T78.0-)

anaphylactic shock due to adverse effect of correct drug or medicament properly administered (T88.6)

anaphylactic shock due to serum (T80.5-)

anesthetic shock (T88.3)

electric shock (T75.4)

obstetric shock (O75.1)

postprocedural shock (T81.1-)

psychic shock (F43.0)

septic shock (R65.21)

shock complicating or following ectopic or molar pregnancy (O00-O07, O08.3)

shock due to lightning (T75.01)

traumatic shock (T79.4)

toxic shock syndrome (A48.3)

R57.0 Cardiogenic shock

R57.1 Hypovolemic shock

R57.8 Other shock

R57.9 Shock, unspecified

Failure of peripheral circulation NOS

R58 Hemorrhage, not elsewhere classified

Hemorrhage NOS

Excludes 1: hemorrhage included with underlying conditions, such as:

acute duodenal ulcer with hemorrhage (K26.0)

acute gastritis with bleeding (K29.01)

ulcerative enterocolitis with rectal bleeding (K51.01)

R59 Enlarged lymph nodes

Includes: swollen glands

Excludes 1: lymphadenitis NOS (I88.9)

acute lymphadenitis (L04.-)

chronic lymphadenitis (I88.1)

mesenteric (acute) (chronic) lymphadenitis (I88.0)

R59.0 Localized enlarged lymph nodes

R59.1 Generalized enlarged lymph nodes

Lymphadenopathy NOS

R59.9 Enlarged lymph nodes, unspecified

R60 Edema, not elsewhere classified

Excludes 1: angioneurotic edema (T78.3)

ascites (R18.-)

cerebral edema (G93.6)

cerebral edema due to birth injury (P11.0)

edema of larynx (J38.4)

edema of nasopharynx (J39.2)

edema of pharynx (J39.2)

gestational edema (O12.0-)

hereditary edema (Q82.0)

hydrops fetalis NOS (P83.2)

hydrothorax (J94.8)

nutritional edema (E40-E46)

hydrops fetalis NOS (P83.2)

newborn edema (P83.3)

pulmonary edema (J81.-)

R60.0 Localized edema

R60.1 Generalized edema

R60.9 Edema, unspecified

Fluid retention NOS

R61 Generalized hyperhidrosis

Excessive sweating

Night sweats

Secondary hyperhidrosis

Code first , if applicable, menopausal and female climacteric states (N95.1)

Excludes 1: focal (primary) (secondary) hyperhidrosis (L74.5-)

Frey's syndrome (L74.52)

localized (primary) (secondary) hyperhidrosis (L74.5-)

R62 Lack of expected normal physiological development in childhood and adults

Excludes 1: delayed puberty (E30.0)

gonadal dysgenesis (Q99.1)

hypopituitarism (E23.0)

R62.0 Delayed milestone in childhood

Delayed attainment of expected physiological developmental stage

Late talker

Late walker

R62.5 Other and unspecified lack of expected normal physiological development in childhood

Excludes 1: HIV disease resulting in failure to thrive (B20)

physical retardation due to malnutrition (E45)

R62.50 Unspecified lack of expected normal physiological development in childhood

Infantilism NOS

R62.51 Failure to thrive (child)

Failure to gain weight

Excludes 1: failure to thrive in child under 28 days old (P92.6)

R62.52 Short stature (child)

Lack of growth

Physical retardation

Short stature NOS

Excludes 1: short stature due to endocrine
disorder (E34.3)

R62.59 Other lack of expected normal physiological
development in childhood

R62.7 Adult failure to thrive

R63 Symptoms and signs concerning food and fluid intake

Excludes 1: bulimia NOS (F50.2)
eating disorders of nonorganic origin (F50.-)
malnutrition (E40-E46)

R63.0 Anorexia
Loss of appetite
Excludes 1: anorexia nervosa (F50.0-)
loss of appetite of nonorganic origin (F50.8)

R63.1 Polydipsia
Excessive thirst

R63.2 Polyphagia
Excessive eating
Hyperalimentation NOS

R63.3 Feeding difficulties
Feeding problem (elderly) (infant) NOS
Excludes 1: feeding problems of newborn (P92.-)
infant feeding disorder of nonorganic origin
(F98.2-)

R63.4 Abnormal weight loss

R63.5 Abnormal weight gain
Excludes 1: excessive weight gain in pregnancy (O26.0-)
obesity (E66.-)

R63.6 Underweight
Use additional code to identify body mass index (BMI), if
known (Z68.-)
Excludes 1: abnormal weight loss (R63.4)
anorexia nervosa (F50.0-)
malnutrition (E40-E46)

R63.8 Other symptoms and signs concerning food and fluid
intake

R64 Cachexia
Wasting syndrome
Code first underlying condition, if known
Excludes 1: abnormal weight loss (R63.4)
nutritional marasmus (E41)

R65 Symptoms and signs specifically associated with systemic
inflammation and infection

R65.1 Systemic inflammatory response syndrome (SIRS) of
non-infectious origin
Code first underlying condition, such as:
heatstroke (T67.0)
injury and trauma (S00-T88)
Excludes 1: sepsis- code to infection
severe sepsis (R65.2)

R65.10 Systemic inflammatory response syndrome
(SIRS) of non-infectious origin without acute
organ dysfunction
Systemic inflammatory response syndrome
(SIRS) NOS

R65.11 Systemic inflammatory response syndrome
(SIRS) of non-infectious origin with acute organ
dysfunction
Use additional code to identify specific acute
organ dysfunction, such as:

acute kidney failure (N17.-)
acute respiratory failure (J96.0-)
critical illness myopathy (G72.81)
critical illness polyneuropathy
(G62.81)
disseminated intravascular
coagulopathy [DIC] (D65)
encephalopathy (metabolic) (septic)
(G93.41)
hepatic failure (K72.0-)

R65.2 Severe sepsis
Infection with associated acute organ dysfunction
Sepsis with acute organ dysfunction
Sepsis with multiple organ dysfunction
Systemic inflammatory response syndrome due to
infectious process with acute organ dysfunction
Code first underlying infection, such as:
infection following a procedure (T81.4)
infections following infusion, transfusion and therapeutic
injection (T80.2-)
puerperal sepsis (O85)
sepsis following complete or unspecified spontaneous
abortion (O03.87)
sepsis following ectopic and molar pregnancy (O08.82)
sepsis following incomplete spontaneous abortion
(O03.37)
sepsis following (induced) termination of pregnancy
(O04.87)
sepsis NOS A41.9
Use additional code to identify specific acute organ
dysfunction, such as:
acute kidney failure (N17.-)
acute respiratory failure (J96.0-)
critical illness myopathy (G72.81)
critical illness polyneuropathy (G62.81)
disseminated intravascular coagulopathy [DIC] (D65)
encephalopathy (metabolic) (septic) (G93.41)
hepatic failure (K72.0-)

R65.20 Severe sepsis without septic shock
Severe sepsis NOS

R65.21 Severe sepsis with septic shock

R68 Other general symptoms and signs

R68.0 Hypothermia, not associated with low environmental
temperature
Excludes 1: hypothermia NOS (accidental) (T68)
hypothermia due to anesthesia (T88.51)
hypothermia due to low environmental
temperature (T68)
newborn hypothermia (P80.-)

R68.1 Nonspecific symptoms peculiar to infancy
Excludes 1: colic, infantile (R10.83)
neonatal cerebral irritability (P91.3)
teething syndrome (K00.7)

R68.11 Excessive crying of infant (baby)
Excludes 1: excessive crying of child,
adolescent, or adult (R45.83)

R68.12 Fussy infant (baby)
Irritable infant

R68.13 Apparent life threatening event in infant (ALTE)

Apparent life threatening event in newborn

Code first confirmed diagnosis, if known

Use additional code(s) for associated signs and symptoms if no confirmed diagnosis established, or if signs and symptoms are not associated routinely with confirmed diagnosis, or provide additional information for cause of ALTE

R68.19   Other nonspecific symptoms peculiar to infancy

R68.2   Dry mouth, unspecified

Excludes 1: dry mouth due to dehydration (E86.0)

dry mouth due to sicca syndrome [Sjögren] (M35.0-)

salivary gland hyposecretion (K11.7)

R68.3   Clubbing of fingers

Clubbing of nails

Excludes 1: congenital clubfinger (Q68.1)

R68.8   Other general symptoms and signs

R68.81   Early satiety

R68.82   Decreased libido

Decreased sexual desire

R68.83   Chills (without fever)

Chills NOS

Excludes 1: chills with fever (R50.9)

R68.84   Jaw pain

Mandibular pain

Maxilla pain

Excludes 1: temporomandibular joint arthralgia (M26.62)

R68.89   Other general symptoms and signs

R69   Illness, unspecified

Unknown and unspecified cases of morbidity

ABNORMAL FINDINGS ON EXAMINATION OF BLOOD, WITHOUT DIAGNOSIS (R70-R79)

Excludes 1: abnormalities (of)(on):

abnormal findings on antenatal screening of mother (O28.-)

coagulation hemorrhagic disorders (D65-D68)

lipids (E78.-)

platelets and thrombocytes (D69.-)

white blood cells classified elsewhere (D70-D72)

diagnostic abnormal findings classified elsewhere - see Alphabetical Index

hemorrhagic and hematological disorders of newborn (P50-P61)

R70   Elevated erythrocyte sedimentation rate and abnormality of plasma viscosity

R70.0   Elevated erythrocyte sedimentation rate

R70.1   Abnormal plasma viscosity

R71   Abnormality of red blood cells

Excludes 1: anemias (D50-D64)

anemia of premature infant (P61.2)

benign (familial) polycythemia (D75.0)

congenital anemias (P61.2-P61.4)

newborn anemia due to isoimmunization (P55.-)

polycythemia neonatorum (P61.1)

polycythemia NOS (D75.1)

polycythemia vera (D45)

secondary polycythemia (D75.1)

R71.0   Precipitous drop in hematocrit

Drop (precipitous) in hemoglobin

Drop in hematocrit

R71.8   Other abnormality of red blood cells

Abnormal red-cell morphology NOS

Abnormal red-cell volume NOS

Anisocytosis

Poikilocytosis

R73   Elevated blood glucose level

Excludes 1: diabetes mellitus (E08-E13)

diabetes mellitus in pregnancy, childbirth and the puerperium (O24.-)

neonatal disorders (P70.0-P70.2)

postsurgical hypoinsulinemia (E89.1)

R73.0   Abnormal glucose

Excludes 1: abnormal glucose in pregnancy (O99.81-)

diabetes mellitus (E08-E13)

dysmetabolic syndrome X (E88.81)

gestational diabetes (O24.4-)

glycosuria (R81)

hypoglycemia (E16.2)

R73.01   Impaired fasting glucose

Elevated fasting glucose

R73.02   Impaired glucose tolerance (oral)

Elevated glucose tolerance

R73.09   Other abnormal glucose

Abnormal glucose NOS

Abnormal non-fasting glucose tolerance

Latent diabetes

Prediabetes

R73.9   Hyperglycemia, unspecified

R74   Abnormal serum enzyme levels

R74.0   Nonspecific elevation of levels of transaminase and lactic acid dehydrogenase [LDH]

R74.8   Abnormal levels of other serum enzymes

Abnormal level of acid phosphatase

Abnormal level of alkaline phosphatase

Abnormal level of amylase

Abnormal level of lipase [triacylglycerol lipase]

R74.9   Abnormal serum enzyme level, unspecified

R75   Inconclusive laboratory evidence of human immunodeficiency virus [HIV]

Nonconclusive HIV-test finding in infants

Excludes 1: asymptomatic human immunodeficiency virus [HIV] infection status (Z21)

human immunodeficiency virus [HIV] disease (B20)

R76   Other abnormal immunological findings in serum

R76.0   Raised antibody titer

Excludes 1: Isoimmunization in pregnancy (O36.0-O36.1)

isoimmunization affecting newborn (P55.-)

R76.1   Nonspecific reaction to test for tuberculosis

R76.11   Nonspecific reaction to tuberculin skin test without active tuberculosis

Abnormal result of Mantoux test

PPD positive

Tuberculin (skin test) positive

Tuberculin (skin test) reactor

Excludes 1: nonspecific reaction to cell mediated immunity measurement of gamma interferon antigen response without active tuberculosis (R76.12)

R76.12   Nonspecific reaction to cell mediated immunity measurement of gamma interferon antigen response without active tuberculosis

Nonspecific reaction to QuantiFERON-TB test (QFT) without active tuberculosis

Excludes 1: nonspecific reaction to tuberculin skin test without active tuberculosis (R76.11)

positive tuberculin skin test (R76.11)

R76.8   Other specified abnormal immunological findings in serum

Raised level of immunoglobulins NOS

R76.9   Abnormal immunological finding in serum, unspecified

R77 Other abnormalities of plasma proteins

Excludes 1: disorders of plasma-protein metabolism (E88.0)

R77.0   Abnormality of albumin

R77.1   Abnormality of globulin

Hyperglobulinemia NOS

R77.2   Abnormality of alphafetoprotein

R77.8   Other specified abnormalities of plasma proteins

R77.9   Abnormality of plasma protein, unspecified

R78 Findings of drugs and other substances, not normally found in blood

Use additional code to identify the any retained foreign body, if applicable (Z18.-)

Excludes 1: mental or behavioral disorders due to psychoactive substance use (F10-F19)

R78.0   Finding of alcohol in blood

Use additional external cause code (Y90.-), for detail regarding alcohol level.

R78.1   Finding of opiate drug in blood

R78.2   Finding of cocaine in blood

R78.3   Finding of hallucinogen in blood

R78.4   Finding of other drugs of addictive potential in blood

R78.5   Finding of other psychotropic drug in blood

R78.6   Finding of steroid agent in blood

R78.7   Finding of abnormal level of heavy metals in blood

R78.71   Abnormal lead level in blood

Excludes 1: lead poisoning (T56.0-)

R78.79   Finding of abnormal level of heavy metals in blood

R78.8   Finding of other specified substances, not normally found in blood

R78.81   Bacteremia

Excludes 1: sepsis-code to specified infection (A00-B99)

R78.89   Finding of other specified substances, not normally found in blood

Finding of abnormal level of lithium in blood

R78.9   Finding of unspecified substance, not normally found in blood

R79 Other abnormal findings of blood chemistry

Use additional code to identify any retained foreign body, if applicable (Z18.-)

Excludes 1: abnormality of fluid, electrolyte or acid-base balance (E86-E87)

asymptomatic hyperuricemia (E79.0)

hyperglycemia NOS (R73.9)

hypoglycemia NOS (E16.2)

neonatal hypoglycemia (P70.3-P70.4)

specific findings indicating disorder of:

amino-acid metabolism (E70-E72)

carbohydrate metabolism (E73-E74)

lipid metabolism (E75.-)

R79.0   Abnormal level of blood mineral

Abnormal blood level of cobalt

Abnormal blood level of copper

Abnormal blood level of iron

Abnormal blood level of magnesium

Abnormal blood level of mineral NEC

Abnormal blood level of zinc

Excludes 1: abnormal level of lithium (R78.89)

disorders of mineral metabolism (E83.-)

neonatal hypomagnesemia (P71.2)

nutritional mineral deficiency (E58-E61)

R79.1   Abnormal coagulation profile

Abnormal or prolonged bleeding time

Abnormal or prolonged coagulation time

Abnormal or prolonged partial thromboplastin time [PTT]

Abnormal or prolonged prothrombin time [PT]

Excludes 1: coagulation defects (D68.-)

R79.8   Other specified abnormal findings of blood chemistry

R79.81   Abnormal blood-gas level

R79.82   Elevated C-reactive protein (CRP)

R79.89   Other specified abnormal findings of blood chemistry

R79.9   Abnormal finding of blood chemistry, unspecified

ABNORMAL FINDINGS ON EXAMINATION OF URINE, WITHOUT DIAGNOSIS (R80-R82)

Excludes 1: abnormal findings on antenatal screening of mother (O28.-)

diagnostic abnormal findings classified elsewhere - see Alphabetical Index

specific findings indicating disorder of:

amino-acid metabolism (E70-E72)

carbohydrate metabolism (E73-E74)

R80 Proteinuria

Excludes 1: gestational proteinuria (O12.1-)

R80.0   Isolated proteinuria

Idiopathic proteinuria

Excludes 1: isolated proteinuria with specific morphological lesion (N06.-)

R80.1   Persistent proteinuria, unspecified

R80.2   Orthostatic proteinuria, unspecified

Postural proteinuria

R80.3   Bence Jones proteinuria

R80.8   Other proteinuria

R80.9   Proteinuria, unspecified

Albuminuria NOS

R81 Glycosuria

Excludes 1: renal glycosuria (E74.8)

R82 Other and unspecified abnormal findings in urine

Includes: chromoabnormalities in urine

Use additional code to identify any retained foreign body, if applicable (Z18.-)

Excludes 2: hematuria (R31.-)

R82.0 Chyluria

Excludes 1: filarial chyluria (B74.-)

R82.1 Myoglobinuria

R82.2 Biliuria

R82.3 Hemoglobinuria

Excludes 1: hemoglobinuria due to hemolysis from external causes NEC (D59.6)

hemoglobinuria due to paroxysmal nocturnal [Marchiafava-Micheli] (D59.5)

R82.4 Acetonuria

Ketonuria

R82.5 Elevated urine levels of drugs, medicaments and biological substances

Elevated urine levels of catecholamines

Elevated urine levels of indoleacetic acid

Elevated urine levels of 17-ketosteroids

Elevated urine levels of steroids

R82.6 Abnormal urine levels of substances chiefly nonmedicinal as to source

Abnormal urine level of heavy metals

R82.7 Abnormal findings on microbiological examination of urine

Positive culture findings of urine

Excludes 1: colonization status (Z22.-)

R82.8 Abnormal findings on cytological and histological examination of urine

R82.9 Other and unspecified abnormal findings in urine

R82.90 Unspecified abnormal findings in urine

R82.91 Other chromoabnormalities of urine

Chromoconversion (dipstick)

Idiopathic dipstick converts positive for blood with no cellular forms in sediment

Excludes 1: hemoglobinuria (R82.3)

myoglobinuria (R82.1)

R82.99 Other abnormal findings in urine

Cells and casts in urine

Crystalluria

Melanuria

ABNORMAL FINDINGS ON EXAMINATION OF OTHER BODY FLUIDS, SUBSTANCES AND TISSUES, WITHOUT DIAGNOSIS (R83-R89)

Excludes 1: abnormal findings on antenatal screening of mother (O28.-)

diagnostic abnormal findings classified elsewhere - see Alphabetical Index

Excludes 2: abnormal findings on examination of blood, without diagnosis (R70-R79)

abnormal findings on examination of urine, without diagnosis (R80-R82)

abnormal tumor markers (R97.-)

R83 Abnormal findings in cerebrospinal fluid

R83.0 Abnormal level of enzymes in cerebrospinal fluid

R83.1 Abnormal level of hormones in cerebrospinal fluid

R83.2 Abnormal level of other drugs, medicaments and biological substances in cerebrospinal fluid

R83.3 Abnormal level of substances chiefly nonmedicinal as to source in cerebrospinal fluid

R83.4 Abnormal immunological findings in cerebrospinal fluid

R83.5 Abnormal microbiological findings in cerebrospinal fluid

Positive culture findings in cerebrospinal fluid

Excludes 1: colonization status (Z22.-)

R83.6 Abnormal cytological findings in cerebrospinal fluid

R83.8 Other abnormal findings in cerebrospinal fluid

Abnormal chromosomal findings in cerebrospinal fluid

R83.9 Unspecified abnormal finding in cerebrospinal fluid

R84 Abnormal findings in specimens from respiratory organs and thorax

Includes: abnormal findings in bronchial washings

abnormal findings in nasal secretions

abnormal findings in pleural fluid

abnormal findings in sputum

abnormal findings in throat scrapings

Excludes 1: blood-stained sputum (R04.2)

R84.0 Abnormal level of enzymes in specimens from respiratory organs and thorax

R84.1 Abnormal level of hormones in specimens from respiratory organs and thorax

R84.2 Abnormal level of other drugs, medicaments and biological substances in specimens from respiratory organs and thorax

R84.3 Abnormal level of substances chiefly nonmedicinal as to source in specimens from respiratory organs and thorax

R84.4 Abnormal immunological findings in specimens from respiratory organs and thorax

R84.5 Abnormal microbiological findings in specimens from respiratory organs and thorax

Positive culture findings in specimens from respiratory organs and thorax

Excludes 1: colonization status (Z22.-)

R84.6 Abnormal cytological findings in specimens from respiratory organs and thorax

R84.7 Abnormal histological findings in specimens from respiratory organs and thorax

R84.8 Other abnormal findings in specimens from respiratory organs and thorax

Abnormal chromosomal findings in specimens from respiratory organs and thorax

R84.9 Unspecified abnormal finding in specimens from respiratory organs and thorax

R85 Abnormal findings in specimens from digestive organs and abdominal cavity

Includes: abnormal findings in peritoneal fluid

abnormal findings in saliva

Excludes 1: cloudy peritoneal dialysis effluent (R88.0)

fecal abnormalities (R19.5)

R85.0 Abnormal level of enzymes in specimens from digestive organs and abdominal cavity

R85.1 Abnormal level of hormones in specimens from digestive organs and abdominal cavity

R85.2 Abnormal level of other drugs, medicaments and biological substances in specimens from digestive organs and abdominal cavity

R85.3 Abnormal level of substances chiefly nonmedicinal as to source in specimens from digestive organs and abdominal cavity

R85.4 Abnormal immunological findings in specimens from digestive organs and abdominal cavity

R85.5 Abnormal microbiological findings in specimens from digestive organs and abdominal cavity

Positive culture findings in specimens from digestive organs and abdominal cavity

Excludes 1: colonization status (Z22.-)

R85.6 Abnormal cytological findings in specimens from digestive organs and abdominal cavity

R85.61 Abnormal cytologic smear of anus

Excludes 1: abnormal cytological findings in specimens from other digestive organs and abdominal cavity (R85.69)

carcinoma in situ of anus (histologically confirmed) (D01.3)

anal intraepithelial neoplasia I [AIN I] (K62.82)

anal intraepithelial neoplasia II [AIN II] (K62.82)

anal intraepithelial neoplasia III [AIN III] (D01.3)

dysplasia (mild) (moderate) of anus (histologically confirmed) (K62.82)

severe dysplasia of anus (histologically confirmed) (D01.3)

Excludes 2: anal high risk human papillomavirus (HPV) DNA test positive (R85.81)

anal low risk human papillomavirus (HPV) DNA test positive (R85.82)

R85.610 Atypical squamous cells of undetermined significance on cytologic smear of anus (ASC-US)

R85.611 Atypical squamous cells cannot exclude high grade squamous intraepithelial lesion on cytologic smear of anus (ASC-H)

R85.612 Low grade squamous intraepithelial lesion on cytologic smear of anus (LGSIL)

R85.613 High grade squamous intraepithelial lesion on cytologic smear of anus (HGSIL)

R85.614 Cytologic evidence of malignancy on smear of anus

R85.615 Unsatisfactory cytologic smear of anus

Inadequate sample of cytologic smear of anus

R85.616 Satisfactory anal smear but lacking transformation zone

R85.618 Other abnormal cytological findings on specimens from anus

R85.619 Unspecified abnormal cytological findings in specimens from anus

Abnormal anal cytology NOS

Atypical glandular cells of anus NOS

R85.69 Abnormal cytological findings in specimens from other digestive organs and abdominal cavity

R85.7 Abnormal histological findings in specimens from digestive organs and abdominal cavity

R85.8 Other abnormal findings in specimens from digestive organs and abdominal cavity

R85.81 Anal high risk human papillomavirus (HPV) DNA test positive

Excludes 1: anogenital warts due to human papillomavirus (HPV) (A63.0)

condyloma acuminatum (A63.0)

R85.82 Anal low risk human papillomavirus (HPV) DNA test positive

Use additional code for associated human papillomavirus (B97.7)

R85.89 Other abnormal findings in specimens from digestive organs and abdominal cavity

Abnormal chromosomal findings in specimens from digestive organs and abdominal cavity

R85.9 Unspecified abnormal finding in specimens from digestive organs and abdominal cavity

R86 Abnormal findings in specimens from male genital organs

Includes: abnormal findings in prostatic secretions

abnormal findings in semen, seminal fluid

abnormal spermatozoa

Excludes 1: azoospermia (N46.0-)

oligospermia (N46.1-)

R86.0 Abnormal level of enzymes in specimens from male genital organs

R86.1 Abnormal level of hormones in specimens from male genital organs

R86.2 Abnormal level of other drugs, medicaments and biological substances in specimens from male genital organs

R86.3 Abnormal level of substances chiefly nonmedicinal as to source in specimens from male genital organs

R86.4 Abnormal immunological findings in specimens from male genital organs

R86.5 Abnormal microbiological findings in specimens from male genital organs

Positive culture findings in specimens from male genital organs

Excludes 1: colonization status (Z22.-)

R86.6 Abnormal cytological findings in specimens from male genital organs

R86.7 Abnormal histological findings in specimens from male genital organs

R86.8 Other abnormal findings in specimens from male genital organs

Abnormal chromosomal findings in specimens from male genital organs

R86.9 Unspecified abnormal finding in specimens from male genital organs

R87 Abnormal findings in specimens from female genital organs

Includes: abnormal findings in secretion and smears from cervix uteri

abnormal findings in secretion and smears from vagina

abnormal findings in secretion and smears from vulva

R87.0 Abnormal level of enzymes in specimens from female genital organs

R87.1 Abnormal level of hormones in specimens from female genital organs

R87.2 Abnormal level of other drugs, medicaments and biological substances in specimens from female genital organs

● New code   ▲ Revised code   ⑦ 7th digit required   ⊗ Placeholder required

R87.3 Abnormal level of substances chiefly nonmedicinal as to source in specimens from female genital organs

R87.4 Abnormal immunological findings in specimens from female genital organs

R87.5 Abnormal microbiological findings in specimens from female genital organs

Positive culture findings in specimens from female genital organs

Excludes 1: colonization status (Z22.-)

R87.6 Abnormal cytological findings in specimens from female genital organs

  R87.61 Abnormal cytological findings in specimens from cervix uteri

Excludes 1: abnormal cytological findings in specimens from other female genital organs (R87.69)

abnormal cytological findings in specimens from vagina (R87.62-)

carcinoma in situ of cervix uteri (histologically confirmed) (D06.-)

cervical intraepithelial neoplasia I [CIN I] (N87.0)

cervical intraepithelial neoplasia II [CIN II] (N87.1)

cervical intraepithelial neoplasia III [CIN III] (D06.-)

dysplasia (mild) (moderate) of cervix uteri (histologically confirmed) (N87.-)

severe dysplasia of cervix uteri (histologically confirmed) (D06.-)

Excludes 2: cervical high risk human papillomavirus (HPV) DNA test positive (R87.810)

cervical low risk human papillomavirus (HPV) DNA test positive (R87.820)

    R87.610 Atypical squamous cells of undetermined significance on cytologic smear of cervix (ASC-US)

    R87.611 Atypical squamous cells cannot exclude high grade squamous intraepithelial lesion on cytologic smear of cervix (ASC-H)

    R87.612 Low grade squamous intraepithelial lesion on cytologic smear of cervix (LGSIL)

    R87.613 High grade squamous intraepithelial lesion on cytologic smear of cervix (HGSIL)

    R87.614 Cytologic evidence of malignancy on smear of cervix

    R87.615 Unsatisfactory cytologic smear of cervix

Inadequate sample of cytologic smear of cervix

    R87.616 Satisfactory cervical smear but lacking transformation zone

    R87.618 Other abnormal cytological findings on specimens from cervix uteri

    R87.619 Unspecified abnormal cytological findings in specimens from cervix uteri

Abnormal cervical cytology NOS

Abnormal Papanicolaou smear of cervix NOS

Abnormal thin preparation smear of cervix NOS

Atypical endocervical cells of cervix NOS

Atypical endometrial cells of cervix NOS

Atypical glandular cells of cervix NOS

  R87.62 Abnormal cytological findings in specimens from vagina

Use additional code to identify acquired absence of uterus and cervix, if applicable (Z90.71-)

Excludes 1: abnormal cytological findings in specimens from cervix uteri (R87.61-)

abnormal cytological findings in specimens from other female genital organs (R87.69)

carcinoma in situ of vagina (histologically confirmed) (D07.2)

vaginal intraepithelial neoplasia I [VAIN I] (N89.0)

vaginal intraepithelial neoplasia II [VAIN II] (N89.1)

vaginal intraepithelial neoplasia III [VAIN III] (D07.2)

dysplasia (mild) (moderate) of vagina (histologically confirmed) (N89.-)

severe dysplasia of vagina (histologically confirmed) (D07.2)

Excludes 2: vaginal high risk human papillomavirus (HPV) DNA test positive (R87.811)

vaginal low risk human papillomavirus (HPV) DNA test positive (R87.821)

    R87.620 Atypical squamous cells of undetermined significance on cytologic smear of vagina (ASC-US)

    R87.621 Atypical squamous cells cannot exclude high grade squamous intraepithelial lesion on cytologic smear of vagina (ASC-H)

    R87.622 Low grade squamous intraepithelial lesion on cytologic smear of vagina (LGSIL)

    R87.623 High grade squamous intraepithelial lesion on cytologic smear of vagina (HGSIL)

    R87.624 Cytologic evidence of malignancy on smear of vagina

    R87.625 Unsatisfactory cytologic smear of vagina

Inadequate sample of cytologic smear of vagina

R87.628 Other abnormal cytological findings on specimens from vagina

R87.629 Unspecified abnormal cytological findings in specimens from vagina

Abnormal Papanicolaou smear of vagina NOS

Abnormal thin preparation smear of vagina NOS

Abnormal vaginal cytology NOS

Atypical endocervical cells of vagina NOS

Atypical endometrial cells of vagina NOS

Atypical glandular cells of vagina NOS

R87.69 Abnormal cytological findings in specimens from other female genital organs

Abnormal cytological findings in specimens from female genital organs NOS

Excludes 1: dysplasia of vulva (histologically confirmed) (N90.0-N90.3)

R87.7 Abnormal histological findings in specimens from female genital organs

Excludes 1: carcinoma in situ (histologically confirmed) of female genital organs (D06-D07.3)

cervical intraepithelial neoplasia I [CIN I] (N87.0)

cervical intraepithelial neoplasia II [CIN II] (N87.1)

cervical intraepithelial neoplasia III [CIN III] (D06.-)

dysplasia (mild) (moderate) of cervix uteri (histologically confirmed) (N87.-)

dysplasia (mild) (moderate) of vagina (histologically confirmed) (N89.-)

vaginal intraepithelial neoplasia I [VAIN I] (N89.0)

vaginal intraepithelial neoplasia II [VAIN II] (N89.1)

vaginal intraepithelial neoplasia III [VAIN III] (D07.2)

severe dysplasia of cervix uteri (histologically confirmed) (D06.-)

severe dysplasia of vagina (histologically confirmed) (D07.2)

R87.8 Other abnormal findings in specimens from female genital organs

R87.81 High risk human papillomavirus (HPV) DNA test positive from female genital organs

Excludes 1: anogenital warts due to human papillomavirus (HPV) (A63.0) condyloma acuminatum (A63.0)

R87.810 Cervical high risk human papillomavirus (HPV) DNA test positive

R87.811 Vaginal high risk human papillomavirus (HPV) DNA test positive

R87.82 Low risk human papillomavirus (HPV) DNA test positive from female genital organs

Use additional code for associated human

papillomavirus (B97.7)

R87.820 Cervical low risk human papillomavirus (HPV) DNA test positive

R87.821 Vaginal low risk human papillomavirus (HPV) DNA test positive

R87.89 Other abnormal findings in specimens from female genital organs

Abnormal chromosomal findings in specimens from female genital organs

R87.9 Unspecified abnormal finding in specimens from female genital organs

R88 Abnormal findings in other body fluids and substances

R88.0 Cloudy (hemodialysis) (peritoneal) dialysis effluent

R88.8 Abnormal findings in other body fluids and substances

R89 Abnormal findings in specimens from other organs, systems and tissues

Includes: abnormal findings in nipple discharge

abnormal findings in synovial fluid

abnormal findings in wound secretions

R89.0 Abnormal level of enzymes in specimens from other organs, systems and tissues

R89.1 Abnormal level of hormones in specimens from other organs, systems and tissues

R89.2 Abnormal level of other drugs, medicaments and biological substances in specimens from other organs, systems and tissues

R89.3 Abnormal level of substances chiefly nonmedicinal as to source in specimens from other organs, systems and tissues

R89.4 Abnormal immunological findings in specimens from other organs, systems and tissues

R89.5 Abnormal microbiological findings in specimens from other organs, systems and tissues

Positive culture findings in specimens from other organs, systems and tissues

Excludes 1: colonization status (Z22.-)

R89.6 Abnormal cytological findings in specimens from other organs, systems and tissues

R89.7 Abnormal histological findings in specimens from other organs, systems and tissues

R89.8 Other abnormal findings in specimens from other organs, systems and tissues

Abnormal chromosomal findings in specimens from other organs, systems and tissues

R89.9 Unspecified abnormal finding in specimens from other organs, systems and tissues

ABNORMAL FINDINGS ON DIAGNOSTIC IMAGING AND IN FUNCTION STUDIES, WITHOUT DIAGNOSIS (R90-R94)

Includes: nonspecific abnormal findings on diagnostic imaging by computerized axial tomography [CAT scan]

nonspecific abnormal findings on diagnostic imaging by magnetic resonance imaging [MRI][NMR]

nonspecific abnormal findings on diagnostic imaging by positron emission tomography [PET scan]

nonspecific abnormal findings on diagnostic imaging by thermography

nonspecific abnormal findings on diagnostic imaging by ultrasound [echogram] nonspecific abnormal findings on diagnostic imaging by X-ray examination

Excludes 1: abnormal findings on antenatal screening of mother (O28.-)
diagnostic abnormal findings classified elsewhere - see Alphabetical Index

R90 Abnormal findings on diagnostic imaging of central nervous system

R90.0 Intracranial space-occupying lesion found on diagnostic imaging of central nervous system

R90.8 Other abnormal findings on diagnostic imaging of central nervous system

    R90.81 Abnormal echoencephalogram

    R90.82 White matter disease, unspecified

    R90.89 Other abnormal findings on diagnostic imaging of central nervous system

       Other cerebrovascular abnormality found on diagnostic imaging of central nervous system

R91 Abnormal findings on diagnostic imaging of lung

R91.1 Solitary pulmonary nodule

    Coin lesion lung

    Solitary pulmonary nodule, subsegmental branch of the bronchial tree

R91.8 Other nonspecific abnormal finding of lung field

    Lung mass NOS found on diagnostic imaging of lung

    Pulmonary infiltrate NOS

    Shadow, lung

R92 Abnormal and inconclusive findings on diagnostic imaging of breast

R92.0 Mammographic microcalcification found on diagnostic imaging of breast

    Excludes 2: mammographic calcification (calculus) found on diagnostic imaging of breast (R92.1)

R92.1 Mammographic calcification found on diagnostic imaging of breast

    Mammographic calculus found on diagnostic imaging of breast

R92.2 Inconclusive mammogram

    Dense breasts NOS

    Inconclusive mammogram NEC

    Inconclusive mammography due to dense breasts

    Inconclusive mammography NEC

R92.8 Other abnormal and inconclusive findings on diagnostic imaging of breast

R93 Abnormal findings on diagnostic imaging of other body structures

R93.0 Abnormal findings on diagnostic imaging of skull and head, not elsewhere classified

    Excludes 1: intracranial space-occupying lesion found on diagnostic imaging (R90.0)

R93.1 Abnormal findings on diagnostic imaging of heart and coronary circulation

    Abnormal echocardiogram NOS

    Abnormal heart shadow

R93.2 Abnormal findings on diagnostic imaging of liver and biliary tract

    Nonvisualization of gallbladder

R93.3 Abnormal findings on diagnostic imaging of other parts of digestive tract

R93.4 Abnormal findings on diagnostic imaging of urinary organs

    Filling defect of bladder found on diagnostic imaging

    Filling defect of kidney found on diagnostic imaging

Filling defect of ureter found on diagnostic imaging

Excludes 1: hypertrophy of kidney (N28.81)

R93.5 Abnormal findings on diagnostic imaging of other abdominal regions, including retroperitoneum

R93.6 Abnormal findings on diagnostic imaging of limbs

Excludes 2: abnormal finding in skin and subcutaneous tissue (R93.8)

R93.7 Abnormal findings on diagnostic imaging of other parts of musculoskeletal system

Excludes 2: abnormal findings on diagnostic imaging of skull (R93.0)

R93.8 Abnormal findings on diagnostic imaging of other specified body structures

    Abnormal finding by radioisotope localization of placenta

    Abnormal radiological finding in skin and subcutaneous tissue

    Mediastinal shift

R93.9 Diagnostic imaging inconclusive due to excess body fat of patient

R94 Abnormal results of function studies

Includes: abnormal results of radionuclide [radioisotope] uptake studies

abnormal results of scintigraphy

R94.0 Abnormal results of function studies of central nervous system

    R94.01 Abnormal electroencephalogram [EEG]

    R94.02 Abnormal brain scan

    R94.09 Abnormal results of other function studies of central nervous system

R94.1 Abnormal results of function studies of peripheral nervous system and special senses

    R94.11 Abnormal results of function studies of eye

        R94.110 Abnormal electro-oculogram [EOG]

        R94.111 Abnormal electroretinogram [ERG]

            Abnormal retinal function study

        R94.112 Abnormal visually evoked potential [VEP]

        R94.113 Abnormal oculomotor study

        R94.118 Abnormal results of other function studies of eye

    R94.12 Abnormal results of function studies of ear and other special senses

        R94.120 Abnormal auditory function study

        R94.121 Abnormal vestibular function study

        R94.128 Abnormal results of other function studies of ear and other special senses

    R94.13 Abnormal results of function studies of peripheral nervous system

        R94.130 Abnormal response to nerve stimulation, unspecified

        R94.131 Abnormal electromyogram [EMG]

            Excludes 1: electromyogram of eye (R94.113)

        R94.138 Abnormal results of other function studies of peripheral nervous system

R94.2 Abnormal results of pulmonary function studies

    Reduced ventilatory capacity

    Reduced vital capacity

R94.3 Abnormal results of cardiovascular function studies

R94.30 Abnormal result of cardiovascular function study, unspecified

R94.31 Abnormal electrocardiogram [ECG] [EKG]

Excludes 1: long QT syndrome (I45.81)

R94.39 Abnormal result of other cardiovascular function study

Abnormal electrophysiological intracardiac studies

Abnormal phonocardiogram

Abnormal vectorcardiogram

R94.4 Abnormal results of kidney function studies

Abnormal renal function test

R94.5 Abnormal results of liver function studies

R94.6 Abnormal results of thyroid function studies

R94.7 Abnormal results of other endocrine function studies

Excludes 2: abnormal glucose (R73.0-)

R94.8 Abnormal results of function studies of other organs and systems

Abnormal basal metabolic rate [BMR]

Abnormal bladder function test

Abnormal splenic function test

ABNORMAL TUMOR MARKERS (R97)

 Abnormal tumor markers

Elevated tumor associated antigens [TAA]

Elevated tumor specific antigens [TSA]

R97.0 Elevated carcinoembryonic antigen [CEA]

R97.1 Elevated cancer antigen 125   [CA 125]

R97.2 Elevated prostate specific antigen [PSA]

R97.8 Other abnormal tumor markers

Ill-defined and unknown cause of mortality (R99)

R99 Ill-defined and unknown cause of mortality

Death (unexplained) NOS

Unspecified cause of mortality

Chapter 19: Injury, Poisoning And Certain Other Consequences Of External Causes (S00-T88)

Note: Use secondary code(s) from Chapter 20, External causes of morbidity, to indicate cause of injury. Codes within the T section that include the external cause do not require an additional external cause code

Use additional code to identify any retained foreign body, if applicable (Z18.-)

Excludes 1: birth trauma (P10-P15)

obstetric trauma (O70-O71)

Note: The chapter uses the S-section for coding different types of injuries related to single body regions and the T-section to cover injuries to unspecified body regions as well as poisoning and certain other consequences of external causes.

This chapter contains the following blocks:

S00-S09	Injuries to the head
S10-S19	Injuries to the neck
S20-S29	Injuries to the thorax
S30-S39	Injuries to the abdomen, lower back, lumbar spine, pelvis and external genitals
S40-S49	Injuries to the shoulder and upper arm
S50-S59	Injuries to the elbow and forearm
S60-S69	Injuries to the wrist, hand and fingers
S70-S79	Injuries to the hip and thigh
S80-S89	Injuries to the knee and lower leg
S90-S99	Injuries to the ankle and foot
T07	Injuries involving multiple body regions
T14	Injury of unspecified body region
T15-T19	Effects of foreign body entering through natural orifice
T20-T32	Burns and corrosions
T20-T25	Burns and corrosions of external body surface, specified by site
T26-T28	Burns and corrosions confined to eye and internal organs
T30-T32	Burns and corrosions of multiple and unspecified body regions
T33-T34	Frostbite
T36-T50	Poisoning by, adverse effect of and underdosing of drugs, medicaments and biological substances
T51-T65	Toxic effects of substances chiefly nonmedicinal as to source
T66-T78	Other and unspecified effects of external causes
T79	Certain early complications of trauma
T80-T88	Complications of surgical and medical care, not elsewhere classified

INJURIES TO THE HEAD (S00-S09)

Includes: injuries of ear

injuries of eye

injuries of face [any part]

injuries of gum

injuries of jaw

injuries of oral cavity

injuries of palate

injuries of periocular area

injuries of scalp

injuries of temporomandibular joint area

injuries of tongue

injuries of tooth

Code also for any associated infection

Excludes 2: burns and corrosions (T20-T32)

effects of foreign body in ear (T16)

effects of foreign body in larynx (T17.3)

effects of foreign body in mouth NOS (T18.0)

effects of foreign body in nose (T17.0-T17.1)

effects of foreign body in pharynx (T17.2)

effects of foreign body on external eye (T15.-)

frostbite (T33-T34)

insect bite or sting, venomous (T63.4)

S00 Superficial injury of head

Excludes 1: diffuse cerebral contusion (S06.2-)

focal cerebral contusion (S06.3-)

injury of eye and orbit (S05.-)

open wound of head (S01.-)

The appropriate 7th character is to be added to each code from category S00

A - initial encounter

D - subsequent encounter

S - sequela

S00.0   Superficial injury of scalp

⊗⑦**S00.00**   Unspecified superficial injury of scalp

⊗⑦**S00.01**   Abrasion of scalp

⊗⑦**S00.02**   Blister (nonthermal) of scalp

⊗⑦**S00.03**   Contusion of scalp

Bruise of scalp

Hematoma of scalp

⊗⑦**S00.04**   External constriction of part of scalp

⊗⑦**S00.05**   Superficial foreign body of scalp

Splinter in the scalp

⊗⑦**S00.06**   Insect bite (nonvenomous) of scalp

⊗⑦**S00.07**   Other superficial bite of scalp

Excludes 1: open bite of scalp (S01.05)

S00.1   Contusion of eyelid and periocular area

Black eye

Excludes 2: contusion of eyeball and orbital tissues (S05.1)

⊗⑦**S00.10**   Contusion of unspecified eyelid and periocular area

⊗⑦**S00.11**   Contusion of right eyelid and periocular area

⊗⑦**S00.12**   Contusion of left eyelid and periocular area

S00.2   Other and unspecified superficial injuries of eyelid and periocular area

Excludes 2: superficial injury of conjunctiva and cornea (S05.0-)

S00.20   Unspecified superficial injury of eyelid and periocular area

⑦**S00.201**   Unspecified superficial injury of right eyelid and periocular area

⑦**S00.202**   Unspecified superficial injury of left eyelid and periocular area

⑦**S00.209**   Unspecified superficial injury of unspecified eyelid and periocular area

S00.21   Abrasion of eyelid and periocular area

⑦**S00.211**   Abrasion of right eyelid and periocular area

⑦S00.212 Abrasion of left eyelid and periocular area

⑦S00.219 Abrasion of unspecified eyelid and periocular area

S00.22 Blister (nonthermal) of eyelid and periocular area

⑦S00.221 Blister (nonthermal) of right eyelid and periocular area

⑦S00.222 Blister (nonthermal) of left eyelid and periocular area

⑦S00.229 Blister (nonthermal) of unspecified eyelid and periocular area

S00.24 External constriction of eyelid and periocular area

⑦S00.241 External constriction of right eyelid and periocular area

⑦S00.242 External constriction of left eyelid and periocular area

⑦S00.249 External constriction of unspecified eyelid and periocular area

S00.25 Superficial foreign body of eyelid and periocular area

Splinter of eyelid and periocular area

Excludes 2: retained foreign body in eyelid (H02.81-)

⑦S00.251 Superficial foreign body of right eyelid and periocular area

⑦S00.252 Superficial foreign body of left eyelid and periocular area

⑦S00.259 Superficial foreign body of unspecified eyelid and periocular area

S00.26 Insect bite (nonvenomous) of eyelid and periocular area

⑦S00.261 Insect bite (nonvenomous) of right eyelid and periocular area

⑦S00.262 Insect bite (nonvenomous) of left eyelid and periocular area

⑦S00.269 Insect bite (nonvenomous) of unspecified eyelid and periocular area

S00.27 Other superficial bite of eyelid and periocular area

Excludes 1: open bite of eyelid and periocular area (S01.15)

⑦S00.271 Other superficial bite of right eyelid and periocular area

⑦S00.272 Other superficial bite of left eyelid and periocular area

⑦S00.279 Other superficial bite of unspecified eyelid and periocular area

S00.3 Superficial injury of nose

⊗⑦S00.30 Unspecified superficial injury of nose

⊗⑦S00.31 Abrasion of nose

⊗⑦S00.32 Blister (nonthermal) of nose

⊗⑦S00.33 Contusion of nose

Bruise of nose

Hematoma of nose

⊗⑦S00.34 External constriction of nose

⊗⑦S00.35 Superficial foreign body of nose

Splinter in the nose

⊗⑦S00.36 Insect bite (nonvenomous) of nose

⊗⑦S00.37 Other superficial bite of nose

Excludes 1: open bite of nose (S01.25)

S00.4 Superficial injury of ear

S00.40 Unspecified superficial injury of ear

⑦S00.401 Unspecified superficial injury of right ear

⑦S00.402 Unspecified superficial injury of left ear

⑦S00.409 Unspecified superficial injury of unspecified ear

S00.41 Abrasion of ear

⑦S00.411 Abrasion of right ear

⑦S00.412 Abrasion of left ear

⑦S00.419 Abrasion of unspecified ear

S00.42 Blister (nonthermal) of ear

⑦S00.421 Blister (nonthermal) of right ear

⑦S00.422 Blister (nonthermal) of left ear

⑦S00.429 Blister (nonthermal) of unspecified ear

S00.43 Contusion of ear

Bruise of ear

Hematoma of ear

⑦S00.431 Contusion of right ear

⑦S00.432 Contusion of left ear

⑦S00.439 Contusion of unspecified ear

S00.44 External constriction of ear

⑦S00.441 External constriction of right ear

⑦S00.442 External constriction of left ear

⑦S00.449 External constriction of unspecified ear

S00.45 Superficial foreign body of ear

Splinter in the ear

⑦S00.451 Superficial foreign body of right ear

⑦S00.452 Superficial foreign body of left ear

⑦S00.459 Superficial foreign body of unspecified ear

S00.46 Insect bite (nonvenomous) of ear

⑦S00.461 Insect bite (nonvenomous) of right ear

⑦S00.462 Insect bite (nonvenomous) of left ear

⑦S00.469 Insect bite (nonvenomous) of unspecified ear

S00.47 Other superficial bite of ear

Excludes 1: open bite of ear (S01.35)

⑦S00.471 Other superficial bite of right ear

⑦S00.472 Other superficial bite of left ear

⑦S00.479 Other superficial bite of unspecified ear

S00.5 Superficial injury of lip and oral cavity

S00.50 Unspecified superficial injury of lip and oral cavity

⑦S00.501 Unspecified superficial injury of lip

⑦S00.502 Unspecified superficial injury of oral cavity

S00.51 Abrasion of lip and oral cavity

⑦**S00.511**   Abrasion of lip

⑦**S00.512**   Abrasion of oral cavity

S00.52   Blister (nonthermal) of lip and oral cavity

⑦**S00.521**   Blister (nonthermal) of lip

⑦**S00.522**   Blister (nonthermal) of oral cavity

S00.53   Contusion of lip and oral cavity

⑦**S00.531**   Contusion of lip

Bruise of lip

Hematoma of oral cavity

⑦**S00.532**   Contusion of oral cavity

Bruise of lip

Hematoma of oral cavity

S00.54   External constriction of lip and oral cavity

⑦**S00.541**   External constriction of lip

⑦**S00.542**   External constriction of oral cavity

S00.55   Superficial foreign body of lip and oral cavity

⑦**S00.551**   Superficial foreign body of lip

Splinter of lip and oral cavity

⑦**S00.552**   Superficial foreign body of oral cavity

Splinter of lip and oral cavity

S00.56   Insect bite (nonvenomous) of lip and oral cavity

⑦**S00.561**   Insect bite (nonvenomous) of lip

⑦**S00.562**   Insect bite (nonvenomous) of oral cavity

S00.57   Other superficial bite of lip and oral cavity

⑦**S00.571**   Other superficial bite of lip

Excludes 1: open bite of lip (S01.551)

⑦**S00.572**   Other superficial bite of oral cavity

Excludes 1: open bite of oral cavity (S01.552)

S00.8   Superficial injury of other parts of head

⊗⑦**S00.80**   Unspecified superficial injury of other part of head

⊗⑦**S00.81**   Abrasion of other part of head

⊗⑦**S00.82**   Blister (nonthermal) of other part of head

⊗⑦**S00.83**   Contusion of other part of head

Bruise of other part of head

Hematoma of other part of head

⊗⑦**S00.84**   External constriction of other part of head

⊗⑦**S00.85**   Superficial foreign body of other part of head

Splinter in other part of head

⊗⑦**S00.86**   Insect bite (nonvenomous) of other part of head

⊗⑦**S00.87**   Other superficial bite of other part of head

Excludes 1: open bite of other part of head (S01.85)

S00.9   Superficial injury of unspecified part of head

⊗⑦**S00.90**   Unspecified superficial injury of unspecified part of head

⊗⑦**S00.91**   Abrasion of unspecified part of head

⊗⑦**S00.92**   Blister (nonthermal) of unspecified part of head

⊗⑦**S00.93**   Contusion of unspecified part of head

Bruise of head

Hematoma of head

⊗⑦**S00.94**   External constriction of unspecified part of head

⊗⑦**S00.95**   Superficial foreign body of unspecified part of head

Splinter of head

⊗⑦**S00.96**   Insect bite (nonvenomous) of unspecified part of head

⊗⑦**S00.97**   Other superficial bite of unspecified part of head

Excludes 1: open bite of head (S01.95)

S01   Open wound of head

Code also any associated:

injury of cranial nerve (S04.-)

injury of muscle and tendon of head (S09.1-)

intracranial injury (S06.-)

wound infection

Excludes 1: open skull fracture (S02.- with 7th character B)

Excludes 2: injury of eye and orbit (S05.-)

traumatic amputation of part of head (S08.-)

The appropriate 7th character is to be added to each code from category S01

A - initial encounter

D - subsequent encounter

S - sequela

S01.0   Open wound of scalp

Excludes 1: avulsion of scalp (S08.0)

⊗⑦**S01.00**   Unspecified open wound of scalp

⊗⑦**S01.01**   Laceration without foreign body of scalp

⊗⑦**S01.02**   Laceration with foreign body of scalp

⊗⑦**S01.03**   Puncture wound without foreign body of scalp

⊗⑦**S01.04**   Puncture wound with foreign body of scalp

⊗⑦**S01.05**   Open bite of scalp

Bite of scalp NOS

Excludes 1: superficial bite of scalp (S00.06, S00.07-)

S01.1   Open wound of eyelid and periocular area

Open wound of eyelid and periocular area with or without involvement of lacrimal passages

S01.10   Unspecified open wound of eyelid and periocular area

⑦**S01.101**   Unspecified open wound of right eyelid and periocular area

⑦**S01.102**   Unspecified open wound of left eyelid and periocular area

⑦**S01.109**   Unspecified open wound of unspecified eyelid and periocular area

S01.11   Laceration without foreign body of eyelid and periocular area

⑦**S01.111**   Laceration without foreign body of right eyelid and periocular area

⑦**S01.112**   Laceration without foreign body of left eyelid and periocular area

⑦**S01.119**   Laceration without foreign body of unspecified eyelid and periocular area

S01.12   Laceration with foreign body of eyelid and periocular area

⑦**S01.121**   Laceration with foreign body of right eyelid and periocular area

⑦**S01.122**   Laceration with foreign body of left eyelid and periocular area

⑦ **S01.129** Laceration with foreign body of unspecified eyelid and periocular area

S01.13 Puncture wound without foreign body of eyelid and periocular area

⑦ **S01.131** Puncture wound without foreign body of right eyelid and periocular area

⑦ **S01.132** Puncture wound without foreign body of left eyelid and periocular area

⑦ **S01.139** Puncture wound without foreign body of unspecified eyelid and periocular area

S01.14 Puncture wound with foreign body of eyelid and periocular area

⑦ **S01.141** Puncture wound with foreign body of right eyelid and periocular area

⑦ **S01.142** Puncture wound with foreign body of left eyelid and periocular area

⑦ **S01.149** Puncture wound with foreign body of unspecified eyelid and periocular area

S01.15 Open bite of eyelid and periocular area
Bite of eyelid and periocular area NOS
Excludes 1: superficial bite of eyelid and periocular area (S00.26, S00.27)

⑦ **S01.151** Open bite of right eyelid and periocular area

⑦ **S01.152** Open bite of left eyelid and periocular area

⑦ **S01.159** Open bite of unspecified eyelid and periocular area

S01.2 Open wound of nose

⊗⑦ **S01.20** Unspecified open wound of nose

⊗⑦ **S01.21** Laceration without foreign body of nose

⊗⑦ **S01.22** Laceration with foreign body of nose

⊗⑦ **S01.23** Puncture wound without foreign body of nose

⊗⑦ **S01.24** Puncture wound with foreign body of nose

⊗⑦ **S01.25** Open bite of nose
Bite of nose NOS
Excludes 1: superficial bite of nose (S00.36, S00.37)

S01.3 Open wound of ear

S01.30 Unspecified open wound of ear

⑦ **S01.301** Unspecified open wound of right ear

⑦ **S01.302** Unspecified open wound of left ear

⑦ **S01.309** Unspecified open wound of unspecified ear

S01.31 Laceration without foreign body of ear

⑦ **S01.311** Laceration without foreign body of right ear

⑦ **S01.312** Laceration without foreign body of left ear

⑦ **S01.319** Laceration without foreign body of unspecified ear

S01.32 Laceration with foreign body of ear

⑦ **S01.321** Laceration with foreign body of right ear

⑦ **S01.322** Laceration with foreign body of left ear

⑦ **S01.329** Laceration with foreign body of unspecified ear

S01.33 Puncture wound without foreign body of ear

⑦ **S01.331** Puncture wound without foreign body of right ear

⑦ **S01.332** Puncture wound without foreign body of left ear

⑦ **S01.339** Puncture wound without foreign body of unspecified ear

S01.34 Puncture wound with foreign body of ear

⑦ **S01.341** Puncture wound with foreign body of right ear

⑦ **S01.342** Puncture wound with foreign body of left ear

⑦ **S01.349** Puncture wound with foreign body of unspecified ear

S01.35 Open bite of ear
Bite of ear NOS
Excludes 1: superficial bite of ear (S00.46, S00.47)

⑦ **S01.351** Open bite of right ear

⑦ **S01.352** Open bite of left ear

⑦ **S01.359** Open bite of unspecified ear

S01.4 Open wound of cheek and temporomandibular area

S01.40 Unspecified open wound of cheek and temporomandibular area

⑦ **S01.401** Unspecified open wound of right cheek and temporomandibular area

⑦ **S01.402** Unspecified open wound of left cheek and temporomandibular area

⑦ **S01.409** Unspecified open wound of unspecified cheek and temporomandibular area

S01.41 Laceration without foreign body of cheek and temporomandibular area

⑦ **S01.411** Laceration without foreign body of right cheek and temporomandibular area

⑦ **S01.412** Laceration without foreign body of left cheek and temporomandibular area

⑦ **S01.419** Laceration without foreign body of unspecified cheek and temporomandibular area

S01.42 Laceration with foreign body of cheek and temporomandibular area

⑦ **S01.421** Laceration with foreign body of right cheek and temporomandibular area

⑦ **S01.422** Laceration with foreign body of left cheek and temporomandibular area

⑦ **S01.429** Laceration with foreign body of unspecified cheek and temporomandibular area

S01.43 Puncture wound without foreign body of cheek and temporomandibular area

● New code ▲ Revised code ⑦ 7ᵗʰ digit required ⊗ Placeholder required

⑦**S01.431**   Puncture wound without foreign body of right cheek and temporomandibular area

⑦**S01.432**   Puncture wound without foreign body of left cheek and temporomandibular area

⑦**S01.439**   Puncture wound without foreign body of unspecified cheek and temporomandibular area

S01.44   Puncture wound with foreign body of cheek and temporomandibular area

⑦**S01.441**   Puncture wound with foreign body of right cheek and temporomandibular area

⑦**S01.442**   Puncture wound with foreign body of left cheek and temporomandibular area

⑦**S01.449**   Puncture wound with foreign body of unspecified cheek and temporomandibular area

S01.45   Open bite of cheek and temporomandibular area

Bite of cheek and temporomandibular area NOS

Excludes 2: superficial bite of cheek and temporomandibular area (S00.86, S00.87)

⑦**S01.451**   Open bite of right cheek and temporomandibular area

⑦**S01.452**   Open bite of left cheek and temporomandibular area

⑦**S01.459**   Open bite of unspecified cheek and temporomandibular area

S01.5   Open wound of lip and oral cavity

Excludes 2: tooth dislocation (S03.2)

tooth fracture (S02.5)

S01.50   Unspecified open wound of lip and oral cavity

⑦**S01.501**   Unspecified open wound of lip

⑦**S01.502**   Unspecified open wound of oral cavity

S01.51   Laceration of lip and oral cavity without foreign body

⑦**S01.511**   Laceration without foreign body of lip

⑦**S01.512**   Laceration without foreign body of oral cavity

S01.52   Laceration of lip and oral cavity with foreign body

⑦**S01.521**   Laceration with foreign body of lip

⑦**S01.522**   Laceration with foreign body of oral cavity

S01.53   Puncture wound of lip and oral cavity without foreign body

⑦**S01.531**   Puncture wound without foreign body of lip

⑦**S01.532**   Puncture wound without foreign body of oral cavity

S01.54   Puncture wound of lip and oral cavity with foreign body

⑦**S01.541**   Puncture wound with foreign body of lip

⑦**S01.542**   Puncture wound with foreign body of oral cavity

S01.55   Open bite of lip and oral cavity

⑦**S01.551**   Open bite of lip

Bite of lip NOS

Excludes 1: superficial bite of lip (S00.571)

⑦**S01.552**   Open bite of oral cavity

Bite of oral cavity NOS

Excludes 1: superficial bite of oral cavity (S00.572)

S01.8   Open wound of other parts of head

⊗⑦**S01.80**   Unspecified open wound of other part of head

⊗⑦**S01.81**   Laceration without foreign body of other part of head

⊗⑦**S01.82**   Laceration with foreign body of other part of head

⊗⑦**S01.83**   Puncture wound without foreign body of other part of head

⊗⑦**S01.84**   Puncture wound with foreign body of other part of head

⊗⑦**S01.85**   Open bite of other part of head

Bite of other part of head NOS

Excludes 1: superficial bite of other part of head (S00.85)

S01.9   Open wound of unspecified part of head

⊗⑦**S01.90**   Unspecified open wound of unspecified part of head

⊗⑦**S01.91**   Laceration without foreign body of unspecified part of head

⊗⑦**S01.92**   Laceration with foreign body of unspecified part of head

⊗⑦**S01.93**   Puncture wound without foreign body of unspecified part of head

⊗⑦**S01.94**   Puncture wound with foreign body of unspecified part of head

⊗⑦**S01.95**   Open bite of unspecified part of head

Bite of head NOS

Excludes 1: superficial bite of head NOS (S00.97)

S02   Fracture of skull and facial bones

Note: A fracture not indicated as open or closed should be coded to closed

Code also any associated intracranial injury (S06.-)

The appropriate 7th character is to be added to each code from category S02

A - initial encounter for closed fracture

B - initial encounter for open fracture

D - subsequent encounter for fracture with routine healing

G - subsequent encounter for fracture with delayed healing

K - subsequent encounter for fracture with nonunion

S - sequela

⊗⑦**S02.0**   Fracture of vault of skull

Fracture of frontal bone

Fracture of parietal bone

⊗⑦**S02.1**   Fracture of base of skull

Excludes 1: orbit NOS (S02.8)

Excludes 2: orbital floor (S02.3-)

⊗⑦**S02.10**   Unspecified fracture of base of skull

S02.11 Fracture of occiput
- ⑦ **S02.110** Type I occipital condyle fracture
- ⑦ **S02.111** Type II occipital condyle fracture
- ⑦ **S02.112** Type III occipital condyle fracture
- ⑦ **S02.113** Unspecified occipital condyle fracture
- ⑦ **S02.118** Other fracture of occiput
- ⑦ **S02.119** Unspecified fracture of occiput

⊗⑦ **S02.19** Other fracture of base of skull
Fracture of anterior fossa of base of skull
Fracture of ethmoid sinus
Fracture of frontal sinus
Fracture of middle fossa of base of skull
Fracture of orbital roof
Fracture of posterior fossa of base of skull
Fracture of sphenoid
Fracture of temporal bone

⊗⑦ **S02.2** Fracture of nasal bones

⊗⑦ **S02.3** Fracture of orbital floor
Excludes 1: orbit NOS (S02.8)
Excludes 2: orbital roof (S02.1-)

S02.4 Fracture of malar, maxillary and zygoma bones
Fracture of superior maxilla
Fracture of upper jaw (bone)
Fracture of zygomatic process of temporal bone
- **S02.40** Fracture of malar, maxillary and zygoma bones, unspecified
  - ⑦ **S02.400** Malar fracture unspecified
  - ⑦ **S02.401** Maxillary fracture, unspecified
  - ⑦ **S02.402** Zygomatic fracture, unspecified
- **S02.41** LeFort fracture
  - ⑦ **S02.411** LeFort I fracture
  - ⑦ **S02.412** LeFort II fracture
  - ⑦ **S02.413** LeFort III fracture
- ⊗⑦ **S02.42** Fracture of alveolus of maxilla

S02.5 Fracture of tooth (traumatic)
Broken tooth
Excludes 1: cracked tooth (nontraumatic) (K03.81)

S02.6 Fracture of mandible
Fracture of lower jaw (bone)
- **S02.60** Fracture of mandible, unspecified
  - ⑦ **S02.600** Fracture of unspecified part of body of mandible
  - ⑦ **S02.609** Fracture of mandible, unspecified
- ⊗⑦ **S02.61** Fracture of condylar process of mandible
- ⊗⑦ **S02.62** Fracture of subcondylar process of mandible
- ⊗⑦ **S02.63** Fracture of coronoid process of mandible
- ⊗⑦ **S02.64** Fracture of ramus of mandible
- ⊗⑦ **S02.65** Fracture of angle of mandible
- ⊗⑦ **S02.66** Fracture of symphysis of mandible
- ⊗⑦ **S02.67** Fracture of alveolus of mandible
- ⊗⑦ **S02.69** Fracture of mandible of other specified site

⊗⑦ **S02.8** Fractures of other specified skull and facial bones
Fracture of orbit NOS
Fracture of palate
Excludes 1: fracture of orbital floor (S02.3-)

fracture of orbital roof (S02.1-)

S02.9 Fracture of unspecified skull and facial bones
- ⊗⑦ **S02.91** Unspecified fracture of skull
- ⊗⑦ **S02.92** Unspecified fracture of facial bones

S03 Dislocation and sprain of joints and ligaments of head
Includes: avulsion of joint (capsule) or ligament of head
laceration of cartilage, joint (capsule) or ligament of head
sprain of cartilage, joint (capsule) or ligament of head
traumatic hemarthrosis of joint or ligament of head
traumatic rupture of joint or ligament of head
traumatic subluxation of joint or ligament of head
traumatic tear of joint or ligament of head
Code also any associated open wound
Excludes 2: Strain of muscle or tendon of head (S09.1)
The appropriate 7th character is to be added to each code from category S03
A - initial encounter
D - subsequent encounter
S - sequela

⊗⑦ **S03.0** Dislocation of jaw
Dislocation of jaw (cartilage) (meniscus)
Dislocation of mandible
Dislocation of temporomandibular (joint)

⊗⑦ **S03.1** Dislocation of septal cartilage of nose

⊗⑦ **S03.2** Dislocation of tooth

⊗⑦ **S03.4** Sprain of jaw
Sprain of temporomandibular (joint) (ligament)

⊗⑦ **S03.8** Sprain of joints and ligaments of other parts of head

⊗⑦ **S03.9** Sprain of joints and ligaments of unspecified parts of head

S04 Injury of cranial nerve
The selection of side should be based on the side of the body being affected
Code first any associated intracranial injury (S06.-)
Code also any associated:
open wound of head (S01.-)
skull fracture (S02.-)
The appropriate 7th character is to be added to each code from category S04
A - initial encounter
D - subsequent encounter
S - sequela

S04.0 Injury of optic nerve and pathways
Use additional code to identify any visual field defect or blindness (H53.4-, H54)
- **S04.01** Injury of optic nerve
  Injury of 2nd cranial nerve
  - ⑦ **S04.011** Injury of optic nerve, right eye
  - ⑦ **S04.012** Injury of optic nerve, left eye
  - ⑦ **S04.019** Injury of optic nerve, unspecified eye
    Injury of optic nerve NOS
- ⊗⑦ **S04.02** Injury of optic chiasm
- **S04.03** Injury of optic tract and pathways
  Injury of optic radiation
  - ⑦ **S04.031** Injury of optic tract and pathways, right eye
  - ⑦ **S04.032** Injury of optic tract and pathways, left eye

● New code   ▲ Revised code   ⑦ 7th digit required   ⊗ Placeholder required

⑦S04.039　Injury of optic tract and pathways, unspecified eye
　　　　　Injury of optic tract and pathways NOS
S04.04　Injury of visual cortex
　　⑦S04.041　Injury of visual cortex, right eye
　　⑦S04.042　Injury of visual cortex, left eye
　　⑦S04.049　Injury of visual cortex, unspecified eye
　　　　　Injury of visual cortex NOS
S04.1　Injury of oculomotor nerve
　　Injury of 3rd cranial nerve
　　⊗⑦S04.10　Injury of oculomotor nerve, unspecified side
　　⊗⑦S04.11　Injury of oculomotor nerve, right side
　　⊗⑦S04.12　Injury of oculomotor nerve, left side
S04.2　Injury of trochlear nerve
　　Injury of 4th cranial nerve
　　⊗⑦S04.20　Injury of trochlear nerve, unspecified side
　　⊗⑦S04.21　Injury of trochlear nerve, right side
　　⊗⑦S04.22　Injury of trochlear nerve, left side
S04.3　Injury of trigeminal nerve
　　Injury of 5th cranial nerve
　　⊗⑦S04.30　Injury of trigeminal nerve, unspecified side
　　⊗⑦S04.31　Injury of trigeminal nerve, right side
　　⊗⑦S04.32　Injury of trigeminal nerve, left side
S04.4　Injury of abducent nerve
　　Injury of 6th cranial nerve
　　⊗⑦S04.40　Injury of abducent nerve, unspecified side
　　⊗⑦S04.41　Injury of abducent nerve, right side
　　⊗⑦S04.42　Injury of abducent nerve, left side
S04.5　Injury of facial nerve
　　Injury of 7th cranial nerve
　　⊗⑦S04.50　Injury of facial nerve, unspecified side
　　⊗⑦S04.51　Injury of facial nerve, right side
　　⊗⑦S04.52　Injury of facial nerve, left side
S04.6　Injury of acoustic nerve
　　Injury of auditory nerve
　　Injury of 8th cranial nerve
　　⊗⑦S04.60　Injury of acoustic nerve, unspecified side
　　⊗⑦S04.61　Injury of acoustic nerve, right side
　　⊗⑦S04.62　Injury of acoustic nerve, left side
S04.7　Injury of accessory nerve
　　Injury of 11th cranial nerve
　　⊗⑦S04.70　Injury of accessory nerve, unspecified side
　　⊗⑦S04.71　Injury of accessory nerve, right side
　　⊗⑦S04.72　Injury of accessory nerve, left side
S04.8　Injury of other cranial nerves
　　S04.81　Injury of olfactory [1st] nerve
　　　　⑦S04.811　Injury of olfactory [1st] nerve, right side
　　　　⑦S04.812　Injury of olfactory [1st] nerve, left side
　　　　⑦S04.819　Injury of olfactory [1st] nerve, unspecified side
　　S04.89　Injury of other cranial nerves
　　　　Injury of vagus [10th] nerve
　　　　⑦S04.891　Injury of other cranial nerves, right side

⑦S04.892　Injury of other cranial nerves, left side
⑦S04.899　Injury of other cranial nerves, unspecified side
⊗⑦S04.9　Injury of unspecified cranial nerve
S05　Injury of eye and orbit
Includes: open wound of eye and orbit
Excludes 2: 2nd cranial [optic] nerve injury (S04.0-)
　　　　3rd cranial [oculomotor] nerve injury (S04.1-)
　　　　open wound of eyelid and periocular area (S01.1-)
　　　　orbital bone fracture (S02.1-, S02.3-, S02.8-)
　　　　superficial injury of eyelid (S00.1-S00.2)
The appropriate 7th character is to be added to each code from category S05
A - initial encounter
D - subsequent encounter
S - sequela
S05.0　Injury of conjunctiva and corneal abrasion without foreign body
　　Excludes 1: foreign body in conjunctival sac (T15.1)
　　　　　foreign body in cornea (T15.0)
　　⊗⑦S05.00　Injury of conjunctiva and corneal abrasion without foreign body, unspecified eye
　　⊗⑦S05.01　Injury of conjunctiva and corneal abrasion without foreign body, right eye
　　⊗⑦S05.02　Injury of conjunctiva and corneal abrasion without foreign body, left eye
S05.1　Contusion of eyeball and orbital tissues
　　Traumatic hyphema
　　Excludes 2: black eye NOS (S00.1)
　　　　　contusion of eyelid and periocular area (S00.1)
　　⊗⑦S05.10　Contusion of eyeball and orbital tissues, unspecified eye
　　⊗⑦S05.11　Contusion of eyeball and orbital tissues, right eye
　　⊗⑦S05.12　Contusion of eyeball and orbital tissues, left eye
S05.2　Ocular laceration and rupture with prolapse or loss of intraocular tissue
　　⊗⑦S05.20　Ocular laceration and rupture with prolapse or loss of intraocular tissue, unspecified eye
　　⊗⑦S05.21　Ocular laceration and rupture with prolapse or loss of intraocular tissue, right eye
　　⊗⑦S05.22　Ocular laceration and rupture with prolapse or loss of intraocular tissue, left eye
S05.3　Ocular laceration without prolapse or loss of intraocular tissue
　　Laceration of eye NOS
　　⊗⑦S05.30　Ocular laceration without prolapse or loss of intraocular tissue, unspecified eye
　　⊗⑦S05.31　Ocular laceration without prolapse or loss of intraocular tissue, right eye
　　⊗⑦S05.32　Ocular laceration without prolapse or loss of intraocular tissue, left eye
S05.4　Penetrating wound of orbit with or without foreign body
　　Excludes 2: retained (old) foreign body following penetrating wound in orbit (H05.5-)
　　⊗⑦S05.40　Penetrating wound of orbit with or without foreign body, unspecified eye

⊗⑦**S05.41** Penetrating wound of orbit with or without foreign body, right eye

⊗⑦**S05.42** Penetrating wound of orbit with or without foreign body, left eye

S05.5 Penetrating wound with foreign body of eyeball

Excludes 2: retained (old) intraocular foreign body (H44.6-, H44.7)

⊗⑦**S05.50** Penetrating wound with foreign body of unspecified eyeball

⊗⑦**S05.51** Penetrating wound with foreign body of right eyeball

⊗⑦**S05.52** Penetrating wound with foreign body of left eyeball

S05.6 Penetrating wound without foreign body of eyeball

Ocular penetration NOS

⊗⑦**S05.60** Penetrating wound without foreign body of unspecified eyeball

⊗⑦**S05.61** Penetrating wound without foreign body of right eyeball

⊗⑦**S05.62** Penetrating wound without foreign body of left eyeball

S05.7 Avulsion of eye

Traumatic enucleation

⊗⑦**S05.70** Avulsion of unspecified eye

⊗⑦**S05.71** Avulsion of right eye

⊗⑦**S05.72** Avulsion of left eye

S05.8 Other injuries of eye and orbit

Lacrimal duct injury

S05.8X Other injuries of eye and orbit

⑦**S05.8X1** Other injuries of right eye and orbit

⑦**S05.8X2** Other injuries of left eye and orbit

⑦**S05.8X9** Other injuries of unspecified eye and orbit

S05.9 Unspecified injury of eye and orbit

Injury of eye NOS

⊗⑦**S05.90** Unspecified injury of unspecified eye and orbit

⊗⑦**S05.91** Unspecified injury of right eye and orbit

⊗⑦**S05.92** Unspecified injury of left eye and orbit

S06 Intracranial injury

Includes: traumatic brain injury

Code also any associated:

open wound of head (S01.-)

skull fracture (S02.-)

Excludes 1: head injury NOS (S09.90)

The appropriate 7th character is to be added to each code from category S06

A - initial encounter

D - subsequent encounter

S - sequela

S06.0 Concussion

Commotio cerebri

Excludes 1: concussion with other intracranial injuries classified in category S06- code to specified intracranial injury

S06.0X Concussion

⑦**S06.0X0** Concussion without loss of consciousness

⑦**S06.0X1** Concussion with loss of consciousness of 30 minutes or less

⑦**S06.0X2** Concussion with loss of consciousness of 31 minutes to 59 minutes

⑦**S06.0X3** Concussion with loss of consciousness of 1 hour to 5 hours 59 minutes

⑦**S06.0X4** Concussion with loss of consciousness of 6 hours to 24 hours

⑦**S06.0X5** Concussion with loss of consciousness greater than 24 hours with return to pre-existing conscious level

⑦**S06.0X6** Concussion with loss of consciousness greater than 24 hours without return to pre-existing conscious level with patient surviving

⑦**S06.0X7** Concussion with loss of consciousness of any duration with death due to brain injury prior to regaining consciousness

⑦**S06.0X8** Concussion with loss of consciousness of any duration with death due to other cause prior to regaining consciousness

⑦**S06.0X9** Concussion with loss of consciousness of unspecified duration

Concussion NOS

S06.1 Traumatic cerebral edema

Diffuse traumatic cerebral edema

Focal traumatic cerebral edema

S06.1X Traumatic cerebral edema

⑦**S06.1X0** Traumatic cerebral edema without loss of consciousness

⑦**S06.1X1** Traumatic cerebral edema with loss of consciousness of 30 minutes or less

⑦**S06.1X2** Traumatic cerebral edema with loss of consciousness of 31 minutes to 59 minutes

⑦**S06.1X3** Traumatic cerebral edema with loss of consciousness of 1 hour to 5 hours 59 minutes

⑦**S06.1X4** Traumatic cerebral edema with loss of consciousness of 6 hours to 24 hours

⑦**S06.1X5** Traumatic cerebral edema with loss of consciousness greater than 24 hours with return to pre-existing conscious level

⑦**S06.1X6** Traumatic cerebral edema with loss of consciousness greater than 24 hours without return to pre-existing conscious level with patient surviving

⑦**S06.1X7** Traumatic cerebral edema with loss of consciousness of any duration with death due to brain injury prior to regaining consciousness

⑦S06.1X8 Traumatic cerebral edema with loss of consciousness of any duration with death due to other cause prior to regaining consciousness

⑦S06.1X9 Traumatic cerebral edema with loss of consciousness of unspecified duration

Traumatic cerebral edema NOS

S06.2 Diffuse traumatic brain injury
Diffuse axonal brain injury
Excludes 1: traumatic diffuse cerebral edema (S06.1x-)

S06.2X Diffuse traumatic brain injury

⑦S06.2X0 Diffuse traumatic brain injury without loss of consciousness

⑦S06.2X1 Diffuse traumatic brain injury with loss of consciousness of 30 minutes or less

⑦S06.2X2 Diffuse traumatic brain injury with loss of consciousness of 31 minutes to 59 minutes

⑦S06.2X3 Diffuse traumatic brain injury with loss of consciousness of 1 hour to 5 hours 59 minutes

⑦S06.2X4 Diffuse traumatic brain injury with loss of consciousness of 6 hours to 24 hours

⑦S06.2X5 Diffuse traumatic brain injury with loss of consciousness greater than 24 hours with return to pre-existing conscious levels

⑦S06.2X6 Diffuse traumatic brain injury with loss of consciousness greater than 24 hours without return to pre-existing conscious level with patient surviving

⑦S06.2X7 Diffuse traumatic brain injury with loss of consciousness of any duration with death due to brain injury prior to regaining consciousness

⑦S06.2X8 Diffuse traumatic brain injury with loss of consciousness of any duration with death due to other cause prior to regaining consciousness

⑦S06.2X9 Diffuse traumatic brain injury with loss of consciousness of unspecified duration

Diffuse traumatic brain injury NOS

S06.3 Focal traumatic brain injury
Excludes 1: any condition classifiable to S06.4-S06.6
focal cerebral edema (S06.1)

S06.30 Unspecified focal traumatic brain injury

⑦S06.300 Unspecified focal traumatic brain injury without loss of consciousness

⑦S06.301 Unspecified focal traumatic brain injury with loss of consciousness of 30 minutes or less

⑦S06.302 Unspecified focal traumatic brain injury with loss of consciousness of 31 minutes to 59 minutes

⑦S06.303 Unspecified focal traumatic brain injury with loss of consciousness of 1 hour to 5 hours 59 minutes

⑦S06.304 Unspecified focal traumatic brain injury with loss of consciousness of 6 hours to 24 hours

⑦S06.305 Unspecified focal traumatic brain injury with loss of consciousness greater than 24 hours with return to pre-existing conscious level

⑦S06.306 Unspecified focal traumatic brain injury with loss of consciousness greater than 24 hours without return to pre-existing conscious level with patient surviving

⑦S06.307 Unspecified focal traumatic brain injury with loss of consciousness of any duration with death due to brain injury prior to regaining consciousness

⑦S06.308 Unspecified focal traumatic brain injury with loss of consciousness of any duration with death due to other cause prior to regaining consciousness

⑦S06.309 Unspecified focal traumatic brain injury with loss of consciousness of unspecified duration

Unspecified focal traumatic brain injury NOS

S06.31 Contusion and laceration of right cerebrum

⑦S06.310 Contusion and laceration of right cerebrum without loss of consciousness

⑦S06.311 Contusion and laceration of right cerebrum with loss of consciousness of 30 minutes or less

⑦S06.312 Contusion and laceration of right cerebrum with loss of consciousness of 31 minutes to 59 minutes

⑦S06.313 Contusion and laceration of right cerebrum with loss of consciousness of 1 hour to 5 hours 59 minutes

⑦S06.314 Contusion and laceration of right cerebrum with loss of consciousness of 6 hours to 24 hours

⑦S06.315 Contusion and laceration of right cerebrum with loss of consciousness greater than 24 hours with return to pre-existing conscious level

⑦S06.316 Contusion and laceration of right cerebrum with loss of consciousness greater than 24 hours without return to pre-existing conscious level with patient surviving

⑦S06.317 Contusion and laceration of right cerebrum with loss of consciousness of any duration with death due to brain injury prior to regaining consciousness

⑦S06.318   Contusion and laceration of right cerebrum with loss of consciousness of any duration with death due to other cause prior to regaining consciousness

⑦S06.319   Contusion and laceration of right cerebrum with loss of consciousness of unspecified duration

Contusion and laceration of right cerebrum NOS

S06.32   Contusion and laceration of left cerebrum

⑦S06.320   Contusion and laceration of left cerebrum without loss of consciousness

⑦S06.321   Contusion and laceration of left cerebrum with loss of consciousness of 30 minutes or less

⑦S06.322   Contusion and laceration of left cerebrum with loss of consciousness of 31 minutes to 59 minutes

⑦S06.323   Contusion and laceration of left cerebrum with loss of consciousness of 1 hour to 5 hours 59 minutes

⑦S06.324   Contusion and laceration of left cerebrum with loss of consciousness of 6 hours to 24 hours

⑦S06.325   Contusion and laceration of left cerebrum with loss of consciousness greater than 24 hours with return to pre-existing conscious level

⑦S06.326   Contusion and laceration of left cerebrum with loss of consciousness greater than 24 hours without return to pre-existing conscious level with patient surviving

⑦S06.327   Contusion and laceration of left cerebrum with loss of consciousness of any duration with death due to brain injury prior to regaining consciousness

⑦S06.328   Contusion and laceration of left cerebrum with loss of consciousness of any duration with death due to other cause prior to regaining consciousness

⑦S06.329   Contusion and laceration of left cerebrum with loss of consciousness of unspecified duration

Contusion and laceration of left cerebrum NOS

S06.33   Contusion and laceration of cerebrum, unspecified

⑦S06.330   Contusion and laceration of cerebrum, unspecified, without loss of consciousness

⑦S06.331   Contusion and laceration of cerebrum, unspecified, with loss of consciousness of 30 minutes or less

⑦S06.332   Contusion and laceration of cerebrum, unspecified, with loss of consciousness of 31 minutes to 59 minutes

⑦S06.333   Contusion and laceration of cerebrum, unspecified, with loss of consciousness of 1 hour to 5 hours 59 minutes

⑦S06.334   Contusion and laceration of cerebrum, unspecified, with loss of consciousness of 6 hours to 24 hours

⑦S06.335   Contusion and laceration of cerebrum, unspecified, with loss of consciousness greater than 24 hours with return to pre-existing conscious level

⑦S06.336   Contusion and laceration of cerebrum, unspecified, with loss of consciousness greater than 24 hours without return to pre-existing conscious level with patient surviving

⑦S06.337   Contusion and laceration of cerebrum, unspecified, with loss of consciousness of any duration with death due to brain injury prior to regaining consciousness

⑦S06.338   Contusion and laceration of cerebrum, unspecified, with loss of consciousness of any duration with death due to other cause prior to regaining consciousness

⑦S06.339   Contusion and laceration of cerebrum, unspecified, with loss of consciousness of unspecified duration

Contusion and laceration of cerebrum NOS

S06.34   Traumatic hemorrhage of right cerebrum

Traumatic intracerebral hemorrhage and hematoma of right cerebrum

⑦S06.340   Traumatic hemorrhage of right cerebrum without loss of consciousness

⑦S06.341   Traumatic hemorrhage of right cerebrum with loss of consciousness of 30 minutes or less

⑦S06.342   Traumatic hemorrhage of right cerebrum with loss of consciousness of 31 minutes to 59 minutes

⑦S06.343   Traumatic hemorrhage of right cerebrum with loss of consciousness of 1 hours to 5 hours 59 minutes

⑦S06.344   Traumatic hemorrhage of right cerebrum with loss of consciousness of 6 hours to 24 hours

⑦S06.345   Traumatic hemorrhage of right cerebrum with loss of consciousness greater than 24 hours with return to pre-existing conscious level

⑦S06.346   Traumatic hemorrhage of right cerebrum with loss of consciousness greater than 24 hours without return to pre-existing conscious level with patient surviving

⑦S06.347   Traumatic hemorrhage of right cerebrum with loss of consciousness of any duration with death due to brain injury prior to regaining consciousness

⑦S06.348   Traumatic hemorrhage of right cerebrum with loss of consciousness of any duration with death due to other cause prior to regaining consciousness

⑦S06.349   Traumatic hemorrhage of right cerebrum with loss of consciousness of unspecified duration

Traumatic hemorrhage of right cerebrum NOS

S06.35   Traumatic hemorrhage of left cerebrum

Traumatic intracerebral hemorrhage and hematoma of left cerebrum

⑦S06.350   Traumatic hemorrhage of left cerebrum without loss of consciousness

⑦S06.351   Traumatic hemorrhage of left cerebrum with loss of consciousness of 30 minutes or less

⑦S06.352   Traumatic hemorrhage of left cerebrum with loss of consciousness of 31 minutes to 59 minutes

⑦S06.353   Traumatic hemorrhage of left cerebrum with loss of consciousness of 1 hours to 5 hours 59 minutes

⑦S06.354   Traumatic hemorrhage of left cerebrum with loss of consciousness of 6 hours to 24 hours

⑦S06.355   Traumatic hemorrhage of left cerebrum with loss of consciousness greater than 24 hours with return to pre-existing conscious level

⑦S06.356   Traumatic hemorrhage of left cerebrum with loss of consciousness greater than 24 hours without return to pre-existing conscious level with patient surviving

⑦S06.357   Traumatic hemorrhage of left cerebrum with loss of consciousness of any duration with death due to brain injury prior to regaining consciousness

⑦S06.358   Traumatic hemorrhage of left cerebrum with loss of consciousness of any duration with death due to other cause prior to regaining consciousness

⑦S06.359   Traumatic hemorrhage of left cerebrum with loss of consciousness of unspecified duration

Traumatic hemorrhage of left cerebrum NOS

S06.36   Traumatic hemorrhage of cerebrum, unspecified

Traumatic intracerebral hemorrhage and hematoma, unspecified

⑦S06.360   Traumatic hemorrhage of cerebrum, unspecified, without loss of consciousness

⑦S06.361   Traumatic hemorrhage of cerebrum, unspecified, with loss of consciousness of 30 minutes or less

⑦S06.362   Traumatic hemorrhage of cerebrum, unspecified, with loss of consciousness of 31 minutes to 59 minutes

⑦S06.363   Traumatic hemorrhage of cerebrum, unspecified, with loss of consciousness of 1 hours to 5 hours 59 minutes

⑦S06.364   Traumatic hemorrhage of cerebrum, unspecified, with loss of consciousness of 6 hours to 24 hours

⑦S06.365   Traumatic hemorrhage of cerebrum, unspecified, with loss of consciousness greater than 24 hours with return to pre-existing conscious level

⑦S06.366   Traumatic hemorrhage of cerebrum, unspecified, with loss of consciousness greater than 24 hours without return to pre-existing conscious level with patient surviving

⑦S06.367   Traumatic hemorrhage of cerebrum, unspecified, with loss of consciousness of any duration with death due to brain injury prior to regaining consciousness

⑦S06.368   Traumatic hemorrhage of cerebrum, unspecified, with loss of consciousness of any duration with death due to other cause prior to regaining consciousness

⑦S06.369   Traumatic hemorrhage of cerebrum, unspecified, with loss of consciousness of unspecified duration

Traumatic hemorrhage of cerebrum NOS

S06.37   Contusion, laceration, and hemorrhage of cerebellum

⑦S06.370   Contusion, laceration, and hemorrhage of cerebellum without loss of consciousness

⑦S06.371   Contusion, laceration, and hemorrhage of cerebellum with loss of consciousness of 30 minutes or less

⑦S06.372   Contusion, laceration, and hemorrhage of cerebellum with loss of consciousness of 31 minutes to 59 minutes

⑦S06.373   Contusion, laceration, and hemorrhage of cerebellum with loss of consciousness of 1 hour to 5 hours 59 minutes

⑦S06.374 Contusion, laceration, and hemorrhage of cerebellum with loss of consciousness of 6 hours to 24 hours

⑦S06.375 Contusion, laceration, and hemorrhage of cerebellum with loss of consciousness greater than 24 hours with return to pre-existing conscious level

⑦S06.376 Contusion, laceration, and hemorrhage of cerebellum with loss of consciousness greater than 24 hours without return to pre-existing conscious level with patient surviving

⑦S06.377 Contusion, laceration, and hemorrhage of cerebellum with loss of consciousness of any duration with death due to brain injury prior to regaining consciousness

⑦S06.378 Contusion, laceration, and hemorrhage of cerebellum with loss of consciousness of any duration with death due to other cause prior to regaining consciousness

⑦S06.379 Contusion, laceration, and hemorrhage of cerebellum with loss of consciousness of unspecified duration

Contusion, laceration, and hemorrhage of cerebellum NOS

S06.38 Contusion, laceration, and hemorrhage of brainstem

⑦S06.380 Contusion, laceration, and hemorrhage of brainstem without loss of consciousness

⑦S06.381 Contusion, laceration, and hemorrhage of brainstem with loss of consciousness of 30 minutes or less

⑦S06.382 Contusion, laceration, and hemorrhage of brainstem with loss of consciousness of 31 minutes to 59 minutes

⑦S06.383 Contusion, laceration, and hemorrhage of brainstem with loss of consciousness of 1 hour to 5 hours 59 minutes

⑦S06.384 Contusion, laceration, and hemorrhage of brainstem with loss of consciousness of 6 hours to 24 hours

⑦S06.385 Contusion, laceration, and hemorrhage of brainstem with loss of consciousness greater than 24 hours with return to pre-existing conscious level

⑦S06.386 Contusion, laceration, and hemorrhage of brainstem with loss of consciousness greater than 24

hours without return to pre-existing conscious level with patient surviving

⑦S06.387 Contusion, laceration, and hemorrhage of brainstem with loss of consciousness of any duration with death due to brain injury prior to regaining consciousness

⑦S06.388 Contusion, laceration, and hemorrhage of brainstem with loss of consciousness of any duration with death due to other cause prior to regaining consciousness

⑦S06.389 Contusion, laceration, and hemorrhage of brainstem with loss of consciousness of unspecified duration

Contusion, laceration, and hemorrhage of brainstem NOS

S06.4 Epidural hemorrhage

Extradural hemorrhage NOS

Extradural hemorrhage (traumatic)

S06.4X Epidural hemorrhage

⑦S06.4X0 Epidural hemorrhage without loss of consciousness

⑦S06.4X1 Epidural hemorrhage with loss of consciousness of 30 minutes or less

⑦S06.4X2 Epidural hemorrhage with loss of consciousness of 31 minutes to 59 minutes

⑦S06.4X3 Epidural hemorrhage with loss of consciousness of 1 hour to 5 hours 59 minutes

⑦S06.4X4 Epidural hemorrhage with loss of consciousness of 6 hours to 24 hours

⑦S06.4X5 Epidural hemorrhage with loss of consciousness greater than 24 hours with return to pre-existing conscious level

⑦S06.4X6 Epidural hemorrhage with loss of consciousness greater than 24 hours without return to pre-existing conscious level with patient surviving

⑦S06.4X7 Epidural hemorrhage with loss of consciousness of any duration with death due to brain injury prior to regaining consciousness

⑦S06.4X8 Epidural hemorrhage with loss of consciousness of any duration with death due to other causes prior to regaining consciousness

⑦S06.4X9 Epidural hemorrhage with loss of consciousness of unspecified duration

Epidural hemorrhage NOS

S06.5 Traumatic subdural hemorrhage

S06.5X Traumatic subdural hemorrhage

⑦S06.5X0 Traumatic subdural hemorrhage without loss of consciousness

⑦S06.5X1 Traumatic subdural hemorrhage with loss of consciousness of 30 minutes or less

⑦S06.5X2 Traumatic subdural hemorrhage with loss of consciousness of 31 minutes to 59 minutes

⑦S06.5X3 Traumatic subdural hemorrhage with loss of consciousness of 1 hour to 5 hours 59 minutes

⑦S06.5X4 Traumatic subdural hemorrhage with loss of consciousness of 6 hours to 24 hours

⑦S06.5X5 Traumatic subdural hemorrhage with loss of consciousness greater than 24 hours with return to pre-existing conscious level

⑦S06.5X6 Traumatic subdural hemorrhage with loss of consciousness greater than 24 hours without return to pre-existing conscious level with patient surviving

⑦S06.5X7 Traumatic subdural hemorrhage with loss of consciousness of any duration with death due to brain injury before regaining consciousness

⑦S06.5X8 Traumatic subdural hemorrhage with loss of consciousness of any duration with death due to other cause before regaining consciousness

⑦S06.5X9 Traumatic subdural hemorrhage with loss of consciousness of unspecified duration
Traumatic subdural hemorrhage NOS

S06.6   Traumatic subarachnoid hemorrhage
     S06.6X Traumatic subarachnoid hemorrhage

⑦S06.6X0 Traumatic subarachnoid hemorrhage without loss of consciousness

⑦S06.6X1 Traumatic subarachnoid hemorrhage with loss of consciousness of 30 minutes or less

⑦S06.6X2 Traumatic subarachnoid hemorrhage with loss of consciousness of 31 minutes to 59 minutes

⑦S06.6X3 Traumatic subarachnoid hemorrhage with loss of consciousness of 1 hour to 5 hours 59 minutes

⑦S06.6X4 Traumatic subarachnoid hemorrhage with loss of consciousness of 6 hours to 24 hours

⑦S06.6X5 Traumatic subarachnoid hemorrhage with loss of consciousness greater than 24 hours with return to pre-existing conscious level

⑦S06.6X6 Traumatic subarachnoid hemorrhage with loss of consciousness greater than 24 hours without return to pre-existing conscious level with patient surviving

⑦S06.6X7 Traumatic subarachnoid hemorrhage with loss of consciousness of any duration with death due to brain injury prior to regaining consciousness

⑦S06.6X8 Traumatic subarachnoid hemorrhage with loss of consciousness of any duration with death due to other cause prior to regaining consciousness

⑦S06.6X9 Traumatic subarachnoid hemorrhage with loss of consciousness of unspecified duration
Traumatic subarachnoid hemorrhage NOS

S06.8   Other specified intracranial injuries
     S06.81 Injury of right internal carotid artery, intracranial portion, not elsewhere classified

⑦S06.810 Injury of right internal carotid artery, intracranial portion, not elsewhere classified without loss of consciousness

⑦S06.811 Injury of right internal carotid artery, intracranial portion, not elsewhere classified with loss of consciousness of 30 minutes or less

⑦S06.812 Injury of right internal carotid artery, intracranial portion, not elsewhere classified with loss of consciousness of 31 minutes to 59 minutes

⑦S06.813 Injury of right internal carotid artery, intracranial portion, not elsewhere classified with loss of consciousness of 1 hour to 5 hours 59 minutes

⑦S06.814 Injury of right internal carotid artery, intracranial portion, not elsewhere classified with loss of consciousness of 6 hours to 24 hours

⑦S06.815 Injury of right internal carotid artery, intracranial portion, not elsewhere classified with loss of consciousness greater than 24 hours with return to pre-existing conscious level

⑦S06.816 Injury of right internal carotid artery, intracranial portion, not elsewhere classified with loss of consciousness greater than 24 hours without return to pre-existing conscious level with patient surviving

⑦S06.817 Injury of right internal carotid artery, intracranial portion, not elsewhere classified with loss of consciousness of any duration with death due to brain injury prior to regaining consciousness

⑦S06.818 Injury of right internal carotid artery, intracranial portion, not elsewhere classified with loss of consciousness of any duration with death due to other cause prior to regaining consciousness

⑦ S06.819 Injury of right internal carotid artery, intracranial portion, not elsewhere classified with loss of consciousness of unspecified duration

Injury of right internal carotid artery, intracranial portion, not elsewhere classified NOS

S06.82 Injury of left internal carotid artery, intracranial portion, not elsewhere classified

⑦ S06.820 Injury of left internal carotid artery, intracranial portion, not elsewhere classified without loss of consciousness

⑦ S06.821 Injury of left internal carotid artery, intracranial portion, not elsewhere classified with loss of consciousness of 30 minutes or less

⑦ S06.822 Injury of left internal carotid artery, intracranial portion, not elsewhere classified with loss of consciousness of 31 minutes to 59 minutes

⑦ S06.823 Injury of left internal carotid artery, intracranial portion, not elsewhere classified with loss of consciousness of 1 hour to 5 hours 59 minutes

⑦ S06.824 Injury of left internal carotid artery, intracranial portion, not elsewhere classified with loss of consciousness of 6 hours to 24 hours

⑦ S06.825 Injury of left internal carotid artery, intracranial portion, not elsewhere classified with loss of consciousness greater than 24 hours with return to pre-existing conscious level

⑦ S06.826 Injury of left internal carotid artery, intracranial portion, not elsewhere classified with loss of consciousness greater than 24 hours without return to pre-existing conscious level with patient surviving

⑦ S06.827 Injury of left internal carotid artery, intracranial portion, not elsewhere classified with loss of consciousness of any duration with death due to brain injury prior to regaining consciousness

⑦ S06.828 Injury of left internal carotid artery, intracranial portion, not elsewhere classified with loss of consciousness of any duration with death due to other cause prior to regaining consciousness

⑦ S06.829 Injury of left internal carotid artery, intracranial portion, not elsewhere classified with loss of consciousness of unspecified duration

Injury of left internal carotid artery, intracranial portion, not elsewhere classified NOS

S06.89 Other specified intracranial injury

⑦ S06.890 Other specified intracranial injury without loss of consciousness

⑦ S06.891 Other specified intracranial injury with loss of consciousness of 30 minutes or less

⑦ S06.892 Other specified intracranial injury with loss of consciousness of 31 minutes to 59 minutes

⑦ S06.893 Other specified intracranial injury with loss of consciousness of 1 hour to 5 hours 59 minutes

⑦ S06.894 Other specified intracranial injury with loss of consciousness of 6 hours to 24 hours

⑦ S06.895 Other specified intracranial injury with loss of consciousness greater than 24 hours with return to pre-existing conscious level

⑦ S06.896 Other specified intracranial injury with loss of consciousness greater than 24 hours without return to pre-existing conscious level with patient surviving

⑦ S06.897 Other specified intracranial injury with loss of consciousness of any duration with death due to brain injury prior to regaining consciousness

⑦ S06.898 Other specified intracranial injury with loss of consciousness of any duration with death due to other cause prior to regaining consciousness

⑦ S06.899 Other specified intracranial injury with loss of consciousness of unspecified duration

S06.9 Unspecified intracranial injury
Brain injury NOS
Head injury NOS with loss of consciousness
Excludes 1: head injury NOS (S09.90)
S06.9X Unspecified intracranial injury

⑦ S06.9X0 Unspecified intracranial injury without loss of consciousness

⑦ S06.9X1 Unspecified intracranial injury with loss of consciousness of 30 minutes or less

⑦ S06.9X2 Unspecified intracranial injury with loss of consciousness of 31 minutes to 59 minutes

⑦ S06.9X3 Unspecified intracranial injury with loss of consciousness of 1 hour to 5 hours 59 minutes

⑦ S06.9X4 Unspecified intracranial injury with loss of consciousness of 6 hours to 24 hours

⑦ S06.9X5 Unspecified intracranial injury with loss of consciousness greater than 24

● New code   ▲ Revised code   ⑦ 7th digit required   ⊗ Placeholder required

⑦S06.9X6 Unspecified intracranial injury with loss of consciousness greater than 24 hours without return to pre-existing conscious level with patient surviving

⑦S06.9X7 Unspecified intracranial injury with loss of consciousness of any duration with death due to brain injury prior to regaining consciousness

⑦S06.9X8 Unspecified intracranial injury with loss of consciousness of any duration with death due to other cause prior to regaining consciousness

⑦S06.9X9 Unspecified intracranial injury with loss of consciousness of unspecified duration

S07 Crushing injury of head

Use additional code for all associated injuries, such as:

intracranial injuries (S06-)

skull fractures (S02.-)

The appropriate 7th character is to be added to each code from category S07

A - initial encounter

D - subsequent encounter

S - sequela

⊗⑦S07.0 Crushing injury of face

⊗⑦S07.1 Crushing injury of skull

⊗⑦S07.8 Crushing injury of other parts of head

⊗⑦S07.9 Crushing injury of head, part unspecified

S08 Avulsion and traumatic amputation of part of head

An amputation not identified as partial or complete should be coded to complete

The appropriate 7th character is to be added to each code from category S08

A - initial encounter

D - subsequent encounter

S - sequela

⊗⑦S08.0 Avulsion of scalp

S08.1 Traumatic amputation of ear

    S08.11 Complete traumatic amputation of ear

        ⑦S08.111 Complete traumatic amputation of right ear

        ⑦S08.112 Complete traumatic amputation of left ear

        ⑦S08.119 Complete traumatic amputation of unspecified ear

    S08.12 Partial traumatic amputation of ear

        ⑦S08.121 Partial traumatic amputation of right ear

        ⑦S08.122 Partial traumatic amputation of left ear

        ⑦S08.129 Partial traumatic amputation of unspecified ear

S08.8 Traumatic amputation of other parts of head

    S08.81 Traumatic amputation of nose

        ⑦S08.811 Complete traumatic amputation of nose

        ⑦S08.812 Partial traumatic amputation of nose

    S08.89 Traumatic amputation of other parts of head

S09 Other and unspecified injuries of head

The appropriate 7th character is to be added to each code from category S09

A - initial encounter

D - subsequent encounter

S - sequela

⊗⑦S09.0 Injury of blood vessels of head, not elsewhere classified

    Excludes 1: injury of cerebral blood vessels (S06.-)

        injury of precerebral blood vessels (S15.-)

S09.1 Injury of muscle and tendon of head

Code also any associated open wound (S01.-)

    Excludes 2: sprain to joints and ligament of head (S03.9)

⊗⑦S09.10 Unspecified injury of muscle and tendon of head

Injury of muscle and tendon of head NOS

⊗⑦S09.11 Strain of muscle and tendon of head

⊗⑦S09.12 Laceration of muscle and tendon of head

⊗⑦S09.19 Other specified injury of muscle and tendon of head

S09.2 Traumatic rupture of ear drum

    Excludes 1: traumatic rupture of ear drum due to blast injury (S09.31-)

⊗⑦S09.20 Traumatic rupture of unspecified ear drum

⊗⑦S09.21 Traumatic rupture of right ear drum

⊗⑦S09.22 Traumatic rupture of left ear drum

S09.3 Other specified and unspecified injury of middle and inner ear

    Excludes 1: injury to ear NOS (S09.91-)

    Excludes 2: injury to external ear (S00.4-, S01.3-, S08.1-)

    S09.30 Unspecified injury of middle and inner ear

        ⑦S09.301 Unspecified injury of right middle and inner ear

        ⑦S09.302 Unspecified injury of left middle and inner ear

        ⑦S09.309 Unspecified injury of unspecified middle and inner ear

    S09.31 Primary blast injury of ear

    Blast injury of ear NOS

        ⑦S09.311 Primary blast injury of right ear

        ⑦S09.312 Primary blast injury of left ear

        ⑦S09.313 Primary blast injury of ear, bilateral

        ⑦S09.319 Primary blast injury of unspecified ear

    S09.39 Other specified injury of middle and inner ear

    Secondary blast injury to ear

        ⑦S09.391 Other specified injury of right middle and inner ear

        ⑦S09.392 Other specified injury of left middle and inner ear

        ⑦S09.399 Other specified injury of unspecified middle and inner ear

⊗⑦S09.8 Other specified injuries of head

S09.9 Unspecified injury of face and head

⊗⑦S09.90 Unspecified injury of head

Head injury NOS

Excludes 1: brain injury NOS (S06.9-)
    head injury NOS with loss of
    consciousness (S06.9-)
    intracranial injury NOS (S06.9-)

⊗⑦**S09.91** Unspecified injury of ear
     Injury of ear NOS

⊗⑦**S09.92** Unspecified injury of nose
     Injury of nose NOS

⊗⑦**S09.93** Unspecified injury of face
     Injury of face NOS

INJURIES TO THE NECK (S10-S19)

Includes: injuries of nape
   injuries of supraclavicular region
   injuries of throat

Excludes 2: burns and corrosions (T20-T32)
  effects of foreign body in esophagus (T18.1)
  effects of foreign body in larynx (T17.3)
  effects of foreign body in pharynx (T17.2)
  effects of foreign body in trachea (T17.4)
  frostbite (T33-T34)
  insect bite or sting, venomous (T63.4)

S10 Superficial injury of neck

The appropriate 7th character is to be added to each code from category S10

A - initial encounter
D - subsequent encounter
S - sequela

⊗⑦**S10.0** Contusion of throat
    Contusion of cervical esophagus
    Contusion of larynx
    Contusion of pharynx
    Contusion of trachea

S10.1 Other and unspecified superficial injuries of throat

 ⊗⑦**S10.10** Unspecified superficial injuries of throat

 ⊗⑦**S10.11** Abrasion of throat

 ⊗⑦**S10.12** Blister (nonthermal) of throat

 ⊗⑦**S10.14** External constriction of part of throat

 ⊗⑦**S10.15** Superficial foreign body of throat
      Splinter in the throat

 ⊗⑦**S10.16** Insect bite (nonvenomous) of throat

 ⊗⑦**S10.17** Other superficial bite of throat
     Excludes 1: open bite of throat (S11.85)

S10.8 Superficial injury of other specified parts of neck

 ⊗⑦**S10.80** Unspecified superficial injury of other specified part of neck

 ⊗⑦**S10.81** Abrasion of other specified part of neck

 ⊗⑦**S10.82** Blister (nonthermal) of other specified part of neck

 ⊗⑦**S10.83** Contusion of other specified part of neck

 ⊗⑦**S10.84** External constriction of other specified part of neck

 ⊗⑦**S10.85** Superficial foreign body of other specified part of neck
      Splinter in other specified part of neck

 ⊗⑦**S10.86** Insect bite of other specified part of neck

 ⊗⑦**S10.87** Other superficial bite of other specified part of neck
     Excludes 1: open bite of other specified parts of neck (S11.85)

S10.9 Superficial injury of unspecified part of neck

 ⊗⑦**S10.90** Unspecified superficial injury of unspecified part of neck

 ⊗⑦**S10.91** Abrasion of unspecified part of neck

 ⊗⑦**S10.92** Blister (nonthermal) of unspecified part of neck

 ⊗⑦**S10.93** Contusion of unspecified part of neck

 ⊗⑦**S10.94** External constriction of unspecified part of neck

 ⊗⑦**S10.95** Superficial foreign body of unspecified part of neck

 ⊗⑦**S10.96** Insect bite of unspecified part of neck

 ⊗⑦**S10.97** Other superficial bite of unspecified part of neck

S11 Open wound of neck

Code also any associated:
  spinal cord injury (S14.0, S14.1-)
  wound infection

Excludes 2: open fracture of vertebra (S12.- with 7th character B)

The appropriate 7th character is to be added to each code from category S11

A - initial encounter
D - subsequent encounter
S - sequela

S11.0 Open wound of larynx and trachea

 S11.01 Open wound of larynx
    Excludes 2: open wound of vocal cord (S11.03)

  ⑦**S11.011** Laceration without foreign body of larynx

  ⑦**S11.012** Laceration with foreign body of larynx

  ⑦**S11.013** Puncture wound without foreign body of larynx

  ⑦**S11.014** Puncture wound with foreign body of larynx

  ⑦**S11.015** Open bite of larynx
       Bite of larynx NOS

  ⑦**S11.019** Unspecified open wound of larynx

 S11.02 Open wound of trachea
    Open wound of cervical trachea
    Open wound of trachea NOS
    Excludes 2: open wound of thoracic trachea (S27.5-)

  ⑦**S11.021** Laceration without foreign body of trachea

  ⑦**S11.022** Laceration with foreign body of trachea

  ⑦**S11.023** Puncture wound without foreign body of trachea

  ⑦**S11.024** Puncture wound with foreign body of trachea

  ⑦**S11.025** Open bite of trachea
       Bite of trachea NOS

  ⑦**S11.029** Unspecified open wound of trachea

 S11.03 Open wound of vocal cord

  ⑦**S11.031** Laceration without foreign body of vocal cord

⑦S11.032　Laceration with foreign body of vocal cord

⑦S11.033　Puncture wound without foreign body of vocal cord

⑦S11.034　Puncture wound with foreign body of vocal cord

⑦S11.035　Open bite of vocal cord
　　　　　　Bite of vocal cord NOS

⑦S11.039　Unspecified open wound of vocal cord

S11.1　Open wound of thyroid gland

⊗⑦S11.10　Unspecified open wound of thyroid gland

⊗⑦S11.11　Laceration without foreign body of thyroid gland

⊗⑦S11.12　Laceration with foreign body of thyroid gland

⊗⑦S11.13　Puncture wound without foreign body of thyroid gland

⊗⑦S11.14　Puncture wound with foreign body of thyroid gland

⊗⑦S11.15　Open bite of thyroid gland
　　　　　　Bite of thyroid gland NOS

S11.2　Open wound of pharynx and cervical esophagus
　　　　Excludes 1: open wound of esophagus NOS (S27.8-)

⊗⑦S11.20　Unspecified open wound of pharynx and cervical esophagus

⊗⑦S11.21　Laceration without foreign body of pharynx and cervical esophagus

⊗⑦S11.22　Laceration with foreign body of pharynx and cervical esophagus

⊗⑦S11.23　Puncture wound without foreign body of pharynx and cervical esophagus

⊗⑦S11.24　Puncture wound with foreign body of pharynx and cervical esophagus

⊗⑦S11.25　Open bite of pharynx and cervical esophagus
　　　　　　Bite of pharynx and cervical esophagus NOS

S11.8　Open wound of other specified parts of neck

⊗⑦S11.80　Unspecified open wound of other specified part of neck

⊗⑦S11.81　Laceration without foreign body of other specified part of neck

⊗⑦S11.82　Laceration with foreign body of other specified part of neck

⊗⑦S11.83　Puncture wound without foreign body of other specified part of neck

⊗⑦S11.84　Puncture wound with foreign body of other specified part of neck

⊗⑦S11.85　Open bite of other specified part of neck
　　　　　　Bite of other specified part of neck NOS
　　　　　　Excludes 1: superficial bite of other specified part of neck (S10.87)

⊗⑦S11.89　Other open wound of other specified part of neck

S11.9　Open wound of unspecified part of neck

⊗⑦S11.90　Unspecified open wound of unspecified part of neck

⊗⑦S11.91　Laceration without foreign body of unspecified part of neck

⊗⑦S11.92　Laceration with foreign body of unspecified part of neck

⊗⑦S11.93　Puncture wound without foreign body of unspecified part of neck

⊗⑦S11.94　Puncture wound with foreign body of unspecified part of neck

⊗⑦S11.95　Open bite of unspecified part of neck
　　　　　　Bite of neck NOS
　　　　　　Excludes 1: superficial bite of neck (S10.97)

S12　Fracture of cervical vertebra and other parts of neck

Note:　A fracture not indicated as displaced or nondisplaced should be coded to displaced
　　　　A fracture not indicated as open or closed should be coded to closed

Includes: fracture of cervical neural arch
　　　　　　fracture of cervical spine
　　　　　　fracture of cervical spinous process
　　　　　　fracture of cervical transverse process
　　　　　　fracture of cervical vertebral arch
　　　　　　fracture of neck

Code also any associated cervical spinal cord injury (S14.0, S14.1-)

The appropriate 7th character is to be added to all codes from subcategories S12.0-S12.6

A - initial encounter for closed fracture

B - initial encounter for open fracture

D - subsequent encounter for fracture with routine healing

G - subsequent encounter for fracture with delayed healing

K - subsequent encounter for fracture with nonunion

S - sequela

S12.0　Fracture of first cervical vertebra
　　　　Atlas

　　S12.00　Unspecified fracture of first cervical vertebra

　　　　⑦S12.000　Unspecified displaced fracture of first cervical vertebra

　　　　⑦S12.001　Unspecified nondisplaced fracture of first cervical vertebra

⊗⑦S12.01　Stable burst fracture of first cervical vertebra

⊗⑦S12.02　Unstable burst fracture of first cervical vertebra

　　S12.03　Posterior arch fracture of first cervical vertebra

　　　　⑦S12.030　Displaced posterior arch fracture of first cervical vertebra

　　　　⑦S12.031　Nondisplaced posterior arch fracture of first cervical vertebra

　　S12.04　Lateral mass fracture of first cervical vertebra

　　　　⑦S12.040　Displaced lateral mass fracture of first cervical vertebra

　　　　⑦S12.041　Nondisplaced lateral mass fracture of first cervical vertebra

　　S12.09　Other fracture of first cervical vertebra

　　　　⑦S12.090　Other displaced fracture of first cervical vertebra

　　　　⑦S12.091　Other nondisplaced fracture of first cervical vertebra

S12.1　Fracture of second cervical vertebra
　　　　Axis

　　S12.10　Unspecified fracture of second cervical vertebra

　　　　⑦S12.100　Unspecified displaced fracture of second cervical vertebra

　　　　⑦S12.101　Unspecified nondisplaced fracture of second cervical vertebra

S12.11   Type II dens fracture

   ⑦S12.110   Anterior displaced Type II dens fracture

   ⑦S12.111   Posterior displaced Type II dens fracture

   ⑦S12.112   Nondisplaced Type II dens fracture

S12.12   Other dens fracture

   ⑦S12.120   Other displaced dens fracture

   ⑦S12.121   Other nondisplaced dens fracture

S12.13   Unspecified traumatic spondylolisthesis of second cervical vertebra

   ⑦S12.130   Unspecified traumatic displaced spondylolisthesis of second cervical vertebra

   ⑦S12.131   Unspecified traumatic nondisplaced spondylolisthesis of second cervical vertebra

⊗⑦S12.14   Type III traumatic spondylolisthesis of second cervical vertebra

S12.15   Other traumatic spondylolisthesis of second cervical vertebra

   ⑦S12.150   Other traumatic displaced spondylolisthesis of second cervical vertebra

   ⑦S12.151   Other traumatic nondisplaced spondylolisthesis of second cervical vertebra

S12.19   Other fracture of second cervical vertebra

   ⑦S12.190   Other displaced fracture of second cervical vertebra

   ⑦S12.191   Other nondisplaced fracture of second cervical vertebra

S12.2   Fracture of third cervical vertebra

   S12.20   Unspecified fracture of third cervical vertebra

     ⑦S12.200   Unspecified displaced fracture of third cervical vertebra

     ⑦S12.201   Unspecified nondisplaced fracture of third cervical vertebra

   S12.23   Unspecified traumatic spondylolisthesis of third cervical vertebra

     ⑦S12.230   Unspecified traumatic displaced spondylolisthesis of third cervical vertebra

     ⑦S12.231   Unspecified traumatic nondisplaced spondylolisthesis of third cervical vertebra

  ⊗⑦S12.24   Type III traumatic spondylolisthesis of third cervical vertebra

   S12.25   Other traumatic spondylolisthesis of third cervical vertebra

     ⑦S12.250   Other traumatic displaced spondylolisthesis of third cervical vertebra

     ⑦S12.251   Other traumatic nondisplaced spondylolisthesis of third cervical vertebra

   S12.29   Other fracture of third cervical vertebra

     ⑦S12.290   Other displaced fracture of third cervical vertebra

     ⑦S12.291   Other nondisplaced fracture of third cervical vertebra

S12.3   Fracture of fourth cervical vertebra

   S12.30   Unspecified fracture of fourth cervical vertebra

     ⑦S12.300   Unspecified displaced fracture of fourth cervical vertebra

     ⑦S12.301   Unspecified nondisplaced fracture of fourth cervical vertebra

   S12.33   Unspecified traumatic spondylolisthesis of fourth cervical vertebra

     ⑦S12.330   Unspecified traumatic displaced spondylolisthesis of fourth cervical vertebra

     ⑦S12.331   Unspecified traumatic nondisplaced spondylolisthesis of fourth cervical vertebra

  ⊗⑦S12.34   Type III traumatic spondylolisthesis of fourth cervical vertebra

   S12.35   Other traumatic spondylolisthesis of fourth cervical vertebra

     ⑦S12.350   Other traumatic displaced spondylolisthesis of fourth cervical vertebra

     ⑦S12.351   Other traumatic nondisplaced spondylolisthesis of fourth cervical vertebra

   S12.39   Other fracture of fourth cervical vertebra

     ⑦S12.390   Other displaced fracture of fourth cervical vertebra

     ⑦S12.391   Other nondisplaced fracture of fourth cervical vertebra

S12.4   Fracture of fifth cervical vertebra

   S12.40   Unspecified fracture of fifth cervical vertebra

     ⑦S12.400   Unspecified displaced fracture of fifth cervical vertebra

     ⑦S12.401   Unspecified nondisplaced fracture of fifth cervical vertebra

   S12.43   Unspecified traumatic spondylolisthesis of fifth cervical vertebra

     ⑦S12.430   Unspecified traumatic displaced spondylolisthesis of fifth cervical vertebra

     ⑦S12.431   Unspecified traumatic nondisplaced spondylolisthesis of fifth cervical vertebra

  ⊗⑦S12.44   Type III traumatic spondylolisthesis of fifth cervical vertebra

   S12.45   Other traumatic spondylolisthesis of fifth cervical vertebra

     ⑦S12.450   Other traumatic displaced spondylolisthesis of fifth cervical vertebra

     ⑦S12.451   Other traumatic nondisplaced spondylolisthesis of fifth cervical vertebra

   S12.49   Other fracture of fifth cervical vertebra

     ⑦S12.490   Other displaced fracture of fifth cervical vertebra

     ⑦S12.491   Other nondisplaced fracture of fifth cervical vertebra

   ● New code   ▲ Revised code   ⑦ 7th digit required   ⊗ Placeholder required

S12.5 Fracture of sixth cervical vertebra
    S12.50 Unspecified fracture of sixth cervical vertebra
        ⑦S12.500 Unspecified displaced fracture of sixth cervical vertebra
        ⑦S12.501 Unspecified nondisplaced fracture of sixth cervical vertebra
    S12.53 Unspecified traumatic spondylolisthesis of sixth cervical vertebra
        ⑦S12.530 Unspecified traumatic displaced spondylolisthesis of sixth cervical vertebra
        ⑦S12.531 Unspecified traumatic nondisplaced spondylolisthesis of sixth cervical vertebra
  ⊗⑦S12.54 Type III traumatic spondylolisthesis of sixth cervical vertebra
    S12.55 Other traumatic spondylolisthesis of sixth cervical vertebra
        ⑦S12.550 Other traumatic displaced spondylolisthesis of sixth cervical vertebra
        ⑦S12.551 Other traumatic nondisplaced spondylolisthesis of sixth cervical vertebra
    S12.59 Other fracture of sixth cervical vertebra
        ⑦S12.590 Other displaced fracture of sixth cervical vertebra
        ⑦S12.591 Other nondisplaced fracture of sixth cervical vertebra
S12.6 Fracture of seventh cervical vertebra
    S12.60 Unspecified fracture of seventh cervical vertebra
        ⑦S12.600 Unspecified displaced fracture of seventh cervical vertebra
        ⑦S12.601 Unspecified nondisplaced fracture of seventh cervical vertebra
    S12.63 Unspecified traumatic spondylolisthesis of seventh cervical vertebra
        ⑦S12.630 Unspecified traumatic displaced spondylolisthesis of seventh cervical vertebra
        ⑦S12.631 Unspecified traumatic nondisplaced spondylolisthesis of seventh cervical vertebra
    S12.64 Type III traumatic spondylolisthesis of seventh cervical vertebra
    S12.65 Other traumatic spondylolisthesis of seventh cervical vertebra
        ⑦S12.650 Other traumatic displaced spondylolisthesis of seventh cervical vertebra
        ⑦S12.651 Other traumatic nondisplaced spondylolisthesis of seventh cervical vertebra
    S12.69 Other fracture of seventh cervical vertebra
        ⑦S12.690 Other displaced fracture of seventh cervical vertebra
        ⑦S12.691 Other nondisplaced fracture of seventh cervical vertebra
⊗⑦S12.8 Fracture of other parts of neck
  The appropriate 7th character is to be added to code S12.8

A - initial encounter
D - subsequent encounter
S - sequela
Hyoid bone
Larynx
Thyroid cartilage
Trachea
⊗⑦S12.9 Fracture of neck, unspecified
  The appropriate 7th character is to be added to code S12.9
A - initial encounter
D - subsequent encounter
S - sequela
Fracture of neck NOS
Fracture of cervical spine NOS
Fracture of cervical vertebra NOS

S13 Dislocation and sprain of joints and ligaments at neck level
Includes: avulsion of joint or ligament at neck level
    laceration of cartilage, joint or ligament at neck level
    sprain of cartilage, joint or ligament at neck level
    traumatic hemarthrosis of joint or ligament at neck level
    traumatic rupture of joint or ligament at neck level
    traumatic subluxation of joint or ligament at neck level
    traumatic tear of joint or ligament at neck level
Code also any associated open wound
Excludes 2: strain of muscle or tendon at neck level (S16.1)
The appropriate 7th character is to be added to each code from category S13
A - initial encounter
D - subsequent encounter
S - sequela
⊗⑦S13.0 Traumatic rupture of cervical intervertebral disc
    Excludes 1: rupture or displacement (nontraumatic) of cervical intervertebral disc NOS (M50.-)
  S13.1 Subluxation and dislocation of cervical vertebrae
    Code also any associated:
      open wound of neck (S11.-)
      spinal cord injury (S14.1-)
    Excludes 2: fracture of cervical vertebrae (S12.0-S12.3)
    S13.10 Subluxation and dislocation of unspecified cervical vertebrae
        ⑦S13.100 Subluxation of unspecified cervical vertebrae
        ⑦S13.101 Dislocation of unspecified cervical vertebrae
    S13.11 Subluxation and dislocation of C0/C1 cervical vertebrae
      Subluxation and dislocation of atlantooccipital joint
      Subluxation and dislocation of atloidooccipital joint
      Subluxation and dislocation of occipitoatloid joint
        ⑦S13.110 Subluxation of C0/C1 cervical vertebrae
        ⑦S13.111 Dislocation of C0/C1 cervical vertebrae
    S13.12 Subluxation and dislocation of C1/C2 cervical vertebrae
      Subluxation and dislocation of atlantoaxial joint

⑦S13.120 Subluxation of C1/C2 cervical vertebrae

⑦S13.121 Dislocation of C1/C2 cervical vertebrae

S13.13 Subluxation and dislocation of C2/C3 cervical vertebrae

⑦S13.130 Subluxation of C2/C3 cervical vertebrae

⑦S13.131 Dislocation of C2/C3 cervical vertebrae

S13.14 Subluxation and dislocation of C3/C4 cervical vertebrae

⑦S13.140 Subluxation of C3/C4 cervical vertebrae

⑦S13.141 Dislocation of C3/C4 cervical vertebrae

S13.15 Subluxation and dislocation of C4/C5 cervical vertebrae

⑦S13.150 Subluxation of C4/C5 cervical vertebrae

⑦S13.151 Dislocation of C4/C5 cervical vertebrae

S13.16 Subluxation and dislocation of C5/C6 cervical vertebrae

⑦S13.160 Subluxation of C5/C6 cervical vertebrae

⑦S13.161 Dislocation of C5/C6 cervical vertebrae

S13.17 Subluxation and dislocation of C6/C7 cervical vertebrae

⑦S13.170 Subluxation of C6/C7 cervical vertebrae

⑦S13.171 Dislocation of C6/C7 cervical vertebrae

S13.18 Subluxation and dislocation of C7/T1 cervical vertebrae

⑦S13.180 Subluxation of C7/T1 cervical vertebrae

⑦S13.181 Dislocation of C7/T1 cervical vertebrae

S13.2 Dislocation of other and unspecified parts of neck

⊗⑦S13.20 Dislocation of unspecified parts of neck

⊗⑦S13.29 Dislocation of other parts of neck

⊗⑦S13.4 Sprain of ligaments of cervical spine
Sprain of anterior longitudinal (ligament), cervical
Sprain of atlanto-axial (joints)
Sprain of atlanto-occipital (joints)
Whiplash injury of cervical spine

⊗⑦S13.5 Sprain of thyroid region
Sprain of cricoarytenoid (joint) (ligament)
Sprain of cricothyroid (joint) (ligament)
Sprain of thyroid cartilage

⊗⑦S13.8 Sprain of joints and ligaments of other parts of neck

⊗⑦S13.9 Sprain of joints and ligaments of unspecified parts of neck

S14 Injury of nerves and spinal cord at neck level
Note: Code to highest level of cervical cord injury
Code also any associated:
fracture of cervical vertebra (S12.0--S12.6.-)
open wound of neck (S11-)

transient paralysis (R29.5)
The appropriate 7th character is to be added to each code from category S14
A - initial encounter
D - subsequent encounter
S - sequela

⊗⑦S14.0 Concussion and edema of cervical spinal cord

S14.1 Other and unspecified injuries of cervical spinal cord

S14.10 Unspecified injury of cervical spinal cord

⑦S14.101 Unspecified injury at C1 level of cervical spinal cord

⑦S14.102 Unspecified injury at C2 level of cervical spinal cord

⑦S14.103 Unspecified injury at C3 level of cervical spinal cord

⑦S14.104 Unspecified injury at C4 level of cervical spinal cord

⑦S14.105 Unspecified injury at C5 level of cervical spinal cord

⑦S14.106 Unspecified injury at C6 level of cervical spinal cord

⑦S14.107 Unspecified injury at C7 level of cervical spinal cord

⑦S14.108 Unspecified injury at C8 level of cervical spinal cord

⑦S14.109 Unspecified injury at unspecified level of cervical spinal cord
Injury of cervical spinal cord NOS

S14.11 Complete lesion of cervical spinal cord

⑦S14.111 Complete lesion at C1 level of cervical spinal cord

⑦S14.112 Complete lesion at C2 level of cervical spinal cord

⑦S14.113 Complete lesion at C3 level of cervical spinal cord

⑦S14.114 Complete lesion at C4 level of cervical spinal cord

⑦S14.115 Complete lesion at C5 level of cervical spinal cord

⑦S14.116 Complete lesion at C6 level of cervical spinal cord

⑦S14.117 Complete lesion at C7 level of cervical spinal cord

⑦S14.118 Complete lesion at C8 level of cervical spinal cord

⑦S14.119 Complete lesion at unspecified level of cervical spinal cord

S14.12 Central cord syndrome of cervical spinal cord

⑦S14.121 Central cord syndrome at C1 level of cervical spinal cord

⑦S14.122 Central cord syndrome at C2 level of cervical spinal cord

⑦S14.123 Central cord syndrome at C3 level of cervical spinal cord

⑦S14.124 Central cord syndrome at C4 level of cervical spinal cord

⑦S14.125 Central cord syndrome at C5 level of cervical spinal cord

● New code ▲ Revised code ⑦ 7th digit required ⊗ Placeholder required

⑦S14.126   Central cord syndrome at C6 level of cervical spinal cord

⑦S14.127   Central cord syndrome at C7 level of cervical spinal cord

⑦S14.128   Central cord syndrome at C8 level of cervical spinal cord

⑦S14.129   Central cord syndrome at unspecified level of cervical spinal cord

S14.13   Anterior cord syndrome of cervical spinal cord

⑦S14.131   Anterior cord syndrome at C1 level of cervical spinal cord

⑦S14.132   Anterior cord syndrome at C2 level of cervical spinal cord

⑦S14.133   Anterior cord syndrome at C3 level of cervical spinal cord

⑦S14.134   Anterior cord syndrome at C4 level of cervical spinal cord

⑦S14.135   Anterior cord syndrome at C5 level of cervical spinal cord

⑦S14.136   Anterior cord syndrome at C6 level of cervical spinal cord

⑦S14.137   Anterior cord syndrome at C7 level of cervical spinal cord

⑦S14.138   Anterior cord syndrome at C8 level of cervical spinal cord

⑦S14.139   Anterior cord syndrome at unspecified level of cervical spinal cord

S14.14   Brown-Sequard syndrome of cervical spinal cord

⑦S14.141   Brown-Sequard syndrome at C1 level of cervical spinal cord

⑦S14.142   Brown-Sequard syndrome at C2 level of cervical spinal cord

⑦S14.143   Brown-Sequard syndrome at C3 level of cervical spinal cord

⑦S14.144   Brown-Sequard syndrome at C4 level of cervical spinal cord

⑦S14.145   Brown-Sequard syndrome at C5 level of cervical spinal cord

⑦S14.146   Brown-Sequard syndrome at C6 level of cervical spinal cord

⑦S14.147   Brown-Sequard syndrome at C7 level of cervical spinal cord

⑦S14.148   Brown-Sequard syndrome at C8 level of cervical spinal cord

⑦S14.149   Brown-Sequard syndrome at unspecified level of cervical spinal cord

S14.15   Other incomplete lesions of cervical spinal cord

Incomplete lesion of cervical spinal cord NOS

Posterior cord syndrome of cervical spinal cord

⑦S14.151   Other incomplete lesion at C1 level of cervical spinal cord

⑦S14.152   Other incomplete lesion at C2 level of cervical spinal cord

⑦S14.153   Other incomplete lesion at C3 level of cervical spinal cord

⑦S14.154   Other incomplete lesion at C4 level of cervical spinal cord

⑦S14.155   Other incomplete lesion at C5 level of cervical spinal cord

⑦S14.156   Other incomplete lesion at C6 level of cervical spinal cord

⑦S14.157   Other incomplete lesion at C7 level of cervical spinal cord

⑦S14.158   Other incomplete lesion at C8 level of cervical spinal cord

⑦S14.159   Other incomplete lesion at unspecified level of cervical spinal cord

⊗⑦S14.2   Injury of nerve root of cervical spine

⊗⑦S14.3   Injury of brachial plexus

⊗⑦S14.4   Injury of peripheral nerves of neck

⊗⑦S14.5   Injury of cervical sympathetic nerves

⊗⑦S14.8   Injury of other specified nerves of neck

⊗⑦S14.9   Injury of unspecified nerves of neck

S15   Injury of blood vessels at neck level

Code also any associated open wound (S11.-)

The appropriate 7th character is to be added to each code from category S15

A - initial encounter

D - subsequent encounter

S - sequela

S15.0   Injury of carotid artery of neck

Injury of carotid artery (common) (external) (internal, extracranial portion)

Injury of carotid artery NOS

Excludes 1: injury of internal carotid artery, intracranial portion (S06.8)

S15.00   Unspecified injury of carotid artery

⑦S15.001   Unspecified injury of right carotid artery

⑦S15.002   Unspecified injury of left carotid artery

⑦S15.009   Unspecified injury of unspecified carotid artery

S15.01   Minor laceration of carotid artery

Incomplete transection of carotid artery

Laceration of carotid artery NOS

Superficial laceration of carotid artery

⑦S15.011   Minor laceration of right carotid artery

⑦S15.012   Minor laceration of left carotid artery

⑦S15.019   Minor laceration of unspecified carotid artery

S15.02   Major laceration of carotid artery

Complete transection of carotid artery

Traumatic rupture of carotid artery

⑦S15.021   Major laceration of right carotid artery

⑦S15.022   Major laceration of left carotid artery

⑦S15.029   Major laceration of unspecified carotid artery

S15.09   Other specified injury of carotid artery

⑦**S15.091** Other specified injury of right carotid artery

⑦**S15.092** Other specified injury of left carotid artery

⑦**S15.099** Other specified injury of unspecified carotid artery

S15.1 Injury of vertebral artery

    S15.10 Unspecified injury of vertebral artery

       ⑦**S15.101** Unspecified injury of right vertebral artery

       ⑦**S15.102** Unspecified injury of left vertebral artery

       ⑦**S15.109** Unspecified injury of unspecified vertebral artery

    S15.11 Minor laceration of vertebral artery

       Incomplete transection of vertebral artery

       Laceration of vertebral artery NOS

       Superficial laceration of vertebral artery

       ⑦**S15.111** Minor laceration of right vertebral artery

       ⑦**S15.112** Minor laceration of left vertebral artery

       ⑦**S15.119** Minor laceration of unspecified vertebral artery

    S15.12 Major laceration of vertebral artery

       Complete transection of vertebral artery

       Traumatic rupture of vertebral artery

       ⑦**S15.121** Major laceration of right vertebral artery

       ⑦**S15.122** Major laceration of left vertebral artery

       ⑦**S15.129** Major laceration of unspecified vertebral artery

    S15.19 Other specified injury of vertebral artery

       ⑦**S15.191** Other specified injury of right vertebral artery

       ⑦**S15.192** Other specified injury of left vertebral artery

       ⑦**S15.199** Other specified injury of unspecified vertebral artery

S15.2 Injury of external jugular vein

    S15.20 Unspecified injury of external jugular vein

       ⑦**S15.201** Unspecified injury of right external jugular vein

       ⑦**S15.202** Unspecified injury of left external jugular vein

       ⑦**S15.209** Unspecified injury of unspecified external jugular vein

    S15.21 Minor laceration of external jugular vein

       Incomplete transection of external jugular vein

       Laceration of external jugular vein NOS

       Superficial laceration of external jugular vein

       ⑦**S15.211** Minor laceration of right external jugular vein

       ⑦**S15.212** Minor laceration of left external jugular vein

       ⑦**S15.219** Minor laceration of unspecified external jugular vein

    S15.22 Major laceration of external jugular vein

       Complete transection of external jugular vein

       Traumatic rupture of external jugular vein

       ⑦**S15.221** Major laceration of right external jugular vein

       ⑦**S15.222** Major laceration of left external jugular vein

       ⑦**S15.229** Major laceration of unspecified external jugular vein

    S15.29 Other specified injury of external jugular vein

       ⑦**S15.291** Other specified injury of right external jugular vein

       ⑦**S15.292** Other specified injury of left external jugular vein

       ⑦**S15.299** Other specified injury of unspecified external jugular vein

S15.3 Injury of internal jugular vein

    S15.30 Unspecified injury of internal jugular vein

       ⑦**S15.301** Unspecified injury of right internal jugular vein

       ⑦**S15.302** Unspecified injury of left internal jugular vein

       ⑦**S15.309** Unspecified injury of unspecified internal jugular vein

    S15.31 Minor laceration of internal jugular vein

       Incomplete transection of internal jugular vein

       Laceration of internal jugular vein NOS

       Superficial laceration of internal jugular vein

       ⑦**S15.311** Minor laceration of right internal jugular vein

       ⑦**S15.312** Minor laceration of left internal jugular vein

       ⑦**S15.319** Minor laceration of unspecified internal jugular vein

    S15.32 Major laceration of internal jugular vein

       Complete transection of internal jugular vein

       Traumatic rupture of internal jugular vein

       ⑦**S15.321** Major laceration of right internal jugular vein

       ⑦**S15.322** Major laceration of left internal jugular vein

       ⑦**S15.329** Major laceration of unspecified internal jugular vein

    S15.39 Other specified injury of internal jugular vein

       ⑦**S15.391** Other specified injury of right internal jugular vein

       ⑦**S15.392** Other specified injury of left internal jugular vein

       ⑦**S15.399** Other specified injury of unspecified internal jugular vein

⊗⑦**S15.8** Injury of other specified blood vessels at neck level

⊗⑦**S15.9** Injury of unspecified blood vessel at neck level

S16 Injury of muscle, fascia and tendon at neck level

Code also any associated open wound (S11.-)

Excludes 2: sprain of joint or ligament at neck level (S13.9)

The appropriate 7th character is to be added to each code from category S16

A - initial encounter

D - subsequent encounter

S - sequela

⊗⑦S16.1   Strain of muscle, fascia and tendon at neck level

⊗⑦S16.2   Laceration of muscle, fascia and tendon at neck level

⊗⑦S16.8   Other specified injury of muscle, fascia and tendon at neck level

⊗⑦S16.9   Unspecified injury of muscle, fascia and tendon at neck level

S17   Crushing injury of neck

Use additional code for all associated injuries, such as:

     injury of blood vessels (S15.-)

     open wound of neck (S11.-)

     spinal cord injury (S14.0, S14.1-)

     vertebral fracture (S12.0--S12.3-)

The appropriate 7th character is to be added to each code from category S17

A - initial encounter

D - subsequent encounter

S - sequela

⊗⑦S17.0   Crushing injury of larynx and trachea

⊗⑦S17.8   Crushing injury of other specified parts of neck

⊗⑦S17.9   Crushing injury of neck, part unspecified

S19   Other specified and unspecified injuries of neck

The appropriate 7th character is to be added to each code from category S19

A - initial encounter

D - subsequent encounter

S - sequela

S19.8   Other specified injuries of neck

⊗⑦S19.80   Other specified injuries of unspecified part of neck

⊗⑦S19.81   Other specified injuries of larynx

⊗⑦S19.82   Other specified injuries of cervical trachea

       Excludes 2: other specified injury of thoracic trachea (S27.5-)

⊗⑦S19.83   Other specified injuries of vocal cord

⊗⑦S19.84   Other specified injuries of thyroid gland

⊗⑦S19.85   Other specified injuries of pharynx and cervical esophagus

⊗⑦S19.89   Other specified injuries of other specified part of neck

⊗⑦S19.9   Unspecified injury of neck

INJURIES TO THE THORAX (S20-S29)

Includes: injuries of breast

     injuries of chest (wall)

     injuries of interscapular area

Excludes 2: burns and corrosions (T20-T32)

     effects of foreign body in bronchus (T17.5)

     effects of foreign body in esophagus (T18.1)

     effects of foreign body in lung (T17.8)

     effects of foreign body in trachea (T17.4)

     frostbite (T33-T34)

     injuries of axilla

     injuries of clavicle

     injuries of scapular region

     injuries of shoulder

     insect bite or sting, venomous (T63.4)

S20   Superficial injury of thorax

The appropriate 7th character is to be added to each code from category S20

A - initial encounter

D - subsequent encounter

S - sequela

S20.0   Contusion of breast

⊗⑦S20.00   Contusion of breast, unspecified breast

⊗⑦S20.01   Contusion of right breast

⊗⑦S20.02   Contusion of left breast

S20.1   Other and unspecified superficial injuries of breast

S20.10   Unspecified superficial injuries of breast

⑦S20.101   Unspecified superficial injuries of breast, right breast

⑦S20.102   Unspecified superficial injuries of breast, left breast

⑦S20.109   Unspecified superficial injuries of breast, unspecified breast

S20.11   Abrasion of breast

⑦S20.111   Abrasion of breast, right breast

⑦S20.112   Abrasion of breast, left breast

⑦S20.119   Abrasion of breast, unspecified breast

S20.12   Blister (nonthermal) of breast

⑦S20.121   Blister (nonthermal) of breast, right breast

⑦S20.122   Blister (nonthermal) of breast, left breast

⑦S20.129   Blister (nonthermal) of breast, unspecified breast

S20.14   External constriction of part of breast

⑦S20.141   External constriction of part of breast, right breast

⑦S20.142   External constriction of part of breast, left breast

⑦S20.149   External constriction of part of breast, unspecified breast

S20.15   Superficial foreign body of breast

Splinter in the breast

⑦S20.151   Superficial foreign body of breast, right breast

⑦S20.152   Superficial foreign body of breast, left breast

⑦S20.159   Superficial foreign body of breast, unspecified breast

S20.16   Insect bite (nonvenomous) of breast

⑦S20.161   Insect bite (nonvenomous) of breast, right breast

⑦S20.162   Insect bite (nonvenomous) of breast, left breast

⑦S20.169   Insect bite (nonvenomous) of breast, unspecified breast

S20.17   Other superficial bite of breast

       Excludes 1: open bite of breast (S21.05-)

⑦S20.171   Other superficial bite of breast, right breast

⑦S20.172   Other superficial bite of breast, left breast

⑦ **S20.179** Other superficial bite of breast, unspecified breast

S20.2 Contusion of thorax

⊗⑦**S20.20** Contusion of thorax, unspecified

S20.21 Contusion of front wall of thorax

⑦S20.211 Contusion of right front wall of thorax

⑦S20.212 Contusion of left front wall of thorax

⑦S20.219 Contusion of unspecified front wall of thorax

S20.22 Contusion of back wall of thorax

⑦S20.221 Contusion of right back wall of thorax

⑦S20.222 Contusion of left back wall of thorax

⑦S20.229 Contusion of unspecified back wall of thorax

S20.3 Other and unspecified superficial injuries of front wall of thorax

S20.30 Unspecified superficial injuries of front wall of thorax

⑦S20.301 Unspecified superficial injuries of right front wall of thorax

⑦S20.302 Unspecified superficial injuries of left front wall of thorax

⑦S20.309 Unspecified superficial injuries of unspecified front wall of thorax

S20.31 Abrasion of front wall of thorax

⑦S20.311 Abrasion of right front wall of thorax

⑦S20.312 Abrasion of left front wall of thorax

⑦S20.319 Abrasion of unspecified front wall of thorax

S20.32 Blister (nonthermal) of front wall of thorax

⑦S20.321 Blister (nonthermal) of right front wall of thorax

⑦S20.322 Blister (nonthermal) of left front wall of thorax

⑦S20.329 Blister (nonthermal) of unspecified front wall of thorax

S20.34 External constriction of front wall of thorax

⑦S20.341 External constriction of right front wall of thorax

⑦S20.342 External constriction of left front wall of thorax

⑦S20.349 External constriction of unspecified front wall of thorax

S20.35 Superficial foreign body of front wall of thorax

Splinter in front wall of thorax

⑦S20.351 Superficial foreign body of right front wall of thorax

⑦S20.352 Superficial foreign body of left front wall of thorax

⑦S20.359 Superficial foreign body of unspecified front wall of thorax

S20.36 Insect bite (nonvenomous) of front wall of thorax

⑦S20.361 Insect bite (nonvenomous) of right front wall of thorax

⑦S20.362 Insect bite (nonvenomous) of left front wall of thorax

⑦S20.369 Insect bite (nonvenomous) of unspecified front wall of thorax

S20.37 Other superficial bite of front wall of thorax

Excludes 1: open bite of front wall of thorax (S21.14)

⑦**S20.371** Other superficial bite of right front wall of thorax

⑦**S20.372** Other superficial bite of left front wall of thorax

⑦**S20.379** Other superficial bite of unspecified front wall of thorax

S20.4 Other and unspecified superficial injuries of back wall of thorax

S20.40 Unspecified superficial injuries of back wall of thorax

⑦S20.401 Unspecified superficial injuries of right back wall of thorax

⑦S20.402 Unspecified superficial injuries of left back wall of thorax

⑦S20.409 Unspecified superficial injuries of unspecified back wall of thorax

S20.41 Abrasion of back wall of thorax

⑦S20.411 Abrasion of right back wall of thorax

⑦S20.412 Abrasion of left back wall of thorax

⑦S20.419 Abrasion of unspecified back wall of thorax

S20.42 Blister (nonthermal) of back wall of thorax

⑦S20.421 Blister (nonthermal) of right back wall of thorax

⑦S20.422 Blister (nonthermal) of left back wall of thorax

⑦S20.429 Blister (nonthermal) of unspecified back wall of thorax

S20.44 External constriction of back wall of thorax

⑦S20.441 External constriction of right back wall of thorax

⑦S20.442 External constriction of left back wall of thorax

⑦S20.449 External constriction of unspecified back wall of thorax

S20.45 Superficial foreign body of back wall of thorax

Splinter of back wall of thorax

⑦S20.451 Superficial foreign body of right back wall of thorax

⑦S20.452 Superficial foreign body of left back wall of thorax

⑦S20.459 Superficial foreign body of unspecified back wall of thorax

S20.46 Insect bite (nonvenomous) of back wall of thorax

⑦S20.461 Insect bite (nonvenomous) of right back wall of thorax

⑦S20.462 Insect bite (nonvenomous) of left back wall of thorax

⑦S20.469 Insect bite (nonvenomous) of unspecified back wall of thorax

● New code   ▲ Revised code   ⑦ 7th digit required   ⊗ Placeholder required

S20.47   Other superficial bite of back wall of thorax
> **Excludes 1:** open bite of back wall of thorax (S21.24)

⑦S20.471   Other superficial bite of right back wall of thorax

⑦S20.472   Other superficial bite of left back wall of thorax

⑦S20.479   Other superficial bite of unspecified back wall of thorax

S20.9   Superficial injury of unspecified parts of thorax
> **Excludes 1:** contusion of thorax NOS (S20.20)

⊗⑦S20.90   Unspecified superficial injury of unspecified parts of thorax
Superficial injury of thoracic wall NOS

⊗⑦S20.91   Abrasion of unspecified parts of thorax

⊗⑦S20.92   Blister (nonthermal) of unspecified parts of thorax

⊗⑦S20.94   External constriction of unspecified parts of thorax

⊗⑦S20.95   Superficial foreign body of unspecified parts of thorax
Splinter in thorax NOS

⊗⑦S20.96   Insect bite (nonvenomous) of unspecified parts of thorax

⊗⑦S20.97   Other superficial bite of unspecified parts of thorax
> **Excludes 1:** open bite of thorax NOS (S21.95)

S21   **Open wound of thorax**
Code also any associated injury (to) (such as) :
> heart (S26.-)
> intrathoracic organs (S27.-)
> rib fracture (S22.3-, S22.4-)
> spinal cord injury (S24.0-, S24.1-)
> traumatic hemothorax (S27.1)
> traumatic hemopneumothorax (S27.3)
> traumatic pneumothorax (S27.0)
> wound infection

Excludes 1: traumatic amputation (partial) of thorax (S28.1)

The appropriate 7th character is to be added to each code from category S21
A - initial encounter
D - subsequent encounter
S - sequela

S21.0   Open wound of breast

S21.00   Unspecified open wound of breast

⑦S21.001   Unspecified open wound of right breast

⑦S21.002   Unspecified open wound of left breast

⑦S21.009   Unspecified open wound of unspecified breast

S21.01   Laceration without foreign body of breast

⑦S21.011   Laceration without foreign body of right breast

⑦S21.012   Laceration without foreign body of left breast

⑦S21.019   Laceration without foreign body of unspecified breast

S21.02   Laceration with foreign body of breast

⑦S21.021   Laceration with foreign body of right breast

⑦S21.022   Laceration with foreign body of left breast

⑦S21.029   Laceration with foreign body of unspecified breast

S21.03   Puncture wound without foreign body of breast

⑦S21.031   Puncture wound without foreign body of right breast

⑦S21.032   Puncture wound without foreign body of left breast

⑦S21.039   Puncture wound without foreign body of unspecified breast

S21.04   Puncture wound with foreign body of breast

⑦S21.041   Puncture wound with foreign body of right breast

⑦S21.042   Puncture wound with foreign body of left breast

⑦S21.049   Puncture wound with foreign body of unspecified breast

S21.05   Open bite of breast
Bite of breast NOS
> **Excludes 1:** superficial bite of breast (S20.17)

⑦S21.051   Open bite of right breast

⑦S21.052   Open bite of left breast

⑦S21.059   Open bite of unspecified breast

S21.1   Open wound of front wall of thorax without penetration into thoracic cavity
Open wound of chest without penetration into thoracic cavity

S21.10   Unspecified open wound of front wall of thorax without penetration into thoracic cavity

⑦S21.101   Unspecified open wound of right front wall of thorax without penetration into thoracic cavity

⑦S21.102   Unspecified open wound of left front wall of thorax without penetration into thoracic cavity

⑦S21.109   Unspecified open wound of unspecified front wall of thorax without penetration into thoracic cavity

⊗⑦S21.11   Laceration without foreign body of front wall of thorax without penetration into thoracic cavity

S21.111   Laceration without foreign body of right front wall of thorax without penetration into thoracic cavity

⑦S21.112   Laceration without foreign body of left front wall of thorax without penetration into thoracic cavity

⑦S21.119   Laceration without foreign body of unspecified front wall of thorax without penetration into thoracic cavity

S21.12   Laceration with foreign body of front wall of thorax without penetration into thoracic cavity

⑦**S21.121**   Laceration with foreign body of right front wall of thorax without penetration into thoracic cavity

⑦**S21.122**   Laceration with foreign body of left front wall of thorax without penetration into thoracic cavity

⑦**S21.129**   Laceration with foreign body of unspecified front wall of thorax without penetration into thoracic cavity

S21.13   Puncture wound without foreign body of front wall of thorax without penetration into thoracic cavity

⑦**S21.131**   Puncture wound without foreign body of right front wall of thorax without penetration into thoracic cavity

⑦**S21.132**   Puncture wound without foreign body of left front wall of thorax without penetration into thoracic cavity

⑦**S21.139**   Puncture wound without foreign body of unspecified front wall of thorax without penetration into thoracic cavity

S21.14   Puncture wound with foreign body of front wall of thorax without penetration into thoracic cavity

⑦**S21.141**   Puncture wound with foreign body of right front wall of thorax without penetration into thoracic cavity

⑦**S21.142**   Puncture wound with foreign body of left front wall of thorax without penetration into thoracic cavity

⑦**S21.149**   Puncture wound with foreign body of unspecified front wall of thorax without penetration into thoracic cavity

S21.15   Open bite of front wall of thorax without penetration into thoracic cavity
Bite of front wall of thorax NOS
Excludes 1: superficial bite of front wall of thorax (S20.37)

⑦**S21.151**   Open bite of right front wall of thorax without penetration into thoracic cavity

⑦**S21.152**   Open bite of left front wall of thorax without penetration into thoracic cavity

⑦**S21.159**   Open bite of unspecified front wall of thorax without penetration into thoracic cavity

S21.2   Open wound of back wall of thorax without penetration into thoracic cavity

S21.20   Unspecified open wound of back wall of thorax without penetration into thoracic cavity

⑦**S21.201**   Unspecified open wound of right back wall of thorax without penetration into thoracic cavity

⑦**S21.202**   Unspecified open wound of left back wall of thorax without penetration into thoracic cavity

⑦**S21.209**   Unspecified open wound of unspecified back wall of thorax without penetration into thoracic cavity

S21.21   Laceration without foreign body of back wall of thorax without penetration into thoracic cavity

⑦**S21.211**   Laceration without foreign body of right back wall of thorax without penetration into thoracic cavity

⑦**S21.212**   Laceration without foreign body of left back wall of thorax without penetration into thoracic cavity

⑦**S21.219**   Laceration without foreign body of unspecified back wall of thorax without penetration into thoracic cavity

S21.22   Laceration with foreign body of back wall of thorax without penetration into thoracic cavity

⑦**S21.221**   Laceration with foreign body of right back wall of thorax without penetration into thoracic cavity

⑦**S21.222**   Laceration with foreign body of left back wall of thorax without penetration into thoracic cavity

⑦**S21.229**   Laceration with foreign body of unspecified back wall of thorax without penetration into thoracic cavity

S21.23   Puncture wound without foreign body of back wall of thorax without penetration into thoracic cavity

⑦**S21.231**   Puncture wound without foreign body of right back wall of thorax without penetration into thoracic cavity

⑦**S21.232**   Puncture wound without foreign body of left back wall of thorax without penetration into thoracic cavity

⑦**S21.239**   Puncture wound without foreign body of unspecified back wall of thorax without penetration into thoracic cavity

S21.24   Puncture wound with foreign body of back wall of thorax without penetration into thoracic cavity

⑦**S21.241**   Puncture wound with foreign body of right back wall of thorax without penetration into thoracic cavity

⑦**S21.242**   Puncture wound with foreign body of left back wall of thorax without penetration into thoracic cavity

⑦**S21.249**   Puncture wound with foreign body of unspecified back wall of thorax without penetration into thoracic cavity

S21.25   Open bite of back wall of thorax without penetration into thoracic cavity
Bite of back wall of thorax NOS
Excludes 1: superficial bite of back wall of thorax (S20.47)

⑦S21.251 Open bite of right back wall of thorax without penetration into thoracic cavity

⑦S21.252 Open bite of left back wall of thorax without penetration into thoracic cavity

⑦S21.259 Open bite of unspecified back wall of thorax without penetration into thoracic cavity

S21.3 Open wound of front wall of thorax with penetration into thoracic cavity
Open wound of chest with penetration into thoracic cavity

S21.30 Unspecified open wound of front wall of thorax with penetration into thoracic cavity

⑦S21.301 Unspecified open wound of right front wall of thorax with penetration into thoracic cavity

⑦S21.302 Unspecified open wound of left front wall of thorax with penetration into thoracic cavity

⑦S21.309 Unspecified open wound of unspecified front wall of thorax with penetration into thoracic cavity

S21.31 Laceration without foreign body of front wall of thorax with penetration into thoracic cavity

⑦S21.311 Laceration without foreign body of right front wall of thorax with penetration into thoracic cavity

⑦S21.312 Laceration without foreign body of left front wall of thorax with penetration into thoracic cavity

⑦S21.319 Laceration without foreign body of unspecified front wall of thorax with penetration into thoracic cavity

S21.32 Laceration with foreign body of front wall of thorax with penetration into thoracic cavity

⑦S21.321 Laceration with foreign body of right front wall of thorax with penetration into thoracic cavity

⑦S21.322 Laceration with foreign body of left front wall of thorax with penetration into thoracic cavity

⑦S21.329 Laceration with foreign body of unspecified front wall of thorax with penetration into thoracic cavity

S21.33 Puncture wound without foreign body of front wall of thorax with penetration into thoracic cavity

⑦S21.331 Puncture wound without foreign body of right front wall of thorax with penetration into thoracic cavity

⑦S21.332 Puncture wound without foreign body of left front wall of thorax with penetration into thoracic cavity

⑦S21.339 Puncture wound without foreign body of unspecified front wall of thorax with penetration into thoracic cavity

⑦S21.34 Puncture wound with foreign body of front wall of thorax with penetration into thoracic cavity

⑦S21.341 Puncture wound with foreign body of right front wall of thorax with penetration into thoracic cavity

⑦S21.342 Puncture wound with foreign body of left front wall of thorax with penetration into thoracic cavity

⑦S21.349 Puncture wound with foreign body of unspecified front wall of thorax with penetration into thoracic cavity

S21.35 Open bite of front wall of thorax with penetration into thoracic cavity
Excludes 1: superficial bite of front wall of thorax (S20.37)

⑦S21.351 Open bite of right front wall of thorax with penetration into thoracic cavity

⑦S21.352 Open bite of left front wall of thorax with penetration into thoracic cavity

⑦S21.359 Open bite of unspecified front wall of thorax with penetration into thoracic cavity

S21.4 Open wound of back wall of thorax with penetration into thoracic cavity

S21.40 Unspecified open wound of back wall of thorax with penetration into thoracic cavity

⑦S21.401 Unspecified open wound of right back wall of thorax with penetration into thoracic cavity

⑦S21.402 Unspecified open wound of left back wall of thorax with penetration into thoracic cavity

⑦S21.409 Unspecified open wound of unspecified back wall of thorax with penetration into thoracic cavity

S21.41 Laceration without foreign body of back wall of thorax with penetration into thoracic cavity

⑦S21.411 Laceration without foreign body of right back wall of thorax with penetration into thoracic cavity

⑦S21.412 Laceration without foreign body of left back wall of thorax with penetration into thoracic cavity

⑦S21.419 Laceration without foreign body of unspecified back wall of thorax with penetration into thoracic cavity

S21.42 Laceration with foreign body of back wall of thorax with penetration into thoracic cavity

⑦S21.421 Laceration with foreign body of right back wall of thorax with penetration into thoracic cavity

⑦S21.422 Laceration with foreign body of left back wall of thorax with penetration into thoracic cavity

⑦S21.429 Laceration with foreign body of unspecified back wall of thorax with penetration into thoracic cavity

S21.43 Puncture wound without foreign body of back wall of thorax with penetration into thoracic cavity

⑦**S21.431** Puncture wound without foreign body of right back wall of thorax with penetration into thoracic cavity

⑦**S21.432** Puncture wound without foreign body of left back wall of thorax with penetration into thoracic cavity

⑦**S21.439** Puncture wound without foreign body of unspecified back wall of thorax with penetration into thoracic cavity

⑦**S21.44** Puncture wound with foreign body of back wall of thorax with penetration into thoracic cavity

⑦**S21.441** Puncture wound with foreign body of right back wall of thorax with penetration into thoracic cavity

⑦**S21.442** Puncture wound with foreign body of left back wall of thorax with penetration into thoracic cavity

⑦**S21.449** Puncture wound with foreign body of unspecified back wall of thorax with penetration into thoracic cavity

S21.45 Open bite of back wall of thorax with penetration into thoracic cavity

Bite of back wall of thorax NOS

Excludes 1: superficial bite of back wall of thorax (S20.47)

⑦**S21.451** Open bite of right back wall of thorax with penetration into thoracic cavity

⑦**S21.452** Open bite of left back wall of thorax with penetration into thoracic cavity

⑦**S21.459** Open bite of unspecified back wall of thorax with penetration into thoracic cavity

S21.9 Open wound of unspecified part of thorax

Open wound of thoracic wall NOS

⊗⑦**S21.90** Unspecified open wound of unspecified part of thorax

⊗⑦**S21.91** Laceration without foreign body of unspecified part of thorax

⊗⑦**S21.92** Laceration with foreign body of unspecified part of thorax

⊗⑦**S21.93** Puncture wound without foreign body of unspecified part of thorax

⊗⑦**S21.94** Puncture wound with foreign body of unspecified part of thorax

⊗⑦**S21.95** Open bite of unspecified part of thorax

Excludes 1: superficial bite of thorax (S20.97)

S22 Fracture of rib(s), sternum and thoracic spine

Note: A fracture not indicated as displaced or nondisplaced should be coded to displaced

A fracture not indicated as open or closed should be coded to closed

Includes: fracture of thoracic neural arch

fracture of thoracic spinous process

fracture of thoracic transverse process

fracture of thoracic vertebra

fracture of thoracic vertebral arch

Code first any associated:

injury of intrathoracic organ (S27.-)

spinal cord injury (S24.0-, S24.1-)

Excludes 1: transection of thorax (S28.1)

Excludes 2: fracture of clavicle (S42.0-)

fracture of scapula (S42.1-)

The appropriate 7th character is to be added to each code from category S22

A - initial encounter for closed fracture

B - initial encounter for open fracture

D - subsequent encounter for fracture with routine healing

G - subsequent encounter for fracture with delayed healing

K - subsequent encounter for fracture with nonunion

S - sequela

S22.0 Fracture of thoracic vertebra

S22.00 Fracture of unspecified thoracic vertebra

⑦**S22.000** Wedge compression fracture of unspecified thoracic vertebra

⑦**S22.001** Stable burst fracture of unspecified thoracic vertebra

⑦**S22.002** Unstable burst fracture of unspecified thoracic vertebra

⑦**S22.008** Other fracture of unspecified thoracic vertebra

⑦**S22.009** Unspecified fracture of unspecified thoracic vertebra

S22.01 Fracture of first thoracic vertebra

⑦**S22.010** Wedge compression fracture of first thoracic vertebra

⑦**S22.011** Stable burst fracture of first thoracic vertebra

⑦**S22.012** Unstable burst fracture of first thoracic vertebra

⑦**S22.018** Other fracture of first thoracic vertebra

⑦**S22.019** Unspecified fracture of first thoracic vertebra

S22.02 Fracture of second thoracic vertebra

⑦**S22.020** Wedge compression fracture of second thoracic vertebra

⑦**S22.021** Stable burst fracture of second thoracic vertebra

⑦**S22.022** Unstable burst fracture of second thoracic vertebra

⑦**S22.028** Other fracture of second thoracic vertebra

⑦**S22.029** Unspecified fracture of second thoracic vertebra

S22.03 Fracture of third thoracic vertebra

⑦**S22.030** Wedge compression fracture of third thoracic vertebra

⑦**S22.031** Stable burst fracture of third thoracic vertebra

⑦**S22.032** Unstable burst fracture of third thoracic vertebra

⑦**S22.038** Other fracture of third thoracic vertebra

● New code   ▲ Revised code   ⑦ 7ᵗʰ digit required   ⊗ Placeholder required

⑦S22.039   Unspecified fracture of third thoracic vertebra

S22.04   Fracture of fourth thoracic vertebra

⑦S22.040   Wedge compression fracture of fourth thoracic vertebra

⑦S22.041   Stable burst fracture of fourth thoracic vertebra

⑦S22.042   Unstable burst fracture of fourth thoracic vertebra

⑦S22.048   Other fracture of fourth thoracic vertebra

⑦S22.049   Unspecified fracture of fourth thoracic vertebra

S22.05   Fracture of T5-T6 vertebra

⑦S22.050   Wedge compression fracture of T5-T6 vertebra

⑦S22.051   Stable burst fracture of T5-T6 vertebra

⑦S22.052   Unstable burst fracture of T5-T6 vertebra

⑦S22.058   Other fracture of T5-T6 vertebra

⑦S22.059   Unspecified fracture of T5-T6 vertebra

S22.06   Fracture of T7-T8 vertebra

⑦S22.060   Wedge compression fracture of T7-T8 vertebra

⑦S22.061   Stable burst fracture of T7-T8 vertebra

⑦S22.062   Unstable burst fracture of T7-T8 vertebra

⑦S22.068   Other fracture of T7-T8 thoracic vertebra

⑦S22.069   Unspecified fracture of T7-T8 vertebra

S22.07   Fracture of T9-T10 vertebra

⑦S22.070   Wedge compression fracture of T9-T10 vertebra

⑦S22.071   Stable burst fracture of T9-T10 vertebra

⑦S22.072   Unstable burst fracture of T9-T10 vertebra

⑦S22.078   Other fracture of T9-T10 vertebra

⑦S22.079   Unspecified fracture of T9-T10 vertebra

S22.08   Fracture of T11-T12 vertebra

⑦S22.080   Wedge compression fracture of T11-T12 vertebra

⑦S22.081   Stable burst fracture of T11-T12 vertebra

⑦S22.082   Unstable burst fracture of T11-T12 vertebra

⑦S22.088   Other fracture of T11-T12 vertebra

⑦S22.089   Unspecified fracture of T11-T12 vertebra

S22.2   Fracture of sternum

⊗⑦S22.20   Unspecified fracture of sternum

⊗⑦S22.21   Fracture of manubrium

⊗⑦S22.22   Fracture of body of sternum

⊗⑦S22.23   Sternal manubrial dissociation

⊗⑦S22.24   Fracture of xiphoid process

S22.3   Fracture of one rib

⊗⑦S22.31   Fracture of one rib, right side

⊗⑦S22.32   Fracture of one rib, left side

⊗⑦S22.39   Fracture of one rib, unspecified side

S22.4   Multiple fractures of ribs

Fractures of two or more ribs

Excludes 1: flail chest (S22.5-)

⊗⑦S22.41   Multiple fractures of ribs, right side

⊗⑦S22.42   Multiple fractures of ribs, left side

⊗⑦S22.43   Multiple fractures of ribs, bilateral

⊗⑦S22.49   Multiple fractures of ribs, unspecified side

⊗⑦S22.5   Flail chest

⊗⑦S22.9   Fracture of bony thorax, part unspecified

S23   Dislocation and sprain of joints and ligaments of thorax

Includes: avulsion of joint or ligament of thorax

laceration of cartilage, joint or ligament of thorax

sprain of cartilage, joint or ligament of thorax

traumatic hemarthrosis of joint or ligament of thorax

traumatic rupture of joint or ligament of thorax

traumatic subluxation of joint or ligament of thorax

traumatic tear of joint or ligament of thorax

Code also any associated open wound

Excludes 2: dislocation, sprain of sternoclavicular joint (S43.2, S43.6)

strain of muscle or tendon of thorax (S29.01-)

The appropriate 7th character is to be added to each code from category S23

A - initial encounter

D - subsequent encounter

S - sequela

⊗⑦S23.0   Traumatic rupture of thoracic intervertebral disc

Excludes 1: rupture or displacement (nontraumatic) of thoracic intervertebral disc NOS (M51.- with fifth character 4)

S23.1   Subluxation and dislocation of thoracic vertebra

Code also any associated

open wound of thorax (S21.-)

spinal cord injury (S24.0-, S24.1-)

Excludes 2: fracture of thoracic vertebrae (S22.0-)

S23.10   Subluxation and dislocation of unspecified thoracic vertebra

⑦S23.100   Subluxation of unspecified thoracic vertebra

⑦S23.101   Dislocation of unspecified thoracic vertebra

S23.11   Subluxation and dislocation of T1/T2 thoracic vertebra

⑦S23.110   Subluxation of T1/T2 thoracic vertebra

⑦S23.111   Dislocation of T1/T2 thoracic vertebra

S23.12   Subluxation and dislocation of T2/T3-T3/T4 thoracic vertebra

⑦S23.120   Subluxation of T2/T3 thoracic vertebra

⑦S23.121 Dislocation of T2/T3 thoracic vertebra

⑦S23.122 Subluxation of T3/T4 thoracic vertebra

⑦S23.123 Dislocation of T3/T4 thoracic vertebra

S23.13 Subluxation and dislocation of T4/T5-T5/T6 thoracic vertebra

⑦S23.130 Subluxation of T4/T5 thoracic vertebra

⑦S23.131 Dislocation of T4/T5 thoracic vertebra

⑦S23.132 Subluxation of T5/T6 thoracic vertebra

⑦S23.133 Dislocation of T5/T6 thoracic vertebra

S23.14 Subluxation and dislocation of T6/T7-T7/T8 thoracic vertebra

⑦S23.140 Subluxation of T6/T7 thoracic vertebra

⑦S23.141 Dislocation of T6/T7 thoracic vertebra

⑦S23.142 Subluxation of T7/T8 thoracic vertebra

⑦S23.143 Dislocation of T7/T8 thoracic vertebra

S23.15 Subluxation and dislocation of T8/T9-T9/T10 thoracic vertebra

⑦S23.150 Subluxation of T8/T9 thoracic vertebra

⑦S23.151 Dislocation of T8/T9 thoracic vertebra

⑦S23.152 Subluxation of T9/T10 thoracic vertebra

⑦S23.153 Dislocation of T9/T10 thoracic vertebra

S23.16 Subluxation and dislocation of T10/T11-T11/T12 thoracic vertebra

⑦S23.160 Subluxation of T10/T11 thoracic vertebra

⑦S23.161 Dislocation of T10/T11 thoracic vertebra

⑦S23.162 Subluxation of T11/T12 thoracic vertebra

⑦S23.163 Dislocation of T11/T12 thoracic vertebra

S23.17 Subluxation and dislocation of T12/L1 thoracic vertebra

⑦S23.170 Subluxation of T12/L1 thoracic vertebra

⑦S23.171 Dislocation of T12/L1 thoracic vertebra

S23.2 Dislocation of other and unspecified parts of thorax

⊗⑦S23.20 Dislocation of unspecified part of thorax

⊗⑦S23.29 Dislocation of other parts of thorax

⊗⑦S23.3 Sprain of ligaments of thoracic spine

S23.4 Sprain of ribs and sternum

⊗⑦S23.41 Sprain of ribs

S23.42 Sprain of sternum

⑦S23.420 Sprain of sternoclavicular (joint) (ligament)

⑦S23.421 Sprain of chondrosternal joint

⑦S23.428 Other sprain of sternum

⑦S23.429 Unspecified sprain of sternum

⊗⑦S23.8 Sprain of other specified parts of thorax

⊗⑦S23.9 Sprain of unspecified parts of thorax

S24 Injury of nerves and spinal cord at thorax level

Note: Code to highest level of thoracic spinal cord injury

Code also any associated:

fracture of thoracic vertebra (S22.0-)

open wound of thorax (S21.-)

transient paralysis (R29.5)

Excludes 2: injury of brachial plexus (S14.3)

The appropriate 7th character is to be added to each code from category S24

A - initial encounter

D - subsequent encounter

S - sequela

⊗⑦S24.0 Concussion and edema of thoracic spinal cord

S24.1 Other and unspecified injuries of thoracic spinal cord

S24.10 Unspecified injury of thoracic spinal cord

⑦S24.101 Unspecified injury at T1 level of thoracic spinal cord

⑦S24.102 Unspecified injury at T2-T6 level of thoracic spinal cord

⑦S24.103 Unspecified injury at T7-T10 level of thoracic spinal cord

⑦S24.104 Unspecified injury at T11-T12 level of thoracic spinal cord

⑦S24.109 Unspecified injury at unspecified level of thoracic spinal cord

Injury of thoracic spinal cord NOS

S24.11 Complete lesion of thoracic spinal cord

⑦S24.111 Complete lesion at T1 level of thoracic spinal cord

⑦S24.112 Complete lesion at T2-T6 level of thoracic spinal cord

⑦S24.113 Complete lesion at T7-T10 level of thoracic spinal cord

⑦S24.114 Complete lesion at T11-T12 level of thoracic spinal cord

⑦S24.119 Complete lesion at unspecified level of thoracic spinal cord

S24.13 Anterior cord syndrome of thoracic spinal cord

⑦S24.131 Anterior cord syndrome at T1 level of thoracic spinal cord

⑦S24.132 Anterior cord syndrome at T2-T6 level of thoracic spinal cord

⑦S24.133 Anterior cord syndrome at T7-T10 level of thoracic spinal cord

⑦S24.134 Anterior cord syndrome at T11-T12 level of thoracic spinal cord

⑦S24.139 Anterior cord syndrome at unspecified level of thoracic spinal cord

S24.14 Brown-Sequard syndrome of thoracic spinal cord

● New code   ▲ Revised code   ⑦ 7th digit required   ⊗ Placeholder required

⑦S24.141   Brown-Sequard syndrome at T1 level of thoracic spinal cord

⑦S24.142   Brown-Sequard syndrome at T2-T6 level of thoracic spinal cord

⑦S24.143   Brown-Sequard syndrome at T7-T10 level of thoracic spinal cord

⑦S24.144   Brown-Sequard syndrome at T11-T12 level of thoracic spinal cord

⑦S24.149   Brown-Sequard syndrome at unspecified level of thoracic spinal cord

S24.15   Other incomplete lesions of thoracic spinal cord
Incomplete lesion of thoracic spinal cord NOS
Posterior cord syndrome of thoracic spinal cord

⑦S24.151   Other incomplete lesion at T1 level of thoracic spinal cord

⑦S24.152   Other incomplete lesion at T2-T6 level of thoracic spinal cord

⑦S24.153   Other incomplete lesion at T7-T10 level of thoracic spinal cord

⑦S24.154   Other incomplete lesion at T11-T12 level of thoracic spinal cord

⑦S24.159   Other incomplete lesion at unspecified level of thoracic spinal cord

⊗⑦S24.2   Injury of nerve root of thoracic spine

⊗⑦S24.3   Injury of peripheral nerves of thorax

⊗⑦S24.4   Injury of thoracic sympathetic nervous system
Injury of cardiac plexus
Injury of esophageal plexus
Injury of pulmonary plexus
Injury of stellate ganglion
Injury of thoracic sympathetic ganglion

⊗⑦S24.8   Injury of other specified nerves of thorax

⊗⑦S24.9   Injury of unspecified nerve of thorax

S25   Injury of blood vessels of thorax
Code also any associated open wound (S21.-)
The appropriate 7th character is to be added to each code from category S25
A - initial encounter
D - subsequent encounter
S - sequela

S25.0   Injury of thoracic aorta
Injury of aorta NOS

⊗⑦S25.00   Unspecified injury of thoracic aorta

⊗⑦S25.01   Minor laceration of thoracic aorta
Incomplete transection of thoracic aorta
Laceration of thoracic aorta NOS
Superficial laceration of thoracic aorta

⊗⑦S25.02   Major laceration of thoracic aorta
Complete transection of thoracic aorta
Traumatic rupture of thoracic aorta

⊗⑦S25.09   Other specified injury of thoracic aorta

S25.1   Injury of innominate or subclavian artery

S25.10   Unspecified injury of innominate or subclavian artery

⑦S25.101   Unspecified injury of right innominate or subclavian artery

⑦S25.102   Unspecified injury of left innominate or subclavian artery

⑦S25.109   Unspecified injury of unspecified innominate or subclavian artery

S25.11   Minor laceration of innominate or subclavian artery
Incomplete transection of innominate or subclavian artery
Laceration of innominate or subclavian artery NOS
Superficial laceration of innominate or subclavian artery

⑦S25.111   Minor laceration of right innominate or subclavian artery

⑦S25.112   Minor laceration of left innominate or subclavian artery

⑦S25.119   Minor laceration of unspecified innominate or subclavian artery

S25.12   Major laceration of innominate or subclavian artery
Complete transection of innominate or subclavian artery
Traumatic rupture of innominate or subclavian artery

⑦S25.121   Major laceration of right innominate or subclavian artery

⑦S25.122   Major laceration of left innominate or subclavian artery

⑦S25.129   Major laceration of unspecified innominate or subclavian artery

S25.19   Other specified injury of innominate or subclavian artery

⑦S25.191   Other specified injury of right innominate or subclavian artery

⑦S25.192   Other specified injury of left innominate or subclavian artery

⑦S25.199   Other specified injury of unspecified innominate or subclavian artery

S25.2   Injury of superior vena cava
Injury of vena cava NOS

⊗⑦S25.20   Unspecified injury of superior vena cava

⊗⑦S25.21   Minor laceration of superior vena cava
Incomplete transection of superior vena cava
Laceration of superior vena cava NOS
Superficial laceration of superior vena cava

⊗⑦S25.22   Major laceration of superior vena cava
Complete transection of superior vena cava
Traumatic rupture of superior vena cava

⊗⑦S25.29   Other specified injury of superior vena cava

S25.3   Injury of innominate or subclavian vein

S25.30   Unspecified injury of innominate or subclavian vein

⑦S25.301   Unspecified injury of right innominate or subclavian vein

⑦S25.302   Unspecified injury of left innominate or subclavian vein

⑦S25.309   Unspecified injury of unspecified innominate or subclavian vein

S25.31   Minor laceration of innominate or subclavian vein

Incomplete transection of innominate or subclavian vein

Laceration of innominate or subclavian vein NOS

Superficial laceration of innominate or subclavian vein

⑦S25.311   Minor laceration of right innominate or subclavian vein

⑦S25.312   Minor laceration of left innominate or subclavian vein

⑦S25.319   Minor laceration of unspecified innominate or subclavian vein

S25.32   Major laceration of innominate or subclavian vein

Complete transection of innominate or subclavian vein

Traumatic rupture of innominate or subclavian vein

⑦S25.321   Major laceration of right innominate or subclavian vein

⑦S25.322   Major laceration of left innominate or subclavian vein

⑦S25.329   Major laceration of unspecified innominate or subclavian vein

S25.39   Other specified injury of innominate or subclavian vein

⑦S25.391   Other specified injury of right innominate or subclavian vein

⑦S25.392   Other specified injury of left innominate or subclavian vein

⑦S25.399   Other specified injury of unspecified innominate or subclavian vein

S25.4   Injury of pulmonary blood vessels

S25.40   Unspecified injury of pulmonary blood vessels

⑦S25.401   Unspecified injury of right pulmonary blood vessels

⑦S25.402   Unspecified injury of left pulmonary blood vessels

⑦S25.409   Unspecified injury of unspecified pulmonary blood vessels

S25.41   Minor laceration of pulmonary blood vessels

Incomplete transection of pulmonary blood vessels

Laceration of pulmonary blood vessels NOS

Superficial laceration of pulmonary blood vessels

⑦S25.411   Minor laceration of right pulmonary blood vessels

⑦S25.412   Minor laceration of left pulmonary blood vessels

⑦S25.419   Minor laceration of unspecified pulmonary blood vessels

S25.42   Major laceration of pulmonary blood vessels

Complete transection of pulmonary blood vessels

Traumatic rupture of pulmonary blood vessels

⑦S25.421   Major laceration of right pulmonary blood vessels

⑦S25.422   Major laceration of left pulmonary blood vessels

⑦S25.429   Major laceration of unspecified pulmonary blood vessels

S25.49   Other specified injury of pulmonary blood vessels

⑦S25.491   Other specified injury of right pulmonary blood vessels

⑦S25.492   Other specified injury of left pulmonary blood vessels

⑦S25.499   Other specified injury of unspecified pulmonary blood vessels

S25.5   Injury of intercostal blood vessels

S25.50   Unspecified injury of intercostal blood vessels

⑦S25.501   Unspecified injury of intercostal blood vessels, right side

⑦S25.502   Unspecified injury of intercostal blood vessels, left side

⑦S25.509   Unspecified injury of intercostal blood vessels, unspecified side

S25.51   Laceration of intercostal blood vessels

⑦S25.511   Laceration of intercostal blood vessels, right side

⑦S25.512   Laceration of intercostal blood vessels, left side

⑦S25.519   Laceration of intercostal blood vessels, unspecified side

S25.59   Other specified injury of intercostal blood vessels

⑦S25.591   Other specified injury of intercostal blood vessels, right side

⑦S25.592   Other specified injury of intercostal blood vessels, left side

⑦S25.599   Other specified injury of intercostal blood vessels, unspecified side

S25.8   Injury of other blood vessels of thorax

Injury of azygos vein

Injury of mammary artery or vein

S25.80   Unspecified injury of other blood vessels of thorax

⑦S25.801   Unspecified injury of other blood vessels of thorax, right side

⑦S25.802   Unspecified injury of other blood vessels of thorax, left side

⑦S25.809   Unspecified injury of other blood vessels of thorax, unspecified side

S25.81   Laceration of other blood vessels of thorax

⑦S25.811   Laceration of other blood vessels of thorax, right side

⑦S25.812   Laceration of other blood vessels of thorax, left side

⑦S25.819   Laceration of other blood vessels of thorax, unspecified side

S25.89   Other specified injury of other blood vessels of thorax

⑦S25.891   Other specified injury of other blood vessels of thorax, right side

⑦S25.892   Other specified injury of other blood vessels of thorax, left side

⑦S25.899   Other specified injury of other blood vessels of thorax, unspecified side

S25.9   Injury of unspecified blood vessel of thorax

    ⊗⑦ **S25.90**   Unspecified injury of unspecified blood vessel of thorax

    ⊗⑦ **S25.91**   Laceration of unspecified blood vessel of thorax

    ⊗⑦ **S25.99**   Other specified injury of unspecified blood vessel of thorax

S26 Injury of heart

Code also any associated:

       open wound of thorax (S21.-)

       traumatic hemopneumothorax (S27.2)

       traumatic hemothorax (S27.1)

       traumatic pneumothorax (S27.0)

The appropriate 7th character is to be added to each code from category S26

A - initial encounter

D - subsequent encounter

S - sequela

S26.0   Injury of heart with hemopericardium

    ⊗⑦ **S26.00**   Unspecified injury of heart with hemopericardium

    ⊗⑦ **S26.01**   Contusion of heart with hemopericardium

    S26.02   Laceration of heart with hemopericardium

        ⑦ **S26.020**   Mild laceration of heart with hemopericardium

             Laceration of heart without penetration of heart chamber

        ⑦ **S26.021**   Moderate laceration of heart with hemopericardium

             Laceration of heart with penetration of heart chamber

        ⑦ **S26.022**   Major laceration of heart with hemopericardium

             Laceration of heart with penetration of multiple heart chambers

    ⊗⑦ **S26.09**   Other injury of heart with hemopericardium

S26.1   Injury of heart without hemopericardium

    ⊗⑦ **S26.10**   Unspecified injury of heart without hemopericardium

    ⊗⑦ **S26.11**   Contusion of heart without hemopericardium

    ⊗⑦ **S26.12**   Laceration of heart without hemopericardium

    ⊗⑦ **S26.19**   Other injury of heart without hemopericardium

S26.9   Injury of heart, unspecified with or without hemopericardium

    ⊗⑦ **S26.90**   Unspecified injury of heart, unspecified with or without hemopericardium

    ⊗⑦ **S26.91**   Contusion of heart, unspecified with or without hemopericardium

    ⊗⑦ **S26.92**   Laceration of heart, unspecified with or without hemopericardium

             Laceration of heart NOS

    ⊗⑦ **S26.99**   Other injury of heart, unspecified with or without hemopericardium

S27 Injury of other and unspecified intrathoracic organs

Code also any associated open wound of thorax (S21.-)

Excludes 2: injury of cervical esophagus (S10-S19)

         injury of trachea (cervical) (S10-S19)

The appropriate 7th character is to be added to each code from category S27

A - initial encounter

D - subsequent encounter

S - sequela

  ⊗⑦ **S27.0**   Traumatic pneumothorax

         Excludes 1: spontaneous pneumothorax (J93.-)

  ⊗⑦ **S27.1**   Traumatic hemothorax

  ⊗⑦ **S27.2**   Traumatic hemopneumothorax

  S27.3   Other and unspecified injuries of lung

    S27.30   Unspecified injury of lung

        ⑦ **S27.301**   Unspecified injury of lung, unilateral

        ⑦ **S27.302**   Unspecified injury of lung, bilateral

        ⑦ **S27.309**   Unspecified injury of lung, unspecified

    S27.31   Primary blast injury of lung

         Blast injury of lung NOS

        ⑦ **S27.311**   Primary blast injury of lung, unilateral

        ⑦ **S27.312**   Primary blast injury of lung, bilateral

        ⑦ **S27.319**   Primary blast injury of lung, unspecified

    S27.32   Contusion of lung

        ⑦ **S27.321**   Contusion of lung, unilateral

        ⑦ **S27.322**   Contusion of lung, bilateral

        ⑦ **S27.329**   Contusion of lung, unspecified

    S27.33   Laceration of lung

        ⑦ **S27.331**   Laceration of lung, unilateral

        ⑦ **S27.332**   Laceration of lung, bilateral

        ⑦ **S27.339**   Laceration of lung, unspecified

    S27.39   Other injuries of lung

         Secondary blast injury of lung

        ⑦ **S27.391**   Other injuries of lung, unilateral

        ⑦ **S27.392**   Other injuries of lung, bilateral

        ⑦ **S27.399**   Other injuries of lung, unspecified

  S27.4   Injury of bronchus

    S27.40   Unspecified injury of bronchus

        ⑦ **S27.401**   Unspecified injury of bronchus, unilateral

        ⑦ **S27.402**   Unspecified injury of bronchus, bilateral

        ⑦ **S27.409**   Unspecified injury of bronchus, unspecified

    S27.41   Primary blast injury of bronchus

         Blast injury of bronchus NOS

        ⑦ **S27.411**   Primary blast injury of bronchus, unilateral

        ⑦ **S27.412**   Primary blast injury of bronchus, bilateral

        ⑦ **S27.419**   Primary blast injury of bronchus, unspecified

    S27.42   Contusion of bronchus

        ⑦ **S27.421**   Contusion of bronchus, unilateral

        ⑦ **S27.422**   Contusion of bronchus, bilateral

        ⑦ **S27.429**   Contusion of bronchus, unspecified

    S27.43   Laceration of bronchus

        ⑦ **S27.431**   Laceration of bronchus, unilateral

        ⑦ **S27.432**   Laceration of bronchus, bilateral

---

⑦**S27.439**   Laceration of bronchus, unspecified

S27.49   Other injury of bronchus
             Secondary blast injury of bronchus
⑦**S27.491**   Other injury of bronchus, unilateral
⑦**S27.492**   Other injury of bronchus, bilateral
⑦**S27.499**   Other injury of bronchus,
                  unspecified

S27.5   Injury of thoracic trachea
⊗⑦**S27.50**   Unspecified injury of thoracic trachea
⊗⑦**S27.51**   Primary blast injury of thoracic trachea
             Blast injury of thoracic trachea NOS
⊗⑦**S27.52**   Contusion of thoracic trachea
⊗⑦**S27.53**   Laceration of thoracic trachea
⊗⑦**S27.59**   Other injury of thoracic trachea
             Secondary blast injury of thoracic trachea

S27.6   Injury of pleura
⊗⑦**S27.60**   Unspecified injury of pleura
⊗⑦**S27.63**   Laceration of pleura
⊗⑦**S27.69**   Other injury of pleura

S27.8   Injury of other specified intrathoracic organs
    S27.80   Injury of diaphragm
⑦**S27.802**   Contusion of diaphragm
⑦**S27.803**   Laceration of diaphragm
⑦**S27.808**   Other injury of diaphragm
⑦**S27.809**   Unspecified injury of diaphragm
    S27.81   Injury of esophagus (thoracic part)
⑦**S27.812**   Contusion of esophagus (thoracic
                  part)
⑦**S27.813**   Laceration of esophagus (thoracic
                  part)
⑦**S27.818**   Other injury of esophagus (thoracic
                  part)
⑦**S27.819**   Unspecified injury of esophagus
                  (thoracic part)
    S27.89   Injury of other specified intrathoracic organs
             Injury of lymphatic thoracic duct
             Injury of thymus gland
⑦**S27.892**   Contusion of other specified
                  intrathoracic organs
⑦**S27.893**   Laceration of other specified
                  intrathoracic organs
⑦**S27.898**   Other injury of other specified
                  intrathoracic organs
⑦**S27.899**   Unspecified injury of other specified
                  intrathoracic organs

S27.9   Injury of unspecified intrathoracic organ
S28 Crushing injury of thorax, and traumatic amputation of part of
       thorax
       The appropriate 7th character is to be added to each code from
       category S28
       A - initial encounter
       D - subsequent encounter
       S - sequela
⊗⑦**S28.0**   Crushed chest
             Use additional code for all associated injuries
             Excludes 1: flail chest (S22.5)

⊗⑦**S28.1**   Traumatic amputation (partial) of part of thorax, except
             breast
S28.2   Traumatic amputation of breast
    S28.21   Complete traumatic amputation of breast
             Traumatic amputation of breast NOS
⑦**S28.211**   Complete traumatic amputation of
                  right breast
⑦**S28.212**   Complete traumatic amputation of
                  left breast
⑦**S28.219**   Complete traumatic amputation of
                  unspecified breast
    S28.22   Partial traumatic amputation of breast
⑦**S28.221**   Partial traumatic amputation of right
                  breast
⑦**S28.222**   Partial traumatic amputation of left
                  breast
⑦**S28.229**   Partial traumatic amputation of
                  unspecified breast
S29 Other and unspecified injuries of thorax
       Code also any associated open wound (S21.-)
       The appropriate 7th character is to be added to each code from
       category S29
       A - initial encounter
       D - subsequent encounter
       S - sequela
S29.0   Injury of muscle and tendon at thorax level
    S29.00   Unspecified injury of muscle and tendon of
             thorax
⑦**S29.001**   Unspecified injury of muscle and
                  tendon of front wall of thorax
⑦**S29.002**   Unspecified injury of muscle and
                  tendon of back wall of thorax
⑦**S29.009**   Unspecified injury of muscle and
                  tendon of unspecified wall of thorax
    S29.01   Strain of muscle and tendon of thorax
⑦**S29.011**   Strain of muscle and tendon of front
                  wall of thorax
⑦**S29.012**   Strain of muscle and tendon of back
                  wall of thorax
⑦**S29.019**   Strain of muscle and tendon of
                  unspecified wall of thorax
    S29.02   Laceration of muscle and tendon of thorax
⑦**S29.021**   Laceration of muscle and tendon of
                  front wall of thorax
⑦**S29.022**   Laceration of muscle and tendon of
                  back wall of thorax
⑦**S29.029**   Laceration of muscle and tendon of
                  unspecified wall of thorax
    S29.09   Other injury of muscle and tendon of thorax
⑦**S29.091**   Other injury of muscle and tendon
                  of front wall of thorax
⑦**S29.092**   Other injury of muscle and tendon
                  of back wall of thorax
⑦**S29.099**   Other injury of muscle and tendon
                  of unspecified wall of thorax
⊗⑦**S29.8**   Other specified injuries of thorax
⊗⑦**S29.9**   Unspecified injury of thorax

INJURIES TO THE ABDOMEN, LOWER BACK, LUMBAR SPINE, PELVIS AND EXTERNAL GENITALS (S30-S39)

Includes: injuries to the abdominal wall
    injuries to the anus
    injuries to the buttock
    injuries to the external genitalia
    injuries to the flank
    injuries to the groin

Excludes 2: burns and corrosions (T20-T32)
    effects of foreign body in anus and rectum (T18.5)
    effects of foreign body in genitourinary tract (T19.-)
    effects of foreign body in stomach, small intestine and colon (T18.2-T18.4)
    frostbite (T33-T34)
    insect bite or sting, venomous (T63.4)

S30   Superficial injury of abdomen, lower back, pelvis and external genitals

    Excludes 2: superficial injury of hip (S70.-)

    The appropriate 7th character is to be added to each code from category S30
    A - initial encounter
    D - subsequent encounter
    S - sequela

⊗⑦ **S30.0**   Contusion of lower back and pelvis
    Contusion of buttock

⊗⑦ **S30.1**   Contusion of abdominal wall
    Contusion of flank
    Contusion of groin

S30.2   Contusion of external genital organs

    S30.20   Contusion of unspecified external genital organ

        ⑦ **S30.201**   Contusion of unspecified external genital organ, male

        ⑦ **S30.202**   Contusion of unspecified external genital organ, female

    ⊗⑦ **S30.21**   Contusion of penis

    ⊗⑦ **S30.22**   Contusion of scrotum and testes

    ⊗⑦ **S30.23**   Contusion of vagina and vulva

⊗⑦ **S30.3**   Contusion of anus

S30.8   Other superficial injuries of abdomen, lower back, pelvis and external genitals

    S30.81   Abrasion of abdomen, lower back, pelvis and external genitals

        ⑦ **S30.810**   Abrasion of lower back and pelvis

        ⑦ **S30.811**   Abrasion of abdominal wall

        ⑦ **S30.812**   Abrasion of penis

        ⑦ **S30.813**   Abrasion of scrotum and testes

        ⑦ **S30.814**   Abrasion of vagina and vulva

        ⑦ **S30.815**   Abrasion of unspecified external genital organs, male

        ⑦ **S30.816**   Abrasion of unspecified external genital organs, female

        ⑦ **S30.817**   Abrasion of anus

    S30.82   Blister (nonthermal) of abdomen, lower back, pelvis and external genitals

        ⑦ **S30.820**   Blister (nonthermal) of lower back and pelvis

        ⑦ **S30.821**   Blister (nonthermal) of abdominal wall

        ⑦ **S30.822**   Blister (nonthermal) of penis

        ⑦ **S30.823**   Blister (nonthermal) of scrotum and testes

        ⑦ **S30.824**   Blister (nonthermal) of vagina and vulva

        ⑦ **S30.825**   Blister (nonthermal) of unspecified external genital organs, male

        ⑦ **S30.826**   Blister (nonthermal) of unspecified external genital organs, female

        ⑦ **S30.827**   Blister (nonthermal) of anus

    S30.84   External constriction of abdomen, lower back, pelvis and external genitals

        ⑦ **S30.840**   External constriction of lower back and pelvis

        ⑦ **S30.841**   External constriction of abdominal wall

        ⑦ **S30.842**   External constriction of penis
            Hair tourniquet syndrome of penis
            Use additional cause code to identify the constricting item (W49.0-)

        ⑦ **S30.843**   External constriction of scrotum and testes

        ⑦ **S30.844**   External constriction of vagina and vulva

        ⑦ **S30.845**   External constriction of unspecified external genital organs, male

        ⑦ **S30.846**   External constriction of unspecified external genital organs, female

    S30.85   Superficial foreign body of abdomen, lower back, pelvis and external genitals
        Splinter in the abdomen, lower back, pelvis and external genitals

        ⑦ **S30.850**   Superficial foreign body of lower back and pelvis

        ⑦ **S30.851**   Superficial foreign body of abdominal wall

        ⑦ **S30.852**   Superficial foreign body of penis

        ⑦ **S30.853**   Superficial foreign body of scrotum and testes

        ⑦ **S30.854**   Superficial foreign body of vagina and vulva

        ⑦ **S30.855**   Superficial foreign body of unspecified external genital organs, male

        ⑦ **S30.856**   Superficial foreign body of unspecified external genital organs, female

        ⑦ **S30.857**   Superficial foreign body of anus

    S30.86   Insect bite (nonvenomous) of abdomen, lower back, pelvis and external genitals

        ⑦ **S30.860**   Insect bite (nonvenomous) of lower back and pelvis

        ⑦ **S30.861**   Insect bite (nonvenomous) of abdominal wall

        ⑦ **S30.862**   Insect bite (nonvenomous) of penis

        ⑦ **S30.863**   Insect bite (nonvenomous) of scrotum and testes

---

⑦**S30.864** Insect bite (nonvenomous) of vagina and vulva

⑦**S30.865** Insect bite (nonvenomous) of unspecified external genital organs, male

⑦**S30.866** Insect bite (nonvenomous) of unspecified external genital organs, female

⑦**S30.867** Insect bite (nonvenomous) of anus

S30.87 Other superficial bite of abdomen, lower back, pelvis and external genitals

> **Excludes 1:** open bite of abdomen, lower back, pelvis and external genitals (S31.05, S31.15, S31.25, S31.35, S31.45, S31.55)

⑦**S30.870** Other superficial bite of lower back and pelvis

⑦**S30.871** Other superficial bite of abdominal wall

⑦**S30.872** Other superficial bite of penis

⑦**S30.873** Other superficial bite of scrotum and testes

⑦**S30.874** Other superficial bite of vagina and vulva

⑦**S30.875** Other superficial bite of unspecified external genital organs, male

⑦**S30.876** Other superficial bite of unspecified external genital organs, female

⑦**S30.877** Other superficial bite of anus

S30.9 Unspecified superficial injury of abdomen, lower back, pelvis and external genitals

⊗⑦**S30.91** Unspecified superficial injury of lower back and pelvis

⊗⑦**S30.92** Unspecified superficial injury of abdominal wall

⊗⑦**S30.93** Unspecified superficial injury of penis

⊗⑦**S30.94** Unspecified superficial injury of scrotum and testes

⊗⑦**S30.95** Unspecified superficial injury of vagina and vulva

⊗⑦**S30.96** Unspecified superficial injury of unspecified external genital organs, male

⊗⑦**S30.97** Unspecified superficial injury of unspecified external genital organs, female

⊗⑦**S30.98** Unspecified superficial injury of anus

S31 Open wound of abdomen, lower back, pelvis and external genitals

Code also any associated:
> spinal cord injury (S24.0, S24.1-, S34.0-, S34.1-)
> wound infection

> **Excludes 1:** traumatic amputation of part of abdomen, lower back and pelvis (S38.2-, S38.3)

> **Excludes 2:** open wound of hip (S71.00-S71.02)
> open fracture of pelvis (S32.1--S32.9 with 7th character B)

The appropriate 7th character is to be added to each code from category S31

A - initial encounter
D - subsequent encounter
S - sequela

S31.0 Open wound of lower back and pelvis

S31.00 Unspecified open wound of lower back and pelvis

⑦**S31.000** Unspecified open wound of lower back and pelvis without penetration into retroperitoneum
Unspecified open wound of lower back and pelvis NOS

⑦**S31.001** Unspecified open wound of lower back and pelvis with penetration into retroperitoneum

S31.01 Laceration without foreign body of lower back and pelvis

⑦**S31.010** Laceration without foreign body of lower back and pelvis without penetration into retroperitoneum
Laceration without foreign body of lower back and pelvis NOS

⑦**S31.011** Laceration without foreign body of lower back and pelvis with penetration into retroperitoneum

S31.02 Laceration with foreign body of lower back and pelvis

⑦**S31.020** Laceration with foreign body of lower back and pelvis without penetration into retroperitoneum
Laceration with foreign body of lower back and pelvis NOS

⑦**S31.021** Laceration with foreign body of lower back and pelvis with penetration into retroperitoneum

S31.03 Puncture wound without foreign body of lower back and pelvis

⑦**S31.030** Puncture wound without foreign body of lower back and pelvis without penetration into retroperitoneum
Puncture wound without foreign body of lower back and pelvis NOS

⑦**S31.031** Puncture wound without foreign body of lower back and pelvis with penetration into retroperitoneum

S31.04 Puncture wound with foreign body of lower back and pelvis

⑦**S31.040** Puncture wound with foreign body of lower back and pelvis without penetration into retroperitoneum
Puncture wound with foreign body of lower back and pelvis NOS

⑦**S31.041** Puncture wound with foreign body of lower back and pelvis with penetration into retroperitoneum

S31.05 Open bite of lower back and pelvis
Bite of lower back and pelvis NOS

> **Excludes 1:** superficial bite of lower back and pelvis (S30.860, S30.870)

⑦**S31.050** Open bite of lower back and pelvis without penetration into retroperitoneum
Open bite of lower back and pelvis NOS

● New code   ▲ Revised code   ⑦ 7ᵗʰ digit required   ⊗ Placeholder required

⑦S31.051   Open bite of lower back and pelvis with penetration into retroperitoneum

S31.1   Open wound of abdominal wall without penetration into peritoneal cavity

Open wound of abdominal wall NOS

Excludes 2: open wound of abdominal wall with penetration into peritoncal cavity (S31.6-)

    S31.10   Unspecified open wound of abdominal wall without penetration into peritoneal cavity

⑦S31.100   Unspecified open wound of abdominal wall, right upper quadrant without penetration into peritoneal cavity

⑦S31.101   Unspecified open wound of abdominal wall, left upper quadrant without penetration into peritoneal cavity

⑦S31.102   Unspecified open wound of abdominal wall, epigastric region without penetration into peritoneal cavity

⑦S31.103   Unspecified open wound of abdominal wall, right lower quadrant without penetration into peritoneal cavity

⑦S31.104   Unspecified open wound of abdominal wall, left lower quadrant without penetration into peritoneal cavity

⑦S31.105   Unspecified open wound of abdominal wall, periumbilic region without penetration into peritoneal cavity

⑦S31.109   Unspecified open wound of abdominal wall, unspecified quadrant without penetration into peritoneal cavity

Unspecified open wound of abdominal wall NOS

    S31.11   Laceration without foreign body of abdominal wall without penetration into peritoneal cavity

⑦S31.110   Laceration without foreign body of abdominal wall, right upper quadrant without penetration into peritoneal cavity

⑦S31.111   Laceration without foreign body of abdominal wall, left upper quadrant without penetration into peritoneal cavity

⑦S31.112   Laceration without foreign body of abdominal wall, epigastric region without penetration into peritoneal cavity

⑦S31.113   Laceration without foreign body of abdominal wall, right lower quadrant without penetration into peritoneal cavity

⑦S31.114   Laceration without foreign body of abdominal wall, left lower quadrant

without penetration into peritoneal cavity

⑦S31.115   Laceration without foreign body of abdominal wall, periumbilic region without penetration into peritoneal cavity

⑦S31.119   Laceration without foreign body of abdominal wall, unspecified quadrant without penetration into peritoneal cavity

    S31.12   Laceration with foreign body of abdominal wall without penetration into peritoneal cavity

⑦S31.120   Laceration of abdominal wall with foreign body, right upper quadrant without penetration into peritoneal cavity

⑦S31.121   Laceration of abdominal wall with foreign body, left upper quadrant without penetration into peritoneal cavity

⑦S31.122   Laceration of abdominal wall with foreign body, epigastric region without penetration into peritoneal cavity

⑦S31.123   Laceration of abdominal wall with foreign body, right lower quadrant without penetration into peritoneal cavity

⑦S31.124   Laceration of abdominal wall with foreign body, left lower quadrant without penetration into peritoneal cavity

⑦S31.125   Laceration of abdominal wall with foreign body, periumbilic region without penetration into peritoneal cavity

⑦S31.129   Laceration of abdominal wall with foreign body, unspecified quadrant without penetration into peritoneal cavity

    S31.13   Puncture wound of abdominal wall without foreign body without penetration into peritoneal cavity

⑦S31.130   Puncture wound of abdominal wall without foreign body, right upper quadrant without penetration into peritoneal cavity

⑦S31.131   Puncture wound of abdominal wall without foreign body, left upper quadrant without penetration into peritoneal cavity

⑦S31.132   Puncture wound of abdominal wall without foreign body, epigastric region without penetration into peritoneal cavity

⑦S31.133   Puncture wound of abdominal wall without foreign body, right lower quadrant without penetration into peritoneal cavity

⑦S31.134   Puncture wound of abdominal wall without foreign body, left lower quadrant without penetration into peritoneal cavity

⑦S31.135   Puncture wound of abdominal wall without foreign body, periumbilic region without penetration into peritoneal cavity

⑦S31.139   Puncture wound of abdominal wall without foreign body, unspecified quadrant without penetration into peritoneal cavity

S31.14   Puncture wound of abdominal wall with foreign body without penetration into peritoneal cavity

⑦S31.140   Puncture wound of abdominal wall with foreign body, right upper quadrant without penetration into peritoneal cavity

⑦S31.141   Puncture wound of abdominal wall with foreign body, left upper quadrant without penetration into peritoneal cavity

⑦S31.142   Puncture wound of abdominal wall with foreign body, epigastric region without penetration into peritoneal cavity

⑦S31.143   Puncture wound of abdominal wall with foreign body, right lower quadrant without penetration into peritoneal cavity

⑦S31.144   Puncture wound of abdominal wall with foreign body, left lower quadrant without penetration into peritoneal cavity

⑦S31.145   Puncture wound of abdominal wall with foreign body, periumbilic region without penetration into peritoneal cavity

⑦S31.149   Puncture wound of abdominal wall with foreign body, unspecified quadrant without penetration into peritoneal cavity

S31.15   Open bite of abdominal wall without penetration into peritoneal cavity

Bite of abdominal wall NOS

Excludes 1: superficial bite of abdominal wall (S30.871)

⑦S31.150   Open bite of abdominal wall, right upper quadrant without penetration into peritoneal cavity

⑦S31.151   Open bite of abdominal wall, left upper quadrant without penetration into peritoneal cavity

⑦S31.152   Open bite of abdominal wall, epigastric region without penetration into peritoneal cavity

⑦S31.153   Open bite of abdominal wall, right lower quadrant without penetration into peritoneal cavity

⑦S31.154   Open bite of abdominal wall, left lower quadrant without penetration into peritoneal cavity

⑦S31.155   Open bite of abdominal wall, periumbilic region without penetration into peritoneal cavity

⑦S31.159   Open bite of abdominal wall, unspecified quadrant without penetration into peritoneal cavity

S31.2   Open wound of penis

⊗⑦S31.20   Unspecified open wound of penis

⊗⑦S31.21   Laceration without foreign body of penis

⊗⑦S31.22   Laceration with foreign body of penis

⊗⑦S31.23   Puncture wound without foreign body of penis

⊗⑦S31.24   Puncture wound with foreign body of penis

⊗⑦S31.25   Open bite of penis

Bite of penis NOS

Excludes 1: superficial bite of penis (S30.862, S30.872)

S31.3   Open wound of scrotum and testes

⊗⑦S31.30   Unspecified open wound of scrotum and testes

⊗⑦S31.31   Laceration without foreign body of scrotum and testes

⊗⑦S31.32   Laceration with foreign body of scrotum and testes

⊗⑦S31.33   Puncture wound without foreign body of scrotum and testes

⊗⑦S31.34   Puncture wound with foreign body of scrotum and testes

⊗⑦S31.35   Open bite of scrotum and testes

Bite of scrotum and testes NOS

Excludes 1: superficial bite of scrotum and testes (S30.863, S30.873)

S31.4   Open wound of vagina and vulva

Excludes 1: injury to vagina and vulva during delivery (O70.-, O71.4)

⊗⑦S31.40   Unspecified open wound of vagina and vulva

⊗⑦S31.41   Laceration without foreign body of vagina and vulva

⊗⑦S31.42   Laceration with foreign body of vagina and vulva

⊗⑦S31.43   Puncture wound without foreign body of vagina and vulva

⊗⑦S31.44   Puncture wound with foreign body of vagina and vulva

⊗⑦S31.45   Open bite of vagina and vulva

Bite of vagina and vulva NOS

Excludes 1: superficial bite of vagina and vulva (S30.864, S30.874)

S31.5   Open wound of unspecified external genital organs

Excludes 1: traumatic amputation of external genital organs (S38.21, S38.22)

S31.50   Unspecified open wound of unspecified external genital organs

⑦S31.501   Unspecified open wound of unspecified external genital organs, male

⑦S31.502   Unspecified open wound of unspecified external genital organs, female

S31.51   Laceration without foreign body of unspecified external genital organs

⑦S31.511 Laceration without foreign body of unspecified external genital organs, male

⑦S31.512 Laceration without foreign body of unspecified external genital organs, female

S31.52 Laceration with foreign body of unspecified external genital organs

⑦S31.521 Laceration with foreign body of unspecified external genital organs, male

⑦S31.522 Laceration with foreign body of unspecified external genital organs, female

S31.53 Puncture wound without foreign body of unspecified external genital organs

⑦S31.531 Puncture wound without foreign body of unspecified external genital organs, male

⑦S31.532 Puncture wound without foreign body of unspecified external genital organs, female

S31.54 Puncture wound with foreign body of unspecified external genital organs

⑦S31.541 Puncture wound with foreign body of unspecified external genital organs, male

⑦S31.542 Puncture wound with foreign body of unspecified external genital organs, female

S31.55 Open bite of unspecified external genital organs
Bite of unspecified external genital organs NOS
Excludes 1: superficial bite of unspecified external genital organs (S30.865, S30.866, S30.875, S30.876)

⑦S31.551 Open bite of unspecified external genital organs, male

⑦S31.552 Open bite of unspecified external genital organs, female

S31.6 Open wound of abdominal wall with penetration into peritoneal cavity

S31.60 Unspecified open wound of abdominal wall with penetration into peritoneal cavity

⑦S31.600 Unspecified open wound of abdominal wall, right upper quadrant with penetration into peritoneal cavity

⑦S31.601 Unspecified open wound of abdominal wall, left upper quadrant with penetration into peritoneal cavity

⑦S31.602 Unspecified open wound of abdominal wall, epigastric region with penetration into peritoneal cavity

⑦S31.603 Unspecified open wound of abdominal wall, right lower quadrant with penetration into peritoneal cavity

⑦S31.604 Unspecified open wound of abdominal wall, left lower quadrant

with penetration into peritoneal cavity

⑦S31.605 Unspecified open wound of abdominal wall, periumbilic region with penetration into peritoneal cavity

⑦S31.609 Unspecified open wound of abdominal wall, unspecified quadrant with penetration into peritoneal cavity

S31.61 Laceration without foreign body of abdominal wall with penetration into peritoneal cavity

⑦S31.610 Laceration without foreign body of abdominal wall, right upper quadrant with penetration into peritoneal cavity

⑦S31.611 Laceration without foreign body of abdominal wall, left upper quadrant with penetration into peritoneal cavity

⑦S31.612 Laceration without foreign body of abdominal wall, epigastric region with penetration into peritoneal cavity

⑦S31.613 Laceration without foreign body of abdominal wall, right lower quadrant with penetration into peritoneal cavity

⑦S31.614 Laceration without foreign body of abdominal wall, left lower quadrant with penetration into peritoneal cavity

⑦S31.615 Laceration without foreign body of abdominal wall, periumbilic region with penetration into peritoneal cavity

⑦S31.619 Laceration without foreign body of abdominal wall, unspecified quadrant with penetration into peritoneal cavity

S31.62 Laceration with foreign body of abdominal wall with penetration into peritoneal cavity

⑦S31.620 Laceration with foreign body of abdominal wall, right upper quadrant with penetration into peritoneal cavity

⑦S31.621 Laceration with foreign body of abdominal wall, left upper quadrant with penetration into peritoneal cavity

⑦S31.622 Laceration with foreign body of abdominal wall, epigastric region with penetration into peritoneal cavity

⑦S31.623 Laceration with foreign body of abdominal wall, right lower quadrant with penetration into peritoneal cavity

⑦S31.624 Laceration with foreign body of abdominal wall, left lower quadrant with penetration into peritoneal cavity

⑦**S31.625**   Laceration with foreign body of abdominal wall, periumbilic region with penetration into peritoneal cavity

⑦**S31.629**   Laceration with foreign body of abdominal wall, unspecified quadrant with penetration into peritoneal cavity

S31.63   Puncture wound without foreign body of abdominal wall with penetration into peritoneal cavity

⑦**S31.630**   Puncture wound without foreign body of abdominal wall, right upper quadrant with penetration into peritoneal cavity

⑦**S31.631**   Puncture wound without foreign body of abdominal wall, left upper quadrant with penetration into peritoneal cavity

⑦**S31.632**   Puncture wound without foreign body of abdominal wall, epigastric region with penetration into peritoneal cavity

⑦**S31.633**   Puncture wound without foreign body of abdominal wall, right lower quadrant with penetration into peritoneal cavity

⑦**S31.634**   Puncture wound without foreign body of abdominal wall, left lower quadrant with penetration into peritoneal cavity

⑦**S31.635**   Puncture wound without foreign body of abdominal wall, periumbilic region with penetration into peritoneal cavity

⑦**S31.639**   Puncture wound without foreign body of abdominal wall, unspecified quadrant with penetration into peritoneal cavity

⑦**S31.64**   Puncture wound with foreign body of abdominal wall with penetration into peritoneal cavity

⑦**S31.640**   Puncture wound with foreign body of abdominal wall, right upper quadrant with penetration into peritoneal cavity

⑦**S31.641**   Puncture wound with foreign body of abdominal wall, left upper quadrant with penetration into peritoneal cavity

⑦**S31.642**   Puncture wound with foreign body of abdominal wall, epigastric region with penetration into peritoneal cavity

⑦**S31.643**   Puncture wound with foreign body of abdominal wall, right lower quadrant with penetration into peritoneal cavity

⑦**S31.644**   Puncture wound with foreign body of abdominal wall, left lower quadrant with penetration into peritoneal cavity

⑦**S31.645**   Puncture wound with foreign body of abdominal wall, periumbilic region with penetration into peritoneal cavity

⑦**S31.649**   Puncture wound with foreign body of abdominal wall, unspecified quadrant with penetration into peritoneal cavity

S31.65   Open bite of abdominal wall with penetration into peritoneal cavity

Excludes 1: superficial bite of abdominal wall (S30.861, S30.871)

⑦**S31.650**   Open bite of abdominal wall, right upper quadrant with penetration into peritoneal cavity

⑦**S31.651**   Open bite of abdominal wall, left upper quadrant with penetration into peritoneal cavity

⑦**S31.652**   Open bite of abdominal wall, epigastric region with penetration into peritoneal cavity

⑦**S31.653**   Open bite of abdominal wall, right lower quadrant with penetration into peritoneal cavity

⑦**S31.654**   Open bite of abdominal wall, left lower quadrant with penetration into peritoneal cavity

⑦**S31.655**   Open bite of abdominal wall, periumbilic region with penetration into peritoneal cavity

⑦**S31.659**   Open bite of abdominal wall, unspecified quadrant with penetration into peritoneal cavity

S31.8   Open wound of other parts of abdomen, lower back and pelvis

S31.80   Open wound of unspecified buttock

⑦**S31.801**   Laceration without foreign body of unspecified buttock

⑦**S31.802**   Laceration with foreign body of unspecified buttock

⑦**S31.803**   Puncture wound without foreign body of unspecified buttock

⑦**S31.804**   Puncture wound with foreign body of unspecified buttock

⑦**S31.805**   Open bite of unspecified buttock

Bite of buttock NOS

Excludes 1: superficial bite of buttock (S30.870)

⑦**S31.809**   Unspecified open wound of unspecified buttock

S31.81   Open wound of right buttock

⑦**S31.811**   Laceration without foreign body of right buttock

⑦**S31.812**   Laceration with foreign body of right buttock

⑦**S31.813**   Puncture wound without foreign body of right buttock

⑦**S31.814**   Puncture wound with foreign body of right buttock

⑦**S31.815**   Open bite of right buttock

Bite of right buttock NOS

Excludes 1: superficial bite of buttock (S30.870)

⑦S31.819 Unspecified open wound of right buttock

S31.82 Open wound of left buttock

⑦S31.821 Laceration without foreign body of left buttock

⑦S31.822 Laceration with foreign body of left buttock

⑦S31.823 Puncture wound without foreign body of left buttock

⑦S31.824 Puncture wound with foreign body of left buttock

⑦S31.825 Open bite of left buttock

Bite of left buttock NOS

Excludes 1: superficial bite of buttock (S30.870)

⑦S31.829 Unspecified open wound of left buttock

S31.83 Open wound of anus

⑦S31.831 Laceration without foreign body of anus

⑦S31.832 Laceration with foreign body of anus

⑦S31.833 Puncture wound without foreign body of anus

⑦S31.834 Puncture wound with foreign body of anus

⑦S31.835 Open bite of anus

Bite of anus NOS

Excludes 1: superficial bite of anus (S30.877)

⑦S31.839 Unspecified open wound of anus

S32 Fracture of lumbar spine and pelvis

Note: A fracture not indicated as displaced or nondisplaced should be coded to displaced

A fracture not indicated as opened or closed should be coded to closed

Includes: fracture of lumbosacral neural arch

fracture of lumbosacral spinous process

fracture of lumbosacral transverse process

fracture of lumbosacral vertebra

fracture of lumbosacral vertebral arch

Code first any associated spinal cord and spinal nerve injury (S34-)

Excludes 1: transection of abdomen (S38.3)

Excludes 2: fracture of hip NOS (S72.0-)

The appropriate 7th character is to be added to each code from category S32

A - initial encounter for closed fracture

B - initial encounter for open fracture

D - subsequent encounter for fracture with routine healing

G - subsequent encounter for fracture with delayed healing

K - subsequent encounter for fracture with nonunion

S - sequela

S32.0 Fracture of lumbar vertebra

Fracture of lumbar spine NOS

S32.00 Fracture of unspecified lumbar vertebra

⑦S32.000 Wedge compression fracture of unspecified lumbar vertebra

⑦S32.001 Stable burst fracture of unspecified lumbar vertebra

⑦S32.002 Unstable burst fracture of unspecified lumbar vertebra

⑦S32.008 Other fracture of unspecified lumbar vertebra

⑦S32.009 Unspecified fracture of unspecified lumbar vertebra

S32.01 Fracture of first lumbar vertebra

⑦S32.010 Wedge compression fracture of first lumbar vertebra

⑦S32.011 Stable burst fracture of first lumbar vertebra

⑦S32.012 Unstable burst fracture of first lumbar vertebra

⑦S32.018 Other fracture of first lumbar vertebra

⑦S32.019 Unspecified fracture of first lumbar vertebra

S32.02 Fracture of second lumbar vertebra

⑦S32.020 Wedge compression fracture of second lumbar vertebra

⑦S32.021 Stable burst fracture of second lumbar vertebra

⑦S32.022 Unstable burst fracture of second lumbar vertebra

⑦S32.028 Other fracture of second lumbar vertebra

⑦S32.029 Unspecified fracture of second lumbar vertebra

S32.03 Fracture of third lumbar vertebra

⑦S32.030 Wedge compression fracture of third lumbar vertebra

⑦S32.031 Stable burst fracture of third lumbar vertebra

⑦S32.032 Unstable burst fracture of third lumbar vertebra

⑦S32.038 Other fracture of third lumbar vertebra

⑦S32.039 Unspecified fracture of third lumbar vertebra

S32.04 Fracture of fourth lumbar vertebra

⑦S32.040 Wedge compression fracture of fourth lumbar vertebra

⑦S32.041 Stable burst fracture of fourth lumbar vertebra

⑦S32.042 Unstable burst fracture of fourth lumbar vertebra

⑦S32.048 Other fracture of fourth lumbar vertebra

⑦S32.049 Unspecified fracture of fourth lumbar vertebra

S32.05 Fracture of fifth lumbar vertebra

⑦S32.050 Wedge compression fracture of fifth lumbar vertebra

⑦S32.051 Stable burst fracture of fifth lumbar vertebra

⑦S32.052   Unstable burst fracture of fifth lumbar vertebra

⑦S32.058   Other fracture of fifth lumbar vertebra

⑦S32.059   Unspecified fracture of fifth lumbar vertebra

S32.1   Fracture of sacrum

For vertical fractures, code to most medial fracture extension

Use two codes if both a vertical and transverse fracture are present

Code also any associated fracture of pelvic ring (S32.8-)

⊗⑦S32.10   Unspecified fracture of sacrum

S32.11   Zone I fracture of sacrum

Vertical sacral ala fracture of sacrum

⑦S32.110   Nondisplaced Zone I fracture of sacrum

⑦S32.111   Minimally displaced Zone I fracture of sacrum

⑦S32.112   Severely displaced Zone I fracture of sacrum

⑦S32.119   Unspecified Zone I fracture of sacrum

S32.12   Zone II fracture of sacrum

Vertical foraminal region fracture of sacrum

⑦S32.120   Nondisplaced Zone II fracture of sacrum

⑦S32.121   Minimally displaced Zone II fracture of sacrum

⑦S32.122   Severely displaced Zone II fracture of sacrum

⑦S32.129   Unspecified Zone II fracture of sacrum

S32.13   Zone III fracture of sacrum

Vertical fracture into spinal canal region of sacrum

⑦S32.130   Nondisplaced Zone III fracture of sacrum

⑦S32.131   Minimally displaced Zone III fracture of sacrum

⑦S32.132   Severely displaced Zone III fracture of sacrum

⑦S32.139   Unspecified Zone III fracture of sacrum

S32.14   Type 1 fracture of sacrum

Transverse flexion fracture of sacrum without displacement

⊗⑦S32.15   Type 2 fracture of sacrum

Transverse flexion fracture of sacrum with posterior displacement

⊗⑦S32.16   Type 3 fracture of sacrum

Transverse extension fracture of sacrum with anterior displacement

⊗⑦S32.17   Type 4 fracture of sacrum

Transverse segmental comminution of upper sacrum

⊗⑦S32.19   Other fracture of sacrum

S32.2   Fracture of coccyx

S32.3   Fracture of ilium

Excludes 1: fracture of ilium with associated disruption of pelvic ring (S32.8-)

S32.30   Unspecified fracture of ilium

⑦S32.301   Unspecified fracture of right ilium

⑦S32.302   Unspecified fracture of left ilium

⑦S32.309   Unspecified fracture of unspecified ilium

S32.31   Avulsion fracture of ilium

⑦S32.311   Displaced avulsion fracture of right ilium

⑦S32.312   Displaced avulsion fracture of left ilium

⑦S32.313   Displaced avulsion fracture of unspecified ilium

⑦S32.314   Nondisplaced avulsion fracture of right ilium

⑦S32.315   Nondisplaced avulsion fracture of left ilium

⑦S32.316   Nondisplaced avulsion fracture of unspecified ilium

S32.39   Other fracture of ilium

⑦S32.391   Other fracture of right ilium

⑦S32.392   Other fracture of left ilium

⑦S32.399   Other fracture of unspecified ilium

S32.4   Fracture of acetabulum

Code also any associated fracture of pelvic ring (S32.8-)

S32.40   Unspecified fracture of acetabulum

⑦S32.401   Unspecified fracture of right acetabulum

⑦S32.402   Unspecified fracture of left acetabulum

⑦S32.409   Unspecified fracture of unspecified acetabulum

S32.41   Fracture of anterior wall of acetabulum

⑦S32.411   Displaced fracture of anterior wall of right acetabulum

⑦S32.412   Displaced fracture of anterior wall of left acetabulum

⑦S32.413   Displaced fracture of anterior wall of unspecified acetabulum

⑦S32.414   Nondisplaced fracture of anterior wall of right acetabulum

⑦S32.415   Nondisplaced fracture of anterior wall of left acetabulum

⑦S32.416   Nondisplaced fracture of anterior wall of unspecified acetabulum

S32.42   Fracture of posterior wall of acetabulum

⑦S32.421   Displaced fracture of posterior wall of right acetabulum

⑦S32.422   Displaced fracture of posterior wall of left acetabulum

⑦S32.423   Displaced fracture of posterior wall of unspecified acetabulum

⑦S32.424   Nondisplaced fracture of posterior wall of right acetabulum

⑦S32.425   Nondisplaced fracture of posterior wall of left acetabulum

● New code   ▲ Revised code   ⑦ 7th digit required   ⊗ Placeholder required

⑦S32.426   Nondisplaced fracture of posterior wall of unspecified acetabulum

S32.43   Fracture of anterior column [iliopubic] of acetabulum

⑦S32.431   Displaced fracture of anterior column [iliopubic] of right acetabulum

⑦S32.432   Displaced fracture of anterior column [iliopubic] of left acetabulum

⑦S32.433   Displaced fracture of anterior column [iliopubic] of unspecified acetabulum

⑦S32.434   Nondisplaced fracture of anterior column [iliopubic] of right acetabulum

⑦S32.435   Nondisplaced fracture of anterior column [iliopubic] of left acetabulum

⑦S32.436   Nondisplaced fracture of anterior column [iliopubic] of unspecified acetabulum

S32.44   Fracture of posterior column [ilioischial] of acetabulum

⑦S32.441   Displaced fracture of posterior column [ilioischial] of right acetabulum

⑦S32.442   Displaced fracture of posterior column [ilioischial] of left acetabulum

⑦S32.443   Displaced fracture of posterior column [ilioischial] of unspecified acetabulum

⑦S32.444   Nondisplaced fracture of posterior column [ilioischial] of right acetabulum

⑦S32.445   Nondisplaced fracture of posterior column [ilioischial] of left acetabulum

⑦S32.446   Nondisplaced fracture of posterior column [ilioischial] of unspecified acetabulum

S32.45   Transverse fracture of acetabulum

⑦S32.451   Displaced transverse fracture of right acetabulum

⑦S32.452   Displaced transverse fracture of left acetabulum

⑦S32.453   Displaced transverse fracture of unspecified acetabulum

⑦S32.454   Nondisplaced transverse fracture of right acetabulum

⑦S32.455   Nondisplaced transverse fracture of left acetabulum

⑦S32.456   Nondisplaced transverse fracture of unspecified acetabulum

S32.46   Associated transverse-posterior fracture of acetabulum

⑦S32.461   Displaced associated transverse-posterior fracture of right acetabulum

⑦S32.462   Displaced associated transverse-posterior fracture of left acetabulum

⑦S32.463   Displaced associated transverse-posterior fracture of unspecified acetabulum

⑦S32.464   Nondisplaced associated transverse-posterior fracture of right acetabulum

⑦S32.465   Nondisplaced associated transverse-posterior fracture of left acetabulum

⑦S32.466   Nondisplaced associated transverse-posterior fracture of unspecified acetabulum

S32.47   Fracture of medial wall of acetabulum

⑦S32.471   Displaced fracture of medial wall of right acetabulum

⑦S32.472   Displaced fracture of medial wall of left acetabulum

⑦S32.473   Displaced fracture of medial wall of unspecified acetabulum

⑦S32.474   Nondisplaced fracture of medial wall of right acetabulum

⑦S32.475   Nondisplaced fracture of medial wall of left acetabulum

⑦S32.476   Nondisplaced fracture of medial wall of unspecified acetabulum

S32.48   Dome fracture of acetabulum

⑦S32.481   Displaced dome fracture of right acetabulum

⑦S32.482   Displaced dome fracture of left acetabulum

⑦S32.483   Displaced dome fracture of unspecified acetabulum

⑦S32.484   Nondisplaced dome fracture of right acetabulum

⑦S32.485   Nondisplaced dome fracture of left acetabulum

⑦S32.486   Nondisplaced dome fracture of unspecified acetabulum

S32.49   Other specified fracture of acetabulum

⑦S32.491   Other specified fracture of right acetabulum

⑦S32.492   Other specified fracture of left acetabulum

⑦S32.499   Other specified fracture of unspecified acetabulum

S32.5   Fracture of pubis

Excludes 1: fracture of pubis with associated disruption of pelvic ring (S32.8-)

S32.50   Unspecified fracture of pubis

⑦S32.501   Unspecified fracture of right pubis

⑦S32.502   Unspecified fracture of left pubis

⑦S32.509   Unspecified fracture of unspecified pubis

S32.51   Fracture of superior rim of pubis

⑦S32.511   Fracture of superior rim of right pubis

⑦S32.512   Fracture of superior rim of left pubis

⑦**S32.519**   Fracture of superior rim of unspecified pubis

S32.59   Other specified fracture of pubis

⑦**S32.591**   Other specified fracture of right pubis

⑦**S32.592**   Other specified fracture of left pubis

⑦**S32.599**   Other specified fracture of unspecified pubis

S32.6   Fracture of ischium

Excludes 1: fracture of ischium with associated disruption of pelvic ring (S32.8-)

S32.60   Unspecified fracture of ischium

⑦**S32.601**   Unspecified fracture of right ischium

⑦**S32.602**   Unspecified fracture of left ischium

⑦**S32.609**   Unspecified fracture of unspecified ischium

S32.61   Avulsion fracture of ischium

⑦**S32.611**   Displaced avulsion fracture of right ischium

⑦**S32.612**   Displaced avulsion fracture of left ischium

⑦**S32.613**   Displaced avulsion fracture of unspecified ischium

⑦**S32.614**   Nondisplaced avulsion fracture of right ischium

⑦**S32.615**   Nondisplaced avulsion fracture of left ischium

⑦**S32.616**   Nondisplaced avulsion fracture of unspecified ischium

S32.69   Other specified fracture of ischium

⑦**S32.691**   Other specified fracture of right ischium

⑦**S32.692**   Other specified fracture of left ischium

⑦**S32.699**   Other specified fracture of unspecified ischium

S32.8   Fracture of other parts of pelvis

Code also any associated:

   fracture of acetabulum (S32.4-)

   sacral fracture (S32.1-)

S32.81   Multiple fractures of pelvis with disruption of pelvic ring

Multiple pelvic fractures with disruption of pelvic circle

⑦**S32.810**   Multiple fractures of pelvis with stable disruption of pelvic ring

⑦**S32.811**   Multiple fractures of pelvis with unstable disruption of pelvic ring

S32.82   Multiple fractures of pelvis without disruption of pelvic ring

Multiple pelvic fractures without disruption of pelvic circle

⊗⑦**S32.89**   Fracture of other parts of pelvis

⊗⑦**S32.9**   Fracture of unspecified parts of lumbosacral spine and pelvis

Fracture of lumbosacral spine NOS

Fracture of pelvis NOS

S33   Dislocation and sprain of joints and ligaments of lumbar spine and pelvis

Includes: avulsion of joint or ligament of lumbar spine and pelvis

laceration of cartilage, joint or ligament of lumbar spine and pelvis

sprain of cartilage, joint or ligament of lumbar spine and pelvis

traumatic hemarthrosis of joint or ligament of lumbar spine and pelvis

traumatic rupture of joint or ligament of lumbar spine and pelvis

traumatic subluxation of joint or ligament of lumbar spine and pelvis

traumatic tear of joint or ligament of lumbar spine and pelvis

Code also any associated open wound

Excludes 1: nontraumatic rupture or displacement of lumbar intervertebral disc NOS (M51.-)

obstetric damage to pelvic joints and ligaments (O71.6)

Excludes 2: dislocation and sprain of joints and ligaments of hip (S73.-)

strain of muscle of lower back and pelvis (S39.01-)

The appropriate 7th character is to be added to each code from category S33

A - initial encounter

D - subsequent encounter

S - sequela

⊗⑦**S33.0**   Traumatic rupture of lumbar intervertebral disc

Excludes 1: rupture or displacement (nontraumatic) of lumbar intervertebral disc NOS (M51.- with fifth character 6)

S33.1   Subluxation and dislocation of lumbar vertebra

Code also any associated:

   open wound of abdomen, lower back and pelvis (S31)

   spinal cord injury (S24.0, S24.1-, S34.0-, S34.1-)

Excludes 2: fracture of lumbar vertebrae (S32.0-)

S33.10   Subluxation and dislocation of unspecified lumbar vertebra

⑦**S33.100**   Subluxation of unspecified lumbar vertebra

⑦**S33.101**   Dislocation of unspecified lumbar vertebra

S33.11   Subluxation and dislocation of L1/L2 lumbar vertebra

⑦**S33.110**   Subluxation of L1/L2 lumbar vertebra

⑦**S33.111**   Dislocation of L1/L2 lumbar vertebra

S33.12   Subluxation and dislocation of L2/L3 lumbar vertebra

⑦**S33.120**   Subluxation of L2/L3 lumbar vertebra

⑦**S33.121**   Dislocation of L2/L3 lumbar vertebra

S33.13   Subluxation and dislocation of L3/L4 lumbar vertebra

⑦**S33.130**   Subluxation of L3/L4 lumbar vertebra

● New code   ▲ Revised code   ⑦ 7ᵗʰ digit required   ⊗ Placeholder required

⑦S33.131 Dislocation of L3/L4 lumbar vertebra

S33.14 Subluxation and dislocation of L4/L5 lumbar vertebra

    ⑦S33.140 Subluxation of L4/L5 lumbar vertebra

    ⑦S33.141 Dislocation of L4/L5 lumbar vertebra

⊗⑦S33.2 Dislocation of sacroiliac and sacrococcygeal joint

S33.3 Dislocation of other and unspecified parts of lumbar spine and pelvis

    ⊗⑦S33.30 Dislocation of unspecified parts of lumbar spine and pelvis

    ⊗⑦S33.39 Dislocation of other parts of lumbar spine and pelvis

⊗⑦S33.4 Traumatic rupture of symphysis pubis

⊗⑦S33.5 Sprain of ligaments of lumbar spine

⊗⑦S33.6 Sprain of sacroiliac joint

⊗⑦S33.8 Sprain of other parts of lumbar spine and pelvis

⊗⑦S33.9 Sprain of unspecified parts of lumbar spine and pelvis

S34 Injury of lumbar and sacral spinal cord and nerves at abdomen, lower back and pelvis level

Note: Code to highest level of lumbar cord injury

Code also any associated:

    fracture of vertebra (S22.0-, S32.0-)

    open wound of abdomen, lower back and pelvis (S31.-)

    transient paralysis (R29.5)

The appropriate 7th character is to be added to each code from category S34

A - initial encounter

D - subsequent encounter

S - sequela

S34.0 Concussion and edema of lumbar and sacral spinal cord

    ⊗⑦S34.01 Concussion and edema of lumbar spinal cord

    ⊗⑦S34.02 Concussion and edema of sacral spinal cord

    Concussion and edema of conus medullaris

S34.1 Other and unspecified injury of lumbar and sacral spinal cord

    S34.10 Unspecified injury to lumbar spinal cord

        ⑦S34.101 Unspecified injury to L1 level of lumbar spinal cord

        ⑦S34.102 Unspecified injury to L2 level of lumbar spinal cord

        ⑦S34.103 Unspecified injury to L3 level of lumbar spinal cord

        ⑦S34.104 Unspecified injury to L4 level of lumbar spinal cord

        ⑦S34.105 Unspecified injury to L5 level of lumbar spinal cord

        ⑦S34.109 Unspecified injury to unspecified level of lumbar spinal cord

    S34.11 Complete lesion of lumbar spinal cord

        ⑦S34.111 Complete lesion of L1 level of lumbar spinal cord

        ⑦S34.112 Complete lesion of L2 level of lumbar spinal cord

        ⑦S34.113 Complete lesion of L3 level of lumbar spinal cord

        ⑦S34.114 Complete lesion of L4 level of lumbar spinal cord

        ⑦S34.115 Complete lesion of L5 level of lumbar spinal cord

        ⑦S34.119 Complete lesion of unspecified level of lumbar spinal cord

    S34.12 Incomplete lesion of lumbar spinal cord

        ⑦S34.121 Incomplete lesion of L1 level of lumbar spinal cord

        ⑦S34.122 Incomplete lesion of L2 level of lumbar spinal cord

        ⑦S34.123 Incomplete lesion of L3 level of lumbar spinal cord

        ⑦S34.124 Incomplete lesion of L4 level of lumbar spinal cord

        ⑦S34.125 Incomplete lesion of L5 level of lumbar spinal cord

        ⑦S34.129 Incomplete lesion of unspecified level of lumbar spinal cord

    S34.13 Other and unspecified injury to sacral spinal cord

    Other injury to conus medullaris

        ⑦S34.131 Complete lesion of sacral spinal cord

        Complete lesion of conus medullaris

        ⑦S34.132 Incomplete lesion of sacral spinal cord

        Incomplete lesion of conus medullaris

        ⑦S34.139 Unspecified injury to sacral spinal cord

        Unspecified injury of conus medullaris

S34.2 Injury of nerve root of lumbar and sacral spine

    ⊗⑦S34.21 Injury of nerve root of lumbar spine

    ⊗⑦S34.22 Injury of nerve root of sacral spine

⊗⑦S34.3 Injury of cauda equina

⊗⑦S34.4 Injury of lumbosacral plexus

⊗⑦S34.5 Injury of lumbar, sacral and pelvic sympathetic nerves

    Injury of celiac ganglion or plexus

    Injury of hypogastric plexus

    Injury of mesenteric plexus (inferior) (superior)

    Injury of splanchnic nerve

⊗⑦S34.6 Injury of peripheral nerve(s) at abdomen, lower back and pelvis level

⊗⑦S34.8 Injury of other nerves at abdomen, lower back and pelvis level

⊗⑦S34.9 Injury of unspecified nerves at abdomen, lower back and pelvis level

S35 Injury of blood vessels at abdomen, lower back and pelvis level

Code also any associated open wound (S31.-)

The appropriate 7th character is to be added to each code from category S35

A - initial encounter

D - subsequent encounter

S - sequela

S35.0 Injury of abdominal aorta

    Excludes 1: injury of aorta NOS (S25.0)

    ⊗⑦S35.00 Unspecified injury of abdominal aorta

    ⊗⑦S35.01 Minor laceration of abdominal aorta

Incomplete transection of abdominal aorta
Laceration of abdominal aorta NOS
Superficial laceration of abdominal aorta

⊗ ⑦ S35.02　Major laceration of abdominal aorta
Complete transection of abdominal aorta
Traumatic rupture of abdominal aorta

⊗ ⑦ S35.09　Other injury of abdominal aorta

S35.1　Injury of inferior vena cava
Injury of hepatic vein
Excludes 1: injury of vena cava NOS (S25.2)

⊗ ⑦ S35.10　Unspecified injury of inferior vena cava

⊗ ⑦ S35.11　Minor laceration of inferior vena cava
Incomplete transection of inferior vena cava
Laceration of inferior vena cava NOS
Superficial laceration of inferior vena cava

⊗ ⑦ S35.12　Major laceration of inferior vena cava
Complete transection of inferior vena cava
Traumatic rupture of inferior vena cava

⊗ ⑦ S35.19　Other injury of inferior vena cava

S35.2　Injury of celiac or mesenteric artery and branches

S35.21　Injury of celiac artery

⑦ S35.211　Minor laceration of celiac artery
Incomplete transection of celiac artery
Laceration of celiac artery NOS
Superficial laceration of celiac artery

⑦ S35.212　Major laceration of celiac artery
Complete transection of celiac artery
Traumatic rupture of celiac artery

⑦ S35.218　Other injury of celiac artery

⑦ S35.219　Unspecified injury of celiac artery

S35.22　Injury of superior mesenteric artery

⑦ S35.221　Minor laceration of superior mesenteric artery
Incomplete transection of superior mesenteric artery
Laceration of superior mesenteric artery NOS
Superficial laceration of superior mesenteric artery

⑦ S35.222　Major laceration of superior mesenteric artery
Complete transection of superior mesenteric artery
Traumatic rupture of superior mesenteric artery

⑦ S35.228　Other injury of superior mesenteric artery

⑦ S35.229　Unspecified injury of superior mesenteric artery

S35.23　Injury of inferior mesenteric artery

⑦ S35.231　Minor laceration of inferior mesenteric artery
Incomplete transection of inferior mesenteric artery
Laceration of inferior mesenteric artery NOS

Superficial laceration of inferior mesenteric artery

⑦ S35.232　Major laceration of inferior mesenteric artery
Complete transection of inferior mesenteric artery
Traumatic rupture of inferior mesenteric artery

⑦ S35.238　Other injury of inferior mesenteric artery

⑦ S35.239　Unspecified injury of inferior mesenteric artery

S35.29　Injury of branches of celiac and mesenteric artery
Injury of gastric artery
Injury of gastroduodenal artery
Injury of hepatic artery
Injury of splenic artery

⑦ S35.291　Minor laceration of branches of celiac and mesenteric artery
Incomplete transection of branches of celiac and mesenteric artery
Laceration of branches of celiac and mesenteric artery NOS
Superficial laceration of branches of celiac and mesenteric artery

⑦ S35.292　Major laceration of branches of celiac and mesenteric artery
Complete transection of branches of celiac and mesenteric artery
Traumatic rupture of branches of celiac and mesenteric artery

⑦ S35.298　Other injury of branches of celiac and mesenteric artery

⑦ S35.299　Unspecified injury of branches of celiac and mesenteric artery

S35.3　Injury of portal or splenic vein and branches

S35.31　Injury of portal vein

⑦ S35.311　Laceration of portal vein

⑦ S35.318　Other specified injury of portal vein

⑦ S35.319　Unspecified injury of portal vein

S35.32　Injury of splenic vein

⑦ S35.321　Laceration of splenic vein

⑦ S35.328　Other specified injury of splenic vein

⑦ S35.329　Unspecified injury of splenic vein

S35.33　Injury of superior mesenteric vein

⑦ S35.331　Laceration of superior mesenteric vein

⑦ S35.338　Other specified injury of superior mesenteric vein

⑦ S35.339　Unspecified injury of superior mesenteric vein

S35.34　Injury of inferior mesenteric vein

⑦ S35.341　Laceration of inferior mesenteric vein

⑦ S35.348　Other specified injury of inferior mesenteric vein

⑦ S35.349　Unspecified injury of inferior mesenteric vein

　● New code　　　　▲ Revised code　　　　⑦ 7th digit required　　　　⊗ Placeholder required

S35.4   Injury of renal blood vessels
    S35.40   Unspecified injury of renal blood vessel
        ⑦S35.401   Unspecified injury of right renal artery
        ⑦S35.402   Unspecified injury of left renal artery
        ⑦S35.403   Unspecified injury of unspecified renal artery
        ⑦S35.404   Unspecified injury of right renal vein
        ⑦S35.405   Unspecified injury of left renal vein
        ⑦S35.406   Unspecified injury of unspecified renal vein
    S35.41   Laceration of renal blood vessel
        ⑦S35.411   Laceration of right renal artery
        ⑦S35.412   Laceration of left renal artery
        ⑦S35.413   Laceration of unspecified renal artery
        ⑦S35.414   Laceration of right renal vein
        ⑦S35.415   Laceration of left renal vein
        ⑦S35.416   Laceration of unspecified renal vein
    S35.49   Other specified injury of renal blood vessel
        ⑦S35.491   Other specified injury of right renal artery
        ⑦S35.492   Other specified injury of left renal artery
        ⑦S35.493   Other specified injury of unspecified renal artery
        ⑦S35.494   Other specified injury of right renal vein
        ⑦S35.495   Other specified injury of left renal vein
        ⑦S35.496   Other specified injury of unspecified renal vein
S35.5   Injury of iliac blood vessels
    ⊗⑦S35.50   Injury of unspecified iliac blood vessel(s)
    S35.51   Injury of iliac artery or vein
        Injury of hypogastric artery or vein
        ⑦S35.511   Injury of right iliac artery
        ⑦S35.512   Injury of left iliac artery
        ⑦S35.513   Injury of unspecified iliac artery
        ⑦S35.514   Injury of right iliac vein
        ⑦S35.515   Injury of left iliac vein
        ⑦S35.516   Injury of unspecified iliac vein
    S35.53   Injury of uterine artery or vein
        ⑦S35.531   Injury of right uterine artery
        ⑦S35.532   Injury of left uterine artery
        ⑦S35.533   Injury of unspecified uterine artery
        ⑦S35.534   Injury of right uterine vein
        ⑦S35.535   Injury of left uterine vein
        ⑦S35.536   Injury of unspecified uterine vein
    S35.59   Injury of other iliac blood vessels
S35.8   Injury of other blood vessels at abdomen, lower back and pelvis level
    Injury of ovarian artery or vein
    S35.8X   Injury of other blood vessels at abdomen, lower back and pelvis level

⑦S35.8X1   Laceration of other blood vessels at abdomen, lower back and pelvis level
⑦S35.8X8   Other specified injury of other blood vessels at abdomen, lower back and pelvis level
⑦S35.8X9   Unspecified injury of other blood vessels at abdomen, lower back and pelvis level
S35.9   Injury of unspecified blood vessel at abdomen, lower back and pelvis level
    ⊗⑦S35.90   Unspecified injury of unspecified blood vessel at abdomen, lower back and pelvis level
    ⊗⑦S35.91   Laceration of unspecified blood vessel at abdomen, lower back and pelvis level
    ⊗⑦S35.99   Other specified injury of unspecified blood vessel at abdomen, lower back and pelvis level

S36   Injury of intra-abdominal organs
Code also any associated open wound (S31.-)
The appropriate 7th character is to be added to each code from category S36
A - initial encounter
D - subsequent encounter
S - sequela
S36.0   Injury of spleen
    ⊗⑦S36.00   Unspecified injury of spleen
    S36.02   Contusion of spleen
        ⑦S36.020   Minor contusion of spleen
                Contusion of spleen less than 2 cm
        ⑦S36.021   Major contusion of spleen
                Contusion of spleen greater than 2 cm
        ⑦S36.029   Unspecified contusion of spleen
    S36.03   Laceration of spleen
        ⑦S36.030   Superficial (capsular) laceration of spleen
                Laceration of spleen less than 1 cm
                Minor laceration of spleen
        ⑦S36.031   Moderate laceration of spleen
                Laceration of spleen 1 to 3 cm
        ⑦S36.032   Major laceration of spleen
                Avulsion of spleen
                Laceration of spleen greater than 3 cm
                Massive laceration of spleen
                Multiple moderate lacerations of spleen
                Stellate laceration of spleen
        ⑦S36.039   Unspecified laceration of spleen
    S36.09   Other injury of spleen
S36.1   Injury of liver and gallbladder and bile duct
    S36.11   Injury of liver
        ⑦S36.112   Contusion of liver
        ⑦S36.113   Laceration of liver, unspecified degree
        ⑦S36.114   Minor laceration of liver
                Laceration involving capsule only, or, without significant involvement

of hepatic parenchyma [i.e., less than 1 cm deep]

⑦S36.115   Moderate laceration of liver
Laceration involving parenchyma but without major disruption of parenchyma [i.e., less than 10 cm long and less than 3 cm deep]

⑦S36.116   Major laceration of liver
Laceration with significant disruption of hepatic parenchyma [i.e., greater than 10 cm long and 3 cm deep]
Multiple moderate lacerations, with or without hematoma
Stellate laceration of liver

⑦S36.118   Other injury of liver
⑦S36.119   Unspecified injury of liver

S36.12   Injury of gallbladder
    ⑦S36.122   Contusion of gallbladder
    ⑦S36.123   Laceration of gallbladder
    ⑦S36.128   Other injury of gallbladder
    ⑦S36.129   Unspecified injury of gallbladder

S36.13   Injury of bile duct

S36.2   Injury of pancreas
   S36.20   Unspecified injury of pancreas
     ⑦S36.200   Unspecified injury of head of pancreas
     ⑦S36.201   Unspecified injury of body of pancreas
     ⑦S36.202   Unspecified injury of tail of pancreas
     ⑦S36.209   Unspecified injury of unspecified part of pancreas

   S36.22   Contusion of pancreas
     ⑦S36.220   Contusion of head of pancreas
     ⑦S36.221   Contusion of body of pancreas
     ⑦S36.222   Contusion of tail of pancreas
     ⑦S36.229   Contusion of unspecified part of pancreas

   S36.23   Laceration of pancreas, unspecified degree
     ⑦S36.230   Laceration of head of pancreas, unspecified degree
     ⑦S36.231   Laceration of body of pancreas, unspecified degree
     ⑦S36.232   Laceration of tail of pancreas, unspecified degree
     ⑦S36.239   Laceration of unspecified part of pancreas, unspecified degree

   S36.24   Minor laceration of pancreas
     ⑦S36.240   Minor laceration of head of pancreas
     ⑦S36.241   Minor laceration of body of pancreas
     ⑦S36.242   Minor laceration of tail of pancreas
     ⑦S36.249   Minor laceration of unspecified part of pancreas

   S36.25   Moderate laceration of pancreas
     ⑦S36.250   Moderate laceration of head of pancreas

⑦S36.251   Moderate laceration of body of pancreas
⑦S36.252   Moderate laceration of tail of pancreas
⑦S36.259   Moderate laceration of unspecified part of pancreas

   S36.26   Major laceration of pancreas
     ⑦S36.260   Major laceration of head of pancreas
     ⑦S36.261   Major laceration of body of pancreas
     ⑦S36.262   Major laceration of tail of pancreas
     ⑦S36.269   Major laceration of unspecified part of pancreas

   S36.29   Other injury of pancreas
     ⑦S36.290   Other injury of head of pancreas
     ⑦S36.291   Other injury of body of pancreas
     ⑦S36.292   Other injury of tail of pancreas
     ⑦S36.299   Other injury of unspecified part of pancreas

S36.3   Injury of stomach
   ⊗⑦S36.30   Unspecified injury of stomach
   ⊗⑦S36.32   Contusion of stomach
   ⊗⑦S36.33   Laceration of stomach
   ⊗⑦S36.39   Other injury of stomach

S36.4   Injury of small intestine
   S36.40   Unspecified injury of small intestine
     ⑦S36.400   Unspecified injury of duodenum
     ⑦S36.408   Unspecified injury of other part of small intestine
     ⑦S36.409   Unspecified injury of unspecified part of small intestine

   S36.41   Primary blast injury of small intestine
Blast injury of small intestine NOS
     ⑦S36.410   Primary blast injury of duodenum
     ⑦S36.418   Primary blast injury of other part of small intestine
     ⑦S36.419   Primary blast injury of unspecified part of small intestine

   S36.42   Contusion of small intestine
     ⑦S36.420   Contusion of duodenum
     ⑦S36.428   Contusion of other part of small intestine
     ⑦S36.429   Contusion of unspecified part of small intestine

   S36.43   Laceration of small intestine
     ⑦S36.430   Laceration of duodenum
     ⑦S36.438   Laceration of other part of small intestine
     ⑦S36.439   Laceration of unspecified part of small intestine

   S36.49   Other injury of small intestine
     ⑦S36.490   Other injury of duodenum
     ⑦S36.498   Other injury of other part of small intestine
     ⑦S36.499   Other injury of unspecified part of small intestine

S36.5   Injury of colon

Excludes 2: injury of rectum (S36.6-)

S36.50   Unspecified injury of colon

⑦S36.500   Unspecified injury of ascending [right] colon

⑦S36.501   Unspecified injury of transverse colon

⑦S36.502   Unspecified injury of descending [left] colon

⑦S36.503   Unspecified injury of sigmoid colon

⑦S36.508   Unspecified injury of other part of colon

⑦S36.509   Unspecified injury of unspecified part of colon

S36.51   Primary blast injury of colon
Blast injury of colon NOS

⑦S36.510   Primary blast injury of ascending [right] colon

⑦S36.511   Primary blast injury of transverse colon

⑦S36.512   Primary blast injury of descending [left] colon

⑦S36.513   Primary blast injury of sigmoid colon

⑦S36.518   Primary blast injury of other part of colon

⑦S36.519   Primary blast injury of unspecified part of colon

S36.52   Contusion of colon

⑦S36.520   Contusion of ascending [right] colon

⑦S36.521   Contusion of transverse colon

⑦S36.522   Contusion of descending [left] colon

⑦S36.523   Contusion of sigmoid colon

⑦S36.528   Contusion of other part of colon

⑦S36.529   Contusion of unspecified part of colon

S36.53   Laceration of colon

⑦S36.530   Laceration of ascending [right] colon

⑦S36.531   Laceration of transverse colon

⑦S36.532   Laceration of descending [left] colon

⑦S36.533   Laceration of sigmoid colon

⑦S36.538   Laceration of other part of colon

⑦S36.539   Laceration of unspecified part of colon

S36.59   Other injury of colon
Secondary blast injury of colon

⑦S36.590   Other injury of ascending [right] colon

⑦S36.591   Other injury of transverse colon

⑦S36.592   Other injury of descending [left] colon

⑦S36.593   Other injury of sigmoid colon

⑦S36.598   Other injury of other part of colon

⑦S36.599   Other injury of unspecified part of colon

S36.6   Injury of rectum

⊗⑦S36.60   Unspecified injury of rectum

⊗⑦S36.61   Primary blast injury of rectum
Blast injury of rectum NOS

⊗⑦S36.62   Contusion of rectum

⊗⑦S36.63   Laceration of rectum

⊗⑦S36.69   Other injury of rectum
Secondary blast injury of rectum

S36.8   Injury of other intra-abdominal organs

⊗⑦S36.81   Injury of peritoneum

S36.89   Injury of other intra-abdominal organs
Injury of retroperitoneum

⑦S36.892   Contusion of other intra-abdominal organs

⑦S36.893   Laceration of other intra-abdominal organs

⑦S36.898   Other injury of other intra-abdominal organs

⑦S36.899   Unspecified injury of other intra-abdominal organs

S36.9   Injury of unspecified intra-abdominal organ

⊗⑦S36.90   Unspecified injury of unspecified intra-abdominal organ

⊗⑦S36.92   Contusion of unspecified intra-abdominal organ

⊗⑦S36.93   Laceration of unspecified intra-abdominal organ

⊗⑦S36.99   Other injury of unspecified intra-abdominal organ

S37   Injury of urinary and pelvic organs
Code also any associated open wound (S31.-)
Excludes 1: obstetric trauma to pelvic organs (O71-)
Excludes 2: injury of peritoneum (S36.81)
injury of retroperitoneum (S36.89-)
The appropriate 7th character is to be added to each code from category S37
A - initial encounter
D - subsequent encounter
S - sequela

S37.0   Injury of kidney
Excludes 2: acute kidney injury (nontraumatic) (N17.9)

S37.00   Unspecified injury of kidney

⑦S37.001   Unspecified injury of right kidney

⑦S37.002   Unspecified injury of left kidney

⑦S37.009   Unspecified injury of unspecified kidney

S37.01   Minor contusion of kidney
Contusion of kidney less than 2 cm
Contusion of kidney NOS

⑦S37.011   Minor contusion of right kidney

⑦S37.012   Minor contusion of left kidney

⑦S37.019   Minor contusion of unspecified kidney

S37.02   Major contusion of kidney
Contusion of kidney greater than 2 cm

⑦S37.021   Major contusion of right kidney

⑦S37.022   Major contusion of left kidney

⑦S37.029   Major contusion of unspecified kidney

S37.03   Laceration of kidney, unspecified degree

⑦S37.031   Laceration of right kidney, unspecified degree

⑦**S37.032** Laceration of left kidney,
            unspecified degree

⑦**S37.039** Laceration of unspecified kidney,
            unspecified degree

S37.04 Minor laceration of kidney
          Laceration of kidney less than 1 cm

⑦**S37.041** Minor laceration of right kidney

⑦**S37.042** Minor laceration of left kidney

⑦**S37.049** Minor laceration of unspecified
            kidney

S37.05 Moderate laceration of kidney
          Laceration of kidney 1 to 3 cm

⑦**S37.051** Moderate laceration of right kidney

⑦**S37.052** Moderate laceration of left kidney

⑦**S37.059** Moderate laceration of unspecified
            kidney

S37.06 Major laceration of kidney
          Avulsion of kidney
          Laceration of kidney greater than 3 cm
          Massive laceration of kidney
          Multiple moderate lacerations of kidney
          Stellate laceration of kidney

⑦**S37.061** Major laceration of right kidney

⑦**S37.062** Major laceration of left kidney

⑦**S37.069** Major laceration of unspecified
            kidney

S37.09 Other injury of kidney

⑦**S37.091** Other injury of right kidney

⑦**S37.092** Other injury of left kidney

⑦**S37.099** Other injury of unspecified kidney

S37.1 Injury of ureter

⊗⑦**S37.10** Unspecified injury of ureter

⊗⑦**S37.12** Contusion of ureter

⊗⑦**S37.13** Laceration of ureter

⊗⑦**S37.19** Other injury of ureter

S37.2 Injury of bladder

⊗⑦**S37.20** Unspecified injury of bladder

⊗⑦**S37.22** Contusion of bladder

⊗⑦**S37.23** Laceration of bladder

⊗⑦**S37.29** Other injury of bladder

S37.3 Injury of urethra

⊗⑦**S37.30** Unspecified injury of urethra

⊗⑦**S37.32** Contusion of urethra

⊗⑦**S37.33** Laceration of urethra

⊗⑦**S37.39** Other injury of urethra

S37.4 Injury of ovary

S37.40 Unspecified injury of ovary

⑦**S37.401** Unspecified injury of ovary,
            unilateral

⑦**S37.402** Unspecified injury of ovary,
            bilateral

⑦**S37.409** Unspecified injury of ovary,
            unspecified

S37.42 Contusion of ovary

⑦**S37.421** Contusion of ovary, unilateral

⑦**S37.422** Contusion of ovary, bilateral

⑦**S37.429** Contusion of ovary, unspecified

S37.43 Laceration of ovary

⑦**S37.431** Laceration of ovary, unilateral

⑦**S37.432** Laceration of ovary, bilateral

⑦**S37.439** Laceration of ovary, unspecified

S37.49 Other injury of ovary

⑦**S37.491** Other injury of ovary, unilateral

⑦**S37.492** Other injury of ovary, bilateral

⑦**S37.499** Other injury of ovary, unspecified

S37.5 Injury of fallopian tube

S37.50 Unspecified injury of fallopian tube

⑦**S37.501** Unspecified injury of fallopian tube,
            unilateral

⑦**S37.502** Unspecified injury of fallopian tube,
            bilateral

⑦**S37.509** Unspecified injury of fallopian tube,
            unspecified

S37.51 Primary blast injury of fallopian tube
          Blast injury of fallopian tube NOS

⑦**S37.511** Primary blast injury of fallopian
            tube, unilateral

⑦**S37.512** Primary blast injury of fallopian
            tube, bilateral

⑦**S37.519** Primary blast injury of fallopian
            tube, unspecified

S37.52 Contusion of fallopian tube

⑦**S37.521** Contusion of fallopian tube,
            unilateral

⑦**S37.522** Contusion of fallopian tube, bilateral

⑦**S37.529** Contusion of fallopian tube,
            unspecified

S37.53 Laceration of fallopian tube

⑦**S37.531** Laceration of fallopian tube,
            unilateral

⑦**S37.532** Laceration of fallopian tube,
            bilateral

⑦**S37.539** Laceration of fallopian tube,
            unspecified

S37.59 Other injury of fallopian tube
          Secondary blast injury of fallopian tube

⑦**S37.591** Other injury of fallopian tube,
            unilateral

⑦**S37.592** Other injury of fallopian tube,
            bilateral

⑦**S37.599** Other injury of fallopian tube,
            unspecified

S37.6 Injury of uterus

Excludes 1: injury to gravid uterus (O9A.2-)
              injury to uterus during delivery (O71.-)

⊗⑦**S37.60** Unspecified injury of uterus

⊗⑦**S37.62** Contusion of uterus

⊗⑦**S37.63** Laceration of uterus

⊗⑦**S37.69** Other injury of uterus

S37.8 Injury of other urinary and pelvic organs

S37.81 Injury of adrenal gland

⑦**S37.812** Contusion of adrenal gland

⑦S37.813   Laceration of adrenal gland

⑦S37.818   Other injury of adrenal gland

⑦S37.819   Unspecified injury of adrenal gland

S37.82   Injury of prostate

⑦S37.822   Contusion of prostate

⑦S37.823   Laceration of prostate

⑦S37.828   Other injury of prostate

⑦S37.829   Unspecified injury of prostate

S37.89   Injury of other urinary and pelvic organ

⑦S37.892   Contusion of other urinary and pelvic organ

⑦S37.893   Laceration of other urinary and pelvic organ

⑦S37.898   Other injury of other urinary and pelvic organ

⑦S37.899   Unspecified injury of other urinary and pelvic organ

S37.9   Injury of unspecified urinary and pelvic organ

⊗⑦S37.90   Unspecified injury of unspecified urinary and pelvic organ

⊗⑦S37.92   Contusion of unspecified urinary and pelvic organ

⊗⑦S37.93   Laceration of unspecified urinary and pelvic organ

⊗⑦S37.99   Other injury of unspecified urinary and pelvic organ

S38 Crushing injury and traumatic amputation of abdomen, lower back, pelvis and external genitals

An amputation not identified as partial or complete should be coded to complete

The appropriate 7th character is to be added to each code from category S38

A - initial encounter

D - subsequent encounter

S - sequela

S38.0   Crushing injury of external genital organs

Use additional code for any associated injuries

S38.00   Crushing injury of unspecified external genital organs

⑦S38.001   Crushing injury of unspecified external genital organs, male

⑦S38.002   Crushing injury of unspecified external genital organs, female

⊗⑦S38.01   Crushing injury of penis

⊗⑦S38.02   Crushing injury of scrotum and testis

⊗⑦S38.03   Crushing injury of vulva

⊗⑦S38.1   Crushing injury of abdomen, lower back, and pelvis

Use additional code for all associated injuries, such as:

fracture of thoracic or lumbar spine and pelvis (S22.0-, S32.-)

injury to intra-abdominal organs (S36.-)

injury to urinary and pelvic organs (S37.-)

open wound of abdominal wall (S31-)

spinal cord injury (S34.0, S34.1-)

Excludes 2: crushing injury of external genital organs (S38.2-)

S38.2   Traumatic amputation of external genital organs

S38.21   Traumatic amputation of female external genital organs

Traumatic amputation of clitoris

Traumatic amputation of labium (majus) (minus)

Traumatic amputation of vulva

⑦S38.211   Complete traumatic amputation of female external genital organs

⑦S38.212   Partial traumatic amputation of female external genital organs

S38.22   Traumatic amputation of penis

⑦S38.221   Complete traumatic amputation of penis

⑦S38.222   Partial traumatic amputation of penis

S38.23   Traumatic amputation of scrotum and testis

⑦S38.231   Complete traumatic amputation of scrotum and testis

⑦S38.232   Partial traumatic amputation of scrotum and testis

S38.3   Transection (partial) of abdomen

S39 Other and unspecified injuries of abdomen, lower back, pelvis and external genitals

Code also any associated open wound (S31.-)

Excludes 2: sprain of joints and ligaments of lumbar spine and pelvis (S33.-)

The appropriate 7th character is to be added to each code from category S39

A - initial encounter

D - subsequent encounter

S - sequela

S39.0   Injury of muscle, fascia and tendon of abdomen, lower back and pelvis

S39.00   Unspecified injury of muscle, fascia and tendon of abdomen, lower back and pelvis

⑦S39.001   Unspecified injury of muscle, fascia and tendon of abdomen

⑦S39.002   Unspecified injury of muscle, fascia and tendon of lower back

⑦S39.003   Unspecified injury of muscle, fascia and tendon of pelvis

S39.01   Strain of muscle, fascia and tendon of abdomen, lower back and pelvis

⑦S39.011   Strain of muscle, fascia and tendon of abdomen

⑦S39.012   Strain of muscle, fascia and tendon of lower back

⑦S39.013   Strain of muscle, fascia and tendon of pelvis

S39.02   Laceration of muscle, fascia and tendon of abdomen, lower back and pelvis

⑦S39.021   Laceration of muscle, fascia and tendon of abdomen

⑦S39.022   Laceration of muscle, fascia and tendon of lower back

⑦S39.023   Laceration of muscle, fascia and tendon of pelvis

S39.09   Other injury of muscle, fascia and tendon of abdomen, lower back and pelvis

⑦S39.091   Other injury of muscle, fascia and tendon of abdomen

⑦S39.092   Other injury of muscle, fascia and tendon of lower back

⑦S39.093   Other injury of muscle, fascia and tendon of pelvis

S39.8   Other specified injuries of abdomen, lower back, pelvis and external genitals

⊗⑦S39.81   Other specified injuries of abdomen

⊗⑦S39.82   Other specified injuries of lower back

⊗⑦S39.83   Other specified injuries of pelvis

S39.84   Other specified injuries of external genitals

⑦S39.840   Fracture of corpus cavernosum penis

⑦S39.848   Other specified injuries of external genitals

S39.9   Unspecified injury of abdomen, lower back, pelvis and external genitals

⊗⑦S39.91   Unspecified injury of abdomen

⊗⑦S39.92   Unspecified injury of lower back

⊗⑦S39.93   Unspecified injury of pelvis

⊗⑦S39.94   Unspecified injury of external genitals

INJURIES TO THE SHOULDER AND UPPER ARM (S40-S49)

Includes: injuries of axilla

injuries of scapular region

Excludes 2: burns and corrosions (T20-T32)

frostbite (T33-T34)

injuries of elbow (S50-S59)

insect bite or sting, venomous (T63.4)

S40   Superficial injury of shoulder and upper arm

The appropriate 7th character is to be added to each code from category S40

A - initial encounter

D - subsequent encounter

S - sequela

S40.0   Contusion of shoulder and upper arm

S40.01   Contusion of shoulder

⑦S40.011   Contusion of right shoulder

⑦S40.012   Contusion of left shoulder

⑦S40.019   Contusion of unspecified shoulder

S40.02   Contusion of upper arm

⑦S40.021   Contusion of right upper arm

⑦S40.022   Contusion of left upper arm

⑦S40.029   Contusion of unspecified upper arm

S40.2   Other superficial injuries of shoulder

S40.21   Abrasion of shoulder

⑦S40.211   Abrasion of right shoulder

⑦S40.212   Abrasion of left shoulder

⑦S40.219   Abrasion of unspecified shoulder

S40.22   Blister (nonthermal) of shoulder

⑦S40.221   Blister (nonthermal) of right shoulder

⑦S40.222   Blister (nonthermal) of left shoulder

⑦S40.229   Blister (nonthermal) of unspecified shoulder

S40.24   External constriction of shoulder

⑦S40.241   External constriction of right shoulder

⑦S40.242   External constriction of left shoulder

⑦S40.249   External constriction of unspecified shoulder

S40.25   Superficial foreign body of shoulder

Splinter in the shoulder

⑦S40.251   Superficial foreign body of right shoulder

⑦S40.252   Superficial foreign body of left shoulder

⑦S40.259   Superficial foreign body of unspecified shoulder

S40.26   Insect bite (nonvenomous) of shoulder

⑦S40.261   Insect bite (nonvenomous) of right shoulder

⑦S40.262   Insect bite (nonvenomous) of left shoulder

⑦S40.269   Insect bite (nonvenomous) of unspecified shoulder

S40.27   Other superficial bite of shoulder

Excludes 1: open bite of shoulder (S41.05)

⑦S40.271   Other superficial bite of right shoulder

⑦S40.272   Other superficial bite of left shoulder

⑦S40.279   Other superficial bite of unspecified shoulder

S40.8   Other superficial injuries of upper arm

S40.81   Abrasion of upper arm

⑦S40.811   Abrasion of right upper arm

⑦S40.812   Abrasion of left upper arm

⑦S40.819   Abrasion of unspecified upper arm

S40.82   Blister (nonthermal) of upper arm

⑦S40.821   Blister (nonthermal) of right upper arm

⑦S40.822   Blister (nonthermal) of left upper arm

⑦S40.829   Blister (nonthermal) of unspecified upper arm

S40.84   External constriction of upper arm

⑦S40.841   External constriction of right upper arm

⑦S40.842   External constriction of left upper arm

⑦S40.849   External constriction of unspecified upper arm

S40.85   Superficial foreign body of upper arm

Splinter in the upper arm

⑦S40.851   Superficial foreign body of right upper arm

⑦S40.852   Superficial foreign body of left upper arm

⑦S40.859   Superficial foreign body of unspecified upper arm

S40.86   Insect bite (nonvenomous) of upper arm

⑦S40.861   Insect bite (nonvenomous) of right upper arm

⑦S40.862　Insect bite (nonvenomous) of left upper arm

⑦S40.869　Insect bite (nonvenomous) of unspecified upper arm

S40.87　Other superficial bite of upper arm
Excludes 1: open bite of upper arm (S41.14)
Excludes 2: other superficial bite of shoulder (S40.27-)

⑦S40.871　Other superficial bite of right upper arm

⑦S40.872　Other superficial bite of left upper arm

⑦S40.879　Other superficial bite of unspecified upper arm

S40.9　Unspecified superficial injury of shoulder and upper arm

S40.91　Unspecified superficial injury of shoulder

⑦S40.911　Unspecified superficial injury of right shoulder

⑦S40.912　Unspecified superficial injury of left shoulder

⑦S40.919　Unspecified superficial injury of unspecified shoulder

S40.92　Unspecified superficial injury of upper arm

⑦S40.921　Unspecified superficial injury of right upper arm

⑦S40.922　Unspecified superficial injury of left upper arm

⑦S40.929　Unspecified superficial injury of unspecified upper arm

S41　Open wound of shoulder and upper arm
Code also any associated wound infection
Excludes 1: traumatic amputation of shoulder and upper arm (S48.-)
Excludes 2: open fracture of shoulder and upper arm (S42.- with 7th character B or C)
The appropriate 7th character is to be added to each code from category S41
A - initial encounter
D - subsequent encounter
S - sequela

S41.0　Open wound of shoulder

S41.00　Unspecified open wound of shoulder

⑦S41.001　Unspecified open wound of right shoulder

⑦S41.002　Unspecified open wound of left shoulder

⑦S41.009　Unspecified open wound of unspecified shoulder

S41.01　Laceration without foreign body of shoulder

⑦S41.011　Laceration without foreign body of right shoulder

⑦S41.012　Laceration without foreign body of left shoulder

⑦S41.019　Laceration without foreign body of unspecified shoulder

S41.02　Laceration with foreign body of shoulder

⑦S41.021　Laceration with foreign body of right shoulder

⑦S41.022　Laceration with foreign body of left shoulder

⑦S41.029　Laceration with foreign body of unspecified shoulder

S41.03　Puncture wound without foreign body of shoulder

⑦S41.031　Puncture wound without foreign body of right shoulder

⑦S41.032　Puncture wound without foreign body of left shoulder

⑦S41.039　Puncture wound without foreign body of unspecified shoulder

S41.04　Puncture wound with foreign body of shoulder

⑦S41.041　Puncture wound with foreign body of right shoulder

⑦S41.042　Puncture wound with foreign body of left shoulder

⑦S41.049　Puncture wound with foreign body of unspecified shoulder

S41.05　Open bite of shoulder
Bite of shoulder NOS
Excludes 1: superficial bite of shoulder (S40.27)

⑦S41.051　Open bite of right shoulder

⑦S41.052　Open bite of left shoulder

⑦S41.059　Open bite of unspecified shoulder

S41.1　Open wound of upper arm

S41.10　Unspecified open wound of upper arm

⑦S41.101　Unspecified open wound of right upper arm

⑦S41.102　Unspecified open wound of left upper arm

⑦S41.109　Unspecified open wound of unspecified upper arm

S41.11　Laceration without foreign body of upper arm

⑦S41.111　Laceration without foreign body of right upper arm

⑦S41.112　Laceration without foreign body of left upper arm

⑦S41.119　Laceration without foreign body of unspecified upper arm

S41.12　Laceration with foreign body of upper arm

⑦S41.121　Laceration with foreign body of right upper arm

⑦S41.122　Laceration with foreign body of left upper arm

⑦S41.129　Laceration with foreign body of unspecified upper arm

S41.13　Puncture wound without foreign body of upper arm

⑦S41.131　Puncture wound without foreign body of right upper arm

⑦S41.132　Puncture wound without foreign body of left upper arm

⑦S41.139　Puncture wound without foreign body of unspecified upper arm

S41.14　Puncture wound with foreign body of upper arm

⑦S41.141　Puncture wound with foreign body of right upper arm

⑦S41.142   Puncture wound with foreign body of left upper arm

⑦S41.149   Puncture wound with foreign body of unspecified upper arm

S41.15   Open bite of upper arm

Bite of upper arm NOS

Excludes 1: superficial bite of upper arm (S40.87)

⑦S41.151   Open bite of right upper arm

⑦S41.152   Open bite of left upper arm

⑦S41.159   Open bite of unspecified upper arm

S42 Fracture of shoulder and upper arm

Note: A fracture not indicated as displaced or nondisplaced should be coded to displaced

A fracture not indicated as open or closed should be coded to closed

Excludes 1: traumatic amputation of shoulder and upper arm (S48.-)

The appropriate 7th character is to be added to all codes from category S42

A - initial encounter for closed fracture

B - initial encounter for open fracture

D - subsequent encounter for fracture with routine healing

G - subsequent encounter for fracture with delayed healing

K - subsequent encounter for fracture with nonunion

P - subsequent encounter for fracture with malunion

S - sequela

S42.0   Fracture of clavicle

S42.00   Fracture of unspecified part of clavicle

⑦S42.001   Fracture of unspecified part of right clavicle

⑦S42.002   Fracture of unspecified part of left clavicle

⑦S42.009   Fracture of unspecified part of unspecified clavicle

S42.01   Fracture of sternal end of clavicle

⑦S42.011   Anterior displaced fracture of sternal end of right clavicle

⑦S42.012   Anterior displaced fracture of sternal end of left clavicle

⑦S42.013   Anterior displaced fracture of sternal end of unspecified clavicle

Displaced fracture of sternal end of clavicle NOS

⑦S42.014   Posterior displaced fracture of sternal end of right clavicle

⑦S42.015   Posterior displaced fracture of sternal end of left clavicle

⑦S42.016   Posterior displaced fracture of sternal end of unspecified clavicle

⑦S42.017   Nondisplaced fracture of sternal end of right clavicle

⑦S42.018   Nondisplaced fracture of sternal end of left clavicle

⑦S42.019   Nondisplaced fracture of sternal end of unspecified clavicle

S42.02   Fracture of shaft of clavicle

⑦S42.021   Displaced fracture of shaft of right clavicle

⑦S42.022   Displaced fracture of shaft of left clavicle

⑦S42.023   Displaced fracture of shaft of unspecified clavicle

⑦S42.024   Nondisplaced fracture of shaft of right clavicle

⑦S42.025   Nondisplaced fracture of shaft of left clavicle

⑦S42.026   Nondisplaced fracture of shaft of unspecified clavicle

S42.03   Fracture of lateral end of clavicle

Fracture of acromial end of clavicle

⑦S42.031   Displaced fracture of lateral end of right clavicle

⑦S42.032   Displaced fracture of lateral end of left clavicle

⑦S42.033   Displaced fracture of lateral end of unspecified clavicle

⑦S42.034   Nondisplaced fracture of lateral end of right clavicle

⑦S42.035   Nondisplaced fracture of lateral end of left clavicle

⑦S42.036   Nondisplaced fracture of lateral end of unspecified clavicle

S42.1   Fracture of scapula

S42.10   Fracture of unspecified part of scapula

⑦S42.101   Fracture of unspecified part of scapula, right shoulder

⑦S42.102   Fracture of unspecified part of scapula, left shoulder

⑦S42.109   Fracture of unspecified part of scapula, unspecified shoulder

S42.11   Fracture of body of scapula

⑦S42.111   Displaced fracture of body of scapula, right shoulder

⑦S42.112   Displaced fracture of body of scapula, left shoulder

⑦S42.113   Displaced fracture of body of scapula, unspecified shoulder

⑦S42.114   Nondisplaced fracture of body of scapula, right shoulder

⑦S42.115   Nondisplaced fracture of body of scapula, left shoulder

⑦S42.116   Nondisplaced fracture of body of scapula, unspecified shoulder

S42.12   Fracture of acromial process

⑦S42.121   Displaced fracture of acromial process, right shoulder

⑦S42.122   Displaced fracture of acromial process, left shoulder

⑦S42.123   Displaced fracture of acromial process, unspecified shoulder

⑦S42.124   Nondisplaced fracture of acromial process, right shoulder

⑦S42.125   Nondisplaced fracture of acromial process, left shoulder

⑦S42.126   Nondisplaced fracture of acromial process, unspecified shoulder

S42.13   Fracture of coracoid process

⑦S42.131   Displaced fracture of coracoid process, right shoulder

⑦S42.132   Displaced fracture of coracoid process, left shoulder

⑦S42.133   Displaced fracture of coracoid process, unspecified shoulder

⑦S42.134   Nondisplaced fracture of coracoid process, right shoulder

⑦S42.135   Nondisplaced fracture of coracoid process, left shoulder

⑦S42.136   Nondisplaced fracture of coracoid process, unspecified shoulder

S42.14   Fracture of glenoid cavity of scapula

⑦S42.141   Displaced fracture of glenoid cavity of scapula, right shoulder

⑦S42.142   Displaced fracture of glenoid cavity of scapula, left shoulder

⑦S42.143   Displaced fracture of glenoid cavity of scapula, unspecified shoulder

⑦S42.144   Nondisplaced fracture of glenoid cavity of scapula, right shoulder

⑦S42.145   Nondisplaced fracture of glenoid cavity of scapula, left shoulder

⑦S42.146   Nondisplaced fracture of glenoid cavity of scapula, unspecified shoulder

S42.15   Fracture of neck of scapula

⑦S42.151   Displaced fracture of neck of scapula, right shoulder

⑦S42.152   Displaced fracture of neck of scapula, left shoulder

⑦S42.153   Displaced fracture of neck of scapula, unspecified shoulder

⑦S42.154   Nondisplaced fracture of neck of scapula, right shoulder

⑦S42.155   Nondisplaced fracture of neck of scapula, left shoulder

⑦S42.156   Nondisplaced fracture of neck of scapula, unspecified shoulder

S42.19   Fracture of other part of scapula

⑦S42.191   Fracture of other part of scapula, right shoulder

⑦S42.192   Fracture of other part of scapula, left shoulder

⑦S42.199   Fracture of other part of scapula, unspecified shoulder

S42.2   Fracture of upper end of humerus
Fracture of proximal end of humerus
Excludes 2: fracture of shaft of humerus (S42.3-)
physeal fracture of upper end of humerus (S49.0-)

S42.20   Unspecified fracture of upper end of humerus

⑦S42.201   Unspecified fracture of upper end of right humerus

⑦S42.202   Unspecified fracture of upper end of left humerus

⑦S42.209   Unspecified fracture of upper end of unspecified humerus

S42.21   Unspecified fracture of surgical neck of humerus
Fracture of neck of humerus NOS

⑦S42.211   Unspecified displaced fracture of surgical neck of right humerus

⑦S42.212   Unspecified displaced fracture of surgical neck of left humerus

⑦S42.213   Unspecified displaced fracture of surgical neck of unspecified humerus

⑦S42.214   Unspecified nondisplaced fracture of surgical neck of right humerus

⑦S42.215   Unspecified nondisplaced fracture of surgical neck of left humerus

⑦S42.216   Unspecified nondisplaced fracture of surgical neck of unspecified humerus

S42.22   2-part fracture of surgical neck of humerus

⑦S42.221   2-part displaced fracture of surgical neck of right humerus

⑦S42.222   2-part displaced fracture of surgical neck of left humerus

⑦S42.223   2-part displaced fracture of surgical neck of unspecified humerus

⑦S42.224   2-part nondisplaced fracture of surgical neck of right humerus

⑦S42.225   2-part nondisplaced fracture of surgical neck of left humerus

⑦S42.226   2-part nondisplaced fracture of surgical neck of unspecified humerus

S42.23   3-part fracture of surgical neck of humerus

⑦S42.231   3-part fracture of surgical neck of right humerus

⑦S42.232   3-part fracture of surgical neck of left humerus

⑦S42.239   3-part fracture of surgical neck of unspecified humerus

S42.24   4-part fracture of surgical neck of humerus

⑦S42.241   4-part fracture of surgical neck of right humerus

⑦S42.242   4-part fracture of surgical neck of left humerus

⑦S42.249   4-part fracture of surgical neck of unspecified humerus

S42.25   Fracture of greater tuberosity of humerus

⑦S42.251   Displaced fracture of greater tuberosity of right humerus

⑦S42.252   Displaced fracture of greater tuberosity of left humerus

⑦S42.253   Displaced fracture of greater tuberosity of unspecified humerus

⑦S42.254   Nondisplaced fracture of greater tuberosity of right humerus

⑦S42.255   Nondisplaced fracture of greater tuberosity of left humerus

⑦S42.256   Nondisplaced fracture of greater tuberosity of unspecified humerus

S42.26   Fracture of lesser tuberosity of humerus

⑦S42.261   Displaced fracture of lesser tuberosity of right humerus

⑦S42.262   Displaced fracture of lesser tuberosity of left humerus

⑦S42.263   Displaced fracture of lesser tuberosity of unspecified humerus

⑦S42.264   Nondisplaced fracture of lesser tuberosity of right humerus

⑦S42.265   Nondisplaced fracture of lesser tuberosity of left humerus

⑦S42.266   Nondisplaced fracture of lesser tuberosity of unspecified humerus

S42.27   Torus fracture of upper end of humerus

The appropriate 7th character is to be added to all codes in subcategory S42.27

A - initial encounter for closed fracture

D - subsequent encounter for fracture with routine healing

G - subsequent encounter for fracture with delayed healing

K - subsequent encounter for fracture with nonunion

P - subsequent encounter for fracture with malunion

S - sequela

⑦S42.271   Torus fracture of upper end of right humerus

⑦S42.272   Torus fracture of upper end of left humerus

⑦S42.279   Torus fracture of upper end of unspecified humerus

S42.29   Other fracture of upper end of humerus

Fracture of anatomical neck of humerus

Fracture of articular head of humerus

⑦S42.291   Other displaced fracture of upper end of right humerus

⑦S42.292   Other displaced fracture of upper end of left humerus

⑦S42.293   Other displaced fracture of upper end of unspecified humerus

⑦S42.294   Other nondisplaced fracture of upper end of right humerus

⑦S42.295   Other nondisplaced fracture of upper end of left humerus

⑦S42.296   Other nondisplaced fracture of upper end of unspecified humerus

S42.3   Fracture of shaft of humerus

Fracture of humerus NOS

Fracture of upper arm NOS

Excludes 2: physeal fractures of upper end of humerus (S49.0-)

physeal fractures of lower end of humerus (S49.1-)

S42.30   Unspecified fracture of shaft of humerus

⑦S42.301   Unspecified fracture of shaft of humerus, right arm

⑦S42.302   Unspecified fracture of shaft of humerus, left arm

⑦S42.309   Unspecified fracture of shaft of humerus, unspecified arm

S42.31   Greenstick fracture of shaft of humerus

The appropriate 7th character is to be added to all codes in subcategory S42.31

A - initial encounter for closed fracture

D - subsequent encounter for fracture with routine healing

G - subsequent encounter for fracture with delayed healing

K - subsequent encounter for fracture with nonunion

P - subsequent encounter for fracture with malunion

S - sequela

⑦S42.311   Greenstick fracture of shaft of humerus, right arm

⑦S42.312   Greenstick fracture of shaft of humerus, left arm

⑦S42.319   Greenstick fracture of shaft of humerus, unspecified arm

S42.32   Transverse fracture of shaft of humerus

⑦S42.321   Displaced transverse fracture of shaft of humerus, right arm

⑦S42.322   Displaced transverse fracture of shaft of humerus, left arm

⑦S42.323   Displaced transverse fracture of shaft of humerus, unspecified arm

⑦S42.324   Nondisplaced transverse fracture of shaft of humerus, right arm

⑦S42.325   Nondisplaced transverse fracture of shaft of humerus, left arm

⑦S42.326   Nondisplaced transverse fracture of shaft of humerus, unspecified arm

S42.33   Oblique fracture of shaft of humerus

⑦S42.331   Displaced oblique fracture of shaft of humerus, right arm

⑦S42.332   Displaced oblique fracture of shaft of humerus, left arm

⑦S42.333   Displaced oblique fracture of shaft of humerus, unspecified arm

⑦S42.334   Nondisplaced oblique fracture of shaft of humerus, right arm

⑦S42.335   Nondisplaced oblique fracture of shaft of humerus, left arm

⑦S42.336   Nondisplaced oblique fracture of shaft of humerus, unspecified arm

S42.34   Spiral fracture of shaft of humerus

⑦S42.341   Displaced spiral fracture of shaft of humerus, right arm

⑦S42.342   Displaced spiral fracture of shaft of humerus, left arm

⑦S42.343   Displaced spiral fracture of shaft of humerus, unspecified arm

⑦S42.344   Nondisplaced spiral fracture of shaft of humerus, right arm

⑦S42.345   Nondisplaced spiral fracture of shaft of humerus, left arm

⑦S42.346   Nondisplaced spiral fracture of shaft of humerus, unspecified arm

S42.35   Comminuted fracture of shaft of humerus

⑦S42.351   Displaced comminuted fracture of shaft of humerus, right arm

⑦S42.352   Displaced comminuted fracture of shaft of humerus, left arm

⑦S42.353   Displaced comminuted fracture of shaft of humerus, unspecified arm

⑦S42.354   Nondisplaced comminuted fracture of shaft of humerus, right arm

⑦S42.355   Nondisplaced comminuted fracture of shaft of humerus, left arm

⑦S42.356   Nondisplaced comminuted fracture of shaft of humerus, unspecified arm

S42.36   Segmental fracture of shaft of humerus

⑦S42.361   Displaced segmental fracture of shaft of humerus, right arm

⑦S42.362   Displaced segmental fracture of shaft of humerus, left arm

⑦S42.363   Displaced segmental fracture of shaft of humerus, unspecified arm

⑦S42.364   Nondisplaced segmental fracture of shaft of humerus, right arm

⑦S42.365   Nondisplaced segmental fracture of shaft of humerus, left arm

⑦S42.366   Nondisplaced segmental fracture of shaft of humerus, unspecified arm

S42.39   Other fracture of shaft of humerus

⑦S42.391   Other fracture of shaft of right humerus

⑦S42.392   Other fracture of shaft of left humerus

⑦S42.399   Other fracture of shaft of unspecified humerus

S42.4   Fracture of lower end of humerus

Fracture of distal end of humerus

Excludes 2:   fracture of shaft of humerus (S42.3-)

physeal fracture of lower end of humerus (S49.1-)

S42.40   Unspecified fracture of lower end of humerus

Fracture of elbow NOS

⑦S42.401   Unspecified fracture of lower end of right humerus

⑦S42.402   Unspecified fracture of lower end of left humerus

⑦S42.409   Unspecified fracture of lower end of unspecified humerus

S42.41   Simple supracondylar fracture without intercondylar fracture of humerus

⑦S42.411   Displaced simple supracondylar fracture without intercondylar fracture of right humerus

⑦S42.412   Displaced simple supracondylar fracture without intercondylar fracture of left humerus

⑦S42.413   Displaced simple supracondylar fracture without intercondylar fracture of unspecified humerus

⑦S42.414   Nondisplaced simple supracondylar fracture without intercondylar fracture of right humerus

⑦S42.415   Nondisplaced simple supracondylar fracture without intercondylar fracture of left humerus

⑦S42.416   Nondisplaced simple supracondylar fracture without intercondylar fracture of unspecified humerus

⑦S42.42   Comminuted supracondylar fracture without intercondylar fracture of humerus

⑦S42.421   Displaced comminuted supracondylar fracture without intercondylar fracture of right humerus

⑦S42.422   Displaced comminuted supracondylar fracture without intercondylar fracture of left humerus

⑦S42.423   Displaced comminuted supracondylar fracture without intercondylar fracture of unspecified humerus

⑦S42.424   Nondisplaced comminuted supracondylar fracture without intercondylar fracture of right humerus

⑦S42.425   Nondisplaced comminuted supracondylar fracture without intercondylar fracture of left humerus

⑦S42.426   Nondisplaced comminuted supracondylar fracture without intercondylar fracture of unspecified humerus

S42.43   Fracture (avulsion) of lateral epicondyle of humerus

⑦S42.431   Displaced fracture (avulsion) of lateral epicondyle of right humerus

⑦S42.432   Displaced fracture (avulsion) of lateral epicondyle of left humerus

⑦S42.433   Displaced fracture (avulsion) of lateral epicondyle of unspecified humerus

⑦S42.434   Nondisplaced fracture (avulsion) of lateral epicondyle of right humerus

⑦S42.435   Nondisplaced fracture (avulsion) of lateral epicondyle of left humerus

⑦S42.436   Nondisplaced fracture (avulsion) of lateral epicondyle of unspecified humerus

S42.44   Fracture (avulsion) of medial epicondyle of humerus

⑦S42.441   Displaced fracture (avulsion) of medial epicondyle of right humerus

⑦S42.442   Displaced fracture (avulsion) of medial epicondyle of left humerus

⑦S42.443   Displaced fracture (avulsion) of medial epicondyle of unspecified humerus

⑦S42.444   Nondisplaced fracture (avulsion) of medial epicondyle of right humerus

⑦S42.445   Nondisplaced fracture (avulsion) of medial epicondyle of left humerus

⑦S42.446   Nondisplaced fracture (avulsion) of medial epicondyle of unspecified humerus

⑦S42.447   Incarcerated fracture (avulsion) of medial epicondyle of right humerus

⑦S42.448   Incarcerated fracture (avulsion) of medial epicondyle of left humerus

⑦S42.449   Incarcerated fracture (avulsion) of medial epicondyle of unspecified humerus

S42.45   Fracture of lateral condyle of humerus
Fracture of capitellum of humerus

⑦S42.451   Displaced fracture of lateral condyle of right humerus

⑦S42.452   Displaced fracture of lateral condyle of left humerus

⑦S42.453   Displaced fracture of lateral condyle of unspecified humerus

⑦S42.454   Nondisplaced fracture of lateral condyle of right humerus

⑦S42.455   Nondisplaced fracture of lateral condyle of left humerus

⑦S42.456   Nondisplaced fracture of lateral condyle of unspecified humerus

S42.46   Fracture of medial condyle of humerus
Trochlea fracture of humerus

⑦S42.461   Displaced fracture of medial condyle of right humerus

⑦S42.462   Displaced fracture of medial condyle of left humerus

⑦S42.463   Displaced fracture of medial condyle of unspecified humerus

⑦S42.464   Nondisplaced fracture of medial condyle of right humerus

⑦S42.465   Nondisplaced fracture of medial condyle of left humerus

⑦S42.466   Nondisplaced fracture of medial condyle of unspecified humerus

S42.47   Transcondylar fracture of humerus

⑦S42.471   Displaced transcondylar fracture of right humerus

⑦S42.472   Displaced transcondylar fracture of left humerus

⑦S42.473   Displaced transcondylar fracture of unspecified humerus

⑦S42.474   Nondisplaced transcondylar fracture of right humerus

⑦S42.475   Nondisplaced transcondylar fracture of left humerus

⑦S42.476   Nondisplaced transcondylar fracture of unspecified humerus

S42.48   Torus fracture of lower end of humerus

The appropriate 7th character is to be added to all codes in subcategory S42.48
A - initial encounter for closed fracture
D - subsequent encounter for fracture with routine healing
G - subsequent encounter for fracture with delayed healing
K - subsequent encounter for fracture with nonunion
P - subsequent encounter for fracture with malunion
S - sequela

⑦S42.481   Torus fracture of lower end of right humerus

⑦S42.482   Torus fracture of lower end of left humerus

⑦S42.489   Torus fracture of lower end of unspecified humerus

S42.49   Other fracture of lower end of humerus

⑦S42.491   Other displaced fracture of lower end of right humerus

⑦S42.492   Other displaced fracture of lower end of left humerus

⑦S42.493   Other displaced fracture of lower end of unspecified humerus

⑦S42.494   Other nondisplaced fracture of lower end of right humerus

⑦S42.495   Other nondisplaced fracture of lower end of left humerus

⑦S42.496   Other nondisplaced fracture of lower end of unspecified humerus

S42.9   Fracture of shoulder girdle, part unspecified
Fracture of shoulder NOS

S42.90   Fracture of unspecified shoulder girdle, part unspecified

S42.91   Fracture of right shoulder girdle, part unspecified

S42.92   Fracture of left shoulder girdle, part unspecified

S43   Dislocation and sprain of joints and ligaments of shoulder girdle

Includes: avulsion of joint or ligament of shoulder girdle
laceration of cartilage, joint or ligament of shoulder girdle
sprain of cartilage, joint or ligament of shoulder girdle
traumatic hemarthrosis of joint or ligament of shoulder girdle
traumatic rupture of joint or ligament of shoulder girdle
traumatic subluxation of joint or ligament of shoulder girdle
traumatic tear of joint or ligament of shoulder girdle

Code also any associated open wound

Excludes 2: strain of muscle, fascia and tendon of shoulder and upper arm (S46.-)

The appropriate 7th character is to be added to each code from category S43
A - initial encounter
D - subsequent encounter
S - sequela

S43.0   Subluxation and dislocation of shoulder joint
Dislocation of glenohumeral joint
Subluxation of glenohumeral joint

  ● New code   ▲ Revised code   ⑦ 7th digit required   ⊗ Placeholder required

S43.00   Unspecified subluxation and dislocation of shoulder joint
           Dislocation of humerus NOS
           Subluxation of humerus NOS

⑦S43.001   Unspecified subluxation of right shoulder joint

⑦S43.002   Unspecified subluxation of left shoulder joint

⑦S43.003   Unspecified subluxation of unspecified shoulder joint

⑦S43.004   Unspecified dislocation of right shoulder joint

⑦S43.005   Unspecified dislocation of left shoulder joint

⑦S43.006   Unspecified dislocation of unspecified shoulder joint

S43.01   Anterior subluxation and dislocation of humerus

⑦S43.011   Anterior subluxation of right humerus

⑦S43.012   Anterior subluxation of left humerus

⑦S43.013   Anterior subluxation of unspecified humerus

⑦S43.014   Anterior dislocation of right humerus

⑦S43.015   Anterior dislocation of left humerus

⑦S43.016   Anterior dislocation of unspecified humerus

S43.02   Posterior subluxation and dislocation of humerus

⑦S43.021   Posterior subluxation of right humerus

⑦S43.022   Posterior subluxation of left humerus

⑦S43.023   Posterior subluxation of unspecified humerus

⑦S43.024   Posterior dislocation of right humerus

⑦S43.025   Posterior dislocation of left humerus

⑦S43.026   Posterior dislocation of unspecified humerus

S43.03   Inferior subluxation and dislocation of humerus

⑦S43.031   Inferior subluxation of right humerus

⑦S43.032   Inferior subluxation of left humerus

⑦S43.033   Inferior subluxation of unspecified humerus

⑦S43.034   Inferior dislocation of right humerus

⑦S43.035   Inferior dislocation of left humerus

⑦S43.036   Inferior dislocation of unspecified humerus

S43.08   Other subluxation and dislocation of shoulder joint

⑦S43.081   Other subluxation of right shoulder joint

⑦S43.082   Other subluxation of left shoulder joint

⑦S43.083   Other subluxation of unspecified shoulder joint

⑦S43.084   Other dislocation of right shoulder joint

⑦S43.085   Other dislocation of left shoulder joint

⑦S43.086   Other dislocation of unspecified shoulder joint

S43.1   Subluxation and dislocation of acromioclavicular joint

S43.10   Unspecified dislocation of acromioclavicular joint

⑦S43.101   Unspecified dislocation of right acromioclavicular joint

⑦S43.102   Unspecified dislocation of left acromioclavicular joint

⑦S43.109   Unspecified dislocation of unspecified acromioclavicular joint

S43.11   Subluxation of acromioclavicular joint

⑦S43.111   Subluxation of right acromioclavicular joint

⑦S43.112   Subluxation of left acromioclavicular joint

⑦S43.119   Subluxation of unspecified acromioclavicular joint

S43.12   Dislocation of acromioclavicular joint, 100%-200% displacement

⑦S43.121   Dislocation of right acromioclavicular joint, 100%-200% displacement

⑦S43.122   Dislocation of left acromioclavicular joint, 100%-200% displacement

⑦S43.129   Dislocation of unspecified acromioclavicular joint, 100%-200% displacement

S43.13   Dislocation of acromioclavicular joint, greater than 200% displacement

⑦S43.131   Dislocation of right acromioclavicular joint, greater than 200% displacement

⑦S43.132   Dislocation of left acromioclavicular joint, greater than 200% displacement

⑦S43.139   Dislocation of unspecified acromioclavicular joint, greater than 200% displacement

S43.14   Inferior dislocation of acromioclavicular joint

⑦S43.141   Inferior dislocation of right acromioclavicular joint

⑦S43.142   Inferior dislocation of left acromioclavicular joint

⑦S43.149   Inferior dislocation of unspecified acromioclavicular joint

S43.15   Posterior dislocation of acromioclavicular joint

⑦S43.151   Posterior dislocation of right acromioclavicular joint

⑦S43.152   Posterior dislocation of left acromioclavicular joint

⑦S43.159   Posterior dislocation of unspecified acromioclavicular joint

S43.2   Subluxation and dislocation of sternoclavicular joint

S43.20   Unspecified subluxation and dislocation of sternoclavicular joint

⑦S43.201   Unspecified subluxation of right sternoclavicular joint

| ■ Add 4th-7th digits | 3 digit reportable | Nonspecific code | Unspecified code | Manifestation code | 641 |

⑦S43.202   Unspecified subluxation of left sternoclavicular joint

⑦S43.203   Unspecified subluxation of unspecified sternoclavicular joint

⑦S43.204   Unspecified dislocation of right sternoclavicular joint

⑦S43.205   Unspecified dislocation of left sternoclavicular joint

⑦S43.206   Unspecified dislocation of unspecified sternoclavicular joint

S43.21   Anterior subluxation and dislocation of sternoclavicular joint

⑦S43.211   Anterior subluxation of right sternoclavicular joint

⑦S43.212   Anterior subluxation of left sternoclavicular joint

⑦S43.213   Anterior subluxation of unspecified sternoclavicular joint

⑦S43.214   Anterior dislocation of right sternoclavicular joint

⑦S43.215   Anterior dislocation of left sternoclavicular joint

⑦S43.216   Anterior dislocation of unspecified sternoclavicular joint

S43.22   Posterior subluxation and dislocation of sternoclavicular joint

⑦S43.221   Posterior subluxation of right sternoclavicular joint

⑦S43.222   Posterior subluxation of left sternoclavicular joint

⑦S43.223   Posterior subluxation of unspecified sternoclavicular joint

⑦S43.224   Posterior dislocation of right sternoclavicular joint

⑦S43.225   Posterior dislocation of left sternoclavicular joint

⑦S43.226   Posterior dislocation of unspecified sternoclavicular joint

S43.3   Subluxation and dislocation of other and unspecified parts of shoulder girdle

S43.30   Subluxation and dislocation of unspecified parts of shoulder girdle

Dislocation of shoulder girdle NOS

Subluxation of shoulder girdle NOS

⑦S43.301   Subluxation of unspecified parts of right shoulder girdle

⑦S43.302   Subluxation of unspecified parts of left shoulder girdle

⑦S43.303   Subluxation of unspecified parts of unspecified shoulder girdle

⑦S43.304   Dislocation of unspecified parts of right shoulder girdle

⑦S43.305   Dislocation of unspecified parts of left shoulder girdle

⑦S43.306   Dislocation of unspecified parts of unspecified shoulder girdle

S43.31   Subluxation and dislocation of scapula

⑦S43.311   Subluxation of right scapula

⑦S43.312   Subluxation of left scapula

⑦S43.313   Subluxation of unspecified scapula

⑦S43.314   Dislocation of right scapula

⑦S43.315   Dislocation of left scapula

⑦S43.316   Dislocation of unspecified scapula

S43.39   Subluxation and dislocation of other parts of shoulder girdle

⑦S43.391   Subluxation of other parts of right shoulder girdle

⑦S43.392   Subluxation of other parts of left shoulder girdle

⑦S43.393   Subluxation of other parts of unspecified shoulder girdle

⑦S43.394   Dislocation of other parts of right shoulder girdle

⑦S43.395   Dislocation of other parts of left shoulder girdle

⑦S43.396   Dislocation of other parts of unspecified shoulder girdle

S43.4   Sprain of shoulder joint

S43.40   Unspecified sprain of shoulder joint

⑦S43.401   Unspecified sprain of right shoulder joint

⑦S43.402   Unspecified sprain of left shoulder joint

⑦S43.409   Unspecified sprain of unspecified shoulder joint

S43.41   Sprain of coracohumeral (ligament)

⑦S43.411   Sprain of right coracohumeral (ligament)

⑦S43.412   Sprain of left coracohumeral (ligament)

⑦S43.419   Sprain of unspecified coracohumeral (ligament)

S43.42   Sprain of rotator cuff capsule

Excludes 1: rotator cuff syndrome (complete) (incomplete), not specified as traumatic (M75.1-)

Excludes 2: injury of tendon of rotator cuff (S46.0-)

⑦S43.421   Sprain of right rotator cuff capsule

⑦S43.422   Sprain of left rotator cuff capsule

⑦S43.429   Sprain of unspecified rotator cuff capsule

S43.43   Superior glenoid labrum lesion

SLAP lesion

⑦S43.431   Superior glenoid labrum lesion of right shoulder

⑦S43.432   Superior glenoid labrum lesion of left shoulder

⑦S43.439   Superior glenoid labrum lesion of unspecified shoulder

S43.49   Other sprain of shoulder joint

⑦S43.491   Other sprain of right shoulder joint

⑦S43.492   Other sprain of left shoulder joint

⑦S43.499   Other sprain of unspecified shoulder joint

S43.5   Sprain of acromioclavicular joint

Sprain of acromioclavicular ligament

   • New code   ▲ Revised code   ⑦ 7th digit required   ⊗ Placeholder required

⊗ ⑦S43.50   Sprain of unspecified acromioclavicular joint

⊗ ⑦S43.51   Sprain of right acromioclavicular joint

⊗ ⑦S43.52   Sprain of left acromioclavicular joint

S43.6   Sprain of sternoclavicular joint

⊗ ⑦S43.60   Sprain of unspecified sternoclavicular joint

⊗ ⑦S43.61   Sprain of right sternoclavicular joint

⊗ ⑦S43.62   Sprain of left sternoclavicular joint

S43.8   Sprain of other specified parts of shoulder girdle

⊗ ⑦S43.80   Sprain of other specified parts of unspecified shoulder girdle

⊗ ⑦S43.81   Sprain of other specified parts of right shoulder girdle

⊗ ⑦S43.82   Sprain of other specified parts of left shoulder girdle

S43.9   Sprain of unspecified parts of shoulder girdle

⊗ ⑦S43.90   Sprain of unspecified parts of unspecified shoulder girdle
Sprain of shoulder girdle NOS

⊗ ⑦S43.91   Sprain of unspecified parts of right shoulder girdle

⊗ ⑦S43.92   Sprain of unspecified parts of left shoulder girdle

S44   Injury of nerves at shoulder and upper arm level
Code also any associated open wound (S41.-)
Excludes 2: injury of brachial plexus (S14.3-)
The appropriate 7th character is to be added to each code from category S44
A - initial encounter
D - subsequent encounter
S - sequela

S44.0   Injury of ulnar nerve at upper arm level
Excludes 1: ulnar nerve NOS (S54.0)

⊗ ⑦S44.00   Injury of ulnar nerve at upper arm level, unspecified arm

⊗ ⑦S44.01   Injury of ulnar nerve at upper arm level, right arm

S44.02   Injury of ulnar nerve at upper arm level, left arm

S44.1   Injury of median nerve at upper arm level
Excludes 1: median nerve NOS (S54.1)

⊗ ⑦S44.10   Injury of median nerve at upper arm level, unspecified arm

⊗ ⑦S44.11   Injury of median nerve at upper arm level, right arm

⊗ ⑦S44.12   Injury of median nerve at upper arm level, left arm

S44.2   Injury of radial nerve at upper arm level
Excludes 1: radial nerve NOS (S54.2)

⊗ ⑦S44.20   Injury of radial nerve at upper arm level, unspecified arm

⊗ ⑦S44.21   Injury of radial nerve at upper arm level, right arm

⊗ ⑦S44.22   Injury of radial nerve at upper arm level, left arm

S44.3   Injury of axillary nerve

⊗ ⑦S44.30   Injury of axillary nerve, unspecified arm

⊗ ⑦S44.31   Injury of axillary nerve, right arm

⊗ ⑦S44.32   Injury of axillary nerve, left arm

S44.4   Injury of musculocutaneous nerve

⊗ ⑦S44.40   Injury of musculocutaneous nerve, unspecified arm

⊗ ⑦S44.41   Injury of musculocutaneous nerve, right arm

⊗ ⑦S44.42   Injury of musculocutaneous nerve, left arm

S44.5   Injury of cutaneous sensory nerve at shoulder and upper arm level

⊗ ⑦S44.50   Injury of cutaneous sensory nerve at shoulder and upper arm level, unspecified arm

⊗ ⑦S44.51   Injury of cutaneous sensory nerve at shoulder and upper arm level, right arm

⊗ ⑦S44.52   Injury of cutaneous sensory nerve at shoulder and upper arm level, left arm

S44.8   Injury of other nerves at shoulder and upper arm level

S44.8X   Injury of other nerves at shoulder and upper arm level

⑦S44.8X1   Injury of other nerves at shoulder and upper arm level, right arm

⑦S44.8X2   Injury of other nerves at shoulder and upper arm level, left arm

⑦S44.8X9   Injury of other nerves at shoulder and upper arm level, unspecified arm

S44.9   Injury of unspecified nerve at shoulder and upper arm level

⊗ ⑦S44.90   Injury of unspecified nerve at shoulder and upper arm level, unspecified arm

⊗ ⑦S44.91   Injury of unspecified nerve at shoulder and upper arm level, right arm

⊗ ⑦S44.92   Injury of unspecified nerve at shoulder and upper arm level, left arm

S45   Injury of blood vessels at shoulder and upper arm level
Code also any associated open wound (S41.-)
Excludes 2: injury of subclavian artery (S25.1)
injury of subclavian vein (S25.3)
The appropriate 7th character is to be added to each code from category S45
A - initial encounter
D - subsequent encounter
S - sequela

S45.0   Injury of axillary artery

S45.00   Unspecified injury of axillary artery

⑦S45.001   Unspecified injury of axillary artery, right side

⑦S45.002   Unspecified injury of axillary artery, left side

⑦S45.009   Unspecified injury of axillary artery, unspecified side

S45.01   Laceration of axillary artery

⑦S45.011   Laceration of axillary artery, right side

⑦S45.012   Laceration of axillary artery, left side

⑦S45.019   Laceration of axillary artery, unspecified side

S45.09   Other specified injury of axillary artery

⑦S45.091   Other specified injury of axillary artery, right side

⑦S45.092   Other specified injury of axillary artery, left side

⑦S45.099   Other specified injury of axillary artery, unspecified side

S45.1   Injury of brachial artery

    S45.10   Unspecified injury of brachial artery

        ⑦**S45.101**   Unspecified injury of brachial artery, right side

        ⑦**S45.102**   Unspecified injury of brachial artery, left side

        ⑦**S45.109**   Unspecified injury of brachial artery, unspecified side

    S45.11   Laceration of brachial artery

        ⑦**S45.111**   Laceration of brachial artery, right side

        ⑦**S45.112**   Laceration of brachial artery, left side

        ⑦**S45.119**   Laceration of brachial artery, unspecified side

    S45.19   Other specified injury of brachial artery

        ⑦**S45.191**   Other specified injury of brachial artery, right side

        ⑦**S45.192**   Other specified injury of brachial artery, left side

        ⑦**S45.199**   Other specified injury of brachial artery, unspecified side

S45.2   Injury of axillary or brachial vein

    S45.20   Unspecified injury of axillary or brachial vein

        ⑦**S45.201**   Unspecified injury of axillary or brachial vein, right side

        ⑦**S45.202**   Unspecified injury of axillary or brachial vein, left side

        ⑦**S45.209**   Unspecified injury of axillary or brachial vein, unspecified side

    S45.21   Laceration of axillary or brachial vein

        ⑦**S45.211**   Laceration of axillary or brachial vein, right side

        ⑦**S45.212**   Laceration of axillary or brachial vein, left side

        ⑦**S45.219**   Laceration of axillary or brachial vein, unspecified side

    S45.29   Other specified injury of axillary or brachial vein

        ⑦**S45.291**   Other specified injury of axillary or brachial vein, right side

        ⑦**S45.292**   Other specified injury of axillary or brachial vein, left side

        ⑦**S45.299**   Other specified injury of axillary or brachial vein, unspecified side

S45.3   Injury of superficial vein at shoulder and upper arm level

    S45.30   Unspecified injury of superficial vein at shoulder and upper arm level

        ⑦**S45.301**   Unspecified injury of superficial vein at shoulder and upper arm level, right arm

        ⑦**S45.302**   Unspecified injury of superficial vein at shoulder and upper arm level, left arm

        ⑦**S45.309**   Unspecified injury of superficial vein at shoulder and upper arm level, unspecified arm

    S45.31   Laceration of superficial vein at shoulder and upper arm level

        ⑦**S45.311**   Laceration of superficial vein at shoulder and upper arm level, right arm

        ⑦**S45.312**   Laceration of superficial vein at shoulder and upper arm level, left arm

        ⑦**S45.319**   Laceration of superficial vein at shoulder and upper arm level, unspecified arm

    S45.39   Other specified injury of superficial vein at shoulder and upper arm level

        ⑦**S45.391**   Other specified injury of superficial vein at shoulder and upper arm level, right arm

        ⑦**S45.392**   Other specified injury of superficial vein at shoulder and upper arm level, left arm

        ⑦**S45.399**   Other specified injury of superficial vein at shoulder and upper arm level, unspecified arm

S45.8   Injury of other specified blood vessels at shoulder and upper arm level

    S45.80   Unspecified injury of other specified blood vessels at shoulder and upper arm level

        ⑦**S45.801**   Unspecified injury of other specified blood vessels at shoulder and upper arm level, right arm

        ⑦**S45.802**   Unspecified injury of other specified blood vessels at shoulder and upper arm level, left arm

        ⑦**S45.809**   Unspecified injury of other specified blood vessels at shoulder and upper arm level, unspecified arm

    S45.81   Laceration of other specified blood vessels at shoulder and upper arm level

        ⑦**S45.811**   Laceration of other specified blood vessels at shoulder and upper arm level, right arm

        ⑦**S45.812**   Laceration of other specified blood vessels at shoulder and upper arm level, left arm

        ⑦**S45.819**   Laceration of other specified blood vessels at shoulder and upper arm level, unspecified arm

    S45.89   Other specified injury of other specified blood vessels at shoulder and upper arm level

        ⑦**S45.891**   Other specified injury of other specified blood vessels at shoulder and upper arm level, right arm

        ⑦**S45.892**   Other specified injury of other specified blood vessels at shoulder and upper arm level, left arm

        ⑦**S45.899**   Other specified injury of other specified blood vessels at shoulder and upper arm level, unspecified arm

S45.9   Injury of unspecified blood vessel at shoulder and upper arm level

    S45.90   Unspecified injury of unspecified blood vessel at shoulder and upper arm level

● New code   ▲ Revised code   ⑦ 7ᵗʰ digit required   ⊗ Placeholder required

⑦**S45.901**   Unspecified injury of unspecified blood vessel at shoulder and upper arm level, right arm

⑦**S45.902**   Unspecified injury of unspecified blood vessel at shoulder and upper arm level, left arm

⑦**S45.909**   Unspecified injury of unspecified blood vessel at shoulder and upper arm level, unspecified arm

S45.91   Laceration of unspecified blood vessel at shoulder and upper arm level

⑦**S45.911**   Laceration of unspecified blood vessel at shoulder and upper arm level, right arm

⑦**S45.912**   Laceration of unspecified blood vessel at shoulder and upper arm level, left arm

⑦**S45.919**   Laceration of unspecified blood vessel at shoulder and upper arm level, unspecified arm

S45.99   Other specified injury of unspecified blood vessel at shoulder and upper arm level

⑦**S45.991**   Other specified injury of unspecified blood vessel at shoulder and upper arm level, right arm

⑦**S45.992**   Other specified injury of unspecified blood vessel at shoulder and upper arm level, left arm

⑦**S45.999**   Other specified injury of unspecified blood vessel at shoulder and upper arm level, unspecified arm

S46   Injury of muscle, fascia and tendon at shoulder and upper arm level
Code also any associated open wound (S41.-)
Excludes 2: injury of muscle, fascia and tendon at elbow (S56.-)
sprain of joints and ligaments of shoulder girdle (S43.9)
The appropriate 7th character is to be added to each code from category S46
A - initial encounter
D - subsequent encounter
S - sequela

S46.0   Injury of muscle(s) and tendon(s) of the rotator cuff of shoulder

S46.00   Unspecified injury of muscle(s) and tendon(s) of the rotator cuff of shoulder

⑦**S46.001**   Unspecified injury of muscle(s) and tendon(s) of the rotator cuff of right shoulder

⑦**S46.002**   Unspecified injury of muscle(s) and tendon(s) of the rotator cuff of left shoulder

⑦**S46.009**   Unspecified injury of muscle(s) and tendon(s) of the rotator cuff of unspecified shoulder

S46.01   Strain of muscle(s) and tendon(s) of the rotator cuff of shoulder

⑦**S46.011**   Strain of muscle(s) and tendon(s) of the rotator cuff of right shoulder

⑦**S46.012**   Strain of muscle(s) and tendon(s) of the rotator cuff of left shoulder

⑦**S46.019**   Strain of muscle(s) and tendon(s) of the rotator cuff of unspecified shoulder

S46.02   Laceration of muscle(s) and tendon(s) of the rotator cuff of shoulder

⑦**S46.021**   Laceration of muscle(s) and tendon(s) of the rotator cuff of right shoulder

⑦**S46.022**   Laceration of muscle(s) and tendon(s) of the rotator cuff of left shoulder

⑦**S46.029**   Laceration of muscle(s) and tendon(s) of the rotator cuff of unspecified shoulder

S46.09   Other injury of muscle(s) and tendon(s) of the rotator cuff of shoulder

⑦**S46.091**   Other injury of muscle(s) and tendon(s) of the rotator cuff of right shoulder

⑦**S46.092**   Other injury of muscle(s) and tendon(s) of the rotator cuff of left shoulder

⑦**S46.099**   Other injury of muscle(s) and tendon(s) of the rotator cuff of unspecified shoulder

S46.1   Injury of muscle, fascia and tendon of long head of biceps

S46.10   Unspecified injury of muscle, fascia and tendon of long head of biceps

⑦**S46.101**   Unspecified injury of muscle, fascia and tendon of long head of biceps, right arm

⑦**S46.102**   Unspecified injury of muscle, fascia and tendon of long head of biceps, left arm

⑦**S46.109**   Unspecified injury of muscle, fascia and tendon of long head of biceps, unspecified arm

S46.11   Strain of muscle, fascia and tendon of long head of biceps

⑦**S46.111**   Strain of muscle, fascia and tendon of long head of biceps, right arm

⑦**S46.112**   Strain of muscle, fascia and tendon of long head of biceps, left arm

⑦**S46.119**   Strain of muscle, fascia and tendon of long head of biceps, unspecified arm

S46.12   Laceration of muscle, fascia and tendon of long head of biceps

⑦**S46.121**   Laceration of muscle, fascia and tendon of long head of biceps, right arm

⑦**S46.122**   Laceration of muscle, fascia and tendon of long head of biceps, left arm

⑦**S46.129**   Laceration of muscle, fascia and tendon of long head of biceps, unspecified arm

S46.19   Other injury of muscle, fascia and tendon of long head of biceps

⑦S46.191   Other injury of muscle, fascia and tendon of long head of biceps, right arm

⑦S46.192   Other injury of muscle, fascia and tendon of long head of biceps, left arm

⑦S46.199   Other injury of muscle, fascia and tendon of long head of biceps, unspecified arm

S46.2   Injury of muscle, fascia and tendon of other parts of biceps

   S46.20   Unspecified injury of muscle, fascia and tendon of other parts of biceps

      ⑦S46.201   Unspecified injury of muscle, fascia and tendon of other parts of biceps, right arm

      ⑦S46.202   Unspecified injury of muscle, fascia and tendon of other parts of biceps, left arm

      ⑦S46.209   Unspecified injury of muscle, fascia and tendon of other parts of biceps, unspecified arm

   S46.21   Strain of muscle, fascia and tendon of other parts of biceps

      ⑦S46.211   Strain of muscle, fascia and tendon of other parts of biceps, right arm

      ⑦S46.212   Strain of muscle, fascia and tendon of other parts of biceps, left arm

      ⑦S46.219   Strain of muscle, fascia and tendon of other parts of biceps, unspecified arm

   S46.22   Laceration of muscle, fascia and tendon of other parts of biceps

      ⑦S46.221   Laceration of muscle, fascia and tendon of other parts of biceps, right arm

      ⑦S46.222   Laceration of muscle, fascia and tendon of other parts of biceps, left arm

      ⑦S46.229   Laceration of muscle, fascia and tendon of other parts of biceps, unspecified arm

   S46.29   Other injury of muscle, fascia and tendon of other parts of biceps

      ⑦S46.291   Other injury of muscle, fascia and tendon of other parts of biceps, right arm

      ⑦S46.292   Other injury of muscle, fascia and tendon of other parts of biceps, left arm

      ⑦S46.299   Other injury of muscle, fascia and tendon of other parts of biceps, unspecified arm

S46.3   Injury of muscle, fascia and tendon of triceps

   S46.30   Unspecified injury of muscle, fascia and tendon of triceps

      ⑦S46.301   Unspecified injury of muscle, fascia and tendon of triceps, right arm

      ⑦S46.302   Unspecified injury of muscle, fascia and tendon of triceps, left arm

      ⑦S46.309   Unspecified injury of muscle, fascia and tendon of triceps, unspecified arm

   S46.31   Strain of muscle, fascia and tendon of triceps

      ⑦S46.311   Strain of muscle, fascia and tendon of triceps, right arm

      ⑦S46.312   Strain of muscle, fascia and tendon of triceps, left arm

      ⑦S46.319   Strain of muscle, fascia and tendon of triceps, unspecified arm

   S46.32   Laceration of muscle, fascia and tendon of triceps

      ⑦S46.321   Laceration of muscle, fascia and tendon of triceps, right arm

      ⑦S46.322   Laceration of muscle, fascia and tendon of triceps, left arm

      ⑦S46.329   Laceration of muscle, fascia and tendon of triceps, unspecified arm

   S46.39   Other injury of muscle, fascia and tendon of triceps

      ⑦S46.391   Other injury of muscle, fascia and tendon of triceps, right arm

      ⑦S46.392   Other injury of muscle, fascia and tendon of triceps, left arm

      ⑦S46.399   Other injury of muscle, fascia and tendon of triceps, unspecified arm

S46.8   Injury of other muscles, fascia and tendons at shoulder and upper arm level

   S46.80   Unspecified injury of other muscles, fascia and tendons at shoulder and upper arm level

      ⑦S46.801   Unspecified injury of other muscles, fascia and tendons at shoulder and upper arm level, right arm

      ⑦S46.802   Unspecified injury of other muscles, fascia and tendons at shoulder and upper arm level, left arm

      ⑦S46.809   Unspecified injury of other muscles, fascia and tendons at shoulder and upper arm level, unspecified arm

   S46.81   Strain of other muscles, fascia and tendons at shoulder and upper arm level

      ⑦S46.811   Strain of other muscles, fascia and tendons at shoulder and upper arm level, right arm

      ⑦S46.812   Strain of other muscles, fascia and tendons at shoulder and upper arm level, left arm

      ⑦S46.819   Strain of other muscles, fascia and tendons at shoulder and upper arm level, unspecified arm

      ⑦S46.82   Laceration of other muscles, fascia and tendons at shoulder and upper arm level

      ⑦S46.821   Laceration of other muscles, fascia and tendons at shoulder and upper arm level, right arm

      ⑦S46.822   Laceration of other muscles, fascia and tendons at shoulder and upper arm level, left arm

⑦S46.829 Laceration of other muscles, fascia and tendons at shoulder and upper arm level, unspecified arm

⑦S46.89 Other injury of other muscles, fascia and tendons at shoulder and upper arm level

⑦S46.891 Other injury of other muscles, fascia and tendons at shoulder and upper arm level, right arm

⑦S46.892 Other injury of other muscles, fascia and tendons at shoulder and upper arm level, left arm

⑦S46.899 Other injury of other muscles, fascia and tendons at shoulder and upper arm level, unspecified arm

S46.9 Injury of unspecified muscle, fascia and tendon at shoulder and upper arm level

S46.90 Unspecified injury of unspecified muscle, fascia and tendon at shoulder and upper arm level

⑦S46.901 Unspecified injury of unspecified muscle, fascia and tendon at shoulder and upper arm level, right arm

⑦S46.902 Unspecified injury of unspecified muscle, fascia and tendon at shoulder and upper arm level, left arm

⑦S46.909 Unspecified injury of unspecified muscle, fascia and tendon at shoulder and upper arm level, unspecified arm

S46.91 Strain of unspecified muscle, fascia and tendon at shoulder and upper arm level

⑦S46.911 Strain of unspecified muscle, fascia and tendon at shoulder and upper arm level, right arm

⑦S46.912 Strain of unspecified muscle, fascia and tendon at shoulder and upper arm level, left arm

⑦S46.919 Strain of unspecified muscle, fascia and tendon at shoulder and upper arm level, unspecified arm

S46.92 Laceration of unspecified muscle, fascia and tendon at shoulder and upper arm level

⑦S46.921 Laceration of unspecified muscle, fascia and tendon at shoulder and upper arm level, right arm

⑦S46.922 Laceration of unspecified muscle, fascia and tendon at shoulder and upper arm level, left arm

⑦S46.929 Laceration of unspecified muscle, fascia and tendon at shoulder and upper arm level, unspecified arm

S46.99 Other injury of unspecified muscle, fascia and tendon at shoulder and upper arm level

⑦S46.991 Other injury of unspecified muscle, fascia and tendon at shoulder and upper arm level, right arm

⑦S46.992 Other injury of unspecified muscle, fascia and tendon at shoulder and upper arm level, left arm

⑦S46.999 Other injury of unspecified muscle, fascia and tendon at shoulder and upper arm level, unspecified arm

S47 Crushing injury of shoulder and upper arm
Use additional code for all associated injuries
Excludes 2: crushing injury of elbow (S57.0-)
The appropriate 7th character is to be added to each code from category S47
A - initial encounter
D - subsequent encounter
S - sequela
S47.1 Crushing injury of right shoulder and upper arm
S47.2 Crushing injury of left shoulder and upper arm
S47.9 Crushing injury of shoulder and upper arm, unspecified arm

S48 Traumatic amputation of shoulder and upper arm
An amputation not identified as partial or complete should be coded to complete
Excludes 1: traumatic amputation at elbow level (S58.0)
The appropriate 7th character is to be added to each code from category S48
A - initial encounter
D - subsequent encounter
S - sequela
S48.0 Traumatic amputation at shoulder joint
S48.01 Complete traumatic amputation at shoulder joint
⑦S48.011 Complete traumatic amputation at right shoulder joint
⑦S48.012 Complete traumatic amputation at left shoulder joint
⑦S48.019 Complete traumatic amputation at unspecified shoulder joint
S48.02 Partial traumatic amputation at shoulder joint
⑦S48.021 Partial traumatic amputation at right shoulder joint
⑦S48.022 Partial traumatic amputation at left shoulder joint
⑦S48.029 Partial traumatic amputation at unspecified shoulder joint
S48.1 Traumatic amputation at level between shoulder and elbow
S48.11 Complete traumatic amputation at level between shoulder and elbow
⑦S48.111 Complete traumatic amputation at level between right shoulder and elbow
⑦S48.112 Complete traumatic amputation at level between left shoulder and elbow
⑦S48.119 Complete traumatic amputation at level between unspecified shoulder and elbow
S48.12 Partial traumatic amputation at level between shoulder and elbow
⑦S48.121 Partial traumatic amputation at level between right shoulder and elbow
⑦S48.122 Partial traumatic amputation at level between left shoulder and elbow
⑦S48.129 Partial traumatic amputation at level between unspecified shoulder and elbow

S48.9   Traumatic amputation of shoulder and upper arm, level unspecified

    S48.91   Complete traumatic amputation of shoulder and upper arm, level unspecified

       ⑦S48.911   Complete traumatic amputation of right shoulder and upper arm, level unspecified

       ⑦S48.912   Complete traumatic amputation of left shoulder and upper arm, level unspecified

       ⑦S48.919   Complete traumatic amputation of unspecified shoulder and upper arm, level unspecified

    S48.92   Partial traumatic amputation of shoulder and upper arm, level unspecified

       ⑦S48.921   Partial traumatic amputation of right shoulder and upper arm, level unspecified

       ⑦S48.922   Partial traumatic amputation of left shoulder and upper arm, level unspecified

       ⑦S48.929   Partial traumatic amputation of unspecified shoulder and upper arm, level unspecified

S49   Other and unspecified injuries of shoulder and upper arm

The appropriate 7th character is to be added to each code from subcategories S49.0 and S49.1

A - initial encounter for closed fracture

D - subsequent encounter for fracture with routine healing

G - subsequent encounter for fracture with delayed healing

K - subsequent encounter for fracture with nonunion

P - subsequent encounter for fracture with malunion

S - sequela

S49.0   Physeal fracture of upper end of humerus

    S49.00   Unspecified physeal fracture of upper end of humerus

       ⑦S49.001   Unspecified physeal fracture of upper end of humerus, right arm

       ⑦S49.002   Unspecified physeal fracture of upper end of humerus, left arm

       ⑦S49.009   Unspecified physeal fracture of upper end of humerus, unspecified arm

    S49.01   Salter-Harris Type I physeal fracture of upper end of humerus

       ⑦S49.011   Salter-Harris Type I physeal fracture of upper end of humerus, right arm

       ⑦S49.012   Salter-Harris Type I physeal fracture of upper end of humerus, left arm

       ⑦S49.019   Salter-Harris Type I physeal fracture of upper end of humerus, unspecified arm

    S49.02   Salter-Harris Type II physeal fracture of upper end of humerus

       ⑦S49.021   Salter-Harris Type II physeal fracture of upper end of humerus, right arm

       ⑦S49.022   Salter-Harris Type II physeal fracture of upper end of humerus, left arm

       ⑦S49.029   Salter-Harris Type II physeal fracture of upper end of humerus, unspecified arm

    S49.03   Salter-Harris Type III physeal fracture of upper end of humerus

       ⑦S49.031   Salter Harris Type III physeal fracture of upper end of humerus, right arm

       ⑦S49.032   Salter Harris Type III physeal fracture of upper end of humerus, left arm

       ⑦S49.039   Salter Harris Type III physeal fracture of upper end of humerus, unspecified arm

    S49.04   Salter-Harris Type IV physeal fracture of upper end of humerus

       ⑦S49.041   Salter-Harris Type IV physeal fracture of upper end of humerus, right arm

       ⑦S49.042   Salter-Harris Type IV physeal fracture of upper end of humerus, left arm

       ⑦S49.049   Salter-Harris Type IV physeal fracture of upper end of humerus, unspecified arm

    S49.09   Other physeal fracture of upper end of humerus

       ⑦S49.091   Other physeal fracture of upper end of humerus, right arm

       ⑦S49.092   Other physeal fracture of upper end of humerus, left arm

       ⑦S49.099   Other physeal fracture of upper end of humerus, unspecified arm

S49.1   Physeal fracture of lower end of humerus

    S49.10   Unspecified physeal fracture of lower end of humerus

       ⑦S49.101   Unspecified physeal fracture of lower end of humerus, right arm

       ⑦S49.102   Unspecified physeal fracture of lower end of humerus, left arm

       ⑦S49.109   Unspecified physeal fracture of lower end of humerus, unspecified arm

    S49.11   Salter-Harris Type I physeal fracture of lower end of humerus

       ⑦S49.111   Salter-Harris Type I physeal fracture of lower end of humerus, right arm

       ⑦S49.112   Salter-Harris Type I physeal fracture of lower end of humerus, left arm

       ⑦S49.119   Salter-Harris Type I physeal fracture of lower end of humerus, unspecified arm

    S49.12   Salter-Harris Type II physeal fracture of lower end of humerus

       ⑦S49.121   Salter-Harris Type II physeal fracture of lower end of humerus, right arm

       ⑦S49.122   Salter-Harris Type II physeal fracture of lower end of humerus, left arm

● New code   ▲ Revised code   ⑦ 7ᵗʰ digit required   ⊗ Placeholder required

⑦**S49.129** Salter-Harris Type II physeal fracture of lower end of humerus, unspecified arm

S49.13 Salter Harris Type III physeal fracture of lower end of humerus

⑦**S49.131** Salter Harris Type III physeal fracture of lower end of humerus, right arm

⑦**S49.132** Salter Harris Type III physeal fracture of lower end of humerus, left arm

⑦**S49.139** Salter Harris Type III physeal fracture of lower end of humerus, unspecified arm

S49.14 Salter-Harris Type IV physeal fracture of lower end of humerus

⑦**S49.141** Salter-Harris Type IV physeal fracture of lower end of humerus, right arm

⑦**S49.142** Salter-Harris Type IV physeal fracture of lower end of humerus, left arm

⑦**S49.149** Salter-Harris Type IV physeal fracture of lower end of humerus, unspecified arm

S49.19 Other physeal fracture of lower end of humerus

⑦**S49.191** Other physeal fracture of lower end of humerus, right arm

⑦**S49.192** Other physeal fracture of lower end of humerus, left arm

⑦**S49.199** Other physeal fracture of lower end of humerus, unspecified arm

S49.8 Other specified injuries of shoulder and upper arm

The appropriate 7th character is to be added to each code in subcategory S49.8

A - initial encounter
D - subsequent encounter
S - sequela

⊗⑦**S49.80** Other specified injuries of shoulder and upper arm, unspecified arm

⊗⑦**S49.81** Other specified injuries of right shoulder and upper arm

⊗⑦**S49.82** Other specified injuries of left shoulder and upper arm

S49.9 Unspecified injury of shoulder and upper arm

The appropriate 7th character is to be added to each code in subcategory S49.9

A - initial encounter
D - subsequent encounter
S - sequela

⊗⑦**S49.90** Unspecified injury of shoulder and upper arm, unspecified arm

⊗⑦**S49.91** Unspecified injury of right shoulder and upper arm

⊗⑦**S49.92** Unspecified injury of left shoulder and upper arm

INJURIES TO THE ELBOW AND FOREARM (S50-S59)

Excludes 2: burns and corrosions (T20-T32)
frostbite (T33-T34)

injuries of wrist and hand (S60-S69)
insect bite or sting, venomous (T63.4)

S50 Superficial injury of elbow and forearm
Excludes 2: superficial injury of wrist and hand (S60.-)

The appropriate 7th character is to be added to each code from category S50

A - initial encounter
D - subsequent encounter
S - sequela

S50.0 Contusion of elbow

⊗⑦**S50.00** Contusion of unspecified elbow
⊗⑦**S50.01** Contusion of right elbow
⊗⑦**S50.02** Contusion of left elbow

S50.1 Contusion of forearm

⊗⑦**S50.10** Contusion of unspecified forearm
⊗⑦**S50.11** Contusion of right forearm
⊗⑦**S50.12** Contusion of left forearm

S50.3 Other superficial injuries of elbow

S50.31 Abrasion of elbow

⑦**S50.311** Abrasion of right elbow
⑦**S50.312** Abrasion of left elbow
⑦**S50.319** Abrasion of unspecified elbow

S50.32 Blister (nonthermal) of elbow

⑦**S50.321** Blister (nonthermal) of right elbow
⑦**S50.322** Blister (nonthermal) of left elbow
⑦**S50.329** Blister (nonthermal) of unspecified elbow

S50.34 External constriction of elbow

⑦**S50.341** External constriction of right elbow
⑦**S50.342** External constriction of left elbow
⑦**S50.349** External constriction of unspecified elbow

S50.35 Superficial foreign body of elbow
Splinter in the elbow

⑦**S50.351** Superficial foreign body of right elbow
⑦**S50.352** Superficial foreign body of left elbow
⑦**S50.359** Superficial foreign body of unspecified elbow

S50.36 Insect bite (nonvenomous) of elbow

⑦**S50.361** Insect bite (nonvenomous) of right elbow
⑦**S50.362** Insect bite (nonvenomous) of left elbow
⑦**S50.369** Insect bite (nonvenomous) of unspecified elbow

S50.37 Other superficial bite of elbow
Excludes 1: open bite of elbow (S51.04)

⑦**S50.371** Other superficial bite of right elbow
⑦**S50.372** Other superficial bite of left elbow
⑦**S50.379** Other superficial bite of unspecified elbow

S50.8 Other superficial injuries of forearm

S50.81 Abrasion of forearm

⑦**S50.811** Abrasion of right forearm
⑦**S50.812** Abrasion of left forearm

⑦S50.819   Abrasion of unspecified forearm

S50.82   Blister (nonthermal) of forearm

    ⑦S50.821   Blister (nonthermal) of right forearm

    ⑦S50.822   Blister (nonthermal) of left forearm

    ⑦S50.829   Blister (nonthermal) of unspecified forearm

S50.84   External constriction of forearm

    ⑦S50.841   External constriction of right forearm

    ⑦S50.842   External constriction of left forearm

    ⑦S50.849   External constriction of unspecified forearm

S50.85   Superficial foreign body of forearm

     Splinter in the forearm

    ⑦S50.851   Superficial foreign body of right forearm

    ⑦S50.852   Superficial foreign body of left forearm

    ⑦S50.859   Superficial foreign body of unspecified forearm

S50.86   Insect bite (nonvenomous) of forearm

    ⑦S50.861   Insect bite (nonvenomous) of right forearm

    ⑦S50.862   Insect bite (nonvenomous) of left forearm

    ⑦S50.869   Insect bite (nonvenomous) of unspecified forearm

S50.87   Other superficial bite of forearm

    Excludes 1: open bite of forearm (S51.84)

    ⑦S50.871   Other superficial bite of right forearm

    ⑦S50.872   Other superficial bite of left forearm

    ⑦S50.879   Other superficial bite of unspecified forearm

S50.9   Unspecified superficial injury of elbow and forearm

   S50.90   Unspecified superficial injury of elbow

     ⑦S50.901   Unspecified superficial injury of right elbow

     ⑦S50.902   Unspecified superficial injury of left elbow

     ⑦S50.909   Unspecified superficial injury of unspecified elbow

   S50.91   Unspecified superficial injury of forearm

     ⑦S50.911   Unspecified superficial injury of right forearm

     ⑦S50.912   Unspecified superficial injury of left forearm

     ⑦S50.919   Unspecified superficial injury of unspecified forearm

S51   Open wound of elbow and forearm

Code also any associated wound infection

Excludes 1: open fracture of elbow and forearm (S52.- with open fracture 7th character)

    traumatic amputation of elbow and forearm (S58.-)

Excludes 2: open wound of wrist and hand (S61.-)

The appropriate 7th character is to be added to each code from category S51

A - initial encounter

D - subsequent encounter

S - sequela

S51.0   Open wound of elbow

   S51.00   Unspecified open wound of elbow

     ⑦S51.001   Unspecified open wound of right elbow

     ⑦S51.002   Unspecified open wound of left elbow

     ⑦S51.009   Unspecified open wound of unspecified elbow

      Open wound of elbow NOS

   S51.01   Laceration without foreign body of elbow

     ⑦S51.011   Laceration without foreign body of right elbow

     ⑦S51.012   Laceration without foreign body of left elbow

     ⑦S51.019   Laceration without foreign body of unspecified elbow

   S51.02   Laceration with foreign body of elbow

     ⑦S51.021   Laceration with foreign body of right elbow

     ⑦S51.022   Laceration with foreign body of left elbow

     ⑦S51.029   Laceration with foreign body of unspecified elbow

   S51.03   Puncture wound without foreign body of elbow

     ⑦S51.031   Puncture wound without foreign body of right elbow

     ⑦S51.032   Puncture wound without foreign body of left elbow

     ⑦S51.039   Puncture wound without foreign body of unspecified elbow

   S51.04   Puncture wound with foreign body of elbow

     ⑦S51.041   Puncture wound with foreign body of right elbow

     ⑦S51.042   Puncture wound with foreign body of left elbow

     ⑦S51.049   Puncture wound with foreign body of unspecified elbow

   S51.05   Open bite of elbow

     Bite of elbow NOS

     Excludes 1: superficial bite of elbow (S50.36, S50.37)

     ⑦S51.051   Open bite, right elbow

     ⑦S51.052   Open bite, left elbow

     ⑦S51.059   Open bite, unspecified elbow

S51.8   Open wound of forearm

Excludes 2: open wound of elbow (S51.0-)

   S51.80   Unspecified open wound of forearm

     ⑦S51.801   Unspecified open wound of right forearm

     ⑦S51.802   Unspecified open wound of left forearm

     ⑦S51.809   Unspecified open wound of unspecified forearm

      Open wound of forearm NOS

   ● New code   ▲ Revised code   ⑦ 7th digit required   ⊗ Placeholder required

S51.81   Laceration without foreign body of forearm
    ⑦ S51.811   Laceration without foreign body of right forearm
    ⑦ S51.812   Laceration without foreign body of left forearm
    ⑦ S51.819   Laceration without foreign body of unspecified forearm

S51.82   Laceration with foreign body of forearm
    ⑦ S51.821   Laceration with foreign body of right forearm
    ⑦ S51.822   Laceration with foreign body of left forearm
    ⑦ S51.829   Laceration with foreign body of unspecified forearm

S51.83   Puncture wound without foreign body of forearm
    ⑦ S51.831   Puncture wound without foreign body of right forearm
    ⑦ S51.832   Puncture wound without foreign body of left forearm
    ⑦ S51.839   Puncture wound without foreign body of unspecified forearm

S51.84   Puncture wound with foreign body of forearm
    ⑦ S51.841   Puncture wound with foreign body of right forearm
    ⑦ S51.842   Puncture wound with foreign body of left forearm
    ⑦ S51.849   Puncture wound with foreign body of unspecified forearm

S51.85   Open bite of forearm
    Bite of forearm NOS
    Excludes 1: superficial bite of forearm (S50.86, S50.87)
    ⑦ S51.851   Open bite of right forearm
    ⑦ S51.852   Open bite of left forearm
    ⑦ S51.859   Open bite of unspecified forearm

S52 Fracture of forearm

Note: A fracture not indicated as displaced or nondisplaced should be coded to displaced

A fracture not indicated as open or closed should be coded to closed

The open fracture designations are based on the Gustilo open fracture classification

Excludes 1: traumatic amputation of forearm (S58.-)

Excludes 2: fracture at wrist and hand level (S62.-)

The appropriate 7th character is to be added to all codes from category S52

A - initial encounter for closed fracture

B - initial encounter for open fracture type I or II initial encounter for open fracture NOS

C - initial encounter for open fracture type IIIA, IIIB, or IIIC

D - subsequent encounter for closed fracture with routine healing

E - subsequent encounter for open fracture type I or II with routine healing

F - subsequent encounter for open fracture type IIIA, IIIB, or IIIC with routine healing

G - subsequent encounter for closed fracture with delayed healing

H - subsequent encounter for open fracture type I or II with delayed healing

J - subsequent encounter for open fracture type IIIA, IIIB, or IIIC with delayed healing

K - subsequent encounter for closed fracture with nonunion

M - subsequent encounter for open fracture type I or II with nonunion

N - subsequent encounter for open fracture type IIIA, IIIB, or IIIC with nonunion

P - subsequent encounter for closed fracture with malunion

Q - subsequent encounter for open fracture type I or II with malunion

R - subsequent encounter for open fracture type IIIA, IIIB, or IIIC with malunion

S - sequela

S52.0   Fracture of upper end of ulna
    Fracture of proximal end of ulna
    Excludes 2: fracture of elbow NOS (S42.40-)
        fractures of shaft of ulna (S52.2-)

S52.00   Unspecified fracture of upper end of ulna
    ⑦ S52.001   Unspecified fracture of upper end of right ulna
    ⑦ S52.002   Unspecified fracture of upper end of left ulna
    ⑦ S52.009   Unspecified fracture of upper end of unspecified ulna

S52.01   Torus fracture of upper end of ulna
    The appropriate 7th character is to be added to all codes in subcategory S52.01

A - initial encounter for closed fracture

D - subsequent encounter for fracture with routine healing

G - subsequent encounter for fracture with delayed healing

K - subsequent encounter for fracture with nonunion

P - subsequent encounter for fracture with malunion

S - sequela

    ⑦ S52.011   Torus fracture of upper end of right ulna
    ⑦ S52.012   Torus fracture of upper end of left ulna
    ⑦ S52.019   Torus fracture of upper end of unspecified ulna

S52.02   Fracture of olecranon process without intraarticular extension of ulna
    ⑦ S52.021   Displaced fracture of olecranon process without intraarticular extension of right ulna
    ⑦ S52.022   Displaced fracture of olecranon process without intraarticular extension of left ulna
    ⑦ S52.023   Displaced fracture of olecranon process without intraarticular extension of unspecified ulna
    ⑦ S52.024   Nondisplaced fracture of olecranon process without intraarticular extension of right ulna
    ⑦ S52.025   Nondisplaced fracture of olecranon process without intraarticular extension of left ulna

⑦S52.026   Nondisplaced fracture of olecranon process without intraarticular extension of unspecified ulna

S52.03   Fracture of olecranon process with intraarticular extension of ulna

⑦S52.031   Displaced fracture of olecranon process with intraarticular extension of right ulna

⑦S52.032   Displaced fracture of olecranon process with intraarticular extension of left ulna

⑦S52.033   Displaced fracture of olecranon process with intraarticular extension of unspecified ulna

⑦S52.034   Nondisplaced fracture of olecranon process with intraarticular extension of right ulna

⑦S52.035   Nondisplaced fracture of olecranon process with intraarticular extension of left ulna

⑦S52.036   Nondisplaced fracture of olecranon process with intraarticular extension of unspecified ulna

S52.04   Fracture of coronoid process of ulna

⑦S52.041   Displaced fracture of coronoid process of right ulna

⑦S52.042   Displaced fracture of coronoid process of left ulna

⑦S52.043   Displaced fracture of coronoid process of unspecified ulna

⑦S52.044   Nondisplaced fracture of coronoid process of right ulna

⑦S52.045   Nondisplaced fracture of coronoid process of left ulna

⑦S52.046   Nondisplaced fracture of coronoid process of unspecified ulna

S52.09   Other fracture of upper end of ulna

⑦S52.091   Other fracture of upper end of right ulna

⑦S52.092   Other fracture of upper end of left ulna

⑦S52.099   Other fracture of upper end of unspecified ulna

S52.1   Fracture of upper end of radius
Fracture of proximal end of radius
Excludes 2: physeal fractures of upper end of radius (S59.2-)
fracture of shaft of radius (S52.3-)

S52.10   Unspecified fracture of upper end of radius

⑦S52.101   Unspecified fracture of upper end of right radius

⑦S52.102   Unspecified fracture of upper end of left radius

⑦S52.109   Unspecified fracture of upper end of unspecified radius

S52.11   Torus fracture of upper end of radius
The appropriate 7th character is to be added to all codes in subcategory S52.11
A - initial encounter for closed fracture

D - subsequent encounter for fracture with routine healing

G - subsequent encounter for fracture with delayed healing

K - subsequent encounter for fracture with nonunion

P - subsequent encounter for fracture with malunion

S - sequela

⑦S52.111   Torus fracture of upper end of right radius

⑦S52.112   Torus fracture of upper end of left radius

⑦S52.119   Torus fracture of upper end of unspecified radius

S52.12   Fracture of head of radius

⑦S52.121   Displaced fracture of head of right radius

⑦S52.122   Displaced fracture of head of left radius

⑦S52.123   Displaced fracture of head of unspecified radius

⑦S52.124   Nondisplaced fracture of head of right radius

⑦S52.125   Nondisplaced fracture of head of left radius

⑦S52.126   Nondisplaced fracture of head of unspecified radius

S52.13   Fracture of neck of radius

⑦S52.131   Displaced fracture of neck of right radius

⑦S52.132   Displaced fracture of neck of left radius

⑦S52.133   Displaced fracture of neck of unspecified radius

⑦S52.134   Nondisplaced fracture of neck of right radius

⑦S52.135   Nondisplaced fracture of neck of left radius

⑦S52.136   Nondisplaced fracture of neck of unspecified radius

S52.18   Other fracture of upper end of radius

⑦S52.181   Other fracture of upper end of right radius

⑦S52.182   Other fracture of upper end of left radius

⑦S52.189   Other fracture of upper end of unspecified radius

S52.2   Fracture of shaft of ulna

S52.20   Unspecified fracture of shaft of ulna
Fracture of ulna NOS

⑦S52.201   Unspecified fracture of shaft of right ulna

⑦S52.202   Unspecified fracture of shaft of left ulna

⑦S52.209   Unspecified fracture of shaft of unspecified ulna

S52.21   Greenstick fracture of shaft of ulna

The appropriate 7th character is to be added to all codes in subcategory S52.21

A - initial encounter for closed fracture

D - subsequent encounter for fracture with routine healing

G - subsequent encounter for fracture with delayed healing

K - subsequent encounter for fracture with nonunion

P - subsequent encounter for fracture with malunion

S - sequela

⑦S52.211   Greenstick fracture of shaft of right ulna

⑦S52.212   Greenstick fracture of shaft of left ulna

⑦S52.219   Greenstick fracture of shaft of unspecified ulna

S52.22   Transverse fracture of shaft of ulna

⑦S52.221   Displaced transverse fracture of shaft of right ulna

⑦S52.222   Displaced transverse fracture of shaft of left ulna

⑦S52.223   Displaced transverse fracture of shaft of unspecified ulna

⑦S52.224   Nondisplaced transverse fracture of shaft of right ulna

⑦S52.225   Nondisplaced transverse fracture of shaft of left ulna

⑦S52.226   Nondisplaced transverse fracture of shaft of unspecified ulna

S52.23   Oblique fracture of shaft of ulna

⑦S52.231   Displaced oblique fracture of shaft of right ulna

⑦S52.232   Displaced oblique fracture of shaft of left ulna

⑦S52.233   Displaced oblique fracture of shaft of unspecified ulna

⑦S52.234   Nondisplaced oblique fracture of shaft of right ulna

⑦S52.235   Nondisplaced oblique fracture of shaft of left ulna

⑦S52.236   Nondisplaced oblique fracture of shaft of unspecified ulna

S52.24   Spiral fracture of shaft of ulna

⑦S52.241   Displaced spiral fracture of shaft of ulna, right arm

⑦S52.242   Displaced spiral fracture of shaft of ulna, left arm

⑦S52.243   Displaced spiral fracture of shaft of ulna, unspecified arm

⑦S52.244   Nondisplaced spiral fracture of shaft of ulna, right arm

⑦S52.245   Nondisplaced spiral fracture of shaft of ulna, left arm

⑦S52.246   Nondisplaced spiral fracture of shaft of ulna, unspecified arm

S52.25   Comminuted fracture of shaft of ulna

⑦S52.251   Displaced comminuted fracture of shaft of ulna, right arm

⑦S52.252   Displaced comminuted fracture of shaft of ulna, left arm

⑦S52.253   Displaced comminuted fracture of shaft of ulna, unspecified arm

⑦S52.254   Nondisplaced comminuted fracture of shaft of ulna, right arm

⑦S52.255   Nondisplaced comminuted fracture of shaft of ulna, left arm

⑦S52.256   Nondisplaced comminuted fracture of shaft of ulna, unspecified arm

S52.26   Segmental fracture of shaft of ulna

⑦S52.261   Displaced segmental fracture of shaft of ulna, right arm

⑦S52.262   Displaced segmental fracture of shaft of ulna, left arm

⑦S52.263   Displaced segmental fracture of shaft of ulna, unspecified arm

⑦S52.264   Nondisplaced segmental fracture of shaft of ulna, right arm

⑦S52.265   Nondisplaced segmental fracture of shaft of ulna, left arm

⑦S52.266   Nondisplaced segmental fracture of shaft of ulna, unspecified arm

S52.27   Monteggia's fracture of ulna

Fracture of upper shaft of ulna with dislocation of radial head

⑦S52.271   Monteggia's fracture of right ulna

⑦S52.272   Monteggia's fracture of left ulna

⑦S52.279   Monteggia's fracture of unspecified ulna

S52.28   Bent bone of ulna

⑦S52.281   Bent bone of right ulna

⑦S52.282   Bent bone of left ulna

⑦S52.283   Bent bone of unspecified ulna

S52.29   Other fracture of shaft of ulna

⑦S52.291   Other fracture of shaft of right ulna

⑦S52.292   Other fracture of shaft of left ulna

⑦S52.299   Other fracture of shaft of unspecified ulna

S52.3   Fracture of shaft of radius

S52.30   Unspecified fracture of shaft of radius

⑦S52.301   Unspecified fracture of shaft of right radius

⑦S52.302   Unspecified fracture of shaft of left radius

⑦S52.309   Unspecified fracture of shaft of unspecified radius

S52.31   Greenstick fracture of shaft of radius

The appropriate 7th character is to be added to all codes in subcategory S52.31

A - initial encounter for closed fracture

D - subsequent encounter for fracture with routine healing

G - subsequent encounter for fracture with delayed healing

K - subsequent encounter for fracture with nonunion

P - subsequent encounter for fracture with malunion

S - sequela

⑦S52.311 Greenstick fracture of shaft of radius, right arm

⑦S52.312 Greenstick fracture of shaft of radius, left arm

⑦S52.319 Greenstick fracture of shaft of radius, unspecified arm

S52.32 Transverse fracture of shaft of radius

⑦S52.321 Displaced transverse fracture of shaft of right radius

⑦S52.322 Displaced transverse fracture of shaft of left radius

⑦S52.323 Displaced transverse fracture of shaft of unspecified radius

⑦S52.324 Nondisplaced transverse fracture of shaft of right radius

⑦S52.325 Nondisplaced transverse fracture of shaft of left radius

⑦S52.326 Nondisplaced transverse fracture of shaft of unspecified radius

S52.33 Oblique fracture of shaft of radius

⑦S52.331 Displaced oblique fracture of shaft of right radius

⑦S52.332 Displaced oblique fracture of shaft of left radius

⑦S52.333 Displaced oblique fracture of shaft of unspecified radius

⑦S52.334 Nondisplaced oblique fracture of shaft of right radius

⑦S52.335 Nondisplaced oblique fracture of shaft of left radius

⑦S52.336 Nondisplaced oblique fracture of shaft of unspecified radius

S52.34 Spiral fracture of shaft of radius

⑦S52.341 Displaced spiral fracture of shaft of radius, right arm

⑦S52.342 Displaced spiral fracture of shaft of radius, left arm

⑦S52.343 Displaced spiral fracture of shaft of radius, unspecified arm

⑦S52.344 Nondisplaced spiral fracture of shaft of radius, right arm

⑦S52.345 Nondisplaced spiral fracture of shaft of radius, left arm

⑦S52.346 Nondisplaced spiral fracture of shaft of radius, unspecified arm

S52.35 Comminuted fracture of shaft of radius

⑦S52.351 Displaced comminuted fracture of shaft of radius, right arm

⑦S52.352 Displaced comminuted fracture of shaft of radius, left arm

⑦S52.353 Displaced comminuted fracture of shaft of radius, unspecified arm

⑦S52.354 Nondisplaced comminuted fracture of shaft of radius, right arm

⑦S52.355 Nondisplaced comminuted fracture of shaft of radius, left arm

⑦S52.356 Nondisplaced comminuted fracture of shaft of radius, unspecified arm

S52.36 Segmental fracture of shaft of radius

⑦S52.361 Displaced segmental fracture of shaft of radius, right arm

⑦S52.362 Displaced segmental fracture of shaft of radius, left arm

⑦S52.363 Displaced segmental fracture of shaft of radius, unspecified arm

⑦S52.364 Nondisplaced segmental fracture of shaft of radius, right arm

⑦S52.365 Nondisplaced segmental fracture of shaft of radius, left arm

⑦S52.366 Nondisplaced segmental fracture of shaft of radius, unspecified arm

S52.37 Galeazzi's fracture

Fracture of lower shaft of radius with radioulnar joint dislocation

⑦S52.371 Galeazzi's fracture of right radius

⑦S52.372 Galeazzi's fracture of left radius

⑦S52.379 Galeazzi's fracture of unspecified radius

S52.38 Bent bone of radius

⑦S52.381 Bent bone of right radius

⑦S52.382 Bent bone of left radius

⑦S52.389 Bent bone of unspecified radius

S52.39 Other fracture of shaft of radius

⑦S52.391 Other fracture of shaft of radius, right arm

⑦S52.392 Other fracture of shaft of radius, left arm

⑦S52.399 Other fracture of shaft of radius, unspecified arm

S52.5 Fracture of lower end of radius

Fracture of distal end of radius

Excludes 2: physeal fractures of lower end of radius (S59.2-)

S52.50 Unspecified fracture of the lower end of radius

⑦S52.501 Unspecified fracture of the lower end of right radius

⑦S52.502 Unspecified fracture of the lower end of left radius

⑦S52.509 Unspecified fracture of the lower end of unspecified radius

S52.51 Fracture of radial styloid process

⑦S52.511 Displaced fracture of right radial styloid process

⑦S52.512 Displaced fracture of left radial styloid process

⑦S52.513 Displaced fracture of unspecified radial styloid process

⑦S52.514 Nondisplaced fracture of right radial styloid process

⑦S52.515 Nondisplaced fracture of left radial styloid process

⑦S52.516 Nondisplaced fracture of unspecified radial styloid process

S52.52   Torus fracture of lower end of radius

The appropriate 7th character is to be added to all codes in subcategory S52.52

A - initial encounter for closed fracture

D - subsequent encounter for fracture with routine healing

G - subsequent encounter for fracture with delayed healing

K - subsequent encounter for fracture with nonunion

P - subsequent encounter for fracture with malunion

S - sequela

⑦S52.521   Torus fracture of lower end of right radius

⑦S52.522   Torus fracture of lower end of left radius

⑦S52.529   Torus fracture of lower end of unspecified radius

S52.53   Colles' fracture

⑦S52.531   Colles' fracture of right radius

⑦S52.532   Colles' fracture of left radius

⑦S52.539   Colles' fracture of unspecified radius

S52.54   Smith's fracture

⑦S52.541   Smith's fracture of right radius

⑦S52.542   Smith's fracture of left radius

⑦S52.549   Smith's fracture of unspecified radius

S52.55   Other extraarticular fracture of lower end of radius

⑦S52.551   Other extraarticular fracture of lower end of right radius

⑦S52.552   Other extraarticular fracture of lower end of left radius

⑦S52.559   Other extraarticular fracture of lower end of unspecified radius

S52.56   Barton's fracture

⑦S52.561   Barton's fracture of right radius

⑦S52.562   Barton's fracture of left radius

⑦S52.569   Barton's fracture of unspecified radius

S52.57   Other intraarticular fracture of lower end of radius

⑦S52.571   Other intraarticular fracture of lower end of right radius

⑦S52.572   Other intraarticular fracture of lower end of left radius

⑦S52.579   Other intraarticular fracture of lower end of unspecified radius

S52.59   Other fractures of lower end of radius

⑦S52.591   Other fractures of lower end of right radius

⑦S52.592   Other fractures of lower end of left radius

⑦S52.599   Other fractures of lower end of unspecified radius

S52.6   Fracture of lower end of ulna

S52.60   Unspecified fracture of lower end of ulna

⑦S52.601   Unspecified fracture of lower end of right ulna

⑦S52.602   Unspecified fracture of lower end of left ulna

⑦S52.609   Unspecified fracture of lower end of unspecified ulna

S52.61   Fracture of ulna styloid process

⑦S52.611   Displaced fracture of right ulna styloid process

⑦S52.612   Displaced fracture of left ulna styloid process

⑦S52.613   Displaced fracture of unspecified ulna styloid process

⑦S52.614   Nondisplaced fracture of right ulna styloid process

⑦S52.615   Nondisplaced fracture of left ulna styloid process

⑦S52.616   Nondisplaced fracture of unspecified ulna styloid process

S52.62   Torus fracture of lower end of ulna

The appropriate 7th character is to be added to all codes in subcategory S52.62

A - initial encounter for closed fracture

D - subsequent encounter for fracture with routine healing

G - subsequent encounter for fracture with delayed healing

K - subsequent encounter for fracture with nonunion

P - subsequent encounter for fracture with malunion

S - sequela

⑦S52.621   Torus fracture of lower end of right ulna

⑦S52.622   Torus fracture of lower end of left ulna

⑦S52.629   Torus fracture of lower end of unspecified ulna

S52.69   Other fracture of lower end of ulna

⑦S52.691   Other fracture of lower end of right ulna

⑦S52.692   Other fracture of lower end of left ulna

⑦S52.699   Other fracture of lower end of unspecified ulna

S52.9   Unspecified fracture of forearm

⊗⑦S52.90   Unspecified fracture of unspecified forearm

⊗⑦S52.91   Unspecified fracture of right forearm

⊗⑦S52.92   Unspecified fracture of left forearm

S53   Dislocation and sprain of joints and ligaments of elbow

Includes: avulsion of joint or ligament of elbow

laceration of cartilage, joint or ligament of elbow

sprain of cartilage, joint or ligament of elbow

traumatic hemarthrosis of joint or ligament of elbow

traumatic rupture of joint or ligament of elbow

traumatic subluxation of joint or ligament of elbow

traumatic tear of joint or ligament of elbow

Code also any associated open wound

Excludes 2: strain of muscle, fascia and tendon at forearm level (S56.-)

The appropriate 7th character is to be added to each code from category S53

A - initial encounter

D - subsequent encounter

S - sequela

S53.0   Subluxation and dislocation of radial head

Dislocation of radiohumeral joint

Subluxation of radiohumeral joint

Excludes 1: Monteggia's fracture-dislocation (S52.27-)

S53.00   Unspecified subluxation and dislocation of radial head

⑦**S53.001**   Unspecified subluxation of right radial head

⑦**S53.002**   Unspecified subluxation of left radial head

⑦**S53.003**   Unspecified subluxation of unspecified radial head

⑦**S53.004**   Unspecified dislocation of right radial head

⑦**S53.005**   Unspecified dislocation of left radial head

⑦**S53.006**   Unspecified dislocation of unspecified radial head

S53.01   Anterior subluxation and dislocation of radial head

Anteromedial subluxation and dislocation of radial head

⑦**S53.011**   Anterior subluxation of right radial head

⑦**S53.012**   Anterior subluxation of left radial head

⑦**S53.013**   Anterior subluxation of unspecified radial head

⑦**S53.014**   Anterior dislocation of right radial head

⑦**S53.015**   Anterior dislocation of left radial head

⑦**S53.016**   Anterior dislocation of unspecified radial head

S53.02   Posterior subluxation and dislocation of radial head

Posterolateral subluxation and dislocation of radial head

⑦**S53.021**   Posterior subluxation of right radial head

⑦**S53.022**   Posterior subluxation of left radial head

⑦**S53.023**   Posterior subluxation of unspecified radial head

⑦**S53.024**   Posterior dislocation of right radial head

⑦**S53.025**   Posterior dislocation of left radial head

⑦**S53.026**   Posterior dislocation of unspecified radial head

S53.03   Nursemaid's elbow

⑦**S53.031**   Nursemaid's elbow, right elbow

⑦**S53.032**   Nursemaid's elbow, left elbow

⑦**S53.033**   Nursemaid's elbow, unspecified elbow

S53.09   Other subluxation and dislocation of radial head

⑦**S53.091**   Other subluxation of right radial head

⑦**S53.092**   Other subluxation of left radial head

⑦**S53.093**   Other subluxation of unspecified radial head

⑦**S53.094**   Other dislocation of right radial head

⑦**S53.095**   Other dislocation of left radial head

⑦**S53.096**   Other dislocation of unspecified radial head

S53.1   Subluxation and dislocation of ulnohumeral joint

Subluxation and dislocation of elbow NOS

Excludes 1: dislocation of radial head alone (S53.0-)

S53.10   Unspecified subluxation and dislocation of ulnohumeral joint

⑦**S53.101**   Unspecified subluxation of right ulnohumeral joint

⑦**S53.102**   Unspecified subluxation of left ulnohumeral joint

⑦**S53.103**   Unspecified subluxation of unspecified ulnohumeral joint

⑦**S53.104**   Unspecified dislocation of right ulnohumeral joint

⑦**S53.105**   Unspecified dislocation of left ulnohumeral joint

⑦**S53.106**   Unspecified dislocation of unspecified ulnohumeral joint

S53.11   Anterior subluxation and dislocation of ulnohumeral joint

⑦**S53.111**   Anterior subluxation of right ulnohumeral joint

⑦**S53.112**   Anterior subluxation of left ulnohumeral joint

⑦**S53.113**   Anterior subluxation of unspecified ulnohumeral joint

⑦**S53.114**   Anterior dislocation of right ulnohumeral joint

⑦**S53.115**   Anterior dislocation of left ulnohumeral joint

⑦**S53.116**   Anterior dislocation of unspecified ulnohumeral joint

S53.12   Posterior subluxation and dislocation of ulnohumeral joint

⑦**S53.121**   Posterior subluxation of right ulnohumeral joint

⑦**S53.122**   Posterior subluxation of left ulnohumeral joint

⑦**S53.123**   Posterior subluxation of unspecified ulnohumeral joint

⑦**S53.124**   Posterior dislocation of right ulnohumeral joint

⑦**S53.125**   Posterior dislocation of left ulnohumeral joint

⑦S53.126   Posterior dislocation of unspecified ulnohumeral joint

S53.13   Medial subluxation and dislocation of ulnohumeral joint

⑦S53.131   Medial subluxation of right ulnohumeral joint

⑦S53.132   Medial subluxation of left ulnohumeral joint

⑦S53.133   Medial subluxation of unspecified ulnohumeral joint

⑦S53.134   Medial dislocation of right ulnohumeral joint

⑦S53.135   Medial dislocation of left ulnohumeral joint

⑦S53.136   Medial dislocation of unspecified ulnohumeral joint

S53.14   Lateral subluxation and dislocation of ulnohumeral joint

⑦S53.141   Lateral subluxation of right ulnohumeral joint

⑦S53.142   Lateral subluxation of left ulnohumeral joint

⑦S53.143   Lateral subluxation of unspecified ulnohumeral joint

⑦S53.144   Lateral dislocation of right ulnohumeral joint

⑦S53.145   Lateral dislocation of left ulnohumeral joint

⑦S53.146   Lateral dislocation of unspecified ulnohumeral joint

S53.19   Other subluxation and dislocation of ulnohumeral joint

⑦S53.191   Other subluxation of right ulnohumeral joint

⑦S53.192   Other subluxation of left ulnohumeral joint

⑦S53.193   Other subluxation of unspecified ulnohumeral joint

⑦S53.194   Other dislocation of right ulnohumeral joint

⑦S53.195   Other dislocation of left ulnohumeral joint

⑦S53.196   Other dislocation of unspecified ulnohumeral joint

S53.2   Traumatic rupture of radial collateral ligament

Excludes 1: sprain of radial collateral ligament NOS (S53.43-)

⊗⑦S53.20   Traumatic rupture of unspecified radial collateral ligament

⊗⑦S53.21   Traumatic rupture of right radial collateral ligament

⊗⑦S53.22   Traumatic rupture of left radial collateral ligament

S53.3   Traumatic rupture of ulnar collateral ligament

Excludes 1: sprain of ulnar collateral ligament (S53.44-)

⊗⑦S53.30   Traumatic rupture of unspecified ulnar collateral ligament

⊗⑦S53.31   Traumatic rupture of right ulnar collateral ligament

⊗⑦S53.32   Traumatic rupture of left ulnar collateral ligament

S53.4   Sprain of elbow

Excludes 2: traumatic rupture of radial collateral ligament (S53.2-)

traumatic rupture of ulnar collateral ligament (S53.3-)

S53.40   Unspecified sprain of elbow

⑦S53.401   Unspecified sprain of right elbow

⑦S53.402   Unspecified sprain of left elbow

⑦S53.409   Unspecified sprain of unspecified elbow

Sprain of elbow NOS

S53.41   Radiohumeral (joint) sprain

⑦S53.411   Radiohumeral (joint) sprain of right elbow

⑦S53.412   Radiohumeral (joint) sprain of left elbow

⑦S53.419   Radiohumeral (joint) sprain of unspecified elbow

S53.42   Ulnohumeral (joint) sprain

⑦S53.421   Ulnohumeral (joint) sprain of right elbow

⑦S53.422   Ulnohumeral (joint) sprain of left elbow

⑦S53.429   Ulnohumeral (joint) sprain of unspecified elbow

S53.43   Radial collateral ligament sprain

⑦S53.431   Radial collateral ligament sprain of right elbow

⑦S53.432   Radial collateral ligament sprain of left elbow

⑦S53.439   Radial collateral ligament sprain of unspecified elbow

S53.44   Ulnar collateral ligament sprain

⑦S53.441   Ulnar collateral ligament sprain of right elbow

⑦S53.442   Ulnar collateral ligament sprain of left elbow

⑦S53.449   Ulnar collateral ligament sprain of unspecified elbow

S53.49   Other sprain of elbow

⑦S53.491   Other sprain of right elbow

⑦S53.492   Other sprain of left elbow

⑦S53.499   Other sprain of unspecified elbow

S54   Injury of nerves at forearm level

Code also any associated open wound (S51.-)

Excludes 2: injury of nerves at wrist and hand level (S64.-)

The appropriate 7th character is to be added to each code from category S54

A - initial encounter

D - subsequent encounter

S - sequela

S54.0   Injury of ulnar nerve at forearm level

Injury of ulnar nerve NOS

⊗⑦S54.00   Injury of ulnar nerve at forearm level, unspecified arm

⊗⑦S54.01   Injury of ulnar nerve at forearm level, right arm

⊗⑦**S54.02**   Injury of ulnar nerve at forearm level, left arm

S54.1   Injury of median nerve at forearm level
      Injury of median nerve NOS

⊗⑦**S54.10**   Injury of median nerve at forearm level, unspecified arm

⊗⑦**S54.11**   Injury of median nerve at forearm level, right arm

⊗⑦**S54.12**   Injury of median nerve at forearm level, left arm

S54.2   Injury of radial nerve at forearm level
      Injury of radial nerve NOS

⊗⑦**S54.20**   Injury of radial nerve at forearm level, unspecified arm

⊗⑦**S54.21**   Injury of radial nerve at forearm level, right arm

⊗⑦**S54.22**   Injury of radial nerve at forearm level, left arm

S54.3   Injury of cutaneous sensory nerve at forearm level

⊗⑦**S54.30**   Injury of cutaneous sensory nerve at forearm level, unspecified arm

⊗⑦**S54.31**   Injury of cutaneous sensory nerve at forearm level, right arm

⊗⑦**S54.32**   Injury of cutaneous sensory nerve at forearm level, left arm

S54.8   Injury of other nerves at forearm level

S54.8X   Injury of other nerves at forearm level

⑦**S54.8X1**   Unspecified injury of other nerves at forearm level, right arm

⑦**S54.8X2**   Unspecified injury of other nerves at forearm level, left arm

⑦**S54.8X9**   Unspecified injury of other nerves at forearm level, unspecified arm

S54.9   Injury of unspecified nerve at forearm level

⊗⑦**S54.90**   Injury of unspecified nerve at forearm level, unspecified arm

⊗⑦**S54.91**   Injury of unspecified nerve at forearm level, right arm

⊗⑦**S54.92**   Injury of unspecified nerve at forearm level, left arm

S55   Injury of blood vessels at forearm level

Code also any associated open wound (S51.-)

Excludes 2: injury of blood vessels at wrist and hand level (S65.-)
      injury of brachial vessels (S45.1-S45.2)

The appropriate 7th character is to be added to each code from category S55

A - initial encounter

D - subsequent encounter

S - sequela

S55.0   Injury of ulnar artery at forearm level

S55.00   Unspecified injury of ulnar artery at forearm level

⑦**S55.001**   Unspecified injury of ulnar artery at forearm level, right arm

⑦**S55.002**   Unspecified injury of ulnar artery at forearm level, left arm

⑦**S55.009**   Unspecified injury of ulnar artery at forearm level, unspecified arm

S55.01   Laceration of ulnar artery at forearm level

⑦**S55.011**   Laceration of ulnar artery at forearm level, right arm

⑦**S55.012**   Laceration of ulnar artery at forearm level, left arm

⑦**S55.019**   Laceration of ulnar artery at forearm level, unspecified arm

S55.09   Other specified injury of ulnar artery at forearm level

⑦**S55.091**   Other specified injury of ulnar artery at forearm level, right arm

⑦**S55.092**   Other specified injury of ulnar artery at forearm level, left arm

⑦**S55.099**   Other specified injury of ulnar artery at forearm level, unspecified arm

S55.1   Injury of radial artery at forearm level

S55.10   Unspecified injury of radial artery at forearm level

⑦**S55.101**   Unspecified injury of radial artery at forearm level, right arm

⑦**S55.102**   Unspecified injury of radial artery at forearm level, left arm

⑦**S55.109**   Unspecified injury of radial artery at forearm level, unspecified arm

S55.11   Laceration of radial artery at forearm level

⑦**S55.111**   Laceration of radial artery at forearm level, right arm

⑦**S55.112**   Laceration of radial artery at forearm level, left arm

⑦**S55.119**   Laceration of radial artery at forearm level, unspecified arm

S55.19   Other specified injury of radial artery at forearm level

⑦**S55.191**   Other specified injury of radial artery at forearm level, right arm

⑦**S55.192**   Other specified injury of radial artery at forearm level, left arm

⑦**S55.199**   Other specified injury of radial artery at forearm level, unspecified arm

S55.2   Injury of vein at forearm level

S55.20   Unspecified injury of vein at forearm level

⑦**S55.201**   Unspecified injury of vein at forearm level, right arm

⑦**S55.202**   Unspecified injury of vein at forearm level, left arm

⑦**S55.209**   Unspecified injury of vein at forearm level, unspecified arm

S55.21   Laceration of vein at forearm level

⑦**S55.211**   Laceration of vein at forearm level, right arm

⑦**S55.212**   Laceration of vein at forearm level, left arm

⑦**S55.219**   Laceration of vein at forearm level, unspecified arm

S55.29   Other specified injury of vein at forearm level

⑦**S55.291**   Other specified injury of vein at forearm level, right arm

⑦**S55.292**   Other specified injury of vein at forearm level, left arm

⑦**S55.299**   Other specified injury of vein at forearm level, unspecified arm

S55.8   Injury of other blood vessels at forearm level

    S55.80   Unspecified injury of other blood vessels at forearm level

        ⑦S55.801   Unspecified injury of other blood vessels at forearm level, right arm

        ⑦S55.802   Unspecified injury of other blood vessels at forearm level, left arm

        ⑦S55.809   Unspecified injury of other blood vessels at forearm level, unspecified arm

    S55.81   Laceration of other blood vessels at forearm level

        ⑦S55.811   Laceration of other blood vessels at forearm level, right arm

        ⑦S55.812   Laceration of other blood vessels at forearm level, left arm

        ⑦S55.819   Laceration of other blood vessels at forearm level, unspecified arm

    S55.89   Other specified injury of other blood vessels at forearm level

        ⑦S55.891   Other specified injury of other blood vessels at forearm level, right arm

        ⑦S55.892   Other specified injury of other blood vessels at forearm level, left arm

        ⑦S55.899   Other specified injury of other blood vessels at forearm level, unspecified arm

S55.9   Injury of unspecified blood vessel at forearm level

    S55.90   Unspecified injury of unspecified blood vessel at forearm level

        ⑦S55.901   Unspecified injury of unspecified blood vessel at forearm level, right arm

        ⑦S55.902   Unspecified injury of unspecified blood vessel at forearm level, left arm

        ⑦S55.909   Unspecified injury of unspecified blood vessel at forearm level, unspecified arm

    S55.91   Laceration of unspecified blood vessel at forearm level

        ⑦S55.911   Laceration of unspecified blood vessel at forearm level, right arm

        ⑦S55.912   Laceration of unspecified blood vessel at forearm level, left arm

        ⑦S55.919   Laceration of unspecified blood vessel at forearm level, unspecified arm

    S55.99   Other specified injury of unspecified blood vessel at forearm level

        ⑦S55.991   Other specified injury of unspecified blood vessel at forearm level, right arm

        ⑦S55.992   Other specified injury of unspecified blood vessel at forearm level, left arm

        ⑦S55.999   Other specified injury of unspecified blood vessel at forearm level, unspecified arm

S56   Injury of muscle, fascia and tendon at forearm level

Code also any associated open wound (S51.-)

Excludes 2:   injury of muscle, fascia and tendon at or below wrist (S66.-)

        sprain of joints and ligaments of elbow (S53.4-)

The appropriate 7th character is to be added to each code from category S56

A - initial encounter

D - subsequent encounter

S - sequela

S56.0   Injury of flexor muscle, fascia and tendon of thumb at forearm level

    S56.00   Unspecified injury of flexor muscle, fascia and tendon of thumb at forearm level

        ⑦S56.001   Unspecified injury of flexor muscle, fascia and tendon of right thumb at forearm level

        ⑦S56.002   Unspecified injury of flexor muscle, fascia and tendon of left thumb at forearm level

        ⑦S56.009   Unspecified injury of flexor muscle, fascia and tendon of unspecified thumb at forearm level

    S56.01   Strain of flexor muscle, fascia and tendon of thumb at forearm level

        ⑦S56.011   Strain of flexor muscle, fascia and tendon of right thumb at forearm level

        ⑦S56.012   Strain of flexor muscle, fascia and tendon of left thumb at forearm level

        ⑦S56.019   Strain of flexor muscle, fascia and tendon of unspecified thumb at forearm level

    S56.02   Laceration of flexor muscle, fascia and tendon of thumb at forearm level

        ⑦S56.021   Laceration of flexor muscle, fascia and tendon of right thumb at forearm level

        ⑦S56.022   Laceration of flexor muscle, fascia and tendon of left thumb at forearm level

        ⑦S56.029   Laceration of flexor muscle, fascia and tendon of unspecified thumb at forearm level

    S56.09   Other injury of flexor muscle, fascia and tendon of thumb at forearm level

        ⑦S56.091   Other injury of flexor muscle, fascia and tendon of right thumb at forearm level

        ⑦S56.092   Other injury of flexor muscle, fascia and tendon of left thumb at forearm level

        ⑦S56.099   Other injury of flexor muscle, fascia and tendon of unspecified thumb at forearm level

S56.1   Injury of flexor muscle, fascia and tendon of other and unspecified finger at forearm level

    S56.10   Unspecified injury of flexor muscle, fascia and tendon of other and unspecified finger at forearm level

        ⑦S56.101   Unspecified injury of flexor muscle, fascia and tendon of right index finger at forearm level

---

| | Add 4th-7th digits | | 3 digit reportable | | Nonspecific code | | Unspecified code | | Manifestation code | 659 |

⑦S56.102   Unspecified injury of flexor muscle, fascia and tendon of left index finger at forearm level

⑦S56.103   Unspecified injury of flexor muscle, fascia and tendon of right middle finger at forearm level

⑦S56.104   Unspecified injury of flexor muscle, fascia and tendon of left middle finger at forearm level

⑦S56.105   Unspecified injury of flexor muscle, fascia and tendon of right ring finger at forearm level

⑦S56.106   Unspecified injury of flexor muscle, fascia and tendon of left ring finger at forearm level

⑦S56.107   Unspecified injury of flexor muscle, fascia and tendon of right little finger at forearm level

⑦S56.108   Unspecified injury of flexor muscle, fascia and tendon of left little finger at forearm level

⑦S56.109   Unspecified injury of flexor muscle, fascia and tendon of unspecified finger at forearm level

S56.11   Strain of flexor muscle, fascia and tendon of other and unspecified finger at forearm level

⑦S56.111   Strain of flexor muscle, fascia and tendon of right index finger at forearm level

⑦S56.112   Strain of flexor muscle, fascia and tendon of left index finger at forearm level

⑦S56.113   Strain of flexor muscle, fascia and tendon of right middle finger at forearm level

⑦S56.114   Strain of flexor muscle, fascia and tendon of left middle finger at forearm level

⑦S56.115   Strain of flexor muscle, fascia and tendon of right ring finger at forearm level

⑦S56.116   Strain of flexor muscle, fascia and tendon of left ring finger at forearm level

⑦S56.117   Strain of flexor muscle, fascia and tendon of right little finger at forearm level

⑦S56.118   Strain of flexor muscle, fascia and tendon of left little finger at forearm level

⑦S56.119   Strain of flexor muscle, fascia and tendon of finger of unspecified finger at forearm level

S56.12   Laceration of flexor muscle, fascia and tendon of other and unspecified finger at forearm level

⑦S56.121   Laceration of flexor muscle, fascia and tendon of right index finger at forearm level

⑦S56.122   Laceration of flexor muscle, fascia and tendon of left index finger at forearm level

⑦S56.123   Laceration of flexor muscle, fascia and tendon of right middle finger at forearm level

⑦S56.124   Laceration of flexor muscle, fascia and tendon of left middle finger at forearm level

⑦S56.125   Laceration of flexor muscle, fascia and tendon of right ring finger at forearm level

⑦S56.126   Laceration of flexor muscle, fascia and tendon of left ring finger at forearm level

⑦S56.127   Laceration of flexor muscle, fascia and tendon of right little finger at forearm level

⑦S56.128   Laceration of flexor muscle, fascia and tendon of left little finger at forearm level

⑦S56.129   Laceration of flexor muscle, fascia and tendon of unspecified finger at forearm level

S56.19   Other injury of flexor muscle, fascia and tendon of other and unspecified finger at forearm level

⑦S56.191   Other injury of flexor muscle, fascia and tendon of right index finger at forearm level

⑦S56.192   Other injury of flexor muscle, fascia and tendon of left index finger at forearm level

⑦S56.193   Other injury of flexor muscle, fascia and tendon of right middle finger at forearm level

⑦S56.194   Other injury of flexor muscle, fascia and tendon of left middle finger at forearm level

⑦S56.195   Other injury of flexor muscle, fascia and tendon of right ring finger at forearm level

⑦S56.196   Other injury of flexor muscle, fascia and tendon of left ring finger at forearm level

⑦S56.197   Other injury of flexor muscle, fascia and tendon of right little finger at forearm level

⑦S56.198   Other injury of flexor muscle, fascia and tendon of left little finger at forearm level

⑦S56.199   Other injury of flexor muscle, fascia and tendon of unspecified finger at forearm level

S56.2   Injury of other flexor muscle, fascia and tendon at forearm level

S56.20   Unspecified injury of other flexor muscle, fascia and tendon at forearm level

⑦S56.201   Unspecified injury of other flexor muscle, fascia and tendon at forearm level, right arm

⑦S56.202   Unspecified injury of other flexor muscle, fascia and tendon at forearm level, left arm

⑦S56.209   Unspecified injury of other flexor muscle, fascia and tendon at forearm level, unspecified arm

S56.21   Strain of other flexor muscle, fascia and tendon at forearm level

⑦S56.211   Strain of other flexor muscle, fascia and tendon at forearm level, right arm

⑦S56.212   Strain of other flexor muscle, fascia and tendon at forearm level, left arm

⑦S56.219   Strain of other flexor muscle, fascia and tendon at forearm level, unspecified arm

S56.22   Laceration of other flexor muscle, fascia and tendon at forearm level

⑦S56.221   Laceration of other flexor muscle, fascia and tendon at forearm level, right arm

⑦S56.222   Laceration of other flexor muscle, fascia and tendon at forearm level, left arm

⑦S56.229   Laceration of other flexor muscle, fascia and tendon at forearm level, unspecified arm

S56.29   Other injury of other flexor muscle, fascia and tendon at forearm level

⑦S56.291   Other injury of other flexor muscle, fascia and tendon at forearm level, right arm

⑦S56.292   Other injury of other flexor muscle, fascia and tendon at forearm level, left arm

⑦S56.299   Other injury of other flexor muscle, fascia and tendon at forearm level, unspecified arm

S56.3   Injury of extensor or abductor muscles, fascia and tendons of thumb at forearm level

S56.30   Unspecified injury of extensor or abductor muscles, fascia and tendons of thumb at forearm level

⑦S56.301   Unspecified injury of extensor or abductor muscles, fascia and tendons of right thumb at forearm level

⑦S56.302   Unspecified injury of extensor or abductor muscles, fascia and tendons of left thumb at forearm level

⑦S56.309   Unspecified injury of extensor or abductor muscles, fascia and tendons of unspecified thumb at forearm level

S56.31   Strain of extensor or abductor muscles, fascia and tendons of thumb at forearm level

⑦S56.311   Strain of extensor or abductor muscles, fascia and tendons of right thumb at forearm level

⑦S56.312   Strain of extensor or abductor muscles, fascia and tendons of left thumb at forearm level

⑦S56.319   Strain of extensor or abductor muscles, fascia and tendons of unspecified thumb at forearm level

S56.32   Laceration of extensor or abductor muscles, fascia and tendons of thumb at forearm level

⑦S56.321   Laceration of extensor or abductor muscles, fascia and tendons of right thumb at forearm level

⑦S56.322   Laceration of extensor or abductor muscles, fascia and tendons of left thumb at forearm level

⑦S56.329   Laceration of extensor or abductor muscles, fascia and tendons of unspecified thumb at forearm level

S56.39   Other injury of extensor or abductor muscles, fascia and tendons of thumb at forearm level

⑦S56.391   Other injury of extensor or abductor muscles, fascia and tendons of right thumb at forearm level

⑦S56.392   Other injury of extensor or abductor muscles, fascia and tendons of left thumb at forearm level

⑦S56.399   Other injury of extensor or abductor muscles, fascia and tendons of unspecified thumb at forearm level

S56.4   Injury of extensor muscle, fascia and tendon of other and unspecified finger at forearm level

S56.40   Unspecified injury of extensor muscle, fascia and tendon of other and unspecified finger at forearm level

⑦S56.401   Unspecified injury of extensor muscle, fascia and tendon of right index finger at forearm level

⑦S56.402   Unspecified injury of extensor muscle, fascia and tendon of left index finger at forearm level

⑦S56.403   Unspecified injury of extensor muscle, fascia and tendon of right middle finger at forearm level

⑦S56.404   Unspecified injury of extensor muscle, fascia and tendon of left middle finger at forearm level

⑦S56.405   Unspecified injury of extensor muscle, fascia and tendon of right ring finger at forearm level

⑦S56.406   Unspecified injury of extensor muscle, fascia and tendon of left ring finger at forearm level

⑦S56.407   Unspecified injury of extensor muscle, fascia and tendon of right little finger at forearm level

⑦S56.408   Unspecified injury of extensor muscle, fascia and tendon of left little finger at forearm level

⑦S56.409   Unspecified injury of extensor muscle, fascia and tendon of unspecified finger at forearm level

S56.41   Strain of extensor muscle, fascia and tendon of other and unspecified finger at forearm level

⑦S56.411   Strain of extensor muscle, fascia and tendon of right index finger at forearm level

⑦S56.412   Strain of extensor muscle, fascia and tendon of left index finger at forearm level

⑦S56.413   Strain of extensor muscle, fascia and tendon of right middle finger at forearm level

⑦S56.414   Strain of extensor muscle, fascia and tendon of left middle finger at forearm level

⑦S56.415   Strain of extensor muscle, fascia and tendon of right ring finger at forearm level

⑦S56.416   Strain of extensor muscle, fascia and tendon of left ring finger at forearm level

⑦S56.417   Strain of extensor muscle, fascia and tendon of right little finger at forearm level

⑦S56.418   Strain of extensor muscle, fascia and tendon of left little finger at forearm level

⑦S56.419   Strain of extensor muscle, fascia and tendon of finger, unspecified finger at forearm level

S56.42   Laceration of extensor muscle, fascia and tendon of other and unspecified finger at forearm level

⑦S56.421   Laceration of extensor muscle, fascia and tendon of right index finger at forearm level

⑦S56.422   Laceration of extensor muscle, fascia and tendon of left index finger at forearm level

⑦S56.423   Laceration of extensor muscle, fascia and tendon of right middle finger at forearm level

⑦S56.424   Laceration of extensor muscle, fascia and tendon of left middle finger at forearm level

⑦S56.425   Laceration of extensor muscle, fascia and tendon of right ring finger at forearm level

⑦S56.426   Laceration of extensor muscle, fascia and tendon of left ring finger at forearm level

⑦S56.427   Laceration of extensor muscle, fascia and tendon of right little finger at forearm level

⑦S56.428   Laceration of extensor muscle, fascia and tendon of left little finger at forearm level

⑦S56.429   Laceration of extensor muscle, fascia and tendon of unspecified finger at forearm level

S56.49   Other injury of extensor muscle, fascia and tendon of other and unspecified finger at forearm level

⑦S56.491   Other injury of extensor muscle, fascia and tendon of right index finger at forearm level

⑦S56.492   Other injury of extensor muscle, fascia and tendon of left index finger at forearm level

⑦S56.493   Other injury of extensor muscle, fascia and tendon of right middle finger at forearm level

⑦S56.494   Other injury of extensor muscle, fascia and tendon of left middle finger at forearm level

⑦S56.495   Other injury of extensor muscle, fascia and tendon of right ring finger at forearm level

⑦S56.496   Other injury of extensor muscle, fascia and tendon of left ring finger at forearm level

⑦S56.497   Other injury of extensor muscle, fascia and tendon of right little finger at forearm level

⑦S56.498   Other injury of extensor muscle, fascia and tendon of left little finger at forearm level

⑦S56.499   Other injury of extensor muscle, fascia and tendon of unspecified finger at forearm level

S56.5   Injury of other extensor muscle, fascia and tendon at forearm level

S56.50   Unspecified injury of other extensor muscle, fascia and tendon at forearm level

⑦S56.501   Unspecified injury of other extensor muscle, fascia and tendon at forearm level, right arm

⑦S56.502   Unspecified injury of other extensor muscle, fascia and tendon at forearm level, left arm

⑦S56.509   Unspecified injury of other extensor muscle, fascia and tendon at forearm level, unspecified arm

S56.51   Strain of other extensor muscle, fascia and tendon at forearm level

⑦S56.511   Strain of other extensor muscle, fascia and tendon at forearm level, right arm

⑦S56.512   Strain of other extensor muscle, fascia and tendon at forearm level, left arm

⑦S56.519   Strain of other extensor muscle, fascia and tendon at forearm level, unspecified arm

S56.52   Laceration of other extensor muscle, fascia and tendon at forearm level

⑦S56.521   Laceration of other extensor muscle, fascia and tendon at forearm level, right arm

⑦S56.522   Laceration of other extensor muscle, fascia and tendon at forearm level, left arm

⑦ S56.529 Laceration of other extensor muscle, fascia and tendon at forearm level, unspecified arm

S56.59 Other injury of other extensor muscle, fascia and tendon at forearm level

⑦ S56.591 Other injury of other extensor muscle, fascia and tendon at forearm level, right arm

⑦ S56.592 Other injury of other extensor muscle, fascia and tendon at forearm level, left arm

⑦ S56.599 Other injury of other extensor muscle, fascia and tendon at forearm level, unspecified arm

S56.8 Injury of other muscles, fascia and tendons at forearm level

S56.80 Unspecified injury of other muscles, fascia and tendons at forearm level

⑦ S56.801 Unspecified injury of other muscles, fascia and tendons at forearm level, right arm

⑦ S56.802 Unspecified injury of other muscles, fascia and tendons at forearm level, left arm

⑦ S56.809 Unspecified injury of other muscles, fascia and tendons at forearm level, unspecified arm

S56.81 Strain of other muscles, fascia and tendons at forearm level

⑦ S56.811 Strain of other muscles, fascia and tendons at forearm level, right arm

⑦ S56.812 Strain of other muscles, fascia and tendons at forearm level, left arm

⑦ S56.819 Strain of other muscles, fascia and tendons at forearm level, unspecified arm

S56.82 Laceration of other muscles, fascia and tendons at forearm level

⑦ S56.821 Laceration of other muscles, fascia and tendons at forearm level, right arm

⑦ S56.822 Laceration of other muscles, fascia and tendons at forearm level, left arm

⑦ S56.829 Laceration of other muscles, fascia and tendons at forearm level, unspecified arm

S56.89 Other injury of other muscles, fascia and tendons at forearm level

⑦ S56.891 Other injury of other muscles, fascia and tendons at forearm level, right arm

⑦ S56.892 Other injury of other muscles, fascia and tendons at forearm level, left arm

⑦ S56.899 Other injury of other muscles, fascia and tendons at forearm level, unspecified arm

S56.9 Injury of unspecified muscles, fascia and tendons at forearm level

S56.90 Unspecified injury of unspecified muscles, fascia and tendons at forearm level

⑦ S56.901 Unspecified injury of unspecified muscles, fascia and tendons at forearm level, right arm

⑦ S56.902 Unspecified injury of unspecified muscles, fascia and tendons at forearm level, left arm

⑦ S56.909 Unspecified injury of unspecified muscles, fascia and tendons at forearm level, unspecified arm

S56.91 Strain of unspecified muscles, fascia and tendons at forearm level

⑦ S56.911 Strain of unspecified muscles, fascia and tendons at forearm level, right arm

⑦ S56.912 Strain of unspecified muscles, fascia and tendons at forearm level, left arm

⑦ S56.919 Strain of unspecified muscles, fascia and tendons at forearm level, unspecified arm

S56.92 Laceration of unspecified muscles, fascia and tendons at forearm level

⑦ S56.921 Laceration of unspecified muscles, fascia and tendons at forearm level, right arm

⑦ S56.922 Laceration of unspecified muscles, fascia and tendons at forearm level, left arm

⑦ S56.929 Laceration of unspecified muscles, fascia and tendons at forearm level, unspecified arm

S56.99 Other injury of unspecified muscles, fascia and tendons at forearm level

⑦ S56.991 Other injury of unspecified muscles, fascia and tendons at forearm level, right arm

⑦ S56.992 Other injury of unspecified muscles, fascia and tendons at forearm level, left arm

⑦ S56.999 Other injury of unspecified muscles, fascia and tendons at forearm level, unspecified arm

S57 Crushing injury of elbow and forearm

Use additional code(s) for all associated injuries

Excludes 2: crushing injury of wrist and hand (S67.-)

The appropriate 7th character is to be added to each code from category S57

A - initial encounter

D - subsequent encounter

S - sequela

S57.0 Crushing injury of elbow

⊗⑦ S57.00 Crushing injury of unspecified elbow

⊗⑦ S57.01 Crushing injury of right elbow

⊗⑦ S57.02 Crushing injury of left elbow

S57.8 Crushing injury of forearm

⊗⑦ S57.80 Crushing injury of unspecified forearm

⊗⑦ S57.81 Crushing injury of right forearm

⊗⑦ S57.82 Crushing injury of left forearm

S58 Traumatic amputation of elbow and forearm

An amputation not identified as partial or complete should be coded to complete

Excludes 1: traumatic amputation of wrist and hand (S68.-)

The appropriate 7th character is to be added to each code from category S58

A - initial encounter

D - subsequent encounter

S - sequela

S58.0   Traumatic amputation at elbow level

    S58.01   Complete traumatic amputation at elbow level

       ⑦**S58.011**   Complete traumatic amputation at elbow level, right arm

       ⑦**S58.012**   Complete traumatic amputation at elbow level, left arm

       ⑦**S58.019**   Complete traumatic amputation at elbow level, unspecified arm

    S58.02   Partial traumatic amputation at elbow level

       ⑦**S58.021**   Partial traumatic amputation at elbow level, right arm

       ⑦**S58.022**   Partial traumatic amputation at elbow level, left arm

       ⑦**S58.029**   Partial traumatic amputation at elbow level, unspecified arm

S58.1   Traumatic amputation at level between elbow and wrist

    S58.11   Complete traumatic amputation at level between elbow and wrist

       ⑦**S58.111**   Complete traumatic amputation at level between elbow and wrist, right arm

       ⑦**S58.112**   Complete traumatic amputation at level between elbow and wrist, left arm

       ⑦**S58.119**   Complete traumatic amputation at level between elbow and wrist, unspecified arm

    S58.12   Partial traumatic amputation at level between elbow and wrist

       ⑦**S58.121**   Partial traumatic amputation at level between elbow and wrist, right arm

       ⑦**S58.122**   Partial traumatic amputation at level between elbow and wrist, left arm

       ⑦**S58.129**   Partial traumatic amputation at level between elbow and wrist, unspecified arm

S58.9   Traumatic amputation of forearm, level unspecified

    Excludes 1: traumatic amputation of wrist (S68.-)

    S58.91   Complete traumatic amputation of forearm, level unspecified

       ⑦**S58.911**   Complete traumatic amputation of right forearm, level unspecified

       ⑦**S58.912**   Complete traumatic amputation of left forearm, level unspecified

       ⑦**S58.919**   Complete traumatic amputation of unspecified forearm, level unspecified

    S58.92   Partial traumatic amputation of forearm, level unspecified

       ⑦**S58.921**   Partial traumatic amputation of right forearm, level unspecified

       ⑦**S58.922**   Partial traumatic amputation of left forearm, level unspecified

       ⑦**S58.929**   Partial traumatic amputation of unspecified forearm, level unspecified

S59   Other and unspecified injuries of elbow and forearm

Excludes 2: other and unspecified injuries of wrist and hand (S69.-)

The appropriate 7th character is to be added to each code from subcategories S59.0, S59.1, and S59.2

A - initial encounter for closed fracture

D - subsequent encounter for fracture with routine healing

G - subsequent encounter for fracture with delayed healing

K - subsequent encounter for fracture with nonunion

P - subsequent encounter for fracture with malunion

S - sequela

S59.0   Physeal fracture of lower end of ulna

    S59.00   Unspecified physeal fracture of lower end of ulna

       ⑦**S59.001**   Unspecified physeal fracture of lower end of ulna, right arm

       ⑦**S59.002**   Unspecified physeal fracture of lower end of ulna, left arm

       ⑦**S59.009**   Unspecified physeal fracture of lower end of ulna, unspecified arm

    S59.01   Salter-Harris Type I physeal fracture of lower end of ulna

       ⑦**S59.011**   Salter-Harris Type I physeal fracture of lower end of ulna, right arm

       ⑦**S59.012**   Salter-Harris Type I physeal fracture of lower end of ulna, left arm

       ⑦**S59.019**   Salter-Harris Type I physeal fracture of lower end of ulna, unspecified arm

    S59.02   Salter-Harris Type II physeal fracture of lower end of ulna

       ⑦**S59.021**   Salter-Harris Type II physeal fracture of lower end of ulna, right arm

       ⑦**S59.022**   Salter-Harris Type II physeal fracture of lower end of ulna, left arm

       ⑦**S59.029**   Salter-Harris Type II physeal fracture of lower end of ulna, unspecified arm

    S59.03   Salter-Harris Type III physeal fracture of lower end of ulna

       ⑦**S59.031**   Salter-Harris Type III physeal fracture of lower end of ulna, right arm

       ⑦**S59.032**   Salter-Harris Type III physeal fracture of lower end of ulna, left arm

       ⑦**S59.039**   Salter-Harris Type III physeal fracture of lower end of ulna, unspecified arm

    S59.04   Salter-Harris Type IV physeal fracture of lower end of ulna

       ⑦**S59.041**   Salter-Harris Type IV physeal fracture of lower end of ulna, right arm

⑦S59.042   Salter-Harris Type IV physeal fracture of lower end of ulna, left arm

⑦S59.049   Salter-Harris Type IV physeal fracture of lower end of ulna, unspecified arm

S59.09   Other physeal fracture of lower end of ulna

     ⑦S59.091   Other physeal fracture of lower end of ulna, right arm

     ⑦S59.092   Other physeal fracture of lower end of ulna, left arm

     ⑦S59.099   Other physeal fracture of lower end of ulna, unspecified arm

S59.1   Physeal fracture of upper end of radius

   S59.10   Unspecified physeal fracture of upper end of radius

     ⑦S59.101   Unspecified physeal fracture of upper end of radius, right arm

     ⑦S59.102   Unspecified physeal fracture of upper end of radius, left arm

     ⑦S59.109   Unspecified physeal fracture of upper end of radius, unspecified arm

   S59.11   Salter-Harris Type I physeal fracture of upper end of radius

     ⑦S59.111   Salter-Harris Type I physeal fracture of upper end of radius, right arm

     ⑦S59.112   Salter-Harris Type I physeal fracture of upper end of radius, left arm

     ⑦S59.119   Salter-Harris Type I physeal fracture of upper end of radius, unspecified arm

   S59.12   Salter-Harris Type II physeal fracture of upper end of radius

     ⑦S59.121   Salter-Harris Type II physeal fracture of upper end of radius, right arm

     ⑦S59.122   Salter-Harris Type II physeal fracture of upper end of radius, left arm

     ⑦S59.129   Salter-Harris Type II physeal fracture of upper end of radius, unspecified arm

   S59.13   Salter-Harris Type III physeal fracture of upper end of radius

     ⑦S59.131   Salter-Harris Type III physeal fracture of upper end of radius, right arm

     ⑦S59.132   Salter-Harris Type III physeal fracture of upper end of radius, left arm

     ⑦S59.139   Salter-Harris Type III physeal fracture of upper end of radius, unspecified arm

   S59.14   Salter-Harris Type IV physeal fracture of upper end of radius

     ⑦S59.141   Salter-Harris Type IV physeal fracture of upper end of radius, right arm

     ⑦S59.142   Salter-Harris Type IV physeal fracture of upper end of radius, left arm

⑦S59.149   Salter-Harris Type IV physeal fracture of upper end of radius, unspecified arm

S59.19   Other physeal fracture of upper end of radius

     ⑦S59.191   Other physeal fracture of upper end of radius, right arm

     ⑦S59.192   Other physeal fracture of upper end of radius, left arm

     ⑦S59.199   Other physeal fracture of upper end of radius, unspecified arm

S59.2   Physeal fracture of lower end of radius

   S59.20   Unspecified physeal fracture of lower end of radius

     ⑦S59.201   Unspecified physeal fracture of lower end of radius, right arm

     ⑦S59.202   Unspecified physeal fracture of lower end of radius, left arm

     ⑦S59.209   Unspecified physeal fracture of lower end of radius, unspecified arm

   S59.21   Salter-Harris Type I physeal fracture of lower end of radius

     ⑦S59.211   Salter-Harris Type I physeal fracture of lower end of radius, right arm

     ⑦S59.212   Salter-Harris Type I physeal fracture of lower end of radius, left arm

     ⑦S59.219   Salter-Harris Type I physeal fracture of lower end of radius, unspecified arm

   S59.22   Salter-Harris Type II physeal fracture of lower end of radius

     ⑦S59.221   Salter-Harris Type II physeal fracture of lower end of radius, right arm

     ⑦S59.222   Salter-Harris Type II physeal fracture of lower end of radius, left arm

     ⑦S59.229   Salter-Harris Type II physeal fracture of lower end of radius, unspecified arm

   S59.23   Salter-Harris Type III physeal fracture of lower end of radius

     ⑦S59.231   Salter-Harris Type III physeal fracture of lower end of radius, right arm

     ⑦S59.232   Salter-Harris Type III physeal fracture of lower end of radius, left arm

     ⑦S59.239   Salter-Harris Type III physeal fracture of lower end of radius, unspecified arm

   S59.24   Salter-Harris Type IV physeal fracture of lower end of radius

     ⑦S59.241   Salter-Harris Type IV physeal fracture of lower end of radius, right arm

     ⑦S59.242   Salter-Harris Type IV physeal fracture of lower end of radius, left arm

     ⑦S59.249   Salter-Harris Type IV physeal fracture of lower end of radius, unspecified arm

S59.29   Other physeal fracture of lower end of radius

   ⑦S59.291   Other physeal fracture of lower end of radius, right arm

   ⑦S59.292   Other physeal fracture of lower end of radius, left arm

   ⑦S59.299   Other physeal fracture of lower end of radius, unspecified arm

S59.8   Other specified injuries of elbow and forearm

The appropriate 7th character is to be added to each code in subcategory S59.8

A - initial encounter

D - subsequent encounter

S - sequela

S59.80   Other specified injuries of elbow

   ⑦S59.801   Other specified injuries of right elbow

   ⑦S59.802   Other specified injuries of left elbow

   ⑦S59.809   Other specified injuries of unspecified elbow

S59.81   Other specified injuries of forearm

   ⑦S59.811   Other specified injuries right forearm

   ⑦S59.812   Other specified injuries left forearm

   ⑦S59.819   Other specified injuries unspecified forearm

S59.9   Unspecified injury of elbow and forearm

The appropriate 7th character is to be added to each code in subcategory S59.9

A - initial encounter

D - subsequent encounter

S - sequela

S59.90   Unspecified injury of elbow

   ⑦S59.901   Unspecified injury of right elbow

   ⑦S59.902   Unspecified injury of left elbow

   ⑦S59.909   Unspecified injury of unspecified elbow

S59.91   Unspecified injury of forearm

   ⑦S59.911   Unspecified injury of right forearm

   ⑦S59.912   Unspecified injury of left forearm

   ⑦S59.919   Unspecified injury of unspecified forearm

INJURIES TO THE WRIST, HAND AND FINGERS (S60-S69)

Excludes 2: burns and corrosions (T20-T32)

frostbite (T33-T34)

insect bite or sting, venomous (T63.4)

S60   Superficial injury of wrist, hand and fingers

The appropriate 7th character is to be added to each code from category S60

A - initial encounter

D - subsequent encounter

S - sequela

S60.0   Contusion of finger without damage to nail

Excludes 1: contusion involving nail (matrix) (S60.1)

⊗⑦S60.00   Contusion of unspecified finger without damage to nail

Contusion of finger(s) NOS

S60.01   Contusion of thumb without damage to nail

   ⑦S60.011   Contusion of right thumb without damage to nail

   ⑦S60.012   Contusion of left thumb without damage to nail

   ⑦S60.019   Contusion of unspecified thumb without damage to nail

S60.02   Contusion of index finger without damage to nail

   ⑦S60.021   Contusion of right index finger without damage to nail

   ⑦S60.022   Contusion of left index finger without damage to nail

   ⑦S60.029   Contusion of unspecified index finger without damage to nail

S60.03   Contusion of middle finger without damage to nail

   ⑦S60.031   Contusion of right middle finger without damage to nail

   ⑦S60.032   Contusion of left middle finger without damage to nail

   ⑦S60.039   Contusion of unspecified middle finger without damage to nail

S60.04   Contusion of ring finger without damage to nail

   ⑦S60.041   Contusion of right ring finger without damage to nail

   ⑦S60.042   Contusion of left ring finger without damage to nail

   ⑦S60.049   Contusion of unspecified ring finger without damage to nail

S60.05   Contusion of little finger without damage to nail

   ⑦S60.051   Contusion of right little finger without damage to nail

   ⑦S60.052   Contusion of left little finger without damage to nail

   ⑦S60.059   Contusion of unspecified little finger without damage to nail

S60.1   Contusion of finger with damage to nail

⊗⑦S60.10   Contusion of unspecified finger with damage to nail

S60.11   Contusion of thumb with damage to nail

   ⑦S60.111   Contusion of right thumb with damage to nail

   ⑦S60.112   Contusion of left thumb with damage to nail

   ⑦S60.119   Contusion of unspecified thumb with damage to nail

S60.12   Contusion of index finger with damage to nail

   ⑦S60.121   Contusion of right index finger with damage to nail

   ⑦S60.122   Contusion of left index finger with damage to nail

   ⑦S60.129   Contusion of unspecified index finger with damage to nail

S60.13   Contusion of middle finger with damage to nail

   ⑦S60.131   Contusion of right middle finger with damage to nail

   ⑦S60.132   Contusion of left middle finger with damage to nail

⑦S60.139　Contusion of unspecified middle finger with damage to nail

S60.14　Contusion of ring finger with damage to nail

⑦S60.141　Contusion of right ring finger with damage to nail

⑦S60.142　Contusion of left ring finger with damage to nail

⑦S60.149　Contusion of unspecified ring finger with damage to nail

S60.15　Contusion of little finger with damage to nail

⑦S60.151　Contusion of right little finger with damage to nail

⑦S60.152　Contusion of left little finger with damage to nail

⑦S60.159　Contusion of unspecified little finger with damage to nail

S60.2　Contusion of wrist and hand

Excludes 2: contusion of fingers (S60.0-, S60.1-)

S60.21　Contusion of wrist

⑦S60.211　Contusion of right wrist

⑦S60.212　Contusion of left wrist

⑦S60.219　Contusion of unspecified wrist

S60.22　Contusion of hand

⑦S60.221　Contusion of right hand

⑦S60.222　Contusion of left hand

⑦S60.229　Contusion of unspecified hand

S60.3　Other superficial injuries of thumb

S60.31　Abrasion of thumb

⑦S60.311　Abrasion of right thumb

⑦S60.312　Abrasion of left thumb

⑦S60.319　Abrasion of unspecified thumb

S60.32　Blister (nonthermal) of thumb

⑦S60.321　Blister (nonthermal) of right thumb

⑦S60.322　Blister (nonthermal) of left thumb

⑦S60.329　Blister (nonthermal) of unspecified thumb

S60.34　External constriction of thumb

Hair tourniquet syndrome of thumb

Use additional cause code to identify the constricting item (W49.0-)

⑦S60.341　External constriction of right thumb

⑦S60.342　External constriction of left thumb

⑦S60.349　External constriction of unspecified thumb

S60.35　Superficial foreign body of thumb

Splinter in the thumb

⑦S60.351　Superficial foreign body of right thumb

⑦S60.352　Superficial foreign body of left thumb

⑦S60.359　Superficial foreign body of unspecified thumb

S60.36　Insect bite (nonvenomous) of thumb

⑦S60.361　Insect bite (nonvenomous) of right thumb

⑦S60.362　Insect bite (nonvenomous) of left thumb

⑦S60.369　Insect bite (nonvenomous) of unspecified thumb

S60.37　Other superficial bite of thumb

Excludes 1: open bite of thumb (S61.05-, S61.15-)

⑦S60.371　Other superficial bite of right thumb

⑦S60.372　Other superficial bite of left thumb

⑦S60.379　Other superficial bite of unspecified thumb

S60.39　Other superficial injuries of thumb

⑦S60.391　Other superficial injuries of right thumb

⑦S60.392　Other superficial injuries of left thumb

⑦S60.399　Other superficial injuries of unspecified thumb

S60.4　Other superficial injuries of other fingers

S60.41　Abrasion of fingers

⑦S60.410　Abrasion of right index finger

⑦S60.411　Abrasion of left index finger

⑦S60.412　Abrasion of right middle finger

⑦S60.413　Abrasion of left middle finger

⑦S60.414　Abrasion of right ring finger

⑦S60.415　Abrasion of left ring finger

⑦S60.416　Abrasion of right little finger

⑦S60.417　Abrasion of left little finger

⑦S60.418　Abrasion of other finger

Abrasion of specified finger with unspecified laterality

⑦S60.419　Abrasion of unspecified finger

S60.42　Blister (nonthermal) of fingers

⑦S60.420　Blister (nonthermal) of right index finger

⑦S60.421　Blister (nonthermal) of left index finger

⑦S60.422　Blister (nonthermal) of right middle finger

⑦S60.423　Blister (nonthermal) of left middle finger

⑦S60.424　Blister (nonthermal) of right ring finger

⑦S60.425　Blister (nonthermal) of left ring finger

⑦S60.426　Blister (nonthermal) of right little finger

⑦S60.427　Blister (nonthermal) of left little finger

⑦S60.428　Blister (nonthermal) of other finger

Blister (nonthermal) of specified finger with unspecified laterality

⑦S60.429　Blister (nonthermal) of unspecified finger

S60.44　External constriction of fingers

Hair tourniquet syndrome of finger

Use additional cause code to identify the constricting item (W49.0-)

⑦S60.440　External constriction of right index finger

⑦S60.441 External constriction of left index finger

⑦S60.442 External constriction of right middle finger

⑦S60.443 External constriction of left middle finger

⑦S60.444 External constriction of right ring finger

⑦S60.445 External constriction of left ring finger

⑦S60.446 External constriction of right little finger

⑦S60.447 External constriction of left little finger

⑦S60.448 External constriction of other finger
External constriction of specified finger with unspecified laterality

⑦S60.449 External constriction of unspecified finger

S60.45 Superficial foreign body of fingers
Splinter in the finger(s)

⑦S60.450 Superficial foreign body of right index finger

⑦S60.451 Superficial foreign body of left index finger

⑦S60.452 Superficial foreign body of right middle finger

⑦S60.453 Superficial foreign body of left middle finger

⑦S60.454 Superficial foreign body of right ring finger

⑦S60.455 Superficial foreign body of left ring finger

⑦S60.456 Superficial foreign body of right little finger

⑦S60.457 Superficial foreign body of left little finger

⑦S60.458 Superficial foreign body of other finger
Superficial foreign body of specified finger with unspecified laterality

⑦S60.459 Superficial foreign body of unspecified finger

S60.46 Insect bite (nonvenomous) of fingers

⑦S60.460 Insect bite (nonvenomous) of right index finger

⑦S60.461 Insect bite (nonvenomous) of left index finger

⑦S60.462 Insect bite (nonvenomous) of right middle finger

⑦S60.463 Insect bite (nonvenomous) of left middle finger

⑦S60.464 Insect bite (nonvenomous) of right ring finger

⑦S60.465 Insect bite (nonvenomous) of left ring finger

⑦S60.466 Insect bite (nonvenomous) of right little finger

⑦S60.467 Insect bite (nonvenomous) of left little finger

⑦S60.468 Insect bite (nonvenomous) of other finger
Insect bite (nonvenomous) of specified finger with unspecified laterality

⑦S60.469 Insect bite (nonvenomous) of unspecified finger

S60.47 Other superficial bite of fingers
Excludes 1: open bite of fingers (S61.25-, S61.35-)

⑦S60.470 Other superficial bite of right index finger

⑦S60.471 Other superficial bite of left index finger

⑦S60.472 Other superficial bite of right middle finger

⑦S60.473 Other superficial bite of left middle finger

⑦S60.474 Other superficial bite of right ring finger

⑦S60.475 Other superficial bite of left ring finger

⑦S60.476 Other superficial bite of right little finger

⑦S60.477 Other superficial bite of left little finger

⑦S60.478 Other superficial bite of other finger
Other superficial bite of specified finger with unspecified laterality

⑦S60.479 Other superficial bite of unspecified finger

S60.5 Other superficial injuries of hand
Excludes 2: superficial injuries of fingers (S60.3-, S60.4-)

S60.51 Abrasion of hand

⑦S60.511 Abrasion of right hand

⑦S60.512 Abrasion of left hand

⑦S60.519 Abrasion of unspecified hand

S60.52 Blister (nonthermal) of hand

⑦S60.521 Blister (nonthermal) of right hand

⑦S60.522 Blister (nonthermal) of left hand

⑦S60.529 Blister (nonthermal) of unspecified hand

S60.54 External constriction of hand

⑦S60.541 External constriction of right hand

⑦S60.542 External constriction of left hand

⑦S60.549 External constriction of unspecified hand

S60.55 Superficial foreign body of hand
Splinter in the hand

⑦S60.551 Superficial foreign body of right hand

⑦S60.552 Superficial foreign body of left hand

⑦S60.559 Superficial foreign body of unspecified hand

S60.56 Insect bite (nonvenomous) of hand

⑦S60.561   Insect bite (nonvenomous) of right hand

⑦S60.562   Insect bite (nonvenomous) of left hand

⑦S60.569   Insect bite (nonvenomous) of unspecified hand

S60.57   Other superficial bite of hand

Excludes 1: open bite of hand (S61.45-)

⑦S60.571   Other superficial bite of hand of right hand

⑦S60.572   Other superficial bite of hand of left hand

⑦S60.579   Other superficial bite of hand of unspecified hand

S60.8   Other superficial injuries of wrist

S60.81   Abrasion of wrist

⑦S60.811   Abrasion of right wrist

⑦S60.812   Abrasion of left wrist

⑦S60.819   Abrasion of unspecified wrist

S60.82   Blister (nonthermal) of wrist

⑦S60.821   Blister (nonthermal) of right wrist

⑦S60.822   Blister (nonthermal) of left wrist

⑦S60.829   Blister (nonthermal) of unspecified wrist

S60.84   External constriction of wrist

⑦S60.841   External constriction of right wrist

⑦S60.842   External constriction of left wrist

⑦S60.849   External constriction of unspecified wrist

S60.85   Superficial foreign body of wrist

Splinter in the wrist

⑦S60.851   Superficial foreign body of right wrist

⑦S60.852   Superficial foreign body of left wrist

⑦S60.859   Superficial foreign body of unspecified wrist

S60.86   Insect bite (nonvenomous) of wrist

⑦S60.861   Insect bite (nonvenomous) of right wrist

⑦S60.862   Insect bite (nonvenomous) of left wrist

⑦S60.869   Insect bite (nonvenomous) of unspecified wrist

S60.87   Other superficial bite of wrist

Excludes 1: open bite of wrist (S61.55)

⑦S60.871   Other superficial bite of right wrist

⑦S60.872   Other superficial bite of left wrist

⑦S60.879   Other superficial bite of unspecified wrist

S60.9   Unspecified superficial injury of wrist, hand and fingers

S60.91   Unspecified superficial injury of wrist

⑦S60.911   Unspecified superficial injury of right wrist

⑦S60.912   Unspecified superficial injury of left wrist

⑦S60.919   Unspecified superficial injury of unspecified wrist

S60.92   Unspecified superficial injury of hand

⑦S60.921   Unspecified superficial injury of right hand

⑦S60.922   Unspecified superficial injury of left hand

⑦S60.929   Unspecified superficial injury of unspecified hand

S60.93   Unspecified superficial injury of thumb

⑦S60.931   Unspecified superficial injury of right thumb

⑦S60.932   Unspecified superficial injury of left thumb

⑦S60.939   Unspecified superficial injury of unspecified thumb

S60.94   Unspecified superficial injury of other fingers

⑦S60.940   Unspecified superficial injury of right index finger

⑦S60.941   Unspecified superficial injury of left index finger

⑦S60.942   Unspecified superficial injury of right middle finger

⑦S60.943   Unspecified superficial injury of left middle finger

⑦S60.944   Unspecified superficial injury of right ring finger

⑦S60.945   Unspecified superficial injury of left ring finger

⑦S60.946   Unspecified superficial injury of right little finger

⑦S60.947   Unspecified superficial injury of left little finger

⑦S60.948   Unspecified superficial injury of other finger

Unspecified superficial injury of specified finger with unspecified laterality

⑦S60.949   Unspecified superficial injury of unspecified finger

S61   Open wound of wrist, hand and fingers

Code also any associated wound infection

Excludes 1: open fracture of wrist, hand and finger (S62.- with 7th character B)

traumatic amputation of wrist and hand (S68.-)

The appropriate 7th character is to be added to each code from category S61

A - initial encounter

D - subsequent encounter

S - sequela

S61.0   Open wound of thumb without damage to nail

Excludes 1: open wound of thumb with damage to nail (S61.1-)

S61.00   Unspecified open wound of thumb without damage to nail

⑦S61.001   Unspecified open wound of right thumb without damage to nail

⑦S61.002   Unspecified open wound of left thumb without damage to nail

⑦S61.009   Unspecified open wound of unspecified thumb without damage to nail

S61.01 Laceration without foreign body of thumb without damage to nail

⑦**S61.011** Laceration without foreign body of right thumb without damage to nail

⑦**S61.012** Laceration without foreign body of left thumb without damage to nail

⑦**S61.019** Laceration without foreign body of unspecified thumb without damage to nail

S61.02 Laceration with foreign body of thumb without damage to nail

⑦**S61.021** Laceration with foreign body of right thumb without damage to nail

⑦**S61.022** Laceration with foreign body of left thumb without damage to nail

⑦**S61.029** Laceration with foreign body of unspecified thumb without damage to nail

S61.03 Puncture wound without foreign body of thumb without damage to nail

⑦**S61.031** Puncture wound without foreign body of right thumb without damage to nail

⑦**S61.032** Puncture wound without foreign body of left thumb without damage to nail

⑦**S61.039** Puncture wound without foreign body of unspecified thumb without damage to nail

S61.04 Puncture wound with foreign body of thumb without damage to nail

⑦**S61.041** Puncture wound with foreign body of right thumb without damage to nail

⑦**S61.042** Puncture wound with foreign body of left thumb without damage to nail

⑦**S61.049** Puncture wound with foreign body of unspecified thumb without damage to nail

S61.05 Open bite of thumb without damage to nail
Bite of thumb NOS
Excludes 1: superficial bite of thumb (S60.36-, S60.37-)

⑦**S61.051** Open bite of right thumb without damage to nail

⑦**S61.052** Open bite of left thumb without damage to nail

⑦**S61.059** Open bite of unspecified thumb without damage to nail

S61.1 Open wound of thumb with damage to nail

S61.10 Unspecified open wound of thumb with damage to nail

⑦**S61.101** Unspecified open wound of right thumb with damage to nail

⑦**S61.102** Unspecified open wound of left thumb with damage to nail

⑦**S61.109** Unspecified open wound of unspecified thumb with damage to nail

S61.11 Laceration without foreign body of thumb with damage to nail

⑦**S61.111** Laceration without foreign body of right thumb with damage to nail

⑦**S61.112** Laceration without foreign body of left thumb with damage to nail

⑦**S61.119** Laceration without foreign body of unspecified thumb with damage to nail

S61.12 Laceration with foreign body of thumb with damage to nail

⑦**S61.121** Laceration with foreign body of right thumb with damage to nail

⑦**S61.122** Laceration with foreign body of left thumb with damage to nail

⑦**S61.129** Laceration with foreign body of unspecified thumb with damage to nail

S61.13 Puncture wound without foreign body of thumb with damage to nail

⑦**S61.131** Puncture wound without foreign body of right thumb with damage to nail

⑦**S61.132** Puncture wound without foreign body of left thumb with damage to nail

⑦**S61.139** Puncture wound without foreign body of unspecified thumb with damage to nail

S61.14 Puncture wound with foreign body of thumb with damage to nail

⑦**S61.141** Puncture wound with foreign body of right thumb with damage to nail

⑦**S61.142** Puncture wound with foreign body of left thumb with damage to nail

⑦**S61.149** Puncture wound with foreign body of unspecified thumb with damage to nail

S61.15 Open bite of thumb with damage to nail
Bite of thumb with damage to nail NOS
Excludes 1: superficial bite of thumb (S60.36-, S60.37-)

⑦**S61.151** Open bite of right thumb with damage to nail

⑦**S61.152** Open bite of left thumb with damage to nail

⑦**S61.159** Open bite of unspecified thumb with damage to nail

S61.2 Open wound of other finger without damage to nail
Excludes 1: open wound of finger involving nail (matrix) (S61.3-)
Excludes 2: open wound of thumb without damage to nail (S61.0-)

S61.20 Unspecified open wound of other finger without damage to nail

⑦**S61.200** Unspecified open wound of right index finger without damage to nail

⑦**S61.201** Unspecified open wound of left index finger without damage to nail

● New code   ▲ Revised code   ⑦ 7th digit required   ⊗ Placeholder required

⑦S61.202 Unspecified open wound of right middle finger without damage to nail

⑦S61.203 Unspecified open wound of left middle finger without damage to nail

⑦S61.204 Unspecified open wound of right ring finger without damage to nail

⑦S61.205 Unspecified open wound of left ring finger without damage to nail

⑦S61.206 Unspecified open wound of right little finger without damage to nail

⑦S61.207 Unspecified open wound of left little finger without damage to nail

⑦S61.208 Unspecified open wound of other finger without damage to nail

Unspecified open wound of specified finger with unspecified laterality without damage to nail

⑦S61.209 Unspecified open wound of unspecified finger without damage to nail

S61.21 Laceration without foreign body of finger without damage to nail

⑦S61.210 Laceration without foreign body of right index finger without damage to nail

⑦S61.211 Laceration without foreign body of left index finger without damage to nail

⑦S61.212 Laceration without foreign body of right middle finger without damage to nail

⑦S61.213 Laceration without foreign body of left middle finger without damage to nail

⑦S61.214 Laceration without foreign body of right ring finger without damage to nail

⑦S61.215 Laceration without foreign body of left ring finger without damage to nail

⑦S61.216 Laceration without foreign body of right little finger without damage to nail

⑦S61.217 Laceration without foreign body of left little finger without damage to nail

⑦S61.218 Laceration without foreign body of other finger without damage to nail

Laceration without foreign body of specified finger with unspecified laterality without damage to nail

⑦S61.219 Laceration without foreign body of unspecified finger without damage to nail

S61.22 Laceration with foreign body of finger without damage to nail

⑦S61.220 Laceration with foreign body of right index finger without damage to nail

⑦S61.221 Laceration with foreign body of left index finger without damage to nail

⑦S61.222 Laceration with foreign body of right middle finger without damage to nail

⑦S61.223 Laceration with foreign body of left middle finger without damage to nail

⑦S61.224 Laceration with foreign body of right ring finger without damage to nail

⑦S61.225 Laceration with foreign body of left ring finger without damage to nail

⑦S61.226 Laceration with foreign body of right little finger without damage to nail

⑦S61.227 Laceration with foreign body of left little finger without damage to nail

⑦S61.228 Laceration with foreign body of other finger without damage to nail

Laceration with foreign body of specified finger with unspecified laterality without damage to nail

⑦S61.229 Laceration with foreign body of unspecified finger without damage to nail

S61.23 Puncture wound without foreign body of finger without damage to nail

⑦S61.230 Puncture wound without foreign body of right index finger without damage to nail

⑦S61.231 Puncture wound without foreign body of left index finger without damage to nail

⑦S61.232 Puncture wound without foreign body of right middle finger without damage to nail

⑦S61.233 Puncture wound without foreign body of left middle finger without damage to nail

⑦S61.234 Puncture wound without foreign body of right ring finger without damage to nail

⑦S61.235 Puncture wound without foreign body of left ring finger without damage to nail

⑦S61.236 Puncture wound without foreign body of right little finger without damage to nail

⑦S61.237 Puncture wound without foreign body of left little finger without damage to nail

⑦S61.238 Puncture wound without foreign body of other finger without damage to nail

Puncture wound without foreign body of specified finger with unspecified laterality without damage to nail

⑦**S61.239** Puncture wound without foreign body of unspecified finger without damage to nail

S61.24 Puncture wound with foreign body of finger without damage to nail

⑦**S61.240** Puncture wound with foreign body of right index finger without damage to nail

⑦**S61.241** Puncture wound with foreign body of left index finger without damage to nail

⑦**S61.242** Puncture wound with foreign body of right middle finger without damage to nail

⑦**S61.243** Puncture wound with foreign body of left middle finger without damage to nail

⑦**S61.244** Puncture wound with foreign body of right ring finger without damage to nail

⑦**S61.245** Puncture wound with foreign body of left ring finger without damage to nail

⑦**S61.246** Puncture wound with foreign body of right little finger without damage to nail

⑦**S61.247** Puncture wound with foreign body of left little finger without damage to nail

⑦**S61.248** Puncture wound with foreign body of other finger without damage to nail
Puncture wound with foreign body of specified finger with unspecified laterality without damage to nail

⑦**S61.249** Puncture wound with foreign body of unspecified finger without damage to nail

S61.25 Open bite of finger without damage to nail
Bite of finger without damage to nail NOS
Excludes 1: superficial bite of finger (S60.46-, S60.47-)

⑦**S61.250** Open bite of right index finger without damage to nail

⑦**S61.251** Open bite of left index finger without damage to nail

⑦**S61.252** Open bite of right middle finger without damage to nail

⑦**S61.253** Open bite of left middle finger without damage to nail

⑦**S61.254** Open bite of right ring finger without damage to nail

⑦**S61.255** Open bite of left ring finger without damage to nail

⑦**S61.256** Open bite of right little finger without damage to nail

⑦**S61.257** Open bite of left little finger without damage to nail

⑦**S61.258** Open bite of other finger without damage to nail

Open bite of specified finger with unspecified laterality without damage to nail

⑦**S61.259** Open bite of unspecified finger without damage to nail

S61.3 Open wound of other finger with damage to nail

S61.30 Unspecified open wound of finger with damage to nail

⑦**S61.300** Unspecified open wound of right index finger with damage to nail

⑦**S61.301** Unspecified open wound of left index finger with damage to nail

⑦**S61.302** Unspecified open wound of right middle finger with damage to nail

⑦**S61.303** Unspecified open wound of left middle finger with damage to nail

⑦**S61.304** Unspecified open wound of right ring finger with damage to nail

⑦**S61.305** Unspecified open wound of left ring finger with damage to nail

⑦**S61.306** Unspecified open wound of right little finger with damage to nail

⑦**S61.307** Unspecified open wound of left little finger with damage to nail

⑦**S61.308** Unspecified open wound of other finger with damage to nail
Unspecified open wound of specified finger with unspecified laterality with damage to nail

⑦**S61.309** Unspecified open wound of unspecified finger with damage to nail

S61.31 Laceration without foreign body of finger with damage to nail

⑦**S61.310** Laceration without foreign body of right index finger with damage to nail

⑦**S61.311** Laceration without foreign body of left index finger with damage to nail

⑦**S61.312** Laceration without foreign body of right middle finger with damage to nail

⑦**S61.313** Laceration without foreign body of left middle finger with damage to nail

⑦**S61.314** Laceration without foreign body of right ring finger with damage to nail

⑦**S61.315** Laceration without foreign body of left ring finger with damage to nail

⑦**S61.316** Laceration without foreign body of right little finger with damage to nail

⑦**S61.317** Laceration without foreign body of left little finger with damage to nail

⑦**S61.318** Laceration without foreign body of other finger with damage to nail
Laceration without foreign body of specified finger with unspecified laterality with damage to nail

⑦**S61.319**   Laceration without foreign body of unspecified finger with damage to nail

S61.32   Laceration with foreign body of finger with damage to nail

⑦**S61.320**   Laceration with foreign body of right index finger with damage to nail

⑦**S61.321**   Laceration with foreign body of left index finger with damage to nail

⑦**S61.322**   Laceration with foreign body of right middle finger with damage to nail

⑦**S61.323**   Laceration with foreign body of left middle finger with damage to nail

⑦**S61.324**   Laceration with foreign body of right ring finger with damage to nail

⑦**S61.325**   Laceration with foreign body of left ring finger with damage to nail

⑦**S61.326**   Laceration with foreign body of right little finger with damage to nail

⑦**S61.327**   Laceration with foreign body of left little finger with damage to nail

⑦**S61.328**   Laceration with foreign body of other finger with damage to nail
Laceration with foreign body of specified finger with unspecified laterality with damage to nail

⑦**S61.329**   Laceration with foreign body of unspecified finger with damage to nail

S61.33   Puncture wound without foreign body of finger with damage to nail

⑦**S61.330**   Puncture wound without foreign body of right index finger with damage to nail

⑦**S61.331**   Puncture wound without foreign body of left index finger with damage to nail

⑦**S61.332**   Puncture wound without foreign body of right middle finger with damage to nail

⑦**S61.333**   Puncture wound without foreign body of left middle finger with damage to nail

⑦**S61.334**   Puncture wound without foreign body of right ring finger with damage to nail

⑦**S61.335**   Puncture wound without foreign body of left ring finger with damage to nail

⑦**S61.336**   Puncture wound without foreign body of right little finger with damage to nail

⑦**S61.337**   Puncture wound without foreign body of left little finger with damage to nail

⑦**S61.338**   Puncture wound without foreign body of other finger with damage to nail

Puncture wound without foreign body of specified finger with unspecified laterality with damage to nail

⑦**S61.339**   Puncture wound without foreign body of unspecified finger with damage to nail

S61.34   Puncture wound with foreign body of finger with damage to nail

⑦**S61.340**   Puncture wound with foreign body of right index finger with damage to nail

⑦**S61.341**   Puncture wound with foreign body of left index finger with damage to nail

⑦**S61.342**   Puncture wound with foreign body of right middle finger with damage to nail

⑦**S61.343**   Puncture wound with foreign body of left middle finger with damage to nail

⑦**S61.344**   Puncture wound with foreign body of right ring finger with damage to nail

⑦**S61.345**   Puncture wound with foreign body of left ring finger with damage to nail

⑦**S61.346**   Puncture wound with foreign body of right little finger with damage to nail

⑦**S61.347**   Puncture wound with foreign body of left little finger with damage to nail

⑦**S61.348**   Puncture wound with foreign body of other finger with damage to nail
Puncture wound with foreign body of specified finger with unspecified laterality with damage to nail

⑦**S61.349**   Puncture wound with foreign body of unspecified finger with damage to nail

S61.35   Open bite of finger with damage to nail
Bite of finger with damage to nail NOS
Excludes 1: superficial bite of finger (S60.46-, S60.47-)

⑦**S61.350**   Open bite of right index finger with damage to nail

⑦**S61.351**   Open bite of left index finger with damage to nail

⑦**S61.352**   Open bite of right middle finger with damage to nail

⑦**S61.353**   Open bite of left middle finger with damage to nail

⑦**S61.354**   Open bite of right ring finger with damage to nail

⑦**S61.355**   Open bite of left ring finger with damage to nail

⑦**S61.356**   Open bite of right little finger with damage to nail

⑦**S61.357**   Open bite of left little finger with damage to nail

⑦S61.358   Open bite of other finger with damage to nail

Open bite of specified finger with unspecified laterality with damage to nail

⑦S61.359   Open bite of unspecified finger with damage to nail

S61.4   Open wound of hand

  S61.40   Unspecified open wound of hand

    ⑦S61.401   Unspecified open wound of right hand

    ⑦S61.402   Unspecified open wound of left hand

    ⑦S61.409   Unspecified open wound of unspecified hand

  S61.41   Laceration without foreign body of hand

    ⑦S61.411   Laceration without foreign body of right hand

    ⑦S61.412   Laceration without foreign body of left hand

    ⑦S61.419   Laceration without foreign body of unspecified hand

  S61.42   Laceration with foreign body of hand

    ⑦S61.421   Laceration with foreign body of right hand

    ⑦S61.422   Laceration with foreign body of left hand

    ⑦S61.429   Laceration with foreign body of unspecified hand

  S61.43   Puncture wound without foreign body of hand

    ⑦S61.431   Puncture wound without foreign body of right hand

    ⑦S61.432   Puncture wound without foreign body of left hand

    ⑦S61.439   Puncture wound without foreign body of unspecified hand

  S61.44   Puncture wound with foreign body of hand

    ⑦S61.441   Puncture wound with foreign body of right hand

    ⑦S61.442   Puncture wound with foreign body of left hand

    ⑦S61.449   Puncture wound with foreign body of unspecified hand

  S61.45   Open bite of hand

    Bite of hand NOS

    Excludes 1: superficial bite of hand (S60.56-, S60.57-)

    ⑦S61.451   Open bite of right hand

    ⑦S61.452   Open bite of left hand

    ⑦S61.459   Open bite of unspecified hand

S61.5   Open wound of wrist

  S61.50   Unspecified open wound of wrist

    ⑦S61.501   Unspecified open wound of right wrist

    ⑦S61.502   Unspecified open wound of left wrist

    ⑦S61.509   Unspecified open wound of unspecified wrist

  S61.51   Laceration without foreign body of wrist

    ⑦S61.511   Laceration without foreign body of right wrist

    ⑦S61.512   Laceration without foreign body of left wrist

    ⑦S61.519   Laceration without foreign body of unspecified wrist

  S61.52   Laceration with foreign body of wrist

    ⑦S61.521   Laceration with foreign body of right wrist

    ⑦S61.522   Laceration with foreign body of left wrist

    ⑦S61.529   Laceration with foreign body of unspecified wrist

  S61.53   Puncture wound without foreign body of wrist

    ⑦S61.531   Puncture wound without foreign body of right wrist

    ⑦S61.532   Puncture wound without foreign body of left wrist

    ⑦S61.539   Puncture wound without foreign body of unspecified wrist

  S61.54   Puncture wound with foreign body of wrist

    ⑦S61.541   Puncture wound with foreign body of right wrist

    ⑦S61.542   Puncture wound with foreign body of left wrist

    ⑦S61.549   Puncture wound with foreign body of unspecified wrist

  S61.55   Open bite of wrist

    Bite of wrist NOS

    Excludes 1: superficial bite of wrist (S60.86-, S60.87-)

    ⑦S61.551   Open bite of right wrist

    ⑦S61.552   Open bite of left wrist

    ⑦S61.559   Open bite of unspecified wrist

S62   Fracture at wrist and hand level

  Note: A fracture not indicated as displaced or nondisplaced should be coded to displaced

      A fracture not indicated as open or closed should be coded to closed

  Excludes 1: traumatic amputation of wrist and hand (S68.-)

  Excludes 2: fracture of distal parts of ulna and radius (S52.-)

The appropriate 7th character is to be added to each code from category S62

A - initial encounter for closed fracture

B - initial encounter for open fracture

D - subsequent encounter for fracture with routine healing

G - subsequent encounter for fracture with delayed healing

K - subsequent encounter for fracture with nonunion

P - subsequent encounter for fracture with malunion

S - sequela

S62.0   Fracture of navicular [scaphoid] bone of wrist

  S62.00   Unspecified fracture of navicular [scaphoid] bone of wrist

    ⑦S62.001   Unspecified fracture of navicular [scaphoid] bone of right wrist

    ⑦S62.002   Unspecified fracture of navicular [scaphoid] bone of left wrist

    ⑦S62.009   Unspecified fracture of navicular [scaphoid] bone of unspecified wrist

S62.01 Fracture of distal pole of navicular [scaphoid] bone of wrist
Fracture of volar tuberosity of navicular [scaphoid] bone of wrist

⑦**S62.011** Displaced fracture of distal pole of navicular [scaphoid] bone of right wrist

⑦**S62.012** Displaced fracture of distal pole of navicular [scaphoid] bone of left wrist

⑦**S62.013** Displaced fracture of distal pole of navicular [scaphoid] bone of unspecified wrist

⑦**S62.014** Nondisplaced fracture of distal pole of navicular [scaphoid] bone of right wrist

⑦**S62.015** Nondisplaced fracture of distal pole of navicular [scaphoid] bone of left wrist

⑦**S62.016** Nondisplaced fracture of distal pole of navicular [scaphoid] bone of unspecified wrist

S62.02 Fracture of middle third of navicular [scaphoid] bone of wrist

⑦**S62.021** Displaced fracture of middle third of navicular [scaphoid] bone of right wrist

⑦**S62.022** Displaced fracture of middle third of navicular [scaphoid] bone of left wrist

⑦**S62.023** Displaced fracture of middle third of navicular [scaphoid] bone of unspecified wrist

⑦**S62.024** Nondisplaced fracture of middle third of navicular [scaphoid] bone of right wrist

⑦**S62.025** Nondisplaced fracture of middle third of navicular [scaphoid] bone of left wrist

⑦**S62.026** Nondisplaced fracture of middle third of navicular [scaphoid] bone of unspecified wrist

S62.03 Fracture of proximal third of navicular [scaphoid] bone of wrist

⑦**S62.031** Displaced fracture of proximal third of navicular [scaphoid] bone of right wrist

⑦**S62.032** Displaced fracture of proximal third of navicular [scaphoid] bone of left wrist

⑦**S62.033** Displaced fracture of proximal third of navicular [scaphoid] bone of unspecified wrist

⑦**S62.034** Nondisplaced fracture of proximal third of navicular [scaphoid] bone of right wrist

⑦**S62.035** Nondisplaced fracture of proximal third of navicular [scaphoid] bone of left wrist

⑦**S62.036** Nondisplaced fracture of proximal third of navicular [scaphoid] bone of unspecified wrist

S62.1 Fracture of other and unspecified carpal bone(s)
Excludes 2: fracture of scaphoid of wrist (S62.0-)

S62.10 Fracture of unspecified carpal bone
Fracture of wrist NOS

⑦**S62.101** Fracture of unspecified carpal bone, right wrist

⑦**S62.102** Fracture of unspecified carpal bone, left wrist

⑦**S62.109** Fracture of unspecified carpal bone, unspecified wrist

S62.11 Fracture of triquetrum [cuneiform] bone of wrist

⑦**S62.111** Displaced fracture of triquetrum [cuneiform] bone, right wrist

⑦**S62.112** Displaced fracture of triquetrum [cuneiform] bone, left wrist

⑦**S62.113** Displaced fracture of triquetrum [cuneiform] bone, unspecified wrist

⑦**S62.114** Nondisplaced fracture of triquetrum [cuneiform] bone, right wrist

⑦**S62.115** Nondisplaced fracture of triquetrum [cuneiform] bone, left wrist

⑦**S62.116** Nondisplaced fracture of triquetrum [cuneiform] bone, unspecified wrist

S62.12 Fracture of lunate [semilunar]

⑦**S62.121** Displaced fracture of lunate [semilunar], right wrist

⑦**S62.122** Displaced fracture of lunate [semilunar], left wrist

⑦**S62.123** Displaced fracture of lunate [semilunar], unspecified wrist

⑦**S62.124** Nondisplaced fracture of lunate [semilunar], right wrist

⑦**S62.125** Nondisplaced fracture of lunate [semilunar], left wrist

⑦**S62.126** Nondisplaced fracture of lunate [semilunar], unspecified wrist

S62.13 Fracture of capitate [os magnum] bone

⑦**S62.131** Displaced fracture of capitate [os magnum] bone, right wrist

⑦**S62.132** Displaced fracture of capitate [os magnum] bone, left wrist

⑦**S62.133** Displaced fracture of capitate [os magnum] bone, unspecified wrist

⑦**S62.134** Nondisplaced fracture of capitate [os magnum] bone, right wrist

⑦**S62.135** Nondisplaced fracture of capitate [os magnum] bone, left wrist

⑦**S62.136** Nondisplaced fracture of capitate [os magnum] bone, unspecified wrist

S62.14 Fracture of body of hamate [unciform] bone
Fracture of hamate [unciform] bone NOS

⑦**S62.141** Displaced fracture of body of hamate [unciform] bone, right wrist

⑦**S62.142** Displaced fracture of body of hamate [unciform] bone, left wrist

⑦ **S62.143** Displaced fracture of body of hamate [unciform] bone, unspecified wrist

⑦ **S62.144** Nondisplaced fracture of body of hamate [unciform] bone, right wrist

⑦ **S62.145** Nondisplaced fracture of body of hamate [unciform] bone, left wrist

⑦ **S62.146** Nondisplaced fracture of body of hamate [unciform] bone, unspecified wrist

S62.15 Fracture of hook process of hamate [unciform] bone

Fracture of unciform process of hamate [unciform] bone

⑦ **S62.151** Displaced fracture of hook process of hamate [unciform] bone, right wrist

⑦ **S62.152** Displaced fracture of hook process of hamate [unciform] bone, left wrist

⑦ **S62.153** Displaced fracture of hook process of hamate [unciform] bone, unspecified wrist

⑦ **S62.154** Nondisplaced fracture of hook process of hamate [unciform] bone, right wrist

⑦ **S62.155** Nondisplaced fracture of hook process of hamate [unciform] bone, left wrist

⑦ **S62.156** Nondisplaced fracture of hook process of hamate [unciform] bone, unspecified wrist

S62.16 Fracture of pisiform

⑦ **S62.161** Displaced fracture of pisiform, right wrist

⑦ **S62.162** Displaced fracture of pisiform, left wrist

⑦ **S62.163** Displaced fracture of pisiform, unspecified wrist

⑦ **S62.164** Nondisplaced fracture of pisiform, right wrist

⑦ **S62.165** Nondisplaced fracture of pisiform, left wrist

⑦ **S62.166** Nondisplaced fracture of pisiform, unspecified wrist

S62.17 Fracture of trapezium [larger multangular]

⑦ **S62.171** Displaced fracture of trapezium [larger multangular], right wrist

⑦ **S62.172** Displaced fracture of trapezium [larger multangular], left wrist

⑦ **S62.173** Displaced fracture of trapezium [larger multangular], unspecified wrist

⑦ **S62.174** Nondisplaced fracture of trapezium [larger multangular], right wrist

⑦ **S62.175** Nondisplaced fracture of trapezium [larger multangular], left wrist

⑦ **S62.176** Nondisplaced fracture of trapezium [larger multangular], unspecified wrist

S62.18 Fracture of trapezoid [smaller multangular]

⑦ **S62.181** Displaced fracture of trapezoid [smaller multangular], right wrist

⑦ **S62.182** Displaced fracture of trapezoid [smaller multangular], left wrist

⑦ **S62.183** Displaced fracture of trapezoid [smaller multangular], unspecified wrist

⑦ **S62.184** Nondisplaced fracture of trapezoid [smaller multangular], right wrist

⑦ **S62.185** Nondisplaced fracture of trapezoid [smaller multangular], left wrist

⑦ **S62.186** Nondisplaced fracture of trapezoid [smaller multangular], unspecified wrist

S62.2 Fracture of first metacarpal bone

S62.20 Unspecified fracture of first metacarpal bone

⑦ **S62.201** Unspecified fracture of first metacarpal bone, right hand

⑦ **S62.202** Unspecified fracture of first metacarpal bone, left hand

⑦ **S62.209** Unspecified fracture of first metacarpal bone, unspecified hand

S62.21 Bennett's fracture

⑦ **S62.211** Bennett's fracture, right hand

⑦ **S62.212** Bennett's fracture, left hand

⑦ **S62.213** Bennett's fracture, unspecified hand

S62.22 Rolando's fracture

⑦ **S62.221** Displaced Rolando's fracture, right hand

⑦ **S62.222** Displaced Rolando's fracture, left hand

⑦ **S62.223** Displaced Rolando's fracture, unspecified hand

⑦ **S62.224** Nondisplaced Rolando's fracture, right hand

⑦ **S62.225** Nondisplaced Rolando's fracture, left hand

⑦ **S62.226** Nondisplaced Rolando's fracture, unspecified hand

S62.23 Other fracture of base of first metacarpal bone

⑦ **S62.231** Other displaced fracture of base of first metacarpal bone, right hand

⑦ **S62.232** Other displaced fracture of base of first metacarpal bone, left hand

⑦ **S62.233** Other displaced fracture of base of first metacarpal bone, unspecified hand

⑦ **S62.234** Other nondisplaced fracture of base of first metacarpal bone, right hand

⑦ **S62.235** Other nondisplaced fracture of base of first metacarpal bone, left hand

⑦ **S62.236** Other nondisplaced fracture of base of first metacarpal bone, unspecified hand

S62.24 Fracture of shaft of first metacarpal bone

⑦ **S62.241** Displaced fracture of shaft of first metacarpal bone, right hand

● New code   ▲ Revised code   ⑦ 7ᵗʰ digit required   ⊗ Placeholder required

⑦S62.242 Displaced fracture of shaft of first metacarpal bone, left hand

⑦S62.243 Displaced fracture of shaft of first metacarpal bone, unspecified hand

⑦S62.244 Nondisplaced fracture of shaft of first metacarpal bone, right hand

⑦S62.245 Nondisplaced fracture of shaft of first metacarpal bone, left hand

⑦S62.246 Nondisplaced fracture of shaft of first metacarpal bone, unspecified hand

S62.25 Fracture of neck of first metacarpal bone

⑦S62.251 Displaced fracture of neck of first metacarpal bone, right hand

⑦S62.252 Displaced fracture of neck of first metacarpal bone, left hand

⑦S62.253 Displaced fracture of neck of first metacarpal bone, unspecified hand

⑦S62.254 Nondisplaced fracture of neck of first metacarpal bone, right hand

⑦S62.255 Nondisplaced fracture of neck of first metacarpal bone, left hand

⑦S62.256 Nondisplaced fracture of neck of first metacarpal bone, unspecified hand

S62.29 Other fracture of first metacarpal bone

⑦S62.291 Other fracture of first metacarpal bone, right hand

⑦S62.292 Other fracture of first metacarpal bone, left hand

⑦S62.299 Other fracture of first metacarpal bone, unspecified hand

S62.3 Fracture of other and unspecified metacarpal bone

Excludes 2: fracture of first metacarpal bone (S62.2-)

S62.30 Unspecified fracture of other metacarpal bone

⑦S62.300 Unspecified fracture of second metacarpal bone, right hand

⑦S62.301 Unspecified fracture of second metacarpal bone, left hand

⑦S62.302 Unspecified fracture of third metacarpal bone, right hand

⑦S62.303 Unspecified fracture of third metacarpal bone, left hand

⑦S62.304 Unspecified fracture of fourth metacarpal bone, right hand

⑦S62.305 Unspecified fracture of fourth metacarpal bone, left hand

⑦S62.306 Unspecified fracture of fifth metacarpal bone, right hand

⑦S62.307 Unspecified fracture of fifth metacarpal bone, left hand

⑦S62.308 Unspecified fracture of other metacarpal bone

Unspecified fracture of specified metacarpal bone with unspecified laterality

⑦S62.309 Unspecified fracture of unspecified metacarpal bone

S62.31 Displaced fracture of base of other metacarpal bone

⑦S62.310 Displaced fracture of base of second metacarpal bone, right hand

⑦S62.311 Displaced fracture of base of second metacarpal bone. left hand

⑦S62.312 Displaced fracture of base of third metacarpal bone, right hand

⑦S62.313 Displaced fracture of base of third metacarpal bone, left hand

⑦S62.314 Displaced fracture of base of fourth metacarpal bone, right hand

⑦S62.315 Displaced fracture of base of fourth metacarpal bone, left hand

⑦S62.316 Displaced fracture of base of fifth metacarpal bone, right hand

⑦S62.317 Displaced fracture of base of fifth metacarpal bone. left hand

⑦S62.318 Displaced fracture of base of other metacarpal bone

Displaced fracture of base of specified metacarpal bone with unspecified laterality

⑦S62.319 Displaced fracture of base of unspecified metacarpal bone

S62.32 Displaced fracture of shaft of other metacarpal bone

⑦S62.320 Displaced fracture of shaft of second metacarpal bone, right hand

⑦S62.321 Displaced fracture of shaft of second metacarpal bone, left hand

⑦S62.322 Displaced fracture of shaft of third metacarpal bone, right hand

⑦S62.323 Displaced fracture of shaft of third metacarpal bone, left hand

⑦S62.324 Displaced fracture of shaft of fourth metacarpal bone, right hand

⑦S62.325 Displaced fracture of shaft of fourth metacarpal bone, left hand

⑦S62.326 Displaced fracture of shaft of fifth metacarpal bone, right hand

⑦S62.327 Displaced fracture of shaft of fifth metacarpal bone, left hand

⑦S62.328 Displaced fracture of shaft of other metacarpal bone

Displaced fracture of shaft of specified metacarpal bone with unspecified laterality

⑦S62.329 Displaced fracture of shaft of unspecified metacarpal bone

S62.33 Displaced fracture of neck of other metacarpal bone

⑦S62.330 Displaced fracture of neck of second metacarpal bone, right hand

⑦S62.331 Displaced fracture of neck of second metacarpal bone, left hand

⑦S62.332 Displaced fracture of neck of third metacarpal bone, right hand

⑦S62.333 Displaced fracture of neck of third metacarpal bone, left hand

⑦S62.334 Displaced fracture of neck of fourth metacarpal bone, right hand

⑦S62.335   Displaced fracture of neck of fourth metacarpal bone, left hand

⑦S62.336   Displaced fracture of neck of fifth metacarpal bone, right hand

⑦S62.337   Displaced fracture of neck of fifth metacarpal bone, left hand

⑦S62.338   Displaced fracture of neck of other metacarpal bone

Displaced fracture of neck of specified metacarpal bone with unspecified laterality

⑦S62.339   Displaced fracture of neck of unspecified metacarpal bone

S62.34   Nondisplaced fracture of base of other metacarpal bone

⑦S62.340   Nondisplaced fracture of base of second metacarpal bone, right hand

⑦S62.341   Nondisplaced fracture of base of second metacarpal bone. left hand

⑦S62.342   Nondisplaced fracture of base of third metacarpal bone, right hand

⑦S62.343   Nondisplaced fracture of base of third metacarpal bone, left hand

⑦S62.344   Nondisplaced fracture of base of fourth metacarpal bone, right hand

⑦S62.345   Nondisplaced fracture of base of fourth metacarpal bone, left hand

⑦S62.346   Nondisplaced fracture of base of fifth metacarpal bone, right hand

⑦S62.347   Nondisplaced fracture of base of fifth metacarpal bone. left hand

⑦S62.348   Nondisplaced fracture of base of other metacarpal bone

Nondisplaced fracture of base of specified metacarpal bone with unspecified laterality

⑦S62.349   Nondisplaced fracture of base of unspecified metacarpal bone

S62.35   Nondisplaced fracture of shaft of other metacarpal bone

⑦S62.350   Nondisplaced fracture of shaft of second metacarpal bone, right hand

⑦S62.351   Nondisplaced fracture of shaft of second metacarpal bone, left hand

⑦S62.352   Nondisplaced fracture of shaft of third metacarpal bone, right hand

⑦S62.353   Nondisplaced fracture of shaft of third metacarpal bone, left hand

⑦S62.354   Nondisplaced fracture of shaft of fourth metacarpal bone, right hand

⑦S62.355   Nondisplaced fracture of shaft of fourth metacarpal bone, left hand

⑦S62.356   Nondisplaced fracture of shaft of fifth metacarpal bone, right hand

⑦S62.357   Nondisplaced fracture of shaft of fifth metacarpal bone, left hand

⑦S62.358   Nondisplaced fracture of shaft of other metacarpal bone

Nondisplaced fracture of shaft of specified metacarpal bone with unspecified laterality

⑦S62.359   Nondisplaced fracture of shaft of unspecified metacarpal bone

S62.36   Nondisplaced fracture of neck of other metacarpal bone

⑦S62.360   Nondisplaced fracture of neck of second metacarpal bone, right hand

⑦S62.361   Nondisplaced fracture of neck of second metacarpal bone, left hand

⑦S62.362   Nondisplaced fracture of neck of third metacarpal bone, right hand

⑦S62.363   Nondisplaced fracture of neck of third metacarpal bone, left hand

⑦S62.364   Nondisplaced fracture of neck of fourth metacarpal bone, right hand

⑦S62.365   Nondisplaced fracture of neck of fourth metacarpal bone, left hand

⑦S62.366   Nondisplaced fracture of neck of fifth metacarpal bone, right hand

⑦S62.367   Nondisplaced fracture of neck of fifth metacarpal bone, left hand

⑦S62.368   Nondisplaced fracture of neck of other metacarpal bone

Nondisplaced fracture of neck of specified metacarpal bone with unspecified laterality

⑦S62.369   Nondisplaced fracture of neck of unspecified metacarpal bone

S62.39   Other fracture of other metacarpal bone

⑦S62.390   Other fracture of second metacarpal bone, right hand

⑦S62.391   Other fracture of second metacarpal bone, left hand

⑦S62.392   Other fracture of third metacarpal bone, right hand

⑦S62.393   Other fracture of third metacarpal bone, left hand

⑦S62.394   Other fracture of fourth metacarpal bone, right hand

⑦S62.395   Other fracture of fourth metacarpal bone, left hand

⑦S62.396   Other fracture of fifth metacarpal bone, right hand

⑦S62.397   Other fracture of fifth metacarpal bone, left hand

⑦S62.398   Other fracture of other metacarpal bone

Other fracture of specified metacarpal bone with unspecified laterality

⑦S62.399   Other fracture of unspecified metacarpal bone

S62.5   Fracture of thumb

S62.50   Fracture of unspecified phalanx of thumb

⑦S62.501   Fracture of unspecified phalanx of right thumb

  ● New code   ▲ Revised code   ⑦ 7th digit required   ⊗ Placeholder required

⑦S62.502   Fracture of unspecified phalanx of left thumb

⑦S62.509   Fracture of unspecified phalanx of unspecified thumb

S62.51   Fracture of proximal phalanx of thumb

⑦S62.511   Displaced fracture of proximal phalanx of right thumb

⑦S62.512   Displaced fracture of proximal phalanx of left thumb

⑦S62.513   Displaced fracture of proximal phalanx of unspecified thumb

⑦S62.514   Nondisplaced fracture of proximal phalanx of right thumb

⑦S62.515   Nondisplaced fracture of proximal phalanx of left thumb

⑦S62.516   Nondisplaced fracture of proximal phalanx of unspecified thumb

S62.52   Fracture of distal phalanx of thumb

⑦S62.521   Displaced fracture of distal phalanx of right thumb

⑦S62.522   Displaced fracture of distal phalanx of left thumb

⑦S62.523   Displaced fracture of distal phalanx of unspecified thumb

⑦S62.524   Nondisplaced fracture of distal phalanx of right thumb

⑦S62.525   Nondisplaced fracture of distal phalanx of left thumb

⑦S62.526   Nondisplaced fracture of distal phalanx of unspecified thumb

S62.6   Fracture of other and unspecified finger(s)

Excludes 2: fracture of thumb (S62.5-)

S62.60   Fracture of unspecified phalanx of finger

⑦S62.600   Fracture of unspecified phalanx of right index finger

⑦S62.601   Fracture of unspecified phalanx of left index finger

⑦S62.602   Fracture of unspecified phalanx of right middle finger

⑦S62.603   Fracture of unspecified phalanx of left middle finger

⑦S62.604   Fracture of unspecified phalanx of right ring finger

⑦S62.605   Fracture of unspecified phalanx of left ring finger

⑦S62.606   Fracture of unspecified phalanx of right little finger

⑦S62.607   Fracture of unspecified phalanx of left little finger

⑦S62.608   Fracture of unspecified phalanx of other finger

Fracture of unspecified phalanx of specified finger with unspecified laterality

⑦S62.609   Fracture of unspecified phalanx of unspecified finger

S62.61   Displaced fracture of proximal phalanx of finger

⑦S62.610   Displaced fracture of proximal phalanx of right index finger

⑦S62.611   Displaced fracture of proximal phalanx of left index finger

⑦S62.612   Displaced fracture of proximal phalanx of right middle finger

⑦S62.613   Displaced fracture of proximal phalanx of left middle finger

⑦S62.614   Displaced fracture of proximal phalanx of right ring finger

⑦S62.615   Displaced fracture of proximal phalanx of left ring finger

⑦S62.616   Displaced fracture of proximal phalanx of right little finger

⑦S62.617   Displaced fracture of proximal phalanx of left little finger

⑦S62.618   Displaced fracture of proximal phalanx of other finger

Displaced fracture of proximal phalanx of specified finger with unspecified laterality

⑦S62.619   Displaced fracture of proximal phalanx of unspecified finger

S62.62   Displaced fracture of medial phalanx of finger

⑦S62.620   Displaced fracture of medial phalanx of right index finger

⑦S62.621   Displaced fracture of medial phalanx of left index finger

⑦S62.622   Displaced fracture of medial phalanx of right middle finger

⑦S62.623   Displaced fracture of medial phalanx of left middle finger

⑦S62.624   Displaced fracture of medial phalanx of right ring finger

⑦S62.625   Displaced fracture of medial phalanx of left ring finger

⑦S62.626   Displaced fracture of medial phalanx of right little finger

⑦S62.627   Displaced fracture of medial phalanx of left little finger

⑦S62.628   Displaced fracture of medial phalanx of other finger

Displaced fracture of medial phalanx of specified finger with unspecified laterality

⑦S62.629   Displaced fracture of medial phalanx of unspecified finger

S62.63   Displaced fracture of distal phalanx of finger

⑦S62.630   Displaced fracture of distal phalanx of right index finger

⑦S62.631   Displaced fracture of distal phalanx of left index finger

⑦S62.632   Displaced fracture of distal phalanx of right middle finger

⑦S62.633   Displaced fracture of distal phalanx of left middle finger

⑦S62.634   Displaced fracture of distal phalanx of right ring finger

⑦S62.635   Displaced fracture of distal phalanx of left ring finger

⑦**S62.636** Displaced fracture of distal phalanx of right little finger

⑦**S62.637** Displaced fracture of distal phalanx of left little finger

⑦**S62.638** Displaced fracture of distal phalanx of other finger

Displaced fracture of distal phalanx of specified finger with unspecified laterality

⑦**S62.639** Displaced fracture of distal phalanx of unspecified finger

S62.64 Nondisplaced fracture of proximal phalanx of finger

⑦**S62.640** Nondisplaced fracture of proximal phalanx of right index finger

⑦**S62.641** Nondisplaced fracture of proximal phalanx of left index finger

⑦**S62.642** Nondisplaced fracture of proximal phalanx of right middle finger

⑦**S62.643** Nondisplaced fracture of proximal phalanx of left middle finger

⑦**S62.644** Nondisplaced fracture of proximal phalanx of right ring finger

⑦**S62.645** Nondisplaced fracture of proximal phalanx of left ring finger

⑦**S62.646** Nondisplaced fracture of proximal phalanx of right little finger

⑦**S62.647** Nondisplaced fracture of proximal phalanx of left little finger

⑦**S62.648** Nondisplaced fracture of proximal phalanx of other finger

Nondisplaced fracture of proximal phalanx of specified finger with unspecified laterality

⑦**S62.649** Nondisplaced fracture of proximal phalanx of unspecified finger

S62.65 Nondisplaced fracture of medial phalanx of finger

⑦**S62.650** Nondisplaced fracture of medial phalanx of right index finger

⑦**S62.651** Nondisplaced fracture of medial phalanx of left index finger

⑦**S62.652** Nondisplaced fracture of medial phalanx of right middle finger

⑦**S62.653** Nondisplaced fracture of medial phalanx of left middle finger

⑦**S62.654** Nondisplaced fracture of medial phalanx of right ring finger

⑦**S62.655** Nondisplaced fracture of medial phalanx of left ring finger

⑦**S62.656** Nondisplaced fracture of medial phalanx of right little finger

⑦**S62.657** Nondisplaced fracture of medial phalanx of left little finger

⑦**S62.658** Nondisplaced fracture of medial phalanx of other finger

Nondisplaced fracture of medial phalanx of specified finger with unspecified laterality

⑦**S62.659** Nondisplaced fracture of medial phalanx of unspecified finger

S62.66 Nondisplaced fracture of distal phalanx of finger

⑦**S62.660** Nondisplaced fracture of distal phalanx of right index finger

⑦**S62.661** Nondisplaced fracture of distal phalanx of left index finger

⑦**S62.662** Nondisplaced fracture of distal phalanx of right middle finger

⑦**S62.663** Nondisplaced fracture of distal phalanx of left middle finger

⑦**S62.664** Nondisplaced fracture of distal phalanx of right ring finger

⑦**S62.665** Nondisplaced fracture of distal phalanx of left ring finger

⑦**S62.666** Nondisplaced fracture of distal phalanx of right little finger

⑦**S62.667** Nondisplaced fracture of distal phalanx of left little finger

⑦**S62.668** Nondisplaced fracture of distal phalanx of other finger

Nondisplaced fracture of distal phalanx of specified finger with unspecified laterality

⑦**S62.669** Nondisplaced fracture of distal phalanx of unspecified finger

S62.9 Unspecified fracture of wrist and hand

⊗⑦**S62.90** Unspecified fracture of unspecified wrist and hand

⊗⑦**S62.91** Unspecified fracture of right wrist and hand

⊗⑦**S62.92** Unspecified fracture of left wrist and hand

S63 Dislocation and sprain of joints and ligaments at wrist and hand level

Includes: avulsion of joint or ligament at wrist and hand level

laceration of cartilage, joint or ligament at wrist and hand level

sprain of cartilage, joint or ligament at wrist and hand level

traumatic hemarthrosis of joint or ligament at wrist and hand level

traumatic rupture of joint or ligament at wrist and hand level

traumatic subluxation of joint or ligament at wrist and hand level

traumatic tear of joint or ligament at wrist and hand level

Code also any associated open wound

Excludes 2: strain of muscle, fascia and tendon of wrist and hand (S66.-)

The appropriate 7th character is to be added to each code from category S63

A - initial encounter

D - subsequent encounter

S - sequela

S63.0 Subluxation and dislocation of wrist and hand joints

S63.00 Unspecified subluxation and dislocation of wrist and hand

Dislocation of carpal bone NOS

Dislocation of distal end of radius NOS

Subluxation of carpal bone NOS

● New code   ▲ Revised code   ⑦ 7th digit required   ⊗ Placeholder required

Subluxation of distal end of radius NOS

⑦S63.001 Unspecified subluxation of right wrist and hand

⑦S63.002 Unspecified subluxation of left wrist and hand

⑦S63.003 Unspecified subluxation of unspecified wrist and hand

⑦S63.004 Unspecified dislocation of right wrist and hand

⑦S63.005 Unspecified dislocation of left wrist and hand

⑦S63.006 Unspecified dislocation of unspecified wrist and hand

S63.01 Subluxation and dislocation of distal radioulnar joint

⑦S63.011 Subluxation of distal radioulnar joint of right wrist

⑦S63.012 Subluxation of distal radioulnar joint of left wrist

⑦S63.013 Subluxation of distal radioulnar joint of unspecified wrist

⑦S63.014 Dislocation of distal radioulnar joint of right wrist

⑦S63.015 Dislocation of distal radioulnar joint of left wrist

⑦S63.016 Dislocation of distal radioulnar joint of unspecified wrist

S63.02 Subluxation and dislocation of radiocarpal joint

⑦S63.021 Subluxation of radiocarpal joint of right wrist

⑦S63.022 Subluxation of radiocarpal joint of left wrist

⑦S63.023 Subluxation of radiocarpal joint of unspecified wrist

⑦S63.024 Dislocation of radiocarpal joint of right wrist

⑦S63.025 Dislocation of radiocarpal joint of left wrist

⑦S63.026 Dislocation of radiocarpal joint of unspecified wrist

S63.03 Subluxation and dislocation of midcarpal joint

⑦S63.031 Subluxation of midcarpal joint of right wrist

⑦S63.032 Subluxation of midcarpal joint of left wrist

⑦S63.033 Subluxation of midcarpal joint of unspecified wrist

⑦S63.034 Dislocation of midcarpal joint of right wrist

⑦S63.035 Dislocation of midcarpal joint of left wrist

⑦S63.036 Dislocation of midcarpal joint of unspecified wrist

S63.04 Subluxation and dislocation of carpometacarpal joint of thumb

Excludes 2: interphalangeal subluxation and dislocation of thumb (S63.1-)

⑦S63.041 Subluxation of carpometacarpal joint of right thumb

⑦S63.042 Subluxation of carpometacarpal joint of left thumb

⑦S63.043 Subluxation of carpometacarpal joint of unspecified thumb

⑦S63.044 Dislocation of carpometacarpal joint of right thumb

⑦S63.045 Dislocation of carpometacarpal joint of left thumb

⑦S63.046 Dislocation of carpometacarpal joint of unspecified thumb

S63.05 Subluxation and dislocation of other carpometacarpal joint

Excludes 2: subluxation and dislocation of carpometacarpal joint of thumb (S63.04-)

⑦S63.051 Subluxation of other carpometacarpal joint of right hand

⑦S63.052 Subluxation of other carpometacarpal joint of left hand

⑦S63.053 Subluxation of other carpometacarpal joint of unspecified hand

⑦S63.054 Dislocation of other carpometacarpal joint of right hand

⑦S63.055 Dislocation of other carpometacarpal joint of left hand

⑦S63.056 Dislocation of other carpometacarpal joint of unspecified hand

S63.06 Subluxation and dislocation of metacarpal (bone), proximal end

⑦S63.061 Subluxation of metacarpal (bone), proximal end of right hand

⑦S63.062 Subluxation of metacarpal (bone), proximal end of left hand

⑦S63.063 Subluxation of metacarpal (bone), proximal end of unspecified hand

⑦S63.064 Dislocation of metacarpal (bone), proximal end of right hand

⑦S63.065 Dislocation of metacarpal (bone), proximal end of left hand

⑦S63.066 Dislocation of metacarpal (bone), proximal end of unspecified hand

S63.07 Subluxation and dislocation of distal end of ulna

⑦S63.071 Subluxation of distal end of right ulna

⑦S63.072 Subluxation of distal end of left ulna

⑦S63.073 Subluxation of distal end of unspecified ulna

⑦S63.074 Dislocation of distal end of right ulna

⑦S63.075 Dislocation of distal end of left ulna

⑦S63.076 Dislocation of distal end of unspecified ulna

S63.09 Other subluxation and dislocation of wrist and hand

⑦S63.091 Other subluxation of right wrist and hand

⑦S63.092 Other subluxation of left wrist and hand

⑦ **S63.093**   Other subluxation of unspecified wrist and hand

⑦ **S63.094**   Other dislocation of right wrist and hand

⑦ **S63.095**   Other dislocation of left wrist and hand

⑦ **S63.096**   Other dislocation of unspecified wrist and hand

S63.1   Subluxation and dislocation of thumb

   S63.10   Unspecified subluxation and dislocation of thumb

     ⑦ **S63.101**   Unspecified subluxation of right thumb

     ⑦ **S63.102**   Unspecified subluxation of left thumb

     ⑦ **S63.103**   Unspecified subluxation of unspecified thumb

     ⑦ **S63.104**   Unspecified dislocation of right thumb

     ⑦ **S63.105**   Unspecified dislocation of left thumb

     ⑦ **S63.106**   Unspecified dislocation of unspecified thumb

   S63.11   Subluxation and dislocation of metacarpophalangeal joint of thumb

     ⑦ **S63.111**   Subluxation of metacarpophalangeal joint of right thumb

     ⑦ **S63.112**   Subluxation of metacarpophalangeal joint of left thumb

     ⑦ **S63.113**   Subluxation of metacarpophalangeal joint of unspecified thumb

     ⑦ **S63.114**   Dislocation of metacarpophalangeal joint of right thumb

     ⑦ **S63.115**   Dislocation of metacarpophalangeal joint of left thumb

     ⑦ **S63.116**   Dislocation of metacarpophalangeal joint of unspecified thumb

   S63.12   Subluxation and dislocation of unspecified interphalangeal joint of thumb

     ⑦ **S63.121**   Subluxation of unspecified interphalangeal joint of right thumb

     ⑦ **S63.122**   Subluxation of unspecified interphalangeal joint of left thumb

     ⑦ **S63.123**   Subluxation of unspecified interphalangeal joint of unspecified thumb

     ⑦ **S63.124**   Dislocation of unspecified interphalangeal joint of right thumb

     ⑦ **S63.125**   Dislocation of unspecified interphalangeal joint of left thumb

     ⑦ **S63.126**   Dislocation of unspecified interphalangeal joint of unspecified thumb

   S63.13   Subluxation and dislocation of proximal interphalangeal joint of thumb

     ⑦ **S63.131**   Subluxation of proximal interphalangeal joint of right thumb

     ⑦ **S63.132**   Subluxation of proximal interphalangeal joint of left thumb

     ⑦ **S63.133**   Subluxation of proximal interphalangeal joint of unspecified thumb

     ⑦ **S63.134**   Dislocation of proximal interphalangeal joint of right thumb

     ⑦ **S63.135**   Dislocation of proximal interphalangeal joint of left thumb

     ⑦ **S63.136**   Dislocation of proximal interphalangeal joint of unspecified thumb

   S63.14   Subluxation and dislocation of distal interphalangeal joint of thumb

     ⑦ **S63.141**   Subluxation of distal interphalangeal joint of right thumb

     ⑦ **S63.142**   Subluxation of distal interphalangeal joint of left thumb

     ⑦ **S63.143**   Subluxation of distal interphalangeal joint of unspecified thumb

     ⑦ **S63.144**   Dislocation of distal interphalangeal joint of right thumb

     ⑦ **S63.145**   Dislocation of distal interphalangeal joint of left thumb

     ⑦ **S63.146**   Dislocation of distal interphalangeal joint of unspecified thumb

S63.2   Subluxation and dislocation of other finger(s)

   Excludes 2: subluxation and dislocation of thumb (S63.1-)

   S63.20   Unspecified subluxation of other finger

     ⑦ **S63.200**   Unspecified subluxation of right index finger

     ⑦ **S63.201**   Unspecified subluxation of left index finger

     ⑦ **S63.202**   Unspecified subluxation of right middle finger

     ⑦ **S63.203**   Unspecified subluxation of left middle finger

     ⑦ **S63.204**   Unspecified subluxation of right ring finger

     ⑦ **S63.205**   Unspecified subluxation of left ring finger

     ⑦ **S63.206**   Unspecified subluxation of right little finger

     ⑦ **S63.207**   Unspecified subluxation of left little finger

     ⑦ **S63.208**   Unspecified subluxation of other finger

       Unspecified subluxation of specified finger with unspecified laterality

     ⑦ **S63.209**   Unspecified subluxation of unspecified finger

   S63.21   Subluxation of metacarpophalangeal joint of finger

     ⑦ **S63.210**   Subluxation of metacarpophalangeal joint of right index finger

     ⑦ **S63.211**   Subluxation of metacarpophalangeal joint of left index finger

     ⑦ **S63.212**   Subluxation of metacarpophalangeal joint of right middle finger

   ● New code   ▲ Revised code   ⑦ 7th digit required   ⊗ Placeholder required

⑦ S63.213　Subluxation of metacarpophalangeal joint of left middle finger

⑦ S63.214　Subluxation of metacarpophalangeal joint of right ring finger

⑦ S63.215　Subluxation of metacarpophalangeal joint of left ring finger

⑦ S63.216　Subluxation of metacarpophalangeal joint of right little finger

⑦ S63.217　Subluxation of metacarpophalangeal joint of left little finger

⑦ S63.218　Subluxation of metacarpophalangeal joint of other finger
Subluxation of metacarpophalangeal joint of specified finger with unspecified laterality

⑦ S63.219　Subluxation of metacarpophalangeal joint of unspecified finger

S63.22　Subluxation of unspecified interphalangeal joint of finger

⑦ S63.220　Subluxation of unspecified interphalangeal joint of right index finger

⑦ S63.221　Subluxation of unspecified interphalangeal joint of left index finger

⑦ S63.222　Subluxation of unspecified interphalangeal joint of right middle finger

⑦ S63.223　Subluxation of unspecified interphalangeal joint of left middle finger

⑦ S63.224　Subluxation of unspecified interphalangeal joint of right ring finger

⑦ S63.225　Subluxation of unspecified interphalangeal joint of left ring finger

⑦ S63.226　Subluxation of unspecified interphalangeal joint of right little finger

⑦ S63.227　Subluxation of unspecified interphalangeal joint of left little finger

⑦ S63.228　Subluxation of unspecified interphalangeal joint of other finger
Subluxation of unspecified interphalangeal joint of specified finger with unspecified laterality

⑦ S63.229　Subluxation of unspecified interphalangeal joint of unspecified finger

S63.23　Subluxation of proximal interphalangeal joint of finger

⑦ S63.230　Subluxation of proximal interphalangeal joint of right index finger

⑦ S63.231　Subluxation of proximal interphalangeal joint of left index finger

⑦ S63.232　Subluxation of proximal interphalangeal joint of right middle finger

⑦ S63.233　Subluxation of proximal interphalangeal joint of left middle finger

⑦ S63.234　Subluxation of proximal interphalangeal joint of right ring finger

⑦ S63.235　Subluxation of proximal interphalangeal joint of left ring finger

⑦ S63.236　Subluxation of proximal interphalangeal joint of right little finger

⑦ S63.237　Subluxation of proximal interphalangeal joint of left little finger

⑦ S63.238　Subluxation of proximal interphalangeal joint of other finger
Subluxation of proximal interphalangeal joint of specified finger with unspecified laterality

⑦ S63.239　Subluxation of proximal interphalangeal joint of unspecified finger

S63.24　Subluxation of distal interphalangeal joint of finger

⑦ S63.240　Subluxation of distal interphalangeal joint of right index finger

⑦ S63.241　Subluxation of distal interphalangeal joint of left index finger

⑦ S63.242　Subluxation of distal interphalangeal joint of right middle finger

⑦ S63.243　Subluxation of distal interphalangeal joint of left middle finger

⑦ S63.244　Subluxation of distal interphalangeal joint of right ring finger

⑦ S63.245　Subluxation of distal interphalangeal joint of left ring finger

⑦ S63.246　Subluxation of distal interphalangeal joint of right little finger

⑦ S63.247　Subluxation of distal interphalangeal joint of left little finger

⑦ S63.248　Subluxation of distal interphalangeal joint of other finger
Subluxation of distal interphalangeal joint of specified finger with unspecified laterality

⑦ S63.249　Subluxation of distal interphalangeal joint of unspecified finger

S63.25　Unspecified dislocation of other finger

⑦ S63.250　Unspecified dislocation of right index finger

⑦ S63.251　Unspecified dislocation of left index finger

⑦ S63.252　Unspecified dislocation of right middle finger

⑦ S63.253　Unspecified dislocation of left middle finger

⑦S63.254 Unspecified dislocation of right ring finger

⑦S63.255 Unspecified dislocation of left ring finger

⑦S63.256 Unspecified dislocation of right little finger

⑦S63.257 Unspecified dislocation of left little finger

⑦S63.258 Unspecified dislocation of other finger

Unspecified dislocation of specified finger with unspecified laterality

⑦S63.259 Unspecified dislocation of unspecified finger

Unspecified dislocation of specified finger with unspecified laterality

S63.26 Dislocation of metacarpophalangeal joint of finger

⑦S63.260 Dislocation of metacarpophalangeal joint of right index finger

⑦S63.261 Dislocation of metacarpophalangeal joint of left index finger

⑦S63.262 Dislocation of metacarpophalangeal joint of right middle finger

⑦S63.263 Dislocation of metacarpophalangeal joint of left middle finger

⑦S63.264 Dislocation of metacarpophalangeal joint of right ring finger

⑦S63.265 Dislocation of metacarpophalangeal joint of left ring finger

⑦S63.266 Dislocation of metacarpophalangeal joint of right little finger

⑦S63.267 Dislocation of metacarpophalangeal joint of left little finger

⑦S63.268 Dislocation of metacarpophalangeal joint of other finger

Dislocation of metacarpophalangeal joint of specified finger with unspecified laterality

⑦S63.269 Dislocation of metacarpophalangeal joint of unspecified finger

S63.27 Dislocation of unspecified interphalangeal joint of finger

⑦S63.270 Dislocation of unspecified interphalangeal joint of right index finger

⑦S63.271 Dislocation of unspecified interphalangeal joint of left index finger

⑦S63.272 Dislocation of unspecified interphalangeal joint of right middle finger

⑦S63.273 Dislocation of unspecified interphalangeal joint of left middle finger

⑦S63.274 Dislocation of unspecified interphalangeal joint of right ring finger

⑦S63.275 Dislocation of unspecified interphalangeal joint of left ring finger

⑦S63.276 Dislocation of unspecified interphalangeal joint of right little finger

⑦S63.277 Dislocation of unspecified interphalangeal joint of left little finger

⑦S63.278 Dislocation of unspecified interphalangeal joint of other finger

Dislocation of unspecified interphalangeal joint of specified finger with unspecified laterality

⑦S63.279 Dislocation of unspecified interphalangeal joint of unspecified finger

Dislocation of unspecified interphalangeal joint of specified finger without specified laterality

S63.28 Dislocation of proximal interphalangeal joint of finger

⑦S63.280 Dislocation of proximal interphalangeal joint of right index finger

⑦S63.281 Dislocation of proximal interphalangeal joint of left index finger

⑦S63.282 Dislocation of proximal interphalangeal joint of right middle finger

⑦S63.283 Dislocation of proximal interphalangeal joint of left middle finger

⑦S63.284 Dislocation of proximal interphalangeal joint of right ring finger

⑦S63.285 Dislocation of proximal interphalangeal joint of left ring finger

⑦S63.286 Dislocation of proximal interphalangeal joint of right little finger

⑦S63.287 Dislocation of proximal interphalangeal joint of left little finger

⑦S63.288 Dislocation of proximal interphalangeal joint of other finger

Dislocation of proximal interphalangeal joint of specified finger with unspecified laterality

⑦S63.289 Dislocation of proximal interphalangeal joint of unspecified finger

S63.29 Dislocation of distal interphalangeal joint of finger

⑦S63.290 Dislocation of distal interphalangeal joint of right index finger

⑦S63.291 Dislocation of distal interphalangeal joint of left index finger

● New code   ▲ Revised code   ⑦ 7th digit required   ⊗ Placeholder required

⑦S63.292 Dislocation of distal interphalangeal joint of right middle finger

⑦S63.293 Dislocation of distal interphalangeal joint of left middle finger

⑦S63.294 Dislocation of distal interphalangeal joint of right ring finger

⑦S63.295 Dislocation of distal interphalangeal joint of left ring finger

⑦S63.296 Dislocation of distal interphalangeal joint of right little finger

⑦S63.297 Dislocation of distal interphalangeal joint of left little finger

⑦S63.298 Dislocation of distal interphalangeal joint of other finger
Dislocation of distal interphalangeal joint of specified finger with unspecified laterality

⑦S63.299 Dislocation of distal interphalangeal joint of unspecified finger

S63.3 Traumatic rupture of ligament of wrist

S63.30 Traumatic rupture of unspecified ligament of wrist

⑦S63.301 Traumatic rupture of unspecified ligament of right wrist

⑦S63.302 Traumatic rupture of unspecified ligament of left wrist

⑦S63.309 Traumatic rupture of unspecified ligament of unspecified wrist

S63.31 Traumatic rupture of collateral ligament of wrist

⑦S63.311 Traumatic rupture of collateral ligament of right wrist

⑦S63.312 Traumatic rupture of collateral ligament of left wrist

⑦S63.319 Traumatic rupture of collateral ligament of unspecified wrist

S63.32 Traumatic rupture of radiocarpal ligament

⑦S63.321 Traumatic rupture of right radiocarpal ligament

⑦S63.322 Traumatic rupture of left radiocarpal ligament

⑦S63.329 Traumatic rupture of unspecified radiocarpal ligament

S63.33 Traumatic rupture of ulnocarpal (palmar) ligament

⑦S63.331 Traumatic rupture of right ulnocarpal (palmar) ligament

⑦S63.332 Traumatic rupture of left ulnocarpal (palmar) ligament

⑦S63.339 Traumatic rupture of unspecified ulnocarpal (palmar) ligament

S63.39 Traumatic rupture of other ligament of wrist

⑦S63.391 Traumatic rupture of other ligament of right wrist

⑦S63.392 Traumatic rupture of other ligament of left wrist

⑦S63.399 Traumatic rupture of other ligament of unspecified wrist

S63.4 Traumatic rupture of ligament of finger at metacarpophalangeal and interphalangeal joint(s)

S63.40 Traumatic rupture of unspecified ligament of finger at metacarpophalangeal and interphalangeal joint

⑦S63.400 Traumatic rupture of unspecified ligament of right index finger at metacarpophalangeal and interphalangeal joint

⑦S63.401 Traumatic rupture of unspecified ligament of left index finger at metacarpophalangeal and interphalangeal joint

⑦S63.402 Traumatic rupture of unspecified ligament of right middle finger at metacarpophalangeal and interphalangeal joint

⑦S63.403 Traumatic rupture of unspecified ligament of left middle finger at metacarpophalangeal and interphalangeal joint

⑦S63.404 Traumatic rupture of unspecified ligament of right ring finger at metacarpophalangeal and interphalangeal joint

⑦S63.405 Traumatic rupture of unspecified ligament of left ring finger at metacarpophalangeal and interphalangeal joint

⑦S63.406 Traumatic rupture of unspecified ligament of right little finger at metacarpophalangeal and interphalangeal joint

⑦S63.407 Traumatic rupture of unspecified ligament of left little finger at metacarpophalangeal and interphalangeal joint

⑦S63.408 Traumatic rupture of unspecified ligament of other finger at metacarpophalangeal and interphalangeal joint
Traumatic rupture of unspecified ligament of specified finger with unspecified laterality at metacarpophalangeal and interphalangeal joint

⑦S63.409 Traumatic rupture of unspecified ligament of unspecified finger at metacarpophalangeal and interphalangeal joint

S63.41 Traumatic rupture of collateral ligament of finger at metacarpophalangeal and interphalangeal joint

⑦S63.410 Traumatic rupture of collateral ligament of right index finger at metacarpophalangeal and interphalangeal joint

⑦S63.411 Traumatic rupture of collateral ligament of left index finger at metacarpophalangeal and interphalangeal joint

⑦S63.412 Traumatic rupture of collateral ligament of right middle finger at metacarpophalangeal and interphalangeal joint

⑦**S63.413** Traumatic rupture of collateral ligament of left middle finger at metacarpophalangeal and interphalangeal joint

⑦**S63.414** Traumatic rupture of collateral ligament of right ring finger at metacarpophalangeal and interphalangeal joint

⑦**S63.415** Traumatic rupture of collateral ligament of left ring finger at metacarpophalangeal and interphalangeal joint

⑦**S63.416** Traumatic rupture of collateral ligament of right little finger at metacarpophalangeal and interphalangeal joint

⑦**S63.417** Traumatic rupture of collateral ligament of left little finger at metacarpophalangeal and interphalangeal joint

⑦**S63.418** Traumatic rupture of collateral ligament of other finger at metacarpophalangeal and interphalangeal joint

Traumatic rupture of collateral ligament of specified finger with unspecified laterality at metacarpophalangeal and interphalangeal joint

⑦**S63.419** Traumatic rupture of collateral ligament of unspecified finger at metacarpophalangeal and interphalangeal joint

S63.42 Traumatic rupture of palmar ligament of finger at metacarpophalangeal and interphalangeal joint

⑦**S63.420** Traumatic rupture of palmar ligament of right index finger at metacarpophalangeal and interphalangeal joint

⑦**S63.421** Traumatic rupture of palmar ligament of left index finger at metacarpophalangeal and interphalangeal joint

⑦**S63.422** Traumatic rupture of palmar ligament of right middle finger at metacarpophalangeal and interphalangeal joint

⑦**S63.423** Traumatic rupture of palmar ligament of left middle finger at metacarpophalangeal and interphalangeal joint

⑦**S63.424** Traumatic rupture of palmar ligament of right ring finger at metacarpophalangeal and interphalangeal joint

⑦**S63.425** Traumatic rupture of palmar ligament of left ring finger at metacarpophalangeal and interphalangeal joint

⑦**S63.426** Traumatic rupture of palmar ligament of right little finger at

metacarpophalangeal and interphalangeal joint

⑦**S63.427** Traumatic rupture of palmar ligament of left little finger at metacarpophalangeal and interphalangeal joint

⑦**S63.428** Traumatic rupture of palmar ligament of other finger at metacarpophalangeal and interphalangeal joint

Traumatic rupture of palmar ligament of specified finger with unspecified laterality at metacarpophalangeal and interphalangeal joint

⑦**S63.429** Traumatic rupture of palmar ligament of unspecified finger at metacarpophalangeal and interphalangeal joint

S63.43 Traumatic rupture of volar plate of finger at metacarpophalangeal and interphalangeal joint

⑦**S63.430** Traumatic rupture of volar plate of right index finger at metacarpophalangeal and interphalangeal joint

⑦**S63.431** Traumatic rupture of volar plate of left index finger at metacarpophalangeal and interphalangeal joint

⑦**S63.432** Traumatic rupture of volar plate of right middle finger at metacarpophalangeal and interphalangeal joint

⑦**S63.433** Traumatic rupture of volar plate of left middle finger at metacarpophalangeal and interphalangeal joint

⑦**S63.434** Traumatic rupture of volar plate of right ring finger at metacarpophalangeal and interphalangeal joint

⑦**S63.435** Traumatic rupture of volar plate of left ring finger at metacarpophalangeal and interphalangeal joint

⑦**S63.436** Traumatic rupture of volar plate of right little finger at metacarpophalangeal and interphalangeal joint

⑦**S63.437** Traumatic rupture of volar plate of left little finger at metacarpophalangeal and interphalangeal joint

⑦**S63.438** Traumatic rupture of volar plate of other finger at metacarpophalangeal and interphalangeal joint

Traumatic rupture of volar plate of specified finger with unspecified laterality at metacarpophalangeal and interphalangeal joint

⑦**S63.439** Traumatic rupture of volar plate of unspecified finger at metacarpophalangeal and interphalangeal joint

S63.49   Traumatic rupture of other ligament of finger at metacarpophalangeal and interphalangeal joint

⑦S63.490   Traumatic rupture of other ligament of right index finger at metacarpophalangeal and interphalangeal joint

⑦S63.491   Traumatic rupture of other ligament of left index finger at metacarpophalangeal and interphalangeal joint

⑦S63.492   Traumatic rupture of other ligament of right middle finger at metacarpophalangeal and interphalangeal joint

⑦S63.493   Traumatic rupture of other ligament of left middle finger at metacarpophalangeal and interphalangeal joint

⑦S63.494   Traumatic rupture of other ligament of right ring finger at metacarpophalangeal and interphalangeal joint

⑦S63.495   Traumatic rupture of other ligament of left ring finger at metacarpophalangeal and interphalangeal joint

⑦S63.496   Traumatic rupture of other ligament of right little finger at metacarpophalangeal and interphalangeal joint

⑦S63.497   Traumatic rupture of other ligament of left little finger at metacarpophalangeal and interphalangeal joint

⑦S63.498   Traumatic rupture of other ligament of other finger at metacarpophalangeal and interphalangeal joint

Traumatic rupture of ligament of specified finger with unspecified laterality at metacarpophalangeal and interphalangeal joint

⑦S63.499   Traumatic rupture of other ligament of unspecified finger at metacarpophalangeal and interphalangeal joint

S63.5   Other and unspecified sprain of wrist

S63.50   Unspecified sprain of wrist

⑦S63.501   Unspecified sprain of right wrist

⑦S63.502   Unspecified sprain of left wrist

⑦S63.509   Unspecified sprain of unspecified wrist

S63.51   Sprain of carpal (joint)

⑦S63.511   Sprain of carpal joint of right wrist

⑦S63.512   Sprain of carpal joint of left wrist

⑦S63.519   Sprain of carpal joint of unspecified wrist

S63.52   Sprain of radiocarpal joint

Excludes 1: traumatic rupture of radiocarpal ligament (S63.32-)

⑦S63.521   Sprain of radiocarpal joint of right wrist

⑦S63.522   Sprain of radiocarpal joint of left wrist

⑦S63.529   Sprain of radiocarpal joint of unspecified wrist

S63.59   Other specified sprain of wrist

⑦S63.591   Other specified sprain of right wrist

⑦S63.592   Other specified sprain of left wrist

⑦S63.599   Other specified sprain of unspecified wrist

S63.6   Other and unspecified sprain of finger(s)

Excludes 1: traumatic rupture of ligament of finger at metacarpophalangeal and interphalangeal joint(s) (S63.4-)

S63.60   Unspecified sprain of thumb

⑦S63.601   Unspecified sprain of right thumb

⑦S63.602   Unspecified sprain of left thumb

⑦S63.609   Unspecified sprain of unspecified thumb

S63.61   Unspecified sprain of other and unspecified finger(s)

⑦S63.610   Unspecified sprain of right index finger

⑦S63.611   Unspecified sprain of left index finger

⑦S63.612   Unspecified sprain of right middle finger

⑦S63.613   Unspecified sprain of left middle finger

⑦S63.614   Unspecified sprain of right ring finger

⑦S63.615   Unspecified sprain of left ring finger

⑦S63.616   Unspecified sprain of right little finger

⑦S63.617   Unspecified sprain of left little finger

⑦S63.618   Unspecified sprain of other finger

Unspecified sprain of specified finger with unspecified laterality

⑦S63.619   Unspecified sprain of unspecified finger

S63.62   Sprain of interphalangeal joint of thumb

⑦S63.621   Sprain of interphalangeal joint of right thumb

⑦S63.622   Sprain of interphalangeal joint of left thumb

⑦S63.629   Sprain of interphalangeal joint of unspecified thumb

S63.63   Sprain of interphalangeal joint of other and unspecified finger(s)

⑦S63.630   Sprain of interphalangeal joint of right index finger

⑦S63.631   Sprain of interphalangeal joint of left index finger

⑦S63.632   Sprain of interphalangeal joint of right middle finger

⑦S63.633   Sprain of interphalangeal joint of left middle finger

⑦S63.634   Sprain of interphalangeal joint of right ring finger

⑦S63.635   Sprain of interphalangeal joint of left ring finger

⑦S63.636   Sprain of interphalangeal joint of right little finger

⑦S63.637   Sprain of interphalangeal joint of left little finger

⑦S63.638   Sprain of interphalangeal joint of other finger

⑦S63.639   Sprain of interphalangeal joint of unspecified finger

S63.64   Sprain of metacarpophalangeal joint of thumb

⑦S63.641   Sprain of metacarpophalangeal joint of right thumb

⑦S63.642   Sprain of metacarpophalangeal joint of left thumb

⑦S63.649   Sprain of metacarpophalangeal joint of unspecified thumb

S63.65   Sprain of metacarpophalangeal joint of other and unspecified finger(s)

⑦S63.650   Sprain of metacarpophalangeal joint of right index finger

⑦S63.651   Sprain of metacarpophalangeal joint of left index finger

⑦S63.652   Sprain of metacarpophalangeal joint of right middle finger

⑦S63.653   Sprain of metacarpophalangeal joint of left middle finger

⑦S63.654   Sprain of metacarpophalangeal joint of right ring finger

⑦S63.655   Sprain of metacarpophalangeal joint of left ring finger

⑦S63.656   Sprain of metacarpophalangeal joint of right little finger

⑦S63.657   Sprain of metacarpophalangeal joint of left little finger

⑦S63.658   Sprain of metacarpophalangeal joint of other finger

Sprain of metacarpophalangeal joint of specified finger with unspecified laterality

⑦S63.659   Sprain of metacarpophalangeal joint of unspecified finger

S63.68   Other sprain of thumb

⑦S63.681   Other sprain of right thumb

⑦S63.682   Other sprain of left thumb

⑦S63.689   Other sprain of unspecified thumb

S63.69   Other sprain of other and unspecified finger(s)

⑦S63.690   Other sprain of right index finger

⑦S63.691   Other sprain of left index finger

⑦S63.692   Other sprain of right middle finger

⑦S63.693   Other sprain of left middle finger

⑦S63.694   Other sprain of right ring finger

⑦S63.695   Other sprain of left ring finger

⑦S63.696   Other sprain of right little finger

⑦S63.697   Other sprain of left little finger

⑦S63.698   Other sprain of other finger

Other sprain of specified finger with unspecified laterality

⑦S63.699   Other sprain of unspecified finger

S63.8   Sprain of other part of wrist and hand

S63.8X   Sprain of other part of wrist and hand

⑦S63.8X1   Sprain of other part of right wrist and hand

⑦S63.8X2   Sprain of other part of left wrist and hand

⑦S63.8X9   Sprain of other part of unspecified wrist and hand

S63.9   Sprain of unspecified part of wrist and hand

⊗⑦S63.90   Sprain of unspecified part of unspecified wrist and hand

⊗⑦S63.91   Sprain of unspecified part of right wrist and hand

⊗⑦S63.92   Sprain of unspecified part of left wrist and hand

S64   Injury of nerves at wrist and hand level

Code also any associated open wound (S61.-)

The appropriate 7th character is to be added to each code from category S64

A - initial encounter

D - subsequent encounter

S - sequela

S64.0   Injury of ulnar nerve at wrist and hand level

⊗⑦S64.00   Injury of ulnar nerve at wrist and hand level of unspecified arm

⊗⑦S64.01   Injury of ulnar nerve at wrist and hand level of right arm

⊗⑦S64.02   Injury of ulnar nerve at wrist and hand level of left arm

S64.1   Injury of median nerve at wrist and hand level

⊗⑦S64.10   Injury of median nerve at wrist and hand level of unspecified arm

⊗⑦S64.11   Injury of median nerve at wrist and hand level of right arm

⊗⑦S64.12   Injury of median nerve at wrist and hand level of left arm

S64.2   Injury of radial nerve at wrist and hand level

⊗⑦S64.20   Injury of radial nerve at wrist and hand level of unspecified arm

⊗⑦S64.21   Injury of radial nerve at wrist and hand level of right arm

⊗⑦S64.22   Injury of radial nerve at wrist and hand level of left arm

S64.3   Injury of digital nerve of thumb

⊗⑦S64.30   Injury of digital nerve of unspecified thumb

⊗⑦S64.31   Injury of digital nerve of right thumb

⊗⑦S64.32   Injury of digital nerve of left thumb

S64.4   Injury of digital nerve of other and unspecified finger

⊗⑦S64.40   Injury of digital nerve of unspecified finger

S64.49   Injury of digital nerve of other finger

⑦S64.490   Injury of digital nerve of right index finger

⑦S64.491   Injury of digital nerve of left index finger

● New code   ▲ Revised code   ⑦ 7th digit required   ⊗ Placeholder required

⑦S64.492   Injury of digital nerve of right middle finger

⑦S64.493   Injury of digital nerve of left middle finger

⑦S64.494   Injury of digital nerve of right ring finger

⑦S64.495   Injury of digital nerve of left ring finger

⑦S64.496   Injury of digital nerve of right little finger

⑦S64.497   Injury of digital nerve of left little finger

⑦S64.498   Injury of digital nerve of other finger

Injury of digital nerve of specified finger with unspecified laterality

S64.8   Injury of other nerves at wrist and hand level

    S64.8X   Injury of other nerves at wrist and hand level

⑦S64.8X1   Injury of other nerves at wrist and hand level of right arm

⑦S64.8X2   Injury of other nerves at wrist and hand level of left arm

⑦S64.8X9   Injury of other nerves at wrist and hand level of unspecified arm

S64.9   Injury of unspecified nerve at wrist and hand level

⊗⑦S64.90   Injury of unspecified nerve at wrist and hand level of unspecified arm

⊗⑦S64.91   Injury of unspecified nerve at wrist and hand level of right arm

⊗⑦S64.92   Injury of unspecified nerve at wrist and hand level of left arm

S65   Injury of blood vessels at wrist and hand level

Code also any associated open wound (S61.-)

The appropriate 7th character is to be added to each code from category S65

A - initial encounter

D - subsequent encounter

S - sequela

S65.0   Injury of ulnar artery at wrist and hand level

    S65.00   Unspecified injury of ulnar artery at wrist and hand level

⑦S65.001   Unspecified injury of ulnar artery at wrist and hand level of right arm

⑦S65.002   Unspecified injury of ulnar artery at wrist and hand level of left arm

⑦S65.009   Unspecified injury of ulnar artery at wrist and hand level of unspecified arm

    S65.01   Laceration of ulnar artery at wrist and hand level

⑦S65.011   Laceration of ulnar artery at wrist and hand level of right arm

⑦S65.012   Laceration of ulnar artery at wrist and hand level of left arm

⑦S65.019   Laceration of ulnar artery at wrist and hand level of unspecified arm

    S65.09   Other specified injury of ulnar artery at wrist and hand level

⑦S65.091   Other specified injury of ulnar artery at wrist and hand level of right arm

⑦S65.092   Other specified injury of ulnar artery at wrist and hand level of left arm

⑦S65.099   Other specified injury of ulnar artery at wrist and hand level of unspecified arm

S65.1   Injury of radial artery at wrist and hand level

    S65.10   Unspecified injury of radial artery at wrist and hand level

⑦S65.101   Unspecified injury of radial artery at wrist and hand level of right arm

⑦S65.102   Unspecified injury of radial artery at wrist and hand level of left arm

⑦S65.109   Unspecified injury of radial artery at wrist and hand level of unspecified arm

    S65.11   Laceration of radial artery at wrist and hand level

⑦S65.111   Laceration of radial artery at wrist and hand level of right arm

⑦S65.112   Laceration of radial artery at wrist and hand level of left arm

⑦S65.119   Laceration of radial artery at wrist and hand level of unspecified arm

    S65.19   Other specified injury of radial artery at wrist and hand level

⑦S65.191   Other specified injury of radial artery at wrist and hand level of right arm

⑦S65.192   Other specified injury of radial artery at wrist and hand level of left arm

⑦S65.199   Other specified injury of radial artery at wrist and hand level of unspecified arm

S65.2   Injury of superficial palmar arch

    S65.20   Unspecified injury of superficial palmar arch

⑦S65.201   Unspecified injury of superficial palmar arch of right hand

⑦S65.202   Unspecified injury of superficial palmar arch of left hand

⑦S65.209   Unspecified injury of superficial palmar arch of unspecified hand

    S65.21   Laceration of superficial palmar arch

⑦S65.211   Laceration of superficial palmar arch of right hand

⑦S65.212   Laceration of superficial palmar arch of left hand

⑦S65.219   Laceration of superficial palmar arch of unspecified hand

    S65.29   Other specified injury of superficial palmar arch

⑦S65.291   Other specified injury of superficial palmar arch of right hand

⑦S65.292   Other specified injury of superficial palmar arch of left hand

⑦S65.299   Other specified injury of superficial palmar arch of unspecified hand

S65.3   Injury of deep palmar arch

    S65.30   Unspecified injury of deep palmar arch

⑦S65.301   Unspecified injury of deep palmar arch of right hand

⑦S65.302 Unspecified injury of deep palmar arch of left hand

⑦S65.309 Unspecified injury of deep palmar arch of unspecified hand

S65.31 Laceration of deep palmar arch

⑦S65.311 Laceration of deep palmar arch of right hand

⑦S65.312 Laceration of deep palmar arch of left hand

⑦S65.319 Laceration of deep palmar arch of unspecified hand

S65.39 Other specified injury of deep palmar arch

⑦S65.391 Other specified injury of deep palmar arch of right hand

⑦S65.392 Other specified injury of deep palmar arch of left hand

⑦S65.399 Other specified injury of deep palmar arch of unspecified hand

S65.4 Injury of blood vessel of thumb

S65.40 Unspecified injury of blood vessel of thumb

⑦S65.401 Unspecified injury of blood vessel of right thumb

⑦S65.402 Unspecified injury of blood vessel of left thumb

⑦S65.409 Unspecified injury of blood vessel of unspecified thumb

S65.41 Laceration of blood vessel of thumb

⑦S65.411 Laceration of blood vessel of right thumb

⑦S65.412 Laceration of blood vessel of left thumb

⑦S65.419 Laceration of blood vessel of unspecified thumb

S65.49 Other specified injury of blood vessel of thumb

⑦S65.491 Other specified injury of blood vessel of right thumb

⑦S65.492 Other specified injury of blood vessel of left thumb

⑦S65.499 Other specified injury of blood vessel of unspecified thumb

S65.5 Injury of blood vessel of other and unspecified finger

S65.50 Unspecified injury of blood vessel of other and unspecified finger

⑦S65.500 Unspecified injury of blood vessel of right index finger

⑦S65.501 Unspecified injury of blood vessel of left index finger

⑦S65.502 Unspecified injury of blood vessel of right middle finger

⑦S65.503 Unspecified injury of blood vessel of left middle finger

⑦S65.504 Unspecified injury of blood vessel of right ring finger

⑦S65.505 Unspecified injury of blood vessel of left ring finger

⑦S65.506 Unspecified injury of blood vessel of right little finger

⑦S65.507 Unspecified injury of blood vessel of left little finger

⑦S65.508 Unspecified injury of blood vessel of other finger

Unspecified injury of blood vessel of specified finger with unspecified laterality

⑦S65.509 Unspecified injury of blood vessel of unspecified finger

S65.51 Laceration of blood vessel of other and unspecified finger

⑦S65.510 Laceration of blood vessel of right index finger

⑦S65.511 Laceration of blood vessel of left index finger

⑦S65.512 Laceration of blood vessel of right middle finger

⑦S65.513 Laceration of blood vessel of left middle finger

⑦S65.514 Laceration of blood vessel of right ring finger

⑦S65.515 Laceration of blood vessel of left ring finger

⑦S65.516 Laceration of blood vessel of right little finger

⑦S65.517 Laceration of blood vessel of left little finger

⑦S65.518 Laceration of blood vessel of other finger

Laceration of blood vessel of specified finger with unspecified laterality

⑦S65.519 Laceration of blood vessel of unspecified finger

S65.59 Other specified injury of blood vessel of other and unspecified finger

⑦S65.590 Other specified injury of blood vessel of right index finger

⑦S65.591 Other specified injury of blood vessel of left index finger

⑦S65.592 Other specified injury of blood vessel of right middle finger

⑦S65.593 Other specified injury of blood vessel of left middle finger

⑦S65.594 Other specified injury of blood vessel of right ring finger

⑦S65.595 Other specified injury of blood vessel of left ring finger

⑦S65.596 Other specified injury of blood vessel of right little finger

⑦S65.597 Other specified injury of blood vessel of left little finger

⑦S65.598 Other specified injury of blood vessel of other finger

Other specified injury of blood vessel of specified finger with unspecified laterality

⑦S65.599 Other specified injury of blood vessel of unspecified finger

S65.8 Injury of other blood vessels at wrist and hand level

● New code ▲ Revised code ⑦ 7th digit required ⊗ Placeholder required

S65.80 Unspecified injury of other blood vessels at wrist and hand level

⑦**S65.801** Unspecified injury of other blood vessels at wrist and hand level of right arm

⑦**S65.802** Unspecified injury of other blood vessels at wrist and hand level of left arm

⑦**S65.809** Unspecified injury of other blood vessels at wrist and hand level of unspecified arm

S65.81 Laceration of other blood vessels at wrist and hand level

⑦**S65.811** Laceration of other blood vessels at wrist and hand level of right arm

⑦**S65.812** Laceration of other blood vessels at wrist and hand level of left arm

⑦**S65.819** Laceration of other blood vessels at wrist and hand level of unspecified arm

S65.89 Other specified injury of other blood vessels at wrist and hand level

⑦**S65.891** Other specified injury of other blood vessels at wrist and hand level of right arm

⑦**S65.892** Other specified injury of other blood vessels at wrist and hand level of left arm

⑦**S65.899** Other specified injury of other blood vessels at wrist and hand level of unspecified arm

S65.9 Injury of unspecified blood vessel at wrist and hand level

S65.90 Unspecified injury of unspecified blood vessel at wrist and hand level

⑦**S65.901** Unspecified injury of unspecified blood vessel at wrist and hand level of right arm

⑦**S65.902** Unspecified injury of unspecified blood vessel at wrist and hand level of left arm

⑦**S65.909** Unspecified injury of unspecified blood vessel at wrist and hand level of unspecified arm

S65.91 Laceration of unspecified blood vessel at wrist and hand level

⑦**S65.911** Laceration of unspecified blood vessel at wrist and hand level of right arm

⑦**S65.912** Laceration of unspecified blood vessel at wrist and hand level of left arm

⑦**S65.919** Laceration of unspecified blood vessel at wrist and hand level of unspecified arm

S65.99 Other specified injury of unspecified blood vessel at wrist and hand level

⑦**S65.991** Other specified injury of unspecified blood vessel at wrist and hand of right arm

⑦**S65.992** Other specified injury of unspecified blood vessel at wrist and hand of left arm

⑦**S65.999** Other specified injury of unspecified blood vessel at wrist and hand of unspecified arm

S66 Injury of muscle, fascia and tendon at wrist and hand level

Code also any associated open wound (S61.-)

Excludes 2: sprain of joints and ligaments of wrist and hand (S63.-)

The appropriate 7th character is to be added to each code from category S66

A - initial encounter

D - subsequent encounter

S - sequela

S66.0 Injury of long flexor muscle, fascia and tendon of thumb at wrist and hand level

S66.00 Unspecified injury of long flexor muscle, fascia and tendon of thumb at wrist and hand level

⑦**S66.001** Unspecified injury of long flexor muscle, fascia and tendon of right thumb at wrist and hand level

⑦**S66.002** Unspecified injury of long flexor muscle, fascia and tendon of left thumb at wrist and hand level

⑦**S66.009** Unspecified injury of long flexor muscle, fascia and tendon of unspecified thumb at wrist and hand level

S66.01 Strain of long flexor muscle, fascia and tendon of thumb at wrist and hand level

⑦**S66.011** Strain of long flexor muscle, fascia and tendon of right thumb at wrist and hand level

⑦**S66.012** Strain of long flexor muscle, fascia and tendon of left thumb at wrist and hand level

⑦**S66.019** Strain of long flexor muscle, fascia and tendon of unspecified thumb at wrist and hand level

S66.02 Laceration of long flexor muscle, fascia and tendon of thumb at wrist and hand level

⑦**S66.021** Laceration of long flexor muscle, fascia and tendon of right thumb at wrist and hand level

⑦**S66.022** Laceration of long flexor muscle, fascia and tendon of left thumb at wrist and hand level

⑦**S66.029** Laceration of long flexor muscle, fascia and tendon of unspecified thumb at wrist and hand level

S66.09 Other specified injury of long flexor muscle, fascia and tendon of thumb at wrist and hand level

⑦**S66.091** Other specified injury of long flexor muscle, fascia and tendon of right thumb at wrist and hand level

⑦**S66.092** Other specified injury of long flexor muscle, fascia and tendon of left thumb at wrist and hand level

⑦ S66.099   Other specified injury of long flexor muscle, fascia and tendon of unspecified thumb at wrist and hand level

S66.1   Injury of flexor muscle, fascia and tendon of other and unspecified finger at wrist and hand level

Excludes 2: Injury of long flexor muscle, fascia and tendon of thumb at wrist and hand level (S66.0-)

S66.10   Unspecified injury of flexor muscle, fascia and tendon of other and unspecified finger at wrist and hand level

⑦ S66.100   Unspecified injury of flexor muscle, fascia and tendon of right index finger at wrist and hand level

⑦ S66.101   Unspecified injury of flexor muscle, fascia and tendon of left index finger at wrist and hand level

⑦ S66.102   Unspecified injury of flexor muscle, fascia and tendon of right middle finger at wrist and hand level

⑦ S66.103   Unspecified injury of flexor muscle, fascia and tendon of left middle finger at wrist and hand level

⑦ S66.104   Unspecified injury of flexor muscle, fascia and tendon of right ring finger at wrist and hand level

⑦ S66.105   Unspecified injury of flexor muscle, fascia and tendon of left ring finger at wrist and hand level

⑦ S66.106   Unspecified injury of flexor muscle, fascia and tendon of right little finger at wrist and hand level

⑦ S66.107   Unspecified injury of flexor muscle, fascia and tendon of left little finger at wrist and hand level

⑦ S66.108   Unspecified injury of flexor muscle, fascia and tendon of other finger at wrist and hand level

Unspecified injury of flexor muscle, fascia and tendon of specified finger with unspecified laterality at wrist and hand level

⑦ S66.109   Unspecified injury of flexor muscle, fascia and tendon of unspecified finger at wrist and hand level

S66.11   Strain of flexor muscle, fascia and tendon of other and unspecified finger at wrist and hand level

⑦ S66.110   Strain of flexor muscle, fascia and tendon of right index finger at wrist and hand level

⑦ S66.111   Strain of flexor muscle, fascia and tendon of left index finger at wrist and hand level

⑦ S66.112   Strain of flexor muscle, fascia and tendon of right middle finger at wrist and hand level

⑦ S66.113   Strain of flexor muscle, fascia and tendon of left middle finger at wrist and hand level

⑦ S66.114   Strain of flexor muscle, fascia and tendon of right ring finger at wrist and hand level

⑦ S66.115   Strain of flexor muscle, fascia and tendon of left ring finger at wrist and hand level

⑦ S66.116   Strain of flexor muscle, fascia and tendon of right little finger at wrist and hand level

⑦ S66.117   Strain of flexor muscle, fascia and tendon of left little finger at wrist and hand level

⑦ S66.118   Strain of flexor muscle, fascia and tendon of other finger at wrist and hand level

Strain of flexor muscle, fascia and tendon of specified finger with unspecified laterality at wrist and hand level

⑦ S66.119   Strain of flexor muscle, fascia and tendon of unspecified finger at wrist and hand level

S66.12   Laceration of flexor muscle, fascia and tendon of other and unspecified finger at wrist and hand level

⑦ S66.120   Laceration of flexor muscle, fascia and tendon of right index finger at wrist and hand level

⑦ S66.121   Laceration of flexor muscle, fascia and tendon of left index finger at wrist and hand level

⑦ S66.122   Laceration of flexor muscle, fascia and tendon of right middle finger at wrist and hand level

⑦ S66.123   Laceration of flexor muscle, fascia and tendon of left middle finger at wrist and hand level

⑦ S66.124   Laceration of flexor muscle, fascia and tendon of right ring finger at wrist and hand level

⑦ S66.125   Laceration of flexor muscle, fascia and tendon of left ring finger at wrist and hand level

⑦ S66.126   Laceration of flexor muscle, fascia and tendon of right little finger at wrist and hand level

⑦ S66.127   Laceration of flexor muscle, fascia and tendon of left little finger at wrist and hand level

⑦ S66.128   Laceration of flexor muscle, fascia and tendon of other finger at wrist and hand level

Laceration of flexor muscle, fascia and tendon of specified finger with unspecified laterality at wrist and hand level

⑦ S66.129   Laceration of flexor muscle, fascia and tendon of unspecified finger at wrist and hand level

S66.19 Other injury of flexor muscle, fascia and tendon of other and unspecified finger at wrist and hand level

⑦**S66.190** Other injury of flexor muscle, fascia and tendon of right index finger at wrist and hand level

⑦**S66.191** Other injury of flexor muscle, fascia and tendon of left index finger at wrist and hand level

⑦**S66.192** Other injury of flexor muscle, fascia and tendon of right middle finger at wrist and hand level

⑦**S66.193** Other injury of flexor muscle, fascia and tendon of left middle finger at wrist and hand level

⑦**S66.194** Other injury of flexor muscle, fascia and tendon of right ring finger at wrist and hand level

⑦**S66.195** Other injury of flexor muscle, fascia and tendon of left ring finger at wrist and hand level

⑦**S66.196** Other injury of flexor muscle, fascia and tendon of right little finger at wrist and hand level

⑦**S66.197** Other injury of flexor muscle, fascia and tendon of left little finger at wrist and hand level

⑦**S66.198** Other injury of flexor muscle, fascia and tendon of other finger at wrist and hand level

Other injury of flexor muscle, fascia and tendon of specified finger with unspecified laterality at wrist and hand level

⑦**S66.199** Other injury of flexor muscle, fascia and tendon of unspecified finger at wrist and hand level

S66.2 Injury of extensor muscle, fascia and tendon of thumb at wrist and hand level

S66.20 Unspecified injury of extensor muscle, fascia and tendon of thumb at wrist and hand level

⑦**S66.201** Unspecified injury of extensor muscle, fascia and tendon of right thumb at wrist and hand level

⑦**S66.202** Unspecified injury of extensor muscle, fascia and tendon of left thumb at wrist and hand level

⑦**S66.209** Unspecified injury of extensor muscle, fascia and tendon of unspecified thumb at wrist and hand level

S66.21 Strain of extensor muscle, fascia and tendon of thumb at wrist and hand level

⑦**S66.211** Strain of extensor muscle, fascia and tendon of right thumb at wrist and hand level

⑦**S66.212** Strain of extensor muscle, fascia and tendon of left thumb at wrist and hand level

⑦**S66.219** Strain of extensor muscle, fascia and tendon of unspecified thumb at wrist and hand level

S66.22 Laceration of extensor muscle, fascia and tendon of thumb at wrist and hand level

⑦**S66.221** Laceration of extensor muscle, fascia and tendon of right thumb at wrist and hand level

⑦**S66.222** Laceration of extensor muscle, fascia and tendon of left thumb at wrist and hand level

⑦**S66.229** Laceration of extensor muscle, fascia and tendon of unspecified thumb at wrist and hand level

S66.29 Other specified injury of extensor muscle, fascia and tendon of thumb at wrist and hand level

⑦**S66.291** Other specified injury of extensor muscle, fascia and tendon of right thumb at wrist and hand level

⑦**S66.292** Other specified injury of extensor muscle, fascia and tendon of left thumb at wrist and hand level

⑦**S66.299** Other specified injury of extensor muscle, fascia and tendon of unspecified thumb at wrist and hand level

S66.3 Injury of extensor muscle, fascia and tendon of other and unspecified finger at wrist and hand level

Excludes 2: Injury of extensor muscle, fascia and tendon of thumb at wrist and hand level (S66.2-)

S66.30 Unspecified injury of extensor muscle, fascia and tendon of other and unspecified finger at wrist and hand level

⑦**S66.300** Unspecified injury of extensor muscle, fascia and tendon of right index finger at wrist and hand level

⑦**S66.301** Unspecified injury of extensor muscle, fascia and tendon of left index finger at wrist and hand level

⑦**S66.302** Unspecified injury of extensor muscle, fascia and tendon of right middle finger at wrist and hand level

⑦**S66.303** Unspecified injury of extensor muscle, fascia and tendon of left middle finger at wrist and hand level

⑦**S66.304** Unspecified injury of extensor muscle, fascia and tendon of right ring finger at wrist and hand level

⑦**S66.305** Unspecified injury of extensor muscle, fascia and tendon of left ring finger at wrist and hand level

⑦**S66.306** Unspecified injury of extensor muscle, fascia and tendon of right little finger at wrist and hand level

⑦**S66.307** Unspecified injury of extensor muscle, fascia and tendon of left little finger at wrist and hand level

⑦**S66.308** Unspecified injury of extensor muscle, fascia and tendon of other finger at wrist and hand level

Unspecified injury of extensor muscle, fascia and tendon of specified finger with unspecified laterality at wrist and hand level

⑦**S66.309** Unspecified injury of extensor muscle, fascia and tendon of unspecified finger at wrist and hand level

S66.31 Strain of extensor muscle, fascia and tendon of other and unspecified finger at wrist and hand level

⑦**S66.310** Strain of extensor muscle, fascia and tendon of right index finger at wrist and hand level

⑦**S66.311** Strain of extensor muscle, fascia and tendon of left index finger at wrist and hand level

⑦**S66.312** Strain of extensor muscle, fascia and tendon of right middle finger at wrist and hand level

⑦**S66.313** Strain of extensor muscle, fascia and tendon of left middle finger at wrist and hand level

⑦**S66.314** Strain of extensor muscle, fascia and tendon of right ring finger at wrist and hand level

⑦**S66.315** Strain of extensor muscle, fascia and tendon of left ring finger at wrist and hand level

⑦**S66.316** Strain of extensor muscle, fascia and tendon of right little finger at wrist and hand level

⑦**S66.317** Strain of extensor muscle, fascia and tendon of left little finger at wrist and hand level

⑦**S66.318** Strain of extensor muscle, fascia and tendon of other finger at wrist and hand level

Strain of extensor muscle, fascia and tendon of specified finger with unspecified laterality at wrist and hand level

⑦**S66.319** Strain of extensor muscle, fascia and tendon of unspecified finger at wrist and hand level

S66.32 Laceration of extensor muscle, fascia and tendon of other and unspecified finger at wrist and hand level

⑦**S66.320** Laceration of extensor muscle, fascia and tendon of right index finger at wrist and hand level

⑦**S66.321** Laceration of extensor muscle, fascia and tendon of left index finger at wrist and hand level

⑦**S66.322** Laceration of extensor muscle, fascia and tendon of right middle finger at wrist and hand level

⑦**S66.323** Laceration of extensor muscle, fascia and tendon of left middle finger at wrist and hand level

⑦**S66.324** Laceration of extensor muscle, fascia and tendon of right ring finger at wrist and hand level

⑦**S66.325** Laceration of extensor muscle, fascia and tendon of left ring finger at wrist and hand level

⑦**S66.326** Laceration of extensor muscle, fascia and tendon of right little finger at wrist and hand level

⑦**S66.327** Laceration of extensor muscle, fascia and tendon of left little finger at wrist and hand level

⑦**S66.328** Laceration of extensor muscle, fascia and tendon of other finger at wrist and hand level

Laceration of extensor muscle, fascia and tendon of specified finger with unspecified laterality at wrist and hand level

⑦**S66.329** Laceration of extensor muscle, fascia and tendon of unspecified finger at wrist and hand level

S66.39 Other injury of extensor muscle, fascia and tendon of other and unspecified finger at wrist and hand level

⑦**S66.390** Other injury of extensor muscle, fascia and tendon of right index finger at wrist and hand level

⑦**S66.391** Other injury of extensor muscle, fascia and tendon of left index finger at wrist and hand level

⑦**S66.392** Other injury of extensor muscle, fascia and tendon of right middle finger at wrist and hand level

⑦**S66.393** Other injury of extensor muscle, fascia and tendon of left middle finger at wrist and hand level

⑦**S66.394** Other injury of extensor muscle, fascia and tendon of right ring finger at wrist and hand level

⑦**S66.395** Other injury of extensor muscle, fascia and tendon of left ring finger at wrist and hand level

⑦**S66.396** Other injury of extensor muscle, fascia and tendon of right little finger at wrist and hand level

⑦**S66.397** Other injury of extensor muscle, fascia and tendon of left little finger at wrist and hand level

⑦**S66.398** Other injury of extensor muscle, fascia and tendon of other finger at wrist and hand level

Other injury of extensor muscle, fascia and tendon of specified finger with unspecified laterality at wrist and hand level

⑦**S66.399** Other injury of extensor muscle, fascia and tendon of unspecified finger at wrist and hand level

S66.4 Injury of intrinsic muscle, fascia and tendon of thumb at wrist and hand level

● New code   ▲ Revised code   ⑦ 7th digit required   ⊗ Placeholder required

S66.40 Unspecified injury of intrinsic muscle, fascia and tendon of thumb at wrist and hand level

⑦**S66.401** Unspecified injury of intrinsic muscle, fascia and tendon of right thumb at wrist and hand level

⑦**S66.402** Unspecified injury of intrinsic muscle, fascia and tendon of left thumb at wrist and hand level

⑦**S66.409** Unspecified injury of intrinsic muscle, fascia and tendon of unspecified thumb at wrist and hand level

S66.41 Strain of intrinsic muscle, fascia and tendon of thumb at wrist and hand level

⑦**S66.411** Strain of intrinsic muscle, fascia and tendon of right thumb at wrist and hand level

⑦**S66.412** Strain of intrinsic muscle, fascia and tendon of left thumb at wrist and hand level

⑦**S66.419** Strain of intrinsic muscle, fascia and tendon of unspecified thumb at wrist and hand level

S66.42 Laceration of intrinsic muscle, fascia and tendon of thumb at wrist and hand level

⑦**S66.421** Laceration of intrinsic muscle, fascia and tendon of right thumb at wrist and hand level

⑦**S66.422** Laceration of intrinsic muscle, fascia and tendon of left thumb at wrist and hand level

⑦**S66.429** Laceration of intrinsic muscle, fascia and tendon of unspecified thumb at wrist and hand level

S66.49 Other specified injury of intrinsic muscle, fascia and tendon of thumb at wrist and hand level

⑦**S66.491** Other specified injury of intrinsic muscle, fascia and tendon of right thumb at wrist and hand level

⑦**S66.492** Other specified injury of intrinsic muscle, fascia and tendon of left thumb at wrist and hand level

⑦**S66.499** Other specified injury of intrinsic muscle, fascia and tendon of unspecified thumb at wrist and hand level

S66.5 Injury of intrinsic muscle, fascia and tendon of other and unspecified finger at wrist and hand level

Excludes 2: injury of intrinsic muscle, fascia and tendon of thumb at wrist and hand level (S66.4-)

S66.50 Unspecified injury of intrinsic muscle, fascia and tendon of other and unspecified finger at wrist and hand level

⑦**S66.500** Unspecified injury of intrinsic muscle, fascia and tendon of right index finger at wrist and hand level

⑦**S66.501** Unspecified injury of intrinsic muscle, fascia and tendon of left index finger at wrist and hand level

⑦**S66.502** Unspecified injury of intrinsic muscle, fascia and tendon of right middle finger at wrist and hand level

⑦**S66.503** Unspecified injury of intrinsic muscle, fascia and tendon of left middle finger at wrist and hand level

⑦**S66.504** Unspecified injury of intrinsic muscle, fascia and tendon of right ring finger at wrist and hand level

⑦**S66.505** Unspecified injury of intrinsic muscle, fascia and tendon of left ring finger at wrist and hand level

⑦**S66.506** Unspecified injury of intrinsic muscle, fascia and tendon of right little finger at wrist and hand level

⑦**S66.507** Unspecified injury of intrinsic muscle, fascia and tendon of left little finger at wrist and hand level

⑦**S66.508** Unspecified injury of intrinsic muscle, fascia and tendon of other finger at wrist and hand level

Unspecified injury of intrinsic muscle, fascia and tendon of specified finger with unspecified laterality at wrist and hand level

⑦**S66.509** Unspecified injury of intrinsic muscle, fascia and tendon of unspecified finger at wrist and hand level

S66.51 Strain of intrinsic muscle, fascia and tendon of other and unspecified finger at wrist and hand level

⑦**S66.510** Strain of intrinsic muscle, fascia and tendon of right index finger at wrist and hand level

⑦**S66.511** Strain of intrinsic muscle, fascia and tendon of left index finger at wrist and hand level

⑦**S66.512** Strain of intrinsic muscle, fascia and tendon of right middle finger at wrist and hand level

⑦**S66.513** Strain of intrinsic muscle, fascia and tendon of left middle finger at wrist and hand level

⑦**S66.514** Strain of intrinsic muscle, fascia and tendon of right ring finger at wrist and hand level

⑦**S66.515** Strain of intrinsic muscle, fascia and tendon of left ring finger at wrist and hand level

⑦**S66.516** Strain of intrinsic muscle, fascia and tendon of right little finger at wrist and hand level

⑦**S66.517** Strain of intrinsic muscle, fascia and tendon of left little finger at wrist and hand Level

⑦**S66.518** Strain of intrinsic muscle, fascia and tendon of other finger at wrist and hand level

Strain of intrinsic muscle, fascia and tendon of specified finger with

⑦S66.519   Strain of intrinsic muscle, fascia and tendon of unspecified finger at wrist and hand level

S66.52   Laceration of intrinsic muscle, fascia and tendon of other and unspecified finger at wrist and hand level

⑦S66.520   Laceration of intrinsic muscle, fascia and tendon of right index finger at wrist and hand level

⑦S66.521   Laceration of intrinsic muscle, fascia and tendon of left index finger at wrist and hand level

⑦S66.522   Laceration of intrinsic muscle, fascia and tendon of right middle finger at wrist and hand level

⑦S66.523   Laceration of intrinsic muscle, fascia and tendon of left middle finger at wrist and hand level

⑦S66.524   Laceration of intrinsic muscle, fascia and tendon of right ring finger at wrist and hand level

⑦S66.525   Laceration of intrinsic muscle, fascia and tendon of left ring finger at wrist and hand level

⑦S66.526   Laceration of intrinsic muscle, fascia and tendon of right little finger at wrist and hand level

⑦S66.527   Laceration of intrinsic muscle, fascia and tendon of left little finger at wrist and hand level

⑦S66.528   Laceration of intrinsic muscle, fascia and tendon of other finger at wrist and hand level

Laceration of intrinsic muscle, fascia and tendon of specified finger with unspecified laterality at wrist and hand level

⑦S66.529   Laceration of intrinsic muscle, fascia and tendon of unspecified finger at wrist and hand level

S66.59   Other injury of intrinsic muscle, fascia and tendon of other and unspecified finger at wrist and hand level

⑦S66.590   Other injury of intrinsic muscle, fascia and tendon of right index finger at wrist and hand level

⑦S66.591   Other injury of intrinsic muscle, fascia and tendon of left index finger at wrist and hand level

⑦S66.592   Other injury of intrinsic muscle, fascia and tendon of right middle finger at wrist and hand level

⑦S66.593   Other injury of intrinsic muscle, fascia and tendon of left middle finger at wrist and hand level

⑦S66.594   Other injury of intrinsic muscle, fascia and tendon of right ring finger at wrist and hand level

⑦S66.595   Other injury of intrinsic muscle, fascia and tendon of left ring finger at wrist and hand level

⑦S66.596   Other injury of intrinsic muscle, fascia and tendon of right little finger at wrist and hand level

⑦S66.597   Other injury of intrinsic muscle, fascia and tendon of left little finger at wrist and hand level

⑦S66.598   Other injury of intrinsic muscle, fascia and tendon of other finger at wrist and hand level

Other injury of intrinsic muscle, fascia and tendon of specified finger with unspecified laterality at wrist and hand level

⑦S66.599   Other injury of intrinsic muscle, fascia and tendon of unspecified finger at wrist and hand level

S66.8   Injury of other specified muscles, fascia and tendons at wrist and hand level

⊗⑦S66.80   Unspecified injury of other specified muscles, fascia and tendons at wrist and hand level

⑦S66.801   Unspecified injury of other specified muscles, fascia and tendons at wrist and hand level, right hand

⑦S66.802   Unspecified injury of other specified muscles, fascia and tendons at wrist and hand level, left hand

⑦S66.809   Unspecified injury of other specified muscles, fascia and tendons at wrist and hand level, unspecified hand

S66.81   Strain of other specified muscles, fascia and tendons at wrist and hand level

⑦S66.811   Strain of other specified muscles, fascia and tendons at wrist and hand level, right hand

⑦S66.812   Strain of other specified muscles, fascia and tendons at wrist and hand level, left hand

⑦S66.819   Strain of other specified muscles, fascia and tendons at wrist and hand level, unspecified hand

⑦S66.82   Laceration of other specified muscles, fascia and tendons at wrist and hand level

⑦S66.821   Laceration of other specified muscles, fascia and tendons at wrist and hand level, right hand

⑦S66.822   Laceration of other specified muscles, fascia and tendons at wrist and hand level, left hand

⑦S66.829   Laceration of other specified muscles, fascia and tendons at wrist and hand level, unspecified hand

⑦S66.89   Other injury of other specified muscles, fascia and tendons at wrist and hand level

⑦S66.891   Other injury of other specified muscles, fascia and tendons at wrist and hand level, right hand

⑦S66.892   Other injury of other specified muscles, fascia and tendons at wrist and hand level, left hand

⑦S66.899   Other injury of other specified muscles, fascia and tendons at wrist and hand level, unspecified hand

S66.9   Injury of unspecified muscle, fascia and tendon at wrist and hand level

   S66.90   Unspecified injury of unspecified muscle, fascia and tendon at wrist and hand level

     ⑦S66.901   Unspecified injury of unspecified muscle, fascia and tendon at wrist and hand level, right hand

     ⑦S66.902   Unspecified injury of unspecified muscle, fascia and tendon at wrist and hand level, left hand

     ⑦S66.909   Unspecified injury of unspecified muscle, fascia and tendon at wrist and hand level, unspecified hand

   S66.91   Strain of unspecified muscle, fascia and tendon at wrist and hand level

     ⑦S66.911   Strain of unspecified muscle, fascia and tendon at wrist and hand level, right hand

     ⑦S66.912   Strain of unspecified muscle, fascia and tendon at wrist and hand level, left hand

     ⑦S66.919   Strain of unspecified muscle, fascia and tendon at wrist and hand level, unspecified hand

   S66.92   Laceration of unspecified muscle, fascia and tendon at wrist and hand level

     ⑦S66.921   Laceration of unspecified muscle, fascia and tendon at wrist and hand level, right hand

     ⑦S66.922   Laceration of unspecified muscle, fascia and tendon at wrist and hand level, left hand

     ⑦S66.929   Laceration of unspecified muscle, fascia and tendon at wrist and hand level, unspecified hand

   S66.99   Other injury of unspecified muscle, fascia and tendon at wrist and hand level

     ⑦S66.991   Other injury of unspecified muscle, fascia and tendon at wrist and hand level, right hand

     ⑦S66.992   Other injury of unspecified muscle, fascia and tendon at wrist and hand level, left hand

     ⑦S66.999   Other injury of unspecified muscle, fascia and tendon at wrist and hand level, unspecified hand

S67   Crushing injury of wrist, hand and fingers

Use additional code for all associated injuries, such as:

   fracture of wrist and hand (S62.-)

   open wound of wrist and hand (S61.-)

The appropriate 7th character is to be added to each code from category S67

A - initial encounter

D - subsequent encounter

S - sequela

S67.0   Crushing injury of thumb

   ⊗⑦S67.00   Crushing injury of unspecified thumb

   ⊗⑦S67.01   Crushing injury of right thumb

   ⊗⑦S67.02   Crushing injury of left thumb

S67.1   Crushing injury of other and unspecified finger(s)

   Excludes 2: crushing injury of thumb (S67.0-)

   ⊗⑦S67.10   Crushing injury of unspecified finger(s)

   S67.19   Crushing injury of other finger(s)

     ⑦S67.190   Crushing injury of right index finger

     ⑦S67.191   Crushing injury of left index finger

     ⑦S67.192   Crushing injury of right middle finger

     ⑦S67.193   Crushing injury of left middle finger

     ⑦S67.194   Crushing injury of right ring finger

     ⑦S67.195   Crushing injury of left ring finger

     ⑦S67.196   Crushing injury of right little finger

     ⑦S67.197   Crushing injury of left little finger

     ⑦S67.198   Crushing injury of other finger

       Crushing injury of specified finger with unspecified laterality

S67.2   Crushing injury of hand

   Excludes 2: crushing injury of fingers (S67.1-)

       crushing injury of thumb (S67.0-)

   ⊗⑦S67.20   Crushing injury of unspecified hand

   ⊗⑦S67.21   Crushing injury of right hand

   ⊗⑦S67.22   Crushing injury of left hand

S67.3   Crushing injury of wrist

   ⊗⑦S67.30   Crushing injury of unspecified wrist

   ⊗⑦S67.31   Crushing injury of right wrist

   ⊗⑦S67.32   Crushing injury of left wrist

S67.4   Crushing injury of wrist and hand

   Excludes 1: crushing injury of hand alone (S67.2-)

       crushing injury of wrist alone (S67.3-)

   Excludes 2: crushing injury of fingers (S67.1-)

       crushing injury of thumb (S67.0-)

   ⊗⑦S67.40   Crushing injury of unspecified wrist and hand

   ⊗⑦S67.41   Crushing injury of right wrist and hand

   ⊗⑦S67.42   Crushing injury of left wrist and hand

S67.9   Crushing injury of unspecified part(s) of wrist, hand and fingers

   ⊗⑦S67.90   Crushing injury of unspecified part(s) of unspecified wrist, hand and fingers

   ⊗⑦S67.91   Crushing injury of unspecified part(s) of right wrist, hand and fingers

   ⊗⑦S67.92   Crushing injury of unspecified part(s) of left wrist, hand and fingers

S68   Traumatic amputation of wrist, hand and fingers

An amputation not identified as partial or complete should be coded to complete

The appropriate 7th character is to be added to each code from category S68

A - initial encounter

D - subsequent encounter

S - sequela

   S68.0   Traumatic metacarpophalangeal amputation of thumb

     Traumatic amputation of thumb NOS

S68.01 Complete traumatic metacarpophalangeal amputation of thumb

⑦**S68.011** Complete traumatic metacarpophalangeal amputation of right thumb

⑦**S68.012** Complete traumatic metacarpophalangeal amputation of left thumb

⑦**S68.019** Complete traumatic metacarpophalangeal amputation of unspecified thumb

S68.02 Partial traumatic metacarpophalangeal amputation of thumb

⑦**S68.021** Partial traumatic metacarpophalangeal amputation of right thumb

⑦**S68.022** Partial traumatic metacarpophalangeal amputation of left thumb

⑦**S68.029** Partial traumatic metacarpophalangeal amputation of unspecified thumb

S68.1 Traumatic metacarpophalangeal amputation of other and unspecified finger

Traumatic amputation of finger NOS

Excludes 2: traumatic metacarpophalangeal amputation of thumb (S68.0-)

S68.11 Complete traumatic metacarpophalangeal amputation of other and unspecified finger

⑦**S68.110** Complete traumatic metacarpophalangeal amputation of right index finger

⑦**S68.111** Complete traumatic metacarpophalangeal amputation of left index finger

⑦**S68.112** Complete traumatic metacarpophalangeal amputation of right middle finger

⑦**S68.113** Complete traumatic metacarpophalangeal amputation of left middle finger

⑦**S68.114** Complete traumatic metacarpophalangeal amputation of right ring finger

⑦**S68.115** Complete traumatic metacarpophalangeal amputation of left ring finger

⑦**S68.116** Complete traumatic metacarpophalangeal amputation of right little finger

⑦**S68.117** Complete traumatic metacarpophalangeal amputation of left little finger

⑦**S68.118** Complete traumatic metacarpophalangeal amputation of other finger

Complete traumatic metacarpophalangeal amputation of specified finger with unspecified laterality

⑦**S68.119** Complete traumatic metacarpophalangeal amputation of unspecified finger

S68.12 Partial traumatic metacarpophalangeal amputation of other and unspecified finger

⑦**S68.120** Partial traumatic metacarpophalangeal amputation of right index finger

⑦**S68.121** Partial traumatic metacarpophalangeal amputation of left index finger

⑦**S68.122** Partial traumatic metacarpophalangeal amputation of right middle finger

⑦**S68.123** Partial traumatic metacarpophalangeal amputation of left middle finger

⑦**S68.124** Partial traumatic metacarpophalangeal amputation of right ring finger

⑦**S68.125** Partial traumatic metacarpophalangeal amputation of left ring finger

⑦**S68.126** Partial traumatic metacarpophalangeal amputation of right little finger

⑦**S68.127** Partial traumatic metacarpophalangeal amputation of left little finger

⑦**S68.128** Partial traumatic metacarpophalangeal amputation of other finger

Partial traumatic metacarpophalangeal amputation of specified finger with unspecified laterality

⑦**S68.129** Partial traumatic metacarpophalangeal amputation of unspecified finger

S68.4 Traumatic amputation of hand at wrist level

Traumatic amputation of hand NOS

Traumatic amputation of wrist

S68.41 Complete traumatic amputation of hand at wrist level

⑦**S68.411** Complete traumatic amputation of right hand at wrist level

⑦**S68.412** Complete traumatic amputation of left hand at wrist level

⑦**S68.419** Complete traumatic amputation of unspecified hand at wrist level

S68.42 Partial traumatic amputation of hand at wrist level

⑦**S68.421** Partial traumatic amputation of right hand at wrist level

⑦**S68.422** Partial traumatic amputation of left hand at wrist level

⑦**S68.429** Partial traumatic amputation of unspecified hand at wrist level

S68.5 Traumatic transphalangeal amputation of thumb

Traumatic interphalangeal joint amputation of thumb

● New code   ▲ Revised code   ⑦ 7th digit required   ⊗ Placeholder required

S68.51　Complete traumatic transphalangeal amputation of thumb

⑦S68.511　Complete traumatic transphalangeal amputation of right thumb

⑦S68.512　Complete traumatic transphalangeal amputation of left thumb

⑦S68.519　Complete traumatic transphalangeal amputation of unspecified thumb

S68.52　Partial traumatic transphalangeal amputation of thumb

⑦S68.521　Partial traumatic transphalangeal amputation of right thumb

⑦S68.522　Partial traumatic transphalangeal amputation of left thumb

⑦S68.529　Partial traumatic transphalangeal amputation of unspecified thumb

S68.6　Traumatic transphalangeal amputation of other and unspecified finger

S68.61　Complete traumatic transphalangeal amputation of other and unspecified finger(s)

⑦S68.610　Complete traumatic transphalangeal amputation of right index finger

⑦S68.611　Complete traumatic transphalangeal amputation of left index finger

⑦S68.612　Complete traumatic transphalangeal amputation of right middle finger

⑦S68.613　Complete traumatic transphalangeal amputation of left middle finger

⑦S68.614　Complete traumatic transphalangeal amputation of right ring finger

⑦S68.615　Complete traumatic transphalangeal amputation of left ring finger

⑦S68.616　Complete traumatic transphalangeal amputation of right little finger

⑦S68.617　Complete traumatic transphalangeal amputation of left little finger

⑦S68.618　Complete traumatic transphalangeal amputation of other finger

Complete traumatic transphalangeal amputation of specified finger with unspecified laterality

⑦S68.619　Complete traumatic transphalangeal amputation of unspecified finger

S68.62　Partial traumatic transphalangeal amputation of other and unspecified finger

⑦S68.620　Partial traumatic transphalangeal amputation of right index finger

⑦S68.621　Partial traumatic transphalangeal amputation of left index finger

⑦S68.622　Partial traumatic transphalangeal amputation of right middle finger

⑦S68.623　Partial traumatic transphalangeal amputation of left middle finger

⑦S68.624　Partial traumatic transphalangeal amputation of right ring finger

⑦S68.625　Partial traumatic transphalangeal amputation of left ring finger

⑦S68.626　Partial traumatic transphalangeal amputation of right little finger

⑦S68.627　Partial traumatic transphalangeal amputation of left little finger

⑦S68.628　Partial traumatic transphalangeal amputation of other finger

Partial traumatic transphalangeal amputation of specified finger with unspecified laterality

⑦S68.629　Partial traumatic transphalangeal amputation of unspecified finger

S68.7　Traumatic transmetacarpal amputation of hand

S68.71　Complete traumatic transmetacarpal amputation of hand

⑦S68.711　Complete traumatic transmetacarpal amputation of right hand

⑦S68.712　Complete traumatic transmetacarpal amputation of left hand

⑦S68.719　Complete traumatic transmetacarpal amputation of unspecified hand

S68.72　Partial traumatic transmetacarpal amputation of hand

⑦S68.721　Partial traumatic transmetacarpal amputation of right hand

⑦S68.722　Partial traumatic transmetacarpal amputation of left hand

⑦S68.729　Partial traumatic transmetacarpal amputation of unspecified hand

S69　Other and unspecified injuries of wrist, hand and finger(s)

The appropriate 7th character is to be added to each code from category S69

A - initial encounter

D - subsequent encounter

S - sequela

S69.8　Other specified injuries of wrist, hand and finger(s)

⊗⑦S69.80　Other specified injuries of unspecified wrist, hand and finger(s)

⊗⑦S69.81　Other specified injuries of right wrist, hand and finger(s)

⊗⑦S69.82　Other specified injuries of left wrist, hand and finger(s)

S69.9　Unspecified injury of wrist, hand and finger(s)

⊗⑦S69.90　Unspecified injury of unspecified wrist, hand and finger(s)

⊗⑦S69.91　Unspecified injury of right wrist, hand and finger(s)

⊗⑦S69.92　Unspecified injury of left wrist, hand and finger(s)

INJURIES TO THE HIP AND THIGH (S70-S79)

Excludes 2: burns and corrosions (T20-T32)

frostbite (T33-T34)

snake bite (T63.0-)

venomous insect bite or sting (T63.4-)

S70　Superficial injury of hip and thigh

The appropriate 7th character is to be added to each code from category S70

A - initial encounter

D - subsequent encounter

S - sequela

S70.0　Contusion of hip

⊗⑦**S70.00**   Contusion of unspecified hip

⊗⑦**S70.01**   Contusion of right hip

⊗⑦**S70.02**   Contusion of left hip

S70.1   Contusion of thigh

⊗⑦**S70.10**   Contusion of unspecified thigh

⊗⑦**S70.11**   Contusion of right thigh

⊗⑦**S70.12**   Contusion of left thigh

S70.2   Other superficial injuries of hip

S70.21   Abrasion of hip

⑦**S70.211**   Abrasion, right hip

⑦**S70.212**   Abrasion, left hip

⑦**S70.219**   Abrasion, unspecified hip

S70.22   Blister (nonthermal) of hip

⑦**S70.221**   Blister (nonthermal), right hip

⑦**S70.222**   Blister (nonthermal), left hip

⑦**S70.229**   Blister (nonthermal), unspecified hip

S70.24   External constriction of hip

⑦**S70.241**   External constriction, right hip

⑦**S70.242**   External constriction, left hip

⑦**S70.249**   External constriction, unspecified hip

S70.25   Superficial foreign body of hip
Splinter in the hip

⑦**S70.251**   Superficial foreign body, right hip

⑦**S70.252**   Superficial foreign body, left hip

⑦**S70.259**   Superficial foreign body, unspecified hip

S70.26   Insect bite (nonvenomous) of hip

⑦**S70.261**   Insect bite (nonvenomous), right hip

⑦**S70.262**   Insect bite (nonvenomous), left hip

⑦**S70.269**   Insect bite (nonvenomous), unspecified hip

S70.27   Other superficial bite of hip

Excludes 1: open bite of hip (S71.05-)

⑦**S70.271**   Other superficial bite of hip, right hip

⑦**S70.272**   Other superficial bite of hip, left hip

⑦**S70.279**   Other superficial bite of hip, unspecified hip

S70.3   Other superficial injuries of thigh

S70.31   Abrasion of thigh

⑦**S70.311**   Abrasion, right thigh

⑦**S70.312**   Abrasion, left thigh

⑦**S70.319**   Abrasion, unspecified thigh

S70.32   Blister (nonthermal) of thigh

⑦**S70.321**   Blister (nonthermal), right thigh

⑦**S70.322**   Blister (nonthermal), left thigh

⑦**S70.329**   Blister (nonthermal), unspecified thigh

S70.34   External constriction of thigh

⑦**S70.341**   External constriction, right thigh

⑦**S70.342**   External constriction, left thigh

⑦**S70.349**   External constriction, unspecified thigh

S70.35   Superficial foreign body of thigh
Splinter in the thigh

⑦**S70.351**   Superficial foreign body, right thigh

⑦**S70.352**   Superficial foreign body, left thigh

⑦**S70.359**   Superficial foreign body, unspecified thigh

S70.36   Insect bite (nonvenomous) of thigh

⑦**S70.361**   Insect bite (nonvenomous), right thigh

⑦**S70.362**   Insect bite (nonvenomous), left thigh

⑦**S70.369**   Insect bite (nonvenomous), unspecified thigh

S70.37   Other superficial bite of thigh

Excludes 1: open bite of thigh (S71.15)

⑦**S70.371**   Other superficial bite of right thigh

⑦**S70.372**   Other superficial bite of left thigh

⑦**S70.379**   Other superficial bite of unspecified thigh

S70.9   Unspecified superficial injury of hip and thigh

S70.91   Unspecified superficial injury of hip

⑦**S70.911**   Unspecified superficial injury of right hip

⑦**S70.912**   Unspecified superficial injury of left hip

⑦**S70.919**   Unspecified superficial injury of unspecified hip

S70.92   Unspecified superficial injury of thigh

⑦**S70.921**   Unspecified superficial injury of right thigh

⑦**S70.922**   Unspecified superficial injury of left thigh

⑦**S70.929**   Unspecified superficial injury of unspecified thigh

S71   Open wound of hip and thigh
Code also any associated wound infection

Excludes 1: open fracture of hip and thigh (S72.-)
traumatic amputation of hip and thigh (S78.-)

Excludes 2: bite of venomous animal (T63.-)
open wound of ankle, foot and toes (S91.-)
open wound of knee and lower leg (S81.-)

The appropriate 7th character is to be added to each code from category S71

A - initial encounter

D - subsequent encounter

S - sequela

S71.0   Open wound of hip

S71.00   Unspecified open wound of hip

⑦**S71.001**   Unspecified open wound, right hip

⑦**S71.002**   Unspecified open wound, left hip

⑦**S71.009**   Unspecified open wound, unspecified hip

S71.01   Laceration without foreign body of hip

⑦**S71.011**   Laceration without foreign body, right hip

⑦**S71.012**   Laceration without foreign body, left hip

⑦**S71.019**   Laceration without foreign body, unspecified hip

S71.02   Laceration with foreign body of hip
   ⑦S71.021   Laceration with foreign body, right hip
   ⑦S71.022   Laceration with foreign body, left hip
   ⑦S71.029   Laceration with foreign body, unspecified hip

S71.03   Puncture wound without foreign body of hip
   ⑦S71.031   Puncture wound without foreign body, right hip
   ⑦S71.032   Puncture wound without foreign body, left hip
   ⑦S71.039   Puncture wound without foreign body, unspecified hip

S71.04   Puncture wound with foreign body of hip
   ⑦S71.041   Puncture wound with foreign body, right hip
   ⑦S71.042   Puncture wound with foreign body, left hip
   ⑦S71.049   Puncture wound with foreign body, unspecified hip

S71.05   Open bite of hip
   Bite of hip NOS
   Excludes 1: superficial bite of hip (S70.26, S70.27)
   ⑦S71.051   Open bite, right hip
   ⑦S71.052   Open bite, left hip
   ⑦S71.059   Open bite, unspecified hip

S71.1   Open wound of thigh
  S71.10   Unspecified open wound of thigh
   ⑦S71.101   Unspecified open wound, right thigh
   ⑦S71.102   Unspecified open wound, left thigh
   ⑦S71.109   Unspecified open wound, unspecified thigh

  S71.11   Laceration without foreign body of thigh
   ⑦S71.111   Laceration without foreign body, right thigh
   ⑦S71.112   Laceration without foreign body, left thigh
   ⑦S71.119   Laceration without foreign body, unspecified thigh

  S71.12   Laceration with foreign body of thigh
   ⑦S71.121   Laceration with foreign body, right thigh
   ⑦S71.122   Laceration with foreign body, left thigh
   ⑦S71.129   Laceration with foreign body, unspecified thigh

  S71.13   Puncture wound without foreign body of thigh
   ⑦S71.131   Puncture wound without foreign body, right thigh
   ⑦S71.132   Puncture wound without foreign body, left thigh
   ⑦S71.139   Puncture wound without foreign body, unspecified thigh

  S71.14   Puncture wound with foreign body of thigh
   ⑦S71.141   Puncture wound with foreign body, right thigh
   ⑦S71.142   Puncture wound with foreign body, left thigh
   ⑦S71.149   Puncture wound with foreign body, unspecified thigh

  S71.15   Open bite of thigh
   Bite of thigh NOS
   Excludes 1: superficial bite of thigh (S70.37-)
   ⑦S71.151   Open bite, right thigh
   ⑦S71.152   Open bite, left thigh
   ⑦S71.159   Open bite, unspecified thigh

S72 Fracture of femur

Note: A fracture not indicated as displaced or nondisplaced should be coded to displaced

A fracture not indicated as open or closed should be coded to closed

The open fracture designations are based on the Gustilo open fracture classification

Excludes 1: traumatic amputation of hip and thigh (S78.-)

Excludes 2: fracture of lower leg and ankle (S82.-)

fracture of foot (S92.-)

periprosthetic fracture of prosthetic implant of hip (T84.040, T84.041)

The appropriate 7th character is to be added to all codes from category S72

A - initial encounter for closed fracture

B - initial encounter for open fracture type I or II initial encounter for open fracture NOS

C - initial encounter for open fracture type IIIA, IIIB, or IIIC

D - subsequent encounter for closed fracture with routine healing

E - subsequent encounter for open fracture type I or II with routine healing

F - subsequent encounter for open fracture type IIIA, IIIB, or IIIC with routine healing

G - subsequent encounter for closed fracture with delayed healing

H - subsequent encounter for open fracture type I or II with delayed healing

J - subsequent encounter for open fracture type IIIA, IIIB, or IIIC with delayed healing

K - subsequent encounter for closed fracture with nonunion

M - subsequent encounter for open fracture type I or II with nonunion

N - subsequent encounter for open fracture type IIIA, IIIB, or IIIC with nonunion

P - subsequent encounter for closed fracture with malunion

Q - subsequent encounter for open fracture type I or II with malunion

R - subsequent encounter for open fracture type IIIA, IIIB, or IIIC with malunion

S - sequela

S72.0   Fracture of head and neck of femur
  Excludes 2: physeal fracture of upper end of femur (S79.0-)
  S72.00   Fracture of unspecified part of neck of femur
   Fracture of hip NOS
   Fracture of neck of femur NOS
   ⑦S72.001   Fracture of unspecified part of neck of right femur
   ⑦S72.002   Fracture of unspecified part of neck of left femur

⑦**S72.009**   Fracture of unspecified part of neck of unspecified femur

S72.01   Unspecified intracapsular fracture of femur

Subcapital fracture of femur

⑦**S72.011**   Unspecified intracapsular fracture of right femur

⑦**S72.012**   Unspecified intracapsular fracture of left femur

⑦**S72.019**   Unspecified intracapsular fracture of unspecified femur

S72.02   Fracture of epiphysis (separation) (upper) of femur

Transepiphyseal fracture of femur

Excludes 1: capital femoral epiphyseal fracture (pediatric) of femur (S79.01-)

Salter-Harris Type I physeal fracture of upper end of femur (S79.01-)

⑦**S72.021**   Displaced fracture of epiphysis (separation) (upper) of right femur

⑦**S72.022**   Displaced fracture of epiphysis (separation) (upper) of left femur

⑦**S72.023**   Displaced fracture of epiphysis (separation) (upper) of unspecified femur

⑦**S72.024**   Nondisplaced fracture of epiphysis (separation) (upper) of right femur

⑦**S72.025**   Nondisplaced fracture of epiphysis (separation) (upper) of left femur

⑦**S72.026**   Nondisplaced fracture of epiphysis (separation) (upper) of unspecified femur

S72.03   Midcervical fracture of femur

Transcervical fracture of femur NOS

⑦**S72.031**   Displaced midcervical fracture of right femur

⑦**S72.032**   Displaced midcervical fracture of left femur

⑦**S72.033**   Displaced midcervical fracture of unspecified femur

⑦**S72.034**   Nondisplaced midcervical fracture of right femur

⑦**S72.035**   Nondisplaced midcervical fracture of left femur

⑦**S72.036**   Nondisplaced midcervical fracture of unspecified femur

S72.04   Fracture of base of neck of femur

Cervicotrochanteric fracture of femur

⑦**S72.041**   Displaced fracture of base of neck of right femur

⑦**S72.042**   Displaced fracture of base of neck of left femur

⑦**S72.043**   Displaced fracture of base of neck of unspecified femur

⑦**S72.044**   Nondisplaced fracture of base of neck of right femur

⑦**S72.045**   Nondisplaced fracture of base of neck of left femur

⑦**S72.046**   Nondisplaced fracture of base of neck of unspecified femur

S72.05   Unspecified fracture of head of femur

Fracture of head of femur NOS

⑦**S72.051**   Unspecified fracture of head of right femur

⑦**S72.052**   Unspecified fracture of head of left femur

⑦**S72.059**   Unspecified fracture of head of unspecified femur

S72.06   Articular fracture of head of femur

⑦**S72.061**   Displaced articular fracture of head of right femur

⑦**S72.062**   Displaced articular fracture of head of left femur

⑦**S72.063**   Displaced articular fracture of head of unspecified femur

⑦**S72.064**   Nondisplaced articular fracture of head of right femur

⑦**S72.065**   Nondisplaced articular fracture of head of left femur

⑦**S72.066**   Nondisplaced articular fracture of head of unspecified femur

S72.09   Other fracture of head and neck of femur

⑦**S72.091**   Other fracture of head and neck of right femur

⑦**S72.092**   Other fracture of head and neck of left femur

⑦**S72.099**   Other fracture of head and neck of unspecified femur

S72.1   Pertrochanteric fracture

S72.10   Unspecified trochanteric fracture of femur

Fracture of trochanter NOS

⑦**S72.101**   Unspecified trochanteric fracture of right femur

⑦**S72.102**   Unspecified trochanteric fracture of left femur

⑦**S72.109**   Unspecified trochanteric fracture of unspecified femur

S72.11   Fracture of greater trochanter of femur

⑦**S72.111**   Displaced fracture of greater trochanter of right femur

⑦**S72.112**   Displaced fracture of greater trochanter of left femur

⑦**S72.113**   Displaced fracture of greater trochanter of unspecified femur

⑦**S72.114**   Nondisplaced fracture of greater trochanter of right femur

⑦**S72.115**   Nondisplaced fracture of greater trochanter of left femur

⑦**S72.116**   Nondisplaced fracture of greater trochanter of unspecified femur

S72.12   Fracture of lesser trochanter of femur

⑦**S72.121**   Displaced fracture of lesser trochanter of right femur

⑦**S72.122**   Displaced fracture of lesser trochanter of left femur

⑦**S72.123**   Displaced fracture of lesser trochanter of unspecified femur

⑦**S72.124**   Nondisplaced fracture of lesser trochanter of right femur

⑦S72.125   Nondisplaced fracture of lesser trochanter of left femur

⑦S72.126   Nondisplaced fracture of lesser trochanter of unspecified femur

S72.13   Apophyseal fracture of femur

Excludes 1: chronic (nontraumatic) slipped upper femoral epiphysis (M93.0-)

⑦S72.131   Displaced apophyseal fracture of right femur

⑦S72.132   Displaced apophyseal fracture of left femur

⑦S72.133   Displaced apophyseal fracture of unspecified femur

⑦S72.134   Nondisplaced apophyseal fracture of right femur

⑦S72.135   Nondisplaced apophyseal fracture of left femur

⑦S72.136   Nondisplaced apophyseal fracture of unspecified femur

S72.14   Intertrochanteric fracture of femur

⑦S72.141   Displaced intertrochanteric fracture of right femur

⑦S72.142   Displaced intertrochanteric fracture of left femur

⑦S72.143   Displaced intertrochanteric fracture of unspecified femur

⑦S72.144   Nondisplaced intertrochanteric fracture of right femur

⑦S72.145   Nondisplaced intertrochanteric fracture of left femur

⑦S72.146   Nondisplaced intertrochanteric fracture of unspecified femur

S72.2   Subtrochanteric fracture of femur

⊗⑦S72.21   Displaced subtrochanteric fracture of right femur

⊗⑦S72.22   Displaced subtrochanteric fracture of left femur

⊗⑦S72.23   Displaced subtrochanteric fracture of unspecified femur

⊗⑦S72.24   Nondisplaced subtrochanteric fracture of right femur

⊗⑦S72.25   Nondisplaced subtrochanteric fracture of left femur

⊗⑦S72.26   Nondisplaced subtrochanteric fracture of unspecified femur

S72.3   Fracture of shaft of femur

S72.30   Unspecified fracture of shaft of femur

⑦S72.301   Unspecified fracture of shaft of right femur

⑦S72.302   Unspecified fracture of shaft of left femur

⑦S72.309   Unspecified fracture of shaft of unspecified femur

S72.32   Transverse fracture of shaft of femur

⑦S72.321   Displaced transverse fracture of shaft of right femur

⑦S72.322   Displaced transverse fracture of shaft of left femur

⑦S72.323   Displaced transverse fracture of shaft of unspecified femur

⑦S72.324   Nondisplaced transverse fracture of shaft of right femur

⑦S72.325   Nondisplaced transverse fracture of shaft of left femur

⑦S72.326   Nondisplaced transverse fracture of shaft of unspecified femur

S72.33   Oblique fracture of shaft of femur

⑦S72.331   Displaced oblique fracture of shaft of right femur

⑦S72.332   Displaced oblique fracture of shaft of left femur

⑦S72.333   Displaced oblique fracture of shaft of unspecified femur

⑦S72.334   Nondisplaced oblique fracture of shaft of right femur

⑦S72.335   Nondisplaced oblique fracture of shaft of left femur

⑦S72.336   Nondisplaced oblique fracture of shaft of unspecified femur

S72.34   Spiral fracture of shaft of femur

⑦S72.341   Displaced spiral fracture of shaft of right femur

⑦S72.342   Displaced spiral fracture of shaft of left femur

⑦S72.343   Displaced spiral fracture of shaft of unspecified femur

⑦S72.344   Nondisplaced spiral fracture of shaft of right femur

⑦S72.345   Nondisplaced spiral fracture of shaft of left femur

⑦S72.346   Nondisplaced spiral fracture of shaft of unspecified femur

S72.35   Comminuted fracture of shaft of femur

⑦S72.351   Displaced comminuted fracture of shaft of right femur

⑦S72.352   Displaced comminuted fracture of shaft of left femur

⑦S72.353   Displaced comminuted fracture of shaft of unspecified femur

⑦S72.354   Nondisplaced comminuted fracture of shaft of right femur

⑦S72.355   Nondisplaced comminuted fracture of shaft of left femur

⑦S72.356   Nondisplaced comminuted fracture of shaft of unspecified femur

S72.36   Segmental fracture of shaft of femur

⑦S72.361   Displaced segmental fracture of shaft of right femur

⑦S72.362   Displaced segmental fracture of shaft of left femur

⑦S72.363   Displaced segmental fracture of shaft of unspecified femur

⑦S72.364   Nondisplaced segmental fracture of shaft of right femur

⑦S72.365   Nondisplaced segmental fracture of shaft of left femur

⑦S72.366   Nondisplaced segmental fracture of shaft of unspecified femur

S72.39   Other fracture of shaft of femur

⑦S72.391 Other fracture of shaft of right femur

⑦S72.392 Other fracture of shaft of left femur

⑦S72.399 Other fracture of shaft of unspecified femur

S72.4 Fracture of lower end of femur

Fracture of distal end of femur

Excludes 2: fracture of shaft of femur (S72.3-)

physeal fracture of lower end of femur (S79.1-)

S72.40 Unspecified fracture of lower end of femur

⑦S72.401 Unspecified fracture of lower end of right femur

⑦S72.402 Unspecified fracture of lower end of left femur

⑦S72.409 Unspecified fracture of lower end of unspecified femur

S72.41 Unspecified condyle fracture of lower end of femur

Condyle fracture of femur NOS

⑦S72.411 Displaced unspecified condyle fracture of lower end of right femur

⑦S72.412 Displaced unspecified condyle fracture of lower end of left femur

⑦S72.413 Displaced unspecified condyle fracture of lower end of unspecified femur

⑦S72.414 Nondisplaced unspecified condyle fracture of lower end of right femur

⑦S72.415 Nondisplaced unspecified condyle fracture of lower end of left femur

⑦S72.416 Nondisplaced unspecified condyle fracture of lower end of unspecified femur

S72.42 Fracture of lateral condyle of femur

⑦S72.421 Displaced fracture of lateral condyle of right femur

⑦S72.422 Displaced fracture of lateral condyle of left femur

⑦S72.423 Displaced fracture of lateral condyle of unspecified femur

⑦S72.424 Nondisplaced fracture of lateral condyle of right femur

⑦S72.425 Nondisplaced fracture of lateral condyle of left femur

⑦S72.426 Nondisplaced fracture of lateral condyle of unspecified femur

S72.43 Fracture of medial condyle of femur

⑦S72.431 Displaced fracture of medial condyle of right femur

⑦S72.432 Displaced fracture of medial condyle of left femur

⑦S72.433 Displaced fracture of medial condyle of unspecified femur

⑦S72.434 Nondisplaced fracture of medial condyle of right femur

⑦S72.435 Nondisplaced fracture of medial condyle of left femur

⑦S72.436 Nondisplaced fracture of medial condyle of unspecified femur

S72.44 Fracture of lower epiphysis (separation) of femur

Excludes 1: Salter-Harris Type I physeal fracture of lower end of femur (S79.11-)

⑦S72.441 Displaced fracture of lower epiphysis (separation) of right femur

⑦S72.442 Displaced fracture of lower epiphysis (separation) of left femur

⑦S72.443 Displaced fracture of lower epiphysis (separation) of unspecified femur

⑦S72.444 Nondisplaced fracture of lower epiphysis (separation) of right femur

⑦S72.445 Nondisplaced fracture of lower epiphysis (separation) of left femur

⑦S72.446 Nondisplaced fracture of lower epiphysis (separation) of unspecified femur

S72.45 Supracondylar fracture without intracondylar extension of lower end of femur

Supracondylar fracture of lower end of femur NOS

Excludes 1: supracondylar fracture with intracondylar extension of lower end of femur (S72.46-)

⑦S72.451 Displaced supracondylar fracture without intracondylar extension of lower end of right femur

⑦S72.452 Displaced supracondylar fracture without intracondylar extension of lower end of left femur

⑦S72.453 Displaced supracondylar fracture without intracondylar extension of lower end of unspecified femur

⑦S72.454 Nondisplaced supracondylar fracture without intracondylar extension of lower end of right femur

⑦S72.455 Nondisplaced supracondylar fracture without intracondylar extension of lower end of left femur

⑦S72.456 Nondisplaced supracondylar fracture without intracondylar extension of lower end of unspecified femur

S72.46 Supracondylar fracture with intracondylar extension of lower end of femur

Excludes 1: supracondylar fracture without intracondylar extension of lower end of femur (S72.45-)

⑦S72.461 Displaced supracondylar fracture with intracondylar extension of lower end of right femur

⑦S72.462 Displaced supracondylar fracture with intracondylar extension of lower end of left femur

⑦S72.463 Displaced supracondylar fracture with intracondylar extension of lower end of unspecified femur

⑦S72.464 Nondisplaced supracondylar fracture with intracondylar extension of lower end of right femur

● New code ▲ Revised code ⑦ 7th digit required ⊗ Placeholder required

⑦S72.465 Nondisplaced supracondylar fracture with intracondylar extension of lower end of left femur

⑦S72.466 Nondisplaced supracondylar fracture with intracondylar extension of lower end of unspecified femur

S72.47 Torus fracture of lower end of femur

The appropriate 7th character is to be added to all codes in subcategory S72.47

A - initial encounter for closed fracture

D - subsequent encounter for fracture with routine healing

G - subsequent encounter for fracture with delayed healing

K - subsequent encounter for fracture with nonunion

P - subsequent encounter for fracture with malunion

S - sequela

⑦S72.471 Torus fracture of lower end of right femur

⑦S72.472 Torus fracture of lower end of left femur

⑦S72.479 Torus fracture of lower end of unspecified femur

S72.49 Other fracture of lower end of femur

⑦S72.491 Other fracture of lower end of right femur

⑦S72.492 Other fracture of lower end of left femur

⑦S72.499 Other fracture of lower end of unspecified femur

S72.8 Other fracture of femur

S72.8X Other fracture of femur

⑦S72.8X1 Other fracture of right femur

⑦S72.8X2 Other fracture of left femur

⑦S72.8X9 Other fracture of unspecified femur

S72.9 Unspecified fracture of femur

Fracture of thigh NOS

Fracture of upper leg NOS

Excludes 1: fracture of hip NOS (S72.00-, S72.01-)

⊗⑦**S72.90** Unspecified fracture of unspecified femur

⊗⑦**S72.91** Unspecified fracture of right femur

⊗⑦**S72.92** Unspecified fracture of left femur

S73 Dislocation and sprain of joint and ligaments of hip

Includes: avulsion of joint or ligament of hip

laceration of cartilage, joint or ligament of hip

sprain of cartilage, joint or ligament of hip

traumatic hemarthrosis of joint or ligament of hip

traumatic rupture of joint or ligament of hip

traumatic subluxation of joint or ligament of hip

traumatic tear of joint or ligament of hip

Code also any associated open wound

Excludes 2: strain of muscle, fascia and tendon of hip and thigh (S76.-)

The appropriate 7th character is to be added to each code from category S73

A - initial encounter

D - subsequent encounter

S - sequela

S73.0 Subluxation and dislocation of hip

Excludes 2: dislocation and subluxation of hip prosthesis (T84.020, T84.021)

S73.00 Unspecified subluxation and dislocation of hip

Dislocation of hip NOS

Subluxation of hip NOS

⑦S73.001 Unspecified subluxation of right hip

⑦S73.002 Unspecified subluxation of left hip

⑦S73.003 Unspecified subluxation of unspecified hip

⑦S73.004 Unspecified dislocation of right hip

⑦S73.005 Unspecified dislocation of left hip

⑦S73.006 Unspecified dislocation of unspecified hip

S73.01 Posterior subluxation and dislocation of hip

⑦S73.011 Posterior subluxation of right hip

⑦S73.012 Posterior subluxation of left hip

⑦S73.013 Posterior subluxation of unspecified hip

⑦S73.014 Posterior dislocation of right hip

⑦S73.015 Posterior dislocation of left hip

⑦S73.016 Posterior dislocation of unspecified hip

S73.02 Obturator subluxation and dislocation of hip

⑦S73.021 Obturator subluxation of right hip

⑦S73.022 Obturator subluxation of left hip

⑦S73.023 Obturator subluxation of unspecified hip

⑦S73.024 Obturator dislocation of right hip

⑦S73.025 Obturator dislocation of left hip

⑦S73.026 Obturator dislocation of unspecified hip

S73.03 Other anterior dislocation of hip

⑦S73.031 Other anterior subluxation of right hip

⑦S73.032 Other anterior subluxation of left hip

⑦S73.033 Other anterior subluxation of unspecified hip

⑦S73.034 Other anterior dislocation of right hip

⑦S73.035 Other anterior dislocation of left hip

⑦S73.036 Other anterior dislocation of unspecified hip

S73.04 Central dislocation of hip

⑦S73.041 Central subluxation of right hip

⑦S73.042 Central subluxation of left hip

⑦S73.043 Central subluxation of unspecified hip

⑦S73.044 Central dislocation of right hip

⑦S73.045 Central dislocation of left hip

⑦S73.046 Central dislocation of unspecified hip

S73.1 Sprain of hip

S73.10 Unspecified sprain of hip

⑦S73.101 Unspecified sprain of right hip

⑦S73.102 Unspecified sprain of left hip

⑦**S73.109**   Unspecified sprain of unspecified hip

S73.11   Iliofemoral ligament sprain of hip

⑦**S73.111**   Iliofemoral ligament sprain of right hip

⑦**S73.112**   Iliofemoral ligament sprain of left hip

⑦**S73.119**   Iliofemoral ligament sprain of unspecified hip

S73.12   Ischiocapsular (ligament) sprain of hip

⑦**S73.121**   Ischiocapsular ligament sprain of right hip

⑦**S73.122**   Ischiocapsular ligament sprain of left hip

⑦**S73.129**   Ischiocapsular ligament sprain of unspecified hip

S73.19   Other sprain of hip

⑦**S73.191**   Other sprain of right hip

⑦**S73.192**   Other sprain of left hip

⑦**S73.199**   Other sprain of unspecified hip

S74 Injury of nerves at hip and thigh level

Code also any associated open wound (S71.-)

Excludes 2: injury of nerves at ankle and foot level (S94.-)

injury of nerves at lower leg level (S84.-)

The appropriate 7th character is to be added to each code from category S74

A - initial encounter

D - subsequent encounter

S - sequela

S74.0   Injury of sciatic nerve at hip and thigh level

⊗⑦**S74.00**   Injury of sciatic nerve at hip and thigh level, unspecified leg

⊗⑦**S74.01**   Injury of sciatic nerve at hip and thigh level, right leg

⊗⑦**S74.02**   Injury of sciatic nerve at hip and thigh level, left leg

S74.1   Injury of femoral nerve at hip and thigh level

⊗⑦**S74.10**   Injury of femoral nerve at hip and thigh level, unspecified leg

⊗⑦**S74.11**   Injury of femoral nerve at hip and thigh level, right leg

⊗⑦**S74.12**   Injury of femoral nerve at hip and thigh level, left leg

S74.2   Injury of cutaneous sensory nerve at hip and thigh level

⊗⑦**S74.20**   Injury of cutaneous sensory nerve at hip and thigh level, unspecified leg

⊗⑦**S74.21**   Injury of cutaneous sensory nerve at hip and high level, right leg

⊗⑦**S74.22**   Injury of cutaneous sensory nerve at hip and thigh level, left leg

S74.8   Injury of other nerves at hip and thigh level

S74.8X   Injury of other nerves at hip and thigh level

⑦**S74.8X1**   Injury of other nerves at hip and thigh level, right leg

⑦**S74.8X2**   Injury of other nerves at hip and thigh level, left leg

⑦**S74.8X9**   Injury of other nerves at hip and thigh level, unspecified leg

S74.9   Injury of unspecified nerve at hip and thigh level

⊗⑦**S74.90**   Injury of unspecified nerve at hip and thigh level, unspecified leg

⊗⑦**S74.91**   Injury of unspecified nerve at hip and thigh level, right leg

⊗⑦**S74.92**   Injury of unspecified nerve at hip and thigh level, left leg

S75 Injury of blood vessels at hip and thigh level

Code also any associated open wound (S71.-)

Excludes 2: injury of blood vessels at lower leg level (S85.-)

injury of popliteal artery (S85.0)

The appropriate 7th character is to be added to each code from category S75

A - initial encounter

D - subsequent encounter

S - sequela

S75.0   Injury of femoral artery

S75.00   Unspecified injury of femoral artery

⑦**S75.001**   Unspecified injury of femoral artery, right leg

⑦**S75.002**   Unspecified injury of femoral artery, left leg

⑦**S75.009**   Unspecified injury of femoral artery, unspecified leg

S75.01   Minor laceration of femoral artery

Incomplete transection of femoral artery

Laceration of femoral artery NOS

Superficial laceration of femoral artery

⑦**S75.011**   Minor laceration of femoral artery, right leg

⑦**S75.012**   Minor laceration of femoral artery, left leg

⑦**S75.019**   Minor laceration of femoral artery, unspecified leg

S75.02   Major laceration of femoral artery

Complete transection of femoral artery

Traumatic rupture of femoral artery

⑦**S75.021**   Major laceration of femoral artery, right leg

⑦**S75.022**   Major laceration of femoral artery, left leg

⑦**S75.029**   Major laceration of femoral artery, unspecified leg

S75.09   Other specified injury of femoral artery

⑦**S75.091**   Other specified injury of femoral artery, right leg

⑦**S75.092**   Other specified injury of femoral artery, left leg

⑦**S75.099**   Other specified injury of femoral artery, unspecified leg

S75.1   Injury of femoral vein at hip and thigh level

S75.10   Unspecified injury of femoral vein at hip and thigh level

⑦**S75.101**   Unspecified injury of femoral vein at hip and thigh level, right leg

⑦**S75.102**   Unspecified injury of femoral vein at hip and thigh level, left leg

⑦S75.109   Unspecified injury of femoral vein at hip and thigh level, unspecified leg

S75.11   Minor laceration of femoral vein at hip and thigh level

Incomplete transection of femoral vein at hip and thigh level

Laceration of femoral vein at hip and thigh level NOS

Superficial laceration of femoral vein at hip and thigh level

⑦S75.111   Minor laceration of femoral vein at hip and thigh level, right leg

⑦S75.112   Minor laceration of femoral vein at hip and thigh level, left leg

⑦S75.119   Minor laceration of femoral vein at hip and thigh level, unspecified leg

S75.12   Major laceration of femoral vein at hip and thigh level

Complete transection of femoral vein at hip and thigh level

Traumatic rupture of femoral vein at hip and thigh level

⑦S75.121   Major laceration of femoral vein at hip and thigh level, right leg

⑦S75.122   Major laceration of femoral vein at hip and thigh level, left leg

⑦S75.129   Major laceration of femoral vein at hip and thigh level, unspecified leg

S75.19   Other specified injury of femoral vein at hip and thigh level

⑦S75.191   Other specified injury of femoral vein at hip and thigh level, right leg

⑦S75.192   Other specified injury of femoral vein at hip and thigh level, left leg

⑦S75.199   Other specified injury of femoral vein at hip and thigh level, unspecified leg

S75.2   Injury of greater saphenous vein at hip and thigh level

Excludes 1: greater saphenous vein NOS (S85.3)

S75.20   Unspecified injury of greater saphenous vein at hip and thigh level

⑦S75.201   Unspecified injury of greater saphenous vein at hip and thigh level, right leg

⑦S75.202   Unspecified injury of greater saphenous vein at hip and thigh level, left leg

⑦S75.209   Unspecified injury of greater saphenous vein at hip and thigh level, unspecified leg

S75.21   Minor laceration of greater saphenous vein at hip and thigh level

Incomplete transection of greater saphenous vein at hip and thigh level

Laceration of greater saphenous vein at hip and thigh level NOS

Superficial laceration of greater saphenous vein at hip and thigh level

⑦S75.211   Minor laceration of greater saphenous vein at hip and thigh level, right leg

⑦S75.212   Minor laceration of greater saphenous vein at hip and thigh level, left leg

⑦S75.219   Minor laceration of greater saphenous vein at hip and thigh level, unspecified leg

S75.22   Major laceration of greater saphenous vein at hip and thigh level

Complete transection of greater saphenous vein at hip and thigh level

Traumatic rupture of greater saphenous vein at hip and thigh level

⑦S75.221   Major laceration of greater saphenous vein at hip and thigh level, right leg

⑦S75.222   Major laceration of greater saphenous vein at hip and thigh level, left leg

⑦S75.229   Major laceration of greater saphenous vein at hip and thigh level, unspecified leg

S75.29   Other specified injury of greater saphenous vein at hip and thigh level

⑦S75.291   Other specified injury of greater saphenous vein at hip and thigh level, right leg

⑦S75.292   Other specified injury of greater saphenous vein at hip and thigh level, left leg

⑦S75.299   Other specified injury of greater saphenous vein at hip and thigh level, unspecified leg

S75.8   Injury of other blood vessels at hip and thigh level

S75.80   Unspecified injury of other blood vessels at hip and thigh level

⑦S75.801   Unspecified injury of other blood vessels at hip and thigh level, right leg

⑦S75.802   Unspecified injury of other blood vessels at hip and thigh level, left leg

⑦S75.809   Unspecified injury of other blood vessels at hip and thigh level, unspecified leg

S75.81   Laceration of other blood vessels at hip and thigh level

⑦S75.811   Laceration of other blood vessels at hip and thigh level, right leg

⑦S75.812   Laceration of other blood vessels at hip and thigh level, left leg

⑦S75.819   Laceration of other blood vessels at hip and thigh level, unspecified leg

S75.89   Other specified injury of other blood vessels at hip and thigh level

⑦S75.891   Other specified injury of other blood vessels at hip and thigh level, right leg

⑦S75.892   Other specified injury of other blood vessels at hip and thigh level, left leg

⑦ S75.899   Other specified injury of other blood vessels at hip and thigh level, unspecified leg

S75.9   Injury of unspecified blood vessel at hip and thigh level

    S75.90   Unspecified injury of unspecified blood vessel at hip and thigh level

      ⑦ S75.901   Unspecified injury of unspecified blood vessel at hip and thigh level, right leg

      ⑦ S75.902   Unspecified injury of unspecified blood vessel at hip and thigh level, left leg

      ⑦ S75.909   Unspecified injury of unspecified blood vessel at hip and thigh level, unspecified leg

    S75.91   Laceration of unspecified blood vessel at hip and thigh level

      ⑦ S75.911   Laceration of unspecified blood vessel at hip and thigh level, right leg

      ⑦ S75.912   Laceration of unspecified blood vessel at hip and thigh level, left leg

      ⑦ S75.919   Laceration of unspecified blood vessel at hip and thigh level, unspecified leg

    S75.99   Other specified injury of unspecified blood vessel at hip and thigh level

      ⑦ S75.991   Other specified injury of unspecified blood vessel at hip and thigh level, right leg

      ⑦ S75.992   Other specified injury of unspecified blood vessel at hip and thigh level, left leg

      ⑦ S75.999   Other specified injury of unspecified blood vessel at hip and thigh level, unspecified leg

S76   Injury of muscle, fascia and tendon at hip and thigh level

Code also any associated open wound (S71.-)

Excludes 2: injury of muscle, fascia and tendon at lower leg level (S86)

    sprain of joint and ligament of hip (S73.1)

The appropriate 7th character is to be added to each code from category S76

A - initial encounter

D - subsequent encounter

S - sequela

S76.0   Injury of muscle, fascia and tendon of hip

    S76.00   Unspecified injury of muscle, fascia and tendon of hip

      ⑦ S76.001   Unspecified injury of muscle, fascia and tendon of right hip

      ⑦ S76.002   Unspecified injury of muscle, fascia and tendon of left hip

      ⑦ S76.009   Unspecified injury of muscle, fascia and tendon of unspecified hip

    S76.01   Strain of muscle, fascia and tendon of hip

      ⑦ S76.011   Strain of muscle, fascia and tendon of right hip

      ⑦ S76.012   Strain of muscle, fascia and tendon of left hip

      ⑦ S76.019   Strain of muscle, fascia and tendon of unspecified hip

    S76.02   Laceration of muscle, fascia and tendon of hip

      ⑦ S76.021   Laceration of muscle, fascia and tendon of right hip

      ⑦ S76.022   Laceration of muscle, fascia and tendon of left hip

      ⑦ S76.029   Laceration of muscle, fascia and tendon of unspecified hip

    S76.09   Other specified injury of muscle, fascia and tendon of hip

      ⑦ S76.091   Other specified injury of muscle, fascia and tendon of right hip

      ⑦ S76.092   Other specified injury of muscle, fascia and tendon of left hip

      ⑦ S76.099   Other specified injury of muscle, fascia and tendon of unspecified hip

S76.1   Injury of quadriceps muscle, fascia and tendon

Injury of patellar ligament (tendon)

    S76.10   Unspecified injury of quadriceps muscle, fascia and tendon

      ⑦ S76.101   Unspecified injury of right quadriceps muscle, fascia and tendon

      ⑦ S76.102   Unspecified injury of left quadriceps muscle, fascia and tendon

      ⑦ S76.109   Unspecified injury of unspecified quadriceps muscle, fascia and tendon

    S76.11   Strain of quadriceps muscle, fascia and tendon

      ⑦ S76.111   Strain of right quadriceps muscle, fascia and tendon

      ⑦ S76.112   Strain of left quadriceps muscle, fascia and tendon

      ⑦ S76.119   Strain of unspecified quadriceps muscle, fascia and tendon

    S76.12   Laceration of quadriceps muscle, fascia and tendon

      ⑦ S76.121   Laceration of right quadriceps muscle, fascia and tendon

      ⑦ S76.122   Laceration of left quadriceps muscle, fascia and tendon

      ⑦ S76.129   Laceration of unspecified quadriceps muscle, fascia and tendon

    S76.19   Other specified injury of quadriceps muscle, fascia and tendon

      ⑦ S76.191   Other specified injury of right quadriceps muscle, fascia and tendon

      ⑦ S76.192   Other specified injury of left quadriceps muscle, fascia and tendon

      ⑦ S76.199   Other specified injury of unspecified quadriceps muscle, fascia and tendon

S76.2   Injury of adductor muscle, fascia and tendon of thigh

    S76.20   Unspecified injury of adductor muscle, fascia and tendon of thigh

⑦S76.201   Unspecified injury of adductor muscle, fascia and tendon of right thigh

⑦S76.202   Unspecified injury of adductor muscle, fascia and tendon of left thigh

⑦S76.209   Unspecified injury of adductor muscle, fascia and tendon of unspecified thigh

S76.21   Strain of adductor muscle, fascia and tendon of thigh

⑦S76.211   Strain of adductor muscle, fascia and tendon of right thigh

⑦S76.212   Strain of adductor muscle, fascia and tendon of left thigh

⑦S76.219   Strain of adductor muscle, fascia and tendon of unspecified thigh

S76.22   Laceration of adductor muscle, fascia and tendon of thigh

⑦S76.221   Laceration of adductor muscle, fascia and tendon of right thigh

⑦S76.222   Laceration of adductor muscle, fascia and tendon of left thigh

⑦S76.229   Laceration of adductor muscle, fascia and tendon of unspecified thigh

S76.29   Other injury of adductor muscle, fascia and tendon of thigh

⑦S76.291   Other injury of adductor muscle, fascia and tendon of right thigh

⑦S76.292   Other injury of adductor muscle, fascia and tendon of left thigh

⑦S76.299   Other injury of adductor muscle, fascia and tendon of unspecified thigh

S76.3   Injury of muscle, fascia and tendon of the posterior muscle group at thigh level

S76.30   Unspecified injury of muscle, fascia and tendon of the posterior muscle group at thigh level

⑦S76.301   Unspecified injury of muscle, fascia and tendon of the posterior muscle group at thigh level, right thigh

⑦S76.302   Unspecified injury of muscle, fascia and tendon of the posterior muscle group at thigh level, left thigh

⑦S76.309   Unspecified injury of muscle, fascia and tendon of the posterior muscle group at thigh level, unspecified thigh

S76.31   Strain of muscle, fascia and tendon of the posterior muscle group at thigh level

⑦S76.311   Strain of muscle, fascia and tendon of the posterior muscle group at thigh level, right thigh

⑦S76.312   Strain of muscle, fascia and tendon of the posterior muscle group at thigh level, left thigh

⑦S76.319   Strain of muscle, fascia and tendon of the posterior muscle group at thigh level, unspecified thigh

S76.32   Laceration of muscle, fascia and tendon of the posterior muscle group at thigh level

⑦S76.321   Laceration of muscle, fascia and tendon of the posterior muscle group at thigh level, right thigh

⑦S76.322   Laceration of muscle, fascia and tendon of the posterior muscle group at thigh level, left thigh

⑦S76.329   Laceration of muscle, fascia and tendon of the posterior muscle group at thigh level, unspecified thigh

S76.39   Other specified injury of muscle, fascia and tendon of the posterior muscle group at thigh level

⑦S76.391   Other specified injury of muscle, fascia and tendon of the posterior muscle group at thigh level, right thigh

⑦S76.392   Other specified injury of muscle, fascia and tendon of the posterior muscle group at thigh level, left thigh

⑦S76.399   Other specified injury of muscle, fascia and tendon of the posterior muscle group at thigh level, unspecified thigh

S76.8   Injury of other specified muscles, fascia and tendons at thigh level

S76.80   Unspecified injury of other specified muscles, fascia and tendons at thigh level

⑦S76.801   Unspecified injury of other specified muscles, fascia and tendons at thigh level, right thigh

⑦S76.802   Unspecified injury of other specified muscles, fascia and tendons at thigh level, left thigh

⑦S76.809   Unspecified injury of other specified muscles, fascia and tendons at thigh level, unspecified thigh

S76.81   Strain of other specified muscles, fascia and tendons at thigh level

⑦S76.811   Strain of other specified muscles, fascia and tendons at thigh level, right thigh

⑦S76.812   Strain of other specified muscles, fascia and tendons at thigh level, left thigh

⑦S76.819   Strain of other specified muscles, fascia and tendons at thigh level, unspecified thigh

S76.82   Laceration of other specified muscles, fascia and tendons at thigh level

⑦S76.821   Laceration of other specified muscles, fascia and tendons at thigh level, right thigh

⑦S76.822   Laceration of other specified muscles, fascia and tendons at thigh level, left thigh

⑦S76.829   Laceration of other specified muscles, fascia and tendons at thigh level, unspecified thigh

S76.89   Other injury of other specified muscles, fascia and tendons at thigh level

⑦**S76.891**   Other injury of other specified muscles, fascia and tendons at thigh level, right thigh

⑦**S76.892**   Other injury of other specified muscles, fascia and tendons at thigh level, left thigh

⑦**S76.899**   Other injury of other specified muscles, fascia and tendons at thigh level, unspecified thigh

S76.9   Injury of unspecified muscles, fascia and tendons at thigh level

S76.90   Unspecified injury of unspecified muscles, fascia and tendons at thigh level

⑦**S76.901**   Unspecified injury of unspecified muscles, fascia and tendons at thigh level, right thigh

⑦**S76.902**   Unspecified injury of unspecified muscles, fascia and tendons at thigh level, left thigh

⑦**S76.909**   Unspecified injury of unspecified muscles, fascia and tendons at thigh level, unspecified thigh

S76.91   Strain of unspecified muscles, fascia and tendons at thigh level

⑦**S76.911**   Strain of unspecified muscles, fascia and tendons at thigh level, right thigh

⑦**S76.912**   Strain of unspecified muscles, fascia and tendons at thigh level, left thigh

⑦**S76.919**   Strain of unspecified muscles, fascia and tendons at thigh level, unspecified thigh

S76.92   Laceration of unspecified muscles, fascia and tendons at thigh level

⑦**S76.921**   Laceration of unspecified muscles, fascia and tendons at thigh level, right thigh

⑦**S76.922**   Laceration of unspecified muscles, fascia and tendons at thigh level, left thigh

⑦**S76.929**   Laceration of unspecified muscles, fascia and tendons at thigh level, unspecified thigh

S76.99   Other specified injury of unspecified muscles, fascia and tendons at thigh level

⑦**S76.991**   Other specified injury of unspecified muscles, fascia and tendons at thigh level, right thigh

⑦**S76.992**   Other specified injury of unspecified muscles, fascia and tendons at thigh level, left thigh

⑦**S76.999**   Other specified injury of unspecified muscles, fascia and tendons at thigh level, unspecified thigh

S77   Crushing injury of hip and thigh

Use additional code(s) for all associated injuries

Excludes 2: crushing injury of ankle and foot (S97.-)

crushing injury of lower leg (S87.-)

The appropriate 7th character is to be added to each code from category S77

A - initial encounter

D - subsequent encounter

S û sequela

S77.0   Crushing injury of hip

⊗⑦**S77.00**   Crushing injury of unspecified hip

⊗⑦**S77.01**   Crushing injury of right hip

⊗⑦**S77.02**   Crushing injury of left hip

S77.1   Crushing injury of thigh

⊗⑦**S77.10**   Crushing injury of unspecified thigh

⊗⑦**S77.11**   Crushing injury of right thigh

⊗⑦**S77.12**   Crushing injury of left thigh

S77.2   Crushing injury of hip with thigh

⊗⑦**S77.20**   Crushing injury of unspecified hip with thigh

⊗⑦**S77.21**   Crushing injury of right hip with thigh

⊗⑦**S77.22**   Crushing injury of left hip with thigh

S78   Traumatic amputation of hip and thigh

An amputation not identified as partial or complete should be coded to complete

Excludes 1: traumatic amputation of knee (S88.0-)

The appropriate 7th character is to be added to each code from category S78

A - initial encounter

D - subsequent encounter

S - sequela

S78.0   Traumatic amputation at hip joint

S78.01   Complete traumatic amputation at hip joint

⑦**S78.011**   Complete traumatic amputation at right hip joint

⑦**S78.012**   Complete traumatic amputation at left hip joint

⑦**S78.019**   Complete traumatic amputation at unspecified hip joint

S78.02   Partial traumatic amputation at hip joint

⑦**S78.021**   Partial traumatic amputation at right hip joint

⑦**S78.022**   Partial traumatic amputation at left hip joint

⑦**S78.029**   Partial traumatic amputation at unspecified hip joint

S78.1   Traumatic amputation at level between hip and knee

Excludes 1: traumatic amputation of knee (S88.0-)

S78.11   Complete traumatic amputation at level between hip and knee

⑦**S78.111**   Complete traumatic amputation at level between right hip and knee

⑦**S78.112**   Complete traumatic amputation at level between left hip and knee

⑦**S78.119**   Complete traumatic amputation at level between unspecified hip and knee

S78.12   Partial traumatic amputation at level between hip and knee

⑦**S78.121**   Partial traumatic amputation at level between right hip and knee

⑦S78.122   Partial traumatic amputation at level between left hip and knee

⑦S78.129   Partial traumatic amputation at level between unspecified hip and knee

S78.9   Traumatic amputation of hip and thigh, level unspecified

    S78.91   Complete traumatic amputation of hip and thigh, level unspecified

        ⑦S78.911   Complete traumatic amputation of right hip and thigh, level unspecified

        ⑦S78.912   Complete traumatic amputation of left hip and thigh, level unspecified

        ⑦S78.919   Complete traumatic amputation of unspecified hip and thigh, level unspecified

    S78.92   Partial traumatic amputation of hip and thigh, level unspecified

        ⑦S78.921   Partial traumatic amputation of right hip and thigh, level unspecified

        ⑦S78.922   Partial traumatic amputation of left hip and thigh, level unspecified

        ⑦S78.929   Partial traumatic amputation of unspecified hip and thigh, level unspecified

S79   Other and unspecified injuries of hip and thigh

Note: A fracture not indicated as open or closed should be coded to closed

The appropriate 7th character is to be added to each code from subcategories S79.0 and S79.1

A - initial encounter for closed fracture

D - subsequent encounter for fracture with routine healing

G - subsequent encounter for fracture with delayed healing

K - subsequent encounter for fracture with nonunion

P - subsequent encounter for fracture with malunion

S - sequela

S79.0   Physeal fracture of upper end of femur

    Excludes 1: apophyseal fracture of upper end of femur (S72.13-)

    nontraumatic slipped upper femoral epiphysis (M93.0-)

    S79.00   Unspecified physeal fracture of upper end of femur

        ⑦S79.001   Unspecified physeal fracture of upper end of right femur

        ⑦S79.002   Unspecified physeal fracture of upper end of left femur

        ⑦S79.009   Unspecified physeal fracture of upper end of unspecified femur

    S79.01   Salter-Harris Type I physeal fracture of upper end of femur

    Acute on chronic slipped capital femoral epiphysis (traumatic)

    Acute slipped capital femoral epiphysis (traumatic)

    Capital femoral epiphyseal fracture

    Excludes 1: chronic slipped upper femoral epiphysis (nontraumatic) (M93.02-)

        ⑦S79.011   Salter-Harris Type I physeal fracture of upper end of right femur

        ⑦S79.012   Salter-Harris Type I physeal fracture of upper end of left femur

        ⑦S79.019   Salter-Harris Type I physeal fracture of upper end of unspecified femur

    S79.09   Other physeal fracture of upper end of femur

        ⑦S79.091   Other physeal fracture of upper end of right femur

        ⑦S79.092   Other physcal fracture of upper end of left femur

        ⑦S79.099   Other physeal fracture of upper end of unspecified femur

S79.1   Physeal fracture of lower end of femur

    S79.10   Unspecified physeal fracture of lower end of femur

        ⑦S79.101   Unspecified physeal fracture of lower end of right femur

        ⑦S79.102   Unspecified physeal fracture of lower end of left femur

        ⑦S79.109   Unspecified physeal fracture of lower end of unspecified femur

    S79.11   Salter-Harris Type I physeal fracture of lower end of femur

        ⑦S79.111   Salter-Harris Type I physeal fracture of lower end of right femur

        ⑦S79.112   Salter-Harris Type I physeal fracture of lower end of left femur

        ⑦S79.119   Salter-Harris Type I physeal fracture of lower end of unspecified femur

    S79.12   Salter-Harris Type II physeal fracture of lower end of femur

        ⑦S79.121   Salter-Harris Type II physeal fracture of lower end of right femur

        ⑦S79.122   Salter-Harris Type II physeal fracture of lower end of left femur

        ⑦S79.129   Salter-Harris Type II physeal fracture of lower end of unspecified femur

    S79.13   Salter-Harris Type III physeal fracture of lower end of femur

        ⑦S79.131   Salter-Harris Type III physeal fracture of lower end of right femur

        ⑦S79.132   Salter-Harris Type III physeal fracture of lower end of left femur

        ⑦S79.139   Salter-Harris Type III physeal fracture of lower end of unspecified femur

    S79.14   Salter-Harris Type IV physeal fracture of lower end of femur

        ⑦S79.141   Salter-Harris Type IV physeal fracture of lower end of right femur

        ⑦S79.142   Salter-Harris Type IV physeal fracture of lower end of left femur

        ⑦S79.149   Salter-Harris Type IV physeal fracture of lower end of unspecified femur

    S79.19   Other physeal fracture of lower end of femur

        ⑦S79.191   Other physeal fracture of lower end of right femur

        ⑦S79.192   Other physeal fracture of lower end of left femur

⑦S79.199　　Other physeal fracture of lower end of unspecified femur

S79.8　　Other specified injuries of hip and thigh

The appropriate 7th character is to be added to each code in subcategory S79.8

A - initial encounter

D - subsequent encounter

S - sequela

S79.81　　Other specified injuries of hip

⑦S79.811　　Other specified injuries of right hip

⑦S79.812　　Other specified injuries of left hip

⑦S79.819　　Other specified injuries of unspecified hip

S79.82　　Other specified injuries of thigh

⑦S79.821　　Other specified injuries of right thigh

⑦S79.822　　Other specified injuries of left thigh

⑦S79.829　　Other specified injuries of unspecified thigh

S79.9　　Unspecified injury of hip and thigh

The appropriate 7th character is to be added to each code in subcategory S79.9

A - initial encounter

D - subsequent encounter

S - sequela

S79.91　　Unspecified injury of hip

⑦S79.911　　Unspecified injury of right hip

⑦S79.912　　Unspecified injury of left hip

⑦S79.919　　Unspecified injury of unspecified hip

S79.92　　Unspecified injury of thigh

⑦S79.921　　Unspecified injury of right thigh

⑦S79.922　　Unspecified injury of left thigh

⑦S79.929　　Unspecified injury of unspecified thigh

INJURIES TO THE KNEE AND LOWER LEG (S80-S89)

Excludes 2:　　burns and corrosions (T20-T32)

frostbite (T33-T34)

injuries of ankle and foot, except fracture of ankle and malleolus (S90-S99)

insect bite or sting, venomous (T63.4)

S80　　Superficial injury of knee and lower leg

Excludes 2: superficial injury of ankle and foot (S90.-)

The appropriate 7th character is to be added to each code from category S80

A - initial encounter

D - subsequent encounter

S - sequela

S80.0　　Contusion of knee

⊗⑦S80.00　　Contusion of unspecified knee

⊗⑦S80.01　　Contusion of right knee

⊗⑦S80.02　　Contusion of left knee

S80.1　　Contusion of lower leg

⊗⑦S80.10　　Contusion of unspecified lower leg

⊗⑦S80.11　　Contusion of right lower leg

⊗⑦S80.12　　Contusion of left lower leg

S80.2　　Other superficial injuries of knee

S80.21　　Abrasion of knee

⑦S80.211　　Abrasion, right knee

⑦S80.212　　Abrasion, left knee

⑦S80.219　　Abrasion, unspecified knee

S80.22　　Blister (nonthermal) of knee

⑦S80.221　　Blister (nonthermal), right knee

⑦S80.222　　Blister (nonthermal), left knee

⑦S80.229　　Blister (nonthermal), unspecified knee

S80.24　　External constriction of knee

⑦S80.241　　External constriction, right knee

⑦S80.242　　External constriction, left knee

⑦S80.249　　External constriction, unspecified knee

S80.25　　Superficial foreign body of knee

Splinter in the knee

⑦S80.251　　Superficial foreign body, right knee

⑦S80.252　　Superficial foreign body, left knee

⑦S80.259　　Superficial foreign body, unspecified knee

S80.26　　Insect bite (nonvenomous) of knee

⑦S80.261　　Insect bite (nonvenomous), right knee

⑦S80.262　　Insect bite (nonvenomous), left knee

⑦S80.269　　Insect bite (nonvenomous), unspecified knee

S80.27　　Other superficial bite of knee

Excludes 1: open bite of knee (S81.05-)

⑦S80.271　　Other superficial bite of right knee

⑦S80.272　　Other superficial bite of left knee

⑦S80.279　　Other superficial bite of unspecified knee

S80.8　　Other superficial injuries of lower leg

S80.81　　Abrasion of lower leg

⑦S80.811　　Abrasion, right lower leg

⑦S80.812　　Abrasion, left lower leg

⑦S80.819　　Abrasion, unspecified lower leg

S80.82　　Blister (nonthermal) of lower leg

⑦S80.821　　Blister (nonthermal), right lower leg

⑦S80.822　　Blister (nonthermal), left lower leg

⑦S80.829　　Blister (nonthermal), unspecified lower leg

S80.84　　External constriction of lower leg

⑦S80.841　　External constriction, right lower leg

⑦S80.842　　External constriction, left lower leg

⑦S80.849　　External constriction, unspecified lower leg

S80.85　　Superficial foreign body of lower leg

Splinter in the lower leg

⑦S80.851　　Superficial foreign body, right lower leg

⑦S80.852　　Superficial foreign body, left lower leg

⑦S80.859　　Superficial foreign body, unspecified lower leg

S80.86　　Insect bite (nonvenomous) of lower leg

⑦ S80.861   Insect bite (nonvenomous), right lower leg

⑦ S80.862   Insect bite (nonvenomous), left lower leg

⑦ S80.869   Insect bite (nonvenomous), unspecified lower leg

S80.87   Other superficial bite of lower leg

> Excludes 1: open bite of lower leg (S81.85-)

⑦ S80.871   Other superficial bite, right lower leg

⑦ S80.872   Other superficial bite, left lower leg

⑦ S80.879   Other superficial bite, unspecified lower leg

S80.9   Unspecified superficial injury of knee and lower leg

S80.91   Unspecified superficial injury of knee

⑦ S80.911   Unspecified superficial injury of right knee

⑦ S80.912   Unspecified superficial injury of left knee

⑦ S80.919   Unspecified superficial injury of unspecified knee

S80.92   Unspecified superficial injury of lower leg

⑦ S80.921   Unspecified superficial injury of right lower leg

⑦ S80.922   Unspecified superficial injury of left lower leg

⑦ S80.929   Unspecified superficial injury of unspecified lower leg

S81   Open wound of knee and lower leg

Code also any associated wound infection

> Excludes 1: open fracture of knee and lower leg (S82.-)
> traumatic amputation of lower leg (S88.-)

> Excludes 2: open wound of ankle and foot (S91.-)

The appropriate 7th character is to be added to each code from category S81

A - initial encounter

D - subsequent encounter

S - sequela

S81.0   Open wound of knee

S81.00   Unspecified open wound of knee

⑦ S81.001   Unspecified open wound, right knee

⑦ S81.002   Unspecified open wound, left knee

⑦ S81.009   Unspecified open wound, unspecified knee

S81.01   Laceration without foreign body of knee

⑦ S81.011   Laceration without foreign body, right knee

⑦ S81.012   Laceration without foreign body, left knee

⑦ S81.019   Laceration without foreign body, unspecified knee

S81.02   Laceration with foreign body of knee

⑦ S81.021   Laceration with foreign body, right knee

⑦ S81.022   Laceration with foreign body, left knee

⑦ S81.029   Laceration with foreign body, unspecified knee

S81.03   Puncture wound without foreign body of knee

⑦ S81.031   Puncture wound without foreign body, right knee

⑦ S81.032   Puncture wound without foreign body, left knee

⑦ S81.039   Puncture wound without foreign body, unspecified knee

S81.04   Puncture wound with foreign body of knee

⑦ S81.041   Puncture wound with foreign body, right knee

⑦ S81.042   Puncture wound with foreign body, left knee

⑦ S81.049   Puncture wound with foreign body, unspecified knee

S81.05   Open bite of knee

Bite of knee NOS

> Excludes 1: superficial bite of knee (S80.27-)

⑦ S81.051   Open bite, right knee

⑦ S81.052   Open bite, left knee

⑦ S81.059   Open bite, unspecified knee

S81.8   Open wound of lower leg

S81.80   Unspecified open wound of lower leg

⑦ S81.801   Unspecified open wound, right lower leg

⑦ S81.802   Unspecified open wound, left lower leg

⑦ S81.809   Unspecified open wound, unspecified lower leg

S81.81   Laceration without foreign body of lower leg

⑦ S81.811   Laceration without foreign body, right lower leg

⑦ S81.812   Laceration without foreign body, left lower leg

⑦ S81.819   Laceration without foreign body, unspecified lower leg

S81.82   Laceration with foreign body of lower leg

⑦ S81.821   Laceration with foreign body, right lower leg

⑦ S81.822   Laceration with foreign body, left lower leg

⑦ S81.829   Laceration with foreign body, unspecified lower leg

S81.83   Puncture wound without foreign body of lower leg

⑦ S81.831   Puncture wound without foreign body, right lower leg

⑦ S81.832   Puncture wound without foreign body, left lower leg

⑦ S81.839   Puncture wound without foreign body, unspecified lower leg

S81.84   Puncture wound with foreign body of lower leg

⑦ S81.841   Puncture wound with foreign body, right lower leg

⑦ S81.842   Puncture wound with foreign body, left lower leg

⑦ S81.849   Puncture wound with foreign body, unspecified lower leg

S81.85   Open bite of lower leg

Bite of lower leg NOS

Excludes 1: superficial bite of lower leg
(S80.86-, S80.87-)

⑦**S81.851**   Open bite, right lower leg

⑦**S81.852**   Open bite, left lower leg

⑦**S81.859**   Open bite, unspecified lower leg

S82 Fracture of lower leg, including ankle

Note: A fracture not indicated as displaced or nondisplaced should be coded to displaced

A fracture not indicated as open or closed should be coded to closed

The open fracture designations are based on the Gustilo open fracture classification

Includes: fracture of malleolus

Excludes 1: traumatic amputation of lower leg (S88.-)

Excludes 2: fracture of foot, except ankle (S92.-)

periprosthetic fracture of prosthetic implant of knee (T84.042, T84.043)

The appropriate 7th character is to be added to all codes from category S82

A - initial encounter for closed fracture

B - initial encounter for open fracture type I or II initial encounter for open fracture NOS

C - initial encounter for open fracture type IIIA, IIIB, or IIIC

D - subsequent encounter for closed fracture with routine healing

E - subsequent encounter for open fracture type I or II with routine healing

F - subsequent encounter for open fracture type IIIA, IIIB, or IIIC with routine healing

G - subsequent encounter for closed fracture with delayed healing

H - subsequent encounter for open fracture type I or II with delayed healing

J - subsequent encounter for open fracture type IIIA, IIIB, or IIIC with delayed healing

K - subsequent encounter for closed fracture with nonunion

M - subsequent encounter for open fracture type I or II with nonunion

N - subsequent encounter for open fracture type IIIA, IIIB, or IIIC with nonunion

P - subsequent encounter for closed fracture with malunion

Q - subsequent encounter for open fracture type I or II with malunion

R - subsequent encounter for open fracture type IIIA, IIIB, or IIIC with malunion

S - sequela

S82.0 Fracture of patella

Knee cap

S82.00 Unspecified fracture of patella

⑦**S82.001**   Unspecified fracture of right patella

⑦**S82.002**   Unspecified fracture of left patella

⑦**S82.009**   Unspecified fracture of unspecified patella

S82.01 Osteochondral fracture of patella

⑦**S82.011**   Displaced osteochondral fracture of right patella

⑦**S82.012**   Displaced osteochondral fracture of left patella

⑦**S82.013**   Displaced osteochondral fracture of unspecified patella

⑦**S82.014**   Nondisplaced osteochondral fracture of right patella

⑦**S82.015**   Nondisplaced osteochondral fracture of left patella

⑦**S82.016**   Nondisplaced osteochondral fracture of unspecified patella

S82.02 Longitudinal fracture of patella

⑦**S82.021**   Displaced longitudinal fracture of right patella

⑦**S82.022**   Displaced longitudinal fracture of left patella

⑦**S82.023**   Displaced longitudinal fracture of unspecified patella

⑦**S82.024**   Nondisplaced longitudinal fracture of right patella

⑦**S82.025**   Nondisplaced longitudinal fracture of left patella

⑦**S82.026**   Nondisplaced longitudinal fracture of unspecified patella

S82.03 Transverse fracture of patella

⑦**S82.031**   Displaced transverse fracture of right patella

⑦**S82.032**   Displaced transverse fracture of left patella

⑦**S82.033**   Displaced transverse fracture of unspecified patella

⑦**S82.034**   Nondisplaced transverse fracture of right patella

⑦**S82.035**   Nondisplaced transverse fracture of left patella

⑦**S82.036**   Nondisplaced transverse fracture of unspecified patella

S82.04 Comminuted fracture of patella

⑦**S82.041**   Displaced comminuted fracture of right patella

⑦**S82.042**   Displaced comminuted fracture of left patella

⑦**S82.043**   Displaced comminuted fracture of unspecified patella

⑦**S82.044**   Nondisplaced comminuted fracture of right patella

⑦**S82.045**   Nondisplaced comminuted fracture of left patella

⑦**S82.046**   Nondisplaced comminuted fracture of unspecified patella

S82.09 Other fracture of patella

⑦**S82.091**   Other fracture of right patella

⑦**S82.092**   Other fracture of left patella

⑦**S82.099**   Other fracture of unspecified patella

S82.1 Fracture of upper end of tibia

Fracture of proximal end of tibia

Excludes 2: fracture of shaft of tibia (S82.2-)

physeal fracture of upper end of tibia (S89.0-)

S82.10 Unspecified fracture of upper end of tibia

⑦**S82.101**   Unspecified fracture of upper end of right tibia

⑦**S82.102**   Unspecified fracture of upper end of left tibia

● New code   ▲ Revised code   ⑦ 7ᵗʰ digit required   ⊗ Placeholder required

⑦ S82.109   Unspecified fracture of upper end of unspecified tibia

S82.11   Fracture of tibial spine

   ⑦ S82.111   Displaced fracture of right tibial spine

   ⑦ S82.112   Displaced fracture of left tibial spine

   ⑦ S82.113   Displaced fracture of unspecified tibial spine

   ⑦ S82.114   Nondisplaced fracture of right tibial spine

   ⑦ S82.115   Nondisplaced fracture of left tibial spine

   ⑦ S82.116   Nondisplaced fracture of unspecified tibial spine

S82.12   Fracture of lateral condyle of tibia

   ⑦ S82.121   Displaced fracture of lateral condyle of right tibia

   ⑦ S82.122   Displaced fracture of lateral condyle of left tibia

   ⑦ S82.123   Displaced fracture of lateral condyle of unspecified tibia

   ⑦ S82.124   Nondisplaced fracture of lateral condyle of right tibia

   ⑦ S82.125   Nondisplaced fracture of lateral condyle of left tibia

   ⑦ S82.126   Nondisplaced fracture of lateral condyle of unspecified tibia

S82.13   Fracture of medial condyle of tibia

   ⑦ S82.131   Displaced fracture of medial condyle of right tibia

   ⑦ S82.132   Displaced fracture of medial condyle of left tibia

   ⑦ S82.133   Displaced fracture of medial condyle of unspecified tibia

   ⑦ S82.134   Nondisplaced fracture of medial condyle of right tibia

   ⑦ S82.135   Nondisplaced fracture of medial condyle of left tibia

   ⑦ S82.136   Nondisplaced fracture of medial condyle of unspecified tibia

S82.14   Bicondylar fracture of tibia

   Fracture of tibial plateau NOS

   ⑦ S82.141   Displaced bicondylar fracture of right tibia

   ⑦ S82.142   Displaced bicondylar fracture of left tibia

   ⑦ S82.143   Displaced bicondylar fracture of unspecified tibia

   ⑦ S82.144   Nondisplaced bicondylar fracture of right tibia

   ⑦ S82.145   Nondisplaced bicondylar fracture of left tibia

   ⑦ S82.146   Nondisplaced bicondylar fracture of unspecified tibia

S82.15   Fracture of tibial tuberosity

   ⑦ S82.151   Displaced fracture of right tibial tuberosity

   ⑦ S82.152   Displaced fracture of left tibial tuberosity

   ⑦ S82.153   Displaced fracture of unspecified tibial tuberosity

   ⑦ S82.154   Nondisplaced fracture of right tibial tuberosity

   ⑦ S82.155   Nondisplaced fracture of left tibial tuberosity

   ⑦ S82.156   Nondisplaced fracture of unspecified tibial tuberosity

S82.16   Torus fracture of upper end of tibia

The appropriate 7th character is to be added to all codes in subcategory S82.16

A - initial encounter for closed fracture

D - subsequent encounter for fracture with routine healing

G - subsequent encounter for fracture with delayed healing

K - subsequent encounter for fracture with nonunion

P - subsequent encounter for fracture with malunion

S - sequela

   ⑦ S82.161   Torus fracture of upper end of right tibia

   ⑦ S82.162   Torus fracture of upper end of left tibia

   ⑦ S82.169   Torus fracture of upper end of unspecified tibia

S82.19   Other fracture of upper end of tibia

   ⑦ S82.191   Other fracture of upper end of right tibia

   ⑦ S82.192   Other fracture of upper end of left tibia

   ⑦ S82.199   Other fracture of upper end of unspecified tibia

S82.2   Fracture of shaft of tibia

S82.20   Unspecified fracture of shaft of tibia

   Fracture of tibia NOS

   ⑦ S82.201   Unspecified fracture of shaft of right tibia

   ⑦ S82.202   Unspecified fracture of shaft of left tibia

   ⑦ S82.209   Unspecified fracture of shaft of unspecified tibia

S82.22   Transverse fracture of shaft of tibia

   ⑦ S82.221   Displaced transverse fracture of shaft of right tibia

   ⑦ S82.222   Displaced transverse fracture of shaft of left tibia

   ⑦ S82.223   Displaced transverse fracture of shaft of unspecified tibia

   ⑦ S82.224   Nondisplaced transverse fracture of shaft of right tibia

   ⑦ S82.225   Nondisplaced transverse fracture of shaft of left tibia

   ⑦ S82.226   Nondisplaced transverse fracture of shaft of unspecified tibia

S82.23   Oblique fracture of shaft of tibia

   ⑦ S82.231   Displaced oblique fracture of shaft of right tibia

⑦S82.232   Displaced oblique fracture of shaft of left tibia

⑦S82.233   Displaced oblique fracture of shaft of unspecified tibia

⑦S82.234   Nondisplaced oblique fracture of shaft of right tibia

⑦S82.235   Nondisplaced oblique fracture of shaft of left tibia

⑦S82.236   Nondisplaced oblique fracture of shaft of unspecified tibia

S82.24   Spiral fracture of shaft of tibia
         Toddler fracture

⑦S82.241   Displaced spiral fracture of shaft of right tibia

⑦S82.242   Displaced spiral fracture of shaft of left tibia

⑦S82.243   Displaced spiral fracture of shaft of unspecified tibia

⑦S82.244   Nondisplaced spiral fracture of shaft of right tibia

⑦S82.245   Nondisplaced spiral fracture of shaft of left tibia

⑦S82.246   Nondisplaced spiral fracture of shaft of unspecified tibia

S82.25   Comminuted fracture of shaft of tibia

⑦S82.251   Displaced comminuted fracture of shaft of right tibia

⑦S82.252   Displaced comminuted fracture of shaft of left tibia

⑦S82.253   Displaced comminuted fracture of shaft of unspecified tibia

⑦S82.254   Nondisplaced comminuted fracture of shaft of right tibia

⑦S82.255   Nondisplaced comminuted fracture of shaft of left tibia

⑦S82.256   Nondisplaced comminuted fracture of shaft of unspecified tibia

S82.26   Segmental fracture of shaft of tibia

⑦S82.261   Displaced segmental fracture of shaft of right tibia

⑦S82.262   Displaced segmental fracture of shaft of left tibia

⑦S82.263   Displaced segmental fracture of shaft of unspecified tibia

⑦S82.264   Nondisplaced segmental fracture of shaft of right tibia

⑦S82.265   Nondisplaced segmental fracture of shaft of left tibia

⑦S82.266   Nondisplaced segmental fracture of shaft of unspecified tibia

S82.29   Other fracture of shaft of tibia

⑦S82.291   Other fracture of shaft of right tibia

⑦S82.292   Other fracture of shaft of left tibia

⑦S82.299   Other fracture of shaft of unspecified tibia

S82.3   Fracture of lower end of tibia
      Excludes 1: bimalleolar fracture of lower leg (S82.84-)
                  fracture of medial malleolus alone (S82.5-)

                  Maisonneuve's fracture (S82.86-)
                  pilon fracture of distal tibia (S82.87-)
                  trimalleolar fractures of lower leg (S82.85-)

S82.30   Unspecified fracture of lower end of tibia

⑦S82.301   Unspecified fracture of lower end of right tibia

⑦S82.302   Unspecified fracture of lower end of left tibia

⑦S82.309   Unspecified fracture of lower end of unspecified tibia

S82.31   Torus fracture of lower end of tibia

The appropriate 7th character is to be added to all codes in subcategory S82.31

A -   initial encounter for closed fracture

D -   subsequent encounter for fracture with routine healing

G -   subsequent encounter for fracture with delayed healing

K -   subsequent encounter for fracture with nonunion

P -   subsequent encounter for fracture with malunion

S -   sequela

⑦S82.311   Torus fracture of lower end of right tibia

⑦S82.312   Torus fracture of lower end of left tibia

⑦S82.319   Torus fracture of lower end of unspecified tibia

S82.39   Other fracture of lower end of tibia

⑦S82.391   Other fracture of lower end of right tibia

⑦S82.392   Other fracture of lower end of left tibia

⑦S82.399   Other fracture of lower end of unspecified tibia

S82.4   Fracture of shaft of fibula
      Excludes 2: fracture of lateral malleolus alone (S82.6-)

S82.40   Unspecified fracture of shaft of fibula

⑦S82.401   Unspecified fracture of shaft of right fibula

⑦S82.402   Unspecified fracture of shaft of left fibula

⑦S82.409   Unspecified fracture of shaft of unspecified fibula

S82.42   Transverse fracture of shaft of fibula

⑦S82.421   Displaced transverse fracture of shaft of right fibula

⑦S82.422   Displaced transverse fracture of shaft of left fibula

⑦S82.423   Displaced transverse fracture of shaft of unspecified fibula

⑦S82.424   Nondisplaced transverse fracture of shaft of right fibula

⑦S82.425   Nondisplaced transverse fracture of shaft of left fibula

⑦S82.426   Nondisplaced transverse fracture of shaft of unspecified fibula

S82.43   Oblique fracture of shaft of fibula

⑦S82.431 Displaced oblique fracture of shaft of right fibula

⑦S82.432 Displaced oblique fracture of shaft of left fibula

⑦S82.433 Displaced oblique fracture of shaft of unspecified fibula

⑦S82.434 Nondisplaced oblique fracture of shaft of right fibula

⑦S82.435 Nondisplaced oblique fracture of shaft of left fibula

⑦S82.436 Nondisplaced oblique fracture of shaft of unspecified fibula

S82.44 Spiral fracture of shaft of fibula

⑦S82.441 Displaced spiral fracture of shaft of right fibula

⑦S82.442 Displaced spiral fracture of shaft of left fibula

⑦S82.443 Displaced spiral fracture of shaft of unspecified fibula

⑦S82.444 Nondisplaced spiral fracture of shaft of right fibula

⑦S82.445 Nondisplaced spiral fracture of shaft of left fibula

⑦S82.446 Nondisplaced spiral fracture of shaft of unspecified fibula

S82.45 Comminuted fracture of shaft of fibula

⑦S82.451 Displaced comminuted fracture of shaft of right fibula

⑦S82.452 Displaced comminuted fracture of shaft of left fibula

⑦S82.453 Displaced comminuted fracture of shaft of unspecified fibula

⑦S82.454 Nondisplaced comminuted fracture of shaft of right fibula

⑦S82.455 Nondisplaced comminuted fracture of shaft of left fibula

⑦S82.456 Nondisplaced comminuted fracture of shaft of unspecified fibula

S82.46 Segmental fracture of shaft of fibula

⑦S82.461 Displaced segmental fracture of shaft of right fibula

⑦S82.462 Displaced segmental fracture of shaft of left fibula

⑦S82.463 Displaced segmental fracture of shaft of unspecified fibula

⑦S82.464 Nondisplaced segmental fracture of shaft of right fibula

⑦S82.465 Nondisplaced segmental fracture of shaft of left fibula

⑦S82.466 Nondisplaced segmental fracture of shaft of unspecified fibula

S82.49 Other fracture of shaft of fibula

⑦S82.491 Other fracture of shaft of right fibula

⑦S82.492 Other fracture of shaft of left fibula

⑦S82.499 Other fracture of shaft of unspecified fibula

S82.5 Fracture of medial malleolus

Excludes 1: pilon fracture of distal tibia (S82.87-)

Salter-Harris type III of lower end of tibia (S89.13-)

Salter-Harris type IV of lower end of tibia (S89.14-)

⊗⑦S82.51 Displaced fracture of medial malleolus of right tibia

⊗⑦S82.52 Displaced fracture of medial malleolus of left tibia

⊗⑦S82.53 Displaced fracture of medial malleolus of unspecified tibia

⊗⑦S82.54 Nondisplaced fracture of medial malleolus of right tibia

⊗⑦S82.55 Nondisplaced fracture of medial malleolus of left tibia

⊗⑦S82.56 Nondisplaced fracture of medial malleolus of unspecified tibia

S82.6 Fracture of lateral malleolus

Excludes 1: pilon fracture of distal tibia (S82.87-)

⊗⑦S82.61 Displaced fracture of lateral malleolus of right fibula

⊗⑦S82.62 Displaced fracture of lateral malleolus of left fibula

⊗⑦S82.63 Displaced fracture of lateral malleolus of unspecified fibula

⊗⑦S82.64 Nondisplaced fracture of lateral malleolus of right fibula

⊗⑦S82.65 Nondisplaced fracture of lateral malleolus of left fibula

⊗⑦S82.66 Nondisplaced fracture of lateral malleolus of unspecified fibula

S82.8 Other fractures of lower leg

S82.81 Torus fracture of upper end of fibula

The appropriate 7th character is to be added to all codes in subcategory S82.81

A - initial encounter for closed fracture

D - subsequent encounter for fracture with routine healing

G - subsequent encounter for fracture with delayed healing

K - subsequent encounter for fracture with nonunion

P - subsequent encounter for fracture with malunion

S - sequela

⑦S82.811 Torus fracture of upper end of right fibula

⑦S82.812 Torus fracture of upper end of left fibula

⑦S82.819 Torus fracture of upper end of unspecified fibula

S82.82 Torus fracture of lower end of fibula

The appropriate 7th character is to be added to all codes in subcategory S82.82

A - initial encounter for closed fracture

D - subsequent encounter for fracture with routine healing

G - subsequent encounter for fracture with delayed healing

K - subsequent encounter for fracture with nonunion

P - subsequent encounter for fracture with malunion

S - sequela

⑦ S82.821 Torus fracture of lower end of right fibula

⑦ S82.822 Torus fracture of lower end of left fibula

⑦ S82.829 Torus fracture of lower end of unspecified fibula

S82.83 Other fracture of upper and lower end of fibula

⑦ S82.831 Other fracture of upper and lower end of right fibula

⑦ S82.832 Other fracture of upper and lower end of left fibula

⑦ S82.839 Other fracture of upper and lower end of unspecified fibula

S82.84 Bimalleolar fracture of lower leg

⑦ S82.841 Displaced bimalleolar fracture of right lower leg

⑦ S82.842 Displaced bimalleolar fracture of left lower leg

⑦ S82.843 Displaced bimalleolar fracture of unspecified lower leg

⑦ S82.844 Nondisplaced bimalleolar fracture of right lower leg

⑦ S82.845 Nondisplaced bimalleolar fracture of left lower leg

⑦ S82.846 Nondisplaced bimalleolar fracture of unspecified lower leg

S82.85 Trimalleolar fracture of lower leg

⑦ S82.851 Displaced trimalleolar fracture of right lower leg

⑦ S82.852 Displaced trimalleolar fracture of left lower leg

⑦ S82.853 Displaced trimalleolar fracture of unspecified lower leg

⑦ S82.854 Nondisplaced trimalleolar fracture of right lower leg

⑦ S82.855 Nondisplaced trimalleolar fracture of left lower leg

⑦ S82.856 Nondisplaced trimalleolar fracture of unspecified lower leg

S82.86 Maisonneuve's fracture

⑦ S82.861 Displaced Maisonneuve's fracture of right leg

⑦ S82.862 Displaced Maisonneuve's fracture of left leg

⑦ S82.863 Displaced Maisonneuve's fracture of unspecified leg

⑦ S82.864 Nondisplaced Maisonneuve's fracture of right leg

⑦ S82.865 Nondisplaced Maisonneuve's fracture of left leg

⑦ S82.866 Nondisplaced Maisonneuve's fracture of unspecified leg

S82.87 Pilon fracture of tibia

⑦ S82.871 Displaced pilon fracture of right tibia

⑦ S82.872 Displaced pilon fracture of left tibia

⑦ S82.873 Displaced pilon fracture of unspecified tibia

⑦ S82.874 Nondisplaced pilon fracture of right tibia

⑦ S82.875 Nondisplaced pilon fracture of left tibia

⑦ S82.876 Nondisplaced pilon fracture of unspecified tibia

S82.89 Other fractures of lower leg
Fracture of ankle NOS

⑦ S82.891 Other fracture of right lower leg

⑦ S82.892 Other fracture of left lower leg

⑦ S82.899 Other fracture of unspecified lower leg

S82.9 Unspecified fracture of lower leg

⊗⑦ S82.90 Unspecified fracture of unspecified lower leg

⊗⑦ S82.91 Unspecified fracture of right lower leg

⊗⑦ S82.92 Unspecified fracture of left lower leg

S83 Dislocation and sprain of joints and ligaments of knee

Includes: avulsion of joint or ligament of knee

laceration of cartilage, joint or ligament of knee

sprain of cartilage, joint or ligament of knee

traumatic hemarthrosis of joint or ligament of knee

traumatic rupture of joint or ligament of knee

traumatic subluxation of joint or ligament of knee

traumatic tear of joint or ligament of knee

Code also any associated open wound

Excludes 1: derangement of patella (M22.0-M22.3)

injury of patellar ligament (tendon) (S76.1-)

internal derangement of knee (M23.-)

old dislocation of knee (M24.36)

pathological dislocation of knee (M24.36)

recurrent dislocation of knee (M22.0)

Excludes 2: strain of muscle, fascia and tendon of lower leg (S86.-)

The appropriate 7th character is to be added to each code from category S83

A - initial encounter

D - subsequent encounter

S - sequela

S83.0 Subluxation and dislocation of patella

S83.00 Unspecified subluxation and dislocation of patella

⑦ S83.001 Unspecified subluxation of right patella

⑦ S83.002 Unspecified subluxation of left patella

⑦ S83.003 Unspecified subluxation of unspecified patella

⑦ S83.004 Unspecified dislocation of right patella

⑦ S83.005 Unspecified dislocation of left patella

⑦ S83.006 Unspecified dislocation of unspecified patella

S83.01 Lateral subluxation and dislocation of patella

⑦ S83.011   Lateral subluxation of right patella

⑦ S83.012   Lateral subluxation of left patella

⑦ S83.013   Lateral subluxation of unspecified patella

⑦ S83.014   Lateral dislocation of right patella

⑦ S83.015   Lateral dislocation of left patella

⑦ S83.016   Lateral dislocation of unspecified patella

S83.09   Other subluxation and dislocation of patella

    ⑦ S83.091   Other subluxation of right patella

    ⑦ S83.092   Other subluxation of left patella

    ⑦ S83.093   Other subluxation of unspecified patella

    ⑦ S83.094   Other dislocation of right patella

    ⑦ S83.095   Other dislocation of left patella

    ⑦ S83.096   Other dislocation of unspecified patella

S83.1   Subluxation and dislocation of knee

    Excludes 2: instability of knee prosthesis (T84.022, T84.023)

S83.10   Unspecified subluxation and dislocation of knee

    ⑦ S83.101   Unspecified subluxation of right knee

    ⑦ S83.102   Unspecified subluxation of left knee

    ⑦ S83.103   Unspecified subluxation of unspecified knee

    ⑦ S83.104   Unspecified dislocation of right knee

    ⑦ S83.105   Unspecified dislocation of left knee

    ⑦ S83.106   Unspecified dislocation of unspecified knee

S83.11   Anterior subluxation and dislocation of proximal end of tibia

    Posterior subluxation and dislocation of distal end of femur

    ⑦ S83.111   Anterior subluxation of proximal end of tibia, right knee

    ⑦ S83.112   Anterior subluxation of proximal end of tibia, left knee

    ⑦ S83.113   Anterior subluxation of proximal end of tibia, unspecified knee

    ⑦ S83.114   Anterior dislocation of proximal end of tibia, right knee

    ⑦ S83.115   Anterior dislocation of proximal end of tibia, left knee

    ⑦ S83.116   Anterior dislocation of proximal end of tibia, unspecified knee

S83.12   Posterior subluxation and dislocation of proximal end of tibia

    Anterior dislocation of distal end of femur

    ⑦ S83.121   Posterior subluxation of proximal end of tibia, right knee

    ⑦ S83.122   Posterior subluxation of proximal end of tibia, left knee

    ⑦ S83.123   Posterior subluxation of proximal end of tibia, unspecified knee

⑦ S83.124   Posterior dislocation of proximal end of tibia, right knee

⑦ S83.125   Posterior dislocation of proximal end of tibia, left knee

⑦ S83.126   Posterior dislocation of proximal end of tibia, unspecified knee

S83.13   Medial subluxation and dislocation of proximal end of tibia

    ⑦ S83.131   Medial subluxation of proximal end of tibia, right knee

    ⑦ S83.132   Medial subluxation of proximal end of tibia, left knee

    ⑦ S83.133   Medial subluxation of proximal end of tibia, unspecified knee

    ⑦ S83.134   Medial dislocation of proximal end of tibia, right knee

    ⑦ S83.135   Medial dislocation of proximal end of tibia, left knee

    ⑦ S83.136   Medial dislocation of proximal end of tibia, unspecified knee

S83.14   Lateral subluxation and dislocation of proximal end of tibia

    ⑦ S83.141   Lateral subluxation of proximal end of tibia, right knee

    ⑦ S83.142   Lateral subluxation of proximal end of tibia, left knee

    ⑦ S83.143   Lateral subluxation of proximal end of tibia, unspecified knee

    ⑦ S83.144   Lateral dislocation of proximal end of tibia, right knee

    ⑦ S83.145   Lateral dislocation of proximal end of tibia, left knee

    ⑦ S83.146   Lateral dislocation of proximal end of tibia, unspecified knee

S83.19   Other subluxation and dislocation of knee

    ⑦ S83.191   Other subluxation of right knee

    ⑦ S83.192   Other subluxation of left knee

    ⑦ S83.193   Other subluxation of unspecified knee

    ⑦ S83.194   Other dislocation of right knee

    ⑦ S83.195   Other dislocation of left knee

    ⑦ S83.196   Other dislocation of unspecified knee

S83.2   Tear of meniscus, current injury

    Excludes 1: old bucket-handle tear (M23.2)

S83.20   Tear of unspecified meniscus, current injury

    Tear of meniscus of knee NOS

    ⑦ S83.200   Bucket-handle tear of unspecified meniscus, current injury, right knee

    ⑦ S83.201   Bucket-handle tear of unspecified meniscus, current injury, left knee

    ⑦ S83.202   Bucket-handle tear of unspecified meniscus, current injury, unspecified knee

    ⑦ S83.203   Other tear of unspecified meniscus, current injury, right knee

    ⑦ S83.204   Other tear of unspecified meniscus, current injury, left knee

⑦S83.205 Other tear of unspecified meniscus, current injury, unspecified knee

⑦S83.206 Unspecified tear of unspecified meniscus, current injury, right knee

⑦S83.207 Unspecified tear of unspecified meniscus, current injury, left knee

⑦S83.209 Unspecified tear of unspecified meniscus, current injury, unspecified knee

S83.21 Bucket-handle tear of medial meniscus, current injury

  ⑦S83.211 Bucket-handle tear of medial meniscus, current injury, right knee

  ⑦S83.212 Bucket-handle tear of medial meniscus, current injury, left knee

  ⑦S83.219 Bucket-handle tear of medial meniscus, current injury, unspecified knee

S83.22 Peripheral tear of medial meniscus, current injury

  ⑦S83.221 Peripheral tear of medial meniscus, current injury, right knee

  ⑦S83.222 Peripheral tear of medial meniscus, current injury, left knee

  ⑦S83.229 Peripheral tear of medial meniscus, current injury, unspecified knee

S83.23 Complex tear of medial meniscus, current injury

  ⑦S83.231 Complex tear of medial meniscus, current injury, right knee

  ⑦S83.232 Complex tear of medial meniscus, current injury, left knee

  ⑦S83.239 Complex tear of medial meniscus, current injury, unspecified knee

S83.24 Other tear of medial meniscus, current injury

  ⑦S83.241 Other tear of medial meniscus, current injury, right knee

  ⑦S83.242 Other tear of medial meniscus, current injury, left knee

  ⑦S83.249 Other tear of medial meniscus, current injury, unspecified knee

S83.25 Bucket-handle tear of lateral meniscus, current injury

  ⑦S83.251 Bucket-handle tear of lateral meniscus, current injury, right knee

  ⑦S83.252 Bucket-handle tear of lateral meniscus, current injury, left knee

  ⑦S83.259 Bucket-handle tear of lateral meniscus, current injury, unspecified knee

S83.26 Peripheral tear of lateral meniscus, current injury

  ⑦S83.261 Peripheral tear of lateral meniscus, current injury, right knee

  ⑦S83.262 Peripheral tear of lateral meniscus, current injury, left knee

  ⑦S83.269 Peripheral tear of lateral meniscus, current injury, unspecified knee

S83.27 Complex tear of lateral meniscus, current injury

  ⑦S83.271 Complex tear of lateral meniscus, current injury, right knee

⑦S83.272 Complex tear of lateral meniscus, current injury, left knee

⑦S83.279 Complex tear of lateral meniscus, current injury, unspecified knee

S83.28 Other tear of lateral meniscus, current injury

  ⑦S83.281 Other tear of lateral meniscus, current injury, right knee

  ⑦S83.282 Other tear of lateral meniscus, current injury, left knee

  ⑦S83.289 Other tear of lateral meniscus, current injury, unspecified knee

S83.3 Tear of articular cartilage of knee, current

  ⊗⑦S83.30 Tear of articular cartilage of unspecified knee, current

  ⊗⑦S83.31 Tear of articular cartilage of right knee, current

  ⊗⑦S83.32 Tear of articular cartilage of left knee, current

S83.4 Sprain of collateral ligament of knee

  S83.40 Sprain of unspecified collateral ligament of knee

    ⑦S83.401 Sprain of unspecified collateral ligament of right knee

    ⑦S83.402 Sprain of unspecified collateral ligament of left knee

    ⑦S83.409 Sprain of unspecified collateral ligament of unspecified knee

  S83.41 Sprain of medial collateral ligament of knee

  Sprain of tibial collateral ligament

    ⑦S83.411 Sprain of medial collateral ligament of right knee

    ⑦S83.412 Sprain of medial collateral ligament of left knee

    ⑦S83.419 Sprain of medial collateral ligament of unspecified knee

  S83.42 Sprain of lateral collateral ligament of knee

  Sprain of fibular collateral ligament

    ⑦S83.421 Sprain of lateral collateral ligament of right knee

    ⑦S83.422 Sprain of lateral collateral ligament of left knee

    ⑦S83.429 Sprain of lateral collateral ligament of unspecified knee

S83.5 Sprain of cruciate ligament of knee

  S83.50 Sprain of unspecified cruciate ligament of knee

    ⑦S83.501 Sprain of unspecified cruciate ligament of right knee

    ⑦S83.502 Sprain of unspecified cruciate ligament of left knee

    ⑦S83.509 Sprain of unspecified cruciate ligament of unspecified knee

  S83.51 Sprain of anterior cruciate ligament of knee

    ⑦S83.511 Sprain of anterior cruciate ligament of right knee

    ⑦S83.512 Sprain of anterior cruciate ligament of left knee

    ⑦S83.519 Sprain of anterior cruciate ligament of unspecified knee

  S83.52 Sprain of posterior cruciate ligament of knee

    ⑦S83.521 Sprain of posterior cruciate ligament of right knee

⑦**S83.522**   Sprain of posterior cruciate ligament of left knee

⑦**S83.529**   Sprain of posterior cruciate ligament of unspecified knee

S83.6   Sprain of the superior tibiofibular joint and ligament

⊗⑦**S83.60**   Sprain of the superior tibiofibular joint and ligament, unspecified knee

⊗⑦**S83.61**   Sprain of the superior tibiofibular joint and ligament, right knee

⊗⑦**S83.62**   Sprain of the superior tibiofibular joint and ligament, left knee

S83.8   Sprain of other specified parts of knee

S83.8X   Sprain of other specified parts of knee

⑦**S83.8X1**   Sprain of other specified parts of right knee

⑦**S83.8X2**   Sprain of other specified parts of left knee

⑦**S83.8X9**   Sprain of other specified parts of unspecified knee

S83.9   Sprain of unspecified site of knee

⊗⑦**S83.90**   Sprain of unspecified site of unspecified knee

⊗⑦**S83.91**   Sprain of unspecified site of right knee

⊗⑦**S83.92**   Sprain of unspecified site of left knee

S84   Injury of nerves at lower leg level

Code also any associated open wound (S81.-)

Excludes 2: injury of nerves at ankle and foot level (S94.-)

The appropriate 7th character is to be added to each code from category S84

A - initial encounter

D - subsequent encounter

S - sequela

S84.0   Injury of tibial nerve at lower leg level

⊗⑦**S84.00**   Injury of tibial nerve at lower leg level, unspecified leg

⊗⑦**S84.01**   Injury of tibial nerve at lower leg level, right leg

⊗⑦**S84.02**   Injury of tibial nerve at lower leg level, left leg

S84.1   Injury of peroneal nerve at lower leg level

⊗⑦**S84.10**   Injury of peroneal nerve at lower leg level, unspecified leg

⊗⑦**S84.11**   Injury of peroneal nerve at lower leg level, right leg

⊗⑦**S84.12**   Injury of peroneal nerve at lower leg level, left leg

S84.2   Injury of cutaneous sensory nerve at lower leg level

⊗⑦**S84.20**   Injury of cutaneous sensory nerve at lower leg level, unspecified leg

⊗⑦**S84.21**   Injury of cutaneous sensory nerve at lower leg level, right leg

⊗⑦**S84.22**   Injury of cutaneous sensory nerve at lower leg level, left leg

S84.8   Injury of other nerves at lower leg level

S84.80   Injury of other nerves at lower leg level

⑦**S84.801**   Injury of other nerves at lower leg level, right leg

⑦**S84.802**   Injury of other nerves at lower leg level, left leg

⑦**S84.809**   Injury of other nerves at lower leg level, unspecified leg

S84.9   Injury of unspecified nerve at lower leg level

⊗⑦**S84.90**   Injury of unspecified nerve at lower leg level, unspecified leg

⊗⑦**S84.91**   Injury of unspecified nerve at lower leg level, right leg

⊗⑦**S84.92**   Injury of unspecified nerve at lower leg level, left leg

S85   Injury of blood vessels at lower leg level

Code also any associated open wound (S81.-)

Excludes 2: injury of blood vessels at ankle and foot level (S95.-)

The appropriate 7th character is to be added to each code from category S85

A - initial encounter

D - subsequent encounter

S - sequela

S85.0   Injury of popliteal artery

S85.00   Unspecified injury of popliteal artery

⑦**S85.001**   Unspecified injury of popliteal artery, right leg

⑦**S85.002**   Unspecified injury of popliteal artery, left leg

⑦**S85.009**   Unspecified injury of popliteal artery, unspecified leg

S85.01   Laceration of popliteal artery

⑦**S85.011**   Laceration of popliteal artery, right leg

⑦**S85.012**   Laceration of popliteal artery, left leg

⑦**S85.019**   Laceration of popliteal artery, unspecified leg

S85.09   Other specified injury of popliteal artery

⑦**S85.091**   Other specified injury of popliteal artery, right leg

⑦**S85.092**   Other specified injury of popliteal artery, left leg

⑦**S85.099**   Other specified injury of popliteal artery, unspecified leg

S85.1   Injury of tibial artery

S85.10   Unspecified injury of unspecified tibial artery

Injury of tibial artery NOS

⑦**S85.101**   Unspecified injury of unspecified tibial artery, right leg

⑦**S85.102**   Unspecified injury of unspecified tibial artery, left leg

⑦**S85.109**   Unspecified injury of unspecified tibial artery, unspecified leg

S85.11   Laceration of unspecified tibial artery

⑦**S85.111**   Laceration of unspecified tibial artery, right leg

⑦**S85.112**   Laceration of unspecified tibial artery, left leg

⑦**S85.119**   Laceration of unspecified tibial artery, unspecified leg

S85.12   Other specified injury of unspecified tibial artery

⑦**S85.121**   Other specified injury of unspecified tibial artery, right leg

⑦**S85.122**   Other specified injury of unspecified tibial artery, left leg

⑦**S85.129**   Other specified injury of unspecified tibial artery, unspecified leg

S85.13　Unspecified injury of anterior tibial artery
   ⑦ S85.131　Unspecified injury of anterior tibial artery, right leg
   ⑦ S85.132　Unspecified injury of anterior tibial artery, left leg
   ⑦ S85.139　Unspecified injury of anterior tibial artery, unspecified leg

S85.14　Laceration of anterior tibial artery
   ⑦ S85.141　Laceration of anterior tibial artery, right leg
   ⑦ S85.142　Laceration of anterior tibial artery, left leg
   ⑦ S85.149　Laceration of anterior tibial artery, unspecified leg

S85.15　Other specified injury of anterior tibial artery
   ⑦ S85.151　Other specified injury of anterior tibial artery, right leg
   ⑦ S85.152　Other specified injury of anterior tibial artery, left leg
   ⑦ S85.159　Other specified injury of anterior tibial artery, unspecified leg

S85.16　Unspecified injury of posterior tibial artery
   ⑦ S85.161　Unspecified injury of posterior tibial artery, right leg
   ⑦ S85.162　Unspecified injury of posterior tibial artery, left leg
   ⑦ S85.169　Unspecified injury of posterior tibial artery, unspecified leg

S85.17　Laceration of posterior tibial artery
   ⑦ S85.171　Laceration of posterior tibial artery, right leg
   ⑦ S85.172　Laceration of posterior tibial artery, left leg
   ⑦ S85.179　Laceration of posterior tibial artery, unspecified leg

S85.18　Other specified injury of posterior tibial artery
   ⑦ S85.181　Other specified injury of posterior tibial artery, right leg
   ⑦ S85.182　Other specified injury of posterior tibial artery, left leg
   ⑦ S85.189　Other specified injury of posterior tibial artery, unspecified leg

S85.2　Injury of peroneal artery
  S85.20　Unspecified injury of peroneal artery
   ⑦ S85.201　Unspecified injury of peroneal artery, right leg
   ⑦ S85.202　Unspecified injury of peroneal artery, left leg
   ⑦ S85.209　Unspecified injury of peroneal artery, unspecified leg

  S85.21　Laceration of peroneal artery
   ⑦ S85.211　Laceration of peroneal artery, right leg
   ⑦ S85.212　Laceration of peroneal artery, left leg
   ⑦ S85.219　Laceration of peroneal artery, unspecified leg

  S85.29　Other specified injury of peroneal artery
   ⑦ S85.291　Other specified injury of peroneal artery, right leg
   ⑦ S85.292　Other specified injury of peroneal artery, left leg
   ⑦ S85.299　Other specified injury of peroneal artery, unspecified leg

S85.3　Injury of greater saphenous vein at lower leg level
Injury of greater saphenous vein NOS
Injury of saphenous vein NOS
  S85.30　Unspecified injury of greater saphenous vein at lower leg level
   ⑦ S85.301　Unspecified injury of greater saphenous vein at lower leg level, right leg
   ⑦ S85.302　Unspecified injury of greater saphenous vein at lower leg level, left leg
   ⑦ S85.309　Unspecified injury of greater saphenous vein at lower leg level, unspecified leg

  S85.31　Laceration of greater saphenous vein at lower leg level
   ⑦ S85.311　Laceration of greater saphenous vein at lower leg level, right leg
   ⑦ S85.312　Laceration of greater saphenous vein at lower leg level, left leg
   ⑦ S85.319　Laceration of greater saphenous vein at lower leg level, unspecified leg

  S85.39　Other specified injury of greater saphenous vein at lower leg level
   ⑦ S85.391　Other specified injury of greater saphenous vein at lower leg level, right leg
   ⑦ S85.392　Other specified injury of greater saphenous vein at lower leg level, left leg
   ⑦ S85.399　Other specified injury of greater saphenous vein at lower leg level, unspecified leg

S85.4　Injury of lesser saphenous vein at lower leg level
  S85.40　Unspecified injury of lesser saphenous vein at lower leg level
   ⑦ S85.401　Unspecified injury of lesser saphenous vein at lower leg level, right leg
   ⑦ S85.402　Unspecified injury of lesser saphenous vein at lower leg level, left leg
   ⑦ S85.409　Unspecified injury of lesser saphenous vein at lower leg level, unspecified leg

  S85.41　Laceration of lesser saphenous vein at lower leg level
   ⑦ S85.411　Laceration of lesser saphenous vein at lower leg level, right leg
   ⑦ S85.412　Laceration of lesser saphenous vein at lower leg level, left leg
   ⑦ S85.419　Laceration of lesser saphenous vein at lower leg level, unspecified leg

S85.49　Other specified injury of lesser saphenous vein at lower leg level

⑦S85.491　Other specified injury of lesser saphenous vein at lower leg level, right leg

⑦S85.492　Other specified injury of lesser saphenous vein at lower leg level, left leg

⑦S85.499　Other specified injury of lesser saphenous vein at lower leg level, unspecified leg

S85.5　Injury of popliteal vein

S85.50　Unspecified injury of popliteal vein

⑦S85.501　Unspecified injury of popliteal vein, right leg

⑦S85.502　Unspecified injury of popliteal vein, left leg

⑦S85.509　Unspecified injury of popliteal vein, unspecified leg

S85.51　Laceration of popliteal vein

⑦S85.511　Laceration of popliteal vein, right leg

⑦S85.512　Laceration of popliteal vein, left leg

⑦S85.519　Laceration of popliteal vein, unspecified leg

S85.59　Other specified injury of popliteal vein

⑦S85.591　Other specified injury of popliteal vein, right leg

⑦S85.592　Other specified injury of popliteal vein, left leg

⑦S85.599　Other specified injury of popliteal vein, unspecified leg

S85.8　Injury of other blood vessels at lower leg level

S85.80　Unspecified injury of other blood vessels at lower leg level

⑦S85.801　Unspecified injury of other blood vessels at lower leg level, right leg

⑦S85.802　Unspecified injury of other blood vessels at lower leg level, left leg

⑦S85.809　Unspecified injury of other blood vessels at lower leg level, unspecified leg

S85.81　Laceration of other blood vessels at lower leg level

⑦S85.811　Laceration of other blood vessels at lower leg level, right leg

⑦S85.812　Laceration of other blood vessels at lower leg level, left leg

⑦S85.819　Laceration of other blood vessels at lower leg level, unspecified leg

S85.89　Other specified injury of other blood vessels at lower leg level

⑦S85.891　Other specified injury of other blood vessels at lower leg level, right leg

⑦S85.892　Other specified injury of other blood vessels at lower leg level, left leg

⑦S85.899　Other specified injury of other blood vessels at lower leg level, unspecified leg

S85.9　Injury of unspecified blood vessel at lower leg level

S85.90　Unspecified injury of unspecified blood vessel at lower leg level

⑦S85.901　Unspecified injury of unspecified blood vessel at lower leg level, right leg

⑦S85.902　Unspecified injury of unspecified blood vessel at lower leg level, left leg

⑦S85.909　Unspecified injury of unspecified blood vessel at lower leg level, unspecified leg

S85.91　Laceration of unspecified blood vessel at lower leg level

⑦S85.911　Laceration of unspecified blood vessel at lower leg level, right leg

⑦S85.912　Laceration of unspecified blood vessel at lower leg level, left leg

⑦S85.919　Laceration of unspecified blood vessel at lower leg level, unspecified leg

S85.99　Other specified injury of unspecified blood vessel at lower leg level

⑦S85.991　Other specified injury of unspecified blood vessel at lower leg level, right leg

⑦S85.992　Other specified injury of unspecified blood vessel at lower leg level, left leg

⑦S85.999　Other specified injury of unspecified blood vessel at lower leg level, unspecified leg

S86　Injury of muscle, fascia and tendon at lower leg level

Code also any associated open wound (S81.-)

Excludes 2: injury of muscle, fascia and tendon at ankle (S96.-)

injury of patellar ligament (tendon) (S76.1-)

sprain of joints and ligaments of knee (S83.-)

The appropriate 7th character is to be added to each code from category S86

A - initial encounter

D - subsequent encounter

S - sequela

S86.0　Injury of Achilles tendon

S86.00　Unspecified injury of Achilles tendon

⑦S86.001　Unspecified injury of right Achilles tendon

⑦S86.002　Unspecified injury of left Achilles tendon

⑦S86.009　Unspecified injury of unspecified Achilles tendon

S86.01　Strain of Achilles tendon

⑦S86.011　Strain of right Achilles tendon

⑦S86.012　Strain of left Achilles tendon

⑦S86.019　Strain of unspecified Achilles tendon

S86.02　Laceration of Achilles tendon

⑦S86.021　Laceration of right Achilles tendon

⑦S86.022　Laceration of left Achilles tendon

⑦S86.029　Laceration of unspecified Achilles tendon

S86.09　Other specified injury of Achilles tendon

---

⑦ **S86.091** Other specified injury of right Achilles tendon

⑦ **S86.092** Other specified injury of left Achilles tendon

⑦ **S86.099** Other specified injury of unspecified Achilles tendon

S86.1 Injury of other muscle(s) and tendon(s) of posterior muscle group at lower leg level

  S86.10 Unspecified injury of other muscle(s) and tendon(s) of posterior muscle group at lower leg level

    ⑦ **S86.101** Unspecified injury of other muscle(s) and tendon(s) of posterior muscle group at lower leg level, right leg

    ⑦ **S86.102** Unspecified injury of other muscle(s) and tendon(s) of posterior muscle group at lower leg level, left leg

    ⑦ **S86.109** Unspecified injury of other muscle(s) and tendon(s) of posterior muscle group at lower leg level, unspecified leg

  S86.11 Strain of other muscle(s) and tendon(s) of posterior muscle group at lower leg level

    ⑦ **S86.111** Strain of other muscle(s) and tendon(s) of posterior muscle group at lower leg level, right leg

    ⑦ **S86.112** Strain of other muscle(s) and tendon(s) of posterior muscle group at lower leg level, left leg

    ⑦ **S86.119** Strain of other muscle(s) and tendon(s) of posterior muscle group at lower leg level, unspecified leg

  S86.12 Laceration of other muscle(s) and tendon(s) of posterior muscle group at lower leg level

    ⑦ **S86.121** Laceration of other muscle(s) and tendon(s) of posterior muscle group at lower leg level, right leg

    ⑦ **S86.122** Laceration of other muscle(s) and tendon(s) of posterior muscle group at lower leg level, left leg

    ⑦ **S86.129** Laceration of other muscle(s) and tendon(s) of posterior muscle group at lower leg level, unspecified leg

  S86.19 Other injury of other muscle(s) and tendon(s) of posterior muscle group at lower leg level

    ⑦ **S86.191** Other injury of other muscle(s) and tendon(s) of posterior muscle group at lower leg level, right leg

    ⑦ **S86.192** Other injury of other muscle(s) and tendon(s) of posterior muscle group at lower leg level, left leg

    ⑦ **S86.199** Other injury of other muscle(s) and tendon(s) of posterior muscle group at lower leg level, unspecified leg

S86.2 Injury of muscle(s) and tendon(s) of anterior muscle group at lower leg level

  S86.20 Unspecified injury of muscle(s) and tendon(s) of anterior muscle group at lower leg level

    ⑦ **S86.201** Unspecified injury of muscle(s) and tendon(s) of anterior muscle group at lower leg level, right leg

    ⑦ **S86.202** Unspecified injury of muscle(s) and tendon(s) of anterior muscle group at lower leg level, left leg

    ⑦ **S86.209** Unspecified injury of muscle(s) and tendon(s) of anterior muscle group at lower leg level, unspecified leg

  S86.21 Strain of muscle(s) and tendon(s) of anterior muscle group at lower leg level

    ⑦ **S86.211** Strain of muscle(s) and tendon(s) of anterior muscle group at lower leg level, right leg

    ⑦ **S86.212** Strain of muscle(s) and tendon(s) of anterior muscle group at lower leg level, left leg

    ⑦ **S86.219** Strain of muscle(s) and tendon(s) of anterior muscle group at lower leg level, unspecified leg

  S86.22 Laceration of muscle(s) and tendon(s) of anterior muscle group at lower leg level

    ⑦ **S86.221** Laceration of muscle(s) and tendon(s) of anterior muscle group at lower leg level, right leg

    ⑦ **S86.222** Laceration of muscle(s) and tendon(s) of anterior muscle group at lower leg level, left leg

    ⑦ **S86.229** Laceration of muscle(s) and tendon(s) of anterior muscle group at lower leg level, unspecified leg

  S86.29 Other injury of muscle(s) and tendon(s) of anterior muscle group at lower leg level

    ⑦ **S86.291** Other injury of muscle(s) and tendon(s) of anterior muscle group at lower leg level, right leg

    ⑦ **S86.292** Other injury of muscle(s) and tendon(s) of anterior muscle group at lower leg level, left leg

    ⑦ **S86.299** Other injury of muscle(s) and tendon(s) of anterior muscle group at lower leg level, unspecified leg

S86.3 Injury of muscle(s) and tendon(s) of peroneal muscle group at lower leg level

  S86.30 Unspecified injury of muscle(s) and tendon(s) of peroneal muscle group at lower leg level

    ⑦ **S86.301** Unspecified injury of muscle(s) and tendon(s) of peroneal muscle group at lower leg level, right leg

    ⑦ **S86.302** Unspecified injury of muscle(s) and tendon(s) of peroneal muscle group at lower leg level, left leg

    ⑦ **S86.309** Unspecified injury of muscle(s) and tendon(s) of peroneal muscle group at lower leg level, unspecified leg

  S86.31 Strain of muscle(s) and tendon(s) of peroneal muscle group at lower leg level

    ⑦ **S86.311** Strain of muscle(s) and tendon(s) of peroneal muscle group at lower leg level, right leg

● New code   ▲ Revised code   ⑦ 7th digit required   ⊗ Placeholder required

⑦S86.312   Strain of muscle(s) and tendon(s) of peroneal muscle group at lower leg level, left leg

⑦S86.319   Strain of muscle(s) and tendon(s) of peroneal muscle group at lower leg level, unspecified leg

S86.32   Laceration of muscle(s) and tendon(s) of peroneal muscle group at lower leg level

⑦S86.321   Laceration of muscle(s) and tendon(s) of peroneal muscle group at lower leg level, right leg

⑦S86.322   Laceration of muscle(s) and tendon(s) of peroneal muscle group at lower leg level, left leg

⑦S86.329   Laceration of muscle(s) and tendon(s) of peroneal muscle group at lower leg level, unspecified leg

S86.39   Other injury of muscle(s) and tendon(s) of peroneal muscle group at lower leg level

⑦S86.391   Other injury of muscle(s) and tendon(s) of peroneal muscle group at lower leg level, right leg

⑦S86.392   Other injury of muscle(s) and tendon(s) of peroneal muscle group at lower leg level, left leg

⑦S86.399   Other injury of muscle(s) and tendon(s) of peroneal muscle group at lower leg level, unspecified leg

S86.8   Injury of other muscles and tendons at lower leg level

S86.80   Unspecified injury of other muscles and tendons at lower leg level

⑦S86.801   Unspecified injury of other muscle(s) and tendon(s) at lower leg level, right leg

⑦S86.802   Unspecified injury of other muscle(s) and tendon(s) at lower leg level, left leg

⑦S86.809   Unspecified injury of other muscle(s) and tendon(s) at lower leg level, unspecified leg

S86.81   Strain of other muscles and tendons at lower leg level

⑦S86.811   Strain of other muscle(s) and tendon(s) at lower leg level, right leg

⑦S86.812   Strain of other muscle(s) and tendon(s) at lower leg level, left leg

⑦S86.819   Strain of other muscle(s) and tendon(s) at lower leg level, unspecified leg

S86.82   Laceration of other muscles and tendons at lower leg level

⑦S86.821   Laceration of other muscle(s) and tendon(s) at lower leg level, right leg

⑦S86.822   Laceration of other muscle(s) and tendon(s) at lower leg level, left leg

⑦S86.829   Laceration of other muscle(s) and tendon(s) at lower leg level, unspecified leg

S86.89   Other injury of other muscles and tendons at lower leg level

⑦S86.891   Other injury of other muscle(s) and tendon(s) at lower leg level, right leg

⑦S86.892   Other injury of other muscle(s) and tendon(s) at lower leg level, left leg

⑦S86.899   Other injury of other muscle(s) and tendon(s) at lower leg level, unspecified leg

S86.9   Injury of unspecified muscle and tendon at lower leg level

S86.90   Unspecified injury of unspecified muscle and tendon at lower leg level

⑦S86.901   Unspecified injury of unspecified muscle(s) and tendon(s) at lower leg level, right leg

⑦S86.902   Unspecified injury of unspecified muscle(s) and tendon(s) at lower leg level, left leg

⑦S86.909   Unspecified injury of unspecified muscle(s) and tendon(s) at lower leg level, unspecified leg

S86.91   Strain of unspecified muscle and tendon at lower leg level

⑦S86.911   Strain of unspecified muscle(s) and tendon(s) at lower leg level, right leg

⑦S86.912   Strain of unspecified muscle(s) and tendon(s) at lower leg level, left leg

⑦S86.919   Strain of unspecified muscle(s) and tendon(s) at lower leg level, unspecified leg

S86.92   Laceration of unspecified muscle and tendon at lower leg level

⑦S86.921   Laceration of unspecified muscle(s) and tendon(s) at lower leg level, right leg

⑦S86.922   Laceration of unspecified muscle(s) and tendon(s) at lower leg level, left leg

⑦S86.929   Laceration of unspecified muscle(s) and tendon(s) at lower leg level, unspecified leg

S86.99   Other injury of unspecified muscle and tendon at lower leg level

⑦S86.991   Other injury of unspecified muscle(s) and tendon(s) at lower leg level, right leg

⑦S86.992   Other injury of unspecified muscle(s) and tendon(s) at lower leg level, left leg

⑦S86.999   Other injury of unspecified muscle(s) and tendon(s) at lower leg level, unspecified leg

S87   Crushing injury of lower leg

Use additional code(s) for all associated injuries

Excludes 2: crushing injury of ankle and foot (S97.-)

The appropriate 7th character is to be added to each code from category S87

A - initial encounter

D - subsequent encounter

S - sequela

S87.0   Crushing injury of knee

⊗⑦S87.00   Crushing injury of unspecified knee

⊗⑦**S87.01**   Crushing injury of right knee

⊗⑦**S87.02**   Crushing injury of left knee

S87.8   Crushing injury of lower leg

⊗⑦**S87.80**   Crushing injury of unspecified lower leg

⊗⑦**S87.81**   Crushing injury of right lower leg

⊗⑦**S87.82**   Crushing injury of left lower leg

S88   Traumatic amputation of lower leg

An amputation not identified as partial or complete should be coded to complete

Excludes 1: traumatic amputation of ankle and foot (S98.-)

The appropriate 7th character is to be added to each code from category S88

A - initial encounter

D - subsequent encounter

S - sequela

S88.0   Traumatic amputation at knee level

S88.01   Complete traumatic amputation at knee level

⑦**S88.011**   Complete traumatic amputation at knee level, right lower leg

⑦**S88.012**   Complete traumatic amputation at knee level, left lower leg

⑦**S88.019**   Complete traumatic amputation at knee level, unspecified lower leg

S88.02   Partial traumatic amputation at knee level

⑦**S88.021**   Partial traumatic amputation at knee level, right lower leg

⑦**S88.022**   Partial traumatic amputation at knee level, left lower leg

⑦**S88.029**   Partial traumatic amputation at knee level, unspecified lower leg

S88.1   Traumatic amputation at level between knee and ankle

S88.11   Complete traumatic amputation at level between knee and ankle

⑦**S88.111**   Complete traumatic amputation at level between knee and ankle, right lower leg

⑦**S88.112**   Complete traumatic amputation at level between knee and ankle, left lower leg

⑦**S88.119**   Complete traumatic amputation at level between knee and ankle, unspecified lower leg

S88.12   Partial traumatic amputation at level between knee and ankle

⑦**S88.121**   Partial traumatic amputation at level between knee and ankle, right lower leg

⑦**S88.122**   Partial traumatic amputation at level between knee and ankle, left lower leg

⑦**S88.129**   Partial traumatic amputation at level between knee and ankle, unspecified lower leg

S88.9   Traumatic amputation of lower leg, level unspecified

S88.91   Complete traumatic amputation of lower leg, level unspecified

⑦**S88.911**   Complete traumatic amputation of right lower leg, level unspecified

⑦**S88.912**   Complete traumatic amputation of left lower leg, level unspecified

⑦**S88.919**   Complete traumatic amputation of unspecified lower leg, level unspecified

S88.92   Partial traumatic amputation of lower leg, level unspecified

⑦**S88.921**   Partial traumatic amputation of right lower leg, level unspecified

⑦**S88.922**   Partial traumatic amputation of left lower leg, level unspecified

⑦**S88.929**   Partial traumatic amputation of unspecified lower leg, level unspecified

S89   Other and unspecified injuries of lower leg

Note: A fracture not indicated as open or closed should be coded to closed

Excludes 2: other and unspecified injuries of ankle and foot (S99.-)

The appropriate 7th character is to be added to each code from subcategories S89.0, S89.1, S89.2, and S89.3

A - initial encounter for closed fracture

D - subsequent encounter for fracture with routine healing

G - subsequent encounter for fracture with delayed healing

K - subsequent encounter for fracture with nonunion

P - subsequent encounter for fracture with malunion

S - sequela

S89.0   Physeal fracture of upper end of tibia

S89.00   Unspecified physeal fracture of upper end of tibia

⑦**S89.001**   Unspecified physeal fracture of upper end of right tibia

⑦**S89.002**   Unspecified physeal fracture of upper end of left tibia

⑦**S89.009**   Unspecified physeal fracture of upper end of unspecified tibia

S89.01   Salter-Harris Type I physeal fracture of upper end of tibia

⑦**S89.011**   Salter-Harris Type I physeal fracture of upper end of right tibia

⑦**S89.012**   Salter-Harris Type I physeal fracture of upper end of left tibia

⑦**S89.019**   Salter-Harris Type I physeal fracture of upper end of unspecified tibia

S89.02   Salter-Harris Type II physeal fracture of upper end of tibia

⑦**S89.021**   Salter-Harris Type II physeal fracture of upper end of right tibia

⑦**S89.022**   Salter-Harris Type II physeal fracture of upper end of left tibia

⑦**S89.029**   Salter-Harris Type II physeal fracture of upper end of unspecified tibia

S89.03   Salter-Harris Type III physeal fracture of upper end of tibia

⑦**S89.031**   Salter-Harris Type III physeal fracture of upper end of right tibia

⑦**S89.032**   Salter-Harris Type III physeal fracture of upper end of left tibia

● New code   ▲ Revised code   ⑦ 7th digit required   ⊗ Placeholder required

⑦S89.039   Salter-Harris Type III physeal fracture of upper end of unspecified tibia

S89.04   Salter-Harris Type IV physeal fracture of upper end of tibia

⑦S89.041   Salter-Harris Type IV physeal fracture of upper end of right tibia

⑦S89.042   Salter-Harris Type IV physeal fracture of upper end of left tibia

⑦S89.049   Salter-Harris Type IV physeal fracture of upper end of unspecified tibia

S89.09   Other physeal fracture of upper end of tibia

⑦S89.091   Other physeal fracture of upper end of right tibia

⑦S89.092   Other physeal fracture of upper end of left tibia

⑦S89.099   Other physeal fracture of upper end of unspecified tibia

S89.1   Physeal fracture of lower end of tibia

S89.10   Unspecified physeal fracture of lower end of tibia

⑦S89.101   Unspecified physeal fracture of lower end of right tibia

⑦S89.102   Unspecified physeal fracture of lower end of left tibia

⑦S89.109   Unspecified physeal fracture of lower end of unspecified tibia

S89.11   Salter-Harris Type I physeal fracture of lower end of tibia

⑦S89.111   Salter-Harris Type I physeal fracture of lower end of right tibia

⑦S89.112   Salter-Harris Type I physeal fracture of lower end of left tibia

⑦S89.119   Salter-Harris Type I physeal fracture of lower end of unspecified tibia

S89.12   Salter-Harris Type II physeal fracture of lower end of tibia

⑦S89.121   Salter-Harris Type II physeal fracture of lower end of right tibia

⑦S89.122   Salter-Harris Type II physeal fracture of lower end of left tibia

⑦S89.129   Salter-Harris Type II physeal fracture of lower end of unspecified tibia

S89.13   Salter-Harris Type III physeal fracture of lower end of tibia

Excludes 1: fracture of medial malleolus (adult) (S82.5-)

⑦S89.131   Salter-Harris Type III physeal fracture of lower end of right tibia

⑦S89.132   Salter-Harris Type III physeal fracture of lower end of left tibia

⑦S89.139   Salter-Harris Type III physeal fracture of lower end of unspecified tibia

S89.14   Salter-Harris Type IV physeal fracture of lower end of tibia

Excludes 1: fracture of medial malleolus (adult) (S82.5-)

⑦S89.141   Salter-Harris Type IV physeal fracture of lower end of right tibia

⑦S89.142   Salter-Harris Type IV physeal fracture of lower end of left tibia

⑦S89.149   Salter-Harris Type IV physeal fracture of lower end of unspecified tibia

S89.19   Other physeal fracture of lower end of tibia

⑦S89.191   Other physeal fracture of lower end of right tibia

⑦S89.192   Other physeal fracture of lower end of left tibia

⑦S89.199   Other physeal fracture of lower end of unspecified tibia

S89.2   Physeal fracture of upper end of fibula

S89.20   Unspecified physeal fracture of upper end of fibula

⑦S89.201   Unspecified physeal fracture of upper end of right fibula

⑦S89.202   Unspecified physeal fracture of upper end of left fibula

⑦S89.209   Unspecified physeal fracture of upper end of unspecified fibula

S89.21   Salter-Harris Type I physeal fracture of upper end of fibula

⑦S89.211   Salter-Harris Type I physeal fracture of upper end of right fibula

⑦S89.212   Salter-Harris Type I physeal fracture of upper end of left fibula

⑦S89.219   Salter-Harris Type I physeal fracture of upper end of unspecified fibula

S89.22   Salter-Harris Type II physeal fracture of upper end of fibula

⑦S89.221   Salter-Harris Type II physeal fracture of upper end of right fibula

⑦S89.222   Salter-Harris Type II physeal fracture of upper end of left fibula

⑦S89.229   Salter-Harris Type II physeal fracture of upper end of unspecified fibula

S89.29   Other physeal fracture of upper end of fibula

⑦S89.291   Other physeal fracture of upper end of right fibula

⑦S89.292   Other physeal fracture of upper end of left fibula

⑦S89.299   Other physeal fracture of upper end of unspecified fibula

S89.3   Physeal fracture of lower end of tibula

S89.30   Unspecified physeal fracture of lower end of fibula

⑦S89.301   Unspecified physeal fracture of lower end of right fibula

⑦S89.302   Unspecified physeal fracture of lower end of left fibula

⑦S89.309   Unspecified physeal fracture of lower end of unspecified fibula

S89.31   Salter-Harris Type I physeal fracture of lower end of fibula

⑦ S89.311   Salter-Harris Type I physeal fracture of lower end of right fibula

⑦ S89.312   Salter-Harris Type I physeal fracture of lower end of left fibula

⑦ S89.319   Salter-Harris Type I physeal fracture of lower end of unspecified fibula

S89.32   Salter-Harris Type II physeal fracture of lower end of fibula

⑦ S89.321   Salter-Harris Type II physeal fracture of lower end of right fibula

⑦ S89.322   Salter-Harris Type II physeal fracture of lower end of left fibula

⑦ S89.329   Salter-Harris Type II physeal fracture of lower end of unspecified fibula

S89.39   Other physeal fracture of lower end of fibula

⑦ S89.391   Other physeal fracture of lower end of right fibula

⑦ S89.392   Other physeal fracture of lower end of left fibula

⑦ S89.399   Other physeal fracture of lower end of unspecified fibula

S89.8   Other specified injuries of lower leg

The appropriate 7th character is to be added to each code in subcategory S89.8

A - initial encounter

D - subsequent encounter

S - sequela

⊗⑦ S89.80   Other specified injuries of unspecified lower leg

⊗⑦ S89.81   Other specified injuries of right lower leg

⊗⑦ S89.82   Other specified injuries of left lower leg

S89.9   Unspecified injury of lower leg

The appropriate 7th character is to be added to each code in subcategory S89.9

A - initial encounter

D - subsequent encounter

S - sequela

⊗⑦ S89.90   Unspecified injury of unspecified lower leg

⊗⑦ S89.91   Unspecified injury of right lower leg

⊗⑦ S89.92   Unspecified injury of left lower leg

INJURIES TO THE ANKLE AND FOOT (S90-S99)

Excludes 2:   burns and corrosions (T20-T32)

fracture of ankle and malleolus (S82.-)

frostbite (T33-T34)

insect bite or sting, venomous (T63.4)

S90   Superficial injury of ankle, foot and toes

The appropriate 7th character is to be added to each code from category S90

A - initial encounter

D - subsequent encounter

S - sequela

S90.0   Contusion of ankle

⊗⑦ S90.00   Contusion of unspecified ankle

⊗⑦ S90.01   Contusion of right ankle

⊗⑦ S90.02   Contusion of left ankle

S90.1   Contusion of toe without damage to nail

S90.11   Contusion of great toe without damage to nail

⑦ S90.111   Contusion of right great toe without damage to nail

⑦ S90.112   Contusion of left great toe without damage to nail

⑦ S90.119   Contusion of unspecified great toe without damage to nail

S90.12   Contusion of lesser toe without damage to nail

⑦ S90.121   Contusion of right lesser toe(s) without damage to nail

⑦ S90.122   Contusion of left lesser toe(s) without damage to nail

⑦ S90.129   Contusion of unspecified lesser toe(s) without damage to nail

Contusion of toe NOS

S90.2   Contusion of toe with damage to nail

S90.21   Contusion of great toe with damage to nail

⑦ S90.211   Contusion of right great toe with damage to nail

⑦ S90.212   Contusion of left great toe with damage to nail

⑦ S90.219   Contusion of unspecified great toe with damage to nail

S90.22   Contusion of lesser toe with damage to nail

⑦ S90.221   Contusion of right lesser toe(s) with damage to nail

⑦ S90.222   Contusion of left lesser toe(s) with damage to nail

⑦ S90.229   Contusion of unspecified lesser toe(s) with damage to nail

S90.3   Contusion of foot

Excludes 2: contusion of toes (S90.1-, S90.2-)

⊗⑦ S90.30   Contusion of unspecified foot

Contusion of foot NOS

⊗⑦ S90.31   Contusion of right foot

⊗⑦ S90.32   Contusion of left foot

S90.4   Other superficial injuries of toe

S90.41   Abrasion of toe

⑦ S90.411   Abrasion, right great toe

⑦ S90.412   Abrasion, left great toe

⑦ S90.413   Abrasion, unspecified great toe

⑦ S90.414   Abrasion, right lesser toe(s)

⑦ S90.415   Abrasion, left lesser toe(s)

⑦ S90.416   Abrasion, unspecified lesser toe(s)

S90.42   Blister (nonthermal) of toe

⑦ S90.421   Blister (nonthermal), right great toe

⑦ S90.422   Blister (nonthermal), left great toe

⑦ S90.423   Blister (nonthermal), unspecified great toe

⑦ S90.424   Blister (nonthermal), right lesser toe(s)

⑦ S90.425   Blister (nonthermal), left lesser toe(s)

⑦ S90.426   Blister (nonthermal), unspecified lesser toe(s)

S90.44   External constriction of toe

Hair tourniquet syndrome of toe

⑦S90.441   External constriction, right great toe

⑦S90.442   External constriction, left great toe

⑦S90.443   External constriction, unspecified great toe

⑦S90.444   External constriction, right lesser toe(s)

⑦S90.445   External constriction, left lesser toe(s)

⑦S90.446   External constriction, unspecified lesser toe(s)

S90.45   Superficial foreign body of toe
     Splinter in the toe

⑦S90.451   Superficial foreign body, right great toe

⑦S90.452   Superficial foreign body, left great toe

⑦S90.453   Superficial foreign body, unspecified great toe

⑦S90.454   Superficial foreign body, right lesser toe(s)

⑦S90.455   Superficial foreign body, left lesser toe(s)

⑦S90.456   Superficial foreign body, unspecified lesser toe(s)

S90.46   Insect bite (nonvenomous) of toe

⑦S90.461   Insect bite (nonvenomous), right great toe

⑦S90.462   Insect bite (nonvenomous), left great toe

⑦S90.463   Insect bite (nonvenomous), unspecified great toe

⑦S90.464   Insect bite (nonvenomous), right lesser toe(s)

⑦S90.465   Insect bite (nonvenomous), left lesser toe(s)

⑦S90.466   Insect bite (nonvenomous), unspecified lesser toe(s)

S90.47   Other superficial bite of toe
     Excludes 1: open bite of toe (S91.15-, S91.25-)

⑦S90.471   Other superficial bite of right great toe

⑦S90.472   Other superficial bite of left great toe

⑦S90.473   Other superficial bite of unspecified great toe

⑦S90.474   Other superficial bite of right lesser toe(s)

⑦S90.475   Other superficial bite of left lesser toe(s)

⑦S90.476   Other superficial bite of unspecified lesser toe(s)

S90.5   Other superficial injuries of ankle

S90.51   Abrasion of ankle

⑦S90.511   Abrasion, right ankle

⑦S90.512   Abrasion, left ankle

⑦S90.519   Abrasion, unspecified ankle

S90.52   Blister (nonthermal) of ankle

⑦S90.521   Blister (nonthermal), right ankle

⑦S90.522   Blister (nonthermal), left ankle

⑦S90.529   Blister (nonthermal), unspecified ankle

S90.54   External constriction of ankle

⑦S90.541   External constriction, right ankle

⑦S90.542   External constriction, left ankle

⑦S90.549   External constriction, unspecified ankle

S90.55   Superficial foreign body of ankle
     Splinter in the ankle

⑦S90.551   Superficial foreign body, right ankle

⑦S90.552   Superficial foreign body, left ankle

⑦S90.559   Superficial foreign body, unspecified ankle

S90.56   Insect bite (nonvenomous) of ankle

⑦S90.561   Insect bite (nonvenomous), right ankle

⑦S90.562   Insect bite (nonvenomous), left ankle

⑦S90.569   Insect bite (nonvenomous), unspecified ankle

S90.57   Other superficial bite of ankle
     Excludes 1: open bite of ankle (S91.05-)

⑦S90.571   Other superficial bite of ankle, right ankle

⑦S90.572   Other superficial bite of ankle, left ankle

⑦S90.579   Other superficial bite of ankle, unspecified ankle

S90.8   Other superficial injuries of foot

S90.81   Abrasion of foot

⑦S90.811   Abrasion, right foot

⑦S90.812   Abrasion, left foot

⑦S90.819   Abrasion, unspecified foot

S90.82   Blister (nonthermal) of foot

⑦S90.821   Blister (nonthermal), right foot

⑦S90.822   Blister (nonthermal), left foot

⑦S90.829   Blister (nonthermal), unspecified foot

S90.84   External constriction of foot

⑦S90.841   External constriction, right foot

⑦S90.842   External constriction, left foot

⑦S90.849   External constriction, unspecified foot

S90.85   Superficial foreign body of foot
     Splinter in the foot

⑦S90.851   Superficial foreign body, right foot

⑦S90.852   Superficial foreign body, left foot

⑦S90.859   Superficial foreign body, unspecified foot

S90.86   Insect bite (nonvenomous) of foot

⑦S90.861   Insect bite (nonvenomous), right foot

⑦S90.862   Insect bite (nonvenomous), left foot

⑦S90.869   Insect bite (nonvenomous), unspecified foot

S90.87   Other superficial bite of foot
     Excludes 1: open bite of foot (S91.35-)

Add 4th-7th digits   3 digit reportable   Nonspecific code   Unspecified code   Manifestation code

⑦S90.871   Other superficial bite of right foot

⑦S90.872   Other superficial bite of left foot

⑦S90.879   Other superficial bite of unspecified foot

S90.9   Unspecified superficial injury of ankle, foot and toe

    S90.91   Unspecified superficial injury of ankle

      ⑦S90.911   Unspecified superficial injury of right ankle

      ⑦S90.912   Unspecified superficial injury of left ankle

      ⑦S90.919   Unspecified superficial injury of unspecified ankle

    S90.92   Unspecified superficial injury of foot

      ⑦S90.921   Unspecified superficial injury of right foot

      ⑦S90.922   Unspecified superficial injury of left foot

      ⑦S90.929   Unspecified superficial injury of unspecified foot

    S90.93   Unspecified superficial injury of toes

      ⑦S90.931   Unspecified superficial injury of right great toe

      ⑦S90.932   Unspecified superficial injury of left great toe

      ⑦S90.933   Unspecified superficial injury of unspecified great toe

      ⑦S90.934   Unspecified superficial injury of right lesser toe(s)

      ⑦S90.935   Unspecified superficial injury of left lesser toe(s)

      ⑦S90.936   Unspecified superficial injury of unspecified lesser toe(s)

S91   Open wound of ankle, foot and toes

Code also any associated wound infection

Excludes 1: open fracture of ankle, foot and toes (S92.-with 7th character B)

    traumatic amputation of ankle and foot (S98.-)

The appropriate 7th character is to be added to each code from category S91

A - initial encounter

D - subsequent encounter

S - sequela

S91.0   Open wound of ankle

    S91.00   Unspecified open wound of ankle

      ⑦S91.001   Unspecified open wound, right ankle

      ⑦S91.002   Unspecified open wound, left ankle

      ⑦S91.009   Unspecified open wound, unspecified ankle

    S91.01   Laceration without foreign body of ankle

      ⑦S91.011   Laceration without foreign body, right ankle

      ⑦S91.012   Laceration without foreign body, left ankle

      ⑦S91.019   Laceration without foreign body, unspecified ankle

    S91.02   Laceration with foreign body of ankle

⑦S91.021   Laceration with foreign body, right ankle

⑦S91.022   Laceration with foreign body, left ankle

⑦S91.029   Laceration with foreign body, unspecified ankle

    S91.03   Puncture wound without foreign body of ankle

      ⑦S91.031   Puncture wound without foreign body, right ankle

      ⑦S91.032   Puncture wound without foreign body, left ankle

      ⑦S91.039   Puncture wound without foreign body, unspecified ankle

    S91.04   Puncture wound with foreign body of ankle

      ⑦S91.041   Puncture wound with foreign body, right ankle

      ⑦S91.042   Puncture wound with foreign body, left ankle

      ⑦S91.049   Puncture wound with foreign body, unspecified ankle

    S91.05   Open bite of ankle

    Excludes 1: superficial bite of ankle (S90.56-, S90.57-)

      ⑦S91.051   Open bite, right ankle

      ⑦S91.052   Open bite, left ankle

      ⑦S91.059   Open bite, unspecified ankle

S91.1   Open wound of toe without damage to nail

    S91.10   Unspecified open wound of toe without damage to nail

      ⑦S91.101   Unspecified open wound of right great toe without damage to nail

      ⑦S91.102   Unspecified open wound of left great toe without damage to nail

      ⑦S91.103   Unspecified open wound of unspecified great toe without damage to nail

      ⑦S91.104   Unspecified open wound of right lesser toe(s) without damage to nail

      ⑦S91.105   Unspecified open wound of left lesser toe(s) without damage to nail

      ⑦S91.106   Unspecified open wound of unspecified lesser toe(s) without damage to nail

      ⑦S91.109   Unspecified open wound of unspecified toe(s) without damage to nail

    S91.11   Laceration without foreign body of toe without damage to nail

      ⑦S91.111   Laceration without foreign body of right great toe without damage to nail

      ⑦S91.112   Laceration without foreign body of left great toe without damage to nail

      ⑦S91.113   Laceration without foreign body of unspecified great toe without damage to nail

      ⑦S91.114   Laceration without foreign body of right lesser toe(s) without damage to nail

⑦S91.115 Laceration without foreign body of left lesser toe(s) without damage to nail

⑦S91.116 Laceration without foreign body of unspecified lesser toe(s) without damage to nail

⑦S91.119 Laceration without foreign body of unspecified toe without damage to nail

S91.12 Laceration with foreign body of toe without damage to nail

⑦S91.121 Laceration with foreign body of right great toe without damage to nail

⑦S91.122 Laceration with foreign body of left great toe without damage to nail

⑦S91.123 Laceration with foreign body of unspecified great toe without damage to nail

⑦S91.124 Laceration with foreign body of right lesser toe(s) without damage to nail

⑦S91.125 Laceration with foreign body of left lesser toe(s) without damage to nail

⑦S91.126 Laceration with foreign body of unspecified lesser toe(s) without damage to nail

⑦S91.129 Laceration with foreign body of unspecified toe(s) without damage to nail

S91.13 Puncture wound without foreign body of toe without damage to nail

⑦S91.131 Puncture wound without foreign body of right great toe without damage to nail

⑦S91.132 Puncture wound without foreign body of left great toe without damage to nail

⑦S91.133 Puncture wound without foreign body of unspecified great toe without damage to nail

⑦S91.134 Puncture wound without foreign body of right lesser toe(s) without damage to nail

⑦S91.135 Puncture wound without foreign body of left lesser toe(s) without damage to nail

⑦S91.136 Puncture wound without foreign body of unspecified lesser toe(s) without damage to nail

⑦S91.139 Puncture wound without foreign body of unspecified toe(s) without damage to nail

S91.14 Puncture wound with foreign body of toe without damage to nail

⑦S91.141 Puncture wound with foreign body of right great toe without damage to nail

⑦S91.142 Puncture wound with foreign body of left great toe without damage to nail

⑦S91.143 Puncture wound with foreign body of unspecified great toe without damage to nail

⑦S91.144 Puncture wound with foreign body of right lesser toe(s) without damage to nail

⑦S91.145 Puncture wound with foreign body of left lesser toe(s) without damage to nail

⑦S91.146 Puncture wound with foreign body of unspecified lesser toe(s) without damage to nail

⑦S91.149 Puncture wound with foreign body of unspecified toe(s) without damage to nail

S91.15 Open bite of toe without damage to nail
Bite of toe NOS
Excludes 1: superficial bite of toe (S90.46-, S90.47-)

⑦S91.151 Open bite of right great toe without damage to nail

⑦S91.152 Open bite of left great toe without damage to nail

⑦S91.153 Open bite of unspecified great toe without damage to nail

⑦S91.154 Open bite of right lesser toe(s) without damage to nail

⑦S91.155 Open bite of left lesser toe(s) without damage to nail

⑦S91.156 Open bite of unspecified lesser toe(s) without damage to nail

⑦S91.159 Open bite of unspecified toe(s) without damage to nail

S91.2 Open wound of toe with damage to nail
S91.20 Unspecified open wound of toe with damage to nail

⑦S91.201 Unspecified open wound of right great toe with damage to nail

⑦S91.202 Unspecified open wound of left great toe with damage to nail

⑦S91.203 Unspecified open wound of unspecified great toe with damage to nail

⑦S91.204 Unspecified open wound of right lesser toe(s) with damage to nail

⑦S91.205 Unspecified open wound of left lesser toe(s) with damage to nail

⑦S91.206 Unspecified open wound of unspecified lesser toe(s) with damage to nail

⑦S91.209 Unspecified open wound of unspecified toe(s) with damage to nail

S91.21 Laceration without foreign body of toe with damage to nail

⑦S91.211 Laceration without foreign body of right great toe with damage to nail

⑦S91.212 Laceration without foreign body of left great toe with damage to nail

⑦**S91.213** Laceration without foreign body of unspecified great toe with damage to nail

⑦**S91.214** Laceration without foreign body of right lesser toe(s) with damage to nail

⑦**S91.215** Laceration without foreign body of left lesser toe(s) with damage to nail

⑦**S91.216** Laceration without foreign body of unspecified lesser toe(s) with damage to nail

⑦**S91.219** Laceration without foreign body of unspecified toe(s) with damage to nail

S91.22 Laceration with foreign body of toe with damage to nail

⑦**S91.221** Laceration with foreign body of right great toe with damage to nail

⑦**S91.222** Laceration with foreign body of left great toe with damage to nail

⑦**S91.223** Laceration with foreign body of unspecified great toe with damage to nail

⑦**S91.224** Laceration with foreign body of right lesser toe(s) with damage to nail

⑦**S91.225** Laceration with foreign body of left lesser toe(s) with damage to nail

⑦**S91.226** Laceration with foreign body of unspecified lesser toe(s) with damage to nail

⑦**S91.229** Laceration with foreign body of unspecified toe(s) with damage to nail

S91.23 Puncture wound without foreign body of toe with damage to nail

⑦**S91.231** Puncture wound without foreign body of right great toe with damage to nail

⑦**S91.232** Puncture wound without foreign body of left great toe with damage to nail

⑦**S91.233** Puncture wound without foreign body of unspecified great toe with damage to nail

⑦**S91.234** Puncture wound without foreign body of right lesser toe(s) with damage to nail

⑦**S91.235** Puncture wound without foreign body of left lesser toe(s) with damage to nail

⑦**S91.236** Puncture wound without foreign body of unspecified lesser toe(s) with damage to nail

⑦**S91.239** Puncture wound without foreign body of unspecified toe(s) with damage to nail

S91.24 Puncture wound with foreign body of toe with damage to nail

⑦**S91.241** Puncture wound with foreign body of right great toe with damage to nail

⑦**S91.242** Puncture wound with foreign body of left great toe with damage to nail

⑦**S91.243** Puncture wound with foreign body of unspecified great toe with damage to nail

⑦**S91.244** Puncture wound with foreign body of right lesser toe(s) with damage to nail

⑦**S91.245** Puncture wound with foreign body of left lesser toe(s) with damage to nail

⑦**S91.246** Puncture wound with foreign body of unspecified lesser toe(s) with damage to nail

⑦**S91.249** Puncture wound with foreign body of unspecified toe(s) with damage to nail

S91.25 Open bite of toe with damage to nail

Bite of toe with damage to nail NOS

Excludes 1: superficial bite of toe (S90.46-, S90.47-)

⑦**S91.251** Open bite of right great toe with damage to nail

⑦**S91.252** Open bite of left great toe with damage to nail

⑦**S91.253** Open bite of unspecified great toe with damage to nail

⑦**S91.254** Open bite of right lesser toe(s) with damage to nail

⑦**S91.255** Open bite of left lesser toe(s) with damage to nail

⑦**S91.256** Open bite of unspecified lesser toe(s) with damage to nail

⑦**S91.259** Open bite of unspecified toe(s) with damage to nail

S91.3 Open wound of foot

S91.30 Unspecified open wound of foot

⑦**S91.301** Unspecified open wound, right foot

⑦**S91.302** Unspecified open wound, left foot

⑦**S91.309** Unspecified open wound, unspecified foot

S91.31 Laceration without foreign body of foot

⑦**S91.311** Laceration without foreign body, right foot

⑦**S91.312** Laceration without foreign body, left foot

⑦**S91.319** Laceration without foreign body, unspecified foot

S91.32 Laceration with foreign body of foot

⑦**S91.321** Laceration with foreign body, right foot

⑦**S91.322** Laceration with foreign body, left foot

⑦**S91.329** Laceration with foreign body, unspecified foot

S91.33 Puncture wound without foreign body of foot

⑦S91.331   Puncture wound without foreign body, right foot

⑦S91.332   Puncture wound without foreign body, left foot

⑦S91.339   Puncture wound without foreign body, unspecified foot

S91.34   Puncture wound with foreign body of foot

     ⑦S91.341   Puncture wound with foreign body, right foot

     ⑦S91.342   Puncture wound with foreign body, left foot

     ⑦S91.349   Puncture wound with foreign body, unspecified foot

S91.35   Open bite of foot

     Excludes 1: superficial bite of foot (S90.86-, S90.87-)

     ⑦S91.351   Open bite, right foot

     ⑦S91.352   Open bite, left foot

     ⑦S91.359   Open bite, unspecified foot

S92   Fracture of foot and toe, except ankle

Note: A fracture not indicated as displaced or nondisplaced should be coded to displaced

A fracture not indicated as open or closed should be coded to closed

Excludes 1: traumatic amputation of ankle and foot (S98.-)

Excludes 2: fracture of ankle (S82.-)

fracture of malleolus (S82.-)

The appropriate 7th character is to be added to each code from category S92

A - initial encounter for closed fracture

B - initial encounter for open fracture

D - subsequent encounter for fracture with routine healing

G - subsequent encounter for fracture with delayed healing

K - subsequent encounter for fracture with nonunion

P - subsequent encounter for fracture with malunion

S - sequela

S92.0   Fracture of calcaneus

Heel bone

Os calcis

S92.00   Unspecified fracture of calcaneus

     ⑦S92.001   Unspecified fracture of right calcaneus

     ⑦S92.002   Unspecified fracture of left calcaneus

     ⑦S92.009   Unspecified fracture of unspecified calcaneus

S92.01   Fracture of body of calcaneus

     ⑦S92.011   Displaced fracture of body of right calcaneus

     ⑦S92.012   Displaced fracture of body of left calcaneus

     ⑦S92.013   Displaced fracture of body of unspecified calcaneus

     ⑦S92.014   Nondisplaced fracture of body of right calcaneus

     ⑦S92.015   Nondisplaced fracture of body of left calcaneus

     ⑦S92.016   Nondisplaced fracture of body of unspecified calcaneus

S92.02   Fracture of anterior process of calcaneus

     ⑦S92.021   Displaced fracture of anterior process of right calcaneus

     ⑦S92.022   Displaced fracture of anterior process of left calcaneus

     ⑦S92.023   Displaced fracture of anterior process of unspecified calcaneus

     ⑦S92.024   Nondisplaced fracture of anterior process of right calcaneus

     ⑦S92.025   Nondisplaced fracture of anterior process of left calcaneus

     ⑦S92.026   Nondisplaced fracture of anterior process of unspecified calcaneus

S92.03   Avulsion fracture of tuberosity of calcaneus

     ⑦S92.031   Displaced avulsion fracture of tuberosity of right calcaneus

     ⑦S92.032   Displaced avulsion fracture of tuberosity of left calcaneus

     ⑦S92.033   Displaced avulsion fracture of tuberosity of unspecified calcaneus

     ⑦S92.034   Nondisplaced avulsion fracture of tuberosity of right calcaneus

     ⑦S92.035   Nondisplaced avulsion fracture of tuberosity of left calcaneus

     ⑦S92.036   Nondisplaced avulsion fracture of tuberosity of unspecified calcaneus

S92.04   Other fracture of tuberosity of calcaneus

     ⑦S92.041   Displaced other fracture of tuberosity of right calcaneus

     ⑦S92.042   Displaced other fracture of tuberosity of left calcaneus

     ⑦S92.043   Displaced other fracture of tuberosity of unspecified calcaneus

     ⑦S92.044   Nondisplaced other fracture of tuberosity of right calcaneus

     ⑦S92.045   Nondisplaced other fracture of tuberosity of left calcaneus

     ⑦S92.046   Nondisplaced other fracture of tuberosity of unspecified calcaneus

S92.05   Other extraarticular fracture of calcaneus

     ⑦S92.051   Displaced other extraarticular fracture of right calcaneus

     ⑦S92.052   Displaced other extraarticular fracture of left calcaneus

     ⑦S92.053   Displaced other extraarticular fracture of unspecified calcaneus

     ⑦S92.054   Nondisplaced other extraarticular fracture of right calcaneus

     ⑦S92.055   Nondisplaced other extraarticular fracture of left calcaneus

     ⑦S92.056   Nondisplaced other extraarticular fracture of unspecified calcaneus

S92.06   Intraarticular fracture of calcaneus

     ⑦S92.061   Displaced intraarticular fracture of right calcaneus

     ⑦S92.062   Displaced intraarticular fracture of left calcaneus

     ⑦S92.063   Displaced intraarticular fracture of unspecified calcaneus

⑦ **S92.064** Nondisplaced intraarticular fracture of right calcaneus

⑦ **S92.065** Nondisplaced intraarticular fracture of left calcaneus

⑦ **S92.066** Nondisplaced intraarticular fracture of unspecified calcaneus

S92.1 Fracture of talus
Astragalus

S92.10 Unspecified fracture of talus

⑦ **S92.101** Unspecified fracture of right talus

⑦ **S92.102** Unspecified fracture of left talus

⑦ **S92.109** Unspecified fracture of unspecified talus

S92.11 Fracture of neck of talus

⑦ **S92.111** Displaced fracture of neck of right talus

⑦ **S92.112** Displaced fracture of neck of left talus

⑦ **S92.113** Displaced fracture of neck of unspecified talus

⑦ **S92.114** Nondisplaced fracture of neck of right talus

⑦ **S92.115** Nondisplaced fracture of neck of left talus

⑦ **S92.116** Nondisplaced fracture of neck of unspecified talus

S92.12 Fracture of body of talus

⑦ **S92.121** Displaced fracture of body of right talus

⑦ **S92.122** Displaced fracture of body of left talus

⑦ **S92.123** Displaced fracture of body of unspecified talus

⑦ **S92.124** Nondisplaced fracture of body of right talus

⑦ **S92.125** Nondisplaced fracture of body of left talus

⑦ **S92.126** Nondisplaced fracture of body of unspecified talus

S92.13 Fracture of posterior process of talus

⑦ **S92.131** Displaced fracture of posterior process of right talus

⑦ **S92.132** Displaced fracture of posterior process of left talus

⑦ **S92.133** Displaced fracture of posterior process of unspecified talus

⑦ **S92.134** Nondisplaced fracture of posterior process of right talus

⑦ **S92.135** Nondisplaced fracture of posterior process of left talus

⑦ **S92.136** Nondisplaced fracture of posterior process of unspecified talus

S92.14 Dome fracture of talus

Excludes 1: osteochondritis dissecans (M93.2)

⑦ **S92.141** Displaced dome fracture of right talus

⑦ **S92.142** Displaced dome fracture of left talus

⑦ **S92.143** Displaced dome fracture of unspecified talus

⑦ **S92.144** Nondisplaced dome fracture of right talus

⑦ **S92.145** Nondisplaced dome fracture of left talus

⑦ **S92.146** Nondisplaced dome fracture of unspecified talus

S92.15 Avulsion fracture (chip fracture) of talus

⑦ **S92.151** Displaced avulsion fracture (chip fracture) of right talus

⑦ **S92.152** Displaced avulsion fracture (chip fracture) of left talus

⑦ **S92.153** Displaced avulsion fracture (chip fracture) of unspecified talus

⑦ **S92.154** Nondisplaced avulsion fracture (chip fracture) of right talus

⑦ **S92.155** Nondisplaced avulsion fracture (chip fracture) of left talus

⑦ **S92.156** Nondisplaced avulsion fracture (chip fracture) of unspecified talus

S92.19 Other fracture of talus

⑦ **S92.191** Other fracture of right talus

⑦ **S92.192** Other fracture of left talus

⑦ **S92.199** Other fracture of unspecified talus

S92.2 Fracture of other and unspecified tarsal bone(s)

S92.20 Fracture of unspecified tarsal bone(s)

⑦ **S92.201** Fracture of unspecified tarsal bone(s) of right foot

⑦ **S92.202** Fracture of unspecified tarsal bone(s) of left foot

⑦ **S92.209** Fracture of unspecified tarsal bone(s) of unspecified foot

S92.21 Fracture of cuboid bone

⑦ **S92.211** Displaced fracture of cuboid bone of right foot

⑦ **S92.212** Displaced fracture of cuboid bone of left foot

⑦ **S92.213** Displaced fracture of cuboid bone of unspecified foot

⑦ **S92.214** Nondisplaced fracture of cuboid bone of right foot

⑦ **S92.215** Nondisplaced fracture of cuboid bone of left foot

⑦ **S92.216** Nondisplaced fracture of cuboid bone of unspecified foot

S92.22 Fracture of lateral cuneiform

⑦ **S92.221** Displaced fracture of lateral cuneiform of right foot

⑦ **S92.222** Displaced fracture of lateral cuneiform of left foot

⑦ **S92.223** Displaced fracture of lateral cuneiform of unspecified foot

⑦ **S92.224** Nondisplaced fracture of lateral cuneiform of right foot

⑦ **S92.225** Nondisplaced fracture of lateral cuneiform of left foot

● New code ▲ Revised code ⑦ 7th digit required ⊗ Placeholder required

⑦S92.226   Nondisplaced fracture of lateral cuneiform of unspecified foot

S92.23   Fracture of intermediate cuneiform

⑦S92.231   Displaced fracture of intermediate cuneiform of right foot

⑦S92.232   Displaced fracture of intermediate cuneiform of left foot

⑦S92.233   Displaced fracture of intermediate cuneiform of unspecified foot

⑦S92.234   Nondisplaced fracture of intermediate cuneiform of right foot

⑦S92.235   Nondisplaced fracture of intermediate cuneiform of left foot

⑦S92.236   Nondisplaced fracture of intermediate cuneiform of unspecified foot

S92.24   Fracture of medial cuneiform

⑦S92.241   Displaced fracture of medial cuneiform of right foot

⑦S92.242   Displaced fracture of medial cuneiform of left foot

⑦S92.243   Displaced fracture of medial cuneiform of unspecified foot

⑦S92.244   Nondisplaced fracture of medial cuneiform of right foot

⑦S92.245   Nondisplaced fracture of medial cuneiform of left foot

⑦S92.246   Nondisplaced fracture of medial cuneiform of unspecified foot

S92.25   Fracture of navicular [scaphoid] of foot

⑦S92.251   Displaced fracture of navicular [scaphoid] of right foot

⑦S92.252   Displaced fracture of navicular [scaphoid] of left foot

⑦S92.253   Displaced fracture of navicular [scaphoid] of unspecified foot

⑦S92.254   Nondisplaced fracture of navicular [scaphoid] of right foot

⑦S92.255   Nondisplaced fracture of navicular [scaphoid] of left foot

⑦S92.256   Nondisplaced fracture of navicular [scaphoid] of unspecified foot

S92.3   Fracture of metatarsal bone(s)

S92.30   Fracture of unspecified metatarsal bone(s)

⑦S92.301   Fracture of unspecified metatarsal bone(s), right foot

⑦S92.302   Fracture of unspecified metatarsal bone(s), left foot

⑦S92.309   Fracture of unspecified metatarsal bone(s), unspecified foot

S92.31   Fracture of first metatarsal bone

⑦S92.311   Displaced fracture of first metatarsal bone, right foot

⑦S92.312   Displaced fracture of first metatarsal bone, left foot

⑦S92.313   Displaced fracture of first metatarsal bone, unspecified foot

⑦S92.314   Nondisplaced fracture of first metatarsal bone, right foot

⑦S92.315   Nondisplaced fracture of first metatarsal bone, left foot

⑦S92.316   Nondisplaced fracture of first metatarsal bone, unspecified foot

S92.32   Fracture of second metatarsal bone

⑦S92.321   Displaced fracture of second metatarsal bone, right foot

⑦S92.322   Displaced fracture of second metatarsal bone, left foot

⑦S92.323   Displaced fracture of second metatarsal bone, unspecified foot

⑦S92.324   Nondisplaced fracture of second metatarsal bone, right foot

⑦S92.325   Nondisplaced fracture of second metatarsal bone, left foot

⑦S92.326   Nondisplaced fracture of second metatarsal bone, unspecified foot

S92.33   Fracture of third metatarsal bone

⑦S92.331   Displaced fracture of third metatarsal bone, right foot

⑦S92.332   Displaced fracture of third metatarsal bone, left foot

⑦S92.333   Displaced fracture of third metatarsal bone, unspecified foot

⑦S92.334   Nondisplaced fracture of third metatarsal bone, right foot

⑦S92.335   Nondisplaced fracture of third metatarsal bone, left foot

⑦S92.336   Nondisplaced fracture of third metatarsal bone, unspecified foot

S92.34   Fracture of fourth metatarsal bone

⑦S92.341   Displaced fracture of fourth metatarsal bone, right foot

⑦S92.342   Displaced fracture of fourth metatarsal bone, left foot

⑦S92.343   Displaced fracture of fourth metatarsal bone, unspecified foot

⑦S92.344   Nondisplaced fracture of fourth metatarsal bone, right foot

⑦S92.345   Nondisplaced fracture of fourth metatarsal bone, left foot

⑦S92.346   Nondisplaced fracture of fourth metatarsal bone, unspecified foot

S92.35   Fracture of fifth metatarsal bone

⑦S92.351   Displaced fracture of fifth metatarsal bone, right foot

⑦S92.352   Displaced fracture of fifth metatarsal bone, left foot

⑦S92.353   Displaced fracture of fifth metatarsal bone, unspecified foot

⑦S92.354   Nondisplaced fracture of fifth metatarsal bone, right foot

⑦S92.355   Nondisplaced fracture of fifth metatarsal bone, left foot

⑦S92.356   Nondisplaced fracture of fifth metatarsal bone, unspecified foot

S92.4   Fracture of great toe

S92.40   Unspecified fracture of great toe

⑦S92.401 Displaced unspecified fracture of right great toe

⑦S92.402 Displaced unspecified fracture of left great toe

⑦S92.403 Displaced unspecified fracture of unspecified great toe

⑦S92.404 Nondisplaced unspecified fracture of right great toe

⑦S92.405 Nondisplaced unspecified fracture of left great toe

⑦S92.406 Nondisplaced unspecified fracture of unspecified great toe

S92.41 Fracture of proximal phalanx of great toe

⑦S92.411 Displaced fracture of proximal phalanx of right great toe

⑦S92.412 Displaced fracture of proximal phalanx of left great toe

⑦S92.413 Displaced fracture of proximal phalanx of unspecified great toe

⑦S92.414 Nondisplaced fracture of proximal phalanx of right great toe

⑦S92.415 Nondisplaced fracture of proximal phalanx of left great toe

⑦S92.416 Nondisplaced fracture of proximal phalanx of unspecified great toe

S92.42 Fracture of distal phalanx of great toe

⑦S92.421 Displaced fracture of distal phalanx of right great toe

⑦S92.422 Displaced fracture of distal phalanx of left great toe

⑦S92.423 Displaced fracture of distal phalanx of unspecified great toe

⑦S92.424 Nondisplaced fracture of distal phalanx of right great toe

⑦S92.425 Nondisplaced fracture of distal phalanx of left great toe

⑦S92.426 Nondisplaced fracture of distal phalanx of unspecified great toe

S92.49 Other fracture of great toe

⑦S92.491 Other fracture of right great toe

⑦S92.492 Other fracture of left great toe

⑦S92.499 Other fracture of unspecified great toe

S92.5 Fracture of lesser toe(s)

S92.50 Unspecified fracture of lesser toe(s)

⑦S92.501 Displaced unspecified fracture of right lesser toe(s)

⑦S92.502 Displaced unspecified fracture of left lesser toe(s)

⑦S92.503 Displaced unspecified fracture of unspecified lesser toe(s)

⑦S92.504 Nondisplaced unspecified fracture of right lesser toe(s)

⑦S92.505 Nondisplaced unspecified fracture of left lesser toe(s)

⑦S92.506 Nondisplaced unspecified fracture of unspecified lesser toe(s)

S92.51 Fracture of proximal phalanx of lesser toe(s)

⑦S92.511 Displaced fracture of proximal phalanx of right lesser toe(s)

⑦S92.512 Displaced fracture of proximal phalanx of left lesser toe(s)

⑦S92.513 Displaced fracture of proximal phalanx of unspecified lesser toe(s)

⑦S92.514 Nondisplaced fracture of proximal phalanx of right lesser toe(s)

⑦S92.515 Nondisplaced fracture of proximal phalanx of left lesser toe(s)

⑦S92.516 Nondisplaced fracture of proximal phalanx of unspecified lesser toe(s)

S92.52 Fracture of medial phalanx of lesser toe(s)

⑦S92.521 Displaced fracture of medial phalanx of right lesser toe(s)

⑦S92.522 Displaced fracture of medial phalanx of left lesser toe(s)

⑦S92.523 Displaced fracture of medial phalanx of unspecified lesser toe(s)

⑦S92.524 Nondisplaced fracture of medial phalanx of right lesser toe(s)

⑦S92.525 Nondisplaced fracture of medial phalanx of left lesser toe(s)

⑦S92.526 Nondisplaced fracture of medial phalanx of unspecified lesser toe(s)

S92.53 Fracture of distal phalanx of lesser toe(s)

⑦S92.531 Displaced fracture of distal phalanx of right lesser toe(s)

⑦S92.532 Displaced fracture of distal phalanx of left lesser toe(s)

⑦S92.533 Displaced fracture of distal phalanx of unspecified lesser toe(s)

⑦S92.534 Nondisplaced fracture of distal phalanx of right lesser toe(s)

⑦S92.535 Nondisplaced fracture of distal phalanx of left lesser toe(s)

⑦S92.536 Nondisplaced fracture of distal phalanx of unspecified lesser toe(s)

S92.59 Other fracture of lesser toe(s)

⑦S92.591 Other fracture of right lesser toe(s)

⑦S92.592 Other fracture of left lesser toe(s)

⑦S92.599 Other fracture of unspecified lesser toe(s)

S92.9 Unspecified fracture of foot and toe

S92.90 Unspecified fracture of foot

⑦S92.901 Unspecified fracture of right foot

⑦S92.902 Unspecified fracture of left foot

⑦S92.909 Unspecified fracture of unspecified foot

S92.91 Unspecified fracture of toe

⑦S92.911 Unspecified fracture of right toe(s)

⑦S92.912 Unspecified fracture of left toe(s)

⑦S92.919 Unspecified fracture of unspecified toe(s)

S93 Dislocation and sprain of joints and ligaments at ankle, foot and toe level

Includes: avulsion of joint or ligament of ankle, foot and toe laceration of cartilage, joint or ligament of ankle, foot and toe

sprain of cartilage, joint or ligament of ankle, foot and toe

traumatic hemarthrosis of joint or ligament of ankle, foot and toe

traumatic rupture of joint or ligament of ankle, foot and toe

traumatic subluxation of joint or ligament of ankle, foot and toe

traumatic tear of joint or ligament of ankle, foot and toe

Code also any associated open wound

Excludes 2: strain of muscle and tendon of ankle and foot (S96.-)

The appropriate 7th character is to be added to each code from category S93

A - initial encounter

D - subsequent encounter

S - sequela

S93.0 Subluxation and dislocation of ankle joint

Subluxation and dislocation of astragalus

Subluxation and dislocation of fibula, lower end

Subluxation and dislocation of talus

Subluxation and dislocation of tibia, lower end

⊗⑦**S93.01** Subluxation of right ankle joint

⊗⑦**S93.02** Subluxation of left ankle joint

⊗⑦**S93.03** Subluxation of unspecified ankle joint

⊗⑦**S93.04** Dislocation of right ankle joint

⊗⑦**S93.05** Dislocation of left ankle joint

⊗⑦**S93.06** Dislocation of unspecified ankle joint

S93.1 Subluxation and dislocation of toe

S93.10 Unspecified subluxation and dislocation of toe

Dislocation of toe NOS

Subluxation of toe NOS

⑦**S93.101** Unspecified subluxation of right toe(s)

⑦**S93.102** Unspecified subluxation of left toe(s)

⑦**S93.103** Unspecified subluxation of unspecified toe(s)

⑦**S93.104** Unspecified dislocation of right toe(s)

⑦**S93.105** Unspecified dislocation of left toe(s)

⑦**S93.106** Unspecified dislocation of unspecified toe(s)

S93.11 Dislocation of interphalangeal joint

⑦**S93.111** Dislocation of interphalangeal joint of right great toe

⑦**S93.112** Dislocation of interphalangeal joint of left great toe

⑦**S93.113** Dislocation of interphalangeal joint of unspecified great toe

⑦**S93.114** Dislocation of interphalangeal joint of right lesser toe(s)

⑦**S93.115** Dislocation of interphalangeal joint of left lesser toe(s)

⑦**S93.116** Dislocation of interphalangeal joint of unspecified lesser toe(s)

⑦**S93.119** Dislocation of interphalangeal joint of unspecified toe(s)

S93.12 Dislocation of metatarsophalangeal joint

⑦**S93.121** Dislocation of metatarsophalangeal joint of right great toe

⑦**S93.122** Dislocation of metatarsophalangeal joint of left great toe

⑦**S93.123** Dislocation of metatarsophalangeal joint of unspecified great toe

⑦**S93.124** Dislocation of metatarsophalangeal joint of right lesser toe(s)

⑦**S93.125** Dislocation of metatarsophalangeal joint of left lesser toe(s)

⑦**S93.126** Dislocation of metatarsophalangeal joint of unspecified lesser toe(s)

⑦**S93.129** Dislocation of metatarsophalangeal joint of unspecified toe(s)

S93.13 Subluxation of interphalangeal joint

⑦**S93.131** Subluxation of interphalangeal joint of right great toe

⑦**S93.132** Subluxation of interphalangeal joint of left great toe

⑦**S93.133** Subluxation of interphalangeal joint of unspecified great toe

⑦**S93.134** Subluxation of interphalangeal joint of right lesser toe(s)

⑦**S93.135** Subluxation of interphalangeal joint of left lesser toe(s)

⑦**S93.136** Subluxation of interphalangeal joint of unspecified lesser toe(s)

⑦**S93.139** Subluxation of interphalangeal joint of unspecified toe(s)

S93.14 Subluxation of metatarsophalangeal joint

⑦**S93.141** Subluxation of metatarsophalangeal joint of right great toe

⑦**S93.142** Subluxation of metatarsophalangeal joint of left great toe

⑦**S93.143** Subluxation of metatarsophalangeal joint of unspecified great toe

⑦**S93.144** Subluxation of metatarsophalangeal joint of right lesser toe(s)

⑦**S93.145** Subluxation of metatarsophalangeal joint of left lesser toe(s)

⑦**S93.146** Subluxation of metatarsophalangeal joint of unspecified lesser toe(s)

⑦**S93.149** Subluxation of metatarsophalangeal joint of unspecified toe(s)

S93.3 Subluxation and dislocation of foot

Excludes 2: dislocation of toe (S93.1-)

S93.30 Unspecified subluxation and dislocation of foot

Dislocation of foot NOS

Subluxation of foot NOS

⑦**S93.301** Unspecified subluxation of right foot

⑦**S93.302** Unspecified subluxation of left foot

⑦**S93.303** Unspecified subluxation of unspecified foot

⑦**S93.304** Unspecified dislocation of right foot

⑦**S93.305** Unspecified dislocation of left foot

⑦**S93.306** Unspecified dislocation of unspecified foot

S93.31   Subluxation and dislocation of tarsal joint
    ⑦S93.311   Subluxation of tarsal joint of right foot
    ⑦S93.312   Subluxation of tarsal joint of left foot
    ⑦S93.313   Subluxation of tarsal joint of unspecified foot
    ⑦S93.314   Dislocation of tarsal joint of right foot
    ⑦S93.315   Dislocation of tarsal joint of left foot
    ⑦S93.316   Dislocation of tarsal joint of unspecified foot

S93.32   Subluxation and dislocation of tarsometatarsal joint
    ⑦S93.321   Subluxation of tarsometatarsal joint of right foot
    ⑦S93.322   Subluxation of tarsometatarsal joint of left foot
    ⑦S93.323   Subluxation of tarsometatarsal joint of unspecified foot
    ⑦S93.324   Dislocation of tarsometatarsal joint of right foot
    ⑦S93.325   Dislocation of tarsometatarsal joint of left foot
    ⑦S93.326   Dislocation of tarsometatarsal joint of unspecified foot

S93.33   Other subluxation and dislocation of foot
    ⑦S93.331   Other subluxation of right foot
    ⑦S93.332   Other subluxation of left foot
    ⑦S93.333   Other subluxation of unspecified foot
    ⑦S93.334   Other dislocation of right foot
    ⑦S93.335   Other dislocation of left foot
    ⑦S93.336   Other dislocation of unspecified foot

S93.4   Sprain of ankle
  Excludes 2: injury of Achilles tendon (S86.0-)

S93.40   Sprain of unspecified ligament of ankle
    Sprain of ankle NOS
    Sprained ankle NOS
    ⑦S93.401   Sprain of unspecified ligament of right ankle
    ⑦S93.402   Sprain of unspecified ligament of left ankle
    ⑦S93.409   Sprain of unspecified ligament of unspecified ankle

S93.41   Sprain of calcaneofibular ligament
    ⑦S93.411   Sprain of calcaneofibular ligament of right ankle
    ⑦S93.412   Sprain of calcaneofibular ligament of left ankle
    ⑦S93.419   Sprain of calcaneofibular ligament of unspecified ankle

S93.42   Sprain of deltoid ligament
    ⑦S93.421   Sprain of deltoid ligament of right ankle
    ⑦S93.422   Sprain of deltoid ligament of left ankle
    ⑦S93.429   Sprain of deltoid ligament of unspecified ankle

S93.43   Sprain of tibiofibular ligament
    ⑦S93.431   Sprain of tibiofibular ligament of right ankle
    ⑦S93.432   Sprain of tibiofibular ligament of left ankle
    ⑦S93.439   Sprain of tibiofibular ligament of unspecified ankle

S93.49   Sprain of other ligament of ankle
    Sprain of internal collateral ligament
    Sprain of talofibular ligament
    ⑦S93.491   Sprain of other ligament of right ankle
    ⑦S93.492   Sprain of other ligament of left ankle
    ⑦S93.499   Sprain of other ligament of unspecified ankle

S93.5   Sprain of toe
S93.50   Unspecified sprain of toe
    ⑦S93.501   Unspecified sprain of right great toe
    ⑦S93.502   Unspecified sprain of left great toe
    ⑦S93.503   Unspecified sprain of unspecified great toe
    ⑦S93.504   Unspecified sprain of right lesser toe(s)
    ⑦S93.505   Unspecified sprain of left lesser toe(s)
    ⑦S93.506   Unspecified sprain of unspecified lesser toe(s)
    ⑦S93.509   Unspecified sprain of unspecified toe(s)

S93.51   Sprain of interphalangeal joint of toe
    ⑦S93.511   Sprain of interphalangeal joint of right great toe
    ⑦S93.512   Sprain of interphalangeal joint of left great toe
    ⑦S93.513   Sprain of interphalangeal joint of unspecified great toe
    ⑦S93.514   Sprain of interphalangeal joint of right lesser toe(s)
    ⑦S93.515   Sprain of interphalangeal joint of left lesser toe(s)
    ⑦S93.516   Sprain of interphalangeal joint of unspecified lesser toe(s)
    ⑦S93.519   Sprain of interphalangeal joint of unspecified toe(s)

S93.52   Sprain of metatarsophalangeal joint of toe
    ⑦S93.521   Sprain of metatarsophalangeal joint of right great toe
    ⑦S93.522   Sprain of metatarsophalangeal joint of left great toe
    ⑦S93.523   Sprain of metatarsophalangeal joint of unspecified great toe
    ⑦S93.524   Sprain of metatarsophalangeal joint of right lesser toe(s)
    ⑦S93.525   Sprain of metatarsophalangeal joint of left lesser toe(s)

⑦S93.526   Sprain of metatarsophalangeal joint of unspecified lesser toe(s)

⑦S93.529   Sprain of metatarsophalangeal joint of unspecified toe(s)

S93.6   Sprain of foot

Excludes 2: sprain of metatarsophalangeal joint of toe (S93.52-)

      sprain of toe (S93.5-)

S93.60   Unspecified sprain of foot

⑦S93.601   Unspecified sprain of right foot

⑦S93.602   Unspecified sprain of left foot

⑦S93.609   Unspecified sprain of unspecified foot

S93.61   Sprain of tarsal ligament of foot

⑦S93.611   Sprain of tarsal ligament of right foot

⑦S93.612   Sprain of tarsal ligament of left foot

⑦S93.619   Sprain of tarsal ligament of unspecified foot

S93.62   Sprain of tarsometatarsal ligament of foot

⑦S93.621   Sprain of tarsometatarsal ligament of right foot

⑦S93.622   Sprain of tarsometatarsal ligament of left foot

⑦S93.629   Sprain of tarsometatarsal ligament of unspecified foot

S93.69   Other sprain of foot

⑦S93.691   Other sprain of right foot

⑦S93.692   Other sprain of left foot

⑦S93.699   Other sprain of unspecified foot

S94   Injury of nerves at ankle and foot level

Code also any associated open wound (S91.-)

The appropriate 7th character is to be added to each code from category S94

A - initial encounter

D - subsequent encounter

S - sequela

S94.0   Injury of lateral plantar nerve

⊗⑦S94.00   Injury of lateral plantar nerve, unspecified leg

⊗⑦S94.01   Injury of lateral plantar nerve, right leg

⊗⑦S94.02   Injury of lateral plantar nerve, left leg

S94.1   Injury of medial plantar nerve

⊗⑦S94.10   Injury of medial plantar nerve, unspecified leg

⊗⑦S94.11   Injury of medial plantar nerve, right leg

⊗⑦S94.12   Injury of medial plantar nerve, left leg

S94.2   Injury of deep peroneal nerve at ankle and foot level

Injury of terminal, lateral branch of deep peroneal nerve

⊗⑦S94.20   Injury of deep peroneal nerve at ankle and foot level, unspecified leg

⊗⑦S94.21   Injury of deep peroneal nerve at ankle and foot level, right leg

⊗⑦S94.22   Injury of deep peroneal nerve at ankle and foot level, left leg

S94.3   Injury of cutaneous sensory nerve at ankle and foot level

⊗⑦S94.30   Injury of cutaneous sensory nerve at ankle and foot level, unspecified leg

⊗⑦S94.31   Injury of cutaneous sensory nerve at ankle and foot level, right leg

⊗⑦S94.32   Injury of cutaneous sensory nerve at ankle and foot level, left leg

S94.8   Injury of other nerves at ankle and foot level

S94.8X   Injury of other nerves at ankle and foot level

⑦S94.8X1   Injury of other nerves at ankle and foot level, right leg

⑦S94.8X2   Injury of other nerves at ankle and foot level, left leg

⑦S94.8X9   Injury of other nerves at ankle and foot level, unspecified leg

S94.9   Injury of unspecified nerve at ankle and foot level

⊗⑦S94.90   Injury of unspecified nerve at ankle and foot level, unspecified leg

⊗⑦S94.91   Injury of unspecified nerve at ankle and foot level, right leg

⊗⑦S94.92   Injury of unspecified nerve at ankle and foot level, left leg

S95   Injury of blood vessels at ankle and foot level

Code also any associated open wound (S91.-)

Excludes 2: injury of posterior tibial artery and vein (S85.1-, S85.8-)

The appropriate 7th character is to be added to each code from category S95

A - initial encounter

D - subsequent encounter

S - sequela

S95.0   Injury of dorsal artery of foot

S95.00   Unspecified injury of dorsal artery of foot

⑦S95.001   Unspecified injury of dorsal artery of right foot

⑦S95.002   Unspecified injury of dorsal artery of left foot

⑦S95.009   Unspecified injury of dorsal artery of unspecified foot

S95.01   Laceration of dorsal artery of foot

⑦S95.011   Laceration of dorsal artery of right foot

⑦S95.012   Laceration of dorsal artery of left foot

⑦S95.019   Laceration of dorsal artery of unspecified foot

S95.09   Other specified injury of dorsal artery of foot

⑦S95.091   Other specified injury of dorsal artery of right foot

⑦S95.092   Other specified injury of dorsal artery of left foot

⑦S95.099   Other specified injury of dorsal artery of unspecified foot

S95.1   Injury of plantar artery of foot

S95.10   Unspecified injury of plantar artery of foot

⑦S95.101   Unspecified injury of plantar artery of right foot

⑦S95.102   Unspecified injury of plantar artery of left foot

⑦S95.109   Unspecified injury of plantar artery of unspecified foot

S95.11   Laceration of plantar artery of foot

⑦S95.111   Laceration of plantar artery of right foot

⑦S95.112　Laceration of plantar artery of left foot

⑦S95.119　Laceration of plantar artery of unspecified foot

S95.19　Other specified injury of plantar artery of foot

⑦S95.191　Other specified injury of plantar artery of right foot

⑦S95.192　Other specified injury of plantar artery of left foot

⑦S95.199　Other specified injury of plantar artery of unspecified foot

S95.2　Injury of dorsal vein of foot

S95.20　Unspecified injury of dorsal vein of foot

⑦S95.201　Unspecified injury of dorsal vein of right foot

⑦S95.202　Unspecified injury of dorsal vein of left foot

⑦S95.209　Unspecified injury of dorsal vein of unspecified foot

S95.21　Laceration of dorsal vein of foot

⑦S95.211　Laceration of dorsal vein of right foot

⑦S95.212　Laceration of dorsal vein of left foot

⑦S95.219　Laceration of dorsal vein of unspecified foot

S95.29　Other specified injury of dorsal vein of foot

⑦S95.291　Other specified injury of dorsal vein of right foot

⑦S95.292　Other specified injury of dorsal vein of left foot

⑦S95.299　Other specified injury of dorsal vein of unspecified foot

S95.8　Injury of other blood vessels at ankle and foot level

S95.80　Unspecified injury of other blood vessels at ankle and foot level

⑦S95.801　Unspecified injury of other blood vessels at ankle and foot level, right leg

⑦S95.802　Unspecified injury of other blood vessels at ankle and foot level, left leg

⑦S95.809　Unspecified injury of other blood vessels at ankle and foot level, unspecified leg

S95.81　Laceration of other blood vessels at ankle and foot level

⑦S95.811　Laceration of other blood vessels at ankle and foot level, right leg

⑦S95.812　Laceration of other blood vessels at ankle and foot level, left leg

⑦S95.819　Laceration of other blood vessels at ankle and foot level, unspecified leg

S95.89　Other specified injury of other blood vessels at ankle and foot level

⑦S95.891　Other specified injury of other blood vessels at ankle and foot level, right leg

⑦S95.892　Other specified injury of other blood vessels at ankle and foot level, left leg

⑦S95.899　Other specified injury of other blood vessels at ankle and foot level, unspecified leg

S95.9　Injury of unspecified blood vessel at ankle and foot level

S95.90　Unspecified injury of unspecified blood vessel at ankle and foot level

⑦S95.901　Unspecified injury of unspecified blood vessel at ankle and foot level, right leg

⑦S95.902　Unspecified injury of unspecified blood vessel at ankle and foot level, left leg

⑦S95.909　Unspecified injury of unspecified blood vessel at ankle and foot level, unspecified leg

S95.91　Laceration of unspecified blood vessel at ankle and foot level

⑦S95.911　Laceration of unspecified blood vessel at ankle and foot level, right leg

⑦S95.912　Laceration of unspecified blood vessel at ankle and foot level, left leg

⑦S95.919　Laceration of unspecified blood vessel at ankle and foot level, unspecified leg

S95.99　Other specified injury of unspecified blood vessel at ankle and foot level

⑦S95.991　Other specified injury of unspecified blood vessel at ankle and foot level, right leg

⑦S95.992　Other specified injury of unspecified blood vessel at ankle and foot level, left leg

⑦S95.999　Other specified injury of unspecified blood vessel at ankle and foot level, unspecified leg

S96　Injury of muscle and tendon at ankle and foot level

Code also any associated open wound (S91.-)

Excludes 2: injury of Achilles tendon (S86.0-)

sprain of joints and ligaments of ankle and foot (S93.-)

The appropriate 7th character is to be added to each code from category S96

A - initial encounter

D - subsequent encounter

S û sequela

S96.0　Injury of muscle and tendon of long flexor muscle of toe at ankle and foot level

S96.00　Unspecified injury of muscle and tendon of long flexor muscle of toe at ankle and foot level

⑦S96.001　Unspecified injury of muscle and tendon of long flexor muscle of toe at ankle and foot level, right foot

⑦S96.002　Unspecified injury of muscle and tendon of long flexor muscle of toe at ankle and foot level, left foot

● New code　　　▲ Revised code　　　⑦ 7th digit required　　　⊗ Placeholder required

⑦S96.009   Unspecified injury of muscle and tendon of long flexor muscle of toe at ankle and foot level, unspecified foot

⑦S96.01   Strain of muscle and tendon of long flexor muscle of toe at ankle and foot level

⑦S96.011   Strain of muscle and tendon of long flexor muscle of toe at ankle and foot level, right foot

⑦S96.012   Strain of muscle and tendon of long flexor muscle of toe at ankle and foot level, left foot

⑦S96.019   Strain of muscle and tendon of long flexor muscle of toe at ankle and foot level, unspecified foot

S96.02   Laceration of muscle and tendon of long flexor muscle of toe at ankle and foot level

⑦S96.021   Laceration of muscle and tendon of long flexor muscle of toe at ankle and foot level, right foot

⑦S96.022   Laceration of muscle and tendon of long flexor muscle of toe at ankle and foot level, left foot

⑦S96.029   Laceration of muscle and tendon of long flexor muscle of toe at ankle and foot level, unspecified foot

S96.09   Other injury of muscle and tendon of long flexor muscle of toe at ankle and foot level

⑦S96.091   Other injury of muscle and tendon of long flexor muscle of toe at ankle and foot level, right foot

⑦S96.092   Other injury of muscle and tendon of long flexor muscle of toe at ankle and foot level, left foot

⑦S96.099   Other injury of muscle and tendon of long flexor muscle of toe at ankle and foot level, unspecified foot

S96.1   Injury of muscle and tendon of long extensor muscle of toe at ankle and foot level

S96.10   Unspecified injury of muscle and tendon of long extensor muscle of toe at ankle and foot level

⑦S96.101   Unspecified injury of muscle and tendon of long extensor muscle of toe at ankle and foot level, right foot

⑦S96.102   Unspecified injury of muscle and tendon of long extensor muscle of toe at ankle and foot level, left foot

⑦S96.109   Unspecified injury of muscle and tendon of long extensor muscle of toe at ankle and foot level, unspecified foot

S96.11   Strain of muscle and tendon of long extensor muscle of toe at ankle and foot level

⑦S96.111   Strain of muscle and tendon of long extensor muscle of toe at ankle and foot level, right foot

⑦S96.112   Strain of muscle and tendon of long extensor muscle of toe at ankle and foot level, left foot

⑦S96.119   Strain of muscle and tendon of long extensor muscle of toe at ankle and foot level, unspecified foot

S96.12   Laceration of muscle and tendon of long extensor muscle of toe at ankle and foot level

⑦S96.121   Laceration of muscle and tendon of long extensor muscle of toe at ankle and foot level, right foot

⑦S96.122   Laceration of muscle and tendon of long extensor muscle of toe at ankle and foot level, left foot

⑦S96.129   Laceration of muscle and tendon of long extensor muscle of toe at ankle and foot level, unspecified foot

S96.19   Other specified injury of muscle and tendon of long extensor muscle of toe at ankle and foot level

⑦S96.191   Other specified injury of muscle and tendon of long extensor muscle of toe at ankle and foot level, right foot

⑦S96.192   Other specified injury of muscle and tendon of long extensor muscle of toe at ankle and foot level, left foot

⑦S96.199   Other specified injury of muscle and tendon of long extensor muscle of toe at ankle and foot level, unspecified foot

S96.2   Injury of intrinsic muscle and tendon at ankle and foot level

S96.20   Unspecified injury of intrinsic muscle and tendon at ankle and foot level

⑦S96.201   Unspecified injury of intrinsic muscle and tendon at ankle and foot level, right foot

⑦S96.202   Unspecified injury of intrinsic muscle and tendon at ankle and foot level, left foot

⑦S96.209   Unspecified injury of intrinsic muscle and tendon at ankle and foot level, unspecified foot

S96.21   Strain of intrinsic muscle and tendon at ankle and foot level

⑦S96.211   Strain of intrinsic muscle and tendon at ankle and foot level, right foot

⑦S96.212   Strain of intrinsic muscle and tendon at ankle and foot level, left foot

⑦S96.219   Strain of intrinsic muscle and tendon at ankle and foot level, unspecified foot

S96.22   Laceration of intrinsic muscle and tendon at ankle and foot level

⑦S96.221   Laceration of intrinsic muscle and tendon at ankle and foot level, right foot

⑦S96.222   Laceration of intrinsic muscle and tendon at ankle and foot level, left foot

⑦S96.229   Laceration of intrinsic muscle and tendon at ankle and foot level, unspecified foot

S96.29   Other specified injury of intrinsic muscle and tendon at ankle and foot level

⑦S96.291   Other specified injury of intrinsic muscle and tendon at ankle and foot level, right foot

⑦S96.292   Other specified injury of intrinsic muscle and tendon at ankle and foot level, left foot

⑦S96.299   Other specified injury of intrinsic muscle and tendon at ankle and foot level, unspecified foot

S96.8   Injury of other specified muscles and tendons at ankle and foot level

S96.80   Unspecified injury of other specified muscles and tendons at ankle and foot level

⑦S96.801   Unspecified injury of other specified muscles and tendons at ankle and foot level, right foot

⑦S96.802   Unspecified injury of other specified muscles and tendons at ankle and foot level, left foot

⑦S96.809   Unspecified injury of other specified muscles and tendons at ankle and foot level, unspecified foot

S96.81   Strain of other specified muscles and tendons at ankle and foot level

⑦S96.811   Strain of other specified muscles and tendons at ankle and foot level, right foot

⑦S96.812   Strain of other specified muscles and tendons at ankle and foot level, left foot

⑦S96.819   Strain of other specified muscles and tendons at ankle and foot level, unspecified foot

S96.82   Laceration of other specified muscles and tendons at ankle and foot level

⑦S96.821   Laceration of other specified muscles and tendons at ankle and foot level, right foot

⑦S96.822   Laceration of other specified muscles and tendons at ankle and foot level, left foot

⑦S96.829   Laceration of other specified muscles and tendons at ankle and foot level, unspecified foot

S96.89   Other specified injury of other specified muscles and tendons at ankle and foot level

⑦S96.891   Other specified injury of other specified muscles and tendons at ankle and foot level, right foot

⑦S96.892   Other specified injury of other specified muscles and tendons at ankle and foot level, left foot

⑦S96.899   Other specified injury of other specified muscles and tendons at ankle and foot level, unspecified foot

S96.9   Injury of unspecified muscle and tendon at ankle and foot level

S96.90   Unspecified injury of unspecified muscle and tendon at ankle and foot level

⑦S96.901   Unspecified injury of unspecified muscle and tendon at ankle and foot level, right foot

⑦S96.902   Unspecified injury of unspecified muscle and tendon at ankle and foot level, left foot

⑦S96.909   Unspecified injury of unspecified muscle and tendon at ankle and foot level, unspecified foot

S96.91   Strain of unspecified muscle and tendon at ankle and foot level

⑦S96.911   Strain of unspecified muscle and tendon at ankle and foot level, right foot

⑦S96.912   Strain of unspecified muscle and tendon at ankle and foot level, left foot

⑦S96.919   Strain of unspecified muscle and tendon at ankle and foot level, unspecified foot

S96.92   Laceration of unspecified muscle and tendon at ankle and foot level

⑦S96.921   Laceration of unspecified muscle and tendon at ankle and foot level, right foot

⑦S96.922   Laceration of unspecified muscle and tendon at ankle and foot level, left foot

⑦S96.929   Laceration of unspecified muscle and tendon at ankle and foot level, unspecified foot

S96.99   Other specified injury of unspecified muscle and tendon at ankle and foot level

⑦S96.991   Other specified injury of unspecified muscle and tendon at ankle and foot level, right foot

⑦S96.992   Other specified injury of unspecified muscle and tendon at ankle and foot level, left foot

⑦S96.999   Other specified injury of unspecified muscle and tendon at ankle and foot level, unspecified foot

S97   Crushing injury of ankle and foot

Use additional code(s) for all associated injuries

The appropriate 7th character is to be added to each code from category S97

A - initial encounter

D - subsequent encounter

S - sequela

S97.0   Crushing injury of ankle

⊗⑦S97.00   Crushing injury of unspecified ankle

⊗⑦S97.01   Crushing injury of right ankle

⊗⑦S97.02   Crushing injury of left ankle

S97.1   Crushing injury of toe

S97.10   Crushing injury of unspecified toe(s)

● New code   ▲ Revised code   ⑦ 7th digit required   ⊗ Placeholder required

⑦**S97.101** Crushing injury of unspecified right toe(s)

⑦**S97.102** Crushing injury of unspecified left toe(s)

⑦**S97.109** Crushing injury of unspecified toe(s)
Crushing injury of toe NOS

S97.11 Crushing injury of great toe

⑦**S97.111** Crushing injury of right great toe

⑦**S97.112** Crushing injury of left great toe

⑦**S97.119** Crushing injury of unspecified great toe

S97.12 Crushing injury of lesser toe(s)

⑦**S97.121** Crushing injury of right lesser toe(s)

⑦**S97.122** Crushing injury of left lesser toe(s)

⑦**S97.129** Crushing injury of unspecified lesser toe(s)

S97.8 Crushing injury of foot

⊗⑦**S97.80** Crushing injury of unspecified foot
Crushing injury of foot NOS

⊗⑦**S97.81** Crushing injury of right foot

⊗⑦**S97.82** Crushing injury of left foot

S98 Traumatic amputation of ankle and foot

An amputation not identified as partial or complete should be coded to complete

The appropriate 7th character is to be added to each code from category S98

A - initial encounter

D - subsequent encounter

S - sequela

S98.0 Traumatic amputation of foot at ankle level

S98.01 Complete traumatic amputation of foot at ankle level

⑦**S98.011** Complete traumatic amputation of right foot at ankle level

⑦**S98.012** Complete traumatic amputation of left foot at ankle level

⑦**S98.019** Complete traumatic amputation of unspecified foot at ankle level

S98.02 Partial traumatic amputation of foot at ankle level

⑦**S98.021** Partial traumatic amputation of right foot at ankle level

⑦**S98.022** Partial traumatic amputation of left foot at ankle level

⑦**S98.029** Partial traumatic amputation of unspecified foot at ankle level

S98.1 Traumatic amputation of one toe

S98.11 Complete traumatic amputation of great toe

⑦**S98.111** Complete traumatic amputation of right great toe

⑦**S98.112** Complete traumatic amputation of left great toe

⑦**S98.119** Complete traumatic amputation of unspecified great toe

S98.12 Partial traumatic amputation of great toe

⑦**S98.121** Partial traumatic amputation of right great toe

⑦**S98.122** Partial traumatic amputation of left great toe

⑦**S98.129** Partial traumatic amputation of unspecified great toe

S98.13 Complete traumatic amputation of one lesser toe
Traumatic amputation of toe NOS

⑦**S98.131** Complete traumatic amputation of one right lesser toe

⑦**S98.132** Complete traumatic amputation of one left lesser toe

⑦**S98.139** Complete traumatic amputation of one unspecified lesser toe

S98.14 Partial traumatic amputation of one lesser toe

⑦**S98.141** Partial traumatic amputation of one right lesser toe

⑦**S98.142** Partial traumatic amputation of one left lesser toe

⑦**S98.149** Partial traumatic amputation of one unspecified lesser toe

S98.2 Traumatic amputation of two or more lesser toes

S98.21 Complete traumatic amputation of two or more lesser toes

⑦**S98.211** Complete traumatic amputation of two or more right lesser toes

⑦**S98.212** Complete traumatic amputation of two or more left lesser toes

⑦**S98.219** Complete traumatic amputation of two or more unspecified lesser toes

S98.22 Partial traumatic amputation of two or more lesser toes

⑦**S98.221** Partial traumatic amputation of two or more right lesser toes

⑦**S98.222** Partial traumatic amputation of two or more left lesser toes

⑦**S98.229** Partial traumatic amputation of two or more unspecified lesser toes

S98.3 Traumatic amputation of midfoot

S98.31 Complete traumatic amputation of midfoot

⑦**S98.311** Complete traumatic amputation of right midfoot

⑦**S98.312** Complete traumatic amputation of left midfoot

⑦**S98.319** Complete traumatic amputation of unspecified midfoot

S98.32 Partial traumatic amputation of midfoot

⑦**S98.321** Partial traumatic amputation of right midfoot

⑦**S98.322** Partial traumatic amputation of left midfoot

⑦**S98.329** Partial traumatic amputation of unspecified midfoot

S98.9 Traumatic amputation of foot, level unspecified

S98.91 Complete traumatic amputation of foot, level unspecified

⑦**S98.911** Complete traumatic amputation of right foot, level unspecified

⑦**S98.912** Complete traumatic amputation of left foot, level unspecified

⑦**S98.919** Complete traumatic amputation of unspecified foot, level unspecified

S98.92 Partial traumatic amputation of foot, level unspecified

⑦**S98.921** Partial traumatic amputation of right foot, level unspecified

⑦**S98.922** Partial traumatic amputation of left foot, level unspecified

⑦**S98.929** Partial traumatic amputation of unspecified foot, level unspecified

S09 Other and unspecified injuries of ankle and foot

The appropriate 7th character is to be added to each code from category S99

A - initial encounter

D - subsequent encounter

S - sequela

S99.8 Other specified injuries of ankle and foot

S99.81 Other specified injuries of ankle

⑦**S99.811** Other specified injuries of right ankle

⑦**S99.812** Other specified injuries of left ankle

⑦**S99.819** Other specified injuries of unspecified ankle

S99.82 Other specified injuries of foot

⑦**S99.821** Other specified injuries of right foot

⑦**S99.822** Other specified injuries of left foot

⑦**S99.829** Other specified injuries of unspecified foot

S99.9 Unspecified injury of ankle and foot

S99.91 Unspecified injury of ankle

⑦**S99.911** Unspecified injury of right ankle

⑦**S99.912** Unspecified injury of left ankle

⑦**S99.919** Unspecified injury of unspecified ankle

S99.92 Unspecified injury of foot

⑦**S99.921** Unspecified injury of right foot

⑦**S99.922** Unspecified injury of left foot

⑦**S99.929** Unspecified injury of unspecified foot

INJURY, POISONING AND CERTAIN OTHER CONSEQUENCES OF EXTERNAL CAUSES (T07-T88)

INJURIES INVOLVING MULTIPLE BODY REGIONS (T07)

Excludes 1: burns and corrosions (T20-T32)

frostbite (T33-T34)

insect bite or sting, venomous (T63.4)

sunburn (L55.-)

T07 Unspecified multiple injuries

Excludes 1: injury NOS (T14)

INJURY OF UNSPECIFIED BODY REGION (T14)

T14 Injury of unspecified body region

Excludes 1: multiple unspecified injuries (T07)

⊗⑦**T14.8** Other injury of unspecified body region

Abrasion NOS

Contusion NOS

Crush injury NOS

Fracture NOS

Skin injury NOS

Vascular injury NOS

T14.9 Unspecified injury

⊗⑦**T14.90** Injury, unspecified

Injury NOS

⊗⑦**T14.91** Suicide attempt

Attempted suicide NOS

EFFECTS OF FOREIGN BODY ENTERING THROUGH NATURAL ORIFICE (T15-T19)

Excludes 2: foreign body accidentally left in operation wound (T81.5-)

foreign body in penetrating wound - See open wound by body region

residual foreign body in soft tissue (M79.5)

splinter, without open wound - See superficial injury by body region

T15 Foreign body on external eye

Excludes 2: foreign body in penetrating wound of orbit and eye ball (S05.4-, S05.5-)

open wound of eyelid and periocular area (S01.1-)

retained foreign body in eyelid (H02.8-)

retained (old) foreign body in penetrating wound of orbit and eye ball (H05.5-, H44.6-, H44.7-)

superficial foreign body of eyelid and periocular area (S00.25-)

The appropriate 7th character is to be added to each code from category T15

A - initial encounter

D - subsequent encounter

S - sequela

T15.0 Foreign body in cornea

⊗⑦**T15.00** Foreign body in cornea, unspecified eye

⊗⑦**T15.01** Foreign body in cornea, right eye

⊗⑦**T15.02** Foreign body in cornea, left eye

T15.1 Foreign body in conjunctival sac

⊗⑦**T15.10** Foreign body in conjunctival sac, unspecified eye

⊗⑦**T15.11** Foreign body in conjunctival sac, right eye

⊗⑦**T15.12** Foreign body in conjunctival sac, left eye

T15.8 Foreign body in other and multiple parts of external eye

Foreign body in lacrimal punctum

⊗⑦**T15.80** Foreign body in other and multiple parts of external eye, unspecified eye

⊗⑦**T15.81** Foreign body in other and multiple parts of external eye, right eye

⊗⑦**T15.82** Foreign body in other and multiple parts of external eye, left eye

T15.9 Foreign body on external eye, part unspecified

⊗⑦**T15.90** Foreign body on external eye, part unspecified, unspecified eye

⊗⑦**T15.91** Foreign body on external eye, part unspecified, right eye

⊗⑦**T15.92** Foreign body on external eye, part unspecified, left eye

T16 Foreign body in ear

Includes: foreign body in auditory canal

The appropriate 7th character is to be added to each code from category T16

A - initial encounter

D - subsequent encounter

S - sequela

⊗⑦**T16.1** Foreign body in right ear

⊗⑦**T16.2** Foreign body in left ear

⊗⑦**T16.9** Foreign body in ear, unspecified ear

T17 Foreign body in respiratory tract

The appropriate 7th character is to be added to each code from category T17

A - initial encounter

D - subsequent encounter

S - sequela

⊗⑦**T17.0** Foreign body in nasal sinus

⊗⑦**T17.1** Foreign body in nostril

Foreign body in nose NOS

T17.2 Foreign body in pharynx

Foreign body in nasopharynx

Foreign body in throat NOS

    T17.20 Unspecified foreign body in pharynx

      ⑦**T17.200** Unspecified foreign body in pharynx causing asphyxiation

      ⑦**T17.208** Unspecified foreign body in pharynx causing other injury

    T17.21 Gastric contents in pharynx

Aspiration of gastric contents into pharynx

Vomitus in pharynx

      ⑦**T17.210** Gastric contents in pharynx causing asphyxiation

      ⑦**T17.218** Gastric contents in pharynx causing other injury

    T17.22 Food in pharynx

Bones in pharynx

Seeds in pharynx

      ⑦**T17.220** Food in pharynx causing asphyxiation

      ⑦**T17.228** Food in pharynx causing other injury

    T17.29 Other foreign object in pharynx

      ⑦**T17.290** Other foreign object in pharynx causing asphyxiation

      ⑦**T17.298** Other foreign object in pharynx causing other injury

T17.3 Foreign body in larynx

    T17.30 Unspecified foreign body in larynx

      ⑦**T17.300** Unspecified foreign body in larynx causing asphyxiation

      ⑦**T17.308** Unspecified foreign body in larynx causing other injury

    T17.31 Gastric contents in larynx

Aspiration of gastric contents into larynx

Vomitus in larynx

      ⑦**T17.310** Gastric contents in larynx causing asphyxiation

      ⑦**T17.318** Gastric contents in larynx causing other injury

    T17.32 Food in larynx

ones in larynx

Seeds in larynx

      ⑦**T17.320** Food in larynx causing asphyxiation

      ⑦**T17.328** Food in larynx causing other injury

    T17.39 Other foreign object in larynx

      ⑦**T17.390** Other foreign object in larynx causing asphyxiation

      ⑦**T17.398** Other foreign object in larynx causing other injury

T17.4 Foreign body in trachea

    T17.40 Unspecified foreign body in trachea

      ⑦**T17.400** Unspecified foreign body in trachea causing asphyxiation

      ⑦**T17.408** Unspecified foreign body in trachea causing other injury

    T17.41 Gastric contents in trachea

Aspiration of gastric contents into trachea

Vomitus in trachea

      ⑦**T17.410** Gastric contents in trachea causing asphyxiation

      ⑦**T17.418** Gastric contents in trachea causing other injury

    T17.42 Food in trachea

Bones in trachea

Seeds in trachea

      ⑦**T17.420** Food in trachea causing asphyxiation

      ⑦**T17.428** Food in trachea causing other injury

    T17.49 Other foreign object in trachea

      ⑦**T17.490** Other foreign object in trachea causing asphyxiation

      ⑦**T17.498** Other foreign object in trachea causing other injury

T17.5 Foreign body in bronchus

    T17.50 Unspecified foreign body in bronchus

      ⑦**T17.500** Unspecified foreign body in bronchus causing asphyxiation

      ⑦**T17.508** Unspecified foreign body in bronchus causing other injury

    T17.51 Gastric contents in bronchus

Aspiration of gastric contents into bronchus

Vomitus in bronchus

      ⑦**T17.510** Gastric contents in bronchus causing asphyxiation

      ⑦**T17.518** Gastric contents in bronchus causing other injury

    T17.52 Food in bronchus

Bones in bronchus

Seeds in bronchus

      ⑦**T17.520** Food in bronchus causing asphyxiation

      ⑦**T17.528** Food in bronchus causing other injury

    T17.59 Other foreign object in bronchus

      ⑦**T17.590** Other foreign object in bronchus causing asphyxiation

      ⑦**T17.598** Other foreign object in bronchus causing other injury

T17.8 Foreign body in other parts of respiratory tract
Foreign body in bronchioles
Foreign body in lung

   T17.80 Unspecified foreign body in other parts of respiratory tract

     ⑦**T17.800** Unspecified foreign body in other parts of respiratory tract causing asphyxiation

     ⑦**T17.808** Unspecified foreign body in other parts of respiratory tract causing other injury

   T17.81 Gastric contents in other parts of respiratory tract
Aspiration of gastric contents into other parts of respiratory tract
Vomitus in other parts of respiratory tract

     ⑦**T17.810** Gastric contents in other parts of respiratory tract causing asphyxiation

     ⑦**T17.818** Gastric contents in other parts of respiratory tract causing other injury

   T17.82 Food in other parts of respiratory tract
Bones in other parts of respiratory tract
Seeds in other parts of respiratory tract

     ⑦**T17.820** Food in other parts of respiratory tract causing asphyxiation

     ⑦**T17.828** Food in other parts of respiratory tract causing other injury

   T17.89 Other foreign object in other parts of respiratory tract

     ⑦**T17.890** Other foreign object in other parts of respiratory tract causing asphyxiation

     ⑦**T17.898** Other foreign object in other parts of respiratory tract causing other injury

T17.9 Foreign body in respiratory tract, part unspecified

   T17.90 Unspecified foreign body in respiratory tract, part unspecified

     ⑦**T17.900** Unspecified foreign body in respiratory tract, part unspecified causing asphyxiation

     ⑦**T17.908** Unspecified foreign body in respiratory tract, part unspecified causing other injury

   T17.91 Gastric contents in respiratory tract, part unspecified
Aspiration of gastric contents into respiratory tract, part unspecified
Vomitus in trachea respiratory tract, part unspecified

     ⑦**T17.910** Gastric contents in respiratory tract, part unspecified causing asphyxiation

     ⑦**T17.918** Gastric contents in respiratory tract, part unspecified causing other injury

   T17.92 Food in respiratory tract, part unspecified
Bones in respiratory tract, part unspecified
Seeds in respiratory tract, part unspecified

     ⑦**T17.920** Food in respiratory tract, part unspecified causing asphyxiation

     ⑦**T17.928** Food in respiratory tract, part unspecified causing other injury

   T17.99 Other foreign object in respiratory tract, part unspecified

     ⑦**T17.990** Other foreign object in respiratory tract, part unspecified in causing asphyxiation

     ⑦**T17.998** Other foreign object in respiratory tract, part unspecified causing other injury

T18 Foreign body in alimentary tract

Excludes 2: foreign body in pharynx (T17.2-)

The appropriate 7th character is to be added to each code from category T18

A - initial encounter
D - subsequent encounter
S - sequela

⊗⑦**T18.0** Foreign body in mouth

T18.1 Foreign body in esophagus

Excludes 2: foreign body in respiratory tract (T17.-)

   T18.10 Unspecified foreign body in esophagus

     ⑦**T18.100** Unspecified foreign body in esophagus causing compression of trachea
Unspecified foreign body in esophagus causing obstruction of respiration

     ⑦**T18.108** Unspecified foreign body in esophagus causing other injury

   T18.11 Gastric contents in esophagus
Vomitus in esophagus

     ⑦**T18.110** Gastric contents in esophagus causing compression of trachea
Gastric contents in esophagus causing obstruction of respiration

     ⑦**T18.118** Gastric contents in esophagus causing other injury

   T18.12 Food in esophagus
Bones in esophagus
Seeds in esophagus

     ⑦**T18.120** Food in esophagus causing compression of trachea
Food in esophagus causing obstruction of respiration

     ⑦**T18.128** Food in esophagus causing other injury

   T18.19 Other foreign object in esophagus

     ⑦**T18.190** Other foreign object in esophagus causing compression of trachea
Other foreign body in esophagus causing obstruction of respiration

     ⑦**T18.198** Other foreign object in esophagus causing other injury

⊗⑦**T18.2** Foreign body in stomach

⊗⑦**T18.3** Foreign body in small intestine

⊗⑦**T18.4** Foreign body in colon

⊗⑦**T18.5** Foreign body in anus and rectum
Foreign body in rectosigmoid (junction)

⊗⑦**T18.8** Foreign body in other parts of alimentary tract

● New code   ▲ Revised code   ⑦ 7th digit required   ⊗ Placeholder required

⊗⑦**T18.9** Foreign body of alimentary tract, part unspecified

Foreign body in digestive system NOS

Swallowed foreign body NOS

T19 Foreign body in genitourinary tract

Excludes 2: complications due to implanted mesh (T83.7-)

mechanical complications of contraceptive device (intrauterine) (vaginal) (T83.3-)

presence of contraceptive device (intrauterine) (vaginal) (Z97.5)

The appropriate 7th character is to be added to each code from category T19

A - initial encounter

D - subsequent encounter

S - sequela

⊗⑦**T19.0** Foreign body in urethra

⊗⑦**T19.1** Foreign body in bladder

⊗⑦**T19.2** Foreign body in vulva and vagina

⊗⑦**T19.3** Foreign body in uterus

⊗⑦**T19.4** Foreign body in penis

⊗⑦**T19.8** Foreign body in other parts of genitourinary tract

⊗⑦**T19.9** Foreign body in genitourinary tract, part unspecified

BURNS AND CORROSIONS (T20-T32)

Includes: burns (thermal) from electrical heating appliances

burns (thermal) from electricity

burns (thermal) from flame

burns (thermal) from friction

burns (thermal) from hot air and hot gases

burns (thermal) from hot objects

burns (thermal) from lightning

burns (thermal) from radiation

chemical burn [corrosion] (external) (internal)

scalds

Excludes 2: erythema [dermatitis] ab igne (L59.0)

radiation-related disorders of the skin and subcutaneous tissue (L55-L59)

sunburn (L55.-)

BURNS AND CORROSIONS OF EXTERNAL BODY SURFACE, SPECIFIED BY SITE (T20-T25)

Includes: burns and corrosions of first degree [erythema]

burns and corrosions of second degree [blisters][epidermal loss]

burns and corrosions of third degree [deep necrosis of underlying tissue] [full- thickness skin loss]

Use additional code from category T31 or T32 to identify extent of body surface involved

T20 Burn and corrosion of head, face, and neck

Excludes 2: burn and corrosion of ear drum (T28.41, T28.91)

burn and corrosion of eye and adnexa (T26.-)

burn and corrosion of mouth and pharynx (T28.0)

The appropriate 7th character is to be added to each code from category T20

A - initial encounter

D - subsequent encounter

S - sequela

T20.0 Burn of unspecified degree of head, face, and neck

Use additional external cause code to identify the source, place and intent of the burn (X00-X19, X75-X77, X96-X98, Y92)

⊗⑦**T20.00** Burn of unspecified degree of head, face, and neck, unspecified site

T20.01 Burn of unspecified degree of ear [any part, except ear drum]

Excludes 2: burn of ear drum (T28.41-)

⑦**T20.011** Burn of unspecified degree of right ear [any part, except ear drum]

⑦**T20.012** Burn of unspecified degree of left ear [any part, except ear drum]

⑦**T20.019** Burn of unspecified degree of unspecified ear [any part, except ear drum]

⊗⑦**T20.02** Burn of unspecified degree of lip(s)

⊗⑦**T20.03** Burn of unspecified degree of chin

⊗⑦**T20.04** Burn of unspecified degree of nose (septum)

⊗⑦**T20.05** Burn of unspecified degree of scalp [any part]

⊗⑦**T20.06** Burn of unspecified degree of forehead and cheek

⊗⑦**T20.07** Burn of unspecified degree of neck

⊗⑦**T20.09** Burn of unspecified degree of multiple sites of head, face, and neck

T20.1 Burn of first degree of head, face, and neck

Use additional external cause code to identify the source, place and intent of the burn (X00-X19, X75-X77, X96-X98, Y92)

⊗⑦**T20.10** Burn of first degree of head, face, and neck, unspecified site

T20.11 Burn of first degree of ear [any part, except ear drum]

Excludes 2: burn of ear drum (T28.41-)

⑦**T20.111** Burn of first degree of right ear [any part, except ear drum]

⑦**T20.112** Burn of first degree of left ear [any part, except ear drum]

⑦**T20.119** Burn of first degree of unspecified ear [any part, except ear drum]

⊗⑦**T20.12** Burn of first degree of lip(s)

⊗⑦**T20.13** Burn of first degree of chin

⊗⑦**T20.14** Burn of first degree of nose (septum)

⊗⑦**T20.15** Burn of first degree of scalp [any part]

⊗⑦**T20.16** Burn of first degree of forehead and cheek

⊗⑦**T20.17** Burn of first degree of neck

⊗⑦**T20.19** Burn of first degree of multiple sites of head, face, and neck

T20.2 Burn of second degree of head, face, and neck

Use additional external cause code to identify the source, place and intent of the burn (X00-X19, X75-X77, X96-X98, Y92)

⊗⑦**T20.20** Burn of second degree of head, face, and neck, unspecified site

T20.21 Burn of second degree of ear [any part, except ear drum]

Excludes 2: burn of ear drum (T28.41-)

⑦**T20.211** Burn of second degree of right ear [any part, except ear drum]

⑦**T20.212**   Burn of second degree of left ear [any part, except ear drum]

⑦**T20.219**   Burn of second degree of unspecified ear [any part, except ear drum]

⊗⑦**T20.22**   Burn of second degree of lip(s)

⊗⑦**T20.23**   Burn of second degree of chin

⊗⑦**T20.24**   Burn of second degree of nose (septum)

⊗⑦**T20.25**   Burn of second degree of scalp [any part]

⊗⑦**T20.26**   Burn of second degree of forehead and cheek

⊗⑦**T20.27**   Burn of second degree of neck

⊗⑦**T20.29**   Burn of second degree of multiple sites of head, face, and neck

T20.3   Burn of third degree of head, face, and neck

   Use additional external cause code to identify the source, place and intent of the burn (X00-X19, X75-X77, X96-X98, Y92)

⊗⑦**T20.30**   Burn of third degree of head, face, and neck, unspecified site

T20.31   Burn of third degree of ear [any part, except ear drum]

   Excludes 2: burn of ear drum (T28.41-)

⑦**T20.311**   Burn of third degree of right ear [any part, except ear drum]

⑦**T20.312**   Burn of third degree of left ear [any part, except ear drum]

⑦**T20.319**   Burn of third degree of unspecified ear [any part, except ear drum]

⊗⑦**T20.32**   Burn of third degree of lip(s)

⊗⑦**T20.33**   Burn of third degree of chin

⊗⑦**T20.34**   Burn of third degree of nose (septum)

⊗⑦**T20.35**   Burn of third degree of scalp [any part]

⊗⑦**T20.36**   Burn of third degree of forehead and cheek

⊗⑦**T20.37**   Burn of third degree of neck

⊗⑦**T20.39**   Burn of third degree of multiple sites of head, face, and neck

T20.4   Corrosion of unspecified degree of head, face, and neck

   Code first (T51-T65) to identify chemical and intent

   Use additional external cause code to identify place (Y92)

⊗⑦**T20.40**   Corrosion of unspecified degree of head, face, and neck, unspecified site

T20.41   Corrosion of unspecified degree of ear [any part, except ear drum]

   Excludes 2: corrosion of ear drum (T28.91-)

⑦**T20.411**   Corrosion of unspecified degree of right ear [any part, except ear drum]

⑦**T20.412**   Corrosion of unspecified degree of left ear [any part, except ear drum]

⑦**T20.419**   Corrosion of unspecified degree of unspecified ear [any part, except ear drum]

⊗⑦**T20.42**   Corrosion of unspecified degree of lip(s)

⊗⑦**T20.43**   Corrosion of unspecified degree of chin

⊗⑦**T20.44**   Corrosion of unspecified degree of nose (septum)

⊗⑦**T20.45**   Corrosion of unspecified degree of scalp [any part]

⊗⑦**T20.46**   Corrosion of unspecified degree of forehead and cheek

⊗⑦**T20.47**   Corrosion of unspecified degree of neck

⊗⑦**T20.49**   Corrosion of unspecified degree of multiple sites of head, face, and neck

T20.5   Corrosion of first degree of head, face, and neck

   Code first (T51-T65) to identify chemical and intent

   Use additional external cause code to identify place (Y92)

⊗⑦**T20.50**   Corrosion of first degree of head, face, and neck, unspecified site

T20.51   Corrosion of first degree of ear [any part, except ear drum]

   Excludes 2: corrosion of ear drum (T28.91-)

⑦**T20.511**   Corrosion of first degree of right ear [any part, except ear drum]

⑦**T20.512**   Corrosion of first degree of left ear [any part, except ear drum]

⑦**T20.519**   Corrosion of first degree of unspecified ear [any part, except ear drum]

⊗⑦**T20.52**   Corrosion of first degree of lip(s)

⊗⑦**T20.53**   Corrosion of first degree of chin

⊗⑦**T20.54**   Corrosion of first degree of nose (septum)

⊗⑦**T20.55**   Corrosion of first degree of scalp [any part]

⊗⑦**T20.56**   Corrosion of first degree of cheek

⊗⑦**T20.57**   Corrosion of first degree of neck

⊗⑦**T20.59**   Corrosion of first degree of multiple sites of head, face, and neck

T20.6   Corrosion of second degree of head, face, and neck

   Code first (T51-T65) to identify chemical and intent

   Use additional external cause code to identify place (Y92)

⊗⑦**T20.60**   Corrosion of second degree of head, face, and neck, unspecified site

T20.61   Corrosion of second degree of ear [any part, except ear drum]

   Excludes 2: corrosion of ear drum (T28.91-)

⑦**T20.611**   Corrosion of second degree of right ear [any part, except ear drum]

⑦**T20.612**   Corrosion of second degree of left ear [any part, except ear drum]

⑦**T20.619**   Corrosion of second degree of unspecified ear [any part, except ear drum]

⊗⑦**T20.62**   Corrosion of second degree of lip(s)

⊗⑦**T20.63**   Corrosion of second degree of chin

⊗⑦**T20.64**   Corrosion of second degree of nose (septum)

⊗⑦**T20.65**   Corrosion of second degree of scalp [any part]

⊗⑦**T20.66**   Corrosion of second degree of forehead and cheek

⊗⑦**T20.67**   Corrosion of second degree of neck

⊗⑦**T20.69**   Corrosion of second degree of multiple sites of head, face, and neck

T20.7   Corrosion of third degree of head, face, and neck

   Code first (T51-T65) to identify chemical and intent

   Use additional external cause code to identify place (Y92)

⊗⑦**T20.70**   Corrosion of third degree of head, face, and neck, unspecified site

T20.71   Corrosion of third degree of ear [any part, except ear drum]

   Excludes 2: corrosion of ear drum (T28.91-)

   ● New code   ▲ Revised code   ⑦ 7ᵗʰ digit required   ⊗ Placeholder required

⑦T20.711   Corrosion of third degree of right ear [any part, except ear drum]

⑦T20.712   Corrosion of third degree of left ear [any part, except ear drum]

⑦T20.719   Corrosion of third degree of unspecified ear [any part, except ear drum]

⊗⑦T20.72   Corrosion of third degree of lip(s)

⊗⑦T20.73   Corrosion of third degree of chin

⊗⑦T20.74   Corrosion of third degree of nose (septum)

⊗⑦T20.75   Corrosion of third degree of scalp [any part]

⊗⑦T20.76   Corrosion of third degree of forehead and cheek

⊗⑦T20.77   Corrosion of third degree of neck

⊗⑦T20.79   Corrosion of third degree of multiple sites of head, face, and neck

T21   Burn and corrosion of trunk

Includes: burns and corrosion of hip region

Excludes 2: burns and corrosion of axilla (T22.- with fifth character 4)

burns and corrosion of scapular region (T22.- with fifth character 6)

burns and corrosion of shoulder (T22.- with fifth character 5)

The appropriate 7th character is to be added to each code from category T21

A - initial encounter

D - subsequent encounter

S - sequela

T21.0   Burn of unspecified degree of trunk

Use additional external cause code to identify the source, place and intent of the burn (X00-X19, X75-X77, X96-X98, Y92)

⊗⑦T21.00   Burn of unspecified degree of trunk, unspecified site

⊗⑦T21.01   Burn of unspecified degree of chest wall

Burn of unspecified degree of breast

⊗⑦T21.02   Burn of unspecified degree of abdominal wall

Burn of unspecified degree of flank

Burn of unspecified degree of groin

⊗⑦T21.03   Burn of unspecified degree of upper back

Burn of unspecified degree of interscapular region

⊗⑦T21.04   Burn of unspecified degree of lower back

⊗⑦T21.05   Burn of unspecified degree of buttock

Burn of unspecified degree of anus

⊗⑦T21.06   Burn of unspecified degree of male genital region

Burn of unspecified degree of penis

Burn of unspecified degree of scrotum

Burn of unspecified degree of testis

⊗⑦T21.07   Burn of unspecified degree of female genital region

Burn of unspecified degree of labium (majus) (minus)

Burn of unspecified degree of perineum

Burn of unspecified degree of vulva

Excludes 2: burn of vagina (T28.3)

⊗⑦T21.09   Burn of unspecified degree of other site of trunk

T21.1   Burn of first degree of trunk

Use additional external cause code to identify the source, place and intent of the burn (X00-X19, X75-X77, X96-X98, Y92)

⊗⑦T21.10   Burn of first degree of trunk, unspecified site

⊗⑦T21.11   Burn of first degree of chest wall

Burn of first degree of breast

⊗⑦T21.12   Burn of first degree of abdominal wall

Burn of first degree of flank

Burn of first degree of groin

⊗⑦T21.13   Burn of first degree of upper back

Burn of first degree of interscapular region

⊗⑦T21.14   Burn of first degree of lower back

⊗⑦T21.15   Burn of first degree of buttock

Burn of first degree of anus

⊗⑦T21.16   Burn of first degree of male genital region

Burn of first degree of penis

Burn of first degree of scrotum

Burn of first degree of testis

⊗⑦T21.17   Burn of first degree of female genital region

Burn of first degree of labium (majus) (minus)

Burn of first degree of perineum

Burn of first degree of vulva

Excludes 2: burn of vagina (T28.3)

⊗⑦T21.19   Burn of first degree of other site of trunk

T21.2   Burn of second degree of trunk

Use additional external cause code to identify the source, place and intent of the burn (X00-X19, X75-X77, X96-X98, Y92)

⊗⑦T21.20   Burn of second degree of trunk, unspecified site

⊗⑦T21.21   Burn of second degree of chest wall

Burn of second degree of breast

⊗⑦T21.22   Burn of second degree of abdominal wall

Burn of second degree of flank

Burn of second degree of groin

⊗⑦T21.23   Burn of second degree of upper back

Burn of second degree of interscapular region

⊗⑦T21.24   Burn of second degree of lower back

⊗⑦T21.25   Burn of second degree of buttock

Burn of second degree of anus

⊗⑦T21.26   Burn of second degree of male genital region

Burn of second degree of penis

Burn of second degree of scrotum

Burn of second degree of testis

⊗⑦T21.27   Burn of second degree of female genital region

Burn of second degree of labium (majus) (minus)

Burn of second degree of perineum

Burn of second degree of vulva

Excludes 2: burn of vagina (T28.3)

⊗⑦T21.29   Burn of second degree of other site of trunk

T21.3   Burn of third degree of trunk

Use additional external cause code to identify the source, place and intent of the burn (X00-X19, X75-X77, X96-X98, Y92)

⊗⑦T21.30   Burn of third degree of trunk, unspecified site

⊗⑦T21.31   Burn of third degree of chest wall

Burn of third degree of breast

⊗⑦T21.32   Burn of third degree of abdominal wall

Burn of third degree of flank

Burn of third degree of groin

⊗⑦**T21.33**   Burn of third degree of upper back

Burn of third degree of interscapular region

⊗⑦**T21.34**   Burn of third degree of lower back

⊗⑦**T21.35**   Burn of third degree of buttock

Burn of third degree of anus

⊗⑦**T21.36**   Burn of third degree of male genital region

Burn of third degree of penis

Burn of third degree of scrotum

Burn of third degree of testis

⊗⑦**T21.37**   Burn of third degree of female genital region

Burn of third degree of labium (majus) (minus)

Burn of third degree of perineum

Burn of third degree of vulva

Excludes 2: burn of vagina (T28.3)

⊗⑦**T21.39**   Burn of third degree of other site of trunk

T21.4   Corrosion of unspecified degree of trunk

Code first (T51-T65) to identify chemical and intent

Use additional external cause code to identify place (Y92)

⊗⑦**T21.40**   Corrosion of unspecified degree of trunk, unspecified site

⊗⑦**T21.41**   Corrosion of unspecified degree of chest wall

Corrosion of unspecified degree of breast

⊗⑦**T21.42**   Corrosion of unspecified degree of abdominal wall

Corrosion of unspecified degree of flank

Corrosion of unspecified degree of groin

⊗⑦**T21.43**   Corrosion of unspecified degree of upper back

Corrosion of unspecified degree of interscapular region

⊗⑦**T21.44**   Corrosion of unspecified degree of lower back

⊗⑦**T21.45**   Corrosion of unspecified degree of buttock

Corrosion of unspecified degree of anus

⊗⑦**T21.46**   Corrosion of unspecified degree of male genital region

Corrosion of unspecified degree of penis

Corrosion of unspecified degree of scrotum

Corrosion of unspecified degree of testis

⊗⑦**T21.47**   Corrosion of unspecified degree of female genital region

Corrosion of unspecified degree of labium (majus) (minus)

Corrosion of unspecified degree of perineum

Corrosion of unspecified degree of vulva

Excludes 2: corrosion of vagina (T28.8)

⊗⑦**T21.49**   Corrosion of unspecified degree of other site of trunk

T21.5   Corrosion of first degree of trunk

Code first (T51-T65) to identify chemical and intent

Use additional external cause code to identify place (Y92)

⊗⑦**T21.50**   Corrosion of first degree of trunk, unspecified site

⊗⑦**T21.51**   Corrosion of first degree of chest wall

Corrosion of first degree of breast

⊗⑦**T21.52**   Corrosion of first degree of abdominal wall

Corrosion of first degree of flank

Corrosion of first degree of groin

⊗⑦**T21.53**   Corrosion of first degree of upper back

Corrosion of first degree of interscapular region

⊗⑦**T21.54**   Corrosion of first degree of lower back

⊗⑦**T21.55**   Corrosion of first degree of buttock

Corrosion of first degree of anus

⊗⑦**T21.56**   Corrosion of first degree of male genital region

Corrosion of first degree of penis

Corrosion of first degree of scrotum

Corrosion of first degree of testis

⊗⑦**T21.57**   Corrosion of first degree of female genital region

Corrosion of first degree of labium (majus) (minus)

Corrosion of first degree of perineum

Corrosion of first degree of vulva

Excludes 2: corrosion of vagina (T28.8)

⊗⑦**T21.59**   Corrosion of first degree of other site of trunk

T21.6   Corrosion of second degree of trunk

Code first (T51-T65) to identify chemical and intent

Use additional external cause code to identify place (Y92)

⊗⑦**T21.60**   Corrosion of second degree of trunk, unspecified site

⊗⑦**T21.61**   Corrosion of second degree of chest wall

Corrosion of second degree of breast

⊗⑦**T21.62**   Corrosion of second degree of abdominal wall

Corrosion of second degree of flank

Corrosion of second degree of groin

⊗⑦**T21.63**   Corrosion of second degree of upper back

Corrosion of second degree of interscapular region

⊗⑦**T21.64**   Corrosion of second degree of lower back

⊗⑦**T21.65**   Corrosion of second degree of buttock

Corrosion of second degree of anus

⊗⑦**T21.66**   Corrosion of second degree of male genital region

Corrosion of second degree of penis

Corrosion of second degree of scrotum

Corrosion of second degree of testis

⊗⑦**T21.67**   Corrosion of second degree of female genital region

Corrosion of second degree of labium (majus) (minus)

Corrosion of second degree of perineum

Corrosion of second degree of vulva

Excludes 2: corrosion of vagina (T28.8)

⊗⑦**T21.69**   Corrosion of second degree of other site of trunk

T21.7   Corrosion of third degree of trunk

Code first (T51-T65) to identify chemical and intent

Use additional external cause code to identify place (Y92)

⊗⑦**T21.70**   Corrosion of third degree of trunk, unspecified site

⊗⑦**T21.71**   Corrosion of third degree of chest wall

Corrosion of third degree of breast

⊗⑦**T21.72**   Corrosion of third degree of abdominal wall

Corrosion of third degree of flank

Corrosion of third degree of groin

⊗⑦**T21.73**   Corrosion of third degree of upper back

Corrosion of third degree of interscapular region

⊗⑦**T21.74**   Corrosion of third degree of lower back

⊗⑦**T21.75** Corrosion of third degree of buttock
Corrosion of third degree of anus

⊗⑦**T21.76** Corrosion of third degree of male genital region
Corrosion of third degree of penis
Corrosion of third degree of scrotum
Corrosion of third degree of testis

⊗⑦**T21.77** Corrosion of third degree of female genital region
Corrosion of third degree of labium (majus) (minus)
Corrosion of third degree of perineum
Corrosion of third degree of vulva
Excludes 2: corrosion of vagina (T28.8)

⊗⑦**T21.79** Corrosion of third degree of other site of trunk

T22 Burn and corrosion of shoulder and upper limb, except wrist and hand
Excludes 2: burn and corrosion of interscapular region (T21.)
burn and corrosion of wrist and hand (T23.-)

The appropriate 7th character is to be added to each code from category T22
A - initial encounter
D - subsequent encounter
S - sequela

T22.0 Burn of unspecified degree of shoulder and upper limb, except wrist and hand
Use additional external cause code to identify the source, place and intent of the burn (X00-X19, X75-X77, X96-X98, Y92)

⊗⑦**T22.00** Burn of unspecified degree of shoulder and upper limb, except wrist and hand, unspecified site

T22.01 Burn of unspecified degree of forearm

⑦**T22.011** Burn of unspecified degree of right forearm

⑦**T22.012** Burn of unspecified degree of left forearm

⑦**T22.019** Burn of unspecified degree of unspecified forearm

T22.02 Burn of unspecified degree of elbow

⑦**T22.021** Burn of unspecified degree of right elbow

⑦**T22.022** Burn of unspecified degree of left elbow

⑦**T22.029** Burn of unspecified degree of unspecified elbow

T22.03 Burn of unspecified degree of upper arm

⑦**T22.031** Burn of unspecified degree of right upper arm

⑦**T22.032** Burn of unspecified degree of left upper arm

⑦**T22.039** Burn of unspecified degree of unspecified upper arm

T22.04 Burn of unspecified degree of axilla

⑦**T22.041** Burn of unspecified degree of right axilla

⑦**T22.042** Burn of unspecified degree of left axilla

⑦**T22.049** Burn of unspecified degree of unspecified axilla

T22.05 Burn of unspecified degree of shoulder

⑦**T22.051** Burn of unspecified degree of right shoulder

⑦**T22.052** Burn of unspecified degree of left shoulder

⑦**T22.059** Burn of unspecified degree of unspecified shoulder

T22.06 Burn of unspecified degree of scapular region

⑦**T22.061** Burn of unspecified degree of right scapular region

⑦**T22.062** Burn of unspecified degree of left scapular region

⑦**T22.069** Burn of unspecified degree of unspecified scapular region

T22.09 Burn of unspecified degree of multiple sites of shoulder and upper limb, except wrist and hand

⑦**T22.091** Burn of unspecified degree of multiple sites of right shoulder and upper limb, except wrist and hand

⑦**T22.092** Burn of unspecified degree of multiple sites of left shoulder and upper limb, except wrist and hand

⑦**T22.099** Burn of unspecified degree of multiple sites of unspecified shoulder and upper limb, except wrist and hand

T22.1 Burn of first degree of shoulder and upper limb, except wrist and hand
Use additional external cause code to identify the source, place and intent of the burn (X00-X19, X75-X77, X96-X98, Y92)

⊗⑦**T22.10** Burn of first degree of shoulder and upper limb, except wrist and hand, unspecified site

T22.11 Burn of first degree of forearm

⑦**T22.111** Burn of first degree of right forearm

⑦**T22.112** Burn of first degree of left forearm

⑦**T22.119** Burn of first degree of unspecified forearm

T22.12 Burn of first degree of elbow

⑦**T22.121** Burn of first degree of right elbow

⑦**T22.122** Burn of first degree of left elbow

⑦**T22.129** Burn of first degree of unspecified elbow

T22.13 Burn of first degree of upper arm

⑦**T22.131** Burn of first degree of right upper arm

⑦**T22.132** Burn of first degree of left upper arm

⑦**T22.139** Burn of first degree of unspecified upper arm

T22.14 Burn of first degree of axilla

⑦**T22.141** Burn of first degree of right axilla

⑦**T22.142** Burn of first degree of left axilla

⑦**T22.149** Burn of first degree of unspecified axilla

T22.15 Burn of first degree of shoulder

⑦**T22.151** Burn of first degree of right shoulder

⑦**T22.152** Burn of first degree of left shoulder

■ Add 4th-7th digits   ▨ 3 digit reportable   ▨ Nonspecific code   ▨ Unspecified code   ▨ Manifestation code   751

⑦**T22.159**   Burn of first degree of unspecified shoulder

T22.16   Burn of first degree of scapular region

    ⑦**T22.161**   Burn of first degree of right scapular region

    ⑦**T22.162**   Burn of first degree of left scapular region

    ⑦**T22.169**   Burn of first degree of unspecified scapular region

T22.19   Burn of first degree of multiple sites of shoulder and upper limb, except wrist and hand

    ⑦**T22.191**   Burn of first degree of multiple sites of right shoulder and upper limb, except wrist and hand

    ⑦**T22.192**   Burn of first degree of multiple sites of left shoulder and upper limb, except wrist and hand

    ⑦**T22.199**   Burn of first degree of multiple sites of unspecified shoulder and upper limb, except wrist and hand

T22.2   Burn of second degree of shoulder and upper limb, except wrist and hand

    Use additional external cause code to identify the source, place and intent of the burn (X00-X19, X75-X77, X96-X98, Y92)

⊗⑦**T22.20**   Burn of second degree of shoulder and upper limb, except wrist and hand, unspecified site

T22.21   Burn of second degree of forearm

    ⑦**T22.211**   Burn of second degree of right forearm

    ⑦**T22.212**   Burn of second degree of left forearm

    ⑦**T22.219**   Burn of second degree of unspecified forearm

T22.22   Burn of second degree of elbow

    ⑦**T22.221**   Burn of second degree of right elbow

    ⑦**T22.222**   Burn of second degree of left elbow

    ⑦**T22.229**   Burn of second degree of unspecified elbow

T22.23   Burn of second degree of upper arm

    ⑦**T22.231**   Burn of second degree of right upper arm

    ⑦**T22.232**   Burn of second degree of left upper arm

    ⑦**T22.239**   Burn of second degree of unspecified upper arm

T22.24   Burn of second degree of axilla

    ⑦**T22.241**   Burn of second degree of right axilla

    ⑦**T22.242**   Burn of second degree of left axilla

    ⑦**T22.249**   Burn of second degree of unspecified axilla

T22.25   Burn of second degree of shoulder

    ⑦**T22.251**   Burn of second degree of right shoulder

    ⑦**T22.252**   Burn of second degree of left shoulder

    ⑦**T22.259**   Burn of second degree of unspecified shoulder

T22.26   Burn of second degree of scapular region

    ⑦**T22.261**   Burn of second degree of right scapular region

    ⑦**T22.262**   Burn of second degree of left scapular region

    ⑦**T22.269**   Burn of second degree of unspecified scapular region

T22.29   Burn of second degree of multiple sites of shoulder and upper limb, except wrist and hand

    ⑦**T22.291**   Burn of second degree of multiple sites of right shoulder and upper limb, except wrist and hand

    ⑦**T22.292**   Burn of second degree of multiple sites of left shoulder and upper limb, except wrist and hand

    ⑦**T22.299**   Burn of second degree of multiple sites of unspecified shoulder and upper limb, except wrist and hand

T22.3   Burn of third degree of shoulder and upper limb, except wrist and hand

    Use additional external cause code to identify the source, place and intent of the burn (X00-X19, X75-X77, X96-X98, Y92)

⊗⑦**T22.30**   Burn of third degree of shoulder and upper limb, except wrist and hand, unspecified site

T22.31   Burn of third degree of forearm

    ⑦**T22.311**   Burn of third degree of right forearm

    ⑦**T22.312**   Burn of third degree of left forearm

    ⑦**T22.319**   Burn of third degree of unspecified forearm

T22.32   Burn of third degree of elbow

    ⑦**T22.321**   Burn of third degree of right elbow

    ⑦**T22.322**   Burn of third degree of left elbow

    ⑦**T22.329**   Burn of third degree of unspecified elbow

T22.33   Burn of third degree of upper arm

    ⑦**T22.331**   Burn of third degree of right upper arm

    ⑦**T22.332**   Burn of third degree of left upper arm

    ⑦**T22.339**   Burn of third degree of unspecified upper arm

T22.34   Burn of third degree of axilla

    ⑦**T22.341**   Burn of third degree of right axilla

    ⑦**T22.342**   Burn of third degree of left axilla

    ⑦**T22.349**   Burn of third degree of unspecified axilla

T22.35   Burn of third degree of shoulder

    ⑦**T22.351**   Burn of third degree of right shoulder

    ⑦**T22.352**   Burn of third degree of left shoulder

    ⑦**T22.359**   Burn of third degree of unspecified shoulder

T22.36   Burn of third degree of scapular region

    ⑦**T22.361**   Burn of third degree of right scapular region

    ⑦**T22.362**   Burn of third degree of left scapular region

⑦T22.369   Burn of third degree of unspecified scapular region

T22.39   Burn of third degree of multiple sites of shoulder and upper limb, except wrist and hand

    ⑦T22.391   Burn of third degree of multiple sites of right shoulder and upper limb, except wrist and hand

    ⑦T22.392   Burn of third degree of multiple sites of left shoulder and upper limb, except wrist and hand

    ⑦T22.399   Burn of third degree of multiple sites of unspecified shoulder and upper limb, except wrist and hand

T22.4   Corrosion of unspecified degree of shoulder and upper limb, except wrist and hand

Code first (T51-T65) to identify chemical and intent

Use additional external cause code to identify place (Y92)

   ⊗⑦T22.40   Corrosion of unspecified degree of shoulder and upper limb, except wrist and hand, unspecified site

T22.41   Corrosion of unspecified degree of forearm

    ⑦T22.411   Corrosion of unspecified degree of right forearm

    ⑦T22.412   Corrosion of unspecified degree of left forearm

    ⑦T22.419   Corrosion of unspecified degree of unspecified forearm

T22.42   Corrosion of unspecified degree of elbow

    ⑦T22.421   Corrosion of unspecified degree of right elbow

    ⑦T22.422   Corrosion of unspecified degree of left elbow

    ⑦T22.429   Corrosion of unspecified degree of unspecified elbow

T22.43   Corrosion of unspecified degree of upper arm

    ⑦T22.431   Corrosion of unspecified degree of right upper arm

    ⑦T22.432   Corrosion of unspecified degree of left upper arm

    ⑦T22.439   Corrosion of unspecified degree of unspecified upper arm

T22.44   Corrosion of unspecified degree of axilla

    ⑦T22.441   Corrosion of unspecified degree of right axilla

    ⑦T22.442   Corrosion of unspecified degree of left axilla

    ⑦T22.449   Corrosion of unspecified degree of unspecified axilla

T22.45   Corrosion of unspecified degree of shoulder

    ⑦T22.451   Corrosion of unspecified degree of right shoulder

    ⑦T22.452   Corrosion of unspecified degree of left shoulder

    ⑦T22.459   Corrosion of unspecified degree of unspecified shoulder

T22.46   Corrosion of unspecified degree of scapular region

    ⑦T22.461   Corrosion of unspecified degree of right scapular region

⑦T22.462   Corrosion of unspecified degree of left scapular region

⑦T22.469   Corrosion of unspecified degree of unspecified scapular region

T22.49   Corrosion of unspecified degree of multiple sites of shoulder and upper limb, except wrist and hand

    ⑦T22.491   Corrosion of unspecified degree of multiple sites of right shoulder and upper limb, except wrist and hand

    ⑦T22.492   Corrosion of unspecified degree of multiple sites of left shoulder and upper limb, except wrist and hand

    ⑦T22.499   Corrosion of unspecified degree of multiple sites of unspecified shoulder and upper limb, except wrist and hand

T22.5   Corrosion of first degree of shoulder and upper limb, except wrist and hand

Code first (T51-T65) to identify chemical and intent

Use additional external cause code to identify place (Y92)

   ⊗⑦T22.50   Corrosion of first degree of shoulder and upper limb, except wrist and hand unspecified site

T22.51   Corrosion of first degree of forearm

    ⑦T22.511   Corrosion of first degree of right forearm

    ⑦T22.512   Corrosion of first degree of left forearm

    ⑦T22.519   Corrosion of first degree of unspecified forearm

T22.52   Corrosion of first degree of elbow

    ⑦T22.521   Corrosion of first degree of right elbow

    ⑦T22.522   Corrosion of first degree of left elbow

    ⑦T22.529   Corrosion of first degree of unspecified elbow

T22.53   Corrosion of first degree of upper arm

    ⑦T22.531   Corrosion of first degree of right upper arm

    ⑦T22.532   Corrosion of first degree of left upper arm

    ⑦T22.539   Corrosion of first degree of unspecified upper arm

T22.54   Corrosion of first degree of axilla

    ⑦T22.541   Corrosion of first degree of right axilla

    ⑦T22.542   Corrosion of first degree of left axilla

    ⑦T22.549   Corrosion of first degree of unspecified axilla

T22.55   Corrosion of first degree of shoulder

    ⑦T22.551   Corrosion of first degree of right shoulder

    ⑦T22.552   Corrosion of first degree of left shoulder

    ⑦T22.559   Corrosion of first degree of unspecified shoulder

T22.56   Corrosion of first degree of scapular region

⑦**T22.561** Corrosion of first degree of right scapular region

⑦**T22.562** Corrosion of first degree of left scapular region

⑦**T22.569** Corrosion of first degree of unspecified scapular region

T22.59 Corrosion of first degree of multiple sites of shoulder and upper limb, except wrist and hand

⑦**T22.591** Corrosion of first degree of multiple sites of right shoulder and upper limb, except wrist and hand

⑦**T22.592** Corrosion of first degree of multiple sites of left shoulder and upper limb, except wrist and hand

⑦**T22.599** Corrosion of first degree of multiple sites of unspecified shoulder and upper limb, except wrist and hand

T22.6 Corrosion of second degree of shoulder and upper limb, except wrist and hand

Code first (T51-T65) to identify chemical and intent

Use additional external cause code to identify place (Y92)

⊗⑦**T22.60** Corrosion of second degree of shoulder and upper limb, except wrist and hand, unspecified site

T22.61 Corrosion of second degree of forearm

⑦**T22.611** Corrosion of second degree of right forearm

⑦**T22.612** Corrosion of second degree of left forearm

⑦**T22.619** Corrosion of second degree of unspecified forearm

T22.62 Corrosion of second degree of elbow

⑦**T22.621** Corrosion of second degree of right elbow

⑦**T22.622** Corrosion of second degree of left elbow

⑦**T22.629** Corrosion of second degree of unspecified elbow

T22.63 Corrosion of second degree of upper arm

⑦**T22.631** Corrosion of second degree of right upper arm

⑦**T22.632** Corrosion of second degree of left upper arm

⑦**T22.639** Corrosion of second degree of unspecified upper arm

T22.64 Corrosion of second degree of axilla

⑦**T22.641** Corrosion of second degree of right axilla

⑦**T22.642** Corrosion of second degree of left axilla

⑦**T22.649** Corrosion of second degree of unspecified axilla

T22.65 Corrosion of second degree of shoulder

⑦**T22.651** Corrosion of second degree of right shoulder

⑦**T22.652** Corrosion of second degree of left shoulder

⑦**T22.659** Corrosion of second degree of unspecified shoulder

T22.66 Corrosion of second degree of scapular region

⑦**T22.661** Corrosion of second degree of right scapular region

⑦**T22.662** Corrosion of second degree of left scapular region

⑦**T22.669** Corrosion of second degree of unspecified scapular region

T22.69 Corrosion of second degree of multiple sites of shoulder and upper limb, except wrist and hand

⑦**T22.691** Corrosion of second degree of multiple sites of right shoulder and upper limb, except wrist and hand

⑦**T22.692** Corrosion of second degree of multiple sites of left shoulder and upper limb, except wrist and hand

⑦**T22.699** Corrosion of second degree of multiple sites of unspecified shoulder and upper limb, except wrist and hand

T22.7 Corrosion of third degree of shoulder and upper limb, except wrist and hand

Code first (T51-T65) to identify chemical and intent

Use additional external cause code to identify place (Y92)

⊗⑦**T22.70** Corrosion of third degree of shoulder and upper limb, except wrist and hand, unspecified site

T22.71 Corrosion of third degree of forearm

⑦**T22.711** Corrosion of third degree of right forearm

⑦**T22.712** Corrosion of third degree of left forearm

⑦**T22.719** Corrosion of third degree of unspecified forearm

T22.72 Corrosion of third degree of elbow

⑦**T22.721** Corrosion of third degree of right elbow

⑦**T22.722** Corrosion of third degree of left elbow

⑦**T22.729** Corrosion of third degree of unspecified elbow

T22.73 Corrosion of third degree of upper arm

⑦**T22.731** Corrosion of third degree of right upper arm

⑦**T22.732** Corrosion of third degree of left upper arm

⑦**T22.739** Corrosion of third degree of unspecified upper arm

T22.74 Corrosion of third degree of axilla

⑦**T22.741** Corrosion of third degree of right axilla

⑦**T22.742** Corrosion of third degree of left axilla

⑦**T22.749** Corrosion of third degree of unspecified axilla

T22.75 Corrosion of third degree of shoulder

⑦**T22.751** Corrosion of third degree of right shoulder

⑦**T22.752** Corrosion of third degree of left shoulder

● New code   ▲ Revised code   ⑦ 7ᵗʰ digit required   ⊗ Placeholder required

⑦**T22.759** Corrosion of third degree of unspecified shoulder

T22.76 Corrosion of third degree of scapular region

⑦**T22.761** Corrosion of third degree of right scapular region

⑦**T22.762** Corrosion of third degree of left scapular region

⑦**T22.769** Corrosion of third degree of unspecified scapular region

T22.79 Corrosion of third degree of multiple sites of shoulder and upper limb, except wrist and hand

⑦**T22.791** Corrosion of third degree of multiple sites of right shoulder and upper limb, except wrist and hand

⑦**T22.792** Corrosion of third degree of multiple sites of left shoulder and upper limb, except wrist and hand

⑦**T22.799** Corrosion of third degree of multiple sites of unspecified shoulder and upper limb, except wrist and hand

T23 Burn and corrosion of wrist and hand

The appropriate 7th character is to be added to each code from category T23

A - initial encounter

D - subsequent encounter

S - sequela

T23.0 Burn of unspecified degree of wrist and hand

Use additional external cause code to identify the source, place and intent of the burn (X00-X19, X75-X77, X96-X98, Y92)

T23.00 Burn of unspecified degree of hand, unspecified site

⑦**T23.001** Burn of unspecified degree of right hand, unspecified site

⑦**T23.002** Burn of unspecified degree of left hand, unspecified site

⑦**T23.009** Burn of unspecified degree of unspecified hand, unspecified site

T23.01 Burn of unspecified degree of thumb (nail)

⑦**T23.011** Burn of unspecified degree of right thumb (nail)

⑦**T23.012** Burn of unspecified degree of left thumb (nail)

⑦**T23.019** Burn of unspecified degree of unspecified thumb (nail)

T23.02 Burn of unspecified degree of single finger (nail) except thumb

⑦**T23.021** Burn of unspecified degree of single right finger (nail) except thumb

⑦**T23.022** Burn of unspecified degree of single left finger (nail) except thumb

⑦**T23.029** Burn of unspecified degree of unspecified single finger (nail) except thumb

T23.03 Burn of unspecified degree of multiple fingers (nail), not including thumb

⑦**T23.031** Burn of unspecified degree of multiple right fingers (nail), not including thumb

⑦**T23.032** Burn of unspecified degree of multiple left fingers (nail), not including thumb

⑦**T23.039** Burn of unspecified degree of unspecified multiple fingers (nail), not including thumb

T23.04 Burn of unspecified degree of multiple fingers (nail), including thumb

⑦**T23.041** Burn of unspecified degree of multiple right fingers (nail), including thumb

⑦**T23.042** Burn of unspecified degree of multiple left fingers (nail), including thumb

⑦**T23.049** Burn of unspecified degree of unspecified multiple fingers (nail), including thumb

T23.05 Burn of unspecified degree of palm

⑦**T23.051** Burn of unspecified degree of right palm

⑦**T23.052** Burn of unspecified degree of left palm

⑦**T23.059** Burn of unspecified degree of unspecified palm

T23.06 Burn of unspecified degree of back of hand

⑦**T23.061** Burn of unspecified degree of back of right hand

⑦**T23.062** Burn of unspecified degree of back of left hand

⑦**T23.069** Burn of unspecified degree of back of unspecified hand

T23.07 Burn of unspecified degree of wrist

⑦**T23.071** Burn of unspecified degree of right wrist

⑦**T23.072** Burn of unspecified degree of left wrist

⑦**T23.079** Burn of unspecified degree of unspecified wrist

T23.09 Burn of unspecified degree of multiple sites of wrist and hand

⑦**T23.091** Burn of unspecified degree of multiple sites of right wrist and hand

⑦**T23.092** Burn of unspecified degree of multiple sites of left wrist and hand

⑦**T23.099** Burn of unspecified degree of multiple sites of unspecified wrist and hand

T23.1 Burn of first degree of wrist and hand

Use additional external cause code to identify the source, place and intent of the burn (X00-X19, X75-X77, X96-X98, Y92)

T23.10 Burn of first degree of hand, unspecified site

⑦**T23.101** Burn of first degree of right hand, unspecified site

⑦**T23.102** Burn of first degree of left hand, unspecified site

⑦**T23.109** Burn of first degree of unspecified hand, unspecified site

T23.11 Burn of first degree of thumb (nail)

⑦**T23.111**   Burn of first degree of right thumb (nail)

⑦**T23.112**   Burn of first degree of left thumb (nail)

⑦**T23.119**   Burn of first degree of unspecified thumb (nail)

T23.12   Burn of first degree of single finger (nail) except thumb

⑦**T23.121**   Burn of first degree of single right finger (nail) except thumb

⑦**T23.122**   Burn of first degree of single left finger (nail) except thumb

⑦**T23.129**   Burn of first degree of unspecified single finger (nail) except thumb

T23.13   Burn of first degree of multiple fingers (nail), not including thumb

⑦**T23.131**   Burn of first degree of multiple right fingers (nail), not including thumb

⑦**T23.132**   Burn of first degree of multiple left fingers (nail), not including thumb

⑦**T23.139**   Burn of first degree of unspecified multiple fingers (nail), not including thumb

T23.14   Burn of first degree of multiple fingers (nail), including thumb

⑦**T23.141**   Burn of first degree of multiple right fingers (nail), including thumb

⑦**T23.142**   Burn of first degree of multiple left fingers (nail), including thumb

⑦**T23.149**   Burn of first degree of unspecified multiple fingers (nail), including thumb

T23.15   Burn of first degree of palm

⑦**T23.151**   Burn of first degree of right palm

⑦**T23.152**   Burn of first degree of left palm

⑦**T23.159**   Burn of first degree of unspecified palm

T23.16   Burn of first degree of back of hand

⑦**T23.161**   Burn of first degree of back of right hand

⑦**T23.162**   Burn of first degree of back of left hand

⑦**T23.169**   Burn of first degree of back of unspecified hand

T23.17   Burn of first degree of wrist

⑦**T23.171**   Burn of first degree of right wrist

⑦**T23.172**   Burn of first degree of left wrist

⑦**T23.179**   Burn of first degree of unspecified wrist

T23.19   Burn of first degree of multiple sites of wrist and hand

⑦**T23.191**   Burn of first degree of multiple sites of right wrist and hand

⑦**T23.192**   Burn of first degree of multiple sites of left wrist and hand

⑦**T23.199**   Burn of first degree of multiple sites of unspecified wrist and hand

T23.2   Burn of second degree of wrist and hand

Use additional external cause code to identify the source, place and intent of the burn (X00-X19, X75-X77, X96-X98, Y92)

T23.20   Burn of second degree of hand, unspecified site

⑦**T23.201**   Burn of second degree of right hand, unspecified site

⑦**T23.202**   Burn of second degree of left hand, unspecified site

⑦**T23.209**   Burn of second degree of unspecified hand, unspecified site

T23.21   Burn of second degree of thumb (nail)

⑦**T23.211**   Burn of second degree of right thumb (nail)

⑦**T23.212**   Burn of second degree of left thumb (nail)

⑦**T23.219**   Burn of second degree of unspecified thumb (nail)

T23.22   Burn of second degree of single finger (nail) except thumb

⑦**T23.221**   Burn of second degree of single right finger (nail) except thumb

⑦**T23.222**   Burn of second degree of single left finger (nail) except thumb

⑦**T23.229**   Burn of second degree of unspecified single finger (nail) except thumb

T23.23   Burn of second degree of multiple fingers (nail), not including thumb

⑦**T23.231**   Burn of second degree of multiple right fingers (nail), not including thumb

⑦**T23.232**   Burn of second degree of multiple left fingers (nail), not including thumb

⑦**T23.239**   Burn of second degree of unspecified multiple fingers (nail), not including thumb

T23.24   Burn of second degree of multiple fingers (nail), including thumb

⑦**T23.241**   Burn of second degree of multiple right fingers (nail), including thumb

⑦**T23.242**   Burn of second degree of multiple left fingers (nail), including thumb

⑦**T23.249**   Burn of second degree of unspecified multiple fingers (nail), including thumb

T23.25   Burn of second degree of palm

⑦**T23.251**   Burn of second degree of right palm

⑦**T23.252**   Burn of second degree of left palm

⑦**T23.259**   Burn of second degree of unspecified palm

T23.26   Burn of second degree of back of hand

⑦**T23.261**   Burn of second degree of back of right hand

⑦**T23.262**   Burn of second degree of back of left hand

⑦**T23.269**   Burn of second degree of back of unspecified hand

T23.27   Burn of second degree of wrist

● New code   ▲ Revised code   ⑦ 7th digit required   ⊗ Placeholder required

⑦T23.271   Burn of second degree of right wrist

⑦T23.272   Burn of second degree of left wrist

⑦T23.279   Burn of second degree of unspecified wrist

T23.29   Burn of second degree of multiple sites of wrist and hand

⑦T23.291   Burn of second degree of multiple sites of right wrist and hand

⑦T23.292   Burn of second degree of multiple sites of left wrist and hand

⑦T23.299   Burn of second degree of multiple sites of unspecified wrist and hand

T23.3   Burn of third degree of wrist and hand

Use additional external cause code to identify the source, place and intent of the burn (X00-X19, X75-X77, X96-X98, Y92)

T23.30   Burn of third degree of hand, unspecified site

⑦T23.301   Burn of third degree of right hand, unspecified site

⑦T23.302   Burn of third degree of left hand, unspecified site

⑦T23.309   Burn of third degree of unspecified hand, unspecified site

T23.31   Burn of third degree of thumb (nail)

⑦T23.311   Burn of third degree of right thumb (nail)

⑦T23.312   Burn of third degree of left thumb (nail)

⑦T23.319   Burn of third degree of unspecified thumb (nail)

T23.32   Burn of third degree of single finger (nail) except thumb

⑦T23.321   Burn of third degree of single right finger (nail) except thumb

⑦T23.322   Burn of third degree of single left finger (nail) except thumb

⑦T23.329   Burn of third degree of unspecified single finger (nail) except thumb

T23.33   Burn of third degree of multiple fingers (nail), not including thumb

⑦T23.331   Burn of third degree of multiple right fingers (nail), not including thumb

⑦T23.332   Burn of third degree of multiple left fingers (nail), not including thumb

⑦T23.339   Burn of third degree of unspecified multiple fingers (nail), not including thumb

T23.34   Burn of third degree of multiple fingers (nail), including thumb

⑦T23.341   Burn of third degree of multiple right fingers (nail), including thumb

⑦T23.342   Burn of third degree of multiple left fingers (nail), including thumb

⑦T23.349   Burn of third degree of unspecified multiple fingers (nail), including thumb

T23.35   Burn of third degree of palm

⑦T23.351   Burn of third degree of right palm

⑦T23.352   Burn of third degree of left palm

⑦T23.359   Burn of third degree of unspecified palm

T23.36   Burn of third degree of back of hand

⑦T23.361   Burn of third degree of back of right hand

⑦T23.362   Burn of third degree of back of left hand

⑦T23.369   Burn of third degree of back of unspecified hand

T23.37   Burn of third degree of wrist

⑦T23.371   Burn of third degree of right wrist

⑦T23.372   Burn of third degree of left wrist

⑦T23.379   Burn of third degree of unspecified wrist

T23.39   Burn of third degree of multiple sites of wrist and hand

⑦T23.391   Burn of third degree of multiple sites of right wrist and hand

⑦T23.392   Burn of third degree of multiple sites of left wrist and hand

⑦T23.399   Burn of third degree of multiple sites of unspecified wrist and hand

T23.4   Corrosion of unspecified degree of wrist and hand

Code first (T51-T65) to identify chemical and intent

Use additional external cause code to identify place (Y92)

T23.40   Corrosion of unspecified degree of hand, unspecified site

⑦T23.401   Corrosion of unspecified degree of right hand, unspecified site

⑦T23.402   Corrosion of unspecified degree of left hand, unspecified site

⑦T23.409   Corrosion of unspecified degree of unspecified hand, unspecified site

T23.41   Corrosion of unspecified degree of thumb (nail)

⑦T23.411   Corrosion of unspecified degree of right thumb (nail)

⑦T23.412   Corrosion of unspecified degree of left thumb (nail)

⑦T23.419   Corrosion of unspecified degree of unspecified thumb (nail)

T23.42   Corrosion of unspecified degree of single finger (nail) except thumb

⑦T23.421   Corrosion of unspecified degree of single right finger (nail) except thumb

⑦T23.422   Corrosion of unspecified degree of single left finger (nail) except thumb

⑦T23.429   Corrosion of unspecified degree of unspecified single finger (nail) except thumb

T23.43   Corrosion of unspecified degree of multiple fingers (nail), not including thumb

⑦T23.431   Corrosion of unspecified degree of multiple right fingers (nail), not including thumb

⑦T23.432   Corrosion of unspecified degree of multiple left fingers (nail), not including thumb

⑦**T23.439** Corrosion of unspecified degree of unspecified multiple fingers (nail), not including thumb

T23.44 Corrosion of unspecified degree of multiple fingers (nail), including thumb

⑦**T23.441** Corrosion of unspecified degree of multiple right fingers (nail), including thumb

⑦**T23.442** Corrosion of unspecified degree of multiple left fingers (nail), including thumb

⑦**T23.449** Corrosion of unspecified degree of unspecified multiple fingers (nail), including thumb

T23.45 Corrosion of unspecified degree of palm

⑦**T23.451** Corrosion of unspecified degree of right palm

⑦**T23.452** Corrosion of unspecified degree of left palm

⑦**T23.459** Corrosion of unspecified degree of unspecified palm

T23.46 Corrosion of unspecified degree of back of hand

⑦**T23.461** Corrosion of unspecified degree of back of right hand

⑦**T23.462** Corrosion of unspecified degree of back of left hand

⑦**T23.469** Corrosion of unspecified degree of back of unspecified hand

T23.47 Corrosion of unspecified degree of wrist

⑦**T23.471** Corrosion of unspecified degree of right wrist

⑦**T23.472** Corrosion of unspecified degree of left wrist

⑦**T23.479** Corrosion of unspecified degree of unspecified wrist

T23.49 Corrosion of unspecified degree of multiple sites of wrist and hand

⑦**T23.491** Corrosion of unspecified degree of multiple sites of right wrist and hand

⑦**T23.492** Corrosion of unspecified degree of multiple sites of left wrist and hand

⑦**T23.499** Corrosion of unspecified degree of multiple sites of unspecified wrist and hand

T23.5 Corrosion of first degree of wrist and hand
Code first (T51-T65) to identify chemical and intent
Use additional external cause code to identify place (Y92)

T23.50 Corrosion of first degree of hand, unspecified site

⑦**T23.501** Corrosion of first degree of right hand, unspecified site

⑦**T23.502** Corrosion of first degree of left hand, unspecified site

⑦**T23.509** Corrosion of first degree of unspecified hand, unspecified site

T23.51 Corrosion of first degree of thumb (nail)

⑦**T23.511** Corrosion of first degree of right thumb (nail)

⑦**T23.512** Corrosion of first degree of left thumb (nail)

⑦**T23.519** Corrosion of first degree of unspecified thumb (nail)

T23.52 Corrosion of first degree of single finger (nail) except thumb

⑦**T23.521** Corrosion of first degree of single right finger (nail) except thumb

⑦**T23.522** Corrosion of first degree of single left finger (nail) except thumb

⑦**T23.529** Corrosion of first degree of unspecified single finger (nail) except thumb

T23.53 Corrosion of first degree of multiple fingers (nail), not including thumb

⑦**T23.531** Corrosion of first degree of multiple right fingers (nail), not including thumb

⑦**T23.532** Corrosion of first degree of multiple left fingers (nail), not including thumb

⑦**T23.539** Corrosion of first degree of unspecified multiple fingers (nail), not including thumb

T23.54 Corrosion of first degree of multiple fingers (nail), including thumb

⑦**T23.541** Corrosion of first degree of multiple right fingers (nail), including thumb

⑦**T23.542** Corrosion of first degree of multiple left fingers (nail), including thumb

⑦**T23.549** Corrosion of first degree of unspecified multiple fingers (nail), including thumb

T23.55 Corrosion of first degree of palm

⑦**T23.551** Corrosion of first degree of right palm

⑦**T23.552** Corrosion of first degree of left palm

⑦**T23.559** Corrosion of first degree of unspecified palm

T23.56 Corrosion of first degree of back of hand

⑦**T23.561** Corrosion of first degree of back of right hand

⑦**T23.562** Corrosion of first degree of back of left hand

⑦**T23.569** Corrosion of first degree of back of unspecified hand

T23.57 Corrosion of first degree of wrist

⑦**T23.571** Corrosion of first degree of right wrist

⑦**T23.572** Corrosion of first degree of left wrist

⑦**T23.579** Corrosion of first degree of unspecified wrist

T23.59 Corrosion of first degree of multiple sites of wrist and hand

⑦**T23.591** Corrosion of first degree of multiple sites of right wrist and hand

⑦**T23.592** Corrosion of first degree of multiple sites of left wrist and hand

⑦T23.599 Corrosion of first degree of multiple sites of unspecified wrist and hand

T23.6 Corrosion of second degree of wrist and hand
Code first (T51-T65) to identify chemical and intent
Use additional external cause code to identify place (Y92)

T23.60 Corrosion of second degree of hand, unspecified site

⑦T23.601 Corrosion of second degree of right hand, unspecified site

⑦T23.602 Corrosion of second degree of left hand, unspecified site

⑦T23.609 Corrosion of second degree of unspecified hand, unspecified site

T23.61 Corrosion of second degree of thumb (nail)

⑦T23.611 Corrosion of second degree of right thumb (nail)

⑦T23.612 Corrosion of second degree of left thumb (nail)

⑦T23.619 Corrosion of second degree of unspecified thumb (nail)

T23.62 Corrosion of second degree of single finger (nail) except thumb

⑦T23.621 Corrosion of second degree of single right finger (nail) except thumb

⑦T23.622 Corrosion of second degree of single left finger (nail) except thumb

⑦T23.629 Corrosion of second degree of unspecified single finger (nail) except thumb

T23.63 Corrosion of second degree of multiple fingers (nail), not including thumb

⑦T23.631 Corrosion of second degree of multiple right fingers (nail), not including thumb

⑦T23.632 Corrosion of second degree of multiple left fingers (nail), not including thumb

⑦T23.639 Corrosion of second degree of unspecified multiple fingers (nail), not including thumb

T23.64 Corrosion of second degree of multiple fingers (nail), including thumb

⑦T23.641 Corrosion of second degree of multiple right fingers (nail), including thumb

⑦T23.642 Corrosion of second degree of multiple left fingers (nail), including thumb

⑦T23.649 Corrosion of second degree of unspecified multiple fingers (nail), including thumb

T23.65 Corrosion of second degree of palm

⑦T23.651 Corrosion of second degree of right palm

⑦T23.652 Corrosion of second degree of left palm

⑦T23.659 Corrosion of second degree of unspecified palm

T23.66 Corrosion of second degree of back of hand

⑦T23.661 Corrosion of second degree back of right hand

⑦T23.662 Corrosion of second degree back of left hand

⑦T23.669 Corrosion of second degree back of unspecified hand

T23.67 Corrosion of second degree of wrist

⑦T23.671 Corrosion of second degree of right wrist

⑦T23.672 Corrosion of second degree of left wrist

⑦T23.679 Corrosion of second degree of unspecified wrist

T23.69 Corrosion of second degree of multiple sites of wrist and hand

⑦T23.691 Corrosion of second degree of multiple sites of right wrist and hand

⑦T23.692 Corrosion of second degree of multiple sites of left wrist and hand

⑦T23.699 Corrosion of second degree of multiple sites of unspecified wrist and hand

T23.7 Corrosion of third degree of wrist and hand
Code first (T51-T65) to identify chemical and intent
Use additional external cause code to identify place (Y92)

T23.70 Corrosion of third degree of hand, unspecified site

⑦T23.701 Corrosion of third degree of right hand, unspecified site

⑦T23.702 Corrosion of third degree of left hand, unspecified site

⑦T23.709 Corrosion of third degree of unspecified hand, unspecified site

T23.71 Corrosion of third degree of thumb (nail)

⑦T23.711 Corrosion of third degree of right thumb (nail)

⑦T23.712 Corrosion of third degree of left thumb (nail)

⑦T23.719 Corrosion of third degree of unspecified thumb (nail)

T23.72 Corrosion of third degree of single finger (nail) except thumb

⑦T23.721 Corrosion of third degree of single right finger (nail) except thumb

⑦T23.722 Corrosion of third degree of single left finger (nail) except thumb

⑦T23.729 Corrosion of third degree of unspecified single finger (nail) except thumb

T23.73 Corrosion of third degree of multiple fingers (nail), not including thumb

⑦T23.731 Corrosion of third degree of multiple right fingers (nail), not including thumb

⑦T23.732 Corrosion of third degree of multiple left fingers (nail), not including thumb

⑦T23.739 Corrosion of third degree of unspecified multiple fingers (nail), not including thumb

T23.74 Corrosion of third degree of multiple fingers (nail), including thumb

⑦T23.741 Corrosion of third degree of multiple right fingers (nail), including thumb

⑦T23.742 Corrosion of third degree of multiple left fingers (nail), including thumb

⑦T23.749 Corrosion of third degree of unspecified multiple fingers (nail), including thumb

T23.75 Corrosion of third degree of palm

⑦T23.751 Corrosion of third degree of right palm

⑦T23.752 Corrosion of third degree of left palm

⑦T23.759 Corrosion of third degree of unspecified palm

T23.76 Corrosion of third degree of back of hand

⑦T23.761 Corrosion of third degree of back of right hand

⑦T23.762 Corrosion of third degree of back of left hand

⑦T23.769 Corrosion of third degree back of unspecified hand

T23.77 Corrosion of third degree of wrist

⑦T23.771 Corrosion of third degree of right wrist

⑦T23.772 Corrosion of third degree of left wrist

⑦T23.779 Corrosion of third degree of unspecified wrist

T23.79 Corrosion of third degree of multiple sites of wrist and hand

⑦T23.791 Corrosion of third degree of multiple sites of right wrist and hand

⑦T23.792 Corrosion of third degree of multiple sites of left wrist and hand

⑦T23.799 Corrosion of third degree of multiple sites of unspecified wrist and hand

T24 Burn and corrosion of lower limb, except ankle and foot

Excludes 2: burn and corrosion of ankle and foot (T25.-)

burn and corrosion of hip region (T21.-)

The appropriate 7th character is to be added to each code from category T24

A - initial encounter

D - subsequent encounter

S - sequela

T24.0 Burn of unspecified degree of lower limb, except ankle and foot

Use additional external cause code to identify the source, place and intent of the burn (X00-X19, X75-X77, X96-X98, Y92)

T24.00 Burn of unspecified degree of unspecified site of lower limb, except ankle and foot

⑦T24.001 Burn of unspecified degree of unspecified site of right lower limb, except ankle and foot

⑦T24.002 Burn of unspecified degree of unspecified site of left lower limb, except ankle and foot

⑦T24.009 Burn of unspecified degree of unspecified site of unspecified lower limb, except ankle and foot

T24.01 Burn of unspecified degree of thigh

⑦T24.011 Burn of unspecified degree of right thigh

⑦T24.012 Burn of unspecified degree of left thigh

⑦T24.019 Burn of unspecified degree of unspecified thigh

T24.02 Burn of unspecified degree of knee

⑦T24.021 Burn of unspecified degree of right knee

⑦T24.022 Burn of unspecified degree of left knee

⑦T24.029 Burn of unspecified degree of unspecified knee

T24.03 Burn of unspecified degree of lower leg

⑦T24.031 Burn of unspecified degree of right lower leg

⑦T24.032 Burn of unspecified degree of left lower leg

⑦T24.039 Burn of unspecified degree of unspecified lower leg

T24.09 Burn of unspecified degree of multiple sites of lower limb, except ankle and foot

⑦T24.091 Burn of unspecified degree of multiple sites of right lower limb, except ankle and foot

⑦T24.092 Burn of unspecified degree of multiple sites of left lower limb, except ankle and foot

⑦T24.099 Burn of unspecified degree of multiple sites of unspecified lower limb, except ankle and foot

T24.1 Burn of first degree of lower limb, except ankle and foot

Use additional external cause code to identify the source, place and intent of the burn (X00-X19, X75-X77, X96-X98, Y92)

T24.10 Burn of first degree of unspecified site of lower limb, except ankle and foot

⑦T24.101 Burn of first degree of unspecified site of right lower limb, except ankle and foot

⑦T24.102 Burn of first degree of unspecified site of left lower limb, except ankle and foot

⑦T24.109 Burn of first degree of unspecified site of unspecified lower limb, except ankle and foot

T24.11 Burn of first degree of thigh

⑦T24.111 Burn of first degree of right thigh

⑦T24.112 Burn of first degree of left thigh

⑦T24.119 Burn of first degree of unspecified thigh

T24.12 Burn of first degree of knee

⑦T24.121 Burn of first degree of right knee

⑦T24.122 Burn of first degree of left knee

● New code   ▲ Revised code   ⑦ 7th digit required   ⊗ Placeholder required

⑦**T24.129** Burn of first degree of unspecified knee

T24.13 Burn of first degree of lower leg

⑦**T24.131** Burn of first degree of right lower leg

⑦**T24.132** Burn of first degree of left lower leg

⑦**T24.139** Burn of first degree of unspecified lower leg

T24.19 Burn of first degree of multiple sites of lower limb, except ankle and foot

⑦**T24.191** Burn of first degree of multiple sites of right lower limb, except ankle and foot

⑦**T24.192** Burn of first degree of multiple sites of left lower limb, except ankle and foot

⑦**T24.199** Burn of first degree of multiple sites of unspecified lower limb, except ankle and foot

T24.2 Burn of second degree of lower limb, except ankle and foot

Use additional external cause code to identify the source, place and intent of the burn (X00-X19, X75-X77, X96-X98, Y92)

T24.20 Burn of second degree of unspecified site of lower limb, except ankle and foot

⑦**T24.201** Burn of second degree of unspecified site of right lower limb, except ankle and foot

⑦**T24.202** Burn of second degree of unspecified site of left lower limb, except ankle and foot

⑦**T24.209** Burn of second degree of unspecified site of unspecified lower limb, except ankle and foot

T24.21 Burn of second degree of thigh

⑦**T24.211** Burn of second degree of right thigh

⑦**T24.212** Burn of second degree of left thigh

⑦**T24.219** Burn of second degree of unspecified thigh

T24.22 Burn of second degree of knee

⑦**T24.221** Burn of second degree of right knee

⑦**T24.222** Burn of second degree of left knee

⑦**T24.229** Burn of second degree of unspecified knee

T24.23 Burn of second degree of lower leg

⑦**T24.231** Burn of second degree of right lower leg

⑦**T24.232** Burn of second degree of left lower leg

⑦**T24.239** Burn of second degree of unspecified lower leg

T24.29 Burn of second degree of multiple sites of lower limb, except ankle and foot

⑦**T24.291** Burn of second degree of multiple sites of right lower limb, except ankle and foot

⑦**T24.292** Burn of second degree of multiple sites of left lower limb, except ankle and foot

⑦**T24.299** Burn of second degree of multiple sites of unspecified lower limb, except ankle and foot

T24.3 Burn of third degree of lower limb, except ankle and foot

Use additional external cause code to identify the source, place and intent of the burn (X00-X19, X75-X77, X96-X98, Y92)

T24.30 Burn of third degree of unspecified site of lower limb, except ankle and foot

⑦**T24.301** Burn of third degree of unspecified site of right lower limb, except ankle and foot

⑦**T24.302** Burn of third degree of unspecified site of left lower limb, except ankle and foot

⑦**T24.309** Burn of third degree of unspecified site of unspecified lower limb, except ankle and foot

T24.31 Burn of third degree of thigh

⑦**T24.311** Burn of third degree of right thigh

⑦**T24.312** Burn of third degree of left thigh

⑦**T24.319** Burn of third degree of unspecified thigh

T24.32 Burn of third degree of knee

⑦**T24.321** Burn of third degree of right knee

⑦**T24.322** Burn of third degree of left knee

⑦**T24.329** Burn of third degree of unspecified knee

T24.33 Burn of third degree of lower leg

⑦**T24.331** Burn of third degree of right lower leg

⑦**T24.332** Burn of third degree of left lower leg

⑦**T24.339** Burn of third degree of unspecified lower leg

T24.39 Burn of third degree of multiple sites of lower limb, except ankle and foot

⑦**T24.391** Burn of third degree of multiple sites of right lower limb, except ankle and foot

⑦**T24.392** Burn of third degree of multiple sites of left lower limb, except ankle and foot

⑦**T24.399** Burn of third degree of multiple sites of unspecified lower limb, except ankle and foot

T24.4 Corrosion of unspecified degree of lower limb, except ankle and foot

Code first (T51-T65) to identify chemical and intent

Use additional external cause code to identify place (Y92)

T24.40 Corrosion of unspecified degree of unspecified site of lower limb, except ankle and foot

⑦**T24.401** Corrosion of unspecified degree of unspecified site of right lower limb, except ankle and foot

⑦**T24.402** Corrosion of unspecified degree of unspecified site of left lower limb, except ankle and foot

⑦**T24.409** Corrosion of unspecified degree of unspecified site of unspecified lower limb, except ankle and foot

T24.41   Corrosion of unspecified degree of thigh
  ⑦**T24.411**   Corrosion of unspecified degree of right thigh
  ⑦**T24.412**   Corrosion of unspecified degree of left thigh
  ⑦**T24.419**   Corrosion of unspecified degree of unspecified thigh
T24.42   Corrosion of unspecified degree of knee
  ⑦**T24.421**   Corrosion of unspecified degree of right knee
  ⑦**T24.422**   Corrosion of unspecified degree of left knee
  ⑦**T24.429**   Corrosion of unspecified degree of unspecified knee
T24.43   Corrosion of unspecified degree of lower leg
  ⑦**T24.431**   Corrosion of unspecified degree of right lower leg
  ⑦**T24.432**   Corrosion of unspecified degree of left lower leg
  ⑦**T24.439**   Corrosion of unspecified degree of unspecified lower leg
T24.49   Corrosion of unspecified degree of multiple sites of lower limb, except ankle and foot
  ⑦**T24.491**   Corrosion of unspecified degree of multiple sites of right lower limb, except ankle and foot
  ⑦**T24.492**   Corrosion of unspecified degree of multiple sites of left lower limb, except ankle and foot
  ⑦**T24.499**   Corrosion of unspecified degree of multiple sites of unspecified lower limb, except ankle and foot

T24.5   Corrosion of first degree of lower limb, except ankle and foot
Code first (T51-T65) to identify chemical and intent
Use additional external cause code to identify place (Y92)
T24.50   Corrosion of first degree of unspecified site of lower limb, except ankle and foot
  ⑦**T24.501**   Corrosion of first degree of unspecified site of right lower limb, except ankle and foot
  ⑦**T24.502**   Corrosion of first degree of unspecified site of left lower limb, except ankle and foot
  ⑦**T24.509**   Corrosion of first degree of unspecified site of unspecified lower limb, except ankle and foot
T24.51   Corrosion of first degree of thigh
  ⑦**T24.511**   Corrosion of first degree of right thigh
  ⑦**T24.512**   Corrosion of first degree of left thigh
  ⑦**T24.519**   Corrosion of first degree of unspecified thigh
T24.52   Corrosion of first degree of knee
  ⑦**T24.521**   Corrosion of first degree of right knee
  ⑦**T24.522**   Corrosion of first degree of left knee
  ⑦**T24.529**   Corrosion of first degree of unspecified knee

T24.53   Corrosion of first degree of lower leg
  ⑦**T24.531**   Corrosion of first degree of right lower leg
  ⑦**T24.532**   Corrosion of first degree of left lower leg
  ⑦**T24.539**   Corrosion of first degree of unspecified lower leg
T24.59   Corrosion of first degree of multiple sites of lower limb, except ankle and foot
  ⑦**T24.591**   Corrosion of first degree of multiple sites of right lower limb, except ankle and foot
  ⑦**T24.592**   Corrosion of first degree of multiple sites of left lower limb, except ankle and foot
  ⑦**T24.599**   Corrosion of first degree of multiple sites of unspecified lower limb, except ankle and foot

T24.6   Corrosion of second degree of lower limb, except ankle and foot
Code first (T51-T65) to identify chemical and intent
Use additional external cause code to identify place (Y92)
T24.60   Corrosion of second degree of unspecified site of lower limb, except ankle and foot
  ⑦**T24.601**   Corrosion of second degree of unspecified site of right lower limb, except ankle and foot
  ⑦**T24.602**   Corrosion of second degree of unspecified site of left lower limb, except ankle and foot
  ⑦**T24.609**   Corrosion of second degree of unspecified site of unspecified lower limb, except ankle and foot
T24.61   Corrosion of second degree of thigh
  ⑦**T24.611**   Corrosion of second degree of right thigh
  ⑦**T24.612**   Corrosion of second degree of left thigh
  ⑦**T24.619**   Corrosion of second degree of unspecified thigh
T24.62   Corrosion of second degree of knee
  ⑦**T24.621**   Corrosion of second degree of right knee
  ⑦**T24.622**   Corrosion of second degree of left knee
  ⑦**T24.629**   Corrosion of second degree of unspecified knee
T24.63   Corrosion of second degree of lower leg
  ⑦**T24.631**   Corrosion of second degree of right lower leg
  ⑦**T24.632**   Corrosion of second degree of left lower leg
  ⑦**T24.639**   Corrosion of second degree of unspecified lower leg
T24.69   Corrosion of second degree of multiple sites of lower limb, except ankle and foot
  ⑦**T24.691**   Corrosion of second degree of multiple sites of right lower limb, except ankle and foot

⑦**T24.692**   Corrosion of second degree of multiple sites of left lower limb, except ankle and foot

⑦**T24.699**   Corrosion of second degree of multiple sites of unspecified lower limb, except ankle and foot

T24.7   Corrosion of third degree of lower limb, except ankle and foot

Code first (T51-T65) to identify chemical and intent
Use additional external cause code to identify place (Y92)

T24.70   Corrosion of third degree of unspecified site of lower limb, except ankle and foot

⑦**T24.701**   Corrosion of third degree of unspecified site of right lower limb, except ankle and foot

⑦**T24.702**   Corrosion of third degree of unspecified site of left lower limb, except ankle and foot

⑦**T24.709**   Corrosion of third degree of unspecified site of unspecified lower limb, except ankle and foot

T24.71   Corrosion of third degree of thigh

⑦**T24.711**   Corrosion of third degree of right thigh

⑦**T24.712**   Corrosion of third degree of left thigh

⑦**T24.719**   Corrosion of third degree of unspecified thigh

T24.72   Corrosion of third degree of knee

⑦**T24.721**   Corrosion of third degree of right knee

⑦**T24.722**   Corrosion of third degree of left knee

⑦**T24.729**   Corrosion of third degree of unspecified knee

T24.73   Corrosion of third degree of lower leg

⑦**T24.731**   Corrosion of third degree of right lower leg

⑦**T24.732**   Corrosion of third degree of left lower leg

⑦**T24.739**   Corrosion of third degree of unspecified lower leg

T24.79   Corrosion of third degree of multiple sites of lower limb, except ankle and foot

⑦**T24.791**   Corrosion of third degree of multiple sites of right lower limb, except ankle and foot

⑦**T24.792**   Corrosion of third degree of multiple sites of left lower limb, except ankle and foot

⑦**T24.799**   Corrosion of third degree of multiple sites of unspecified lower limb, except ankle and foot

T25   Burn and corrosion of ankle and foot

The appropriate 7th character is to be added to each code from category T25
A - initial encounter
D - subsequent encounter
S - sequela

T25.0   Burn of unspecified degree of ankle and foot

Use additional external cause code to identify the source, place and intent of the burn (X00-X19, X75-X77, X96-X98, Y92)

T25.01   Burn of unspecified degree of ankle

⑦**T25.011**   Burn of unspecified degree of right ankle

⑦**T25.012**   Burn of unspecified degree of left ankle

⑦**T25.019**   Burn of unspecified degree of unspecified ankle

T25.02   Burn of unspecified degree of foot

Excludes 2: burn of unspecified degree of toe(s) (nail) (T25.03-)

⑦**T25.021**   Burn of unspecified degree of right foot

⑦**T25.022**   Burn of unspecified degree of left foot

⑦**T25.029**   Burn of unspecified degree of unspecified foot

T25.03   Burn of unspecified degree of toe(s) (nail)

⑦**T25.031**   Burn of unspecified degree of right toe(s) (nail)

⑦**T25.032**   Burn of unspecified degree of left toe(s) (nail)

⑦**T25.039**   Burn of unspecified degree of unspecified toe(s) (nail)

T25.09   Burn of unspecified degree of multiple sites of ankle and foot

⑦**T25.091**   Burn of unspecified degree of multiple sites of right ankle and foot

⑦**T25.092**   Burn of unspecified degree of multiple sites of left ankle and foot

⑦**T25.099**   Burn of unspecified degree of multiple sites of unspecified ankle and foot

T25.1   Burn of first degree of ankle and foot

Use additional external cause code to identify the source, place and intent of the burn (X00-X19, X75-X77, X96-X98, Y92)

T25.11   Burn of first degree of ankle

⑦**T25.111**   Burn of first degree of right ankle

⑦**T25.112**   Burn of first degree of left ankle

⑦**T25.119**   Burn of first degree of unspecified ankle

T25.12   Burn of first degree of foot

Excludes 2: burn of first degree of toe(s) (nail) (T25.13-)

⑦**T25.121**   Burn of first degree of right foot

⑦**T25.122**   Burn of first degree of left foot

⑦**T25.129**   Burn of first degree of unspecified foot

T25.13   Burn of first degree of toe(s) (nail)

⑦**T25.131**   Burn of first degree of right toe(s) (nail)

⑦**T25.132**   Burn of first degree of left toe(s) (nail)

⑦**T25.139**   Burn of first degree of unspecified toe(s) (nail)

T25.19   Burn of first degree of multiple sites of ankle and foot

⑦ **T25.191**   Burn of first degree of multiple sites of right ankle and foot

⑦ **T25.192**   Burn of first degree of multiple sites of left ankle and foot

⑦ **T25.199**   Burn of first degree of multiple sites of unspecified ankle and foot

T25.2   Burn of second degree of ankle and foot

Use additional external cause code to identify the source, place and intent of the burn (X00-X19, X75-X77, X96-X98, Y92)

T25.21   Burn of second degree of ankle

⑦ **T25.211**   Burn of second degree of right ankle

⑦ **T25.212**   Burn of second degree of left ankle

⑦ **T25.219**   Burn of second degree of unspecified ankle

T25.22   Burn of second degree of foot

Excludes 2: burn of second degree of toe(s) (nail) (T25.23-)

⑦ **T25.221**   Burn of second degree of right foot

⑦ **T25.222**   Burn of second degree of left foot

⑦ **T25.229**   Burn of second degree of unspecified foot

T25.23   Burn of second degree of toe(s) (nail)

⑦ **T25.231**   Burn of second degree of right toe(s) (nail)

⑦ **T25.232**   Burn of second degree of left toe(s) (nail)

⑦ **T25.239**   Burn of second degree of unspecified toe(s) (nail)

T25.29   Burn of second degree of multiple sites of ankle and foot

⑦ **T25.291**   Burn of second degree of multiple sites of right ankle and foot

⑦ **T25.292**   Burn of second degree of multiple sites of left ankle and foot

⑦ **T25.299**   Burn of second degree of multiple sites of unspecified ankle and foot

T25.3   Burn of third degree of ankle and foot

Use additional external cause code to identify the source, place and intent of the burn (X00-X19, X75-X77, X96-X98, Y92)

T25.31   Burn of third degree of ankle

⑦ **T25.311**   Burn of third degree of right ankle

⑦ **T25.312**   Burn of third degree of left ankle

⑦ **T25.319**   Burn of third degree of unspecified ankle

T25.32   Burn of third degree of foot

Excludes 2: burn of third degree of toe(s) (nail) (T25.33-)

⑦ **T25.321**   Burn of third degree of right foot

⑦ **T25.322**   Burn of third degree of left foot

⑦ **T25.329**   Burn of third degree of unspecified foot

T25.33   Burn of third degree of toe(s) (nail)

⑦ **T25.331**   Burn of third degree of right toe(s) (nail)

⑦ **T25.332**   Burn of third degree of left toe(s) (nail)

⑦ **T25.339**   Burn of third degree of unspecified toe(s) (nail)

T25.39   Burn of third degree of multiple sites of ankle and foot

⑦ **T25.391**   Burn of third degree of multiple sites of right ankle and foot

⑦ **T25.392**   Burn of third degree of multiple sites of left ankle and foot

⑦ **T25.399**   Burn of third degree of multiple sites of unspecified ankle and foot

T25.4   Corrosion of unspecified degree of ankle and foot

Code first (T51-T65) to identify chemical and intent

Use additional external cause code to identify place (Y92)

T25.41   Corrosion of unspecified degree of ankle

⑦ **T25.411**   Corrosion of unspecified degree of right ankle

⑦ **T25.412**   Corrosion of unspecified degree of left ankle

⑦ **T25.419**   Corrosion of unspecified degree of unspecified ankle

T25.42   Corrosion of unspecified degree of foot

Excludes 2: corrosion of unspecified degree of toe(s) (nail) (T25.43-)

⑦ **T25.421**   Corrosion of unspecified degree of right foot

⑦ **T25.422**   Corrosion of unspecified degree of left foot

⑦ **T25.429**   Corrosion of unspecified degree of unspecified foot

T25.43   Corrosion of unspecified degree of toe(s) (nail)

⑦ **T25.431**   Corrosion of unspecified degree of right toe(s) (nail)

⑦ **T25.432**   Corrosion of unspecified degree of left toe(s) (nail)

⑦ **T25.439**   Corrosion of unspecified degree of unspecified toe(s) (nail)

T25.49   Corrosion of unspecified degree of multiple sites of ankle and foot

⑦ **T25.491**   Corrosion of unspecified degree of multiple sites of right ankle and foot

⑦ **T25.492**   Corrosion of unspecified degree of multiple sites of left ankle and foot

⑦ **T25.499**   Corrosion of unspecified degree of multiple sites of unspecified ankle and foot

T25.5   Corrosion of first degree of ankle and foot

Code first (T51-T65) to identify chemical and intent

Use additional external cause code to identify place (Y92)

T25.51   Corrosion of first degree of ankle

⑦ **T25.511**   Corrosion of first degree of right ankle

⑦ **T25.512**   Corrosion of first degree of left ankle

⑦ **T25.519**   Corrosion of first degree of unspecified ankle

T25.52   Corrosion of first degree of foot

● New code   ▲ Revised code   ⑦ 7th digit required   ⊗ Placeholder required

Excludes 2: corrosion of first degree of toe(s) (nail) (T25.53-)

⑦T25.521 Corrosion of first degree of right foot

⑦T25.522 Corrosion of first degree of left foot

⑦T25.529 Corrosion of first degree of unspecified foot

T25.53 Corrosion of first degree of toe(s) (nail)

⑦T25.531 Corrosion of first degree of right toe(s) (nail)

⑦T25.532 Corrosion of first degree of left toe(s) (nail)

⑦T25.539 Corrosion of first degree of unspecified toe(s) (nail)

T25.59 Corrosion of first degree of multiple sites of ankle and foot

⑦T25.591 Corrosion of first degree of multiple sites of right ankle and foot

⑦T25.592 Corrosion of first degree of multiple sites of left ankle and foot

⑦T25.599 Corrosion of first degree of multiple sites of unspecified ankle and foot

T25.6 Corrosion of second degree of ankle and foot
Code first (T51-T65) to identify chemical and intent
Use additional external cause code to identify place (Y92)

T25.61 Corrosion of second degree of ankle

⑦T25.611 Corrosion of second degree of right ankle

⑦T25.612 Corrosion of second degree of left ankle

⑦T25.619 Corrosion of second degree of unspecified ankle

T25.62 Corrosion of second degree of foot

Excludes 2: corrosion of second degree of toe(s) (nail) (T25.63-)

⑦T25.621 Corrosion of second degree of right foot

⑦T25.622 Corrosion of second degree of left foot

⑦T25.629 Corrosion of second degree of unspecified foot

T25.63 Corrosion of second degree of toe(s) (nail)

⑦T25.631 Corrosion of second degree of right toe(s) (nail)

⑦T25.632 Corrosion of second degree of left toe(s) (nail)

⑦T25.639 Corrosion of second degree of unspecified toe(s) (nail)

T25.69 Corrosion of second degree of multiple sites of ankle and foot

⑦T25.691 Corrosion of second degree of right ankle and foot

⑦T25.692 Corrosion of second degree of left ankle and foot

⑦T25.699 Corrosion of second degree of unspecified ankle and foot

T25.7 Corrosion of third degree of ankle and foot
Code first (T51-T65) to identify chemical and intent
Use additional external cause code to identify place (Y92)

T25.71 Corrosion of third degree of ankle

⑦T25.711 Corrosion of third degree of right ankle

⑦T25.712 Corrosion of third degree of left ankle

⑦T25.719 Corrosion of third degree of unspecified ankle

T25.72 Corrosion of third degree of foot

Excludes 2: corrosion of third degree of toe(s) (nail) (T25.73-)

⑦T25.721 Corrosion of third degree of right foot

⑦T25.722 Corrosion of third degree of left foot

⑦T25.729 Corrosion of third degree of unspecified foot

T25.73 Corrosion of third degree of toe(s) (nail)

⑦T25.731 Corrosion of third degree of right toe(s) (nail)

⑦T25.732 Corrosion of third degree of left toe(s) (nail)

⑦T25.739 Corrosion of third degree of unspecified toe(s) (nail)

T25.79 Corrosion of third degree of multiple sites of ankle and foot

⑦T25.791 Corrosion of third degree of multiple sites of right ankle and foot

⑦T25.792 Corrosion of third degree of multiple sites of left ankle and foot

⑦T25.799 Corrosion of third degree of multiple sites of unspecified ankle and foot

BURNS AND CORROSIONS CONFINED TO EYE AND INTERNAL ORGANS (T26-T28)

T26 Burn and corrosion confined to eye and adnexa
The appropriate 7th character is to be added to each code from category T26
A - initial encounter
D - subsequent encounter
S - sequela

T26.0 Burn of eyelid and periocular area
Use additional external cause code to identify the source, place and intent of the burn (X00-X19, X75-X77, X96-X98, Y92)

⊗⑦T26.00 Burn of unspecified eyelid and periocular area

⊗⑦T26.01 Burn of right eyelid and periocular area

⊗⑦T26.02 Burn of left eyelid and periocular area

T26.1 Burn of cornea and conjunctival sac
Use additional external cause code to identify the source, place and intent of the burn (X00-X19, X75-X77, X96-X98, Y92)

⊗⑦T26.10 Burn of cornea and conjunctival sac, unspecified eye

⊗⑦T26.11 Burn of cornea and conjunctival sac, right eye

⊗⑦T26.12 Burn of cornea and conjunctival sac, left eye

T26.2 Burn with resulting rupture and destruction of eyeball
Use additional external cause code to identify the source, place and intent of the burn (X00-X19, X75-X77, X96-X98, Y92)

⊗⑦**T26.20** Burn with resulting rupture and destruction of unspecified eyeball

⊗⑦**T26.21** Burn with resulting rupture and destruction of right eyeball

⊗⑦**T26.22** Burn with resulting rupture and destruction of left eyeball

T26.3 Burns of other specified parts of eye and adnexa
Use additional external cause code to identify the source, place and intent of the burn (X00-X19, X75-X77, X96-X98, Y92)

⊗⑦**T26.30** Burns of other specified parts of unspecified eye and adnexa

⊗⑦**T26.31** Burns of other specified parts of right eye and adnexa

⊗⑦**T26.32** Burns of other specified parts of left eye and adnexa

T26.4 Burn of eye and adnexa, part unspecified
Use additional external cause code to identify the source, place and intent of the burn (X00-X19, X75-X77, X96-X98, Y92)

⊗⑦**T26.40** Burn of unspecified eye and adnexa, part unspecified

⊗⑦**T26.41** Burn of right eye and adnexa, part unspecified

⊗⑦**T26.42** Burn of left eye and adnexa, part unspecified

T26.5 Corrosion of eyelid and periocular area
Code first (T51-T65) to identify chemical and intent
Use additional external cause code to identify place (Y92)

⊗⑦**T26.50** Corrosion of unspecified eyelid and periocular area

⊗⑦**T26.51** Corrosion of right eyelid and periocular area

⊗⑦**T26.52** Corrosion of left eyelid and periocular area

T26.6 Corrosion of cornea and conjunctival sac
Code first (T51-T65) to identify chemical and intent
Use additional external cause code to identify place (Y92)

⊗⑦**T26.60** Corrosion of cornea and conjunctival sac, unspecified eye

⊗⑦**T26.61** Corrosion of cornea and conjunctival sac, right eye

⊗⑦**T26.62** Corrosion of cornea and conjunctival sac, left eye

T26.7 Corrosion with resulting rupture and destruction of eyeball
Code first (T51-T65) to identify chemical and intent
Use additional external cause code to identify place (Y92)

⊗⑦**T26.70** Corrosion with resulting rupture and destruction of unspecified eyeball

⊗⑦**T26.71** Corrosion with resulting rupture and destruction of right eyeball

⊗⑦**T26.72** Corrosion with resulting rupture and destruction of left eyeball

T26.8 Corrosions of other specified parts of eye and adnexa
Code first (T51-T65) to identify chemical and intent
Use additional external cause code to identify place (Y92)

⊗⑦**T26.80** Corrosions of other specified parts of unspecified eye and adnexa

⊗⑦**T26.81** Corrosions of other specified parts of right eye and adnexa

⊗⑦**T26.82** Corrosions of other specified parts of left eye and adnexa

T26.9 Corrosion of eye and adnexa, part unspecified
Code first (T51-T65) to identify chemical and intent

Use additional external cause code to identify place (Y92)

⊗⑦**T26.90** Corrosion of unspecified eye and adnexa, part unspecified

⊗⑦**T26.91** Corrosion of right eye and adnexa, part unspecified

⊗⑦**T26.92** Corrosion of left eye and adnexa, part unspecified

T27 Burn and corrosion of respiratory tract
Use additional external cause code to identify the source and intent of the burn (X00- X19, X75-X77, X96-X98)
external cause code to identify place (Y92)
The appropriate 7th character is to be added to each code from category T27
A - initial encounter
D - subsequent encounter
S - sequela

⊗⑦**T27.0** Burn of larynx and trachea

⊗⑦**T27.1** Burn involving larynx and trachea with lung

⊗⑦**T27.2** Burn of other parts of respiratory tract
Burn of thoracic cavity

⊗⑦**T27.3** Burn of respiratory tract, part unspecified
Code first (T51-T65) to identify chemical and intent for codes T27.4-T27.7

⊗⑦**T27.4** Corrosion of larynx and trachea

⊗⑦**T27.5** Corrosion involving larynx and trachea with lung

⊗⑦**T27.6** Corrosion of other parts of respiratory tract

⊗⑦**T27.7** Corrosion of respiratory tract, part unspecified

T28 Burn and corrosion of other internal organs
Use additional external cause code to identify the source and intent of the burn (X00- X19, X75-X77, X96-X98)
external cause code to identify place (Y92)
The appropriate 7th character is to be added to each code from category T28
A - initial encounter
D - subsequent encounter
S - sequela

⊗⑦**T28.0** Burn of mouth and pharynx

⊗⑦**T28.1** Burn of esophagus

⊗⑦**T28.2** Burn of other parts of alimentary tract

⊗⑦**T28.3** Burn of internal genitourinary organs

T28.4 Burns of other and unspecified internal organs

⊗⑦**T28.40** Burn of unspecified internal organ

T28.41 Burn of ear drum

⑦**T28.411** Burn of right ear drum

⑦**T28.412** Burn of left ear drum

⑦**T28.419** Burn of unspecified ear drum

⊗⑦**T28.49** Burn of other internal organ
Code first (T51-T65) to identify chemical and intent for T28.5-T28.9-

⊗⑦**T28.5** Corrosion of mouth and pharynx

⊗⑦**T28.6** Corrosion of esophagus

⊗⑦**T28.7** Corrosion of other parts of alimentary tract

⊗⑦**T28.8** Corrosion of internal genitourinary organs

T28.9 Corrosions of other and unspecified internal organs

⊗⑦**T28.90** Corrosions of unspecified internal organs

T28.91 Corrosions of ear drum

⑦**T28.911** Corrosions of right ear drum

● New code   ▲ Revised code   ⑦ 7th digit required   ⊗ Placeholder required

⑦T28.912   Corrosions of left ear drum

⑦T28.919   Corrosions of unspecified ear drum

⊗⑦T28.99   Corrosions of other internal organs

BURNS AND CORROSIONS OF MULTIPLE AND UNSPECIFIED BODY REGIONS (T30-T32)

T30   Burn and corrosion, body region unspecified

T30.0   Burn of unspecified body region, unspecified degree
This code is not for inpatient use. Code to specified site and degree of burns
Burn NOS
Multiple burns NOS

T30.4   Corrosion of unspecified body region, unspecified degree
This code is not for inpatient use. Code to specified site and degree of corrosion
Corrosion NOS
Multiple corrosion NOS

T31   Burns classified according to extent of body surface involved
This category is to be used as the primary code only when the site of the burn is unspecified. It should be used as a supplementary code with categories T20-T25 when the site is specified.

T31.0   Burns involving less than 10% of body surface

T31.1   Burns involving 10-19% of body surface

     T31.10   Burns involving 10-19% of body surface with 0% to 9% third degree burns
Burns involving 10-19% of body surface NOS

     T31.11   Burns involving 10-19% of body surface with 10-19% third degree burns

T31.2   Burns involving 20-29% of body surface

     T31.20   Burns involving 20-29% of body surface with 0% to 9% third degree burns
Burns involving 20-29% of body surface NOS

     T31.21   Burns involving 20-29% of body surface with 10-19% third degree burns

     T31.22   Burns involving 20-29% of body surface with 20-29% third degree burns

T31.3   Burns involving 30-39% of body surface

     T31.30   Burns involving 30-39% of body surface with 0% to 9% third degree burns
Burns involving 30-39% of body surface NOS

     T31.31   Burns involving 30-39% of body surface with 10-19% third degree burns

     T31.32   Burns involving 30-39% of body surface with 20-29% third degree burns

     T31.33   Burns involving 30-39% of body surface with 30-39% third degree burns

T31.4   Burns involving 40-49% of body surface

     T31.40   Burns involving 40-49% of body surface with 0% to 9% third degree burns
Burns involving 40-49% of body surface NOS

     T31.41   Burns involving 40-49% of body surface with 10-19% third degree burns

     T31.42   Burns involving 40-49% of body surface with 20-29% third degree burns

     T31.43   Burns involving 40-49% of body surface with 30-39% third degree burns

     T31.44   Burns involving 40-49% of body surface with 40-49% third degree burns

T31.5   Burns involving 50-59% of body surface

     T31.50   Burns involving 50-59% of body surface with 0% to 9% third degree burns
Burns involving 50-59% of body surface NOS

     T31.51   Burns involving 50-59% of body surface with 10-19% third degree burns

     T31.52   Burns involving 50-59% of body surface with 20-29% third degree burns

     T31.53   Burns involving 50-59% of body surface with 30-39% third degree burns

     T31.54   Burns involving 50-59% of body surface with 40-49% third degree burns

     T31.55   Burns involving 50-59% of body surface with 50-59% third degree burns

T31.6   Burns involving 60-69% of body surface

     T31.60   Burns involving 60-69% of body surface with 0% to 9% third degree burns
Burns involving 60-69% of body surface NOS

     T31.61   Burns involving 60-69% of body surface with 10-19% third degree burns

     T31.62   Burns involving 60-69% of body surface with 20-29% third degree burns

     T31.63   Burns involving 60-69% of body surface with 30-39% third degree burns

     T31.64   Burns involving 60-69% of body surface with 40-49% third degree burns

     T31.65   Burns involving 60-69% of body surface with 50-59% third degree burns

     T31.66   Burns involving 60-69% of body surface with 60-69% third degree burns

T31.7   Burns involving 70-79% of body surface

     T31.70   Burns involving 70-79% of body surface with 0% to 9% third degree burns
Burns involving 70-79% of body surface NOS

     T31.71   Burns involving 70-79% of body surface with 10-19% third degree burns

     T31.72   Burns involving 70-79% of body surface with 20-29% third degree burns

     T31.73   Burns involving 70-79% of body surface with 30-39% third degree burns

     T31.74   Burns involving 70-79% of body surface with 40-49% third degree burns

     T31.75   Burns involving 70-79% of body surface with 50-59% third degree burns

     T31.76   Burns involving 70-79% of body surface with 60-69% third degree burns

     T31.77   Burns involving 70-79% of body surface with 70-79% third degree burns

T31.8   Burns involving 80-89% of body surface

     T31.80   Burns involving 80-89% of body surface with 0% to 9% third degree burns
Burns involving 80-89% of body surface NOS

     T31.81   Burns involving 80-89% of body surface with 10-19% third degree burns

     T31.82   Burns involving 80-89% of body surface with 20-29% third degree burns

     T31.83   Burns involving 80-89% of body surface with 30-39% third degree burns

     T31.84   Burns involving 80-89% of body surface with 40-49% third degree burns

T31.85 Burns involving 80-89% of body surface with 50-59% third degree burns

T31.86 Burns involving 80-89% of body surface with 60-69% third degree burns

T31.87 Burns involving 80-89% of body surface with 70-79% third degree burns

T31.88 Burns involving 80-89% of body surface with 80-89% third degree burns

T31.9 Burns involving 90% or more of body surface

T31.90 Burns involving 90% or more of body surface with 0% to 9% third degree burns

Burns involving 90% or more of body surface NOS

T31.91 Burns involving 90% or more of body surface with 10-19% third degree burns

T31.92 Burns involving 90% or more of body surface with 20-29% third degree burns

T31.93 Burns involving 90% or more of body surface with 30-39% third degree burns

T31.94 Burns involving 90% or more of body surface with 40-49% third degree burns

T31.95 Burns involving 90% or more of body surface with 50-59% third degree burns

T31.96 Burns involving 90% or more of body surface with 60-69% third degree burns

T31.97 Burns involving 90% or more of body surface with 70-79% third degree burns

T31.98 Burns involving 90% or more of body surface with 80-89% third degree burns

T31.99 Burns involving 90% or more of body surface with 90% or more third degree burns

T32 Corrosions classified according to extent of body surface involved

Note: This category is to be used as the primary code only when the site of the corrosion is unspecified. It may be used as a supplementary code with categories T20-T25 when the site is specified.

T32.0 Corrosions involving less than 10% of body surface

T32.1 Corrosions involving 10-19% of body surface

T32.10 Corrosions involving 10-19% of body surface with 0% to 9% third degree corrosion

Corrosions involving 10-19% of body surface NOS

T32.11 Corrosions involving 10-19% of body surface with 10-19% third degree corrosion

T32.2 Corrosions involving 20-29% of body surface

T32.20 Corrosions involving 20-29% of body surface with 0% to 9% third degree corrosion

T32.21 Corrosions involving 20-29% of body surface with 10-19% third degree corrosion

T32.22 Corrosions involving 20-29% of body surface with 20-29% third degree corrosion

T32.3 Corrosions involving 30-39% of body surface

T32.30 Corrosions involving 30-39% of body surface with 0% to 9% third degree corrosion

T32.31 Corrosions involving 30-39% of body surface with 10-19% third degree corrosion

T32.32 Corrosions involving 30-39% of body surface with 20-29% third degree corrosion

T32.33 Corrosions involving 30-39% of body surface with 30-39% third degree corrosion

T32.4 Corrosions involving 40-49% of body surface

T32.40 Corrosions involving 40-49% of body surface with 0% to 9% third degree corrosion

T32.41 Corrosions involving 40-49% of body surface with 10-19% third degree corrosion

T32.42 Corrosions involving 40-49% of body surface with 20-29% third degree corrosion

T32.43 Corrosions involving 40-49% of body surface with 30-39% third degree corrosion

T32.44 Corrosions involving 40-49% of body surface with 40-49% third degree corrosion

T32.5 Corrosions involving 50-59% of body surface

T32.50 Corrosions involving 50-59% of body surface with 0% to 9% third degree corrosion

T32.51 Corrosions involving 50-59% of body surface with 10-19% third degree corrosion

T32.52 Corrosions involving 50-59% of body surface with 20-29% third degree corrosion

T32.53 Corrosions involving 50-59% of body surface with 30-39% third degree corrosion

T32.54 Corrosions involving 50-59% of body surface with 40-49% third degree corrosion

T32.55 Corrosions involving 50-59% of body surface with 50-59% third degree corrosion

T32.6 Corrosions involving 60-69% of body surface

T32.60 Corrosions involving 60-69% of body surface with 0% to 9% third degree corrosion

T32.61 Corrosions involving 60-69% of body surface with 10-19% third degree corrosion

T32.62 Corrosions involving 60-69% of body surface with 20-29% third degree corrosion

T32.63 Corrosions involving 60-69% of body surface with 30-39% third degree corrosion

T32.64 Corrosions involving 60-69% of body surface with 40-49% third degree corrosion

T32.65 Corrosions involving 60-69% of body surface with 50-59% third degree corrosion

T32.66 Corrosions involving 60-69% of body surface with 60-69% third degree corrosion

T32.7 Corrosions involving 70-79% of body surface

T32.70 Corrosions involving 70-79% of body surface with 0% to 9% third degree corrosion

T32.71 Corrosions involving 70-79% of body surface with 10-19% third degree corrosion

T32.72 Corrosions involving 70-79% of body surface with 20-29% third degree corrosion

T32.73 Corrosions involving 70-79% of body surface with 30-39% third degree corrosion

T32.74 Corrosions involving 70-79% of body surface with 40-49% third degree corrosion

T32.75 Corrosions involving 70-79% of body surface with 50-59% third degree corrosion

T32.76 Corrosions involving 70-79% of body surface with 60-69% third degree corrosion

T32.77 Corrosions involving 70-79% of body surface with 70-79% third degree corrosion

T32.8 Corrosions involving 80-89% of body surface

● New code ▲ Revised code ⑦ 7th digit required ⊗ Placeholder required

T32.80   Corrosions involving 80-89% of body surface with 0% to 9% third degree corrosion

T32.81   Corrosions involving 80-89% of body surface with 10-19% third degree corrosion

T32.82   Corrosions involving 80-89% of body surface with 20-29% third degree corrosion

T32.83   Corrosions involving 80-89% of body surface with 30-39% third degree corrosion

T32.84   Corrosions involving 80-89% of body surface with 40-49% third degree corrosion

T32.85   Corrosions involving 80-89% of body surface with 50-59% third degree corrosion

T32.86   Corrosions involving 80-89% of body surface with 60-69% third degree corrosion

T32.87   Corrosions involving 80-89% of body surface with 70-79% third degree corrosion

T32.88   Corrosions involving 80-89% of body surface with 80-89% third degree corrosion

T32.9   Corrosions involving 90% or more of body surface

T32.90   Corrosions involving 90% or more of body surface with 0% to 9% third degree corrosion

T32.91   Corrosions involving 90% or more of body surface with 10-19% third degree corrosion

T32.92   Corrosions involving 90% or more of body surface with 20-29% third degree corrosion

T32.93   Corrosions involving 90% or more of body surface with 30-39% third degree corrosion

T32.94   Corrosions involving 90% or more of body surface with 40-49% third degree corrosion

T32.95   Corrosions involving 90% or more of body surface with 50-59% third degree corrosion

T32.96   Corrosions involving 90% or more of body surface with 60-69% third degree corrosion

T32.97   Corrosions involving 90% or more of body surface with 70-79% third degree corrosion

T32.98   Corrosions involving 90% or more of body surface with 80-89% third degree corrosion

T32.99   Corrosions involving 90% or more of body surface with 90% or more third degree corrosion

FROSTBITE (T33-T34)

Excludes 2: hypothermia and other effects of reduced temperature (T68, T69.-)

T33   Superficial frostbite

Includes: frostbite with partial thickness skin loss

The appropriate 7th character is to be added to each code from category T33

A - initial encounter

D - subsequent encounter

S - sequela

T33.0   Superficial frostbite of head

T33.01   Superficial frostbite of ear

⑦T33.011   Superficial frostbite of right ear

⑦T33.012   Superficial frostbite of left ear

⑦T33.019   Superficial frostbite of unspecified ear

⊗⑦T33.02   Superficial frostbite of nose

⊗⑦T33.09   Superficial frostbite of other part of head

⊗⑦T33.1   Superficial frostbite of neck

⊗⑦T33.2   Superficial frostbite of thorax

⊗⑦T33.3   Superficial frostbite of abdominal wall, lower back and pelvis

T33.4   Superficial frostbite of arm

Excludes 2: superficial frostbite of wrist and hand (T33.5-)

⊗⑦T33.40   Superficial frostbite of unspecified arm

⊗⑦T33.41   Superficial frostbite of right arm

⊗⑦T33.42   Superficial frostbite of left arm

T33.5   Superficial frostbite of wrist, hand, and fingers

T33.51   Superficial frostbite of wrist

⑦T33.511   Superficial frostbite of right wrist

⑦T33.512   Superficial frostbite of left wrist

⑦T33.519   Superficial frostbite of unspecified wrist

T33.52   Superficial frostbite of hand

Excludes 2: superficial frostbite of fingers (T33.53-)

⑦T33.521   Superficial frostbite of right hand

⑦T33.522   Superficial frostbite of left hand

⑦T33.529   Superficial frostbite of unspecified hand

T33.53   Superficial frostbite of finger(s)

⑦T33.531   Superficial frostbite of right finger(s)

⑦T33.532   Superficial frostbite of left finger(s)

⑦T33.539   Superficial frostbite of unspecified finger(s)

T33.6   Superficial frostbite of hip and thigh

⊗⑦T33.60   Superficial frostbite of unspecified hip and thigh

⊗⑦T33.61   Superficial frostbite of right hip and thigh

⊗⑦T33.62   Superficial frostbite of left hip and thigh

T33.7   Superficial frostbite of knee and lower leg

Excludes 2: superficial frostbite of ankle and foot (T33.8-)

⊗⑦T33.70   Superficial frostbite of unspecified knee and lower leg

⊗⑦T33.71   Superficial frostbite of right knee and lower leg

⊗⑦T33.72   Superficial frostbite of left knee and lower leg

T33.8   Superficial frostbite of ankle, foot, and toe(s)

T33.81   Superficial frostbite of ankle

⑦T33.811   Superficial frostbite of right ankle

⑦T33.812   Superficial frostbite of left ankle

⑦T33.819   Superficial frostbite of unspecified ankle

T33.82   Superficial frostbite of foot

⑦T33.821   Superficial frostbite of right foot

⑦T33.822   Superficial frostbite of left foot

⑦T33.829   Superficial frostbite of unspecified foot

T33.83   Superficial frostbite of toe(s)

⑦T33.831   Superficial frostbite of right toe(s)

⑦T33.832   Superficial frostbite of left toe(s)

⑦T33.839   Superficial frostbite of unspecified toe(s)

T33.9   Superficial frostbite of other and unspecified sites

⊗⑦T33.90   Superficial frostbite of unspecified sites
Superficial frostbite NOS

⊗⑦T33.99   Superficial frostbite of other sites

Superficial frostbite of leg NOS
Superficial frostbite of trunk NOS

T34 Frostbite with tissue necrosis

The appropriate 7th character is to be added to each code from category T34

A - initial encounter

D - subsequent encounter

S - sequela

T34.0 Frostbite with tissue necrosis of head

T34.01 Frostbite with tissue necrosis of ear

⑦**T34.011** Frostbite with tissue necrosis of right ear

⑦**T34.012** Frostbite with tissue necrosis of left ear

⑦**T34.019** Frostbite with tissue necrosis of unspecified ear

⊗⑦**T34.02** Frostbite with tissue necrosis of nose

⊗⑦**T34.09** Frostbite with tissue necrosis of other part of head

⊗⑦**T34.1** Frostbite with tissue necrosis of neck

⊗⑦**T34.2** Frostbite with tissue necrosis of thorax

⊗⑦**T34.3** Frostbite with tissue necrosis of abdominal wall, lower back and pelvis

T34.4 Frostbite with tissue necrosis of arm

Excludes 2: frostbite with tissue necrosis of wrist and hand (T34.5-)

⊗⑦**T34.40** Frostbite with tissue necrosis of unspecified arm

⊗⑦**T34.41** Frostbite with tissue necrosis of right arm

⊗⑦**T34.42** Frostbite with tissue necrosis of left arm

T34.5 Frostbite with tissue necrosis of wrist, hand, and finger(s)

T34.51 Frostbite with tissue necrosis of wrist

⑦**T34.511** Frostbite with tissue necrosis of right wrist

⑦**T34.512** Frostbite with tissue necrosis of left wrist

⑦**T34.519** Frostbite with tissue necrosis of unspecified wrist

T34.52 Frostbite with tissue necrosis of hand

Excludes 2: frostbite with tissue necrosis of finger(s) (T34.53-)

⑦**T34.521** Frostbite with tissue necrosis of right hand

⑦**T34.522** Frostbite with tissue necrosis of left hand

⑦**T34.529** Frostbite with tissue necrosis of unspecified hand

T34.53 Frostbite with tissue necrosis of finger(s)

⑦**T34.531** Frostbite with tissue necrosis of right finger(s)

⑦**T34.532** Frostbite with tissue necrosis of left finger(s)

⑦**T34.539** Frostbite with tissue necrosis of unspecified finger(s)

T34.6 Frostbite with tissue necrosis of hip and thigh

⊗⑦**T34.60** Frostbite with tissue necrosis of unspecified hip and thigh

⊗⑦**T34.61** Frostbite with tissue necrosis of right hip and thigh

⊗⑦**T34.62** Frostbite with tissue necrosis of left hip and thigh

T34.7 Frostbite with tissue necrosis of knee and lower leg

Excludes 2: frostbite with tissue necrosis of ankle and foot (T34.8-)

⊗⑦**T34.70** Frostbite with tissue necrosis of unspecified knee and lower leg

⊗⑦**T34.71** Frostbite with tissue necrosis of right knee and lower leg

⊗⑦**T34.72** Frostbite with tissue necrosis of left knee and lower leg

T34.8 Frostbite with tissue necrosis of ankle, foot, and toe(s)

T34.81 Frostbite with tissue necrosis of ankle

⑦**T34.811** Frostbite with tissue necrosis of right ankle

⑦**T34.812** Frostbite with tissue necrosis of left ankle

⑦**T34.819** Frostbite with tissue necrosis of unspecified ankle

T34.82 Frostbite with tissue necrosis of foot

⑦**T34.821** Frostbite with tissue necrosis of right foot

⑦**T34.822** Frostbite with tissue necrosis of left foot

⑦**T34.829** Frostbite with tissue necrosis of unspecified foot

T34.83 Frostbite with tissue necrosis of toe(s)

⑦**T34.831** Frostbite with tissue necrosis of right toe(s)

⑦**T34.832** Frostbite with tissue necrosis of left toe(s)

⑦**T34.839** Frostbite with tissue necrosis of unspecified toe(s)

T34.9 Frostbite with tissue necrosis of other and unspecified sites

⊗⑦**T34.90** Frostbite with tissue necrosis of unspecified sites
Frostbite with tissue necrosis NOS

⊗⑦**T34.99** Frostbite with tissue necrosis of other sites
Frostbite with tissue necrosis of leg NOS
Frostbite with tissue necrosis of trunk NOS

POISONING BY, ADVERSE EFFECTS OF AND UNDERDOSING OF DRUGS, MEDICAMENTS AND BIOLOGICAL SUBSTANCES (T36-T50)

Includes: adverse effect of correct substance properly administered
poisoning by overdose of substance
poisoning by wrong substance given or taken in error
underdosing by (inadvertently) (deliberately) taking less substance than prescribed or instructed

Code first , for adverse effects, the nature of the adverse effect, such as:
adverse effect NOS (T88.7)
aspirin gastritis (K29.-)
blood disorders (D56-D76)
contact dermatitis (L23-L25)
dermatitis due to substances taken internally (L27.-)
nephropathy (N14.0-N14.2)

Note: The drug giving rise to the adverse effect should be identified by use of codes from categories T36-T50 with fifth or sixth character 5.

Use additional code(s) to specify:
manifestations of poisoning

---

underdosing or failure in dosage during medical and surgical care (Y63.6, Y63.8-Y63.9)

underdosing of medication regimen (Z91.12-, Z91.13-)

Excludes 1: toxic reaction to local anesthesia in pregnancy (O29.3-)

Excludes 2: abuse and dependence of psychoactive substances (F10-F19)

abuse of non-dependence-producing substances (F55.-)

drug reaction and poisoning affecting newborn (P00-P96)

pathological drug intoxication (inebriation) (F10-F19)

T36 Poisoning by, adverse effect of and underdosing of systemic antibiotics

Excludes 1: antineoplastic antibiotics (T45.1-)

locally applied antibiotic NEC (T49.0)

topically used antibiotic for ear, nose and throat (T49.6)

topically used antibiotic for eye (T49.5)

The appropriate 7th character is to be added to each code from category T36

A - initial encounter

D - subsequent encounter

S - sequela

T36.0 Poisoning by, adverse effect of and underdosing of penicillins

   T36.0X Poisoning by, adverse effect of and underdosing of penicillins

      ⑦**T36.0X1** Poisoning by penicillins, accidental (unintentional)

Poisoning by penicillins NOS

      ⑦**T36.0X2** Poisoning by penicillins, intentional self-harm

      ⑦**T36.0X3** Poisoning by penicillins, assault

      ⑦**T36.0X4** Poisoning by penicillins, undetermined

      ⑦**T36.0X5** Adverse effect of penicillins

      ⑦**T36.0X6** Underdosing of penicillins

T36.1 Poisoning by, adverse effect of and underdosing of cephalosporins and other beta-lactam antibiotics

   T36.1X Poisoning by, adverse effect of and underdosing of cephalosporins and other beta-lactam antibiotics

      ⑦**T36.1X1** Poisoning by cephalosporins and other beta-lactam antibiotics, accidental (unintentional)

Poisoning by cephalosporins and other beta-lactam antibiotics NOS

      ⑦**T36.1X2** Poisoning by cephalosporins and other beta-lactam antibiotics, intentional self-harm

      ⑦**T36.1X3** Poisoning by cephalosporins and other beta-lactam antibiotics, assault

      ⑦**T36.1X4** Poisoning by cephalosporins and other beta-lactam antibiotics, undetermined

      ⑦**T36.1X5** Adverse effect of cephalosporins and other beta-lactam antibiotics

      ⑦**T36.1X6** Underdosing of cephalosporins and other beta-lactam antibiotics

T36.2 Poisoning by, adverse effect of and underdosing of chloramphenicol group

   T36.2X Poisoning by, adverse effect of and underdosing of chloramphenicol group

      ⑦**T36.2X1** Poisoning by chloramphenicol group, accidental (unintentional)

Poisoning by chloramphenicol group NOS

      ⑦**T36.2X2** Poisoning by chloramphenicol group, intentional self-harm

      ⑦**T36.2X3** Poisoning by chloramphenicol group, assault

      ⑦**T36.2X4** Poisoning by chloramphenicol group, undetermined

      ⑦**T36.2X5** Adverse effect of chloramphenicol group

      ⑦**T36.2X6** Underdosing of chloramphenicol group

T36.3 Poisoning by, adverse effect of and underdosing of macrolides

   T36.3X Poisoning by, adverse effect of and underdosing of macrolides

      ⑦**T36.3X1** Poisoning by macrolides, accidental (unintentional)

Poisoning by macrolides NOS

      ⑦**T36.3X2** Poisoning by macrolides, intentional self-harm

      ⑦**T36.3X3** Poisoning by macrolides, assault

      ⑦**T36.3X4** Poisoning by macrolides, undetermined

      ⑦**T36.3X5** Adverse effect of macrolides

      ⑦**T36.3X6** Underdosing of macrolides

T36.4 Poisoning by, adverse effect of and underdosing of tetracyclines

   T36.4X Poisoning by, adverse effect of and underdosing of tetracyclines

      ⑦**T36.4X1** Poisoning by tetracyclines, accidental (unintentional)

Poisoning by tetracyclines NOS

      ⑦**T36.4X2** Poisoning by tetracyclines, intentional self-harm

      ⑦**T36.4X3** Poisoning by tetracyclines, assault

      ⑦**T36.4X4** Poisoning by tetracyclines, undetermined

      ⑦**T36.4X5** Adverse effect of tetracyclines

      ⑦**T36.4X6** Underdosing of tetracyclines

T36.5 Poisoning by, adverse effect of and underdosing of aminoglycosides

Poisoning by, adverse effect of and underdosing of streptomycin

   T36.5X Poisoning by, adverse effect of and underdosing of aminoglycosides

      ⑦**T36.5X1** Poisoning by aminoglycosides, accidental (unintentional)

Poisoning by aminoglycosides NOS

      ⑦**T36.5X2** Poisoning by aminoglycosides, intentional self-harm

      ⑦**T36.5X3** Poisoning by aminoglycosides, assault

      ⑦**T36.5X4** Poisoning by aminoglycosides, undetermined

⑦**T36.5X5**   Adverse effect of aminoglycosides

⑦**T36.5X6**   Underdosing of aminoglycosides

T36.6   Poisoning by, adverse effect of and underdosing of rifampicins

    T36.6X   Poisoning by, adverse effect of and underdosing of rifampicins

      ⑦**T36.6X1**   Poisoning by rifampicins, accidental (unintentional)

                 Poisoning by rifampicins NOS

      ⑦**T36.6X2**   Poisoning by rifampicins, intentional self-harm

      ⑦**T36.6X3**   Poisoning by rifampicins, assault

      ⑦**T36.6X4**   Poisoning by rifampicins, undetermined

      ⑦**T36.6X5**   Adverse effect of rifampicins

      ⑦**T36.6X6**   Underdosing of rifampicins

T36.7   Poisoning by, adverse effect of and underdosing of antifungal antibiotics, systemically used

    T36.7X   Poisoning by, adverse effect of and underdosing of antifungal antibiotics, systemically used

      ⑦**T36.7X1**   Poisoning by antifungal antibiotics, systemically used, accidental (unintentional)

                 Poisoning by antifungal antibiotics, systemically used NOS

      ⑦**T36.7X2**   Poisoning by antifungal antibiotics, systemically used, intentional self-harm

      ⑦**T36.7X3**   Poisoning by antifungal antibiotics, systemically used, assault

      ⑦**T36.7X4**   Poisoning by antifungal antibiotics, systemically used, undetermined

      ⑦**T36.7X5**   Adverse effect of antifungal antibiotics, systemically used

      ⑦**T36.7X6**   Underdosing of antifungal antibiotics, systemically used

T36.8   Poisoning by, adverse effect of and underdosing of other systemic antibiotics

    T36.8X   Poisoning by, adverse effect of and underdosing of other systemic antibiotics

      ⑦**T36.8X1**   Poisoning by other systemic antibiotics, accidental (unintentional)

                 Poisoning by other systemic antibiotics NOS

      ⑦**T36.8X2**   Poisoning by other systemic antibiotics, intentional self-harm

      ⑦**T36.8X3**   Poisoning by other systemic antibiotics, assault

      ⑦**T36.8X4**   Poisoning by other systemic antibiotics, undetermined

      ⑦**T36.8X5**   Adverse effect of other systemic antibiotics

      ⑦**T36.8X6**   Underdosing of other systemic antibiotics

T36.9   Poisoning by, adverse effect of and underdosing of unspecified systemic antibiotic

    T36.91   Poisoning by unspecified systemic antibiotic, accidental (unintentional)

           Poisoning by systemic antibiotic NOS

    T36.92   Poisoning by unspecified systemic antibiotic, intentional self-harm

    T36.93   Poisoning by unspecified systemic antibiotic, assault

    T36.94   Poisoning by unspecified systemic antibiotic, undetermined

    T36.95   Adverse effect of unspecified systemic antibiotic

    T36.96   Underdosing of unspecified systemic antibiotic

T37   Poisoning by, adverse effect of and underdosing of other systemic anti- infectives and antiparasitics

    Excludes 1:   anti-infectives topically used for ear, nose and throat (T49.6-)

              anti-infectives topically used for eye (T49.5-)

              locally applied anti-infectives NEC (T49.0-)

The appropriate 7th character is to be added to each code from category T37

A - initial encounter

D - subsequent encounter

S - sequela

T37.0   Poisoning by, adverse effect of and underdosing of sulfonamides

    T37.0X   Poisoning by, adverse effect of and underdosing of sulfonamides

      ⑦**T37.0X1**   Poisoning by sulfonamides, accidental (unintentional)

                 Poisoning by sulfonamides NOS

      ⑦**T37.0X2**   Poisoning by sulfonamides, intentional self-harm

      ⑦**T37.0X3**   Poisoning by sulfonamides, assault

      ⑦**T37.0X4**   Poisoning by sulfonamides, undetermined

      ⑦**T37.0X5**   Adverse effect of sulfonamides

      ⑦**T37.0X6**   Underdosing of sulfonamides

T37.1   Poisoning by, adverse effect of and underdosing of antimycobacterial drugs

    Excludes 1:   rifampicins (T36.6-)

              streptomycin (T36.5-)

    T37.1X   Poisoning by, adverse effect of and underdosing of antimycobacterial drugs

      ⑦**T37.1X1**   Poisoning by antimycobacterial drugs, accidental (unintentional)

                 Poisoning by antimycobacterial drugs NOS

      ⑦**T37.1X2**   Poisoning by antimycobacterial drugs, intentional self-harm

      ⑦**T37.1X3**   Poisoning by antimycobacterial drugs, assault

      ⑦**T37.1X4**   Poisoning by antimycobacterial drugs, undetermined

      ⑦**T37.1X5**   Adverse effect of antimycobacterial drugs

      ⑦**T37.1X6**   Underdosing of antimycobacterial drugs

T37.2   Poisoning by, adverse effect of and underdosing of antimalarials and drugs acting on other blood protozoa

    Excludes 1: hydroxyquinoline derivatives (T37.8-)

    T37.2X   Poisoning by, adverse effect of and underdosing of antimalarials and drugs acting on other blood protozoa

   ● New code   ▲ Revised code   ⑦ 7th digit required   ⊗ Placeholder required

⑦T37.2X1 Poisoning by antimalarials and drugs acting on other blood protozoa, accidental (unintentional)

Poisoning by antimalarials and drugs acting on other blood protozoa NOS

⑦T37.2X2 Poisoning by antimalarials and drugs acting on other blood protozoa, intentional self-harm

⑦T37.2X3 Poisoning by antimalarials and drugs acting on other blood protozoa, assault

⑦T37.2X4 Poisoning by antimalarials and drugs acting on other blood protozoa, undetermined

⑦T37.2X5 Adverse effect of antimalarials and drugs acting on other blood protozoa

⑦T37.2X6 Underdosing of antimalarials and drugs acting on other blood protozoa

T37.3 Poisoning by, adverse effect of and underdosing of other antiprotozoal drugs

  T37.3X Poisoning by, adverse effect of and underdosing of other antiprotozoal drugs

⑦T37.3X1 Poisoning by other antiprotozoal drugs, accidental (unintentional)

Poisoning by other antiprotozoal drugs NOS

⑦T37.3X2 Poisoning by other antiprotozoal drugs, intentional self-harm

⑦T37.3X3 Poisoning by other antiprotozoal drugs, assault

⑦T37.3X4 Poisoning by other antiprotozoal drugs, undetermined

⑦T37.3X5 Adverse effect of other antiprotozoal drugs

⑦T37.3X6 Underdosing of other antiprotozoal drugs

T37.4 Poisoning by, adverse effect of and underdosing of anthelminthics

  T37.4X Poisoning by, adverse effect of and underdosing of anthelminthics

⑦T37.4X1 Poisoning by anthelminthics, accidental (unintentional)

Poisoning by anthelminthics NOS

⑦T37.4X2 Poisoning by anthelminthics, intentional self-harm

⑦T37.4X3 Poisoning by anthelminthics, assault

⑦T37.4X4 Poisoning by anthelminthics, undetermined

⑦T37.4X5 Adverse effect of anthelminthics

⑦T37.4X6 Underdosing of anthelminthics

T37.5 Poisoning by, adverse effect of and underdosing of antiviral drugs

Excludes 1: amantadine (T42.8-)

          cytarabine (T45.1-)

  T37.5X Poisoning by, adverse effect of and underdosing of antiviral drugs

⑦T37.5X1 Poisoning by antiviral drugs, accidental (unintentional)

Poisoning by antiviral drugs NOS

⑦T37.5X2 Poisoning by antiviral drugs, intentional self-harm

⑦T37.5X3 Poisoning by antiviral drugs, assault

⑦T37.5X4 Poisoning by antiviral drugs, undetermined

⑦T37.5X5 Adverse effect of antiviral drugs

⑦T37.5X6 Underdosing of antiviral drugs

T37.8 Poisoning by, adverse effect of and underdosing of other specified systemic anti-infectives and antiparasitics

Poisoning by, adverse effect of and underdosing of hydroxyquinoline derivatives

Excludes 1: antimalarial drugs (T37.2-)

  T37.8X Poisoning by, adverse effect of and underdosing of other specified systemic anti-infectives and antiparasitics

⑦T37.8X1 Poisoning by other specified systemic anti-infectives and antiparasitics, accidental (unintentional)

Poisoning by other specified systemic anti-infectives and antiparasitics NOS

⑦T37.8X2 Poisoning by other specified systemic anti-infectives and antiparasitics, intentional self-harm

⑦T37.8X3 Poisoning by other specified systemic anti-infectives and antiparasitics, assault

⑦T37.8X4 Poisoning by other specified systemic anti-infectives and antiparasitics, undetermined

⑦T37.8X5 Adverse effect of other specified systemic anti-infectives and antiparasitics

⑦T37.8X6 Underdosing of other specified systemic anti-infectives and antiparasitics

T37.9 Poisoning by, adverse effect of and underdosing of unspecified systemic anti-infective and antiparasitics

⊗⑦T37.91 Poisoning by unspecified systemic anti-infective and antiparasitics, accidental (unintentional)

Poisoning by, adverse effect of and underdosing of systemic anti-infective and antiparasitics NOS

⊗⑦T37.92 Poisoning by unspecified systemic anti-infective and antiparasitics, intentional self-harm

⊗⑦T37.93 Poisoning by unspecified systemic anti-infective and antiparasitics, assault

⊗⑦T37.94 Poisoning by unspecified systemic anti-infective and antiparasitics, undetermined

⊗⑦T37.95 Adverse effect of unspecified systemic anti-infective and antiparasitic

⊗⑦T37.96 Underdosing of unspecified systemic anti-infectives and antiparasitics

T38 Poisoning by, adverse effect of and underdosing of hormones and their synthetic substitutes and antagonists, not elsewhere classified

Excludes 1: mineralocorticoids and their antagonists (T50.0-)

          oxytocic hormones (T48.0-)

          parathyroid hormones and derivatives (T50.9-)

The appropriate 7th character is to be added to each code from category T38

A - initial encounter
D - subsequent encounter
S - sequela

T38.0 Poisoning by, adverse effect of and underdosing of glucocorticoids and synthetic analogues

Excludes 1: glucocorticoids, topically used (T49.-)

T38.0X Poisoning by, adverse effect of and underdosing of glucocorticoids and synthetic analogues

⑦**T38.0X1** Poisoning by glucocorticoids and synthetic analogues, accidental (unintentional)

Poisoning by glucocorticoids and synthetic analogues NOS

⑦**T38.0X2** Poisoning by glucocorticoids and synthetic analogues, intentional self-harm

⑦**T38.0X3** Poisoning by glucocorticoids and synthetic analogues, assault

⑦**T38.0X4** Poisoning by glucocorticoids and synthetic analogues, undetermined

⑦**T38.0X5** Adverse effect of glucocorticoids and synthetic analogues

⑦**T38.0X6** Underdosing of glucocorticoids and synthetic analogues

T38.1 Poisoning by, adverse effect of and underdosing of thyroid hormones and substitutes

T38.1X Poisoning by, adverse effect of and underdosing of thyroid hormones and substitutes

⑦**T38.1X1** Poisoning by thyroid hormones and substitutes, accidental (unintentional)

Poisoning by thyroid hormones and substitutes NOS

⑦**T38.1X2** Poisoning by thyroid hormones and substitutes, intentional self-harm

⑦**T38.1X3** Poisoning by thyroid hormones and substitutes, assault

⑦**T38.1X4** Poisoning by thyroid hormones and substitutes, undetermined

⑦**T38.1X5** Adverse effect of thyroid hormones and substitutes

⑦**T38.1X6** Underdosing of thyroid hormones and substitutes

T38.2 Poisoning by, adverse effect of and underdosing of antithyroid drugs

T38.2X Poisoning by, adverse effect of and underdosing of antithyroid drugs

⑦**T38.2X1** Poisoning by antithyroid drugs, accidental (unintentional)

Poisoning by antithyroid drugs NOS

⑦**T38.2X2** Poisoning by antithyroid drugs, intentional self-harm

⑦**T38.2X3** Poisoning by antithyroid drugs, assault

⑦**T38.2X4** Poisoning by antithyroid drugs, undetermined

⑦**T38.2X5** Adverse effect of antithyroid drugs

⑦**T38.2X6** Underdosing of antithyroid drugs

T38.3 Poisoning by, adverse effect of and underdosing of insulin and oral hypoglycemic [antidiabetic] drugs

T38.3X Poisoning by, adverse effect of and underdosing of insulin and oral hypoglycemic [antidiabetic] drugs

⑦**T38.3X1** Poisoning by insulin and oral hypoglycemic [antidiabetic] drugs, accidental (unintentional)

Poisoning by insulin and oral hypoglycemic [antidiabetic] drugs NOS

⑦**T38.3X2** Poisoning by insulin and oral hypoglycemic [antidiabetic] drugs, intentional self-harm

⑦**T38.3X3** Poisoning by insulin and oral hypoglycemic [antidiabetic] drugs, assault

⑦**T38.3X4** Poisoning by insulin and oral hypoglycemic [antidiabetic] drugs, undetermined

⑦**T38.3X5** Adverse effect of insulin and oral hypoglycemic [antidiabetic] drugs

⑦**T38.3X6** Underdosing of insulin and oral hypoglycemic [antidiabetic] drugs

T38.4 Poisoning by, adverse effect of and underdosing of oral contraceptives

Poisoning by, adverse effect of and underdosing of multiple- and single-ingredient oral contraceptive preparations

T38.4X Poisoning by, adverse effect of and underdosing of oral contraceptives

⑦**T38.4X1** Poisoning by oral contraceptives, accidental (unintentional)

Poisoning by oral contraceptives NOS

⑦**T38.4X2** Poisoning by oral contraceptives, intentional self-harm

⑦**T38.4X3** Poisoning by oral contraceptives, assault

⑦**T38.4X4** Poisoning by oral contraceptives, undetermined

⑦**T38.4X5** Adverse effect of oral contraceptives

⑦**T38.4X6** Underdosing of oral contraceptives

T38.5 Poisoning by, adverse effect of and underdosing of other estrogens and progestogens

Poisoning by, adverse effect of and underdosing of estrogens and progestogens mixtures and substitutes

T38.5X Poisoning by, adverse effect of and underdosing of other estrogens and progestogens

⑦**T38.5X1** Poisoning by other estrogens and progestogens, accidental (unintentional)

Poisoning by other estrogens and progestogens NOS

⑦**T38.5X2** Poisoning by other estrogens and progestogens, intentional self-harm

⑦**T38.5X3** Poisoning by other estrogens and progestogens, assault

⑦**T38.5X4** Poisoning by other estrogens and progestogens, undetermined

⑦**T38.5X5** Adverse effect of other estrogens and progestogens

● New code   ▲ Revised code   ⑦ 7ᵗʰ digit required   ⊗ Placeholder required

⑦ **T38.5X6** Underdosing of other estrogens and progestogens

T38.6 Poisoning by, adverse effect of and underdosing of antigonadotrophins, antiestrogens, antiandrogens, not elsewhere classified

Poisoning by, adverse effect of and underdosing of tamoxifen

⑦ **T38.6X** Poisoning by, adverse effect of and underdosing of antigonadotrophins, antiestrogens, antiandrogens, not elsewhere classified

⑦ **T38.6X1** Poisoning by antigonadotrophins, antiestrogens, antiandrogens, not elsewhere classified, accidental (unintentional)

Poisoning by antigonadotrophins, antiestrogens, antiandrogens, not elsewhere classified NOS

⑦ **T38.6X2** Poisoning by antigonadotrophins, antiestrogens, antiandrogens, not elsewhere classified, intentional self-harm

⑦ **T38.6X3** Poisoning by antigonadotrophins, antiestrogens, antiandrogens, not elsewhere classified, assault

⑦ **T38.6X4** Poisoning by antigonadotrophins, antiestrogens, antiandrogens, not elsewhere classified, undetermined

⑦ **T38.6X5** Adverse effect of antigonadotrophins, antiestrogens, antiandrogens, not elsewhere classified

⑦ **T38.6X6** Underdosing of antigonadotrophins, antiestrogens, antiandrogens, not elsewhere classified

T38.7 Poisoning by, adverse effect of and underdosing of androgens and anabolic congeners

T38.7X Poisoning by, adverse effect of and underdosing of androgens and anabolic congeners

⑦ **T38.7X1** Poisoning by androgens and anabolic congeners, accidental (unintentional)

Poisoning by androgens and anabolic congeners NOS

⑦ **T38.7X2** Poisoning by androgens and anabolic congeners, intentional self-harm

⑦ **T38.7X3** Poisoning by androgens and anabolic congeners, assault

⑦ **T38.7X4** Poisoning by androgens and anabolic congeners, undetermined

⑦ **T38.7X5** Adverse effect of androgens and anabolic congeners

⑦ **T38.7X6** Underdosing of androgens and anabolic congeners

T38.8 Poisoning by, adverse effect of and underdosing of other and unspecified hormones and synthetic substitutes

T38.80 Poisoning by, adverse effect of and underdosing of unspecified hormones and synthetic substitutes

⑦ **T38.801** Poisoning by unspecified hormones and synthetic substitutes, accidental (unintentional)

Poisoning by unspecified hormones and synthetic substitutes NOS

⑦ **T38.802** Poisoning by unspecified hormones and synthetic substitutes, intentional self-harm

⑦ **T38.803** Poisoning by unspecified hormones and synthetic substitutes, assault

⑦ **T38.804** Poisoning by unspecified hormones and synthetic substitutes, undetermined

⑦ **T38.805** Adverse effect of unspecified hormones and synthetic substitutes

⑦ **T38.806** Underdosing of unspecified hormones and synthetic substitutes

T38.81 Poisoning by, adverse effect of and underdosing of anterior pituitary [adenohypophyseal] hormones

⑦ **T38.811** Poisoning by anterior pituitary [adenohypophyseal] hormones, accidental (unintentional)

Poisoning by anterior pituitary [adenohypophyseal] hormones NOS

⑦ **T38.812** Poisoning by anterior pituitary [adenohypophyseal] hormones, intentional self-harm

⑦ **T38.813** Poisoning by anterior pituitary [adenohypophyseal] hormones, assault

⑦ **T38.814** Poisoning by anterior pituitary [adenohypophyseal] hormones, undetermined

⑦ **T38.815** Adverse effect of anterior pituitary [adenohypophyseal] hormones

⑦ **T38.816** Underdosing of anterior pituitary [adenohypophyseal] hormones

T38.89 Poisoning by, adverse effect of and underdosing of other hormones and synthetic substitutes

⑦ **T38.891** Poisoning by other hormones and synthetic substitutes, accidental (unintentional)

Poisoning by other hormones and synthetic substitutes NOS

⑦ **T38.892** Poisoning by other hormones and synthetic substitutes, intentional self-harm

⑦ **T38.893** Poisoning by other hormones and synthetic substitutes, assault

⑦ **T38.894** Poisoning by other hormones and synthetic substitutes, undetermined

⑦ **T38.895** Adverse effect of other hormones and synthetic substitutes

⑦ **T38.896** Underdosing of other hormones and synthetic substitutes

T38.9 Poisoning by, adverse effect of and underdosing of other and unspecified hormone antagonists

T38.90 Poisoning by, adverse effect of and underdosing of unspecified hormone antagonists

⑦**T38.901** Poisoning by unspecified hormone antagonists, accidental (unintentional)

Poisoning by unspecified hormone antagonists NOS

⑦**T38.902** Poisoning by unspecified hormone antagonists, intentional self-harm

⑦**T38.903** Poisoning by unspecified hormone antagonists, assault

⑦**T38.904** Poisoning by unspecified hormone antagonists, undetermined

⑦**T38.905** Adverse effect of unspecified hormone antagonists

⑦**T38.906** Underdosing of unspecified hormone antagonists

T38.99 Poisoning by, adverse effect of and underdosing of other hormone antagonists

⑦**T38.991** Poisoning by other hormone antagonists, accidental (unintentional)

Poisoning by other hormone antagonists NOS

⑦**T38.992** Poisoning by other hormone antagonists, intentional self-harm

⑦**T38.993** Poisoning by other hormone antagonists, assault

⑦**T38.994** Poisoning by other hormone antagonists, undetermined

⑦**T38.995** Adverse effect of other hormone antagonists

⑦**T38.996** Underdosing of other hormone antagonists

T39 Poisoning by, adverse effect of and underdosing of nonopioid analgesics, antipyretics and antirheumatics

The appropriate 7th character is to be added to each code from category T39

A - initial encounter

D - subsequent encounter

S - sequela

T39.0 Poisoning by, adverse effect of and underdosing of salicylates

T39.01 Poisoning by, adverse effect of and underdosing of aspirin

Poisoning by, adverse effect of and underdosing of acetylsalicylic acid

⑦**T39.011** Poisoning by aspirin, accidental (unintentional)

⑦**T39.012** Poisoning by aspirin, intentional self-harm

⑦**T39.013** Poisoning by aspirin, assault

⑦**T39.014** Poisoning by aspirin, undetermined

⑦**T39.015** Adverse effect of aspirin

⑦**T39.016** Underdosing of aspirin

T39.09 Poisoning by, adverse effect of and underdosing of other salicylates

⑦**T39.091** Poisoning by salicylates, accidental (unintentional)

Poisoning by salicylates NOS

⑦**T39.092** Poisoning by salicylates, intentional self-harm

⑦**T39.093** Poisoning by salicylates, assault

⑦**T39.094** Poisoning by salicylates, undetermined

⑦**T39.095** Adverse effect of salicylates

⑦**T39.096** Underdosing of salicylates

T39.1 Poisoning by, adverse effect of and underdosing of 4-Aminophenol derivatives

T39.1X Poisoning by, adverse effect of and underdosing of 4-Aminophenol derivatives

⑦**T39.1X1** Poisoning by 4-Aminophenol derivatives, accidental (unintentional)

Poisoning by 4-Aminophenol derivatives NOS

⑦**T39.1X2** Poisoning by 4-Aminophenol derivatives, intentional self-harm

⑦**T39.1X3** Poisoning by 4-Aminophenol derivatives, assault

⑦**T39.1X4** Poisoning by 4-Aminophenol derivatives, undetermined

⑦**T39.1X5** Adverse effect of 4-Aminophenol derivatives

⑦**T39.1X6** Underdosing of 4-Aminophenol derivatives

T39.2 Poisoning by, adverse effect of and underdosing of pyrazolone derivatives

T39.2X Poisoning by, adverse effect of and underdosing of pyrazolone derivatives

⑦**T39.2X1** Poisoning by pyrazolone derivatives, accidental (unintentional)

Poisoning by pyrazolone derivatives NOS

⑦**T39.2X2** Poisoning by pyrazolone derivatives, intentional self-harm

⑦**T39.2X3** Poisoning by pyrazolone derivatives, assault

⑦**T39.2X4** Poisoning by pyrazolone derivatives, undetermined

⑦**T39.2X5** Adverse effect of pyrazolone derivatives

⑦**T39.2X6** Underdosing of pyrazolone derivatives

T39.3 Poisoning by, adverse effect of and underdosing of other nonsteroidal anti-inflammatory drugs [NSAID]

T39.31 Poisoning by, adverse effect of and underdosing of propionic acid derivatives

Poisoning by, adverse effect of and underdosing of fenoprofen

Poisoning by, adverse effect of and underdosing of flurbiprofen

Poisoning by, adverse effect of and underdosing of ibuprofen

Poisoning by, adverse effect of and underdosing of ketoprofen

Poisoning by, adverse effect of and underdosing of naproxen

Poisoning by, adverse effect of and underdosing of oxaprozin

⑦ **T39.311** Poisoning by propionic acid derivatives, accidental (unintentional)

⑦ **T39.312** Poisoning by propionic acid derivatives, intentional self-harm

⑦ **T39.313** Poisoning by propionic acid derivatives, assault

⑦ **T39.314** Poisoning by propionic acid derivatives, undetermined

⑦ **T39.315** Adverse effect of propionic acid derivatives

⑦ **T39.316** Underdosing of propionic acid derivatives

T39.39 Poisoning by, adverse effect of and underdosing of other nonsteroidal anti-inflammatory drugs [NSAID]

⑦ **T39.391** Poisoning by other nonsteroidal anti-inflammatory drugs [NSAID], accidental (unintentional)

Poisoning by other nonsteroidal anti-inflammatory drugs NOS

⑦ **T39.392** Poisoning by other nonsteroidal anti-inflammatory drugs [NSAID], intentional self-harm

⑦ **T39.393** Poisoning by other nonsteroidal anti-inflammatory drugs [NSAID], assault

⑦ **T39.394** Poisoning by other nonsteroidal anti-inflammatory drugs [NSAID], undetermined

⑦ **T39.395** Adverse effect of other nonsteroidal anti-inflammatory drugs [NSAID]

⑦ **T39.396** Underdosing of other nonsteroidal anti-inflammatory drugs [NSAID]

T39.4 Poisoning by, adverse effect of and underdosing of antirheumatics, not elsewhere classified

Excludes 1: poisoning by, adverse effect of and underdosing of glucocorticoids (T38.0-)

poisoning by, adverse effect of and underdosing of salicylates (T39.0)

T39.4X Poisoning by, adverse effect of and underdosing of antirheumatics, not elsewhere classified

⑦ **T39.4X1** Poisoning by antirheumatics, not elsewhere classified, accidental (unintentional)

Poisoning by antirheumatics, not elsewhere classified NOS

⑦ **T39.4X2** Poisoning by antirheumatics, not elsewhere classified, intentional self-harm

⑦ **T39.4X3** Poisoning by antirheumatics, not elsewhere classified, assault

⑦ **T39.4X4** Poisoning by antirheumatics, not elsewhere classified, undetermined

⑦ **T39.4X5** Adverse effect of antirheumatics, not elsewhere classified

⑦ **T39.4X6** Underdosing of antirheumatics, not elsewhere classified

T39.8 Poisoning by, adverse effect of and underdosing of other nonopioid analgesics and antipyretics, not elsewhere classified

T39.8X Poisoning by, adverse effect of and underdosing of other nonopioid analgesics and antipyretics, not elsewhere classified

⑦ **T39.8X1** Poisoning by other nonopioid analgesics and antipyretics, not elsewhere classified, accidental (unintentional)

Poisoning by other nonopioid analgesics and antipyretics, not elsewhere classified NOS

⑦ **T39.8X2** Poisoning by other nonopioid analgesics and antipyretics, not elsewhere classified, intentional self-harm

⑦ **T39.8X3** Poisoning by other nonopioid analgesics and antipyretics, not elsewhere classified, assault

⑦ **T39.8X4** Poisoning by other nonopioid analgesics and antipyretics, not elsewhere classified, undetermined

⑦ **T39.8X5** Adverse effect of other nonopioid analgesics and antipyretics, not elsewhere classified

⑦ **T39.8X6** Underdosing of other nonopioid analgesics and antipyretics, not elsewhere classified

T39.9 Poisoning by, adverse effect of and underdosing of unspecified nonopioid analgesic, antipyretic and antirheumatic

⊗⑦ **T39.91** Poisoning by unspecified nonopioid analgesic, antipyretic and antirheumatic, accidental (unintentional)

Poisoning by nonopioid analgesic, antipyretic and antirheumatic NOS

⊗⑦ **T39.92** Poisoning by unspecified nonopioid analgesic, antipyretic and antirheumatic, intentional self-harm

⊗⑦ **T39.93** Poisoning by unspecified nonopioid analgesic, antipyretic and antirheumatic, assault

⊗⑦ **T39.94** Poisoning by unspecified nonopioid analgesic, antipyretic and antirheumatic, undetermined

⊗⑦ **T39.95** Adverse effect of unspecified nonopioid analgesic, antipyretic and antirheumatic

⊗⑦ **T39.96** Underdosing of unspecified nonopioid analgesic, antipyretic and antirheumatic

T40 Poisoning by, adverse effect of and underdosing of narcotics and psychodysleptics [hallucinogens]

Excludes 2: drug dependence and related mental and behavioral disorders due to psychoactive substance use (F10.-F19.-)

The appropriate 7th character is to be added to each code from category T40

A - initial encounter

D - subsequent encounter

S - sequela

T40.0 Poisoning by, adverse effect of and underdosing of opium

T40.0X Poisoning by, adverse effect of and underdosing of opium

⑦ **T40.0X1** Poisoning by opium, accidental (unintentional)

Poisoning by opium NOS

⑦ **T40.0X2** Poisoning by opium, intentional self-harm

⑦ **T40.0X3** Poisoning by opium, assault

⑦ **T40.0X4** Poisoning by opium, undetermined

⑦ **T40.0X5** Adverse effect of opium

⑦ **T40.0X6** Underdosing of opium

T40.1 Poisoning by and adverse effect of heroin

  T40.1X Poisoning by and adverse effect of heroin

⑦ **T40.1X1** Poisoning by heroin, accidental (unintentional)

Poisoning by heroin NOS

⑦ **T40.1X2** Poisoning by heroin, intentional self-harm

⑦ **T40.1X3** Poisoning by heroin, assault

⑦ **T40.1X4** Poisoning by heroin, undetermined

⑦ **T40.1X5** Adverse effect of heroin (deleted 2014)

T40.2 Poisoning by, adverse effect of and underdosing of other opioids

  T40.2X Poisoning by, adverse effect of and underdosing of other opioids

⑦ **T40.2X1** Poisoning by other opioids, accidental (unintentional)

Poisoning by other opioids NOS

⑦ **T40.2X2** Poisoning by other opioids, intentional self-harm

⑦ **T40.2X3** Poisoning by other opioids, assault

⑦ **T40.2X4** Poisoning by other opioids, undetermined

⑦ **T40.2X5** Adverse effect of other opioids

⑦ **T40.2X6** Underdosing of other opioids

T40.3 Poisoning by, adverse effect of and underdosing of methadone

  T40.3X Poisoning by, adverse effect of and underdosing of methadone

⑦ **T40.3X1** Poisoning by methadone, accidental (unintentional)

Poisoning by methadone NOS

⑦ **T40.3X2** Poisoning by methadone, intentional self-harm

⑦ **T40.3X3** Poisoning by methadone, assault

⑦ **T40.3X4** Poisoning by methadone, undetermined

⑦ **T40.3X5** Adverse effect of methadone

⑦ **T40.3X6** Underdosing of methadone

T40.4 Poisoning by, adverse effect of and underdosing of other synthetic narcotics

  T40.4X Poisoning by, adverse effect of and underdosing of other synthetic narcotics

⑦ **T40.4X1** Poisoning by other synthetic narcotics, accidental (unintentional)

Poisoning by other synthetic narcotics NOS

⑦ **T40.4X2** Poisoning by other synthetic narcotics, intentional self-harm

⑦ **T40.4X3** Poisoning by other synthetic narcotics, assault

⑦ **T40.4X4** Poisoning by other synthetic narcotics, undetermined

⑦ **T40.4X5** Adverse effect of other synthetic narcotics

⑦ **T40.4X6** Underdosing of other synthetic narcotics

T40.5 Poisoning by, adverse effect of and underdosing of cocaine

  T40.5X Poisoning by, adverse effect of and underdosing of cocaine

⑦ **T40.5X1** Poisoning by cocaine, accidental (unintentional)

Poisoning by cocaine NOS

⑦ **T40.5X2** Poisoning by cocaine, intentional self-harm

⑦ **T40.5X3** Poisoning by cocaine, assault

⑦ **T40.5X4** Poisoning by cocaine, undetermined

⑦ **T40.5X5** Adverse effect of cocaine

⑦ **T40.5X6** Underdosing of cocaine

T40.6 Poisoning by, adverse effect of and underdosing of other and unspecified narcotics

  T40.60 Poisoning by, adverse effect of and underdosing of unspecified narcotics

⑦ **T40.601** Poisoning by unspecified narcotics, accidental (unintentional)

Poisoning by narcotics NOS

⑦ **T40.602** Poisoning by unspecified narcotics, intentional self-harm

⑦ **T40.603** Poisoning by unspecified narcotics, assault

⑦ **T40.604** Poisoning by unspecified narcotics, undetermined

⑦ **T40.605** Adverse effect of unspecified narcotics

⑦ **T40.606** Underdosing of unspecified narcotics

  T40.69 Poisoning by, adverse effect of and underdosing of other narcotics

⑦ **T40.691** Poisoning by other narcotics, accidental (unintentional)

Poisoning by other narcotics NOS

⑦ **T40.692** Poisoning by other narcotics, intentional self-harm

⑦ **T40.693** Poisoning by other narcotics, assault

⑦ **T40.694** Poisoning by other narcotics, undetermined

⑦ **T40.695** Adverse effect of other narcotics

⑦ **T40.696** Underdosing of other narcotics

T40.7 Poisoning by, adverse effect of and underdosing of cannabis (derivatives)

  T40.7X Poisoning by, adverse effect of and underdosing of cannabis (derivatives)

⑦ **T40.7X1** Poisoning by cannabis (derivatives), accidental (unintentional)

Poisoning by cannabis NOS

⑦ **T40.7X2** Poisoning by cannabis (derivatives), intentional self-harm

⑦**T40.7X3** Poisoning by cannabis (derivatives), assault

⑦**T40.7X4** Poisoning by cannabis (derivatives), undetermined

⑦**T40.7X5** Adverse effect of cannabis (derivatives)

⑦**T40.7X6** Underdosing of cannabis (derivatives)

T40.8 Poisoning by and adverse effect of lysergide [LSD]

T40.8X Poisoning by and adverse effect of lysergide [LSD]

⑦**T40.8X1** Poisoning by lysergide [LSD], accidental (unintentional)
Poisoning by lysergide [LSD]NOS

⑦**T40.8X2** Poisoning by lysergide [LSD], intentional self-harm

⑦**T40.8X3** Poisoning by lysergide [LSD], assault

⑦**T40.8X4** Poisoning by lysergide [LSD], undetermined

⑦**T40.8X5** Adverse effect of lysergide [LSD]

T40.9 Poisoning by, adverse effect of and underdosing of other and unspecified psychodysleptics [hallucinogens]

T40.90 Poisoning by, adverse effect of and underdosing of unspecified psychodysleptics [hallucinogens]

⑦**T40.901** Poisoning by unspecified psychodysleptics [hallucinogens], accidental (unintentional)

⑦**T40.902** Poisoning by unspecified psychodysleptics [hallucinogens], intentional self-harm

⑦**T40.903** Poisoning by unspecified psychodysleptics [hallucinogens], assault

⑦**T40.904** Poisoning by unspecified psychodysleptics [hallucinogens], undetermined

⑦**T40.905** Adverse effect of unspecified psychodysleptics [hallucinogens]

⑦**T40.906** Underdosing of unspecified psychodysleptics

T40.99 Poisoning by, adverse effect of and underdosing of other psychodysleptics [hallucinogens]

⑦**T40.991** Poisoning by other psychodysleptics [hallucinogens], accidental (unintentional)
Poisoning by other psychodysleptics [hallucinogens] NOS

⑦**T40.992** Poisoning by other psychodysleptics [hallucinogens], intentional self-harm

⑦**T40.993** Poisoning by other psychodysleptics [hallucinogens], assault

⑦**T40.994** Poisoning by other psychodysleptics [hallucinogens], undetermined

⑦**T40.995** Adverse effect of other psychodysleptics [hallucinogens]

⑦**T40.996** Underdosing of other psychodysleptics

T41 Poisoning by, adverse effect of and underdosing of anesthetics and therapeutic gases

Excludes 1: benzodiazepines (T42.4-)
cocaine (T40.5-)
complications of anesthesia during pregnancy (O29.-)
complications of anesthesia during labor and delivery (O74.-)
complications of anesthesia during the puerperium (O89.-)
opioids (T40.0-T40.2-)

The appropriate 7th character is to be added to each code from category T41

A - initial encounter

D - subsequent encounter

S - sequela

T41.0 Poisoning by, adverse effect of and underdosing of inhaled anesthetics

Excludes 1: oxygen (T41.5-)

T41.0X Poisoning by, adverse effect of and underdosing of inhaled anesthetics

⑦**T41.0X1** Poisoning by inhaled anesthetics, accidental (unintentional)
Poisoning by inhaled anesthetics NOS

⑦**T41.0X2** Poisoning by inhaled anesthetics, intentional self-harm

⑦**T41.0X3** Poisoning by inhaled anesthetics, assault

⑦**T41.0X4** Poisoning by inhaled anesthetics, undetermined

⑦**T41.0X5** Adverse effect of inhaled anesthetics

⑦**T41.0X6** Underdosing of inhaled anesthetics

T41.1 Poisoning by, adverse effect of and underdosing of intravenous anesthetics
Poisoning by, adverse effect of and underdosing of thiobarbiturates

T41.1X Poisoning by, adverse effect of and underdosing of intravenous anesthetics

⑦**T41.1X1** Poisoning by intravenous anesthetics, accidental (unintentional)
Poisoning by intravenous anesthetics NOS

⑦**T41.1X2** Poisoning by intravenous anesthetics, intentional self-harm

⑦**T41.1X3** Poisoning by intravenous anesthetics, assault

⑦**T41.1X4** Poisoning by intravenous anesthetics, undetermined

⑦**T41.1X5** Adverse effect of intravenous anesthetics

⑦**T41.1X6** Underdosing of intravenous anesthetics

T41.2 Poisoning by, adverse effect of and underdosing of other and unspecified general anesthetics

T41.20 Poisoning by, adverse effect of and underdosing of unspecified general anesthetics

⑦**T41.201** Poisoning by unspecified general anesthetics, accidental (unintentional)

Poisoning by general anesthetics NOS

⑦**T41.202** Poisoning by unspecified general anesthetics, intentional self-harm

⑦**T41.203** Poisoning by unspecified general anesthetics, assault

⑦**T41.204** Poisoning by unspecified general anesthetics, undetermined

⑦**T41.205** Adverse effect of unspecified general anesthetics

⑦**T41.206** Underdosing of unspecified general anesthetics

T41.29 Poisoning by, adverse effect of and underdosing of other general anesthetics

⑦**T41.291** Poisoning by other general anesthetics, accidental (unintentional)

Poisoning by other general anesthetics NOS

⑦**T41.292** Poisoning by other general anesthetics, intentional self-harm

⑦**T41.293** Poisoning by other general anesthetics, assault

⑦**T41.294** Poisoning by other general anesthetics, undetermined

⑦**T41.295** Adverse effect of other general anesthetics

⑦**T41.296** Underdosing of other general anesthetics

T41.3 Poisoning by, adverse effect of and underdosing of local anesthetics

Cocaine (topical)

Excludes 2: poisoning by cocaine used as a central nervous system stimulant (T40.5x1-T40.5x4)

T41.3X Poisoning by, adverse effect of and underdosing of local anesthetics

⑦**T41.3X1** Poisoning by local anesthetics, accidental (unintentional)

Poisoning by local anesthetics NOS

⑦**T41.3X2** Poisoning by local anesthetics, intentional self-harm

⑦**T41.3X3** Poisoning by local anesthetics, assault

⑦**T41.3X4** Poisoning by local anesthetics, undetermined

⑦**T41.3X5** Adverse effect of local anesthetics

⑦**T41.3X6** Underdosing of local anesthetics

T41.4 Poisoning by, adverse effect of and underdosing of unspecified anesthetic

⊗⑦**T41.41** Poisoning by unspecified anesthetic, accidental (unintentional)

Poisoning by anesthetic NOS

⊗⑦**T41.42** Poisoning by unspecified anesthetic, intentional self-harm

⊗⑦**T41.43** Poisoning by unspecified anesthetic, assault

⊗⑦**T41.44** Poisoning by unspecified anesthetic, undetermined

⊗⑦**T41.45** Adverse effect of unspecified anesthetic

⊗⑦**T41.46** Underdosing of unspecified anesthetics

T41.5 Poisoning by, adverse effect of and underdosing of therapeutic gases

T41.5X Poisoning by, adverse effect of and underdosing of therapeutic gases

⑦**T41.5X1** Poisoning by therapeutic gases, accidental (unintentional)

Poisoning by therapeutic gases NOS

⑦**T41.5X2** Poisoning by therapeutic gases, intentional self-harm

⑦**T41.5X3** Poisoning by therapeutic gases, assault

⑦**T41.5X4** Poisoning by therapeutic gases, undetermined

⑦**T41.5X5** Adverse effect of therapeutic gases

⑦**T41.5X6** Underdosing of therapeutic gases

T42 Poisoning by, adverse effect of and underdosing of antiepileptic, sedative- hypnotic and antiparkinsonism drugs

Excludes 2: drug dependence and related mental and behavioral disorders due to psychoactive substance use (F10.--F19.-)

The appropriate 7th character is to be added to each code from category T42

A - initial encounter

D - subsequent encounter

S - sequela

T42.0 Poisoning by, adverse effect of and underdosing of hydantoin derivatives

T42.0X Poisoning by, adverse effect of and underdosing of hydantoin derivatives

⑦**T42.0X1** Poisoning by hydantoin derivatives, accidental (unintentional)

Poisoning by hydantoin derivatives NOS

⑦**T42.0X2** Poisoning by hydantoin derivatives, intentional self-harm

⑦**T42.0X3** Poisoning by hydantoin derivatives, assault

⑦**T42.0X4** Poisoning by hydantoin derivatives, undetermined

⑦**T42.0X5** Adverse effect of hydantoin derivatives

⑦**T42.0X6** Underdosing of hydantoin derivatives

T42.1 Poisoning by, adverse effect of and underdosing of iminostilbenes

Poisoning by, adverse effect of and underdosing of carbamazepine

T42.1X Poisoning by, adverse effect of and underdosing of iminostilbenes

⑦**T42.1X1** Poisoning by iminostilbenes, accidental (unintentional)

Poisoning by iminostilbenes NOS

⑦**T42.1X2** Poisoning by iminostilbenes, intentional self-harm

⑦**T42.1X3** Poisoning by iminostilbenes, assault

⑦**T42.1X4** Poisoning by iminostilbenes, undetermined

⑦**T42.1X5** Adverse effect of iminostilbenes

⑦**T42.1X6** Underdosing of iminostilbenes

● New code   ▲ Revised code   ⑦ 7ᵗʰ digit required   ⊗ Placeholder required

T42.2 Poisoning by, adverse effect of and underdosing of succinimides and oxazolidinediones

    T42.2X Poisoning by, adverse effect of and underdosing of succinimides and oxazolidinediones

        ⑦**T42.2X1** Poisoning by succinimides and oxazolidinediones, accidental (unintentional)

                Poisoning by succinimides and oxazolidinediones NOS

        ⑦**T42.2X2** Poisoning by succinimides and oxazolidinediones, intentional self-harm

        ⑦**T42.2X3** Poisoning by succinimides and oxazolidinediones, assault

        ⑦**T42.2X4** Poisoning by succinimides and oxazolidinediones, undetermined

        ⑦**T42.2X5** Adverse effect of succinimides and oxazolidinediones

        ⑦**T42.2X6** Underdosing of succinimides and oxazolidinediones

T42.3 Poisoning by, adverse effect of and underdosing of barbiturates

    Excludes 1: poisoning by, adverse effect of and underdosing of thiobarbiturates (T41.1-)

    T42.3X Poisoning by, adverse effect of and underdosing of barbiturates

        ⑦**T42.3X1** Poisoning by barbiturates, accidental (unintentional)

                Poisoning by barbiturates NOS

        ⑦**T42.3X2** Poisoning by barbiturates, intentional self-harm

        ⑦**T42.3X3** Poisoning by barbiturates, assault

        ⑦**T42.3X4** Poisoning by barbiturates, undetermined

        ⑦**T42.3X5** Adverse effect of barbiturates

        ⑦**T42.3X6** Underdosing of barbiturates

T42.4 Poisoning by, adverse effect of and underdosing of benzodiazepines

    T42.4X Poisoning by, adverse effect of and underdosing of benzodiazepines

        ⑦**T42.4X1** Poisoning by benzodiazepines, accidental (unintentional)

                Poisoning by benzodiazepines NOS

        ⑦**T42.4X2** Poisoning by benzodiazepines, intentional self-harm

        ⑦**T42.4X3** Poisoning by benzodiazepines, assault

        ⑦**T42.4X4** Poisoning by benzodiazepines, undetermined

        ⑦**T42.4X5** Adverse effect of benzodiazepines

        ⑦**T42.4X6** Underdosing of benzodiazepines

T42.5 Poisoning by, adverse effect of and underdosing of mixed antiepileptics

    T42.5X Poisoning by, adverse effect of and underdosing of antiepileptics

        ⑦**T42.5X1** Poisoning by mixed antiepileptics, accidental (unintentional)

                Poisoning by mixed antiepileptics NOS

        ⑦**T42.5X2** Poisoning by mixed antiepileptics, intentional self-harm

        ⑦**T42.5X3** Poisoning by mixed antiepileptics, assault

        ⑦**T42.5X4** Poisoning by mixed antiepileptics, undetermined

        ⑦**T42.5X5** Adverse effect of mixed antiepileptics

        ⑦**T42.5X6** Underdosing of mixed antiepileptics

T42.6 Poisoning by, adverse effect of and underdosing of other antiepileptic and sedative-hypnotic drugs

    Poisoning by, adverse effect of and underdosing of methaqualone

    Poisoning by, adverse effect of and underdosing of valproic acid

    Excludes 1: poisoning by, adverse effect of and underdosing of carbamazepine (T42.1-)

    T42.6X Poisoning by, adverse effect of and underdosing of other antiepileptic and sedative-hypnotic drugs

        ⑦**T42.6X1** Poisoning by other antiepileptic and sedative-hypnotic drugs, accidental (unintentional)

                Poisoning by other antiepileptic and sedative-hypnotic drugs NOS

        ⑦**T42.6X2** Poisoning by other antiepileptic and sedative-hypnotic drugs, intentional self-harm

        ⑦**T42.6X3** Poisoning by other antiepileptic and sedative-hypnotic drugs, assault

        ⑦**T42.6X4** Poisoning by other antiepileptic and sedative-hypnotic drugs, undetermined

        ⑦**T42.6X5** Adverse effect of other antiepileptic and sedative-hypnotic drugs

        ⑦**T42.6X6** Underdosing of other antiepileptic and sedative-hypnotic drugs

T42.7 Poisoning by, adverse effect of and underdosing of unspecified antiepileptic and sedative-hypnotic drugs

    ⊗⑦**T42.71** Poisoning by unspecified antiepileptic and sedative-hypnotic drugs, accidental (unintentional)

        Poisoning by antiepileptic and sedative-hypnotic drugs NOS

    ⊗⑦**T42.72** Poisoning by unspecified antiepileptic and sedative-hypnotic drugs, intentional self-harm

    ⊗⑦**T42.73** Poisoning by unspecified antiepileptic and sedative-hypnotic drugs, assault

    ⊗⑦**T42.74** Poisoning by unspecified antiepileptic and sedative-hypnotic drugs, undetermined

    ⊗⑦**T42.75** Adverse effect of unspecified antiepileptic and sedative-hypnotic drugs

    ⊗⑦**T42.76** Underdosing of unspecified antiepileptic and sedative-hypnotic drugs

T42.8 Poisoning by, adverse effect of and underdosing of antiparkinsonism drugs and other central muscle-tone depressants

    Poisoning by, adverse effect of and underdosing of amantadine

T42.8X Poisoning by, adverse effect of and underdosing of antiparkinsonism drugs and other central muscle-tone depressants

⑦**T42.8X1** Poisoning by antiparkinsonism drugs and other central muscle-tone depressants, accidental (unintentional)

Poisoning by antiparkinsonism drugs and other central muscle-tone depressants NOS

⑦**T42.8X2** Poisoning by antiparkinsonism drugs and other central muscle-tone depressants, intentional self-harm

⑦**T42.8X3** Poisoning by antiparkinsonism drugs and other central muscle-tone depressants, assault

⑦**T42.8X4** Poisoning by antiparkinsonism drugs and other central muscle-tone depressants, undetermined

⑦**T42.8X5** Adverse effect of antiparkinsonism drugs and other central muscle-tone depressants

⑦**T42.8X6** Underdosing of antiparkinsonism drugs and other central muscle-tone depressants

T43 Poisoning by, adverse effect of and underdosing of psychotropic drugs, not elsewhere classified

Excludes 1: appetite depressants (T50.5-)
barbiturates (T42.3-)
benzodiazepines (T42.4-)
methaqualone (T42.6-)
psychodysleptics [hallucinogens] (T40.7-T40.9-)

Excludes 2: drug dependence and related mental and behavioral disorders due to psychoactive substance use (F10.--F19.-)

The appropriate 7th character is to be added to each code from category T43

A - initial encounter
D - subsequent encounter
S - sequela

T43.0 Poisoning by, adverse effect of and underdosing of tricyclic and tetracyclic antidepressants

T43.01 Poisoning by, adverse effect of and underdosing of tricyclic antidepressants

⑦**T43.011** Poisoning by tricyclic antidepressants, accidental (unintentional)

Poisoning by tricyclic antidepressants NOS

⑦**T43.012** Poisoning by tricyclic antidepressants, intentional self-harm

⑦**T43.013** Poisoning by tricyclic antidepressants, assault

⑦**T43.014** Poisoning by tricyclic antidepressants, undetermined

⑦**T43.015** Adverse effect of tricyclic antidepressants

⑦**T43.016** Underdosing of tricyclic antidepressants

T43.02 Poisoning by, adverse effect of and underdosing of tetracyclic antidepressants

⑦**T43.021** Poisoning by tetracyclic antidepressants, accidental (unintentional)

Poisoning by tetracyclic antidepressants NOS

⑦**T43.022** Poisoning by tetracyclic antidepressants, intentional self-harm

⑦**T43.023** Poisoning by tetracyclic antidepressants, assault

⑦**T43.024** Poisoning by tetracyclic antidepressants, undetermined

⑦**T43.025** Adverse effect of tetracyclic antidepressants

⑦**T43.026** Underdosing of tetracyclic antidepressants

T43.1 Poisoning by, adverse effect of and underdosing of monoamine-oxidase-inhibitor antidepressants

T43.1X Poisoning by, adverse effect of and underdosing of monoamine-oxidase-inhibitor antidepressants

⑦**T43.1X1** Poisoning by monoamine-oxidase-inhibitor antidepressants, accidental (unintentional)

Poisoning by monoamine-oxidase-inhibitor antidepressants NOS

⑦**T43.1X2** Poisoning by monoamine-oxidase-inhibitor antidepressants, intentional self-harm

⑦**T43.1X3** Poisoning by monoamine-oxidase-inhibitor antidepressants, assault

⑦**T43.1X4** Poisoning by monoamine-oxidase-inhibitor antidepressants, undetermined

⑦**T43.1X5** Adverse effect of monoamine-oxidase-inhibitor antidepressants

⑦**T43.1X6** Underdosing of monoamine-oxidase-inhibitor antidepressants

T43.2 Poisoning by, adverse effect of and underdosing of other and unspecified antidepressants

T43.20 Poisoning by, adverse effect of and underdosing of unspecified antidepressants

⑦**T43.201** Poisoning by unspecified antidepressants, accidental (unintentional)

Poisoning by antidepressants NOS

⑦**T43.202** Poisoning by unspecified antidepressants, intentional self-harm

⑦**T43.203** Poisoning by unspecified antidepressants, assault

⑦**T43.204** Poisoning by unspecified antidepressants, undetermined

⑦**T43.205** Adverse effect of unspecified antidepressants

⑦**T43.206** Underdosing of unspecified antidepressants

● New code   ▲ Revised code   ⑦ 7ᵗʰ digit required   ⊗ Placeholder required

T43.21 Poisoning by, adverse effect of and underdosing of selective serotonin and norepinephrine reuptake inhibitors
Poisoning by, adverse effect of and underdosing of SSNRI antidepressants
⑦ T43.211 Poisoning by selective serotonin and norepinephrine reuptake inhibitors, accidental (unintentional)
⑦ T43.212 Poisoning by selective serotonin and norepinephrine reuptake inhibitors, intentional self-harm
⑦ T43.213 Poisoning by selective serotonin and norepinephrine reuptake inhibitors, assault
⑦ T43.214 Poisoning by selective serotonin and norepinephrine reuptake inhibitors, undetermined
⑦ T43.215 Adverse effect of selective serotonin and norepinephrine reuptake inhibitors
⑦ T43.216 Underdosing of selective serotonin and norepinephrine reuptake inhibitors
T43.22 Poisoning by, adverse effect of and underdosing of selective serotonin reuptake inhibitors
Poisoning by, adverse effect of and underdosing of SSRI antidepressants
⑦ T43.221 Poisoning by selective serotonin reuptake inhibitors, accidental (unintentional)
⑦ T43.222 Poisoning by selective serotonin reuptake inhibitors, intentional self-harm
⑦ T43.223 Poisoning by selective serotonin reuptake inhibitors, assault
⑦ T43.224 Poisoning by selective serotonin reuptake inhibitors, undetermined
⑦ T43.225 Adverse effect of selective serotonin reuptake inhibitors
⑦ T43.226 Underdosing of selective serotonin reuptake inhibitors
T43.29 Poisoning by, adverse effect of and underdosing of other antidepressants
⑦ T43.291 Poisoning by other antidepressants, accidental (unintentional)
Poisoning by other antidepressants NOS
⑦ T43.292 Poisoning by other antidepressants, intentional self-harm
⑦ T43.293 Poisoning by other antidepressants, assault
⑦ T43.294 Poisoning by other antidepressants, undetermined
⑦ T43.295 Adverse effect of other antidepressants
⑦ T43.296 Underdosing of other antidepressants
T43.3 Poisoning by, adverse effect of and underdosing of phenothiazine antipsychotics and neuroleptics
T43.3X Poisoning by, adverse effect of and underdosing of phenothiazine antipsychotics and neuroleptics

⑦ T43.3X1 Poisoning by phenothiazine antipsychotics and neuroleptics, accidental (unintentional)
Poisoning by phenothiazine antipsychotics and neuroleptics NOS
⑦ T43.3X2 Poisoning by phenothiazine antipsychotics and neuroleptics, intentional self-harm
⑦ T43.3X3 Poisoning by phenothiazine antipsychotics and neuroleptics, assault
⑦ T43.3X4 Poisoning by phenothiazine antipsychotics and neuroleptics, undetermined
⑦ T43.3X5 Adverse effect of phenothiazine antipsychotics and neuroleptics
⑦ T43.3X6 Underdosing of phenothiazine antipsychotics and neuroleptics
T43.4 Poisoning by, adverse effect of and underdosing of butyrophenone and thiothixene neuroleptics
T43.4X Poisoning by, adverse effect of and underdosing of butyrophenone and thiothixene neuroleptics
⑦ T43.4X1 Poisoning by butyrophenone and thiothixene neuroleptics, accidental (unintentional)
Poisoning by butyrophenone and thiothixene neuroleptics NOS
⑦ T43.4X2 Poisoning by butyrophenone and thiothixene neuroleptics, intentional self-harm
⑦ T43.4X3 Poisoning by butyrophenone and thiothixene neuroleptics, assault
⑦ T43.4X4 Poisoning by butyrophenone and thiothixene neuroleptics, undetermined
⑦ T43.4X5 Adverse effect of butyrophenone and thiothixene neuroleptics
⑦ T43.4X6 Underdosing of butyrophenone and thiothixene neuroleptics
T43.5 Poisoning by, adverse effect of and underdosing of other and unspecified antipsychotics and neuroleptics
Excludes 1: poisoning by, adverse effect of and underdosing of rauwolfia (T46.5-)
T43.50 Poisoning by, adverse effect of and underdosing of unspecified antipsychotics and neuroleptics
⑦ T43.501 Poisoning by unspecified antipsychotics and neuroleptics, accidental (unintentional)
Poisoning by antipsychotics and neuroleptics NOS
⑦ T43.502 Poisoning by unspecified antipsychotics and neuroleptics, intentional self-harm
⑦ T43.503 Poisoning by unspecified antipsychotics and neuroleptics, assault
⑦ T43.504 Poisoning by unspecified antipsychotics and neuroleptics, undetermined
⑦ T43.505 Adverse effect of unspecified antipsychotics and neuroleptics

⑦ **T43.506** Underdosing of unspecified antipsychotics and neuroleptics

T43.59 Poisoning by, adverse effect of and underdosing of other antipsychotics and neuroleptics

⑦ **T43.591** Poisoning by other antipsychotics and neuroleptics, accidental (unintentional)

Poisoning by other antipsychotics and neuroleptics NOS

⑦ **T43.592** Poisoning by other antipsychotics and neuroleptics, intentional self-harm

⑦ **T43.593** Poisoning by other antipsychotics and neuroleptics, assault

⑦ **T43.594** Poisoning by other antipsychotics and neuroleptics, undetermined

⑦ **T43.595** Adverse effect of other antipsychotics and neuroleptics

⑦ **T43.596** Underdosing of other antipsychotics and neuroleptics

T43.6 Poisoning by, adverse effect of and underdosing of psychostimulants

Excludes 1: poisoning by, adverse effect of and underdosing of cocaine (T40.5-)

T43.60 Poisoning by, adverse effect of and underdosing of unspecified psychostimulant

⑦ **T43.601** Poisoning by unspecified psychostimulants, accidental (unintentional)

Poisoning by psychostimulants NOS

⑦ **T43.602** Poisoning by unspecified psychostimulants, intentional self-harm

⑦ **T43.603** Poisoning by unspecified psychostimulants, assault

⑦ **T43.604** Poisoning by unspecified psychostimulants, undetermined

⑦ **T43.605** Adverse effect of unspecified psychostimulants

⑦ **T43.606** Underdosing of unspecified psychostimulants

T43.61 Poisoning by, adverse effect of and underdosing of caffeine

⑦ **T43.611** Poisoning by caffeine, accidental (unintentional)

Poisoning by caffeine NOS

⑦ **T43.612** Poisoning by caffeine, intentional self-harm

⑦ **T43.613** Poisoning by caffeine, assault

⑦ **T43.614** Poisoning by caffeine, undetermined

⑦ **T43.615** Adverse effect of caffeine

⑦ **T43.616** Underdosing of caffeine

T43.62 Poisoning by, adverse effect of and underdosing of amphetamines

Poisoning by, adverse effect of and underdosing of methamphetamines

⑦ **T43.621** Poisoning by amphetamines, accidental (unintentional)

Poisoning by amphetamines NOS

⑦ **T43.622** Poisoning by amphetamines, intentional self-harm

⑦ **T43.623** Poisoning by amphetamines, assault

⑦ **T43.624** Poisoning by amphetamines, undetermined

⑦ **T43.625** Adverse effect of amphetamines

⑦ **T43.626** Underdosing of amphetamines

T43.63 Poisoning by, adverse effect of and underdosing of methylphenidate

⑦ **T43.631** Poisoning by methylphenidate, accidental (unintentional)

Poisoning by methylphenidate NOS

⑦ **T43.632** Poisoning by methylphenidate, intentional self-harm

⑦ **T43.633** Poisoning by methylphenidate, assault

⑦ **T43.634** Poisoning by methylphenidate, undetermined

⑦ **T43.635** Adverse effect of methylphenidate

⑦ **T43.636** Underdosing of methylphenidate

T43.69 Poisoning by, adverse effect of and underdosing of other psychostimulants

⑦ **T43.691** Poisoning by other psychostimulants, accidental (unintentional)

Poisoning by other psychostimulants NOS

⑦ **T43.692** Poisoning by other psychostimulants, intentional self-harm

⑦ **T43.693** Poisoning by other psychostimulants, assault

⑦ **T43.694** Poisoning by other psychostimulants, undetermined

⑦ **T43.695** Adverse effect of other psychostimulants

⑦ **T43.696** Underdosing of other psychostimulants

T43.8 Poisoning by, adverse effect of and underdosing of other psychotropic drugs

T43.8X Poisoning by, adverse effect of and underdosing of other psychotropic drugs

⑦ **T43.8X1** Poisoning by other psychotropic drugs, accidental (unintentional)

Poisoning by other psychotropic drugs NOS

⑦ **T43.8X2** Poisoning by other psychotropic drugs, intentional self-harm

⑦ **T43.8X3** Poisoning by other psychotropic drugs, assault

⑦ **T43.8X4** Poisoning by other psychotropic drugs, undetermined

⑦ **T43.8X5** Adverse effect of other psychotropic drugs

⑦ **T43.8X6** Underdosing of other psychotropic drugs

T43.9 Poisoning by, adverse effect of and underdosing of unspecified psychotropic drug

⊗⑦**T43.91** Poisoning by unspecified psychotropic drug, accidental (unintentional)
Poisoning by psychotropic drug NOS

⊗⑦**T43.92** Poisoning by unspecified psychotropic drug, intentional self-harm

⊗⑦**T43.93** Poisoning by unspecified psychotropic drug, assault

⊗⑦**T43.94** Poisoning by unspecified psychotropic drug, undetermined

⊗⑦**T43.95** Adverse effect of unspecified psychotropic drug

⊗⑦**T43.96** Underdosing of unspecified psychotropic drug

T44 Poisoning by, adverse effect of and underdosing of drugs primarily affecting the autonomic nervous system

The appropriate 7th character is to be added to each code from category T44

A - initial encounter

D - subsequent encounter

S - sequela

T44.0 Poisoning by, adverse effect of and underdosing of anticholinesterase agents

    T44.0X Poisoning by, adverse effect of and underdosing of anticholinesterase agents

      ⑦**T44.0X1** Poisoning by anticholinesterase agents, accidental (unintentional)
Poisoning by anticholinesterase agents NOS

      ⑦**T44.0X2** Poisoning by anticholinesterase agents, intentional self-harm

      ⑦**T44.0X3** Poisoning by anticholinesterase agents, assault

      ⑦**T44.0X4** Poisoning by anticholinesterase agents, undetermined

      ⑦**T44.0X5** Adverse effect of anticholinesterase agents

      ⑦**T44.0X6** Underdosing of anticholinesterase agents

T44.1 Poisoning by, adverse effect of and underdosing of other parasympathomimetics [cholinergics]

    T44.1X Poisoning by, adverse effect of and underdosing of other parasympathomimetics [cholinergics]

      ⑦**T44.1X1** Poisoning by other parasympathomimetics [cholinergics], accidental (unintentional)
Poisoning by other parasympathomimetics [cholinergics] NOS

      ⑦**T44.1X2** Poisoning by other parasympathomimetics [cholinergics], intentional self-harm

      ⑦**T44.1X3** Poisoning by other parasympathomimetics [cholinergics], assault

      ⑦**T44.1X4** Poisoning by other parasympathomimetics [cholinergics], undetermined

      ⑦**T44.1X5** Adverse effect of other parasympathomimetics [cholinergics]

⑦**T44.1X6** Underdosing of other parasympathomimetics

T44.2 Poisoning by, adverse effect of and underdosing of ganglionic blocking drugs

    T44.2X Poisoning by, adverse effect of and underdosing of ganglionic blocking drugs

      ⑦**T44.2X1** Poisoning by ganglionic blocking drugs, accidental (unintentional)
Poisoning by ganglionic blocking drugs NOS

      ⑦**T44.2X2** Poisoning by ganglionic blocking drugs, intentional self-harm

      ⑦**T44.2X3** Poisoning by ganglionic blocking drugs, assault

      ⑦**T44.2X4** Poisoning by ganglionic blocking drugs, undetermined

      ⑦**T44.2X5** Adverse effect of ganglionic blocking drugs

      ⑦**T44.2X6** Underdosing of ganglionic blocking drugs

T44.3 Poisoning by, adverse effect of and underdosing of other parasympatholytics [anticholinergics and antimuscarinics] and spasmolytics
Poisoning by, adverse effect of and underdosing of papaverine

    T44.3X Poisoning by, adverse effect of and underdosing of other parasympatholytics [anticholinergics and antimuscarinics] and spasmolytics

      ⑦**T44.3X1** Poisoning by other parasympatholytics [anticholinergics and antimuscarinics] and spasmolytics, accidental (unintentional)
Poisoning by other parasympatholytics [anticholinergics and antimuscarinics] and spasmolytics NOS

      ⑦**T44.3X2** Poisoning by other parasympatholytics [anticholinergics and antimuscarinics] and spasmolytics, intentional self-harm

      ⑦**T44.3X3** Poisoning by other parasympatholytics [anticholinergics and antimuscarinics] and spasmolytics, assault

      ⑦**T44.3X4** Poisoning by other parasympatholytics [anticholinergics and antimuscarinics] and spasmolytics, undetermined

      ⑦**T44.3X5** Adverse effect of other parasympatholytics [anticholinergics and antimuscarinics] and spasmolytics

      ⑦**T44.3X6** Underdosing of other parasympatholytics [anticholinergics and antimuscarinics] and spasmolytics

T44.4 Poisoning by, adverse effect of and underdosing of predominantly alpha-adrenoreceptor agonists

Poisoning by, adverse effect of and underdosing of
metaraminol

T44.4X Poisoning by, adverse effect of and underdosing
of predominantly alpha-adrenoreceptor agonists

⑦ T44.4X1 Poisoning by predominantly
alpha-adrenoreceptor agonists,
accidental (unintentional)
Poisoning by predominantly
alpha-adrenoreceptor agonists NOS

⑦ T44.4X2 Poisoning by predominantly
alpha-adrenoreceptor agonists,
intentional self-harm

⑦ T44.4X3 Poisoning by predominantly
alpha-adrenoreceptor agonists,
assault

⑦ T44.4X4 Poisoning by predominantly
alpha-adrenoreceptor agonists,
undetermined

⑦ T44.4X5 Adverse effect of predominantly
alpha-adrenoreceptor agonists

⑦ T44.4X6 Underdosing of predominantly
alpha-adrenoreceptor agonists

T44.5 Poisoning by, adverse effect of and underdosing of
predominantly beta-adrenoreceptor agonists

Excludes 1: poisoning by, adverse effect of and
underdosing of beta-adrenoreceptor agonists
used in asthma therapy (T48.6-)

T44.5X Poisoning by, adverse effect of and underdosing
of predominantly beta-adrenoreceptor agonists

⑦ T44.5X1 Poisoning by predominantly
beta-adrenoreceptor agonists,
accidental (unintentional)
Poisoning by predominantly
beta-adrenoreceptor agonists NOS

⑦ T44.5X2 Poisoning by predominantly
beta-adrenoreceptor agonists,
intentional self-harm

⑦ T44.5X3 Poisoning by predominantly
beta-adrenoreceptor agonists, assault

⑦ T44.5X4 Poisoning by predominantly
beta-adrenoreceptor agonists,
undetermined

⑦ T44.5X5 Adverse effect of predominantly
beta-adrenoreceptor agonists

⑦ T44.5X6 Underdosing of predominantly
beta-adrenoreceptor agonists

T44.6 Poisoning by, adverse effect of and underdosing of
alpha-adrenoreceptor antagonists

Excludes 1: poisoning by, adverse effect of and
underdosing of ergot alkaloids (T48.0)

T44.6X Poisoning by, adverse effect of and underdosing
of alpha-adrenoreceptor antagonists

⑦ T44.6X1 Poisoning by alpha-adrenoreceptor
antagonists, accidental
(unintentional)
Poisoning by alpha-adrenoreceptor
antagonists NOS

⑦ T44.6X2 Poisoning by alpha-adrenoreceptor
antagonists, intentional self-harm

⑦ T44.6X3 Poisoning by alpha-adrenoreceptor
antagonists, assault

⑦ T44.6X4 Poisoning by alpha-adrenoreceptor
antagonists, undetermined

⑦ T44.6X5 Adverse effect of alpha-
adrenoreceptor antagonists

⑦ T44.6X6 Underdosing of
alpha-adrenoreceptor antagonists

T44.7 Poisoning by, adverse effect of and underdosing of
beta-adrenoreceptor antagonists

T44.7X Poisoning by, adverse effect of and underdosing
of beta-adrenoreceptor antagonists

⑦ T44.7X1 Poisoning by beta-adrenoreceptor
antagonists, accidental
(unintentional)
Poisoning by beta-adrenoreceptor
antagonists NOS

⑦ T44.7X2 Poisoning by beta-adrenoreceptor
antagonists, intentional self-harm

⑦ T44.7X3 Poisoning by beta-adrenoreceptor
antagonists, assault

⑦ T44.7X4 Poisoning by beta-adrenoreceptor
antagonists, undetermined

⑦ T44.7X5 Adverse effect of
beta-adrenoreceptor antagonists

⑦ T44.7X6 Underdosing of beta-adrenoreceptor
antagonists

T44.8 Poisoning by, adverse effect of and underdosing of
centrally-acting and adrenergic-neuron- blocking agents

Excludes 1: poisoning by, adverse effect of and
underdosing of clonidine (T46.5)
poisoning by, adverse effect of and
underdosing of guanethidine (T46.5)

T44.8X Poisoning by, adverse effect of and underdosing
of centrally-acting and adrenergic-neuron-
blocking agents

⑦ T44.8X1 Poisoning by centrally-acting and
adrenergic-neuron-blocking agents,
accidental (unintentional)
Poisoning by centrally-acting and
adrenergic-neuron-blocking agents
NOS

⑦ T44.8X2 Poisoning by centrally-acting and
adrenergic-neuron-blocking agents,
intentional self-harm

⑦ T44.8X3 Poisoning by centrally-acting and
adrenergic-neuron-blocking agents,
assault

⑦ T44.8X4 Poisoning by centrally-acting and
adrenergic-neuron-blocking agents,
undetermined

⑦ T44.8X5 Adverse effect of centrally-acting
and adrenergic-neuron-blocking
agents

⑦ T44.8X6 Underdosing of centrally-acting and
adrenergic-neuron-blocking agents

T44.9 Poisoning by, adverse effect of and underdosing of other
and unspecified drugs primarily affecting the autonomic
nervous system

Poisoning by, adverse effect of and underdosing of drug stimulating both alpha and beta-adrenoreceptors

T44.90 Poisoning by, adverse effect of and underdosing of unspecified drugs primarily affecting the autonomic nervous system

⑦**T44.901** Poisoning by unspecified drugs primarily affecting the autonomic nervous system, accidental (unintentional)

Poisoning by unspecified drugs primarily affecting the autonomic nervous system NOS

⑦**T44.902** Poisoning by unspecified drugs primarily affecting the autonomic nervous system, intentional self-harm

⑦**T44.903** Poisoning by unspecified drugs primarily affecting the autonomic nervous system, assault

⑦**T44.904** Poisoning by unspecified drugs primarily affecting the autonomic nervous system, undetermined

⑦**T44.905** Adverse effect of unspecified drugs primarily affecting the autonomic nervous system

⑦**T44.906** Underdosing of unspecified drugs primarily affecting the autonomic nervous system

T44.99 Poisoning by, adverse effect of and underdosing of other drugs primarily affecting the autonomic nervous system

⑦**T44.991** Poisoning by other drug primarily affecting the autonomic nervous system, accidental (unintentional)

Poisoning by other drugs primarily affecting the autonomic nervous system NOS

⑦**T44.992** Poisoning by other drug primarily affecting the autonomic nervous system, intentional self-harm

⑦**T44.993** Poisoning by other drug primarily affecting the autonomic nervous system, assault

⑦**T44.994** Poisoning by other drug primarily affecting the autonomic nervous system, undetermined

⑦**T44.995** Adverse effect of other drug primarily affecting the autonomic nervous system

⑦**T44.996** Underdosing of other drug primarily affecting the autonomic nervous system

T45 Poisoning by, adverse effect of and underdosing of primarily systemic and hematological agents, not elsewhere classified

The appropriate 7th character is to be added to each code from category T45

A - initial encounter

D - subsequent encounter

S - sequela

T45.0 Poisoning by, adverse effect of and underdosing of antiallergic and antiemetic drugs

Excludes 1: poisoning by, adverse effect of and underdosing of phenothiazine-based neuroleptics (T43.3)

T45.0X Poisoning by, adverse effect of and underdosing of antiallergic and antiemetic drugs

⑦**T45.0X1** Poisoning by antiallergic and antiemetic drugs, accidental (unintentional)

Poisoning by antiallergic and antiemetic drugs NOS

⑦**T45.0X2** Poisoning by antiallergic and antiemetic drugs, intentional self-harm

⑦**T45.0X3** Poisoning by antiallergic and antiemetic drugs, assault

⑦**T45.0X4** Poisoning by antiallergic and antiemetic drugs, undetermined

⑦**T45.0X5** Adverse effect of antiallergic and antiemetic drugs

⑦**T45.0X6** Underdosing of antiallergic and antiemetic drugs

T45.1 Poisoning by, adverse effect of and underdosing of antineoplastic and immunosuppressive drugs

Excludes 1: poisoning by, adverse effect of and underdosing of tamoxifen (T38.6)

T45.1X Poisoning by, adverse effect of and underdosing of antineoplastic and immunosuppressive drugs

⑦**T45.1X1** Poisoning by antineoplastic and immunosuppressive drugs, accidental (unintentional)

Poisoning by antineoplastic and immunosuppressive drugs NOS

⑦**T45.1X2** Poisoning by antineoplastic and immunosuppressive drugs, intentional self-harm

⑦**T45.1X3** Poisoning by antineoplastic and immunosuppressive drugs, assault

⑦**T45.1X4** Poisoning by antineoplastic and immunosuppressive drugs, undetermined

⑦**T45.1X5** Adverse effect of antineoplastic and immunosuppressive drugs

⑦**T45.1X6** Underdosing of antineoplastic and immunosuppressive drugs

T45.2 Poisoning by, adverse effect of and underdosing of vitamins

Excludes 2: poisoning by, adverse effect of and underdosing of nicotinic acid (derivatives) (T46.7)

poisoning by, adverse effect of and underdosing of iron (T45.4)

poisoning by, adverse effect of and underdosing of vitamin K (T45.7)

T45.2X Poisoning by, adverse effect of and underdosing of vitamins

⑦**T45.2X1** Poisoning by vitamins, accidental (unintentional)

Poisoning by vitamins NOS

⑦**T45.2X2** Poisoning by vitamins, intentional self-harm

⑦ **T45.2X3** Poisoning by vitamins, assault

⑦ **T45.2X4** Poisoning by vitamins, undetermined

⑦ **T45.2X5** Adverse effect of vitamins

⑦ **T45.2X6** Underdosing of vitamins

Excludes 1: vitamin deficiencies (E50-E56)

T45.3 Poisoning by, adverse effect of and underdosing of enzymes

   T45.3X Poisoning by, adverse effect of and underdosing of enzymes

      ⑦ **T45.3X1** Poisoning by enzymes, accidental (unintentional)

            Poisoning by enzymes NOS

      ⑦ **T45.3X2** Poisoning by enzymes, intentional self-harm

      ⑦ **T45.3X3** Poisoning by enzymes, assault

      ⑦ **T45.3X4** Poisoning by enzymes, undetermined

      ⑦ **T45.3X5** Adverse effect of enzymes

      ⑦ **T45.3X6** Underdosing of enzymes

T45.4 Poisoning by, adverse effect of and underdosing of iron and its compounds

   T45.4X Poisoning by, adverse effect of and underdosing of iron and its compounds

      ⑦ **T45.4X1** Poisoning by iron and its compounds, accidental (unintentional)

            Poisoning by iron and its compounds NOS

      ⑦ **T45.4X2** Poisoning by iron and its compounds, intentional self-harm

      ⑦ **T45.4X3** Poisoning by iron and its compounds, assault

      ⑦ **T45.4X4** Poisoning by iron and its compounds, undetermined

      ⑦ **T45.4X5** Adverse effect of iron and its compounds

      ⑦ **T45.4X6** Underdosing of iron and its compounds

Excludes 1: iron deficiency (E61.1)

T45.5 Poisoning by, adverse effect of and underdosing of anticoagulants and antithrombotic drugs

   T45.51 Poisoning by, adverse effect of and underdosing of anticoagulants

      ⑦ **T45.511** Poisoning by anticoagulants, accidental (unintentional)

            Poisoning by anticoagulants NOS

      ⑦ **T45.512** Poisoning by anticoagulants, intentional self-harm

      ⑦ **T45.513** Poisoning by anticoagulants, assault

      ⑦ **T45.514** Poisoning by anticoagulants, undetermined

      ⑦ **T45.515** Adverse effect of anticoagulants

      ⑦ **T45.516** Underdosing of anticoagulants

   T45.52 Poisoning by, adverse effect of and underdosing of antithrombotic drugs

      Poisoning by, adverse effect of and underdosing of antiplatelet drugs

Excludes 2: poisoning by, adverse effect of and underdosing of aspirin (T39.01-)

poisoning by, adverse effect of and underdosing of acetylsalicylic acid (T39.01-)

      ⑦ **T45.521** Poisoning by antithrombotic drugs, accidental (unintentional)

            Poisoning by antithrombotic drug NOS

      ⑦ **T45.522** Poisoning by antithrombotic drugs, intentional self-harm

      ⑦ **T45.523** Poisoning by antithrombotic drugs, assault

      ⑦ **T45.524** Poisoning by antithrombotic drugs, undetermined

      ⑦ **T45.525** Adverse effect of antithrombotic drugs

      ⑦ **T45.526** Underdosing of antithrombotic drugs

T45.6 Poisoning by, adverse effect of and underdosing of fibrinolysis-affecting drugs

   T45.60 Poisoning by, adverse effect of and underdosing of unspecified fibrinolysis-affecting drugs

      ⑦ **T45.601** Poisoning by unspecified fibrinolysis-affecting drugs, accidental (unintentional)

            Poisoning by fibrinolysis-affecting drug NOS

      ⑦ **T45.602** Poisoning by unspecified fibrinolysis-affecting drugs, intentional self-harm

      ⑦ **T45.603** Poisoning by unspecified fibrinolysis-affecting drugs, assault

      ⑦ **T45.604** Poisoning by unspecified fibrinolysis-affecting drugs, undetermined

      ⑦ **T45.605** Adverse effect of unspecified fibrinolysis-affecting drugs

      ⑦ **T45.606** Underdosing of unspecified fibrinolysis-affecting drugs

   T45.61 Poisoning by, adverse effect of and underdosing of thrombolytic drugs

      ⑦ **T45.611** Poisoning by thrombolytic drug, accidental (unintentional)

            Poisoning by thrombolytic drug NOS

      ⑦ **T45.612** Poisoning by thrombolytic drug, intentional self-harm

      ⑦ **T45.613** Poisoning by thrombolytic drug, assault

      ⑦ **T45.614** Poisoning by thrombolytic drug, undetermined

      ⑦ **T45.615** Adverse effect of thrombolytic drugs

      ⑦ **T45.616** Underdosing of thrombolytic drugs

   T45.62 Poisoning by, adverse effect of and underdosing of hemostatic drugs

      ⑦ **T45.621** Poisoning by hemostatic drug, accidental (unintentional)

            Poisoning by hemostatic drug NOS

● New code   ▲ Revised code   ⑦ 7ᵗʰ digit required   ⊗ Placeholder required

⑦T45.622 Poisoning by hemostatic drug, intentional self-harm

⑦T45.623 Poisoning by hemostatic drug, assault

⑦T45.624 Poisoning by hemostatic drug, undetermined

⑦T45.625 Adverse effect of hemostatic drug

⑦T45.626 Underdosing of hemostatic drugs

T45.69 Poisoning by, adverse effect of and underdosing of other fibrinolysis-affecting drugs

⑦T45.691 Poisoning by other fibrinolysis-affecting drugs, accidental (unintentional)

Poisoning by other fibrinolysis-affecting drug NOS

⑦T45.692 Poisoning by other fibrinolysis-affecting drugs, intentional self-harm

⑦T45.693 Poisoning by other fibrinolysis-affecting drugs, assault

⑦T45.694 Poisoning by other fibrinolysis-affecting drugs, undetermined

⑦T45.695 Adverse effect of other fibrinolysis-affecting drugs

⑦T45.696 Underdosing of other fibrinolysis-affecting drugs

T45.7 Poisoning by, adverse effect of and underdosing of anticoagulant antagonists, vitamin K and other coagulants

T45.7X Poisoning by, adverse effect of and underdosing of anticoagulant antagonists, vitamin K and other coagulants

⑦T45.7X1 Poisoning by anticoagulant antagonists, vitamin K and other coagulants, accidental (unintentional)

Poisoning by anticoagulant antagonists, vitamin K and other coagulants NOS

⑦T45.7X2 Poisoning by anticoagulant antagonists, vitamin K and other coagulants, intentional self-harm

⑦T45.7X3 Poisoning by anticoagulant antagonists, vitamin K and other coagulants, assault

⑦T45.7X4 Poisoning by anticoagulant antagonists, vitamin K and other coagulants, undetermined

⑦T45.7X5 Adverse effect of anticoagulant antagonists, vitamin K and other coagulants

⑦T45.7X6 Underdosing of anticoagulant antagonist, vitamin K and other coagulants

Excludes 1: vitamin K deficiency (E56.1)

T45.8 Poisoning by, adverse effect of and underdosing of other primarily systemic and hematological agents

Poisoning by, adverse effect of and underdosing of liver preparations and other antianemic agents

Poisoning by, adverse effect of and underdosing of natural blood and blood products

Poisoning by, adverse effect of and underdosing of plasma substitute

Excludes 2: poisoning by, adverse effect of and underdosing of immunoglobulin (T50.Z1)

poisoning by, adverse effect of and underdosing of iron (T45.4)

transfusion reactions (T80.-)

T45.8X Poisoning by, adverse effect of and underdosing of other primarily systemic and hematological agents

⑦T45.8X1 Poisoning by other primarily systemic and hematological agents, accidental (unintentional)

Poisoning by other primarily systemic and hematological agents NOS

⑦T45.8X2 Poisoning by other primarily systemic and hematological agents, intentional self-harm

⑦T45.8X3 Poisoning by other primarily systemic and hematological agents, assault

⑦T45.8X4 Poisoning by other primarily systemic and hematological agents, undetermined

⑦T45.8X5 Adverse effect of other primarily systemic and hematological agents

⑦T45.8X6 Underdosing of other primarily systemic and hematological agents

T45.9 Poisoning by, adverse effect of and underdosing of unspecified primarily systemic and hematological agent

⊗⑦T45.91 Poisoning by unspecified primarily systemic and hematological agent, accidental (unintentional)

Poisoning by primarily systemic and hematological agent NOS

⊗⑦T45.92 Poisoning by unspecified primarily systemic and hematological agent, intentional self-harm

⊗⑦T45.93 Poisoning by unspecified primarily systemic and hematological agent, assault

⊗⑦T45.94 Poisoning by unspecified primarily systemic and hematological agent, undetermined

⊗⑦T45.95 Adverse effect of unspecified primarily systemic and hematological agent

⊗⑦T45.96 Underdosing of unspecified primarily systemic and hematological agent

T46 Poisoning by, adverse effect of and underdosing of agents primarily affecting the cardiovascular system

Excludes 1: poisoning by, adverse effect of and underdosing of metaraminol (T44.4)

The appropriate 7th character is to be added to each code from category T46

A - initial encounter

D - subsequent encounter

S - sequela

T46.0 Poisoning by, adverse effect of and underdosing of cardiac-stimulant glycosides and drugs of similar action

⑦T46.0X Poisoning by, adverse effect of and underdosing of cardiac-stimulant glycosides and drugs of similar action

⑦**T46.0X1** Poisoning by cardiac-stimulant glycosides and drugs of similar action, accidental (unintentional)

Poisoning by cardiac-stimulant glycosides and drugs of similar action NOS

⑦**T46.0X2** Poisoning by cardiac-stimulant glycosides and drugs of similar action, intentional self-harm

⑦**T46.0X3** Poisoning by cardiac-stimulant glycosides and drugs of similar action, assault

⑦**T46.0X4** Poisoning by cardiac-stimulant glycosides and drugs of similar action, undetermined

⑦**T46.0X5** Adverse effect of cardiac-stimulant glycosides and drugs of similar action

⑦**T46.0X6** Underdosing of cardiac-stimulant glycosides and drugs of similar action

T46.1 Poisoning by, adverse effect of and underdosing of calcium-channel blockers

T46.1X Poisoning by, adverse effect of and underdosing of calcium-channel blockers

⑦**T46.1X1** Poisoning by calcium-channel blockers, accidental (unintentional)

Poisoning by calcium-channel blockers NOS

⑦**T46.1X2** Poisoning by calcium-channel blockers, intentional self-harm

⑦**T46.1X3** Poisoning by calcium-channel blockers, assault

⑦**T46.1X4** Poisoning by calcium-channel blockers, undetermined

⑦**T46.1X5** Adverse effect of calcium-channel blockers

⑦**T46.1X6** Underdosing of calcium-channel blockers

T46.2 Poisoning by, adverse effect of and underdosing of other antidysrhythmic drugs, not elsewhere classified

Excludes 1: poisoning by, adverse effect of and underdosing of beta-adrenoreceptor antagonists (T44.7-)

T46.2X Poisoning by, adverse effect of and underdosing of other antidysrhythmic drugs

⑦**T46.2X1** Poisoning by other antidysrhythmic drugs, accidental (unintentional)

Poisoning by other antidysrhythmic drugs NOS

⑦**T46.2X2** Poisoning by other antidysrhythmic drugs, intentional self-harm

⑦**T46.2X3** Poisoning by other antidysrhythmic drugs, assault

⑦**T46.2X4** Poisoning by other antidysrhythmic drugs, undetermined

⑦**T46.2X5** Adverse effect of other antidysrhythmic drugs

⑦**T46.2X6** Underdosing of other antidysrhythmic drugs

T46.3 Poisoning by, adverse effect of and underdosing of coronary vasodilators

Poisoning by, adverse effect of and underdosing of dipyridamole

Excludes 1: poisoning by, adverse effect of and underdosing of calcium-channel blockers (T46.1)

T46.3X Poisoning by, adverse effect of and underdosing of coronary vasodilators

⑦**T46.3X1** Poisoning by coronary vasodilators, accidental (unintentional)

Poisoning by coronary vasodilators NOS

⑦**T46.3X2** Poisoning by coronary vasodilators, intentional self-harm

⑦**T46.3X3** Poisoning by coronary vasodilators, assault

⑦**T46.3X4** Poisoning by coronary vasodilators, undetermined

⑦**T46.3X5** Adverse effect of coronary vasodilators

⑦**T46.3X6** Underdosing of coronary vasodilators

T46.4 Poisoning by, adverse effect of and underdosing of angiotensin-converting-enzyme inhibitors

T46.4X Poisoning by, adverse effect of and underdosing of angiotensin-converting-enzyme inhibitors

⑦**T46.4X1** Poisoning by angiotensin-converting-enzyme inhibitors, accidental (unintentional)

Poisoning by angiotensin-converting-enzyme inhibitors NOS

⑦**T46.4X2** Poisoning by angiotensin-converting- enzyme inhibitors, intentional self-harm

⑦**T46.4X3** Poisoning by angiotensin-converting-enzyme inhibitors, assault

⑦**T46.4X4** Poisoning by angiotensin-converting-enzyme inhibitors, undetermined

⑦**T46.4X5** Adverse effect of angiotensin-converting-enzyme inhibitors

⑦**T46.4X6** Underdosing of angiotensin-converting-enzyme inhibitors

T46.5 Poisoning by, adverse effect of and underdosing of other antihypertensive drugs

Excludes 2: poisoning by, adverse effect of and underdosing of beta-adrenoreceptor antagonists (T44.7)

poisoning by, adverse effect of and underdosing of calcium-channel blockers (T46.1)

poisoning by, adverse effect of and underdosing of diuretics (T50.0-T50.2)

T46.5X Poisoning by, adverse effect of and underdosing of other antihypertensive drugs

⑦**T46.5X1** Poisoning by other antihypertensive drugs, accidental (unintentional)

Poisoning by other antihypertensive drugs NOS

● New code   ▲ Revised code   ⑦ 7ᵗʰ digit required   ⊗ Placeholder required

⑦T46.5X2 Poisoning by other antihypertensive drugs, intentional self-harm

⑦T46.5X3 Poisoning by other antihypertensive drugs, assault

⑦T46.5X4 Poisoning by other antihypertensive drugs, undetermined

⑦T46.5X5 Adverse effect of other antihypertensive drugs

⑦T46.5X6 Underdosing of other antihypertensive drugs

T46.6 Poisoning by, adverse effect of and underdosing of antihyperlipidemic and antiarteriosclerotic drugs

    T46.6X Poisoning by, adverse effect of and underdosing of antihyperlipidemic and antiarteriosclerotic drugs

        ⑦T46.6X1 Poisoning by antihyperlipidemic and antiarteriosclerotic drugs, accidental (unintentional)

            Poisoning by antihyperlipidemic and antiarteriosclerotic drugs NOS

        ⑦T46.6X2 Poisoning by antihyperlipidemic and antiarteriosclerotic drugs, intentional self-harm

        ⑦T46.6X3 Poisoning by antihyperlipidemic and antiarteriosclerotic drugs, assault

        ⑦T46.6X4 Poisoning by antihyperlipidemic and antiarteriosclerotic drugs, undetermined

        ⑦T46.6X5 Adverse effect of antihyperlipidemic and antiarteriosclerotic drugs

        ⑦T46.6X6 Underdosing of antihyperlipidemic and antiarteriosclerotic drugs

T46.7 Poisoning by, adverse effect of and underdosing of peripheral vasodilators

Poisoning by, adverse effect of and underdosing of nicotinic acid (derivatives)

Excludes 1: poisoning by, adverse effect of and underdosing of papaverine (T44.3)

    T46.7X Poisoning by, adverse effect of and underdosing of peripheral vasodilators

        ⑦T46.7X1 Poisoning by peripheral vasodilators, accidental (unintentional)

            Poisoning by peripheral vasodilators NOS

        ⑦T46.7X2 Poisoning by peripheral vasodilators, intentional self-harm

        ⑦T46.7X3 Poisoning by peripheral vasodilators, assault

        ⑦T46.7X4 Poisoning by peripheral vasodilators, undetermined

        ⑦T46.7X5 Adverse effect of peripheral vasodilators

        ⑦T46.7X6 Underdosing of peripheral vasodilators

T46.8 Poisoning by, adverse effect of and underdosing of antivaricose drugs, including sclerosing agents

    T46.8X Poisoning by, adverse effect of and underdosing of antivaricose drugs, including sclerosing agents

        ⑦T46.8X1 Poisoning by antivaricose drugs, including sclerosing agents, accidental (unintentional)

            Poisoning by antivaricose drugs, including sclerosing agents NOS

        ⑦T46.8X2 Poisoning by antivaricose drugs, including sclerosing agents, intentional self-harm

        ⑦T46.8X3 Poisoning by antivaricose drugs, including sclerosing agents, assault

        ⑦T46.8X4 Poisoning by antivaricose drugs, including sclerosing agents, undetermined

        ⑦T46.8X5 Adverse effect of antivaricose drugs, including sclerosing agents

        ⑦T46.8X6 Underdosing of antivaricose drugs, including sclerosing agents

T46.9 Poisoning by, adverse effect of and underdosing of other and unspecified agents primarily affecting the cardiovascular system

    T46.90 Poisoning by, adverse effect of and underdosing of unspecified agents primarily affecting the cardiovascular system

        ⑦T46.901 Poisoning by unspecified agents primarily affecting the cardiovascular system, accidental (unintentional)

        ⑦T46.902 Poisoning by unspecified agents primarily affecting the cardiovascular system, intentional self-harm

        ⑦T46.903 Poisoning by unspecified agents primarily affecting the cardiovascular system, assault

        ⑦T46.904 Poisoning by unspecified agents primarily affecting the cardiovascular system, undetermined

        ⑦T46.905 Adverse effect of unspecified agents primarily affecting the cardiovascular system

        ⑦T46.906 Underdosing of unspecified agents primarily affecting the cardiovascular system

    T46.99 Poisoning by, adverse effect of and underdosing of other agents primarily affecting the cardiovascular system

        ⑦T46.991 Poisoning by other agents primarily affecting the cardiovascular system, accidental (unintentional)

        ⑦T46.992 Poisoning by other agents primarily affecting the cardiovascular system, intentional self-harm

        ⑦T46.993 Poisoning by other agents primarily affecting the cardiovascular system, assault

        ⑦T46.994 Poisoning by other agents primarily affecting the cardiovascular system, undetermined

        ⑦T46.995 Adverse effect of other agents primarily affecting the cardiovascular system

---

⑦**T46.996**   Underdosing of other agents primarily affecting the cardiovascular system

T47 Poisoning by, adverse effect of and underdosing of agents primarily affecting the gastrointestinal system

The appropriate 7th character is to be added to each code from category T47

A - initial encounter

D - subsequent encounter

S - sequela

T47.0   Poisoning by, adverse effect of and underdosing of histamine H2-receptor blockers

T47.0X   Poisoning by, adverse effect of and underdosing of histamine H2-receptor blockers

⑦**T47.0X1**   Poisoning by histamine H2-receptor blockers, accidental (unintentional)

Poisoning by histamine H2-receptor blockers NOS

⑦**T47.0X2**   Poisoning by histamine H2-receptor blockers, intentional self-harm

⑦**T47.0X3**   Poisoning by histamine H2-receptor blockers, assault

⑦**T47.0X4**   Poisoning by histamine H2-receptor blockers, undetermined

⑦**T47.0X5**   Adverse effect of histamine H2-receptor blockers

⑦**T47.0X6**   Underdosing of histamine H2-receptor blockers

T47.1   Poisoning by, adverse effect of and underdosing of other antacids and anti-gastric-secretion drugs

T47.1X   Poisoning by, adverse effect of and underdosing of other antacids and anti-gastric-secretion drugs

⑦**T47.1X1**   Poisoning by other antacids and anti-gastric-secretion drugs, accidental (unintentional)

Poisoning by other antacids and anti-gastric-secretion drugs NOS

⑦**T47.1X2**   Poisoning by other antacids and anti-gastric-secretion drugs, intentional self-harm

⑦**T47.1X3**   Poisoning by other antacids and anti-gastric-secretion drugs, assault

⑦**T47.1X4**   Poisoning by other antacids and anti-gastric-secretion drugs, undetermined

⑦**T47.1X5**   Adverse effect of other antacids and anti-gastric-secretion drugs

⑦**T47.1X6**   Underdosing of other antacids and anti-gastric-secretion drugs

T47.2   Poisoning by, adverse effect of and underdosing of stimulant laxatives

T47.2X   Poisoning by, adverse effect of and underdosing of stimulant laxatives

⑦**T47.2X1**   Poisoning by stimulant laxatives, accidental (unintentional)

Poisoning by stimulant laxatives NOS

⑦**T47.2X2**   Poisoning by stimulant laxatives, intentional self-harm

⑦**T47.2X3**   Poisoning by stimulant laxatives, assault

⑦**T47.2X4**   Poisoning by stimulant laxatives, undetermined

⑦**T47.2X5**   Adverse effect of stimulant laxatives

⑦**T47.2X6**   Underdosing of stimulant laxatives

T47.3   Poisoning by, adverse effect of and underdosing of saline and osmotic laxatives

T47.3X   Poisoning by and adverse effect of saline and osmotic laxatives

⑦**T47.3X1**   Poisoning by saline and osmotic laxatives, accidental (unintentional)

Poisoning by saline and osmotic laxatives NOS

⑦**T47.3X2**   Poisoning by saline and osmotic laxatives, intentional self-harm

⑦**T47.3X3**   Poisoning by saline and osmotic laxatives, assault

⑦**T47.3X4**   Poisoning by saline and osmotic laxatives, undetermined

⑦**T47.3X5**   Adverse effect of saline and osmotic laxatives

⑦**T47.3X6**   Underdosing of saline and osmotic laxatives

T47.4   Poisoning by, adverse effect of and underdosing of other laxatives

T47.4X   Poisoning by, adverse effect of and underdosing of other laxatives

⑦**T47.4X1**   Poisoning by other laxatives, accidental (unintentional)

Poisoning by other laxatives NOS

⑦**T47.4X2**   Poisoning by other laxatives, intentional self-harm

⑦**T47.4X3**   Poisoning by other laxatives, assault

⑦**T47.4X4**   Poisoning by other laxatives, undetermined

⑦**T47.4X5**   Adverse effect of other laxatives

⑦**T47.4X6**   Underdosing of other laxatives

T47.5   Poisoning by, adverse effect of and underdosing of digestants

T47.5X   Poisoning by, adverse effect of and underdosing of digestants

⑦**T47.5X1**   Poisoning by digestants, accidental (unintentional)

Poisoning by digestants NOS

⑦**T47.5X2**   Poisoning by digestants, intentional self-harm

⑦**T47.5X3**   Poisoning by digestants, assault

⑦**T47.5X4**   Poisoning by digestants, undetermined

⑦**T47.5X5**   Adverse effect of digestants

⑦**T47.5X6**   Underdosing of digestants

T47.6   Poisoning by, adverse effect of and underdosing of antidiarrheal drugs

Excludes 2: poisoning by, adverse effect of and underdosing of systemic antibiotics and other anti-infectives (T36-T37)

T47.6X   Poisoning by, adverse effect of and underdosing of antidiarrheal drugs

⑦**T47.6X1** Poisoning by antidiarrheal drugs, accidental (unintentional)

Poisoning by antidiarrheal drugs NOS

⑦**T47.6X2** Poisoning by antidiarrheal drugs, intentional self-harm

⑦**T47.6X3** Poisoning by antidiarrheal drugs, assault

⑦**T47.6X4** Poisoning by antidiarrheal drugs, undetermined

⑦**T47.6X5** Adverse effect of antidiarrheal drugs

⑦**T47.6X6** Underdosing of antidiarrheal drugs

T47.7 Poisoning by, adverse effect of and underdosing of emetics

T47.7X Poisoning by, adverse effect of and underdosing of emetics

⑦**T47.7X1** Poisoning by emetics, accidental (unintentional)

Poisoning by emetics NOS

⑦**T47.7X2** Poisoning by emetics, intentional self-harm

⑦**T47.7X3** Poisoning by emetics, assault

⑦**T47.7X4** Poisoning by emetics, undetermined

⑦**T47.7X5** Adverse effect of emetics

⑦**T47.7X6** Underdosing of emetics

T47.8 Poisoning by, adverse effect of and underdosing of other agents primarily affecting gastrointestinal system

T47.8X Poisoning by, adverse effect of and underdosing of other agents primarily affecting gastrointestinal system

⑦**T47.8X1** Poisoning by other agents primarily affecting gastrointestinal system, accidental (unintentional)

Poisoning by other agents primarily affecting gastrointestinal system NOS

⑦**T47.8X2** Poisoning by other agents primarily affecting gastrointestinal system, intentional self-harm

⑦**T47.8X3** Poisoning by other agents primarily affecting gastrointestinal system, assault

⑦**T47.8X4** Poisoning by other agents primarily affecting gastrointestinal system, undetermined

⑦**T47.8X5** Adverse effect of other agents primarily affecting gastrointestinal system

⑦**T47.8X6** Underdosing of other agents primarily affecting gastrointestinal system

T47.9 Poisoning by, adverse effect of and underdosing of unspecified agents primarily affecting the gastrointestinal system

⊗⑦**T47.91** Poisoning by unspecified agents primarily affecting the gastrointestinal system, accidental (unintentional)

Poisoning by agents primarily affecting the gastrointestinal system NOS

⊗⑦**T47.92** Poisoning by unspecified agents primarily affecting the gastrointestinal system, intentional self-harm

⊗⑦**T47.93** Poisoning by unspecified agents primarily affecting the gastrointestinal system, assault

⊗⑦**T47.94** Poisoning by unspecified agents primarily affecting the gastrointestinal system, undetermined

⊗⑦**T47.95** Adverse effect of unspecified agents primarily affecting the gastrointestinal system

⊗⑦**T47.96** Underdosing of unspecified agents primarily affecting the gastrointestinal system

T48 Poisoning by, adverse effect of and underdosing of agents primarily acting on smooth and skeletal muscles and the respiratory system

The appropriate 7th character is to be added to each code from category T48

A - initial encounter

D - subsequent encounter

S - sequela

T48.0 Poisoning by, adverse effect of and underdosing of oxytocic drugs

Excludes 1: poisoning by, adverse effect of and underdosing of estrogens, progestogens and antagonists (T38.4-T38.6)

T48.0X Poisoning by, adverse effect of and underdosing of oxytocic drugs

⑦**T48.0X1** Poisoning by oxytocic drugs, accidental (unintentional)

Poisoning by oxytocic drugs NOS

⑦**T48.0X2** Poisoning by oxytocic drugs, intentional self-harm

⑦**T48.0X3** Poisoning by oxytocic drugs, assault

⑦**T48.0X4** Poisoning by oxytocic drugs, undetermined

⑦**T48.0X5** Adverse effect of oxytocic drugs

⑦**T48.0X6** Underdosing of oxytocic drugs

T48.1 Poisoning by, adverse effect of and underdosing of skeletal muscle relaxants [neuromuscular blocking agents]

T48.1X Poisoning by, adverse effect of and underdosing of skeletal muscle relaxants [neuromuscular blocking agents]

⑦**T48.1X1** Poisoning by skeletal muscle relaxants [neuromuscular blocking agents], accidental (unintentional)

Poisoning by skeletal muscle relaxants [neuromuscular blocking agents] NOS

⑦**T48.1X2** Poisoning by skeletal muscle relaxants [neuromuscular blocking agents], intentional self-harm

⑦**T48.1X3** Poisoning by skeletal muscle relaxants [neuromuscular blocking agents], assault

⑦**T48.1X4** Poisoning by skeletal muscle relaxants [neuromuscular blocking agents], undetermined

⑦**T48.1X5** Adverse effect of skeletal muscle relaxants [neuromuscular blocking agents]

⑦**T48.1X6**   Underdosing of skeletal muscle relaxants [neuromuscular blocking agents]

T48.2   Poisoning by, adverse effect of and underdosing of other and unspecified drugs acting on muscles

    T48.20   Poisoning by, adverse effect of and underdosing of unspecified drugs acting on muscles

        ⑦**T48.201**   Poisoning by unspecified drugs acting on muscles, accidental (unintentional)

                        Poisoning by unspecified drugs acting on muscles NOS

        ⑦**T48.202**   Poisoning by unspecified drugs acting on muscles, intentional self-harm

        ⑦**T48.203**   Poisoning by unspecified drugs acting on muscles, assault

        ⑦**T48.204**   Poisoning by unspecified drugs acting on muscles, undetermined

        ⑦**T48.205**   Adverse effect of unspecified drugs acting on muscles

        ⑦**T48.206**   Underdosing of unspecified drugs acting on muscles

    T48.29   Poisoning by, adverse effect of and underdosing of other drugs acting on muscles

        ⑦**T48.291**   Poisoning by other drugs acting on muscles, accidental (unintentional)

                        Poisoning by other drugs acting on muscles NOS

        ⑦**T48.292**   Poisoning by other drugs acting on muscles, intentional self-harm

        ⑦**T48.293**   Poisoning by other drugs acting on muscles, assault

        ⑦**T48.294**   Poisoning by other drugs acting on muscles, undetermined

        ⑦**T48.295**   Adverse effect of other drugs acting on muscles

        ⑦**T48.296**   Underdosing of other drugs acting on muscles

T48.3   Poisoning by, adverse effect of and underdosing of antitussives

    T48.3X   Poisoning by, adverse effect of and underdosing of antitussives

        ⑦**T48.3X1**   Poisoning by antitussives, accidental (unintentional)

                        Poisoning by antitussives NOS

        ⑦**T48.3X2**   Poisoning by antitussives, intentional self-harm

        ⑦**T48.3X3**   Poisoning by antitussives, assault

        ⑦**T48.3X4**   Poisoning by antitussives, undetermined

        ⑦**T48.3X5**   Adverse effect of antitussives

        ⑦**T48.3X6**   Underdosing of antitussives

T48.4   Poisoning by, adverse effect of and underdosing of expectorants

    T48.4X   Poisoning by, adverse effect of and underdosing of expectorants

        ⑦**T48.4X1**   Poisoning by expectorants, accidental (unintentional)

                        Poisoning by expectorants NOS

        ⑦**T48.4X2**   Poisoning by expectorants, intentional self-harm

        ⑦**T48.4X3**   Poisoning by expectorants, assault

        ⑦**T48.4X4**   Poisoning by expectorants, undetermined

        ⑦**T48.4X5**   Adverse effect of expectorants

        ⑦**T48.4X6**   Underdosing of expectorants

T48.5   Poisoning by, adverse effect of and underdosing of other anti-common-cold drugs

    Poisoning by, adverse effect of and underdosing of decongestants

    Excludes 2: poisoning by, adverse effect of and underdosing of antipyretics, NEC (T39.9-)

                  poisoning by, adverse effect of and underdosing of non-steroidal antiinflammatory drugs (T39.3-)

                  poisoning by, adverse effect of and underdosing of salicylates (T39.0-)

    T48.5X   Poisoning by, adverse effect of and underdosing of other anti-common-cold drugs

        ⑦**T48.5X1**   Poisoning by other anti-common-cold drugs, accidental (unintentional)

                        Poisoning by other anti-common-cold drugs NOS

        ⑦**T48.5X2**   Poisoning by other anti-common-cold drugs, intentional self-harm

        ⑦**T48.5X3**   Poisoning by other anti-common-cold drugs, assault

        ⑦**T48.5X4**   Poisoning by other anti-common-cold drugs, undetermined

        ⑦**T48.5X5**   Adverse effect of other anti-common-cold drugs

        ⑦**T48.5X6**   Underdosing of other anti-common-cold drugs

T48.6   Poisoning by, adverse effect of and underdosing of antiasthmatics, not elsewhere classified

    Poisoning by, adverse effect of and underdosing of beta-adrenoreceptor agonists used in asthma therapy

    Excludes 1: poisoning by, adverse effect of and underdosing of beta-adrenoreceptor agonists not used in asthma therapy (T44.5)

                  poisoning by, adverse effect of and underdosing of anterior pituitary [adenohypophyseal] hormones (T38.8)

    T48.6X   Poisoning by, adverse effect of and underdosing of antiasthmatics

        ⑦**T48.6X1**   Poisoning by antiasthmatics, accidental (unintentional)

                        Poisoning by antiasthmatics NOS

        ⑦**T48.6X2**   Poisoning by antiasthmatics, intentional self-harm

        ⑦**T48.6X3**   Poisoning by antiasthmatics, assault

        ⑦**T48.6X4**   Poisoning by antiasthmatics, undetermined

        ⑦**T48.6X5**   Adverse effect of antiasthmatics

        ⑦**T48.6X6**   Underdosing of antiasthmatics

T48.9 Poisoning by, adverse effect of and underdosing of other and unspecified agents primarily acting on the respiratory system

    T48.90 Poisoning by, adverse effect of and underdosing of unspecified agents primarily acting on the respiratory system

        ⑦ T48.901 Poisoning by unspecified agents primarily acting on the respiratory system, accidental (unintentional)

        ⑦ T48.902 Poisoning by unspecified agents primarily acting on the respiratory system, intentional self-harm

        ⑦ T48.903 Poisoning by unspecified agents primarily acting on the respiratory system, assault

        ⑦ T48.904 Poisoning by unspecified agents primarily acting on the respiratory system, undetermined

        ⑦ T48.905 Adverse effect of unspecified agents primarily acting on the respiratory system

        ⑦ T48.906 Underdosing of unspecified agents primarily acting on the respiratory system

    T48.99 Poisoning by, adverse effect of and underdosing of other agents primarily acting on the respiratory system

        ⑦ T48.991 Poisoning by other agents primarily acting on the respiratory system, accidental (unintentional)

        ⑦ T48.992 Poisoning by other agents primarily acting on the respiratory system, intentional self-harm

        ⑦ T48.993 Poisoning by other agents primarily acting on the respiratory system, assault

        ⑦ T48.994 Poisoning by other agents primarily acting on the respiratory system, undetermined

        ⑦ T48.995 Adverse effect of other agents primarily acting on the respiratory system

        ⑦ T48.996 Underdosing of other agents primarily acting on the respiratory system

T49 Poisoning by, adverse effect of and underdosing of topical agents primarily affecting skin and mucous membrane and by ophthalmological, otorhinolaryngological and dental drugs

Includes: poisoning by, adverse effect of and underdosing of glucocorticoids, topically used

The appropriate 7th character is to be added to each code from category T49

A - initial encounter

D - subsequent encounter

S - sequela

T49.0 Poisoning by, adverse effect of and underdosing of local antifungal, anti-infective and anti-inflammatory drugs

    T49.0X Poisoning by, adverse effect of and underdosing of local antifungal, anti-infective and anti-inflammatory drugs

        ⑦ T49.0X1 Poisoning by local antifungal, anti-infective and anti-inflammatory drugs, accidental (unintentional)

            Poisoning by local antifungal, anti-infective and anti-inflammatory drugs NOS

        ⑦ T49.0X2 Poisoning by local antifungal, anti-infective and anti-inflammatory drugs, intentional self-harm

        ⑦ T49.0X3 Poisoning by local antifungal, anti-infective and anti-inflammatory drugs, assault

        ⑦ T49.0X4 Poisoning by local antifungal, anti-infective and anti-inflammatory drugs, undetermined

        ⑦ T49.0X5 Adverse effect of local antifungal, anti-infective and anti-inflammatory drugs

        ⑦ T49.0X6 Underdosing of local antifungal, anti-infective and anti-inflammatory drugs

T49.1 Poisoning by, adverse effect of and underdosing of antipruritics

    T49.1X Poisoning by, adverse effect of and underdosing of antipruritics

        ⑦ T49.1X1 Poisoning by antipruritics, accidental (unintentional)

            Poisoning by antipruritics NOS

        ⑦ T49.1X2 Poisoning by antipruritics, intentional self-harm

        ⑦ T49.1X3 Poisoning by antipruritics, assault

        ⑦ T49.1X4 Poisoning by antipruritics, undetermined

        ⑦ T49.1X5 Adverse effect of antipruritics

        ⑦ T49.1X6 Underdosing of antipruritics

T49.2 Poisoning by, adverse effect of and underdosing of local astringents and local detergents

    T49.2X Poisoning by, adverse effect of and underdosing of local astringents and local detergents

        ⑦ T49.2X1 Poisoning by local astringents and local detergents, accidental (unintentional)

            Poisoning by local astringents and local detergents NOS

        ⑦ T49.2X2 Poisoning by local astringents and local detergents, intentional self-harm

        ⑦ T49.2X3 Poisoning by local astringents and local detergents, assault

        ⑦ T49.2X4 Poisoning by local astringents and local detergents, undetermined

        ⑦ T49.2X5 Adverse effect of local astringents and local detergents

        ⑦ T49.2X6 Underdosing of local astringents and local detergents

T49.3 Poisoning by, adverse effect of and underdosing of emollients, demulcents and protectants

    T49.3X Poisoning by, adverse effect of and underdosing of emollients, demulcents and protectants

⑦**T49.3X1** Poisoning by emollients, demulcents and protectants, accidental (unintentional)

Poisoning by emollients, demulcents and protectants NOS

⑦**T49.3X2** Poisoning by emollients, demulcents and protectants, intentional self-harm

⑦**T49.3X3** Poisoning by emollients, demulcents and protectants, assault

⑦**T49.3X4** Poisoning by emollients, demulcents and protectants, undetermined

⑦**T49.3X5** Adverse effect of emollients, demulcents and protectants

⑦**T49.3X6** Underdosing of emollients, demulcents and protectants

T49.4 Poisoning by, adverse effect of and underdosing of keratolytics, keratoplastics, and other hair treatment drugs and preparations

T49.4X Poisoning by, adverse effect of and underdosing of keratolytics, keratoplastics, and other hair treatment drugs and preparations

⑦**T49.4X1** Poisoning by keratolytics, keratoplastics, and other hair treatment drugs and preparations, accidental (unintentional)

Poisoning by keratolytics, keratoplastics, and other hair treatment drugs and preparations NOS

⑦**T49.4X2** Poisoning by keratolytics, keratoplastics, and other hair treatment drugs and preparations, intentional self-harm

⑦**T49.4X3** Poisoning by keratolytics, keratoplastics, and other hair treatment drugs and preparations, assault

⑦**T49.4X4** Poisoning by keratolytics, keratoplastics, and other hair treatment drugs and preparations, undetermined

⑦**T49.4X5** Adverse effect of keratolytics, keratoplastics, and other hair treatment drugs and preparations

⑦**T49.4X6** Underdosing of keratolytics, keratoplastics, and other hair treatment drugs and preparations

T49.5 Poisoning by, adverse effect of and underdosing of ophthalmological drugs and preparations

T49.5X Poisoning by, adverse effect of and underdosing of ophthalmological drugs and preparations

⑦**T49.5X1** Poisoning by ophthalmological drugs and preparations, accidental (unintentional)

Poisoning by ophthalmological drugs and preparations NOS

⑦**T49.5X2** Poisoning by ophthalmological drugs and preparations, intentional self-harm

⑦**T49.5X3** Poisoning by ophthalmological drugs and preparations, assault

⑦**T49.5X4** Poisoning by ophthalmological drugs and preparations, undetermined

⑦**T49.5X5** Adverse effect of ophthalmological drugs and preparations

⑦**T49.5X6** Underdosing of ophthalmological drugs and preparations

T49.6 Poisoning by, adverse effect of and underdosing of otorhinolaryngological drugs and preparations

T49.6X Poisoning by, adverse effect of and underdosing of otorhinolaryngological drugs and preparations

⑦**T49.6X1** Poisoning by otorhinolaryngological drugs and preparations, accidental (unintentional)

Poisoning by otorhinolaryngological drugs and preparations NOS

⑦**T49.6X2** Poisoning by otorhinolaryngological drugs and preparations, intentional self-harm

⑦**T49.6X3** Poisoning by otorhinolaryngological drugs and preparations, assault

⑦**T49.6X4** Poisoning by otorhinolaryngological drugs and preparations, undetermined

⑦**T49.6X5** Adverse effect of otorhinolaryngological drugs and preparations

⑦**T49.6X6** Underdosing of otorhinolaryngological drugs and preparations

T49.7 Poisoning by, adverse effect of and underdosing of dental drugs, topically applied

T49.7X Poisoning by, adverse effect of and underdosing of dental drugs, topically applied

⑦**T49.7X1** Poisoning by dental drugs, topically applied, accidental (unintentional)

Poisoning by dental drugs, topically applied NOS

⑦**T49.7X2** Poisoning by dental drugs, topically applied, intentional self-harm

⑦**T49.7X3** Poisoning by dental drugs, topically applied, assault

⑦**T49.7X4** Poisoning by dental drugs, topically applied, undetermined

⑦**T49.7X5** Adverse effect of dental drugs, topically applied

⑦**T49.7X6** Underdosing of dental drugs, topically applied

T49.8 Poisoning by, adverse effect of and underdosing of other topical agents

Poisoning by, adverse effect of and underdosing of spermicides

T49.8X Poisoning by, adverse effect of and underdosing of other topical agents

⑦**T49.8X1** Poisoning by other topical agents, accidental (unintentional)

Poisoning by other topical agents NOS

⑦ **T49.8X2** Poisoning by other topical agents, intentional self-harm

⑦ **T49.8X3** Poisoning by other topical agents, assault

⑦ **T49.8X4** Poisoning by other topical agents, undetermined

⑦ **T49.8X5** Adverse effect of other topical agents

⑦ **T49.8X6** Underdosing of other topical agents

T49.9 Poisoning by, adverse effect of and underdosing of unspecified topical agent

⊗⑦ **T49.91** Poisoning by unspecified topical agent, accidental (unintentional)

⊗⑦ **T49.92** Poisoning by unspecified topical agent, intentional self-harm

⊗⑦ **T49.93** Poisoning by unspecified topical agent, assault

⊗⑦ **T49.94** Poisoning by unspecified topical agent, undetermined

⊗⑦ **T49.95** Adverse effect of unspecified topical agent

⊗⑦ **T49.96** Underdosing of unspecified topical agent

T50 Poisoning by, adverse effect of and underdosing of diuretics and other and unspecified drugs, medicaments and biological substances

The appropriate 7th character is to be added to each code from category T50

A - initial encounter

D - subsequent encounter

S - sequela

T50.0 Poisoning by, adverse effect of and underdosing of mineralocorticoids and their antagonists

T50.0X Poisoning by, adverse effect of and underdosing of mineralocorticoids and their antagonists

⑦ **T50.0X1** Poisoning by mineralocorticoids and their antagonists, accidental (unintentional)

Poisoning by mineralocorticoids and their antagonists NOS

⑦ **T50.0X2** Poisoning by mineralocorticoids and their antagonists, intentional self-harm

⑦ **T50.0X3** Poisoning by mineralocorticoids and their antagonists, assault

⑦ **T50.0X4** Poisoning by mineralocorticoids and their antagonists, undetermined

⑦ **T50.0X5** Adverse effect of mineralocorticoids and their antagonists

⑦ **T50.0X6** Underdosing of mineralocorticoids and their antagonists

T50.1 Poisoning by, adverse effect of and underdosing of loop [high-ceiling] diuretics

T50.1X Poisoning by, adverse effect of and underdosing of loop [high-ceiling] diuretics

⑦ **T50.1X1** Poisoning by loop [high-ceiling] diuretics, accidental (unintentional)

Poisoning by loop [high-ceiling] diuretics NOS

⑦ **T50.1X2** Poisoning by loop [high-ceiling] diuretics, intentional self-harm

⑦ **T50.1X3** Poisoning by loop [high-ceiling] diuretics, assault

⑦ **T50.1X4** Poisoning by loop [high-ceiling] diuretics, undetermined

⑦ **T50.1X5** Adverse effect of loop [high-ceiling] diuretics

⑦ **T50.1X6** Underdosing of loop [high-ceiling] diuretics

T50.2 Poisoning by, adverse effect of and underdosing of carbonic-anhydrase inhibitors, benzothiadiazides and other diuretics

Poisoning by, adverse effect of and underdosing of acetazolamide

⑦ **T50.2X** Poisoning by, adverse effect of and underdosing of carbonic-anhydrase inhibitors, benzothiadiazides and other diuretics

⑦ **T50.2X1** Poisoning by carbonic-anhydrase inhibitors, benzothiadiazides and other diuretics, accidental (unintentional)

Poisoning by carbonic-anhydrase inhibitors, benzothiadiazides and other diuretics NOS

⑦ **T50.2X2** Poisoning by carbonic-anhydrase inhibitors, benzothiadiazides and other diuretics, intentional self-harm

⑦ **T50.2X3** Poisoning by carbonic-anhydrase inhibitors, benzothiadiazides and other diuretics, assault

⑦ **T50.2X4** Poisoning by carbonic-anhydrase inhibitors, benzothiadiazides and other diuretics, undetermined

⑦ **T50.2X5** Adverse effect of carbonic-anhydrase inhibitors, benzothiadiazides and other diuretics

⑦ **T50.2X6** Underdosing of carbonic-anhydrase inhibitors, benzothiadiazides and other diuretics

T50.3 Poisoning by, adverse effect of and underdosing of electrolytic, caloric and water-balance agents

Poisoning by, adverse effect of and underdosing of oral rehydration salts

T50.3X Poisoning by, adverse effect of and underdosing of electrolytic, caloric and water-balance agents

⑦ **T50.3X1** Poisoning by electrolytic, caloric and water-balance agents, accidental (unintentional)

Poisoning by electrolytic, caloric and water-balance agents NOS

⑦ **T50.3X2** Poisoning by electrolytic, caloric and water-balance agents, intentional self-harm

⑦ **T50.3X3** Poisoning by electrolytic, caloric and water-balance agents, assault

⑦ **T50.3X4** Poisoning by electrolytic, caloric and water-balance agents, undetermined

⑦ **T50.3X5** Adverse effect of electrolytic, caloric and water-balance agents

⑦ **T50.3X6** Underdosing of electrolytic, caloric and water-balance agents

T50.4 Poisoning by, adverse effect of and underdosing of drugs affecting uric acid metabolism

    T50.4X Poisoning by, adverse effect of and underdosing of drugs affecting uric acid metabolism

        ⑦**T50.4X1** Poisoning by drugs affecting uric acid metabolism, accidental (unintentional)

                Poisoning by drugs affecting uric acid metabolism NOS

        ⑦**T50.4X2** Poisoning by drugs affecting uric acid metabolism, intentional self-harm

        ⑦**T50.4X3** Poisoning by drugs affecting uric acid metabolism, assault

        ⑦**T50.4X4** Poisoning by drugs affecting uric acid metabolism, undetermined

        ⑦**T50.4X5** Adverse effect of drugs affecting uric acid metabolism

        ⑦**T50.4X6** Underdosing of drugs affecting uric acid metabolism

T50.5 Poisoning by, adverse effect of and underdosing of appetite depressants

    T50.5X Poisoning by, adverse effect of and underdosing of appetite depressants

        ⑦**T50.5X1** Poisoning by appetite depressants, accidental (unintentional)

                Poisoning by appetite depressants NOS

        ⑦**T50.5X2** Poisoning by appetite depressants, intentional self-harm

        ⑦**T50.5X3** Poisoning by appetite depressants, assault

        ⑦**T50.5X4** Poisoning by appetite depressants, undetermined

        ⑦**T50.5X5** Adverse effect of appetite depressants

        ⑦**T50.5X6** Underdosing of appetite depressants

T50.6 Poisoning by, adverse effect of and underdosing of antidotes and chelating agents

    Poisoning by, adverse effect of and underdosing of alcohol deterrents

    T50.6X Poisoning by, adverse effect of and underdosing of antidotes and chelating agents

        ⑦**T50.6X1** Poisoning by antidotes and chelating agents, accidental (unintentional)

                Poisoning by antidotes and chelating agents NOS

        ⑦**T50.6X2** Poisoning by antidotes and chelating agents, intentional self-harm

        ⑦**T50.6X3** Poisoning by antidotes and chelating agents, assault

        ⑦**T50.6X4** Poisoning by antidotes and chelating agents, undetermined

        ⑦**T50.6X5** Adverse effect of antidotes and chelating agents

        ⑦**T50.6X6** Underdosing of antidotes and chelating agents

T50.7 Poisoning by, adverse effect of and underdosing of analeptics and opioid receptor antagonists

T50.7X Poisoning by, adverse effect of and underdosing of analeptics and opioid receptor antagonists

        ⑦**T50.7X1** Poisoning by analeptics and opioid receptor antagonists, accidental (unintentional)

                Poisoning by analeptics and opioid receptor antagonists NOS

        ⑦**T50.7X2** Poisoning by analeptics and opioid receptor antagonists, intentional self-harm

        ⑦**T50.7X3** Poisoning by analeptics and opioid receptor antagonists, assault

        ⑦**T50.7X4** Poisoning by analeptics and opioid receptor antagonists, undetermined

        ⑦**T50.7X5** Adverse effect of analeptics and opioid receptor antagonists

        ⑦**T50.7X6** Underdosing of analeptics and opioid receptor antagonists

T50.8 Poisoning by, adverse effect of and underdosing of diagnostic agents

    T50.8X Poisoning by, adverse effect of and underdosing of diagnostic agents

        ⑦**T50.8X1** Poisoning by diagnostic agents, accidental (unintentional)

                Poisoning by diagnostic agents NOS

        ⑦**T50.8X2** Poisoning by diagnostic agents, intentional self-harm

        ⑦**T50.8X3** Poisoning by diagnostic agents, assault

        ⑦**T50.8X4** Poisoning by diagnostic agents, undetermined

        ⑦**T50.8X5** Adverse effect of diagnostic agents

        ⑦**T50.8X6** Underdosing of diagnostic agents

T50.A Poisoning by, adverse effect of and underdosing of bacterial vaccines

    T50.A1 Poisoning by, adverse effect of and underdosing of pertussis vaccine, including combinations with a pertussis component

        ⑦**T50.A11** Poisoning by pertussis vaccine, including combinations with a pertussis component, accidental (unintentional)

        ⑦**T50.A12** Poisoning by pertussis vaccine, including combinations with a pertussis component, intentional self-harm

        ⑦**T50.A13** Poisoning by pertussis vaccine, including combinations with a pertussis component, assault

        ⑦**T50.A14** Poisoning by pertussis vaccine, including combinations with a pertussis component, undetermined

        ⑦**T50.A15** Adverse effect of pertussis vaccine, including combinations with a pertussis component

        ⑦**T50.A16** Underdosing of pertussis vaccine, including combinations with a pertussis component

● New code   ▲ Revised code   ⑦ 7ᵗʰ digit required   ⊗ Placeholder required

T50.A2 Poisoning by, adverse effect of and underdosing of mixed bacterial vaccines without a pertussis component

⑦**T50.A21** Poisoning by mixed bacterial vaccines without a pertussis component, accidental (unintentional)

⑦**T50.A22** Poisoning by mixed bacterial vaccines without a pertussis component, intentional self-harm

⑦**T50.A23** Poisoning by mixed bacterial vaccines without a pertussis component, assault

⑦**T50.A24** Poisoning by mixed bacterial vaccines without a pertussis component, undetermined

⑦**T50.A25** Adverse effect of mixed bacterial vaccines without a pertussis component

⑦**T50.A26** Underdosing of mixed bacterial vaccines without a pertussis component

T50.A9 Poisoning by, adverse effect of and underdosing of other bacterial vaccines

⑦**T50.A91** Poisoning by other bacterial vaccines, accidental (unintentional)

⑦**T50.A92** Poisoning by other bacterial vaccines, intentional self-harm

⑦**T50.A93** Poisoning by other bacterial vaccines, assault

⑦**T50.A94** Poisoning by other bacterial vaccines, undetermined

⑦**T50.A95** Adverse effect of other bacterial vaccines

⑦**T50.A96** Underdosing of other bacterial vaccines

T50.B Poisoning by, adverse effect of and underdosing of viral vaccines

T50.B1 Poisoning by, adverse effect of and underdosing of smallpox vaccines

⑦**T50.B11** Poisoning by smallpox vaccines, accidental (unintentional)

⑦**T50.B12** Poisoning by smallpox vaccines, intentional self-harm

⑦**T50.B13** Poisoning by smallpox vaccines, assault

⑦**T50.B14** Poisoning by smallpox vaccines, undetermined

⑦**T50.B15** Adverse effect of smallpox vaccines

⑦**T50.B16** Underdosing of smallpox vaccines

T50.B9 Poisoning by, adverse effect of and underdosing of other viral vaccines

⑦**T50.B91** Poisoning by other viral vaccines, accidental (unintentional)

⑦**T50.B92** Poisoning by other viral vaccines, intentional self-harm

⑦**T50.B93** Poisoning by other viral vaccines, assault

⑦**T50.B94** Poisoning by other viral vaccines, undetermined

⑦**T50.B95** Adverse effect of other viral vaccines

⑦**T50.B96** Underdosing of other viral vaccines

T50.Z Poisoning by, adverse effect of and underdosing of other vaccines and biological substances

T50.Z1 Poisoning by, adverse effect of and underdosing of immunoglobulin

⑦**T50.Z11** Poisoning by immunoglobulin, accidental (unintentional)

⑦**T50.Z12** Poisoning by immunoglobulin, intentional self-harm

⑦**T50.Z13** Poisoning by immunoglobulin, assault

⑦**T50.Z14** Poisoning by immunoglobulin, undetermined

⑦**T50.Z15** Adverse effect of immunoglobulin

⑦**T50.Z16** Underdosing of immunoglobulin

T50.Z9 Poisoning by, adverse effect of and underdosing of other vaccines and biological substances

⑦**T50.Z91** Poisoning by other vaccines and biological substances, accidental (unintentional)

⑦**T50.Z92** Poisoning by other vaccines and biological substances, intentional self-harm

⑦**T50.Z93** Poisoning by other vaccines and biological substances, assault

⑦**T50.Z94** Poisoning by other vaccines and biological substances, undetermined

⑦**T50.Z95** Adverse effect of other vaccines and biological substances

⑦**T50.Z96** Underdosing of other vaccines and biological substances

T50.9 Poisoning by, adverse effect of and underdosing of other and unspecified drugs, medicaments and biological substances

T50.90 Poisoning by, adverse effect of and underdosing of unspecified drugs, medicaments and biological substances

⑦**T50.901** Poisoning by unspecified drugs, medicaments and biological substances, accidental (unintentional)

⑦**T50.902** Poisoning by unspecified drugs, medicaments and biological substances, intentional self-harm

⑦**T50.903** Poisoning by unspecified drugs, medicaments and biological substances, assault

⑦**T50.904** Poisoning by unspecified drugs, medicaments and biological substances, undetermined

⑦**T50.905** Adverse effect of unspecified drugs, medicaments and biological substances

⑦**T50.906** Underdosing of unspecified drugs, medicaments and biological substances

T50.99 Poisoning by, adverse effect of and underdosing of other drugs, medicaments and biological substances

---

■ Add 4th-7th digits ■ 3 digit reportable ■ Nonspecific code □ Unspecified code ■ Manifestation code

⑦ **T50.991**   Poisoning by other drugs, medicaments and biological substances, accidental (unintentional)

⑦ **T50.992**   Poisoning by other drugs, medicaments and biological substances, intentional self-harm

⑦ **T50.993**   Poisoning by other drugs, medicaments and biological substances, assault

⑦ **T50.994**   Poisoning by other drugs, medicaments and biological substances, undetermined

⑦ **T50.995**   Adverse effect of other drugs, medicaments and biological substances

⑦ **T50.996**   Underdosing of other drugs, medicaments and biological substances

TOXIC EFFECTS OF SUBSTANCES CHIEFLY NONMEDICINAL AS TO SOURCE (T51-T65)

Note: When no intent is indicated code to accidental. Undetermined intent is only for use when there is specific documentation in the record that the intent of the toxic effect cannot be determined

Use additional code(s):

for all associated manifestations of toxic effect, such as:

respiratory conditions due to external agents (J60-J70)

personal history of foreign body fully removed (Z87.821)

to identify any retained foreign body, if applicable (Z18.-)

Excludes 1: contact with and (suspected) exposure to toxic substances (Z77.-)

 T51   Toxic effect of alcohol

The appropriate 7th character is to be added to each code from category T51

A - initial encounter

D - subsequent encounter

S - sequela

T51.0   Toxic effect of ethanol

Toxic effect of ethyl alcohol

Excludes 2: acute alcohol intoxication or 'hangover' effects (F10.129, F10.229, F10.929)

drunkenness (F10.129, F10.229, F10.929)

pathological alcohol intoxication (F10.129, F10.229, F10.929)

T51.0X   Toxic effect of ethanol

⑦ **T51.0X1**   Toxic effect of ethanol, accidental (unintentional)

Toxic effect of ethanol NOS

⑦ **T51.0X2**   Toxic effect of ethanol, intentional self-harm

⑦ **T51.0X3**   Toxic effect of ethanol, assault

⑦ **T51.0X4**   Toxic effect of ethanol, undetermined

T51.1   Toxic effect of methanol

Toxic effect of methyl alcohol

T51.1X   Toxic effect of methanol

⑦ **T51.1X1**   Toxic effect of methanol, accidental (unintentional)

Toxic effect of methanol NOS

⑦ **T51.1X2**   Toxic effect of methanol, intentional self-harm

⑦ **T51.1X3**   Toxic effect of methanol, assault

⑦ **T51.1X4**   Toxic effect of methanol, undetermined

T51.2   Toxic effect of 2-Propanol

Toxic effect of isopropyl alcohol

T51.2X   Toxic effect of 2-Propanol

⑦ **T51.2X1**   Toxic effect of 2-Propanol, accidental (unintentional)

Toxic effect of 2-Propanol NOS

⑦ **T51.2X2**   Toxic effect of 2-Propanol, intentional self-harm

⑦ **T51.2X3**   Toxic effect of 2-Propanol, assault

⑦ **T51.2X4**   Toxic effect of 2-Propanol, undetermined

T51.3   Toxic effect of fusel oil

Toxic effect of amyl alcohol

Toxic effect of butyl [1-butanol] alcohol

Toxic effect of propyl [1-propanol] alcohol

T51.3X   Toxic effect of fusel oil

⑦ **T51.3X1**   Toxic effect of fusel oil, accidental (unintentional)

Toxic effect of fusel oil NOS

⑦ **T51.3X2**   Toxic effect of fusel oil, intentional self-harm

⑦ **T51.3X3**   Toxic effect of fusel oil, assault

⑦ **T51.3X4**   Toxic effect of fusel oil, undetermined

T51.8   Toxic effect of other alcohols

T51.8X   Toxic effect of other alcohols

⑦ **T51.8X1**   Toxic effect of other alcohols, accidental (unintentional)

Toxic effect of other alcohols NOS

⑦ **T51.8X2**   Toxic effect of other alcohols, intentional self-harm

⑦ **T51.8X3**   Toxic effect of other alcohols, assault

⑦ **T51.8X4**   Toxic effect of other alcohols, undetermined

T51.9   Toxic effect of unspecified alcohol

⊗⑦ **T51.91**   Toxic effect of unspecified alcohol, accidental (unintentional)

⊗⑦ **T51.92**   Toxic effect of unspecified alcohol, intentional self-harm

⊗⑦ **T51.93**   Toxic effect of unspecified alcohol, assault

⊗⑦ **T51.94**   Toxic effect of unspecified alcohol, undetermined

T52   Toxic effect of organic solvents

Excludes 1: halogen derivatives of aliphatic and aromatic hydrocarbons (T53.-)

The appropriate 7th character is to be added to each code from category T52

A - initial encounter

D - subsequent encounter

S - sequela

T52.0   Toxic effects of petroleum products

Toxic effects of gasoline [petrol]

Toxic effects of kerosene [paraffin oil]
Toxic effects of paraffin wax
Toxic effects of ether petroleum
Toxic effects of naphtha petroleum
Toxic effects of spirit petroleum

T52.0X　Toxic effects of petroleum products

⑦**T52.0X1**　Toxic effect of petroleum products, accidental (unintentional)
Toxic effects of petroleum products NOS

⑦**T52.0X2**　Toxic effect of petroleum products, intentional self-harm

⑦**T52.0X3**　Toxic effect of petroleum products, assault

⑦**T52.0X4**　Toxic effect of petroleum products, undetermined

T52.1　Toxic effects of benzene

Excludes 1: homologues of benzene (T52.2)
nitroderivatives and aminoderivatives of benzene and its homologues (T65.3)

T52.1X　Toxic effects of benzene

⑦**T52.1X1**　Toxic effect of benzene, accidental (unintentional)
Toxic effects of benzene NOS

⑦**T52.1X2**　Toxic effect of benzene, intentional self-harm

⑦**T52.1X3**　Toxic effect of benzene, assault

⑦**T52.1X4**　Toxic effect of benzene, undetermined

T52.2　Toxic effects of homologues of benzene
Toxic effects of toluene [methylbenzene]
Toxic effects of xylene [dimethylbenzene]

T52.2X　Toxic effects of homologues of benzene

⑦**T52.2X1**　Toxic effect of homologues of benzene, accidental (unintentional)
Toxic effects of homologues of benzene NOS

⑦**T52.2X2**　Toxic effect of homologues of benzene, intentional self-harm

⑦**T52.2X3**　Toxic effect of homologues of benzene, assault

⑦**T52.2X4**　Toxic effect of homologues of benzene, undetermined

T52.3　Toxic effects of glycols

T52.3X　Toxic effects of glycols

⑦**T52.3X1**　Toxic effect of glycols, accidental (unintentional)
Toxic effects of glycols NOS

⑦**T52.3X2**　Toxic effect of glycols, intentional self-harm

⑦**T52.3X3**　Toxic effect of glycols, assault

⑦**T52.3X4**　Toxic effect of glycols, undetermined

T52.4　Toxic effects of ketones

T52.4X　Toxic effects of ketones

⑦**T52.4X1**　Toxic effect of ketones, accidental (unintentional)
Toxic effects of ketones NOS

⑦**T52.4X2**　Toxic effect of ketones, intentional self-harm

⑦**T52.4X3**　Toxic effect of ketones, assault

⑦**T52.4X4**　Toxic effect of ketones, undetermined

T52.8　Toxic effects of other organic solvents

T52.8X　Toxic effects of other organic solvents

⑦**T52.8X1**　Toxic effect of other organic solvents, accidental (unintentional)
Toxic effects of other organic solvents NOS

⑦**T52.8X2**　Toxic effect of other organic solvents, intentional self-harm

⑦**T52.8X3**　Toxic effect of other organic solvents, assault

⑦**T52.8X4**　Toxic effect of other organic solvents, undetermined

T52.9　Toxic effects of unspecified organic solvent

⊗⑦**T52.91**　Toxic effect of unspecified organic solvent, accidental (unintentional)

⊗⑦**T52.92**　Toxic effect of unspecified organic solvent, intentional self-harm

⊗⑦**T52.93**　Toxic effect of unspecified organic solvent, assault

⊗⑦**T52.94**　Toxic effect of unspecified organic solvent, undetermined

T53　Toxic effect of halogen derivatives of aliphatic and aromatic hydrocarbons

The appropriate 7th character is to be added to each code from category T53

A - initial encounter

D - subsequent encounter

S - sequela

T53.0　Toxic effects of carbon tetrachloride
Toxic effects of tetrachloromethane

T53.0X　Toxic effects of carbon tetrachloride

⑦**T53.0X1**　Toxic effect of carbon tetrachloride, accidental (unintentional)
Toxic effects of carbon tetrachloride NOS

⑦**T53.0X2**　Toxic effect of carbon tetrachloride, intentional self-harm

⑦**T53.0X3**　Toxic effect of carbon tetrachloride, assault

⑦**T53.0X4**　Toxic effect of carbon tetrachloride, undetermined

T53.1　Toxic effects of chloroform
Toxic effects of trichloromethane

T53.1X　Toxic effects of chloroform

⑦**T53.1X1**　Toxic effect of chloroform, accidental (unintentional)
Toxic effects of chloroform NOS

⑦**T53.1X2**　Toxic effect of chloroform, intentional self-harm

⑦**T53.1X3**　Toxic effect of chloroform, assault

⑦**T53.1X4**　Toxic effect of chloroform, undetermined

T53.2　Toxic effects of trichloroethylene
Toxic effects of trichloroethene

T53.2X Toxic effects of trichloroethylene

⑦**T53.2X1** Toxic effect of trichloroethylene, accidental (unintentional)

Toxic effects of trichloroethylene NOS

⑦**T53.2X2** Toxic effect of trichloroethylene, intentional self-harm

⑦**T53.2X3** Toxic effect of trichloroethylene, assault

⑦**T53.2X4** Toxic effect of trichloroethylene, undetermined

T53.3 Toxic effects of tetrachloroethylene

Toxic effects of perchloroethylene

Toxic effect of tetrachloroethane

T53.3X Toxic effects of tetrachloroethylene

⑦**T53.3X1** Toxic effect of tetrachloroethylene, accidental (unintentional)

Toxic effects of tetrachloroethylene NOS

⑦**T53.3X2** Toxic effect of tetrachloroethylene, intentional self-harm

⑦**T53.3X3** Toxic effect of tetrachloroethylene, assault

⑦**T53.3X4** Toxic effect of tetrachloroethylene, undetermined

T53.4 Toxic effects of dichloromethane

Toxic effects of methylene chloride

T53.4X Toxic effects of dichloromethane

⑦**T53.4X1** Toxic effect of dichloromethane, accidental (unintentional)

Toxic effects of dichloromethane NOS

⑦**T53.4X2** Toxic effect of dichloromethane, intentional self-harm

⑦**T53.4X3** Toxic effect of dichloromethane, assault

⑦**T53.4X4** Toxic effect of dichloromethane, undetermined

T53.5 Toxic effects of chlorofluorocarbons

T53.5X Toxic effects of chlorofluorocarbons

⑦**T53.5X1** Toxic effect of chlorofluorocarbons, accidental (unintentional)

Toxic effects of chlorofluorocarbons NOS

⑦**T53.5X2** Toxic effect of chlorofluorocarbons, intentional self-harm

⑦**T53.5X3** Toxic effect of chlorofluorocarbons, assault

⑦**T53.5X4** Toxic effect of chlorofluorocarbons, undetermined

T53.6 Toxic effects of other halogen derivatives of aliphatic hydrocarbons

T53.6X Toxic effects of other halogen derivatives of aliphatic hydrocarbons

⑦**T53.6X1** Toxic effect of other halogen derivatives of aliphatic hydrocarbons, accidental (unintentional)

Toxic effects of other halogen derivatives of aliphatic hydrocarbons NOS

⑦**T53.6X2** Toxic effect of other halogen derivatives of aliphatic hydrocarbons, intentional self-harm

⑦**T53.6X3** Toxic effect of other halogen derivatives of aliphatic hydrocarbons, assault

⑦**T53.6X4** Toxic effect of other halogen derivatives of aliphatic hydrocarbons, undetermined

T53.7 Toxic effects of other halogen derivatives of aromatic hydrocarbons

T53.7X Toxic effects of other halogen derivatives of aromatic hydrocarbons

⑦**T53.7X1** Toxic effect of other halogen derivatives of aromatic hydrocarbons, accidental (unintentional)

Toxic effects of other halogen derivatives of aromatic hydrocarbons NOS

⑦**T53.7X2** Toxic effect of other halogen derivatives of aromatic hydrocarbons, intentional self-harm

⑦**T53.7X3** Toxic effect of other halogen derivatives of aromatic hydrocarbons, assault

⑦**T53.7X4** Toxic effect of other halogen derivatives of aromatic hydrocarbons, undetermined

T53.9 Toxic effects of unspecified halogen derivatives of aliphatic and aromatic hydrocarbons

⑦**T53.91** Toxic effect of unspecified halogen derivatives of aliphatic and aromatic hydrocarbons, accidental (unintentional)

⑦**T53.92** Toxic effect of unspecified halogen derivatives of aliphatic and aromatic hydrocarbons, intentional self-harm

⑦**T53.93** Toxic effect of unspecified halogen derivatives of aliphatic and aromatic hydrocarbons, assault

⑦**T53.94** Toxic effect of unspecified halogen derivatives of aliphatic and aromatic hydrocarbons, undetermined

T54 Toxic effect of corrosive substances

The appropriate 7th character is to be added to each code from category T54

A - initial encounter

D - subsequent encounter

S - sequela

T54.0 Toxic effects of phenol and phenol homologues

T54.0X Toxic effects of phenol and phenol homologues

⑦**T54.0X1** Toxic effect of phenol and phenol homologues, accidental (unintentional)

Toxic effects of phenol and phenol homologues NOS

⑦**T54.0X2** Toxic effect of phenol and phenol homologues, intentional self-harm

● New code   ▲ Revised code   ⑦ 7ᵗʰ digit required   ⊗ Placeholder required

⑦**T54.0X3**   Toxic effect of phenol and phenol homologues, assault

⑦**T54.0X4**   Toxic effect of phenol and phenol homologues, undetermined

T54.1   Toxic effects of other corrosive organic compounds

    T54.1X   Toxic effects of other corrosive organic compounds

      ⑦**T54.1X1**   Toxic effect of other corrosive organic compounds, accidental (unintentional)

           Toxic effects of other corrosive organic compounds NOS

      ⑦**T54.1X2**   Toxic effect of other corrosive organic compounds, intentional self-harm

      ⑦**T54.1X3**   Toxic effect of other corrosive organic compounds, assault

      ⑦**T54.1X4**   Toxic effect of other corrosive organic compounds, undetermined

T54.2   Toxic effects of corrosive acids and acid-like substances

Toxic effects of hydrochloric acid

Toxic effects of sulfuric acid

    T54.2X   Toxic effects of corrosive acids and acid-like substances

      ⑦**T54.2X1**   Toxic effect of corrosive acids and acid-like substances, accidental (unintentional)

           Toxic effects of corrosive acids and acid-like substances NOS

      ⑦**T54.2X2**   Toxic effect of corrosive acids and acid-like substances, intentional self-harm

      ⑦**T54.2X3**   Toxic effect of corrosive acids and acid-like substances, assault

      ⑦**T54.2X4**   Toxic effect of corrosive acids and acid-like substances, undetermined

T54.3   Toxic effects of corrosive alkalis and alkali-like substances

Toxic effects of potassium hydroxide

Toxic effects of sodium hydroxide

    T54.3X   Toxic effects of corrosive alkalis and alkali-like substances

      ⑦**T54.3X1**   Toxic effect of corrosive alkalis and alkali-like substances, accidental (unintentional)

           Toxic effects of corrosive alkalis and alkali-like substances NOS

      ⑦**T54.3X2**   Toxic effect of corrosive alkalis and alkali-like substances, intentional self-harm

      ⑦**T54.3X3**   Toxic effect of corrosive alkalis and alkali-like substances, assault

      ⑦**T54.3X4**   Toxic effect of corrosive alkalis and alkali-like substances, undetermined

T54.9   Toxic effects of unspecified corrosive substance

    ⊗⑦**T54.91**   Toxic effect of unspecified corrosive substance, accidental (unintentional)

    ⊗⑦**T54.92**   Toxic effect of unspecified corrosive substance, intentional self-harm

    ⊗⑦**T54.93**   Toxic effect of unspecified corrosive substance, assault

    ⊗⑦**T54.94**   Toxic effect of unspecified corrosive substance, undetermined

T55   Toxic effect of soaps and detergents

The appropriate 7th character is to be added to each code from category T55

A - initial encounter

D - subsequent encounter

S - sequela

    T55.0   Toxic effect of soaps

      T55.0X   Toxic effect of soaps

        ⑦**T55.0X1**   Toxic effect of soaps, accidental (unintentional)

             Toxic effect of soaps NOS

        ⑦**T55.0X2**   Toxic effect of soaps, intentional self-harm

        ⑦**T55.0X3**   Toxic effect of soaps, assault

        ⑦**T55.0X4**   Toxic effect of soaps, undetermined

    T55.1   Toxic effect of detergents

      T55.1X   Toxic effect of detergents

        ⑦**T55.1X1**   Toxic effect of detergents, accidental (unintentional)

             Toxic effect of detergents NOS

        ⑦**T55.1X2**   Toxic effect of detergents, intentional self-harm

        ⑦**T55.1X3**   Toxic effect of detergents, assault

        ⑦**T55.1X4**   Toxic effect of detergents, undetermined

T56   Toxic effect of metals

Includes: toxic effects of fumes and vapors of metals

             toxic effects of metals from all sources, except medicinal substances

Use additional code to identify any retained metal foreign body, if applicable (Z18.0-, T18.1-)

Excludes 1: arsenic and its compounds (T57.0)

             manganese and its compounds (T57.2)

The appropriate 7th character is to be added to each code from category T56

A - initial encounter

D - subsequent encounter

S - sequela

    T56.0   Toxic effects of lead and its compounds

      T56.0X   Toxic effects of lead and its compounds

        ⑦**T56.0X1**   Toxic effect of lead and its compounds, accidental (unintentional)

             Toxic effects of lead and its compounds NOS

        ⑦**T56.0X2**   Toxic effect of lead and its compounds, intentional self-harm

        ⑦**T56.0X3**   Toxic effect of lead and its compounds, assault

        ⑦**T56.0X4**   Toxic effect of lead and its compounds, undetermined

    T56.1   Toxic effects of mercury and its compounds

      T56.1X   Toxic effects of mercury and its compounds

        ⑦**T56.1X1**   Toxic effect of mercury and its compounds, accidental (unintentional)

Toxic effects of mercury and its compounds NOS

⑦ **T56.1X2** Toxic effect of mercury and its compounds, intentional self-harm

⑦ **T56.1X3** Toxic effect of mercury and its compounds, assault

⑦ **T56.1X4** Toxic effect of mercury and its compounds, undetermined

T56.2 Toxic effects of chromium and its compounds

T56.2X Toxic effects of chromium and its compounds

⑦ **T56.2X1** Toxic effect of chromium and its compounds, accidental (unintentional)

Toxic effects of chromium and its compounds NOS

⑦ **T56.2X2** Toxic effect of chromium and its compounds, intentional self-harm

⑦ **T56.2X3** Toxic effect of chromium and its compounds, assault

⑦ **T56.2X4** Toxic effect of chromium and its compounds, undetermined

T56.3 Toxic effects of cadmium and its compounds

T56.3X Toxic effects of cadmium and its compounds

⑦ **T56.3X1** Toxic effect of cadmium and its compounds, accidental (unintentional)

Toxic effects of cadmium and its compounds NOS

⑦ **T56.3X2** Toxic effect of cadmium and its compounds, intentional self-harm

⑦ **T56.3X3** Toxic effect of cadmium and its compounds, assault

⑦ **T56.3X4** Toxic effect of cadmium and its compounds, undetermined

T56.4 Toxic effects of copper and its compounds

T56.4X Toxic effects of copper and its compounds

⑦ **T56.4X1** Toxic effect of copper and its compounds, accidental (unintentional)

Toxic effects of copper and its compounds NOS

⑦ **T56.4X2** Toxic effect of copper and its compounds, intentional self-harm

⑦ **T56.4X3** Toxic effect of copper and its compounds, assault

⑦ **T56.4X4** Toxic effect of copper and its compounds, undetermined

T56.5 Toxic effects of zinc and its compounds

T56.5X Toxic effects of zinc and its compounds

⑦ **T56.5X1** Toxic effect of zinc and its compounds, accidental (unintentional)

Toxic effects of zinc and its compounds NOS

⑦ **T56.5X2** Toxic effect of zinc and its compounds, intentional self-harm

⑦ **T56.5X3** Toxic effect of zinc and its compounds, assault

⑦ **T56.5X4** Toxic effect of zinc and its compounds, undetermined

T56.6 Toxic effects of tin and its compounds

T56.6X Toxic effects of tin and its compounds

⑦ **T56.6X1** Toxic effect of tin and its compounds, accidental (unintentional)

Toxic effects of tin and its compounds NOS

⑦ **T56.6X2** Toxic effect of tin and its compounds, intentional self-harm

⑦ **T56.6X3** Toxic effect of tin and its compounds, assault

⑦ **T56.6X4** Toxic effect of tin and its compounds, undetermined

T56.7 Toxic effects of beryllium and its compounds

T56.7X Toxic effects of beryllium and its compounds

⑦ **T56.7X1** Toxic effect of beryllium and its compounds, accidental (unintentional)

Toxic effects of beryllium and its compounds NOS

⑦ **T56.7X2** Toxic effect of beryllium and its compounds, intentional self-harm

⑦ **T56.7X3** Toxic effect of beryllium and its compounds, assault

⑦ **T56.7X4** Toxic effect of beryllium and its compounds, undetermined

T56.8 Toxic effects of other metals

T56.81 Toxic effect of thallium

⑦ **T56.811** Toxic effect of thallium, accidental (unintentional)

Toxic effect of thallium NOS

⑦ **T56.812** Toxic effect of thallium, intentional self-harm

⑦ **T56.813** Toxic effect of thallium, assault

⑦ **T56.814** Toxic effect of thallium, undetermined

T56.89 Toxic effects of other metals

⑦ **T56.891** Toxic effect of other metals, accidental (unintentional)

Toxic effects of other metals NOS

⑦ **T56.892** Toxic effect of other metals, intentional self-harm

⑦ **T56.893** Toxic effect of other metals, assault

⑦ **T56.894** Toxic effect of other metals, undetermined

T56.9 Toxic effects of unspecified metal

⊗⑦ **T56.91** Toxic effect of unspecified metal, accidental (unintentional)

⊗⑦ **T56.92** Toxic effect of unspecified metal, intentional self-harm

⊗⑦ **T56.93** Toxic effect of unspecified metal, assault

⊗⑦ **T56.94** Toxic effect of unspecified metal, undetermined

T57 Toxic effect of other inorganic substances

The appropriate 7th character is to be added to each code from category T57

A - initial encounter

D - subsequent encounter

● New code   ▲ Revised code   ⑦ 7th digit required   ⊗ Placeholder required

S - sequela

T57.0 Toxic effect of arsenic and its compounds

    T57.0X Toxic effect of arsenic and its compounds

        ⑦**T57.0X1** Toxic effect of arsenic and its compounds, accidental (unintentional)

                Toxic effect of arsenic and its compounds NOS

        ⑦**T57.0X2** Toxic effect of arsenic and its compounds, intentional self-harm

        ⑦**T57.0X3** Toxic effect of arsenic and its compounds, assault

        ⑦**T57.0X4** Toxic effect of arsenic and its compounds, undetermined

T57.1 Toxic effect of phosphorus and its compounds

    Excludes 1: organophosphate insecticides (T60.0)

    T57.1X Toxic effect of phosphorus and its compounds

        ⑦**T57.1X1** Toxic effect of phosphorus and its compounds, accidental (unintentional)

                Toxic effect of phosphorus and its compounds NOS

        ⑦**T57.1X2** Toxic effect of phosphorus and its compounds, intentional self-harm

        ⑦**T57.1X3** Toxic effect of phosphorus and its compounds, assault

        ⑦**T57.1X4** Toxic effect of phosphorus and its compounds, undetermined

T57.2 Toxic effect of manganese and its compounds

    T57.2X Toxic effect of manganese and its compounds

        ⑦**T57.2X1** Toxic effect of manganese and its compounds, accidental (unintentional)

                Toxic effect of manganese and its compounds NOS

        ⑦**T57.2X2** Toxic effect of manganese and its compounds, intentional self-harm

        ⑦**T57.2X3** Toxic effect of manganese and its compounds, assault

        ⑦**T57.2X4** Toxic effect of manganese and its compounds, undetermined

T57.3 Toxic effect of hydrogen cyanide

    T57.3X Toxic effect of hydrogen cyanide

        ⑦**T57.3X1** Toxic effect of hydrogen cyanide, accidental (unintentional)

                Toxic effect of hydrogen cyanide NOS

        ⑦**T57.3X2** Toxic effect of hydrogen cyanide, intentional self-harm

        ⑦**T57.3X3** Toxic effect of hydrogen cyanide, assault

        ⑦**T57.3X4** Toxic effect of hydrogen cyanide, undetermined

T57.8 Toxic effect of other specified inorganic substances

    T57.8X Toxic effect of other specified inorganic substances

        ⑦**T57.8X1** Toxic effect of other specified inorganic substances, accidental (unintentional)

                Toxic effect of other specified inorganic substances NOS

        ⑦**T57.8X2** Toxic effect of other specified inorganic substances, intentional self-harm

        ⑦**T57.8X3** Toxic effect of other specified inorganic substances, assault

        ⑦**T57.8X4** Toxic effect of other specified inorganic substances, undetermined

T57.9 Toxic effect of unspecified inorganic substance

    ⊗⑦**T57.91** Toxic effect of unspecified inorganic substance, accidental (unintentional)

    ⊗⑦**T57.92** Toxic effect of unspecified inorganic substance, intentional self-harm

    ⊗⑦**T57.93** Toxic effect of unspecified inorganic substance, assault

    ⊗⑦**T57.94** Toxic effect of unspecified inorganic substance, undetermined

T58 Toxic effect of carbon monoxide

    Includes: asphyxiation from carbon monoxide

            toxic effect of carbon monoxide from all sources

The appropriate 7th character is to be added to each code from category T58

A - initial encounter

D - subsequent encounter

S - sequela

T58.0 Toxic effect of carbon monoxide from motor vehicle exhaust

    Toxic effect of exhaust gas from gas engine

    Toxic effect of exhaust gas from motor pump

    ⊗⑦**T58.01** Toxic effect of carbon monoxide from motor vehicle exhaust, accidental (unintentional)

    ⊗⑦**T58.02** Toxic effect of carbon monoxide from motor vehicle exhaust, intentional self-harm

    ⊗⑦**T58.03** Toxic effect of carbon monoxide from motor vehicle exhaust, assault

    ⊗⑦**T58.04** Toxic effect of carbon monoxide from motor vehicle exhaust, undetermined

T58.1 Toxic effect of carbon monoxide from utility gas

    Toxic effect of acetylene

    Toxic effect of gas NOS used for lighting, heating, cooking

    Toxic effect of water gas

    ⊗⑦**T58.11** Toxic effect of carbon monoxide from utility gas, accidental (unintentional)

    ⊗⑦**T58.12** Toxic effect of carbon monoxide from utility gas, intentional self-harm

    ⊗⑦**T58.13** Toxic effect of carbon monoxide from utility gas, assault

    ⊗⑦**T58.14** Toxic effect of carbon monoxide from utility gas, undetermined

T58.2 Toxic effect of carbon monoxide from incomplete combustion of other domestic fuels

    Toxic effect of carbon monoxide from incomplete combustion of coal, coke, kerosene, wood

    T58.2X Toxic effect of carbon monoxide from incomplete combustion of other domestic fuels

        ⑦**T58.2X1** Toxic effect of carbon monoxide from incomplete combustion of other domestic fuels, accidental (unintentional)

■ Add 4th-7th digits   ■ 3 digit reportable   Nonspecific code   Unspecified code   Manifestation code   805

⑦ **T58.2X2** Toxic effect of carbon monoxide from incomplete combustion of other domestic fuels, intentional self-harm

⑦ **T58.2X3** Toxic effect of carbon monoxide from incomplete combustion of other domestic fuels, assault

⑦ **T58.2X4** Toxic effect of carbon monoxide from incomplete combustion of other domestic fuels, undetermined

T58.8 Toxic effect of carbon monoxide from other source
Toxic effect of carbon monoxide from blast furnace gas
Toxic effect of carbon monoxide from fuels in industrial use
Toxic effect of carbon monoxide from kiln vapor

T58.8X Toxic effect of carbon monoxide from other source

⑦ **T58.8X1** Toxic effect of carbon monoxide from other source, accidental (unintentional)

⑦ **T58.8X2** Toxic effect of carbon monoxide from other source, intentional self-harm

⑦ **T58.8X3** Toxic effect of carbon monoxide from other source, assault

⑦ **T58.8X4** Toxic effect of carbon monoxide from other source, undetermined

T58.9 Toxic effect of carbon monoxide from unspecified source

⊗⑦ **T58.91** Toxic effect of carbon monoxide from unspecified source, accidental (unintentional)

⊗⑦ **T58.92** Toxic effect of carbon monoxide from unspecified source, intentional self-harm

⊗⑦ **T58.93** Toxic effect of carbon monoxide from unspecified source, assault

⊗⑦ **T58.94** Toxic effect of carbon monoxide from unspecified source, undetermined

T59 Toxic effect of other gases, fumes and vapors

Includes: aerosol propellants

Excludes 1: chlorofluorocarbons (T53.5)

The appropriate 7th character is to be added to each code from category T59

A - initial encounter
D - subsequent encounter
S - sequela

T59.0 Toxic effect of nitrogen oxides

T59.0X Toxic effect of nitrogen oxides

⑦ **T59.0X1** Toxic effect of nitrogen oxides, accidental (unintentional)
Toxic effect of nitrogen oxides NOS

⑦ **T59.0X2** Toxic effect of nitrogen oxides, intentional self-harm

⑦ **T59.0X3** Toxic effect of nitrogen oxides, assault

⑦ **T59.0X4** Toxic effect of nitrogen oxides, undetermined

T59.1 Toxic effect of sulfur dioxide

T59.1X Toxic effect of sulfur dioxide

⑦ **T59.1X1** Toxic effect of sulfur dioxide, accidental (unintentional)
Toxic effect of sulfur dioxide NOS

⑦ **T59.1X2** Toxic effect of sulfur dioxide, intentional self-harm

⑦ **T59.1X3** Toxic effect of sulfur dioxide, assault

⑦ **T59.1X4** Toxic effect of sulfur dioxide, undetermined

T59.2 Toxic effect of formaldehyde

T59.2X Toxic effect of formaldehyde

⑦ **T59.2X1** Toxic effect of formaldehyde, accidental (unintentional)
Toxic effect of formaldehyde NOS

⑦ **T59.2X2** Toxic effect of formaldehyde, intentional self-harm

⑦ **T59.2X3** Toxic effect of formaldehyde, assault

⑦ **T59.2X4** Toxic effect of formaldehyde, undetermined

T59.3 Toxic effect of lacrimogenic gas
Toxic effect of tear gas

T59.3X Toxic effect of lacrimogenic gas

⑦ **T59.3X1** Toxic effect of lacrimogenic gas, accidental (unintentional)
Toxic effect of lacrimogenic gas NOS

⑦ **T59.3X2** Toxic effect of lacrimogenic gas, intentional self-harm

⑦ **T59.3X3** Toxic effect of lacrimogenic gas, assault

⑦ **T59.3X4** Toxic effect of lacrimogenic gas, undetermined

T59.4 Toxic effect of chlorine gas

T59.4X Toxic effect of chlorine gas

⑦ **T59.4X1** Toxic effect of chlorine gas, accidental (unintentional)
Toxic effect of chlorine gas NOS

⑦ **T59.4X2** Toxic effect of chlorine gas, intentional self-harm

⑦ **T59.4X3** Toxic effect of chlorine gas, assault

⑦ **T59.4X4** Toxic effect of chlorine gas, undetermined

T59.5 Toxic effect of fluorine gas and hydrogen fluoride

T59.5X Toxic effect of fluorine gas and hydrogen fluoride

⑦ **T59.5X1** Toxic effect of fluorine gas and hydrogen fluoride, accidental (unintentional)
Toxic effect of fluorine gas and hydrogen fluoride NOS

⑦ **T59.5X2** Toxic effect of fluorine gas and hydrogen fluoride, intentional self-harm

⑦ **T59.5X3** Toxic effect of fluorine gas and hydrogen fluoride, assault

⑦ **T59.5X4** Toxic effect of fluorine gas and hydrogen fluoride, undetermined

T59.6 Toxic effect of hydrogen sulfide

T59.6X Toxic effect of hydrogen sulfide

● New code   ▲ Revised code   ⑦ 7th digit required   ⊗ Placeholder required

⑦ **T59.6X1** Toxic effect of hydrogen sulfide, accidental (unintentional)
Toxic effect of hydrogen sulfide NOS

⑦ **T59.6X2** Toxic effect of hydrogen sulfide, intentional self-harm

⑦ **T59.6X3** Toxic effect of hydrogen sulfide, assault

⑦ **T59.6X4** Toxic effect of hydrogen sulfide, undetermined

T59.7 Toxic effect of carbon dioxide

  T59.7X Toxic effect of carbon dioxide

    ⑦ **T59.7X1** Toxic effect of carbon dioxide, accidental (unintentional)
Toxic effect of carbon dioxide NOS

    ⑦ **T59.7X2** Toxic effect of carbon dioxide, intentional self-harm

    ⑦ **T59.7X3** Toxic effect of carbon dioxide, assault

    ⑦ **T59.7X4** Toxic effect of carbon dioxide, undetermined

T59.8 Toxic effect of other specified gases, fumes and vapors

  T59.81 Toxic effect of smoke
Smoke inhalation
Excludes 2: toxic effect of cigarette (tobacco) smoke (T65.22-)

    ⑦ **T59.811** Toxic effect of smoke, accidental (unintentional)
Toxic effect of smoke NOS

    ⑦ **T59.812** Toxic effect of smoke, intentional self-harm

    ⑦ **T59.813** Toxic effect of smoke, assault

    ⑦ **T59.814** Toxic effect of smoke, undetermined

  T59.89 Toxic effect of other specified gases, fumes and vapors

    ⑦ **T59.891** Toxic effect of other specified gases, fumes and vapors, accidental (unintentional)

    ⑦ **T59.892** Toxic effect of other specified gases, fumes and vapors, intentional self-harm

    ⑦ **T59.893** Toxic effect of other specified gases, fumes and vapors, assault

    ⑦ **T59.894** Toxic effect of other specified gases, fumes and vapors, undetermined

T59.9 Toxic effect of unspecified gases, fumes and vapors

  ⊗⑦ **T59.91** Toxic effect of unspecified gases, fumes and vapors, accidental (unintentional)

  ⊗⑦ **T59.92** Toxic effect of unspecified gases, fumes and vapors, intentional self-harm

  ⊗⑦ **T59.93** Toxic effect of unspecified gases, fumes and vapors, assault

  ⊗⑦ **T59.94** Toxic effect of unspecified gases, fumes and vapors, undetermined

T60 Toxic effect of pesticides
Includes: toxic effect of wood preservatives
The appropriate 7th character is to be added to each code from category T60
A - initial encounter

D - subsequent encounter
S - sequela

T60.0 Toxic effect of organophosphate and carbamate insecticides

  T60.0X Toxic effect of organophosphate and carbamate insecticides

    ⑦ **T60.0X1** Toxic effect of organophosphate and carbamate insecticides, accidental (unintentional)
Toxic effect of organophosphate and carbamate insecticides NOS

    ⑦ **T60.0X2** Toxic effect of organophosphate and carbamate insecticides, intentional self-harm

    ⑦ **T60.0X3** Toxic effect of organophosphate and carbamate insecticides, assault

    ⑦ **T60.0X4** Toxic effect of organophosphate and carbamate insecticides, undetermined

T60.1 Toxic effect of halogenated insecticides
Excludes 1: chlorinated hydrocarbon (T53.-)

  T60.1X Toxic effect of halogenated insecticides

    ⑦ **T60.1X1** Toxic effect of halogenated insecticides, accidental (unintentional)
Toxic effect of halogenated insecticides NOS

    ⑦ **T60.1X2** Toxic effect of halogenated insecticides, intentional self-harm

    ⑦ **T60.1X3** Toxic effect of halogenated insecticides, assault

    ⑦ **T60.1X4** Toxic effect of halogenated insecticides, undetermined

T60.2 Toxic effect of other insecticides

  T60.2X Toxic effect of other insecticides

    ⑦ **T60.2X1** Toxic effect of other insecticides, accidental (unintentional)
Toxic effect of other insecticides NOS

    ⑦ **T60.2X2** Toxic effect of other insecticides, intentional self-harm

    ⑦ **T60.2X3** Toxic effect of other insecticides, assault

    ⑦ **T60.2X4** Toxic effect of other insecticides, undetermined

T60.3 Toxic effect of herbicides and fungicides

  T60.3X Toxic effect of herbicides and fungicides

    ⑦ **T60.3X1** Toxic effect of herbicides and fungicides, accidental (unintentional)
Toxic effect of herbicides and fungicides NOS

    ⑦ **T60.3X2** Toxic effect of herbicides and fungicides, intentional self-harm

    ⑦ **T60.3X3** Toxic effect of herbicides and fungicides, assault

    ⑦ **T60.3X4** Toxic effect of herbicides and fungicides, undetermined

T60.4 Toxic effect of rodenticides
Excludes 1: strychnine and its salts (T65.1)

---

thallium (T56.81-)

T60.4X Toxic effect of rodenticides

⑦**T60.4X1** Toxic effect of rodenticides, accidental (unintentional)

Toxic effect of rodenticides NOS

⑦**T60.4X2** Toxic effect of rodenticides, intentional self-harm

⑦**T60.4X3** Toxic effect of rodenticides, assault

⑦**T60.4X4** Toxic effect of rodenticides, undetermined

T60.8 Toxic effect of other pesticides

T60.8X Toxic effect of other pesticides

⑦**T60.8X1** Toxic effect of other pesticides, accidental (unintentional)

Toxic effect of other pesticides NOS

⑦**T60.8X2** Toxic effect of other pesticides, intentional self-harm

⑦**T60.8X3** Toxic effect of other pesticides, assault

⑦**T60.8X4** Toxic effect of other pesticides, undetermined

T60.9 Toxic effect of unspecified pesticide

⊗⑦**T60.91** Toxic effect of unspecified pesticide, accidental (unintentional)

⊗⑦**T60.92** Toxic effect of unspecified pesticide, intentional self-harm

⊗⑦**T60.93** Toxic effect of unspecified pesticide, assault

⊗⑦**T60.94** Toxic effect of unspecified pesticide, undetermined

T61 Toxic effect of noxious substances eaten as seafood

Excludes 1: allergic reaction to food, such as:

anaphylactic reaction or shock due to adverse food reaction (T78.0-)

dermatitis (L23.6, L25.4, L27.2)

gastroenteritis (noninfective) (K52.2)

anaphylactic shock (T78.02, T78.05)

bacterial foodborne intoxications (A05.-)

toxic effect of food contaminants, such as:

aflatoxin and other mycotoxins (T64)

cyanides (T65.0-)

harmful algae bloom (T65.82-)

hydrogen cyanide (T57.3-)

mercury (T56.1-)

red tide (T65.82-)

The appropriate 7th character is to be added to each code from category T61

A - initial encounter

D - subsequent encounter

S - sequela

T61.0 Ciguatera fish poisoning

⊗⑦**T61.01** Ciguatera fish poisoning, accidental (unintentional)

⊗⑦**T61.02** Ciguatera fish poisoning, intentional self-harm

⊗⑦**T61.03** Ciguatera fish poisoning, assault

⊗⑦**T61.04** Ciguatera fish poisoning, undetermined

T61.1 Scombroid fish poisoning

Histamine-like syndrome

⊗⑦**T61.11** Scombroid fish poisoning, accidental (unintentional)

⊗⑦**T61.12** Scombroid fish poisoning, intentional self-harm

⊗⑦**T61.13** Scombroid fish poisoning, assault

⊗⑦**T61.14** Scombroid fish poisoning, undetermined

T61.7 Other fish and shellfish poisoning

T61.77 Other fish poisoning

⑦**T61.771** Other fish poisoning, accidental (unintentional)

⑦**T61.772** Other fish poisoning, intentional self-harm

⑦**T61.773** Other fish poisoning, assault

⑦**T61.774** Other fish poisoning, undetermined

T61.78 Other shellfish poisoning

⑦**T61.781** Other shellfish poisoning, accidental (unintentional)

⑦**T61.782** Other shellfish poisoning, intentional self-harm

⑦**T61.783** Other shellfish poisoning, assault

⑦**T61.784** Other shellfish poisoning, undetermined

T61.8 Toxic effect of other seafood

T61.8X Toxic effect of other seafood

⑦**T61.8X1** Toxic effect of other seafood, accidental (unintentional)

⑦**T61.8X2** Toxic effect of other seafood, intentional self-harm

⑦**T61.8X3** Toxic effect of other seafood, assault

⑦**T61.8X4** Toxic effect of other seafood, undetermined

T61.9 Toxic effect of unspecified seafood

⊗⑦**T61.91** Toxic effect of unspecified seafood, accidental (unintentional)

⊗⑦**T61.92** Toxic effect of unspecified seafood, intentional self-harm

⊗⑦**T61.93** Toxic effect of unspecified seafood, assault

⊗⑦**T61.94** Toxic effect of unspecified seafood, undetermined

T62 Toxic effect of other noxious substances eaten as food

Excludes 1: allergic reaction to food, such as:

anaphylactic shock (reaction) due to adverse food reaction (T78.0-)

dermatitis (L23.6, L25.4, L27.2)

gastroenteritis (noninfective) (K52.2)

bacterial food borne intoxications (A05.-)

toxic effect of food contaminants, such as:

aflatoxin and other mycotoxins (T64)

cyanides (T65.0-)

hydrogen cyanide (T57.3-)

mercury (T56.1-)

The appropriate 7th character is to be added to each code from category T62

A - initial encounter

D - subsequent encounter

S - sequela

T62.0 Toxic effect of ingested mushrooms

T62.0X Toxic effect of ingested mushrooms

⑦ **T62.0X1**   Toxic effect of ingested mushrooms, accidental (unintentional)
Toxic effect of ingested mushrooms NOS

⑦ **T62.0X2**   Toxic effect of ingested mushrooms, intentional self-harm

⑦ **T62.0X3**   Toxic effect of ingested mushrooms, assault

⑦ **T62.0X4**   Toxic effect of ingested mushrooms, undetermined

T62.1   Toxic effect of ingested berries

　T62.1X   Toxic effect of ingested berries

　　⑦ **T62.1X1**   Toxic effect of ingested berries, accidental (unintentional)
Toxic effect of ingested berries NOS

　　⑦ **T62.1X2**   Toxic effect of ingested berries, intentional self-harm

　　⑦ **T62.1X3**   Toxic effect of ingested berries, assault

　　⑦ **T62.1X4**   Toxic effect of ingested berries, undetermined

T62.2   Toxic effect of other ingested (parts of) plant(s)

　T62.2X   Toxic effect of other ingested (parts of) plant(s)

　　⑦ **T62.2X1**   Toxic effect of other ingested (parts of) plant(s), accidental (unintentional)
Toxic effect of other ingested (parts of) plant(s) NOS

　　⑦ **T62.2X2**   Toxic effect of other ingested (parts of) plant(s), intentional self-harm

　　⑦ **T62.2X3**   Toxic effect of other ingested (parts of) plant(s), assault

　　⑦ **T62.2X4**   Toxic effect of other ingested (parts of) plant(s), undetermined

T62.8   Toxic effect of other specified noxious substances eaten as food

　T62.8X   Toxic effect of other specified noxious substances eaten as food

　　⑦ **T62.8X1**   Toxic effect of other specified noxious substances eaten as food, accidental (unintentional)
Toxic effect of other specified noxious substances eaten as food NOS

　　⑦ **T62.8X2**   Toxic effect of other specified noxious substances eaten as food, intentional self-harm

　　⑦ **T62.8X3**   Toxic effect of other specified noxious substances eaten as food, assault

　　⑦ **T62.8X4**   Toxic effect of other specified noxious substances eaten as food, undetermined

T62.9   Toxic effect of unspecified noxious substance eaten as food

　T62.91   Toxic effect of unspecified noxious substance eaten as food, accidental (unintentional)
Toxic effect of unspecified noxious substance eaten as food NOS

T62.92   Toxic effect of unspecified noxious substance eaten as food, intentional self-harm

T62.93   Toxic effect of unspecified noxious substance eaten as food, assault

T62.94   Toxic effect of unspecified noxious substance eaten as food, undetermined

T63   Toxic effect of contact with venomous animals and plants

Includes: bite or touch of venomous animal
pricked or stuck by thorn or leaf

Excludes 2: ingestion of toxic animal or plant (T61.-, T62.-)

The appropriate 7th character is to be added to each code from category T63

A - initial encounter

D - subsequent encounter

S - sequela

T63.0   Toxic effect of snake venom

　T63.00   Toxic effect of unspecified snake venom

　　⑦ **T63.001**   Toxic effect of unspecified snake venom, accidental (unintentional)
Toxic effect of unspecified snake venom NOS

　　⑦ **T63.002**   Toxic effect of unspecified snake venom, intentional self-harm

　　⑦ **T63.003**   Toxic effect of unspecified snake venom, assault

　　⑦ **T63.004**   Toxic effect of unspecified snake venom, undetermined

　T63.01   Toxic effect of rattlesnake venom

　　⑦ **T63.011**   Toxic effect of rattlesnake venom, accidental (unintentional)
Toxic effect of rattlesnake venom NOS

　　⑦ **T63.012**   Toxic effect of rattlesnake venom, intentional self-harm

　　⑦ **T63.013**   Toxic effect of rattlesnake venom, assault

　　⑦ **T63.014**   Toxic effect of rattlesnake venom, undetermined

　T63.02   Toxic effect of coral snake venom

　　⑦ **T63.021**   Toxic effect of coral snake venom, accidental (unintentional)
Toxic effect of coral snake venom NOS

　　⑦ **T63.022**   Toxic effect of coral snake venom, intentional self-harm

　　⑦ **T63.023**   Toxic effect of coral snake venom, assault

　　⑦ **T63.024**   Toxic effect of coral snake venom, undetermined

　T63.03   Toxic effect of taipan venom

　　⑦ **T63.031**   Toxic effect of taipan venom, accidental (unintentional)
Toxic effect of taipan venom NOS

　　⑦ **T63.032**   Toxic effect of taipan venom, intentional self-harm

　　⑦ **T63.033**   Toxic effect of taipan venom, assault

　　⑦ **T63.034**   Toxic effect of taipan venom, undetermined

　T63.04   Toxic effect of cobra venom

⑦T63.041   Toxic effect of cobra venom, accidental (unintentional)

Toxic effect of cobra venom NOS

⑦T63.042   Toxic effect of cobra venom, intentional self-harm

⑦T63.043   Toxic effect of cobra venom, assault

⑦T63.044   Toxic effect of cobra venom, undetermined

T63.06   Toxic effect of venom of other North and South American snake

⑦T63.061   Toxic effect of venom of other North and South American snake, accidental (unintentional)

Toxic effect of venom of other North and South American snake NOS

⑦T63.062   Toxic effect of venom of other North and South American snake, intentional self-harm

⑦T63.063   Toxic effect of venom of other North and South American snake, assault

⑦T63.064   Toxic effect of venom of other North and South American snake, undetermined

T63.07   Toxic effect of venom of other Australian snake

⑦T63.071   Toxic effect of venom of other Australian snake, accidental (unintentional)

Toxic effect of venom of other Australian snake NOS

⑦T63.072   Toxic effect of venom of other Australian snake, intentional self-harm

⑦T63.073   Toxic effect of venom of other Australian snake, assault

⑦T63.074   Toxic effect of venom of other Australian snake, undetermined

T63.08   Toxic effect of venom of other African and Asian snake

⑦T63.081   Toxic effect of venom of other African and Asian snake, accidental (unintentional)

Toxic effect of venom of other African and Asian snake NOS

⑦T63.082   Toxic effect of venom of other African and Asian snake, intentional self-harm

⑦T63.083   Toxic effect of venom of other African and Asian snake, assault

⑦T63.084   Toxic effect of venom of other African and Asian snake, undetermined

T63.09   Toxic effect of venom of other snake

⑦T63.091   Toxic effect of venom of other snake, accidental (unintentional)

Toxic effect of venom of other snake NOS

⑦T63.092   Toxic effect of venom of other snake, intentional self-harm

⑦T63.093   Toxic effect of venom of other snake, assault

⑦T63.094   Toxic effect of venom of other snake, undetermined

T63.1   Toxic effect of venom of other reptiles

T63.11   Toxic effect of venom of gila monster

⑦T63.111   Toxic effect of venom of gila monster, accidental (unintentional)

Toxic effect of venom of gila monster NOS

⑦T63.112   Toxic effect of venom of gila monster, intentional self-harm

⑦T63.113   Toxic effect of venom of gila monster, assault

⑦T63.114   Toxic effect of venom of gila monster, undetermined

T63.12   Toxic effect of venom of other venomous lizard

⑦T63.121   Toxic effect of venom of other venomous lizard, accidental (unintentional)

Toxic effect of venom of other venomous lizard NOS

⑦T63.122   Toxic effect of venom of other venomous lizard, intentional self-harm

⑦T63.123   Toxic effect of venom of other venomous lizard, assault

⑦T63.124   Toxic effect of venom of other venomous lizard, undetermined

T63.19   Toxic effect of venom of other reptiles

⑦T63.191   Toxic effect of venom of other reptiles, accidental (unintentional)

Toxic effect of venom of other reptiles NOS

⑦T63.192   Toxic effect of venom of other reptiles, intentional self-harm

⑦T63.193   Toxic effect of venom of other reptiles, assault

⑦T63.194   Toxic effect of venom of other reptiles, undetermined

T63.2   Toxic effect of venom of scorpion

T63.2X   Toxic effect of venom of scorpion

⑦T63.2X1   Toxic effect of venom of scorpion, accidental (unintentional)

Toxic effect of venom of scorpion NOS

⑦T63.2X2   Toxic effect of venom of scorpion, intentional self-harm

⑦T63.2X3   Toxic effect of venom of scorpion, assault

⑦T63.2X4   Toxic effect of venom of scorpion, undetermined

T63.3   Toxic effect of venom of spider

T63.30   Toxic effect of unspecified spider venom

⑦T63.301   Toxic effect of unspecified spider venom, accidental (unintentional)

⑦T63.302   Toxic effect of unspecified spider venom, intentional self-harm

● New code   ▲ Revised code   ⑦ 7th digit required   ⊗ Placeholder required

⑦T63.303 Toxic effect of unspecified spider venom, assault

⑦T63.304 Toxic effect of unspecified spider venom, undetermined

T63.31 Toxic effect of venom of black widow spider

⑦T63.311 Toxic effect of venom of black widow spider, accidental (unintentional)

⑦T63.312 Toxic effect of venom of black widow spider, intentional self-harm

⑦T63.313 Toxic effect of venom of black widow spider, assault

⑦T63.314 Toxic effect of venom of black widow spider, undetermined

T63.32 Toxic effect of venom of tarantula

⑦T63.321 Toxic effect of venom of tarantula, accidental (unintentional)

⑦T63.322 Toxic effect of venom of tarantula, intentional self-harm

⑦T63.323 Toxic effect of venom of tarantula, assault

⑦T63.324 Toxic effect of venom of tarantula, undetermined

T63.33 Toxic effect of venom of brown recluse spider

⑦T63.331 Toxic effect of venom of brown recluse spider, accidental (unintentional)

⑦T63.332 Toxic effect of venom of brown recluse spider, intentional self-harm

⑦T63.333 Toxic effect of venom of brown recluse spider, assault

⑦T63.334 Toxic effect of venom of brown recluse spider, undetermined

T63.39 Toxic effect of venom of other spider

⑦T63.391 Toxic effect of venom of other spider, accidental (unintentional)

⑦T63.392 Toxic effect of venom of other spider, intentional self-harm

⑦T63.393 Toxic effect of venom of other spider, assault

⑦T63.394 Toxic effect of venom of other spider, undetermined

T63.4 Toxic effect of venom of other arthropods

T63.41 Toxic effect of venom of centipedes and venomous millipedes

⑦T63.411 Toxic effect of venom of centipedes and venomous millipedes, accidental (unintentional)

⑦T63.412 Toxic effect of venom of centipedes and venomous millipedes, intentional self-harm

⑦T63.413 Toxic effect of venom of centipedes and venomous millipedes, assault

⑦T63.414 Toxic effect of venom of centipedes and venomous millipedes, undetermined

T63.42 Toxic effect of venom of ants

⑦T63.421 Toxic effect of venom of ants, accidental (unintentional)

⑦T63.422 Toxic effect of venom of ants, intentional self-harm

⑦T63.423 Toxic effect of venom of ants, assault

⑦T63.424 Toxic effect of venom of ants, undetermined

T63.43 Toxic effect of venom of caterpillars

⑦T63.431 Toxic effect of venom of caterpillars, accidental (unintentional)

⑦T63.432 Toxic effect of venom of caterpillars, intentional self-harm

⑦T63.433 Toxic effect of venom of caterpillars, assault

⑦T63.434 Toxic effect of venom of caterpillars, undetermined

T63.44 Toxic effect of venom of bees

⑦T63.441 Toxic effect of venom of bees, accidental (unintentional)

⑦T63.442 Toxic effect of venom of bees, intentional self-harm

⑦T63.443 Toxic effect of venom of bees, assault

⑦T63.444 Toxic effect of venom of bees, undetermined

T63.45 Toxic effect of venom of hornets

⑦T63.451 Toxic effect of venom of hornets, accidental (unintentional)

⑦T63.452 Toxic effect of venom of hornets, intentional self-harm

⑦T63.453 Toxic effect of venom of hornets, assault

⑦T63.454 Toxic effect of venom of hornets, undetermined

T63.46 Toxic effect of venom of wasps
Toxic effect of yellow jacket

⑦T63.461 Toxic effect of venom of wasps, accidental (unintentional)

⑦T63.462 Toxic effect of venom of wasps, intentional self-harm

⑦T63.463 Toxic effect of venom of wasps, assault

⑦T63.464 Toxic effect of venom of wasps, undetermined

T63.48 Toxic effect of venom of other arthropod

⑦T63.481 Toxic effect of venom of other arthropod, accidental (unintentional)

⑦T63.482 Toxic effect of venom of other arthropod, intentional self-harm

⑦T63.483 Toxic effect of venom of other arthropod, assault

⑦T63.484 Toxic effect of venom of other arthropod, undetermined

T63.5 Toxic effect of contact with venomous fish

Excludes 2: poisoning by ingestion of fish (T61-)

T63.51 Toxic effect of contact with stingray

⑦T63.511 Toxic effect of contact with stingray, accidental (unintentional)

⑦T63.512 Toxic effect of contact with stingray, intentional self-harm

⑦T63.513 Toxic effect of contact with stingray, assault

⑦T63.514 Toxic effect of contact with stingray, undetermined

T63.59 Toxic effect of contact with other venomous fish

⑦T63.591 Toxic effect of contact with other venomous fish, accidental (unintentional)

⑦T63.592 Toxic effect of contact with other venomous fish, intentional self-harm

⑦T63.593 Toxic effect of contact with other venomous fish, assault

⑦T63.594 Toxic effect of contact with other venomous fish, undetermined

T63.6 Toxic effect of contact with other venomous marine animals

Excludes 1: sea-snake venom (T63.09)

Excludes 2: poisoning by ingestion of shellfish (T61.78-)

T63.61 Toxic effect of contact with Portugese Man-o-war

Toxic effect of contact with bluebottle

⑦T63.611 Toxic effect of contact with Portuguese Man-o-war, accidental (unintentional)

⑦T63.612 Toxic effect of contact with Portuguese Man-o-war, intentional self-harm

⑦T63.613 Toxic effect of contact with Portuguese Man-o-war, assault

⑦T63.614 Toxic effect of contact with Portuguese Man-o-war, undetermined

T63.62 Toxic effect of contact with other jellyfish

⑦T63.621 Toxic effect of contact with other jellyfish, accidental (unintentional)

⑦T63.622 Toxic effect of contact with other jellyfish, intentional self-harm

⑦T63.623 Toxic effect of contact with other jellyfish, assault

⑦T63.624 Toxic effect of contact with other jellyfish, undetermined

T63.63 Toxic effect of contact with sea anemone

⑦T63.631 Toxic effect of contact with sea anemone, accidental (unintentional)

⑦T63.632 Toxic effect of contact with sea anemone, intentional self-harm

⑦T63.633 Toxic effect of contact with sea anemone, assault

⑦T63.634 Toxic effect of contact with sea anemone, undetermined

T63.69 Toxic effect of contact with other venomous marine animals

⑦T63.691 Toxic effect of contact with other venomous marine animals, accidental (unintentional)

⑦T63.692 Toxic effect of contact with other venomous marine animals, intentional self-harm

⑦T63.693 Toxic effect of contact with other venomous marine animals, assault

⑦T63.694 Toxic effect of contact with other venomous marine animals, undetermined

T63.7 Toxic effect of contact with venomous plant

T63.71 Toxic effect of contact with venomous marine plant

⑦T63.711 Toxic effect of contact with venomous marine plant, accidental (unintentional)

⑦T63.712 Toxic effect of contact with venomous marine plant, intentional self-harm

⑦T63.713 Toxic effect of contact with venomous marine plant, assault

⑦T63.714 Toxic effect of contact with venomous marine plant, undetermined

T63.79 Toxic effect of contact with other venomous plant

⑦T63.791 Toxic effect of contact with other venomous plant, accidental (unintentional)

⑦T63.792 Toxic effect of contact with other venomous plant, intentional self-harm

⑦T63.793 Toxic effect of contact with other venomous plant, assault

⑦T63.794 Toxic effect of contact with other venomous plant, undetermined

T63.8 Toxic effect of contact with other venomous animals

T63.81 Toxic effect of contact with venomous frog

Excludes 1: contact with nonvenomous frog (W62.0)

⑦T63.811 Toxic effect of contact with venomous frog, accidental (unintentional)

⑦T63.812 Toxic effect of contact with venomous frog, intentional self-harm

⑦T63.813 Toxic effect of contact with venomous frog, assault

⑦T63.814 Toxic effect of contact with venomous frog, undetermined

T63.82 Toxic effect of contact with venomous toad

Excludes 1: contact with nonvenomous toad (W62.1)

⑦T63.821 Toxic effect of contact with venomous toad, accidental (unintentional)

⑦T63.822 Toxic effect of contact with venomous toad, intentional self-harm

⑦T63.823 Toxic effect of contact with venomous toad, assault

⑦T63.824   Toxic effect of contact with venomous toad, undetermined

T63.83   Toxic effect of contact with other venomous amphibian

     Excludes 1: contact with nonvenomous amphibian (W62.9)

⑦T63.831   Toxic effect of contact with other venomous amphibian, accidental (unintentional)

⑦T63.832   Toxic effect of contact with other venomous amphibian, intentional self-harm

⑦T63.833   Toxic effect of contact with other venomous amphibian, assault

⑦T63.834   Toxic effect of contact with other venomous amphibian, undetermined

T63.89   Toxic effect of contact with other venomous animals

⑦T63.891   Toxic effect of contact with other venomous animals, accidental (unintentional)

⑦T63.892   Toxic effect of contact with other venomous animals, intentional self-harm

⑦T63.893   Toxic effect of contact with other venomous animals, assault

⑦T63.894   Toxic effect of contact with other venomous animals, undetermined

T63.9   Toxic effect of contact with unspecified venomous animal

⊗⑦T63.91   Toxic effect of contact with unspecified venomous animal, accidental (unintentional)

⊗⑦T63.92   Toxic effect of contact with unspecified venomous animal, intentional self-harm

⊗⑦T63.93   Toxic effect of contact with unspecified venomous animal, assault

⊗⑦T63.94   Toxic effect of contact with unspecified venomous animal, undetermined

T64   Toxic effect of aflatoxin and other mycotoxin food contaminants

The appropriate 7th character is to be added to each code from category T64

A - initial encounter

D - subsequent encounter

S - sequela

T64.0   Toxic effect of aflatoxin

⊗⑦T64.01   Toxic effect of aflatoxin, accidental (unintentional)

⊗⑦T64.02   Toxic effect of aflatoxin, intentional self-harm

⊗⑦T64.03   Toxic effect of aflatoxin, assault

⊗⑦T64.04   Toxic effect of aflatoxin, undetermined

T64.8   Toxic effect of other mycotoxin food contaminants

⊗⑦T64.81   Toxic effect of other mycotoxin food contaminants, accidental (unintentional)

⊗⑦T64.82   Toxic effect of other mycotoxin food contaminants, intentional self-harm

⊗⑦T64.83   Toxic effect of other mycotoxin food contaminants, assault

⊗⑦T64.84   Toxic effect of other mycotoxin food contaminants, undetermined

T65   Toxic effect of other and unspecified substances

The appropriate 7th character is to be added to each code from category T65

A - initial encounter

D - subsequent encounter

S - sequela

T65.0   Toxic effect of cyanides

     Excludes 1: hydrogen cyanide (T57.3-)

T65.0X   Toxic effect of cyanides

⑦T65.0X1   Toxic effect of cyanides, accidental (unintentional)

     Toxic effect of cyanides NOS

⑦T65.0X2   Toxic effect of cyanides, intentional self-harm

⑦T65.0X3   Toxic effect of cyanides, assault

⑦T65.0X4   Toxic effect of cyanides, undetermined

T65.1   Toxic effect of strychnine and its salts

T65.1X   Toxic effect of strychnine and its salts

⑦T65.1X1   Toxic effect of strychnine and its salts, accidental (unintentional)

     Toxic effect of strychnine and its salts NOS

⑦T65.1X2   Toxic effect of strychnine and its salts, intentional self-harm

⑦T65.1X3   Toxic effect of strychnine and its salts, assault

⑦T65.1X4   Toxic effect of strychnine and its salts, undetermined

T65.2   Toxic effect of tobacco and nicotine

     Excludes 2: nicotine dependence (F17.)

T65.21   Toxic effect of chewing tobacco

⑦T65.211   Toxic effect of chewing tobacco, accidental (unintentional)

     Toxic effect of chewing tobacco NOS

⑦T65.212   Toxic effect of chewing tobacco, intentional self-harm

⑦T65.213   Toxic effect of chewing tobacco, assault

⑦T65.214   Toxic effect of chewing tobacco, undetermined

T65.22   Toxic effect of tobacco cigarettes

     Toxic effect of tobacco smoke

     Use additional code for exposure to second hand tobacco smoke (Z57.31, Z77.22)

⑦T65.221   Toxic effect of tobacco cigarettes, accidental (unintentional)

     Toxic effect of tobacco cigarettes NOS

⑦T65.222   Toxic effect of tobacco cigarettes, intentional self-harm

⑦T65.223   Toxic effect of tobacco cigarettes, assault

⑦T65.224   Toxic effect of tobacco cigarettes, undetermined

T65.29   Toxic effect of other tobacco and nicotine

⑦T65.291   Toxic effect of other tobacco and nicotine, accidental (unintentional)

Toxic effect of other tobacco and
nicotine NOS

⑦ T65.292   Toxic effect of other tobacco and
nicotine, intentional self-harm

⑦ T65.293   Toxic effect of other tobacco and
nicotine, assault

⑦ T65.294   Toxic effect of other tobacco and
nicotine, undetermined

T65.3   Toxic effect of nitroderivatives and aminoderivatives of
benzene and its homologues

Toxic effect of anilin [benzeneamine]

Toxic effect of nitrobenzene

Toxic effect of trinitrotoluene

T65.3X   Toxic effect of nitroderivatives and
aminoderivatives of benzene and its homologues

⑦ T65.3X1   Toxic effect of nitroderivatives and
aminoderivatives of benzene and its
homologues, accidental
(unintentional)

Toxic effect of nitroderivatives and
aminoderivatives of benzene and its
homologues NOS

⑦ T65.3X2   Toxic effect of nitroderivatives and
aminoderivatives of benzene and its
homologues, intentional self-harm

⑦ T65.3X3   Toxic effect of nitroderivatives and
aminoderivatives of benzene and its
homologues, assault

⑦ T65.3X4   Toxic effect of nitroderivatives and
aminoderivatives of benzene and its
homologues, undetermined

T65.4   Toxic effect of carbon disulfide

T65.4X   Toxic effect of carbon disulfide

⑦ T65.4X1   Toxic effect of carbon disulfide,
accidental (unintentional)

Toxic effect of carbon disulfide
NOS

⑦ T65.4X2   Toxic effect of carbon disulfide,
intentional self-harm

⑦ T65.4X3   Toxic effect of carbon disulfide,
assault

⑦ T65.4X4   Toxic effect of carbon disulfide,
undetermined

T65.5   Toxic effect of nitroglycerin and other nitric acids and
esters

Toxic effect of 1,2,3-Propanetriol trinitrate

T65.5X   Toxic effect of nitroglycerin and other nitric
acids and esters

⑦ T65.5X1   Toxic effect of nitroglycerin and
other nitric acids and esters,
accidental (unintentional)

Toxic effect of nitroglycerin and
other nitric acids and esters NOS

⑦ T65.5X2   Toxic effect of nitroglycerin and
other nitric acids and esters,
intentional self-harm

⑦ T65.5X3   Toxic effect of nitroglycerin and
other nitric acids and esters, assault

⑦ T65.5X4   Toxic effect of nitroglycerin and
other nitric acids and esters,
undetermined

T65.6   Toxic effect of paints and dyes, not elsewhere classified

T65.6X   Toxic effect of paints and dyes, not elsewhere
classified

⑦ T65.6X1   Toxic effect of paints and dyes, not
elsewhere classified, accidental
(unintentional)

Toxic effect of paints and dyes NOS

⑦ T65.6X2   Toxic effect of paints and dyes, not
elsewhere classified, intentional
self-harm

⑦ T65.6X3   Toxic effect of paints and dyes, not
elsewhere classified, assault

⑦ T65.6X4   Toxic effect of paints and dyes, not
elsewhere classified, undetermined

T65.8   Toxic effect of other specified substances

T65.81   Toxic effect of latex

⑦ T65.811   Toxic effect of latex, accidental
(unintentional)

Toxic effect of latex NOS

⑦ T65.812   Toxic effect of latex, intentional
self-harm

⑦ T65.813   Toxic effect of latex, assault

⑦ T65.814   Toxic effect of latex, undetermined

T65.82   Toxic effect of harmful algae and algae toxins

Toxic effect of (harmful) algae bloom NOS

Toxic effect of blue-green algae bloom

Toxic effect of brown tide

Toxic effect of cyanobacteria bloom

Toxic effect of Florida red tide

Toxic effect of pfiesteria piscicida

Toxic effect of red tide

⑦ T65.821   Toxic effect of harmful algae and
algae toxins, accidental
(unintentional)

Toxic effect of harmful algae and
algae toxins NOS

⑦ T65.822   Toxic effect of harmful algae and
algae toxins, intentional self-harm

⑦ T65.823   Toxic effect of harmful algae and
algae toxins, assault

⑦ T65.824   Toxic effect of harmful algae and
algae toxins, undetermined

T65.83   Toxic effect of fiberglass

⑦ T65.831   Toxic effect of fiberglass, accidental
(unintentional)

Toxic effect of fiberglass NOS

⑦ T65.832   Toxic effect of fiberglass,
intentional self-harm

⑦ T65.833   Toxic effect of fiberglass, assault

⑦ T65.834   Toxic effect of fiberglass,
undetermined

T65.89   Toxic effect of other specified substances

⑦ T65.891   Toxic effect of other specified
substances, accidental
(unintentional)

Toxic effect of other specified substances NOS

⑦**T65.892** Toxic effect of other specified substances, intentional self-harm

⑦**T65.893** Toxic effect of other specified substances, assault

⑦**T65.894** Toxic effect of other specified substances, undetermined

T65.9 Toxic effect of unspecified substance

⊗⑦**T65.91** Toxic effect of unspecified substance, accidental (unintentional)
Poisoning NOS

⊗⑦**T65.92** Toxic effect of unspecified substance, intentional self-harm

⊗⑦**T65.93** Toxic effect of unspecified substance, assault

⊗⑦**T65.94** Toxic effect of unspecified substance, undetermined

OTHER AND UNSPECIFIED EFFECTS OF EXTERNAL CAUSES (T66-T78)

T66 Radiation sickness, unspecified

Excludes 1: specified adverse effects of radiation, such as:
burns (T20-T31)
leukemia (C91-C95)
radiation gastroenteritis and colitis (K52.0)
radiation pneumonitis (J70.0)
radiation related disorders of the skin and subcutaneous tissue (L55-L59)
sunburn (L55.-)

The appropriate 7th character is to be added to code T66

A - initial encounter

D - subsequent encounter

S - sequela

T67 Effects of heat and light

Excludes 1: erythema [dermatitis] ab igne (L59.0)
malignant hyperpyrexia due to anesthesia (T88.3)
radiation-related disorders of the skin and subcutaneous tissue (L55-L59)

Excludes 2: burns (T20-T31)
sunburn (L55.-)
sweat disorder due to heat (L74-L75)

The appropriate 7th character is to be added to each code from category T67

A - initial encounter

D - subsequent encounter

S - sequela

⊗⑦**T67.0** Heatstroke and sunstroke
Heat apoplexy
Heat pyrexia
Siriasis
Thermoplegia
Use additional code(s) to identify any associated complications of heatstroke, such as:
coma and stupor (R40.-)
systemic inflammatory response syndrome (R65.1-)

⊗⑦**T67.1** Heat syncope
Heat collapse

⊗⑦**T67.2** Heat cramp

⊗⑦**T67.3** Heat exhaustion, anhydrotic

Heat prostration due to water depletion
Excludes 1: heat exhaustion due to salt depletion (T67.4)

⊗⑦**T67.4** Heat exhaustion due to salt depletion
Heat prostration due to salt (and water) depletion

⊗⑦**T67.5** Heat exhaustion, unspecified
Heat prostration NOS

⊗⑦**T67.6** Heat fatigue, transient

⊗⑦**T67.7** Heat edema

⊗⑦**T67.8** Other effects of heat and light

⊗⑦**T67.9** Effect of heat and light, unspecified

T68 Hypothermia
Accidental hypothermia
Hypothermia NOS
Use additional code to identify source of exposure:
Exposure to excessive cold of man-made origin (W93)
Exposure to excessive cold of natural origin (X31)
Excludes 1: hypothermia following anesthesia (T88.51)
hypothermia not associated with low environmental temperature (R68.0)
hypothermia of newborn (P80.-)
Excludes 2: frostbite (T33-T34)

The appropriate 7th character is to be added to code T68

A - initial encounter

D - subsequent encounter

S - sequela

T69 Other effects of reduced temperature
Use additional code to identify source of exposure:
Exposure to excessive cold of man-made origin (W93)
Exposure to excessive cold of natural origin (X31)
Excludes 2: frostbite (T33-T34)

The appropriate 7th character is to be added to each code from category T69

A - initial encounter

D - subsequent encounter

S - sequela

T69.0 Immersion hand and foot

T69.01 Immersion hand

⑦**T69.011** Immersion hand, right hand

⑦**T69.012** Immersion hand, left hand

⑦**T69.019** Immersion hand, unspecified hand

T69.02 Immersion foot
Trench foot

⑦**T69.021** Immersion foot, right foot

⑦**T69.022** Immersion foot, left foot

⑦**T69.029** Immersion foot, unspecified foot

⊗⑦**T69.1** Chilblains

⊗⑦**T69.8** Other specified effects of reduced temperature

⊗⑦**T69.9** Effect of reduced temperature, unspecified

T70 Effects of air pressure and water pressure

The appropriate 7th character is to be added to each code from category T70

A - initial encounter

D - subsequent encounter

S - sequela

⊗⑦**T70.0** Otitic barotrauma
Aero-otitis media
Effects of change in ambient atmospheric pressure or water pressure on ears

⊗⑦**T70.1** Sinus barotrauma
Aerosinusitis
Effects of change in ambient atmospheric pressure on sinuses

T70.2 Other and unspecified effects of high altitude
Excludes 2: polycythemia due to high altitude (D75.1)

⊗⑦**T70.20** Unspecified effects of high altitude

⊗⑦**T70.29** Other effects of high altitude
Alpine sickness
Anoxia due to high altitude
Barotrauma NOS
Hypobaropathy
Mountain sickness

⊗⑦**T70.3** Caisson disease [decompression sickness]
Compressed-air disease
Diver's palsy or paralysis

⊗⑦**T70.4** Effects of high-pressure fluids
Hydraulic jet injection (industrial)
Pneumatic jet injection (industrial)
Traumatic jet injection (industrial)

⊗⑦**T70.8** Other effects of air pressure and water pressure

⊗⑦**T70.9** Effect of air pressure and water pressure, unspecified

T71 Asphyxiation
Mechanical suffocation
Traumatic suffocation
Excludes 1: acute respiratory distress (syndrome) (J80)
anoxia due to high altitude (T70.2)
asphyxia NOS (R09.01)
asphyxia from carbon monoxide (T58.-)
asphyxia from inhalation of food or foreign body (T17.-)
asphyxia from other gases, fumes and vapors (T59.-)
respiratory distress (syndrome) in newborn (P22.-)

The appropriate 7th character is to be added to each code from category T71

A - initial encounter

D - subsequent encounter

S - sequela

T71.1 Asphyxiation due to mechanical threat to breathing
Suffocation due to mechanical threat to breathing

T71.11 Asphyxiation due to smothering under pillow

⑦**T71.111** Asphyxiation due to smothering under pillow, accidental
Asphyxiation due to smothering under pillow NOS

⑦**T71.112** Asphyxiation due to smothering under pillow, intentional self-harm

⑦**T71.113** Asphyxiation due to smothering under pillow, assault

⑦**T71.114** Asphyxiation due to smothering under pillow, undetermined

T71.12 Asphyxiation due to plastic bag

⑦**T71.121** Asphyxiation due to plastic bag, accidental
Asphyxiation due to plastic bag NOS

⑦**T71.122** Asphyxiation due to plastic bag, intentional self-harm

⑦**T71.123** Asphyxiation due to plastic bag, assault

⑦**T71.124** Asphyxiation due to plastic bag, undetermined

T71.13 Asphyxiation due to being trapped in bed linens

⑦**T71.131** Asphyxiation due to being trapped in bed linens, accidental
Asphyxiation due to being trapped in bed linens NOS

⑦**T71.132** Asphyxiation due to being trapped in bed linens, intentional self-harm

⑦**T71.133** Asphyxiation due to being trapped in bed linens, assault

⑦**T71.134** Asphyxiation due to being trapped in bed linens, undetermined

T71.14 Asphyxiation due to smothering under another person's body (in bed)

⑦**T71.141** Asphyxiation due to smothering under another person's body (in bed), accidental
Asphyxiation due to smothering under another person's body (in bed) NOS

⑦**T71.143** Asphyxiation due to smothering under another person's body (in bed), assault

⑦**T71.144** Asphyxiation due to smothering under another person's body (in bed), undetermined

T71.15 Asphyxiation due to smothering in furniture

⑦**T71.151** Asphyxiation due to smothering in furniture, accidental
Asphyxiation due to smothering in furniture NOS

⑦**T71.152** Asphyxiation due to smothering in furniture, intentional self-harm

⑦**T71.153** Asphyxiation due to smothering in furniture, assault

⑦**T71.154** Asphyxiation due to smothering in furniture, undetermined

T71.16 Asphyxiation due to hanging
Hanging by window shade cord
Use additional code for any associated injuries, such as:
crushing injury of neck (S17.-)
fracture of cervical vertebrae (S12.0-S12.2-)
open wound of neck (S11.-)

⑦**T71.161** Asphyxiation due to hanging, accidental
Asphyxiation due to hanging NOS
Hanging NOS

⑦**T71.162** Asphyxiation due to hanging, intentional self-harm

⑦**T71.163** Asphyxiation due to hanging, assault

⑦**T71.164** Asphyxiation due to hanging, undetermined

T71.19 Asphyxiation due to mechanical threat to breathing due to other causes

⑦**T71.191** Asphyxiation due to mechanical threat to breathing due to other causes, accidental
Asphyxiation due to other causes NOS

⑦**T71.192** Asphyxiation due to mechanical threat to breathing due to other causes, intentional self-harm

⑦**T71.193** Asphyxiation due to mechanical threat to breathing due to other causes, assault

⑦**T71.194** Asphyxiation due to mechanical threat to breathing due to other causes, undetermined

T71.2 Asphyxiation due to systemic oxygen deficiency due to low oxygen content in ambient air
Suffocation due to systemic oxygen deficiency due to low oxygen content in ambient air

T71.20 Asphyxiation due to systemic oxygen deficiency due to low oxygen content in ambient air due to unspecified cause

T71.21 Asphyxiation due to cave-in or falling earth
Use additional code for any associated cataclysm (X34-X38)

T71.22 Asphyxiation due to being trapped in a car trunk

⑦**T71.221** Asphyxiation due to being trapped in a car trunk, accidental

⑦**T71.222** Asphyxiation due to being trapped in a car trunk, intentional self-harm

⑦**T71.223** Asphyxiation due to being trapped in a car trunk, assault

⑦**T71.224** Asphyxiation due to being trapped in a car trunk, undetermined

T71.23 Asphyxiation due to being trapped in a (discarded) refrigerator

⑦**T71.231** Asphyxiation due to being trapped in a (discarded) refrigerator, accidental

⑦**T71.232** Asphyxiation due to being trapped in a (discarded) refrigerator, intentional self-harm

⑦**T71.233** Asphyxiation due to being trapped in (discarded) refrigerator, assault

⑦**T71.234** Asphyxiation due to being trapped in a (discarded) refrigerator, undetermined

T71.29 Asphyxiation due to being trapped in other low oxygen environment

T71.9 Asphyxiation due to unspecified cause
Suffocation (by strangulation) due to unspecified cause
Suffocation NOS
Systemic oxygen deficiency due to low oxygen content in ambient air due to unspecified cause
Systemic oxygen deficiency due to mechanical threat to breathing due to unspecified cause
Traumatic asphyxia NOS

T73 Effects of other deprivation
The appropriate 7th character is to be added to each code from category T73
A - initial encounter

D - subsequent encounter
S - sequela

⊗⑦**T73.0** Starvation
Deprivation of food

⊗⑦**T73.1** Deprivation of water

⊗⑦**T73.2** Exhaustion due to exposure

⊗⑦**T73.3** Exhaustion due to excessive exertion
Exhaustion due to overexertion

⊗⑦**T73.8** Other effects of deprivation

⊗⑦**T73.9** Effect of deprivation, unspecified

T74 Adult and child abuse, neglect and other maltreatment, confirmed
Use additional code, if applicable, to identify any associated current injury external cause code to identify perpetrator, if known (Y07.-)
Excludes 1: abuse and maltreatment in pregnancy (O9A.3-, O9A.4-, O9A.5-)
adult and child maltreatment, suspected (T76.-)
The appropriate 7th character is to be added to each code from category T74
A - initial encounter
D - subsequent encounter
S - sequela

T74.0 Neglect or abandonment, confirmed

⊗⑦**T74.01** Adult neglect or abandonment, confirmed

⊗⑦**T74.02** Child neglect or abandonment, confirmed

T74.1 Physical abuse, confirmed
Excludes 2: sexual abuse (T74.2-)

⊗⑦**T74.11** Adult physical abuse, confirmed

⊗⑦**T74.12** Child physical abuse, confirmed
Excludes 2: shaken infant syndrome (T74.4)

T74.2 Sexual abuse, confirmed
Rape, confirmed
Sexual assault, confirmed

⊗⑦**T74.21** Adult sexual abuse, confirmed

⊗⑦**T74.22** Child sexual abuse, confirmed

T74.3 Psychological abuse, confirmed

⊗⑦**T74.31** Adult psychological abuse, confirmed

⊗⑦**T74.32** Child psychological abuse, confirmed

T74.4 Shaken infant syndrome

T74.9 Unspecified maltreatment, confirmed

⊗⑦**T74.91** Unspecified adult maltreatment, confirmed

⊗⑦**T74.92** Unspecified child maltreatment, confirmed

T75 Other and unspecified effects of other external causes
Excludes 1: adverse effects NEC (T78.-)
Excludes 2: burns (electric) (T20-T31)
The appropriate 7th character is to be added to each code from category T75
A - initial encounter
D - subsequent encounter
S - sequela

T75.0 Effects of lightning
Struck by lightning

⊗⑦**T75.00** Unspecified effects of lightning
Struck by lightning NOS

⊗⑦**T75.01** Shock due to being struck by lightning

⊗⑦**T75.09** Other effects of lightning
Use additional code for other effects of lightning

T75.1 Unspecified effects of drowning and nonfatal submersion
Immersion

Excludes 1: specified effects of drowning- code to effects

T75.2   Effects of vibration

   ⊗⑦**T75.20**   Unspecified effects of vibration

   ⊗⑦**T75.21**   Pneumatic hammer syndrome

   ⊗⑦**T75.22**   Traumatic vasospastic syndrome

   ⊗⑦**T75.23**   Vertigo from infrasound

       Excludes 1: vertigo NOS (R42)

   ⊗⑦**T75.29**   Other effects of vibration

⊗⑦**T75.3**   Motion sickness

   Airsickness

   Seasickness

   Travel sickness

   Use additional external cause code to identify vehicle or type of motion (Y92.81-, Y93.5-)

⊗⑦**T75.4**   Electrocution

   Shock from electric current

   Shock from electroshock gun (taser)

T75.8   Other specified effects of external causes

   ⊗⑦**T75.81**   Effects of abnormal gravitation [G] forces

   ⊗⑦**T75.82**   Effects of weightlessness

   ⊗⑦**T75.89**   Other specified effects of external causes

T76   Adult and child abuse, neglect and other maltreatment, suspected

Use additional code, if applicable, to identify any associated current injury

Excludes 1: adult and child maltreatment, confirmed (T74.-)

       suspected abuse and maltreatment in pregnancy (O9A.3-, O9A.4-, O9A.5-)

       suspected adult physical abuse, ruled out (Z04.71)

       suspected adult sexual abuse, ruled out (Z04.41)

       suspected child physical abuse, ruled out (Z04.72)

       suspected child sexual abuse, ruled out (Z04.42)

The appropriate 7th character is to be added to each code from category T76

A - initial encounter

D - subsequent encounter

S - sequela

T76.0   Neglect or abandonment, suspected

   ⊗⑦**T76.01**   Adult neglect or abandonment, suspected

   ⊗⑦**T76.02**   Child neglect or abandonment, suspected

T76.1   Physical abuse, suspected

   ⊗⑦**T76.11**   Adult physical abuse, suspected

   ⊗⑦**T76.12**   Child physical abuse, suspected

T76.2   Sexual abuse, suspected

   Rape, suspected

   Sexual abuse, suspected

   Excludes 1: alleged abuse, ruled out (Z04.7)

   ⊗⑦**T76.21**   Adult sexual abuse, suspected

   ⊗⑦**T76.22**   Child sexual abuse, suspected

T76.3   Psychological abuse, suspected

   ⊗⑦**T76.31**   Adult psychological abuse, suspected

   ⊗⑦**T76.32**   Child psychological abuse, suspected

T76.9   Unspecified maltreatment, suspected

   ⊗⑦**T76.91**   Unspecified adult maltreatment, suspected

   ⊗⑦**T76.92**   Unspecified child maltreatment, suspected

T78   Adverse effects, not elsewhere classified

Excludes 2: complications of surgical and medical care NEC (T80-T88)

The appropriate 7th character is to be added to each code from category T78

A - initial encounter

D - subsequent encounter

S - sequela

T78.0   Anaphylactic reaction due to food

   Anaphylactic reaction due to adverse food reaction

   Anaphylactic shock or reaction due to nonpoisonous foods

   Anaphylactoid reaction due to food

   ⊗⑦**T78.00**   Anaphylactic reaction due to unspecified food

   ⊗⑦**T78.01**   Anaphylactic reaction due to peanuts

   ⊗⑦**T78.02**   Anaphylactic reaction due to shellfish (crustaceans)

   ⊗⑦**T78.03**   Anaphylactic reaction due to other fish

   ⊗⑦**T78.04**   Anaphylactic reaction due to fruits and vegetables

   ⊗⑦**T78.05**   Anaphylactic reaction due to tree nuts and seeds

       Excludes 1: anaphylactic reaction due to peanuts (T78.01)

   ⊗⑦**T78.06**   Anaphylactic reaction due to food additives

   ⊗⑦**T78.07**   Anaphylactic reaction due to milk and dairy products

   ⊗⑦**T78.08**   Anaphylactic reaction due to eggs

   ⊗⑦**T78.09**   Anaphylactic reaction due to other food products

T78.1   Other adverse food reactions, not elsewhere classified

Use additional code to identify the type of reaction

Excludes 1: anaphylactic reaction or shock due to adverse food reaction (T78.0-)

       anaphylactic reaction due to food (T78.0-)

       bacterial food borne intoxications (A05.-)

Excludes 2: allergic and dietetic gastroenteritis and colitis (K52.2)

       allergic rhinitis due to food (J30.5)

       dermatitis due to food in contact with skin (L23.6, L24.6, L25.4)

       dermatitis due to ingested food (L27.2)

⊗⑦**T78.2**   Anaphylactic shock, unspecified

   Allergic shock

   Anaphylactic reaction

   Anaphylaxis

   Excludes 1: anaphylactic reaction or shock due to adverse effect of correct medicinal substance properly administered (T88.6)

       anaphylactic reaction or shock due to adverse food reaction (T78.0-)

       anaphylactic reaction or shock due to serum (T80.5-)

⊗⑦**T78.3**   Angioneurotic edema

   Allergic angioedema

   Giant urticaria

   Quincke's edema

   Excludes 1: serum urticaria (T80.6-)

       urticaria (L50.-)

T78.4   Other and unspecified allergy

   Excludes 1: specified types of allergic reaction such as:

       allergic diarrhea (K52.2)

       allergic gastroenteritis and colitis (K52.2)

       dermatitis (L23-L25, L27.-)

hay fever (J30.1)

⊗⑦**T78.40** Allergy, unspecified

Allergic reaction NOS

Hypersensitivity NOS

⊗⑦**T78.41** Arthus phenomenon

Arthus reaction

⊗⑦**T78.49** Other allergy

T78.8 Other adverse effects, not elsewhere classified

CERTAIN EARLY COMPLICATIONS OF TRAUMA (T79)

T79 Certain early complications of trauma, not elsewhere classified

Excludes 2: acute respiratory distress syndrome (J80)

complications occurring during or following medical procedures (T80-T88)

complications of surgical and medical care NEC (T80-T88)

newborn respiratory distress syndrome (P22.0)

The appropriate 7th character is to be added to each code from category T79

A - initial encounter

D - subsequent encounter

S - sequela

⊗⑦**T79.0** Air embolism (traumatic)

Excludes 1: air embolism complicating:

abortion or ectopic or molar pregnancy (O00-O07, O08.2)

pregnancy, childbirth and the puerperium (O88.0)

air embolism following:

infusion, transfusion, and therapeutic injection (T80.0)

procedure NEC (T81.7-)

⊗⑦**T79.1** Fat embolism (traumatic)

Excludes 1: fat embolism complicating:

abortion or ectopic or molar pregnancy (O00-O07, O08.2)

pregnancy, childbirth and the puerperium (O88.8)

⊗⑦**T79.2** Traumatic secondary and recurrent hemorrhage and seroma

⊗⑦**T79.4** Traumatic shock

Shock (immediate) (delayed) following injury

Excludes 1: anaphylactic shock due to adverse food reaction (T78.0-)

anaphylactic shock due to correct medicinal substance properly administered (T88.6)

anaphylactic shock due to serum (T80.5-)

anaphylactic shock NOS (T78.2)

anesthetic shock (T88.2)

electric shock (T75.4)

nontraumatic shock NEC (R57.-)

obstetric shock (O75.1)

postprocedural shock (T81.1-)

septic shock (R65.21)

shock complicating abortion or ectopic or molar pregnancy (O00-O07, O08.3)

shock due to lightning (T75.01)

shock NOS (R57.9)

⊗⑦**T79.5** Traumatic anuria

Crush syndrome

Renal failure following crushing

⊗⑦**T79.6** Traumatic ischemia of muscle

Traumatic rhabdomyolysis

Volkmann's ischemic contracture

Excludes 2: anterior tibial syndrome (M76.8)

compartment syndrome (traumatic) (T79.A-)

nontraumatic ischemia of muscle (M62.2-)

⊗⑦**T79.7** Traumatic subcutaneous emphysema

Excludes 1: emphysema NOS (J43)

emphysema (subcutaneous) resulting from a procedure (T81.82)

⊗⑦**T79.A** Traumatic compartment syndrome

Excludes 1: fibromyalgia (M79.7)

nontraumatic compartment syndrome (M79.A-)

traumatic ischemic infarction of muscle (T79.6)

⊗⑦**T79.A0** Compartment syndrome, unspecified

Compartment syndrome NOS

⊗⑦**T79.A1** Traumatic compartment syndrome of upper extremity

Traumatic compartment syndrome of shoulder, arm, forearm, wrist, hand, and fingers

⑦**T79.A11** Traumatic compartment syndrome of right upper extremity

⑦**T79.A12** Traumatic compartment syndrome of left upper extremity

⑦**T79.A19** Traumatic compartment syndrome of unspecified upper extremity

⊗⑦**T79.A2** Traumatic compartment syndrome of lower extremity

Traumatic compartment syndrome of hip, buttock, thigh, leg, foot, and toes

⑦**T79.A21** Traumatic compartment syndrome of right lower extremity

⑦**T79.A22** Traumatic compartment syndrome of left lower extremity

⑦**T79.A29** Traumatic compartment syndrome of unspecified lower extremity

⊗⑦**T79.A3** Traumatic compartment syndrome of abdomen

⊗⑦**T79.A9** Traumatic compartment syndrome of other sites

⊗⑦**T79.8** Other early complications of trauma

⊗⑦**T79.9** Unspecified early complication of trauma

COMPLICATIONS OF SURGICAL AND MEDICAL CARE, NOT ELSEWHERE CLASSIFIED (T80-T88)

Use additional code for adverse effect, if applicable, to identify drug (T36-T50 with fifth or sixth character 5)

Use additional code(s) to identify the specified condition resulting from the complication

Use additional code to identify devices involved and details of circumstances (Y62-Y82)

Excludes 2: any encounters with medical care for postprocedural conditions in which no complications are present, such as:

artificial opening status (Z93.-)

closure of external stoma (Z43.-)

fitting and adjustment of external prosthetic device (Z44.-)

burns and corrosions from local applications and irradiation (T20-T32)

Add 4th-7th digits	3 digit reportable	Nonspecific code	Unspecified code	Manifestation code

complications of surgical procedures during pregnancy, childbirth and the puerperium (O00-O9A)

mechanical complication of respirator [ventilator] (J95.850)

poisoning and toxic effects of drugs and chemicals (T36-T65 with fifth or sixth character 1-4 or 6)

postprocedural fever (R50.82)

specified complications classified elsewhere, such as:

  cerebrospinal fluid leak from spinal puncture (G97.0)

  colostomy malfunction (K94.0-)

  disorders of fluid and electrolyte imbalance (E86- E87)

  functional disturbances following cardiac surgery (I97.0-I97.1)

  intraoperative and postprocedural complications of specified body systems (D78.-, E36.-, E89.-, G97.3-, G97.4, H59.3-, H59.-, H95.2-, H95.3, I97.4-, I97.5, J95.6-, J95.7, K91.6-, L76.-, M96.-, N99.-)

  ostomy complications (J95.0-, K94-, N99.5-)

  postgastric surgery syndromes (K91.1)

  postlaminectomy syndrome NEC (M96.1)

  postmastectomy lymphedema syndrome (I97.2)

  postsurgical blind-loop syndrome (K91.2)

  ventilator associated pneumonia (J95.851)

T80 Complications following infusion, transfusion and therapeutic injection

Includes: complications following perfusion

Excludes 2: bone marrow transplant rejection (T86.01)

        febrile nonhemolytic transfusion reaction (R50.84)

        fluid overload due to transfusion (E87.71)

        posttransfusion purpura (D69.51)

        transfusion associated circulatory overload (TACO) (E87.71)

        transfusion (red blood cell) associated hemochromatosis (E83.111)

        transfusion related acute lung injury (TRALI) (J95.84)

The appropriate 7th character is to be added to each code from category T80

A - initial encounter

D - subsequent encounter

S - sequela

⊗⑦ **T80.0** Air embolism following infusion, transfusion and therapeutic injection

⊗⑦ **T80.1** Vascular complications following infusion, transfusion and therapeutic injection

Use additional code to identify the vascular complication

Excludes 2: extravasation of vesicant agent (T80.81-)

        infiltration of vesicant agent (T80.81-)

        vascular complications specified as due to prosthetic devices, implants and grafts (T82.8-, T83.8, T84.8-, T85.8)

        postprocedural vascular complications (T81.7-)

⊗⑦ **T80.2** Infections following infusion, transfusion and therapeutic injection

Use additional code to identify the specific infection, such as:

  sepsis (A41.9)

Use additional code (R65.2-) to identify severe sepsis, if applicable

Excludes 2: infections specified as due to prosthetic devices, implants and grafts (T82.6-T82.7, T83.5-T83.6, T84.5-T84.7, T85.7)

postprocedural infections (T81.4)

⊗⑦ **T80.21** Infection due to central venous catheter

⑦ **T80.211** Bloodstream infection due to central venous catheter

Catheter-related bloodstream infection (CRBSI) NOS

Central line-associated bloodstream infection (CLABSI)

Bloodstream infection due to Hickman catheter

Bloodstream infection due to peripherally inserted central catheter (PICC)

Bloodstream infection due to portacath (port-a-cath)

Bloodstream infection due to triple lumen catheter

Bloodstream infection due to umbilical venous catheter

⑦ **T80.212** Local infection due to central venous catheter

Exit or insertion site infection

Local infection due to Hickman catheter

Local infection due to peripherally inserted central catheter (PICC)

Local infection due to portacath (port-a-cath)

Local infection due to triple lumen catheter

Local infection due to umbilical venous catheter

Port or reservoir infection

Tunnel infection

⑦ **T80.218** Other infection due to central venous catheter

Other central line-associated infection

Other infection due to Hickman catheter

Other infection due to peripherally inserted central catheter (PICC)

Other infection due to portacath (port-a-cath)

Other infection due to triple lumen catheter

Other infection due to umbilical venous catheter

⑦ **T80.219** Unspecified infection due to central venous catheter

Central line-associated infection NOS

Unspecified infection due to Hickman catheter

Unspecified infection due to peripherally inserted central catheter (PICC)

Unspecified infection due to portacath (port-a-cath)

Unspecified infection due to triple lumen catheter

● New code   ▲ Revised code   ⑦ 7th digit required   ⊗ Placeholder required

Unspecified infection due to umbilical venous catheter

⊗⑦**T80.22** Acute infection following transfusion, infusion, or injection of blood and blood products

⊗⑦**T80.29** Infection following other infusion, transfusion and therapeutic injection

⊗⑦**T80.3** ABO incompatibility reaction due to transfusion of blood or blood products

Excludes 1: minor blood group antigens reactions (Duffy) (E) (K(ell)) (Kidd) (Lewis) (M) (N) (P) (S) (T80.A)

⊗⑦**T80.30** ABO incompatibility reaction due to transfusion of blood or blood products, unspecified

ABO incompatibility blood transfusion NOS

Reaction to ABO incompatibility from transfusion NOS

⑦**T80.31** ABO incompatibility with hemolytic transfusion reaction

⑦**T80.310** ABO incompatibility with acute hemolytic transfusion reaction

ABO incompatibility with hemolytic transfusion reaction less than 24 hours after transfusion

Acute hemolytic transfusion reaction (AHTR) due to ABO incompatibility

⑦**T80.311** ABO incompatibility with delayed hemolytic transfusion reaction

ABO incompatibility with hemolytic transfusion reaction 24 hours or more after transfusion

Delayed hemolytic transfusion reaction (DHTR) due to ABO incompatibility

⑦**T80.319** ABO incompatibility with hemolytic transfusion reaction, unspecified

ABO incompatibility with hemolytic transfusion reaction at unspecified time after transfusion

Hemolytic transfusion reaction (HTR) due to ABO incompatibility NOS

⊗⑦**T80.39** Other ABO incompatibility reaction due to transfusion of blood or blood products

Delayed serologic transfusion reaction (DSTR) from ABO incompatibility

Other ABO incompatible blood transfusion

Other reaction to ABO incompatible blood transfusion

T80.4 Rh incompatibility reaction due to transfusion of blood or blood products

Reaction due to incompatibility of Rh antigens (C) (c) (D) (E) (e)

⊗⑦**T80.40** Rh incompatibility reaction due to transfusion of blood or blood products, unspecified

Reaction due to Rh factor in transfusion NOS

Rh incompatible blood transfusion NOS

T80.41 Rh incompatibility with hemolytic transfusion reaction

⑦**T80.410** Rh incompatibility with acute hemolytic transfusion reaction

Acute hemolytic transfusion reaction (AHTR) due to Rh incompatibility

Rh incompatibility with hemolytic transfusion reaction less than 24 hours after transfusion

⑦**T80.411** Rh incompatibility with delayed hemolytic transfusion reaction

Delayed hemolytic transfusion reaction (DHTR) due to Rh incompatibility

Rh incompatibility with hemolytic transfusion reaction 24 hours or more after transfusion

⑦**T80.419** Rh incompatibility with hemolytic transfusion reaction, unspecified

Rh incompatibility with hemolytic transfusion reaction at unspecified time after transfusion

Hemolytic transfusion reaction (HTR) due to Rh incompatibility NOS

⊗⑦**T80.49** Other Rh incompatibility reaction due to transfusion of blood or blood products

Delayed serologic transfusion reaction (DSTR) from Rh incompatibility

Other reaction to Rh incompatible blood transfusion

T80.A Non-ABO incompatibility reaction due to transfusion of blood or blood products

Reaction due to incompatibility of minor antigens (Duffy) (Kell) (Kidd) (Lewis) (M) (N) (P) (S)

⊗⑦**T80.A0** Non-ABO incompatibility reaction due to transfusion of blood or blood products, unspecified

Non-ABO antigen incompatibility reaction from transfusion NOS

T80.A1 Non-ABO incompatibility with hemolytic transfusion reaction

⑦**T80.A10** Non-ABO incompatibility with acute hemolytic transfusion reaction

Acute hemolytic transfusion reaction (AHTR) due to non-ABO incompatibility

Non-ABO incompatibility with hemolytic transfusion reaction less than 24 hours after transfusion

⑦**T80.A11** Non-ABO incompatibility with delayed hemolytic transfusion reaction

Delayed hemolytic transfusion reaction (DHTR) due to non-ABO incompatibility

Non-ABO incompatibility with hemolytic transfusion reaction 24 or more hours after transfusion

⑦**T80.A19** Non-ABO incompatibility with hemolytic transfusion reaction, unspecified

Hemolytic transfusion reaction (HTR) due to non-ABO incompatibility NOS

Non-ABO incompatibility with hemolytic transfusion reaction at unspecified time after transfusion

⊗⑦**T80.A9** Other non-ABO incompatibility reaction due to transfusion of blood or blood products

Delayed serologic transfusion reaction (DSTR) from non-ABO incompatibility

Other reaction to non-ABO incompatible blood transfusion

T80.5 Anaphylactic reaction due to serum

Allergic shock due to serum

Anaphylactic shock due to serum

Anaphylactoid reaction due to serum

Anaphylaxis due to serum

Excludes 1: ABO incompatibility reaction due to transfusion of blood or blood products (T80.3-)

allergic reaction or shock NOS (T78.2)

anaphylactic reaction or shock NOS (T78.2)

anaphylactic reaction or shock due to adverse effect of correct medicinal substance properly administered (T88.6)

other serum reaction (T80.6-)

⊗⑦**T80.51** Anaphylactic reaction due to administration of blood and blood products

⊗⑦**T80.52** Anaphylactic reaction due to vaccination

⊗⑦**T80.59** Anaphylactic reaction due to other serum

T80.6 Other serum reactions

Intoxication by serum

Protein sickness

Serum rash

Serum sickness

Serum urticaria

Excludes 2: serum hepatitis (B16.-)

⊗⑦**T80.61** Other serum reaction due to administration of blood and blood products

⊗⑦**T80.62** Other serum reaction due to vaccination

⊗⑦**T80.69** Other serum reaction due to other serum

T80.8 Other complications following infusion, transfusion and therapeutic injection

T80.81 Extravasation of vesicant agent

Infiltration of vesicant agent

⑦**T80.810** Extravasation of vesicant antineoplastic chemotherapy

Infiltration of vesicant antineoplastic chemotherapy

⑦**T80.818** Extravasation of other vesicant agent

Infiltration of other vesicant agent

⊗⑦**T80.89** Other complications following infusion, transfusion and therapeutic injection

Delayed serologic transfusion reaction (DSTR), unspecified incompatibility

Use additional code to identify graft-versus-host reaction, if applicable, (D89.81-)

T80.9 Unspecified complication following infusion, transfusion and therapeutic injection

⊗⑦**T80.90** Unspecified complication following infusion and therapeutic injection

T80.91 Hemolytic transfusion reaction, unspecified incompatibility

Excludes 1: ABO incompatibility with hemolytic transfusion reaction (T80.31-)

Non-ABO incompatibility with hemolytic transfusion reaction (T80.A1-)

Rh incompatibility with hemolytic transfusion reaction (T80.41-)

⑦**T80.910** Acute hemolytic transfusion reaction, unspecified incompatibility

⑦**T80.911** Delayed hemolytic transfusion reaction, unspecified incompatibility

⑦**T80.919** Hemolytic transfusion reaction, unspecified incompatibility, unspecified as acute or delayed

Hemolytic transfusion reaction NOS

⊗⑦**T80.92** Unspecified transfusion reaction

Transfusion reaction NOS

T81 Complications of procedures, not elsewhere classified

Use additional code for adverse effect, if applicable, to identify drug (T36-T50 with fifth or sixth character 5)

Excludes 2: complications following immunization (T88.0-T88.1)

complications following infusion, transfusion and therapeutic injection (T80.-)

complications of transplanted organs and tissue (T86.-)

specified complications classified elsewhere, such as:

complication of prosthetic devices, implants and grafts (T82-T85)

dermatitis due to drugs and medicaments (L23.3, L24.4, L25.1, L27.0-L27.1)

endosseous dental implant failure (M27.6-)

floppy iris syndrome (IFIS) (intraoperative) H21.81

intraoperative and postprocedural complications of specific body system (D78.-, E36.-, E89.-, G97.3-, G97.4, H59.3-, H59.-, H95.2-, H95.3, I97.4-, I97.5, J95, K91-, L76.-, M96.-, N99.-)

ostomy complications (J95.0-, K94.-, N99.5-)

plateau iris syndrome (post-iridectomy) (postprocedural) H21.82

poisoning and toxic effects of drugs and chemicals (T36-T65 with fifth or sixth character 1-4or 6)

The appropriate 7th character is to be added to each code from category T81

A - initial encounter

D - subsequent encounter

S - sequela

T81.1 Postprocedural shock

Shock during or resulting from a procedure, not elsewhere classified

Excludes 1: anaphylactic shock NOS (T78.2)

anaphylactic shock due to correct substance properly administered (T88.6)

anaphylactic shock due to serum (T80.5-)

anesthetic shock (T88.2)

electric shock (T75.4)

obstetric shock (O75.1)

septic shock (R65.21)

shock following abortion or ectopic or molar pregnancy (O00-O07, O08.3) traumatic shock (T79.4)

⊗⑦**T81.10** Postprocedural shock unspecified

Collapse NOS during or resulting from a procedure, not elsewhere classified

Postprocedural failure of peripheral circulation

Postprocedural shock NOS

⊗⑦**T81.11** Postprocedural cardiogenic shock

⊗⑦**T81.12** Postprocedural septic shock

Postprocedural endotoxic shock during or resulting from a procedure, not elsewhere classified

Postprocedural gram-negative shock during or resulting from a procedure, not elsewhere classified

Code first underlying infection

Use additional code, to identify any associated acute organ dysfunction, if applicable

⊗⑦**T81.19** Other postprocedural shock

Postprocedural hypovolemic shock

T81.3 Disruption of wound, not elsewhere classified

Disruption of any suture materials or other closure methods

Excludes 1: breakdown (mechanical) of permanent sutures (T85.612)

displacement of permanent sutures (T85.622)

disruption of cesarean delivery wound (O90.0)

disruption of perineal obstetric wound (O90.1)

mechanical complication of permanent sutures NEC (T85.692)

⊗⑦**T81.30** Disruption of wound, unspecified

Disruption of wound NOS

⊗⑦**T81.31** Disruption of external operation (surgical) wound, not elsewhere classified

Dehiscence of operation wound NOS

Disruption of operation wound NOS

Disruption or dehiscence of closure of cornea

Disruption or dehiscence of closure of mucosa

Disruption or dehiscence of closure of skin and subcutaneous tissue

Full-thickness skin disruption or dehiscence

Superficial disruption or dehiscence of operation wound

Excludes 1: dehiscence of amputation stump (T87.81)

⊗⑦**T81.32** Disruption of internal operation (surgical) wound, not elsewhere classified

Deep disruption or dehiscence of operation wound NOS

Disruption or dehiscence of closure of internal organ or other internal tissue

Disruption or dehiscence of closure of muscle or muscle flap

Disruption or dehiscence of closure of ribs or rib cage

Disruption or dehiscence of closure of skull or craniotomy

Disruption or dehiscence of closure of sternum or sternotomy

Disruption or dehiscence of closure of tendon or ligament

Disruption or dehiscence of closure of superficial or muscular fascia

⊗⑦**T81.33** Disruption of traumatic injury wound repair

Disruption or dehiscence of closure of traumatic laceration (external) (internal)

⊗⑦**T81.4** Infection following a procedure

Intra-abdominal abscess following a procedure

Postprocedural infection, not elsewhere classified

Sepsis following a procedure

Stitch abscess following a procedure

Subphrenic abscess following a procedure

Wound abscess following a procedure

Use additional code to identify infection

Use additional code (R65.2-) to identify severe sepsis, if applicable

Excludes 1: obstetric surgical wound infection (O86.0)

postprocedural fever NOS (R50.82)

postprocedural retroperitoneal abscess (K68.11)

Excludes 2: bleb associated endophthalmitis (H59.4-)

infection due to infusion, transfusion and therapeutic injection (T80.2-)

infection due to prosthetic devices, implants and grafts (T82.6-T82.7, T83.5-T83.6, T84.5-T84.7, T85.7)

T81.5 Complications of foreign body accidentally left in body following procedure

T81.50 Unspecified complication of foreign body accidentally left in body following procedure

⑦**T81.500** Unspecified complication of foreign body accidentally left in body following surgical operation

⑦**T81.501** Unspecified complication of foreign body accidentally left in body following infusion or transfusion

⑦**T81.502** Unspecified complication of foreign body accidentally left in body following kidney dialysis

⑦**T81.503** Unspecified complication of foreign body accidentally left in body following injection or immunization

⑦**T81.504** Unspecified complication of foreign body accidentally left in body following endoscopic examination

⑦**T81.505** Unspecified complication of foreign body accidentally left in body following heart catheterization

⑦**T81.506** Unspecified complication of foreign body accidentally left in body following aspiration, puncture or other catheterization

⑦**T81.507** Unspecified complication of foreign body accidentally left in body following removal of catheter or packing

⑦**T81.508** Unspecified complication of foreign body accidentally left in body following other procedure

⑦**T81.509** Unspecified complication of foreign body accidentally left in body following unspecified procedure

T81.51   Adhesions due to foreign body accidentally left in body following procedure

⑦T81.510   Adhesions due to foreign body accidentally left in body following surgical operation

⑦T81.511   Adhesions due to foreign body accidentally left in body following infusion or transfusion

⑦T81.512   Adhesions due to foreign body accidentally left in body following kidney dialysis

⑦T81.513   Adhesions due to foreign body accidentally left in body following injection or immunization

⑦T81.514   Adhesions due to foreign body accidentally left in body following endoscopic examination

⑦T81.515   Adhesions due to foreign body accidentally left in body following heart catheterization

⑦T81.516   Adhesions due to foreign body accidentally left in body following aspiration, puncture or other catheterization

⑦T81.517   Adhesions due to foreign body accidentally left in body following removal of catheter or packing

⑦T81.518   Adhesions due to foreign body accidentally left in body following other procedure

⑦T81.519   Adhesions due to foreign body accidentally left in body following unspecified procedure

T81.52   Obstruction due to foreign body accidentally left in body following procedure

⑦T81.520   Obstruction due to foreign body accidentally left in body following surgical operation

⑦T81.521   Obstruction due to foreign body accidentally left in body following infusion or transfusion

⑦T81.522   Obstruction due to foreign body accidentally left in body following kidney dialysis

⑦T81.523   Obstruction due to foreign body accidentally left in body following injection or immunization

⑦T81.524   Obstruction due to foreign body accidentally left in body following endoscopic examination

⑦T81.525   Obstruction due to foreign body accidentally left in body following heart catheterization

⑦T81.526   Obstruction due to foreign body accidentally left in body following aspiration, puncture or other catheterization

⑦T81.527   Obstruction due to foreign body accidentally left in body following removal of catheter or packing

⑦T81.528   Obstruction due to foreign body accidentally left in body following other procedure

⑦T81.529   Obstruction due to foreign body accidentally left in body following unspecified procedure

T81.53   Perforation due to foreign body accidentally left in body following procedure

⑦T81.530   Perforation due to foreign body accidentally left in body following surgical operation

⑦T81.531   Perforation due to foreign body accidentally left in body following infusion or transfusion

⑦T81.532   Perforation due to foreign body accidentally left in body following kidney dialysis

⑦T81.533   Perforation due to foreign body accidentally left in body following injection or immunization

⑦T81.534   Perforation due to foreign body accidentally left in body following endoscopic examination

⑦T81.535   Perforation due to foreign body accidentally left in body following heart catheterization

⑦T81.536   Perforation due to foreign body accidentally left in body following aspiration, puncture or other catheterization

⑦T81.537   Perforation due to foreign body accidentally left in body following removal of catheter or packing

⑦T81.538   Perforation due to foreign body accidentally left in body following other procedure

⑦T81.539   Perforation due to foreign body accidentally left in body following unspecified procedure

T81.59   Other complications of foreign body accidentally left in body following procedure

Excludes 2: obstruction or perforation due to prosthetic devices and implants intentionally left in body (T82.0-T82.5, T83.0-T83.4, T83.7, T84.0-T84.4, T85.0-T85.6)

⑦T81.590   Other complications of foreign body accidentally left in body following surgical operation

⑦T81.591   Other complications of foreign body accidentally left in body following infusion or transfusion

⑦T81.592   Other complications of foreign body accidentally left in body following kidney dialysis

⑦T81.593   Other complications of foreign body accidentally left in body following injection or immunization

⑦T81.594   Other complications of foreign body accidentally left in body following endoscopic examination

⑦**T81.595** Other complications of foreign body accidentally left in body following heart catheterization

⑦**T81.596** Other complications of foreign body accidentally left in body following aspiration, puncture or other catheterization

⑦**T81.597** Other complications of foreign body accidentally left in body following removal of catheter or packing

⑦**T81.598** Other complications of foreign body accidentally left in body following other procedure

⑦**T81.599** Other complications of foreign body accidentally left in body following unspecified procedure

T81.6 Acute reaction to foreign substance accidentally left during a procedure

Excludes 2: complications of foreign body accidentally left in body cavity or operation wound following procedure (T81.5-)

⊗⑦**T81.60** Unspecified acute reaction to foreign substance accidentally left during a procedure

⊗⑦**T81.61** Aseptic peritonitis due to foreign substance accidentally left during a procedure
Chemical peritonitis

⊗⑦**T81.69** Other acute reaction to foreign substance accidentally left during a procedure

T81.7 Vascular complications following a procedure, not elsewhere classified
Air embolism following procedure NEC
Phlebitis or thrombophlebitis resulting from a procedure

Excludes 1: embolism complicating abortion or ectopic or molar pregnancy (O00-O07, O08.2)
embolism complicating pregnancy, childbirth and the puerperium (O88.-)
traumatic embolism (T79.0)

Excludes 2: embolism due to prosthetic devices, implants and grafts (T82.8-, T83.8, T84.8-, T85.8)
embolism following infusion, transfusion and therapeutic injection (T80.0)

T81.71 Complication of artery following a procedure, not elsewhere classified

⑦**T81.710** Complication of mesenteric artery following a procedure, not elsewhere classified

⑦**T81.711** Complication of renal artery following a procedure, not elsewhere classified

⑦**T81.718** Complication of other artery following a procedure, not elsewhere classified

⑦**T81.719** Complication of unspecified artery following a procedure, not elsewhere classified

T81.72 Complication of vein following a procedure, not elsewhere classified

T81.8 Other complications of procedures, not elsewhere classified

Excludes 2: hypothermia following anesthesia (T88.51)

malignant hyperpyrexia due to anesthesia (T88.3)

⊗⑦**T81.81** Complication of inhalation therapy

⊗⑦**T81.82** Emphysema (subcutaneous) resulting from a procedure

⊗⑦**T81.83** Persistent postprocedural fistula

⊗⑦**T81.89** Other complications of procedures, not elsewhere classified
Use additional code to specify complication, such as:
postprocedural delirium (F05)

⊗⑦**T81.9** Unspecified complication of procedure

T82 Complications of cardiac and vascular prosthetic devices, implants and grafts

Excludes 2: failure and rejection of transplanted organs and tissue (T86.-)

The appropriate 7th character is to be added to each code from category T82
A - initial encounter
D - subsequent encounter
S - sequela

T82.0 Mechanical complication of heart valve prosthesis
Mechanical complication of artificial heart valve
Excludes 1: mechanical complication of biological heart valve graft (T82.22-)

⊗⑦**T82.01** Breakdown (mechanical) of heart valve prosthesis

⊗⑦**T82.02** Displacement of heart valve prosthesis
Malposition of heart valve prosthesis

⊗⑦**T82.03** Leakage of heart valve prosthesis

⊗⑦**T82.09** Other mechanical complication of heart valve prosthesis
Obstruction (mechanical) of heart valve prosthesis
Perforation of heart valve prosthesis
Protrusion of heart valve prosthesis

T82.1 Mechanical complication of cardiac electronic device

T82.11 Breakdown (mechanical) of cardiac electronic device

⑦**T82.110** Breakdown (mechanical) of cardiac electrode

⑦**T82.111** Breakdown (mechanical) of cardiac pulse generator (battery)

⑦**T82.118** Breakdown (mechanical) of other cardiac electronic device

⑦**T82.119** Breakdown (mechanical) of unspecified cardiac electronic device

T82.12 Displacement of cardiac electronic device
Malposition of cardiac electronic device

⑦**T82.120** Displacement of cardiac electrode

⑦**T82.121** Displacement of cardiac pulse generator (battery)

⑦**T82.128** Displacement of other cardiac electronic device

⑦**T82.129** Displacement of unspecified cardiac electronic device

T82.19 Other mechanical complication of cardiac electronic device
Leakage of cardiac electronic device

Obstruction of cardiac electronic device
Perforation of cardiac electronic device
Protrusion of cardiac electronic device

⑦T82.190   Other mechanical complication of cardiac electrode

⑦T82.191   Other mechanical complication of cardiac pulse generator (battery)

⑦T82.198   Other mechanical complication of other cardiac electronic device

⑦T82.199   Other mechanical complication of unspecified cardiac device

T82.2   Mechanical complication of coronary artery bypass graft and biological heart valve graft

Excludes 1: mechanical complication of artificial heart valve prosthesis (T82.0-)

T82.21   Mechanical complication of coronary artery bypass graft

⑦T82.211   Breakdown (mechanical) of coronary artery bypass graft

⑦T82.212   Displacement of coronary artery bypass graft

Malposition of coronary artery bypass graft

⑦T82.213   Leakage of coronary artery bypass graft

⑦T82.218   Other mechanical complication of coronary artery bypass graft

Obstruction, mechanical of coronary artery bypass graft

Perforation of coronary artery bypass graft

Protrusion of coronary artery bypass graft

T82.22   Mechanical complication of biological heart valve graft

⑦T82.221   Breakdown (mechanical) of biological heart valve graft

⑦T82.222   Displacement of biological heart valve graft

Malposition of biological heart valve graft

⑦T82.223   Leakage of biological heart valve graft

⑦T82.228   Other mechanical complication of biological heart valve graft

Obstruction of biological heart valve graft

Perforation of biological heart valve graft

Protrusion of biological heart valve graft

T82.3   Mechanical complication of other vascular grafts

T82.31   Breakdown (mechanical) of other vascular grafts

⑦T82.310   Breakdown (mechanical) of aortic (bifurcation) graft (replacement)

⑦T82.311   Breakdown (mechanical) of carotid arterial graft (bypass)

⑦T82.312   Breakdown (mechanical) of femoral arterial graft (bypass)

⑦T82.318   Breakdown (mechanical) of other vascular grafts

⑦T82.319   Breakdown (mechanical) of unspecified vascular grafts

T82.32   Displacement of other vascular grafts

Malposition of other vascular grafts

⑦T82.320   Displacement of aortic (bifurcation) graft (replacement)

⑦T82.321   Displacement of carotid arterial graft (bypass)

⑦T82.322   Displacement of femoral arterial graft (bypass)

⑦T82.328   Displacement of other vascular grafts

⑦T82.329   Displacement of unspecified vascular grafts

T82.33   Leakage of other vascular grafts

⑦T82.330   Leakage of aortic (bifurcation) graft (replacement)

⑦T82.331   Leakage of carotid arterial graft (bypass)

⑦T82.332   Leakage of femoral arterial graft (bypass)

⑦T82.338   Leakage of other vascular grafts

⑦T82.339   Leakage of unspecified vascular graft

T82.39   Other mechanical complication of other vascular grafts

Obstruction (mechanical) of other vascular grafts

Perforation of other vascular grafts

Protrusion of other vascular grafts

⑦T82.390   Other mechanical complication of aortic (bifurcation) graft (replacement)

⑦T82.391   Other mechanical complication of carotid arterial graft (bypass)

⑦T82.392   Other mechanical complication of femoral arterial graft (bypass)

⑦T82.398   Other mechanical complication of other vascular grafts

⑦T82.399   Other mechanical complication of unspecified vascular grafts

T82.4   Mechanical complication of vascular dialysis catheter

Mechanical complication of hemodialysis catheter

Excludes 1: mechanical complication of intraperitoneal dialysis catheter (T85.62)

⊗⑦T82.41   Breakdown (mechanical) of vascular dialysis catheter

⊗⑦T82.42   Displacement of vascular dialysis catheter

Malposition of vascular dialysis catheter

⊗⑦T82.43   Leakage of vascular dialysis catheter

⊗⑦T82.49   Other complication of vascular dialysis catheter

Obstruction (mechanical) of vascular dialysis catheter

Perforation of vascular dialysis catheter

Protrusion of vascular dialysis catheter

T82.5   Mechanical complication of other cardiac and vascular devices and implants

Excludes 2: mechanical complication of epidural and subdural infusion catheter (T85.61)

T82.51 Breakdown (mechanical) of other cardiac and vascular devices and implants

⑦ **T82.510** Breakdown (mechanical) of surgically created arteriovenous fistula

⑦ **T82.511** Breakdown (mechanical) of surgically created arteriovenous shunt

⑦ **T82.512** Breakdown (mechanical) of artificial heart

⑦ **T82.513** Breakdown (mechanical) of balloon (counterpulsation) device

⑦ **T82.514** Breakdown (mechanical) of infusion catheter

⑦ **T82.515** Breakdown (mechanical) of umbrella device

⑦ **T82.518** Breakdown (mechanical) of other cardiac and vascular devices and implants

⑦ **T82.519** Breakdown (mechanical) of unspecified cardiac and vascular devices and implants

T82.52 Displacement of other cardiac and vascular devices and implants

Malposition of other cardiac and vascular devices and implants

⑦ **T82.520** Displacement of surgically created arteriovenous fistula

⑦ **T82.521** Displacement of surgically created arteriovenous shunt

⑦ **T82.522** Displacement of artificial heart

⑦ **T82.523** Displacement of balloon (counterpulsation) device

⑦ **T82.524** Displacement of infusion catheter

⑦ **T82.525** Displacement of umbrella device

⑦ **T82.528** Displacement of other cardiac and vascular devices and implants

⑦ **T82.529** Displacement of unspecified cardiac and vascular devices and implants

T82.53 Leakage of other cardiac and vascular devices and implants

⑦ **T82.530** Leakage of surgically created arteriovenous fistula

⑦ **T82.531** Leakage of surgically created arteriovenous shunt

⑦ **T82.532** Leakage of artificial heart

⑦ **T82.533** Leakage of balloon (counterpulsation) device

⑦ **T82.534** Leakage of infusion catheter

⑦ **T82.535** Leakage of umbrella device

⑦ **T82.538** Leakage of other cardiac and vascular devices and implants

⑦ **T82.539** Leakage of unspecified cardiac and vascular devices and implants

T82.59 Other mechanical complication of other cardiac and vascular devices and implants

Obstruction (mechanical) of other cardiac and vascular devices and implants

Perforation of other cardiac and vascular devices and implants

Protrusion of other cardiac and vascular devices and implants

⑦ **T82.590** Other mechanical complication of surgically created arteriovenous fistula

⑦ **T82.591** Other mechanical complication of surgically created arteriovenous shunt

⑦ **T82.592** Other mechanical complication of artificial heart

⑦ **T82.593** Other mechanical complication of balloon (counterpulsation) device

⑦ **T82.594** Other mechanical complication of infusion catheter

⑦ **T82.595** Other mechanical complication of umbrella device

⑦ **T82.598** Other mechanical complication of other cardiac and vascular devices and implants

⑦ **T82.599** Other mechanical complication of unspecified cardiac and vascular devices and implants

⊗⑦ **T82.6** Infection and inflammatory reaction due to cardiac valve prosthesis

Use additional code to identify infection

⊗⑦ **T82.7** Infection and inflammatory reaction due to other cardiac and vascular devices, implants and grafts

Use additional code to identify infection

T82.8 Other specified complications of cardiac and vascular prosthetic devices, implants and grafts

T82.81 Embolism of cardiac and vascular prosthetic devices, implants and grafts

⑦ **T82.817** Embolism of cardiac prosthetic devices, implants and grafts

⑦ **T82.818** Embolism of vascular prosthetic devices, implants and grafts

T82.82 Fibrosis of cardiac and vascular prosthetic devices, implants and grafts

⑦ **T82.827** Fibrosis of cardiac prosthetic devices, implants and grafts

⑦ **T82.828** Fibrosis of vascular prosthetic devices, implants and grafts

T82.83 Hemorrhage of cardiac and vascular prosthetic devices, implants and grafts

⑦ **T82.837** Hemorrhage of cardiac prosthetic devices, implants and grafts

⑦ **T82.838** Hemorrhage of vascular prosthetic devices, implants and grafts

T82.84 Pain from cardiac and vascular prosthetic devices, implants and grafts

⑦ **T82.847** Pain from cardiac prosthetic devices, implants and grafts

⑦ **T82.848** Pain from vascular prosthetic devices, implants and grafts

T82.85 Stenosis of cardiac and vascular prosthetic devices, implants and grafts

⑦ **T82.857** Stenosis of cardiac prosthetic devices, implants and grafts

⑦ **T82.858** Stenosis of vascular prosthetic devices, implants and grafts

T82.86 Thrombosis of cardiac and vascular prosthetic devices, implants and grafts

⑦ **T82.867** Thrombosis of cardiac prosthetic devices, implants and grafts

⑦ **T82.868** Thrombosis of vascular prosthetic devices, implants and grafts

T82.89 Other specified complication of cardiac and vascular prosthetic devices, implants and grafts

⑦ **T82.897** Other specified complication of cardiac prosthetic devices, implants and grafts

⑦ **T82.898** Other specified complication of vascular prosthetic devices, implants and grafts

T82.9 Unspecified complication of cardiac and vascular prosthetic device, implant and graft

T83 Complications of genitourinary prosthetic devices, implants and grafts

Excludes 2: failure and rejection of transplanted organs and tissue (T86.-)

The appropriate 7th character is to be added to each code from ` category T83

A - initial encounter

D - subsequent encounter

S - sequela

T83.0 Mechanical complication of urinary (indwelling) catheter

Excludes 2: complications of stoma of urinary tract (N99.5-)

T83.01 Breakdown (mechanical) of urinary (indwelling) catheter

⑦ **T83.010** Breakdown (mechanical) of cystostomy catheter

⑦ **T83.018** Breakdown (mechanical) of other indwelling urethral catheter

T83.02 Displacement of urinary (indwelling) catheter

Malposition of urinary (indwelling) catheter

⑦ **T83.020** Displacement of cystostomy catheter

⑦ **T83.028** Displacement of other indwelling urethral catheter

T83.03 Leakage of urinary (indwelling) catheter

⑦ **T83.030** Leakage of cystostomy catheter

⑦ **T83.038** Leakage of other indwelling urethral catheter

T83.09 Other mechanical complication of urinary (indwelling) catheter

Obstruction (mechanical) of urinary (indwelling) catheter

Perforation of urinary (indwelling) catheter

Protrusion of urinary (indwelling) catheter

⑦ **T83.090** Other mechanical complication of cystostomy catheter

⑦ **T83.098** Other mechanical complication of other indwelling urethral catheter

T83.1 Mechanical complication of other urinary devices and implants

T83.11 Breakdown (mechanical) of other urinary devices and implants

⑦ **T83.110** Breakdown (mechanical) of urinary electronic stimulator device

⑦ **T83.111** Breakdown (mechanical) of urinary sphincter implant

⑦ **T83.112** Breakdown (mechanical) of urinary stent

⑦ **T83.118** Breakdown (mechanical) of other urinary devices and implants

T83.12 Displacement of other urinary devices and implants

Malposition of other urinary devices and implants

⑦ **T83.120** Displacement of urinary electronic stimulator device

⑦ **T83.121** Displacement of urinary sphincter implant

⑦ **T83.122** Displacement of urinary stent

⑦ **T83.128** Displacement of other urinary devices and implants

T83.19 Other mechanical complication of other urinary devices and implants

Leakage of other urinary devices and implants

Obstruction (mechanical) of other urinary devices and implants

Perforation of other urinary devices and implants

Protrusion of other urinary devices and implants

⑦ **T83.190** Other mechanical complication of urinary electronic stimulator device

⑦ **T83.191** Other mechanical complication of urinary sphincter implant

⑦ **T83.192** Other mechanical complication of urinary stent

⑦ **T83.198** Other mechanical complication of other urinary devices and implants

T83.2 Mechanical complication of graft of urinary organ

⊗⑦ **T83.21** Breakdown (mechanical) of graft of urinary organ

⊗⑦ **T83.22** Displacement of graft of urinary organ

Malposition of graft of urinary organ

⊗⑦ **T83.23** Leakage of graft of urinary organ

⊗⑦ **T83.29** Other mechanical complication of graft of urinary organ

Obstruction (mechanical) of graft of urinary organ

Perforation of graft of urinary organ

Protrusion of graft of urinary organ

T83.3 Mechanical complication of intrauterine contraceptive device

⊗⑦ **T83.31** Breakdown (mechanical) of intrauterine contraceptive device

⊗⑦ **T83.32** Displacement of intrauterine contraceptive device

Malposition of intrauterine contraceptive device

⊗⑦ **T83.39** Other mechanical complication of intrauterine contraceptive device

Leakage of intrauterine contraceptive device

Obstruction (mechanical) of intrauterine contraceptive device

Perforation of intrauterine contraceptive device

Protrusion of intrauterine contraceptive device

● New code   ▲ Revised code   ⑦ 7ᵗʰ digit required   ⊗ Placeholder required

T83.4 Mechanical complication of other prosthetic devices, implants and grafts of genital tract

    T83.41 Breakdown (mechanical) of other prosthetic devices, implants and grafts of genital tract

        ⑦**T83.410** Breakdown (mechanical) of penile (implanted) prosthesis

        ⑦**T83.418** Breakdown (mechanical) of other prosthetic devices, implants and grafts of genital tract

    T83.42 Displacement of other prosthetic devices, implants and grafts of genital tract

    Malposition of other prosthetic devices, implants and grafts of genital tract

        ⑦**T83.420** Displacement of penile (implanted) prosthesis

        ⑦**T83.428** Displacement of other prosthetic devices, implants and grafts of genital tract

    T83.49 Other mechanical complication of other prosthetic devices, implants and grafts of genital tract

    Leakage of other prosthetic devices, implants and grafts of genital tract

    Obstruction, mechanical of other prosthetic devices, implants and grafts of genital tract

    Perforation of other prosthetic devices, implants and grafts of genital tract

    Protrusion of other prosthetic devices, implants and grafts of genital tract

        ⑦**T83.490** Other mechanical complication of penile (implanted) prosthesis

        ⑦**T83.498** Other mechanical complication of other prosthetic devices, implants and grafts of genital tract

T83.5 Infection and inflammatory reaction due to prosthetic device, implant and graft in urinary system

    Use additional code to identify infection

    ⊗⑦**T83.51** Infection and inflammatory reaction due to indwelling urinary catheter

        Excludes 2: complications of stoma of urinary tract (N99.5-)

    ⊗⑦**T83.59** Infection and inflammatory reaction due to prosthetic device, implant and graft in urinary system

⊗⑦T83.6 Infection and inflammatory reaction due to prosthetic device, implant and graft in genital tract

    Use additional code to identify infection

T83.7 Complications due to implanted mesh and other prosthetic materials

    T83.71 Erosion of implanted mesh and other prosthetic materials to surrounding organ or tissue

        ⑦**T83.711** Erosion of implanted vaginal mesh and other prosthetic materials to surrounding organ or tissue

        Erosion of implanted vaginal mesh and other prosthetic materials into pelvic floor muscles

        ⑦**T83.718** Erosion of other implanted mesh and other prosthetic materials to surrounding organ or tissue

T83.72 Exposure of implanted mesh and other prosthetic materials into surrounding organ or tissue

    ⑦**T83.721** Exposure of implanted vaginal mesh and other prosthetic materials into vagina

    Exposure of implanted vaginal mesh and other prosthetic materials through vaginal wall

    ⑦**T83.728** Exposure of other implanted mesh and other prosthetic materials to surrounding organ or tissue

T83.8 Other specified complications of genitourinary prosthetic devices, implants and grafts

    ⊗⑦**T83.81** Embolism of genitourinary prosthetic devices, implants and grafts

    ⊗⑦**T83.82** Fibrosis of genitourinary prosthetic devices, implants and grafts

    ⊗⑦**T83.83** Hemorrhage of genitourinary prosthetic devices, implants and grafts

    ⊗⑦**T83.84** Pain from genitourinary prosthetic devices, implants and grafts

    ⊗⑦**T83.85** Stenosis of genitourinary prosthetic devices, implants and grafts

    ⊗⑦**T83.86** Thrombosis of genitourinary prosthetic devices, implants and grafts

    ⊗⑦**T83.89** Other specified complication of genitourinary prosthetic devices, implants and grafts

⊗⑦T83.9 Unspecified complication of genitourinary prosthetic device, implant and graft

T84 Complications of internal orthopedic prosthetic devices, implants and grafts

> **Excludes 2:** failure and rejection of transplanted organs and tissues (T86.-)
>
> fracture of bone following insertion of orthopedic implant, joint prosthesis or bone plate (M96.6)

The appropriate 7th character is to be added to each code from category T84

A - initial encounter

D - subsequent encounter

S - sequela

T84.0 Mechanical complication of internal joint prosthesis

    T84.01 Broken internal joint prosthesis

    Breakage (fracture) of prosthetic joint

    Broken prosthetic joint implant

        Excludes 1: periprosthetic joint implant fracture (T84.04)

        ⑦**T84.010** Broken internal right hip prosthesis

        ⑦**T84.011** Broken internal left hip prosthesis

        ⑦**T84.012** Broken internal right knee prosthesis

        ⑦**T84.013** Broken internal left knee prosthesis

        ⑦**T84.018** Broken internal joint prosthesis, other site

        Use additional code to identify the joint (Z96.6-)

        ⑦**T84.019** Broken internal joint prosthesis, unspecified site

    T84.02 Dislocation of internal joint prosthesis

    Instability of internal joint prosthesis

    Subluxation of internal joint prosthesis

⑦**T84.020** Dislocation of internal right hip prosthesis

⑦**T84.021** Dislocation of internal left hip prosthesis

⑦**T84.022** Instability of internal right knee prosthesis

⑦**T84.023** Instability of internal left knee prosthesis

⑦**T84.028** Dislocation of other internal joint prosthesis

Use additional code to identify the joint (Z96.6-)

⑦**T84.029** Dislocation of unspecified internal joint prosthesis

T84.03 Mechanical loosening of internal prosthetic joint
Aseptic loosening of prosthetic joint

⑦**T84.030** Mechanical loosening of internal right hip prosthetic joint

⑦**T84.031** Mechanical loosening of internal left hip prosthetic joint

⑦**T84.032** Mechanical loosening of internal right knee prosthetic joint

⑦**T84.033** Mechanical loosening of internal left knee prosthetic joint

⑦**T84.038** Mechanical loosening of other internal prosthetic joint

Use additional code to identify the joint (Z96.6-)

⑦**T84.039** Mechanical loosening of unspecified internal prosthetic joint

T84.04 Periprosthetic fracture around internal prosthetic joint

Excludes 2: breakage (fracture) of prosthetic joint (T84.01)

⑦**T84.040** Periprosthetic fracture around internal prosthetic right hip joint

⑦**T84.041** Periprosthetic fracture around internal prosthetic left hip joint

⑦**T84.042** Periprosthetic fracture around internal prosthetic right knee joint

⑦**T84.043** Periprosthetic fracture around internal prosthetic left knee joint

⑦**T84.048** Periprosthetic fracture around other internal prosthetic joint

Use additional code to identify the joint (Z96.6-)

⑦**T84.049** Periprosthetic fracture around unspecified internal prosthetic joint

T84.05 Periprosthetic osteolysis of internal prosthetic joint

Use additional code to identify major osseous defect, if applicable (M89.7-)

⑦**T84.050** Periprosthetic osteolysis of internal prosthetic right hip joint

⑦**T84.051** Periprosthetic osteolysis of internal prosthetic left hip joint

⑦**T84.052** Periprosthetic osteolysis of internal prosthetic right knee joint

⑦**T84.053** Periprosthetic osteolysis of internal prosthetic left knee joint

⑦**T84.058** Periprosthetic osteolysis of other internal prosthetic joint

Use additional code to identify the joint (Z96.6-)

⑦**T84.059** Periprosthetic osteolysis of unspecified internal prosthetic joint

T84.06 Wear of articular bearing surface of internal prosthetic joint

⑦**T84.060** Wear of articular bearing surface of internal prosthetic right hip joint

⑦**T84.061** Wear of articular bearing surface of internal prosthetic left hip joint

⑦**T84.062** Wear of articular bearing surface of internal prosthetic right knee joint

⑦**T84.063** Wear of articular bearing surface of internal prosthetic left knee joint

⑦**T84.068** Wear of articular bearing surface of other internal prosthetic joint

Use additional code to identify the joint (Z96.6-)

⑦**T84.069** Wear of articular bearing surface of unspecified internal prosthetic joint

T84.09 Other mechanical complication of internal joint prosthesis
Prosthetic joint implant failure NOS

⑦**T84.090** Other mechanical complication of internal right hip prosthesis

⑦**T84.091** Other mechanical complication of internal left hip prosthesis

⑦**T84.092** Other mechanical complication of internal right knee prosthesis

⑦**T84.093** Other mechanical complication of internal left knee prosthesis

⑦**T84.098** Other mechanical complication of other internal joint prosthesis

Use additional code to identify the joint (Z96.6-)

⑦**T84.099** Other mechanical complication of unspecified internal joint prosthesis

T84.1 Mechanical complication of internal fixation device of bones of limb

Excludes 2: mechanical complication of internal fixation device of bones of feet (T84.2-)
mechanical complication of internal fixation device of bones of fingers (T84.2-)
mechanical complication of internal fixation device of bones of hands (T84.2-)
mechanical complication of internal fixation device of bones of toes (T84.2-)

T84.11 Breakdown (mechanical) of internal fixation device of bones of limb

⑦**T84.110** Breakdown (mechanical) of internal fixation device of right humerus

⑦**T84.111** Breakdown (mechanical) of internal fixation device of left humerus

⑦**T84.112** Breakdown (mechanical) of internal fixation device of bone of right forearm

● New code   ▲ Revised code   ⑦ 7ᵗʰ digit required   ⊗ Placeholder required

⑦T84.113   Breakdown (mechanical) of internal fixation device of bone of left forearm

⑦T84.114   Breakdown (mechanical) of internal fixation device of right femur

⑦T84.115   Breakdown (mechanical) of internal fixation device of left femur

⑦T84.116   Breakdown (mechanical) of internal fixation device of bone of right lower leg

⑦T84.117   Breakdown (mechanical) of internal fixation device of bone of left lower leg

⑦T84.119   Breakdown (mechanical) of internal fixation device of unspecified bone of limb

T84.12   Displacement of internal fixation device of bones of limb

Malposition of internal fixation device of bones of limb

⑦T84.120   Displacement of internal fixation device of right humerus

⑦T84.121   Displacement of internal fixation device of left humerus

⑦T84.122   Displacement of internal fixation device of bone of right forearm

⑦T84.123   Displacement of internal fixation device of bone of left forearm

⑦T84.124   Displacement of internal fixation device of right femur

⑦T84.125   Displacement of internal fixation device of left femur

⑦T84.126   Displacement of internal fixation device of bone of right lower leg

⑦T84.127   Displacement of internal fixation device of bone of left lower leg

⑦T84.129   Displacement of internal fixation device of unspecified bone of limb

T84.19   Other mechanical complication of internal fixation device of bones of limb

Obstruction (mechanical) of internal fixation device of bones of limb

Perforation of internal fixation device of bones of limb

Protrusion of internal fixation device of bones of limb

⑦T84.190   Other mechanical complication of internal fixation device of right humerus

⑦T84.191   Other mechanical complication of internal fixation device of left humerus

⑦T84.192   Other mechanical complication of internal fixation device of bone of right forearm

⑦T84.193   Other mechanical complication of internal fixation device of bone of left forearm

⑦T84.194   Other mechanical complication of internal fixation device of right femur

⑦T84.195   Other mechanical complication of internal fixation device of left femur

⑦T84.196   Other mechanical complication of internal fixation device of bone of right lower leg

⑦T84.197   Other mechanical complication of internal fixation device of bone of left lower leg

⑦T84.199   Other mechanical complication of internal fixation device of unspecified bone of limb

T84.2   Mechanical complication of internal fixation device of other bones

T84.21   Breakdown (mechanical) of internal fixation device of other bones

⑦T84.210   Breakdown (mechanical) of internal fixation device of bones of hand and fingers

⑦T84.213   Breakdown (mechanical) of internal fixation device of bones of foot and toes

⑦T84.216   Breakdown (mechanical) of internal fixation device of vertebrae

⑦T84.218   Breakdown (mechanical) of internal fixation device of other bones

T84.22   Displacement of internal fixation device of other bones

Malposition of internal fixation device of other bones

⑦T84.220   Displacement of internal fixation device of bones of hand and fingers

⑦T84.223   Displacement of internal fixation device of bones of foot and toes

⑦T84.226   Displacement of internal fixation device of vertebrae

⑦T84.228   Displacement of internal fixation device of other bones

T84.29   Other mechanical complication of internal fixation device of other bones

Obstruction (mechanical) of internal fixation device of other bones

Perforation of internal fixation device of other bones

Protrusion of internal fixation device of other bones

⑦T84.290   Other mechanical complication of internal fixation device of bones of hand and fingers

⑦T84.293   Other mechanical complication of internal fixation device of bones of foot and toes

⑦T84.296   Other mechanical complication of internal fixation device of vertebrae

⑦T84.298   Other mechanical complication of internal fixation device of other bones

T84.3   Mechanical complication of other bone devices, implants and grafts

Excludes 2: other complications of bone graft (T86.83-)

T84.31   Breakdown (mechanical) of other bone devices, implants and grafts

⑦T84.310   Breakdown (mechanical) of electronic bone stimulator

⑦T84.318   Breakdown (mechanical) of other bone devices, implants and grafts

T84.32   Displacement of other bone devices, implants and grafts

Malposition of other bone devices, implants and grafts

⑦T84.320   Displacement of electronic bone stimulator

⑦T84.328   Displacement of other bone devices, implants and grafts

T84.39   Other mechanical complication of other bone devices, implants and grafts

Obstruction (mechanical) of other bone devices, implants and grafts

Perforation of other bone devices, implants and grafts

Protrusion of other bone devices, implants and grafts

⑦T84.390   Other mechanical complication of electronic bone stimulator

⑦T84.398   Other mechanical complication of other bone devices, implants and grafts

T84.4   Mechanical complication of other internal orthopedic devices, implants and grafts

T84.41   Breakdown (mechanical) of other internal orthopedic devices, implants and grafts

⑦T84.410   Breakdown (mechanical) of muscle and tendon graft

⑦T84.418   Breakdown (mechanical) of other internal orthopedic devices, implants and grafts

T84.42   Displacement of other internal orthopedic devices, implants and grafts

Malposition of other internal orthopedic devices, implants and grafts

⑦T84.420   Displacement of muscle and tendon graft

⑦T84.428   Displacement of other internal orthopedic devices, implants and grafts

T84.49   Other mechanical complication of other internal orthopedic devices, implants and grafts

Mechanical complication of other internal orthopedic devices, implants and grafts NOS

Obstruction (mechanical) of other internal orthopedic devices, implants and grafts

Perforation of other internal orthopedic devices, implants and grafts

Protrusion of other internal orthopedic devices, implants and grafts

⑦T84.490   Other mechanical complication of muscle and tendon graft

⑦T84.498   Other mechanical complication of other internal orthopedic devices, implants and grafts

T84.5   Infection and inflammatory reaction due to internal joint prosthesis

Use additional code to identify infection

⊗⑦T84.50   Infection and inflammatory reaction due to unspecified internal joint prosthesis

⊗⑦T84.51   Infection and inflammatory reaction due to internal right hip prosthesis

⊗⑦T84.52   Infection and inflammatory reaction due to internal left hip prosthesis

⊗⑦T84.53   Infection and inflammatory reaction due to internal right knee prosthesis

⊗⑦T84.54   Infection and inflammatory reaction due to internal left knee prosthesis

⊗⑦T84.59   Infection and inflammatory reaction due to other internal joint prosthesis

T84.6   Infection and inflammatory reaction due to internal fixation device

Use additional code to identify infection

⊗⑦T84.60   Infection and inflammatory reaction due to internal fixation device of unspecified site

T84.61   Infection and inflammatory reaction due to internal fixation device of arm

⑦T84.610   Infection and inflammatory reaction due to internal fixation device of right humerus

⑦T84.611   Infection and inflammatory reaction due to internal fixation device of left humerus

⑦T84.612   Infection and inflammatory reaction due to internal fixation device of right radius

⑦T84.613   Infection and inflammatory reaction due to internal fixation device of left radius

⑦T84.614   Infection and inflammatory reaction due to internal fixation device of right ulna

⑦T84.615   Infection and inflammatory reaction due to internal fixation device of left ulna

⑦T84.619   Infection and inflammatory reaction due to internal fixation device of unspecified bone of arm

T84.62   Infection and inflammatory reaction due to internal fixation device of leg

⑦T84.620   Infection and inflammatory reaction due to internal fixation device of right femur

⑦T84.621   Infection and inflammatory reaction due to internal fixation device of left femur

⑦T84.622   Infection and inflammatory reaction due to internal fixation device of right tibia

⑦T84.623   Infection and inflammatory reaction due to internal fixation device of left tibia

⑦T84.624   Infection and inflammatory reaction due to internal fixation device of right fibula

● New code   ▲ Revised code   ⑦ 7ᵗʰ digit required   ⊗ Placeholder required

⑦**T84.625** Infection and inflammatory reaction due to internal fixation device of left fibula

⑦**T84.629** Infection and inflammatory reaction due to internal fixation device of unspecified bone of leg

⊗⑦**T84.63** Infection and inflammatory reaction due to internal fixation device of spine

⊗⑦**T84.69** Infection and inflammatory reaction due to internal fixation device of other site

⊗⑦**T84.7** Infection and inflammatory reaction due to other internal orthopedic prosthetic devices, implants and grafts
Use additional code to identify infection

T84.8 Other specified complications of internal orthopedic prosthetic devices, implants and grafts

⊗⑦**T84.81** Embolism due to internal orthopedic prosthetic devices, implants and grafts

⊗⑦**T84.82** Fibrosis due to internal orthopedic prosthetic devices, implants and grafts

⊗⑦**T84.83** Hemorrhage due to internal orthopedic prosthetic devices, implants and grafts

⊗⑦**T84.84** Pain due to internal orthopedic prosthetic devices, implants and grafts

⊗⑦**T84.85** Stenosis due to internal orthopedic prosthetic devices, implants and grafts

⊗⑦**T84.86** Thrombosis due to internal orthopedic prosthetic devices, implants and grafts

⊗⑦**T84.89** Other specified complication of internal orthopedic prosthetic devices, implants and grafts

T84.9 Unspecified complication of internal orthopedic prosthetic device, implant and graft

T85 Complications of other internal prosthetic devices, implants and grafts

Excludes 2: failure and rejection of transplanted organs and tissue (T86.-)

The appropriate 7th character is to be added to each code from category T85

A - initial encounter

D - subsequent encounter

S - sequela

T85.0 Mechanical complication of ventricular intracranial (communicating) shunt

⊗⑦**T85.01** Breakdown (mechanical) of ventricular intracranial (communicating) shunt

⊗⑦**T85.02** Displacement of ventricular intracranial (communicating) shunt
Malposition of ventricular intracranial (communicating) shunt

⊗⑦**T85.03** Leakage of ventricular intracranial (communicating) shunt

⊗⑦**T85.09** Other mechanical complication of ventricular intracranial (communicating) shunt
Obstruction (mechanical) of ventricular intracranial (communicating) shunt
Perforation of ventricular intracranial (communicating) shunt
Protrusion of ventricular intracranial (communicating) shunt

T85.1 Mechanical complication of implanted electronic stimulator of nervous system

T85.11 Breakdown (mechanical) of implanted electronic stimulator of nervous system

⑦**T85.110** Breakdown (mechanical) of implanted electronic neurostimulator (electrode) of brain

⑦**T85.111** Breakdown (mechanical) of implanted electronic neurostimulator (electrode) of peripheral nerve

⑦**T85.112** Breakdown (mechanical) of implanted electronic neurostimulator (electrode) of spinal cord

⑦**T85.118** Breakdown (mechanical) of other implanted electronic stimulator of nervous system

T85.12 Displacement of implanted electronic stimulator of nervous system
Malposition of implanted electronic stimulator of nervous system

⑦**T85.120** Displacement of implanted electronic neurostimulator (electrode) of brain

⑦**T85.121** Displacement of implanted electronic neurostimulator (electrode) of peripheral nerve

⑦**T85.122** Displacement of implanted electronic neurostimulator (electrode) of spinal cord

⑦**T85.128** Displacement of other implanted electronic stimulator of nervous system

T85.19 Other mechanical complication of implanted electronic stimulator of nervous system
Leakage of implanted electronic stimulator of nervous system
Obstruction (mechanical) of implanted electronic stimulator of nervous system
Perforation of implanted electronic stimulator of nervous system
Protrusion of implanted electronic stimulator of nervous system

⑦**T85.190** Other mechanical complication of implanted electronic neurostimulator (electrode) of brain

⑦**T85.191** Other mechanical complication of implanted electronic neurostimulator (electrode) of peripheral nerve

⑦**T85.192** Other mechanical complication of implanted electronic neurostimulator (electrode) of spinal cord

⑦**T85.199** Other mechanical complication of other implanted electronic stimulator of nervous system

T85.2 Mechanical complication of intraocular lens

⊗⑦**T85.21** Breakdown (mechanical) of intraocular lens

⊗⑦**T85.22** Displacement of intraocular lens
Malposition of intraocular lens

⊗⑦**T85.29** Other mechanical complication of intraocular lens
Obstruction (mechanical) of intraocular lens
Perforation of intraocular lens
Protrusion of intraocular lens

T85.3 Mechanical complication of other ocular prosthetic devices, implants and grafts

Excludes 2: other complications of corneal graft (T86.84-)

T85.31 Breakdown (mechanical) of other ocular prosthetic devices, implants and grafts

⑦ **T85.310** Breakdown (mechanical) of prosthetic orbit of right eye

⑦ **T85.311** Breakdown (mechanical) of prosthetic orbit of left eye

⑦ **T85.318** Breakdown (mechanical) of other ocular prosthetic devices, implants and grafts

T85.32 Displacement of other ocular prosthetic devices, implants and grafts

Malposition of other ocular prosthetic devices, implants and grafts

⑦ **T85.320** Displacement of prosthetic orbit of right eye

⑦ **T85.321** Displacement of prosthetic orbit of left eye

⑦ **T85.328** Displacement of other ocular prosthetic devices, implants and grafts

T85.39 Other mechanical complication of other ocular prosthetic devices, implants and grafts

Obstruction (mechanical) of other ocular prosthetic devices, implants and grafts

Perforation of other ocular prosthetic devices, implants and grafts

Protrusion of other ocular prosthetic devices, implants and grafts

⑦ **T85.390** Other mechanical complication of prosthetic orbit of right eye

⑦ **T85.391** Other mechanical complication of prosthetic orbit of left eye

⑦ **T85.398** Other mechanical complication of other ocular prosthetic devices, implants and grafts

T85.4 Mechanical complication of breast prosthesis and implant

⊗⑦ **T85.41** Breakdown (mechanical) of breast prosthesis and implant

⊗⑦ **T85.42** Displacement of breast prosthesis and implant

Malposition of breast prosthesis and implant

⊗⑦ **T85.43** Leakage of breast prosthesis and implant

⊗⑦ **T85.44** Capsular contracture of breast implant

⊗⑦ **T85.49** Other mechanical complication of breast prosthesis and implant

Obstruction (mechanical) of breast prosthesis and implant

Perforation of breast prosthesis and implant

Protrusion of breast prosthesis and implant

T85.5 Mechanical complication of gastrointestinal prosthetic devices, implants and grafts

T85.51 Breakdown (mechanical) of gastrointestinal prosthetic devices, implants and grafts

⑦ **T85.510** Breakdown (mechanical) of bile duct prosthesis

⑦ **T85.511** Breakdown (mechanical) of esophageal anti-reflux device

⑦ **T85.518** Breakdown (mechanical) of other gastrointestinal prosthetic devices, implants and grafts

T85.52 Displacement of gastrointestinal prosthetic devices, implants and grafts

Malposition of gastrointestinal prosthetic devices, implants and grafts

⑦ **T85.520** Displacement of bile duct prosthesis

⑦ **T85.521** Displacement of esophageal anti-reflux device

⑦ **T85.528** Displacement of other gastrointestinal prosthetic devices, implants and grafts

T85.59 Other mechanical complication of gastrointestinal prosthetic devices, implants and

Obstruction, mechanical of gastrointestinal prosthetic devices, implants and grafts

Perforation of gastrointestinal prosthetic devices, implants and grafts

Protrusion of gastrointestinal prosthetic devices, implants and grafts

⑦ **T85.590** Other mechanical complication of bile duct prosthesis

⑦ **T85.591** Other mechanical complication of esophageal anti-reflux device

⑦ **T85.598** Other mechanical complication of other gastrointestinal prosthetic devices, implants and grafts

T85.6 Mechanical complication of other specified internal and external prosthetic devices, implants and grafts

T85.61 Breakdown (mechanical) of other specified internal prosthetic devices, implants and grafts

⑦ **T85.610** Breakdown (mechanical) of epidural and subdural infusion catheter

⑦ **T85.611** Breakdown (mechanical) of intraperitoneal dialysis catheter

Excludes 1: mechanical complication of vascular dialysis catheter (T82.4-)

⑦ **T85.612** Breakdown (mechanical) of permanent sutures

Excludes 1: mechanical complication of permanent (wire) suture used in bone repair (T84.1-T84.2)

⑦ **T85.613** Breakdown (mechanical) of artificial skin graft and decellularized allodermis

Failure of artificial skin graft and decellularized allodermis

Poor incorporation of artificial skin graft and decellularized allodermis

Shearing of artificial skin graft and decellularized allodermis

⑦ **T85.614** Breakdown (mechanical) of insulin pump

⑦ **T85.618** Breakdown (mechanical) of other specified internal prosthetic devices, implants and grafts

● New code ▲ Revised code ⑦ 7th digit required ⊗ Placeholder required

T85.62   Displacement of other specified internal prosthetic devices, implants and grafts
> Malposition of other specified internal prosthetic devices, implants and grafts

⑦**T85.620**   Displacement of epidural and subdural infusion catheter

⑦**T85.621**   Displacement of intraperitoneal dialysis catheter
> **Excludes 1:** mechanical complication of vascular dialysis catheter (T82.4-)

⑦**T85.622**   Displacement of permanent sutures
> **Excludes 1:** mechanical complication of permanent (wire) suture used in bone repair (T84.1-T84.2)

⑦**T85.623**   Displacement of artificial skin graft and decellularized allodermis
> Dislodgement of artificial skin graft and decellularized allodermis
> Displacement of artificial skin graft and decellularized allodermis

⑦**T85.624**   Displacement of insulin pump

⑦**T85.628**   Displacement of other specified internal prosthetic devices, implants and grafts

T85.63   Leakage of other specified internal prosthetic devices, implants and grafts

⑦**T85.630**   Leakage of epidural and subdural infusion catheter

⑦**T85.631**   Leakage of intraperitoneal dialysis catheter
> **Excludes 1:** mechanical complication of vascular dialysis catheter (T82.4)

⑦**T85.633**   Leakage of insulin pump

⑦**T85.638**   Leakage of other specified internal prosthetic devices, implants and grafts

T85.69   Other mechanical complication of other specified internal prosthetic devices, implants and grafts
> Obstruction, mechanical of other specified internal prosthetic devices, implants and grafts
> Perforation of other specified internal prosthetic devices, implants and grafts
> Protrusion of other specified internal prosthetic devices, implants and grafts

⑦**T85.690**   Other mechanical complication of epidural and subdural infusion catheter

⑦**T85.691**   Other mechanical complication of intraperitoneal dialysis catheter
> **Excludes 1:** mechanical complication of vascular dialysis catheter (T82.4)

⑦**T85.692**   Other mechanical complication of permanent sutures
> **Excludes 1:** mechanical complication of permanent (wire) suture

used in bone repair (T84.1-T84.2)

⑦**T85.693**   Other mechanical complication of artificial skin graft and decellularized allodermis

⑦**T85.694**   Other mechanical complication of insulin pump

⑦**T85.698**   Other mechanical complication of other specified internal prosthetic devices, implants and grafts
> Mechanical complication of nonabsorbable surgical material NOS

T85.7   Infection and inflammatory reaction due to other internal prosthetic devices, implants and grafts
> Use additional code to identify infection

⊗⑦**T85.71**   Infection and inflammatory reaction due to peritoneal dialysis catheter

⊗⑦**T85.72**   Infection and inflammatory reaction due to insulin pump

⊗⑦**T85.79**   Infection and inflammatory reaction due to other internal prosthetic devices, implants and grafts

T85.8   Other specified complications of internal prosthetic devices, implants and grafts, not elsewhere classified

⊗⑦**T85.81**   Embolism due to internal prosthetic devices, implants and grafts, not elsewhere classified

⊗⑦**T85.82**   Fibrosis due to internal prosthetic devices, implants and grafts, not elsewhere classified

⊗⑦**T85.83**   Hemorrhage due to internal prosthetic devices, implants and grafts, not elsewhere classified

⊗⑦**T85.84**   Pain due to internal prosthetic devices, implants and grafts, not elsewhere classified

⊗⑦**T85.85**   Stenosis due to internal prosthetic devices, implants and grafts, not elsewhere classified

⊗⑦**T85.86**   Thrombosis due to internal prosthetic devices, implants and grafts, not elsewhere classified

⊗⑦**T85.89**   Other specified complication of internal prosthetic devices, implants and grafts, not elsewhere classified

⊗⑦**T85.9**   Unspecified complication of internal prosthetic device, implant and graft
> Complication of internal prosthetic device, implant and graft NOS

T86   Complications of transplanted organs and tissue
> Use additional code to identify other transplant complications, such as:
> graft-versus-host disease (D89.81-)
> malignancy associated with organ transplant (C80.2)
> post-transplant lymphoproliferative disorders (PTLD) (D47.Z1)

T86.0   Complications of bone marrow transplant

T86.00   Unspecified complication of bone marrow transplant

T86.01   Bone marrow transplant rejection

T86.02   Bone marrow transplant failure

T86.03   Bone marrow transplant infection

T86.09   Other complications of bone marrow transplant

T86.1   Complications of kidney transplant

T86.10   Unspecified complication of kidney transplant

T86.11   Kidney transplant rejection

T86.12	Kidney transplant failure
T86.13	Kidney transplant infection
	Use additional code to specify infection
T86.19	Other complication of kidney transplant

T86.2 Complications of heart transplant

Excludes 1: complication of:
artificial heart device (T82.5)
heart-lung transplant (T86.3)

T86.20	Unspecified complication of heart transplant
T86.21	Heart transplant rejection
T86.22	Heart transplant failure
T86.23	Heart transplant infection
	Use additional code to specify infection
T86.29	Other complications of heart transplant

T86.290 Cardiac allograft vasculopathy
Excludes 1: atherosclerosis of coronary arteries (I25.75-, I25.76-, I25.81-)

T86.298 Other complications of heart transplant

T86.3 Complications of heart-lung transplant

T86.30	Unspecified complication of heart-lung transplant
T86.31	Heart-lung transplant rejection
T86.32	Heart-lung transplant failure
T86.33	Heart-lung transplant infection
	Use additional code to specify infection
T86.39	Other complications of heart-lung transplant

T86.4 Complications of liver transplant

T86.40	Unspecified complication of liver transplant
T86.41	Liver transplant rejection
T86.42	Liver transplant failure
T86.43	Liver transplant infection

Use additional code to identify infection, such as:
Cytomegalovirus (CMV) infection (B25.-)

T86.49	Other complications of liver transplant

T86.5 Complications of stem cell transplant
Complications from stem cells from peripheral blood
Complications from stem cells from umbilical cord

T86.8 Complications of other transplanted organs and tissues

T86.81 Complications of lung transplant
Excludes 1: complication of heart-lung transplant (T86.3-)

T86.810	Lung transplant rejection
T86.811	Lung transplant failure
T86.812	Lung transplant infection
	Use additional code to specify infection
T86.818	Other complications of lung transplant
T86.819	Unspecified complication of lung transplant

T86.82 Complications of skin graft (allograft) (autograft)
Excludes 2: complication of artificial skin graft (T85.64)

T86.820 Skin graft (allograft) rejection

T86.821 Skin graft (allograft) (autograft) failure

T86.822 Skin graft (allograft) (autograft) infection
Use additional code to specify infection

T86.828 Other complications of skin graft (allograft) (autograft)

T86.829 Unspecified complication of skin graft (allograft) (autograft)

T86.83 Complications of bone graft
Excludes 2: mechanical complications of bone graft (T84.3-)

T86.830	Bone graft rejection
T86.831	Bone graft failure
T86.832	Bone graft infection
	Use additional code to specify infection
T86.838	Other complications of bone graft
T86.839	Unspecified complication of bone graft

T86.84 Complications of corneal transplant
Excludes 2: mechanical complications of corneal graft (T85.3-)

T86.840	Corneal transplant rejection
T86.841	Corneal transplant failure
T86.842	Corneal transplant infection
	Use additional code to specify infection
T86.848	Other complications of corneal transplant
T86.849	Unspecified complication of corneal transplant

T86.85 Complication of intestine transplant

T86.850	Intestine transplant rejection
T86.851	Intestine transplant failure
T86.852	Intestine transplant infection
	Use additional code to specify infection
T86.858	Other complications of intestine transplant
T86.859	Unspecified complication of intestine transplant

T86.89 Complications of other transplanted tissue
Transplant failure or rejection of pancreas

T86.890	Other transplanted tissue rejection
T86.891	Other transplanted tissue failure
T86.892	Other transplanted tissue infection
	Use additional code to specify infection
T86.898	Other complications of other transplanted tissue
T86.899	Unspecified complication of other transplanted tissue

T86.9 Complication of unspecified transplanted organ and tissue

T86.90 Unspecified complication of unspecified transplanted organ and tissue

T86.91 Unspecified transplanted organ and tissue rejection

T86.92 Unspecified transplanted organ and tissue failure

T86.93 Unspecified transplanted organ and tissue infection

Use additional code to specify infection

T86.99 Other complications of unspecified transplanted organ and tissue

T87 Complications peculiar to reattachment and amputation

T87.0 Complications of reattached (part of) upper extremity

T87.0X Complications of reattached (part of) upper extremity

T87.0X1 Complications of reattached (part of) right upper extremity

T87.0X2 Complications of reattached (part of) left upper extremity

T87.0X9 Complications of reattached (part of) unspecified upper extremity

T87.1 Complications of reattached (part of) lower extremity

T87.1X Complications of reattached (part of) lower extremity

T87.1X1 Complications of reattached (part of) right lower extremity

T87.1X2 Complications of reattached (part of) left lower extremity

T87.1X9 Complications of reattached (part of) unspecified lower extremity

T87.2 Complications of other reattached body part

T87.3 Neuroma of amputation stump

T87.30 Neuroma of amputation stump, unspecified extremity

T87.31 Neuroma of amputation stump, right upper extremity

T87.32 Neuroma of amputation stump, left upper extremity

T87.33 Neuroma of amputation stump, right lower extremity

T87.34 Neuroma of amputation stump, left lower extremity

T87.4 Infection of amputation stump

T87.40 Infection of amputation stump, unspecified extremity

T87.41 Infection of amputation stump, right upper extremity

T87.42 Infection of amputation stump, left upper extremity

T87.43 Infection of amputation stump, right lower extremity

T87.44 Infection of amputation stump, left lower extremity

T87.5 Necrosis of amputation stump

T87.50 Necrosis of amputation stump, unspecified extremity

T87.51 Necrosis of amputation stump, right upper extremity

T87.52 Necrosis of amputation stump, left upper extremity

T87.53 Necrosis of amputation stump, right lower extremity

T87.54 Necrosis of amputation stump, left lower extremity

T87.8 Other complications of amputation stump

T87.81 Dehiscence of amputation stump

T87.89 Other complications of amputation stump

Amputation stump contracture

Amputation stump contracture of next proximal joint

Amputation stump flexion

Amputation stump edema

Amputation stump hematoma

Excludes 2: phantom limb syndrome (G54.6-G54.7)

T87.9 Unspecified complications of amputation stump

T88 Other complications of surgical and medical care, not elsewhere classified

Excludes 2: complication following infusion, transfusion and therapeutic injection (T80.-)

complication following procedure NEC (T81.-)

complications of anesthesia in labor and delivery (O74.-)

complications of anesthesia in pregnancy (O29.-)

complications of anesthesia in puerperium (O89.-)

complications of devices, implants and grafts (T82-T85)

complications of obstetric surgery and procedure (O75.4)

dermatitis due to drugs and medicaments (L23.3, L24.4, L25.1, L27.0-L27.1)

poisoning and toxic effects of drugs and chemicals (T36-T65 with fifth or sixth character 1-4 or 6)

specified complications classified elsewhere

The appropriate 7th character is to be added to each code from category T88

A - initial encounter

D - subsequent encounter

S - sequela

T88.0 Infection following immunization

Sepsis following immunization

T88.1 Other complications following immunization, not elsewhere classified

Generalized vaccinia

Rash following immunization

Excludes 1: vaccinia not from vaccine (B08.011)

Excludes 2: anaphylactic shock due to serum (T80.5-)

other serum reactions (T80.6-)

postimmunization arthropathy (M02.2)

postimmunization encephalitis (G04.02)

postimmunization fever (R50.83)

T88.2 Shock due to anesthesia

Use additional code for adverse effect, if applicable, to identify drug (T41.- with fifth or sixth character 5)

Excludes 1: complications of anesthesia (in):

labor and delivery (O74.-)

pregnancy (O29.-)

puerperium (O89.-)

postprocedural shock NOS (T81.1-)

T88.3 Malignant hyperthermia due to anesthesia

Use additional code for adverse effect, if applicable, to identify drug (T41.- with fifth or sixth character 5)

⊗⑦**T88.4**   Failed or difficult intubation

    T88.5   Other complications of anesthesia

Use additional code for adverse effect, if applicable, to identify drug (T41.- with fifth or sixth character 5)

⊗⑦**T88.51**   Hypothermia following anesthesia

⊗⑦**T88.52**   Failed moderate sedation during procedure

Failed conscious sedation during procedure

Excludes 2: personal history of failed moderate sedation (Z92.83)

⊗⑦**T88.59**   Other complications of anesthesia

⊗⑦**T88.6**   Anaphylactic reaction due to adverse effect of correct drug or medicament properly administered

Anaphylactic shock due to adverse effect of correct drug or medicament properly administered

Anaphylactoid reaction NOS

Use additional code for adverse effect, if applicable, to identify drug (T36-T50 with fifth or sixth character 5)

Excludes 1: anaphylactic reaction due to serum (T80.5-)

anaphylactic shock or reaction due to adverse food reaction (T78.0-)

⊗⑦**T88.7**   Unspecified adverse effect of drug or medicament

Drug hypersensitivity NOS

Drug reaction NOS

Use additional code for adverse effect, if applicable, to identify drug (T36-T50 with fifth or sixth character 5)

Excludes 1: specified adverse effects of drugs and medicaments (A00-R94and T80-T88.6, T88.8)

⊗⑦**T88.8**   Other specified complications of surgical and medical care, not elsewhere classified

Use additional code to identify the complication

⊗⑦**T88.9**   Complication of surgical and medical care, unspecified

● New code   ▲ Revised code   ⑦ 7th digit required   ⊗ Placeholder required

Chapter 20: External Causes Of Morbidity (V00-Y99)

Note: This chapter permits the classification of environmental events and circumstances as the cause of injury, and other adverse effects. Where a code from this section is applicable, it is intended that it shall be used secondary to a code from another chapter of the Classification indicating the nature of the condition. Most often, the condition will be classifiable to Chapter 19, Injury, poisoning and certain other consequences of external causes (S00-T88). Other conditions that may be stated to be due to external causes are classified in Chapters I to XVIII. For these conditions, codes from Chapter 20 should be used to provide additional information as to the cause of the condition.

This chapter contains the following blocks:

V00-X58	Accidents
V00-V99	Transport accidents
V00-V09	Pedestrian injured in transport accident
V10-V19	Pedal cycle rider injured in transport accident
V20-V29	Motorcycle rider injured in transport accident
V30-V39	Occupant of three-wheeled motor vehicle injured in transport accident
V40-V49	Car occupant injured in transport accident
V50-V59	Occupant of pick-up truck or van injured in transport accident
V60-V69	Occupant of heavy transport vehicle injured in transport accident
V70-V79	Bus occupant injured in transport accident
V80-V89	Other land transport accidents
V90-V94	Water transport accidents
V95-V97	Air and space transport accidents
V98-V99	Other and unspecified transport accidents
W00-X58	Other external causes of accidental injury
W00-W19	Slipping, tripping, stumbling and falls
W20-W49	Exposure to inanimate mechanical forces
W50-W64	Exposure to animate mechanical forces
W65-W74	Accidental non-transport drowning and submersion
W85-W99	Exposure to electric current, radiation and extreme ambient air temperature and pressure
X00-X08	Exposure to smoke, fire and flames
X10-X19	Contact with heat and hot substances
X30-X39	Exposure to forces of nature
X52-X58	Accidental exposure to other specified factors
X71-X83	Intentional self-harm
X92-Y08	Assault
Y21-Y33	Event of undetermined intent
Y35 Y38	Legal intervention, operations of war, military operations, and terrorism
Y62-Y84	Complications of medical and surgical care
Y62-Y69	Misadventures to patients during surgical and medical care
Y70-Y82	Medical devices associated with adverse incidents in diagnostic and therapeutic use
Y83-Y84	Surgical and other medical procedures as the cause of abnormal reaction of the patient, or of later complication, without mention of misadventure at the time of the procedure
Y90-Y99	Supplementary factors related to causes of morbidity classified elsewhere

ACCIDENTS (V00-X58)

TRANSPORT ACCIDENTS (V00-V99)

Note: This section is structured in 12 groups. Those relating to land transport accidents (V01- V89) reflect the victim's mode of transport and are subdivided to identify the victim's 'counterpart' or the type of event. The vehicle of which the injured person is an occupant is identified in the first two characters since it is seen as the most important factor to identify for prevention purposes. A transport accident is one in which the vehicle involved must be moving or running or in use for transport purposes at the time of the accident.

Use additional code to identify:

Airbag injury (W22.1)

Type of street or road (Y92.4-)

Use of cellular telephone and other electronic equipment at the time of the transport accident (Y93.C-)

Excludes 1: agricultural vehicles in stationary use or maintenance (W31.-)

assault by crashing of motor vehicle (Y03.-)

automobile or motor cycle in stationary use or maintenance- code to type of accident

crashing of motor vehicle, undetermined intent (Y32)

intentional self-harm by crashing of motor vehicle (X82)

Excludes 2: transport accidents due to cataclysm (X34-X38)

Note: Definitions of transport vehicles:

(a) A transport accident is any accident involving a device designed primarily for, or used at the time primarily for, conveying persons or good from one place to another.

(b) A public highway [traffic way] or street is the entire width between property lines (or other boundary lines) of land open to the public as a matter of right or custom for purposes of moving persons or property from one place to another. A roadway is that part of the public highway designed, improved and customarily used for vehicular traffic.

(c) A traffic accident is any vehicle accident occurring on the public highway [i.e. originating on, terminating on, or involving a vehicle partially on the highway]. A vehicle accident is assumed to have occurred on the public highway unless another place is specified, except in the case of accidents involving only off-road motor vehicles, which are classified as nontraffic accidents unless the contrary is stated.

(d) A nontraffic accident is any vehicle accident that occurs entirely in any place other than a public highway.

(e) A pedestrian is any person involved in an accident who was not at the time of the accident riding in or on a motor vehicle, railway train, streetcar or animal-drawn or other vehicle, or on a pedal cycle or animal. This includes, a person changing a tire or working on a parked car. It also includes the use of a pedestrian conveyance such as a baby carriage, ice-skates, roller skates, a skateboard, nonmotorized or motorized wheelchair, motorized mobility scooter, or nonmotorized scooter.

(f) A driver is an occupant of a transport vehicle who is operating or intending to operate it.

(g) A passenger is any occupant of a transport vehicle other than the driver, except a person traveling on the outside of the vehicle.

(h) A person on the outside of a vehicle is any person being transported by a vehicle but not occupying the space normally reserved for the driver or

passengers, or the space intended for the transport of property. This includes the body, bumper, fender, roof, running board or step of a vehicle.

(i) A pedal cycle is any land transport vehicle operated solely by nonmotorized pedals including a bicycle or tricycle.

(j) A pedal cyclist is any person riding a pedal cycle or in a sidecar or trailer attached to a pedal cycle.

(k) A motorcycle is a two-wheeled motor vehicle with one or two riding saddles and sometimes with a third wheel for the support of a sidecar. The

sidecar is considered part of the motorcycle.

(l) A motorcycle rider is any person riding a motorcycle or in a sidecar or trailer attached to the motorcycle.

(m) A three-wheeled motor vehicle is a motorized tricycle designed primarily for on-road use. This includes a motor-driven tricycle, a motorized

rickshaw, or a three-wheeled motor car.

(n) A car [automobile] is a four-wheeled motor vehicle designed primarily for carrying up to 7persons. A trailer being towed by the car is considered part of the car.

(o) A pick-up truck or van is a four or six-wheeled motor vehicle designed for carrying passengers as well as property or cargo weighing less than the local limit for classification as a heavy goods vehicle, and not requiring a special driver's license. This includes a minivan and a sport-utility vehicle (SUV).

(p) A heavy transport vehicle is a motor vehicle designed primarily for carrying property, meeting local criteria for classification as a heavy goods

vehicle in terms of weight and requiring a special driver's license.

(q) A bus (coach) is a motor vehicle designed or adapted primarily for carrying more than 10 passengers, and requiring a special driver's license.

(r) A railway train or railway vehicle is any device, with or without freight or passenger cars couple to it, designed for traffic on a railway track. This includes subterranean (subways) or elevated trains.

(s) A streetcar, is a device designed and used primarily for transporting passengers within a municipality, running on rails, usually subject to normal traffic control signals, and operated principally on a right-of-way that forms part of the roadway. This includes a tram or trolley that runs on rails. A trailer being towed by a streetcar is considered part of the streetcar.

(t) A special vehicle mainly used on industrial premises is a motor vehicle designed primarily for use within the buildings and premises of industrial or commercial establishments. This includes battery-powered trucks, forklifts, coal-cars in a coal mine, logging cars and trucks used in mines or quarries.

(u) A special vehicle mainly used in agriculture is a motor vehicle designed specifically for use in farming and agriculture (horticulture), to work the

land, tend and harvest crops and transport materials on the farm. This includes harvesters, farm machinery and tractor and trailers.

(v) A special construction vehicle is a motor vehicle designed specifically for use on construction and demolition sites. This includes bulldozers, diggers, earth levellers, dump trucks. backhoes, front-end loaders, pavers, and mechanical shovels.

(w) A special all-terrain vehicle is a motor vehicle of special design to enable it to negotiate over rough or soft terrain , snow or sand. This includes snow mobiles, All-terrain vehicles (ATV), and dune buggies. It does not include passenger vehicle designated as Sport Utility Vehicles. (SUV)

(x) A watercraft is any device designed for transporting passengers or goods on water. This includes motor or sail boats, ships, and hovercraft.

(y) An aircraft is any device for transporting passengers or goods in the air. This includes hot-air balloons, gliders, helicopters and airplanes.

(z) A military vehicle is any motorized vehicle operating on a public roadway owned by the military and being operated by a member of the military.

PEDESTRIAN INJURED IN TRANSPORT ACCIDENT (V00-V09)

Includes: person changing tire on transport vehicle

person examining engine of vehicle broken down in (on side of) road

Excludes 1: fall due to non-transport collision with other person (W03)

pedestrian on foot falling (slipping) on ice and snow (W00.-)

struck or bumped by another person (W51)

V00 Pedestrian conveyance accident

Use additional place of occurrence and activity external cause codes, if known (Y92.-, Y93.-)

Excludes 1: collision with another person without fall (W51)

fall due to person on foot colliding with another person on foot (W03)

fall from non-moving wheelchair, nonmotorized scooter and motorized mobility scooter without collision (W05.-)

pedestrian (conveyance) collision with other land transport vehicle (V01-V09)

pedestrian on foot falling (slipping) on ice and snow (W00.-)

The appropriate 7th character is to be added to each code from category V00

A - initial encounter

D - subsequent encounter

S - sequela

V00.0 Pedestrian on foot injured in collision with pedestrian conveyance

⊗⑦**V00.01** Pedestrian on foot injured in collision with roller-skater

⊗⑦**V00.02** Pedestrian on foot injured in collision with skateboarder

⊗⑦**V00.09** Pedestrian on foot injured in collision with other pedestrian conveyance

V00.1 Rolling-type pedestrian conveyance accident

Excludes 1: accident with babystroller (V00.82-)

accident with wheelchair (powered) (V00.81-)

accident with motorized mobility scooter (V00.83-)

V00.11 In-line roller-skate accident

⑦**V00.111** Fall from in-line roller-skates

⑦**V00.112** In-line roller-skater colliding with stationary object

⑦**V00.118** Other in-line roller-skate accident

Excludes 1: roller-skater collision with other land transport vehicle (V01-V09 with 5th character 1)

V00.12 Non-in- line roller-skate accident

⑦**V00.121** Fall from non-in-line roller-skates

⑦**V00.122** Non-in-line roller-skater colliding with stationary object

⑦**V00.128** Other non-in-line roller-skating accident

● New code   ▲ Revised code   ⑦ 7th digit required   ⊗ Placeholder required

Excludes 1: roller-skater collision with other land transport vehicle (V01-V09 with 5th character 1)

V00.13 Skateboard accident

⑦ **V00.131** Fall from skateboard

⑦ **V00.132** Skateboarder colliding with stationary object

⑦ **V00.138** Other skateboard accident

Excludes 1: skateboarder collision with other land transport vehicle (V01-V09 with 5th character 2)

V00.14 Scooter (nonmotorized) accident

Excludes 1: motorscooter accident (V20-V29)

⑦ **V00.141** Fall from scooter (nonmotorized)

⑦ **V00.142** Scooter (nonmotorized) colliding with stationary object

⑦ **V00.148** Other scooter (nonmotorized) accident

Excludes 1: scooter (nonmotorized) collision with other land transport vehicle (V01-V09 with fifth character 9)

V00.15 Heelies accident

Rolling shoe

Wheeled shoe

Wheelies accident

⑦ **V00.151** Fall from heelies

⑦ **V00.152** Heelies colliding with stationary object

⑦ **V00.158** Other heelies accident

V00.18 Accident on other rolling-type pedestrian conveyance

⑦ **V00.181** Fall from other rolling-type pedestrian conveyance

⑦ **V00.182** Pedestrian on other rolling-type pedestrian conveyance colliding with stationary object

⑦ **V00.188** Other accident on other rolling-type pedestrian conveyance

V00.2 Gliding-type pedestrian conveyance accident

V00.21 Ice-skates accident

⑦ **V00.211** Fall from ice-skates

⑦ **V00.212** Ice-skater colliding with stationary object

⑦ **V00.218** Other ice-skates accident

Excludes 1: ice-skater collision with other land transport vehicle (V01-V09 with 5th digit 9)

V00.22 Sled accident

⑦ **V00.221** Fall from sled

⑦ **V00.222** Sledder colliding with stationary object

⑦ **V00.228** Other sled accident

Excludes 1: sled collision with other land transport vehicle

(V01-V09 with 5th digit 9)

V00.28 Other gliding-type pedestrian conveyance accident

⑦ **V00.281** Fall from other gliding-type pedestrian conveyance

⑦ **V00.282** Pedestrian on other gliding-type pedestrian conveyance colliding with stationary object

⑦ **V00.288** Other accident on other gliding-type pedestrian conveyance

Excludes 1: gliding-type pedestrian conveyance collision with other land transport vehicle (V01-V09 with 5th digit 9)

V00.3 Flat-bottomed pedestrian conveyance accident

V00.31 Snowboard accident

⑦ **V00.311** Fall from snowboard

⑦ **V00.312** Snowboarder colliding with stationary object

⑦ **V00.318** Other snowboard accident

Excludes 1: snowboarder collision with other land transport vehicle (V01-V09 with 5th digit 9)

V00.32 Snow-ski accident

⑦ **V00.321** Fall from snow-skis

⑦ **V00.322** Snow-skier colliding with stationary object

⑦ **V00.328** Other snow-ski accident

Excludes 1: snow-skier collision with other land transport vehicle (V01-V09 with 5th digit 9)

V00.38 Other flat-bottomed pedestrian conveyance accident

⑦ **V00.381** Fall from other flat-bottomed pedestrian conveyance

⑦ **V00.382** Pedestrian on other flat-bottomed pedestrian conveyance colliding with stationary object

⑦ **V00.388** Other accident on other flat-bottomed pedestrian conveyance

V00.8 Accident on other pedestrian conveyance

V00.81 Accident with wheelchair (powered)

⑦ **V00.811** Fall from moving wheelchair (powered)

Excludes 1: fall from non moving wheelchair (W05.0)

⑦ **V00.812** Wheelchair (powered) colliding with stationary object

⑦ **V00.818** Other accident with wheelchair (powered)

V00.82 Accident with babystroller

⑦ **V00.821** Fall from babystroller

⑦ **V00.822** Babystroller colliding with stationary object

⑦ **V00.828** Other accident with babystroller

V00.83 Accident with motorized mobility scooter

■ Add 4th-7th digits   ■ 3 digit reportable   ■ Nonspecific code   ■ Unspecified code   ■ Manifestation code

⑦**V00.831** Fall from motorized mobility scooter
Excludes 1: fall from non-moving motorized mobility scooter (W05.2)

⑦**V00.832** Motorized mobility scooter colliding with stationary object

⑦**V00.838** Other accident with motorized mobility scooter

V00.89 Accident on other pedestrian conveyance

⑦**V00.891** Fall from other pedestrian conveyance

⑦**V00.892** Pedestrian on other pedestrian conveyance colliding with stationary object

⑦**V00.898** Other accident on other pedestrian conveyance
Excludes 1: other pedestrian (conveyance) collision with other land transport vehicle (V01-V09 with 5th digit 9)

V01 Pedestrian injured in collision with pedal cycle
The appropriate 7th character is to be added to each code from category V01
A - initial encounter
D - subsequent encounter
S - sequela

V01.0 Pedestrian injured in collision with pedal cycle in nontraffic accident

⊗⑦**V01.00** Pedestrian on foot injured in collision with pedal cycle in nontraffic accident
Pedestrian NOS injured in collision with pedal cycle in nontraffic accident

⊗⑦**V01.01** Pedestrian on roller-skates injured in collision with pedal cycle in nontraffic accident

⊗⑦**V01.02** Pedestrian on skateboard injured in collision with pedal cycle in nontraffic accident

⊗⑦**V01.09** Pedestrian with other conveyance injured in collision with pedal cycle in nontraffic accident
Pedestrian with babystroller injured in collision with pedal cycle in nontraffic accident
Pedestrian on ice-skates injured in collision with pedal cycle in nontraffic accident
Pedestrian on nonmotorized scooter injured in collision with pedal cycle in nontraffic accident
Pedestrian on sled injured in collision with pedal cycle in nontraffic accident
Pedestrian on snowboard injured in collision with pedal cycle in nontraffic accident
Pedestrian on snow-skis injured in collision with pedal cycle in nontraffic accident
Pedestrian in wheelchair (powered) injured in collision with pedal cycle in nontraffic accident
Pedestrian in motorized mobility scooter injured in collision with pedal cycle in nontraffic accident

V01.1 Pedestrian injured in collision with pedal cycle in traffic accident

⊗⑦**V01.10** Pedestrian on foot injured in collision with pedal cycle in traffic accident

Pedestrian NOS injured in collision with pedal cycle in traffic accident

⊗⑦**V01.11** Pedestrian on roller-skates injured in collision with pedal cycle in traffic accident

⊗⑦**V01.12** Pedestrian on skateboard injured in collision with pedal cycle in traffic accident

⊗⑦**V01.19** Pedestrian with other conveyance injured in collision with pedal cycle in traffic accident
Pedestrian with babystroller injured in collision with pedal cycle in traffic accident
Pedestrian on ice-skates injured in collision with pedal cycle in traffic accident
Pedestrian on nonmotorized scooter injured in collision with pedal cycle in traffic accident
Pedestrian on sled injured in collision with pedal cycle in traffic accident
Pedestrian on snowboard injured in collision with pedal cycle in traffic accident
Pedestrian on snow-skis injured in collision with pedal cycle in traffic accident
Pedestrian in wheelchair (powered) injured in collision with pedal cycle in traffic accident
Pedestrian in motorized mobility scooter injured in collision with pedal cycle in traffic accident

V01.9 Pedestrian injured in collision with pedal cycle, unspecified whether traffic or nontraffic accident

⊗⑦**V01.90** Pedestrian on foot injured in collision with pedal cycle, unspecified whether traffic or nontraffic accident
Pedestrian NOS injured in collision with pedal cycle, unspecified whether traffic or nontraffic accident

⊗⑦**V01.91** Pedestrian on roller-skates injured in collision with pedal cycle, unspecified whether traffic or nontraffic accident

⊗⑦**V01.92** Pedestrian on skateboard injured in collision with pedal cycle, unspecified whether traffic or nontraffic accident

⊗⑦**V01.99** Pedestrian with other conveyance injured in collision with pedal cycle, unspecified whether traffic or nontraffic accident
Pedestrian with babystroller injured in collision with pedal cycle, unspecified whether traffic or nontraffic accident
Pedestrian on ice-skates injured in collision with pedal cycle unspecified, whether traffic or nontraffic accident
Pedestrian on nonmotorized scooter injured in collision with pedal cycle, unspecified whether traffic or nontraffic accident
Pedestrian on sled injured in collision with pedal cycle unspecified, whether traffic or nontraffic accident
Pedestrian on snowboard injured in collision with pedal cycle, unspecified whether traffic or nontraffic accident
Pedestrian on snow-skis injured in collision with pedal cycle, unspecified whether traffic or nontraffic accident

Pedestrian in wheelchair (powered) injured in collision with pedal cycle, unspecified whether traffic or nontraffic accident

Pedestrian in motorized mobility scooter injured in collision with pedal cycle, unspecified whether traffic or nontraffic accident

V02 Pedestrian injured in collision with two- or three-wheeled motor vehicle

The appropriate 7th character is to be added to each code from category V02

A - initial encounter

D - subsequent encounter

S - sequela

V02.0 Pedestrian injured in collision with two- or three-wheeled motor vehicle in nontraffic accident

⊗⑦**V02.00** Pedestrian on foot injured in collision with two- or three-wheeled motor vehicle in nontraffic accident

Pedestrian NOS injured in collision with two- or three-wheeled motor vehicle in nontraffic accident

⊗⑦**V02.01** Pedestrian on roller-skates injured in collision with two- or three-wheeled motor vehicle in nontraffic accident

⊗⑦**V02.02** Pedestrian on skateboard injured in collision with two- or three-wheeled motor vehicle in nontraffic accident

⊗⑦**V02.09** Pedestrian with other conveyance injured in collision with two- or three-wheeled motor vehicle in nontraffic accident

Pedestrian with babystroller injured in collision with two- or three-wheeled motor vehicle in nontraffic accident

Pedestrian on ice-skates injured in collision with two- or three-wheeled motor vehicle in nontraffic accident

Pedestrian on nonmotorized scooter injured in collision with two- or three-wheeled motor vehicle in nontraffic accident

Pedestrian on sled injured in collision with two- or three-wheeled motor vehicle in nontraffic accident

Pedestrian on snowboard injured in collision with two- or three-wheeled motor vehicle in nontraffic accident

Pedestrian on snow-skis injured in collision with two- or three-wheeled motor vehicle in nontraffic accident

Pedestrian in wheelchair (powered) injured in collision with two- or three-wheeled motor vehicle in nontraffic accident

Pedestrian in motorized mobility scooter injured in collision with two- or three-wheeled motor vehicle in nontraffic accident

V02.1 Pedestrian injured in collision with two- or three-wheeled motor vehicle in traffic accident

⊗⑦**V02.10** Pedestrian on foot injured in collision with two- or three-wheeled motor vehicle in traffic accident

Pedestrian NOS injured in collision with two- or three-wheeled motor vehicle in traffic accident

⊗⑦**V02.11** Pedestrian on roller-skates injured in collision with two- or three-wheeled motor vehicle in traffic accident

⊗⑦**V02.12** Pedestrian on skateboard injured in collision with two- or three-wheeled motor vehicle in traffic accident

⊗⑦**V02.19** Pedestrian with other conveyance injured in collision with two- or three-wheeled motor vehicle in traffic accident

Pedestrian with babystroller injured in collision with two- or three-wheeled motor vehicle in traffic accident

Pedestrian on ice-skates injured in collision with two- or three-wheeled motor vehicle in traffic accident

Pedestrian on nonmotorized scooter injured in collision with two- or three-wheeled motor vehicle in traffic accident

Pedestrian on sled injured in collision with two- or three-wheeled motor vehicle in traffic accident

Pedestrian on snowboard injured in collision with two- or three-wheeled motor vehicle in traffic accident

Pedestrian on snow-skis injured in collision with two- or three-wheeled motor vehicle in traffic accident

Pedestrian in wheelchair (powered) injured in collision with two- or three-wheeled motor vehicle in traffic accident

Pedestrian in motorized mobility scooter injured in collision with two- or three-wheeled motor vehicle in traffic accident

V02.9 Pedestrian injured in collision with two- or three-wheeled motor vehicle, unspecified whether traffic or nontraffic accident

V02.90 Pedestrian on foot injured in collision with two- or three-wheeled motor vehicle, unspecified whether traffic or nontraffic accident

Pedestrian NOS injured in collision with two- or three-wheeled motor vehicle, unspecified whether traffic or nontraffic accident

⊗⑦**V02.91** Pedestrian on roller-skates injured in collision with two- or three-wheeled motor vehicle, unspecified whether traffic or nontraffic accident

⊗⑦**V02.92** Pedestrian on skateboard injured in collision with two- or three-wheeled motor vehicle, unspecified whether traffic or nontraffic accident

⊗⑦**V02.99** Pedestrian with other conveyance injured in collision with two- or three-wheeled motor vehicle, unspecified whether traffic or nontraffic accident

Pedestrian with babystroller injured in collision with two- or three-wheeled motor vehicle, unspecified whether traffic or nontraffic accident

Pedestrian on ice-skates injured in collision with two- or three-wheeled motor vehicle, unspecified whether traffic or nontraffic accident

Pedestrian on nonmotorized scooter injured in collision with two- or three-wheeled motor vehicle, unspecified whether traffic or nontraffic accident

Pedestrian on sled injured in collision with two- or three-wheeled motor vehicle, unspecified whether traffic or nontraffic accident

Pedestrian on snowboard injured in collision with two- or three-wheeled motor vehicle, unspecified whether traffic or nontraffic accident

Pedestrian on snow-skis injured in collision with two- or three-wheeled motor vehicle, unspecified whether traffic or nontraffic accident

Pedestrian in wheelchair (powered) injured in collision with two- or three-wheeled motor vehicle, unspecified whether traffic or nontraffic accident

Pedestrian in motorized mobility scooter injured in collision with two- or three-wheeled motor vehicle, unspecified whether traffic or nontraffic accident

V03 Pedestrian injured in collision with car, pick-up truck or van

The appropriate 7th character is to be added to each code from category V03

A - initial encounter

D - subsequent encounter

S - sequela

V03.0 Pedestrian injured in collision with car, pick-up truck or van in nontraffic accident

⊗⑦**V03.00** Pedestrian on foot injured in collision with car, pick-up truck or van in nontraffic accident

Pedestrian NOS injured in collision with car, pick-up truck or van in nontraffic accident

⊗⑦**V03.01** Pedestrian on roller-skates injured in collision with car, pick-up truck or van in nontraffic accident

⊗⑦**V03.02** Pedestrian on skateboard injured in collision with car, pick-up truck or van in nontraffic accident

⊗⑦**V03.09** Pedestrian with other conveyance injured in collision with car, pick-up truck or van in nontraffic accident

Pedestrian with babystroller injured in collision with car, pick-up truck or van in nontraffic accident

Pedestrian on ice-skates injured in collision with car, pick-up truck or van in nontraffic accident

Pedestrian on nonmotorized scooter injured in collision with car, pick-up truck or van in nontraffic accident

Pedestrian on sled injured in collision with car, pick-up truck or van in nontraffic accident

Pedestrian on snowboard injured in collision with car, pick-up truck or van in nontraffic accident

Pedestrian on snow-skis injured in collision with car, pick-up truck or van in nontraffic accident

Pedestrian in wheelchair (powered) injured in collision with car, pick-up truck or van in nontraffic accident

Pedestrian in motorized mobility scooter injured in collision with car, pick-up truck or van in nontraffic accident

V03.1 Pedestrian injured in collision with car, pick-up truck or van in traffic accident

⊗⑦**V03.10** Pedestrian on foot injured in collision with car, pick-up truck or van in traffic accident

Pedestrian NOS injured in collision with car, pick-up truck or van in traffic accident

⊗⑦**V03.11** Pedestrian on roller-skates injured in collision with car, pick-up truck or van in traffic accident

⊗⑦**V03.12** Pedestrian on skateboard injured in collision with car, pick-up truck or van in traffic accident

⊗⑦**V03.19** Pedestrian with other conveyance injured in collision with car, pick-up truck or van in traffic accident

Pedestrian with babystroller injured in collision with car, pick-up truck or van in traffic accident

Pedestrian on ice-skates injured in collision with car, pick-up truck or van in traffic accident

Pedestrian on nonmotorized scooter injured in collision with car, pick-up truck or van in traffic accident

Pedestrian on sled injured in collision with car, pick-up truck or van in traffic accident

Pedestrian on snowboard injured in collision with car, pick-up truck or van in traffic accident

Pedestrian on snow-skis injured in collision with car, pick-up truck or van in traffic accident

Pedestrian in wheelchair (powered) injured in collision with car, pick-up truck or van in traffic accident

Pedestrian in motorized mobility scooter injured in collision with car, pick-up truck or van in traffic accident

V03.9 Pedestrian injured in collision with car, pick-up truck or van, unspecified whether traffic or nontraffic accident

⊗⑦**V03.90** Pedestrian on foot injured in collision with car, pick-up truck or van, unspecified whether traffic or nontraffic accident

Pedestrian NOS injured in collision with car, pick-up truck or van, unspecified whether traffic or nontraffic accident

⊗⑦**V03.91** Pedestrian on roller-skates injured in collision with car, pick-up truck or van, unspecified whether traffic or nontraffic accident

⊗⑦**V03.92** Pedestrian on skateboard injured in collision with car, pick-up truck or van, unspecified whether traffic or nontraffic accident

⊗⑦**V03.99** Pedestrian with other conveyance injured in collision with car, pick-up truck or van, unspecified whether traffic or nontraffic accident

Pedestrian with babystroller injured in collision with car, pick-up truck or van, unspecified whether traffic or nontraffic accident

Pedestrian on ice-skates injured in collision with car, pick-up truck or van, unspecified whether traffic or nontraffic accident

Pedestrian on nonmotorized scooter injured in collision with car, pick-up truck or van, unspecified whether traffic or nontraffic accident

Pedestrian on sled injured in collision with car, pick-up truck or van in nontraffic accident

Pedestrian on snowboard injured in collision with car, pick-up truck or van, unspecified whether traffic or nontraffic accident

Pedestrian on snow-skis injured in collision with car, pick-up truck or van, unspecified whether traffic or nontraffic accident

● New code   ▲ Revised code   ⑦ 7ᵗʰ digit required   ⊗ Placeholder required

Pedestrian in wheelchair (powered) injured in collision with car, pick-up truck or van, unspecified whether traffic or nontraffic accident

Pedestrian in motorized mobility scooter injured in collision with car, pick-up truck or van, unspecified whether traffic or nontraffic accident

V04 Pedestrian injured in collision with heavy transport vehicle or bus

Excludes 1: pedestrian injured in collision with military vehicle (V09.01, V09.21)

The appropriate 7th character is to be added to each code from category V04

A - initial encounter

D - subsequent encounter

S - sequela

V04.0 Pedestrian injured in collision with heavy transport vehicle or bus in nontraffic accident

⊗⑦**V04.00** Pedestrian on foot injured in collision with heavy transport vehicle or bus in nontraffic accident

Pedestrian NOS injured in collision with heavy transport vehicle or bus in nontraffic accident

⊗⑦**V04.01** Pedestrian on roller-skates injured in collision with heavy transport vehicle or bus in nontraffic accident

⊗⑦**V04.02** Pedestrian on skateboard injured in collision with heavy transport vehicle or bus in nontraffic accident

⊗⑦**V04.09** Pedestrian with other conveyance injured in collision with heavy transport vehicle or bus in nontraffic accident

Pedestrian with babystroller injured in collision with heavy transport vehicle or bus in nontraffic accident

Pedestrian on ice-skates injured in collision with heavy transport vehicle or bus in nontraffic accident

Pedestrian on nonmotorized scooter injured in collision with heavy transport vehicle or bus in nontraffic accident

Pedestrian on sled injured in collision with heavy transport vehicle or bus in nontraffic accident

Pedestrian on snowboard injured in collision with heavy transport vehicle or bus in nontraffic accident

Pedestrian on snow-skis injured in collision with heavy transport vehicle or bus in nontraffic accident

Pedestrian in wheelchair (powered) injured in collision with heavy transport vehicle or bus in nontraffic accident

Pedestrian in motorized mobility scooter injured in collision with heavy transport vehicle or bus in nontraffic accident

V04.1 Pedestrian injured in collision with heavy transport vehicle or bus in traffic accident

⊗⑦**V04.10** Pedestrian on foot injured in collision with heavy transport vehicle or bus in traffic accident

Pedestrian NOS injured in collision with heavy transport vehicle or bus in traffic accident

⊗⑦**V04.11** Pedestrian on roller-skates injured in collision with heavy transport vehicle or bus in traffic accident

⊗⑦**V04.12** Pedestrian on skateboard injured in collision with heavy transport vehicle or bus in traffic accident

⊗⑦**V04.19** Pedestrian with other conveyance injured in collision with heavy transport vehicle or bus in traffic accident

Pedestrian with babystroller injured in collision with heavy transport vehicle or bus in traffic accident

Pedestrian on ice-skates injured in collision with heavy transport vehicle or bus in traffic accident

Pedestrian on nonmotorized scooter injured in collision with heavy transport vehicle or bus inn traffic accident

Pedestrian on sled injured in collision with heavy transport vehicle or bus in traffic accident

Pedestrian on snowboard injured in collision with heavy transport vehicle or bus in traffic accident

Pedestrian on snow-skis injured in collision with heavy transport vehicle or bus in traffic accident

Pedestrian in wheelchair (powered) injured in collision with heavy transport vehicle or bus in traffic accident

Pedestrian in motorized mobility scooter injured in collision with heavy transport vehicle or bus in traffic accident

V04.9 Pedestrian injured in collision with heavy transport vehicle or bus, unspecified whether traffic or nontraffic accident

⊗⑦**V04.90** Pedestrian on foot injured in collision with heavy transport vehicle or bus, unspecified whether traffic or nontraffic accident

Pedestrian NOS injured in collision with heavy transport vehicle or bus, unspecified whether traffic or nontraffic accident

⊗⑦**V04.91** Pedestrian on roller-skates injured in collision with heavy transport vehicle or bus, unspecified whether traffic or nontraffic accident

⊗⑦**V04.92** Pedestrian on skateboard injured in collision with heavy transport vehicle or bus, unspecified whether traffic or nontraffic accident

⊗⑦**V04.99** Pedestrian with other conveyance injured in collision with heavy transport vehicle or bus, unspecified whether traffic or nontraffic accident

Pedestrian with babystroller injured in collision with heavy transport vehicle or bus, unspecified whether traffic or nontraffic accident

Pedestrian on ice-skates injured in collision with heavy transport vehicle or bus, unspecified whether traffic or nontraffic accident

Pedestrian on nonmotorized scooter injured in collision with heavy transport vehicle or bus, unspecified whether traffic or nontraffic accident

Pedestrian on sled injured in collision with heavy transport vehicle or bus, unspecified whether traffic or nontraffic accident

Pedestrian on snowboard injured in collision with heavy transport vehicle or bus, unspecified whether traffic or nontraffic accident

Pedestrian on snow-skis injured in collision with heavy transport vehicle or bus, unspecified whether traffic or nontraffic accident

Pedestrian in wheelchair (powered) injured in collision with heavy transport vehicle or bus, unspecified whether traffic or nontraffic accident

Pedestrian in motorized mobility scooter injured in collision with heavy transport vehicle or bus, unspecified whether traffic or nontraffic accident

V05 Pedestrian injured in collision with railway train or railway vehicle

The appropriate 7th character is to be added to each code from category V05

A - initial encounter

D - subsequent encounter

S - sequela

V05.0 Pedestrian injured in collision with railway train or railway vehicle in nontraffic accident

⊗⑦ **V05.00** Pedestrian on foot injured in collision with railway train or railway vehicle in nontraffic accident

Pedestrian NOS injured in collision with railway train or railway vehicle in nontraffic accident

⊗⑦ **V05.01** Pedestrian on roller-skates injured in collision with railway train or railway vehicle in nontraffic accident

⊗⑦ **V05.02** Pedestrian on skateboard injured in collision with railway train or railway vehicle in nontraffic accident

⊗⑦ **V05.09** Pedestrian with other conveyance injured in collision with railway train or railway vehicle in nontraffic accident

Pedestrian with babystroller injured in collision with railway train or railway vehicle in nontraffic accident

Pedestrian on ice-skates injured in collision with railway train or railway vehicle in nontraffic accident

Pedestrian on nonmotorized scooter injured in collision with railway train or railway vehicle in nontraffic accident

Pedestrian on sled injured in collision with railway train or railway vehicle in nontraffic accident

Pedestrian on snowboard injured in collision with railway train or railway vehicle in nontraffic accident

Pedestrian on snow-skis injured in collision with railway train or railway vehicle in nontraffic accident

Pedestrian in wheelchair (powered) injured in collision with railway train or railway vehicle in nontraffic accident

Pedestrian in motorized mobility scooter injured in collision with railway train or railway vehicle in nontraffic accident

V05.1 Pedestrian injured in collision with railway train or railway vehicle in traffic accident

⊗⑦ **V05.10** Pedestrian on foot injured in collision with railway train or railway vehicle in traffic accident

Pedestrian NOS injured in collision with railway train or railway vehicle in traffic accident

⊗⑦ **V05.11** Pedestrian on roller-skates injured in collision with railway train or railway vehicle in traffic accident

⊗⑦ **V05.12** Pedestrian on skateboard injured in collision with railway train or railway vehicle in traffic accident

⊗⑦ **V05.19** Pedestrian with other conveyance injured in collision with railway train or railway vehicle in traffic accident

Pedestrian with babystroller injured in collision with railway train or railway vehicle in traffic accident

Pedestrian on ice-skates injured in collision with railway train or railway vehicle in traffic accident

Pedestrian on nonmotorized scooter injured in collision with railway train or railway vehicle in traffic accident

Pedestrian on sled injured in collision with railway train or railway vehicle in traffic accident

Pedestrian on snowboard injured in collision with railway train or railway vehicle in traffic accident

Pedestrian on snow-skis injured in collision with railway train or railway vehicle in traffic accident

Pedestrian in wheelchair (powered) injured in collision with railway train or railway vehicle in traffic accident

Pedestrian in motorized mobility scooter injured in collision with railway train or railway vehicle in traffic accident

V05.9 Pedestrian injured in collision with railway train or railway vehicle, unspecified whether traffic or nontraffic accident

⊗⑦ **V05.90** Pedestrian on foot injured in collision with railway train or railway vehicle, unspecified whether traffic or nontraffic accident

Pedestrian NOS injured in collision with railway train or railway vehicle, unspecified whether traffic or nontraffic accident

⊗⑦ **V05.91** Pedestrian on roller-skates injured in collision with railway train or railway vehicle, unspecified whether traffic or nontraffic accident

⊗⑦ **V05.92** Pedestrian on skateboard injured in collision with railway train or railway vehicle, unspecified whether traffic or nontraffic accident

⊗⑦ **V05.99** Pedestrian with other conveyance injured in collision with railway train or railway vehicle, unspecified whether traffic or nontraffic accident

Pedestrian with babystroller injured in collision with railway train or railway vehicle, unspecified whether traffic or nontraffic

Pedestrian on ice-skates injured in collision with railway train or railway vehicle, unspecified whether traffic or nontraffic

Pedestrian on nonmotorized scooter injured in collision with railway train or railway vehicle, unspecified whether traffic or nontraffic

Pedestrian on sled injured in collision with railway train or railway vehicle, unspecified whether traffic or nontraffic

Pedestrian on snowboard injured in collision with railway train or railway vehicle, unspecified whether traffic or nontraffic

Pedestrian on snow-skis injured in collision with railway train or railway vehicle, unspecified whether traffic or nontraffic

Pedestrian in wheelchair (powered) injured in collision with railway train or railway vehicle, unspecified whether traffic or nontraffic

Pedestrian in motorized mobility scooter injured in collision with railway train or railway vehicle, unspecified whether traffic or nontraffic

V06 Pedestrian injured in collision with other nonmotor vehicle

Includes: collision with animal-drawn vehicle, animal being ridden, nonpowered streetcar

Excludes 1: pedestrian injured in collision with pedestrian conveyance (V00.0-)

The appropriate 7th character is to be added to each code from category V06

A - initial encounter

D - subsequent encounter

S - sequela

V06.0 Pedestrian injured in collision with other nonmotor vehicle in nontraffic accident

⊗⑦**V06.00** Pedestrian on foot injured in collision with other nonmotor vehicle in nontraffic accident

Pedestrian NOS injured in collision with other nonmotor vehicle in nontraffic accident

⊗⑦**V06.01** Pedestrian on roller-skates injured in collision with other nonmotor vehicle in nontraffic accident

⊗⑦**V06.02** Pedestrian on skateboard injured in collision with other nonmotor vehicle in nontraffic accident

⊗⑦**V06.09** Pedestrian with other conveyance injured in collision with other nonmotor vehicle in nontraffic accident

Pedestrian with babystroller injured in collision with other nonmotor vehicle in nontraffic accident

Pedestrian on ice-skates injured in collision with other nonmotor vehicle in nontraffic accident

Pedestrian on nonmotorized scooter injured in collision with other nonmotor vehicle in nontraffic accident

Pedestrian on sled injured in collision with other nonmotor vehicle in nontraffic accident

Pedestrian on snowboard injured in collision with other nonmotor vehicle in nontraffic accident

Pedestrian on snow-skis injured in collision with other nonmotor vehicle in nontraffic accident

Pedestrian in wheelchair (powered) injured in collision with other nonmotor vehicle in nontraffic accident

Pedestrian in motorized mobility scooter injured in collision with other nonmotor vehicle in nontraffic accident

V06.1 Pedestrian injured in collision with other nonmotor vehicle in traffic accident

⊗⑦**V06.10** Pedestrian on foot injured in collision with other nonmotor vehicle in traffic accident

Pedestrian NOS injured in collision with other nonmotor vehicle in traffic accident

⊗⑦**V06.11** Pedestrian on roller-skates injured in collision with other nonmotor vehicle in traffic accident

⊗⑦**V06.12** Pedestrian on skateboard injured in collision with other nonmotor vehicle in traffic accident

⊗⑦**V06.19** Pedestrian with other conveyance injured in collision with other nonmotor vehicle in traffic accident

Pedestrian with babystroller injured in collision with other nonmotor vehicle in nontraffic accident

Pedestrian on ice-skates injured in collision with other nonmotor vehicle in traffic accident

Pedestrian on nonmotorized scooter injured in collision with other nonmotor vehicle in traffic accident

Pedestrian on sled injured in collision with other nonmotor vehicle in traffic accident

Pedestrian on snowboard injured in collision with other nonmotor vehicle in traffic accident

Pedestrian on snow-skis injured in collision with other nonmotor vehicle in traffic accident

Pedestrian in wheelchair (powered) injured in collision with other nonmotor vehicle in traffic accident

Pedestrian in motorized mobility scooter injured in collision with other nonmotor vehicle in traffic accident

V06.9 Pedestrian injured in collision with other nonmotor vehicle, unspecified whether traffic or nontraffic accident

⊗⑦**V06.90** Pedestrian on foot injured in collision with other nonmotor vehicle, unspecified whether traffic or nontraffic accident

Pedestrian NOS injured in collision with other nonmotor vehicle, unspecified whether traffic or nontraffic accident

⊗⑦**V06.91** Pedestrian on roller-skates injured in collision with other nonmotor vehicle, unspecified whether traffic or nontraffic accident

⊗⑦**V06.92** Pedestrian on skateboard injured in collision with other nonmotor vehicle, unspecified whether traffic or nontraffic accident

⊗⑦**V06.99** Pedestrian with other conveyance injured in collision with other nonmotor vehicle, unspecified whether traffic or nontraffic accident

Pedestrian with babystroller injured in collision with other nonmotor vehicle, unspecified whether traffic or nontraffic accident

Pedestrian on ice-skates injured in collision with other nonmotor vehicle, unspecified whether traffic or nontraffic accident

Pedestrian on nonmotorized scooter injured in collision with other nonmotor vehicle, unspecified whether traffic or nontraffic accident

Pedestrian on sled injured in collision with other nonmotor vehicle, unspecified whether traffic or nontraffic accident

Pedestrian on snowboard injured in collision with other nonmotor vehicle, unspecified whether traffic or nontraffic accident

Pedestrian on snow-skis injured in collision with other nonmotor vehicle, unspecified whether traffic or nontraffic accident

Pedestrian in wheelchair (powered) injured in collision with other nonmotor vehicle, unspecified whether traffic or nontraffic accident

Pedestrian in motorized mobility scooter injured in collision with other nonmotor vehicle, unspecified whether traffic or nontraffic accident

V09 Pedestrian injured in other and unspecified transport accidents

The appropriate 7th character is to be added to each code from category V09

A - initial encounter

D - subsequent encounter

S - sequela

V09.0 Pedestrian injured in nontraffic accident involving other and unspecified motor vehicles

⊗⑦**V09.00** Pedestrian injured in nontraffic accident involving unspecified motor vehicles

⊗⑦**V09.01** Pedestrian injured in nontraffic accident involving military vehicle

⊗⑦**V09.09** Pedestrian injured in nontraffic accident involving other motor vehicles

Pedestrian injured in nontraffic accident by special vehicle

V09.1 Pedestrian injured in unspecified nontraffic accident

V09.2 Pedestrian injured in traffic accident involving other and unspecified motor vehicles

⊗⑦**V09.20** Pedestrian injured in traffic accident involving unspecified motor vehicles

⊗⑦**V09.21** Pedestrian injured in traffic accident involving military vehicle

⊗⑦**V09.29** Pedestrian injured in traffic accident involving other motor vehicles

⊗⑦**V09.3** Pedestrian injured in unspecified traffic accident

⊗⑦**V09.9** Pedestrian injured in unspecified transport accident

PEDAL CYCLE RIDER INJURED IN TRANSPORT ACCIDENT (V10-V19)

Includes: any non-motorized vehicle, excluding an animal-drawn vehicle, or a sidecar or trailer attached to the pedal cycle

Excludes 2: rupture of pedal cycle tire (W37.0)

V10 Pedal cycle rider injured in collision with pedestrian or animal

Excludes 1: pedal cycle rider collision with animal-drawn vehicle or animal being ridden (Vl6.-)

The appropriate 7th character is to be added to each code from category V10

A - initial encounter

D - subsequent encounter

S - sequela

⊗⑦**V10.0** Pedal cycle driver injured in collision with pedestrian or animal in nontraffic accident

⊗⑦**V10.1** Pedal cycle passenger injured in collision with pedestrian or animal in nontraffic accident

⊗⑦**V10.2** Unspecified pedal cyclist injured in collision with pedestrian or animal in nontraffic accident

⊗⑦**V10.3** Person boarding or alighting a pedal cycle injured in collision with pedestrian or animal

⊗⑦**V10.4** Pedal cycle driver injured in collision with pedestrian or animal in traffic accident

⊗⑦**V10.5** Pedal cycle passenger injured in collision with pedestrian or animal in traffic accident

⊗⑦**V10.9** Unspecified pedal cyclist injured in collision with pedestrian or animal in traffic accident

V11 Pedal cycle rider injured in collision with other pedal cycle

The appropriate 7th character is to be added to each code from category V11

A - initial encounter

D - subsequent encounter

S - sequela

⊗⑦**V11.0** Pedal cycle driver injured in collision with other pedal cycle in nontraffic accident

⊗⑦**V11.1** Pedal cycle passenger injured in collision with other pedal cycle in nontraffic accident

⊗⑦**V11.2** Unspecified pedal cyclist injured in collision with other pedal cycle in nontraffic accident

⊗⑦**V11.3** Person boarding or alighting a pedal cycle injured in collision with other pedal cycle

⊗⑦**V11.4** Pedal cycle driver injured in collision with other pedal cycle in traffic accident

⊗⑦**V11.5** Pedal cycle passenger injured in collision with other pedal cycle in traffic accident

⊗⑦**V11.9** Unspecified pedal cyclist injured in collision with other pedal cycle in traffic accident

V12 Pedal cycle rider injured in collision with two- or three-wheeled motor vehicle

The appropriate 7th character is to be added to each code from category V12

A - initial encounter

D - subsequent encounter

S - sequela

⊗⑦**V12.0** Pedal cycle driver injured in collision with two- or three-wheeled motor vehicle in nontraffic accident

⊗⑦**V12.1** Pedal cycle passenger injured in collision with two- or three-wheeled motor vehicle in nontraffic accident

⊗⑦**V12.2** Unspecified pedal cyclist injured in collision with two- or three-wheeled motor vehicle in nontraffic accident

⊗⑦**V12.3** Person boarding or alighting a pedal cycle injured in collision with two- or three-wheeled motor vehicle

⊗⑦**V12.4** Pedal cycle driver injured in collision with two- or three-wheeled motor vehicle in traffic accident

⊗⑦**V12.5** Pedal cycle passenger injured in collision with two- or three-wheeled motor vehicle in traffic accident

⊗⑦**V12.9** Unspecified pedal cyclist injured in collision with two- or three-wheeled motor vehicle in traffic accident

V13 Pedal cycle rider injured in collision with car, pick-up truck or van

The appropriate 7th character is to be added to each code from category V13

A - initial encounter

D - subsequent encounter

S - sequela

⊗⑦**V13.0** Pedal cycle driver injured in collision with car, pick-up truck or van in nontraffic accident

⊗⑦**V13.1** Pedal cycle passenger injured in collision with car, pick-up truck or van in nontraffic accident

⊗⑦**V13.2** Unspecified pedal cyclist injured in collision with car, pick-up truck or van in nontraffic accident

⊗⑦**V13.3** Person boarding or alighting a pedal cycle injured in collision with car, pick-up truck or van

⊗⑦**V13.4** Pedal cycle driver injured in collision with car, pick-up truck or van in traffic accident

⊗⑦**V13.5** Pedal cycle passenger injured in collision with car, pick-up truck or van in traffic accident

⊗⑦**V13.9** Unspecified pedal cyclist injured in collision with car, pick-up truck or van in traffic accident

V14 Pedal cycle rider injured in collision with heavy transport vehicle or bus

Excludes 1: pedal cycle rider injured in collision with military vehicle (V19.81)

The appropriate 7th character is to be added to each code from category V14

A - initial encounter

D - subsequent encounter

S - sequela

⊗⑦**V14.0** Pedal cycle driver injured in collision with heavy transport vehicle or bus in nontraffic accident

⊗⑦**V14.1** Pedal cycle passenger injured in collision with heavy transport vehicle or bus in nontraffic accident

⊗⑦**V14.2** Unspecified pedal cyclist injured in collision with heavy transport vehicle or bus in nontraffic accident

⊗⑦**V14.3** Person boarding or alighting a pedal cycle injured in collision with heavy transport vehicle or bus

⊗⑦**V14.4** Pedal cycle driver injured in collision with heavy transport vehicle or bus in traffic accident

⊗⑦**V14.5** Pedal cycle passenger injured in collision with heavy transport vehicle or bus in traffic accident

⊗⑦**V14.9** Unspecified pedal cyclist injured in collision with heavy transport vehicle or bus in traffic accident

V15 Pedal cycle rider injured in collision with railway train or railway vehicle

The appropriate 7th character is to be added to each code from category V15

A - initial encounter

D - subsequent encounter

S - sequela

⊗⑦**V15.0** Pedal cycle driver injured in collision with railway train or railway vehicle in nontraffic accident

⊗⑦**V15.1** Pedal cycle passenger injured in collision with railway train or railway vehicle in nontraffic accident

⊗⑦**V15.2** Unspecified pedal cyclist injured in collision with railway train or railway vehicle in nontraffic accident

⊗⑦**V15.3** Person boarding or alighting a pedal cycle injured in collision with railway train or railway vehicle

⊗⑦**V15.4** Pedal cycle driver injured in collision with railway train or railway vehicle in traffic accident

⊗⑦**V15.5** Pedal cycle passenger injured in collision with railway train or railway vehicle in traffic accident

⊗⑦**V15.9** Unspecified pedal cyclist injured in collision with railway train or railway vehicle in traffic accident

V16 Pedal cycle rider injured in collision with other nonmotor vehicle

Includes: collision with animal-drawn vehicle, animal being ridden, streetcar

The appropriate 7th character is to be added to each code from category V16

A - initial encounter

D - subsequent encounter

S - sequela

⊗⑦**V16.0** Pedal cycle driver injured in collision with other nonmotor vehicle in nontraffic accident

⊗⑦**V16.1** Pedal cycle passenger injured in collision with other nonmotor vehicle in nontraffic accident

⊗⑦**V16.2** Unspecified pedal cyclist injured in collision with other nonmotor vehicle in nontraffic accident

⊗⑦**V16.3** Person boarding or alighting a pedal cycle injured in collision with other nonmotor vehicle in nontraffic accident

⊗⑦**V16.4** Pedal cycle driver injured in collision with other nonmotor vehicle in traffic accident

⊗⑦**V16.5** Pedal cycle passenger injured in collision with other nonmotor vehicle in traffic accident

⊗⑦**V16.9** Unspecified pedal cyclist injured in collision with other nonmotor vehicle in traffic accident

V17 Pedal cycle rider injured in collision with fixed or stationary object

The appropriate 7th character is to be added to each code from category V17

A - initial encounter

D - subsequent encounter

S - sequela

⊗⑦**V17.0** Pedal cycle driver injured in collision with fixed or stationary object in nontraffic accident

⊗⑦**V17.1** Pedal cycle passenger injured in collision with fixed or stationary object in nontraffic accident

⊗⑦**V17.2** Unspecified pedal cyclist injured in collision with fixed or stationary object in nontraffic accident

⊗⑦**V17.3** Person boarding or alighting a pedal cycle injured in collision with fixed or stationary object

⊗⑦**V17.4** Pedal cycle driver injured in collision with fixed or stationary object in traffic accident

⊗⑦**V17.5** Pedal cycle passenger injured in collision with fixed or stationary object in traffic accident

⊗⑦**V17.9** Unspecified pedal cyclist injured in collision with fixed or stationary object in traffic accident

V18 Pedal cycle rider injured in noncollision transport accident

Includes: fall or thrown from pedal cycle (without antecedent collision)

overturning pedal cycle NOS

overturning pedal cycle without collision

The appropriate 7th character is to be added to each code from category V18

A - initial encounter

D - subsequent encounter

S - sequela

⊗⑦**V18.0** Pedal cycle driver injured in noncollision transport accident in nontraffic accident

⊗⑦**V18.1** Pedal cycle passenger injured in noncollision transport accident in nontraffic accident

⊗⑦**V18.2** Unspecified pedal cyclist injured in noncollision transport accident in nontraffic accident

⊗⑦**V18.3** Person boarding or alighting a pedal cycle injured in noncollision transport accident

⊗⑦**V18.4** Pedal cycle driver injured in noncollision transport accident in traffic accident

⊗⑦**V18.5** Pedal cycle passenger injured in noncollision transport accident in traffic accident

⊗⑦**V18.9** Unspecified pedal cyclist injured in noncollision transport accident in traffic accident

V19 Pedal cycle rider injured in other and unspecified transport accidents

The appropriate 7th character is to be added to each code from category V19

A - initial encounter

D - subsequent encounter

S - sequela

V19.0 Pedal cycle driver injured in collision with other and unspecified motor vehicles in nontraffic accident

⊗⑦**V19.00** Pedal cycle driver injured in collision with unspecified motor vehicles in nontraffic accident

⊗⑦**V19.09** Pedal cycle driver injured in collision with other motor vehicles in nontraffic accident

V19.1 Pedal cycle passenger injured in collision with other and unspecified motor vehicles in nontraffic accident

⊗⑦**V19.10** Pedal cycle passenger injured in collision with unspecified motor vehicles in nontraffic accident

⊗⑦**V19.19** Pedal cycle passenger injured in collision with other motor vehicles in nontraffic accident

⊗⑦**V19.2** Unspecified pedal cyclist injured in collision with other and unspecified motor vehicles in nontraffic accident

⊗⑦**V19.20** Unspecified pedal cyclist injured in collision with unspecified motor vehicles in nontraffic accident

Pedal cycle collision NOS, nontraffic

⊗⑦**V19.29** Unspecified pedal cyclist injured in collision with other motor vehicles in nontraffic accident

V19.3 Pedal cyclist (driver) (passenger) injured in unspecified nontraffic accident

Pedal cycle accident NOS, nontraffic

Pedal cyclist injured in nontraffic accident NOS

V19.4 Pedal cycle driver injured in collision with other and unspecified motor vehicles in traffic accident

⊗⑦**V19.40** Pedal cycle driver injured in collision with unspecified motor vehicles in traffic accident

⊗⑦**V19.49** Pedal cycle driver injured in collision with other motor vehicles in traffic accident

V19.5 Pedal cycle passenger injured in collision with other and unspecified motor vehicles in traffic accident

⊗⑦**V19.50** Pedal cycle passenger injured in collision with unspecified motor vehicles in traffic accident

⊗⑦**V19.59** Pedal cycle passenger injured in collision with other motor vehicles in traffic accident

V19.6 Unspecified pedal cyclist injured in collision with other and unspecified motor vehicles in traffic accident

⊗⑦**V19.60** Unspecified pedal cyclist injured in collision with unspecified motor vehicles in traffic accident

Pedal cycle collision NOS (traffic)

⊗⑦**V19.69** Unspecified pedal cyclist injured in collision with other motor vehicles in traffic accident

V19.8 Pedal cyclist (driver) (passenger) injured in other specified transport accidents

⊗⑦**V19.81** Pedal cyclist (driver) (passenger) injured in transport accident with military vehicle

⊗⑦**V19.88** Pedal cyclist (driver) (passenger) injured in other specified transport accidents

V19.9 Pedal cyclist (driver) (passenger) injured in unspecified traffic accident

Pedal cycle accident NOS

MOTORCYCLE RIDER INJURED IN TRANSPORT ACCIDENT (V20-V29)

Includes: moped

motorcycle with sidecar

motorized bicycle

motor scooter

Excludes 1: three-wheeled motor vehicle (V30-V39)

V20 Motorcycle rider injured in collision with pedestrian or animal

Excludes 1: motorcycle rider collision with animal-drawn vehicle or animal being ridden (V26.-)

The appropriate 7th character is to be added to each code from category V20

A - initial encounter

D - subsequent encounter

S - sequela

⊗⑦**V20.0** Motorcycle driver injured in collision with pedestrian or animal in nontraffic accident

⊗⑦**V20.1** Motorcycle passenger injured in collision with pedestrian or animal in nontraffic accident

⊗⑦**V20.2** Unspecified motorcycle rider injured in collision with pedestrian or animal in nontraffic accident

⊗⑦**V20.3** Person boarding or alighting a motorcycle injured in collision with pedestrian or animal

⊗⑦**V20.4** Motorcycle driver injured in collision with pedestrian or animal in traffic accident

⊗⑦**V20.5** Motorcycle passenger injured in collision with pedestrian or animal in traffic accident

⊗⑦**V20.9** Unspecified motorcycle rider injured in collision with pedestrian or animal in traffic accident

V21 Motorcycle rider injured in collision with pedal cycle

The appropriate 7th character is to be added to each code from category V21

A - initial encounter

D - subsequent encounter

S - sequela

⊗⑦**V21.0** Motorcycle driver injured in collision with pedal cycle in nontraffic accident

⊗⑦**V21.1** Motorcycle passenger injured in collision with pedal cycle in nontraffic accident

⊗⑦**V21.2** Unspecified motorcycle rider injured in collision with pedal cycle in nontraffic accident

⊗⑦**V21.3** Person boarding or alighting a motorcycle injured in collision with pedal cycle

⊗⑦**V21.4** Motorcycle driver injured in collision with pedal cycle in traffic accident

⊗⑦**V21.5** Motorcycle passenger injured in collision with pedal cycle in traffic accident

⊗⑦**V21.9** Unspecified motorcycle rider injured in collision with pedal cycle in traffic accident

V22 Motorcycle rider injured in collision with two- or three-wheeled motor vehicle

The appropriate 7th character is to be added to each code from category V22

A - initial encounter

D - subsequent encounter

S - sequela

⊗⑦**V22.0** Motorcycle driver injured in collision with two- or three-wheeled motor vehicle in nontraffic accident

⊗⑦**V22.1** Motorcycle passenger injured in collision with two- or three-wheeled motor vehicle in nontraffic accident

⊗⑦**V22.2** Unspecified motorcycle rider injured in collision with two- or three-wheeled motor vehicle in nontraffic accident

⊗⑦**V22.3** Person boarding or alighting a motorcycle injured in collision with two- or three-wheeled motor vehicle

⊗⑦**V22.4** Motorcycle driver injured in collision with two- or three-wheeled motor vehicle in traffic accident

⊗⑦**V22.5** Motorcycle passenger injured in collision with three-wheeled motor vehicle in traffic accident

⊗⑦**V22.9** Unspecified motorcycle rider injured in collision with two- or three-wheeled motor vehicle in traffic accident

V23 Motorcycle rider injured in collision with car, pick-up truck or van

The appropriate 7th character is to be added to each code from category V23

A - initial encounter

D - subsequent encounter

S - sequela

⊗⑦**V23.0** Motorcycle driver injured in collision with car, pick-up truck or van in nontraffic accident

⊗⑦**V23.1** Motorcycle passenger injured in collision with car, pick-up truck or van in nontraffic accident

⊗⑦**V23.2** Unspecified motorcycle rider injured in collision with car, pick-up truck or van in nontraffic accident

⊗⑦**V23.3** Person boarding or alighting a motorcycle injured in collision with car, pick-up truck or van

⊗⑦**V23.4** Motorcycle driver injured in collision with car, pick-up truck or van in traffic accident

⊗⑦**V23.5** Motorcycle passenger injured in collision with car, pick-up truck or van in traffic accident

⊗⑦**V23.9** Unspecified motorcycle rider injured in collision with car, pick-up truck or van in traffic accident

V24 Motorcycle rider injured in collision with heavy transport vehicle or bus

Excludes 1: motorcycle rider injured in collision with military vehicle (V29.81)

The appropriate 7th character is to be added to each code from category V24

A - initial encounter

D - subsequent encounter

S - sequela

⊗⑦**V24.0** Motorcycle driver injured in collision with heavy transport vehicle or bus in nontraffic accident

⊗⑦**V24.1** Motorcycle passenger injured in collision with heavy transport vehicle or bus in nontraffic accident

⊗⑦**V24.2** Unspecified motorcycle rider injured in collision with heavy transport vehicle or bus in nontraffic accident

⊗⑦**V24.3** Person boarding or alighting a motorcycle injured in collision with heavy transport vehicle or bus

⊗⑦**V24.4** Motorcycle driver injured in collision with heavy transport vehicle or bus in traffic accident

⊗⑦**V24.5** Motorcycle passenger injured in collision with heavy transport vehicle or bus in traffic accident

⊗⑦**V24.9** Unspecified motorcycle rider injured in collision with heavy transport vehicle or bus in traffic accident

V25 Motorcycle rider injured in collision with railway train or railway vehicle

The appropriate 7th character is to be added to each code from category V25

A - initial encounter

D - subsequent encounter

S - sequela

⊗⑦**V25.0** Motorcycle driver injured in collision with railway train or railway vehicle in nontraffic accident

⊗⑦**V25.1** Motorcycle passenger injured in collision with railway train or railway vehicle in nontraffic accident

⊗⑦**V25.2** Unspecified motorcycle rider injured in collision with railway train or railway vehicle in nontraffic accident

⊗⑦**V25.3** Person boarding or alighting a motorcycle injured in collision with railway train or railway vehicle

⊗⑦**V25.4** Motorcycle driver injured in collision with railway train or railway vehicle in traffic accident

⊗⑦**V25.5** Motorcycle passenger injured in collision with railway train or railway vehicle in traffic accident

⊗⑦**V25.9** Unspecified motorcycle rider injured in collision with railway train or railway vehicle in traffic accident

V26 Motorcycle rider injured in collision with other nonmotor vehicle

Includes: collision with animal-drawn vehicle, animal being ridden, streetcar

The appropriate 7th character is to be added to each code from category V26

A - initial encounter

D - subsequent encounter

S - sequela

⊗⑦**V26.0** Motorcycle driver injured in collision with other nonmotor vehicle in nontraffic accident

⊗⑦**V26.1** Motorcycle passenger injured in collision with other nonmotor vehicle in nontraffic accident

⊗⑦**V26.2** Unspecified motorcycle rider injured in collision with other nonmotor vehicle in nontraffic accident

⊗⑦**V26.3** Person boarding or alighting a motorcycle injured in collision with other nonmotor vehicle

⊗⑦**V26.4** Motorcycle driver injured in collision with other nonmotor vehicle in traffic accident

⊗⑦**V26.5** Motorcycle passenger injured in collision with other nonmotor vehicle in traffic accident

⊗⑦**V26.9** Unspecified motorcycle rider injured in collision with other nonmotor vehicle in traffic accident

V27 Motorcycle rider injured in collision with fixed or stationary object

The appropriate 7th character is to be added to each code from category V27

A - initial encounter

D - subsequent encounter

S - sequela

⊗⑦**V27.0** Motorcycle driver injured in collision with fixed or stationary object in nontraffic accident

⊗⑦**V27.1** Motorcycle passenger injured in collision with fixed or stationary object in nontraffic accident

⊗⑦**V27.2** Unspecified motorcycle rider injured in collision with fixed or stationary object in nontraffic accident

⊗⑦**V27.3** Person boarding or alighting a motorcycle injured in collision with fixed or stationary object

⊗⑦**V27.4** Motorcycle driver injured in collision with fixed or stationary object in traffic accident

⊗⑦**V27.5** Motorcycle passenger injured in collision with fixed or stationary object in traffic accident

⊗⑦**V27.9** Unspecified motorcycle rider injured in collision with fixed or stationary object in traffic accident

V28 Motorcycle rider injured in noncollision transport accident

Includes: fall or thrown from motorcycle (without antecedent collision)

overturning motorcycle NOS

overturning motorcycle without collision

The appropriate 7th character is to be added to each code from category V28

A - initial encounter

D - subsequent encounter

S - sequela

⊗⑦ **V28.0** Motorcycle driver injured in noncollision transport accident in nontraffic accident

⊗⑦ **V28.1** Motorcycle passenger injured in noncollision transport accident in nontraffic accident

⊗⑦ **V28.2** Unspecified motorcycle rider injured in noncollision transport accident in nontraffic accident

⊗⑦ **V28.3** Person boarding or alighting a motorcycle injured in noncollision transport accident

⊗⑦ **V28.4** Motorcycle driver injured in noncollision transport accident in traffic accident

⊗⑦ **V28.5** Motorcycle passenger injured in noncollision transport accident in traffic accident

⊗⑦ **V28.9** Unspecified motorcycle rider injured in noncollision transport accident in traffic accident

V29 Motorcycle rider injured in other and unspecified transport accidents

The appropriate 7th character is to be added to each code from category V29

A - initial encounter

D - subsequent encounter

S - sequela

V29.0 Motorcycle driver injured in collision with other and unspecified motor vehicles in nontraffic accident

⊗⑦ **V29.00** Motorcycle driver injured in collision with unspecified motor vehicles in nontraffic accident

⊗⑦ **V29.09** Motorcycle driver injured in collision with other motor vehicles in nontraffic accident

V29.1 Motorcycle passenger injured in collision with other and unspecified motor vehicles in nontraffic accident

⊗⑦ **V29.10** Motorcycle passenger injured in collision with unspecified motor vehicles in nontraffic accident

⊗⑦ **V29.19** Motorcycle passenger injured in collision with other motor vehicles in nontraffic accident

V29.2 Unspecified motorcycle rider injured in collision with other and unspecified motor vehicles in nontraffic accident

⊗⑦ **V29.20** Unspecified motorcycle rider injured in collision with unspecified motor vehicles in nontraffic accident

Motorcycle collision NOS, nontraffic

⊗⑦ **V29.29** Unspecified motorcycle rider injured in collision with other motor vehicles in nontraffic accident

V29.3 Motorcycle rider (driver) (passenger) injured in unspecified nontraffic accident

Motorcycle accident NOS, nontraffic

Motorcycle rider injured in nontraffic accident NOS

V29.4 Motorcycle driver injured in collision with other and unspecified motor vehicles in traffic accident

⊗⑦ **V29.40** Motorcycle driver injured in collision with unspecified motor vehicles in traffic accident

⊗⑦ **V29.49** Motorcycle driver injured in collision with other motor vehicles in traffic accident

V29.5 Motorcycle passenger injured in collision with other and unspecified motor vehicles in traffic accident

⊗⑦ **V29.50** Motorcycle passenger injured in collision with unspecified motor vehicles in traffic accident

⊗⑦ **V29.59** Motorcycle passenger injured in collision with other motor vehicles in traffic accident

V29.6 Unspecified motorcycle rider injured in collision with other and unspecified motor vehicles in traffic accident

⊗⑦ **V29.60** Unspecified motorcycle rider injured in collision with unspecified motor vehicles in traffic accident

Motorcycle collision NOS (traffic)

⊗⑦ **V29.69** Unspecified motorcycle rider injured in collision with other motor vehicles in traffic accident

V29.8 Motorcycle rider (driver) (passenger) injured in other specified transport accidents

⊗⑦ **V29.81** Motorcycle rider (driver) (passenger) injured in transport accident with military vehicle

⊗⑦ **V29.88** Motorcycle rider (driver) (passenger) injured in other specified transport accidents

V29.9 Motorcycle rider (driver) (passenger) injured in unspecified traffic accident

Motorcycle accident NOS

OCCUPANT OF THREE-WHEELED MOTOR VEHICLE INJURED IN TRANSPORT ACCIDENT (V30-V39)

Includes: motorized tricycle

motorized rickshaw

three-wheeled motor car

Excludes 1: all-terrain vehicles (V86.-)

motorcycle with sidecar (V20-V29)

vehicle designed primarily for off-road use (V86.-)

V30 Occupant of three-wheeled motor vehicle injured in collision with pedestrian or animal

Excludes 1: three-wheeled motor vehicle collision with animal-drawn vehicle or animal being ridden (V36.-)

The appropriate 7th character is to be added to each code from category V30

A - initial encounter

D - subsequent encounter

S - sequela

⊗⑦ **V30.0** Driver of three-wheeled motor vehicle injured in collision with pedestrian or animal in nontraffic accident

⊗⑦ **V30.1** Passenger in three-wheeled motor vehicle injured in collision with pedestrian or animal in nontraffic accident

⊗⑦ **V30.2** Person on outside of three-wheeled motor vehicle injured in collision with pedestrian or animal in nontraffic accident

⊗⑦ **V30.3** Unspecified occupant of three-wheeled motor vehicle injured in collision with pedestrian or animal in nontraffic accident

⊗⑦ **V30.4** Person boarding or alighting a three-wheeled motor vehicle injured in collision with pedestrian or animal

⊗⑦ **V30.5** Driver of three-wheeled motor vehicle injured in collision with pedestrian or animal in traffic accident

⊗⑦ **V30.6** Passenger in three-wheeled motor vehicle injured in collision with pedestrian or animal in traffic accident

⊗⑦ **V30.7** Person on outside of three-wheeled motor vehicle injured in collision with pedestrian or animal in traffic accident

⊗⑦ **V30.9** Unspecified occupant of three-wheeled motor vehicle injured in collision with pedestrian or animal in traffic accident

V31 Occupant of three-wheeled motor vehicle injured in collision with pedal cycle

The appropriate 7th character is to be added to each code from category V31

A - initial encounter

● New code   ▲ Revised code   ⑦ 7th digit required   ⊗ Placeholder required

D - subsequent encounter

S - sequela

⊗⑦**V31.0** Driver of three-wheeled motor vehicle injured in collision with pedal cycle in nontraffic accident

⊗⑦**V31.1** Passenger in three-wheeled motor vehicle injured in collision with pedal cycle in nontraffic accident

⊗⑦**V31.2** Person on outside of three-wheeled motor vehicle injured in collision with pedal cycle in nontraffic accident

⊗⑦**V31.3** Unspecified occupant of three-wheeled motor vehicle injured in collision with pedal cycle in nontraffic accident

⊗⑦**V31.4** Person boarding or alighting a three-wheeled motor vehicle injured in collision with pedal cycle

⊗⑦**V31.5** Driver of three-wheeled motor vehicle injured in collision with pedal cycle in traffic accident

⊗⑦**V31.6** Passenger in three-wheeled motor vehicle injured in collision with pedal cycle in traffic accident

⊗⑦**V31.7** Person on outside of three-wheeled motor vehicle injured in collision with pedal cycle in traffic accident

⊗⑦**V31.9** Unspecified occupant of three-wheeled motor vehicle injured in collision with pedal cycle in traffic accident

V32 Occupant of three-wheeled motor vehicle injured in collision with two- or three-wheeled motor vehicle

The appropriate 7th character is to be added to each code from category V32

A - initial encounter

D - subsequent encounter

S - sequela

⊗⑦**V32.0** Driver of three-wheeled motor vehicle injured in collision with two- or three-wheeled motor vehicle in nontraffic accident

⊗⑦**V32.1** Passenger in three-wheeled motor vehicle injured in collision with two- or three-wheeled motor vehicle in nontraffic accident

⊗⑦**V32.2** Person on outside of three-wheeled motor vehicle injured in collision with two- or three-wheeled motor vehicle in nontraffic accident

⊗⑦**V32.3** Unspecified occupant of three-wheeled motor vehicle injured in collision with two- or three-wheeled motor vehicle in nontraffic accident

⊗⑦**V32.4** Person boarding or alighting a three-wheeled motor vehicle injured in collision with two- or three-wheeled motor vehicle

⊗⑦**V32.5** Driver of three-wheeled motor vehicle injured in collision with two- or three-wheeled motor vehicle in traffic accident

⊗⑦**V32.6** Passenger in three-wheeled motor vehicle injured in collision with two- or three-wheeled motor vehicle in traffic accident

⊗⑦**V32.7** Person on outside of three-wheeled motor vehicle injured in collision with two- or three-wheeled motor vehicle in traffic accident

⊗⑦**V32.9** Unspecified occupant of three-wheeled motor vehicle injured in collision with two- or three-wheeled motor vehicle in traffic accident

V33 Occupant of three-wheeled motor vehicle injured in collision with car, pick-up truck or van

The appropriate 7th character is to be added to each code from category V33

A - initial encounter

D - subsequent encounter

S - sequela

⊗⑦**V33.0** Driver of three-wheeled motor vehicle injured in collision with car, pick-up truck or van in nontraffic accident

⊗⑦**V33.1** Passenger in three-wheeled motor vehicle injured in collision with car, pick-up truck or van in nontraffic accident

⊗⑦**V33.2** Person on outside of three-wheeled motor vehicle injured in collision with car, pick-up truck or van in nontraffic accident

⊗⑦**V33.3** Unspecified occupant of three-wheeled motor vehicle injured in collision with car, pick-up truck or van in nontraffic accident

⊗⑦**V33.4** Person boarding or alighting a three-wheeled motor vehicle injured in collision with car, pick-up truck or van

⊗⑦**V33.5** Driver of three-wheeled motor vehicle injured in collision with car, pick-up truck or van in traffic accident

⊗⑦**V33.6** Passenger in three-wheeled motor vehicle injured in collision with car, pick-up truck or van in traffic accident

⊗⑦**V33.7** Person on outside of three-wheeled motor vehicle injured in collision with car, pick-up truck or van in traffic accident

⊗⑦**V33.9** Unspecified occupant of three-wheeled motor vehicle injured in collision with car, pick-up truck or van in traffic accident

V34 Occupant of three-wheeled motor vehicle injured in collision with heavy transport vehicle or bus

Excludes 1: occupant of three-wheeled motor vehicle injured in collision with military vehicle (V39.81)

The appropriate 7th character is to be added to each code from category V34

A - initial encounter

D - subsequent encounter

S - sequela

⊗⑦**V34.0** Driver of three-wheeled motor vehicle injured in collision with heavy transport vehicle or bus in nontraffic accident

⊗⑦**V34.1** Passenger in three-wheeled motor vehicle injured in collision with heavy transport vehicle or bus in nontraffic accident

⊗⑦**V34.2** Person on outside of three-wheeled motor vehicle injured in collision with heavy transport vehicle or bus in nontraffic accident

⊗⑦**V34.3** Unspecified occupant of three-wheeled motor vehicle injured in collision with heavy transport vehicle or bus in nontraffic accident

⊗⑦**V34.4** Person boarding or alighting a three-wheeled motor vehicle injured in collision with heavy transport vehicle or bus

⊗⑦**V34.5** Driver of three-wheeled motor vehicle injured in collision with heavy transport vehicle or bus in traffic accident

⊗⑦**V34.6** Passenger in three-wheeled motor vehicle injured in collision with heavy transport vehicle or bus in traffic accident

⊗⑦**V34.7** Person on outside of three-wheeled motor vehicle injured in collision with heavy transport vehicle or bus in traffic accident

⊗⑦**V34.9** Unspecified occupant of three-wheeled motor vehicle injured in collision with heavy transport vehicle or bus in traffic accident

V35 Occupant of three-wheeled motor vehicle injured in collision with railway train or railway vehicle

The appropriate 7th character is to be added to each code from category V35

A - initial encounter
D - subsequent encounter
S - sequela

⊗⑦**V35.0** Driver of three-wheeled motor vehicle injured in collision with railway train or railway vehicle in nontraffic accident

⊗⑦**V35.1** Passenger in three-wheeled motor vehicle injured in collision with railway train or railway vehicle in nontraffic accident

⊗⑦**V35.2** Person on outside of three-wheeled motor vehicle injured in collision with railway train or railway vehicle in nontraffic accident

⊗⑦**V35.3** Unspecified occupant of three-wheeled motor vehicle injured in collision with railway train or railway vehicle in nontraffic accident

⊗⑦**V35.4** Person boarding or alighting a three-wheeled motor vehicle injured in collision with railway train or railway vehicle

⊗⑦**V35.5** Driver of three-wheeled motor vehicle injured in collision with railway train or railway vehicle in traffic accident

⊗⑦**V35.6** Passenger in three-wheeled motor vehicle injured in collision with railway train or railway vehicle in traffic accident

⊗⑦**V35.7** Person on outside of three-wheeled motor vehicle injured in collision with railway train or railway vehicle in traffic accident

⊗⑦**V35.9** Unspecified occupant of three-wheeled motor vehicle injured in collision with railway train or railway vehicle in traffic accident

V36 Occupant of three-wheeled motor vehicle injured in collision with other nonmotor vehicle
   Includes: collision with animal-drawn vehicle, animal being ridden, streetcar

The appropriate 7th character is to be added to each code from category V36
   A - initial encounter
   D - subsequent encounter
   S - sequela

⊗⑦**V36.0** Driver of three-wheeled motor vehicle injured in collision with other nonmotor vehicle in nontraffic accident

⊗⑦**V36.1** Passenger in three-wheeled motor vehicle injured in collision with other nonmotor vehicle in nontraffic accident

⊗⑦**V36.2** Person on outside of three-wheeled motor vehicle injured in collision with other nonmotor vehicle in nontraffic accident

⊗⑦**V36.3** Unspecified occupant of three-wheeled motor vehicle injured in collision with other nonmotor vehicle in nontraffic accident

⊗⑦**V36.4** Person boarding or alighting a three-wheeled motor vehicle injured in collision with other nonmotor vehicle

⊗⑦**V36.5** Driver of three-wheeled motor vehicle injured in collision with other nonmotor vehicle in traffic accident

⊗⑦**V36.6** Passenger in three-wheeled motor vehicle injured in collision with other nonmotor vehicle in traffic accident

⊗⑦**V36.7** Person on outside of three-wheeled motor vehicle injured in collision with other nonmotor vehicle in traffic accident

⊗⑦**V36.9** Unspecified occupant of three-wheeled motor vehicle injured in collision with other nonmotor vehicle in traffic accident

V37 Occupant of three-wheeled motor vehicle injured in collision with fixed or stationary object

The appropriate 7th character is to be added to each code from category V37
   A - initial encounter
   D - subsequent encounter
   S - sequela

⊗⑦**V37.0** Driver of three-wheeled motor vehicle injured in collision with fixed or stationary object in nontraffic accident

⊗⑦**V37.1** Passenger in three-wheeled motor vehicle injured in collision with fixed or stationary object in nontraffic accident

⊗⑦**V37.2** Person on outside of three-wheeled motor vehicle injured in collision with fixed or stationary object in nontraffic accident

⊗⑦**V37.3** Unspecified occupant of three-wheeled motor vehicle injured in collision with fixed or stationary object in nontraffic accident

⊗⑦**V37.4** Person boarding or alighting a three-wheeled motor vehicle injured in collision with fixed or stationary object

⊗⑦**V37.5** Driver of three-wheeled motor vehicle injured in collision with fixed or stationary object in traffic accident

⊗⑦**V37.6** Passenger in three-wheeled motor vehicle injured in collision with fixed or stationary object in traffic accident

⊗⑦**V37.7** Person on outside of three-wheeled motor vehicle injured in collision with fixed or stationary object in traffic accident

⊗⑦**V37.9** Unspecified occupant of three-wheeled motor vehicle injured in collision with fixed or stationary object in traffic accident

V38 Occupant of three-wheeled motor vehicle injured in noncollision transport accident
   Includes: fall or thrown from three-wheeled motor vehicle
      overturning of three-wheeled motor vehicle NOS
      overturning of three-wheeled motor vehicle without collision

The appropriate 7th character is to be added to each code from category V38
   A - initial encounter
   D - subsequent encounter
   S - sequela

⊗⑦**V38.0** Driver of three-wheeled motor vehicle injured in noncollision transport accident in nontraffic accident

⊗⑦**V38.1** Passenger in three-wheeled motor vehicle injured in noncollision transport accident in nontraffic accident

⊗⑦**V38.2** Person on outside of three-wheeled motor vehicle injured in noncollision transport accident in nontraffic accident

⊗⑦**V38.3** Unspecified occupant of three-wheeled motor vehicle injured in noncollision transport accident in nontraffic accident

⊗⑦**V38.4** Person boarding or alighting a three-wheeled motor vehicle injured in noncollision transport accident

⊗⑦**V38.5** Driver of three-wheeled motor vehicle injured in noncollision transport accident in traffic accident

⊗⑦**V38.6** Passenger in three-wheeled motor vehicle injured in noncollision transport accident in traffic accident

⊗⑦**V38.7** Person on outside of three-wheeled motor vehicle injured in noncollision transport accident in traffic accident

⊗⑦**V38.9** Unspecified occupant of three-wheeled motor vehicle injured in noncollision transport accident in traffic accident

V39 Occupant of three-wheeled motor vehicle injured in other and unspecified transport accidents

● New code   ▲ Revised code   ⑦ 7th digit required   ⊗ Placeholder required

The appropriate 7th character is to be added to each code from category V39

A - initial encounter

D - subsequent encounter

S - sequela

V39.0 Driver of three-wheeled motor vehicle injured in collision with other and unspecified motor vehicles in nontraffic accident

⊗⑦**V39.00** Driver of three-wheeled motor vehicle injured in collision with unspecified motor vehicles in nontraffic accident

⊗⑦**V39.09** Driver of three-wheeled motor vehicle injured in collision with other motor vehicles in nontraffic accident

V39.1 Passenger in three-wheeled motor vehicle injured in collision with other and unspecified motor vehicles in nontraffic accident

⊗⑦**V39.10** Passenger in three-wheeled motor vehicle injured in collision with unspecified motor vehicles in nontraffic accident

⊗⑦**V39.19** Passenger in three-wheeled motor vehicle injured in collision with other motor vehicles in nontraffic accident

V39.2 Unspecified occupant of three-wheeled motor vehicle injured in collision with other and unspecified motor vehicles in nontraffic accident

⊗⑦**V39.20** Unspecified occupant of three-wheeled motor vehicle injured in collision with unspecified motor vehicles in nontraffic accident

Collision NOS involving three-wheeled motor vehicle, nontraffic

⊗⑦**V39.29** Unspecified occupant of three-wheeled motor vehicle injured in collision with other motor vehicles in nontraffic accident

V39.3 Occupant (driver) (passenger) of three-wheeled motor vehicle injured in unspecified nontraffic accident

Accident NOS involving three-wheeled motor vehicle, nontraffic

Occupant of three-wheeled motor vehicle injured in nontraffic accident NOS

V39.4 Driver of three-wheeled motor vehicle injured in collision with other and unspecified motor vehicles in traffic accident

⊗⑦**V39.40** Driver of three-wheeled motor vehicle injured in collision with unspecified motor vehicles in traffic accident

⊗⑦**V39.49** Driver of three-wheeled motor vehicle injured in collision with other motor vehicles in traffic accident

V39.5 Passenger in three-wheeled motor vehicle injured in collision with other and unspecified motor vehicles in traffic accident

⊗⑦**V39.50** Passenger in three-wheeled motor vehicle injured in collision with unspecified motor vehicles in traffic accident

⊗⑦**V39.59** Passenger in three-wheeled motor vehicle injured in collision with other motor vehicles in traffic accident

V39.6 Unspecified occupant of three-wheeled motor vehicle injured in collision with other and unspecified motor vehicles in traffic accident

⊗⑦**V39.60** Unspecified occupant of three-wheeled motor vehicle injured in collision with unspecified motor vehicles in traffic accident

Collision NOS involving three-wheeled motor vehicle (traffic)

⊗⑦**V39.69** Unspecified occupant of three-wheeled motor vehicle injured in collision with other motor vehicles in traffic accident

V39.8 Occupant (driver) (passenger) of three-wheeled motor vehicle injured in other specified transport accidents

⊗⑦**V39.81** Occupant (driver) (passenger) of three-wheeled motor vehicle injured in transport accident with military vehicle

⊗⑦**V39.89** Occupant (driver) (passenger) of three-wheeled motor vehicle injured in other specified transport accidents

V39.9 Occupant (driver) (passenger) of three-wheeled motor vehicle injured in unspecified traffic accident

Accident NOS involving three-wheeled motor vehicle

CAR OCCUPANT INJURED IN TRANSPORT ACCIDENT (V40-V49)

Includes: a four-wheeled motor vehicle designed primarily for carrying passengers

automobile (pulling a trailer or camper)

Excludes 1: bus (V50-V59)

minibus (V50-V59)

minivan (V50-V59)

motorcoach (V70-V79)

pick-up truck (V50-V59)

sport utility vehicle (SUV) (V50-V59)

V40 Car occupant injured in collision with pedestrian or animal

Excludes 1: car collision with animal-drawn vehicle or animal being ridden (V46.-)

The appropriate 7th character is to be added to each code from category V40

A - initial encounter

D - subsequent encounter

S - sequela

⊗⑦**V40.0** Car driver injured in collision with pedestrian or animal in nontraffic accident

⊗⑦**V40.1** Car passenger injured in collision with pedestrian or animal in nontraffic accident

⊗⑦**V40.2** Person on outside of car injured in collision with pedestrian or animal in nontraffic accident

⊗⑦**V40.3** Unspecified car occupant injured in collision with pedestrian or animal in nontraffic accident

⊗⑦**V40.4** Person boarding or alighting a car injured in collision with pedestrian or animal

⊗⑦**V40.5** Car driver injured in collision with pedestrian or animal in traffic accident

⊗⑦**V40.6** Car passenger injured in collision with pedestrian or animal in traffic accident

⊗⑦**V40.7** Person on outside of car injured in collision with pedestrian or animal in traffic accident

⊗⑦**V40.9** Unspecified car occupant injured in collision with pedestrian or animal in traffic accident

V41 Car occupant injured in collision with pedal cycle

The appropriate 7th character is to be added to each code from category V41

A - initial encounter

D - subsequent encounter

S - sequela

⊗⑦**V41.0** Car driver injured in collision with pedal cycle in nontraffic accident

⊗⑦**V41.1** Car passenger injured in collision with pedal cycle in nontraffic accident

⊗⑦**V41.2** Person on outside of car injured in collision with pedal cycle in nontraffic accident

⊗⑦**V41.3** Unspecified car occupant injured in collision with pedal cycle in nontraffic accident

⊗⑦**V41.4** Person boarding or alighting a car injured in collision with pedal cycle

⊗⑦**V41.5** Car driver injured in collision with pedal cycle in traffic accident

⊗⑦**V41.6** Car passenger injured in collision with pedal cycle in traffic accident

⊗⑦**V41.7** Person on outside of car injured in collision with pedal cycle in traffic accident

⊗⑦**V41.9** Unspecified car occupant injured in collision with pedal cycle in traffic accident

V42 Car occupant injured in collision with two- or three-wheeled motor vehicle

The appropriate 7th character is to be added to each code from category V42

A - initial encounter

D - subsequent encounter

S - sequela

⊗⑦**V42.0** Car driver injured in collision with two- or three-wheeled motor vehicle in nontraffic accident

⊗⑦**V42.1** Car passenger injured in collision with two- or three-wheeled motor vehicle in nontraffic accident

⊗⑦**V42.2** Person on outside of car injured in collision with two- or three-wheeled motor vehicle in nontraffic accident

⊗⑦**V42.3** Unspecified car occupant injured in collision with two- or three-wheeled motor vehicle in nontraffic accident

⊗⑦**V42.4** Person boarding or alighting a car injured in collision with two- or three-wheeled motor vehicle

⊗⑦**V42.5** Car driver injured in collision with two- or three-wheeled motor vehicle in traffic accident

⊗⑦**V42.6** Car passenger injured in collision with two- or three-wheeled motor vehicle in traffic accident

⊗⑦**V42.7** Person on outside of car injured in collision with two- or three-wheeled motor vehicle in traffic accident

⊗⑦**V42.9** Unspecified car occupant injured in collision with two- or three-wheeled motor vehicle in traffic accident

V43 Car occupant injured in collision with car, pick-up truck or van

The appropriate 7th character is to be added to each code from category V43

A - initial encounter

D - subsequent encounter

S - sequela

V43.0 Car driver injured in collision with car, pick-up truck or van in nontraffic accident

⊗⑦**V43.01** Car driver injured in collision with sport utility vehicle in nontraffic accident

⊗⑦**V43.02** Car driver injured in collision with other type car in nontraffic accident

⊗⑦**V43.03** Car driver injured in collision with pick-up truck in nontraffic accident

⊗⑦**V43.04** Car driver injured in collision with van in nontraffic accident

V43.1 Car passenger injured in collision with car, pick-up truck or van in nontraffic accident

⊗⑦**V43.11** Car passenger injured in collision with sport utility vehicle in nontraffic accident

⊗⑦**V43.12** Car passenger injured in collision with other type car in nontraffic accident

⊗⑦**V43.13** Car passenger injured in collision with pick-up in nontraffic accident

⊗⑦**V43.14** Car passenger injured in collision with van in nontraffic accident

V43.2 Person on outside of car injured in collision with car, pick-up truck or van in nontraffic accident

⊗⑦**V43.21** Person on outside of car injured in collision with sport utility vehicle in nontraffic accident

⊗⑦**V43.22** Person on outside of car injured in collision with other type car in nontraffic accident

⊗⑦**V43.23** Person on outside of car injured in collision with pick-up truck in nontraffic accident

⊗⑦**V43.24** Person on outside of car injured in collision with van in nontraffic accident

V43.3 Unspecified car occupant injured in collision with car, pick-up truck or van in nontraffic accident

⊗⑦**V43.31** Unspecified car occupant injured in collision with sport utility vehicle in nontraffic accident

⊗⑦**V43.32** Unspecified car occupant injured in collision with other type car in nontraffic accident

⊗⑦**V43.33** Unspecified car occupant injured in collision with pick-up truck in nontraffic accident

⊗⑦**V43.34** Unspecified car occupant injured in collision with van in nontraffic accident

V43.4 Person boarding or alighting a car injured in collision with car, pick-up truck or van

⊗⑦**V43.41** Person boarding or alighting a car injured in collision with sport utility vehicle

⊗⑦**V43.42** Person boarding or alighting a car injured in collision with other type car

⊗⑦**V43.43** Person boarding or alighting a car injured in collision with pick-up truck

⊗⑦**V43.44** Person boarding or alighting a car injured in collision with van

V43.5 Car driver injured in collision with car, pick-up truck or van in traffic accident

⊗⑦**V43.51** Car driver injured in collision with sport utility vehicle in traffic accident

⊗⑦**V43.52** Car driver injured in collision with other type car in traffic accident

⊗⑦**V43.53** Car driver injured in collision with pick-up truck in traffic accident

⊗⑦**V43.54** Car driver injured in collision with van in traffic accident

V43.6 Car passenger injured in collision with car, pick-up truck or van in traffic accident

⊗⑦**V43.61** Car passenger injured in collision with sport utility vehicle in traffic accident

● New code ▲ Revised code ⑦ 7th digit required ⊗ Placeholder required

⊗⑦**V43.62** Car passenger injured in collision with other type car in traffic accident

⊗⑦**V43.63** Car passenger injured in collision with pick-up truck in traffic accident

⊗⑦**V43.64** Car passenger injured in collision with van in traffic accident

V43.7 Person on outside of car injured in collision with car, pick-up truck or van in traffic accident

⊗⑦**V43.71** Person on outside of car injured in collision with sport utility vehicle in traffic accident

⊗⑦**V43.72** Person on outside of car injured in collision with other type car in traffic accident

⊗⑦**V43.73** Person on outside of car injured in collision with pick-up truck in traffic accident

⊗⑦**V43.74** Person on outside of car injured in collision with van in traffic accident

V43.9 Unspecified car occupant injured in collision with car, pick-up truck or van in traffic accident

⊗⑦**V43.91** Unspecified car occupant injured in collision with sport utility vehicle in traffic accident

⊗⑦**V43.92** Unspecified car occupant injured in collision with other type car in traffic accident

⊗⑦**V43.93** Unspecified car occupant injured in collision with pick-up truck in traffic accident

⊗⑦**V43.94** Unspecified car occupant injured in collision with van in traffic accident

V44 Car occupant injured in collision with heavy transport vehicle or bus

Excludes 1: car occupant injured in collision with military vehicle (V49.81)

The appropriate 7th character is to be added to each code from category V44

A - initial encounter

D - subsequent encounter

S - sequela

⊗⑦**V44.0** Car driver injured in collision with heavy transport vehicle or bus in nontraffic accident

⊗⑦**V44.1** Car passenger injured in collision with heavy transport vehicle or bus in nontraffic accident

⊗⑦**V44.2** Person on outside of car injured in collision with heavy transport vehicle or bus in nontraffic accident

⊗⑦**V44.3** Unspecified car occupant injured in collision with heavy transport vehicle or bus in nontraffic accident

⊗⑦**V44.4** Person boarding or alighting a car injured in collision with heavy transport vehicle or bus

⊗⑦**V44.5** Car driver injured in collision with heavy transport vehicle or bus in traffic accident

⊗⑦**V44.6** Car passenger injured in collision with heavy transport vehicle or bus in traffic accident

⊗⑦**V44.7** Person on outside of car injured in collision with heavy transport vehicle or bus in traffic accident

⊗⑦**V44.9** Unspecified car occupant injured in collision with heavy transport vehicle or bus in traffic accident

V45 Car occupant injured in collision with railway train or railway vehicle

The appropriate 7th character is to be added to each code from category V45

A - initial encounter

D - subsequent encounter

S - sequela

⊗⑦**V45.0** Car driver injured in collision with railway train or railway vehicle in nontraffic accident

⊗⑦**V45.1** Car passenger injured in collision with railway train or railway vehicle in nontraffic accident

⊗⑦**V45.2** Person on outside of car injured in collision with railway train or railway vehicle in nontraffic accident

⊗⑦**V45.3** Unspecified car occupant injured in collision with railway train or railway vehicle in nontraffic accident

⊗⑦**V45.4** Person boarding or alighting a car injured in collision with railway train or railway vehicle

⊗⑦**V45.5** Car driver injured in collision with railway train or railway vehicle in traffic accident

⊗⑦**V45.6** Car passenger injured in collision with railway train or railway vehicle in traffic accident

⊗⑦**V45.7** Person on outside of car injured in collision with railway train or railway vehicle in traffic accident

⊗⑦**V45.9** Unspecified car occupant injured in collision with railway train or railway vehicle in traffic accident

V46 Car occupant injured in collision with other nonmotor vehicle

Includes: collision with animal-drawn vehicle, animal being ridden, streetcar

The appropriate 7th character is to be added to each code from category V46

A - initial encounter

D - subsequent encounter

S - sequela

⊗⑦**V46.0** Car driver injured in collision with other nonmotor vehicle in nontraffic accident

⊗⑦**V46.1** Car passenger injured in collision with other nonmotor vehicle in nontraffic accident

⊗⑦**V46.2** Person on outside of car injured in collision with other nonmotor vehicle in nontraffic accident

⊗⑦**V46.3** Unspecified car occupant injured in collision with other nonmotor vehicle in nontraffic accident

⊗⑦**V46.4** Person boarding or alighting a car injured in collision with other nonmotor vehicle

⊗⑦**V46.5** Car driver injured in collision with other nonmotor vehicle in traffic accident

⊗⑦**V46.6** Car passenger injured in collision with other nonmotor vehicle in traffic accident

⊗⑦**V46.7** Person on outside of car injured in collision with other nonmotor vehicle in traffic accident

⊗⑦**V46.9** Unspecified car occupant injured in collision with other nonmotor vehicle in traffic accident

V47 Car occupant injured in collision with fixed or stationary object

The appropriate 7th character is to be added to each code from category V47

A - initial encounter

D - subsequent encounter

S - sequela

V47.0 Car driver injured in collision with fixed or stationary object in nontraffic accident

⊗⑦**V47.01** Driver of sport utility vehicle injured in collision with fixed or stationary object in nontraffic accident

⊗⑦**V47.02** Driver of other type car injured in collision with fixed or stationary object in nontraffic accident

V47.1 Car passenger injured in collision with fixed or stationary object in nontraffic accident

⊗⑦**V47.11**   Passenger of sport utility vehicle injured in collision with fixed or stationary object in nontraffic accident

⊗⑦**V47.12**   Passenger of other type car injured in collision with fixed or stationary object in nontraffic accident

V47.2   Person on outside of car injured in collision with fixed or stationary object in nontraffic accident

V47.3   Unspecified car occupant injured in collision with fixed or stationary object in nontraffic accident

⊗⑦**V47.31**   Unspecified occupant of sport utility vehicle injured in collision with fixed or stationary object in nontraffic accident

⊗⑦**V47.32**   Unspecified occupant of other type car injured in collision with fixed or stationary object in nontraffic accident

V47.4   Person boarding or alighting a car injured in collision with fixed or stationary object

V47.5   Car driver injured in collision with fixed or stationary object in traffic accident

⊗⑦**V47.51**   Driver of sport utility vehicle injured in collision with fixed or stationary object in traffic accident

⊗⑦**V47.52**   Driver of other type car injured in collision with fixed or stationary object in traffic accident

V47.6   Car passenger injured in collision with fixed or stationary object in traffic accident

⊗⑦**V47.61**   Passenger of sport utility vehicle injured in collision with fixed or stationary object in traffic accident

⊗⑦**V47.62**   Passenger of other type car injured in collision with fixed or stationary object in traffic accident

⊗⑦**V47.7**   Person on outside of car injured in collision with fixed or stationary object in traffic accident

V47.9   Unspecified car occupant injured in collision with fixed or stationary object in traffic accident

⊗⑦**V47.91**   Unspecified occupant of sport utility vehicle injured in collision with fixed or stationary object in traffic accident

⊗⑦**V47.92**   Unspecified occupant of other type car injured in collision with fixed or stationary object in traffic accident

V48   Car occupant injured in noncollision transport accident

Includes: overturning car NOS
overturning car without collision

The appropriate 7th character is to be added to each code from category V48

A - initial encounter

D - subsequent encounter

S - sequela

⊗⑦**V48.0**   Car driver injured in noncollision transport accident in nontraffic accident

⊗⑦**V48.1**   Car passenger injured in noncollision transport accident in nontraffic accident

⊗⑦**V48.2**   Person on outside of car injured in noncollision transport accident in nontraffic accident

⊗⑦**V48.3**   Unspecified car occupant injured in noncollision transport accident in nontraffic accident

⊗⑦**V48.4**   Person boarding or alighting a car injured in noncollision transport accident

⊗⑦**V48.5**   Car driver injured in noncollision transport accident in traffic accident

⊗⑦**V48.6**   Car passenger injured in noncollision transport accident in traffic accident

⊗⑦**V48.7**   Person on outside of car injured in noncollision transport accident in traffic accident

⊗⑦**V48.9**   Unspecified car occupant injured in noncollision transport accident in traffic accident

V49   Car occupant injured in other and unspecified transport accidents

The appropriate 7th character is to be added to each code from category V49

A - initial encounter

D - subsequent encounter

S - sequela

V49.0   Driver injured in collision with other and unspecified motor vehicles in nontraffic accident

⊗⑦**V49.00**   Driver injured in collision with unspecified motor vehicles in nontraffic accident

⊗⑦**V49.09**   Driver injured in collision with other motor vehicles in nontraffic accident

V49.1   Passenger injured in collision with other and unspecified motor vehicles in nontraffic accident

⊗⑦**V49.10**   Passenger injured in collision with unspecified motor vehicles in nontraffic accident

⊗⑦**V49.19**   Passenger injured in collision with other motor vehicles in nontraffic accident

V49.2   Unspecified car occupant injured in collision with other and unspecified motor vehicles in nontraffic accident

⊗⑦**V49.20**   Unspecified car occupant injured in collision with unspecified motor vehicles in nontraffic accident

Car collision NOS, nontraffic

⊗⑦**V49.29**   Unspecified car occupant injured in collision with other motor vehicles in nontraffic accident

⊗⑦**V49.3**   Car occupant (driver) (passenger) injured in unspecified nontraffic accident

Car accident NOS, nontraffic

Car occupant injured in nontraffic accident NOS

V49.4   Driver injured in collision with other and unspecified motor vehicles in traffic accident

⊗⑦**V49.40**   Driver injured in collision with unspecified motor vehicles in traffic accident

⊗⑦**V49.49**   Driver injured in collision with other motor vehicles in traffic accident

V49.5   Passenger injured in collision with other and unspecified motor vehicles in traffic accident

⊗⑦**V49.50**   Passenger injured in collision with unspecified motor vehicles in traffic accident

⊗⑦**V49.59**   Passenger injured in collision with other motor vehicles in traffic accident

V49.6   Unspecified car occupant injured in collision with other and unspecified motor vehicles in traffic accident

⊗⑦**V49.60**   Unspecified car occupant injured in collision with unspecified motor vehicles in traffic accident

Car collision NOS (traffic)

⊗⑦**V49.69**   Unspecified car occupant injured in collision with other motor vehicles in traffic accident

V49.8   Car occupant (driver) (passenger) injured in other specified transport accidents

● New code   ▲ Revised code   ⑦ 7ᵗʰ digit required   ⊗ Placeholder required

⊗⑦ **V49.81** Car occupant (driver) (passenger) injured in transport accident with military vehicle

⊗⑦ **V49.88** Car occupant (driver) (passenger) injured in other specified transport accidents

V49.9 Car occupant (driver) (passenger) injured in unspecified traffic accident

Car accident NOS

OCCUPANT OF PICK-UP TRUCK OR VAN INJURED IN TRANSPORT ACCIDENT (V50-V59)

Includes: a four or six wheel motor vehicle designed primarily for carrying passengers and property but weighing less than the local limit for classification as a heavy goods vehicle

minibus

minivan

sport utility vehicle (SUV)

truck

van

Excludes 1: heavy transport vehicle (V60-V69)

V50 Occupant of pick-up truck or van injured in collision with pedestrian or animal

Excludes 1: pick-up truck or van collision with animal-drawn vehicle or animal being ridden (V56.-)

The appropriate 7th character is to be added to each code from category V50

A - initial encounter

D - subsequent encounter

S - sequela

⊗⑦ **V50.0** Driver of pick-up truck or van injured in collision with pedestrian or animal in nontraffic accident

⊗⑦ **V50.1** Passenger in pick-up truck or van injured in collision with pedestrian or animal in nontraffic accident

⊗⑦ **V50.2** Person on outside of pick-up truck or van injured in collision with pedestrian or animal in nontraffic accident

⊗⑦ **V50.3** Unspecified occupant of pick-up truck or van injured in collision with pedestrian or animal in nontraffic accident

⊗⑦ **V50.4** Person boarding or alighting a pick-up truck or van injured in collision with pedestrian or animal

⊗⑦ **V50.5** Driver of pick-up truck or van injured in collision with pedestrian or animal in traffic accident

⊗⑦ **V50.6** Passenger in pick-up truck or van injured in collision with pedestrian or animal in traffic accident

⊗⑦ **V50.7** Person on outside of pick-up truck or van injured in collision with pedestrian or animal in traffic accident

⊗⑦ **V50.9** Unspecified occupant of pick-up truck or van injured in collision with pedestrian or animal in traffic accident

V51 Occupant of pick-up truck or van injured in collision with pedal cycle

The appropriate 7th character is to be added to each code from category V51

A - initial encounter

D - subsequent encounter

S - sequela

⊗⑦ **V51.0** Driver of pick-up truck or van injured in collision with pedal cycle in nontraffic accident

⊗⑦ **V51.1** Passenger in pick-up truck or van injured in collision with pedal cycle in nontraffic accident

⊗⑦ **V51.2** Person on outside of pick-up truck or van injured in collision with pedal cycle in nontraffic accident

⊗⑦ **V51.3** Unspecified occupant of pick-up truck or van injured in collision with pedal cycle in nontraffic accident

⊗⑦ **V51.4** Person boarding or alighting a pick-up truck or van injured in collision with pedal cycle

⊗⑦ **V51.5** Driver of pick-up truck or van injured in collision with pedal cycle in traffic accident

⊗⑦ **V51.6** Passenger in pick-up truck or van injured in collision with pedal cycle in traffic accident

⊗⑦ **V51.7** Person on outside of pick-up truck or van injured in collision with pedal cycle in traffic accident

⊗⑦ **V51.9** Unspecified occupant of pick-up truck or van injured in collision with pedal cycle in traffic accident

V52 Occupant of pick-up truck or van injured in collision with two- or three-wheeled motor vehicle

The appropriate 7th character is to be added to each code from category V52

A - initial encounter

D - subsequent encounter

S - sequela

⊗⑦ **V52.0** Driver of pick-up truck or van injured in collision with two- or three-wheeled motor vehicle in nontraffic accident

⊗⑦ **V52.1** Passenger in pick-up truck or van injured in collision with two- or three-wheeled motor vehicle in nontraffic accident

⊗⑦ **V52.2** Person on outside of pick-up truck or van injured in collision with two- or three-wheeled motor vehicle in nontraffic accident

⊗⑦ **V52.3** Unspecified occupant of pick-up truck or van injured in collision with two- or three-wheeled motor vehicle in nontraffic accident

⊗⑦ **V52.4** Person boarding or alighting a pick-up truck or van injured in collision with two- or three-wheeled motor vehicle

⊗⑦ **V52.5** Driver of pick-up truck or van injured in collision with two- or three-wheeled motor vehicle in traffic accident

⊗⑦ **V52.6** Passenger in pick-up truck or van injured in collision with two- or three-wheeled motor vehicle in traffic accident

⊗⑦ **V52.7** Person on outside of pick-up truck or van injured in collision with two- or three-wheeled motor vehicle in traffic accident

⊗⑦ **V52.9** Unspecified occupant of pick-up truck or van injured in collision with two- or three-wheeled motor vehicle in traffic accident

V53 Occupant of pick-up truck or van injured in collision with car, pick-up truck or van

The appropriate 7th character is to be added to each code from category V53

A - initial encounter

D - subsequent encounter

S - sequela

⊗⑦ **V53.0** Driver of pick-up truck or van injured in collision with car, pick-up truck or van in nontraffic accident

⊗⑦ **V53.1** Passenger in pick-up truck or van injured in collision with car, pick-up truck or van in nontraffic accident

⊗⑦ **V53.2** Person on outside of pick-up truck or van injured in collision with car, pick-up truck or van in nontraffic accident

⊗⑦ **V53.3** Unspecified occupant of pick-up truck or van injured in collision with car, pick-up truck or van in nontraffic accident

⊗⑦ **V53.4** Person boarding or alighting a pick-up truck or van injured in collision with car, pick-up truck or van

⊗⑦**V53.5** Driver of pick-up truck or van injured in collision with car, pick-up truck or van in traffic accident

⊗⑦**V53.6** Passenger in pick-up truck or van injured in collision with car, pick-up truck or van in traffic accident

⊗⑦**V53.7** Person on outside of pick-up truck or van injured in collision with car, pick-up truck or van in traffic accident

⊗⑦**V53.9** Unspecified occupant of pick-up truck or van injured in collision with car, pick-up truck or van in traffic accident

V54 Occupant of pick-up truck or van injured in collision with heavy transport vehicle or bus

Excludes 1: occupant of pick-up truck or van injured in collision with military vehicle (V59.81)

The appropriate 7th character is to be added to each code from category V54

A - initial encounter

D - subsequent encounter

S - sequela

⊗⑦**V54.0** Driver of pick-up truck or van injured in collision with heavy transport vehicle or bus in nontraffic accident

⊗⑦**V54.1** Passenger in pick-up truck or van injured in collision with heavy transport vehicle or bus in nontraffic accident

⊗⑦**V54.2** Person on outside of pick-up truck or van injured in collision with heavy transport vehicle or bus in nontraffic accident

⊗⑦**V54.3** Unspecified occupant of pick-up truck or van injured in collision with heavy transport vehicle or bus in nontraffic accident

⊗⑦**V54.4** Person boarding or alighting a pick-up truck or van injured in collision with heavy transport vehicle or bus

⊗⑦**V54.5** Driver of pick-up truck or van injured in collision with heavy transport vehicle or bus in traffic accident

⊗⑦**V54.6** Passenger in pick-up truck or van injured in collision with heavy transport vehicle or bus in traffic accident

⊗⑦**V54.7** Person on outside of pick-up truck or van injured in collision with heavy transport vehicle or bus in traffic accident

⊗⑦**V54.9** Unspecified occupant of pick-up truck or van injured in collision with heavy transport vehicle or bus in traffic accident

V55 Occupant of pick-up truck or van injured in collision with railway train or railway vehicle

The appropriate 7th character is to be added to each code from category V55

A - initial encounter

D - subsequent encounter

S - sequela

⊗⑦**V55.0** Driver of pick-up truck or van injured in collision with railway train or railway vehicle in nontraffic accident

⊗⑦**V55.1** Passenger in pick-up truck or van injured in collision with railway train or railway vehicle in nontraffic accident

⊗⑦**V55.2** Person on outside of pick-up truck or van injured in collision with railway train or railway vehicle in nontraffic accident

⊗⑦**V55.3** Unspecified occupant of pick-up truck or van injured in collision with railway train or railway vehicle in nontraffic accident

⊗⑦**V55.4** Person boarding or alighting a pick-up truck or van injured in collision with railway train or railway vehicle

⊗⑦**V55.5** Driver of pick-up truck or van injured in collision with railway train or railway vehicle in traffic accident

⊗⑦**V55.6** Passenger in pick-up truck or van injured in collision with railway train or railway vehicle in traffic accident

⊗⑦**V55.7** Person on outside of pick-up truck or van injured in collision with railway train or railway vehicle in traffic accident

⊗⑦**V55.9** Unspecified occupant of pick-up truck or van injured in collision with railway train or railway vehicle in traffic accident

V56 Occupant of pick-up truck or van injured in collision with other nonmotor vehicle

Includes: collision with animal-drawn vehicle, animal being ridden, streetcar

The appropriate 7th character is to be added to each code from category V56

A - initial encounter

D - subsequent encounter

S - sequela

⊗⑦**V56.0** Driver of pick-up truck or van injured in collision with other nonmotor vehicle in nontraffic accident

⊗⑦**V56.1** Passenger in pick-up truck or van injured in collision with other nonmotor vehicle in nontraffic accident

⊗⑦**V56.2** Person on outside of pick-up truck or van injured in collision with other nonmotor vehicle in nontraffic accident

⊗⑦**V56.3** Unspecified occupant of pick-up truck or van injured in collision with other nonmotor vehicle in nontraffic accident

⊗⑦**V56.4** Person boarding or alighting a pick-up truck or van injured in collision with other nonmotor vehicle

⊗⑦**V56.5** Driver of pick-up truck or van injured in collision with other nonmotor vehicle in traffic accident

⊗⑦**V56.6** Passenger in pick-up truck or van injured in collision with other nonmotor vehicle in traffic accident

⊗⑦**V56.7** Person on outside of pick-up truck or van injured in collision with other nonmotor vehicle in traffic accident

⊗⑦**V56.9** Unspecified occupant of pick-up truck or van injured in collision with other nonmotor vehicle in traffic accident

V57 Occupant of pick-up truck or van injured in collision with fixed or stationary object

The appropriate 7th character is to be added to each code from category V57

A - initial encounter

D - subsequent encounter

S - sequela

⊗⑦**V57.0** Driver of pick-up truck or van injured in collision with fixed or stationary object in nontraffic accident

⊗⑦**V57.1** Passenger in pick-up truck or van injured in collision with fixed or stationary object in nontraffic accident

⊗⑦**V57.2** Person on outside of pick-up truck or van injured in collision with fixed or stationary object in nontraffic accident

⊗⑦**V57.3** Unspecified occupant of pick-up truck or van injured in collision with fixed or stationary object in nontraffic accident

⊗⑦**V57.4** Person boarding or alighting a pick-up truck or van injured in collision with fixed or stationary object

⊗⑦**V57.5** Driver of pick-up truck or van injured in collision with fixed or stationary object in traffic accident

⊗⑦**V57.6** Passenger in pick-up truck or van injured in collision with fixed or stationary object in traffic accident

⊗⑦**V57.7** Person on outside of pick-up truck or van injured in collision with fixed or stationary object in traffic accident

⊗⑦V57.9 Unspecified occupant of pick-up truck or van injured in collision with fixed or stationary object in traffic accident

V58 Occupant of pick-up truck or van injured in noncollision transport accident

Includes: overturning pick-up truck or van NOS
overturning pick-up truck or van without collision

The appropriate 7th character is to be added to each code from category V58

A - initial encounter

D - subsequent encounter

S - sequela

⊗⑦V58.0 Driver of pick-up truck or van injured in noncollision transport accident in nontraffic accident

⊗⑦V58.1 Passenger in pick-up truck or van injured in noncollision transport accident in nontraffic accident

⊗⑦V58.2 Person on outside of pick-up truck or van injured in noncollision transport accident in nontraffic accident

⊗⑦V58.3 Unspecified occupant of pick-up truck or van injured in noncollision transport accident in nontraffic accident

⊗⑦V58.4 Person boarding or alighting a pick-up truck or van injured in noncollision transport accident

⊗⑦V58.5 Driver of pick-up truck or van injured in noncollision transport accident in traffic accident

⊗⑦V58.6 Passenger in pick-up truck or van injured in noncollision transport accident in traffic accident

⊗⑦V58.7 Person on outside of pick-up truck or van injured in noncollision transport accident in traffic accident

⊗⑦V58.9 Unspecified occupant of pick-up truck or van injured in noncollision transport accident in traffic accident

V59 Occupant of pick-up truck or van injured in other and unspecified transport accidents

The appropriate 7th character is to be added to each code from category V59

A - initial encounter

D - subsequent encounter

S - sequela

V59.0 Driver of pick-up truck or van injured in collision with other and unspecified motor vehicles in nontraffic accident

⊗⑦V59.00 Driver of pick-up truck or van injured in collision with unspecified motor vehicles in nontraffic accident

⊗⑦V59.09 Driver of pick-up truck or van injured in collision with other motor vehicles in nontraffic accident

V59.1 Passenger in pick-up truck or van injured in collision with other and unspecified motor vehicles in nontraffic accident

⊗⑦V59.10 Passenger in pick-up truck or van injured in collision with unspecified motor vehicles in nontraffic accident

⊗⑦V59.19 Passenger in pick-up truck or van injured in collision with other motor vehicles in nontraffic accident

V59.2 Unspecified occupant of pick-up truck or van injured in collision with other and unspecified motor vehicles in nontraffic accident

⊗⑦V59.20 Unspecified occupant of pick-up truck or van injured in collision with unspecified motor vehicles in nontraffic accident
Collision NOS involving pick-up truck or van, nontraffic

⊗⑦V59.29 Unspecified occupant of pick-up truck or van injured in collision with other motor vehicles in nontraffic accident

⊗⑦V59.3 Occupant (driver) (passenger) of pick-up truck or van injured in unspecified nontraffic accident
Accident NOS involving pick-up truck or van, nontraffic
Occupant of pick-up truck or van injured in nontraffic accident NOS

V59.4 Driver of pick-up truck or van injured in collision with other and unspecified motor vehicles in traffic accident

⊗⑦V59.40 Driver of pick-up truck or van injured in collision with unspecified motor vehicles in traffic accident

⊗⑦V59.49 Driver of pick-up truck or van injured in collision with other motor vehicles in traffic accident

V59.5 Passenger in pick-up truck or van injured in collision with other and unspecified motor vehicles in traffic accident

⊗⑦V59.50 Passenger in pick-up truck or van injured in collision with unspecified motor vehicles in traffic accident

⊗⑦V59.59 Passenger in pick-up truck or van injured in collision with other motor vehicles in traffic accident

V59.6 Unspecified occupant of pick-up truck or van injured in collision with other and unspecified motor vehicles in traffic accident

⊗⑦V59.60 Unspecified occupant of pick-up truck or van injured in collision with unspecified motor vehicles in traffic accident
Collision NOS involving pick-up truck or van (traffic)

⊗⑦V59.69 Unspecified occupant of pick-up truck or van injured in collision with other motor vehicles in traffic accident

V59.8 Occupant (driver) (passenger) of pick-up truck or van injured in other specified transport accidents

⊗⑦V59.81 Occupant (driver) (passenger) of pick-up truck or van injured in transport accident with military vehicle

⊗⑦V59.88 Occupant (driver) (passenger) of pick-up truck or van injured in other specified transport accidents

V59.9 Occupant (driver) (passenger) of pick-up truck or van injured in unspecified traffic accident
Accident NOS involving pick-up truck or van

OCCUPANT OF HEAVY TRANSPORT VEHICLE INJURED IN TRANSPORT ACCIDENT (V60-V69)

Includes: 18 wheeler
armored car
panel truck

Excludes 1: bus
motorcoach

V60 Occupant of heavy transport vehicle injured in collision with pedestrian or animal

Excludes 1: heavy transport vehicle collision with animal-drawn vehicle or animal being ridden (V66.-)

The appropriate 7th character is to be added to each code from category V60

A - initial encounter

D - subsequent encounter

S - sequela

⊗⑦**V60.0** Driver of heavy transport vehicle injured in collision with pedestrian or animal in nontraffic accident

⊗⑦**V60.1** Passenger in heavy transport vehicle injured in collision with pedestrian or animal in nontraffic accident

⊗⑦**V60.2** Person on outside of heavy transport vehicle injured in collision with pedestrian or animal in nontraffic accident

⊗⑦**V60.3** Unspecified occupant of heavy transport vehicle injured in collision with pedestrian or animal in nontraffic accident

⊗⑦**V60.4** Person boarding or alighting a heavy transport vehicle injured in collision with pedestrian or animal

⊗⑦**V60.5** Driver of heavy transport vehicle injured in collision with pedestrian or animal in traffic accident

⊗⑦**V60.6** Passenger in heavy transport vehicle injured in collision with pedestrian or animal in traffic accident

⊗⑦**V60.7** Person on outside of heavy transport vehicle injured in collision with pedestrian or animal in traffic accident

⊗⑦**V60.9** Unspecified occupant of heavy transport vehicle injured in collision with pedestrian or animal in traffic accident

V61 Occupant of heavy transport vehicle injured in collision with pedal cycle

The appropriate 7th character is to be added to each code from category V61

A - initial encounter

D - subsequent encounter

S - sequela

⊗⑦**V61.0** Driver of heavy transport vehicle injured in collision with pedal cycle in nontraffic accident

⊗⑦**V61.1** Passenger in heavy transport vehicle injured in collision with pedal cycle in nontraffic accident

⊗⑦**V61.2** Person on outside of heavy transport vehicle injured in collision with pedal cycle in nontraffic accident

⊗⑦**V61.3** Unspecified occupant of heavy transport vehicle injured in collision with pedal cycle in nontraffic accident

⊗⑦**V61.4** Person boarding or alighting a heavy transport vehicle injured in collision with pedal cycle while boarding or alighting

⊗⑦**V61.5** Driver of heavy transport vehicle injured in collision with pedal cycle in traffic accident

⊗⑦**V61.6** Passenger in heavy transport vehicle injured in collision with pedal cycle in traffic accident

⊗⑦**V61.7** Person on outside of heavy transport vehicle injured in collision with pedal cycle in traffic accident

⊗⑦**V61.9** Unspecified occupant of heavy transport vehicle injured in collision with pedal cycle in traffic accident

V62 Occupant of heavy transport vehicle injured in collision with two- or three-wheeled motor vehicle

The appropriate 7th character is to be added to each code from category V62

A - initial encounter

D - subsequent encounter

S - sequela

⊗⑦**V62.0** Driver of heavy transport vehicle injured in collision with two- or three-wheeled motor vehicle in nontraffic accident

⊗⑦**V62.1** Passenger in heavy transport vehicle injured in collision with two- or three-wheeled motor vehicle in nontraffic accident

⊗⑦**V62.2** Person on outside of heavy transport vehicle injured in collision with two- or three-wheeled motor vehicle in nontraffic accident

⊗⑦**V62.3** Unspecified occupant of heavy transport vehicle injured in collision with two- or three-wheeled motor vehicle in nontraffic accident

⊗⑦**V62.4** Person boarding or alighting a heavy transport vehicle injured in collision with two- or three-wheeled motor vehicle

⊗⑦**V62.5** Driver of heavy transport vehicle injured in collision with two- or three-wheeled motor vehicle in traffic accident

⊗⑦**V62.6** Passenger in heavy transport vehicle injured in collision with two- or three-wheeled motor vehicle in traffic accident

⊗⑦**V62.7** Person on outside of heavy transport vehicle injured in collision with two- or three-wheeled motor vehicle in traffic accident

⊗⑦**V62.9** Unspecified occupant of heavy transport vehicle injured in collision with two- or three-wheeled motor vehicle in traffic accident

V63 Occupant of heavy transport vehicle injured in collision with car, pick-up truck or van

The appropriate 7th character is to be added to each code from category V63

A - initial encounter

D - subsequent encounter

S - sequela

⊗⑦**V63.0** Driver of heavy transport vehicle injured in collision with car, pick-up truck or van in nontraffic accident

⊗⑦**V63.1** Passenger in heavy transport vehicle injured in collision with car, pick-up truck or van in nontraffic accident

⊗⑦**V63.2** Person on outside of heavy transport vehicle injured in collision with car, pick-up truck or van in nontraffic accident

⊗⑦**V63.3** Unspecified occupant of heavy transport vehicle injured in collision with car, pick-up truck or van in nontraffic accident

⊗⑦**V63.4** Person boarding or alighting a heavy transport vehicle injured in collision with car, pick-up truck or van

⊗⑦**V63.5** Driver of heavy transport vehicle injured in collision with car, pick-up truck or van in traffic accident

⊗⑦**V63.6** Passenger in heavy transport vehicle injured in collision with car, pick-up truck or van in traffic accident

⊗⑦**V63.7** Person on outside of heavy transport vehicle injured in collision with car, pick-up truck or van in traffic accident

⊗⑦**V63.9** Unspecified occupant of heavy transport vehicle injured in collision with car, pick-up truck or van in traffic accident

V64 Occupant of heavy transport vehicle injured in collision with heavy transport vehicle or bus

Excludes 1: occupant of heavy transport vehicle injured in collision with military vehicle (V69.81)

The appropriate 7th character is to be added to each code from category V64

A - initial encounter

D - subsequent encounter

S - sequela

⊗⑦**V64.0** Driver of heavy transport vehicle injured in collision with heavy transport vehicle or bus in nontraffic accident

⊗⑦**V64.1** Passenger in heavy transport vehicle injured in collision with heavy transport vehicle or bus in nontraffic accident

⊗⑦**V64.2** Person on outside of heavy transport vehicle injured in collision with heavy transport vehicle or bus in nontraffic accident

● New code ▲ Revised code ⑦ 7th digit required ⊗ Placeholder required

⊗⑦**V64.3**   Unspecified occupant of heavy transport vehicle injured in collision with heavy transport vehicle or bus in nontraffic accident

⊗⑦**V64.4**   Person boarding or alighting a heavy transport vehicle injured in collision with heavy transport vehicle or bus while boarding or alighting

⊗⑦**V64.5**   Driver of heavy transport vehicle injured in collision with heavy transport vehicle or bus in traffic accident

⊗⑦**V64.6**   Passenger in heavy transport vehicle injured in collision with heavy transport vehicle or bus in traffic accident

⊗⑦**V64.7**   Person on outside of heavy transport vehicle injured in collision with heavy transport vehicle or bus in traffic accident

⊗⑦**V64.9**   Unspecified occupant of heavy transport vehicle injured in collision with heavy transport vehicle or bus in traffic accident

V65   Occupant of heavy transport vehicle injured in collision with railway train or railway vehicle

The appropriate 7th character is to be added to each code from category V65

A - initial encounter

D - subsequent encounter

S - sequela

⊗⑦**V65.0**   Driver of heavy transport vehicle injured in collision with railway train or railway vehicle in nontraffic accident

⊗⑦**V65.1**   Passenger in heavy transport vehicle injured in collision with railway train or railway vehicle in nontraffic accident

⊗⑦**V65.2**   Person on outside of heavy transport vehicle injured in collision with railway train or railway vehicle in nontraffic accident

⊗⑦**V65.3**   Unspecified occupant of heavy transport vehicle injured in collision with railway train or railway vehicle in nontraffic accident

⊗⑦**V65.4**   Person boarding or alighting a heavy transport vehicle injured in collision with railway train or railway vehicle

⊗⑦**V65.5**   Driver of heavy transport vehicle injured in collision with railway train or railway vehicle in traffic accident

⊗⑦**V65.6**   Passenger in heavy transport vehicle injured in collision with railway train or railway vehicle in traffic accident

⊗⑦**V65.7**   Person on outside of heavy transport vehicle injured in collision with railway train or railway vehicle in traffic accident

⊗⑦**V65.9**   Unspecified occupant of heavy transport vehicle injured in collision with railway train or railway vehicle in traffic accident

V66   Occupant of heavy transport vehicle injured in collision with other nonmotor vehicle

Includes: collision with animal-drawn vehicle, animal being ridden, streetcar

The appropriate 7th character is to be added to each code from category V66

A - initial encounter

D - subsequent encounter

S - sequela

⊗⑦**V66.0**   Driver of heavy transport vehicle injured in collision with other nonmotor vehicle in nontraffic accident

⊗⑦**V66.1**   Passenger in heavy transport vehicle injured in collision with other nonmotor vehicle in nontraffic accident

⊗⑦**V66.2**   Person on outside of heavy transport vehicle injured in collision with other nonmotor vehicle in nontraffic accident

⊗⑦**V66.3**   Unspecified occupant of heavy transport vehicle injured in collision with other nonmotor vehicle in nontraffic accident

⊗⑦**V66.4**   Person boarding or alighting a heavy transport vehicle injured in collision with other nonmotor vehicle

⊗⑦**V66.5**   Driver of heavy transport vehicle injured in collision with other nonmotor vehicle in traffic accident

⊗⑦**V66.6**   Passenger in heavy transport vehicle injured in collision with other nonmotor vehicle in traffic accident

⊗⑦**V66.7**   Person on outside of heavy transport vehicle injured in collision with other nonmotor vehicle in traffic accident

⊗⑦**V66.9**   Unspecified occupant of heavy transport vehicle injured in collision with other nonmotor vehicle in traffic accident

V67   Occupant of heavy transport vehicle injured in collision with fixed or stationary object

The appropriate 7th character is to be added to each code from category V67

A - initial encounter

D - subsequent encounter

S - sequela

⊗⑦**V67.0**   Driver of heavy transport vehicle injured in collision with fixed or stationary object in nontraffic accident

⊗⑦**V67.1**   Passenger in heavy transport vehicle injured in collision with fixed or stationary object in nontraffic accident

⊗⑦**V67.2**   Person on outside of heavy transport vehicle injured in collision with fixed or stationary object in nontraffic accident

⊗⑦**V67.3**   Unspecified occupant of heavy transport vehicle injured in collision with fixed or stationary object in nontraffic accident

⊗⑦**V67.4**   Person boarding or alighting a heavy transport vehicle injured in collision with fixed or stationary object

⊗⑦**V67.5**   Driver of heavy transport vehicle injured in collision with fixed or stationary object in traffic accident

⊗⑦**V67.6**   Passenger in heavy transport vehicle injured in collision with fixed or stationary object in traffic accident

⊗⑦**V67.7**   Person on outside of heavy transport vehicle injured in collision with fixed or stationary object in traffic accident

⊗⑦**V67.9**   Unspecified occupant of heavy transport vehicle injured in collision with fixed or stationary object in traffic accident

V68   Occupant of heavy transport vehicle injured in noncollision transport accident

Includes: overturning heavy transport vehicle NOS
overturning heavy transport vehicle without collision

The appropriate 7th character is to be added to each code from category V68

A - initial encounter

D - subsequent encounter

S - sequela

⊗⑦**V68.0**   Driver of heavy transport vehicle injured in noncollision transport accident in nontraffic accident

⊗⑦**V68.1**   Passenger in heavy transport vehicle injured in noncollision transport accident in nontraffic accident

⊗⑦**V68.2**   Person on outside of heavy transport vehicle injured in noncollision transport accident in nontraffic accident

⊗⑦**V68.3**   Unspecified occupant of heavy transport vehicle injured in noncollision transport accident in nontraffic accident

⊗⑦**V68.4**   Person boarding or alighting a heavy transport vehicle injured in noncollision transport accident

---

⊗⑦V68.5   Driver of heavy transport vehicle injured in noncollision transport accident in traffic accident

⊗⑦V68.6   Passenger in heavy transport vehicle injured in noncollision transport accident in traffic accident

⊗⑦V68.7   Person on outside of heavy transport vehicle injured in noncollision transport accident in traffic accident

⊗⑦V68.9   Unspecified occupant of heavy transport vehicle injured in noncollision transport accident in traffic accident

V69 Occupant of heavy transport vehicle injured in other and unspecified transport accidents

The appropriate 7th character is to be added to each code from category V69

A - initial encounter

D - subsequent encounter

S - sequela

V69.0   Driver of heavy transport vehicle injured in collision with other and unspecified motor vehicles in nontraffic accident

⊗⑦V69.00   Driver of heavy transport vehicle injured in collision with unspecified motor vehicles in nontraffic accident

⊗⑦V69.09   Driver of heavy transport vehicle injured in collision with other motor vehicles in nontraffic accident

V69.1   Passenger in heavy transport vehicle injured in collision with other and unspecified motor vehicles in nontraffic accident

⊗⑦V69.10   Passenger in heavy transport vehicle injured in collision with unspecified motor vehicles in nontraffic accident

⊗⑦V69.19   Passenger in heavy transport vehicle injured in collision with other motor vehicles in nontraffic accident

V69.2   Unspecified occupant of heavy transport vehicle injured in collision with other and unspecified motor vehicles in nontraffic accident

⊗⑦V69.20   Unspecified occupant of heavy transport vehicle injured in collision with unspecified motor vehicles in nontraffic accident

Collision NOS involving heavy transport vehicle, nontraffic

⊗⑦V69.29   Unspecified occupant of heavy transport vehicle injured in collision with other motor vehicles in nontraffic accident

⊗⑦V69.3   Occupant (driver) (passenger) of heavy transport vehicle injured in unspecified nontraffic accident

Accident NOS involving heavy transport vehicle, nontraffic

Occupant of heavy transport vehicle injured in nontraffic accident NOS

V69.4   Driver of heavy transport vehicle injured in collision with other and unspecified motor vehicles in traffic accident

⊗⑦V69.40   Driver of heavy transport vehicle injured in collision with unspecified motor vehicles in traffic accident

⊗⑦V69.49   Driver of heavy transport vehicle injured in collision with other motor vehicles in traffic accident

V69.5   Passenger in heavy transport vehicle injured in collision with other and unspecified motor vehicles in traffic accident

⊗⑦V69.50   Passenger in heavy transport vehicle injured in collision with unspecified motor vehicles in traffic accident

⊗⑦V69.59   Passenger in heavy transport vehicle injured in collision with other motor vehicles in traffic accident

V69.6   Unspecified occupant of heavy transport vehicle injured in collision with other and unspecified motor vehicles in traffic accident

⊗⑦V69.60   Unspecified occupant of heavy transport vehicle injured in collision with unspecified motor vehicles in traffic accident

Collision NOS involving heavy transport vehicle (traffic)

⊗⑦V69.69   Unspecified occupant of heavy transport vehicle injured in collision with other motor vehicles in traffic accident

V69.8   Occupant (driver) (passenger) of heavy transport vehicle injured in other specified transport accidents

⊗⑦V69.81   Occupant (driver) (passenger) of heavy transport vehicle injured in transport accidents with military vehicle

⊗⑦V69.88   Occupant (driver) (passenger) of heavy transport vehicle injured in other specified transport accidents

V69.9   Occupant (driver) (passenger) of heavy transport vehicle injured in unspecified traffic accident

Accident NOS involving heavy transport vehicle

BUS OCCUPANT INJURED IN TRANSPORT ACCIDENT (V70-V79)

Includes: motorcoach

Excludes 1: minibus (V50-V59)

V70 Bus occupant injured in collision with pedestrian or animal

The appropriate 7th character is to be added to each code from category V70

A - initial encounter

D - subsequent encounter

S - sequela

Excludes 1: bus collision with animal-drawn vehicle or animal being ridden (V76.-)

⊗⑦V70.0   Driver of bus injured in collision with pedestrian or animal in nontraffic accident

⊗⑦V70.1   Passenger on bus injured in collision with pedestrian or animal in nontraffic accident

⊗⑦V70.2   Person on outside of bus injured in collision with pedestrian or animal in nontraffic accident

⊗⑦V70.3   Unspecified occupant of bus injured in collision with pedestrian or animal in nontraffic accident

⊗⑦V70.4   Person boarding or alighting from bus injured in collision with pedestrian or animal

⊗⑦V70.5   Driver of bus injured in collision with pedestrian or animal in traffic accident

⊗⑦V70.6   Passenger on bus injured in collision with pedestrian or animal in traffic accident

⊗⑦V70.7   Person on outside of bus injured in collision with pedestrian or animal in traffic accident

⊗⑦V70.9   Unspecified occupant of bus injured in collision with pedestrian or animal in traffic accident

V71 Bus occupant injured in collision with pedal cycle

The appropriate 7th character is to be added to each code from category V71

A - initial encounter

D - subsequent encounter

S - sequela

⊗⑦**V71.0** Driver of bus injured in collision with pedal cycle in nontraffic accident

⊗⑦**V71.1** Passenger on bus injured in collision with pedal cycle in nontraffic accident

⊗⑦**V71.2** Person on outside of bus injured in collision with pedal cycle in nontraffic accident

⊗⑦**V71.3** Unspecified occupant of bus injured in collision with pedal cycle in nontraffic accident

⊗⑦**V71.4** Person boarding or alighting from bus injured in collision with pedal cycle

⊗⑦**V71.5** Driver of bus injured in collision with pedal cycle in traffic accident

⊗⑦**V71.6** Passenger on bus injured in collision with pedal cycle in traffic accident

⊗⑦**V71.7** Person on outside of bus injured in collision with pedal cycle in traffic accident

⊗⑦**V71.9** Unspecified occupant of bus injured in collision with pedal cycle in traffic accident

V72 Bus occupant injured in collision with two- or three-wheeled motor vehicle

The appropriate 7th character is to be added to each code from category V72

A - initial encounter

D - subsequent encounter

S - sequela

⊗⑦**V72.0** Driver of bus injured in collision with two- or three-wheeled motor vehicle in nontraffic accident

⊗⑦**V72.1** Passenger on bus injured in collision with two- or three-wheeled motor vehicle in nontraffic accident

⊗⑦**V72.2** Person on outside of bus injured in collision with two- or three-wheeled motor vehicle in nontraffic accident

⊗⑦**V72.3** Unspecified occupant of bus injured in collision with two- or three-wheeled motor vehicle in nontraffic accident

⊗⑦**V72.4** Person boarding or alighting from bus injured in collision with two- or three-wheeled motor vehicle

⊗⑦**V72.5** Driver of bus injured in collision with two- or three-wheeled motor vehicle in traffic accident

⊗⑦**V72.6** Passenger on bus injured in collision with two- or three-wheeled motor vehicle in traffic accident

⊗⑦**V72.7** Person on outside of bus injured in collision with two- or three-wheeled motor vehicle in traffic accident

⊗⑦**V72.9** Unspecified occupant of bus injured in collision with two- or three-wheeled motor vehicle in traffic accident

V73 Bus occupant injured in collision with car, pick-up truck or van

The appropriate 7th character is to be added to each code from category V73

A - initial encounter

D - subsequent encounter

S - sequela

⊗⑦**V73.0** Driver of bus injured in collision with car, pick-up truck or van in nontraffic accident

⊗⑦**V73.1** Passenger on bus injured in collision with car, pick-up truck or van in nontraffic accident

⊗⑦**V73.2** Person on outside of bus injured in collision with car, pick-up truck or van in nontraffic accident

⊗⑦**V73.3** Unspecified occupant of bus injured in collision with car, pick-up truck or van in nontraffic accident

⊗⑦**V73.4** Person boarding or alighting from bus injured in collision with car, pick-up truck or van

⊗⑦**V73.5** Driver of bus injured in collision with car, pick-up truck or van in traffic accident

⊗⑦**V73.6** Passenger on bus injured in collision with car, pick-up truck or van in traffic accident

⊗⑦**V73.7** Person on outside of bus injured in collision with car, pick-up truck or van in traffic accident

⊗⑦**V73.9** Unspecified occupant of bus injured in collision with car, pick-up truck or van in traffic accident

V74 Bus occupant injured in collision with heavy transport vehicle or bus

Excludes 1: bus occupant injured in collision with military vehicle (V79.81)

The appropriate 7th character is to be added to each code from category V74

A - initial encounter

D - subsequent encounter

S - sequela

⊗⑦**V74.0** Driver of bus injured in collision with heavy transport vehicle or bus in nontraffic accident

⊗⑦**V74.1** Passenger on bus injured in collision with heavy transport vehicle or bus in nontraffic accident

⊗⑦**V74.2** Person on outside of bus injured in collision with heavy transport vehicle or bus in nontraffic accident

⊗⑦**V74.3** Unspecified occupant of bus injured in collision with heavy transport vehicle or bus in nontraffic accident

⊗⑦**V74.4** Person boarding or alighting from bus injured in collision with heavy transport vehicle or bus

⊗⑦**V74.5** Driver of bus injured in collision with heavy transport vehicle or bus in traffic accident

⊗⑦**V74.6** Passenger on bus injured in collision with heavy transport vehicle or bus in traffic accident

⊗⑦**V74.7** Person on outside of bus injured in collision with heavy transport vehicle or bus in traffic accident

⊗⑦**V74.9** Unspecified occupant of bus injured in collision with heavy transport vehicle or bus in traffic accident

V75 Bus occupant injured in collision with railway train or railway vehicle

The appropriate 7th character is to be added to each code from category V75

A - initial encounter

D - subsequent encounter

S - sequela

⊗⑦**V75.0** Driver of bus injured in collision with railway train or railway vehicle in nontraffic accident

⊗⑦**V75.1** Passenger on bus injured in collision with railway train or railway vehicle in nontraffic accident

⊗⑦**V75.2** Person on outside of bus injured in collision with railway train or railway vehicle in nontraffic accident

⊗⑦**V75.3** Unspecified occupant of bus injured in collision with railway train or railway vehicle in nontraffic accident

⊗⑦**V75.4** Person boarding or alighting from bus injured in collision with railway train or railway vehicle

⊗⑦**V75.5** Driver of bus injured in collision with railway train or railway vehicle in traffic accident

⊗⑦**V75.6** Passenger on bus injured in collision with railway train or railway vehicle in traffic accident

⊗⑦**V75.7** Person on outside of bus injured in collision with railway train or railway vehicle in traffic accident

⊗⑦**V75.9** Unspecified occupant of bus injured in collision with railway train or railway vehicle in traffic accident

V76 Bus occupant injured in collision with other nonmotor vehicle

Includes: collision with animal-drawn vehicle, animal being ridden, streetcar

The appropriate 7th character is to be added to each code from category V76

A - initial encounter

D - subsequent encounter

S - sequela

⊗⑦**V76.0** Driver of bus injured in collision with other nonmotor vehicle in nontraffic accident

⊗⑦**V76.1** Passenger on bus injured in collision with other nonmotor vehicle in nontraffic accident

⊗⑦**V76.2** Person on outside of bus injured in collision with other nonmotor vehicle in nontraffic accident

⊗⑦**V76.3** Unspecified occupant of bus injured in collision with other nonmotor vehicle in nontraffic accident

⊗⑦**V76.4** Person boarding or alighting from bus injured in collision with other nonmotor vehicle

⊗⑦**V76.5** Driver of bus injured in collision with other nonmotor vehicle in traffic accident

⊗⑦**V76.6** Passenger on bus injured in collision with other nonmotor vehicle in traffic accident

⊗⑦**V76.7** Person on outside of bus injured in collision with other nonmotor vehicle in traffic accident

⊗⑦**V76.9** Unspecified occupant of bus injured in collision with other nonmotor vehicle in traffic accident

V77 Bus occupant injured in collision with fixed or stationary object

The appropriate 7th character is to be added to each code from category V77

A - initial encounter

D - subsequent encounter

S - sequela

⊗⑦**V77.0** Driver of bus injured in collision with fixed or stationary object in nontraffic accident

⊗⑦**V77.1** Passenger on bus injured in collision with fixed or stationary object in nontraffic accident

⊗⑦**V77.2** Person on outside of bus injured in collision with fixed or stationary object in nontraffic accident

⊗⑦**V77.3** Unspecified occupant of bus injured in collision with fixed or stationary object in nontraffic accident

⊗⑦**V77.4** Person boarding or alighting from bus injured in collision with fixed or stationary object

⊗⑦**V77.5** Driver of bus injured in collision with fixed or stationary object in traffic accident

⊗⑦**V77.6** Passenger on bus injured in collision with fixed or stationary object in traffic accident

⊗⑦**V77.7** Person on outside of bus injured in collision with fixed or stationary object in traffic accident

⊗⑦**V77.9** Unspecified occupant of bus injured in collision with fixed or stationary object in traffic accident

V78 Bus occupant injured in noncollision transport accident

Includes: overturning bus NOS

overturning bus without collision

The appropriate 7th character is to be added to each code from category V78

A - initial encounter

D - subsequent encounter

S - sequela

⊗⑦**V78.0** Driver of bus injured in noncollision transport accident in nontraffic accident

⊗⑦**V78.1** Passenger on bus injured in noncollision transport accident in nontraffic accident

⊗⑦**V78.2** Person on outside of bus injured in noncollision transport accident in nontraffic accident

⊗⑦**V78.3** Unspecified occupant of bus injured in noncollision transport accident in nontraffic accident

⊗⑦**V78.4** Person boarding or alighting from bus injured in noncollision transport accident

⊗⑦**V78.5** Driver of bus injured in noncollision transport accident in traffic accident

⊗⑦**V78.6** Passenger on bus injured in noncollision transport accident in traffic accident

⊗⑦**V78.7** Person on outside of bus injured in noncollision transport accident in traffic accident

⊗⑦**V78.9** Unspecified occupant of bus injured in noncollision transport accident in traffic accident

V79 Bus occupant injured in other and unspecified transport accidents

The appropriate 7th character is to be added to each code from category V79

A - initial encounter

D - subsequent encounter

S - sequela

V79.0 Driver of bus injured in collision with other and unspecified motor vehicles in nontraffic accident

⊗⑦**V79.00** Driver of bus injured in collision with unspecified motor vehicles in nontraffic accident

⊗⑦**V79.09** Driver of bus injured in collision with other motor vehicles in nontraffic accident

V79.1 Passenger on bus injured in collision with other and unspecified motor vehicles in nontraffic accident

⊗⑦**V79.10** Passenger on bus injured in collision with unspecified motor vehicles in nontraffic accident

⊗⑦**V79.19** Passenger on bus injured in collision with other motor vehicles in nontraffic accident

V79.2 Unspecified bus occupant injured in collision with other and unspecified motor vehicles in nontraffic accident

⊗⑦**V79.20** Unspecified bus occupant injured in collision with unspecified motor vehicles in nontraffic accident

Bus collision NOS, nontraffic

⊗⑦**V79.29** Unspecified bus occupant injured in collision with other motor vehicles in nontraffic accident

⊗⑦**V79.3** Bus occupant (driver) (passenger) injured in unspecified nontraffic accident

Bus accident NOS, nontraffic

Bus occupant injured in nontraffic accident NOS

V79.4 Driver of bus injured in collision with other and unspecified motor vehicles in traffic accident

⊗⑦**V79.40** Driver of bus injured in collision with unspecified motor vehicles in traffic accident

⊗⑦**V79.49** Driver of bus injured in collision with other motor vehicles in traffic accident

● New code   ▲ Revised code   ⑦ 7th digit required   ⊗ Placeholder required

V79.5   Passenger on bus injured in collision with other and unspecified motor vehicles in traffic accident

⊗⑦V79.50   Passenger on bus injured in collision with unspecified motor vehicles in traffic accident

⊗⑦V79.59   Passenger on bus injured in collision with other motor vehicles in traffic accident

V79.6   Unspecified bus occupant injured in collision with other and unspecified motor vehicles in traffic accident

⊗⑦V79.60   Unspecified bus occupant injured in collision with unspecified motor vehicles in traffic accident
Bus collision NOS (traffic)

⊗⑦V79.69   Unspecified bus occupant injured in collision with other motor vehicles in traffic accident

V79.8   Bus occupant (driver) (passenger) injured in other specified transport accidents

⊗⑦V79.81   Bus occupant (driver) (passenger) injured in transport accidents with military vehicle

⊗⑦V79.88   Bus occupant (driver) (passenger) injured in other specified transport accidents

⊗⑦V79.9   Bus occupant (driver) (passenger) injured in unspecified traffic accident
Bus accident NOS

OTHER LAND TRANSPORT ACCIDENTS (V80-V89)

V80   Animal-rider or occupant of animal-drawn vehicle injured in transport accident

The appropriate 7th character is to be added to each code from category V80

A - initial encounter

D - subsequent encounter

S - sequela

V80.0   Animal-rider or occupant of animal drawn vehicle injured by fall from or being thrown from animal or animal-drawn vehicle in noncollision accident

⊗⑦V80.01   Animal-rider injured by fall from or being thrown from animal in noncollision accident

⑦V80.010   Animal-rider injured by fall from or being thrown from horse in noncollision accident

⑦V80.018   Animal-rider injured by fall from or being thrown from other animal in noncollision accident

⊗⑦V80.02   Occupant of animal-drawn vehicle injured by fall from or being thrown from animal-drawn vehicle in noncollision accident
Overturning animal-drawn vehicle NOS
Overturning animal-drawn vehicle without collision

V80.1   Animal-rider or occupant of animal-drawn vehicle injured in collision with pedestrian or animal

Excludes 1: animal-rider or animal-drawn vehicle collision with animal-drawn vehicle or animal being ridden (V80.7)

⊗⑦V80.11   Animal-rider injured in collision with pedestrian or animal

⊗⑦V80.12   Occupant of animal-drawn vehicle injured in collision with pedestrian or animal

V80.2   Animal-rider or occupant of animal-drawn vehicle injured in collision with pedal cycle

⊗⑦V80.21   Animal-rider injured in collision with pedal cycle

⊗⑦V80.22   Occupant of animal-drawn vehicle injured in collision with pedal cycle

V80.3   Animal-rider or occupant of animal-drawn vehicle injured in collision with two- or three-wheeled motor vehicle

⊗⑦V80.31   Animal-rider injured in collision with two- or three-wheeled motor vehicle

⊗⑦V80.32   Occupant of animal-drawn vehicle injured in collision with two- or three-wheeled motor vehicle

⊗⑦V80.4   Animal-rider or occupant of animal-drawn vehicle injured in collision with car, pick-up truck, van, heavy transport vehicle or bus

Excludes 1: animal-rider injured in collision with military vehicle (V80.910)
occupant of animal-drawn vehicle injured in collision with military vehicle (V80.920)

⊗⑦V80.41   Animal-rider injured in collision with car, pick-up truck, van, heavy transport vehicle or bus

⊗⑦V80.42   Occupant of animal-drawn vehicle injured in collision with car, pick-up truck, van, heavy transport vehicle or bus

V80.5   Animal-rider or occupant of animal-drawn vehicle injured in collision with other specified motor vehicle

⊗⑦V80.51   Animal-rider injured in collision with other specified motor vehicle

⊗⑦V80.52   Occupant of animal-drawn vehicle injured in collision with other specified motor vehicle

V80.6   Animal-rider or occupant of animal-drawn vehicle injured in collision with railway train or railway vehicle

⊗⑦V80.61   Animal-rider injured in collision with railway train or railway vehicle

⊗⑦V80.62   Occupant of animal-drawn vehicle injured in collision with railway train or railway vehicle

V80.7   Animal-rider or occupant of animal-drawn vehicle injured in collision with other nonmotor vehicles

V80.71   Animal-rider or occupant of animal-drawn vehicle injured in collision with animal being ridden

⑦V80.710   Animal-rider injured in collision with other animal being ridden

⑦V80.711   Occupant of animal-drawn vehicle injured in collision with animal being ridden

V80.72   Animal-rider or occupant of animal-drawn vehicle injured in collision with other animal-drawn vehicle

⑦V80.720   Animal-rider injured in collision with animal-drawn vehicle

⑦V80.721   Occupant of animal-drawn vehicle injured in collision with other animal-drawn vehicle

V80.73   Animal-rider or occupant of animal-drawn vehicle injured in collision with streetcar

⑦V80.730   Animal-rider injured in collision with streetcar

⑦V80.731   Occupant of animal-drawn vehicle injured in collision with streetcar

V80.79   Animal-rider or occupant of animal-drawn vehicle injured in collision with other nonmotor vehicles

⑦**V80.790** Animal-rider injured in collision with other nonmotor vehicles

⑦**V80.791** Occupant of animal-drawn vehicle injured in collision with other nonmotor vehicles

V80.8 Animal-rider or occupant of animal-drawn vehicle injured in collision with fixed or stationary object

⊗⑦**V80.81** Animal-rider injured in collision with fixed or stationary object

⊗⑦**V80.82** Occupant of animal-drawn vehicle injured in collision with fixed or stationary object

V80.9 Animal-rider or occupant of animal-drawn vehicle injured in other and unspecified transport accidents

V80.91 Animal-rider injured in other and unspecified transport accidents

⑦**V80.910** Animal-rider injured in transport accident with military vehicle

⑦**V80.918** Animal-rider injured in other transport accident

⑦**V80.919** Animal-rider injured in unspecified transport accident

Animal rider accident NOS

V80.92 Occupant of animal-drawn vehicle injured in other and unspecified transport accidents

⑦**V80.920** Occupant of animal-drawn vehicle injured in transport accident with military vehicle

⑦**V80.928** Occupant of animal-drawn vehicle injured in other transport accident

⑦**V80.929** Occupant of animal-drawn vehicle injured in unspecified transport accident

Animal-drawn vehicle accident NOS

V81 Occupant of railway train or railway vehicle injured in transport accident

Includes: derailment of railway train or railway vehicle

person on outside of train

Excludes 1: streetcar (V82.-)

The appropriate 7th character is to be added to each code from category V81

A - initial encounter

D - subsequent encounter

S - sequela

⊗⑦**V81.0** Occupant of railway train or railway vehicle injured in collision with motor vehicle in nontraffic accident

Excludes 1: Occupant of railway train or railway vehicle injured due to collision with military vehicle (V81.83)

⊗⑦**V81.1** Occupant of railway train or railway vehicle injured in collision with motor vehicle in traffic accident

Excludes 1: Occupant of railway train or railway vehicle injured due to collision with military vehicle (V81.83)

⊗⑦**V81.2** Occupant of railway train or railway vehicle injured in collision with or hit by rolling stock

⊗⑦**V81.3** Occupant of railway train or railway vehicle injured in collision with other object

Railway collision NOS

⊗⑦**V81.4** Person injured while boarding or alighting from railway train or railway vehicle

⊗⑦**V81.5** Occupant of railway train or railway vehicle injured by fall in railway train or railway vehicle

⊗⑦**V81.6** Occupant of railway train or railway vehicle injured by fall from railway train or railway vehicle

⊗⑦**V81.7** Occupant of railway train or railway vehicle injured in derailment without antecedent collision

V81.8 Occupant of railway train or railway vehicle injured in other specified railway accidents

⊗⑦**V81.81** Occupant of railway train or railway vehicle injured due to explosion or fire on train

⊗⑦**V81.82** Occupant of railway train or railway vehicle injured due to object falling onto train

Occupant of railway train or railway vehicle injured due to falling earth onto train

Occupant of railway train or railway vehicle injured due to falling rocks onto train

Occupant of railway train or railway vehicle injured due to falling snow onto train

Occupant of railway train or railway vehicle injured due to falling trees onto train

⊗⑦**V81.83** Occupant of railway train or railway vehicle injured due to collision with military vehicle

⊗⑦**V81.89** Occupant of railway train or railway vehicle injured due to other specified railway accident

⊗⑦**V81.9** Occupant of railway train or railway vehicle injured in unspecified railway accident

Railway accident NOS

V82 Occupant of powered streetcar injured in transport accident

Includes: interurban electric car

person on outside of streetcar

tram (car)

trolley (car)

Excludes 1: bus (V70-V79)

motorcoach (V70-V79)

nonpowered streetcar (V76.-)

train (V81.-)

The appropriate 7th character is to be added to each code from category V82

A - initial encounter

D - subsequent encounter

S - sequela

⊗⑦**V82.0** Occupant of streetcar injured in collision with motor vehicle in nontraffic accident

⊗⑦**V82.1** Occupant of streetcar injured in collision with motor vehicle in traffic accident

⊗⑦**V82.2** Occupant of streetcar injured in collision with or hit by rolling stock

⊗⑦**V82.3** Occupant of streetcar injured in collision with other object

Excludes 1: collision with animal-drawn vehicle or animal being ridden (V82.8)

⊗⑦**V82.4** Person injured while boarding or alighting from streetcar

⊗⑦**V82.5** Occupant of streetcar injured by fall in streetcar

Excludes 1: fall in streetcar:

while boarding or alighting (V82.4)

with antecedent collision (V82.0-V82.3)

⊗⑦**V82.6** Occupant of streetcar injured by fall from streetcar

Excludes 1: fall from streetcar:

while boarding or alighting (V82.4)

with antecedent collision (V82.0-V82.3)

⊗⑦**V82.7** Occupant of streetcar injured in derailment without antecedent collision

Excludes 1: occupant of streetcar injured in derailment with antecedent collision (V82.0-V82.3)

⊗⑦**V82.8** Occupant of streetcar injured in other specified transport accidents

Streetcar collision with military vehicle

Streetcar collision with train or nonmotor vehicles

⊗⑦**V82.9** Occupant of streetcar injured in unspecified traffic accident

Streetcar accident NOS

V83 Occupant of special vehicle mainly used on industrial premises injured in transport accident

Includes: battery-powered airport passenger vehicle

battery-powered truck (baggage) (mail)

coal-car in mine

forklift (truck)

logging car

self-propelled industrial truck

station baggage truck (powered)

tram, truck, or tub (powered) in mine or quarry

Excludes 1: special construction vehicles (V85.-)

special industrial vehicle in stationary use or maintenance (W31.-)

The appropriate 7th character is to be added to each code from category V83

A - initial encounter

D - subsequent encounter

S - sequela

⊗⑦**V83.0** Driver of special industrial vehicle injured in traffic accident

⊗⑦**V83.1** Passenger of special industrial vehicle injured in traffic accident

⊗⑦**V83.2** Person on outside of special industrial vehicle injured in traffic accident

⊗⑦**V83.3** Unspecified occupant of special industrial vehicle injured in traffic accident

⊗⑦**V83.4** Person injured while boarding or alighting from special industrial vehicle

⊗⑦**V83.5** Driver of special industrial vehicle injured in nontraffic accident

⊗⑦**V83.6** Passenger of special industrial vehicle injured in nontraffic accident

⊗⑦**V83.7** Person on outside of special industrial vehicle injured in nontraffic accident

⊗⑦**V83.9** Unspecified occupant of special industrial vehicle injured in nontraffic accident

Special-industrial-vehicle accident NOS

V84 Occupant of special vehicle mainly used in agriculture injured in transport accident

Includes: self-propelled farm machinery

tractor (and trailer)

Excludes 1: animal-powered farm machinery accident (W30.8-)

contact with combine harvester (W30.0)

special agricultural vehicle in stationary use or maintenance (W30.-)

The appropriate 7th character is to be added to each code from category V84

A - initial encounter

D - subsequent encounter

S - sequela

⊗⑦**V84.0** Driver of special agricultural vehicle injured in traffic accident

⊗⑦**V84.1** Passenger of special agricultural vehicle injured in traffic accident

⊗⑦**V84.2** Person on outside of special agricultural vehicle injured in traffic accident

⊗⑦**V84.3** Unspecified occupant of special agricultural vehicle injured in traffic accident

⊗⑦**V84.4** Person injured while boarding or alighting from special agricultural vehicle

⊗⑦**V84.5** Driver of special agricultural vehicle injured in nontraffic accident

⊗⑦**V84.6** Passenger of special agricultural vehicle injured in nontraffic accident

⊗⑦**V84.7** Person on outside of special agricultural vehicle injured in nontraffic accident

⊗⑦**V84.9** Unspecified occupant of special agricultural vehicle injured in nontraffic accident

Special-agricultural vehicle accident NOS

V85 Occupant of special construction vehicle injured in transport accident

Includes: bulldozer

digger

dump truck

earth-leveller

mechanical shovel

road-roller

Excludes 1: special industrial vehicle (V83.-)

special construction vehicle in stationary use or maintenance (W31.-)

The appropriate 7th character is to be added to each code from category V85

A - initial encounter

D - subsequent encounter

S - sequela

⊗⑦**V85.0** Driver of special construction vehicle injured in traffic accident

⊗⑦**V85.1** Passenger of special construction vehicle injured in traffic accident

⊗⑦**V85.2** Person on outside of special construction vehicle injured in traffic accident

⊗⑦**V85.3** Unspecified occupant of special construction vehicle injured in traffic accident

⊗⑦**V85.4** Person injured while boarding or alighting from special construction vehicle

⊗⑦**V85.5** Driver of special construction vehicle injured in nontraffic accident

⊗⑦**V85.6** Passenger of special construction vehicle injured in nontraffic accident

⊗⑦**V85.7** Person on outside of special construction vehicle injured in nontraffic accident

⊗⑦**V85.9** Unspecified occupant of special construction vehicle injured in nontraffic accident

Special-construction-vehicle accident NOS

V86 Occupant of special all-terrain or other off-road motor vehicle, injured in transport accident

Excludes 1: special all-terrain vehicle in stationary use or maintenance (W31.-)

sport-utility vehicle (V50-V59)

three-wheeled motor vehicle designed for on-road use (V30-V39)

The appropriate 7th character is to be added to each code from category V86

A - initial encounter

D - subsequent encounter

S - sequela

V86.0   Driver of special all-terrain or other off-road motor vehicle injured in traffic accident

⊗⑦**V86.01**   Driver of ambulance or fire engine injured in traffic accident

⊗⑦**V86.02**   Driver of snowmobile injured in traffic accident

⊗⑦**V86.03**   Driver of dune buggy injured in traffic accident

⊗⑦**V86.04**   Driver of military vehicle injured in traffic accident

⊗⑦**V86.09**   Driver of other special all-terrain or other off-road motor vehicle injured in traffic accident

Driver of dirt bike injured in traffic accident

Driver of go cart injured in traffic accident

Driver of golf cart injured in traffic accident

V86.1   Passenger of special all-terrain or other off-road motor vehicle injured in traffic accident

⊗⑦**V86.11**   Passenger of ambulance or fire engine injured in traffic accident

⊗⑦**V86.12**   Passenger of snowmobile injured in traffic accident

⊗⑦**V86.13**   Passenger of dune buggy injured in traffic accident

⊗⑦**V86.14**   Passenger of military vehicle injured in traffic accident

⊗⑦**V86.19**   Passenger of other special all-terrain or other off-road motor vehicle injured in traffic accident

Passenger of dirt bike injured in traffic accident

Passenger of go cart injured in traffic accident

Passenger of golf cart injured in traffic accident

V86.2   Person on outside of special all-terrain or other off-road motor vehicle injured in traffic accident

⊗⑦**V86.21**   Person on outside of ambulance or fire engine injured in traffic accident

⊗⑦**V86.22**   Person on outside of snowmobile injured in traffic accident

⊗⑦**V86.23**   Person on outside of dune buggy injured in traffic accident

⊗⑦**V86.24**   Person on outside of military vehicle injured in traffic accident

⊗⑦**V86.29**   Person on outside of other special all-terrain or other off-road motor vehicle injured in traffic accident

Person on outside of dirt bike injured in traffic accident

Person on outside of go cart in traffic accident

Person on outside of golf cart injured in traffic accident

V86.3   Unspecified occupant of special all-terrain or other off-road motor vehicle injured in traffic accident

⊗⑦**V86.31**   Unspecified occupant of ambulance or fire engine injured in traffic accident

⊗⑦**V86.32**   Unspecified occupant of snowmobile injured in traffic accident

⊗⑦**V86.33**   Unspecified occupant of dune buggy injured in traffic accident

⊗⑦**V86.34**   Unspecified occupant of military vehicle injured in traffic accident

⊗⑦**V86.39**   Unspecified occupant of other special all-terrain or other off-road motor vehicle injured in traffic accident

Unspecified occupant of dirt bike injured in traffic accident

Unspecified occupant of go cart injured in traffic accident

Unspecified occupant of golf cart injured in traffic accident

V86.4   Person injured while boarding or alighting from special all-terrain or other off-road motor vehicle

⊗⑦**V86.41**   Person injured while boarding or alighting from ambulance or fire engine

⊗⑦**V86.42**   Person injured while boarding or alighting from snowmobile

⊗⑦**V86.43**   Person injured while boarding or alighting from dune buggy

⊗⑦**V86.44**   Person injured while boarding or alighting from military vehicle

⊗⑦**V86.49**   Person injured while boarding or alighting from other special all-terrain or other off-road motor vehicle

Person injured while boarding or alighting from dirt bike

Person injured while boarding or alighting from go cart

Person injured while boarding or alighting from golf cart

V86.5   Driver of special all-terrain or other off-road motor vehicle injured in nontraffic accident

⊗⑦**V86.51**   Driver of ambulance or fire engine injured in nontraffic accident

⊗⑦**V86.52**   Driver of snowmobile injured in nontraffic accident

⊗⑦**V86.53**   Driver of dune buggy injured in nontraffic accident

⊗⑦**V86.54**   Driver of military vehicle injured in nontraffic accident

⊗⑦**V86.59**   Driver of other special all-terrain or other off-road motor vehicle injured in nontraffic accident

Driver of dirt bike injured in nontraffic accident

Driver of go cart injured in nontraffic accident

Driver of golf cart injured in nontraffic accident

V86.6   Passenger of special all-terrain or other off-road motor vehicle injured in nontraffic accident

⊗⑦**V86.61**   Passenger of ambulance or fire engine injured in nontraffic accident

⊗⑦**V86.62**   Passenger of snowmobile injured in nontraffic accident

⊗⑦**V86.63**   Passenger of dune buggy injured in nontraffic accident

⊗⑦**V86.64**   Passenger of military vehicle injured in nontraffic accident

● New code   ▲ Revised code   ⑦ 7ᵗʰ digit required   ⊗ Placeholder required

⊗⑦**V86.69** Passenger of other special all-terrain or other off-road motor vehicle injured in nontraffic accident

Passenger of dirt bike injured in nontraffic accident

Passenger of go cart injured in nontraffic accident

Passenger of golf cart injured in nontraffic accident

V86.7 Person on outside of special all-terrain or other off-road motor vehicle injured in nontraffic accident

⊗⑦**V86.71** Person on outside of ambulance or fire engine injured in nontraffic accident

⊗⑦**V86.72** Person on outside of snowmobile injured in nontraffic accident

⊗⑦**V86.73** Person on outside of dune buggy injured in nontraffic accident

⊗⑦**V86.74** Person on outside of military vehicle injured in nontraffic accident

⊗⑦**V86.79** Person on outside of other special all-terrain or other off-road motor vehicles injured in nontraffic accident

Person on outside of dirt bike injured in nontraffic accident

Person on outside of go cart injured in nontraffic accident

Person on outside of golf cart injured in nontraffic accident

V86.9 Unspecified occupant of special all-terrain or other off-road motor vehicle injured in nontraffic accident

⊗⑦**V86.91** Unspecified occupant of ambulance or fire engine injured in nontraffic accident

⊗⑦**V86.92** Unspecified occupant of snowmobile injured in nontraffic accident

⊗⑦**V86.93** Unspecified occupant of dune buggy injured in nontraffic accident

⊗⑦**V86.94** Unspecified occupant of military vehicle injured in nontraffic accident

⊗⑦**V86.99** Unspecified occupant of other special all-terrain or other off-road motor vehicle injured in nontraffic accident

All-terrain motor-vehicle accident NOS

Off-road motor-vehicle accident NOS

Other motor-vehicle accident NOS

Unspecified occupant of dirt bike injured in nontraffic accident

Unspecified occupant of go cart injured in nontraffic accident

Unspecified occupant of golf cart injured in nontraffic accident

V87 Traffic accident of specified type but victim's mode of transport unknown

Excludes 1: collision involving:

pedal cycle (V10-V19)

pedestrian (V01-V09)

The appropriate 7th character is to be added to each code from category V87

A - initial encounter

D - subsequent encounter

S - sequela

⊗⑦**V87.0** Person injured in collision between car and two- or three-wheeled powered vehicle (traffic)

⊗⑦**V87.1** Person injured in collision between other motor vehicle and two- or three-wheeled motor vehicle (traffic)

⊗⑦**V87.2** Person injured in collision between car and pick-up truck or van (traffic)

⊗⑦**V87.3** Person injured in collision between car and bus (traffic)

⊗⑦**V87.4** Person injured in collision between car and heavy transport vehicle (traffic)

⊗⑦**V87.5** Person injured in collision between heavy transport vehicle and bus (traffic)

⊗⑦**V87.6** Person injured in collision between railway train or railway vehicle and car (traffic)

⊗⑦**V87.7** Person injured in collision between other specified motor vehicles (traffic)

⊗⑦**V87.8** Person injured in other specified noncollision transport accidents involving motor vehicle (traffic)

⊗⑦**V87.9** Person injured in other specified (collision)(noncollision) transport accidents involving nonmotor vehicle (traffic)

V88 Nontraffic accident of specified type but victim's mode of transport unknown

Excludes 1: collision involving:

pedal cycle (V10-V19)

pedestrian (V01-V09)

The appropriate 7th character is to be added to each code from category V88

A - initial encounter

D - subsequent encounter

S - sequela

⊗⑦**V88.0** Person injured in collision between car and two- or three-wheeled motor vehicle, nontraffic

⊗⑦**V88.1** Person injured in collision between other motor vehicle and two- or three-wheeled motor vehicle, nontraffic

⊗⑦**V88.2** Person injured in collision between car and pick-up truck or van, nontraffic

⊗⑦**V88.3** Person injured in collision between car and bus, nontraffic

⊗⑦**V88.4** Person injured in collision between car and heavy transport vehicle, nontraffic

⊗⑦**V88.5** Person injured in collision between heavy transport vehicle and bus, nontraffic

⊗⑦**V88.6** Person injured in collision between railway train or railway vehicle and car, nontraffic

⊗⑦**V88.7** Person injured in collision between other specified motor vehicle, nontraffic

⊗⑦**V88.8** Person injured in other specified noncollision transport accidents involving motor vehicle, nontraffic

⊗⑦**V88.9** Person injured in other specified (collision)(noncollision) transport accidents involving nonmotor vehicle, nontraffic

V89 Motor- or nonmotor-vehicle accident, type of vehicle unspecified

The appropriate 7th character is to be added to each code from category V89

A - initial encounter

D - subsequent encounter

S - sequela

⊗⑦**V89.0** Person injured in unspecified motor-vehicle accident, nontraffic

Motor-vehicle accident NOS, nontraffic

⊗⑦**V89.1** Person injured in unspecified nonmotor-vehicle accident, nontraffic

Nonmotor-vehicle accident NOS (nontraffic)

⊗⑦**V89.2** Person injured in unspecified motor-vehicle accident, traffic

Motor-vehicle accident [MVA] NOS

Road (traffic) accident [RTA] NOS

⊗⑦**V89.3** Person injured in unspecified nonmotor-vehicle accident, traffic

Nonmotor-vehicle traffic accident NOS

⊗⑦**V89.9** Person injured in unspecified vehicle accident

Collision NOS

WATER TRANSPORT ACCIDENTS (V90-V94)

V94 Drowning and submersion due to accident to watercraft

Excludes 1: civilian water transport accident involving military watercraft (V94.81-)

fall into water not from watercraft (W16.-)

military watercraft accident in military or war operations (Y36.0-, Y37.0-)

water-transport-related drowning or submersion without accident to watercraft (V92.-)

The appropriate 7th character is to be added to each code from category V90

A - initial encounter

D - subsequent encounter

S - sequela

V90.0 Drowning and submersion due to watercraft overturning

⊗⑦**V90.00** Drowning and submersion due to merchant ship overturning

⊗⑦**V90.01** Drowning and submersion due to passenger ship overturning

Drowning and submersion due to Ferry-boat overturning

Drowning and submersion due to Liner overturning

⊗⑦**V90.02** Drowning and submersion due to fishing boat overturning

⊗⑦**V90.03** Drowning and submersion due to other powered watercraft overturning

Drowning and submersion due to Hovercraft (on open water) overturning

Drowning and submersion due to Jet ski overturning

⊗⑦**V90.04** Drowning and submersion due to sailboat overturning

⊗⑦**V90.05** Drowning and submersion due to canoe or kayak overturning

⊗⑦**V90.06** Drowning and submersion due to (nonpowered) inflatable craft overturning

⊗⑦**V90.08** Drowning and submersion due to other unpowered watercraft overturning

Drowning and submersion due to windsurfer overturning

⊗⑦**V90.09** Drowning and submersion due to unspecified watercraft overturning

Drowning and submersion due to boat NOS overturning

Drowning and submersion due to ship NOS overturning

Drowning and submersion due to watercraft NOS overturning

V90.1 Drowning and submersion due to watercraft sinking

⊗⑦**V90.10** Drowning and submersion due to merchant ship sinking

⊗⑦**V90.11** Drowning and submersion due to passenger ship sinking

Drowning and submersion due to Ferry-boat sinking

Drowning and submersion due to Liner sinking

⊗⑦**V90.12** Drowning and submersion due to fishing boat sinking

⊗⑦**V90.13** Drowning and submersion due to other powered watercraft sinking

Drowning and submersion due to Hovercraft (on open water) sinking

Drowning and submersion due to Jet ski sinking

⊗⑦**V90.14** Drowning and submersion due to sailboat sinking

⊗⑦**V90.15** Drowning and submersion due to canoe or kayak sinking

⊗⑦**V90.16** Drowning and submersion due to (nonpowered) inflatable craft sinking

⊗⑦**V90.18** Drowning and submersion due to other unpowered watercraft sinking

⊗⑦**V90.19** Drowning and submersion due to unspecified watercraft sinking

Drowning and submersion due to boat NOS sinking

Drowning and submersion due to ship NOS sinking

Drowning and submersion due to watercraft NOS sinking

V90.2 Drowning and submersion due to falling or jumping from burning watercraft

⊗⑦**V90.20** Drowning and submersion due to falling or jumping from burning merchant ship

⊗⑦**V90.21** Drowning and submersion due to falling or jumping from burning passenger ship

Drowning and submersion due to falling or jumping from burning Ferry-boat

Drowning and submersion due to falling or jumping from burning Liner

⊗⑦**V90.22** Drowning and submersion due to falling or jumping from burning fishing boat

⊗⑦**V90.23** Drowning and submersion due to falling or jumping from other burning powered watercraft

Drowning and submersion due to falling and jumping from burning Hovercraft (on open water)

Drowning and submersion due to falling and jumping from burning Jet ski

⊗⑦**V90.24** Drowning and submersion due to falling or jumping from burning sailboat

⊗⑦**V90.25** Drowning and submersion due to falling or jumping from burning canoe or kayak

⊗⑦**V90.26** Drowning and submersion due to falling or jumping from burning (nonpowered) inflatable craft

⊗⑦**V90.27** Drowning and submersion due to falling or jumping from burning water-skis

● New code ▲ Revised code ⑦ 7th digit required ⊗ Placeholder required

⊗⑦**V90.28** Drowning and submersion due to falling or jumping from other burning unpowered watercraft

Drowning and submersion due to falling and jumping from burning surf-board

Drowning and submersion due to falling and jumping from burning windsurfer

⊗⑦**V90.29** Drowning and submersion due to falling or jumping from unspecified burning watercraft

Drowning and submersion due to falling or jumping from burning boat NOS

Drowning and submersion due to falling or jumping from burning ship NOS

Drowning and submersion due to falling or jumping from burning watercraft NOS

V90.3 Drowning and submersion due to falling or jumping from crushed watercraft

⊗⑦**V90.30** Drowning and submersion due to falling or jumping from crushed merchant ship

⊗⑦**V90.31** Drowning and submersion due to falling or jumping from crushed passenger ship

Drowning and submersion due to falling and jumping from crushed Ferry boat

Drowning and submersion due to falling and jumping from crushed Liner

⊗⑦**V90.32** Drowning and submersion due to falling or jumping from crushed fishing boat

⊗⑦**V90.33** Drowning and submersion due to falling or jumping from other crushed powered watercraft

Drowning and submersion due to falling and jumping from crushed Hovercraft

Drowning and submersion due to falling and jumping from crushed Jet ski

⊗⑦**V90.34** Drowning and submersion due to falling or jumping from crushed sailboat

⊗⑦**V90.35** Drowning and submersion due to falling or jumping from crushed canoe or kayak

⊗⑦**V90.36** Drowning and submersion due to falling or jumping from crushed (nonpowered) inflatable craft

⊗⑦**V90.37** Drowning and submersion due to falling or jumping from crushed water-skis

⊗⑦**V90.38** Drowning and submersion due to falling or jumping from other crushed unpowered watercraft

Drowning and submersion due to falling and jumping from crushed surf-board

Drowning and submersion due to falling and jumping from crushed windsurfer

⊗⑦**V90.39** Drowning and submersion due to falling or jumping from crushed unspecified watercraft

Drowning and submersion due to falling and jumping from crushed boat NOS

Drowning and submersion due to falling and jumping from crushed ship NOS

Drowning and submersion due to falling and jumping from crushed watercraft NOS

V90.8 Drowning and submersion due to other accident to watercraft

⊗⑦**V90.80** Drowning and submersion due to other accident to merchant ship

⊗⑦**V90.81** Drowning and submersion due to other accident to passenger ship

Drowning and submersion due to other accident to Ferry-boat

Drowning and submersion due to other accident to Liner

⊗⑦**V90.82** Drowning and submersion due to other accident to fishing boat

⊗⑦**V90.83** Drowning and submersion due to other accident to other powered watercraft

Drowning and submersion due to other accident to Hovercraft (on open water)

Drowning and submersion due to other accident to Jet ski

⊗⑦**V90.84** Drowning and submersion due to other accident to sailboat

⊗⑦**V90.85** Drowning and submersion due to other accident to canoe or kayak

⊗⑦**V90.86** Drowning and submersion due to other accident to (nonpowered) inflatable craft

⊗⑦**V90.87** Drowning and submersion due to other accident to water-skis

⊗⑦**V90.88** Drowning and submersion due to other accident to other unpowered watercraft

Drowning and submersion due to other accident to surf-board

Drowning and submersion due to other accident to windsurfer

⊗⑦**V90.89** Drowning and submersion due to other accident to unspecified watercraft

Drowning and submersion due to other accident to boat NOS

Drowning and submersion due to other accident to ship NOS

Drowning and submersion due to other accident to watercraft NOS

V91 Other injury due to accident to watercraft

Includes: any injury except drowning and submersion as a result of an accident to watercraft

Excludes 1: civilian water transport accident involving military watercraft (V94.81-)

military watercraft accident in military or war operations (Y36, Y37-)

Excludes 2: drowning and submersion due to accident to watercraft (V90.-)

The appropriate 7th character is to be added to each code from category V91

A - initial encounter

D - subsequent encounter

S - sequela

V91.0 Burn due to watercraft on fire

Excludes 1: burn from localized fire or explosion on board ship without accident to watercraft (V93.-)

⊗⑦**V91.00** Burn due to merchant ship on fire

⊗⑦**V91.01** Burn due to passenger ship on fire

Burn due to Ferry-boat on fire

Burn due to Liner on fire

⊗⑦**V91.02** Burn due to fishing boat on fire

⊗⑦**V91.03** Burn due to other powered watercraft on fire

Burn due to Hovercraft (on open water) on fire

Burn due to Jet ski on fire

⊗⑦**V91.04** Burn due to sailboat on fire

⊗⑦**V91.05** Burn due to canoe or kayak on fire

⊗⑦**V91.06** Burn due to (nonpowered) inflatable craft on fire

⊗⑦**V91.07** Burn due to water-skis on fire

⊗⑦**V91.08** Burn due to other unpowered watercraft on fire

⊗⑦**V91.09** Burn due to unspecified watercraft on fire

Burn due to boat NOS on fire

Burn due to ship NOS on fire

Burn due to watercraft NOS on fire

V91.1 Crushed between watercraft and other watercraft or other object due to collision

Crushed by lifeboat after abandoning ship in a collision

Note: select the specified type of watercraft that the victim was on at the time of the collision

⊗⑦**V91.10** Crushed between merchant ship and other watercraft or other object due to collision

⊗⑦**V91.11** Crushed between passenger ship and other watercraft or other object due to collision

Crushed between Ferry-boat and other watercraft or other object due to collision

Crushed between Liner and other watercraft or other object due to collision

⊗⑦**V91.12** Crushed between fishing boat and other watercraft or other object due to collision

⊗⑦**V91.13** Crushed between other powered watercraft and other watercraft or other object due to collision

Crushed between Hovercraft (on open water) and other watercraft or other object due to collision

Crushed between Jet ski and other watercraft or other object due to collision

⊗⑦**V91.14** Crushed between sailboat and other watercraft or other object due to collision

⊗⑦**V91.15** Crushed between canoe or kayak and other watercraft or other object due to collision

⊗⑦**V91.16** Crushed between (nonpowered) inflatable craft and other watercraft or other object due to collision

⊗⑦**V91.18** Crushed between other unpowered watercraft and other watercraft or other object due to collision

Crushed between surfboard and other watercraft or other object due to collision

Crushed between windsurfer and other watercraft or other object due to collision

⊗⑦**V91.19** Crushed between unspecified watercraft and other watercraft or other object due to collision

Crushed between boat NOS and other watercraft or other object due to collision

Crushed between ship NOS and other watercraft or other object due to collision

Crushed between watercraft NOS and other watercraft or other object due to collision

V91.2 Fall due to collision between watercraft and other watercraft or other object

Fall while remaining on watercraft after collision

Note: select the specified type of watercraft that the victim was on at the time of the collision

Excludes 1: crushed between watercraft and other watercraft and other object due to collision (V91.1-)

drowning and submersion due to falling from crushed watercraft (V90.3-)

⊗⑦**V91.20** Fall due to collision between merchant ship and other watercraft or other object

⊗⑦**V91.21** Fall due to collision between passenger ship and other watercraft or other object

Fall due to collision between Ferry-boat and other watercraft or other object

Fall due to collision between Liner and other watercraft or other object

⊗⑦**V91.22** Fall due to collision between fishing boat and other watercraft or other object

⊗⑦**V91.23** Fall due to collision between other powered watercraft and other watercraft or other object

Fall due to collision between Hovercraft (on open water) and other watercraft or other object

Fall due to collision between Jet ski and other watercraft or other object

⊗⑦**V91.24** Fall due to collision between sailboat and other watercraft or other object

⊗⑦**V91.25** Fall due to collision between canoe or kayak and other watercraft or other object

⊗⑦**V91.26** Fall due to collision between (nonpowered) inflatable craft and other watercraft or other object

⊗⑦**V91.29** Fall due to collision between unspecified watercraft and other watercraft or other object

Fall due to collision between boat NOS and other watercraft or other object

Fall due to collision between ship NOS and other watercraft or other object

Fall due to collision between watercraft NOS and other watercraft or other object

V91.3 Hit or struck by falling object due to accident to watercraft

Hit or struck by falling object (part of damaged watercraft or other object) after falling or jumping from damaged watercraft

Excludes 2: drowning or submersion due to fall or jumping from damaged watercraft (V90.2-, V90.3-)

⊗⑦**V91.30** Hit or struck by falling object due to accident to merchant ship

⊗⑦**V91.31** Hit or struck by falling object due to accident to passenger ship

Hit or struck by falling object due to accident to Ferry-boat

Hit or struck by falling object due to accident to Liner

⊗⑦**V91.32** Hit or struck by falling object due to accident to fishing boat

⊗⑦**V91.33** Hit or struck by falling object due to accident to other powered watercraft

Hit or struck by falling object due to accident to Hovercraft (on open water)

Hit or struck by falling object due to accident to Jet ski

⊗⑦**V91.34** Hit or struck by falling object due to accident to sailboat

⊗⑦**V91.35** Hit or struck by falling object due to accident to canoe or kayak

⊗⑦**V91.36** Hit or struck by falling object due to accident to (nonpowered) inflatable craft

⊗⑦**V91.37** Hit or struck by falling object due to accident to water-skis

Hit by water-skis after jumping off of waterskis

⊗⑦**V91.38** Hit or struck by falling object due to accident to other unpowered watercraft

Hit or struck by surf-board after falling off damaged surf-board

Hit or struck by object after falling off damaged windsurfer

⊗⑦**V91.39** Hit or struck by falling object due to accident to unspecified watercraft

Hit or struck by falling object due to accident to boat NOS

Hit or struck by falling object due to accident to ship NOS

Hit or struck by falling object due to accident to watercraft NOS

V91.8 Other injury due to other accident to watercraft

⊗⑦**V91.80** Other injury due to other accident to merchant ship

⊗⑦**V91.81** Other injury due to other accident to passenger ship

Other injury due to other accident to Ferry-boat

Other injury due to other accident to Liner

⊗⑦**V91.82** Other injury due to other accident to fishing boat

⊗⑦**V91.83** Other injury due to other accident to other powered watercraft

Other injury due to other accident to Hovercraft (on open water)

Other injury due to other accident to Jet ski

⊗⑦**V91.84** Other injury due to other accident to sailboat

⊗⑦**V91.85** Other injury due to other accident to canoe or kayak

⊗⑦**V91.86** Other injury due to other accident to (nonpowered) inflatable craft

⊗⑦**V91.87** Other injury due to other accident to water-skis

⊗⑦**V91.88** Other injury due to other accident to other unpowered watercraft

Other injury due to other accident to surf-board

Other injury due to other accident to windsurfer

⊗⑦**V91.89** Other injury due to other accident to unspecified watercraft

Other injury due to other accident to boat NOS

Other injury due to other accident to ship NOS

Other injury due to other accident to watercraft NOS

V92 Drowning and submersion due to accident on board watercraft, without accident to watercraft

Excludes 1: civilian water transport accident involving military watercraft (V94.81-)

drowning or submersion due to accident to watercraft (V90-V91)

drowning or submersion of diver who voluntarily jumps from boat not involved in an accident (W16.711, W16.721)

fall into water without watercraft (W16.-)

military watercraft accident in military or war operations (Y36, Y37)

The appropriate 7th character is to be added to each code from category V92

A - initial encounter

D - subsequent encounter

S - sequela

V92.0 Drowning and submersion due to fall off watercraft

Drowning and submersion due to fall from gangplank of watercraft

Drowning and submersion due to fall overboard watercraft

Excludes 2: hitting head on object or bottom of body of water due to fall from watercraft (V94.0-)

⊗⑦**V92.00** Drowning and submersion due to fall off merchant ship

⊗⑦**V92.01** Drowning and submersion due to fall off passenger ship

Drowning and submersion due to fall off Ferry-boat

Drowning and submersion due to fall off Liner

⊗⑦**V92.02** Drowning and submersion due to fall off fishing boat

⊗⑦**V92.03** Drowning and submersion due to fall off other powered watercraft

Drowning and submersion due to fall off Hovercraft (on open water)

Drowning and submersion due to fall off Jet ski

⊗⑦**V92.04** Drowning and submersion due to fall off sailboat

⊗⑦**V92.05** Drowning and submersion due to fall off canoe or kayak

⊗⑦**V92.06** Drowning and submersion due to fall off (nonpowered) inflatable craft

⊗⑦**V92.07** Drowning and submersion due to fall off water-skis

Excludes 1: drowning and submersion due to falling off burning water-skis (V90.27)

drowning and submersion due to falling off crushed water-skis (V90.37)

hit by boat while water-skiing NOS (V94.x)

⊗⑦**V92.08** Drowning and submersion due to fall off other unpowered watercraft

Drowning and submersion due to fall off surf-board

Drowning and submersion due to fall off windsurfer

Excludes 1: drowning and submersion due to fall off burning unpowered watercraft (V90.28)

drowning and submersion due to fall off crushed unpowered watercraft (V90.38)

drowning and submersion due to fall off damaged unpowered watercraft (V90.88)

drowning and submersion due to rider of nonpowered watercraft being hit by other watercraft (V94...)

Add 4th-7th digits	3 digit reportable	Nonspecific code	Unspecified code	Manifestation code

873

other injury due to rider of
nonpowered watercraft being hit by
other watercraft (V94...)

⊗⑦**V92.09** Drowning and submersion due to fall off
unspecified watercraft

Drowning and submersion due to fall off boat
NOS

Drowning and submersion due to fall off ship

Drowning and submersion due to fall off
watercraft NOS

V92.1 Drowning and submersion due to being thrown overboard
by motion of watercraft

Excludes 1: drowning and submersion due to fall off
surf-board (V92.08)

drowning and submersion due to fall off
water-skis (V92.07)

drowning and submersion due to fall off
windsurfer (V92.08)

⊗⑦**V92.10** Drowning and submersion due to being thrown
overboard by motion of merchant ship

⊗⑦**V92.11** Drowning and submersion due to being thrown
overboard by motion of passenger ship

Drowning and submersion due to being thrown
overboard by motion of Ferry-boat

Drowning and submersion due to being thrown
overboard by motion of Liner

⊗⑦**V92.12** Drowning and submersion due to being thrown
overboard by motion of fishing boat

⊗⑦**V92.13** Drowning and submersion due to being thrown
overboard by motion of other powered watercraft

Drowning and submersion due to being thrown
overboard by motion of Hovercraft

⊗⑦**V92.14** Drowning and submersion due to being thrown
overboard by motion of sailboat

⊗⑦**V92.15** Drowning and submersion due to being thrown
overboard by motion of canoe or kayak

⊗⑦**V92.16** Drowning and submersion due to being thrown
overboard by motion of (nonpowered) inflatable
craft

⊗⑦**V92.19** Drowning and submersion due to being thrown
overboard by motion of unspecified watercraft

Drowning and submersion due to being thrown
overboard by motion of boat NOS

Drowning and submersion due to being thrown
overboard by motion of ship NOS

Drowning and submersion due to being thrown
overboard by motion of watercraft NOS

V92.2 Drowning and submersion due to being washed overboard
from watercraft

Code first any associated cataclysm (X37.0-)

⊗⑦**V92.20** Drowning and submersion due to being washed
overboard from merchant ship

⊗⑦**V92.21** Drowning and submersion due to being washed
overboard from passenger ship

Drowning and submersion due to being washed
overboard from Ferry-boat

Drowning and submersion due to being washed
overboard from Liner

⊗⑦**V92.22** Drowning and submersion due to being washed
overboard from fishing boat

⊗⑦**V92.23** Drowning and submersion due to being washed
overboard from other powered watercraft

Drowning and submersion due to being washed
overboard from Hovercraft (on open water)

Drowning and submersion due to being washed
overboard from Jet ski

⊗⑦**V92.24** Drowning and submersion due to being washed
overboard from sailboat

⊗⑦**V92.25** Drowning and submersion due to being washed
overboard from canoe or kayak

⊗⑦**V92.26** Drowning and submersion due to being washed
overboard from (nonpowered) inflatable craft

⊗⑦**V92.27** Drowning and submersion due to being washed
overboard from water-skis

Excludes 1: drowning and submersion due to fall
off water-skis (V92.07)

⊗⑦**V92.28** Drowning and submersion due to being washed
overboard from other unpowered watercraft

Drowning and submersion due to being washed
overboard from surf-board

Drowning and submersion due to being washed
overboard from windsurfer

⊗⑦**V92.29** Drowning and submersion due to being washed
overboard from unspecified watercraft

Drowning and submersion due to being washed
overboard from boat NOS

Drowning and submersion due to being washed
overboard from ship NOS

Drowning and submersion due to being washed
overboard from watercraft NOS

V93 Other injury due to accident on board watercraft, without accident
to watercraft

Excludes 1: civilian water transport accident involving military
watercraft (V94.81-)

other injury due to accident to watercraft (V91.-)

military watercraft accident in military or war operations (
Y36, Y37-)

Excludes 2: drowning and submersion due to accident on board
watercraft, without accident to watercraft (V92.-)

The appropriate 7th character is to be added to each code from
category V93

A - initial encounter

D - subsequent encounter

S - sequela

V93.0 Burn due to localized fire on board watercraft

Excludes 1: burn due to watercraft on fire (V91.0-)

⊗⑦**V93.00** Burn due to localized fire on board merchant
vessel

⊗⑦**V93.01** Burn due to localized fire on board passenger
vessel

Burn due to localized fire on board Ferry-boat

Burn due to localized fire on board Liner

⊗⑦**V93.02** Burn due to localized fire on board fishing boat

⊗⑦**V93.03** Burn due to localized fire on board other
powered watercraft

Burn due to localized fire on board Hovercraft

Burn due to localized fire on board Jet ski

⊗⑦**V93.04** Burn due to localized fire on board sailboat

⊗⑦**V93.09** Burn due to localized fire on board unspecified
watercraft

● New code   ▲ Revised code   ⑦ 7th digit required   ⊗ Placeholder required

Burn due to localized fire on board boat NOS

Burn due to localized fire on board ship NOS

Burn due to localized fire on board watercraft NOS

V93.1 Other burn on board watercraft

Burn due to source other than fire on board watercraft

Excludes 1: burn due to watercraft on fire (V91.0-)

⊗⑦ **V93.10** Other burn on board merchant vessel

⊗⑦ **V93.11** Other burn on board passenger vessel

Other burn on board Ferry-boat

Other burn on board Liner

⊗⑦ **V93.12** Other burn on board fishing boat

⊗⑦ **V93.13** Other burn on board other powered watercraft

Other burn on board Hovercraft

Other burn on board Jet ski

⊗⑦ **V93.14** Other burn on board sailboat

⊗⑦ **V93.19** Other burn on board unspecified watercraft

Other burn on board boat NOS

Other burn on board ship NOS

Other burn on board watercraft NOS

V93.2 Heat exposure on board watercraft

Excludes 1: exposure to man-made heat not aboard watercraft (W92)

exposure to natural heat while on board watercraft (X30)

exposure to sunlight while on board watercraft (X32)

Excludes 2: burn due to fire on board watercraft (V93.0-)

⊗⑦ **V93.20** Heat exposure on board merchant ship

⊗⑦ **V93.21** Heat exposure on board passenger ship

Heat exposure on board Ferry-boat

Heat exposure on board Liner

⊗⑦ **V93.22** Heat exposure on board fishing boat

⊗⑦ **V93.23** Heat exposure on board other powered watercraft

Heat exposure on board hovercraft

⊗⑦ **V93.24** Heat exposure on board sailboat

⊗⑦ **V93.29** Heat exposure on board unspecified watercraft

Heat exposure on board boat NOS

Heat exposure on board ship NOS

Heat exposure on board watercraft NOS

V93.3 Fall on board watercraft

Excludes 1: fall due to collision of watercraft (V91.2-)

⊗⑦ **V93.30** Fall on board merchant ship

⊗⑦ **V93.31** Fall on board passenger ship

Fall on board Ferry-boat

Fall on board Liner

⊗⑦ **V93.32** Fall on board fishing boat

⊗⑦ **V93.33** Fall on board other powered watercraft

Fall on board Hovercraft (on open water)

Fall on board Jet ski

⊗⑦ **V93.34** Fall on board sailboat

⊗⑦ **V93.35** Fall on board canoe or kayak

⊗⑦ **V93.36** Fall on board (nonpowered) inflatable craft

⊗⑦ **V93.38** Fall on board other unpowered watercraft

⊗⑦ **V93.39** Fall on board unspecified watercraft

Fall on board boat NOS

Fall on board ship NOS

Fall on board watercraft NOS

V93.4 Struck by falling object on board watercraft

Hit by falling object on board watercraft

Excludes 1: struck by falling object due to accident to watercraft (V91.3)

⊗⑦ **V93.40** Struck by falling object on merchant ship

⊗⑦ **V93.41** Struck by falling object on passenger ship

Struck by falling object on Ferry-boat

Struck by falling object on Liner

⊗⑦ **V93.42** Struck by falling object on fishing boat

⊗⑦ **V93.43** Struck by falling object on other powered watercraft

Struck by falling object on Hovercraft

⊗⑦ **V93.44** Struck by falling object on sailboat

⊗⑦ **V93.48** Struck by falling object on other unpowered watercraft

⊗⑦ **V93.49** Struck by falling object on unspecified watercraft

V93.5 Explosion on board watercraft

Boiler explosion on steamship

Excludes 2: fire on board watercraft (V93.0-)

⊗⑦ **V93.50** Explosion on board merchant ship

⊗⑦ **V93.51** Explosion on board passenger ship

Explosion on board Ferry-boat

Explosion on board Liner

⊗⑦ **V93.52** Explosion on board fishing boat

⊗⑦ **V93.53** Explosion on board other powered watercraft

Explosion on board Hovercraft

Explosion on board Jet ski

⊗⑦ **V93.54** Explosion on board sailboat

⊗⑦ **V93.59** Explosion on board unspecified watercraft

Explosion on board boat NOS

Explosion on board ship NOS

Explosion on board watercraft NOS

V93.6 Machinery accident on board watercraft

Excludes 1: machinery explosion on board watercraft (V93.4-)

machinery fire on board watercraft (V93.0-)

⊗⑦ **V93.60** Machinery accident on board merchant ship

⊗⑦ **V93.61** Machinery accident on board passenger ship

Machinery accident on board Ferry-boat

Machinery accident on board Liner

⊗⑦ **V93.62** Machinery accident on board fishing boat

⊗⑦ **V93.63** Machinery accident on board other powered watercraft

Machinery accident on board Hovercraft

⊗⑦ **V93.64** Machinery accident on board sailboat

⊗⑦ **V93.69** Machinery accident on board unspecified watercraft

Machinery accident on board boat NOS

Machinery accident on board ship NOS

Machinery accident on board watercraft NOS

V93.8 Other injury due to other accident on board watercraft

Accidental poisoning by gases or fumes on watercraft

⊗⑦ **V93.80** Other injury due to other accident on board merchant ship

⊗⑦ **V93.81** Other injury due to other accident on board passenger ship

Other injury due to other accident on board Ferry-boat

Other injury due to other accident on board Liner

⊗⑦**V93.82** Other injury due to other accident on board fishing boat

⊗⑦**V93.83** Other injury due to other accident on board other powered watercraft

Other injury due to other accident on board Hovercraft

Other injury due to other accident on board Jet ski

⊗⑦**V93.84** Other injury due to other accident on board sailboat

⊗⑦**V93.85** Other injury due to other accident on board canoe or kayak

⊗⑦**V93.86** Other injury due to other accident on board (nonpowered) inflatable craft

⊗⑦**V93.87** Other injury due to other accident on board water-skis

Hit or struck by object while waterskiing

⊗⑦**V93.88** Other injury due to other accident on board other unpowered watercraft

Hit or struck by object while surfing

Hit or struck by object while on board windsurfer

⊗⑦**V93.89** Other injury due to other accident on board unspecified watercraft

Other injury due to other accident on board boat NOS

Other injury due to other accident on board ship NOS

Other injury due to other accident on board watercraft NOS

V94 Other and unspecified water transport accidents

Excludes 1: military watercraft accidents in military or war operations (Y36, Y37)

The appropriate 7th character is to be added to each code from category V94

A - initial encounter

D - subsequent encounter

S - sequela

⊗⑦**V94.0** Hitting object or bottom of body of water due to fall from watercraft

Excludes 2: drowning and submersion due to fall from watercraft (V92.0-)

V94.1 Bather struck by watercraft

Swimmer hit by watercraft

⊗⑦**V94.11** Bather struck by powered watercraft

⊗⑦**V94.12** Bather struck by nonpowered watercraft

V94.2 Rider of nonpowered watercraft struck by other watercraft

⊗⑦**V94.21** Rider of nonpowered watercraft struck by other nonpowered watercraft

Canoer hit by other nonpowered watercraft

Surfer hit by other nonpowered watercraft

Windsurfer hit by other nonpowered watercraft

⊗⑦**V94.22** Rider of nonpowered watercraft struck by powered watercraft

Canoer hit by motorboat

Surfer hit by motorboat

Windsurfer hit by motorboat

V94.3 Injury to rider of (inflatable) watercraft being pulled behind other watercraft

⊗⑦**V94.31** Injury to rider of (inflatable) recreational watercraft being pulled behind other watercraft

Injury to rider of inner-tube pulled behind motor boat

⊗⑦**V94.32** Injury to rider of non-recreational watercraft being pulled behind other watercraft

Injury to occupant of dingy being pulled behind boat or ship

Injury to occupant of life-raft being pulled behind boat or ship

⊗⑦**V94.4** Injury to barefoot water-skier

Injury to person being pulled behind boat or ship

V94.8 Other water transport accident

V94.81 Water transport accident involving military watercraft

⑦**V94.810** Civilian watercraft involved in water transport accident with military watercraft

Passenger on civilian watercraft injured due to accident with military watercraft

⑦**V94.811** Civilian in water injured by military watercraft

⑦**V94.818** Other water transport accident involving military watercraft

⊗⑦**V94.89** Other water transport accident

⊗⑦**V94.9** Unspecified water transport accident

Water transport accident NOS

AIR AND SPACE TRANSPORT ACCIDENTS (V95-V97)

Excludes 1: military aircraft accidents in military or war operations (Y36, Y37)

V95 Accident to powered aircraft causing injury to occupant

The appropriate 7th character is to be added to each code from category V95

A - initial encounter

D - subsequent encounter

S - sequela

V95.0 Helicopter accident injuring occupant

⊗⑦**V95.00** Unspecified helicopter accident injuring occupant

⊗⑦**V95.01** Helicopter crash injuring occupant

⊗⑦**V95.02** Forced landing of helicopter injuring occupant

⊗⑦**V95.03** Helicopter collision injuring occupant

Helicopter collision with any object, fixed, movable or moving

⊗⑦**V95.04** Helicopter fire injuring occupant

⊗⑦**V95.05** Helicopter explosion injuring occupant

⊗⑦**V95.09** Other helicopter accident injuring occupant

V95.1 Ultralight, microlight or powered-glider accident injuring occupant

⊗⑦**V95.10** Unspecified ultralight, microlight or powered-glider accident injuring occupant

⊗⑦**V95.11** Ultralight, microlight or powered-glider crash injuring occupant

⊗⑦**V95.12** Forced landing of ultralight, microlight or powered-glider injuring occupant

⊗⑦**V95.13**   Ultralight, microlight or powered-glider collision injuring occupant

Ultralight, microlight or powered-glider collision with any object, fixed, movable or moving

⊗⑦**V95.14**   Ultralight, microlight or powered-glider fire injuring occupant

⊗⑦**V95.15**   Ultralight, microlight or powered-glider explosion injuring occupant

⊗⑦**V95.19**   Other ultralight, microlight or powered-glider accident injuring occupant

V95.2   Other private fixed-wing aircraft accident injuring occupant

⊗⑦**V95.20**   Unspecified accident to other private fixed-wing aircraft, injuring occupant

⊗⑦**V95.21**   Other private fixed-wing aircraft crash injuring occupant

⊗⑦**V95.22**   Forced landing of other private fixed-wing aircraft injuring occupant

⊗⑦**V95.23**   Other private fixed-wing aircraft collision injuring occupant

Other private fixed-wing aircraft collision with any object, fixed, movable or moving

⊗⑦**V95.24**   Other private fixed-wing aircraft fire injuring occupant

⊗⑦**V95.25**   Other private fixed-wing aircraft explosion injuring occupant

⊗⑦**V95.29**   Other accident to other private fixed-wing aircraft injuring occupant

V95.3   Commercial fixed-wing aircraft accident injuring occupant

⊗⑦**V95.30**   Unspecified accident to commercial fixed-wing aircraft injuring occupant

⊗⑦**V95.31**   Commercial fixed-wing aircraft crash injuring occupant

⊗⑦**V95.32**   Forced landing of commercial fixed-wing aircraft injuring occupant

⊗⑦**V95.33**   Commercial fixed-wing aircraft collision injuring occupant

Commercial fixed-wing aircraft collision with any object, fixed, movable or moving

⊗⑦**V95.34**   Commercial fixed-wing aircraft fire injuring occupant

⊗⑦**V95.35**   Commercial fixed-wing aircraft explosion injuring occupant

⊗⑦**V95.39**   Other accident to commercial fixed-wing aircraft injuring occupant

V95.4   Spacecraft accident injuring occupant

⊗⑦**V95.40**   Unspecified spacecraft accident injuring occupant

⊗⑦**V95.41**   Spacecraft crash injuring occupant

⊗⑦**V95.42**   Forced landing of spacecraft injuring occupant

⊗⑦**V95.43**   Spacecraft collision injuring occupant

Spacecraft collision with any object, fixed, moveable or moving

⊗⑦**V95.44**   Spacecraft fire injuring occupant

⊗⑦**V95.45**   Spacecraft explosion injuring occupant

⊗⑦**V95.49**   Other spacecraft accident injuring occupant

⊗⑦**V95.8**   Other powered aircraft accidents injuring occupant

⊗⑦**V95.9**   Unspecified aircraft accident injuring occupant

Aircraft accident NOS

Air transport accident NOS

V96   Accident to nonpowered aircraft causing injury to occupant

The appropriate 7th character is to be added to each code from category V96

A - initial encounter

D - subsequent encounter

S - sequela

V96.0   Balloon accident injuring occupant

⊗⑦**V96.00**   Unspecified balloon accident injuring occupant

⊗⑦**V96.01**   Balloon crash injuring occupant

⊗⑦**V96.02**   Forced landing of balloon injuring occupant

⊗⑦**V96.03**   Balloon collision injuring occupant

Balloon collision with any object, fixed, moveable or moving

⊗⑦**V96.04**   Balloon fire injuring occupant

⊗⑦**V96.05**   Balloon explosion injuring occupant

⊗⑦**V96.09**   Other balloon accident injuring occupant

V96.1   Hang-glider accident injuring occupant

⊗⑦**V96.10**   Unspecified hang-glider accident injuring occupant

⊗⑦**V96.11**   Hang-glider crash injuring occupant

⊗⑦**V96.12**   Forced landing of hang-glider injuring occupant

⊗⑦**V96.13**   Hang-glider collision injuring occupant

Hang-glider collision with any object, fixed, moveable or moving

⊗⑦**V96.14**   Hang-glider fire injuring occupant

⊗⑦**V96.15**   Hang-glider explosion injuring occupant

⊗⑦**V96.19**   Other hang-glider accident injuring occupant

V96.2   Glider (nonpowered) accident injuring occupant

⊗⑦**V96.20**   Unspecified glider (nonpowered) accident injuring occupant

⊗⑦**V96.21**   Glider (nonpowered) crash injuring occupant

⊗⑦**V96.22**   Forced landing of glider (nonpowered) injuring occupant

⊗⑦**V96.23**   Glider (nonpowered) collision injuring occupant

Glider (nonpowered) collision with any object, fixed, moveable or moving

⊗⑦**V96.24**   Glider (nonpowered) fire injuring occupant

⊗⑦**V96.25**   Glider (nonpowered) explosion injuring occupant

⊗⑦**V96.29**   Other glider (nonpowered) accident injuring occupant

⊗⑦**V96.8**   Other nonpowered-aircraft accidents injuring occupant

Kite carrying a person accident injuring occupant

⊗⑦**V96.9**   Unspecified nonpowered-aircraft accident injuring occupant

Nonpowered-aircraft accident NOS

V97   Other specified air transport accidents

The appropriate 7th character is to be added to each code from category V97

A - initial encounter

D - subsequent encounter

S - sequela

⊗⑦**V97.0**   Occupant of aircraft injured in other specified air transport accidents

Fall in, on or from aircraft in air transport accident

Excludes 1: accident while boarding or alighting aircraft (V97.1)

⊗⑦**V97.1**   Person injured while boarding or alighting from aircraft

V97.2   Parachutist accident

⊗⑦**V97.21**   Parachutist entangled in object

Parachutist landing in tree

⊗⑦**V97.22**   Parachutist injured on landing

⊗⑦**V97.29**   Other parachutist accident

V97.3   Person on ground injured in air transport accident

⊗⑦**V97.31**   Hit by object falling from aircraft

Hit by crashing aircraft

Injured by aircraft hitting house

Injured by aircraft hitting car

⊗⑦**V97.32**   Injured by rotating propeller

⊗⑦**V97.33**   Sucked into jet engine

⊗⑦**V97.39**   Other injury to person on ground due to air transport accident

V97.8   Other air transport accidents, not elsewhere classified

Excludes 1: aircraft accident NOS (V95.9)

exposure to changes in air pressure during ascent or descent (W94.-)

V97.81   Air transport accident involving military aircraft

⑦**V97.810**   Civilian aircraft involved in air transport accident with military aircraft

Passenger in civilian aircraft injured due to accident with military aircraft

⑦**V97.811**   Civilian injured by military aircraft

⑦**V97.818**   Other air transport accident involving military aircraft

V97.89   Other air transport accidents, not elsewhere classified

Injury from machinery on aircraft

OTHER AND UNSPECIFIED TRANSPORT ACCIDENTS (V98-V99)

Excludes 1: vehicle accident, type of vehicle unspecified (V89.-)

V98   Other specified transport accidents

The appropriate 7th character is to be added to each code from category V98

A - initial encounter

D - subsequent encounter

S - sequela

⊗⑦**V98.0**   Accident to, on or involving cable-car, not on rails

Caught or dragged by cable-car, not on rails

Fall or jump from cable-car, not on rails

Object thrown from or in cable-car, not on rails

⊗⑦**V98.1**   Accident to, on or involving land-yacht

⊗⑦**V98.2**   Accident to, on or involving ice yacht

⊗⑦**V98.3**   Accident to, on or involving ski lift

Accident to, on or involving ski chair-lift

Accident to, on or involving ski-lift with gondola

⊗⑦**V98.8**   Other specified transport accidents

V99   Unspecified transport accident

The appropriate 7th character is to be added to code V99

A - initial encounter

D - subsequent encounter

S - sequela

OTHER EXTERNAL CAUSES OF ACCIDENTAL INJURY (W00-X58)

Slipping, tripping, stumbling and falls (W00-W19)

Excludes 1: assault involving a fall (Y01-Y02)

fall (in) (from):

animal (V80.-)

machinery (in operation) (W28-W31)

transport vehicle (V01-V99)

intentional self-harm involving a fall (X80-X81)

Excludes 2: at risk for fall (history of fall) Z91.81

fall (in) (from):

burning building (X00.-)

into fire (X00-X04, X08-X09)

W00   Fall due to ice and snow

Includes: pedestrian on foot falling (slipping) on ice and snow

Excludes 1: fall on (from) ice and snow involving pedestrian conveyance (V00.-)

fall from stairs and steps not due to ice and snow (W10.-)

The appropriate 7th character is to be added to each code from category W00

A - initial encounter

D - subsequent encounter

S - sequela

⊗⑦**W00.0**   Fall on same level due to ice and snow

⊗⑦**W00.1**   Fall from stairs and steps due to ice and snow

⊗⑦**W00.2**   Other fall from one level to another due to ice and snow

⊗⑦**W00.9**   Unspecified fall due to ice and snow

W01   Fall on same level from slipping, tripping and stumbling

Includes: fall on moving sidewalk

Excludes 1: fall due to bumping (striking) against object (W18.0-)

fall in shower or bathtub (W18.2-)

fall on same level NOS (W18.30)

fall on same level from slipping, tripping and stumbling due to ice or snow (W00.0)

fall off or from toilet (W18.1-)

slipping, tripping and stumbling NOS (W18.40)

slipping, tripping and stumbling without falling (W18.4-)

The appropriate 7th character is to be added to each code from category W01

A - initial encounter

D - subsequent encounter

S - sequela

⊗⑦**W01.0**   Fall on same level from slipping, tripping and stumbling without subsequent striking against object

Falling over animal

W01.1   Fall on same level from slipping, tripping and stumbling with subsequent striking against object

⊗⑦**W01.10**   Fall on same level from slipping, tripping and stumbling with subsequent striking against unspecified object

W01.11   Fall on same level from slipping, tripping and stumbling with subsequent striking against sharp object

⑦**W01.110**   Fall on same level from slipping, tripping and stumbling with subsequent striking against sharp glass

⑦**W01.111**   Fall on same level from slipping, tripping and stumbling with

● New code   ▲ Revised code   ⑦ 7th digit required   ⊗ Placeholder required

subsequent striking against power tool or machine

⑦**W01.118** Fall on same level from slipping, tripping and stumbling with subsequent striking against other sharp object

⑦**W01.119** Fall on same level from slipping, tripping and stumbling with subsequent striking against unspecified sharp object

W01.19 Fall on same level from slipping, tripping and stumbling with subsequent striking against other object

⑦**W01.190** Fall on same level from slipping, tripping and stumbling with subsequent striking against furniture

⑦**W01.198** Fall on same level from slipping, tripping and stumbling with subsequent striking against other object

W03 Other fall on same level due to collision with another person
Fall due to non-transport collision with other person
Excludes 1: collision with another person without fall (W51)
crushed or pushed by a crowd or human stampede (W52)
fall involving pedestrian conveyance (V00-V09)
fall due to ice or snow (W00)
fall on same level NOS (W18.30)
The appropriate 7th character is to be added to code W03
A - initial encounter
D - subsequent encounter
S - sequela

W04 Fall while being carried or supported by other persons
Accidentally dropped while being carried
The appropriate 7th character is to be added to code W04
A - initial encounter
D - subsequent encounter
S - sequela

W05 Fall from non-moving wheelchair, nonmotorized scooter and motorized mobility scooter
Excludes 1: fall from moving wheelchair (powered) (V00.811)
fall from moving motorized mobility scooter (V00.831)
fall from nonmotorized scooter (V00.141)
The appropriate 7th character is to be added to each code from category W05
A - initial encounter
D - subsequent encounter
S - sequela

⊗⑦**W05.0** Fall from non-moving wheelchair
⊗⑦**W05.1** Fall from non-moving nonmotorized scooter
⊗⑦**W05.2** Fall from non-moving motorized mobility scooter

W06 Fall from bed
The appropriate 7th character is to be added to code W06
A - initial encounter
D - subsequent encounter
S - sequela

W07 Fall from chair
The appropriate 7th character is to be added to code W07
A - initial encounter
D - subsequent encounter
S - sequela

W08 Fall from other furniture
The appropriate 7th character is to be added to code W08
A - initial encounter
D - subsequent encounter
S - sequela

W09 Fall on and from playground equipment
Excludes 1: fall involving recreational machinery (W31)
The appropriate 7th character is to be added to each code from category W09
A - initial encounter
D - subsequent encounter
S - sequela

⊗⑦**W09.0** Fall on or from playground slide
⊗⑦**W09.1** Fall from playground swing
⊗⑦**W09.2** Fall on or from jungle gym
⊗⑦**W09.8** Fall on or from other playground equipment

W10 Fall on and from stairs and steps
Excludes 1: Fall from stairs and steps due to ice and snow (W00.1)
The appropriate 7th character is to be added to each code from category W10
A - initial encounter
D - subsequent encounter
S - sequela

⊗⑦**W10.0** Fall (on)(from) escalator
⊗⑦**W10.1** Fall (on)(from) sidewalk curb
⊗⑦**W10.2** Fall (on)(from) incline
Fall (on) (from) ramp
⊗⑦**W10.8** Fall (on) (from) other stairs and steps
⊗⑦**W10.9** Fall (on) (from) unspecified stairs and steps

W11 Fall on and from ladder
The appropriate 7th character is to be added to code W11
A - initial encounter
D - subsequent encounter
S - sequela

W12 Fall on and from scaffolding
The appropriate 7th character is to be added to code W12
A - initial encounter
D - subsequent encounter
S - sequela

W13 Fall from, out of or through building or structure
The appropriate 7th character is to be added to each code from category W13
A - initial encounter
D - subsequent encounter
S - sequela

⊗⑦**W13.0** Fall from, out of or through balcony
Fall from, out of or through railing
⊗⑦**W13.1** Fall from, out of or through bridge
⊗⑦**W13.2** Fall from, out of or through roof
⊘⑦**W13.3** Fall through floor
⊗⑦**W13.4** Fall from, out of or through window
Excludes 2: fall with subsequent striking against sharp glass (W01.110)
⊗⑦**W13.8** Fall from, out of or through other building or structure
Fall from, out of or through viaduct
Fall from, out of or through wall
Fall from, out of or through flag-pole

⊗⑦**W13.9** Fall from, out of or through building, not otherwise specified

Excludes 1: collapse of a building or structure (W20.-)

fall or jump from burning building or structure (X00.-)

W14 Fall from tree

The appropriate 7th character is to be added to code W14

A - initial encounter

D - subsequent encounter

S - sequela

W15 Fall from cliff

The appropriate 7th character is to be added to code W15

A - initial encounter

D - subsequent encounter

S - sequela

W16 Fall, jump or diving into water

Excludes 1: accidental non-watercraft drowning and submersion not involving fall (W65-W74)

effects of air pressure from diving (W94.-)

fall into water from watercraft (V90-V94)

hitting an object or against bottom when falling from watercraft (V94.0)

Excludes 2: striking or hitting diving board (W21.3)

The appropriate 7th character is to be added to each code from category W16

A - initial encounter

D - subsequent encounter

S - sequela

W16.0 Fall into swimming pool

Fall into swimming pool NOS

Excludes 1: fall into empty swimming pool (W17.3)

W16.01 Fall into swimming pool striking water surface

⑦**W16.011** Fall into swimming pool striking water surface causing drowning and submersion

Excludes 1: drowning and submersion while in swimming pool without fall (W67)

⑦**W16.012** Fall into swimming pool striking water surface causing other injury

W16.02 Fall into swimming pool striking bottom

⑦**W16.021** Fall into swimming pool striking bottom causing drowning and submersion

Excludes 1: drowning and submersion while in swimming pool without fall (W67)

⑦**W16.022** Fall into swimming pool striking bottom causing other injury

W16.03 Fall into swimming pool striking wall

⑦**W16.031** Fall into swimming pool striking wall causing drowning and submersion

Excludes 1: drowning and submersion while in swimming pool without fall (W67)

⑦**W16.032** Fall into swimming pool striking wall causing other injury

W16.1 Fall into natural body of water

Fall into lake

Fall into open sea

Fall into river

Fall into stream

W16.11 Fall into natural body of water striking water surface

⑦**W16.111** Fall into natural body of water striking water surface causing drowning and submersion

Excludes 1: drowning and submersion while in natural body of water without fall (W69)

⑦**W16.112** Fall into natural body of water striking water surface causing other injury

W16.12 Fall into natural body of water striking bottom

⑦**W16.121** Fall into natural body of water striking bottom causing drowning and submersion

Excludes 1: drowning and submersion while in natural body of water without fall (W69)

⑦**W16.122** Fall into natural body of water striking bottom causing other injury

W16.13 Fall into natural body of water striking side

⑦**W16.131** Fall into natural body of water striking side causing drowning and submersion

Excludes 1: drowning and submersion while in natural body of water without fall (W69)

⑦**W16.132** Fall into natural body of water striking side causing other injury

W16.2 Fall in (into) filled bathtub or bucket of water

W16.21 Fall in (into) filled bathtub

Excludes 1: fall into empty bathtub (W18.2)

⑦**W16.211** Fall in (into) filled bathtub causing drowning and submersion

Excludes 1: drowning and submersion while in filled bathtub without fall (W65)

⑦**W16.212** Fall in (into) filled bathtub causing other injury

W16.22 Fall in (into) bucket of water

⑦**W16.221** Fall in (into) bucket of water causing drowning and submersion

⑦**W16.222** Fall in (into) bucket of water causing other injury

W16.3 Fall into other water

Fall into fountain

Fall into reservoir

W16.31 Fall into other water striking water surface

⑦**W16.311** Fall into other water striking water surface causing drowning and submersion

Excludes 1: drowning and submersion while in other water without fall (W73)

⑦**W16.312** Fall into other water striking water surface causing other injury

W16.32 Fall into other water striking bottom

● New code   ▲ Revised code   ⑦ 7th digit required   ⊗ Placeholder required

⑦**W16.321** Fall into other water striking bottom causing drowning and submersion

Excludes 1: drowning and submersion while in other water without fall (W73)

⑦**W16.322** Fall into other water striking bottom causing other injury

W16.33 Fall into other water striking wall

⑦**W16.331** Fall into other water striking wall causing drowning and submersion

Excludes 1: drowning and submersion while in other water without fall (W73)

⑦**W16.332** Fall into other water striking wall causing other injury

W16.4 Fall into unspecified water

W16.41 Fall into unspecified water causing drowning and submersion

W16.42 Fall into unspecified water causing other injury

W16.5 Jumping or diving into swimming pool

W16.51 Jumping or diving into swimming pool striking water surface

⑦**W16.511** Jumping or diving into swimming pool striking water surface causing drowning and submersion

Excludes 1: drowning and submersion while in swimming pool without jumping or diving (W67)

⑦**W16.512** Jumping or diving into swimming pool striking water surface causing other injury

W16.52 Jumping or diving into swimming pool striking bottom

⑦**W16.521** Jumping or diving into swimming pool striking bottom causing drowning and submersion

Excludes 1: drowning and submersion while in swimming pool without jumping or diving (W67)

⑦**W16.522** Jumping or diving into swimming pool striking bottom causing other injury

W16.53 Jumping or diving into swimming pool striking wall

⑦**W16.531** Jumping or diving into swimming pool striking wall causing drowning and submersion

Excludes 1: drowning and submersion while in swimming pool without jumping or diving (W67)

⑦**W16.532** Jumping or diving into swimming pool striking wall causing other injury

W16.6 Jumping or diving into natural body of water

Jumping or diving into lake

Jumping or diving into open sea

Jumping or diving into river

Jumping or diving into stream

W16.61 Jumping or diving into natural body of water striking water surface

⑦**W16.611** Jumping or diving into natural body of water striking water surface causing drowning and submersion

Excludes 1: drowning and submersion while in natural body of water without jumping or diving (W69)

⑦**W16.612** Jumping or diving into natural body of water striking water surface causing other injury

W16.62 Jumping or diving into natural body of water striking bottom

⑦**W16.621** Jumping or diving into natural body of water striking bottom causing drowning and submersion

Excludes 1: drowning and submersion while in natural body of water without jumping or diving (W69)

⑦**W16.622** Jumping or diving into natural body of water striking bottom causing other injury

W16.7 Jumping or diving from boat

Excludes 1: Fall from boat into water -see watercraft accident (V90-V94)

W16.71 Jumping or diving from boat striking water surface

⑦**W16.711** Jumping or diving from boat striking water surface causing drowning and submersion

⑦**W16.712** Jumping or diving from boat striking water surface causing other injury

W16.72 Jumping or diving from boat striking bottom

⑦**W16.721** Jumping or diving from boat striking bottom causing drowning and submersion

⑦**W16.722** Jumping or diving from boat striking bottom causing other injury

W16.8 Jumping or diving into other water

Jumping or diving into fountain

Jumping or diving into reservoir

W16.81 Jumping or diving into other water striking water surface

⑦**W16.811** Jumping or diving into other water striking water surface causing drowning and submersion

Excludes 1: drowning and submersion while in other water without jumping or diving (W73)

⑦**W16.812** Jumping or diving into other water striking water surface causing other injury

W16.82 Jumping or diving into other water striking bottom

⑦**W16.821** Jumping or diving into other water striking bottom causing drowning and submersion

Excludes 1: drowning and submersion while in other water without jumping or diving (W73)

⑦**W16.822** Jumping or diving into other water striking bottom causing other injury

W16.83 Jumping or diving into other water striking wall

⑦**W16.831** Jumping or diving into other water striking wall causing drowning and submersion

> **Excludes 1:** drowning and submersion while in other water without jumping or diving (W73)

⑦**W16.832** Jumping or diving into other water striking wall causing other injury

W16.9 Jumping or diving into unspecified water

⊗⑦**W16.91** Jumping or diving into unspecified water causing drowning and submersion

⊗⑦**W16.92** Jumping or diving into unspecified water causing other injury

W17 Other fall from one level to another

The appropriate 7th character is to be added to each code from category W17

A - initial encounter

D - subsequent encounter

S - sequela

⊗⑦**W17.0** Fall into well

⊗⑦**W17.1** Fall into storm drain or manhole

⊗⑦**W17.2** Fall into hole

Fall into pit

⊗⑦**W17.3** Fall into empty swimming pool

> **Excludes 1:** fall into filled swimming pool (W16.0-)

⊗⑦**W17.4** Fall from dock

W17.8 Other fall from one level to another

⊗⑦**W17.81** Fall down embankment (hill)

⊗⑦**W17.82** Fall from (out of) grocery cart

Fall due to grocery cart tipping over

⊗⑦**W17.89** Other fall from one level to another

Fall from cherry picker

Fall from lifting device

Fall from mobile elevated work platform [MEWP]

Fall from sky lift

W18 Other slipping, tripping and stumbling and falls

The appropriate 7th character is to be added to each code from category W18

A - initial encounter

D - subsequent encounter

S - sequela

W18.0 Fall due to bumping against object

Striking against object with subsequent fall

> **Excludes 1:** fall on same level due to slipping, tripping, or stumbling with subsequent striking against object (W01.1-)

⊗⑦**W18.00** Striking against unspecified object with subsequent fall

⊗⑦**W18.01** Striking against sports equipment with subsequent fall

⊗⑦**W18.02** Striking against glass with subsequent fall

⊗⑦**W18.09** Striking against other object with subsequent fall

W18.1 Fall from or off toilet

⊗⑦**W18.11** Fall from or off toilet without subsequent striking against object

Fall from (off) toilet NOS

⊗⑦**W18.12** Fall from or off toilet with subsequent striking against object

⊗⑦**W18.2** Fall in (into) shower or empty bathtub

> **Excludes 1:** fall in full bathtub causing drowning or submersion (W16.21-)

W18.3 Other and unspecified fall on same level

⊗⑦**W18.30** Fall on same level, unspecified

⊗⑦**W18.31** Fall on same level due to stepping on an object

Fall on same level due to stepping on an animal

> **Excludes 1:** slipping, tripping and stumbling without fall due to stepping on animal (W18.41)

⊗⑦**W18.39** Other fall on same level

W18.4 Slipping, tripping and stumbling without falling

> **Excludes 1:** collision with another person without fall (W51)

⊗⑦**W18.40** Slipping, tripping and stumbling without falling, unspecified

⊗⑦**W18.41** Slipping, tripping and stumbling without falling due to stepping on object

Slipping, tripping and stumbling without falling due to stepping on animal

> **Excludes 1:** slipping, tripping and stumbling with fall due to stepping on animal (W18.31)

⊗⑦**W18.42** Slipping, tripping and stumbling without falling due to stepping into hole or opening

⊗⑦**W18.43** Slipping, tripping and stumbling without falling due to stepping from one level to another

⊗⑦**W18.49** Other slipping, tripping and stumbling without falling

W19 Unspecified fall

Accidental fall NOS

The appropriate 7th character is to be added to code W19

A - initial encounter

D - subsequent encounter

S - sequela

EXPOSURE TO INANIMATE MECHANICAL FORCES (W20-W49)

> **Excludes 1:** assault (X92-Y08)
>
> contact or collision with animals or persons (W50-W64)
>
> exposure to inanimate mechanical forces involving military or war operations (Y36.-, Y37.-)
>
> intentional self-harm (X71-X83)

W20 Struck by thrown, projected or falling object

Code first any associated:

cataclysm (X34-X39)

lightning strike (T75.00)

> **Excludes 1:** falling object in:
>
> machinery accident (W24, W28-W31)
>
> transport accident (V01-V99)
>
> object set in motion by:
>
> explosion (W35-W40)
>
> firearm (W32-W34)
>
> struck by thrown sports equipment (W21.-)

The appropriate 7th character is to be added to each code from category W20

A - initial encounter

D - subsequent encounter

S - sequela

⊗⑦**W20.0** Struck by falling object in cave-in

Excludes 2: asphyxiation due to cave-in (T71.21)

⊗⑦**W20.1** Struck by object due to collapse of building

Excludes 1: struck by object due to collapse of burning building (X00.2, X02.2)

⊗⑦**W20.8** Other cause of strike by thrown, projected or falling object

Excludes 1: struck by thrown sports equipment (W21.-)

W21 Striking against or struck by sports equipment

Excludes 1: assault with sports equipment (Y08.0-)

striking against or struck by sports equipment with subsequent fall (W18.01)

The appropriate 7th character is to be added to each code from category W21

A - initial encounter

D - subsequent encounter

S - sequela

W21.0 Struck by hit or thrown ball

⊗⑦**W21.00** Struck by hit or thrown ball, unspecified type

⊗⑦**W21.01** Struck by football

⊗⑦**W21.02** Struck by soccer ball

⊗⑦**W21.03** Struck by baseball

⊗⑦**W21.04** Struck by golf ball

⊗⑦**W21.05** Struck by basketball

⊗⑦**W21.06** Struck by volleyball

⊗⑦**W21.07** Struck by softball

⊗⑦**W21.09** Struck by other hit or thrown ball

W21.1 Struck by bat, racquet or club

⊗⑦**W21.11** Struck by baseball bat

⊗⑦**W21.12** Struck by tennis racquet

⊗⑦**W21.13** Struck by golf club

⊗⑦**W21.19** Struck by other bat, racquet or club

W21.2 Struck by hockey stick or puck

W21.21 Struck by hockey stick

⑦**W21.210** Struck by ice hockey stick

⑦**W21.211** Struck by field hockey stick

W21.22 Struck by hockey puck

⑦**W21.220** Struck by ice hockey puck

⑦**W21.221** Struck by field hockey puck

W21.3 Struck by sports foot wear

⊗⑦**W21.31** Struck by shoe cleats

Stepped on by shoe cleats

⊗⑦**W21.32** Struck by skate blades

Skated over by skate blades

⊗⑦**W21.39** Struck by other sports foot wear

⊗⑦**W21.4** Striking against diving board

Use additional code for subsequent falling into water, if applicable (W16.-)

W21.8 Striking against or struck by other sports equipment

⊗⑦**W21.81** Striking against or struck by football helmet

⊗⑦**W21.89** Striking against or struck by other sports equipment

⊗⑦**W21.9** Striking against or struck by unspecified sports equipment

W22 Striking against or struck by other objects

Excludes 1: striking against or struck by object with subsequent fall (W18.09)

The appropriate 7th character is to be added to each code from category W22

A - initial encounter

D - subsequent encounter

S - sequela

W22.0 Striking against stationary object

Excludes 1: striking against stationary sports equipment (W21.8)

⊗⑦**W22.01** Walked into wall

⊗⑦**W22.02** Walked into lamppost

⊗⑦**W22.03** Walked into furniture

W22.04 Striking against wall of swimming pool

⑦**W22.041** Striking against wall of swimming pool causing drowning and submersion

Excludes 1: drowning and submersion while swimming without striking against wall (W67)

⑦**W22.042** Striking against wall of swimming pool causing other injury

⊗⑦**W22.09** Striking against other stationary object

W22.1 Striking against or struck by automobile airbag

⊗⑦**W22.10** Striking against or struck by unspecified automobile airbag

⊗⑦**W22.11** Striking against or struck by driver side automobile airbag

⊗⑦**W22.12** Striking against or struck by front passenger side automobile airbag

⊗⑦**W22.19** Striking against or struck by other automobile airbag

⊗⑦**W22.8** Striking against or struck by other objects

Striking against or struck by object NOS

Excludes 1: struck by thrown, projected or falling object (W20.-)

W23 Caught, crushed, jammed or pinched in or between objects

Excludes 1: injury caused by cutting or piercing instruments (W25-W27)

injury caused by firearms malfunction (W32.1, W33.1-, W34.1-)

injury caused by lifting and transmission devices (W24.-)

injury caused by machinery (W28-W31)

injury caused by nonpowered hand tools (W27.-)

injury caused by transport vehicle being used as a means of transportation (V01-V99)

injury caused by struck by thrown, projected or falling object (W20.-)

The appropriate 7th character is to be added to each code from category W23

A - initial encounter

D - subsequent encounter

S - sequela

⊗⑦**W23.0** Caught, crushed, jammed, or pinched between moving objects

⊗⑦**W23.1** Caught, crushed, jammed, or pinched between stationary objects

W24 Contact with lifting and transmission devices, not elsewhere classified

Excludes 1: transport accidents (V01-V99)

The appropriate 7th character is to be added to each code from category W24

A - initial encounter

D - subsequent encounter

S - sequela

⊗⑦ **W24.0** Contact with lifting devices, not elsewhere classified

Contact with chain hoist

Contact with drive belt

Contact with pulley (block)

⊗⑦ **W24.1** Contact with transmission devices, not elsewhere classified

Contact with transmission belt or cable

W25 Contact with sharp glass

Code first any associated:

injury due to flying glass from explosion or firearm discharge (W32-W40)

transport accident (V00-V99)

Excludes 1: fall on same level due to slipping, tripping and stumbling with subsequent striking against sharp glass (W01.10)

striking against sharp glass with subsequent fall (W18.02)

The appropriate 7th character is to be added to code W25

A - initial encounter

D - subsequent encounter

S - sequela

W26 Contact with knife, sword or dagger

The appropriate 7th character is to be added to each code from category W26

A - initial encounter

D - subsequent encounter

S - sequela

⊗⑦ **W26.0** Contact with knife

Excludes 1: contact with electric knife (W29.1)

⊗⑦ **W26.1** Contact with sword or dagger

W27 Contact with nonpowered hand tool

The appropriate 7th character is to be added to each code from category W27

A - initial encounter

D - subsequent encounter

S - sequela

⊗⑦ **W27.0** Contact with workbench tool

Contact with auger

Contact with axe

Contact with chisel

Contact with handsaw

Contact with screwdriver

⊗⑦ **W27.1** Contact with garden tool

Contact with hoe

Contact with nonpowered lawn mower

Contact with pitchfork

Contact with rake

⊗⑦ **W27.2** Contact with scissors

⊗⑦ **W27.3** Contact with needle (sewing)

Excludes 1: contact with hypodermic needle (W46.-)

⊗⑦ **W27.4** Contact with kitchen utensil

Contact with fork

Contact with ice-pick

Contact with can-opener NOS

⊗⑦ **W27.5** Contact with paper-cutter

⊗⑦ **W27.8** Contact with other nonpowered hand tool

Contact with nonpowered sewing machine

Contact with shovel

W28 Contact with powered lawn mower

Powered lawn mower (commercial) (residential)

Excludes 1: contact with nonpowered lawn mower (W27.1)

Excludes 2: exposure to electric current (W86.-)

The appropriate 7th character is to be added to code W28

A - initial encounter

D - subsequent encounter

S - sequela

W29 Contact with other powered hand tools and household machinery

Excludes 1: contact with commercial machinery (W31.82)

contact with hot household appliance (X15)

contact with nonpowered hand tool (W27.-)

exposure to electric current (W86)

The appropriate 7th character is to be added to each code from category W29

A - initial encounter

D - subsequent encounter

S - sequela

⊗⑦ **W29.0** Contact with powered kitchen appliance

Contact with blender

Contact with can-opener

Contact with garbage disposal

Contact with mixer

⊗⑦ **W29.1** Contact with electric knife

⊗⑦ **W29.2** Contact with other powered household machinery

Contact with electric fan

Contact with powered dryer (clothes) (powered) (spin)

Contact with washing-machine

Contact with sewing machine

⊗⑦ **W29.3** Contact with powered garden and outdoor hand tools and machinery

Contact with chainsaw

Contact with edger

Contact with garden cultivator (tiller)

Contact with hedge trimmer

Contact with other powered garden tool

Excludes 1: contact with powered lawn mower (W28)

⊗⑦ **W29.4** Contact with nail gun

⊗⑦ **W29.8** Contact with other powered powered hand tools and household machinery

Contact with do-it-yourself tool NOS

W30 Contact with agricultural machinery

Includes: animal-powered farm machine

Excludes 1: agricultural transport vehicle accident (V01-V99)

explosion of grain store (W40.8)

exposure to electric current (W86.-)

The appropriate 7th character is to be added to each code from category W30

A - initial encounter

D - subsequent encounter

S - sequela

⊗⑦ **W30.0** Contact with combine harvester

Contact with reaper

Contact with thresher

⊗⑦ **W30.1** Contact with power take-off devices (PTO)

⊗⑦ **W30.2** Contact with hay derrick

⊗⑦ **W30.3** Contact with grain storage elevator

Excludes 1: explosion of grain store (W40.8)

W30.8 Contact with other specified agricultural machinery

⊗⑦ **W30.81** Contact with agricultural transport vehicle in stationary use

Contact with agricultural transport vehicle under repair, not on public roadway

Excludes 1: agricultural transport vehicle accident (V01-V99)

⊗⑦ **W30.89** Contact with other specified agricultural machinery

⊗⑦ **W30.9** Contact with unspecified agricultural machinery

Contact with farm machinery NOS

W31 Contact with other and unspecified machinery

Excludes 1: contact with agricultural machinery (W30.-)

contact with machinery in transport under own power or being towed by a vehicle (V01-V99)

exposure to electric current (W86)

The appropriate 7th character is to be added to each code from category W31

A - initial encounter

D - subsequent encounter

S - sequela

⊗⑦ **W31.0** Contact with mining and earth-drilling machinery

Contact with bore or drill (land) (seabed)

Contact with shaft hoist

Contact with shaft lift

Contact with undercutter

⊗⑦ **W31.1** Contact with metalworking machines

Contact with abrasive wheel

Contact with forging machine

Contact with lathe

Contact with mechanical shears

Contact with metal drilling machine

Contact with milling machine

Contact with power press

Contact with rolling-mill

Contact with metal sawing machine

⊗⑦ **W31.2** Contact with powered woodworking and forming machines

Contact with band saw

Contact with bench saw

Contact with circular saw

Contact with molding machine

Contact with overhead plane

Contact with powered saw

Contact with radial saw

Contact with sander

Excludes 1: nonpowered woodworking tools (W27.0)

⊗⑦ **W31.3** Contact with prime movers

Contact with gas turbine

Contact with internal combustion engine

Contact with steam engine

Contact with water driven turbine

W31.8 Contact with other specified machinery

⊗⑦ **W31.81** Contact with recreational machinery

Contact with roller coaster

⊗⑦ **W31.82** Contact with other commercial machinery

Contact with commercial electric fan

Contact with commercial kitchen appliances

Contact with commercial powered dryer (clothes) (powered) (spin)

Contact with commercial washing-machine

Contact with commercial sewing machine

Excludes 1: contact with household machinery (W29.-)

contact with powered lawn mower (W28)

⊗⑦ **W31.83** Contact with special construction vehicle in stationary use

Contact with special construction vehicle under repair, not on public roadway

Excludes 1: special construction vehicle accident (V01-V99)

⊗⑦ **W31.89** Contact with other specified machinery

⊗⑦ **W31.9** Contact with unspecified machinery

Contact with machinery NOS

W32 Accidental handgun discharge and malfunction

Includes: accidental discharge and malfunction of gun for single hand use

accidental discharge and malfunction of pistol

accidental discharge and malfunction of revolver

Handgun discharge and malfunction NOS

Excludes 1: accidental airgun discharge and malfunction (W34.010, W34.110)

accidental BB gun discharge and malfunction (W34.010, W34.110)

accidental pellet gun discharge and malfunction (W34.010, W34.110)

accidental shotgun discharge and malfunction (W33.01, W33.11)

assault by handgun discharge (X93)

handgun discharge involving legal intervention (Y35.0-)

handgun discharge involving military or war operations (Y36.4-)

intentional self-harm by handgun discharge (X72)

Very pistol discharge and malfunction (W34.09, W34.19)

The appropriate 7th character is to be added to each code from category W32

A - initial encounter

D - subsequent encounter

S - sequela

⊗⑦ **W32.0** Accidental handgun discharge

⊗⑦ **W32.1** Accidental handgun malfunction

Injury due to explosion of handgun (parts)

Injury due to malfunction of mechanism or component of handgun

Injury due to recoil of handgun

Powder burn from handgun

W33 Accidental rifle, shotgun and larger firearm discharge and malfunction

Includes: rifle, shotgun and larger firearm discharge and malfunction NOS

Excludes 1: accidental airgun discharge and malfunction (W34.010, W34.110)

accidental BB gun discharge and malfunction (W34.010, W34.110) accidental handgun discharge and malfunction (W32-)

accidental pellet gun discharge and malfunction (W34.010, W34.110)

assault by rifle, shotgun and larger firearm discharge (X94)

firearm discharge involving legal intervention (Y35.0-)

firearm discharge involving military or war operations (Y36.4-)

intentional self-harm by rifle, shotgun and larger firearm discharge (X73)

The appropriate 7th character is to be added to each code from category W33

A - initial encounter

D - subsequent encounter

S - sequela

W33.0 Accidental rifle, shotgun and larger firearm discharge

⊗⑦**W33.00** Accidental discharge of unspecified larger firearm

Discharge of unspecified larger firearm NOS

⊗⑦**W33.01** Accidental discharge of shotgun

Discharge of shotgun NOS

⊗⑦**W33.02** Accidental discharge of hunting rifle

Discharge of hunting rifle NOS

⊗⑦**W33.03** Accidental discharge of machine gun

Discharge of machine gun NOS

⊗⑦**W33.09** Accidental discharge of other larger firearm

Discharge of other larger firearm NOS

W33.1 Accidental rifle, shotgun and larger firearm malfunction

Injury due to explosion of rifle, shotgun and larger firearm (parts)

Injury due to malfunction of mechanism or component of rifle, shotgun and larger firearm

Injury due to piercing, cutting, crushing or pinching due to (by) slide trigger mechanism, scope or other gun part

Injury due to recoil of rifle, shotgun and larger firearm

Powder burn from rifle, shotgun and larger firearm

⊗⑦**W33.10** Accidental malfunction of unspecified larger firearm

Malfunction of unspecified larger firearm NOS

⊗⑦**W33.11** Accidental malfunction of shotgun

Malfunction of shotgun NOS

⊗⑦**W33.12** Accidental malfunction of hunting rifle

Malfunction of hunting rifle NOS

⊗⑦**W33.13** Accidental malfunction of machine gun

Malfunction of machine gun NOS

⊗⑦**W33.19** Accidental malfunction of other larger firearm

Malfunction of other larger firearm NOS

W34 Accidental discharge and malfunction from other and unspecified firearms and guns

The appropriate 7th character is to be added to each code from category W34

A - initial encounter

D - subsequent encounter

S - sequela

W34.0 Accidental discharge from other and unspecified firearms and guns

⊗⑦**W34.00** Accidental discharge from unspecified firearms or gun

Discharge from firearm NOS

Gunshot wound NOS

Shot NOS

W34.01 Accidental discharge of gas, air or spring-operated guns

⑦**W34.010** Accidental discharge of airgun

Accidental discharge of BB gun

Accidental discharge of pellet gun

⑦**W34.011** Accidental discharge of paintball gun

Accidental injury due to paintball discharge

⑦**W34.018** Accidental discharge of other gas, air or spring-operated gun

⊗⑦**W34.09** Accidental discharge from other specified firearms

Accidental discharge from Very pistol [flare]

W34.1 Accidental malfunction from other and unspecified firearms and guns

⊗⑦**W34.10** Accidental malfunction from unspecified firearms or gun

Firearm malfunction NOS

W34.11 Accidental malfunction of gas, air or spring-operated guns

⑦**W34.110** Accidental malfunction of airgun

Accidental malfunction of BB gun

Accidental malfunction of pellet gun

⑦**W34.111** Accidental malfunction of paintball gun

Accidental injury due to paintball gun malfunction

⑦**W34.118** Accidental malfunction of other gas, air or spring-operated gun

⊗⑦**W34.19** Accidental malfunction from other specified firearms

Accidental malfunction from Very pistol [flare]

W35 Explosion and rupture of boiler

Excludes 1: explosion and rupture of boiler on watercraft (V93.4)

The appropriate 7th character is to be added to code W35

A - initial encounter

D - subsequent encounter

S - sequela

W36 Explosion and rupture of gas cylinder

The appropriate 7th character is to be added to each code from category W36

A - initial encounter

D - subsequent encounter

S - sequela

⊗⑦**W36.1** Explosion and rupture of aerosol can

⊗⑦**W36.2** Explosion and rupture of air tank

⊗⑦**W36.3** Explosion and rupture of pressurized-gas tank

⊗⑦**W36.8** Explosion and rupture of other gas cylinder

⊗⑦**W36.9** Explosion and rupture of unspecified gas cylinder

W37 Explosion and rupture of pressurized tire, pipe or hose

The appropriate 7th character is to be added to each code from category W37

A - initial encounter

D - subsequent encounter

S - sequela

⊗⑦**W37.0** Explosion of bicycle tire

● New code　　　▲ Revised code　　　⑦ 7ᵗʰ digit required　　　⊗ Placeholder required

⊗⑦**W37.8** Explosion and rupture of other pressurized tire, pipe or
hose

W38 Explosion and rupture of other specified pressurized devices

The appropriate 7th character is to be added to code W38

A - initial encounter

D - subsequent encounter

S - sequela

W39 Discharge of firework

The appropriate 7th character is to be added to code W39

A - initial encounter

D - subsequent encounter

S - sequela

W40 Explosion of other materials

Excludes 1: assault by explosive material (X96)

explosion involving legal intervention (Y35.1-)

explosion involving military or war operations (Y36.0-,
Y36.2-)

intentional self-harm by explosive material (X75)

The appropriate 7th character is to be added to each code from
category W40

A - initial encounter

D - subsequent encounter

S - sequela

⊗⑦**W40.0** Explosion of blasting material

Explosion of blasting cap

Explosion of detonator

Explosion of dynamite

Explosion of explosive (any) used in blasting operations

⊗⑦**W40.1** Explosion of explosive gases

Explosion of acetylene

Explosion of butane

Explosion of coal gas

Explosion in mine NOS

Explosion of explosive gas

Explosion of fire damp

Explosion of gasoline fumes

Explosion of methane

Explosion of propane

⊗⑦**W40.8** Explosion of other specified explosive materials

Explosion in dump NOS

Explosion in factory NOS

Explosion in grain store

Explosion in munitions

Excludes 1: explosion involving legal intervention
(Y35.1-)

explosion involving military or war operations
(Y36.0-, Y36.2-)

⊗⑦**W40.9** Explosion of unspecified explosive materials

Explosion NOS

W42 Exposure to noise

The appropriate 7th character is to be added to each code from
category W42

A - initial encounter

D - subsequent encounter

S - sequela

⊗⑦**W42.0** Exposure to supersonic waves

⊗⑦**W42.9** Exposure to other noise

Exposure to sound waves NOS

W45 Foreign body or object entering through skin

Excludes 2: contact with hand tools (nonpowered) (powered)
(W27-W29)

contact with knife, sword or dagger (W26.-)

contact with sharp glass (W25.-)

struck by objects (W20-W22)

The appropriate 7th character is to be added to each code from
category W45

A - initial encounter

D - subsequent encounter

S - sequela

⊗⑦**W45.0** Nail entering through skin

⊗⑦**W45.1** Paper entering through skin

Paper cut

⊗⑦**W45.2** Lid of can entering through skin

⊗⑦**W45.8** Other foreign body or object entering through skin

Splinter in skin NOS

W46 Contact with hypodermic needle

The appropriate 7th character is to be added to each code from
category W46

A - initial encounter

D - subsequent encounter

S - sequela

⊗⑦**W46.0** Contact with hypodermic needle

Hypodermic needle stick NOS

⊗⑦**W46.1** Contact with contaminated hypodermic needle

W49 Exposure to other inanimate mechanical forces

Includes: exposure to abnormal gravitational [G] forces

exposure to inanimate mechanical forces NEC

Excludes 1: exposure to inanimate mechanical forces involving
military or war operations (Y36.-, Y37.-)

The appropriate 7th character is to be added to each code
from category W49

A - initial encounter

D - subsequent encounter

S - sequela

W49.0 Item causing external constriction

⊗⑦**W49.01** Hair causing external constriction

⊗⑦**W49.02** String or thread causing external constriction

⊗⑦**W49.03** Rubber band causing external constriction

⊗⑦**W49.04** Ring or other jewelry causing external
constriction

⊗⑦**W49.09** Other specified item causing external constriction

⊗⑦**W49.9** Exposure to other inanimate mechanical forces

EXPOSURE TO ANIMATE MECHANICAL FORCES (W50-W64)

Excludes 1: Toxic effect of contact with venomous animals and plants
(T63.-)

W50 Accidental hit, strike, kick, twist, bite or scratch by another person

Includes: hit, strike, kick, twist, bite, or scratch by another person
NOS

Excludes 1: assault by bodily force (Y04)

struck by objects (W20-W22)

The appropriate 7th character is to be added to each code from
category W50

A - initial encounter

D - subsequent encounter

S - sequela

⊗⑦**W50.0** Accidental hit or strike by another person

Hit or strike by another person NOS

⊗⑦**W50.1** Accidental kick by another person
    Kick by another person NOS

⊗⑦**W50.2** Accidental twist by another person
    Twist by another person NOS

⊗⑦**W50.3** Accidental bite by another person
    Human bite
    Bite by another person NOS

⊗⑦**W50.4** Accidental scratch by another person
    Scratch by another person NOS

W51 Accidental striking against or bumped into by another person

    Excludes 1: assault by striking against or bumping into by another person (Y04.2)
        fall due to collision with another person (W03)

    The appropriate 7th character is to be added to code W51

    A - initial encounter
    D - subsequent encounter
    S - sequela

W52 Crushed, pushed or stepped on by crowd or human stampede
    Crushed, pushed or stepped on by crowd or human stampede with or without fall

    The appropriate 7th character is to be added to code W52

    A - initial encounter
    D - subsequent encounter
    S - sequela

W53 Contact with rodent

    Includes: contact with saliva, feces or urine of rodent

    The appropriate 7th character is to be added to each code from category W53

    A - initial encounter
    D - subsequent encounter
    S - sequela

    W53.0 Contact with mouse

      ⊗⑦**W53.01** Bitten by mouse
      ⊗⑦**W53.09** Other contact with mouse

    W53.1 Contact with rat

      ⊗⑦**W53.11** Bitten by rat
      ⊗⑦**W53.19** Other contact with rat

    W53.2 Contact with squirrel

      ⊗⑦**W53.21** Bitten by squirrel
      ⊗⑦**W53.29** Other contact with squirrel

    W53.8 Contact with other rodent

      ⊗⑦**W53.81** Bitten by other rodent
      ⊗⑦**W53.89** Other contact with other rodent

W54 Contact with dog

    Includes: contact with saliva, feces or urine of dog

    The appropriate 7th character is to be added to each code from category W54

    A - initial encounter
    D - subsequent encounter
    S - sequela

⊗⑦**W54.0** Bitten by dog

⊗⑦**W54.1** Struck by dog
    Knocked over by dog

⊗⑦**W54.8** Other contact with dog

W55 Contact with other mammals

    Includes: contact with saliva, feces or urine of mammal

    Excludes 1: animal being ridden- see transport accidents

        bitten or struck by dog (W54)
        bitten or struck by rodent (W53.-)
        contact with marine mammals (W56.x-)

The appropriate 7th character is to be added to each code from category W55

A - initial encounter
D - subsequent encounter
S - sequela

W55.0 Contact with cat

    ⊗⑦**W55.01** Bitten by cat
    ⊗⑦**W55.03** Scratched by cat
    ⊗⑦**W55.09** Other contact with cat

W55.1 Contact with horse

    ⊗⑦**W55.11** Bitten by horse
    ⊗⑦**W55.12** Struck by horse
    ⊗⑦**W55.19** Other contact with horse

W55.2 Contact with cow
    Contact with bull

    ⊗⑦**W55.21** Bitten by cow
    ⊗⑦**W55.22** Struck by cow
        Gored by bull
    ⊗⑦**W55.29** Other contact with cow

W55.3 Contact with other hoof stock
    Contact with goats
    Contact with sheep

    ⊗⑦**W55.31** Bitten by other hoof stock
    ⊗⑦**W55.32** Struck by other hoof stock
        Gored by goat
        Gored by ram
    ⊗⑦**W55.39** Other contact with other hoof stock

W55.4 Contact with pig

    ⊗⑦**W55.41** Bitten by pig
    ⊗⑦**W55.42** Struck by pig
    ⊗⑦**W55.49** Other contact with pig

W55.5 Contact with raccoon

    ⊗⑦**W55.51** Bitten by raccoon
    ⊗⑦**W55.52** Struck by raccoon
    ⊗⑦**W55.59** Other contact with raccoon

W55.8 Contact with other mammals

    ⊗⑦**W55.81** Bitten by other mammals
    ⊗⑦**W55.82** Struck by other mammals
    ⊗⑦**W55.89** Other contact with other mammals

W56 Contact with nonvenomous marine animal

    Excludes 1: contact with venomous marine animal (T63.-)

The appropriate 7th character is to be added to each code from category W56

A - initial encounter
D - subsequent encounter
S - sequela

W56.0 Contact with dolphin

    ⊗⑦**W56.01** Bitten by dolphin
    ⊗⑦**W56.02** Struck by dolphin
    ⊗⑦**W56.09** Other contact with dolphin

W56.1 Contact with sea lion

    ⊗⑦**W56.11** Bitten by sea lion
    ⊗⑦**W56.12** Struck by sea lion

● New code   ▲ Revised code   ⑦ 7th digit required   ⊗ Placeholder required

⊗⑦**W56.19** Other contact with sea lion

W56.2 Contact with orca
    Contact with killer whale

⊗⑦**W56.21** Bitten by orca

⊗⑦**W56.22** Struck by orca

⊗⑦**W56.29** Other contact with orca

W56.3 Contact with other marine mammals

⊗⑦**W56.31** Bitten by other marine mammals

⊗⑦**W56.32** Struck by other marine mammals

⊗⑦**W56.39** Other contact with other marine mammals

W56.4 Contact with shark

⊗⑦**W56.41** Bitten by shark

⊗⑦**W56.42** Struck by shark

⊗⑦**W56.49** Other contact with shark

W56.5 Contact with other fish

⊗⑦**W56.51** Bitten by other fish

⊗⑦**W56.52** Struck by other fish

⊗⑦**W56.59** Other contact with other fish

W56.8 Contact with other nonvenomous marine animals

⊗⑦**W56.81** Bitten by other nonvenomous marine animals

⊗⑦**W56.82** Struck by other nonvenomous marine animals

⊗⑦**W56.89** Other contact with other nonvenomous marine animals

W57 Bitten or stung by nonvenomous insect and other nonvenomous arthropods

Excludes 1: contact with venomous insects and arthropods (T63.2-, T63.3-, T63.4-)

The appropriate 7th character is to be added to code W57

A - initial encounter

D - subsequent encounter

S - sequela

W58 Contact with crocodile or alligator

The appropriate 7th character is to be added to each code from category W58

A - initial encounter

D - subsequent encounter

S - sequela

W58.0 Contact with alligator

⊗⑦**W58.01** Bitten by alligator

⊗⑦**W58.02** Struck by alligator

⊗⑦**W58.03** Crushed by alligator

⊗⑦**W58.09** Other contact with alligator

W58.1 Contact with crocodile

⊗⑦**W58.11** Bitten by crocodile

⊗⑦**W58.12** Struck by crocodile

⊗⑦**W58.13** Crushed by crocodile

⊗⑦**W58.19** Other contact with crocodile

W59 Contact with other nonvenomous reptiles

Excludes 1: contact with venomous reptile (T63.0-, T63.1-)

The appropriate 7th character is to be added to each code from category W59

A - initial encounter

D - subsequent encounter

S - sequela

W59.0 Contact with nonvenomous lizards

⊗⑦**W59.01** Bitten by nonvenomous lizards

⊗⑦**W59.02** Struck by nonvenomous lizards

⊗⑦**W59.09** Other contact with nonvenomous lizards
    Exposure to nonvenomous lizards

W59.1 Contact with nonvenomous snakes

⊗⑦**W59.11** Bitten by nonvenomous snake

⊗⑦**W59.12** Struck by nonvenomous snake

⊗⑦**W59.13** Crushed by nonvenomous snake

⊗⑦**W59.19** Other contact with nonvenomous snake

W59.2 Contact with turtles

    Excludes 1: contact with tortoises (W59.8-)

⊗⑦**W59.21** Bitten by turtle

⊗⑦**W59.22** Struck by turtle

⊗⑦**W59.29** Other contact with turtle
    Exposure to turtles

W59.8 Contact with other nonvenomous reptiles

⊗⑦**W59.81** Bitten by other nonvenomous reptiles

⊗⑦**W59.82** Struck by other nonvenomous reptiles

⊗⑦**W59.83** Crushed by other nonvenomous reptiles

⊗⑦**W59.89** Other contact with other nonvenomous reptiles

W60 Contact with nonvenomous plant thorns and spines and sharp leaves

Excludes 1: Contact with venomous plants (T63.x-)

The appropriate 7th character is to be added to code W60

A - initial encounter

D - subsequent encounter

S - sequela

W61 Contact with birds (domestic) (wild)

Includes: contact with excreta of birds

The appropriate 7th character is to be added to each code from category W61

A - initial encounter

D - subsequent encounter

S - sequela

W61.0 Contact with parrot

⊗⑦**W61.01** Bitten by parrot

⊗⑦**W61.02** Struck by parrot

⊗⑦**W61.09** Other contact with parrot
    Exposure to parrots

W61.1 Contact with macaw

⊗⑦**W61.11** Bitten by macaw

⊗⑦**W61.12** Struck by macaw

⊗⑦**W61.19** Other contact with macaw
    Exposure to macaws

W61.2 Contact with other psittacines

⊗⑦**W61.21** Bitten by other psittacines

⊗⑦**W61.22** Struck by other psittacines

⊗⑦**W61.29** Other contact with other psittacines
    Exposure to other psittacines

W61.3 Contact with chicken

⊗⑦**W61.32** Struck by chicken

⊗⑦**W61.33** Pecked by chicken

⊗⑦**W61.39** Other contact with chicken
    Exposure to chickens

W61.4 Contact with turkey

⊗⑦**W61.42** Struck by turkey

⊗⑦**W61.43** Pecked by turkey

⊗⑦**W61.49** Other contact with turkey

W61.5 Contact with goose

⊗⑦**W61.51**   Bitten by goose

⊗⑦**W61.52**   Struck by goose

⊗⑦**W61.59**   Other contact with goose

W61.6   Contact with duck

⊗⑦**W61.61**   Bitten by duck

⊗⑦**W61.62**   Struck by duck

⊗⑦**W61.69**   Other contact with duck

W61.9   Contact with other birds

⊗⑦**W61.91**   Bitten by other birds

⊗⑦**W61.92**   Struck by other birds

⊗⑦**W61.99**   Other contact with other birds
Contact with bird NOS

W62 Contact with nonvenomous amphibians

Excludes 1: contact with venomous amphibians (T63.81-R63.83)

The appropriate 7th character is to be added to each code from category W62

A - initial encounter

D - subsequent encounter

S - sequela

⊗⑦**W62.0**   Contact with nonvenomous frogs

⊗⑦**W62.1**   Contact with nonvenomous toads

⊗⑦**W62.9**   Contact with other nonvenomous amphibians

W64 Exposure to other animate mechanical forces

Includes: exposure to nonvenomous animal NOS

Excludes 1: contact with venomous animal (T63.-)

The appropriate 7th character is to be added to code W64

A - initial encounter

D - subsequent encounter

S - sequela

ACCIDENTAL NON-TRANSPORT DROWNING AND SUBMERSION (W65-W74)

Excludes 1: accidental drowning and submersion due to fall into water (W16.-)

accidental drowning and submersion due to water transport accident (V90.-, V92.-)

Excludes 2: accidental drowning and submersion due to cataclysm (X34-X39)

W65 Accidental drowning and submersion while in bath-tub

Excludes 1: accidental drowning and submersion due to fall in (into) bathtub (W16.211)

The appropriate 7th character is to be added to code W65

A - initial encounter

D - subsequent encounter

S - sequela

W67 Accidental drowning and submersion while in swimming-pool

Excludes 1: accidental drowning and submersion due to fall into swimming pool (W16.011, W16.021, W16.031)

accidental drowning and submersion due to striking into wall of swimming pool (W22.041)

The appropriate 7th character is to be added to code W67

A - initial encounter

D - subsequent encounter

S - sequela

W69 Accidental drowning and submersion while in natural water

Accidental drowning and submersion while in lake

Accidental drowning and submersion while in open sea

Accidental drowning and submersion while in river

Accidental drowning and submersion while in stream

Excludes 1: accidental drowning and submersion due to fall into natural body of water (W16.111, W16.121, W16.131)

The appropriate 7th character is to be added to code W69

A - initial encounter

D - subsequent encounter

S - sequela

W73 Other specified cause of accidental non-transport drowning and submersion

Accidental drowning and submersion while in quenching tank

Accidental drowning and submersion while in reservoir

Excludes 1: accidental drowning and submersion due to fall into other water (W16.311, W16.321, W16.331)

The appropriate 7th character is to be added to code W73

A - initial encounter

D - subsequent encounter

S - sequela

W74 Unspecified cause of accidental drowning and submersion

Drowning NOS

The appropriate 7th character is to be added to code W74

A - initial encounter

D - subsequent encounter

S - sequela

EXPOSURE TO ELECTRIC CURRENT, RADIATION AND EXTREME AMBIENT AIR TEMPERATURE AND PRESSURE (W85-W99)

Excludes 1: exposure to:

failure in dosage of radiation or temperature during surgical and medical care (Y63.2-Y63.5)

lightning (T75.0-)

natural cold (X31)

natural heat (X30)

natural radiation NOS (X39)

radiological procedure and radiotherapy (Y84.2)

sunlight (X32)

W85 Exposure to electric transmission lines

Broken power line

The appropriate 7th character is to be added to code W85

A - initial encounter

D - subsequent encounter

S - sequela

W86 Exposure to other specified electric current

The appropriate 7th character is to be added to each code from category W86

A - initial encounter

D - subsequent encounter

S - sequela

⊗⑦**W86.0**   Exposure to domestic wiring and appliances

⊗⑦**W86.1**   Exposure to industrial wiring, appliances and electrical machinery

Exposure to conductors

Exposure to control apparatus

Exposure to electrical equipment and machinery

Exposure to transformers

⊗⑦**W86.8**   Exposure to other electric current

Exposure to wiring and appliances in or on farm (not farmhouse)

Exposure to wiring and appliances outdoors

Exposure to wiring and appliances in or on public building
Exposure to wiring and appliances in or on residential institutions
Exposure to wiring and appliances in or on schools

W88 Exposure to ionizing radiation
Excludes 1: exposure to sunlight (X32)
The appropriate 7th character is to be added to each code from category W88
A - initial encounter
D - subsequent encounter
S - sequela

⊗⑦ **W88.0** Exposure to X-rays
⊗⑦ **W88.1** Exposure to radioactive isotopes
⊗⑦ **W88.8** Exposure to other ionizing radiation

W89 Exposure to man-made visible and ultraviolet light
Includes: exposure to welding light (arc)
Excludes 2: exposure to sunlight (X32)
The appropriate 7th character is to be added to each code from category W89
A - initial encounter
D - subsequent encounter
S - sequela

⊗⑦ **W89.0** Exposure to welding light (arc)
⊗⑦ **W89.1** Exposure to tanning bed
⊗⑦ **W89.8** Exposure to other man-made visible and ultraviolet light
⊗⑦ **W89.9** Exposure to unspecified man-made visible and ultraviolet light

W90 Exposure to other nonionizing radiation
Excludes 1: exposure to sunlight (X32)
The appropriate 7th character is to be added to each code from category W90
A - initial encounter
D - subsequent encounter
S - sequela

⊗⑦ **W90.0** Exposure to radiofrequency
⊗⑦ **W90.1** Exposure to infrared radiation
⊗⑦ **W90.2** Exposure to laser radiation
⊗⑦ **W90.8** Exposure to other nonionizing radiation

W92 Exposure to excessive heat of man-made origin
The appropriate 7th character is to be added to code W92
A - initial encounter
D - subsequent encounter
S - sequela

W93 Exposure to excessive cold of man-made origin
The appropriate 7th character is to be added to each code from category W93
A - initial encounter
D - subsequent encounter
S - sequela

W93.0 Contact with or inhalation of dry ice
⊗⑦ **W93.01** Contact with dry ice
⊗⑦ **W93.02** Inhalation of dry ice

W93.1 Contact with or inhalation of liquid air
⊗⑦ **W93.11** Contact with liquid air
Contact with liquid hydrogen
Contact with liquid nitrogen
⊗⑦ **W93.12** Inhalation of liquid air
Inhalation of liquid hydrogen

Inhalation of liquid nitrogen
⊗⑦ **W93.2** Prolonged exposure in deep freeze unit or refrigerator
⊗⑦ **W93.8** Exposure to other excessive cold of man-made origin

W94 Exposure to high and low air pressure and changes in air pressure
The appropriate 7th character is to be added to each code from category W94
A - initial encounter
D - subsequent encounter
S - sequela

⊗⑦ **W94.0** Exposure to prolonged high air pressure
W94.1 Exposure to prolonged low air pressure
⊗⑦ **W94.11** Exposure to residence or prolonged visit at high altitude
⊗⑦ **W94.12** Exposure to other prolonged low air pressure
W94.2 Exposure to rapid changes in air pressure during ascent
⊗⑦ **W94.21** Exposure to reduction in atmospheric pressure while surfacing from deep-water diving
⊗⑦ **W94.22** Exposure to reduction in atmospheric pressure while surfacing from underground
⊗⑦ **W94.23** Exposure to sudden change in air pressure in aircraft during ascent
⊗⑦ **W94.29** Exposure to other rapid changes in air pressure during ascent
W94.3 Exposure to rapid changes in air pressure during descent
▲⊗⑦ **W94.31** Exposure to sudden change in air pressure in aircraft during descent
⊗⑦ **W94.32** Exposure to high air pressure from rapid descent in water
⊗⑦ **W94.39** Exposure to other rapid changes in air pressure during descent

W99 Exposure to other man-made environmental factors
The appropriate 7th character is to be added to code W99
A - initial encounter
D - subsequent encounter
S - sequela

EXPOSURE TO SMOKE, FIRE AND FLAMES (X00-X08)

Excludes 1: arson (X97)
Excludes 2: explosions (W35-W40)
lightning (T75.0-)
transport accident (V01-V99)

X00 Exposure to uncontrolled fire in building or structure
Includes: conflagration in building or structure
Code first any associated cataclysm
Excludes 2: Exposure to ignition or melting of nightwear (X05)
Exposure to ignition or melting of other clothing and apparel (X06-)
Exposure to other specified smoke, fire and flames (X08.-)
The appropriate 7th character is to be added to each code from category X00
A - initial encounter
D - subsequent encounter
S - sequela

⊗⑦ **X00.0** Exposure to flames in uncontrolled fire in building or structure
⊗⑦ **X00.1** Exposure to smoke in uncontrolled fire in building or structure
⊗⑦ **X00.2** Injury due to collapse of burning building or structure in uncontrolled fire

⊗① **Excludes 1:** injury due to collapse of building not on fire (W20.1)

⊗①**X00.3** Fall from burning building or structure in uncontrolled fire

⊗①**X00.4** Hit by object from burning building or structure in uncontrolled fire

⊗①**X00.5** Jump from burning building or structure in uncontrolled fire

⊗①**X00.8** Other exposure to uncontrolled fire in building or structure

X01 Exposure to uncontrolled fire, not in building or structure

Includes: exposure to forest fire

The appropriate 7th character is to be added to each code from category X01

A - initial encounter

D - subsequent encounter

S - sequela

⊗①**X01.0** Exposure to flames in uncontrolled fire, not in building or structure

⊗①**X01.1** Exposure to smoke in uncontrolled fire, not in building or structure

⊗①**X01.3** Fall due to uncontrolled fire, not in building or structure

⊗①**X01.4** Hit by object due to uncontrolled fire, not in building or structure

⊗①**X01.8** Other exposure to uncontrolled fire, not in building or structure

X02 Exposure to controlled fire in building or structure

Includes: exposure to fire in fireplace

exposure to fire in stove

The appropriate 7th character is to be added to each code from category X02

A - initial encounter

D - subsequent encounter

S - sequela

⊗①**X02.0** Exposure to flames in controlled fire in building or structure

⊗①**X02.1** Exposure to smoke in controlled fire in building or structure

⊗①**X02.2** Injury due to collapse of burning building or structure in controlled fire

Excludes 1: injury due to collapse of building not on fire (W20.1)

⊗①**X02.3** Fall from burning building or structure in controlled fire

⊗①**X02.4** Hit by object from burning building or structure in controlled fire

⊗①**X02.5** Jump from burning building or structure in controlled fire

⊗①**X02.8** Other exposure to controlled fire in building or structure

X03 Exposure to controlled fire, not in building or structure

Includes: exposure to bon fire

exposure to camp-fire

exposure to trash fire

The appropriate 7th character is to be added to each code from category X03

A - initial encounter

D - subsequent encounter

S - sequela

⊗①**X03.0** Exposure to flames in controlled fire, not in building or structure

⊗①**X03.1** Exposure to smoke in controlled fire, not in building or structure

⊗①**X03.3** Fall due to controlled fire, not in building or structure

⊗①**X03.4** Hit by object due to controlled fire, not in building or structure

⊗①**X03.8** Other exposure to controlled fire, not in building or structure

X04 Exposure to ignition of highly flammable material

Exposure to ignition of gasoline

Exposure to ignition of kerosene

Exposure to ignition of petrol

Excludes 2: exposure to ignition or melting of nightwear (X05)

exposure to ignition or melting of other clothing and apparel (X06)

The appropriate 7th character is to be added to code X04

A - initial encounter

D - subsequent encounter

S - sequela

X05 Exposure to ignition or melting of nightwear

Excludes 2: exposure to uncontrolled fire in building or structure (X00.-)

exposure to uncontrolled fire, not in building or structure (X01.-)

exposure to controlled fire in building or structure (X02.-)

exposure to controlled fire, not in building or structure (X03.-)

exposure to ignition of highly flammable materials (X04.-)

The appropriate 7th character is to be added to code X05

A - initial encounter

D - subsequent encounter

S - sequela

X06 Exposure to ignition or melting of other clothing and apparel

Excludes 2: exposure to uncontrolled fire in building or structure (X00.-)

exposure to uncontrolled fire, not in building or structure (X01.-)

exposure to controlled fire in building or structure (X02.-)

exposure to controlled fire, not in building or structure (X03.-)

exposure to ignition of highly flammable materials (X04.-)

The appropriate 7th character is to be added to each code from category X06

A - initial encounter

D - subsequent encounter

S - sequela

⊗①**X06.0** Exposure to ignition of plastic jewelry

⊗①**X06.1** Exposure to melting of plastic jewelry

⊗①**X06.2** Exposure to ignition of other clothing and apparel

⊗①**X06.3** Exposure to melting of other clothing and apparel

X08 Exposure to other specified smoke, fire and flames

The appropriate 7th character is to be added to each code from category X08

A - initial encounter

D - subsequent encounter

S - sequela

X08.0 Exposure to bed fire

Exposure to mattress fire

⊗①**X08.00** Exposure to bed fire due to unspecified burning material

⊗①**X08.01** Exposure to bed fire due to burning cigarette

⊗⑦**X08.09**   Exposure to bed fire due to other burning material

X08.1   Exposure to sofa fire

⊗⑦**X08.10**   Exposure to sofa fire due to unspecified burning material

⊗⑦**X08.11**   Exposure to sofa fire due to burning cigarette

⊗⑦**X08.19**   Exposure to sofa fire due to other burning material

X08.2   Exposure to other furniture fire

⊗⑦**X08.20**   Exposure to other furniture fire due to unspecified burning material

⊗⑦**X08.21**   Exposure to other furniture fire due to burning cigarette

⊗⑦**X08.29**   Exposure to other furniture fire due to other burning material

⊗⑦**X08.8**   Exposure to other specified smoke, fire and flames

CONTACT WITH HEAT AND HOT SUBSTANCES (X10-X19)

Excludes 1: exposure to excessive natural heat (X30)

exposure to fire and flames (X00-X09)

X10   Contact with hot drinks, food, fats and cooking oils

The appropriate 7th character is to be added to each code from category X10

A - initial encounter

D - subsequent encounter

S - sequela

⊗⑦**X10.0**   Contact with hot drinks

⊗⑦**X10.1**   Contact with hot food

⊗⑦**X10.2**   Contact with fats and cooking oils

X11   Contact with hot tap-water

Includes: contact with boiling tap-water

contact with boiling water NOS

Excludes 1: contact with water heated on stove (X12)

The appropriate 7th character is to be added to each code from category X11

A - initial encounter

D - subsequent encounter

S - sequela

⊗⑦**X11.0**   Contact with hot water in bath or tub

Excludes 1: contact with running hot water in bath or tub (X11.1)

⊗⑦**X11.1**   Contact with running hot water

Contact with hot water running out of hose

Contact with hot water running out of tap

⊗⑦**X11.8**   Contact with other hot tap-water

Contact with hot water in bucket

Contact with hot tap-water NOS

X12   Contact with other hot fluids

Contact with water heated on stove

Excludes 1: hot (liquid) metals (X18)

The appropriate 7th character is to be added to code X12

A - initial encounter

D - subsequent encounter

S - sequela

X13   Contact with steam and other hot vapors

The appropriate 7th character is to be added to each code from category X13

A - initial encounter

D - subsequent encounter

S - sequela

⊗⑦**X13.0**   Inhalation of steam and other hot vapors

⊗⑦**X13.1**   Other contact with steam and other hot vapors

X14   Contact with hot air and other hot gases

The appropriate 7th character is to be added to each code from category X14

A - initial encounter

D - subsequent encounter

S - sequela

⊗⑦**X14.0**   Inhalation of hot air and gases

⊗⑦**X14.1**   Other contact with hot air and other hot gases

X15   Contact with hot household appliances

Excludes 1: contact with heating appliances (X16)

contact with powered household appliances (W29.-)

exposure to controlled fire in building or structure due to household appliance (X02.8)

exposure to household appliances electrical current (W86.0)

The appropriate 7th character is to be added to each code from category X15

A - initial encounter

D - subsequent encounter

S - sequela

⊗⑦**X15.0**   Contact with hot stove (kitchen)

⊗⑦**X15.1**   Contact with hot toaster

⊗⑦**X15.2**   Contact with hotplate

⊗⑦**X15.3**   Contact with hot saucepan or skillet

⊗⑦**X15.8**   Contact with other hot household appliances

Contact with cooker

Contact with kettle

Contact with light bulbs

X16   Contact with hot heating appliances, radiators and pipes

Excludes 1: contact with powered appliances (W29.-)

exposure to controlled fire in building or structure due to appliance (X02.8)

exposure to industrial appliances electrical current (W86.1)

The appropriate 7th character is to be added to code X16

A - initial encounter

D - subsequent encounter

S - sequela

X17   Contact with hot engines, machinery and tools

Excludes 1: contact with hot heating appliances, radiators and pipes (X16)

contact with hot household appliances (X15)

The appropriate 7th character is to be added to code X17

A - initial encounter

D - subsequent encounter

S - sequela

X18   Contact with other hot metals

Contact with liquid metal

The appropriate 7th character is to be added to code X18

A - initial encounter

D - subsequent encounter

S - sequela

X19   Contact with other heat and hot substances

Excludes 1: objects that are not normally hot, e.g., an object made hot by a house fire (X00-X09)

The appropriate 7th character is to be added to code X19

A - initial encounter

D - subsequent encounter
S - sequela

EXPOSURE TO FORCES OF NATURE (X30-X39)

X30 Exposure to excessive natural heat
Exposure to excessive heat as the cause of sunstroke
Exposure to heat NOS
Excludes 1: excessive heat of man-made origin (W92)
  exposure to man-made radiation (W89)
  exposure to sunlight (X32)
  exposure to tanning bed (W89)
The appropriate 7th character is to be added to code X30
A - initial encounter
D - subsequent encounter
S - sequela

X31 Exposure to excessive natural cold
Excessive cold as the cause of chilblains NOS
Excessive cold as the cause of immersion foot or hand
Exposure to cold NOS
Exposure to weather conditions
Excludes 1: cold of man-made origin (W93.-)
  contact with or inhalation of:
  dry ice (W93.-)
  liquefied gas (W93.-)
The appropriate 7th character is to be added to code X31
A - initial encounter
D - subsequent encounter
S - sequela

X32 Exposure to sunlight
Excludes 1: radiation-related disorders of the skin and
  subcutaneous tissue (L55-L59)
  man-made radiation (tanning bed) (W89)
The appropriate 7th character is to be added to code X32
A - initial encounter
D - subsequent encounter
S - sequela

X34 Earthquake
Excludes 2: tidal wave (tsunami) due to earthquake (X37.41)
The appropriate 7th character is to be added to code X34
A - initial encounter
D - subsequent encounter
S - sequela

X35 Volcanic eruption
Excludes 2: tidal wave (tsunami) due to volcanic eruption (X37.41)
The appropriate 7th character is to be added to code X35
A - initial encounter
D - subsequent encounter
S - sequela

X36 Avalanche, landslide and other earth movements
Includes: victim of mudslide of cataclysmic nature
Excludes 1: earthquake (X34)
Excludes 2: transport accident involving collision with avalanche
  or landslide not in motion (V01-V99)
The appropriate 7th character is to be added to each code from
category X36
A - initial encounter
D - subsequent encounter
S - sequela

⊗⑦**X36.0** Collapse of dam or man-made structure causing earth
  movement
⊗⑦**X36.1** Avalanche, landslide, or mudslide
X37 Cataclysmic storm
The appropriate 7th character is to be added to each code from
category X37
A - initial encounter
D - subsequent encounter
S - sequela

⊗⑦**X37.0** Hurricane
  Storm surge
  Typhoon
⊗⑦**X37.1** Tornado
  Cyclone
  Twister
⊗⑦**X37.2** Blizzard (snow)(ice)
⊗⑦**X37.3** Dust storm
X37.4 Tidalwave
⊗⑦**X37.41** Tidal wave due to earthquake or volcanic
  eruption
  Tidal wave NOS
  Tsunami
⊗⑦**X37.42** Tidal wave due to storm
⊗⑦**X37.43** Tidal wave due to landslide
⊗⑦**X37.8** Other cataclysmic storms
  Cloudburst
  Torrential rain
  Excludes 2: flood (X38)
⊗⑦**X37.9** Unspecified cataclysmic storm
  Storm NOS
  Excludes 1: collapse of dam or man-made structure
    causing earth movement (X39.0)

X38 Flood
Flood arising from remote storm
Flood of cataclysmic nature arising from melting snow
Flood resulting directly from storm
Excludes 1: collapse of dam or man-made structure causing earth
  movement (X39.0)
  tidal wave NOS (X37.41)
  tidal wave caused by storm (X37.2)
The appropriate 7th character is to be added to code X38
A - initial encounter
D - subsequent encounter
S - sequela

X39 Exposure to other forces of nature
The appropriate 7th character is to be added to each code from
category X39
A - initial encounter
D - subsequent encounter
S - sequela
X39.0 Exposure to natural radiation
  Excludes 1: contact with and (suspected) exposure to
    radon and other naturally occuring radiation
    (Z77.122)
    exposure to man-made radiation (W88-W90)
    exposure to sunlight (X32)
⊗⑦**X39.01** Exposure to radon
⊗⑦**X39.08** Exposure to other natural radiation

⊗⑦**X39.8**   Other exposure to forces of nature

ACCIDENTAL EXPOSURE TO OTHER SPECIFIED FACTORS (X52-X58)

X52   Prolonged stay in weightless environment
Weightlessness in spacecraft (simulator)
The appropriate 7th character is to be added to code X52
A - initial encounter
D - subsequent encounter
S - sequela

X58   Exposure to other specified factors
Accident NOS
Exposure NOS
The appropriate 7th character is to be added to code X58
A - initial encounter
D - subsequent encounter
S - sequela

INTENTIONAL SELF-HARM (X71-X83)

Purposely self-inflicted injury
Suicide (attempted)

X71   Intentional self-harm by drowning and submersion
The appropriate 7th character is to be added to each code from category X71
A - initial encounter
D - subsequent encounter
S - sequela

⊗⑦**X71.0**   Intentional self-harm by drowning and submersion while in bathtub

⊗⑦**X71.1**   Intentional self-harm by drowning and submersion while in swimming pool

⊗⑦**X71.2**   Intentional self-harm by drowning and submersion after jump into swimming pool

⊗⑦**X71.3**   Intentional self-harm by drowning and submersion in natural water

⊗⑦**X71.8**   Other intentional self-harm by drowning and submersion

⊗⑦**X71.9**   Intentional self-harm by drowning and submersion, unspecified

X72   Intentional self-harm by handgun discharge
Intentional self-harm by gun for single hand use
Intentional self-harm by pistol
Intentional self-harm by revolver
Excludes 1: Very pistol (X74.8)
The appropriate 7th character is to be added to code X72
A - initial encounter
D - subsequent encounter
S - sequela

X73   Intentional self-harm by rifle, shotgun and larger firearm discharge
Excludes 1: airgun (X74.01)
The appropriate 7th character is to be added to each code from category X73
A - initial encounter
D - subsequent encounter
S - sequela

⊗⑦**X73.0**   Intentional self-harm by shotgun discharge

⊗⑦**X73.1**   Intentional self-harm by hunting rifle discharge

⊗⑦**X73.2**   Intentional self-harm by machine gun discharge

⊗⑦**X73.8**   Intentional self-harm by other larger firearm discharge

⊗⑦**X73.9**   Intentional self-harm by unspecified larger firearm discharge

X74   Intentional self-harm by other and unspecified firearm and gun discharge
The appropriate 7th character is to be added to each code from category X74
A - initial encounter
D - subsequent encounter
S - sequela

X74.0   Intentional self-harm by gas, air or spring-operated guns

⊗⑦**X74.01**   Intentional self-harm by airgun
Intentional self-harm by BB gun discharge
Intentional self-harm by pellet gun discharge

⊗⑦**X74.02**   Intentional self-harm by paintball gun

⊗⑦**X74.09**   Intentional self-harm by other gas, air or spring-operated gun

⊗⑦**X74.8**   Intentional self-harm by other firearm discharge
Intentional self-harm by Very pistol [flare] discharge

⊗⑦**X74.9**   Intentional self-harm by unspecified firearm discharge

X75   Intentional self-harm by explosive material
The appropriate 7th character is to be added to code X75
A - initial encounter
D - subsequent encounter
S - sequela

X76   Intentional self-harm by smoke, fire and flames
The appropriate 7th character is to be added to code X76
A - initial encounter
D - subsequent encounter
S - sequela

X77   Intentional self-harm by steam, hot vapors and hot objects
The appropriate 7th character is to be added to each code from category X77
A - initial encounter
D - subsequent encounter
S - sequela

⊗⑦**X77.0**   Intentional self-harm by steam or hot vapors

⊗⑦**X77.1**   Intentional self-harm by hot tap water

⊗⑦**X77.2**   Intentional self-harm by other hot fluids

⊗⑦**X77.3**   Intentional self-harm by hot household appliances

⊗⑦**X77.8**   Intentional self-harm by other hot objects

⊗⑦**X77.9**   Intentional self-harm by unspecified hot objects

X78   Intentional self-harm by sharp object
The appropriate 7th character is to be added to each code from category X78
A - initial encounter
D - subsequent encounter
S - sequela

⊗⑦**X78.0**   Intentional self-harm by sharp glass

⊗⑦**X78.1**   Intentional self-harm by knife

⊗⑦**X78.2**   Intentional self-harm by sword or dagger

⊗⑦**X78.8**   Intentional self-harm by other sharp object

⊗⑦**X78.9**   Intentional self-harm by unspecified sharp object

X79   Intentional self-harm by blunt object
The appropriate 7th character is to be added to code X79
A - initial encounter
D - subsequent encounter
S - sequela

X80   Intentional self-harm by jumping from a high place

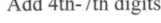   Add 4th-7th digits   ▢ 3 digit reportable   ▢ Nonspecific code   ▢ Unspecified code   ▢ Manifestation code   895

Intentional fall from one level to another

The appropriate 7th character is to be added to code X80

A - initial encounter

D - subsequent encounter

S - sequela

X81 Intentional self-harm by jumping or lying in front of moving object

The appropriate 7th character is to be added to each code from category X81

A - initial encounter

D - subsequent encounter

S - sequela

⊗⑦**X81.0**   Intentional self-harm by jumping or lying in front of motor vehicle

⊗⑦**X81.1**   Intentional self-harm by jumping or lying in front of (subway) train

⊗⑦**X81.8**   Intentional self-harm by jumping or lying in front of other moving object

X82 Intentional self-harm by crashing of motor vehicle

The appropriate 7th character is to be added to each code from category X82

A - initial encounter

D - subsequent encounter

S - sequela

⊗⑦**X82.0**   Intentional collision of motor vehicle with other motor vehicle

⊗⑦**X82.1**   Intentional collision of motor vehicle with train

⊗⑦**X82.2**   Intentional collision of motor vehicle with tree

⊗⑦**X82.8**   Other intentional self-harm by crashing of motor vehicle

X83 Intentional self-harm by other specified means

Excludes 1: intentional self-harm by poisoning or contact with toxic substance- See Table of Drugs and Chemicals

The appropriate 7th character is to be added to each code from category X83

A - initial encounter

D - subsequent encounter

S - sequela

⊗⑦**X83.0**   Intentional self-harm by crashing of aircraft

⊗⑦**X83.1**   Intentional self-harm by electrocution

⊗⑦**X83.2**   Intentional self-harm by exposure to extremes of cold

⊗⑦**X83.8**   Intentional self-harm by other specified means

ASSAULT (X92-Y08)

Includes: homicide

injuries inflicted by another person with intent to injure or kill, by any means

Excludes 1: injuries due to legal intervention (Y35.-)

injuries due to operations of war (Y36.-)

injuries due to terrorism (Y38.-)

X92 Assault by drowning and submersion

The appropriate 7th character is to be added to each code from category X92

A - initial encounter

D - subsequent encounter

S - sequela

⊗⑦**X92.0**   Assault by drowning and submersion while in bathtub

⊗⑦**X92.1**   Assault by drowning and submersion while in swimming pool

⊗⑦**X92.2**   Assault by drowning and submersion after push into swimming pool

⊗⑦**X92.3**   Assault by drowning and submersion in natural water

⊗⑦**X92.8**   Other assault by drowning and submersion

⊗⑦**X92.9**   Assault by drowning and submersion, unspecified

X93 Assault by handgun discharge

Assault by discharge of gun for single hand use

Assault by discharge of pistol

Assault by discharge of revolver

Excludes 1: Very pistol (X95.8)

The appropriate 7th character is to be added to code X93

A - initial encounter

D - subsequent encounter

S - sequela

X94 Assault by rifle, shotgun and larger firearm discharge

Excludes 1: airgun (X95.01)

The appropriate 7th character is to be added to each code from category X94

A - initial encounter

D - subsequent encounter

S - sequela

⊗⑦**X94.0**   Assault by shotgun

⊗⑦**X94.1**   Assault by hunting rifle

⊗⑦**X94.2**   Assault by machine gun

⊗⑦**X94.8**   Assault by other larger firearm discharge

⊗⑦**X94.9**   Assault by unspecified larger firearm discharge

X95 Assault by other and unspecified firearm and gun discharge

The appropriate 7th character is to be added to each code from category X95

A - initial encounter

D - subsequent encounter

S - sequela

X95.0   Assault by gas, air or spring-operated guns

⊗⑦**X95.01**   Assault by airgun discharge

Assault by BB gun discharge

Assault by pellet gun discharge

⊗⑦**X95.02**   Assault by paintball gun discharge

⊗⑦**X95.09**   Assault by other gas, air or spring-operated gun

⊗⑦**X95.8**   Assault by other firearm discharge

Assault by very pistol [flare] discharge

⊗⑦**X95.9**   Assault by unspecified firearm discharge

X96 Assault by explosive material

Excludes 1: incendiary device (X97)

terrorism involving explosive material (Y38.2-)

The appropriate 7th character is to be added to each code from category X96

A - initial encounter

D - subsequent encounter

S - sequela

⊗⑦**X96.0**   Assault by antipersonnel bomb

Excludes 1: antipersonnel bomb use in military or war (Y36.2-)

⊗⑦**X96.1**   Assault by gasoline bomb

⊗⑦**X96.2**   Assault by letter bomb

⊗⑦**X96.3**   Assault by fertilizer bomb

⊗⑦**X96.4**   Assault by pipe bomb

⊗⑦**X96.8**   Assault by other specified explosive

⊗⑦**X96.9**   Assault by unspecified explosive

X97 Assault by smoke, fire and flames

Assault by arson

Assault by cigarettes

Assault by incendiary device

The appropriate 7th character is to be added to code X97

A - initial encounter

D - subsequent encounter

S - sequela

X98 Assault by steam, hot vapors and hot objects

The appropriate 7th character is to be added to each code from category X98

A - initial encounter

D - subsequent encounter

S - sequela

⊗⑦**X98.0**   Assault by steam or hot vapors

⊗⑦**X98.1**   Assault by hot tap water

⊗⑦**X98.2**   Assault by hot fluids

⊗⑦**X98.3**   Assault by hot household appliances

⊗⑦**X98.8**   Assault by other hot objects

⊗⑦**X98.9**   Assault by unspecified hot objects

X99 Assault by sharp object

Excludes 1: assault by strike by sports equipment (Y08.0-)

The appropriate 7th character is to be added to each code from category X99

A - initial encounter

D - subsequent encounter

S - sequela

⊗⑦**X99.0**   Assault by sharp glass

⊗⑦**X99.1**   Assault by knife

⊗⑦**X99.2**   Assault by sword or dagger

⊗⑦**X99.8**   Assault by other sharp object

⊗⑦**X99.9**   Assault by unspecified sharp object

Assault by stabbing NOS

Y00 Assault by blunt object

Excludes 1: assault by strike by sports equipment (Y08.0-)

The appropriate 7th character is to be added to code Y00

A - initial encounter

D - subsequent encounter

S - sequela

Y01 Assault by pushing from high place

The appropriate 7th character is to be added to code Y01

A - initial encounter

D - subsequent encounter

S - sequela

Y02 Assault by pushing or placing victim in front of moving object

The appropriate 7th character is to be added to each code from category Y02

A - initial encounter

D - subsequent encounter

S - sequela

⊗⑦**Y02.0**   Assault by pushing or placing victim in front of motor vehicle

⊗⑦**Y02.1**   Assault by pushing or placing victim in front of (subway) train

⊗⑦**Y02.8**   Assault by pushing or placing victim in front of other moving object

Y03 Assault by crashing of motor vehicle

The appropriate 7th character is to be added to each code from category Y03

A - initial encounter

D - subsequent encounter

S - sequela

⊗⑦**Y03.0**   Assault by being hit or run over by motor vehicle

⊗⑦**Y03.8**   Other assault by crashing of motor vehicle

Y04 Assault by bodily force

Excludes 1: assault by:

submersion (X92.-)

use of weapon (X93-X95, X99, Y00)

The appropriate 7th character is to be added to each code from category Y04

A - initial encounter

D - subsequent encounter

S - sequela

⊗⑦**Y04.0**   Assault by unarmed brawl or fight

⊗⑦**Y04.1**   Assault by human bite

⊗⑦**Y04.2**   Assault by strike against or bumped into by another person

⊗⑦**Y04.8**   Assault by other bodily force

Assault by bodily force NOS

Y07 Perpetrator of assault, maltreatment and neglect

Note: Codes from this category are for use only in cases of confirmed abuse (T74.-)

Selection of the correct perpetrator code is based on the relationship between the perpetrator and the victim

Includes: perpetrator of abandonment

perpetrator of emotional neglect

perpetrator of mental cruelty

perpetrator of physical abuse

perpetrator of physical neglect

perpetrator of sexual abuse

perpetrator of torture

Y07.0 Spouse or partner, perpetrator of maltreatment and neglect

Spouse or partner, perpetrator of maltreatment and neglect against spouse or partner

Y07.01 Husband, perpetrator of maltreatment and neglect

Y07.02 Wife, perpetrator of maltreatment and neglect

Y07.03 Male partner, perpetrator of maltreatment and neglect

Y07.04 Female partner, perpetrator of maltreatment and neglect

Y07.1 Parent (adoptive) (biological), perpetrator of maltreatment and neglect

Y07.11 Biological father, perpetrator of maltreatment and neglect

Y07.12 Biological mother, perpetrator of maltreatment and neglect

Y07.13 Adoptive father, perpetrator of maltreatment and neglect

Y07.14 Adoptive mother, perpetrator of maltreatment and neglect

Y07.4 Other family member, perpetrator of maltreatment and neglect

Y07.41 Sibling, perpetrator of maltreatment and neglect

Excludes 1: stepsibling, perpetrator of maltreatment and neglect (Y07.435, Y07.436)

Y07.410 Brother, perpetrator of maltreatment and neglect

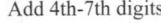

Y07.411 Sister, perpetrator of maltreatment and neglect

Y07.42 Foster parent, perpetrator of maltreatment and neglect

 Y07.420 Foster father, perpetrator of maltreatment and neglect

 Y07.421 Foster mother, perpetrator of maltreatment and neglect

Y07.43 Stepparent or stepsibling, perpetrator of maltreatment and neglect

 Y07.430 Stepfather, perpetrator of maltreatment and neglect

 Y07.432 Male friend of parent (co-residing in household), perpetrator of maltreatment and neglect

 Y07.433 Stepmother, perpetrator of maltreatment and neglect

 Y07.434 Female friend of parent (co-residing in household), perpetrator of maltreatment and neglect

 Y07.435 Stepbrother, perpetrator or maltreatment and neglect

 Y07.436 Stepsister, perpetrator of maltreatment and neglect

Y07.49 Other family member, perpetrator of maltreatment and neglect

 Y07.490 Male cousin, perpetrator of maltreatment and neglect

 Y07.491 Female cousin, perpetrator of maltreatment and neglect

 Y07.499 Other family member, perpetrator of maltreatment and neglect

Y07.5 Non-family member, perpetrator of maltreatment and neglect

 Y07.50 Unspecified non-family member, perpetrator of maltreatment and neglect

 Y07.51 Daycare provider, perpetrator of maltreatment and neglect

  Y07.510 At-home childcare provider, perpetrator of maltreatment and neglect

  Y07.511 Daycare center childcare provider, perpetrator of maltreatment and neglect

  Y07.512 At-home adultcare provider, perpetrator of maltreatment and neglect

  Y07.513 Adultcare center provider, perpetrator of maltreatment and neglect

  Y07.519 Unspecified daycare provider, perpetrator of maltreatment and neglect

 Y07.52 Healthcare provider, perpetrator of maltreatment and neglect

  Y07.521 Mental health provider, perpetrator of maltreatment and neglect

  Y07.528 Other therapist or healthcare provider, perpetrator of maltreatment and neglect

   Nurse perpetrator of maltreatment and neglect

   Occupational therapist perpetrator of maltreatment and neglect

   Physical therapist perpetrator of maltreatment and neglect

   Speech therapist perpetrator of maltreatment and neglect

  Y07.529 Unspecified healthcare provider, perpetrator of maltreatment and neglect

 Y07.53 Teacher or instructor, perpetrator of maltreatment and neglect

   Coach, perpetrator of maltreatment and neglect

 Y07.59 Other non-family member, perpetrator of maltreatment and neglect

Y07.9 Unspecified perpetrator of maltreatment and neglect

Y08 Assault by other specified means

The appropriate 7th character is to be added to each code from category Y08

A - initial encounter

D - subsequent encounter

S - sequela

Y08.0 Assault by strike by sport equipment

 Y08.01 Assault by strike by hockey stick

 Y08.02 Assault by strike by baseball bat

 Y08.09 Assault by strike by other specified type of sport equipment

Y08.8 Assault by other specified means

 Y08.81 Assault by crashing of aircraft

 Y08.89 Assault by other specified means

Y09 Assault by unspecified means

Assassination (attempted) NOS

Homicide (attempted) NOS

Manslaughter (attempted) NOS

Murder (attempted) NOS

EVENT OF UNDETERMINED INTENT (Y21-Y33)

Undetermined intent is only for use when there is specific documentation in the record that the intent of the injury cannot be determined. If no such documentation is present, code to accidental (unintentional)

Y21 Drowning and submersion, undetermined intent

The appropriate 7th character is to be added to each code from category Y21

A - initial encounter

D - subsequent encounter

S - sequela

⊗⑦**Y21.0** Drowning and submersion while in bathtub, undetermined intent

⊗⑦**Y21.1** Drowning and submersion after fall into bathtub, undetermined intent

⊗⑦**Y21.2** Drowning and submersion while in swimming pool, undetermined intent

⊗⑦**Y21.3** Drowning and submersion after fall into swimming pool, undetermined intent

⊗⑦**Y21.4** Drowning and submersion in natural water, undetermined intent

⊗⑦**Y21.8** Other drowning and submersion, undetermined intent

⊗⑦**Y21.9** Unspecified drowning and submersion, undetermined intent

Y22 Handgun discharge, undetermined intent

 ● New code   ▲ Revised code   ⑦ 7th digit required   ⊗ Placeholder required

Discharge of gun for single hand use, undetermined intent
Discharge of pistol, undetermined intent
Discharge of revolver, undetermined intent
Excludes 2: very pistol (Y24.8)
The appropriate 7th character is to be added to code Y22
A - initial encounter
D - subsequent encounter
S - sequela

Y23 Rifle, shotgun and larger firearm discharge, undetermined intent
Excludes 2: airgun (Y24.0)
The appropriate 7th character is to be added to each code from category Y23
A - initial encounter
D - subsequent encounter
S - sequela

⊗⑦**Y23.0** Shotgun discharge, undetermined intent
⊗⑦**Y23.1** Hunting rifle discharge, undetermined intent
⊗⑦**Y23.2** Military firearm discharge, undetermined intent
⊗⑦**Y23.3** Machine gun discharge, undetermined intent
⊗⑦**Y23.8** Other larger firearm discharge, undetermined intent
⊗⑦**Y23.9** Unspecified larger firearm discharge, undetermined intent

Y24 Other and unspecified firearm discharge, undetermined intent
The appropriate 7th character is to be added to each code from category Y24
A - initial encounter
D - subsequent encounter
S - sequela

⊗⑦**Y24.0** Airgun discharge, undetermined intent
BB gun discharge, undetermined intent
Pellet gun discharge, undetermined intent
⊗⑦**Y24.8** Other firearm discharge, undetermined intent
Paintball gun discharge, undetermined intent
Very pistol [flare] discharge, undetermined intent
⊗⑦**Y24.9** Unspecified firearm discharge, undetermined intent

Y25 Contact with explosive material, undetermined intent
The appropriate 7th character is to be added to code Y25
A - initial encounter
D - subsequent encounter
S - sequela

Y26 Exposure to smoke, fire and flames, undetermined intent
The appropriate 7th character is to be added to code Y26
A - initial encounter
D - subsequent encounter
S - sequela

Y27 Contact with steam, hot vapors and hot objects, undetermined intent
The appropriate 7th character is to be added to each code from category Y27
A - initial encounter
D - subsequent encounter
S - sequela

⊗⑦**Y27.0** Contact with steam and hot vapors, undetermined intent
⊗⑦**Y27.1** Contact with hot tap water, undetermined intent
⊗⑦**Y27.2** Contact with hot fluids, undetermined intent
⊗⑦**Y27.3** Contact with hot household appliance, undetermined intent
⊗⑦**Y27.8** Contact with other hot objects, undetermined intent
⊗⑦**Y27.9** Contact with unspecified hot objects, undetermined intent

Y28 Contact with sharp object, undetermined intent
The appropriate 7th character is to be added to each code from category Y28
A - initial encounter
D - subsequent encounter
S - sequela

⊗⑦**Y28.0** Contact with sharp glass, undetermined intent
⊗⑦**Y28.1** Contact with knife, undetermined intent
⊗⑦**Y28.2** Contact with sword or dagger, undetermined intent
⊗⑦**Y28.8** Contact with other sharp object, undetermined intent
⊗⑦**Y28.9** Contact with unspecified sharp object, undetermined intent

Y29 Contact with blunt object, undetermined intent
The appropriate 7th character is to be added to code Y29
A - initial encounter
D - subsequent encounter
S - sequela

Y30 Falling, jumping or pushed from a high place, undetermined intent
Victim falling from one level to another, undetermined intent
The appropriate 7th character is to be added to code Y30
A - initial encounter
D - subsequent encounter
S - sequela

Y31 Falling, lying or running before or into moving object, undetermined intent
The appropriate 7th character is to be added to code Y31
A - initial encounter
D - subsequent encounter
S - sequela

Y32 Crashing of motor vehicle, undetermined intent
The appropriate 7th character is to be added to code Y32
A - initial encounter
D - subsequent encounter
S - sequela

Y33 Other specified events, undetermined intent
The appropriate 7th character is to be added to code Y33
A - initial encounter
D - subsequent encounter
S - sequela

LEGAL INTERVENTION, OPERATIONS OF WAR, MILITARY OPERATIONS, AND TERRORISM (Y35-Y38)

Y35 Legal intervention
Includes: any injury sustained as a result of an encounter with any law enforcement official, serving in any capacity at the time of the encounter, whether on-duty or off-duty. Includes injury to law enforcement official, suspect and bystander
The appropriate 7th character is to be added to each code from category Y35
A - initial encounter
D - subsequent encounter
S - sequela

Y35.0 Legal intervention involving firearm discharge
Y35.00 Legal intervention involving unspecified firearm discharge
Legal intervention involving gunshot wound
Legal intervention involving shot NOS
⑦**Y35.001** Legal intervention involving unspecified firearm discharge, law enforcement official injured

⑦**Y35.002** Legal intervention involving unspecified firearm discharge, bystander injured

⑦**Y35.003** Legal intervention involving unspecified firearm discharge, suspect injured

Y35.01 Legal intervention involving injury by machine gun

⑦**Y35.011** Legal intervention involving injury by machine gun, law enforcement official injured

⑦**Y35.012** Legal intervention involving injury by machine gun, bystander injured

⑦**Y35.013** Legal intervention involving injury by machine gun, suspect injured

Y35.02 Legal intervention involving injury by handgun

⑦**Y35.021** Legal intervention involving injury by handgun, law enforcement official injured

⑦**Y35.022** Legal intervention involving injury by handgun, bystander injured

⑦**Y35.023** Legal intervention involving injury by handgun, suspect injured

Y35.03 Legal intervention involving injury by rifle pellet

⑦**Y35.031** Legal intervention involving injury by rifle pellet, law enforcement official injured

⑦**Y35.032** Legal intervention involving injury by rifle pellet, bystander injured

⑦**Y35.033** Legal intervention involving injury by rifle pellet, suspect injured

Y35.04 Legal intervention involving injury by rubber bullet

⑦**Y35.041** Legal intervention involving injury by rubber bullet, law enforcement official injured

⑦**Y35.042** Legal intervention involving injury by rubber bullet, bystander injured

⑦**Y35.043** Legal intervention involving injury by rubber bullet, suspect injured

Y35.09 Legal intervention involving other firearm discharge

⑦**Y35.091** Legal intervention involving other firearm discharge, law enforcement official injured

⑦**Y35.092** Legal intervention involving other firearm discharge, bystander injured

⑦**Y35.093** Legal intervention involving other firearm discharge, suspect injured

Y35.1 Legal intervention involving explosives

Y35.10 Legal intervention involving unspecified explosives

⑦**Y35.101** Legal intervention involving unspecified explosives, law enforcement official injured

⑦**Y35.102** Legal intervention involving unspecified explosives, bystander injured

⑦**Y35.103** Legal intervention involving unspecified explosives, suspect injured

Y35.11 Legal intervention involving injury by dynamite

⑦**Y35.111** Legal intervention involving injury by dynamite, law enforcement official injured

⑦**Y35.112** Legal intervention involving injury by dynamite, bystander injured

⑦**Y35.113** Legal intervention involving injury by dynamite, suspect injured

Y35.12 Legal intervention involving injury by explosive shell

⑦**Y35.121** Legal intervention involving injury by explosive shell, law enforcement official injured

⑦**Y35.122** Legal intervention involving injury by explosive shell, bystander injured

⑦**Y35.123** Legal intervention involving injury by explosive shell, suspect injured

Y35.19 Legal intervention involving other explosives

Legal intervention involving injury by grenade

Legal intervention involving injury by mortar bomb

⑦**Y35.191** Legal intervention involving other explosives, law enforcement official injured

⑦**Y35.192** Legal intervention involving other explosives, bystander injured

⑦**Y35.193** Legal intervention involving other explosives, suspect injured

Y35.2 Legal intervention involving gas

Legal intervention involving asphyxiation by gas

Legal intervention involving poisoning by gas

Y35.20 Legal intervention involving unspecified gas

⑦**Y35.201** Legal intervention involving unspecified gas, law enforcement official injured

⑦**Y35.202** Legal intervention involving unspecified gas, bystander injured

⑦**Y35.203** Legal intervention involving unspecified gas, suspect injured

Y35.21 Legal intervention involving injury by tear gas

⑦**Y35.211** Legal intervention involving injury by tear gas, law enforcement official injured

⑦**Y35.212** Legal intervention involving injury by tear gas, bystander injured

⑦**Y35.213** Legal intervention involving injury by tear gas, suspect injured

Y35.29 Legal intervention involving other gas

⑦**Y35.291** Legal intervention involving other gas, law enforcement official injured

⑦**Y35.292** Legal intervention involving other gas, bystander injured

⑦**Y35.293** Legal intervention involving other gas, suspect injured

Y35.3 Legal intervention involving blunt objects

● New code   ▲ Revised code   ⑦ 7th digit required   ⊗ Placeholder required

Legal intervention involving being hit or struck by blunt object

Y35.30 Legal intervention involving unspecified blunt objects

⑦**Y35.301** Legal intervention involving unspecified blunt objects, law enforcement official injured

⑦**Y35.302** Legal intervention involving unspecified blunt objects, bystander injured

⑦**Y35.303** Legal intervention involving unspecified blunt objects, suspect injured

Y35.31 Legal intervention involving baton

⑦**Y35.311** Legal intervention involving baton, law enforcement official injured

⑦**Y35.312** Legal intervention involving baton, bystander injured

⑦**Y35.313** Legal intervention involving baton, suspect injured

Y35.39 Legal intervention involving other blunt objects

⑦**Y35.391** Legal intervention involving other blunt objects, law enforcement official injured

⑦**Y35.392** Legal intervention involving other blunt objects, bystander injured

⑦**Y35.393** Legal intervention involving other blunt objects, suspect injured

Y35.4 Legal intervention involving sharp objects

Legal intervention involving being cut by sharp objects

Legal intervention involving being stabbed by sharp objects

Y35.40 Legal intervention involving unspecified sharp objects

⑦**Y35.401** Legal intervention involving unspecified sharp objects, law enforcement official injured

⑦**Y35.402** Legal intervention involving unspecified sharp objects, bystander injured

⑦**Y35.403** Legal intervention involving unspecified sharp objects, suspect injured

Y35.41 Legal intervention involving bayonet

⑦**Y35.411** Legal intervention involving bayonet, law enforcement official injured

⑦**Y35.412** Legal intervention involving bayonet, bystander injured

⑦**Y35.413** Legal intervention involving bayonet, suspect injured

Y35.49 Legal intervention involving other sharp objects

⑦**Y35.491** Legal intervention involving other sharp objects, law enforcement official injured

⑦**Y35.492** Legal intervention involving other sharp objects, bystander injured

⑦**Y35.493** Legal intervention involving other sharp objects, suspect injured

Y35.8 Legal intervention involving other specified means

Y35.81 Legal intervention involving manhandling

⑦**Y35.811** Legal intervention involving manhandling, law enforcement official injured

⑦**Y35.812** Legal intervention involving manhandling, bystander injured

⑦**Y35.813** Legal intervention involving manhandling, suspect injured

Y35.89 Legal intervention involving other specified means

⑦**Y35.891** Legal intervention involving other specified means, law enforcement official injured

⑦**Y35.892** Legal intervention involving other specified means, bystander injured

⑦**Y35.893** Legal intervention involving other specified means, suspect injured

Y35.9 Legal intervention, means unspecified

Y35.91 Legal intervention, means unspecified, law enforcement official injured

Y35.92 Legal intervention, means unspecified, bystander injured

Y35.93 Legal intervention, means unspecified, suspect injured

Y36 Operations of war

Includes: injuries to military personnel and civilians caused by war, civil insurrection, and peacekeeping missions

Excludes 1: injury to military personnel occurring during peacetime military operations (Y37.-)

military vehicles involved in transport accidents with non-military vehicle during peacetime (V09.01, V09.21, V19.81, V29.81, V39.81, V49.81, V59.81, V69.81, V79.81)

The appropriate 7th character is to be added to each code from category Y36

A - initial encounter

D - subsequent encounter

S - sequela

Y36.0 War operations involving explosion of marine weapons

Y36.00 War operations involving explosion of unspecified marine weapon

War operations involving underwater blast NOS

⑦**Y36.000** War operations involving explosion of unspecified marine weapon, militarypersonnel

⑦**Y36.001** War operations involving explosion of unspecified marine weapon, civilian

Y36.01 War operations involving explosion of depth-charge

⑦**Y36.010** War operations involving explosion of depth-charge, military personnel

⑦**Y36.011** War operations involving explosion of depth-charge, civilian

Y36.02 War operations involving explosion of marine mine

War operations involving explosion of marine mine, at sea or in harbor

⑦**Y36.020** War operations involving explosion of marine mine, military personnel

⑦**Y36.021**   War operations involving explosion of marine mine, civilian

Y36.03   War operations involving explosion of sea-based artillery shell

⑦**Y36.030**   War operations involving explosion of sea-based artillery shell, military personnel

⑦**Y36.031**   War operations involving explosion of sea-based artillery shell, civilian

Y36.04   War operations involving explosion of torpedo

⑦**Y36.040**   War operations involving explosion of torpedo, military personnel

⑦**Y36.041**   War operations involving explosion of torpedo, civilian

Y36.05   War operations involving accidental detonation of onboard marine weapons

⑦**Y36.050**   War operations involving accidental detonation of onboard marine weapons, military personnel

⑦**Y36.051**   War operations involving accidental detonation of onboard marine weapons, civilian

Y36.09   War operations involving explosion of other marine weapons

⑦**Y36.090**   War operations involving explosion of other marine weapons, military personnel

⑦**Y36.091**   War operations involving explosion of other marine weapons, civilian

Y36.1   War operations involving destruction of aircraft

Y36.10   War operations involving unspecified destruction of aircraft

⑦**Y36.100**   War operations involving unspecified destruction of aircraft, military personnel

⑦**Y36.101**   War operations involving unspecified destruction of aircraft, civilian

Y36.11   War operations involving destruction of aircraft due to enemy fire or explosives

War operations involving destruction of aircraft due to air to air missile

War operations involving destruction of aircraft due to explosive placed on aircraft

War operations involving destruction of aircraft due to rocket propelled grenade [RPG]

War operations involving destruction of aircraft due to small arms fire

War operations involving destruction of aircraft due to surface to air missile

⑦**Y36.110**   War operations involving destruction of aircraft due to enemy fire or explosives, military personnel

⑦**Y36.111**   War operations involving destruction of aircraft due to enemy fire or explosives, civilian

Y36.12   War operations involving destruction of aircraft due to collision with other aircraft

⑦**Y36.120**   War operations involving destruction of aircraft due to

collision with other aircraft, military personnel

⑦**Y36.121**   War operations involving destruction of aircraft due to collision with other aircraft, civilian

Y36.13   War operations involving destruction of aircraft due to onboard fire

⑦**Y36.130**   War operations involving destruction of aircraft due to onboard fire, military personnel

⑦**Y36.131**   War operations involving destruction of aircraft due to onboard fire, civilian

Y36.14   War operations involving destruction of aircraft due to accidental detonation of onboard munitions and explosives

⑦**Y36.140**   War operations involving destruction of aircraft due to accidental detonation of onboard munitions and explosives, military personnel

⑦**Y36.141**   War operations involving destruction of aircraft due to accidental detonation of onboard munitions and explosives, civilian

Y36.19   War operations involving other destruction of aircraft

⑦**Y36.190**   War operations involving other destruction of aircraft, military personnel

⑦**Y36.191**   War operations involving other destruction of aircraft, civilian

Y36.2   War operations involving other explosions and fragments

Excludes 1: war operations involving explosion of aircraft (Y36.1-)

war operations involving explosion of marine weapons (Y36.0-)

war operations involving explosion of nuclear weapons (Y36.5-)

war operations involving explosion occurring after cessation of hostilities (Y36.8-)

Y36.20   War operations involving unspecified explosion and fragments

War operations involving air blast NOS

War operations involving blast NOS

War operations involving blast fragments NOS

War operations involving blast wave NOS

War operations involving blast wind NOS

War operations involving explosion NOS

War operations involving explosion of bomb NOS

⑦**Y36.200**   War operations involving unspecified explosion and fragments, military personnel

⑦**Y36.201**   War operations involving unspecified explosion and fragments, civilian

Y36.21   War operations involving explosion of aerial bomb

⑦**Y36.210**   War operations involving explosion of aerial bomb, military personnel

● New code   ▲ Revised code   ⑦ 7ᵗʰ digit required   ⊗ Placeholder required

⑦**Y36.211** War operations involving explosion of aerial bomb, civilian

Y36.22 War operations involving explosion of guided missile

⑦**Y36.220** War operations involving explosion of guided missile, military personnel

⑦**Y36.221** War operations involving explosion of guided missile, civilian

Y36.23 War operations involving explosion of improvised explosive device [IED]

War operations involving explosion of person-borne improvised explosive device [IED]

War operations involving explosion of vehicle-borne improvised explosive device [IED]

War operations involving explosion of roadside improvised explosive device [IED]

⑦**Y36.230** War operations involving explosion of improvised explosive device [IED], military personnel

⑦**Y36.231** War operations involving explosion of improvised explosive device [IED], civilian

Y36.24 War operations involving explosion due to accidental detonation and discharge of own munitions or munitions launch device

⑦**Y36.240** War operations involving explosion due to accidental detonation and discharge of own munitions or munitions launch device, military personnel

⑦**Y36.241** War operations involving explosion due to accidental detonation and discharge of own munitions or munitions launch device, civilian

Y36.25 War operations involving fragments from munitions

⑦**Y36.250** War operations involving fragments from munitions, military personnel

⑦**Y36.251** War operations involving fragments from munitions, civilian

Y36.26 War operations involving fragments of improvised explosive device [IED]

War operations involving fragments of person-borne improvised explosive device [IED]

War operations involving fragments of vehicle-borne improvised explosive device [IED]

War operations involving fragments of roadside improvised explosive device [IED]

⑦**Y36.260** War operations involving fragments of improvised explosive device [IED], military personnel

⑦**Y36.261** War operations involving fragments of improvised explosive device [IED], civilian

Y36.27 War operations involving fragments from weapons

⑦**Y36.270** War operations involving fragments from weapons, military personnel

⑦**Y36.271** War operations involving fragments from weapons, civilian

Y36.29 War operations involving other explosions and fragments

War operations involving explosion of grenade

War operations involving explosions of land mine

War operations involving shrapnel NOS

⑦**Y36.290** War operations involving other explosions and fragments, military personnel

⑦**Y36.291** War operations involving other explosions and fragments, civilian

Y36.3 War operations involving fires, conflagrations and hot substances

War operations involving smoke, fumes, and heat from fires, conflagrations and hot substances

Excludes 1: war operations involving fires and conflagrations aboard military aircraft (Y36.1-)

war operations involving fires and conflagrations aboard military watercraft (Y36.0-)

war operations involving fires and conflagrations caused indirectly by conventional weapons (Y36.2-)

war operations involving fires and thermal effects of nuclear weapons (Y36.53-)

Y36.30 War operations involving unspecified fire, conflagration and hot substance

⑦**Y36.300** War operations involving unspecified fire, conflagration and hot substance, military personnel

⑦**Y36.301** War operations involving unspecified fire, conflagration and hot substance, civilian

Y36.31 War operations involving gasoline bomb

War operations involving incendiary bomb

War operations involving petrol bomb

⑦**Y36.310** War operations involving gasoline bomb, military personnel

⑦**Y36.311** War operations involving gasoline bomb, civilian

Y36.32 War operations involving incendiary bullet

⑦**Y36.320** War operations involving incendiary bullet, military personnel

⑦**Y36.321** War operations involving incendiary bullet, civilian

Y36.33 War operations involving flamethrower

⑦**Y36.330** War operations involving flamethrower, military personnel

⑦**Y36.331** War operations involving flamethrower, civilian

Y36.39 War operations involving other fires, conflagrations and hot substances

⑦**Y36.390** War operations involving other fires, conflagrations and hot substances, military personnel

⑦**Y36.391** War operations involving other fires, conflagrations and hot substances, civilian

Y36.4 War operations involving firearm discharge and other forms of conventional warfare

Y36.41 War operations involving rubber bullets

⑦Y36.410 War operations involving rubber bullets, military personnel

⑦Y36.411 War operations involving rubber bullets, civilian

Y36.42 War operations involving firearms pellets

⑦Y36.420 War operations involving firearms pellets, military personnel

⑦Y36.421 War operations involving firearms pellets, civilian

Y36.43 War operations involving other firearms discharge
War operations involving bullets NOS
Excludes 1: war operations involving munitions fragments (Y36.25-)
war operations involving incendiary bullets (Y36.32-)

⑦Y36.430 War operations involving other firearms discharge, military personnel

⑦Y36.431 War operations involving other firearms discharge, civilian

Y36.44 War operations involving unarmed hand to hand combat
Excludes 1: war operations involving combat using blunt or piercing object (Y36.45-)
war operations involving intentional restriction of air and airway (Y36.46-)
war operations involving unintentional restriction of air and airway (Y36.47-)

⑦Y36.440 War operations involving unarmed hand to hand combat, military personnel

⑦Y36.441 War operations involving unarmed hand to hand combat, civilian

Y36.45 War operations involving combat using blunt or piercing object

⑦Y36.450 War operations involving combat using blunt or piercing object, military personnel

⑦Y36.451 War operations involving combat using blunt or piercing object, civilian

Y36.46 War operations involving intentional restriction of air and airway

⑦Y36.460 War operations involving intentional restriction of air and airway, military personnel

⑦Y36.461 War operations involving intentional restriction of air and airway, civilian

Y36.47 War operations involving unintentional restriction of air and airway

⑦Y36.470 War operations involving unintentional restriction of air and airway, military personnel

⑦Y36.471 War operations involving unintentional restriction of air and airway, civilian

Y36.49 War operations involving other forms of conventional warfare

⑦Y36.490 War operations involving other forms of conventional warfare, military personnel

⑦Y36.491 War operations involving other forms of conventional warfare, civilian

Y36.5 War operations involving nuclear weapons
War operations involving dirty bomb NOS

Y36.50 War operations involving unspecified effect of nuclear weapon

⑦Y36.500 War operations involving unspecified effect of nuclear weapon, military personnel

⑦Y36.501 War operations involving unspecified effect of nuclear weapon, civilian

Y36.51 War operations involving direct blast effect of nuclear weapon
War operations involving blast pressure of nuclear weapon

⑦Y36.510 War operations involving direct blast effect of nuclear weapon, military personnel

⑦Y36.511 War operations involving direct blast effect of nuclear weapon, civilian

Y36.52 War operations involving indirect blast effect of nuclear weapon
War operations involving being thrown by blast of nuclear weapon
War operations involving being struck or crushed by blast debris of nuclear weapon

⑦Y36.520 War operations involving indirect blast effect of nuclear weapon, military personnel

⑦Y36.521 War operations involving indirect blast effect of nuclear weapon, civilian

Y36.53 War operations involving thermal radiation effect of nuclear weapon
War operations involving direct heat from nuclear weapon
War operation involving fireball effects from nuclear weapon

⑦Y36.530 War operations involving thermal radiation effect of nuclear weapon, military personnel

⑦Y36.531 War operations involving thermal radiation effect of nuclear weapon, civilian

Y36.54 War operation involving nuclear radiation effects of nuclear weapon
War operation involving acute radiation exposure from nuclear weapon
War operation involving exposure to immediate ionizing radiation from nuclear weapon
War operation involving fallout exposure from nuclear weapon

● New code   ▲ Revised code   ⑦ 7th digit required   ⊗ Placeholder required

War operation involving secondary effects of nuclear weapons

⑦Y36.540   War operation involving nuclear radiation effects of nuclear weapon, military personnel

⑦Y36.541   War operation involving nuclear radiation effects of nuclear weapon, civilian

Y36.59   War operation involving other effects of nuclear weapons

⑦Y36.590   War operation involving other effects of nuclear weapons, military personnel

⑦Y36.591   War operation involving other effects of nuclear weapons, civilian

Y36.6   War operations involving biological weapons

Y36.6X   War operations involving biological weapons

⑦Y36.6X0   War operations involving biological weapons, military personnel

⑦Y36.6X1   War operations involving biological weapons, civilian

Y36.7   War operations involving chemical weapons and other forms of unconventional warfare

Excludes 1: war operations involving incendiary devices (Y36.3-, Y36.5-)

Y36.7X   War operations involving chemical weapons and other forms of unconventional warfare

⑦Y36.7X0   War operations involving chemical weapons and other forms of unconventional warfare, military personnel

⑦Y36.7X1   War operations involving chemical weapons and other forms of unconventional warfare, civilian

Y36.8   War operations occurring after cessation of hostilities

War operations classifiable to categories Y36.0-Y36.8 but occurring after cessation of hostilities

Y36.81   Explosion of mine placed during war operations but exploding after cessation of hostilities

⑦Y36.810   Explosion of mine placed during war operations but exploding after cessation of hostilities, military personnel

⑦Y36.811   Explosion of mine placed during war operations but exploding after cessation of hostilities, civilian

Y36.82   Explosion of bomb placed during war operations but exploding after cessation of hostilities

⑦Y36.820   Explosion of bomb placed during war operations but exploding after cessation of hostilities, military personnel

⑦Y36.821   Explosion of bomb placed during war operations but exploding after cessation of hostilities, civilian

Y36.88   Other war operations occurring after cessation of hostilities

⑦Y36.880   Other war operations occurring after cessation of hostilities, military personnel

⑦Y36.881   Other war operations occurring after cessation of hostilities, civilian

Y36.89   Unspecified war operations occurring after cessation of hostilities

⑦Y36.890   Unspecified war operations occurring after cessation of hostilities, military personnel

⑦Y36.891   Unspecified war operations occurring after cessation of hostilities, civilian

Y36.9   Other and unspecified war operations

Y36.90   War operations, unspecified

Y36.91   War operations involving unspecified weapon of mass destruction [WMD]

Y36.92   War operations involving friendly fire

Y37   Military operations

Includes: injuries to military personnel and civilians occurring during peacetime on military property and during routine military exercises and operations

Excludes 1: military aircraft involved in aircraft accident with civilian aircraft (V97.81-)

military vehicles involved in transport accident with civilian vehicle (V09.01, V09.21, V19.81, V29.81, V39.81, V49.81, V59.81, V69.81, V79.81)

military watercraft involved in water transport accident with civilian watercraft (V94.81-)

war operations (Y36.-)

The appropriate 7th character is to be added to each code from category Y37

A - initial encounter

D - subsequent encounter

S - sequela

Y37.0   Military operations involving explosion of marine weapons

Y37.00   Military operations involving explosion of unspecified marine weapon

Military operations involving underwater blast NOS

⑦Y37.000   Military operations involving explosion of unspecified marine weapon, military personnel

⑦Y37.001   Military operations involving explosion of unspecified marine weapon, civilian

Y37.01   Military operations involving explosion of depth-charge

⑦Y37.010   Military operations involving explosion of depth-charge, military personnel

⑦Y37.011   Military operations involving explosion of depth-charge, civilian

Y37.02   Military operations involving explosion of marine mine

Military operations involving explosion of marine mine, at sea or in harbor

⑦Y37.020   Military operations involving explosion of marine mine, military personnel

⑦Y37.021   Military operations involving explosion of marine mine, civilian

Y37.03 Military operations involving explosion of sea-based artillery shell

⑦ **Y37.030** Military operations involving explosion of sea-based artillery shell, military personnel

⑦ **Y37.031** Military operations involving explosion of sea-based artillery shell, civilian

Y37.04 Military operations involving explosion of torpedo

⑦ **Y37.040** Military operations involving explosion of torpedo, military personnel

⑦ **Y37.041** Military operations involving explosion of torpedo, civilian

Y37.05 Military operations involving accidental detonation of onboard marine weapons

⑦ **Y37.050** Military operations involving accidental detonation of onboard marine weapons, military personnel

⑦ **Y37.051** Military operations involving accidental detonation of onboard marine weapons, civilian

Y37.09 Military operations involving explosion of other marine weapons

⑦ **Y37.090** Military operations involving explosion of other marine weapons, military personnel

⑦ **Y37.091** Military operations involving explosion of other marine weapons, civilian

Y37.1 Military operations involving destruction of aircraft

Y37.10 Military operations involving unspecified destruction of aircraft

⑦ **Y37.100** Military operations involving unspecified destruction of aircraft, military personnel

⑦ **Y37.101** Military operations involving unspecified destruction of aircraft, civilian

Y37.11 Military operations involving destruction of aircraft due to enemy fire or explosives

Military operations involving destruction of aircraft due to air to air missile

Military operations involving destruction of aircraft due to explosive placed on aircraft

Military operations involving destruction of aircraft due to rocket propelled grenade [RPG]

Military operations involving destruction of aircraft due to small arms fire

Military operations involving destruction of aircraft due to surface to air missile

⑦ **Y37.110** Military operations involving destruction of aircraft due to enemy fire or explosives, military personnel

⑦ **Y37.111** Military operations involving destruction of aircraft due to enemy fire or explosives, civilian

Y37.12 Military operations involving destruction of aircraft due to collision with other aircraft

⑦ **Y37.120** Military operations involving destruction of aircraft due to collision with other aircraft, military personnel

⑦ **Y37.121** Military operations involving destruction of aircraft due to collision with other aircraft, civilian

Y37.13 Military operations involving destruction of aircraft due to onboard fire

⑦ **Y37.130** Military operations involving destruction of aircraft due to onboard fire, military personnel

⑦ **Y37.131** Military operations involving destruction of aircraft due to onboard fire, civilian

Y37.14 Military operations involving destruction of aircraft due to accidental detonation of onboard munitions and explosives

⑦ **Y37.140** Military operations involving destruction of aircraft due to accidental detonation of onboard munitions and explosives, military personnel

⑦ **Y37.141** Military operations involving destruction of aircraft due to accidental detonation of onboard munitions and explosives, civilian

Y37.19 Military operations involving other destruction of aircraft

⑦ **Y37.190** Military operations involving other destruction of aircraft, military personnel

⑦ **Y37.191** Military operations involving other destruction of aircraft, civilian

Y37.2 Military operations involving other explosions and fragments

Excludes 1: military operations involving explosion of aircraft (Y37.1-)

military operations involving explosion of marine weapons (Y37.0-)

military operations involving explosion of nuclear weapons (Y37.5-)

Y37.20 Military operations involving unspecified explosion and fragments

Military operations involving air blast NOS

Military operations involving blast NOS

Military operations involving blast fragments NOS

Military operations involving blast wave NOS

Military operations involving blast wind NOS

Military operations involving explosion NOS

Military operations involving explosion of bomb NOS

⑦ **Y37.200** Military operations involving unspecified explosion and fragments, military personnel

⑦ **Y37.201** Military operations involving unspecified explosion and fragments, civilian

Y37.21 Military operations involving explosion of aerial bomb

● New code   ▲ Revised code   ⑦ 7ᵗʰ digit required   ⊗ Placeholder required

⑦ **Y37.210** Military operations involving explosion of aerial bomb, military personnel

⑦ **Y37.211** Military operations involving explosion of aerial bomb, civilian

Y37.22 Military operations involving explosion of guided missile

⑦ **Y37.220** Military operations involving explosion of guided missile, military personnel

⑦ **Y37.221** Military operations involving explosion of guided missile, civilian

Y37.23 Military operations involving explosion of improvised explosive device [IED]

Military operations involving explosion of person-borne improvised explosive device [IED]

Military operations involving explosion of vehicle-borne improvised explosive device [IED]

Military operations involving explosion of roadside improvised explosive device [IED]

⑦ **Y37.230** Military operations involving explosion of improvised explosive device [IED], military personnel

⑦ **Y37.231** Military operations involving explosion of improvised explosive device [IED], civilian

Y37.24 Military operations involving explosion due to accidental detonation and discharge of own munitions or munitions launch device

⑦ **Y37.240** Military operations involving explosion due to accidental detonation and discharge of own munitions or munitions launch device, military personnel

⑦ **Y37.241** Military operations involving explosion due to accidental detonation and discharge of own munitions or munitions launch device, civilian

Y37.25 Military operations involving fragments from munitions

⑦ **Y37.250** Military operations involving fragments from munitions, military personnel

⑦ **Y37.251** Military operations involving fragments from munitions, civilian

Y37.26 Military operations involving fragments of improvised explosive device [IED]

Military operations involving fragments of person-borne improvised explosive device [IED]

Military operations involving fragments of vehicle-borne improvised explosive device [IED]

Military operations involving fragments of roadside improvised explosive device [IED]

⑦ **Y37.260** Military operations involving fragments of improvised explosive device [IED], military personnel

⑦ **Y37.261** Military operations involving fragments of improvised explosive device [IED], civilian

Y37.27 Military operations involving fragments from weapons

⑦ **Y37.270** Military operations involving fragments from weapons, military personnel

⑦ **Y37.271** Military operations involving fragments from weapons, civilian

Y37.29 Military operations involving other explosions and fragments

Military operations involving explosion of grenade

Military operations involving explosions of land mine

Military operations involving shrapnel NOS

⑦ **Y37.290** Military operations involving other explosions and fragments, military personnel

⑦ **Y37.291** Military operations involving other explosions and fragments, civilian

Y37.3 Military operations involving fires, conflagrations and hot substances

Military operations involving smoke, fumes, and heat from fires, conflagrations and hot substances

Excludes 1: military operations involving fires and conflagrations aboard military aircraft (Y37.1-)

military operations involving fires and conflagrations aboard military watercraft (Y37.0-)

military operations involving fires and conflagrations caused indirectly by conventional weapons (Y37.2-)

military operations involving fires and thermal effects of nuclear weapons (Y36.53-)

Y37.30 Military operations involving unspecified fire, conflagration and hot substance

⑦ **Y37.300** Military operations involving unspecified fire, conflagration and hot substance, military personnel

⑦ **Y37.301** Military operations involving unspecified fire, conflagration and hot substance, civilian

Y37.31 Military operations involving gasoline bomb

Military operations involving incendiary bomb

Military operations involving petrol bomb

⑦ **Y37.310** Military operations involving gasoline bomb, military personnel

⑦ **Y37.311** Military operations involving gasoline bomb, civilian

Y37.32 Military operations involving incendiary bullet

⑦ **Y37.320** Military operations involving incendiary bullet, military personnel

⑦ **Y37.321** Military operations involving incendiary bullet, civilian

Y37.33 Military operations involving flamethrower

⑦ **Y37.330** Military operations involving flamethrower, military personnel

⑦ **Y37.331** Military operations involving flamethrower, civilian

Y37.39 Military operations involving other fires, conflagrations and hot substances

⑦Y37.390   Military operations involving other fires, conflagrations and hot substances, military personnel

⑦Y37.391   Military operations involving other fires, conflagrations and hot substances, civilian

Y37.4   Military operations involving firearm discharge and other forms of conventional warfare

   Y37.41   Military operations involving rubber bullets

     ⑦Y37.410   Military operations involving rubber bullets, military personnel

     ⑦Y37.411   Military operations involving rubber bullets, civilian

   Y37.42   Military operations involving firearms pellets

     ⑦Y37.420   Military operations involving firearms pellets, military personnel

     ⑦Y37.421   Military operations involving firearms pellets, civilian

   Y37.43   Military operations involving other firearms discharge

     Military operations involving bullets NOS

     Excludes 1: military operations involving munitions fragments (Y37.25-)

           military operations involving incendiary bullets (Y37.32-)

     ⑦Y37.430   Military operations involving other firearms discharge, military personnel

     ⑦Y37.431   Military operations involving other firearms discharge, civilian

   Y37.44   Military operations involving unarmed hand to hand combat

     Excludes 1: military operations involving combat using blunt or piercing object (Y37.45-)

           military operations involving intentional restriction of air and airway (Y37.46-)

           military operations involving unintentional restriction of air and airway (Y37.47-)

     ⑦Y37.440   Military operations involving unarmed hand to hand combat, military personnel

     ⑦Y37.441   Military operations involving unarmed hand to hand combat, civilian

   Y37.45   Military operations involving combat using blunt or piercing object

     ⑦Y37.450   Military operations involving combat using blunt or piercing object, military personnel

     ⑦Y37.451   Military operations involving combat using blunt or piercing object, civilian

   Y37.46   Military operations involving intentional restriction of air and airway

     ⑦Y37.460   Military operations involving intentional restriction of air and airway, military personnel

     ⑦Y37.461   Military operations involving intentional restriction of air and airway, civilian

   Y37.47   Military operations involving unintentional restriction of air and airway

     ⑦Y37.470   Military operations involving unintentional restriction of air and airway, military personnel

     ⑦Y37.471   Military operations involving unintentional restriction of air and airway, civilian

   Y37.49   Military operations involving other forms of conventional warfare

     ⑦Y37.490   Military operations involving other forms of conventional warfare, military personnel

     ⑦Y37.491   Military operations involving other forms of conventional warfare, civilian

Y37.5   Military operations involving nuclear weapons

   Military operation involving dirty bomb NOS

   Y37.50   Military operations involving unspecified effect of nuclear weapon

     ⑦Y37.500   Military operations involving unspecified effect of nuclear weapon, military personnel

     ⑦Y37.501   Military operations involving unspecified effect of nuclear weapon, civilian

   Y37.51   Military operations involving direct blast effect of nuclear weapon

     Military operations involving blast pressure of nuclear weapon

     ⑦Y37.510   Military operations involving direct blast effect of nuclear weapon, military personnel

     ⑦Y37.511   Military operations involving direct blast effect of nuclear weapon, civilian

   Y37.52   Military operations involving indirect blast effect of nuclear weapon

     Military operations involving being thrown by blast of nuclear weapon

     Military operations involving being struck or crushed by blast debris of nuclear weapon

     ⑦Y37.520   Military operations involving indirect blast effect of nuclear weapon, military personnel

     ⑦Y37.521   Military operations involving indirect blast effect of nuclear weapon, civilian

   Y37.53   Military operations involving thermal radiation effect of nuclear weapon

     Military operations involving direct heat from nuclear weapon

     Military operation involving fireball effects from nuclear weapon

     ⑦Y37.530   Military operations involving thermal radiation effect of nuclear weapon, military personnel

⑦**Y37.531**   Military operations involving thermal radiation effect of nuclear weapon, civilian

Y37.54   Military operation involving nuclear radiation effects of nuclear weapon
Military operation involving acute radiation exposure from nuclear weapon
Military operation involving exposure to immediate ionizing radiation from nuclear weapon
Military operation involving fallout exposure from nuclear weapon
Military operation involving secondary effects of nuclear weapons

⑦**Y37.540**   Military operation involving nuclear radiation effects of nuclear weapon, military personnel

⑦**Y37.541**   Military operation involving nuclear radiation effects of nuclear weapon, civilian

Y37.59   Military operation involving other effects of nuclear weapons

⑦**Y37.590**   Military operation involving other effects of nuclear weapons, military personnel

⑦**Y37.591**   Military operation involving other effects of nuclear weapons, civilian

Y37.6   Military operations involving biological weapons

Y37.6X   Military operations involving biological weapons

⑦**Y37.6X0**   Military operations involving biological weapons, military personnel

⑦**Y37.6X1**   Military operations involving biological weapons, civilian

Y37.7   Military operations involving chemical weapons and other forms of unconventional warfare

Excludes 1: military operations involving incendiary devices (Y36.3-, Y36.5-)

Y37.7X   Military operations involving chemical weapons and other forms of unconventional warfare

⑦**Y37.7X0**   Military operations involving chemical weapons and other forms of unconventional warfare, military personnel

⑦**Y37.7X1**   Military operations involving chemical weapons and other forms of unconventional warfare, civilian

Y37.9   Other and unspecified military operations

Y37.90   Military operations, unspecified

Y37.91   Military operations involving unspecified weapon of mass destruction [WMD]

Y37.92   Military operations involving friendly fire

Y38 Terrorism

These codes are for use to identify injuries resulting from the unlawful use of force or violence against persons or property to intimidate or coerce a Government, the civilian population, or any segment thereof, in furtherance of political or social objective

Use additional code for place of occurrence (Y92.-)

The appropriate 7th character is to be added to each code from category Y38

A - initial encounter

D - subsequent encounter

S - sequela

Y38.0   Terrorism involving explosion of marine weapons
Terrorism involving depth-charge
Terrorism involving marine mine
Terrorism involving mine NOS, at sea or in harbor
Terrorism involving sea-based artillery shell
Terrorism involving torpedo
Terrorism involving underwater blast

Y38.0X   Terrorism involving explosion of marine weapons

⑦**Y38.0X1**   Terrorism involving explosion of marine weapons, public safety official injured

⑦**Y38.0X2**   Terrorism involving explosion of marine weapons, civilian injured

⑦**Y38.0X3**   Terrorism involving explosion of marine weapons, terrorist injured

Y38.1   Terrorism involving destruction of aircraft
Terrorism involving aircraft burned
Terrorism involving aircraft exploded
Terrorism involving aircraft being shot down
Terrorism involving aircraft used as a weapon

Y38.1X   Terrorism involving destruction of aircraft

⑦**Y38.1X1**   Terrorism involving destruction of aircraft, public safety official injured

⑦**Y38.1X2**   Terrorism involving destruction of aircraft, civilian injured

⑦**Y38.1X3**   Terrorism involving destruction of aircraft, terrorist injured

Y38.2   Terrorism involving other explosions and fragments
Terrorism involving antipersonnel (fragments) bomb
Terrorism involving blast NOS
Terrorism involving explosion NOS
Terrorism involving explosion of breech block
Terrorism involving explosion of cannon block
Terrorism involving explosion (fragments) of artillery shell
Terrorism involving explosion (fragments) of bomb
Terrorism involving explosion (fragments) of grenade
Terrorism involving explosion (fragments) of guided missile
Terrorism involving explosion (fragments) of land mine
Terrorism involving explosion of mortar bomb
Terrorism involving explosion of munitions
Terrorism involving explosion (fragments) of rocket
Terrorism involving explosion (fragments) of shell
Terrorism involving shrapnel
Terrorism involving mine NOS, on land

Excludes 1: terrorism involving explosion of nuclear weapon (Y38.5)
terrorism involving suicide bomber (Y38.81)

Y38.2X   Terrorism involving other explosions and fragments

⑦**Y38.2X1**   Terrorism involving other explosions and fragments, public safety official injured

⑦**Y38.2X2**   Terrorism involving other explosions and fragments, civilian injured

---

⑦ **Y38.2X3** Terrorism involving other explosions and fragments, terrorist injured

Y38.3 Terrorism involving fires, conflagration and hot substances
Terrorism involving conflagration NOS
Terrorism involving fire NOS
Terrorism involving petrol bomb
Excludes 1: terrorism involving fire or heat of nuclear weapon (Y38.5)

Y38.3X Terrorism involving fires, conflagration and hot substances

⑦ **Y38.3X1** Terrorism involving fires, conflagration and hot substances, public safety official injured

⑦ **Y38.3X2** Terrorism involving fires, conflagration and hot substances, civilian injured

⑦ **Y38.3X3** Terrorism involving fires, conflagration and hot substances, terrorist injured

Y38.4 Terrorism involving firearms
Terrorism involving carbine bullet
Terrorism involving machine gun bullet
Terrorism involving pellets (shotgun)
Terrorism involving pistol bullet
Terrorism involving rifle bullet
Terrorism involving rubber (rifle) bullet

Y38.4X Terrorism involving firearms

⑦ **Y38.4X1** Terrorism involving firearms, public safety official injured

⑦ **Y38.4X2** Terrorism involving firearms, civilian injured

⑦ **Y38.4X3** Terrorism involving firearms, terrorist injured

Y38.5 Terrorism involving nuclear weapons
Terrorism involving blast effects of nuclear weapon
Terrorism involving exposure to ionizing radiation from nuclear weapon
Terrorism involving fireball effect of nuclear weapon
Terrorism involving heat from nuclear weapon

Y38.5X Terrorism involving nuclear weapons

⑦ **Y38.5X1** Terrorism involving nuclear weapons, public safety official injured

⑦ **Y38.5X2** Terrorism involving nuclear weapons, civilian injured

⑦ **Y38.5X3** Terrorism involving nuclear weapons, terrorist injured

Y38.6 Terrorism involving biological weapons
Terrorism involving anthrax
Terrorism involving cholera
Terrorism involving smallpox

Y38.6X Terrorism involving biological weapons

⑦ **Y38.6X1** Terrorism involving biological weapons, public safety official injured

⑦ **Y38.6X2** Terrorism involving biological weapons, civilian injured

⑦ **Y38.6X3** Terrorism involving biological weapons, terrorist injured

Y38.7 Terrorism involving chemical weapons
Terrorism involving gases, fumes, chemicals
Terrorism involving hydrogen cyanide
Terrorism involving phosgene
Terrorism involving sarin

Y38.7X Terrorism involving chemical weapons

⑦ **Y38.7X1** Terrorism involving chemical weapons, public safety official injured

⑦ **Y38.7X2** Terrorism involving chemical weapons, civilian injured

⑦ **Y38.7X3** Terrorism involving chemical weapons, terrorist injured

Y38.8 Terrorism involving other and unspecified means

Y38.80 Terrorism involving unspecified means
Terrorism NOS

Y38.81 Terrorism involving suicide bomber

⑦ **Y38.811** Terrorism involving suicide bomber, public safety official injured

⑦ **Y38.812** Terrorism involving suicide bomber, civilian injured

Y38.89 Terrorism involving other means
Terrorism involving drowning and submersion
Terrorism involving lasers
Terrorism involving piercing or stabbing instruments

⑦ **Y38.891** Terrorism involving other means, public safety official injured

⑦ **Y38.892** Terrorism involving other means, civilian injured

⑦ **Y38.893** Terrorism involving other means, terrorist injured

Y38.9 Terrorism, secondary effects
Note: This code is for use to identify conditions occurring subsequent to a terrorist attack not those that are due to the initial terrorist attack

Y38.9X Terrorism, secondary effects

⑦ **Y38.9X1** Terrorism, secondary effects, public safety official injured

⑦ **Y38.9X2** Terrorism, secondary effects, civilian injured

COMPLICATIONS OF MEDICAL AND SURGICAL CARE (Y62-Y84)
Includes: complications of medical devices
surgical and medical procedures as the cause of abnormal reaction of the patient, or of later complication, without mention of misadventure at the time of the procedure

MISADVENTURES TO PATIENTS DURING SURGICAL AND MEDICAL CARE (Y62-Y69)
Excludes 2: breakdown or malfunctioning of medical device (during procedure) (after implantation) (ongoing use) (Y70-Y82)
surgical and medical procedures as the cause of abnormal reaction of the patient, without mention of misadventure at the time of the procedure (Y83-Y84)

 Failure of sterile precautions during surgical and medical care

Y62.0 Failure of sterile precautions during surgical operation

Y62.1 Failure of sterile precautions during infusion or transfusion

Y62.2 Failure of sterile precautions during kidney dialysis and other perfusion

Y62.3 Failure of sterile precautions during injection or immunization

Y62.4 Failure of sterile precautions during endoscopic examination

Y62.5 Failure of sterile precautions during heart catheterization

Y62.6 Failure of sterile precautions during aspiration, puncture and other catheterization

Y62.8 Failure of sterile precautions during other surgical and medical care

Y62.9 Failure of sterile precautions during unspecified surgical and medical care

Y63 Failure in dosage during surgical and medical care

Excludes 2: accidental overdose of drug or wrong drug given in error (T36-T50)

Y63.0 Excessive amount of blood or other fluid given during transfusion or infusion

Y63.1 Incorrect dilution of fluid used during infusion

Y63.2 Overdose of radiation given during therapy

Y63.3 Inadvertent exposure of patient to radiation during medical care

Y63.4 Failure in dosage in electroshock or insulin-shock therapy

Y63.5 Inappropriate temperature in local application and packing

Y63.6 Underdosing and nonadministration of necessary drug, medicament or biological substance

Y63.8 Failure in dosage during other surgical and medical care

Y63.9 Failure in dosage during unspecified surgical and medical care

Y64 Contaminated medical or biological substances

Y64.0 Contaminated medical or biological substance, transfused or infused

Y64.1 Contaminated medical or biological substance, injected or used for immunization

Y64.8 Contaminated medical or biological substance administered by other means

Y64.9 Contaminated medical or biological substance administered by unspecified means

Administered contaminated medical or biological substance NOS

Y65 Other misadventures during surgical and medical care

Y65.0 Mismatched blood in transfusion

Y65.1 Wrong fluid used in infusion

Y65.2 Failure in suture or ligature during surgical operation

Y65.3 Endotracheal tube wrongly placed during anesthetic procedure

Y65.4 Failure to introduce or to remove other tube or instrument

Y65.5 Performance of wrong procedure (operation)

  Y65.51 Performance of wrong procedure (operation) on correct patient

  Wrong device implanted into correct surgical site

  Excludes 1: performance of correct procedure (operation) on wrong side or body part (Y65.53)

  Y65.52 Performance of procedure (operation) on patient not scheduled for surgery

  Performance of procedure (operation) intended for another patient

Performance of procedure (operation) on wrong patient

  Y65.53 Performance of correct procedure (operation) on wrong side or body part

  Performance of correct procedure (operation) on wrong side

  Performance of correct procedure (operation) on wrong site

Y65.8 Other specified misadventures during surgical and medical care

Y66 Nonadministration of surgical and medical care

Premature cessation of surgical and medical care

Excludes 1: DNR status (Z66)

palliative care (Z51.5)

Y69 Unspecified misadventure during surgical and medical care

MEDICAL DEVICES ASSOCIATED WITH ADVERSE INCIDENTS IN DIAGNOSTIC AND THERAPEUTIC USE (Y70-Y82)

Includes: breakdown or malfunction of medical devices (during use) (after implantation) (ongoing use)

Excludes 1: misadventure to patients during surgical and medical care, classifiable to (Y62-Y69)

later complications following use of medical devices without breakdown or malfunctioning of device (Y83-Y84)

Y70 Anesthesiology devices associated with adverse incidents

Y70.0 Diagnostic and monitoring anesthesiology devices associated with adverse incidents

Y70.1 Therapeutic (nonsurgical) and rehabilitative anesthesiology devices associated with adverse incidents

Y70.2 Prosthetic and other implants, materials and accessory anesthesiology devices associated with adverse incidents

Y70.3 Surgical instruments, materials and anesthesiology devices (including sutures) associated with adverse incidents

Y70.8 Miscellaneous anesthesiology devices associated with adverse incidents, not elsewhere classified

Y71 Cardiovascular devices associated with adverse incidents

Y71.0 Diagnostic and monitoring cardiovascular devices associated with adverse incidents

Y71.1 Therapeutic (nonsurgical) and rehabilitative cardiovascular devices associated with adverse incidents

Y71.2 Prosthetic and other implants, materials and accessory cardiovascular devices associated with adverse incidents

Y71.3 Surgical instruments, materials and cardiovascular devices (including sutures) associated with adverse incidents

Y71.8 Miscellaneous cardiovascular devices associated with adverse incidents, not elsewhere classified

Y72 Otorhinolaryngological devices associated with adverse incidents

Y72.0 Diagnostic and monitoring otorhinolaryngological devices associated with adverse incidents

Y72.1 Therapeutic (nonsurgical) and rehabilitative otorhinolaryngological devices associated with adverse incidents

Y72.2 Prosthetic and other implants, materials and accessory otorhinolaryngological devices associated with adverse incidents

Y72.3 Surgical instruments, materials and otorhinolaryngological devices (including sutures) associated with adverse incidents

Y72.8 Miscellaneous otorhinolaryngological devices associated with adverse incidents, not elsewhere classified

Y73 Gastroenterology and urology devices associated with adverse incidents

Y73.0 Diagnostic and monitoring gastroenterology and urology devices associated with adverse incidents

Y73.1 Therapeutic (nonsurgical) and rehabilitative gastroenterology and urology devices associated with adverse incidents

Y73.2 Prosthetic and other implants, materials and accessory gastroenterology and urology devices associated with adverse incidents

Y73.3 Surgical instruments, materials and gastroenterology and urology devices (including sutures) associated with adverse incidents

Y73.8 Miscellaneous gastroenterology and urology devices associated with adverse incidents, not elsewhere classified

Y74 General hospital and personal-use devices associated with adverse incidents

Y74.0 Diagnostic and monitoring general hospital and personal-use devices associated with adverse incidents

Y74.1 Therapeutic (nonsurgical) and rehabilitative general hospital and personal-use devices associated with adverse incidents

Y74.2 Prosthetic and other implants, materials and accessory general hospital and personal-use devices associated with adverse incidents

Y74.3 Surgical instruments, materials and general hospital and personal-use devices (including sutures) associated with adverse incidents

Y74.8 Miscellaneous general hospital and personal-use devices associated with adverse incidents, not elsewhere classified

Y75 Neurological devices associated with adverse incidents

Y75.0 Diagnostic and monitoring neurological devices associated with adverse incidents

Y75.1 Therapeutic (nonsurgical) and rehabilitative neurological devices associated with adverse incidents

Y75.2 Prosthetic and other implants, materials and neurological devices associated with adverse incidents

Y75.3 Surgical instruments, materials and neurological devices (including sutures) associated with adverse incidents

Y75.8 Miscellaneous neurological devices associated with adverse incidents, not elsewhere classified

Y76 Obstetric and gynecological devices associated with adverse incidents

Y76.0 Diagnostic and monitoring obstetric and gynecological devices associated with adverse incidents

Y76.1 Therapeutic (nonsurgical) and rehabilitative obstetric and gynecological devices associated with adverse incidents

Y76.2 Prosthetic and other implants, materials and accessory obstetric and gynecological devices associated with adverse incidents

Y76.3 Surgical instruments, materials and obstetric and gynecological devices (including sutures) associated with adverse incidents

Y76.8 Miscellaneous obstetric and gynecological devices associated with adverse incidents, not elsewhere classified

Y77 Ophthalmic devices associated with adverse incidents

Y77.0 Diagnostic and monitoring ophthalmic devices associated with adverse incidents

Y77.1 Therapeutic (nonsurgical) and rehabilitative ophthalmic devices associated with adverse incidents

Y77.2 Prosthetic and other implants, materials and accessory ophthalmic devices associated with adverse incidents

Y77.3 Surgical instruments, materials and ophthalmic devices (including sutures) associated with adverse incidents

Y77.8 Miscellaneous ophthalmic devices associated with adverse incidents, not elsewhere classified

Y78 Radiological devices associated with adverse incidents

Y78.0 Diagnostic and monitoring radiological devices associated with adverse incidents

Y78.1 Therapeutic (nonsurgical) and rehabilitative radiological devices associated with adverse incidents

Y78.2 Prosthetic and other implants, materials and accessory radiological devices associated with adverse incidents

Y78.3 Surgical instruments, materials and radiological devices (including sutures) associated with adverse incidents

Y78.8 Miscellaneous radiological devices associated with adverse incidents, not elsewhere classified

Y79 Orthopedic devices associated with adverse incidents

Y79.0 Diagnostic and monitoring orthopedic devices associated with adverse incidents

Y79.1 Therapeutic (nonsurgical) and rehabilitative orthopedic devices associated with adverse incidents

Y79.2 Prosthetic and other implants, materials and accessory orthopedic devices associated with adverse incidents

Y79.3 Surgical instruments, materials and orthopedic devices (including sutures) associated with adverse incidents

Y79.8 Miscellaneous orthopedic devices associated with adverse incidents, not elsewhere classified

Y80 Physical medicine devices associated with adverse incidents

Y80.0 Diagnostic and monitoring physical medicine devices associated with adverse incidents

Y80.1 Therapeutic (nonsurgical) and rehabilitative physical medicine devices associated with adverse incidents

Y80.2 Prosthetic and other implants, materials and accessory physical medicine devices associated with adverse incidents

Y80.3 Surgical instruments, materials and physical medicine devices (including sutures) associated with adverse incidents

Y80.8 Miscellaneous physical medicine devices associated with adverse incidents, not elsewhere classified

Y81 General- and plastic-surgery devices associated with adverse incidents

Y81.0 Diagnostic and monitoring general- and plastic-surgery devices associated with adverse incidents

Y81.1 Therapeutic (nonsurgical) and rehabilitative general- and plastic-surgery devices associated with adverse incidents

Y81.2 Prosthetic and other implants, materials and accessory general- and plastic-surgery devices associated with adverse incidents

Y81.3 Surgical instruments, materials and general- and plastic-surgery devices (including sutures) associated with adverse incidents

Y81.8 Miscellaneous general- and plastic-surgery devices associated with adverse incidents, not elsewhere classified

Y82 Other and unspecified medical devices associated with adverse incidents

Y82.8 Other medical devices associated with adverse incidents

Y82.9 Unspecified medical devices associated with adverse incidents

SURGICAL AND OTHER MEDICAL PROCEDURES AS THE CAUSE OF ABNORMAL REACTION OF THE PATIENT, OR OF LATER COMPLICATION, WITHOUT MENTION OF MISADVENTURE AT THE TIME OF THE PROCEDURE (Y83-Y84)

Excludes 1: misadventures to patients during surgical and medical care, classifiable to (Y62-Y69)

Y83 Surgical operation and other surgical procedures as the cause of abnormal reaction of the patient, or of later complication, without mention of misadventure at the time of the procedure

Y83.0 Surgical operation with transplant of whole organ as the cause of abnormal reaction of the patient, or of later complication, without mention of misadventure at the time of the procedure

Y83.1 Surgical operation with implant of artificial internal device as the cause of abnormal reaction of the patient, or of later complication, without mention of misadventure at the time of the procedure

Y83.2 Surgical operation with anastomosis, bypass or graft as the cause of abnormal reaction of the patient, or of later complication, without mention of misadventure at the time of the procedure

Y83.3 Surgical operation with formation of external stoma as the cause of abnormal reaction of the patient, or of later complication, without mention of misadventure at the time of the procedure

Y83.4 Other reconstructive surgery as the cause of abnormal reaction of the patient, or of later complication, without mention of misadventure at the time of the procedure

Y83.5 Amputation of limb(s) as the cause of abnormal reaction of the patient, or of later complication, without mention of misadventure at the time of the procedure

Y83.6 Removal of other organ (partial) (total) as the cause of abnormal reaction of the patient, or of later complication, without mention of misadventure at the time of the procedure

Y83.8 Other surgical procedures as the cause of abnormal reaction of the patient, or of later complication, without mention of misadventure at the time of the procedure

Y83.9 Surgical procedure, unspecified as the cause of abnormal reaction of the patient, or of later complication, without mention of misadventure at the time of the procedure

Y84 Other medical procedures as the cause of abnormal reaction of the patient, or of later complication, without mention of misadventure at the time of the procedure

Y84.0 Cardiac catheterization as the cause of abnormal reaction of the patient, or of later complication, without mention of misadventure at the time of the procedure

Y84.1 Kidney dialysis as the cause of abnormal reaction of the patient, or of later complication, without mention of misadventure at the time of the procedure

Y84.2 Radiological procedure and radiotherapy as the cause of abnormal reaction of the patient, or of later complication, without mention of misadventure at the time of the procedure

Y84.3 Shock therapy as the cause of abnormal reaction of the patient, or of later complication, without mention of misadventure at the time of the procedure

Y84.4 Aspiration of fluid as the cause of abnormal reaction of the patient, or of later complication, without mention of misadventure at the time of the procedure

Y84.5 Insertion of gastric or duodenal sound as the cause of abnormal reaction of the patient, or of later complication,

without mention of misadventure at the time of the procedure

Y84.6 Urinary catheterization as the cause of abnormal reaction of the patient, or of later complication, without mention of misadventure at the time of the procedure

Y84.7 Blood-sampling as the cause of abnormal reaction of the patient, or of later complication, without mention of misadventure at the time of the procedure

Y84.8 Other medical procedures as the cause of abnormal reaction of the patient, or of later complication, without mention of misadventure at the time of the procedure

Y84.9 Medical procedure, unspecified as the cause of abnormal reaction of the patient, or of later complication, without mention of misadventure at the time of the procedure

SUPPLEMENTARY FACTORS RELATED TO CAUSES OF MORBIDITY CLASSIFIED ELSEWHERE (Y90-Y99)

Note: These categories may be used to provide supplementary information concerning causes of morbidity. They are not to be used for single-condition coding.

Y90 Evidence of alcohol involvement determined by blood alcohol level
Code first any associated alcohol related disorders (F10)

Y90.0 Blood alcohol level of less than 20 mg/100 ml

Y90.1 Blood alcohol level of 20-39 mg/100 ml

Y90.2 Blood alcohol level of 40-59 mg/100 ml

Y90.3 Blood alcohol level of 60-79 mg/100 ml

Y90.4 Blood alcohol level of 80-99 mg/100 ml

Y90.5 Blood alcohol level of 100-119 mg/100 ml

Y90.6 Blood alcohol level of 120-199 mg/100 ml

Y90.7 Blood alcohol level of 200-239 mg/100 ml

Y90.8 Blood alcohol level of 240 mg/100 ml or more

Y90.9 Presence of alcohol in blood, level not specified

Y92 Place of occurrence of the external cause

The following category is for use, when relevant, to identify the place of occurrence of the external cause. Use in conjunction with an activity code.

Place of occurrence should be recorded only at the initial encounter for treatment

Y92.0 Non-institutional (private) residence as the place of occurrence of the external cause

Excludes 1: abandoned or derelict house (Y92.89)
home under construction but not yet occupied (Y92.6-)
institutional place of residence (Y92.1-)

Y92.00 Unspecified non-institutional (private) residence as the place of occurrence of the external cause

Y92.000 Kitchen of unspecified non-institutional (private) residence as the place of occurrence of the external cause

Y92.001 Dining room of unspecified non-institutional (private) residence as the place of occurrence of the external cause

▲ Y92.002 Bathroom of unspecified non-institutional (private) residence single-family (private) house as the place of occurrence of the external cause

Y92.003 Bedroom of unspecified non-institutional (private) residence as the place of occurrence of the external cause

Y92.007 Garden or yard of unspecified non-institutional (private) residence as the place of occurrence of the external cause

Y92.008 Other place in unspecified non-institutional (private) residence as the place of occurrence of the external cause

Y92.009 Unspecified place in unspecified non-institutional (private) residence as the place of occurrence of the external cause

Home (NOS) as the place of occurrence of the external cause

Y92.01 Single-family non-institutional (private) house as the place of occurrence of the external cause

Farmhouse as the place of occurrence of the external cause

Excludes 1: barn (Y92.71)

chicken coop or hen house (Y92.72)

farm field (Y92.73)

orchard (Y92.74)

single family mobile home or trailer (Y92.02-)

slaughter house (Y92.86)

Y92.010 Kitchen of single-family (private) house as the place of occurrence of the external cause

Y92.011 Dining room of single-family (private) house as the place of occurrence of the external cause

Y92.012 Bathroom of single-family (private) house as the place of occurrence of the external cause

Y92.013 Bedroom of single-family (private) house as the place of occurrence of the external cause

Y92.014 Private driveway to single-family (private) house as the place of occurrence of the external cause

Y92.015 Private garage of single-family (private) house as the place of occurrence of the external cause

Y92.016 Swimming-pool in single-family (private) house or garden as the place of occurrence of the external cause

Y92.017 Garden or yard in single-family (private) house as the place of occurrence of the external cause

Y92.018 Other place in single-family (private) house as the place of occurrence of the external cause

Y92.019 Unspecified place in single-family (private) house as the place of occurrence of the external cause

Y92.02 Mobile home as the place of occurrence of the external cause

Y92.020 Kitchen in mobile home as the place of occurrence of the external cause

Y92.021 Dining room in mobile home as the place of occurrence of the external cause

Y92.022 Bathroom in mobile home as the place of occurrence of the external cause

Y92.023 Bedroom in mobile home as the place of occurrence of the external cause

Y92.024 Driveway of mobile home as the place of occurrence of the external cause

Y92.025 Garage of mobile home as the place of occurrence of the external cause

Y92.026 Swimming-pool of mobile home as the place of occurrence of the external cause

Y92.027 Garden or yard of mobile home as the place of occurrence of the external cause

Y92.028 Other place in mobile home as the place of occurrence of the external cause

Y92.029 Unspecified place in mobile home as the place of occurrence of the external cause

Y92.03 Apartment as the place of occurrence of the external cause

Condominium as the place of occurrence of the external cause

Co-op apartment as the place of occurrence of the external cause

Y92.030 Kitchen in apartment as the place of occurrence of the external cause

Y92.031 Bathroom in apartment as the place of occurrence of the external cause

Y92.032 Bedroom in apartment as the place of occurrence of the external cause

Y92.038 Other place in apartment as the place of occurrence of the external cause

Y92.039 Unspecified place in apartment as the place of occurrence of the external cause

Y92.04 Boarding-house as the place of occurrence of the external cause

Y92.040 Kitchen in boarding-house as the place of occurrence of the external cause

Y92.041 Bathroom in boarding-house as the place of occurrence of the external cause

Y92.042 Bedroom in boarding-house as the place of occurrence of the external cause

Y92.043 Driveway of boarding-house as the place of occurrence of the external cause

Y92.044 Garage of boarding-house as the place of occurrence of the external cause

Y92.045 Swimming-pool of boarding-house as the place of occurrence of the external cause

Y92.046 Garden or yard of boarding-house as the place of occurrence of the external cause

Y92.048 Other place in boarding-house as the place of occurrence of the external cause

Y92.049 Unspecified place in boarding-house as the place of occurrence of the external cause

Y92.09 Other non-institutional residence as the place of occurrence of the external cause

Y92.090 Kitchen in other non-institutional residence as the place of occurrence of the external cause

Y92.091 Bathroom in other non-institutional residence as the place of occurrence of the external cause

Y92.092 Bedroom in other non-institutional residence as the place of occurrence of the external cause

Y92.093 Driveway of other non-institutional residence as the place of occurrence of the external cause

Y92.094 Garage of other non-institutional residence as the place of occurrence of the external cause

Y92.095 Swimming-pool of other non-institutional residence as the place of occurrence of the external cause

Y92.096 Garden or yard of other non-institutional residence as the place of occurrence of the external cause

Y92.098 Other place in other non-institutional residence as the place of occurrence of the external cause

Y92.099 Unspecified place in other non-institutional residence as the place of occurrence of the external cause

Y92.1 Institutional (nonprivate) residence as the place of occurrence of the external cause

Y92.10 Unspecified residential institution as the place of occurrence of the external cause

Y92.11 Children's home and orphanage as the place of occurrence of the external cause

Y92.110 Kitchen in children's home and orphanage as the place of occurrence of the external cause

Y92.111 Bathroom in children's home and orphanage as the place of occurrence of the external cause

Y92.112 Bedroom in children's home and orphanage as the place of occurrence of the external cause

Y92.113 Driveway of children's home and orphanage as the place of occurrence of the external cause

Y92.114 Garage of children's home and orphanage as the place of occurrence of the external cause

Y92.115 Swimming-pool of children's home and orphanage as the place of occurrence of the external cause

Y92.116 Garden or yard of children's home and orphanage as the place of occurrence of the external cause

Y92.118 Other place in children's home and orphanage as the place of occurrence of the external cause

Y92.119 Unspecified place in children's home and orphanage as the place of occurrence of the external cause

Y92.12 Nursing home as the place of occurrence of the external cause

Home for the sick as the place of occurrence of the external cause

Hospice as the place of occurrence of the external cause

Y92.120 Kitchen in nursing home as the place of occurrence of the external cause

Y92.121 Bathroom in nursing home as the place of occurrence of the external cause

Y92.122 Bedroom in nursing home as the place of occurrence of the external cause

Y92.123 Driveway of nursing home as the place of occurrence of the external cause

Y92.124 Garage of nursing home as the place of occurrence of the external cause

Y92.125 Swimming-pool of nursing home as the place of occurrence of the external cause

Y92.126 Garden or yard of nursing home as the place of occurrence of the external cause

Y92.128 Other place in nursing home as the place of occurrence of the external cause

Y92.129 Unspecified place in nursing home as the place of occurrence of the external cause

Y92.13 Military base as the place of occurrence of the external cause

Excludes 1: military training grounds (Y92.83)

Y92.130 Kitchen on military base as the place of occurrence of the external cause

Y92.131 Mess hall on military base as the place of occurrence of the external cause

Y92.133 Barracks on military base as the place of occurrence of the external cause

Y92.135 Garage on military base as the place of occurrence of the external cause

Y92.136 Swimming-pool on military base as the place of occurrence of the external cause

Y92.137 Garden or yard on military base as the place of occurrence of the external cause

Y92.138 Other place on military base as the place of occurrence of the external cause

Y92.139 Unspecified place military base as the place of occurrence of the external cause

Y92.14 Prison as the place of occurrence of the external cause

Y92.140 Kitchen in prison as the place of occurrence of the external cause

Y92.141 Dining room in prison as the place of occurrence of the external cause

Y92.142 Bathroom in prison as the place of occurrence of the external cause

Y92.143 Cell of prison as the place of occurrence of the external cause

Y92.146 Swimming-pool of prison as the place of occurrence of the external cause

Y92.147 Courtyard of prison as the place of occurrence of the external cause

Y92.148 Other place in prison as the place of occurrence of the external cause

Y92.149 Unspecified place in prison as the place of occurrence of the external cause

Y92.15 Reform school as the place of occurrence of the external cause

Y92.150 Kitchen in reform school as the place of occurrence of the external cause

Y92.151 Dining room in reform school as the place of occurrence of the external cause

Y92.152 Bathroom in reform school as the place of occurrence of the external cause

Y92.153 Bedroom in reform school as the place of occurrence of the external cause

Y92.154 Driveway of reform school as the place of occurrence of the external cause

Y92.155 Garage of reform school as the place of occurrence of the external cause

Y92.156 Swimming-pool of reform school as the place of occurrence of the external cause

Y92.157 Garden or yard of reform school as the place of occurrence of the external cause

Y92.158 Other place in reform school as the place of occurrence of the external cause

Y92.159 Unspecified place in reform school as the place of occurrence of the external cause

Y92.16 School dormitory as the place of occurrence of the external cause

Excludes 1: reform school as the place of occurrence of the external cause (Y92.15-)

school buildings and grounds as the place of occurrence of the external cause (Y92.2-)

school sports and athletic areas as the place of occurrence of the external cause (Y92.3-)

Y92.160 Kitchen in school dormitory as the place of occurrence of the external cause

Y92.161 Dining room in school dormitory as the place of occurrence of the external cause

Y92.162 Bathroom in school dormitory as the place of occurrence of the external cause

Y92.163 Bedroom in school dormitory as the place of occurrence of the external cause

Y92.168 Other place in school dormitory as the place of occurrence of the external cause

Y92.169 Unspecified place in school dormitory as the place of occurrence of the external cause

Y92.19 Other specified residential institution as the place of occurrence of the external cause

Y92.190 Kitchen in other specified residential institution as the place of occurrence of the external cause

Y92.191 Dining room in other specified residential institution as the place of occurrence of the external cause

Y92.192 Bathroom in other specified residential institution as the place of occurrence of the external cause

Y92.193 Bedroom in other specified residential institution as the place of occurrence of the external cause

Y92.194 Driveway of other specified residential institution as the place of occurrence of the external cause

Y92.195 Garage of other specified residential institution as the place of occurrence of the external cause

Y92.196 Pool of other specified residential institution as the place of occurrence of the external cause

Y92.197 Garden or yard of other specified residential institution as the place of occurrence of the external cause

Y92.198 Other place in other specified residential institution as the place of occurrence of the external cause

Y92.199 Unspecified place in other specified residential institution as the place of occurrence of the external cause

Y92.2 School, other institution and public administrative area as the place of occurrence of the external cause

● New code ▲ Revised code ⑦ 7th digit required ⊗ Placeholder required

Building and adjacent grounds used by the general public or by a particular group of the public

Excludes 1: building under construction as the place of occurrence of the external cause (Y92.6)

residential institution as the place of occurrence of the external cause (Y92.1)

school dormitory as the place of occurrence of the external cause (Y92.16-)

sports and athletics area of schools as the place of occurrence of the external cause (Y92.3-)

Y92.21 School (private) (public) (state) as the place of occurrence of the external cause

Y92.210 Daycare center as the place of occurrence of the external cause

Y92.211 Elementary school as the place of occurrence of the external cause

Kindergarten as the place of occurrence of the external cause

Y92.212 Middle school as the place of occurrence of the external cause

Y92.213 High school as the place of occurrence of the external cause

Y92.214 College as the place of occurrence of the external cause

University as the place of occurrence of the external cause

Y92.215 Trade school as the place of occurrence of the external cause

Y92.218 Other school as the place of occurrence of the external cause

Y92.219 Unspecified school as the place of occurrence of the external cause

Y92.22 Religious institution as the place of occurrence of the external cause

Church as the place of occurrence of the external cause

Mosque as the place of occurrence of the external cause

Synagogue as the place of occurrence of the external cause

Y92.23 Hospital as the place of occurrence of the external cause

Excludes 1: ambulatory (outpatient) health services establishments (Y92.53-)

home for the sick as the place of occurrence of the external cause (Y92.12-)

hospice as the place of occurrence of the external cause (Y92.12-)

nursing home as the place of occurrence of the external cause (Y92.12-)

Y92.230 Patient room in hospital as the place of occurrence of the external cause

Y92.231 Patient bathroom in hospital as the place of occurrence of the external cause

Y92.232 Corridor of hospital as the place of occurrence of the external cause

Y92.233 Cafeteria of hospital as the place of occurrence of the external cause

Y92.234 Operating room of hospital as the place of occurrence of the external cause

Y92.238 Other place in hospital as the place of occurrence of the external cause

Y92.239 Unspecified place in hospital as the place of occurrence of the external cause

Y92.24 Public administrative building as the place of occurrence of the external cause

Y92.240 Courthouse as the place of occurrence of the external cause

Y92.241 Library as the place of occurrence of the external cause

Y92.242 Post office as the place of occurrence of the external cause

Y92.243 City hall as the place of occurrence of the external cause

Y92.248 Other public administrative building as the place of occurrence of the external cause

Y92.25 Cultural building as the place of occurrence of the external cause

Y92.250 Art Gallery as the place of occurrence of the external cause

Y92.251 Museum as the place of occurrence of the external cause

Y92.252 Music hall as the place of occurrence of the external cause

Y92.253 Opera house as the place of occurrence of the external cause

Y92.254 Theater (live) as the place of occurrence of the external cause

Y92.258 Other cultural public building as the place of occurrence of the external cause

Y92.26 Movie house or cinema as the place of occurrence of the external cause

Y92.29 Other specified public building as the place of occurrence of the external cause

Assembly hall as the place of occurrence of the external cause

Clubhouse as the place of occurrence of the external cause

Y92.3 Sports and athletics area as the place of occurrence of the external cause

Y92.31 Athletic court as the place of occurrence of the external cause

Excludes 1: tennis court in private home or garden (Y92.09)

Y92.310 Basketball court as the place of occurrence of the external cause

Y92.311 Squash court as the place of occurrence of the external cause

Y92.312 Tennis court as the place of occurrence of the external cause

Y92.318 Other athletic court as the place of occurrence of the external cause

Y92.32 Athletic field as the place of occurrence of the external cause

Y92.320 Baseball field as the place of occurrence of the external cause

Y92.321 Football field as the place of occurrence of the external cause

Y92.322 Soccer field as the place of occurrence of the external cause

Y92.328 Other athletic field as the place of occurrence of the external cause

Cricket field as the place of occurrence of the external cause

Hockey field as the place of occurrence of the external cause

Y92.33 Skating rink as the place of occurrence of the external cause

Y92.330 Ice skating rink (indoor) (outdoor) as the place of occurrence of the external cause

Y92.331 Roller skating rink as the place of occurrence of the external cause

Y92.34 Swimming pool (public) as the place of occurrence of the external cause

Excludes 1: swimming pool in private home or garden (Y92.016)

Y92.39 Other specified sports and athletic area as the place of occurrence of the external cause

Golf-course as the place of occurrence of the external cause

Gymnasium as the place of occurrence of the external cause

Riding-school as the place of occurrence of the external cause

Stadium as the place of occurrence of the external cause

Y92.4 Street , highway and other paved roadways as the place of occurrence of the external cause

Excludes 1: private driveway of residence (Y92.0x4, Y92.1x3)

Y92.41 Street and highway as the place of occurrence of the external cause

Y92.410 Unspecified street and highway as the place of occurrence of the external cause

Road NOS as the place of occurrence of the external cause

Y92.411 Interstate highway as the place of occurrence of the external cause

Freeway as the place of occurrence of the external cause

Motorway as the place of occurrence of the external cause

Y92.412 Parkway as the place of occurrence of the external cause

Y92.413 State road as the place of occurrence of the external cause

Y92.414 Local residential or business street as the place of occurrence of the external cause

Y92.415 Exit ramp or entrance ramp of street or highway as the place of occurrence of the external cause

Y92.48 Other paved roadways as the place of occurrence of the external cause

Y92.480 Sidewalk as the place of occurrence of the external cause

Y92.481 Parking lot as the place of occurrence of the external cause

Y92.482 Bike path as the place of occurrence of the external cause

Y92.488 Other paved roadways as the place of occurrence of the external cause

Y92.5 Trade and service area as the place of occurrence of the external cause

Excludes 1: garage in private home (Y92.015)

schools and other public administration buildings (Y92.2-)

Y92.51 Private commercial establishments as the place of occurrence of the external cause

Y92.510 Bank as the place of occurrence of the external cause

Y92.511 Restaurant or cafΘ as the place of occurrence of the external cause

Y92.512 Supermarket, store or market as the place of occurrence of the external cause

Y92.513 Shop (commercial) as the place of occurrence of the external cause

Y92.52 Service areas as the place of occurrence of the external cause

Y92.520 Airport as the place of occurrence of the external cause

Y92.521 Bus station as the place of occurrence of the external cause

Y92.522 Railway station as the place of occurrence of the external cause

Y92.523 Highway rest stop as the place of occurrence of the external cause

Y92.524 Gas station as the place of occurrence of the external cause

Petroleum station as the place of occurrence of the external cause

Service station as the place of occurrence of the external cause

Y92.53 Ambulatory health services establishments as the place of occurrence of the external cause

Y92.530 Ambulatory surgery center as the place of occurrence of the external cause

Outpatient surgery center, including that connected with a hospital as the place of occurrence of the external cause

Same day surgery center, including that connected with a hospital as the place of occurrence of the external cause

Y92.531 Health care provider office as the place of occurrence of the external cause

Physician office as the place of occurrence of the external cause

Y92.532 Urgent care center as the place of occurrence of the external cause

● New code ▲ Revised code ⑦ 7ᵗʰ digit required ⊗ Placeholder required

Y92.538 Other ambulatory health services establishments as the place of occurrence of the external cause

Y92.59 Other trade areas as the place of occurrence of the external cause

Office building as the place of occurrence of the external cause

Casino as the place of occurrence of the external cause

Garage (commercial) as the place of occurrence of the external cause

Hotel as the place of occurrence of the external cause

Radio or television station as the place of occurrence of the external cause

Shopping mall as the place of occurrence of the external cause

Warehouse as the place of occurrence of the external cause

Y92.6 Industrial and construction area as the place of occurrence of the external cause

Y92.61 Building [any] under construction as the place of occurrence of the external cause

Y92.62 Dock or shipyard as the place of occurrence of the external cause

Dockyard as the place of occurrence of the external cause

Dry dock as the place of occurrence of the external cause

Shipyard as the place of occurrence of the external cause

Y92.63 Factory as the place of occurrence of the external cause

Factory building as the place of occurrence of the external cause

Factory premises as the place of occurrence of the external cause

Industrial yard as the place of occurrence of the external cause

Y92.64 Mine or pit as the place of occurrence of the external cause

Mine as the place of occurrence of the external cause

Y92.65 Oil rig as the place of occurrence of the external cause

Pit (coal) (gravel) (sand) as the place of occurrence of the external cause

Y92.69 Other specified industrial and construction area as the place of occurrence of the external cause

Gasworks as the place of occurrence of the external cause

Power-station (coal) (nuclear) (oil) as the place of occurrence of the external cause

Tunnel under construction as the place of occurrence of the external cause

Workshop as the place of occurrence of the external cause

Y92.7 Farm as the place of occurrence of the external cause

Ranch as the place of occurrence of the external cause

Excludes 1: farmhouse and home premises of farm (Y92.01-)

Y92.71 Barn as the place of occurrence of the external cause

Y92.72 Chicken coop as the place of occurrence of the external cause

Hen house as the place of occurrence of the external cause

Y92.73 Farm field as the place of occurrence of the external cause

Y92.74 Orchard as the place of occurrence of the external cause

Y92.79 Other farm location as the place of occurrence of the external cause

Y92.8 Other places as the place of occurrence of the external cause

Y92.81 Transport vehicle as the place of occurrence of the external cause

Excludes 1: transport accidents (V00-V99)

Y92.810 Car as the place of occurrence of the external cause

Y92.811 Bus as the place of occurrence of the external cause

Y92.812 Truck as the place of occurrence of the external cause

Y92.813 Airplane as the place of occurrence of the external cause

Y92.814 Boat as the place of occurrence of the external cause

Y92.815 Train as the place of occurrence of the external cause

Y92.816 Subway car as the place of occurrence of the external cause

Y92.818 Other transport vehicle as the place of occurrence of the external cause

Y92.82 Wilderness area

Y92.820 Desert as the place of occurrence of the external cause

Y92.821 Forest as the place of occurrence of the external cause

Y92.828 Other wilderness area as the place of occurrence of the external cause

Swamp as the place of occurrence of the external cause

Mountain as the place of occurrence of the external cause

Marsh as the place of occurrence of the external cause

Prairie as the place of occurrence of the external cause

Y92.83 Recreation area as the place of occurrence of the external cause

Y92.830 Public park as the place of occurrence of the external cause

Y92.831 Amusement park as the place of occurrence of the external cause

Y92.832 Beach as the place of occurrence of the external cause

Seashore as the place of occurrence of the external cause

Y92.833 Campsite as the place of occurrence of the external cause

Y92.834 Zoological garden (Zoo) as the place of occurrence of the external cause

Y92.838 Other recreation area as the place of occurrence of the external cause

Y92.84 Military training ground as the place of occurrence of the external cause

Y92.85 Railroad track as the place of occurrence of the external cause

Y92.86 Slaughter house as the place of occurrence of the external cause

Y92.89 Other specified places as the place of occurrence of the external cause

Derelict house as the place of occurrence of the external cause

Y92.9 Unspecified place or not applicable

Y93 Activity codes

Note: Category Y93 is provided for use to indicate the activity of the person seeking healthcare for an injury or health condition, such as a heart attack while shoveling snow, which resulted from, or was contributed to, by the activity. These codes are appropriate for use for both acute injuries, such as those from chapter 19, and conditions that are due to the long-term, cumulative effects of an activity, such as those from chapter 13. They are also appropriate for use with external cause codes for cause and intent if identifying the activity provides additional information on the event. These codes should be used in conjunction with codes for external cause status (Y99) and place of occurrence (Y92).

This section contains the following broad activity categories:

Y93.0 Activities involving walking and running

Y93.1 Activities involving water and water craft

Y93.2 Activities involving ice and snow

Y93.3 Activities involving climbing, rappelling, and jumping off

Y93.4 Activities involving dancing and other rhythmic movement

Y93.5 Activities involving other sports and athletics played individually

Y93.6 Activities involving other sports and athletics played as a team or group

Y93.7 Activities involving other specified sports and athletics

Y93.A Activities involving other cardiorespiratory exercise

Y93.B Activities involving other muscle strengthening exercises

Y93.C Activities involving computer technology and electronic devices

Y93.D Activities involving arts and handcrafts

Y93.E Activities involving personal hygiene and interior property and clothing maintenance

Y93.F Activities involving caregiving

Y93.G Activities involving food preparation, cooking and grilling

Y93.H Activities involving exterior property and land maintenance, building and construction

Y93.I Activities involving roller coasters and other types of external motion

Y93.J Activities involving playing musical instrument

Y93.K Activities involving animal care

Y93.8 Activities, other specified

Y93.9 Activity, unspecified

Y93.0 Activities involving walking and running

Excludes 1: activity, walking an animal (Y93.K1)

activity, walking or running on a treadmill (Y93.A1)

Y93.01 Activity, walking, marching and hiking

Activity, walking, marching and hiking on level or elevated terrain

Excludes 1: activity, mountain climbing (Y93.31)

Y93.02 Activity, running

Y93.1 Activities involving water and water craft

Excludes 1: activities involving ice (Y93.2-)

Y93.11 Activity, swimming

Y93.12 Activity, springboard and platform diving

Y93.13 Activity, water polo

Y93.14 Activity, water aerobics and water exercise

Y93.15 Activity, underwater diving and snorkeling

Activity, SCUBA diving

Y93.16 Activity, rowing, canoeing, kayaking, rafting and tubing

Activity, canoeing, kayaking, rafting and tubing in calm and turbulent water

Y93.17 Activity, water skiing and wake boarding

Y93.18 Activity, surfing, windsurfing and boogie boarding

Activity, water sliding

Y93.19 Activity, other involving water and watercraft

Activity involving water NOS

Activity, parasailing

Activity, water survival training and testing

Y93.2 Activities involving ice and snow

Excludes 1: activity, shoveling ice and snow (Y93.H1)

Y93.21 Activity, ice skating

Activity, figure skating (singles) (pairs)

Activity, ice dancing

Excludes 1: activity, ice hockey (Y93.22)

Y93.22 Activity, ice hockey

Y93.23 Activity, snow (alpine) (downhill) skiing, snow boarding, sledding, tobogganing and snow tubing

Excludes 1: activity, cross country skiing (Y93.24)

Y93.24 Activity, cross country skiing

Activity, nordic skiing

Y93.29 Activity, other involving ice and snow

Activity involving ice and snow NOS

Y93.3 Activities involving climbing, rappelling and jumping off

Excludes 1: activity, hiking on level or elevated terrain (Y93.01)

activity, jumping rope (Y93.56)

activity, trampoline jumping (Y93.44)

Y93.31 Activity, mountain climbing, rock climbing and wall climbing

Y93.32 Activity, rappelling

Y93.33 Activity, BASE jumping

Activity, Building, Antenna, Span, Earth jumping

Y93.34 Activity, bungee jumping

Y93.35 Activity, hang gliding

Y93.39 Activity, other involving climbing, rappelling and jumping off

Y93.4 Activities involving dancing and other rhythmic movement

Excludes 1: activity, martial arts (Y93.75)

Y93.41 Activity, dancing

Y93.42 Activity, yoga

Y93.43 Activity, gymnastics

Activity, rhythmic gymnastics
> **Excludes 1:** activity, trampolining (Y93.44)

Y93.44 Activity, trampolining

Y93.45 Activity, cheerleading

Y93.49 Activity, other involving dancing and other rhythmic movements

Y93.5 Activities involving other sports and athletics played individually
> **Excludes 1:** activity, dancing (Y93.41)
> activity, gymnastic (Y93.43)
> activity, trampolining (Y93.44)
> activity, yoga (Y93.42)

Y93.51 Activity, roller skating (inline) and skateboarding

Y93.52 Activity, horseback riding

Y93.53 Activity, golf

Y93.54 Activity, bowling

Y93.55 Activity, bike riding

Y93.56 Activity, jumping rope

Y93.57 Activity, non-running track and field events
> **Excludes 1:** activity, running (any form) (Y93.02)

Y93.59 Activity, other involving other sports and athletics played individually
> **Excludes 1:** activities involving climbing, rappelling, and jumping (Y93.3-)
> activities involving ice and snow (Y93.2-)
> activities involving walking and running (Y93.0-)
> activities involving water and watercraft (Y93.1-)

Y93.6 Activities involving other sports and athletics played as a team or group
> **Excludes 1:** activity, ice hockey (Y93.22)
> activity, water polo (Y93.13)

Y93.61 Activity, american tackle football
Activity, football NOS

Y93.62 Activity, american flag or touch football

Y93.63 Activity, rugby

Y93.64 Activity, baseball
Activity, softball

Y93.65 Activity, lacrosse and field hockey

Y93.66 Activity, soccer

Y93.67 Activity, basketball

Y93.68 Activity, volleyball (beach) (court)

Y93.6A Activity, physical games generally associated with school recess, summer camp and children
Activity, capture the flag
Activity, dodge ball
Activity, four square
Activity, kickball

Y93.69 Activity, other involving other sports and athletics played as a team or group
Activity, cricket

Y93.7 Activities involving other specified sports and athletics

Y93.71 Activity, boxing

Y93.72 Activity, wrestling

Y93.73 Activity, racquet and hand sports
Activity, handball
Activity, racquetball

Activity, squash
Activity, tennis

Y93.74 Activity, frisbee
Activity, ultimate frisbee

Y93.75 Activity, martial arts
Activity, combatives

Y93.79 Activity, other specified sports and athletics
> **Excludes 1:** sports and athletics activities specified in categories Y93.0-Y93.6

Y93.A Activities involving other cardiorespiratory exercise
Activities involving physical training

Y93.A1 Activity, exercise machines primarily for cardiorespiratory conditioning
Activity, elliptical and stepper machines
Activity, stationary bike
Activity, treadmill

Y93.A2 Activity, calisthenics
Activity, jumping jacks
Activity, warm up and cool down

Y93.A3 Activity, aerobic and step exercise

Y93.A4 Activity, circuit training

Y93.A5 Activity, obstacle course
Activity, challenge course
Activity, confidence course

Y93.A6 Activity, grass drills
Activity, guerilla drills

Y93.A9 Activity, other involving cardiorespiratory exercise
> **Excludes 1:** activities involving cardiorespiratory exercise specified in categories Y93.0-Y93.7

Y93.B Activities involving other muscle strengthening exercises

Y93.B1 Activity, exercise machines primarily for muscle strengthening

Y93.B2 Activity, push-ups, pull-ups, sit-ups

Y93.B3 Activity, free weights
Activity, barbells
Activity, dumbbells

Y93.B4 Activity, pilates

Y93.B9 Activity, other involving muscle strengthening exercises
> **Excludes 1:** activities involving muscle strengthening specified in categories Y93.0-Y93.A

Y93.C Activities involving computer technology and electronic devices
> **Excludes 1:** activity, electronic musical keyboard or instruments (Y93.J-)

Y93.C1 Activity, computer keyboarding
Activity, electronic game playing using keyboard or other stationary device

Y93.C2 Activity, hand held interactive electronic device
Activity, cellular telephone and communication device
Activity, electronic game playing using interactive device
> **Excludes 1:** activity, electronic game playing using keyboard or other stationary device (Y93.C1)

Add 4th-7th digits   3 digit reportable   Nonspecific code   Unspecified code   Manifestation code   921 alleged rape

Encounter for examination and observation of victim following alleged rape

Encounter for examination and observation of victim following alleged sexual abuse

- **Z04.41** Encounter for examination and observation following alleged adult rape

  Suspected adult rape, ruled out

  Suspected adult sexual abuse, ruled out

- **Z04.42** Encounter for examination and observation following alleged child rape

  Suspected child rape, ruled out

  Suspected child sexual abuse, ruled out

Z04.6 Encounter for general psychiatric examination, requested by authority

Z04.7 Encounter for examination and observation following alleged physical abuse

- **Z04.71** Encounter for examination and observation following alleged adult physical abuse

  Suspected adult physical abuse, ruled out

  Excludes 1: confirmed case of adult physical abuse (T74.-)

  encounter for examination and observation following alleged adult sexual abuse (Z04.41)

  suspected case of adult physical abuse, not ruled out (T76.-)

- **Z04.72** Encounter for examination and observation following alleged child physical abuse

  Suspected child physical abuse, ruled out

  Excludes 1: confirmed case of child physical abuse (T74.-)

  encounter for examination and observation following alleged child sexual abuse (Z04.42)

  suspected case of child physical abuse, not ruled out (T76.-)

Z04.8 Encounter for examination and observation for other specified reasons

Encounter for examination and observation for request for expert evidence

Z04.9 Encounter for examination and observation for unspecified reason

Encounter for observation NOS

Z08 Encounter for follow-up examination after completed treatment for malignant neoplasm

Medical surveillance following completed treatment

Use additional code to identify any acquired absence of organs (Z90.-)

Use additional code to identify the personal history of malignant neoplasm (Z85.-)

Excludes 1: aftercare following medical care (Z43-Z49, Z51)

Z09 Encounter for follow-up examination after completed treatment for conditions other than malignant neoplasm

Medical surveillance following completed treatment

Use additional code to identify any applicable history of disease code (Z86.-. Z87.-)

Excludes 1: aftercare following medical care (Z43-Z49, Z51)

surveillance of contraception (Z30.4-)

surveillance of prosthetic and other medical devices

(Z44-Z46)

Z11 Encounter for screening for infectious and parasitic diseases

Screening is the testing for disease or disease precursors in asymptomatic individuals so that early detection and treatment can be provided for those who test positive for the disease.

Excludes 1: encounter for diagnostic examination-code to sign or symptom

Z11.0 Encounter for screening for intestinal infectious diseases

Z11.1 Encounter for screening for respiratory tuberculosis

Z11.2 Encounter for screening for other bacterial diseases

Z11.3 Encounter for screening for infections with a predominantly sexual mode of transmission

Excludes 2: encounter for screening for human immunodeficiency virus [HIV] (Z11.4)

encounter for screening for human papillomavirus (Z11.51)

Z11.4 Encounter for screening for human immunodeficiency virus [HIV]

Z11.5 Encounter for screening for other viral diseases

Excludes 2: encounter for screening for viral intestinal disease (Z11.0)

- **Z11.51** Encounter for screening for human papillomavirus (HPV)

- **Z11.59** Encounter for screening for other viral diseases

Z11.6 Encounter for screening for other protozoal diseases and helminthiases

Excludes 2: encounter for screening for protozoal intestinal disease (Z11.0)

Z11.8 Encounter for screening for other infectious and parasitic diseases

Encounter for screening for chlamydia

Encounter for screening for rickettsial

Encounter for screening for spirochetal

Encounter for screening for mycoses

Z11.9 Encounter for screening for infectious and parasitic diseases, unspecified

Z12 Encounter for screening for malignant neoplasms

Screening is the testing for disease or disease precursors in asymptomatic individuals so that early detection and treatment can be provided for those who test positive for the disease.

Use additional code to identify any family history of malignant neoplasm (Z80.-)

Excludes 1: encounter for diagnostic examination-code to sign or symptom

Z12.0 Encounter for screening for malignant neoplasm of stomach

Z12.1 Encounter for screening for malignant neoplasm of intestinal tract

- **Z12.10** Encounter for screening for malignant neoplasm of intestinal tract, unspecified

- **Z12.11** Encounter for screening for malignant neoplasm of colon

  Encounter for screening colonoscopy NOS

- **Z12.12** Encounter for screening for malignant neoplasm of rectum

- **Z12.13** Encounter for screening for malignant neoplasm of small intestine

Z12.2 Encounter for screening for malignant neoplasm of respiratory organs

Z12.3 Encounter for screening for malignant neoplasm of breast

    Z12.31 Encounter for screening mammogram for malignant neoplasm of breast
        Excludes 1: inconclusive mammogram (R92.2)

    Z12.39 Encounter for other screening for malignant neoplasm of breast

Z12.4 Encounter for screening for malignant neoplasm of cervix
Encounter for screening pap smear for malignant neoplasm of cervix
    Excludes 1: encounter for screening for human papillomavirus (Z11.51)
    when screening is part of general gynecological examination (Z01.4-)

Z12.5 Encounter for screening for malignant neoplasm of prostate

Z12.6 Encounter for screening for malignant neoplasm of bladder

Z12.7 Encounter for screening for malignant neoplasm of other genitourinary organs

    Z12.71 Encounter for screening for malignant neoplasm of testis

    Z12.72 Encounter for screening for malignant neoplasm of vagina
    Vaginal pap smear status-post hysterectomy for non-malignant condition
    Use additional code to identify acquired absence of uterus (Z90.71-)
        Excludes 1: vaginal pap smear status-post hysterectomy for malignant conditions (Z08)

    Z12.73 Encounter for screening for malignant neoplasm of ovary

    Z12.79 Encounter for screening for malignant neoplasm of other genitourinary organs

Z12.8 Encounter for screening for malignant neoplasm of other sites

    Z12.81 Encounter for screening for malignant neoplasm of oral cavity

    Z12.82 Encounter for screening for malignant neoplasm of nervous system

    Z12.83 Encounter for screening for malignant neoplasm of skin

    Z12.89 Encounter for screening for malignant neoplasm of other sites

Z12.9 Encounter for screening for malignant neoplasm, site unspecified

Z13 Encounter for screening for other diseases and disorders
Screening is the testing for disease or disease precursors in asymptomatic individuals so that early detection and treatment can be provided for those who test positive for the disease.
    Excludes 1: encounter for diagnostic examination-code to sign or symptom

Z13.0 Encounter for screening for diseases of the blood and blood-forming organs and certain disorders involving the immune mechanism

Z13.1 Encounter for screening for diabetes mellitus

Z13.2 Encounter for screening for nutritional, metabolic and other endocrine disorders

    Z13.21 Encounter for screening for nutritional disorder

    Z13.22 Encounter for screening for metabolic disorder

        Z13.220 Encounter for screening for lipoid disorders
        Encounter for screening for cholesterol level
        Encounter for screening for hypercholesterolemia
        Encounter for screening for hyperlipidemia

        Z13.228 Encounter for screening for other metabolic disorders

    Z13.29 Encounter for screening for other suspected endocrine disorder
        Excludes 1: encounter for screening for diabetes mellitus (Z13.1)

Z13.4 Encounter for screening for certain developmental disorders in childhood
Encounter for screening for developmental handicaps in early childhood
    Excludes 1: routine development testing of infant or child (Z00.1-)

Z13.5 Encounter for screening for eye and ear disorders
    Excludes 2: encounter for general hearing examination (Z01.1-)
    encounter for general vision examination (Z01.0-)

Z13.6 Encounter for screening for cardiovascular disorders

Z13.7 Encounter for screening for genetic and chromosomal anomalies
    Excludes 1: genetic testing for procreative management (Z31.4-)

    Z13.71 Encounter for nonprocreative screening for genetic disease carrier status

    Z13.79 Encounter for other screening for genetic and chromosomal anomalies

Z13.8 Encounter for screening for other specified diseases and disorders
    Excludes 2: screening for malignant neoplasms (Z12.-)

    Z13.81 Encounter for screening for digestive system disorders

        Z13.810 Encounter for screening for upper gastrointestinal disorder

        Z13.811 Encounter for screening for lower gastrointestinal disorder
            Excludes 1: encounter for screening for intestinal infectious disease (Z11.0)

        Z13.818 Encounter for screening for other digestive system disorders

    Z13.82 Encounter for screening for musculoskeletal disorder

        Z13.820 Encounter for screening for osteoporosis

        Z13.828 Encounter for screening for other musculoskeletal disorder

    Z13.83 Encounter for screening for respiratory disorder NEC
        Excludes 1: encounter for screening for respiratory tuberculosis (Z11.1)

    Z13.84 Encounter for screening for dental disorders

    Z13.85 Encounter for screening for nervous system

disorders

Z13.850   Encounter for screening for traumatic brain injury

Z13.858   Encounter for screening for other nervous system disorders

Z13.88   Encounter for screening for disorder due to exposure to contaminants

Excludes 1: those exposed to contaminants without suspected disorders (Z57.-, Z77.-)

Z13.89   Encounter for screening for other disorder

Encounter for screening for genitourinary disorders

Z13.9   Encounter for screening, unspecified

GENETIC CARRIER AND GENETIC SUSCEPTIBILITY TO DISEASE (Z14-Z15)

Z14   Genetic carrier

Z14.0   Hemophilia A carrier

Z14.01   Asymptomatic hemophilia A carrier

Z14.02   Symptomatic hemophilia A carrier

Z14.1   Cystic fibrosis carrier

Z14.8   Genetic carrier of other disease

Z15   Genetic susceptibility to disease

Includes: confirmed abnormal gene

Use additional code, if applicable, for any associated family history of the disease (Z80-Z84)

Excludes 1: chromosomal anomalies (Q90-Q99)

Z15.0   Genetic susceptibility to malignant neoplasm

Code first , if applicable, any current malignant neoplasm (C00-C75, C81-C96)

Use additional code, if applicable, for any personal history of malignant neoplasm (Z85.-)

Z15.01   Genetic susceptibility to malignant neoplasm of breast

Z15.02   Genetic susceptibility to malignant neoplasm of ovary

Z15.03   Genetic susceptibility to malignant neoplasm of prostate

Z15.04   Genetic susceptibility to malignant neoplasm of endometrium

Z15.09   Genetic susceptibility to other malignant neoplasm

Z15.8   Genetic susceptibility to other disease

Z15.81   Genetic susceptibility to multiple endocrine neoplasia [MEN]

Excludes 1: multiple endocrine neoplasia [MEN] syndromes (E31.2-)

Z15.89   Genetic susceptibility to other disease

RESISTANCE TO ANTIMICROBIAL DRUGS (Z16)

Z16   Resistance to antimicrobial drugs

Note: The codes in this category are provided for use as additional codes to identify the resistance and non-responsiveness of a condition to antimicrobial drugs.

Code first the infection

Excludes 1: Methicillin resistant Staphylococcus aureus infection (A49.02)

Methicillin resistant Staphylococcus aureus infection in

diseases classified elsewhere (B95.62)

Methicillin resistant Staphylococcus aureus pneumonia (J15.212)

Sepsis due to Methicillin resistant Staphylococcus aureus (A41.02)

Z16.1   Resistance to beta lactam antibiotics

Z16.10   Resistance to unspecified beta lactam antibiotics

Z16.11   Resistance to penicillins

Resistance to amoxicillin

Resistance to ampicillin

Z16.12   Extended spectrum beta lactamase (ESBL) resistance

Z16.19   Resistance to other specified beta lactam antibiotics

Resistance to cephalosporins

Z16.2   Resistance to other antibiotics

Z16.20   Resistance to unspecified antibiotic

Resistance to antibiotics NOS

Z16.21   Resistance to vancomycin

Z16.22   Resistance to vancomycin related antibiotics

Z16.23   Resistance to quinolones and fluoroquinolones

Z16.24   Resistance to multiple antibiotics

Z16.29   Resistance to other single specified antibiotic

Resistance to aminoglycosides

Resistance to macrolides

Resistance to sulfonamides

Resistance to tetracyclines

Z16.3   Resistance to other antimicrobial drugs

Excludes 1: resistance to antibiotics (Z16.1-, Z16.2-)

Z16.30   Resistance to unspecified antimicrobial drugs

Drug resistance NOS

Z16.31   Resistance to antiparasitic drug(s)

Resistance to quinine and related compounds

Z16.32   Resistance to antifungal drug(s)

Z16.33   Resistance to antiviral drug(s)

Z16.34   Resistance to antimycobacterial drug(s)

Resistance to tuberculostatics

Z16.341   Resistance to single antimycobacterial drug

Resistance to antimycobacterial drug NOS

Z16.342   Resistance to multiple antimycobacterial drugs

Z16.35   Resistance to multiple antimicrobial drugs

Excludes 1: Resistance to multiple antibiotics only (Z16.24)

Z16.39   Resistance to other specified antimicrobial drug

ESTROGEN RECEPTOR STATUS (Z17)

Z17   Estrogen receptor status

Code first malignant neoplasm of breast (C50.-)

Z17.0   Estrogen receptor positive status [ER+]

Z17.1   Estrogen receptor negative status [ER-]

Retained foreign body fragments (Z18)

Z18   Retained foreign body fragments

Includes: embedded fragment (status)

embedded splinter (status)

● New code   ▲ Revised code   ⑦ 7th digit required   ⊗ Placeholder required

retained foreign body status

Excludes 1: artificial joint prosthesis status (Z96.6-)

foreign body accidentally left during a procedure (T81.5-)

foreign body entering through orifice (T15-T19)

in situ cardiac device (Z95.-)

organ or tissue replaced by means other than transplant (Z96.-, Z97.-)

organ or tissue replaced by transplant (Z94.-)

personal history of retained foreign body fully removed Z87.821

superficial foreign body (non-embedded splinter) - code to superficial foreign body, by site

Z18.0 Retained radioactive fragments

  Z18.01 Retained depleted uranium fragments

  Z18.09 Other retained radioactive fragments

  Other retained depleted isotope fragments

  Retained nontherapeutic radioactive fragments

Z18.1 Retained metal fragments

  Excludes 1: retained radioactive metal fragments (Z18.01-Z18.09)

  Z18.10 Retained metal fragments, unspecified

  Retained metal fragment NOS

  Z18.11 Retained magnetic metal fragments

  Z18.12 Retained nonmagnetic metal fragments

Z18.2 Retained plastic fragments

  Acrylics fragments

  Diethylhexylphthalates fragments

  Isocyanate fragments

Z18.3 Retained organic fragments

  Z18.31 Retained animal quills or spines

  Z18.32 Retained tooth

  Z18.33 Retained wood fragments

  Z18.39 Other retained organic fragments

Z18.8 Other specified retained foreign body

  Z18.81 Retained glass fragments

  Z18.83 Retained stone or crystalline fragments

  Retained concrete or cement fragments

  Z18.89 Other specified retained foreign body fragments

Z18.9 Retained foreign body fragments, unspecified material

PERSONS WITH POTENTIAL HEALTH HAZARDS RELATED TO COMMUNICABLE DISEASES (Z20-Z28)

Z20 Contact with and (suspected) exposure to communicable diseases

  Excludes 1: carrier of infectious disease (Z22.-)

  diagnosed current infectious or parasitic disease -see Alphabetic Index

  Excludes 2: personal history of infectious and parasitic diseases (Z86.1-)

  Z20.0 Contact with and (suspected) exposure to intestinal infectious diseases

    Z20.01 Contact with and (suspected) exposure to intestinal infectious diseases due to Escherichia coli (E. coli)

    Z20.09 Contact with and (suspected) exposure to other intestinal infectious diseases

  Z20.1 Contact with and (suspected) exposure to tuberculosis

    Z20.2 Contact with and (suspected) exposure to infections with a predominantly sexual mode of transmission

Z20.3 Contact with and (suspected) exposure to rabies

Z20.4 Contact with and (suspected) exposure to rubella

Z20.5 Contact with and (suspected) exposure to viral hepatitis

Z20.6 Contact with and (suspected) exposure to human immunodeficiency virus [HIV]

  Excludes 1: asymptomatic human immunodeficiency virus [HIV]

  HIV infection status (Z21)

Z20.7 Contact with and (suspected) exposure to pediculosis, acariasis and other infestations

Z20.8 Contact with and (suspected) exposure to other communicable diseases

  Z20.81 Contact with and (suspected) exposure to other bacterial communicable diseases

    Z20.810 Contact with and (suspected) exposure to anthrax

    Z20.811 Contact with and (suspected) exposure to meningococcus

    Z20.818 Contact with and (suspected) exposure to other bacterial communicable diseases

  Z20.82 Contact with and (suspected) exposure to other viral communicable diseases

    Z20.820 Contact with and (suspected) exposure to varicella

    Z20.828 Contact with and (suspected) exposure to other viral communicable diseases

  Z20.89 Contact with and (suspected) exposure to other communicable diseases

Z20.9 Contact with and (suspected) exposure to unspecified communicable disease

Z21 Asymptomatic human immunodeficiency virus [HIV] infection status

HIV positive NOS

Code first Human immunodeficiency virus [HIV] disease complicating pregnancy, childbirth and the puerperium, if applicable (O98.7-)

Excludes 1: acquired immunodeficiency syndrome (B20)

contact with human immunodeficiency virus [HIV] (Z20.6)

exposure to human immunodeficiency virus [HIV] (Z20.6)

human immunodeficiency virus [HIV] disease (B20)

inconclusive laboratory evidence of human immunodeficiency virus [HIV] (R75)

Z22 Carrier of infectious disease

Includes: colonization status

suspected carrier

Z22.0 Carrier of typhoid

Z22.1 Carrier of other intestinal infectious diseases

Z22.2 Carrier of diphtheria

Z22.3 Carrier of other specified bacterial diseases

  Z22.31 Carrier of bacterial disease due to meningococci

  Z22.32 Carrier of bacterial disease due to staphylococci

    Z22.321 Carrier or suspected carrier of Methicillin susceptible Staphylococcus aureus

    MSSA colonization

    Z22.322 Carrier or suspected carrier of Methicillin resistant Staphylococcus aureus

MRSA colonization

Z22.33 Carrier of bacterial disease due to streptococci

   Z22.330 Carrier of Group B streptococcus

   Z22.338 Carrier of other streptococcus

Z22.39 Carrier of other specified bacterial diseases

Z22.4 Carrier of infections with a predominantly sexual mode of transmission

Z22.5 Carrier of viral hepatitis

   Z22.50 Carrier of unspecified viral hepatitis

   Z22.51 Carrier of viral hepatitis B

   Hepatitis B surface antigen [HBsAg] carrier

   Z22.52 Carrier of viral hepatitis C

   Z22.59 Carrier of other viral hepatitis

Z22.6 Carrier of human T-lymphotropic virus type-1[HTLV-1] infection

Z22.8 Carrier of other infectious diseases

Z22.9 Carrier of infectious disease, unspecified

Z23 Encounter for immunization

Code first any routine childhood examination

Note: procedure codes are required to identify the types of immunizations given

Z28 Immunization not carried out and underimmunization status

Includes: vaccination not carried out

Z28.0 Immunization not carried out because of contraindication

   Z28.01 Immunization not carried out because of acute illness of patient

   Z28.02 Immunization not carried out because of chronic illness or condition of patient

   Z28.03 Immunization not carried out because of immune compromised state of patient

   Z28.04 Immunization not carried out because of patient allergy to vaccine or component

   Z28.09 Immunization not carried out because of other contraindication

Z28.1 Immunization not carried out because of patient decision for reasons of belief or group pressure

   Immunization not carried out because of religious belief

Z28.2 Immunization not carried out because of patient decision for other and unspecified reason

   Z28.20 Immunization not carried out because of patient decision for unspecified reason

   Z28.21 Immunization not carried out because of patient refusal

   Z28.29 Immunization not carried out because of patient decision for other reason

Z28.3 Underimmunization status

Delinquent immunization status

Lapsed immunization schedule status

Z28.8 Immunization not carried out for other reason

   Z28.81 Immunization not carried out due to patient having had the disease

   Z28.82 Immunization not carried out because of caregiver refusal

   Immunization not carried out because of guardian refusal

   Immunization not carried out because of parent refusal

Excludes 1: immunization not carried out because of caregiver refusal because of religious belief (Z28.1)

   Z28.89 Immunization not carried out for other reason

Z28.9 Immunization not carried out for unspecified reason

PERSONS ENCOUNTERING HEALTH SERVICES IN CIRCUMSTANCES RELATED TO REPRODUCTION (Z30-Z39)

Z30 Encounter for contraceptive management

Z30.0 Encounter for general counseling and advice on contraception

   Z30.01 Encounter for initial prescription of contraceptives

   Excludes 1: encounter for surveillance of contraceptives (Z30.4-)

      Z30.011 Encounter for initial prescription of contraceptive pills

      Z30.012 Encounter for prescription of emergency contraception

      Encounter for postcoital contraception

      Z30.013 Encounter for initial prescription of injectable contraceptive

      Z30.014 Encounter for initial prescription of intrauterine contraceptive device

      Excludes 1: encounter for insertion of intrauterine contraceptive device (Z30.430, Z30.432)

      Z30.018 Encounter for initial prescription of other contraceptives

      Z30.019 Encounter for initial prescription of contraceptives, unspecified

   Z30.02 Counseling and instruction in natural family planning to avoid pregnancy

   Z30.09 Encounter for other general counseling and advice on contraception

   Encounter for family planning advice NOS

Z30.2 Encounter for sterilization

Z30.4 Encounter for surveillance of contraceptives

   Z30.40 Encounter for surveillance of contraceptives, unspecified

   Z30.41 Encounter for surveillance of contraceptive pills

   Encounter for repeat prescription for contraceptive pill

   Z30.42 Encounter for surveillance of injectable contraceptive

   Z30.43 Encounter for surveillance of intrauterine contraceptive device

      Z30.430 Encounter for insertion of intrauterine contraceptive device

      Z30.431 Encounter for routine checking of intrauterine contraceptive device

      Z30.432 Encounter for removal of intrauterine contraceptive device

      Z30.433 Encounter for removal and reinsertion of intrauterine contraceptive device

      Encounter for replacement of

Z30.49 Encounter for surveillance of other contraceptives

Z30.8 Encounter for other contraceptive management

Encounter for postvasectomy sperm count

Encounter for routine examination for contraceptive maintenance

Excludes 1: sperm count following sterilization reversal (Z31.42)

sperm count for fertility testing (Z31.41)

Z30.9 Encounter for contraceptive management, unspecified

Z31 Encounter for procreative management

Excludes 1: complications associated with artificial fertilization (N98.-)

female infertility (N97.-)

male infertility (N46.-)

Z31.0 Encounter for reversal of previous sterilization

Z31.4 Encounter for procreative investigation and testing

Excludes 1: postvasectomy sperm count (Z30.8)

Z31.41 Encounter for fertility testing

Encounter for fallopian tube patency testing

Encounter for sperm count for fertility testing

Z31.42 Aftercare following sterilization reversal

Sperm count following sterilization reversal

Z31.43 Encounter for genetic testing of female for procreative management

Use additional code for recurrent pregnancy loss, if applicable (N96, O26.2-)

Excludes 1: nonprocreative genetic testing (Z13.7-)

Z31.430 Encounter of female for testing for genetic disease carrier status for procreative management

Z31.438 Encounter for other genetic testing of female for procreative management

Z31.44 Encounter for genetic testing of male for procreative management

Excludes 1: nonprocreative genetic testing (Z13.7-)

Z31.440 Encounter of male for testing for genetic disease carrier status for procreative management

Z31.441 Encounter for testing of male partner of patient with recurrent pregnancy loss

Z31.448 Encounter for other genetic testing of male for procreative management

Z31.49 Encounter for other procreative investigation and testing

Z31.5 Encounter for genetic counseling

Z31.6 Encounter for general counseling and advice on procreation

Z31.61 Procreative counseling and advice using natural family planning

Z31.62 Encounter for fertility preservation counseling

Encounter for fertility preservation counseling prior to cancer therapy

Encounter for fertility preservation counseling prior to surgical removal of gonads

Z31.69 Encounter for other general counseling and advice on procreation

Z31.8 Encounter for other procreative management

Z31.81 Encounter for male factor infertility in female patient

Z31.82 Encounter for Rh incompatibility status

Z31.83 Encounter for assisted reproductive fertility procedure cycle

Patient undergoing in vitro fertilization cycle

Use additional code to identify the type of infertility

Excludes 1: pre-cycle diagnosis and testing - code to reason for encounter

Z31.84 Encounter for fertility preservation procedure

Encounter for fertility preservation procedure prior to cancer therapy

Encounter for fertility preservation procedure prior to surgical removal of gonads

Z31.89 Encounter for other procreative management

Z31.9 Encounter for procreative management, unspecified

Z32 Encounter for pregnancy test and childbirth and childcare instruction

Z32.0 Encounter for pregnancy test

Z32.00 Encounter for pregnancy test, result unknown

Encounter for pregnancy test NOS

Z32.01 Encounter for pregnancy test, result positive

Z32.02 Encounter for pregnancy test, result negative

Z32.2 Encounter for childbirth instruction

Z32.3 Encounter for childcare instruction

Encounter for prenatal or postpartum childcare instruction

Z33 Pregnant state

Z33.1 Pregnant state, incidental

Pregnant state NOS

Excludes 1: complications of pregnancy (O00-O9A)

Z33.2 Encounter for elective termination of pregnancy

Excludes 1: early fetal death with retention of dead fetus (O02.1)

late fetal death (O36.4)

spontaneous abortion (O03)

Z34 Encounter for supervision of normal pregnancy

Excludes 1: any complication of pregnancy (O00-O9A)

encounter for pregnancy test (Z32.0-)

encounter for supervision of high risk pregnancy (O09.-)

Z34.0 Encounter for supervision of normal first pregnancy

Z34.00 Encounter for supervision of normal first pregnancy, unspecified trimester

Z34.01 Encounter for supervision of normal first pregnancy, first trimester

Z34.02 Encounter for supervision of normal first pregnancy, second trimester

Z34.03 Encounter for supervision of normal first pregnancy, third trimester

Z34.8 Encounter for supervision of other normal pregnancy

Z34.80 Encounter for supervision of other normal pregnancy, unspecified trimester

Z34.81 Encounter for supervision of other normal pregnancy, first trimester

Z34.82 Encounter for supervision of other normal pregnancy, second trimester

Z34.83 Encounter for supervision of other normal pregnancy, third trimester

Z34.9 Encounter for supervision of normal pregnancy, unspecified

Z34.90 Encounter for supervision of normal pregnancy, unspecified, unspecified trimester

Z34.91 Encounter for supervision of normal pregnancy, unspecified, first trimester

Z34.92 Encounter for supervision of normal pregnancy, unspecified, second trimester

Z34.93 Encounter for supervision of normal pregnancy, unspecified, third trimester

Z36 Encounter for antenatal screening of mother

Excludes 1: abnormal findings on antenatal screening of mother (O28.-)

diagnostic examination- code to sign or symptom

encounter for suspected maternal and fetal conditions ruled out (Z03.7-)

suspected fetal condition affecting management of pregnancy - code to condition in Chapter 15

Excludes 2: genetic counseling and testing (Z31.43-, Z31.5)

routine prenatal care (Z34)

Z3A **Weeks of gestation**

Note: Codes from category Z3A are for use, only on the maternal record, to indicate the weeks of gestation of the pregnancy.

Code first complications of pregnancy, childbirth and the puerperium (O00-O9A)

Z3A.0 Weeks of gestation of pregnancy, unspecified or less than 10 weeks

Z3A.00 weeks of gestation of pregnancy not specified

Z3A.01 Less than 8 weeks gestation of pregnancy

Z3A.08 8 weeks gestation of pregnancy

Z3A.09 9 weeks gestation of pregnancy

Z3A.1 Weeks of gestation of pregnancy, weeks 10-19

Z3A.10 10 weeks gestation of pregnancy

Z3A.11 11 weeks gestation of pregnancy

Z3A.12 12 weeks gestation of pregnancy

Z3A.13 13 weeks gestation of pregnancy

Z3A.14 14 weeks gestation of pregnancy

Z3A.15 15 weeks gestation of pregnancy

Z3A.16 16 weeks gestation of pregnancy

Z3A.17 17 weeks gestation of pregnancy

Z3A.18 18 weeks gestation of pregnancy

Z3A.19 19 weeks gestation of pregnancy

Z3A.2 Weeks of gestation of pregnancy, weeks 20-29

Z3A.20 20 weeks gestation of pregnancy

Z3A.21 21 weeks gestation of pregnancy

Z3A.22 22 weeks gestation of pregnancy

Z3A.23 23 weeks gestation of pregnancy

Z3A.24 24 weeks gestation of pregnancy

Z3A.25 25 weeks gestation of pregnancy

Z3A.26 26 weeks gestation of pregnancy

Z3A.27 27 weeks gestation of pregnancy

Z3A.28 28 weeks gestation of pregnancy

Z3A.29 29 weeks gestation of pregnancy

Z3A.3 Weeks of gestation of pregnancy, weeks 30-39

Z3A.30 30 weeks gestation of pregnancy

Z3A.31 31 weeks gestation of pregnancy

Z3A.32 32 weeks gestation of pregnancy

Z3A.33 33 weeks gestation of pregnancy

Z3A.34 34 weeks gestation of pregnancy

Z3A.35 35 weeks gestation of pregnancy

Z3A.36 36 weeks gestation of pregnancy

Z3A.37 37 weeks gestation of pregnancy

Z3A.38 38 weeks gestation of pregnancy

Z3A.39 39 weeks gestation of pregnancy

Z3A.4 Weeks of gestation of pregnancy, weeks 40 or greater

Z3A.40 40 weeks gestation of pregnancy

Z3A.41 41 weeks gestation of pregnancy

Z3A.42 42 weeks gestation of pregnancy

Z3A.49 Greater than 42 weeks gestation of pregnancy

Z37 Outcome of delivery

This category is intended for use as an additional code to identify the outcome of delivery on the mother's record. It is not for use on the newborn record.

Excludes 1: stillbirth (P95)

Z37.0 Single live birth

Z37.1 Single stillbirth

Z37.2 Twins, both liveborn

Z37.3 Twins, one liveborn and one stillborn

Z37.4 Twins, both stillborn

Z37.5 Other multiple births, all liveborn

Z37.50 Multiple births, unspecified, all liveborn

Z37.51 Triplets, all liveborn

Z37.52 Quadruplets, all liveborn

Z37.53 Quintuplets, all liveborn

Z37.54 Sextuplets, all liveborn

Z37.59 Other multiple births, all liveborn

Z37.6 Other multiple births, some liveborn

Z37.60 Multiple births, unspecified, some liveborn

Z37.61 Triplets, some liveborn

Z37.62 Quadruplets, some liveborn

Z37.63 Quintuplets, some liveborn

Z37.64 Sextuplets, some liveborn

Z37.69 Other multiple births, some liveborn

Z37.7 Other multiple births, all stillborn

Z37.9 Outcome of delivery, unspecified

Multiple birth NOS

Single birth NOS

Z38 Liveborn infants according to place of birth and type of delivery

This category is for use as the principal code on the initial record of a newborn baby. It is to be used for the initial birth record only. It is not to be used on the mother's record.

Z38.0 Single liveborn infant, born in hospital

Single liveborn infant, born in birthing center or other health care facility

Z38.00 Single liveborn infant, delivered vaginally

Z38.01 Single liveborn infant, delivered by cesarean

Z38.1 Single liveborn infant, born outside hospital

Z38.2 Single liveborn infant, unspecified as to place of birth

Single liveborn infant NOS

Z38.3 Twin liveborn infant, born in hospital

Z38.30 Twin liveborn infant, delivered vaginally

Z38.31 Twin liveborn infant, delivered by cesarean

Z38.4 Twin liveborn infant, born outside hospital

Z38.5 Twin liveborn infant, unspecified as to place of birth

Z38.6 Other multiple liveborn infant, born in hospital

Z38.61 Triplet liveborn infant, delivered vaginally

Z38.62 Triplet liveborn infant, delivered by cesarean

Z38.63 Quadruplet liveborn infant, delivered vaginally

Z38.64 Quadruplet liveborn infant, delivered by cesarean

Z38.65 Quintuplet liveborn infant, delivered vaginally

Z38.66 Quintuplet liveborn infant, delivered by cesarean

Z38.68 Other multiple liveborn infant, delivered vaginally

Z38.69 Other multiple liveborn infant, delivered by cesarean

Z38.7 Other multiple liveborn infant, born outside hospital

Z38.8 Other multiple liveborn infant, unspecified as to place of birth

Z39 Encounter for maternal postpartum care and examination

Z39.0 Encounter for care and examination of mother immediately after delivery

Care and observation in uncomplicated cases when the delivery occurs outside a healthcare facility

Excludes 1: care for postpartum complication- see Alphabetic index

Z39.1 Encounter for care and examination of lactating mother

Encounter for supervision of lactation

Excludes 1: disorders of lactation (O92.-)

Z39.2 Encounter for routine postpartum follow-up

ENCOUNTERS FOR OTHER SPECIFIC HEALTH CARE (Z40-Z53)

Categories Z40-Z53 are intended for use to indicate a reason for care. They may be used for patients who have already been treated for a disease or injury, but who are receiving aftercare or prophylactic care, or care to consolidate the treatment, or to deal with a residual state

Excludes 2: follow-up examination for medical surveillance after treatment (Z08-Z09)

Z40 Encounter for prophylactic surgery

Excludes 1: organ donations (Z52.-)

therapeutic organ removal-code to condition

Z40.0 Encounter for prophylactic surgery for risk factors related to malignant neoplasms

Admission for prophylactic organ removal

Use additional code to identify risk factor

Z40.00 Encounter for prophylactic removal of unspecified organ

Z40.01 Encounter for prophylactic removal of breast

Z40.02 Encounter for prophylactic removal of ovary

Z40.09 Encounter for prophylactic removal of other organ

Z40.8 Encounter for other prophylactic surgery

Z40.9 Encounter for prophylactic surgery, unspecified

Z41 Encounter for procedures for purposes other than remedying health state

Z41.1 Encounter for cosmetic surgery

Encounter for cosmetic breast implant

Encounter for cosmetic procedure

Excludes 1: encounter for plastic and reconstructive

surgery following medical procedure or healed injury (Z42.-)

encounter for post-mastectomy breast implantation (Z42.1)

Z41.2 Encounter for routine and ritual male circumcision

Z41.3 Encounter for ear piercing

Z41.8 Encounter for other procedures for purposes other than remedying health state

Z41.9 Encounter for procedure for purposes other than remedying health state, unspecified

Z42 Encounter for plastic and reconstructive surgery following medical procedure or healed injury

Excludes 1: encounter for cosmetic plastic surgery (Z41.1)

encounter for plastic surgery for treatment of current injury - code to relevant injury

Z42.1 Encounter for breast reconstruction following mastectomy

Excludes 1: deformity and disproportion of reconstructed breast (N65.1-)

Z42.8 Encounter for other plastic and reconstructive surgery following medical procedure or healed injury

Z43 Encounter for attention to artificial openings

Includes: closure of artificial openings

passage of sounds or bougies through artificial openings

reforming artificial openings

removal of catheter from artificial openings

toilet or cleansing of artificial openings

Excludes 1: artificial opening status only, without need for care (Z93.-)

complications of external stoma (J95.0-, K94.-, N99.5-)

Excludes 2: fitting and adjustment of prosthetic and other devices (Z44-Z46)

Z43.0 Encounter for attention to tracheostomy

Z43.1 Encounter for attention to gastrostomy

Z43.2 Encounter for attention to ileostomy

Z43.3 Encounter for attention to colostomy

Z43.4 Encounter for attention to other artificial openings of digestive tract

Z43.5 Encounter for attention to cystostomy

Z43.6 Encounter for attention to other artificial openings of urinary tract

Encounter for attention to nephrostomy

Encounter for attention to ureterostomy

Encounter for attention to urethrostomy

Z43.7 Encounter for attention to artificial vagina

Z43.8 Encounter for attention to other artificial openings

Z43.9 Encounter for attention to unspecified artificial opening

Z44 Encounter for fitting and adjustment of external prosthetic device

Includes: removal or replacement of external prosthetic device

Excludes 1: malfunction or other complications of device - see Alphabetical Index

presence of prosthetic device (Z97.-)

Z44.0 Encounter for fitting and adjustment of artificial arm

Z44.00 Encounter for fitting and adjustment of unspecified artificial arm

Z44.001 Encounter for fitting and adjustment of unspecified right artificial arm

Z44.002 Encounter for fitting and adjustment of unspecified left artificial arm

Z44.009 Encounter for fitting and adjustment

---

of unspecified artificial arm, unspecified arm

Z44.01 Encounter for fitting and adjustment of complete artificial arm

   Z44.011 Encounter for fitting and adjustment of complete right artificial arm

   Z44.012 Encounter for fitting and adjustment of complete left artificial arm

   Z44.019 Encounter for fitting and adjustment of complete artificial arm, unspecified arm

Z44.02 Encounter for fitting and adjustment of partial artificial arm

   Z44.021 Encounter for fitting and adjustment of partial artificial right arm

   Z44.022 Encounter for fitting and adjustment of partial artificial left arm

   Z44.029 Encounter for fitting and adjustment of partial artificial arm, unspecified arm

Z44.1 Encounter for fitting and adjustment of artificial leg

  Z44.10 Encounter for fitting and adjustment of unspecified artificial leg

   Z44.101 Encounter for fitting and adjustment of unspecified right artificial leg

   Z44.102 Encounter for fitting and adjustment of unspecified left artificial leg

   Z44.109 Encounter for fitting and adjustment of unspecified artificial leg, unspecified leg

  Z44.11 Encounter for fitting and adjustment of complete artificial leg

   Z44.111 Encounter for fitting and adjustment of complete right artificial leg

   Z44.112 Encounter for fitting and adjustment of complete left artificial leg

   Z44.119 Encounter for fitting and adjustment of complete artificial leg, unspecified leg

  Z44.12 Encounter for fitting and adjustment of partial artificial leg

   Z44.121 Encounter for fitting and adjustment of partial artificial right leg

   Z44.122 Encounter for fitting and adjustment of partial artificial left leg

   Z44.129 Encounter for fitting and adjustment of partial artificial leg, unspecified leg

Z44.2 Encounter for fitting and adjustment of artificial eye
  Excludes 1: mechanical complication of ocular prosthesis (T85.3)

  Z44.20 Encounter for fitting and adjustment of artificial eye, unspecified

  Z44.21 Encounter for fitting and adjustment of artificial right eye

  Z44.22 Encounter for fitting and adjustment of artificial left eye

Z44.3 Encounter for fitting and adjustment of external breast prosthesis
  Excludes 1: complications of breast implant (T85.4-)

encounter for adjustment or removal of breast implant (Z45.81-)
encounter for initial breast implant insertion for cosmetic breast augmentation (Z41.1)
encounter for breast reconstruction following mastectomy (Z42.1)

  Z44.30 Encounter for fitting and adjustment of external breast prosthesis, unspecified breast

  Z44.31 Encounter for fitting and adjustment of external right breast prosthesis

  Z44.32 Encounter for fitting and adjustment of external left breast prosthesis

Z44.8 Encounter for fitting and adjustment of other external prosthetic devices

Z44.9 Encounter for fitting and adjustment of unspecified external prosthetic device

Z45 Encounter for adjustment and management of implanted device
  Includes: removal or replacement of implanted device
  Excludes 1: malfunction or other complications of device - see Alphabetical Index
   presence of prosthetic and other devices (Z95-Z97)
  Excludes 2: encounter for fitting and adjustment of non-implanted device (Z46.-)

Z45.0 Encounter for adjustment and management of cardiac device

  Z45.01 Encounter for adjustment and management of cardiac pacemaker
   Excludes 1: encounter for adjustment and management of automatic implantable cardiac defibrillator with synchronous cardiac pacemaker (Z45.02)

   Z45.010 Encounter for checking and testing of cardiac pacemaker pulse generator [battery]
    Encounter for replacing cardiac pacemaker pulse generator [battery]

   Z45.018 Encounter for adjustment and management of other part of cardiac pacemaker

  Z45.02 Encounter for adjustment and management of automatic implantable cardiac defibrillator
   Encounter for adjustment and management of automatic implantable cardiac defibrillator with synchronous cardiac pacemaker

  Z45.09 Encounter for adjustment and management of other cardiac device

Z45.1 Encounter for adjustment and management of infusion pump

Z45.2 Encounter for adjustment and management of vascular access device
  Encounter for adjustment and management of vascular catheters
  Excludes 1: encounter for adjustment and management of renal dialysis catheter (Z49.01)

Z45.3 Encounter for adjustment and management of implanted devices of the special senses

  Z45.31 Encounter for adjustment and management of implanted visual substitution device

  Z45.32 Encounter for adjustment and management of

implanted hearing device

Excludes 1: Encounter for fitting and adjustment of hearing aide (Z46.1)

Z45.320 Encounter for adjustment and management of bone conduction device

Z45.321 Encounter for adjustment and management of cochlear device

Z45.328 Encounter for adjustment and management of other implanted hearing device

Z45.4 Encounter for adjustment and management of implanted nervous system device

   Z45.41 Encounter for adjustment and management of cerebrospinal fluid drainage device

   Encounter for adjustment and management of cerebral ventricular (communicating) shunt

   Z45.42 Encounter for adjustment and management of neuropacemaker (brain) (peripheral nerve) (spinal cord)

   Z45.49 Encounter for adjustment and management of other implanted nervous system device

Z45.8 Encounter for adjustment and management of other implanted devices

   Z45.81 Encounter for adjustment or removal of breast implant

   Encounter for elective implant exchange (different material) (different size)

   Encounter removal of tissue expander without synchronous insertion of permanent implant

   Excludes 1: complications of breast implant (T85.4-)

      encounter for initial breast implant insertion for cosmetic breast augmentation (Z41.1)

      encounter for breast reconstruction following mastectomy (Z42.1)

      Z45.811 Encounter for adjustment or removal of right breast implant

      Z45.812 Encounter for adjustment or removal of left breast implant

      Z45.819 Encounter for adjustment or removal of unspecified breast implant

   Z45.82 Encounter for adjustment or removal of myringotomy device (stent) (tube)

   Z45.89 Encounter for adjustment and management of other implanted devices

Z45.9 Encounter for adjustment and management of unspecified implanted device

Z46 Encounter for fitting and adjustment of other devices

Includes: removal or replacement of other device

Excludes 1: malfunction or other complications of device - see Alphabetical Index

Excludes 2: encounter for fitting and management of implanted devices (Z45.-)

   issue of repeat prescription only (Z76.0)

   presence of prosthetic and other devices (Z95-Z97)

Z46.0 Encounter for fitting and adjustment of spectacles and contact lenses

Z46.1 Encounter for fitting and adjustment of hearing aid

Excludes 1: encounter for adjustment and management of implanted hearing device (Z45.32-)

Z46.2 Encounter for fitting and adjustment of other devices related to nervous system and special senses

Excludes 2: encounter for adjustment and management of implanted nervous system device (Z45.4-)

   encounter for adjustment and management of implanted visual substitution device (Z45.31)

Z46.3 Encounter for fitting and adjustment of dental prosthetic device

   Encounter for fitting and adjustment of dentures

Z46.4 Encounter for fitting and adjustment of orthodontic device

Z46.5 Encounter for fitting and adjustment of other gastrointestinal appliance and device

Excludes 1: encounter for attention to artificial openings of digestive tract (Z43.1-Z43.4)

   Z46.51 Encounter for fitting and adjustment of gastric lap band

   Z46.59 Encounter for fitting and adjustment of other gastrointestinal appliance and device

Z46.6 Encounter for fitting and adjustment of urinary device

Excludes 2: attention to artificial openings of urinary tract (Z43.5, Z43.6)

Z46.8 Encounter for fitting and adjustment of other specified devices

   Z46.81 Encounter for fitting and adjustment of insulin pump

   Encounter for insulin pump titration

   Encounter for insulin pump instruction and training

   Z46.82 Encounter for fitting and adjustment of non-vascular catheter

   Z46.89 Encounter for fitting and adjustment of other specified devices

   Encounter for fitting and adjustment of wheelchair

Z46.9 Encounter for fitting and adjustment of unspecified device

Z47 Orthopedic aftercare

Excludes 1: aftercare for healing fracture code to fracture with 7th character D

Z47.1 Aftercare following joint replacement surgery

   Use additional code to identify the joint (Z96.6-)

Z47.2 Encounter for removal of internal fixation device

Excludes 1: encounter for adjustment of internal fixation device for fracture treatment- code to fracture with appropriate 7th

   Character encounter for removal of external fixation device- code to fracture with 7th character D infection or inflammatory reaction to internal fixation device (T84.6-) mechanical complication of internal fixation device (T84.1-)

Z47.3 Aftercare following explanation of joint prosthesis

   Aftercare following explanation of joint prosthesis, staged procedure

   Encounter for joint prosthesis insertion following prior explanation of joint prosthesis

   Z47.31 Aftercare following explanation of shoulder joint prosthesis

      Excludes 1: acquired absence of shoulder joint following prior explanation of

---

shoulder joint
prosthesis (Z89.23-)
shoulder joint prosthesis
explantation status (Z89.23-)

Z47.32 Aftercare following explantation of hip joint
prosthesis
Excludes 1: acquired absence of hip joint
following prior explantation of hip
joint prosthesis (Z89.62-)
hip joint prosthesis explantation
status (Z89.62-)

Z47.33 Aftercare following explantation of knee joint
prosthesis
Excludes 1: acquired absence of knee joint
following prior explantation of knee
prosthesis (Z89.52-
knee joint prosthesis explantation
status (Z89.52-)

Z47.8 Encounter for other orthopedic aftercare

Z47.81 Encounter for orthopedic aftercare following
surgical amputation
Use additional code to identify the limb
amputated (Z89.-)

Z47.82 Encounter for orthopedic aftercare following
scoliosis surgery

Z47.89 Encounter for other orthopedic aftercare

Z48 Encounter for other postprocedural aftercare
Excludes 1: encounter for follow-up examination after completed
treatment (Z08-Z09)
Excludes 2: encounter for attention to artificial openings (Z43.-)
encounter for fitting and adjustment of prosthetic and other
devices (Z44-Z46)

Z48.0 Encounter for attention to dressings, sutures and drains
Excludes 1: encounter for planned postprocedural wound
closure (Z48.1)

Z48.00 Encounter for change or removal of nonsurgical
wound dressing
Encounter for change or removal of wound
dressing NOS

Z48.01 Encounter for change or removal of surgical
wound dressing

Z48.02 Encounter for removal of sutures
Encounter for removal of staples

Z48.03 Encounter for change or removal of drains

Z48.1 Encounter for planned postprocedural wound closure
Excludes 1: encounter for attention to dressings and
sutures (Z48.0-)

Z48.2 Encounter for aftercare following organ transplant

Z48.21 Encounter for aftercare following heart transplant

Z48.22 Encounter for aftercare following kidney
transplant

Z48.23 Encounter for aftercare following liver transplant

Z48.24 Encounter for aftercare following lung transplant

Z48.28 Encounter for aftercare following multiple organ
transplant

Z48.280 Encounter for aftercare following
heart-lung transplant

Z48.288 Encounter for aftercare following
multiple organ transplant

Z48.29 Encounter for aftercare following other organ
transplant

Z48.290 Encounter for aftercare following
bone marrow transplant

Z48.298 Encounter for aftercare following
other organ transplant

Z48.3 Aftercare following surgery for neoplasm
Use additional code to identify the neoplasm

Z48.8 Encounter for other specified postprocedural aftercare

Z48.81 Encounter for surgical aftercare following
surgery on specified body systems
These codes identify the body system requiring
aftercare. They are for use in conjunction with
other aftercare codes to fully explain the aftercare
encounter. The condition treated should also be
coded if still present.
Excludes 1: aftercare for injury- code the injury
with 7th character D
aftercare following surgery for
neoplasm (Z48.3)
Excludes 2: aftercare following organ transplant
(Z48.2-)
orthopedic aftercare (Z47.-)

Z48.810 Encounter for surgical aftercare
following surgery on the sense
organs

Z48.811 Encounter for surgical aftercare
following surgery on the nervous
system
Excludes 2: encounter for surgical
aftercare following
surgery on the sense
organs (Z48.810)

Z48.812 Encounter for surgical aftercare
following surgery on the circulatory
system

Z48.813 Encounter for surgical aftercare
following surgery on the respiratory
system

Z48.814 Encounter for surgical aftercare
following surgery on the teeth or
oral cavity

Z48.815 Encounter for surgical aftercare
following surgery on the digestive
system

Z48.816 Encounter for surgical aftercare
following surgery on the
genitourinary system
Excludes 1: encounter for aftercare
following sterilization
reversal (Z31.42)

Z48.817 Encounter for surgical aftercare
following surgery on the skin and
subcutaneous tissue

Z48.89 Encounter for other specified surgical aftercare

Z49 Encounter for care involving renal dialysis
Code also associated end stage renal disease (N18.6)

Z49.0 Preparatory care for renal dialysis
Encounter for dialysis instruction and training

Z49.01 Encounter for fitting and adjustment of

extracorporeal dialysis catheter
Removal or replacement of renal dialysis catheter
Toilet or cleansing of renal dialysis catheter

Z49.02 Encounter for fitting and adjustment of peritoneal dialysis catheter

Z49.3 Encounter for adequacy testing for dialysis

Z49.31 Encounter for adequacy testing for hemodialysis

Z49.32 Encounter for adequacy testing for peritoneal dialysis
Encounter for peritoneal equilibration test

Z51 Encounter for other aftercare
Code also condition requiring care
Excludes 1: follow-up examination after treatment (Z08-Z09)

Z51.0 Encounter for antineoplastic radiation therapy

Z51.1 Encounter for antineoplastic chemotherapy and immunotherapy
Excludes 2: encounter for chemotherapy and immunotherapy for nonneoplastic condition - code to condition

Z51.11 Encounter for antineoplastic chemotherapy

Z51.12 Encounter for antineoplastic immunotherapy

Z51.5 Encounter for palliative care

Z51.8 Encounter for other specified aftercare
Excludes 1: holiday relief care (Z75.5)

Z51.81 Encounter for therapeutic drug level monitoring
Code also any long-term (current) drug therapy (Z79.-)
Excludes 1: encounter for blood-drug test for administrative or medicolegal reasons (Z02.83)

Z51.89 Encounter for other specified aftercare

Z52 Donors of organs and tissues
Includes: autologous and other living donors
Excludes 1: cadaveric donor - omit code
examination of potential donor (Z00.5)

Z52.0 Blood donor

Z52.00 Unspecified blood donor

Z52.000 Unspecified donor, whole blood

Z52.001 Unspecified donor, stem cells

Z52.008 Unspecified donor, other blood

Z52.01 Autologous blood donor

Z52.010 Autologous donor, whole blood

Z52.011 Autologous donor, stem cells

Z52.018 Autologous donor, other blood

Z52.09 Other blood donor
Volunteer donor

Z52.090 Other blood donor, whole blood

Z52.091 Other blood donor, stem cells

Z52.098 Other blood donor, other blood

Z52.1 Skin donor

Z52.10 Skin donor, unspecified

Z52.11 Skin donor, autologous

Z52.19 Skin donor, other

Z52.2 Bone donor

Z52.20 Bone donor, unspecified

Z52.21 Bone donor, autologous

Z52.29 Bone donor, other

Z52.3 Bone marrow donor

Z52.4 Kidney donor

Z52.5 Cornea donor

Z52.6 Liver donor

Z52.8 Donor of other specified organs or tissues

Z52.81 Egg (Oocyte) donor

Z52.810 Egg (Oocyte) donor under age 35, anonymous recipient
Egg donor under age 35 NOS

Z52.811 Egg (Oocyte) donor under age 35, designated recipient

Z52.812 Egg (Oocyte) donor age 35 and over, anonymous recipient
Egg donor age 35 and over NOS

Z52.813 Egg (Oocyte) donor age 35 and over, designated recipient

Z52.819 Egg (Oocyte) donor, unspecified

Z52.89 Donor of other specified organs or tissues

Z52.9 Donor of unspecified organ or tissue
Donor NOS

Z53 Persons encountering health services for specific procedures and treatment, not carried out

Z53.0 Procedure and treatment not carried out because of contraindication

Z53.01 Procedure and treatment not carried out due to patient smoking

Z53.09 Procedure and treatment not carried out because of other contraindication

Z53.1 Procedure and treatment not carried out because of patient's decision for reasons of belief and group pressure

Z53.2 Procedure and treatment not carried out because of patient's decision for other and unspecified reasons

Z53.20 Procedure and treatment not carried out because of patient's decision for unspecified reasons

Z53.21 Procedure and treatment not carried out due to patient leaving prior to being seen by health care provider

Z53.29 Procedure and treatment not carried out because of patient's decision for other reasons

Z53.8 Procedure and treatment not carried out for other reasons

Z53.9 Procedure and treatment not carried out, unspecified reason

PERSONS WITH POTENTIAL HEALTH HAZARDS RELATED TO SOCIOECONOMIC AND PSYCHOSOCIAL CIRCUMSTANCES (Z55-Z65)

Z55 Problems related to education and literacy
Excludes 1: disorders of psychological development (F80-F89)

Z55.0 Illiteracy and low-level literacy

Z55.1 Schooling unavailable and unattainable

Z55.2 Failed school examinations

Z55.3 Underachievement in school

Z55.4 Educational maladjustment and discord with teachers and classmates

Z55.8 Other problems related to education and literacy
Problems related to inadequate teaching

Z55.9 Problems related to education and literacy, unspecified
Academic problems NOS

Z56 Problems related to employment and unemployment

Excludes 2: occupational exposure to risk factors (Z57.-)
problems related to housing and economic circumstances (Z59.-)

Z56.0 Unemployment, unspecified
Z56.1 Change of job
Z56.2 Threat of job loss
Z56.3 Stressful work schedule
Z56.4 Discord with boss and workmates
Z56.5 Uncongenial work environment
Difficult conditions at work
Z56.6 Other physical and mental strain related to work
Z56.8 Other problems related to employment
  Z56.81 Sexual harassment on the job
  Z56.82 Military deployment status
Individual (civilian or military) currently deployed in theater or in support of military war, peacekeeping and humanitarian operations
  Z56.89 Other problems related to employment
Z56.9 Unspecified problems related to employment
Occupational problems NOS

Z57 Occupational exposure to risk factors
Z57.0 Occupational exposure to noise
Z57.1 Occupational exposure to radiation
Z57.2 Occupational exposure to dust
Z57.3 Occupational exposure to other air contaminants
  Z57.31 Occupational exposure to environmental tobacco smoke
    Excludes 2: exposure to environmental tobacco smoke (Z77.22)
  Z57.39 Occupational exposure to other air contaminants
Z57.4 Occupational exposure to toxic agents in agriculture
Occupational exposure to solids, liquids, gases or vapors in agriculture
Z57.5 Occupational exposure to toxic agents in other industries
Occupational exposure to solids, liquids, gases or vapors in other industries
Z57.6 Occupational exposure to extreme temperature
Z57.7 Occupational exposure to vibration
Z57.8 Occupational exposure to other risk factors
Z57.9 Occupational exposure to unspecified risk factor

Z59 Problems related to housing and economic circumstances
Excludes 2: problems related to upbringing (Z62.-)
Z59.0 Homelessness
Z59.1 Inadequate housing
Lack of heating
Restriction of space
Technical defects in home preventing adequate care
Unsatisfactory surroundings
Excludes 1: problems related to the natural and physical environment (Z77.1-)
Z59.2 Discord with neighbors, lodgers and landlord
Z59.3 Problems related to living in residential institution
Boarding-school resident
Excludes 1: institutional upbringing (Z62.2)
Z59.4 Lack of adequate food and safe drinking water
Inadequate drinking water supply
Excludes 1: effects of hunger (T73.0)

inappropriate diet or eating habits (Z72.4)
malnutrition (E40-E46)

Z59.5 Extreme poverty
Z59.6 Low income
Z59.7 Insufficient social insurance and welfare support
Z59.8 Other problems related to housing and economic circumstances
Foreclosure on loan
Isolated dwelling
Problems with creditors
Z59.9 Problem related to housing and economic circumstances, unspecified

Z60 Problems related to social environment
Z60.0 Problems of adjustment to life-cycle transitions
Empty nest syndrome
Phase of life problem
Problem with adjustment to retirement [pension]
Z60.2 Problems related to living alone
Z60.3 Acculturation difficulty
Problem with migration
Problem with social transplantation
Z60.4 Social exclusion and rejection
Exclusion and rejection on the basis of personal characteristics, such as unusual physical appearance, illness or behavior.
Excludes 1: target of adverse discrimination such as for racial or religious reasons (Z60.5)
Z60.5 Target of (perceived) adverse discrimination and persecution
Excludes 1: social exclusion and rejection (Z60.4)
Z60.8 Other problems related to social environment
Z60.9 Problem related to social environment, unspecified

Z62 Problems related to upbringing
Includes: current and past negative life events in childhood
current and past problems of a child related to upbringing
Excludes 2: maltreatment syndrome (T74.-)
problems related to housing and economic circumstances (Z59.-)
Z62.0 Inadequate parental supervision and control
Z62.1 Parental overprotection
Z62.2 Upbringing away from parents
Excludes 1: problems with boarding school (Z59.3)
  Z62.21 Child in welfare custody
Child in care of non-parental family member
Child in foster care
    Excludes 2: problem for parent due to child in welfare custody (Z63.5)
  Z62.22 Institutional upbringing
Child living in orphanage or group home
  Z62.29 Other upbringing away from parents
Z62.3 Hostility towards and scapegoating of child
Z62.6 Inappropriate (excessive) parental pressure
Z62.8 Other specified problems related to upbringing
  Z62.81 Personal history of abuse in childhood
    Z62.810 Personal history of physical and sexual abuse in childhood
      Excludes 1: current child physical abuse (T74.12, T76.12)

● New code   ▲ Revised code   ⑦ 7th digit required   ⊗ Placeholder required

current child sexual
abuse (T74.22, T76.22)

Z62.811 Personal history of psychological
abuse in childhood
Excludes 1: current child
psychological abuse
(T74.32, T76.32)

Z62.812 Personal history of neglect in
childhood
Excludes 1: current child neglect
(T74.02, T76.02)

Z62.819 Personal history of unspecified
abuse in childhood
Excludes 1: current child abuse
NOS (T74.92, T76.92)

Z62.82 Parent-child conflict

Z62.820 Parent-biological child conflict
Parent-child problem NOS

Z62.821 Parent-adopted child conflict

Z62.822 Parent-foster child conflict

Z62.89 Other specified problems related to upbringing

Z62.890 Parent-child estrangement NEC

Z62.891 Sibling rivalry

Z62.898 Other specified problems related to
upbringing

Z62.9 Problem related to upbringing, unspecified

Z63 Other problems related to primary support group, including family
circumstances
Excludes 2: maltreatment syndrome (T74.-, T76)
parent-child problems (Z62.-)
problems related to negative life events in childhood
(Z62.-)
problems related to upbringing (Z62.-)

Z63.0 Problems in relationship with spouse or partner
Excludes 1: counseling for spousal or partner abuse
problems (Z69.1)
counseling related to sexual attitude, behavior,
and orientation (Z70.-)

Z63.1 Problems in relationship with in-laws

Z63.3 Absence of family member
Excludes 1: absence of family member due to
disappearance and death (Z63.4)
absence of family member due to separation and
divorce (Z63.5)

Z63.31 Absence of family member due to military
deployment
Individual or family affected by other family
member being on military deployment
Excludes 1: family disruption due to return of
family member from military
deployment (Z63.71)

Z63.32 Other absence of family member

Z63.4 Disappearance and death of family member
Assumed death of family member
Bereavement

Z63.5 Disruption of family by separation and divorce
Marital estrangement

Z63.6 Dependent relative needing care at home

Z63.7 Other stressful life events affecting family and household

Z63.71 Stress on family due to return of family member
from military deployment
Individual or family affected by family member
having returned from military deployment
(current or
past conflict)

Z63.72 Alcoholism and drug addiction in family

Z63.79 Other stressful life events affecting family and
household
Anxiety (normal) about sick person in family
Health problems within family
Ill or disturbed family member
Isolated family

Z63.8 Other specified problems related to primary support group
Family discord NOS
Family estrangement NOS
High expressed emotional level within family
Inadequate family support NOS
Inadequate or distorted communication within family

Z63.9 Problem related to primary support group, unspecified
Relationship disorder NOS

Z64 Problems related to certain psychosocial circumstances

Z64.0 Problems related to unwanted pregnancy

Z64.1 Problems related to multiparity

Z64.4 Discord with counselors
Discord with probation officer
Discord with social worker

Z65 Problems related to other psychosocial circumstances

Z65.0 Conviction in civil and criminal proceedings without
imprisonment

Z65.1 Imprisonment and other incarceration

Z65.2 Problems related to release from prison

Z65.3 Problems related to other legal circumstances
Arrest
Child custody or support proceedings
Litigation
Prosecution

Z65.4 Victim of crime and terrorism
Victim of torture

Z65.5 Exposure to disaster, war and other hostilities
Excludes 1: target of perceived discrimination or
persecution (Z60.5)

Z65.8 Other specified problems related to psychosocial
circumstances

Z65.9 Problem related to unspecified psychosocial circumstances

DO NOT RESUSCITATE STATUS (Z66)

Z66 Do not resuscitate
DNR status

BLOOD TYPE (Z67)

Z67 Blood type

Z67.1 Type A blood

Z67.10 Type A blood, Rh positive

Z67.11 Type A blood, Rh negative

Z67.2 Type B blood

Z67.20 Type B blood, Rh positive

Z67.21 Type B blood, Rh negative

Z67.3   Type AB blood

    Z67.30   Type AB blood, Rh positive

    Z67.31   Type AB blood, Rh negative

Z67.4   Type O blood

    Z67.40   Type O blood, Rh positive

    Z67.41   Type O blood, Rh negative

Z67.9   Unspecified blood type

    Z67.90   Unspecified blood type, Rh positive

    Z67.91   Unspecified blood type, Rh negative

BODY MASS INDEX [BMI] (Z68)

Z68 Body mass index [BMI]

Kilograms per meters squared

Note: BMI adult codes are for use for persons 21 years of age or older

BMI pediatric codes are for use for persons 2-20 years of age. These percentiles are based on the growth charts published by the Centers for Disease Control and Prevention (CDC)

Z68.1   Body mass index (BMI) 19 or less, adult

Z68.2   Body mass index (BMI) 20-29, adult

    Z68.20   Body mass index (BMI) 20.0-20.9, adult

    Z68.21   Body mass index (BMI) 21.0-21.9, adult

    Z68.22   Body mass index (BMI) 22.0-22.9, adult

    Z68.23   Body mass index (BMI) 23.0-23.9, adult

    Z68.24   Body mass index (BMI) 24.0-24.9, adult

    Z68.25   Body mass index (BMI) 25.0-25.9, adult

    Z68.26   Body mass index (BMI) 26.0-26.9, adult

    Z68.27   Body mass index (BMI) 27.0-27.9, adult

    Z68.28   Body mass index (BMI) 28.0-28.9, adult

    Z68.29   Body mass index (BMI) 29.0-29.9, adult

Z68.3   Body mass index (BMI) 30-39, adult

    Z68.30   Body mass index (BMI) 30.0-30.9, adult

    Z68.31   Body mass index (BMI) 31.0-31.9, adult

    Z68.32   Body mass index (BMI) 32.0-32.9, adult

    Z68.33   Body mass index (BMI) 33.0-33.9, adult

    Z68.34   Body mass index (BMI) 34.0-34.9, adult

    Z68.35   Body mass index (BMI) 35.0-35.9, adult

    Z68.36   Body mass index (BMI) 36.0-36.9, adult

    Z68.37   Body mass index (BMI) 37.0-37.9, adult

    Z68.38   Body mass index (BMI) 38.0-38.9, adult

    Z68.39   Body mass index (BMI) 39.0-39.9, adult

Z68.4   Body mass index (BMI) 40 or greater, adult

    Z68.41   Body mass index (BMI) 40.0-44.9, adult

    Z68.42   Body mass index (BMI) 45.0-49.9, adult

    Z68.43   Body mass index (BMI) 50-59.9, adult

    Z68.44   Body mass index (BMI) 60.0-69.9, adult

    Z68.45   Body mass index (BMI) 70 or greater, adult

Z68.5   Body mass index (BMI) pediatric

    Z68.51   Body mass index (BMI) pediatric, less than 5th percentile for age

    Z68.52   Body mass index (BMI) pediatric, 5th percentile to less than 85th percentile for age

    Z68.53   Body mass index (BMI) pediatric, 85th percentile to less than 95th percentile for age

    Z68.54   Body mass index (BMI) pediatric, greater than or equal to 95th percentile for age

PERSONS ENCOUNTERING HEALTH SERVICES IN OTHER CIRCUMSTANCES (Z69-Z76)

Z69 Encounter for mental health services for victim and perpetrator of abuse

Includes: counseling for victims and perpetrators of abuse

Z69.0   Encounter for mental health services for child abuse problems

    Z69.01   Encounter for mental health services for parental child abuse

        Z69.010   Encounter for mental health services for victim of parental child abuse

        Z69.011   Encounter for mental health services for perpetrator of parental child abuse

            Excludes 1: encounter for mental health services for non-parental child abuse (Z69.02-)

    Z69.02   Encounter for mental health services for non-parental child abuse

        Z69.020   Encounter for mental health services for victim of non-parental child abuse

        Z69.021   Encounter for mental health services for perpetrator of non-parental child abuse

Z69.1   Encounter for mental health services for spousal or partner abuse problems

    Z69.11   Encounter for mental health services for victim of spousal or partner abuse

    Z69.12   Encounter for mental health services for perpetrator of spousal or partner abuse

Z69.8   Encounter for mental health services for victim or perpetrator of other abuse

    Z69.81   Encounter for mental health services for victim of other abuse

        Encounter for rape victim counseling

    Z69.82   Encounter for mental health services for perpetrator of other abuse

Z70 Counseling related to sexual attitude, behavior and orientation

Includes: encounter for mental health services for sexual attitude, behavior and orientation

Excludes 2: contraceptive or procreative counseling (Z30-Z31)

Z70.0   Counseling related to sexual attitude

Z70.1   Counseling related to patient's sexual behavior and orientation

    Patient concerned regarding impotence

    Patient concerned regarding non-responsiveness

    Patient concerned regarding promiscuity

    Patient concerned regarding sexual orientation

Z70.2   Counseling related to sexual behavior and orientation of third party

    Advice sought regarding sexual behavior and orientation of child

    Advice sought regarding sexual behavior and orientation of partner

    Advice sought regarding sexual behavior and orientation of spouse

Z70.3   Counseling related to combined concerns regarding sexual attitude, behavior and orientation

Z70.8 Other sex counseling

Encounter for sex education

Z70.9 Sex counseling, unspecified

Z71 Persons encountering health services for other counseling and medical advice, not elsewhere classified

Excludes 2: contraceptive or procreation counseling (Z30-Z31)

sex counseling (Z70.-)

Z71.0 Person encountering health services to consult on behalf of another person

Person encountering health services to seek advice or treatment for non-attending third party

Excludes 2: anxiety (normal) about sick person in family (Z63.7)

expectant (adoptive) parent(s) pre-birth pediatrician visit (Z76.81)

Z71.1 Person with feared health complaint in whom no diagnosis is made

Person encountering health services with feared condition which was not demonstrated

Person encountering health services in which problem was normal state

'Worried well'

Excludes 1: medical observation for suspected diseases and conditions proven not to exist (Z03.-)

Z71.2 Person consulting for explanation of examination or test findings

Z71.3 Dietary counseling and surveillance

Use additional code for any associated underlying medical condition

Use additional code to identify body mass index (BMI), if known (Z68.-)

Z71.4 Alcohol abuse counseling and surveillance

Use additional code for alcohol abuse or dependence (F10.-)

Z71.41 Alcohol abuse counseling and surveillance of alcoholic

Z71.42 Counseling for family member of alcoholic

Counseling for significant other, partner, or friend of alcoholic

Z71.5 Drug abuse counseling and surveillance

Use additional code for drug abuse or dependence (F11-F16, F18-F19)

Z71.51 Drug abuse counseling and surveillance of drug abuser

Z71.52 Counseling for family member of drug abuser

Counseling for significant other, partner, or friend of drug abuser

Z71.6 Tobacco abuse counseling

Use additional code for nicotine dependence (F17.-)

Z71.7 Human immunodeficiency virus [HIV] counseling

Z71.8 Other specified counseling

Excludes 2: counseling for contraception (Z30.0-)

counseling for genetics (Z31.5)

counseling for procreative management (Z31.6-)

Z71.81 Spiritual or religious counseling

Z71.89 Other specified counseling

Z71.9 Counseling, unspecified

Encounter for medical advice NOS

Z72 Problems related to lifestyle

Excludes 2: problems related to life-management difficulty (Z73.-)

problems related to socioeconomic and psychosocial circumstances (Z55-Z65)

Z72.0 Tobacco use

Tobacco use NOS

Excludes 1: history of tobacco dependence (Z87.891)

nicotine dependence (F17.2-)

tobacco dependence (F17.2-)

tobacco use during pregnancy (O99.33-)

Z72.3 Lack of physical exercise

Z72.4 Inappropriate diet and eating habits

Excludes 1: behavioral eating disorders of infancy or childhood (F98.2.- F98.3)

eating disorders (F50.-)

lack of adequate food (Z59.4)

malnutrition and other nutritional deficiencies (E40-E64)

Z72.5 High risk sexual behavior

Promiscuity

Excludes 1: paraphilias (F65)

Z72.51 High risk heterosexual behavior

Z72.52 High risk homosexual behavior

Z72.53 High risk bisexual behavior

Z72.6 Gambling and betting

Excludes 1: compulsive or pathological gambling (F63.0)

Z72.8 Other problems related to lifestyle

Z72.81 Antisocial behavior

Excludes 1: conduct disorders (F91.-)

Z72.810 Child and adolescent antisocial behavior

Antisocial behavior (child) (adolescent) without manifest psychiatric disorder

Delinquency NOS

Group delinquency

Offenses in the context of gang membership

Stealing in company with others

Truancy from school

Z72.811 Adult antisocial behavior

Adult antisocial behavior without manifest psychiatric disorder

Z72.82 Problems related to sleep

Z72.820 Sleep deprivation

Lack of adequate sleep

Excludes 1: insomnia (G47.0-)

Z72.821 Inadequate sleep hygiene

Bad sleep habits

Irregular sleep habits

Unhealthy sleep wake schedule

Excludes 1: insomnia (F51.0-, G47.0-)

Z72.89 Other problems related to lifestyle

Self-damaging behavior

Z72.9 Problem related to lifestyle, unspecified

Z73 Problems related to life management difficulty

Excludes 2: problems related to socioeconomic and psychosocial circumstances (Z55-Z65)

Z73.0   Burn-out

Z73.1   Type A behavior pattern

Z73.2   Lack of relaxation and leisure

Z73.3   Stress, not elsewhere classified
        Physical and mental strain NOS
        Excludes 1: stress related to employment or unemployment (Z56.-)

Z73.4   Inadequate social skills, not elsewhere classified

Z73.5   Social role conflict, not elsewhere classified

Z73.6   Limitation of activities due to disability
        Excludes 1: care-provider dependency (Z74.-)

Z73.8   Other problems related to life management difficulty

      Z73.81   Behavioral insomnia of childhood

          Z73.810   Behavioral insomnia of childhood, sleep-onset association type

          Z73.811   Behavioral insomnia of childhood, limit setting type

          Z73.812   Behavioral insomnia of childhood, combined type

          Z73.819   Behavioral insomnia of childhood, unspecified type

      Z73.82   Dual sensory impairment

      Z73.89   Other problems related to life management difficulty

Z73.9   Problem related to life management difficulty, unspecified

Z74   Problems related to care provider dependency
      Excludes 2: dependence on enabling machines or devices NEC (Z99.-)

Z74.0   Reduced mobility

      Z74.01   Bed confinement status
          Bedridden

      Z74.09   Other reduced mobility
          Chair ridden
          Reduced mobility NOS
          Excludes 2: wheelchair dependence (Z99.3)

Z74.1   Need for assistance with personal care

Z74.2   Need for assistance at home and no other household member able to render care

Z74.3   Need for continuous supervision

Z74.8   Other problems related to care provider dependency

Z74.9   Problem related to care provider dependency, unspecified

Z75   Problems related to medical facilities and other health care

Z75.0   Medical services not available in home
      Excludes 1: no other household member able to render care (Z74.2)

Z75.1   Person awaiting admission to adequate facility elsewhere

Z75.2   Other waiting period for investigation and treatment

Z75.3   Unavailability and inaccessibility of health-care facilities
      Excludes 1: bed unavailable (Z75.1)

Z75.4   Unavailability and inaccessibility of other helping agencies

Z75.5   Holiday relief care

Z75.8   Other problems related to medical facilities and other health care

Z75.9   Unspecified problem related to medical facilities and other health care

Z76   Persons encountering health services in other circumstances

Z76.0   Encounter for issue of repeat prescription
      Encounter for issue of repeat prescription for appliance
      Encounter for issue of repeat prescription for medicaments
      Encounter for issue of repeat prescription for spectacles
      Excludes 2: issue of medical certificate (Z02.7)
          repeat prescription for contraceptive (Z30.4-)

Z76.1   Encounter for health supervision and care of foundling

Z76.2   Encounter for health supervision and care of other healthy infant and child
      Encounter for medical or nursing care or supervision of healthy infant under circumstances such as adverse socioeconomic conditions at home
      Encounter for medical or nursing care or supervision of healthy infant under circumstances such as awaiting foster or adoptive placement
      Encounter for medical or nursing care or supervision of healthy infant under circumstances such as maternal illness
      Encounter for medical or nursing care or supervision of healthy infant under circumstances such as number of children at home preventing or interfering with normal care

Z76.3   Healthy person accompanying sick person

Z76.4   Other boarder to healthcare facility
      Excludes 1: homelessness (Z59.0)

Z76.5   Malingerer [conscious simulation]
      Person feigning illness (with obvious motivation)
      Excludes 1: factitious disorder (F68.1-)
          peregrinating patient (F68.1-)

Z76.8   Persons encountering health services in other specified circumstances

      Z76.81   Expectant parent(s) prebirth pediatrician visit
          Pre-adoption pediatrician visit for adoptive parent(s)

      Z76.82   Awaiting organ transplant status
          Patient waiting for organ availability

      Z76.89   Persons encountering health services in other specified circumstances
          Persons encountering health services NOS

PERSONS WITH POTENTIAL HEALTH HAZARDS RELATED TO FAMILY AND PERSONAL HISTORY AND CERTAIN CONDITIONS INFLUENCING HEALTH STATUS (Z77-Z99)

Code also any follow-up examination (Z08-Z09)

Z77   Other contact with and (suspected) exposures hazardous to health
      Includes: contact with and (suspected) exposures to potential hazards to health
      Excludes 2: contact with and (suspected) exposure to communicable diseases (Z20.-)
          exposure to (parental) (environmental) tobacco smoke in the perinatal period (P96.81)
          newborn (suspected to be) affected by noxious substances transmitted via placenta or breast milk (P04.-)
          occupational exposure to risk factors (Z57.-)
          retained foreign body (Z18.-)
          retained foreign body fully removed (Z87.821)
          toxic effects of substances chiefly nonmedicinal as to source (T51-T65)

Z77.0   Contact with and (suspected) exposure to hazardous, chiefly nonmedicinal, chemicals

      Z77.01   Contact with and (suspected) exposure to hazardous metals

Z77.010 Contact with and (suspected) exposure to arsenic

Z77.011 Contact with and (suspected) exposure to lead

Z77.012 Contact with and (suspected) exposure to uranium

> **Excludes 1:** retained depleted uranium fragments (Z18.01)

Z77.018 Contact with and (suspected) exposure to other hazardous metals

Contact with and (suspected) exposure to chromium compounds

Contact with and (suspected) exposure to nickel dust

Z77.02 Contact with and (suspected) exposure to hazardous aromatic compounds

Z77.020 Contact with and (suspected) exposure to aromatic amines

Z77.021 Contact with and (suspected) exposure to benzene

Z77.028 Contact with and (suspected) exposure to other hazardous aromatic compounds

Aromatic dyes NOS

Polycyclic aromatic hydrocarbons

Z77.09 Contact with and (suspected) exposure to other hazardous, chiefly nonmedicinal, chemicals

Z77.090 Contact with and (suspected) exposure to asbestos

Z77.098 Contact with and (suspected) exposure to other hazardous, chiefly nonmedicinal, chemicals

Dyes NOS

Z77.1 Contact with and (suspected) exposure to environmental pollution and hazards in the physical environment

Z77.11 Contact with and (suspected) exposure to environmental pollution

Z77.110 Contact with and (suspected) exposure to air pollution

Z77.111 Contact with and (suspected) exposure to water pollution

Z77.112 Contact with and (suspected) exposure to soil pollution

Z77.118 Contact with and (suspected) exposure to other environmental pollution

Z77.12 Contact with and (suspected) exposure to hazards in the physical environment

Z77.120 Contact with and (suspected) exposure to mold (toxic)

Z77.121 Contact with and (suspected) exposure to harmful algae and algae toxins

Contact with and (suspected) exposure to (harmful) algae bloom NOS

Contact with and (suspected) exposure to blue-green algae bloom

Contact with and (suspected) exposure to brown tide

Contact with and (suspected) exposure to cyanobacteria bloom

Contact with and (suspected) exposure to Florida red tide

Contact with and (suspected) exposure to pfiesteria piscicida

Contact with and (suspected) exposure to red tide

Z77.122 Contact with and (suspected) exposure to noise

Z77.123 Contact with and (suspected) exposure to radon and other naturally occurring radiation

> **Excludes 2:** radiation exposure as the cause of a confirmed condition (W88-W90, X39.0-)
>
> radiation sickness NOS (T66)

Z77.128 Contact with and (suspected) exposure to other hazards in the physical environment

Z77.2 Contact with and (suspected) exposure to other hazardous substances

Z77.21 Contact with and (suspected) exposure to potentially hazardous body fluids

Z77.22 Contact with and (suspected) exposure to environmental tobacco smoke (acute) (chronic)

Exposure to second hand tobacco smoke (acute) (chronic)

Passive smoking (acute) (chronic)

> **Excludes 1:** nicotine dependence (F17.-)
>
> tobacco use (Z72.0)

> **Excludes 2:** occupational exposure to environmental tobacco smoke (Z57.31)

Z77.29 Contact with and (suspected) exposure to other hazardous substances

Z77.9 Other contact with and (suspected) exposures hazardous to health

Z78 Other specified health status

> **Excludes 2:** asymptomatic human immunodeficiency virus [HIV] infection status (Z21)
>
> postprocedural status (Z93- Z99)
>
> sex reassignment status (Z87.890)

Z78.0 Asymptomatic menopausal state

Menopausal state NOS

Postmenopausal status NOS

> **Excludes 2:** symptomatic menopausal state (N95.1)

Z78.1 Physical restraint status

> **Excludes 1:** physical restraint due to a procedure - omit code

Z78.9 Other specified health status

Z79 Long term (current) drug therapy

> **Includes:** long term (current) drug use for prophylactic purposes

Code also any therapeutic drug level monitoring (Z51.81)

> **Excludes 2:** drug abuse and dependence (F11-F19)
>
> drug use complicating pregnancy, childbirth, and the puerperium (O99.32-)

Z79.0 Long term (current) use of anticoagulants and antithrombotics/antiplatelets

Excludes 2: long term (current) use of aspirin (Z79.82)

Z79.01 Long term (current) use of anticoagulants

Z79.02 Long term (current) use of antithrombotics/antiplatelets

Z79.1 Long term (current) use of non-steroidal anti-inflammatories (NSAID)

Excludes 2: long term (current) use of aspirin (Z79.82)

Z79.2 Long term (current) use of antibiotics

Z79.3 Long term (current) use of hormonal contraceptives

Long term (current) use of birth control pill or patch

Z79.4 Long term (current) use of insulin

Z79.5 Long term (current) use of steroids

Z79.51 Long term (current) use of inhaled steroids

Z79.52 Long term (current) use of systemic steroids

Z79.8 Other long term (current) drug therapy

Z79.81 Long term (current) use of agents affecting estrogen receptors and estrogen levels

Code first , if applicable:

malignant neoplasm of breast (C50.-)

malignant neoplasm of prostate (C61)

Use additional code, if applicable, to identify:

estrogen receptor positive status (Z17.0)

family history of breast cancer (Z80.3)

genetic susceptibility to malignant neoplasm (cancer) (Z15.0-)

personal history of breast cancer (Z85.3)

personal history of prostate cancer (Z85.46)

postmenopausal status (Z78.0)

Excludes 1: hormone replacement therapy (postmenopausal) (Z79.890)

Z79.810 Long term (current) use of selective estrogen receptor modulators (SERMs)

Long term (current) use of raloxifene (Evista)

Long term (current) use of tamoxifen (Nolvadex)

Long term (current) use of toremifene (Fareston)

Z79.811 Long term (current) use of aromatase inhibitors

Long term (current) use of anastrozole (Arimidex)

Long term (current) use of exemestane (Aromasin)

Long term (current) use of letrozole (Femara)

Z79.818 Long term (current) use of other agents affecting estrogen receptors and estrogen levels

Long term (current) use of estrogen receptor down regulators

Long term (current) use of fulvestrant (Faslodex)

Long term (current) use of gonadotropin-releasing hormone (GnRH) agonist

Long term (current) use of goserelin acetate (Zoladex)

Long term (current) use of

leuprolide acetate (leuprorelin) (Lupron)

Long term (current) use of megestrol acetate (Megace)

Z79.82 Long term (current) use of aspirin

Z79.83 Long term (current) use of bisphosphonates

Z79.89 Other long term (current) drug therapy

Z79.890 Hormone replacement therapy (postmenopausal)

Z79.891 Long term (current) use of opiate analgesic

Long term (current) use of methadone for pain management

Excludes 1: methadone use NOS (F11.2-)

use of methadone for treatment of heroin addiction (F11.2-)

Z79.899 Other long term (current) drug therapy

Z80 Family history of primary malignant neoplasm

Z80.0 Family history of malignant neoplasm of digestive organs

Conditions classifiable to C15-C26

Z80.1 Family history of malignant neoplasm of trachea, bronchus and lung

Conditions classifiable to C33-C34

Z80.2 Family history of malignant neoplasm of other respiratory and intrathoracic organs

Conditions classifiable to C30-C32, C37-C39

Z80.3 Family history of malignant neoplasm of breast

Conditions classifiable to C50.-

Z80.4 Family history of malignant neoplasm of genital organs

Conditions classifiable to C51-C63

Z80.41 Family history of malignant neoplasm of ovary

Z80.42 Family history of malignant neoplasm of prostate

Z80.43 Family history of malignant neoplasm of testis

Z80.49 Family history of malignant neoplasm of other genital organs

Z80.5 Family history of malignant neoplasm of urinary tract

Conditions classifiable to C64-C68

Z80.51 Family history of malignant neoplasm of kidney

Z80.52 Family history of malignant neoplasm of bladder

Z80.59 Family history of malignant neoplasm of other urinary tract organ

Z80.6 Family history of leukemia

Conditions classifiable to C91-C95

Z80.7 Family history of other malignant neoplasms of lymphoid, hematopoietic and related tissues

Conditions classifiable to C81-C90, C96.-

Z80.8 Family history of malignant neoplasm of other organs or systems

Conditions classifiable to C00-C14, C40-C49, C69-C79

Z80.9 Family history of malignant neoplasm, unspecified

Conditions classifiable to C80.1

Z81 Family history of mental and behavioral disorders

Z81.0 Family history of intellectual disabilities

Conditions classifiable to F70-F79

Z81.1 Family history of alcohol abuse and dependence

Conditions classifiable to F10.-

Z81.2 Family history of tobacco abuse and dependence
Conditions classifiable to F17.-

Z81.3 Family history of other psychoactive substance abuse and dependence
Conditions classifiable to F11-F16, F18-F19

Z81.4 Family history of other substance abuse and dependence
Conditions classifiable to F55

Z81.8 Family history of other mental and behavioral disorders
Conditions classifiable elsewhere in F01-F99

Z82 Family history of certain disabilities and chronic diseases (leading to disablement)

Z82.0 Family history of epilepsy and other diseases of the nervous system
Conditions classifiable to G00-G99

Z82.1 Family history of blindness and visual loss
Conditions classifiable to H54.-

Z82.2 Family history of deafness and hearing loss
Conditions classifiable to H90-H91

Z82.3 Family history of stroke
Conditions classifiable to I60-I64

Z82.4 Family history of ischemic heart disease and other diseases of the circulatory system
Conditions classifiable to I00-I52, I65-I99

    Z82.41 Family history of sudden cardiac death

    Z82.49 Family history of ischemic heart disease and other diseases of the circulatory system

Z82.5 Family history of asthma and other chronic lower respiratory diseases
Conditions classifiable to J40-J47
Excludes 2: family history of other diseases of the respiratory system (Z83.6)

Z82.6 Family history of arthritis and other diseases of the musculoskeletal system and connective tissue
Conditions classifiable to M00-M99

    Z82.61 Family history of arthritis

    Z82.62 Family history of osteoporosis

    Z82.69 Family history of other diseases of the musculoskeletal system and connective tissue

Z82.7 Family history of congenital malformations, deformations and chromosomal abnormalities
Conditions classifiable to Q00-Q99

    Z82.71 Family history of polycystic kidney

    Z82.79 Family history of other congenital malformations, deformations and chromosomal abnormalities

Z82.8 Family history of other disabilities and chronic diseases leading to disablement, not elsewhere classified

Z83 Family history of other specific disorders
Excludes 2: contact with and (suspected) exposure to communicable disease in the family (Z20.-)

Z83.0 Family history of human immunodeficiency virus [HIV] disease
Conditions classifiable to B20

Z83.1 Family history of other infectious and parasitic diseases
Conditions classifiable to A00-B19, B25-B94, B99

Z83.2 Family history of diseases of the blood and blood-forming organs and certain disorders involving the immune mechanism

Conditions classifiable to D50-D89

Z83.3 Family history of diabetes mellitus
Conditions classifiable to E08-E13

Z83.4 Family history of other endocrine, nutritional and metabolic diseases
Conditions classifiable to E00-E07, E15-E88

    Z83.41 Family history of multiple endocrine neoplasia [MEN] syndrome

    Z83.49 Family history of other endocrine, nutritional and metabolic diseases

Z83.5 Family history of eye and ear disorders

    Z83.51 Family history of eye disorders
    Conditions classifiable to H00-H53, H55-H59
    Excludes 2: family history of blindness and visual loss (Z82.1)

        Z83.511 Family history of glaucoma

        Z83.518 Family history of other specified eye disorder

    Z83.52 Family history of ear disorders
    Conditions classifiable to H60-H83, H92-H95
    Excludes 2: family history of deafness and hearing loss (Z82.2)

Z83.6 Family history of other diseases of the respiratory system
Conditions classifiable to J00-J39, J60-J99
Excludes 2: family history of asthma and other chronic lower respiratory diseases (Z82.5)

Z83.7 Family history of diseases of the digestive system
Conditions classifiable to K00-K93

    Z83.71 Family history of colonic polyps
    Excludes 1: family history of malignant neoplasm of digestive organs (Z80.0)

    Z83.79 Family history of other diseases of the digestive system

Z84 Family history of other conditions

Z84.0 Family history of diseases of the skin and subcutaneous tissue
Conditions classifiable to L00-L99

Z84.1 Family history of disorders of kidney and ureter
Conditions classifiable to N00-N29

Z84.2 Family history of other diseases of the genitourinary system
Conditions classifiable to N30-N99

Z84.3 Family history of consanguinity

Z84.8 Family history of other specified conditions

    Z84.81 Family history of carrier of genetic disease

    Z84.89 Family history of other specified conditions

Z85 Personal history of malignant neoplasm
Code first any follow-up examination after treatment of malignant neoplasm (Z08)
Use additional code to identify:
alcohol use and dependence (F10.-)
exposure to environmental tobacco smoke (Z77.22)
history of tobacco use (Z87.891)
occupational exposure to environmental tobacco smoke (Z57.31)
tobacco dependence (F17.-)
tobacco use (Z72.0)
Excludes 2: personal history of benign neoplasm (Z86.01-)
personal history of carcinoma-in-situ (Z86.00-)

Z85.0 Personal history of malignant neoplasm of digestive organs

Z85.00 Personal history of malignant neoplasm of unspecified digestive organ

Z85.01 Personal history of malignant neoplasm of esophagus
Conditions classifiable to C15

Z85.02 Personal history of malignant neoplasm of stomach

Z85.020 Personal history of malignant carcinoid tumor of stomach
Conditions classifiable to C7A.092

Z85.028 Personal history of other malignant neoplasm of stomach
Conditions classifiable to C16

Z85.03 Personal history of malignant neoplasm of large intestine

Z85.030 Personal history of malignant carcinoid tumor of large intestine
Conditions classifiable to C7A.022-C7A.025, C7A.029

Z85.038 Personal history of other malignant neoplasm of large intestine
Conditions classifiable to C18

Z85.04 Personal history of malignant neoplasm of rectum, rectosigmoid junction, and anus

Z85.040 Personal history of malignant carcinoid tumor of rectum
Conditions classifiable to C7A.026

Z85.048 Personal history of other malignant neoplasm of rectum, rectosigmoid junction, and anus
Conditions classifiable to C19-C21

Z85.05 Personal history of malignant neoplasm of liver
Conditions classifiable to C22

Z85.06 Personal history of malignant neoplasm of small intestine

Z85.060 Personal history of malignant carcinoid tumor of small intestine
Conditions classifiable to C7A.01-

Z85.068 Personal history of other malignant neoplasm of small intestine
Conditions classifiable to C17

Z85.07 Personal history of malignant neoplasm of pancreas
Conditions classifiable to C25

Z85.09 Personal history of malignant neoplasm of other digestive organs

Z85.1 Personal history of malignant neoplasm of trachea, bronchus and lung

Z85.11 Personal history of malignant neoplasm of bronchus and lung

Z85.110 Personal history of malignant carcinoid tumor of bronchus and lung
Conditions classifiable to C7A.090

Z85.118 Personal history of other malignant neoplasm of bronchus and lung
Conditions classifiable to C34

Z85.12 Personal history of malignant neoplasm of trachea
Conditions classifiable to C33

Z85.2 Personal history of malignant neoplasm of other respiratory and intrathoracic organs

Z85.20 Personal history of malignant neoplasm of unspecified respiratory organ

Z85.21 Personal history of malignant neoplasm of larynx
Conditions classifiable to C32

Z85.22 Personal history of malignant neoplasm of nasal cavities, middle ear, and accessory sinuses
Conditions classifiable to C30-C31

Z85.23 Personal history of malignant neoplasm of thymus

⑦**Z85.230** Personal history of malignant carcinoid tumor of thymus
Conditions classifiable to C7A.091

⑦**Z85.238** Personal history of other malignant neoplasm of thymus
Conditions classifiable to C37

Z85.29 Personal history of malignant neoplasm of other respiratory and intrathoracic organs

Z85.3 Personal history of malignant neoplasm of breast
Conditions classifiable to C50.-

Z85.4 Personal history of malignant neoplasm of genital organs
Conditions classifiable to C51-C63

Z85.40 Personal history of malignant neoplasm of unspecified female genital organ

Z85.41 Personal history of malignant neoplasm of cervix uteri

Z85.42 Personal history of malignant neoplasm of other parts of uterus

Z85.43 Personal history of malignant neoplasm of ovary

Z85.44 Personal history of malignant neoplasm of other female genital organs

Z85.45 Personal history of malignant neoplasm of unspecified male genital organ

Z85.46 Personal history of malignant neoplasm of prostate

Z85.47 Personal history of malignant neoplasm of testis

Z85.48 Personal history of malignant neoplasm of epididymis

Z85.49 Personal history of malignant neoplasm of other male genital organs

Z85.5 Personal history of malignant neoplasm of urinary tract
Conditions classifiable to C64-C68

Z85.50 Personal history of malignant neoplasm of unspecified urinary tract organ

Z85.51 Personal history of malignant neoplasm of bladder

Z85.52 Personal history of malignant neoplasm of kidney
Excludes 1: personal history of malignant neoplasm of renal pelvis (Z85.53)

Z85.520 Personal history of malignant carcinoid tumor of kidney
Conditions classifiable to C7A.093

Z85.528 Personal history of other malignant neoplasm of kidney
Conditions classifiable to C64

● New code   ▲ Revised code   ⑦ 7ᵗʰ digit required   ⊗ Placeholder required

Z85.53 Personal history of malignant neoplasm of renal pelvis

Z85.54 Personal history of malignant neoplasm of ureter

Z85.59 Personal history of malignant neoplasm of other urinary tract organ

Z85.6 Personal history of leukemia
Conditions classifiable to C91-C95
Excludes 1: leukemia in remission C91.0-C95.9 with 5th character 1

Z85.7 Personal history of other malignant neoplasms of lymphoid, hematopoietic and related tissues

Z85.71 Personal history of Hodgkin lymphoma
Conditions classifiable to C81

Z85.72 Personal history of non-Hodgkin lymphomas
Conditions classifiable to C82-C85

Z85.79 Personal history of other malignant neoplasms of lymphoid, hematopoietic and related tissues
Conditions classifiable to C88-C90, C96
Excludes 1: multiple myeloma in remission (C90.01)
plasma cell leukemia in remission (C90.11)
plasmacytoma in remission (C90.21)

Z85.8 Personal history of malignant neoplasms of other organs and systems
Conditions classifiable to C00-C14, C40-C49, C69-C79, C7A.098

Z85.81 Personal history of malignant neoplasm of lip, oral cavity, and pharynx

Z85.810 Personal history of malignant neoplasm of tongue

Z85.818 Personal history of malignant neoplasm of other sites of lip, oral cavity, and pharynx

Z85.819 Personal history of malignant neoplasm of unspecified site of lip, oral cavity, and pharynx

Z85.82 Personal history of malignant neoplasm of skin

Z85.820 Personal history of malignant melanoma of skin
Conditions classifiable to C43

Z85.821 Personal history of Merkel cell carcinoma
Conditions classifiable to C4A

Z85.828 Personal history of other malignant neoplasm of skin
Conditions classifiable to C44

Z85.83 Personal history of malignant neoplasm of bone and soft tissue

Z85.830 Personal history of malignant neoplasm of bone

Z85.831 Personal history of malignant neoplasm of soft tissue
Excludes 2: personal history of malignant neoplasm of skin (Z85.82-)

Z85.84 Personal history of malignant neoplasm of eye and nervous tissue

Z85.840 Personal history of malignant neoplasm of eye

Z85.841 Personal history of malignant neoplasm of brain

Z85.848 Personal history of malignant neoplasm of other parts of nervous tissue

Z85.85 Personal history of malignant neoplasm of endocrine glands

Z85.850 Personal history of malignant neoplasm of thyroid

Z85.858 Personal history of malignant neoplasm of other endocrine glands

Z85.89 Personal history of malignant neoplasm of other organs and systems

Z85.9 Personal history of malignant neoplasm, unspecified
Conditions classifiable to C7A.00, C80.1

Z86 Personal history of certain other diseases
Code first any follow-up examination after treatment (Z09)

Z86.0 Personal history of in-situ and benign neoplasms and neoplasms of uncertain behavior
Excludes 2: personal history of malignant neoplasms (Z85.-)

Z86.00 Personal history of in-situ neoplasm

Z86.000 Personal history of in-situ neoplasm of breast

Z86.001 Personal history of in-situ neoplasm of cervix uteri

Z86.008 Personal history of in-situ neoplasm of other site

Z86.01 Personal history of benign neoplasm

Z86.010 Personal history of colonic polyps

Z86.011 Personal history of benign neoplasm of the brain

Z86.012 Personal history of benign carcinoid tumor

Z86.018 Personal history of other benign neoplasm

Z86.03 Personal history of neoplasm of uncertain behavior

Z86.1 Personal history of infectious and parasitic diseases
Conditions classifiable to A00-B89, B99
Excludes 1: personal history of infectious diseases specific to a body system
sequelae of infectious and parasitic diseases (B90-B94)

Z86.11 Personal history of tuberculosis

Z86.12 Personal history of poliomyelitis

Z86.13 Personal history of malaria

Z86.14 Personal history of Methicillin resistant Staphylococcus aureus infection
Personal history of MRSA infection

Z86.19 Personal history of other infectious and parasitic diseases

⊗⑦**Z86.2** Personal history of diseases of the blood and blood-forming organs and certain disorders involving the immune mechanism
Conditions classifiable to D50-D89

Z86.3 Personal history of endocrine, nutritional and metabolic diseases
Conditions classifiable to E00-E88

Z86.31 Personal history of diabetic foot ulcer
> **Excludes 2:** current diabetic foot ulcer (E08.621, E09.621, E10.621, E11.621, E13.621)

Z86.32 Personal history of gestational diabetes
Personal history of conditions classifiable to O24.4-
> **Excludes 1:** gestational diabetes mellitus in current pregnancy (O24.4-)

Z86.39 Personal history of other endocrine, nutritional and metabolic disease

Z86.5 Personal history of mental and behavioral disorders
Conditions classifiable to F40-F59

Z86.51 Personal history of combat and operational stress reaction

Z86.59 Personal history of other mental and behavioral disorders

Z86.6 Personal history of diseases of the nervous system and sense organs
Conditions classifiable to G00-G99, H00-H95

Z86.61 Personal history of infections of the central nervous system
Personal history of encephalitis
Personal history of meningitis

Z86.69 Personal history of other diseases of the nervous system and sense organs

Z86.7 Personal history of diseases of the circulatory system
Conditions classifiable to I00-I99
> **Excludes 2:** old myocardial infarction (I25.2)
> personal history of anaphylactic shock (Z87.892)
> postmyocardial infarction syndrome (I24.1)

Z86.71 Personal history of venous thrombosis and embolism

Z86.711 Personal history of pulmonary embolism

Z86.718 Personal history of other venous thrombosis and embolism

Z86.72 Personal history of thrombophlebitis

Z86.73 Personal history of transient ischemic attack (TIA), and cerebral infarction without residual deficits
Personal history of prolonged reversible ischemic neurological deficit (PRIND)
Personal history of stroke NOS without residual deficits
> **Excludes 1:** personal history of traumatic brain injury (Z87.820)
> sequelae of cerebrovascular disease (I69.-)

Z86.74 Personal history of sudden cardiac arrest
Personal history of sudden cardiac death successfully resuscitated

Z86.79 Personal history of other diseases of the circulatory system

Z87 Personal history of other diseases and conditions
Code first any follow-up examination after treatment (Z09)

Z87.0 Personal history of diseases of the respiratory system
Conditions classifiable to J00-J99

Z87.01 Personal history of pneumonia (recurrent)

Z87.09 Personal history of other diseases of the respiratory system

Z87.1 Personal history of diseases of the digestive system
Conditions classifiable to K00-K93

Z87.11 Personal history of peptic ulcer disease

Z87.19 Personal history of other diseases of the digestive system

Z87.2 Personal history of diseases of the skin and subcutaneous tissue
Conditions classifiable to L00-L99
> **Excludes 2:** personal history of diabetic foot ulcer (Z86.31)

Z87.3 Personal history of diseases of the musculoskeletal system and connective tissue
Conditions classifiable to M00-M99
> **Excludes 2:** personal history of (healed) traumatic fracture (Z87.81)

Z87.31 Personal history of (healed) nontraumatic fracture

Z87.310 Personal history of (healed) osteoporosis fracture
Personal history of (healed) fragility fracture
Personal history of (healed) collapsed vertebra due to osteoporosis

Z87.311 Personal history of (healed) other pathological fracture
Personal history of (healed) collapsed vertebra NOS
> **Excludes 2:** personal history of osteoporosis fracture (Z87.310)

Z87.312 Personal history of (healed) stress fracture
Personal history of (healed) fatigue fracture

⑦ **Z87.39** Personal history of other diseases of the musculoskeletal system and connective tissue

Z87.4 Personal history of diseases of genitourinary system
Conditions classifiable to N00-N99

Z87.41 Personal history of dysplasia of the female genital tract
> **Excludes 1:** personal history of malignant neoplasm of female genital tract (Z85.40-Z85.44)

Z87.410 Personal history of cervical dysplasia

Z87.411 Personal history of vaginal dysplasia

Z87.412 Personal history of vulvar dysplasia

⑦ **Z87.42** Personal history of other diseases of the female genital tract

Z87.43 Personal history of diseases of male genital organs

Z87.430 Personal history of prostatic dysplasia
> **Excludes 1:** personal history of malignant neoplasm of prostate (Z85.46)

Z87.438 Personal history of other diseases of male genital organs

Z87.44 Personal history of diseases of urinary system
>
> **Excludes 1:** personal history of malignant neoplasm of cervix uteri (Z85.41)

> **Z87.440** Personal history of urinary (tract) infections

> **Z87.441** Personal history of nephrotic syndrome

> **Z87.442** Personal history of urinary calculi
> Personal history of kidney stones

> **Z87.448** Personal history of other diseases of urinary system

Z87.5 Personal history of complications of pregnancy, childbirth and the puerperium
Conditions classifiable to O00-O9A
>
> **Excludes 2:** recurrent pregnancy loss (N96)

> **Z87.51** Personal history of pre-term labor
> >
> > **Excludes 1:** current pregnancy with history of pre-term labor (O09.21-)

> **Z87.59** Personal history of other complications of pregnancy, childbirth and the puerperium
> Personal history of trophoblastic disease

Z87.7 Personal history of (corrected) congenital malformations
Conditions classifiable to Q00-Q89 that have been repaired or corrected
>
> **Excludes 1:** congenital malformations that have been partially corrected or repair but which still require
> medical treatment - code to condition
>
> **Excludes 2:** other postprocedural states (Z98.-)
> personal history of medical treatment (Z92.-)
> presence of cardiac and vascular implants and grafts (Z95.-)
> presence of other devices (Z97.-)
> presence of other functional implants (Z96.-)
> transplanted organ and tissue status (Z94.-)

> **Z87.71** Personal history of (corrected) congenital malformations of genitourinary system

> > **Z87.710** Personal history of (corrected) hypospadias

> > **Z87.718** Personal history of other specified (corrected) congenital malformations of genitourinary system

> **Z87.72** Personal history of (corrected) congenital malformations of nervous system and sense organs

> > **Z87.720** Personal history of (corrected) congenital malformations of eye

> > **Z87.721** Personal history of (corrected) congenital malformations of ear

> > **Z87.728** Personal history of other specified (corrected) congenital malformations of nervous system and sense organs

> **Z87.73** Personal history of (corrected) congenital malformations of digestive system

> > **Z87.730** Personal history of (corrected) cleft lip and palate

> > **Z87.738** Personal history of other specified (corrected) congenital malformations of digestive system

> **Z87.74** Personal history of (corrected) congenital malformations of heart and circulatory system

> **Z87.75** Personal history of (corrected) congenital malformations of respiratory system

> **Z87.76** Personal history of (corrected) congenital malformations of integument, limbs and musculoskeletal system

> **Z87.79** Personal history of other (corrected) congenital malformations

> > **Z87.790** Personal history of (corrected) congenital malformations of face and neck

> > **Z87.798** Personal history of other (corrected) congenital malformations

Z87.8 Personal history of other specified conditions
>
> **Excludes 2:** personal history of self harm (Z91.5)

> **Z87.81** Personal history of (healed) traumatic fracture
> >
> > **Excludes 2:** personal history of (healed) nontraumatic fracture (Z87.31-)

> **Z87.82** Personal history of other (healed) physical injury and trauma
> Conditions classifiable to S00-T88, except traumatic fractures

> > **Z87.820** Personal history of traumatic brain injury
> > >
> > > **Excludes 1:** personal history of transient ischemic attack (TIA), and cerebral infarction without residual deficits (Z86.73)

> > **Z87.821** Personal history of retained foreign body fully removed

> > **Z87.828** Personal history of other (healed) physical injury and trauma

> **Z87.89** Personal history of other specified conditions

> > **Z87.890** Personal history of sex reassignment

> > **Z87.891** Personal history of nicotine dependence
> > >
> > > **Excludes 1:** current nicotine dependence (F17.2-)

> > **Z87.892** Personal history of anaphylaxis
> > Code also allergy status such as:
> > allergy status to drugs, medicaments and biological substances (Z88.-)
> > allergy status, other than to drugs and biological substances (Z91.0-)

> > **Z87.898** Personal history of other specified conditions

Z88 Allergy status to drugs, medicaments and biological substances
>
> **Excludes 2:** Allergy status, other than to drugs and biological substances (Z91.0-)

Z88.0 Allergy status to penicillin

Z88.1 Allergy status to other antibiotic agents status

Z88.2 Allergy status to sulfonamides status

Z88.3 Allergy status to other anti-infective agents status

Z88.4 Allergy status to anesthetic agent status

Z88.5 Allergy status to narcotic agent status

Z88.6 Allergy status to analgesic agent status

Z88.7 Allergy status to serum and vaccine status

Z88.8 Allergy status to other drugs, medicaments and biological substances status

Z88.9 Allergy status to unspecified drugs, medicaments and biological substances status

Z89 Acquired absence of limb

Includes: amputation status

postprocedural loss of limb

post-traumatic loss of limb

Excludes 1: acquired deformities of limbs (M20-M21)

congenital absence of limbs (Q71-Q73)

Z89.0 Acquired absence of thumb and other finger(s)

Z89.01 Acquired absence of thumb

Z89.011 Acquired absence of right thumb

Z89.012 Acquired absence of left thumb

Z89.019 Acquired absence of unspecified thumb

Z89.02 Acquired absence of other finger(s)

Excludes 2: acquired absence of thumb (Z89.01-)

Z89.021 Acquired absence of right finger(s)

Z89.022 Acquired absence of left finger(s)

Z89.029 Acquired absence of unspecified finger(s)

Z89.1 Acquired absence of hand and wrist

Z89.11 Acquired absence of hand

Z89.111 Acquired absence of right hand

Z89.112 Acquired absence of left hand

Z89.119 Acquired absence of unspecified hand

Z89.12 Acquired absence of wrist

Disarticulation at wrist

Z89.121 Acquired absence of right wrist

Z89.122 Acquired absence of left wrist

Z89.129 Acquired absence of unspecified wrist

Z89.2 Acquired absence of upper limb above wrist

Z89.20 Acquired absence of upper limb, unspecified level

Z89.201 Acquired absence of right upper limb, unspecified level

Z89.202 Acquired absence of left upper limb, unspecified level

Z89.209 Acquired absence of unspecified upper limb, unspecified level

Acquired absence of arm NOS

Z89.21 Acquired absence of upper limb below elbow

Z89.211 Acquired absence of right upper limb below elbow

Z89.212 Acquired absence of left upper limb below elbow

Z89.219 Acquired absence of unspecified upper limb below elbow

Z89.22 Acquired absence of upper limb above elbow

Disarticulation at elbow

Z89.221 Acquired absence of right upper limb above elbow

Z89.222 Acquired absence of left upper limb above elbow

Z89.229 Acquired absence of unspecified

upper limb above elbow

Z89.23 Acquired absence of shoulder

Acquired absence of shoulder joint following explantation of shoulder joint prosthesis, with or without

presence of antibiotic-impregnated cement spacer

Z89.231 Acquired absence of right shoulder

Z89.232 Acquired absence of left shoulder

Z89.239 Acquired absence of unspecified shoulder

Z89.4 Acquired absence of toe(s), foot, and ankle

Z89.41 Acquired absence of great toe

Z89.411 Acquired absence of right great toe

Z89.412 Acquired absence of left great toe

Z89.419 Acquired absence of unspecified great toe

Z89.42 Acquired absence of other toe(s)

Excludes 2: acquired absence of great toe (Z89.41-)

Z89.421 Acquired absence of other right toe(s)

Z89.422 Acquired absence of other left toe(s)

Z89.429 Acquired absence of other toe(s), unspecified side

Z89.43 Acquired absence of foot

Z89.431 Acquired absence of right foot

Z89.432 Acquired absence of left foot

Z89.439 Acquired absence of unspecified foot

Z89.44 Acquired absence of ankle

Disarticulation of ankle

Z89.441 Acquired absence of right ankle

Z89.442 Acquired absence of left ankle

Z89.449 Acquired absence of unspecified ankle

Z89.5 Acquired absence of leg below knee

Z89.51 Acquired absence of leg below knee

Z89.511 Acquired absence of right leg below knee

Z89.512 Acquired absence of left leg below knee

Z89.519 Acquired absence of unspecified leg below knee

Z89.52 Acquired absence of knee

Acquired absence of knee joint following explantation of knee joint prosthesis, with or without presence of antibiotic-impregnated cement spacer

Z89.521 Acquired absence of right knee

Z89.522 Acquired absence of left knee

Z89.529 Acquired absence of unspecified knee

Z89.6 Acquired absence of leg above knee

Z89.61 Acquired absence of leg above knee

Acquired absence of leg NOS

Disarticulation at knee

Z89.611 Acquired absence of right leg above knee

● New code   ▲ Revised code   ⑦ 7th digit required   ⊗ Placeholder required

Z89.612 Acquired absence of left leg above knee

Z89.619 Acquired absence of unspecified leg above knee

Z89.62 Acquired absence of hip
Acquired absence of hip joint following explantation of hip joint prosthesis, with or without presence of antibiotic-impregnated cement spacer
Disarticulation at hip

Z89.621 Acquired absence of right hip joint

Z89.622 Acquired absence of left hip joint

Z89.629 Acquired absence of unspecified hip joint

Z89.9 Acquired absence of limb, unspecified

Z90 Acquired absence of organs, not elsewhere classified
Includes: postprocedural or post-traumatic loss of body part NEC
Excludes 1: congenital absence - see Alphabetical Index
Excludes 2: postprocedural absence of endocrine glands (E89.-)

Z90.0 Acquired absence of part of head and neck

Z90.01 Acquired absence of eye

Z90.02 Acquired absence of larynx

Z90.09 Acquired absence of other part of head and neck
Acquired absence of nose
Excludes 2: teeth (K08.1)

Z90.1 Acquired absence of breast and nipple

Z90.10 Acquired absence of unspecified breast and nipple

Z90.11 Acquired absence of right breast and nipple

Z90.12 Acquired absence of left breast and nipple

Z90.13 Acquired absence of bilateral breasts and nipples

Z90.2 Acquired absence of lung [part of]

Z90.3 Acquired absence of stomach [part of]

Z90.4 Acquired absence of other specified parts of digestive tract

Z90.41 Acquired absence of pancreas
Use additional code to identify any associated:
insulin use (Z79.4)
diabetes mellitus, post pancreatectomy (E13.-)

Z90.410 Acquired total absence of pancreas
Acquired absence of pancreas NOS

Z90.411 Acquired partial absence of pancreas

Z90.49 Acquired absence of other specified parts of digestive tract

Z90.5 Acquired absence of kidney

Z90.6 Acquired absence of other parts of urinary tract
Acquired absence of bladder

Z90.7 Acquired absence of genital organ(s)
Excludes 1: personal history of sex reassignment (Z87.890)
Excludes 2: female genital mutilation status (N90.81-)

Z90.71 Acquired absence of cervix and uterus

Z90.710 Acquired absence of both cervix and uterus
Acquired absence of uterus NOS
Status post total hysterectomy

Z90.711 Acquired absence of uterus with remaining cervical stump
Status post partial hysterectomy with remaining cervical stump

Z90.712 Acquired absence of cervix with remaining uterus

Z90.72 Acquired absence of ovaries

Z90.721 Acquired absence of ovaries, unilateral

Z90.722 Acquired absence of ovaries, bilateral

Z90.79 Acquired absence of other genital organ(s)

Z90.8 Acquired absence of other organs

Z90.81 Acquired absence of spleen

Z90.89 Acquired absence of other organs

Z91 Personal risk factors, not elsewhere classified
Excludes 2: contact with and (suspected) exposures hazardous to health (Z77.-)
exposure to pollution and other problems related to physical environment (Z77.1-)
personal history of physical injury and trauma (Z87.81, Z87.82-)
occupational exposure to risk factors (Z57.-)

Z91.0 Allergy status, other than to drugs and biological substances
Excludes 2: Allergy status to drugs, medicaments, and biological substances (Z88.-)

Z91.01 Food allergy status
Excludes 2: food additives allergy status (Z91.02)

Z91.010 Allergy to peanuts

Z91.011 Allergy to milk products
Excludes 1: lactose intolerance (E73.-)

Z91.012 Allergy to eggs

Z91.013 Allergy to seafood
Allergy to shellfish
Allergy to octopus or squid ink

Z91.018 Allergy to other foods
Allergy to nuts other than peanuts

Z91.02 Food additives allergy status

Z91.03 Insect allergy status

Z91.030 Bee allergy status

Z91.038 Other insect allergy status

Z91.04 Nonmedicinal substance allergy status

Z91.040 Latex allergy status
Latex sensitivity status

Z91.041 Radiographic dye allergy status
Allergy status to contrast media used for diagnostic X-ray procedure

Z91.048 Other nonmedicinal substance allergy status

Z91.09 Other allergy status, other than to drugs and biological substances

Z91.1 Patient's noncompliance with medical treatment and regimen

Z91.11 Patient's noncompliance with dietary regimen

Z91.12 Patient's intentional underdosing of medication regimen
Code first underdosing of medication (T36-T50) with fifth or sixth character 6
Excludes 1: adverse effect of prescribed drug

taken as directed- code to adverse effect

poisoning (overdose) -code to poisoning

Z91.120 Patient's intentional underdosing of medication regimen due to financial hardship

Z91.128 Patient's intentional underdosing of medication regimen for other reason

Z91.13 Patient's unintentional underdosing of medication regimen

Code first underdosing of medication (T36-T50) with fifth or sixth character 6

Excludes 1: adverse effect of prescribed drug taken as directed- code to adverse effect

poisoning (overdose) -code to poisoning

Z91.130 Patient's unintentional underdosing of medication regimen due to age-related debility

Z91.138 Patient's unintentional underdosing of medication regimen for other reason

Z91.14 Patient's other noncompliance with medication regimen

Patient's underdosing of medication NOS

Z91.15 Patient's noncompliance with renal dialysis

Z91.19 Patient's noncompliance with other medical treatment and regimen

Z91.4 Personal history of psychological trauma, not elsewhere classified

Z91.41 Personal history of adult abuse

Excludes 2: personal history of abuse in childhood (Z62.81-)

Z91.410 Personal history of adult physical and sexual abuse

Excludes 1: current adult physical abuse (T74.11, T76.11)

current adult sexual abuse (T74. 21, T76.11)

Z91.411 Personal history of adult psychological abuse

Z91.412 Personal history of adult neglect

Excludes 1: current adult neglect (T74.01, T76.01)

Z91.419 Personal history of unspecified adult abuse

Z91.49 Other personal history of psychological trauma, not elsewhere classified

Z91.5 Personal history of self-harm

Personal history of parasuicide

Personal history of self-poisoning

Personal history of suicide attempt

Z91.8 Other specified personal risk factors, not elsewhere classified

Z91.81 History of falling

At risk for falling

Z91.82 Personal history of military deployment

Individual (civilian or military) with past history

of military war, peacekeeping and humanitarian deployment (current or past conflict)

Returned from military deployment

Z91.83 Wandering in diseases classified elsewhere

Code first underlying disorder such as:

Alzheimer's disease (G30-)

autism or pervasive developmental disorder (F84-)

intellectual disabilities (F70-F79)

unspecified dementia with behavioral disturbance (F03.9-)

Z91.89 Other specified personal risk factors, not elsewhere classified

Z92 Personal history of medical treatment

Excludes 2: postprocedural states (Z98.-)

Z92.0 Personal history of contraception

Excludes 1: counseling or management of current contraceptive practices (Z30.-)

long term (current) use of contraception (Z79.3)

presence of (intrauterine) contraceptive device (Z97.5)

Z92.2 Personal history of drug therapy

Excludes 2: long term (current) drug therapy (Z79.-)

Z92.21 Personal history of antineoplastic chemotherapy

Z92.22 Personal history of monoclonal drug therapy

Z92.23 Personal history of estrogen therapy

Z92.24 Personal history of steroid therapy

Z92.240 Personal history of inhaled steroid therapy

Z92.241 Personal history of systemic steroid therapy

Personal history of steroid therapy NOS

Z92.25 Personal history of immunosupression therapy

Excludes 2: personal history of steroid therapy (Z92.24)

Z92.29 Personal history of other drug therapy

Z92.3 Personal history of irradiation

Personal history of exposure to therapeutic radiation

Excludes 1: exposure to radiation in the physical environment (Z77.12)

occupational exposure to radiation (Z57.1)

Z92.8 Personal history of other medical treatment

Z92.81 Personal history of extracorporeal membrane oxygenation (ECMO)

Z92.82 Status post administration of tPA (rtPA) in a different facility within the last 24 hours prior to admission to current facility

Code first condition requiring tPA administration, such as:

acute cerebral infarction (I63.-)

acute myocardial infarction (I21.-, I22.-)

Z92.83 Personal history of failed moderate sedation

Personal history of failed conscious sedation

Excludes 2: failed moderate sedation during procedure (T88.52)

Z92.89 Personal history of other medical treatment

Z93 Artificial opening status

Excludes 1: artificial openings requiring attention or management

● New code   ▲ Revised code   ⑦ 7ᵗʰ digit required   ⊗ Placeholder required

(Z43.-)

complications of external stoma (J95.0-, K94.-, N99.5-)

Z93.0 Tracheostomy status

Z93.1 Gastrostomy status

Z93.2 Ileostomy status

Z93.3 Colostomy status

Z93.4 Other artificial openings of gastrointestinal tract status

Z93.5 Cystostomy status

    Z93.50 Unspecified cystostomy status

    Z93.51 Cutaneous-vesicostomy status

    Z93.52 Appendico-vesicostomy status

    Z93.59 Other cystostomy status

Z93.6 Other artificial openings of urinary tract status

Nephrostomy status

Ureterostomy status

Urethrostomy status

Z93.8 Other artificial opening status

Z93.9 Artificial opening status, unspecified

Z94 Transplanted organ and tissue status

Includes: organ or tissue replaced by heterogenous or homogenous transplant

Excludes 1: complications of transplanted organ or tissue - see Alphabetical Index

Excludes 2: presence of vascular grafts (Z95.-)

Z94.0 Kidney transplant status

Z94.1 Heart transplant status

    Excludes 1: artificial heart status (Z95.811)

        heart-valve replacement status (Z95.2-Z95.4)

Z94.2 Lung transplant status

Z94.3 Heart and lungs transplant status

Z94.4 Liver transplant status

Z94.5 Skin transplant status

Autogenous skin transplant status

Z94.6 Bone transplant status

Z94.7 Corneal transplant status

Z94.8 Other transplanted organ and tissue status

    Z94.81 Bone marrow transplant status

    Z94.82 Intestine transplant status

    Z94.83 Pancreas transplant status

    Z94.84 Stem cells transplant status

    Z94.89 Other transplanted organ and tissue status

Z94.9 Transplanted organ and tissue status, unspecified

Z95 Presence of cardiac and vascular implants and grafts

Excludes 1: complications of cardiac and vascular devices, implants and grafts (T82.-)

Z95.0 Presence of cardiac pacemaker

    Excludes 1: adjustment or management of cardiac pacemaker (Z45.0)

        presence of automatic (implantable) cardiac defibrillator with synchronous cardiac pacemaker Z95.810

Z95.1 Presence of aortocoronary bypass graft

Z95.2 Presence of prosthetic heart valve

Presence of heart valve NOS

Z95.3 Presence of xenogenic heart valve

Z95.4 Presence of other heart-valve replacement

Z95.5 Presence of coronary angioplasty implant and graft

    Excludes 1: coronary angioplasty status without implant and graft (Z98.61)

Z95.8 Presence of other cardiac and vascular implants and grafts

    Z95.81 Presence of other cardiac implants and grafts

        Z95.810 Presence of automatic (implantable) cardiac defibrillator

            Presence of automatic (implantable) cardiac defibrillator with synchronous cardiac pacemaker

        Z95.811 Presence of heart assist device

        Z95.812 Presence of fully implantable artificial heart

        Z95.818 Presence of other cardiac implants and grafts

    Z95.82 Presence of other vascular implants and grafts

        Z95.820 Peripheral vascular angioplasty status with implants and grafts

            Excludes 1: peripheral vascular angioplasty without implant and graft (Z98.62)

        Z95.828 Presence of other vascular implants and grafts

            Presence of intravascular prosthesis NEC

Z95.9 Presence of cardiac and vascular implant and graft, unspecified

Z96 Presence of other functional implants

Excludes 2: complications of internal prosthetic devices, implants and grafts (T82-T85)

fitting and adjustment of prosthetic and other devices (Z44-Z46)

Z96.0 Presence of urogenital implants

Z96.1 Presence of intraocular lens

Presence of pseudophakia

Z96.2 Presence of otological and audiological implants

    Z96.20 Presence of otological and audiological implant, unspecified

    Z96.21 Cochlear implant status

    Z96.22 Myringotomy tube(s) status

    Z96.29 Presence of other otological and audiological implants

        Presence of bone-conduction hearing device

        Presence of eustachian tube stent

        Stapes replacement

Z96.3 Presence of artificial larynx

Z96.4 Presence of endocrine implants

    Z96.41 Presence of insulin pump (external) (internal)

    Z96.49 Presence of other endocrine implants

Z96.5 Presence of tooth-root and mandibular implants

Z96.6 Presence of orthopedic joint implants

    Z96.60 Presence of unspecified orthopedic joint implant

    Z96.61 Presence of artificial shoulder joint

        Z96.611 Presence of right artificial shoulder joint

        Z96.612 Presence of left artificial shoulder joint

        Z96.619 Presence of unspecified artificial shoulder joint

---

Z96.62 Presence of artificial elbow joint

    Z96.621 Presence of right artificial elbow joint

    Z96.622 Presence of left artificial elbow joint

    Z96.629 Presence of unspecified artificial elbow joint

Z96.63 Presence of artificial wrist joint

    Z96.631 Presence of right artificial wrist joint

    Z96.632 Presence of left artificial wrist joint

    Z96.639 Presence of unspecified artificial wrist joint

Z96.64 Presence of artificial hip joint

Hip-joint replacement (partial) (total)

    Z96.641 Presence of right artificial hip joint

    Z96.642 Presence of left artificial hip joint

    Z96.643 Presence of artificial hip joint, bilateral

    Z96.649 Presence of unspecified artificial hip joint

Z96.65 Presence of artificial knee joint

    Z96.651 Presence of right artificial knee joint

    Z96.652 Presence of left artificial knee joint

    Z96.653 Presence of artificial knee joint, bilateral

    Z96.659 Presence of unspecified artificial knee joint

Z96.66 Presence of artificial ankle joint

    Z96.661 Presence of right artificial ankle joint

    Z96.662 Presence of left artificial ankle joint

    Z96.669 Presence of unspecified artificial ankle joint

Z96.69 Presence of other orthopedic joint implants

    Z96.691 Finger-joint replacement of right hand

    Z96.692 Finger-joint replacement of left hand

    Z96.693 Finger-joint replacement, bilateral

    Z96.698 Presence of other orthopedic joint implants

Z96.7 Presence of other bone and tendon implants

Presence of skull plate

Z96.8 Presence of other specified functional implants

    Z96.81 Presence of artificial skin

    Z96.89 Presence of other specified functional implants

Z96.9 Presence of functional implant, unspecified

Z97 Presence of other devices

Excludes 1: complications of internal prosthetic devices, implants and grafts (T82-T85)

fitting and adjustment of prosthetic and other devices (Z44-Z46)

Excludes 2: presence of cerebrospinal fluid drainage device (Z98.2)

Z97.0 Presence of artificial eye

Z97.1 Presence of artificial limb (complete) (partial)

    Z97.10 Presence of artificial limb (complete) (partial), unspecified

    Z97.11 Presence of artificial right arm (complete)

    (partial)

    Z97.12 Presence of artificial left arm (complete) (partial)

    Z97.13 Presence of artificial right leg (complete) (partial)

    Z97.14 Presence of artificial left leg (complete) (partial)

    Z97.15 Presence of artificial arms, bilateral (complete) (partial)

    Z97.16 Presence of artificial legs, bilateral (complete) (partial)

Z97.2 Presence of dental prosthetic device (complete) (partial)

Presence of dentures (complete) (partial)

Z97.3 Presence of spectacles and contact lenses

Z97.4 Presence of external hearing-aid

Z97.5 Presence of (intrauterine) contraceptive device

Excludes 1: checking, reinsertion or removal of contraceptive device (Z30.43)

Z97.8 Presence of other specified devices

Z98 Other postprocedural states

Excludes 2: aftercare (Z43-Z49, Z51)

follow-up medical care (Z08-Z09)

postprocedural complication - see Alphabetical Index

Z98.0 Intestinal bypass and anastomosis status

Excludes 2: bariatric surgery status (Z98.84)

gastric bypass status (Z98.84)

obesity surgery status (Z98.84)

Z98.1 Arthrodesis status

Z98.2 Presence of cerebrospinal fluid drainage device

Presence of CSF shunt

Z98.3 Post therapeutic collapse of lung status

Code first underlying disease

Z98.4 Cataract extraction status

Use additional code to identify intraocular lens implant status (Z96.1)

Excludes 1: aphakia (H27.0)

    Z98.41 Cataract extraction status, right eye

    Z98.42 Cataract extraction status, left eye

    Z98.49 Cataract extraction status, unspecified eye

Z98.5 Sterilization status

Excludes 1: female infertility (N97.-)

male infertility (N46.-)

    Z98.51 Tubal ligation status

    Z98.52 Vasectomy status

Z98.6 Angioplasty status

    Z98.61 Coronary angioplasty status

    Excludes 1: coronary angioplasty status with implant and graft (Z95.5)

    Z98.62 Peripheral vascular angioplasty status

    Excludes 1: peripheral vascular angioplasty status with implant and graft (Z95.820)

Z98.8 Other specified postprocedural states

    Z98.81 Dental procedure status

        Z98.810 Dental sealant status

        Z98.811 Dental restoration status

Dental crown status

Dental fillings status

        Z98.818 Other dental procedure status

    Z98.82 Breast implant status

● New code   ▲ Revised code   ⑦ 7th digit required   ⊗ Placeholder required

Excludes 1: breast implant removal status (Z98.86)

Z98.83 Filtering (vitreous) bleb after glaucoma surgery status

Excludes 1: Inflammation (infection) of postprocedural bleb (H59.4-)

Z98.84 Bariatric surgery status

Gastric banding status

Gastric bypass status for obesity

Obesity surgery status

Excludes 1: bariatric surgery status complicating pregnancy, childbirth, or the puerperium (O99.84)

Excludes 2: intestinal bypass and anastomosis status (Z98.0)

Z98.85 Transplanted organ removal status

Transplanted organ previously removed due to complication, failure, rejection or infection

Excludes 1: encounter for removal of transplanted organ -code to complication of transplanted organ (T86.-)

Z98.86 Personal history of breast implant removal

Z98.87 Personal history of in utero procedure

Z98.870 Personal history of in utero procedure during pregnancy

Excludes 2: complications from in utero procedure for current pregnancy (O35.7)

supervision of current pregnancy with history of in utero procedure during previous pregnancy (O09.82-)

Z98.871 Personal history of in utero procedure while a fetus

Z98.89 Other specified postprocedural states

Personal history of surgery, not elsewhere classified

Z99 Dependence on enabling machines and devices, not elsewhere classified

Excludes 1: cardiac pacemaker status (Z95.0)

Z99.0 Dependence on aspirator

Z99.1 Dependence on respirator

Dependence on ventilator

Z99.11 Dependence on respirator [ventilator] status

Z99.12 Encounter for respirator [ventilator] dependence during power failure

Excludes 1: mechanical complication of respirator [ventilator] (J95.850)

Z99.2 Dependence on renal dialysis

Hemodialysis status

Peritoneal dialysis status

Presence of arteriovenous shunt for dialysis

Renal dialysis status NOS

Excludes 1: encounter for fitting and adjustment of dialysis catheter (Z49.0-)

noncompliance with renal dialysis (Z91.15)

Z99.3 Dependence on wheelchair

Wheelchair confinement status

Code first cause of dependence, such as:

muscular dystrophy (G71.0)

obesity (E66.-)

Z99.8 Dependence on other enabling machines and devices

Z99.81 Dependence on supplemental oxygen

Dependence on long-term oxygen

Z99.89 Dependence on other enabling machines and devices

Dependence on machine or device NOS

● New code   ▲ Revised code   ⑦ 7th digit required   ⊗ Placeholder required

A

Aarskog's syndrome Q87.1
Abandonment —*see* Maltreatment
Abasia (-astasia) (hysterical) F44.4
Abderhalden-Kaufmann-Lignac syndrome
(cystinosis) E72.04
Abdomen, abdominal —*see also* condition
acute R10.0
angina K55.1
muscle deficiency syndrome Q79.4
Abdominalgia —*see* Pain, abdominal
Abduction contracture, hip or other joint —
see Contraction, joint
Aberrant (congenital) —*see also* Malposition,
congenital
adrenal gland Q89.1
artery (peripheral) Q27.8
basilar NEC Q28.1
cerebral Q28.3
coronary Q24.5
digestive system Q27.8
eye Q15.8
lower limb Q27.8
precerebral Q28.1
pulmonary Q25.79
renal Q27.2
retina Q14.1
specified site NEC Q27.8
subclavian Q27.8
upper limb Q27.8
vertebral Q28.1
breast Q83.8
endocrine gland NEC Q89.2
hepatic duct Q44.5
pancreas Q45.3
parathyroid gland Q89.2
pituitary gland Q89.2
sebaceous glands, mucous membrane, mouth,
congenital Q38.6
spleen Q89.09
subclavian artery Q27.8
thymus (gland) Q89.2
thyroid gland Q89.2
vein (peripheral) NEC Q27.8
cerebral Q28.3
digestive system Q27.8
lower limb Q27.8
precerebral Q28.1
specified site NEC Q27.8
upper limb Q27.8
Aberration
distantial —*see* Disturbance, visual
mental F99
Abetalipoproteinemia E78.6
Abiotrophy R68.89
Ablatio, ablation
retinae —*see* Detachment, retina
Ablepharia, ablepharon Q10.3
Abnormal, abnormality, abnormalities —*see*
also Anomaly
acid-base balance (mixed) E87.4
albumin R77.0
alphafetoprotein R77.2
alveolar ridge K08.9
anatomical relationship Q89.9
apertures, congenital, diaphragm Q79.1
auditory perception H93.29
diplacusis —*see* Diplacusis
hyperacusis —*see* Hyperacusis
recruitment —*see* Recruitment, auditory
threshold shift —*see* Shift, auditory
threshold

Abnormal, abnormality, abnormalities -
continued
autosomes Q99.9
fragile site Q95.5
basal metabolic rate R94.8
biosynthesis, testicular androgen E29.1
bleeding time R79.1
blood-gas level R79.81
blood level (of)
cobalt R79.0
copper R79.0
iron R79.0
lithium R78.89
magnesium R79.0
mineral NEC R79.0
zinc R79.0
blood pressure
elevated R03.0
low reading (nonspecific) R03.1
blood sugar R73.09
bowel sounds R19.15
absent R19.11
hyperactive R19.12
brain scan R94.02
breathing R06.9
caloric test R94.138
cerebrospinal fluid R83.9
cytology R83.6
drug level R83.2
enzyme level R83.0
hormones R83.1
immunology R83.4
microbiology R83.5
nonmedicinal level R83.3
specified type NEC R83.8
chemistry, blood R79.9
C-reactive protein R79.82
drugs —*see* Findings, abnormal, in blood
gas level R79.81
minerals R79.0
pancytopenia D61.818
PTT R79.1
specified NEC R79.89
toxins —*see* Findings, abnormal, in blood
chest sounds (friction) (rales) R09.89
chromosome, chromosomal Q99.9
with more than three X chromosomes,
female Q97.1
analysis result R89.8
bronchial washings R84.8
cerebrospinal fluid R83.8
cervix uteri NEC R87.89
nasal secretions R84.8
nipple discharge R89.8
peritoneal fluid R85.89
pleural fluid R84.8
prostatic secretions R86.8
saliva R85.89
seminal fluid R86.8
sputum R84.8
synovial fluid R89.8
throat scrapings R84.8
vagina R87.89
vulva R87.89
wound secretions R89.8
dicentric replacement Q93.2
ring replacement Q93.2
sex Q99.8
female phenotype Q97.9
specified NEC Q97.8
male phenotype Q98.9
specified NEC Q98.8
structural male Q98.6

Abnormal, abnormality, abnormalities -
continued
specified NEC Q99.8
clinical findings NEC R68.89
coagulation D68.9
newborn, transient P61.6
profile R79.1
time R79.1
communication —*see* Fistula
conjunctiva, vascular H11.41
coronary artery Q24.5
cortisol-binding globulin E27.8
course, eustachian tube Q17.8
creatinine clearance R94.4
cytology
anus R85.619
atypical squamous cells cannot exclude
high grade squamous intraepithelial lesion
(ASC-H) R85.611
atypical squamous cells of undetermined
significance (ASC-US) R85.610
cytologic evidence of malignancy R85.614
high grade squamous intraepithelial lesion
(HGSIL) R85.613
human papillomavirus (HPV) DNA test
high risk positive R85.81
low risk positive R85.82
inadequate smear R85.615
low grade squamous intraepithelial lesion
(LGSIL) R85.612
satisfactory anal smear but lacking
transformation zone R85.616
specified NEC R85.618
unsatisfactory smear R85.615
female genital organs —*see* Abnormal,
Papanicolaou (smear)
dark adaptation curve H53.61
dentofacial NEC —*see* Anomaly, dentofacial
development, developmental Q89.9
central nervous system Q07.9
diagnostic imaging
abdomen, abdominal region NEC R93.5
biliary tract R93.2
breast R92.8
central nervous system NEC R90.89
cerebrovascular NEC R90.89
coronary circulation R93.1
digestive tract NEC R93.3
gastrointestinal (tract) R93.3
genitourinary organs R93.8
head R93.0
heart R93.1
intrathoracic organ NEC R93.8
limbs R93.6
liver R93.2
lung (field) R91.8
musculoskeletal system NEC R93.7
retroperitoneum R93.5
site specified NEC R93.8
skin and subcutaneous tissue R93.8
skull R93.0
urinary organs R93.4
direction, teeth, fully erupted M26.30
ear ossicles, acquired NEC H74.39
ankylosis —*see* Ankylosis, ear ossicles
discontinuity —*see* Discontinuity, ossicles,
ear
partial loss —*see* Loss, ossicles, ear (partial)
Ebstein Q22.5
echocardiogram R93.1
echoencephalogram R90.81
echogram —*see* Abnormal, diagnostic
imaging

Abnormal, abnormality, abnormalities - *continued*

electrocardiogram -ECG -EKG R94.31

electroencephalogram -EEG R94.01

electrolyte —*see* Imbalance, electrolyte

electromyogram -EMG R94.131

electro-oculogram -EOG] R94.110

electrophysiological intracardiac studies R94.39

electroretinogram -ERG] R94.111

erythrocytes

  congenital, with perinatal jaundice D58.9

feces (color) (contents) (mucus) R19.5

finding —*see* Findings, abnormal, without diagnosis

fluid

  amniotic —*see* Abnormal, specimen, specified

  cerebrospinal —*see* Abnormal, cerebrospinal fluid

  peritoneal —*see* Abnormal, specimen, digestive organs

  pleural —*see* Abnormal, specimen, respiratory organs

  synovial —*see* Abnormal, specimen, specified

  thorax (bronchial washings) (pleural fluid) —*see* Abnormal, specimen, respiratory organs

  vaginal —*see* Abnormal, specimen, female genital organs

form

  teeth K00.2

  uterus —*see* Anomaly, uterus

function studies

  auditory R94.120

  bladder R94.8

  brain R94.09

  cardiovascular R94.30

  ear R94.128

  endocrine NEC R94.7

  eye NEC R94.118

  kidney R94.4

  liver R94.5

  nervous system

    central NEC R94.09

    peripheral NEC R94.138

  pancreas R94.8

  placenta R94.8

  pulmonary R94.2

  special senses NEC R94.128

  spleen R94.8

  thyroid R94.6

  vestibular R94.121

gait —*see* Gait

  hysterical F44.4

gastrin secretion E16.4

globulin R77.1

  cortisol-binding E27.8

  thyroid-binding E07.89

glomerular, minor (*see also* N00-N07 with fourth character .0) N05.0

glucagon secretion E16.3

glucose tolerance (test) (non-fasting) R73.09

gravitational (G) forces or states (effect of) T75.81

hair (color) (shaft) L67.9

  specified NEC L67.8

hard tissue formation in pulp (dental) K04.3

head movement R25.0

heart

  rate R00.9

    specified NEC R00.8

  shadow R93.1

Abnormal, abnormality, abnormalities - *continued*

  sounds NEC R01.2

hemoglobin (disease) (*see also* Disease, hemoglobin) D58.2

  trait —*see* Trait, hemoglobin, abnormal

histology NEC R89.7

immunological findings R89.4

  in serum R76.9

    specified NEC R76.8

increase in appetite R63.2

involuntary movement —*see* Abnormal, movement, involuntary

jaw closure M26.51

karyotype R89.8

kidney function test R94.4

knee jerk R29.2

leukocyte (cell) (differential) NEC D72.9

liver

  loss of

    height R29.890

    weight R63.4

mammogram NEC R92.8

  calcification (calculus) R92.1

  microcalcification R92.0

Mantoux test R76.11

movement (disorder) —*see also* Disorder, movement

  head R25.0

  involuntary R25.9

    fasciculation R25.3

    of head R25.0

    spasm R25.2

    specified type NEC R25.8

    tremor R25.1

myoglobin (Aberdeen) (Annapolis) R89.7

neonatal screening P09

oculomotor study R94.113

palmar creases Q82.8

Papanicolaou (smear)

  anus R85.619

    atypical squamous cells cannot exclude high grade squamous intraepithelial lesion (ASC-H) R85.611

    atypical squamous cells of undetermined significance (ASC-US) R85.610

      cytologic evidence of malignancy R85.614

      high grade squamous intraepithelial lesion (HGSIL) R85.613

      human papillomavirus (HPV) DNA test

        high risk positive R85.81

        low risk positive R85.82

      inadequate smear R85.615

      low grade squamous intraepithelial lesion (LGSIL) R85.612

    satisfactory anal smear but lacking transformation zone R85.616

      specified NEC R85.618

      unsatisfactory smear R85.615

  bronchial washings R84.6

  cerebrospinal fluid R83.6

  cervix R87.619

    atypical squamous cells cannot exclude high grade squamous intraepithelial lesion (ASC-H) R87.611

    atypical squamous cells of undetermined significance (ASC-US) R87.610

      cytologic evidence of malignancy R87.614

      high grade squamous intraepithelial lesion (HGSIL) R87.613

        inadequate smear R87.615

        low grade squamous intraepithelial lesion (LGSIL) R87.612

Abnormal, abnormality, abnormalities - *continued*

    non-atypical endometrial cells R87.618

    satisfactory cervical smear but lacking transformation zone R87.616

      specified NEC R87.618

      thin preparation R87.619

      unsatisfactory smear R87.615

  nasal secretions R84.6

  nipple discharge R89.6

  peritoneal fluid R85.69

  pleural fluid R84.6

  prostatic secretions R86.6

  saliva R85.69

  seminal fluid R86.6

  sites NEC R89.6

  sputum R84.6

  synovial fluid R89.6

  throat scrapings R84.6

  vagina R87.629

    atypical squamous cells cannot exclude high grade squamous intraepithelial lesion (ASC-H) R87.621

    atypical squamous cells of undetermined significance (ASC-US) R87.620

      cytologic evidence of malignancy R87.624

      high grade squamous intraepithelial lesion (HGSIL) R87.623

        inadequate smear R87.625

        low grade squamous intraepithelial lesion (LGSIL) R87.622

        specified NEC R87.628

        thin preparation R87.629

        unsatisfactory smear R87.625

  vulva R87.69

  wound secretions R89.6

partial thromboplastin time (PTT) R79.1

pelvis (bony) —*see* Deformity, pelvis

percussion, chest (tympany) R09.89

periods (grossly) —*see* Menstruation

phonocardiogram R94.39

plantar reflex R29.2

plasma

  protein R77.9

    specified NEC R77.8

  viscosity R70.1

pleural (folds) Q34.0

posture R29.3

product of conception O02.9

  specified type NEC O02.89

prothrombin time (PT) R79.1

pulmonary

  artery, congenital Q25.79

  function, newborn P28.89

  test results R94.2

pulsations in neck R00.2

pupillary H21.56

  function (reaction) (reflex) —*see* Anomaly, pupil, function

radiological examination —*see* Abnormal, diagnostic imaging

red blood cell (s) (morphology) (volume) R71.8

reflex —*see* Reflex

renal function test R94.4

response to nerve stimulation R94.130

retinal correspondence H53.31

retinal function study R94.111

rhythm, heart —*see also* Arrhythmia

saliva —*see* Abnormal, specimen, digestive organs

scan

  kidney R94.4

Abnormal, abnormality, abnormalities - *continued*
- liver R93.2
- thyroid R94.6
- secretion
  - gastrin E16.4
  - glucagon E16.3
- semen, seminal fluid —*see* Abnormal, specimen, male genital organs
- serum level (of)
  - acid phosphatase R74.8
  - alkaline phosphatase R74.8
  - amylase R74.8
  - enzymes R74.9
    - specified NEC R74.8
  - lipase R74.8
  - triacylglycerol lipase R74.8
- shape
  - gravid uterus —*see* Anomaly, uterus
- sinus venosus Q21.1
- size, tooth, teeth K00.2
- spacing, tooth, teeth, fully erupted M26.30
- specimen
  - digestive organs (peritoneal fluid) (saliva) R85.9
    - cytology R85.69
    - drug level R85.2
    - enzyme level R85.0
    - histology R85.7
    - hormones R85.1
    - immunology R85.4
    - microbiology R85.5
    - nonmedicinal level R85.3
    - specified type NEC R85.89
  - female genital organs (secretions) (smears) R87.9
    - cytology R87.69
      - cervix R87.619
        - human papillomavirus (HPV) DNA test
          - high risk positive R87.810
          - low risk positive R87.820
        - inadequate (unsatisfactory) smear R87.615
        - non-atypical endometrial cells R87.618
        - specified NEC R87.618
      - vagina R87.629
        - human papillomavirus (HPV) DNA test
          - high risk positive R87.811
          - low risk positive R87.821
        - inadequate (unsatisfactory) smear R87.625
        - vulva R87.69
    - drug level R87.2
    - enzyme level R87.0
    - histological R87.7
    - hormones R87.1
    - immunology R87.4
    - microbiology R87.5
    - nonmedicinal level R87.3
    - specified type NEC R87.89
  - male genital organs (prostatic secretions) (semen) R86.9
    - cytology R86.6
    - drug level R86.2
    - enzyme level R86.0
    - histological R86.7
    - hormones R86.1
    - immunology R86.4
    - microbiology R86.5
    - nonmedicinal level R86.3
    - specified type NEC R86.8
  - nipple discharge —*see* Abnormal, specimen, specified

Abnormal, abnormality, abnormalities - *continued*
  - respiratory organs (bronchial washings) (nasal secretions) (pleural fluid) (sputum) R84.9
    - cytology R84.6
    - drug level R84.2
    - enzyme level R84.0
    - histology R84.7
    - hormones R84.1
    - immunology R84.4
    - microbiology R84.5
    - nonmedicinal level R84.3
    - specified type NEC R84.8
  - specified organ, system and tissue NOS R89.9
    - cytology R89.6
    - drug level R89.2
    - enzyme level R89.0
    - histology R89.7
    - hormones R89.1
    - immunology R89.4
    - microbiology R89.5
    - nonmedicinal level R89.3
    - specified type NEC R89.8
  - synovial fluid —*see* Abnormal, specimen, specified
    - thorax (bronchial washings) (pleural fluids) —*see* Abnormal, specimen, respiratory organs
    - vagina (secretion) (smear) R87.629
    - vulva (secretion) (smear) R87.69
    - wound secretion —*see* Abnormal, specimen, specified
  - spermatozoa —*see* Abnormal, specimen, male genital organs
- sputum (amount) (color) (odor) R09.3
- stool (color) (contents) (mucus) R19.5
  - bloody K92.1
  - guaiac positive R19.5
- synchondrosis Q78.8
- thermography (*see also* Abnormal, diagnostic imaging) R93.8
- thyroid-binding globulin E07.89
- tooth, teeth (form) (size) K00.2
- toxicology (findings) R78.9
- transport protein E88.09
- tumor marker NEC R97.8
- ultrasound results —*see* Abnormal, diagnostic imaging
- umbilical cord complicating delivery O69.9
- urination NEC R39.19
- urine (constituents) R82.90
  - bile R82.2
  - cytological examination R82.8
  - drugs R82.5
  - fat R82.0
  - glucose R81
  - heavy metals R82.6
  - hemoglobin R82.3
  - histological examination R82.8
  - ketones R82.4
  - microbiological examination (culture) R82.7
  - myoglobin R82.1
  - positive culture R82.7
  - protein —*see* Proteinuria
  - specified substance NEC R82.99
    - chromoabnormality NEC R82.91
  - substances nonmedical R82.6
- uterine hemorrhage —*see* Hemorrhage, uterus
- vectorcardiogram R94.39
- visually evoked potential (VEP) R94.112
- white blood cells D72.9
  - specified NEC D72.89

Abnormal, abnormality, abnormalities - *continued*
  - X-ray examination —*see* Abnormal, diagnostic imaging
Abnormity (any organ or part) —*see* Anomaly
Abocclusion M26.29
- hemolytic disease (newborn) P55.1
- incompatibility reaction ABO —*see* Complication(s) , transfusion, incompatibility reaction, ABO
Abolition, language R48.8
Aborter, habitual or recurrent —*see* Loss (of) , pregnancy, recurrent
Abortion (complete) (spontaneous) O03.9
- with
  - retained products of conception —*see* Abortion, incomplete
- attempted (elective) (failed) O07.4
  - complicated by O07.30
    - afibrinogenemia O07.1
    - cardiac arrest O07.36
    - chemical damage of pelvic organ (s) O07.34
    - circulatory collapse O07.31
    - cystitis O07.38
    - defibrination syndrome O07.1
    - electrolyte imbalance O07.33
    - embolism (air) (amniotic fluid) (blood clot) (fat) (pulmonary) (septic) (soap) O07.2
    - endometritis O07.0
    - genital tract and pelvic infection O07.0
    - hemolysis O07.1
    - hemorrhage (delayed) (excessive) O07.1
    - infection
      - genital tract or pelvic O07.0
      - urinary tract O07.38
    - intravascular coagulation O07.1
    - laceration of pelvic organ (s) O07.34
    - metabolic disorder O07.33
    - oliguria O07.32
    - oophoritis O07.0
    - parametritis O07.0
    - pelvic peritonitis O07.0
    - perforation of pelvic organ (s) O07.34
    - renal failure or shutdown O07.32
    - salpingitis or salpingo-oophoritis O07.0
    - sepsis O07.37
    - shock O07.31
    - specified condition NEC O07.39
    - tubular necrosis (renal) O07.32
    - uremia O07.32
    - urinary tract infection O07.38
    - venous complication NEC O07.35
      - embolism (air) (amniotic fluid) (blood clot) (fat) (pulmonary) (septic) (soap) O07.2
- complicated (by) (following) O03.80
  - afibrinogenemia O03.6
  - cardiac arrest O03.86
  - chemical damage of pelvic organ (s) O03.84
  - circulatory collapse O03.81
  - cystitis O03.88
  - defibrination syndrome O03.6
  - electrolyte imbalance O03.83
  - embolism (air) (amniotic fluid) (blood clot) (fat) (pulmonary) (septic) (soap) O03.7
  - endometritis O03.5
  - genital tract and pelvic infection O03.5
  - hemolysis O03.6
  - hemorrhage (delayed) (excessive) O03.6
  - infection
    - genital tract or pelvic O03.5
    - urinary tract O03.88
  - intravascular coagulation O03.6

Abortion - *continued*
- laceration of pelvic organ (s) O03.84
- metabolic disorder O03.83
- oliguria O03.82
- oophoritis O03.5
- parametritis O03.5
- pelvic peritonitis O03.5
- perforation of pelvic organ (s) O03.84
- renal failure or shutdown O03.82
- salpingitis or salpingo-oophoritis O03.5
- sepsis O03.87
- shock O03.81
- specified condition NEC O03.89
- tubular necrosis (renal) O03.82
- uremia O03.82
- urinary tract infection O03.88
- venous complication NEC O03.85
  - embolism (air) (amniotic fluid) (blood clot) (fat) (pulmonary) (septic) (soap) O03.7
- failed —*see* Abortion, attempted
- habitual or recurrent N96
  - with current abortion —*see* categories O03-O06
  - without current pregnancy N96
  - care in current pregnancy O26.2
- incomplete (spontaneous) O03.4
  - complicated (by) (following) O03.30
    - afibrinogenemia O03.1
    - cardiac arrest O03.36
    - chemical damage of pelvic organ (s) O03.34
    - circulatory collapse O03.31
    - cystitis O03.38
    - defibrination syndrome O03.1
    - electrolyte imbalance O03.33
    - embolism (air) (amniotic fluid) (blood clot) (fat) (pulmonary) (septic) (soap) O03.2
    - endometritis O03.0
    - genital tract and pelvic infection O03.0
    - hemolysis O03.1
    - hemorrhage (delayed) (excessive) O03.1
    - infection
      - genital tract or pelvic O03.0
      - urinary tract O03.38
    - intravascular coagulation O03.1
    - laceration of pelvic organ (s) O03.34
    - metabolic disorder O03.33
    - oliguria O03.32
    - oophoritis O03.0
    - parametritis O03.0
    - pelvic peritonitis O03.0
    - perforation of pelvic organ (s) O03.34
    - renal failure or shutdown O03.32
    - salpingitis or salpingo-oophoritis O03.0
    - sepsis O03.37
    - shock O03.31
    - specified condition NEC O03.39
    - tubular necrosis (renal) O03.32
    - uremia O03.32
    - urinary infection O03.38
    - venous complication NEC O03.35
      - embolism (air) (amniotic fluid) (blood clot) (fat) (pulmonary) (septic) (soap) O03.2
- induced (encounter for) Z33.2
  - complicated by O04.80
    - afibrinogenemia O04.6
    - cardiac arrest O04.86
    - chemical damage of pelvic organ (s) O04.84
    - circulatory collapse O04.81
    - cystitis O04.88
    - defibrination syndrome O04.6
    - electrolyte imbalance O04.83

Abortion - *continued*
- embolism (air) (amniotic fluid) (blood clot) (fat) (pulmonary) (septic) (soap) O04.7
  - endometritis O04.5
  - genital tract and pelvic infection O04.5
  - hemolysis O04.6
  - hemorrhage (delayed) (excessive) O04.6
  - infection
    - genital tract or pelvic O04.5
    - urinary tract O04.88
  - intravascular coagulation O04.6
  - laceration of pelvic organ (s) O04.84
  - metabolic disorder O04.83
  - oliguria O04.82
  - oophoritis O04.5
  - parametritis O04.5
  - pelvic peritonitis O04.5
  - perforation of pelvic organ (s) O04.84
  - renal failure or shutdown O04.82
  - salpingitis or salpingo-oophoritis O04.5
  - sepsis O04.87
  - shock O04.81
  - specified condition NEC O04.89
  - tubular necrosis (renal) O04.82
  - uremia O04.82
  - urinary tract infection O04.88
  - venous complication NEC O04.85
    - embolism (air) (amniotic fluid) (blood clot) (fat) (pulmonary) (septic) (soap) O04.7
- missed O02.1
- spontaneous —*see* Abortion (complete) (spontaneous)
  - threatened O20.0
- threatened (spontaneous) O20.0
- tubal O00.1

Abortus fever A23.1
Aboulomania F60.7
Abrami's disease D59.8
Abramov-Fiedler myocarditis (acute isolated myocarditis) I40.1
Abrasion T14.8
- abdomen, abdominal (wall) S30.811
- alveolar process S00.512
- ankle S90.51
- antecubital space —*see* Abrasion, elbow
- anus S30.817
- arm (upper) S40.81
- auditory canal —*see* Abrasion, ear
- auricle —*see* Abrasion, ear
- axilla —*see* Abrasion, arm
- back, lower S30.810
- breast S20.11
- brow S00.81
- buttock S30.810
- calf —*see* Abrasion, leg
- canthus —*see* Abrasion, eyelid
- cheek S00.81
  - internal S00.512
- chest wall —*see* Abrasion, thorax
- chin S00.81
- clitoris S30.814
- cornea S05.0
- costal region —*see* Abrasion, thorax
- dental K03.1
- digit (s)
  - foot —*see* Abrasion, toe
  - hand —*see* Abrasion, finger
- ear S00.41
- elbow S50.31
- epididymis S30.813
- epigastric region S30.811
- epiglottis S10.11
- esophagus (thoracic) S27.818

Abrasion - *continued*
- cervical S10.11
- eyebrow —*see* Abrasion, eyelid
- eyelid S00.21
- face S00.81
- finger (s) S60.41
  - index S60.41
  - little S60.41
  - middle S60.41
  - ring S60.41
- flank S30.811
- foot (except toe(s) alone) S90.81
  - toe —*see* Abrasion, toe
- forearm S50.81
  - elbow only —*see* Abrasion, elbow
- forehead S00.81
- genital organs, external
  - female S30.816
  - male S30.815
- groin S30.811
- gum S00.512
- hand S60.51
- head S00.91
  - ear —*see* Abrasion, ear
  - eyelid —*see* Abrasion, eyelid
  - lip S00.511
  - nose S00.31
  - oral cavity S00.512
  - scalp S00.01
  - specified site NEC S00.81
- heel —*see* Abrasion, foot
- hip S70.21
- inguinal region S30.811
- interscapular region S20.419
- jaw S00.81
- knee S80.21
- labium (majus) (minus) S30.814
- larynx S10.11
- leg (lower) S80.81
  - knee —*see* Abrasion, knee
  - upper —*see* Abrasion, thigh
- lip S00.511
- lower back S30.810
- lumbar region S30.810
- malar region S00.81
- mammary —*see* Abrasion, breast
- mastoid region S00.81
- mouth S00.512
- nail
  - finger —*see* Abrasion, finger
  - toe —*see* Abrasion, toe
- nape S10.81
- nasal S00.31
- neck S10.91
  - specified site NEC S10.81
  - throat S10.11
- nose S00.31
- occipital region S00.01
- oral cavity S00.512
- orbital region —*see* Abrasion, eyelid
- palate S00.512
- palm —*see* Abrasion, hand
- parietal region S00.01
- pelvis S30.810
- penis S30.812
- perineum
  - female S30.814
  - male S30.810
- periocular area —*see* Abrasion, eyelid
- phalanges
  - finger —*see* Abrasion, finger
  - toe —*see* Abrasion, toe
- pharynx S10.11

Abrasion - *continued*
pinna —*see* Abrasion, ear
popliteal space —*see* Abrasion, knee
prepuce S30.812
pubic region S30.810
pudendum
  female S30.816
  male S30.815
sacral region S30.810
scalp S00.01
scapular region —*see* Abrasion, shoulder
scrotum S30.813
shin —*see* Abrasion, leg
shoulder S40.21
skin NEC T14.8
sternal region S20.319
submaxillary region S00.81
submental region S00.81
subungual
  finger (s) —*see* Abrasion, finger
  toe (s) —*see* Abrasion, toe
supraclavicular fossa S10.81
supraorbital S00.81
temple S00.81
temporal region S00.81
testis S30.813
thigh S70.31
thorax, thoracic (wall) S20.91
  back S20.41
  front S20.31
throat S10.11
thumb S60.31
toe (s) (lesser) S90.416
  great S90.41
tongue S00.512
tooth, teeth (dentifrice) (habitual) (hard
tissues) (occupational) (ritual) (traditional)
K03.1
trachea S10 11
tunica vaginalis S30.813
tympanum, tympanic membrane —*see*
Abrasion, ear
uvula S00.512
vagina S30.814
vocal cords S10.11
vulva S30.814
wrist S60.81
Abrism —*see* Poisoning, food, noxious, plant
Abruptio placentae O45.9
with
  afibrinogenemia O45.01
  coagulation defect O45.00
    specified NEC O45.09
  disseminated intravascular coagulation
O45.02
  hypofibrinogenemia O45.01
  specified NEC O45.8
Abruption, placenta —*see* Abruptio placentae
Abscess (connective tissue) (embolic)
(fistulous) (infective) (metastatic) (multiple)
(pernicious) (pyogenic) (septic) L02.91
with
  diverticular disease (intestine) K57.80
    with bleeding K57.81
    large intestine K57.20
      with
        bleeding K57.21
        small intestine K57.40
          with bleeding K57.41
    small intestine K57.00
      with
        bleeding K57.01
        large intestine K57.40

Abscess - *continued*
    with bleeding K57.41
  lymphangitis
code by site under Abscess
abdomen, abdominal
  cavity K65.1
  wall L02.211
abdominopelvic K65.1
accessory sinus —*see* Sinusitis
adrenal (capsule) (gland) E27.8
alveolar K04.7
  with sinus K04.6
amebic A06.4
  brain (and liver or lung abscess) A06.6
  genitourinary tract A06.82
  liver (without mention of brain or lung
abscess) A06.4
  lung (and liver) (without mention of brain
abscess) A06.5
  specified site NEC A06.89
  spleen A06.89
anaerobic A48.0
ankle —*see* Abscess, lower limb
anorectal K61.2
antecubital space —*see* Abscess, upper limb
antrum (chronic) (Highmore) —*see* Sinusitis,
maxillary
anus K61.0
apical (tooth) K04.7
  with sinus (alveolar) K04.6
appendix K35.3
areola (acute) (chronic) (nonpuerperal) N61
  puerperal, postpartum or gestational —*see*
Infection, nipple
arm (any part) —*see* Abscess, upper limb
artery (wall) I77.89
atheromatous I77.2
auricle, ear —*see* Abscess, ear, external
axilla (region) L02.41
  lymph gland or node L04.2
back (any part, except buttock) L02.212
Bartholin's gland N75.1
  with
    abortion —*see* Abortion, by type
  complicated by, sepsis
    ectopic or molar pregnancy O08.0
    following ectopic or molar pregnancy O08.0
Bezold's —*see* Mastoiditis, acute
bilharziasis B65.1
bladder (wall) —*see* Cystitis, specified type
NEC
bone (subperiosteal) —*see also*
Osteomyelitis, specified type NEC
  accessory sinus (chronic) —*see* Sinusitis
  chronic or old —*see* Osteomyelitis, chronic
  jaw (lower) (upper) M27.2
  mastoid —*see* Mastoiditis, acute,
subperiosteal
  petrous —*see* Petrositis
  spinal (tuberculous) A18.01
    nontuberculous —*see* Osteomyelitis,
vertebra
bowel K63.0
brain (any part) (cystic) (otogenic) G06.0
  amebic (with abscess of any other site)
A06.6
  gonococcal A54.82
  pheomycotic (chromomycotic) B43.1
  tuberculous A17.81
breast (acute) (chronic) (nonpuerperal) N61
  newborn P39.0
  puerperal, postpartum, gestational —*see*
Mastitis, obstetric, purulent

Abscess - *continued*
broad ligament N73.2
  acute N73.0
  chronic N73.1
Brodie's (localized) (chronic) M86.8X
bronchi J98.09
buccal cavity K12.2
bulbourethral gland N34.0
bursa M71.00
  ankle M71.07
  elbow M71.02
  foot M71.07
  hand M71.04
  hip M71.05
  knee M71.06
  multiple sites M71.09
  pharyngeal J39.1
  shoulder M71.01
  specified site NEC M71.08
  wrist M71.03
buttock L02.31
canthus —*see* Blepharoconjunctivitis
cartilage —*see* Disorder, cartilage, specified
type NEC
cecum K35.3
cerebellum, cerebellar G06.0
  sequelae G09
cerebral (embolic) G06.0
  sequelae G09
cervical (meaning neck) L02.11
  lymph gland or node L04.0
cervix (stump) (uteri) —*see* Cervicitis
cheek (external) L02.01
  inner K12.2
chest J86.9
  with fistula J86.0
  wall L02.213
chin L02.01
choroid —*see* Inflammation, chorioretinal
circumtonsillar J36
cold (lung) (tuberculous) —*see also*
Tuberculosis, abscess, lung
  articular —*see* Tuberculosis, joint
colon (wall) K63.0
colostomy K94.02
conjunctiva —*see* Conjunctivitis, acute
cornea H16.31
corpus
  cavernosum N48.21
  luteum —*see* Oophoritis
Cowper's gland N34.0
cranium G06.0
cul-de-sac (Douglas') (posterior) —*see*
Peritonitis, pelvic, female
cutaneous —*see* Abscess, by site
dental K04.7
  with sinus (alveolar) K04.6
dentoalveolar K04.7
  with sinus K04.6
diaphragm, diaphragmatic K65.1
Douglas' cul-de-sac or pouch —*see*
Peritonitis, pelvic, female
Dubois A50.59
ear (middle) —*see also* Otitis, media,
suppurative
  acute —*see* Otitis, media, suppurative, acute
  external H60.0
entamebic —*see* Abscess, amebic
enterostomy K94.12
epididymis N45.4
epidural G06.2
  brain G06.0
  spinal cord G06.1

Abscess — *continued*
  epiglottis J38.7
  epiploon, epiploic K65.1
  erysipelatous —*see* Erysipelas
  esophagus K20.8
  ethmoid (bone) (chronic) (sinus) J32.2
  external auditory canal —*see* Abscess, ear, external
  extradural G06.2
    brain G06.0
      sequelae G09
    spinal cord G06.1
  extraperitoneal K68.19
  eye —*see* Endophthalmitis, purulent
  eyelid H00.03
  face (any part, except ear, eye and nose) L02.01
  fallopian tube —*see* Salpingitis
  fascia M72.8
  fauces J39.1
  fecal K63.0
  femoral (region) —*see* Abscess, lower limb
  filaria, filarial —*see* Infestation, filarial
  finger (any) —*see also* Abscess, hand
    nail —*see* Cellulitis, finger
  foot L02.61
  forehead L02.01
  frontal sinus (chronic) J32.1
  gallbladder K81.0
  genital organ or tract
    female (external) N76.4
    male N49.9
      multiple sites N49.8
      specified NEC N49.8
  gestational mammary O91.11
  gestational subareolar O91.11
  gingival K05.21
  gland, glandular (lymph) (acute) —*see* Lymphadenitis, acute
  gluteal (region) L02.31
  gonorrheal —*see* Gonococcus
  groin L02.214
  gum K05.21
  hand L02.51
  head NEC L02.811
    face (any part, except ear, eye and nose) L02.01
  heart —*see* Carditis
  heel —*see* Abscess, foot
  helminthic —*see* Infestation, helminth
  hepatic (cholangitic) (hematogenic) (lymphogenic) (pylephlebitic) K75.0
    amebic A06.4
  hip (region) —*see* Abscess, lower limb
  ileocecal K35.3
  ileostomy (bud) K94.12
  iliac (region) L02.214
    fossa K35.3
  infraclavicular (fossa) —*see* Abscess, upper limb
  inguinal (region) L02.214
    lymph gland or node L04.1
  intestine, intestinal NEC K63.0
    rectal K61.1
  intra-abdominal (*see also* Abscess, peritoneum) K65.1
    postoperative T81.4
      retroperitoneal K68.11
  intracranial G06.0
  intramammary —*see* Abscess, breast
  intraorbital —*see* Abscess, orbit
  intraperitoneal K65.1
  intrasphincteric (anus) K61.4

Abscess — *continued*
  intraspinal G06.1
  intratonsillar J36
  ischiorectal (fossa) K61.3
  jaw (bone) (lower) (upper) M27.2
  joint —*see* Arthritis, pyogenic or pyemic
    spine (tuberculous) A18.01
      nontuberculous —*see* Spondylopathy, infective
  kidney N15.1
    with calculus N20.0
      with hydronephrosis N13.6
    puerperal (postpartum) O86.21
  knee —*see also* Abscess, lower limb
    joint M00.9
  labium (majus) (minus) N76.4
  lacrimal
    caruncle —*see* Inflammation, lacrimal, passages, acute
    gland —*see* Dacryoadenitis
    passages (duct) (sac) —*see* Inflammation, lacrimal, passages, acute
  lacunar N34.0
  larynx J38.7
  lateral (alveolar) K04.7
    with sinus K04.6
  leg (any part) —*see* Abscess, lower limb
  lens H27.8
  lingual K14.0
    tonsil J36
  lip K13.0
  Littre's gland N34.0
  liver (cholangitic) (hematogenic) (lymphogenic) (pylephlebitic) (pyogenic) K75.0
    amebic (due to Entamoeba histolytica) (dysenteric) (tropical) A06.4
      with
        brain abscess (and liver or lung abscess) A06.6
          lung abscess A06.5
  loin (region) L02.211
  lower limb L02.41
  lumbar (tuberculous) A18.01
    nontuberculous L02.212
  lung (miliary) (putrid) J85.2
    with pneumonia J85.1
      due to specified organism (see Pneumonia, in (due to))
    amebic (with liver abscess) A06.5
      with
        brain abscess A06.6
        pneumonia A06.5
  lymph, lymphatic, gland or node (acute) —*see also* Lymphadenitis, acute
    mesentery I88.0
  malar M27.2
  mammary gland —*see* Abscess, breast
  marginal, anus K61.0
  mastoid —*see* Mastoiditis, acute
  maxilla, maxillary M27.2
    molar (tooth) K04.7
      with sinus K04.6
    premolar K04.7
    sinus (chronic) J32.0
  mediastinum J85.3
  meibomian gland —*see* Hordeolum
  meninges G06.2
  mesentery, mesenteric K65.1
  mesosalpinx —*see* Salpingitis
  mons pubis L02.215
  mouth (floor) K12.2
  muscle —*see* Myositis, infective

Abscess — *continued*
  myocardium I40.0
  nabothian (follicle) —*see* Cervicitis
  nasal J32.9
  nasopharyngeal J39.1
  navel L02.216
    newborn P38.9
      with mild hemorrhage P38.1
      without hemorrhage P38.9
  neck (region) L02.11
    lymph gland or node L04.0
  nephritic —*see* Abscess, kidney
  nipple N61
    associated with
      lactation —*see* Pregnancy, complicated by, pregnancy —*see* Pregnancy, complicated by
  nose (external) (fossa) (septum) J34.0
    sinus (chronic) —*see* Sinusitis
  omentum K65.1
  operative wound T81.4
  orbit, orbital —*see* Cellulitis, orbit
  otogenic G06.0
  ovary, ovarian (corpus luteum) —*see* Oophoritis
  oviduct —*see* Oophoritis
  palate (soft) K12.2
    hard M27.2
  palmar (space) —*see* Abscess, hand
  pancreas (duct) —*see* Pancreatitis, acute
  parafrenal N48.21
  parametric, parametrium N73.2
    acute N73.0
    chronic N73.1
  paranephric N15.1
  parapancreatic —*see* Pancreatitis, acute
  parapharyngeal J39.0
  pararectal K61.1
  parasinus —*see* Sinusitis
  parauterine (*see also* Disease, pelvis, inflammatory) N73.2
  paravaginal —*see* Vaginitis
  parietal region (scalp) L02.811
  parodontal K05.21
  parotid (duct) (gland) K11.3
    region K12.2
  pectoral (region) L02.213
  pelvis, pelvic
    female —*see* Disease, pelvis, inflammatory
    male, peritoneal K65.1
  penis N48.21
    gonococcal (accessory gland) (periurethral) A54.1
  perianal K61.0
  periapical K04.7
    with sinus (alveolar) K04.6
  periappendicular K35.3
  pericardial I30.1
  pericecal K35.3
  pericemental K05.21
  pericholecystic —*see* Cholecystitis, acute
  pericoronal K05.21
  peridental K05.21
  perimetric (*see also* Disease, pelvis, inflammatory) N73.2
  perinephric, perinephritic —*see* Abscess, kidney
  perineum, perineal (superficial) L02.215
    urethra N34.0
  periodontal (parietal) K05.21
    apical K04.7
  periosteum, periosteal —*see also* Osteomyelitis, specified type NEC

Abscess - *continued*
with osteomyelitis —*see also* Osteomyelitis, specified type NEC
  acute —*see* Osteomyelitis, acute
  chronic —*see* Osteomyelitis, chronic
peripharyngeal J39.0
peripleuritic J86.9
  with fistula J86.0
periprostatic N41.2
perirectal K61.1
perirenal (tissue) —*see* Abscess, kidney
perisinuous (nose) —*see* Sinusitis
peritoneum, peritoneal (perforated) (ruptured) K65.1
  with appendicitis K35.3
  pelvic
    female —*see* Peritonitis, pelvic, female
    male K65.1
  postoperative T81.4
  puerperal, postpartum, childbirth O85
  tuberculous A18.31
peritonsillar J36
perityphlic K35.3
periureteral N28.89
periurethral N34.0
  gonococcal (accessory gland) (periurethral) A54.1
periuterine (*see also* Disease, pelvis, inflammatory) N73.2
perivesical —*see* Cystitis, specified type NEC
petrous bone —*see* Petrositis
phagedenic NOS L02.91
  chancroid A57
pharynx, pharyngeal (lateral) J39.1
pilonidal L05.01
pituitary (gland) E23.6
pleura J86.9
  with fistula J86.0
popliteal —*see* Abscess, lower limb
postcecal K35.3
postlaryngeal J38.7
postnasal J34.0
postoperative (any site) T81.4
  retroperitoneal K68.11
postpharyngeal J39.0
posttonsillar J36
post-typhoid A01.09
pouch of Douglas —*see* Peritonitis, pelvic, female
premammary —*see* Abscess, breast
prepatellar —*see* Abscess, lower limb
prostate N41.2
  gonococcal (acute) (chronic) A54.22
psoas muscle K68.12
puerperal
  code by site under Puerperal, abscess
pulmonary —*see* Abscess, lung
pulp, pulpal (dental) K04.0
rectovaginal septum K63.0
rectovesical —*see* Cystitis, specified type NEC
rectum K61.1
renal —*see* Abscess, kidney
retina —*see* Inflammation, chorioretinal
retrobulbar —*see* Abscess, orbit
retrocecal K65.1
retrolaryngeal J38.7
retromammary —*see* Abscess, breast
retroperitoneal NEC K68.19
  postprocedural K68.11
retropharyngeal J39.0
retrouterine —*see* Peritonitis, pelvic, female

Abscess - *continued*
retrovesical —*see* Cystitis, specified type NEC
root, tooth K04.7
  with sinus (alveolar) K04.6
round ligament (*see also* Disease, pelvis, inflammatory) N73.2
rupture (spontaneous) NOS L02.91
sacrum (tuberculous) A18.01
  nontuberculous M46.28
salivary (duct) (gland) K11.3
scalp (any part) L02.811
scapular —*see* Osteomyelitis, specified type NEC
sclera —*see* Scleritis
scrofulous (tuberculous) A18.2
scrotum N49.2
seminal vesicle N49.0
septal, dental K04.7
  with sinus (alveolar) K04.6
serous —*see* Periostitis
shoulder (region) —*see* Abscess, upper limb
sigmoid K63.0
sinus (accessory) (chronic) (nasal) —*see also* Sinusitis
  intracranial venous (any) G06.0
Skene's duct or gland N34.0
skin —*see* Abscess, by site
specified site NEC L02.818
spermatic cord N49.1
sphenoidal (sinus) (chronic) J32.3
spinal cord (any part) (staphylococcal) G06.1
  tuberculous A17.81
spine (column) (tuberculous) A18.01
  epidural G06.1
  nontuberculous —*see* Osteomyelitis, vertebra
spleen D73.3
  amebic A06.89
stitch T81.4
subarachnoid G06.2
  brain G06.0
  spinal cord G06.1
subareolar —*see* Abscess, breast
subcecal K35.3
subcutaneous —*see also* Abscess, by site
  pheomycotic (chromomycotic) B43.2
subdiaphragmatic K65.1
subdural G06.2
  brain G06.0
    sequelae G09
  spinal cord G06.1
subgaleal L02.811
subhepatic K65.1
sublingual K12.2
  gland K11.3
submammary —*see* Abscess, breast
submandibular (region) (space) (triangle) K12.2
  gland K11.3
submaxillary (region) L02.01
  gland K11.3
submental L02.01
  gland K11.3
subperiosteal —*see* Osteomyelitis, specified type NEC
subphrenic K65.1
  postoperative T81.4
suburethral N34.0
sudoriparous L75.8
supraclavicular (fossa) —*see* Abscess, upper limb
suprapelvic, acute N73.0

Abscess - *continued*
suprarenal (capsule) (gland) E27.8
sweat gland L74.8
tear duct —*see* Inflammation, lacrimal, passages, acute
temple L02.01
temporal region L02.01
temporosphenoidal G06.0
tendon (sheath) M65.00
  ankle M65.07
  foot M65.07
  forearm M65.03
  hand M65.04
  lower leg M65.06
  pelvic region M65.05
  shoulder region M65.01
  specified site NEC M65.08
  thigh M65.05
  upper arm M65.02
testis N45.4
thigh —*see* Abscess, lower limb
thorax J86.9
  with fistula J86.0
throat J39.1
thumb —*see also* Abscess, hand
  nail —*see* Cellulitis, finger
thymus (gland) E32.1
thyroid (gland) E06.0
toe (any) —*see also* Abscess, foot
  nail —*see* Cellulitis, toe
tongue (staphylococcal) K14.0
tonsil (s) (lingual) J36
tonsillopharyngeal J36
tooth, teeth (root) K04.7
  with sinus (alveolar) K04.6
  supporting structures NEC K05.21
trachea J39.8
trunk L02.219
  abdominal wall L02.211
  back L02.212
  chest wall L02.213
  groin L02.214
  perineum L02.215
  umbilicus L02.216
tubal —*see* Salpingitis
tuberculous —*see* Tuberculosis, abscess
tubo-ovarian —*see* Salpingo-oophoritis
tunica vaginalis N49.1
umbilicus L02.216
upper
  limb L02.41
  respiratory J39.8
urethral (gland) N34.0
urinary N34.0
uterus, uterine (wall) —*see also* Endometritis
  ligament (*see also* Disease, pelvis, inflammatory) N73.2
  neck —*see* Cervicitis
uvula K12.2
vagina (wall) —*see* Vaginitis
vaginorectal —*see* Vaginitis
vas deferens N49.1
vermiform appendix K35.3
vertebra (column) (tuberculous) A18.01
  nontuberculous —*see* Osteomyelitis, vertebra
vesical —*see* Cystitis, specified type NEC
vesico-uterine pouch —*see* Peritonitis, pelvic, female
vitreous (humor) —*see* Endophthalmitis, purulent
vocal cord J38.3
von Bezold's —*see* Mastoiditis, acute

Abscess - *continued*
vulva N76.4
vulvovaginal gland N75.1
web space —*see* Abscess, hand
wound T81.4
wrist —*see* Abscess, upper limb
Absence (of) (organ or part) (complete or partial)
adrenal (gland) (congenital) Q89.1
acquired E89.6
albumin in blood E88.09
alimentary tract (congenital) Q45.8
upper Q40.8
alveolar process (acquired) —*see* Anomaly, alveolar
ankle (acquired) Z89.44
anus (congenital) Q42.3
with fistula Q42.2
aorta (congenital) Q25.4
appendix, congenital Q42.8
arm (acquired) Z89.20
above elbow Z89.22
congenital (with hand present) —*see* Agenesis, arm, with hand present
and hand —*see* Agenesis, forearm, and hand
below elbow Z89.21
congenital (with hand present) —*see* Agenesis, arm, with hand present
and hand —*see* Agenesis, forearm, and hand
congenital —*see* Defect, reduction, upper limb
shoulder (following explanation of shoulder joint prosthesis) (joint) (with or without presence of antibiotic-impregnated cement spacer) Z89.23
congenital (with hand present) —*see* Agenesis, arm, with hand present
artery (congenital) (peripheral) Q27.8
brain Q28.3
coronary Q24.5
pulmonary Q25.79
specified NEC Q27.8
umbilical Q27.0
atrial septum (congenital) Q21.1
auditory canal (congenital) (external) Q16.1
auricle (ear) , congenital Q16.0
bile, biliary duct, congenital Q44.5
bladder (acquired) Z90.6
congenital Q64.5
bowel sounds R19.11
brain Q00.0
part of Q04.3
breast (s) (and nipple(s)) (acquired) Z90.1
congenital Q83.8
broad ligament Q50.6
bronchus (congenital) Q32.4
canaliculus lacrimalis, congenital Q10.4
cerebellum (vermis) Q04.3
cervix (acquired) (with uterus) Z90.710
with remaining uterus Z90.712
congenital Q51.5
chin, congenital Q18.8
cilia (congenital) Q10.3
acquired —*see* Madarosis
clitoris (congenital) Q52.6
coccyx, congenital Q76.49
cold sense R20.8
congenital
lumen —*see* Atresia
organ or site NEC —*see* Agenesis
septum —*see* Imperfect, closure

Absence - *continued*
corpus callosum Q04.0
cricoid cartilage, congenital Q31.8
diaphragm (with hernia) , congenital Q79.1
digestive organ (s) or tract, congenital Q45.8
acquired NEC Z90.49
upper Q40.8
ductus arteriosus Q28.8
duodenum (acquired) Z90.49
congenital Q41.0
ear, congenital Q16.9
acquired H93.8
auricle Q16.0
external Q16.0
inner Q16.5
lobe, lobule Q17.8
middle, except ossicles Q16.4
ossicles Q16.3
ossicles Q16.3
ejaculatory duct (congenital) Q55.4
endocrine gland (congenital) NEC Q89.2
acquired E89.89
epididymis (congenital) Q55.4
acquired Z90.79
epiglottis, congenital Q31.8
esophagus (congenital) Q39.8
acquired (partial) Z90.49
eustachian tube (congenital) Q16.2
extremity (acquired) Z89.9
congenital Q73.0
knee (following explanation of knee joint prosthesis) (joint) (with or without presence of antibiotic-impregnated cement spacer) Z89.52
lower (above knee) Z89.619
below knee Z89.51
upper —*see* Absence, arm
eye (acquired) Z90.01
congenital Q11.1
muscle (congenital) Q10.3
eyeball (acquired) Z90.01
eyelid (fold) (congenital) Q10.3
acquired Z90.01
face, specified part NEC Q18.8
fallopian tube (s) (acquired) Z90.79
congenital Q50.6
family member (causing problem in home) NEC (*see also* Disruption, family) Z63.32
femur, congenital —*see* Defect, reduction, lower limb, longitudinal, femur
fibrinogen (congenital) D68.2
acquired D65
finger (s) (acquired) Z89.02
congenital —*see* Agenesis, hand
foot (acquired) Z89.43
congenital —*see* Agenesis, foot
forearm (acquired) —*see* Absence, arm, below elbow
gallbladder (acquired) Z90.49
congenital Q44.0
gamma globulin in blood D80.1
hereditary D80.0
genital organs
acquired (female) (male) Z90.79
female, congenital Q52.8
external Q52.71
internal NEC Q52.8
male, congenital Q55.8
genitourinary organs, congenital NEC
female Q52.8
male Q55.8
globe (acquired) Z90.01
congenital Q11.1

Absence - *continued*
glottis, congenital Q31.8
hand and wrist (acquired) Z89.11
congenital —*see* Agenesis, hand
head, part (acquired) NEC Z90.09
heat sense R20.8
hip (following explanation of hip joint prosthesis) (joint) (with or without presence of antibiotic-impregnated cement spacer) Z89.62
hymen (congenital) Q52.4
ileum (acquired) Z90.49
congenital Q41.2
immunoglobulin, isolated NEC D80.3
IgA D80.2
IgG D80.3
IgM D80.4
incus (acquired) —*see* Loss, ossicles, ear
congenital Q16.3
inner ear, congenital Q16.5
intestine (acquired) (small) Z90.49
congenital Q41.9
specified NEC Q41.8
large Z90.49
congenital Q42.9
specified NEC Q42.8
iris, congenital Q13.1
jejunum (acquired) Z90.49
congenital Q41.1
joint
acquired
hip (following explanation of hip joint prosthesis) (with or without presence of antibiotic-impregnated cement spacer) Z89.62
knee (following explanation of knee joint prosthesis) (with or without presence of antibiotic-impregnated cement spacer) Z89.52
shoulder (following explanation of shoulder joint prosthesis) (with or without presence of antibiotic-impregnated cement spacer) Z89.23
congenital NEC Q74.8
kidney (s) (acquired) Z90.5
congenital Q60.2
bilateral Q60.1
unilateral Q60.0
knee (following explanation of knee joint prosthesis) (joint) (with or without presence of antibiotic-impregnated cement spacer) Z89.52
labyrinth, membranous Q16.5
larynx (congenital) Q31.8
acquired Z90.02
leg (acquired) (above knee) Z89.61
below knee (acquired) Z89.51
congenital —*see* Defect, reduction, lower limb
lens (acquired) —*see also* Aphakia
congenital Q12.3
post cataract extraction Z98.4
limb (acquired) —*see* Absence, extremity
lip Q38.6
liver (congenital) Q44.7
lung (fissure) (lobe) (bilateral) (unilateral) (congenital) Q33.3
acquired (any part) Z90.2
menstruation —*see* Amenorrhea
muscle (congenital) (pectoral) Q79.8
ocular Q10.3
neck, part Q18.8
neutrophil —*see* Agranulocytosis
nipple (s) (with breast(s)) (acquired) Z90.1
congenital Q83.2

Absence - *continued*
  nose (congenital) Q30.1
    acquired Z90.09
  organ
    of Corti, congenital Q16.5
    or site, congenital NEC Q89.8
      acquired NEC Z90.89
  osseous meatus (ear) Q16.4
  ovary (acquired)
    bilateral Z90.722
    congenital
      bilateral Q50.02
      unilateral Q50.01
    unilateral Z90.721
  oviduct (acquired)
    bilateral Z90.722
    congenital Q50.6
    unilateral Z90.721
  pancreas (congenital) Q45.0
    acquired Z90.410
      complete Z90.410
      partial Z90.411
      total Z90.410
  parathyroid gland (acquired) E89.2
    congenital Q89.2
  patella, congenital Q74.1
  penis (congenital) Q55.5
    acquired Z90.79
  pericardium (congenital) Q24.8
  pituitary gland (congenital) Q89.2
    acquired E89.3
  prostate (acquired) Z90.79
    congenital Q55.4
  pulmonary valve Q22.0
  punctum lacrimale (congenital) Q10.4
  radius, congenital —*see* Defect, reduction,
  upper limb, longitudinal, radius
  rectum (congenital) Q42.1
    with fistula Q42.0
    acquired Z90.49
  respiratory organ NOS Q34.9
  rib (acquired) Z90.89
    congenital Q76.6
  sacrum, congenital Q76.49
  salivary gland (s) , congenital Q38.4
  scrotum, congenital Q55.29
  seminal vesicles (congenital) Q55.4
    acquired Z90.79
  septum
    atrial (congenital) Q21.1
    between aorta and pulmonary artery Q21.4
    ventricular (congenital) Q20.4
  sex chromosome
    female phenotype Q97.8
    male phenotype Q98.8
  skull bone (congenital) Q75.8
    with
      anencephaly Q00.0
      encephalocele —*see* Encephalocele
      hydrocephalus Q03.9
        with spina bifida   *see* Spina bifida, by
  site, with hydrocephalus
      microcephaly Q02
  spermatic cord, congenital Q55.4
  spine, congenital Q76.49
  spleen (congenital) Q89.01
    acquired Z90.81
  sternum, congenital Q76.7
  stomach (acquired) (partial) Z90.3
    congenital Q40.2
  superior vena cava, congenital Q26.8
  teeth, tooth (congenital) K00.0
    acquired (complete) K08.109

Absence - *continued*
  class I K08.101
  class II K08.102
  class III K08.103
  class IV K08.104
  due to
    caries K08.139
      class I K08.131
      class II K08.132
      class III K08.133
      class IV K08.134
    periodontal disease K08.129
      class I K08.121
      class II K08.122
      class III K08.123
      class IV K08.124
    specified NEC K08.199
      class I K08.191
      class II K08.192
      class III K08.193
      class IV K08.194
    trauma K08.119
      class I K08.111
      class II K08.112
      class III K08.113
      class IV K08.114
  partial K08.409
    class I K08.401
    class II K08.402
    class III K08.403
    class IV K08.404
    due to
      caries K08.439
        class I K08.431
        class II K08.432
        class III K08.433
        class IV K08.434
      periodontal disease K08.429
        class I K08.421
        class II K08.422
        class III K08.423
        class IV K08.424
      specified NEC K08.499
        class I K08.491
        class II K08.492
        class III K08.493
        class IV K08.494
      trauma K08.419
        class I K08.411
        class II K08.412
        class III K08.413
        class IV K08.414
  tendon (congenital) Q79.8
  testis (congenital) Q55.0
    acquired Z90.79
  thumb (acquired) Z89.01
    congenital —*see* Agenesis, hand
  thymus gland Q89.2
  thyroid (gland) (acquired) E89.0
    cartilage, congenital Q31.8
    congenital E03.1
  toe (s) (acquired) Z89.42
    with foot —*see* Absence, foot and ankle
    congenital —*see* Agenesis, foot
    great Z89.41
  tongue, congenital Q38.3
  trachea (cartilage) , congenital Q32.1
  transverse aortic arch, congenital Q25.4
  tricuspid valve Q22.4
  umbilical artery, congenital Q27.0
  upper arm and forearm with hand present,
  congenital —*see* Agenesis, arm, with hand
  present

Absence - *continued*
  ureter (congenital) Q62.4
    acquired Z90.6
  urethra, congenital Q64.5
  uterus (acquired) Z90.710
    with cervix Z90.710
    with remaining cervical stump Z90.711
    congenital Q51.0
  uvula, congenital Q38.5
  vagina, congenital Q52.0
  vas deferens (congenital) Q55.4
    acquired Z90.79
  vein (peripheral) congenital NEC Q27.8
    cerebral Q28.3
    digestive system Q27.8
    great Q26.8
    lower limb Q27.8
    portal Q26.5
    precerebral Q28.1
    specified site NEC Q27.8
    upper limb Q27.8
  vena cava (inferior) (superior) , congenital
  Q26.8
  ventricular septum Q20.4
  vertebra, congenital Q76.49
  vulva, congenital Q52.71
  wrist (acquired) Z89.12
Absorbent system disease I87.8
Absorption
  carbohydrate, disturbance K90.4
  chemical —*see* Table of Drugs and Chemicals
    through placenta (newborn) P04.9
      environmental substance P04.6
      nutritional substance P04.5
      obstetric anesthetic or analgesic drug P04.0
  drug NEC —*see* Table of Drugs and
  Chemicals
    addictive
      through placenta (newborn) P04.49
        cocaine P04.41
    medicinal
      through placenta (newborn) P04.1
      through placenta (newborn) P04.1
      obstetric anesthetic or analgesic drug P04.0
  fat, disturbance K90.4
    pancreatic K90.3
  noxious substance —*see* Table of Drugs and
  Chemicals
  protein, disturbance K90.4
  starch, disturbance K90.4
  toxic substance —*see* Table of Drugs and
  Chemicals
  uremic —*see* Uremia
Abstinence symptoms, syndrome
  alcohol F10.239
    with delirium F10.231
  cocaine F14.23
  neonatal P96.1
  nicotine —*see* Dependence, drug, nicotine,
  with, withdrawal
  opioid F11.93
    with dependence F11.23
  psychoactive NEC F19.939
    with
      delirium F19.931
      dependence F19.239
        with
          delirium F19.231
          perceptual disturbance F19.232
          uncomplicated F19.230
      perceptual disturbance F19.932
    uncomplicated F19.930

Abstinence symptoms *- continued*
  sedative F13.939
    with
      delirium F13.931
      dependence F13.239
        with
          delirium F13.231
          perceptual disturbance F13.232
        uncomplicated F13.230
      perceptual disturbance F13.932
      uncomplicated F13.930
  stimulant NEC F15.93
    with dependence F15.23
Abulia R68.89
Abulomania F60.7
Abuse
  adult —*see* Maltreatment, adult
  as reason for
    couple seeking advice (including offender)
    Z63.0
  alcohol (non-dependent) F10.10
    with
      anxiety disorder F10.180
      intoxication F10.129
        with delirium F10.121
        uncomplicated F10.120
      mood disorder F10.14
      other specified disorder F10.188
      psychosis F10.159
        delusions F10.150
        hallucinations F10.151
      sexual dysfunction F10.181
      sleep disorder F10.182
      unspecified disorder F10.19
    counseling and surveillance Z71.41
  amphetamine (or related substance) —*see*
  Abuse, drug, stimulant NEC
  analgesics (non-prescribed) (over the counter)
  F55.8
  antacids F55.0
  antidepressants —*see* Abuse, drug,
  psychoactive NEC
  anxiolytic —*see* Abuse, drug, sedative
  barbiturates —*see* Abuse, drug, sedative
  caffeine —*see* Abuse, drug, stimulant NEC
  cannabis, cannabinoids —*see* Abuse, drug,
  cannabis
  child —*see* Maltreatment, child
  cocaine —*see* Abuse, drug, cocaine
  drug NEC (non-dependent) F19.10
    with sleep disorder F19.182
    amphetamine type —*see* Abuse, drug,
    stimulant NEC
    analgesics (non-prescribed) (over the
    counter) F55.8
    antacids F55.0
    antidepressants —*see* Abuse, drug,
    psychoactive NEC
    anxiolytics —*see* Abuse, drug, sedative
    barbiturates —*see* Abuse, drug, sedative
    caffeine —*see* Abuse, drug, stimulant NEC
    cannabis F12.10
      with
        anxiety disorder F12.180
        intoxication F12.129
          with
            delirium F12.121
            perceptual disturbance F12.122
          uncomplicated F12.120
        other specified disorder F12.188
        psychosis F12.159
          delusions F12.150
          hallucinations F12.151

Abuse *- continued*
    unspecified disorder F12.19
  cocaine F14.10
    with
      anxiety disorder F14.180
      intoxication F14.129
        with
          delirium F14.121
          perceptual disturbance F14.122
        uncomplicated F14.120
      mood disorder F14.14
      other specified disorder F14.188
      psychosis F14.159
        delusions F14.150
        hallucinations F14.151
      sexual dysfunction F14.181
      sleep disorder F14.182
      unspecified disorder F14.19
    counseling and surveillance Z71.51
  hallucinogen F16.10
    with
      anxiety disorder F16.180
      flashbacks F16.183
      intoxication F16.129
        with
          delirium F16.121
          perceptual disturbance F16.122
        uncomplicated F16.120
      mood disorder F16.14
      other specified disorder F16.188
      perception disorder, persisting F16.183
      psychosis F16.159
        delusions F16.150
        hallucinations F16.151
      unspecified disorder F16.19
  hashish —*see* Abuse, drug, cannabis
  herbal or folk remedies F55.1
  hormones F55.3
  hypnotics —*see* Abuse, drug, sedative
  inhalant F18.10
    with
      anxiety disorder F18.180
      dementia, persisting F18.17
      intoxication F18.129
        with delirium F18.121
        uncomplicated F18.120
      mood disorder F18.14
      other specified disorder F18.188
      psychosis F18.159
        delusions F18.150
        hallucinations F18.151
      unspecified disorder F18.19
  laxatives F55.2
  LSD —*see* Abuse, drug, hallucinogen
  marihuana —*see* Abuse, drug, cannabis
  morphine type (opioids) —*see* Abuse, drug,
  opioid
  opioid F11.10
    with
      intoxication F11.129
        with
          delirium F11.121
          perceptual disturbance F11.122
        uncomplicated F11.120
      mood disorder F11.14
      other specified disorder F11.188
      psychosis F11.159
        delusions F11.150
        hallucinations F11.151
      sexual dysfunction F11.181
      sleep disorder F11.182
      unspecified disorder F11.19

Abuse *- continued*
  PCP (phencyclidine) (or related substance)
  —*see* Abuse, drug, hallucinogen
  psychoactive NEC F19.10
    with
      amnestic disorder F19.16
      anxiety disorder F19.180
      dementia F19.17
      intoxication F19.129
        with
          delirium F19.121
          perceptual disturbance F19.122
        uncomplicated F19.120
      mood disorder F19.14
      other specified disorder F19.188
      psychosis F19.159
        delusions F19.150
        hallucinations F19.151
      sexual dysfunction F19.181
      sleep disorder F19.182
      unspecified disorder F19.19
  sedative, hypnotic or anxiolytic F13.10
    with
      anxiety disorder F13.180
      intoxication F13.129
        with delirium F13.121
        uncomplicated F13.120
      mood disorder F13.14
      other specified disorder F13.188
      psychosis F13.159
        delusions F13.150
        hallucinations F13.151
      sexual dysfunction F13.181
      sleep disorder F13.182
      unspecified disorder F13.19
  solvent —*see* Abuse, drug, inhalant
  steroids F55.3
  stimulant NEC F15.10
    with
      anxiety disorder F15.180
      intoxication F15.129
        with
          delirium F15.121
          perceptual disturbance F15.122
        uncomplicated F15.120
      mood disorder F15.14
      other specified disorder F15.188
      psychosis F15.159
        delusions F15.150
        hallucinations F15.151
      sexual dysfunction F15.181
      sleep disorder F15.182
      unspecified disorder F15.19
  tranquilizers —*see* Abuse, drug, sedative
  vitamins F55.4
  hallucinogens —*see* Abuse, drug,
  hallucinogen
  hashish —*see* Abuse, drug, cannabis
  herbal or folk remedies F55.1
  hormones F55.3
  hypnotic —*see* Abuse, drug, sedative
  inhalant —*see* Abuse, drug, inhalant
  laxatives F55.2
  LSD —*see* Abuse, drug, hallucinogen
  marihuana —*see* Abuse, drug, cannabis
  morphine type (opioids) —*see* Abuse, drug,
  opioid
  non-psychoactive substance NEC F55.8
    antacids F55.0
    folk remedies F55.1
    herbal remedies F55.1
    hormones F55.3
    laxatives F55.2

Abuse - *continued*
 steroids F55.3
 vitamins F55.4
 opioids —*see* Abuse, drug, opioid
 PCP (phencyclidine) (or related substance) —
 see Abuse, drug, hallucinogen
 physical (adult) (child) —*see* Maltreatment
 psychoactive substance —*see* Abuse, drug,
 psychoactive NEC
 psychological (adult) (child) —*see*
 Maltreatment
 sedative —*see* Abuse, drug, sedative
 sexual —*see* Maltreatment
 solvent —*see* Abuse, drug, inhalant
 steroids F55.3
 vitamins F55.4
Acalculia R48.8
 developmental F81.2
Acanthamebiasis (with) B60.10
 conjunctiva B60.12
 keratoconjunctivitis B60.13
 meningoencephalitis B60.11
 other specified B60.19
Acanthocephaliasis B83.8
Acanthocheilonemiasis B74.4
Acanthocytosis E78.6
Acantholysis L11.9
Acanthosis (acquired) (nigricans) L83
 benign Q82.8
 congenital Q82.8
 seborrheic L82.1
 inflamed L82.0
 tongue K14.3
Acapnia E87.3
Acarbia E87.2
Acardia, acardius Q89.8
Acardiacus amorphus Q89.8
Acardiotrophia I51.4
Acariasis B88.0
 scabies B86
Acarodermatitis (urticarioides) B88.0
Acarophobia F40.218
Acatalasemia, acatalasia E80.3
Acathisia (drug induced) G25.71
Accelerated atrioventricular conduction
 I45.6
Accentuation of personality traits (type A)
 Z73.1
Accessory (congenital)
 adrenal gland Q89.1
 anus Q43.4
 appendix Q43.4
 atrioventricular conduction I45.6
 auditory ossicles Q16.3
 auricle (ear) Q17.0
 biliary duct or passage Q44.5
 bladder Q64.79
 blood vessels NEC Q27.9
 coronary Q24.5
 bone NEC Q79.8
 breast tissue, axilla Q83.1
 carpal bones Q74.0
 cecum Q43.4
 chromosome (s) NEC (nonsex) Q92.9
 with complex rearrangements NEC Q92.5
 seen only at prometaphase Q92.8
 partial Q92.9
 sex
 female phenotype Q97.8
 13 —*see* Trisomy, 13
 18 —*see* Trisomy, 18
 21 —*see* Trisomy, 21

Accessory - *continued*
 coronary artery Q24.5
 cusp (s), heart valve NEC Q24.8
 pulmonary Q22.3
 cystic duct Q44.5
 digit (s) Q69.9
 ear (auricle) (lobe) Q17.0
 endocrine gland NEC Q89.2
 eye muscle Q10.3
 eyelid Q10.3
 face bone (s) Q75.8
 fallopian tube (fimbria) (ostium) Q50.6
 finger (s) Q69.0
 foreskin N47.8
 frontonasal process Q75.8
 gallbladder Q44.1
 genital organ (s)
 female Q52.8
 external Q52.79
 internal NEC Q52.8
 male Q55.8
 genitourinary organs NEC Q89.8
 female Q52.8
 male Q55.8
 hallux Q69.2
 heart Q24.8
 valve NEC Q24.8
 pulmonary Q22.3
 hepatic ducts Q44.5
 hymen Q52.4
 intestine (large) (small) Q43.4
 kidney Q63.0
 lacrimal canal Q10.6
 leaflet, heart valve NEC Q24.8
 ligament, broad Q50.6
 liver Q44.7
 duct Q44.5
 lobule (ear) Q17.0
 lung (lobe) Q33.1
 muscle Q79.8
 navicular of carpus Q74.0
 nervous system, part NEC Q07.8
 nipple Q83.3
 nose Q30.8
 organ or site not listed —*see* Anomaly, by site
 ovary Q50.31
 oviduct Q50.6
 pancreas Q45.3
 parathyroid gland Q89.2
 parotid gland (and duct) Q38.4
 pituitary gland Q89.2
 preauricular appendage Q17.0
 prepuce N47.8
 renal arteries (multiple) Q27.2
 rib Q76.6
 cervical Q76.5
 roots (teeth) K00.2
 salivary gland Q38.4
 sesamoid bones Q74.8
 foot Q74.2
 hand Q74.0
 skin tags Q82.8
 spleen Q89.09
 sternum Q76.7
 submaxillary gland Q38.4
 tarsal bones Q74.2
 teeth, tooth K00.1
 tendon Q79.8
 thumb Q69.1
 thymus gland Q89.2
 thyroid gland Q89.2
 toes Q69.2
 tongue Q38.3

Accessory - *continued*
 tooth, teeth K00.1
 tragus Q17.0
 ureter Q62.5
 urethra Q64.79
 urinary organ or tract NEC Q64.8
 uterus Q51.2
 vagina Q52.10
 valve, heart NEC Q24.8
 pulmonary Q22.3
 vertebra Q76.49
 vocal cords Q31.8
 vulva Q52.79
Accident
 birth —*see* Birth, injury
 cardiac —*see* Infarct, myocardium
 cerebral I63.9
 cerebrovascular (embolic) (ischemic)
 (thrombotic) I63.9
 aborted I63.9
 hemorrhagic —*see* Hemorrhage,
 intracranial, intracerebral
 old (without sequelae) Z86.73
 with sequelae (of) —*see* Sequelae,
 infarction, cerebral
 coronary —*see* Infarct, myocardium
 craniovascular I63.9
 vascular, brain I63.9
Accidental —*see* condition
Accommodation (disorder) —*see also*
 condition
 hysterical paralysis of F44.89
 insufficiency of H52.4
 paresis —*see* Paresis, of accommodation
 spasm —*see* Spasm, of accommodation
Accouchement —*see* Delivery
Accreta placenta O43.21
Accretio cordis (nonrheumatic) I31.0
Accretions, tooth, teeth K03.6
Acculturation difficulty Z60.3
Accumulation secretion, prostate N42.89
Acephalia, acephalism, acephalus, acephaly
 Q00.0
Acephalobrachia monster Q89.8
Acephalochirus monster Q89.8
Acephalogaster Q89.8
Acephalostomus monster Q89.8
Acephalothorax Q89.8
Acerophobia F40.298
Acetonemia R79.89
 in Type 1 diabetes E10.10
 with coma E10.11
Acetonuria R82.4
Achalasia (cardia) (esophagus) K22.0
 congenital Q39.5
 pylorus Q40.0
 sphincteral NEC K59.8
Ache (s) —*see* Pain
Acheilia Q38.6
Achillobursitis —*see* Tendinitis, Achilles
Achillodynia *see* Tendinitis, Achilles
Achlorhydria, achlorhydric (neurogenic)
 K31.83
 anemia D50.8
 diarrhea K31.83
 psychogenic F45.8
 secondary to vagotomy K91.1
Achluophobia F40.228
Acholia K82.8
Acholuric jaundice (familial) (splenomegalic)
 —*see also* Spherocytosis
 acquired D59.8
Achondrogenesis Q77.0

Achondroplasia (osteosclerosis congenita) Q77.4

Achroma, cutis L80

Achromat (ism) , achromatopsia (acquired) (congenital) H53.51

Achromia, congenital —*see* Albinism

Achromia parasitica B36.0

Achylia gastrica K31.89

  psychogenic F45.8

Acid

  burn —*see* Corrosion

  deficiency

    amide nicotinic E52

    ascorbic E54

    folic E53.8

    nicotinic E52

    pantothenic E53.8

  intoxication E87.2

  peptic disease K30

  phosphatase deficiency E83.39

  stomach K30

    psychogenic F45.8

Acidemia E87.2

  argininosuccinic E72.22

  isovaleric E71.110

  metabolic (newborn) P19.9

    first noted before onset of labor P19.0

    first noted during labor P19.1

    noted at birth P19.2

  methylmalonic E71.120

  pipecolic E72.3

  propionic E71.121

Acidity, gastric (high) K30

  psychogenic F45.8

Acidocytopenia —*see* Agranulocytosis

Acidocytosis D72.1

Acidopenia —*see* Agranulocytosis

Acidosis (lactic) (respiratory) E87.2

  in Type 1 diabetes E10.10

    with coma E10.11

  kidney, tubular N25.89

  lactic E87.2

  metabolic NEC E87.2

    with respiratory acidosis E87.4

    late, of newborn P74.0

  mixed metabolic and respiratory, newborn P84

  newborn P84

  renal (hyperchloremic) (tubular) N25.89

  respiratory E87.2

    complicated by

      metabolic

        acidosis E87.4

        alkalosis E87.4

Aciduria

  argininosuccinic E72.22

  glutaric (type I) E72.3

    type II E71.313

    type III E71.5

  orotic (congenital) (hereditary) (pyrimidine deficiency) E79.8

    anemia D53.0

Acladiosis (skin) B36.0

Aclasis, diaphyseal Q78.6

Acleistocardia Q21.1

Aclusion —*see* Anomaly, dentofacial, malocclusion

Acne L70.9

  artificialis L70.8

  atrophica L70.2

  cachecticorum (Hebra) L70.8

  conglobata L70.1

  cystic L70.0

Acne - *continued*

  decalvans L66.2

  excoriée des jeunes filles L70.5

  frontalis L70.2

  indurata L70.0

  infantile L70.4

  keloid L73.0

  lupoid L70.2

  necrotic, necrotica (miliaris) L70.2

  neonatal L70.4

  nodular L70.0

  occupational L70.8

  picker's L70.5

  pustular L70.0

  rodens L70.2

  rosacea L71.9

  specified NEC L70.8

  tropica L70.3

  varioliformis L70.2

  vulgaris L70.0

Acnitis (primary) A18.4

Acosta's disease T70.29

Acoustic —*see* condition

Acousticophobia F40.298

Acquired —*see also* condition

  immunodeficiency syndrome (AIDS) B20

Acrania Q00.0

Acroangiodermatitis I78.9

Acroasphyxia, chronic I73.89

Acrobystitis N47.7

Acrocephalopolysyndactyly Q87.0

Acrocephalosyndactyly Q87.0

Acrocephaly Q75.0

Acrochondrohyperplasia —*see* Syndrome, Marfan's

Acrocyanosis I73.8

  newborn P28.2

    meaning transient blue hands and feet omit code

Acrodermatitis L30.8

  atrophicans (chronica) L90.4

  continua (Hallopeau) L40.2

  enteropathica (hereditary) E83.2

  Hallopeau's L40.2

  infantile papular L44.4

  perstans L40.2

  pustulosa continua L40.2

  recalcitrant pustular L40.2

Acrodynia —*see* Poisoning, mercury

Acromegaly, acromegalia E22.0

Acromelalgia I73.81

Acromicria, acromicria Q79.8

Acronyx L60.0

Acropachy, thyroid —*see* Thyrotoxicosis

Acroparesthesia (simple) (vasomotor) I73.89

Acropathy, thyroid —*see* Thyrotoxicosis

Acrophobia F40.241

Acroposthitis N47.7

Acroscleriasis, acroscleroderma, acrosclerosis —*see* Sclerosis, systemic

Acrosphacelus I96

Acrospiroma, eccrine —*see* Neoplasm, skin, benign

Acrostealgia —*see* Osteochondropathy

Acrotrophodynia —*see* Immersion

ACTH ectopic syndrome E24.3

Actinic —*see* condition

Actinobacillosis, actinobacillus A28.8

  mallei A24.0

  muris A25.1

Actinomyces israelii (infection) —*see* Actinomycosis

Actinomycetoma (foot) B47.1

Actinomycosis, actinomycotic A42.9

  with pneumonia A42.0

  abdominal A42.1

  cervicofacial A42.2

  cutaneous A42.89

  gastrointestinal A42.1

  pulmonary A42.0

  sepsis A42.7

  specified site NEC A42.89

Actinoneuritis G62.82

Action, heart

  disorder I49.9

  irregular I49.9

    psychogenic F45.8

Activated protein C resistance D68.51

Active —*see* condition

Acute —*see also* condition

  abdomen R10.0

  gallbladder —*see* Cholecystitis, acute

Acyanotic heart disease (congenital) Q24.9

Acystia Q64.5

Adair-Dighton syndrome (brittle bones and blue sclera, deafness) Q78.0

Adamantinoblastoma —*see* Ameloblastoma

Adamantinoma —*see also* Cyst, calcifying odontogenic

  long bones C40.90

    lower limb C40.2

    upper limb C40.0

  malignant C41.1

    jaw (bone) (lower) C41.1

      upper C41.0

  tibial C40.2

Adamantoblastoma —*see* Ameloblastoma

Adams-Stokes (-Morgagni) disease or syndrome I45.9

Adaption reaction —*see* Disorder, adjustment

Addiction (see also Dependence) F19.20

  alcohol, alcoholic (ethyl) (methyl) (wood) (without remission) F10.20

    with remission F10.21

  drug —*see* Dependence, drug

  ethyl alcohol (without remission) F10.20

    with remission F10.21

  heroin —*see* Dependence, drug, opioid

  methyl alcohol (without remission) F10.20

    with remission F10.21

  methylated spirit (without remission) F10.20

    with remission F10.21

  morphine (-like substances) —*see* Dependence, drug, opioid

  nicotine —*see* Dependence, drug, nicotine

  opium and opioids —*see* Dependence, drug, opioid

  tobacco —*see* Dependence, drug, nicotine

Addisonian crisis E27.2

Addison's

  anemia (pernicious) D51.0

  disease (bronze) or syndrome E27.1

    tuberculous A18.7

  keloid L94.0

Addison-Biermer anemia (pernicious) D51.0

Addison-Schilder complex E71.528

Additional —*see also* Accessory

  chromosome (s) Q99.8

    sex —*see* Abnormal, chromosome, sex

    21 —*see* Trisomy, 21

Adduction contracture, hip or other joint — *see* Contraction, joint

Adenitis —*see also* Lymphadenitis

  acute, unspecified site L04.9

  axillary I88.9

    acute L04.2

Adenitis *- continued*
  chronic or subacute I88.1
  Bartholin's gland N75.8
  bulbourethral gland —*see* Urethritis
  cervical I88.9
    acute L04.0
    chronic or subacute I88.1
  chancroid (Hemophilus ducreyi) A57
  chronic, unspecified site I88.1
  Cowper's gland —*see* Urethritis
  due to Pasteurella multocida (p. septica)
  A28.0
  epidemic, acute B27.09
  gangrenous L04.9
  gonorrheal NEC A54.89
  groin I88.9
    acute L04.1
    chronic or subacute I88.1
  infectious (acute) (epidemic) B27.09
  inguinal I88.9
    acute L04.1
    chronic or subacute I88.1
  lymph gland or node, except mesenteric I88.9
    acute —*see* Lymphadenitis, acute
    chronic or subacute I88.1
  mesenteric (acute) (chronic) (nonspecific)
  (subacute) I88.0
  parotid gland (suppurative) —*see*
  Sialoadenitis
  salivary gland (any) (suppurative) —*see*
  Sialoadenitis
  scrofulous (tuberculous) A18.2
  Skene's duct or gland —*see* Urethritis
  strumous, tuberculous A18.2
  subacute, unspecified site I88.1
  sublingual gland (suppurative) —*see*
  Sialoadenitis
  submandibular gland (suppurative) —*see*
  Sialoadenitis
  submaxillary gland (suppurative) —*see*
  Sialoadenitis
  tuberculous —*see* Tuberculosis, lymph gland
  urethral gland —*see* Urethritis
  Wharton's duct (suppurative) —*see*
  Sialoadenitis
Adenoacanthoma —*see* Neoplasm, malignant,
  by site
Adenoameloblastoma —*see* Cyst, calcifying
  odontogenic
Adenocarcinoid (tumor) —*see* Neoplasm,
  malignant, by site
Adenocarcinoma —*see also* Neoplasm,
  malignant, by site
  acidophil
    specified site —*see* Neoplasm, malignant,
    by site
    unspecified site C75.1
  adrenal cortical C74.0
  alveolar —*see* Neoplasm, lung, malignant
  apocrine
    breast —*see* Neoplasm, breast, malignant
    in situ
      breast D05.8
      specified site NEC —*see* Neoplasm, skin,
  in situ
      unspecified site D04.9
    specified site NEC —*see* Neoplasm, skin,
  malignant
    unspecified site C44.99
  basal cell
    specified site —*see* Neoplasm, skin,
  malignant
    unspecified site C08.9

Adenocarcinoma *- continued*
  basophil
    specified site —*see* Neoplasm, malignant,
  by site
    unspecified site C75.1
  bile duct type C22.1
    liver C22.1
    specified site NEC —*see* Neoplasm,
  malignant, by site
    unspecified site C22.1
  bronchiolar —*see* Neoplasm, lung, malignant
  bronchioloalveolar —*see* Neoplasm, lung,
  malignant
  ceruminous C44.29
  cervix, in situ (*see also* Carcinoma, cervix
  uteri, in situ) D06.9
  chromophobe
    specified site —*see* Neoplasm, malignant,
  by site
    unspecified site C75.1
  diffuse type
    specified site —*see* Neoplasm, malignant,
  by site
    unspecified site C16.9
  duct
    infiltrating
      with Paget's disease —*see* Neoplasm,
  breast, malignant
      specified site —*see* Neoplasm, malignant,
  by site
      unspecified site (female) C50.91
        male C50.92
    specified site —*see* Neoplasm, malignant,
  by site
    unspecified site
      female C56.9
      male C61
  eosinophil
    specified site —*see* Neoplasm, malignant,
  by site
    unspecified site C75.1
  follicular
    with papillary C73
    moderately differentiated C73
    specified site —*see* Neoplasm, malignant,
  by site
    trabecular C73
    unspecified site C73
    well differentiated C73
  Hürthle cell C73
  in
    adenomatous
      polyposis coli C18.9
  infiltrating duct
    with Paget's disease —*see* Neoplasm, breast,
  malignant
    specified site —*see* Neoplasm, by site,
  malignant
    unspecified site (female) C50.91
      male C50.92
  inflammatory
    specified site —*see* Neoplasm, by site,
  malignant
    unspecified site (female) C50.91
      male C50.92
  intestinal type
    specified site —*see* Neoplasm, by site,
  malignant
    unspecified site C16.9
  intracystic papillary
  intraductal
    breast D05.1
    noninfiltrating

Adenocarcinoma *- continued*
  breast D05.1
  papillary
    with invasion
      specified site —*see* Neoplasm, by site,
  malignant
      unspecified site (female) C50.91
        male C50.92
    breast D05.1
    specified site NEC —*see* Neoplasm, in
  situ, by site
    unspecified site D05.1
    specified site NEC —*see* Neoplasm, in
  situ, by site
    unspecified site D05.1
  papillary
    with invasion
      specified site —*see* Neoplasm, malignant,
  by site
      unspecified site (female) C50.91
        male C50.92
    breast D05.1
    specified site —*see* Neoplasm, in situ, by
  site
    unspecified site D05.1
    specified site NEC —*see* Neoplasm, in situ,
  by site
    unspecified site D05.1
  islet cell
    with exocrine, mixed
      specified site —*see* Neoplasm, malignant,
  by site
      unspecified site C25.9
    pancreas C25.4
    specified site NEC —*see* Neoplasm,
  malignant, by site
    unspecified site C25.4
  lobular
    in situ
      breast D05.0
      specified site NEC —*see* Neoplasm, in
  situ, by site
      unspecified site D05.0
    specified site —*see* Neoplasm, malignant,
  by site
    unspecified site (female) C50.91
      male C50.92
  mucoid —*see also* Neoplasm, malignant, by
  site
    cell
      specified site —*see* Neoplasm, malignant,
  by site
      unspecified site C75.1
  nonencapsulated sclerosing C73
  papillary
    with follicular C73
    follicular variant C73
    intraductal (noninfiltrating)
      with invasion
        specified site —*see* Neoplasm, malignant,
  by site
        unspecified site (female) C50.91
          male C50.92
      breast D05.1
      specified site NEC —*see* Neoplasm, in
  situ, by site
      unspecified site D05.1
    serous
      specified site —*see* Neoplasm, malignant,
  by site
      unspecified site C56.9

Adenocarcinoma - *continued*
  papillocystic
    specified site —*see* Neoplasm, malignant, by site
    unspecified site C56.9
  pseudomucinous
    specified site —*see* Neoplasm, malignant, by site
    unspecified site C56.9
  renal cell C64
  sebaceous —*see* Neoplasm, skin, malignant
  serous —*see also* Neoplasm, malignant, by site
    papillary
      specified site —*see* Neoplasm, malignant, by site
      unspecified site C56.9
  sweat gland —*see* Neoplasm, skin, malignant
  water-clear cell C75.0
Adenocarcinoma-in-situ —*see also* Neoplasm, in situ, by site
  breast D05.9
Adenofibroma
  clear cell —*see* Neoplasm, benign, by site
  endometrioid D27.9
    borderline malignancy D39.10
    malignant C56
  mucinous
    specified site —*see* Neoplasm, benign, by site
    unspecified site D27.9
  papillary
    specified site —*see* Neoplasm, benign, by site
    unspecified site D27.9
  prostate —*see* Enlargement, enlarged, prostate
  serous
    specified site —*see* Neoplasm, benign, by site
    unspecified site D27.9
  specified site —*see* Neoplasm, benign, by site
  unspecified site D27.9
Adenofibrosis
  breast —*see* Fibroadenosis, breast
  endometrioid N80.0
Adenoiditis (chronic) J35.02
  with tonsillitis J35.03
  acute J03.90
    recurrent J03.91
    specified organism NEC J03.80
      recurrent J03.81
    staphylococcal J03.80
      recurrent J03.81
    streptococcal J03.00
      recurrent J03.01
Adenoids —*see* condition
Adenolipoma —*see* Neoplasm, benign, by site
Adenolipomatosis, Launois-Bensaude E88.89
Adenolymphoma
  specified site —*see* Neoplasm, benign, by site
  unspecified site D11.9
Adenoma —*see also* Neoplasm, benign, by site
  acidophil
    specified site —*see* Neoplasm, benign, by site
    unspecified site D35.2
  acidophil-basophil, mixed
    specified site —*see* Neoplasm, benign, by site
    unspecified site D35.2

Adenoma - *continued*
  adrenal (cortical) D35.00
    clear cell D35.00
    compact cell D35.00
    glomerulosa cell D35.00
    heavily pigmented variant D35.00
    mixed cell D35.00
  alpha-cell
    pancreas D13.7
    specified site NEC —*see* Neoplasm, benign, by site
    unspecified site D13.7
  alveolar D14.30
  apocrine
    breast D24
    specified site NEC —*see* Neoplasm, skin, benign, by site
    unspecified site D23.9
  basal cell D11.9
  basophil
    specified site —*see* Neoplasm, benign, by site
    unspecified site D35.2
  basophil-acidophil, mixed
    specified site —*see* Neoplasm, benign, by site
    unspecified site D35.2
  beta-cell
    pancreas D13.7
    specified site NEC —*see* Neoplasm, benign, by site
    unspecified site D13.7
  bile duct D13.4
    common D13.5
    extrahepatic D13.5
    intrahepatic D13.4
    specified site NEC —*see* Neoplasm, benign, by site
    unspecified site D13.4
  black D35.00
  bronchial D38.1
    cylindroid type —*see* Neoplasm, lung, malignant
  ceruminous D23.2
  chief cell D35.1
  chromophobe
    specified site —*see* Neoplasm, benign, by site
    unspecified site D35.2
  colloid
    specified site —*see* Neoplasm, benign, by site
    unspecified site D34
  duct
  eccrine, papillary —*see* Neoplasm, skin, benign
  endocrine, multiple
    single specified site —*see* Neoplasm, uncertain behavior, by site
    two or more specified sites D44
    unspecified site D44.9
  endometrioid —*see also* Neoplasm, benign
    borderline malignancy —*see* Neoplasm, uncertain behavior, by site
  eosinophil
    specified site —*see* Neoplasm, benign, by site
    unspecified site D35.2
  fetal
    specified site —*see* Neoplasm, benign, by site
    unspecified site D34

Adenoma - *continued*
  follicular
    specified site —*see* Neoplasm, benign, by site
    unspecified site D34
  hepatocellular D13.4
  Hürthle cell D34
  islet cell
    pancreas D13.7
    specified site NEC —*see* Neoplasm, benign, by site
    unspecified site D13.7
  liver cell D13.4
  macrofollicular
    specified site —*see* Neoplasm, benign, by site
    unspecified site D34
  malignant, malignum —*see* Neoplasm, malignant, by site
  microcystic
    pancreas D13.7
    specified site NEC —*see* Neoplasm, benign, by site
    unspecified site D13.7
  microfollicular
    specified site —*see* Neoplasm, benign, by site
    unspecified site D34
  mucoid cell
    specified site —*see* Neoplasm, benign, by site
    unspecified site D35.2
  multiple endocrine
    single specified site —*see* Neoplasm, uncertain behavior, by site
    two or more specified sites D44
    unspecified site D44.9
  nipple D24
  papillary —*see also* Neoplasm, benign, by site
    eccrine —*see* Neoplasm, skin, benign, by site
  Pick's tubular
    specified site —*see* Neoplasm, benign, by site
    unspecified site
      female D27.9
      male D29.20
  pleomorphic
    carcinoma in —*see* Neoplasm, salivary gland, malignant
      specified site —*see* Neoplasm, malignant, by site
      unspecified site C08.9
  polypoid —*see also* Neoplasm, benign
    adenocarcinoma in —*see* Neoplasm, malignant, by site
    adenocarcinoma in situ —*see* Neoplasm, in situ, by site
  prostate —*see* Neoplasm, benign, prostate
  rete cell D29.20
  sebaceous —*see* Neoplasm, skin, benign
  Sertoli cell
    specified site —*see* Neoplasm, benign, by site
    unspecified site
      female D27.9
      male D29.20
  skin appendage —*see* Neoplasm, skin, benign
  sudoriferous gland —*see* Neoplasm, skin, benign
  sweat gland —*see* Neoplasm, skin, benign

Adenoma - *continued*
testicular
  specified site —*see* Neoplasm, benign, by
  site
    unspecified site
      female D27.9
      male D29.20
tubular —*see also* Neoplasm, benign, by site
  adenocarcinoma in —*see* Neoplasm,
  malignant, by site
  adenocarcinoma in situ —*see* Neoplasm, in
  situ, by site
  Pick's
    specified site —*see* Neoplasm, benign, by
    site
      unspecified site
        female D27.9
        male D29.20
tubulovillous —*see also* Neoplasm, benign,
by site
  adenocarcinoma in —*see* Neoplasm,
  malignant, by site
  adenocarcinoma in situ —*see* Neoplasm, in
  situ, by site
  villous —*see* Neoplasm, uncertain behavior,
  by site
  adenocarcinoma in —*see* Neoplasm,
  malignant, by site
  adenocarcinoma in situ —*see* Neoplasm, in
  situ, by site
water-clear cell D35.1
Adenomatosis
endocrine (multiple) E31.20
  single specified site —*see* Neoplasm,
  uncertain behavior, by site
erosive of nipple D24
pluriendocrine —*see* Adenomatosis,
endocrine
pulmonary D38.1
  malignant —*see* Neoplasm, lung, malignant
specified site —*see* Neoplasm, benign, by site
unspecified site D12.6
Adenomatous
goiter (nontoxic) E04.9
  with hyperthyroidism —*see*
Hyperthyroidism, with, goiter, nodular
  toxic —*see* Hyperthyroidism, with, goiter,
  nodular
Adenomyoma —*see also* Neoplasm, benign,
by site
prostate —*see* Enlarged, prostate
Adenomyometritis N80.0
Adenomyosis N80.0
Adenopathy (lymph gland) R59.9
generalized R59.1
inguinal R59.0
localized R59.0
mediastinal R59.0
mesentery R59.0
syphilitic (secondary) A51.49
tracheobronchial R59.0
  tuberculous A15.4
    primary (progressive) A15.7
tuberculous —*see also* Tuberculosis, lymph
gland
  tracheobronchial A15.4
    primary (progressive) A15.7
Adenosalpingitis —*see* Salpingitis
Adenosarcoma —*see* Neoplasm, malignant,
by site
Adenosclerosis I88.8

Adenosis (sclerosing) **breast** —*see*
Fibroadenosis, breast
**Adenovirus, as cause of disease classified
elsewhere** B97.0
Adentia (complete) (partial) —*see* Absence,
teeth
Adherent —*see also* Adhesions
labia (minora) N90.89
pericardium (nonrheumatic) I31.0
  rheumatic I09.2
placenta (with hemorrhage) O72.0
  without hemorrhage O73.0
prepuce, newborn N47.0
scar (skin) L90.5
tendon in scar L90.5
Adhesions, adhesive (postinfective) K66.0
with intestinal obstruction K56.5
abdominal (wall) —*see* Adhesions,
peritoneum
appendix K38.8
bile duct (common) (hepatic) K83.8
bladder (sphincter) N32.89
bowel —*see* Adhesions, peritoneum
cardiac I31.0
  rheumatic I09.2
cecum —*see* Adhesions, peritoneum
cervicovaginal N88.1
  congenital Q52.8
  postpartal O90.89
  old N88.1
cervix N88.1
ciliary body NEC —*see* Adhesions, iris
clitoris N90.89
colon —*see* Adhesions, peritoneum
common duct K83.8
congenital —*see also* Anomaly, by site
  fingers —*see* Syndactylism, complex,
  fingers
  omental, anomalous Q43.3
  peritoneal Q43.3
  tongue (to gum or roof of mouth) Q38.3
conjunctiva (acquired) H11.21
  congenital Q15.8
cystic duct K82.8
diaphragm —*see* Adhesions, peritoneum
due to foreign body —*see* Foreign body
duodenum —*see* Adhesions, peritoneum
ear
  middle H74.1
epididymis N50.8
epidural —*see* Adhesions, meninges
epiglottis J38.7
eyelid H02.59
female pelvis N73.6
gallbladder K82.8
globe H44.89
heart I31.0
  rheumatic I09.2
ileocecal (coil) —*see* Adhesions, peritoneum
ileum —*see* Adhesions, peritoneum
intestine —*see also* Adhesions, peritoneum
  with obstruction K56.5
intra-abdominal —*see* Adhesions, peritoneum
iris H21.50
  anterior H21.51
  goniosynechiae H21.52
  posterior H21.54
  to corneal graft T85.89
joint —*see* Ankylosis
  knee M23.8X
  temporomandibular M26.61
labium (majus) (minus) , congenital Q52.5
liver —*see* Adhesions, peritoneum

Adhesions, adhesive - *continued*
lung J98.4
mediastinum J98.5
meninges (cerebral) (spinal) G96.12
  congenital Q07.8
  tuberculous (cerebral) (spinal) A17.0
mesenteric —*see* Adhesions, peritoneum
nasal (septum) (to turbinates) J34.89
ocular muscle —*see* Strabismus, mechanical
omentum —*see* Adhesions, peritoneum
ovary N73.6
  congenital (to cecum, kidney or omentum)
  Q50.39
paraovarian N73.6
pelvic (peritoneal)
  female N73.6
    postprocedural N99.4
  male —*see* Adhesions, peritoneum
  postpartal (old) N73.6
  tuberculous A18.17
penis to scrotum (congenital) Q55.8
periappendiceal —*see also* Adhesions,
peritoneum
pericardium (nonrheumatic) I31.0
  focal I31.8
  rheumatic I09.2
  tuberculous A18.84
pericholecystic K82.8
perigastric —*see* Adhesions, peritoneum
periovarian N73.6
periprostatic N42.89
perirectal —*see* Adhesions, peritoneum
perirenal N28.89
peritoneum, peritoneal (postinfective)
(postprocedural) K66.0
  with obstruction (intestinal) K56.5
  congenital Q43.3
  pelvic, female N73.6
    postprocedural N99.4
  postpartal, pelvic N73.6
  to uterus N73.6
peritubal N73.6
periureteral N28.89
periuterine N73.6
perivesical N32.89
perivesicular (seminal vesicle) N50.8
pleura, pleuritic J94.8
  tuberculous NEC A15.6
pleuropericardial J94.8
postoperative (gastrointestinal tract) K66.0
  with obstruction K91.3
  due to foreign body accidentally left in
wound —*see* Foreign body, accidentally left
during a procedure
  pelvic peritoneal N99.4
  urethra —*see* Stricture, urethra,
postprocedural
  vagina N99.2
postpartal, old (vulva or perineum) N90.89
preputial, prepuce N47.5
pulmonary J98.4
pylorus —*see* Adhesions, peritoneum
sciatic nerve —*see* Lesion, nerve, sciatic
seminal vesicle N50.8
shoulder (joint) —*see* Capsulitis, adhesive
sigmoid flexure —*see* Adhesions, peritoneum
spermatic cord (acquired) N50.8
  congenital Q55.4
spinal canal G96.12
stomach —*see* Adhesions, peritoneum
subscapular —*see* Capsulitis, adhesive
temporomandibular M26.61

Adhesions, adhesive - *continued*
tendinitis —*see also* Tenosynovitis, specified type NEC
  shoulder —*see* Capsulitis, adhesive
testis N44.8
tongue, congenital (to gum or roof of mouth) Q38.3
  acquired K14.8
trachea J39.8
tubo-ovarian N73.6
tunica vaginalis N44.8
uterus N73.6
  internal N85.6
  to abdominal wall N73.6
vagina (chronic) N89.5
  postoperative N99.2
vitreomacular H43.82
vitreous H43.89
vulva N90.89
Adiaspiromycosis B48.8
Adie (-Holmes) **pupil or syndrome** —*see* Anomaly, pupil, function, tonic pupil
Adiponecrosis neonatorum P83.8
Adiposis —*see also* Obesity
cerebralis E23.6
dolorosa E88.2
Adiposity —*see also* Obesity
heart —*see* Degeneration, myocardial
localized E65
Adiposogenital dystrophy E23.6
Adjustment
disorder —*see* Disorder, adjustment
implanted device —*see* Encounter (for), adjustment (of)
prosthesis, external —*see* Fitting
reaction —*see* Disorder, adjustment
Administration of tPA (rtPA) **in a different facility within the last 24 hours prior to admission to current facility** Z92.82
Admission (for) —*see also* Encounter (for)
adjustment (of)
  artificial
    arm Z44.00
      complete Z44.01
      partial Z44.02
    eye Z44.2
    leg Z44.10
      complete Z44.11
      partial Z44.12
  brain neuropacemaker Z46.2
    implanted Z45.42
  breast
    implant Z45.81
    prosthesis (external) Z44.3
  colostomy belt Z46.89
  contact lenses Z46.0
  cystostomy device Z46.6
  dental prosthesis Z46.3
  device NEC
    abdominal Z46.89
    implanted Z45.89
      cardiac Z45.09
        defibrillator (with synchronous cardiac pacemaker) Z45.02
        pacemaker Z45.018
          pulse generator Z45.010
      hearing device Z45.328
        bone conduction Z45.320
        cochlear Z45.321
      infusion pump Z45.1
      nervous system Z45.49
        CSF drainage Z45.41

Admission (for) - *continued*
  hearing device —*see* Admission, adjustment, device, implanted, hearing device
    neuropacemaker Z45.42
      visual substitution Z45.31
    specified NEC Z45.89
    vascular access Z45.2
    visual substitution Z45.31
    nervous system Z46.2
      implanted —*see* Admission, adjustment, device, implanted, nervous system
    orthodontic Z46.4
    prosthetic Z44.9
      arm —*see* Admission, adjustment, artificial, arm
      breast Z44.3
      dental Z46.3
      eye Z44.2
      leg —*see* Admission, adjustment, artificial, leg
      specified type NEC Z44.8
    substitution
      auditory Z46.2
        implanted —*see* Admission, adjustment, device, implanted, hearing device
      nervous system Z46.2
        implanted —*see* Admission, adjustment, device, implanted, nervous system
      visual Z46.2
        implanted Z45.31
      urinary Z46.6
    hearing aid Z46.1
      implanted —*see* Admission, adjustment, device, implanted, hearing device
    ileostomy device Z46.89
    intestinal appliance or device NEC Z46.89
    neuropacemaker (brain) (peripheral nerve) (spinal cord) Z46.2
      implanted Z45.42
    orthodontic device Z46.4
    orthopedic (brace) (cast) (device) (shoes) Z46.89
    pacemaker
      cardiac Z45.018
        pulse generator Z45.010
      nervous system Z46.2
        implanted Z45.42
    portacath (port-a-cath) Z45.2
    prosthesis Z44.9
      arm —*see* Admission, adjustment, artificial, arm
      breast Z44.3
      dental Z46.3
      eye Z44.2
      leg —*see* Admission, adjustment, artificial, leg
      specified NEC Z44.8
    spectacles Z46.0
  aftercare (*see also* Aftercare) Z51.89
    postpartum
      immediately after delivery Z39.0
      routine follow-up Z39.2
    radiation therapy (antineoplastic) Z51.0
  attention to artificial opening (of) Z43.9
    artificial vagina Z43.7
    colostomy Z43.3
    cystostomy Z43.5
    enterostomy Z43.4
    gastrostomy Z43.1
    ileostomy Z43.2
    jejunostomy Z43.4
    nephrostomy Z43.6

Admission (for) - *continued*
    specified site NEC Z43.8
    intestinal tract Z43.4
    urinary tract Z43.6
    tracheostomy Z43.0
    ureterostomy Z43.6
    urethrostomy Z43.6
  breast augmentation or reduction Z41.1
  breast reconstruction following mastectomy Z42.1
  change of
    dressing (nonsurgical) Z48.00
    neuropacemaker device (brain) (peripheral nerve) (spinal cord) Z46.2
      implanted Z45.42
    surgical dressing Z48.01
  circumcision, ritual or routine (in absence of diagnosis) Z41.2
  clinical research investigation (control) (normal comparison) (participant) Z00.6
  contraceptive management Z30.9
  cosmetic surgery NEC Z41.1
  counseling —*see also* Counseling
    dietary Z71.3
    HIV Z71.7
    human immunodeficiency virus Z71.7
    nonattending third party Z71.0
    procreative management NEC Z31.69
  delivery, full-term, uncomplicated O80
    cesarean, without indication O82
  dietary surveillance and counseling Z71.3
  ear piercing Z41.3
  examination at health care facility (adult) (*see also* Examination) Z00.00
    with abnormal findings Z00.01
    clinical research investigation (control) (normal comparison) (participant) Z00.6
    dental Z01.20
      with abnormal findings Z01.21
    donor (potential) Z00.5
    ear Z01.10
      with abnormal findings NEC Z01.118
    eye Z01.00
      with abnormal findings Z01.01
    general, specified reason NEC Z00.8
    hearing Z01.10
      with abnormal findings NEC Z01.118
    postpartum checkup Z39.2
    psychiatric (general) Z00.8
      requested by authority Z04.6
    vision Z01.00
      with abnormal findings Z01.01
  fitting (of)
    artificial
      arm —*see* Admission, adjustment, artificial, arm
      eye Z44.2
      leg —*see* Admission, adjustment, artificial, leg
    brain neuropacemaker Z46.2
      implanted Z45.42
    breast prosthesis (external) Z44.3
    colostomy belt Z46.89
    contact lenses Z46.0
    cystostomy device Z46.6
    dental prosthesis Z46.3
    dentures Z46.3
    device NEC
      abdominal Z46.89
      nervous system Z46.2
        implanted —*see* Admission, adjustment, device, implanted, nervous system

Admission (for) - *continued*
    orthodontic Z46.4
    prosthetic Z44.9
        breast Z44.3
        dental Z46.3
        eye Z44.2
        substitution
            auditory Z46.2
                implanted —*see* Admission, adjustment, device, implanted, hearing device
            nervous system Z46.2
                implanted —*see* Admission, adjustment, device, implanted, nervous system
            visual Z46.2
                implanted Z45.31
        hearing aid Z46.1
        ileostomy device Z46.89
        intestinal appliance or device NEC Z46.89
        neuropacemaker (brain) (peripheral nerve) (spinal cord) Z46.2
            implanted Z45.42
        orthodontic device Z46.4
        orthopedic device (brace) (cast) (shoes) Z46.89
        prosthesis Z44.9
            arm —*see* Admission, adjustment, artificial, arm
            breast Z44.3
            dental Z46.3
            eye Z44.2
            leg —*see* Admission, adjustment, artificial, leg
            specified type NEC Z44.8
        spectacles Z46.0
    follow-up examination Z09
    intrauterine device management Z30.431
        initial prescription Z30.014
    mental health evaluation Z00.8
        requested by authority Z04.6
    observation —*see* Observation
    Papanicolaou smear, cervix Z12.4
        for suspected malignant neoplasm Z12.4
    plastic and reconstructive surgery following medical procedure or healed injury NEC Z42.8
    plastic surgery, cosmetic NEC Z41.1
    postpartum observation
        immediately after delivery Z39.0
        routine follow-up Z39.2
    poststerilization (for restoration) Z31.0
        aftercare Z31.42
    procreative management Z31.9
    prophylactic (measure)
        organ removal Z40.00
            breast Z40.01
            ovary Z40.02
            specified organ NEC Z40.09
            testes Z40.09
        vaccination Z23
    psychiatric examination (general) Z00.8
        requested by authority Z04.6
    radiation therapy (antineoplastic) Z51.0
    reconstructive surgery following medical procedure or healed injury NEC Z42.8
    removal of
        cystostomy catheter Z43.5
        drains Z48.03
        dressing (nonsurgical) Z48.00
        intrauterine contraceptive device Z30.432
        neuropacemaker (brain) (peripheral nerve) (spinal cord) Z46.2
            implanted Z45.42

Admission (for) - *continued*
        staples Z48.02
        surgical dressing Z48.01
        sutures Z48.02
        ureteral stent Z46.6
    respirator -ventilator] use during power failure Z99.12
    restoration of organ continuity (poststerilization) Z31.0
        aftercare Z31.42
    sensitivity test —*see also* Test, skin
        allergy NEC Z01.82
        Mantoux Z11.1
    tuboplasty following previous sterilization Z31.0
        aftercare Z31.42
    vasoplasty following previous sterilization Z31.0
        aftercare Z31.42
    vision examination Z01.00
        with abnormal findings Z01.01
    waiting period for admission to other facility Z75.1
Adnexitis (suppurative) —*see* Salpingo-oophoritis
Adolescent X-linked adrenoleukodystrophy E71.521
Adrenal (gland) —*see* condition
Adrenalism, tuberculous A18.7
Adrenalitis, adrenitis E27.8
    autoimmune E27.1
    meningococcal, hemorrhagic A39.1
Adrenarche, premature E27.0
Adrenocortical syndrome —*see* Cushing's, syndrome
Adrenogenital syndrome E25.9
    acquired E25.8
    congenital E25.0
    salt loss E25.0
Adrenogenitalism, congenital E25.0
Adrenoleukodystrophy E71.529
    neonatal E71.511
    X-linked E71.529
        Addison only phenotype E71.528
        Addison-Schilder E71.528
        adolescent E71.521
        adrenomyeloneuropathy E71.522
        childhood cerebral E71.520
        other specified E71.528
Adrenomyeloneuropathy E71.522
Adventitious bursa —*see* Bursopathy, specified type NEC
Adverse effect —*see* Table of Drugs and Chemicals, categories T36-T50, with 6th character 5
Advice —*see* Counseling
Adynamia (episodica) (hereditary) (periodic) G72.3
Aeration lung imperfect, newborn —*see* Atelectasis
Aerobullosis T70.3
Aerocele —*see* Embolism, air
Aerodermectasia
    subcutaneous (traumatic) T79.7
Aerodontalgia T70.29
Aeroembolism T70.3
Aerogenes capsulatus infection A48.0
Aero-otitis media T70.0
Aerophagy, aerophagia (psychogenic) F45.8
Aerophobia F40.228
Aerosinusitis T70.1
Aerotitis T70.0

Affection —*see* Disease
Afibrinogenemia (*see also* Defect, coagulation) D68.8
    acquired D65
    congenital D68.2
    following ectopic or molar pregnancy O08.1
    in abortion —*see* Abortion, by type, complicated by, afibrinogenemia
    puerperal O72.3
African
    sleeping sickness B56.9
    tick fever A68.1
    trypanosomiasis B56.9
        Gambian B56.0
        Rhodesian B56.1
Aftercare (*see also* Care) Z51.89
    following surgery (for) (on)
        amputation Z47.81
        attention to
            drains Z48.03
            dressings (nonsurgical) Z48.00
                surgical Z48.01
            sutures Z48.02
        circulatory system Z48.812
        delayed (planned) wound closure Z48.1
        digestive system Z48.815
        explantation of joint prosthesis (staged procedure)
            hip Z47.32
            knee Z47.33
            shoulder Z47.31
        genitourinary system Z48.816
        joint replacement Z47.1
        neoplasm Z48.3
        nervous system Z48.811
        oral cavity Z48.814
        organ transplant
            bone marrow Z48.290
            heart Z48.21
            heart-lung Z48.280
            kidney Z48.22
            liver Z48.23
            lung Z48.24
            multiple organs NEC Z48.288
            specified NEC Z48.298
        orthopedic NEC Z47.89
        planned wound closure Z48.1
        removal of internal fixation device Z47.2
        respiratory system Z48.813
        scoliosis Z47.82
        sense organs Z48.810
        skin and subcutaneous tissue Z48.817
        specified body system
            circulatory Z48.812
            digestive Z48.815
            genitourinary Z48.816
            nervous Z48.811
            oral cavity Z48.814
            respiratory Z48.813
            sense organs Z48.810
            skin and subcutaneous tissue Z48.817
            teeth Z48.814
            specified NEC Z48.89
        spinal Z48.89
        teeth Z48.814
    fracture
    code to fracture with seventh character D
    involving
        removal of
            drains Z48.03
            dressings (nonsurgical) Z48.00
            staples Z48.02

Aftercare - *continued*
surgical dressings Z48.01
sutures Z48.02
neuropacemaker (brain) (peripheral nerve) (spinal cord) Z46.2
implanted Z45.42
orthopedic NEC Z47.89
postprocedural —*see* Aftercare, following surgery
After-cataract —*see* Cataract, secondary
Agalactia (primary) O92.3
elective, secondary or therapeutic O92.5
Agammaglobulinemia (acquired (secondary)) (nonfamilial) D80.1
with
immunoglobulin-bearing B-lymphocytes D80.1
lymphopenia D81.9
autosomal recessive (Swiss type) D80.0
Bruton's X-linked D80.0
common variable (CVA gamma) D80.1
congenital sex-linked D80.0
hereditary D80.0
lymphopenic D81.9
Swiss type (autosomal recessive) D80.0
X-linked (with growth hormone deficiency) (Bruton) D80.0
Aganglionosis (bowel) (colon) Q43.1
Age (old) —*see* Senility
Agenesis
adrenal (gland) Q89.1
alimentary tract (complete) (partial) NEC Q45.8
upper Q40.8
anus, anal (canal) Q42.3
with fistula Q42.2
aorta Q25.4
appendix Q42.8
arm (complete) Q71.0
with hand present Q71.1
artery (peripheral) Q27.9
brain Q28.3
coronary Q24.5
pulmonary Q25.79
specified NEC Q27.8
umbilical Q27.0
auditory (canal) (external) Q16.1
auricle (ear) Q16.0
bile duct or passage Q44.5
bladder Q64.5
bone Q79.9
brain Q00.0
part of Q04.3
breast (with nipple present) Q83.8
with absent nipple Q83.0
bronchus Q32.4
canaliculus lacrimalis Q10.4
carpus —*see* Agenesis, hand
cartilage Q79.9
cecum Q42.8
cerebellum Q04.3
cervix Q51.5
chin Q18.8
cilia Q10.3
circulatory system, part NOS Q28.9
clavicle Q74.0
clitoris Q52.6
coccyx Q76.49
colon Q42.9
specified NEC Q42.8
corpus callosum Q04.0
cricoid cartilage Q31.8

Agenesis - *continued*
diaphragm (with hernia) Q79.1
digestive organ (s) or tract (complete) (partial) NEC Q45.8
upper Q40.8
ductus arteriosus Q28.8
duodenum Q41.0
ear Q16.9
auricle Q16.0
lobe Q17.8
ejaculatory duct Q55.4
endocrine (gland) NEC Q89.2
epiglottis Q31.8
esophagus Q39.8
eustachian tube Q16.2
eye Q11.1
adnexa Q15.8
eyelid (fold) Q10.3
face
bones NEC Q75.8
specified part NEC Q18.8
fallopian tube Q50.6
femur —*see* Defect, reduction, lower limb, longitudinal, femur
fibula —*see* Defect, reduction, lower limb, longitudinal, fibula
finger (complete) (partial) —*see* Agenesis, hand
foot (and toes) (complete) (partial) Q72.3
forearm (with hand present) —*see* Agenesis, arm, with hand present
and hand Q71.2
gallbladder Q44.0
gastric Q40.2
genitalia, genital (organ(s))
female Q52.8
external Q52.71
internal NEC Q52.8
male Q55.8
glottis Q31.8
hair Q84.0
hand (and fingers) (complete) (partial) Q71.3
heart Q24.8
valve NEC Q24.8
pulmonary Q22.0
hepatic Q44.7
humerus —*see* Defect, reduction, upper limb
hymen Q52.4
ileum Q41.2
incus Q16.3
intestine (small) Q41.9
large Q42.9
specified NEC Q42.8
iris (dilator fibers) Q13.1
jaw M26.09
jejunum Q41.1
kidney (s) (partial) Q60.2
bilateral Q60.1
unilateral Q60.0
labium (majus) (minus) Q52.71
labyrinth, membranous Q16.5
lacrimal apparatus Q10.4
larynx Q31.8
leg (complete) Q72.0
with foot present Q72.1
lower leg (with foot present) —*see* Agenesis, leg, with foot present
and foot Q72.2
lens Q12.3
limb (complete) Q73.0
lower —*see* Agenesis, leg
upper —*see* Agenesis, arm

Agenesis - *continued*
lip Q38.0
liver Q44.7
lung (fissure) (lobe) (bilateral) (unilateral) Q33.3
mandible, maxilla M26.09
metacarpus —*see* Agenesis, hand
metatarsus —*see* Agenesis, foot
muscle Q79.8
eyelid Q10.3
ocular Q15.8
musculoskeletal system NEC Q79.8
nail (s) Q84.3
neck, part Q18.8
nerve Q07.8
nervous system, part NEC Q07.8
nipple Q83.2
nose Q30.1
nuclear Q07.8
organ
of Corti Q16.5
or site not listed —*see* Anomaly, by site
osseous meatus (ear) Q16.1
ovary
bilateral Q50.02
unilateral Q50.01
oviduct Q50.6
pancreas Q45.0
parathyroid (gland) Q89.2
parotid gland (s) Q38.4
patella Q74.1
pelvic girdle (complete) (partial) Q74.2
penis Q55.5
pericardium Q24.8
pituitary (gland) Q89.2
prostate Q55.4
punctum lacrimale Q10.4
radioulnar —*see* Defect, reduction, upper limb
radius —*see* Defect, reduction, upper limb, longitudinal, radius
rectum Q42.1
with fistula Q42.0
renal Q60.2
bilateral Q60.1
unilateral Q60.0
respiratory organ NEC Q34.8
rib Q76.6
roof of orbit Q75.8
round ligament Q52.8
sacrum Q76.49
salivary gland Q38.4
scapula Q74.0
scrotum Q55.29
seminal vesicles Q55.4
septum
atrial Q21.1
between aorta and pulmonary artery Q21.4
ventricular Q20.4
shoulder girdle (complete) (partial) Q74.0
skull (bone) Q75.8
with
anencephaly Q00.0
encephalocele —*see* Encephalocele
hydrocephalus Q03.9
with spina bifida —*see* Spina bifida, by site, with hydrocephalus
microcephaly Q02
spermatic cord Q55.4
spinal cord Q06.0
spine Q76.49
spleen Q89.01

Agenesis - *continued*
  sternum Q76.7
  stomach Q40.2
  submaxillary gland (s) (congenital) Q38.4
  tarsus —*see* Agenesis, foot
  tendon Q79.8
  testicle Q55.0
  thymus (gland) Q89.2
  thyroid (gland) E03.1
    cartilage Q31.8
  tibia —*see* Defect, reduction, lower limb, longitudinal, tibia
  tibiofibular —*see* Defect, reduction, lower limb, specified type NEC
  toe (and foot) (complete) (partial) —*see* Agenesis, foot
  tongue Q38.3
  trachea (cartilage) Q32.1
  ulna —*see* Defect, reduction, upper limb, longitudinal, ulna
  upper limb —*see* Agenesis, arm
  ureter Q62.4
  urethra Q64.5
  urinary tract NEC Q64.8
  uterus Q51.0
  uvula Q38.5
  vagina Q52.0
  vas deferens Q55.4
  vein (s) (peripheral) Q27.9
    brain Q28.3
    great NEC Q26.8
    portal Q26.5
  vena cava (inferior) (superior) Q26.8
  vermis of cerebellum Q04.3
  vertebra Q76.49
  vulva Q52.71
Ageusia R43.2
Agitated —*see* condition
Agitation R45.1
Aglossia (congenital) Q38.3
Aglossia-adactylia syndrome Q87.0
Aglycogenosis E74.00
Agnosia (body image) (other senses) (tactile) R48.1
  developmental F88
  verbal R48.1
    auditory R48.1
      developmental F80.2
    developmental F80.2
  visual (object) R48.3
Agoraphobia F40.00
  with panic disorder F40.01
  without panic disorder F40.02
Agrammatism R48.8
Agranulocytopenia — *see* Agranulocytosis
Agranulocytosis (chronic) (cyclical) (genetic) (infantile) (periodic) (pernicious) (*see also* Neutropenia) D70.9
  congenital D70.0
  cytoreductive cancer chemotherapy sequela D70.1
  drug-induced D70.2
    due to cytoreductive cancer chemotherapy D70.1
  due to infection D70.3
  secondary D70.4
    drug-induced D70.2
      due to cytoreductive cancer chemotherapy D70.1
Agraphia (absolute) R48.8
  with alexia R48.0
  developmental F81.81

Ague (dumb) —*see* Malaria
Agyria Q04.3
Ahumada-del Castillo syndrome E23.0
Aichmophobia F40.298
AIDS (related complex) B20
Ailment heart —*see* Disease, heart
Ailurophobia F40.218
Ainhum (disease) L94.6
AIPHI (acute idiopathic pulmonary hemorrhage in infants (over 28 days old)) R04.81
Air
  anterior mediastinum J98.2
  compressed, disease T70.3
  conditioner lung or pneumonitis J67.7
  embolism (artery) (cerebral) (any site) T79.0
    with ectopic or molar pregnancy O08.2
    due to implanted device NEC —*see* Complications, by site and type, specified NEC
    following
      abortion —*see* Abortion by type, complicated by, embolism
      ectopic or molar pregnancy O08.2
    infusion, therapeutic injection or transfusion T80.0
    in pregnancy, childbirth or puerperium — *see* Embolism, obstetric
    traumatic T79.0
  hunger, psychogenic F45.8
  rarefied, effects of *see* Effect, adverse, high altitude
  sickness T75.3
Airplane sickness T75.3
Akathisia (drug-induced) (treatment-induced) G25.71
  neuroleptic induced (acute) G25.71
Akinesia R29.898
Akinetic mutism R41.89
Akureyri's disease G93.3
Alactasia, congenital E73.0
Alagille's syndrome Q44.7
Alastrim B03
Albers-Schönberg syndrome Q78.2
Albert's syndrome —*see* Tendinitis, Achilles
Albinism, albino E70.30
  with hematologic abnormality E70.339
    Chédiak-Higashi syndrome E70.330
    Hermansky-Pudlak syndrome E70.331
    other specified E70.338
  I E70.320
  II E70.321
  ocular E70.319
    autosomal recessive E70.311
    other specified E70.318
    X-linked E70.310
  oculocutaneous E70.329
    other specified E70.328
    tyrosinase (ty) negative E70.320
    tyrosinase (ty) positive E70.321
  other specified E70.39
Albinismus E70.30
Albright (-McCune) (-Sternberg) syndrome Q78.1
Albuminous —*see* condition
Albuminuria, albuminuric (acute) (chronic) (subacute) (*see also* Proteinuria) R80.9
  complicating pregnancy —*see* Proteinuria, gestational
    with
      gestational hypertension —*see* Pre-eclampsia

Albuminuria, albuminuric - *continued*
  pre-existing hypertension —*see* Hypertension, complicating pregnancy, pre-existing, with, pre-eclampsia
  gestational —*see* Proteinuria, gestational
    with
      gestational hypertension —*see* Pre-eclampsia
      pre-existing hypertension —*see* Hypertension, complicating pregnancy, pre-existing, with, pre-eclampsia
  orthostatic R80.2
  postural R80.2
  pre-eclamptic —*see* Pre-eclampsia
  scarlatinal A38.8
Albuminurophobia F40.298
Alcaptonuria E70.29
Alcohol, alcoholic, alcohol-induced
  addiction (without remission) F10.20
    with remission F10.21
  amnestic disorder, persisting F10.96
    with dependence F10.26
  brain syndrome, chronic F10.97
    with dependence F10.27
  cardiopathy I42.6
  counseling and surveillance Z71.41
    family member Z71.42
  delirium (acute) (tremens) (withdrawal) F10.231
    with intoxication F10.921
    in
      abuse F10.121
      dependence F10.221
  dementia F10.97
    with dependence F10.27
  deterioration F10.97
    with dependence F10.27
  hallucinosis (acute) F10.951
    in
      abuse F10.151
      dependence F10.251
  insanity F10.959
  intoxication (acute) (without dependence) F10.129
    with
      delirium F10.121
      dependence F10.229
        with delirium F10.221
      uncomplicated F10.220
    uncomplicated F10.120
  jealousy F10.988
  Korsakoff's, Korsakov's, Korsakov's F10.26
  liver K70.9
    acute —*see* Disease, liver, alcoholic, hepatitis
  mania (acute) (chronic) F10.959
  paranoia, paranoid (type) psychosis F10.950
  pellagra E52
  poisoning, accidental (acute) NEC —*see* Table of Drugs and Chemicals, alcohol, poisoning
  psychosis —*see* Psychosis, alcoholic
  withdrawal (without convulsions) F10.239
    with delirium F10.231
  with
    psychosis —*see* Psychosis, alcoholic
    remission F10.21
  Korsakov's F10.96
    with dependence F10.26
Alder (-Reilly) anomaly or syndrome (leukocyte granulation) D72.0

Aldosteronism E26.9
  familial (type I) E26.02
  glucocorticoid-remediable E26.02
  primary (due to (bilateral) adrenal
    hyperplasia) E26.09
  primary NEC E26.09
  secondary E26.1
  specified NEC E26.89
Aldosteronoma D44.10
Aldrich (-Wiskott) syndrome (eczema-
  thrombocytopenia) D82.0
Alektorophobia F40.218
Aleppo boil B55.1
Aleukemic —*see* condition
Aleukia
  congenital D70.0
  hemorrhagica D61.9
    congenital D61.09
  splenica D73.1
Alexia R48.0
  developmental F81.0
  secondary to organic lesion R48.0
Algoneurodystrophy M89.00
  ankle M89.07
  foot M89.07
  forearm M89.03
  hand M89.04
  lower leg M89.06
  multiple sites M89.0
  shoulder M89.01
  specified site NEC M89.08
  thigh M89.05
  upper arm M89.02
Algophobia F40.298
Alienation, mental —*see* Psychosis
Alkalemia E87.3
Alkalosis E87.3
  metabolic E87.3
    with respiratory acidosis E87.4
  respiratory E87.3
Alkaptonuria E70.29
Allen-Masters syndrome N83.8
Allergy, allergic (reaction) (to) T78.40
  air-borne substance NEC (rhinitis) J30.89
  alveolitis (extrinsic) J67.9
    due to
      Aspergillus clavatus J67.4
      Cryptostroma corticale J67.6
      organisms (fungal, thermophilic
    actinomycete) growing in ventilation (air
    conditioning) systems J67.7
      specified type NEC J67.8
  anaphylactic reaction or shock T78.2
  angioneurotic edema T78.3
  animal (dander) (epidermal) (hair) (rhinitis)
    J30.81
  bee sting (anaphylactic shock) —*see* Toxicity,
    venom, arthropod, bee
  biological —*see* Allergy, drug
  colitis K52.2
  dander (animal) (rhinitis) J30.81
  dandruff (rhinitis) J30.81
  dental restorative material (existing) K08.55
  dermatitis —*see* Dermatitis, contact, allergic
  diathesis —*see* History, allergy
  drug, medicament & biological (any)
    (external) (internal) T78.40
    correct substance properly administered —
  see Table of Drugs and Chemicals, by drug,
    adverse effect
    wrong substance given or taken NEC (by
  accident) —*see* Table of Drugs and
  Chemicals, by drug, poisoning

Allergy, allergic - *continued*
  due to pollen J30.1
  dust (house) (stock) (rhinitis) J30.89
    with asthma —*see* Asthma, allergic extrinsic
  eczema —*see* Dermatitis, contact, allergic
  epidermal (animal) (rhinitis) J30.81
  feathers (rhinitis) J30.89
  food (any) (ingested) NEC T78.1
    anaphylactic shock —*see* Shock,
  anaphylactic, due to food
    dermatitis —*see* Dermatitis, due to, food
    dietary counseling and surveillance Z71.3
    in contact with skin L23.6
    rhinitis J30.5
    status (without reaction) Z91.018
      eggs Z91.012
      milk products Z91.011
      peanuts Z91.010
      seafood Z91.013
      specified NEC Z91.018
  gastrointestinal K52.2
  grain J30.1
  grass (hay fever) (pollen) J30.1
    asthma —*see* Asthma, allergic extrinsic
  hair (animal) (rhinitis) J30.81
  history (of) —*see* History, allergy
  horse serum —*see* Allergy, serum
  inhalant (rhinitis) J30.89
    pollen J30.1
  kapok (rhinitis) J30.89
  medicine —*see* Allergy, drug
  milk protein K52.2
  nasal, seasonal due to pollen J30.1
  pneumonia J82
  pollen (any) (hay fever) J30.1
    asthma —*see* Asthma, allergic extrinsic
  primrose J30.1
  primula J30.1
  purpura D69.0
  ragweed (hay fever) (pollen) J30.1
    asthma —*see* Asthma, allergic extrinsic
  rose (pollen) J30.1
  seasonal NEC J30.2
  Senecio jacobae (pollen) J30.1
  serum (*see also* Reaction, serum) T80.69
    anaphylactic shock T80.59
  shock (anaphylactic) T78.2
    due to
      administration of blood and blood products
    T80.51
      adverse effect of correct medicinal
    substance properly administered T88.6
        immunization T80.52
        serum NEC T80.59
        vaccination T80.52
    specific NEC T78.49
  tree (any) (hay fever) (pollen) J30.1
    asthma —*see* Asthma, allergic extrinsic
  upper respiratory J30.9
  urticaria L50.0
  vaccine —*see* Allergy, serum
  wheat —*see* Allergy, food
Allescheriasis B48.2
Alligator skin disease Q80.9
Allocheiria, allochiria R20.8
Almeida's disease —*see*
  Paracoccidioidomycosis
Alopecia (hereditaria) (seborrheica) L65.9
  androgenic L64.9
    drug-induced L64.0
    specified NEC L64.8
  areata L63.9

Alopecia - *continued*
  ophiasis L63.2
  specified NEC L63.8
  totalis L63.0
  universalis L63.1
  cicatricial L66.9
    specified NEC L66.8
  circumscripta L63.9
  congenital, congenitalis Q84.0
  due to cytotoxic drugs NEC L65.8
  mucinosa L65.2
  postinfective NEC L65.8
  postpartum L65.0
  premature L64.8
  specific (syphilitic) A51.32
  specified NEC L65.8
  syphilitic (secondary) A51.32
  totalis (capitis) L63.0
  universalis (entire body) L63.1
  X-ray L58.1
Alpers' disease G31.81
Alpine sickness T70.29
Alport syndrome Q87.81
ALTE (apparent life threatening event) in
  newborn and infant R68.13
Alteration (of) , **Altered**
  awareness, transient R40.4
  mental status R41.82
  pattern of family relationships affecting child
    Z62.898
  sensation
    following
      cerebrovascular disease I69.998
        cerebral infarction I69.398
        intracerebral hemorrhage I69.198
        nontraumatic intracranial hemorrhage
      NEC I69.298
          specified disease NEC I69.898
          subarachnoid hemorrhage I69.098
Alternating —*see* condition
Altitude, high (effects) —*see* Effect, adverse,
  high altitude
Aluminosis (of lung) J63.0
Alveolitis
  allergic (extrinsic) —*see* Pneumonitis,
  hypersensitivity
  due to
    Aspergillus clavatus J67.4
    Cryptostroma corticale J67.6
  fibrosing (cryptogenic) (idiopathic) J84.112
  jaw M27.3
  sicca dolorosa M27.3
Alveolus, alveolar —*see* condition
Alymphocytosis D72.810
  thymic (with immunodeficiency) D82.1
Alymphoplasia, thymic D82.1
Alzheimer's disease or sclerosis —*see*
  Disease, Alzheimer's
Amastia (with nipple present) Q83.8
  with absent nipple Q83.0
Amathophobia F40.228
Amaurosis (acquired) (congenital) —*see also*
  Blindness
  fugax G45.3
  hysterical F44.6
  Leber's congenital H35.50
  uremic —*see* Uremia
Amaurotic idiocy (infantile) (juvenile) (late)
  E75.4
Amaxophobia F40.248
Ambiguous genitalia Q56.4
Amblyopia (congenital) (ex anopsia) (partial)
  (suppression) H53.00

Amblyopia - *continued*
anisometropic —*see* Amblyopia, refractive
deprivation H53.01
hysterical F44.6
nocturnal —*see also* Blindness, night
   vitamin A deficiency E50.5
refractive H53.02
strabismic H53.03
tobacco H53.8
toxic NEC H53.8
uremic —*see* Uremia
Ameba, amebic (histolytica) —*see also*
Amebiasis
abscess (liver) A06.4
Amebiasis A06.9
with abscess —*see* Abscess, amebic
acute A06.0
chronic (intestine) A06.1
   with abscess —*see* Abscess, amebic
cutaneous A06.7
cutis A06.7
cystitis A06.81
genitourinary tract NEC A06.82
hepatic —*see* Abscess, liver, amebic
intestine A06.0
nondysenteric colitis A06.2
skin A06.7
specified site NEC A06.89
Ameboma (of intestine) A06.3
Amelia Q73.0
lower limb —*see* Agenesis, leg
upper limb —*see* Agenesis, arm
Ameloblastoma —*see also* Cyst, calcifying
odontogenic
long bones C40.9
   lower limb C40.2
   upper limb C40.0
malignant C41.1
   jaw (bone) (lower) C41.1
      upper C41.0
tibial C40.2
Amelogenesis imperfecta K00.5
nonhereditaria (segmentalis) K00.4
Amenorrhea N91.2
hyperhormonal E28.8
primary N91.0
secondary N91.1
Amentia —*see* Disability, intellectual
Meynert's (nonalcoholic) F04
American
leishmaniasis B55.2
mountain tick fever A93.2
Ametropia —*see* Disorder, refraction
Amianthosis J61
Amimia R48.8
Amino-acid disorder E72.9
anemia D53.0
Aminoacidopathy E72.9
Aminoaciduria E72.9
Amnes (t) ic syndrome (post-traumatic) F04
induced by
   alcohol F10.96
      with dependence F10.26
   psychoactive NEC F19.96
      with
         abuse F19.16
         dependence F19.26
   sedative F13.96
      with dependence F13.26
Amnesia R41.3
anterograde R41.1
auditory R48.8

Amnesia - *continued*
dissociative F44.0
hysterical F44.0
postictal in epilepsy —*see* Epilepsy
psychogenic F44.0
retrograde R41.2
transient global G45.4
Amnion, amniotic —*see* condition
Amnionitis —*see* Pregnancy, complicated by
Amok F68.8
Amoral traits F60.89
Ampulla
lower esophagus K22.8
phrenic K22.8
Amputation —*see also* Absence, by site,
acquired
neuroma (postoperative) (traumatic) —*see*
Complications, amputation stump, neuroma
stump (surgical)
   abnormal, painful, or with complication
(late) —*see* Complications, amputation stump
   healed or old NOS Z89.9
traumatic (complete) (partial)
   arm (upper) (complete) S48.91
      at
         elbow S58.01
           partial S58.02
         shoulder joint (complete) S48.01
           partial S48.02
      between
         elbow and wrist (complete) S58.11
           partial S58.12
         shoulder and elbow (complete) S48.11
           partial S48.12
      partial S48.92
   breast (complete) S28.21
      partial S28.22
   clitoris (complete) S38.211
      partial S38.212
   ear (complete) S08.11
      partial S08.12
   finger (complete) (metacarpophalangeal)
S68.11
      index S68.11
      little S68.11
      middle S68.11
      partial S68.12
         index S68.12
         little S68.12
         middle S68.12
         ring S68.12
      ring S68.11
      thumb —*see* Amputation, traumatic, thumb
      transphalangeal (complete) S68.61
         index S68.61
         little S68.61
         middle S68.61
         partial S68.62
           index S68.62
           little S68.62
           middle S68.62
           ring S68.62
         ring S68.61
   foot (complete) S98.91
      at ankle level S98.01
      partial S98.02
      midfoot S98.31
         partial S98.32
      partial S98.92
   forearm (complete) S58.91
      at elbow level (complete) S58.01
      partial S58.02

Amputation - *continued*
between elbow and wrist (complete)
S58.11
   partial S58.12
   partial S58.92
genital organ (s) (external)
   female (complete) S38.211
      partial S38.212
   male
      penis (complete) S38.221
         partial S38.222
      scrotum (complete) S38.231
         partial S38.232
      testes (complete) S38.231
         partial S38.232
hand (complete) (wrist level) S68.41
   finger (s) alone —*see* Amputation,
traumatic, finger
   partial S68.42
   thumb alone —*see* Amputation, traumatic,
thumb
   transmetacarpal (complete) S68.71
      partial S68.72
head
   ear —*see* Amputation, traumatic, ear
   nose (partial) S08.812
      complete S08.811
   part S08.89
      scalp S08.0
hip (and thigh) (complete) S78.91
   at hip joint (complete) S78.01
      partial S78.02
   between hip and knee (complete) S78.11
      partial S78.12
      partial S78.92
labium (majus) (minus) (complete) S38.21
   partial S38.21
leg (lower) S88.91
   at knee level S88.01
      partial S88.02
   between knee and ankle S88.11
      partial S88.12
      partial S88.92
nose (partial) S08.812
   complete S08.811
penis (complete) S38.221
   partial S38.222
scrotum (complete) S38.231
   partial S38.232
shoulder —*see* Amputation, traumatic, arm
   at shoulder joint —*see* Amputation,
traumatic, arm, at shoulder joint
testes (complete) S38.231
   partial S38.232
thigh —*see* Amputation, traumatic, hip
thorax, part of S28.1
   breast —*see* Amputation, traumatic, breast
thumb (complete) (metacarpophalangeal)
S68.01
   partial S68.02
   transphalangeal (complete) S68.51
      partial S68.52
toe (lesser) S98.13
   great S98.11
      partial S98.12
   more than one S98.21
      partial S98.22
      partial S98.14
vulva (complete) S38.211
   partial S38.212
Amputee (bilateral) (old) Z89.9
Amsterdam dwarfism Q87.1

Amusia R48.8
  developmental F80.89
Amyelencephalus, amyelencephaly Q00.0
Amyelia Q06.0
Amygdalitis —*see* Tonsillitis
Amygdalolith J35.8
Amyloid heart (disease) E85.4 *[I43]*
Amyloidosis (generalized) (primary) E85.9
  with lung involvement E85.4 *[J99]*
  familial E85.2
  genetic E85.2
  heart E85.4 *[I43]*
  hemodialysis-associated E85.3
  liver E85.4 *[K77]*
  localized E85.4
  neuropathic heredofamilial E85.1
  non-neuropathic heredofamilial E85.0
  organ limited E85.4
  Portuguese E85.1
  pulmonary E85.4 *[J99]*
  secondary systemic E85.3
  skin (lichen) (macular) E85.4 *[L99]*
  specified NEC E85.8
  subglottic E85.4 *[J99]*
Amylopectinosis (brancher enzyme deficiency)
    E74.03
Amylophagia —*see* Pica
Amyoplasia congenita Q79.8
Amyotonia M62.89
  congenita G70.2
Amyotrophia, amyotrophy, amyotrophic
    G71.8
  congenita Q79.8
  diabetic —*see* Diabetes, amyotrophy
  lateral sclerosis G12.21
  neuralgic G54.5
  spinal progressive G12.21
Anacidity, gastric K31.83
  psychogenic F45.8
Anaerosis of newborn P28.89
Analbuminemia E88.09
Analgesia —*see* Anesthesia
Analphalipoproteinemia E78.6
Anaphylactic
  purpura D69.0
  shock or reaction —*see* Shock, anaphylactic
Anaphylactoid shock or reaction —*see*
    Shock, anaphylactic
Anaphylactoid syndrome of pregnancy
    O88.01
Anaphylaxis —*see* Shock, anaphylactic
Anaplasia cervix (*see also* Dysplasia, cervix)
    N87.9
Anaplasmosis, human A77.49
Anarthria R47.1
Anasarca R60.1
  cardiac —*see* Failure, heart, congestive
  lung J18.2
  newborn P83.2
  nutritional E43
  pulmonary J18.2
  renal N04.9
Anastomosis
  aneurysmal —*see* Aneurysm
  arteriovenous ruptured brain I60.8
  intestinal K63.89
    complicated NEC K91.89
      involving urinary tract N99.89
  retinal and choroidal vessels (congenital)
    Q14.8
Anatomical narrow angle H40.03

Ancylostoma, ancylostomiasis (braziliense)
    (caninum) (ceylanicum) (duodenale) B76.0
    Necator americanus B76.1
Andersen's disease (glycogen storage) E74.09
Anderson-Fabry disease E75.21
Andes disease T70.29
Andrews' disease (bacterid) L08.89
Androblastoma
  benign
    specified site —*see* Neoplasm, benign, by
    site
    unspecified site
      female D27.9
      male D29.20
  malignant
    specified site —*see* Neoplasm, malignant,
    by site
    unspecified site
      female C56.9
      male C62.90
  specified site —*see* Neoplasm, uncertain
  behavior, by site
  tubular
    with lipid storage
      specified site —*see* Neoplasm, benign, by
      site
      unspecified site
        female D27.9
        male D29.20
    specified site —*see* Neoplasm, benign, by
    site
    unspecified site
      female D27.9
      male D29.20
    unspecified site
      female D39.10
      male D40.10
Androgen insensitivity syndrome (*see also*
    Syndrome, androgen insensitivity) E34.50
Androgen resistance syndrome (*see also*
    Syndrome, androgen insensitivity) E34.50
Android pelvis Q74.2
  with disproportion (fetopelvic) O33.3
    causing obstructed labor O65.3
Androphobia F40.290
Anectasis, pulmonary (newborn) —*see*
    Atelectasis
Anemia (essential) (general) (hemoglobin
    deficiency) (infantile) (primary) (profound)
    D64.9
  with (due to) (in)
    disorder of
      anaerobic glycolysis D55.2
      pentose phosphate pathway D55.1
    koilonychia D50.9
  achlorhydric D50.8
  achrestic D53.1
  Addison (-Biermer) (pernicious) D51.0
  agranulocytic —*see* Agranulocytosis
  amino-acid-deficiency D53.0
  aplastic D61.9
    congenital D61.09
    drug-induced D61.1
    due to
      drugs D61.1
      external agents NEC D61.2
      infection D61.2
      radiation D61.2
    idiopathic D61.3
    red cell (pure) D60.9
      chronic D60.0
      congenital D61.01

Anemia - *continued*
  specified type NEC D60.8
    transient D60.1
  specified type NEC D61.89
    toxic D61.2
  aregenerative
    congenital D61.09
  asiderotic D50.9
  atypical (primary) D64.9
  Baghdad spring D55.0
  Balantidium coli A07.0
  Biermer's (pernicious) D51.0
  blood loss (chronic) D50.0
    acute D62
  bothriocephalus B70.0 *[D63.8]*
  brickmaker's B76.9 *[D63.8]*
  cerebral I67.89
  childhood D58.9
  chlorotic D50.8
  chronic
    blood loss D50.0
    hemolytic D58.9
      idiopathic D59.9
    simple D53.9
  chronica congenita aregenerativa D61.09
  combined system disease NEC D51.0 *[G32.0]*
    due to dietary vitamin B12 deficiency D51.3
    [G32.0]
  complicating pregnancy, childbirth or
    puerperium —*see* Pregnancy, complicated by
    (management affected by), anemia
  congenital P61.4
    aplastic D61.09
    due to isoimmunization NOS P55.9
    dyserythropoietic, dyshematopoietic D64.4
    following fetal blood loss P61.3
    Heinz body D58.2
    hereditary hemolytic NOS D58.9
    pernicious D51.0
    spherocytic D58.0
  Cooley's (erythroblastic) D56.1
  cytogenic D51.0
  deficiency D53.9
    2, 3 diphosphoglycerate mutase D55.2
    2, 3 PG D55.2
    6 phosphogluconate dehydrogenase D55.1
    6-PGD D55.1
    amino-acid D53.0
    combined B12 and folate D53.1
    enzyme D55.9
      drug-induced (hemolytic) D59.2
      glucose 6-phosphate dehydrogenase
      (G6PD) D55.0
      glycolytic D55.2
      nucleotide metabolism D55.3
      related to hexose monophosphate (HMP)
  shunt pathway NEC D55.1
      specified type NEC D55.8
    erythrocytic glutathione D55.1
    folate D52.9
      dietary D52.0
      drug-induced D52.1
    folic acid D52.9
      dietary D52.0
      drug-induced D52.1
    G SH D55.1
    GGS-R D55.1
    glucose 6-phosphate dehydrogenase D55.0
    glutathione reductase D55.1
    glyceraldehyde phosphate dehydrogenase
    D55.2
    G6PD D55.0
    hexokinase D55.2

Anemia - *continued*
iron D50.9
  secondary to blood loss (chronic) D50.0
nutritional D53.9
  with
    poor iron absorption D50.8
    specified deficiency NEC D53.8
phosphofructo-aldolase D55.2
phosphoglycerate kinase D55.2
PK D55.2
protein D53.0
pyruvate kinase D55.2
transcobalamin II D51.2
triose-phosphate isomerase D55.2
vitamin B12 NOS D51.9
  dietary D51.3
  due to
    intrinsic factor deficiency D51.0
    selective vitamin B12 malabsorption with
proteinuria D51.1
  pernicious D51.0
  specified type NEC D51.8
Diamond-Blackfan (congenital hypoplastic)
D61.01
Dibothriocephalus B70.0 *[D63.8]*
dimorphic D53.1
diphasic D53.1
Diphyllobothrium (Dibothriocephalus) B70.0
[D63.8]
due to (in) (with)
  antineoplastic chemotherapy D64.81
  blood loss (chronic) D50.0
    acute D62
  chemotherapy, antineoplastic D64.81
  chronic disease classified elsewhere NEC
D63.8
  chronic kidney disease D63.1
  deficiency
    amino-acid D53.0
    copper D53.8
    folate (folic acid) D52.9
      dietary D52.0
      drug-induced D52.1
    molybdenum D53.8
    protein D53.0
    zinc D53.8
  dietary vitamin B12 deficiency D51.3
  disorder of
    glutathione metabolism D55.1
    nucleotide metabolism D55.3
  drug —*see* Anemia, by type —*see also*
Table of Drugs and Chemicals
  end stage renal disease D63.1
  enzyme disorder D55.9
  fetal blood loss P61.3
  fish tapeworm (D. Latum) infestation B70.0
[D63.8]
  hemorrhage (chronic) D50.0
    acute D62
  impaired absorption D50.9
  loss of blood (chronic) D50.0
    acute D62
  myxedema E03.9 *[D63.8]*
  Necator americanus B76.1 *[D63.8]*
  prematurity P61.2
  selective vitamin B12 malabsorption with
proteinuria D51.1
  transcobalamin II deficiency D51.2
Dyke-Young type (secondary) (symptomatic)
D59.1
dyserythropoietic (congenital) D64.4
dyshematopoietic (congenital) D64.4

Anemia - *continued*
Egyptian B76.9 *[D63.8]*
elliptocytosis —*see* Elliptocytosis
enzyme-deficiency, drug-induced D59.2
epidemic (*see also* Ancylostomiasis) B76.9
[D63.8]
erythroblastic
  familial D56.1
  newborn (*see also* Disease, hemolytic) P55.9
  of childhood D56.1
erythrocytic glutathione deficiency D55.1
erythropoietin-resistant anemia (EPO resistant
anemia) D63.1
Faber's (achlorhydric anemia) D50.9
factitious (self-induced bloodletting) D50.0
familial erythroblastic D56.1
Fanconi's (congenital pancytopenia) D61.09
favism D55.0
fish tapeworm (D. latum) infestation B70.0
[D63.8]
folate (folic acid) deficiency D52.9
glucose 6-phosphate dehydrogenase (G6PD)
deficiency D55.0
glutathione-reductase deficiency D55.1
goat's milk D52.0
granulocytic —*see* Agranulocytosis
Heinz body, congenital D58.2
hemolytic D58.9
  acquired D59.9
    with hemoglobinuria NEC D59.6
    autoimmune NEC D59.1
    infectious D59.4
    specified type NEC D59.8
    toxic D59.4
  acute D59.9
    due to enzyme deficiency specified type
NEC D55.8
    Lederer's D59.1
  autoimmune D59.1
    drug-induced D59.0
  chronic D58.9
    idiopathic D59.9
  cold type (secondary) (symptomatic) D59.1
  congenital (spherocytic) —*see*
Spherocytosis
  due to
    cardiac conditions D59.4
    drugs (nonautoimmune) D59.2
      autoimmune D59.0
    enzyme disorder D55.9
      drug-induced D59.2
    presence of shunt or other internal
prosthetic device D59.4
  familial D58.9
  hereditary D58.9
    due to enzyme disorder D55.9
      specified type NEC D55.8
    specified type NEC D58.8
  idiopathic (chronic) D59.9
  mechanical D59.4
  microangiopathic D59.4
  nonautoimmune D59.4
    drug-induced D59.2
  nonspherocytic
    congenital or hereditary NEC D55.8
    glucose 6-phosphate dehydrogenase
deficiency D55.0
    pyruvate kinase deficiency D55.2
    type
      I D55.1
      II D55.2

Anemia - *continued*
type
  I D55.1
  II D55.2
secondary D59.4
  autoimmune D59.1
specified (hereditary) type NEC D58.8
Stransky-Regala type (*see also*
Hemoglobinopathy) D58.8
symptomatic D59.4
  autoimmune D59.1
  toxic D59.4
  warm type (secondary) (symptomatic) D59.1
hemorrhagic (chronic) D50.0
  acute D62
Herrick's D57.1
hexokinase deficiency D55.2
hookworm B76.9 *[D63.8]*
hypochromic (idiopathic) (microcytic)
(normoblastic) D50.9
  due to blood loss (chronic) D50.0
    acute D62
  familial sex-linked D64.0
  pyridoxine-responsive D64.3
  sideroblastic, sex-linked D64.0
hypoplasia, red blood cells D61.9
  congenital or familial D61.01
hypoplastic (idiopathic) D61.9
  congenital or familial (of childhood) D61.01
hypoproliferative (refractive) D61.9
idiopathic D64.9
  aplastic D61.3
  hemolytic, chronic D59.9
in (due to) (with)
  chronic kidney disease D63.1
  end stage renal disease D63.1
  failure, kidney (renal) D63.1
  neoplastic disease (*see also* Neoplasm)
D63.0
intertropical (*see also* Ancylostomiasis)
D63.8
iron deficiency D50.9
  secondary to blood loss (chronic) D50.0
    acute D62
  specified type NEC D50.8
Joseph-Diamond-Blackfan (congenital
hypoplastic) D61.01
Lederer's (hemolytic) D59.1
leukoerythroblastic D61.82
macrocytic D53.9
  nutritional D52.0
  tropical D52.8
malarial (*see also* Malaria) B54 *[D63.8]*
malignant (progressive) D51.0
malnutrition D53.9
marsh (*see also* Malaria) B54 *[D63.8]*
Mediterranean (with other hemoglobinopathy)
D56.9
megaloblastic D53.1
  combined B12 and folate deficiency D53.1
  hereditary D51.1
  nutritional D52.0
  orotic aciduria D53.0
  refractory D53.1
  specified type NEC D53.1
megalocytic D53.1
microcytic (hypochromic) D50.9
  due to blood loss (chronic) D50.0
    acute D62
  familial D56.8
microdrepanocytosis D57.40
microelliptopoikilocytic (Rietti-Greppi
Micheli) D56.9

Anemia - *continued*
  miner's B76.9 *[D63.8]*
  myelodysplastic D46.9
  myelofibrosis D75.81
  myelogenous D64.89
  myelopathic D64.89
  myelophthisic D61.82
  myeloproliferative D47.Z9
  newborn P61.4
    due to
      ABO (antibodies, isoimmunization, maternal/fetal incompatibility) P55.1
      Rh (antibodies, isoimmunization, maternal/fetal incompatibility) P55.0
    following fetal blood loss P61.3
    posthemorrhagic (fetal) P61.3
  nonspherocytic hemolytic —*see* Anemia, hemolytic, nonspherocytic
  normocytic (infectional) D64.9
    due to blood loss (chronic) D50.0
      acute D62
    myelophthisic D61.82
  nutritional (deficiency) D53.9
    with
      poor iron absorption D50.8
      specified deficiency NEC D53.8
    megaloblastic D52.0
  of prematurity P61.2
  orotaciduric (congenital) (hereditary) D53.0
  osteosclerotic D64.89
  ovalocytosis (hereditary) —*see* Elliptocytosis
  paludal (*see also* Malaria) B54 *[D63.8]*
  pernicious (congenital) (malignant) (progressive) D51.0
  pleochromic D64.89
    of sprue D52.8
  posthemorrhagic (chronic) D50.0
    acute D62
    newborn P61.3
  postoperative (postprocedural)
    due to (acute) blood loss D62
      chronic blood loss D50.0
    specified NEC D64.9
  postpartum O90.81
  pressure D64.89
  progressive D64.9
    malignant D51.0
    pernicious D51.0
  protein-deficiency D53.0
  pseudoleukemica infantum D64.89
  pure red cell D60.9
    congenital D61.01
  pyridoxine-responsive D64.3
  pyruvate kinase deficiency D55.2
  refractory D46.4
    with
      excess of blasts D46.20
        1 (RAEB 1) D46.21
        2 (RAEB 2) D46.22
        in transformation (RAEB T) —*see* Leukemia, acute myeloblastic
    hemochromatosis D46.1
    sideroblasts (ring) (RARS) D46.1
    megaloblastic D53.1
    sideroblastic D46.1
    sideropenic D50.9
    without ring sideroblasts, so stated D46.0
    without sideroblasts without excess of blasts D46.0
  Rietti-Greppi-Micheli D56.9
  scorbutic D53.2

Anemia - *continued*
  secondary to
    blood loss (chronic) D50.0
      acute D62
    hemorrhage (chronic) D50.0
      acute D62
  semiplastic D61.89
  sickle-cell —*see* Disease, sickle-cell
  sideroblastic D64.3
    hereditary D64.0
    hypochromic, sex-linked D64.0
    pyridoxine-responsive NEC D64.3
    refractory D46.1
    secondary (due to)
      disease D64.1
      drugs and toxins D64.2
    specified type NEC D64.3
  sideropenic (refractory) D50.9
    due to blood loss (chronic) D50.0
      acute D62
  simple chronic D53.9
  specified type NEC D64.89
  spherocytic (hereditary) —*see* Spherocytosis
  splenic D64.89
  splenomegalic D64.89
  stomatocytosis D58.8
  syphilitic (acquired) (late) A52.79 *[D63.8]*
  target cell D64.89
  thalassemia D56.9
  thrombocytopenic —*see* Thrombocytopenia
  toxic D61.2
  tropical B76.9 *[D63.8]*
    macrocytic D52.8
  tuberculous A18.89 *[D63.8]*
  vegan D51.3
  vitamin
    B6-responsive D64.3
    B12 deficiency (dietary) pernicious D51.0
  von Jaksch's D64.89
  Witts' (achlorhydric anemia) D50.8
Anemophobia F40.228
Anencephalus, anencephaly Q00.0
Anergasia —*see* Psychosis, organic
Anesthesia, anesthetic R20.0
  complication or reaction NEC (*see also* Complications, anesthesia) T88.59
    due to
      correct substance properly administered —*see* Table of Drugs and Chemicals, by drug, adverse effect
      overdose or wrong substance given —*see* Table of Drugs and Chemicals, by drug, poisoning
  cornea H18.81
  dissociative F44.6
  functional (hysterical) F44.6
  hyperesthetic, thalamic G89.0
  hysterical F44.6
  local skin lesion R20.0
  sexual (psychogenic) F52.1
  shock (due to) T88.2
  skin R20.0
  testicular N50.9
Anetoderma (maculosum) (of) L90.8
  Jadassohn-Pellizzari L90.2
  Schweninger-Buzzi L90.1
Aneurin deficiency E51.9
Aneurysm (anastomotic) (artery) (cirsoid) (diffuse) (false) (fusiform) (multiple) (saccular) I72.9
  abdominal (aorta) I71.4
    ruptured I71.3

Aneurysm - *continued*
  syphilitic A52.01
  aorta, aortic (nonsyphilitic) I71.9
    abdominal I71.4
      ruptured I71.3
    arch I71.2
      ruptured I71.1
    arteriosclerotic I71.9
      ruptured I71.8
    ascending I71.2
      ruptured I71.1
    congenital Q25.4
    descending I71.9
      abdominal I71.4
        ruptured I71.3
      ruptured I71.8
      thoracic I71.2
        ruptured I71.1
    ruptured I71.8
    sinus, congenital Q25.4
    syphilitic A52.01
    thoracic I71.2
      ruptured I71.1
    thoracoabdominal I71.6
      ruptured I71.5
    thorax, thoracic (arch) I71.2
      ruptured I71.1
    transverse I71.2
      ruptured I71.1
    valve (heart) (*see also* Endocarditis, aortic) I35.8
  arteriosclerotic I72.9
    cerebral I67.1
      ruptured —*see* Hemorrhage, intracranial, subarachnoid
  arteriovenous (congenital) —*see also* Malformation, arteriovenous
    acquired I77.0
    brain I67.1
    coronary I25.41
    pulmonary I28.0
  brain Q28.2
    ruptured I60.8
    peripheral —*see* Malformation, arteriovenous, peripheral
    precerebral vessels Q28.0
    specified site NEC —*see also* Malformation, arteriovenous
      acquired I77.0
  basal —*see* Aneurysm, brain
  berry (congenital) (nonruptured) I67.1
    ruptured I60.7
  brain I67.1
    arteriosclerotic I67.1
      ruptured —*see* Hemorrhage, intracranial, subarachnoid
    arteriovenous (congenital) (nonruptured) Q28.2
      acquired I67.1
        ruptured I60.8
      ruptured I60.8
    berry (congenital) (nonruptured) I67.1
      ruptured (*see also* Hemorrhage, intracranial, subarachnoid) I60.7
    congenital Q28.3
      ruptured I60.7
    meninges I67.1
      ruptured I60.8
    miliary (congenital) (nonruptured) I67.1
      ruptured (*see also* Hemorrhage, intracranial, subarachnoid) I60.7
    mycotic I33.0

Aneurysm - *continued*
ruptured —*see* Hemorrhage, intracranial, subarachnoid
syphilitic (hemorrhage) A52.05
cardiac (false) (*see also* Aneurysm, heart) I25.3
carotid artery (common) (external) I72.0
internal (intracranial) I67.1
extracranial portion I72.0
ruptured into brain I60.0
syphilitic A52.09
intracranial A52.05
cavernous sinus I67.1
arteriovenous (congenital) (nonruptured) Q28.3
ruptured I60.8
celiac I72.8
central nervous system, syphilitic A52.05
cerebral —*see* Aneurysm, brain
chest —*see* Aneurysm, thorax
circle of Willis I67.1
congenital Q28.3
ruptured I60.6
ruptured I60.6
common iliac artery I72.3
congenital (peripheral) Q27.8
brain Q28.3
ruptured I60.7
coronary Q24.5
digestive system Q27.8
lower limb Q27.8
pulmonary Q25.79
retina Q14.1
specified site NEC Q27.8
upper limb Q27.8
conjunctiva —*see* Abnormality, conjunctiva, vascular
conus arteriosus —*see* Aneurysm, heart
coronary (arteriosclerotic) (artery) I25.41
arteriovenous, congenital Q24.5
congenital Q24.5
ruptured —*see* Infarct, myocardium
syphilitic A52.06
vein I25.89
cylindroid (aorta) I71.9
ruptured I71.8
syphilitic A52.01
ductus arteriosus Q25.0
endocardial, infective (any valve) I33.0
femoral (artery) (ruptured) I72.4
gastroduodenal I72.8
gastroepiploic I72.8
heart (wall) (chronic or with a stated duration of over 4 weeks) I25.3
valve —*see* Endocarditis
hepatic I72.8
iliac (common) (artery) (ruptured) I72.3
infective I72.9
endocardial (any valve) I33.0
innominate (nonsyphilitic) I72.8
syphilitic A52.09
interauricular septum —*see* Aneurysm, heart
interventricular septum —*see* Aneurysm, heart
intrathoracic (nonsyphilitic) I71.2
ruptured I71.1
syphilitic A52.01
lower limb I72.4
lung (pulmonary artery) I28.1
mediastinal (nonsyphilitic) I72.8
syphilitic A52.09
miliary (congenital) I67.1

Aneurysm - *continued*
ruptured —*see* Hemorrhage, intracerebral, subarachnoid, intracranial
mitral (heart) (valve) I34.8
mural —*see* Aneurysm, heart
mycotic I72.9
endocardial (any valve) I33.0
ruptured, brain —*see* Hemorrhage, intracerebral, subarachnoid
myocardium —*see* Aneurysm, heart
neck I72.0
pancreaticoduodenal I72.8
patent ductus arteriosus Q25.0
peripheral NEC I72.8
congenital Q27.8
digestive system Q27.8
lower limb Q27.8
specified site NEC Q27.8
upper limb Q27.8
popliteal (artery) (ruptured) I72.4
precerebral, congenital (nonruptured) Q28.1
pulmonary I28.1
arteriovenous Q25.72
acquired I28.0
syphilitic A52.09
valve (heart) —*see* Endocarditis, pulmonary
racemose (peripheral) I72.9
congenital —*see* Aneurysm, congenital
radial I72.1
Rasmussen NEC A15.0
renal (artery) I72.2
retina —*see also* Disorder, retina, microaneurysms
congenital Q14.1
diabetic —*see* Diabetes, microaneurysms, retinal
sinus of Valsalva Q25.4
specified NEC I72.8
spinal (cord) I72.8
syphilitic (hemorrhage) A52.09
splenic I72.8
subclavian (artery) (ruptured) I72.8
syphilitic A52.09
superior mesenteric I72.8
syphilitic (aorta) A52.01
central nervous system A52.05
congenital (late) A50.54 *[I79.0]*
spine, spinal A52.09
thoracoabdominal (aorta) I71.6
ruptured I71.5
syphilitic A52.01
thorax, thoracic (aorta) (arch) (nonsyphilitic) I71.2
ruptured I71.1
syphilitic A52.01
traumatic (complication) (early) , specified site —*see* Injury, blood vessel
tricuspid (heart) (valve) I07.8
ulnar I72.1
upper limb (ruptured) I72.1
valve, valvular —*see* Endocarditis
venous (*see also* Varix) I86.8
congenital Q27.8
digestive system Q27.8
lower limb Q27.8
specified site NEC Q27.8
upper limb Q27.8
ventricle —*see* Aneurysm, heart
visceral NEC I72.8
Angelman syndrome Q93.5
Anger R45.4
Angiectasis, angiectopia I99.8

Angiitis I77.6
allergic granulomatous M30.1
hypersensitivity M31.0
necrotizing M31.9
specified NEC M31.8
nervous system, granulomatous I67.7
Angina (attack) (cardiac) (chest) (heart) (pectoris) (syndrome) (vasomotor) I20.9
with
atherosclerotic heart disease —*see* Arteriosclerosis, coronary (artery)
documented spasm I20.1
abdominal K55.1
accelerated —*see* Angina, unstable
agranulocytic —*see* Agranulocytosis
angiospastic —*see* Angina, with documented spasm
aphthous B08.5
crescendo —*see* Angina, unstable
croupous J05.0
cruris I73.9
de novo effort —*see* Angina, unstable
diphtheritic, membranous A36.0
equivalent I20.8
exudative, chronic J37.0
following acute myocardial infarction I23.7
gangrenous diphtheritic A36.0
intestinal K55.1
Ludovici K12.2
Ludwig's K12.2
malignant diphtheritic A36.0
membranous J05.0
diphtheritic A36.0
Vincent's A69.1
mesenteric K55.1
monocytic —*see* Mononucleosis, infectious
of effort —*see* Angina, specified NEC
phlegmonous J36
diphtheritic A36.0
post-infarctional I23.7
pre-infarctional —*see* Angina, unstable
Prinzmetal —*see* Angina, with documented spasm
progressive —*see* Angina, unstable
pseudomembranous A69.1
pultaceous, diphtheritic A36.0
spasm-induced —*see* Angina, with documented spasm
specified NEC I20.8
stable I20.9
stenocardia —*see* Angina, specified NEC
stridulous, diphtheritic A36.2
tonsil J36
trachealis J05.0
unstable I20.0
variant —*see* Angina, with documented spasm
Vincent's A69.1
worsening effort —*see* Angina, unstable
Angioblastoma —*see* Neoplasm, connective tissue, uncertain behavior
Angiocholecystitis —*see* Cholecystitis, acute
Angiocholitis (*see also* Cholecystitis, acute) K83.0
Angiodysgenesis spinalis G95.19
Angiodysplasia (cecum) (colon) K55.20
with bleeding K55.21
duodenum (and stomach) K31.819
with bleeding K31.811
stomach (and duodenum) K31.819
with bleeding K31.811

Angioedema (allergic) (any site) (with urticaria) T78.3
  hereditary D84.1
Angioendothelioma —*see* Neoplasm, uncertain behavior, by site
  benign D18.00
    intra-abdominal D18.03
    intracranial D18.02
    skin D18.01
    specified site NEC D18.09
  bone —*see* Neoplasm, bone, malignant
  Ewing's —*see* Neoplasm, bone, malignant
Angioendotheliomatosis C85.8
Angiofibroma —*see also* Neoplasm, benign, by site
  juvenile
    specified site —*see* Neoplasm, benign, by site
    unspecified site D10.6
Angiohemophilia (A) (B) D68.0
Angioid streaks (choroid) (macula) (retina) H35.33
Angiokeratoma —*see* Neoplasm, skin, benign
  corporis diffusum E75.21
Angioleiomyoma —*see* Neoplasm, connective tissue, benign
Angiolipoma —*see also* Lipoma
  infiltrating —*see* Lipoma
Angioma —*see also* Hemangioma, by site
  capillary I78.1
  hemorrhagicum hereditaria I78.0
  intra-abdominal D18.03
  intracranial D18.02
  malignant —*see* Neoplasm, connective tissue, malignant
  plexiform D18.00
    intra-abdominal D18.03
    intracranial D18.02
    skin D18.01
    specified site NEC D18.09
  senile I78.1
  serpiginosum L81.7
  skin D18.01
  specified site NEC D18.09
  spider I78.1
  stellate I78.1
  venous Q28.3
Angiomatosis Q82.8
  bacillary A79.89
  encephalotrigeminal Q85.8
  hemorrhagic familial I78.0
  hereditary familial I78.0
  liver K76.4
Angiomyolipoma —*see* Lipoma
Angiomyoliposarcoma —*see* Neoplasm, connective tissue, malignant
Angiomyoma —*see* Neoplasm, connective tissue, benign
Angiomyosarcoma —*see* Neoplasm, connective tissue, malignant
Angiomyxoma —*see* Neoplasm, connective tissue, uncertain behavior
Angioneurosis F45.8
Angioneurotic edema (allergic) (any site) (with urticaria) T78.3
  hereditary D84.1
Angiopathia, angiopathy I99.9
  cerebral I67.9
    amyloid E85.4 *[I68.0]*
  diabetic (peripheral) —*see* Diabetes, angiopathy
  peripheral I73.9

Angiopathia, angiopathy - *continued*
  diabetic —*see* Diabetes, angiopathy
  specified type NEC I73.89
  retinae syphilitica A52.05
  retinalis (juvenilis)
    diabetic —*see* Diabetes, retinopathy
    proliferative —*see* Retinopathy, proliferative
Angiosarcoma —*see also* Neoplasm, connective tissue, malignant
  liver C22.3
Angiosclerosis —*see* Arteriosclerosis
Angiospasm (peripheral) (traumatic) (vessel) I73.9
  brachial plexus G54.0
  cerebral G45.9
  cervical plexus G54.2
  nerve
    arm —*see* Mononeuropathy, upper limb
      axillary G54.0
      median —*see* Lesion, nerve, median
      ulnar —*see* Lesion, nerve, ulnar
    axillary G54.0
    leg —*see* Mononeuropathy, lower limb
    median —*see* Lesion, nerve, median
    plantar —*see* Lesion, nerve, plantar
    ulnar —*see* Lesion, nerve, ulnar
Angiospastic disease or edema I73.9
Angiostrongyliasis
  due to
    Parastrongylus
      cantonensis B83.2
      costaricensis B81.3
  intestinal B81.3
Anguillulosis —*see* Strongyloidiasis
Angulation
  cecum —*see* Obstruction, intestine
  coccyx (acquired) (*see also* subcategory) M43.8
    congenital NEC Q76.49
  femur (acquired) —*see also* Deformity, limb, specified type NEC, thigh
    congenital Q74.2
  intestine (large) (small) —*see* Obstruction, intestine
  sacrum (acquired) (*see also* subcategory) M43.8
    congenital NEC Q76.49
  sigmoid (flexure) —*see* Obstruction, intestine
  spine —*see* Dorsopathy, deforming, specified NEC
  tibia (acquired) —*see also* Deformity, limb, specified type NEC, lower leg
    congenital Q74.2
  ureter N13.5
    with infection N13.6
  wrist (acquired) —*see also* Deformity, limb, specified type NEC, forearm
    congenital Q74.0
Angulus infectiosus (lips) K13.0
Anhedonia R45.84
Anhidrosis L74.4
Anhydration, anhydremia E86.0
  with
    hypernatremia E87.0
    hyponatremia E87.1
Anhydremia E86.0
  with
    hypernatremia E87.0
    hyponatremia E87.1
Anidrosis L74.4
Aniridia (congenital) Q13.1
Anisakiasis (infection) (infestation) B81.0

Anisakis larvae infestation B81.0
Aniseikonia H52.32
Anisocoria (pupil) H57.02
  congenital Q13.2
Anisocytosis R71.8
Anisometropia (congenital) H52.31
Ankle —*see* condition
Ankyloblepharon (eyelid) (acquired) —*see also* Blepharophimosis
  filiforme (adnatum) (congenital) Q10.3
  total Q10.3
Ankyloglossia Q38.1
Ankylosis (fibrous) (osseous) (joint) M24.60
  ankle M24.67
  arthrodesis status Z98.1
  cricoarytenoid (cartilage) (joint) (larynx) J38.7
  dental K03.5
  ear ossicles H74.31
  elbow M24.62
  foot M24.67
  hand M24.64
  hip M24.65
  incostapedial joint (infectional) —*see* Ankylosis, ear ossicles
  jaw (temporomandibular) M26.61
  knee M24.66
  lumbosacral (joint) M43.27
  postoperative (status) Z98.1
  produced by surgical fusion, status Z98.1
  sacro-iliac (joint) M43.28
  shoulder M24.61
  spine (joint) —*see also* Fusion, spine
    spondylitic —*see* Spondylitis, ankylosing
  surgical Z98.1
  temporomandibular M26.61
  tooth, teeth (hard tissues) K03.5
  wrist M24.63
Ankylostoma —*see* Ancylostoma
Ankylostomiasis —*see* Ancylostomiasis
Ankylurethria —*see* Stricture, urethra
Annular —*see also* condition
  detachment, cervix N88.8
  organ or site, congenital NEC —*see* Distortion
  pancreas (congenital) Q45.1
Anodontia (complete) (partial) (vera) K00.0
  acquired K08.10
Anomaly, anomalous (congenital) (unspecified type) Q89.9
  abdominal wall NEC Q79.59
  acoustic nerve Q07.8
  adrenal (gland) Q89.1
  Alder (-Reilly) (leukocyte granulation) D72.0
  alimentary tract Q45.9
    upper Q40.9
  alveolar M26.70
    hyperplasia M26.79
      mandibular M26.72
      maxillary M26.71
    hypoplasia M26.79
      mandibular M26.74
      maxillary M26.73
    ridge (process) M26.79
    specified NEC M26.79
  ankle (joint) Q74.2
  anus Q43.9
  aorta (arch) NEC Q25.4
    coarctation (preductal) (postductal) Q25.1
  aortic cusp or valve Q23.9
  appendix Q43.8
  apple peel syndrome Q41.1
  aqueduct of Sylvius Q03.0

Anomaly, anomalous - *continued*

with spina bifida —*see* Spina bifida, with hydrocephalus
arm Q74.0
arteriovenous NEC
coronary Q24.5
gastrointestinal Q27.33
acquired —*see* Angiodysplasia
artery (peripheral) Q27.9
basilar NEC Q28.1
cerebral Q28.3
coronary Q24.5
digestive system Q27.8
eye Q15.8
great Q25.9
specified NEC Q25.8
lower limb Q27.8
peripheral Q27.9
specified NEC Q27.8
pulmonary NEC Q25.79
renal Q27.2
retina Q14.1
specified site NEC Q27.8
subclavian Q27.8
umbilical Q27.0
upper limb Q27.8
vertebral NEC Q28.1
aryteno-epiglottic folds Q31.8
atrial
bands or folds Q20.8
septa Q21.1
atrioventricular
excitation I45.6
septum Q21.0
auditory canal Q17.8
auricle
ear Q17.8
causing impairment of hearing Q16.9
heart Q20.8
Axenfeld's Q15.0
back Q89.9
band
atrial Q20.8
heart Q24.8
ventricular Q24.8
Bartholin's duct Q38.4
biliary duct or passage Q44.5
bladder Q64.70
absence Q64.5
diverticulum Q64.6
exstrophy Q64.10
cloacal Q64.12
extroversion Q64.19
specified type NEC Q64.19
supravesical fissure Q64.11
neck obstruction Q64.31
specified type NEC Q64.79
bone Q79.9
arm Q74.0
face Q75.9
leg Q74.2
pelvic girdle Q74.2
shoulder girdle Q74.0
skull Q75.9
with
anencephaly Q00.0
encephalocele —*see* Encephalocele
hydrocephalus Q03.9
with spina bifida —*see* Spina bifida, by site, with hydrocephalus
microcephaly Q02

brain (multiple) Q04.9
vessel Q28.3
breast Q83.9
broad ligament Q50.6
bronchus Q32.4
bulbus cordis Q21.9
bursa Q79.9
canal of Nuck Q52.4
canthus Q10.3
capillary Q27.9
cardiac Q24.9
chambers Q20.9
specified NEC Q20.8
septal closure Q21.9
specified NEC Q21.8
valve NEC Q24.8
pulmonary Q22.3
cardiovascular system Q28.8
carpus Q74.0
caruncle, lacrimal Q10.6
cascade stomach Q40.2
cauda equina Q06.3
cecum Q43.9
cerebral Q04.9
vessels Q28.3
cervix Q51.9
Chédiak-Higashi (-Steinbrinck) (congenital gigantism of peroxidase granules) E70.330
cheek Q18.9
chest wall Q67.8
bones Q76.9
chin Q18.9
chordae tendineae Q24.8
choroid Q14.3
plexus Q07.8
chromosomes, chromosomal Q99.9
D (1) —*see* condition, chromosome 13
E (3) —*see* condition, chromosome 18
G —*see* condition, chromosome 21
sex
female phenotype Q97.8
gonadal dysgenesis (pure) Q99.1
Klinefelter's Q98.4
male phenotype Q98.9
Turner's Q96.9
specified NEC Q99.8
cilia Q10.3
circulatory system Q28.9
clavicle Q74.0
clitoris Q52.6
coccyx Q76.49
colon Q43.9
common duct Q44.5
communication
coronary artery Q24.5
left ventricle with right atrium Q21.0
concha (ear) Q17.3
connection
portal vein Q26.5
pulmonary venous Q26.4
partial Q26.3
total Q26.2
renal artery with kidney Q27.2
cornea (shape) Q13.4
coronary artery or vein Q24.5
cranium —*see* Anomaly, skull
cricoid cartilage Q31.8
cystic duct Q44.5
dental
alveolar —*see* Anomaly, alveolar
arch relationship M26.20
specified NEC M26.29

dentofacial M26.9
alveolar —*see* Anomaly, alveolar
dental arch relationship M26.20
specified NEC M26.29
functional M26.50
specified NEC M26.59
jaw-cranial base relationship M26.10
asymmetry M26.12
maxillary M26.11
specified type NEC M26.19
jaw size M26.00
macrogenia M26.05
mandibular
hyperplasia M26.03
hypoplasia M26.04
maxillary
hyperplasia M26.01
hypoplasia M26.02
microgenia M26.06
specified type NEC M26.09
malocclusion M26.4
dental arch relationship NEC M26.29
jaw-cranial base relationship —*see* Anomaly, dentofacial, jaw-cranial base relationship
jaw size —*see* Anomaly, dentofacial, jaw size
specified type NEC M26.89
temporomandibular joint M26.60
adhesions M26.61
ankylosis M26.61
arthralgia M26.62
articular disc M26.63
specified type NEC M26.69
tooth position, fully erupted M26.30
specified NEC M26.39
dermatoglyphic Q82.8
diaphragm (apertures) NEC Q79.1
digestive organ (s) or tract Q45.9
lower Q43.9
upper Q40.9
distance, interarch (excessive) (inadequate) M26.25
distribution, coronary artery Q24.5
ductus
arteriosus Q25.0
botalli Q25.0
duodenum Q43.9
dura (brain) Q04.9
spinal cord Q06.9
ear (external) Q17.9
causing impairment of hearing Q16.9
inner Q16.5
middle (causing impairment of hearing) Q16.4
ossicles Q16.3
Ebstein's (heart) (tricuspid valve) Q22.5
ectodermal Q82.9
Eisenmenger's (ventricular septal defect) Q21.8
ejaculatory duct Q55.4
elbow Q74.0
endocrine gland NEC Q89.2
epididymis Q55.4
epiglottis Q31.8
esophagus Q39.9
eustachian tube Q17.8
eye Q15.9
anterior segment Q13.9
specified NEC Q13.89
posterior segment Q14.9
specified NEC Q14.8

Anomaly, anomalous - *continued*
  ptosis (eyelid) Q10.0
    specified NEC Q15.8
  eyebrow Q18.8
  eyelid Q10.3
    ptosis Q10.0
  face Q18.9
    bone (s) Q75.9
  fallopian tube Q50.6
  fascia Q79.9
  femur NEC Q74.2
  fibula NEC Q74.2
  finger Q74.0
  fixation, intestine Q43.3
  flexion (joint) NOS Q74.9
    hip or thigh Q65.89
  foot NEC Q74.2
    varus (congenital) Q66.3
  foramen
    Botalli Q21.1
    ovale Q21.1
  forearm Q74.0
  forehead Q75.8
  form, teeth K00.2
  fovea centralis Q14.1
  frontal bone —*see* Anomaly, skull
  gallbladder (position) (shape) (size) Q44.1
  Gartner's duct Q52.4
  gastrointestinal tract Q45.9
  genitalia, genital organ (s) or system
    female Q52.9
      external Q52.70
      internal NOS Q52.9
    male Q55.9
      hydrocele P83.5
      specified NEC Q55.8
  genitourinary NEC
    female Q52.9
    male Q55.9
  Gerbode Q21.0
  glottis Q31.8
  granulation or granulocyte, genetic (constitutional) (leukocyte) D72.0
  gum Q38.6
  gyri Q07.9
  hair Q84.2
  hand Q74.0
  hard tissue formation in pulp K04.3
  head —*see* Anomaly, skull
  heart Q24.9
    auricle Q20.8
    bands or folds Q24.8
    fibroelastosis cordis I42.4
    obstructive NEC Q22.6
    patent ductus arteriosus (Botalli) Q25.0
    septum Q21.9
      auricular Q21.1
      interatrial Q21.1
      interventricular Q21.0
        with pulmonary stenosis or atresia, dextroposition of aorta and hypertrophy of right ventricle Q21.3
      specified NEC Q21.8
      ventricular Q21.0
        with pulmonary stenosis or atresia, dextroposition of aorta and hypertrophy of right ventricle Q21.3
      tetralogy of Fallot Q21.3
    valve NEC Q24.8
      aortic
        bicuspid valve Q23.1
        insufficiency Q23.1

Anomaly, anomalous - *continued*
    stenosis Q23.0
      subaortic Q24.4
    mitral
      insufficiency Q23.3
      stenosis Q23.2
    pulmonary Q22.3
      atresia Q22.0
      insufficiency Q22.2
      stenosis Q22.1
        infundibular Q24.3
        subvalvular Q24.3
    tricuspid
      atresia Q22.4
      stenosis Q22.4
    ventricle Q20.8
  heel NEC Q74.2
  Hegglin's D72.0
  hemianencephaly Q00.0
  hemicephaly Q00.0
  hemicrania Q00.0
  hepatic duct Q44.5
  hip NEC Q74.2
  hourglass stomach Q40.2
  humerus Q74.0
  hydatid of Morgagni
    female Q50.5
    male (epididymal) Q55.4
      testicular Q55.29
  hymen Q52.4
  hypersegmentation of neutrophils, hereditary D72.0
  hypophyseal Q89.2
  ileocecal (coil) (valve) Q43.9
  ileum Q43.9
  ilium NEC Q74.2
  integument Q84.9
    specified NEC Q84.8
  interarch distance (excessive) (inadequate) M26.25
  intervertebral cartilage or disc Q76.49
  intestine (large) (small) Q43.9
    with anomalous adhesions, fixation or malrotation Q43.3
  iris Q13.2
  ischium NEC Q74.2
  jaw —*see* Anomaly, dentofacial
    alveolar —*see* Anomaly, alveolar
  jaw-cranial base relationship —*see* Anomaly, dentofacial, jaw-cranial base relationship
  jejunum Q43.8
  joint Q74.9
    specified NEC Q74.8
  Jordan's D72.0
  kidney (s) (calyx) (pelvis) Q63.9
    artery Q27.2
    specified NEC Q63.8
  Klippel-Feil (brevicollis) Q76.1
  knee Q74.1
  labium (majus) (minus) Q52.70
  labyrinth, membranous Q16.5
  lacrimal apparatus or duct Q10.6
  larynx, laryngeal (muscle) Q31.9
    web (bed) Q31.0
  lens Q12.9
  leukocytes, genetic D72.0
    granulation (constitutional) D72.0
  lid (fold) Q10.3
  ligament Q79.9
    broad Q50.6
    round Q52.8

Anomaly, anomalous - *continued*
  limb Q74.9
    lower NEC Q74.2
      reduction deformity —*see* Defect, reduction, lower limb
    upper Q74.0
  lip Q38.0
  liver Q44.7
    duct Q44.5
  lower limb NEC Q74.2
  lumbosacral (joint) (region) Q76.49
    kyphosis —*see* Kyphosis, congenital
    lordosis —*see* Lordosis, congenital
  lung (fissure) (lobe) Q33.9
  mandible —*see* Anomaly, dentofacial
  maxilla —*see* Anomaly, dentofacial
  May (-Hegglin) D72.0
  meatus urinarius NEC Q64.79
  meningeal bands or folds Q07.9
    constriction of Q07.8
    spinal Q06.9
  meninges Q07.9
    cerebral Q04.8
    spinal Q06.9
  meningocele Q05.9
  mesentery Q45.9
  metacarpus Q74.0
  metatarsus NEC Q74.2
  middle ear Q16.4
    ossicles Q16.3
  mitral (leaflets) (valve) Q23.9
    insufficiency Q23.3
    specified NEC Q23.8
    stenosis Q23.2
  mouth Q38.6
  Müllerian —*see also* Anomaly, by site
    uterus NEC Q51.818
  multiple NEC Q89.7
  muscle Q79.9
    eyelid Q10.3
  musculoskeletal system, except limbs Q79.9
  myocardium Q24.8
  nail Q84.6
  narrowness, eyelid Q10.3
  nasal sinus (wall) Q30.8
  neck (any part) Q18.9
  nerve Q07.9
    acoustic Q07.8
    optic Q07.8
  nervous system (central) Q07.9
  nipple Q83.9
  nose, nasal (bones) (cartilage) (septum) (sinus) Q30.9
    specified NEC Q30.8
  ocular muscle Q15.8
  omphalomesenteric duct Q43.0
  opening, pulmonary veins Q26.4
  optic
    disc Q14.2
    nerve Q07.8
  opticociliary vessels Q13.2
  orbit (eye) Q10.7
  organ Q89.9
    of Corti Q16.5
  origin
    artery
      innominate Q25.8
      pulmonary Q25.79
      renal Q27.2
      subclavian Q25.8
  osseous meatus (ear) Q16.1
  ovary Q50.39

Anomaly, anomalous - *continued*
oviduct Q50.6
palate (hard) (soft) NEC Q38.5
pancreas or pancreatic duct Q45.3
papillary muscles Q24.8
parathyroid gland Q89.2
paraurethral ducts Q64.79
parotid (gland) Q38.4
patella Q74.1
Pelger-Huët (hereditary hyposegmentation)
D72.0
pelvic girdle NEC Q74.2
pelvis (bony) NEC Q74.2
   rachitic E64.3
penis (glans) Q55.69
pericardium Q24.8
peripheral vascular system Q27.9
Peter's Q13.4
pharynx Q38.8
pigmentation L81.9
   congenital Q82.8
pituitary (gland) Q89.2
pleural (folds) Q34.0
portal vein Q26.5
   connection Q26.5
position, tooth, teeth, fully erupted M26.30
   specified NEC M26.39
precerebral vessel Q28.1
prepuce Q55.69
prostate Q55.4
pulmonary Q33.9
   artery NEC Q25.79
   valve Q22.3
      atresia Q22.0
      insufficiency Q22.2
      specified type NEC Q22.3
      stenosis Q22.1
         infundibular Q24.3
         subvalvular Q24.3
   venous connection Q26.4
      partial Q26.3
      total Q26.2
pupil Q13.2
   function H57.00
      anisocoria H57.02
      Argyll Robertson pupil H57.01
      miosis H57.03
      mydriasis H57.04
      specified type NEC H57.09
      tonic pupil H57.05
pylorus Q40.3
radius Q74.0
rectum Q43.9
reduction (extremity) (limb)
   femur (longitudinal) —*see* Defect,
   reduction, lower limb, longitudinal, femur
   fibula (longitudinal) —*see* Defect,
   reduction, lower limb, longitudinal, fibula
   lower limb —*see* Defect, reduction, lower
   limb
   radius (longitudinal) —*see* Defect,
   reduction, upper limb, longitudinal, radius
   tibia (longitudinal) —*see* Defect, reduction,
   lower limb, longitudinal, tibia
   ulna (longitudinal) —*see* Defect, reduction,
   upper limb, longitudinal, ulna
   upper limb —*see* Defect, reduction, upper
   limb
refraction —*see* Disorder, refraction
renal Q63.9
   artery Q27.2
   pelvis Q63.9

Anomaly, anomalous - *continued*
   specified NEC Q63.8
respiratory system Q34.9
   specified NEC Q34.8
retina Q14.1
rib Q76.6
   cervical Q76.5
Rieger's Q13.81
rotation —*see* Malrotation
   hip or thigh Q65.89
round ligament Q52.8
sacroiliac (joint) NEC Q74.2
sacrum NEC Q76.49
   kyphosis —*see* Kyphosis, congenital
   lordosis —*see* Lordosis, congenital
saddle nose, syphilitic A50.57
salivary duct or gland Q38.4
scapula Q74.0
scrotum —*see* Malformation, testis and
scrotum
sebaceous gland Q82.9
seminal vesicles Q55.4
sense organs NEC Q07.8
sex chromosomes NEC —*see also* Anomaly,
chromosomes
   female phenotype Q97.8
   male phenotype Q98.9
shoulder (girdle) (joint) Q74.0
sigmoid (flexure) Q43.9
simian crease Q82.8
sinus of Valsalva Q25.4
skeleton generalized Q78.9
skin (appendage) Q82.9
skull Q75.9
   with
      anencephaly Q00.0
      encephalocele —*see* Encephalocele
      hydrocephalus Q03.9
         with spina bifida —*see* Spina bifida, by
site, with hydrocephalus
      microcephaly Q02
specified organ or site NEC Q89.8
spermatic cord Q55.4
spine, spinal NEC Q76.49
   column NEC Q76.49
      kyphosis —*see* Kyphosis, congenital
      lordosis —*see* Lordosis, congenital
   cord Q06.9
   nerve root Q07.8
spleen Q89.09
   agenesis Q89.01
stenonian duct Q38.4
sternum NEC Q76.7
stomach Q40.3
submaxillary gland Q38.4
tarsus NEC Q74.2
tendon Q79.9
testis —*see* Malformation, testis and scrotum
thigh NEC Q74.2
thorax (wall) Q67.8
   bony Q76.9
throat Q38.8
thumb Q74.0
thymus gland Q89.2
thyroid (gland) Q89.2
   cartilage Q31.8
tibia NEC Q74.2
   saber A50.56
toe Q74.2
tongue Q38.3
tooth, teeth K00.9
   eruption K00.6

Anomaly, anomalous - *continued*
   position, fully erupted M26.30
   spacing, fully erupted M26.30
trachea (cartilage) Q32.1
tragus Q17.9
tricuspid (leaflet) (valve) Q22.9
   atresia or stenosis Q22.4
   Ebstein's Q22.5
Uhl's (hypoplasia of myocardium, right
ventricle) Q24.8
ulna Q74.0
umbilical artery Q27.0
union
   cricoid cartilage and thyroid cartilage Q31.8
   thyroid cartilage and hyoid bone Q31.8
   trachea with larynx Q31.8
upper limb Q74.0
urachus Q64.4
ureter Q62.8
   obstructive NEC Q62.39
      cecoureterocele Q62.32
      orthotopic ureterocele Q62.31
urethra Q64.70
   absence Q64.5
   double Q64.74
   fistula to rectum Q64.73
   obstructive Q64.39
      stricture Q64.32
   prolapse Q64.71
   specified type NEC Q64.79
urinary tract Q64.9
uterus Q51.9
   with only one functioning horn Q51.4
uvula Q38.5
vagina Q52.4
valleculae Q31.8
valve (heart) NEC Q24.8
   coronary sinus Q24.5
   inferior vena cava Q24.8
   pulmonary Q22.3
   sinus coronario Q24.5
   venae cavae inferioris Q24.8
vas deferens Q55.4
vascular Q27.9
   brain Q28.3
   ring Q25.4
vein (s) (peripheral) Q27.9
   brain Q28.3
   cerebral Q28.3
   coronary Q24.5
   developmental Q28.3
   great Q26.9
      specified NEC Q26.8
vena cava (inferior) (superior) Q26.9
venous —*see* Anomaly, vein(s)
venous return Q26.8
ventricular
   bands or folds Q24.8
   septa Q21.0
vertebra Q76.49
   kyphosis —*see* Kyphosis, congenital
   lordosis —*see* Lordosis, congenital
vesicourethral orifice Q64.79
vessel (s) Q27.9
   optic papilla Q14.2
   precerebral Q28.1
vitelline duct Q43.0
vitreous body or humor Q14.0
vulva Q52.70
wrist (joint) Q74.0
Anomia R48.8
Anonychia (congenital) Q84.3
   acquired L60.8

Anophthalmos, anophthalmus (congenital)
(globe) Q11.1
acquired Z90.01
Anopia, anopsia H53.46
quadrant H53.46
Anorchia, anorchism, anorchidism Q55.0
Anorexia R63.0
hysterical F44.89
nervosa F50.00
atypical F50.9
binge-eating type F50.2
with purging F50.02
restricting type F50.01
Anorgasmy, psychogenic (female) F52.31
male F52.32
Anosmia R43.0
hysterical F44.6
postinfectional J39.8
Anosognosia R41.89
Anosteoplasia Q78.9
Anovulatory cycle N97.0
Anoxemia R09.02
newborn P84
Anoxia (pathological) R09.02
altitude T70.29
cerebral G93.1
complicating
anesthesia (general) (local) or other
sedation T88.59
in labor and delivery O74.3
in pregnancy O29.21
postpartum, puerperal O89.2
delivery (cesarean) (instrumental) O75.4
during a procedure G97.81
newborn P84
resulting from a procedure G97.82
due to
drowning T75.1
high altitude T70.29
heart —*see* Insufficiency, coronary
intrauterine P84
myocardial —*see* Insufficiency, coronary
newborn P84
spinal cord G95.11
systemic (by suffocation) (low content in
atmosphere) —*see* Asphyxia, traumatic
Anteflexion —*see* Anteversion
Antenatal
care (normal pregnancy) Z34.90
screening (encounter for) of mother Z36
Antepartum —*see* condition
Anterior —*see* condition
Antero-occlusion M26.220
Anteversion
cervix —*see* Anteversion, uterus
femur (neck) , congenital Q65.89
uterus, uterine (cervix) (postinfectional)
(postpartal, old) N85.4
congenital Q51.818
in pregnancy or childbirth —*see* Pregnancy,
complicated by
Anthophobia F40.228
Anthracosilicosis J60
Anthracosis (lung) (occupational) J60
lingua K14.3
Anthrax A22.9
with pneumonia A22.1
cerebral A22.8
colitis A22.2
cutaneous A22.0
gastrointestinal A22.2
inhalation A22.1

Anthrax - *continued*
intestinal A22.2
meningitis A22.8
pulmonary A22.1
respiratory A22.1
sepsis A22.7
specified manifestation NEC A22.8
Anthropoid pelvis Q74.2
with disproportion (fetopelvic) O33.0
Anthropophobia F40.10
generalized F40.11
Antibodies, maternal (blood group) —*see*
Isoimmunization, affecting management of
pregnancy
anti-D —*see* Isoimmunization, affecting
management of pregnancy, Rh
newborn P55.0
Antibody
anticardiolipin R76.0
with
hemorrhagic disorder D68.312
hypercoagulable state D68.61
antiphosphatidylglycerol R76.0
with
hemorrhagic disorder D68.312
hypercoagulable state D68.61
antiphosphatidylinositol R76.0
with
hemorrhagic disorder D68.312
hypercoagulable state D68.61
antiphosphatidylserine R76.0
with
hemorrhagic disorder D68.312
hypercoagulable state D68.61
antiphospholipid R76.0
with
hemorrhagic disorder D68.312
hypercoagulable state D68.61
Anticardiolipin syndrome D68.61
Anticoagulant, circulating (intrinsic) (*see also*
Disorder, hemorrhagic) D68.318
drug-induced (extrinsic) (*see also*
Disorder, hemorrhagic) D68.32
Antidiuretic hormone syndrome E22.2
Antimonial cholera —*see* Poisoning,
antimony
Antiphospholipid
antibody
with hemorrhagic disorder D68.312
syndrome D68.61
Antisocial personality F60.2
Antithrombinemia —*see* Circulating
anticoagulants
Antithromboplastinemia D68.318
Antithromboplastinogenemia D68.318
Antitoxin complication or reaction —*see*
Complications, vaccination
Antlophobia F40.228
Antritis J32.0
maxilla J32.0
acute J01.00
recurrent J01.01
stomach K29.60
with bleeding K29.61
Antrum, antral —*see* condition
Anuria R34
calculous (impacted) (recurrent) (*see also*
Calculus, urinary) N20.9
following
abortion —*see* Abortion by type
complicated by, renal failure
ectopic or molar pregnancy O08.4

Anuria – - *continued*
newborn P96.0
postprocedural N99.0
postrenal N13.8
traumatic (following crushing) T79.5
Anus, anal —*see* condition
Anusitis K62.89
Anxiety F41.9
depression F41.8
episodic paroxysmal F41.0
generalized F41.1
hysteria F41.8
neurosis F41.1
panic type F41.0
reaction F41.1
separation, abnormal (of childhood) F93.0
specified NEC F41.8
state F41.1
Aorta, aortic —*see* condition
Aortectasia —*see* Ectasia, aorta
with aneurysm —*see* Aneurysm, aorta
Aortitis (nonsyphilitic) (calcific) I77.6
arteriosclerotic I70.0
Doehle-Heller A52.02
luetic A52.02
rheumatic —*see* Endocarditis, acute,
rheumatic
specific (syphilitic) A52.02
syphilitic A52.02
congenital A50.54 *[I79.1]*
Apathetic thyroid storm —*see* Thyrotoxicosis
Apathy R45.3
Apeirophobia F40.228
Apepsia K30
psychogenic F45.8
Aperistalsis, esophagus K22.0
Apertognathia M26.29
Apert's syndrome Q87.0
Aphagia R13.0
psychogenic F50.9
Aphakia (acquired) (postoperative) H27.0
congenital Q12.3
Aphasia (amnestic) (global) (nominal)
(semantic) (syntactic) R47.01
acquired, with epilepsy (Landau-Kleffner
syndrome) —*see* Epilepsy, specified NEC
auditory (developmental) F80.2
developmental (receptive type) F80.2
expressive type F80.1
Wernicke's F80.2
following
cerebrovascular disease I69.920
cerebral infarction I69.320
intracerebral hemorrhage I69.120
nontraumatic intracranial hemorrhage NEC
I69.220
specified disease NEC I69.820
subarachnoid hemorrhage I69.020
primary progressive G31.01 *[F02.80]*
with behavioral disturbance G31.01
[F02.81]
progressive isolated G31.01 *[F02.80]*
with behavioral disturbance G31.01
[F02.81]
sensory F80.2
syphilis, tertiary A52.19
Wernicke's (developmental) F80.2
Aphonia (organic) R49.1
hysterical F44.4
psychogenic F44.4
Aphthae, aphthous —*see also* condition
Bednar's K12.0
cachectic K14.0

Aphthae, aphthous - *continued*
epizootic B08.8
fever B08.8
oral (recurrent) K12.0
stomatitis (major) (minor) K12.0
thrush B37.0
ulcer (oral) (recurrent) K12.0
genital organ (s) NEC
female N76.6
male N50.8
larynx J38.7
Apical —*see* condition
Apiphobia F40.218
Aplasia —*see also* Agenesis
abdominal muscle syndrome Q79.4
alveolar process (acquired) —*see* Anomaly, alveolar
congenital Q38.6
aorta (congenital) Q25.4
axialis extracorticalis (congenita) E75.29
bone marrow (myeloid) D61.9
congenital D61.01
brain Q00.0
part of Q04.3
bronchus Q32.4
cementum K00.4
cerebellum Q04.3
cervix (congenital) Q51.5
congenital pure red cell D61.01
corpus callosum Q04.0
cutis congenita Q84.8
erythrocyte congenital D61.01
extracortical axial E75.29
eye Q11.1
fovea centralis (congenital) Q14.1
gallbladder, congenital Q44.0
iris Q13.1
labyrinth, membranous Q16.5
limb (congenital) Q73.8
lower —*see* Defect, reduction, lower limb
upper —*see* Agenesis, arm
lung, congenital (bilateral) (unilateral) Q33.3
pancreas Q45.0
parathyroid-thymic D82.1
Pelizaeus-Merzbacher E75.29
penis Q55.5
prostate Q55.4
red cell (with thymoma) D60.9
acquired D60.9
due to drugs D60.9
adult D60.9
chronic D60.0
congenital D61.01
constitutional D61.01
due to drugs D60.9
hereditary D61.01
of infants D61.01
primary D61.01
pure D61.01
due to drugs D60.9
specified type NEC D60.8
transient D60.1
round ligament Q52.8
skin Q84.8
spermatic cord Q55.4
spleen Q89.01
testicle Q55.0
thymic, with immunodeficiency D82.1
thyroid (congenital) (with myxedema) E03.1
uterus Q51.0
ventral horn cell Q06.1

Apnea, apneic (of) (spells) R06.81
newborn NEC P28.4
obstructive P28.4
sleep (central) (obstructive) (primary) P28.3
prematurity P28.4
sleep G47.30
central (primary) G47.31
in conditions classified elsewhere G47.37
obstructive (adult) (pediatric) G47.33
primary central G47.31
specified NEC G47.39
Apneumatosis, newborn P28.0
Apocrine metaplasia (breast) —*see* Dysplasia, mammary, specified type NEC
Apophysitis (bone) —*see also* Osteochondropathy
calcaneus M92.8
juvenile M92.9
Apoplectiform convulsions (cerebral ischemia) I67.82
Apoplexia, apoplexy, apoplectic
adrenal A39.1
heart (auricle) (ventricle) —*see* Infarct, myocardium
heat T67.0
hemorrhagic (stroke) —*see* Hemorrhage, intracranial
meninges, hemorrhagic —*see* Hemorrhage, intracranial, subarachnoid
uremic N18.9 *[I68.8]*
Appearance
bizarre R46.1
specified NEC R46.89
very low level of personal hygiene R46.0
Appendage
epididymal (organ of Morgagni) Q55.4
intestine (epiploic) Q43.8
preauricular Q17.0
testicular (organ of Morgagni) Q55.29
Appendicitis (pneumococcal) (retrocecal) K37
with
perforation or rupture K35.2
peritoneal abscess K35.3
peritonitis NEC K35.3
generalized (with perforation or rupture) K35.2
localized (with perforation or rupture) K35.3
acute (catarrhal) (fulminating) (gangrenous) (obstructive) (retrocecal) (suppurative) K35.80
with
peritoneal abscess K35.3
peritonitis NEC K35.3
generalized (with perforation or rupture) K35.2
localized (with perforation or rupture) K35.3
specified NEC K35.89
amebic A06.89
chronic (recurrent) K36
exacerbation —*see* Appendicitis, acute
gangrenous —*see* Appendicitis, acute
healed (obliterative) K36
interval K36
neurogenic K36
obstructive K36
recurrent K36
relapsing K36
subacute (adhesive) K36
subsiding K36
suppurative —*see* Appendicitis, acute
tuberculous A18.32

Appendicopathia oxyurica B80
Appendix, appendicular —*see also* condition
epididymis Q55.4
Morgagni
female Q50.5
male (epididymal) Q55.4
testicular Q55.29
testis Q55.29
Appetite
depraved —*see* Pica
excessive R63.2
lack or loss (*see also* Anorexia) R63.0
nonorganic origin F50.8
psychogenic F50.8
perverted (hysterical) —*see* Pica
Apple peel syndrome Q41.1
Apprehension state F41.1
Apprehensiveness, abnormal F41.9
Approximal wear K03.0
Apraxia (classic) (ideational) (ideokinetic) (ideomotor) (motor) (verbal) R48.2
following
cerebrovascular disease I69.990
cerebral infarction I69.390
intracerebral hemorrhage I69.190
nontraumatic intracranial hemorrhage NEC I69.290
specified disease NEC I69.890
subarachnoid hemorrhage I69.090
oculomotor, congenital H51.8
Aptyalism K11.7
Apudoma —*see* Neoplasm, uncertain behavior, by site
Aqueous misdirection H40.83
Arabicum elephantiasis —*see* Infestation, filarial
Arachnitis —*see* Meningitis
Arachnodactyly —*see* Syndrome, Marfan's
Arachnoiditis (acute) (adhesive) (basal) (brain) (cerebrospinal) —*see* Meningitis
Arachnophobia F40.210
Arboencephalitis, Australian A83.4
Arborization block (heart) I45.5
ARC (AIDS-related complex) B20
Arches —*see* condition
Arcuate uterus Q51.810
Arcuatus uterus Q51.810
Arcus (cornea) **senilis** —*see* Degeneration, cornea, senile
Arc-welder's lung J63.4
Areflexia R29.2
Areola —*see* condition
Argentaffinoma —*see also* Neoplasm, uncertain behavior, by site
malignant —*see* Neoplasm, malignant, by site
syndrome E34.0
Argininemia E72.21
Arginosuccinic aciduria E72.22
Argyll Robertson phenomenon, pupil or syndrome (syphilitic) A52.19
atypical H57.09
nonsyphilitic H57.09
Argyria, argyriasis
conjunctival H11.13
from drug or medicament —*see* Table of Drugs and Chemicals, by substance
Argyrosis, conjunctival H11.13
Arhinencephaly Q04.1
Ariboflavinosis E53.0
Arm —*see* condition

Arnold-Chiari disease, obstruction or syndrome (type II) Q07.00
  with
    hydrocephalus Q07.02
      with spina bifida Q07.03
    spina bifida Q07.01
      with hydrocephalus Q07.03
  type III —*see* Encephalocele
  type IV Q04.8
Aromatic amino-acid metabolism disorder E70.9
  specified NEC E70.8
Arousals, confusional G47.51
Arrest, arrested
  cardiac I46.9
    complicating
      abortion —*see* Abortion, by type, complicated by, cardiac arrest
      anesthesia (general) (local) or other sedation —*see* Table of Drugs and Chemicals, by drug
        in labor and delivery O74.2
        in pregnancy O29.11
        postpartum, puerperal O89.1
      delivery (cesarean) (instrumental) O75.4
    due to
      cardiac condition I46.2
      specified condition NEC I46.8
    intraoperative I97.71
    newborn P29.81
    postprocedural I97.12
      obstetric procedure O75.4
  cardiorespiratory —*see* Arrest, cardiac
  circulatory —*see* Arrest, cardiac
  deep transverse O64.0
  development or growth
    bone —*see* Disorder, bone, development or growth
    child R62.50
    tracheal rings Q32.1
  epiphyseal
    complete
      femur M89.15
      humerus M89.12
      tibia M89.16
      ulna M89.13
      forearm M89.13
        specified NEC M89.13
      ulna —*see* Arrest, epiphyseal, by type,
    ulna
      lower leg M89.16
        specified NEC M89.168
      tibia —*see* Arrest, epiphyseal, by type,
    tibia
      partial
        femur M89.15
        humerus M89.12
        tibia M89.16
        ulna M89.13
        specified NEC M89.18
  granulopoiesis —*see* Agranulocytosis
  growth plate —*see* Arrest, epiphyseal
  heart —*see* Arrest, cardiac
  legal, anxiety concerning Z65.3
  physeal —*see* Arrest, epiphyseal
  respiratory R09.2
    newborn P28.81
  sinus I45.5
  spermatogenesis (complete) —*see* Azoospermia
    incomplete —*see* Oligospermia
  transverse (deep) O64.0

Arrhenoblastoma
  benign
    specified site —*see* Neoplasm, benign, by site
    unspecified site
      female D27.9
      male D29.20
  malignant
    specified site —*see* Neoplasm, malignant, by site
    unspecified site
      female C56.9
      male C62.90
  specified site —*see* Neoplasm, uncertain behavior, by site
  unspecified site
    female D39.10
    male D40.10
Arrhythmia (auricle) (cardiac) (juvenile) (nodal) (reflex) (sinus) (supraventricular) (transitory) (ventricle) I49.9
  block I45.9
  extrasystolic I49.49
  newborn
    bradycardia P29.12
    occurring before birth P03.819
      before onset of labor P03.810
      during labor P03.811
    tachycardia P29.11
  psychogenic F45.8
  specified NEC I49.8
  vagal R55
  ventricular re-entry I47.0
Arrillaga-Ayerza syndrome (pulmonary sclerosis with pulmonary hypertension) I27.0
Arsenical pigmentation L81.8
  from drug or medicament —*see* Table of Drugs and Chemicals
Arsenism —*see* Poisoning, arsenic
Arterial —*see* condition
Arteriofibrosis —*see* Arteriosclerosis
Arteriolar sclerosis —*see* Arteriosclerosis
Arteriolith —*see* Arteriosclerosis
Arteriolitis I77.6
  necrotizing, kidney I77.5
  renal —*see* Hypertension, kidney
Arteriolosclerosis —*see* Arteriosclerosis
Arterionephrosclerosis —*see* Hypertension, kidney
Arteriopathy I77.9
Arteriosclerosis, arteriosclerotic (diffuse) (obliterans) (of) (senile) (with calcification) I70.90
  aorta I70.0
  arteries of extremities —*see* Arteriosclerosis, extremities
  brain I67.2
  bypass graft
    coronary —*see* Arteriosclerosis, coronary, bypass graft
    extremities —*see* Arteriosclerosis, extremities, bypass graft
  cardiac —*see* Disease, heart, ischemic, atherosclerotic
  cardiopathy —*see* Disease, heart, ischemic, atherosclerotic
  cardiorenal —*see* Hypertension, cardiorenal
  cardiovascular —*see* Disease, heart, ischemic, atherosclerotic
  carotid (*see also* Occlusion, artery, carotid) I65.2
  central nervous system I67.2

  cerebral I67.2
  cerebrovascular I67.2
  coronary (artery) I25.10
    due to
      calcified coronary lesion (severely) I25.84
      lipid rich plaque I25.83
    bypass graft I25.810
      with
        angina pectoris I25.709
          with documented spasm I25.701
          specified type NEC I25.708
          unstable I25.700
        ischemic chest pain I25.709
    autologous artery I25.810
      with
        angina pectoris I25.729
          with documented spasm I25.721
          specified type I25.728
          unstable I25.720
        ischemic chest pain I25.729
    autologous vein I25.810
      with
        angina pectoris I25.719
          with documented spasm I25.711
          specified type I25.718
          unstable I25.710
        ischemic chest pain I25.719
    nonautologous biological I25.810
      with
        angina pectoris I25.739
          with documented spasm I25.731
          specified type I25.738
          unstable I25.730
        ischemic chest pain I25.739
    specified type NEC I25.810
      with
        angina pectoris I25.799
          with documented spasm I25.791
          specified type I25.798
          unstable I25.790
        ischemic chest pain I25.799
    native vessel
      with
        angina pectoris I25.119
          with documented spasm I25.111
          specified type NEC I25.118
          unstable I25.110
        ischemic chest pain I25.119
    transplanted heart I25.811
      bypass graft I25.812
        with
          angina pectoris I25.769
            with documented spasm I25.761
            specified type I25.768
            unstable I25.760
          ischemic chest pain I25.769
      native coronary artery I25.811
        with
          angina pectoris I25.759
            with documented spasm I25.751
            specified type I25.758
            unstable I25.750
          ischemic chest pain I25.759
  extremities (native arteries) I70.209
    bypass graft I70.309
      autologous vein graft I70.409
        leg I70.409
          with
            gangrene (and intermittent claudication, rest pain and ulcer) I70.469
            intermittent claudication I70.419

Arteriosclerosis, arteriosclerotic - *continued*
    rest pain (and intermittent
       claudication) I70.429
      bilateral I70.403
        with
          gangrene (and intermittent
        claudication, rest pain and ulcer) I70.463
            intermittent claudication I70.413
            rest pain (and intermittent
        claudication) I70.423
            specified type NEC I70.493
      left I70.402
        with
          gangrene (and intermittent
        claudication, rest pain and ulcer) I70.462
            intermittent claudication I70.412
            rest pain (and intermittent
        claudication) I70.422
            ulceration (and intermittent
        claudication and rest pain) I70.449
          ankle I70.443
          calf I70.442
          foot site NEC I70.445
          heel I70.444
          lower leg NEC I70.448
          midfoot I70.444
          thigh I70.441
        specified type NEC I70.492
      right I70.401
        with
          gangrene (and intermittent
        claudication, rest pain and ulcer) I70.461
            intermittent claudication I70.411
            rest pain (and intermittent
        claudication) I70.421
            ulceration (and intermittent
        claudication and rest pain) I70.439
          ankle I70.433
          calf I70.432
          foot site NEC I70.435
          heel I70.434
          lower leg NEC I70.438
          midfoot I70.434
          thigh I70.431
        specified type NEC I70.491
      specified type NEC I70.499
    specified NEC I70.408
      with
        gangrene (and intermittent
      claudication, rest pain and ulcer) I70.468
          intermittent claudication I70.418
          rest pain (and intermittent
      claudication) I70.428
          ulceration (and intermittent
      claudication and rest pain) I70.45
        specified type NEC I70.498
    leg I70.309
      with
        gangrene (and intermittent claudication,
    rest pain and ulcer) I70.369
        intermittent claudication I70.319
        rest pain (and intermittent claudication)
    I70.329
      bilateral I70.303
        with
          gangrene (and intermittent
        claudication, rest pain and ulcer) I70.363
            intermittent claudication I70.313
            rest pain (and intermittent
        claudication) I70.323
            specified type NEC I70.393
      left I70.302

Arteriosclerosis, arteriosclerotic - *continued*
      with
        gangrene (and intermittent
      claudication, rest pain and ulcer) I70.362
          intermittent claudication I70.312
          rest pain (and intermittent
      claudication) I70.322
          ulceration (and intermittent
      claudication and rest pain) I70.349
        ankle I70.343
        calf I70.342
        foot site NEC I70.345
        heel I70.344
        lower leg NEC I70.348
        midfoot I70.344
        thigh I70.341
      specified type NEC I70.392
    right I70.301
      with
        gangrene (and intermittent
      claudication, rest pain and ulcer) I70.361
          intermittent claudication I70.311
          rest pain (and intermittent
      claudication) I70.321
          ulceration (and intermittent
      claudication and rest pain) I70.339
        ankle I70.333
        calf I70.332
        foot site NEC I70.335
        heel I70.334
        lower leg NEC I70.338
        midfoot I70.334
        thigh I70.331
      specified type NEC I70.391
    specified type NEC I70.399
    nonautologous biological graft I70.509
    leg I70.509
      with
        gangrene (and intermittent
      claudication, rest pain and ulcer) I70.569
          intermittent claudication I70.519
          rest pain (and intermittent
      claudication) I70.529
      bilateral I70.503
        with
          gangrene (and intermittent
        claudication, rest pain and ulcer) I70.563
            intermittent claudication I70.513
            rest pain (and intermittent
        claudication) I70.523
            specified type NEC I70.593
      left I70.502
        with
          gangrene (and intermittent
        claudication, rest pain and ulcer) I70.562
            intermittent claudication I70.512
            rest pain (and intermittent
        claudication) I70.522
            ulceration (and intermittent
        claudication and rest pain) I70.549
          ankle I70.543
          calf I70.542
          foot site NEC I70.545
          heel I70.544
          lower leg NEC I70.548
          midfoot I70.544
          thigh I70.541
        specified type NEC I70.592
      right I70.501
        with
          gangrene (and intermittent
        claudication, rest pain and ulcer) I70.561

Arteriosclerosis, arteriosclerotic - *continued*
      intermittent claudication I70.511
      rest pain (and intermittent
    claudication) I70.521
      ulceration (and intermittent
    claudication and rest pain) I70.539
      ankle I70.533
      calf I70.532
      foot site NEC I70.535
      heel I70.534
      lower leg NEC I70.538
      midfoot I70.534
      thigh I70.531
    specified type NEC I70.591
    specified type NEC I70.599
    specified NEC I70.508
      with
        gangrene (and intermittent
      claudication, rest pain and ulcer) I70.568
          intermittent claudication I70.518
          rest pain (and intermittent
      claudication) I70.528
          ulceration (and intermittent
      claudication and rest pain) I70.55
        specified type NEC I70.598
    nonbiological graft I70.609
    leg I70.609
      with
        gangrene (and intermittent
      claudication, rest pain and ulcer) I70.669
          intermittent claudication I70.619
          rest pain (and intermittent
      claudication) I70.629
      bilateral I70.603
        with
          gangrene (and intermittent
        claudication, rest pain and ulcer) I70.663
            intermittent claudication I70.613
            rest pain (and intermittent
        claudication) I70.623
            specified type NEC I70.693
      left I70.602
        with
          gangrene (and intermittent
        claudication, rest pain and ulcer) I70.662
            intermittent claudication I70.612
            rest pain (and intermittent
        claudication) I70.622
            ulceration (and intermittent
        claudication and rest pain) I70.649
          ankle I70.643
          calf I70.642
          foot site NEC I70.645
          heel I70.644
          lower leg NEC I70.648
          midfoot I70.644
          thigh I70.641
        specified type NEC I70.692
      right I70.601
        with
          gangrene (and intermittent
        claudication, rest pain and ulcer) I70.661
            intermittent claudication I70.611
            rest pain (and intermittent
        claudication) I70.621
            ulceration (and intermittent
        claudication and rest pain) I70.639
          ankle I70.633
          calf I70.632
          foot site NEC I70.635
          heel I70.634
          lower leg NEC I70.638
          midfoot I70.634

Arteriosclerosis, arteriosclerotic *- continued*
  thigh I70.631
    specified type NEC I70.691
    specified type NEC I70.699
  specified NEC I70.608
    with
      gangrene (and intermittent
    claudication, rest pain and ulcer) I70.668
      intermittent claudication I70.618
      rest pain (and intermittent
    claudication) I70.628
      ulceration (and intermittent
    claudication and rest pain) I70.65
      specified type NEC I70.698
  specified graft NEC I70.709
    leg I70.709
      with
        gangrene (and intermittent
    claudication, rest pain and ulcer) I70.769
        intermittent claudication I70.719
        rest pain (and intermittent
    claudication) I70.729
      bilateral I70.703
        with
          gangrene (and intermittent
    claudication, rest pain and ulcer) I70.763
          intermittent claudication I70.713
          rest pain (and intermittent
    claudication) I70.723
        specified type NEC I70.793
      left I70.702
        with
          gangrene (and intermittent
    claudication, rest pain and ulcer) I70.762
          intermittent claudication I70.712
          rest pain (and intermittent
    claudication) I70.722
        ulceration (and intermittent
    claudication and rest pain) I70.749
          ankle I70.743
          calf I70.742
          foot site NEC I70.745
          heel I70.744
          lower leg NEC I70.748
          midfoot I70.744
          thigh I70.741
        specified type NEC I70.792
      right I70.701
        with
          gangrene (and intermittent
    claudication, rest pain and ulcer) I70.761
          intermittent claudication I70.711
          rest pain (and intermittent
    claudication) I70.721
        ulceration (and intermittent
    claudication and rest pain) I70.739
          ankle I70.733
          calf I70.732
          foot site NEC I70.735
          heel I70.734
          lower leg NEC I70.738
          midfoot I70.734
          thigh I70.731
        specified type NEC I70.791
      specified type NEC I70.799
    specified NEC I70.708
      with
        gangrene (and intermittent
    claudication, rest pain and ulcer) I70.768
        intermittent claudication I70.718
        rest pain (and intermittent
    claudication) I70.728

Arteriosclerosis, arteriosclerotic *- continued*
    ulceration (and intermittent
  claudication and rest pain) I70.75
      specified type NEC I70.798
    specified NEC I70.308
      with
        gangrene (and intermittent claudication,
  rest pain and ulcer) I70.368
        intermittent claudication I70.318
        rest pain (and intermittent claudication)
  I70.328
        ulceration (and intermittent claudication
  and rest pain) I70.35
        specified type NEC I70.398
    leg I70.209
      with
        gangrene (and intermittent claudication,
  rest pain and ulcer) I70.269
        intermittent claudication I70.219
        rest pain (and intermittent claudication)
  I70.229
      bilateral I70.203
        with
          gangrene (and intermittent claudication,
  rest pain and ulcer) I70.263
          intermittent claudication I70.213
          rest pain (and intermittent claudication)
  I70.223
        specified type NEC I70.293
      left I70.202
        with
          gangrene (and intermittent claudication,
  rest pain and ulcer) I70.262
          intermittent claudication I70.212
          rest pain (and intermittent claudication)
  I70.222
          ulceration (and intermittent claudication
  and rest pain) I70.249
          ankle I70.243
          calf I70.242
          foot site NEC I70.245
          heel I70.244
          lower leg NEC I70.248
          midfoot I70.244
          thigh I70.241
        specified type NEC I70.292
      right I70.201
        with
          gangrene (and intermittent claudication,
  rest pain and ulcer) I70.261
          intermittent claudication I70.211
          rest pain (and intermittent claudication)
  I70.221
          ulceration (and intermittent claudication
  and rest pain) I70.239
          ankle I70.233
          calf I70.232
          foot site NEC I70.235
          heel I70.234
          lower leg NEC I70.238
          midfoot I70.234
          thigh I70.231
        specified type NEC I70.291
      specified type NEC I70.299
    specified site NEC I70.208
      with
        gangrene (and intermittent claudication,
  rest pain and ulcer) I70.268
        intermittent claudication I70.218
        rest pain (and intermittent claudication)
  I70.228

Arteriosclerosis, arteriosclerotic *- continued*
    ulceration (and intermittent claudication
  and rest pain) I70.25
      specified type NEC I70.298
  generalized I70.91
  heart (disease) —*see* Arteriosclerosis,
  coronary (artery)
  kidney —*see* Hypertension, kidney
  medial —*see* Arteriosclerosis, extremities
  mesenteric (artery) K55.1
  Mönckeberg's —*see* Arteriosclerosis,
  extremities
  myocarditis I51.4
  peripheral (of extremities) —*see*
  Arteriosclerosis, extremities
  pulmonary (idiopathic) I27.0
  renal (arterioles) —*see also* Hypertension,
  kidney
    artery I70.1
  retina (vascular) I70.8 *[H35.0]*
  specified artery NEC I70.8
  spinal (cord) G95.19
  vertebral (artery) I67.2
Arteriospasm I73.9
Arteriovenous —*see* condition
Arteritis I77.6
  allergic M31.0
  aorta (nonsyphilitic) I77.6
    syphilitic A52.02
  aortic arch M31.4
  brachiocephalic M31.4
  brain I67.7
    syphilitic A52.04
  cerebral I67.7
    in
      diseases classified elsewhere I68.2
      systemic lupus erythematosus M32.19
    listerial A32.89
    syphilitic A52.04
    tuberculous A18.89
  coronary (artery) I25.89
    rheumatic I01.8
      chronic I09.89
    syphilitic A52.06
  cranial (left) (right) , giant cell M31.6
  deformans —*see* Arteriosclerosis
  giant cell NEC M31.6
    with polymyalgia rheumatica M31.5
  necrosing or necrotizing M31.9
    specified NEC M31.8
  nodosa M30.0
  obliterans —*see* Arteriosclerosis
  pulmonary I28.8
  rheumatic —*see* Fever, rheumatic
  senile —*see* Arteriosclerosis
  suppurative I77.2
  syphilitic (general) A52.09
    brain A52.04
    coronary A52.06
    spinal A52.09
  temporal, giant cell M31.6
  young female aortic arch syndrome M31.4
Artery, arterial —*see also* condition
  abscess I77.89
  single umbilical Q27.0
Arthralgia (allergic) —*see also* Pain, joint
  in caisson disease T70.3
  temporomandibular M26.62
Arthritis, arthritic (acute) (chronic)
  (nonpyogenic) (subacute) M19.90
  allergic —*see* Arthritis, specified form NEC
  ankylosing (crippling) (spine) —*see also*
  Spondylitis, ankylosing

Arthritis, arthritic - *continued*
  sites other than spine —*see* Arthritis, specified form NEC
  atrophic —*see* Osteoarthritis
    spine —*see* Spondylitis, ankylosing
  back —*see* Spondylopathy, inflammatory
  blennorrhagic (gonococcal) A54.42
  Charcot's —*see* Arthropathy, neuropathic
    diabetic —*see* Diabetes, arthropathy, neuropathic
    syringomyelic G95.0
  chylous (filarial) (*see also* category M01) B74.9
  climacteric (any site) NEC —*see* Arthritis, specified form NEC
  crystal (-induced) —*see* Arthritis, in, crystals
  deformans —*see* Osteoarthritis
  degenerative —*see* Osteoarthritis
  due to or associated with
    acromegaly E22.0
    brucellosis —*see* Brucellosis
    caisson disease T70.3
    diabetes —*see* Diabetes, arthropathy
    dracontiasis (*see also* category M01) B72
    enteritis NEC
      regional —*see* Enteritis, regional
    erysipelas (*see also* category M01) A46
    erythema
      epidemic A25.1
      nodosum L52
    filariasis NOS B74.9
    glanders A24.0
    helminthiasis (*see also* category M01) B83.9
    hemophilia D66 *[M36.2]*
    Henoch (Schönlein) purpura D69.0 *[M36.4]*
    human parvovirus (*see also* category M01) B97.6
    infectious disease NEC —see category M01
    leprosy (see also category M01) (*see also* Leprosy) A30.9
    Lyme disease A69.23
    mycobacteria (*see also* category M01) A31.8
    parasitic disease NEC (*see also* category M01) B89
    paratyphoid fever (see also category M01) (*see also* Fever, paratyphoid) A01.4
    rat bite fever (*see also* category M01) A25.1
    regional enteritis —*see* Enteritis, regional
    respiratory disorder NOS J98.9
    serum sickness (*see also* Reaction, serum) T80.69
    syringomyelia G95.0
    typhoid fever A01.04
  epidemic erythema A25.1
  febrile —*see* Fever, rheumatic
  gonococcal A54.42
  gouty (acute) —*see* Gout, idiopathic
  in (due to)
    acromegaly (*see also* subcategory M14.8) E22.0
    amyloidosis (*see also* subcategory M14.8) E85.4
    bacterial disease (*see also* subcategory M01) A49.9
      Behçet's syndrome M35.2
    caisson disease (*see also* subcategory M14.8) T70.3
    coliform bacilli (Escherichia coli) —*see* Arthritis, in, pyogenic organism NEC
    crystals M11.9

Arthritis, arthritic - *continued*
    dicalcium phosphate —*see* Arthritis, in, crystals, specified type NEC
      hydroxyapatite M11.0
    pyrophosphate —*see* Arthritis, in, crystals, specified type NEC
      specified type NEC M11.80
        ankle M11.87
        elbow M11.82
        foot joint M11.87
        hand joint M11.84
        hip M11.85
        knee M11.86
        multiple sites M11.8
        shoulder M11.81
        vertebrae M11.88
        wrist M11.83
    dermatoarthritis, lipoid E78.81
    dracontiasis (dracunculiasis) (*see also* category M01) B72
    endocrine disorder NEC (*see also* subcategory M14.8) E34.9
    enteritis, infectious NEC (*see also* category M01) A09
      specified organism NEC (*see also* category M01) A08.8
    erythema
      multiforme (*see also* subcategory M14.8) L51.9
      nodosum (*see also* subcategory M14.8) L52
    gout —*see* Gout, idiopathic
    helminthiasis NEC (*see also* category M01) B83.9
    hemochromatosis (*see also* subcategory M14.8) E83.118
    hemoglobinopathy NEC D58.2 *[M36.3]*
    hemophilia NEC D66 *[M36.2]*
    Hemophilus influenzae M00.8 *[B96.3]*
    Henoch (-Schönlein) purpura D69.0 *[M36.4]*
    hyperparathyroidism NEC (*see also* subcategory M14.8) E21.3
    hypersensitivity reaction NEC T78.49 *[M36.4]*
    hypogammaglobulinemia (*see also* subcategory M14.8) D80.1
    hypothyroidism NEC (*see also* subcategory M14.8) E03.9
    infection —*see* Arthritis, pyogenic or pyemic
      spine —*see* Spondylopathy, infective
    infectious disease NEC —see category M01
    leprosy (*see also* category M01) A30.9
    leukemia NEC C95.9 *[M36.1]*
    lipoid dermatoarthritis E78.81
    Lyme disease A69.23
    Mediterranean fever, familial (*see also* subcategory M14.8) E85.0
    Meningococcus A39.83
    metabolic disorder NEC (*see also* subcategory M14.8) E88.9
    multiple myelomatosis C90.0 *[M36.1]*
    mumps B26.85
    mycosis NEC (*see also* category M01) B49
    myelomatosis (multiple) C90.0 *[M36.1]*
    neurological disorder NEC G98.0
    ochronosis (*see also* subcategory M14.8) E70.29
    O'nyong-nyong (*see also* category M01) A92.1

Arthritis, arthritic - *continued*
    parasitic disease NEC (*see also* category M01) B89
    paratyphoid fever (*see also* category M01) A01.4
    Pseudomonas —*see* Arthritis, pyogenic, bacterial NEC
    psoriasis L40.50
    pyogenic organism NEC —*see* Arthritis, pyogenic, bacterial NEC
    Reiter's disease —*see* Reiter's disease
    respiratory disorder NEC (*see also* subcategory M14.8) J98.9
    reticulosis, malignant (*see also* subcategory M14.8) C86.0
    rubella B06.82
    Salmonella (arizonae) (cholerae-suis) (enteritidis) (typhimurium) A02.23
    sarcoidosis D86.86
    specified bacteria NEC —*see* Arthritis, pyogenic, bacterial NEC
    sporotrichosis B42.82
    syringomyelia G95.0
    thalassemia NEC D56.9 *[M36.3]*
    tuberculosis —*see* Tuberculosis, arthritis
    typhoid fever A01.04
    urethritis, Reiter's —*see* Reiter's disease
    viral disease NEC (*see also* category M01) B34.9
  infectious or infective —*see also* Arthritis, pyogenic or pyemic
    spine —*see* Spondylopathy, infective
  juvenile M08.90
    with systemic onset —*see* Still's disease
    ankle M08.97
    elbow M08.92
    foot joint M08.97
    hand joint M08.94
    hip M08.95
    knee M08.96
    multiple site M08.99
    pauciarticular M08.40
      ankle M08.47
      elbow M08.42
      foot joint M08.47
      hand joint M08.44
      hip M08.45
      knee M08.46
      shoulder M08.41
      vertebrae M08.48
      wrist M08.43
    psoriatic L40.54
    rheumatoid —*see* Arthritis, rheumatoid, juvenile
    shoulder M08.91
    vertebra M08.98
    specified type NEC M08.80
      ankle M08.87
      elbow M08.82
      foot joint M08.87
      hand joint M08.84
      hip M08.85
      knee M08.86
      multiple site M08.89
      shoulder M08.81
      specified joint NEC M08.88
      vertebrae M08.88
      wrist M08.83
    wrist M08.93
  meaning osteoarthritis —*see* Osteoarthritis
  meningococcal A39.83
  menopausal (any site) NEC —*see* Arthritis, specified form NEC

Arthritis, arthritic - *continued*
mutilans (psoriatic) L40.52
mycotic NEC (*see also* category M01) B49
neuropathic (Charcot) —*see* Arthropathy,
neuropathic
diabetic —*see* Diabetes, arthropathy,
neuropathic
nonsyphilitic NEC G98.0
syringomyelic G95.0
ochronotic (*see also* subcategory M14.8)
E70.29
palindromic (any site) —*see* Rheumatism,
palindromic
pneumococcal M00.10
ankle M00.17
elbow M00.12
foot joint —*see* Arthritis, pneumococcal,
ankle
hand joint M00.14
hip M00.15
knee M00.16
multiple site M00.19
shoulder M00.11
vertebra M00.18
wrist M00.13
postdysenteric —*see* Arthropathy,
postdysenteric
postmeningococcal A39.84
postrheumatic, chronic —*see* Arthropathy,
postrheumatic, chronic
primary progressive —*see also* Arthritis,
specified form NEC
spine —*see* Spondylitis, ankylosing
psoriatic L40.50
purulent (any site except spine) —*see*
Arthritis, pyogenic or pyemic
spine —*see* Spondylopathy, infective
pyogenic or pyemic (any site except spine)
M00.9
bacterial NEC M00.80
ankle M00.87
elbow M00.82
foot joint —*see* Arthritis, pyogenic,
bacterial NEC, ankle
hand joint M00.84
hip M00.85
knee M00.86
multiple site M00.89
shoulder M00.81
vertebra M00.88
wrist M00.83
pneumococcal —*see* Arthritis,
pneumococcal
spine —*see* Spondylopathy, infective
staphylococcal —*see* Arthritis,
staphylococcal
streptococcal —*see* Arthritis, streptococcal
NEC
pneumococcal —*see* Arthritis,
pneumococcal
reactive —*see* Reiter's disease
rheumatic —*see also* Arthritis, rheumatoid
acute or subacute —*see* Fever, rheumatic
rheumatoid M06.9
with
carditis —*see* Rheumatoid, carditis
endocarditis —*see* Rheumatoid, carditis
heart involvement NEC —*see* Rheumatoid,
carditis
lung involvement —*see* Rheumatoid, lung
myocarditis —*see* Rheumatoid, carditis
myopathy —*see* Rheumatoid, myopathy

Arthritis, arthritic - *continued*
pericarditis —*see* Rheumatoid, carditis
polyneuropathy —*see* Rheumatoid,
polyneuropathy
rheumatoid factor —*see* Arthritis,
rheumatoid, seropositive
splenoadenomegaly and leukopenia —*see*
Felty's syndrome
vasculitis —*see* Rheumatoid, vasculitis
visceral involvement NEC —*see*
Rheumatoid, arthritis, with involvement of
organs NEC
juvenile (with or without rheumatoid factor)
M08.00
ankle M08.07
elbow M08.02
foot joint M08.07
hand joint M08.04
hip M08.05
knee M08.06
multiple site M08.09
shoulder M08.01
vertebra M08.08
wrist M08.03
seronegative M06.00
ankle M06.07
elbow M06.02
foot joint M06.07
hand joint M06.04
hip M06.05
knee M06.06
multiple site M06.09
shoulder M06.01
vertebra M06.08
wrist M06.03
seropositive M05.9
specified NEC M05.80
ankle M05.87
elbow M05.82
foot joint M05.87
hand joint M05.84
hip M05.85
knee M05.86
multiple sites M05.89
shoulder M05.81
vertebra —*see* Spondylitis, ankylosing
wrist M05.83
without organ involvement M05.70
ankle M05.77
elbow M05.72
foot joint M05.77
hand joint M05.74
hip M05.75
knee M05.76
multiple sites M05.79
shoulder M05.71
vertebra —*see* Spondylitis, ankylosing
wrist M05.73
specified type NEC M06.80
ankle M06.87
elbow M06.82
foot joint M06.87
hand joint M06.84
hip M06.85
knee M06.86
multiple site M06.89
shoulder M06.81
vertebra M06.88
wrist M06.83
spine —*see* Spondylitis, ankylosing
rubella B06.82
scorbutic (*see also* subcategory M14.8) E54

Arthritis, arthritic - *continued*
senile or senescent —*see* Osteoarthritis
septic (any site except spine) —*see* Arthritis,
pyogenic or pyemic
spine —*see* Spondylopathy, infective
serum (nontherapeutic) (therapeutic) —*see*
Arthropathy, postimmunization
specified form NEC M13.80
ankle M13.87
elbow M13.82
foot joint M13.87
hand joint M13.84
hip M13.85
knee M13.86
multiple site M13.89
shoulder M13.81
specified joint NEC M13.88
wrist M13.83
spine —*see also* Spondylopathy,
inflammatory
infectious or infective NEC —*see*
Spondylopathy, infective
Marie-Strümpell —*see* Spondylitis,
ankylosing
pyogenic —*see* Spondylopathy, infective
rheumatoid —*see* Spondylitis, ankylosing
traumatic (old) —*see* Spondylopathy,
traumatic
tuberculous A18.01
staphylococcal M00.00
ankle M00.07
elbow M00.02
foot joint —*see* Arthritis, staphylococcal,
ankle
hand joint M00.04
hip M00.05
knee M00.06
multiple site M00.09
shoulder M00.01
vertebra M00.08
wrist M00.03
streptococcal NEC M00.20
ankle M00.27
elbow M00.22
foot joint —*see* Arthritis, streptococcal,
ankle
hand joint M00.24
hip M00.25
knee M00.26
multiple site M00.29
shoulder M00.21
vertebra M00.28
wrist M00.23
suppurative —*see* Arthritis, pyogenic or
pyemic
syphilitic (late) A52.16
congenital A50.55 *[M12.80]*
syphilitica deformans (Charcot) A52.16
temporomandibular M26.69
toxic of menopause (any site) —*see* Arthritis,
specified form NEC
transient —*see* Arthropathy, specified form
NEC
traumatic (chronic) —*see* Arthropathy,
traumatic
tuberculous A18.02
spine A18.01
uratic —*see* Gout, idiopathic
urethritica (Reiter's) —*see* Reiter's disease
vertebral —*see* Spondylopathy, inflammatory
villous (any site) —*see* Arthropathy, specified
form NEC

Arthrocele —*see* Effusion, joint
Arthrodesis status Z98.1
Arthrodynia —*see also* Pain, joint
Arthrodysplasia Q74.9
Arthrofibrosis, joint —*see* Ankylosis
Arthrogryposis (congenital) Q68.8
  multiplex congenita Q74.3
Arthrokatadysis M24.7
Arthropathy (*see also* Arthritis) M12.9
  Charcot's —*see* Arthropathy, neuropathic
    diabetic —*see* Diabetes, arthropathy,
    neuropathic
      syringomyelic G95.0
  cricoarytenoid J38.7
  crystal (-induced) —*see* Arthritis, in, crystals
  diabetic NEC —*see* Diabetes, arthropathy
  distal interphalangeal, psoriatic L40.51
  enteropathic M07.60
    ankle M07.67
    elbow M07.62
    foot joint M07.67
    hand joint M07.64
    hip M07.65
    knee M07.66
    multiple site M07.69
    shoulder M07.61
    vertebra M07.68
    wrist M07.63
  following intestinal bypass M02.00
    ankle M02.07
    elbow M02.02
    foot joint M02.07
    hand joint M02.04
    hip M02.05
    knee M02.06
    multiple site M02.09
    shoulder M02.01
    vertebra M02.08
    wrist M02.03
  gouty —*see also* Gout, idiopathic
    in (due to)
      Lesch-Nyhan syndrome E79.1 *[M14.8]*
      sickle-cell disorders D57 *[M14.8]*
  hemophilic NEC D66 *[M36.2]*
    in (due to)
      hyperparathyroidism NEC E21.3 *[M14.8]*
      metabolic disease NOS E88.9 *[M14.8]*
  in (due to)
    acromegaly E22.0 *[M14.8]*
    amyloidosis E85.4 *[M14.8]*
    blood disorder NOS D75.9 *[M36.3]*
    diabetes —*see* Diabetes, arthropathy
    endocrine disease NOS E34.9 *[M14.8]*
    erythema
      multiforme L51.9 *[M14.8]*
      nodosum L52 *[M14.8]*
    hemochromatosis E83.118 *[M14.8]*
    hemoglobinopathy NEC D58.2 *[M36.3]*
    hemophilia NEC D66 *[M36.2]*
    Henoch-Schönlein purpura D69.0 *[M36.4]*
    hyperthyroidism E05.90 *[M14.8]*
    hypothyroidism E03.9 *[M14.8]*
    infective endocarditis I33.0 *[M12.80]*
    leukemia NEC C95.9 *[M36.1]*
    malignant histiocytosis C96.A *[M36.1]*
    metabolic disease NOS E88.9 *[M14.8]*
    multiple myeloma C90.0 *[M36.1]*
    neoplastic disease NOS (see also Neoplasm)
    D49.9 *[M36.1]*
    nutritional deficiency (*see also* subcategory
    M14.8) E63.9
      psoriasis NOS L40.50

Arthropathy - *continued*
  sarcoidosis D86.86
  syphilis (late) A52.77
    congenital A50.55 *[M12.80]*
  thyrotoxicosis (*see also* subcategory M14.8
) E05.90
    ulcerative colitis K51.90 *[M07.60]*
    viral hepatitis (postinfectious) NEC B19.9
  [M12.80]
    Whipple's disease (*see also* subcategory
  M14.8) K90.81
  Jaccoud —*see* Arthropathy, postrheumatic,
  chronic
  juvenile —*see* Arthritis, juvenile
    psoriatic L40.54
  mutilans (psoriatic) L40.52
  neuropathic (Charcot) M14.60
    ankle M14.67
    diabetic —*see* Diabetes, arthropathy,
    neuropathic
    elbow M14.62
    foot joint M14.67
    hand joint M14.64
    hip M14.65
    knee M14.66
    multiple site M14.69
    nonsyphilitic NEC G98.0
    shoulder M14.61
    syringomyelic G95.0
    vertebra M14.68
    wrist M14.63
  osteopulmonary —*see* Osteoarthropathy,
  hypertrophic, specified NEC
  postdysenteric M02.10
    ankle M02.17
    elbow M02.12
    foot joint M02.17
    hand joint M02.14
    hip M02.15
    knee M02.16
    multiple site M02.19
    shoulder M02.11
    vertebra M02.18
    wrist M02.13
  postimmunization M02.20
    ankle M02.27
    elbow M02.22
    foot joint M02.27
    hand joint M02.24
    hip M02.25
    knee M02.26
    multiple site M02.29
    shoulder M02.21
    vertebra M02.28
    wrist M02.23
  postinfectious NEC B99 *[M12.80]*
    in (due to)
      enteritis due to Yersinia enterocolitica
    A04.6 *[M12.80]*
      syphilis A52.77
      viral hepatitis NEC B19.9 *[M12.80]*
  postrheumatic, chronic (Jaccoud) M12.00
    ankle M12.07
    elbow M12.02
    foot joint M12.07
    hand joint M12.04
    hip M12.05
    knee M12.06
    multiple site M12.09
    shoulder M12.01
    specified joint NEC M12.08
    vertebrae M12.08

Arthropathy - *continued*
  wrist M12.03
  psoriatic NEC L40.59
    interphalangeal, distal L40.51
  reactive M02.9
    in (due to)
      infective endocarditis I33.0 *[M02.9]*
    specified type NEC M02.80
      ankle M02.87
      elbow M02.82
      foot joint M02.87
      hand joint M02.84
      hip M02.85
      knee M02.86
      multiple site M02.89
      shoulder M02.81
      vertebra M02.88
      wrist M02.83
  specified form NEC M12.80
    ankle M12.87
    elbow M12.82
    foot joint M12.87
    hand joint M12.84
    hip M12.85
    knee M12.86
    multiple site M12.89
    shoulder M12.81
    specified joint NEC M12.88
    vertebrae M12.88
    wrist M12.83
  syringomyelic G95.0
  tabes dorsalis A52.16
  tabetic A52.16
  transient —*see* Arthropathy, specified form
  NEC
  traumatic M12.50
    ankle M12.57
    elbow M12.52
    foot joint M12.57
    hand joint M12.54
    hip M12.55
    knee M12.56
    multiple site M12.59
    shoulder M12.51
    specified joint NEC M12.58
    vertebrae M12.58
    wrist M12.53
Arthropyosis —*see* Arthritis, pyogenic or
pyemic
Arthrosis (deformans) (degenerative)
(localized) (*see also* Osteoarthritis) M19.90
  spine —*see* Spondylosis
Arthus' phenomenon or reaction T78.41
  due to
    drug —*see* Table of Drugs and Chemicals,
  by drug
Articular —*see* condition
Articulation, reverse (teeth) M26.24
Artificial
  insemination complication —*see*
  Complications, artificial, fertilization
  opening status (functioning) (without
  complication) Z93.9
    anus (colostomy) Z93.3
    colostomy Z93.3
    cystostomy Z93.50
      appendico-vesicostomy Z93.52
      cutaneous Z93.51
      specified NEC Z93.59
    enterostomy Z93.4
    gastrostomy Z93.1
    ileostomy Z93.2
    intestinal tract NEC Z93.4

Artificial - *continued*
jejunostomy Z93.4
nephrostomy Z93.6
specified site NEC Z93.8
tracheostomy Z93.0
ureterostomy Z93.6
urethrostomy Z93.6
urinary tract NEC Z93.6
vagina Z93.8
vagina status Z93.8
Arytenoid —*see* condition
Asbestosis (occupational) J61
ASC-H (atypical squamous cells cannot
exclude high grade squamous intraepithelial
lesion on cytologic smear)
anus R85.611
cervix R87.611
vagina R87.621
ASC-US (atypical squamous cells of
undetermined significance on cytologic
smear)
anus R85.610
cervix R87.610
vagina R87.620
Ascariasis B77.9
with
complications NEC B77.89
intestinal complications B77.0
pneumonia, pneumonitis B77.81
Ascaridosis, ascaridiasis —*see* Ascariasis
Ascaris (infection) (infestation) (lumbricoides)
—*see* Ascariasis
Ascending —*see* condition
Aschoff's bodies —*see* Myocarditis, rheumatic
Ascites (abdominal) R18.8
cardiac I50.9
chylous (nonfilarial) I89.8
filarial —*see* Infestation, filarial
due to
cirrhosis, alcoholic K70.31
hepatitis
alcoholic K70.11
chronic active K71.51
S. japonicum B65.2
heart I50.9
malignant R18.0
pseudochylous R18.8
syphilitic A52.74
tuberculous A18.31
Aseptic —*see* condition
Asherman's syndrome N85.6
Asialia K11.7
Asiatic cholera —*see* Cholera
Asimultagnosia (simultanagnosia) R48.3
Askin's tumor —*see* Neoplasm, connective
tissue, malignant
Asocial personality F60.2
Asomatognosia R41.4
Aspartylglucosaminuria E77.1
Asperger's disease or syndrome F84.5
Aspergilloma —*see* Aspergillosis
Aspergillosis (with pneumonia) B44.9
bronchopulmonary, allergic B44.81
disseminated B44.7
generalized B44.7
pulmonary NEC B44.1
allergic B44.81
invasive B44.0
specified NEC B44.89
tonsillar B44.2
Aspergillus (flavus) (fumigatus) (infection)
(terreus) —*see* Aspergillosis
Aspermatogenesis —*see* Azoospermia

Aspermia (testis) —*see* Azoospermia
Asphyxia, asphyxiation (by) R09.01
antenatal P84
birth P84
bunny bag —*see* Asphyxia, due to,
mechanical threat to breathing, trapped in bed
clothes
crushing S28.0
drowning T75.1
gas, fumes, or vapor —*see* Table of Drugs
and Chemicals
inhalation —*see* Inhalation
intrauterine P84
local I73.00
with gangrene I73.01
mucus —*see also* Foreign body, respiratory
tract, causing asphyxia
newborn P84
pathological R09.01
postnatal P84
mechanical —*see* Asphyxia, due to,
mechanical threat to breathing
prenatal P84
reticularis R23.1
strangulation —*see* Asphyxia, due to,
mechanical threat to breathing
submersion T75.1
traumatic T71.9
due to
crushed chest S28.0
foreign body (in) —*see* Foreign body,
respiratory tract, causing asphyxia
low oxygen content of ambient air T71.20
due to
being trapped in
low oxygen environment T71.29
in car trunk T71.221
circumstances undetermined
T71.224
done with intent to harm by
another person T71.223
self T71.222
in refrigerator T71.231
circumstances undetermined
T71.234
done with intent to harm by
another person T71.233
self T71.232
cave-in T71.21
mechanical threat to breathing (accidental)
T71.191
circumstances undetermined T71.194
done with intent to harm by
another person T71.193
self T71.192
hanging T71.161
circumstances undetermined T71.164
done with intent to harm by
another person T71.163
self T71.162
plastic bag T71.121
circumstances undetermined T71.124
done with intent to harm by
another person T71.123
self T71.122
smothering
in furniture T71.151
circumstances undetermined T71.154
done with intent to harm by
another person T71.153
self T71.152

Asphyxia, asphyxiation - *continued*
under
another person's body T71.141
circumstances undetermined T71.144
done with intent to harm T71.143
pillow T71.111
circumstances undetermined T71.114
done with intent to harm by
another person T71.113
self T71.112
trapped in bed clothes T71.131
circumstances undetermined T71.134
done with intent to harm by
another person T71.133
self T71.132
vomiting, vomitus —*see* Foreign body,
respiratory tract, causing asphyxia
Aspiration
amniotic (clear) fluid (newborn) P24.10
with
pneumonia (pneumonitis) P24.11
respiratory symptoms P24.11
blood
newborn (without respiratory symptoms)
P24.20
with
pneumonia (pneumonitis) P24.21
respiratory symptoms P24.21
specified age NEC —*see* Foreign body,
respiratory tract
bronchitis J69.0
food or foreign body (with asphyxiation) —
see Asphyxia, food
liquor (amnii) (newborn) P24.10
with
pneumonia (pneumonitis) P24.11
respiratory symptoms P24.11
meconium (newborn) (without respiratory
symptoms) P24.00
with
pneumonitis (pneumonitis) P24.01
respiratory symptoms P24.01
milk (newborn) (without respiratory
symptoms) P24.30
with
pneumonia (pneumonitis) P24.31
respiratory symptoms P24.31
specified age NEC —*see* Foreign body,
respiratory tract
mucus —*see also* Foreign body, by site,
causing asphyxia
newborn P24.10
with
pneumonia (pneumonitis) P24.11
respiratory symptoms P24.11
neonatal P24.9
specific NEC (without respiratory
symptoms) P24.80
with
pneumonia (pneumonitis) P24.81
respiratory symptoms P24.81
newborn P24.9
specific NEC (without respiratory
symptoms) P24.80
with
pneumonia (pneumonitis) P24.81
respiratory symptoms P24.81
pneumonia J69.0
pneumonitis J69.0
syndrome of newborn —*see* Aspiration, by
substance, with pneumonia
vernix caseosa (newborn) P24.80
with pneumonia (pneumonitis) P24.81

Aspiration - *continued*
    respiratory symptoms P24.81
  vomitus —*see also* Foreign body, respiratory
  tract
  newborn (without respiratory symptoms)
  P24.30
    with
      pneumonia (pneumonitis) P24.31
      respiratory symptoms P24.31
Asplenia (congenital) Q89.01
  postsurgical Z90.81
Assam fever B55.0
Assault, sexual —*see* Maltreatment
Assmann's focus NEC A15.0
Astasia (-abasia) (hysterical) F44.4
Asteatosis cutis L85.3
Astereognosia, astereognosis R48.1
Asterixis R27.8
  in liver disease K71.3
Asteroid hyalitis —*see* Deposit, crystalline
Asthenia, asthenic R53.1
  cardiac (*see also* Failure, heart) I50.9
    psychogenic F45.8
  cardiovascular (*see also* Failure, heart) I50.9
    psychogenic F45.8
  heart (*see also* Failure, heart) I50.9
    psychogenic F45.8
  hysterical F44.4
  myocardial (*see also* Failure, heart) I50.9
    psychogenic F45.8
  nervous F48.8
  neurocirculatory F45.8
  neurotic F48.8
  psychogenic F48.8
  psychoneurotic F48.8
  psychophysiologic F48.8
  reaction (psychophysiologic) F48.8
  senile R54
Asthenopia —*see also* Discomfort, visual
  hysterical F44.6
  psychogenic F44.6
Asthenospermia —*see* Abnormal, specimen,
male genital organs
Asthma, asthmatic (bronchial) (catarrh)
(spasmodic) J45.909
  with
    chronic obstructive bronchitis J44.9
      with
        acute lower respiratory infection J44.0
        exacerbation (acute) J44.1
    chronic obstructive pulmonary disease J44.9
      with
        acute lower respiratory infection J44.0
        exacerbation (acute) J44.1
    exacerbation (acute) J45.901
  hay fever —*see* Asthma, allergic extrinsic
  rhinitis, allergic —*see* Asthma, allergic
  extrinsic
    status asthmaticus J45.902
  allergic extrinsic J45.909
    with
      exacerbation (acute) J45.901
      status asthmaticus J45.902
  atopic —*see* Asthma, allergic extrinsic
  cardiac —*see* Failure, ventricular, left
  cardiobronchial I50.1
  childhood J45.909
    with
      exacerbation (acute) J45.901
      status asthmaticus J45.902

Asthma, asthmatic – *continued*
  chronic obstructive J44.9
    with
      acute lower respiratory infection J44.0
      exacerbation (acute) J44.1
  collier's J60
  cough variant J45.991
  detergent J69.8
  due to
    detergent J69.8
    inhalation of fumes J68.3
  eosinophilic J82
  extrinsic, allergic —*see* Asthma, allergic
  extrinsic
  grinder's J62.8
  hay —*see* Asthma, allergic extrinsic
  heart I50.1
  idiosyncratic —*see* Asthma, nonallergic
  intermittent (mild) J45.20
    with
      exacerbation (acute) J45.21
      status asthmaticus J45.22
  intrinsic, nonallergic —*see* Asthma,
  nonallergic
  Kopp's E32.8
  late-onset J45.909
    with
      exacerbation (acute) J45.901
      status asthmaticus J45.902
  mild intermittent J45.20
    with
      exacerbation (acute) J45.21
      status asthmaticus J45.22
  mild persistent J45.30
    with
      exacerbation (acute) J45.31
      status asthmaticus J45.32
  Millar's (laryngismus stridulus) J38.5
  miner's J60
  mixed J45.909
    with
      exacerbation (acute) J45.901
      status asthmaticus J45.902
  moderate persistent J45.40
    with
      exacerbation (acute) J45.41
      status asthmaticus J45.42
  nervous —*see* Asthma, nonallergic
  nonallergic (intrinsic) J45.909
    with
      exacerbation (acute) J45.901
      status asthmaticus J45.902
  persistent
    mild J45.30
      with
        exacerbation (acute) J45.31
        status asthmaticus J45.32
    moderate J45.40
      with
        exacerbation (acute) J45.41
        status asthmaticus J45.42
    severe J45.50
      with
        exacerbation (acute) J45.51
        status asthmaticus J45.52
  platinum J45.998
  pneumoconiotic NEC J64
  potter's J62.8
  predominantly allergic J45.909
  psychogenic F54
  pulmonary eosinophilic J82
  red cedar J67.8

Asthma, asthmatic – *continued*
  Rostan's I50.1
  sandblaster's J62.8
  sequoiosis J67.8
  severe persistent J45.50
    with
      exacerbation (acute) J45.51
      status asthmaticus J45.52
  specified NEC J45.998
  stonemason's J62.8
  thymic E32.8
  tuberculous —*see* Tuberculosis, pulmonary
  Wichmann's (laryngismus stridulus) J38.5
  wood J67.8
Astigmatism (compound) (congenital) H52.20
  irregular H52.21
  regular H52.22
Astraphobia F40.220
Astroblastoma
  specified site —*see* Neoplasm, malignant, by
  site
  unspecified site C71.9
Astrocytoma (cystic)
  anaplastic
    specified site —*see* Neoplasm, malignant,
    by site
    unspecified site C71.9
  fibrillary
    specified site —*see* Neoplasm, malignant,
    by site
    unspecified site C71.9
  fibrous
    specified site —*see* Neoplasm, malignant,
    by site
    unspecified site C71.9
  gemistocytic
    specified site —*see* Neoplasm, malignant,
    by site
    unspecified site C71.9
  juvenile
    specified site —*see* Neoplasm, malignant,
    by site
    unspecified site C71.9
  pilocytic
    specified site —*see* Neoplasm, malignant,
    by site
    unspecified site C71.9
  piloid
    specified site —*see* Neoplasm, malignant,
    by site
    unspecified site C71.9
  protoplasmic
    specified site —*see* Neoplasm, malignant,
    by site
    unspecified site C71.9
  specified site NEC —*see* Neoplasm,
  malignant, by site
  subependymal D43.2
    giant cell
      specified site —*see* Neoplasm, uncertain
  behavior, by site
      unspecified site D43.2
    specified site —*see* Neoplasm, uncertain
  behavior, by site
    unspecified site D43.2
  unspecified site C71.9
Astroglioma
  specified site —*see* Neoplasm, malignant, by
  site
  unspecified site C71.9
Asymbolia R48.8

Asymmetry —*see also* Distortion
between native and reconstructed breast N65.1
face Q67.0
jaw (lower) —*see* Anomaly, dentofacial, jaw-cranial base relationship, asymmetry
Asynergia, asynergy R27.8
ventricular I51.89
Asystole (heart) —*see* Arrest, cardiac
At risk
for falling Z91.81
Ataxia, ataxy, ataxic R27.0
acute R27.8
brain (hereditary) G11.9
cerebellar (hereditary) G11.9
with defective DNA repair G11.3
alcoholic G31.2
early-onset G11.1
in
alcoholism G31.2
myxedema E03.9 *[G13.2]*
neoplastic disease (*see also* Neoplasm) D49.9 *[G13.1]*
specified disease NEC G32.81
late-onset (Marie's) G11.2
cerebral (hereditary) G11.9
congenital nonprogressive G11.0
family, familial —*see* Ataxia, hereditary
following
cerebrovascular disease I69.993
cerebral infarction I69.393
intracerebral hemorrhage I69.193
nontraumatic intracranial hemorrhage NEC I69.293
specified disease NEC I69.893
subarachnoid hemorrhage I69.093
Friedreich's (heredofamilial) (cerebellar) (spinal) G11.1
gait R26.0
hysterical F44.4
general R27.8
gluten M35.9 *[G32.81]*
with celiac disease K90.0 *[G32.81]*
hereditary G11.9
with neuropathy G60.2
cerebellar —*see* Ataxia, cerebellar
spastic G11.4
specified NEC G11.8
spinal (Friedreich's) G11.1
heredofamilial —*see* Ataxia, hereditary
Hunt's G11.1
hysterical F44.4
locomotor (progressive) (syphilitic) (partial) (spastic) A52.11
diabetic —*see* Diabetes, ataxia
Marie's (cerebellar) (heredofamilial) (late onset) G11.2
nonorganic origin F44.4
nonprogressive, congenital G11.0
psychogenic F44.4
Roussy-Lévy G60.0
Sanger-Brown's (hereditary) G11.2
spastic hereditary G11.4
spinal
hereditary (Friedreich's) G11.1
progressive (syphilitic) A52.11
spinocerebellar, X-linked recessive G11.1
telangiectasia (Louis-Bar) G11.3
Ataxia-telangiectasia (Louis-Bar) G11.3
Atelectasis (massive) (partial) (pressure) (pulmonary) J98.11

Atelectasis - *continued*
newborn P28.10
due to resorption P28.11
partial P28.19
primary P28.0
secondary P28.19
primary (newborn) P28.0
tuberculous —*see* Tuberculosis, pulmonary
Atelocardia Q24.9
Atelomyelia Q06.1
Atheroembolism
of
extremities
lower I75.02
upper I75.01
kidney I75.81
specified NEC I75.89
Atheroma, atheromatous (*see also* Arteriosclerosis) I70.90
aorta, aortic I70.0
valve (*see also* Endocarditis, aortic) I35.8
aorto-iliac I70.0
artery —*see* Arteriosclerosis
basilar (artery) I67.2
carotid (artery) (common) (internal) I67.2
cerebral (arteries) I67.2
coronary (artery) I25.10
with angina pectoris —*see* Arteriosclerosis, coronary (artery) ,
degeneration —*see* Arteriosclerosis
heart, cardiac —*see* Disease, heart, ischemic, atherosclerotic
mitral (valve) I34.8
myocardium, myocardial —*see* Disease, heart, ischemic, atherosclerotic
pulmonary valve (heart) (*see also* Endocarditis, pulmonary) I37.8
tricuspid (heart) (valve) I36.8
valve, valvular —*see* Endocarditis
vertebral (artery) I67.2
Atheromatosis —*see* Arteriosclerosis
Atherosclerosis —*see also* Arteriosclerosis
coronary
artery I25.10
with angina pectoris —*see* Arteriosclerosis, coronary (artery)
due to
calcified coronary lesion (severely) I25.84
lipid rich plaque I25.83
transplanted heart I25.811
bypass graft I25.812
with angina pectoris —*see* Arteriosclerosis, coronary (artery)
native coronary artery I25.811
with angina pectoris —*see* Arteriosclerosis, coronary (artery) ,
Athetosis (acquired) R25.8
bilateral (congenital) G80.3
congenital (bilateral) (double) G80.3
double (congenital) G80.3
unilateral R25.8
Athlete's
foot B35.3
heart I51.7
Athrepsia E41
Athyrea (acquired) —*see also* Hypothyroidism
congenital E03.1
Atonia, atony, atonic
bladder (sphincter) (neurogenic) N31.2
capillary I78.8
cecum K59.8

Atonia, atony, atonic - *continued*
psychogenic F45.8
colon —*see* Atony, intestine
congenital P94.2
esophagus K22.8
intestine K59.8
psychogenic F45.8
stomach K31.89
neurotic or psychogenic F45.8
uterus (during labor) O62.2
with hemorrhage (postpartum) O72.1
postpartum (with hemorrhage) O72.1
without hemorrhage O75.89
Atopy —*see* History, allergy
Atransferrinemia, congenital E88.09
Atresia, atretic
alimentary organ or tract NEC Q45.8
upper Q40.8
ani, anus, anal (canal) Q42.3
with fistula Q42.2
aorta (arch) (ring) Q25.2
aortic (orifice) (valve) Q23.0
arch Q25.2
congenital with hypoplasia of ascending aorta and defective development of left ventricle (with mitral stenosis) Q23.4
in hypoplastic left heart syndrome Q23.4
aqueduct of Sylvius Q03.0
with spina bifida —*see* Spina bifida, with hydrocephalus
artery NEC Q27.8
cerebral Q28.3
coronary Q24.5
digestive system Q27.8
eye Q15.8
lower limb Q27.8
pulmonary Q25.5
specified site NEC Q27.8
umbilical Q27.0
upper limb Q27.8
auditory canal (external) Q16.1
bile duct (common) (congenital) (hepatic) Q44.2
acquired —*see* Obstruction, bile duct
bladder (neck) Q64.39
obstruction Q64.31
bronchus Q32.4
cecum Q42.8
cervix (acquired) N88.2
congenital Q51.828
in pregnancy or childbirth —*see* Anomaly, cervix, in pregnancy or childbirth
causing obstructed labor O65.5
choana Q30.0
colon Q42.9
specified NEC Q42.8
common duct Q44.2
cricoid cartilage Q31.8
cystic duct Q44.2
acquired K82.8
with obstruction K82.0
digestive organs NEC Q45.8
duodenum Q41.0
ear canal Q16.1
ejaculatory duct Q55.4
epiglottis Q31.8
esophagus Q39.0
with tracheoesophageal fistula Q39.1
eustachian tube Q17.8
fallopian tube (congenital) Q50.6
acquired N97.1
follicular cyst N83.0

Atresia, atretic - *continued*
  foramen of
    Luschka Q03.1
      with spina bifida —*see* Spina bifida, with
  hydrocephalus
    Magendie Q03.1
      with spina bifida —*see* Spina bifida, with
  hydrocephalus
  gallbladder Q44.1
  genital organ
    external
      female Q52.79
      male Q55.8
    internal
      female Q52.8
      male Q55.8
  glottis Q31.8
  gullet Q39.0
    with tracheoesophageal fistula Q39.1
  heart valve NEC Q24.8
    pulmonary Q22.0
    tricuspid Q22.4
  hymen Q52.3
    acquired (postinfective) N89.6
  ileum Q41.2
  intestine (small) Q41.9
    large Q42.9
      specified NEC Q42.8
  iris, filtration angle Q15.0
  jejunum Q41.1
  lacrimal apparatus Q10.4
  larynx Q31.8
  meatus urinarius Q64.33
  mitral valve Q23.2
    in hypoplastic left heart syndrome Q23.4
  nares (anterior) (posterior) Q30.0
  nasopharynx Q34.8
  nose, nostril Q30.0
    acquired J34.89
  organ or site NEC Q89.8
  osseous meatus (ear) Q16.1
  oviduct (congenital) Q50.6
    acquired N97.1
  parotid duct Q38.4
    acquired K11.8
  pulmonary (artery) Q25.5
    valve Q22.0
  pulmonic Q22.0
  pupil Q13.2
  rectum Q42.1
    with fistula Q42.0
  salivary duct Q38.4
    acquired K11.8
  sublingual duct Q38.4
    acquired K11.8
  submandibular duct Q38.4
    acquired K11.8
  submaxillary duct Q38.4
    acquired K11.8
  thyroid cartilage Q31.8
  trachea Q32.1
  tricuspid valve Q22.4
  ureter Q62.10
    pelvic junction Q62.11
    vesical orifice Q62.12
  ureteropelvic junction Q62.11
  ureterovesical orifice Q62.12
  urethra (valvular) Q64.39
    stricture Q64.32
  urinary tract NEC Q64.8
  uterus Q51.818
    acquired N85.8

Atresia, atretic   - *continued*
  vagina (congenital) Q52.4
    acquired (postinfectional) (senile) N89.5
  vas deferens Q55.3
  vascular NEC Q27.8
    cerebral Q28.3
    digestive system Q27.8
    lower limb Q27.8
    specified site NEC Q27.8
    upper limb Q27.8
  vein NEC Q27.8
    digestive system Q27.8
    great Q26.8
    lower limb Q27.8
    portal Q26.5
    pulmonary Q26.3
    specified site NEC Q27.8
    upper limb Q27.8
  vena cava (inferior) (superior) Q26.8
  vesicourethral orifice Q64.31
  vulva Q52.79
    acquired N90.5
Atrichia, atrichosis —*see* Alopecia
Atrophia —*see also* Atrophy
  cutis senilis L90.8
    due to radiation L57.8
  gyrata of choroid and retina H31.23
  senilis R54
    dermatological L90.8
      due to radiation (nonionizing) (solar) L57.8
  unguium L60.3
    congenita Q84.6
Atrophie blanche (en plaque) (de Milian)
L95.0
Atrophoderma, atrophoderma (of) L90.9
  diffusum (idiopathic) L90.4
  maculatum L90.8
    et striatum L90.8
      due to syphilis A52.79
    syphilitic A51.39
  neuriticum L90.8
  Pasini and Pierini L90.3
  pigmentosum Q82.1
  reticulatum symmetricum faciei L66.4
  senile L90.8
    due to radiation (nonionizing) (solar) L57.8
  vermiculata (cheeks) L66.4
Atrophy, atrophic (of)
  adrenal (capsule) (gland) E27.49
    primary (autoimmune) E27.1
  alveolar process or ridge (edentulous) K08.20
  anal sphincter (disuse) N81.84
  appendix K38.8
  arteriosclerotic —*see* Arteriosclerosis
  bile duct (common) (hepatic) K83.8
  bladder N32.89
    neurogenic N31.8
  blanche (en plaque) (of Milian) L95.0
  bone (senile) NEC —*see also* Disorder, bone,
  specified type NEC
    due to
      tabes dorsalis (neurogenic) A52.11
  brain (cortex) (progressive) G31.9
    frontotemporal circumscribed G31.01
  [F02.80]
      with behavioral disturbance G31.01
  [F02.81]
    senile NEC G31.1
  breast N64.2
    obstetric —*see* Disorder, breast, specified
  type NEC
  buccal cavity K13.79

Atrophy, atrophic (of)   - *continued*
  cardiac —*see* Degeneration, myocardial
  cartilage (infectional) (joint) —*see* Disorder,
  cartilage, specified NEC
  cerebellar —*see* Atrophy, brain
  cerebral —*see* Atrophy, brain
  cervix (mucosa) (senile) (uteri) N88.8
    menopausal N95.8
  Charcot-Marie-Tooth G60.0
  choroid (central) (macular) (myopic) (retina)
  H31.10
    diffuse secondary H31.12
      gyrate H31.23
      senile H31.11
  ciliary body —*see* Atrophy, iris
  conjunctiva (senile) H11.89
  corpus cavernosum N48.89
  cortical —*see* Atrophy, brain
  cystic duct K82.8
  Déjérine-Thomas G23.8
  disuse NEC —*see* Atrophy, muscle
  Duchenne-Aran G12.21
  ear H93.8
  edentulous alveolar ridge K08.20
  endometrium (senile) N85.8
    cervix N88.8
  enteric K63.89
  epididymis N50.8
  eyeball —*see* Disorder, globe, degenerated
  condition, atrophy
  eyelid (senile) —*see* Disorder, eyelid,
  degenerative
  facial (skin) L90.9
  fallopian tube (senile) N83.32
    with ovary N83.33
  fascioscapulohumeral (Landouzy Déjérine)
  G71.0
  fatty, thymus (gland) E32.8
  gallbladder K82.8
  gastric K29.40
    with bleeding K29.41
  gastrointestinal K63.89
  glandular I89.8
  globe H44.52
  gum K06.0
  hair L67.8
  heart (brown) —*see* Degeneration,
  myocardial
  hemifacial Q67.4
    Romberg G51.8
  infantile E41
    paralysis, acute —*see* Poliomyelitis,
  paralytic
  intestine K63.89
  iris (essential) (progressive) H21.26
    specified NEC H21.29
  kidney (senile) (terminal) (*see also* Sclerosis,
  renal) N26.1
    congenital or infantile Q60.5
      bilateral Q60.4
      unilateral Q60.3
    hydronephrotic —*see* Hydronephrosis
  lacrimal gland (primary) H04.14
    secondary H04.15
  Landouzy-Déjérine G71.0
  laryngitis, infective J37.0
  larynx J38.7
  Leber's optic (hereditary) H47.22
  lip K13.0
  liver (yellow) K72.90
    with coma K72.91
    acute, subacute K72.00
      with coma K72.01

Atrophy, atrophic (of)

chronic K72.10
  with coma K72.11
lung (senile) J98.4
macular (dermatological) L90.8
  syphilitic, skin A51.39
   striated A52.79
mandible (edentulous) K08.20
  minimal K08.21
  moderate K08.22
  severe K08.23
maxilla K08.20
  minimal K08.24
  moderate K08.25
  severe K08.26
muscle, muscular (diffuse) (general)
(idiopathic) (primary) M62.50
  ankle M62.57
  Duchenne-Aran G12.21
  foot M62.57
  forearm M62.53
  hand M62.54
  infantile spinal G12.0
  lower leg M62.56
  multiple sites M62.59
  myelopathic —*see* Atrophy, muscle, spinal
  myotonic G71.11
  neuritic G58.9
  neuropathic (peroneal) (progressive) G60.0
  pelvic (disuse) N81.84
  peroneal G60.0
  progressive (bulbar) G12.21
   adult G12.1
   infantile (spinal) G12.0
   spinal G12.9
    adult G12.1
    infantile G12.0
  pseudohypertrophic G71.0
  shoulder region M62.51
  specified site NEC M62.58
  spinal G12.9
   adult form G12.1
   Aran-Duchenne G12.21
   childhood form, type II G12.1
   distal G12.1
   hereditary NEC G12.1
   infantile, type I (Werdnig-Hoffmann)
G12.0
   juvenile form, type III (Kugelberg
Welander) G12.1
   progressive G12.21
   scapuloperoneal form G12.1
   specified NEC G12.8
  syphilitic A52.78
  thigh M62.55
  upper arm M62.52
myocardium —*see* Degeneration, myocardial
myometrium (senile) N85.8
  cervix N88.8
myopathic NEC —*see* Atrophy, muscle
myotonia G71.11
nail L60.3
nasopharynx J31.1
nerve —*see also* Disorder, nerve
  abducens —*see* Strabismus, paralytic, sixth
nerve
  accessory G52.8
  acoustic or auditory —see subcategory
H93.3
  cranial G52.9
   eighth (auditory) —see subcategory H93.3
   eleventh (accessory) G52.8

Atrophy, atrophic (of)

fifth (trigeminal) G50.8
first (olfactory) G52.0
fourth (trochlear) —*see* Strabismus,
paralytic, fourth nerve
  second (optic) H47.20
  sixth (abducens) —*see* Strabismus,
paralytic, sixth nerve
   tenth (pneumogastric) (vagus) G52.2
   third (oculomotor) —*see* Strabismus,
paralytic, third nerve
   twelfth (hypoglossal) G52.3
hypoglossal G52.3
oculomotor —*see* Strabismus, paralytic,
third nerve
olfactory G52.0
optic (papillomacular bundle)
  syphilitic (late) A52.15
   congenital A50.44
pneumogastric G52.2
trigeminal G50.8
trochlear —*see* Strabismus, paralytic, fourth
nerve
vagus (pneumogastric) G52.2
neurogenic, bone, tabetic A52.11
nutritional E41
old age R54
olivopontocerebellar G23.8
optic (nerve) H47.20
  glaucomatous H47.23
  hereditary H47.22
  primary H47.21
  specified type NEC H47.29
  syphilitic (late) A52.15
   congenital A50.44
orbit H05.31
ovary (senile) N83.31
  with fallopian tube N83.33
oviduct (senile) —*see* Atrophy, fallopian tube
palsy, diffuse (progressive) G12.22
pancreas (duct) (senile) K86.8
parotid gland K11.0
pelvic muscle N81.84
penis N48.89
pharynx J39.2
pluriglandular E31.8
  autoimmune E31.0
polyarthritis M15.9
prostate N42.89
pseudohypertrophic (muscle) G71.0
renal (*see also* Sclerosis, renal) N26.1
retina, retinal (postinfectional) H35.89
rhinitis J31.0
salivary gland K11.0
scar L90.5
sclerosis, lobar (of brain) G31.09 *[F02.80]*
  with behavioral disturbance G31.09
[F02.81]
scrotum N50.8
seminal vesicle N50.8
senile R54
  due to radiation (nonionizing) (solar) L57.8
skin (patches) (spots) L90.9
  degenerative (senile) L90.8
  due to radiation (nonionizing) (solar) L57.8
  senile L90.8
spermatic cord N50.8
spinal (acute) (cord) G95.89
  muscular —*see* Atrophy, muscle, spinal
  paralysis G12.20
   acute —*see* Poliomyelitis, paralytic

Atrophy, atrophic (of)

meaning progressive muscular atrophy
G12.21
spine (column) —*see* Spondylopathy,
specified NEC
spleen (senile) D73.0
stomach K29.40
  with bleeding K29.41
striate (skin) L90.6
  syphilitic A52.79
subcutaneous L90.9
sublingual gland K11.0
submandibular gland K11.0
submaxillary gland K11.0
Sudeck's —*see* Algoneurodystrophy
suprarenal (capsule) (gland) E27.49
  primary E27.1
systemic affecting central nervous system
in
  myxedema E03.9 *[G13.2]*
  neoplastic disease (*see also* Neoplasm)
D49.9 *[G13.1]*
   specified disease NEC G13.8
tarso-orbital fascia, congenital Q10.3
testis N50.0
thenar, partial —*see* Syndrome, carpal tunnel
thymus (fatty) E32.8
thyroid (gland) (acquired) E03.4
  with cretinism E03.1
  congenital (with myxedema) E03.1
tongue (senile) K14.8
  papillae K14.4
trachea J39.8
tunica vaginalis N50.8
turbinate J34.89
tympanic membrane (nonflaccid) H73.82
  flaccid H73.81
upper respiratory tract J39.8
uterus, uterine (senile) N85.8
  cervix N88.8
  due to radiation (intended effect) N85.8
   adverse effect or misadventure N99.89
vagina (senile) N95.2
vas deferens N50.8
vascular I99.8
vertebra (senile) —*see* Spondylopathy,
specified NEC
vulva (senile) N90.5
Werdnig-Hoffmann G12.0
yellow —*see* Failure, hepatic

Attack, attacks

with alteration of consciousness (with
automatisms) —*see* Epilepsy, localization-
related, symptomatic, with complex partial
seizures
Adams-Stokes I45.9
akinetic —*see* Epilepsy, generalized,
specified NEC
angina —*see* Angina
atonic —*see* Epilepsy, generalized, specified
NEC
benign shuddering G25.83
cataleptic —*see* Catalepsy
coronary —*see* Infarct, myocardium
cyanotic, newborn P28.2
drop NEC R55
epileptic —*see* Epilepsy
heart —*see* infarct, myocardium
hysterical F44.9
jacksonian —*see* Epilepsy, localization-
related, symptomatic, with simple partial
seizures

Attack, attacks - *continued*
  myocardium, myocardial —*see* Infarct, myocardium
  myoclonic —*see* Epilepsy, generalized, specified NEC
  panic F41.0
  psychomotor —*see* Epilepsy, localization-related, symptomatic, with complex partial seizures
  salaam —*see* Epilepsy, spasms
  schizophreniform, brief F23
  shuddering, benign G25.83
  Stokes-Adams I45.9
  syncope R55
  transient ischemic (TIA) G45.9
    specified NEC G45.8
  unconsciousness R55
    hysterical F44.89
  vasomotor R55
  vasovagal (paroxysmal) (idiopathic) R55
  without alteration of consciousness —*see* Epilepsy, localization-related, symptomatic, with simple partial seizures
Attention (to)
  artificial
    opening (of) Z43.9
      digestive tract NEC Z43.4
        colon Z43.3
        ilium Z43.2
        stomach Z43.1
      specified NEC Z43.8
      trachea Z43.0
      urinary tract NEC Z43.6
        cystostomy Z43.5
        nephrostomy Z43.6
        ureterostomy Z43.6
        urethrostomy Z43.6
      vagina Z43.7
    colostomy Z43.3
    cystostomy Z43.5
  deficit disorder or syndrome F98.8
    with hyperactivity —*see* Disorder, attention-deficit hyperactivity
  gastrostomy Z43.1
  ileostomy Z43.2
  jejunostomy Z43.4
  nephrostomy Z43.6
  surgical dressings Z48.01
  sutures Z48.02
  tracheostomy Z43.0
  ureterostomy Z43.6
  urethrostomy Z43.6
Attrition
  gum K06.0
  tooth, teeth (excessive) (hard tissues) K03.0
Atypical, atypism —*see also* condition
  cells (on cytological smear) (endocervical) (endometrial) (glandular)
    cervix R87.619
    vagina R87.629
  cervical N87.9
  endometrium N85.9
    hyperplasia N85.00
  parenting situation Z62.9
Auditory —*see* condition
Aujeszky's disease B33.8
Aurantiasis, cutis E67.1
Auricle, auricular —*see also* condition
  cervical Q18.2
Auriculotemporal syndrome G50.8
Austin Flint murmur (aortic insufficiency) I35.1

Australian
  Q fever A78
  X disease A83.4
Autism, autistic (childhood) (infantile) F84.0
  atypical F84.9
Autodigestion R68.89
Autoerythrocyte sensitization (syndrome) D69.2
Autographism L50.3
Autoimmune
  disease (systemic) M35.9
  inhibitors to clotting factors D68.311
  lymphoproliferative syndrome -ALPS] D89.82
  thyroiditis E06.3
Autointoxication R68.89
Automatism G93.89
  with temporal sclerosis G93.81
  epileptic —*see* Epilepsy, localization-related, symptomatic, with complex partial seizures
  paroxysmal, idiopathic —*see* Epilepsy, localization-related, symptomatic, with complex partial seizures
Autonomic, autonomous
  bladder (neurogenic) N31.2
  hysteria seizure F44.5
Autosensitivity, erythrocyte D69.2
Autosensitization, cutaneous L30.2
Autosome —*see* condition by chromosome involved
Autotopagnosia R48.1
Autotoxemia R68.89
Autumn —*see* condition
Avellis' syndrome G46.8
Aversion
  oral R63.3
    newborn P92.
    nonorganic origin F98.2
  sexual F52.1
Aviator's
  disease or sickness —*see* Effect, adverse, high altitude
  ear T70.0
Avitaminosis (multiple) (*see also* Deficiency, vitamin) E56.9
  B E53.9
    with
      beriberi E51.11
      pellagra E52
    B2 E53.0
    B6 E53.1
    B12 E53.8
    D E55.9
      with rickets E55.0
    G E53.0
    K E56.1
  nicotinic acid E52
AVNRT (atrioventricular nodal re-entrant tachycardia) I47.1
AVRT (atrioventricular nodal re-entrant tachycardia) I47.1
Avulsion (traumatic)
  blood vessel —*see* Injury, blood vessel
  bone —*see* Fracture, by site
  cartilage —*see also* Dislocation, by site
    symphyseal (inner) , complicating delivery O71.6
  external site other than limb —*see* Wound, open, by site
  eye S05.7
  head (intracranial)
    external site NEC S08.89

Avulsion - *continued*
  scalp S08.0
  internal organ or site —*see* Injury, by site
  joint —*see also* Dislocation, by site
    capsule —*see* Sprain, by site
  kidney S37.06
  ligament —*see* Sprain, by site
  limb —*see also* Amputation, traumatic, by site
    skin and subcutaneous tissue —*see* Wound, open, by site
  muscle —*see* Injury, muscle
  nerve (root) —*see* Injury, nerve
  scalp S08.0
  skin and subcutaneous tissue —*see* Wound, open, by site
  spleen S36.032
  symphyseal cartilage (inner) , complicating delivery O71.6
  tendon —*see* Injury, muscle
  tooth S03.2
Awareness of heart beat R00.2
Axenfeld's
  anomaly or syndrome Q15.0
  degeneration (calcareous) Q13.4
Axilla, axillary —*see also* condition
  breast Q83.1
Axonotmesis —*see* Injury, nerve
Ayerza's disease or syndrome (pulmonary artery sclerosis with pulmonary hypertension) I27.0
Azoospermia (organic) N46.01
  due to
    drug therapy N46.021
    efferent duct obstruction N46.023
    infection N46.022
    radiation N46.024
    specified cause NEC N46.029
    systemic disease N46.025
Azotemia R79.89
  meaning uremia N19
Aztec ear Q17.3
Azygos
  continuation inferior vena cava Q26.8
  lobe (lung) Q33.1

B

Baastrup's disease —*see* Kissing spine
Babesiosis B60.0
Babington's disease (familial hemorrhagic telangiectasia) I78.0
Babinski's syndrome A52.79
Baby
  crying constantly R68.11
  floppy (syndrome) P94.2
Bacillary —*see* condition
Bacilluria N39.0
Bacillus —*see also* Infection, bacillus
  abortus infection A23.1
  anthracis infection A22.9
  coli infection (*see also* Escherichia coli) B96.20
  Flexner's A03.1
  mallei infection A24.0
  Shiga's A03.0
  suipestifer infection —*see* Infection, salmonella
Back —*see* condition
Backache (postural) M54.9
  sacroiliac M53.3
  specified NEC M54.89
Backflow —*see* Reflux
Backward reading (dyslexia) F81.0

Bacteremia R78.81
  with sepsis —*see* Sepsis
Bactericholia —*see* Cholecystitis, acute
Bacterid, bacteride (pustular) L40.3
Bacterium, bacteria, bacterial
  agent NEC, as cause of disease classified
  elsewhere B96.89
  in blood —*see* Bacteremia
  in urine —*see* Bacteriuria
Bacteriuria, bacteruria N39.0
  asymptomatic N39.0
Bacteroides
  fragilis, as cause of disease classified
  elsewhere B96.6
Bad
  heart —*see* Disease, heart
  trip
    due to drug abuse —*see* Abuse, drug,
    hallucinogen
    due to drug dependence —*see* Dependence,
    drug, hallucinogen
Baelz's disease (cheilitis glandularis
  apostematosa) K13.0
Baerensprung's disease (eczema marginatum)
  B35.6
Bagasse disease or pneumonitis J67.1
Bagassosis J67.1
Baker's cyst —*see* Cyst, Baker's
Bakwin-Krida syndrome (craniometaphyseal
  dysplasia) Q78.5
Balancing side interference M26.56
Balanitis (circinata) (erosiva) (gangrenosa)
  (phagedenic) (vulgaris) N48.1
  amebic A06.82
  candidal B37.42
  due to Haemophilus ducreyi A57
  gonococcal (acute) (chronic) A54.09
  xerotica obliterans N48.0
Balanoposthitis N47.6
  gonococcal (acute) (chronic) A54.09
  ulcerative (specific) A63.8
Balanorrhagia —*see* Balanitis
Balantidiasis, balantidiosis A07.0
Bald tongue K14.4
Baldness —*see also* Alopecia
  male-pattern —*see* Alopecia, androgenic
Balkan grippe A78
Balloon disease —*see* Effect, adverse, high
  altitude
Balo's disease (concentric sclerosis) G37.5
Bamberger-Marie disease —*see*
  Osteoarthropathy, hypertrophic, specified type
  NEC
Bancroft's filariasis B74.0
Band (s)
  adhesive —*see* Adhesions, peritoneum
  anomalous or congenital —*see also* Anomaly,
  by site
    heart (atrial) (ventricular) Q24.8
    intestine Q43.3
    omentum Q43.3
  cervix N88.1
  constricting, congenital Q79.8
  gallbladder (congenital) Q44.1
  intestinal (adhesive) —*see* Adhesions,
  peritoneum
  obstructive
    intestine K56.5
    peritoneum K56.5
  periappendiceal, congenital Q43.3
  peritoneal (adhesive) —*see* Adhesions,
  peritoneum

Band(s) – *continued*
  uterus N73.6
    internal N85.6
    vagina N89.5
Bandemia D72.825
Bandl's ring (contraction) , **complicating
  delivery** O62.4
Bangkok hemorrhagic fever A91
Bang's disease (brucella abortus) A23.1
Bankruptcy, anxiety concerning Z59.8
Bannister's disease T78.3
  hereditary D84.1
Banti's disease or syndrome (with cirrhosis)
  (with portal hypertension) K76.6
Bar, median, prostate —*see* Enlargement,
  enlarged, prostate
Barcoo disease or rot —*see* Ulcer, skin
Barlow's disease E54
Barodontalgia T70.29
Baron Münchausen syndrome —*see*
  Disorder, factitious
Barosinusitis T70.1
Barotitis T70.0
Barotrauma T70.29
  odontalgia T70.29
  otitic T70.0
  sinus T70.1
Barraquer (-Simons) disease or syndrome
  (progressive lipodystrophy) E88.1
Barré-Guillain disease or syndrome G61.0
Barré-Liéou syndrome (posterior cervical
  sympathetic) M53.0
Barrel chest M95.4
Barrett's
  disease —*see* Barrett's, esophagus
  esophagus K22.70
    with dysplasia K22.719
      high grade K22.711
      low grade K22.710
    without dysplasia K22.70
  syndrome —*see* Barrett's, esophagus
  ulcer K22.10
    with bleeding K22.11
    without bleeding K22.10
Bársony (-Polgár) (-Teschendorf) syndrome
  (corkscrew esophagus) K22.4
Bartholinitis (suppurating) N75.8
  gonococcal (acute) (chronic) (with abscess)
  A54.1
Barth syndrome E78.71
Bartonellosis A44.9
  cutaneous A44.1
  mucocutaneous A44.1
  specified NEC A44.8
  systemic A44.0
Barton's fracture S52.56
Bartter's syndrome E26.81
Basal —*see* condition
Basan's (hidrotic) **ectodermal dysplasia**
  Q82.4
Baseball finger —*see* Dislocation, finger
Basedow's disease (exophthalmic goiter) —*see*
  Hyperthyroidism, with, goiter
Basic —*see* condition
Basilar —*see* condition
Bason's (hidrotic) **ectodermal dysplasia**
  Q82.4
Basopenia —*see* Agranulocytosis
Basophilia D72.824
Basophilism (cortico-adrenal) (Cushing's)
  (pituitary) E24.0
Bassen-Kornzweig disease or syndrome
  E78.6

Bat ear Q17.5
Bateman's
  disease B08.1
  purpura (senile) D69.2
Bathing cramp T75.1
Bathophobia F40.248
Batten (-Mayou) **disease** E75.4
  retina E75.4 *[H36]*
Batten-Steinert syndrome G71.11
Battered —*see* Maltreatment
Battey Mycobacterium infection A31.0
Battle exhaustion F43.0
Battledore placenta O43.19
**Baumgarten-Cruveilhier cirrhosis, disease
  or syndrome** K74.69
Bauxite fibrosis (of lung) J63.1
Bayle's disease (general paresis) A52.17
Bazin's disease (primary) (tuberculous) A18.4
Beach ear —*see* Swimmer's, ear
Beaded hair (congenital) Q84.1
Béal conjunctivitis or syndrome B30.2
Beard's disease (neurasthenia) F48.8
Beat (s)
  atrial, premature I49.1
  ectopic I49.49
  elbow —*see* Bursitis, elbow
  escaped, heart I49.49
  hand —*see* Bursitis, hand
  knee —*see* Bursitis, knee
  premature I49.40
    atrial I49.1
    auricular I49.1
    supraventricular I49.1
Beau's
  disease or syndrome —*see* Degeneration,
  myocardial
  lines (transverse furrows on fingernails) L60.4
Bechterew's syndrome —*see* Spondylitis,
  ankylosing
Beck's syndrome (anterior spinal artery
  occlusion) I65.8
Becker's
  cardiomyopathy I42.8
  disease
    idiopathic mural endomyocardial disease
    I42.3
    myotonia congenita, recessive form G71.12
  dystrophy G71.0
  pigmented hairy nevus D22.5
Beckwith-Wiedemann syndrome Q87.3
Bed confinement status Z74.01
Bed sore —*see* Ulcer, pressure, by site
Bedbug bite (s) —*see* Bite(s) , by site,
  superficial, insect
Bedclothes, asphyxiation or suffocation by
  —*see* Asphyxia, traumatic, due to,
  mechanical, trapped
Bednar's
  aphthae K12.0
  tumor —*see* Neoplasm, malignant, by site
Bedridden Z74.01
Bedsore —*see* Ulcer, pressure, by site
Bedwetting —*see* Enuresis
Bee sting (with allergic or anaphylactic shock)
  —*see* Toxicity, venom, arthropod, bee
Beer drinker's heart (disease) I42.6
Begbie's disease (exophthalmic goiter) —*see*
  Hyperthyroidism, with, goiter
Behavior
  antisocial
    adult Z72.811
    child or adolescent Z72.810

Behavior - *continued*
 disorder, disturbance —*see* Disorder, conduct
 disruptive —*see* Disorder, conduct
 drug seeking Z72.89
 inexplicable R46.2
 marked evasiveness R46.5
 obsessive-compulsive R46.81
 overactivity R46.3
 poor responsiveness R46.4
 self-damaging (life-style) Z72.89
 sleep-incompatible Z72.821
 slowness R46.4
 specified NEC R46.89
 strange (and inexplicable) R46.2
 suspiciousness R46.5
 type A pattern Z73.1
 undue concern or preoccupation with stressful
 events R46.6
 verbosity and circumstantial detail obscuring
 reason for contact R46.7
Behçet's disease or syndrome M35.2
Behr's disease —*see* Degeneration, macula
Beigel's disease or morbus (white piedra)
 B36.2
Bejel A65
Bekhterev's syndrome —*see* Spondylitis,
 ankylosing
Belching —*see* Eructation
Bell's
 mania F30.8
 palsy, paralysis G51.0
 infant or newborn P11.3
 spasm G51.3
Bence Jones albuminuria or proteinuria
 NEC R80.3
Bends T70.3
Benedikt's paralysis or syndrome G46.3
Benign —*see also* condition
 prostatic hyperplasia —*see* Hyperplasia,
 prostate
Bennett's fracture (displaced) S62.21
Benson's disease —*see* Deposit, crystalline
Bent
 back (hysterical) F44.4
 nose M95.0
 congenital Q67.4
Bereavement (uncomplicated) Z63.4
Bergeron's disease (hysterical chorea) F44.4
Berger's disease —*see* Nephropathy, IgA
Beriberi (dry) E51.11
 heart (disease) E51.12
 polyneuropathy E51.11
 wet E51.12
 involving circulatory system E51.11
Berlin's disease or edema (traumatic) S05.8X
Berlock (berloque) **dermatitis** L56.2
Bernard-Horner syndrome G90.2
Bernard-Soulier disease or thrombopathia
 D69.1
Bernhardt (-Roth) **disease** —*see*
 Mononeuropathy, lower limb, meralgia
 paresthetica
Bernheim's syndrome —*see* Failure, heart,
 congestive
Bertielliasis B71.8
Berylliosis (lung) J63.2
Besnier-Boeck (-Schaumann) **disease** —*see*
 Sarcoidosis
Besnier's
 lupus pernio D86.3
 prurigo L20.0
Bestiality F65.89

Best's disease H35.50
Beta-mercaptolactate-cysteine disulfiduria
 E72.09
Betalipoproteinemia, broad or floating E78.2
Betting and gambling Z72.6
 pathological (compulsive) F63.0
Bezoar T18.9
 intestine T18.3
 stomach T18.2
Bezold's abscess —*see* Mastoiditis, acute
Bianchi's syndrome R48.8
Bicornate or bicornis uterus Q51.3
 in pregnancy or childbirth O34.59
 causing obstructed labor O65.5
Bicuspid aortic valve Q23.1
Biedl-Bardet syndrome Q87.89
Bielschowsky (-Jansky) **disease** E75.4
Biermer's (pernicious) **anemia or disease**
 D51.0
Biett's disease L93.0
Bifid (congenital)
 apex, heart Q24.8
 clitoris Q52.6
 kidney Q63.8
 nose Q30.2
 patella Q74.1
 scrotum Q55.29
 toe NEC Q74.2
 tongue Q38.3
 ureter Q62.8
 uterus Q51.3
 uvula Q35.7
Biforis uterus (suprasimplex) Q51.3
Bifurcation (congenital)
 gallbladder Q44.1
 kidney pelvis Q63.8
 renal pelvis Q63.8
 rib Q76.6
 tongue, congenital Q38.3
 trachea Q32.1
 ureter Q62.8
 urethra Q64.74
 vertebra Q76.49
Big spleen syndrome D73.1
Bigeminal pulse R00.8
Bilateral —*see* condition
Bile
 duct —*see* condition
 pigments in urine R82.2
Bilharziasis —*see also* Schistosomiasis
 chyluria B65.0
 cutaneous B65.3
 galacturia B65.0
 hematochyluria B65.0
 intestinal B65.1
 lipemia B65.9
 lipuria B65.0
 oriental B65.2
 piarhemia B65.9
 pulmonary NOS B65.9 *[J99]*
 pneumonia B65.9 *[J17]*
 tropical hematuria B65.0
 vesical B65.0
Biliary —*see* condition
Bilirubin metabolism disorder E80.7
 specified NEC E80.6
Bilirubinemia, familial nonhemolytic E80.4
Bilirubinuria R82.2
Biliuria R82.2
Bilocular stomach K31.2
Binswanger's disease I67.3

Biparta, bipartite
 carpal scaphoid Q74.0
 patella Q74.1
 vagina Q52.10
Bird
 face Q75.8
 fancier's disease or lung J67.2
Birt-Hogg-Dube syndrome Q87.89
Birth
 complications in mother —*see* Delivery,
 complicated
 compression during NOS P15.9
 defect —*see* Anomaly
 immature (less than 37 completed weeks) —
 see Preterm, newborn
 extremely (less than 28 completed weeks)
 —*see* Immaturity, extreme
 inattention, at or after —*see* Maltreatment,
 child, neglect
 injury NOS P15.9
 basal ganglia P11.1
 brachial plexus NEC P14.3
 brain (compression) (pressure) P11.2
 central nervous system NOS P11.9
 cerebellum P11.1
 cerebral hemorrhage P10.1
 external genitalia P15.5
 eye P15.3
 face P15.4
 fracture
 bone P13.9
 specified NEC P13.8
 clavicle P13.4
 femur P13.2
 humerus P13.3
 long bone, except femur P13.3
 radius and ulna P13.3
 skull P13.0
 spine P11.5
 tibia and fibula P13.3
 intracranial P11.2
 laceration or hemorrhage P10.9
 specified NEC P10.8
 intraventricular hemorrhage P10.2
 laceration
 brain P10.1
 by scalpel P15.8
 peripheral nerve P14.9
 liver P15.0
 meninges
 brain P11.1
 spinal cord P11.5
 nerve
 brachial plexus P14.3
 cranial NEC (except facial) P11.4
 facial P11.3
 peripheral P14.9
 phrenic (paralysis) P14.2
 paralysis
 facial nerve P11.3
 spinal P11.5
 penis P15.5
 rupture
 spinal cord P11.5
 scalp P12.9
 scalpel wound P15.8
 scrotum P15.5
 skull NEC P13.1
 fracture P13.0
 specified type NEC P15.8
 spinal cord P11.5
 spine P11.5
 spleen P15.1

Birth - *continued*
  sternomastoid (hematoma) P15.2
  subarachnoid hemorrhage P10.3
  subcutaneous fat necrosis P15.6
  subdural hemorrhage P10.0
  tentorial tear P10.4
  testes P15.5
  vulva P15.5
 lack of care, at or after —*see* Maltreatment, child, neglect
 neglect, at or after —*see* Maltreatment, child, neglect
 palsy or paralysis, newborn, NOS (birth injury) P14.9
 premature (infant) —*see* Preterm, newborn
 shock, newborn P96.89
 trauma —*see* Birth, injury
 weight
   low (2499 grams or less) —*see* Low, birthweight
     extremely (999 grams or less) —*see* Low, birthweight, extreme
   4000 grams to 4499 grams P08.1
   4500 grams or more P08.0
Birthmark Q82.5
Bisalbuminemia E88.09
Biskra's button B55.1
Bite (s) (animal) (human)
 abdomen, abdominal
   wall S31.159
     with penetration into peritoneal cavity S31.659
     epigastric region S31.152
       with penetration into peritoneal cavity S31.652
       left
         lower quadrant S31.154
           with penetration into peritoneal cavity S31.654
         upper quadrant S31.151
           with penetration into peritoneal cavity S31.651
         periumbilic region S31.155
           with penetration into peritoneal cavity S31.655
         right
           lower quadrant S31.153
             with penetration into peritoneal cavity S31.653
           upper quadrant S31.150
             with penetration into peritoneal cavity S31.650
         superficial NEC S30.871
           insect S30.861
 alveolar (process) —*see* Bite, oral cavity
 amphibian (venomous) —*see* Venom, bite, amphibian
 animal —*see also* Bite, by site
   venomous —*see* Venom
 ankle S91.05
   superficial NEC S90.57
     insect S90.56
 antecubital space —*see* Bite, elbow
 anus S31.835
   superficial NEC S30.877
     insect S30.867
 arm (upper) S41.15
   lower —*see* Bite, forearm
   superficial NEC S40.87
     insect S40.86
 arthropod NEC —*see* Venom, bite, arthropod

Bite(s) – *continued*
 auditory canal (external) (meatus) —*see* Bite, ear
 auricle, ear —*see* Bite, ear
 axilla —*see* Bite, arm
 back —*see also* Bite, thorax, back
   lower S31.050
     with penetration into retroperitoneal space S31.051
     superficial NEC S30.870
       insect S30.860
 bedbug —*see* Bite(s) , by site, superficial, insect
 breast S21.05
   superficial NEC S20.17
     insect S20.16
 brow —*see* Bite, head, specified site NEC
 buttock S31.805
   left S31.825
   right S31.815
   superficial NEC S30.870
     insect S30.860
 calf —*see* Bite, leg
 canaliculus lacrimalis —*see* Bite, eyelid
 canthus, eye —*see* Bite, eyelid
 centipede —*see* Toxicity, venom, arthropod, centipede
 cheek (external) S01.45
   superficial NEC S00.87
     insect S00.86
   internal —*see* Bite, oral cavity
 chest wall —*see* Bite, thorax
 chigger B88.0
 chin —*see* Bite, head, specified site NEC
 clitoris —*see* Bite, vulva
 costal region —*see* Bite, thorax
 digit (s)
   hand —*see* Bite, finger
   toe —*see* Bite, toe
 ear (canal) (external) S01.35
   superficial NEC S00.47
     insect S00.46
 elbow S51.05
   superficial NEC S50.37
     insect S50.36
 epididymis —*see* Bite, testis
 epigastric region —*see* Bite, abdomen
 epiglottis —*see* Bite, neck, specified site NEC
 esophagus, cervical S11.25
   superficial NEC S10.17
     insect S10.16
 eyebrow —*see* Bite, eyelid
 eyelid S01.15
   superficial NEC S00.27
     insect S00.26
 face NEC —*see* Bite, head, specified site NEC
 finger (s) S61.259
   with
     damage to nail S61.359
   index S61.258
     with
       damage to nail S61.358
     left S61.251
       with
         damage to nail S61.351
     right S61.250
       with
         damage to nail S61.350
     superficial NEC S60.478
       insect S60.46

Bite(s) – *continued*
   little S61.25
     with
       damage to nail S61.35
     superficial NEC S60.47
       insect S60.46
   middle S61.25
     with
       damage to nail S61.35
     superficial NEC S60.47
       insect S60.46
   ring S61.25
     with
       damage to nail S61.35
     superficial NEC S60.47
       insect S60.46
   superficial NEC S60.479
     insect S60.469
   thumb —*see* Bite, thumb
 flank —*see* Bite, abdomen, wall
 flea —*see* Bite, by site, superficial, insect
 foot (except toe(s) alone) S91.35
   superficial NEC S90.87
     insect S90.86
   toe —*see* Bite, toe
 forearm S51.85
   elbow only —*see* Bite, elbow
   superficial NEC S50.87
     insect S50.86
 forehead —*see* Bite, head, specified site NEC
 genital organs, external
   female S31.552
     superficial NEC S30.876
       insect S30.866
     vagina and vulva —*see* Bite, vulva
   male S31.551
     penis —*see* Bite, penis
     scrotum —*see* Bite, scrotum
     superficial NEC S30.875
       insect S30.865
     testes —*see* Bite, testis
 groin —*see* Bite, abdomen, wall
 gum —*see* Bite, oral cavity
 hand S61.45
   finger —*see* Bite, finger
   superficial NEC S60.57
     insect S60.56
   thumb —*see* Bite, thumb
 head S01.95
   cheek —*see* Bite, cheek
   ear —*see* Bite, ear
   eyelid —*see* Bite, eyelid
   lip —*see* Bite, lip
   nose —*see* Bite, nose
   oral cavity —*see* Bite, oral cavity
   scalp —*see* Bite, scalp
   specified site NEC S01.85
     superficial NEC S00.87
       insect S00.86
   superficial NEC S00.97
     insect S00.96
   temporomandibular area —*see* Bite, cheek
 heel —*see* Bite, foot
 hip S71.05
   superficial NEC S70.27
     insect S70.26
 hymen S31.45
 hypochondrium —*see* Bite, abdomen, wall
 hypogastric region —*see* Bite, abdomen, wall
 inguinal region —*see* Bite, abdomen, wall
 insect —*see* Bite, by site, superficial, insect
 instep —*see* Bite, foot

Bite(s) – *continued*
  interscapular region —*see* Bite, thorax, back
  jaw —*see* Bite, head, specified site NEC
  knee S81.05
    superficial NEC S80.27
      insect S80.26
  labium (majus) (minus) —*see* Bite, vulva
  lacrimal duct —*see* Bite, eyelid
  larynx S11.015
    superficial NEC S10.17
      insect S10.16
  leg (lower) S81.85
    ankle —*see* Bite, ankle
    foot —*see* Bite, foot
    knee —*see* Bite, knee
    superficial NEC S80.87
      insect S80.86
    toe —*see* Bite, toe
    upper —*see* Bite, thigh
  lip S01.551
    superficial NEC S00.571
      insect S00.561
  lizard (venomous) —*see* Venom, bite, reptile
  loin —*see* Bite, abdomen, wall
  lower back —*see* Bite, back, lower
  lumbar region —*see* Bite, back, lower
  malar region —*see* Bite, head, specified site NEC
  mammary —*see* Bite, breast
  marine animals (venomous) —*see* Toxicity, venom, marine animal
  mastoid region —*see* Bite, head, specified site NEC
  mouth —*see* Bite, oral cavity
  nail
    finger —*see* Bite, finger
    toe —*see* Bite, toe
  nape —*see* Bite, neck, specified site NEC
  nasal (septum) (sinus) —*see* Bite, nose
  nasopharynx —*see* Bite, head, specified site NEC
  neck S11.95
    involving
      cervical esophagus —*see* Bite, esophagus, cervical
    larynx —*see* Bite, larynx
    pharynx —*see* Bite, pharynx
    thyroid gland S11.15
    trachea —*see* Bite, trachea
    specified site NEC S11.85
      superficial NEC S10.87
        insect S10.86
    superficial NEC S10.97
      insect S10.96
    throat S11.85
      superficial NEC S10.17
        insect S10.16
  nose (septum) (sinus) S01.25
    superficial NEC S00.37
      insect S00.36
  occipital region —*see* Bite, scalp
  oral cavity S01.552
    superficial NEC S00.572
      insect S00.562
  orbital region —*see* Bite, eyelid
  palate —*see* Bite, oral cavity
  palm —*see* Bite, hand
  parietal region —*see* Bite, scalp
  pelvis S31.050
    with penetration into retroperitoneal space S31.051

Bite(s) – *continued*
    superficial NEC S30.870
      insect S30.860
  penis S31.25
    superficial NEC S30.872
      insect S30.862
  perineum
    female —*see* Bite, vulva
    male —*see* Bite, pelvis
  periocular area (with or without lacrimal passages) —*see* Bite, eyelid
  phalanges
    finger —*see* Bite, finger
    toe —*see* Bite, toe
  pharynx S11.25
    superficial NEC S10.17
      insect S10.16
  pinna —*see* Bite, ear
  poisonous —*see* Venom
  popliteal space —*see* Bite, knee
  prepuce —*see* Bite, penis
  pubic region —*see* Bite, abdomen, wall
  rectovaginal septum —*see* Bite, vulva
  red bug B88.0
  reptile NEC —*see also* Venom, bite, reptile
    nonvenomous —*see* Bite, by site
    snake —*see* Venom, bite, snake
  sacral region —*see* Bite, back, lower
  sacroiliac region —*see* Bite, back, lower
  salivary gland —*see* Bite, oral cavity
  scalp S01.05
    superficial NEC S00.07
      insect S00.06
  scapular region —*see* Bite, shoulder
  scrotum S31.35
    superficial NEC S30.873
      insect S30.863
  sea-snake (venomous) —*see* Toxicity, venom, snake, sea snake
  shin —*see* Bite, leg
  shoulder S41.05
    superficial NEC S40.27
      insect S40.26
  snake —*see also* Venom, bite, snake
    nonvenomous —*see* Bite, by site
  spermatic cord —*see* Bite, testis
  spider (venomous) —*see* Toxicity, venom, spider
    nonvenomous —*see* Bite, by site, superficial, insect
  sternal region —*see* Bite, thorax, front
  submaxillary region —*see* Bite, head, specified site NEC
  submental region —*see* Bite, head, specified site NEC
  subungual
    finger (s) —*see* Bite, finger
    toe —*see* Bite, toe
  superficial —*see* Bite, by site, superficial
  supraclavicular fossa S11.85
  supraorbital —*see* Bite, head, specified site NEC
  temple, temporal region —*see* Bite, head, specified site NEC
  temporomandibular area —*see* Bite, cheek
  testis S31.35
    superficial NEC S30.873
      insect S30.863
  thigh S71.15
    superficial NEC S70.37
      insect S70.36

Bite(s) – *continued*
  thorax, thoracic (wall) S21.95
    back S21.25
      with penetration into thoracic cavity S21.45
    breast —*see* Bite, breast
    front S21.15
      with penetration into thoracic cavity S21.35
    superficial NEC S20.97
      back S20.47
      front S20.37
      insect S20.96
        back S20.46
        front S20.36
  throat —*see* Bite, neck, throat
  thumb S61.05
    with
      damage to nail S61.15
    superficial NEC S60.37
      insect S60.36
  thyroid S11.15
    superficial NEC S10.87
      insect S10.86
  toe (s) S91.15
    with
      damage to nail S91.25
    great S91.15
      with
        damage to nail S91.25
    lesser S91.15
      with
        damage to nail S91.25
    superficial NEC S90.47
      great S90.47
      insect S90.46
        great S90.46
  tongue S01.552
  trachea S11.025
    superficial NEC S10.17
      insect S10.16
  tunica vaginalis —*see* Bite, testis
  tympanum, tympanic membrane —*see* Bite, ear
  umbilical region S31.155
  uvula —*see* Bite, oral cavity
  vagina —*see* Bite, vulva
  venomous —*see* Venom
  vocal cords S11.035
    superficial NEC S10.17
      insect S10.16
  vulva S31.45
    superficial NEC S30.874
      insect S30.864
  wrist S61.55
    superficial NEC S60.87
      insect S60.86
Biting, cheek or lip K13.1
Biventricular failure (heart) I50.9
Björck (-Thorson) syndrome (malignant carcinoid) E34.0
Black
  death A20.9
  eye S00.1
  hairy tongue K14.3
  heel (foot) S90.3
  lung (disease) J60
  palm (hand) S60.22
Blackfan-Diamond anemia or syndrome (congenital hypoplastic anemia) D61.01
Blackhead L70.0
Blackout R55
Bladder —*see* condition

Blast (air) (hydraulic) (immersion)
(underwater)
blindness S05.8X
injury
abdomen or thorax —*see* Injury, by site
ear (acoustic nerve trauma) —*see* Injury,
nerve, acoustic, specified type NEC
syndrome NEC T70.8
Blastoma —*see* Neoplasm, malignant, by site
pulmonary —*see* Neoplasm, lung, malignant
Blastomycosis, blastomycotic B40.9
Brazilian —*see* Paracoccidioidomycosis
cutaneous B40.3
disseminated B40.7
European —*see* Cryptococcosis
generalized B40.7
keloidal B48.0
North American B40.9
primary pulmonary B40.0
pulmonary B40.2
acute B40.0
chronic B40.1
skin B40.3
South American —*see*
Paracoccidioidomycosis
specified NEC B40.89
Bleb (s) R23.8
emphysematous (lung) (solitary) J43.9
endophthalmitis H59.43
filtering (vitreous) , after glaucoma surgery
Z98.83
inflamed (infected) , postprocedural H59.40
stage 1 H59.41
stage 2 H59.42
stage 3 H59.43
lung (ruptured) J43.9
congenital —*see* Atelectasis
newborn P25.8
subpleural (emphysematous) J43.9
Blebitis, postprocedural H59.40
stage 1 H59.41
stage 2 H59.42
stage 3 H59.43
Bleeder (familial) (hereditary) —*see*
Hemophilia
Bleeding —*see also* Hemorrhage
anal K62.5
anovulatory N97.0
atonic, following delivery O72.1
capillary I78.8
puerperal O72.2
contact (postcoital) N93.0
due to uterine subinvolution N85.3
ear —*see* Otorrhagia
excessive, associated with menopausal onset
N92.4
familial —*see* Defect, coagulation
following intercourse N93.0
gastrointestinal K92.2
hemorrhoids —*see* Hemorrhoids
intermenstrual (regular) N92.3
irregular N92.1
intraoperative —*see* Complication,
intraoperative, hemorrhage
irregular N92.6
menopausal N92.4
newborn, intraventricular —*see* Newborn,
affected by, hemorrhage, intraventricular
nipple N64.59
nose R04.0
ovulation N92.3
postclimacteric N95.0

Bleeding - *continued*
postcoital N93.0
postmenopausal N95.0
postoperative —*see* Complication,
postprocedural, hemorrhage
preclimacteric N92.4
puberty (excessive, with onset of menstrual
periods) N92.2
rectum, rectal K62.5
newborn P54.2
tendencies —*see* Defect, coagulation
throat R04.1
tooth socket (post-extraction) K91.840
umbilical stump P51.9
uterus, uterine NEC N93.9
climacteric N92.4
dysfunctional of functional N93.8
menopausal N92.4
preclimacteric or premenopausal N92.4
unrelated to menstrual cycle N93.9
vagina, vaginal (abnormal) N93.9
dysfunctional or functional N93.8
newborn P54.6
vicarious N94.89
Blennorrhagia, blennorrhagic —*see*
Gonorrhea
Blennorrhea (acute) (chronic) —*see also*
Gonorrhea
inclusion (neonatal) (newborn) P39.1
lower genitourinary tract (gonococcal)
A54.00
neonatorum (gonococcal ophthalmia) A54.31
Blepharelosis —*see* Entropion
Blepharitis (angularis) (ciliaris) (eyelid)
(marginal) (nonulcerative) H01.009
herpes zoster B02.39
left H01.006
lower H01.005
upper H01.004
right H01.003
lower H01.002
upper H01.001
squamous H01.029
left H01.026
lower H01.025
upper H01.024
right H01.023
lower H01.022
upper H01.021
ulcerative H01.019
left H01.016
lower H01.015
upper H01.014
right H01.013
lower H01.012
upper H01.011
Blepharochalasis H02.30
congenital Q10.0
left H02.36
lower H02.35
upper H02.34
right H02.33
lower H02.32
upper H02.31
Blepharoclonus H02.59
Blepharoconjunctivitis H10.50
angular H10.52
contact H10.53
ligneous H10.51
Blepharophimosis (eyelid) H02.529
congenital Q10.3
left H02.526

Blepharophimosis - *continued*
lower H02.525
upper H02.524
right H02.523
lower H02.522
upper H02.521
Blepharoptosis H02.40
congenital Q10.0
mechanical H02.41
myogenic H02.42
neurogenic H02.43
paralytic H02.43
Blepharopyorrhea, gonococcal A54.39
Blepharospasm G24.5
drug induced G24.01
Blighted ovum O02.0
Blind —*see also* Blindness
bronchus (congenital) Q32.4
loop syndrome K90.2
congenital Q43.8
sac, fallopian tube (congenital) Q50.6
spot, enlarged —*see* Defect, visual field,
localized, scotoma, blind spot area
tract or tube, congenital NEC —*see* Atresia,
by site
Blindness (acquired) (congenital) (both eyes)
H54.0
blast S05.8X
color —*see* Deficiency, color vision
concussion S05.8X
cortical H47.619
left brain H47.612
right brain H47.611
day H53.11
due to injury (current episode) S05.9
sequelae
code to injury with seventh character S
eclipse (total) —*see* Retinopathy, solar
emotional (hysterical) F44.6
face H53.16
hysterical F44.6
legal (both eyes) (USA definition) H54.8
mind R48.8
night H53.60
abnormal dark adaptation curve H53.61
acquired H53.62
congenital H53.63
specified type NEC H53.69
vitamin A deficiency E50.5
one eye (other eye normal) H54.40
left (normal vision on right) H54.42
low vision on right H54.12
low vision, other eye H54.10
right (normal vision on left) H54.41
low vision on left H54.11
psychic R48.8
river B73.01
snow —*see* Photokeratitis
sun, solar —*see* Retinopathy, solar
transient —*see* Disturbance, vision,
subjective, loss, transient
traumatic (current episode) S05.9
word (developmental) F81.0
acquired R48.0
secondary to organic lesion R48.0
Blister (nonthermal)
abdominal wall S30.821
alveolar process S00.522
ankle S90.52
antecubital space —*see* Blister, elbow
anus S30.827
arm (upper) S40.82
auditory canal —*see* Blister, ear

Blister – *continued*
auricle —*see* Blister, ear
axilla —*see* Blister, arm
back, lower S30.820
beetle dermatitis L24.89
breast S20.12
brow S00.82
calf —*see* Blister, leg
canthus —*see* Blister, eyelid
cheek S00.82
  internal S00.522
chest wall —*see* Blister, thorax
chin S00.82
costal region —*see* Blister, thorax
digit (s)
  foot —*see* Blister, toe
  hand —*see* Blister, finger
due to burn —*see* Burn, by site, second
degree
ear S00.42
elbow S50.32
epiglottis S10.12
esophagus, cervical S10.12
eyebrow —*see* Blister, eyelid
eyelid S00.22
face S00.82
fever B00.1
finger (s) S60.429
  index S60.42
  little S60.42
  middle S60.42
  ring S60.42
foot (except toe(s) alone) S90.82
  toe —*see* Blister, toe
forearm S50.82
  elbow only —*see* Blister, elbow
forehead S00.82
fracture
omit code
genital organ
  female S30.826
  male S30.825
gum S00.522
hand S60.52
head S00.92
  ear —*see* Blister, ear
  eyelid —*see* Blister, eyelid
  lip S00.521
  nose S00.32
  oral cavity S00.522
  scalp S00.02
  specified site NEC S00.82
heel —*see* Blister, foot
hip S70.22
interscapular region S20.429
jaw S00.82
knee S80.22
larynx S10.12
leg (lower) S80.82
  knee —*see* Blister, knee
  upper —*see* Blister, thigh
lip S00.521
malar region S00.82
mammary —*see* Blister, breast
mastoid region S00.82
mouth S00.522
multiple, skin, nontraumatic R23.8
nail
  finger —*see* Blister, finger
  toe —*see* Blister, toe
nasal S00.32

Blister – *continued*
neck S10.92
  specified site NEC S10.82
  throat S10.12
nose S00.32
occipital region S00.02
oral cavity S00.522
orbital region —*see* Blister, eyelid
palate S00.522
palm —*see* Blister, hand
parietal region S00.02
pelvis S30.820
penis S30.822
periocular area —*see* Blister, eyelid
phalanges
  finger —*see* Blister, finger
  toe —*see* Blister, toe
pharynx S10.12
pinna —*see* Blister, ear
popliteal space —*see* Blister, knee
scalp S00.02
scapular region —*see* Blister, shoulder
scrotum S30.823
shin —*see* Blister, leg
shoulder S40.22
sternal region S20.329
submaxillary region S00.82
submental region S00.82
subungual
  finger (s) —*see* Blister, finger
  toe (s) —*see* Blister, toe
supraclavicular fossa S10.82
supraorbital S00.82
temple S00.82
temporal region S00.82
testis S30.823
thermal —*see* Burn, second degree, by site
thigh S70.32
thorax, thoracic (wall) S20.92
  back S20.42
  front S20.32
throat S10.12
thumb S60.32
toe (s) S90.42
  great S90.42
tongue S00.522
trachea S10.12
tympanum, tympanic membrane —*see*
Blister, ear
upper arm —*see* Blister, arm (upper)
uvula S00.522
vagina S30.824
vocal cords S10.12
vulva S30.824
wrist S60.82
Bloating R14.0
Bloch-Sulzberger disease or syndrome Q82.3
Block, blocked
alveolocapillary J84.10
arborization (heart) I45.5
arrhythmic I45.9
atrioventricular (incomplete) (partial) I44.30
  with atrioventricular dissociation I44.2
  complete I44.2
    congenital Q24.6
  congenital Q24.6
  first degree I44.0
  second degree (types I and II) I44.1
  specified NEC I44.39
  third degree I44.2
  types I and II I44.1

Block, blocked – *continued*
auriculoventricular —*see* Block,
atrioventricular
bifascicular (cardiac) I45.2
bundle-branch (complete) (false) (incomplete)
I45.4
  bilateral I45.2
  left I44.7
    with right bundle branch block I45.2
    hemiblock I44.60
      anterior I44.4
      posterior I44.5
    incomplete I44.7
      with right bundle branch block I45.2
  right I45.10
    with
      left bundle branch block I45.2
      left fascicular block I45.2
    specified NEC I45.19
  Wilson's type I45.19
cardiac I45.9
conduction I45.9
  complete I44.2
fascicular (left) I44.60
  anterior I44.4
  posterior I44.5
  right I45.0
  specified NEC I44.69
foramen Magendie (acquired) G91.1
  congenital Q03.1
    with spina bifida —*see* Spina bifida, by
site, with hydrocephalus
heart I45.9
  bundle branch I45.4
    bilateral I45.2
  complete (atrioventricular) I44.2
  congenital Q24.6
  first degree (atrioventricular) I44.0
  second degree (atrioventricular) I44.1
  specified type NEC I45.5
  third degree (atrioventricular) I44.2
hepatic vein I82.0
intraventricular (nonspecific) I45.4
  bundle branch
    bilateral I45.2
kidney N28.9
  postcystoscopic or postprocedural N99.0
Mobitz (types I and II) I44.1
myocardial —*see* Block, heart
nodal I45.5
organ or site, congenital NEC —*see* Atresia,
by site
portal (vein) I81
second degree (types I and II) I44.1
sinoatrial I45.5
sinoauricular I45.5
third degree I44.2
trifascicular I45.3
tubal N97.1
vein NOS I82.90
Wenckebach (types I and II) I44.1
Blockage —*see* Obstruction
Blocq's disease F44.4
Blood
constituents, abnormal R78.9
disease D75.9
donor —*see* Donor, blood
dyscrasia D75.9
  with
    abortion —*see* Abortion, by type,
    complicated by, hemorrhage
    ectopic pregnancy O08.1
    molar pregnancy O08.1

Blood – *continued*
following ectopic or molar pregnancy O08.1
newborn P61.9
puerperal, postpartum O72.3
flukes NEC —*see* Schistosomiasis
in
feces K92.1
occult R19.5
urine —*see* Hematuria
mole O02.0
occult in feces R19.5
pressure
decreased, due to shock following injury T79.4
examination only Z01.30
fluctuating I99.8
high —*see* Hypertension
borderline R03.0
incidental reading, without diagnosis of hypertension R03.0
low —*see also* Hypotension
incidental reading, without diagnosis of hypotension R03.1
spitting —*see* Hemoptysis
staining cornea —*see* Pigmentation, cornea, stromal
transfusion
reaction or complication —*see* Complications, transfusion
type
A (Rh positive) Z67.10
Rh negative Z67.11
AB (Rh positive) Z67.30
Rh negative Z67.31
B (Rh positive) Z67.20
Rh negative Z67.21
O (Rh positive) Z67.40
Rh negative Z67.41
Rh (positive) Z67.90
negative Z67.91
vessel rupture —*see* Hemorrhage
vomiting —*see* Hematemesis
Blood-forming organs, disease D75.9
Bloodgood's disease —*see* Mastopathy, cystic
Bloom (-Machacek) (-Torre) **syndrome** Q82.8
Blount's disease or osteochondrosis —*see* Osteochondrosis, juvenile, tibia
Blue
baby Q24.9
diaper syndrome E72.09
dome cyst (breast) —*see* Cyst, breast
dot cataract Q12.0
nevus D22.9
sclera Q13.5
with fragility of bone and deafness Q78.0
toe syndrome I75.02
Blueness —*see* Cyanosis
Blues, postpartal O90.6
baby O90.6
Blurring, visual H53.8
Blushing (abnormal) (excessive) R23.2
BMI —*see* Body, mass index
Boarder, hospital NEC Z76.4
accompanying sick person Z76.3
healthy infant or child Z76.2
foundling Z76.1
Bockhart's impetigo L01.02
Bodechtel-Guttman disease (subacute sclerosing panencephalitis) A81.1
Boder-Sedgwick syndrome (ataxia-telangiectasia) G11.3

Body, bodies
Aschoff's —*see* Myocarditis, rheumatic
asteroid, vitreous —*see* Deposit, crystalline
cytoid (retina) —*see* Occlusion, artery, retina
drusen (degenerative) (macula) (retinal) —*see also* Degeneration, macula, drusen
optic disc —*see* Drusen, optic disc
foreign —*see* Foreign body
loose
joint, except knee —*see* Loose, body, joint
knee M23.4
sheath, tendon —*see* Disorder, tendon, specified type NEC
mass index (BMI)
adult
19 or less Z68.1
20.0 20.9 Z68.20
21.0 21.9 Z68.21
22.0 22.9 Z68.22
23.0 23.9 Z68.23
24.0 24.9 Z68.24
25.0 25.9 Z68.25
26.0 26.9 Z68.26
27.0 27.9 Z68.27
28.0 28.9 Z68.28
29.0 29.9 Z68.29
30.0 30.9 Z68.30
31.0 31.9 Z68.31
32.0 32.9 Z68.32
33.0 33.9 Z68.33
34.0 34.9 Z68.34
35.0 35.9 Z68.35
36.0 36.9 Z68.36
37.0 37.9 Z68.37
38.0 38.9 Z68.38
39.0 39.9 Z68.39
40.0 44.9 Z68.41
45.0 49.9 Z68.42
50.0 59.9 Z68.43
60.0 69.9 Z68.44
70 and over Z68.45
pediatric
5th percentile to less than 85th percentile for age Z68.52
85th percentile to less than 95th percentile for age Z68.53
greater than or equal to ninety-fifth percentile for age Z68.54
less than fifth percentile for age Z68.51
Mooser's A75.2
rice —*see also* Loose, body, joint
knee M23.4
rocking F98.4
Boeck's
disease or sarcoid —*see* Sarcoidosis
lupoid (miliary) D86.3
Boerhaave's syndrome (spontaneous esophageal rupture) K22.3
Boggy
cervix N88.8
uterus N85.8
Boil —*see also* Furuncle, by site
Aleppo B55.1
Baghdad B55.1
Delhi B55.1
lacrimal
gland —*see* Dacryoadenitis
passages (duct) (sac) —*see* Inflammation, lacrimal, passages, acute
Natal B55.1
orbit, orbital —*see* Abscess, orbit
tropical B55.1
Bold hives —*see* Urticaria

Bombé, iris —*see* Membrane, pupillary
Bone —*see* condition
Bonnevie-Ullrich syndrome Q87.1
Bonnier's syndrome —*see* subcategory H81.8
Bonvale dam fever T73.3
Bony block of joint —*see* Ankylosis
BOOP (bronchiolitis obliterans organized pneumonia) J84.89
Borderline
diabetes mellitus R73.09
hypertension R03.0
osteopenia M85.8
pelvis, with obstruction during labor O65.1
personality F60.3
Borna disease A83.9
Bornholm disease B33.0
Boston exanthem A88.0
Botalli, ductus (patent) (persistent) Q25.0
Bothriocephalus latus infestation B70.0
Botulism (foodborne intoxication) A05.1
infant A48.51
non-foodborne A48.52
wound A48.52
Bouba —*see* Yaws
Bouchard's nodes (with arthropathy) M15.2
Bouffée délirante F23
Bouillaud's disease or syndrome (rheumatic heart disease) I01.9
Bourneville's disease Q85.1
Boutonniere deformity (finger) —*see* Deformity, finger, boutonniere
Bouveret (-Hoffmann) **syndrome** (paroxysmal tachycardia) I47.9
Bovine heart —*see* Hypertrophy, cardiac
Bowel —*see* condition
Bowen's
dermatosis (precancerous) —*see* Neoplasm, skin, in situ
disease —*see* Neoplasm, skin, in situ
epithelioma —*see* Neoplasm, skin, in situ
type
epidermoid carcinoma-in-situ —*see* Neoplasm, skin, in situ
intraepidermal squamous cell carcinoma —*see* Neoplasm, skin, in situ
Bowing
femur —*see also* Deformity, limb, specified type NEC, thigh
congenital Q68.3
fibula —*see also* Deformity, limb, specified type NEC, lower leg
congenital Q68.4
forearm —*see* Deformity, limb, specified type NEC, forearm
leg (s) , long bones, congenital Q68.5
radius —*see* Deformity, limb, specified type NEC, forearm
tibia —*see also* Deformity, limb, specified type NEC, lower leg
congenital Q68.4
Bowleg (s) (acquired) M21.16
congenital Q68.5
rachitic E64.3
Boyd's dysentery A03.2
Brachial —*see* condition
Brachycardia R00.1
Brachycephaly Q75.0
Bradley's disease A08.19
Bradyarrhythmia, cardiac I49.8
Bradycardia (sinoatrial) (sinus) (vagal) R00.1
neonatal P29.12
reflex G90.09
tachycardia syndrome I49.5

Bradykinesia R25.8
Bradypnea R06.89
Bradytachycardia I49.5
Brailsford's disease or osteochondrosis —*see*
Osteochondrosis, juvenile, radius
Brain —*see also* condition
death G93.82
syndrome —*see* Syndrome, brain
Branched-chain amino-acid disorder E71.2
Branchial —*see* condition
cartilage, congenital Q18.2
Branchiogenic remnant (in neck) Q18.0
Brandt's syndrome (acrodermatitis
enteropathica) E83.2
Brash (water) R12
Bravais-jacksonian epilepsy —*see* Epilepsy,
localization-related, symptomatic, with simple
partial seizures
Braxton Hicks contractions —*see* False, labor
Brazilian leishmaniasis B55.2
BRBPR K62.5
Break, retina (without detachment) H33.30
with retinal detachment —*see* Detachment,
retina
horseshoe tear H33.31
multiple H33.33
round hole H33.32
Breakdown
device, graft or implant (*see also*
Complications, by site and type, mechanical)
T85.618
arterial graft NEC —*see* Complication,
cardiovascular device, mechanical, vascular
breast (implant) T85.41
catheter NEC T85.618
cystostomy T83.010
dialysis (renal) T82.41
intraperitoneal T85.611
infusion NEC T82.514
spinal (epidural) (subdural) T85.610
urinary (indwelling) T83.018
electronic (electrode) (pulse generator)
(stimulator)
bone T84.310
cardiac T82.119
electrode T82.110
pulse generator T82.111
specified type NEC T82.118
nervous system —*see* Complication,
prosthetic device, mechanical, electronic
nervous system stimulator
urinary —*see* Complication, genitourinary,
device, urinary, mechanical
fixation, internal (orthopedic) NEC —*see*
Complication, fixation device, mechanical
gastrointestinal —*see* Complications,
prosthetic device, mechanical, gastrointestinal
device
genital NEC T83.418
intrauterine contraceptive device T83.31
penile prosthesis T83.410
heart NEC —*see* Complication,
cardiovascular device, mechanical
joint prosthesis —*see* Complications..., joint
prosthesis, internal, mechanical, by site
ocular NEC —*see* Complications, prosthetic
device, mechanical, ocular device
orthopedic NEC —*see* Complication,
orthopedic, device, mechanical
specified NEC T85.618
sutures, permanent T85.612

Breakdown – *continued*
used in bone repair —*see* Complications,
fixation device, internal (orthopedic) ,
mechanical
urinary NEC —*see also* Complication,
genitourinary, device, urinary, mechanical
graft T83.21
vascular NEC —*see* Complication,
cardiovascular device, mechanical
ventricular intracranial shunt T85.01
nervous F48.8
perineum O90.1
respirator J95.850
specified NEC J95.859
ventilator J95.850
specified NEC J95.859
Breast —*see also* condition
buds E30.1
in newborn P96.89
dense R92.2
nodule N63
Breath
foul R19.6
holder, child R06.89
holding spell R06.89
shortness R06.02
Breathing
labored —*see* Hyperventilation
mouth R06.5
causing malocclusion M26.5
periodic R06.3
high altitude G47.32
Breathlessness R06.81
Breda's disease —*see* Yaws
Breech presentation (mother) O32.1
causing obstructed labor O64.1
footling O32.8
causing obstructed labor O64.8
incomplete O32.8
causing obstructed labor O64.8
Breisky's disease N90.4
Brennemann's syndrome I88.0
Brenner
tumor (benign) D27.9
borderline malignancy D39.1
malignant C56
proliferating D39.1
Bretonneau's disease or angina A36.0
Breus' mole O02.0
Brevicollis Q76.49
Brickmakers' anemia B76.9 [D63.8]
Bridge, myocardial Q24.5
Bright red blood per rectum (BRBPR) K62.5
Bright's disease —*see also* Nephritis
arteriosclerotic —*see* Hypertension, kidney
Brill (-Zinsser) disease (recrudescent typhus)
A75.1
flea-borne A75.2
louse-borne A75.1
Brill-Symmers' disease C82.90
Brion-Kayser disease —*see* Fever,
parathyroid
Briquet's disorder or syndrome F45.0
Brissaud's
infantilism or dwarfism E23.0
motor-verbal tic F95.2
Brittle
bones disease Q78.0
nails L60.3
congenital Q84.6
Broad —*see also* condition
beta disease E78.2
ligament laceration syndrome N83.8

Broad or floating-betalipoproteinemia
E78.2
Brock's syndrome (atelectasis due to enlarged
lymph nodes) J98.19
Brocq-Duhring disease (dermatitis
herpetiformis) L13.0
Brodie's abscess or disease M86.8X
Broken
arches —*see also* Deformity, limb, flat foot
arm (meaning upper limb) —*see* Fracture,
arm
back —*see* Fracture, vertebra
bone —*see* Fracture
implant or internal device —*see*
Complications, by site and type, mechanical
leg (meaning lower limb) —*see* Fracture, leg
nose S02.2
tooth, teeth —*see* Fracture, tooth
Bromhidrosis, bromidrosis L75.0
Bromidism, bromism G92
due to
correct substance properly administered —
see Table of Drugs and Chemicals, by drug,
adverse effect
overdose or wrong substance given or taken
—*see* Table of Drugs and Chemicals, by drug,
poisoning
chronic (dependence) F13.20
Bromidrosiphobia F40.298
Bronchi, bronchial —*see* condition
Bronchiectasis (cylindrical) (diffuse)
(fusiform) (localized) (saccular) J47.9
with
acute
bronchitis J47.0
lower respiratory infection J47.0
exacerbation (acute) J47.1
congenital Q33.4
tuberculous NEC —*see* Tuberculosis,
pulmonary
Bronchiolectasis —*see* Bronchiectasis
Bronchiolitis (acute) (infective) (subacute)
J21.9
with
bronchospasm or obstruction J21.9
influenza, flu or grippe —*see* Influenza,
with, respiratory manifestations NEC
chemical (chronic) J68.4
acute J68.0
chronic (fibrosing) (obliterative) J44.9
due to
external agent —*see* Bronchitis, acute, due
to
human metapneumovirus J21.1
respiratory syncytial virus J21.0
specified organism NEC J21.8
fibrosa obliterans J44.9
influenzal —*see* Influenza, with, respiratory
manifestations NEC
obliterans J42
with organizing pneumonia (BOOP) J84.89
obliterative (chronic) (subacute) J44.9
due to fumes or vapors J68.4
due to chemicals, gases, fumes or vapors
(inhalation) J68.4
respiratory, interstitial lung disease J84.115
Bronchitis (diffuse) (fibrinous) (hypostatic)
(infective) (membranous) J40
with
influenza, flu or grippe —*see* Influenza,
with, respiratory manifestations NEC
obstruction (airway) (lung) J44.9
tracheitis (15 years of age and above) J40

Bronchitis - *continued*
  acute or subacute J20.9
    chronic J42
    under l5 years of age J20.9
  acute or subacute (with bronchospasm or
    obstruction) J20.9
    with
      bronchiectasis J47.0
      chronic obstructive pulmonary disease
        J44.0
      chemical (due to gases, fumes or vapors)
        J68.0
      due to
        fumes or vapors J68.0
        Haemophilus influenzae J20.1
        Mycoplasma pneumoniae J20.0
        radiation J70.0
        specified organism NEC J20.8
        Streptococcus J20.2
        virus
          coxsackie J20.3
          echovirus J20.7
          parainfluenzae J20.4
          respiratory syncytial J20.5
          rhinovirus J20.6
      viral NEC J20.8
  allergic (acute) J45.909
    with
      exacerbation (acute) J45.901
      status asthmaticus J45.902
  arachidic T17.528
  aspiration (due to fumes or vapors) J68.0
  asthmatic J45.9
    chronic J44.9
      with
        acute lower respiratory infection J44.0
        exacerbation (acute) J44.1
  capillary —*see* Pneumonia, broncho
  caseous (tuberculous) A15.5
  Castellani's A69.8
  catarrhal (l5 years of age and above) J40
    acute —*see* Bronchitis, acute
    chronic J41.0
    under l5 years of age J20.9
  chemical (acute) (subacute) J68.0
    chronic J68.4
    due to fumes or vapors J68.0
      chronic J68.4
  chronic J42
    with
      airways obstruction J44.9
      tracheitis (chronic) J42
      asthmatic (obstructive) J44.9
      catarrhal J41.0
      chemical (due to fumes or vapors) J68.4
    due to
      chemicals, gases, fumes or vapors
        (inhalation) J68.4
        radiation J70.1
        tobacco smoking J41.0
    emphysematous J44.9
    mucopurulent J41.1
    non-obstructive J41.0
    obliterans J44.9
    obstructive J44.9
    purulent J41.1
    simple J41.0
  croupous —*see* Bronchitis, acute
  due to gases, fumes or vapors (chemical)
    J68.0
  emphysematous (obstructive) J44.9
  exudative —*see* Bronchitis, acute

Bronchitis - *continued*
  fetid J41.1
  grippal —*see* Influenza, with, respiratory
    manifestations NEC
  in those under l5 years age —*see* Bronchitis,
    acute
    chronic —*see* Bronchitis, chronic
  influenzal —*see* Influenza, with, respiratory
    manifestations NEC
  mixed simple and mucopurulent J41.8
  moulder's J62.8
  mucopurulent (chronic) (recurrent) J41.1
    acute or subacute J20.9
    simple (mixed) J41.8
  obliterans (chronic) J44.9
  obstructive (chronic) (diffuse) J44.9
  pituitous J41.1
  pneumococcal, acute or subacute J20.2
  pseudomembranous, acute or subacute —*see*
    Bronchitis, acute
  purulent (chronic) (recurrent) J41.1
    acute or subacute —*see* Bronchitis, acute
  putrid J41.1
  senile (chronic) J42
  simple and mucopurulent (mixed) J41.8
  smokers' J41.0
  spirochetal NEC A69.8
  subacute —*see* Bronchitis, acute
  suppurative (chronic) J41.1
    acute or subacute —*see* Bronchitis, acute
  tuberculous A15.5
  under l5 years of age —*see* Bronchitis, acute
    chronic —*see* Bronchitis, chronic
  viral NEC, acute or subacute (see also
    Bronchitis, acute) J20.8
Bronchoalveolitis J18.0
Bronchoaspergillosis B44.1
Bronchocele meaning goiter E04.0
Broncholithiasis J98.09
  tuberculous NEC A15.5
Bronchomalacia J98.09
  congenital Q32.2
Bronchomycosis NOS B49 *[J99]*
  candidal B37.1
Bronchopleuropneumonia —*see* Pneumonia,
  broncho
Bronchopneumonia —*see* Pneumonia,
  broncho
Bronchopneumonitis —*see* Pneumonia,
  broncho
Bronchopulmonary —*see* condition
Bronchopulmonitis —*see* Pneumonia,
  broncho
Bronchorrhagia (see Hemoptysis)
Bronchorrhea J98.09
  acute J20.9
  chronic (infective) (purulent) J42 ·
Bronchospasm (acute) J98.01
  with
    bronchiolitis, acute J21.9
    bronchitis, acute (conditions in J20) —*see*
      Bronchitis, acute
  due to external agent —*see* condition,
    respiratory, acute, due to
  exercise induced J45.990
Bronchospirochetosis A69.8
  Castellani A69.8
Bronchostenosis J98.09
Bronchus —*see* condition
Brontophobia F40.220
Bronze baby syndrome P83.8
Brooke's tumor —*see* Neoplasm, skin, benign
Brown enamel of teeth (hereditary) K00.5

Brown's sheath syndrome H50.61
Brown-Séquard disease, paralysis or
  syndrome G83.81
Bruce sepsis A23.0
Brucellosis (infection) A23.9
  abortus A23.1
  canis A23.3
  dermatitis A23.9
  melitensis A23.0
  mixed A23.8
  sepsis A23.9
    melitensis A23.0
    specified NEC A23.8
  suis A23.2
Bruck-de Lange disease Q87.1
Bruck's disease —*see* Deformity, limb
Brugsch's syndrome Q82.8
Bruise (skin surface intact) —*see also*
  Contusion
  with
    open wound —*see* Wound, open
    internal organ —*see* Injury, by site
  newborn P54.5
  scalp, due to birth injury, newborn P12.3
  umbilical cord O69.5
Bruit (arterial) R09.89
  cardiac R01.1
Brush burn —*see* Abrasion, by site
Bruton's X-linked agammaglobulinemia
  D80.0
Bruxism
  psychogenic F45.8
  sleep related G47.63
Bubbly lung syndrome P27.0
Bubo I88.8
  blennorrhagic (gonococcal) A54.89
  chancroidal A57
  climatic A55
  due to Haemophilus ducreyi A57
  gonococcal A54.89
  indolent (nonspecific) I88.8
  inguinal (nonspecific) I88.8
    chancroidal A57
    climatic A55
    due to H. ducreyi A57
    infective I88.8
  scrofulous (tuberculous) A18.2
  soft chancre A57
  suppurating —*see* Lymphadenitis, acute
  syphilitic (primary) A51.0
    congenital A50.07
  tropical A55
  virulent (chancroidal) A57
Bubonic plague A20.0
Bubonocele —*see* Hernia, inguinal
Buccal —*see* condition
Buchanan's disease or osteochondrosis
  M91.0
Buchem's syndrome (hyperostosis corticalis)
  M85.2
Bucket-handle fracture or tear (semilunar
  cartilage) —*see* Tear, meniscus
Budd-Chiari syndrome (hepatic vein
  thrombosis) I82.0
Budgerigar fancier's disease or lung J67.2
Buds
  breast E30.1
    in newborn P96.89
Buerger's disease (thromboangiitis obliterans)
  I73.1
Bulbar —*see* condition
Bulbus cordis (left ventricle) (persistent)
  Q21.8

Bulimia (nervosa) F50.2
 atypical F50.9
 normal weight F50.9
Bulky
 stools R19.5
 uterus N85.2
Bulla (e) R23.8
 lung (emphysematous) (solitary) J43.9
 newborn P25.8
Bullet wound —*see also* Wound, open
 fracture
 code as Fracture, by site
 internal organ —*see* Injury, by site
Bundle
 branch block (complete) (false) (incomplete)
 —*see* Block, bundle-branch
 of His —*see* condition
Bunion —*see* Deformity, toe, hallux valgus
Buphthalmia, buphthalmos (congenital)
 Q15.0
Burdwan fever B55.0
Bürger-Grütz disease or syndrome E78.3
Buried
 penis (congenital) Q55.64
 acquired N48.83
 roots K08.3
Burke's syndrome K86.8
Burkitt
 cell leukemia C91.0
 lymphoma (malignant) C83.7
 small noncleaved, diffuse C83.7
 spleen C83.77
 undifferentiated C83.7
 tumor C83.7
 type
 acute lymphoblastic leukemia C91.0
 undifferentiated C83.7
Burn (electricity) (flame) (hot gas, liquid or
 hot object) (radiation) (steam) (thermal) T30.0
 abdomen, abdominal (muscle) (wall) T21.02
 first degree T21.12
 second degree T21.22
 third degree T21.32
 above elbow T22.039
 first degree T22.139
 left T22.032
 first degree T22.132
 second degree T22.232
 third degree T22.332
 right T22.031
 first degree T22.131
 second degree T22.231
 third degree T22.331
 second degree T22.239
 third degree T22.339
 acid (caustic) (external) (internal) —*see*
 Corrosion, by site
 alimentary tract NEC T28.2
 esophagus T28.1
 mouth T28.0
 pharynx T28.0
 alkaline (caustic) (external) (internal) —*see*
 Corrosion, by site
 ankle T25.019
 first degree T25.119
 left T25.012
 first degree T25.112
 second degree T25.212
 third degree T25.312
 multiple with foot —*see* Burn, lower, limb,
 multiple, ankle and foot
 right T25.011

Burn – *continued*
 first degree T25.111
 second degree T25.211
 third degree T25.311
 second degree T25.219
 third degree T25.319
 anus —*see* Burn, buttock
 arm (lower) (upper) —*see* Burn, upper, limb
 axilla T22.049
 first degree T22.149
 left T22.042
 first degree T22.142
 second degree T22.242
 third degree T22.342
 right T22.041
 first degree T22.141
 second degree T22.241
 third degree T22.341
 second degree T22.249
 third degree T22.349
 back (lower) T21.04
 first degree T21.14
 second degree T21.24
 third degree T21.34
 upper T21.03
 first degree T21.13
 second degree T21.23
 third degree T21.33
 blisters
 code as Burn, second degree, by site
 breast (s) —*see* Burn, chest wall
 buttock (s) T21.05
 first degree T21.15
 second degree T21.25
 third degree T21.35
 calf T24.039
 first degree T24.139
 left T24.032
 first degree T24.132
 second degree T24.232
 third degree T24.332
 right T24.031
 first degree T24.131
 second degree T24.231
 third degree T24.331
 second degree T24.239
 third degree T24.339
 canthus (eye) —*see* Burn, eyelid
 caustic acid or alkaline —*see* Corrosion, by
 site
 cervix T28.3
 cheek T20.06
 first degree T20.16
 second degree T20.26
 third degree T20.36
 chemical (acids) (alkalines) (caustics)
 (external) (internal) —*see* Corrosion, by site
 chest wall T21.01
 first degree T21.11
 second degree T21.21
 third degree T21.31
 chin T20.03
 first degree T20.13
 second degree T20.23
 third degree T20.33
 colon T28.2
 conjunctiva (and cornea) —*see* Burn, cornea
 cornea (and conjunctiva) T26.1
 chemical —*see* Corrosion, cornea
 corrosion (external) (internal) —*see*
 Corrosion, by site
 deep necrosis of underlying tissue

Burn – *continued*
 code as Burn, third degree, by site
 dorsum of hand T23.069
 first degree T23.169
 left T23.062
 first degree T23.162
 second degree T23.262
 third degree T23.362
 right T23.061
 first degree T23.161
 second degree T23.261
 third degree T23.361
 second degree T23.269
 third degree T23.369
 due to ingested chemical agent —*see*
 Corrosion, by site
 ear (auricle) (external) (canal) T20.01
 first degree T20.11
 second degree T20.21
 third degree T20.31
 elbow T22.029
 first degree T22.129
 left T22.022
 first degree T22.122
 second degree T22.222
 third degree T22.322
 right T22.021
 first degree T22.121
 second degree T22.221
 third degree T22.321
 second degree T22.229
 third degree T22.329
 epidermal loss
 code as Burn, second degree, by site
 erythema, erythematous
 code as Burn, first degree, by site
 esophagus T28.1
 extent (percentage of body surface)
 less than 10 percent T31.0
 10 19 percent T31.10
 with 0 9 percent third degree burns T31.10
 with 10 19 percent third degree burns
 T31.11
 20 29 percent T31.20
 with 0 9 percent third degree burns T31.20
 with 10 19 percent third degree burns
 T31.21
 with 20 29 percent third degree burns
 T31.22
 30 39 percent T31.30
 with 0 9 percent third degree burns T31.30
 with 10 19 percent third degree burns
 T31.31
 with 20 29 percent third degree burns
 T31.32
 with 30 39 percent third degree burns
 T31.33
 40 49 percent T31.40
 with 0 9 percent third degree burns T31.40
 with 10 19 percent third degree burns
 T31.41
 with 20 29 percent third degree burns
 T31.42
 with 30 39 percent third degree burns
 T31.43
 with 40 49 percent third degree burns
 T31.44
 50 59 percent T31.50
 with 0 9 percent third degree burns T31.50
 with 10 19 percent third degree burns
 T31.51
 with 20 29 percent third degree burns
 T31.52

Burn – *continued*

  with 30 39 percent third degree burns T31.53

  with 40 49 percent third degree burns T31.54

  with 50 59 percent third degree burns T31.55

 60 69 percent T31.60

  with 0 9 percent third degree burns T31.60

  with 10 19 percent third degree burns T31.61

  with 20 29 percent third degree burns T31.62

  with 30 39 percent third degree burns T31.63

  with 40 49 percent third degree burns T31.64

  with 50 59 percent third degree burns T31.65

  with 60 69 percent third degree burns T31.66

 70 79 percent T31.70

  with 0 9 percent third degree burns T31.70

  with 10 19 percent third degree burns T31.71

  with 20 29 percent third degree burns T31.72

  with 30 39 percent third degree burns T31.73

  with 40 49 percent third degree burns T31.74

  with 50 59 percent third degree burns T31.75

  with 60 69 percent third degree burns T31.76

  with 70 79 percent third degree burns T31.77

 80 89 percent T31.80

  with 0 9 percent third degree burns T31.80

  with 10 19 percent third degree burns T31.81

  with 20 29 percent third degree burns T31.82

  with 30 39 percent third degree burns T31.83

  with 40 49 percent third degree burns T31.84

  with 50 59 percent third degree burns T31.85

  with 60 69 percent third degree burns T31.86

  with 70 79 percent third degree burns T31.87

  with 80 89 percent third degree burns T31.88

 90 percent or more T31.90

  with 0 9 percent third degree burns T31.90

  with 10 19 percent third degree burns T31.91

  with 20 29 percent third degree burns T31.92

  with 30 39 percent third degree burns T31.93

  with 40 49 percent third degree burns T31.94

  with 50 59 percent third degree burns T31.95

  with 60 69 percent third degree burns T31.96

  with 70 79 percent third degree burns T31.97

Burn – *continued*

  with 80 89 percent third degree burns T31.98

  with 90 percent or more third degree burns T31.99

extremity —*see* Burn, limb

eye (s) and adnexa T26.4

 with resulting rupture and destruction of eyeball T26.2

 conjunctival sac —*see* Burn, cornea

 cornea —*see* Burn, cornea

 lid —*see* Burn, eyelid

 periocular area —*see* Burn, eyelid

 specified site NEC T26.3

eyeball —*see* Burn, eye

eyelid (s) T26.0

 chemical —*see* Corrosion, eyelid

face —*see* Burn, head

finger T23.029

 first degree T23.129

 left T23.022

  first degree T23.122

  second degree T23.222

  third degree T23.322

 multiple sites (without thumb) T23.039

  with thumb T23.049

   first degree T23.149

   left T23.042

    first degree T23.142

    second degree T23.242

    third degree T23.342

   right T23.041

    first degree T23.141

    second degree T23.241

    third degree T23.341

   second degree T23.249

   third degree T23.349

  first degree T23.139

  left T23.032

   first degree T23.132

   second degree T23.232

   third degree T23.332

  right T23.031

   first degree T23.131

   second degree T23.231

   third degree T23.331

  second degree T23.239

  third degree T23.339

 right T23.021

  first degree T23.121

  second degree T23.221

  third degree T23.321

 second degree T23.229

 third degree T23.329

flank —*see* Burn, abdominal wall

foot T25.029

 first degree T25.129

 left T25.022

  first degree T25.122

  second degree T25.222

  third degree T25.322

 multiple with ankle —*see* Burn, lower, limb, multiple, ankle and foot

 right T25.021

  first degree T25.121

  second degree T25.221

  third degree T25.321

 second degree T25.229

 third degree T25.329

forearm T22.019

 first degree T22.119

Burn – *continued*

 left T22.012

  first degree T22.112

  second degree T22.212

  third degree T22.312

 right T22.011

  first degree T22.111

  second degree T22.211

  third degree T22.311

 second degree T22.219

 third degree T22.319

forehead T20.06

 first degree T20.16

 second degree T20.26

 third degree T20.36

fourth degree

 code as Burn, third degree, by site

friction —*see* Burn, by site

from swallowing caustic or corrosive substance NEC —*see* Corrosion, by site

full thickness skin loss

 code as Burn, third degree, by site

gastrointestinal tract NEC T28.2

 from swallowing caustic or corrosive substance T28.7

genital organs

 external

  female T21.07

   first degree T21.17

   second degree T21.27

   third degree T21.37

  male T21.06

   first degree T21.16

   second degree T21.26

   third degree T21.36

 internal T28.3

  from caustic or corrosive substance T28.8

groin —*see* Burn, abdominal wall

hand (s) T23.009

 back —*see* Burn, dorsum of hand

 finger —*see* Burn, finger

 first degree T23.109

 left T23.002

  first degree T23.102

  second degree T23.202

  third degree T23.302

 multiple sites with wrist T23.099

  first degree T23.199

  left T23.092

   first degree T23.192

   second degree T23.292

   third degree T23.392

  right T23.091

   first degree T23.191

   second degree T23.291

   third degree T23.391

  second degree T23.299

  third degree T23.399

 palm —*see* Burn, palm

 right T23.001

  first degree T23.101

  second degree T23.201

  third degree T23.301

 second degree T23.209

 third degree T23.309

 thumb —*see* Burn, thumb

head (and face) (and neck) T20.00

 cheek —*see* Burn, cheek

 chin —*see* Burn, chin

 ear —*see* Burn, ear

 eye (s) only —*see* Burn, eye

 first degree T20.10

 forehead —*see* Burn, forehead

Burn —*continued*
  lip —*see* Burn, lip
  multiple sites T20.09
    first degree T20.19
    second degree T20.29
    third degree T20.39
  neck —*see* Burn, neck
  nose —*see* Burn, nose
  scalp —*see* Burn, scalp
  second degree T20.20
  third degree T20.30
  hip (s) —*see* Burn, lower, limb
  inhalation —*see* Burn, respiratory tract
    caustic or corrosive substance (fumes) —*see*
Corrosion, respiratory tract
  internal organ (s) T28.40
    alimentary tract T28.2
      esophagus T28.1
    eardrum T28.41
    esophagus T28.1
    from caustic or corrosive substance
(swallowing) NEC —*see* Corrosion, by site
    genitourinary T28.3
    mouth T28.0
    pharynx T28.0
    respiratory tract —*see* Burn, respiratory tract
    specified organ NEC T28.49
  interscapular region —*see* Burn, back, upper
  intestine (large) (small) T28.2
  knee T24.029
    first degree T24.129
    left T24.022
      first degree T24.122
      second degree T24.222
      third degree T24.322
    right T24.021
      first degree T24.121
      second degree T24.221
      third degree T24.321
    second degree T24.229
    third degree T24.329
  labium (majus) (minus) —*see* Burn, genital
organs, external, female
  lacrimal apparatus, duct, gland or sac —*see*
Burn, eye, specified site NEC
  larynx T27.0
    with lung T27.1
  leg (s) (lower) (upper) —*see* Burn, lower,
limb
  lightning —*see* Burn, by site
  limb (s)
    lower (except ankle or foot alone) —*see*
Burn, lower, limb
    upper —*see* Burn, upper limb
  lip (s) T20.02
    first degree T20.12
    second degree T20.22
    third degree T20.32
  lower
    back —*see* Burn, back
    limb T24.009
      ankle —*see* Burn, ankle
      calf —*see* Burn, calf
      first degree T24.109
      foot —*see* Burn, foot
      hip —*see* Burn, thigh
      knee —*see* Burn, knee
      left T24.002
        first degree T24.102
        second degree T24.202
        third degree T24.302

Burn —*continued*
  multiple sites, except ankle and foot
T24.099
    ankle and foot T25.099
      first degree T25.199
      left T25.092
        first degree T25.192
        second degree T25.292
        third degree T25.392
      right T25.091
        first degree T25.191
        second degree T25.291
        third degree T25.391
      second degree T25.299
      third degree T25.399
    first degree T24.199
    left T24.092
      first degree T24.192
      second degree T24.292
      third degree T24.392
    right T24.091
      first degree T24.191
      second degree T24.291
      third degree T24.391
    second degree T24.299
    third degree T24.399
    right T24.001
      first degree T24.101
      second degree T24.201
      third degree T24.301
    second degree T24.209
    thigh —*see* Burn, thigh
    third degree T24.309
    toe —*see* Burn, toe
  lung (with larynx and trachea) T27.1
  mouth T28.0
  neck T20.07
    first degree T20.17
    second degree T20.27
    third degree T20.37
  nose (septum) T20.04
    first degree T20.14
    second degree T20.24
    third degree T20.34
  ocular adnexa —*see* Burn, eye
  orbit region —*see* Burn, eyelid
  palm T23.059
    first degree T23.159
    left T23.052
      first degree T23.152
      second degree T23.252
      third degree T23.352
    right T23.051
      first degree T23.151
      second degree T23.251
      third degree T23.351
    second degree T23.259
    third degree T23.359
  partial thickness
    code as Burn, unspecified degree, by site
  pelvis —*see* Burn, trunk
  penis —*see* Burn, genital organs, external,
male
  perineum
    female —*see* Burn, genital organs, external,
female
    male —*see* Burn, genital organs, external,
male
  periocular area —*see* Burn, eyelid
  pharynx T28.0
  rectum T28.2

Burn —*continued*
  respiratory tract T27.3
    larynx —*see* Burn, larynx
    specified part NEC T27.2
    trachea —*see* Burn, trachea
  sac, lacrimal —*see* Burn, eye, specified site
NEC
  scalp T20.05
    first degree T20.15
    second degree T20.25
    third degree T20.35
  scapular region T22.069
    first degree T22.169
    left T22.062
      first degree T22.162
      second degree T22.262
      third degree T22.362
    right T22.061
      first degree T22.161
      second degree T22.261
      third degree T22.361
    second degree T22.269
    third degree T22.369
  sclera —*see* Burn, eye, specified site NEC
  scrotum —*see* Burn, genital organs, external,
male
  shoulder T22.059
    first degree T22.159
    left T22.052
      first degree T22.152
      second degree T22.252
      third degree T22.352
    right T22.051
      first degree T22.151
      second degree T22.251
      third degree T22.351
    second degree T22.259
    third degree T22.359
  stomach T28.2
  temple —*see* Burn, head
  testis —*see* Burn, genital organs, external,
male
  thigh T24.019
    first degree T24.119
    left T24.012
      first degree T24.112
      second degree T24.212
      third degree T24.312
    right T24.011
      first degree T24.111
      second degree T24.211
      third degree T24.311
    second degree T24.219
    third degree T24.319
  thorax (external) —*see* Burn, trunk
  throat (meaning pharynx) T28.0
  thumb (s) T23.019
    first degree T23.119
    left T23.012
      first degree T23.112
      second degree T23.212
      third degree T23.312
    multiple sites with fingers T23.049
      first degree T23.149
      left T23.042
        first degree T23.142
        second degree T23.242
        third degree T23.342
      right T23.041
        first degree T23.141
        second degree T23.241
        third degree T23.341
      second degree T23.249

Burn – *continued*

    third degree T23.349
   right T23.011
    first degree T23.111
    second degree T23.211
    third degree T23.311
   second degree T23.219
   third degree T23.319
  toe T25.039
   first degree T25.139
   left T25.032
    first degree T25.132
    second degree T25.232
    third degree T25.332
   right T25.031
    first degree T25.131
    second degree T25.231
    third degree T25.331
   second degree T25.239
   third degree T25.339
  tongue T28.0
  tonsil (s) T28.0
  trachea T27.0
   with lung T27.1
  trunk T21.00
   abdominal wall —*see* Burn, abdominal wall
   anus —*see* Burn, buttock
   axilla —*see* Burn, upper limb
   back —*see* Burn, back
   breast —*see* Burn, chest wall
   buttock —*see* Burn, buttock
   chest wall —*see* Burn, chest wall
   first degree T21.10
   flank —*see* Burn, abdominal wall
   genital
    female —*see* Burn, genital organs, external, female
    male —*see* Burn, genital organs, external, male
   groin —*see* Burn, abdominal wall
   interscapular region —*see* Burn, back, upper
   labia —*see* Burn, genital organs, external, female
   lower back —*see* Burn, back
   penis —*see* Burn, genital organs, external, male
   perineum
    female —*see* Burn, genital organs, external, female
    male —*see* Burn, genital organs, external, male
   scapula region —*see* Burn, scapular region
   scrotum —*see* Burn, genital organs, external, male
   second degree T21.20
   specified site NEC T21.09
    first degree T21.19
    second degree T21.29
    third degree T21.39
   testes —*see* Burn, genital organs, external, male
   third degree T21.30
   upper back —*see* Burn, back, upper
   vulva —*see* Burn, genital organs, external, female
  unspecified site with extent of body surface involved specified
   less than 10 per cent T31.0
   10 19 per cent (0 9 percent third degree) T31.10
    with 10 19 percent third degree T31.11

Burn – *continued*

  20 29 per cent (0 9 percent third degree) T31.20
   with
    10 19 percent third degree T31.21
    20 29 percent third degree T31.22
  30 39 per cent (0 9 percent third degree) T31.30
   with
    10 19 percent third degree T31.31
    20 29 percent third degree T31.32
    30 39 percent third degree T31.33
  40 49 per cent (0 9 percent third degree) T31.40
   with
    10 19 percent third degree T31.41
    20 29 percent third degree T31.42
    30 39 percent third degree T31.43
    40 49 percent third degree T31.44
  50 59 per cent (0 9 percent third degree) T31.50
   with
    10 19 percent third degree T31.51
    20 29 percent third degree T31.52
    30 39 percent third degree T31.53
    40 49 percent third degree T31.54
    50 59 percent third degree T31.55
  60 69 per cent (0 9 percent third degree) T31.60
   with
    10 19 percent third degree T31.61
    20 29 percent third degree T31.62
    30 39 percent third degree T31.63
    40 49 percent third degree T31.64
    50 59 percent third degree T31.65
    60 69 percent third degree T31.66
  70 79 per cent (0 9 percent third degree) T31.70
   with
    10 19 percent third degree T31.71
    20 29 percent third degree T31.72
    30 39 percent third degree T31.73
    40 49 percent third degree T31.74
    50 59 percent third degree T31.75
    60 69 percent third degree T31.76
    70 79 percent third degree T31.77
  80 89 per cent (0 9 percent third degree) T31.80
   with
    10 19 percent third degree T31.81
    20 29 percent third degree T31.82
    30 39 percent third degree T31.83
    40 49 percent third degree T31.84
    50 59 percent third degree T31.85
    60 69 percent third degree T31.86
    70 79 percent third degree T31.87
    80 89 percent third degree T31.88
  90 per cent or more (0 9 percent third degree) T31.90
   with
    10 19 percent third degree T31.91
    20 29 percent third degree T31.92
    30 39 percent third degree T31.93
    40 49 percent third degree T31.94
    50 59 percent third degree T31.95
    60 69 percent third degree T31.96
    70 79 percent third degree T31.97
    80 89 percent third degree T31.98
    90 99 percent third degree T31.99
  upper limb T22.00
   above elbow —*see* Burn, above elbow
   axilla —*see* Burn, axilla

Burn – *continued*

   elbow —*see* Burn, elbow
   first degree T22.10
   forearm —*see* Burn, forearm
   hand —*see* Burn, hand
   interscapular region —*see* Burn, back, upper
   multiple sites T22.099
    first degree T22.199
    left T22.092
     first degree T22.192
     second degree T22.292
     third degree T22.392
    right T22.091
     first degree T22.191
     second degree T22.291
     third degree T22.391
    second degree T22.299
    third degree T22.399
   scapular region —*see* Burn, scapular region
   second degree T22.20
   shoulder —*see* Burn, shoulder
   third degree T22.30
   wrist —*see* Burn, wrist
  uterus T28.3
  vagina T28.3
  vulva —*see* Burn, genital organs, external, female
  wrist T23.079
   first degree T23.179
   left T23.072
    first degree T23.172
    second degree T23.272
    third degree T23.372
   multiple sites with hand T23.099
    first degree T23.199
    left T23.092
     first degree T23.192
     second degree T23.292
     third degree T23.392
    right T23.091
     first degree T23.191
     second degree T23.291
     third degree T23.391
    second degree T23.299
    third degree T23.399
   right T23.071
    first degree T23.171
    second degree T23.271
    third degree T23.371
   second degree T23.279
   third degree T23.379

Burnett's syndrome E83.52

Burning
  feet syndrome E53.9
  sensation R20.8
  tongue K14.6

Burn-out (state) Z73.0

Burns' disease or osteochondrosis —*see* Osteochondrosis, juvenile, ulna

Bursa —*see* condition

Bursitis M71.9
  Achilles —*see* Tendinitis, Achilles
  adhesive —*see* Bursitis, specified NEC
  ankle —*see* Enthesopathy, lower limb, ankle, specified type NEC
  calcaneal —*see* Enthesopathy, foot, specified type NEC
  collateral ligament, tibial —*see* Bursitis, tibial collateral
  due to use, overuse, pressure —*see also* Disorder, soft tissue, due to use, specified type NEC

Bursitis - *continued*

specified NEC —*see* Disorder, soft tissue, due to use, specified NEC

Duplay's M75.0

elbow NEC M70.3

olecranon M70.2

finger —*see* Disorder, soft tissue, due to use, specified type NEC, hand

foot —*see* Enthesopathy, foot, specified type NEC

gonococcal A54.49

gouty —*see* Gout, idiopathic

hand M70.1

hip NEC M70.7

trochanteric M70.6

infective NEC M71.10

abscess —*see* Abscess, bursa

ankle M71.17

elbow M71.12

foot M71.17

hand M71.14

hip M71.15

knee M71.16

multiple sites M71.19

shoulder M71.11

specified site NEC M71.18

wrist M71.13

ischial —*see* Bursitis, hip

knee NEC M70.5

prepatellar M70.4

occupational NEC — *see also* Disorder, soft tissue, due to, use

olecranon —*see* Bursitis, elbow, olecranon

pharyngeal J39.1

popliteal —*see* Bursitis, knee

prepatellar M70.4

radiohumeral M77.8

rheumatoid M06.20

ankle M06.27

elbow M06.22

foot joint M06.27

hand joint M06.24

hip M06.25

knee M06.26

multiple site M06.29

shoulder M06.21

vertebra M06.28

wrist M06.23

scapulohumeral —*see* Bursitis, shoulder

semimembranous muscle (knee) —*see* Bursitis, knee

shoulder M75.5

adhesive —*see* Capsulitis, adhesive

specified NEC M71.50

ankle M71.57

due to use, overuse or pressure —*see* Disorder, soft tissue, due to, use

elbow M71.52

foot M71.57

hand M71.54

hip M71.55

knee M71.56

shoulder —*see* Bursitis, shoulder

specified site NEC M71.58

tibial collateral M76.4

wrist M71.53

subacromial —*see* Bursitis, shoulder

subcoracoid —*see* Bursitis, shoulder

subdeltoid —*see* Bursitis, shoulder

syphilitic A52.78

Thornwaldt, Tornwaldt J39.2

tibial collateral —*see* Bursitis, tibial collateral

Bursitis - *continued*

toe —*see* Enthesopathy, foot, specified type NEC

trochanteric (area) —*see* Bursitis, hip, trochanteric

wrist —*see* Bursitis, hand

Bursopathy M71.9

specified type NEC M71.80

ankle M71.87

elbow M71.82

foot M71.87

hand M71.84

hip M71.85

knee M71.86

multiple sites M71.89

shoulder M71.81

specified site NEC M71.88

wrist M71.83

Burst stitches or sutures (complication of surgery) T81.31

external operation wound T81.31

internal operation wound T81.32

Buruli ulcer A31.1

Bury's disease L95.1

Buschke's

disease B45.3

scleredema —*see* Sclerosis, systemic

Busse-Buschke disease B45.3

Buttock —*see* condition

Button

Biskra B55.1

Delhi B55.1

oriental B55.1

Buttonhole deformity (finger) —*see* Deformity, finger, boutonniere

Bwamba fever A92.8

Byssinosis J66.0

Bywaters' syndrome T79.5

C

Cachexia R64

cancerous R64

cardiac —*see* Disease, heart

dehydration E86.0

with

hypernatremia E87.0

hyponatremia E87.1

due to malnutrition R64

exophthalmic —*see* Hyperthyroidism

heart —*see* Disease, heart

hypophyseal E23.0

hypopituitary E23.0

lead —*see* Poisoning, lead

malignant R64

marsh —*see* Malaria

nervous F48.8

old age R54

paludal —*see* Malaria

pituitary E23.0

renal N28.9

saturnine —*see* Poisoning, lead

senile R54

Simmonds' E23.0

splenica D73.0

strumipriva E03.4

tuberculous NEC —*see* Tuberculosis

Café, au lait spots L81.3

Caffey's syndrome Q78.8

Caisson disease T70.3

Cake kidney Q63.1

Caked breast (puerperal, postpartum) O92.79

Calabar swelling B74.3

Calcaneal spur —*see* Spur, bone, calcaneal

Calcaneo-apophysitis M92.8

Calcareous —*see* condition

Calcicosis J62.8

Calciferol (vitamin D) **deficiency** E55.9

with rickets E55.0

Calcification

adrenal (capsule) (gland) E27.49

tuberculous E35 *[B90.8]*

aorta I70.0

artery (annular) —*see* Arteriosclerosis

auricle (ear) —*see* Disorder, pinna, specified type NEC

basal ganglia G23.8

bladder N32.89

due to Schistosoma hematobium B65.0

brain (cortex) —*see* Calcification, cerebral

bronchus J98.09

bursa M71.40

ankle M71.47

elbow M71.42

foot M71.47

hand M71.44

hip M71.45

knee M71.46

multiple sites M71.49

shoulder M75.3

specified site NEC M71.48

wrist M71.43

cardiac —*see* Degeneration, myocardial

cerebral (cortex) G93.89

artery I67.2

cervix (uteri) N88.8

choroid plexus G93.89

conjunctiva —*see* Concretion, conjunctiva

corpora cavernosa (penis) N48.89

cortex (brain) —*see* Calcification, cerebral

dental pulp (nodular) K04.2

dentinal papilla K00.4

fallopian tube N83.8

falx cerebri G96.19

gallbladder K82.8

general E83.59

heart —*see also* Degeneration, myocardial

valve —*see* Endocarditis

idiopathic infantile arterial (IIAC) Q28.8

intervertebral cartilage or disc (postinfective) —*see* Disorder, disc, specified NEC

intracranial —*see* Calcification, cerebral

joint —*see* Disorder, joint, specified type NEC

kidney N28.89

tuberculous N29 *[B90.1]*

larynx (senile) J38.7

lens —*see* Cataract, specified NEC

lung (active) (postinfectional) J98.4

tuberculous B90.9

lymph gland or node (postinfectional) I89.8

tuberculous (*see also* Tuberculosis, lymph gland) B90.8

mammographic R92.1

massive (paraplegic) —*see* Myositis, ossificans, in, quadriplegia

medial —*see* Arteriosclerosis, extremities

meninges (cerebral) (spinal) G96.19

metastatic E83.59

Mönckeberg's —*see* Arteriosclerosis, extremities

muscle M61.9

due to burns —*see* Myositis, ossificans, in, burns

paralytic —*see* Myositis, ossificans, in, quadriplegia

specified type NEC M61.40

Calcification - *continued*
ankle M61.47
foot M61.47
forearm M61.43
hand M61.44
lower leg M61.46
multiple sites M61.49
pelvic region M61.45
shoulder region M61.41
specified site NEC M61.48
thigh M61.45
upper arm M61.42
myocardium, myocardial —*see* Degeneration, myocardial
ovary N83.8
pancreas K86.8
penis N48.89
periarticular —*see* Disorder, joint, specified type NEC
pericardium (*see also* Pericarditis) I31.1
pineal gland E34.8
pleura J94.8
postinfectional J94.8
tuberculous NEC B90.9
pulpal (dental) (nodular) K04.2
sclera H15.89
spleen D73.89
subcutaneous L94.2
suprarenal (capsule) (gland) E27.49
tendon (sheath) —*see also* Tenosynovitis, specified type NEC
with bursitis, synovitis or tenosynovitis —*see* Tendinitis, calcific
trachea J39.8
ureter N28.89
uterus N85.8
vitreous —*see* Deposit, crystalline
Calcified —*see* Calcification
Calcinosis (interstitial) (tumoral) (universalis) E83.59
with Raynaud's phenomenon, esophageal dysfunction, sclerodactyly, telangiectasia (CREST syndrome) M34.1
circumscripta (skin) L94.2
cutis L94.2
Calciphylaxis (*see also* Calcification, by site) E83.59
Calcium
deposits —*see* Calcification, by site
metabolism disorder E83.50
salts or soaps in vitreous —*see* Deposit, crystalline
Calciuria R82.99
Calculi —*see* Calculus
Calculosis, intrahepatic —*see* Calculus, bile duct
Calculus, calculi, calculous
ampulla of Vater —*see* Calculus, bile duct
anuria (impacted) (recurrent) (*see also* Calculus, urinary) N20.9
appendix K38.1
bile duct (common) (hepatic) K80.50
with
calculus of gallbladder —*see* Calculus, gallbladder and bile duct
cholangitis K80.30
with
cholecystitis —*see* Calculus, bile duct, with cholecystitis
obstruction K80.31
acute K80.32
with

Calculus, calculi, calculous - *continued*
chronic cholangitis K80.36
with obstruction K80.37
obstruction K80.33
chronic K80.34
with
acute cholangitis K80.36
with obstruction K80.37
obstruction K80.35
cholecystitis (with cholangitis) K80.40
with obstruction K80.41
acute K80.42
with
chronic cholecystitis K80.46
with obstruction K80.47
obstruction K80.43
chronic K80.44
with
acute cholecystitis K80.46
with obstruction K80.47
obstruction K80.45
obstruction K80.51
biliary —*see also* Calculus, gallbladder
specified NEC K80.80
with obstruction K80.81
bilirubin, multiple —*see* Calculus, gallbladder
bladder (encysted) (impacted) (urinary) (diverticulum) N21.0
bronchus J98.09
calyx (kidney) (renal) —*see* Calculus, kidney
cholesterol (pure) (solitary) —*see* Calculus, gallbladder
common duct (bile) —*see* Calculus, bile duct
conjunctiva —*see* Concretion, conjunctiva
cystic N21.0
duct —*see* Calculus, gallbladder
dental (subgingival) (supragingival) K03.6
diverticulum
bladder N21.0
kidney N20.0
epididymis N50.8
gallbladder K80.20
with
bile duct calculus —*see* Calculus, gallbladder and bile duct
cholecystitis K80.10
with obstruction K80.11
acute K80.00
with
chronic cholecystitis K80.12
with obstruction K80.13
obstruction K80.01
chronic K80.10
with
acute cholecystitis K80.12
with obstruction K80.13
obstruction K80.11
specified NEC K80.18
with obstruction K80.19
obstruction K80.21
gallbladder and bile duct K80.70
with
cholecystitis K80.60
with obstruction K80.61
acute K80.62
with
chronic cholecystitis K80.66
with obstruction K80.67
obstruction K80.63
chronic K80.64
with
acute cholecystitis K80.66

Calculus, calculi, calculous - *continued*
with obstruction K80.67
obstruction K80.65
obstruction K80.71
hepatic (duct) —*see* Calculus, bile duct
hepatobiliary K80.80
with obstruction K80.81
ileal conduit N21.8
intestinal (impaction) (obstruction) K56.49
kidney (impacted) (multiple) (pelvis) (recurrent) (staghorn) N20.0
with calculus, ureter N20.2
congenital Q63.8
lacrimal passages —*see* Dacryolith
liver (impacted) —*see* Calculus, bile duct
lung J98.4
mammographic R92.1
nephritic (impacted) (recurrent) —*see* Calculus, kidney
nose J34.89
pancreas (duct) K86.8
parotid duct or gland K11.5
pelvis, encysted —*see* Calculus, kidney
prostate N42.0
pulmonary J98.4
pyelitis (impacted) (recurrent) N20.0
with hydronephrosis N13.2
pyelonephritis (impacted) (recurrent) —*see* category N20
with hydronephrosis N13.2
renal (impacted) (recurrent) —*see* Calculus, kidney
salivary (duct) (gland) K11.5
seminal vesicle N50.8
staghorn —*see* Calculus, kidney
Stensen's duct K11.5
stomach K31.89
sublingual duct or gland K11.5
congenital Q38.4
submandibular duct, gland or region K11.5
submaxillary duct, gland or region K11.5
suburethral N21.8
tonsil J35.8
tooth, teeth (subgingival) (supragingival) K03.6
tunica vaginalis N50.8
ureter (impacted) (recurrent) N20.1
with calculus, kidney N20.2
with hydronephrosis N13.2
with infection N13.6
urethra (impacted) N21.1
urinary (duct) (impacted) (passage) (tract) N20.9
with hydronephrosis N13.2
with infection N13.6
in (due to)
lower N21.9
specified NEC N21.8
vagina N89.8
vesical (impacted) N21.0
Wharton's duct K11.5
xanthine E79.8 *[N22]*
Calicectasis N28.89
Caliectasis N28.89
California
disease B38.9
encephalitis A83.5
Caligo cornea —*see* Opacity, cornea, central
Callositas, callosity (infected) L84
Callus (infected) L84
bone —*see* Osteophyte
excessive, following fracture
code as Sequelae of fracture

Calorie deficiency or malnutrition (*see also* Malnutrition) E46

Calvé-Perthes disease —*see* Legg-Calvé-Perthes disease

Calvé's disease —*see* Osteochondrosis, juvenile, spine

Calvities —*see* Alopecia, androgenic

Cameroon fever —*see* Malaria

Camptocormia (hysterical) F44.4

Camurati-Engelmann syndrome Q78.3

Canal —*see also* condition
  atrioventricular common Q21.2

Canaliculitis (lacrimal) (acute) (subacute) H04.33
  Actinomyces A42.89
  chronic H04.42

Canavan's disease E75.29

Canceled procedure (surgical) Z53.9
  because of
    contraindication Z53.09
      smoking Z53.01
    left against medical advice (AMA) Z53.21
    patient's decision Z53.20
      for reasons of belief or group pressure Z53.1
        specified reason NEC Z53.29
      specified reason NEC Z53.8

Cancer —*see also* Neoplasm, by site, malignant
  bile duct type liver C22.1
  blood —*see* Leukemia
  breast (*see also* Neoplasm, breast, malignant) C50.91
  hepatocellular C22.0
  lung (*see also* Neoplasm, lung, malignant) C34.90
  ovarian (*see also* Neoplasm ovary, malignant) C56.9
  unspecified site (primary) C80.1

Cancer (o) **phobia** F45.29

Cancerous —*see* Neoplasm, malignant, by site

Cancrum oris A69.0

Candidiasis, candidal B37.9
  balanitis B37.42
  bronchitis B37.1
  cheilitis B37.83
  congenital P37.5
  cystitis B37.41
  disseminated B37.7
  endocarditis B37.6
  enteritis B37.82
  esophagitis B37.81
  intertrigo B37.2
  lung B37.1
  meningitis B37.5
  mouth B37.0
  nails B37.2
  neonatal P37.5
  onychia B37.2
  oral B37.0
  osteomyelitis B37.89
  otitis externa B37.84
  paronychia B37.2
  perionyxis B37.2
  pneumonia B37.1
  proctitis B37.82
  pulmonary B37.1
  pyelonephritis B37.49
  sepsis B37.7
  skin B37.2
  specified site NEC B37.89
  stomatitis B37.0

Candidiasis, candidal - *continued*
  systemic B37.7
  urethritis B37.41
  urogenital site NEC B37.49
  vagina B37.3
  vulva B37.3
  vulvovaginitis B37.3

Candidid L30.2

Candidosis —*see* Candidiasis

Candiru infection or infestation B88.8

Canities (premature) L67.1
  congenital Q84.2

Canker (mouth) (sore) K12.0
  rash A38.9

Cannabinosis J66.2

Canton fever A75.9

Cantrell's syndrome Q87.89

Capillariasis (intestinal) B81.1
  hepatic B83.8

Capillary —*see* condition

Caplan's syndrome —*see* Rheumatoid, lung

Capsule —*see* condition

Capsulitis (joint) —*see also* Enthesopathy
  adhesive (shoulder) M75.0
  hepatic K65.8
  labyrinthine —*see* Otosclerosis, specified NEC
  thyroid E06.9

Caput
  crepitus Q75.8
  medusae I86.8
  succedaneum P12.81

Car sickness T75.3

Carapata (disease) A68.0

Carate —*see* Pinta

Carbon lung J60

Carbuncle L02.93
  abdominal wall L02.231
  anus K61.0
  auditory canal, external —*see* Abscess, ear, external
  auricle ear —*see* Abscess, ear, external
  axilla L02.43
  back (any part) L02.232
  breast N61
  buttock L02.33
  cheek (external) L02.03
  chest wall L02.233
  chin L02.03
  corpus cavernosum N48.21
  ear (any part) (external) (middle) —*see* Abscess, ear, external
  external auditory canal —*see* Abscess, ear, external
  eyelid —*see* Abscess, eyelid
  face NEC L02.03
  femoral (region) —*see* Carbuncle, lower limb
  finger —*see* Carbuncle, hand
  flank L02.231
  foot L02.63
  forehead L02.03
  genital —*see* Abscess, genital
  gluteal (region) L02.33
  groin L02.234
  hand L02.53
  head NEC L02.831
  heel —*see* Carbuncle, foot
  hip —*see* Carbuncle, lower limb
  kidney —*see* Abscess, kidney
  knee —*see* Carbuncle, lower limb
  labium (majus) (minus) N76.4

Carbuncle - *continued*
  lacrimal
    gland —*see* Dacryoadenitis
    passages (duct) (sac) —*see* Inflammation, lacrimal, passages, acute
  leg —*see* Carbuncle, lower limb
  lower limb L02.43
  malignant A22.0
  navel L02.236
  neck L02.13
  nose (external) (septum) J34.0
  orbit, orbital —*see* Abscess, orbit
  palmar (space) —*see* Carbuncle, hand
  partes posteriores L02.33
  pectoral region L02.233
  penis N48.21
  perineum L02.235
  pinna —*see* Abscess, ear, external
  popliteal —*see* Carbuncle, lower limb
  scalp L02.831
  seminal vesicle N49.0
  shoulder —*see* Carbuncle, upper limb
  specified site NEC L02.838
  temple (region) L02.03
  thumb —*see* Carbuncle, hand
  toe —*see* Carbuncle, foot
  trunk L02.239
    abdominal wall L02.231
    back L02.232
    chest wall L02.233
    groin L02.234
    perineum L02.235
    umbilicus L02.236
  umbilicus L02.236
  upper limb L02.43
  urethra N34.0
  vulva N76.4

Carbunculus —*see* Carbuncle

Carcinoid (tumor) —*see* Tumor, carcinoid

Carcinoidosis E34.0

Carcinoma (malignant) —*see also* Neoplasm, by site, malignant
  acidophil
    specified site —*see* Neoplasm, malignant, by site
    unspecified site C75.1
  acidophil-basophil, mixed
    specified site —*see* Neoplasm, malignant, by site
    unspecified site C75.1
  adnexal (skin) —*see* Neoplasm, skin, malignant
  adrenal cortical C74.0
  alveolar —*see* Neoplasm, lung, malignant
    cell —*see* Neoplasm, lung, malignant
  ameloblastic C41.1
    upper jaw (bone) C41.0
  apocrine
    breast —*see* Neoplasm, breast, malignant
    specified site NEC —*see* Neoplasm, skin, malignant
    unspecified site C44.99
  basal cell (pigmented) (see also Neoplasm, skin, malignant) C44.91
    fibro-epithelial —*see* Neoplasm, skin, malignant
    morphea —*see* Neoplasm, skin, malignant
    multicentric —*see* Neoplasm, skin, malignant
  basaloid
  basal-squamous cell, mixed —*see* Neoplasm, skin, malignant

Carcinoma (malignant) - *continued*
  basophil
    specified site —*see* Neoplasm, malignant,
    by site
      unspecified site C75.1
  basophil-acidophil, mixed
    specified site —*see* Neoplasm, malignant,
    by site
      unspecified site C75.1
  basosquamous —*see* Neoplasm, skin,
  malignant
  bile duct
    with hepatocellular, mixed C22.0
    liver C22.1
    specified site NEC —*see* Neoplasm,
  malignant, by site
    unspecified site C22.1
  branchial or branchiogenic C10.4
  bronchial or bronchogenic —*see* Neoplasm,
  lung, malignant
  bronchiolar —*see* Neoplasm, lung, malignant
  bronchioloalveolar —*see* Neoplasm, lung,
  malignant
  C cell
    specified site —*see* Neoplasm, malignant,
    by site
      unspecified site C73
  ceruminous C44.29
  cervix uteri
    in situ D06.9
      endocervix D06.0
      exocervix D06.1
      specified site NEC D06.7
  chorionic
    specified site —*see* Neoplasm, malignant,
    by site
      unspecified site
        female C58
        male C62.90
  chromophobe
    specified site —*see* Neoplasm, malignant,
    by site
      unspecified site C75.1
  cloacogenic
    specified site —*see* Neoplasm, malignant,
    by site
      unspecified site C21.2
  diffuse type
    specified site —*see* Neoplasm, malignant,
    by site
      unspecified site C16.9
  duct (cell)
    with Paget's disease —*see* Neoplasm, breast,
  malignant
    infiltrating
      with lobular carcinoma (in situ)
        specified site —*see* Neoplasm, malignant,
        by site
          unspecified site (female) C50.91
            male C50.92
        specified site —*see* Neoplasm, malignant,
        by site
          unspecified site (female) C50.91
            male C50.92
  ductal
    with lobular
      specified site —*see* Neoplasm, malignant,
      by site
        unspecified site (female) C50.91
          male C50.92
  ductular, infiltrating

Carcinoma (malignant) - *continued*
    specified site —*see* Neoplasm, malignant,
    by site
      unspecified site (female) C50.91
        male C50.92
  embryonal
    liver C22.7
  endometrioid
    specified site —*see* Neoplasm, malignant,
    by site
      unspecified site
        female C56.9
        male C61
  eosinophil
    specified site —*see* Neoplasm, malignant,
    by site
      unspecified site C75.1
  epidermoid —*see also* Neoplasm, skin
  malignant
    in situ, Bowen's type —*see* Neoplasm, skin,
  in situ
    fibroepithelial, basal cell —*see* Neoplasm,
  skin, malignant
  follicular
    with papillary (mixed) C73
    moderately differentiated C73
    pure follicle C73
    specified site —*see* Neoplasm, malignant,
    by site
    trabecular C73
    unspecified site C73
    well differentiated C73
  generalized, with unspecified primary site
  C80.0
  glycogen-rich —*see* Neoplasm, breast,
  malignant
  granulosa cell C56
  hepatic cell C22.0
  hepatocellular C22.0
    with bile duct, mixed C22.0
    fibrolamellar C22.0
  hepatocholangiolitic C22.0
  Hürthle cell C73
  in
    adenomatous
      polyposis coli C18.9
    pleomorphic adenoma —*see* Neoplasm,
  salivary glands, malignant
    situ —*see* Carcinoma-in-situ
  infiltrating
    duct
      with lobular
        specified site —*see* Neoplasm, malignant,
      by site
        unspecified site (female) C50.91
          male C50.92
      with Paget's disease —*see* Neoplasm,
  breast, malignant
        specified site —*see* Neoplasm, malignant
        unspecified site (female) C50.91
          male C50.92
    ductular
      specified site —*see* Neoplasm, malignant
      unspecified site (female) C50.91
        male C50.92
    lobular
      specified site —*see* Neoplasm, malignant
      unspecified site (female) C50.91
        male C50.92
  inflammatory
    specified site —*see* Neoplasm, malignant
    unspecified site (female) C50.91

Carcinoma (malignant) - *continued*
    male C50.92
  intestinal type
    specified site —*see* Neoplasm, malignant,
    by site
      unspecified site C16.9
  intracystic
    noninfiltrating —*see* Neoplasm, in situ, by
  site
  intraductal (noninfiltrating)
    with Paget's disease —*see* Neoplasm, breast,
  malignant
    breast D05.1
    papillary
      with invasion
        specified site —*see* Neoplasm, malignant,
  by site
        unspecified site (female) C50.91
          male C50.92
      breast D05.1
      specified site NEC —*see* Neoplasm, in
  situ, by site
        unspecified site (female) D05.1
    specified site NEC —*see* Neoplasm, in situ,
    by site
      unspecified site (female) D05.1
  intraepidermal —*see* Neoplasm, in situ
    squamous cell, Bowen's type —*see*
  Neoplasm, skin, in situ
  intraepithelial —*see* Neoplasm, in situ, by site
    squamous cell —*see* Neoplasm, in situ, by
  site
  intraosseous C41.1
    upper jaw (bone) C41.0
  islet cell
    with exocrine, mixed
      specified site —*see* Neoplasm, malignant,
      by site
        unspecified site C25.9
    pancreas C25.4
    specified site NEC —*see* Neoplasm,
  malignant, by site
      unspecified site C25.4
  juvenile, breast —*see* Neoplasm, breast,
  malignant
  large cell
    small cell
      specified site —*see* Neoplasm, malignant,
    by site
      unspecified site C34.90
  Leydig cell (testis)
    specified site —*see* Neoplasm, malignant,
    by site
      unspecified site
        female C56.9
        male C62.90
  lipid-rich (female) C50.91
    male C50.92
  liver cell C22.0
  liver NEC C22.7
  lobular (infiltrating)
    with intraductal
      specified site —*see* Neoplasm, malignant,
      by site
        unspecified site (female) C50.91
          male C50.92
    noninfiltrating
      breast D05.0
      specified site NEC —*see* Neoplasm, in
  situ, by site
        unspecified site D05.0
      specified site —*see* Neoplasm, malignant,
      by site

Carcinoma (malignant) - *continued*
   unspecified site (female) C50.91
     male C50.92
   medullary
     with
       amyloid stroma
         specified site —*see* Neoplasm, malignant, by site
         unspecified site C73
       lymphoid stroma
         specified site —*see* Neoplasm, malignant, by site
         unspecified site (female) C50.91
          male C50.92
   Merkel cell C4A.9
     anal margin C4A.51
     anal skin C4A.51
     canthus C4A.1
     ear and external auricular canal C4A.2
     external auricular canal C4A.2
     eyelid, including canthus C4A.1
     face C4A.30
       specificd NEC C4A.39
     hip C4A.7
     lip C4A.0
     lower limb, including hip C4A.7
     neck C4A.4
     nodal presentation C7B.1
     nose C4A.31
     overlapping sites C4A.8
     perianal skin C4A.51
     scalp C4A.4
     secondary C7B.1
     shoulder C4A.6
     skin of breast C4A.52
     trunk NEC C4A.59
     upper limb, including shoulder C4A.6
     visceral metastatic C7B.1
   metastatic —*see* Neoplasm, secondary, by site
   metatypical —*see* Neoplasm, skin, malignant
   morphea, basal cell —*see* Neoplasm, skin, malignant
   mucoid
     cell
       specified site —*see* Neoplasm, malignant, by site
       unspecified site C75.1
   neuroendocrine —*see also* Tumor, neuroendocrine
     high grade, any site C7A.1
     poorly differentiated, any site C7A.1
   nonencapsulated sclerosing C73
   noninfiltrating
     intracystic —*see* Neoplasm, in situ, by site
     intraductal
       breast D05.1
       papillary
         breast D05.1
         specified site NEC —*see* Neoplasm, in situ, by site
         unspccified sitc D05.1
       specified site —*see* Neoplasm, in situ, by site
       unspecified site D05.1
     lobular
       breast D05.0
       specified site NEC —*see* Neoplasm, in situ, by site
       unspecified site (female) D05.0
   oat cell
     specified site —*see* Neoplasm, malignant, by site

Carcinoma (malignant) - *continued*
   unspecified site C34.90
   odontogenic C41.1
     upper jaw (bone) C41.0
   papillary
     with follicular (mixed) C73
     follicular variant C73
     intraductal (noninfiltrating)
       with invasion
         specified site —*see* Neoplasm, malignant, by site
         unspecified site (female) C50.91
          male C50.92
       breast D05.1
       specified site NEC —*see* Neoplasm, in situ, by site
       unspecified site D05.1
     serous
       specified site —*see* Neoplasm, malignant, by site
       surface
         specified site —*see* Neoplasm, malignant, by sitc
         unspecified site C56.9
       unspecified site C56.9
   papillocystic
     specified site —*see* Neoplasm, malignant, by site
     unspecified site C56.9
   parafollicular cell
     specified site —*see* Neoplasm, malignant, by site
     unspecified site C73
   pilomatrix —*see* Neoplasm, skin, malignant
   pseudomucinous
     specified site —*see* Neoplasm, malignant, by site
     unspecified site C56.9
   renal cell C64
   Schmincke —*see* Neoplasm, nasopharynx, malignant
   Schneiderian
     specified site —*see* Neoplasm, malignant, by site
     unspecified site C30.0
   sebaceous —*see* Neoplasm, skin, malignant
   secondary —*see also* Neoplasm, secondary, by site
     Merkel cell C7B.1
   secretory, breast —*see* Neoplasm, breast, malignant
   serous
     papillary
       specified site —*see* Neoplasm, malignant, by site
       unspecified site C56.9
     surface, papillary
       specified site —*see* Neoplasm, malignant, by site
       unspecified site C56.9
   Sertoli cell
     specified site —*see* Neoplasm, malignant, by site
     unspecified site C62.90
       female C56.9
       male C62.90
   skin appendage —*see* Neoplasm, skin, malignant
   small cell
     fusiform cell
       specified site —*see* Neoplasm, malignant, by site

Carcinoma (malignant) - *continued*
   unspecified site C34.90
   intermediate cell
     specified site —*see* Neoplasm, malignant, by site
     unspecified site C34.90
   large cell
     specified site —*see* Neoplasm, malignant, by site
     unspecified site C34.90
   solid
     with amyloid stroma
       specified site —*see* Neoplasm, malignant, by site
       unspecified site C73
     microinvasive
       specified site —*see* Neoplasm, malignant, by site
       unspecified site C53.9
   sweat gland —*see* Neoplasm, skin, malignant
   theca cell C56.
   thymic C37
   unspccified sitc (primary) C80.1
   water-clear cell C75.0
Carcinoma-in-situ —*see also* Neoplasm, in situ, by site
   breast NOS D05.9
     specified type NEC D05.8
   epidermoid —*see also* Neoplasm, in situ, by site
     with questionable stromal invasion
       cervix D06.9
       specified site NEC —*see* Neoplasm, in situ, by site
       unspecified site D06.9
   Bowen's type —*see* Neoplasm, skin, in situ
   intraductal
     breast D05.1
     specified site NEC —*see* Neoplasm, in situ, by site
     unspecified site D05.1
   lobular
     with
       infiltrating duct
         breast (female) C50.91
          male C50.92
         specified site NEC —*see* Neoplasm, malignant
         unspecified site (female) C50.91
          male C50.92
     intraductal
       breast D05.8
       specified site NEC —*see* Neoplasm, in situ, by site
       unspecified site (female) D05.8
     breast D05.0
     specified site NEC —*see* Neoplasm, in situ, by site
     unspecified site D05.0
   squamous cell —*see also* Neoplasm, in situ, by sitc
     with questionable stromal invasion
       cervix D06.9
       specified site NEC —*see* Neoplasm, in situ, by site
       unspecified site D06.9
Carcinomaphobia F45.29
Carcinomatosis C80.0
   peritonei C78.6
   unspecified site (primary) (secondary) C80.0

Carcinosarcoma —*see* Neoplasm, malignant, by site
  embryonal —*see* Neoplasm, malignant, by site
Cardia, cardial —*see* condition
Cardiac —*see also* condition
  death, sudden —*see* Arrest, cardiac
  pacemaker
    in situ Z95.0
      management or adjustment Z45.018
  tamponade I31.4
Cardialgia —*see* Pain, precordial
Cardiectasis —*see* Hypertrophy, cardiac
Cardiochalasia K21.9
Cardiomalacia I51.5
Cardiomegalia glycogenica diffusa E74.02 *[I43]*
Cardiomegaly —*see also* Hypertrophy, cardiac
  congenital Q24.8
  glycogen E74.02 *[I43]*
  idiopathic I51.7
Cardiomyoliposis I51.5
Cardiomyopathy (familial) (idiopathic) I42.9
  alcoholic I42.6
  amyloid E85.4 *[I43]*
  arteriosclerotic —*see* Disease, heart, ischemic, atherosclerotic
  beriberi E51.12
  cobalt-beer I42.6
  congenital I42.4
  congestive I42.0
  constrictive NOS I42.5
  dilated I42.0
  due to
    alcohol I42.6
    beriberi E51.12
    cardiac glycogenosis E74.02 *[I43]*
    drugs I42.7
    external agents NEC I42.7
    Friedreich's ataxia G11.1
    myotonia atrophica G71.11 *[I43]*
    progressive muscular dystrophy G71.0
  glycogen storage E74.02 *[I43]*
  hypertensive —*see* Hypertension, heart
  hypertrophic (nonobstructive) I42.2
    obstructive I42.1
      congenital Q24.8
  in
    Chagas' disease (chronic) B57.2
      acute B57.0
    sarcoidosis D86.85
  ischemic I25.5
  metabolic E88.9 *[I43]*
    thyrotoxic E05.90 *[I43]*
      with thyroid storm E05.91 *[I43]*
  newborn I42.8
    congenital I42.4
  nutritional E63.9 *[I43]*
    beriberi E51.12
  obscure of Africa I42.8
  peripartum O90.3
  postpartum O90.3
  restrictive NEC I42.5
  rheumatic I09.0
  secondary I42.9
  stress induced I51.81
  takotsubo I51.81
  thyrotoxic E05.90 *[I43]*
    with thyroid storm E05.91 *[I43]*
  toxic NEC I42.7
  tuberculous A18.84
  viral B33.24

Cardionephritis —*see* Hypertension, cardiorenal
Cardionephropathy —*see* Hypertension, cardiorenal
Cardionephrosis —*see* Hypertension, cardiorenal
Cardiopathia nigra I27.0
Cardiopathy (*see also* Disease, heart) I51.9
  idiopathic I42.9
  mucopolysaccharidosis E76.3 *[I52]*
Cardiopericarditis —*see* Pericarditis
Cardiophobia F45.29
Cardiorenal —*see* condition
Cardiorrhexis —*see* Infarct, myocardium
Cardiosclerosis —*see* Disease, heart, ischemic, atherosclerotic
Cardiosis —*see* Disease, heart
Cardiospasm (esophagus) (reflex) (stomach) K22.0
  congenital Q39.5
    with megaesophagus Q39.5
Cardiostenosis —*see* Disease, heart
Cardiosymphysis I31.0
Cardiovascular —*see* condition
Carditis (acute) (bacterial) (chronic) (subacute) I51.89
  meningococcal A39.50
  rheumatic —*see* Disease, heart, rheumatic
  rheumatoid —*see* Rheumatoid, carditis
  viral B33.20
Care (of) (for) (following)
  child (routine) Z76.2
  family member (handicapped) (sick)
    creating problem for family Z63.6
    provided away from home for holiday relief Z75.5
    unavailable, due to
      absence (person rendering care) (sufferer) Z74.2
      inability (any reason) of person rendering care Z74.2
  foundling Z76.1
  holiday relief Z75.5
  improper —*see* Maltreatment
  lack of (at or after birth) (infant) —*see* Maltreatment, child, neglect
  lactating mother Z39.1
  palliative Z51.5
  postpartum
    immediately after delivery Z39.0
    routine follow-up Z39.2
  respite Z75.5
  unavailable, due to
    absence of person rendering care Z74.2
    inability (any reason) of person rendering care Z74.2
  well-baby Z76.2
Caries
  bone NEC A18.03
  dental K02.9
    arrested (coronal) (root) K02.3
    chewing surface
      limited to enamel K02.51
      penetrating into dentin K02.52
      penetrating into pulp K02.53
    coronal surface
      chewing surface
        limited to enamel K02.51
        penetrating into dentin K02.52
        penetrating into pulp K02.53
      pit and fissure surface
        limited to enamel K02.51

Caries - *continued*
        penetrating into dentin K02.52
        penetrating into pulp K02.53
      smooth surface
        limited to enamel K02.61
        penetrating into dentin K02.62
        penetrating into pulp K02.63
    pit and fissure surface
      limited to enamel K02.51
      penetrating into dentin K02.52
      penetrating into pulp K02.53
    root K02.7
    smooth surface
      limited to enamel K02.61
      penetrating into dentin K02.62
      penetrating into pulp K02.63
  external meatus —*see* Disorder, ear, external, specified type NEC
  hip (tuberculous) A18.02
  initial (tooth)
    chewing surface K02.51
    pit and fissure surface K02.51
    smooth surface K02.61
  knee (tuberculous) A18.02
  labyrinth —*see* subcategory H83.8
  limb NEC (tuberculous) A18.03
  mastoid process (chronic) —*see* Mastoiditis, chronic
    tuberculous A18.03
  middle ear —*see* subcategory H74.8
  nose (tuberculous) A18.03
  orbit (tuberculous) A18.03
  ossicles, ear —*see* Abnormal, ear ossicles
  petrous bone —*see* Petrositis
  root (dental) (tooth) K02.7
  sacrum (tuberculous) A18.01
  spine, spinal (column) (tuberculous) A18.01
  syphilitic A52.77
    congenital (early) A50.02 *[M90.80]*
  tooth, teeth —*see* Caries, dental
  tuberculous A18.03
  vertebra (column) (tuberculous) A18.01
Carious teeth —*see* Caries, dental
Carneous mole O02.0
Carnitine insufficiency E71.40
Carotid body or sinus syndrome G90.01
Carotidynia G90.01
Carotinemia (dietary) E67.1
Carotinosis (cutis) (skin) E67.1
Carpal tunnel syndrome —*see* Syndrome, carpal tunnel
Carpenter's syndrome Q87.0
Carpopedal spasm —*see* Tetany
Carr-Barr-Plunkett syndrome Q97.1
Carrier (suspected) of
  amebiasis Z22.1
  bacterial disease NEC Z22.39
    diphtheria Z22.2
    intestinal infectious NEC Z22.1
      typhoid Z22.0
    meningococcal Z22.31
    sexually transmitted Z22.4
    specified NEC Z22.39
    staphylococcal (Methicillin susceptible) Z22.321
      Methicillin resistant Z22.322
    streptococcal Z22.338
      group B Z22.330
    typhoid Z22.0
  cholera Z22.1
  diphtheria Z22.2
  gastrointestinal pathogens NEC Z22.1
  genetic Z14.8

Carrier (suspected) **of** - *continued*
  cystic fibrosis Z14.1
  hemophilia A (asymptomatic) Z14.01
    symptomatic Z14.02
  gonorrhea Z22.4
  HAA (hepatitis Australian-antigen) Z22.59
  HB (c) (s) -AG Z22.51
  hepatitis (viral) Z22.50
    Australia-antigen (HAA) Z22.59
    B surface antigen (HBsAg) Z22.51
      with acute delta (super) infection B17.0
    C Z22.52
    specified NEC Z22.59
  human T-cell lymphotropic virus type 1
  (HTLV 1) infection Z22.6
  infectious organism Z22.9
    specified NEC Z22.8
  meningococci Z22.31
  Salmonella typhosa Z22.0
  serum hepatitis —*see* Carrier, hepatitis
  staphylococci (Methicillin susceptible)
  Z22.321
    Methicillin resistant Z22.322
  streptococci Z22.338
    group B Z22.330
  syphilis Z22.4
  typhoid Z22.0
  venereal disease NEC Z22.4
Carrion's disease A44.0
Carter's relapsing fever (Asiatic) A68.1
Cartilage —*see* condition
Caruncle (inflamed)
  conjunctiva (acute) —*see* Conjunctivitis,
  acute
  labium (majus) (minus) N90.89
  lacrimal —*see* Inflammation, lacrimal,
  passages
  myrtiform N89.8
  urethral (benign) N36.2
Cascade stomach K31.2
Caseation lymphatic gland (tuberculous)
  A18.2
Cassidy (-Scholte) **syndrome** (malignant
  carcinoid) E34.0
Castellani's disease A69.8
Castration, traumatic, male S38.231
Casts in urine R82.99
Cat
  cry syndrome Q93.4
  ear Q17.3
  eye syndrome Q92.8
Catabolism, senile R54
Catalepsy (hysterical) F44.2
  schizophrenic F20.2
Cataplexy (idiopathic) —*see*
  Narcolepsy
Cataract (cortical) (immature) (incipient)
  H26.9
  with
    neovascularization —*see* Cataract,
  complicated
  age-related —*see* Cataract, senile
  anterior
    and posterior axial embryonal Q12.0
    pyramidal Q12.0
  associated with
    galactosemia E74.21 *[H28]*
    myotonic disorders G71.19 *[H28]*
  blue Q12.0
  central Q12.0
  cerulean Q12.0

Cataract – *continued*
  complicated H26.20
    with
      neovascularization H26.21
      ocular disorder H26.22
      glaucomatous flecks H26.23
  congenital Q12.0
  coralliform Q12.0
  coronary Q12.0
  crystalline Q12.0
  diabetic —*see* Diabetes, cataract
  drug-induced H26.3
  due to
    ocular disorder —*see* Cataract, complicated
    radiation H26.8
  electric H26.8
  extraction status Z98.4
  glass-blower's H26.8
  heat ray H26.8
  heterochromic —*see* Cataract, complicated
  hypermature —*see* Cataract, senile,
  morgagnian type
  in (due to)
    chronic iridocyclitis —*see* Cataract,
  complicated
    diabetes —*see* Diabetes, cataract
    endocrine disease E34.9 *[H28]*
    eye disease —*see* Cataract, complicated
    hypoparathyroidism E20.9 *[H28]*
    malnutrition-dehydration E46 *[H28]*
    metabolic disease E88.9 *[H28]*
    myotonic disorders G71.19 *[H28]*
    nutritional disease E63.9 *[H28]*
  infantile —*see* Cataract, presenile
  irradiational —*see* Cataract, specified NEC
  juvenile —*see* Cataract, presenile
  malnutrition-dehydration E46 *[H28]*
  morgagnian —*see* Cataract, senile,
  morgagnian type
  myotonic G71.19 *[H28]*
  myxedema E03.9 *[H28]*
  nuclear
    embryonal Q12.0
    sclerosis —*see* Cataract, senile, nuclear
  presenile H26.00
    combined forms H26.06
    cortical H26.01
    lamellar —*see* Cataract, presenile, cortical
    nuclear H26.03
    specified NEC H26.09
    subcapsular polar (anterior) H26.04
      posterior H26.05
    zonular —*see* Cataract, presenile, cortical
  secondary H26.40
    Soemmering's ring H26.41
    specified NEC H26.49
    to eye disease —*see* Cataract, complicated
  senile H25.9
    brunescens —*see* Cataract, senile, nuclear
    combined forms H25.81
    coronary —*see* Cataract, senile, incipient
    cortical H25.01
    hypermature —*see* Cataract, senile,
    morgagnian type
    incipient (mature) (total) H25.09
      cortical —*see* Cataract, senile, cortical
      subcapsular —*see* Cataract, senile,
    subcapsular
    morgagnian type (hypermature) H25.2
    nuclear (sclerosis) H25.1
    polar subcapsular (anterior) (posterior) —
  see Cataract, senile, incipient

Cataract – *continued*
  punctate —*see* Cataract, senile, incipient
  specified NEC H25.89
  subcapsular polar (anterior) H25.03
    posterior H25.04
  snowflake —*see* Diabetes, cataract
  specified NEC H26.8
  toxic —*see* Cataract, drug-induced
  traumatic H26.10
    localized H26.11
    partially resolved H26.12
    total H26.13
  zonular (perinuclear) Q12.0
Cataracta —*see also* Cataract
  brunescens —*see* Cataract, senile, nuclear
  centralis pulverulenta Q12.0
  cerulea Q12.0
  complicata —*see* Cataract, complicated
  congenita Q12.0
  coralliformis Q12.0
  coronaria Q12.0
  diabetic —*see* Diabetes, cataract
  membranacea
    accreta —*see* Cataract, secondary
    congenita Q12.0
  nigra —*see* Cataract, senile, nuclear
  sunflower —*see* Cataract, complicated
Catarrh, catarrhal (acute) (febrile)
  (infectious) (inflammation) (*see also*
  condition) J00
  bronchial —*see* Bronchitis
  chest —*see* Bronchitis
  chronic J31.0
  due to congenital syphilis A50.03
  enteric —*see* Enteritis
  eustachian H68.009
  fauces —*see* Pharyngitis
  gastrointestinal —*see* Enteritis
  gingivitis K05.00
    nonplaque induced K05.01
    plaque induced K05.00
  hay —*see* Fever, hay
  intestinal —*see* Enteritis
  larynx, chronic J37.0
  liver B15.9
    with hepatic coma B15.0
  lung —*see* Bronchitis
  middle ear, chronic —*see* Otitis, media,
  nonsuppurative, chronic, serous
  mouth K12.1
  nasal (chronic) —*see* Rhinitis
  nasobronchial J31.1
  nasopharyngeal (chronic) J31.1
    acute J00
  pulmonary —*see* Bronchitis
  spring (eye) (vernal) —*see* Conjunctivitis,
  acute, atopic
  summer (hay) —*see* Fever, hay
  throat J31.2
  tubotympanal —*see also* Otitis, media,
  nonsuppurative
    chronic —*see* Otitis, media, nonsuppurative,
  chronic, serous
Catatonia (schizophrenic) F20.2
Catatonic
  disorder due to known physiologic condition
  F06.1
  schizophrenia F20.2
  stupor R40.1
Cat-scratch —*see also* Abrasion
  disease or fever A28.1
Cauda equina —*see* condition
Cauliflower ear M95.1

Causalgia (upper limb) G56.4
  lower limb G57.7
Cause
  external, general effects T75.89
Caustic burn —*see* Corrosion, by site
Cavare's disease (familial periodic paralysis)
  G72.3
Cave-in, injury
  crushing (severe) —*see* Crush
  suffocation —*see* Asphyxia, traumatic, due to
  low oxygen, due to cave-in
Cavernitis (penis) N48.29
Cavernositis N48.29
Cavernous —*see* condition
Cavitation of lung —*see also* Tuberculosis,
  pulmonary
  nontuberculous J98.4
Cavities, dental —*see* Caries, dental
Cavity
  lung —*see* Cavitation of lung
  optic papilla Q14.2
  pulmonary —*see* Cavitation of lung
Cavovarus foot, congenital Q66.1
Cavus foot (congenital) Q66.7
  acquired —*see* Deformity, limb, foot,
  specified NEC
Cazenave's disease L10.2
Cecitis K52.9
  with perforation, peritonitis, or rupture K65.8
Cecum —*see* condition
Celiac
  artery compression syndrome I77.4
  disease K90.0
  infantilism K90.0
Cell (s) , **cellular** —*see also* condition
  in urine R82.99
Cellulitis (diffuse) (phlegmonous) (septic)
  (suppurative) L03.90
  abdominal wall L03.311
  anaerobic A48.0
  ankle —*see* Cellulitis, lower limb
  anus K61.0
  arm —*see* Cellulitis, upper limb
  auricle (ear) —*see* Cellulitis, ear
  axilla L03.11
  back (any part) L03.312
  broad ligament
    acute N73.0
  buttock L03.317
  cervical (meaning neck) L03.221
  cervix (uteri) —*see* Cervicitis
  cheek (external) L03.211
    internal K12.2
  chest wall L03.313
  chronic L03.90
  clostridial A48.0
  corpus cavernosum N48.22
  digit
    finger —*see* Cellulitis, finger
    toe —*see* Cellulitis, toe
  Douglas' cul-de-sac or pouch
    acute N73.0
  drainage site (following operation) T81.4
  ear (external) H60.1
  eosinophilic (granulomatous) L98.3
  erysipelatous —*see* Erysipelas
  external auditory canal —*see* Cellulitis, ear
  eyelid —*see* Abscess, eyelid
  face NEC L03.211
  finger (intrathecal) (periosteal)
  (subcutaneous) (subcuticular) L03.01
  foot —*see* Cellulitis, lower limb

Cellulitis – *continued*
  gangrenous —*see* Gangrene
  genital organ NEC
    female (external) N76.4
    male N49.9
      multiple sites N49.8
      specified NEC N49.8
  gluteal (region) L03.317
  gonococcal A54.89
  groin L03.314
  hand —*see* Cellulitis, upper limb
  head NEC L03.811
    face (any part, except ear, eye and nose)
    L03.211
  heel —*see* Cellulitis, lower limb
  hip —*see* Cellulitis, lower limb
  jaw (region) L03.211
  knee —*see* Cellulitis, lower limb
  labium (majus) (minus) —*see* Vulvitis
  lacrimal passages —*see* Inflammation,
  lacrimal, passages
  larynx J38.7
  leg —*see* Cellulitis, lower limb
  lip K13.0
  lower limb L03.11
    toe —*see* Cellulitis, toe
  mouth (floor) K12.2
  multiple sites, so stated L03.90
  nasopharynx J39.1
  navel L03.316
    newborn P38.9
      with mild hemorrhage P38.1
      without hemorrhage P38.9
  neck (region) L03.221
  nose (septum) (external) J34.0
  orbit, orbital H05.01
  palate (soft) K12.2
  pectoral (region) L03.313
  pelvis, pelvic (chronic)
    female (*see also* Disease, pelvis,
  inflammatory) N73.2
      acute N73.0
      following ectopic or molar pregnancy O08.0
    male K65.0
  penis N48.22
  perineal, perineum L03.315
  perirectal K61.1
  peritonsillar J36
  periurethral N34.0
  periuterine (*see also* Disease, pelvis,
  inflammatory) N73.2
    acute N73.0
  pharynx J39.1
  rectum K61.1
  retroperitoneal K68.9
  round ligament
    acute N73.0
  scalp (any part) L03.811
  scrotum N49.2
  seminal vesicle N49.0
  shoulder —*see* Cellulitis, upper limb
  specified site NEC L03.818
  submandibular (region) (space) (triangle)
  K12.2
    gland K11.3
  submaxillary (region) K12.2
    gland K11.3
  thigh —*see* Cellulitis, lower limb
  thumb (intrathecal) (periosteal)
  (subcutaneous) (subcuticular) —*see* Cellulitis,
  finger
  toe (intrathecal) (periosteal) (subcutaneous)
  (subcuticular) L03.03

Cellulitis – *continued*
  tonsil J36
  trunk L03.319
    abdominal wall L03.311
    back (any part) L03.312
    buttock L03.317
    chest wall L03.313
    groin L03.314
    perineal, perineum L03.315
    umbilicus L03.316
  tuberculous (primary) A18.4
  umbilicus L03.316
  upper limb L03.11
    axilla —*see* Cellulitis, axilla
    finger —*see* Cellulitis, finger
    thumb —*see* Cellulitis, finger
  vaccinal T88.0
  vocal cord J38.3
  vulva —*see* Vulvitis
  wrist —*see* Cellulitis, upper limb
Cementoblastoma, benign —*see* Cyst,
  calcifying odontogenic
Cementoma —*see* Cyst, calcifying
  odontogenic
Cementoperiostitis —*see* Periodontitis
Cementosis K03.4
Central auditory processing disorder H93.25
Central pain syndrome G89.0
Cephalematocele, cephal (o) **hematocele**
  newborn P52.8
    birth injury P10.8
  traumatic —*see* Hematoma, brain
Cephalematoma, cephalhematoma (calcified)
  newborn (birth injury) P12.0
  traumatic —*see* Hematoma, brain
Cephalgia, cephalalgia —*see also* Headache
  histamine G44.009
    intractable G44.001
    not intractable G44.009
  trigeminal autonomic (TAC) NEC G44.099
    intractable G44.091
    not intractable G44.099
Cephalic —*see* condition
Cephalitis —*see* Encephalitis
Cephalocele —*see* Encephalocele
Cephalomenia N94.89
Cephalopelvic —*see* condition
Cerclage (with cervical incompetence) **in**
  pregnancy —*see* Incompetence, cervix, in
  pregnancy
Cerebellitis —*see* Encephalitis
Cerebellum, cerebellar —*see* condition
Cerebral —*see* condition
Cerebritis —*see* Encephalitis
Cerebro-hepato-renal syndrome Q87.89
Cerebromalacia —*see* Softening, brain
  sequelae of cerebrovascular disease I69.398
Cerebroside lipidosis E75.22
Cerebrospasticity (congenital) G80.1
Cerebrospinal —*see* condition
Cerebrum —*see* condition
Ceroid-lipofuscinosis, neuronal E75.4
Cerumen (accumulation) (impacted) H61.2
Cervical —*see also* condition
  auricle Q18.2
  dysplasia in pregnancy —*see* Abnormal,
  cervix, in pregnancy or childbirth
  erosion in pregnancy —*see* Abnormal, cervix,
  in pregnancy or childbirth
  fibrosis in pregnancy —*see* Abnormal, cervix,
  in pregnancy or childbirth
  fusion syndrome Q76.1
  rib Q76.5

Cervical - *continued*
  shortening (complicating pregnancy) O26.87
Cervicalgia M54.2
Cervicitis (acute) (chronic) (nonvenereal)
  (senile (atrophic)) (subacute) (with
  ulceration) N72
  with
    abortion —*see* Abortion, by type
  complicated by genital tract and pelvic
  infection
    ectopic pregnancy O08.0
    molar pregnancy O08.0
  chlamydial A56.09
  gonococcal A54.03
  herpesviral A60.03
  puerperal (postpartum) O86.11
  syphilitic A52.76
  trichomonal A59.09
  tuberculous A18.16
Cervicocolpitis (emphysematosa) (see also
  Cervicitis) N72
Cervix —*see* condition
Cesarean delivery, previous, affecting
  management of pregnancy O34.21
Céstan (-Chenais) **paralysis or syndrome**
  G46.3
Céstan-Raymond syndrome I65.8
Cestode infestation B71.9
  specified type NEC B71.8
Cestodiasis B71.9
Chabert's disease A22.9
Chacaleh E53.8
Chafing L30.4
Chagas' (-Mazza) **disease** (chronic) B57.2
  with
    cardiovascular involvement NEC B57.2
    digestive system involvement B57.30
      megacolon B57.32
      megaesophagus B57.31
      other specified B57.39
    megacolon B57.32
    megaesophagus B57.31
    myocarditis B57.2
    nervous system involvement B57.40
      meningitis B57.41
      meningoencephalitis B57.42
      other specified B57.49
    specified organ involvement NEC B57.5
  acute (with) B57.1
    cardiovascular NEC B57.0
    myocarditis B57.0
Chagres fever B50.9
Chair ridden Z74.09
Chalasia (cardiac sphincter) K21.9
Chalazion H00.19
  left H00.16
    lower H00.15
    upper H00.14
  right H00.13
    lower H00.12
    upper H00.11
Chalcosis —*see also* Disorder, globe,
  degenerative, chalcosis
  cornea —*see* Deposit, cornea
  crystalline lens —*see* Cataract, complicated
  retina H35.89
Chalicosis (pulmonum) J62.8
Chancre (any genital site) (hard) (hunterian)
  (mixed) (primary) (seronegative)
  (seropositive) (syphilitic) A51.0
  congenital A50.07
  conjunctiva NEC A51.2

Chancre - *continued*
  Ducrey's A57
  extragenital A51.2
  eyelid A51.2
  lip A51.2
  nipple A51.2
  Nisbet's A57
  of
    carate A67.0
    pinta A67.0
    yaws A66.0
  palate, soft A51.2
  phagedenic A57
  simple A57
  soft A57
    bubo A57
    palate A51.2
  urethra A51.0
  yaws A66.0
Chancroid (anus) (genital) (penis) (perineum)
  (rectum) (urethra) (vulva) A57
Chandler's disease (osteochondritis dissecans,
  hip) —*see* Osteochondritis, dissecans, hip
Change (s) (in) (of) —*see also* Removal
  arteriosclerotic —*see* Arteriosclerosis
  bone —*see also* Disorder, bone
    diabetic —*see* Diabetes, bone change
  bowel habit R19.4
  cardiorenal (vascular) — *see* Hypertension,
  cardiorenal
  cardiovascular —*see* Disease, cardiovascular
  circulatory I99.9
  cognitive (mild) (organic) R41.89
  color, tooth, teeth
    during formation K00.8
    posteruptive K03.7
  contraceptive device Z30.433
  corneal membrane H18.30
    Bowman's membrane fold or rupture H18.31
    Descemet's membrane
      fold H18.32
      rupture H18.33
  coronary —*see* Disease, heart, ischemic
  degenerative, spine or vertebra —*see*
  Spondylosis
  dental pulp, regressive K04.2
  dressing (nonsurgical) Z48.00
    surgical Z48.01
  heart —*see* Disease, heart
  hip joint —*see* Derangement, joint, hip
  hyperplastic larynx J38.7
  hypertrophic
    nasal sinus J34.89
    turbinate, nasal J34.3
    upper respiratory tract J39.8
  indwelling catheter Z46.6
  inflammatory —*see also* Inflammation
    sacroiliac M46.1
  job, anxiety concerning Z56.1
  joint —*see* Derangement, joint
  life —*see* Menopause
  mental status R41.82
  minimal (glomerular) (*see also* N00-N07 with
  fourth character .0) N05.0
  myocardium, myocardial —*see* Degeneration,
  myocardial
  of life —*see* Menopause
  pacemaker Z45.018
    pulse generator Z45.010
  personality (enduring) F68.8
    due to (secondary to)
      general medical condition F07.0

Change(s) (in) (of) – *continued*
  secondary (nonspecific) F60.89
  regressive, dental pulp K04.2
  renal —*see* Disease, renal
  retina H35.9
    myopic H44.2
  sacroiliac joint M53.3
  senile (*see also* condition) R54
  sensory R20.8
  skin R23.9
    acute, due to ultraviolet radiation L56.9
      specified NEC L56.8
    chronic, due to nonionizing radiation L57.9
      specified NEC L57.8
    cyanosis R23.0
    flushing R23.2
    pallor R23.1
    petechiae R23.3
    specified change NEC R23.8
    swelling —*see* Mass, localized
    texture R23.4
  trophic
    arm —*see* Mononeuropathy, upper limb
    leg —*see* Mononeuropathy, lower limb
  vascular I99.9
  vasomotor I73.9
  voice R49.9
    psychogenic F44.4
    specified NEC R49.8
Changing sleep-work schedule, affecting
  sleep G47.26
Changuinola fever A93.1
Chapping skin T69.8
Charcot-Marie-Tooth disease, paralysis or
  syndrome G60.0
Charcot's
  arthropathy —*see* Arthropathy, neuropathic
  cirrhosis K74.3
  disease (tabetic arthropathy) A52.16
  joint (disease) (tabetic) A52.16
    diabetic —*see* Diabetes, with, arthropathy
    syringomyelic G95.0
  syndrome (intermittent claudication) I73.9
CHARGE association Q89.8
Charley-horse (quadriceps) M62.831
  traumatic (quadriceps) S76.11
Charlouis' disease —*see* Yaws
Cheadle's disease E54
Checking (of)
  cardiac pacemaker (battery) (electrode(s))
  Z45.018
    pulse generator Z45.010
  intrauterine contraceptive device Z30.431
Check-up —*see* Examination
Chédiak-Higashi (-Steinbrinck) syndrome
  (congenital gigantism of peroxidase granules)
  E70.330
Cheek —*see* condition
Cheese itch B88.0
Cheese-washer's lung J67.8
Cheese-worker's lung J67.8
Cheilitis (acute) (angular) (catarrhal) (chronic)
  (exfoliative) (gangrenous) (glandular)
  (infectional) (suppurative) (ulcerative)
  (vesicular) K13.0
  actinic (due to sun) L56.8
    other than from sun L59.8
  candidal B37.83
Cheilodynia K13.0
Cheiloschisis —*see* Cleft, lip

Cheilosis (angular) K13.0
  with pellagra E52
  due to
    vitamin B2 (riboflavin) deficiency E53.0
Cheiromegaly M79.89
Cheiropompholyx L30.1
Cheloid —see Keloid
Chemical burn —see Corrosion, by site
Chemodectoma —see Paraganglioma, nonchromaffin
Chemosis, conjunctiva —see Edema, conjunctiva
Chemotherapy (session) (for)
  cancer Z51.11
  neoplasm Z51.11
Cherubism M27.8
Chest —see condition
Cheyne-Stokes breathing (respiration) R06.3
Chiari's
  disease or syndrome (hepatic vein thrombosis) I82.0
  malformation
    type I G93.5
    type II —see Spina bifida
  net Q24.8
Chicago disease B40.9
Chickenpox —see Varicella
Chiclero ulcer or sore B55.1
Chigger (infestation) B88.0
Chignon (disease) B36.8
  newborn (from vacuum extraction) (birth injury) P12.1
Chilaiditi's syndrome (subphrenic displacement, colon) Q43.3
Chilblain (s) (lupus) T69.1
Child
  custody dispute Z65.3
Childbirth —see Delivery
Childhood
  cerebral X-linked adrenoleukodystrophy E71.520
  period of rapid growth Z00.2
Chill (s) R68.83
  with fever R50.9
  congestive in malarial regions B54
  without fever R68.83
Chilomastigiasis A07.8
Chimera 46,XX/46,XY Q99.0
Chin —see condition
Chinese dysentery A03.9
Chionophobia F40.228
Chitral fever A93.1
Chlamydia, chlamydial A74.9
  cervicitis A56.09
  conjunctivitis A74.0
  cystitis A56.01
  endometritis A56.11
  epididymitis A56.19
  female
    pelvic inflammatory disease A56.11
    pelviperitonitis A56.11
  orchitis A56.19
  peritonitis A74.81
  pharyngitis A56.4
  proctitis A56.3
  psittaci (infection) A70
  salpingitis A56.11
  sexually-transmitted infection NEC A56.8
  specified NEC A74.89
  urethritis A56.01
  vulvovaginitis A56.02
Chlamydiosis —see Chlamydia

Chloasma (skin) (idiopathic) (symptomatic) L81.1
  eyelid H02.719
    hyperthyroid E05.90 [H02.719]
      with thyroid storm E05.91 [H02.719]
    left H02.716
      lower H02.715
      upper H02.714
    right H02.713
      lower H02.712
      upper H02.711
Chloroma C92.3
Chlorosis D50.9
  Egyptian B76.9 [D63.8]
  miner's B76.9 [D63.8]
Chlorotic anemia D50.8
Chocolate cyst (ovary) N80.1
Choked
  disc or disk —see Papilledema
  on food, phlegm, or vomitus NOS —see Foreign body, by site
  while vomiting NOS —see Foreign body, by site
Chokes (resulting from bends) T70.3
Choking sensation R09.89
Cholangiectasis K83.8
Cholangiocarcinoma
  with hepatocellular carcinoma, combined C22.0
  liver C22.1
  specified site NEC —see Neoplasm, malignant, by site
  unspecified site C22.1
Cholangiohepatitis K83.8
  due to fluke infestation B66.1
Cholangiohepatoma C22.0
Cholangiolitis (acute) (chronic) (extrahepatic) (gangrenous) (intrahepatic) K83.0
  paratyphoidal —see Fever, paratyphoid
  typhoidal A01.09
Cholangioma D13.4
  malignant —see Cholangiocarcinoma
Cholangitis (ascending) (primary) (recurrent) (sclerosing) (secondary) (stenosing) (suppurative) K83.0
  with calculus, bile duct —see Calculus, bile duct, with cholangitis
  chronic nonsuppurative destructive K74.3
Cholecystectasia K82.8
Cholecystitis K81.9
  with
    calculus, stones in
      bile duct (common) (hepatic) —see Calculus, bile duct, with cholecystitis
      cystic duct —see Calculus, gallbladder, with cholecystitis
      gallbladder —see Calculus, gallbladder, with cholecystitis
    choledocholithiasis —see Calculus, bile duct, with cholecystitis
    cholelithiasis —see Calculus, gallbladder, with cholecystitis
  acute (emphysematous) (gangrenous) (suppurative) K81.0
    with
      calculus, stones in
        cystic duct —see Calculus, gallbladder, with cholecystitis, acute
        gallbladder —see Calculus, gallbladder, with cholecystitis, acute
      choledocholithiasis —see Calculus, bile duct, with cholecystitis, acute

Cholecystitis - continued
    cholelithiasis —see Calculus, gallbladder, with cholecystitis, acute
    chronic cholecystitis K81.2
      with gallbladder calculus K80.12
        with obstruction K80.13
  chronic K81.1
    with acute cholecystitis K81.2
      with gallbladder calculus K80.12
        with obstruction K80.13
  emphysematous (acute) —see Cholecystitis, acute
  gangrenous —see Cholecystitis, acute
  paratyphoidal, current A01.4
  suppurative —see Cholecystitis, acute
  typhoidal A01.09
Cholecystolithiasis —see Calculus, gallbladder
Choledochitis (suppurative) K83.0
Choledocholith —see Calculus, bile duct
Choledocholithiasis (common duct) (hepatic duct) —see Calculus, bile duct
  cystic —see Calculus, gallbladder
  typhoidal A01.09
Cholelithiasis (cystic duct) (gallbladder) (impacted) (multiple) —see Calculus, gallbladder
  bile duct (common) (hepatic) —see Calculus, bile duct
  hepatic duct —see Calculus, bile duct
  specified NEC K80.80
    with obstruction K80.81
Cholemia —see also Jaundice
  familial (simple) (congenital) E80.4
  Gilbert's E80.4
Choleperitoneum, choleperitonitis K65.3
Cholera (Asiatic) (epidemic) (malignant) A00.9
  antimonial —see Poisoning, antimony
  classical A00.0
  due to Vibrio cholerae 01 A00.9
    biovar cholerae A00.0
    biovar eltor A00.1
  el tor A00.1
Cholerine —see Cholera
Cholestasis NEC K83.1
  with hepatocyte injury K71.0
  due to total parenteral nutrition (TPN) K76.89
  pure K71.0
Cholesteatoma (ear) (middle) (with reaction) H71.9
  attic H71.0
  external ear (canal) H60.4
  mastoid H71.2
  postmastoidectomy cavity (recurrent) —see Complications, postmastoidectomy, recurrent cholesteatoma
  recurrent (postmastoidectomy) —see Complications, postmastoidectomy, recurrent cholesteatoma
  tympanum H71.1
Cholesteatosis, diffuse H71.3
Cholesteremia E78.0
Cholesterin in vitreous —see Deposit, crystalline
Cholesterol
  deposit
    retina H35.89
    vitreous —see Deposit, crystalline
  elevated (high) E78.0
    with elevated (high) triglycerides E78.2
  screening for Z13.220

Cholesterol - *continued*
imbibition of gallbladder K82.4
Cholesterolemia (essential) (familial)
(hereditary) (pure) E78.0
Cholesterolosis, cholesterosis (gallbladder)
K82.4
cerebrotendinous E75.5
Cholocolic fistula K82.3
Choluria R82.2
Chondritis M94.8X9
auricle H61.03
costal (Tietze's) M94.0
external ear H61.03
patella, posttraumatic —*see* Chondromalacia,
patella
pinna H61.03
purulent M94.8X
tuberculous NEC A18.02
intervertebral A18.01
Chondroblastoma —*see also* Neoplasm, bone,
benign
malignant —*see* Neoplasm, bone, malignant
Chondrocalcinosis M11.20
ankle M11.27
elbow M11.22
familial M11.10
ankle M11.17
elbow M11.12
foot joint M11.17
hand joint M11.14
hip M11.15
knee M11.16
multiple site M11.19
shoulder M11.11
vertebrae M11.18
wrist M11.13
foot joint M11.27
hand joint M11.24
hip M11.25
knee M11.26
multiple site M11.29
shoulder M11.21
vertebrae M11.28
specified type NEC M11.20
ankle M11.27
elbow M11.22
foot joint M11.27
hand joint M11.24
hip M11.25
knee M11.26
multiple site M11.29
shoulder M11.21
vertebrae M11.28
wrist M11.23
wrist M11.23
Chondrodermatitis nodularis helicis or
anthelicis —*see* Perichondritis, ear
Chondrodysplasia Q78.9
with hemangioma Q78.4
calcificans congenita Q77.3
fetalis Q77.4
metaphyseal (Jansen's) (McKusick's)
(Schmid's) Q78.5
punctata Q77.3
Chondrodystrophy, chondrodystrophia
(familial) (fetalis) (hypoplastic) Q78.9
calcificans congenita Q77.3
myotonic (congenital) G71.13
punctata Q77.3
Chondroectodermal dysplasia Q77.6
Chondrogenesis imperfecta Q77.4
Chondrolysis M94.35

Chondroma —*see also* Neoplasm, cartilage,
benign
juxtacortical —*see* Neoplasm, bone, benign
periosteal —*see* Neoplasm, bone, benign
Chondromalacia (systemic) M94.20
acromioclavicular joint M94.21
ankle M94.27
elbow M94.22
foot joint M94.27
glenohumeral joint M94.21
hand joint M94.24
hip M94.25
knee M94.26
patella M22.4
multiple sites M94.29
patella M22.4
rib M94.28
sacroiliac joint M94.259
shoulder M94.21
sternoclavicular joint M94.21
vertebral joint M94.28
wrist M94.23
Chondromatosis —*see also* Neoplasm,
cartilage, uncertain behavior
internal Q78.4
Chondromyxosarcoma —*see* Neoplasm,
cartilage, malignant
Chondro-osteodysplasia (Morquio-Brailsford
type) E76.219
Chondro-osteodystrophy E76.29
Chondro-osteoma —*see* Neoplasm, bone,
benign
Chondropathia tuberosa M94.0
Chondrosarcoma —*see* Neoplasm, cartilage,
malignant
juxtacortical —*see* Neoplasm, bone,
malignant
mesenchymal —*see* Neoplasm, connective
tissue, malignant
myxoid —*see* Neoplasm, cartilage, malignant
Chordee (nonvenereal) N48.89
congenital Q54.4
gonococcal A54.09
Chorditis (fibrinous) (nodosa) (tuberosa) J38.2
Chordoma —*see* Neoplasm, vertebral
(column) , malignant
Chorea (chronic) (gravis) (posthemiplegic)
(senile) (spasmodic) G25.5
with
heart involvement I02.0
active or acute (conditions in I01) I02.0
rheumatic I02.9
with valvular disorder I02.0
rheumatic heart disease (chronic) (inactive)
(quiescent)
code to rheumatic heart condition involved
drug-induced G25.4
habit F95.8
hereditary G10
Huntington's G10
hysterical F44.4
minor I02.9
with heart involvement I02.0
progressive G25.5
hereditary G10
rheumatic (chronic) I02.9
with heart involvement I02.0
Sydenham's I02.9
with heart involvement —*see* Chorea, with
rheumatic heart disease
nonrheumatic G25.5
Choreoathetosis (paroxysmal) G25.5
Chorioadenoma (destruens) D39.2

Chorioamnionitis O41.12
Chorioangioma D26.7
Choriocarcinoma —*see* Neoplasm, malignant,
by site
combined with
embryonal carcinoma —*see* Neoplasm,
malignant, by site
other germ cell elements —*see* Neoplasm,
malignant, by site
teratoma —*see* Neoplasm, malignant, by site
specified site —*see* Neoplasm, malignant, by
site
unspecified site
female C58
male C62.90
Chorioencephalitis (acute) (lymphocytic)
(serous) A87.2
Chorioepithelioma —*see* Choriocarcinoma
Choriomeningitis (acute) (lymphocytic)
(serous) A87.2
Chorionepithelioma —*see* Choriocarcinoma
Chorioretinitis —*see also* Inflammation,
chorioretinal
disseminated —*see also* Inflammation,
chorioretinal, disseminated
in neurosyphilis A52.19
Egyptian B76.9 *[D63.8]*
focal —*see also* Inflammation, chorioretinal,
focal
histoplasmic B39.9 *[H32]*
in (due to)
histoplasmosis B39.9 *[H32]*
syphilis (secondary) A51.43
late A52.71
toxoplasmosis (acquired) B58.01
congenital (active) P37.1 *[H32]*
tuberculosis A18.53
juxtapapillary, juxtapapillaris —*see*
Inflammation, chorioretinal, focal,
juxtapapillary
leprous A30.9 *[H32]*
minor's B76.9 *[D63.8]*
progressive myopia (degeneration) H44.2
syphilitic (secondary) A51.43
congenital (early) A50.01 *[H32]*
late A50.32
late A52.71
tuberculous A18.53
Chorioretinopathy, central serous H35.71
Choroid —*see* condition
Choroideremia H31.21
Choroiditis —*see* Chorioretinitis
Choroidopathy —*see* Disorder, choroid
Choroidoretinitis —*see* Chorioretinitis
Choroidoretinopathy, central serous —*see*
Chorioretinopathy, central serous
Christian-Weber disease M35.6
Christmas disease D67
Chromaffinoma —*see also* Neoplasm, benign,
by site
malignant —*see* Neoplasm, malignant, by site
Chromatopsia —*see* Deficiency, color vision
Chromhidrosis, chromidrosis L75.1
Chromoblastomycosis —*see* Chromomycosis
Chromoconversion R82.91
Chromomycosis B43.9
brain abscess B43.1
cerebral B43.1
cutaneous B43.0
skin B43.0
specified NEC B43.8
subcutaneous abscess or cyst B43.2

Chromophytosis B36.0
Chromosome —*see* condition by chromosome
  involved
  D (1) —*see* condition, chromosome 13
  E (3) —*see* condition, chromosome 18
  G —*see* condition, chromosome 21
Chromotrichomycosis B36.8
Chronic —*see* condition
  fracture —*see* Fracture, pathological
Churg-Strauss syndrome M30.1
Chyle cyst, mesentery I89.8
Chylocele (nonfilarial) I89.8
  filarial (*see also* Infestation, filarial) B74.9
  [N51]
  tunica vaginalis N50.8
    filarial (*see also* Infestation, filarial) B74.9
    [N51]
Chylomicronemia (fasting) (with
  hyperprebetalipoproteinemia) E78.3
Chylopericardium I31.3
  acute I30.9
Chylothorax (nonfilarial) I89.8
  filarial (*see also* Infestation, filarial) B74.9
  [J91.8]
Chylous —*see* condition
Chyluria (nonfilarial) R82.0
  due to
    bilharziasis B65.0
    Brugia (malayi) B74.1
      timori B74.2
    schistosomiasis (bilharziasis) B65.0
    Wuchereria (bancrofti) B74.0
  filarial —*see* Infestation, filarial
Cicatricial (deformity) —*see* Cicatrix
Cicatrix (adherent) (contracted) (painful)
  (vicious) (*see also* Scar) L90.5
  adenoid (and tonsil) J35.8
  alveolar process M26.79
  anus K62.89
  auricle —*see* Disorder, pinna, specified type
  NEC
  bile duct (common) (hepatic) K83.8
  bladder N32.89
  bone —*see* Disorder, bone, specified type
  NEC
  brain G93.89
  cervix (postoperative) (postpartal) N88.1
  common duct K83.8
  cornea H17.9
    tuberculous A18.59
  duodenum (bulb) , obstructive K31.5
  esophagus K22.2
  eyelid —*see* Disorder, eyelid function
  hypopharynx J39.2
  lacrimal passages —*see* Obstruction, lacrimal
  larynx J38.7
  lung J98.4
  middle ear —see subcategory H74.8
  mouth K13.79
  muscle M62.89
    with contracture —*see* Contraction, muscle
  NEC
  nasopharynx J39.2
  palate (soft) K13.79
  penis N48.89
  pharynx J39.2
  prostate N42.89
  rectum K62.89
  retina —*see* Scar, chorioretinal
  semilunar cartilage —*see* Derangement,
  meniscus
  seminal vesicle N50.8

Cicatrix – *continued*
  skin L90.5
    infected L08.89
    postinfective L90.5
    tuberculous B90.8
  specified site NEC L90.5
  throat J39.2
  tongue K14.8
  tonsil (and adenoid) J35.8
  trachea J39.8
  tuberculous NEC B90.9
  urethra N36.8
  uterus N85.8
  vagina N89.8
    postoperative N99.2
  vocal cord J38.3
  wrist, constricting (annular) L90.5
CIDP (chronic inflammatory demyelinating
  polyneuropathy) G61.81
CIN —*see* Neoplasia, intraepithelial, cervix
Cinchonism —*see* Deafness, ototoxic
  correct substance properly administered —*see*
  Table of Drugs and Chemicals, by drug,
  adverse effect
  overdose or wrong substance given or taken
  —*see* Table of Drugs and Chemicals, by drug,
  poisoning
Circle of Willis —*see* condition
Circular —*see* condition
Circulating anticoagulants (*see also*
  Disorder, hemorrhagic) D68.318
  due to drugs (*see also*
  Disorder, hemorrhagic) D68.32
  following childbirth O72.3
Circulation
  collateral, any site I99.8
  defective (lower extremity) I99.8
    congenital Q28.9
  embryonic Q28.9
  failure (peripheral) R57.9
    newborn P29.89
  fetal, persistent P29.3
  heart, incomplete Q28.9
Circulatory system —*see* condition
Circulus senilis (cornea) —*see* Degeneration,
  cornea, senile
Circumcision (in absence of medical
  indication) (ritual) (routine) Z41.2
Circumscribed —*see* condition
Circumvallate placenta O43.11
Cirrhosis, cirrhotic (hepatic) (liver) K74.60
  alcoholic K70.30
    with ascites K70.31
  atrophic —*see* Cirrhosis, liver
  Baumgarten-Cruveilhier K74.69
  biliary (cholangiolitic) (cholangitic)
  (hypertrophic) (obstructive)
  (pericholangiolitic) K74.5
    due to
      Clonorchiasis B66.1
      flukes B66.3
    primary K74.3
    secondary K74.4
  cardiac (of liver) K76.1
  Charcot's K74.3
  cholangiolitic, cholangitic, cholestatic
  (primary) K74.3
  congestive K76.1
  Cruveilhier-Baumgarten K74.69
  cryptogenic (liver) K74.69
  due to
    hepatolenticular degeneration E83.01

Cirrhosis, cirrhotic - *continued*
  Wilson's disease E83.01
  xanthomatosis E78.2
  fatty K76.0
    alcoholic K70.0
  Hanot's (hypertrophic) K74.3
  hepatic —*see* Cirrhosis, liver
  hypertrophic K74.3
  Indian childhood K74.69
  kidney —*see* Sclerosis, renal
  Laennec's K70.30
    with ascites K70.31
    alcoholic K70.30
      with ascites K70.31
    nonalcoholic K74.69
  liver K74.60
    alcoholic K70.30
      with ascites K70.31
      fatty K70.0
    congenital P78.81
    syphilitic A52.74
  lung (chronic) J84.10
  macronodular K74.69
    alcoholic K70.30
      with ascites K70.31
  micronodular K74.69
    alcoholic K70.30
      with ascites K70.31
  mixed type K74.69
  monolobular K74.3
  nephritis —*see* Sclerosis, renal
  nutritional K74.69
    alcoholic K70.30
      with ascites K70.31
  obstructive —*see* Cirrhosis, biliary
  ovarian N83.8
  pancreas (duct) K86.8
  pigmentary E83.110
  portal K74.69
    alcoholic K70.30
      with ascites K70.31
  postnecrotic K74.69
    alcoholic K70.30
      with ascites K70.31
  pulmonary J84.10
  renal —*see* Sclerosis, renal
  spleen D73.2
  stasis K76.1
  Todd's K74.3
  unilobar K74.3
  xanthomatous (biliary) K74.5
    due to xanthomatosis (familial) (metabolic)
    (primary) E78.2
Cistern, subarachnoid R93.0
Citrullinemia E72.23
Citrullinuria E72.23
Civatte's disease or poikiloderma L57.3
Clam digger's itch B65.3
Clammy skin R23.1
Clap —*see* Gonorrhea
Clarke-Hadfield syndrome (pancreatic
  infantilism) K86.8
Clark's paralysis G80.9
Clastothrix L67.8
Claude Bernard-Horner syndrome G90.2
  traumatic —*see* Injury, nerve, cervical
  sympathetic
Claude's disease or syndrome G46.3
Claudication, intermittent I73.9
  cerebral (artery) G45.9
  spinal cord (arteriosclerotic) G95.19
    syphilitic A52.09
  venous (axillary) I87.8

Claudication venosa intermittens I87.8
Claustrophobia F40.240
Clavus (infected) L84
Clawfoot (congenital) Q66.89
  acquired —*see* Deformity, limb, clawfoot
Clawhand (acquired) —*see also* Deformity,
  limb, clawhand
  congenital Q68.1
Claw toe (congenital) Q66.89
  acquired —*see* Deformity, toe, specified NEC
Clay eating —*see* Pica
Cleansing of artificial opening —*see*
  Attention to, artificial, opening
Cleft (congenital) —*see also* Imperfect, closure
  alveolar process M26.79
  branchial (cyst) (persistent) Q18.2
  cricoid cartilage, posterior Q31.8
  lip (unilateral) Q36.9
    with cleft palate Q37.9
      hard Q37.1
        with soft Q37.5
      soft Q37.3
        with hard Q37.5
    bilateral Q36.0
      with cleft palate Q37.8
        hard Q37.0
          with soft Q37.4
        soft Q37.2
          with hard Q37.4
    median Q36.1
  nose Q30.2
  palate Q35.9
    with cleft lip (unilateral) Q37.9
      bilateral Q37.8
    hard Q35.1
      with
        cleft lip (unilateral) Q37.1
          bilateral Q37.0
        soft Q35.5
          with cleft lip (unilateral) Q37.5
            bilateral Q37.4
    medial Q35.5
    soft Q35.3
      with
        cleft lip (unilateral) Q37.3
          bilateral Q37.2
        hard Q35.5
          with cleft lip (unilateral) Q37.5
            bilateral Q37.4
  penis Q55.69
  scrotum Q55.29
  thyroid cartilage Q31.8
  uvula Q35.7
Cleidocranial dysostosis Q74.0
Cleptomania F63.2
Clicking hip (newborn) R29.4
Climacteric (female) —*see also* Menopause
  arthritis (any site) NEC —*see* Arthritis,
  specified form NEC
  depression (single episode) F32.8
  male (symptoms) (syndrome) NEC N50.8
  paranoid state F22
  polyarthritis NEC —*see* Arthritis, specified
  form NEC
  symptoms (female) N95.1
Clinical research investigation (clinical trial)
  (control subject) (normal comparison)
  (participant) Z00.6
Clitoris —*see* condition
Cloaca (persistent) Q43.7
Clonorchiasis, clonorchis infection (liver)
  B66.1
Clonus R25.8

Closed bite M26.29
Clostridium (C.) **perfringens, as cause of**
  disease classified elsewhere B96.7
Closure
  congenital, nose Q30.0
  cranial sutures, premature Q75.0
  defective or imperfect NEC —*see* Imperfect,
  closure
  fistula, delayed —*see* Fistula
  foramen ovale, imperfect Q21.1
  hymen N89.6
  interauricular septum, defective Q21.1
  interventricular septum, defective Q21.0
  lacrimal duct —*see also* Stenosis, lacrimal,
  duct
    congenital Q10.5
  nose (congenital) Q30.0
    acquired M95.0
  of artificial opening —*see* Attention to,
  artificial, opening
  primary angle, without glaucoma damage
  H40.06
  vagina N89.5
  valve —*see* Endocarditis
  vulva N90.5
Clot (blood) —*see also* Embolism
  artery (obstruction) (occlusion) —*see*
  Embolism
  bladder N32.89
  brain (intradural or extradural) —*see*
  Occlusion, artery, cerebral
  circulation I74.9
  heart —*see also* Infarct, myocardium
    not resulting in infarction I24.0
  vein —*see* Thrombosis
Clouded state R40.1
  epileptic —*see* Epilepsy, specified NEC
  paroxysmal —*see* Epilepsy, specified NEC
Cloudy antrum, antra J32.0
Clouston's (hidrotic) **ectodermal dysplasia**
  Q82.4
Clubbed nail pachydermoperiostosis M89.40
  [L62]
Clubbing of finger (s) (nails) R68.3
Club finger R68.3
  congenital Q68.1
Clubfoot (congenital) Q66.89
  acquired —*see* Deformity, limb, clubfoot
  equinovarus Q66.0
  paralytic —*see* Deformity, limb, clubfoot
Clubhand (congenital) (radial) Q71.4
  acquired —*see* Deformity, limb, clubhand
Club nail R68.3
  congenital Q84.6
Clump, kidney Q63.1
Clumsiness, clumsy child syndrome F82
Cluttering F80.81
Clutton's joints A50.51 [M12.80]
Coagulation, intravascular (diffuse)
  (disseminated) —*see also* Defibrination
  syndrome
  complicating abortion —*see* Abortion, by
  type, complicated by, intravascular
  coagulation
  following ectopic or molar pregnancy O08.1
Coagulopathy —*see also* Defect, coagulation
  consumption D65
  intravascular D65
  newborn P60
Coalition
  calcaneo-scaphoid Q66.89
  tarsal Q66.89

Coalminer's
  elbow —*see* Bursitis, elbow, olecranon
  lung or pneumoconiosis J60
Coalworker's lung or pneumoconiosis J60
Coarctation
  aorta (preductal) (postductal) Q25.1
  pulmonary artery Q25.71
Coated tongue K14.3
Coats' disease (exudative retinopathy) —*see*
  Retinopathy, exudative
Cocainism —*see* Dependence, drug, cocaine
Coccidioidomycosis B38.9
  cutaneous B38.3
  disseminated B38.7
  generalized B38.7
  meninges B38.4
  prostate B38.81
  pulmonary B38.2
    acute B38.0
    chronic B38.1
  skin B38.3
  specified NEC B38.89
Coccidioidosis —*see* Coccidioidomycosis
Coccidiosis (intestinal) A07.3
Coccydynia, coccygodynia M53.3
Coccyx —*see* condition
Cochin-China diarrhea K90.1
Cockayne's syndrome Q87.1
Cocked up toe —*see* Deformity, toe, specified
  NEC
Cock's peculiar tumor L72.3
Codman's tumor —*see* Neoplasm, bone,
  benign
Coenurosis B71.8
Coffee-worker's lung J67.8
Cogan's syndrome H16.32
  oculomotor apraxia H51.8
Coitus, painful (female) N94.1
  male N53.12
  psychogenic F52.6
Cold J00
  with influenza, flu, or grippe —*see* Influenza,
  with, respiratory manifestations NEC
  agglutinin disease or hemoglobinuria
  (chronic) D59.1
  bronchial —*see* Bronchitis
  chest —*see* Bronchitis
  common (head) J00
  effects of T69.9
    specified effect NEC T69.8
  excessive, effects of T69.9
    specified effect NEC T69.8
  exhaustion from T69.8
  exposure to T69.9
    specified effect NEC T69.8
  head J00
  injury syndrome (newborn) P80.0
  on lung —*see* Bronchitis
  rose J30.1
  sensitivity, auto-immune D59.1
  virus J00
Cold sore B00.1
Colibacillosis A49.8
  as the cause of other disease (*see also*
  Escherichia coli) B96.20
  generalized A41.50
Colic (bilious) (infantile) (intestinal)
  (recurrent) (spasmodic) R10.83
  abdomen R10.83
    psychogenic F45.8
  appendix, appendicular K38.8
  bile duct —*see* Calculus, bile duct
  biliary —*see* Calculus, bile duct

Colic - *continued*
common duct —*see* Calculus, bile duct
cystic duct —*see* Calculus, gallbladder
Devonshire NEC —*see* Poisoning, lead
gallbladder —*see* Calculus, gallbladder
gallstone —*see* Calculus, gallbladder
 gallbladder or cystic duct —*see* Calculus,
gallbladder
hepatic (duct) —*see* Calculus, bile duct
hysterical F45.8
kidney N23
lead NEC —*see* Poisoning, lead
mucous K58.9
 with diarrhea K58.0
 psychogenic F54
nephritic N23
painter's NEC —*see* Poisoning, lead
pancreas K86.8
psychogenic F45.8
renal N23
saturnine NEC —*see* Poisoning, lead
ureter N23
urethral N36.8
 due to calculus N21.1
uterus NEC N94.89
 menstrual —*see* Dysmenorrhea
worm NOS B83.9
Colicystitis —*see* Cystitis
Colitis (acute) (catarrhal) (chronic)
 (noninfective) (hemorrhagic) (*see also*
 Enteritis) K52.9
allergic K52.2
amebic (acute) (*see also* Amebiasis) A06.0
 nondysenteric A06.2
anthrax A22.2
bacillary —*see* Infection, Shigella
balantidial A07.0
Clostridium difficile A04.7
coccidial A07.3
collagenous K52.89
cystica superficialis K52.89
dietary counseling and surveillance (for)
 Z71.3
dietetic K52.2
drug-induced K52.1
due to radiation K52.0
eosinophilic K52.82
food hypersensitivity K52.2
giardial A07.1
granulomatous —*see* Enteritis, regional, large
 intestine
infectious —*see* Enteritis, infectious
ischemic K55.9
 acute (fulminant) (subacute) K55.0
 chronic K55.1
 due to mesenteric artery insufficiency K55.1
 fulminant (acute) K55.0
left sided K51.50
 with
 abscess K51.514
 complication K51.519
 specified NEC K51.518
 fistula K51.513
 obstruction K51.512
 rectal bleeding K51.511
lymphocytic K52.89
membranous
 psychogenic F54
microscopic (collagenous) (lymphocytic)
 K52.89
mucous —*see* Syndrome, irritable, bowel
 psychogenic F54

Colitis - *continued*
noninfective K52.9
 specified NEC K52.89
polyposa —*see* Polyp, colon, inflammatory
protozoal A07.9
pseudomembranous A04.7
pseudomucinous —*see* Syndrome, irritable,
bowel
regional —*see* Enteritis, regional, large
intestine
segmental —*see* Enteritis, regional, large
intestine
septic —*see* Enteritis, infectious
spastic K58.9
 with diarrhea K58.0
 psychogenic F54
staphylococcal A04.8
 foodborne A05.0
subacute ischemic K55.0
thromboulcerative K55.0
toxic NEC K52.1
 due to Clostridium difficile A04.7
transmural —*see* Enteritis, regional, large
intestine
trichomonal A07.8
tuberculous (ulcerative) A18.32
ulcerative (chronic) K51.90
 with
 complication K51.919
 abscess K51.914
 fistula K51.913
 obstruction K51.912
 rectal bleeding K51.911
 specified complication NEC K51.918
 enterocolitis —*see* Enterocolitis, ulcerative
 ileocolitis —*see* Ileocolitis, ulcerative
 mucosal proctocolitis —*see* Proctocolitis,
mucosal
 proctitis —*see* Proctitis, ulcerative
 pseudopolyposis —*see* Polyp, colon,
inflammatory
 psychogenic F54
 rectosigmoiditis —*see* Rectosigmoiditis,
ulcerative
 specified type NEC K51.80
 with
 complication K51.819
 abscess K51.814
 fistula K51.813
 obstruction K51.812
 rectal bleeding K51.811
 specified complication NEC K51.818
Collagenosis, collagen disease (nonvascular)
 (vascular) M35.9
cardiovascular I42.8
reactive perforating L87.1
specified NEC M35.8
Collapse R55
adrenal E27.2
cardiorespiratory R57.0
cardiovascular R57.0
 newborn P29.89
circulatory (peripheral) R57.9
 during or after labor and delivery O75.1
 following ectopic or molar pregnancy O08.3
 newborn P29.89
during or
 after labor and delivery O75.1
 resulting from a procedure, not elsewhere
classified T81.10
external ear canal —*see* Stenosis, external ear
canal

Collapse – *continued*
general R55
heart —*see* Disease, heart
heat T67.1
hysterical F44.89
labyrinth, membranous (congenital) Q16.5
lung (massive) (*see also* Atelectasis) J98.19
 pressure due to anesthesia (general) (local)
or other sedation T88.2
 during labor and delivery O74.1
 in pregnancy O29.02
 postpartum, puerperal O89.09
myocardial —*see* Disease, heart
nervous F48.8
neurocirculatory F45.8
nose M95.0
postoperative T81.10
pulmonary (*see also* Atelectasis) J98.19
 newborn —*see* Atelectasis
trachea J39.8
tracheobronchial J98.09
valvular —*see* Endocarditis
vascular (peripheral) R57.9
 during or after labor and delivery O75.1
 following ectopic or molar pregnancy O08.3
 newborn P29.89
vertebra M48.50
 cervical region M48.52
 cervicothoracic region M48.53
 in (due to)
 metastasis —*see* Collapse, vertebra, in,
specified disease NEC
 osteoporosis (*see also* Osteoporosis)
M80.88
 cervical region M80.88
 cervicothoracic region M80.88
 lumbar region M80.88
 lumbosacral region M80.88
 multiple sites M80.88
 occipito-atlanto-axial region M80.88
 sacrococcygeal region M80.88
 thoracic region M80.88
 thoracolumbar region M80.88
 specified disease NEC M48.50
 cervical region M48.52
 cervicothoracic region M48.53
 lumbar region M48.56
 lumbosacral region M48.57
 occipito-atlanto-axial region M48.51
 sacrococcygeal region M48.58
 thoracic region M48.54
 thoracolumbar region M48.55
 lumbar region M48.56
 lumbosacral region M48.57
 occipito-atlanto-axial region M48.51
 sacrococcygeal region M48.58
 thoracic region M48.54
 thoracolumbar region M48.55
Collateral —*see also* condition
circulation (venous) I87.8
dilation, veins I87.8
Colles' fracture S52.53
Collet (-Sicard) **syndrome** G52.7
Collier's asthma or lung J60
Collodion baby Q80.2
Colloid nodule (of thyroid) (cystic) E04.1
Coloboma (iris) Q13.0
eyelid Q10.3
fundus Q14.8
lens Q12.2
optic disc (congenital) Q14.2
 acquired H47.31
Coloenteritis —*see* Enteritis

Colon —*see* condition
Colonization
  MRSA (Methicillin resistant Staphylococcus aureus) Z22.322
  MSSA (Methicillin susceptible Staphylococcus aureus) Z22.321
  status —*see* Carrier (suspected) of
Coloptosis K63.4
Color blindness —*see* Deficiency, color vision
Colostomy
  attention to Z43.3
  fitting or adjustment Z46.89
  malfunctioning K94.03
  status Z93.3
Colpitis (acute) —*see* Vaginitis
Colpocele N81.5
Colpocystitis —*see* Vaginitis
Colpospasm N94.2
Column, spinal, vertebral —*see* condition
Coma R40.20
  with
    motor response (none) R40.231
      abnormal R40.233
      extension R40.232
      flexion withdrawal R40.234
      localizes pain R40.235
      obeys commands R40.236
    opening of eyes (never) R40.211
      in response to
        pain R40.212
        sound R40.213
      spontaneous R40.214
    verbal response (none) R40.221
      confused conversation R40.224
      inappropriate words R40.223
      incomprehensible words R40.222
      oriented R40.225
  eclamptic —*see* Eclampsia
  epileptic —*see* Epilepsy
  Glasgow, scale score —*see* Glasgow coma scale
  hepatic —*see* Failure, hepatic, by type, with coma
  hyperglycemic (diabetic) —*see* Diabetes, coma
  hyperosmolar (diabetic) —*see* Diabetes, coma
  hypoglycemic (diabetic) —*see* Diabetes, coma, hypoglycemic
    nondiabetic E15
  in diabetes —*see* Diabetes, coma
  insulin-induced —*see* Coma, hypoglycemic
  myxedematous E03.5
  newborn P91.5
  persistent vegetative state R40.3
  specified NEC, without documented Glasgow coma scale score, or with partial Glasgow coma scale score reported R40.244
Comatose —*see* Coma
Combat fatigue F43.0
Combined —*see* condition
Comedo, comedones (giant) L70.0
Comedocarcinoma —*see also* Neoplasm, breast, malignant
  noninfiltrating
    breast D05.8
    specified site —*see* Neoplasm, in situ, by site
    unspecified site D05.8
Comedomastitis —*see* Ectasia, mammary duct
Comminuted fracture
  code as Fracture, closed Common
  arterial trunk Q20.0

Comminuted fracture - *continued*
  atrioventricular canal Q21.2
  atrium Q21.1
  cold (head) J00
  truncus (arteriosus) Q20.0
  variable immunodeficiency —*see* Immunodeficiency, common variable
  ventricle Q20.4
Commotio, commotion (current)
  brain —*see* Injury, intracranial, concussion
  cerebri —*see* Injury, intracranial, concussion
  retinae S05.8X
  spinal cord —*see* Injury, spinal cord, by region
  spinalis —*see* Injury, spinal cord, by region
Communication
  between
    base of aorta and pulmonary artery Q21.4
    left ventricle and right atrium Q20.5
    pericardial sac and pleural sac Q34.8
    pulmonary artery and pulmonary vein, congenital Q25.72
    congenital between uterus and digestive or urinary tract Q51.7
Compartment syndrome (deep) (posterior) (traumatic) T79.A0
  abdomen T79.A3
  lower extremity (hip, buttock, thigh, leg, foot, toes) T79.A2
  nontraumatic
    abdomen M79.A3
    lower extremity (hip, buttock, thigh, leg, foot, toes) M79.A2
    specified site NEC M79.A9
    upper extremity (shoulder, arm, forearm, wrist, hand, fingers) M79.A1
  specified site NEC T79.A9
  upper extremity (shoulder, arm, forearm, wrist, hand, fingers) T79.A1
Compensation
  failure —*see* Disease, heart
  neurosis, psychoneurosis —*see* Disorder, factitious
Complaint —*see also* Disease
  bowel, functional K59.9
    psychogenic F45.8
  intestine, functional K59.9
    psychogenic F45.8
  kidney —*see* Disease, renal
  miners' J60
Complete —*see* condition
Complex
  Addison-Schilder E71.528
  cardiorenal —*see* Hypertension, cardiorenal
  Costen's M26.69
  disseminated mycobacterium avium intracellulare (DMAC) A31.2
  Eisenmenger's (ventricular septal defect) I27.89
  hypersexual F52.8
  jumped process, spine —*see* Dislocation, vertebra
  primary, tuberculous A15.7
  Schilder-Addison E71.528
  subluxation (vertebral) M99.19
    abdomen M99.19
    acromioclavicular M99.17
    cervical region M99.11
    cervicothoracic M99.11
    costochondral M99.18
    costovertebral M99.18
    head region M99.10

Complex – *continued*
    hip M99.15
    lower extremity M99.16
    lumbar region M99.13
    lumbosacral M99.13
    occipitocervical M99.10
    pelvic region M99.15
    pubic M99.15
    rib cage M99.18
    sacral region M99.14
    sacrococcygeal M99.14
    sacroiliac M99.14
    specified NEC M99.19
    sternochondral M99.18
    sternoclavicular M99.17
    thoracic region M99.12
    thoracolumbar M99.12
    upper extremity M99.17
  Taussig-Bing (transposition, aorta and overriding pulmonary artery) Q20.1
Complication (s) (from) (of)
  accidental puncture or laceration during a procedure (of) —*see* Complications, intraoperative (intraprocedural), puncture or laceration
  amputation stump (surgical) (late) NEC T87.9
    dehiscence T87.81
    infection or inflammation T87.40
      lower limb T87.4
      upper limb T87.4
    necrosis T87.50
      lower limb T87.5
      upper limb T87.5
    neuroma T87.30
      lower limb T87.3
      upper limb T87.3
    specified type NEC T87.89
  anastomosis (and bypass) —*see also* Complications, prosthetic device or implant
    intestinal (internal) NEC K91.89
      involving urinary tract N99.89
    urinary tract (involving intestinal tract) N99.89
    vascular —*see* Complications, cardiovascular device or implant
  anesthesia, anesthetic (*see also* Anesthesia, complication) T88.59
    brain, postpartum, puerperal O89.2
    cardiac
      in
        labor and delivery O74.2
        pregnancy O29.19
      postpartum, puerperal O89.1
    central nervous system
      in
        labor and delivery O74.3
        pregnancy O29.29
      postpartum, puerperal O89.2
    difficult or failed intubation T88.4
      in pregnancy O29.6
    failed sedation (conscious) (moderate) during procedure T88.52
    hyperthermia, malignant T88.3
    hypothermia T88.51
    intubation failure T88.4
    malignant hyperthermia T88.3
    pulmonary
      in
        labor and delivery O74.1
        pregnancy NEC O29.09
      postpartum, puerperal O89.09
    shock T88.2
    spinal and epidural

Complication - *continued*

in

labor and delivery NEC O74.6

headache O74.5

pregnancy NEC O29.5X

postpartum, puerperal NEC O89.5

headache O89.4

anti-reflux device —*see* Complications, esophageal anti-reflux device

aortic (bifurcation) graft —*see* Complications, graft, vascular

aortocoronary (bypass) graft —*see* Complications, coronary artery (bypass) graft

aortofemoral (bypass) graft —*see* Complications, extremity artery (bypass) graft

arteriovenous

fistula, surgically created T82.9

embolism T82.818

fibrosis T82.828

hemorrhage T82.838

infection or inflammation T82.7

mechanical

breakdown T82.510

displacement T82.520

leakage T82.530

malposition T82.520

obstruction T82.590

perforation T82.590

protrusion T82.590

pain T82.848

specified type NEC T82.898

stenosis T82.858

thrombosis T82.868

shunt, surgically created T82.9

embolism T82.818

fibrosis T82.828

hemorrhage T82.838

infection or inflammation T82.7

mechanical

breakdown T82.511

displacement T82.521

leakage T82.531

malposition T82.521

obstruction T82.591

perforation T82.591

protrusion T82.591

pain T82.848

specified type NEC T82.898

stenosis T82.858

thrombosis T82.868

arthroplasty —*see* Complications, joint prosthesis

artificial

fertilization or insemination N98.9

attempted introduction (of)

embryo in embryo transfer N98.3

ovum following in vitro fertilization N98.2

hyperstimulation of ovaries N98.1

infection N98.0

specified NEC N98.8

heart T82.9

embolism T82.817

fibrosis T82.827

hemorrhage T82.837

infection or inflammation T82.7

mechanical

breakdown T82.512

displacement T82.522

leakage T82.532

malposition T82.522

obstruction T82.592

Complication - *continued*

perforation T82.592

protrusion T82.592

pain T82.847

specified type NEC T82.897

stenosis T82.857

thrombosis T82.867

opening

cecostomy —*see* Complications, colostomy

colostomy —*see* Complications, colostomy

cystostomy —*see* Complications, cystostomy

enterostomy —*see* Complications, enterostomy

gastrostomy —*see* Complications, gastrostomy

ileostomy —*see* Complications, enterostomy

jejunostomy —*see* Complications, enterostomy

nephrostomy —*see* Complications, stoma, urinary tract

tracheostomy —*see* Complications, tracheostomy

ureterostomy —*see* Complications, stoma, urinary tract

urethrostomy —*see* Complications, stoma, urinary tract

balloon implant or device

gastrointestinal T85.9

embolism T85.81

fibrosis T85.82

hemorrhage T85.83

infection and inflammation T85.79

pain T85.84

specified type NEC T85.89

stenosis T85.85

thrombosis T85.86

vascular (counterpulsation) T82.9

embolism T82.818

fibrosis T82.828

hemorrhage T82.838

infection or inflammation T82.7

mechanical

breakdown T82.513

displacement T82.523

leakage T82.533

malposition T82.523

obstruction T82.593

perforation T82.593

protrusion T82.593

pain T82.848

specified type NEC T82.898

stenosis T82.858

thrombosis T82.868

bariatric procedure

gastric band procedure K95.09

infection K95.01

specified procedure NEC K95.89

infection K95.81

bile duct implant (prosthetic) T85.9

embolism T85.81

fibrosis T85.82

hemorrhage T85.83

infection and inflammation T85.79

mechanical

breakdown T85.510

displacement T85.520

malfunction T85.510

malposition T85.520

obstruction T85.590

Complication - *continued*

perforation T85.590

protrusion T85.590

specified NEC T85.590

pain T85.84

specified type NEC T85.89

stenosis T85.85

thrombosis T85.86

bladder device (auxiliary) —*see* Complications, genitourinary, device or implant, urinary system

bleeding (postoperative) —*see* Complication, postoperative, hemorrhage

intraoperative —*see* Complication, intraoperative, hemorrhage

blood vessel graft —*see* Complications, graft, vascular

bone

device NEC T84.9

embolism T84.81

fibrosis T84.82

hemorrhage T84.83

infection or inflammation T84.7

mechanical

breakdown T84.318

displacement T84.328

malposition T84.328

obstruction T84.398

perforation T84.398

protrusion T84.398

pain T84.84

specified type NEC T84.89

stenosis T84.85

thrombosis T84.86

graft —*see* Complications, graft, bone

growth stimulator (electrode) —*see* Complications, electronic stimulator device, bone

marrow transplant —*see* Complications, transplant, bone, marrow

brain neurostimulator (electrode) —*see* Complications, electronic stimulator device, brain

breast implant (prosthetic) T85.9

capsular contracture T85.44

embolism T85.81

fibrosis T85.82

hemorrhage T85.83

infection and inflammation T85.79

mechanical

breakdown T85.41

displacement T85.42

leakage T85.43

malposition T85.42

obstruction T85.49

perforation T85.49

protrusion T85.49

specified NEC T85.49

pain T85.84

specified type NEC T85.89

stenosis T85.85

thrombosis T85.86

bypass —*see also* Complications, prosthetic device or implant

aortocoronary —*see* Complications, coronary artery (bypass) graft

arterial —*see also* Complications, graft, vascular

extremity —*see* Complications, extremity artery (bypass) graft

cardiac —*see also* Disease, heart

device, implant or graft T82.9

embolism T82.817

Complication - *continued*

fibrosis T82.827
hemorrhage T82.837
infection or inflammation T82.7
valve prosthesis T82.6
mechanical
breakdown T82.519
specified device NEC T82.518
displacement T82.529
specified device NEC T82.528
leakage T82.539
specified device NEC T82.538
malposition T82.529
specified device NEC T82.528
obstruction T82.599
specified device NEC T82.598
perforation T82.599
specified device NEC T82.598
protrusion T82.599
specified device NEC T82.598
pain T82.847
specified type NEC T82.897
stenosis T82.857
thrombosis T82.867
cardiovascular device, graft or implant T82.9
aortic graft —*see* Complications, graft,
vascular
arteriovenous
fistula, artificial —*see* Complication,
arteriovenous, fistula, surgically created
shunt —*see* Complication, arteriovenous,
shunt, surgically created
artificial heart —*see* Complication, artificial,
heart
balloon (counterpulsation) device —*see*
Complication, balloon implant, vascular
carotid artery graft —*see* Complications,
graft, vascular
coronary bypass graft —*see* Complication,
coronary artery (bypass) graft
dialysis catheter (vascular) —*see*
Complication, catheter, dialysis
electronic T82.9
electrode T82.9
embolism T82.817
fibrosis T82.827
hemorrhage T82.837
infection T82.7
mechanical
breakdown T82.110
displacement T82.120
leakage T82.190
obstruction T82.190
perforation T82.190
protrusion T82.190
specified type NEC T82.190
pain T82.847
specified NEC T82.897
stenosis T82.857
thrombosis T82.867
embolism T82.817
fibrosis T82.827
hemorrhage T82.837
infection T82.7
mechanical
breakdown T82.119
displacement T82.129
leakage T82.199
obstruction T82.199
perforation T82.199
protrusion T82.199
specified type NEC T82.199

Complication - *continued*

pain T82.847
pulse generator T82.9
embolism T82.817
fibrosis T82.827
hemorrhage T82.837
infection T82.7
mechanical
breakdown T82.111
displacement T82.121
leakage T82.191
obstruction T82.191
perforation T82.191
protrusion T82.191
specified type NEC T82.191
pain T82.847
specified NEC T82.897
stenosis T82.857
thrombosis T82.867
specified condition NEC T82.897
specified device NEC T82.9
embolism T82.817
fibrosis T82.827
hemorrhage T82.837
infection T82.7
mechanical
breakdown T82.118
displacement T82.128
leakage T82.198
obstruction T82.198
perforation T82.198
protrusion T82.198
specified type NEC T82.198
pain T82.847
specified NEC T82.897
stenosis T82.857
thrombosis T82.867
stenosis T82.857
thrombosis T82.867
extremity artery graft —*see* Complication,
extremity artery (bypass) graft
femoral artery graft —*see* Complication,
extremity artery (bypass) graft
heart-lung transplant —*see* Complication,
transplant, heart, with lung
heart
transplant —*see* Complication, transplant,
heart
valve —*see* Complication, prosthetic
device, heart valve
graft —*see* Complication, heart, valve,
graft
infection or inflammation T82.7
umbrella device —*see* Complication,
umbrella device, vascular
vascular graft (or anastomosis) —*see*
Complication, graft, vascular
carotid artery (bypass) graft —*see*
Complications, graft, vascular
catheter (device) NEC —*see also*
Complications, prosthetic device or implant
cystostomy T83.9
embolism T83.81
fibrosis T83.82
hemorrhage T83.83
infection and inflammation T83.59
mechanical
breakdown T83.010
displacement T83.020
leakage T83.030
malposition T83.020
obstruction T83.090

Complication - *continued*

perforation T83.090
protrusion T83.090
specified NEC T83.090
pain T83.84
specified type NEC T83.89
stenosis T83.85
thrombosis T83.86
dialysis (vascular) T82.9
embolism T82.818
fibrosis T82.828
hemorrhage T82.838
infection and inflammation T82.7
intraperitoneal —*see* Complications,
catheter, intraperitoneal
mechanical
breakdown T82.41
displacement T82.42
leakage T82.43
malposition T82.42
obstruction T82.49
perforation T82.49
protrusion T82.49
pain T82.848
specified type NEC T82.898
stenosis T82.858
thrombosis T82.868
epidural infusion T85.9
embolism T85.81
fibrosis T85.82
hemorrhage T85.83
infection and inflammation T85.79
mechanical
breakdown T85.610
displacement T85.620
leakage T85.630
malfunction T85.610
malposition T85.620
obstruction T85.690
perforation T85.690
protrusion T85.690
specified NEC T85.690
pain T85.84
specified type NEC T85.89
stenosis T85.85
thrombosis T85.86
intraperitoneal dialysis T85.9
embolism T85.81
fibrosis T85.82
hemorrhage T85.83
infection and inflammation T85.71
mechanical
breakdown T85.611
displacement T85.621
leakage T85.631
malfunction T85.611
malposition T85.621
obstruction T85.691
perforation T85.691
protrusion T85.691
specified NEC T85.691
pain T85.84
specified type NEC T85.89
stenosis T85.85
thrombosis T85.86
intravenous infusion T82.9
embolism T82.818
fibrosis T82.828
hemorrhage T82.838
infection or inflammation T82.7
mechanical
breakdown T82.514
displacement T82.524

Complication - *continued*
- leakage T82.534
- malposition T82.524
- obstruction T82.594
- perforation T82.594
- protrusion T82.594
- pain T82.848
- specified type NEC T82.898
- stenosis T82.858
- thrombosis T82.868
- subdural infusion T85.9
  - embolism T85.81
  - fibrosis T85.82
  - hemorrhage T85.83
  - infection and inflammation T85.79
  - mechanical
    - breakdown T85.610
    - displacement T85.620
    - leakage T85.630
    - malfunction T85.610
    - malposition T85.620
    - obstruction T85.690
    - perforation T85.690
    - protrusion T85.690
    - specified NEC T85.690
  - pain T85.84
  - specified type NEC T85.89
  - stenosis T85.85
  - thrombosis T85.86
- urethral, indwelling T83.9
  - displacement T83.028
  - embolism T83.81
  - fibrosis T83.82
  - hemorrhage T83.83
  - infection and inflammation T83.51
  - leakage T83.038
  - malposition T83.028
  - mechanical
    - breakdown T83.018
  - obstruction (mechanical) T83.098
  - pain T83.84
  - perforation T83.098
  - protrusion T83.098
  - specified type NEC T83.098
  - stenosis T83.85
  - thrombosis T83.86
- urinary (indwelling) —*see* Complications, catheter, urethral, indwelling
- cecostomy (stoma) —*see* Complications, colostomy
- cesarean delivery wound NEC O90.89
  - disruption O90.0
  - hematoma O90.2
  - infection (following delivery) O86.0
- chemotherapy (antineoplastic) NEC T88.7
- chin implant (prosthetic) —*see* Complication, prosthetic device or implant, specified NEC
- circulatory system I99.8
  - intraoperative I97.88
  - postprocedural I97.89
    - following cardiac surgery I97.19
      - postcardiotomy syndrome I97.0
    - hypertension I97.3
    - lymphedema after mastectomy I97.2
    - postcardiotomy syndrome I97.0
    - specified NEC I97.89
- colostomy (stoma) K94.00
  - hemorrhage K94.01
  - infection K94.02
  - malfunction K94.03
  - mechanical K94.03
  - specified complication NEC K94.09

Complication - *continued*
- contraceptive device, intrauterine —*see* Complications, intrauterine, contraceptive device
- cord (umbilical) —*see* Complications, umbilical cord
- corneal graft —*see* Complications, graft, cornea
- coronary artery (bypass) graft T82.9
  - atherosclerosis —*see* Arteriosclerosis, coronary (artery)
  - embolism T82.818
  - fibrosis T82.828
  - hemorrhage T82.838
  - infection and inflammation T82.7
  - mechanical
    - breakdown T82.211
    - displacement T82.212
    - leakage T82.213
    - malposition T82.212
    - obstruction T82.218
    - perforation T82.218
    - protrusion T82.218
    - specified NEC T82.218
  - pain T82.848
  - specified type NEC T82.897
  - stenosis T82.858
  - thrombosis T82.868
- counterpulsation device (balloon) , intra aortic —*see* Complications, balloon implant, vascular
- cystostomy (stoma) N99.518
  - catheter —*see* Complications, catheter, cystostomy
  - hemorrhage N99.510
  - infection N99.511
  - malfunction N99.512
  - specified type NEC N99.518
- delivery (*see also* Complications, obstetric) O75.9
  - procedure (instrumental) (manual) (surgical) O75.4
  - specified NEC O75.89
- dialysis (peritoneal) (renal) —*see also* Complications, infusion
  - catheter (vascular) —*see* Complication, catheter, dialysis
    - peritoneal, intraperitoneal —*see* Complications, catheter, intraperitoneal
- dorsal column (spinal) neurostimulator —*see* Complications, electronic stimulator device, spinal cord
- drug NEC T88.7
- ear procedure —*see also* Disorder, ear
  - intraoperative H95.88
    - hematoma —*see* Complications, intraoperative, hemorrhage (hematoma) (of) , ear
    - hemorrhage —*see* Complications, intraoperative, hemorrhage (hematoma) (of) , ear
    - laceration —*see* Complications, intraoperative, puncture or laceration..., ear
  - specified NEC H95.88
  - postoperative H95.89
    - external ear canal stenosis H95.81
    - hematoma —*see* Complications, postprocedural, hemorrhage (hematoma) (of) , ear
    - hemorrhage —*see* Complications, postprocedural, hemorrhage (hematoma) (of) , ear

Complication - *continued*
- postmastoidectomy —*see* Complications, postmastoidectomy
  - specified NEC H95.89
- ectopic pregnancy O08.9
  - damage to pelvic organs O08.6
  - embolism O08.2
  - genital infection O08.0
  - hemorrhage (delayed) (excessive) O08.1
  - metabolic disorder O08.5
  - renal failure O08.4
  - shock O08.3
  - specified type NEC O08.0
  - venous complication NEC O08.7
- electronic stimulator device
  - bladder (urinary) —*see* Complications, electronic stimulator device, urinary
  - bone T84.9
    - breakdown T84.310
    - displacement T84.320
    - embolism T84.81
    - fibrosis T84.82
    - hemorrhage T84.83
    - infection or inflammation T84.7
    - malfunction T84.310
    - malposition T84.320
    - mechanical NEC T84.390
    - obstruction T84.390
    - pain T84.84
    - perforation T84.390
    - protrusion T84.390
    - specified type NEC T84.89
    - stenosis T84.85
    - thrombosis T84.86
  - brain T85.9
    - embolism T85.81
    - fibrosis T85.82
    - hemorrhage T85.83
    - infection and inflammation T85.79
    - mechanical
      - breakdown T85.110
      - displacement T85.120
      - leakage T85.190
      - malposition T85.120
      - obstruction T85.190
      - perforation T85.190
      - protrusion T85.190
      - specified NEC T85.190
    - pain T85.84
    - specified type NEC T85.89
    - stenosis T85.85
    - thrombosis T85.86
  - cardiac (defibrillator) (pacemaker) —*see* Complications, cardiovascular device or implant, electronic
  - muscle T84.9
    - breakdown T84.418
    - displacement T84.428
    - embolism T84.81
    - fibrosis T84.82
    - hemorrhage T84.83
    - infection or inflammation T84.7
    - mechanical NEC T84.498
    - pain T84.84
    - specified type NEC T84.89
    - stenosis T84.85
    - thrombosis T84.86
  - nervous system T85.9
    - brain —*see* Complications, electronic stimulator device, brain
    - embolism T85.81
    - fibrosis T85.82
    - hemorrhage T85.83

Complication - *continued*
  infection and inflammation T85.79
  mechanical
    breakdown T85.118
    displacement T85.128
    leakage T85.199
    malposition T85.128
    obstruction T85.199
    perforation T85.199
    protrusion T85.199
    specified NEC T85.199
  pain T85.84
  peripheral nerve —*see* Complications,
electronic stimulator device, peripheral nerve
  specified type NEC T85.89
  spinal cord —*see* Complications,
electronic stimulator device, spinal cord
  stenosis T85.85
  thrombosis T85.86
  peripheral nerve T85.9
    embolism T85.81
    fibrosis T85.82
    hemorrhage T85.83
    infection and inflammation T85.79
    mechanical
      breakdown T85.111
      displacement T85.121
      leakage T85.191
      malposition T85.121
      obstruction T85.191
      perforation T85.191
      protrusion T85.191
      specified NEC T85.191
    pain T85.84
    specified type NEC T85.89
    stenosis T85.85
    thrombosis T85.86
  spinal cord T85.9
    embolism T85.81
    fibrosis T85.82
    hemorrhage T85.83
    infection and inflammation T85.79
    mechanical
      breakdown T85.112
      displacement T85.122
      leakage T85.192
      malposition T85.122
      obstruction T85.192
      perforation T85.192
      protrusion T85.192
      specified NEC T85.192
    pain T85.84
    specified type NEC T85.89
    stenosis T85.85
    thrombosis T85.86
  urinary T83.9
    embolism T83.81
    fibrosis T83.82
    hemorrhage T83.83
    infection and inflammation T83.59
    mechanical
      breakdown T83.110
      displacement T83.120
      malposition T83.120
      perforation T83.190
      protrusion T83.190
      specified NEC T83.190
    pain T83.84
    specified type NEC T83.89
    stenosis T83.85
    thrombosis T83.86

Complication - *continued*
  electroshock therapy T88.9
    specified NEC T88.8
  endocrine E34.9
    postprocedural
      adrenal hypofunction E89.6
      hypoinsulinemia E89.1
      hypoparathyroidism E89.2
      hypopituitarism E89.3
      hypothyroidism E89.0
      ovarian failure E89.40
        asymptomatic E89.40
        symptomatic E89.41
      specified NEC E89.89
      testicular hypofunction E89.5
  endodontic treatment NEC M27.59
  enterostomy (stoma) K94.10
    hemorrhage K94.11
    infection K94.12
    malfunction K94.13
    mechanical K94.13
    specified complication NEC K94.19
  episiotomy, disruption O90.1
  esophageal anti-reflux device T85.9
    embolism T85.81
    fibrosis T85.82
    hemorrhage T85.83
    infection and inflammation T85.79
    mechanical
      breakdown T85.511
      displacement T85.521
      malfunction T85.511
      malposition T85.521
      obstruction T85.591
      perforation T85.591
      protrusion T85.591
      specified NEC T85.591
    pain T85.84
    specified type NEC T85.89
    stenosis T85.85
    thrombosis T85.86
  esophagostomy K94.30
    hemorrhage K94.31
    infection K94.32
    malfunction K94.33
    mechanical K94.33
    specified complication NEC K94.39
  extracorporeal circulation T80.90
  extremity artery (bypass) graft T82.9
    arteriosclerosis —*see* Arteriosclerosis,
extremities, bypass graft
    embolism T82.818
    fibrosis T82.828
    hemorrhage T82.838
    infection and inflammation T82.7
    mechanical
      breakdown T82.318
        femoral artery T82.312
      displacement T82.328
        femoral artery T82.322
      leakage T82.338
        femoral artery T82.332
      malposition T82.328
        femoral artery T82.322
      obstruction T82.398
        femoral artery T82.392
      perforation T82.398
        femoral artery T82.392
      protrusion T82.398
        femoral artery T82.392
    pain T82.848
    specified type NEC T82.898

Complication - *continued*
    stenosis T82.858
    thrombosis T82.868
  eye H57.9
    corneal graft —*see* Complications, graft,
cornea
    implant (prosthetic) T85.9
      embolism T85.81
      fibrosis T85.82
      hemorrhage T85.83
      infection and inflammation T85.79
      mechanical
        breakdown T85.318
        displacement T85.328
        leakage T85.398
        malposition T85.328
        obstruction T85.398
        perforation T85.398
        protrusion T85.398
        specified NEC T85.398
      pain T85.84
      specified type NEC T85.89
      stenosis T85.85
      thrombosis T85.86
    intraocular lens —*see* Complications,
intraocular lens
    orbital prosthesis —*see* Complications,
orbital prosthesis
  female genital N94.9
    device, implant or graft NEC —*see*
Complications, genitourinary, device or
implant, genital tract
  femoral artery (bypass) graft —*see*
Complication, extremity artery (bypass) graft
  fixation device, internal (orthopedic) T84.9
    infection and inflammation T84.60
      arm T84.61
        humerus T84.61
        radius T84.61
        ulna T84.61
      leg T84.629
        femur T84.62
        fibula T84.62
        tibia T84.62
      specified site NEC T84.69
      spine T84.63
    mechanical
      breakdown
        limb T84.119
          carpal T84.210
          femur T84.11
          fibula T84.11
          humerus T84.11
          metacarpal T84.210
          metatarsal T84.213
          phalanx
            foot T84.213
            hand T84.210
          radius T84.11
          tarsal T84.213
          tibia T84.11
          ulna T84.11
        specified bone NEC T84.218
        spine T84.216
      displacement
        limb T84.129
          carpal T84.220
          femur T84.12
          fibula T84.12
          humerus T84.12
          metacarpal T84.220
          metatarsal T84.223
          phalanx

Complication - *continued*
      foot T84.223
      hand T84.220
      radius T84.12
      tarsal T84.223
      tibia T84.12
      ulna T84.12
     specified bone NEC T84.228
     spine T84.226
    malposition —*see* Complications, fixation device, internal, mechanical, displacement
    obstruction —*see* Complications, fixation device, internal, mechanical, specified type NEC
    perforation —*see* Complications, fixation device, internal, mechanical, specified type NEC
    protrusion —*see* Complications, fixation device, internal, mechanical, specified type NEC
     specified type NEC
      limb T84.199
       carpal T84.290
       femur T84.19
       fibula T84.19
       humerus T84.19
       metacarpal T84.290
       metatarsal T84.293
       phalanx
        foot T84.293
        hand T84.290
       radius T84.19
       tarsal T84.293
       tibia T84.19
       ulna T84.19
      specified bone NEC T84.298
      vertebra T84.296
    specified type NEC T84.89
     embolism T84.81
     fibrosis T84.82
     hemorrhage T84.83
     pain T84.84
     specified complication NEC T84.89
     stenosis T84.85
     thrombosis T84.86
  following
   acute myocardial infarction NEC I23.8
   aneurysm (false) (of cardiac wall) (of heart wall) (ruptured) I23.3
   angina I23.7
   atrial
    septal defect I23.1
    thrombosis I23.6
   cardiac wall rupture I23.3
   chordae tendinae rupture I23.4
   defect
    septal
     atrial (heart) I23.1
     ventricular (heart) I23.2
   hemopericardium I23.0
   papillary muscle rupture I23.5
   rupture
    cardiac wall I23.3
     with hemopericardium I23.0
    chordae tendineae I23.4
    papillary muscle I23.5
   specified NEC I23.8
   thrombosis
    atrium I23.6
    auricular appendage I23.6
    ventricle (heart) I23.6
   ventricular

Complication - *continued*
    septal defect I23.2
    thrombosis I23.6
  ectopic or molar pregnancy O08.9
   cardiac arrest O08.81
   sepsis O08.82
   specified type NEC O08.89
   urinary tract infection O08.83
  termination of pregnancy —*see* Abortion
  gastrointestinal K92.9
   bile duct prosthesis —*see* Complications, bile duct implant
   esophageal anti-reflux device —*see* Complications, esophageal anti-reflux device
   postoperative
    colostomy —*see* Complications, colostomy
    dumping syndrome K91.1
    enterostomy —*see* Complications, enterostomy
    gastrostomy —*see* Complications, gastrostomy
    malabsorption NEC K91.2
    obstruction K91.3
    postcholecystectomy syndrome K91.5
    specified NEC K91.89
    vomiting after GI surgery K91.0
   prosthetic device or implant
    bile duct prosthesis —*see* Complications, bile duct implant
    esophageal anti-reflux device —*see* Complications, esophageal anti-reflux device
    specified type NEC
     embolism T85.81
     fibrosis T85.82
     hemorrhage T85.83
     mechanical
      breakdown T85.518
      displacement T85.528
      malfunction T85.518
      malposition T85.528
      obstruction T85.598
      perforation T85.598
      protrusion T85.598
      specified NEC T85.598
     pain T85.84
     specified complication NEC T85.89
     stenosis T85.85
     thrombosis T85.86
  gastrostomy (stoma) K94.20
   hemorrhage K94.21
   infection K94.22
   malfunction K94.23
   mechanical K94.23
   specified complication NEC K94.29
  genitourinary
   device or implant T83.9
    genital tract T83.9
     infection or inflammation T83.6
     intrauterine contraceptive device —*see* Complications, intrauterine, contraceptive device
     mechanical —*see* Complications, by device, mechanical
     mesh —*see* Complications, mesh
     penile prosthesis —*see* Complications, prosthetic device, penile
     specified type NEC T83.89
      embolism T83.81
      fibrosis T83.82
      hemorrhage T83.83
      pain T83.84
      specified complication NEC T83.89

Complication - *continued*
      stenosis T83.85
      thrombosis T83.86
    vaginal mesh —*see* Complications, mesh
   urinary system T83.9
    cystostomy catheter —*see* Complication, catheter, cystostomy
    electronic stimulator —*see* Complications, electronic stimulator device, urinary
    indwelling urethral catheter —*see* Complications, catheter, urethral, indwelling
    infection or inflammation T83.59
     indwelling urinary catheter T83.51
    kidney transplant —*see* Complication, transplant, kidney
    organ graft —*see* Complication, graft, urinary organ
    specified type NEC T83.89
     embolism T83.81
     fibrosis T83.82
     hemorrhage T83.83
     mechanical T83.198
      breakdown T83.118
      displacement T83.128
      malfunction T83.118
      malposition T83.128
      obstruction T83.198
      perforation T83.198
      protrusion T83.198
      specified NEC T83.198
     pain T83.84
     specified complication NEC T83.89
     stenosis T83.85
     thrombosis T83.86
    sphincter implant —*see* Complications, implant, urinary sphincter
   postprocedural
    pelvic peritoneal adhesions N99.4
    renal failure N99.0
    specified NEC N99.89
    stoma —*see* Complications, stoma, urinary tract
    urethral stricture —*see* Stricture, urethra, postprocedural
    vaginal
     adhesions N99.2
     vault prolapse N99.3
  graft (bypass) (patch) —*see also* Complications, prosthetic device or implant
   aorta —*see* Complications, graft, vascular
   arterial —*see* Complication, graft, vascular
   bone T86.839
    failure T86.831
    infection T86.832
    mechanical T84.318
     breakdown T84.318
     displacement T84.328
     protrusion T84.398
     specified type NEC T84.398
    rejection T86.830
    specified type NEC T86.838
   carotid artery —*see* Complications, graft, vascular
   cornea T86.849
    failure T86.841
    infection T86.842
    mechanical T85.398
     breakdown T85.318
     displacement T85.328
     protrusion T85.398
     specified type NEC T85.398
    rejection T86.840

Complication - *continued*

retroprosthetic membrane T85.398
specified type NEC T86.848
femoral artery (bypass) —*see* Complication, extremity artery (bypass) graft
genital organ or tract —*see* Complications, genitourinary, device or implant, genital tract
muscle T84.9
breakdown T84.410
displacement T84.420
embolism T84.81
fibrosis T84.82
hemorrhage T84.83
infection and inflammation T84.7
mechanical NEC T84.490
pain T84.84
specified type NEC T84.89
stenosis T84.85
thrombosis T84.86
nerve —*see* Complication, prosthetic device or implant, specified NEC
skin —*see* Complications, prosthetic device or implant, skin graft
tendon T84.9
breakdown T84.410
displacement T84.420
embolism T84.81
fibrosis T84.82
hemorrhage T84.83
infection and inflammation T84.7
mechanical NEC T84.490
pain T84.84
specified type NEC T84.89
stenosis T84.85
thrombosis T84.86
urinary organ T83.9
embolism T83.81
fibrosis T83.82
hemorrhage T83.83
infection and inflammation T83.59
indwelling urinary catheter T83.51
mechanical
breakdown T83.21
displacement T83.22
leakage T83.23
malposition T83.22
obstruction T83.29
perforation T83.29
protrusion T83.29
specified NEC T83.29
pain T83.84
specified type NEC T83.89
stenosis T83.85
thrombosis T83.86
vascular T82.9
embolism T82.818
femoral artery —*see* Complication, extremity artery (bypass) graft
fibrosis T82.828
hemorrhage T82.838
mechanical
breakdown T82.319
aorta (bifurcation) T82.310
carotid artery T82.311
specified vessel NEC T82.318
displacement T82.329
aorta (bifurcation) T82.320
carotid artery T82.321
specified vessel NEC T82.328
leakage T82.339
aorta (bifurcation) T82.330
carotid artery T82.331

Complication - *continued*

specified vessel NEC T82.338
malposition T82.329
aorta (bifurcation) T82.320
carotid artery T82.321
specified vessel NEC T82.328
obstruction T82.399
aorta (bifurcation) T82.390
carotid artery T82.391
specified vessel NEC T82.398
perforation T82.399
aorta (bifurcation) T82.390
carotid artery T82.391
specified vessel NEC T82.398
protrusion T82.399
aorta (bifurcation) T82.390
carotid artery T82.391
specified vessel NEC T82.398
pain T82.848
specified complication NEC T82.898
stenosis T82.858
thrombosis T82.868
heart I51.9
assist device
infection and inflammation T82.7
following acute myocardial infarction —*see* Complications, following, acute myocardial infarction
postoperative —*see* Complications, circulatory system
transplant —*see* Complication, transplant, heart
and lung (s) —*see* Complications, transplant, heart, with lung
valve
graft (biological) T82.9
embolism T82.817
fibrosis T82.827
hemorrhage T82.837
infection and inflammation T82.7
mechanical T82.228
breakdown T82.221
displacement T82.222
leakage T82.223
malposition T82.222
obstruction T82.228
perforation T82.228
protrusion T82.228
pain T82.847
specified type NEC T82.897
stenosis T82.857
thrombosis T82.867
prosthesis T82.9
embolism T82.817
fibrosis T82.827
hemorrhage T82.837
infection or inflammation T82.6
mechanical T82.09
breakdown T82.01
displacement T82.02
leakage T82.03
malposition T82.02
obstruction T82.09
perforation T82.09
protrusion T82.09
pain T82.847
specified type NEC T82.897
mechanical T82.09
stenosis T82.857
thrombosis T82.867

Complication - *continued*

hematoma
intraoperative —*see* Complication, intraoperative, hemorrhage
postprocedural —*see* Complication, postprocedural, hemorrhage
hemodialysis —*see* Complications, dialysis
hemorrhage
intraoperative —*see* Complication, intraoperative, hemorrhage
postprocedural —*see* Complication, postprocedural, hemorrhage
ileostomy (stoma) —*see* Complications, enterostomy
immunization (procedure) —*see* Complications, vaccination
implant —*see also* Complications, by site and type
urinary sphincter T83.9
embolism T83.81
fibrosis T83.82
hemorrhage T83.83
infection and inflammation T83.59
mechanical
breakdown T83.111
displacement T83.121
leakage T83.191
malposition T83.121
obstruction T83.191
perforation T83.191
protrusion T83.191
specified NEC T83.191
pain T83.84
specified type NEC T83.89
stenosis T83.85
thrombosis T83.86
infusion (procedure) T80.90
air embolism T80.0
blood —*see* Complications, transfusion
catheter —*see* Complications, catheter
infection T80.29
pump —*see* Complications, cardiovascular, device or implant
sepsis T80.29
serum reaction (*see also* Reaction, serum) T80.69
anaphylactic shock (*see also* Shock, anaphylactic) T80.59
specified type NEC T80.89
inhalation therapy NEC T81.81
injection (procedure) T80.90
drug reaction —*see* Reaction, drug
infection T80.29
sepsis T80.29
serum (prophylactic) (therapeutic) —*see* Complications, vaccination
specified type NEC T80.89
vaccine (any) —*see* Complications, vaccination
inoculation (any) —*see* Complications, vaccination
insulin pump
infection and inflammation T85.72
mechanical
breakdown T85.614
displacement T85.624
leakage T85.633
malposition T85.624
obstruction T85.694
perforation T85.694
protrusion T85.694
specified NEC T85.694

Complication - *continued*
intestinal pouch NEC K91.858
intraocular lens (prosthetic) T85.9
  embolism T85.81
  fibrosis T85.82
  hemorrhage T85.83
  infection and inflammation T85.79
  mechanical
    breakdown T85.21
    displacement T85.22
    malposition T85.22
    obstruction T85.29
    perforation T85.29
    protrusion T85.29
    specified NEC T85.29
  pain T85.84
  specified type NEC T85.89
  stenosis T85.85
  thrombosis T85.86
intraoperative (intraprocedural)
  cardiac arrest
    during cardiac surgery I97.710
    during other surgery I97.711
  cardiac functional disturbance NEC
    during cardiac surgery I97.790
    during other surgery I97.791
  hemorrhage (hematoma) (of)
    circulatory system organ or structure
      during cardiac bypass I97.411
      during cardiac catheterization I97.410
      during other circulatory system procedure
    I97.418
      during other procedure I97.42
    digestive system organ
      during procedure on digestive system
    K91.61
      during procedure on other organ K91.62
    ear
      during procedure on ear and mastoid
    process H95.21
      during procedure on other organ H95.22
    endocrine system organ or structure
      during procedure on endocrine system
    organ or structure E36.01
      during procedure on other organ E36.02
    eye and adnexa
      during ophthalmic procedure H59.11
      during other procedure H59.12
    genitourinary organ or structure
      during procedure on genitourinary organ
    or structure N99.61
      during procedure on other organ N99.62
    mastoid process
      during procedure on ear and mastoid
    process H95.21
      during procedure on other organ H95.22
    musculoskeletal structure
      during musculoskeletal surgery M96.810
      during non-orthopedic surgery M96.811
      during orthopedic surgery M96.810
    nervous system
      during a nervous system procedure
    G97.31
      during other procedure G97.32
    respiratory system
      during other procedure J95.62
      during procedure on respiratory system
    organ or structure J95.61
    skin and subcutaneous tissue
      during a dermatologic procedure L76.01
      during a procedure on other organ L76.02
    spleen

Complication - *continued*
      during a procedure on other organ D78.02
      during a procedure on the spleen D78.01
    puncture or laceration (accidental)
  (unintentional) (of)
    brain
      during a nervous system procedure
    G97.48
      during other procedure G97.49
    circulatory system organ or structure
      during circulatory system procedure
    I97.51
      during other procedure I97.52
    digestive system
      during procedure on digestive system
    K91.71
      during procedure on other organ K91.72
    ear
      during procedure on ear and mastoid
    process H95.31
      during procedure on other organ H95.32
    endocrine system organ or structure
      during procedure on endocrine system
    organ or structure E36.11
      during procedure on other organ E36.12
    eye and adnexa
      during ophthalmic procedure H59.21
      during other procedure H59.22
    genitourinary organ or structure
      during procedure on genitourinary organ
    or structure N99.71
      during procedure on other organ N99.72
    mastoid process
      during procedure on ear and mastoid
    process H95.31
      during procedure on other organ H95.32
    musculoskeletal structure
      during musculoskeletal surgery M96.820
      during non-orthopedic surgery M96.821
      during orthopedic surgery M96.820
    nervous system
      during a nervous system procedure
    G97.48
      during other procedure G97.49
    respiratory system
      during other procedure J95.72
      during procedure on respiratory system
    organ or structure J95.71
    skin and subcutaneous tissue
      during a dermatologic procedure L76.11
      during a procedure on other organ L76.12
    spleen
      during a procedure on other organ D78.12
      during a procedure on the spleen D78.11
  specified NEC
    circulatory system I97.88
    digestive system K91.81
    ear H95.88
    endocrine system E36.8
    eye and adnexa H59.88
    genitourinary system N99.81
    mastoid process H95.88
    musculoskeletal structure M96.89
    nervous system G97.81
    respiratory system J95.88
    skin and subcutaneous tissue L76.81
    spleen D78.81
intraperitoneal catheter (dialysis) (infusion)
  —*see* Complications, catheter, intraperitoneal
intrauterine
  contraceptive device
    embolism T83.81

Complication - *continued*
  fibrosis T83.82
  hemorrhage T83.83
  infection and inflammation T83.6
  mechanical
    breakdown T83.31
    displacement T83.32
    malposition T83.32
    obstruction T83.39
    perforation T83.39
    protrusion T83.39
    specified NEC T83.39
  pain T83.84
  specified type NEC T83.89
  stenosis T83.85
  thrombosis T83.86
  procedure (fetal) , to newborn P96.5
jejunostomy (stoma) —*see* Complications,
  enterostomy
joint prosthesis, internal T84.9
  breakage (fracture) T84.01
  dislocation T84.02
  fracture T84.01
  infection or inflammation T84.50
    hip T84.5
    knee T84.5
    specified joint NEC T84.59
  instability T84.02
  malposition —*see* Complications, joint
prosthesis, mechanical, displacement
  mechanical
    breakage, broken T84.01
    dislocation T84.02
    fracture T84.01
    instability T84.02
    leakage —*see* Complications, joint
  prosthesis, mechanical, specified NEC
    loosening T84.039
      hip T84.03
      knee T84.03
      specified joint NEC T84.038
    obstruction —*see* Complications, joint
  prosthesis, mechanical, specified NEC
    perforation —*see* Complications, joint
  prosthesis, mechanical, specified NEC
    periprosthetic
      fracture T84.049
        hip T84.04
        knee T84.04
        other specified joint T84.048
      osteolysis T84.059
        hip T84.05
        knee T84.05
        other specified joint T84.058
    protrusion —*see* Complications, joint
  prosthesis, mechanical, specified NEC
    specified complication NEC T84.099
      hip T84.09
      knee T84.09
      other specified joint T84.098
    subluxation T84.02
    wear of articular bearing surface T84.069
      hip T84.06
      knee T84.06
      other specified joint T84.068
  specified joint NEC T84.89
    embolism T84.81
    fibrosis T84.82
    hemorrhage T84.83
    pain T84.84
    specified complication NEC T84.89
    stenosis T84.85
    thrombosis T84.86

Complication - *continued*
  subluxation T84.02
  kidney transplant —*see* Complications, transplant, kidney
  labor O75.9
    specified NEC O75.89
  liver transplant (immune or nonimmune) — *see* Complications, transplant, liver
  lumbar puncture G97.1
    cerebrospinal fluid leak G97.0
    headache or reaction G97.1
  lung transplant —*see* Complications, transplant, lung
    and heart —*see* Complications, transplant, lung, with heart
  male genital N50.9
    device, implant or graft —*see* Complications, genitourinary, device or implant, genital tract
    postprocedural or postoperative —*see* Complications, genitourinary, postprocedural
      specified NEC N99.89
  mastoid (process) procedure
    intraoperative H95.88
      hematoma —*see* Complications, intraoperative, hemorrhage (hematoma) (of) , mastoid process
      hemorrhage —*see* Complications, intraoperative, hemorrhage (hematoma) (of) , mastoid process
      laceration —*see* Complications, intraoperative, puncture or laceration..., mastoid process
        specified NEC H95.88
    postmastoidectomy —*see* Complications, postmastoidectomy
    postoperative H95.89
      external ear canal stenosis H95.81
      hematoma —*see* Complications..., postprocedural, hemorrhage (hematoma) (of) , mastoid process
      hemorrhage —*see* Complications..., postprocedural, hemorrhage (hematoma) (of) , mastoid process
        postmastoidectomy —*see* Complications, postmastoidectomy
        specified NEC H95.89
  mastoidectomy cavity —*see* Complications, postmastoidectomy
  mechanical —*see* Complications, by site and type, mechanical
  medical procedures (*see also* Complication(s) , intraoperative) T88.9
  metabolic E88.9
    postoperative E89.89
      specified NEC E89.89
  molar pregnancy NOS O08.9
    damage to pelvic organs O08.6
    embolism O08.2
    genital infection O08.0
    hemorrhage (delayed) (excessive) O08.1
    metabolic disorder O08.5
    renal failure O08.4
    shock O08.3
    specified type NEC O08.0
    venous complication NEC O08.7
  musculoskeletal system —*see also* Complication, intraoperative (intraprocedural), by site
    device, implant or graft NEC —*see* Complications, orthopedic, device or implant
    internal fixation (nail) (plate) (rod) —*see* Complications, fixation device, internal

Complication - *continued*
  joint prosthesis —*see* Complications, joint prosthesis
    postoperative (postprocedural) M96.89
      with osteoporosis —*see* Osteoporosis
      fracture following insertion of device —*see* Fracture, following insertion of orthopedic implant, joint prosthesis or bone plate
      joint instability after prosthesis removal M96.89
      lordosis M96.4
      postlaminectomy syndrome NEC M96.1
        kyphosis M96.3
      pseudarthrosis M96.0
      specified complication NEC M96.89
    post radiation M96.89
      kyphosis M96.3
      scoliosis M96.5
      specified complication NEC M96.89
  nephrostomy (stoma) —*see* Complications, stoma, urinary tract, external NEC
  nervous system G98.8
    central G96.9
      device, implant or graft —*see also* Complication, prosthetic device or implant, specified NEC
        electronic stimulator (electrode(s)) —*see* Complications, electronic stimulator device
        ventricular shunt —*see* Complications, ventricular shunt
      electronic stimulator (electrode(s)) —*see* Complications, electronic stimulator device
      postprocedural G97.82
        intracranial hypotension G97.2
        specified NEC G97.82
        spinal fluid leak G97.0
  newborn, due to intrauterine (fetal) procedure P96.5
  nonabsorbable (permanent) sutures —*see* Complication, sutures, permanent
  obstetric O75.9
    procedure (instrumental) (manual) (surgical) specified NEC O75.4
      specified NEC O75.89
    surgical wound NEC O90.89
      hematoma O90.2
      infection O86.0
  ocular lens implant —*see* Complications, intraocular lens
  ophthalmologic
    postprocedural bleb —*see* Blebitis
  orbital prosthesis T85.9
    embolism T85.81
    fibrosis T85.82
    hemorrhage T85.83
    infection and inflammation T85.79
    mechanical
      breakdown T85.31
      displacement T85.32
      malposition T85.32
      obstruction T85.39
      perforation T85.39
      protrusion T85.39
      specified NEC T85.39
    pain T85.84
    specified type NEC T85.89
    stenosis T85.85
    thrombosis T85.86
  organ or tissue transplant (partial) (total) —*see* Complications, transplant
  orthopedic —*see also* Disorder, soft tissue
    device or implant T84.9

Complication - *continued*
  bone
    device or implant —*see* Complication, bone, device NEC
      graft —*see* Complication, graft, bone
    breakdown T84.418
    displacement T84.428
    electronic bone stimulator —*see* Complications, electronic stimulator device, bone
    embolism T84.81
    fibrosis T84.82
    fixation device —*see* Complication, fixation device, internal
    hemorrhage T84.83
    infection or inflammation T84.7
    joint prosthesis —*see* Complication, joint prosthesis, internal
    malfunction T84.418
    malposition T84.428
    mechanical NEC T84.498
    muscle graft —*see* Complications, graft, muscle
    obstruction T84.498
    pain T84.84
    perforation T84.498
    protrusion T84.498
    specified complication NEC T84.89
    stenosis T84.85
    tendon graft —*see* Complications, graft, tendon
    thrombosis T84.86
  fracture (following insertion of device) —*see* Fracture, following insertion of orthopedic implant, joint prosthesis or bone plate
    postprocedural M96.89
    fracture —*see* Fracture, following insertion of orthopedic implant, joint prosthesis or bone plate
    postlaminectomy syndrome NEC M96.1
      kyphosis M96.3
      lordosis M96.4
    postradiation
      kyphosis M96.2
      scoliosis M96.5
    pseudarthrosis post-fusion M96.0
    specified type NEC M96.89
  pacemaker (cardiac) —*see* Complications, cardiovascular device or implant, electronic
  pancreas transplant —*see* Complications, transplant, pancreas
  penile prosthesis (implant) —*see* Complications, prosthetic device, penile
  perfusion NEC T80.90
  perineal repair (obstetrical) NEC O90.89
    disruption O90.1
    hematoma O90.2
    infection (following delivery) O86.0
  phototherapy T88.9
    specified NEC T88.8
  postmastoidectomy NEC H95.19
    cyst, mucosal H95.13
    granulation H95.12
    inflammation, chronic H95.11
    recurrent cholesteatoma H95.0
  postoperative —*see* Complications, postprocedural
    circulatory —*see* Complications, circulatory system
    ear —*see* Complications, ear
    endocrine —*see* Complications, endocrine
    eye —*see* Complications, eye
    lumbar puncture G97.1

Complication - *continued*
  cerebrospinal fluid leak G97.0
  nervous system (central) (peripheral) —*see* Complications, nervous system
  respiratory system —*see* Complications, respiratory system
  postprocedural —*see also* Complications, surgical procedure
    cardiac arrest
      following cardiac surgery I97.120
      following other surgery I97.121
    cardiac functional disturbance NEC
      following cardiac surgery I97.190
      following other surgery I97.191
    cardiac insufficiency
      following cardiac surgery I97.110
      following other surgery I97.111
    chorioretinal scars following retinal surgery H59.81
    following cataract surgery
      cataract (lens) fragments H59.02
      cystoid macular edema H59.03
      specified NEC H59.09
      vitreous (touch) syndrome H59.01
    heart failure
      following cardiac surgery I97.130
      following other surgery I97.131
    hemorrhage (hematoma) (of)
      circulatory system organ or structure
        following a cardiac bypass I97.611
        following a cardiac catheterization I97.610
        following other circulatory system procedure I97.618
        following other procedure I97.62
      digestive system
        following procedure on digestive system K91.840
        following procedure on other organ K91.841
      ear
        following other procedure H95.42
        following procedure on ear and mastoid process H95.41
      endocrine system
        following endocrine system procedure E89.810
        following other procedure E89.811
      eye and adnexa
        following ophthalmic procedure H59.31
        following other procedure H59.32
      genitourinary organ or structure
        following procedure on genitourinary organ or structure N99.820
        following procedure on other organ N99.821
      mastoid process
        following other procedure H95.42
        following procedure on ear and mastoid process H95.41
      musculoskeletal structure
        following musculoskeletal surgery M96.830
        following non-orthopedic surgery M96.831
        following orthopedic surgery M96.830
      nervous system
        following a nervous system procedure G97.51
        following other procedure G97.52
      respiratory system

Complication - *continued*
      following other procedure J95.831
      following procedure on respiratory system organ or structure J95.830
      skin and subcutaneous tissue
        following a dermatologic procedure L76.21
        following a procedure on other organ L76.22
      spleen
        following procedure on other organ D78.22
        following procedure on the spleen D78.21
    specified NEC
      circulatory system I97.89
      digestive K91.89
      ear H95.89
      endocrine E89.89
      eye and adnexa H59.89
      genitourinary N99.89
      mastoid process H95.89
      metabolic E89.89
      musculoskeletal structure M96.89
      nervous system G97.82
      respiratory system J95.89
      skin and subcutaneous tissue L76.82
      spleen D78.89
  pregnancy NEC —*see* Pregnancy, complicated by
  prosthetic device or implant T85.9
    bile duct —*see* Complications, bile duct implant
    breast —*see* Complications, breast implant
    cardiac and vascular NEC —*see* Complications, cardiovascular device or implant
    corneal transplant —*see* Complications, graft, cornea
    electronic nervous system stimulator —*see* Complications, electronic stimulator device
    epidural infusion catheter —*see* Complications, catheter, epidural
    esophageal anti-reflux device —*see* Complications, esophageal anti-reflux device
    genital organ or tract —*see* Complications, genitourinary, device or implant, genital tract
    heart valve —*see* Complications, heart, valve, prosthesis
    infection or inflammation T85.79
      intestine transplant T86.892
      liver transplant T86.43
      lung transplant T86.812
      pancreas transplant T86.892
      skin graft T86.822
    intraocular lens —*see* Complications, intraocular lens
    intraperitoneal (dialysis) catheter —*see* Complications, catheter, intraperitoneal
    joint —*see* Complications, joint prosthesis, internal
    mechanical NEC T85.698
      dialysis catheter (vascular) —*see also* Complication, catheter, dialysis, mechanical
      peritoneal —*see* Complication, catheter, intraperitoneal, mechanical
      gastrointestinal device T85.598
      ocular device T85.398
      subdural (infusion) catheter T85.690
      suture, permanent T85.692
        that for bone repair —*see* Complications, fixation device, internal (orthopedic), mechanical

Complication - *continued*
    ventricular shunt
      breakdown T85.01
      displacement T85.02
      leakage T85.03
      malposition T85.02
      obstruction T85.09
      perforation T85.09
      protrusion T85.09
      specified NEC T85.09
    mesh
      erosion (to surrounding organ or tissue) T83.718
        vaginal (into pelvic floor muscles) T83.711
      exposure (into surrounding organ or tissue) T83.728
        vaginal (into vagina) (through vaginal wall) T83.721
    orbital —*see* Complications, orbital prosthesis
    penile T83.9
      embolism T83.81
      fibrosis T83.82
      hemorrhage T83.83
      infection and inflammation T83.6
      mechanical
        breakdown T83.410
        displacement T83.420
        leakage T83.490
        malposition T83.420
        obstruction T83.490
        perforation T83.490
        protrusion T83.490
        specified NEC T83.490
      pain T83.84
      specified type NEC T83.89
      stenosis T83.85
      thrombosis T83.86
    prosthetic materials NEC
      erosion (to surrounding organ or tissue) T83.718
        vaginal (into pelvic floor muscles) T83.711
      exposure (into surrounding organ or tissue) T83.728
        vaginal (into vagina) (through vaginal wall) T83.721
    skin graft T86.829
      artificial skin or decellularized allodermis
        embolism T85.81
        fibrosis T85.82
        hemorrhage T85.83
        infection and inflammation T85.79
        mechanical
          breakdown T85.613
          displacement T85.623
          malfunction T85.613
          malposition T85.623
          obstruction T85.693
          perforation T85.693
          protrusion T85.693
          specified NEC T85.693
        pain T85.84
        specified type NEC T85.89
        stenosis T85.85
        thrombosis T85.86
      failure T86.821
      infection T86.822
      rejection T86.820
      specified NEC T86.828
    specified NEC T85.9
      embolism T85.81

Complication - *continued*
  fibrosis T85.82
  hemorrhage T85.83
  infection and inflammation T85.79
  mechanical
    breakdown T85.618
    displacement T85.628
    leakage T85.638
    malfunction T85.618
    malposition T85.628
    obstruction T85.698
    perforation T85.698
    protrusion T85.698
    specified NEC T85.698
  pain T85.84
  specified type NEC T85.89
  stenosis T85.85
  thrombosis T85.86
  subdural infusion catheter —*see*
  Complications, catheter, subdural
    sutures —*see* Complications, sutures
    urinary organ or tract NEC —*see*
  Complications, genitourinary, device or
  implant, urinary system
    vascular —*see* Complications,
  cardiovascular device or implant
    ventricular shunt —*see* Complications,
  ventricular shunt (device)
  puerperium —*see* Puerperal
  puncture, spinal G97.1
    cerebrospinal fluid leak G97.0
    headache or reaction G97.1
  pyelogram N99.89
  radiation
    kyphosis M96.2
    scoliosis M96.5
  reattached
    extremity (infection) (rejection)
      lower T87.1X
      upper T87.0X
    specified body part NEC T87.2
  reconstructed breast
    asymmetry between native and
  reconstructed breast N65.1
    deformity N65.0
    disproportion between native and
  reconstructed breast N65.1
    excess tissue N65.0
    misshapen N65.0
  reimplant NEC —*see also* Complications,
  prosthetic device or implant
    limb (infection) (rejection) —*see*
  Complications, reattached, extremity
    organ (partial) (total) —*see* Complications,
  transplant
    prosthetic device NEC —*see* Complications,
  prosthetic device
  renal N28.9
    allograft —*see* Complications, transplant,
  kidney
    dialysis —*see* Complications, dialysis
  respirator
    mechanical J95.850
    specified NEC J95.859
  respiratory system J98.9
    device, implant or graft —*see* Complication,
  prosthetic device or implant, specified NEC
    lung transplant —*see* Complications,
  prosthetic device or implant, lung transplant
    postoperative J95.89
      air leak J95.812

Complication - *continued*
    Mendelson's syndrome (chemical
  pneumonitis) J95.4
      pneumothorax J95.811
      pulmonary insufficiency (acute) (after
  nonthoracic surgery) J95.2
        chronic J95.3
          following thoracic surgery J95.1
      respiratory failure (acute) J95.821
        acute and chronic J95.822
      specified NEC J95.89
      subglottic stenosis J95.5
      trachcostomy complication —*see*
  Complications, tracheostomy
    therapy T81.89
  sedation during labor and delivery O74.9
    cardiac O74.2
    central nervous system O74.3
    pulmonary NEC O74.1
  shunt —*see also* Complications, prosthetic
  device or implant
    arteriovenous —*see* Complications,
  arteriovenous, shunt
    ventricular (communicating) —*see*
  Complications, ventricular shunt
  skin
    graft T86.829
      failure T86.821
      infection T86.822
      rejection T86.820
      specified type NEC T86.828
  spinal
    anesthesia —*see* Complications, anesthesia,
  spinal
    catheter (epidural) (subdural) —*see*
  Complications, catheter
    puncture or tap G97.1
      cerebrospinal fluid leak G97.0
      headache or reaction G97.1
  stent
    bile duct —*see* Complications, bile duct
  prosthesis
    urinary T83.9
      embolism T83.81
      fibrosis T83.82
      hemorrhage T83.83
      infection and inflammation T83.59
      mechanical
        breakdown T83.112
        displacement T83.122
        leakage T83.192
        malposition T83.122
        obstruction T83.192
        perforation T83.192
        protrusion T83.192
        specified NEC T83.192
      pain T83.84
      specified type NEC T83.89
      stenosis T83.85
      thrombosis T83.86
  stoma
    digestive tract
      colostomy —*see* Complications, colostomy
      enterostomy —*see* Complications,
  enterostomy
      esophagostomy —*see* Complications,
  esophagostomy
      gastrostomy —*see* Complications,
  gastrostomy
    urinary tract N99.538
      cystostomy —*see* Complications,
  cystostomy

Complication - *continued*
    external NOS N99.528
      hemorrhage N99.520
      infection N99.521
      malfunction N99.522
      specified type NEC N99.528
    hemorrhage N99.530
    infection N99.531
    malfunction N99.532
    specified type NEC N99.538
  stomach banding —*see* Complication(s) ,
  bariatric procedure
  stomach stapling —*see* Complication(s) ,
  bariatric procedure
  surgical material, nonabsorbable —*see*
  Complication, suture, permanent
  surgical procedure (on) T81.9
    amputation stump (late) —*see*
  Complications, amputation stump
    cardiac —*see* Complications, circulatory
  system
    cholesteatoma, recurrent —*see*
  Complications, postmastoidectomy, recurrent
  cholesteatoma
    circulatory (early) —*see* Complications,
  circulatory system
    digestive system —*see* Complications,
  gastrointestinal
    dumping syndrome (postgastrectomy) K91.1
    ear —*see* Complications, ear
    elephantiasis or lymphedema I97.89
      postmastectomy I97.2
    emphysema (surgical) T81.82
    endocrine —*see* Complications, endocrine
    eye —*see* Complications, eye
    fistula (persistent postoperative) T81.83
    foreign body inadvertently left in wound
  (sponge) (suture) (swab) —*see* Foreign body,
  accidentally left during a procedure
    gastrointestinal —*see* Complications,
  gastrointestinal
    genitourinary NEC N99.89
    hematoma
      intraoperative —*see* Complication,
  intraoperative, hemorrhage
      postprocedural —*see* Complication,
  postprocedural, hemorrhage
    hemorrhage
      intraoperative —*see* Complication,
  intraoperative, hemorrhage
      postprocedural —*see* Complication,
  postprocedural, hemorrhage
    hepatic failure K91.82
    hyperglycemia (postpancreatectomy) E89.1
    hypoinsulinemia (postpancreatectomy)
  E89.1
    hypoparathyroidism
  (postparathyroidectomy) E89.2
    hypopituitarism (posthypophysectomy)
  E89.3
    hypothyroidism (post-thyroidectomy) E89.0
    intestinal obstruction K91.3
    intracranial hypotension following
  ventricular shunting (ventriculostomy) G97.2
    lymphedema I97.89
      postmastectomy I97.2
    malabsorption (postsurgical) NEC K91.2
    osteoporosis —*see* Osteoporosis,
  postsurgical malabsorption
    mastoidectomy cavity NEC —*see*
  Complications, postmastoidectomy
    metabolic E89.89
      specified NEC E89.89

Complication *- continued*
  musculoskeletal —*see* Complications, musculoskeletal system
  nervous system (central) (peripheral) —*see* Complications, nervous system
  ovarian failure E89.40
    asymptomatic E89.40
    symptomatic E89.41
  peripheral vascular —*see* Complications, surgical procedure, vascular
  postcardiotomy syndrome I97.0
  postcholecystectomy syndrome K91.5
  postcommissurotomy syndrome I97.0
  postgastrectomy dumping syndrome K91.1
  postlaminectomy syndrome NEC M96.1
    kyphosis M96.3
  postmastectomy lymphedema syndrome I97.2
  postmastoidectomy cholesteatoma —*see* Complications, postmastoidectomy, recurrent cholesteatoma
  postvagotomy syndrome K91.1
  postvalvulotomy syndrome I97.0
  pulmonary insufficiency (acute) J95.2
    chronic J95.3
    following thoracic surgery J95.1
  reattached body part —*see* Complications, reattached
  respiratory —*see* Complications, respiratory system
    shock (hypovolemic) T81.19
    spleen (postoperative) D78.89
      intraoperative D78.81
    stitch abscess T81.4
    subglottic stenosis (postsurgical) J95.5
    testicular hypofunction E89.5
  transplant —*see* Complications, organ or tissue transplant
    urinary NEC N99.89
    vaginal vault prolapse (posthysterectomy) N99.3
    vascular (peripheral)
      artery T81.719
        mesenteric T81.710
        renal T81.711
        specified NEC T81.718
      vein T81.72
    wound infection T81.4
  suture, permanent (wire) NEC T85.9
  with repair of bone —*see* Complications, fixation device, internal
    embolism T85.81
    fibrosis T85.82
    hemorrhage T85.83
    infection and inflammation T85.79
    mechanical
      breakdown T85.612
      displacement T85.622
      malfunction T85.612
      malposition T85.622
      obstruction T85.692
      perforation T85.692
      protrusion T85.692
      specified NEC T85.692
    pain T85.84
    specified type NEC T85.89
    stenosis T85.85
    thrombosis T85.86
  tracheostomy J95.00
    granuloma J95.09
    hemorrhage J95.01
    infection J95.02

Complication *- continued*
    malfunction J95.03
    mechanical J95.03
    obstruction J95.03
    specified type NEC J95.09
    tracheo-esophageal fistula J95.04
  transfusion (blood) (lymphocytes) (plasma) T80.92
    air embolism T80.0
    circulatory overload E87.71
    febrile nonhemolytic transfusion reaction R50.84
    hemolysis T80.89
    hemochromatosis E83.111
    hemolytic reaction (antigen unspecified) T80.919
    incompatibility reaction (antigen unspecified) T80.919
      ABO T80.30
        delayed serologic (DSTR) T80.39
        hemolytic transfusion reaction (HTR) (unspecified time after transfusion) T80.319
          acute (AHTR) (less than 24 hours after transfusion) T80.310
          delayed (DHTR) (24 hours or more after transfusion) T80.311
        specified NEC T80.39
      acute (antigen unspecified) T80.910
      delayed (antigen unspecified) T80.911
      delayed serologic (DSTR) T80.89
      Non-ABO (minor antigens (Duffy) (Kell) (Kidd) (Lewis) (M) (N) (P) (S)) T80.A0
        delayed serologic (DSTR) T80.A9
        hemolytic transfusion reaction (HTR) (unspecified time after transfusion) T80.A19
          acute (AHTR) (less than 24 hours after transfusion) T80.A10
          delayed (DHTR) (24 hours or more after transfusion) T80.A11
        specified NEC T80.A9
      Rh (antigens (C) (c) (D) (E) (e)) (factor) T80.40
        delayed serologic (DSTR) T80.49
        hemolytic transfusion reaction (HTR) (unspecified time after transfusion) T80.419
          acute (AHTR) (less than 24 hours after transfusion) T80.410
          delayed (DHTR) (24 hours or more after transfusion) T80.411
        specified NEC T80.49
    infection T80.29
      acute T80.22
    reaction NEC T80.89
    sepsis T80.29
    shock T80.89
  transplant T86.90
    bone T86.839
      failure T86.831
      infection T86.832
      rejection T86.830
      specified type NEC T86.838
    bone marrow T86.00
      failure T86.02
      infection T86.03
      rejection T86.01
      specified type NEC T86.09
    cornea T86.849
      failure T86.841
      infection T86.842
      rejection T86.840
      specified type NEC T86.848
    failure T86.92

Complication *- continued*
    heart T86.20
      with lung T86.30
      cardiac allograft vasculopathy T86.290
        failure T86.32
        infection T86.33
        rejection T86.31
        specified type NEC T86.39
      failure T86.22
      infection T86.23
      rejection T86.21
      specified type NEC T86.298
    infection T86.93
    intestine T86.859
      failure T86.851
      infection T86.852
      rejection T86.850
      specified type NEC T86.858
    kidney T86.10
      failure T86.12
      infection T86.13
      rejection T86.11
      specified type NEC T86.19
    liver T86.40
      failure T86.42
      infection T86.43
      rejection T86.41
      specified type NEC T86.49
    lung T86.819
      with heart T86.30
        failure T86.32
        infection T86.33
        rejection T86.31
        specified type NEC T86.39
      failure T86.811
      infection T86.812
      rejection T86.810
      specified type NEC T86.818
    malignant neoplasm C80.2
    pancreas T86.899
      failure T86.891
      infection T86.892
      rejection T86.890
      specified type NEC T86.898
    peripheral blood stem cells T86.5
    post-transplant lymphoproliferative disorder (PTLD) D47.Z1
    rejection T86.91
    skin T86.829
      failure T86.821
      infection T86.822
      rejection T86.820
      specified type NEC T86.828
    specified
      tissue T86.899
        failure T86.891
        infection T86.892
        rejection T86.890
        specified type NEC T86.898
      type NEC T86.99
    stem cell (from peripheral blood) (from umbilical cord) T86.5
    umbilical cord stem cells T86.5
  trauma (early) T79.9
    specified NEC T79.8
  ultrasound therapy NEC T88.9
  umbilical cord NEC
    complicating delivery O69.9
      specified NEC O69.89
  umbrella device, vascular T82.9
    embolism T82.818
    fibrosis T82.828
    hemorrhage T82.838

Complication - *continued*
  infection or inflammation T82.7
  mechanical
    breakdown T82.515
    displacement T82.525
    leakage T82.535
    malposition T82.525
    obstruction T82.595
    perforation T82.595
    protrusion T82.595
  pain T82.848
  specified type NEC T82.898
  stenosis T82.858
  thrombosis T82.868
  urethral catheter —*see* Complications, catheter, urethral, indwelling
  vaccination T88.1
    anaphylaxis NEC T80.52
    arthropathy —*see* Arthropathy, postimmunization
    cellulitis T88.0
    encephalitis or encephalomyelitis G04.02
    infection (general) (local) NEC T88.0
    meningitis G03.8
    myelitis G04.89
    protein sickness T80.62
    rash T88.1
    reaction (allergic) T88.1
      serum T80.62
    sepsis T88.0
    serum intoxication, sickness, rash, or other serum reaction NEC T80.62
      anaphylactic shock T80.52
    shock (allergic) (anaphylactic) T80.52
    vaccinia (generalized) (localized) T88.1
  vas deferens device or implant —*see* Complications, genitourinary, device or implant, genital tract
  vascular I99.9
    device or implant T82.9
      embolism T82.818
      fibrosis T82.828
      hemorrhage T82.838
      infection or inflammation T82.7
      mechanical
        breakdown T82.519
          specified device NEC T82.518
        displacement T82.529
          specified device NEC T82.528
        leakage T82.539
          specified device NEC T82.538
        malposition T82.529
          specified device NEC T82.528
        obstruction T82.599
          specified device NEC T82.598
        perforation T82.599
          specified device NEC T82.598
        protrusion T82.599
          specified device NEC T82.598
      pain T82.848
      specified type NEC T82.898
      stenosis T82.858
      thrombosis T82.868
    dialysis catheter —*see* Complication, catheter, dialysis
    following infusion, therapeutic injection or transfusion T80.1
    graft T82.9
      embolism T82.818
      fibrosis T82.828
      hemorrhage T82.838
      mechanical

Complication - *continued*
    breakdown T82.319
      aorta (bifurcation) T82.310
      carotid artery T82.311
      specified vessel NEC T82.318
    displacement T82.329
      aorta (bifurcation) T82.320
      carotid artery T82.321
      specified vessel NEC T82.328
    leakage T82.339
      aorta (bifurcation) T82.330
      carotid artery T82.331
      specified vessel NEC T82.338
    malposition T82.329
      aorta (bifurcation) T82.320
      carotid artery T82.321
      specified vessel NEC T82.328
    obstruction T82.399
      aorta (bifurcation) T82.390
      carotid artery T82.391
      specified vessel NEC T82.398
    perforation T82.399
      aorta (bifurcation) T82.390
      carotid artery T82.391
      specified vessel NEC T82.398
    protrusion T82.399
      aorta (bifurcation) T82.390
      carotid artery T82.391
      specified vessel NEC T82.398
    pain T82.848
    specified complication NEC T82.898
    stenosis T82.858
    thrombosis T82.868
  postoperative —*see* Complications, postoperative, circulatory
  vena cava device (filter) (sieve) (umbrella) —*see* Complications, umbrella device, vascular
  ventilation therapy NEC T81.81
  ventilator
    mechanical J95.850
      specified NEC J95.859
  ventricular (communicating) shunt (device) T85.9
    embolism T85.81
    fibrosis T85.82
    hemorrhage T85.83
    infection and inflammation T85.79
    mechanical
      breakdown T85.01
      displacement T85.02
      leakage T85.03
      malposition T85.02
      obstruction T85.09
      perforation T85.09
      protrusion T85.09
      specified NEC T85.09
    pain T85.84
    specified type NEC T85.89
    stenosis T85.85
    thrombosis T85.86
  wire suture, permanent (implanted) —*see* Complications, suture, permanent

Compressed air disease T70.3
Compression
  with injury
  code by Nature of injury
  artery I77.1
    celiac, syndrome I77.4
  brachial plexus G54.0

Compression - *continued*
  brain (stem) G93.5
    due to
      contusion (diffuse) —*see* Injury, intracranial, diffuse
        focal —*see* Injury, intracranial, focal
      injury NEC —*see* Injury, intracranial, diffuse
      traumatic —*see* Injury, intracranial, diffuse
  bronchus J98.09
  cauda equina G83.4
  celiac (artery) (axis) I77.4
  cerebral —*see* Compression, brain
  cervical plexus G54.2
  cord
    spinal —*see* Compression, spinal
    umbilical —*see* Compression, umbilical cord
  cranial nerve G52.9
    eighth —see subcategory H93.3
    eleventh G52.8
    fifth G50.8
    first G52.0
    fourth —*see* Strabismus, paralytic, fourth nerve
    ninth G52.1
    second —*see* Disorder, nerve, optic
    seventh G52.8
    sixth —*see* Strabismus, paralytic, sixth nerve
    tenth G52.2
    third —*see* Strabismus, paralytic, third nerve
    twelfth G52.3
  diver's squeeze T70.3
  during birth (newborn) P15.9
  esophagus K22.2
  eustachian tube —*see* Obstruction, eustachian tube, cartilaginous
  facies Q67.1
  fracture —*see* Fracture
  heart —*see* Disease, heart
  intestine —*see* Obstruction, intestine
  laryngeal nerve, recurrent G52.2
    with paralysis of vocal cords and larynx J38.00
      bilateral J38.02
      unilateral J38.01
  lumbosacral plexus G54.1
  lung J98.4
  lymphatic vessel I89.0
  medulla —*see* Compression, brain
  nerve (*see also* Disorder, nerve) G58.9
    arm NEC —*see* Mononeuropathy, upper limb
    axillary G54.0
    cranial —*see* Compression, cranial nerve
    leg NEC —*see* Mononeuropathy, lower limb
    median (in carpal tunnel) —*see* Syndrome, carpal tunnel
    optic —*see* Disorder, nerve, optic
    plantar —*see* Lesion, nerve, plantar
    posterior tibial (in tarsal tunnel) —*see* Syndrome, tarsal tunnel
    root or plexus NOS (in) G54.9
      intervertebral disc disorder NEC —*see* Disorder, disc, with, radiculopathy
      with myelopathy —*see* Disorder, disc, with, myelopathy
      neoplastic disease (*see also* Neoplasm) D49.9 *[G55]*
      spondylosis —*see* Spondylosis, with radiculopathy
      sciatic (acute) —*see* Lesion, nerve, sciatic

Compression - *continued*
  sympathetic G90.8
  traumatic —*see* Injury, nerve
  ulnar —*see* Lesion, nerve, ulnar
  upper extremity NEC —*see*
  Mononeuropathy, upper limb
  spinal (cord) G95.20
    by displacement of intervertebral disc NEC
    —*see also* Disorder, disc, with, myelopathy
    nerve root NOS G54.9
      due to displacement of intervertebral disc
  NEC —*see* Disorder, disc, with,
  radiculopathy
     with myelopathy —*see* Disorder, disc,
  with, myelopathy
    specified NEC G95.29
    spondylogenic (cervical) (lumbar,
  lumbosacral) (thoracic) —*see* Spondylosis,
  with myelopathy NEC
     anterior —*see* Syndrome, anterior, spinal
  artery, compression
     traumatic —*see* Injury, spinal cord, by
  region
  subcostal nerve (syndrome) —*see*
  Mononeuropathy, upper limb, specified NEC
  sympathetic nerve NEC G90.8
  syndrome T79.5
  trachea J39.8
  ulnar nerve (by scar tissue) —*see* Lesion,
  nerve, ulnar
  umbilical cord
    complicating delivery O69.2
      cord around neck O69.1
      prolapse O69.0
      specified NEC O69.2
  ureter N13.5
  vein I87.1
  vena cava (inferior) (superior) I87.1
Compulsion, compulsive
  gambling F63.0
  neurosis F42
  personality F60.5
  states F42
  swearing F42
    in Gilles de la Tourette's syndrome F95.2
  tics and spasms F95.9
Concato's disease (pericardial polyserositis)
  A19.9
  nontubercular I31.1
  pleural —*see* Pleurisy, with effusion
Concavity chest wall M95.4
Concealed penis Q55.69
Concern (normal) **about sick person in
family** Z63.6
Concrescence (teeth) K00.2
Concretio cordis I31.1
  rheumatic I09.2
Concretion —*see also* Calculus
  appendicular K38.1
  canaliculus —*see* Dacryolith
  clitoris N90.89
  conjunctiva H11.12
  eyelid —*see* Disorder, eyelid, specified type
  NEC
  lacrimal passages —*see* Dacryolith
  prepuce (male) N47.8
  salivary gland (any) K11.5
  seminal vesicle N50.8
  tonsil J35.8

Concussion (brain) (cerebral) (current) S06.0X
  blast (air) (hydraulic) (immersion)
  (underwater)
    abdomen or thorax —*see* Injury, blast, by
  site
    ear with acoustic nerve injury —*see* Injury,
  nerve, acoustic, specified type NEC
  cauda equina S34.3
  conus medullaris S34.02
  ocular S05.8X
  spinal (cord)
    cervical S14.0
    lumbar S34.01
    sacral S34.02
    thoracic S24.0
  syndrome F07.81
Condition —*see* Disease
Conditions arising in the perinatal period —
  see Newborn, affected by
Conduct disorder —*see* Disorder, conduct
Condyloma A63.0
  acuminatum A63.0
  gonorrheal A54.09
  latum A51.31
  syphilitic A51.31
    congenital A50.07
  venereal, syphilitic A51.31
Conflagration —*see also* Burn
  asphyxia (by inhalation of gases, fumes or
  vapors) (*see also* Table of Drugs and
  Chemicals) T59.9
Conflict (with) —*see also* Discord
  family Z73.9
  marital Z63.0
    involving divorce or estrangement Z63.5
  parent-child Z62.820
    parent-adopted child Z62.821
    parent-biological child Z62.820
    parent-foster child Z62.822
  social role NEC Z73.5
Confluent —*see* condition
Confusion, confused R41.0
  epileptic F05
  mental state (psychogenic) F44.89
  psychogenic F44.89
  reactive (from emotional stress, psychological
  trauma) F44.89
Confusional arousals G47.51
Congelation T69.9
Congenital —*see also* condition
  aortic septum Q25.4
  intrinsic factor deficiency D51.0
  malformation —*see* Anomaly
Congestion, congestive
  bladder N32.89
  bowel K63.89
  brain G93.89
  breast N64.59
  bronchial J98.09
  catarrhal J31.0
  chest R09.89
  chill, malarial —*see* Malaria
  circulatory NEC I99.8
  duodenum K31.89
  eye —*see* Hyperemia, conjunctiva
  facial, due to birth injury P15.4
  general R68.89
  glottis J37.0
  heart —*see* Failure, heart, congestive
  hepatic K76.1
  hypostatic (lung) —*see* Edema, lung
  intestine K63.89

Congestion, congestive - *continued*
  kidney N28.89
  labyrinth —*see* subcategory H83.8
  larynx J37.0
  liver K76.1
  lung R09.89
    active or acute —*see* Pneumonia
  malaria, malarial —*see* Malaria
  nasal R09.81
  nose R09.81
  orbit, orbital —*see also* Exophthalmos
    inflammatory (chronic) —*see* Inflammation,
  orbit
  ovary N83.8
  pancreas K86.8
  pelvic, female N94.89
  pleural J94.8
  prostate (active) N42.1
  pulmonary —*see* Congestion, lung
  renal N28.89
  retina H35.81
  seminal vesicle N50.1
  spinal cord G95.19
  spleen (chronic) D73.2
  stomach K31.89
  trachea —*see* Tracheitis
  urethra N36.8
  uterus N85.8
    with subinvolution N85.3
  venous (passive) I87.8
  viscera R68.89
Congestive —*see* Congestion
Conical
  cervix (hypertrophic elongation) N88.4
  cornea —*see* Keratoconus
  teeth K00.2
Conjoined twins Q89.4
Conjugal maladjustment Z63.0
  involving divorce or estrangement Z63.5
Conjunctiva —*see* condition
Conjunctivitis (staphylococcal) (streptococcal)
  NOS H10.9
  Acanthamoeba B60.12
  acute H10.3
    atopic H10.1
    mucopurulent H10.02
     follicular H10.01
    chemical (*see also* Corrosion, cornea)
  H10.21
    pseudomembranous H10.22
    serous except viral H10.23
    viral —*see* Conjunctivitis, viral
    toxic H10.21
  adenoviral (acute) (follicular) B30.1
  allergic (acute) —*see* Conjunctivitis, acute,
  atopic
    chronic H10.45
     vernal H10.44
  anaphylactic —*see* Conjunctivitis, acute,
  atopic
  Apollo B30.3
  atopic (acute) —*see* Conjunctivitis, acute,
  atopic
  Béal's B30.2
  blennorrhagic (gonococcal) (neonatorum)
  A54.31
  chemical (acute) (*see also* Corrosion, cornea)
  H10.21
  chlamydial A74.0
    due to trachoma A71.1
    neonatal P39.1
  chronic (nodosa) (petrificans) (phlyctenular)
  H10.40

Conjunctivitis - *continued*
  allergic H10.45
    vernal H10.44
  follicular H10.43
  giant papillary H10.41
  simple H10.42
  vernal H10.44
  coxsackievirus 24 B30.3
  diphtheritic A36.86
  due to
    dust —*see* Conjunctivitis, acute, atopic
    filariasis B74.9
    mucocutaneous leishmaniasis B55.2
  enterovirus type 70 (hemorrhagic) B30.3
  epidemic (viral) B30.9
    hemorrhagic B30.3
  gonococcal (neonatorum) A54.31
  granular (trachomatous) A71.1
    sequelae (late effect) B94.0
  hemorrhagic (acute) (epidemic) B30.3
  herpes zoster B02.31
  in (due to)
    Acanthamoeba B60.12
    adenovirus (acute) (follicular) B30.1
    Chlamydia A74.0
    coxsackievirus 24 B30.3
    diphtheria A36.86
    enterovirus type 70 (hemorrhagic) B30.3
    filariasis B74.9
    gonococci A54.31
    herpes (simplex) virus B00.53
      zoster B02.31
    infectious disease NEC B99
    meningococci A39.89
    mucocutaneous leishmaniasis B55.2
    rosacea L71.9
    syphilis (late) A52.71
    zoster B02.31
  inclusion A74.0
  infantile P39.1
    gonococcal A54.31
  Koch-Weeks' —*see* Conjunctivitis, acute, mucopurulent
  light —*see* Conjunctivitis, acute, atopic
  ligneous —*see* Blepharoconjunctivitis, ligneous
  meningococcal A39.89
  mucopurulent —*see* Conjunctivitis, acute, mucopurulent
  neonatal P39.1
    gonococcal A54.31
  Newcastle B30.8
  of Béal B30.2
  parasitic
    filariasis B74.9
    mucocutaneous leishmaniasis B55.2
  Parinaud's H10.89
  petrificans H10.89
  rosacea L71.9
  specified NEC H10.89
  swimming-pool B30.1
  trachomatous A71.1
    acute A71.0
    sequelae (late effect) B94.0
  traumatic NEC H10.89
  tuberculous A18.59
  tularemic A21.1
  tularensis A21.1
  viral B30.9
    due to
      adenovirus B30.1
      enterovirus B30.3
    specified NEC B30.8

Conjunctivochalasis H11.82
Connective tissue —*see* condition
Conn's syndrome E26.01
Conradi (-Hunermann) **disease** Q77.3
Consanguinity Z84.3
  counseling Z71.89
Conscious simulation (of illness) Z76.5
Consecutive —*see* condition
Consolidation lung (base) —*see* Pneumonia, lobar
Constipation (atonic) (neurogenic) (simple) (spastic) K59.00
  drug-induced —*see* Table of Drugs and Chemicals
  outlet dysfunction K59.02
  psychogenic F45.8
  slow transit K59.01
  specified NEC K59.09
Constitutional —*see also* condition
  substandard F60.7
Constitutionally substandard F60.7
Constriction —*see also* Stricture
  auditory canal —*see* Stenosis, external ear canal
  bronchial J98.09
  duodenum K31.5
  esophagus K22.2
  external
    abdomen, abdominal (wall) S30.841
    alveolar process S00.542
    ankle S90.54
    antecubital space —*see* Constriction, external, forearm
    arm (upper) S40.84
    auricle —*see* Constriction, external, ear
    axilla —*see* Constriction, external, arm
    back, lower S30.840
    breast S20.14
    brow S00.84
    buttock S30.840
    calf —*see* Constriction, external, leg
    canthus —*see* Constriction, external, eyelid
    cheek S00.84
      internal S00.542
    chest wall —*see* Constriction, external, thorax
    chin S00.84
    clitoris S30.844
    costal region —*see* Constriction, external, thorax
    digit (s)
      foot —*see* Constriction, external, toe
      hand —*see* Constriction, external, finger
    ear S00.44
    elbow S50.34
    epididymis S30.843
    epigastric region S30.841
    esophagus, cervical S10.14
    eyebrow —*see* Constriction, external, eyelid
    eyelid S00.24
    face S00.84
    finger (s) S60.44
      index S60.44
      little S60.44
      middle S60.44
      ring S60.44
    flank S30.841
    foot (except toe(s) alone) S90.84
      toe —*see* Constriction, external, toe
    forearm S50.84
      elbow only —*see* Constriction, external, elbow

Constriction - *continued*
    forehead S00.84
    genital organs, external
      female S30.846
      male S30.845
    groin S30.841
    gum S00.542
    hand S60.54
    head S00.94
      ear —*see* Constriction, external, ear
      eyelid —*see* Constriction, external, eyelid
      lip S00.541
      nose S00.34
      oral cavity S00.542
      scalp S00.04
      specified site NEC S00.84
    heel —*see* Constriction, external, foot
    hip S70.24
    inguinal region S30.841
    interscapular region S20.449
    jaw S00.84
    knee S80.24
    labium (majus) (minus) S30.844
    larynx S10.14
    leg (lower) S80.84
      knee —*see* Constriction, external, knee
      upper —*see* Constriction, external, thigh
    lip S00.541
    lower back S30.840
    lumbar region S30.840
    malar region S00.84
    mammary —*see* Constriction, external, breast
    mastoid region S00.84
    mouth S00.542
    nail
      finger —*see* Constriction, external, finger
      toe —*see* Constriction, external, toe
    nasal S00.34
    neck S10.94
      specified site NEC S10.84
      throat S10.14
    nose S00.34
    occipital region S00.04
    oral cavity S00.542
    orbital region —*see* Constriction, external, eyelid
    palate S00.542
    palm —*see* Constriction, external, hand
    parietal region S00.04
    pelvis S30.840
    penis S30.842
    perineum
      female S30.844
      male S30.840
    periocular area —*see* Constriction, external, eyelid
    phalanges
      finger —*see* Constriction, external, finger
      toe —*see* Constriction, external, toe
    pharynx S10.14
    pinna —*see* Constriction, external, ear
    popliteal space —*see* Constriction, external, knee
    prepuce S30.842
    pubic region S30.840
    pudendum
      female S30.846
      male S30.845
    sacral region S30.840
    scalp S00.04
    scapular region —*see* Constriction, external, shoulder

Constriction - *continued*
  scrotum S30.843
  shin —*see* Constriction, external, leg
  shoulder S40.24
  sternal region S20.349
  submaxillary region S00.84
  submental region S00.84
  subungual
    finger (s) —*see* Constriction, external, finger
    toe (s) —*see* Constriction, external, toe
  supraclavicular fossa S10.84
  supraorbital S00.84
  temple S00.84
  temporal region S00.84
  testis S30.843
  thigh S70.34
  thorax, thoracic (wall) S20.94
    back S20.44
    front S20.34
  throat S10.14
  thumb S60.34
  toe (s) (lesser) S90.44
    great S90.44
  tongue S00.542
  trachea S10.14
  tunica vaginalis S30.843
  uvula S00.542
  vagina S30.844
  vulva S30.844
  wrist S60.84
  gallbladder —*see* Obstruction, gallbladder
  intestine —*see* Obstruction, intestine
  larynx J38.6
    congenital Q31.8
      specified NEC Q31.8
      subglottic Q31.1
  organ or site, congenital NEC —*see* Atresia, by site
  prepuce (acquired) (congenital) N47.1
  pylorus (adult hypertrophic) K31.1
    congenital or infantile Q40.0
    newborn Q40.0
  ring dystocia (uterus) O62.4
  spastic —*see also* Spasm
    ureter N13.5
  ureter N13.5
    with infection N13.6
  urethra —*see* Stricture, urethra
  visual field (peripheral) (functional) —*see* Defect, visual field
Constrictive —*see* condition
Consultation
  medical —*see* Counseling, medical
  religious Z71.81
  specified reason NEC Z71.89
  spiritual Z71.81
  without complaint or sickness Z71.9
    feared complaint unfounded Z71.1
    specified reason NEC Z71.89
Consumption —*see* Tuberculosis
Contact (with) —*see also* Exposure (to)
  acariasis Z20.7
  AIDS virus Z20.6
  air pollution Z77.110
  algae and algae toxins Z77.121
  algae bloom Z77.121
  anthrax Z20.810
  aromatic amines Z77.020
  aromatic (hazardous) compounds NEC Z77.028
  aromatic dyes NOS Z77.028

Contact (with) – *continued*
  arsenic Z77.010
  asbestos Z77.090
  bacterial disease NEC Z20.818
  benzene Z77.021
  blue-green algae bloom Z77.121
  body fluids (potentially hazardous) Z77.21
  brown tide Z77.121
  chemicals (chiefly nonmedicinal) (hazardous) NEC Z77.098
  cholera Z20.09
  chromium compounds Z77.018
  communicable disease Z20.9
    bacterial NEC Z20.818
    specified NEC Z20.89
    viral NEC Z20.828
  cyanobacteria bloom Z77.121
  dyes Z77.098
  Escherichia coli (E. coli) Z20.01
  fiberglass —*see* Table of Drugs and Chemicals, fiberglass
  German measles Z20.4
  gonorrhea Z20.2
  hazardous metals NEC Z77.018
  hazardous substances NEC Z77.29
  hazards in the physical environment NEC Z77.128
  hazards to health NEC Z77.9
  HIV Z20.6
  HTLV-III/LAV Z20.6
  human immunodeficiency virus (HIV) Z20.6
  infection Z20.9
    specified NEC Z20.89
  infestation (parasitic) NEC Z20.7
  intestinal infectious disease NEC Z20.09
    Escherichia coli (E. coli) Z20.01
  lead Z77.011
  meningococcus Z20.811
  mold (toxic) Z77.120
  nickel dust Z77.018
  noise Z77.122
  parasitic disease Z20.7
  pediculosis Z20.7
  pfiesteria piscicida Z77.121
  poliomyelitis Z20.89
  pollution
    air Z77.110
    environmental NEC Z77.118
    soil Z77.112
    water Z77.111
  polycyclic aromatic hydrocarbons Z77.028
  rabies Z20.3
  radiation, naturally occurring NEC Z77.123
  radon Z77.123
  red tide (Florida) Z77.121
  rubella Z20.4
  sexually-transmitted disease Z20.2
  smallpox (laboratory) Z20.89
  syphilis Z20.2
  tuberculosis Z20.1
  uranium Z77.012
  varicella Z20.820
  venereal disease Z20.2
  viral disease NEC Z20.828
  viral hepatitis Z20.5
  water pollution Z77.111
Contamination, food —*see* Intoxication, foodborne
Contraception, contraceptive
  advice Z30.09
  counseling Z30.09

Contraception, contraceptive - *continued*
  device (intrauterine) (in situ) Z97.5
    causing menorrhagia T83.83
    checking Z30.431
    complications —*see* Complications, intrauterine, contraceptive device
    in place Z97.5
    initial prescription Z30.014
    reinsertion Z30.433
    removal Z30.432
    replacement Z30.433
  emergency (postcoital) Z30.012
  initial prescription Z30.019
    injectable Z30.013
    intrauterine device Z30.014
    pills Z30.011
    postcoital (emergency) Z30.012
    specified type NEC Z30.018
    subdermal implantable Z30.019
  maintenance Z30.40
    examination Z30.8
    injectable Z30.42
    intrauterine device Z30.431
    pills Z30.41
    specified type NEC Z30.49
    subdermal implantable Z30.49
  management Z30.9
    specified NEC Z30.8
  postcoital (emergency) Z30.012
  prescription Z30.019
    repeat Z30.40
  sterilization Z30.2
  surveillance (drug) —*see* Contraception, maintenance
Contraction (s) , contracture, contracted
  Achilles tendon —*see also* Short, tendon, Achilles
    congenital Q66.89
  amputation stump (surgical) (flexion) (late) (next proximal joint) T87.89
  anus K59.8
  bile duct (common) (hepatic) K83.8
  bladder N32.89
    neck or sphincter N32.0
  bowel, cecum, colon or intestine, any part — *see* Obstruction, intestine
  Braxton Hicks —*see* False, labor
  breast implant, capsular T85.44
  bronchial J98.09
  burn (old) —*see* Cicatrix
  cervix —*see* Stricture, cervix
  cicatricial —*see* Cicatrix
  conjunctiva, trachomatous, active A71.1
    sequelae (late effect) B94.0
  Dupuytren's M72.0
  eyelid —*see* Disorder, eyelid function
  fascia (lata) (postural) M72.8
    Dupuytren's M72.0
    palmar M72.0
    plantar M72.2
  finger NEC —*see also* Deformity, finger
    congenital Q68.1
    joint —*see* Contraction, joint, hand
  flaccid —*see* Contraction, paralytic
  gallbladder K82.0
  heart valve —*see* Endocarditis
  hip —*see* Contraction, joint, hip
  hourglass
    bladder N32.89
      congenital Q64.79
    gallbladder K82.0
      congenital Q44.1
    stomach K31.89

Contraction (s) - *continued*
    congenital Q40.2
      psychogenic F45.8
    uterus (complicating delivery) O62.4
  hysterical F44.4
  internal os —*see* Stricture, cervix
  joint (abduction) (acquired) (adduction)
  (flexion) (rotation) M24.50
    ankle M24.57
    congenital NEC Q68.8
      hip Q65.89
    elbow M24.52
    foot joint M24.57
    hand joint M24.54
    hip M24.55
      congenital Q65.89
    hysterical F44.4
    knee M24.56
    shoulder M24.51
    wrist M24.53
  kidney (granular) (secondary) N26.9
    congenital Q63.8
    hydronephrotic —*see* Hydronephrosis
    Page N26.2
    pyelonephritic —*see* Pyelitis, chronic
    tuberculous A18.11
  ligament —*see also* Disorder, ligament
    congenital Q79.8
  muscle (postinfective) (postural) NEC
  M62.40
    with contracture of joint —*see* Contraction,
  joint
    ankle M62.47
    congenital Q79.8
      sternocleidomastoid Q68.0
    extraocular —*see* Strabismus
    eye (extrinsic) —*see* Strabismus
    foot M62.47
    forearm M62.43
    hand M62.44
    hysterical F44.4
    ischemic (Volkmann's) T79.6
    lower leg M62.46
    multiple sites M62.49
    pelvic region M62.45
    posttraumatic —*see* Strabismus, paralytic
    psychogenic F45.8
      conversion reaction F44.4
    shoulder region M62.41
    specified site NEC M62.48
    thigh M62.45
    upper arm M62.42
  neck —*see* Torticollis
  ocular muscle —*see* Strabismus
  organ or site, congenital NEC —*see* Atresia,
  by site
  outlet (pelvis) —*see* Contraction, pelvis
  palmar fascia M72.0
  paralytic
    joint —*see* Contraction, joint
    muscle —*see also* Contraction, muscle NEC
    ocular —*see* Strabismus, paralytic
  pelvis (acquired) (general) M95.5
    with disproportion (fetopelvic) O33.1
      causing obstructed labor O65.1
      inlet O33.2
      mid-cavity O33.3
      outlet O33.3
  plantar fascia M72.2
  premature
    atrium I49.1
    auriculoventricular I49.49

Contraction (s) - *continued*
    heart I49.49
    junctional I49.2
    supraventricular I49.1
    ventricular I49.3
  prostate N42.89
  pylorus NEC —*see also* Pylorospasm
    psychogenic F45.8
  rectum, rectal (sphincter) K59.8
  ring (Bandl's) (complicating delivery) O62.4
  scar —*see* Cicatrix
  spine —*see* Dorsopathy, deforming
  sternocleidomastoid (muscle) , congenital
  Q68.0
  stomach K31.89
    hourglass K31.89
      congenital Q40.2
      psychogenic F45.8
    psychogenic F45.8
  tendon (sheath) M62.40
    with contracture of joint —*see* Contraction,
  joint
    Achilles —*see* Short, tendon, Achilles
    ankle M62.47
      Achilles —*see* Short, tendon, Achilles
    foot M62.47
    forearm M62.43
    hand M62.44
    lower leg M62.46
    multiple sites M62.49
    neck M62.48
    pelvic region M62.45
    shoulder region M62.41
    specified site NEC M62.48
    thigh M62.45
    thorax M62.48
    trunk M62.48
    upper arm M62.42
  toe —*see* Deformity, toe, specified NEC
  ureterovesical orifice (postinfectional) N13.5
    with infection N13.6
  urethra —*see also* Stricture, urethra
    orifice N32.0
  uterus N85.8
    abnormal NEC O62.9
    clonic (complicating delivery) O62.4
    dyscoordinate (complicating delivery) O62.4
    hourglass (complicating delivery) O62.4
    hypertonic O62.4
    hypotonic NEC O62.2
    inadequate
      primary O62.0
      secondary O62.1
    incoordinate (complicating delivery) O62.4
    poor O62.2
    tetanic (complicating delivery) O62.4
  vagina (outlet) N89.5
  vesical N32.89
    neck or urethral orifice N32.0
  visual field —*see* Defect, visual field,
  generalized
  Volkmann's (ischemic) T79.6
Contusion (skin surface intact) T14.8
  abdomen, abdominal (muscle) (wall) S30.1
  adnexa, eye NEC S05.8X
  adrenal gland S37.812
  alveolar process S00.532
  ankle S90.0
  antecubital space —*see* Contusion, forearm
  anus S30.3

Contusion – *continued*
  arm (upper) S40.02
    lower (with elbow) —*see* Contusion,
    forearm
  auditory canal —*see* Contusion, ear
  auricle —*see* Contusion, ear
  axilla —*see* Contusion, arm, upper
  back —*see also* Contusion, thorax, back
    lower S30.0
  bile duct S36.13
  bladder S37.22
  bone NEC T14.8
  brain (diffuse) —*see* Injury, intracranial,
  diffuse
    focal —*see* Injury, intracranial, focal
  brainstem S06.38
  breast S20.0
  broad ligament S37.892
  brow S00.83
  buttock S30.0
  canthus, eye S00.1
  cauda equina S34.3
  cerebellar, traumatic S06.37
  cerebral S06.33
    left side S06.32
    right side S06.31
  cheek S00.83
    internal S00.532
  chest (wall) —*see* Contusion, thorax
  chin S00.83
  clitoris S30.23
  colon —*see* Injury, intestine, large, contusion
  common bile duct S36.13
  conjunctiva S05.1
    with foreign body (in conjunctival sac) —
  see Foreign body, conjunctival sac
  conus medullaris (spine) S34.139
  cornea —*see* Contusion, eyeball
    with foreign body —*see* Foreign body,
  cornea
  corpus cavernosum S30.21
  cortex (brain) (cerebral) —*see* Injury,
  intracranial, diffuse
    focal —*see* Injury, intracranial, focal
  costal region —*see* Contusion, thorax
  cystic duct S36.13
  diaphragm S27.802
  duodenum S36.420
  ear S00.43
  elbow S50.0
    with forearm —*see* Contusion, forearm
  epididymis S30.22
  epigastric region S30.1
  epiglottis S10.0
  esophagus (thoracic) S27.812
    cervical S10.0
  eyeball S05.1
  eyebrow S00.1
  eyelid (and periocular area) S00.1
  face NEC S00.83
  fallopian tube S37.529
    bilateral S37.522
    unilateral S37.521
  femoral triangle S30.1
  finger (s) S60.00
    with damage to nail (matrix) S60.10
    index S60.02
      with damage to nail S60.12
    little S60.05
      with damage to nail S60.15
    middle S60.03
      with damage to nail S60.13
    ring S60.04

Contusion – *continued*

   with damage to nail S60.14

    thumb —*see* Contusion, thumb

  flank S30.1

  foot (except toe(s) alone) S90.3

   toe —*see* Contusion, toe

  forearm S50.1

   elbow only —*see* Contusion, elbow

  forehead S00.83

  gallbladder S36.122

  genital organs, external

   female S30.202

   male S30.201

  globe (eye) —*see* Contusion, eyeball

  groin S30.1

  gum S00.532

  hand S60.22

   finger (s) —*see* Contusion, finger

   wrist —*see* Contusion, wrist

  head S00.93

   ear —*see* Contusion, ear

   eyelid —*see* Contusion, eyelid

   lip S00.531

   nose S00.33

   oral cavity S00.532

   scalp S00.03

   specified part NEC S00.83

  heel —*see* Contusion, foot

  hepatic duct S36.13

  hip S70.0

  ileum S36.428

  iliac region S30.1

  inguinal region S30.1

  interscapular region S20.229

  intra-abdominal organ S36.92

   colon —*see* Injury, intestine, large, contusion

   liver S36.112

   pancreas —*see* Contusion, pancreas

   rectum S36.62

   small intestine —*see* Injury, intestine, small, contusion

   specified organ NEC S36.892

   spleen —*see* Contusion, spleen

   stomach S36.32

  iris (eye) —*see* Contusion, eyeball

  jaw S00.83

  jejunum S36.428

  kidney S37.01

   major (greater than 2 cm) S37.02

   minor (less than 2 cm) S37.01

  knee S80.0

  labium (majus) (minus) S30.23

  lacrimal apparatus, gland or sac S05.8X

  larynx S10.0

  leg (lower) S80.1

   knee —*see* Contusion, knee

  lens —*see* Contusion, eyeball

  lip S00.531

  liver S36.112

  lower back S30.0

  lumbar region S30.0

  lung S27.329

   bilateral S27.322

   unilateral S27.321

  malar region S00.83

  mastoid region S00.83

  membrane, brain —*see* Injury, intracranial, diffuse

   focal —*see* Injury, intracranial, focal

  mesentery S36.892

  mesosalpinx S37.892

Contusion – *continued*

  mouth S00.532

  muscle —*see* Contusion, by site

  nail

   finger —*see* Contusion, finger, with damage to nail

   toe —*see* Contusion, toe, with damage to nail

  nasal S00.33

  neck S10.93

   specified site NEC S10.83

   throat S10.0

  nerve —*see* Injury, nerve

  newborn P54.5

  nose S00.33

  occipital

   lobe (brain) —*see* Injury, intracranial, diffuse

    focal —*see* Injury, intracranial, focal

   region (scalp) S00.03

  orbit (region) (tissues) S05.1

  ovary S37.429

   bilateral S37.422

   unilateral S37.421

  palate S00.532

  pancreas S36.229

   body S36.221

   head S36.220

   tail S36.222

  parietal

   lobe (brain) —*see* Injury, intracranial, diffuse

    focal —*see* Injury, intracranial, focal

   region (scalp) S00.03

  pelvic organ S37.92

   adrenal gland S37.812

   bladder S37.22

   fallopian tube —*see* Contusion, fallopian tube

   kidney —*see* Contusion, kidney

   ovary —*see* Contusion, ovary

   prostate S37.822

   specified organ NEC S37.892

   ureter S37.12

   urethra S37.32

   uterus S37.62

  pelvis S30.0

  penis S30.21

  perineum

   female S30.23

   male S30.0

  periocular area S00.1

  peritoneum S36.81

  periurethral tissue —*see* Contusion, urethra

  pharynx S10.0

  pinna —*see* Contusion, ear

  popliteal space —*see* Contusion, knee

  prepuce S30.21

  prostate S37.822

  pubic region S30.1

  pudendum

   female S30.202

   male S30.201

  quadriceps femoris —*see* Contusion, thigh

  rectum S36.62

  retroperitoneum S36.892

  round ligament S37.892

  sacral region S30.0

  scalp S00.03

   due to birth injury P12.3

  scapular region —*see* Contusion, shoulder

  sclera —*see* Contusion, eyeball

Contusion – *continued*

  scrotum S30.22

  seminal vesicle S37.892

  shoulder S40.01

  skin NEC T14.8

  small intestine —*see* Injury, intestine, small, contusion

  spermatic cord S30.22

  spinal cord —*see* Injury, spinal cord, by region

   cauda equina S34.3

   conus medullaris S34.139

  spleen S36.029

   major S36.021

   minor S36.020

  sternal region S20.219

  stomach S36.32

  subconjunctival S05.1

  subcutaneous NEC T14.8

  submaxillary region S00.83

  submental region S00.83

  subperiosteal NEC T14.8

  subungual

   finger —*see* Contusion, finger, with damage to nail

   toe —*see* Contusion, toe, with damage to nail

  supraclavicular fossa S10.83

  supraorbital S00.83

  suprarenal gland S37.812

  temple (region) S00.83

  temporal

   lobe (brain) —*see* Injury, intracranial, diffuse

    focal —*see* Injury, intracranial, focal

   region S00.83

  testis S30.22

  thigh S70.1

  thorax (wall) S20.20

   back S20.22

   front S20.21

  throat S10.0

  thumb S60.01

   with damage to nail S60.11

  toe (s) (lesser) S90.12

   with damage to nail S90.22

   great S90.11

    with damage to nail S90.21

    specified type NEC S90.221

  tongue S00.532

  trachea (cervical) S10.0

   thoracic S27.52

  tunica vaginalis S30.22

  tympanum, tympanic membrane —*see* Contusion, ear

  ureter S37.12

  urethra S37.32

  urinary organ NEC S37.892

  uterus S37.62

  uvula S00.532

  vagina S30.23

  vas deferens S37.892

  vesical S37.22

  vocal cord (s) S10.0

  vulva S30.23

  wrist S60.21

Conus (congenital) (any type) Q14.8

  cornea —*see* Keratoconus

  medullaris syndrome G95.81

Conversion hysteria, neurosis or reaction F44.9

Converter, tuberculosis (test reaction) R76.11

Conviction (legal) **, anxiety concerning** Z65.0
  with imprisonment Z65.1
Convulsions (idiopathic) (*see also* Seizure(s))
  R56.9
  apoplectiform (cerebral ischemia) I67.82
  benign neonatal (familial) —*see* Epilepsy,
  generalized, idiopathic
  dissociative F44.5
  epileptic —*see* Epilepsy
  epileptiform, epileptoid —*see* Seizure,
  epileptiform
  ether (anesthetic) —*see* Table of Drugs and
  Chemicals, by drug
  febrile R56.00
    with status epilepticus G40.901
    complex R56.01
      with status epilepticus G40.901
    simple R56.00
  hysterical F44.5
  infantile P90
    epilepsy —*see* Epilepsy
  jacksonian —*see* Epilepsy, localization-
  related, symptomatic, with simple partial
  seizures
  myoclonic G25.3
  neonatal, benign (familial) —*see* Epilepsy,
  generalized, idiopathic
  newborn P90
  obstetrical (nephritic) (uremic) —*see*
  Eclampsia
  paretic A52.17
  post traumatic R56.1
  psychomotor —*see* Epilepsy, localization-
  related, symptomatic, with complex partial
  seizures
  recurrent R56.9
  reflex R25.8
  scarlatinal A38.8
  tetanus, tetanic —*see* Tetanus
  thymic E32.8
Convulsive —*see also* Convulsions
Cooley's anemia D56.1
Coolie itch B76.9
Cooper's
  disease —*see* Mastopathy, cystic
  hernia —*see* Hernia, abdomen, specified site
  NEC
Copra itch B88.0
Coprophagy F50.8
Coprophobia F40.298
Coproporphyria, hereditary E80.29
Cor
  biloculare Q20.8
  bovis, bovinum —*see* Hypertrophy, cardiac
  pulmonale (chronic) I27.81
    acute I26.09
  triatriatum, triatrium Q24.2
  triloculare Q20.8
    biatrium Q20.4
    biventriculare Q21.1
Corbus' disease (gangrenous balanitis) N48.1
Cord —*see also* condition
  around neck (tightly) (with compression)
    complicating delivery O69.1
  bladder G95.89
  tabetic A52.19
Cordis ectopia Q24.8
Corditis (spermatic) N49.1
Corectopia Q13.2
Cori's disease (glycogen storage) E74.03
Cork handler's disease or lung J67.3
Corkscrew esophagus K22.4
Cork worker's disease or lung J67.3

Corn (infected) L84
Cornea —*see also* condition
  donor Z52.5
  plana Q13.4
Cornelia de Lange syndrome Q87.1
Cornu cutaneum L85.8
Cornual gestation or pregnancy O00.8
Coronary (artery) —*see* condition
Coronavirus, as cause of disease classified
  elsewhere B97.29
  SARS-associated B97.21
Corpora —*see also* condition
  amylacea, prostate N42.89
  cavernosa —*see* condition
Corpulence —*see* Obesity
Corpus —*see* condition
Corrected transposition Q20.5
Corrosion (injury) (acid) (caustic) (chemical)
  (lime) (external) (internal) T30.4
  abdomen, abdominal (muscle) (wall) T21.42
    first degree T21.52
    second degree T21.62
    third degree T21.72
  above elbow T22.439
    first degree T22.539
    left T22.432
      first degree T22.532
      second degree T22.632
      third degree T22.732
    right T22.431
      first degree T22.531
      second degree T22.631
      third degree T22.731
    second degree T22.639
    third degree T22.739
  alimentary tract NEC T28.7
  ankle T25.419
    first degree T25.519
    left T25.412
      first degree T25.512
      second degree T25.612
      third degree T25.712
    multiple with foot —*see* Corrosion, lower,
  limb, multiple, ankle and foot
    right T25.411
      first degree T25.511
      second degree T25.611
      third degree T25.711
    second degree T25.619
    third degree T25.719
  anus —*see* Corrosion, buttock
  arm (s) (meaning upper limb(s)) —*see*
  Corrosion, upper limb
  axilla T22.449
    first degree T22.549
    left T22.442
      first degree T22.542
      second degree T22.642
      third degree T22.742
    right T22.441
      first degree T22.541
      second degree T22.641
      third degree T22.741
    second degree T22.649
    third degree T22.749
  back (lower) T21.44
    first degree T21.54
    second degree T21.64
    third degree T21.74
    upper T21.43
      first degree T21.53
      second degree T21.63

Corrosion – *continued*
  third degree T21.73
  blisters
  code as Corrosion, second degree, by site
  breast (s) —*see* Corrosion, chest wall
  buttock (s) T21.45
    first degree T21.55
    second degree T21.65
    third degree T21.75
  calf T24.439
    first degree T24.539
    left T24.432
      first degree T24.532
      second degree T24.632
      third degree T24.732
    right T24.431
      first degree T24.531
      second degree T24.631
      third degree T24.731
    second degree T24.639
    third degree T24.739
  canthus (eye) —*see* Corrosion, eyelid
  cervix T28.8
  cheek T20.46
    first degree T20.56
    second degree T20.66
    third degree T20.76
  chest wall T21.41
    first degree T21.51
    second degree T21.61
    third degree T21.71
  chin T20.43
    first degree T20.53
    second degree T20.63
    third degree T20.73
  colon T28.7
  conjunctiva (and cornea) —*see* Corrosion,
  cornea
  cornea (and conjunctiva) T26.6
  deep necrosis of underlying tissue
  code as Corrosion, third degree, by site
  dorsum of hand T23.469
    first degree T23.569
    left T23.462
      first degree T23.562
      second degree T23.662
      third degree T23.762
    right T23.461
      first degree T23.561
      second degree T23.661
      third degree T23.761
    second degree T23.669
    third degree T23.769
  ear (auricle) (external) (canal) T20.41
    drum T28.91
    first degree T20.51
    second degree T20.61
    third degree T20.71
  elbow T22.429
    first degree T22.529
    left T22.422
      first degree T22.522
      second degree T22.622
      third degree T22.722
    right T22.421
      first degree T22.521
      second degree T22.621
      third degree T22.721
    second degree T22.629
    third degree T22.729
  entire body —*see* Corrosion, multiple body
  regions

Corrosion – *continued*
epidermal loss
code as Corrosion, second degree, by site
epiglottis T27.4
erythema, erythematous
code as Corrosion, first degree, by site
esophagus T28.6
extent (percentage of body surface)
  less than 10 per cent T32.0
  10 19 per cent (0 9 percent third degree)
    T32.10
    with 10 19 percent third degree T32.11
  20 29 per cent (0 9 percent third degree)
    T32.20
    with
      10 19 percent third degree T32.21
      20 29 percent third degree T32.22
  30 39 per cent (0 9 percent third degree)
    T32.30
    with
      10 19 percent third degree T32.31
      20 29 percent third degree T32.32
      30 39 percent third degree T32.33
  40 49 per cent (0 9 percent third degree)
    T32.40
    with
      10 19 percent third degree T32.41
      20 29 percent third degree T32.42
      30 39 percent third degree T32.43
      40 49 percent third degree T32.44
  50 59 per cent (0 9 percent third degree)
    T32.50
    with
      10 19 percent third degree T32.51
      20 29 percent third degree T32.52
      30 39 percent third degree T32.53
      40 49 percent third degree T32.54
      50 59 percent third degree T32.55
  60 69 per cent (0 9 percent third degree)
    T32.60
    with
      10 19 percent third degree T32.61
      20 29 percent third degree T32.62
      30 39 percent third degree T32.63
      40 49 percent third degree T32.64
      50 59 percent third degree T32.65
      60 69 percent third degree T32.66
  70 79 per cent (0 9 percent third degree)
    T32.70
    with
      10 19 percent third degree T32.71
      20 29 percent third degree T32.72
      30 39 percent third degree T32.73
      40 49 percent third degree T32.74
      50 59 percent third degree T32.75
      60 69 percent third degree T32.76
      70 79 percent third degree T32.77
  80 89 per cent (0 9 percent third degree)
    T32.80
    with
      10 19 percent third degree T32.81
      20 29 percent third degree T32.82
      30 39 percent third degree T32.83
      40 49 percent third degree T32.84
      50 59 percent third degree T32.85
      60 69 percent third degree T32.86
      70 79 percent third degree T32.87
      80 89 percent third degree T32.88
  90 per cent or more (0 9 percent third
    degree) T32.90
    with
      10 19 percent third degree T32.91

Corrosion – *continued*
      20 29 percent third degree T32.92
      30 39 percent third degree T32.93
      40 49 percent third degree T32.94
      50 59 percent third degree T32.95
      60 69 percent third degree T32.96
      70 79 percent third degree T32.97
      80 89 percent third degree T32.98
      90 99 percent third degree T32.99
extremity —*see* Corrosion, limb
eye (s) and adnexa T26.9
  with resulting rupture and destruction of
eyeball T26.7
  conjunctival sac —*see* Corrosion, cornea
  cornea —*see* Corrosion, cornea
  lid —*see* Corrosion, eyelid
  periocular area —*see* Corrosion eyelid
  specified site NEC T26.8
eyeball —*see* Corrosion, eye
eyelid (s) T26.5
face —*see* Corrosion, head
finger T23.429
  first degree T23.529
  left T23.422
    first degree T23.522
    second degree T23.622
    third degree T23.722
  multiple sites (without thumb) T23.439
    with thumb T23.449
      first degree T23.549
      left T23.442
        first degree T23.542
        second degree T23.642
        third degree T23.742
      right T23.441
        first degree T23.541
        second degree T23.641
        third degree T23.741
      second degree T23.649
      third degree T23.749
    first degree T23.539
    left T23.432
      first degree T23.532
      second degree T23.632
      third degree T23.732
    right T23.431
      first degree T23.531
      second degree T23.631
      third degree T23.731
    second degree T23.639
    third degree T23.739
  right T23.421
    first degree T23.521
    second degree T23.621
    third degree T23.721
  second degree T23.629
  third degree T23.729
flank —*see* Corrosion, abdomen
foot T25.429
  first degree T25.529
  left T25.422
    first degree T25.522
    second degree T25.622
    third degree T25.722
  multiple with ankle —*see* Corrosion, lower,
limb, multiple, ankle and foot
  right T25.421
    first degree T25.521
    second degree T25.621
    third degree T25.721
  second degree T25.629
  third degree T25.729

Corrosion – *continued*
forearm T22.419
  first degree T22.519
  left T22.412
    first degree T22.512
    second degree T22.612
    third degree T22.712
  right T22.411
    first degree T22.511
    second degree T22.611
    third degree T22.711
  second degree T22.619
  third degree T22.719
forehead T20.46
  first degree T20.56
  second degree T20.66
  third degree T20.76
fourth degree
code as Corrosion, third degree, by site
full thickness skin loss
code as Corrosion, third degree, by site
gastrointestinal tract NEC T28.7
genital organs
  external
    female T21.47
      first degree T21.57
      second degree T21.67
      third degree T21.77
    male T21.46
      first degree T21.56
      second degree T21.66
      third degree T21.76
  internal T28.8
groin —*see* Corrosion, abdominal wall
hand (s) T23.409
  back —*see* Corrosion, dorsum of hand
  finger —*see* Corrosion, finger
  first degree T23.509
  left T23.402
    first degree T23.502
    second degree T23.602
    third degree T23.702
  multiple sites with wrist T23.499
    first degree T23.599
    left T23.492
      first degree T23.592
      second degree T23.692
      third degree T23.792
    right T23.491
      first degree T23.591
      second degree T23.691
      third degree T23.791
    second degree T23.699
    third degree T23.799
  palm —*see* Corrosion, palm
  right T23.401
    first degree T23.501
    second degree T23.601
    third degree T23.701
  second degree T23.609
  third degree T23.709
  thumb —*see* Corrosion, thumb
head (and face) (and neck) T20.40
  cheek —*see* Corrosion, cheek
  chin —*see* Corrosion, chin
  ear —*see* Corrosion, ear
  eye (s) only —*see* Corrosion, eye
  first degree T20.50
  forehead —*see* Corrosion, forehead
  lip —*see* Corrosion, lip
  multiple sites T20.49
    first degree T20.59
    second degree T20.69

Corrosion – *continued*

third degree T20.79
neck —*see* Corrosion, neck
nose —*see* Corrosion, nose
scalp —*see* Corrosion, scalp
second degree T20.60
third degree T20.70
hip (s) —*see* Corrosion, lower, limb
inhalation —*see* Corrosion, respiratory tract
internal organ (s) (*see also* Corrosion, by site) T28.90
  alimentary tract T28.7
    esophagus T28.6
  esophagus T28.6
  genitourinary T28.8
  mouth T28.5
  pharynx T28.5
  specified organ NEC T28.99
interscapular region —*see* Corrosion, back, upper
intestine (large) (small) T28.7
knee T24.429
  first degree T24.529
  left T24.422
    first degree T24.522
    second degree T24.622
    third degree T24.722
  right T24.421
    first degree T24.521
    second degree T24.621
    third degree T24.721
  second degree T24.629
  third degree T24.729
labium (majus) (minus) —*see* Corrosion, genital organs, external, female
lacrimal apparatus, duct, gland or sac —*see* Corrosion, eye, specified site NEC
larynx T27.4
  with lung T27.5
leg (s) (meaning lower limb(s)) —*see* Corrosion, lower limb
limb (s)
  lower —*see* Corrosion, lower, limb
  upper —*see* Corrosion, upper limb
lip (s) T20.42
  first degree T20.52
  second degree T20.62
  third degree T20.72
lower
  back —*see* Corrosion, back
  limb T24.409
    ankle —*see* Corrosion, ankle
    calf —*see* Corrosion, calf
    first degree T24.509
    foot —*see* Corrosion, foot
    knee —*see* Corrosion, knee
    left T24.402
      first degree T24.502
      second degree T24.602
      third degree T24.702
    multiple sites, except ankle and foot T24.499
      ankle and foot T25.499
        first degree T25.599
        left T25.492
          first degree T25.592
          second degree T25.692
          third degree T25.792
        right T25.491
          first degree T25.591
          second degree T25.691
          third degree T25.791

Corrosion – *continued*

      second degree T25.699
      third degree T25.799
    first degree T24.599
    left T24.492
      first degree T24.592
      second degree T24.692
      third degree T24.792
    right T24.491
      first degree T24.591
      second degree T24.691
      third degree T24.791
    second degree T24.699
    third degree T24.799
  right T24.401
    first degree T24.501
    second degree T24.601
    third degree T24.701
  second degree T24.609
  hip —*see* Corrosion, thigh
  thigh —*see* Corrosion, thigh
  third degree T24.709
lung (with larynx and trachea) T27.5
mouth T28.5
neck T20.47
  first degree T20.57
  second degree T20.67
  third degree T20.77
nose (septum) T20.44
  first degree T20.54
  second degree T20.64
  third degree T20.74
ocular adnexa —*see* Corrosion, eye
orbit region —*see* Corrosion, eyelid
palm T23.459
  first degree T23.559
  left T23.452
    first degree T23.552
    second degree T23.652
    third degree T23.752
  right T23.451
    first degree T23.551
    second degree T23.651
    third degree T23.751
  second degree T23.659
  third degree T23.759
partial thickness
code as Corrosion, unspecified degree, by site
pelvis —*see* Corrosion, trunk
penis —*see* Corrosion, genital organs, external, male
perineum
  female —*see* Corrosion, genital organs, external, female
  male —*see* Corrosion, genital organs, external, male
periocular area —*see* Corrosion, eyelid
pharynx T28.5
rectum T28.7
respiratory tract T27.7
  larynx —*see* Corrosion, larynx
  specified part NEC T27.6
  trachea —*see* Corrosion, larynx
sac, lacrimal —*see* Corrosion, eye, specified site NEC
scalp T20.45
  first degree T20.55
  second degree T20.65
  third degree T20.75
scapular region T22.469
  first degree T22.569
  left T22.462

Corrosion – *continued*

    first degree T22.562
    second degree T22.662
    third degree T22.762
  right T22.461
    first degree T22.561
    second degree T22.661
    third degree T22.761
  second degree T22.669
  third degree T22.769
sclera —*see* Corrosion, eye, specified site NEC
scrotum —*see* Corrosion, genital organs, external, male
shoulder T22.459
  first degree T22.559
  left T22.452
    first degree T22.552
    second degree T22.652
    third degree T22.752
  right T22.451
    first degree T22.551
    second degree T22.651
    third degree T22.751
  second degree T22.659
  third degree T22.759
stomach T28.7
temple —*see* Corrosion, head
testis —*see* Corrosion, genital organs, external, male
thigh T24.419
  first degree T24.519
  left T24.412
    first degree T24.512
    second degree T24.612
    third degree T24.712
  right T24.411
    first degree T24.511
    second degree T24.611
    third degree T24.711
  second degree T24.619
  third degree T24.719
thorax (external) —*see* Corrosion, trunk
throat (meaning pharynx) T28.5
thumb (s) T23.419
  first degree T23.519
  left T23.412
    first degree T23.512
    second degree T23.612
    third degree T23.712
  multiple sites with fingers T23.449
    first degree T23.549
    left T23.442
      first degree T23.542
      second degree T23.642
      third degree T23.742
    right T23.441
      first degree T23.541
      second degree T23.641
      third degree T23.741
    second degree T23.649
    third degree T23.749
  right T23.411
    first degree T23.511
    second degree T23.611
    third degree T23.711
  second degree T23.619
  third degree T23.719
toe T25.439
  first degree T25.539
  left T25.432
    first degree T25.532
    second degree T25.632

Corrosion – *continued*
   third degree T25.732
  right T25.431
   first degree T25.531
   second degree T25.631
   third degree T25.731
  second degree T25.639
  third degree T25.739
 tongue T28.5
 tonsil (s) T28.5
 total body —*see* Corrosion, multiple body regions
 trachea T27.4
  with lung T27.5
 trunk T21.40
  abdominal wall —*see* Corrosion, abdominal wall
  anus —*see* Corrosion, buttock
  axilla —*see* Corrosion, upper limb
  back —*see* Corrosion, back
  breast —*see* Corrosion, chest wall
  buttock —*see* Corrosion, buttock
  chest wall —*see* Corrosion, chest wall
  first degree T21.50
  flank —*see* Corrosion, abdominal wall
  genital
   female —*see* Corrosion, genital organs, external, female
   male —*see* Corrosion, genital organs, external, male
  groin —*see* Corrosion, abdominal wall
  interscapular region —*see* Corrosion, back, upper
  labia —*see* Corrosion, genital organs, external, female
  lower back —*see* Corrosion, back
  penis —*see* Corrosion, genital organs, external, male
  perineum
   female —*see* Corrosion, genital organs, external, female
   male —*see* Corrosion, genital organs, external, male
  scapular region —*see* Corrosion, upper limb
  scrotum —*see* Corrosion, genital organs, external, male
  second degree T21.60
  shoulder —*see* Corrosion, upper limb
  specified site NEC T21.49
   first degree T21.59
   second degree T21.69
   third degree T21.79
  testes —*see* Corrosion, genital organs, external, male
  third degree T21.70
  upper back —*see* Corrosion, back, upper
  vagina T28.8
  vulva —*see* Corrosion, genital organs, external, female
 unspecified site with extent of body surface involved specified
  less than 10 per cent T32.0
  10 19 per cent (0 9 percent third degree) T32.10
   with 10 19 percent third degree T32.11
  20 29 per cent (0 9 percent third degree) T32.20
   with
    10 19 percent third degree T32.21
    20 29 percent third degree T32.22
  30 39 per cent (0 9 percent third degree) T32.30

Corrosion – *continued*
  with
   10 19 percent third degree T32.31
   20 29 percent third degree T32.32
   30 39 percent third degree T32.33
  40 49 per cent (0 9 percent third degree) T32.40
   with
    10 19 percent third degree T32.41
    20 29 percent third degree T32.42
    30 39 percent third degree T32.43
    40 49 percent third degree T32.44
  50 59 per cent (0 9 percent third degree) T32.50
   with
    10 19 percent third degree T32.51
    20 29 percent third degree T32.52
    30 39 percent third degree T32.53
    40 49 percent third degree T32.54
    50 59 percent third degree T32.55
  60 69 per cent (0 9 percent third degree) T32.60
   with
    10 19 percent third degree T32.61
    20 29 percent third degree T32.62
    30 39 percent third degree T32.63
    40 49 percent third degree T32.64
    50 59 percent third degree T32.65
    60 69 percent third degree T32.66
  70 79 per cent (0 9 percent third degree) T32.70
   with
    10 19 percent third degree T32.71
    20 29 percent third degree T32.72
    30 39 percent third degree T32.73
    40 49 percent third degree T32.74
    50 59 percent third degree T32.75
    60 69 percent third degree T32.76
    70 79 percent third degree T32.77
  80 89 per cent (0 9 percent third degree) T32.80
   with
    10 19 percent third degree T32.81
    20 29 percent third degree T32.82
    30 39 percent third degree T32.83
    40 49 percent third degree T32.84
    50 59 percent third degree T32.85
    60 69 percent third degree T32.86
    70 79 percent third degree T32.87
    80 89 percent third degree T32.88
  90 per cent or more (0 9 percent third degree) T32.90
   with
    10 19 percent third degree T32.91
    20 29 percent third degree T32.92
    30 39 percent third degree T32.93
    40 49 percent third degree T32.94
    50 59 percent third degree T32.95
    60 69 percent third degree T32.96
    70 79 percent third degree T32.97
    80 89 percent third degree T32.98
    90 99 percent third degree T32.99
 upper limb (axilla) (scapular region) T22.40
  above elbow —*see* Corrosion, above elbow
  axilla —*see* Corrosion, axilla
  elbow —*see* Corrosion, elbow
  first degree T22.50
  forearm —*see* Corrosion, forearm
  hand —*see* Corrosion, hand
  interscapular region —*see* Corrosion, back, upper
  multiple sites T22.499

Corrosion – *continued*
  first degree T22.599
  left T22.492
   first degree T22.592
   second degree T22.692
   third degree T22.792
  right T22.491
   first degree T22.591
   second degree T22.691
   third degree T22.791
  second degree T22.699
  third degree T22.799
  scapular region —*see* Corrosion, scapular region
  second degree T22.60
  shoulder —*see* Corrosion, shoulder
  third degree T22.70
  wrist —*see* Corrosion, hand
 uterus T28.8
 vagina T28.8
 vulva —*see* Corrosion, genital organs, external, female
 wrist T23.479
  first degree T23.579
  left T23.472
   first degree T23.572
   second degree T23.672
   third degree T23.772
  multiple sites with hand T23.499
   first degree T23.599
   left T23.492
    first degree T23.592
    second degree T23.692
    third degree T23.792
   right T23.491
    first degree T23.591
    second degree T23.691
    third degree T23.791
   second degree T23.699
   third degree T23.799
  right T23.471
   first degree T23.571
   second degree T23.671
   third degree T23.771
  second degree T23.679
  third degree T23.779
Corrosive burn —*see* Corrosion
Corsican fever —*see* Malaria
Cortical —*see* condition
Cortico-adrenal —*see* condition
Coryza (acute) J00
 with grippe or influenza —*see* Influenza, with, respiratory manifestations NEC
 syphilitic
  congenital (chronic) A50.05
Costen's syndrome or complex M26.69
Costiveness —*see* Constipation
Costochondritis M94.0
Cotard's syndrome F22
Cot death R99
Cotia virus B08.8
Cotton wool spots (retinal) H35.81
Cotungo's disease —*see* Sciatica
Cough (affected) (chronic) (epidemic) (nervous) R05
 with hemorrhage —*see* Hemoptysis
 bronchial R05
  with grippe or influenza —*see* Influenza, with, respiratory manifestations NEC
 functional F45.8
 hysterical F45.8
 laryngeal, spasmodic R05
 psychogenic F45.8

Cough - *continued*
  smokers' J41.0
  tea taster's B49
Counseling (for) Z71.9
  abuse NEC
    perpetrator Z69.82
    victim Z69.81
  alcohol abuser Z71.41
    family Z71.42
  child abuse
    nonparental
      perpetrator Z69.021
      victim Z69.020
    parental
      perpetrator Z69.011
      victim Z69.010
  consanguinity Z71.89
  contraceptive Z30.09
  dietary Z71.3
  drug abuser Z71.51
    family member Z71.52
  family Z71.89
  fertility preservation (prior to cancer therapy) (prior to removal of gonads) Z31.62
  for non-attending third party Z71.0
    related to sexual behavior or orientation Z70.2
  genetic NEC Z31.5
  health (advice) (education) (instruction) —*see* Counseling, medical
  human immunodeficiency virus (HIV) Z71.7
  impotence Z70.1
  insulin pump use Z46.81
  medical (for) Z71.9
    boarding school resident Z59.3
    consanguinity Z71.89
    feared complaint and no disease found Z71.1
    human immunodeficiency virus (HIV) Z71.7
    institutional resident Z59.3
    on behalf of another Z71.0
      related to sexual behavior or orientation Z70.2
    person living alone Z60.2
    specified reason NEC Z71.89
  natural family planning
    procreative Z31.61
    to avoid pregnancy Z30.02
  perpetrator (of)
    abuse NEC Z69.82
    child abuse
      non-parental Z69.021
      parental Z69.011
    rape NEC Z69.82
    spousal abuse Z69.12
  procreative NEC Z31.69
    fertility preservation (prior to cancer therapy) (prior to removal of gonads) Z31.62
    using natural family planning Z31.61
  promiscuity Z70.1
  rape victim Z69.81
  religious Z71.81
  sex, sexual (related to) Z70.9
    attitude (s) Z70.0
    behavior or orientation Z70.1
    combined concerns Z70.3
    non-responsiveness Z70.1
    on behalf of third party Z70.2
    specified reason NEC Z70.8
  specified reason NEC Z71.89
  spiritual Z71.81
  spousal abuse (perpetrator) Z69.12
    victim Z69.11

Counseling - *continued*
  substance abuse Z71.89
    alcohol Z71.41
    drug Z71.51
    tobacco Z71.6
  tobacco use Z71.6
  use (of)
    insulin pump Z46.81
  victim (of)
    abuse Z69.81
    child abuse
      by parent Z69.010
      non-parental Z69.020
    rape NEC Z69.81
Coupled rhythm R00.8
Couvelaire syndrome or uterus (complicating delivery) O45.8X
Cowperitis —*see* Urethritis
Cowper's gland —*see* condition
Cowpox B08.010
  due to vaccination T88.1
Coxa
  magna M91.4
  plana M91.2
  valga (acquired) —*see also* Deformity, limb, specified type NEC, thigh
    congenital Q65.81
    sequelae (late effect) of rickets E64.3
  vara (acquired) —*see also* Deformity, limb, specified type NEC, thigh
    congenital Q65.82
    sequelae (late effect) of rickets E64.3
Coxalgia, coxalgic (nontuberculous) —*see also* Pain, joint, hip
  tuberculous A18.02
Coxitis —*see* Monoarthritis, hip
Coxsackie (virus) (infection) B34.1
  as cause of disease classified elsewhere B97.11
  carditis B33.20
  central nervous system NEC A88.8
  endocarditis B33.21
  enteritis A08.39
  meningitis (aseptic) A87.0
  myocarditis B33.22
  pericarditis B33.23
  pharyngitis B08.5
  pleurodynia B33.0
  specific disease NEC B33.8
Crabs, meaning pubic lice B85.3
Crack baby P04.41
Cracked nipple N64.0
  associated with
    lactation O92.13
    pregnancy O92.11
    puerperium O92.12
Cracked tooth K03.81
Cradle cap L21.0
Craft neurosis F48.8
Cramp (s) R25.2
  abdominal —*see* Pain, abdominal
  bathing T75.1
  colic R10.83
    psychogenic F45.8
  due to immersion T75.1
  fireman T67.2
  heat T67.2
  immersion T75.1
  intestinal —*see* Pain, abdominal
    psychogenic F45.8
  leg, sleep related G47.62

Cramp – *continued*
  limb (lower) (upper) NEC R25.2
    sleep related G47.62
  linotypist's F48.8
    organic G25.89
  muscle (limb) (general) R25.2
    due to immersion T75.1
    psychogenic F45.8
  occupational (hand) F48.8
    organic G25.89
  salt-depletion E87.1
  sleep related, leg G47.62
  stoker's T67.2
  swimmer's T75.1
  telegrapher's F48.8
    organic G25.89
  typist's F48.8
    organic G25.89
  uterus N94.89
    menstrual —*see* Dysmenorrhea
  writer's F48.8
    organic G25.89
Cranial —*see* condition
Craniocleidodysostosis Q74.0
Craniofenestria (skull) Q75.8
Craniolacunia (skull) Q75.8
Craniopagus Q89.4
Craniopathy, metabolic M85.2
Craniopharyngeal —*see* condition
Craniopharyngioma D44.4
Craniorachischisis (totalis) Q00.1
Cranioschisis Q75.8
Craniostenosis Q75.0
Craniosynostosis Q75.0
Craniotabes (cause unknown) M83.8
  neonatal P96.3
  rachitic E64.3
  syphilitic A50.56
Cranium —*see* condition
Craw-craw —*see* Onchocerciasis
Creaking joint —*see* Derangement, joint, specified type NEC
Creeping
  eruption B76.9
  palsy or paralysis G12.22
Crenated tongue K14.8
Creotoxism A05.9
Crepitus
  caput Q75.8
  joint —*see* Derangement, joint, specified type NEC
Crescent or conus choroid, congenital Q14.3
CREST syndrome M34.1
Cretin, cretinism (congenital) (endemic) (nongoitrous) (sporadic) E00.9
  pelvis
    with disproportion (fetopelvic) O33.0
      causing obstructed labor O65.0
  type
    hypothyroid E00.1
    mixed E00.2
    myxedematous E00.1
    neurological E00.0
Creutzfeldt-Jakob disease or syndrome (with dementia) A81.00
  familial A81.09
  iatrogenic A81.09
  specified NEC A81.09
  sporadic A81.09
  variant (vCJD) A81.01
Crib death R99
Cribriform hymen Q52.3
Cri-du-chat syndrome Q93.4

Crigler-Najjar disease or syndrome E80.5
Crime, victim of Z65.4
Crimean hemorrhagic fever A98.0
Criminalism F60.2
Crisis
  abdomen R10.0
  acute reaction F43.0
  addisonian E27.2
  adrenal (cortical) E27.2
  celiac K90.0
  Dietl's N13.8
  emotional —*see also* Disorder, adjustment
    acute reaction to stress F43.0
    specific to childhood and adolescence F93.8
  glaucomatocyclitic —*see* Glaucoma,
  secondary, inflammation
  heart —*see* Failure, heart
  nitritoid I95.2
    correct substance properly administered —
  see Table of Drugs and Chemicals, by drug,
  adverse effect
    overdose or wrong substance given or taken
  —*see* Table of Drugs and Chemicals, by drug,
  poisoning
  oculogyric H51.8
    psychogenic F45.8
  Pel's (tabetic) A52.11
  psychosexual identity F64.2
  renal N28.0
  sickle-cell D57.00
    with
      acute chest syndrome D57.01
      splenic sequestration D57.02
  state (acute reaction) F43.0
  tabetic A52.11
  thyroid —*see* Thyrotoxicosis with thyroid
  storm
  thyrotoxic —*see* Thyrotoxicosis with thyroid
  storm
Crocq's disease (acrocyanosis) I73.89
Crohn's disease —*see* Enteritis, regional
Crooked septum, nasal J34.2
Cross syndrome E70.328
Crossbite (anterior) (posterior) M26.24
Cross-eye —*see* Strabismus, convergent
  concomitant
Croup, croupous (catarrhal) (infectious)
  (inflammatory) (nondiphtheritic) J05.0
  bronchial J20.9
  diphtheritic A36.2
  false J38.5
  spasmodic J38.5
    diphtheritic A36.2
  stridulous J38.5
    diphtheritic A36.2
Crouzon's disease Q75.1
Crowding, tooth, teeth, fully erupted M26.31
CRST syndrome M34.1
Cruchet's disease A85.8
Cruelty in children —*see also* Disorder,
  conduct
Crural ulcer —*see* Ulcer, lower limb
Crush, crushed, crushing T14.8
  abdomen S38.1
  ankle S97.0
  arm (upper) (and shoulder) S47.
  axilla —*see* Crush, arm
  back, lower S38.1
  buttock S38.1
  cheek S07.0
  chest S28.0
  cranium S07.1

Crush, crushed, crushing – *continued*
  ear S07.0
  elbow S57.0
  extremity
    lower
      ankle —*see* Crush, ankle
      below knee —*see* Crush, leg
      foot —*see* Crush, foot
      hip —*see* Crush, hip
      knee —*see* Crush, knee
      thigh —*see* Crush, thigh
      toe —*see* Crush, toe
    upper
      below elbow S67.9
      elbow —*see* Crush, elbow
      finger —*see* Crush, finger
      forearm —*see* Crush, forearm
      hand —*see* Crush, hand
      thumb —*see* Crush, thumb
      upper arm —*see* Crush, arm
      wrist —*see* Crush, wrist
  face S07.0
  finger (s) S67.1
    with hand (and wrist) —*see* Crush, hand,
  specified site NEC
    index S67.19
    little S67.19
    middle S67.19
    ring S67.19
    thumb —*see* Crush, thumb
  foot S97.8
    toe —*see* Crush, toe
  forearm S57.8
  genitalia, external
    female S38.002
      vagina S38.03
      vulva S38.03
    male S38.001
      penis S38.01
      scrotum S38.02
      testis S38.02
  hand (except fingers alone) S67.2
    with wrist S67.4
  head S07.9
    specified NEC S07.8
  heel —*see* Crush, foot
  hip S77.0
    with thigh S77.2
  internal organ (abdomen, chest, or pelvis)
  NEC T14.8
  knee S87.0
  labium (majus) (minus) S38.03
  larynx S17.0
  leg (lower) S87.8
    knee —*see* Crush, knee
  lip S07.0
  lower
    back S38.1
    leg —*see* Crush, leg
  neck S17.9
  nerve —*see* Injury, nerve
  nose S07.0
  pelvis S38.1
  penis S38.01
  scalp S07.8
  scapular region —*see* Crush, arm
  scrotum S38.02
  severe, unspecified site T14.8
  shoulder (and upper arm) —*see* Crush, arm
  skull S07.1
  syndrome (complication of trauma) T79.5
  testis S38.02

Crush, crushed, crushing – *continued*
  thigh S77.1
    with hip S77.2
  throat S17.8
  thumb S67.0
    with hand (and wrist) —*see* Crush, hand,
  specified site NEC
  toe (s) S97.10
    great S97.11
    lesser S97.12
  trachea S17.0
  vagina S38.03
  vulva S38.03
  wrist S67.3
    with hand S67.4
Crusta lactea L21.0
Crusts R23.4
Crutch paralysis —*see* Injury, brachial plexus
Cruveilhier-Baumgarten cirrhosis, disease
  or syndrome K74.69
Cruveilhier's atrophy or disease G12.8
Crying (constant) (continuous) (excessive)
  child, adolescent, or adult R45.83
  infant (baby) (newborn) R68.11
Cryofibrinogenemia D89.2
Cryoglobulinemia (essential) (idiopathic)
  (mixed) (primary) (purpura) (secondary)
  (vasculitis) D89.1
  with lung involvement D89.1 *[J99]*
Cryptitis (anal) (rectal) K62.89
Cryptococcosis, cryptococcus (infection)
  (neoformans) B45.9
  bone B45.3
  cerebral B45.1
  cutaneous B45.2
  disseminated B45.7
  generalized B45.7
  meningitis B45.1
  meningocerebralis B45.1
  osseous B45.3
  pulmonary B45.0
  skin B45.2
  specified NEC B45.8
Cryptopapillitis (anus) K62.89
Cryptophthalmos Q11.2
  syndrome Q87.0
Cryptorchid, cryptorchism, cryptorchidism
  Q53.9
  bilateral Q53.20
    abdominal Q53.21
    perineal Q53.22
  unilateral Q53.10
    abdominal Q53.11
    perineal Q53.12
Cryptosporidiosis A07.2
  hepatobiliary B88.8
  respiratory B88.8
Cryptostromosis J67.6
Crystalluria R82.99
Cubitus
  congenital Q68.8
  valgus (acquired) M21.0
    congenital Q68.8
    sequelae (late effect) of rickets E64.3
  varus (acquired) M21.1
    congenital Q68.8
    sequelae (late effect) of rickets E64.3
Cultural deprivation or shock Z60.3
Curling esophagus K22.4
Curling's ulcer —*see* Ulcer, peptic, acute
Curschmann (-Batten) (-Steinert) **disease or**
  syndrome G71.11
Curse, Ondine's —*see* Apnea, sleep

Curvature
  organ or site, congenital NEC —*see*
    Distortion
  penis (lateral) Q55.61
  Pott's (spinal) A18.01
  radius, idiopathic, progressive (congenital)
    Q74.0
  spine (acquired) (angular) (idiopathic)
    (incorrect) (postural) —*see* Dorsopathy,
    deforming
    congenital Q67.5
    due to or associated with
      Charcot-Marie-Tooth disease (*see also*
    subcategory M49.8) G60.0
      osteitis
        deformans M88.88
        fibrosa cystica (*see also* subcategory
    M49.8) E21.0
        tuberculosis (Pott's curvature) A18.01
      sequelae (late effect) of rickets E64.3
      tuberculous A18.01
Cushingoid due to steroid therapy E24.2
  correct substance properly administered — *see*
  Table of Drugs and Chemicals, by drug,
  adverse effect
  overdose or wrong substance given or taken
  —*see* Table of Drugs and Chemicals, by drug,
  poisoning
Cushing's
  syndrome or disease E24.9
    drug-induced E24.2
    iatrogenic E24.2
    pituitary-dependent E24.0
    specified NEC E24.8
  ulcer —*see* Ulcer, peptic, acute
Cusp, Carabelli omit code
Cut (external) —*see also* Laceration
  muscle —*see* Injury, muscle
Cutaneous —*see also* condition
  hemorrhage R23.3
  larva migrans B76.9
Cutis —*see also* condition
  hyperelastica Q82.8
    acquired L57.4
  laxa (hyperelastica) —*see* Dermatolysis
  marmorata R23.8
  osteosis L94.2
  pendula —*see* Dermatolysis
  rhomboidalis nuchae L57.2
  verticis gyrata Q82.8
    acquired L91.8
Cyanosis R23.0
  due to
    patent foramen botalli Q21.1
    persistent foramen ovale Q21.1
  enterogenous D74.8
  paroxysmal digital —*see* Raynaud's disease
    with gangrene I73.01
  retina, retinal H35.89
Cyanotic heart disease I24.9
  congenital Q24.9
Cycle
  anovulatory N97.0
  menstrual, irregular N92.6
Cyclencephaly Q04.9
Cyclical vomiting (*see also* Vomiting,
  cyclical) G43.A0
  psychogenic F50.8
Cyclitis (*see also* Iridocyclitis) H20.9
  chronic —*see* Iridocyclitis, chronic
  Fuchs' heterochromic H20.81
  granulomatous —*see* Iridocyclitis, chronic

Cyclitis - *continued*
  lens-induced —*see* Iridocyclitis, lens-induced
  posterior H30.2
Cycloid personality F34.0
Cyclophoria H50.54
Cyclopia, cyclops Q87.0
Cyclopism Q87.0
Cyclosporiasis A07.4
Cyclothymia F34.0
Cyclothymic personality F34.0
Cyclotropia H50.41
Cylindroma —*see also* Neoplasm, malignant,
  by site
  eccrine dermal —*see* Neoplasm, skin, benign
  skin —*see* Neoplasm, skin, benign
Cylindruria R82.99
Cynanche
  diphtheritic A36.2
  tonsillaris J36
Cynophobia F40.218
Cynorexia R63.2
Cyphosis —*see* Kyphosis
Cyprus fever —*see* Brucellosis
Cyst (colloid) (mucous) (simple) (retention)
  adenoid (infected) J35.8
  adrenal gland E27.8
    congenital Q89.1
  air, lung J98.4
  allantoic Q64.4
  alveolar process (jaw bone) M27.40
  amnion, amniotic O41.8X
  anterior
    chamber (eye) —*see* Cyst, iris
    nasopalatine K09.1
  antrum J34.1
  anus K62.89
  apical (tooth) (periodontal) K04.8
  appendix K38.8
  arachnoid, brain (acquired) G93.0
    congenital Q04.6
  arytenoid J38.7
  Baker's M71.2
    ruptured M66.0
    tuberculous A18.02
  Bartholin's gland N75.0
  bile duct (common) (hepatic) K83.5
  bladder (multiple) (trigone) N32.89
  blue dome (breast) —*see* Cyst, breast
  bone (local) NEC M85.60
    aneurysmal M85.50
      ankle M85.57
      foot M85.57
      forearm M85.53
      hand M85.54
      jaw M27.49
      lower leg M85.56
      multiple site M85.59
      neck M85.58
      rib M85.58
      shoulder M85.51
      skull M85.58
      specified site NEC M85.58
      thigh M85.55
      toe M85.57
      upper arm M85.52
      vertebra M85.58
    solitary M85.40
      ankle M85.47
      fibula M85.46
      foot M85.47
      hand M85.44
      humerus M85.42

Cyst – *continued*
      jaw M27.49
      neck M85.48
      pelvis M85.45
      radius M85.43
      rib M85.48
      shoulder M85.41
      skull M85.48
      specified site NEC M85.48
      tibia M85.46
      toe M85.47
      ulna M85.43
      vertebra M85.48
    specified type NEC M85.60
      ankle M85.67
      foot M85.67
      forearm M85.63
      hand M85.64
      jaw M27.40
        developmental (nonodontogenic) K09.1
          odontogenic K09.0
        latent M27.0
      lower leg M85.66
      multiple site M85.69
      neck M85.68
      rib M85.68
      shoulder M85.61
      skull M85.68
      specified site NEC M85.68
      thigh M85.65
      toe M85.67
      upper arm M85.62
      vertebra M85.68
  brain (acquired) G93.0
    congenital Q04.6
    hydatid B67.99 *[G94]*
    third ventricle (colloid) , congenital Q04.6
  branchial (cleft) Q18.0
  branchiogenic Q18.0
  breast (benign) (blue dome) (pedunculated)
  (solitary) N60.0
    involution —*see* Dysplasia, mammary,
    specified type NEC
    sebaceous —*see* Dysplasia, mammary,
    specified type NEC
  broad ligament (benign) N83.8
  bronchogenic (mediastinal) (sequestration)
  J98.4
    congenital Q33.0
  buccal K09.8
  bulbourethral gland N36.8
  bursa, bursal NEC M71.30
    with rupture —*see* Rupture, synovium
    ankle M71.37
    elbow M71.32
    foot M71.37
    hand M71.34
    hip M71.35
    multiple sites M71.39
    pharyngeal J39.2
    popliteal space —*see* Cyst, Baker's
    shoulder M71.31
    specified site NEC M71.38
    wrist M71.33
  calcifying odontogenic D16.5
    upper jaw (bone) (maxilla) D16.4
  canal of Nuck (female) N94.89
    congenital Q52.4
  canthus —*see* Cyst, conjunctiva
  carcinomatous —*see* Neoplasm, malignant,
  by site
  cauda equina G95.89
  cavum septi pellucidi —*see* Cyst, brain

Cyst – *continued*
celomic (pericardium) Q24.8
cerebellopontine (angle) —*see* Cyst, brain
cerebellum —*see* Cyst, brain
cerebral —*see* Cyst, brain
cervical lateral Q18.1
cervix NEC N88.8
  embryonic Q51.6
  nabothian N88.8
chiasmal optic NEC —*see* Disorder, optic, chiasm
chocolate (ovary) N80.1
choledochus, congenital Q44.4
chorion O41.8X
choroid plexus G93.0
ciliary body —*see* Cyst, iris
clitoris N90.7
colon K63.89
common (bile) duct K83.5
congenital NEC Q89.8
  adrenal gland Q89.1
  epiglottis Q31.8
  esophagus Q39.8
  fallopian tube Q50.4
  kidney Q61.00
    more than one (multiple) Q61.02
      specified as polycystic Q61.3
        adult type Q61.2
        infantile type NEC Q61.19
          collecting duct dilation Q61.11
    solitary Q61.01
  larynx Q31.8
  liver Q44.6
  lung Q33.0
  mediastinum Q34.1
  ovary Q50.1
  oviduct Q50.4
  periurethral (tissue) Q64.79
  prepuce Q55.69
  salivary gland (any) Q38.4
  sublingual Q38.6
  submaxillary gland Q38.6
  thymus (gland) Q89.2
  tongue Q38.3
  ureterovesical orifice Q62.8
  vulva Q52.79
conjunctiva H11.44
cornea H18.89
corpora quadrigemina G93.0
corpus
  albicans N83.29
  luteum (hemorrhagic) (ruptured) N83.1
Cowper's gland (benign) (infected) N36.8
cranial meninges G93.0
craniobuccal pouch E23.6
craniopharyngeal pouch E23.6
cystic duct K82.8
Cysticercus —*see* Cysticercosis
Dandy-Walker Q03.1
  with spina bifida —*see* Spina bifida
dental (root) K04.8
  developmental K09.0
  eruption K09.0
  primordial K09.0
dentigerous (mandible) (maxilla) K09.0
dermoid —*see* Neoplasm, benign, by site
  with malignant transformation C56.
  implantation
    external area or site (skin) NEC L72.0
    iris —*see* Cyst, iris, implantation
    vagina N89.8
    vulva N90.7

Cyst – *continued*
  mouth K09.8
  oral soft tissue K09.8
  sacrococcygeal —*see* Cyst, pilonidal
developmental K09.1
  odontogenic K09.0
  oral region (nonodontogenic) K09.1
  ovary, ovarian Q50.1
dura (cerebral) G93.0
  spinal G96.19
ear (external) Q18.1
echinococcal —*see* Echinococcus
embryonic
  cervix uteri Q51.6
  fallopian tube Q50.4
  vagina Q51.6
endometrium, endometrial (uterus) N85.8
  ectopic —*see* Endometriosis
enterogenous Q43.8
epidermal, epidermoid (inclusion) (see also Cyst, skin) L72.0
  mouth K09.8
  oral soft tissue K09.8
epididymis N50.3
epiglottis J38.7
epiphysis cerebri E34.8
epithelial (inclusion) L72.0
epoophoron Q50.5
eruption K09.0
esophagus K22.8
ethmoid sinus J34.1
external female genital organs NEC N90.7
eye NEC H57.8
  congenital Q15.8
eyelid (sebaceous) H02.829
  infected —*see* Hordeolum
  left H02.826
    lower H02.825
    upper H02.824
  right H02.823
    lower H02.822
    upper H02.821
fallopian tube N83.8
  congenital Q50.4
fimbrial (twisted) Q50.4
fissural (oral region) K09.1
follicle (graafian) (hemorrhagic) N83.0
  nabothian N88.8
follicular (atretic) (hemorrhagic) (ovarian) N83.0
  dentigerous K09.0
  odontogenic K09.0
  skin L72.9
    specified NEC L72.8
frontal sinus J34.1
gallbladder K82.8
ganglion —*see* Ganglion
Gartner's duct Q52.4
gingiva K09.0
gland of Moll —*see* Cyst, eyelid
globulomaxillary K09.1
graafian follicle (hemorrhagic) N83.0
granulosal lutein (hemorrhagic) N83.1
hemangiomatous D18.00
  intra-abdominal D18.03
  intracranial D18.02
  skin D18.01
  specified site NEC D18.09
hydatid (*see also* Echinococcus) B67.90
  brain B67.99 *[G94]*
  liver (*see also* Cyst, liver, hydatid) B67.8
  lung NEC B67.99 *[J99]*

Cyst – *continued*
  Morgagni
    female Q50.5
    male (epididymal) Q55.4
    testicular Q55.29
  specified site NEC B67.99
  hymen N89.8
    embryonic Q52.4
  hypopharynx J39.2
  hypophysis, hypophyseal (duct) (recurrent) E23.6
    cerebri E23.6
  implantation (dermoid)
    external area or site (skin) NEC L72.0
    iris —*see* Cyst, iris, implantation
    vagina N89.8
    vulva N90.7
  incisive canal K09.1
  inclusion (epidermal) (epithelial) (epidermoid) (squamous) L72.0
    not of skin
  code under Cyst, by site
  intestine (large) (small) K63.89
  intracranial —*see* Cyst, brain
  intraligamentous —*see also* Disorder, ligament
    knee —*see* Derangement, knee
  intrasellar E23.6
  iris H21.309
    exudative H21.31
    idiopathic H21.30
    implantation H21.32
    parasitic H21.33
    pars plana (primary) H21.34
      exudative H21.35
  jaw (bone) M27.40
    aneurysmal M27.49
    hemorrhagic M27.49
    traumatic M27.49
    developmental (odontogenic) K09.0
    fissural K09.1
  joint NEC —*see* Disorder, joint, specified type NEC
  kidney (acquired) N28.1
    calyceal —*see* Hydronephrosis
    congenital Q61.00
      more than one (multiple) Q61.02
        specified as polycystic Q61.3
          adult type (autosomal dominant) Q61.2
          infantile type (autosomal recessive) NEC Q61.19
            collecting duct dilation Q61.11
    pyelogenic —*see* Hydronephrosis
    simple N28.1
    solitary (single) Q61.01
      acquired N28.1
  labium (majus) (minus) N90.7
    sebaceous N90.7
  lacrimal —*see also* Disorder, lacrimal system, specified NEC
    gland H04.13
    passages or sac —*see* Disorder, lacrimal system, specified NEC
  larynx J38.7
  lateral periodontal K09.0
  lens H27.8
    congenital Q12.8
  lip (gland) K13.0
  liver (idiopathic) (simple) K76.89
    congenital Q44.6
    hydatid B67.8
      granulosus B67.0
      multilocularis B67.5

Cyst – *continued*
lung J98.4
  congenital Q33.0
  giant bullous J43.9
lutein N83.1
lymphangiomatous D18.1
lymphoepithelial, oral soft tissue K09.8
macula —*see* Degeneration, macula, hole
malignant —*see* Neoplasm, malignant, by site
mammary gland —*see* Cyst, breast
mandible M27.40
  dentigerous K09.0
  radicular K04.8
maxilla M27.40
  dentigerous K09.0
  radicular K04.8
medial, face and neck Q18.8
median
  anterior maxillary K09.1
  palatal K09.1
mediastinum, congenital Q34.1
meibomian (gland) —*see* Chalazion
  infected —*see* Hordeolum
membrane, brain G93.0
meninges (cerebral) G93.0
  spinal G96.19
meniscus, knee —*see* Derangement, knee,
meniscus, cystic
mesentery, mesenteric K66.8
  chyle I89.8
mesonephric duct
  female Q50.5
  male Q55.4
milk N64.89
Morgagni (hydatid)
  female Q50.5
  male (epididymal) Q55.4
    testicular Q55.29
mouth K09.8
Müllerian duct Q50.4
  appendix testis Q55.29
  cervix Q51.6
  fallopian tube Q50.4
  female Q50.4
  male Q55.29
  prostatic utricle Q55.4
  vagina (embryonal) Q52.4
multilocular (ovary) D39.10
  benign —*see* Neoplasm, benign, by site
myometrium N85.8
nabothian (follicle) (ruptured) N88.8
nasoalveolar K09.1
nasolabial K09.1
nasopalatine (anterior) (duct) K09.1
nasopharynx J39.2
neoplastic —*see* Neoplasm, uncertain
behavior, by site
  benign —*see* Neoplasm, benign, by site
nervous system NEC G96.8
neuroenteric (congenital) Q06.8
nipple —*see* Cyst, breast
nose (turbinates) J34.1
  sinus J34.1
odontogenic, developmental K09.0
omentum (lesser) K66.8
  congenital Q45.8
ora serrata —*see* Cyst, retina, ora serrata
oral
  region K09.9
    developmental (nonodontogenic) K09.1
    specified NEC K09.8
  soft tissue K09.9

Cyst – *continued*
  specified NEC K09.8
orbit H05.81
ovary, ovarian (twisted) N83.20
  adherent N83.20
  chocolate N80.1
  corpus
    albicans N83.29
    luteum (hemorrhagic) N83.1
  dermoid D27.9
  developmental Q50.1
  due to failure of involution NEC N83.20
  endometrial N80.1
  follicular (graafian) (hemorrhagic) N83.0
  hemorrhagic N83.20
  in pregnancy or childbirth O34.8
    with obstructed labor O65.5
  multilocular D39.10
  pseudomucinous D27.9
  retention N83.29
  serous N83.20
  specified NEC N83.29
  theca lutein (hemorrhagic) N83.1
  tuberculous A18.18
oviduct N83.8
palate (median) (fissural) K09.1
palatine papilla (jaw) K09.1
pancreas, pancreatic (hemorrhagic) (true)
K86.2
  congenital Q45.2
  false K86.3
paralabral
  hip M24.85
  shoulder S43.43
paramesonephric duct Q50.4
  female Q50.4
  male Q55.29
paranephric N28.1
paraphysis, cerebri, congenital Q04.6
parasitic B89
parathyroid (gland) E21.4
paratubal N83.8
paraurethral duct N36.8
paroophoron Q50.5
parotid gland K11.6
parovarian Q50.5
pelvis, female N94.89
  in pregnancy or childbirth O34.8
    causing obstructed labor O65.5
penis (sebaceous) N48.89
periapical K04.8
pericardial (congenital) Q24.8
  acquired (secondary) I31.8
pericoronal K09.0
periodontal K04.8
  lateral K09.0
peripelvic (lymphatic) N28.1
peritoneum K66.8
  chylous I89.8
periventricular, acquired, newborn P91.1
pharynx (wall) J39.2
pilar L72.11
pilonidal (infected) (rectum) L05.91
  with abscess L05.01
  malignant C44.59
pituitary (duct) (gland) E23.6
placenta O43.19
pleura J94.8
popliteal —*see* Cyst, Baker's
porencephalic Q04.6
  acquired G93.0
postanal (infected) —*see* Cyst, pilonidal

Cyst – *continued*
postmastoidectomy cavity (mucosal) —*see*
Complications, postmastoidectomy, cyst
preauricular Q18.1
prepuce N47.4
  congenital Q55.69
primordial (jaw) K09.0
prostate N42.83
pseudomucinous (ovary) D27.9
pupillary, miotic H21.27
radicular (residual) K04.8
radiculodental K04.8
ranular K11.8
Rathke's pouch E23.6
rectum (epithelium) (mucous) K62.89
renal —*see* Cyst, kidney
residual (radicular) K04.8
retention (ovary) N83.29
  salivary gland K11.6
retina H33.19
  ora serrata H33.11
  parasitic H33.12
retroperitoneal K68.9
sacrococcygeal (dermoid) —*see* Cyst,
pilonidal
salivary gland or duct (mucous extravasation
or retention) K11.6
Sampson's N80.1
sclera H15.89
scrotum L72.9
  sebaceous L72.3
sebaceous (duct) (gland) L72.3
  breast —*see* Dysplasia, mammary, specified
type NEC
  eyelid —*see* Cyst, eyelid
  genital organ NEC
    female N94.89
    male N50.8
  scrotum L72.3
semilunar cartilage (knee) (multiple) —*see*
Derangement, knee, meniscus, cystic
seminal vesicle N50.8
serous (ovary) N83.20
sinus (accessory) (nasal) J34.1
Skene's gland N36.8
skin L72.9
  breast —*see* Dysplasia, mammary, specified
type NEC
  epidermal, epidermoid L72.0
  epithelial L72.0
  eyelid —*see* Cyst, eyelid
  genital organ NEC
    female N90.7
    male N50.8
  inclusion L72.0
  scrotum L72.9
  sebaceous L72.3
  sweat gland or duct L74.8
solitary
  bone —*see* Cyst, bone, solitary
  jaw M27.40
  kidney N28.1
spermatic cord N50.8
sphenoid sinus J34.1
spinal meninges G96.19
spleen NEC D73.4
  congenital Q89.09
  hydatid (*see also* Echinococcus) B67.99
[D77]
Stafne's M27.0
subarachnoid intrasellar R93.0
subcutaneous, pheomycotic (chromomycotic)
B43.2

Cyst – *continued*
  subdural (cerebral) G93.0
    spinal cord G96.19
  sublingual gland K11.6
  submandibular gland K11.6
  submaxillary gland K11.6
  suburethral N36.8
  suprarenal gland E27.8
  suprasellar —*see* Cyst, brain
  sweat gland or duct L74.8
  synovial —*see also* Cyst, bursa
    ruptured —*see* Rupture, synovium
  tarsal —*see* Chalazion
  tendon (sheath) —*see* Disorder, tendon,
  specified type NEC
  testis N44.2
    tunica albuginea N44.1
  theca lutein (ovary) N83.1
  Thornwaldt's J39.2
  thymus (gland) E32.8
  thyroglossal duct (infected) (persistent) Q89.2
  thyrolingual duct (infected) (persistent) Q89.2
  thyroid (gland) E04.1
  tongue K14.8
  tonsil J35.8
  tooth —*see* Cyst, dental
  Tornwaldt's J39.2
  trichilemmal (proliferating) L72.12
  trichodermal L72.12
  tubal (fallopian) N83.8
    inflammatory —*see* Salpingitis, chronic
  tubo-ovarian N83.8
    inflammatory N70.13
  tunica
    albuginea testis N44.1
    vaginalis N50.8
  turbinate (nose) J34.1
  Tyson's gland N48.89
  urachus, congenital Q64.4
  ureter N28.89
  ureterovesical orifice N28.89
  urethra, urethral (gland) N36.8
  uterine ligament N83.8
  uterus (body) (corpus) (recurrent) N85.8
    embryonic Q51.818
      cervix Q51.6
  vagina, vaginal (implantation) (inclusion)
  (squamous cell) (wall) N89.8
    embryonic Q52.4
  vallecula, vallecular (epiglottis) J38.7
  vesical (orifice) N32.89
  vitreous body H43.89
  vulva (implantation) (inclusion) N90.7
    congenital Q52.79
    sebaceous gland N90.7
  vulvovaginal gland N90.7
  wolffian
    female Q50.5
    male Q55.4
Cystadenocarcinoma —*see* Neoplasm,
malignant, by site
  bile duct C22.1
  endometrioid —*see* Neoplasm, malignant, by
site
    specified site —*see* Neoplasm, malignant,
      by site
    unspecified site
      female C56.9
      male C61
  mucinous
    papillary

Cystadenocarcinoma   - *continued*
    specified site —*see* Neoplasm, malignant,
    by site
      unspecified site C56.9
    specified site —*see* Neoplasm, malignant,
    by site
    unspecified site C56.9
  papillary
    mucinous
      specified site —*see* Neoplasm, malignant,
      by site
      unspecified site C56.9
    pseudomucinous
      specified site —*see* Neoplasm, malignant,
      by site
      unspecified site C56.9
    serous
      specified site —*see* Neoplasm, malignant,
      by site
      unspecified site C56.9
    specified site —*see* Neoplasm, malignant,
    by site
    unspecified site C56.9
  pseudomucinous
    papillary
      specified site —*see* Neoplasm, malignant,
      by site
      unspecified site C56.9
    specified site —*see* Neoplasm, malignant,
    by site
    unspecified site C56.9
  serous
    papillary
      specified site —*see* Neoplasm, malignant,
      by site
      unspecified site C56.9
    specified site —*see* Neoplasm, malignant,
    by site
    unspecified site C56.9
Cystadenofibroma
  clear cell —*see* Neoplasm, benign, by site
  endometrioid D27.9
    borderline malignancy D39.1
    malignant C56.
  mucinous
    specified site —*see* Neoplasm, benign, by
    site
    unspecified site D27.9
  serous
    specified site —*see* Neoplasm, benign, by
    site
    unspecified site D27.9
  specified site —*see* Neoplasm, benign, by site
  unspecified site D27.9
Cystadenoma —*see also* Neoplasm, benign,
by site
  bile duct D13.4
  endometrioid —*see* Neoplasm, benign, by site
    borderline malignancy —*see* Neoplasm,
  uncertain behavior, by site
  malignant —*see* Neoplasm, malignant, by site
  mucinous
    borderline malignancy
      ovary C56.
      specified site NEC —*see* Neoplasm,
  uncertain behavior, by site
      unspecified site C56.9
    papillary
      borderline malignancy
        ovary C56.
        specified site NEC —*see* Neoplasm,
  uncertain behavior, by site

Cystadenoma   - *continued*
    unspecified site C56.9
      specified site —*see* Neoplasm, benign, by
      site
      unspecified site D27.9
    specified site —*see* Neoplasm, benign, by
    site
    unspecified site D27.9
  papillary
    borderline malignancy
      ovary C56
      specified site NEC —*see* Neoplasm,
  uncertain behavior, by site
      unspecified site C56.9
    lymphomatosum
      specified site —*see* Neoplasm, benign, by
      site
      unspecified site D11.9
    mucinous
      borderline malignancy
        ovary C56.
        specified site NEC —*see* Neoplasm,
  uncertain behavior, by site
        unspecified site C56.9
      specified site —*see* Neoplasm, benign, by
      site
      unspecified site D27.9
    pseudomucinous
      borderline malignancy
        ovary C56.
        specified site NEC —*see* Neoplasm,
  uncertain behavior, by site
        unspecified site C56.9
      specified site —*see* Neoplasm, benign, by
      site
      unspecified site D27.9
    serous
      borderline malignancy
        ovary C56.
        specified site NEC —*see* Neoplasm,
  uncertain behavior, by site
        unspecified site C56.9
      specified site —*see* Neoplasm, benign, by
      site
      unspecified site D27.9
    specified site —*see* Neoplasm, benign, by
    site
    unspecified site D27.9
  pseudomucinous
    borderline malignancy
      ovary C56.
      specified site NEC —*see* Neoplasm,
  uncertain behavior, by site
      unspecified site C56.9
    papillary
      borderline malignancy
        ovary C56.
        specified site NEC —*see* Neoplasm,
  uncertain behavior, by site
        unspecified site C56.9
      specified site —*see* Neoplasm, benign, by
      site
      unspecified site D27.9
    specified site —*see* Neoplasm, benign, by
    site
    unspecified site D27.9
  serous
    borderline malignancy
      ovary C56.
      specified site NEC —*see* Neoplasm,
  uncertain behavior, by site
      unspecified site C56.9

Cystadenoma - *continued*
  papillary
    borderline malignancy
      ovary C56.
        specified site NEC —*see* Neoplasm,
  uncertain behavior, by site
        unspecified site C56.9
      specified site —*see* Neoplasm, benign, by
      site
      unspecified site D27.9
    specified site —*see* Neoplasm, benign, by
    site
    unspecified site D27.9
Cystathionine synthase deficiency E72.11
Cystathioninemia E72.19
Cystathioninuria E72.19
Cystic —*see also* condition
  breast (chronic) —*see* Mastopathy, cystic
  corpora lutea (hemorrhagic) N83.1
  duct —*see* condition
  eyeball (congenital) Q11.0
  fibrosis —*see* Fibrosis, cystic
  kidney (congenital) Q61.9
    adult type Q61.2
    infantile type NEC Q61.19
      collecting duct dilatation Q61.11
    medullary Q61.5
  liver, congenital Q44.6
  lung disease J98.4
    congenital Q33.0
  mastitis, chronic —*see* Mastopathy, cystic
  medullary, kidney Q61.5
  meniscus —*see* Derangement, knee,
  meniscus, cystic
  ovary N83.20
Cysticercosis, cysticerciasis B69.9
  with
    epileptiform fits B69.0
    myositis B69.81
  brain B69.0
  central nervous system B69.0
  cerebral B69.0
  ocular B69.1
  specified NEC B69.89
Cysticercus cellulose infestation —*see*
Cysticercosis
Cystinosis (malignant) E72.04
Cystinuria E72.01
Cystitis (exudative) (hemorrhagic) (septic)
(suppurative) N30.90
  with
    fibrosis —*see* Cystitis, chronic, interstitial
    hematuria N30.91
    leukoplakia —*see* Cystitis, chronic,
    interstitial
    malakoplakia —*see* Cystitis, chronic,
    interstitial
    metaplasia —*see* Cystitis, chronic,
    interstitial
    prostatitis N41.3
  acute N30.00
    with hematuria N30.01
    of trigone N30.30
      with hematuria N30.31
  allergic —*see* Cystitis, specified type NEC
  amebic A06.81
  bilharzial B65.9 *[N33]*
  blennorrhagic (gonococcal) A54.01
  bullous —*see* Cystitis, specified type NEC
  calculous N21.0
  chlamydial A56.01

Cystitis – *continued*
  chronic N30.20
    with hematuria N30.21
    interstitial N30.10
      with hematuria N30.11
    of trigone N30.30
      with hematuria N30.31
    specified NEC N30.20
      with hematuria N30.21
  cystic (a) —*see* Cystitis, specified type NEC
  diphtheritic A36.85
  echinococcal
    granulosus B67.39
    multilocularis B67.69
  emphysematous —*see* Cystitis, specified type
NEC
  encysted —*see* Cystitis, specified type NEC
  eosinophilic —*see* Cystitis, specified type
NEC
  follicular —*see* Cystitis, of trigone
  gangrenous —*see* Cystitis, specified type
NEC
  glandularis —*see* Cystitis, specified type NEC
  gonococcal A54.01
  incrusted —*see* Cystitis, specified type NEC
  interstitial (chronic) —*see* Cystitis, chronic,
  interstitial
  irradiation N30.40
    with hematuria N30.41
  irritation —*see* Cystitis, specified type NEC
  malignant —*see* Cystitis, specified type NEC
  of trigone N30.30
    with hematuria N30.31
  panmural —*see* Cystitis, chronic, interstitial
  polyposa —*see* Cystitis, specified type NEC
  prostatic N41.3
  puerperal (postpartum) O86.22
  radiation —*see* Cystitis, irradiation
  specified type NEC N30.80
    with hematuria N30.81
  subacute —*see* Cystitis, chronic
  submucous —*see* Cystitis, chronic, interstitial
  syphilitic (late) A52.76
  trichomonal A59.03
  tuberculous A18.12
  ulcerative —*see* Cystitis, chronic, interstitial
Cystocele (-urethrocele)
  female N81.10
    with prolapse of uterus —*see* Prolapse,
  uterus
    lateral N81.12
    midline N81.11
    paravaginal N81.12
  in pregnancy or childbirth O34.8
    causing obstructed labor O65.5
  male N32.89
Cystolithiasis N21.0
Cystoma —*see also* Neoplasm, benign, by site
  endometrial, ovary N80.1
  mucinous
    specified site —*see* Neoplasm, benign, by
  site
    unspecified site D27.9
  serous
    specified site —*see* Neoplasm, benign, by
  site
    unspecified site D27.9
  simple (ovary) N83.29
Cystoplegia N31.2
Cystoptosis N32.89
Cystopyelitis —*see* Pyelonephritis
Cystorrhagia N32.89

Cystosarcoma phyllodes D48.6
  benign D24
  malignant —*see* Neoplasm, breast, malignant
Cystostomy
  attention to Z43.5
  complication —*see* Complications,
  cystostomy
  status Z93.50
    appendico-vesicostomy Z93.52
    cutaneous Z93.51
    specified NEC Z93.59
Cystourethritis —*see* Urethritis
Cystourethrocele —*see also* Cystocele
  female N81.10
    with uterine prolapse —*see* Prolapse, uterus
    lateral N81.12
    midline N81.11
    paravaginal N81.12
  male N32.89
Cytomegalic inclusion disease
  congenital P35.1
Cytomegalovirus infection B25.9
Cytomycosis (reticuloendothelial) B39.4
Cytopenia D75.9
  refractory
    with multilineage dysplasia D46.A
    and ring sideroblasts (RCMD RS) D46.B
Czerny's disease (periodic hydrarthrosis of the
knee) —*see* Effusion, joint, knee

D

Daae (-Finsen) disease (epidemic pleurodynia)
B33.0
Da Costa's syndrome F45.8
Dabney's grip B33.0
Dacryoadenitis, dacryadenitis H04.00
  acute H04.01
  chronic H04.02
Dacryocystitis H04.30
  acute H04.32
  chronic H04.41
  neonatal P39.1
  phlegmonous H04.31
  syphilitic A52.71
    congenital (early) A50.01
  trachomatous, active A71.1
    sequelae (late effect) B94.0
Dacryocystoblennorrhea —*see* Inflammation,
lacrimal, passages, chronic
Dacryocystocele —*see* Disorder, lacrimal
system, changes
Dacryolith, dacryolithiasis H04.51
Dacryoma —*see* Disorder, lacrimal system,
changes
Dacryopericystitis —*see* Dacryocystitis
Dacryops H04.11
Dacryostenosis —*see also* Stenosis, lacrimal
  congenital Q10.5
Dactylitis
  bone —*see* Osteomyelitis
  sickle-cell D57.00
    Hb C D57.219
    Hb SS D57.00
    specified NEC D57.819
  skin L08.9
  syphilitic A52.77
  tuberculous A18.03
Dactylolysis spontanea (ainhum) L94.6
Dactylosymphysis Q70.9
  fingers —*see* Syndactylism, complex, fingers
  toes —*see* Syndactylism, complex, toes

Damage
  arteriosclerotic —*see* Arteriosclerosis
  brain (nontraumatic) G93.9
    anoxic, hypoxic G93.1
      resulting from a procedure G97.82
    child NEC G80.9
    due to birth injury P11.2
  cardiorenal (vascular) —*see* Hypertension,
    cardiorenal
  cerebral NEC —*see* Damage, brain
  coccyx, complicating delivery O71.6
  coronary —*see* Disease, heart, ischemic
  eye, birth injury P15.3
  liver (nontraumatic) K76.9
    alcoholic K70.9
    due to drugs —*see* Disease, liver, toxic
    toxic —*see* Disease, liver, toxic
  medication T88.7
  pelvic
    joint or ligament, during delivery O71.6
    organ NEC
      during delivery O71.5
      following ectopic or molar pregnancy
      O08.6
  renal —*see* Disease, renal
  subendocardium, subendocardial —*see*
    Degeneration, myocardial
  vascular I99.9
Dana-Putnam syndrome (subacute combined
  sclerosis with pernicious anemia) —*see*
  Degeneration, combined
Danbolt (-Cross) **syndrome** (acrodermatitis
  enteropathica) E83.2
Dandruff L21.0
Dandy-Walker syndrome Q03.1
  with spina bifida —*see* Spina bifida
Danlos' syndrome Q79.6
Darier (-White) **disease** (congenital) Q82.8
  meaning erythema annulare centrifugum
  L53.1
Darier-Roussy sarcoid D86.3
Darling's disease or histoplasmosis B39.4
Darwin's tubercle Q17.8
Dawson's (inclusion body) **encephalitis** A81.1
De Beurmann (-Gougerot) **disease** B42.1
De la Tourette's syndrome F95.2
De Lange's syndrome Q87.1
De Morgan's spots (senile angiomas) I78.1
De Quervain's
  disease (tendon sheath) M65.4
  syndrome E34.51
  thyroiditis (subacute granulomatous
    thyroiditis) E06.1
De Toni-Fanconi (-Debré) **syndrome** E72.09
  with cystinosis E72.04
Dead
  fetus, retained (mother) O36.4
    early pregnancy O02.1
  labyrinth —*see* subcategory H83.2
  ovum, retained O02.0
Deaf nonspeaking NEC H91.3
Deafmutism (acquired) (congenital) **NEC**
  H91.3
  hysterical F44.6
  syphilitic, congenital (*see also* subcategory
    H94.8) A50.09
Deafness (acquired) (complete) (hereditary)
  (partial) H91.9
-with blue sclera and fragility of bone Q78.0
  auditory fatigue —*see* Deafness, specified
    type NEC

Deafness - *continued*
  aviation T70.0
    nerve injury —*see* Injury, nerve, acoustic,
    specified type NEC
  boilermaker's —*see* subcategory H83.3
  central —*see* Deafness, sensorineural
  conductive H90.2
    and sensorineural, mixed H90.8
      bilateral H90.6
    bilateral H90.0
    unilateral H90.1
-congenital H90.5
    with blue sclera and fragility of bone Q78.0
  due to toxic agents —*see* Deafness, ototoxic
  emotional (hysterical) F44.6
  functional (hysterical) F44.6
  high frequency H91.9
  hysterical F44.6
  low frequency H91.9
-mental R48.8
  mixed conductive and sensorineural H90.8
    bilateral H90.6
    unilateral H90.7
  nerve —*see* Deafness, sensorineural
  neural —*see* Deafness, sensorineural
  noise-induced (*see also* subcategory) H83.3
    nerve injury —*see* Injury, nerve, acoustic,
    specified type NEC
  nonspeaking H91.3
  ototoxic —*see* subcategory H91.0
  perceptive —*see* Deafness, sensorineural
  psychogenic (hysterical) F44.6
  sensorineural H90.5
    and conductive, mixed H90.8
      bilateral H90.6
    bilateral H90.3
    unilateral H90.4
  sensory —*see* Deafness, sensorineural
  specified type NEC —*see* subcategory H91.8
  sudden (idiopathic) H91.2
  syphilitic A52.15
  transient ischemic H93.01
  traumatic —*see* Injury, nerve, acoustic,
    specified type NEC
  word (developmental) H93.25
Death (cause unknown) (of) (unexplained)
  (unspecified cause) R99
  brain G93.82
  cardiac (sudden) (with successful
    resuscitation)
  code to underlying disease
    family history of Z82.41
    personal history of Z86.74
  family member (assumed) Z63.4
Debility (chronic) (general) (nervous) R53.81
  congenital or neonatal NOS P96.9
  nervous R53.81
  old age R54
  senile R54
Débove's disease (splenomegaly) R16.1
Decalcification
  bone —*see* Osteoporosis
  teeth K03.89
Decapsulation, kidney N28.89
Decay
  dental —*see* Caries, dental
  senile R54
  tooth, teeth —*see* Caries, dental
Deciduitis (acute)
  following ectopic or molar pregnancy O08.0
Decline (general) —*see* Debility
  cognitive, age-associated R41.81

Decompensation
  cardiac (acute) (chronic) —*see* Disease, heart
  cardiovascular —*see* Disease, cardiovascular
  heart —*see* Disease, heart
  hepatic —*see* Failure, hepatic
  myocardial (acute) (chronic) —*see* Disease,
    heart
  respiratory J98.8
Decompression sickness T70.3
Decrease (d)
  absolute neutrophile count —*see* Neutropenia
  blood
    platelets —*see* Thrombocytopenia
    pressure R03.1
      due to shock following
        injury T79.4
        operation T81.19
  estrogen E28.39
    postablative E89.40
      asymptomatic E89.40
      symptomatic E89.41
  fragility of erythrocytes D58.8
  function
    lipase (pancreatic) K90.3
    ovary in hypopituitarism E23.0
    parenchyma of pancreas K86.8
    pituitary (gland) (anterior) (lobe) E23.0
      posterior (lobe) E23.0
  functional activity R68.89
  glucose R73.09
  hematocrit R71.0
  hemoglobin R71.0
  leukocytes D72.819
    specified NEC D72.818
  libido R68.82
  lymphocytes D72.810
  platelets D69.6
  respiration, due to shock following injury
    T79.4
  sexual desire R68.82
  tear secretion NEC —*see* Syndrome, dry eye
  tolerance
    fat K90.4
    glucose R73.09
    pancreatic K90.3
  salt and water E87.8
  vision NEC H54.7
  white blood cell count D72.819
    specified NEC D72.818
Decubitus (ulcer) —*see* Ulcer, pressure, by site
  cervix N86
Deepening acetabulum —*see* Derangement,
  joint, specified type NEC, hip
Defect, defective Q89.9
  3-beta-hydroxysteroid dehydrogenase E25.0
  11-hydroxylase E25.0
  21-hydroxylase E25.0
  abdominal wall, congenital Q79.59
  antibody immunodeficiency D80.9
  aorticopulmonary septum Q21.4
  atrial septal (ostium secundum type) Q21.1
    following acute myocardial infarction
    (current complication) I23.1
    ostium primum type Q21.2
  atrioventricular
    canal Q21.2
    septum Q21.2
  auricular septal Q21.1
  bilirubin excretion NEC E80.6
  biosynthesis, androgen (testicular) E29.1
  bulbar septum Q21.0
  catalase E80.3
  cell membrane receptor complex (CR3) D71

Defect, defective - *continued*
circulation I99.9
  congenital Q28.9
  newborn Q28.9
coagulation (factor) (*see also* Deficiency, factor) D68.9
  with
    ectopic pregnancy O08.1
    molar pregnancy O08.1
  acquired D68.4
  antepartum with hemorrhage —*see* Hemorrhage, antepartum, with coagulation defect
  due to
    liver disease D68.4
    vitamin K deficiency D68.4
  hereditary NEC D68.2
  intrapartum O67.0
  newborn, transient P61.6
  postpartum O72.3
  specified type NEC D68.8
complement system D84.1
conduction (heart) I45.9
  bone —*see* Deafness, conductive
congenital, organ or site not listed —*see* Anomaly, by site
coronary sinus Q21.1
cushion, endocardial Q21.2
degradation, glycoprotein E77.1
dental bridge, crown, fillings —*see* Defect, dental restoration
dental restoration K08.50
  specified NEC K08.59
dentin (hereditary) K00.5
Descemet's membrane, congenital Q13.89
developmental —*see also* Anomaly
  cauda equina Q06.3
diaphragm
  with elevation, eventration or hernia —*see* Hernia, diaphragm
  congenital Q79.1
    with hernia Q79.0
    gross (with hernia) Q79.0
ectodermal, congenital Q82.9
Eisenmenger's Q21.8
enzyme
  catalase E80.3
  peroxidase E80.3
esophagus, congenital Q39.9
extensor retinaculum M62.89
fibrin polymerization D68.2
filling
  bladder R93.4
  kidney R93.4
  stomach R93.3
  ureter R93.4
Gerbode Q21.0
glycoprotein degradation E77.1
Hageman (factor) D68.2
hearing —*see* Deafness
high grade F70
interatrial septal Q21.1
interauricular septal Q21.1
interventricular septal Q21.0
  with dextroposition of aorta, pulmonary stenosis and hypertrophy of right ventricle Q21.3
    in tetralogy of Fallot Q21.3
learning (specific) —*see* Disorder, learning
lymphocyte function antigen 1 (LFA 1) D84.0

Defect, defective - *continued*
lysosomal enzyme, post-translational modification E77.0
major osseous M89.70
  ankle M89.77
  carpus M89.74
  clavicle M89.71
  femur M89.75
  fibula M89.76
  fingers M89.74
  foot M89.77
  forearm M89.73
  hand M89.74
  humerus M89.72
  lower leg M89.76
  metacarpus M89.74
  metatarsus M89.77
  multiple sites M89.79
  pelvic region M89.75
  pelvis M89.75
  radius M89.73
  scapula M89.71
  shoulder region M89.71
  specified NEC M89.78
  tarsus M89.77
  thigh M89.75
  tibia M89.76
  toes M89.77
  ulna M89.73
mental —*see* Disability, intellectual
modification, lysosomal enzymes, post-translational E77.0
obstructive, congenital
  renal pelvis Q62.39
  ureter Q62.39
    atresia —*see* Atresia, ureter
    cecoureterocele Q62.32
    megaureter Q62.2
    orthotopic ureterocele Q62.31
osseous, major M89.70
  ankle M89.77
  carpus M89.74
  clavicle M89.71
  femur M89.75
  fibula M89.76
  fingers M89.74
  foot M89.77
  forearm M89.73
  hand M89.74
  humerus M89.72
  lower leg M89.76
  metacarpus M89.74
  metatarsus M89.77
  multiple sites M89.9
  pelvic region M89.75
  pelvis M89.75
  radius M89.73
  scapula M89.71
  shoulder region M89.71
  specified NEC M89.78
  tarsus M89.77
  thigh M89.75
  tibia M89.76
  toes M89.77
  ulna M89.73
osteochondral NEC (*see also* Deformity) M95.8
ostium
  primum Q21.2
  secundum Q21.1
peroxidase E80.3
placental blood supply —*see* Insufficiency, placental

Defect, defective - *continued*
platelets, qualitative D69.1
  constitutional D68.0
postural NEC, spine —*see* Dorsopathy, deforming
reduction
  limb Q73.8
    lower Q72.9
      absence —*see* Agenesis, leg
      foot —*see* Agenesis, foot
      longitudinal
        femur Q72.4
        fibula Q72.6
        tibia Q72.5
      specified type NEC Q72.89
      split foot Q72.7
    specified type NEC Q73.8
    upper Q71.9
      absence —*see* Agenesis, arm
      forearm —*see* Agenesis, forearm
      hand —*see* Agenesis, hand
      lobster-claw hand Q71.6
      longitudinal
        radius Q71.4
        ulna Q71.5
      specified type NEC Q71.89
renal pelvis Q63.8
  obstructive Q62.39
respiratory system, congenital Q34.9
restoration, dental K08.50
  specified NEC K08.59
retinal nerve bundle fibers H35.89
septal (heart) NOS Q21.9
  acquired (atrial) (auricular) (ventricular) (old) I51.0
  atrial Q21.1
    concurrent with acute myocardial infarction —*see* Infarct, myocardium
    following acute myocardial infarction (current complication) I23.1
  ventricular (*see also* Defect, ventricular septal) Q21.0
sinus venosus Q21.1
speech R47.9
  developmental F80.9
  specified NEC R47.89
Taussig-Bing (aortic transposition and overriding pulmonary artery) Q20.1
teeth, wedge K03.1
vascular (local) I99.9
  congenital Q27.9
ventricular septal Q21.0
  concurrent with acute myocardial infarction —*see* Infarct, myocardium
  following acute myocardial infarction (current complication) I23.2
  in tetralogy of Fallot Q21.3
vision NEC H54.7
visual field H53.40
  bilateral
    heteronymous H53.47
    homonymous H53.46
  generalized contraction H53.48
  localized
    arcuate H53.43
    scotoma (central area) H53.41
      blind spot area H53.42
    sector H53.43
    specified type NEC H53.45
voice R49.9
  specified NEC R49.8
wedge, tooth, teeth (abrasion) K03.1

Deferentitis N49.1
  gonorrheal (acute) (chronic) A54.23
Defibrination (syndrome) D65
  antepartum —see Hemorrhage, antepartum,
  with coagulation defect, disseminated
  intravascular coagulation
  following ectopic or molar pregnancy O08.1
  intrapartum O67.0
  newborn P60
  postpartum O72.3
Deficiency, deficient
  3-beta hydroxysteroid dehydrogenase E25.0
  5-alpha reductase (with male
  pseudohermaphroditism) E29.1
  11-hydroxylase E25.0
  21-hydroxylase E25.0
  abdominal muscle syndrome Q79.4
  accelerator globulin (Ac G) (blood) D68.2
  AC globulin (congenital) (hereditary) D68.2
    acquired D68.4
  acid phosphatase E83.39
  activating factor (blood) D68.2
  adenosine deaminase (ADA) D81.3
  aldolase (hereditary) E74.19
  alpha 1-antitrypsin E88.01
  amino-acids E72.9
  anemia —see Anemia
  aneurin E51.9
  antibody with
    hyperimmunoglobulinemia D80.6
    near-normal immunoglobins D80.6
  antidiuretic hormone E23.2
  anti-hemophilic
    factor (A) D66
      B D67
      C D68.1
    globulin (AHG) NEC D66
  antithrombin (antithrombin III) D68.59
  ascorbic acid E54
  attention (disorder) (syndrome) F98.8
    with hyperactivity —see Disorder, attention-
  deficit hyperactivity
  autoprothrombin
    I D68.2
    II D67
    C D68.2
  beta-glucuronidase E76.29
  biotin E53.8
  biotin-dependent carboxylase D81.819
  biotinidase D81.810
  brancher enzyme (amylopectinosis) E74.03
  calciferol E55.9
    with
      adult osteomalacia M83.8
      rickets —see Rickets
  calcium (dietary) E58
  calorie, severe E43
    with marasmus E41
      and kwashiorkor E42
  cardiac —see Insufficiency, myocardial
  carnitine E71.40
    due to
      hemodialysis E71.43
      inborn errors of metabolism E71.42
      Valproic acid therapy E71.43
    iatrogenic E71.43
    muscle palmitoyltransferase E71.314
    primary E71.41
    secondary E71.448
  carotene E50.9
  central nervous system G96.8
  ceruloplasmin (Wilson) E83.01

Deficiency, deficient - continued
  choline E53.8
  Christmas factor D67
  chromium E61.4
  clotting (blood) (see also Deficiency,
  coagulation factor) D68.9
  clotting factor NEC (hereditary) (see also
  Deficiency, factor) D68.2
  coagulation NOS D68.9
    with
      ectopic pregnancy O08.1
      molar pregnancy O08.1
    acquired (any) D68.4
    antepartum hemorrhage —see Hemorrhage,
  antepartum, with coagulation defect
    clotting factor NEC (see also Deficiency,
  factor) D68.2
    due to
      hyperprothrombinemia D68.4
      liver disease D68.4
      vitamin K deficiency D68.4
    newborn, transient P61.6
    postpartum O72.3
    specified NEC D68.8
  cognitive F09
  color vision H53.50
    achromatopsia H53.51
    acquired H53.52
    deuteranomaly H53.53
    protanomaly H53.54
    specified type NEC H53.59
    tritanomaly H53.55
  combined glucocorticoid and
  mineralocorticoid E27.49
  contact factor D68.2
  copper (nutritional) E61.0
  corticoadrenal E27.40
    primary E27.1
  craniofacial axis Q75.0
  cyanocobalamin E53.8
  C1 esterase inhibitor (C1-INH) D84.1
  debrancher enzyme (limit dextrinosis) E74.03
  dehydrogenase
    long chain/very long chain acyl CoA
  E71.310
      medium chain acyl CoA E71.311
      short chain acyl CoA E71.312
  diet E63.9
  dihydropyrimidine dehydrogenase (DPD)
  E88.89
  disaccharidase E73.9
  edema —see Malnutrition, severe
  endocrine E34.9
  energy-supply —see Malnutrition
  enzymes, circulating NEC E88.09
  ergosterol E55.9
    with
      adult osteomalacia M83.8
      rickets —see Rickets
  essential fatty acid (EFA) E63.0
  factor —see also Deficiency, coagulation
    Hageman D68.2
    I (congenital) (hereditary) D68.2
    II (congenital) (hereditary) D68.2
    IX (congenital) (functional) (hereditary)
  (with functional defect) D67
    multiple (congenital) D68.8
      acquired D68.4
    V (congenital) (hereditary) D68.2
    VII (congenital) (hereditary) D68.2
    VIII (congenital) (functional) (hereditary)
  (with functional defect) D66

Deficiency, deficient - continued
    with vascular defect D68.0
    X (congenital) (hereditary) D68.2
    XI (congenital) (hereditary) D68.1
    XII (congenital) (hereditary) D68.2
    XIII (congenital) (hereditary) D68.2
  femoral, proximal focal (congenital) —see
  Defect, reduction, lower limb, longitudinal,
  femur
  fibrin-stabilizing factor (congenital)
  (hereditary) D68.2
    acquired D68.4
  fibrinase D68.2
  fibrinogen (congenital) (hereditary) D68.2
    acquired D65
  folate E53.8
  folic acid E53.8
  foreskin N47.3
  fructokinase E74.11
  fructose 1,6-diphosphatase E74.19
  fructose 1-phosphate aldolase E74.19
  galactokinase E74.29
  galactose 1-phosphate uridyl transferase
  E74.29
  gammaglobulin in blood D80.1
    hereditary D80.0
  glass factor D68.2
  glucocorticoid E27.49
    mineralocorticoid E27.49
  glucose 6-phosphatase E74.01
  glucose 6-phosphate dehydrogenase anemia
  D55.0
  glucuronyl transferase E80.5
  glycogen synthetase E74.09
  gonadotropin (isolated) E23.0
  growth hormone (idiopathic) (isolated) E23.0
  Hageman factor D68.2
  hemoglobin D64.9
  hepatophosphorylase E74.09
  homogentisate 1,2-dioxygenase E70.29
  hormone
    anterior pituitary (partial) NEC E23.0
      growth E23.0
    growth (isolated) E23.0
    pituitary E23.0
    testicular E29.1
  hypoxanthine (guanine) -
  phosphoribosyltransferase (HG PRT) (total
  H-PRT) E79.1
  immunity D84.9
    cell-mediated D84.8
      with thrombocytopenia and eczema D82.0
    combined D81.9
    humoral D80.9
    IgA (secretory) D80.2
    IgG D80.3
    IgM D80.4
  immuno —see Immunodeficiency
  immunoglobulin, selective
    A (IgA) D80.2
    G (IgG) (subclasses) D80.3
    M (IgM) D80.4
  inositol (B complex) E53.8
  intrinsic
    factor (congenital) D51.0
    sphincter N36.42
      with urethral hypermobility N36.43
  iodine E61.8
    congenital syndrome —see Syndrome,
  iodine-deficiency, congenital
  iron E61.1
    anemia D50.9

Deficiency, deficient - *continued*
  kalium E87.6
  kappa-light chain D80.8
  labile factor (congenital) (hereditary) D68.2
    acquired D68.4
  lacrimal fluid (acquired) —*see also*
  Syndrome, dry eye
    congenital Q10.6
  lactase
    congenital E73.0
    secondary E73.1
  Laki-Lorand factor D68.2
  lecithin cholesterol acyltransferase E78.6
  lipocaic K86.8
  lipoprotein (familial) (high density) E78.6
  liver phosphorylase E74.09
  lysosomal alpha 1, 4 glucosidase E74.02
  magnesium E61.2
  major histocompatibility complex
    class I D81.6
    class II D81.7
  manganese E61.3
  menadione (vitamin K) E56.1
    newborn P53
  mental (familial) (hereditary) —*see*
  Disability, intellectual
  methylenetetrahydrofolate reductase
    (MTHFR) E72.12
  mineral NEC E61.8
  mineralocorticoid E27.49
    with glucocorticoid E27.49
  molybdenum (nutritional) E61.5
  moral F60.2
  multiple nutrient elements E61.7
  muscle
    carnitine (palmitoyltransferase) E71.314
    phosphofructokinase E74.09
  myoadenylate deaminase E79.2
  myocardial —*see* Insufficiency, myocardial
  myophosphorylase E74.04
  NADH diaphorase or reductase (congenital)
    D74.0
  NADH-methemoglobin reductase (congenital)
    D74.0
  natrium E87.1
  niacin (amide) (-tryptophan) E52
  nicotinamide E52
  nicotinic acid E52
  number of teeth —*see* Anodontia
  nutrient element E61.9
    multiple E61.7
    specified NEC E61.8
  nutrition, nutritional E63.9
    sequelae —*see* Sequelae, nutritional
  deficiency
    specified NEC E63.8
  ornithine transcarbamylase E72.4
  ovarian E28.39
  oxygen —*see* Anoxia
  pantothenic acid E53.8
  parathyroid (gland) E20.9
  perineum (female) N81.89
  phenylalanine hydroxylase E70.1
  phosphoenolpyruvate carboxykinase E74.4
  phosphofructokinase E74.19
  phosphomannomutase E74.8
  phosphomannose isomerase E74.8
  phosphomannosyl mutase E74.8
  phosphorylase kinase, liver E74.09
  pituitary hormone (isolated) E23.0
  plasma thromboplastin
    antecedent (PTA) D68.1

Deficiency, deficient - *continued*
    component (PTC) D67
  platelet NEC D69.1
    constitutional D68.0
  polyglandular E31.8
    autoimmune E31.0
  potassium (K) E87.6
  prepuce N47.3
  proaccelerin (congenital) (hereditary) D68.2
    acquired D68.4
  proconvertin factor (congenital) (hereditary)
    D68.2
    acquired D68.4
  protein (*see also* Malnutrition) E46
    anemia D53.0
    C D68.59
    S D68.59
  prothrombin (congenital) (hereditary) D68.2
    acquired D68.4
  Prower factor D68.2
  pseudocholinesterase E88.09
  PTA (plasma thromboplastin antecedent)
    D68.1
  PTC (plasma thromboplastin component) D67
  purine nucleoside phosphorylase (PNP) D81.5
  pyracin (alpha) (beta) E53.1
  pyridoxal E53.1
  pyridoxamine E53.1
  pyridoxine (derivatives) E53.1
  pyruvate
    carboxylase E74.4
    dehydrogenase E74.4
  riboflavin (vitamin B2) E53.0
  salt E87.1
  secretion
    ovary E28.39
    salivary gland (any) K11.7
    urine R34
  selenium (dietary) E59
  serum antitrypsin, familial E88.01
  short stature homeobox gene (SHOX)
    with
      dyschondrosteosis Q78.8
      short stature (idiopathic) E34.3
      Turner's syndrome Q96.9
  sodium (Na) E87.1
  SPCA (factor VII) D68.2
  sphincter, intrinsic N36.42
    with urethral hypermobility N36.43
  stable factor (congenital) (hereditary) D68.2
    acquired D68.4
  Stuart-Prower (factor X) D68.2
  sucrase E74.39
  sulfatase E75.29
  sulfite oxidase E72.19
  thiamin, thiaminic (chloride) E51.9
    beriberi (dry) E51.11
    wet E51.12
  thrombokinase D68.2
    newborn P53
  thyroid (gland) —*see* Hypothyroidism
  tocopherol E56.0
  tooth bud K00.0
  transcobalamine II (anemia) D51.2
  vanadium E61.6
  vascular I99.9
  vasopressin E23.2
  viosterol —*see* Deficiency, calciferol
  vitamin (multiple) NOS E56.9
    A E50.9
      with
        Bitot's spot (corneal) E50.1
        follicular keratosis E50.8

Deficiency, deficient - *continued*
    keratomalacia E50.4
    manifestations NEC E50.8
    night blindness E50.5
    scar of cornea, xerophthalmic E50.6
    xeroderma E50.8
    xerophthalmia E50.7
    xerosis
      conjunctival E50.0
        and Bitot's spot E50.1
      cornea E50.2
        and ulceration E50.3
    sequelae E64.1
    B (complex) NOS E53.9
      with
        beriberi (dry) E51.11
          wet E51.12
        pellagra E52
    B1 NOS E51.9
      beriberi (dry) E51.11
        with circulatory system manifestations
    E51.11
          wet E51.12
    B12 E53.8
    B2 (riboflavin) E53.0
    B6 E53.1
    C E54
      sequelae E64.2
    D E55.9
      with
        adult osteomalacia M83.8
        rickets —*see* Rickets
      25-hydroxylase E83.32
    E E56.0
    folic acid E53.8
    G E53.0
    group B E53.9
      specified NEC E53.8
    H (biotin) E53.8
    K E56.1
      of newborn P53
    nicotinic E52
    P E56.8
    PP (pellagra-preventing) E52
    specified NEC E56.8
    thiamin E51.9
      beriberi —*see* Beriberi
    zinc, dietary E60
Deficit —*see also* Deficiency
  attention and concentration R41.840
    disorder —*see* Attention, deficit
  cognitive communication R41.841
  cognitive NEC R41.89
    following
      cerebral infarction I69.31
      cerebrovascular disease I69.91
        specified disease NEC I69.81
      intracerebral hemorrhage I69.11
      nontraumatic intracranial hemorrhage NEC
    I69.21
      subarachnoid hemorrhage I69.01
  concentration R41.840
  executive function R41.844
  frontal lobe R41.844
  neurologic NEC R29.818
    ischemic
      reversible (RIND) I63.9
      prolonged (PRIND) I63.9
  oxygen R09.02
  prolonged reversible ischemic neurologic
    (PRIND) I63.9
  psychomotor R41.843
  visuospatial R41.842

Deflection
radius —*see* Deformity, limb, specified type NEC, forearm
septum (acquired) (nasal) (nose) J34.2
spine —*see* Curvature, spine
turbinate (nose) J34.2
Defluvium
capillorum —*see* Alopecia
ciliorum —*see* Madarosis
unguium L60.8
Deformity Q89.9
abdomen, congenital Q89.9
abdominal wall
acquired M95.8
congenital Q79.59
acquired (unspecified site) M95.9
adrenal gland Q89.1
alimentary tract, congenital Q45.9
upper Q40.9
ankle (joint) (acquired) —*see also* Deformity, limb, lower leg
abduction —*see* Contraction, joint, ankle
congenital Q68.8
contraction —*see* Contraction, joint, ankle
specified type NEC —*see* Deformity, limb, foot, specified NEC
anus (acquired) K62.89
congenital Q43.9
aorta (arch) (congenital) Q25.4
acquired I77.89
aortic
arch, acquired I77.89
cusp or valve (congenital) Q23.8
acquired (*see also* Endocarditis, aortic) I35.8
arm (acquired) (upper) —*see also* Deformity, limb, upper arm
congenital Q68.8
forearm —*see* Deformity, limb, forearm
artery (congenital) (peripheral) NOS Q27.9
acquired I77.89
coronary (acquired) I25.9
congenital Q24.5
umbilical Q27.0
atrial septal Q21.1
auditory canal (external) (congenital) —*see also* Malformation, ear, external
acquired —*see* Disorder, ear, external, specified type NEC
auricle
ear (congenital) —*see also* Malformation, ear, external
acquired —*see* Disorder, pinna, deformity
back —*see* Dorsopathy, deforming
bile duct (common) (congenital) (hepatic) Q44.5
acquired K83.8
biliary duct or passage (congenital) Q44.5
acquired K83.8
bladder (neck) (trigone) (sphincter) (acquired) N32.89
congenital Q64.79
bone (acquired) NOS M95.9
congenital Q79.9
turbinate M95.0
brain (congenital) Q04.9
acquired G93.89
reduction Q04.3
breast (acquired) N64.89
congenital Q83.9
reconstructed N65.0

Deformity - *continued*
bronchus (congenital) Q32.4
acquired NEC J98.09
bursa, congenital Q79.9
canaliculi (lacrimalis) (acquired) —*see also* Disorder, lacrimal system, changes
congenital Q10.6
canthus, acquired —*see* Disorder, eyelid, specified type NEC
capillary (acquired) I78.8
cardiovascular system, congenital Q28.9
caruncle, lacrimal (acquired) —*see also* Disorder, lacrimal system, changes
congenital Q10.6
cascade, stomach K31.2
cecum (congenital) Q43.9
acquired K63.89
cerebral, acquired G93.89
congenital Q04.9
cervix (uterus) (acquired) NEC N88.8
congenital Q51.9
cheek (acquired) M95.2
congenital Q18.9
chest (acquired) (wall) M95.4
congenital Q67.8
sequelae (late effect) of rickets E64.3
chin (acquired) M95.2
congenital Q18.9
choroid (congenital) Q14.3
acquired H31.8
plexus Q07.8
acquired G96.19
cicatricial —*see* Cicatrix
cilia, acquired —*see* Disorder, eyelid, specified type NEC
clavicle (acquired) M95.8
congenital Q68.8
clitoris (congenital) Q52.6
acquired N90.89
clubfoot —*see* Clubfoot
coccyx (acquired) —*see* subcategory M43.8
colon (congenital) Q43.9
acquired K63.89
concha (ear) , congenital —*see also* Malformation, ear, external
acquired —*see* Disorder, pinna, deformity
cornea (acquired) H18.70
congenital Q13.4
descemetocele —*see* Descemetocele
ectasia —*see* Ectasia, cornea
specified NEC H18.79
staphyloma —*see* Staphyloma, cornea
coronary artery (acquired) I25.9
congenital Q24.5
cranium (acquired) —*see* Deformity, skull
cricoid cartilage (congenital) Q31.8
acquired J38.7
cystic duct (congenital) Q44.5
acquired K82.8
Dandy-Walker Q03.1
with spina bifida —*see* Spina bifida
diaphragm (congenital) Q79.1
acquired J98.6
digestive organ NOS Q45.9
ductus arteriosus Q25.0
duodenal bulb K31.89
duodenum (congenital) Q43.9
acquired K31.89
dura —*see* Deformity, meninges
ear (acquired) —*see also* Disorder, pinna, deformity
congenital (external) Q17.9

Deformity - *continued*
internal Q16.5
middle Q16.4
ossicles Q16.3
ossicles Q16.3
ectodermal (congenital) NEC Q84.9
ejaculatory duct (congenital) Q55.4
acquired N50.8
elbow (joint) (acquired) —*see also* Deformity, limb, upper arm
congenital Q68.8
contraction —*see* Contraction, joint, elbow
endocrine gland NEC Q89.2
epididymis (congenital) Q55.4
acquired N50.8
epiglottis (congenital) Q31.8
acquired J38.7
esophagus (congenital) Q39.9
acquired K22.8
eustachian tube (congenital) NEC Q17.8
eye, congenital Q15.9
eyebrow (congenital) Q18.8
eyelid (acquired) —*see also* Disorder, eyelid, specified type NEC
congenital Q10.3
face (acquired) M95.2
congenital Q18.9
fallopian tube, acquired N83.8
femur (acquired) —*see* Deformity, limb, specified type NEC, thigh
fetal
with fetopelvic disproportion O33.7
causing obstructed labor O66.3
finger (acquired) M20.00
boutonniere M20.02
congenital Q68.1
flexion contracture —*see* Contraction, joint, hand
mallet finger M20.01
specified NEC M20.09
swan-neck M20.03
flexion (joint) (acquired) (*see also* Deformity, limb, flexion) M21.20
congenital NOS Q74.9
hip Q65.89
foot (acquired) —*see also* Deformity, limb, lower leg
cavovarus (congenital) Q66.1
congenital NOS Q66.9
specified type NEC Q66.89
specified type NEC —*see* Deformity, limb, foot, specified NEC
valgus (congenital) Q66.6
acquired —*see* Deformity, valgus, ankle
varus (congenital) NEC Q66.3
acquired —*see* Deformity, varus, ankle
forearm (acquired) —*see also* Deformity, limb, forearm
congenital Q68.8
forehead (acquired) M95.2
congenital Q75.8
frontal bone (acquired) M95.2
congenital Q75.8
gallbladder (congenital) Q44.1
acquired K82.8
gastrointestinal tract (congenital) NOS Q45.9
acquired K63.89
genitalia, genital organ (s) or system NEC
female (congenital) Q52.9
acquired N94.89
external Q52.70
male (congenital) Q55.9
acquired N50.8

Deformity *- continued*
- globe (eye) (congenital) Q15.8
  - acquired H44.89
- gum, acquired NEC K06.8
- hand (acquired) —*see* Deformity, limb, hand
  - congenital Q68.1
- head (acquired) M95.2
  - congenital Q75.8
- heart (congenital) Q24.9
  - septum Q21.9
    - auricular Q21.1
    - ventricular Q21.0
  - valve (congenital) NEC Q24.8
    - acquired —*see* Endocarditis
- heel (acquired) —*see* Deformity, foot
- hepatic duct (congenital) Q44.5
  - acquired K83.8
- hip (joint) (acquired) —*see also* Deformity, limb, thigh
  - congenital Q65.9
  - due to (previous) juvenile osteochondrosis —*see* Coxa, plana
  - flexion —*see* Contraction, joint, hip
- hourglass —*see* Contraction, hourglass
- humerus (acquired) M21.82
  - congenital Q74.0
- hypophyseal (congenital) Q89.2
- ileocecal (coil) (valve) (acquired) K63.89
  - congenital Q43.9
- ileum (congenital) Q43.9
  - acquired K63.89
- ilium (acquired) M95.5
  - congenital Q74.2
- integument (congenital) Q84.9
- intervertebral cartilage or disc (acquired) — *see* Disorder, disc, specified NEC
- intestine (large) (small) (congenital) NOS Q43.9
  - acquired K63.89
- intrinsic minus or plus (hand) —*see* Deformity, limb, specified type NEC, forearm
- iris (acquired) H21.89
  - congenital Q13.2
- ischium (acquired) M95.5
  - congenital Q74.2
- jaw (acquired) (congenital) M26.9
- joint (acquired) NEC M21.90
  - congenital Q68.8
  - elbow M21.92
  - hand M21.94
  - hip M21.95
  - knee M21.96
  - shoulder M21.92
  - wrist M21.93
- kidney (s) (calyx) (pelvis) (congenital) Q63.9
  - acquired N28.89
  - artery (congenital) Q27.2
    - acquired I77.89
- Klippel-Feil (brevicollis) Q76.1
- knee (acquired) NEC —*see also* Deformity, limb, lower leg
  - congenital Q68.2
- labium (majus) (minus) (congenital) Q52.79
  - acquired N90.89
- lacrimal passages or duct (congenital) NEC Q10.6
  - acquired —*see* Disorder, lacrimal system, changes
- larynx (muscle) (congenital) Q31.8
  - acquired J38.7
  - web (glottic) Q31.0

Deformity *- continued*
- leg (upper) (acquired) NEC —*see also* Deformity, limb, thigh
  - congenital Q68.8
  - lower leg —*see* Deformity, limb, lower leg
- lens (acquired) H27.8
  - congenital Q12.9
- lid (fold) (acquired) —*see also* Disorder, eyelid, specified type NEC
  - congenital Q10.3
- ligament (acquired) —*see* Disorder, ligament
  - congenital Q79.9
- limb (acquired) M21.90
  - clawfoot M21.53
  - clawhand M21.51
  - clubfoot M21.54
  - clubhand M21.52
  - congenital, except reduction deformity Q74.9
  - flat foot M21.4
  - flexion M21.20
    - ankle M21.27
    - elbow M21.22
    - finger M21.24
    - hip M21.25
    - knee M21.26
    - shoulder M21.21
    - toe M21.27
    - wrist M21.23
  - foot
    - claw —*see* Deformity, limb, clawfoot
    - club —*see* Deformity, limb, clubfoot
    - drop M21.37
    - flat —*see* Deformity, limb, flat foot
    - specified NEC M21.6X
  - forearm M21.93
  - hand M21.94
  - lower leg M21.96
  - specified type NEC M21.80
    - forearm M21.83
    - lower leg M21.86
    - thigh M21.85
    - upper arm M21.82
  - thigh M21.95
  - unequal length M21.70
    - short site is
      - femur M21.75
      - fibula M21.76
      - humerus M21.72
      - radius M21.73
      - tibia M21.76
      - ulna M21.73
    - upper arm M21.92
  - valgus —*see* Deformity, valgus
  - varus —*see* Deformity, varus
  - wrist drop M21.33
- lip (acquired) NEC K13.0
  - congenital Q38.0
- liver (congenital) Q44.7
  - acquired K76.89
- lumbosacral (congenital) (joint) (region) Q76.49
  - acquired —*see* subcategory M43.8
  - kyphosis —*see* Kyphosis, congenital
  - lordosis —*see* Lordosis, congenital
- lung (congenital) Q33.9
  - acquired J98.4
- lymphatic system, congenital Q89.9
- Madelung's (radius) Q74.0
- mandible (acquired) (congenital) M26.9
- maxilla (acquired) (congenital) M26.9

Deformity *- continued*
- meninges or membrane (congenital) Q07.9
  - cerebral Q04.8
    - acquired G96.19
  - spinal cord (congenital) G96.19
    - acquired G96.19
- metacarpus (acquired) —*see* Deformity, limb, forearm
  - congenital Q74.0
- metatarsus (acquired) —*see* Deformity, foot
  - congenital Q66.9
- middle ear (congenital) Q16.4
  - ossicles Q16.3
- mitral (leaflets) (valve) I05.8
  - parachute Q23.2
  - stenosis, congenital Q23.2
- mouth (acquired) K13.79
  - congenital Q38.6
- multiple, congenital NEC Q89.7
- muscle (acquired) M62.89
  - congenital Q79.9
    - sternocleidomastoid Q68.0
- musculoskeletal system (acquired) M95.9
  - congenital Q79.9
  - specified NEC M95.8
- nail (acquired) L60.8
  - congenital Q84.6
- nasal —*see* Deformity, nose
- neck (acquired) M95.3
  - congenital Q18.9
    - sternocleidomastoid Q68.0
- nervous system (congenital) Q07.9
- nipple (congenital) Q83.9
  - acquired N64.89
- nose (acquired) (cartilage) M95.0
  - bone (turbinate) M95.0
  - congenital Q30.9
    - bent or squashed Q67.4
  - saddle M95.0
    - syphilitic A50.57
  - septum (acquired) J34.2
    - congenital Q30.8
  - sinus (wall) (congenital) Q30.8
    - acquired M95.0
  - syphilitic (congenital) A50.57
    - late A52.73
- ocular muscle (congenital) Q10.3
  - acquired —*see* Strabismus, mechanical
- opticociliary vessels (congenital) Q13.2
- orbit (eye) (acquired) H05.30
  - atrophy —*see* Atrophy, orbit
  - congenital Q10.7
  - due to
    - bone disease NEC H05.32
    - trauma or surgery H05.33
  - enlargement —*see* Enlargement, orbit
  - exostosis —*see* Exostosis, orbit
- organ of Corti (congenital) Q16.5
- ovary (congenital) Q50.39
  - acquired N83.8
- oviduct, acquired N83.8
- palate (congenital) Q38.5
  - acquired M27.8
  - cleft (congenital) —*see* Cleft, palate
- pancreas (congenital) Q45.3
  - acquired K86.8
- parathyroid (gland) Q89.2
- parotid (gland) (congenital) Q38.4
  - acquired K11.8
- patella (acquired) —*see* Disorder, patella, specified NEC

Deformity - *continued*

pelvis, pelvic (acquired) (bony) M95.5
  with disproportion (fetopelvic) O33.0
    causing obstructed labor O65.0
  congenital Q74.2
  rachitic sequelae (late effect) E64.3
penis (glans) (congenital) Q55.69
  acquired N48.89
pericardium (congenital) Q24.8
  acquired —*see* Pericarditis
pharynx (congenital) Q38.8
  acquired J39.2
pinna, acquired —*see also* Disorder, pinna, deformity
  congenital Q17.9
pituitary (congenital) Q89.2
posture —*see* Dorsopathy, deforming
prepuce (congenital) Q55.69
  acquired N47.8
prostate (congenital) Q55.4
  acquired N42.89
pupil (congenital) Q13.2
  acquired —*see* Abnormality, pupillary
pylorus (congenital) Q40.3
  acquired K31.89
rachitic (acquired) , old or healed E64.3
radius (acquired) —*see also* Deformity, limb, forearm
  congenital Q68.8
rectum (congenital) Q43.9
  acquired K62.89
reduction (extremity) (limb) , congenital (*see also* condition and site) Q73.8
  brain Q04.3
  lower —*see* Defect, reduction, lower limb
  upper —*see* Defect, reduction, upper limb
renal —*see* Deformity, kidney
respiratory system (congenital) Q34.9
rib (acquired) M95.4
  congenital Q76.6
    cervical Q76.5
rotation (joint) (acquired) —*see* Deformity, limb, specified site NEC
  congenital Q74.9
  hip —*see* Deformity, limb, specified type NEC, thigh
    congenital Q65.89
sacroiliac joint (congenital) Q74.2
  acquired —see subcategory M43.8
sacrum (acquired) —see subcategory M43.8
saddle
  back —*see* Lordosis
  nose M95.0
    syphilitic A50.57
salivary gland or duct (congenital) Q38.4
  acquired K11.8
scapula (acquired) M95.8
  congenital Q68.8
scrotum (congenital) —*see also* Malformation, testis and scrotum
  acquired N50.8
seminal vesicles (congenital) Q55.4
  acquired N50.8
septum, nasal (acquired) J34.2
shoulder (joint) (acquired) —*see* Deformity, limb, upper arm
  congenital Q74.0
  contraction —*see* Contraction, joint, shoulder
sigmoid (flexure) (congenital) Q43.9
  acquired K63.89
skin (congenital) Q82.9

Deformity - *continued*

skull (acquired) M95.2
  congenital Q75.8
    with
      anencephaly Q00.0
      encephalocele —*see* Encephalocele
      hydrocephalus Q03.9
        with spina bifida —*see* Spina bifida, by site, with hydrocephalus
      microcephaly Q02
soft parts, organs or tissues (of pelvis)
  in pregnancy or childbirth NEC O34.8
    causing obstructed labor O65.5
spermatic cord (congenital) Q55.4
  acquired N50.8
  torsion —*see* Torsion, spermatic cord
spinal —*see* Dorsopathy, deforming
  column (acquired) —*see* Dorsopathy, deforming
    congenital Q67.5
  cord (congenital) Q06.9
    acquired G95.89
  nerve root (congenital) Q07.9
spine (acquired) —*see also* Dorsopathy, deforming
  congenital Q67.5
  rachitic E64.3
  specified NEC —*see* Dorsopathy, deforming, specified NEC
spleen
  acquired D73.89
  congenital Q89.09
Sprengel's (congenital) Q74.0
sternocleidomastoid (muscle) , congenital Q68.0
sternum (acquired) M95.4
  congenital NEC Q76.7
stomach (congenital) Q40.3
  acquired K31.89
submandibular gland (congenital) Q38.4
submaxillary gland (congenital) Q38.4
  acquired K11.8
talipes —*see* Talipes
testis (congenital) —*see also* Malformation, testis and scrotum
  acquired N44.8
  torsion —*see* Torsion, testis
thigh (acquired) —*see also* Deformity, limb, thigh
  congenital NEC Q68.8
thorax (acquired) (wall) M95.4
  congenital Q67.8
  sequelae of rickets E64.3
thumb (acquired) —*see also* Deformity, finger
  congenital NEC Q68.1
thymus (tissue) (congenital) Q89.2
thyroid (gland) (congenital) Q89.2
  cartilage Q31.8
  acquired J38.7
tibia (acquired) —*see also* Deformity, limb, specified type NEC, lower leg
  congenital NEC Q68.8
  saber (syphilitic) A50.56
toe (acquired) M20.6
  congenital Q66.9
  hallux rigidus M20.2
  hallux valgus M20.1
  hallux varus M20.3
  hammer toe M20.4
  specified NEC M20.5X

Deformity - *continued*

tongue (congenital) Q38.3
  acquired K14.8
tooth, teeth K00.2
trachea (rings) (congenital) Q32.1
  acquired J39.8
transverse aortic arch (congenital) Q25.4
tricuspid (leaflets) (valve) I07.8
  atresia or stenosis Q22.4
  Ebstein's Q22.5
trunk (acquired) M95.8
  congenital Q89.9
ulna (acquired) —*see also* Deformity, limb, forearm
  congenital NEC Q68.8
urachus, congenital Q64.4
ureter (opening) (congenital) Q62.8
  acquired N28.89
urethra (congenital) Q64.79
  acquired N36.8
urinary tract (congenital) Q64.9
  urachus Q64.4
uterus (congenital) Q51.9
  acquired N85.8
uvula (congenital) Q38.5
vagina (acquired) N89.8
  congenital Q52.4
valgus NEC M21.00
  ankle M21.07
  elbow M21.02
  hip M21.05
  knee M21.06
valve, valvular (congenital) (heart) Q24.8
  acquired —*see* Endocarditis
varus NEC M21.10
  ankle M21.17
  elbow M21.12
  hip M21.15
  knee M21.16
  tibia —*see* Osteochondrosis, juvenile, tibia
vas deferens (congenital) Q55.4
  acquired N50.8
vein (congenital) Q27.9
  great Q26.9
vertebra —*see* Dorsopathy, deforming
vertical talus (congenital) Q66.80
  left foot Q66.82
  right foot Q66.81
vesicourethral orifice (acquired) N32.89
  congenital NEC Q64.79
vessels of optic papilla (congenital) Q14.2
visual field (contraction) —*see* Defect, visual field
vitreous body, acquired H43.89
vulva (congenital) Q52.79
  acquired N90.89
wrist (joint) (acquired) —*see also* Deformity, limb, forearm
  congenital Q68.8
  contraction —*see* Contraction, joint, wrist
Degeneration, degenerative
adrenal (capsule) (fatty) (gland) (hyaline) (infectional) E27.8
amyloid (*see also* Amyloidosis) E85.9
anterior cornua, spinal cord G12.29
anterior labral S43.49
aorta, aortic I70.0
  fatty I77.89
aortic valve (heart) —*see* Endocarditis, aortic
arteriovascular —*see* Arteriosclerosis

Degeneration, degenerative - *continued*
artery, arterial (atheromatous) (calcareous) —
see also Arteriosclerosis
  cerebral, amyloid E85.4 *[I68.0]*
  medial —*see* Arteriosclerosis, extremities
articular cartilage NEC —*see* Derangement,
joint, articular cartilage, by site
atheromatous —*see* Arteriosclerosis
basal nuclei or ganglia G23.9
  specified NEC G23.8
bone NEC —*see* Disorder, bone, specified
type NEC
brachial plexus G54.0
brain (cortical) (progressive) G31.9
  alcoholic G31.2
  arteriosclerotic I67.2
  childhood G31.9
    specified NEC G31.89
  cystic G31.89
    congenital Q04.6
  in
    alcoholism G31.2
    beriberi E51.2
    cerebrovascular disease I67.9
    congenital hydrocephalus Q03.9
      with spina bifida —*see also* Spina bifida
    Fabry-Anderson disease E75.21
    Gaucher's disease E75.22
    Hunter's syndrome E76.1
    lipidosis
      cerebral E75.4
      generalized E75.6
    mucopolysaccharidosis —*see*
Mucopolysaccharidosis
    myxedema E03.9 *[G32.89]*
    neoplastic disease (*see also* Neoplasm)
D49.6 *[G32.89]*
    Niemann-Pick disease E75.249 *[G32.89]*
    sphingolipidosis E75.3 *[G32.89]*
    vitamin B12 deficiency E53.8 *[G32.89]*
  senile NEC G31.1
breast N64.89
Bruch's membrane —*see* Degeneration,
choroid
capillaries (fatty) I78.8
  amyloid E85.8 *[I79.8]*
cardiac —*see also* Degeneration, myocardial
  valve, valvular —*see* Endocarditis
cardiorenal —*see* Hypertension, cardiorenal
cardiovascular —*see also* Disease,
cardiovascular
  renal —*see* Hypertension, cardiorenal
cerebellar NOS G31.9
  alcoholic G31.2
  primary (hereditary) (sporadic) G11.9
cerebral —*see* Degeneration, brain
cerebrovascular I67.9
  due to hypertension I67.4
cervical plexus G54.2
cervix N88.8
  due to radiation (intended effect) N88.8
    adverse effect or misadventure N99.89
chamber angle H21.21
changes, spine or vertebra —*see* Spondylosis
chorioretinal —*see also* Degeneration,
choroid
  hereditary H31.20
choroid (colloid) (drusen) H31.10
  atrophy —*see* Atrophy, choroidal
  hereditary —*see* Dystrophy, choroidal,
hereditary
ciliary body H21.22

Degeneration, degenerative - *continued*
cochlear —*see* subcategory H83.8
combined (spinal cord) (subacute) E53.8
[G32.0]
  with anemia (pernicious) D51.0 *[G32.0]*
  due to dietary vitamin B12 deficiency
D51.3 *[G32.0]*
  in (due to)
    vitamin B12 deficiency E53.8 *[G32.0]*
      anemia D51.9 *[G32.0]*
conjunctiva H11.10
  concretions —*see* Concretion, conjunctiva
  deposits —*see* Deposit, conjunctiva
  pigmentations —*see* Pigmentation,
conjunctiva
  pinguecula —*see* Pinguecula
  xerosis —*see* Xerosis, conjunctiva
cornea H18.40
  calcereous H18.43
    band keratopathy H18.42
  familial, hereditary —*see* Dystrophy, cornea
  hyaline (of old scars) H18.49
  keratomalacia —*see* Keratomalacia
  nodular H18.45
  peripheral H18.46
  senile H18.41
  specified type NEC H18.49
cortical (cerebellar) (parenchymatous) G31.89
  alcoholic G31.2
  diffuse, due to arteriopathy I67.2
corticobasal G31.85
cutis L98.8
  amyloid E85.4 *[L99]*
dental pulp K04.2
disc disease —*see* Degeneration,
intervertebral disc NEC
dorsolateral (spinal cord) —*see* Degeneration,
combined
extrapyramidal G25.9
eye, macular —*see also* Degeneration, macula
  congenital or hereditary —*see* Dystrophy,
retina
facet joints —*see* Spondylosis
fatty
  liver NEC K76.0
    alcoholic K70.0
grey matter (brain) (Alpers') G31.81
heart —*see also* Degeneration, myocardial
  amyloid E85.4 *[I43]*
  atheromatous —*see* Disease, heart,
ischemic, atherosclerotic
  ischemic —*see* Disease, heart, ischemic
hepatolenticular (Wilson's) E83.01
hepatorenal K76.7
hyaline (diffuse) (generalized)
  localized —*see* Degeneration, by site
infrapatellar fat pad M79.4
intervertebral disc NOS
  with
    myelopathy —*see* Disorder, disc, with,
myelopathy
    radiculitis or radiculopathy —*see* Disorder,
disc, with, radiculopathy
  cervical, cervicothoracic —*see* Disorder,
disc, cervical, degeneration
    with
      myelopathy —*see* Disorder, disc,
cervical, with myelopathy
      neuritis, radiculitis or radiculopathy —*see*
Disorder, disc, cervical, with neuritis
  lumbar region M51.36
    with

Degeneration, degenerative - *continued*
      myelopathy M51.06
      neuritis, radiculitis, radiculopathy or
sciatica M51.16
  lumbosacral region M51.37
    with
      neuritis, radiculitis, radiculopathy or
sciatica M51.17
  sacrococcygeal region M53.3
  thoracic region M51.34
    with
      myelopathy M51.04
      neuritis, radiculitis, radiculopathy
M51.14
  thoracolumbar region M51.35
    with
      myelopathy M51.05
      neuritis, radiculitis, radiculopathy
M51.15
intestine, amyloid E85.4
iris (pigmentary) H21.23
ischemic —*see* Ischemia
joint disease —*see* Osteoarthritis
kidney N28.89
  amyloid E85.4 *[N29]*
  cystic, congenital Q61.9
  fatty N28.89
  polycystic Q61.3
    adult type (autosomal dominant) Q61.2
    infantile type (autosomal recessive) NEC
Q61.19
      collecting duct dilatation Q61.11
Kuhnt-Junius (*see also* Degeneration, macula)
H35.32
lens —*see* Cataract
lenticular (familial) (progressive) (Wilson's)
(with cirrhosis of liver) E83.01
liver (diffuse) NEC K76.89
  amyloid E85.4 *[K77]*
  cystic K76.89
    congenital Q44.6
  fatty NEC K76.0
    alcoholic K70.0
  hypertrophic K76.89
  parenchymatous, acute or subacute K72.00
    with coma K72.01
  pigmentary K76.89
  toxic (acute) K71.9
lung J98.4
lymph gland I89.8
  hyaline I89.8
macula, macular (acquired) (age-related)
(senile) H35.30
  angioid streaks H35.33
  atrophic age-related H35.31
  congenital or hereditary —*see* Dystrophy,
retina
  cystoid H35.35
  drusen H35.36
  exudative H35.32
  hole H35.34
  nonexudative H35.31
  puckering H35.37
  toxic H35.38
membranous labyrinth, congenital (causing
impairment of hearing) Q16.5
meniscus —*see* Derangement, meniscus
mitral —*see* Insufficiency, mitral
Mönckeberg's —*see* Arteriosclerosis,
extremities
motor centers, senile G31.1
multi-system G90.3
mural —*see* Degeneration, myocardial

Degeneration, degenerative - *continued*
muscle (fatty) (fibrous) (hyaline)
(progressive) M62.89
  heart —*see* Degeneration, myocardial
myelin, central nervous system G37.9
myocardial, myocardium (fatty) (hyaline)
(senile) I51.5
  with rheumatic fever (conditions in I00)
  I09.0
    active, acute or subacute I01.2
      with chorea I02.0
    inactive or quiescent (with chorea) I09.0
  hypertensive —*see* Hypertension, heart
  rheumatic —*see* Degeneration, myocardial,
  with rheumatic fever
    syphilitic A52.06
nasal sinus (mucosa) J32.9
  frontal J32.1
  maxillary J32.0
nerve —*see* Disorder, nerve
nervous system G31.9
  alcoholic G31.2
  amyloid E85.4 *[G99.8]*
  autonomic G90.9
  fatty G31.89
  specified NEC G31.89
nipple N64.89
olivopontocerebellar (hereditary) (familial)
G23.8
osseous labyrinth —see subcategory H83.8
ovary N83.8
  cystic N83.20
  microcystic N83.20
pallidal pigmentary (progressive) G23.0
pancreas K86.8
  tuberculous A18.83
penis N48.89
pigmentary (diffuse) (general)
  localized —*see* Degeneration, by site
  pallidal (progressive) G23.0
pineal gland E34.8
pituitary (gland) E23.6
popliteal fat pad M79.4
posterolateral (spinal cord) —*see*
Degeneration, combined
pulmonary valve (heart) I37.8
pulp (tooth) K04.2
pupillary margin H21.24
renal —*see* Degeneration, kidney
retina H35.9
  hereditary (cerebroretinal) (congenital)
  (juvenile) (macula) (peripheral) (pigmentary)
  —*see* Dystrophy, retina
  Kuhnt-Junius (*see also* Degeneration,
  macula) H35.32
  macula (cystic) (exudative) (hole)
  (nonexudative) (pseudohole) (senile) (toxic)
  —*see* Degeneration, macula
  peripheral H35.40
    lattice H35.41
    microcystoid H35.42
    paving stone H35.43
    secondary
      pigmentary H35.45
      vitreoretinal H35.46
    senile reticular H35.44
  pigmentary (primary) —*see also* Dystrophy,
retina
    secondary —*see* Degeneration, retina,
peripheral, secondary
    posterior pole —*see* Degeneration, macula

Degeneration, degenerative - *continued*
saccule, congenital (causing impairment of
hearing) Q16.5
senile R54
  brain G31.1
  cardiac, heart or myocardium —*see*
Degeneration, myocardial
    motor centers G31.1
    vascular —*see* Arteriosclerosis
sinus (cystic) —*see also* Sinusitis
    polypoid J33.1
skin L98.8
    amyloid E85.4 *[L99]*
    colloid L98.8
spinal (cord) G31.89
    amyloid E85.4 *[G32.89]*
    combined (subacute) —*see* Degeneration,
combined
    dorsolateral —*see* Degeneration, combined
    familial NEC G31.89
    fatty G31.89
    funicular —*see* Degeneration, combined
    posterolateral —*see* Degeneration,
combined
    subacute combined —*see* Degeneration,
combined
    tuberculous A17.81
spleen D73.0
    amyloid E85.4 *[D77]*
stomach K31.89
striatonigral G23.2
suprarenal (capsule) (gland) E27.8
synovial membrane (pulpy) —*see* Disorder,
synovium, specified type NEC
tapetoretinal —*see* Dystrophy, retina
thymus (gland) E32.8
    fatty E32.8
thyroid (gland) E07.89
tricuspid (heart) (valve) I07.9
tuberculous NEC —*see* Tuberculosis
turbinate J34.89
uterus (cystic) N85.8
vascular (senile) —*see* Arteriosclerosis
    hypertensive —*see* Hypertension
vitreoretinal, secondary —*see* Degeneration,
retina, peripheral, secondary, vitreoretinal
vitreous (body) H43.81
Wallerian —*see* Disorder, nerve
Wilson's hepatolenticular E83.01
Deglutition
paralysis R13.0
    hysterical F44.4
    pneumonia J69.0
Degos' disease I77.89
Dehiscence (of)
amputation stump T87.81
cesarean wound O90.0
closure of
    cornea T81.31
    craniotomy T81.32
    fascia (muscular) (superficial) T81.32
    internal organ or tissue T81.32
    laceration (external) (internal) T81.33
    ligament T81.32
    mucosa T81.31
    muscle or muscle flap T81.32
    ribs or rib cage T81.32
    skin and subcutaneous tissue (full-thickness)
    (superficial) T81.31
    skull T81.32
    sternum (sternotomy) T81.32
    tendon T81.32

Dehiscence (of) - *continued*
traumatic laceration (external) (internal)
T81.33
    episiotomy O90.1
    operation wound NEC T81.31
      external operation wound (superficial)
      T81.31
      internal operation wound (deep) T81.32
    perineal wound (postpartum) O90.1
    traumatic injury wound repair T81.33
    wound T81.30
      traumatic repair T81.33
Dehydration E86.0
    hypertonic E87.0
    hypotonic E87.1
    newborn P74.1
Déjérine-Roussy syndrome G89.0
Déjérine-Sottas disease or neuropathy
(hypertrophic) G60.0
Déjérine-Thomas atrophy G23.8
Delay, delayed
any plane in pelvis
    complicating delivery O66.9
    birth or delivery NOS O63.9
    closure, ductus arteriosus (Botalli) P29.3
    coagulation —*see* Defect, coagulation
    conduction (cardiac) (ventricular) I45.9
    delivery, second twin, triplet, etc O63.2
    development R62.50
      global F88
      intellectual (specific) F81.9
      language F80.9
        due to hearing loss F80.4
      learning F81.9
      pervasive F84.9
      physiological R62.50
        specified stage NEC R62.0
      reading F81.0
      sexual E30.0
      speech F80.9
        due to hearing loss F80.4
      spelling F81.81
    gastric emptying K30
    menarche E30.0
    menstruation (cause unknown) N91.0
    milestone R62.0
    passage of meconium (newborn) P76.0
    primary respiration P28.9
    puberty (constitutional) E30.0
    separation of umbilical cord P96.82
    sexual maturation, female E30.0
    sleep phase syndrome G47.21
    union, fracture —*see* Fracture, by site
    vaccination Z28.9
Deletion (s)
autosome Q93.9
    identified by fluorescence in situ
    hybridization (FISH) Q93.89
    identified by in situ hybridization (ISH)
    Q93.89
chromosome
    with complex rearrangements NEC Q93.7
    part of NEC Q93.5
    seen only at prometaphase Q93.89
    short arm
      4 Q93.3
      5p Q93.4
      22q11.2 Q93.81
    specified NEC Q93.89
    long arm chromosome 18 or 21 Q93.89
      with complex rearrangements NEC Q93.7
    microdeletions NEC Q93.88
Delhi boil or button B55.1

Delinquency (juvenile) (neurotic) F91.8
  group Z72.810
Delinquent immunization status Z28.3
Delirium, delirious (acute or subacute) (not
  alcohol or drug-induced) (with dementia)
  R41.0
  alcoholic (acute) (tremens) (withdrawal)
  F10.921
    with intoxication F10.921
      in
        abuse F10.121
        dependence F10.221
  due to (secondary to)
    alcohol
      intoxication F10.921
        in
          abuse F10.121
          dependence F10.221
      withdrawal F10.231
    amphetamine intoxication F15.921
      in
        abuse F15.121
        dependence F15.221
    anxiolytic
      intoxication F13.921
        in
          abuse F13.121
          dependence F13.221
      withdrawal F13.231
    cannabis intoxication (acute) F12.921
      in
        abuse F12.121
        dependence F12.221
    cocaine intoxication (acute) F14.921
      in
        abuse F14.121
        dependence F14.221
    general medical condition F05
    hallucinogen intoxication F16.921
      in
        abuse F16.121
        dependence F16.221
    hypnotic
      intoxication F13.921
        in
          abuse F13.121
          dependence F13.221
      withdrawal F13.231
    inhalant intoxication (acute) F18.921
      in
        abuse F18.121
        dependence F18.221
    multiple etiologies F05
    opioid intoxication (acute) F11.921
      in
        abuse F11.121
        dependence F11.221
    phencyclidine intoxication (acute) F16.921
      in
        abuse F16.121
        dependence F16.221
    psychoactive substance NEC intoxication
    (acute) F19.921
      in
        abuse F19.121
        dependence F19.221
    sedative
      intoxication F13.921
        in
          abuse F13.121
          dependence F13.221
      withdrawal F13.231

Delirium, delirious   - *continued*
  unknown etiology F05
  exhaustion F43.0
  hysterical F44.89
  postprocedural (postoperative) F05
  puerperal F05
  thyroid —*see* Thyrotoxicosis with thyroid
  storm
  traumatic —*see* Injury, intracranial
  tremens (alcohol-induced) F10.231
  sedative-induced F13.231
Delivery (childbirth) (labor)
  arrested active phase O62.1
  cesarean (for)
    abnormal
      pelvis (bony) (deformity) (major) NEC
  with disproportion (fetopelvic) O33.0
    with obstructed labor O65.0
    presentation or position O32.9
  abruptio placentae (*see also* Abruptio
  placentae) O45.9
  acromion presentation O32.2
  atony, uterus O62.2
  breech presentation O32.1
    incomplete O32.8
  brow presentation O32.3
  cephalopelvic disproportion O33.9
  cerclage O34.3
  chin presentation O32.3
  cicatrix of cervix O34.4
  contracted pelvis (general)
    inlet O33.2
    outlet O33.3
  cord presentation or prolapse O69.0
  cystocele O34.8
  deformity (acquired) (congenital)
    pelvic organs or tissues NEC O34.8
    pelvis (bony) NEC O33.0
  disproportion NOS O33.9
  eclampsia —*see* Eclampsia
  face presentation O32.3
  failed
    forceps O66.5
    induction of labor O61.9
      instrumental O61.1
      mechanical O61.1
      medical O61.0
      specified NEC O61.8
      surgical O61.1
    trial of labor NOS O66.40
      following previous cesarean delivery
  O66.41
    vacuum extraction O66.5
    ventouse O66.5
  fetal-maternal hemorrhage O43.01
  hemorrhage (intrapartum) O67.9
    with coagulation defect O67.0
    specified cause NEC O67.8
  high head at term O32.4
  hydrocephalic fetus O33.6
  incarceration of uterus O34.51
  incoordinate uterine action O62.4
  increased size, fetus O33.5
  inertia, uterus O62.2
    primary O62.0
    secondary O62.1
  lateroversion, uterus O34.59
  mal lie O32.9
  malposition
    fetus O32.9
    pelvic organs or tissues NEC O34.8
    uterus NEC O34.59

Delivery   - *continued*
  malpresentation NOS O32.9
  oblique presentation O32.2
  occurring after 37 completed weeks of
  gestation but before 39 completed weeks
  gestation due to (spontaneous) onset of labor
  O75.82
  oversize fetus O33.5
  pelvic tumor NEC O34.8
  placenta previa O44.1
    without hemorrhage O44.0
  placental insufficiency O36.51
  planned, occurring after 37 completed weeks
  of gestation but before 39 completed weeks
  gestation due to (spontaneous) onset of labor
  O75.82
  polyp, cervix O34.4
    causing obstructed labor O65.5
  poor dilatation, cervix O62.0
  pre-eclampsia O14.9
    mild O14.0
    moderate O14.0
    severe
      with hemolysis, elevated liver enzymes
  and low platelet count (HELLP) O14.2
  previous
    cesarean delivery O34.21
    surgery (to)
      cervix O34.4
      gynecological NEC O34.8
      rectum O34.7
      uterus O34.29
      vagina O34.6
  prolapse
    arm or hand O32.2
    uterus O34.52
  prolonged labor NOS O63.9
  rectocele O34.8
  retroversion
    uterus O34.53
  rigid
    cervix O34.4
    pelvic floor O34.8
    perineum O34.7
    vagina O34.6
    vulva O34.7
  sacculation, pregnant uterus O34.59
  scar (s)
    cervix O34.4
    cesarean delivery O34.21
    uterus O34.29
  Shirodkar suture in situ O34.3
  shoulder presentation O32.2
  stenosis or stricture, cervix O34.4
  streptococcus B carrier state O99.824
  transverse presentation or lie O32.2
  tumor, pelvic organs or tissues NEC O34.8
    cervix O34.4
  umbilical cord presentation or prolapse
  O69.0
  without indication O82
  completely normal case O80
  complicated O75.9
    by
      abnormal, abnormality (of)
        forces of labor O62.9
          specified type NEC O62.8
        glucose O99.814
        uterine contractions NOS O62.9
      abruptio placentae (*see also* Abruptio
    placentae) O45.9
      abuse
        physical O9A.32

Delivery - *continued*
    psychological O9A.52
    sexual O9A.42
  adherent placenta O72.0
    without hemorrhage O73.0
  alcohol use O99.314
  anemia (pre-existing) O99.02
  anesthetic death O74.8
  annular detachment of cervix O71.3
  atony, uterus O62.2
  attempted vacuum extraction and forceps O66.5
  Bandl's ring O62.4
  bariatric surgery status O99.844
  biliary tract disorder O26.62
  bleeding —*see* Delivery, complicated by, hemorrhage
  blood disorder NEC O99.12
  cervical dystocia (hypotonic) O62.2
    primary O62.0
    secondary O62.1
  circulatory system disorder O99.42
  compression of cord (umbilical) NEC O69.2
  condition NEC O99.89
  contraction, contracted ring O62.4
  cord (umbilical)
    around neck
      with compression O69.1
      without compression O69.81
    bruising O69.5
    complication O69.9
      specified NEC O69.89
    compression NEC O69.2
    entanglement O69.2
      without compression O69.82
    hematoma O69.5
    presentation O69.0
    prolapse O69.0
    short O69.3
    thrombosis (vessels) O69.5
    vascular lesion O69.5
  Couvelaire uterus O45.8X
  damage to (injury to) NEC
    perineum O71.82
    periurethral tissue O71.82
    vulva O71.82
  delay following rupture of membranes (spontaneous) —*see* Pregnancy, complicated by, premature rupture of membranes
  depressed fetal heart tones O76
  diabetes O24.92
    gestational O24.429
      diet controlled O24.420
      insulin controlled O24.424
    pre-existing O24.32
      specified NEC O24.82
      type 1 O24.02
      type 2 O24.12
  diastasis recti (abdominis) O71.89
  dilatation
    bladder O66.8
    cervix incomplete, poor or slow O62.0
  disease NEC O99.89
  disruptio uteri —*see* Delivery, complicated by, rupture, uterus
  drug use O99.324
  dysfunction, uterus NOS O62.9
    hypertonic O62.4
    hypotonic O62.2
      primary O62.0
      secondary O62.1

Delivery - *continued*
  incoordinate O62.4
  eclampsia O15.1
  embolism (pulmonary) —*see* Embolism, obstetric
  endocrine, nutritional or metabolic disease NEC O99.284
  failed
    attempted vaginal birth after previous cesarean delivery O66.41
    induction of labor O61.9
      instrumental O61.1
      mechanical O61.1
      medical O61.0
      specified NEC O61.8
      surgical O61.1
    trial of labor O66.40
  female genital mutilation O65.5
  fetal
    abnormal acid-base balance O68
    acidemia O68
    acidosis O68
    alkalosis O68
    death, early O02.1
    deformity O66.3
    heart rate or rhythm (abnormal) (non-reassuring) O76
    hypoxia O77.8
    stress O77.9
      due to drug administration O77.1
      electrocardiographic evidence of O77.8
      specified NEC O77.8
      ultrasound evidence of O77.8
  fever during labor O75.2
  gastric banding status O99.844
  gastric bypass status O99.844
  gastrointestinal disease NEC O99.62
  gestational diabetes O24.429
    diet controlled O24.420
    insulin (and diet) controlled O24.424
  gonorrhea O98.22
  hematoma O71.7
    ischial spine O71.7
    pelvic O71.7
    vagina O71.7
    vulva or perineum O71.7
  hemorrhage (uterine) O67.9
    associated with
      afibrinogenemia O67.0
      coagulation defect O67.0
      hyperfibrinolysis O67.0
      hypofibrinogenemia O67.0
    due to
      low-lying placenta O44.1
      placenta previa O44.1
      premature separation of placenta (normally implanted) (*see also* Abruptio placentae) O45.9
      retained placenta O72.0
      uterine leiomyoma O67.8
    placenta NEC O67.8
    postpartum NEC (atonic) (immediate) O72.1
      with retained or trapped placenta O72.0
      delayed O72.2
      secondary O72.2
      third stage O72.0
  hourglass contraction, uterus O62.4
  hypertension, hypertensive (pre-existing) —*see* Hypertension, complicated by, childbirth (labor)
    hypotension O26.5

Delivery - *continued*
  incomplete dilatation (cervix) O62.0
  incoordinate uterus contractions O62.4
  inertia, uterus O62.2
    during latent phase of labor O62.0
    primary O62.0
    secondary O62.1
  infection (maternal) O98.92
    carrier state NEC O99.834
    gonorrhea O98.22
    human immunodeficiency virus (HIV) O98.72
    sexually transmitted NEC O98.32
    specified NEC O98.82
    syphilis O98.12
    tuberculosis O98.02
    viral hepatitis O98.42
    viral NEC O98.52
  injury (to mother) (*see also* Delivery, complicated, by, damage to) O71.9
    nonobstetric O9A.22
    caused by abuse —*see* Delivery, complicated by, abuse
  intrauterine fetal death, early O02.1
  inversion, uterus O71.2
  laceration (perineal) O70.9
    anus (sphincter) O70.4
      with third degree laceration O70.2
        with mucosa O70.3
      without third degree laceration O70.4
    bladder (urinary) O71.5
    bowel O71.5
    cervix (uteri) O71.3
    fourchette O70.0
    hymen O70.0
    labia O70.0
    pelvic
      floor O70.1
      organ NEC O71.5
    perineum, perineal O70.9
      first degree O70.0
      fourth degree O70.3
      muscles O70.1
      second degree O70.1
      skin O70.0
      slight O70.0
      third degree O70.2
    peritoneum (pelvic) O71.5
    rectovaginal (septum) (without perineal laceration) O71.4
      with perineum O70.2
        with anal or rectal mucosa O70.3
    specified NEC O71.89
    sphincter ani —*see* Delivery, complicated, by, laceration, anus (sphincter)
    urethra O71.5
    uterus O71.81
      before labor O71.81
    vagina, vaginal (deep) (high) (without perineal laceration) O71.4
      with perineum O70.0
      muscles, with perineum O70.1
    vulva O70.0
  liver disorder O26.62
  malignancy O9A.12
  malnutrition O25.2
  malposition, malpresentation
    placenta (with hemorrhage) O44.1
      without hemorrhage O44.0
    uterus or cervix O65.5
    without obstruction (*see also* Delivery, complicated by, obstruction) O32.9
      breech O32.1

Delivery - *continued*
  compound O32.6
  face (brow) (chin) O32.3
  footling O32.8
  high head O32.4
  oblique O32.2
  specified NEC O32.8
  transverse O32.2
  unstable lie O32.0
  meconium in amniotic fluid O77.0
  mental disorder NEC O99.344
  metrorrhexis —*see* Delivery, complicated
by, rupture, uterus
  nervous system disorder O99.354
  obesity (pre-existing) O99.214
  obesity surgery status O99.844
  obstetric trauma O71.9
    specified NEC O71.89
  obstructed labor
  due to
    breech (complete) (frank) presentation
O64.1
      incomplete O64.8
    brow presentation O64.3
    buttock presentation O64.1
    chin presentation O64.2
    compound presentation O64.5
    contracted pelvis O65.1
    deep transverse arrest O64.0
    deformed pelvis O65.0
    dystocia (fetal) O66.9
      due to
        conjoined twins O66.3
        fetal
          abnormality NEC O66.3
          ascites O66.3
          hydrops O66.3
          meningomyelocele O66.3
          sacral teratoma O66.3
          tumor O66.3
        hydrocephalic fetus O66.3
        shoulder O66.0
    face presentation O64.2
    fetopelvic disproportion O65.4
    footling presentation O64.8
    impacted shoulders O66.0
    incomplete rotation of fetal head O64.0
    large fetus O66.2
    locked twins O66.1
    malposition O64.9
      specified NEC O64.8
    malpresentation O64.9
      specified NEC O64.8
    multiple fetuses NEC O66.6
    pelvic
      abnormality (maternal) O65.9
        organ O65.5
        specified NEC O65.8
      contraction
        inlet O65.2
        mid cavity O65.3
        outlet O65.3
    persistent (position)
      occipitoiliac O64.0
      occipitoposterior O64.0
      occipitosacral O64.0
      occipitotransverse O64.0
    prolapsed arm O64.4
    shoulder presentation O64.4
    specified NEC O66.8
  pathological retraction ring, uterus O62.4

Delivery - *continued*
  penetration, pregnant uterus by instrument
O71.1
  perforation —*see* Delivery, complicated
by, laceration
  placenta, placental
    ablatio (*see also* Abruptio placentae)
O45.9
      abnormality O43.9
        specified NEC O43.89
      abruptio (*see also* Abruptio placentae)
O45.9
      accreta O43.21
      adherent (with hemorrhage) O72.0
        without hemorrhage O73.0
      detachment (premature) (*see also*
Abruptio placentae) O45.9
      disorder O43.9
        specified NEC O43.89
      hemorrhage NEC O67.8
      increta O43.22
      low (implantation) O44.1
        without hemorrhage O44.0
      malformation O43.10
      malposition O44.1
        without hemorrhage O44.0
      percreta O43.23
      previa (central) (lateral) (low) (marginal)
(partial) (total) O44.1
        without hemorrhage O44.0
      retained (with hemorrhage) O72.0
        without hemorrhage O73.0
      separation (premature) O45.9
        specified NEC O45.8X
      vicious insertion O44.1
    precipitate labor O62.3
    premature rupture, membranes (*see also*
Pregnancy, complicated by, premature rupture
of membranes) O42.90
    prolapse
      arm or hand O32.2
      cord (umbilical) O69.0
      foot or leg O32.8
      uterus O34.52
    prolonged labor O63.9
      first stage O63.0
      second stage O63.1
    protozoal disease (maternal) O98.62
    respiratory disease NEC O99.52
    retained membranes or portions of placenta
O72.2
      without hemorrhage O73.1
    retarded birth O63.9
    retention of secundines (with hemorrhage)
O72.0
      without hemorrhage O73.0
      partial O72.2
        without hemorrhage O73.1
    rupture
      bladder (urinary) O71.5
      cervix O71.3
      pelvic organ NEC O71.5
      urethra O71.5
      uterus (during or after labor) O71.1
        before labor O71.0
    separation, pubic bone (symphysis pubis)
O71.6
    shock O75.1
    shoulder presentation O64.4
    skin disorder NEC O99.72
    spasm, cervix O62.4
    stenosis or stricture, cervix O65.5

Delivery - *continued*
    streptococcus B carrier state O99.824
    subluxation of symphysis (pubis) O26.72
    syphilis (maternal) O98.12
    tear —*see* Delivery, complicated by,
laceration
    tetanic uterus O62.4
    trauma (obstetrical) (*see also* Delivery,
complicated, by, damage to) O71.9
      non-obstetric O9A.22
      periurethral O71.82
      specified NEC O71.89
    tuberculosis (maternal) O98.02
    tumor, pelvic organs or tissues NEC O65.5
    umbilical cord around neck
      with compression O69.1
      without compression O69.81
    uterine inertia O62.2
      during latent phase of labor O62.0
      primary O62.0
      secondary O62.1
    vasa previa O69.4
    velamentous insertion of cord O43.12
    specified complication NEC O75.89
  delayed NOS O63.9
    following rupture of membranes
      artificial O75.5
    second twin, triplet, etc. O63.2
  forceps, low following failed vacuum
extraction O66.5
  missed (at or near term) O36.4
  normal O80
  obstructed —*see* Delivery, complicated by,
obstruction
  precipitate O62.3
  preterm (*see also* Pregnancy, complicated by,
preterm labor) O60.10
  spontaneous O80
  term pregnancy NOS O80
  uncomplicated O80
  vaginal, following previous cesarean delivery
O34.21

Delusions (paranoid) —*see* Disorder,
delusional

Dementia (degenerative (primary)) (old age)
(persisting) F03.90
  with
    aggressive behavior F03.91
    behavioral disturbance F03.91
    combative behavior F03.91
    Lewy bodies G31.83 *[F02.80]*
      with behavioral disturbance G31.83
      [F02.81]
    Parkinsonism G31.83 *[F02.80]*
      with behavioral disturbance G31.83
      [F02.81]
    Parkinson's disease G20 *[F02.80]*
      with behavioral disturbance G20 *[F02.81]*
    violent behavior F03.91
  alcoholic F10.97
    with dependence F10.27
  Alzheimer's type —*see* Disease, Alzheimer's
  arteriosclerotic —*see* Dementia, vascular
  atypical, Alzheimer's type —*see* Disease,
Alzheimer's, specified NEC
  congenital —*see* Disability, intellectual
  frontal (lobe) G31.09 *[F02.80]*
    with behavioral disturbance G31.09
    [F02.81]
  frontotemporal G31.09 *[F02.80]*
    with behavioral disturbance G31.09
    [F02.81]
    specified NEC G31.09 *[F02.80]*

Dementia - *continued*
with behavioral disturbance G31.09
[F02.81]
in (due to)
alcohol F10.97
with dependence F10.27
Alzheimer's disease —*see* Disease,
Alzheimer's
arteriosclerotic brain disease —*see*
Dementia, vascular
cerebral lipidoses E75. [F02.80]
with behavioral disturbance E75. [F02.81]
Creutzfeldt-Jakob disease (*see also*
Creutzfeldt-Jakob disease or syndrome (with
dementia)) A81.00
epilepsy G40. [F02.80]
with behavioral disturbance G40.
[F02.81]
hepatolenticular degeneration E83.01
[F02.80]
with behavioral disturbance E83.01
[F02.81]
human immunodeficiency virus (HIV)
disease B20 [F02.80]
with behavioral disturbance B20 [F02.81]
Huntington's disease or chorea G10
hypercalcemia E83.52 [F02.80]
with behavioral disturbance E83.52
[F02.81]
hypothyroidism, acquired E03.9 [F02.80]
with behavioral disturbance E03.9
[F02.81]
due to iodine deficiency E01.8 [F02.80]
with behavioral disturbance E01.8
[F02.81]
inhalants F18.97
with dependence F18.27
multiple
etiologies F03
sclerosis G35 [F02.80]
with behavioral disturbance G35
[F02.81]
neurosyphilis A52.17 [F02.80]
with behavioral disturbance A52.17
[F02.81]
juvenile A50.49 [F02.80]
with behavioral disturbance A50.49
[F02.81]
niacin deficiency E52 [F02.80]
with behavioral disturbance E52 [F02.81]
paralysis agitans G20 [F02.80]
with behavioral disturbance G20 [F02.81]
Parkinson's disease G20 [F02.80]
pellagra E52 [F02.80]
with behavioral disturbance E52 [F02.81]
Pick's G31.01 [F02.80]
with behavioral disturbance G31.01
[F02.81]
polyarteritis nodosa M30.0 [F02.80]
with behavioral disturbance M30.0
[F02.81]
psychoactive drug F19.97
with dependence F19.27
inhalants F18.97
with dependence F18.27
sedatives, hypnotics or anxiolytics F13.97
with dependence F13.27
sedatives, hypnotics or anxiolytics F13.97
with dependence F13.27
systemic lupus erythematosus M32.
[F02.80]

Dementia - *continued*
with behavioral disturbance M32.
[F02.81]
trypanosomiasis
African B56.9 [F02.80]
with behavioral disturbance B56.9
[F02.81]
unknown etiology F03
vitamin B12 deficiency E53.8 [F02.80]
with behavioral disturbance E53.8
[F02.81]
volatile solvents F18.97
with dependence F18.27
with behavioral disturbance G31.83
[F02.81]
infantile, infantilis F84.3
Lewy body G31.83 [F02.80]
with behavioral disturbance G31.83
[F02.81]
multi-infarct —*see* Dementia, vascular
paralytica, paralytic (syphilitic) A52.17
[F02.80]
with behavioral disturbance A52.17
[F02.81]
juvenilis A50.45
paretic A52.17
praecox —*see* Schizophrenia
presenile F03
Alzheimer's type —*see* Disease,
Alzheimer's, early onset
primary degenerative F03
progressive, syphilitic A52.17
senile F03
with acute confusional state F05
Alzheimer's type —*see* Disease,
Alzheimer's, late onset
depressed or paranoid type F03
vascular (acute onset) (mixed) (multi-infarct)
(subcortical) F01.50
with behavioral disturbance F01.51
Demineralization, bone —*see* Osteoporosis
Demodex folliculorum (infestation) B88.0
Demophobia F40.248
Demoralization R45.3
Demyelination, demyelinization
central nervous system G37.9
specified NEC G37.8
corpus callosum (central) G37.1
disseminated, acute G36.9
specified NEC G36.8
global G35
in optic neuritis G36.0
Dengue (classical) (fever) A90
hemorrhagic A91
sandfly A93.1
Dennie-Marfan syphilitic syndrome A50.45
Dens evaginatus, in dente or invaginatus
K00.2
Dense breasts R92.2
Density
increased, bone (disseminated) (generalized)
(spotted) —*see* Disorder, bone, density and
structure, specified type NEC
lung (nodular) J98.4
Dental —*see also* condition
examination Z01.20
with abnormal findings Z01.21
restoration
aesthetically inadequate or displeasing
K08.56
defective K08.50
specified NEC K08.59

Dental - *continued*
failure of marginal integrity K08.51
failure of periodontal anatomical integrity
K08.54
Dentia praecox K00.6
Denticles (pulp) K04.2
Dentigerous cyst K09.0
Dentin
irregular (in pulp) K04.3
opalescent K00.5
secondary (in pulp) K04.3
sensitive K03.89
Dentinogenesis imperfecta K00.5
Dentinoma —*see* Cyst, calcifying odontogenic
Dentition (syndrome) K00.7
delayed K00.6
difficult K00.7
precocious K00.6
premature K00.6
retarded K00.6
Dependence (on) (syndrome) F19.20
with remission F19.21
alcohol (ethyl) (methyl) (without remission)
F10.20
with
amnestic disorder, persisting F10.26
anxiety disorder F10.280
dementia, persisting F10.27
intoxication F10.229
with delirium F10.221
uncomplicated F10.220
mood disorder F10.24
psychotic disorder F10.259
with
delusions F10.250
hallucinations F10.251
remission F10.21
sexual dysfunction F10.281
sleep disorder F10.282
specified disorder NEC F10.288
withdrawal F10.239
with
delirium F10.231
perceptual disturbance F10.232
uncomplicated F10.230
counseling and surveillance Z71.41
amobarbital —*see* Dependence, drug, sedative
amphetamine (s) (type) —*see* Dependence,
drug, stimulant NEC
amytal (sodium) —*see* Dependence, drug,
sedative
analgesic NEC F55.8
anesthetic (agent) (gas) (general) (local) NEC
—*see* Dependence, drug, psychoactive NEC
anxiolytic NEC —*see* Dependence, drug,
sedative
barbital (s) —*see* Dependence, drug, sedative
barbiturate (s) (compounds) (drugs
classifiable to T42) —*see* Dependence, drug,
sedative
benzedrine —*see* Dependence, drug,
stimulant NEC
bhang —*see* Dependence, drug, cannabis
bromide (s) NEC —*see* Dependence, drug,
sedative
caffeine —*see* Dependence, drug, stimulant
NEC
cannabis (sativa) (indica) (resin) (derivatives)
(type) —*see* Dependence, drug, cannabis
chloral (betaine) (hydrate) —*see* Dependence,
drug, sedative
chlordiazepoxide —*see* Dependence, drug,
sedative

Dependence - *continued*

coca (leaf) (derivatives) —*see* Dependence, drug, cocaine

cocaine —*see* Dependence, drug, cocaine

codeine —*see* Dependence, drug, opioid

combinations of drugs F19.20

dagga —*see* Dependence, drug, cannabis

demerol —*see* Dependence, drug, opioid

dexamphetamine —*see* Dependence, drug, stimulant NEC

dexedrine —*see* Dependence, drug, stimulant NEC

dextromethorphan —*see* Dependence, drug, opioid

dextromoramide —*see* Dependence, drug, opioid

dextro-nor-pseudo-ephedrine —*see* Dependence, drug, stimulant NEC

dextrorphan —*see* Dependence, drug, opioid

diazepam —*see* Dependence, drug, sedative

dilaudid —*see* Dependence, drug, opioid

D-lysergic acid diethylamide —*see* Dependence, drug, hallucinogen

drug NEC F19.20

  with sleep disorder F19.282

  cannabis F12.20

    with

      anxiety disorder F12.280

      intoxication F12.229

        with

          delirium F12.221

          perceptual disturbance F12.222

        uncomplicated F12.220

      other specified disorder F12.288

      psychosis F12.259

        delusions F12.250

        hallucinations F12.251

      unspecified disorder F12.29

    in remission F12.21

  cocaine F14.20

    with

      anxiety disorder F14.280

      intoxication F14.229

        with

          delirium F14.221

          perceptual disturbance F14.222

        uncomplicated F14.220

      mood disorder F14.24

      other specified disorder F14.288

      psychosis F14.259

        delusions F14.250

        hallucinations F14.251

      sexual dysfunction F14.281

      sleep disorder F14.282

      unspecified disorder F14.29

      withdrawal F14.23

    in remission F14.21

    withdrawal symptoms in newborn P96.1

  counseling and surveillance Z71.51

  hallucinogen F16.20

    with

      anxiety disorder F16.280

      flashbacks F16.283

      intoxication F16.229

        with delirium F16.221

        uncomplicated F16.220

      mood disorder F16.24

      other specified disorder F16.288

      perception disorder, persisting F16.283

      psychosis F16.259

        delusions F16.250

        hallucinations F16.251

unspecified disorder F16.29

  in remission F16.21

  in remission F19.21

  inhalant F18.20

    with

      anxiety disorder F18.280

      dementia, persisting F18.27

      intoxication F18.229

        with delirium F18.221

        uncomplicated F18.220

      mood disorder F18.24

      other specified disorder F18.288

      psychosis F18.259

        delusions F18.250

        hallucinations F18.251

      unspecified disorder F18.29

    in remission F18.21

  nicotine F17.200

    with disorder F17.209

      remission F17.201

      specified disorder NEC F17.208

      withdrawal F17.203

    chewing tobacco F17.220

      with disorder F17.229

        remission F17.221

        specified disorder NEC F17.228

        withdrawal F17.223

    cigarettes F17.210

      with disorder F17.219

        remission F17.211

        specified disorder NEC F17.218

        withdrawal F17.213

    specified product NEC F17.290

      with disorder F17.299

        remission F17.291

        specified disorder NEC F17.298

        withdrawal F17.293

  opioid F11.20

    with

      intoxication F11.229

        with

          delirium F11.221

          perceptual disturbance F11.222

        uncomplicated F11.220

      mood disorder F11.24

      other specified disorder F11.288

      psychosis F11.259

        delusions F11.250

        hallucinations F11.251

      sexual dysfunction F11.281

      sleep disorder F11.282

      unspecified disorder F11.29

      withdrawal F11.23

    in remission F11.21

  psychoactive NEC F19.20

    with

      amnestic disorder F19.26

      anxiety disorder F19.280

      dementia F19.27

      intoxication F19.229

        with

          delirium F19.221

          perceptual disturbance F19.222

        uncomplicated F19.220

      mood disorder F19.24

      other specified disorder F19.288

      psychosis F19.259

        delusions F19.250

        hallucinations F19.251

      sexual dysfunction F19.281

      sleep disorder F19.282

unspecified disorder F19.29

    withdrawal F19.239

      with

        delirium F19.231

        perceptual disturbance F19.232

      uncomplicated F19.230

  sedative, hypnotic or anxiolytic F13.20

    with

      amnestic disorder F13.26

      anxiety disorder F13.280

      dementia, persisting F13.27

      intoxication F13.229

        with delirium F13.221

        uncomplicated F13.220

      mood disorder F13.24

      other specified disorder F13.288

      psychosis F13.259

        delusions F13.250

        hallucinations F13.251

      sexual dysfunction F13.281

      sleep disorder F13.282

      unspecified disorder F13.29

    withdrawal F13.239

      with

        delirium F13.231

        perceptual disturbance F13.232

      uncomplicated F13.230

    in remission F13.21

  stimulant NEC F15.20

    with

      anxiety disorder F15.280

      intoxication F15.229

        with

          delirium F15.221

          perceptual disturbance F15.222

        uncomplicated F15.220

      mood disorder F15.24

      other specified disorder F15.288

      psychosis F15.259

        delusions F15.250

        hallucinations F15.251

      sexual dysfunction F15.281

      sleep disorder F15.282

      unspecified disorder F15.29

      withdrawal F15.23

    in remission F15.21

ethyl

  alcohol (without remission) F10.20

    with remission F10.21

  bromide —*see* Dependence, drug, sedative

carbamate F19.20

chloride F19.20

morphine —*see* Dependence, drug, opioid

ganja —*see* Dependence, drug, cannabis

glue (airplane) (sniffing) —*see* Dependence, drug, inhalant

glutethimide —*see* Dependence, drug, sedative

hallucinogenics —*see* Dependence, drug, hallucinogen

hashish —*see* Dependence, drug, cannabis

hemp —*see* Dependence, drug, cannabis

heroin (salt) (any) —*see* Dependence, drug, opioid

hypnotic NEC —*see* Dependence, drug, sedative

Indian hemp —*see* Dependence, drug, cannabis

inhalants —*see* Dependence, drug, inhalant

khat —*see* Dependence, drug, stimulant NEC

laudanum —*see* Dependence, drug, opioid

Dependence - *continued*
LSD (25) (derivatives) —*see* Dependence, drug, hallucinogen
luminal —*see* Dependence, drug, sedative
lysergic acid —*see* Dependence, drug, hallucinogen
maconha —*see* Dependence, drug, cannabis
marihuana —*see* Dependence, drug, cannabis
meprobamate —*see* Dependence, drug, sedative
mescaline —*see* Dependence, drug, hallucinogen
methadone —*see* Dependence, drug, opioid
methamphetamine (s) —*see* Dependence, drug, stimulant NEC
methaqualone —*see* Dependence, drug, sedative
methyl
  alcohol (without remission) F10.20
    with remission F10.21
  bromide —*see* Dependence, drug, sedative
  morphine —*see* Dependence, drug, opioid
  phenidate —*see* Dependence, drug, stimulant NEC
  sulfonal —*see* Dependence, drug, sedative
morphine (sulfate) (sulfite) (type) —*see* Dependence, drug, opioid
narcotic (drug) NEC —*see* Dependence, drug, opioid
nembutal —*see* Dependence, drug, sedative
neraval —*see* Dependence, drug, sedative
neraval —*see* Dependence, drug, sedative
neurobarb —*see* Dependence, drug, sedative
nicotine —*see* Dependence, drug, nicotine
nitrous oxide F19.20
nonbarbiturate sedatives and tranquilizers with similar effect —*see* Dependence, drug, sedative
on
  artificial heart (fully implantable) (mechanical) Z95.812
  aspirator Z99.0
  care provider (because of) Z74.9
    impaired mobility Z74.09
    need for
      assistance with personal care Z74.1
      continuous supervision Z74.3
    no other household member able to render care Z74.2
    specified reason NEC Z74.8
  machine Z99.89
    enabling NEC Z99.89
    specified type NEC Z99.89
  renal dialysis (hemodialysis) (peritoneal) Z99.2
  respirator Z99.11
  ventilator Z99.11
  wheelchair Z99.3
opiate —*see* Dependence, drug, opioid
opioids —*see* Dependence, drug, opioid
opium (alkaloids) (derivatives) (tincture) —*see* Dependence, drug, opioid
oxygen (long-term) (supplemental) Z99.81
paraldehyde —*see* Dependence, drug, sedative
paregoric —*see* Dependence, drug, opioid
PCP (phencyclidine) (*see also* Abuse, drug, hallucinogen) F16.20
pentobarbital —*see* Dependence, drug, sedative
pentobarbitone (sodium) —*see* Dependence, drug, sedative

Dependence - *continued*
pentothal —*see* Dependence, drug, sedative
peyote —*see* Dependence, drug, hallucinogen
phencyclidine (PCP) (and related substances) (*see also* Abuse, drug, hallucinogen) F16.20
phenmetrazine —*see* Dependence, drug, stimulant NEC
phenobarbital —*see* Dependence, drug, sedative
polysubstance F19.20
psilocybin, psilocin, psilocin, psilocyline — *see* Dependence, drug, hallucinogen
psychostimulant NEC —*see* Dependence, drug, stimulant NEC
secobarbital —*see* Dependence, drug, sedative
seconal —*see* Dependence, drug, sedative
sedative NEC —*see* Dependence, drug, sedative
specified drug NEC —*see* Dependence, drug
stimulant NEC —*see* Dependence, drug, stimulant NEC
substance NEC —*see* Dependence, drug
supplemental oxygen Z99.81
tobacco —*see* Dependence, drug, nicotine
  counseling and surveillance Z71.6
tranquilizer NEC —*see* Dependence, drug, sedative
vitamin B6 E53.1
volatile solvents —*see* Dependence, drug, inhalant
Dependency
care-provider Z74.9
passive F60.7
reactions (persistent) F60.7
Depersonalization (in neurotic state) (neurotic) (syndrome) F48.1
Depletion
extracellular fluid E86.9
plasma E86.1
potassium E87.6
  nephropathy N25.89
salt or sodium E87.1
  causing heat exhaustion or prostration T67.4
  nephropathy N28.9
volume NOS E86.9
Deployment (current) (military) **status** Z56.82
in theater or in support of military war, peacekeeping and humanitarian operations Z56.82
personal history of Z91.82
  military war, peacekeeping and humanitarian deployment (current or past conflict) Z91.82
  returned from Z91.82
Depolarization, premature I49.40
atrial I49.1
junctional I49.2
specified NEC I49.49
ventricular I49.3
Deposit
bone in Boeck's sarcoid D86.89
calcareous, calcium —*see* Calcification
cholesterol
  retina H35.89
  vitreous (body) (humor) —*see* Deposit, crystalline
conjunctiva H11.11
cornea H18.00
  argentous H18.02
  due to metabolic disorder H18.03
  Kayser-Fleischer ring H18.04

Deposit – *continued*
  pigmentation —*see* Pigmentation, cornea
  crystalline, vitreous (body) (humor) H43.2
  hemosiderin in old scars of cornea —*see* Pigmentation, cornea, stromal
  metallic in lens —*see* Cataract, specified NEC
  skin R23.8
  tooth, teeth (betel) (black) (green) (materia alba) (orange) (tobacco) K03.6
  urate, kidney —*see* Calculus, kidney
Depraved appetite —*see* Pica
Depressed
HDL cholesterol E78.6
Depression (acute) (mental) F32.9
agitated (single episode) F32.2
anaclitic —*see* Disorder, adjustment
anxiety F41.8
  persistent F34.1
arches —*see also* Deformity, limb, flat foot
atypical (single episode) F32.8
basal metabolic rate R94.8
bone marrow D75.89
central nervous system R09.2
cerebral R29.818
  newborn P91.4
cerebrovascular I67.9
chest wall M95.4
climacteric (single episode) F32.8
endogenous (without psychotic symptoms) F33.2
  with psychotic symptoms F33.3
functional activity R68.89
hysterical F44.89
involutional (single episode) F32.8
major F32.9
  with psychotic symptoms F32.3
  recurrent —*see* Disorder, depressive, recurrent
manic-depressive —*see* Disorder, depressive, recurrent
masked (single episode) F32.8
medullary G93.89
menopausal (single episode) F32.8
metatarsus —*see* Depression, arches
monopolar F33.9
nervous F34.1
neurotic F34.1
nose M95.0
postnatal F53
postpartum F53
post-psychotic of schizophrenia F32.8
post-schizophrenic F32.8
psychogenic (reactive) (single episode) F32.9
psychoneurotic F34.1
psychotic (single episode) F32.3
  recurrent F33.3
reactive (psychogenic) (single episode) F32.9
  psychotic (single episode) F32.3
recurrent —*see* Disorder, depressive, recurrent
respiratory center G93.89
seasonal —*see* Disorder, depressive, recurrent
senile F03
severe, single episode F32.2
situational F43.21
skull Q67.4
specified NEC (single episode) F32.8
sternum M95.4
visual field —*see* Defect, visual field
vital (recurrent) (without psychotic symptoms) F33.2
  with psychotic symptoms F33.3
  single episode F32.2

Deprivation
cultural Z60.3
effects NOS T73.9
  specified NEC T73.8
emotional NEC Z65.8
  affecting infant or child —*see* Maltreatment, child, psychological
food T73.0
protein —*see* Malnutrition
sleep Z72.820
social Z60.4
  affecting infant or child —*see* Maltreatment, child, psychological
specified NEC T73.8
vitamins —*see* Deficiency, vitamin
water T73.1

Derangement
ankle (internal) —*see* Derangement, joint, ankle
cartilage (articular) NEC —*see* Derangement, joint, articular cartilage, by site
  recurrent —*see* Dislocation, recurrent
cruciate ligament, anterior, current injury —*see* Sprain, knee, cruciate, anterior
elbow (internal) —*see* Derangement, joint, elbow
hip (joint) (internal) (old) —*see* Derangement, joint, hip
joint (internal) M24.9
  ankylosis —*see* Ankylosis
  articular cartilage M24.10
    ankle M24.17
    elbow M24.12
    foot M24.17
    hand M24.14
    hip M24.15
    knee NEC M23.9
    loose body —*see* Loose, body
    shoulder M24.11
    wrist M24.13
  contracture —*see* Contraction, joint
  current injury *see also* Dislocation
    knee, meniscus or cartilage —*see* Tear, meniscus
  dislocation
    pathological —*see* Dislocation, pathological
    recurrent —*see* Dislocation, recurrent
  knee —*see* Derangement, knee
  ligament —*see* Disorder, ligament
  loose body —*see* Loose, body
  recurrent —*see* Dislocation, recurrent
  specified type NEC M24.80
    ankle M24.87
    elbow M24.82
    foot joint M24.87
    hand joint M24.84
    hip M24.85
    shoulder M24.81
    wrist M24.83
  temporomandibular M26.69
knee (recurrent) M23.9
  ligament disruption, spontaneous M23.60
    anterior cruciate M23.61
    capsular M23.67
    instability, chronic M23.5
    lateral collateral M23.64
    medial collateral M23.63
    posterior cruciate M23.62
  loose body M23.4
  meniscus M23.30
    cystic M23.00

Derangement - *continued*
  lateral M23.002
    anterior horn M23.04
    posterior horn M23.05
    specified NEC M23.06
    medial M23.005
    anterior horn M23.01
    posterior horn M23.02
    specified NEC M23.03
  degenerate —*see* Derangement, knee, meniscus, specified NEC
  detached —*see* Derangement, knee, meniscus, specified NEC
  due to old tear or injury M23.20
    lateral M23.20
      anterior horn M23.24
      posterior horn M23.25
      specified NEC M23.26
    medial M23.20
      anterior horn M23.21
      posterior horn M23.22
      specified NEC M23.23
  retained —*see* Derangement, knee, meniscus, specified NEC
  specified NEC M23.30
    lateral M23.30
      anterior horn M23.34
      posterior horn M23.35
      specified NEC M23.36
    medial M23.30
      anterior horn M23.31
      posterior horn M23.32
      specified NEC M23.33
  old M23.8X
  specified NEC —*see* subcategory M23.8
low back NEC —*see* Dorsopathy, specified NEC
meniscus —*see* Derangement, knee, meniscus
mental —*see* Psychosis
patella, specified NEC —*see* Disorder, patella, derangement NEC
semilunar cartilage (knee) —*see* Derangement, knee, meniscus, specified NEC
shoulder (internal) —*see* Derangement, joint, shoulder

Dercum's disease E88.2
Derealization (neurotic) F48.1
Dermal —*see* condition
Dermaphytid *see* Dermatophytosis
Dermatitis (eczematous) L30.9
ab igne L59.0
acarine B88.0
actinic (due to sun) L57.8
  other than from sun L59.8
allergic —*see* Dermatitis, contact, allergic
ambustionis, due to burn or scald —*see* Burn
amebic A06.7
ammonia L22
arsenical (ingested) L27.8
artefacta L98.1
  psychogenic F54
atopic L20.9
  psychogenic F54
  specified NEC L20.89
autoimmune progesterone L30.8
berlock, berloque L56.2
blastomycotic B40.3
blister beetle L24.89
bullous, bullosa L13.9
  mucosynechial, atrophic L12.1
  seasonal L30.8
  specified NEC L13.8

Dermatitis – *continued*
calorica L59.0
  due to burn or scald —*see* Burn
caterpillar L24.89
cercarial B65.3
combustionis L59.0
  due to burn or scald —*see* Burn
congelationis T69.1
contact (occupational) L25.9
  allergic L23.9
    due to
      adhesives L23.1
      cement L23.5
      chemical products NEC L23.5
      chromium L23.0
      cosmetics L23.2
      dander (cat) (dog) L23.81
      drugs in contact with skin L23.3
      dyes L23.4
      food in contact with skin L23.6
      hair (cat) (dog) L23.81
      insecticide L23.5
      metals L23.0
      nickel L23.0
      plants, non-food L23.7
      plastic L23.5
      rubber L23.5
      specified agent NEC L23.89
    due to
      cement L25.3
      chemical products NEC L25.3
      cosmetics L25.0
      dander (cat) (dog) L23.81
      drugs in contact with skin L25.1
      dyes L25.2
      food in contact with skin L25.4
      hair (cat) (dog) L23.81
      plants, non-food L25.5
      specified agent NEC L25.8
  irritant L24.9
    due to
      cement L25.3
      chemical products NEC L24.5
      cosmetics L24.3
      detergents L24.0
      drugs in contact with skin L24.4
      food in contact with skin L24.6
      oils and greases L24.1
      plants, non-food L24.7
      solvents L24.2
      specified agent NEC L24.89
contusiformis L52
diabetic —*see* E08-E13 with .620
diaper L22
diphtheritica A36.3
dry skin L85.3
due to
  acetone (contact) (irritant) L24.2
  acids (contact) (irritant) L24.5
  adhesive (s) (allergic) (contact) (plaster) L23.1
    irritant L24.5
  alcohol (irritant) (skin contact) (substances in category T51) L24.2
    taken internally L27.8
  alkalis (contact) (irritant) L24.5
  arsenic (ingested) L27.8
  carbon disulfide (contact) (irritant) L24.2
  caustics (contact) (irritant) L24.5
  cement (contact) L25.3
  cereal (ingested) L27.2
  chemical (s) NEC L25.3

Dermatitis – *continued*
taken internally L27.8
chlorocompounds L24.2
chromium (contact) (irritant) L24.81
coffee (ingested) L27.2
cold weather L30.8
cosmetics (contact) L25.0
allergic L23.2
irritant L24.3
cyclohexanes L24.2
dander (cat) (dog) L23.81
Demodex species B88.0
Dermanyssus gallinae B88.0
detergents (contact) (irritant) L24.0
dichromate L24.81
drugs and medicaments (generalized)
(internal use) L27.0
external —*see* Dermatitis, due to, drugs, in
contact with skin
in contact with skin L25.1
allergic L23.3
irritant L24.4
localized skin eruption L27.1
specified substance —*see* Table of Drugs
and Chemicals
dyes (contact) L25.2
allergic L23.4
irritant L24.89
epidermophytosis —*see* Dermatophytosis
esters L24.2
external irritant NEC L24.9
fish (ingested) L27.2
flour (ingested) L27.2
food (ingested) L27.2
in contact with skin L25.4
fruit (ingested) L27.2
furs (allergic) (contact) L23.81
glues —*see* Dermatitis, due to, adhesives
glycols L24.2
greases NEC (contact) (irritant) L24.1
hair (cat) (dog) L23.81
hot
objects and materials —*see* Burn
weather or places L59.0
hydrocarbons L24.2
infrared rays L59.8
ingestion, ingested substance L27.9
chemical NEC L27.8
drugs and medicaments —*see* Dermatitis,
due to, drugs
food L27.2
specified NEC L27.8
insecticide in contact with skin L24.5
internal agent L27.9
drugs and medicaments (generalized) —
see Dermatitis, due to, drugs
food L27.2
irradiation —*see* Dermatitis, due to,
radioactive substance
ketones L24.2
lacquer tree (allergic) (contact) L23.7
light (sun) NEC L57.8
acute L56.8
other L59.8
Liponyssoides sanguineus B88.0
low temperature L30.8
meat (ingested) L27.2
metals, metal salts (contact) (irritant) L24.81
milk (ingested) L27.2
nickel (contact) (irritant) L24.81
nylon (contact) (irritant) L24.5
oils NEC (contact) (irritant) L24.1

Dermatitis – *continued*
paint solvent (contact) (irritant) L24.2
petroleum products (contact) (irritant)
(substances in T52.0) L24.2
plants NEC (contact) L25.5
allergic L23.7
irritant L24.7
plasters (adhesive) (any) (allergic) (contact)
L23.1
irritant L24.5
plastic (contact) L25.3
preservatives (contact) —*see* Dermatitis, due
to, chemical, in contact with skin
primrose (allergic) (contact) L23.7
primula (allergic) (contact) L23.7
radiation L59.8
nonionizing (chronic exposure) L57.8
sun NEC L57.8
acute L56.8
radioactive substance L58.9
acute L58.0
chronic L58.1
radium L58.9
acute L58.0
chronic L58.1
ragweed (allergic) (contact) L23.7
Rhus (allergic) (contact) (diversiloba)
(radicans) (toxicodendron) (venenata)
(verniciflua) L23.7
rubber (contact) L24.5
Senecio jacobaea (allergic) (contact) L23.7
solvents (contact) (irritant) (substances in
categories T52) L24.2
specified agent NEC (contact) L25.8
allergic L23.89
irritant L24.89
sunshine NEC L57.8
acute L56.8
tetrachlorethylene (contact) (irritant) L24.2
toluene (contact) (irritant) L24.2
turpentine (contact) L24.2
ultraviolet rays (sun NEC) (chronic
exposure) L57.8
acute L56.8
vaccine or vaccination L27.0
specified substance —*see* Table of Drugs
and Chemicals
varicose veins —*see* Varix, leg, with,
inflammation
X-rays L58.9
acute L58.0
chronic L58.1
dyshidrotic L30.1
dysmenorrheica N94.6
escharotica —*see* Burn
exfoliative, exfoliativa (generalized) L26
neonatorum L00
eyelid —*see also* Dermatosis, eyelid
allergic H01.119
left H01.116
lower H01.115
upper H01.114
right H01.113
lower H01.112
upper H01.111
contact —*see* Dermatitis, eyelid, allergic
due to
Demodex species B88.0
herpes (zoster) B02.39
simplex B00.59
eczematous H01.139
left H01.136

Dermatitis – *continued*
lower H01.135
upper H01.134
right H01.133
lower H01.132
upper H01.131
facta, factitia, factitial L98.1
psychogenic F54
flexural NEC L20.82
friction L30.4
fungus B36.9
specified type NEC B36.8
gangrenosa, gangrenous infantum L08.0
harvest mite B88.0
heat L59.0
herpesviral, vesicular (ear) (lip) B00.1
herpetiformis (bullous) (erythematous)
(pustular) (vesicular) L13.0
juvenile L12.2
senile L12.0
hiemalis L30.8
hypostatic, hypostatica —*see* Varix, leg, with,
inflammation
infectious eczematoid L30.3
infective L30.3
irritant —*see* Dermatitis, contact, irritant
Jacquet's (diaper dermatitis) L22
Leptus B88.0
lichenified NEC L28.0
medicamentosa (generalized) (internal use) —
see Dermatitis, due to drugs
mite B88.0
multiformis L13.0
juvenile L12.2
napkin L22
neurotica L13.0
nummular L30.0
papillaris capillitii L73.0
pellagrous E52
perioral L71.0
photocontact L56.2
polymorpha dolorosa L13.0
pruriginosa L13.0
pruritic NEC L30.8
psychogenic F54
purulent L08.0
pustular
contagious B08.02
subcorneal L13.1
pyococcal L08.0
pyogenica L08.0
repens L40.2
Ritter's (exfoliativa) L00
Schamberg's L81.7
schistosome B65.3
seasonal bullous L30.8
seborrheic L21.9
infantile L21.1
specified NEC L21.8
sensitization NOS L23.9
septic L08.0
solare L57.8
specified NEC L30.8
stasis I87.2
with varicose ulcer —*see* Varix, leg, with
ulcer, with inflammation
due to postthrombotic syndrome —*see*
Syndrome, postthrombotic
suppurative L08.0
traumatic NEC L30.4
trophoneurotica L13.0
ultraviolet (sun) (chronic exposure) L57.8
acute L56.8

Dermatitis – *continued*
varicose —*see* Varix, leg, with, inflammation
vegetans L10.1
verrucosa B43.0
vesicular, herpesviral B00.1
Dermatoarthritis, lipoid E78.81
Dermatochalasis, eyelid H02.839
left H02.836
lower H02.835
upper H02.834
right H02.833
lower H02.832
upper H02.831
Dermatofibroma (lenticulare) —*see*
Neoplasm, skin, benign
protuberans —*see* Neoplasm, skin, uncertain
behavior
Dermatofibrosarcoma (pigmented)
(protuberans) —*see* Neoplasm, skin,
malignant
Dermatographia L50.3
Dermatolysis (exfoliativa) (congenital) Q82.8
acquired L57.4
eyelids —*see* Blepharochalasis
palpebrarum —*see* Blepharochalasis
senile L57.4
Dermatomegaly NEC Q82.8
Dermatomucosomyositis M33.10
with
myopathy M33.12
respiratory involvement M33.11
specified organ involvement NEC M33.19
Dermatomycosis B36.9
furfuracea B36.0
specified type NEC B36.8
Dermatomyositis (acute) (chronic) —*see also*
Dermatopolymyositis
in (due to) neoplastic disease (*see also*
Neoplasm) D49.9 *[M36.0]*
Dermatoneuritis of children —*see* Poisoning,
mercury
Dermatophilosis A48.8
Dermatophytid L30.2
Dermatophytid —*see* Dermatophytosis
Dermatophytosis (epidermophyton)
(infection) (Microsporum) (tinea)
(Trichophyton) B35.9
beard B35.0
body B35.4
capitis B35.0
corporis B35.4
deep-seated B35.8
disseminated B35.8
foot B35.3
granulomatous B35.8
groin B35.6
hand B35.2
nail B35.1
perianal (area) B35.6
scalp B35.0
specified NEC B35.8
Dermatopolymyositis M33.90
with
myopathy M33.92
respiratory involvement M33.91
specified organ involvement NEC M33.99
in neoplastic disease (*see also* Neoplasm)
D49.9 *[M36.0]*
juvenile M33.00
with
myopathy M33.02
respiratory involvement M33.01

Dermatopolymyositis - *continued*
specified organ involvement NEC M33.09
specified NEC M33.10
myopathy M33.12
respiratory involvement M33.11
specified organ involvement NEC M33.19
Dermatopolyneuritis —*see* Poisoning,
mercury
Dermatorrhexis Q79.6
acquired L57.4
Dermatosclerosis —*see also* Scleroderma
localized L94.0
Dermatosis L98.9
Andrews' L08.89
Bowen's —*see* Neoplasm, skin, in situ
bullous L13.9
specified NEC L13.8
exfoliativa L26
eyelid (noninfectious)
dermatitis —*see* Dermatitis, eyelid
discoid lupus erythematosus —*see* Lupus,
erythematosus, eyelid
xeroderma —*see* Xeroderma, acquired,
eyelid
factitial L98.1
febrile neutrophilic L98.2
gonococcal A54.89
herpetiformis L13.0
juvenile L12.2
linear IgA L13.8
menstrual NEC L98.8
neutrophilic, febrile L98.2
occupational —*see* Dermatitis, contact
papulosa nigra L82.1
pigmentary L81.9
progressive L81.7
Schamberg's L81.7
psychogenic F54
purpuric, pigmented L81.7
pustular, subcorneal L13.1
transient acantholytic L11.1
Dermographia, dermographism L50.3
Dermoid (cyst) —*see also* Neoplasm, benign,
by site
with malignant transformation C56
due to radiation (nonionizing) L57.8
Dermopathy
infiltrative with thyrotoxicosis —*see*
Thyrotoxicosis
nephrogenic fibrosing L90.8
Dermophytosis —*see* Dermatophytosis
Descemetocele H18.73
Descemet's membrane —*see* condition
Descending —*see* condition
Descensus uteri —*see* Prolapse, uterus
Desert
rheumatism B38.0
sore —*see* Ulcer, skin
Desertion (newborn) —*see* Maltreatment
Desmoid (extra-abdominal) (tumor) —*see*
Neoplasm, connective tissue, uncertain
behavior
abdominal D48.1
Despondency F32.9
Desquamation, skin R23.4
Destruction, destructive —*see also* Damage
articular facet —*see also* Derangement, joint,
specified type NEC
knee M23.8X
vertebra —*see* Spondylosis
bone —*see also* Disorder, bone, specified
type NEC
syphilitic A52.77

Destruction, destructive - *continued*
joint —*see also* Derangement, joint, specified
type NEC
sacroiliac M53.3
rectal sphincter K62.89
septum (nasal) J34.89
tuberculous NEC —*see* Tuberculosis
tympanum, tympanic membrane
(nontraumatic) —*see* Disorder, tympanic
membrane, specified NEC
vertebral disc —*see* Degeneration,
intervertebral disc
Destructiveness —*see also* Disorder, conduct
adjustment reaction —*see* Disorder,
adjustment
Desultory labor O62.2
Detachment
cartilage —*see* Sprain
cervix, annular N88.8
complicating delivery O71.3
choroid (old) (postinfectional) (simple)
(spontaneous) H31.40
hemorrhagic H31.41
serous H31.42
ligament —*see* Sprain
meniscus (knee) —*see also* Derangement,
knee, meniscus, specified NEC
current injury —*see* Tear, meniscus
due to old tear or injury —*see* Derangement,
knee, meniscus, due to old tear
retina (without retinal break) (serous) H33.2
with retinal:
break H33.00
giant H33.03
multiple H33.02
single H33.01
dialysis H33.04
pigment epithelium —*see* Degeneration,
retina, separation of layers, pigment
epithelium detachment
rhegmatogenous —*see* Detachment, retina,
with retinal, break
specified NEC H33.8
total H33.05
traction H33.4
vitreous (body) H43.81
Detergent asthma J69.8
Deterioration
epileptic F06.8
general physical R53.81
heart, cardiac —*see* Degeneration, myocardial
mental —*see* Psychosis
myocardial, myocardium —*see* Degeneration,
myocardial
senile (simple) R54
Deuteranomaly (anomalous trichromat)
H53.53
Deuteranopia (complete) (incomplete) H53.53
Development
abnormal, bone Q79.9
arrested R62.50
bone —*see* Arrest, development or growth,
bone
child R62.50
due to malnutrition E45
defective, congenital —*see also* Anomaly, by
site
cauda equina Q06.3
left ventricle Q24.8
in hypoplastic left heart syndrome Q23.4
valve Q24.8
pulmonary Q22.3

Development - *continued*
delayed (*see also* Delay, development)
R62.50
  arithmetical skills F81.2
  language (skills) (expressive) F80.1
  learning skill F81.9
  mixed skills F88
  motor coordination F82
  reading F81.0
  specified learning skill NEC F81.89
  speech F80.9
  spelling F81.81
  written expression F81.81
imperfect, congenital —*see also* Anomaly, by
site
  heart Q24.9
  lungs Q33.6
incomplete
  bronchial tree Q32.4
  organ or site not listed —*see* Hypoplasia, by
site
  respiratory system Q34.9
sexual, precocious NEC E30.1
tardy, mental (*see also* Disability, intellectual)
F79
Developmental —*see* condition
testing, child —*see* Examination, child
Devergie's disease (pityriasis rubra pilaris)
L44.0
Deviation (in)
conjugate palsy (eye) (spastic) H51.0
esophagus (acquired) K22.8
eye, skew H51.8
midline (jaw) (teeth) (dental arch) M26.29
  specified site NEC —*see* Malposition
nasal septum J34.2
  congenital Q67.4
opening and closing of the mandible M26.53
organ or site, congenital NEC —*see*
Malposition, congenital
septum (nasal) (acquired) J34.2
  congenital Q67.4
sexual F65.9
  bestiality F65.89
  erotomania F52.8
  exhibitionism F65.2
  fetishism, fetishistic F65.0
   transvestism F65.1
  frotteurism F65.81
  masochism F65.51
  multiple F65.89
  necrophilia F65.89
  nymphomania F52.8
  pederosis F65.4
  pedophilia F65.4
  sadism, sadomasochism F65.52
  satyriasis F52.8
  specified type NEC F65.89
  transvestism F64.1
  voyeurism F65.3
teeth, midline M26.29
trachea J39.8
ureter, congenital Q62.61
Device
cerebral ventricle (communicating) in situ
Z98.2
contraceptive —*see* Contraceptive, device
drainage, cerebrospinal fluid, in situ Z98.2
Devic's disease G36.0
Devil's
grip B33.0
pinches (purpura simplex) D69.2
Devitalized tooth K04.99

Devonshire colic —*see* Poisoning, lead
in tetralogy of Fallot Q21.3
Dextrinosis, limit (debrancher enzyme
deficiency) E74.03
Dextrocardia (true) Q24.0
with
  complete transposition of viscera Q89.3
  situs inversus Q89.3
Dextroposition, aorta Q20.3
Dextrotransposition, aorta Q20.3
d-glycericacidemia E72.59
Dhat syndrome F48.8
Dhobi itch B35.6
Di George's syndrome D82.1
Di Guglielmo's disease C94.0
Diabetes, diabetic (mellitus) (sugar) E11.9
with
  amyotrophy E11.44
  arthropathy NEC E11.618
  autonomic (poly) neuropathy E11.43
  cataract E11.36
  Charcot's joints E11.610
  chronic kidney disease E11.22
  circulatory complication NEC E11.59
  complication E11.8
   specified NEC E11.69
  dermatitis E11.620
  foot ulcer E11.621
  gangrene E11.52
  gastroparesis E11.43
  glomerulonephrosis, intracapillary E11.21
  glomerulosclerosis, intercapillary E11.21
  hyperglycemia E11.65
  hyperosmolarity E11.00
   with coma E11.01
  hypoglycemia E11.649
   with coma E11.641
  kidney complications NEC E11.29
  Kimmelstiel-Wilson disease E11.21
  loss of protective sensation (LOPS) —*see*
Diabetes, by type, with neuropathy
  mononeuropathy E11.41
  myasthenia E11.44
  necrobiosis lipoidica E11.620
  nephropathy E11.21
  neuralgia E11.42
  neurologic complication NEC E11.49
  neuropathic arthropathy E11.610
  neuropathy E11.40
  ophthalmic complication NEC E11.39
  oral complication NEC E11.638
  periodontal disease E11.630
  peripheral angiopathy E11.51
   with gangrene E11.52
  polyneuropathy E11.42
  renal complication NEC E11.29
  renal tubular degeneration E11.29
  retinopathy E11.319
   with macular edema E11.311
   nonproliferative E11.329
    with macular edema E11.321
    mild E11.329
     with macular edema E11.321
    moderate E11.339
     with macular edema E11.331
    severe E11.349
     with macular edema E11.341
   proliferative E11.359
    with macular edema E11.351
  skin complication NEC E11.628
  skin ulcer NEC E11.622
bronzed E83.110

Diabetes, diabetic – *continued*
complicating pregnancy —*see* Pregnancy,
complicated by, diabetes
dietary counseling and surveillance Z71.3
due to drug or chemical E09.9
with
  amyotrophy E09.44
  arthropathy NEC E09.618
  autonomic (poly) neuropathy E09.43
  cataract E09.36
  Charcot's joints E09.610
  chronic kidney disease E09.22
  circulatory complication NEC E09.59
  complication E09.8
   specified NEC E09.69
  dermatitis E09.620
  foot ulcer E09.621
  gangrene E09.52
  gastroparesis E09.43
  glomerulonephrosis, intracapillary E09.21
  glomerulosclerosis, intercapillary E09.21
  hyperglycemia E09.65
  hyperosmolarity E09.00
   with coma E09.01
  hypoglycemia E09.649
   with coma E09.641
  ketoacidosis E09.10
   with coma E09.11
  kidney complications NEC E09.29
  Kimmelstiel-Wilson disease E09.21
  mononeuropathy E09.41
  myasthenia E09.44
  necrobiosis lipoidica E09.620
  nephropathy E09.21
  neuralgia E09.42
  neurologic complication NEC E09.49
  neuropathic arthropathy E09.610
  neuropathy E09.40
  ophthalmic complication NEC E09.39
  oral complication NEC E09.638
  periodontal disease E09.630
  peripheral angiopathy E09.51
   with gangrene E09.52
  polyneuropathy E09.42
  renal complication NEC E09.29
  renal tubular degeneration E09.29
  retinopathy E09.319
   with macular edema E09.311
   nonproliferative E09.329
    with macular edema E09.321
    mild E09.329
     with macular edema E09.321
    moderate E09.339
     with macular edema E09.331
    severe E09.349
     with macular edema E09.341
   proliferative E09.359
    with macular edema E09.351
  skin complication NEC E09.628
  skin ulcer NEC E09.622
due to underlying condition E08.9
with
  amyotrophy E08.44
  arthropathy NEC E08.618
  autonomic (poly) neuropathy E08.43
  cataract E08.36
  Charcot's joints E08.610
  chronic kidney disease E08.22
  circulatory complication NEC E08.59
  complication E08.8
   specified NEC E08.69
  dermatitis E08.620
  foot ulcer E08.621

Diabetes, diabetic – *continued*
  gangrene E08.52
  gastroparesis E08.43
  glomerulonephrosis, intracapillary E08.21
  glomerulosclerosis, intercapillary E08.21
  hyperglycemia E08.65
  hyperosmolarity E08.00
   with coma E08.01
  hypoglycemia E08.649
   with coma E08.641
  ketoacidosis E08.10
   with coma E08.11
  kidney complications NEC E08.29
  Kimmelstiel-Wilson disease E08.21
  mononeuropathy E08.41
  myasthenia E08.44
  necrobiosis lipoidica E08.620
  nephropathy E08.21
  neuralgia E08.42
  neurologic complication NEC E08.49
  neuropathic arthropathy E08.610
  neuropathy E08.40
  ophthalmic complication NEC E08.39
  oral complication NEC E08.638
  periodontal disease E08.630
  peripheral angiopathy E08.51
   with gangrene E08.52
  polyneuropathy E08.42
  renal complication NEC E08.29
  renal tubular degeneration E08.29
  retinopathy E08.319
   with macular edema E08.311
   nonproliferative E08.329
    with macular edema E08.321
    mild E08.329
     with macular edema E08.321
    moderate E08.339
     with macular edema E08.331
    severe E08.349
     with macular edema E08.341
   proliferative E08.359
    with macular edema E08.351
  skin complication NEC E08.628
  skin ulcer NEC E08.622
 gestational (in pregnancy) O24.419
  affecting newborn P70.0
  diet controlled O24.410
  in childbirth O24.429
   diet controlled O24.420
   insulin (and diet) controlled O24.424
  insulin (and diet) controlled O24.414
  puerperal O24.439
   diet controlled O24.430
   insulin (and diet) controlled O24.434
 hepatogenous E13.9
 inadequately controlled
 code to Diabetes, by type, with hyperglycemia
 insipidus E23.2
  nephrogenic N25.1
  pituitary E23.2
  vasopressin resistant N25.1
 insulin dependent
 code to type of diabetes
 juvenile-onset —*see* Diabetes, type 1
 ketosis-prone —*see* Diabetes, type 1
 latent R73.09
 neonatal (transient) P70.2
 non-insulin dependent
 code to type of diabetes
 out of control
 code to Diabetes, by type, with hyperglycemia
 phosphate E83.39

Diabetes, diabetic – *continued*
 poorly controlled
 code to Diabetes, by type, with hyperglycemia
 postpancreatectomy —*see* Diabetes, specified type NEC
 postprocedural —*see* Diabetes, specified type NEC
 secondary diabetes mellitus NEC —*see* Diabetes, specified type NEC
 specified type NEC E13.9
  with
   amyotrophy E13.44
   arthropathy NEC E13.618
   autonomic (poly) neuropathy E13.43
   cataract E13.36
   Charcot's joints E13.610
   chronic kidney disease E13.22
   circulatory complication NEC E13.59
   complication E13.8
    specified NEC E13.69
   dermatitis E13.620
   foot ulcer E13.621
   gangrene E13.52
   gastroparesis E13.43
   glomerulonephrosis, intracapillary E13.21
   glomerulosclerosis, intercapillary E13.21
   hyperglycemia E13.65
   hyperosmolarity E13.00
    with coma E13.01
   hypoglycemia E13.649
    with coma E13.641
   ketoacidosis E13.10
    with coma E13.11
   kidney complications NEC E13.29
   Kimmelstiel-Wilson disease E13.21
   mononeuropathy E13.41
   myasthenia E13.44
   necrobiosis lipoidica E13.620
   nephropathy E13.21
   neuralgia E13.42
   neurologic complication NEC E13.49
   neuropathic arthropathy E13.610
   neuropathy E13.40
   ophthalmic complication NEC E13.39
   oral complication NEC E13.638
   periodontal disease E13.630
   peripheral angiopathy E13.51
    with gangrene E13.52
   polyneuropathy E13.42
   renal complication NEC E13.29
   renal tubular degeneration E13.29
   retinopathy E13.319
    with macular edema E13.311
    nonproliferative E13.329
     with macular edema E13.321
     mild E13.329
      with macular edema E13.321
     moderate E13.339
      with macular edema E13.331
     severe E13.349
      with macular edema E13.341
    proliferative E13.359
     with macular edema E13.351
   skin complication NEC E13.628
   skin ulcer NEC E13.622
 steroid-induced —*see* Diabetes, due to, drug or chemical
 type 1 E10.9
  with
   amyotrophy E10.44
   arthropathy NEC E10.618
   autonomic (poly) neuropathy E10.43

Diabetes, diabetic – *continued*
   cataract E10.36
   Charcot's joints E10.610
   chronic kidney disease E10.22
   circulatory complication NEC E10.59
   complication E10.8
    specified NEC E10.69
   dermatitis E10.620
   foot ulcer E10.621
   gangrene E10.52
   gastroparesis E10.43
   glomerulonephrosis, intracapillary E10.21
   glomerulosclerosis, intercapillary E10.21
   hyperglycemia E10.65
   hypoglycemia E10.649
    with coma E10.641
   ketoacidosis E10.10
    with coma E10.11
   kidney complications NEC E10.29
   Kimmelstiel-Wilson disease E10.21
   mononeuropathy E10.41
   myasthenia E10.44
   necrobiosis lipoidica E10.620
   nephropathy E10.21
   neuralgia E10.42
   neurologic complication NEC E10.49
   neuropathic arthropathy E10.610
   neuropathy E10.40
   ophthalmic complication NEC E10.39
   oral complication NEC E10.638
   periodontal disease E10.630
   peripheral angiopathy E10.51
    with gangrene E10.52
   polyneuropathy E10.42
   renal complication NEC E10.29
   renal tubular degeneration E10.29
   retinopathy E10.319
    with macular edema E10.311
    nonproliferative E10.329
     with macular edema E10.321
     mild E10.329
      with macular edema E10.321
     moderate E10.339
      with macular edema E10.331
     severe E10.349
      with macular edema E10.341
    proliferative E10.359
     with macular edema E10.351
   skin complication NEC E10.628
   skin ulcer NEC E10.622
 type 2 E11.9
  with
   amyotrophy E11.44
   arthropathy NEC E11.618
   autonomic (poly) neuropathy E11.43
   cataract E11.36
   Charcot's joints E11.610
   chronic kidney disease E11.22
   circulatory complication NEC E11.59
   complication E11.8
    specified NEC E11.69
   dermatitis E11.620
   foot ulcer E11.621
   gangrene E11.52
   gastroparesis E11.43
   glomerulonephrosis, intracapillary E11.21
   glomerulosclerosis, intercapillary E11.21
   hyperglycemia E11.65
   hyperosmolarity E11.00
    with coma E11.01
   hypoglycemia E11.649
    with coma E11.641

Diabetes, diabetic – *continued*
    kidney complications NEC E11.29
    Kimmelstiel-Wilson disease E11.21
    mononeuropathy E11.41
    myasthenia E11.44
    necrobiosis lipoidica E11.620
    nephropathy E11.21
    neuralgia E11.42
    neurologic complication NEC E11.49
    neuropathic arthropathy E11.610
    neuropathy E11.40
    ophthalmic complication NEC E11.39
    oral complication NEC E11.638
    periodontal disease E11.630
    peripheral angiopathy E11.51
     with gangrene E11.52
    polyneuropathy E11.42
    renal complication NEC E11.29
    renal tubular degeneration E11.29
    retinopathy E11.319
     with macular edema E11.311
     nonproliferative E11.329
      with macular edema E11.321
      mild E11.329
       with macular edema E11.321
      moderate E11.339
       with macular edema E11.331
      severe E11.349
       with macular edema E11.341
     proliferative E11.359
      with macular edema E11.351
    skin complication NEC E11.628
    skin ulcer NEC E11.622
Diacyclothrombopathia D69.1
Diagnosis deferred R69
Dialysis (intermittent) (treatment)
    noncompliance (with) Z91.15
    renal (hemodialysis) (peritoneal) , status Z99.2
    retina, retinal —*see* Detachment, retina, with retinal, dialysis
Diamond-Blackfan anemia (congenital hypoplastic) D61.01
Diamond-Gardener syndrome (autoerythrocyte sensitization) D69.2
Diaper rash L22
Diaphoresis (excessive) R61
Diaphragm —*see* condition
Diaphragmalgia R07.1
Diaphragmatitis, diaphragmitis J98.6
Diaphysial aclasis Q78.6
Diaphysitis —*see* Osteomyelitis, specified type NEC
Diarrhea, diarrheal (disease) (infantile) (inflammatory) R19.7
    achlorhydric K31.83
    allergic K52.2
    amebic (*see also* Amebiasis) A06.0
     with abscess —*see* Abscess, amebic
     acute A06.0
     chronic A06.1
     nondysenteric A06.2
    bacillary —*see* Dysentery, bacillary
    balantidial A07.0
    cachectic NEC K52.89
    Chilomastix A07.8
    choleriformis A00.1
    chronic (noninfectious) K52.9
    coccidial A07.3
    Cochin-China K90.1
     strongyloidiasis B78.0
    Dientamoeba A07.8

Diarrhea, diarrheal - *continued*
    dietetic K52.2
    drug-induced K52.1
    due to
     bacteria A04.9
      specified NEC A04.8
     Campylobacter A04.5
     Capillaria philippinensis B81.1
     Clostridium difficile A04.7
     Clostridium perfringens (C) (F) A04.8
     Cryptosporidium A07.2
     drugs K52.1
     Escherichia coli A04.4
      enteroaggregative A04.4
      enterohemorrhagic A04.3
      enteroinvasive A04.2
      enteropathogenic A04.0
      enterotoxigenic A04.1
      specified NEC A04.4
     food hypersensitivity K52.2
     Necator americanus B76.1
     S. japonicum B65.2
     specified organism NEC A08.8
      bacterial A04.8
      viral A08.39
     Staphylococcus A04.8
     Trichuris trichiura B79
     virus —*see* Enteritis, viral
     Yersinia enterocolitica A04.6
    dysenteric A09
    endemic A09
    epidemic A09
    flagellate A07.9
    Flexner's (ulcerative) A03.1
    functional K59.1
     following gastrointestinal surgery K91.89
     psychogenic F45.8
    Giardia lamblia A07.1
    giardial A07.1
    hill K90.1
    infectious A09
    malarial —*see* Malaria
    mite B88.0
    mycotic NEC B49
    neonatal (noninfectious) P78.3
    nervous F45.8
    neurogenic K59.1
    noninfectious K52.9
    postgastrectomy K91.1
    postvagotomy K91.1
    protozoal A07.9
     specified NEC A07.8
    psychogenic F45.8
    specified
     bacterium NEC A04.8
     virus NEC A08.39
    strongyloidiasis B78.0
    toxic K52.1
    trichomonal A07.8
    tropical K90.1
    tuberculous A18.32
    viral —*see* Enteritis, viral
Diastasis
    cranial bones M84.88
     congenital NEC Q75.8
    joint (traumatic) —*see* Dislocation
    muscle M62.00
     ankle M62.07
     congenital Q79.8
     foot M62.07
     forearm M62.03
     hand M62.04

Diastasis - *continued*
     lower leg M62.06
     pelvic region M62.05
     shoulder region M62.01
     specified site NEC M62.08
     thigh M62.05
     upper arm M62.02
    recti (abdomen)
     complicating delivery O71.89
     congenital Q79.59
Diastema, tooth, teeth, fully erupted M26.32
Diastematomyelia Q06.2
Diataxia, cerebral G80.4
Diathesis
    allergic —*see* History, allergy
    bleeding (familial) D69.9
    cystine (familial) E72.00
    gouty —*see* Gout
    hemorrhagic (familial) D69.9
     newborn NEC P53
    spasmophilic R29.0
Diaz's disease or osteochondrosis (juvenile) (talus) —*see* Osteochondrosis, juvenile, tarsus
Dibothriocephalus, dibothriocephaliasis (latus) (infection) (infestation) B70.0
    larval B70.1
Dicephalus, dicephaly Q89.4
Dichotomy, teeth K00.2
Dichromat, dichromatopsia (congenital) — *see* Deficiency, color vision
Dichuchwa A65
Dicroceliasis B66.2 —*see* Double uterus
Didelphia, didelphys —*see* Double uterus
Didymitis N45.1
    with orchitis N45.3
Dietary
    inadequacy or deficiency E63.9
    surveillance and counseling Z71.3
Dietl's crisis N13.8
Dieulafoy lesion (hemorrhagic)
    duodenum K31.82
    esophagus K22.8
    intestine (colon) K63.81
    stomach K31.82
Difficult, difficulty (in)
    acculturation Z60.3
    feeding R63.3
     newborn P92.9
      breast P92.5
      specified NEC P92.8
     nonorganic (infant or child) F98.29
    intubation, in anesthesia T88.4
    mechanical, gastroduodenal stoma K91.89
     causing obstruction K91.3
    reading (developmental) F81.0
     secondary to emotional disorders F93.9
    spelling (specific) F81.81
     with reading disorder F81.89
     due to inadequate teaching Z55.8
    swallowing —*see* Dysphagia
    walking R26.2
    work
     conditions NEC Z56.5
     schedule Z56.3
Diffuse —*see* condition
Digeorge's syndrome (thymic hypoplasia) D82.1
Digestive —*see* condition
Dihydropyrimidine dehydrogenase disease (DPD) E88.89
Diktyoma —*see* Neoplasm, malignant, by site
Dilaceration, tooth K00.4

Dilatation
anus K59.8
  venule —*see* Hemorrhoids
aorta (focal) (general) —*see* Ectasia, aorta
  with aneurysm —*see* Aneurysm, aorta
artery —*see* Aneurysm
bladder (sphincter) N32.89
  congenital Q64.79
blood vessel I99.8
bronchial J47.9
  with
    exacerbation (acute) J47.1
    lower respiratory infection J47.0
calyx (due to obstruction) —*see*
Hydronephrosis
capillaries I78.8
cardiac (acute) (chronic) —*see also*
Hypertrophy, cardiac
  congenital Q24.8
    valve NEC Q24.8
      pulmonary Q22.3
  valve —*see* Endocarditis
cavum septi pellucidi Q06.8
cervix (uteri) —*see also* Incompetency, cervix
  incomplete, poor, slow complicating
delivery O62.0
colon K59.3
  congenital Q43.1
  psychogenic F45.8
common duct (acquired) K83.8
  congenital Q44.5
cystic duct (acquired) K82.8
  congenital Q44.5
duct, mammary —*see* Ectasia, mammary duct
duodenum K59.8
esophagus K22.8
  congenital Q39.5
  due to achalasia K22.0
eustachian tube, congenital Q17.8
gallbladder K82.8
gastric —*see* Dilatation, stomach
heart (acute) (chronic) —*see also*
Hypertrophy, cardiac
  congenital Q24.8
  valve —*see* Endocarditis
ileum K59.8
  psychogenic F45.8
jejunum K59.8
  psychogenic F45.8
kidney (calyx) (collecting structures) (cystic)
(parenchyma) (pelvis) (idiopathic) N28.89
lacrimal passages or duct —*see* Disorder,
lacrimal system, changes
lymphatic vessel I89.0
mammary duct —*see* Ectasia, mammary duct
Meckel's diverticulum (congenital) Q43.0
  malignant —*see* Table of Neoplasms, small
intestine, malignant
myocardium (acute) (chronic) —*see*
Hypertrophy, cardiac
organ or site, congenital NEC —*see*
Distortion
pancreatic duct K86.8
pericardium —*see* Pericarditis
pharynx J39.2
prostate N42.89
pulmonary
  artery (idiopathic) I28.8
  valve, congenital Q22.3
pupil H57.04
rectum K59.3
saccule, congenital Q16.5

Dilatation – *continued*
salivary gland (duct) K11.8
sphincter ani K62.89
stomach K31.89
  acute K31.0
  psychogenic F45.8
submaxillary duct K11.8
trachea, congenital Q32.1
ureter (idiopathic) N28.82
  congenital Q62.2
  due to obstruction N13.4
urethra (acquired) N36.8
vasomotor I73.9
vein I86.8
ventricular, ventricle (acute) (chronic) —*see*
also Hypertrophy, cardiac
  cerebral, congenital Q04.8
  venule NEC I86.8
vesical orifice N32.89
Dilated, dilation —*see* Dilatation
Diminished, diminution
  hearing (acuity) —*see* Deafness
  sense or sensation (cold) (heat) (tactile)
(vibratory) R20.8
  vision NEC H54.7
  vital capacity R94.2
Diminuta taenia B71.0
Dimitri-Sturge-Weber disease Q85.8
Dimple
  parasacral, pilonidal or postanal —*see* Cyst,
pilonidal
Dioctophyma renalis (infection) (infestation)
B83.8
Dipetalonemiasis B74.4
Diphallus Q55.69
Diphtheria, diphtheritic (gangrenous)
(hemorrhagic) A36.9
  carrier (suspected) Z22.2
  cutaneous A36.3
  faucial A36.0
  infection of wound A36.3
  laryngeal A36.2
  myocarditis A36.81
  nasal, anterior A36.89
  nasopharyngeal A36.1
  neurological complication A36.89
  pharyngeal A36.0
  specified site NEC A36.89
  tonsillar A36.0
Diphyllobothriasis (intestine) B70.0
  larval B70.1
Diplacusis H93.22
Diplegia (upper limbs) G83.0
  congenital (cerebral) G80.8
  facial G51.0
  lower limbs G82.20
  spastic G80.1
Diplococcus, diplococcal —*see* condition
Diplopia H53.2
Dipsomania F10.20
  with
    psychosis —*see* Psychosis, alcoholic
    remission F10.21
Dipylidiasis B71.1
Direction, teeth, abnormal, fully erupted
M26.30
Dirofilariasis B74.8
Dirt-eating child F98.3
Disability, disabilities
  heart —*see* Disease, heart
  intellectual F79
    with
      autistic features F84.9

Disability, disabilities - *continued*
  mild (I.Q.50 69) F70
  moderate (I.Q.35 49) F71
  profound (I.Q. under 20) F73
  severe (I.Q.20 34) F72
  specified level NEC F78
  knowledge acquisition F81.9
  learning F81.9
  limiting activities Z73.6
  spelling, specific F81.81
Disappearance of family member Z63.4
Disarticulation —*see* Amputation
  meaning traumatic amputation —*see*
Amputation, traumatic
Discharge (from)
  abnormal finding in —*see* Abnormal,
specimen
  breast (female) (male) N64.52
  diencephalic autonomic idiopathic —*see*
Epilepsy, specified NEC
  ear — *see also* Otorrhea
    blood —*see* Otorrhagia
  excessive urine R35.8
  nipple N64.52
  penile R36.9
  postnasal R09.82
  prison, anxiety concerning Z65.2
  urethral R36.9
    without blood R36.0
    hematospermia R36.1
  vaginal N89.8
Discitis, diskitis M46.40
  cervical region M46.42
  cervicothoracic region M46.43
  lumbar region M46.46
  lumbosacral region M46.47
  multiple sites M46.49
  occipito-atlanto-axial region M46.41
  pyogenic —*see* Infection, intervertebral disc,
pyogenic
  sacrococcygeal region M46.48
  thoracic region M46.44
  thoracolumbar region M46.45
Discoid
  meniscus (congenital) Q68.6
  semilunar cartilage (congenital) —*see*
Derangement, knee, meniscus, specified NEC
Discoloration
  nails L60.8
  teeth (posteruptive) K03.7
    during formation K00.8
Discomfort
  chest R07.89
  visual H53.14
Discontinuity, ossicles, ear H74.2
Discord (with)
  boss Z56.4
  classmates Z55.4
  counselor Z64.4
  employer Z56.4
  family Z63.8
  fellow employees Z56.4
  in-laws Z63.1
  landlord Z59.2
  lodgers Z59.2
  neighbors Z59.2
  probation officer Z64.4
  social worker Z64.4
  teachers Z55.4
  workmates Z56.4
Discordant connection
  atrioventricular (congenital) Q20.5
  ventriculoarterial Q20.3

Discrepancy
centric occlusion maximum intercuspation
M26.55
leg length (acquired) —*see* Deformity, limb,
unequal length
   congenital —*see* Defect, reduction, lower
limb
uterine size date O26.84
Discrimination
ethnic Z60.5
political Z60.5
racial Z60.5
religious Z60.5
sex Z60.5
Disease, diseased —*see also* Syndrome
absorbent system I87.8
acid-peptic K30
Acosta's T70.29
Adams-Stokes (-Morgagni) (syncope with
heart block) I45.9
Addison's anemia (pernicious) D51.0
adenoids (and tonsils) J35.9
adrenal (capsule) (cortex) (gland) (medullary)
E27.9
  hyperfunction E27.0
  specified NEC E27.8
ainhum L94.6
airway
  obstructive, chronic J44.9
    due to
      cotton dust J66.0
      specific organic dusts NEC J66.8
  reactive —*see* Asthma
akamushi (scrub typhus) A75.3
Albers-Schönberg (marble bones) Q78.2
Albert's —*see* Tendinitis, Achilles
alimentary canal K63.9
alligator-skin Q80.9
  acquired L85.0
alpha heavy chain C88.3
alpine T70.29
altitude T70.20
alveolar ridge
  edentulous K06.9
    specified NEC K06.8
alveoli, teeth K08.9
Alzheimer's G30.9 *[F02.80]*
  with behavioral disturbance G30.9 *[F02.81]*
  early onset G30.0 *[F02.80]*
    with behavioral disturbance G30.0
    [F02.81]
  late onset G30.1 *[F02.80]*
    with behavioral disturbance G30.1
    [F02.81]
  specified NEC G30.8 *[F02.80]*
    with behavioral disturbance G30.8
    [F02.81]
amyloid —*see* Amyloidosis
Andersen's (glycogenosis IV) E74.09
Andes T70.29
Andrews' (bacterid) L08.89
angiospastic I73.9
  cerebral G45.9
  vein I87.8
anterior
  chamber H21.9
  horn cell G12.29
antiglomerular basement membrane (anti
GBM) antibody M31.0
  tubulo-interstitial nephritis N12
antral —*see* Sinusitis, maxillary
anus K62.9
  specified NEC K62.89

Disease, diseased - *continued*
aorta (nonsyphilitic) I77.9
  syphilitic NEC A52.02
aortic (heart) (valve) I35.9
  rheumatic I06.9
Apollo B30.3
aponeuroses —*see* Enthesopathy
appendix K38.9
  specified NEC K38.8
aqueous (chamber) H21.9
Arnold-Chiari —*see* Arnold-Chiari disease
arterial I77.9
  occlusive —*see* Occlusion, by site
  due to stricture or stenosis I77.1
arteriocardiorenal —*see* Hypertension,
cardiorenal
arteriolar (generalized) (obliterative) I77.9
arteriorenal —*see* Hypertension, kidney
arteriosclerotic —*see also* Arteriosclerosis
  cardiovascular —*see* Disease, heart,
ischemic, atherosclerotic
  coronary (artery) —*see* Disease, heart,
ischemic, atherosclerotic
  heart —*see* Disease, heart, ischemic,
atherosclerotic
artery I77.9
  cerebral I67.9
  coronary I25.10
    with angina pectoris —*see*
Arteriosclerosis, coronary (artery) ,
arthropod-borne NOS (viral) A94
  specified type NEC A93.8
atticoantral, chronic H66.20
  left H66.22
    with right H66.23
  right H66.21
    with left H66.23
auditory canal —*see* Disorder, ear, external
auricle, ear NEC —*see* Disorder, pinna
Australian X A83.4
autoimmune (systemic) NOS M35.9
  hemolytic (cold type) (warm type) D59.1
    drug-induced D59.0
  thyroid E06.3
aviator's —*see* Effect, adverse, high altitude
Ayala's Q78.5
Ayerza's (pulmonary artery sclerosis with
pulmonary hypertension) I27.0
Babington's (familial hemorrhagic
telangiectasia) I78.0
bacterial A49.9
  specified NEC A48.8
  zoonotic A28.9
    specified type NEC A28.8
Baelz's (cheilitis glandularis apostematosa)
K13.0
bagasse J67.1
balloon —*see* Effect, adverse, high altitude
Bang's (brucella abortus) A23.1
Bannister's T78.3
barometer makers' —*see* Poisoning, mercury
Barraquer (-Simons') (progressive
lipodystrophy) E88.1
Barrett's —*see* Barrett's, esophagus
Bartholin's gland N75.9
basal ganglia G25.9
  degenerative G23.9
    specified NEC G23.8
  specified NEC G25.89
Basedow's (exophthalmic goiter) —*see*
Hyperthyroidism, with, goiter (diffuse)
Bateman's B08.1

Disease, diseased - *continued*
Batten-Steinert G71.11
Battey A31.0
Beard's (neurasthenia) F48.8
Becker
  idiopathic mural endomyocardial I42.3
  myotonia congenita G71.12
Begbie's (exophthalmic goiter) —*see*
Hyperthyroidism, with, goiter (diffuse)
behavioral, organic F07.9
Beigel's (white piedra) B36.2
Benson's —*see* Deposit, crystalline
Bernard-Soulier (thrombopathy) D69.1
Bernhardt (-Roth) —*see* Mononeuropathy,
lower limb, meralgia paresthetica
Biermer's (pernicious anemia) D51.0
bile duct (common) (hepatic) K83.9
  with calculus, stones —*see* Calculus, bile
duct
  specified NEC K83.8
biliary (tract) K83.9
  specified NEC K83.8
Billroth's —*see* Spina bifida
bird fancier's J67.2
black lung J60
bladder N32.9
  in (due to)
    schistosomiasis (bilharziasis) B65.0 *[N33]*
  specified NEC N32.89
bleeder's D66
blood D75.9
  forming organs D75.9
  vessel I99.9
Bloodgood's —*see* Mastopathy, cystic
Bodechtel-Guttmann (subacute sclerosing
panencephalitis) A81.1
bone —*see also* Disorder, bone
  aluminum M83.4
  fibrocystic NEC
    jaw M27.49
bone-marrow D75.9
Borna A83.9
Bornholm (epidemic pleurodynia) B33.0
Bouchard's (myopathic dilatation of the
stomach) K31.0
Bouillaud's (rheumatic heart disease) I01.9
Bourneville (-Brissaud) (tuberous sclerosis)
Q85.1
Bouveret (-Hoffmann) (paroxysmal
tachycardia) I47.9
bowel K63.9
  functional K59.9
    psychogenic F45.8
brain G93.9
  arterial, artery I67.9
  arteriosclerotic I67.2
  congenital Q04.9
  degenerative —*see* Degeneration, brain
  inflammatory —*see* Encephalitis
  organic G93.9
    arteriosclerotic I67.2
  parasitic NEC B71.9 *[G94]*
  senile NEC G31.1
  specified NEC G93.89
breast (*see also* Disorder, breast) N64.9
  cystic (chronic) —*see* Mastopathy, cystic
  fibrocystic —*see* Mastopathy, cystic
  Paget's
    female, unspecified side C50.91
    male, unspecified side C50.92
  specified NEC N64.89
Breda's —*see* Yaws

Disease, diseased - *continued*
Bretonneau's (diphtheritic malignant angina) A36.0
Bright's —*see* Nephritis
  arteriosclerotic —*see* Hypertension, kidney
Brill's (recrudescent typhus) A75.1
Brill-Zinsser (recrudescent typhus) A75.1
Brion-Kayser —*see* Fever, paratyphoid
broad
  beta E78.2
  ligament (noninflammatory) N83.9
    inflammatory —*see* Disease, pelvis, inflammatory
      specified NEC N83.8
Brocq-Duhring (dermatitis herpetiformis) L13.0
Brocq's
  meaning
    dermatitis herpetiformis L13.0
    prurigo L28.2
bronchopulmonary J98.4
bronchus NEC J98.09
bronze Addison's E27.1
  tuberculous A18.7
budgerigar fancier's J67.2
bullous L13.9
  chronic of childhood L12.2
  specified NEC L13.8
Buerger's (thromboangiitis obliterans) I73.1
Bürger-Grütz (essential familial hyperlipemia) E78.3
bursa —*see* Bursopathy
caisson T70.3
California —*see* Coccidioidomycosis
capillaries I78.9
  specified NEC I78.8
Carapata A68.0
cardiac —*see* Disease, heart
cardiopulmonary, chronic I27.9
cardiorenal (hepatic) (hypertensive) (vascular) —*see* Hypertension, cardiorenal
cardiovascular (atherosclerotic) I25.10
  with angina pectoris —*see* Arteriosclerosis, coronary (artery)
  congenital Q28.9
  newborn P29.9
    specified NEC P29.89
  hypertensive —*see* Hypertension, heart
  renal (hypertensive) —*see* Hypertension, cardiorenal
  syphilitic (asymptomatic) A52.00
cartilage —*see* Disorder, cartilage
Castellani's A69.8
cat-scratch A28.1
Cavare's (familial periodic paralysis) G72.3
cecum K63.9
celiac (adult) (infantile) K90.0
cellular tissue L98.9
central core G71.2
cerebellar, cerebellum —*see* Disease, brain
cerebral —*see also* Disease, brain
  degenerative —*see* Degeneration, brain
cerebrospinal G96.9
cerebrovascular I67.9
  acute I67.89
    embolic I63.4
    thrombotic I63.3
  arteriosclerotic I67.2
  specified NEC I67.89
cervix (uteri) (noninflammatory) N88.9
  inflammatory —*see* Cervicitis
  specified NEC N88.8

Chabert's A22.9
Chandler's (osteochondritis dissecans, hip) —*see* Osteochondritis, dissecans, hip
Charlouis —*see* Yaws
Chédiak-Steinbrinck (-Higashi) (congenital gigantism of peroxidase granules) E70.330
chest J98.9
Chiari's (hepatic vein thrombosis) I82.0
Chicago B40.9
Chignon B36.8
chigo, chigoe B88.1
childhood granulomatous D71
Chinese liver fluke B66.1
chlamydial A74.9
  specified NEC A74.89
cholecystic K82.9
choroid H31.9
  specified NEC H31.8
Christmas D67
chronic bullous of childhood L12.2
chylomicron retention E78.3
ciliary body H21.9
  specified NEC H21.89
circulatory (system) NEC I99.8
  newborn P29.9
  syphilitic A52.00
    congenital A50.54
coagulation factor deficiency (congenital) —*see* Defect, coagulation
coccidioidal —*see* Coccidioidomycosis
cold
  agglutinin or hemoglobinuria D59.1
    paroxysmal D59.6
  hemagglutinin (chronic) D59.1
collagen NOS (nonvascular) (vascular) M35.9
  specified NEC M35.8
colon K63.9
  functional K59.9
    congenital Q43.2
  ischemic K55.0
combined system —*see* Degeneration, combined
compressed air T70.3
Concato's (pericardial polyserositis) A19.9
  nontubercular I31.1
  pleural —*see* Pleurisy, with effusion
conjunctiva H11.9
  chlamydial A74.0
  specified NEC H11.89
  viral B30.9
    specified NEC B30.8
connective tissue, systemic (diffuse) M35.9
  in (due to)
    hypogammaglobulinemia D80.1 *[M36.8]*
    ochronosis E70.29 *[M36.8]*
  specified NEC M35.8
Conor and Bruch's (boutonneuse fever) A77.1
Cooper's —*see* Mastopathy, cystic
Cori's (glycogenosis III) E74.03
cork handler's or cork worker's J67.3
cornea H18.9
  specified NEC H18.89
coronary (artery) —*see* Disease, heart, ischemic, atherosclerotic
  congenital Q24.5
  ostial, syphilitic (aortic) (mitral) (pulmonary) A52.03
corpus cavernosum N48.9
  specified NEC N48.89
Cotugno's —*see* Sciatica
coxsackie (virus) NEC B34.1

cranial nerve NOS G52.9
Creutzfeldt-Jakob —*see* Creutzfeldt-Jakob disease or syndrome
Crocq's (acrocyanosis) I73.89
Crohn's —*see* Enteritis, regional
Curschmann G71.11
cystic
  breast (chronic) —*see* Mastopathy, cystic
  kidney, congenital Q61.9
  liver, congenital Q44.6
  lung J98.4
    congenital Q33.0
cytomegalic inclusion (generalized) B25.9
  with pneumonia B25.0
  congenital P35.1
cytomegaloviral B25.9
  specified NEC B25.8
Czerny's (periodic hydrarthrosis of the knee) —*see* Effusion, joint, knee
Daae (-Finsen) (epidemic pleurodynia) B33.0
Darling's —*see* Histoplasmosis capsulati
Debove's (splenomegaly) R16.1
deer fly —*see* Tularemia
Degos' I77.89
demyelinating, demyelinizating (nervous system) G37.9
  multiple sclerosis G35
  specified NEC G37.8
dense deposit (*see also* N00-N07 with fourth character .6) N05.6
deposition, hydroxyapatite —*see* Disease, hydroxyapatite deposition
de Quervain's (tendon sheath) M65.4
  thyroid (subacute granulomatous thyroiditis) E06.1
Devergie's (pityriasis rubra pilaris) L44.0
Devic's G36.0
diaphorase deficiency D74.0
diaphragm J98.6
diarrheal, infectious NEC A09
digestive system K92.9
  specified NEC K92.89
disc, degenerative —*see* Degeneration, intervertebral disc
discogenic —*see also* Displacement, intervertebral disc NEC
  with myelopathy —*see* Disorder, disc, with, myelopathy
diverticular —*see* Diverticula
Dubois (thymus) A50.59 *[E35]*
Duchenne-Griesinger G71.0
Duchenne's
  muscular dystrophy G71.0
  pseudohypertrophy, muscles G71.0
ductless glands E34.9
Duhring's (dermatitis herpetiformis) L13.0
duodenum K31.9
  specified NEC K31.89
Dupré's (meningism) R29.1
Dupuytren's (muscle contracture) M72.0
Durand-Nicholas-Favre (climatic bubo) A55
Duroziez's (congenital mitral stenosis) Q23.2
ear —*see* Disorder, ear
Eberth's —*see* Fever, typhoid
Ebola (virus) A98.4
Ebstein's heart Q22.5
Echinococcus —*see* Echinococcus
echovirus NEC B34.1
Eddowes' (brittle bones and blue sclera) Q78.0
edentulous (alveolar) ridge K06.9
  specified NEC K06.8

Disease, diseased - *continued*

Edsall's T67.2
Eichstedt's (pityriasis versicolor) B36.0
Ellis-van Creveld (chondroectodermal dysplasia) Q77.6
end stage renal (ESRD) N18.6
  due to hypertension I12.0
endocrine glands or system NEC E34.9
endomyocardial (eosinophilic) I42.3
English (rickets) E55.0
enteroviral, enterovirus NEC B34.1
  central nervous system NEC A88.8
epidemic B99.9
  specified NEC B99.8
epididymis N50.9
Erb (-Landouzy) G71.0
Erdheim-Chester (ECD) E88.89
esophagus K22.9
  functional K22.4
  psychogenic F45.8
  specified NEC K22.8
Eulenburg's (congenital paramyotonia) G71.19
eustachian tube —*see* Disorder, eustachian tube
external
  auditory canal —*see* Disorder, ear, external
  ear —*see* Disorder, ear, external
extrapyramidal G25.9
  specified NEC G25.89
eye H57.9
  anterior chamber H21.9
  inflammatory NEC H57.8
  muscle (external) —*see* Strabismus
  specified NEC H57.8
  syphilitic —*see* Oculopathy, syphilitic
eyeball H44.9
  specified NEC H44.89
eyelid —*see* Disorder, eyelid
  specified NEC —*see* Disorder, eyelid, specified type NEC
eyeworm of Africa B74.3
facial nerve (seventh) G51.9
  newborn (birth injury) P11.3
Fahr (of brain) G23.8
Fahr Volhard (of kidney) I12.
fallopian tube (noninflammatory) N83.9
  inflammatory —*see* Salpingo-oophoritis
  specified NEC N83.8
familial periodic paralysis G72.3
Fanconi's (congenital pancytopenia) D61.09
fascia NEC —*see also* Disorder, muscle
  inflammatory —*see* Myositis
  specified NEC M62.89
Fauchard's (periodontitis) —*see* Periodontitis
Favre-Durand-Nicolas (climatic bubo) A55
Fede's K14.0
Feer's —*see* Poisoning, mercury
female pelvic inflammatory (*see also* Disease, pelvis, inflammatory) N73.9
  syphilitic (secondary) A51.42
  tuberculous A18.17
Fernels' (aortic aneurysm) I71.9
fibrocaseous of lung —*see* Tuberculosis, pulmonary
fibrocystic —*see* Fibrocystic disease
Fiedler's (leptospiral jaundice) A27.0
fifth B08.3
file-cutter's —*see* Poisoning, lead
fish-skin Q80.9
  acquired L85.0

Disease, diseased - *continued*

Flajani (-Basedow) (exophthalmic goiter) — *see* Hyperthyroidism, with, goiter (diffuse)
flax-dresser's J66.1
fluke —*see* Infestation, fluke
foot and mouth B08.8
foot process N04.9
Forbes' (glycogenosis III) E74.03
Fordyce-Fox (apocrine miliaria) L75.2
Fordyce's (ectopic sebaceous glands) (mouth) Q38.6
Forestier's (rhizomelic pseudopolyarthritis) M35.3
  meaning ankylosing hyperostosis —*see* Hyperostosis, ankylosing
Fothergill's
  neuralgia —*see* Neuralgia, trigeminal
  scarlatina anginosa A38.9
Fournier (gangrene) N49.3
  female N76.89
fourth B08.8
Fox (-Fordyce) (apocrine miliaria) L75.2
Francis' —*see* Tularemia
Franklin C88.2
Frei's (climatic bubo) A55
Friedreich's
  combined systemic or ataxia G11.1
  myoclonia G25.3
frontal sinus —*see* Sinusitis, frontal
fungus NEC B49
Gaisböck's (polycythemia hypertonica) D75.1
gallbladder K82.9
  calculus —*see* Calculus, gallbladder
  cholecystitis —*see* Cholecystitis
  cholesterolosis K82.4
  fistula —*see* Fistula, gallbladder
  hydrops K82.1
  obstruction —*see* Obstruction, gallbladder
  perforation K82.2
  specified NEC K82.8
gamma heavy chain C88.2
Gamna's (siderotic splenomegaly) D73.2
Gamstorp's (adynamia episodica hereditaria) G72.3
Gandy-Nanta (siderotic splenomegaly) D73.2
ganister J62.8
gastric —*see* Disease, stomach
gastroesophageal reflux (GERD) K21.9
  with esophagitis K21.0
gastrointestinal (tract) K92.9
  amyloid E85.4
  functional K59.9
    psychogenic F45.8
  specified NEC K92.89
Gee (-Herter) (-Heubner) (-Thaysen) (nontropical sprue) K90.0
genital organs
  female N94.9
  male N50.9
Gerhardt's (erythromelalgia) I73.81
Gibert's (pityriasis rosea) L42
Gierke's (glycogenosis I) E74.01
Gilles de la Tourette's (motor-verbal tic) F95.2
gingiva K06.9
  specified NEC K06.8
gland (lymph) I89.9
Glanzmann's (hereditary hemorrhagic thrombasthenia) D69.1
glass-blower's (cataract) —*see* Cataract, specified NEC
  salivary gland hypertrophy K11.1

Disease, diseased - *continued*

Glisson's —*see* Rickets
globe H44.9
  specified NEC H44.89
glomerular —*see also* Glomerulonephritis
  with edema —*see* Nephrosis
  acute —*see* Nephritis, acute
  chronic —*see* Nephritis, chronic
  minimal change N05.0
  rapidly progressive N01.9
glycogen storage E74.00
  Andersen's E74.09
  Cori's E74.03
  Forbes' E74.03
  generalized E74.00
  glucose 6-phosphatase deficiency E74.01
  heart E74.02 *[143]*
  hepatorenal E74.09
  Hers' E74.09
  liver and kidney E74.09
  McArdlc's E74.04
  muscle phosphofructokinase E74.09
  myocardium E74.02 *[143]*
  Pompe's E74.02
  Tauri's E74.09
  type 0 E74.09
  type I E74.01
  type II E74.02
  type III E74.03
  type IV E74.09
  type V E74.04
  type VI-XI E74.09
  Von Gierke's E74.01
Goldstein's (familial hemorrhagic telangiectasia) I78.0
gonococcal NOS A54.9
graft-versus-host (GVH) D89.813
  acute D89.810
  acute on chronic D89.812
  chronic D89.811
grain handler's J67.8
granulomatous (childhood) (chronic) D71
Graves' (exophthalmic goiter) —*see* Hyperthyroidism, with, goiter (diffuse)
Griesinger's —*see* Ancylostomiasis
Grisel's M43.6
Gruby's (tinea tonsurans) B35.0
Guillain-Barré G61.0
Guinon's (motor-verbal tic) F95.2
gum K06.9
gynecological N94.9
H (Hartnup's) E72.02
Haff —*see* Poisoning, mercury
Hageman (congenital factor XII deficiency) D68.2
hair (color) (shaft) L67.9
  follicles L73.9
    specified NEC L73.8
Hamman's (spontaneous mediastinal emphysema) J98.2
hand, foot and mouth B08.4
Hansen's —*see* Leprosy
Hantavirus, with pulmonary manifestations B33.4
  with renal manifestations A98.5
Harada's H30.81
Hartnup (pellagra-cerebellar ataxia-renal aminoaciduria) E72.02
Hart's (pellagra-cerebellar ataxia-renal aminoaciduria) E72.02
Hashimoto's (struma lymphomatosa) E06.3
Hb —*see* Disease, hemoglobin

Disease, diseased - *continued*

heart (organic) I51.9
  with
    pulmonary edema (acute) (*see also* Failure,
  ventricular, left) I50.1
    rheumatic fever (conditions in I00)
      active I01.9
        with chorea I02.0
        specified NEC I01.8
      inactive or quiescent (with chorea) I09.9
        specified NEC I09.89
  amyloid E85.4 *[I43]*
  aortic (valve) I35.9
  arteriosclerotic or sclerotic (senile) —*see*
  Disease, heart, ischemic, atherosclerotic
  artery, arterial —*see* Disease, heart,
  ischemic, atherosclerotic
  beer drinkers' I42.6
  beriberi (wet) E51.12
  black I27.0
  congenital Q24.9
    cyanotic Q24.9
    specified NEC Q24.8
  coronary —*see* Disease, heart, ischemic
  cryptogenic I51.9
  fibroid —*see* Myocarditis
  functional I51.89
    psychogenic F45.8
  glycogen storage E74.02 *[I43]*
  gonococcal A54.83
  hypertensive —*see* Hypertension, heart
  hyperthyroid (*see also* Hyperthyroidism)
  E05.90 *[I43]*
    with thyroid storm E05.91 *[I43]*
  ischemic (chronic or with a stated duration
  of over 4 weeks) I25.9
    atherosclerotic (of) I25.10
      with angina pectoris —*see*
  Arteriosclerosis, coronary (artery)
      coronary artery bypass graft —*see*
  Arteriosclerosis, coronary (artery)
    cardiomyopathy I25.5
    diagnosed on ECG or other special
  investigation, but currently presenting no
  symptoms I25.6
    silent I25.6
    specified form NEC I25.89
  kyphoscoliotic I27.1
  meningococcal A39.50
    endocarditis A39.51
    myocarditis A39.52
    pericarditis A39.53
  mitral I05.9
    specified NEC I05.8
  muscular —*see* Degeneration, myocardial
  psychogenic (functional) F45.8
  pulmonary (chronic) I27.9
    in schistosomiasis B65.9 *[I52]*
    specified NEC I27.89
  rheumatic (chronic) (inactive) (old)
  (quiescent) (with chorea) I09.9
    active or acute I01.9
      with chorea (acute) (rheumatic)
  (Sydenham's) I02.0
    specified NEC I09.89
  senile —*see* Myocarditis
  syphilitic A52.06
    aortic A52.03
      aneurysm A52.01
    congenital A50.54 *[I52]*
  thyrotoxic (*see also* Thyrotoxicosis) E05.90
  [I43]

Disease, diseased - *continued*

  with thyroid storm E05.91 *[I43]*
  valve, valvular (obstructive) (regurgitant) —
  see also Endocarditis
    congenital NEC Q24.8
      pulmonary Q22.3
  vascular —*see* Disease, cardiovascular
heavy chain NEC C88.2
  alpha C88.3
  gamma C88.2
  mu C88.2
Hebra's
  pityriasis
    maculata et circinata L42
    rubra pilaris L44.0
  prurigo L28.2
hematopoietic organs D75.9
hemoglobin or Hb
  abnormal (mixed) NEC D58.2
    with thalassemia D56.9
  AS genotype D57.3
  Bart's D56.0
  C (Hb-C) D58.2
    with other abnormal hemoglobin NEC
  D58.2
    elliptocytosis D58.1
    Hb-S D57.2
    sickle-cell D57.2
    thalassemia D56.8
  Constant Spring D58.2
  D (Hb-D) D58.2
  E (Hb-E) D58.2
  E-beta thalassemia D56.5
  elliptocytosis D58.1
  H (Hb-H) (thalassemia) D56.0
    with other abnormal hemoglobin NEC
  D56.9
    Constant Spring D56.0
  I thalassemia D56.9
  M D74.0
  S or SS D57.1
  SC D57.2
  SD D57.8
  SE D57.8
  spherocytosis D58.0
  unstable, hemolytic D58.2
hemolytic (newborn) P55.9
  autoimmune (cold type) (warm type) D59.1
  drug-induced D59.0
  due to or with
    incompatibility
      ABO (blood group) P55.1
      blood (group) (Duffy) (K(ell)) (Kidd)
  (Lewis) (M) (S) NEC P55.8
      Rh (blood group) (factor) P55.0
      Rh negative mother P55.0
    specified type NEC P55.8
    unstable hemoglobin D58.2
hemorrhagic D69.9
  newborn P53
  Henoch (-Schönlein) (purpura nervosa) D69.0
hepatic —*see* Disease, liver
hepatobiliary K83.9
  toxic K71.9
hepatolenticular E83.01
heredodegenerative NEC
  spinal cord G95.89
herpesviral, disseminated B00.7
Hers' (glycogenosis VI) E74.09
Herter (-Gee) (-Heubner) (nontropical spruc)
K90.0

Disease, diseased - *continued*

Heubner-Herter (nontropical sprue) K90.
high fetal gene or hemoglobin thalassemia
  D56.9
Hildebrand's —*see* Typhus
hip (joint) M25.9
  congenital Q65.89
  suppurative M00.9
  tuberculous A18.02
His (-Werner) (trench fever) A79.0
Hodgson's I71.2
  ruptured I71.1
Holla —*see* Spherocytosis
hookworm B76.9
  specified NEC B76.8
host-versus-graft D89.813
  acute D89.810
  acute on chronic D89.812
  chronic D89.811
human immunodeficiency virus (HIV) B20
Huntington's G10
Hutchinson's (cheiropompholyx) —*see*
  Hutchinson's disease
hyaline (diffuse) (generalized)
  membrane (lung) (newborn) P22.0
    adult J80
hydatid —*see* Echinococcus
hydroxyapatite deposition M11.00
  ankle M11.07
  elbow M11.02
  foot joint M11.07
  hand joint M11.04
  hip M11.05
  knee M11.06
  multiple site M11.09
  shoulder M11.01
  vertebra M11.08
  wrist M11.03
hyperkinetic —*see* Hyperkinesia
hypertensive —*see* Hypertension
hypophysis E23.7
Iceland G93.3
I-cell E77.0
immune D89.9
immunoproliferative (malignant) C88.9
  small intestinal C88.3
  specified NEC C88.8
inclusion B25.9
  salivary gland B25.9
infectious, infective B99.9
  congenital P37.9
    specified NEC P37.8
    viral P35.9
      specified type NEC P35.8
  specified NEC B99.8
inflammatory
  penis N48.29
    abscess N48.21
    cellulitis N48.22
    prepuce N47.7
      balanoposthitis N47.6
  tubo-ovarian —*see* Salpingo-oophoritis
intervertebral disc —*see also* Disorder, disc
  with myelopathy —*see* Disorder, disc, with,
  myelopathy
  cervical, cervicothoracic —*see* Disorder,
  disc, cervical
    with
      myelopathy —*see* Disorder, disc,
  cervical, with myelopathy
      neuritis, radiculitis or radiculopathy —*see*
  Disorder, disc, cervical, with neuritis

Disease, diseased - *continued*
   specified NEC —*see* Disorder, disc,
cervical, specified type NEC
  lumbar (with)
   myelopathy M51.06
   neuritis, radiculitis, radiculopathy or
sciatica M51.16
    specified NEC M51.86
  lumbosacral (with)
   neuritis, radiculitis, radiculopathy or
sciatica M51.17
    specified NEC M51.87
  specified NEC —*see* Disorder, disc,
specified NEC
  thoracic (with)
   myelopathy M51.04
   neuritis, radiculitis or radiculopathy
M51.14
    specified NEC M51.84
  thoracolumbar (with)
   myelopathy M51.05
   neuritis, radiculitis or radiculopathy
M51.15
    specified NEC M51.85
 intestine K63.9
  functional K59.9
   psychogenic F45.8
   specified NEC K59.8
  organic K63.9
  protozoal A07.9
  specified NEC K63.89
 iris H21.9
  specified NEC H21.89
 iron metabolism or storage E83.10
 island (scrub typhus) A75.3
 itai-itai —*see* Poisoning, cadmium
 Jakob-Creutzfeldt —*see* Creutzfeldt-Jakob
disease or syndrome
 jaw M27.9
  fibrocystic M27.49
  specified NEC M27.8
 jigger B88.1
 joint —*see also* Disorder, joint
  Charcot's —*see* Arthropathy, neuropathic
(Charcot)
  degenerative —*see* Osteoarthritis
   multiple M15.9
   spine —*see* Spondylosis
  hypertrophic —*see* Osteoarthritis
  sacroiliac M53.3
  specified NEC —*see* Disorder, joint,
specified type NEC
  spine NEC —*see* Dorsopathy
  suppurative —*see* Arthritis, pyogenic or
pyemic
 Jourdain's (acute gingivitis) K05.00
  nonplaque induced K05.01
  plaque induced K05.00
 Kaschin-Beck (endemic polyarthritis) M12.10
  ankle M12.17
  elbow M12.12
  foot joint M12.17
  hand joint M12.14
  hip M12.15
  knee M12.16
  multiple site M12.19
  shoulder M12.11
  vertebra M12.18
  wrist M12.13
 Katayama B65.2
 Kedani (scrub typhus) A75.3
 Keshan E59

Disease, diseased - *continued*
 kidney (functional) (pelvis) N28.9
  chronic N18.9
   hypertensive —*see* Hypertension, kidney
   stage 1 N18.1
   stage 2 (mild) N18.2
   stage 3 (moderate) N18.3
   stage 4 (severe) N18.4
   stage 5 N18.5
  complicating pregnancy —*see* Pregnancy,
complicated by, renal disease
  cystic (congenital) Q61.9
  diabetic —*see* E08-E13 with .22
  fibrocystic (congenital) Q61.8
  hypertensive —*see* Hypertension, kidney
  in (due to)
   schistosomiasis (bilharziasis) B65.9 *[N29]*
  multicystic Q61.4
  polycystic Q61.3
   adult type Q61.2
   childhood type NEC Q61.19
    collecting duct dilatation Q61.11
 Kimmelstiel (-Wilson) (intercapillary
polycystic (congenital) glomerulosclerosis) —
see E08-E13 with .21
 Kimura D21.9
  specified site (see Neoplasm, connective
tissue benign)
 Kinnier Wilson's (hepatolenticular
degeneration) E83.01
 kissing —*see* Mononucleosis, infectious
 Klebs' (*see also* Glomerulonephritis) N05.
 Klippel-Feil (brevicollis) Q76.1
 Köhler-Pellegrini-Stieda (calcification, knee
joint) —*see* Bursitis, tibial collateral
 Kok Q89.8
 König's (osteochondritis dissecans) —*see*
Osteochondritis, dissecans
 Korsakoff's (nonalcoholic) F04
  alcoholic F10.96
   with dependence F10.26
 Kostmann's (infantile genetic agranulocytosis)
D70.0
 kuru A81.81
 Kyasanur Forest A98.2
 labyrinth, ear —*see* Disorder, ear, inner
 lacrimal system —*see* Disorder, lacrimal
system
 Lafora's —*see* Epilepsy, generalized,
idiopathic
 Lancereaux-Mathieu (leptospiral jaundice)
A27.0
 Landry's G61.0
 Larrey-Weil (leptospiral jaundice) A27.0
 larynx J38.7
 legionnaires' A48.1
  nonpneumonic A48.2
 Lenègre's I44.2
 lens H27.9
  specified NEC H27.8
 Lev's (acquired complete heart block) I44.2
 Lewy body (dementia) G31.83 *[F02.80]*
  with behavioral disturbance G31.83
[F02.81]
 Lichtheim's (subacute combined sclerosis
with pernicious anemia) D51.0
 Lightwood's (renal tubular acidosis) N25.89
 Lignac's (cystinosis) E72.04
 lip K13.0
 lipid-storage E75.6
  specified NEC E75.5
 Lipschütz's N76.6

Disease, diseased - *continued*
 liver (chronic) (organic) K76.9
  alcoholic (chronic) K70.9
   acute —*see* Disease, liver, alcoholic,
hepatitis
   cirrhosis K70.30
    with ascites K70.31
   failure K70.40
    with coma K70.41
   fatty liver K70.0
   fibrosis K70.2
   hepatitis K70.10
    with ascites K70.11
   sclerosis K70.2
  cystic, congenital Q44.6
  drug-induced (idiosyncratic) (toxic)
(predictable) (unpredictable) —*see* Disease,
liver, toxic
  end stage K72.90
   due to hepatitis —*see* Hepatitis
  fatty, nonalcoholic (NAFLD) K76.0
   alcoholic K70.0
  fibrocystic (congenital) Q44.6
  fluke
   Chinese B66.1
   oriental B66.1
   sheep B66.3
  glycogen storage E74.09 *[K77]*
  in (due to)
   schistosomiasis (bilharziasis) B65.9 *[K77]*
  inflammatory K75.9
   alcoholic K70.1
   specified NEC K75.89
  polycystic (congenital) Q44.6
  toxic K71.9
   with
    cholestasis K71.0
    cirrhosis (liver) K71.7
    fibrosis (liver) K71.7
    focal nodular hyperplasia K71.8
    hepatic granuloma K71.8
    hepatic necrosis K71.10
     with coma K71.11
    hepatitis NEC K71.6
     acute K71.2
     chronic
      active K71.50
       with ascites K71.51
      lobular K71.4
      persistent K71.3
     lupoid K71.50
      with ascites K71.51
    peliosis hepatis K71.8
    veno-occlusive disease (VOD) of liver
K71.8
  veno-occlusive K76.5
 Lobo's (keloid blastomycosis) B48.0
 Lobstein's (brittle bones and blue sclera)
Q78.0
 Ludwig's (submaxillary cellulitis) K12.2
 lumbosacral region M53.87
 lung J98.4
  black J60
  congenital Q33.9
  cystic J98.4
   congenital Q33.0
  fibroid (chronic) —*see* Fibrosis, lung
  fluke B66.4
   oriental B66.4
  in
   amyloidosis E85.4 *[J99]*
   sarcoidosis D86.0
   Sjögren's syndrome M35.02

Disease, diseased - *continued*
systemic
　lupus erythematosus M32.13
　sclerosis M34.81
interstitial J84.9
of childhood, specified NEC J84.848
respiratory bronchiolitis J84.115
specified NEC J84.89
obstructive (chronic) J44.9
　with
　　acute
　　　bronchitis J44.0
　　　exacerbation NEC J44.1
　　　lower respiratory infection J44.0
　　alveolitis, allergic J67.9
　　asthma J44.9
　　bronchiectasis J47.9
　　　with
　　　　exacerbation (acute) J47.1
　　　　lower respiratory infection J47.0
　　bronchitis J44.9
　　　with
　　　　exacerbation (acute) J44.1
　　　　lower respiratory infection J44.0
　　emphysema J44.9
　　hypersensitivity pneumonitis J67.9
decompensated J44.1
　with
　　exacerbation (acute) J44.1
polycystic J98.4
　congenital Q33.0
rheumatoid (diffuse) (interstitial) —*see*
Rheumatoid, lung
Lutembacher's (atrial septal defect with mitral
stenosis) Q21.1
Lyme A69.20
lymphatic (gland) (system) (channel) (vessel)
I89.9
lymphoproliferative D47.9
　specified NEC D47.Z9
　T-gamma D47.Z9
　X-linked D82.3
Magitot's M27.2
malarial —*see* Malaria
malignant —*see also* Neoplasm, malignant,
by site
Manson's B65.1
maple bark J67.6
maple-syrup-urine E71.0
Marburg (virus) A98.3
Marion's (bladder neck obstruction) N32.0
Marsh's (exophthalmic goiter) —*see*
Hyperthyroidism, with, goiter (diffuse)
mastoid (process) —*see* Disorder, ear, middle
Mathieu's (leptospiral jaundice) A27.0
Maxcy's A75.2
McArdle (-Schmid-Pearson) (glycogenosis V)
E74.04
mediastinum J98.5
medullary center (idiopathic) (respiratory)
G93.89
Meige's (chronic hereditary edema) Q82.0
meningococcal —*see* Infection,
meningococcal
mental F99
　organic F09
mesenchymal M35.9
mesenteric embolic K55.0
metabolic, metabolism E88.9
　bilirubin E80.7
metal-polisher's J62.8

Disease, diseased - *continued*
metastatic (*see also* Neoplasm, secondary, by
site) C79.9
microvascular
code to condition
microvillus
　atrophy Q43.8
　inclusion (MVD) Q43.8
middle ear —*see* Disorder, ear, middle
Mikulicz' (dryness of mouth, absent or
decreased lacrimation) K11.8
Milroy's (chronic hereditary edema) Q82.0
Minamata —*see* Poisoning, mercury
minicore G71.2
Minor's G95.19
Minot's (hemorrhagic disease, newborn) P53
Minot-von Willebrand-Jürgens
(angiohemophilia) D68.0
Mitchell's (erythromelalgia) I73.81
mitral (valve) I05.9
　nonrheumatic I34.9
mixed connective tissue M35.1
moldy hay J67.0
Monge's T70.29
Morgagni-Adams-Stokes (syncope with heart
block) I45.9
Morgagni's (syndrome) (hyperostosis frontalis
interna) M85.2
Morton's (with metatarsalgia) —*see* Lesion,
nerve, plantar
Morvan's G60.8
motor neuron (bulbar) (familial) (mixed type)
(spinal) G12.20
　amyotrophic lateral sclerosis G12.21
　progressive bulbar palsy G12.22
　specified NEC G12.29
moyamoya I67.5
mu heavy chain disease C88.2
multicore G71.2
muscle —*see also* Disorder, muscle
　inflammatory —*see* Myositis
　ocular (external) —*see* Strabismus
musculoskeletal system, soft tissue —*see also*
Disorder, soft tissue
　specified NEC —*see* Disorder, soft tissue,
specified type NEC
mushroom workers' J67.5
mycotic B49
myelodysplastic, not classified C94.6
myeloproliferative, not classified C94.6
　chronic D47.1
myocardium, myocardial (*see also*
Degeneration, myocardial) I51.5
　primary (idiopathic) I42.9
myoneural G70.9
Naegeli's D69.1
nails L60.9
　specified NEC L60.8
Nairobi (sheep virus) A93.8
nasal J34.9
nemaline body G71.2
nerve —*see* Disorder, nerve
nervous system G98.8
　autonomic G90.9
　central G96.9
　　specified NEC G96.8
　congenital Q07.9
　parasympathetic G90.9
　specified NEC G98.8
　sympathetic G90.9
　vegetative G90.9
　neuromuscular system G70.9

Disease, diseased - *continued*
Newcastle B30.8
Nicolas (-Durand) -Favre (climatic bubo) A55
nipple N64.9
　Paget's C50.01
　　female C50.01
　　male C50.02
Nishimoto (-Takeuchi) I67.5
nonarthropod-borne NOS (viral) B34.9
　enterovirus NEC B34.1
nonautoimmune hemolytic D59.4
　drug-induced D59.2
Nonne-Milroy-Meige (chronic hereditary
edema) Q82.0
nose J34.9
nucleus pulposus —*see* Disorder, disc
nutritional E63.9
oast-house-urine E72.19
ocular
　herpesviral B00.50
　zoster B02.30
obliterative vascular I77.1
Ohara's —*see* Tularemia
Opitz's (congestive splenomegaly) D73.2
Oppenheim-Urbach (necrobiosis lipoidica
diabeticorum) —*see* E08-E13 with .620
optic nerve NEC —*see* Disorder, nerve, optic
orbit —*see* Disorder, orbit
Oriental liver fluke B66.1
Oriental lung fluke B66.4
Ormond's N13.5
Oropouche virus A93.0
Osler-Rendu (familial hemorrhagic
telangiectasia) I78.0
osteofibrocystic E21.0
Otto's M24.7
outer ear —*see* Disorder, ear, external
ovary (noninflammatory) N83.9
　cystic N83.20
　inflammatory —*see* Salpingo-oophoritis
　polycystic E28.2
　specified NEC N83.8
Owren's (congenital) —*see* Defect,
coagulation
pancreas K86.9
　cystic K86.2
　fibrocystic E84.9
　specified NEC K86.8
panvalvular I08.9
　specified NEC I08.8
parametrium (noninflammatory) N83.9
parasitic B89
　cerebral NEC B71.9 *[G94]*
　intestinal NOS B82.9
　mouth B37.0
　skin NOS B88.9
　specified type —*see* Infestation
　tongue B37.0
parathyroid (gland) E21.5
　specified NEC E21.4
Parkinson's G20
parodontal K05.6
Parrot's (syphilitic osteochondritis) A50.02
Parry's (exophthalmic goiter) —*see*
Hyperthyroidism, with, goiter (diffuse)
Parson's (exophthalmic goiter) —*see*
Hyperthyroidism, with, goiter (diffuse)
Paxton's (white piedra) B36.2
pearl-worker's —*see* Osteomyelitis, specified
type NEC
Pellegrini-Stieda (calcification, knee joint) —
see Bursitis, tibial collateral

Disease, diseased - *continued*
  pelvis, pelvic
    female NOS N94.9
      specified NEC N94.89
    gonococcal (acute) (chronic) A54.24
    inflammatory (female) N73.9
      acute N73.0
      chronic N73.1
      specified NEC N73.8
      syphilitic (secondary) A51.42
        late A52.76
      tuberculous A18.17
    organ, female N94.9
    peritoneum, female NEC N94.89
  penis N48.9
    inflammatory N48.29
      abscess N48.21
      cellulitis N48.22
    specified NEC N48.89
  periapical tissues NOS K04.90
  periodontal K05.6
    specified NEC K05.5
  periosteum —*see* Disorder, bone, specified type NEC
  peripheral
    arterial I73.9
    autonomic nervous system G90.9
    nerves —*see* Polyneuropathy
    vascular NOS I73.9
  peritoneum K66.9
    pelvic, female NEC N94.89
    specified NEC K66.8
  persistent mucosal (middle ear) H66.20
    left H66.22
      with right H66.23
    right H66.21
      with left H66.23
  Petit's —*see* Hernia, abdomen, specified site NEC
  pharynx J39.2
    specified NEC J39.2
  Phocas' —*see* Mastopathy, cystic
  photochromogenic (acid-fast bacilli) (pulmonary) A31.0
    nonpulmonary A31.9
  Pick's G31.01 *[F02.80]*
    with behavioral disturbance G31.01 *[F02.81]*
  pigeon fancier's J67.2
  pineal gland E34.8
  pink —*see* Poisoning, mercury
  Pinkus' (lichen nitidus) L44.1
  pinworm B80
  Piry virus A93.8
  pituitary (gland) E23.7
  pituitary-snuff-taker's J67.8
  pleura (cavity) J94.9
    specified NEC J94.8
  pneumatic drill (hammer) T75.21
  Pollitzer's (hidradenitis suppurativa) L73.2
  polycystic
    kidney or renal Q61.3
      adult type Q61.2
      childhood type NEC Q61.19
        collecting duct dilatation Q61.11
    liver or hepatic Q44.6
    lung or pulmonary J98.4
      congenital Q33.0
    ovary, ovaries E28.2
    spleen Q89.09
  polyethylene T84.05
  Pompe's (glycogenosis II) E74.02

Disease, diseased - *continued*
  Posadas-Wernicke B38.9
  Potain's (pulmonary edema) —*see* Edema, lung
  prepuce N47.8
    inflammatory N47.7
      balanoposthitis N47.6
  Pringle's (tuberous sclerosis) Q85.1
  prion, central nervous system A81.9
    specified NEC A81.89
  prostate N42.9
    specified NEC N42.89
  protozoal B64
    acanthamebiasis —*see* Acanthamebiasis
    African trypanosomiasis —*see* African trypanosomiasis
    babesiosis B60.0
    Chagas disease —*see* Chagas disease
    intestine, intestinal A07.9
    leishmaniasis —*see* Leishmaniasis
    malaria —*see* Malaria
    naegleriasis B60.2
    pneumocystosis B59
    specified organism NEC B60.8
    toxoplasmosis —*see* Toxoplasmosis
  pseudo-Hurler's E77.0
  psychiatric F99
  psychotic —*see* Psychosis
  Puente's (simple glandular cheilitis) K13.0
  puerperal (*see also* Puerperal) O90.89
  pulmonary —*see also* Disease, lung
    artery I28.9
    chronic obstructive J44.9
      with
        acute bronchitis J44.0
        exacerbation (acute) J44.1
        lower respiratory infection (acute) J44.0
      decompensated J44.1
        with
          exacerbation (acute) J44.1
    heart I27.9
      specified NEC I27.89
    hypertensive (vascular) I27.0
    valve I37.9
      rheumatic I09.89
  pulp (dental) NOS K04.90
  pulseless M31.4
  Putnam's (subacute combined sclerosis with pernicious anemia) D51.0
  Pyle (-Cohn) (craniometaphyseal dysplasia) Q78.5
  ragpicker's or ragsorter's A22.1
  Raynaud's —*see* Raynaud's disease
  reactive airway —*see* Asthma
  Reclus' (cystic) —*see* Mastopathy, cystic
  rectum K62.9
    specified NEC K62.89
  Refsum's (heredopathia atactica polyneuritiformis) G60.1
  renal (functional) (pelvis) (*see also* Disease, kidney) N28.9
    with
      edema —*see* Nephrosis
      glomerular lesion —*see* Glomerulonephritis
        with edema —*see* Nephrosis
      interstitial nephritis N12
    acute N28.9
    chronic (*see also* Disease, kidney, chronic) N18.9
    cystic, congenital Q61.9
    diabetic —*see* E08-E13 with .22

Disease, diseased - *continued*
  end-stage (failure) N18.6
    due to hypertension I12.0
  fibrocystic (congenital) Q61.8
  hypertensive —*see* Hypertension, kidney
  lupus M32.14
  phosphate-losing (tubular) N25.0
  polycystic (congenital) Q61.3
    adult type Q61.2
    childhood type NEC Q61.19
      collecting duct dilatation Q61.11
  rapidly progressive N01.9
  subacute N01.9
  Rendu-Osler-Weber (familial hemorrhagic telangiectasia) I78.0
  renovascular (arteriosclerotic) —*see* Hypertension, kidney
  respiratory (tract) J98.9
    acute or subacute NOS J06.9
      due to
        chemicals, gases, fumes or vapors (inhalation) J68.3
        external agent J70.9
          specified NEC J70.8
        radiation J70.0
        smoke inhalation J70.5
      noninfectious J39.8
    chronic NOS J98.9
      due to
        chemicals, gases, fumes or vapors J68.4
        external agent J70.9
          specified NEC J70.8
        radiation J70.1
      newborn P27.9
        specified NEC P27.8
    due to
      chemicals, gases, fumes or vapors J68.9
        acute or subacute NEC J68.3
        chronic J68.4
      external agent J70.9
        specified NEC J70.8
    newborn P28.9
      specified type NEC P28.89
    upper J39.9
      acute or subacute J06.9
      noninfectious NEC J39.8
      specified NEC J39.8
      streptococcal J06.9
  retina, retinal H35.9
    Batten's or Batten-Mayou E75.4 *[H36]*
    specified NEC H35.89
  rheumatoid —*see* Arthritis, rheumatoid
  rickettsial NOS A79.9
    specified type NEC A79.89
  Riga (-Fede) (cachectic aphthae) K14.0
  Riggs' (compound periodontitis) —*see* Periodontitis
  Ritter's L00
  Rivalta's (cervicofacial actinomycosis) A42.2
  Robles' (onchocerciasis) B73.01
  Roger's (congenital interventricular septal defect) Q21.0
  Rosenthal's (factor XI deficiency) D68.1
  Rossbach's (hyperchlorhydria) K30
  Ross River B33.1
  Rotes Quérol —*see* Hyperostosis, ankylosing
  Roth (-Bernhardt) —*see* Mononeuropathy, lower limb, meralgia paresthetica
  Runeberg's (progressive pernicious anemia) D51.0
  sacroiliac NEC M53.3

Disease, diseased - *continued*
salivary gland or duct K11.9
  inclusion B25.9
  specified NEC K11.8
  virus B25.9
sandworm B76.9
Schimmelbusch's —*see* Mastopathy, cystic
Schmorl's —*see* Schmorl's disease or nodes
Schönlein (-Henoch) (purpura rheumatica) D69.0
Schottmüller's —*see* Fever, paratyphoid
Schultz's (agranulocytosis) —*see* Agranulocytosis
Schwalbe-Ziehen-Oppenheim G24.1
Schwartz-Jampel G71.13
sclera H15.9
  specified NEC H15.89
scrofulous (tuberculous) A18.2
scrotum N50.9
sebaceous glands L73.9
semilunar cartilage, cystic —*see also* Derangement, knee, meniscus, cystic
seminal vesicle N50.9
serum NEC (*see also* Reaction, serum) T80.69
sexually transmitted A64
  anogenital
    herpesviral infection —*see* Herpes, anogenital
      warts A63.0
  chancroid A57
  chlamydial infection —*see* Chlamydia
  gonorrhea —*see* Gonorrhea
  granuloma inguinale A58
  specified organism NEC A63.8
  syphilis —*see* Syphilis
  trichomoniasis —*see* Trichomoniasis
Sézary C84.1
shimamushi (scrub typhus) A75.3
shipyard B30.0
sickle-cell D57.1
  with crisis (vasoocclusive pain) D57.00
    with
      acute chest syndrome D57.01
      splenic sequestration D57.02
  elliptocytosis D57.8
  Hb-C D57.20
    with crisis (vasoocclusive pain) D57.219
      with
        acute chest syndrome D57.211
        splenic sequestration D57.212
    without crisis D57.20
  Hb-SD D57.80
    with crisis D57.819
      with
        acute chest syndrome D57.811
        splenic sequestration D57.812
  Hb-SE D57.80
    with crisis D57.819
      with
        acute chest syndrome D57.811
        splenic sequestration D57.812
  specified NEC D57.80
    with crisis D57.819
      with
        acute chest syndrome D57.811
        splenic sequestration D57.812
  spherocytosis D57.80
    with crisis D57.819
      with
        acute chest syndrome D57.811
        splenic sequestration D57.812

thalassemia D57.40
  with crisis (vasoocclusive pain) D57.419
    with
      acute chest syndrome D57.411
      splenic sequestration D57.412
  without crisis D57.40
silo-filler's J68.8
  bronchitis J68.0
  pneumonitis J68.0
  pulmonary edema J68.1
simian B B00.4
Simons' (progressive lipodystrophy) E88.1
sin nombre virus B33.4
sinus —*see* Sinusitis
Sirkari's B55.0
sixth B08.20
  due to human herpesvirus 6 B08.21
  due to human herpesvirus 7 B08.22
skin L98.9
  due to metabolic disorder NEC E88.9 *[L99]*
  specified NEC L98.8
slim (HIV) B20
small vessel I73.9
Sneddon-Wilkinson (subcorneal pustular dermatosis) L13.1
South African creeping B88.0
spinal (cord) G95.9
  congenital Q06.9
  specified NEC G95.89
spine —*see also* Spondylopathy
  joint —*see* Dorsopathy
  tuberculous A18.01
spinocerebellar (hereditary) G11.9
  specified NEC G11.8
spleen D73.9
  amyloid E85.4 *[D77]*
  organic D73.9
  polycystic Q89.09
  postinfectional D73.89
sponge-diver's —*see* Toxicity, venom, marine animal, sea anemone
Startle Q89.8
Steinert's G71.11
Sticker's (erythema infectiosum) B08.3
Stieda's (calcification, knee joint) —*see* Bursitis, tibial collateral
Stokes' (exophthalmic goiter) —*see* Hyperthyroidism, with, goiter (diffuse)
Stokes-Adams (syncope with heart block) I45.9
stomach K31.9
  functional, psychogenic F45.8
  specified NEC K31.89
stonemason's J62.8
storage
  glycogen —*see* Disease, glycogen storage
  mucopolysaccharide —*see* Mucopolysaccharidosis
striatopallidal system NEC G25.89
Stuart-Prower (congenital factor X deficiency) D68.2
Stuart's (congenital factor X deficiency) D68.2
subcutaneous tissue —*see* Disease, skin
supporting structures of teeth K08.9
  specified NEC K08.8
suprarenal (capsule) (gland) E27.9
  hyperfunction E27.0
  specified NEC E27.8
sweat glands L74.9
  specified NEC L74.8

Sweeley-Klionsky E75.21
Swift (-Feer) —*see* Poisoning, mercury
swimming-pool granuloma A31.1
Sylvest's (epidemic pleurodynia) B33.0
sympathetic nervous system G90.9
synovium —*see* Disorder, synovium
syphilitic —*see* Syphilis
systemic tissue mast cell C96.2
tanapox (virus) B08.71
Tangier E78.6
Tarral-Besnier (pityriasis rubra pilaris) L44.0
Tauri's E74.09
tear duct —*see* Disorder, lacrimal system
tendon, tendinous —*see also* Disorder, tendon
  nodular —*see* Trigger finger
terminal vessel I73.9
testis N50.9
thalassemia Hb-S —*see* Disease, sickle-cell, thalassemia
Thaysen-Gee (nontropical sprue) K90.0
Thomsen G71.12
throat J39.2
  septic J02.0
thromboembolic —*see* Embolism
thymus (gland) E32.9
  specified NEC E32.8
thyroid (gland) E07.9
  heart (*see also* Hyperthyroidism) E05.90 *[I43]*
    with thyroid storm E05.91 *[I43]*
  specified NEC E07.89
Tietze's M94.0
tongue K14.9
  specified NEC K14.8
tonsils, tonsillar (and adenoids) J35.9
tooth, teeth K08.9
  hard tissues K03.9
    specified NEC K03.89
  pulp NEC K04.99
  specified NEC K08.8
Tourette's F95.2
trachea NEC J39.8
tricuspid I07.9
  nonrheumatic I36.9
triglyceride-storage E75.5
trophoblastic —*see* Mole, hydatidiform
tsutsugamushi A75.3
tube (fallopian) (noninflammatory) N83.9
  inflammatory —*see* Salpingitis
  specified NEC N83.8
tuberculous NEC —*see* Tuberculosis
tubo-ovarian (noninflammatory) N83.9
  inflammatory —*see* Salpingo-oophoritis
  specified NEC N83.8
tubotympanic, chronic —*see* Otitis, media, suppurative, chronic, tubotympanic
tubulo-interstitial N15.9
  specified NEC N15.8
tympanum —*see* Disorder, tympanic membrane
Uhl's Q24.8
Underwood's (sclerema neonatorum) P83.0
Unverricht (-Lundborg) —*see* Epilepsy, generalized, idiopathic
Urbach-Oppenheim (necrobiosis lipoidica diabeticorum) —*see* E08-E13 with .620
ureter N28.9
  in (due to)
    schistosomiasis (bilharziasis) B65.0 *[N29]*
urethra N36.9
  specified NEC N36.8

Disease, diseased - *continued*

urinary (tract) N39.9
  bladder N32.9
    specified NEC N32.89
  specified NEC N39.8
uterus (noninflammatory) N85.9
  infective —*see* Endometritis
  inflammatory —*see* Endometritis
  specified NEC N85.8
uveal tract (anterior) H21.9
  posterior H31.9
vagabond's B85.1
vagina, vaginal (noninflammatory) N89.9
  inflammatory NEC N76.89
  specified NEC N89.8
valve, valvular I38
  multiple I08.9
    specified NEC I08.8
van Creveld-von Gierke (glycogenosis I)
  E74.01
vas deferens N50.9
vascular I99.9
  arteriosclerotic —*see* Arteriosclerosis
  ciliary body NEC —*see* Disorder, iris,
  vascular
  hypertensive —*see* Hypertension
  iris NEC —*see* Disorder, iris, vascular
  obliterative I77.1
    peripheral I73.9
  occlusive I99.8
  peripheral (occlusive) I73.9
    in diabetes mellitus —*see* E08-E13 with
    .51
vasomotor I73.9
vasospastic I73.9
vein I87.9
venereal (*see also* Disease, sexually
transmitted) A64
  chlamydial NEC A56.8
    anus A56.3
    genitourinary NOS A56.2
    pharynx A56.4
    rectum A56.3
  fifth A55
  sixth A55
  specified nature or type NEC A63.8
vertebra, vertebral —*see also* Spondylopathy
  disc —*see* Disorder, disc
vibration —*see* Vibration, adverse effects
viral, virus (*see also* Disease, by type of virus)
B34.9
  arbovirus NOS A94
  arthropod-borne NOS A94
  congenital P35.9
    specified NEC P35.8
  Hanta (with renal manifestations) (Dobrava)
  (Puumala) (Seoul) A98.5
    with pulmonary manifestations (Andes)
    (Bayou) (Bermejo) (Black Creek Canal)
    (Choclo) (Juquitiba) (Laguna negra)
    (Lechiguanas) (New York) (Oran) (Sin
    nombre) B33.4
    Hantaan (Korean hemorrhagic fever) A98.5
    human immunodeficiency (HIV) B20
    Kunjin A83.4
    nonarthropod-borne NOS B34.9
    Powassan A84.8
    Rocio (encephalitis) A83.6
    Sin nombre (Hantavirus) (cardio)
  -pulmonary syndrome) B33.4
    Tahyna B33.8
    vesicular stomatitis A93.8

Disease, diseased - *continued*

vitreous H43.9
  specified NEC H43.89
vocal cord J38.3
Volkmann's, acquired T79.6
von Eulenburg's (congenital paramyotonia)
G71.19
von Gierke's (glycogenosis I) E74.01
von Graefe's —*see* Strabismus, paralytic,
ophthalmoplegia, progressive
von Willebrand (-Jürgens) (angiohemophilia)
D68.0
Vrolik's (osteogenesis imperfecta) Q78.0
vulva (noninflammatory) N90.9
  inflammatory NEC N76.89
  specified NEC N90.89
Wallgren's (obstruction of splenic vein with
collateral circulation) I87.8
Wassilieff's (leptospiral jaundice) A27.0
wasting NEC R64
  due to malnutrition E41
Waterhouse-Friderichsen A39.1
Wegner's (syphilitic osteochondritis) A50.02
Weil's (leptospiral jaundice of lung) A27.0
Weir Mitchell's (erythromelalgia) I73.81
Werdnig-Hoffmann G12.0
Wermer's E31.21
Werner-His (trench fever) A79.0
Werner-Schultz (neutropenic splenomegaly)
D73.81
Wernicke-Posadas B38.9
whipworm B79
white blood cells D72.9
  specified NEC D72.89
white matter R90.82
white-spot, meaning lichen sclerosus et
atrophicus L90.0
  penis N48.0
  vulva N90.4
Wilkie's K55.1
Wilkinson-Sneddon (subcorneal pustular
dermatosis) L13.1
Willis' —*see* Diabetes
Wilson's (hepatolenticular degeneration)
E83.01
woolsorter's A22.1
yaba monkey tumor B08.72
yaba pox (virus) B08.72
zoonotic, bacterial A28.9
  specified type NEC A28.8

Disfigurement (due to scar) L90.5

Disgerminoma —*see* Dysgerminoma

DISH (diffuse idiopathic skeletal hyperostosis)
—*see* Hyperostosis, ankylosing

Disinsertion, retina —*see* Detachment, retina

Dislocatable hip, congenital Q65.6

Dislocation (articular)

with fracture —*see* Fracture
acromioclavicular (joint) S43.10
  with displacement
    100% 200% S43.12
    more than 200% S43.13
  inferior S43.14
  posterior S43.15
ankle S93.0
astragalus —*see* Dislocation, ankle
atlantoaxial S13.121
atlantooccipital S13.111
atloido-occipital S13.111
breast bone S23.29
capsule, joint
code by site under Dislocation

Dislocation - *continued*

carpal (bone) —*see* Dislocation, wrist
carpometacarpal (joint) NEC S63.05
  thumb S63.04
cartilage (joint)
code by site under Dislocation
cervical spine (vertebra) —*see* Dislocation,
vertebra, cervical
chronic —*see* Dislocation, recurrent
clavicle —*see* Dislocation, acromioclavicular
joint
coccyx S33.2
congenital NEC Q68.8
coracoid —*see* Dislocation, shoulder
costal cartilage S23.29
costochondral S23.29
cricoarytenoid articulation S13.29
cricothyroid articulation S13.29
dorsal vertebra —*see* Dislocation, vertebra,
thoracic
ear ossicle —*see* Discontinuity, ossicles, ear
elbow S53.10
  congenital Q68.8
  pathological —*see* Dislocation, pathological
  NEC, elbow
  radial head alone —*see* Dislocation, radial
  head
  recurrent —*see* Dislocation, recurrent,
  elbow
  traumatic S53.10
    anterior S53.11
    lateral S53.14
    medial S53.13
    posterior S53.12
    specified type NEC S53.19
eye, nontraumatic —*see* Luxation, globe
eyeball, nontraumatic —*see* Luxation, globe
femur
  distal end —*see* Dislocation, knee
  proximal end —*see* Dislocation, hip
fibula
  distal end —*see* Dislocation, ankle
  proximal end —*see* Dislocation, knee
finger S63.25
  index S63.25
  interphalangeal S63.27
    distal S63.29
      index S63.29
      little S63.29
      middle S63.29
      ring S63.29
    index S63.27
    little S63.27
    middle S63.27
    proximal S63.28
      index S63.28
      little S63.28
      middle S63.28
      ring S63.28
    ring S63.27
  little S63.25
  metacarpophalangeal S63.26
    index S63.26
    little S63.26
    middle S63.26
    ring S63.26
  middle S63.25
  recurrent —*see* Dislocation, recurrent, finger
  ring S63.25
  thumb —*see* Dislocation, thumb
foot S93.30
  recurrent —*see* Dislocation, recurrent, foot
  specified site NEC S93.33

Dislocation - *continued*

tarsal joint S93.31
tarsometatarsal joint S93.32
toe —*see* Dislocation, toe
fracture —*see* Fracture
glenohumeral (joint) —*see* Dislocation, shoulder
glenoid —*see* Dislocation, shoulder
habitual —*see* Dislocation, recurrent
hip S73.00
  anterior S73.03
   obturator S73.02
  central S73.04
  congenital (total) Q65.2
   bilateral Q65.1
   partial Q65.5
    bilateral Q65.4
    unilateral Q65.3
   unilateral Q65.0
  developmental M24.85
  pathological —*see* Dislocation, pathological NEC, hip
  posterior S73.01
  recurrent —*see* Dislocation, recurrent, hip
humerus, proximal end —*see* Dislocation, shoulder
incomplete —*see* Subluxation, by site
incus —*see* Discontinuity, ossicles, ear
infracoracoid —*see* Dislocation, shoulder
innominate (pubic junction) (sacral junction) S33.39
  acetabulum —*see* Dislocation, hip
interphalangeal (joint(s))
  finger S63.279
   distal S63.29
    index S63.29
    little S63.29
    middle S63.29
    ring S63.29
   index S63.27
   little S63.27
   middle S63.27
   proximal S63.28
    index S63.28
    little S63.28
    middle S63.28
    ring S63.28
   ring S63.27
  foot or toe —*see* Dislocation, toe
  thumb S63.12
   distal joint S63.14
   proximal joint S63.13
jaw (cartilage) (meniscus) S03.0
joint prosthesis —*see* Complications, joint prosthesis, mechanical, displacement, by site
knee S83.106
  cap —*see* Dislocation, patella
  congenital Q68.2
  old M23.8X
  patella —*see* Dislocation, patella
  pathological —*see* Dislocation, pathological NEC, knee
  proximal tibia
   anteriorly S83.11
   laterally S83.14
   medially S83.13
   posteriorly S83.12
  recurrent —*see also* Derangement, knee, specified NEC
  specified type NEC S83.19
lacrimal gland H04.16

Dislocation - *continued*

lens (complete) H27.10
  anterior H27.12
  congenital Q12.1
  ocular implant —*see* Complications, intraocular lens
  partial H27.11
  posterior H27.13
  traumatic S05.8X
ligament
  code by site under Dislocation
lumbar (vertebra) —*see* Dislocation, vertebra, lumbar
lumbosacral (vertebra) —*see also* Dislocation, vertebra, lumbar
  congenital Q76.49
mandible S03.0
meniscus (knee) —*see* Tear, meniscus
  other sites
  code by site under Dislocation
metacarpal (bone)
  distal end —*see* Dislocation, finger
  proximal end S63.06
metacarpophalangeal (joint)
  finger S63.26
   index S63.26
   little S63.26
   middle S63.26
   ring S63.26
  thumb S63.11
metatarsal (bone) —*see* Dislocation, foot
metatarsophalangeal (joint(s)) —*see* Dislocation, toe
midcarpal (joint) S63.03
midtarsal (joint) —*see* Dislocation, foot
neck S13.20
  specified site NEC S13.29
  vertebra —*see* Dislocation, vertebra, cervical
nose (septal cartilage) S03.1
occipitoatloid S13.111
old —*see* Derangement, joint, specified type NEC
ossicles, ear —*see* Discontinuity, ossicles, ear
partial —*see* Subluxation, by site
patella S83.006
  congenital Q74.1
  lateral S83.01
  recurrent (nontraumatic) M22.0
   incomplete M22.1
  specified type NEC S83.09
pathological NEC M24.30
  ankle M24.37
  elbow M24.32
  foot joint M24.37
  hand joint M24.34
  hip M24.35
  knee M24.36
  lumbosacral joint —*see* subcategory M53.2
  pelvic region —*see* Dislocation, pathological, hip
  sacroiliac —*see* subcategory M53.2
  shoulder M24.31
  wrist M24.33
pelvis NEC S33.30
  specified NEC S33.39
phalanx
  finger or hand —*see* Dislocation, finger
  foot or toe —*see* Dislocation, toe
prosthesis, internal —*see* Complications, prosthetic device, by site, mechanical

Dislocation - *continued*

radial head S53.006
  anterior S53.01
  posterior S53.02
  specified type NEC S53.09
radiocarpal (joint) S63.02
radiohumeral (joint) —*see* Dislocation, radial head
radioulnar (joint)
  distal S63.01
  proximal —*see* Dislocation, elbow
radius
  distal end —*see* Dislocation, wrist
  proximal end —*see* Dislocation, radial head
recurrent M24.40
  ankle M24.47
  elbow M24.42
  finger M24.44
  foot joint M24.47
  hand joint M24.44
  hip M24.45
  knee M24.46
   patella —*see* Dislocation, patella, recurrent
  patella —*see* Dislocation, patella, recurrent
  sacroiliac —*see* subcategory M53.2
  shoulder M24.41
  toe M24.47
  vertebra (*see also* subcategory) M43.5
   atlantoaxial M43.4
   with myelopathy M43.3
  wrist M24.43
rib (cartilage) S23.29
sacrococcygeal S33.2
sacroiliac (joint) (ligament) S33.2
  congenital Q74.2
  recurrent —*see* subcategory M53.2
sacrum S33.2
scaphoid (bone) (hand) (wrist) —*see* Dislocation, wrist
  foot —*see* Dislocation, foot
scapula —*see* Dislocation, shoulder, girdle, scapula
semilunar cartilage, knee —*see* Tear, meniscus
septal cartilage (nose) S03.1
septum (nasal) (old) J34.2
sesamoid bone
  code by site under Dislocation
shoulder (blade) (ligament) (joint) (traumatic) S43.006
  acromioclavicular —*see* Dislocation, acromioclavicular
  chronic —*see* Dislocation, recurrent, shoulder
  congenital Q68.8
  girdle S43.30
   scapula S43.31
   specified site NEC S43.39
  humerus S43.00
   anterior S43.01
   inferior S43.03
   posterior S43.02
  pathological —*see* Dislocation, pathological NEC, shoulder
  recurrent —*see* Dislocation, recurrent, shoulder
  specified type NEC S43.08
spine
  cervical —*see* Dislocation, vertebra, cervical
  congenital Q76.49
  due to birth trauma P11.5
  lumbar —*see* Dislocation, vertebra, lumbar

Dislocation - *continued*
  thoracic —*see* Dislocation, vertebra,
  thoracic
  spontaneous —*see* Dislocation, pathological
  sternoclavicular (joint) S43.206
    anterior S43.21
    posterior S43.22
  sternum S23.29
  subglenoid —*see* Dislocation, shoulder
  symphysis pubis S33.4
  talus —*see* Dislocation, ankle
  tarsal (bone(s)) (joint(s)) —*see* Dislocation,
  foot
  tarsometatarsal (joint(s)) —*see* Dislocation,
  foot
  temporomandibular (joint) S03.0
  thigh, proximal end —*see* Dislocation, hip
  thorax S23.20
    specified site NEC S23.29
    vertebra —*see* Dislocation, vertebra
  thumb S63.10
    interphalangeal joint —*see* Dislocation,
    interphalangeal (joint) , thumb
    metacarpophalangeal joint —*see*
    Dislocation, metacarpophalangeal (joint) ,
    thumb
  thyroid cartilage S13.29
  tibia
    distal end —*see* Dislocation, ankle
    proximal end —*see* Dislocation, knee
  tibiofibular (joint)
    distal —*see* Dislocation, ankle
    superior —*see* Dislocation, knee
  toe (s) S93.106
    great S93.10
      interphalangeal joint S93.11
      metatarsophalangeal joint S93.12
    interphalangeal joint S93.119
    lesser S93.106
      interphalangeal joint S93.11
      metatarsophalangeal joint S93.12
    metatarsophalangeal joint S93.12
  tooth S03.2
  trachea S23.29
  ulna
    distal end S63.07
    proximal end —*see* Dislocation, elbow
  ulnohumeral (joint) —*see* Dislocation, elbow
  vertebra (articular process) (body) (traumatic)
    cervical S13.101
      atlantoaxial joint S13.121
      atlantooccipital joint S13.111
      atloido-occipital joint S13.111
      joint between
        C0 and C1 S13.111
        C1 and C2 S13.121
        C2 and C3 S13.131
        C3 and C4 S13.141
        C4 and C5 S13.151
        C5and C6 S13.161
        C6and C7 S13.171
        C7and T1 S13.181
      occipitoatloid joint S13.111
    congenital Q76.49
    lumbar S33.101
      joint between
        L1and L2 S33.111
        L2and L3 S33.121
        L3 and L4 S33.131
        L4and L5 S33.141
    nontraumatic —*see* Displacement,
  intervertebral disc

Dislocation - *continued*
  partial —*see* Subluxation, by site
  recurrent NEC —*see* subcategory M43.5
  thoracic S23.101
    joint between
      T1 and T2 S23.111
      T2 and T3 S23.121
      T3 and T4 S23.123
      T4 and T5 S23.131
      T5 and T6 S23.133
      T6 and T7 S23.141
      T7 and T8 S23.143
      T8 and T9 S23.151
      T9 and T10 S23.153
      T10 and T11 S23.161
      T11 and T12 S23.163
      T12 and L1 S23.171
  wrist (carpal bone) S63.006
    carpometacarpal joint —*see* Dislocation,
    carpometacarpal (joint)
    distal radioulnar joint —*see* Dislocation,
    radioulnar (joint) , distal
    metacarpal bone, proximal —*see*
    Dislocation, metacarpal (bone) , proximal end
    midcarpal —*see* Dislocation, midcarpal
    (joint)
    radiocarpal joint —*see* Dislocation,
    radiocarpal (joint)
    recurrent —*see* Dislocation, recurrent, wrist
    specified site NEC S63.09
    ulna —*see* Dislocation, ulna, distal end
  xiphoid cartilage S23.29
Disorder (of) —*see also* Disease
  acantholytic L11.9
    specified NEC L11.8
  acute
    psychotic —*see* Psychosis, acute
    stress F43.0
  adjustment (grief) F43.20
    with
      anxiety F43.22
        with depressed mood F43.23
      conduct disturbance F43.24
        with emotional disturbance F43.25
      depressed mood F43.21
        with anxiety F43.23
      other specified symptom F43.29
  adrenal (capsule) (gland) (medullary) E27.9
    specified NEC E27.8
  adrenogenital E25.9
    drug-induced E25.8
    iatrogenic E25.8
    idiopathic E25.8
  adult personality (and behavior) F69
    specified NEC F68.8
  affective (mood) —*see* Disorder, mood
  aggressive, unsocialized F91.1
  alcohol-related F10.99
    with
      amnestic disorder, persisting F10.96
      anxiety disorder F10.980
      dementia, persisting F10.97
      intoxication F10.929
        with delirium F10.921
        uncomplicated F10.920
      mood disorder F10.94
      other specified F10.988
      psychotic disorder F10.959
        with
          delusions F10.950
          hallucinations F10.951
      sexual dysfunction F10.981

Disorder (of) – *continued*
    sleep disorder F10.982
  allergic —*see* Allergy
  alveolar NEC J84.09
  amino-acid
    cystathioninuria E72.19
    cystinosis E72.04
    cystinuria E72.01
    glycinuria E72.09
    homocystinuria E72.11
    metabolism —*see* Disturbance, metabolism,
    amino-acid
      specified NEC E72.8
    neonatal, transitory P74.8
    renal transport NEC E72.09
    transport NEC E72.09
  amnesic, amnestic
    alcohol-induced F10.96
      with dependence F10.26
    due to (secondary to) general medical
  condition F04
    psychoactive NEC-induced F19.96
      with
        abuse F19.16
        dependence F19.26
    sedative, hypnotic or anxiolytic-induced
  F13.96
      with dependence F13.26
  anaerobic glycolysis with anemia D55.2
  anxiety F41.9
    due to (secondary to)
      alcohol F10.980
      amphetamine F15.980
        in
          abuse F15.180
          dependence F15.280
      anxiolytic F13.980
        in
          abuse F13.180
          dependence F13.280
      caffeine F15.980
        in
          abuse F15.180
          dependence F15.280
      cannabis F12.980
        in
          abuse F12.180
          dependence F12.280
      cocaine F14.980
        in
          abuse F14.180
          dependence F14.180
      general medical condition F06.4
      hallucinogen F16.980
        in
          abuse F16.180
          dependence F16.280
      hypnotic F13.980
        in
          abuse F13.180
          dependence F13.280
      inhalant F18.980
        in
          abuse F18.180
          dependence F18.280
      phencyclidine F16.980
        in
          abuse F16.180
          dependence F16.280
      psychoactive substance NEC F19.980
        in
          abuse F19.180
          dependence F19.280

Disorder (of) – *continued*
  sedative F13.980
    in
      abuse F13.180
      dependence F13.280
    volatile solvents F18.980
      in
        abuse F18.180
        dependence F18.280
  generalized F41.1
  mixed
    with depression (mild) F41.8
    specified NEC F41.3
  organic F06.4
  phobic F40.9
    of childhood F40.8
    specified NEC F41.8
  aortic valve —*see* Endocarditis, aortic
  aromatic amino-acid metabolism E70.9
    specified NEC E70.8
  arteriole NEC I77.89
  artery NEC I77.89
  articulation —*see* Disorder, joint
  attachment (childhood)
    disinhibited F94.2
    reactive F94.1
  attention-deficit hyperactivity (adolescent)
  (adult) (child) F90.9
    combined type F90.2
    hyperactive type F90.1
    inattentive type F90.0
    specified type NEC F90.8
  attention-deficit without hyperactivity
  (adolescent) (adult) (child) F90.0
  auditory processing (central) H93.25
  autistic F84.0
  autonomic nervous system G90.9
    specified NEC G90.8
  avoidant, child or adolescent F40.10
  balance
    acid-base E87.8
      mixed E87.4
    electrolyte E87.8
    fluid NEC E87.8
  behavioral (disruptive) —*see* Disorder,
  conduct
  beta-amino-acid metabolism E72.8
  bile acid and cholesterol metabolism E78.70
    Barth syndrome E78.71
    other specified E78.79
    Smith-Lemli-Opitz syndrome E78.72
  bilirubin excretion E80.6
  binocular
    movement H51.9
      convergence
        excess H51.12
        insufficiency H51.11
      internuclear ophthalmoplegia —*see*
  Ophthalmoplegia, internuclear
      palsy of conjugate gaze H51.0
      specified type NEC H51.8
    vision NEC —*see* Disorder, vision,
  binocular
  bipolar (I) F31.9
    current episode
      depressed F31.9
        with psychotic features F31.5
        without psychotic features F31.30
          mild F31.31
          moderate F31.32
          severe (without psychotic features)
  F31.4

Disorder (of) – *continued*
      with psychotic features F31.5
    hypomanic F31.0
    manic F31.9
      with psychotic features F31.2
      without psychotic features F31.10
        mild F31.11
        moderate F31.12
        severe (without psychotic features)
  F31.13
        with psychotic features F31.2
    mixed F31.60
      mild F31.61
      moderate F31.62
      severe (without psychotic features)
  F31.63
        with psychotic features F31.64
      severe depression (without psychotic
  features) F31.4
        with psychotic features F31.5
    in remission (currently) F31.70
      in full remission
        most recent episode
          depressed F31.76
          hypomanic F31.72
          manic F31.74
          mixed F31.78
      in partial remission
        most recent episode
          depressed F31.75
          hypomanic F31.71
          manic F31.73
          mixed F31.77
    specified NEC F31.89
    II F31.81
    organic F06.30
    single manic episode F30.9
      mild F30.11
      moderate F30.12
      severe (without psychotic symptoms)
  F30.13
        with psychotic symptoms F30.2
  bladder N32.9
    functional NEC N31.9
    in schistosomiasis B65.0 *[N33]*
    specified NEC N32.89
  bleeding D68.9
  blood D75.9
    in congenital early syphilis A50.09 *[D77]*
  body dysmorphic F45.22
  bone M89.9
    continuity M84.9
      specified type NEC M84.80
        ankle M84.87
        fibula M84.86
        foot M84.87
        hand M84.84
        humerus M84.82
        neck M84.88
        pelvis M84.859
        radius M84.83
        rib M84.88
        shoulder M84.81
        skull M84.88
        thigh M84.85
        tibia M84.86
        ulna M84.83
        vertebra M84.88
    density and structure M85.9
    cyst —*see also* Cyst, bone, specified type
  NEC
      aneurysmal —*see* Cyst, bone, aneurysmal

Disorder (of) – *continued*
    solitary —*see* Cyst, bone, solitary
    diffuse idiopathic skeletal hyperostosis —
  see Hyperostosis, ankylosing
    fibrous dysplasia (monostotic) —*see*
  Dysplasia, fibrous, bone
    fluorosis —*see* Fluorosis, skeletal
    hyperostosis of skull M85.2
    osteitis condensans —*see* Osteitis,
  condensans
    specified type NEC M85.8
      ankle M85.87
      foot M85.87
      forearm M85.83
      hand M85.84
      lower leg M85.86
      multiple sites M85.89
      neck M85.88
      rib M85.88
      shoulder M85.81
      skull M85.88
      thigh M85.85
      upper arm M85.82
      vertebra M85.88
  development and growth NEC M89.20
    carpus M89.24
    clavicle M89.21
    femur M89.25
    fibula M89.26
    finger M89.24
    humerus M89.22
    ilium M89.259
    ischium M89.259
    metacarpus M89.24
    metatarsus M89.27
    multiple sites M89.29
    neck M89.28
    radius M89.23
    rib M89.28
    scapula M89.21
    skull M89.28
    tarsus M89.27
    tibia M89.26
    toe M89.27
    ulna M89.23
    vertebra M89.28
  specified type NEC M89.8X
  brachial plexus G54.0
  branched-chain amino-acid metabolism E71.2
    specified NEC E71.19
  breast N64.9
    agalactia —*see* Agalactia
    associated with
      lactation O92.70
        specified NEC O92.79
      pregnancy O92.20
        specified NEC O92.29
      puerperium O92.20
        specified NEC O92.29
    cracked nipple —*see* Cracked nipple
    galactorrhea —*see* Galactorrhea
    hypogalactia O92.4
    lactation disorder NEC O92.79
    mastitis —*see* Mastitis
    nipple infection —*see* Infection, nipple
    retracted nipple —*see* Retraction, nipple
    specified type NEC N64.89
  Briquet's F45.0
  bullous, in diseases classified elsewhere L14
  cannabis use
    due to drug abuse —*see* Abuse, drug,
  cannabis

Disorder (of) – *continued*
  due to drug dependence —*see* Dependence, drug, cannabis
  carbohydrate
    absorption, intestinal NEC E74.39
    metabolism (congenital) E74.9
      specified NEC E74.8
  cardiac, functional I51.89
  carnitine metabolism E71.40
  cartilage M94.9
    articular NEC —*see* Derangement, joint, articular cartilage
      chondrocalcinosis —*see* Chondrocalcinosis
    specified type NEC M94.8X
      articular —*see* Derangement, joint, articular cartilage
        multiple sites M94.8X0
  catatonic
    due to (secondary to) known physiological condition F06.1
    organic F06.1
  central auditory processing H93.25
  cervical
    region NEC M53.82
    root (nerve) NEC G54.2
  character NOS F60.9
  childhood disintegrative NEC F84.3
  cholesterol and bile acid metabolism E78.70
    Barth syndrome E78.71
    other specified E78.79
    Smith-Lemli-Opitz syndrome E78.72
  choroid H31.9
    atrophy —*see* Atrophy, choroid
    degeneration —*see* Degeneration, choroid
    detachment —*see* Detachment, choroid
    dystrophy —*see* Dystrophy, choroid
    hemorrhage —*see* Hemorrhage, choroid
    rupture —*see* Rupture, choroid
    scar —*see* Scar, chorioretinal
    solar retinopathy —*see* Retinopathy, solar
    specified type NEC H31.8
  ciliary body —*see* Disorder, iris
    degeneration —*see* Degeneration, ciliary body
  coagulation (factor) (*see also* Defect, coagulation) D68.9
    newborn, transient P61.6
  coccyx NEC M53.3
  cognitive F09
    due to (secondary to) general medical condition F09
    persisting R41.89
      due to
        alcohol F10.97
          with dependence F10.27
        anxiolytics F13.97
          with dependence F13.27
        hypnotics F13.97
          with dependence F13.27
        sedatives F13.97
          with dependence F13.27
        specified substance NEC F19.97
          with
            abuse F19.17
            dependence F19.27
  communication F80.9
  conduct (childhood) F91.9
    adjustment reaction —*see* Disorder, adjustment
    adolescent onset type F91.2
    childhood onset type F91.1
    compulsive F63.9

    confined to family context F91.0
    depressive F91.8
    group type F91.2
    hyperkinetic —*see* Disorder, attention-deficit hyperactivity
    oppositional defiance F91.3
    socialized F91.2
    solitary aggressive type F91.1
    specified NEC F91.8
    unsocialized (aggressive) F91.1
  conduction, heart I45.9
  congenital glycosylation (CDG) E74.8
  conjunctiva H11.9
    infection —*see* Conjunctivitis
  connective tissue, localized L94.9
    specified NEC L94.8
  conversion —*see* Disorder, dissociative
  convulsive (secondary) —*see* Convulsions
  cornea H18.9
    deformity —*see* Deformity, cornea
    degeneration —*see* Degeneration, cornea
    deposits —*see* Deposit, cornea
    due to contact lens H18.82
      specified as edema —*see* Edema, cornea
    edema —*see* Edema, cornea
    keratitis —*see* Keratitis
    keratoconjunctivitis —*see* Keratoconjunctivitis
    membrane change —*see* Change, corneal membrane
    neovascularization —*see* Neovascularization, cornea
    scar —*see* Opacity, cornea
    specified type NEC H18.89
    ulcer —*see* Ulcer, cornea
  corpus cavernosum N48.9
  cranial nerve —*see* Disorder, nerve, cranial
  cyclothymic F34.0
  defiant oppositional F91.3
  delusional (persistent) (systematized) F22
    induced F24
  depersonalization F48.1
  depressive F32.9
    major F32.9
      with psychotic symptoms F32.3
      in remission (full) F32.5
        partial F32.4
      recurrent F33.9
      single episode F32.9
        mild F32.0
        moderate F32.1
        severe (without psychotic symptoms) F32.2
          with psychotic symptoms F32.3
    organic F06.31
    recurrent F33.9
      current episode
        mild F33.0
        moderate F33.1
        severe (without psychotic symptoms) F33.2
          with psychotic symptoms F33.3
      in remission F33.40
        full F33.42
        partial F33.41
      specified NEC F33.8
    single episode —*see* Episode, depressive
  developmental F89
    arithmetical skills F81.2
    coordination (motor) F82
    expressive writing F81.81

  language F80.9
    expressive F80.1
    mixed receptive and expressive F80.2
    receptive type F80.2
    specified NEC F80.89
  learning F81.9
    arithmetical F81.2
    reading F81.0
  mixed F88
  motor coordination or function F82
  pervasive F84.9
    specified NEC F84.8
  phonological F80.0
  reading F81.0
  scholastic skills —*see also* Disorder, learning
    mixed F81.89
    specified NEC F88
  speech F80.9
    articulation F80.0
    specified NEC F80.89
    written expression F81.81
  diaphragm J98.6
  digestive (system) K92.9
    newborn P78.9
      specified NEC P78.89
    postprocedural —*see* Complication, gastrointestinal
    psychogenic F45.8
  disc (intervertebral) M51.9
    with
      myelopathy
        cervical region M50.00
        cervicothoracic region M50.03
        high cervical region M50.01
        lumbar region M51.06
        mid-cervical region M50.02
        sacrococcygeal region M53.3
        thoracic region M51.04
        thoracolumbar region M51.05
      radiculopathy
        cervical region M50.10
        cervicothoracic region M50.13
        high cervical region M50.11
        lumbar region M51.16
        lumbosacral region M51.17
        mid-cervical region M50.12
        sacrococcygeal region M53.3
        thoracic region M51.14
        thoracolumbar region M51.15
    cervical M50.90
      with
        myelopathy M50.00
          C2-C3 M50.01
          C3-C4 M50.01
          C4-C5 M50.02
          C5-C6 M50.02
          C6-C7 M50.02
          C7-T1 M50.03
          cervicothoracic region M50.03
          high cervical region M50.01
          mid-cervical region M50.02
        neuritis, radiculitis or radiculopathy M50.10
          C2-C3 M50.11
          C3-C4 M50.11
          C4-C5 M50.12
          C5-C6 M50.12
          C6-C7 M50.12
          C7-T1 M50.13
          cervicothoracic region M50.13
          high cervical region M50.11

Disorder (of) – *continued*

mid-cervical region M50.12
C2-C3 M50.91
C3-C4 M50.91
C4-C5 M50.92
C5-C6 M50.92
C6-C7 M50.92
C7-T1 M50.93
cervicothoracic region M50.93
degeneration M50.30
  C2-C3 M50.31
  C3-C4 M50.31
  C4-C5 M50.32
  C5-C6 M50.32
  C6-C7 M50.32
  C7-T1 M50.33
  cervicothoracic region M50.33
  high cervical region M50.31
  mid-cervical region M50.32
displacement M50.20
  C2-C3 M50.21
  C3-C4 M50.21
  C4-C5 M50.22
  C5-C6 M50.22
  C6-C7 M50.22
  C7-T1 M50.23
  cervicothoracic region M50.23
  high cervical region M50.21
  mid-cervical region M50.22
high cervical region M50.91
mid-cervical region M50.92
specified type NEC M50.80
  C2-C3 M50.81
  C3-C4 M50.81
  C4-C5 M50.82
  C5-C6 M50.82
  C6-C7 M50.82
  C7-T1 M50.83
  cervicothoracic region M50.83
  high cervical region M50.81
  mid-cervical region M50.82
specified NEC
  lumbar region M51.86
  lumbosacral region M51.87
  sacrococcygeal region M53.3
  thoracic region M51.84
  thoracolumbar region M51.85
disinhibited attachment (childhood) F94.2
disintegrative, childhood NEC F84.3
disruptive behavior F98.9
dissocial personality F60.2
dissociative F44.9
  affecting
    motor function F44.4
    and sensation F44.7
    sensation F44.6
    and motor function F44.7
  brief reactive F43.0
  due to (secondary to) general medical
condition F06.8
    mixed F44.7
    organic F06.8
  other specified NEC F44.89
double heterozygous sickling —*see* Disease,
sickle-cell
dream anxiety F51.5
drug induced hemorrhagic D68.32
drug related F19.99
  abuse —*see* Abuse, drug
  dependence —*see* Dependence, drug
dysmorphic body F45.1
dysthymic F34.1

Disorder (of) – *continued*

ear H93.9
  bleeding —*see* Otorrhagia
  deafness —*see* Deafness
  degenerative H93.09
  discharge —*see* Otorrhea
  external H61.9
    auditory canal stenosis —*see* Stenosis,
external ear canal
    exostosis —*see* Exostosis, external ear
canal
    impacted cerumen —*see* Impaction,
cerumen
    otitis —*see* Otitis, externa
    perichondritis —*see* Perichondritis, ear
    pinna —*see* Disorder, pinna
    specified type NEC H61.89
      in diseases classified elsewhere H62.8X
  inner H83.9
    vestibular dysfunction —*see* Disorder,
vestibular function
  middle H74.9
    adhesive H74.1
    ossicle —*see* Abnormal, ear ossicles
    polyp —*see* Polyp, ear (middle)
    specified NEC, in diseases classified
elsewhere H75.8
  postprocedural —*see* Complications, ear,
procedure
  specified NEC, in diseases classified
elsewhere H94.8
eating (adult) (psychogenic) F50.9
  anorexia —*see* Anorexia
  bulimia F50.2
  child F98.29
    pica F98.3
    rumination disorder F98.21
  pica F50.8
    childhood F98.3
electrolyte (balance) NEC E87.8
  with
    abortion —*see* Abortion by type
  complicated by specified condition NEC
    ectopic pregnancy O08.5
    molar pregnancy O08.5
  acidosis (metabolic) (respiratory) E87.2
  alkalosis (metabolic) (respiratory) E87.3
elimination, transepidermal L87.9
  specified NEC L87.8
emotional (persistent) F34.9
  of childhood F93.9
    specified NEC F93.8
endocrine E34.9
  postprocedural E89.89
  specified NEC E89.89
erectile (male) (organic) (*see also*
Dysfunction, sexual, male, erectile) N52.9
  nonorganic F52.21
erythematous —*see* Erythema
esophagus K22.9
  functional K22.4
  psychogenic F45.8
eustachian tube H69.9
  infection —*see* Salpingitis, eustachian
  obstruction —*see* Obstruction, eustachian
tube
  patulous —*see* Patulous, eustachian tube
  specified NEC H69.8
extrapyramidal G25.9
  in diseases classified elsewhere —*see*
category G26
  specified type NEC G25.89

Disorder (of) – *continued*

eye H57.9
  postprocedural —*see* Complication,
postprocedural, eye
eyelid H02.9
  cyst —*see* Cyst, eyelid
  degenerative H02.70
    chloasma —*see* Chloasma, eyelid
    madarosis —*see* Madarosis
    specified type NEC H02.79
    vitiligo —*see* Vitiligo, eyelid
    xanthelasma —*see* Xanthelasma
  dermatochalasis —*see* Dermatochalasis
  edema —*see* Edema, eyelid
  elephantiasis —*see* Elephantiasis, eyelid
  foreign body, retained —*see* Foreign body,
retained, eyelid
  function H02.59
    abnormal innervation syndrome —*see*
Syndrome, abnormal innervation
    blepharochalasis —*see* Blepharochalasis
    blepharoclonus —*see* Blepharoclonus
    blepharophimosis —*see* Blepharophimosis
    blepharoptosis —*see* Blepharoptosis
    lagophthalmos —*see* Lagophthalmos
    lid retraction —*see* Retraction, lid
    hypertrichosis —*see* Hypertrichosis, eyelid
    specified type NEC H02.89
  vascular H02.879
    left H02.876
      lower H02.875
      upper H02.874
    right H02.873
      lower H02.872
      upper H02.871
factitious F68.10
  with predominantly
    psychological symptoms F68.11
      with physical symptoms F68.13
    physical symptoms F68.12
      with psychological symptoms F68.13
factor, coagulation —*see* Defect, coagulation
fatty acid
  metabolism E71.30
    specified NEC E71.39
  oxidation
    LCAD E71.310
    MCAD E71.311
    SCAD E71.312
    specified deficiency NEC E71.318
feeding (infant or child) (*see also* Disorder,
eating) R63.3
feigned (with obvious motivation) Z76.5
  without obvious motivation —*see* Disorder,
factitious
female
  hypoactive sexual desire F52.0
  orgasmic F52.31
  sexual arousal F52.22
fibroblastic M72.9
  specified NEC M72.8
fluency
  adult onset F98.5
  childhood onset F80.81
  following
    cerebral infarction I69.323
    cerebrovascular disease I69.923
      specified disease NEC I69.823
    intracerebral hemorrhage I69.123
    nontraumatic intracranial hemorrhage NEC
I69.223
    subarachnoid hemorrhage I69.023
  in conditions classified elsewhere R47.82

Disorder (of) – *continued*
fluid balance E87.8
follicular (skin) L73.9
  specified NEC L73.8
fructose metabolism E74.10
  essential fructosuria E74.11
  fructokinase deficiency E74.11
  fructose 1, 6-diphosphatase deficiency
E74.19
  hereditary fructose intolerance E74.12
  other specified E74.19
functional polymorphonuclear neutrophils
D71
gallbladder, biliary tract and pancreas in
diseases classified elsewhere K87
gamma-glutamyl cycle E72.8
gastric (functional) K31.9
  motility K30
  psychogenic F45.8
  secretion K30
gastrointestinal (functional) NOS K92.9
  newborn P78.9
  psychogenic F45.8
gender-identity or -role F64.9
  childhood F64.2
  effect on relationship F66
  of adolescence or adulthood
(nontranssexual) F64.1
  specified NEC F64.8
  uncertainty F66
genitourinary system
  female N94.9
  male N50.9
  psychogenic F45.8
globe H44.9
  degenerated condition H44.50
   absolute glaucoma H44.51
   atrophy H44.52
   leucocoria H44.53
  degenerative H44.30
   chalcosis H44.31
   myopia H44.2
   siderosis H44.32
   specified type NEC H44.39
  endophthalmitis —*see* Endophthalmitis
  foreign body, retained —*see* Foreign body,
intraocular, old, retained
  hemophthalmos —*see* Hemophthalmos
  hypotony H44.40
   due to
    ocular fistula H44.42
    specified disorder NEC H44.43
   flat anterior chamber H44.41
   primary H44.44
  luxation —*see* Luxation, globe
  specified type NEC H44.89
glomerular (in) N05.9
  amyloidosis E85.4 *[N08]*
  cryoglobulinemia D89.1 *[N08]*
  disseminated intravascular coagulation D65
[N08]
  Fabry's disease E75.21 *[N08]*
  familial lecithin cholesterol acyltransferase
deficiency E78.6 *[N08]*
  Goodpasture's syndrome M31.0
  hemolytic-uremic syndrome D59.3
  Henoch (-Schönlein) purpura D69.0 *[N08]*
  malariae malaria B52.0
  microscopic polyangiitis M31.7 *[N08]*
  multiple myeloma C90.0 *[N08]*
  mumps B26.83
  schistosomiasis B65.9 *[N08]*

Disorder (of) – *continued*
  sepsis NEC A41. *[N08]*
   streptococcal A40. *[N08]*
  sickle-cell disorders D57. *[N08]*
  strongyloidiasis B78.9 *[N08]*
  subacute bacterial endocarditis I33.0 *[N08]*
  syphilis A52.75
  systemic lupus erythematosus M32.14
  thrombotic thrombocytopenic purpura
M31.1 *[N08]*
  Waldenström macroglobulinemia C88.0
[N08]
  Wegener's granulomatosis M31.31
gluconeogenesis E74.4
glucosaminoglycan metabolism —*see*
Disorder, metabolism, glucosaminoglycan
glycine metabolism E72.50
  d-glycericacidemia E72.59
  hyperhydroxyprolinemia E72.59
  hyperoxaluria E72.53
  hyperprolinemia E72.59
  non-ketotic hyperglycinemia E72.51
  oxalosis E72.53
  oxaluria E72.53
  sarcosinemia E72.59
  trimethylaminuria E72.52
glycoprotein metabolism E77.9
  specified NEC E77.8
habit (and impulse) F63.9
  involving sexual behavior NEC F65.9
  specified NEC F63.89
heart action I49.9
hematological D75.9
  newborn (transient) P61.9
   specified NEC P61.8
hematopoietic organs D75.9
hemorrhagic NEC D69.9
  drug-induced D68.32
  due to
   extrinsic circulating anticoagulants D68.32
   increase in
    anti-IIa D68.32
    anti-Xa D68.32
   intrinsic
    circulating anticoagulants D68.318
    increase in
     antithrombin D68.318
     anti-VIIIa D68.318
     anti-IXa D68.318
     anti-XIa D68.318
  following childbirth O72.3
hemostasis —*see* Defect, coagulation
histidine metabolism E70.40
  histidinemia E70.41
  other specified E70.49
hyperkinetic —*see* Disorder, attention-deficit
hyperactivity
hyperleucine-isoleucinemia E71.19
hypervalinemia E71.19
hypoactive sexual desire F52.0
hypochondriacal F45.20
  body dysmorphic F45.22
  neurosis F45.21
  other specified F45.29
identity
  dissociative F44.81
  of childhood F93.8
immune mechanism (immunity) D89.9
  specified type NEC D89.89
impaired renal tubular function N25.9
  specified NEC N25.89
impulse (control) F63.9

Disorder (of) – *continued*
inflammatory
  pelvic, in diseases classified elsewhere —
see category N74
penis N48.29
  abscess N48.21
  cellulitis N48.22
integument, newborn P83.9
  specified NEC P83.8
intermittent explosive F63.81
internal secretion pancreas —*see* Increased,
secretion, pancreas, endocrine
intestine, intestinal
  carbohydrate absorption NEC E74.39
   postoperative K91.2
  functional NEC K59.9
   postoperative K91.89
   psychogenic F45.8
  vascular K55.9
   chronic K55.1
   specified NEC K55.8
intraoperative (intraprocedural) —*see*
Complications, intraoperative
involuntary emotional expression (IEED)
F48.2
iris H21.9
  adhesions —*see* Adhesions, iris
  atrophy —*see* Atrophy, iris
  chamber angle recession —*see* Recession,
chamber angle
  cyst —*see* Cyst, iris
  degeneration —*see* Degeneration, iris
  in diseases classified elsewhere H22
  iridodialysis —*see* Iridodialysis
  iridoschisis —*see* Iridoschisis
  miotic pupillary cyst —*see* Cyst, pupillary
  pupillary
   abnormality —*see* Abnormality, pupillary
   membrane —*see* Membrane, pupillary
  specified type NEC H21.89
  vascular NEC H21.1X
iron metabolism E83.10
  specified NEC E83.19
isovaleric acidemia E71.110
jaw, developmental M27.0
  temporomandibular —*see* Anomaly,
dentofacial, temporomandibular joint
joint M25.9
  derangement —*see* Derangement, joint
  effusion —*see* Effusion, joint
  fistula —*see* Fistula, joint
  hemarthrosis —*see* Hemarthrosis
  instability —*see* Instability, joint
  osteophyte —*see* Osteophyte
  pain —*see* Pain, joint
  psychogenic F45.8
  specified type NEC M25.80
   ankle M25.87
   elbow M25.82
   foot joint M25.87
   hand joint M25.84
   hip M25.85
   knee M25.86
   shoulder M25.81
   wrist M25.83
  stiffness —*see* Stiffness, joint
ketone metabolism E71.32
kidney N28.9
  functional (tubular) N25.9
  in
   schistosomiasis B65.9 *[N29]*
  tubular function N25.9
   specified NEC N25.89

Disorder (of) – *continued*
lacrimal system H04.9
  changes H04.69
    fistula —*see* Fistula, lacrimal
  gland H04.19
    atrophy —*see* Atrophy, lacrimal gland
    cyst —*see* Cyst, lacrimal, gland
    dacryops —*see* Dacryops
    dislocation —*see* Dislocation, lacrimal gland
    dry eye syndrome —*see* Syndrome, dry eye
    infection —*see* Dacryoadenitis
    granuloma —*see* Granuloma, lacrimal
    inflammation —*see* Inflammation, lacrimal
    obstruction —*see* Obstruction, lacrimal
    specified NEC H04.89
lactation NEC O92.79
language (developmental) F80.9
  expressive F80.1
  mixed receptive and expressive F80.2
  receptive F80.2
late luteal phase dysphoric N94.89
learning (specific) F81.9
  acalculia R48.8
  alexia R48.0
  mathematics F81.2
  reading F81.0
  specified NEC F81.89
  spelling F81.81
  written expression F81.81
lens H27.9
  aphakia —*see* Aphakia
  cataract —*see* Cataract
  dislocation —*see* Dislocation, lens
  specified type NEC H27.8
ligament M24.20
  ankle M24.27
  attachment, spine —*see* Enthesopathy, spinal
  elbow M24.22
  foot joint M24.27
  hand joint M24.24
  hip M24.25
  knee —*see* Derangement, knee, specified NEC
  shoulder M24.21
  vertebra M24.28
  wrist M24.23
ligamentous attachments —*see also* Enthesopathy
  spine —*see* Enthesopathy, spinal
lipid
  metabolism, congenital E78.9
  storage E75.6
    specified NEC E75.5
lipoprotein
  deficiency (familial) E78.6
  metabolism E78.9
    specified NEC E78.89
liver K76.9
  malarial B54 *[K77]*
low back —*see also* Dorsopathy, specified NEC
lumbosacral
  plexus G54.1
  root (nerve) NEC G54.4
lung, interstitial, drug-induced J70.4
  acute J70.2
  chronic J70.3
lymphoproliferative, post-transplant (PTLD) D47.Z1

Disorder (of) – *continued*
lysine and hydroxylysine metabolism E72.3
male
  erectile (organic) (*see also* Dysfunction, sexual, male, erectile) N52.9
    nonorganic F52.21
  hypoactive sexual desire F52.0
  orgasmic F52.32
manic F30.9
  organic F06.33
mastoid —*see also* Disorder, ear, middle
  postprocedural —*see* Complications, ear, procedure
meniscus —*see* Derangement, knee, meniscus
menopausal N95.9
  specified NEC N95.8
menstrual N92.6
  psychogenic F45.8
  specified NEC N92.5
mental (or behavioral) (nonpsychotic) F99
  due to (secondary to)
    amphetamine
      due to drug abuse —*see* Abuse, drug, stimulant
      due to drug dependence —*see* Dependence, drug, stimulant
    brain disease, damage and dysfunction F09
    caffeine use
      due to drug abuse —*see* Abuse, drug, stimulant
      due to drug dependence —*see* Dependence, drug, stimulant
    cannabis use
      due to drug abuse —*see* Abuse, drug, cannabis
      due to drug dependence —*see* Dependence, drug, cannabis
    general medical condition F09
    sedative or hypnotic use
      due to drug abuse —*see* Abuse, drug, sedative
      due to drug dependence —*see* Dependence, drug, sedative
    tobacco (nicotine) use —*see* Dependence, drug, nicotine
  following organic brain damage F07.9
    frontal lobe syndrome F07.0
    personality change F07.0
    postconcussional syndrome F07.81
    specified NEC F07.89
  infancy, childhood or adolescence F98.9
  neurotic —*see* Neurosis
  organic or symptomatic F09
  presenile, psychotic F03
  problem NEC
  psychoneurotic —*see* Neurosis
  psychotic —*see* Psychosis
  puerperal F53
  senile, psychotic NEC F03
metabolic, amino acid, transitory, newborn P74.8
metabolism NOS E88.9
  amino-acid E72.9
    aromatic E70.9
      albinism —*see* Albinism
      histidine E70.40
        histidinemia E70.41
        other specified E70.49
      hyperphenylalaninemia E70.1
        classical phenylketonuria E70.0
      other specified E70.8
      tryptophan E70.5

Disorder (of) – *continued*
      tyrosine E70.20
        hypertyrosinemia E70.21
        other specified E70.29
    branched chain E71.2
      3-methylglutaconic aciduria E71.111
      hyperleucine-isoleucinemia E71.19
      hypervalinemia E71.19
      isovaleric acidemia E71.110
      maple syrup urine disease E71.0
      methylmalonic acidemia E71.120
      organic aciduria NEC E71.118
      other specified E71.19
      propionate NEC E71.128
      propionic acidemia E71.121
    glycine E72.50
      d-glycericacidemia E72.59
      hyperhydroxyprolinemia E72.59
      hyperoxaluria E72.53
      hyperprolinemia E72.59
      non-ketotic hyperglycinemia E72.51
      other specified E72.59
      sarcosinemia E72.59
      trimethylaminuria E72.52
    hydroxylysine E72.3
    lysine E72.3
    ornithine E72.4
    other specified E72.8
      beta-amino acid E72.8
      gamma-glutamyl cycle E72.8
      straight-chain E72.8
      sulfur-bearing E72.10
        homocystinuria E72.11
        methylenetetrahydrofolate reductase deficiency E72.12
      other specified E72.19
    bile acid and cholesterol metabolism E78.70
    bilirubin E80.7
      specified NEC E80.6
    calcium E83.50
      hypercalcemia E83.52
      hypocalcemia E83.51
      other specified E83.59
    carbohydrate E74.9
      specified NEC E74.8
    cholesterol and bile acid metabolism E78.70
    congenital E88.9
    copper E83.00
      Wilson's disease E83.01
      specified type NEC E83.09
    cystinuria E72.01
    fructose E74.10
    galactose E74.20
    glucosaminoglycan E76.9
      mucopolysaccharidosis —*see* Mucopolysaccharidosis
      specified NEC E76.8
    glutamine E72.8
    glycine E72.50
    glycogen storage (hepatorenal) E74.09
    glycoprotein E77.9
      specified NEC E77.8
    glycosaminoglycan E76.9
      specified NEC E76.8
    in labor and delivery O75.89
    iron E83.10
    isoleucine E71.19
    leucine E71.19
    lipoid E78.9
    lipoprotein E78.9
      specified NEC E78.89

Disorder (of) – *continued*
  magnesium E83.40
    hypermagnesemia E83.41
    hypomagnesemia E83.42
    other specified E83.49
  mineral E83.9
    specified NEC E83.89
  mitochondrial E88.40
    MELAS syndrome E88.41
    MERRF syndrome (myoclonic epilepsy
associated with ragged-red fibers) E88.42
    other specified E88.49
  ornithine E72.4
  phosphatases E83.30
  phosphorus E83.30
    acid phosphatase deficiency E83.39
    hypophosphatasia E83.39
    hypophosphatemia E83.39
      familial E83.31
    other specified E83.39
    pseudovitamin D deficiency E83.32
  plasma protein NEC E88.09
  porphyrin —*see* Porphyria
  postprocedural E89.89
    specified NEC E89.89
  purine E79.9
    specified NEC E79.8
  pyrimidine E79.9
    specified NEC E79.8
  pyruvate E74.4
  serine E72.8
  sodium E87.8
  specified NEC E88.89
  threonine E72.8
  valine E71.19
  zinc E83.2
  methylmalonic acidemia E71.120
  micturition NEC R39.19
    feeling of incomplete emptying R39.14
    hesitancy R39.11
    poor stream R39.12
    psychogenic F45.8
    split stream R39.13
    straining R39.16
    urgency R39.15
  mitochondrial metabolism E88.40
  mitral (valve) —*see* Endocarditis, mitral
  mixed
    anxiety and depressive F41.8
    of scholastic skills (developmental) F81.89
    receptive expressive language F80.2
  mood F39
    bipolar —*see* Disorder, bipolar
    depressive —*see* Disorder, depressive
    due to (secondary to)
      alcohol F10.94
      amphetamine F15.94
        in
          abuse F15.14
          dependence F15.24
      anxiolytic F13.94
        in
          abuse F13.14
          dependence F13.24
      cocaine F14.94
        in
          abuse F14.14
          dependence F14.24
      general medical condition F06.30
      hallucinogen F16.94
        in
          abuse F16.14

Disorder (of) – *continued*
        dependence F16.24
      hypnotic F13.94
        in
          abuse F13.14
          dependence F13.24
      inhalant F18.94
        in
          abuse F18.14
          dependence F18.24
      opioid F11.94
        in
          abuse F11.14
          dependence F11.24
      phencyclidine (PCP) F16.94
        in
          abuse F16.14
          dependence F16.24
      physiological condition F06.30
        with
          depressive features F06.31
          major depressive-like episode F06.32
          manic features F06.33
          mixed features F06.34
      psychoactive substance NEC F19.94
        in
          abuse F19.14
          dependence F19.24
      sedative F13.94
        in
          abuse F13.14
          dependence F13.24
      volatile solvents F18.94
        in
          abuse F18.14
          dependence F18.24
    manic episode F30.9
      with psychotic symptoms F30.2
      in remission (full) F30.4
        partial F30.3
      specified type NEC F30.8
      without psychotic symptoms F30.10
        mild F30.11
        moderate F30.12
        severe F30.13
    organic F06.30
      right hemisphere F07.89
    persistent F34.9
      cyclothymia F34.0
      dysthymia F34.1
      specified type NEC F34.8
    recurrent F39
    right hemisphere organic F07.89
  movement G25.9
    drug-induced G25.70
      akathisia G25.71
      specified NEC G25.79
    hysterical F44.4
    in diseases classified elsewhere —see
category G26
    periodic limb G47.61
      sleep related G47.61
    specified NEC G25.89
    sleep related NEC G47.69
    stereotyped F98.4
    treatment-induced G25.9
  multiple personality F44.81
  muscle M62.9
    attachment, spine —*see* Enthesopathy,
spinal
    in trichinellosis —*see* Trichinellosis, with
muscle disorder

Disorder (of) – *continued*
    psychogenic F45.8
    specified type NEC M62.89
    tone, newborn P94.9
      specified NEC P94.8
  muscular
    attachments —*see also* Enthesopathy
      spine —*see* Enthesopathy, spinal
    urethra N36.44
  musculoskeletal system, soft tissue —*see*
Disorder, soft tissue
    postprocedural M96.89
    psychogenic F45.8
  myoneural G70.9
    due to lead G70.1
    specified NEC G70.89
    toxic G70.1
  myotonic NEC G71.19
  nail, in diseases classified elsewhere L62
  neck region NEC —*see* Dorsopathy, specified
NEC
  nerve G58.9
    abducent NEC —*see* Strabismus, paralytic,
sixth nerve
    accessory G52.8
    acoustic —*see* subcategory H93.3
    auditory —*see* subcategory H93.3
    auriculotemporal G50.8
    axillary G54.0
    cerebral —*see* Disorder, nerve, cranial
    cranial G52.9
      eighth —*see* subcategory H93.3
      eleventh G52.8
      fifth G50.9
      first G52.0
      fourth NEC —*see* Strabismus, paralytic,
fourth nerve
      multiple G52.7
      ninth G52.1
      second NEC —*see* Disorder, nerve, optic
      seventh NEC G51.8
      sixth NEC —*see* Strabismus, paralytic,
sixth nerve
      specified NEC G52.8
      tenth G52.2
      third NEC —*see* Strabismus, paralytic,
third nerve
      twelfth G52.3
    entrapment —*see* Neuropathy, entrapment
    facial G51.9
      specified NEC G51.8
    femoral —*see* Lesion, nerve, femoral
    glossopharyngeal NEC G52.1
    hypoglossal G52.3
    intercostal G58.0
    lateral
      cutaneous of thigh —*see* Mononeuropathy,
lower limb, meralgia paresthetica
      popliteal —*see* Lesion, nerve, popliteal
    lower limb —*see* Mononeuropathy, lower
limb
    medial popliteal —*see* Lesion, nerve,
popliteal, medial
    median NEC —*see* Lesion, nerve, median
    multiple G58.7
    oculomotor NEC —*see* Strabismus,
paralytic, third nerve
    olfactory G52.0
    optic NEC H47.09
      hemorrhage into sheath —*see* Hemorrhage,
optic nerve
      ischemic H47.01

Disorder (of) – *continued*

  peroneal —*see* Lesion, nerve, popliteal

  phrenic G58.8

  plantar —*see* Lesion, nerve, plantar

  pneumogastric G52.2

  posterior tibial —*see* Syndrome, tarsal tunnel

  radial —*see* Lesion, nerve, radial

  recurrent laryngeal G52.2

  root G54.9

    cervical G54.2

    lumbosacral G54.1

    specified NEC G54.8

    thoracic G54.3

  sciatic NEC —*see* Lesion, nerve, sciatic

  specified NEC G58.8

    lower limb —*see* Mononeuropathy, lower limb, specified NEC

    upper limb —*see* Mononeuropathy, upper limb, specified NEC

  sympathetic G90.9

  tibial —*see* Lesion, nerve, popliteal, medial

  trigeminal G50.9

    specified NEC G50.8

  trochlear NEC —*see* Strabismus, paralytic, fourth nerve

  ulnar —*see* Lesion, nerve, ulnar

  upper limb —*see* Mononeuropathy, upper limb

  vagus G52.2

  nervous system G98.8

    autonomic (peripheral) G90.9

      specified NEC G90.8

    central G96.9

      specified NEC G96.8

    parasympathetic G90.9

    specified NEC G98.8

    sympathetic G90.9

    vegetative G90.9

  neurohypophysis NEC E23.3

  neurological NEC R29.818

  neuromuscular G70.9

    hereditary NEC G71.9

    specified NEC G70.89

    toxic G70.1

  neurotic F48.9

    specified NEC F48.8

  neutrophil, polymorphonuclear D71

  nicotine use —*see* Dependence, drug, nicotine

  nightmare F51.5

  nose J34.9

    specified NEC J34.89

  obsessive-compulsive F42

  odontogenesis NOS K00.9

  opioid use

    with

      opioid-induced psychotic disorder F11.959

      with

        delusions F11.950

        hallucinations F11.951

    due to drug abuse —*see* Abuse, drug, opioid

    due to drug dependence —*see* Dependence, drug, opioid

  oppositional defiant F91.3

  optic

    chiasm H47.49

      due to

        inflammatory disorder H47.41

        neoplasm H47.42

        vascular disorder H47.43

    disc H47.39

      coloboma —*see* Coloboma, optic disc

Disorder (of) – *continued*

    drusen —*see* Drusen, optic disc

    pseudopapilledema —*see* Pseudopapilledema

    radiations —*see* Disorder, visual, pathway

    tracts —*see* Disorder, visual, pathway

  orbit H05.9

    cyst —*see* Cyst, orbit

    deformity —*see* Deformity, orbit

    edema —*see* Edema, orbit

    enophthalmos —*see* Enophthalmos

    exophthalmos —*see* Exophthalmos

    hemorrhage —*see* Hemorrhage, orbit

    inflammation —*see* Inflammation, orbit

    myopathy —*see* Myopathy, extraocular muscles

    retained foreign body —*see* Foreign body, orbit, old

    specified type NEC H05.89

  organic

    anxiety F06.4

    catatonic F06.1

    delusional F06.2

    dissociative F06.8

    emotionally labile (asthenic) F06.8

    mood (affective) F06.30

    schizophrenia-like F06.2

  orgasmic (female) F52.31

    male F52.32

  ornithine metabolism E72.4

  overanxious F41.1

    of childhood F93.8

  pain

    with related psychological factors F45.42

    exclusively related to psychological factors F45.41

  pancreatic internal secretion E16.9

    specified NEC E16.8

  panic F41.0

    with agoraphobia F40.01

  papulosquamous L44.9

    in diseases classified elsewhere L45

    specified NEC L44.8

  paranoid F22

    induced F24

    shared F24

  parathyroid (gland) E21.5

    specified NEC E21.4

  parietoalveolar NEC J84.09

  paroxysmal, mixed R56.9

  patella M22.9

    chondromalacia —*see* Chondromalacia, patella

    derangement NEC M22.3X

    recurrent

      dislocation —*see* Dislocation, patella, recurrent

      subluxation —*see* Dislocation, patella, recurrent, incomplete

    specified NEC M22.8X

  patellofemoral M22.2X

  pentose phosphate pathway with anemia D55.1

  perception, due to hallucinogens F16.983

    in

      abuse F16.183

      dependence F16.283

  peripheral nervous system NEC G64

  peroxisomal E71.50

    biogenesis

      neonatal adrenoleukodystrophy E71.511

      specified disorder NEC E71.518

Disorder (of) – *continued*

    Zellweger syndrome E71.510

    rhizomelic chondrodysplasia punctata E71.540

    specified form NEC E71.548

      group 1 E71.518

      group 2 E71.53

      group 3 E71.542

    X-linked adrenoleukodystrophy E71.529

      adolescent E71.521

      adrenomyeloneuropathy E71.522

      childhood E71.520

      specified form NEC E71.528

    Zellweger-like syndrome E71.541

  persistent

    (somatoform) pain F45.41

    affective (mood) F34.9

  personality (*see also* Personality) F60.9

    affective F34.0

    aggressive F60.3

    amoral F60.2

    anankastic F60.5

    antisocial F60.2

    anxious F60.6

    asocial F60.2

    asthenic F60.7

    avoidant F60.6

    borderline F60.3

    change (secondary) due to general medical condition F07.0

    compulsive F60.5

    cyclothymic F34.0

    dependent (passive) F60.7

    depressive F34.1

    dissocial F60.2

    emotional instability F60.3

    expansive paranoid F60.0

    explosive F60.3

    following organic brain damage F07.9

    histrionic F60.4

    hyperthymic F34.0

    hypothymic F34.1

    hysterical F60.4

    immature F60.89

    inadequate F60.7

    labile F60.3

    mixed (nonspecific) F60.89

    moral deficiency F60.2

    narcissistic F60.81

    negativistic F60.89

    obsessional F60.5

    obsessive (-compulsive) F60.5

    organic F07.9

    overconscientious F60.5

    paranoid F60.0

    passive (-dependent) F60.7

    passive-aggressive F60.89

    pathological NEC F60.9

    pseudosocial F60.2

    psychopathic F60.2

    schizoid F60.1

    schizotypal F21

    self-defeating F60.7

    specified NEC F60.89

    type A F60.5

    unstable (emotional) F60.3

  pervasive, developmental F84.9

  phobic anxiety, childhood F40.8

  phosphate-losing tubular N25.0

  pigmentation L81.9

    choroid, congenital Q14.3

    diminished melanin formation L81.6

    iron L81.8

Disorder (of) – *continued*
  specified NEC L81.8
  pinna (noninfective) H61.10
    deformity, acquired H61.11
    hematoma H61.12
    perichondritis —*see* Perichondritis, ear
    specified type NEC H61.19
  pituitary gland E23.7
    iatrogenic (postprocedural) E89.3
    specified NEC E23.6
  platelets D69.1
  plexus G54.9
    specified NEC G54.8
  polymorphonuclear neutrophils D71
  porphyrin metabolism —*see* Porphyria
  postconcussional F07.81
  posthallucinogen perception F16.983
    in
      abuse F16.183
      dependence F16.283
  postmenopausal N95.9
    specified NEC N95.8
  postprocedural (postoperative) —*see*
  Complications, postprocedural
  post-transplant lymphoproliferative D47.Z1
  post-traumatic stress (PTSD) F43.10
    acute F43.11
    chronic F43.12
  premenstrual dysphoric (PMDD) N94.3
  prepuce N47.8
  propionic acidemia E71.121
  prostate N42.9
    specified NEC N42.89
  psychogenic NOS (*see also* condition) F45.9
    anxiety F41.8
    appetite F50.9
    asthenic F48.8
    cardiovascular (system) F45.8
    compulsive F42
    cutaneous F54
    depressive F32.9
    digestive (system) F45.8
    dysmenorrheic F45.8
    dyspneic F45.8
    endocrine (system) F54
    eye NEC F45.8
    feeding —*see* Disorder, eating
    functional NEC F45.8
    gastric F45.8
    gastrointestinal (system) F45.8
    genitourinary (system) F45.8
    heart (function) (rhythm) F45.8
    hyperventilatory F45.8
    hypochondriacal —*see* Disorder,
  hypochondriacal
    intestinal F45.8
    joint F45.8
    learning F81.9
    limb F45.8
    lymphatic (system) F45.8
    menstrual F45.8
    micturition F45.8
    monoplegic NEC F44.4
    motor F44.4
    muscle F45.8
    musculoskeletal F45.8
    neurocirculatory F45.8
    obsessive F42
    occupational F48.8
    organ or part of body NEC F45.8
    paralytic NEC F44.4
    phobic F40.9

Disorder (of) – *continued*
  physical NEC F45.8
  rectal F45.8
  respiratory (system) F45.8
  rheumatic F45.8
  sexual (function) F52.9
  skin (allergic) (eczematous) F54
  sleep F51.9
  specified part of body NEC F45.8
  stomach F45.8
  psychological F99
    associated with
      disease classified elsewhere F54
      sexual
        development F66
        relationship F66
      uncertainty about gender identity F66
  psychomotor NEC F44.4
    hysterical F44.4
  psychoneurotic —*see also* Neurosis
    mixed NEC F48.8
  psychophysiologic —*see* Disorder,
  somatoform
  psychosexual F65.9
    development F66
    identity of childhood F64.2
  psychosomatic NOS —*see* Disorder,
  somatoform
    multiple F45.0
    undifferentiated F45.1
  psychotic —*see* Psychosis
    transient (acute) F23
  puberty E30.9
    specified NEC E30.8
  pulmonary (valve) —*see* Endocarditis,
  pulmonary
  purine metabolism E79.9
  pyrimidine metabolism E79.9
  pyruvate metabolism E74.4
  reactive attachment (childhood) F94.1
  reading R48.0
    developmental (specific) F81.0
  receptive language F80.2
  receptor, hormonal, peripheral (*see also*
  Syndrome, androgen insensitivity) E34.50
  recurrent brief depressive F33.8
  reflex R29.2
  refraction H52.7
    aniseikonia H52.32
    anisometropia H52.31
    astigmatism —*see* Astigmatism
    hypermetropia —*see* Hypermetropia
    myopia —*see* Myopia
    presbyopia H52.4
    specified NEC H52.6
  relationship F68.8
    due to sexual orientation F66
  REM sleep behavior G47.52
  renal function, impaired (tubular) N25.9
  resonance R49.9
    specified NEC R49.8
  respiratory function, impaired —*see also*
  Failure, respiration
    postprocedural —*see* Complication,
  postoperative, respiratory system
    psychogenic F45.8
  retina H35.9
    angioid streaks H35.33
    changes in vascular appearance H35.01
    degeneration —*see* Degeneration, retina
    dystrophy (hereditary) —*see* Dystrophy,
  retina

Disorder (of) – *continued*
  edema H35.81
  hemorrhage —*see* Hemorrhage, retina
  ischemia H35.82
  macular degeneration —*see* Degeneration,
  macula
  microaneurysms H35.04
  microvascular abnormality NEC H35.09
  neovascularization —*see*
  Neovascularization, retina
  retinopathy —*see* Retinopathy
  separation of layers H35.70
    central serous chorioretinopathy H35.71
    pigment epithelium detachment (serous)
  H35.72
      hemorrhagic H35.73
    specified type NEC H35.89
    telangiectasis —*see* Telangiectasis, retina
    vasculitis —*see* Vasculitis, retina
  retroperitoneal K68.9
  right hemisphere organic affective F07.89
  rumination (infant or child) F98.21
  sacrum, sacrococcygeal NEC M53.3
  schizoaffective F25.9
    bipolar type F25.0
    depressive type F25.1
    manic type F25.0
    mixed type F25.0
    specified NEC F25.8
  schizoid of childhood F84.5
  schizophreniform F20.81
    brief F23
  schizotypal (personality) F21
  secretion, thyrocalcitonin E07.0
  seizure (*see also* Epilepsy) G40.909
    intractable G40.919
      with status epilepticus G40.911
  semantic pragmatic F80.89
    with autism F84.0
  sense of smell R43.1
    psychogenic F45.8
  separation anxiety, of childhood F93.0
  sexual
    arousal, female F52.22
    aversion F52.1
    function, psychogenic F52.9
    maturation F66
    nonorganic F52.9
    preference (*see also* Deviation, sexual)
  F65.9
      fetishistic transvestism F65.1
    relationship F66
  shyness, of childhood and adolescence F40.10
  sibling rivalry F93.8
  sickle-cell (sickling) (homozygous) —*see*
  Disease, sickle-cell
    heterozygous D57.3
    specified type NEC D57.8
    trait D57.3
  sinus (nasal) J34.9
    specified NEC J34.89
  skin L98.9
    atrophic L90.9
      specified NEC L90.8
    granulomatous L92.9
      specified NEC L92.8
    hypertrophic L91.9
      specified NEC L91.8
    infiltrative NEC L98.6
    newborn P83.9
      specified NEC P83.8
    psychogenic (allergic) (eczematous) F54

Disorder (of) – *continued*
  sleep G47.9
    breathing-related —*see* Apnea, sleep
    circadian rhythm G47.20
      advance sleep phase type G47.22
      delayed sleep phase type G47.21
      due to
        alcohol
          abuse F10.182
          dependence F10.282
          use F10.982
        amphetamines
          abuse F15.182
          dependence F15.282
          use F15.982
        caffeine
          abuse F15.182
          dependence F15.282
          use F15.982
        cocaine
          abuse F14.182
          dependence F14.282
          use F14.982
        drug NEC
          abuse F19.182
          dependence F19.282
          use F19.982
        opioid
          abuse F11.182
          dependence F11.282
          use F11.982
        psychoactive substance NEC
          abuse F19.182
          dependence F19.282
          use F19.982
        sedative, hypnotic, or anxiolytic
          abuse F13.182
          dependence F13.282
          use F13.982
        stimulant NEC
          abuse F15.182
          dependence F15.282
          use F15.982
      free running type G47.24
      in conditions classified elsewhere G47.27
      irregular sleep wake type G47.23
      jet lag type G47.25
      shift work type G47.26
      specified NEC G47.29
    due to
      alcohol
        abuse F10.182
        dependence F10.282
        use F10.982
      amphetamine
        abuse F15.182
        dependence F15.282
        use F15.982
      anxiolytic
        abuse F13.182
        dependence F13.282
        use F13.982
      caffeine
        abuse F15.182
        dependence F15.282
        use F15.982
      cocaine
        abuse F14.182
        dependence F14.282
        use F14.982
      drug NEC
        abuse F19.182

        dependence F19.282
        use F19.982
      hypnotic
        abuse F13.182
        dependence F13.282
        use F13.982
      opioid
        abuse F11.182
        dependence F11.282
        use F11.982
      psychoactive substance NEC
        abuse F19.182
        dependence F19.282
        use F19.982
      sedative
        abuse F13.182
        dependence F13.282
        use F13.982
      stimulant NEC
        abuse F15.182
        dependence F15.282
        use F15.982
    emotional F51.9
    excessive somnolence —*see* Hypersomnia
    hypersomnia type —*see* Hypersomnia
    initiating or maintaining —*see* Insomnia
    nightmares F51.5
    nonorganic F51.9
      specified NEC F51.8
    parasomnia type G47.50
    specified NEC G47.8
    terrors F51.4
    walking F51.3
  sleep-wake pattern or schedule —*see*
  Disorder, sleep, circadian rhythm
  social
    anxiety of childhood F40.10
    functioning in childhood F94.9
      specified NEC F94.8
  soft tissue M79.9
    ankle M79.9
    due to use, overuse and pressure M70.90
      ankle M70.97
      bursitis —*see* Bursitis
      foot M70.97
      forearm M70.93
      hand M70.94
      lower leg M70.96
      multiple sites M70.99
      pelvic region M70.95
      shoulder region M70.91
      specified site NEC M70.98
      specified type NEC M70.80
        ankle M70.87
        foot M70.87
        forearm M70.83
        hand M70.84
        lower leg M70.86
        multiple sites M70.89
        pelvic region M70.85
        shoulder region M70.81
        specified site NEC M70.88
        thigh M70.85
        upper arm M70.82
      thigh M70.95
      upper arm M70.92
    foot M79.9
    forearm M79.9
    hand M79.9
    lower leg M79.9
    multiple sites M79.9

Disorder (of) – *continued*
  occupational —*see* Disorder, soft tissue, due
  to use, overuse and pressure
    pelvic region M79.9
    shoulder region M79.9
    specified type NEC M79.89
    thigh M79.9
    upper arm M79.9
  somatization F45.0
  somatoform F45.9
    pain (persistent) F45.41
    somatization (multiple) (long-lasting) F45.0
    specified NEC F45.8
    undifferentiated F45.1
  somnolence, excessive —*see* Hypersomnia
  specific
    arithmetical F81.2
    developmental, of motor F82
    reading F81.0
    speech and language F80.9
    spelling F81.81
    written expression F81.81
  speech R47.9
    articulation (functional) (specific) F80.0
    developmental F80.9
    specified NEC R47.89
  spelling (specific) F81.81
  spine —*see also* Dorsopathy
    ligamentous or muscular attachments,
  peripheral —*see* Enthesopathy, spinal
    specified NEC —*see* Dorsopathy, specified
  NEC
  stereotyped, habit or movement F98.4
  stomach (functional) —*see* Disorder, gastric
  stress F43.9
    post-traumatic F43.10
      acute F43.11
      chronic F43.12
  sulfur-bearing amino-acid metabolism E72.10
  sweat gland (eccrine) L74.9
    apocrine L75.9
      specified NEC L75.8
    specified NEC L74.8
  synovium M67.90
    acromioclavicular M67.91
    ankle M67.97
    elbow M67.92
    foot M67.97
    forearm M67.93
    hand M67.94
    hip M67.95
    knee M67.96
    multiple sites M67.99
    rupture —*see* Rupture, synovium
    shoulder M67.91
    specified type NEC M67.80
      acromioclavicular M67.81
      ankle M67.87
      elbow M67.82
      foot M67.87
      hand M67.84
      hip M67.85
      knee M67.86
      multiple sites M67.89
      wrist M67.83
    synovitis —*see* Synovitis
    upper arm M67.92
    wrist M67.93
  temperature regulation, newborn P81.9
    specified NEC P81.8
  temporomandibular joint —*see* Anomaly,
  dentofacial, temporomandibular joint

Disorder (of) – *continued*
- tendon M67.90
  - acromioclavicular M67.91
  - ankle M67.97
  - contracture —*see* Contracture, tendon
  - elbow M67.92
  - foot M67.97
  - forearm M67.93
  - hand M67.94
  - hip M67.95
  - knee M67.96
  - multiple sites M67.99
  - rupture —*see* Rupture, tendon
  - shoulder M67.91
  - specified type NEC M67.80
    - acromioclavicular M67.81
    - ankle M67.87
    - elbow M67.82
    - foot M67.87
    - hand M67.84
    - hip M67.85
    - knee M67.86
    - multiple sites M67.89
    - trunk M67.88
    - wrist M67.83
  - synovitis —*see* Synovitis
  - tendinitis —*see* Tendinitis
  - tenosynovitis —*see* Tenosynovitis
  - trunk M67.98
  - upper arm M67.92
  - wrist M67.93
- thoracic root (nerve) NEC G54.3
- thyrocalcitonin hypersecretion E07.0
- thyroid (gland) E07.9
  - function NEC, neonatal, transitory P72.2
  - iodine-deficiency related E01.8
  - specified NEC E07.89
- tic —*see* Tic
- tooth K08.9
  - development K00.9
    - specified NEC K00.8
  - eruption K00.6
- Tourette's F95.2
- trance and possession F44.89
- tricuspid (valve) —*see* Endocarditis, tricuspid
- tryptophan metabolism E70.5
- tubular, phosphate-losing N25.0
- tubulo-interstitial (in)
  - brucellosis A23.9 *[N16]*
  - cystinosis E72.04
  - diphtheria A36.84
  - glycogen storage disease E74.00 *[N16]*
  - leukemia NEC C95.9 *[N16]*
  - lymphoma NEC C85.9 *[N16]*
  - mixed cryoglobulinemia D89.1 *[N16]*
  - multiple myeloma C90.0 *[N16]*
  - Salmonella infection A02.25
  - sarcoidosis D86.84
  - sepsis A41.9 *[N16]*
    - streptococcal A40.9 *[N16]*
  - systemic lupus erythematosus M32.15
  - toxoplasmosis B58.83
  - transplant rejection T86.91 *[N16]*
  - Wilson's disease E83.01 *[N16]*
- tubulo-renal function, impaired N25.9
  - specified NEC N25.89
- tympanic membrane H73.9
  - atrophy —*see* Atrophy, tympanic membrane
  - infection —*see* Myringitis
  - perforation —*see* Perforation, tympanum
  - specified NEC H73.89
- unsocialized aggressive F91.1

Disorder (of) – *continued*
- urea cycle metabolism E72.20
  - argininemia E72.21
  - arginosuccinic aciduria E72.22
  - citrullinemia E72.23
  - ornithine transcarbamylase deficiency E72.4
  - other specified E72.29
- ureter (in) N28.9
  - schistosomiasis B65.0 *[N29]*
  - tuberculosis A18.11
- urethra N36.9
  - specified NEC N36.8
- urinary system N39.9
  - specified NEC N39.8
- valve, heart
  - aortic —*see* Endocarditis, aortic
  - mitral —*see* Endocarditis, mitral
  - pulmonary —*see* Endocarditis, pulmonary
  - rheumatic
    - aortic —*see* Endocarditis, aortic, rheumatic
    - mitral —*see* Endocarditis, mitral
    - pulmonary —*see* Endocarditis, pulmonary, rheumatic
    - tricuspid —*see* Endocarditis, tricuspid
  - tricuspid —*see* Endocarditis, tricuspid
- vestibular function H81.9
  - specified NEC —*see* subcategory H81.8
  - in diseases classified elsewhere H82.
  - vertigo —*see* Vertigo
- vision, binocular H53.30
  - abnormal retinal correspondence H53.31
  - diplopia H53.2
  - fusion with defective stereopsis H53.32
  - simultaneous perception H53.33
  - suppression H53.34
- visual
  - cortex
    - blindness H47.619
      - left brain H47.612
      - right brain H47.611
    - due to
      - inflammatory disorder H47.629
        - left brain H47.622
        - right brain H47.621
      - neoplasm H47.639
        - left brain H47.632
        - right brain H47.631
      - vascular disorder H47.649
        - left brain H47.642
        - right brain H47.641
  - pathway H47.9
    - due to
      - inflammatory disorder H47.51
      - neoplasm H47.52
      - vascular disorder H47.53
  - optic chiasm —*see* Disorder, optic, chiasm
- vitreous body H43.9
  - crystalline deposits —*see* Deposit, crystalline
  - degeneration —*see* Degeneration, vitreous
  - hemorrhage —*see* Hemorrhage, vitreous
  - opacities —*see* Opacity, vitreous
  - prolapse —*see* Prolapse, vitreous
  - specified type NEC H43.89
- voice R49.9
  - specified type NEC R49.8
- volatile solvent use
  - due to drug abuse —*see* Abuse, drug, inhalant
  - due to drug dependence —*see* Dependence, drug, inhalant

Disorder (of) – *continued*
- white blood cells D72.9
  - specified NEC D72.89
- withdrawing, child or adolescent F40.10

Disorientation R41.0

Displacement, displaced
- acquired traumatic of bone, cartilage, joint, tendon NEC —*see* Dislocation
- adrenal gland (congenital) Q89.1
- appendix, retrocecal (congenital) Q43.8
- auricle (congenital) Q17.4
- bladder (acquired) N32.89
  - congenital Q64.19
- brachial plexus (congenital) Q07.8
- brain stem, caudal (congenital) Q04.8
- canaliculus (lacrimalis) , congenital Q10.6
- cardia through esophageal hiatus (congenital) Q40.1
- cerebellum, caudal (congenital) Q04.8
- cervix —*see* Malposition, uterus
- colon (congenital) Q43.3
- device, implant or graft (*see also* Complications, by site and type, mechanical) T85.628
  - arterial graft NEC —*see* Complication, cardiovascular device, mechanical, vascular
  - breast (implant) T85.42
  - catheter NEC T85.628
    - dialysis (renal) T82.42
      - intraperitoneal T85.621
    - infusion NEC T82.524
      - spinal (epidural) (subdural) T85.620
    - urinary (indwelling) T83.028
      - cystostomy T83.020
  - electronic (electrode) (pulse generator) (stimulator) —*see* Complication, electronic stimulator
  - fixation, internal (orthopedic) NEC —*see* Complication, fixation device, mechanical
  - gastrointestinal —*see* Complications, prosthetic device, mechanical, gastrointestinal device
  - genital NEC T83.428
    - intrauterine contraceptive device T83.32
    - penile prosthesis T83.420
  - heart NEC —*see* Complication, cardiovascular device, mechanical
  - joint prosthesis —*see* Complications, joint prosthesis, mechanical
  - ocular —*see* Complications, prosthetic device, mechanical, ocular device
  - orthopedic NEC —*see* Complication, orthopedic, device or graft, mechanical
  - specified NEC T85.628
  - urinary NEC —*see also* Complication, genitourinary, device, urinary, mechanical
    - graft T83.22
  - vascular NEC —*see* Complication, cardiovascular device, mechanical
  - ventricular intracranial shunt T85.02
- electronic stimulator
  - bone T84.320
  - cardiac —*see* Complications, cardiac device, electronic
  - nervous system —*see* Complication, prosthetic device, mechanical, electronic nervous system stimulator
  - urinary —*see* Complications, electronic stimulator, urinary
- esophageal mucosa into cardia of stomach, congenital Q39.8

Displacement, displaced - *continued*
  esophagus (acquired) K22.8
    congenital Q39.8
  eyeball (acquired) (lateral) (old) —*see*
  Displacement, globe
    congenital Q15.8
    current —*see* Avulsion, eye
  fallopian tube (acquired) N83.4
    congenital Q50.6
    opening (congenital) Q50.6
  gallbladder (congenital) Q44.1
  gastric mucosa (congenital) Q40.2
  globe (acquired) (old) (lateral) H05.21
    current —*see* Avulsion, eye
  heart (congenital) Q24.8
    acquired I51.89
  hymen (upward) (congenital) Q52.4
  intervertebral disc NEC
    with myelopathy —*see* Disorder, disc, with,
    myelopathy
      cervical, cervicothoracic (with) M50.20
        myelopathy —*see* Disorder, disc, cervical,
        with myelopathy
        neuritis, radiculitis or radiculopathy —*see*
    Disorder, disc, cervical, with neuritis
      due to trauma —*see* Dislocation, vertebra
      lumbar region M51.26
        with
          myelopathy M51.06
          neuritis, radiculitis, radiculopathy or
    sciatica M51.16
      lumbosacral region M51.27
        with
          neuritis, radiculitis, radiculopathy or
    sciatica M51.17
      sacrococcygeal region M53.3
      thoracic region M51.24
        with
          myelopathy M51.04
          neuritis, radiculitis, radiculopathy
    M51.14
      thoracolumbar region M51.25
        with
          myelopathy M51.05
          neuritis, radiculitis, radiculopathy
    M51.15
  intrauterine device T83.32
  kidney (acquired) N28.83
    congenital Q63.2
  lachrymal, lacrimal apparatus or duct
  (congenital) Q10.6
  lens, congenital Q12.1
  macula (congenital) Q14.1
  Meckel's diverticulum Q43.0
    malignant —*see* Table of Neoplasms, small
    intestine, malignant
  nail (congenital) Q84.6
    acquired L60.8
  opening of Wharton's duct in mouth Q38.4
  organ or site, congenital NEC —*see*
  Malposition, congenital
  ovary (acquired) N83.4
    congenital Q50.39
    free in peritoneal cavity (congenital) Q50.39
    into hernial sac N83.4
  oviduct (acquired) N83.4
    congenital Q50.6
  parathyroid (gland) E21.4
  parotid gland (congenital) Q38.4
  punctum lacrimale (congenital) Q10.6
  sacro-iliac (joint) (congenital) Q74.2
    current injury S33.2

Displacement, displaced - *continued*
  old —*see* subcategory M53.2
  salivary gland (any) (congenital) Q38.4
  spleen (congenital) Q89.09
  stomach, congenital Q40.2
  sublingual duct Q38.4
  tongue (downward) (congenital) Q38.3
  tooth, teeth, fully erupted M26.30
    horizontal M26.33
    vertical M26.34
  trachea (congenital) Q32.1
  ureter or ureteric opening or orifice
  (congenital) Q62.62
  uterine opening of oviducts or fallopian tubes
  Q50.6
  uterus, uterine —*see* Malposition, uterus
  ventricular septum Q21.0
    with rudimentary ventricle Q20.4
Disproportion
  between native and reconstructed breast
  N65.1
  fiber-type G71.2
Disruptio uteri —*see* Rupture, uterus
Disruption (of)
  ciliary body NEC H21.89
  closure of
    cornea T81.31
    craniotomy T81.32
    fascia (muscular) (superficial) T81.32
    internal organ or tissue T81.32
    laceration (external) (internal) T81.33
    ligament T81.32
    mucosa T81.31
    muscle or muscle flap T81.32
    ribs or rib cage T81.32
    skin and subcutaneous tissue (full-thickness)
  (superficial) T81.31
    skull T81.32
    sternum (sternotomy) T81.32
    tendon T81.32
    traumatic laceration (external) (internal)
  T81.33
  family Z63.8
    due to
      absence of family member due to military
  deployment Z63.31
      absence of family member NEC Z63.32
      alcoholism and drug addiction in family
  Z63.72
      bereavement Z63.4
      death (assumed) or disappearance of
  family member Z63.4
      divorce or separation Z63.5
      drug addiction in family Z63.72
      return of family member from military
  deployment (current or past conflict) Z63.71
      stressful life events NEC Z63.79
  iris NEC H21.89
  ligament (s) —*see also* Sprain
    knee
      current injury —*see* Dislocation, knee
      old (chronic) —*see* Derangement, knee,
  ligament, instability, chronic
      spontaneous NEC —*see* Derangement,
  knee, disruption ligament
  ossicular chain —*see* Discontinuity, ossicles,
  ear
  pelvic ring (stable) S32.810
    unstable S32.811
  wound T81.30
    episiotomy O90.1

Disruption - *continued*
  operation T81.31
    cesarean O90.0
    external operation wound (superficial)
  T81.31
      internal operation wound (deep) T81.32
    perineal (obstetric) O90.1
    traumatic injury repair T81.33
    traumatic injury wound repair T81.33
Dissatisfaction with
  employment Z56.9
  school environment Z55.4
Dissecting —*see* condition
Dissection
  aorta I71.00
    abdominal I71.02
    thoracic I71.01
    thoracoabdominal I71.03
  artery
    carotid I77.71
    cerebral (nonruptured) I67.0
      ruptured —*see* Hemorrhage, intracranial,
  subarachnoid
    coronary I25.42
    iliac I77.72
    renal I77.73
    specified NEC I77.79
    vertebral I77.74
  traumatic —*see* Wound, open, by site
  vascular I99.8
  wound —*see* Wound, open
Disseminated —*see* condition
Dissociation
  auriculoventricular or atrioventricular (AV)
  (any degree) (isorhythmic) I45.89
    with heart block I44.2
  interference I45.89
Dissociative reaction, state F44.9
Dissolution, vertebra —*see* Osteoporosis
Distension, distention
  abdomen R14.0
  bladder N32.89
  cecum K63.89
  colon K63.89
  gallbladder K82.8
  intestine K63.89
  kidney N28.89
  liver K76.89
  seminal vesicle N50.8
  stomach K31.89
    acute K31.0
    psychogenic F45.8
  ureter —*see* Dilatation, ureter
  uterus N85.8
Distoma hepaticum infestation B66.3
Distomiasis B66.9
  bile passages B66.3
  hemic B65.9
  hepatic B66.3
    due to Clonorchis sinensis B66.1
  intestinal B66.5
  liver B66.3
    due to Clonorchis sinensis B66.1
  lung B66.4
  pulmonary B66.4
Distomolar (fourth molar) K00.1
Disto-occlusion (Division I) (Division II)
  M26.212
Distortion (s) (congenital)
  adrenal (gland) Q89.1
  arm NEC Q68.8
  bile duct or passage Q44.5
  bladder Q64.79

Distortion - *continued*
brain Q04.9
cervix (uteri) Q51.9
chest (wall) Q67.8
  bones Q76.8
clavicle Q74.0
clitoris Q52.6
coccyx Q76.49
common duct Q44.5
coronary Q24.5
cystic duct Q44.5
ear (auricle) (external) Q17.3
  inner Q16.5
  middle Q16.4
    ossicles Q16.3
endocrine NEC Q89.2
eustachian tube Q17.8
eye (adnexa) Q15.8
face bone (s) NEC Q75.8
fallopian tube Q50.6
femur NEC Q68.8
fibula NEC Q68.8
finger (s) Q68.1
foot Q66.9
genitalia, genital organ (s)
  female Q52.8
    external Q52.79
    internal NEC Q52.8
gyri Q04.8
hand bone (s) Q68.1
heart (auricle) (ventricle) Q24.8
  valve (cusp) Q24.8
hepatic duct Q44.5
humerus NEC Q68.8
hymen Q52.4
intrafamilial communications Z63.8
jaw NEC M26.89
labium (majus) (minus) Q52.79
leg NEC Q68.8
lens Q12.8
liver Q44.7
lumbar spine Q76.49
  with disproportion O33.8
    causing obstructed labor O65.0
lumbosacral (joint) (region) Q76.49
  kyphosis —*see* Kyphosis, congenital
  lordosis —*see* Lordosis, congenital
nerve Q07.8
nose Q30.8
organ
  of Corti Q16.5
  or site not listed —*see* Anomaly, by site
ossicles, ear Q16.3
oviduct Q50.6
pancreas Q45.3
parathyroid (gland) Q89.2
pituitary (gland) Q89.2
radius NEC Q68.8
sacroiliac joint Q74.2
sacrum Q76.49
scapula Q74.0
shoulder girdle Q74.0
skull bone (s) NEC Q75.8
  with
    anencephalus Q00.0
    encephalocele —*see* Encephalocele
    hydrocephalus Q03.9
      with spina bifida —*see* Spina bifida, with
hydrocephalus
      microcephaly Q02
spinal cord Q06.8

Distortion - *continued*
spine Q76.49
  kyphosis —*see* Kyphosis, congenital
  lordosis —*see* Lordosis, congenital
spleen Q89.09
sternum NEC Q76.7
thorax (wall) Q67.8
  bony Q76.8
thymus (gland) Q89.2
thyroid (gland) Q89.2
tibia NEC Q68.8
toe (s) Q66.9
tongue Q38.3
trachea (cartilage) Q32.1
ulna NEC Q68.8
ureter Q62.8
urethra Q64.79
  causing obstruction Q64.39
uterus Q51.9
vagina Q52.4
vertebra Q76.49
  kyphosis —*see* Kyphosis, congenital
  lordosis —*see* Lordosis, congenital
visual —*see also* Disturbance, vision
  shape and size H53.15
vulva Q52.79
wrist (bones) (joint) Q68.8
Distress
abdomen —*see* Pain, abdominal
acute respiratory (adult) (child) J80
epigastric R10.13
fetal P84
  complicating pregnancy —*see* Stress, fetal
gastrointestinal (functional) K30
  psychogenic F45.8
intestinal (functional) NOS K59.9
  psychogenic F45.8
maternal, during labor and delivery O75.0
respiratory R06.00
  adult J80
  child J80
  newborn P22.9
    specified NEC P22.8
  orthopnea R06.01
  psychogenic F45.8
  shortness of breath R06.02
  specified type NEC R06.09
Distribution vessel, atypical Q27.9
coronary artery Q24.5
precerebral Q28.1
Distichiasis L68.8
Disturbance (s) —*see also* Disease
absorption K90.9
  calcium E58
  carbohydrate K90.4
  fat K90.4
    pancreatic K90.3
  protein K90.4
  starch K90.4
  vitamin —*see* Deficiency, vitamin
acid-base equilibrium E87.8
  mixed E87.4
activity and attention (with hyperkinesis) —
see Disorder, attention-deficit hyperactivity
amino acid transport E72.00
assimilation, food K90.9
auditory nerve, except deafness —*see*
subcategory H93.3
behavior —*see* Disorder, conduct
blood clotting (mechanism) (*see also* Defect,
coagulation) D68.9

Disturbance(s) - *continued*
cerebral
  nerve —*see* Disorder, nerve, cranial
  status, newborn P91.9
    specified NEC P91.8
circulatory I99.9
conduct (*see also* Disorder, conduct) F91.9
  adjustment reaction —*see* Disorder,
adjustment
  compulsive F63.9
  disruptive F91.9
  hyperkinetic —*see* Disorder, attention-
deficit hyperactivity
  socialized F91.2
  specified NEC F91.8
  unsocialized F91.1
coordination R27.8
cranial nerve —*see* Disorder, nerve, cranial
deep sensibility —*see* Disturbance, sensation
digestive K30
  psychogenic F45.8
electrolyte —*see also* Imbalance, electrolyte
  newborn, transitory P74.4
    hyperammonemia P74.6
    potassium balance P74.3
    sodium balance P74.2
    specified type NEC P74.4
emotions specific to childhood and
adolescence F93.9
  with
    anxiety and fearfulness NEC F93.8
    elective mutism F94.0
    oppositional disorder F91.3
    sensitivity (withdrawal) F40.10
    shyness F40.10
    social withdrawal F40.10
  involving relationship problems F93.8
  mixed F93.8
  specified NEC F93.8
endocrine (gland) E34.9
  neonatal, transitory P72.9
    specified NEC P72.8
equilibrium R42
fructose metabolism E74.10
gait —*see* Gait
  hysterical F44.4
  psychogenic F44.4
gastrointestinal (functional) K30
  psychogenic F45.8
habit, child F98.9
hearing, except deafness and tinnitus —*see*
Abnormal, auditory perception
heart, functional (conditions in I44-I50)
  due to presence of (cardiac) prosthesis
I97.19
    postoperative I97.89
      cardiac surgery I97.19
hormones E34.9
innervation uterus (parasympathetic)
(sympathetic) N85.8
keratinization NEC
  gingiva K05.10
    nonplaque induced K05.11
    plaque induced K05.10
  lip K13.0
  oral (mucosa) (soft tissue) K13.29
  tongue K13.29
learning (specific) —*see* Disorder, learning
memory —*see* Amnesia
  mild, following organic brain damage F06.8
mental F99
  associated with diseases classified elsewhere
F54

Disturbance(s) - *continued*
  metabolism E88.9
    with
      abortion —*see* Abortion, by type with
    other specified complication
      ectopic pregnancy O08.5
      molar pregnancy O08.5
    amino-acid E72.9
      aromatic E70.9
      branched-chain E71.2
      straight-chain E72.8
      sulfur-bearing E72.10
    ammonia E72.20
    arginine E72.21
    arginosuccinic acid E72.22
    carbohydrate E74.9
    cholesterol E78.9
    citrulline E72.23
    cystathionine E72.19
    general E88.9
    glutamine E72.8
    histidine E70.40
    homocystine E72.19
    hydroxylysine E72.3
    in labor or delivery O75.89
    iron E83.10
    lipoid E78.9
    lysine E72.3
    methionine E72.19
    neonatal, transitory P74.9
      calcium and magnesium P71.9
        specified type NEC P71.8
      carbohydrate metabolism P70.9
        specified type NEC P70.8
        specified NEC P74.8
    ornithine E72.4
    phosphate E83.39
    sodium NEC E87.8
    threonine E72.8
    tryptophan E70.5
    tyrosine E70.20
    urea cycle E72.20
  motor R29.2
  nervous, functional R45.0
  neuromuscular mechanism (eye) , due to
  syphilis A52.15
  nutritional E63.9
    nail L60.3
  ocular motion H51.9
    psychogenic F45.8
  oculogyric H51.8
    psychogenic F45.8
  oculomotor H51.9
    psychogenic F45.8
  olfactory nerve R43.1
  optic nerve NEC —*see* Disorder, nerve, optic
  oral epithelium, including tongue NEC
  K13.29
  perceptual due to
    alcohol withdrawal F10.232
    amphetamine intoxication F15.922
      in
        abuse F15.122
        dependence F15.222
    anxiolytic withdrawal F13.232
    cannabis intoxication (acute) F12.922
      in
        abuse F12.122
        dependence F12.222
    cocaine intoxication (acute) F14.922
      in
        abuse F14.122

Disturbance(s) - *continued*
      dependence F14.222
    hypnotic withdrawal F13.232
    opioid intoxication (acute) F11.922
      in
        abuse F11.122
        dependence F11.222
    phencyclidine intoxication (acute) F19.922
      in
        abuse F19.122
        dependence F19.222
    sedative withdrawal F13.232
  personality (pattern) (trait) (*see also* Disorder,
  personality) F60.9
    following organic brain damage F07.9
  polyglandular E31.9
    specified NEC E31.8
  potassium balance, newborn P74.3
  psychogenic F45.9
  psychomotor F44.4
  psychophysical visual H53.16
  pupillary —*see* Anomaly, pupil, function
  reflex R29.2
  rhythm, heart I49.9
  salivary secretion K11.7
  sensation (cold) (heat) (localization) (tactile
  discrimination) (texture) (vibratory) NEC
  R20.9
    hysterical F44.6
    skin R20.9
      anesthesia R20.0
      hyperesthesia R20.3
      hypoesthesia R20.1
      paresthesia R20.2
      specified type NEC R20.8
    smell R43.9
      and taste (mixed) R43.8
      anosmia R43.0
      parosmia R43.1
      specified NEC R43.8
    taste R43.9
      and smell (mixed) R43.8
      parageusia R43.2
      specified NEC R43.8
  sensory —*see* Disturbance, sensation
  situational (transient) —*see also* Disorder,
  adjustment
    acute F43.0
  sleep G47.9
    nonorganic origin F51.9
  smell —*see* Disturbance, sensation, smell
  sociopathic F60.2
  sodium balance, newborn P74.2
  speech R47.9
    developmental F80.9
    specified NEC R47.89
  stomach (functional) K31.9
  sympathetic (nerve) G90.9
  taste —*see* Disturbance, sensation, taste
  temperature
    regulation, newborn P81.9
      specified NEC P81.8
    sense R20.8
      hysterical F44.6
  tooth
    eruption K00.6
    formation K00.4
    structure, hereditary NEC K00.5
  touch —*see* Disturbance, sensation
  vascular I99.9
    arteriosclerotic —*see* Arteriosclerosis
  vasomotor I73.9

Disturbance(s) - *continued*
  vasospastic I73.9
  vision, visual H53.9
    following
      cerebral infarction I69.398
      cerebrovascular disease I69.998
        specified NEC I69.898
      intracerebral hemorrhage I69.198
      nontraumatic intracranial hemorrhage NEC
      I69.298
        specified disease NEC I69.898
      subarachnoid hemorrhage I69.098
    psychophysical H53.16
    specified NEC H53.8
    subjective H53.10
      day blindness H53.11
      discomfort H53.14
      distortions of shape and size H53.15
      loss
        sudden H53.13
        transient H53.12
      specified type NEC H53.19
  voice R49.9
    psychogenic F44.4
    specified NEC R49.8
Diuresis R35.8
Diver's palsy, paralysis or squeeze T70.3
Diverticulitis (acute) K57.92
  bladder —*see* Cystitis
  ileum —*see* Diverticulitis, intestine, small
  intestine K57.92
    with
      abscess, perforation or peritonitis K57.80
        with bleeding K57.81
      bleeding K57.93
    congenital Q43.8
    large K57.32
      with
        abscess, perforation or peritonitis K57.20
          with bleeding K57.21
        bleeding K57.33
        small intestine K57.52
          with
            abscess, perforation or peritonitis
            K57.40
              with bleeding K57.41
              bleeding K57.53
    small K57.12
      with
        abscess, perforation or peritonitis K57.00
          with bleeding K57.01
        bleeding K57.13
        large intestine K57.52
          with
            abscess, perforation or peritonitis
            K57.40
              with bleeding K57.41
              bleeding K57.53
Diverticulosis K57.90
  with bleeding K57.91
  large intestine K57.30
    with
      bleeding K57.31
      small intestine K57.50
        with bleeding K57.51
  small intestine K57.10
    with
      bleeding K57.11
      large intestine K57.50
        with bleeding K57.51

Diverticulum, diverticula (multiple) K57.90
appendix (noninflammatory) K38.2
bladder (sphincter) N32.3
congenital Q64.6
bronchus (congenital) Q32.4
acquired J98.09
calyx, calyceal (kidney) N28.89
cardia (stomach) K31.4
cecum —*see* Diverticulosis, intestine, large
congenital Q43.8
colon —*see* Diverticulosis, intestine, large
congenital Q43.8
duodenum —*see* Diverticulosis, intestine, small
congenital Q43.8
epiphrenic (esophagus) K22.5
esophagus (congenital) Q39.6
acquired (epiphrenic) (pulsion) (traction) K22.5
eustachian tube —*see* Disorder, eustachian tube, specified NEC
fallopian tube N83.8
gastric K31.4
heart (congenital) Q24.8
ileum —*see* Diverticulosis, intestine, small
jejunum —*see* Diverticulosis, intestine, small
kidney (pelvis) (calyces) N28.89
with calculus —*see* Calculus, kidney
Meckel's (displaced) (hypertrophic) Q43.0
malignant —*see* Table of Neoplasms, small intestine, malignant
midthoracic K22.5
organ or site, congenital NEC —*see* Distortion
pericardium (congenital) (cyst) Q24.8
acquired I31.8
pharyngoesophageal (congenital) Q39.6
acquired K22.5
pharynx (congenital) Q38.7
rectosigmoid —*see* Diverticulosis, intestine, large
congenital Q43.8
rectum —*see* Diverticulosis, intestine, large
Rokitansky's K22.5
seminal vesicle N50.8
sigmoid —*see* Diverticulosis, intestine, large
congenital Q43.8
stomach (acquired) K31.4
congenital Q40.2
trachea (acquired) J39.8
ureter (acquired) N28.89
congenital Q62.8
ureterovesical orifice N28.89
urethra (acquired) N36.1
congenital Q64.79
ventricle, left (congenital) Q24.8
vesical N32.3
congenital Q64.6
Zenker's (esophagus) K22.5
Division
cervix uteri (acquired) N88.8
glans penis Q55.69
labia minora (congenital) Q52.79
ligament (partial or complete) (current) —*see also* Sprain
with open wound —*see* Wound, open
muscle (partial or complete) (current) —*see also* Injury, muscle
with open wound —*see* Wound, open
nerve (traumatic) —*see* Injury, nerve
spinal cord —*see* Injury, spinal cord, by region
vein I87.8

Divorce, causing family disruption Z63.5
Dix-Hallpike neurolabyrinthitis —*see* Neuronitis, vestibular
Dizziness R42
hysterical F44.89
psychogenic F45.8
DMAC (disseminated mycobacterium avium intracellulare complex) A31.2
DNR (do not resuscitate) Z66
Doan-Wiseman syndrome (primary splenic neutropenia) —*see* Agranulocytosis
Doehle-Heller aortitis A52.02
Dog bite —*see* Bite
Dohle body panmyelopathic syndrome D72.0
Dolichocephaly Q67.2
Dolichocolon Q43.8
Dolichostenomelia —*see* Syndrome, Marfan's
Donohue's syndrome E34.8
Donor (organ or tissue) Z52.9
blood (whole) Z52.000
autologous Z52.010
specified component (lymphocytes) (platelets) NEC Z52.008
autologous Z52.018
specified donor NEC Z52.098
specified donor NEC Z52.090
stem cells Z52.001
autologous Z52.011
specified donor NEC Z52.091
bone Z52.20
autologous Z52.21
marrow Z52.3
specified type NEC Z52.29
cornea Z52.5
egg (Oocyte) Z52.819
age 35 and over Z52.812
anonymous recipient Z52.812
designated recipient Z52.813
under age 35 Z52.810
anonymous recipient Z52.810
designated recipient Z52.811
kidney Z52.4
liver Z52.6
lung Z52.89
lymphocyte —*see* Donor, blood, specified components NEC
Oocyte —*see* Donor, egg
platelets Z52.008
potential, examination of Z00.5
semen Z52.89
skin Z52.10
autologous Z52.11
specified type NEC Z52.19
specified organ or tissue NEC Z52.89
sperm Z52.89
Donovanosis A58
Dorsalgia M54.9
psychogenic F45.41
specified NEC M54.89
Dorsopathy M53.9
deforming M43.9
specified NEC —*see* subcategory M43.8
specified NEC M53.80
cervical region M53.82
cervicothoracic region M53.83
lumbar region M53.86
lumbosacral region M53.87
occipito-atlanto-axial region M53.81
sacrococcygeal region M53.88
thoracic region M53.84
thoracolumbar region M53.85

Double
albumin E88.09
aortic arch Q25.4
auditory canal Q17.8
auricle (heart) Q20.8
bladder Q64.79
cervix Q51.820
with doubling of uterus (and vagina) Q51.10
with obstruction Q51.11
inlet ventricle Q20.4
kidney with double pelvis (renal) Q63.0
meatus urinarius Q64.75
monster Q89.4
outlet
left ventricle Q20.2
right ventricle Q20.1
pelvis (renal) with double ureter Q62.5
tongue Q38.3
ureter (one or both sides) Q62.5
with double pelvis (renal) Q62.5
urethra Q64.74
urinary meatus Q64.75
uterus Q51.2
with
doubling of cervix (and vagina) Q51.10
with obstruction Q51.11
in pregnancy or childbirth O34.59
causing obstructed labor O65.5
vagina Q52.10
with doubling of uterus (and cervix) Q51.10
with obstruction Q51.11
vision H53.2
vulva Q52.79
Douglas' pouch, cul-de-sac —*see* condition
Down syndrome Q90.9
meiotic nondisjunction Q90.0
mitotic nondisjunction Q90.1
mosaicism Q90.1
translocation Q90.2
DPD (dihydropyrimidine dehydrogenase deficiency) E88.89
Dracontiasis B72
Dracunculiasis, dracunculosis B72
Dream state, hysterical F44.89
Dreschlera (hawaiiensis) (infection) B43.8
Drepanocytic anemia —*see* Disease, sickle-cell
Dresbach's syndrome (elliptocytosis) D58.1
Dressler's syndrome I24.1
Drift, ulnar —*see* Deformity, limb, specified type NEC, forearm
Drinking (alcohol)
excessive, to excess NEC (without dependence) F10.10
habitual (continual) (without remission) F10.20
with remission F10.21
Drip, postnasal (chronic) R09.82
due to
allergic rhinitis —*see* Rhinitis, allergic
common cold J00
gastroesophageal reflux —*see* Reflux, gastroesophageal
nasopharyngitis —*see* Nasopharyngitis
other know condition
code to condition
sinusitis —*see* Sinusitis
Droop
facial R29.810
cerebrovascular disease I69.992
cerebral infarction I69.392
intracerebral hemorrhage I69.192

Droop - *continued*
    nontraumatic intracranial hemorrhage NEC
    I69.292
        specified disease NEC I69.892
        subarachnoid hemorrhage I69.092
Drop (in)
    attack NEC R55
    finger —*see* Deformity, finger
    foot —*see* Deformity, limb, foot, drop
    hematocrit (precipitous) R71.0
    hemoglobin R71.0
    toe —*see* Deformity, toe, specified NEC
    wrist —*see* Deformity, limb, wrist drop
Dropped heart beats I45.9
Dropsy, dropsical —*see also* Hydrops
    abdomen R18.8
    brain —*see* Hydrocephalus
    cardiac, heart —*see* Failure, heart, congestive
    gangrenous —*see* Gangrene
    heart —*see* Failure, heart, congestive
    kidney —*see* Nephrosis
    lung —*see* Edema, lung
    newborn due to isoimmunization P56.0
    pericardium —*see* Pericarditis
Drowned, drowning (near) T75.1
Drowsiness R40.0
Drug
    abuse counseling and surveillance Z71.51
    addiction —*see* Dependence
    dependence —*see* Dependence
    habit —*see* Dependence
    harmful use —*see* Abuse, drug
    induced fever R50.2
    overdose —*see* Table of Drugs and
    Chemicals, by drug, poisoning
    poisoning —*see* Table of Drugs and
    Chemicals, by drug, poisoning
    resistant organism infection (*see also*
    Resistant, organism, to, drug) Z16.30
    therapy
        long term (current) (prophylactic) —*see*
    Therapy, drug long-term (current)
    (prophylactic)
        short term
    omit code
    wrong substance given or taken in error —*see*
    Table of Drugs and Chemicals, by drug,
    poisoning
Drunkenness (without dependence) F10.129
    acute in alcoholism F10.229
    chronic (without remission) F10.20
        with remission F10.21
    pathological (without dependence) F10.129
        with dependence F10.229
    sleep F51.9
Drusen
    macula (degenerative) (retina) —*see*
    Degeneration, macula, drusen
    optic disc H47.32
Dry, dryness —*see also* condition
    larynx J38.7
    mouth R68.2
        due to dehydration E86.0
    nose J34.89
    socket (teeth) M27.3
    throat J39.2
DSAP L56.5
Duane's syndrome H50.81
Dubin-Johnson disease or syndrome E80.6
Dubois' disease (thymus gland) A50.59 *[E35]*
Dubowitz' syndrome Q87.1
Duchenne-Aran muscular atrophy G12.21
Duchenne-Griesinger disease G71.0

Duchenne's
    disease or syndrome
        motor neuron disease G12.22
        muscular dystrophy G71.0
    locomotor ataxia (syphilitic) A52.11
    paralysis
        birth injury P14.0
        due to or associated with
            motor neuron disease G12.22
            muscular dystrophy G71.0
Ducrey's chancre A57
Duct, ductus —*see* condition
Duhring's disease (dermatitis herpetiformis)
    L13.0
Dullness, cardiac (decreased) (increased)
    R01.2
Dumb ague —*see* Malaria
Dumbness —*see* Aphasia
Dumdum fever B55.0
Dumping syndrome (postgastrectomy) K91.1
Duodenitis (nonspecific) (peptic) K29.80
    with bleeding K29.81
Duodenocholangitis —*see* Cholangitis
Duodenum, duodenal —*see* condition
Duplay's bursitis or periarthritis —*see*
    Tendinitis, calcific, shoulder
Duplication, duplex —*see also* Accessory
    alimentary tract Q45.8
    anus Q43.4
    appendix (and cecum) Q43.4
    biliary duct (any) Q44.5
    bladder Q64.79
    cecum (and appendix) Q43.4
    cervix Q51.820
    chromosome NEC
        with complex rearrangements NEC Q92.5
        seen only at prometaphase Q92.8
    cystic duct Q44.5
    digestive organs Q45.8
    esophagus Q39.8
    frontonasal process Q75.8
    intestine (large) (small) Q43.4
    kidney Q63.0
    liver Q44.7
    pancreas Q45.3
    penis Q55.69
    respiratory organs NEC Q34.8
    salivary duct Q38.4
    spinal cord (incomplete) Q06.2
    stomach Q40.2
Dupré's disease (meningism) R29.1
Dupuytren's contraction or disease M72.0
Durand-Nicolas-Favre disease A55
Durotomy (inadvertent) (incidental) G97.41
Duroziez's disease (congenital mitral stenosis)
    Q23.2
Dutton's relapsing fever (West African)
    A68.1
Dwarfism E34.3
    achondroplastic Q77.4
    congenital E34.3
    constitutional E34.3
    hypochondroplastic Q77.4
    hypophyseal E23.0
    infantile E34.3
    Laron-type E34.3
    Lorain (-Levi) type E23.0
    metatropic Q77.8
    nephrotic-glycosuric (with hypophosphatemic
    rickets) E72.09
    nutritional E45
    pancreatic K86.8

Dwarfism - *continued*
    pituitary E23.0
    renal N25.0
    thanatophoric Q77.1
Dyke-Young anemia (secondary)
    (symptomatic) D59.1
Dysacusis —*see* Abnormal, auditory
    perception
Dysadrenocortism E27.9
    hyperfunction E27.0
Dysarthria R47.1
    following
        cerebral infarction I69.322
        cerebrovascular disease I69.922
            specified disease NEC I69.822
        intracerebral hemorrhage I69.122
        nontraumatic intracranial hemorrhage NEC
    I69.222
        subarachnoid hemorrhage I69.022
Dysautonomia (familial) G90.1
Dysbarism T70.3
Dysbasia R26.2
    angiosclerotica intermittens I73.9
    hysterical F44.4
    lordotica (progressiva) G24.1
    nonorganic origin F44.4
    psychogenic F44.4
Dysbetalipoproteinemia (familial) E78.2
Dyscalculia R48.8
    developmental F81.2
Dyschezia K59.00
Dyschondroplasia (with hemangiomata)
    Q78.4
Dyschromia (skin) L81.9
Dyscollagenosis M35.9
Dyscranio-pygo-phalangy Q87.0
Dyscrasia
    blood (with) D75.9
        antepartum hemorrhage —*see* Hemorrhage,
    antepartum, with coagulation defect
        newborn P61.9
            specified type NEC P61.8
        intrapartum hemorrhage O67.0
        puerperal, postpartum O72.3
        polyglandular, pluriglandular E31.9
Dysendocrinism E34.9
Dysentery, dysenteric (catarrhal) (diarrhea)
    (epidemic) (hemorrhagic) (infectious)
    (sporadic) (tropical) A09
    abscess, liver A06.4
    amebic (*see also* Amebiasis) A06.0
        with abscess —*see* Abscess, amebic
        acute A06.0
        chronic A06.1
    arthritis (*see also* category M01) A09
    bacillary (*see also* category M01) A03.9
    bacillary A03.9
        arthritis (*see also* category M01) A03.9
        Boyd A03.2
        Flexner A03.1
        Schmitz (-Stutzer) A03.0
        Shiga (-Kruse) A03.0
        Shigella A03.9
            boydii A03.2
            dysenteriae A03.0
            flexneri A03.1
            group A A03.0
            group B A03.1
            group C A03.2
            group D A03.3
            sonnei A03.3
        specified type NEC A03.8

Dysentery, dysenteric - *continued*
   Sonne A03.3
    specified type NEC A03.8
  balantidial A07.0
  Balantidium coli A07.0
  Boyd's A03.2
  candidal B37.82
  Chilomastix A07.8
  Chinese A03.9
  coccidial A07.3
  Dientamoeba (fragilis) A07.8
  Embadomonas A07.8
  Entamoeba, entamebic —*see* Dysentery,
  amebic
  Flexner-Boyd A03.2
  Flexner's A03.1
  Giardia lamblia A07.1
  Hiss-Russell A03.1
  Lamblia A07.1
  leishmanial B55.0
  malarial —*see* Malaria
  metazoal B82.0
  monilial B37.82
  protozoal A07.9
  Salmonella A02.0
  schistosomal B65.1
  Schmitz (-Stutzer) A03.0
  Shiga (-Kruse) A03.0
  Shigella NOS —*see* Dysentery, bacillary
  Sonne A03.3
  strongyloidiasis B78.0
  trichomonal A07.8
  viral (*see also* Enteritis, viral) A08.4
Dysequilibrium R42
Dysesthesia R20.8
  hysterical F44.6
Dysfibrinogenemia (congenital) D68.2
Dysfunction
  adrenal E27.9
   hyperfunction E27.0
  autonomic
   due to alcohol G31.2
   somatoform F45.8
  bladder N31.9
   neurogenic NOS —*see* Dysfunction,
  bladder, neuromuscular
   neuromuscular NOS N31.9
    atonic (motor) (sensory) N31.2
    autonomous N31.2
    flaccid N31.2
    nonreflex N31.2
    reflex N31.1
    specified NEC N31.8
    uninhibited N31.0
  bleeding, uterus N93.8
  cerebral G93.89
  colon K59.9
   psychogenic F45.8
  colostomy K94.03
  cystic duct K82.8
  cystostomy (stoma) —*see* Complications,
  cystostomy
  ejaculatory N53.19
   anejaculatory orgasm N53.13
   painful N53.12
   premature F52.4
   retarded N53.11
  endocrine NOS E34.9
  endometrium N85.8
  enterostomy K94.13
  gallbladder K82.8
  gastrostomy (stoma) K94.23

Dysfunction – *continued*
  gland, glandular NOS E34.9
  heart I51.89
  hemoglobin D75.89
  hepatic K76.89
  hypophysis E23.7
  hypothalamic NEC E23.3
  ileostomy (stoma) K94.13
  jejunostomy (stoma) K94.13
  kidney —*see* Disease, renal
  labyrinthine —see subcategory H83.2
  left ventricular, following sudden emotional
  stress I51.81
  liver K76.89
  male —*see* Dysfunction, sexual, male
  orgasmic (female) F52.31
   male F52.32
  ovary E28.9
   specified NEC E28.8
  papillary muscle I51.89
  parathyroid E21.4
  physiological NEC R68.89
   psychogenic F59
  pineal gland E34.8
  pituitary (gland) E23.3
  platelets D69.1
  polyglandular E31.9
   specified NEC E31.8
  psychophysiologic F59
  psychosexual F52.9
   with
    dyspareunia F52.6
    premature ejaculation F52.4
    vaginismus F52.5
  pylorus K31.9
  rectum K59.9
   psychogenic F45.8
  reflex (sympathetic) —*see* Syndrome, pain,
  complex regional I
  segmental —*see* Dysfunction, somatic
  senile R54
  sexual (due to) R37
   alcohol F10.981
   amphetamine F15.981
    in
     abuse F15.181
     dependence F15.281
   anxiolytic F13.981
    in
     abuse F13.181
     dependence F13.281
   cocaine F14.981
    in
     abuse F14.181
     dependence F14.281
   excessive sexual drive F52.8
   failure of genital response (male) F52.21
    female F52.22
   female N94.9
    aversion F52.1
    dyspareunia N94.1
     psychogenic F52.6
    frigidity F52.22
    nymphomania F52.8
    orgasmic F52.31
    psychogenic F52.9
     aversion F52.1
     dyspareunia F52.6
     frigidity F52.22
     nymphomania F52.8
     orgasmic F52.31
     vaginismus F52.5

Dysfunction – *continued*
    vaginismus N94.2
     psychogenic F52.5
   hypnotic F13.981
    in
     abuse F13.181
     dependence F13.281
   inhibited orgasm (female) F52.31
    male F52.32
   lack
    of sexual enjoyment F52.1
    or loss of sexual desire F52.0
   male N53.9
    anejaculatory orgasm N53.13
    ejaculatory N53.19
     painful N53.12
     premature F52.4
     retarded N53.11
    erectile N52.9
     drug induced N52.2
     due to
      disease classified elsewhere N52.1
      drug N52.2
     postoperative (postprocedural) N52.39
      following
       prostatectomy N52.34
        radical N52.31
       radical cystectomy N52.32
       urethral surgery N52.33
     psychogenic F52.21
     specified cause NEC N52.8
     vasculogenic
      arterial insufficiency N52.01
       with corporo-venous occlusive N52.03
      corporo-venous occlusive N52.02
       with arterial insufficiency N52.03
    impotence —*see* Dysfunction, sexual,
    male, erectile
    psychogenic F52.9
     aversion F52.1
     erectile F52.21
     orgasmic F52.32
     premature ejaculation F52.4
     satyriasis F52.8
     specified type NEC F52.8
    specified type NEC N53.8
   nonorganic F52.9
    specified NEC F52.8
   opioid F11.981
    in
     abuse F11.181
     dependence F11.281
   orgasmic dysfunction (female) F52.31
    male F52.32
   premature ejaculation F52.4
   psychoactive substances NEC F19.981
    in
     abuse F19.181
     dependence F19.281
   psychogenic F52.9
   sedative F13.981
    in
     abuse F13.181
     dependence F13.281
   sexual aversion F52.1
   vaginismus (nonorganic) (psychogenic)
   F52.5
  sinoatrial node I49.5
  somatic M99.09
   abdomen M99.09
   acromioclavicular M99.07
   cervical region M99.01
   cervicothoracic M99.01

Dysfunction – *continued*
  costochondral M99.08
  costovertebral M99.08
  head region M99.00
  hip M99.05
  lower extremity M99.06
  lumbar region M99.03
  lumbosacral M99.03
  occipitocervical M99.00
  pelvic region M99.05
  pubic M99.05
  rib cage M99.08
  sacral region M99.04
  sacrococcygeal M99.04
  sacroiliac M99.04
  specified NEC M99.09
  sternochondral M99.08
  sternoclavicular M99.07
  thoracic region M99.02
  thoracolumbar M99.02
  upper extremity M99.07
 somatoform autonomic F45.8
 stomach K31.89
  psychogenic F45.8
 suprarenal E27.9
  hyperfunction E27.0
 symbolic R48.9
  specified type NEC R48.8
 temporomandibular (joint) M26.69
  joint-pain syndrome M26.62
 testicular (endocrine) E29.9
  specified NEC E29.8
 thymus E32.9
 thyroid E07.9
 ureterostomy (stoma) —*see* Complications, stoma, urinary tract
 urethrostomy (stoma) —*see* Complications, stoma, urinary tract
 uterus, complicating delivery O62.9
  hypertonic O62.4
  hypotonic O62.2
   primary O62.0
   secondary O62.1
 ventricular I51.9
  with congestive heart failure I50.9   left, reversible, following sudden emotional stress I51.81
Dysgenesis
 gonadal (due to chromosomal anomaly) Q96.9
  pure Q99.1
 renal Q60.5
  bilateral Q60.4
  unilateral Q60.3
 reticular D72.0
 tidal platelet D69.3
Dysgerminoma
 specified site —*see* Neoplasm, malignant, by site
 unspecified site
  female C56.9
  male C62.90
Dysgeusia R43.2
Dysgraphia R27.8
Dyshidrosis, dysidrosis L30.1
Dyskaryotic cervical smear R87.619
Dyskeratosis L85.8
 cervix —*see* Dysplasia, cervix
 congenital Q82.8
 uterus NEC N85.8
Dyskinesia G24.9
 biliary (cystic duct or gallbladder) K82.8

Dyskinesia - *continued*
 drug induced
  orofacial G24.01
 esophagus K22.4
 hysterical F44.4
 intestinal K59.8
 nonorganic origin F44.4
 orofacial (idiopathic) G24.4
  drug induced G24.01
 psychogenic F44.4
 subacute, drug induced G24.01
 tardive G24.01
  neuroleptic induced G24.01
 trachea J39.8
 tracheobronchial J98.09
Dyslalia (developmental) F80.0
Dyslexia R48.0
 developmental F81.0
Dyslipidemia E78.5
 depressed HDL cholesterol E78.6
 elevated fasting triglycerides E78.1
Dysmaturity —*see also* Light for dates
 pulmonary (newborn) (Wilson-Mikity) P27.0
Dysmenorrhea (essential) (exfoliative) N94.6
 congestive (syndrome) N94.6
 primary N94.4
 psychogenic F45.8
 secondary N94.5
Dysmetabolic syndrome X E88.81
Dysmetria R27.8
Dysmorphism (due to)
 alcohol Q86.0
 exogenous cause NEC Q86.8
 hydantoin Q86.1
 warfarin Q86.2
Dysmorphophobia (nondelusional) F45.22
 delusional F22
Dysnomia R47.01
Dysorexia R63.0
 psychogenic F50.8
Dysostosis
 cleidocranial, cleidocranialis Q74.0
 craniofacial Q75.1
 Fairbank's (idiopathic familial generalized osteophytosis) Q78.9
 mandibulofacial (incomplete) Q75.4
 multiplex E76.01
 oculomandibular Q75.5
Dyspareunia (female) N94.1
 male N53.12
 nonorganic F52.6
 psychogenic F52.6
 secondary N94.1
Dyspepsia R10.13
 atonic K30
 functional (allergic) (congenital) (gastrointestinal) (occupational) (reflex) K30
 intestinal K59.8
 nervous F45.8
 neurotic F45.8
 psychogenic F45.8
Dysphagia R13.10
 cervical R13.19
 following
  cerebral infarction I69.391
  cerebrovascular disease I69.991
   specified NEC I69.891
  intracerebral hemorrhage I69.191
  nontraumatic intracranial hemorrhage NEC I69.291
   specified disease NEC I69.891
  subarachnoid hemorrhage I69.091

Dysphagia - *continued*
 functional (hysterical) F45.8
 hysterical F45.8
 nervous (hysterical) F45.8
 neurogenic R13.19
 oral phase R13.11
 oropharyngeal phase R13.12
 pharyngeal phase R13.13
 pharyngoesophageal phase R13.14
 psychogenic F45.8
 sideropenic D50.1
 spastica K22.4
 specified NEC R13.19
Dysphagocytosis, congenital D71
Dysphasia R47.02
 developmental
  expressive type F80.1
  receptive type F80.2
 following
  cerebrovascular disease I69.921
   cerebral infarction I69.321
   intracerebral hemorrhage I69.121
   nontraumatic intracranial hemorrhage NEC I69.221
    specified disease NEC I69.821
    subarachnoid hemorrhage I69.021
Dysphonia R49.0
 functional F44.4
 hysterical F44.4
 psychogenic F44.4
 spastica J38.3
Dysphoria, postpartal O90.6
Dyspituitarism E23.3
Dysplasia —*see also* Anomaly
 acetabular, congenital Q65.89
 alveolar capillary, with vein misalignment J84.843
 anus (histologically confirmed) (mild) (moderate) K62.82
  severe D01.3
 arrhythmogenic right ventricular I42.8
 arterial, fibromuscular I77.3
 asphyxiating thoracic (congenital) Q77.2
 brain Q07.9
 bronchopulmonary, perinatal P27.1
 cervix (uteri) N87.9
  mild N87.0
  moderate N87.1
  severe D06.9
 chondroectodermal Q77.6
 colon D12.6
 craniometaphyseal Q78.5
 dentinal K00.5
 diaphyseal, progressive Q78.3
 dystrophic Q77.5
 ectodermal (anhidrotic) (congenital) (hereditary) Q82.4
  hidrotic Q82.8
 epithelial, uterine cervix —*see* Dysplasia, cervix
 eye (congenital) Q11.2
 fibrous
  bone NEC (monostotic) M85.00
   ankle M85.07
   foot M85.07
   forearm M85.03
   hand M85.04
   lower leg M85.06
   multiple site M85.09
   neck M85.08
   rib M85.08
   shoulder M85.01
   skull M85.08

Dysplasia - continued
   specified site NEC M85.08
     thigh M85.05
     toe M85.07
     upper arm M85.02
     vertebra M85.08
   diaphyseal, progressive Q78.3
   jaw M27.8
     polyostotic Q78.1
   florid osseous —see also Cyst, calcifying odontogenic
   high grade, focal D12.6
   hip, congenital Q65.89
   joint, congenital Q74.8
   kidney Q61.4
     multicystic Q61.4
   leg Q74.2
   lung, congenital (not associated with short gestation) Q33.6
   mammary (gland) (benign) N60.9
     cyst (solitary) —see Cyst, breast
     cystic —see Mastopathy, cystic
     duct ectasia —see Ectasia, mammary duct
     fibroadenosis —see Fibroadenosis, breast
     fibrosclerosis —see Fibrosclerosis, breast
     specified type NEC N60.8
   metaphyseal (Jansen's) (McKusick's) (Schmid's) Q78.5
   muscle Q79.8
   oculodentodigital Q87.0
   periapical (cemental) (cemento-osseous) — see Cyst, calcifying odontogenic
   periosteum —see Disorder, bone, specified type NEC
   polyostotic fibrous Q78.1
   prostate (see also Neoplasia, intraepithelial, prostate) N42.3
     severe D07.5
   renal Q61.4
     multicystic Q61.4
   retinal, congenital Q14.1
   right ventricular, arrhythmogenic I42.8
   septo-optic Q04.4
   skin L98.8
   spinal cord Q06.1
   spondyloepiphyseal Q77.7
   thymic, with immunodeficiency D82.1
   vagina N89.3
     mild N89.0
     moderate N89.1
     severe NEC D07.2
   vulva N90.3
     mild N90.0
     moderate N90.1
     severe NEC D07.1
Dyspnea (nocturnal) (paroxysmal) R06.00
   asthmatic (bronchial) J45.909
   with
     exacerbation (acute) J45.901
     bronchitis J45.909
     with
       exacerbation (acute) J45.901
       status asthmaticus J45.902
     chronic J44.9
     status asthmaticus J45.902
   cardiac —see Failure, ventricular, left
   cardiac —see Failure, ventricular, left
   functional F45.8
   hyperventilation R06.4
   hysterical F45.8
   newborn P28.89
   orthopnea R06.01

Dyspnea - continued
   psychogenic F45.8
   shortness of breath R06.02
   specified type NEC R06.09
Dyspraxia R27.8
   developmental (syndrome) F82
Dysproteinemia E88.09
Dysreflexia, autonomic G90.4
Dysrhythmia
   cardiac I49.9
     newborn
       bradycardia P29.12
       occurring before birth P03.819
         before onset of labor P03.810
         during labor P03.811
       tachycardia P29.11
     postoperative I97.89
   cerebral or cortical —see Epilepsy
Dyssomnia —see Disorder, sleep
Dyssynergia
   biliary K83.8
   bladder sphincter N36.44
   cerebellaris myoclonica (Hunt's ataxia) G11.1
Dysthymia F34.1
Dysthyroidism E07.9
Dystocia O66.9
   affecting newborn P03.1
   cervical (hypotonic) O62.2
     affecting newborn P03.6
     primary O62.0
     secondary O62.1
   contraction ring O62.4
   fetal O66.9
     abnormality NEC O66.3
     conjoined twins O66.3
     oversize O66.2
   maternal O66.9
   positional O64.9
   shoulder (girdle) O66.0
     causing obstructed labor O66.0
   uterine NEC O62.4
Dystonia G24.9
   deformans progressiva G24.1
   drug induced NEC G24.09
     acute G24.02
     specified NEC G24.09
   familial G24.1
   idiopathic G24.1
     familial G24.1
     nonfamilial G24.2
     orofacial G24.4
   lenticularis G24.8
   musculorum deformans G24.1
   neuroleptic induced (acute) G24.02
   orofacial (idiopathic) G24.4
   oromandibular G24.4
     due to drug G24.01
   specified NEC G24.8
   torsion (familial) (idiopathic) G24.1
     acquired G24.8
     genetic G24.1
     symptomatic (nonfamilial) G24.2
Dystonic movements R25.8
Dystrophy, dystrophia
   adiposogenital E23.6
   Becker's type G71.0
   cervical sympathetic G90.2
   choroid (hereditary) H31.20
     central areolar H31.22
     choroideremia H31.21
     gyrate atrophy H31.23
     specified type NEC H31.29

Dystrophy, dystrophia - continued
   cornea (hereditary) H18.50
     endothelial H18.51
     epithelial H18.52
     granular H18.53
     lattice H18.54
     macular H18.55
     specified type NEC H18.59
   Duchenne's type G71.0
   due to malnutrition E45
   Erb's G71.0
   Fuchs' H18.51
   Gower's muscular G71.0
   hair L67.8
   infantile neuraxonal G31.89
   Landouzy-Déjérine G71.0
   Leyden-Möbius G71.0
   muscular G71.0
     benign (Becker type) G71.0
     congenital (hereditary) (progressive) (with specific morphological abnormalities of the muscle fiber) G71.0
       myotonic G71.11
     distal G71.0
     Duchenne type G71.0
     Emery-Dreifuss G71.0
     Erb type G71.0
     facioscapulohumeral G71.0
     Gower's G71.0
     hereditary (progressive) G71.0
     Landouzy-Déjérine type G71.0
     limb-girdle G71.0
     myotonic G71.11
     progressive (hereditary) G71.0
       Charcot-Marie (-Tooth) type G60.0
     pseudohypertrophic (infantile) G71.0
     severe (Duchenne type) G71.0
   myocardium, myocardial —see Degeneration, myocardial
   myotonic, myotonica G71.11
   nail L60.3
     congenital Q84.6
   nutritional E45
   ocular G71.0
   oculocerebrorenal E72.03
   oculopharyngeal G71.0
   ovarian N83.8
   polyglandular E31.8
   reflex (neuromuscular) (sympathetic) —see Syndrome, pain, complex regional I
   retinal (hereditary) H35.50
     in
       lipid storage disorders E75.6 [H36]
       systemic lipidoses E75.6 [H36]
     involving
       pigment epithelium H35.54
       sensory area H35.53
     pigmentary H35.52
     vitreoretinal H35.51
   Salzmann's nodular —see Degeneration, cornea, nodular
   scapuloperoneal G71.0
   skin NEC L98.8
   sympathetic (reflex) —see Syndrome, pain, complex regional I
     cervical G90.2
   tapetoretinal H35.54
   thoracic, asphyxiating Q77.2
   unguium L60.3
     congenital Q84.6
   vitreoretinal H35.51
   vulva N90.4
   yellow (liver) —see Failure, hepatic

Dysuria R30.0
  psychogenic F45.8

E

Eales' disease H35.06
Ear —*see also* condition
  piercing Z41.3
  tropical B36.8
  wax (impacted) H61.20
    left H61.22
      with right H61.23
    right H61.21
      with left H61.23
Earache —see subcategory H92.0
Early satiety R68.81
Eaton-Lambert syndrome —*see* Syndrome, Lambert-Eaton
Eberth's disease (typhoid fever) A01.00
Ebola virus disease A98.4
Ebstein's anomaly or syndrome (heart) Q22.5
Eccentro-osteochondrodysplasia E76.29
Ecchondroma —*see* Neoplasm, bone, benign
Ecchondrosis D48.0
Ecchymosis R58
  conjunctiva —*see* Hemorrhage, conjunctiva
  eye (traumatic) —*see* Contusion, eyeball
  eyelid (traumatic) —*see* Contusion, eyelid
  newborn P54.5
  spontaneous R23.3
  traumatic —*see* Contusion
Echinococciasis —*see* Echinococcus
Echinococcosis —*see* Echinococcus
Echinococcus (infection) B67.90
  granulosus B67.4
    bone B67.2
    liver B67.0
    lung B67.1
    multiple sites B67.32
    specified site NEC B67.39
    thyroid B67.31 *[E35]*
  liver NOS B67.8
    granulosus B67.0
    multilocularis B67.5
  lung NEC B67.99
    granulosus B67.1
    multilocularis B67.69
  multilocularis B67.7
    liver B67.5
    multiple sites B67.61
    specified site NEC B67.69
  specified site NEC B67.99
    granulosus B67.39
    multilocularis B67.69
  thyroid NEC B67.99
    granulosus B67.31 *[E35]*
    multilocularis B67.69 *[E35]*
Echinorhynchiasis B83.8
Echinostomiasis B66.8
Echolalia R48.8
Echovirus, as cause of disease classified elsewhere B97.12
Eclampsia, eclamptic (coma) (convulsions) (delirium) (with hypertension) NEC O15.9
  during labor and delivery O15.1
  postpartum O15.2
  pregnancy O15.0
  puerperal O15.2
Economic circumstances affecting care Z59.9
Economo's disease A85.8
Ectasia, ectasis
  annuloaortic I35.8

Ectasia, ectasis - *continued*
  aorta I77.819
    with aneurysm —*see* Aneurysm, aorta
    abdominal I77.811
    thoracic I77.810
    thoracoabdominal I77.812
  breast —*see* Ectasia, mammary duct
  capillary I78.8
  cornea H18.71
  gastric antral vascular (GAVE) K31.819
    with hemorrhage K31.811
    without hemorrhage K31.819
  mammary duct N60.4
  salivary gland (duct) K11.8
  sclera —*see* Sclerectasia
Ecthyma L08.0
  contagiosum B08.02
  gangrenosum L08.0
  infectiosum B08.02
Ectocardia Q24.8
Ectodermal dysplasia (anhidrotic) Q82.4
Ectodermosis erosiva pluriorificialis L51.1
Ectopic, ectopia (congenital)
  abdominal viscera Q45.8
    due to defect in anterior abdominal wall Q79.59
  ACTH syndrome E24.3
  adrenal gland Q89.1
  anus Q43.5
  atrial beats I49.1
  beats I49.49
    atrial I49.1
    ventricular I49.3
  bladder Q64.10
  bone and cartilage in lung Q33.5
  brain Q04.8
  breast tissue Q83.8
  cardiac Q24.8
  cerebral Q04.8
  cordis Q24.8
  endometrium —*see* Endometriosis
  gastric mucosa Q40.2
  gestation —*see* Pregnancy, by site
  heart Q24.8
  hormone secretion NEC E34.2
  kidney (crossed) (pelvis) Q63.2
  lens, lentis Q12.1
  mole —*see* Pregnancy, by site
  organ or site NEC —*see* Malposition, congenital
  pancreas Q45.3
  pregnancy —*see* Pregnancy, ectopic
  pupil —*see* Abnormality, pupillary
  renal Q63.2
  sebaceous glands of mouth Q38.6
  spleen Q89.09
  testis Q53.00
    bilateral Q53.02
    unilateral Q53.01
  thyroid Q89.2
  tissue in lung Q33.5
  ureter Q62.63
  ventricular beats I49.3
  vesicae Q64.10
Ectromelia Q73.8
  lower limb —*see* Defect, reduction, limb, lower, specified type NEC
  upper limb —*see* Defect, reduction, limb, upper, specified type NEC
Ectropion H02.109
  cervix N86
    with cervicitis N72

Ectropion continued
  congenital Q10.1
  eyelid (paralytic) H02.109
    cicatricial H02.119
      left H02.116
        lower H02.115
        upper H02.114
      right H02.113
        lower H02.112
        upper H02.111
    congenital Q10.1
    left H02.106
      lower H02.105
      upper H02.104
    mechanical H02.129
      left H02.126
        lower H02.125
        upper H02.124
      right H02.123
        lower H02.122
        upper H02.121
    right H02.103
      lower H02.102
      upper H02.101
    senile H02.139
      left H02.136
        lower H02.135
        upper H02.134
      right H02.133
        lower H02.132
        upper H02.131
    spastic H02.149
      left H02.146
        lower H02.145
        upper H02.144
      right H02.143
        lower H02.142
        upper H02.141
  iris H21.89
  lip (acquired) K13.0
    congenital Q38.0
  urethra N36.8
  uvea H21.89
Eczema (acute) (chronic) (erythematous) (fissum) (rubrum) (squamous) (*see also* Dermatitis) L30.9
  contact —*see* Dermatitis, contact
  dyshidrotic L30.1
  external ear —*see* Otitis, externa, acute, eczematoid
  flexural L20.82
  herpeticum B00.0
  hypertrophicum L28.0
  hypostatic —*see* Varix, leg, with, inflammation
  impetiginous L01.1
  infantile (due to any substance) L20.83
    intertriginous L21.1
    seborrheic L21.1
  intertriginous NEC L30.4
    infantile L21.1
  intrinsic (allergic) L20.84
  lichenified NEC L28.0
  marginatum (hebrae) B35.6
  pustular L30.3
  stasis —*see* Varix, leg, with, inflammation
  vaccination, vaccinatum T88.1
  varicose —*see* Varix, leg, with, inflammation
Eczematid L30.2
Eddowes (-Spurway) **syndrome** Q78.0
Edema, edematous (infectious) (pitting) (toxic) R60.9
  with nephritis —*see* Nephrosis

Edema, edematous - *continued*
allergic T78.3
amputation stump (surgical) (sequelae (late effect)) T87.89
angioneurotic (allergic) (any site) (with urticaria) T78.3
  hereditary D84.1
angiospastic I73.9
Berlin's (traumatic) S05.8X
brain (cytotoxic) (vasogenic) G93.6
  due to birth injury P11.0
  newborn (anoxia or hypoxia) P52.4
    birth injury P11.0
  traumatic —*see* Injury, intracranial, cerebral edema
cardiac —*see* Failure, heart, congestive
cardiovascular —*see* Failure, heart, congestive
cerebral —*see* Edema, brain
cerebrospinal —*see* Edema, brain
cervix (uteri) (acute) N88.8
  puerperal, postpartum O90.89
chronic hereditary Q82.0
circumscribed, acute T78.3
  hereditary D84.1
conjunctiva H11.42
cornea H18.2
  idiopathic H18.22
  secondary H18.23
    due to contact lens H18.21
due to
  lymphatic obstruction I89.0
  salt retention E87.0
epiglottis —*see* Edema, glottis
essential, acute T78.3
  hereditary D84.1
extremities, lower —*see* Edema, legs
eyelid NEC H02.849
  left H02.846
    lower H02.845
    upper H02.844
  right H02.843
    lower H02.842
    upper H02.841
familial, hereditary Q82.0
famine —*see* Malnutrition, severe
generalized R60.1
glottis, glottic, glottidis (obstructive) (passive) J38.4
  allergic T78.3
    hereditary D84.1
heart —*see* Failure, heart, congestive
heat T67.7
hereditary Q82.0
inanition —*see* Malnutrition, severe
intracranial G93.6
iris H21.89
joint —*see* Effusion, joint
larynx —*see* Edema, glottis
legs R60.0
  due to venous obstruction I87.1
  hereditary Q82.0
localized R60.0
  due to venous obstruction I87.1
lower limbs —*see* Edema, legs
lung J81.1
  with heart condition or failure —*see* Failure, ventricular, left
  acute J81.0
  chemical (acute) J68.1
    chronic J68.1

Edema, edematous - *continued*
chronic J81.1
  due to
    chemicals, gases, fumes or vapors (inhalation) J68.1
      external agent J70.9
        specified NEC J70.8
      radiation J70.1
  due to
    chemicals, fumes or vapors (inhalation) J68.1
      external agent J70.9
        specified NEC J70.8
      high altitude T70.29
      near drowning T75.1
      radiation J70.0
  meaning failure, left ventricle I50.1
lymphatic I89.0
  due to mastectomy I97.2
macula H35.81
  cystoid, following cataract surgery —*see* Complications, postprocedural, following cataract surgery
  diabetic —*see* Diabetes, by type, with, retinopathy, with macular edema
malignant —*see* Gangrene, gas
Milroy's Q82.0
nasopharynx J39.2
newborn P83.30
  hydrops fetalis —*see* Hydrops, fetalis
  specified NEC P83.39
nutritional —*see also* Malnutrition, severe
  with dyspigmentation, skin and hair E40
optic disc or nerve —*see* Papilledema
orbit H05.22
pancreas K86.8
papilla, optic —*see* Papilledema
penis N48.89
periodic T78.3
  hereditary D84.1
pharynx J39.2
pulmonary —*see* Edema, lung
Quincke's T78.3
  hereditary D84.1
renal —*see* Nephrosis
retina H35.81
  diabetic —*see* Diabetes, by type, with, retinopathy, with macular edema
salt E87.0
scrotum N50.8
seminal vesicle N50.8
spermatic cord N50.8
spinal (cord) (vascular) (nontraumatic) G95.19
starvation —*see* Malnutrition, severe
stasis —*see* Hypertension, venous, (chronic)
subglottic —*see* Edema, glottis
supraglottic —*see* Edema, glottis
testis N44.8
tunica vaginalis N50.8
vas deferens N50.8
vulva (acute) N90.89
Edentulism —*see* Absence, teeth, acquired
Edsall's disease T67.2
Educational handicap Z55.9
  specified NEC Z55.8
Edward's syndrome —*see* Trisomy, 18
Effect, adverse
  abnormal gravitational (G) forces or states T75.81
  abuse —*see* Maltreatment

Effect, adverse - *continued*
air pressure T70.9
  specified NEC T70.8
altitude (high) —*see* Effect, adverse, high altitude
anesthesia (*see also* Anesthesia) T88.59
  in labor and delivery O74.9
  in pregnancy NEC O29.3
  local, toxic
    in labor and delivery O74.4
    postpartum, puerperal O89.3
  postpartum, puerperal O89.9
  specified NEC T88.59
    in labor and delivery O74.8
    postpartum, puerperal O89.8
  spinal and epidural T88.59
    headache T88.59
      in labor and delivery O74.5
      postpartum, puerperal O89.4
    specified NEC
      in labor and delivery O74.6
      postpartum, puerperal O89.5
antitoxin —*see* Complications, vaccination
atmospheric pressure T70.9
  due to explosion T70.8
  high T70.3
  low —*see* Effect, adverse, high altitude
  specified effect NEC T70.8
biological, correct substance properly administered —*see* Effect, adverse, drug
blood (derivatives) (serum) (transfusion) — *see* Complications, transfusion
chemical substance —*see* Table of Drugs and Chemicals
cold (temperature) (weather) T69.9
  chilblains T69.1
  frostbite —*see* Frostbite
  specified effect NEC T69.8
drugs and medicaments T88.7
  specified drug —*see* Table of Drugs and Chemicals, by drug, adverse effect
  specified effect
    code to condition
electric current, electricity (shock) T75.4
  burn —*see* Burn
exertion (excessive) T73.3
exposure —*see* Exposure
external cause NEC T75.89
foodstuffs T78.1
  allergic reaction —*see* Allergy, food
  causing anaphylaxis —*see* Shock, anaphylactic, due to food
  noxious —*see* Poisoning, food, noxious
gases, fumes, or vapors T59.9
  specified agent —*see* Table of Drugs and Chemicals
glue (airplane) sniffing
  due to drug abuse —*see* Abuse, drug, inhalant
  due to drug dependence —*see* Dependence, drug, inhalant
heat —*see* Heat
high altitude NEC T70.29
  anoxia T70.29
  on
    ears T70.0
    sinuses T70.1
  polycythemia D75.1
high pressure fluids T70.4
hot weather —*see* Heat
hunger T73.0
immersion, foot —*see* Immersion

Effect, adverse - *continued*
- immunization —*see* Complications, vaccination
- immunological agents —*see* Complications, vaccination
- infrared (radiation) (rays) NOS T66
  - dermatitis or eczema L59.8
- infusion —*see* Complications, infusion
- lack of care of infants —*see* Maltreatment, child
- lightning —*see* Lightning
- medical care T88.9
  - specified NEC T88.8
- medicinal substance, correct, properly administered —*see* Effect, adverse, drug
- motion T75.3
- noise, on inner ear —see subcategory H83.3
- overheated places —*see* Heat
- psychosocial, of work environment Z56.5
- radiation (diagnostic) (infrared) (natural source) (therapeutic) (ultraviolet) (X-ray) NOS T66
  - dermatitis or eczema —*see* Dermatitis, due to, radiation
    - fibrosis of lung J70.1
    - pneumonitis J70.0
    - pulmonary manifestations
      - acute J70.0
      - chronic J70.1
    - skin L59.9
- radioactive substance NOS
  - dermatitis or eczema —*see* Radiodermatitis
- reduced temperature T69.9
  - immersion foot or hand —*see* Immersion
  - specified effect NEC T69.8
- serum NEC (*see also* Reaction, serum) T80.69
- specified NEC T78.8
  - external cause NEC T75.89
- strangulation —*see* Asphyxia, traumatic
- submersion T75.1
- thirst T73.1
- toxic —*see* Toxicity
- transfusion —*see* Complications, transfusion
- ultraviolet (radiation) (rays) NOS T66
  - burn —*see* Burn
  - dermatitis or eczema —*see* Dermatitis, due to, ultraviolet rays
    - acute L56.8
- vaccine (any) —*see* Complications, vaccination
- vibration —*see* Vibration, adverse effects
- water pressure NEC T70.9
  - specified NEC T70.8
- weightlessness T75.82
- whole blood —*see* Complications, transfusion
- work environment Z56.5

Effect (s) (of) (from) —*see* Effect, adverse NEC

Effects, late —*see* Sequelae

Effluvium
- anagen L65.1
- telogen L65.0

Effort syndrome (psychogenic) F45.8

Effusion
- amniotic fluid —*see* Pregnancy, complicated by, premature rupture of membranes
- brain (serous) G93.6
- bronchial —*see* Bronchitis
- cerebral G93.6
- cerebrospinal —*see also* Meningitis
  - vessel G93.6

Effusion - *continued*
- chest —*see* Effusion, pleura
- chylous, chyliform (pleura) J94.0
- intracranial G93.6
- joint M25.40
  - ankle M25.47
  - elbow M25.42
  - foot joint M25.47
  - hand joint M25.44
  - hip M25.45
  - knee M25.46
  - shoulder M25.41
  - specified joint NEC M25.48
  - wrist M25.43
- malignant pleural J91.0
- meninges —*see* Meningitis
- pericardium, pericardial (noninflammatory) I31.3
  - acute —*see* Pericarditis, acute
- peritoneal (chronic) R18.8
- pleura, pleurisy, pleuritic, pleuropericardial J90
  - chylous, chyliform J94.0
  - due to systemic lupus erythematosus M32.13
  - influenzal —*see* Influenza, with, respiratory manifestations NEC
  - malignant J91.0
  - newborn P28.89
  - tuberculous NEC A15.6
    - primary (progressive) A15.7
- spinal —*see* Meningitis
- thorax, thoracic —*see* Effusion, pleura

Egg shell nails L60.3
- congenital Q84.6

Egyptian splenomegaly B65.1

Ehrlichiosis A77.40
- due to
  - E. chafeensis A77.41
  - E. sennetsu A79.81
  - specified organism NEC A77.49

Ehlers-Danlos syndrome Q79.6

Eichstedt's disease B36.0

Eisenmenger's
- complex or syndrome I27.89
- defect Q21.8

Ejaculation
- painful N53.12
- premature F52.4
- retarded N53.11
- retrograde N53.14
- semen, painful N53.12
- psychogenic F52.6

Ekbom's syndrome (restless legs) G25.81

Ekman's syndrome (brittle bones and blue sclera) Q78.0

Elastic skin Q82.8
- acquired L57.4

Elastofibroma —*see* Neoplasm, connective tissue, benign

Elastoma (juvenile) Q82.8
- Miescher's L87.2

Elastomyofibrosis I42.4

Elastosis
- actinic, solar L57.8
- atrophicans (senile) L57.4
- perforans serpiginosa L87.2
- senilis L57.4

Elbow —*see* condition

Electric current, electricity, effects (concussion) (fatal) (nonfatal) (shock) T75.4
- burn —*see* Burn

Electric feet syndrome E53.8

Electrocution T75.4
- from electroshock gun (taser) T75.4

Electrolyte imbalance E87.8
- with
  - abortion —*see* Abortion by type, complicated by, electrolyte imbalance
  - ectopic pregnancy O08.5
  - molar pregnancy O08.5

Elephantiasis (nonfilarial) I89.0
- arabicum —*see* Infestation, filarial
- bancroftian B74.0
- congenital (any site) (hereditary) Q82.0
- due to
  - Brugia (malayi) B74.1
    - timori B74.2
  - mastectomy I97.2
  - Wuchereria (bancrofti) B74.0
- eyelid H02.859
  - left H02.856
    - lower H02.855
    - upper H02.854
  - right H02.853
    - lower H02.852
    - upper H02.851
- filarial, filariensis —*see* Infestation, filarial
- glandular I89.0
- graecorum A30.9
- lymphangiectatic I89.0
- lymphatic vessel I89.0
  - due to mastectomy I97.2
- scrotum (nonfilarial) I89.0
- streptococcal I89.0
- surgical I97.89
  - postmastectomy I97.2
- telangiectodes I89.0
- vulva (nonfilarial) N90.89

Elevated, elevation
- antibody titer R76.0
- basal metabolic rate R94.8
- blood pressure —*see also* Hypertension
  - reading (incidental) (isolated) (nonspecific) , no diagnosis of hypertension R03.0
- blood sugar R73.9
- body temperature (of unknown origin) R50.9
- C-reactive protein (CRP) R79.82
- cancer antigen 125 -CA 125] R97.1
- carcinoembryonic antigen -CEA] R97.0
- cholesterol E78.0
  - with high triglycerides E78.2
- conjugate, eye H51.0
- diaphragm, congenital Q79.1
- erythrocyte sedimentation rate R70.0
- fasting glucose R73.01
- fasting triglycerides E78.1
- finding on laboratory examination —*see* Findings, abnormal, inconclusive, without diagnosis, by type of exam
- GFR (glomerular filtration rate) —*see* Findings, abnormal, inconclusive, without diagnosis, by type of exam
- glucose tolerance (oral) R73.02
- immunoglobulin level R76.8
- indoleacetic acid R82.5
- lactic acid dehydrogenase (LDH) level R74.0
- leukocytes D72.829
- lipoprotein a level E78.8
- liver function
  - study R94.5
  - test R79.89
    - alkaline phosphatase R74.8
    - aminotransferase R74.0
    - bilirubin R17
    - hepatic enzyme R74.8

Elevated, elevation - *continued*
   lactate dehydrogenase R74.0
   lymphocytes D72.820
   prostate specific antigen -PSA] R97.2
   Rh titer —*see* Complication(s) , transfusion,
   incompatibility reaction, Rh (factor)
   scapula, congenital Q74.0
   sedimentation rate R70.0
   SGOT R74.0
   SGPT R74.0
   transaminase level R74.0
   triglycerides E78.1
    with high cholesterol E78.2
   tumor associated antigens -TAA] NEC R97.8
   tumor specific antigens -TSA] NEC R97.8
   urine level of
    catecholamine R82.5
    indoleacetic acid R82.5
    17-ketosteroids R82.5
    steroids R82.5
    vanillylmandelic acid (VMA) R82.5
   venous pressure I87.8
   white blood cell count D72.829
    specified NEC D72.828
Elliptocytosis (congenital) (hereditary) D58.1
   Hb C (disease) D58.1
   hemoglobin disease D58.1
   sickle-cell (disease) D57.8
    trait D57.3
Ellison-Zollinger syndrome E16.4
Ellis-van Creveld syndrome
   (chondroectodermal dysplasia) Q77.6
Elongated, elongation (congenital) —*see also*
   Distortion
   bone Q79.9
   cervix (uteri) Q51.828
    acquired N88.4
    hypertrophic N88.4
   colon Q43.8
   common bile duct Q44.5
   cystic duct Q44.5
   frenulum, penis Q55.69
   labia minora (acquired) N90.6
   ligamentum patellae Q74.1
   petiolus (epiglottidis) Q31.8
   tooth, teeth K00.2
   uvula Q38.6
Eltor cholera A00.1
Emaciation (due to malnutrition) E41
Embadomoniasis A07.8
Embedded tooth, teeth K01.0
   root only K08.3
Embolic —*see* condition
Embolism (multiple) (paradoxical) I74.9
   air (any site) (traumatic) T79.0
    following
     abortion —*see* Abortion by type
    complicated by embolism
     ectopic pregnancy O08.2
     infusion, therapeutic injection or
    transfusion T80.0
     molar pregnancy O08.2
     procedure NEC
      artery T81.719
       mesenteric T81.710
       renal T81.711
       specified NEC T81.718
      vein T81.72
    in pregnancy, childbirth or puerperium —
    see Embolism, obstetric
   amniotic fluid (pulmonary) —*see also*
   Embolism, obstetric

Embolism – *continued*
   following
    abortion —*see* Abortion by type
   complicated by embolism
    ectopic pregnancy O08.2
    molar pregnancy O08.2
   aorta, aortic I74.10
    abdominal I74.09
     saddle I74.01
    bifurcation I74.09
     saddle I74.01
    thoracic I74.11
   artery I74.9
    auditory, internal I65.8
    basilar —*see* Occlusion, artery, basilar
    carotid (common) (internal) —*see*
   Occlusion, artery, carotid
    cerebellar (anterior inferior) (posterior
   inferior) (superior) I66.3
    cerebral —*see* Occlusion, artery, cerebral
    choroidal (anterior) I66.8
    communicating posterior I66.8
    coronary —*see also* Infarct, myocardium
     not resulting in infarction I24.0
    extremity I74.4
     lower I74.3
     upper I74.2
    hypophyseal I66.8
    iliac I74.5
    limb I74.4
     lower I74.3
     upper I74.2
    mesenteric (with gangrene) K55.0
    ophthalmic —*see* Occlusion, artery, retina
    peripheral I74.4
    pontine I66.8
    precerebral —*see* Occlusion, artery,
   precerebral
    pulmonary —*see* Embolism, pulmonary
    renal N28.0
    retinal —*see* Occlusion, artery, retina
    septic I76
    specified NEC I74.8
    vertebral —*see* Occlusion, artery, vertebral
   basilar (artery) I65.1
   blood clot
    following
     abortion —*see* Abortion by type
    complicated by embolism
     ectopic or molar pregnancy O08.2
    in pregnancy, childbirth or puerperium —
   see Embolism, obstetric
   brain —*see also* Occlusion, artery, cerebral
    following
     abortion —*see* Abortion by type
    complicated by embolism
     ectopic or molar pregnancy O08.2
    puerperal, postpartum, childbirth —*see*
   Embolism, obstetric
   capillary I78.8
   cardiac —*see also* Infarct, myocardium
    not resulting in infarction I24.0
   carotid (artery) (common) (internal) —*see*
   Occlusion, artery, carotid
   cavernous sinus (venous) —*see* Embolism,
   intracranial venous sinus
   cerebral —*see* Occlusion, artery, cerebral
   cholesterol —*see* Atheroembolism
   coronary (artery or vein) (systemic) —*see*
   Occlusion, coronary
   due to device, implant or graft —*see also*
   Complications, by site and type, specified
   NEC

Embolism – *continued*
   arterial graft NEC T82.818
   breast (implant) T85.81
   catheter NEC T85.81
    dialysis (renal) T82.818
     intraperitoneal T85.81
    infusion NEC T82.818
     spinal (epidural) (subdural) T85.81
    urinary (indwelling) T83.81
   electronic (electrode) (pulse generator)
   (stimulator)
    bone T84.81
    cardiac T82.817
    nervous system (brain) (peripheral nerve)
   (spinal) T85.81
    urinary T83.81
   fixation, internal (orthopedic) NEC T84.81
   gastrointestinal (bile duct) (esophagus)
   T85.81
   genital NEC T83.81
   heart (graft) (valve) T82.817
   joint prosthesis T84.81
   ocular (corneal graft) (orbital implant)
   T85.81
   orthopedic (bone graft) NEC T86.838
   specified NEC T85.81
   urinary (graft) NEC T83.81
   vascular NEC T82.818
   ventricular intracranial shunt T85.81
   extremities
   lower —*see* Embolism, vein, lower
   extremity
    arterial I74.3
   upper I74.2
   eye H34.9
   fat (cerebral) (pulmonary) (systemic) T79.1
    following
     abortion —*see* Abortion by type
    complicated by embolism
     ectopic or molar pregnancy O08.2
    complicating delivery —*see* Embolism,
   obstetric
    following
     abortion —*see* Abortion by type
    complicated by embolism
     ectopic or molar pregnancy O08.2
     infusion, therapeutic injection or transfusion
     air T80.0
   heart (fatty) —*see also* Infarct, myocardium
    not resulting in infarction I24.0
   hepatic (vein) I82.0
   in pregnancy, childbirth or puerperium —*see*
   Embolism, obstetric
   intestine (artery) (vein) (with gangrene) K55.0
   intracranial —*see also* Occlusion, artery,
   cerebral
    venous sinus (any) G08
     nonpyogenic I67.6
   intraspinal venous sinuses or veins G08
    nonpyogenic G95.19
   kidney (artery) N28.0
   lateral sinus (venous) —*see* Embolism,
   intracranial, venous sinus
   leg —*see* Embolism, vein, lower extremity
    arterial I74.3
   longitudinal sinus (venous) —*see* Embolism,
   intracranial, venous sinus
   lung (massive) —*see* Embolism, pulmonary
   meninges I66.8
   mesenteric (artery) (vein) (with gangrene)
   K55.0
   obstetric (in) (pulmonary)
    childbirth O88.82

Embolism – *continued*
  air O88.02
  amniotic fluid O88.12
  blood clot O88.22
  fat O88.82
  pyemic O88.32
  septic O88.32
  specified type NEC O88.82
  pregnancy O88.81
    air O88.01
    amniotic fluid O88.11
    blood clot O88.21
    fat O88.81
    pyemic O88.31
    septic O88.31
    specified type NEC O88.81
  puerperal O88.83
    air O88.03
    amniotic fluid O88.13
    blood clot O88.23
    fat O88.83
    pyemic O88.33
    septic O88.33
    specified type NEC O88.83
  ophthalmic —*see* Occlusion, artery, retina
  penis N48.81
  peripheral artery NOS I74.4
  pituitary E23.6
  popliteal (artery) I74.3
  portal (vein) I81
  postoperative, postprocedural
    artery T81.719
      mesenteric T81.710
      renal T81.711
      specified NEC T81.718
    vein T81.72
  precerebral artery —*see* Occlusion, artery, precerebral
  puerperal —*see* Embolism, obstetric
  pulmonary (acute) (artery) (vein) I26.99
    with acute cor pulmonale I26.09
    chronic I27.82
    following
      abortion —*see* Abortion by type
    complicated by embolism
      ectopic or molar pregnancy O08.2
    healed or old Z86.711
    in pregnancy, childbirth or puerperium —
    see Embolism, obstetric
    personal history of Z86.711
    saddle I26.92
      with acute cor pulmonale I26.02
    septic I26.90
      with acute cor pulmonale I26.01
  pyemic (multiple) I76
    following
      abortion —*see* Abortion by type
    complicated by embolism
      ectopic or molar pregnancy O08.2
    Hemophilus influenzae A41.3
    pneumococcal A40.3
      with pneumonia J13
    puerperal, postpartum, childbirth (any
    organism) —*see* Embolism, obstetric
    specified organism NEC A41.89
    staphylococcal A41.2
    streptococcal A40.9
  renal (artery) N28.0
    vein I82.3
  retina, retinal   *see* Occlusion, artery, retina
  saddle
    abdominal aorta I74.01

Embolism – *continued*
  pulmonary artery I26.92
    with acute cor pulmonale I26.02
  septic (arterial) I76
    complicating abortion —*see* Abortion, by
    type, complicated by, embolism
  sinus —*see* Embolism, intracranial, venous
  sinus
  soap complicating abortion —*see* Abortion,
  by type, complicated by, embolism
  spinal cord G95.19
    pyogenic origin G06.1
  spleen, splenic (artery) I74.8
  upper extremity I74.2
  vein (acute) I82.90
    antecubital I82.61
      chronic I82.71
    axillary I82.A1
      chronic I82.A2
    basilic I82.61
      chronic I82.71
    brachial I82.62
      chronic I82.72
    brachiocephalic (innominate) I82.290
      chronic I82.291
    cephalic I82.61
      chronic I82.71
    chronic I82.91
    deep (DVT) I82.40
      calf I82.4Z
        chronic I82.5Z
      lower leg I82.4Z
        chronic I82.5Z
      thigh I82.4Y
        chronic I82.5Y
      upper leg I82.4Y
        chronic I82.5y
    femoral I82.41
      chronic I82.51
    iliac (iliofemoral) I82.42
      chronic I82.52
    innominate I82.290
      chronic I82.291
    internal jugular I82.C1
      chronic I82.C2
    lower extremity
      deep I82.40
        chronic I82.50
        specified NEC I82.49
          chronic NEC I82.59
      distal
        deep I82.4Z
      proximal
        deep I82.4Y
          chronic I82.5Y
      superficial I82.81
    popliteal I82.43
      chronic I82.53
    radial I82.62
      chronic I82.72
    renal I82.3
    saphenous (greater) (lesser) I82.81
    specified NEC I82.890
      chronic NEC I82.891
    subclavian I82.B1
      chronic I82.B2
    thoracic NEC I82.290
      chronic I82.291
    tibial I82.44
      chronic I82.54
    ulnar I82.62
      chronic I82.72

Embolism – *continued*
  upper extremity I82.60
    chronic I82.70
    deep I82.62
      chronic I82.72
    superficial I82.61
      chronic I82.71
  vena cava
    inferior (acute) I82.220
      chronic I82.221
    superior (acute) I82.210
      chronic I82.211
  venous sinus G08
  vessels of brain —*see* Occlusion, artery,
  cerebral
Embolus —*see* Embolism
Embryoma —*see also* Neoplasm, uncertain
behavior, by site
  benign —*see* Neoplasm, benign, by site
  kidney C64.
  liver C22.0
  malignant —*see also* Neoplasm, malignant,
  by site
    kidney C64.
    liver C22.0
    testis C62.9
      descended (scrotal) C62.1
      undescended C62.0
  testis C62.9
    descended (scrotal) C62.1
    undescended C62.0
Embryonic
  circulation Q28.9
  heart Q28.9
  vas deferens Q55.4
Embryopathia NOS Q89.9
Embryotoxon Q13.4
Emesis —*see* Vomiting
Emotional lability R45.86
Emotionality, pathological F60.3
Emotogenic disease —*see* Disorder,
psychogenic
Emphysema (atrophic) (bullous) (chronic)
(interlobular) (lung) (obstructive) (pulmonary)
(senile) (vesicular) J43.9
  cellular tissue (traumatic) T79.7
    surgical T81.82
  centrilobular J43.2
  compensatory J98.3
  congenital (interstitial) P25.0
  conjunctiva H11.89
  connective tissue (traumatic) T79.7
    surgical T81.82
  due to chemicals, gases, fumes or vapors
  J68.4
  eyelid (s) —*see* Disorder, eyelid, specified
  type NEC
    surgical T81.82
    traumatic T79.7
  interstitial J98.2
    congenital P25.0
    perinatal period P25.0
  laminated tissue T79.7
    surgical T81.82
  mediastinal J98.2
    newborn P25.2
  orbit, orbital —*see* Disorder, orbit, specified
  type NEC
  panacinar J43.1
  panlobular J43.1
  specified NEC J43.8

Emphysema - *continued*
subcutaneous (traumatic) T79.7
  nontraumatic J98.2
  postprocedural T81.82
  surgical T81.82
surgical T81.82
thymus (gland) (congenital) E32.8
traumatic (subcutaneous) T79.7
unilateral J43.0
Empty nest syndrome Z60.0
Empyema (acute) (chest) (double) (pleura) (supradiaphragmatic) (thorax) J86.9
with fistula J86.0
accessory sinus (chronic) —*see* Sinusitis
antrum (chronic) —*see* Sinusitis, maxillary
brain (any part) —*see* Abscess, brain
ethmoidal (chronic) (sinus) —*see* Sinusitis, ethmoidal
extradural —*see* Abscess, extradural
frontal (chronic) (sinus) —*see* Sinusitis, frontal
gallbladder K81.0
mastoid (process) (acute) —*see* Mastoiditis, acute
maxilla, maxillary M27.2
  sinus (chronic) —*see* Sinusitis, maxillary
nasal sinus (chronic) —*see* Sinusitis
sinus (accessory) (chronic) (nasal) —*see* Sinusitis
sphenoidal (sinus) (chronic) —*see* Sinusitis, sphenoidal
subarachnoid —*see* Abscess, extradural
subdural —*see* Abscess, subdural
tuberculous A15.6
ureter —*see* Ureteritis
ventricular —*see* Abscess, brain
En coup de sabre lesion L94.1
Enamel pearls K00.2
Enameloma K00.2
Enanthema, viral B09
Encephalitis (chronic) (hemorrhagic) (idiopathic) (nonepidemic) (spurious) (subacute) G04.90
acute (*see also* Encephalitis, viral) A86
  disseminated G04.00
    infectious G04.01
    noninfectious G04.81
    postimmunization (postvaccination) G04.02
    postinfectious G04.01
  inclusion body A85.8
  necrotizing hemorrhagic G04.30
    postimmunization G04.32
    postinfectious G04.31
    specified NEC G04.39
arboviral, arbovirus NEC A85.2
arthropod-borne NEC (viral) A85.2
Australian A83.4
California (virus) A83.5
Central European (tick-borne) A84.1
Czechoslovakian A84.1
Dawson's (inclusion body) A81.1
diffuse sclerosing A81.1
disseminated, acute G04.00
due to
  cat scratch disease A28.1
  human immunodeficiency virus (HIV) disease B20 *[G05.3]*
  malaria —*see* Malaria
  rickettsiosis —*see* Rickettsiosis
  smallpox inoculation G04.02
  typhus —*see* Typhus

Encephalitis - *continued*
Eastern equine A83.2
endemic (viral) A86
epidemic NEC (viral) A86
equine (acute) (infectious) (viral) A83.9
  Eastern A83.2
  Venezuelan A92.2
  Western A83.1
Far Eastern (tick-borne) A84.0
following vaccination or other immunization procedure G04.02
herpes zoster B02.0
herpesviral B00.4
  due to herpesvirus 6 B10.01
  due to herpesvirus 7 B10.09
  specified NEC B10.09
Ilheus (virus) A83.8
inclusion body A81.1
in (due to)
  actinomycosis A42.82
  adenovirus A85.1
  African trypanosomiasis B56.9 *[G05.3]*
  Chagas' disease (chronic) B57.42
  cytomegalovirus B25.8
  enterovirus A85.0
  herpes (simplex) virus B00.4
    due to herpesvirus 6 B10.01
    due to herpesvirus 7 B10.09
    specified NEC B10.09
  infectious disease NEC B99 *[G05.3]*
  influenza —*see* Influenza, with, encephalopathy
  listeriosis A32.12
  measles B05.0
  mumps B26.2
  naegleriasis B60.2
  parasitic disease NEC B89 *[G05.3]*
  poliovirus A80.9 *[G05.3]*
  rubella B06.01
  syphilis
    congenital A50.42
    late A52.14
  systemic lupus erythematosus M32.19
  toxoplasmosis (acquired) B58.2
    congenital P37.1
  tuberculosis A17.82
  zoster B02.0
infectious (acute) (virus) NEC A86
Japanese (B type) A83.0
La Crosse A83.5
lead —*see* Poisoning, lead
lethargica (acute) (infectious) A85.8
louping ill A84.8
lupus erythematosus, systemic M32.19
lymphatica A87.2
Mengo A85.8
meningococcal A39.81
Murray Valley A83.4
otitic NEC H66.40 *[G05.3]*
parasitic NOS B71.9
periaxial G37.0
periaxialis (concentrica) (diffuse) G37.5
post chickenpox B01.11
postexanthematous NEC B09
postimmunization G04.02
postinfectious NEC G04.01
postmeasles B05.0
postvaccinal G04.02
post varicella B01.11
postviral NEC A86
Powassan A84.8
Rasmussen G04.81

Encephalitis - *continued*
Rio Bravo A85.8
Russian
  autumnal A83.0
  spring-summer (taiga) A84.0
saturnine —*see* Poisoning, lead
specified NEC G04.81
St. Louis A83.3
subacute sclerosing A81.1
summer A83.0
suppurative G04.81
tick-borne A84.9
Torula, torular (cryptococcal) B45.1
toxic NEC G92
trichinosis B75 *[G05.3]*
type
  B A83.0
  C A83.3
van Bogaert's A81.1
Venezuelan equine A92.2
Vienna A85.8
viral, virus A86
  arthropod-borne NEC A85.2
  mosquito-borne A83.9
    Australian X disease A83.4
    California virus A83.5
    Eastern equine A83.2
    Japanese (B type) A83.0
    Murray Valley A83.4
    specified NEC A83.8
    St. Louis A83.3
    type B A83.0
    type C A83.3
    Western equine A83.1
  tick-borne A84.9
    biundulant A84.1
    central European A84.1
    Czechoslovakian A84.1
    diphasic meningoencephalitis A84.1
    Far Eastern A84.0
    Russian spring-summer (taiga) A84.0
    specified NEC A84.8
  specified type NEC A85.8
Western equine A83.1
Encephalocele Q01.9
frontal Q01.0
nasofrontal Q01.1
occipital Q01.2
specified NEC Q01.8
Encephalocystocele —*see* Encephalocele
Encephaloduroarteriomyosynangiosis (EDAMS) I67.5
Encephalomalacia (brain) (cerebellar) (cerebral) —*see* Softening, brain
Encephalomeningitis —*see* Meningoencephalitis
Encephalomeningocele —*see* Encephalocele
Encephalomeningomyelitis —*see* Meningoencephalitis
Encephalomyelitis (*see also* Encephalitis) G04.90
acute disseminated G04.00
  infectious G04.01
  noninfectious G04.81
  postimmunization G04.02
  postinfectious G04.01
acute necrotizing hemorrhagic G04.30
  postimmunization G04.32
  postinfectious G04.31
  specified NEC G04.39
benign myalgic G93.3
equine A83.9
  Eastern A83.2

Encephalomyelitis - *continued*
    Venezuelan A92.2
    Western A83.1
    in diseases classified elsewhere G05.3
    myalgic, benign G93.3
    post chickenpox B01.11
    postinfectious NEC G04.01
    postmeasles B05.0
    postvaccinal G04.02
    post varicella B01.11
    rubella B06.01
    specified NEC G04.81
    Venezuelan equine A92.2
Encephalomyelocele —*see* Encephalocele
Encephalomyelomeningitis —*see*
    Meningoencephalitis
Encephalomyelopathy G96.9
Encephalomyeloradiculitis (acute) G61.0
Encephalomyeloradiculoneuritis (acute)
    (Guillain-Barré) G61.0
Encephalomyeloradiculopathy G96.9
Encephalopathia hyperbilirubinemia,
newborn P57.9
    due to isoimmunization (conditions in P55)
    P57.0
Encephalopathy (acute) G93.40
    acute necrotizing hemorrhagic G04.30
        postimmunization G04.32
        postinfectious G04.31
        specified NEC G04.39
    alcoholic G31.2
    anoxic —*see* Damage, brain, anoxic
    arteriosclerotic I67.2
    centrolobar progressive (Schilder) G37.0
    congenital Q07.9
    degenerative, in specified disease NEC
    G32.89
    demyelinating callosal G37.1
    due to
      drugs
    (*see also* Table of Drugs and Chemicals) G92
    hepatic —*see* Failure, hepatic
    hyperbilirubinemic, newborn P57.9
      due to isoimmunization (conditions in P55)
    P57.0
    hypertensive I67.4
    hypoglycemic E16.2
    hypoxic —*see* Damage, brain, anoxic
    hypoxic ischemic P91.60
      mild P91.61
      moderate P91.62
      severe P91.63
    in (due to) (with)
      birth injury P11.1
      hyperinsulinism E16.1 *[G94]*
      influenza —*see* Influenza, with,
    encephalopathy
      lack of vitamin (*see also* Deficiency,
    vitamin) E56.9 *[G32.89]*
      neoplastic disease (see also Neoplasm)
    D49.9 *[G13.1]*
      serum (*see also* Reaction, serum) T80.69
      syphilis A52.17
      trauma (postconcussional) F07.81
        current injury —*see* Injury, intracranial
      vaccination G04.02
    lead —*see* Poisoning, lead
    metabolic G93.41
      drug induced G92
      toxic G92
    myoclonic, early, symptomatic —*see*
    Epilepsy, generalized, specified NEC

Encephalopathy - *continued*
    necrotizing, subacute (Leigh) G31.82
    pellagrous E52 *[G32.89]*
    portosystemic —*see* Failure, hepatic
    postcontusional F07.81
      current injury —*see* Injury, intracranial,
    diffuse
    posthypoglycemic (coma) E16.1 *[G94]*
    postradiation G93.89
    saturnine —*see* Poisoning, lead
    septic G93.41
    specified NEC G93.49
    spongiform, subacute (viral) A81.09
    toxic G92
      metabolic G92
    traumatic (postconcussional) F07.81
      current injury —*see* Injury, intracranial
    vitamin B deficiency NEC E53.9 *[G32.89]*
      vitamin B1 E51.2
    Wernicke's E51.2
Encephalorrhagia —*see* Hemorrhage,
    intracranial, intracerebral
Encephalosis, posttraumatic F07.81
Enchondroma —*see also* Neoplasm, bone,
    benign
Enchondromatosis (cartilaginous) (multiple)
    Q78.4
Encopresis R15.9
    functional F98.1
    nonorganic origin F98.1
    psychogenic F98.1
Encounter (with health service) (for) Z76.89
    adjustment and management (of)
      breast implant Z45.81
      implanted device NEC Z45.89
      myringotomy device (stent) (tube) Z45.82
    administrative purpose only Z02.9
      examination for
        adoption Z02.82
        armed forces Z02.3
        disability determination Z02.71
        driving license Z02.4
        employment Z02.1
        insurance Z02.6
        medical certificate NEC Z02.79
        paternity testing Z02.81
        residential institution admission Z02.2
        school admission Z02.0
        sports Z02.5
      specified reason NEC Z02.89
    aftercare —*see* Aftercare
    antenatal screening Z36
    assisted reproductive fertility procedure cycle
    Z31.83
    blood typing Z01.83
      Rh typing Z01.83
    breast augmentation or reduction Z41.1
    breast implant exchange (different material)
    (different size) Z45.81
    breast reconstruction following mastectomy
    Z42.1
    check-up —*see* Examination
    chemotherapy for neoplasm Z51.11
    colonoscopy, screening Z12.11
    counseling —*see* Counseling
    delivery, full-term, uncomplicated O80
      cesarean, without indication O82
    ear piercing Z41.3
    examination —*see* Examination
    expectant parent (s) (adoptive) pre-birth
    pediatrician visit Z76.81

Encounter – *continued*
    fertility preservation procedure (prior to
    cancer therapy) (prior to removal of gonads)
    Z31.84
    fitting (of) —*see* Fitting (and adjustment) (of)
    genetic
      counseling Z31.5
      testing —*see* Test, genetic
    hearing conservation and treatment Z01.12
    immunotherapy for neoplasm Z51.12
    in vitro fertilization cycle Z31.83
    instruction (in)
      childbirth Z32.2
      child care (postpartal) (prenatal) Z32.3
      natural family planning
        procreative Z31.61
        to avoid pregnancy Z30.02
    insulin pump titration Z46.81
    joint prosthesis insertion following prior
    explantation of joint prosthesis (staged
    procedure)
      hip Z47.32
      knee Z47.33
      shoulder Z47.31
    laboratory (as part of a general medical
    examination) Z00.00
      with abnormal findings Z00.01
    mental health services (for)
      abuse NEC
        perpetrator Z69.82
        victim Z69.81
      child abuse
        nonparental
          perpetrator Z69.021
          victim Z69.020
        parental
          perpetrator Z69.011
          victim Z69.010
      spousal or partner abuse
        perpetrator Z69.12
        victim Z69.11
    observation (for) (ruled out)
      exposure to (suspected)
        anthrax Z03.810
        biological agent NEC Z03.818
    pediatrician visit, by expectant parent (s)
    (adoptive) Z76.81
    plastic and reconstructive surgery following
    medical procedure or healed injury NEC
    Z42.8
    pregnancy
      supervision of —*see* Pregnancy, supervision
    of
      test Z32.00
        result negative Z32.02
        result positive Z32.01
    radiation therapy (antineoplastic) Z51.0
    radiological (as part of a general medical
    examination) Z00.00
      with abnormal findings Z00.01
    reconstructive surgery following medical
    procedure or healed injury NEC Z42.8
    removal (of) —*see also* Removal
      artificial
        arm Z44.00
          complete Z44.01
          partial Z44.02
        eye Z44.2
        leg Z44.10
          complete Z44.11
          partial Z44.12

Encounter – *continued*
　breast implant Z45.81
　　tissue expander (without synchronous
　insertion of permanent implant) Z45.81
　device Z46.9
　　specified NEC Z46.89
　external
　fixation device
　code to fracture with seventh character D
　　prosthesis, prosthetic device Z44.9
　　　breast Z44.3
　　　specified NEC Z44.8
　implanted device NEC Z45.89
　insulin pump Z46.81
　internal fixation device Z47.2
　myringotomy device (stent) (tube) Z45.82
　nervous system device NEC Z46.2
　　brain neuropacemaker Z46.2
　　visual substitution device Z46.2
　　　implanted Z45.31
　non-vascular catheter Z46.82
　orthodontic device Z46.4
　stent
　　ureteral Z46.6
　urinary device Z46.6
　repeat cervical smear to confirm findings of
　recent normal smear following initial
　abnormal smear Z01.42
　respirator -ventilator] use during power
　failure Z99.12
　Rh typing Z01.83
　screening —*see* Screening
　specified NEC Z76.89
　sterilization Z30.2
　suspected condition, ruled out
　　amniotic cavity and membrane Z03.71
　　cervical shortening Z03.75
　　fetal anomaly Z03.73
　　fetal growth Z03.74
　　maternal and fetal conditions NEC Z03.79
　　oligohydramnios Z03.71
　　placental problem Z03.72
　　polyhydramnios Z03.71
　suspected exposure (to) , ruled out
　　anthrax Z03.810
　　biological agents NEC Z03.818
　termination of pregnancy, elective Z33.2
　testing —*see* Test
　therapeutic drug level monitoring Z51.81
　titration, insulin pump Z46.81
　to determine fetal viability of pregnancy
　O36.80
　training
　　insulin pump Z46.81
　X-ray of chest (as part of a general medical
　examination) Z00.00
　　with abnormal findings Z00.01
Encystment —*see* Cyst
Endarteritis (bacterial, subacute) (infective)
I77.6
　brain I67.7
　cerebral or cerebrospinal I67.7
　deformans —*see* Arteriosclerosis
　embolic —*see* Embolism
　obliterans —*see also* Arteriosclerosis
　　pulmonary I28.8
　pulmonary I28.8
　retina —*see* Vasculitis, retina
　senile —*see* Arteriosclerosis
　syphilitic A52.09
　　brain or cerebral A52.04
　　congenital A50.54 *[I79.8]*

Endarteritis - *continued*
　tuberculous A18.89
Endemic —*see* condition
Endocarditis (chronic) (marantic)
(nonbacterial) (thrombotic) (valvular) I38
　with rheumatic fever (conditions in I00)
　　active —*see* Endocarditis, acute, rheumatic
　　inactive or quiescent (with chorea) I09.1
　acute or subacute I33.9
　　infective I33.0
　　rheumatic (aortic) (mitral) (pulmonary)
　(tricuspid) I01.1
　　　with chorea (acute) (rheumatic)
　(Sydenham's) I02.0
　aortic (heart) (nonrheumatic) (valve) I35.8
　　with
　　　mitral disease I08.0
　　　　with tricuspid (valve) disease I08.3
　　　　active or acute I01.1
　　　　　with chorea (acute) (rheumatic)
　(Sydenham's) I02.0
　　　rheumatic fever (conditions in I00)
　　　　active —*see* Endocarditis, acute,
　rheumatic
　　　　inactive or quiescent (with chorea) I06.9
　　　tricuspid (valve) disease I08.2
　　　　with mitral (valve) disease I08.3
　　acute or subacute I33.9
　　arteriosclerotic I35.8
　　rheumatic I06.9
　　　with mitral disease I08.0
　　　　with tricuspid (valve) disease I08.3
　　　active or acute I01.1
　　　　with chorea (acute) (rheumatic)
　(Sydenham's) I02.0
　　　active or acute I01.1
　　　　with chorea (acute) (rheumatic)
　(Sydenham's) I02.0
　　　specified NEC I06.8
　　specified cause NEC I35.8
　　syphilitic A52.03
　arteriosclerotic I38
　atypical verrucous (Libman-Sacks) M32.11
　bacterial (acute) (any valve) (subacute) I33.0
　candidal B37.6
　congenital Q24.8
　constrictive I33.0
　Coxiella burnetii A78 *[I39]*
　Coxsackie B33.21
　due to
　　prosthetic cardiac valve T82.6
　　Q fever A78 *[I39]*
　　Serratia marcescens I33.0
　　typhoid (fever) A01.02
　gonococcal A54.83
　infectious or infective (acute) (any valve)
　(subacute) I33.0
　lenta (acute) (any valve) (subacute) I33.0
　Libman-Sacks M32.11
　listerial A32.82
　Löffler's I42.3
　malignant (acute) (any valve) (subacute) I33.0
　meningococcal A39.51
　mitral (chronic) (double) (fibroid) (heart)
　(inactive) (valve) (with chorea) I05.9
　　with
　　　aortic (valve) disease I08.0
　　　　with tricuspid (valve) disease I08.3
　　　active or acute I01.1
　　　　with chorea (acute) (rheumatic)
　(Sydenham's) I02.0
　　　rheumatic fever (conditions in I00)

Endocarditis – *continued*
　active —*see* Endocarditis, acute,
　rheumatic
　　inactive or quiescent (with chorea) I05.9
　　tricuspid (valve) disease I08.1
　　　with aortic (valve) disease I08.3
　　active or acute I01.1
　　　with chorea (acute) (rheumatic)
　(Sydenham's) I02.0
　　　bacterial I33.0
　　arteriosclerotic I34.8
　　nonrheumatic I34.8
　　　acute or subacute I33.9
　　specified NEC I05.8
　monilial B37.6
　multiple valves I08.9
　　specified disorders I08.8
　mycotic (acute) (any valve) (subacute) I33.0
　pneumococcal (acute) (any valve) (subacute)
　I33.0
　pulmonary (chronic) (heart) (valve) I37.8
　　with rheumatic fever (conditions in I00)
　　　active —*see* Endocarditis, acute, rheumatic
　　　inactive or quiescent (with chorea) I09.89
　　　　with aortic, mitral or tricuspid disease
　I08.8
　　acute or subacute I33.9
　　rheumatic I01.1
　　　with chorea (acute) (rheumatic)
　(Sydenham's) I02.0
　　arteriosclerotic I37.8
　　congenital Q22.2
　　rheumatic (chronic) (inactive) (with chorea)
　I09.89
　　　active or acute I01.1
　　　　with chorea (acute) (rheumatic)
　(Sydenham's) I02.0
　　syphilitic A52.03
　purulent (acute) (any valve) (subacute) I33.0
　Q fever A78 *[I39]*
　rheumatic (chronic) (inactive) (with chorea)
　I09.1
　　active or acute (aortic) (mitral) (pulmonary)
　(tricuspid) I01.1
　　　with chorea (acute) (rheumatic)
　(Sydenham's) I02.0
　rheumatoid —*see* Rheumatoid, carditis
　septic (acute) (any valve) (subacute) I33.0
　streptococcal (acute) (any valve) (subacute)
　I33.0
　subacute —*see* Endocarditis, acute
　suppurative (acute) (any valve) (subacute)
　I33.0
　syphilitic A52.03
　toxic I33.9
　tricuspid (chronic) (heart) (inactive)
　(rheumatic) (valve) (with chorea) I07.9
　　with
　　　aortic (valve) disease I08.2
　　　　mitral (valve) disease I08.3
　　　mitral (valve) disease I08.1
　　　　aortic (valve) disease I08.3
　　　rheumatic fever (conditions in I00)
　　　　active —*see* Endocarditis, acute,
　rheumatic
　　　　inactive or quiescent (with chorea) I07.8
　　active or acute I01.1
　　　with chorea (acute) (rheumatic)
　(Sydenham's) I02.0
　　arteriosclerotic I36.8
　　nonrheumatic I36.8
　　　acute or subacute I33.9
　　specified cause, except rheumatic I36.8

Endocarditis – *continued*
tuberculous —*see* Tuberculosis, endocarditis
typhoid A01.02
ulcerative (acute) (any valve) (subacute) I33.0
vegetative (acute) (any valve) (subacute) I33.0
verrucous (atypical) (nonbacterial) (nonrheumatic) M32.11
Endocardium, endocardial —*see also* condition
cushion defect Q21.2
Endocervicitis —*see also* Cervicitis
due to intrauterine (contraceptive) device T83.6
hyperplastic N72
Endocrine —*see* condition
Endocrinopathy, pluriglandular E31.9
Endodontic
overfill M27.52
underfill M27.53
Endodontitis K04.0
Endomastoiditis —*see* Mastoiditis
Endometrioma N80.9
Endometriosis N80.9
appendix N80.5
bladder N80.8
bowel N80.5
broad ligament N80.3
cervix N80.0
colon N80.5
cul-de-sac (Douglas') N80.3
exocervix N80.0
fallopian tube N80.2
female genital organ NEC N80.8
gallbladder N80.8
in scar of skin N80.6
internal N80.0
intestine N80.5
lung N80.8
myometrium N80.0
ovary N80.1
parametrium N80.3
pelvic peritoneum N80.3
peritoneal (pelvic) N80.3
rectovaginal septum N80.4
rectum N80.5
round ligament N80.3
skin (scar) N80.6
specified site NEC N80.8
stromal D39.0
umbilicus N80.8
uterus (internal) N80.0
vagina N80.4
vulva N80.8
Endometritis (decidual) (nonspecific) (purulent) (senile) (atrophic) (suppurative) N71.9
with ectopic pregnancy O08.0
acute N71.0
blenorrhagic (gonococcal) (acute) (chronic) A54.24
cervix, cervical (with erosion or ectropion) —*see also* Cervicitis
hyperplastic N72
chlamydial A56.11
chronic N71.1
following
abortion —*see* Abortion by type
complicated by genital infection
ectopic or molar pregnancy O08.0
gonococcal, gonorrheal (acute) (chronic) A54.24

Endometritis - *continued*
hyperplastic (*see also* Hyperplasia, endometrial) N85.00
cervix N72
puerperal, postpartum, childbirth O86.12
subacute N71.0
tuberculous A18.17
Endometrium —*see* condition
Endomyocardiopathy, South African I42.3
Endomyocarditis —*see* Endocarditis
Endomyofibrosis I42.3
Endomyometritis —*see* Endometritis
Endopericarditis —*see* Endocarditis
Endoperineuritis —*see* Disorder, nerve
Endophlebitis —*see* Phlebitis
Endophthalmia —*see* Endophthalmitis, purulent
Endophthalmitis (acute) (infective) (metastatic) (subacute) H44.009
bleb associated H59.4 —*see also* Bleb, inflamed (infected) , postprocedural
gonorrheal A54.39
in (due to)
cysticercosis B69.1
onchocerciasis B73.01
toxocariasis B83.0
panuveitis —*see* Panuveitis
parasitic H44.12
purulent H44.00
panophthalmitis —*see* Panophthalmitis
vitreous abscess H44.02
specified NEC H44.19
sympathetic —*see* Uveitis, sympathetic
Endosalpingioma D28.2
Endosalpingiosis N94.89
Endosteitis —*see* Osteomyelitis
Endothelioma, bone —*see* Neoplasm, bone, malignant
Endotheliosis (hemorrhagic infectional) D69.8
Endotoxemia
code to condition
Endotrachelitis —*see* Cervicitis
Engelmann (-Camurati) **syndrome** Q78.3
English disease —*see* Rickets
Engman's disease L30.3
Engorgement
breast N64.59
newborn P83.4
puerperal, postpartum O92.79
lung (passive) —*see* Edema, lung
pulmonary (passive) —*see* Edema, lung
stomach K31.89
venous, retina —*see* Occlusion, retina, vein, engorgement
Enlargement, enlarged —*see also* Hypertrophy
adenoids J35.2
with tonsils J35.3
alveolar ridge K08.8
congenital —*see* Anomaly, alveolar
apertures of diaphragm (congenital) Q79.1
gingival K06.1
heart, cardiac —*see* Hypertrophy, cardiac
lacrimal gland, chronic H04.03
liver —*see* Hypertrophy, liver
lymph gland or node R59.9
generalized R59.1
localized R59.0
orbit H05.34
organ or site, congenital NEC —*see* Anomaly, by site
parathyroid (gland) E21.0
pituitary fossa R93.0

Enlargement, enlarged - *continued*
prostate N40.0
with lower urinary tract symptoms (LUTS) N40.1
without lower urinary tract symptoms (LUTS) N40.0
sella turcica R93.0
spleen —*see* Splenomegaly
thymus (gland) (congenital) E32.0
thyroid (gland) —*see* Goiter
tongue K14.8
tonsils J35.1
with adenoids J35.3
uterus N85.2
Enophthalmos H05.40
due to
orbital tissue atrophy H05.41
trauma or surgery H05.42
Enostosis M27.8
Entamebic, entamebiasis —*see* Amebiasis
Entanglement
umbilical cord (s) O69.2
with compression O69.2
without compression O69.82
around neck (with compression) O69.1
without compression O69.81
of twins in monoamniotic sac O69.2
Enteralgia —*see* Pain, abdominal
Enteric —*see* condition
Enteritis (acute) (diarrheal) (hemorrhagic) (noninfective) (septic) K52.9
adenovirus A08.2
aertrycke infection A02.0
allergic K52.2
amebic (acute) A06.0
with abscess —*see* Abscess, amebic
chronic A06.1
with abscess —*see* Abscess, amebic
nondysenteric A06.2
nondysenteric A06.2
astrovirus A08.32
bacillary NOS A03.9
bacterial A04.9
specified NEC A04.8
calicivirus A08.31
candidal B37.82
Chilomastix A07.8
choleriformis A00.1
chronic (noninfectious) K52.9
ulcerative —*see* Colitis, ulcerative
cicatrizing (chronic) —*see* Enteritis, regional, small intestine
Clostridium
botulinum (food poisoning) A05.1
difficile A04.7
coccidial A07.3
coxsackie virus A08.39
dietetic K52.2
drug-induced K52.1
due to
astrovirus A08.32
calicivirus A08.31
coxsackie virus A08.39
drugs K52.1
echovirus A08.39
enterovirus NEC A08.39
food hypersensitivity K52.2
infectious organism (bacterial) (viral) —*see* Enteritis, infectious
torovirus A08.39
Yersinia enterocolitica A04.6
echovirus A08.39
eltor A00.1

Enteritis - *continued*
  enterovirus NEC A08.39
  eosinophilic K52.81
  epidemic (infectious) A09
  fulminant K55.0
  gangrenous —*see* Enteritis, infectious
  giardial A07.1
  infectious NOS A09
    due to
      adenovirus A08.2
      Aerobacter aerogenes A04.8
      Arizona (bacillus) A02.0
      bacteria NOS A04.9
        specified NEC A04.8
      Campylobacter A04.5
      Clostridium difficile A04.7
      Clostridium perfringens A04.8
      Enterobacter aerogenes A04.8
      enterovirus A08.39
      Escherichia coli A04.4
        enteroaggregative A04.4
        enterohemorrhagic A04.3
        enteroinvasive A04.2
        enteropathogenic A04.0
        enterotoxigenic A04.1
        specified NEC A04.4
      specified
        bacteria NEC A04.8
        virus NEC A08.39
      Staphylococcus A04.8
      virus NEC A08.4
        specified type NEC A08.39
      Yersinia enterocolitica A04.6
    specified organism NEC A08.8
  influenzal —*see* Influenza, with, digestive manifestations
  ischemic K55.9
    acute K55.0
    chronic K55.1
  microsporidial A07.8
  mucomembranous, myxomembranous —*see* Syndrome, irritable bowel
  mucous —*see* Syndrome, irritable bowel
  necroticans A05.2
  necrotizing of newborn —*see* Enterocolitis, necrotizing, in newborn
  neurogenic —*see* Syndrome, irritable bowel
  newborn necrotizing —*see* Enterocolitis, necrotizing, in newborn
  noninfectious K52.9
  norovirus A08.11
  parasitic NEC B82.9
  paratyphoid (fever) —*see* Fever, paratyphoid
  protozoal A07.9
    specified NEC A07.8
  radiation K52.0
  regional (of) K50.90
    with
      complication K50.919
        abscess K50.914
        fistula K50.913
        intestinal obstruction K50.912
        rectal bleeding K50.911
        specified complication NEC K50.918
    colon —*see* Enteritis, regional, large intestine
    duodenum —*see* Enteritis, regional, small intestine
    ileum —*see* Enteritis, regional, small intestine
    jejunum —*see* Enteritis, regional, small intestine

Enteritis - *continued*
  large bowel —*see* Enteritis, regional, large intestine
  large intestine (colon) (rectum) K50.10
    with
      complication K50.119
        abscess K50.114
        fistula K50.113
        intestinal obstruction K50.112
        rectal bleeding K50.111
        small intestine (duodenum) (ileum) (jejunum) involvement K50.80
        with
          complication K50.819
            abscess K50.814
            fistula K50.813
            intestinal obstruction K50.812
            rectal bleeding K50.811
            specified complication NEC K50.818
        specified complication NEC K50.118
    rectum —*see* Enteritis, regional, large intestine
    small intestine (duodenum) (ileum) (jejunum) K50.00
      with
        complication K50.019
          abscess K50.014
          fistula K50.013
          intestinal obstruction K50.012
          large intestine (colon) (rectum) involvement K50.80
            with
              complication K50.819
                abscess K50.814
                fistula K50.813
                intestinal obstruction K50.812
                rectal bleeding K50.811
                specified complication NEC K50.818
          rectal bleeding K50.011
          specified complication NEC K50.018
  rotaviral A08.0
  Salmonella, salmonellosis (arizonae) (cholerae-suis) (enteritidis) (typhimurium) A02.0
  segmental —*see* Enteritis, regional
  septic A09
  Shigella —*see* Infection, Shigella
  small round structured NEC A08.19
  spasmodic, spastic —*see* Syndrome, irritable bowel
  staphylococcal A04.8
    due to food A05.0
  torovirus A08.39
  toxic NEC K52.1
    due to Clostridium difficile A04.7
  trichomonal A07.8
  tuberculous A18.32
  typhosa A01.00
  ulcerative (chronic) —*see* Colitis, ulcerative
  viral A08.4
    adenovirus A08.2
    enterovirus A08.39
    Rotavirus A08.0
    small round structured NEC A08.19
    specified NEC A08.39
    virus specified NEC A08.39
Enterobiasis B80
Enterobius vermicularis (infection) (infestation) B80

Enterocele —*see also* Hernia, abdomen
  pelvic, pelvis (acquired) (congenital) N81.5
  vagina, vaginal (acquired) (congenital) NEC N81.5
Enterocolitis (*see also* Enteritis) K52.9
  due to Clostridium difficile A04.7
  fulminant ischemic K55.0
  granulomatous —*see* Enteritis, regional
  hemorrhagic (acute) K55.0
    chronic K55.1
  infectious NEC A09
  ischemic K55.9
  necrotizing
    due to Clostridium difficile A04.7
    in newborn P77.9
    stage 1 (without pneumatosis, without perforation) P77.1
    stage 2 (with pneumatosis, without perforation) P77.2
    stage 3 (with pneumatosis, with perforation) P77.3
  noninfectious K52.9
    newborn —*see* Enterocolitis, necrotizing, in newborn
  pseudomembranous (newborn) A04.7
  radiation K52.0
    newborn —*see* Enterocolitis, necrotizing, in newborn
  ulcerative (chronic) —*see* Pancolitis, ulcerative (chronic)
Enterogastritis —*see* Enteritis
Enteropathy K63.9
  gluten-sensitive K90.0
  hemorrhagic, terminal K55.0
  protein-losing K90.4
Enteroperitonitis —*see* Peritonitis
Enteroptosis K63.4
Enterorrhagia K92.2
Enterospasm —*see also* Syndrome, irritable, bowel
  psychogenic F45.8
Enterostenosis —*see also* Obstruction, intestine K56.69
Enterostomy
  complication —*see* Complication, enterostomy
  status Z93.4
Enterovirus, as cause of disease classified elsewhere B97.10
  coxsackievirus B97.11
  echovirus B97.12
  other specified B97.19
Enthesopathy (peripheral) M77.9
  Achilles tendinitis —*see* Tendinitis, Achilles
  ankle and tarsus M77.9
    specified type NEC —*see* Enthesopathy, foot, specified type NEC
  anterior tibial syndrome M76.81
  calcaneal spur —*see* Spur, bone, calcaneal
  elbow region M77.8
    lateral epicondylitis —*see* Epicondylitis, lateral
    medial epicondylitis —*see* Epicondylitis, medial
  foot NEC M77.9
    metatarsalgia —*see* Metatarsalgia
    specified type NEC M77.5
  forearm M77.9
  gluteal tendinitis —*see* Tendinitis, gluteal
  hand M77.9
  hip —*see* Enthesopathy, lower limb, specified type NEC

Enthesopathy - *continued*
iliac crest spur —*see* Spur, bone, iliac crest
iliotibial band syndrome —*see* Syndrome,
iliotibial band
knee —*see* Enthesopathy, lower limb, lower
leg, specified type NEC
lateral epicondylitis —*see* Epicondylitis,
lateral
lower limb (excluding foot) M76.9
  Achilles tendinitis —*see* Tendinitis, Achilles
  anterior tibial syndrome M76.81
  gluteal tendinitis —*see* Tendinitis, gluteal
  iliac crest spur —*see* Spur, bone, iliac crest
  iliotibial band syndrome —*see* Syndrome,
  iliotibial band
    patellar tendinitis —*see* Tendinitis, patellar
    pelvic region —*see* Enthesopathy, lower
limb, specified type NEC
  peroneal tendinitis —*see* Tendinitis,
peroneal
    posterior tibial syndrome M76.82
    psoas tendinitis —*see* Tendinitis, psoas
    shoulder M77.9
    specified type NEC M76.89
    tibial collateral bursitis —*see* Bursitis, tibial
collateral
medial epicondylitis —*see* Epicondylitis,
medial
metatarsalgia —*see* Metatarsalgia
multiple sites M77.9
patellar tendinitis —*see* Tendinitis, patellar
pelvis M77.9
periarthritis of wrist —*see* Periarthritis, wrist
peroneal tendinitis —*see* Tendinitis, peroneal
posterior tibial syndrome M76.82
psoas tendinitis —*see* Tendinitis, psoas
shoulder region —*see* Lesion, shoulder
specified site NEC M77.9
specified type NEC M77.8
spinal M46.00
  cervical region M46.02
  cervicothoracic region M46.03
  lumbar region M46.06
  lumbosacral region M46.07
  multiple sites M46.09
  occipito-atlanto-axial region M46.01
  sacrococcygeal region M46.08
  thoracic region M46.04
  thoracolumbar region M46.05
tibial collateral bursitis —*see* Bursitis, tibial
collateral
upper arm M77.9
wrist and carpus NEC M77.8
  calcaneal spur —*see* Spur, bone, calcaneal
  periarthritis of wrist —*see* Periarthritis, wrist
Entomophobia F40.218
Entomophthoromycosis B46.8
Entrance, air into vein —*see* Embolism, air
Entrapment, nerve —*see* Neuropathy,
entrapment
Entropion (eyelid) (paralytic) H02.009
cicatricial H02.019
  left H02.016
    lower H02.015
    upper H02.014
  right H02.013
    lower H02.012
    upper H02.011
congenital Q10.2
left H02.006
  lower H02.005
  upper H02.004

Entropion – *continued*
mechanical H02.029
  left H02.026
    lower H02.025
    upper H02.024
  right H02.023
    lower H02.022
    upper H02.021
right H02.003
  lower H02.002
  upper H02.001
senile H02.039
  left H02.036
    lower H02.035
    upper H02.034
  right H02.033
    lower H02.032
    upper H02.031
spastic H02.049
  left H02.046
    lower H02.045
    upper H02.044
  right H02.043
    lower H02.042
    upper H02.041
Enucleated eye (traumatic, current) S05.7
Enuresis R32
functional F98.0
habit disturbance F98.0
nocturnal N39.44
  psychogenic F98.0
nonorganic origin F98.0
psychogenic F98.0
Eosinopenia —*see* Agranulocytosis
Eosinophilia (allergic) (hereditary) (idiopathic)
(secondary) D72.1
with
  angiolymphoid hyperplasia (ALHE) D18.01
infiltrative J82
Löffler's J82
peritoneal —*see* Peritonitis, eosinophilic
pulmonary NEC J82
tropical (pulmonary) J82
Eosinophilia-myalgia syndrome M35.8
Ependymitis (acute) (cerebral) (chronic)
(granular) —*see* Encephalomyelitis
Ependymoblastoma
specified site —*see* Neoplasm, malignant, by
site
unspecified site C71.9
Ependymoma (epithelial) (malignant)
anaplastic
  specified site —*see* Neoplasm, malignant,
by site
  unspecified site C71.9
benign
  specified site —*see* Neoplasm, benign, by
site
  unspecified site D33.2
myxopapillary D43.2
  specified site —*see* Neoplasm, uncertain
behavior, by site
  unspecified site D43.2
papillary D43.2
  specified site —*see* Neoplasm, uncertain
behavior, by site
  unspecified site D43.2
specified site —*see* Neoplasm, malignant, by
site
unspecified site C71.9
Ependymopathy G93.89
Ephelis, ephelides L81.2
Epiblepharon (congenital) Q10.3

Epicanthus, epicanthic fold (eyelid)
(congenital) Q10.3
Epicondylitis (elbow)
lateral M77.1
medial M77.0
Epicystitis —*see* Cystitis
Epidemic —*see* condition
Epidermidalization, cervix —*see* Dysplasia,
cervix
Epidermis, epidermal —*see* condition
Epidermodysplasia verruciformis B07.8
Epidermolysis
bullosa (congenital) Q81.9
  acquired L12.30
    drug-induced L12.31
    specified cause NEC L12.35
  dystrophica Q81.2
  letalis Q81.1
  simplex Q81.0
  specified NEC Q81.8
necroticans combustiformis L51.2
  due to drug —*see* Table of Drugs and
Chemicals, by drug
Epidermophytid —*see* Dermatophytosis
Epidermophytosis (infected) —*see*
Dermatophytosis
Epididymis —*see* condition
Epididymitis (acute) (nonvenereal) (recurrent)
(residual) N45.1
with orchitis N45.3
blennorrhagic (gonococcal) A54.23
caseous (tuberculous) A18.15
chlamydial A56.19
filarial (*see also* Infestation, filarial) B74.9
[N51]
gonococcal A54.23
syphilitic A52.76
tuberculous A18.15
Epididymo-orchitis (*see also* Epididymitis)
N45.3
Epidural —*see* condition
Epigastrium, epigastric —*see* condition
Epigastrocele —*see* Hernia, ventral
Epiglottis —*see* condition
Epiglottitis, epiglottiditis (acute) J05.10
with obstruction J05.11
chronic J37.0
Epignathus Q89.4
Epilepsia partialis continua (*see also*
Kozhevnikov's epilepsy) G40.1
Epilepsy, epileptic, epilepsia (attack)
(cerebral) (convulsion) (fit) (seizure) G40.909
Note: the following terms are to be considered
equivalent to intractable: pharmacoresistant
(pharmacologically resistant) , treatment
resistant, refractory (medically) and poorly
controlled
with
  complex partial seizures —*see* Epilepsy,
localization-related, symptomatic, with
complex partial seizures
  grand mal seizures on awakening —*see*
Epilepsy, generalized, specified NEC
  myoclonic absences —*see* Epilepsy,
generalized, specified NEC
  myoclonic-astatic seizures —*see* Epilepsy,
generalized, specified NEC
  simple partial seizures —*see* Epilepsy,
localization-related, symptomatic, with simple
partial seizures
  akinetic —*see* Epilepsy, generalized,
specified NEC

Epilepsy, epileptic, epilepsia - *continued*
benign childhood with centrotemporal EEG spikes —*see* Epilepsy, localization-related, idiopathic
benign myoclonic in infancy G40.80
Bravais-jacksonian —*see* Epilepsy, localization-related, symptomatic, with simple partial seizures
childhood
  with occipital EEG paroxysms —*see* Epilepsy, localization-related, idiopathic
  absence G40.A09
    intractable G40.A19
     with status epilepticus G40.A11
     without status epilepticus G40.A19
    not intractable G40.A09
     with status epilepticus G40.A01
     without status epilepticus G40.A09
climacteric —*see* Epilepsy, specified NEC
cysticercosis B69.0
deterioration (mental) F06.8
due to syphilis A52.19
focal —*see* Epilepsy, localization-related, symptomatic, with simple partial seizures
generalized
  idiopathic G40.309
    intractable G40.319
     with status epilepticus G40.311
     without status epilepticus G40.319
    not intractable G40.309
     with status epilepticus G40.301
     without status epilepticus G40.309
  specified NEC G40.409
    intractable G40.419
     with status epilepticus G40.411
     without status epilepticus G40.419
    not intractable G40.409
     with status epilepticus G40.401
     without status epilepticus G40.409
impulsive petit mal —*see* Epilepsy, juvenile myoclonic
intractable G40.919
  with status epilepticus G40.911
  without status epilepticus G40.919
juvenile absence G40.A09
  intractable G40.A19
    with status epilepticus G40.A11
    without status epilepticus G40.A19
  not intractable G40.A09
    with status epilepticus G40.A01
    without status epilepticus G40.A09
juvenile myoclonic G40.B09
  intractable G40.B19
    with status epilepticus G40.B11
    without status epilepticus G40.B19
  not intractable G40.B09
    with status epilepticus G40.B01
    without status epilepticus G40.B09
localization-related (focal) (partial)
  idiopathic G40.009
    with seizures of localized onset G40.009
    intractable G40.019
     with status epilepticus G40.011
     without status epilepticus G40.019
    not intractable G40.009
     with status epilepticus G40.001
     without status epilepticus G40.009
  symptomatic
    with complex partial seizures G40.209
    intractable G40.219
     with status epilepticus G40.211
     without status epilepticus G40.219

Epilepsy, epileptic, epilepsia - *continued*
    not intractable G40.209
     with status epilepticus G40.201
     without status epilepticus G40.209
    with simple partial seizures G40.109
    intractable G40.119
     with status epilepticus G40.111
     without status epilepticus G40.119
    not intractable G40.109
     with status epilepticus G40.101
     without status epilepticus G40.109
myoclonus, myoclonic (progressive) —*see* Epilepsy, generalized, specified NEC
not intractable G40.909
  with status epilepticus G40.901
  without status epilepticus G40.909
on awakening —*see* Epilepsy, generalized, specified NEC
parasitic NOS B71.9 *[G94]*
partialis continua (*see also* Kozhevnikov's epilepsy) G40.1
peripheral —*see* Epilepsy, specified NEC
procursiva —*see* Epilepsy, localization-related, symptomatic, with simple partial seizures
progressive (familial) myoclonic —*see* Epilepsy, generalized, idiopathic
reflex —*see* Epilepsy, specified NEC
related to
  alcohol G40.509
    not intractable G40.509
     with status epilepticus G40.501
     without status epilepticus G40.509
  drugs G40.509
    not intractable G40.509
     with status epilepticus G40.501
     without status epilepticus G40.509
  external causes G40.509
    not intractable G40.509
     with status epilepticus G40.501
     without status epilepticus G40.509
  hormonal changes G40.509
    not intractable G40.509
     with status epilepticus G40.501
     without status epilepticus G40.509
  sleep deprivation G40.509
    not intractable G40.509
     with status epilepticus G40.501
     without status epilepticus G40.509
  stress G40.509
    not intractable G40.509
     with status epilepticus G40.501
     without status epilepticus G40.509
somatomotor —*see* Epilepsy, localization-related, symptomatic, with simple partial seizures
somatosensory —*see* Epilepsy, localization-related, symptomatic, with simple partial seizures
spasms G40.822
  intractable G40.824
    with status epilepticus G40.823
    without status epilepticus G40.824
  not intractable G40.822
    with status epilepticus G40.821
    without status epilepticus G40.822
specified NEC G40.802
  intractable G40.804
    with status epilepticus G40.803
    without status epilepticus G40.804
  not intractable G40.802
    with status epilepticus G40.801

Epilepsy, epileptic, epilepsia - *continued*
    without status epilepticus G40.802
syndromes
  generalized
    idiopathic G40.309
     intractable G40.319
      with status epilepticus G40.311
      without status epilepticus G40.319
     not intractable G40.309
      with status epilepticus G40.301
      without status epilepticus G40.309
    specified NEC G40.409
     intractable G40.419
      with status epilepticus G40.411
      without status epilepticus G40.419
     not intractable G40.409
      with status epilepticus G40.401
      without status epilepticus G40.409
  localization-related (focal) (partial)
    idiopathic G40.009
     with seizures of localized onset G40.009
     intractable G40.019
      with status epilepticus G40.011
      without status epilepticus G40.019
     not intractable G40.009
      with status epilepticus G40.001
      without status epilepticus G40.009
    symptomatic
     with complex partial seizures G40.209
     intractable G40.219
      with status epilepticus G40.211
      without status epilepticus G40.219
     not intractable G40.209
      with status epilepticus G40.201
      without status epilepticus G40.209
     with simple partial seizures G40.109
     intractable G40.119
      with status epilepticus G40.111
      without status epilepticus G40.119
     not intractable G40.109
      with status epilepticus G40.101
      without status epilepticus G40.109
  specified NEC G40.802
    intractable G40.804
     with status epilepticus G40.803
     without status epilepticus G40.804
    not intractable G40.802
     with status epilepticus G40.801
     without status epilepticus G40.802
tonic (-clonic) —*see* Epilepsy, generalized, specified NEC
twilight F05
uncinate (gyrus) —*see* Epilepsy, localization-related, symptomatic, with complex partial seizures
Unverricht (-Lundborg) (familial myoclonic) —*see* Epilepsy, generalized, idiopathic
visceral —*see* Epilepsy, specified NEC
visual —*see* Epilepsy, specified NEC
Epiloia Q85.1
Epimenorrhea N92.0
Epipharyngitis —*see* Nasopharyngitis
Epiphora H04.20
due to
  excess lacrimation H04.21
  insufficient drainage H04.22
Epiphyseal arrest —*see* Arrest, epiphyseal
Epiphyseolysis, epiphysiolysis —*see* Osteochondropathy
Epiphysitis —*see also* Osteochondropathy
juvenile M92.9
syphilitic (congenital) A50.02

Epiplocele —*see* Hernia, abdomen
Epiploitis —*see* Peritonitis
Epiplosarcomphalocele —*see* Hernia, umbilicus
Episcleritis (suppurative) H15.10
  in (due to)
    syphilis A52.71
    tuberculosis A18.51
  nodular H15.12
  periodica fugax H15.11
    angioneurotic —*see* Edema, angioneurotic
  syphilitic (late) A52.71
  tuberculous A18.51
Episode
  affective, mixed F39
  depersonalization (in neurotic state) F48.1
  depressive F32.9
    major F32.9
      mild F32.0
      moderate F32.1
      severe (without psychotic symptoms) F32.2
        with psychotic symptoms F32.3
    recurrent F33.9
      brief F33.8
    specified NEC F32.8
  hypomanic F30.8
  manic F30.9
    with
      psychotic symptoms F30.2
      remission (full) F30.4
        partial F30.3
    other specified F30.8
    recurrent F31.89
    without psychotic symptoms F30.10
      mild F30.11
      moderate F30.12
      severe (without psychotic symptoms) F30.13
        with psychotic symptoms F30.2
  psychotic F23
    organic F06.8
  schizophrenic (acute) NEC, brief F23
Epispadias (female) (male) Q64.0
Episplenitis D73.89
Epistaxis (multiple) R04.0
  hereditary I78.0
  vicarious menstruation N94.89
Epithelioma (malignant) —*see also* Neoplasm, malignant, by site
  adenoides cysticum —*see* Neoplasm, skin, benign
  basal cell —*see* Neoplasm, skin, malignant
  benign —*see* Neoplasm, benign, by site
  Bowen's —*see* Neoplasm, skin, in situ
  calcifying, of Malherbe —*see* Neoplasm, skin, benign
  external site —*see* Neoplasm, skin, malignant
  intraepidermal, Jadassohn —*see* Neoplasm, skin, benign
  squamous cell —*see* Neoplasm, malignant, by site
Epitheliomatosis pigmented Q82.1
Epitheliopathy, multifocal placoid pigment H30.14
Epithelium, epithelial —*see* condition
Epituberculosis (with atelectasis) (allergic) A15.7
Eponychia Q84.6
Epstein's
  nephrosis or syndrome —*see* Nephrosis
  pearl K09.8
Epulis (gingiva) (fibrous) (giant cell) K06.8

Equinia A24.0
Equinovarus (congenital) (talipes) Q66.0
  acquired —*see* Deformity, limb, clubfoot
Equivalent
  convulsive (abdominal) —*see* Epilepsy, specified NEC
  epileptic (psychic) —*see* Epilepsy, localization-related, symptomatic, with complex partial seizures
Erb (-Duchenne) paralysis (birth injury) (newborn) P14.0
Erb-Goldflam disease or syndrome G70.00
  with exacerbation (acute) G70.01
  in crisis G70.01
Erb's
  disease G71.0
  palsy, paralysis (brachial) (birth) (newborn) P14.0
    spinal (spastic) syphilitic A52.17
  pseudohypertrophic muscular dystrophy G71.0
Erdheim's syndrome (acromegalic macrospondylitis) E22.0
Erection, painful (persistent) —*see* Priapism
Ergosterol deficiency (vitamin D) E55.9
  with
    adult osteomalacia M83.8
    rickets —*see* Rickets
Ergotism —*see also* Poisoning, food, noxious, plant
  from ergot used as drug (migraine therapy) *see* Table of Drugs and Chemicals
Erosio interdigitalis blastomycetica B37.2
Erosion
  artery I77.2
    without rupture I77.89
  bone —*see* Disorder, bone, density and structure, specified NEC
  bronchus J98.09
  cartilage (joint) —*see* Disorder, cartilage, specified type NEC
  cervix (uteri) (acquired) (chronic) (congenital) N86
    with cervicitis N72
  cornea (nontraumatic) —*see* Ulcer, cornea
    recurrent H18.83
    traumatic —*see* Abrasion, cornea
  dental (idiopathic) (occupational) (due to diet, drugs or vomiting) K03.2
  duodenum, postpyloric —*see* Ulcer, duodenum
  esophagus K22.10
    with bleeding K22.11
  gastric —*see* Ulcer, stomach
  gastrojejunal —*see* Ulcer, gastrojejunal
  implanted mesh —*see* Complications, mesh
  intestine K63.3
  lymphatic vessel I89.8
  pylorus, pyloric (ulcer) —*see* Ulcer, stomach
  spine, aneurysmal A52.09
  stomach —*see* Ulcer, stomach
  teeth (idiopathic) (occupational) (due to diet, drugs or vomiting) K03.2
  urethra N36.8
  uterus N85.8
Erotomania F52.8
Error
  metabolism, inborn se Disorder, metabolism
  refractive —*see* Disorder, refraction
Eructation R14.2
  nervous or psychogenic F45.8

Eruption
  creeping B76.9
  drug (generalized) (taken internally) L27.0
    fixed L27.1
    in contact with skin —*see* Dermatitis, due to drugs
    localized L27.1
  Hutchinson, summer L56.4
  Kaposi's varicelliform B00.0
  napkin L22
  polymorphous light (sun) L56.4
  recalcitrant pustular L13.8
  ringed R23.8
  skin (nonspecific) R21
    creeping (meaning hookworm) B76.9
    due to inoculation/vaccination (generalized) (*see also* Dermatitis, due to, vaccine) L27.0
      localized L27.1
    erysipeloid A26.0
    feigned L98.1
    Kaposi's varicelliform B00.0
    lichenoid L28.0
    meaning dermatitis —*see* Dermatitis
    toxic NEC L53.0
  tooth, teeth, abnormal (incomplete) (late) (premature) (sequence) K00.6
  vesicular R23.8
Erysipelas (gangrenous) (infantile) (newborn) (phlegmonous) (suppurative) A46
  external ear A46 *[H62.40]*
  puerperal, postpartum O86.89
Erysipeloid A26.9
  cutaneous (Rosenbach's) A26.0
  disseminated A26.8
  sepsis A26.7
  specified NEC A26.8
Erythema, erythematous (infectional) (inflammation) L53.9
  ab igne L59.0
  annulare (centrifugum) (rheumaticum) L53.1
  arthriticum epidemicum A25.1
  brucellum —*see* Brucellosis
  chronic figurate NEC L53.3
  chronicum migrans (Borrelia burgdorferi) A69.20
  diaper L22
  due to
    chemical NEC L53.0
      in contact with skin L24.5
    drug (internal use) —*see* Dermatitis, due to, drugs
  elevatum diutinum L95.1
  endemic E52
  epidemic, arthritic A25.1
  figuratum perstans L53.3
  gluteal L22
  heat
    code by site under Burn, first degree
  ichthyosiforme congenitum bullous Q80.3
  in diseases classified elsewhere L54
  induratum (nontuberculous) L52
    tuberculous A18.4
  infectiosum B08.3
  intertrigo L30.4
  iris L51.9
  marginatum L53.2
    in (due to) acute rheumatic fever I00
  medicamentosum —*see* Dermatitis, due to, drugs
  migrans A26.0
    chronicum A69.20
    tongue K14.1
  multiforme (major) (minor) L51.9

Erythema, erythematous - *continued*
  bullous, bullosum L51.1
    conjunctiva L51.1
    nonbullous L51.0
    pemphigoides L12.0
    specified NEC L51.8
  napkin L22
  neonatorum P83.8
    toxic P83.1
  nodosum L52
    tuberculous A18.4
  palmar L53.8
  pernio T69.1
  rash, newborn P83.8
  scarlatiniform (recurrent) (exfoliative) L53.8
  solare L55.0
  specified NEC L53.8
  toxic, toxicum NEC L53.0
    newborn P83.1
  tuberculous (primary) A18.4
Erythematous, erythematosus —*see*
  condition
Erythermalgia (primary) I73.81
Erythralgia I73.81
Erythrasma L08.1
Erythredema (polyneuropathy) —*see*
  Poisoning, mercury
Erythremia (acute) C94.0
  chronic D45
  secondary D75.1
Erythroblastopenia (*see also* Aplasia, red
  cell) D60.9
  congenital D61.01
Erythroblastophthisis D61.09
Erythroblastosis (fetalis) (newborn) P55.9
  due to
    ABO (antibodies) (incompatibility)
      (isoimmunization) P55.1
      Rh (antibodies) (incompatibility)
        (isoimmunization) P55.0
Erythrocyanosis (crurum) I73.89
Erythrocythemia —*see* Erythremia
Erythrocytosis (megalosplenic) (secondary)
  D75.1
  familial D75.0
  oval, hereditary —*see* Elliptocytosis
  secondary D75.1
  stress D75.1
Erythroderma (secondary) (*see also*
  Erythema) L53.9
  bullous ichthyosiform, congenital Q80.3
  desquamativum L21.1
  ichthyosiform, congenital (bullous) Q80.3
  neonatorum P83.8
  psoriaticum L40.8
Erythrodysesthesia, palmar plantar (PPE)
  L27.1
Erythrogenesis imperfecta D61.09
Erythroleukemia C94.0
Erythromelalgia I73.81
Erythrophagocytosis D75.89
Erythrophobia F40.298
Erythroplakia, oral epithelium, and tongue
  K13.29
Erythroplasia (Queyrat) D07.4
  specified site —*see* Neoplasm, skin, in situ
  unspecified site D07.4
Escherichia coli (E. coli) , as cause of disease
  classified elsewhere B96.20
  non-O157 Shiga toxin-producing (with known
    O group) B96.22
  non-Shiga toxin-producing B96.29

Escherichia coli – *continued*
  O157 with confirmation of Shiga toxin when
    H antigen is unknown, or is not H7 B96.21
  O157:H (nonmotile) with confirmation of
    Shiga toxin B96.21
  O157:H7 with or without confirmation of
    Shiga toxin-production B96.21
  Shiga toxin-producing (with unspecified O
    group) (STEC) B96.23
  O157 B96.21
  O157:H7 with or without confirmation of
    Shiga toxin-production B96.21
    specified NEC B96.22
  specified NEC B96.29
Esophagismus K22.4
Esophagitis (acute) (alkaline) (chemical)
  (chronic) (infectional) (necrotic) (peptic)
  (postoperative) K20.9
  candidal B37.81
  due to gastrointestinal reflux disease K21.0
  eosinophilic K20.0
  reflux K21.0
  specified NEC K20.8
  tuberculous A18.83
  ulcerative K22.10
    with bleeding K22.11
Esophagocele K22.5
Esophagomalacia K22.8
Esophagospasm K22.4
Esophagostenosis K22.2
Esophagostomiasis B81.8
Esophagotracheal —*see* condition
Esophagus —*see* condition
Esophoria H50.51
  convergence, excess H51.12
  divergence, insufficiency H51.8
Esotropia —*see* Strabismus, convergent
  concomitant
Espundia B55.2
Essential —*see* condition
Esthesioneuroblastoma C30.0
Esthesioneurocytoma C30.0
Esthesioneuroepithelioma C30.0
Esthiomene A55
Estivo-autumnal malaria (fever) B50.9
Estrangement (marital) Z63.5
  parent-child NEC Z62.890
Estriasis —*see* Myiasis
Ethanolism —*see* Alcoholism
Etherism —*see* Dependence, drug, inhalant
Ethmoid, ethmoidal —*see* condition
Ethmoiditis (chronic) (nonpurulent) (purulent)
  —*see also* Sinusitis, ethmoidal
  influenzal —*see* Influenza, with, respiratory
  manifestations NEC
  Woakes' J33.1
Ethylism —*see* Alcoholism
Eulenburg's disease (congenital
  paramyotonia) G71.19
Eumycetoma B47.0
Eunuchoidism E29.1
  hypogonadotropic E23.0
European blastomycosis —*see*
  Cryptococcosis
Eustachian —*see* condition
Evaluation (for) (of)
  development state
    adolescent Z00.3
    period of
      delayed growth in childhood Z00.70
        with abnormal findings Z00.71
      rapid growth in childhood Z00.2

Evaluation – *continued*
    puberty Z00.3
  growth and developmental state (period of
    rapid growth) Z00.2
    delayed growth Z00.70
      with abnormal findings Z00.71
  mental health (status) Z00.8
    requested by authority Z04.6
  period of
    delayed growth in childhood Z00.70
      with abnormal findings Z00.71
    rapid growth in childhood Z00.2
  suspected condition —*see* Observation
Evans syndrome D69.41
Event, apparent life threatening in newborn
  and infant (ALTE) R68.13
Eventration —*see also* Hernia, ventral
  colon into chest —*see* Hernia, diaphragm
  diaphragm (congenital) Q79.1
Eversion
  bladder N32.89
  cervix (uteri) N86
    with cervicitis N72
  foot NEC —*see also* Deformity, valgus, ankle
    congenital Q66.6
  punctum lacrimale (postinfectional) (senile)
    H04.52
  ureter (meatus) N28.89
  urethra (meatus) N36.8
  uterus N81.4
Evidence
  cytologic
    of malignancy on anal smear R85.614
    of malignancy on cervical smear R87.614
    of malignancy on vaginal smear R87.624
Evisceration
  birth injury P15.8
  traumatic NEC
    eye —*see* Enucleated eye
Evulsion —*see* Avulsion
Ewing's sarcoma or tumor
  —*see* Neoplasm, bone, malignant
Examination (for) (following) (general) (of)
  (routine) Z00.00
  with abnormal findings Z00.01
  abuse, physical (alleged) , ruled out
    adult Z04.71
    child Z04.72
  adolescent (development state) Z00.3
  alleged rape or sexual assault (victim) , ruled
    out
    adult Z04.41
    child Z04.42
  allergy Z01.82
  annual (adult) (periodic) (physical) Z00.00
    with abnormal findings Z00.01
    gynecological Z01.419
      with abnormal findings Z01.411
  antibody response Z01.84
  blood —*see* Examination, laboratory
  blood pressure Z01.30
    with abnormal findings Z01.31
  cancer staging —*see* Neoplasm, malignant, by
    site
  cervical Papanicolaou smear Z12.4
    as part of routine gynecological examination
      Z01.419
      with abnormal findings Z01.411
  child (over 28 days old) Z00.129
    with abnormal findings Z00.121
    under 28 days old —*see* Newborn,
      examination

Examination - *continued*
clinical research control or normal
comparison (control) (participant) Z00.6
contraceptive (drug) maintenance (routine)
Z30.8
  device (intrauterine) Z30.431
dental Z01.20
  with abnormal findings Z01.21
developmental —*see* Examination, child
donor (potential) Z00.5
ear Z01.10
  with abnormal findings NEC Z01.118
eye Z01.00
  with abnormal findings Z01.01
following
  accident NEC Z04.3
    transport Z04.1
    work Z04.2
  assault, alleged, ruled out
    adult Z04.71
    child Z04.72
  motor vehicle accident Z04.1
  treatment (for) Z09
    combined NEC Z09
      fracture Z09
      malignant neoplasm Z08
    malignant neoplasm Z08
    mental disorder Z09
    specified condition NEC Z09
follow-up (routine) (following) Z09
  chemotherapy NEC Z09
    malignant neoplasm Z08
  fracture Z09
  malignant neoplasm Z08
  postpartum Z39.2
  psychotherapy Z09
  radiotherapy NEC Z09
    malignant neoplasm Z08
  surgery NEC Z09
    malignant neoplasm Z08
gynecological Z01.419
  with abnormal findings Z01.411
  for contraceptive maintenance Z30.8
health —*see* Examination, medical
hearing Z01.10
  with abnormal findings NEC Z01.118
  following failed hearing screening Z01.110
immunity status testing Z01.84
laboratory (as part of a general medical
examination) Z00.00
  with abnormal findings Z00.01
  preprocedural Z01.812
lactating mother Z39.1
medical (adult) (for) (of) Z00.00
  with abnormal findings Z00.01
  administrative purpose only Z02.9
    specified NEC Z02.89
  admission to
    armed forces Z02.3
    old age home Z02.2
    prison Z02.89
    residential institution Z02.2
    school Z02.0
      following illness or medical treatment
Z02.0
    summer camp Z02.89
  adoption Z02.82
  blood alcohol or drug level Z02.83
  camp (summer) Z02.89
  clinical research, normal subject (control)
(participant) Z00.6

Examination - *continued*
  control subject in clinical research (normal
comparison (participant) Z00.6
  donor (potential) Z00.5
  driving license Z02.4
  general (adult) Z00.00
    with abnormal findings Z00.01
  immigration Z02.89
  insurance purposes Z02.6
  marriage Z02.89
  medicolegal reasons NEC Z04.8
  naturalization Z02.89
  participation in sport Z02.5
  paternity testing Z02.81
  population survey Z00.8
  pre-employment Z02.1
  pre-operative —*see* Examination, pre-
procedural
  pre-procedural
    cardiovascular Z01.810
    respiratory Z01.811
    specified NEC Z01.818
  preschool children
    for admission to school Z02.0
  prisoners
    for entrance into prison Z02.89
  recruitment for armed forces Z02.3
  specified NEC Z00.8
  sport competition Z02.5
medicolegal reason NEC Z04.8
newborn —*see* Newborn, examination
pelvic (annual) (periodic) Z01.419
  with abnormal findings Z01.411
period of rapid growth in childhood Z00.2
periodic (adult) (annual) (routine) Z00.00
  with abnormal findings Z00.01
physical (adult) —*see also* Examination,
medical Z00.00
  sports Z02.5
postpartum
  immediately after delivery Z39.0
  routine follow-up Z39.2
prenatal (normal pregnancy) (*see also*
Pregnancy, normal) Z34.9
pre-chemotherapy (antineoplastic) Z01.818
pre-procedural (pre-operative)
  cardiovascular Z01.810
  laboratory Z01.812
  respiratory Z01.811
  specified NEC Z01.818
prior to chemotherapy (antineoplastic)
Z01.818
psychiatric NEC Z00.8
  follow-up not needing further care Z09
  requested by authority Z04.6
radiological (as part of a general medical
examination) Z00.00
  with abnormal findings Z00.01
repeat cervical smear to confirm findings of
recent normal smear following initial
abnormal smear Z01.42
skin (hypersensitivity) Z01.82
special (*see also* Examination, by type)
Z01.89
  specified type NEC Z01.89
specified type or reason NEC Z04.8
teeth Z01.20
  with abnormal findings Z01.21
urine —*see* Examination, laboratory
vision Z01.00
  with abnormal findings Z01.01

Exanthem, exanthema —*see also* Rash
with enteroviral vesicular stomatitis B08.4
Boston A88.0
epidemic with meningitis A88.0 *[G02]*
subitum B08.20
  due to human herpesvirus 6 B08.21
  due to human herpesvirus 7 B08.22
viral, virus B09
  specified type NEC B08.8
Excess, excessive, excessively
alcohol level in blood R78.0
androgen (ovarian) E28.1
attrition, tooth, teeth K03.0
carotene, carotin (dietary) E67.1
cold, effects of T69.9
  specified effect NEC T69.8
convergence H51.12
crying
  in child, adolescent, or adult R45.83
  in infant R68.11
development, breast N62
divergence H51.8
drinking (alcohol) NEC (without dependence)
F10.10
  habitual (continual) (without remission)
F10.20
eating R63.2
estrogen E28.0
fat —*see also* Obesity
  in heart —*see* Degeneration, myocardial
  localized E65
foreskin N47.8
gas R14.0
glucagon E16.3
heat —*see* Heat
intermaxillary vertical dimension of fully
erupted teeth M26.37
interocclusal distance of fully erupted teeth
M26.37
kalium E87.5
large
  colon K59.3
    congenital Q43.8
  infant P08.0
  organ or site, congenital NEC —*see*
Anomaly, by site
long
  organ or site, congenital NEC —*see*
Anomaly, by site
menstruation (with regular cycle) N92.0
  with irregular cycle N92.1
napping Z72.821
natrium E87.0
number of teeth K00.1
nutrient (dietary) NEC R63.2
potassium (K) E87.5
salivation K11.7
secretion —*see also* Hypersecretion
  milk O92.6
  sputum R09.3
  sweat R61
sexual drive F52.8
short
  organ or site, congenital NEC —*see*
Anomaly, by site
  umbilical cord in labor or delivery O69.3
skin, eyelid (acquired) —*see* Blepharochalasis
  congenital Q10.3
sodium (Na) E87.0
spacing of fully erupted teeth M26.32
sputum R09.3
sweating R61

Excess, excessive, excessively - *continued*
thirst R63.1
due to deprivation of water T73.1
tuberosity of jaw M26.07
vitamin
A (dietary) E67.0
administered as drug (prolonged intake) —
see Table of Drugs and Chemicals, vitamins,
adverse effect
overdose or wrong substance given or
taken —*see* Table of Drugs and Chemicals,
vitamins, poisoning
D (dietary) E67.3
administered as drug (prolonged intake) —
see Table of Drugs and Chemicals, vitamins,
adverse effect
overdose or wrong substance given or
taken —*see* Table of Drugs and Chemicals,
vitamins, poisoning
weight
gain R63.5
loss R63.4
Excitability, abnormal, under minor stress
(personality disorder) F60.3
Excitation
anomalous atrioventricular I45.6
psychogenic F30.8
reactive (from emotional stress, psychological
trauma) F30.8
Excitement
hypomanic F30.8
manic F30.9
mental, reactive (from emotional stress,
psychological trauma) F30.8
state, reactive (from emotional stress,
psychological trauma) F30.8
Excoriation (traumatic) —*see also* Abrasion
neurotic L98.1
Exfoliation
due to erythematous conditions according to
extent of body surface involved L49.0
10 19 percent of body surface L49.1
20 29 percent of body surface L49.2
30 39 percent of body surface L49.3
40 49 percent of body surface L49.4
50 59 percent of body surface L49.5
60 69 percent of body surface L49.6
70 79 percent of body surface L49.7
80 89 percent of body surface L49.8
90 99 percent of body surface L49.9
less than 10 percent of body surface L49.0
teeth, due to systemic causes K08.0
Exfoliative —*see* condition
Exhaustion, exhaustive (physical NEC)
R53.83
battle F43.0
cardiac —*see* Failure, heart
delirium F43.0
due to
cold T69.8
excessive exertion T73.3
exposure T73.2
neurasthenia F48.8
heart —*see* Failure, heart
heat (*see also* Heat, exhaustion) T67.5
due to
salt depletion T67.4
water depletion T67.3
maternal, complicating delivery O75.81
mental F48.8
myocardium, myocardial —*see* Failure, heart
nervous F48.8

Exhaustion, exhaustive -*continued*
old age R54
psychogenic F48.8
psychosis F43.0
senile R54
vital NEC Z73.0
Exhibitionism F65.2
Exocervicitis —*see* Cervicitis
Exomphalos Q79.2
meaning hernia —*see* Hernia, umbilicus
Exophoria H50.52
convergence, insufficiency H51.11
divergence, excess H51.8
Exophthalmos H05.2
congenital Q15.8
constant NEC H05.24
displacement, globe —*see* Displacement,
globe
due to thyrotoxicosis (hyperthyroidism) —*see*
Hyperthyroidism, with, goiter (diffuse)
dysthyroid —*see* Hyperthyroidism, with,
goiter (diffuse)
goiter —*see* Hyperthyroidism, with, goiter
(diffuse)
intermittent NEC H05.25
malignant —*see* Hyperthyroidism, with,
goiter (diffuse)
orbital
edema —*see* Edema, orbit
hemorrhage —*see* Hemorrhage, orbit
pulsating NEC H05.26
thyrotoxic, thyrotropic —*see*
Hyperthyroidism, with, goiter (diffuse)
Exostosis —*see also* Disorder, bone
cartilaginous —*see* Neoplasm, bone, benign
congenital (multiple) Q78.6
external ear canal H61.81
gonococcal A54.49
jaw (bone) M27.8
multiple, congenital Q78.6
orbit H05.35
osteocartilaginous —*see* Neoplasm, bone,
benign
syphilitic A52.77
Exotropia —*see* Strabismus, divergent
concomitant
Explanation of
investigation finding Z71.2
medication Z71.89
Exposure (to) (*see also* Contact, with) T75.89
acariasis Z20.7
AIDS virus Z20.6
air pollution Z77.110
algae and algae toxins Z77.121
algae bloom Z77.121
anthrax Z20.810
aromatic amines Z77.020
aromatic (hazardous) compounds NEC
Z77.028
aromatic dyes NOS Z77.028
arsenic Z77.010
asbestos Z77.090
bacterial disease NEC Z20.818
benzene Z77.021
blue-green algae bloom Z77.121
body fluids (potentially hazardous) Z77.21
brown tide Z77.121
chemicals (chiefly nonmedicinal) (hazardous)
NEC Z77.098
cholera Z20.09
chromium compounds Z77.018
cold, effects of T69.9
specified effect NEC T69.8

Exposure - *continued*
communicable disease Z20.9
bacterial NEC Z20.818
specified NEC Z20.89
viral NEC Z20.828
cyanobacteria bloom Z77.121
disaster Z65.5
discrimination Z60.5
dyes Z77.098
effects of T73.9
environmental tobacco smoke (acute)
(chronic) Z77.22
Escherichia coli (E. coli) Z20.01
exhaustion due to T73.2
fiberglass —*see* Table of Drugs and
Chemicals, fiberglass
German measles Z20.4
gonorrhea Z20.2
hazardous metals NEC Z77.018
hazardous substances NEC Z77.29
hazards in the physical environment NEC
Z77.128
hazards to health NEC Z77.9
human immunodeficiency virus (HIV) Z20.6
human T-lymphotropic virus type 1 (HTLV
1) Z20.89
implanted
mesh —*see* Complications, mesh
prosthetic materials NEC —*see*
Complications, prosthetic materials NEC
infestation (parasitic) NEC Z20.7
intestinal infectious disease NEC Z20.09
Escherichia coli (E. coli) Z20.01
lead Z77.011
meningococcus Z20.811
mold (toxic) Z77.120
nickel dust Z77.018
noise Z77.122
occupational
air contaminants NEC Z57.39
dust Z57.2
environmental tobacco smoke Z57.31
extreme temperature Z57.6
noise Z57.0
radiation Z57.1
risk factors Z57.9
specified NEC Z57.8
toxic agents (gases) (liquids) (solids)
(vapors) in agriculture Z57.4
toxic agents (gases) (liquids) (solids)
(vapors) in industry NEC Z57.5
vibration Z57.7
parasitic disease NEC Z20.7
pediculosis Z20.7
persecution Z60.5
pfiesteria piscicida Z77.121
poliomyelitis Z20.89
polycyclic aromatic hydrocarbons Z77.028
pollution
air Z77.110
environmental NEC Z77.118
soil Z77.112
water Z77.111
prenatal (drugs) (toxic chemicals) —*see*
Newborn, affected by (suspected to be) ,
noxious substances transmitted via placenta or
breast milk
rabies Z20.3
radiation, naturally occurring NEC Z77.123
radon Z77.123
red tide (Florida) Z77.121
rubella Z20.4

Exposure - *continued*
  second hand tobacco smoke (acute) (chronic) Z77.22
    in the perinatal period P96.81
  sexually-transmitted disease Z20.2
  smallpox (laboratory) Z20.89
  syphilis Z20.2
  terrorism Z65.4
  torture Z65.4
  tuberculosis Z20.1
  uranium Z77.012
  varicella Z20.820
  venereal disease Z20.2
  viral disease NEC Z20.828
  war Z65.5
  water pollution Z77.111
Exsanguination —*see* Hemorrhage
Exstrophy
  abdominal contents Q45.8
  bladder Q64.10
    cloacal Q64.12
    specified type NEC Q64.19
    supravesical fissure Q64.11
Extensive —*see* condition
Extra —*see also* Accessory
  marker chromosomes (normal individual) Q92.61
    in abnormal individual Q92.62
  rib Q76.6
    cervical Q76.5
Extrasystoles (supraventricular) I49.49
  atrial I49.1
  auricular I49.1
  junctional I49.2
  ventricular I49.3
Extrauterine gestation or pregnancy
  —*see* Pregnancy, by site
Extravasation
  blood R58
  chyle into mesentery I89.8
  pelvicalyceal N13.8
  pyelosinus N13.8
  urine (from ureter) R39.0
  vesicant agent
    antineoplastic chemotherapy T80.810
    other agent NEC T80.818
Extremity —*see* condition, limb
Extrophy —*see* Exstrophy
Extroversion
  bladder Q64.19
  uterus N81.4
    complicating delivery O71.2
    postpartal (old) N81.4
Extruded tooth (teeth) M26.34
Extrusion
  breast implant (prosthetic) T85.42
  eye implant (globe) (ball) T85.328
  intervertebral disc —*see* Displacement, intervertebral disc
  ocular lens implant (prosthetic) —*see* Complications, intraocular lens
  vitreous —*see* Prolapse, vitreous
Exudate
  pleural —*see* Effusion, pleura
  retina H35.89
Exudative —*see* condition
Eye, eyeball, eyelid —*see* condition
Eyestrain —*see* Disturbance, vision, subjective
Eyeworm disease of Africa B74.3

F

Faber's syndrome (achlorhydric anemia) D50.9
Fabry (-Anderson) **disease** E75.21
Faciocephalalgia, autonomic (*see also* Neuropathy, peripheral, autonomic) G90.09
Factor (s)
  psychic, associated with diseases classified elsewhere F54
  psychological
    affecting physical conditions F54
    or behavioral
      affecting general medical condition F54
      associated with disorders or diseases classified elsewhere F54
Fahr disease (of brain) G23.8
Fahr Volhard disease (of kidney) I12
Failure, failed
  abortion —*see* Abortion, attempted
  aortic (valve) I35.8
    rheumatic I06.8
  attempted abortion —*see* Abortion, attempted
  biventricular I50.9
  bone marrow —*see* Anemia, aplastic
  cardiac —*see* Failure, heart
  cardiorenal (chronic) I50.9
    hypertensive I13.2
  cardiorespiratory (*see also* Failure, heart) R09.2
  cardiovascular (chronic) — *see* Failure, heart
  cerebrovascular I67.9
  cervical dilatation in labor O62.0
  circulation, circulatory (peripheral) R57.9
    newborn P29.89
  compensation —*see* Disease, heart
  compliance with medical treatment or regimen —*see* Noncompliance
  congestive —*see* Failure, heart, congestive
  dental implant (endosseous) M27.69
    due to
      failure of dental prosthesis M27.63
      lack of attached gingiva M27.62
      occlusal trauma (poor prosthetic design) M27.62
      parafunctional habits M27.62
      periodontal infection (peri-implantitis) M27.62
      poor oral hygiene M27.62
    osseointegration M27.61
      due to
        complications of systemic disease M27.61
        poor bone quality M27.61
      iatrogenic M27.61
      post-osseointegration
      biological M27.62
      due to complications of systemic disease M27.62
      iatrogenic M27.62
      mechanical M27.63
      pre-integration M27.61
      pre osseointegration M27.61
    specified NEC M27.69
  descent of head (at term) of pregnancy (mother) O32.4
  endosseous dental implant —*see* Failure, dental implant
  engagement of head (term of pregnancy) (mother) O32.4
  erection (penile) (*see also* Dysfunction, sexual, male, erectile) N52.9
    nonorganic F52.21

Failure, failed - *continued*
  examination (s) , anxiety concerning Z55.2
  expansion terminal respiratory units (newborn) (primary) P28.0
  forceps NOS (with subsequent cesarean delivery) O66.5
  gain weight (child over 28 days old) R62.51
    adult R62.7
    newborn P92.6
  genital response (male) F52.21
    female F52.22
  heart (acute) (senile) (sudden) I50.9
    with
      acute pulmonary edema —*see* Failure, ventricular, left
      decompensation —*see* Failure, heart, congestive
      dilatation —*see* Disease, heart
    arteriosclerotic I70.90
    biventricular I50.9
    combined left-right sided I50.9
    compensated I50.9
    complicating
      anesthesia (general) (local) or other sedation
        in labor and delivery O74.2
        in pregnancy O29.12
        postpartum, puerperal O89.1
      delivery (cesarean) (instrumental) O75.4
    congestive (compensated) (decompensated) I50.9
      with rheumatic fever (conditions in I00)
        active I01.8
        inactive or quiescent (with chorea) I09.81
      newborn P29.0
      rheumatic (chronic) (inactive) (with chorea) I09.81
        active or acute I01.8
          with chorea I02.0
    decompensated I50.9
    degenerative —*see* Degeneration, myocardial
    diastolic (congestive) I50.30
      acute (congestive) I50.31
        and (on) chronic (congestive) I50.33
      chronic (congestive) I50.32
        and (on) acute (congestive) I50.33
      combined with systolic (congestive) I50.40
        acute (congestive) I50.41
          and (on) chronic (congestive) I50.43
        chronic (congestive) I50.42
          and (on) acute (congestive) I50.43
    due to presence of cardiac prosthesis I97.13
    following cardiac surgery I97.13
    high output NOS I50.9
    hypertensive —*see* Hypertension, heart
    left (ventricular) —*see* Failure, ventricular, left
    low output (syndrome) NOS I50.9
    newborn P29.0
    organic *see* Disease, heart
    peripartum O90.3
    postprocedural I97.13
    rheumatic (chronic) (inactive) I09.9
    right (ventricular) (secondary to left heart failure) —*see* Failure, heart, congestive
    systolic (congestive) I50.20
      acute (congestive) I50.21
        and (on) chronic (congestive) I50.23
      chronic (congestive) I50.22
        and (on) acute (congestive) I50.23
      combined with diastolic (congestive) I50.40

Failure, failed - *continued*
acute (congestive) I50.41
  and (on) chronic (congestive) I50.43
  chronic (congestive) I50.42
    and (on) acute (congestive) I50.43
thyrotoxic (*see also* Thyrotoxicosis) E05.90
[143]
  with thyroid storm E05.91 *[143]*
valvular —*see* Endocarditis
hepatic K72.90
  with coma K72.91
  acute or subacute K72.00
    with coma K72.01
    due to drugs K71.10
      with coma K71.11
  alcoholic (acute) (chronic) (subacute)
  K70.40
    with coma K70.41
  chronic K72.10
    with coma K72.11
    due to drugs (acute) (subacute) (chronic)
    K71.10
      with coma K71.11
    due to drugs (acute) (subacute) (chronic)
    K71.10
      with coma K71.11
  postprocedural K91.82
hepatorenal K76.7
induction (of labor) O61.9
  abortion —*see* Abortion, attempted
  by
    oxytocic drugs O61.0
    prostaglandins O61.0
  instrumental O61.1
  mechanical O61.1
  medical O61.0
  specified NEC O61.8
  surgical O61.1
intubation during anesthesia T88.4
  in pregnancy O29.6
  labor and delivery O74.7
  postpartum, puerperal O89.6
involution, thymus (gland) E32.0
kidney (*see also* Disease, kidney, chronic)
N19
  acute (*see also* Failure, renal, acute) N17.9
  diabetic —*see* E08-E13 with .22
lactation (complete) O92.3
  partial O92.4
Leydig's cell, adult E29.1
liver —*see* Failure, hepatic
menstruation at puberty N91.0
mitral I05.8
myocardial, myocardium (*see also* Failure,
heart) I50.9
  chronic (*see also* Failure, heart, congestive)
  I50.9
  congestive (*see also* Failure, heart,
  congestive) I50.9
orgasm (female) (psychogenic) F52.31
  male F52.32
ovarian (primary) E28.39
  iatrogenic E89.40
    asymptomatic E89.40
    symptomatic E89.41
  postprocedural (postablative)
  (postirradiation) (postsurgical) E89.40
    asymptomatic E89.40
    symptomatic E89.41
ovulation causing infertility N97.0
polyglandular, autoimmune E31.0

Failure, failed - *continued*
prosthetic joint implant —*see* Complications,
joint prosthesis, mechanical, breakdown, by
site
renal N19
  with
    tubular necrosis (acute) N17.0
  acute N17.9
    with
      cortical necrosis N17.1
      medullary necrosis N17.2
      tubular necrosis N17.0
    specified NEC N17.8
  chronic N18.9
    hypertensive —*see* Hypertension, kidney
  congenital P96.0
  end stage (chronic) N18.6
    due to hypertension I12.0
  following
    abortion —*see* Abortion by type
  complicated by specified condition NEC
    crushing T79.5
    ectopic or molar pregnancy O08.4
    labor and delivery (acute) O90.4
  hypertensive —*see* Hypertension, kidney
  postprocedural N99.0
respiration, respiratory J96.90
  with
    hypercapnia J96.92
    hypoxia J96.91
  acute J96.00
    with
      hypercapnia J96.02
      hypoxia J96.01
  center G93.89
  acute and (on) chronic J96.20
    with
      hypercapnia J96.22
      hypoxia J96.21
  chronic J96.10
    with
      hypercapnia J96.12
      hypoxia J96.11
  newborn P28.5
  postprocedural (acute) J95.821
    acute and chronic J95.822
rotation
  cecum Q43.3
  colon Q43.3
  intestine Q43.3
  kidney Q63.2
sedation (conscious) (moderate) during
procedure T88.52
  history of Z92.83
segmentation —*see also* Fusion
  fingers —*see* Syndactylism, complex,
fingers
  vertebra Q76.49
    with scoliosis Q76.3
seminiferous tubule, adult E29.1
senile (general) R54
sexual arousal (male) F52.21
  female F52.22
testicular endocrine function E29.1
to thrive (child over 28 days old) R62.51
  adult R62.7
  newborn P92.6
transplant T86.92
  bone T86.831
    marrow T86.02
  cornea T86.841
  heart T86.22
    with lung (s) T86.32

Failure, failed - *continued*
  intestine T86.851
  kidney T86.12
  liver T86.42
  lung (s) T86.811
    with heart T86.32
  pancreas T86.891
  skin (allograft) (autograft) T86.821
  specified organ or tissue NEC T86.891
  stem cell (peripheral blood) (umbilical cord)
  T86.5
trial of labor (with subsequent cesarean
delivery) O66.40
  following previous cesarean delivery O66.41
tubal ligation N99.89
urinary —*see* Disease, kidney, chronic
vacuum extraction NOS (with subsequent
cesarean delivery) O66.5
vasectomy N99.89
ventouse NOS (with subsequent cesarean
delivery) O66.5
ventricular (*see also* Failure, heart) I50.9
  left I50.1
    with rheumatic fever (conditions in I00)
      active I01.8
        with chorea I02.0
      inactive or quiescent (with chorea) I09.81
    rheumatic (chronic) (inactive) (with
chorea) I09.81
      active or acute I01.8
        with chorea I02.0
  right (*see also* Failure, heart, congestive)
  I50.9
vital centers, newborn P91.8
Fainting (fit) R55
Fallen arches —*see* Deformity, limb, flat foot
Falling, falls (repeated) R29.6
  any organ or part —*see* Prolapse
Fallopian
  insufflation Z31.41
  tube —*see* condition
Fallot's
  pentalogy Q21.8
  tetrad or tetralogy Q21.3
  triad or trilogy Q22.3
False —*see also* condition
  croup J38.5
  joint —*see* Nonunion, fracture
  labor (pains) O47.9
    at or after 37 completed weeks of gestation
O47.1
    before 37 completed weeks of gestation
O47.0
  passage, urethra (prostatic) N36.5
  pregnancy F45.8
Family, familial —*see also* condition
  disruption Z63.8
    involving divorce or separation Z63.5
  Li-Fraumeni (syndrome) Z15.01
  planning advice Z30.09
  problem Z63.9
    specified NEC Z63.8
  retinoblastoma C69.2
Famine (effects of) T73.0
  edema —*see* Malnutrition, severe
Fanconi (-de Toni) (-Debré) **syndrome** E72.09
  with cystinosis E72.04
Fanconi's anemia (congenital pancytopenia)
D61.09
Farber's disease or syndrome E75.29
Farcy A24.0

Farmer's
  lung J67.0
  skin L57.8
Farsightedness —*see* Hypermetropia
Fascia —*see* condition
Fasciculation R25.3
Fasciitis M72.9
  diffuse (eosinophilic) M35.4
  infective M72.8
    necrotizing M72.6
  necrotizing M72.6
  nodular M72.4
  perirenal (with ureteral obstruction) N13.5
    with infection N13.6
  plantar M72.2
  specified NEC M72.8
  traumatic (old) M72.8
    current
  code by site under Sprain
Fascioliasis B66.3
Fasciolopsis, fasciolopsiasis (intestinal) B66.5
Fascioscapulohumeral myopathy G71.0
Fast pulse R00.0
Fat
  embolism —*see* Embolism, fat
  excessive —*see also* Obesity
    in heart —*see* Degeneration, myocardial
  in stool R19.5
  localized (pad) E65
    heart —*see* Degeneration, myocardial
    knee M79.4
    retropatellar M79.4
  necrosis
    breast N64.1
    mesentery K65.4
    omentum K65.4
  pad E65
    knee M79.4
Fatigue R53.83
  auditory deafness —*see* Deafness
  chronic R53.82
  combat F43.0
  general R53.83
    psychogenic F48.8
  heat (transient) T67.6
  muscle M62.89
  myocardium —*see* Failure, heart
  neoplasm-related R53.0
  nervous, neurosis F48.8
  operational F48.8
  psychogenic (general) F48.8
  senile R54
  voice R49.8
Fatness —*see* Obesity
Fatty —*see also* condition
  apron E65
  degeneration —*see* Degeneration, fatty
  heart (enlarged) —*see* Degeneration,
  myocardial
  liver NEC K76.0
    alcoholic K70.0
    nonalcoholic K76.0
  necrosis —*see* Degeneration, fatty
Fauces —*see* condition
Fauchard's disease (periodontitis) —*see*
  Periodontitis
Faucitis J02.9
Favism (anemia) D55.0
Favus —*see* Dermatophytosis
Fazio-Londe disease or syndrome G12.1
Fear complex or reaction F40.9
Fear of —*see* Phobia
Feared complaint unfounded Z71.1

Febris, febrile —*see also* Fever
  flava (*see also* Fever, yellow) A95.9
  melitensis A23.0
  pestis —*see* Plague
  recurrens —*see* Fever, relapsing
  rubra A38.9
Fecal
  incontinence R15.9
  smearing R15.1
  soiling R15.1
  urgency R15.2
Fecalith (impaction) K56.41
  appendix K38.1
  congenital P76.8
Fede's disease K14.0
**Feeble rapid pulse due to shock following
  injury** T79.4
Feeble-minded F70
Feeding
  difficulties R63.3
  problem R63.3
    newborn P92.9
      specified NEC P92.8
    nonorganic (adult) —*see* Disorder, eating
Feeling (of)
  foreign body in throat R09.89
Feer's disease —*see* Poisoning, mercury
Feet —*see* condition
Feigned illness Z76.5
Feil-Klippel syndrome (brevicollis) Q76.1
Feinmesser's (hidrotic) **ectodermal dysplasia**
  Q82.4
Felinophobia F40.218
Felon —*see also* Cellulitis, digit
  with lymphangitis —*see* Lymphangitis, acute,
  digit
Felty's syndrome M05.00
  ankle M05.07
  elbow M05.02
  foot joint M05.07
  hand joint M05.04
  hip M05.05
  knee M05.06
  multiple site M05.09
  shoulder M05.01
  vertebra —*see* Spondylitis, ankylosing
  wrist M05.03
Female genital cutting status —*see* Female
  genital mutilation status (FGM)
Female genital mutilation status (FGM)
  N90.810
  specified NEC N90.818
  type I (clitorectomy status) N90.811
  type II (clitorectomy with excision of labia
  minora status) N90.812
  type III (infibulation status) N90.813
  type IV N90.818
Femur, femoral —*see* condition
Fenestration, fenestrated —*see also*
  Imperfect, closure
  aortico pulmonary Q21.4
  cusps, heart valve NEC Q24.8
    pulmonary Q22.3
  pulmonic cusps Q22.3
Fernell's disease (aortic aneurysm) I71.9
Fertile eunuch syndrome E23.0
Fetid
  breath R19.6
  sweat L75.0
Fetishism F65.0
  transvestic F65.1

Fetus, fetal —*see also* condition
  alcohol syndrome (dysmorphic) Q86.0
  compressus O31.0
  hydantoin syndrome Q86.1
  lung tissue P28.0
  papyraceous O31.0
Fever (inanition) (of unknown origin)
  (persistent) (with chills) (with rigor) R50.9
  abortus A23.1
  Aden (dengue) A90
  African tick-borne A68.1
  American
    mountain (tick) A93.2
    spotted A77.0
  aphthous B08.8
  arbovirus, arboviral A94
    hemorrhagic A94
    specified NEC A93.8
  Argentinian hemorrhagic A96.0
  Assam B55.0
  Australian Q A78
  Bangkok hemorrhagic A91
  Barmah forest A92.8
  Bartonella A44.0
  bilious, hemoglobinuric B50.8
  blackwater B50.8
  blister B00.1
  Bolivian hemorrhagic A96.1
  Bonvale dam T73.3
  boutonneuse A77.1
  brain —*see* Encephalitis
  Brazilian purpuric A48.4
  breakbone A90
  Bullis A77.0
  Bunyamwera A92.8
  Burdwan B55.0
  Bwamba A92.8
  Cameroon —*see* Malaria
  Canton A75.9
  catarrhal (acute) J00
    chronic J31.0
  cat-scratch A28.1
  Central Asian hemorrhagic A98.0
  cerebral —*see* Encephalitis
  cerebrospinal meningococcal A39.0
  Chagres B50.9
  Chandipura A92.8
  Changuinola A93.1
  Charcot's (biliary) (hepatic) (intermittent)
  see Calculus, bile duct
  Chikungunya (viral) (hemorrhagic) A92.0
  Chitral A93.1
  Colombo —*see* Fever, paratyphoid
  Colorado tick (virus) A93.2
  congestive (remittent) —*see* Malaria
  Congo virus A98.0
  continued malarial B50.9
  Corsican —*see* Malaria
  Crimean-Congo hemorrhagic A98.0
  Cyprus —*see* Brucellosis
  dandy A90
  deer fly —*see* Tularemia
  dengue (virus) A90
    hemorrhagic A91
    sandfly A93.1
  desert B38.0
  drug induced R50.2
  due to
    conditions classified elsewhere R50.81
    heat T67.0
  enteric A01.00
  enteroviral exanthematous (Boston exanthem)
  A88.0

Fever - *continued*
  ephemeral (of unknown origin) R50.9
  epidemic hemorrhagic A98.5
  erysipelatous —*see* Erysipelas
  estivo-autumnal (malarial) B50.9
  famine A75.0
  five day A79.0
  following delivery O86.4
  Fort Bragg A27.89
  gastroenteric A01.00
  gastromalarial —*see* Malaria
  Gibraltar —*see* Brucellosis
  glandular —*see* Mononucleosis, infectious
  Guama (viral) A92.8
  Haverhill A25.1
  hay (allergic) J30.1
    with asthma (bronchial) J45.909
      with
        exacerbation (acute) J45.901
        status asthmaticus J45.902
      due to
        allergen other than pollen J30.89
        pollen, any plant or tree J30.1
  heat (effects) T67.0
  hematuric, bilious B50.8
  hemoglobinuric (malarial) (bilious) B50.8
  hemorrhagic (arthropod-borne) NOS A94
    with renal syndrome A98.5
    arenaviral A96.9
      specified NEC A96.8
    Argentinian A96.0
    Bangkok A91
    Bolivian A96.1
    Central Asian A98.0
    Chikungunya A92.0
    Crimean-Congo A98.0
    dengue (virus) A91
    epidemic A98.5
    Junin (virus) A96.0
    Korean A98.5
    Kyasanur forest A98.2
    Machupo (virus) A96.1
    mite-borne A93.8
    mosquito-borne A92.8
    Omsk A98.1
    Philippine A91
    Russian A98.5
    Singapore A91
    Southeast Asia A91
    Thailand A91
    tick-borne NEC A93.8
    viral A99
      specified NEC A98.8
  hepatic —*see* Cholecystitis
  herpetic —*see* Herpes
  icterohemorrhagic A27.0
  Indiana A93.8
  infective B99.9
    specified NEC B99.8
  intermittent (bilious) —*see also* Malaria
    of unknown origin R50.9
    pernicious B50.9
  iodide R50.2
  Japanese river A75.3
  jungle —*see also* Malaria
    yellow A95.0
  Junin (virus) hemorrhagic A96.0
  Katayama B65.2
  kedani A75.3
  Kenya (tick) A77.1
  Kew Garden A79.1
  Korean hemorrhagic A98.5

Fever - *continued*
  Lassa A96.2
  Lone Star A77.0
  Machupo (virus) hemorrhagic A96.1
  malaria, malarial —*see* Malaria
  Malta A23.9
  Marseilles A77.1
  marsh —*see* Malaria
  Mayaro (viral) A92.8
  Mediterranean (*see also* Brucellosis) A23.9
    familial E85.0
    tick A77.1
  meningeal —*see* Meningitis
  Meuse A79.0
  Mexican A75.2
  mianeh A68.1
  miasmatic —*see* Malaria
  mosquito-borne (viral) A92.9
    hemorrhagic A92.8
  mountain —*see also* Brucellosis
    meaning Rocky Mountain spotted fever
      A77.0
    tick (American) (Colorado) (viral) A93.2
  Mucambo (viral) A92.8
  mud A27.9
  Neapolitan —*see* Brucellosis
  neutropenic D70.9
  newborn P81.9
    environmental P81.0
  Nine-Mile A78
  non-exanthematous tick A93.2
  North Asian tick-borne A77.2
  Omsk hemorrhagic A98.1
  O'nyong-nyong (viral) A92.1
  Oropouche (viral) A93.0
  Oroya A44.0
  paludal —*see* Malaria
  Panama (malarial) B50.9
  Pappataci A93.1
  paratyphoid A01.4
    A A01.1
    B A01.2
    C A01.3
  parrot A70
  periodic (Mediterranean) E85.0
  persistent (of unknown origin) R50.9
  petechial A39.0
  pharyngoconjunctival B30.2
  Philippine hemorrhagic A91
  phlebotomus A93.1
  Piry (virus) A93.8
  Pixuna (viral) A92.8
  Plasmodium ovale B53.0
  polioviral (nonparalytic) A80.4
  Pontiac A48.2
  postimmunization R50.83
  postoperative R50.82
    due to infection T81.4
  posttransfusion R50.84
  postvaccination R50.83
  presenting with conditions classified
    elsewhere R50.81
  pretibial A27.89
  puerperal O86.4
  Q A78
  quadrilateral A78
  quartan (malaria) B52.9
  Queensland (coastal) (tick) A77.3
  quintan A79.0
  rabbit —*see* Tularemia
  rat-bite A25.9
    due to

Fever - *continued*
  Spirillum A25.0
  Streptobacillus moniliformis A25.1
  recurrent —*see* Fever, relapsing
  relapsing (Borrelia) A68.9
    Carter's (Asiatic) A68.1
    Dutton's (West African) A68.1
    Koch's A68.9
    louse-borne A68.0
    Novy's
      louse-borne A68.0
      tick-borne A68.1
    Obermeyer's (European) A68.0
    tick-borne A68.1
  remittent (bilious) (congestive) (gastric) —*see*
    Malaria
  rheumatic (active) (acute) (chronic)
    (subacute) I00
    with central nervous system involvement
      I02.9
    active with heart involvement (*see* category)
      I01
    inactive or quiescent with
      cardiac hypertrophy I09.89
      carditis I09.9
      endocarditis I09.1
        aortic (valve) I06.9
          with mitral (valve) disease I08.0
        mitral (valve) I05.9
          with aortic (valve) disease I08.0
        pulmonary (valve) I09.89
        tricuspid (valve) I07.8
      heart disease NEC I09.89
      heart failure (congestive) (conditions in
        I50.9) I09.81
      left ventricular failure (conditions in I50.1)
        I09.81
      myocarditis, myocardial degeneration
        (conditions in I51.4) I09.0
      pancarditis I09.9
      pericarditis I09.2
  Rift Valley (viral) A92.4
  Rocky Mountain spotted A77.0
  rose J30.1
  Ross River B33.1
  Russian hemorrhagic A98.5
  San Joaquin (Valley) B38.0
  sandfly A93.1
  Sao Paulo A77.0
  scarlet A38.9
  seven day (leptospirosis) (autumnal)
    (Japanese) A27.89
    dengue A90
  shin-bone A79.0
  Singapore hemorrhagic A91
  solar A90
  Songo A98.5
  sore B00.1
  South African tick-bite A68.1
  Southeast Asia hemorrhagic A91
  spinal —*see* Meningitis
  spirillary A25.0
  splenic —*see* Anthrax
  spotted A77.9
    American A77.0
    Brazilian A77.0
    cerebrospinal meningitis A39.0
    Colombian A77.0
    due to Rickettsia
      australis A77.3
      conorii A77.1
      rickettsii A77.0
      sibirica A77.2

Fever - *continued*
   specified type NEC A77.8
   Ehrlichiosis A77.40
     due to
      E. chafeensis A77.41
      specified organism NEC A77.49
   Rocky Mountain A77.0
   steroid R50.2
   streptobacillary A25.1
   subtertian B50.9
   Sumatran mite A75.3
   sun A90
   swamp A27.9
   swine A02.8
   sylvatic, yellow A95.0
   Tahyna B33.8
   tertian —*see* Malaria, tertian
   Thailand hemorrhagic A91
   thermic T67.0
   three-day A93.1
   tick
     American mountain A93.2
     Colorado A93.2
     Kemerovo A93.8
     Mediterranean A77.1
     mountain A93.2
     nonexanthematous A93.2
     Quaranfil A93.8
   tick-bite NEC A93.8
   tick-borne (hemorrhagic) NEC A93.8
   trench A79.0
   tsutsugamushi A75.3
   typhogastric A01.00
   typhoid (abortive) (hemorrhagic)
   (intermittent) (malignant) A01.00
     complicated by
      arthritis A01.04
      heart involvement A01.02
      meningitis A01.01
      osteomyelitis A01.05
      pneumonia A01.03
      specified NEC A01.09
   typhomalarial —*see* Malaria
   typhus —*see* Typhus (fever)
   undulant —*see* Brucellosis
   unknown origin R50.9
   uveoparotid D86.89
   valley B38.0
   Venezuelan equine A92.2
   vesicular stomatitis A93.8
   viral hemorrhagic —*see* Fever, hemorrhagic,
   by type of virus
   Volhynian A79.0
   Wesselsbron (viral) A92.8
   West
     African B50.8
     Nile (viral) A92.30
      with
       complications NEC A92.39
       cranial nerve disorders A92.32
       encephalitis A92.31
       encephalomyelitis A92.31
       neurologic manifestation NEC A92.32
       optic neuritis A92.32
       polyradiculitis A92.32
   Whitmore's —*see* Melioidosis
   Wolhynian A79.0
   worm B83.9
   yellow A95.9
     jungle A95.0
     sylvatic A95.0
     urban A95.1
   Zika (viral) A92.8

Fibrillation
   atrial or auricular (established) I48.91
     chronic I48.2
     paroxysmal I48.0
     permanent I48.2
     persistent I48.1
   cardiac I49.8
   heart I49.8
   muscular M62.89
   ventricular I49.01
Fibrin
   ball or bodies, pleural (sac) J94.1
   chamber, anterior (eye) (gelatinous exudate)
   —*see* Iridocyclitis, acute
Fibrinogenolysis —*see* Fibrinolysis
Fibrinogenopenia D68.8
   acquired D65
   congenital D68.2
Fibrinolysis (hemorrhagic) (acquired) D65
   antepartum hemorrhage —*see* Hemorrhage,
   antepartum, with coagulation defect
   following
     abortion —*see* Abortion by type
   complicated by hemorrhage
     ectopic or molar pregnancy O08.1
   intrapartum O67.0
   newborn, transient P60
   postpartum O72.3
Fibrinopenia (hereditary) D68.2
   acquired D68.4
Fibrinopurulent —*see* condition
Fibrinous —*see* condition
Fibroadenoma
   cellular intracanalicular D24
   giant D24
   intracanalicular
     cellular D24
     giant D24
     specified site —*see* Neoplasm, benign, by
   site
     unspecified site D24
   juvenile D24
   pericanalicular
     specified site —*see* Neoplasm, benign, by
   site
     unspecified site D24
   phyllodes D24
   prostate D29.1
   specified site NEC —*see* Neoplasm, benign,
   by site
   unspecified site D24
Fibroadenosis, breast (chronic) (cystic)
(diffuse) (periodic) (segmental) N60.2
Fibroangioma —*see also* Neoplasm, benign,
by site
   juvenile
     specified site —*see* Neoplasm, benign, by
   site
     unspecified site D10.6
Fibrochondrosarcoma —*see* Neoplasm,
cartilage, malignant
Fibrocystic
   disease —*see also* Fibrosis, cystic
     breast —*see* Mastopathy, cystic
     jaw M27.49
     kidney (congenital) Q61.8
     liver Q44.6
     pancreas E84.9
     kidney (congenital) Q61.8
Fibrodysplasia ossificans progressiva —*see*
Myositis, ossificans, progressiva
Fibroelastosis (cordis) (endocardial)
(endomyocardial) I42.4

Fibroid (tumor) —*see also* Neoplasm,
connective tissue, benign
   disease, lung (chronic) —*see* Fibrosis, lung
   heart (disease) —*see* Myocarditis
   in pregnancy or childbirth O34.1
     causing obstructed labor O65.5
   induration, lung (chronic) —*see* Fibrosis, lung
   lung —*see* Fibrosis, lung
   pneumonia (chronic) —*see* Fibrosis, lung
   uterus D25.9
Fibrolipoma —*see* Lipoma
Fibroliposarcoma —*see* Neoplasm,
connective tissue, malignant
Fibroma —*see also* Neoplasm, connective
tissue, benign
   ameloblastic —*see* Cyst, calcifying
odontogenic
   bone (nonossifying) —*see* Disorder, bone,
specified type NEC
     ossifying —*see* Neoplasm, bone, benign
   cementifying —*see* Neoplasm, bone, benign
   chondromyxoid —*see* Neoplasm, bone,
benign
   desmoplastic —*see* Neoplasm, connective
tissue, uncertain behavior
   durum —*see* Neoplasm, connective tissue,
benign
   fascial —*see* Neoplasm, connective tissue,
benign
   invasive —*see* Neoplasm, connective tissue,
uncertain behavior
   molle —*see* Lipoma
   myxoid —*see* Neoplasm, connective tissue,
benign
   nasopharynx, nasopharyngeal (juvenile)
D10.6
   nonosteogenic (nonossifying) —*see*
Dysplasia, fibrous
   odontogenic (central) —*see* Cyst, calcifying
odontogenic
   ossifying —*see* Neoplasm, bone, benign
   periosteal —*see* Neoplasm, bone, benign
   soft —*see* Lipoma
Fibromatosis M72.9
   abdominal —*see* Neoplasm, connective
tissue, uncertain behavior
   aggressive —*see* Neoplasm, connective
tissue, uncertain behavior
   congenital generalized —*see* Neoplasm,
connective tissue, uncertain behavior
   Dupuytren's M72.0
   gingival K06.1
   palmar (fascial) M72.0
   plantar (fascial) M72.2
   pseudosarcomatous (proliferative)
(subcutaneous) M72.4
   retroperitoneal D48.3
   specified NEC M72.8
Fibromyalgia M79.7
Fibromyoma —*see also* Neoplasm, connective
tissue, benign
   uterus (corpus) —*see also* Leiomyoma, uterus
     in pregnancy or childbirth —*see* Fibroid, in
pregnancy or childbirth
     causing obstructed labor O65.5
Fibromyositis M79.7
Fibromyxolipoma D17.9
Fibromyxoma —*see* Neoplasm, connective
tissue, benign
Fibromyxosarcoma —*see* Neoplasm,
connective tissue, malignant
Fibro-odontoma, ameloblastic —*see* Cyst,
calcifying odontogenic

Fibro-osteoma —*see* Neoplasm, bone, benign
Fibroplasia, retrolental H35.17
Fibropurulent —*see* condition
Fibrosarcoma —*see also* Neoplasm,
  connective tissue, malignant
  ameloblastic C41.1
    upper jaw (bone) C41.0
  congenital —*see* Neoplasm, connective tissue,
    malignant
  fascial —*see* Neoplasm, connective tissue,
    malignant
  infantile —*see* Neoplasm, connective tissue,
    malignant
  odontogenic C41.1
    upper jaw (bone) C41.0
  periosteal —*see* Neoplasm, bone, malignant
Fibrosclerosis
  breast N60.3
  multifocal M35.5
  penis (corpora cavernosa) N48.6
Fibrosis, fibrotic
  adrenal (gland) E27.8
  amnion O41.8X
  anal papillae K62.89
  arteriocapillary —*see* Arteriosclerosis
  bladder N32.89
    interstitial —*see* Cystitis, chronic, interstitial
    localized submucosal —*see* Cystitis,
    chronic, interstitial
    panmural —*see* Cystitis, chronic, interstitial
  breast —*see* Fibrosclerosis, breast
  capillary (*see also* Arteriosclerosis) I70.90
    lung (chronic) —*see* Fibrosis, lung
  cardiac —*see* Myocarditis
  cervix N88.8
  chorion O41.8X
  corpus cavernosum (sclerosing) N48.6
  cystic (of pancreas) E84.9
    with
      distal intestinal obstruction syndrome
      E84.19
        fecal impaction E84.19
        intestinal manifestations NEC E84.19
        pulmonary manifestations E84.0
        specified manifestations NEC E84.8
  due to device, implant or graft (*see also*
  Complications, by site and type, specified
  NEC) T85.82
    arterial graft NEC T82.828
    breast (implant) T85.82
    catheter NEC T85.82
      dialysis (renal) T82.828
        intraperitoneal T85.82
      infusion NEC T82.828
        spinal (epidural) (subdural) T85.82
      urinary (indwelling) T83.82
    electronic (electrode) (pulse generator)
    (stimulator)
        bone T84.82
        cardiac T82.827
        nervous system (brain) (peripheral nerve)
    (spinal) T85.82
        urinary T83.82
    fixation, internal (orthopedic) NEC T84.82
    gastrointestinal (bile duct) (esophagus)
    T85.82
      genital NEC T83.82
      heart NEC T82.827
      joint prosthesis T84.82
      ocular (corneal graft) (orbital implant) NEC
    T85.82
      orthopedic NEC T84.82

Fibrosis, fibrotic - *continued*
  specified NEC T85.82
  urinary NEC T83.82
  vascular NEC T82.828
  ventricular intracranial shunt T85.82
  ejaculatory duct N50.8
  endocardium —*see* Endocarditis
  endomyocardial (tropical) I42.3
  epididymis N50.8
  eye muscle —*see* Strabismus, mechanical
  heart —*see* Myocarditis
  hepatic —*see* Fibrosis, liver
  hepatolienal (portal hypertension) K76.6
  hepatosplenic (portal hypertension) K76.6
  infrapatellar fat pad M79.4
  intrascrotal N50.8
  kidney N26.9
  liver K74.0
    with sclerosis K74.2
      alcoholic K70.2
  lung (atrophic) (chronic) (confluent)
  (massive) (perialveolar) (peribronchial)
  J84.10
    with
      anthracosilicosis J60
      anthracosis J60
      asbestosis J61
      bagassosis J67.1
      bauxite J63.1
      berylliosis J63.2
      byssinosis J66.0
      calcicosis J62.8
      chalicosis J62.8
      dust reticulation J64
      farmer's lung J67.0
      ganister disease J62.8
      graphite J63.3
      pneumoconiosis NOS J64
      siderosis J63.4
      silicosis J62.8
    capillary J84.10
    congenital P27.8
    diffuse (idiopathic) J84.10
      chemicals, gases, fumes or vapors
    (inhalation) J68.4
      interstitial J84.10
        acute J84.114
      talc J62.0
    following radiation J70.1
    idiopathic J84.112
    postinflammatory J84.10
    silicotic J62.8
    tuberculous —*see* Tuberculosis, pulmonary
  lymphatic gland I89.8
  median bar —*see* Hyperplasia, prostate
  mediastinum (idiopathic) J98.5
  meninges G96.19
  myocardium, myocardial —*see* Myocarditis
  ovary N83.8
  oviduct N83.8
  pancreas K86.8
  penis NEC N48.6
  pericardium I31.0
  perineum, in pregnancy or childbirth O34.7
    causing obstructed labor O65.5
  pleura J94.1
  popliteal fat pad M79.4
  prostate (chronic) —*see* Hyperplasia, prostate
  pulmonary (*see also* Fibrosis, lung) J84.10
    congenital P27.8
    idiopathic J84.112
  rectal sphincter K62.89

Fibrosis, fibrotic - *continued*
  retroperitoneal, idiopathic (with ureteral
    obstruction) N13.5
    with infection N13.6
  sclerosing mesenteric (idiopathic) K65.4
  scrotum N50.8
  seminal vesicle N50.8
  senile R54
  skin L90.5
  spermatic cord N50.8
  spleen D73.89
    in schistosomiasis (bilharziasis) B65.9
    [D77]
  subepidermal nodular —*see* Neoplasm, skin,
  benign
  submucous (oral) (tongue) K13.5
  testis N44.8
    chronic, due to syphilis A52.76
  thymus (gland) E32.8
  tongue, submucous K13.5
  tunica vaginalis N50.8
  uterus (non-neoplastic) N85.8
  vagina N89.8
  valve, heart —*see* Endocarditis
  vas deferens N50.8
  vein I87.8
Fibrositis (periarticular) M79.7
  nodular, chronic (Jaccoud's) (rheumatoid) —
  see Arthropathy, postrheumatic, chronic
Fibrothorax J94.1
Fibrotic —*see* Fibrosis
Fibrous —*see* condition
Fibroxanthoma —*see also* Neoplasm,
  connective tissue, benign
  atypical —*see* Neoplasm, connective tissue,
    uncertain behavior
  malignant —*see* Neoplasm, connective tissue,
    malignant
Fibroxanthosarcoma —*see* Neoplasm,
  connective tissue, malignant
Fiedler's
  disease (icterohemorrhagic leptospirosis)
  A27.0
  myocarditis (acute) I40.1
Fifth disease B08.3
  venereal A55
Filaria, filarial, filariasis —*see* Infestation,
  filarial
Filatov's disease —*see* Mononucleosis,
  infectious
File-cutter's disease —*see* Poisoning, lead
Filling defect
  biliary tract R93.2
  bladder R93.4
  duodenum R93.3
  gallbladder R93.2
  gastrointestinal tract R93.3
  intestine R93.3
  kidney R93.4
  stomach R93.3
  ureter R93.4
Fimbrial cyst Q50.4
Financial problem affecting care NOS Z59.9
  bankruptcy Z59.8
  foreclosure on loan Z59.8
Findings, abnormal, inconclusive, without
  diagnosis —*see also* Abnormal
  17-ketosteroids, elevated R82.5
  acetonuria R82.4
  alcohol in blood R78.0
  anisocytosis R71.8

Findings *- continued*
  antenatal screening of mother O28.9
    biochemical O28.1
    chromosomal O28.5
    cytological O28.2
    genetic O28.5
    hematological O28.0
    radiological O28.4
    specified NEC O28.8
    ultrasonic O28.3
  antibody titer, elevated R76.0
  anticardiolipin antibody R76.0
  antiphosphatidylglycerol antibody R76.0
  antiphosphatidylinositol antibody R76.0
  antiphosphatidylserine antibody R76.0
  antiphospholipid antibody R76.0
  bacteriuria N39.0
  bicarbonate E87.8
  bile in urine R82.2
  blood sugar R73.09
    high R73.9
    low (transicnt) E16.2
  body fluid or substance, specified NEC R88.8
  casts, urine R82.99
  catecholamines R82.5
  cells, urine R82.99
  chloride E87.8
  cholesterol E78.9
    high E78.0
      with high triglycerides E78.2
  chyluria R82.0
  cloudy
    dialysis effluent R88.0
    urine R82.90
  creatinine clearance R94.4
  crystals, urine R82.99
  culture
    blood R78.81
    positive —*see* Positive, culture
  echocardiogram R93.1
  electrolyte level, urinary R82.99
  function study NEC R94.8
    bladder R94.8
    endocrine NEC R94.7
      thyroid R94.6
    kidney R94.4
    liver R94.5
    pancreas R94.8
    placenta R94.8
    pulmonary R94.2
    spleen R94.8
  gallbladder, nonvisualization R93.2
  glucose (tolerance test) (non-fasting) R73.09
  glycosuria R81
  heart
    shadow R93.1
    sounds R01.2
  hematinuria R82.3
  hematocrit drop (precipitous) R71.0
  hemoglobinuria R82.3
  human papillomavirus (HPV) DNA test
  positive
    cervix
      high risk R87.810
      low risk R87.820
    vagina
      high risk R87.811
      low risk R87.821
  in blood (of substance not normally found in blood) R78.9
    addictive drug NEC R78.4
    alcohol (excessive level) R78.0

Findings *- continued*
    cocaine R78.2
    hallucinogen R78.3
    heavy metals (abnormal level) R78.79
    lead R78.71
    lithium (abnormal level) R78.89
    opiate drug R78.1
    psychotropic drug R78.5
    specified substance NEC R78.89
    steroid agent R78.6
  indoleacetic acid, elevated R82.5
  ketonuria R82.4
  lactic acid dehydrogenase (LDH) R74.0
  liver function test R79.89
  mammogram NEC R92.8
    calcification (calculus) R92.1
    inconclusive result (due to dense breasts) R92.2
    microcalcification R92.0
  mediastinal shift R93.8
  melanin, urine R82.99
  myoglobinuria R82.1
  neonatal screening P09
  nonvisualization of gallbladder R93.2
  odor of urine NOS R82.90
  Papanicolaou cervix R87.619
    non-atypical endometrial cells R87.618
  pneumoencephalogram R93.0
  poikilocytosis R71.8
  potassium (deficiency) E87.6
    excess E87.5
  PPD R76.11
  radiologic (X-ray) R93.8
    abdomen R93.5
    biliary tract R93.2
    breast R92.8
    gastrointestinal tract R93.3
    genitourinary organs R93.8
    head R93.0
    inconclusive due to excess body fat of patient R93.9
    intrathoracic organs NEC R93.1
    placenta R93.8
    retroperitoneum R93.5
    skin R93.8
    skull R93.0
    subcutaneous tissue R93.8
  red blood cell (count) (morphology) (sickling) (volume) R71.8
  scan NEC R94.8
    bladder R94.8
    bone R94.8
    kidney R94.4
    liver R93.2
    lung R94.2
    pancreas R94.8
    placental R94.8
    spleen R94.8
    thyroid R94.6
  sedimentation rate, elevated R70.0
  SGOT R74.0
  SGPT R74.0
  sodium (deficiency) E87.1
    excess E87.0
  specified body fluid NEC R88.8
  stress test R94.39
  thyroid (function) (metabolic rate) (scan) (uptake) R94.6
  transaminase (level) R74.0
  triglycerides E78.9
    high E78.1
      with high cholesterol E78.2

Findings *- continued*
  tuberculin skin test (without active tuberculosis) R76.11
  urine R82.90
    acetone R82.4
    bacteria N39.0
    bile R82.2
    casts or cells R82.99
    chyle R82.0
    culture positive R82.7
    glucose R81
    hemoglobin R82.3
    ketone R82.4
    sugar R81
  vanillylmandelic acid (VMA) , elevated R82.5
  vectorcardiogram (VCG) R94.39
  ventriculogram R93.0
  white blood cell (count) (differential) (morphology) D72.9
  xerography R92.8
Finger —*see* condition
Fire, Saint Anthony's —*see* Erysipelas
Fire-setting
  pathological (compulsive) F63.1
Fish hook stomach K31.89
Fishmeal-worker's lung J67.8
Fissure, fissured
  anus, anal K60.2
    acute K60.0
    chronic K60.1
    congenital Q43.8
  ear, lobule, congenital Q17.8
  epiglottis (congenital) Q31.8
  larynx J38.7
    congenital Q31.8
  lip K13.0
    congenital —*see* Cleft, lip
  nipple N64.0
    associated with
      lactation O92.13
      pregnancy O92.11
      puerperium O92.12
  nose Q30.2
  palate (congenital) —*see* Cleft, palate
  skin R23.4
  spine (congenital) —*see also* Spina bifida
    with hydrocephalus —*see* Spina bifida, by site, with hydrocephalus
  tongue (acquired) K14.5
    congenital Q38.3
Fistula (cutaneous) L98.8
  abdomen (wall) K63.2
    bladder N32.2
    intestine NEC K63.2
    ureter N28.89
    uterus N82.5
  abdominorectal K63.2
  abdominosigmoidal K63.2
  abdominothoracic J86.0
  abdominouterine N82.5
    congenital Q51.7
  abdominovesical N32.2
  accessory sinuses —*see* Sinusitis
  actinomycotic —*see* Actinomycosis
  alveolar antrum —*see* Sinusitis, maxillary
  alveolar process K04.6
  anorectal K60.5
  antrobuccal —*see* Sinusitis, maxillary
  antrum —*see* Sinusitis, maxillary
  anus, anal (recurrent) (infectional) K60.3
    congenital Q43.6

Fistula - *continued*

with absence, atresia and stenosis Q42.2
tuberculous A18.32
aorta-duodenal I77.2
appendix, appendicular K38.3
arteriovenous (acquired) (nonruptured) I77.0
brain I67.1
congenital Q28.2
ruptured I60.8
ruptured I60.8
cerebral —*see* Fistula, arteriovenous, brain
congenital (peripheral) —*see also*
Malformation, arteriovenous
brain Q28.2
ruptured I60.8
coronary Q24.5
pulmonary Q25.72
coronary I25.41
congenital Q24.5
pulmonary I28.0
congenital Q25.72
surgically created (for dialysis) Z99.2
complication —*see* Complication,
arteriovenous, fistula, surgically created
traumatic —*see* Injury, blood vessel
artery I77.2
aural (mastoid) —*see* Mastoiditis, chronic
auricle —*see also* Disorder, pinna, specified
type NEC
congenital Q18.1
Bartholin's gland N82.8
bile duct (common) (hepatic) K83.3
with calculus, stones —*see* Calculus, bile
duct
biliary (tract) —*see* Fistula, bile duct
bladder (sphincter) NEC (*see also* Fistula,
vesico) N32.2
into seminal vesicle N32.2
bone —*see also* Disorder, bone, specified
type NEC
with osteomyelitis, chronic —*see*
Osteomyelitis, chronic, with draining sinus
brain G93.89
arteriovenous (acquired) I67.1
congenital Q28.2
branchial (cleft) Q18.0
branchiogenous Q18.0
breast N61
puerperal, postpartum or gestational, due to
mastitis (purulent) —*see* Mastitis, obstetric,
purulent
bronchial J86.0
bronchocutaneous, bronchomediastinal,
bronchopleural, bronchopleuromediastinal
(infective) J86.0
tuberculous NEC A15.5
bronchoesophageal J86.0
congenital Q39.2
with atresia of esophagus Q39.1
bronchovisceral J86.0
buccal cavity (infective) K12.2
cecosigmoidal K63.2
cecum K63.2
cerebrospinal (fluid) G96.0
cervical, lateral Q18.1
cervicoaural Q18.1
cervicosigmoidal N82.4
cervicovesical N82.1
cervix N82.8
chest (wall) J86.0
cholecystenteric —*see* Fistula, gallbladder
cholecystocolic —*see* Fistula, gallbladder

Fistula - *continued*

cholecystocolonic —*see* Fistula, gallbladder
cholecystoduodenal —*see* Fistula, gallbladder
cholecystogastric —*see* Fistula, gallbladder
cholecystointestinal —*see* Fistula, gallbladder
choledochoduodenal —*see* Fistula, bile duct
cholocolic K82.3
coccyx —*see* Sinus, pilonidal
colon K63.2
colostomy K94.09
common duct —*see* Fistula, bile duct
congenital, site not listed —*see* Anomaly, by
site
coronary, arteriovenous I25.41
congenital Q24.5
costal region J86.0
cul-de-sac, Douglas' N82.8
cystic duct —*see also* Fistula, gallbladder
congenital Q44.5
dental K04.6
diaphragm J86.0
duodenum K31.6
ear (external) (canal) —*see* Disorder, ear,
external, specified type NEC
enterocolic K63.2
enterocutaneous K63.2
enterouterine N82.4
congenital Q51.7
enterovaginal N82.4
congenital Q52.2
large intestine N82.3
small intestine N82.2
enterovesical N32.1
epididymis N50.8
tuberculous A18.15
esophagobronchial J86.0
congenital Q39.2
with atresia of esophagus Q39.1
esophagocutaneous K22.8
esophagopleural-cutaneous J86.0
esophagotracheal J86.0
congenital Q39.2
with atresia of esophagus Q39.1
esophagus K22.8
congenital Q39.2
with atresia of esophagus Q39.1
ethmoid —*see* Sinusitis, ethmoidal
eyeball (cornea) (sclera) —*see* Disorder,
globe, hypotony
eyelid H01.8
fallopian tube, external N82.5
fecal K63.2
congenital Q43.6
from periapical abscess K04.6
frontal sinus —*see* Sinusitis, frontal
gallbladder K82.3
with calculus, cholelithiasis, stones —*see*
Calculus, gallbladder
gastric K31.6
gastrocolic K31.6
congenital Q40.2
tuberculous A18.32
gastroenterocolic K31.6
gastroesophageal K31.6
gastrojejunal K31.6
gastrojejunocolic K31.6
genital tract (female) N82.9
specified NEC N82.8
to intestine NEC N82.4
to skin N82.5
hepatic artery-portal vein, congenital Q26.6
hepatopleural J86.0

Fistula - *continued*

hepatopulmonary J86.0
ileorectal or ileosigmoidal K63.2
ileovaginal N82.2
ileovesical N32.1
ileum K63.2
in ano K60.3
tuberculous A18.32
inner ear (labyrinth) —*see* subcategory H83.1
intestine NEC K63.2
intestinocolonic (abdominal) K63.2
intestinoureteral N28.89
intestinouterine N82.4
intestinovaginal N82.4
large intestine N82.3
small intestine N82.2
intestinovesical N32.1
ischiorectal (fossa) K61.3
jejunum K63.2
joint M25.10
ankle M25.17
elbow M25.12
foot joint M25.17
hand joint M25.14
hip M25.15
knee M25.16
shoulder M25.11
specified joint NEC M25.18
tuberculous —*see* Tuberculosis, joint
vertebrae M25.18
wrist M25.13
kidney N28.89
labium (majus) (minus) N82.8
labyrinth —*see* subcategory H83.1
lacrimal (gland) (sac) H04.61
lacrimonasal duct —*see* Fistula, lacrimal
laryngotracheal, congenital Q34.8
larynx J38.7
lip K13.0
congenital Q38.0
lumbar, tuberculous A18.01
lung J86.0
lymphatic I89.8
mammary (gland) N61
mastoid (process) (region) —*see* Mastoiditis,
chronic
maxillary J32.0
medial, face and neck Q18.8
mediastinal J86.0
mediastinobronchial J86.0
mediastinocutaneous J86.0
middle ear —*see* subcategory H74.8
mouth K12.2
nasal J34.89
sinus —*see* Sinusitis
nasopharynx J39.2
nipple N64.0
nose J34.89
oral (cutaneous) K12.2
maxillary J32.0
nasal (with cleft palate) —*see* Cleft, palate
orbit, orbital —*see* Disorder, orbit, specified
type NEC
oroantral J32.0
oviduct, external N82.5
palate (hard) M27.8
pancreatic K86.8
pancreaticoduodenal K86.8
parotid (gland) K11.4
region K12.2
penis N48.89
perianal K60.3
pericardium (pleura) (sac) —*see* Pericarditis

Fistula - *continued*
  pericecal K63.2
  perineorectal K60.4
  perineosigmoidal K63.2
  perineum, perineal (with urethral
  involvement) NEC N36.0
    tuberculous A18.13
    ureter N28.89
  perirectal K60.4
    tuberculous A18.32
  peritoneum K65.9
  pharyngoesophageal J39.2
  pharynx J39.2
    branchial cleft (congenital) Q18.0
  pilonidal (infected) (rectum) —*see* Sinus,
  pilonidal
  pleura, pleural, pleurocutaneous,
  pleuroperitoneal J86.0
    tuberculous NEC A15.6
  pleuropericardial I31.8
  portal vein-hepatic artery, congenital Q26.6
  postauricular H70.81
  postoperative, persistent T81.83
    specified site —*see* Fistula, by site
  preauricular (congenital) Q18.1
  prostate N42.89
  pulmonary J86.0
    arteriovenous I28.0
      congenital Q25.72
    tuberculous —*see* Tuberculosis, pulmonary
  pulmonoperitoneal J86.0
  rectolabial N82.4
  rectosigmoid (intercommunicating) K63.2
  rectoureteral N28.89
  rectourethral N36.0
    congenital Q64.73
  rectouterine N82.4
    congenital Q51.7
  rectovaginal N82.3
    congenital Q52.2
    tuberculous A18.18
  rectovesical N32.1
    congenital Q64.79
  rectovesicovaginal N82.3
  rectovulval N82.4
    congenital Q52.79
  rectum (to skin) K60.4
    congenital Q43.6
      with absence, atresia and stenosis Q42.0
    tuberculous A18.32
  renal N28.89
  retroauricular —*see* Fistula, postauricular
  salivary duct or gland (any) K11.4
    congenital Q38.4
  scrotum (urinary) N50.8
    tuberculous A18.15
  semicircular canals —see subcategory H83.1
  sigmoid K63.2
    to bladder N32.1
  sinus —*see* Sinusitis
  skin L98.8
    to genital tract (female) N82.5
  splenocolic D73.89
  stercoral K63.2
  stomach K31.6
  sublingual gland K11.4
  submandibular gland K11.4
  submaxillary (gland) K11.4
    region K12.2
  thoracic J86.0
    duct I89.8
  thoracoabdominal J86.0

Fistula - *continued*
  thoracogastric J86.0
  thoracointestinal J86.0
  thorax J86.0
  thyroglossal duct Q89.2
  thyroid E07.89
  trachea, congenital (external) (internal) Q32.1
  tracheoesophageal J86.0
    congenital Q39.2
      with atresia of esophagus Q39.1
    following tracheostomy J95.04
  traumatic arteriovenous —*see* Injury, blood
  vessel, by site
  tuberculous
  code by site under Tuberculosis
  typhoid A01.09
  umbilicourinary Q64.8
  urachus, congenital Q64.4
  ureter (persistent) N28.89
  ureteroabdominal N28.89
  ureterorectal N28.89
  ureterosigmoido-abdominal N28.89
  ureterovaginal N82.1
  ureterovesical N32.2
  urethra N36.0
    congenital Q64.79
    tuberculous A18.13
  urethroperineal N36.0
  urethroperineovesical N32.2
  urethrorectal N36.0
    congenital Q64.73
  urethroscrotal N50.8
  urethrovaginal N82.1
  urethrovesical N32.2
  urinary (tract) (persistent) (recurrent) N36.0
  uteroabdominal N82.5
    congenital Q51.7
  uteroenteric, uterointestinal N82.4
    congenital Q51.7
  uterorectal N82.4
    congenital Q51.7
  uteroureteric N82.1
  uterourethral Q51.7
  uterovaginal N82.8
  uterovesical N82.1
    congenital Q51.7
  uterus N82.8
  vagina (postpartal) (wall) N82.8
  vaginocutaneous (postpartal) N82.5
  vaginointestinal NEC N82.4
    large intestine N82.3
    small intestine N82.2
  vaginoperineal N82.5
  vasocutaneous, congenital Q55.7
  vesical NEC N32.2
  vesicoabdominal N32.2
  vesicocervicovaginal N82.1
  vesicocolic N32.1
  vesicocutaneous N32.2
  vesicoenteric N32.1
  vesicointestinal N32.1
  vesicometrorectal N82.4
  vesicoperineal N32.2
  vesicorectal N32.1
    congenital Q64.79
  vesicosigmoidal N32.1
  vesicosigmoidovaginal N82.3
  vesicoureteral N32.2
  vesicourethrovaginal N82.1
  vesicourethral N32.2
  vesicourethrorectal N32.1
  vesicouterine N82.1

Fistula - *continued*
  congenital Q51.7
  vesicovaginal N82.0
  vulvorectal N82.4
    congenital Q52.79
Fit R56.9
  epileptic —*see* Epilepsy
  fainting R55
  hysterical F44.5
  newborn P90
Fitting (and adjustment) (of)
  artificial
    arm —*see* Admission, adjustment, artificial,
    arm
      breast Z44.3
      eye Z44.2
    leg —*see* Admission, adjustment, artificial,
    leg
  automatic implantable cardiac defibrillator
  (with synchronous cardiac pacemaker) Z45.02
  brain neuropacemaker Z46.2
    implanted Z45.42
  cardiac defibrillator —*see* Fitting (and
  adjustment) (of) , automatic implantable
  cardiac defibrillator
  catheter, non-vascular Z46.82
  colostomy belt Z46.89
  contact lenses Z46.0
  cystostomy device Z46.6
  defibrillator, cardiac —*see* Fitting (and
  adjustment) (of) , automatic implantable
  cardiac defibrillator
  dentures Z46.3
  device NOS Z46.9
    abdominal Z46.89
    gastrointestinal NEC Z46.59
    implanted NEC Z45.89
    nervous system Z46.2
      implanted —*see* Admission, adjustment,
    device, implanted, nervous system
    orthodontic Z46.4
    orthoptic Z46.0
    orthotic Z46.89
    prosthetic (external) Z44.9
      breast Z44.3
      dental Z46.3
      eye Z44.2
      specified NEC Z44.8
    specified NEC Z46.89
    substitution
      auditory Z46.2
        implanted —*see* Admission, adjustment,
      device, implanted, hearing device
      nervous system Z46.2
        implanted —*see* Admission, adjustment,
      device, implanted, nervous system
      visual Z46.2
        implanted Z45.31
    urinary Z46.6
  gastric lap band Z46.51
  gastrointestinal appliance NEC Z46.59
  glasses (reading) Z46.0
  hearing aid Z46.1
  ileostomy device Z46.89
  insulin pump Z46.81
  intestinal appliance NEC Z46.89
  myringotomy device (stent) (tube) Z45.82
  neuropacemaker Z46.2
    implanted Z45.42
  non-vascular catheter Z46.82
  orthodontic device Z46.4
  orthopedic device (brace) (cast) (corset)
  (shoes) Z46.89

Fitting - *continued*
  pacemaker (cardiac) Z45.018
    nervous system (brain) (peripheral nerve)
    (spinal cord) Z46.2
      implanted Z45.42
    pulse generator Z45.010
  portacath (port-a-cath) Z45.2
  prosthesis (external) Z44.9
    arm —*see* Admission, adjustment, artificial,
    arm
      breast Z44.3
      dental Z46.3
      eye Z44.2
      leg —*see* Admission, adjustment, artificial,
      leg
        specified NEC Z44.8
  spectacles Z46.0
  wheelchair Z46.89
Fitzhugh-Curtis syndrome
  due to
    Chlamydia trachomatis A74.81
    Neisseria gonorrhorea (gonococcal
    peritonitis) A54.85
Fitz's syndrome (acute hemorrhagic
  pancreatitis) K85.8
Fixation
  joint —*see* Ankylosis
  larynx J38.7
  stapes —*see* Ankylosis, ear ossicles
    deafness —*see* Deafness, conductive
  uterus (acquired) —*see* Malposition, uterus
  vocal cord J38.3
Flabby ridge K06.8
Flaccid —*see also* condition
  palate, congenital Q38.5
Flail
  chest S22.5
    newborn (birth injury) P13.8
  joint (paralytic) M25.20
    ankle M25.27
    elbow M25.22
    foot joint M25.27
    hand joint M25.24
    hip M25.25
    knee M25.26
    shoulder M25.21
    specified joint NEC M25.28
    wrist M25.23
Flajani's disease —*see* Hyperthyroidism, with,
  goiter (diffuse)
Flap, liver K71.3
Flashbacks (residual to hallucinogen use)
  F16.283
Flat
  chamber (eye) —*see* Disorder, globe,
  hypotony, flat anterior chamber
  chest, congenital Q67.8
  foot (acquired) (fixed type) (painful)
  (postural) —*see also* Deformity, limb, flat
  foot
    congenital (rigid) (spastic (everted)) Q66.5
    rachitic sequelae (late effect) E64.3
  organ or site, congenital NEC —*see*
  Anomaly, by site
  pelvis M95.5
    with disproportion (fetopelvic) O33.0
      causing obstructed labor O65.0
    congenital Q74.2
Flatau-Schilder disease G37.0
Flatback syndrome M40.30
  lumbar region M40.36
  lumbosacral region M40.37
  thoracolumbar region M40.35

Flattening
  head, femur M89.8X5
  hip —*see* Coxa, plana
  lip (congenital) Q18.8
  nose (congenital) Q67.4
    acquired M95.0
Flatulence R14.3
  psychogenic F45.8
Flatus R14.3
  vaginalis N89.8
Flax-dresser's disease J66.1
Flea bite —*see* Injury, bite, by site, superficial,
  insect
Flecks, glaucomatous (subcapsular) —*see*
  Cataract, complicated
Fleischer (-Kayser) ring (cornea) H18.04
Fleshy mole O02.0
Flexibilitas cerea —*see* Catalepsy
Flexion
  amputation stump (surgical) T87.89
  cervix —*see* Malposition, uterus
  contracture, joint —*see* Contraction, joint
  deformity, joint (*see also* Deformity, limb,
  flexion) M21.20
    hip, congenital Q65.89
  uterus —*see also* Malposition, uterus
    lateral —*see* Lateroversion, uterus
Flexner-Boyd dysentery A03.2
Flexner's dysentery A03.1
Flexure —*see* Flexion
Flint murmur (aortic insufficiency) I35.1
Floater, vitreous —*see* Opacity, vitreous
Floating
  cartilage (joint) —*see also* Loose, body, joint
    knee —*see* Derangement, knee, loose body
  gallbladder, congenital Q44.1
  kidney N28.89
    congenital Q63.8
  spleen D73.89
Flooding N92.0
Floor —*see* condition
Floppy
  baby syndrome (nonspecific) P94.2
  iris syndrome (intraoperative) (IFIS) H21.81
  nonrheumatic mitral valve syndrome I34.1
Flu —*see also* Influenza
  avian (*see also* Influenza, due to, identified
  novel influenza A virus) J09.X2
  bird (*see also* Influenza, due to, identified
  novel influenza A virus) J09.X2
  intestinal NEC A08.4
  swine (viruses that normally cause infections
  in pigs) (*see also* Influenza, due to, identified
  novel influenza A virus) J09.X2
Fluctuating blood pressure I99.8
Fluid
  abdomen R18.8
  chest J94.8
  heart —*see* Failure, heart, congestive
  joint —*see* Effusion, joint
  loss (acute) E86.9
    with
      hypernatremia E87.0
      hyponatremia E87.1
  lung —*see* Edema, lung
  overload E87.70
    specified NEC E87.79
  peritoneal cavity R18.8
  pleural cavity J94.8
  retention R60.9
Flukes NEC —*see also* Infestation, fluke
  blood NEC —*see* Schistosomiasis
  liver B66.3

Fluor (vaginalis) N89.8
  trichomonal or due to Trichomonas
  (vaginalis) A59.00
Fluorosis
  dental K00.3
  skeletal M85.10
    ankle M85.17
    foot M85.17
    forearm M85.13
    hand M85.14
    lower leg M85.16
    multiple site M85.19
    neck M85.18
    rib M85.18
    shoulder M85.11
    skull M85.18
    specified site NEC M85.18
    thigh M85.15
    toe M85.17
    upper arm M85.12
    vertebra M85.18
Flush syndrome E34.0
Flushing R23.2
  menopausal N95.1
Flutter
  atrial or auricular I48.92
    atypical I48.4
    type I I48.3
    type II I48.4
    typical I48.3
  heart I49.8
    atrial or auricular I48.92
      atypical I48.4
      type I I48.3
      type II I48.4
      typical I48.3
    ventricular I49.02
  ventricular I49.02
FNHTR (febrile nonhemolytic transfusion
  reaction) R50.84
Fochier's abscess
  code by site under Abscess
Focus, Assmann's —*see* Tuberculosis,
  pulmonary
Fogo selvagem L10.3
Foix-Alajouanine syndrome G95.19
Fold, folds (anomalous) —*see also* Anomaly,
  by site
  Descemet's membrane —*see* Change, corneal
  membrane, Descemet's, fold
  epicanthic Q10.3
  heart Q24.8
Folie à deux F24
Follicle
  cervix (nabothian) (ruptured) N88.8
  graafian, ruptured, with hemorrhage N83.0
  nabothian N88.8
Follicular —*see* condition
Folliculitis (superficial) L73.9
  abscedens et suffodiens L66.3
  cyst N83.0
  decalvans L66.2
  deep —*see* Furuncle, by site
  gonococcal (acute) (chronic) A54.01
  keloid, keloidalis L73.0
  pustular L01.02
  ulerythematosa reticulata L66.4
Folliculome lipidique
  specified site —*see* Neoplasm, benign, by site
  unspecified site
    female D27.9
    male D29.20
Følling's disease E70.0

Follow-up —*see* Examination, follow-up
Fong's syndrome (hereditary osteo-onychodysplasia) Q78.5
Food
  allergy L27.2
  asphyxia (from aspiration or inhalation) —*see* Foreign body, by site
  choked on —*see* Foreign body, by site
  deprivation T73.0
    specified kind of food NEC E63.8
  intoxication —*see* Poisoning, food
  lack of T73.0
  poisoning —*see* Poisoning, food
  rejection NEC —*see* Disorder, eating
  strangulation or suffocation —*see* Foreign body, by site
  toxemia —*see* Poisoning, food
Foot —*see* condition
Foramen ovale (nonclosure) (patent) (persistent) Q21.1
Forbes' glycogen storage disease E74.03
Fordyce-Fox disease L75.2
Fordyce's disease (mouth) Q38.6
Forearm —*see* condition
Foreign body
  with
    laceration —*see* Laceration, by site, with foreign body
    puncture wound —*see* Puncture, by site, with foreign body
  accidentally left following a procedure T81.509
  aspiration T81.506
    resulting in
      adhesions T81.516
      obstruction T81.526
      perforation T81.536
      specified complication NEC T81.596
  cardiac catheterization T81.505
    resulting in
      acute reaction T81.60
        aseptic peritonitis T81.61
        specified NEC T81.69
      adhesions T81.515
      obstruction T81.525
      perforation T81.535
      specified complication NEC T81.595
  causing
    acute reaction T81.60
      aseptic peritonitis T81.61
      specified complication NEC T81.69
    adhesions T81.519
    aseptic peritonitis T81.61
    obstruction T81.529
    perforation T81.539
    specified complication NEC T81.599
  endoscopy T81.504
    resulting in
      adhesions T81.514
      obstruction T81.524
      perforation T81.534
      specified complication NEC T81.594
  immunization T81.503
    resulting in
      adhesions T81.513
      obstruction T81.523
      perforation T81.533
      specified complication NEC T81.593
  infusion T81.501
    resulting in
      adhesions T81.511
      obstruction T81.521
      perforation T81.531

Foreign body – *continued*
      specified complication NEC T81.591
  injection T81.503
    resulting in
      adhesions T81.513
      obstruction T81.523
      perforation T81.533
      specified complication NEC T81.593
  kidney dialysis T81.502
    resulting in
      adhesions T81.512
      obstruction T81.522
      perforation T81.532
      specified complication NEC T81.592
  packing removal T81.507
    resulting in
      acute reaction T81.60
        aseptic peritonitis T81.61
        specified NEC T81.69
      adhesions T81.517
      obstruction T81.527
      perforation T81.537
      specified complication NEC T81.597
  puncture T81.506
    resulting in
      adhesions T81.516
      obstruction T81.526
      perforation T81.536
      specified complication NEC T81.596
  specified procedure NEC T81.508
    resulting in
      acute reaction T81.60
        aseptic peritonitis T81.61
        specified NEC T81.69
      adhesions T81.518
      obstruction T81.528
      perforation T81.538
      specified complication NEC T81.598
  surgical operation T81.500
    resulting in
      acute reaction T81.60
        aseptic peritonitis T81.61
        specified NEC T81.69
      adhesions T81.510
      obstruction T81.520
      perforation T81.530
      specified complication NEC T81.590
  transfusion T81.501
    resulting in
      adhesions T81.511
      obstruction T81.521
      perforation T81.531
      specified complication NEC T81.591
  alimentary tract T18.9
  anus T18.5
  colon T18.4
  esophagus —*see* Foreign body, esophagus
  mouth T18.0
  multiple sites T18.8
  rectosigmoid (junction) T18.5
  rectum T18.5
  small intestine T18.3
  specified site NEC T18.8
  stomach T18.2
  anterior chamber (eye) S05.5
  auditory canal —*see* Foreign body, entering through orifice, ear
  bronchus T17.508
    causing
      asphyxiation T17.500
        food (bone) (seed) T17.520
        gastric contents (vomitus) T17.510
        specified type NEC T17.590

Foreign body – *continued*
  injury NEC T17.508
    food (bone) (seed) T17.528
    gastric contents (vomitus) T17.518
    specified type NEC T17.598
  canthus —*see* Foreign body, conjunctival sac
  ciliary body (eye) S05.5
  conjunctival sac T15.1
  cornea T15.0
  entering through orifice
    accessory sinus T17.0
    alimentary canal T18.9
      multiple parts T18.8
      specified part NEC T18.8
    alveolar process T18.0
    antrum (Highmore's) T17.0
    anus T18.5
    appendix T18.4
    auditory canal —*see* Foreign body, entering through orifice, ear
    auricle —*see* Foreign body, entering through orifice, ear
    bladder T19.1
    bronchioles —*see* Foreign body, respiratory tract, specified site NEC
    bronchus (main) —*see* Foreign body, bronchus
    buccal cavity T18.0
    canthus (inner) —*see* Foreign body, conjunctival sac
    cecum T18.4
    cervix (canal) (uteri) T19.3
    colon T18.4
    conjunctival sac —*see* Foreign body, conjunctival sac
    cornea —*see* Foreign body, cornea
    digestive organ or tract NOS T18.9
      multiple parts T18.8
      specified part NEC T18.8
    duodenum T18.3
    ear (external) T16.
    esophagus —*see* Foreign body, esophagus
    eye (external) NOS T15.9
      conjunctival sac —*see* Foreign body, conjunctival sac
      cornea —*see* Foreign body, cornea
      specified part NEC T15.8
    eyeball —*see also* Foreign body, entering through orifice, eye, specified part NEC
      with penetrating wound —*see* Puncture, eyeball
    eyelid —*see also* Foreign body, conjunctival sac
      with
        laceration —*see* Laceration, eyelid, with foreign body
        puncture —*see* Puncture, eyelid, with foreign body
      superficial injury —*see* Foreign body, superficial, eyelid
    gastrointestinal tract T18.9
      multiple parts T18.8
      specified part NEC T18.8
    genitourinary tract T19.9
      multiple parts T19.8
      specified part NEC T19.8
    globe —*see* Foreign body, entering through orifice, eyeball
    gum T18.0
    Highmore's antrum T17.0
    hypopharynx —*see* Foreign body, pharynx
    ileum T18.3
    intestine (small) T18.3

Foreign body – *continued*
   large T18.4
   lacrimal apparatus (punctum) —*see* Foreign body, entering through orifice, eye, specified part NEC
   large intestine T18.4
   larynx —*see* Foreign body, larynx
   lung —*see* Foreign body, respiratory tract, specified site NEC
    maxillary sinus T17.0
    mouth T18.0
    nasal sinus T17.0
    nasopharynx —*see* Foreign body, pharynx
    nose (passage) T17.1
    nostril T17.1
    oral cavity T18.0
    palate T18.0
    penis T19.4
    pharynx —*see* Foreign body, pharynx
    piriform sinus —*see* Foreign body, pharynx
    rectosigmoid (junction) T18.5
    rectum T18.5
    respiratory tract —*see* Foreign body, respiratory tract
    sinus (accessory) (frontal) (maxillary) (nasal) T17.0
     piriform —*see* Foreign body, pharynx
    small intestine T18.3
    stomach T18.2
    suffocation by —*see* Foreign body, by site
    tear ducts or glands —*see* Foreign body, entering through orifice, eye, specified part NEC
    throat —*see* Foreign body, pharynx
    tongue T18.0
    tonsil, tonsillar (fossa) —*see* Foreign body, pharynx
    trachea —*see* Foreign body, trachea
    ureter T19.8
    urethra T19.0
    uterus (any part) T19.3
    vagina T19.2
    vulva T19.2
   esophagus T18.108
    causing
     injury NEC T18.108
      food (bone) (seed) T18.128
      gastric contents (vomitus) T18.118
      specified type NEC T18.198
     tracheal compression T18.100
      food (bone) (seed) T18.120
      gastric contents (vomitus) T18.110
      specified type NEC T18.190
   felling of, in throat R09.89
   fragment —*see* Retained, foreign body fragments (type of)
   genitourinary tract T19.9
    bladder T19.1
    multiple parts T19.8
    penis T19.4
    specified site NEC T19.8
    urethra T19.0
    uterus T19.3
     IUD Z97.5
    vagina T19.2
     contraceptive device Z97.5
    vulva T19.2
   granuloma (old) (soft tissue) —*see also* Granuloma, foreign body
    skin L92.3
   in

Foreign body – *continued*
   laceration —*see* Laceration, by site, with foreign body
    puncture wound —*see* Puncture, by site, with foreign body
    soft tissue (residual) M79.5
   inadvertently left in operation wound —*see* Foreign body, accidentally left during a procedure
   ingestion, ingested NOS T18.9
   inhalation or inspiration —*see* Foreign body, by site
   internal organ, not entering through a natural orifice
   code as specific injury with foreign body
   intraocular S05.5
    old, retained (nonmagnetic) H44.70
     anterior chamber H44.71
     ciliary body H44.72
     iris H44.72
     lens H44.73
     magnetic H44.60
      anterior chamber H44.61
      ciliary body H44.62
      iris H44.62
      lens H44.63
      posterior wall H44.64
      specified site NEC H44.69
      vitreous body H44.65
     posterior wall H44.74
     specified site NEC H44.79
     vitreous body H44.75
    iris —*see* Foreign body, intraocular
   lacrimal punctum —*see* Foreign body, entering through orifice, eye, specified part NEC
   larynx T17.308
    causing
     asphyxiation T17.300
      food (bone) (seed) T17.320
      gastric contents (vomitus) T17.310
      specified type NEC T17.390
     injury NEC T17.308
      food (bone) (seed) T17.328
      gastric contents (vomitus) T17.318
      specified type NEC T17.398
   lens —*see* Foreign body, intraocular
   ocular muscle S05.4
    old, retained —*see* Foreign body, orbit, old
   old or residual
    soft tissue (residual) M79.5
   operation wound, left accidentally —*see* Foreign body, accidentally left during a procedure
   orbit S05.4
    old, retained H05.5
   pharynx T17.208
    causing
     asphyxiation T17.200
      food (bone) (seed) T17.220
      gastric contents (vomitus) T17.210
      specified type NEC T17.290
     injury NEC T17.208
      food (bone) (seed) T17.228
      gastric contents (vomitus) T17.218
      specified type NEC T17.298
   respiratory tract T17.908
    bronchioles —*see* Foreign body, respiratory tract, specified site NEC
    bronchus —*see* Foreign body, bronchus
    causing
     asphyxiation T17.900

Foreign body – *continued*
      food (bone) (seed) T17.920
      gastric contents (vomitus) T17.910
      specified type NEC T17.990
     injury NEC T17.908
      food (bone) (seed) T17.928
      gastric contents (vomitus) T17.918
      specified type NEC T17.998
    larynx —*see* Foreign body, larynx
    lung —*see* Foreign body, respiratory tract, specified site NEC
    multiple parts —*see* Foreign body, respiratory tract, specified site NEC
    nasal sinus T17.0
    nasopharynx —*see* Foreign body, pharynx
    nose T17.1
    nostril T17.1
    pharynx —*see* Foreign body, pharynx
    specified site NEC T17.808
     causing
      asphyxiation T17.800
       food (bone) (seed) T17.820
       gastric contents (vomitus) T17.810
       specified type NEC T17.890
      injury NEC T17.808
       food (bone) (seed) T17.828
       gastric contents (vomitus) T17.818
       specified type NEC T17.898
    throat —*see* Foreign body, pharynx
    trachea —*see* Foreign body, trachea
   retained (old) (nonmagnetic) (in)
    anterior chamber (eye) —*see* Foreign body, intraocular, old, retained, anterior chamber
     magnetic —*see* Foreign body, intraocular, old, retained, magnetic, anterior chamber
    ciliary body —*see* Foreign body, intraocular, old, retained, ciliary body
     magnetic —*see* Foreign body, intraocular, old, retained, magnetic, ciliary body
    eyelid H02.819
     left H02.816
      lower H02.815
      upper H02.814
     right H02.813
      lower H02.812
      upper H02.811
    fragments —*see* Retained, foreign body fragments (type of)
    globe —*see* Foreign body, intraocular, old, retained
     magnetic —*see* Foreign body, intraocular, old, retained, magnetic
    intraocular —*see* Foreign body, intraocular, old, retained
     magnetic —*see* Foreign body, intraocular, old, retained, magnetic
    iris —*see* Foreign body, intraocular, old, retained, iris
     magnetic —*see* Foreign body, intraocular, old, retained, magnetic, iris
    lens —*see* Foreign body, intraocular, old, retained, lens
     magnetic —*see* Foreign body, intraocular, old, retained, magnetic, lens
    muscle —*see* Foreign body, retained, soft tissue
    orbit —*see* Foreign body, orbit, old
    posterior wall of globe —*see* Foreign body, intraocular, old, retained, posterior wall
     magnetic —*see* Foreign body, intraocular, old, retained, magnetic, posterior wall
    retrobulbar —*see* Foreign body, orbit, old, retrobulbar

Foreign body – *continued*
- soft tissue M79.5
- vitreous —*see* Foreign body, intraocular, old, retained, vitreous body
  - magnetic —*see* Foreign body, intraocular, old, retained, magnetic, vitreous body
- retina S05.5
- superficial, without open wound
  - abdomen, abdominal (wall) S30.851
  - alveolar process S00.552
  - ankle S90.55
  - antecubital space —*see* Foreign body, superficial, forearm
  - anus S30.857
  - arm (upper) S40.85
  - auditory canal —*see* Foreign body, superficial, ear
  - auricle —*see* Foreign body, superficial, ear
  - axilla —*see* Foreign body, superficial, arm
  - back, lower S30.850
  - breast S20.15
  - brow S00.85
  - buttock S30.850
  - calf —*see* Foreign body, superficial, leg
  - canthus —*see* Foreign body, superficial, eyelid
  - cheek S00.85
    - internal S00.552
  - chest wall —*see* Foreign body, superficial, thorax
  - chin S00.85
  - clitoris S30.854
  - costal region —*see* Foreign body, superficial, thorax
  - digit (s)
    - hand —*see* Foreign body, superficial, finger
    - foot —*see* Foreign body, superficial, toe
  - ear S00.45
  - elbow S50.35
  - epididymis S30.853
  - epigastric region S30.851
  - epiglottis S10.15
  - esophagus, cervical S10.15
  - eyebrow —*see* Foreign body, superficial, eyelid
  - eyelid S00.25
  - face S00.85
  - finger (s) S60.459
    - index S60.45
    - little S60.45
    - middle S60.45
    - ring S60.45
  - flank S30.851
  - foot (except toe(s) alone) S90.85
    - toe —*see* Foreign body, superficial, toe
  - forearm S50.85
    - elbow only —*see* Foreign body, superficial, elbow
  - forehead S00.85
  - genital organs, external
    - female S30.856
    - male S30.855
  - groin S30.851
  - gum S00.552
  - hand S60.55
  - head S00.95
    - ear —*see* Foreign body, superficial, ear
    - eyelid —*see* Foreign body, superficial, eyelid
    - lip S00.551
    - nose S00.35

Foreign body – *continued*
- oral cavity S00.552
  - scalp S00.05
  - specified site NEC S00.85
- heel —*see* Foreign body, superficial, foot
- hip S70.25
- inguinal region S30.851
- interscapular region S20.459
- jaw S00.85
- knee S80.25
- labium (majus) (minus) S30.854
- larynx S10.15
- leg (lower) S80.85
  - knee —*see* Foreign body, superficial, knee
  - upper —*see* Foreign body, superficial, thigh
- lip S00.551
- lower back S30.850
- lumbar region S30.850
- malar region S00.85
- mammary —*see* Foreign body, superficial, breast
- mastoid region S00.85
- mouth S00.552
- nail
  - finger —*see* Foreign body, superficial, finger
  - toe —*see* Foreign body, superficial, toe
- nape S10.85
- nasal S00.35
- neck S10.95
  - specified site NEC S10.85
  - throat S10.15
- nose S00.35
- occipital region S00.05
- oral cavity S00.552
- orbital region —*see* Foreign body, superficial, eyelid
- palate S00.552
- palm —*see* Foreign body, superficial, hand
- parietal region S00.05
- pelvis S30.850
- penis S30.852
- perineum
  - female S30.854
  - male S30.850
- periocular area —*see* Foreign body, superficial, eyelid
- phalanges
  - finger —*see* Foreign body, superficial, finger
  - toe —*see* Foreign body, superficial, toe
- pharynx S10.15
- pinna —*see* Foreign body, superficial, ear
- popliteal space —*see* Foreign body, superficial, knee
- prepuce S30.852
- pubic region S30.850
- pudendum
  - female S30.856
  - male S30.855
- sacral region S30.850
- scalp S00.05
- scapular region —*see* Foreign body, superficial, shoulder
- scrotum S30.853
- shin —*see* Foreign body, superficial, leg
- shoulder S40.25
- sternal region S20.359
- submaxillary region S00.85
- submental region S00.85
- subungual

Foreign body – *continued*
- finger (s) —*see* Foreign body, superficial, finger
- toe (s) —*see* Foreign body, superficial, toe
- supraclavicular fossa S10.85
- supraorbital S00.85
- temple S00.85
- temporal region S00.85
- testis S30.853
- thigh S70.35
- thorax, thoracic (wall) S20.95
  - back S20.45
  - front S20.35
- throat S10.15
- thumb S60.35
- toe (s) (lesser) S90.456
  - great S90.45
- tongue S00.552
- trachea S10.15
- tunica vaginalis S30.853
- tympanum, tympanic membrane —*see* Foreign body, superficial, ear
- uvula S00.552
- vagina S30.854
- vocal cords S10.15
- vulva S30.854
- wrist S60.85
- swallowed T18.9
- trachea T17.408
  - causing
    - asphyxiation T17.400
      - food (bone) (seed) T17.420
      - gastric contents (vomitus) T17.410
      - specified type NEC T17.490
    - injury NEC T17.408
      - food (bone) (seed) T17.428
      - gastric contents (vomitus) T17.418
      - specified type NEC T17.498
- type of fragment —*see* Retained, foreign body fragments (type of)
- vitreous (humor) S05.5

Forestier's disease (rhizomelic pseudopolyarthritis) M35.3
- meaning ankylosing hyperostosis —*see* Hyperostosis, ankylosing

Formation
- hyalin in cornea —*see* Degeneration, cornea
- sequestrum in bone (due to infection) —*see* Osteomyelitis, chronic
- valve
  - colon, congenital Q43.8
  - ureter (congenital) Q62.39

Formication R20.2
Fort Bragg fever A27.89
Fossa —*see also* condition
- pyriform —*see* condition
Foster-Kennedy syndrome H47.14
Fothergill's
- disease (trigeminal neuralgia) —*see also* Neuralgia, trigeminal
- scarlatina anginosa A38.9
Foul breath R19.6
Foundling Z76.1
Fournier disease or gangrene N49.3
- female N76.89
Fourth
- cranial nerve —*see* condition
- molar K00.1
Foville's (peduncular) **disease or syndrome** G46.3
Fox (-Fordyce) **disease** (apocrine miliaria) L75.2

Fracture, burst —*see* Fracture, traumatic, by site
Fracture, chronic —*see* Fracture, pathological
Fracture, insufficiency —*see* Fracture, pathologic, by site
Fracture, pathological (pathologic) —*see also* Fracture, traumatic M84.40
  ankle M84.47
  carpus M84.44
  clavicle M84.41
  dental implant M27.63
  dental restorative material K08.539
    with loss of material K08.531
    without loss of material K08.530
  due to
    neoplastic disease NEC (*see also* Neoplasm) M84.50
      ankle M84.57
      carpus M84.54
      clavicle M84.51
      femur M84.55
      fibula M84.56
      finger M84.54
      hip M84.559
      humerus M84.52
      ilium M84.550
      ischium M84.550
      metacarpus M84.54
      metatarsus M84.57
      neck M84.58
      pelvis M84.550
      radius M84.53
      rib M84.58
      scapula M84.51
      skull M84.58
      specified site NEC M84.58
      tarsus M84.57
      tibia M84.56
      toe M84.57
      ulna M84.53
      vertebra M84.58
    osteoporosis M80.80
    disuse —*see* Osteoporosis, specified type NEC, with pathological fracture
    drug-induced —*see* Osteoporosis, drug induced, with pathological fracture
    idiopathic —*see* Osteoporosis, specified type NEC, with pathological fracture
    postmenopausal —*see* Osteoporosis, postmenopausal, with pathological fracture
    postoophorectomy —*see* Osteoporosis, postoophorectomy, with pathological fracture
    postsurgical malabsorption —*see* Osteoporosis, specified type NEC, with pathological fracture
    specified cause NEC —*see* Osteoporosis, specified type NEC, with pathological fracture
  specified disease NEC M84.60
    ankle M84.67
    carpus M84.64
    clavicle M84.61
    femur M84.65
    fibula M84.66
    finger M84.64
    hip M84.65
    humerus M84.62
    ilium M84.650
    ischium M84.650
    metacarpus M84.64
    metatarsus M84.67
    neck M84.68

Fracture, pathological - *continued*
  radius M84.63
  rib M84.68
  scapula M84.61
  skull M84.68
  tarsus M84.67
  tibia M84.66
  toe M84.67
  ulna M84.63
  vertebra M84.68
  femur M84.45
  fibula M84.46
  finger M84.44
  hip M84.459
  humerus M84.42
  ilium M84.454
  ischium M84.454
  joint prosthesis —*see* Complications, joint prosthesis, mechanical, breakdown, by site
    periprosthetic —*see* Complications, joint prosthesis, mechanical, periprosthesis, fracture, by site
  metacarpus M84.44
  metatarsus M84.47
  neck M84.48
  pelvis M84.454
  radius M84.43
  restorative material (dental) K08.539
    with loss of material K08.531
    without loss of material K08.530
  rib M84.48
  scapula M84.41
  skull M84.48
  tarsus M84.47
  tibia M84.46
  toe M84.47
  ulna M84.43
  vertebra M84.48
Fracture, traumatic (abduction) (adduction) (separation) (*see also* Fracture, pathological) T14.8
  acetabulum S32.40
    column
      anterior (displaced) (iliopubic) S32.43
        nondisplaced S32.436
      posterior (displaced) (ilioischial) S32.443
        nondisplaced S32.44
    dome (displaced) S32.48
      nondisplaced S32.48
    specified NEC S32.49
    transverse (displaced) S32.45
      with associated posterior wall fracture (displaced) S32.46
        nondisplaced S32.46
      nondisplaced S32.45
    wall
      anterior (displaced) S32.41
        nondisplaced S32.41
      medial (displaced) S32.47
        nondisplaced S32.47
      posterior (displaced) S32.42
        with associated transverse fracture (displaced) S32.46
          nondisplaced S32.46
        nondisplaced S32.42
  acromion —*see* Fracture, scapula, acromial process
  ankle S82.899
    bimalleolar (displaced) S82.84
      nondisplaced S82.84
    lateral malleolus only (displaced) S82.6
      nondisplaced S82.6

Fracture, traumatic - *continued*
    medial malleolus (displaced) S82.5
      associated with Maisonneuve's fracture —*see* Fracture, Maisonneuve's
      nondisplaced S82.5
    trimalleolar (displaced) S82.85
      nondisplaced S82.85
  arm (upper) —*see also* Fracture, humerus, shaft
    humerus —*see* Fracture, humerus
    radius —*see* Fracture, radius
    ulna —*see* Fracture, ulna
  astragalus —*see* Fracture, tarsal, talus
  atlas —*see* Fracture, neck, cervical vertebra, first
  axis —*see* Fracture, neck, cervical vertebra, second
  back —*see* Fracture, vertebra
  Barton's —*see* Barton's fracture
  base of skull —*see* Fracture, skull, base
  basicervical (basal) (femoral) S72.0
  Bennett's —*see* Bennett's fracture
  bimalleolar —*see* Fracture, ankle, bimalleolar
  blow-out S02.3
  bone NEC T14.8
    birth injury P13.9
    following insertion of orthopedic implant, joint prosthesis or bone plate —*see* Fracture, following insertion of orthopedic implant, joint prosthesis or bone plate
    in (due to) neoplastic disease NEC —*see* Fracture, pathological, due to, neoplastic disease
    pathological (cause unknown) —*see* Fracture, pathological
  breast bone —*see* Fracture, sternum
  bucket handle (semilunar cartilage) —*see* Tear, meniscus
  burst —*see* Fracture, traumatic, by site
  calcaneus —*see* Fracture, tarsal, calcaneus
  carpal bone (s) S62.10
    capitate (displaced) S62.13
      nondisplaced S62.13
    cuneiform —*see* Fracture, carpal bone, triquetrum
    hamate (body) (displaced) S62.143
      hook process (displaced) S62.15
        nondisplaced S62.15
      nondisplaced S62.14
    larger multangular —*see* Fracture, carpal bones, trapezium
    lunate (displaced) S62.12
      nondisplaced S62.12
    navicular S62.00
      distal pole (displaced) S62.01
        nondisplaced S62.01
      middle third (displaced) S62.02
        nondisplaced S62.02
      proximal third (displaced) S62.03
        nondisplaced S62.03
      volar tuberosity —*see* Fracture, carpal bones, navicular, distal pole
    os magnum —*see* Fracture, carpal bones, capitate
    pisiform (displaced) S62.16
      nondisplaced S62.16
    semilunar —*see* Fracture, carpal bones, lunate
    smaller multangular —*see* Fracture, carpal bones, trapezoid
    trapezium (displaced) S62.17
      nondisplaced S62.17

Fracture, traumatic   - continued
proximal phalanx (displaced) S62.61
  nondisplaced S62.64
little S62.60
  distal phalanx (displaced) S62.63
    nondisplaced S62.66
  medial phalanx (displaced) S62.62
    nondisplaced S62.65
  proximal phalanx (displaced) S62.61
    nondisplaced S62.64
medial phalanx (displaced) S62.62
  nondisplaced S62.65
middle S62.60
  distal phalanx (displaced) S62.63
    nondisplaced S62.66
  medial phalanx (displaced) S62.62
    nondisplaced S62.65
  proximal phalanx (displaced) S62.61
    nondisplaced S62.64
proximal phalanx (displaced) S62.61
  nondisplaced S62.64
ring S62.60
  distal phalanx (displaced) S62.63
    nondisplaced S62.66
  medial phalanx (displaced) S62.62
    nondisplaced S62.65
  proximal phalanx (displaced) S62.61
    nondisplaced S62.64
thumb —see Fracture, thumb
following insertion (intraoperative)
(postoperative) of orthopedic implant, joint
prosthesis or bone plate M96.69
  femur M96.66
  fibula M96.67
  humerus M96.62
  pelvis M96.65
  radius M96.63
  specified bone NEC M96.69
  tibia M96.67
  ulna M96.63
foot S92.90
  astragalus —see Fracture, tarsal, talus
  calcaneus —see Fracture, tarsal, calcaneus
  cuboid —see Fracture, tarsal, cuboid
  cuneiform —see Fracture, tarsal, cuneiform
  metatarsal —see Fracture, metatarsal
  navicular —see Fracture, tarsal, navicular
  talus —see Fracture, tarsal, talus
  tarsal —see Fracture, tarsal
  toe —see Fracture, toe
forearm S52.9
  radius —see Fracture, radius
  ulna —see Fracture, ulna
fossa (anterior) (middle) (posterior) S02.19
frontal (bone) (skull) S02.0
  sinus S02.19
glenoid (cavity) (scapula) —see Fracture,
scapula, glenoid cavity
greenstick —see Fracture, by site
hallux —see Fracture, toe, great
hand S62.9
  carpal —see Fracture, carpal bone
  finger (except thumb) —see Fracture, finger
  metacarpal —see Fracture, metacarpal
  navicular (scaphoid) (hand) —see Fracture,
  carpal bone, navicular
  thumb —see Fracture, thumb
healed or old
  with complications
code by Nature of the complication
heel bone —see Fracture, tarsal, calcaneus
Hill-Sachs S42.29

Fracture, traumatic   - continued
hip —see Fracture, femur, neck
humerus S42.30
  anatomical neck —see Fracture, humerus,
  upper end
  articular process —see Fracture, humerus,
  lower end
  capitellum —see Fracture, humerus, lower
  end, condyle, lateral
  distal end —see Fracture, humerus, lower
  end
  epiphysis
    lower —see Fracture, humerus, lower end,
    physeal
    upper —see Fracture, humerus, upper end,
    physeal
  external condyle —see Fracture, humerus,
  lower end, condyle, lateral
  following insertion of implant, prosthesis or
  plate M96.62
  great tuberosity —see Fracture, humerus,
  upper end, greater tuberosity
  intercondylar —see Fracture, humerus,
  lower end
  internal epicondyle —see Fracture, humerus,
  lower end, epicondyle, medial
  lesser tuberosity —see Fracture, humerus,
  upper end, lesser tuberosity
  lower end S42.40
    condyle
      lateral (displaced) S42.45
        nondisplaced S42.45
      medial (displaced) S42.46
        nondisplaced S42.46
    epicondyle
      lateral (displaced) S42.43
        nondisplaced S42.43
      medial (displaced) S42.44
        incarcerated S42.44
        nondisplaced S42.44
    physeal S49.10
      Salter-Harris
        Type I S49.11
        Type II S49.12
        Type III S49.13
        Type IV S49.14
      specified NEC S49.19
    specified NEC (displaced) S42.49
      nondisplaced S42.49
    supracondylar (simple) (displaced) S42.41
      comminuted (displaced) S42.42
        nondisplaced S42.42
      nondisplaced S42.41
    torus S42.48
    transcondylar (displaced) S42.47
      nondisplaced S42.47
  proximal end —see Fracture, humerus,
  upper end
  shaft S42.30
    comminuted (displaced) S42.35
      nondisplaced S42.35
    greenstick S42.31
    oblique (displaced) S42.33
      nondisplaced S42.33
    segmental (displaced) S42.36
      nondisplaced S42.36
    specified NEC S42.39
    spiral (displaced) S42.34
      nondisplaced S42.34
    transverse (displaced) S42.32
      nondisplaced S42.32

Fracture, traumatic   - continued
supracondylar —see Fracture, humerus,
lower end
  surgical neck —see Fracture, humerus,
  upper end, surgical neck
  trochlea —see Fracture, humerus, lower end,
  condyle, medial
  tuberosity —see Fracture, humerus, upper
  end
  upper end S42.20
    anatomical neck —see Fracture, humerus,
    upper end, specified NEC
    articular head —see Fracture, humerus,
    upper end, specified NEC
    epiphysis —see Fracture, humerus, upper
    end, physeal
    greater tuberosity (displaced) S42.25
      nondisplaced S42.25
    lesser tuberosity (displaced) S42.26
      nondisplaced S42.26
    physeal S49.00
      Salter-Harris
        Type I S49.01
        Type II S49.02
        Type III S49.03
        Type IV S49.04
      specified NEC S49.09
    specified NEC (displaced) S42.29
      nondisplaced S42.29
    surgical neck (displaced) S42.21
      four-part S42.24
      nondisplaced S42.21
      three-part S42.23
      two-part (displaced) S42.22
        nondisplaced S42.22
    torus S42.27
    transepiphyseal —see Fracture, humerus,
    upper end, physeal
hyoid bone S12.8
ilium S32.30
  with disruption of pelvic ring —see
  Disruption, pelvic ring
  avulsion (displaced) S32.31
    nondisplaced S32.31
  specified NEC S32.39
impaction, impacted
code as Fracture, by site
innominate bone —see Fracture, ilium
instep —see Fracture, foot
ischium S32.60
  with disruption of pelvic ring —see
  Disruption, pelvic ring
  avulsion (displaced) S32.61
    nondisplaced S32.61
  specified NEC S32.69
jaw (bone) (lower) —see Fracture, mandible
  upper —see Fracture, maxilla
joint prosthesis —see Complications, joint
prosthesis, mechanical, breakdown, by site
  periprosthetic —see Complications, joint
prosthesis, mechanical, periprosthesis,
fracture, by site
knee cap —see Fracture, patella
larynx S12.8
late effects —see Sequelae, fracture
leg (lower) S82.9
  ankle —see Fracture, ankle
  femur —see Fracture, femur
  fibula —see Fracture, fibula
  malleolus —see Fracture, ankle
  patella —see Fracture, patella
  specified site NEC S82.89
  tibia —see Fracture, tibia

Fracture, traumatic - *continued*
lumbar spine —*see* Fracture, vertebra, lumbar
lumbosacral spine S32.9
Maisonneuve's (displaced) S82.86
  nondisplaced S82.86
malar bone (*see also* Fracture, maxilla)
S02.400
malleolus —*see* Fracture, ankle
malunion —*see* Fracture, by site
mandible (lower jaw (bone)) S02.609
  alveolus S02.67
  angle (of jaw) S02.65
  body, unspecified S02.600
  condylar process S02.61
  coronoid process S02.63
  ramus, unspecified S02.64
  specified site NEC S02.69
  subcondylar process S02.62
  symphysis S02.66
manubrium (sterni) S22.21
  dissociation from sternum S22.23
march —*see* Fracture, traumatic, stress, by site
maxilla, maxillary (bone) (sinus) (superior) (upper jaw) S02.401
  alveolus S02.42
  inferior —*see* Fracture, mandible
  LeFort I S02.411
  LeFort II S02.412
  LeFort III S02.413
metacarpal S62.309
  base (displaced) S62.319
    nondisplaced S62.349
  fifth S62.30
    base (displaced) S62.31
      nondisplaced S62.34
    neck (displaced) S62.33
      nondisplaced S62.36
    shaft (displaced) S62.32
      nondisplaced S62.35
    specified NEC S62.398
  first S62.20
    base NEC (displaced) S62.23
      nondisplaced S62.23
    Bennett's —*see* Bennett's fracture
    neck (displaced) S62.25
      nondisplaced S62.25
    shaft (displaced) S62.24
      nondisplaced S62.24
    specified NEC S62.29
  fourth S62.30
    base (displaced) S62.31
      nondisplaced S62.34
    neck (displaced) S62.33
      nondisplaced S62.36
    shaft (displaced) S62.32
      nondisplaced S62.35
    specified NEC S62.39
  neck (displaced) S62.33
    nondisplaced S62.36
  Rolando's —*see* Rolando's fracture
  second S62.30
    base (displaced) S62.31
      nondisplaced S62.34
    neck (displaced) S62.33
      nondisplaced S62.36
    shaft (displaced) S62.32
      nondisplaced S62.35
    specified NEC S62.39
  shaft (displaced) S62.32
    nondisplaced S62.35
  third S62.30

Fracture, traumatic - *continued*
    base (displaced) S62.31
      nondisplaced S62.34
    neck (displaced) S62.33
      nondisplaced S62.36
    shaft (displaced) S62.32
      nondisplaced S62.35
    specified NEC S62.39
  specified NEC S62.399
metastatic —*see* Fracture, pathological, due to, neoplastic disease —*see also* Neoplasm
metatarsal bone S92.30
  fifth (displaced) S92.35
    nondisplaced S92.35
  first (displaced) S92.31
    nondisplaced S92.31
  fourth (displaced) S92.34
    nondisplaced S92.34
  second (displaced) S92.32
    nondisplaced S92.32
  third (displaced) S92.33
    nondisplaced S92.33
Monteggia's —*see* Monteggia's fracture
multiple
  hand (and wrist) NEC —*see* Fracture, by site
  ribs —*see* Fracture, rib, multiple
nasal (bone(s)) S02.2
navicular (scaphoid) (foot) —*see also* Fracture, tarsal, navicular
  hand —*see* Fracture, carpal, navicular
neck S12.9
  cervical vertebra S12.9
    fifth (displaced) S12.400
      nondisplaced S12.401
      specified type NEC (displaced) S12.490
        nondisplaced S12.491
    first (displaced) S12.000
      burst (stable) S12.01
        unstable S12.02
      lateral mass (displaced) S12.040
        nondisplaced S12.041
      nondisplaced S12.001
      posterior arch (displaced) S12.030
        nondisplaced S12.031
      specified type NEC (displaced) S12.090
        nondisplaced S12.091
    fourth (displaced) S12.300
      nondisplaced S12.301
      specified type NEC (displaced) S12.390
        nondisplaced S12.391
    second (displaced) S12.100
      nondisplaced S12.101
      dens (anterior) (displaced) (type II) S12.110
        nondisplaced S12.112
        posterior S12.111
      specified type NEC (displaced) S12.120
        nondisplaced S12.121
      specified type NEC (displaced) S12.190
        nondisplaced S12.191
    seventh (displaced) S12.600
      nondisplaced S12.601
      specified type NEC (displaced) S12.690
        displaced S12.691
    sixth (displaced) S12.500
      nondisplaced S12.501
      specified type NEC (displaced) S12.590
        displaced S12.591
    third (displaced) S12.200
      nondisplaced S12.201
      specified type NEC (displaced) S12.290

Fracture, traumatic - *continued*
      displaced S12.291
  hyoid bone S12.8
  larynx S12.8
  specified site NEC S12.8
  thyroid cartilage S12.8
  trachea S12.8
neoplastic NEC —*see* Fracture, pathological, due to, neoplastic disease
neural arch —*see* Fracture, vertebra
newborn —*see* Birth, injury, fracture
nontraumatic —*see* Fracture, pathological
nonunion —*see* Nonunion, fracture
nose, nasal (bone) (septum) S02.2
occiput —*see* Fracture, skull, base, occiput
odontoid process —*see* Fracture, neck, cervical vertebra, second
olecranon (process) (ulna) —*see* Fracture, ulna, upper end, olecranon process
orbit, orbital (bone) (region) S02.8
  floor (blow-out) S02.3
  roof S02.19
os
  calcis —*see* Fracture, tarsal, calcaneus
  magnum —*see* Fracture, carpal, capitate
  pubis —*see* Fracture, pubis
palate S02.8
parietal bone (skull) S02.0
patella S82.00
  comminuted (displaced) S82.04
    nondisplaced S82.04
  longitudinal (displaced) S82.02
    nondisplaced S82.02
  osteochondral (displaced) S82.01
    nondisplaced S82.01
  specified NEC S82.09
  transverse (displaced) S82.03
    nondisplaced S82.03
pedicle (of vertebral arch) —*see* Fracture, vertebra
pelvis, pelvic (bone) S32.9
  acetabulum —*see* Fracture, acetabulum
  circle —*see* Disruption, pelvic ring
  following insertion of implant, prosthesis or plate M96.65
  ilium —*see* Fracture, ilium
  ischium —*see* Fracture, ischium
  multiple
    with disruption of pelvic ring (circle) —*see* Disruption, pelvic ring
    without disruption of pelvic ring (circle) S32.82
  pubis —*see* Fracture, pubis
  specified site NEC S32.89
  sacrum —*see* Fracture, sacrum
phalanx
  foot —*see* Fracture, toe
  hand —*see* Fracture, finger
pisiform —*see* Fracture, carpal, pisiform
pond —*see* Fracture, skull
prosthetic device, internal —*see* Complications, prosthetic device, by site, mechanical
pubis S32.50
  with disruption of pelvic ring —*see* Disruption, pelvic ring
  specified site NEC S32.59
  superior rim S32.51
radius S52.9
  distal end —*see* Fracture, radius, lower end
  following insertion of implant, prosthesis or plate M96.63

Fracture, traumatic *- continued*
  head —*see* Fracture, radius, upper end, head
  lower end S52.50
    Barton's —*see* Barton's fracture
    Colles' —*see* Colles' fracture
    extraarticular NEC S52.55
    intraarticular NEC S52.57
    physeal S59.20
      Salter-Harris
        Type I S59.21
        Type II S59.22
        Type III S59.23
        Type IV S59.24
      specified NEC S59.29
    Smith's —*see* Smith's fracture
    specified NEC S52.59
    styloid process (displaced) S52.51
      nondisplaced S52.51
    torus S52.52
  neck —*see* Fracture, radius, upper end
  proximal end —*see* Fracture, radius, upper end
  shaft S52.30
    bent bone S52.38
    comminuted (displaced) S52.35
      nondisplaced S52.35
    Galeazzi's —*see* Galeazzi's fracture
    greenstick S52.31
    oblique (displaced) S52.33
      nondisplaced S52.33
    segmental (displaced) S52.36
      nondisplaced S52.36
    specified NEC S52.39
    spiral (displaced) S52.34
      nondisplaced S52.34
    transverse (displaced) S52.32
      nondisplaced S52.32
  upper end S52.10
    head (displaced) S52.12
      nondisplaced S52.12
    neck (displaced) S52.13
      nondisplaced S52.13
    specified NEC S52.18
    physeal S59.10
      Salter-Harris
        Type I S59.11
        Type II S59.12
        Type III S59.13
        Type IV S59.14
      specified NEC S59.19
    torus S52.11
  ramus
    inferior or superior, pubis —*see* Fracture, pubis
    mandible —*see* Fracture, mandible
  restorative material (dental) K08.539
    with loss of material K08.531
    without loss of material K08.530
  rib S22.3
    with flail chest —*see* Flail, chest
    multiple S22.4
      with flail chest —*see* Flail, chest
  root, tooth —*see* Fracture, tooth
  sacrum S32.10
    specified NEC S32.19
    Type
      1 S32.14
      2 S32.15
      3 S32.16
      4 S32.17
    Zone
      I S32.119

Fracture, traumatic *- continued*
    displaced (minimally) S32.111
      severely S32.112
    nondisplaced S32.110
    II S32.129
    displaced (minimally) S32.121
      severely S32.122
    nondisplaced S32.120
    III S32.139
    displaced (minimally) S32.131
      severely S32.132
    nondisplaced S32.130
  scaphoid (hand) —*see also* Fracture, carpal, navicular
    foot —*see* Fracture, tarsal, navicular
  scapula S42.10
    acromial process (displaced) S42.12
      nondisplaced S42.12
    body (displaced) S42.11
      nondisplaced S42.11
    coracoid process (displaced) S42.13
      nondisplaced S42.13
    glenoid cavity (displaced) S42.14
      nondisplaced S42.14
    neck (displaced) S42.15
      nondisplaced S42.15
    specified NEC S42.19
  semilunar bone, wrist —*see* Fracture, carpal, lunate
  sequelae —*see* Sequelae, fracture
  sesamoid bone
    hand —*see* Fracture, carpal
    other
    code by site under Fracture
  shepherd's —*see* Fracture, tarsal, talus
  shoulder (girdle) S42.9
    blade —*see* Fracture, scapula
  sinus (ethmoid) (frontal) S02.19
  skull S02.91
    base S02.10
      occiput S02.119
      condyle S02.113
        type I S02.110
        type II S02.111
        type III S02.112
      specified NEC S02.118
      specified NEC S02.19
    birth injury P13.0
    frontal bone S02.0
    parietal bone S02.0
    specified site NEC S02.8
    temporal bone S02.19
    vault S02.0
  Smith's —*see* Smith's fracture
  sphenoid (bone) (sinus) S02.19
  spine —*see* Fracture, vertebra
  spinous process —*see* Fracture, vertebra
  spontaneous (cause unknown) —*see* Fracture, pathological
  stave (of thumb) —*see* Fracture, metacarpal, first
  sternum S22.20
    with flail chest —*see* Flail, chest
    body S22.22
    manubrium S22.21
    xiphoid (process) S22.24
  stress M84.30
    ankle M84.37
    carpus M84.34
    clavicle M84.31
    femoral neck M84.359
    femur M84.35

Fracture, traumatic *- continued*
    fibula M84.36
    finger M84.34
    hip M84.359
    humerus M84.32
    ilium M84.350
    ischium M84.350
    metacarpus M84.34
    metatarsus M84.37
    neck —*see* Fracture, fatigue, vertebra
    pelvis M84.350
    radius M84.33
    rib M84.38
    scapula M84.31
    skull M84.38
    tarsus M84.37
    tibia M84.36
    toe M84.37
    ulna M84.33
    vertebra —*see* Fracture, fatigue, vertebra
  supracondylar, elbow —*see* Fracture, humerus, lower end, supracondylar
  symphysis pubis —*see* Fracture, pubis
  talus (ankle bone) —*see* Fracture, tarsal, talus
  tarsal bone (s) S92.20
    astragalus —*see* Fracture, tarsal, talus
    calcaneus S92.00
      anterior process (displaced) S92.02
        nondisplaced S92.02
      body (displaced) S92.01
        nondisplaced S92.01
      extraarticular NEC (displaced) S92.05
        nondisplaced S92.05
      intraarticular (displaced) S92.06
        nondisplaced S92.06
      tuberosity (displaced) S92.04
        avulsion (displaced) S92.03
          nondisplaced S92.03
        nondisplaced S92.04
    cuboid (displaced) S92.21
      nondisplaced S92.21
    cuneiform
      intermediate (displaced) S92.23
        nondisplaced S92.23
      lateral (displaced) S92.22
        nondisplaced S92.22
      medial (displaced) S92.24
        nondisplaced S92.24
    navicular (displaced) S92.25
      nondisplaced S92.25
    scaphoid —*see* Fracture, tarsal, navicular
    talus S92.10
      avulsion (displaced) S92.15
        nondisplaced S92.15
      body (displaced) S92.12
        nondisplaced S92.12
      dome (displaced) S92.14
        nondisplaced S92.14
      head (displaced) S92.12
        nondisplaced S92.12
      lateral process (displaced) S92.14
        nondisplaced S92.14
      neck (displaced) S92.11
        nondisplaced S92.11
      posterior process (displaced) S92.13
        nondisplaced S92.13
      specified NEC S92.19
  temporal bone (styloid) S02.19
  thorax (bony) S22.9
    with flail chest —*see* Flail, chest
    rib S22.3
      multiple S22.4

Fracture, traumatic *- continued*
  with flail chest —*see* Flail, chest
  sternum S22.20
    body S22.22
    manubrium S22.21
    xiphoid process S22.24
  vertebra (displaced) S22.009
    burst (stable) S22.001
      unstable S22.002
    eighth S22.069
      burst (stable) S22.061
        unstable S22.062
      specified type NEC S22.068
      wedge compression S22.060
    eleventh S22.089
      burst (stable) S22.081
        unstable S22.082
      specified type NEC S22.088
      wedge compression S22.080
    fifth S22.059
      burst (stable) S22.051
        unstable S22.052
      specified type NEC S22.058
      wedge compression S22.050
    first S22.019
      burst (stable) S22.011
        unstable S22.012
      specified type NEC S22.018
      wedge compression S22.010
    fourth S22.049
      burst (stable) S22.041
        unstable S22.042
      specified type NEC S22.048
      wedge compression S22.040
    ninth S22.079
      burst (stable) S22.071
        unstable S22.072
      specified type NEC S22.078
      wedge compression S22.070
    nondisplaced S22.001
    second S22.029
      burst (stable) S22.021
        unstable S22.022
      specified type NEC S22.028
      wedge compression S22.020
    seventh S22.069
      burst (stable) S22.061
        unstable S22.062
      specified type NEC S22.068
      wedge compression S22.060
    sixth S22.059
      burst (stable) S22.051
        unstable S22.052
      specified type NEC S22.058
      wedge compression S22.050
    specified type NEC S22.008
    tenth S22.079
      burst (stable) S22.071
        unstable S22.072
      specified type NEC S22.078
      wedge compression S22.070
    third S22.039
      burst (stable) S22.031
        unstable S22.032
      specified type NEC S22.038
      wedge compression S22.030
    twelfth S22.089
      burst (stable) S22.081
        unstable S22.082
      specified type NEC S22.088
      wedge compression S22.080
    wedge compression S22.000

Fracture, traumatic *- continued*
  thumb S62.50
    distal phalanx (displaced) S62.52
      nondisplaced S62.52
    proximal phalanx (displaced) S62.51
      nondisplaced S62.51
  thyroid cartilage S12.8
  tibia (shaft) S82.20
    comminuted (displaced) S82.25
      nondisplaced S82.25
    condyles —*see* Fracture, tibia, upper end
    distal end —*see* Fracture, tibia, lower end
    epiphysis
      lower —*see* Fracture, tibia, lower end
      upper —*see* Fracture, tibia, upper end
    following insertion of implant, prosthesis or plate M96.67
    head (involving knee joint) —*see* Fracture, tibia, upper end
    intercondyloid eminence —*see* Fracture, tibia, upper end
    involving ankle or malleolus —*see* Fracture, ankle, medial malleolus
    lower end S82.30
      physeal S89.10
        Salter-Harris
          Type I S89.11
          Type II S89.12
          Type III S89.13
          Type IV S89.14
        specified NEC S89.19
      pilon (displaced) S82.87
        nondisplaced S82.87
      specified NEC S82.39
      torus S82.31
    malleolus —*see* Fracture, ankle, medial malleolus
    oblique (displaced) S82.23
      nondisplaced S82.23
    pilon —*see* Fracture, tibia, lower end, pilon
    proximal end —*see* Fracture, tibia, upper end
    segmental (displaced) S82.26
      nondisplaced S82.26
    specified NEC S82.29
    spine —*see* Fracture, upper end, spine
    spiral (displaced) S82.24
      nondisplaced S82.24
    transverse (displaced) S82.22
      nondisplaced S82.22
    tuberosity —*see* Fracture, tibia, upper end, tuberosity
    upper end S82.10
      bicondylar (displaced) S82.14
        nondisplaced S82.14
      lateral condyle (displaced) S82.12
        nondisplaced S82.12
      medial condyle (displaced) S82.13
        nondisplaced S82.13
      physeal S89.00
        Salter-Harris
          Type I S89.01
          Type II S89.02
          Type III S89.03
          Type IV S89.04
        specified NEC S89.09
      plateau —*see* Fracture, tibia, upper end, bicondylar
      spine (displaced) S82.11
        nondisplaced S82.11
      torus S82.16
      specified NEC S82.19

Fracture, traumatic *- continued*
    tuberosity (displaced) S82.15
      nondisplaced S82.15
  toe S92.91
    great (displaced) S92.40
      distal phalanx (displaced) S92.42
        nondisplaced S92.42
      nondisplaced S92.40
      proximal phalanx (displaced) S92.41
        nondisplaced S92.41
      specified NEC S92.49
    lesser (displaced) S92.50
      distal phalanx (displaced) S92.53
        nondisplaced S92.53
      medial phalanx (displaced) S92.52
        nondisplaced S92.52
      nondisplaced S92.50
      proximal phalanx (displaced) S92.51
        nondisplaced S92.51
      specified NEC S92.59
  tooth (root) S02.5
  trachea (cartilage) S12.8
  transverse process —*see* Fracture, vertebra
  trapezium or trapezoid bone —*see* Fracture, carpal
  trimalleolar —*see* Fracture, ankle, trimalleolar
  triquetrum (cuneiform of carpus) —*see* Fracture, carpal, triquetrum
  trochanter —*see* Fracture, femur, trochanteric
  tuberosity (external)
    code by site under Fracture
  ulna (shaft) S52.20
    bent bone S52.28
    coronoid process —*see* Fracture, ulna, upper end, coronoid process
    distal end —*see* Fracture, ulna, lower end
    following insertion of implant, prosthesis or plate M96.63
    head S52.00
    lower end S52.60
      physeal S59.00
        Salter-Harris
          Type I S59.01
          Type II S59.02
          Type III S59.03
          Type IV S59.04
        specified NEC S59.09
      specified NEC S52.69
      styloid process (displaced) S52.61
        nondisplaced S52.61
      torus S52.62
    proximal end —*see* Fracture, ulna, upper end
    shaft S52.20
      comminuted (displaced) S52.25
        nondisplaced S52.25
      greenstick S52.21
      Monteggia's —*see* Monteggia's fracture
      oblique (displaced) S52.23
        nondisplaced S52.23
      segmental (displaced) S52.26
        nondisplaced S52.26
      specified NEC S52.29
      spiral (displaced) S52.24
        nondisplaced S52.24
      transverse (displaced) S52.22
        nondisplaced S52.22
    upper end S52.00
      coronoid process (displaced) S52.04
        nondisplaced S52.04
      olecranon process (displaced) S52.02
        with intraarticular extension S52.03
        nondisplaced S52.02

Fracture, traumatic *- continued*
   with intraarticular extension S52.03
    specified NEC S52.09
    torus S52.01
  unciform —*see* Fracture, carpal, hamate
  vault of skull S02.0
  vertebra, vertebral (arch) (body) (column) (neural arch) (pedicle) (spinous process) (transverse process)
   atlas —*see* Fracture, neck, cervical vertebra, first
   axis —*see* Fracture, neck, cervical vertebra, second
   cervical (teardrop) S12.9
   axis —*see* Fracture, neck, cervical vertebra, second
   first (atlas) —*see* Fracture, neck, cervical vertebra, first
   second (axis) —*see* Fracture, neck, cervical vertebra, second
   chronic M84.48
   coccyx S32.2
   dorsal —*see* Fracture, thorax, vertebra
   lumbar S32.009
    burst (stable) S32.001
     unstable S32.002
    fifth S32.059
     burst (stable) S32.051
      unstable S32.052
     specified type NEC S32.058
     wedge compression S32.050
    first S32.019
     burst (stable) S32.011
      unstable S32.012
     specified type NEC S32.018
     wedge compression S32.010
    fourth S32.049
     burst (stable) S32.041
      unstable S32.042
     specified type NEC S32.048
     wedge compression S32.040
    second S32.029
     burst (stable) S32.021
      unstable S32.022
     specified type NEC S32.028
     wedge compression S32.020
    specified type NEC S32.008
    third S32.039
     burst (stable) S32.031
      unstable S32.032
     specified type NEC S32.038
     wedge compression S32.030
    wedge compression S32.000
   metastatic —*see* Collapse, vertebra, in, specified disease NEC —*see also* Neoplasm
   newborn (birth injury) P11.5
   sacrum S32.10
    specified NEC S32.19
    Type
     1 S32.14
     2 S32.15
     3 S32.16
     4 S32.17
    Zone
     I S32.119
      displaced (minimally) S32.111
       severely S32.112
      nondisplaced S32.110
     II S32.129
      displaced (minimally) S32.121
       severely S32.122
      nondisplaced S32.120

Fracture, traumatic *- continued*
     III S32.139
      displaced (minimally) S32.131
       severely S32.132
      nondisplaced S32.130
   thoracic —*see* Fracture, thorax, vertebra
  vertex S02.0
  vomer (bone) S02.2
  wrist S62.10
   carpal —*see* Fracture, carpal bone
   navicular (scaphoid) (hand) —*see* Fracture, carpal, navicular
  xiphisternum, xiphoid (process) S22.24
  zygoma S02.402
Fragile, fragility
  autosomal site Q95.5
  bone, congenital (with blue sclera) Q78.0
  capillary (hereditary) D69.8
  hair L67.8
  nails L60.3
  non-sex chromosome site Q95.5
  X chromosome Q99.2
Fragilitas
  crinium L67.8
  ossium (with blue sclerae) (hereditary) Q78.0
  unguium L60.3
   congenital Q84.6
Fragments, cataract (lens) , **following cataract surgery** H59.02
  retained foreign body —*see* Retained, foreign body fragments (type of)
Frailty (frail) R54
  mental R41.81
Frambesia, frambesial (tropica) —*see also* Yaws
  initial lesion or ulcer A66.0
  primary A66.0
Frambeside
  gummatous A66.4
  of early yaws A66.2
Frambesioma A66.1
Franceschetti-Klein (-Wildervanck) **disease or syndrome** Q75.4
Francis' disease —*see* Tularemia
Franklin disease C88.2
Frank's essential thrombocytopenia D69.3
Fraser's syndrome Q87.0
Freckle (s) L81.2
  malignant melanoma in —*see* Melanoma
  melanotic (Hutchinson's) —*see* Melanoma, in situ
  retinal D49.81
Frederickson's hyperlipoproteinemia, type
  I and V E78.3
  IIA E78.0
  IIB and III E78.2
  IV E78.1
Freeman Sheldon syndrome Q87.0
Freezing (*see also* Effect, adverse, cold) T69.9
Freiberg's disease (infraction of metatarsal head or osteochondrosis) —*see* Osteochondrosis, juvenile, metatarsus
Frei's disease A55
Fremitus, friction, cardiac R01.2
Frenum, frenulum
  external os Q51.828
  tongue (shortening) (congenital) Q38.1
Frequency micturition (nocturnal) R35.0
  psychogenic F45.8
Frey's syndrome
  auriculotemporal G50.8
  hyperhidrosis L74.52

Friction
  burn —*see* Burn, by site
  fremitus, cardiac R01.2
  precordial R01.2
  sounds, chest R09.89
Friderichsen-Waterhouse syndrome or disease A39.1
Friedländer's B (bacillus) **NEC** (*see also* condition) A49.8
Friedreich's
  ataxia G11.1
  combined systemic disease G11.1
  facial hemihypertrophy Q67.4
  sclerosis (cerebellum) (spinal cord) G11.1
Frigidity F52.22
Fröhlich's syndrome E23.6
Frontal —*see also* condition
  lobe syndrome F07.0
Frostbite (superficial) T33.90
  with
   partial thickness skin loss —*see* Frostbite (superficial) , by site
   tissue necrosis T34.90
  abdominal wall T33.3
   with tissue necrosis T34.3
  ankle T33.81
   with tissue necrosis T34.81
  arm T33.4
   with tissue necrosis T34.4
   finger (s) —*see* Frostbite, finger
   hand —*see* Frostbite, hand
   wrist —*see* Frostbite, wrist
  ear T33.01
   with tissue necrosis T34.01
  face T33.09
   with tissue necrosis T34.09
  finger T33.53
   with tissue necrosis T34.53
  foot T33.82
   with tissue necrosis T34.82
  hand T33.52
   with tissue necrosis T34.52
  head T33.09
   with tissue necrosis T34.09
   ear —*see* Frostbite, ear
   nose —*see* Frostbite, nose
  hip (and thigh) T33.6
   with tissue necrosis T34.6
  knee T33.7
   with tissue necrosis T34.7
  leg T33.9
   with tissue necrosis T34.9
   ankle —*see* Frostbite, ankle
   foot —*see* Frostbite, foot
   knee —*see* Frostbite, knee
   lower T33.7
    with tissue necrosis T34.7
   thigh —*see* Frostbite, hip
   toe —*see* Frostbite, toe
  limb
   lower T33.99
    with tissue necrosis T34.99
   upper —*see* Frostbite, arm
  neck T33.1
   with tissue necrosis T34.1
  nose T33.02
   with tissue necrosis T34.02
  pelvis T33.3
   with tissue necrosis T34.3
  specified site NEC T33.99
   with tissue necrosis T34.99
  thigh —*see* Frostbite, hip
  thorax T33.2

Frostbite - *continued*
  with tissue necrosis T34.2
  toes T33.83
    with tissue necrosis T34.83
  trunk T33.99
    with tissue necrosis T34.99
  wrist T33.51
    with tissue necrosis T34.51\
Frotteurism F65.81
Frozen (*see also* Effect, adverse, cold) T69.9
  pelvis (female) N94.89
    male K66.8
  shoulder —*see* Capsulitis, adhesive
Fructokinase deficiency E74.11
Fructose 1,6 diphosphatase deficiency
  E74.19
Fructosemia (benign) (essential) E74.12
Fructosuria (benign) (essential) E74.11
Fuchs'
  black spot (myopic) H44.2
  dystrophy (corneal endothelium) II18.51
  heterochromic cyclitis —*see* Cyclitis, Fuchs'
  heterochromic
Fucosidosis E77.1
Fugue R68.89
  dissociative F44.1
  hysterical (dissociative) F44.1
  postictal in epilepsy —*see* Epilepsy
  reaction to exceptional stress (transient) F43.0
Fulminant, fulminating —*see* condition
Functional —*see also* condition
  bleeding (uterus) N93.8
Functioning, intellectual, borderline R41.83
Fundus —*see* condition
Fungemia NOS B49
Fungus, fungous
  cerebral G93.89
  disease NOS B49
  infection —*see* Infection, fungus
Funiculitis (acute) (chronic) (endemic) N49.1
  gonococcal (acute) (chronic) A54.23
  tuberculous A18.15
Funnel
  breast (acquired) M95.4
    congenital Q67.6
    sequelae (late effect) of rickets E64.3
  chest (acquired) M95.4
    congenital Q67.6
    sequelae (late effect) of rickets E64.3
  pelvis (acquired) M95.5
    with disproportion (fetopelvic) O33.3
      causing obstructed labor O65.3
    congenital Q74.2
FUO (fever of unknown origin) R50.9
Furfur L21.0
  microsporon B36.0
Furrier's lung J67.8
Furrowed K14.5
  nail (s) (transverse) L60.4
    congenital Q84.6
  tongue K14.5
    congenital Q38.3
Furuncle L02.92
  abdominal wall L02.221
  ankle —*see* Furuncle, lower limb
  anus K61.0
  antecubital space —*see* Furuncle, upper limb
  arm —*see* Furuncle, upper limb
  auditory canal, external —*see* Abscess, ear,
  external
  auricle (ear) —*see* Abscess, ear, external
  axilla (region) L02.42

Furuncle – *continued*
  back (any part) L02.222
  breast N61
  buttock L02.32
  cheek (external) L02.02
  chest wall L02.223
  chin L02.02
  corpus cavernosum N48.21
  ear, external —*see* Abscess, ear, external
  external auditory canal —*see* Abscess, ear,
  external
  eyelid —*see* Abscess, eyelid
  face L02.02
  femoral (region) —*see* Furuncle, lower limb
  finger —*see* Furuncle, hand
  flank L02.221
  foot L02.62
  forehead L02.02
  gluteal (region) L02.32
  groin L02.224
  hand L02.52
  head L02.821
    face L02.02
  hip —*see* Furuncle, lower limb
  kidney —*see* Abscess, kidney
  knee —*see* Furuncle, lower limb
  labium (majus) (minus) N76.4
  lacrimal
    gland —*see* Dacryoadenitis
    passages (duct) (sac) —*see* Inflammation,
  lacrimal, passages, acute
  leg (any part) —*see* Furuncle, lower limb
  lower limb L02.42
  malignant A22.0
  mouth K12.2
  navel L02.226
  neck L02.12
  nose J34.0
  orbit, orbital —*see* Abscess, orbit
  palmar (space) —*see* Furuncle, hand
  partes posteriores L02.32
  pectoral region L02.223
  penis N48.21
  perineum L02.225
  pinna —*see* Abscess, ear, external
  popliteal —*see* Furuncle, lower limb
  prepatellar —*see* Furuncle, lower limb
  scalp L02.821
  seminal vesicle N49.0
  shoulder —*see* Furuncle, upper limb
  specified site NEC L02.828
  submandibular K12.2
  temple (region) L02.02
  thumb —*see* Furuncle, hand
  toe —*see* Furuncle, foot
  trunk L02.229
    abdominal wall L02.221
    back L02.222
    chest wall L02.223
    groin L02.224
    perineum L02.225
    umbilicus L02.226
    umbilicus L02.226
  upper limb L02.42
  vulva N76.4
Furunculosis —*see* Furuncle
Fused —*see* Fusion, fused
Fusion, fused (congenital)
  astragaloscaphoid Q74.2
  atria Q21.1
  auditory canal Q16.1
  auricles, heart Q21.1

Fusion, fused – *continued*
  binocular with defective stereopsis H53.32
  bone Q79.8
  cervical spine M43.22
  choanal Q30.0
  commissure, mitral valve Q23.2
  cusps, heart valve NEC Q24.8
    mitral Q23.2
    pulmonary Q22.1
    tricuspid Q22.4
  ear ossicles Q16.3
  fingers Q70.0
  hymen Q52.3
  joint (acquired) —*see also* Ankylosis
    congenital Q74.8
  kidneys (incomplete) Q63.1
  labium (majus) (minus) Q52.5
  larynx and trachea Q34.8
  limb, congenital Q74.8
    lower Q74.2
    upper Q74.0
  lobes, lung Q33.8
  lumbosacral (acquired) M43.27
    arthrodesis status Z98.1
    congenital Q76.49
    postprocedural status Z98.1
  nares, nose, nasal, nostril (s) Q30.0
  organ or site not listed —*see* Anomaly, by site
  ossicles Q79.9
    auditory Q16.3
  pulmonic cusps Q22.1
  ribs Q76.6
  sacroiliac (joint) (acquired) M43.28
    arthrodesis status Z98.1
    congenital Q74.2
    postprocedural status Z98.1
  spine (acquired) NEC M43.20
    arthrodesis status Z98.1
    cervical region M43.22
    cervicothoracic region M43.23
    congenital Q76.49
    lumbar M43.26
    lumbosacral region M43.27
    occipito-atlanto-axial region M43.21
    postoperative status Z98.1
    sacrococcygeal region M43.28
    thoracic region M43.24
    thoracolumbar region M43.25
  sublingual duct with submaxillary duct at
  opening in mouth Q38.4
  testes Q55.1
  toes Q70.2
  tooth, teeth K00.2
  trachea and esophagus Q39.8
  twins Q89.4
  vagina Q52.4
  ventricles, heart Q21.0
  vertebra (arch) —*see* Fusion, spine
  vulva Q52.5
Fusospirillosis (mouth) (tongue) (tonsil) A69.1
Fussy baby R68.12

G

Gain in weight (abnormal) (excessive) —*see
also* Weight, gain
Gaisböck's disease (polycythemia
hypertonica) D75.1
Gait abnormality R26.9
  ataxic R26.0
  falling R29.6
  hysterical (ataxic) (staggering) F44.4
  paralytic R26.1
  spastic R26.1

Gait abnormality - *continued*
  specified type NEC R26.89
  staggering R26.0
  unsteadiness R26.81
  walking difficulty NEC R26.2
Galactocele (breast) N64.89
  puerperal, postpartum O92.79
Galactokinase deficiency E74.29
Galactophoritis N61
  gestational, puerperal, postpartum O91.2
Galactorrhea O92.6
  not associated with childbirth N64.3
Galactosemia (classic) (congenital) E74.21
Galactosuria E74.29
Galacturia R82.0
  schistosomiasis (bilharziasis) B65.0
Galeazzi's fracture S52.37
Galen's vein —*see* condition
Galeophobia F40.218
Gall duct —*see* condition
Gallbladder —*see also* condition
  acute K81.0
Gallop rhythm R00.8
Gallstone (colic) (cystic duct) (gallbladder)
  (impacted) (multiple) —*see also* Calculus,
  gallbladder
  with
    cholecystitis —*see* Calculus, gallbladder,
    with cholecystitis
    bile duct (common) (hepatic) —*see* Calculus,
    bile duct
  causing intestinal obstruction K56.3
  specified NEC K80.80
    with obstruction K80.81
Gambling Z72.6
  pathological (compulsive) F63.0
Gammopathy (of undetermined significance -
  MGUS]) D47.2
  associated with lymphoplasmacytic dyscrasia
  D47.2
  monoclonal D47.2
  polyclonal D89.0
Gamna's disease (siderotic splenomegaly)
  D73.1
Gamophobia F40.298
Gampsodactylia (congenital) Q66.7
Gamstorp's disease (adynamia episodica
  hereditaria) G72.3
Gandy-Nanta disease (siderotic
  splenomegaly) D73.1
Gang
  membership offenses Z72.810
Gangliocytoma D36.10
Ganglioglioma —*see* Neoplasm, uncertain
  behavior, by site
Ganglion (compound) (diffuse) (joint) (tendon
  (sheath)) M67.40
  ankle M67.47
  foot M67.47
  forearm M67.43
  hand M67.44
  lower leg M67.46
  multiple sites M67.49
  of yaws (early) (late) A66.6
  pelvic region M67.45
  periosteal —*see* Periostitis
  shoulder region M67.41
  specified site NEC M67.48
  thigh region M67.45
  tuberculous A18.09
  upper arm M67.42
  wrist M67.43

Ganglioneuroblastoma —*see* Neoplasm,
  nerve, malignant
Ganglioneuroma D36.10
  malignant —*see* Neoplasm, nerve, malignant
Ganglioneuromatosis D36.10
Ganglionitis
  fifth nerve —*see* Neuralgia, trigeminal
  gasserian (postherpetic) (postzoster) B02.21
  geniculate G51.1
    newborn (birth injury) P11.3
    postherpetic, postzoster B02.21
  herpes zoster B02.21
  postherpetic geniculate B02.21
Gangliosidosis E75.10
  GM1 E75.19
  GM2 E75.00
    other specified E75.09
    Sandhoff disease E75.01
    Tay-Sachs disease E75.02
  GM3 E75.19
  mucolipidosis IV E75.11
Gangosa A66.5
Gangrene, gangrenous (connective tissue)
  (dropsical) (dry) (moist) (skin) (ulcer) (*see
  also* Necrosis) I96
  with diabetes (mellitus) —*see* Diabetes,
  gangrene
  abdomen (wall) I96
  alveolar M27.3
  appendix K35.80
    with
      perforation or rupture K35.2
      peritoneal abscess K35.3
      peritonitis NEC K35.3
        generalized (with perforation or rupture)
        K35.2
        localized (with perforation or rupture)
        K35.3
  arteriosclerotic (general) (senile) —*see*
  Arteriosclerosis, extremities, with, gangrene
  auricle I96
  Bacillus welchii A48.0
  bladder (infectious) —*see* Cystitis, specified
  type NEC
  bowel, cecum, or colon —*see* Gangrene,
  intestine
  Clostridium perfringens or welchii A48.0
  cornea H18.89
  corpora cavernosa N48.29
    noninfective N48.89
  cutaneous, spreading I96
  decubital —*see* Ulcer, pressure, by site
  diabetic (any site) —*see* Diabetes, gangrene
  epidemic —*see* Poisoning, food, noxious,
  plant
  epididymis (infectional) N45.1
  erysipelas —*see* Erysipelas
  emphysematous —*see* Gangrene, gas
  extremity (lower) (upper) I96
  Fournier N49.3
    female N76.89
  fusospirochetal A69.0
  gallbladder —*see* Cholecystitis, acute
  gas (bacillus) A48.0
    following
      abortion —*see* Abortion by type
    complicated by infection
      ectopic or molar pregnancy O08.0
  glossitis K14.0
  hernia —*see* Hernia, by site, with gangrene
  intestine, intestinal (hemorrhagic) (massive)
  K55.0

Gangrene, gangrenous – *continued*
  with
    mesenteric embolism K55.0
    obstruction —*see* Obstruction, intestine
  laryngitis J04.0
  limb (lower) (upper) I96
  lung J85.0
    spirochetal A69.8
  lymphangitis I89.1
  Meleney's (synergistic) —*see* Ulcer, skin
  mesentery K55.0
    with
      embolism K55.0
      intestinal obstruction —*see* Obstruction,
  intestine
  mouth A69.0
  ovary —*see* Oophoritis
  pancreas K85.9
  penis N48.29
    noninfective N48.89
  perineum I96
  pharynx —*see also* Pharyngitis
    Vincent's A69.1
  presenile I73.1
  progressive synergistic —*see* Ulcer, skin
  pulmonary J85.0
  pulpal (dental) K04.1
  quinsy J36
  Raynaud's (symmetric gangrene) I73.01
  retropharyngeal J39.2
  scrotum N49.3
    noninfective N50.8
  senile (atherosclerotic) —*see* Arteriosclerosis,
  extremities, with, gangrene
  spermatic cord N49.1
    noninfective N50.8
  spine I96
  spirochetal NEC A69.8
  spreading cutaneous I96
  stomatitis A69.0
  symmetrical I73.01
  testis (infectional) N45.2
    noninfective N44.8
  throat —*see also* Pharyngitis
    diphtheritic A36.0
    Vincent's A69.1
  thyroid (gland) E07.89
  tooth (pulp) K04.1
  tuberculous NEC —*see* Tuberculosis
  tunica vaginalis N49.1
    noninfective N50.8
  umbilicus I96
  uterus —*see* Endometritis
  uvulitis K12.2
  vas deferens N49.1
    noninfective N50.8
  vulva N76.89
Ganister disease J62.8
Ganser's syndrome (hysterical) F44.89
Gardner-Diamond syndrome
  (autoerythrocyte sensitization) D69.2
Gargoylism E76.01
Garré's disease, osteitis (sclerosing) ,
  osteomyelitis —*see* Osteomyelitis, specified
  type NEC
Garrod's pad, knuckle M72.1
Gartner's duct
  cyst Q52.4
  persistent Q50.6
Gas R14.3
  asphyxiation, inhalation, poisoning,
  suffocation NEC —*see* Table of Drugs and
  Chemicals

Gas - *continued*
excessive R14.0
gangrene A48.0
following
abortion —*see* Abortion by type
complicated by infection
ectopic or molar pregnancy O08.0
on stomach R14.0
pains R14.1
Gastralgia —*see also* Pain, abdominal
Gastrectasis K31.0
psychogenic F45.8
Gastric —*see* condition
Gastrinoma
malignant
pancreas C25.4
specified site NEC —*see* Neoplasm,
malignant, by site
unspecified site C25.4
specified site —*see* Neoplasm, uncertain
behavior
unspecified site D37.9
Gastritis (simple) K29.70
with bleeding K29.71
acute (erosive) K29.00
with bleeding K29.01
alcoholic K29.20
with bleeding K29.21
allergic K29.60
with bleeding K29.61
atrophic (chronic) K29.40
with bleeding K29.41
chronic (antral) (fundal) K29.50
with bleeding K29.51
atrophic K29.40
with bleeding K29.41
superficial K29.30
with bleeding K29.31
dietary counseling and surveillance Z71.3
due to diet deficiency E63.9
eosinophilic K52.81
giant hypertrophic K29.60
with bleeding K29.61
granulomatous K29.60
with bleeding K29.61
hypertrophic (mucosa) K29.60
with bleeding K29.61
nervous F54
spastic K29.60
with bleeding K29.61
specified NEC K29.60
with bleeding K29.61
superficial chronic K29.30
with bleeding K29.31
tuberculous A18.83
viral NEC A08.4
Gastrocarcinoma —*see* Neoplasm, malignant,
stomach
Gastrocolic —*see* condition
Gastrodisciasis, gastrodiscoidiasis B66.8
Gastroduodenitis K29.90
with bleeding K29.91
virus, viral A08.4
specified type NEC A08.39
Gastrodynia —*see* Pain, abdominal
Gastroenteritis (acute) (chronic)
(noninfectious) (*see also* Enteritis) K52.9
allergic K52.2
dietetic K52.2
drug-induced K52.1
due to
Cryptosporidium A07.2

Gastroenteritis – *continued*
drugs K52.1
food poisoning —*see* Intoxication,
foodborne
radiation K52.0
eosinophilic K52.81
epidemic (infectious) A09
food hypersensitivity K52.2
infectious —*see* Enteritis, infectious
influenzal —*see* Influenza, with
gastroenteritis
noninfectious K52.9
specified NEC K52.89
rotaviral A08.0
Salmonella A02.0
toxic K52.1
viral NEC A08.4
acute infectious A08.39
type Norwalk A08.11
infantile (acute) A08.39
Norwalk agent A08.11
rotaviral A08.0
severe of infants A08.39
specified type NEC A08.39
Gastroenteropathy (*see also* Gastroenteritis)
K52.9
acute, due to Norwalk agent A08.11
acute, due to Norovirus A08.11
infectious A09
Gastroenteroptosis K63.4
Gastroesophageal laceration hemorrhage
syndrome K22.6
Gastrointestinal —*see* condition
Gastrojejunal —*see* condition
Gastrojejunitis (*see also* Enteritis) K52.9
Gastrojejunocolic —*see* condition
Gastroliths K31.89
Gastromalacia K31.89
Gastroparalysis K31.84
diabetic —*see* Diabetes, gastroparalysis
Gastroparesis K31.84
diabetic —*see* Diabetes, by type, with
gastroparesis
Gastropathy K31.9
congestive portal K31.89
erythematous K29.70
exudative K90.89
portal hypertensive K31.89
Gastroptosis K31.89
Gastrorrhagia K92.2
psychogenic F45.8
Gastroschisis (congenital) Q79.3
Gastrospasm (neurogenic) (reflex) K31.89
neurotic F45.8
psychogenic F45.8
Gastrostaxis —*see* Gastritis, with bleeding
Gastrostenosis K31.89
Gastrostomy
attention to Z43.1
status Z93.1
Gastrosuccorrhea (continuous) (intermittent)
K31.89
neurotic F45.8
psychogenic F45.8
Gatophobia F40.218
Gaucher's disease or splenomegaly (adult)
(infantile) E75.22
Gee (-Herter) (-Thaysen) disease (nontropical
sprue) K90.0
Gélineau's syndrome G47.419
with cataplexy G47.411
Gemination, tooth, teeth K00.2

Gemistocytoma
specified site —*see* Neoplasm, malignant, by
site
unspecified site C71.9
General, generalized —*see* condition
Genetic
carrier (status)
cystic fibrosis Z14.1
hemophilia A (asymptomatic) Z14.01
symptomatic Z14.02
specified NEC Z14.8
susceptibility to disease NEC Z15.89
malignant neoplasm Z15.09
breast Z15.01
endometrium Z15.04
ovary Z15.02
prostate Z15.03
specified NEC Z15.09
multiple endocrine neoplasia Z15.81
Genital —*see* condition
Genito-anorectal syndrome A55
Genitourinary system —*see* condition
Genu
congenital Q74.1
extrorsum (acquired) —*see also* Deformity,
varus, knee
congenital Q74.1
sequelae (late effect) of rickets E64.3
introrsum (acquired) —*see also* Deformity,
valgus, knee
congenital Q74.1
sequelae (late effect) of rickets E64.3
rachitic (old) E64.3
recurvatum (acquired) —*see also* Deformity,
limb, specified type NEC, lower leg
congenital Q68.2
sequelae (late effect) of rickets E64.3
valgum (acquired) (knock-knee) M21.06
congenital Q74.1
sequelae (late effect) of rickets E64.3
varum (acquired) (bowleg) M21.16
congenital Q74.1
sequelae (late effect) of rickets E64.3
Geographic tongue K14.1
Geophagia —*see* Pica
Geotrichosis B48.3
stomatitis B48.3
Gephyrophobia F40.242
Gerbode defect Q21.0
GERD (gastroesophageal reflux disease) K21.9
Gerhardt's
disease (erythromelalgia) I73.81
syndrome (vocal cord paralysis) J38.00
bilateral J38.02
unilateral J38.01
German measles —*see also* Rubella
exposure to Z20.4
Germinoblastoma (diffuse) C85.9
follicular C82.9
Germinoma —*see* Neoplasm, malignant, by
site
Gerontoxon —*see* Degeneration, cornea,
senile
Gerstmann-Sträussler-Scheinker syndrome
(GSS) A81.82
Gerstmann's syndrome R48.8
developmental F81.2
Gestation (period) —*see also* Pregnancy
ectopic —*see* Pregnancy, by site
multiple O30.9
greater than quadruplets —*see* Pregnancy,
multiple (gestation) , specified NEC

Gestation – *continued*
  specified NEC —*see* Pregnancy, multiple
  (gestation) , specified NEC
Gestational
  mammary abscess O91.11
  purulent mastitis O91.11
  subareolar abscess O91.11
Ghon tubercle, primary infection A15.7
Ghost
  teeth K00.4
  vessels (cornea) H16.41
Ghoul hand A66.3
Gianotti-Crosti disease L44.4
Giant
  cell
    epulis K06.8
    peripheral granuloma K06.8
  esophagus, congenital Q39.5
  kidney, congenital Q63.3
  urticaria T78.3
    hereditary D84.1
Giardiasis A07.1
Gibert's disease or pityriasis L42
Giddiness R42
  hysterical F44.89
  psychogenic F45.8
Gierke's disease (glycogenosis I) E74.01
Gigantism (cerebral) (hypophyseal) (pituitary)
  E22.0
  constitutional E34.4
Gilbert's disease or syndrome E80.4
Gilchrist's disease B40.9
Gilford-Hutchinson disease E34.8
Gilles de la Tourette's disease or syndrome
  (motor-verbal tic) F95.2
Gingivitis K05.10
  acute (catarrhal) K05.00
    necrotizing A69.1
    nonplaque induced K05.01
    plaque induced K05.00
  chronic (desquamative) (hyperplastic) (simple
  marginal) (ulcerative) K05.10
    nonplaque induced K05.11
    plaque induced K05.10
  expulsiva —*see* Periodontitis
  necrotizing ulcerative (acute) A69.1
  pellagrous E52
    acute necrotizing A69.1
  Vincent's A69.1
Gingivoglossitis K14.0
Gingivopericementitis —*see* Periodontitis
Gingivosis —*see* Gingivitis, chronic
Gingivostomatitis K05.10
  herpesviral B00.2
  necrotizing ulcerative (acute) A69.1
Gland, glandular —*see* condition
Glanders A24.0
Glanzmann (-Naegeli) **disease or**
  thrombasthenia D69.1
Glasgow coma scale
  total score
    3 8 R40.243
    9 12 R40.242
    13 15 R40.241
Glass-blower's disease (cataract) —*see*
  Cataract, specified NEC
Glaucoma H40.9
  with
    increased episcleral venous pressure H40.81
    pseudoexfoliation of lens —*see* Glaucoma,
  open angle, primary, capsular
  absolute H44.51
  angle-closure (primary) H40.20

Glaucoma – *continued*
    acute (attack) (crisis) H40.21
    chronic H40.22
    intermittent H40.23
    residual stage H40.24
  borderline H40.00
  capsular (with pseudoexfoliation of lens) —
  see Glaucoma, open angle, primary, capsular
  childhood Q15.0
  closed angle —*see* Glaucoma, angle-closure
  congenital Q15.0
  corticosteroid-induced —*see* Glaucoma,
  secondary, drugs
  hypersecretion H40.82
  in (due to)
    amyloidosis E85.4 *[H42]*
    aniridia Q13.1 *[H42]*
    concussion of globe —*see* Glaucoma,
  secondary, trauma
    dislocation of lens —*see* Glaucoma,
  secondary
    disorder of lens NEC —*see* Glaucoma,
  secondary
    drugs —*see* Glaucoma, secondary, drugs
    endocrine disease NOS E34.9 *[H42]*
    eye
      inflammation —*see* Glaucoma, secondary,
  inflammation
      trauma —*see* Glaucoma, secondary,
  trauma
    hypermature cataract —*see* Glaucoma,
  secondary
    iridocyclitis —*see* Glaucoma, secondary,
  inflammation
    lens disorder —*see* Glaucoma, secondary,
    Lowe's syndrome E72.03 *[H42]*
    metabolic disease NOS E88.9 *[H42]*
    ocular disorders NEC —*see* Glaucoma,
  secondary
    onchocerciasis B73.02
    pupillary block —*see* Glaucoma, secondary
    retinal vein occlusion —*see* Glaucoma,
  secondary
    Rieger's anomaly Q13.81 *[H42]*
    rubeosis of iris —*see* Glaucoma, secondary
    tumor of globe —*see* Glaucoma, secondary
  infantile Q15.0
  low tension —*see* Glaucoma, open angle,
  primary, low-tension
  malignant H40.83
  narrow angle —*see* Glaucoma, angle-closure
  newborn Q15.0
  noncongestive (chronic) —*see* Glaucoma,
  open angle
  nonobstructive —*see* Glaucoma, open angle
  obstructive —*see also* Glaucoma, angle-
  closure
    due to lens changes —*see* Glaucoma,
  secondary
  open angle H40.10
    primary H40.11
      capsular (with pseudoexfoliation of lens)
  H40.14
      low-tension H40.12
      pigmentary H40.13
      residual stage H40.15
  phacolytic —*see* Glaucoma, secondary
  pigmentary —*see* Glaucoma, open angle,
  primary, pigmentary
  postinfectious —*see* Glaucoma, secondary,
  inflammation
  secondary (to) H40.5

Glaucoma – *continued*
  drugs H40.6
  inflammation H40.4
  trauma H40.3
  simple (chronic) H40.11
  simplex H40.11
  specified type NEC H40.89
  suspect H40.00
  syphilitic A52.71
  traumatic —*see also* Glaucoma, secondary,
  trauma
    newborn (birth injury) P15.3
  tuberculous A18.59
Glaucomatous flecks (subcapsular) —*see*
  Cataract, complicated
Glazed tongue K14.4
Gleet (gonococcal) A54.01
Glénard's disease K63.4
Glioblastoma (multiforme)
  with sarcomatous component
    specified site —*see* Neoplasm, malignant,
  by site
    unspecified site C71.9
  giant cell
    specified site —*see* Neoplasm, malignant,
  by site
    unspecified site C71.9
  specified site —*see* Neoplasm, malignant, by
  site
  unspecified site C71.9
Glioma (malignant)
  astrocytic
    specified site —*see* Neoplasm, malignant,
  by site
    unspecified site C71.9
  mixed
    specified site —*see* Neoplasm, malignant,
  by site
    unspecified site C71.9
  nose Q30.8
  specified site NEC —*see* Neoplasm,
  malignant, by site
  subependymal D43.2
    specified site —*see* Neoplasm, uncertain
  behavior, by site
    unspecified site D43.2
  unspecified site C71.9
Gliomatosis cerebri C71.0
Glioneuroma —*see* Neoplasm, uncertain
  behavior, by site
Gliosarcoma
  specified site —*see* Neoplasm, malignant, by
  site
  unspecified site C71.9
Gliosis (cerebral) G93.89
  spinal G95.89
Glisson's disease —*see* Rickets
Globinuria R82.3
Globus (hystericus) F45.8
Glomangioma D18.00
  intra-abdominal D18.03
  intracranial D18.02
  skin D18.01
  specified site NEC D18.09
Glomangiomyoma D18.00
  intra-abdominal D18.03
  intracranial D18.02
  skin D18.01
  specified site NEC D18.09
Glomangiosarcoma —*see* Neoplasm,
  connective tissue, malignant

Glomerular
disease in syphilis A52.75
nephritis —*see* Glomerulonephritis
Glomerulitis —*see* Glomerulonephritis
Glomerulonephritis (*see also* Nephritis)
N05.9
with
edema —*see* Nephrosis
minimal change N05.0
minor glomerular abnormality N05.0
acute N00.9
chronic N03.9
crescentic (diffuse) NEC (*see also* N00-N07
with fourth character .7) N05.7
dense deposit (*see also* N00-N07 with fourth
character .6) N05.6
diffuse
crescentic (*see also* N00-N07 with fourth
character .7) N05.7
endocapillary proliferative (*see also* N00-
N07 with fourth character .4) N05.4
membranous (*see also* N00-N07 with fourth
character .2) N05.2
mesangial proliferative (*see also* N00-N07
with fourth character .3) N05.3
mesangiocapillary (*see also* N00-N07 with
fourth character .5) N05.5
sclerosing N05.8
endocapillary proliferative (diffuse) NEC (*see
also* N00-N07 with fourth character .4) N05.4
extracapillary NEC (*see also* N00-N07 with
fourth character .7) N05.7
focal (and segmental) (*see also* N00-N07 with
fourth character .1) N05.1
hypocomplementemic —*see*
Glomerulonephritis, membranoproliferative
IgA —*see* Nephropathy, IgA
immune complex (circulating) NEC N05.8
in (due to)
amyloidosis E85.4 *[N08]*
bilharziasis B65.9 *[N08]*
cryoglobulinemia D89.1 *[N08]*
defibrination syndrome D65 *[N08]*
diabetes mellitus —*see* Diabetes,
glomerulosclerosis
disseminated intravascular coagulation D65
[N08]
Fabry (-Anderson) disease E75.21 *[N08]*
Goodpasture's syndrome M31.0
hemolytic-uremic syndrome D59.3
Henoch (-Schönlein) purpura D69.0 *[N08]*
lecithin cholesterol acyltransferase
deficiency E78.6 *[N08]*
microscopic polyangiitis M31.7 *[N08]*
multiple myeloma C90.0 *[N08]*
Plasmodium malariae B52.0
schistosomiasis B65.9 *[N08]*
sepsis A41.9 *[N08]*
streptococcal A40 *[N08]*
sickle-cell disorders D57. *[N08]*
strongyloidiasis B78.9 *[N08]*
subacute bacterial endocarditis I33.0 *[N08]*
syphilis (late) congenital A50.59 *[N08]*
systemic lupus erythematosus M32.14
thrombotic thrombocytopenic purpura
M31.1 *[N08]*
typhoid fever A01.09
Waldenström macroglobulinemia C88.0
[N08]
Wegener's granulomatosis M31.31
latent or quiescent N03.9

Glomerulonephritis – *continued*
lobular, lobulonodular —*see*
Glomerulonephritis, membranoproliferative
membranoproliferative (diffuse) (type 1 or 3)
(*see also* N00-N07 with fourth character .5)
N05.5
dense deposit (type 2) NEC (*see also* N00-
N07 with fourth character .6) N05.6
membranous (diffuse) NEC (*see also* N00-
N07 with fourth character .2) N05.2
mesangial
IgA/IgG —*see* Nephropathy, IgA
proliferative (diffuse) NEC (*see also* N00-
N07 with fourth character .3) N05.3
mesangiocapillary (diffuse) NEC (*see also*
N00-N07 with fourth character .5) N05.5
necrotic, necrotizing NEC (*see also* N00-N07
with fourth character .8) N05.8
nodular —*see* Glomerulonephritis,
membranoproliferative
poststreptococcal NEC N05.9
acute N00.9
chronic N03.9
rapidly progressive N01.9
proliferative NEC (*see also* N00-N07 with
fourth character .8) N05.8
diffuse (lupus) M32.14
rapidly progressive N01.9
sclerosing, diffuse N05.8
specified pathology NEC (*see also* N00-N07
with fourth character .8) N05.8
subacute N01.9
Glomerulopathy —*see* Glomerulonephritis
Glomerulosclerosis —*see also* Sclerosis, renal
intercapillary (nodular) (with diabetes) —*see*
Diabetes, glomerulosclerosis
intracapillary —*see* Diabetes,
glomerulosclerosis
Glossagra K14.6
Glossalgia K14.6
Glossitis (chronic superficial) (gangrenous)
(Moeller's) K14.0
areata exfoliativa K14.1
atrophic K14.4
benign migratory K14.1
cortical superficial, sclerotic K14.0
Hunter's D51.0
interstitial, sclerous K14.0
median rhomboid K14.2
pellagrous E52
superficial, chronic K14.0
Glossocele K14.8
Glossodynia K14.6
exfoliativa K14.4
Glossoncus K14.8
Glossopathy K14.9
Glossophytia K14.3
Glossoplegia K14.8
Glossoptosis K14.8
Glossopyrosis K14.6
Glossotrichia K14.3
Glossy skin L90.8
Glottis —*see* condition
Glottitis (*see also* Laryngitis) J04.0
Glucagonoma
pancreas
benign D13.7
malignant C25.4
uncertain behavior D37.8
specified site NEC
benign —*see* Neoplasm, benign, by site
malignant —*see* Neoplasm, malignant, by
site

Glucagonoma - *continued*
uncertain behavior —*see* Neoplasm,
uncertain behavior, by site
unspecified site
benign D13.7
malignant C25.4
uncertain behavior D37.8
Glucoglycinuria E72.51
Glucose-galactose malabsorption E74.39
Glue
ear —*see* Otitis, media, nonsuppurative,
chronic, mucoid
sniffing (airplane) —*see* Abuse, drug,
inhalant
dependence —*see* Dependence, drug,
inhalant
Glutaric aciduria E72.3
Glycinemia E72.51
Glycinuria (renal) (with ketosis) E72.09
Glycogen
infiltration —*see* Disease, glycogen storage
storage disease —*see* Disease, glycogen
storage
Glycogenosis (diffuse) (generalized) —*see
also* Disease, glycogen storage
cardiac E74.02 *[143]*
diabetic, secondary —*see* Diabetes,
glycogenosis, secondary
pulmonary interstitial J84.842
Glycopenia E16.2
Glycosuria R81
renal E74.8
Gnathostoma spinigerum (infection)
(infestation) , gnathostomiasis (wandering
swelling) B83.1
Goiter (plunging) (substernal) E04.9
with
hyperthyroidism (recurrent) —*see*
Hyperthyroidism, with, goiter
thyrotoxicosis —*see* Hyperthyroidism, with,
goiter
adenomatous —*see* Goiter, nodular
cancerous C73
congenital (nontoxic) E03.0
diffuse E03.0
parenchymatous E03.0
transitory, with normal functioning P72.0
cystic E04.2
due to iodine-deficiency E01.1
due to
enzyme defect in synthesis of thyroid
hormone E07.1
iodine-deficiency (endemic) E01.2
dyshormonogenetic (familial) E07.1
endemic (iodine-deficiency) E01.2
diffuse E01.0
multinodular E01.1
exophthalmic —*see* Hyperthyroidism, with,
goiter
iodine-deficiency (endemic) E01.2
diffuse E01.0
multinodular E01.1
nodular E01.1
lingual Q89.2
lymphadenoid E06.3
malignant C73
multinodular (cystic) (nontoxic) E04.2
toxic or with hyperthyroidism E05.20
with thyroid storm E05.21
neonatal NEC P72.0
nodular (nontoxic) (due to) E04.9
with
hyperthyroidism E05.20

Goiter - *continued*

    with thyroid storm E05.21

   thyrotoxicosis E05.20

    with thyroid storm E05.21

  endemic E01.1

  iodine-deficiency E01.1

  sporadic E04.9

  toxic E05.20

   with thyroid storm E05.21

 nontoxic E04.9

  diffuse (colloid) E04.0

  multinodular E04.2

  simple E04.0

  specified NEC E04.8

  uninodular E04.1

 simple E04.0

 toxic —*see* Hyperthyroidism, with, goiter

 uninodular (nontoxic) E04.1

  toxic or with hyperthyroidism E05.10

   with thyroid storm E05.11

Goiter-deafness syndrome E07.1

Goldberg syndrome Q89.8

Goldberg-Maxwell syndrome E34.51

Goldblatt's hypertension or kidney I70.1

Goldenhar (-Gorlin) **syndrome** Q87.0

Goldflam-Erb disease or syndrome G70.00

 with exacerbation (acute) G70.01

 in crisis G70.01

Goldscheider's disease Q81.8

Goldstein's disease (familial hemorrhagic

 telangiectasia) I78.0

Golfer's elbow —*see* Epicondylitis, medial

Gonadoblastoma

 specified site —*see* Neoplasm, uncertain

 behavior, by site

 unspecified site

  female D39.10

  male D40.10

Gonecystitis —*see* Vesiculitis

Gongylonemiasis B83.8

Goniosynechiae —*see* Adhesions, iris,

 goniosynechiae

Gonococcemia A54.86

Gonococcus, gonococcal (disease) (infection)

 (*see also* condition) A54.9

 anus A54.6

 bursa, bursitis A54.49

 conjunctiva, conjunctivitis (neonatorum)

 A54.31

 endocardium A54.83

 eye A54.30

  conjunctivitis A54.31

  iridocyclitis A54.32

  keratitis A54.33

  newborn A54.31

  other specified A54.39

 fallopian tubes (acute) (chronic) A54.24

 genitourinary (organ) (system) (tract) (acute)

  lower A54.00

   with abscess (accessory gland)

   (periurethral) A54.1

  upper (*see also* condition) A54.29

 heart A54.83

 iridocyclitis A54.32

 joint A54.42

 lymphatic (gland) (node) A54.89

 meninges, meningitis A54.81

 musculoskeletal A54.40

  arthritis A54.42

  osteomyelitis A54.43

  other specified A54.49

  spondylopathy A54.41

Gonococcus, gonococcal – *continued*

 pelviperitonitis A54.24

 pelvis (acute) (chronic) A54.24

 pharynx A54.5

 proctitis A54.6

 pyosalpinx (acute) (chronic) A54.24

 rectum A54.6

 skin A54.89

 specified site NEC A54.89

 tendon sheath A54.49

 throat A54.5

 urethra (acute) (chronic) A54.01

  with abscess (accessory gland) (periurethral)

  A54.1

 vulva (acute) (chronic) A54.02

Gonocytoma

 specified site —*see* Neoplasm, uncertain

 behavior, by site

 unspecified site

  female D39.10

  male D40.10

Gonorrhea (acute) (chronic) A54.9

 Bartholin's gland (acute) (chronic) (purulent)

 A54.02

  with abscess (accessory gland) (periurethral)

  A54.1

 bladder A54.01

 cervix A54.03

 conjunctiva, conjunctivitis (neonatorum)

 A54.31

 contact Z20.2

 Cowper's gland (with abscess) A54.1

 exposure to Z20.2

 fallopian tube (acute) (chronic) A54.24

 kidney (acute) (chronic) A54.21

 lower genitourinary tract A54.00

  with abscess (accessory gland) (periurethral)

  A54.1

 ovary (acute) (chronic) A54.24

 pelvis (acute) (chronic) A54.24

  female pelvic inflammatory disease A54.24

 penis A54.09

 prostate (acute) (chronic) A54.22

 seminal vesicle (acute) (chronic) A54.23

 specified site not listed (*see also* Gonococcus)

 A54.89

 spermatic cord (acute) (chronic) A54.23

 urethra A54.01

  with abscess (accessory gland) (periurethral)

  A54.1

 vagina A54.02

 vas deferens (acute) (chronic) A54.23

 vulva A54.02

Goodall's disease A08.19

Goodpasture's syndrome M31.0

Gopalan's syndrome (burning feet) E53.0

Gorlin-Chaudry-Moss syndrome Q87.0

Gottron's papules L94.4

Gougerot's syndrome (trisymptomatic) L81.7

Gougerot-Blum syndrome (pigmented

 purpuric lichenoid dermatitis) L81.7

Gougerot-Carteaud disease or syndrome

 (confluent reticulate papillomatosis) L83

Gouley's syndrome (constrictive pericarditis)

 I31.1

Goundou A66.6

Gout, gouty (acute) (attack) (flare) (*see also*

 Gout, chronic) M10.9

 drug-induced M10.20

  ankle M10.27

  elbow M10.22

  foot joint M10.27

Gout, gouty – *continued*

  hand joint M10.24

  hip M10.25

  knee M10.26

  multiple site M10.29

  shoulder M10.21

  vertebrae M10.28

  wrist M10.23

 idiopathic M10.00

  ankle M10.07

  elbow M10.02

  foot joint M10.07

  hand joint M10.04

  hip M10.05

  knee M10.06

  multiple site M10.09

  shoulder M10.01

  vertebrae M10.08

  wrist M10.03

 in (due to) renal impairment M10.30

  ankle M10.37

  elbow M10.32

  foot joint M10.37

  hand joint M10.34

  hip M10.35

  knee M10.36

  multiple site M10.39

  shoulder M10.31

  vertebrae M10.38

  wrist M10.33

 lead-induced M10.10

  ankle M10.17

  elbow M10.12

  foot joint M10.17

  hand joint M10.14

  hip M10.15

  knee M10.16

  multiple site M10.19

  shoulder M10.11

  vertebrae M10.18

  wrist M10.13

 primary —*see* Gout, idiopathic

 saturnine —*see* Gout, lead-induced

 secondary NEC M10.40

  ankle M10.47

  elbow M10.42

  foot joint M10.47

  hand joint M10.44

  hip M10.45

  knee M10.46

  multiple site M10.49

  shoulder M10.41

  vertebrae M10.48

  wrist M10.43

 syphilitic (*see also* subcategory M14.8)

 A52.77

 tophi —*see* Gout, chronic

Gout, chronic (*see also* Gout, gouty) M1A.9

 drug-induced M1A.20

  ankle M1A.27

  elbow M1A.22

  foot joint M1A.27

  hand joint M1A.24

  hip M1A.25

  knee M1A.26

  multiple site M1A.29

  shoulder M1A.21

  vertebrae M1A.28

  wrist M1A.23

 idiopathic M1A.00

  ankle M1A.07

  elbow M1A.02

  foot joint M1A.07

Gout, chronic - *continued*
  hand joint M1A.04
  hip M1A.05
  knee M1A.06
  multiple site M1A.09
  shoulder M1A.01
  vertebrae M1A.08
  wrist M1A.03
  in (due to) renal impairment M1A.30
    ankle M1A.37
    elbow M1A.32
    foot joint M1A.37
    hand joint M1A.34
    hip M1A.35
    knee M1A.36
    multiple site M1A.39
    shoulder M1A.31
    vertebrae M1A.38
    wrist M1A.33
  lead-induced M1A.10
    ankle M1A.17
    elbow M1A.12
    foot joint M1A.17
    hand joint M1A.14
    hip M1A.15
    knee M1A.16
    multiple site M1A.19
    shoulder M1A.11
    vertebrae M1A.18
    wrist M1A.13
  primary —*see* Gout, chronic, idiopathic
  saturnine —*see* Gout, chronic, lead-induced
  secondary NEC M1A.40
    ankle M1A.47
    elbow M1A.42
    foot joint M1A.47
    hand joint M1A.44
    hip M1A.45
    knee M1A.46
    multiple site M1A.49
    shoulder M1A.41
    vertebrae M1A.48
    wrist M1A.43
  syphilitic (*see also* subcategory M14.8) A52.77
  tophi M1A.9
Gower's
  muscular dystrophy G71.0
  syndrome (vasovagal attack) R55
Gradenigo's syndrome —*see* Otitis, media, suppurative, acute
Graefe's disease —*see* Strabismus, paralytic, ophthalmoplegia, progressive
Graft-versus-host disease D89.813
  acute D89.810
  acute on chronic D89.812
  chronic D89.811
Grain handler's disease or lung J67.8
Grain mite (itch) B88.0
Grand mal —*see* Epilepsy, generalized, specified NEC
Grand multipara status only (not pregnant) Z64.1
  pregnant —*see* Pregnancy, complicated by, grand multiparity
Granite worker's lung J62.8
Granular —*see also* condition
  inflammation, pharynx J31.2
  kidney (contracting) —*see* Sclerosis, renal
  liver K74.69

Granulation tissue (abnormal) (excessive) L92.9
  postmastoidectomy cavity —*see* Complications, postmastoidectomy, granulation
Granulocytopenia (primary) (malignant) —*see* Agranulocytosis
Granuloma L92.9
  abdomen K66.8
    from residual foreign body L92.3
    pyogenicum L98.0
  actinic L57.5
  annulare (perforating) L92.0
  apical K04.5
  aural —*see* Otitis, externa, specified NEC
  beryllium (skin) L92.3
  bone
    eosinophilic C96.6
    from residual foreign body —*see* Osteomyelitis, specified type NEC
    lung C96.6
  brain (any site) G06.0
    schistosomiasis B65.9 *[G07]*
  canaliculus lacrimalis —*see* Granuloma, lacrimal
  candidal (cutaneous) B37.2
  cerebral (any site) G06.0
  coccidioidal (primary) (progressive) B38.7
    lung B38.1
    meninges B38.4
  colon K63.89
  conjunctiva H11.22
  dental K04.5
  ear, middle —*see* Cholesteatoma
  eosinophilic C96.6
    bone C96.6
    lung C96.6
    oral mucosa K13.4
    skin L92.2
  eyelid H01.8
  facial (e) L92.2
  foreign body (in soft tissue) NEC M60.20
    ankle M60.27
    foot M60.27
    forearm M60.23
    hand M60.24
    in operation wound —*see* Foreign body, accidentally left during a procedure
    lower leg M60.26
    pelvic region M60.25
    shoulder region M60.21
    skin L92.3
    specified site NEC M60.28
    subcutaneous tissue L92.3
    thigh M60.25
    upper arm M60.22
  gangraenescens M31.2
  genito-inguinale A58
  giant cell (central) (reparative) (jaw) M27.1
    gingiva (peripheral) K06.8
  gland (lymph) I88.8
  hepatic NEC K75.3
    in (due to)
      berylliosis J63.2 *[K77]*
      sarcoidosis D86.89
  Hodgkin C81.9
  ileum K63.89
  infectious B99.9
    specified NEC B99.8
  inguinale (Donovan) (venereal) A58
  intestine NEC K63.89
  intracranial (any site) G06.0

Granuloma - *continued*
  intraspinal (any part) G06.1
  iridocyclitis —*see* Iridocyclitis, chronic
  jaw (bone) (central) M27.1
    reparative giant cell M27.1
  kidney (*see also* Infection, kidney) N15.8
  lacrimal H04.81
  larynx J38.7
  lethal midline (faciale(e)) M31.2
  liver NEC —*see* Granuloma, hepatic
  lung (infectious) —*see also* Fibrosis, lung
    coccidioidal B38.1
    eosinophilic C96.6
  Majocchi's B35.8
  malignant (facial(e)) M31.2
  mandible (central) M27.1
  midline (lethal) M31.2
  monilial (cutaneous) B37.2
  nasal sinus —*see* Sinusitis
  operation wound T81.89
    foreign body *see* Foreign body, accidentally left during a procedure
    stitch T81.89
    talc —*see* Foreign body, accidentally left during a procedure
  oral mucosa K13.4
  orbit, orbital H05.11
  paracoccidioidal B41.8
  penis, venereal A58
  periapical K04.5
  peritoneum K66.8
    due to ova of helminths NOS (*see also* Helminthiasis) B83.9 *[K67]*
  postmastoidectomy cavity —*see* Complications, postmastoidectomy, recurrent cholesteatoma
  prostate N42.89
  pudendi (ulcerating) A58
  pulp, internal (tooth) K03.3
  pyogenic, pyogenicum (of) (skin) L98.0
    gingiva K06.8
    maxillary alveolar ridge K04.5
    oral mucosa K13.4
  rectum K62.89
  reticulohistiocytic D76.3
  rubrum nasi L74.8
  Schistosoma —*see* Schistosomiasis
  septic (skin) L98.0
  silica (skin) L92.3
  sinus (accessory) (infective) (nasal) —*see* Sinusitis
  skin L92.9
    from residual foreign body L92.3
    pyogenicum L98.0
  spine
    syphilitic (epidural) A52.19
    tuberculous A18.01
  stitch (postoperative) T81.89
  suppurative (skin) L98.0
  swimming pool A31.1
  talc —*see also* Granuloma, foreign body
    in operation wound —*see* Foreign body, accidentally left during a procedure
  telangiectaticum (skin) L98.0
  tracheostomy J95.09
  trichophyticum B35.8
  tropicum A66.4
  umbilicus L92.9
  urethra N36.8
  uveitis —*see* Iridocyclitis, chronic
  vagina A58
  venereum A58
  vocal cord J38.3

Granulomatosis L92.9
  lymphoid C83.8
  miliary (listerial) A32.89
  necrotizing, respiratory M31.30
  progressive septic D71
  specified NEC L92.8
  Wegener's M31.30
    with renal involvement M31.31
Granulomatous tissue (abnormal) (excessive)
  L92.9
Granulosis rubra nasi L74.8
Graphite fibrosis (of lung) J63.3
Graphospasm F48.8
  organic G25.89
Grating scapula M89.8X1
Gravel (urinary) —*see* Calculus, urinary
Graves' disease —*see* Hyperthyroidism, with,
  goiter
Gravis —*see* condition
Grawitz tumor C64.
Gray syndrome (newborn) P93.0
Grayness, hair (premature) L67.1
  congenital Q84.2
Green sickness D50.8
Greenfield's disease
  meaning
    concentric sclerosis (encephalitis periaxialis
    concentrica) G37.5
    metachromatic leukodystrophy E75.25
Greenstick fracture   code as Fracture, by site
Grey syndrome (newborn) P93.0
Grief F43.21
  prolonged F43.29
  reaction (*see also* Disorder, adjustment)
  F43.20
Griesinger's disease B76.9
Grinder's lung or pneumoconiosis J62.8
Grinding, teeth
  psychogenic F45.8
  sleep related G47.63
Grip
  Dabney's B33.0
  devil's B33.0
Grippe, grippal —*see also* Influenza
  Balkan A78
  summer, of Italy A93.1
Grisel's disease M43.6
Groin —*see* condition
Grooved tongue K14.5
Ground itch B76.9
Grover's disease or syndrome L11.1
Growing pains, children R29.898
Growth (fungoid) (neoplastic) (new) —*see*
  also Neoplasm
  adenoid (vegetative) J35.8
  benign —*see* Neoplasm, benign, by site
  malignant —*see* Neoplasm, malignant, by site
  rapid, childhood Z00.2
  secondary —*see* Neoplasm, secondary, by site
Gruby's disease B35.0
Gubler-Millard paralysis or syndrome G46.3
Guerin-Stern syndrome Q74.3
Guidance, insufficient anterior (occlusal)
  M26.54
Guillain-Barré disease or syndrome G61.0
  sequelae G65.0
Guinea worms (infection) (infestation) B72
Guinon's disease (motor-verbal tic) F95.2
Gull's disease E03.4
Gum —*see* condition
Gumboil K04.7
  with sinus K04.6
Gumma (syphilitic) A52.79
  artery A52.09
    cerebral A52.04

Gumma (syphilitic) - *continued*
  bone A52.77
    of yaws (late) A66.6
  brain A52.19
  cauda equina A52.19
  central nervous system A52.3
  ciliary body A52.71
  congenital A50.59
  eyelid A52.71
  heart A52.06
  intracranial A52.19
  iris A52.71
  kidney A52.75
  larynx A52.73
  leptomeninges A52.19
  liver A52.74
  meninges A52.19
  myocardium A52.06
  nasopharynx A52.73
  neurosyphilitic A52.3
  nose A52.73
  orbit A52.71
  palate (soft) A52.79
  penis A52.76
  pericardium A52.06
  pharynx A52.73
  pituitary A52.79
  scrofulous (tuberculous) A18.4
  skin A52.79
  specified site NEC A52.79
  spinal cord A52.19
  tongue A52.79
  tonsil A52.73
  trachea A52.73
  tuberculous A18.4
  ulcerative due to yaws A66.4
  ureter A52.75
  yaws A66.4
    bone A66.6
Gunn's syndrome Q07.8
Gunshot wound —*see also* Wound, open
  fracture
  code as Fracture, by site
  internal organs —*see* Injury, by site
Gynandrism Q56.0
Gynandroblastoma
  specified site —*see* Neoplasm, uncertain
  behavior, by site
  unspecified site
    female D39.10
    male D40.10
Gynecological examination (periodic)
  (routine) Z01.419
  with abnormal findings Z01.411
Gynecomastia N62
Gynephobia F40.291
Gyrate scalp Q82.8

H

H (Hartnup's) **disease** E72.02
Haas' disease or osteochondrosis (juvenile)
  (head of humerus) —*see* Osteochondrosis,
  juvenile, humerus
Habit, habituation
  bad sleep Z72.821
  chorea F95.8
  disturbance, child F98.9
  drug —*see* Dependence, drug
  irregular sleep Z72.821
  laxative F55.2
  spasm —*see* Tic
  tic —*see* Tic
Haemophilus (H.) **influenzae,** as cause of
  disease classified elsewhere B96.3
Haff disease —*see* Poisoning, mercury

Hageman's factor defect, deficiency or
  disease D68.2
Haglund's disease or osteochondrosis
  (juvenile) (os tibiale externum) —*see*
  Osteochondrosis, juvenile, tarsus
Hailey-Hailey disease Q82.8
Hair —*see also* condition
  plucking F63.3
    in stereotyped movement disorder F98.4
  tourniquet syndrome —*see also* Constriction,
    external, by site
    finger S60.44
    penis S30.842
    thumb S60.34
    toe S90.44
Hairball in stomach T18.2
Hair-pulling, pathological (compulsive) F63.3
Hairy black tongue K14.3
Half vertebra Q76.49
Halitosis R19.6
Hallerman-Streiff syndrome Q87.0
Hallervorden-Spatz disease G23.0
Hallopeau's acrodermatitis or disease L40.2
Hallucination R44.3
  auditory R44.0
  gustatory R44.2
  olfactory R44.2
  specified NEC R44.2
  tactile R44.2
  visual R44.1
Hallucinosis (chronic) F28
  alcoholic (acute) F10.951
    in
      abuse F10.151
      dependence F10.251
  drug-induced F19.951
    cannabis F12.951
    cocaine F14.951
    hallucinogen F16.151
    in
      abuse F19.151
        cannabis F12.151
        cocaine F14.151
        hallucinogen F16.151
        inhalant F18.151
        opioid F11.151
        sedative, anxiolytic or hypnotic F13.151
        stimulant NEC F15.151
      dependence F19.251
        cannabis F12.251
        cocaine F14.251
        hallucinogen F16.251
        inhalant F18.251
        opioid F11.251
        sedative, anxiolytic or hypnotic F13.251
        stimulant NEC F15.251
    inhalant F18.951
    opioid F11.951
    sedative, anxiolytic or hypnotic F13.951
    stimulant NEC F15.951
  organic F06.0
Hallux
  deformity (acquired) NEC M20.5X
  limitus M20.5X
  malleus (acquired) NEC M20.3
  rigidus (acquired) M20.2
    congenital Q74.2
    sequelae (late effect) of rickets E64.3
  valgus (acquired) M20.1
    congenital Q66.6

Hallux - *continued*
 varus (acquired) M20.3
  congenital Q66.3
Halo, visual H53.19
Hamartoma, hamartoblastoma Q85.9
 epithelial (gingival) , odontogenic, central or
 peripheral —*see* Cyst, calcifying odontogenic
Hamartoses Q85.9
Hamman-Rich syndrome J84.114
Hammer toe (acquired) **NEC** —*see also*
 Deformity, toe, hammer toe
 congenital Q66.89
 sequelae (late effect) of rickets E64.3
Hand —*see* condition
Hand-foot syndrome L27.1
Handicap, handicapped
 educational Z55.9
  specified NEC Z55.8
**Hand-Schüller-Christian disease or
 syndrome** C96.5
Hanging (asphyxia) (strangulation)
 (suffocation) —*see* Asphyxia, traumatic, due
 to mechanical threat
Hangnail —*see also* Cellulitis, digit
 with lymphangitis —*see* Lymphangitis, acute,
 digit
Hangover (alcohol) F10.129
Hanhart's syndrome Q87.0
Hanot-Chauffard (-Troisier) **syndrome**
 E83.19
Hanot's cirrhosis or disease K74.3
Hansen's disease —*see* Leprosy
Hantaan virus disease (Korean hemorrhagic
 fever) A98.5
Hantavirus disease (with renal manifestations)
 (Dobrava) (Puumala) (Seoul) A98.5
 with pulmonary manifestations (Andes)
 (Bayou) (Bermejo) (Black Creek Canal)
 (Choclo) (Juquitiba) (Laguna negra)
 (Lechiguanas) (New York) (Oran) (Sin
 nombre) B33.4
Happy puppet syndrome Q93.5
Harada's disease or syndrome H30.81
Hardening
 artery —*see* Arteriosclerosis
 brain G93.89
Harelip (complete) (incomplete) —*see* Cleft,
 lip
Harlequin (newborn) Q80.4
Harley's disease D59.6
Harmful use (of)
 alcohol F10.10
 anxiolytics —*see* Abuse, drug, sedative
 cannabinoids —*see* Abuse, drug, cannabis
 cocaine —*see* Abuse, drug, cocaine
 drug —*see* Abuse, drug
 hallucinogens —*see* Abuse, drug,
 hallucinogen
 hypnotics —*see* Abuse, drug, sedative
 opioids —*see* Abuse, drug, opioid
 PCP (phencyclidine) —*see* Abuse, drug,
 hallucinogen
 sedatives —*see* Abuse, drug, sedative
 stimulants NEC —*see* Abuse, drug, stimulant
Harris' lines —*see* Arrest, epiphyseal
Hartnup's disease E72.02
Harvester's lung J67.0
Harvesting ovum for in vitro fertilization
 Z31.83
Hashimoto's disease or thyroiditis E06.3
Hashitoxicosis (transient) E06.3
Hassal-Henle bodies or warts (cornea)
 H18.49

Haut mal —*see* Epilepsy, generalized,
 specified NEC
Haverhill fever A25.1
Hay fever (*see also* Fever, hay) J30.1
Hayem-Widal syndrome D59.8
Haygarth's nodes M15.8
Haymaker's lung J67.0
Hb (abnormal)
 Bart's disease D56.0
 disease —*see* Disease, hemoglobin
 trait —*see* Trait
Head —*see* condition
Headache R51
 allergic NEC G44.89
 associated with sexual activity G44.82
 chronic daily R51
 cluster G44.009
  chronic G44.029
   intractable G44.021
   not intractable G44.029
  episodic G44.019
   intractable G44.011
   not intractable G44.019
  intractable G44.001
  not intractable G44.009
 cough (primary) G44.83
 daily chronic R51
 drug-induced NEC G44.40
  intractable G44.41
  not intractable G44.40
 exertional (primary) G44.84
 histamine G44.009
  intractable G44.001
  not intractable G44.009
 hypnic G44.81
 lumbar puncture G97.1
 medication overuse G44.40
  intractable G44.41
  not intractable G44.40
 menstrual —*see* Migraine, menstrual
 migraine (type) (*see also* Migraine) G43.909
 nasal septum R51
 neuralgiform, short lasting unilateral, with
 conjunctival injection and tearing (SUNCT)
 G44.059
  intractable G44.051
  not intractable G44.059
 new daily persistent (NDPH) G44.52
 orgasmic G44.82
 periodic syndromes in adults and children
 G43.C0
  with refractory migraine G43.C1
  intractable G43.C1
  not intractable G43.C0
  without refractory migraine G43.C0
 postspinal puncture G97.1
 post-traumatic G44.309
  acute G44.319
   intractable G44.311
   not intractable G44.319
  chronic G44.329
   intractable G44.321
   not intractable G44.329
  intractable G44.301
  not intractable G44.309
 pre-menstrual —*see* Migraine, menstrual
 preorgasmic G44.82
 primary
  cough G44.83
  exertional G44.84
  stabbing G44.85
  thunderclap G44.53

Headache – *continued*
 rebound G44.40
  intractable G44.41
  not intractable G44.40
 short lasting unilateral neuralgiform, with
 conjunctival injection and tearing (SUNCT)
 G44.059
  intractable G44.051
  not intractable G44.059
 specified syndrome NEC G44.89
 spinal and epidural anesthesia
 induced T88.59
  in labor and delivery O74.5
  in pregnancy O29.4
  postpartum, puerperal O89.4
 spinal fluid loss (from puncture) G97.1
 stabbing (primary) G44.85
 tension (-type) G44.209
  chronic G44.229
   intractable G44.221
   not intractable G44.229
  episodic G44.219
   intractable G44.211
   not intractable G44.219
  intractable G44.201
  not intractable G44.209
 thunderclap (primary) G44.53
 vascular NEC G44.1
Healthy
 infant
  accompanying sick mother Z76.3
  receiving care Z76.2
 person accompanying sick person Z76.3
Hearing examination Z01.10
 with abnormal findings NEC Z01.118
 following failed hearing screening Z01.110
 for hearing conservation and treatment Z01.12
Heart —*see* condition
Heart beat
 abnormality R00.9
  specified NEC R00.8
 awareness R00.2
 rapid R00.0
 slow R00.1
Heartburn R12
 psychogenic F45.8
Heat (effects) T67.9
 apoplexy T67.0
 burn (*see also* Burn) L55.9
 collapse T67.1
 cramps T67.2
 dermatitis or eczema L59.0
 edema T67.7
 erythema
 code by site under Burn, first degree
 excessive T67.9
  specified effect NEC T67.8
 exhaustion T67.5
  anhydrotic T67.3
  due to
   salt (and water) depletion T67.4
   water depletion T67.3
    with salt depletion T67.4
 fatigue (transient) T67.6
 fever T67.0
 hyperpyrexia T67.0
 prickly L74.0
 prostration —*see* Heat, exhaustion
 pyrexia T67.0
 rash L74.0
 specified effect NEC T67.8
 stroke T67.0

Heat - *continued*
 sunburn —*see* Sunburn
 syncope T67.1
Heavy-for-dates NEC (infant) (4000g to
 4499g) P08.1
 exceptionally (4500g or more) P08.0
Hebephrenia, hebephrenic (schizophrenia)
 F20.1
Heberden's disease or nodes (with
 arthropathy) M15.1
Hebra's
 pityriasis L26
 prurigo L28.2
Heel —*see* condition
Heerfordt's disease D86.89
Hegglin's anomaly or syndrome D72.0
Heilmeyer-Schoner disease D45
Heine-Medin disease A80.9
Heinz body anemia, congenital D58.2
Heliophobia F40.228
Heller's disease or syndrome F84.3
HELLP syndrome (hemolysis, elevated liver
 enzymes and low platelet count) O14.2
Helminthiasis —*see also* Infestation, helminth
 Ancylostoma B76.0
 intestinal B82.0
  mixed types (types classifiable to more than
  one of the titles B65.0-B81.3 and B81.8)
  B81.4
  specified type NEC B81.8
 mixed types (intestinal) (types classifiable to
 more than one of the titles B65.0-B81.3 and
 B81.8) B81.4
 Necator (americanus) B76.1
 specified type NEC B83.8
Heloma L84
Hemangioblastoma —*see* Neoplasm,
 connective tissue, uncertain behavior
 malignant —*see* Neoplasm, connective tissue,
 malignant
Hemangioendothelioma —*see also* Neoplasm,
 uncertain behavior, by site
 benign D18.00
  intra-abdominal D18.03
  intracranial D18.02
  skin D18.01
  specified site NEC D18.09
 bone (diffuse) —*see* Neoplasm, bone,
 malignant
 epithelioid —*see also* Neoplasm, uncertain
 behavior, by site
  malignant —*see* Neoplasm, malignant, by
 site
 malignant —*see* Neoplasm, connective tissue,
 malignant
Hemangiofibroma —*see* Neoplasm, benign,
 by site
Hemangiolipoma —*see* Lipoma
Hemangioma D18.00
 arteriovenous D18.00
  intra-abdominal D18.03
  intracranial D18.02
  skin D18.01
  specified site NEC D18.09
 capillary D18.00
  intra-abdominal D18.03
  intracranial D18.02
  skin D18.01
  specified site NEC D18.09
 cavernous D18.00
  intra-abdominal D18.03
  intracranial D18.02

Hemangioma - *continued*
 skin D18.01
 specified site NEC D18.09
 epithelioid D18.00
  intra-abdominal D18.03
  intracranial D18.02
  skin D18.01
  specified site NEC D18.09
 histiocytoid D18.00
  intra-abdominal D18.03
  intracranial D18.02
  skin D18.01
  specified site NEC D18.09
 infantile D18.00
  intra-abdominal D18.03
  intracranial D18.02
  skin D18.01
  specified site NEC D18.09
 intra-abdominal D18.03
 intracranial D18.02
 intramuscular D18.00
  intra-abdominal D18.03
  intracranial D18.02
  skin D18.01
  specified site NEC D18.09
 juvenile D18.00
 malignant —*see* Neoplasm, connective tissue,
 malignant
 plexiform D18.00
  intra-abdominal D18.03
  intracranial D18.02
  skin D18.01
  specified site NEC D18.09
 racemose D18.00
  intra-abdominal D18.03
  intracranial D18.02
  skin D18.01
  specified site NEC D18.09
 sclerosing —*see* Neoplasm, skin, benign
 simplex D18.00
  intra-abdominal D18.03
  intracranial D18.02
  skin D18.01
  specified site NEC D18.09
 skin D18.01
 specified site NEC D18.09
 venous D18.00
  intra-abdominal D18.03
  intracranial D18.02
  skin D18.01
  specified site NEC D18.09
 verrucous keratotic D18.00
  intra-abdominal D18.03
  intracranial D18.02
  skin D18.01
  specified site NEC D18.09
Hemangiomatosis (systemic) I78.8
 involving single site —*see* Hemangioma
Hemangiopericytoma —*see also* Neoplasm,
 connective tissue, uncertain behavior
 benign —*see* Neoplasm, connective tissue,
 benign
 malignant —*see* Neoplasm, connective tissue,
 malignant
Hemangiosarcoma —*see* Neoplasm,
 connective tissue, malignant
Hemarthrosis (nontraumatic) M25.00
 ankle M25.07
 elbow M25.02
 foot joint M25.07
 hand joint M25.04
 hip M25.05

Hemarthrosis – *continued*
 in hemophilic arthropathy —*see* Arthropathy,
 hemophilic
 knee M25.06
 shoulder M25.01
 specified joint NEC M25.08
 traumatic —*see* Sprain, by site
 vertebrae M25.08
 wrist M25.03
Hematemesis K92.0
 with ulcer
 code by site under Ulcer, with hemorrhage
 K27.4
 newborn, neonatal P54.0
  due to swallowed maternal blood P78.2
Hematidrosis L74.8
Hematinuria —*see also* Hemoglobinuria
 malarial B50.8
Hematobilia K83.8
Hematocele
 female NEC N94.89
  with ectopic pregnancy O00.9
 ovary N83.8
 male N50.1
Hematochezia (*see also* Melena) K92.1
Hematochyluria —*see also* Infestation, filarial
 schistosomiasis (bilharziasis) B65.0
Hematocolpos (with hematometra or
 hematosalpinx) N89.7
Hematocornea —*see* Pigmentation, cornea,
 stromal
Hematogenous —*see* condition
Hematoma (traumatic) (skin surface intact) —
 see also Contusion
 with
  injury of internal organs —*see* Injury, by
 site
  open wound —*see* Wound, open
 amputation stump (surgical) (late) T87.89
 aorta, dissecting I71.00
  abdominal I71.02
  thoracic I71.01
  thoracoabdominal I71.03
 aortic intramural —*see* Dissection, aorta
 arterial (complicating trauma) —*see* Injury,
 blood vessel, by site
 auricle —*see* Contusion, ear
  nontraumatic —*see* Disorder, pinna,
 hematoma
 birth injury NEC P15.8
 brain (traumatic)
  with
   cerebral laceration or contusion (diffuse)
  —*see* Injury, intracranial, diffuse
   focal —*see* Injury, intracranial, focal
  cerebellar, traumatic S06.37
  newborn NEC P52.4
   birth injury P10.1
  intracerebral, traumatic —*see* Injury,
 intracranial, intracerebral hemorrhage
   nontraumatic —*see* Hemorrhage,
 intracranial
  subarachnoid, arachnoid, traumatic —*see*
 Injury, intracranial, subarachnoid hemorrhage
  subdural, traumatic —*see* Injury,
 intracranial, subdural hemorrhage
 breast (nontraumatic) N64.89
 broad ligament (nontraumatic) N83.7
  traumatic S37.892
 cerebellar, traumatic S06.37
 cerebral —*see* Hematoma, brain
 cerebrum S06.36
  left S06.35

Hematoma - *continued*
   right S06.34
  cesarean delivery wound O90.2
  complicating delivery (perineal) (pelvic)
  (vagina) (vulva) O71.7
  corpus cavernosum (nontraumatic) N48.89
  epididymis (nontraumatic) N50.1
  epidural (traumatic) —*see* Injury, intracranial,
  epidural hemorrhage
    spinal —*see* Injury, spinal cord, by region
  episiotomy O90.2
  face, birth injury P15.4
  genital organ NEC (nontraumatic)
    female (nonobstetric) N94.89
      traumatic S30.202
    male N50.1
      traumatic S30.201
  internal organs —*see* Injury, by site
  intracerebral, traumatic —*see* Injury,
  intracranial, intracerebral hemorrhage
  intraoperative —*see* Complications,
  intraoperative, hemorrhage
  labia (nontraumatic) (nonobstetric) N90.89
  liver (subcapsular) (nontraumatic) K76.89
    birth injury P15.0
  mediastinum —*see* Injury, intrathoracic
  mesosalpinx (nontraumatic) N83.7
    traumatic S37.898
  muscle
  code by site under Contusion
  nontraumatic
    muscle M79.81
    soft tissue M79.81
  obstetrical surgical wound O90.2
  orbit, orbital (nontraumatic) —*see also*
  Hemorrhage, orbit
    traumatic —*see* Contusion, orbit
  pelvis (female) (nontraumatic) (nonobstetric)
  N94.89
    obstetric O71.7
    traumatic —*see* Injury, by site
  penis (nontraumatic) N48.89
    birth injury P15.5
  perianal (nontraumatic) K64.5
  perineal S30.23
    complicating delivery O71.7
  perirenal —*see* Injury, kidney
  pinna —*see* Contusion, ear
    nontraumatic —*see* Disorder, pinna,
  hematoma
  placenta O43.89
  postoperative (postprocedural) —*see*
  Complication, postprocedural, hemorrhage
  retroperitoneal (nontraumatic) K66.1
    traumatic S36.892
  scrotum, superficial S30.22
    birth injury P15.5
  seminal vesicle (nontraumatic) N50.1
    traumatic S37.892
  spermatic cord (traumatic) S37.892
    nontraumatic N50.1
  spinal (cord) (meninges) —*see also* Injury,
  spinal cord, by region
    newborn (birth injury) P11.5
  spleen D73.5
    intraoperative —*see* Complications,
  intraoperative, hemorrhage, spleen
    postprocedural (postoperative) —*see*
  Complications, postprocedural, hemorrhage,
  spleen
  sternocleidomastoid, birth injury P15.2
  sternomastoid, birth injury P15.2

Hematoma - *continued*
  subarachnoid (traumatic) —*see* Injury,
  intracranial, subarachnoid hemorrhage
    newborn (nontraumatic) P52.5
      due to birth injury P10.3
    nontraumatic —*see* Hemorrhage,
  intracranial, subarachnoid
  subdural (traumatic) —*see* Injury,
  intracranial, subdural hemorrhage
    newborn (localized) P52.8
      birth injury P10.0
    nontraumatic —*see* Hemorrhage,
  intracranial, subdural
  superficial, newborn P54.5
  testis (nontraumatic) N50.1
    birth injury P15.5
  tunica vaginalis (nontraumatic) N50.1
  umbilical cord, complicating delivery O69.5
  uterine ligament (broad) (nontraumatic)
  N83.7
    traumatic S37.892
  vagina (ruptured) (nontraumatic) N89.8
    complicating delivery O71.7
  vas deferens (nontraumatic) N50.1
    traumatic S37.892
  vitreous —*see* Hemorrhage, vitreous
  vulva (nontraumatic) (nonobstetric) N90.89
    complicating delivery O71.7
    newborn (birth injury) P15.5
Hematometra N85.7
  with hematocolpos N89.7
Hematomyelia (central) G95.19
  newborn (birth injury) P11.5
  traumatic T14.8
Hematomyelitis G04.90
Hematoperitoneum —*see* Hemoperitoneum
Hematophobia F40.230
Hematopneumothorax (see Hemothorax)
Hematopoiesis, cyclic D70.4
Hematoporphyria —*see* Porphyria
Hematorachis, hematorrhachis G95.19
  newborn (birth injury) P11.5
Hematosalpinx N83.6
  with
    hematocolpos N89.7
    hematometra N85.7
      with hematocolpos N89.7
  infectional —*see* Salpingitis
Hematospermia R36.1
Hematothorax (see Hemothorax)
Hematuria R31.9
  due to sulphonamide, sulfonamide —*see*
  Table of Drugs and Chemicals, by drug
  benign (familial) (of childhood) —*see also*
  Hematuria, idiopathic
    essential microscopic R31.1
  endemic (*see also* Schistosomiasis) B65.0
  gross R31.0
  idiopathic N02.9
    with glomerular lesion
      crescentic (diffuse) glomerulonephritis
  N02.7
      dense deposit disease N02.6
      endocapillary proliferative
  glomerulonephritis N02.4
      focal and segmental hyalinosis or sclerosis
  N02.1
      membranoproliferative (diffuse) N02.5
      membranous (diffuse) N02.2
      mesangial proliferative (diffuse) N02.3
      mesangiocapillary (diffuse) N02.5
      minor abnormality N02.0

Hematuria – *continued*
    proliferative NEC N02.8
    specified pathology NEC N02.8
  intermittent —*see* Hematuria, idiopathic
  malarial B50.8
  microscopic NEC R31.2
    benign essential R31.1
  paroxysmal —*see also* Hematuria, idiopathic
    nocturnal D59.5
  persistent —*see* Hematuria, idiopathic
  recurrent —*see* Hematuria, idiopathic
  tropical (*see also* Schistosomiasis) B65.0
  tuberculous A18.13
Hemeralopia (day blindness) H53.11
  vitamin A deficiency E50.5
Hemi-akinesia R41.4
Hemianalgesia R20.0
Hemianencephaly Q00.0
Hemianesthesia R20.0
Hemianopia, hemianopsia (heteronymous)
H53.47
  homonymous H53.46
  syphilitic A52.71
Hemiathetosis R25.8
Hemiatrophy R68.89
  cerebellar G31.9
  face, facial, progressive (Romberg) G51.8
  tongue K14.8
Hemiballism (us) G25.5
Hemicardia Q24.8
Hemicephalus, hemicephaly Q00.0
Hemichorea G25.5
Hemicolitis, left —*see* Colitis, left sided
Hemicrania
  congenital malformation Q00.0
  continua G44.51
  meaning migraine (*see also* Migraine)
  G43.909
  paroxysmal G44.039
    chronic G44.049
      intractable G44.041
      not intractable G44.049
    episodic G44.039
      intractable G44.031
      not intractable G44.039
    intractable G44.031
    not intractable G44.039
Hemidystrophy —*see* Hemiatrophy
Hemiectromelia Q73.8
Hemihypalgesia R20.8
Hemihypesthesia R20.1
Hemi-inattention R41.4
Hemimelia Q73.8
  lower limb —*see* Defect, reduction, lower
  limb, specified type NEC
  upper limb —*see* Defect, reduction, upper
  limb, specified type NEC
Hemiparalysis —*see* Hemiplegia
Hemiparesis —*see* Hemiplegia
Hemiparesthesia R20.2
Hemiparkinsonism G20
Hemiplegia G81.9
  alternans facialis G83.89
  ascending NEC G81.90
    spinal G95.89
  congenital (cerebral) G80.8
    spastic G80.2
  embolic (current episode) I63.4
  flaccid G81.0
  following
    cerebrovascular disease I69.959
      cerebral infarction I69.35
      intracerebral hemorrhage I69.15

Hemiplegia - *continued*
  nontraumatic intracranial hemorrhage NEC I69.25
    specified disease NEC I69.85
    stroke NOS I69.35
    subarachnoid hemorrhage I69.05
  hysterical F44.4
  newborn NEC P91.8
    birth injury P11.9
  spastic G81.1
    congenital G80.2
  thrombotic (current episode) I63.3
Hemisection, spinal cord —*see* Injury, spinal cord, by region
Hemispasm (facial) R25.2
Hemisporosis B48.8
Hemitremor R25.1
Hemivertebra Q76.49
  failure of segmentation with scoliosis Q76.3
  fusion with scoliosis Q76.3
Hemochromatosis E83.119
  with refractory anemia D46.1
  due to repeated red blood cell transfusion E83.111
  hereditary (primary) E83.110
  primary E83.110
  specified NEC E83.118
Hemoglobin —*see also* condition
  abnormal (disease) —*see* Disease, hemoglobin
  AS genotype D57.3
  Constant Spring D58.2
  E-beta thalassemia D56.5
  fetal, hereditary persistence (HPFH) D56.4
  H Constant Spring D56.0
  low NOS D64.9
  S (Hb S) , heterozygous D57.3
Hemoglobinemia D59.9
  due to blood transfusion T80.89
  paroxysmal D59.6
    nocturnal D59.5
Hemoglobinopathy (mixed) D58.2
  with thalassemia D56.8
  sickle-cell D57.1
    with thalassemia D57.40
      with crisis (vasoocclusive pain) D57.419
        with
          acute chest syndrome D57.411
          splenic sequestration D57.412
      without crisis D57.40
Hemoglobinuria R82.3
  with anemia, hemolytic, acquired (chronic) NEC D59.6
  cold (agglutinin) (paroxysmal) (with Raynaud's syndrome) D59.6
  due to exertion or hemolysis NEC D59.6
  intermittent D59.6
  malarial B50.8
  march D59.6
  nocturnal (paroxysmal) D59.5
  paroxysmal (cold) D59.6
    nocturnal D59.5
Hemolymphangioma D18.1
Hemolysis
  intravascular
    with
      abortion —*see* Abortion, by type, complicated by, hemorrhage
      ectopic or molar pregnancy O08.1
      hemorrhage
        antepartum —*see* Hemorrhage, antepartum, with coagulation defect

Hemolysis – *continued*
    intrapartum (*see also* Hemorrhage, complicating, delivery) O67.0
    postpartum O72.3
  neonatal (excessive) P58.9
    specified NEC P58.8
Hemolytic —*see* condition
Hemopericardium I31.2
  following acute myocardial infarction (current complication) I23.0
  newborn P54.8
  traumatic —*see* Injury, heart, with hemopericardium
Hemoperitoneum K66.1
  infectional K65.9
  traumatic S36.899
    with open wound —*see* Wound, open, with penetration into peritoneal cavity
Hemophilia (classical) (familial) (hereditary) D66
  A D66
  B D67
  C D68.1
  acquired D68.311
  autoimmune D68.311
  calcipriva (*see also* Defect, coagulation) D68.4
  nonfamilial (*see also* Defect, coagulation) D68.4
  secondary D68.311
  vascular D68.0
Hemophthalmos H44.81
Hemopneumothorax —*see also* Hemothorax
  traumatic S27.2
Hemoptysis R04.2
  newborn P26.9
  tuberculous —*see* Tuberculosis, pulmonary
Hemorrhage, hemorrhagic (concealed) R58
  abdomen R58
  accidental antepartum —*see* Hemorrhage, antepartum
  acute idiopathic pulmonary, in infants R04.81
  adenoid J35.8
  adrenal (capsule) (gland) E27.49
    medulla E27.8
    newborn P54.4
  after delivery —*see* Hemorrhage, postpartum
  alveolar
    lung, newborn P26.8
    process K08.8
  alveolus K08.8
  amputation stump (surgical) T87.89
  anemia (chronic) D50.0
    acute D62
  antepartum (with) O46.90
    with coagulation defect O46.00
      afibrinogenemia O46.01
      disseminated intravascular coagulation O46.02
      hypofibrinogenemia O46.01
      specified defect NEC O46.09
    before 20 weeks gestation O20.9
      specified type NEC O20.8
      threatened abortion O20.0
    due to
      abruptio placenta (*see also* Abruptio placentae) O45.9
      leiomyoma, uterus —*see* Hemorrhage, antepartum, specified cause NEC
      placenta previa O44.1
      specified cause NEC —see subcategory O46.8X

Hemorrhage, hemorrhagic – *continued*
  anus (sphincter) K62.5
  apoplexy (stroke) —*see* Hemorrhage, intracranial, intracerebral
  arachnoid —*see* Hemorrhage, intracranial, subarachnoid
  artery R58
  brain —*see* Hemorrhage, intracranial, intracerebral
  basilar (ganglion) I61.0
  bladder N32.89
  bowel K92.2
    newborn P54.3
  brain (miliary) (nontraumatic) —*see* Hemorrhage, intracranial, intracerebral
    due to
      birth injury P10.1
      syphilis A52.05
    epidural or extradural (traumatic) —*see* Injury, intracranial, epidural hemorrhage
    newborn P52.4
      birth injury P10.1
    subarachnoid —*see* Hemorrhage, intracranial, subarachnoid
    subdural —*see* Hemorrhage, intracranial, subdural
  brainstem (nontraumatic) I61.3
    traumatic S06.38
  breast N64.59
  bronchial tube —*see* Hemorrhage, lung
  bronchopulmonary —*see* Hemorrhage, lung
  bronchus —*see* Hemorrhage, lung
  bulbar I61.5
  capillary I78.8
    primary D69.8
  cecum K92.2
  cerebellar, cerebellum (nontraumatic) I61.4
    newborn P52.6
    traumatic S06.37
  cerebral, cerebrum —*see also* Hemorrhage, intracranial, intracerebral
    newborn (anoxic) P52.4
      birth injury P10.1
    lobe I61.1
  cerebromeningeal I61.8
  cerebrospinal —*see* Hemorrhage, intracranial, intracerebral
  cervix (uteri) (stump) NEC N88.8
  chamber, anterior (eye) —*see* Hyphema
  childbirth —*see* Hemorrhage, complicating, delivery
  choroid H31.30
    expulsive H31.31
  ciliary body —*see* Hyphema
  cochlea —see subcategory H83.8
  colon K92.2
  complicating
    abortion —*see* Abortion, by type, complicated by, hemorrhage
    delivery O67.9
      associated with coagulation defect (afibrinogenemia) (DIC) (hyperfibrinolysis) O67.0
      specified cause NEC O67.8
    surgical procedure —*see* Hemorrhage, intraoperative
  conjunctiva H11.3
    newborn P54.8
  cord, newborn (stump) P51.9
  corpus luteum (ruptured) cyst N83.1
  cortical (brain) I61.1
  cranial —*see* Hemorrhage, intracranial
  cutaneous R23.3

Hemorrhage, hemorrhagic - *continued*
    due to autosensitivity, erythrocyte D69.2
      newborn P54.5
    delayed
      following ectopic or molar pregnancy O08.1
      postpartum O72.2
    diathesis (familial) D69.9
    disease D69.9
      newborn P53
      specified type NEC D69.8
    due to or associated with
      afibrinogenemia or other coagulation defect
      (conditions in categories D65-D69)
        antepartum —*see* Hemorrhage,
    antepartum, with coagulation defect
        intrapartum O67.0
      dental implant M27.61
      device, implant or graft (*see also*
    Complications, by site and type, specified
    NEC) T85.83
        arterial graft NEC T82.838
        breast T85.83
        catheter NEC T85.83
          dialysis (renal) T82.838
            intraperitoneal T85.83
          infusion NEC T82.838
            spinal (epidural) (subdural) T85.83
          urinary (indwelling) T83.83
        electronic (electrode) (pulse generator)
    (stimulator)
          bone T84.83
          cardiac T82.837
          nervous system (brain) (peripheral nerve)
    (spinal) T85.83
            urinary T83.83
        fixation, internal (orthopedic) NEC T84.83
        gastrointestinal (bile duct) (esophagus)
    T85.83
        genital NEC T83.83
        heart NEC T82.837
        joint prosthesis T84.83
        ocular (corneal graft) (orbital implant)
    NEC T85.83
        orthopedic NEC T84.83
          bone graft T86.838
        specified NEC T85.83
        urinary NEC T83.83
        vascular NEC T82.838
        ventricular intracranial shunt T85.83
    duodenum, duodenal K92.2
      ulcer —*see* Ulcer, duodenum, with
    hemorrhage
    dura mater —*see* Hemorrhage, intracranial,
    subdural
    endotracheal —*see* Hemorrhage, lung
    epicranial subaponeurotic (massive) , birth
    injury P12.2
    epidural (traumatic) —*see also* Injury,
    intracranial, epidural hemorrhage
      nontraumatic I62.1
    esophagus K22.8
      varix I85.01
        secondary I85.11
    excessive, following ectopic gestation
    (subsequent episode) O08.1
    extradural (traumatic) —*see* Injury,
    intracranial, epidural hemorrhage
      birth injury P10.8
      newborn (anoxic) (nontraumatic) P52.8
      nontraumatic I62.1
    eye NEC H57.8
      fundus —*see* Hemorrhage, retina

Hemorrhage, hemorrhagic - *continued*
    lid —*see* Disorder, eyelid, specified type
    NEC
    fallopian tube N83.6
    fibrinogenolysis —*see* Fibrinolysis
    fibrinolytic (acquired) —*see* Fibrinolysis
    from
      ear (nontraumatic) —*see* Otorrhagia
      tracheostomy stoma J95.01
    fundus, eye —*see* Hemorrhage, retina
    funis —*see* Hemorrhage, umbilicus, cord
    gastric —*see* Hemorrhage, stomach
    gastroenteric K92.2
      newborn P54.3
    gastrointestinal (tract) K92.2
      newborn P54.3
    genital organ, male N50.1
    genitourinary (tract) NOS R31.9
    gingiva K06.8
    globe (eye) —*see* Hemophthalmos
    graafian follicle cyst (ruptured) N83.0
    gum K06.8
    heart I51.89
    hypopharyngeal (throat) R04.1
    intermenstrual (regular) N92.3
      irregular N92.1
    internal (organs) NEC R58
      capsule I61.0
      ear —*see* subcategory H83.8
        newborn P54.8
      intestine K92.2
        newborn P54.3
    intra-abdominal R58
    intra-alveolar (lung) , newborn P26.8
    intracerebral (nontraumatic) —*see*
    Hemorrhage, intracranial, intracerebral
    intracranial (nontraumatic) I62.9
      birth injury P10.9
      epidural, nontraumatic I62.1
      extradural, nontraumatic I62.1
      newborn P52.9
        specified NEC P52.8
      intracerebral (nontraumatic) (in) I61.9
        brain stem I61.3
        cerebellum I61.4
        newborn P52.4
          birth injury P10.1
        hemisphere I61.2
          cortical (superficial) I61.1
          subcortical (deep) I61.0
      intraoperative
        during a nervous system procedure
    G97.31
        during other procedure G97.32
      intraventricular I61.5
      multiple localized I61.6
      postprocedural
        following a nervous system procedure
    G97.51
        following other procedure G97.52
      specified NEC I61.8
      superficial I61.1
      traumatic (diffuse) —*see* Injury,
    intracranial, diffuse
      focal —*see* Injury, intracranial, focal
    subarachnoid (nontraumatic) (from) I60.9
      newborn P52.5
        birth injury P10.3
      intracranial (cerebral) artery I60.7
        anterior communicating I60.2
        basilar I60.4
        carotid siphon and bifurcation I60.0

Hemorrhage, hemorrhagic - *continued*
      communicating I60.7
        anterior I60.2
        posterior I60.3
      middle cerebral I60.1
      posterior communicating I60.3
      specified artery NEC I60.6
      vertebral I60.5
      specified NEC I60.8
      traumatic S06.6X
      subdural (nontraumatic) I62.00
      acute I62.01
      birth injury P10.0
      chronic I62.03
      newborn (anoxic) (hypoxic) P52.8
        birth injury P10.0
      spinal G95.19
      subacute I62.02
      traumatic —*see* Injury, intracranial,
    subdural hemorrhage
      traumatic —*see* Injury, intracranial, focal
    brain injury
    intramedullary NEC G95.19
    intraocular —*see* Hemophthalmos
    intraoperative, intraprocedural —*see*
    Complication, hemorrhage (hematoma) ,
    intraoperative (intraprocedural) , by site
    intrapartum —*see* Hemorrhage, complicating,
    delivery
    intrapelvic
      female N94.89
      male K66.1
    intraperitoneal K66.1
    intrapontine I61.3
    intraprocedural —*see* Complication,
    hemorrhage (hematoma) , intraoperative
    (intraprocedural) , by site
    intrauterine N85.7
      complicating delivery (*see also* Hemorrhage,
    complicating, delivery) O67.9
      postpartum —*see* Hemorrhage, postpartum
    intraventricular I61.5
      newborn (nontraumatic) (*see also* Newborn,
    affected by, hemorrhage) P52.3
        due to birth injury P10.2
        grade
          1 P52.0
          2 P52.1
          3 P52.21
          4 P52.22
    intravesical N32.89
    iris (postinfectional) (postinflammatory)
    (toxic) —*see* Hyphema
    joint (nontraumatic) —*see* Hemarthrosis
    kidney N28.89
    knee (joint) (nontraumatic) —*see*
    Hemarthrosis, knee
    labyrinth —*see* subcategory H83.8
    lenticular striate artery I61.0
    ligature, vessel —*see* Hemorrhage,
    postoperative
    liver K76.89
    lung R04.89
      newborn P26.9
        massive P26.1
        specified NEC P26.8
      tuberculous —*see* Tuberculosis, pulmonary
    massive umbilical, newborn P51.0
    mediastinum —*see* Hemorrhage, lung
    medulla I61.3
    membrane (brain) I60.8
      spinal cord —*see* Hemorrhage, spinal cord

Hemorrhage, hemorrhagic - *continued*
  meninges, meningeal (brain) (middle) I60.8
    spinal cord —*see* Hemorrhage, spinal cord
  mesentery K66.1
  metritis —*see* Endometritis
  mouth K13.79
  mucous membrane NEC R58
    newborn P54.8
  muscle M62.89
  nail (subungual) L60.8
  nasal turbinate R04.0
    newborn P54.8
  navel, newborn P51.9
  newborn P54.9
    specified NEC P54.8
  nipple N64.59
  nose R04.0
    newborn P54.8
  omentum K66.1
  optic nerve (sheath) H47.02
  orbit, orbital H05.23
  ovary NEC N83.8
  oviduct N83.6
  pancreas K86.8
  parathyroid (gland) (spontaneous) E21.4
  parturition —*see* Hemorrhage, complicating, delivery
  penis N48.89
  pericardium, pericarditis I31.2
  peritoneum, peritoneal K66.1
  peritonsillar tissue J35.8
    due to infection J36
  petechial R23.3
    due to autosensitivity, erythrocyte D69.2
  pituitary (gland) E23.6
  pleura —*see* Hemorrhage, lung
  polioencephalitis, superior E51.2
  polymyositis —*see* Polymyositis
  pons, pontine I61.3
  posterior fossa (nontraumatic) I61.8
    newborn P52.6
  postmenopausal N95.0
  postnasal R04.0
  postoperative —*see* Complications, postprocedural, hemorrhage, by site
  postpartum NEC (following delivery of placenta) O72.1
    delayed or secondary O72.2
    retained placenta O72.0
    third stage O72.0
  pregnancy —*see* Hemorrhage, antepartum
  preretinal —*see* Hemorrhage, retina
  prostate N42.1
  puerperal —*see* Hemorrhage, postpartum
    delayed or secondary O72.2
  pulmonary R04.89
    newborn P26.9
      massive P26.1
      specified NEC P26.8
    tuberculous —*see* Tuberculosis, pulmonary
  purpura (primary) D69.3
  rectum (sphincter) K62.5
    newborn P54.2
  recurring, following initial hemorrhage at time of injury T79.2
  renal N28.89
  respiratory passage or tract R04.9
    specified NEC R04.89
  retina, retinal (vessels) H35.6
    diabetic —*see* Diabetes, retinal, hemorrhage
  retroperitoneal R58
  scalp R58

Hemorrhage, hemorrhagic - *continued*
  scrotum N50.1
  secondary (nontraumatic) R58
    following initial hemorrhage at time of injury T79.2
  seminal vesicle N50.1
  skin R23.3
    newborn P54.5
  slipped umbilical ligature P51.8
  spermatic cord N50.1
  spinal (cord) G95.19
    newborn (birth injury) P11.5
  spleen D73.5
    intraoperative —*see* Complications, intraoperative, hemorrhage, spleen
    postprocedural —*see* Complications, postprocedural, hemorrhage, spleen
  stomach K92.2
    newborn P54.3
    ulcer —*see* Ulcer, stomach, with hemorrhage
  subarachnoid (nontraumatic) —*see* Hemorrhage, intracranial, subarachnoid
  subconjunctival —*see also* Hemorrhage, conjunctiva
    birth injury P15.3
  subcortical (brain) I61.0
  subcutaneous R23.3
  subdiaphragmatic R58
  subdural (acute) (nontraumatic) —*see* Hemorrhage, intracranial, subdural
  subependymal
    newborn P52.0
      with intraventricular extension P52.1
        and intracerebral extension P52.22
  subgaleal P12.1
  subhyaloid —*see* Hemorrhage, retina
  subperiosteal —*see* Disorder, bone, specified type NEC
  subretinal —*see* Hemorrhage, retina
  subtentorial —*see* Hemorrhage, intracranial, subdural
  subungual L60.8
  suprarenal (capsule) (gland) E27.49
    newborn P54.4
  tentorium (traumatic) NEC —*see* Hemorrhage, brain
    newborn (birth injury) P10.4
  testis N50.1
  third stage (postpartum) O72.0
  thorax —*see* Hemorrhage, lung
  throat R04.1
  thymus (gland) E32.8
  thyroid (cyst) (gland) E07.89
  tongue K14.8
  tonsil J35.8
  trachea —*see* Hemorrhage, lung
  tracheobronchial R04.89
    newborn P26.0
  traumatic
  code to specific injury
    cerebellar —*see* Hemorrhage, brain
    intracranial —*see* Hemorrhage, brain
    recurring or secondary (following initial hemorrhage at time of injury) T79.2
  tuberculous NEC (*see also* Tuberculosis, pulmonary) A15.0
  tunica vaginalis N50.1
  ulcer
  code by site under Ulcer, with hemorrhage
    K27.4

Hemorrhage, hemorrhagic - *continued*
  umbilicus, umbilical
    cord
      after birth, newborn P51.9
      complicating delivery O69.5
    newborn P51.9
      massive P51.0
      slipped ligature P51.8
    stump P51.9
  urethra (idiopathic) N36.8
  uterus, uterine (abnormal) N93.9
    climacteric N92.4
    complicating delivery —*see* Hemorrhage, complicating, delivery
    dysfunctional or functional N93.8
    intermenstrual (regular) N92.3
      irregular N92.1
    postmenopausal N95.0
    postpartum —*see* Hemorrhage, postpartum
    preclimacteric or premenopausal N92.4
    prepubertal N93.8
    pubertal N92.2
  vagina (abnormal) N93.9
    newborn P54.6
  vas deferens N50.1
  vasa previa O69.4
  ventricular I61.5
  vesical N32.89
  viscera NEC R58
    newborn P54.8
  vitreous (humor) (intraocular) H43.1
  vulva N90.89
Hemorrhoids (bleeding) (without mention of degree) K64.9
  1st degree (grade/stage I) (without prolapse outside of anal canal) K64.0
  2nd degree (grade/stage II) (that prolapse with straining but retract spontaneously) K64.1
  3rd degree (grade/stage III) (that prolapse with straining and require manual replacement back inside anal canal) K64.2
  4th degree (grade/stage IV) (with prolapsed tissue that cannot be manually replaced) K64.3
  complicating
    pregnancy O22.4
    puerperium O87.2
  external K64.4
    with
      thrombosis K64.5
  internal (without mention of degree) K64.8
  prolapsed K64.8
  skin tags
    anus K64.4
    residual K64.4
  specified NEC K64.8
  strangulated (*see also* Hemorrhoids, by degree) K64.8
  thrombosed (*see also* Hemorrhoids, by degree) K64.5
  ulcerated (*see also* Hemorrhoids, by degree) K64.8
Hemosalpinx N83.6
  with
    hematocolpos N89.7
    hematometra N85.7
      with hematocolpos N89.7
Hemosiderosis (dietary) E83.19
  pulmonary, idiopathic E83.1 *[J84.03]*
  transfusion T80.89

Hemothorax (bacterial) (nontuberculous)
J94.2
  newborn P54.8
  traumatic S27.1
    with pneumothorax S27.2
  tuberculous NEC A15.6
Henoch (-Schönlein) disease or syndrome
(purpura) D69.0
Henpue, henpuye A66.6
Hepar lobatum (syphilitic) A52.74
Hepatalgia K76.89
Hepatitis K75.9
  acute B17.9
    with coma K72.01
    with hepatic failure —*see* Failure, hepatic
    alcoholic —*see* Hepatitis, alcoholic
    infectious B15.9
      with hepatic coma B15.0
    viral B17.9
  alcoholic (acute) (chronic) K70.10
    with ascites K70.11
  amebic —*see* Abscess, liver, amebic
  anicteric, (viral) —*see* Hepatitis, viral
  antigen-associated (HAA) —*see* Hepatitis, B
  Australia-antigen (positive) —*see* Hepatitis, B
  autoimmune K75.4
  B B19.10
    with hepatic coma B19.11
    acute B16.9
      with
        delta-agent (coinfection) (without hepatic
coma) B16.1
          with hepatic coma B16.0
        hepatic coma (without delta-agent
coinfection) B16.2
    chronic B18.1
      with delta-agent B18.0
  bacterial NEC K75.89
  C (viral) B19.20
    with hepatic coma B19.21
    acute B17.10
      with hepatic coma B17.11
    chronic B18.2
  catarrhal (acute) B15.9
    with hepatic coma B15.0
  cholangiolitic K75.89
  cholestatic K75.89
  chronic K73.9
    active NEC K73.2
    lobular NEC K73.1
    persistent NEC K73.0
    specified NEC K73.8
  cytomegaloviral B25.1
  due to ethanol (acute) (chronic) —*see*
Hepatitis, alcoholic
  epidemic B15.9
    with hepatic coma B15.0
  fulminant NEC (viral) —*see* Hepatitis, viral
  neonatal giant cell P59.29
  granulomatous NEC K75.3
  herpesviral B00.81
  history of
    B Z86.19
    C Z86.19
  homologous serum —*see* Hepatitis, viral, type
B in (due to)
    mumps B26.81
    toxoplasmosis (acquired) B58.1
      congenital (active) P37.1 *[K77]*
  infectious, infective (acute) (chronic)
(subacute) B15.9
    with hepatic coma B15.0

Hepatitis – *continued*
  inoculation —*see* Hepatitis, viral, type B
  interstitial (chronic) K74.69
  lupoid NEC K75.4
  malignant NEC (with hepatic failure) K72.90
    with coma K72.91
  neonatal (idiopathic) (toxic) P59.29
  newborn P59.29
  postimmunization —*see* Hepatitis, viral, type
B post-transfusion —*see* Hepatitis, viral,
type B
  reactive, nonspecific K75.2
  serum —*see* Hepatitis, viral, type B
  specified type NEC
    with hepatic failure —*see* Failure, hepatic
  syphilitic (late) A52.74
    congenital (early) A50.08 *[K77]*
      late A50.59 *[K77]*
    secondary A51.45
  toxic (*see also* Disease, liver, toxic) K71.6
  tuberculous A18.83
  viral, virus B19.9
    with hepatic coma B19.0
    acute B17.9
    chronic B18.9
      specified NEC B18.8
      type
        B B18.1
          with delta-agent B18.0
        C B18.2
    congenital P35.3
    coxsackie B33.8 *[K77]*
    cytomegalic inclusion B25.1
    in remission, any type
    code to Hepatitis, chronic, by type
    non-A, non-B B17.8
    specified type NEC (with or without coma)
B17.8
    type
      A B15.9
        with hepatic coma B15.0
      B B19.10
        with hepatic coma B19.11
      acute B16.9
        with
          delta-agent (coinfection) (without
hepatic coma) B16.1
            with hepatic coma B16.0
          hepatic coma (without delta-agent
coinfection) B16.2
        chronic B18.1
          with delta-agent B18.0
      C B19.20
        with hepatic coma B19.21
      acute B17.10
        with hepatic coma B17.11
      chronic B18.2
      E B17.2
    non-A, non-B B17.8
Hepatization lung (acute) —*see* Pneumonia,
lobar
Hepatoblastoma C22.2
Hepatocarcinoma C22.0
Hepatocholangiocarcinoma C22.0
Hepatocholangioma, benign D13.4
Hepatocholangitis K75.89
Hepatolenticular degeneration E83.01
Hepatoma (malignant) C22.0
  benign D13.4
  embryonal C22.0
Hepatomegaly —*see also* Hypertrophy, liver
  with splenomegaly R16.2

Hepatomegaly – *continued*
  congenital Q44.7
  in mononucleosis
    gammaherpesviral B27.09
    infectious specified NEC B27.89
Hepatoptosis K76.89
**Hepatorenal syndrome following labor and
delivery** O90.4
Hepatosis K76.89
Hepatosplenomegaly R16.2
  hyperlipemic (Bürger-Grütz type) E78.3
[K77]
Hereditary —*see* condition
Heredodegeneration, macular —*see*
Dystrophy, retina
Heredopathia atactica polyneuritiformis
G60.1
Heredosyphilis —*see* Syphilis, congenital
Herlitz' syndrome Q81.1
Hermansky-Pudlak syndrome E70.331
Hermaphrodite, hermaphroditism (true)
Q56.0
  46,XX with streak gonads Q99.1
  46,XX/46,XY Q99.0
  46,XY with streak gonads Q99.1
  chimera 46,XX/46,XY Q99.0
Hernia, hernial (acquired) (recurrent) K46.9
  with
    gangrene —*see* Hernia, by site, with,
gangrene
    incarceration —*see* Hernia, by site, with,
obstruction
    irreducible —*see* Hernia, by site, with,
obstruction
    obstruction —*see* Hernia, by site, with,
obstruction
    strangulation —*see* Hernia, by site, with,
obstruction
  abdomen, abdominal K46.9
    with
      gangrene (and obstruction) K46.1
      obstruction K46.0
    femoral —*see* Hernia, femoral
    incisional —*see* Hernia, incisional
    inguinal —*see* Hernia, inguinal
    specified site NEC K45.8
      with
        gangrene (and obstruction) K45.1
        obstruction K45.0
    umbilical —*see* Hernia, umbilical
    wall —*see* Hernia, ventral
  appendix —*see* Hernia, abdomen
  bladder (mucosa) (sphincter)
    congenital (female) (male) Q79.51
    female —*see* Cystocele
    male N32.89
  brain, congenital —*see* Encephalocele
  cartilage, vertebra —*see* Displacement,
intervertebral disc
  cerebral, congenital —*see also* Encephalocele
    endaural Q01.8
  ciliary body (traumatic) S05.2
  colon —*see* Hernia, abdomen
  Cooper's —*see* Hernia, abdomen, specified
site NEC
  crural —*see* Hernia, femoral
  diaphragm, diaphragmatic K44.9
    with
      gangrene (and obstruction) K44.1
      obstruction K44.0
    congenital Q79.0
  direct (inguinal) —*see* Hernia, inguinal

Hernia, hernia – *continued*

diverticulum, intestine —*see* Hernia, abdomen
double (inguinal) —*see* Hernia, inguinal, bilateral
due to adhesions (with obstruction) K56.5
epigastric (*see also* Hernia, ventral) K43.9
esophageal hiatus —*see* Hernia, hiatal
external (inguinal) —*see* Hernia, inguinal
fallopian tube N83.4
fascia M62.89
femoral K41.90
  with
    gangrene (and obstruction) K41.40
      not specified as recurrent K41.40
      recurrent K41.41
    obstruction K41.30
      not specified as recurrent K41.30
      recurrent K41.31
  bilateral K41.20
    with
      gangrene (and obstruction) K41.10
        not specified as recurrent K41.10
        recurrent K41.11
      obstruction K41.00
        not specified as recurrent K41.00
        recurrent K41.01
    not specified as recurrent K41.20
    recurrent K41.21
  unilateral K41.90
    with
      gangrene (and obstruction) K41.40
        not specified as recurrent K41.40
        recurrent K41.41
      obstruction K41.30
        not specified as recurrent K41.30
        recurrent K41.31
    not specified as recurrent K41.90
    recurrent K41.91
  not specified as recurrent K41.90
  recurrent K41.91
foramen magnum G93.5
  congenital Q01.8
funicular (umbilical) —*see also* Hernia, umbilicus
  spermatic (cord) —*see* Hernia, inguinal
gastrointestinal tract —*see* Hernia, abdomen
Hesselbach's —*see* Hernia, femoral, specified site NEC
hiatal (esophageal) (sliding) K44.9
  with
    gangrene (and obstruction) K44.1
    obstruction K44.0
  congenital Q40.1
hypogastric —*see* Hernia, ventral
incarcerated —*see also* Hernia, by site, with obstruction
  with gangrene —*see* Hernia, by site, with gangrene
incisional K43.2
  with
    gangrene (and obstruction) K43.1
    obstruction K43.0
indirect (inguinal) —*see* Hernia, inguinal
inguinal (direct) (external) (funicular) (indirect) (internal) (oblique) (scrotal) (sliding) K40.90
  with
    gangrene (and obstruction) K40.40
      not specified as recurrent K40.40
      recurrent K40.41
    obstruction K40.30

Hernia, hernia – *continued*

      not specified as recurrent K40.30
      recurrent K40.31
    not specified as recurrent K40.90
    recurrent K40.91
  bilateral K40.20
    with
      gangrene (and obstruction) K40.10
        not specified as recurrent K40.10
        recurrent K40.11
      obstruction K40.00
        not specified as recurrent K40.00
        recurrent K40.01
    not specified as recurrent K40.20
    recurrent K40.21
  unilateral K40.90
    with
      gangrene (and obstruction) K40.40
        not specified as recurrent K40.40
        recurrent K40.41
      obstruction K40.30
        not specified as recurrent K40.30
        recurrent K40.31
    not specified as recurrent K40.90
    recurrent K40.91
internal —*see also* Hernia, abdomen
  inguinal —*see* Hernia, inguinal
interstitial —*see* Hernia, abdomen
intervertebral cartilage or disc —*see* Displacement, intervertebral disc
intestine, intestinal —*see* Hernia, by site
intra-abdominal —*see* Hernia, abdomen
iris (traumatic) S05.2
irreducible —*see also* Hernia, by site, with obstruction
  with gangrene —*see* Hernia, by site, with gangrene
ischiatic —*see* Hernia, abdomen, specified site NEC
ischiorectal —*see* Hernia, abdomen, specified site NEC
lens (traumatic) S05.2
linea (alba) (semilunaris) —*see* Hernia, ventral
Littre's —*see* Hernia, abdomen
lumbar —*see* Hernia, abdomen, specified site NEC
lung (subcutaneous) J98.4
mediastinum J98.5
mesenteric (internal) —*see* Hernia, abdomen
midline —*see* Hernia, ventral
muscle (sheath) M62.89
nucleus pulposus —*see* Displacement, intervertebral disc
oblique (inguinal) —*see* Hernia, inguinal
obstructive —*see also* Hernia, by site, with obstruction
  with gangrene —*see* Hernia, by site, with gangrene
obturator —*see* Hernia, abdomen, specified site NEC
omental —*see* Hernia, abdomen
ovary N83.4
oviduct N83.4
paraesophageal —*see also* Hernia, diaphragm
  congenital Q40.1
parastomal K43.5
  with
    gangrene (and obstruction) K43.4
    obstruction K43.3
paraumbilical —*see* Hernia, umbilicus

Hernia, hernia – *continued*

perineal —*see* Hernia, abdomen, specified site NEC
Petit's —*see* Hernia, abdomen, specified site NEC
postoperative —*see* Hernia, incisional
pregnant uterus —*see* Abnormal, uterus in pregnancy or childbirth
prevesical N32.89
properitoneal —*see* Hernia, abdomen, specified site NEC
pudendal —*see* Hernia, abdomen, specified site NEC
rectovaginal N81.6
retroperitoneal —*see* Hernia, abdomen, specified site NEC
Richter's —*see* Hernia, abdomen, with obstruction
Rieux's, Riex's —*see* Hernia, abdomen, specified site NEC
sac condition (adhesion) (dropsy) (inflammation) (laceration) (suppuration) code by site under Hernia
sciatic —*see* Hernia, abdomen, specified site NEC
scrotum, scrotal —*see* Hernia, inguinal
sliding (inguinal) —*see also* Hernia, inguinal
  hiatus —*see* Hernia, hiatal
spigelian —*see* Hernia, ventral
spinal —*see* Spina bifida
strangulated —*see also* Hernia, by site, with obstruction
  with gangrene —*see* Hernia, by site, with gangrene
subxiphoid —*see* Hernia, ventral
supra-umbilicus —*see* Hernia, ventral
tendon —*see* Disorder, tendon, specified type NEC
Treitz's (fossa) —*see* Hernia, abdomen, specified site NEC
tunica vaginalis Q55.29
umbilicus, umbilical K42.9
  with
    gangrene (and obstruction) K42.1
    obstruction K42.0
ureter N28.89
urethra, congenital Q64.79
urinary meatus, congenital Q64.79
uterus N81.4
  pregnant —*see* Abnormal, uterus in pregnancy or childbirth
vaginal (anterior) (wall) —*see* Cystocele
Velpeau's —*see* Hernia, femoral
ventral K43.9
  with
    gangrene (and obstruction) K43.7
    obstruction K43.6
  recurrent —*see* Hernia, incisional
  incisional K43.2
    with
      gangrene (and obstruction) K43.1
      obstruction K43.0
  specified NEC K43.9
    with
      gangrene (and obstruction) K43.7
      obstruction K43.6
vesical
  congenital (female) (male) Q79.51
  female —*see* Cystocele
  male N32.89
vitreous (into wound) S05.2
  into anterior chamber —*see* Prolapse, vitreous

Herniation —*see also* Hernia
  brain (stem) G93.5
  cerebral G93.5
  mediastinum J98.5
  nucleus pulposus —*see* Displacement,
  intervertebral disc
Herpangina B08.5
Herpes, herpesvirus, herpetic B00.9
  anogenital A60.9
    perianal skin A60.1
    rectum A60.1
    urogenital tract A60.00
      cervix A60.03
      male genital organ NEC A60.02
      penis A60.01
      specified site NEC A60.09
      vagina A60.04
      vulva A60.04
  blepharitis (zoster) B02.39
    simplex B00.59
  circinatus B35.4
    bullosus L12.0
  conjunctivitis (simplex) B00.53
    zoster B02.31
  cornea B02.33
  encephalitis B00.4
    due to herpesvirus 6 B10.01
    due to herpesvirus 7 B10.09
    specified NEC B10.09
  eye (zoster) B02.30
    simplex B00.50
  eyelid (zoster) B02.39
    simplex B00.59
  facialis B00.1
  febrilis B00.1
  geniculate ganglionitis B02.21
  genital, genitalis A60.00
    female A60.09
    male A60.02
  gestational, gestationis O26.4
  gingivostomatitis B00.2
  human B00.9
    1 —*see* Herpes, simplex
    2 —*see* Herpes, simplex
    3 —*see* Varicella
    4 —*see* Mononucleosis, Epstein-Barr (virus)
    5 —*see* Disease, cytomegalic inclusion
    (generalized)
    6
      encephalitis B10.01
      specified NEC B10.81
    7
      encephalitis B10.09
      specified NEC B10.82
    8 B10.89
  infection NEC B10.89
    Kaposi's sarcoma associated B10.89
  iridocyclitis (simplex) B00.51
    zoster B02.32
  iris (vesicular erythema multiforme) L51.9
  iritis (simplex) B00.51
  Kaposi's sarcoma associated B10.89
  keratitis (simplex) (dendritic) (disciform)
    (interstitial) B00.52
    zoster (interstitial) B02.33
  keratoconjunctivitis (simplex) B00.52
    zoster B02.33
  labialis B00.1
  lip B00.1
  meningitis (simplex) B00.3
    zoster B02.1
  ophthalmicus (zoster) NEC B02.30

Herpes – *continued*
  simplex B00.50
  penis A60.01
  perianal skin A60.1
  pharyngitis, pharyngotonsillitis B00.2
  rectum A60.1
  scrotum A60.02
  sepsis B00.7
  simplex B00.9
    complicated NEC B00.89
    congenital P35.2
    conjunctivitis B00.53
    external ear B00.1
    eyelid B00.59
    hepatitis B00.81
    keratitis (interstitial) B00.52
    myelitis B00.82
    specified complication NEC B00.89
    visceral B00.89
  stomatitis B00.2
  tonsurans B35.0
  visceral B00.89
  vulva A60.04
  whitlow B00.89
  zoster (*see also* condition) B02.9
    auricularis B02.21
    complicated NEC B02.8
    conjunctivitis B02.31
    disseminated B02.7
    encephalitis B02.0
    eye (lid) B02.39
    geniculate ganglionitis B02.21
    keratitis (interstitial) B02.33
    meningitis B02.1
    myelitis B02.24
    neuritis, neuralgia B02.29
    ophthalmicus NEC B02.30
    oticus B02.21
    polyneuropathy B02.23
    specified complication NEC B02.8
    trigeminal neuralgia B02.22
Herpesvirus (human) —*see* Herpes
Herpetophobia F40.218
Herrick's anemia —*see* Disease, sickle-cell
Hers' disease E74.09
Herter-Gee syndrome K90.0
Herxheimer's reaction R68.89
Hesitancy
  of micturition R39.11
  urinary R39.11
Hesselbach's hernia —*see* Hernia, femoral,
specified site NEC
Heterochromia (congenital) Q13.2
  cataract —*see* Cataract, complicated
  cyclitis (Fuchs) —*see* Cyclitis, Fuchs'
  heterochromic
  hair L67.1
  iritis —*see* Cyclitis, Fuchs' heterochromic
  retained metallic foreign body (nonmagnetic)
  —*see* Foreign body, intraocular, old, retained
    magnetic —*see* Foreign body, intraocular,
    old, retained, magnetic
  uveitis —*see* Cyclitis, Fuchs' heterochromic
Heterophoria —*see* Strabismus, heterophoria
Heterophyes, heterophyiasis (small intestine)
B66.8
Heterotopia, heterotopic —*see also*
Malposition, congenital
  cerebralis Q04.8
Heterotropia —*see* Strabismus
Heubner-Herter disease K90.0
Hexadactylism Q69.9

HGSIL (cytology finding) (high grade
squamous intraepithelial lesion on cytologic
smear) (Pap smear finding)
  anus R85.613
  cervix R87.613
    biopsy (histology) finding
    code to CIN II or CIN III
  vagina R87.623
    biopsy (histology) finding
    code to VAIN II or VAIN III
Hibernoma —*see* Lipoma
Hiccup, hiccough R06.6
  epidemic B33.0
  psychogenic F45.8
Hidden penis (congenital) Q55.64
  acquired N48.83
Hidradenitis (axillaris) (suppurative) L73.2
Hidradenoma (nodular) —*see also* Neoplasm,
skin, benign
  clear cell —*see* Neoplasm, skin, benign
  papillary —*see* Neoplasm, skin, benign
Hidrocystoma —*see* Neoplasm, skin, benign
High
  altitude effects T70.20
    anoxia T70.29
    on
      ears T70.0
      sinuses T70.1
    polycythemia D75.1
  arch
    foot Q66.7
    palate, congenital Q38.5
  arterial tension —*see* Hypertension
  basal metabolic rate R94.8
  blood pressure —*see also* Hypertension
    borderline R03.0
    reading (incidental) (isolated) (nonspecific) ,
    without diagnosis of hypertension R03.0
  cholesterol E78.0
    with high triglycerides E78.2
  diaphragm (congenital) Q79.1
  expressed emotional level within family
  Z63.8
  head at term O32.4
  palate, congenital Q38.5
  risk
    infant NEC Z76.2
    sexual behavior (heterosexual) Z72.51
      bisexual Z72.53
      homosexual Z72.52
  temperature (of unknown origin) R50.9
  thoracic rib Q76.6
  triglycerides E78.1
    with high cholesterol E78.2
Hildebrand's disease A75.0
Hilum —*see* condition
Hip —*see* condition
Hippel's disease Q85.8
Hippophobia F40.218
Hippus H57.09
Hirschsprung's disease or megacolon Q43.1
Hirsutism, hirsuties L68.0
Hirudiniasis
  external B88.3
  internal B83.4
Hiss-Russell dysentery A03.1
Histidinemia, histidinuria E70.41
Histiocytoma —*see also* Neoplasm, skin,
benign
  fibrous —*see also* Neoplasm, skin, benign
    atypical —*see* Neoplasm, connective tissue,
    uncertain behavior

Histiocytoma – *continued*
   malignant —*see* Neoplasm, connective tissue, malignant
Histiocytosis D76.3
   acute differentiated progressive C96.0
   Langerhans' cell NEC C96.6
      multifocal X
         multisystemic (disseminated) C96.0
         unisystemic C96.5
      pulmonary, adult (adult PLCH) J84.82
      unifocal (X) C96.6
   lipid, lipoid D76.3
      essential E75.29
   malignant C96.A
   mononuclear phagocytes NEC D76.1
      Langerhans' cells C96.6
   non-Langerhans cell D76.3
   polyostotic sclerosing D76.3
   sinus, with massive lymphadenopathy D76.3
   syndrome NEC D76.3
   X NEC C96.6
      acute (progressive) C96.0
      chronic C96.6
      multifocal C96.5
      multisystemic C96.0
      unifocal C96.6
Histoplasmosis B39.9
   with pneumonia NEC B39.2
   African B39.5
   American —*see* Histoplasmosis, capsulati
   capsulati B39.4
      disseminated B39.3
      generalized B39.3
      pulmonary B39.2
         acute B39.0
         chronic B39.1
   Darling's B39.4
   duboisii B39.5
   lung NEC B39.2
History
   family (of) —*see also* History, personal (of)
      alcohol abuse Z81.1
      allergy NEC Z84.89
      anemia Z83.2
      arthritis Z82.61
      asthma Z82.5
      blindness Z82.1
      cardiac death (sudden) Z82.41
      carrier of genetic disease Z84.81
      chromosomal anomaly Z82.79
      chronic
         disabling disease NEC Z82.8
         lower respiratory disease Z82.5
      colonic polyps Z83.71
      congenital malformations and deformations Z82.79
         polycystic kidney Z82.71
      consanguinity Z84.3
      deafness Z82.2
      diabetes mellitus Z83.3
      disability NEC Z82.8
      disease or disorder (of)
         allergic NEC Z84.89
         behavioral NEC Z81.8
         blood and blood-forming organs Z83.2
         cardiovascular NEC Z82.49
         chronic disabling NEC Z82.8
         digestive Z83.79
         ear NEC Z83.52
         endocrine NEC Z83.49
         eye NEC Z83.518
            glaucoma Z83.511

History – *continued*
      genitourinary NEC Z84.2
      glaucoma Z83.511
      hematological Z83.2
      immune mechanism Z83.2
      infectious NEC Z83.1
      ischemic heart Z82.49
      kidney Z84.1
      mental NEC Z81.8
      metabolic Z83.49
      musculoskeletal NEC Z82.69
      neurological NEC Z82.0
      nutritional Z83.49
      parasitic NEC Z83.1
      psychiatric NEC Z81.8
      respiratory NEC Z83.6
      skin and subcutaneous tissue NEC Z84.0
      specified NEC Z84.89
   drug abuse NEC Z81.3
   epilepsy Z82.0
   genetic disease carrier Z84.81
   glaucoma Z83.511
   hearing loss Z82.2
   human immunodeficiency virus (HIV) infection Z83.0
   Huntington's chorea Z82.0
   intellectual disability Z81.0
   leukemia Z80.6
   malignant neoplasm (of) NOS Z80.9
      bladder Z80.52
      breast Z80.3
      bronchus Z80.1
      digestive organ Z80.0
      gastrointestinal tract Z80.0
      genital organ Z80.49
         ovary Z80.41
         prostate Z80.42
         specified organ NEC Z80.49
         testis Z80.43
      hematopoietic NEC Z80.7
      intrathoracic organ NEC Z80.2
      kidney Z80.51
      lung Z80.1
      lymphatic NEC Z80.7
      ovary Z80.41
      prostate Z80.42
      respiratory organ NEC Z80.2
      specified site NEC Z80.8
      testis Z80.43
      trachea Z80.1
      urinary organ or tract Z80.59
         bladder Z80.52
         kidney Z80.51
   mental
      disorder NEC Z81.8
   multiple endocrine neoplasia (MEN) syndrome Z83.41
   osteoporosis Z82.62
   polycystic kidney Z82.71
   polyps (colon) Z83.71
   psychiatric disorder Z81.8
   psychoactive substance abuse NEC Z81.3
   respiratory condition NEC Z83.6
      asthma and other lower respiratory conditions Z82.5
   self-harmful behavior Z81.8
   skin condition Z84.0
   specified condition NEC Z84.89
   stroke (cerebrovascular) Z82.3
   substance abuse NEC Z81.4
      alcohol Z81.1
      drug NEC Z81.3

History – *continued*
      psychoactive NEC Z81.3
      tobacco Z81.2
   sudden cardiac death Z82.41
   tobacco abuse Z81.2
   violence, violent behavior Z81.8
   visual loss Z82.1
   personal (of) —*see also* History, family (of)
      abuse
         childhood Z62.819
            physical Z62.810
            psychological Z62.811
            sexual Z62.810
         adult Z91.419
            physical and sexual Z91.410
            psychological Z91.411
      alcohol dependence F10.21
      allergy (to) Z88.9
         analgesic agent NEC Z88.6
         anesthetic Z88.4
         antibiotic agent NEC Z88.1
         anti-infective agent NEC Z88.3
         contrast media Z91.041
         drugs, medicaments and biological substances Z88.9
            specified NEC Z88.8
         food Z91.018
            additives Z91.02
            eggs Z91.012
            milk products Z91.011
            peanuts Z91.010
            seafood Z91.013
            specified food NEC Z91.018
         insect Z91.038
            bee Z91.030
         latex Z91.040
         medicinal agents Z88.9
            specified NEC Z88.8
         narcotic agent NEC Z88.5
         nonmedicinal agents Z91.048
         penicillin Z88.0
         serum Z88.7
         specified NEC Z91.09
         sulfonamides Z88.2
         vaccine Z88.7
      anaphylactic shock Z87.892
      anaphylaxis Z87.892
      behavioral disorders Z86.59
      benign carcinoid tumor Z86.012
      benign neoplasm Z86.018
         carcinoid Z86.012
         brain Z86.011
         colonic polyps Z86.010
      brain injury (traumatic) Z87.820
      breast implant removal Z98.86
      calculi, renal Z87.442
      cancer —*see* History, personal (of), malignant neoplasm (of)
      cardiac arrest (death), successfully resuscitated Z86.74
      cerebral infarction without residual deficit Z86.73
      cervical dysplasia Z87.410
      chemotherapy for neoplastic condition Z92.21
      childhood abuse —*see* History, personal (of), abuse
      cleft lip (corrected) Z87.730
      cleft palate (corrected) Z87.730
      collapsed vertebra (healed) Z87.311
         due to osteoporosis Z87.310

History – *continued*
  combat and operational stress reaction Z86.51
  congenital malformation (corrected) Z87.798
    circulatory system (corrected) Z87.74
    digestive system (corrected) NEC Z87.738
    ear (corrected) Z87.720
    eye (corrected) Z87.721
    face and neck (corrected) Z87.790
    genitourinary system (corrected) NEC Z87.718
    heart (corrected) Z87.74
    integument (corrected) Z87.76
    limb (s) (corrected) Z87.76
    musculoskeletal system (corrected) Z87.76
    neck (corrected) Z87.790
    nervous system (corrected) NEC Z87.728
    respiratory system (corrected) Z87.75
    sense organs (corrected) NEC Z87.728
    specified NEC Z87.798
  contraception Z92.0
  deployment (military) Z91.82
  diabetic foot ulcer Z86.31
  disease or disorder (of) Z87.898
    blood and blood-forming organs Z86.2
    circulatory system Z86.79
      specified condition NEC Z86.79
    connective tissue NEC Z87.39
    digestive system Z87.19
      colonic polyp Z86.010
      peptic ulcer disease Z87.11
      specified condition NEC Z87.19
    ear Z86.69
    endocrine Z86.39
      diabetic foot ulcer Z86.31
      gestational diabetes Z86.32
      specified type NEC Z86.39
    eye Z86.69
    genital (track) system NEC
      female Z87.42
      male Z87.438
    hematological Z86.2
    Hodgkin Z85.71
    immune mechanism Z86.2
    infectious Z86.19
      malaria Z86.13
      Methicillin resistant Staphylococcus aureus (MRSA) Z86.14
      poliomyelitis Z86.12
      specified NEC Z86.19
      tuberculosis Z86.11
    mental NEC Z86.59
    metabolic Z86.39
      diabetic foot ulcer Z86.31
      gestational diabetes Z86.32
      specified type NEC Z86.39
    musculoskeletal NEC Z87.39
    nervous system Z86.69
    nutritional Z86.39
    parasitic Z86.19
    respiratory system NEC Z87.09
    sense organs Z86.69
    skin Z87.2
    specified site or type NEC Z87.898
    subcutaneous tissue Z87.2
    trophoblastic Z87.59
    urinary system NEC Z87.448
  drug dependence —*see* Dependence, drug, by type, in remission
  drug therapy
    antineoplastic chemotherapy Z92.21

History – *continued*
    estrogen Z92.23
    immunosuppression Z92.25
    inhaled steroids Z92.240
    monoclonal drug Z92.22
    specified NEC Z92.29
    steroid Z92.241
    systemic steroids Z92.241
  dysplasia
    cervical Z87.410
    prostatic Z87.430
    vaginal Z87.411
    vulvar Z87.412
  embolism (venous) Z86.718
    pulmonary Z86.711
  encephalitis Z86.61
  estrogen therapy Z92.23
  extracorporeal membrane oxygenation (ECMO) Z92.81
  failed moderate sedation Z92.83
  failed conscious sedation Z92.83
  fall, falling Z91.81
  fracture (healed)
    fatigue Z87.312
    fragility Z87.310
    osteoporosis Z87.310
    pathological NEC Z87.311
    stress Z87.312
    traumatic Z87.81
  gestational diabetes Z86.32
  hepatitis
    B Z86.19
    C Z86.19
  Hodgkin disease Z85.71
  hyperthermia, malignant Z88.4
  hypospadias (corrected) Z87.710
  hysterectomy Z90.710
  immunosuppression therapy Z92.25
  in situ neoplasm
    breast Z86.000
    cervix uteri Z86.001
    specified NEC Z86.008
  infection NEC Z86.19
    central nervous system Z86.61
    Methicillin resistant Staphylococcus aureus (MRSA) Z86.14
    urinary (recurrent) (tract) Z87.440
  injury NEC Z87.828
  in utero procedure during pregnancy Z98.870
  in utero procedure while a fetus Z98.871
  irradiation Z92.3
  kidney stones Z87.442
  leukemia Z85.6
  lymphoma (non-Hodgkin) Z85.72
  malignant melanoma (skin) Z85.820
  malignant neoplasm (of) Z85.9
    accessory sinuses Z85.22
    anus NEC Z85.048
      carcinoid Z85.040
    bladder Z85.51
    bone Z85.830
    brain Z85.841
    breast Z85.3
    bronchus NEC Z85.118
      carcinoid Z85.110
    carcinoid —*see* History, personal (of) , malignant neoplasm, by site, carcinoid
    cervix Z85.41
    colon NEC Z85.038
      carcinoid Z85.030
    digestive organ Z85.00

History – *continued*
    specified NEC Z85.09
    endocrine gland NEC Z85.858
    epididymis Z85.48
    esophagus Z85.01
    eye Z85.840
    gastrointestinal tract —*see* History, malignant neoplasm, digestive organ
    genital organ
      female Z85.40
        specified NEC Z85.44
      male Z85.45
        specified NEC Z85.49
    hematopoietic NEC Z85.79
    intrathoracic organ Z85.20
    kidney NEC Z85.528
      carcinoid Z85.520
    large intestine NEC Z85.038
      carcinoid Z85.030
    larynx Z85.21
    liver Z85.05
    lung NEC Z85.118
      carcinoid Z85.110
    mediastinum Z85.29
    Merkel cell Z85.821
    middle ear Z85.22
    nasal cavities Z85.22
    nervous system NEC Z85.848
    oral cavity Z85.819
      specified site NEC Z85.818
    ovary Z85.43
    pancreas Z85.07
    pharynx Z85.819
      specified site NEC Z85.818
    pelvis Z85.53
    pleura Z85.29
    prostate Z85.46
    rectosigmoid junction NEC Z85.048
      carcinoid Z85.040
    rectum NEC Z85.048
      carcinoid Z85.040
    respiratory organ Z85.20
    sinuses, accessory Z85.22
    skin NEC Z85.828
      melanoma Z85.820
      Merkel cell Z85.821
    small intestine NEC Z85.068
      carcinoid Z85.060
    soft tissue Z85.831
    specified site NEC Z85.89
    stomach NEC Z85.028
      carcinoid Z85.020
    testis Z85.47
    thymus NEC Z85.238
      carcinoid Z85.230
    thyroid Z85.850
    tongue Z85.810
    trachea Z85.12
    ureter Z85.54
    urinary organ or tract Z85.50
      specified NEC Z85.59
    uterus Z85.42
  maltreatment Z91.89
  medical treatment NEC Z92.89
  melanoma (malignant) (skin) Z85.820
  meningitis Z86.61
  mental disorder Z86.59
  Merkel cell carcinoma (skin) Z85.821
  Methicillin resistant Staphylococcus aureus (MRSA) Z86.14
  military deployment Z91.82

History – *continued*
  military war, peacekeeping and
  humanitarian deployment (current or past
  conflict) Z91.82
  myocardial infarction (old) I25.2
  neglect (in)
    adult Z91.412
    childhood Z62.812
  neoplasm
    benign Z86.018
      brain Z86.011
      colon polyp Z86.010
    in situ
      breast Z86.000
      cervix uteri Z86.001
      specified NEC Z86.008
    malignant —*see* History of, malignant
  neoplasm
    uncertain behavior Z86.03
  nephrotic syndrome Z87.441
  nicotine dependence Z87.891
  noncompliance with medical treatment or
  regimen —*see* Noncompliance
  nutritional deficiency Z86.39
  obstetric complications Z87.59
    childbirth Z87.59
    pregnancy Z87.59
    pre-term labor Z87.51
    puerperium Z87.59
  osteoporosis fractures Z87.31
  parasuicide (attempt) Z91.5
  physical trauma NEC Z87.828
    self-harm or suicide attempt Z91.5
  poisoning NEC Z91.89
    self-harm or suicide attempt Z91.5
  poor personal hygiene Z91.89
  pneumonia (recurrent) Z87.01
  preterm labor Z87.51
  prolonged reversible ischemic neurologic
  deficit (PRIND) Z86.73
  procedure during pregnancy Z98.870
  procedure while a fetus Z98.871
  prostatic dysplasia Z87.430
  psychological
    abuse
      adult Z91.411
      child Z62.811
    trauma, specified NEC Z91.49
  radiation therapy Z92.3
  removal
    implant
      breast Z98.86
  renal calculi Z87.442
  respiratory condition NEC Z87.09
  retained foreign body fully removed
  Z87.821
  risk factors NEC Z91.89
  self-harm Z91.5
  self-poisoning attempt Z91.5
  sex reassignment Z87.890
  sleep-wake cycle problem Z72.821
  specified NEC Z87.898
  steroid therapy (systemic) Z92.241
    inhaled Z92.240
  stroke without residual deficits Z86.73
  substance abuse NEC F10-F19 with fifth
  character 1
  sudden cardiac arrest Z86.74
  sudden cardiac death successfully
  resuscitated Z86.74
  suicide attempt Z91.5
  surgery NEC Z98.89

History – *continued*
  sex reassignment Z87.890
  transplant —*see* Transplant
  thrombophlebitis Z86.72
  thrombosis (venous) Z86.718
    pulmonary Z86.711
  tobacco dependence Z87.891
  transient ischemic attack (TIA) without
  residual deficits Z86.73
  trauma (physical) NEC Z87.828
    psychological NEC Z91.49
    self-harm Z91.5
  traumatic brain injury Z87.820
  unhealthy sleep-wake cycle Z72.821
  urinary calculi Z87.442
  urinary (recurrent) (tract) infection(s)
  Z87.440
  vaginal dysplasia Z87.411
  venous thrombosis or embolism Z86.718
    pulmonary Z86.711
  vulvar dysplasia Z87.412
His-Werner disease A79.0
HIV (*see also* Human, immunodeficiency
  virus) B20
  laboratory evidence (nonconclusive) R75
  positive, seropositive Z21
  nonconclusive test (in infants) R75
Hives (bold) —*see* Urticaria
Hoarseness R49.0
Hobo Z59.0
Hodgkin disease —*see* Lymphoma, Hodgkin
Hodgson's disease I71.2
  ruptured I71.1
Hoffa-Kastert disease E88.89
Hoffa's disease E88.89
Hoffmann-Bouveret syndrome I47.9
Hoffmann's syndrome E03.9 *[G73.7]*
Hole (round)
  macula H35.34
  retina (without detachment) —*see* Break,
  retina, round hole
    with detachment —*see* Detachment, retina,
  with retinal, break
Holiday relief care Z75.5
Hollenhorst's plaque —*see* Occlusion, artery,
  retina
Hollow foot (congenital) Q66.7
  acquired —*see* Deformity, limb, foot,
  specified NEC
Holoprosencephaly Q04.2
Holt-Oram syndrome Q87.2
Homelessness Z59.0
Homesickness —*see* Disorder, adjustment
Homocystinemia, homocystinuria E72.11
Homogentisate 1,2-dioxygenase deficiency
  E70.29
Homologous serum hepatitis (prophylactic)
  (therapeutic) —*see* Hepatitis, viral, type B
Honeycomb lung J98.4
  congenital Q33.0
Hooded
  clitoris Q52.6
  penis Q55.69
Hookworm (anemia) (disease) (infection)
  (infestation) B76.9
  specified NEC B76.8
Hordeolum (eyelid) (externum) (recurrent)
  H00.019
  internum H00.029
    left H00.026
      lower H00.025
      upper H00.024

Hordeolum – *continued*
    right H00.023
      lower H00.022
      upper H00.021
  left H00.016
    lower H00.015
    upper H00.014
  right H00.013
    lower H00.012
    upper H00.011
Horn
  cutaneous L85.8
  nail L60.2
    congenital Q84.6
Horner (-Claude Bernard) **syndrome** G90.2
  traumatic —*see* Injury, nerve, cervical
  sympathetic
Horseshoe kidney (congenital) Q63.1
Horton's headache or neuralgia G44.099
  intractable G44.091
  not intractable G44.099
Hospital hopper syndrome —*see* Disorder,
  factitious
Hospitalism in children —*see* Disorder,
  adjustment
Hostility R45.5
  towards child Z62.3
Hot flashes
  menopausal N95.1
Hourglass (contracture) —*see also*
  Contraction, hourglass
  stomach K31.89
    congenital Q40.2
    stricture K31.2
**Household, housing circumstance affecting
  care** Z59.9
  specified NEC Z59.8
Housemaid's knee —*see* Bursitis, prepatellar
Hudson (-Stähli) **line** (cornea) —*see*
  Pigmentation, cornea, anterior
Human
  bite (open wound) —*see also* Bite
    intact skin surface —*see* Bite, superficial
  herpesvirus —*see* Herpes
  immunodeficiency virus (HIV) disease
  (infection) B20
    asymptomatic status Z21
    contact Z20.6
    counseling Z71.7
    dementia B20 *[F02.80]*
      with behavioral disturbance B20 *[F02.81]*
    exposure to Z20.6
    laboratory evidence R75
    type 2 (HIV 2) as cause of disease classified
  elsewhere B97.35
  papillomavirus (HPV)
    DNA test positive
      high risk
        cervix R87.810
        vagina R87.811
      low risk
        cervix R87.820
        vagina R87.821
    screening for Z11.51
  T-cell lymphotropic virus
    type 1 (HTLV-I) infection B33.3
      as cause of disease classified elsewhere
  B97.33
      carrier Z22.6
    type 2 (HTLV-II) as cause of disease
  classified elsewhere B97.34
Humidifier lung or pneumonitis J67.7

Humiliation (experience) **in childhood** Z62.898
Humpback (acquired) —*see* Kyphosis
Hunchback (acquired) —*see* Kyphosis
Hunger T73.0
  air, psychogenic F45.8
Hungry bone syndrome E83.81
Hunner's ulcer —*see* Cystitis, chronic, interstitial
Hunter's
  glossitis D51.0
  syndrome E76.1
Huntington's disease or chorea G10
  with dementia G10 *[F02.80]*
    with behavioral disturbance G10 *[F02.81]*
Hunt's
  disease or syndrome (herpetic geniculate ganglionitis) B02.21
    dyssynergia cerebellaris myoclonica G11.1
    neuralgia B02.21
Hurler (-Scheie) **disease or syndrome** E76.02
Hurst's disease G36.1
Hürthle cell
  adcnocarcinoma C73
  adenoma D34
  carcinoma C73
  tumor D34
Hutchinson-Boeck disease or syndrome — *see* Sarcoidosis
Hutchinson-Gilford disease or syndrome E34.8
Hutchinson's
  disease, meaning
    angioma serpiginosum L81.7
    pompholyx (cheiropompholyx) L30.1
    prurigo estivalis L56.4
    summer eruption or summer prurigo L56.4
  melanotic freckle —*see* Melanoma, in situ
    malignant melanoma in — *see* Melanoma
  teeth or incisors (congenital syphilis) A50.52
  triad (congenital syphilis) A50.53
Hyalin plaque, sclera, senile H15.89
Hyaline membrane (disease) (lung) (pulmonary) (newborn) P22.0
Hyalinosis
  cutis (et mucosae) E78.89
  focal and segmental (glomerular) (*see also* N00-N07 with fourth character .1) N05.1
Hyalitis, hyalosis, asteroid —*see also* Deposit, crystalline
  syphilitic (late) A52.71
Hydatid
  cyst or tumor —*see* Echinococcus
  mole —*see* Hydatidiform mole
  Morgagni
    female Q50.5
    male (epididymal) Q55.4
      testicular Q55.29
Hydatidiform mole (benign) (complicating pregnancy) (delivered) (undelivered) O01.9
  classical O01.0
  complete O01.0
  incomplete O01.1
  invasive D39.2
  malignant D39.2
  partial O01.1
Hydatidosis —*see* Echinococcus
Hydradenitis (axillaris) (suppurative) L73.2
Hydradenoma —*see* Hidradenoma
Hydramnios O40.
Hydrancephaly, hydranencephaly Q04.3
  with spina bifida —*see* Spina bifida, with hydrocephalus

Hydrargyrism NEC —*see* Poisoning, mercury
Hydrarthrosis —*see also* Effusion, joint
  gonococcal A54.42
  intermittent M12.40
    ankle M12.47
    elbow M12.42
    foot joint M12.47
    hand joint M12.44
    hip M12.45
    knee M12.46
    multiple site M12.49
    shoulder M12.41
    specified joint NEC M12.48
    wrist M12.43
  of yaws (early) (late) (*see also* subcategory M14.8) A66.6
  syphilitic (late) A52.77
    congenital A50.55 *[M12.80]*
Hydremia D64.89
Hydrencephalocele (congenital) —*see* Encephalocele
Hydrencephalomeningocele (congenital) — *see* Encephalocele
Hydroa R23.8
  aestivale L56.4
  vacciniforme L56.4
Hydroadenitis (axillaris) (suppurative) L73.2
Hydrocalycosis —*see* Hydronephrosis
Hydrocele (spermatic cord) (testis) (tunica vaginalis) N43.3
  canal of Nuck N94.89
  communicating N43.2
    congenital P83.5
  congenital P83.5
  encysted N43.0
  female NEC N94.89
  infected N43.1
  newborn P83.5
  round ligament N94.89
  specified NEC N43.2
  spinalis —*see* Spina bifida
  vulva N90.89
Hydrocephalus (acquired) (external) (internal) (malignant) (recurrent) G91.9
  aqueduct Sylvius stricture Q03.0
  causing disproportion O33.6
    with obstructed labor O66.3
  communicating G91.0
  congenital (external) (internal) Q03.9
    with spina bifida Q05.4
      cervical Q05.0
      dorsal Q05.1
      lumbar Q05.2
      lumbosacral Q05.2
      sacral Q05.3
      thoracic Q05.1
      thoracolumbar Q05.1
    specified NEC Q03.8
  due to toxoplasmosis (congenital) P37.1
  foramen Magendie block (acquired) G91.1
    congenital (*see also* Hydrocephalus, congenital) Q03.1
  in (due to)
    infectious disease NEC B89 *[G91.4]*
    neoplastic disease NEC (see also Neoplasm) G91.4
    parasitic disease B89 *[G91.4]*
  newborn Q03.9
    with spina bifida —*see* Spina bifida, with hydrocephalus
  noncommunicating G91.1
  normal pressure G91.2

Hydrocephalus – *continued*
  secondary G91.0
  obstructive G91.1
  otitic G93.2
  post-traumatic NEC G91.3
  secondary G91.4
    post-traumatic G91.3
  specified NEC G91.8
  syphilitic, congenital A50.49
Hydrocolpos (congenital) N89.8
Hydrocystoma —*see* Neoplasm, skin, benign
Hydroencephalocele (congenital) —*see* Encephalocele
Hydroencephalomeningocele (congenital) — *see* Encephalocele
Hydrohematopneumothorax —*see* Hemothorax
Hydromeningitis —*see* Meningitis
Hydromeningocele (spinal) —*see also* Spina bifida
  cranial —*see* Encephalocele
Hydrometra N85.8
Hydrometrocolpos N89.8
Hydromicrocephaly Q02
Hydromphalos (since birth) Q45.8
Hydromyelia Q06.4
Hydromyelocele —*see* Spina bifida
Hydronephrosis (atrophic) (early) (functionless) (intermittent) (primary) (secondary) NEC N13.30
  with
    infection N13.6
    obstruction (by) (of)
      renal calculus N13.2
        with infection N13.6
      ureteral NEC N13.1
        with infection N13.6
        calculus N13.2
          with infection N13.6
      ureteropelvic junction (congenital) Q62.0
        with infection N13.6
      ureteral stricture NEC N13.1
        with infection N13.6
  congenital Q62.0
  specified type NEC N13.39
  tuberculous A18.11
Hydropericarditis —*see* Pericarditis
Hydropericardium —*see* Pericarditis
Hydroperitoneum R18.8
Hydrophobia —*see* Rabies
Hydrophthalmos Q15.0
Hydropneumohemothorax —*see* Hemothorax
Hydropneumopericarditis —*see* Pericarditis
Hydropneumopericardium —*see* Pericarditis
Hydropneumothorax J94.8
  traumatic —*see* Injury, intrathoracic, lung
  tuberculous NEC A15.6
Hydrops R60.9
  abdominis R18.8
  articulorum intermittens —*see* Hydrarthrosis, intermittent
  cardiac — *see* Failure, heart, congestive
  causing obstructed labor (mother) O66.3
  endolymphatic H81.0
  fetal —*see* Pregnancy, complicated by, hydrops, fetalis
  fetalis P83.2
    due to
      ABO isoimmunization P56.0
      alpha thalassemia D56.0
      hemolytic disease P56.90
        specified NEC P56.99
      isoimmunization (ABO) (Rh) P56.0

Hydrops - *continued*
  other specified nonhemolytic disease NEC
  P83.2
    Rh incompatibility P56.0
  during pregnancy —*see* Pregnancy,
  complicated by, hydrops, fetalis
  gallbladder K82.1
  joint —*see* Effusion, joint
  labyrinth H81.0
  newborn (idiopathic) P83.2
    due to
      ABO isoimmunization P56.0
      alpha thalassemia D56.0
      hemolytic disease P56.90
        specified NEC P56.99
      isoimmunization (ABO) (Rh) P56.0
      Rh incompatibility P56.0
  nutritional —*see* Malnutrition, severe
  pericardium —*see* Pericarditis
  pleura —*see* Hydrothorax
  spermatic cord —*see* Hydrocele
Hydropyonephrosis N13.6
Hydrorachis Q06.4
Hydrorrhea (nasal) J34.89
  pregnancy —*see* Rupture, membranes,
  premature
Hydrosadenitis (axillaris) (suppurative) L73.2
Hydrosalpinx (fallopian tube) (follicularis)
  N70.11
Hydrothorax (double) (pleura) J94.8
  chylous (nonfilarial) I89.8
    filarial (*see also* Infestation, filarial) B74.9
    [J91.8]
  traumatic —*see* Injury, intrathoracic
  tuberculous NEC (non primary) A15.6
Hydroureter (*see also* Hydronephrosis) N13.4
  with infection N13.6
  congenital Q62.39
Hydroureteronephrosis —*see*
  Hydronephrosis
Hydrourethra N36.8
Hydroxykynureninuria E70.8
Hydroxylysinemia E72.3
Hydroxyprolinemia E72.59
Hygiene, sleep
  abuse Z72.821
  inadequate Z72.821
  poor Z72.821
Hygroma (congenital) (cystic) D18.1
  praepatellare, prepatellar —*see* Bursitis,
  prepatellar
Hymen —*see* condition
Hymenolepis, hymenolepiasis (diminuta)
  (infection) (infestation) (nana) B71.0
Hypalgesia R20.8
Hyperacidity (gastric) K31.89
  psychogenic F45.8
Hyperactive, hyperactivity F90.9
  basal cell, uterine cervix —*see* Dysplasia,
  cervix
  bowel sounds R19.12
  cervix epithelial (basal) —*see* Dysplasia,
  cervix
  child F90.9
    attention deficit —*see* Disorder, attention-
    deficit hyperactivity
  detrusor muscle N32.81
  gastrointestinal K31.89
    psychogenic F45.8
  nasal mucous membrane J34.3
  stomach K31.89
  thyroid (gland) —*see* Hyperthyroidism
Hyperacusis H93.23

Hyperadrenalism E27.5
Hyperadrenocorticism E24.9
  congenital E25.0
  iatrogenic E24.2
    correct substance properly administered —
    see Table of Drugs and Chemicals, by drug,
    adverse effect
      overdose or wrong substance given or taken
      —*see* Table of Drugs and Chemicals, by drug,
      poisoning
  not associated with Cushing's syndrome
  E27.0
  pituitary-dependent E24.0
Hyperaldosteronism E26.9
  familial (type I) E26.02
  glucocorticoid-remediable E26.02
  primary (due to (bilateral) adrenal
  hyperplasia) E26.09
  primary NEC E26.09
  secondary E26.1
  specified NEC E26.89
Hyperalgesia R20.8
Hyperalimentation R63.2
  carotene, carotin E67.1
  specified NEC E67.8
  vitamin
    A E67.0
    D E67.3
Hyperaminoaciduria
  arginine E72.21
  cystine E72.01
  lysine E72.3
  ornithine E72.4
Hyperammonemia (congenital) E72.20
Hyperazotemia —*see* Uremia
Hyperbetalipoproteinemia (familial) E78.0
  with prebetalipoproteinemia E78.2
Hyperbilirubinemia
  constitutional E80.6
  familial conjugated E80.6
  neonatal (transient) —*see* Jaundice, newborn
Hypercalcemia, hypocalciuric, familial
  E83.52
Hypercalciuria, idiopathic E83.52
Hypercapnia R06.89
  newborn P84
Hypercarotenemia, hypercarotenemia
  (dietary) E67.1
Hypercementosis K03.4
Hyperchloremia E87.8
Hyperchlorhydria K31.89
  neurotic F45.8
  psychogenic F45.8
Hypercholesterinemia —*see*
  Hypercholesterolemia
Hypercholesterolemia (essential) (familial)
  (hereditary) (primary) (pure) E78.0
  with hyperglyceridemia, endogenous E78.2
  dietary counseling and surveillance Z71.3
Hyperchylia gastrica, psychogenic F45.8
Hyperchylomicronemia (familial) (primary)
  E78.3
  with hyperbetalipoproteinemia E78.3
Hypercoagulable (state) D68.59
  activated protein C resistance D68.51
  antithrombin (III) deficiency D68.59
  factor V Leiden mutation D68.51
  primary NEC D68.59
  protein C deficiency D68.59
  protein S deficiency D68.59
  prothrombin gene mutation D68.52
  secondary D68.69
  specified NEC D68.69

Hypercoagulation (state) D68.59
Hypercorticalism, pituitary-dependent E24.0
Hypercorticosolism —*see* Cushing's,
  syndrome
Hypercorticosteronism E24.2
  correct substance properly administered —*see*
  Table of Drugs and Chemicals, by drug,
  adverse effect
    overdose or wrong substance given or taken
    —*see* Table of Drugs and Chemicals, by drug,
    poisoning
Hypercortisonism E24.2
  correct substance properly administered —*see*
  Table of Drugs and Chemicals, by drug,
  adverse effect
    overdose or wrong substance given or taken
    —*see* Table of Drugs and Chemicals, by drug,
    poisoning
Hyperekplexia Q89.8
Hyperelectrolytemia E87.8
Hyperemesis R11.10
  with nausea R11.2
  gravidarum (mild) O21.0
    with
      carbohydrate depletion O21.1
      dehydration O21.1
      electrolyte imbalance O21.1
      metabolic disturbance O21.1
    severe (with metabolic disturbance) O21.1
  projectile R11.12
  psychogenic F45.8
Hyperemia (acute) (passive) R68.89
  anal mucosa K62.89
  bladder N32.89
  cerebral I67.89
  conjunctiva H11.43
  ear internal, acute —see subcategory H83.0
  enteric K59.8
  eye —*see* Hyperemia, conjunctiva
  eyelid (active) (passive) —*see* Disorder,
  eyelid, specified type NEC
  intestine K59.8
  iris —*see* Disorder, iris, vascular
  kidney N28.89
  labyrinth —see subcategory H83.0
  liver (active) K76.89
  lung (passive) —*see* Edema, lung
  pulmonary (passive) —*see* Edema, lung
  renal N28.89
  retina H35.89
  stomach K31.89
Hyperesthesia (body surface) R20.3
  larynx (reflex) J38.7
    hysterical F44.89
  pharynx (reflex) J39.2
    hysterical F44.89
Hyperestrogenism (drug-induced) (iatrogenic)
  E28.0
Hyperexplexia Q89.8
Hyperfibrinolysis —*see* Fibrinolysis
Hyperfructosemia E74.19
Hyperfunction
  adrenal cortex, not associated with Cushing's
  syndrome E27.0
    medulla E27.5
      adrenomedullary E27.5
    virilism E25.9
      congenital E25.0
  ovarian E28.8
  pancreas K86.8
  parathyroid (gland) E21.3
  pituitary (gland) (anterior) E22.9
    specified NEC E22.8

Hyperfunction - *continued*
polyglandular E31.1
testicular E29.0
Hypergammaglobulinemia D89.2
polyclonal D89.0
Waldenström D89.0
Hypergastrinemia E16.4
Hyperglobulinemia R77.1
Hyperglycemia, hyperglycemic (transient)
R73.9
coma —*see* Diabetes, by type, with coma
postpancreatectomy E89.1
Hyperglyceridemia (endogenous) (essential)
(familial) (hereditary) (pure) E78.1
mixed E78.3
Hyperglycinemia (non-ketotic) E72.51
Hypergonadism
ovarian E28.8
testicular (primary) (infantile) E29.0
Hyperheparinemia D68.32
Hyperhidrosis, hyperidrosis R61
focal
primary L74.519
axilla L74.510
face L74.511
palms L74.512
soles L74.513
secondary L74.52
generalized R61
localized
primary L74.519
axilla L74.510
face L74.511
palms L74.512
soles L74.513
secondary L74.52
psychogenic F45.8
secondary R61
focal L74.52
Hyperhistidinemia E70.41
Hyperhomocysteinemia E72.11
Hyperhydroxyprolinemia E72.59
Hyperinsulinism (functional) E16.1
with
coma (hypoglycemic) E15
encephalopathy E16.1 *[G94]*
ectopic E16.1
therapeutic misadventure (from
administration of insulin) —see subcategory
T38.3
Hyperkalemia E87.5
Hyperkeratosis (*see also* Keratosis) L85.9
cervix N88.0
due to yaws (early) (late) (palmar or plantar)
A66.3
follicularis Q82.8
penetrans (in cutem) L87.0
palmoplantaris climacterica L85.1
pinta A67.1
senile (with pruritus) L57.0
universalis congenita Q80.8
vocal cord J38.3
vulva N90.4
Hyperkinesia, hyperkinetic (disease)
(reaction) (syndrome) (childhood)
(adolescence) —*see also* Disorder, attention-
deficit hyperactivity
heart I51.89
Hyperleucine-isoleucinemia E71.19
Hyperlipemia, hyperlipidemia E78.5
combined E78.2
familial E78.4

Hyperlipemia, hyperlipidemia – *continued*
group
A E78.0
B E78.1
C E78.2
D E78.3
mixed E78.2
specified NEC E78.4
Hyperlipidosis E75.6
hereditary NEC E75.5
Hyperlipoproteinemia E78.5
Fredrickson's type
I E78.3
IIa E78.0
IIb E78.2
III E78.2
IV E78.1
V E78.3
low-density-lipoprotein-type (LDL) E78.0
very-low-density-lipoprotein-type (VLDL)
E78.1
Hyperlucent lung, unilateral J43.0
Hyperlysinemia E72.3
Hypermagnesemia E83.41
neonatal P71.8
Hypermenorrhea N92.0
Hypermethioninemia E72.19
Hypermetropia (congenital) H52.0\
Hypermobility, hypermotility
cecum —*see* Syndrome, irritable bowel
coccyx —see subcategory M53.2
colon —*see* Syndrome, irritable bowel
psychogenic F45.8
ileum K58.9
intestine (*see also* Syndrome, irritable bowel)
K58.9
psychogenic F45.8
meniscus (knee) —*see* Derangement, knee,
meniscus
scapula —*see* Instability, joint, shoulder
stomach K31.89
psychogenic F45.8
syndrome M35.7
urethra N36.41
with intrinsic sphincter deficiency N36.43
Hypernasality R49.21
Hypernatremia E87.0
Hypernephroma C64.
Hyperopia —*see* Hypermetropia
Hyperorexia nervosa F50.2
Hyperornithinemia E72.4
Hyperosmia R43.1
Hyperosmolality E87.0
Hyperostosis (monomelic) —*see also*
Disorder, bone, density and structure,
specified NEC
ankylosing (spine) M48.10
cervical region M48.12
cervicothoracic region M48.13
lumbar region M48.16
lumbosacral region M48.17
multiple sites M48.19
occipito-atlanto-axial region M48.11
sacrococcygeal region M48.18
thoracic region M48.14
thoracolumbar region M48.15
cortical (skull) M85.2
infantile M89.8X
frontal, internal of skull M85.2
interna frontalis M85.2
skeletal, diffuse idiopathic —*see*
Hyperostosis, ankylosing

Hyperostosis – *continued*
skull M85.2
congenital Q75.8
vertebral, ankylosing —*see* Hyperostosis,
ankylosing
Hyperovarism E28.8
Hyperoxaluria (primary) E72.53
Hyperparathyroidism E21.3
primary E21.0
secondary (renal) N25.81
non-renal E21.1
specified NEC E21.2
tertiary E21.2
Hyperpathia R20.8
Hyperperistalsis R19.2
psychogenic F45.8
Hyperpermeability, capillary I78.8
Hyperphagia R63.2
Hyperphenylalaninemia NEC E70.1
Hyperphoria (alternating) H50.53
Hyperphosphatemia E83.39
Hyperpiesis, hyperpiesia —*see* Hypertension
Hyperpigmentation —*see also* Pigmentation
melanin NEC L81.4
postinflammatory L81.0
Hyperpinealism E34.8
Hyperpituitarism E22.9
Hyperplasia, hyperplastic
adenoids J35.2
adrenal (capsule) (cortex) (gland) E27.8
with
sexual precocity (male) E25.9
congenital E25.0
virilism, adrenal E25.9
congenital E25.0
virilization (female) E25.9
congenital E25.0
congenital E25.0
salt-losing E25.0
adrenomedullary E27.5
angiolymphoid, eosinophilia (ALHE) D18.01
appendix (lymphoid) K38.0
artery, fibromuscular I77.3
bone —*see also* Hypertrophy, bone
marrow D75.89
breast —*see also* Hypertrophy, breast
ductal (atypical) N60.9
C-cell, thyroid E07.0
cementation (tooth) (teeth) K03.4
cervical gland R59.0
cervix (uteri) (basal cell) (endometrium)
(polypoid) —*see also* Dysplasia, cervix
congenital Q51.828
clitoris, congenital Q52.6
denture K06.2
endocervicitis N72
endometrium, endometrial (adenomatous)
(benign) (cystic) (glandular) (glandular-
cystic) (polypoid) N85.00
with atypia N85.02
cervix —*see* Dysplasia, cervix
complex (without atypia) N85.01
simple (without atypia) N85.01
epithelial L85.9
focal, oral, including tongue K13.29
nipple N62
skin L85.9
tongue K13.29
vaginal wall N89.3
erythroid D75.89
fibromuscular of artery (carotid) (renal) I77.3

Hyperplasia, hyperplastic – *continued*
  genital
    female NEC N94.89
    male N50.8
  gingiva K06.1
  glandularis cystica uteri (interstitialis) (*see also* Hyperplasia, endometrial) N85.00
  gum K06.1
  hymen, congenital Q52.4
  irritative, edentulous (alveolar) K06.2
  jaw M26.09
    alveolar M26.79
    lower M26.03
      alveolar M26.72
    upper M26.01
      alveolar M26.71
  kidney (congenital) Q63.3
  labia N90.6
    epithelial N90.3
  liver (congenital) Q44.7
    nodular, focal K76.89
  lymph gland or node R59.9
  mandible, mandibular M26.03
    alveolar M26.72
    unilateral condylar M27.8
  maxilla, maxillary M26.01
    alveolar M26.71
  myometrium, myometrial N85.2
  neuroendocrine cell, of infancy J84.841
  nose
    lymphoid J34.89
    polypoid J33.9
  oral mucosa (irritative) K13.6
  organ or site, congenital NEC —*see* Anomaly, by site
  ovary N83.8
  palate, papillary (irritative) K13.6
  pancreatic islet cells E16.9
    alpha E16.8
      with excess
        gastrin E16.4
        glucagon E16.3
    beta E16.1
  parathyroid (gland) E21.0
  pharynx (lymphoid) J39.2
  prostate (adenofibromatous) (nodular) N40.0
    with lower urinary tract symptoms (LUTS) N40.1
    without lower urinary tract symptoms (LUTS) N40.0
  renal artery I77.89
  reticulo-endothelial (cell) D75.89
  salivary gland (any) K11.1
  Schimmelbusch's —*see* Mastopathy, cystic
  suprarenal capsule (gland) E27.8
  thymus (gland) (persistent) E32.0
  thyroid (gland) —*see* Goiter
  tonsils (faucial) (infective) (lingual) (lymphoid) J35.1
    with adenoids J35.3
  unilateral condylar M27.8
  uterus, uterine N85.2
    endometrium (glandular) (*see also* Hyperplasia, endometrial) N85.00
  vulva N90.6
    epithelial N90.3
Hyperpnea —*see* Hyperventilation
Hyperpotassemia E87.5
Hyperprebetalipoproteinemia (familial) E78.1
Hyperprolactinemia E22.1
Hyperprolinemia (type I) (type II) E72.59
Hyperproteinemia E88.09

Hyperprothrombinemia, causing coagulation factor deficiency D68.4
Hyperpyrexia R50.9
  heat (effects) T67.0
  malignant, due to anesthetic T88.3
  rheumatic —*see* Fever, rheumatic
  unknown origin R50.9
Hyper-reflexia R29.2
Hypersalivation K11.7
Hypersecretion
  ACTH (not associated with Cushing's syndrome) E27.0
    pituitary E24.0
  adrenaline E27.5
  adrenomedullary E27.5
  androgen (testicular) E29.0
    ovarian (drug-induced) (iatrogenic) E28.1
  calcitonin E07.0
  catecholamine E27.5
  corticoadrenal E24.9
  cortisol E24.9
  epinephrine E27.5
  estrogen E28.0
  gastric K31.89
    psychogenic F45.8
  gastrin E16.4
  glucagon E16.3
  hormone (s)
    ACTH (not associated with Cushing's syndrome) E27.0
      pituitary E24.0
    antidiuretic E22.2
    growth E22.0
    intestinal NEC E34.1
    ovarian androgen E28.1
    pituitary E22.9
    testicular E29.0
    thyroid stimulating E05.80
      with thyroid storm E05.81
  insulin —*see* Hyperinsulinism
  lacrimal glands —*see* Epiphora
  medulloadrenal E27.5
  milk O92.6
  ovarian androgens E28.1
  salivary gland (any) K11.7
  thyrocalcitonin E07.0
  upper respiratory J39.8
Hypersegmentation, leukocytic, hereditary D72.0
Hypersensitive, hypersensitiveness, hypersensitivity —*see also* Allergy
  carotid sinus G90.01
  colon —*see* Irritable, colon
  drug T88.7
  gastrointestinal K52.2
    psychogenic F45.8
  labyrinth —see subcategory H83.2
  pain R20.8
  pneumonitis —*see* Pneumonitis, allergic
  reaction T78.40
    upper respiratory tract NEC J39.3
Hypersomnia (organic) G47.10
  due to
    alcohol
      abuse F10.182
      dependence F10.282
      use F10.982
    amphetamines
      abuse F15.182
      dependence F15.282
      use F15.982
    caffeine

Hypersomnia – *continued*
    abuse F15.182
    dependence F15.282
    use F15.982
  cocaine
    abuse F14.182
    dependence F14.282
    use F14.982
  drug NEC
    abuse F19.182
    dependence F19.282
    use F19.982
  medical condition G47.14
  mental disorder F51.13
  opioid
    abuse F11.182
    dependence F11.282
    use F11.982
  psychoactive substance NEC
    abuse F19.182
    dependence F19.282
    use F19.982
  sedative, hypnotic, or anxiolytic
    abuse F13.182
    dependence F13.282
    use F13.982
  stimulant NEC
    abuse F15.182
    dependence F15.282
    use F15.982
  idiopathic G47.11
    with long sleep time G47.11
    without long sleep time G47.12
  menstrual related G47.13
  nonorganic origin F51.11
    specified NEC F51.19
  not due to a substance or known physiological condition F51.11
    specified NEC F51.19
  primary F51.11
  recurrent G47.13
  specified NEC G47.19
Hypersplenia, hypersplenism D73.1
Hyperstimulation, ovaries (associated with induced ovulation) N98.1
Hypersusceptibility —*see* Allergy
Hypertelorism (ocular) (orbital) Q75.2
Hypertension, hypertensive (accelerated) (benign) (essential) (idiopathic) (malignant) (systemic) I10
  with
    heart involvement (conditions in I51.4 I51.9 due to hypertension) —*see* Hypertension, heart
    kidney involvement —*see* Hypertension, kidney
  benign, intracranial G93.2
  borderline R03.0
  cardiorenal (disease) I13.10
    with heart failure I13.0
      with stage 1 through stage 4 chronic kidney disease I13.0
      with stage 5 or end stage renal disease I13.2
    without heart failure I13.10
      with stage 1 through stage 4 chronic kidney disease I13.10
      with stage 5 or end stage renal disease I13.11
  cardiovascular
    disease (arteriosclerotic) (sclerotic) —*see* Hypertension, heart

Hypertension, hypertensive – *continued*
  renal (disease) —*see* Hypertension,
  cardiorenal
  chronic venous —*see* Hypertension, venous
  (chronic)
  complicating
    childbirth (labor) O10.92
      with
        heart disease O10.12
          with renal disease O10.32
        renal disease O10.22
          with heart disease O10.32
      essential O10.02
      secondary O10.42
    pregnancy O16.
      with edema (*see also* Pre-eclampsia) O14.9
      gestational (pregnancy induced) (transient)
    (without proteinuria) O13.
      with proteinuria O14.9
        mild pre-eclampsia O14.0
        moderate pre-eclampsia O14.0
        severe pre-eclampsia O14.1
          with hemolysis, elevated liver
  enzymes and low platelet count (HELLP)
  O14.2
      pre-existing O10.91
        with
          heart disease O10.11
            with renal disease O10.31
          pre-eclampsia O11.
          renal disease O10.21
            with heart disease O10.31
        essential O10.01
        secondary O10.41
      puerperium, pre-existing O10.93
        with
          heart disease O10.13
            with renal disease O10.33
          renal disease O10.23
            with heart disease O10.33
        essential O10.03
      pregnancy-induced O13.9
      secondary O10.43
  due to
    endocrine disorders I15.2
    phcochromocytoma I15.2
    renal disorders NEC I15.1
      arterial I15.0
    renovascular disorders I15.0
    specified disease NEC I15.8
  encephalopathy I67.4
  gestational (without significant proteinuria)
  (pregnancy-induced) (transient) O13.
    with significant proteinuria —*see* Pre-
  eclampsia
  Goldblatt's I70.1
  heart (disease) (conditions in I51.4-I51.9 due
  to hypertension) I11.9
    with
      heart failure (congestive) I11.0
      kidney disease (chronic) —*see*
  Hypertension, cardiorenal
  intracranial (benign) G93.2
  kidney I12.9
    with
      heart disease —*see* Hypertension,
  cardiorenal
      stage 5 chronic kidney disease (CKD) or
  end stage renal disease (ESRD) I12.0
      stage 1 through stage 4 chronic kidney
  disease I12.9
  lesser circulation I27.0

Hypertension, hypertensive – *continued*
  newborn P29.2
    pulmonary (persistent) P29.3
  ocular H40.05
  pancreatic duct
  code to underlying condition
    with chronic pancreatitis K86.1
  portal (due to chronic liver disease)
  (idiopathic) K76.6
    gastropathy K31.89
    in (due to) schistosomiasis (bilharziasis)
  B65.9 *[K77]*
  postoperative I97.3
  psychogenic F45.8
  pulmonary (artery) (secondary) NEC I27.2
    with
      cor pulmonale (chronic) I27.2
        acute I26.09
      right heart ventricular strain/failure I27.2
        acute I26.09
    of newborn (persistent) P29.3
    primary (idiopathic) I27.0
  renal —*see* Hypertension, kidney
  renovascular I15.0
  secondary NEC I15.9
    due to
      endocrine disorders I15.2
      pheochromocytoma I15.2
      renal disorders NEC I15.1
        arterial I15.0
      renovascular disorders I15.0
    specified NEC I15.8
  venous (chronic)
    due to
      deep vein thrombosis —*see* Syndrome,
  postthrombotic
    idiopathic I87.309
      with
        inflammation I87.32
          with ulcer I87.33
        specified complication NEC I87.39
        ulcer I87.31
          with inflammation I87.33
      asymptomatic I87.30

Hypertensive urgency —*see* Hypertension
Hyperthecosis ovary E28.8
Hyperthermia (of unknown origin) —*see also*
Hyperpyrexia
malignant, due to anesthesia T88.3
newborn P81.9
  environmental P81.0
Hyperthyroid (recurrent) —*see*
Hyperthyroidism
Hyperthyroidism (latent) (pre-adult)
(recurrent) E05.90
with
  goiter (diffuse) E05.00
    with thyroid storm E05.01
    nodular (multinodular) E05.20
      with thyroid storm E05.21
    uninodular E05.10
      with thyroid storm E05.11
  storm E05.91
due to ectopic thyroid tissue E05.30
  with thyroid storm E05.31
neonatal, transitory P72.1
specified NEC E05.80
  with thyroid storm E05.81
Hypertony, hypertonia, hypertonicity
bladder N31.8
congenital P94.1

Hypertony – *continued*
  stomach K31.89
    psychogenic F45.8
  uterus, uterine (contractions) (complicating
  delivery) O62.4
Hypertrichosis L68.9
congenital Q84.2
eyelid H02.869
  left H02.866
    lower H02.865
    upper H02.864
  right H02.863
    lower H02.862
    upper H02.861
lanuginosa Q84.2
  acquired L68.1
localized L68.2
specified NEC L68.8
Hypertriglyceridemia, essential E78.1
Hypertrophy, hypertrophic
adenofibromatous, prostate —*see*
Enlargement, enlarged, prostate
adenoids (infective) J35.2
  with tonsils J35.3
adrenal cortex E27.8
alveolar process or ridge —*see* Anomaly,
alveolar
anal papillae K62.89
artery I77.89
  congenital NEC Q27.8
    digestive system Q27.8
    lower limb Q27.8
    specified site NEC Q27.8
    upper limb Q27.8
auricular —*see* Hypertrophy, cardiac
Bartholin's gland N75.8
bile duct (common) (hepatic) K83.8
bladder (sphincter) (trigone) N32.89
bone M89.30
  carpus M89.34
  clavicle M89.31
  femur M89.35
  fibula M89.36
  finger M89.34
  humerus M89.32
  ilium M89.359
  ischium M89.359
  metacarpus M89.34
  metatarsus M89.37
  multiple sites M89.39
  neck M89.38
  radius M89.33
  rib M89.38
  scapula M89.31
  skull M89.38
  tarsus M89.37
  tibia M89.36
  toe M89.37
  ulna M89.33
  vertebra M89.38
brain G93.89
breast N62
  cystic —*see* Mastopathy, cystic
  newborn P83.4
  pubertal, massive N62
  puerperal, postpartum —*see* Disorder,
breast, specified type NEC
  senile (parenchymatous) N62
cardiac (chronic) (idiopathic) I51.7
  with rheumatic fever (conditions in I00)
    active I01.8
    inactive or quiescent (with chorea) I09.89
  congenital NEC Q24.8

Hypertrophy, hypertrophic - *continued*
- fatty —*see* Degeneration, myocardial
- hypertensive —*see* Hypertension, heart
- rheumatic (with chorea) I09.89
  - active or acute I01.8
    - with chorea I02.0
  - valve —*see* Endocarditis
- cartilage —*see* Disorder, cartilage, specified type NEC
- cecum —*see* Megacolon
- cervix (uteri) N88.8
  - congenital Q51.828
  - elongation N88.4
- clitoris (cirrhotic) N90.89
  - congenital Q52.6
- colon —*see also* Megacolon
  - congenital Q43.2
- conjunctiva, lymphoid H11.89
- corpora cavernosa N48.89
- cystic duct K82.8
- duodenum K31.89
- endometrium (glandular) (*see also* Hyperplasia, endometrial) N85.00
  - cervix N88.8
- epididymis N50.8
- esophageal hiatus (congenital) Q79.1
  - with hernia —*see* Hernia, hiatal
- eyelid —*see* Disorder, eyelid, specified type NEC
- fat pad E65
  - knee (infrapatellar) (popliteal) (prepatellar) (retropatellar) M79.4
- foot (congenital) Q74.2
- frenulum, frenum (tongue) K14.8
  - lip K13.0
- gallbladder K82.8
- gastric mucosa K29.60
  - with bleeding K29.61
- gland, glandular R59.9
  - generalized R59.1
  - localized R59.0
- gum (mucous membrane) K06.1
- heart (idiopathic) —*see also* Hypertrophy, cardiac
  - valve (*see also* Endocarditis) I38
- hemifacial Q67.4
- hepatic —*see* Hypertrophy, liver
- hiatus (esophageal) Q79.1
- hilus gland R59.0
- hymen, congenital Q52.4
- ileum K63.89
- intestine NEC K63.89
- jejunum K63.89
- kidney (compensatory) N28.81
  - congenital Q63.3
- labium (majus) (minus) N90.6
- ligament —*see* Disorder, ligament
- lingual tonsil (infective) J35.1
  - with adenoids J35.3
- lip K13.0
  - congenital Q18.6
- liver R16.0
  - acute K76.89
  - congenital Q44.7
  - cirrhotic —*see* Cirrhosis, liver
  - fatty —*see* Fatty, liver
- lymph, lymphatic gland R59.9
  - generalized R59.1
  - localized R59.0
  - tuberculous —*see* Tuberculosis, lymph gland
- mammary gland —*see* Hypertrophy, breast

Hypertrophy, hypertrophic – *continued*
- Meckel's diverticulum (congenital) Q43.0
  - malignant —*see* Table of Neoplasms, small intestine, malignant
- median bar —*see* Hyperplasia, prostate
- meibomian gland —*see* Chalazion
- meniscus, knee, congenital Q74.1
- metatarsal head —*see* Hypertrophy, bone, metatarsus
- metatarsus —*see* Hypertrophy, bone, metatarsus
- mucous membrane
  - alveolar ridge K06.2
    - gum K06.1
    - nose (turbinate) J34.3
- muscle M62.89
- muscular coat, artery I77.89
- myocardium —*see also* Hypertrophy, cardiac
  - idiopathic I42.2
- myometrium N85.2
- nail L60.2
  - congenital Q84.5
- nasal J34.89
  - alae J34.89
  - bone J34.89
  - cartilage J34.89
  - mucous membrane (septum) J34.3
  - sinus J34.89
  - turbinate J34.3
- nasopharynx, lymphoid (infectional) (tissue) (wall) J35.2
- nipple N62
- organ or site, congenital NEC —*see* Anomaly, by site
- ovary N83.8
- palate (hard) M27.8
  - soft K13.79
- pancreas, congenital Q45.3
- parathyroid (gland) E21.0
- parotid gland K11.1
- penis N48.89
- pharyngeal tonsil J35.2
- pharynx J39.2
  - lymphoid (infectional) (tissue) (wall) J35.2
- pituitary (anterior) (fossa) (gland) E23.6
- prepuce (congenital) N47.8
  - female N90.89
- prostate —*see* Enlargement, enlarged, prostate
  - congenital Q55.4
- pseudomuscular G71.0
- pylorus (adult) (muscle) (sphincter) K31.1
  - congenital or infantile Q40.0
- rectal, rectum (sphincter) K62.89
- rhinitis (turbinate) J31.0
- salivary gland (any) K11.1
  - congenital Q38.4
- scaphoid (tarsal) —*see* Hypertrophy, bone, tarsus
- scar L91.0
- scrotum N50.8
- seminal vesicle N50.8
- sigmoid —*see* Megacolon
- skin L91.9
  - specified NEC L91.8
- spermatic cord N50.8
- spleen —*see* Splenomegaly
- spondylitis —*see* Spondylosis
- stomach K31.89
- sublingual gland K11.1
- submandibular gland K11.1
- suprarenal cortex (gland) E27.8

Hypertrophy, hypertrophic – *continued*
- synovial NEC M67.20
  - acromioclavicular M67.21
  - ankle M67.27
  - elbow M67.22
  - foot M67.27
  - hand M67.24
  - hip M67.25
  - knee M67.26
  - multiple sites M67.29
  - specified site NEC M67.28
  - wrist M67.23
- tendon —*see* Disorder, tendon, specified type NEC
- testis N44.8
  - congenital Q55.29
- thymic, thymus (gland) (congenital) E32.0
- thyroid (gland) —*see* Goiter
- toe (congenital) Q74.2
  - acquired —*see also* Deformity, toe, specified NEC
- tongue K14.8
  - congenital Q38.2
  - papillae (foliate) K14.3
- tonsils (faucial) (infective) (lingual) (lymphoid) J35.1
  - with adenoids J35.3
- tunica vaginalis N50.8
- ureter N28.89
- urethra N36.8
- uterus N85.2
  - neck (with elongation) N88.4
  - puerperal O90.89
- uvula K13.79
- vagina N89.8
- vas deferens N50.8
- vein I87.8
- ventricle, ventricular (heart) —*see also* Hypertrophy, cardiac
  - congenital Q24.8
  - in tetralogy of Fallot Q21.3
- verumontanum N36.8
- vocal cord J38.3
- vulva N90.6
  - stasis (nonfilarial) N90.6

Hypertropia H50.2\
Hypertyrosinemia E70.21
Hyperuricemia (asymptomatic) E79.0
Hypervalinemia E71.19
Hyperventilation (tetany) R06.4
- hysterical F45.8
- psychogenic F45.8
- syndrome F45.8

Hypervitaminosis (dietary) **NEC** E67.8
- A E67.0
  - administered as drug (prolonged intake) —*see* Table of Drugs and Chemicals, vitamins, adverse effect
  - overdose or wrong substance given or taken —*see* Table of Drugs and Chemicals, vitamins, poisoning
- B6 E67.2
- D E67.3
  - administered as drug (prolonged intake) —*see* Table of Drugs and Chemicals, vitamins, adverse effect
  - overdose or wrong substance given or taken —*see* Table of Drugs and Chemicals, vitamins, poisoning
- K E67.8
  - administered as drug (prolonged intake) —*see* Table of Drugs and Chemicals, vitamins, adverse effect

Hypervitaminosis – *continued*
  overdose or wrong substance given or taken
  —*see* Table of Drugs and Chemicals,
  vitamins, poisoning
Hypervolemia E87.70
  specified NEC E87.79
Hypesthesia R20.1
  cornea —*see* Anesthesia, cornea
Hyphema H21.0
  traumatic S05.1-**Hypoacidity, gastric** K31.89
  psychogenic F45.8
Hypoadrenalism, hypoadrenia E27.40
  primary E27.1
  tuberculous A18.7
Hypoadrenocorticism E27.40
  pituitary E23.0
  primary E27.1
Hypoalbuminemia E88.09
Hypoaldosteronism E27.40
Hypoalphalipoproteinemia E78.6
Hypobarism T70.29
Hypobaropathy T70.29
Hypobetalipoproteinemia (familial) E78.6
Hypocalcemia E83.51
  dietary E58
  neonatal P71.1
    due to cow's milk P71.0
  phosphate-loading (newborn) P71.1
Hypochloremia E87.8
Hypochlorhydria K31.89
  neurotic F45.8
  psychogenic F45.8
Hypochondria, hypochondriac,
  hypochondriasis (reaction) F45.21
  sleep F51.03
Hypochondrogenesis Q77.0
Hypochondroplasia Q77.4
Hypochromasia, blood cells D50.8
Hypodontia —*see* Anodontia
Hypoeosinophilia D72.89
Hypoesthesia R20.1
Hypofibrinogenemia D68.8
  acquired D65
  congenital (hereditary) D68.2
Hypofunction
  adrenocortical E27.40
    drug-induced E27.3
    postprocedural E89.6
    primary E27.1
  adrenomedullary, postprocedural E89.6
  cerebral R29.818
  corticoadrenal NEC E27.40
  intestinal K59.8
  labyrinth —*see* subcategory H83.2
  ovary E28.39
  pituitary (gland) (anterior) E23.0
  testicular E29.1
    postprocedural (postsurgical)
    (postirradiation) (iatrogenic) E89.5
Hypogalactia O92.4
Hypogammaglobulinemia (*see also*
  Agammaglobulinemia) D80.1
  hereditary D80.0
  nonfamilial D80.1
  transient, of infancy D80.7
Hypogenitalism (congenital) —*see*
  Hypogonadism
Hypoglossia Q38.3
Hypoglycemia (spontaneous) E16.2
  coma E15
    diabetic —*see* Diabetes, coma
  diabetic —*see* Diabetes, hypoglycemia

Hypoglycemia – *continued*
  dietary counseling and surveillance Z71.3
  drug-induced E16.0
    with coma (nondiabetic) E15
  due to insulin E16.0
    with coma (nondiabetic) E15
    therapeutic misadventure —*see* subcategory
    T38.3
  functional, nonhyperinsulinemic E16.1
  iatrogenic E16.0
    with coma (nondiabetic) E15
  in infant of diabetic mother P70.1
    gestational diabetes P70.0
  infantile E16.1
  leucine-induced E71.19
  neonatal (transitory) P70.4
    iatrogenic P70.3
  reactive (not drug-induced) E16.1
  transitory neonatal P70.4
Hypogonadism
  female E28.39
  hypogonadotropic E23.0
  male E29.1
  ovarian (primary) E28.39
  pituitary E23.0
  testicular (primary) E29.1
Hypohidrosis, hypoidrosis L74.4
Hypoinsulinemia, postprocedural E89.1
Hypokalemia E87.6
Hypoleukocytosis —*see* Agranulocytosis
Hypolipoproteinemia (alpha) (beta) E78.6
Hypomagnesemia E83.42
  neonatal P71.2
Hypomania, hypomanic reaction F30.8
Hypomenorrhea —*see* Oligomenorrhea
Hypometabolism R63.8
Hypomotility
  gastrointestinal (tract) K31.89
    psychogenic F45.8
  intestine K59.8
    psychogenic F45.8
  stomach K31.89
    psychogenic F45.8
Hyponasality R49.22
Hyponatremia E87.1
Hypo-osmolality E87.1
Hypo-ovarianism, hypo-ovarism E28.39
Hypoparathyroidism E20.9
  familial E20.8
  idiopathic E20.0
  neonatal, transitory P71.4
  postprocedural E89.2
  specified NEC E20.8
Hypoperfusion (in)
  newborn P96.89
Hypopharyngitis —*see* Laryngopharyngitis
Hypophoria H50.53
Hypophosphatemia, hypophosphatasia
  (acquired) (congenital) (renal) E83.39
  familial E83.31
Hypophyseal, hypophysis —*see also*
  condition
  dwarfism E23.0
  gigantism E22.0
Hypopiesis —*see* Hypotension
Hypopinealism E34.8
Hypopituitarism (juvenile) E23.0
  drug-induced E23.1
  due to
    hypophysectomy E89.3
    radiotherapy E89.3
  iatrogenic NEC E23.1

Hypopituitarism – *continued*
  postirradiation E89.3
  postpartum E23.0
  postprocedural E89.3
Hypoplasia, hypoplastic
  adrenal (gland) , congenital Q89.1
  alimentary tract, congenital Q45.8
    upper Q40.8
  anus, anal (canal) Q42.3
    with fistula Q42.2
  aorta, aortic Q25.4
    ascending, in hypoplastic left heart
    syndrome Q23.4
    valve Q23.1
      in hypoplastic left heart syndrome Q23.4
  areola, congenital Q83.8
  arm (congenital) —*see* Defect, reduction,
  upper limb
  artery (peripheral) Q27.8
    brain (congenital) Q28.3
    coronary Q24.5
    digestive system Q27.8
    lower limb Q27.8
    pulmonary Q25.79
      functional, unilateral J43.0
    retinal (congenital) Q14.1
    specified site NEC Q27.8
    umbilical Q27.0
    upper limb Q27.8
  auditory canal Q17.8
    causing impairment of hearing Q16.9
  biliary duct or passage Q44.5
  bone NOS Q79.9
    face Q75.8
    marrow D61.9
      megakaryocytic D69.49
    skull —*see* Hypoplasia, skull
  brain Q02
    gyri Q04.3
    part of Q04.3
  breast (areola) N64.82
  bronchus Q32.4
  cardiac Q24.8
  carpus —*see* Defect, reduction, upper limb,
  specified type NEC
  cartilage hair Q78.5
  cecum Q42.8
  cementum K00.4
  cephalic Q02
  cerebellum Q04.3
  cervix (uteri) , congenital Q51.821
  clavicle (congenital) Q74.0
  coccyx Q76.49
  colon Q42.9
    specified NEC Q42.8
  corpus callosum Q04.0
  cricoid cartilage Q31.2
  digestive organ (s) or tract NEC Q45.8
    upper (congenital) Q40.8
  ear (auricle) (lobe) Q17.2
    middle Q16.4
  enamel of teeth (neonatal) (postnatal)
    (prenatal) K00.4
  endocrine (gland) NEC Q89.2
  endometrium N85.8
  epididymis (congenital) Q55.4
  epiglottis Q31.2
  erythroid, congenital D61.01
  esophagus (congenital) Q39.8
  eustachian tube Q17.8
  eye Q11.2
  eyelid (congenital) Q10.3
  face Q18.8

Hypoplasia, hypoplastic - *continued*
  bone (s) Q75.8
  femur (congenital) —*see* Defect, reduction, lower limb, specified type NEC
  fibula (congenital) —*see* Defect, reduction, lower limb, specified type NEC
  finger (congenital) —*see* Defect, reduction, upper limb, specified type NEC
  focal dermal Q82.8
  foot —*see* Defect, reduction, lower limb, specified type NEC
  gallbladder Q44.0
  genitalia, genital organ (s)
    female, congenital Q52.8
      external Q52.79
      internal NEC Q52.8
    in adiposogenital dystrophy E23.6
  glottis Q31.2
  hair Q84.2
  hand (congenital) —*see* Defect, reduction, upper limb, specified type NEC
  heart Q24.8
  humerus (congenital) —*see* Defect, reduction, upper limb, specified type NEC
  intestine (small) Q41.9
    large Q42.9
      specified NEC Q42.8
  jaw M26.09
    alveolar M26.79
    lower M26.04
      alveolar M26.74
    upper M26.02
      alveolar M26.73
  kidney (s) Q60.5
    bilateral Q60.4
    unilateral Q60.3
  labium (majus) (minus) , congenital Q52.79
  larynx Q31.2
  left heart syndrome Q23.4
  leg (congenital) —*see* Defect, reduction, lower limb
  limb Q73.8
    lower (congenital) —*see* Defect, reduction, lower limb
    upper (congenital) —*see* Defect, reduction, upper limb
  liver Q44.7
  lung (lobe) (not associated with short gestation) Q33.6
    associated with immaturity, low birth weight, prematurity, or short gestation P28.0
  mammary (areola) , congenital Q83.8
  mandible, mandibular M26.04
    alveolar M26.74
    unilateral condylar M27.8
  maxillary M26.02
    alveolar M26.73
  medullary D61.9
  megakaryocytic D69.49
  metacarpus —*see* Defect, reduction, upper limb, specified type NEC
  metatarsus —*see* Defect, reduction, lower limb, specified type NEC
  muscle Q79.8
  nail (s) Q84.6
  nose, nasal Q30.1
  optic nerve H47.03
  osseous meatus (ear) Q17.8
  ovary, congenital Q50.39
  pancreas Q45.0
  parathyroid (gland) Q89.2
  parotid gland Q38.4

Hypoplasia, hypoplastic - *continued*
  patella Q74.1
  pelvis, pelvic girdle Q74.2
  penis (congenital) Q55.62
  peripheral vascular system Q27.8
    digestive system Q27.8
    lower limb Q27.8
    specified site NEC Q27.8
    upper limb Q27.8
  pituitary (gland) (congenital) Q89.2
  pulmonary (not associated with short gestation) Q33.6
    artery, functional J43.0
    associated with short gestation P28.0
  radioulnar —*see* Defect, reduction, upper limb, specified type NEC
  radius —*see* Defect, reduction, upper limb
  rectum Q42.1
    with fistula Q42.0
  respiratory system NEC Q34.8
  rib Q76.6
  right heart syndrome Q22.6
  sacrum Q76.49
  scapula Q74.0
  scrotum Q55.1
  shoulder girdle Q74.0
  skin Q82.8
  skull (bone) Q75.8
    with
      anencephaly Q00.0
      encephalocele —*see* Encephalocele
      hydrocephalus Q03.9
        with spina bifida —*see* Spina bifida, by site, with hydrocephalus
      microcephaly Q02
  spinal (cord) (ventral horn cell) Q06.1
  spine Q76.49
  sternum Q76.7
  tarsus —*see* Defect, reduction, lower limb, specified type NEC
  testis Q55.1
  thymic, with immunodeficiency D82.1
  thymus (gland) Q89.2
    with immunodeficiency D82.1
  thyroid (gland) E03.1
    cartilage Q31.2
  tibiofibular (congenital) —*see* Defect, reduction, lower limb, specified type NEC
  toe —*see* Defect, reduction, lower limb, specified type NEC
  tongue Q38.3
  Turner's K00.4
  ulna (congenital) —*see* Defect, reduction, upper limb
  umbilical artery Q27.0
  unilateral condylar M27.8
  ureter Q62.8
  uterus, congenital Q51.811
  vagina Q52.4
  vascular NEC peripheral Q27.8
    brain Q28.3
    digestive system Q27.8
    lower limb Q27.8
    specified site NEC Q27.8
    upper limb Q27.8
  vein (s) (peripheral) Q27.8
    brain Q28.3
    digestive system Q27.8
    great Q26.8
    lower limb Q27.8
    specified site NEC Q27.8
    upper limb Q27.8

Hypoplasia, hypoplastic - *continued*
  vena cava (inferior) (superior) Q26.8
  vertebra Q76.49
  vulva, congenital Q52.79
  zonule (ciliary) Q12.8
Hypopotassemia E87.6
Hypoproconvertinemia, congenital (hereditary) D68.2
Hypoproteinemia E77.8
Hypoprothrombinemia (congenital) (hereditary) (idiopathic) D68.2
  acquired D68.4
  newborn, transient P61.6
Hypoptyalism K11.7
Hypopyon (eye) (anterior chamber) —*see* Iridocyclitis, acute, hypopyon
Hypopyrexia R68.0
Hyporeflexia R29.2
Hyposecretion
  ACTH E23.0
  antidiuretic hormone E23.2
  ovary E28.39
  salivary gland (any) K11.7
  vasopressin E23.2
Hyposegmentation, leukocytic, hereditary D72.0
Hyposiderinemia D50.9
Hypospadias Q54.9
  balanic Q54.0
  coronal Q54.0
  glandular Q54.0
  penile Q54.1
  penoscrotal Q54.2
  perineal Q54.3
  specified NEC Q54.8
Hypospermatogenesis —*see* Oligospermia
Hyposplenism D73.0
Hypostasis pulmonary, passive —*see* Edema, lung
Hypostatic —*see* condition
Hyposthenuria N28.89
Hypotension (arterial) (constitutional) I95.9
  chronic I95.89
  due to (of) hemodialysis I95.3
  drug-induced I95.2
  iatrogenic I95.89
  idiopathic (permanent) I95.0
  intracranial, following ventricular shunting (ventriculostomy) G97.2
  intra-dialytic I95.3
  maternal, syndrome (following labor and delivery) O26.5
  neurogenic, orthostatic G90.3
  orthostatic (chronic) I95.1
    due to drugs I95.2
    neurogenic G90.3
  postoperative I95.81
  postural I95.1
  specified NEC I95.89
Hypothermia (accidental) T68
  due to anesthesia, anesthetic T88.51
  low environmental temperature T68
  neonatal P80.9
    environmental (mild) NEC P80.8
    mild P80.8
    severe (chronic) (cold injury syndrome) P80.0
    specified NEC P80.8
  not associated with low environmental temperature R68.0

Hypothyroidism (acquired) E03.9
  congenital (without goiter) E03.1
    with goiter (diffuse) E03.0
  due to
    exogenous substance NEC E03.2
    iodine-deficiency, acquired E01.8
      subclinical E02
    irradiation therapy E89.0
    medicament NEC E03.2
    P-aminosalicylic acid (PAS) E03.2
    phenylbutazone E03.2
    resorcinol E03.2
    sulfonamide E03.2
    surgery E89.0
    thiourea group drugs E03.2
  iatrogenic NEC E03.2
  iodine-deficiency (acquired) E01.8
    congenital —see Syndrome, iodine
  deficiency, congenital
    subclinical E02
  neonatal, transitory P72.2
  postinfectious E03.3
  postirradiation E89.0
  postprocedural E89.0
  postsurgical E89.0
  specified NEC E03.8
  subclinical, iodine-deficiency related E02
Hypotonia, hypotonicity, hypotony
  bladder N31.2
  congenital (benign) P94.2
  eye —see Disorder, globe, hypotony
Hypotrichosis see Alopecia
Hypotropia H50.2
Hypoventilation R06.89
  congenital central alveolar G47.35
  sleep related
    idiopathic nonobstructive alveolar G47.34
    in conditions classified elsewhere G47.36
Hypovitaminosis —see Deficiency, vitamin
Hypovolemia E86.1
  surgical shock T81.19
  traumatic (shock) T79.4
Hypoxemia R09.02
  newborn P84
  sleep related, in conditions classified
  elsewhere G47.36
Hypoxia (see also Anoxia) R09.02
  cerebral, during a procedure NEC G97.81
    postprocedural NEC G97.82
  intrauterine P84
  myocardial see Insufficiency, coronary
  newborn P84
  sleep-related G47.34
Hypsarhythmia —see Epilepsy, generalized,
  specified NEC
Hysteralgia, pregnant uterus O26.89
Hysteria, hysterical (conversion) (dissociative
  state) F44.9
  anxiety F41.8
  convulsions F44.5
  psychosis, acute F44.9
Hysteroepilepsy F44.5

I

Ichthyoparasitism due to Vandellia cirrhosa
  B88.8
Ichthyosis (congenital) Q80.9
  acquired L85.0
  fetalis Q80.4
  hystrix Q80.8
  lamellar Q80.2
  lingual K13.29

Ichthyosis – continued
  palmaris and plantaris Q82.8
  simplex Q80.0
  vera Q80.8
  vulgaris Q80.0
  X-linked Q80.1
Ichthyotoxism —see Poisoning, fish
  bacterial —see Intoxication, foodborne
Icteroanemia, hemolytic (acquired) D59.9
  congenital —see Spherocytosis
Icterus —see also Jaundice
  conjunctiva R17
  newborn P59.9
  gravis, newborn P55.0
  hematogenous (acquired) D59.9
  hemolytic (acquired) D59.9
    congenital —see Spherocytosis
  hemorrhagic (acute) (leptospiral) (spirochetal)
  A27.0
    newborn P53
  infectious B15.9
    with hepatic coma B15.0
    leptospiral A27.0
    spirochetal A27.0
  neonatorum —see Jaundice, newborn
  spirochetal A27.0
Ictus solaris, solis T67.0
Ideation
  homicidal R45.850
  suicidal R45.851
Identity disorder (child) F64.9
  gender role F64.2
  psychosexual F64.2
Id reaction (due to bacteria) L30.2
Idioglossia F80.0
Idiopathic —see condition
Idiot, idiocy (congenital) F73
  amaurotic (Bielschowsky(-Jansky)) (family)
  (infantile (late)) (juvenile (late)) (Vogt-
  Spielmeyer) E75.4
  microcephalic Q02
IgE asthma J45.909
IIAC (idiopathic infantile arterial calcification)
  Q28.8
Ileitis (chronic) (noninfectious) (see also
  Enteritis) K52.9
  backwash —see Pancolitis, ulcerative
  (chronic)
  infectious A09
  regional (ulcerative) —see Enteritis, regional,
  small intestine
  segmental —see Enteritis, regional
  terminal (ulcerative) —see Enteritis, regional,
  small intestine
Ileocolitis (see also Enteritis) K52.9
  regional —see Enteritis, regional
  infectious A09
Ileostomy
  attention to Z43.2
  malfunctioning K94.13
  status Z93.2
    with complication —see Complications,
    enterostomy
Ileotyphus —see Typhoid
Ileum —see condition
Ileus (bowel) (colon) (inhibitory) (intestine)
  K56.7
  adynamic K56.0
  due to gallstone (in intestine) K56.3
  duodenal (chronic) K31.5
  gallstone K56.3
  mechanical NEC K56.69

Ileus – continued
  meconium P76.0
    in cystic fibrosis E84.11
    meaning meconium plug (without cystic
    fibrosis) P76.0
  myxedema K59.8
  neurogenic K56.0
    Hirschsprung's disease or megacolon Q43.1
  newborn
    due to meconium P76.0
    in cystic fibrosis E84.11
    meaning meconium plug (without cystic
    fibrosis) P76.0
    transitory P76.1
  obstructive K56.69
  paralytic K56.0
Iliac —see condition
Iliotibial band syndrome M76.3
Illiteracy Z55.0
Illness (see also Disease) R69
  manic-depressive —see Disorder, bipolar
Imbalance R26.89
  autonomic G90.8
  constituents of food intake E63.1
  electrolyte E87.8
    with
      abortion —see Abortion by type,
    complicated by, electrolyte imbalance
      molar pregnancy O08.5
    due to hyperemesis gravidarum O21.1
    following ectopic or molar pregnancy O08.5
    neonatal, transitory NEC P74.4
      potassium P74.3
      sodium P74.2
  endocrine E34.9
  eye muscle NOS H50.9
  hormone E34.9
  hysterical F44.4
  labyrinth —see subcategory H83.2
  posture R29.3
  protein-energy —see Malnutrition
  sympathetic G90.8
Imbecile, imbecility (I.Q.35 49) F71
Imbedding, intrauterine device T83.39
Imbibition, cholesterol (gallbladder) K82.4
Imbrication, teeth,, fully erupted M26.30
Imerslund (-Gräsbeck) **syndrome** D51.1
Immature —see also Immaturity
  birth (less than 37 completed weeks) —see
  Preterm, newborn
    extremely (less than 28 completed weeks)
    —see Immaturity, extreme
  personality F60.89
Immaturity (less than 37 completed weeks) —
  see also Preterm, newborn
  extreme of newborn (less than 28 completed
  weeks of gestation) (less than 196 completed
  days of gestation) (unspecified weeks of
  gestation) P07.20
    gestational age
      23 completed weeks (23 weeks, 0 days
      through 23 weeks, 6 days) P07.22
      24 completed weeks (24 weeks, 0 days
      through 24 weeks, 6 days) P07.23
      25 completed weeks (25 weeks, 0 days
      through 25 weeks, 6 days) P07.24
      26 completed weeks (26 weeks, 0 days
      through 26 weeks, 6 days) P07.25
      27 completed weeks (27 weeks, 0 days
      through 27 weeks, 6 days) P07.26
      less than 23 completed weeks P07.21
  fetus or infant light-for-dates —see Light-for-
  dates

Immaturity - *continued*
lung, newborn P28.0
organ or site NEC —*see* Hypoplasia
pulmonary, newborn P28.0
reaction F60.89
sexual (female) (male) , after puberty E30.0
Immersion T75.1
hand T69.01
foot T69.02
Immobile, immobility
complete, due to severe physical disability or
frailty R53.2
intestine K59.8
syndrome (paraplegic) M62.3
Immune reconstitution (inflammatory)
syndrome -IRIS] D89.3
Immunization —*see also* Vaccination
ABO —*see* Incompatibility, ABO
in newborn P55.1
complication —*see* Complications,
vaccination
encounter for Z23
not done (not carried out) Z28.9
because (of)
acute illness of patient Z28.01
allergy to vaccine (or component) Z28.04
caregiver refusal Z28.82
chronic illness of patient Z28.02
contraindication NEC Z28.09
group pressure Z28.1
guardian refusal Z28.82
immune compromised state of patient
Z28.03
parent refusal Z28.82
patient's belief Z28.1
patient had disease being vaccinated
against Z28.81
patient refusal Z28.21
religious beliefs of patient Z28.1
specified reason NEC Z28.89
of patient Z28.29
unspecified patient reason Z28.20
Rh factor
affecting management of pregnancy NEC
O36.09
anti-D antibody O36.01
from transfusion —*see* Complication(s) ,
transfusion, incompatibility reaction, Rh
(factor)
Immunocytoma C83.0
Immunodeficiency D84.9
with
adenosine-deaminase deficiency D81.3
antibody defects D80.9
specified type NEC D80.8
hyperimmunoglobulinemia D80.6
increased immunoglobulin M (IgM) D80.5
major defect D82.9
specified type NEC D82.8
partial albinism D82.8
short-limbed stature D82.2
thrombocytopenia and eczema D82.0
antibody with
hyperimmunoglobulinemia D80.6
near-normal immunoglobulins D80.6
autosomal recessive, Swiss type D80.0
combined D81.9
biotin-dependent carboxylase D81.819
biotinidase D81.810
holocarboxylase synthetase D81.818
specified type NEC D81.818
severe (SCID) D81.9

Immunodeficiency – *continued*
with
low or normal B-cell numbers D81.2
low T and B-cell numbers D81.1
reticular dysgenesis D81.0
specified type NEC D81.89
common variable D83.9
with
abnormalities of B-cell numbers and
function D83.0
autoantibodies to B or T-cells D83.2
immunoregulatory T-cell disorders D83.1
specified type NEC D83.8
following hereditary defective response to
Epstein-Barr virus (EBV) D82.3
selective, immunoglobulin
A (IgA) D80.2
G (IgG) (subclasses) D80.3
M (IgM) D80.4
severe combined (SCID) D81.9
specified type NEC D84.8
X-linked, with increased IgM D80.5
Immunotherapy (encounter for)
antineoplastic Z51.12
Impaction, impacted
bowel, colon, rectum (*see also* Impaction,
fecal) K56.49
by gallstone K56.3
calculus —*see* Calculus
cerumen (ear) (external) H61.2
cuspid —*see* Impaction, tooth
dental (same or adjacent tooth) K01.1
fecal, feces K56.41
fracture —*see* Fracture, by site
gallbladder —*see* Calculus, gallbladder
gallstone (s) —*see* Calculus, gallbladder
bile duct (common) (hepatic) —*see*
Calculus, bile duct
cystic duct —*see* Calculus, gallbladder
in intestine, with obstruction (any part)
K56.3
intestine (calculous) NEC (*see also*
Impaction, fecal) K56.49
gallstone, with ileus K56.3
intrauterine device (IUD) T83.39
molar —*see* Impaction, tooth
shoulder, causing obstructed labor O66.0
tooth, teeth K01.1
turbinate J34.89
Impaired, impairment (function)
auditory discrimination —*see* Abnormal,
auditory perception
cognitive, mild, so stated G31.84
dual sensory Z73.82
fasting glucose R73.01
glucose tolerance (oral) R73.02
hearing —*see* Deafness
heart —*see* Disease, heart
kidney N28.9
disorder resulting from N25.9
specified NEC N25.89
liver K72.90
with coma K72.91
mastication K08.8
mild cognitive, so stated G31.84
mobility
ear ossicles —*see* Ankylosis, ear ossicles
requiring care provider Z74.09
myocardium, myocardial —*see* Insufficiency,
myocardial
rectal sphincter R19.8
renal (acute) (chronic) N28.9

Impaired, impairment – *continued*
disorder resulting from N25.9
specified NEC N25.89
vision NEC H54.7
both eyes H54.3
Impediment, speech R47.9
psychogenic (childhood) F98.8
slurring R47.81
specified NEC R47.89
Impending
coronary syndrome I20.0
delirium tremens F10.239
myocardial infarction I20.0
Imperception auditory (acquired) —*see also*
Deafness
congenital H93.25
Imperfect
aeration, lung (newborn) NEC —*see*
Atelectasis
closure (congenital)
alimentary tract NEC Q45.8
lower Q43.8
upper Q40.8
atrioventricular ostium Q21.2
atrium (secundum) Q21.1
branchial cleft or sinus Q18.0
choroid Q14.3
cricoid cartilage Q31.8
cusps, heart valve NEC Q24.8
pulmonary Q22.3
ductus
arteriosus Q25.0
Botalli Q25.0
ear drum (causing impairment of hearing)
Q16.4
esophagus with communication to bronchus
or trachea Q39.1
eyelid Q10.3
foramen
botalli Q21.1
ovale Q21.1
genitalia, genital organ (s) or system
female Q52.8
external Q52.79
internal NEC Q52.8
male Q55.8
glottis Q31.8
interatrial ostium or septum Q21.1
interauricular ostium or septum Q21.1
interventricular ostium or septum Q21.0
larynx Q31.8
lip —*see* Cleft, lip
nasal septum Q30.3
nose Q30.2
omphalomesenteric duct Q43.0
optic nerve entry Q14.2
organ or site not listed —*see* Anomaly, by
site
ostium
interatrial Q21.1
interauricular Q21.1
interventricular Q21.0
palate —*see* Cleft, palate
preauricular sinus Q18.1
retina Q14.1
roof of orbit Q75.8
sclera Q13.5
septum
aorticopulmonary Q21.4
atrial (secundum) Q21.1
between aorta and pulmonary artery Q21.4
heart Q21.9
interatrial (secundum) Q21.1

Imperfect - *continued*
  interauricular (secundum) Q21.1
  interventricular Q21.0
    in tetralogy of Fallot Q21.3
  nasal Q30.3
  ventricular Q21.0
    with pulmonary stenosis or atresia,
dextroposition of aorta, and hypertrophy of
right ventricle Q21.3
      in tetralogy of Fallot Q21.3
  skull Q75.0
    with
      anencephaly Q00.0
      encephalocele —*see* Encephalocele
      hydrocephalus Q03.9
        with spina bifida —*see* Spina bifida, by
site, with hydrocephalus
      microcephaly Q02
  spine (with meningocele) —*see* Spina bifida
  trachea Q32.1
  tympanic membrane (causing impairment of
hearing) Q16.4
  uterus Q51.818
  vitelline duct Q43.0
  erection —*see* Dysfunction, sexual, male,
erectile
  fusion —*see* Imperfect, closure
  inflation, lung (newborn) —*see* Atelectasis
  posture R29.3
  rotation, intestine Q43.3
  septum, ventricular Q21.0
Imperfectly descended testis — *see*
Cryptorchid
Imperforate (congenital) —*see also* Atresia
  anus Q42.3
    with fistula Q42.2
  cervix (uteri) Q51.828
  esophagus Q39.0
    with tracheoesophageal fistula Q39.1
  hymen Q52.3
  jejunum Q41.1
  pharynx Q38.8
  rectum Q42.1
    with fistula Q42.0
  urethra Q64.39
  vagina Q52.4
Impervious (congenital) —*see also* Atresia
  anus Q42.3
    with fistula Q42.2
  bile duct Q44.2
  esophagus Q39.0
    with tracheoesophageal fistula Q39.1
  intestine (small) Q41.9
    large Q42.9
      specified NEC Q42.8
  rectum Q42.1
    with fistula Q42.0
  ureter —*see* Atresia, ureter
  urethra Q64.39
Impetiginization of dermatoses L01.1
Impetigo (any organism) (any site) (circinate)
(contagiosa) (simplex) (vulgaris) L01.00
  Bockhart's L01.02
  bullous, bullosa L01.03
  external ear L01.00 *[H62.40]*
  follicularis L01.02
  furfuracea L30.5
  herpetiformis L40.1
    nonobstetrical L40.1
  neonatorum L01.03
  nonbullous L01.01
  specified type NEC L01.09
  ulcerative L01.09

Impingement (on teeth)
  soft tissue
    anterior M26.81
    posterior M26.82
Implant, endometrial N80.9
Implantation
  anomalous —*see* Anomaly, by site
    ureter Q62.63
  cyst
    external area or site (skin) NEC L72.0
    iris —*see* Cyst, iris, implantation
    vagina N89.8
    vulva N90.7
  dermoid (cyst) —*see* Implantation, cyst
Impotence (sexual) N52.9
  counseling Z70.1
  organic origin (*see also* Dysfunction, sexual,
male, erectile) N52.9
  psychogenic F52.21
Impression, basilar Q75.8
Imprisonment, anxiety concerning Z65.1
Improper care (child) (newborn) —*see*
Maltreatment
Improperly tied umbilical cord (causing
hemorrhage) P51.8
Impulsiveness (impulsive) R45.87
Inability to swallow —*see* Aphagia
Inaccessible, inaccessibility
  health care NEC Z75.3
    due to
      waiting period Z75.2
        for admission to facility elsewhere Z75.1
  other helping agencies Z75.4
Inactive —*see* condition
Inadequate, inadequacy
  aesthetics of dental restoration K08.56
  biologic, constitutional, functional, or social
F60.7
  development
    child R62.50
    genitalia
      after puberty NEC E30.0
      congenital
        female Q52.8
          external Q52.79
          internal Q52.8
        male Q55.8
    lungs Q33.6
      associated with short gestation P28.0
    organ or site not listed —*see* Anomaly, by
site
  diet (causing nutritional deficiency) E63.9
  eating habits Z72.4
  environment, household Z59.1
  family support Z63.8
  food (supply) NEC Z59.4
    hunger effects T73.0
  functional F60.7
  household care, due to
    family member
      handicapped or ill Z74.2
      on vacation Z75.5
      temporarily away from home Z74.2
    technical defects in home Z59.1
    temporary absence from home of person
rendering care Z74.2
  housing (heating) (space) Z59.1
  income (financial) Z59.6
  intrafamilial communication Z63.8
  material resources Z59.9
  mental —*see* Disability, intellectual
  parental supervision or control of child Z62.0
  personality F60.7

Inadequate, inadequacy – *continued*
  pulmonary
    function R06.89
      newborn P28.5
    ventilation, newborn P28.5
  sample of cytologic smear
    anus R85.615
    cervix R87.615
    vagina R87.625
  social F60.7
    insurance Z59.7
    skills NEC Z73.4
  supervision of child by parent Z62.0
  teaching affecting education Z55.8
  welfare support Z59.7
Inanition R64
  with edema —*see* Malnutrition, severe
  due to
    deprivation of food T73.0
    malnutrition —*see* Malnutrition
  fever R50.9
Inappropriate
  change in quantitative human chorionic
gonadotropin (hCG) in early pregnancy
O02.81
  diet or eating habits Z72.4
  level of quantitative human chorionic
gonadotropin (hCG) for gestational age in
early pregnancy O02.81
  secretion
    antidiuretic hormone (ADH) (excessive)
E22.2
      deficiency E23.2
    pituitary (posterior) E22.2
Inattention at or after birth —*see* Neglect
Incarceration, incarcerated
  enterocele K46.0
    gangrenous K46.1
  epiplocele K46.0
    gangrenous K46.1
  exophthalmos K42.0
    gangrenous K42.1
  hernia —*see also* Hernia, by site, with
obstruction
    with gangrene —*see* Hernia, by site, with
gangrene
  iris, in wound —*see* Injury, eye, laceration,
with prolapse
  lens, in wound —*see* Injury, eye, laceration,
with prolapse
  omphalocele K42.0
  prison, anxiety concerning Z65.1
  rupture —*see* Hernia, by site
  sarcoepiplocele K46.0
    gangrenous K46.1
  sarcoepiplomphalocele K42.0
    with gangrene K42.1
  uterus N85.8
    gravid O34.51
      causing obstructed labor O65.5
Incised wound
  external —*see* Laceration
  internal organs —*see* Injury, by site
Incision, incisional
  hernia K43.2
    with
      gangrene (and obstruction) K43.1
      obstruction K43.0
  surgical, complication —*see* Complications,
surgical procedure
  traumatic
    external —*see* Laceration
    internal organs —*see* Injury, by site

Inclusion
azurophilic leukocytic D72.0
blennorrhea (neonatal) (newborn) P39.1
gallbladder in liver (congenital) Q44.1
Incompatibility
ABO
affecting management of pregnancy O36.11
anti-A sensitization O36.11
anti-B sensitization O36.19
specified NEC O36.19
infusion or transfusion reaction —see
Complication(s) , transfusion, incompatibility
reaction, ABO
newborn P55.1
blood (group) (Duffy) (K(ell)) (Kidd)
(Lewis) (M) (S) NEC
affecting management of pregnancy O36.11
anti-A sensitization O36.11
anti-B sensitization O36.19
infusion or transfusion reaction T80.89
newborn P55.8
divorce or estrangement Z63.5
Rh (blood group) (factor) Z31.82
affecting management of pregnancy NEC
O36.09
anti-D antibody O36.01
infusion or transfusion reaction —see
Complication(s) , transfusion, incompatibility
reaction, Rh (factor)
newborn P55.0
rhesus —see Incompatibility, Rh
Incompetency, incompetent, incompetence
annular
aortic (valve) —see Insufficiency, aortic
mitral (valve) I34.0
pulmonary valve (heart) I37.1
aortic (valve) —see Insufficiency, aortic
cardiac valve —see Endocarditis
cervix, cervical (os) N88.3
in pregnancy O34.3
chronotropic I45.89
with
autonomic dysfunction G90.8
ischemic heart disease I25.89
left ventricular dysfunction I51.89
sinus node dysfunction I49.8
esophagogastric (junction) (sphincter) K22.0
mitral (valve) —see Insufficiency, mitral
pelvic fundus N81.89
pubocervical tissue N81.82
pulmonary valve (heart) I37.1
congenital Q22.3
rectovaginal tissue N81.83
tricuspid (annular) (valve) —see
Insufficiency, tricuspid
valvular —see Endocarditis
congenital Q24.8
vein, venous (saphenous) (varicose) —see
Varix, leg
Incomplete —see also condition
bladder, emptying R33.9
defecation R15.0
expansion lungs (newborn) NEC —see
Atelectasis
rotation, intestine Q43.3
Inconclusive
diagnostic imaging due to excess body fat of
patient R93.9
findings on diagnostic imaging of breast NEC
R92.8
mammogram (due to dense breasts) R92.2

Incontinence R32
anal sphincter R15.9
feces R15.9
nonorganic origin F98.1
overflow N39.490
psychogenic F45.8
rectal R15.9
reflex N39.498
stress (female) (male) N39.3
and urge N39.46
urethral sphincter R32
urge N39.41
and stress (female) (male) N39.46
urine (urinary) R32
continuous N39.45
due to cognitive impairment, or severe
physical disability or immobility R39.81
functional R39.81
mixed (stress and urge) N39.46
nocturnal N39.44
nonorganic origin F98.0
overflow N39.490
post dribbling N39.43
reflex N39.498
specified NEC N39.498
stress (female) (male) N39.3
and urge N39.46
total N39.498
unaware N39.42
urge N39.41
and stress (female) (male) N39.46
Incontinentia pigmenti Q82.3
Incoordinate, incoordination
esophageal-pharyngeal (newborn) —see
Dysphagia
muscular R27.8
uterus (action) (contractions) (complicating
delivery) O62.4
Increase, increased
abnormal, in development R63.8
androgens (ovarian) E28.1
anticoagulants (antithrombin) (anti-VIIIa)
(anti-IXa) (anti-Xa) (anti-XIa) —see
Circulating anticoagulants
cold sense R20.8
estrogen E28.0
function
adrenal
cortex —see Cushing's, syndrome
medulla E27.5
pituitary (gland) (anterior) (lobe) E22.9
posterior E22.2
heat sense R20.8
intracranial pressure (benign) G93.2
permeability, capillaries I78.8
pressure, intracranial G93.2
secretion
gastrin E16.4
glucagon E16.3
pancreas, endocrine E16.9
growth hormone-releasing hormone E16.8
pancreatic polypeptide E16.8
somatostatin E16.8
vasoactive-intestinal polypeptide E16.8
sphericity, lens Q12.4
splenic activity D73.1
venous pressure I87.8
portal K76.6
Increta placenta O43.22
Incrustation, cornea, foreign body (lead)
(zinc) —see Foreign body, cornea
Incyclophoria H50.54
Incyclotropia —see Cyclotropia

Indeterminate sex Q56.4
India rubber skin Q82.8
Indigestion (acid) (bilious) (functional) K30
catarrhal K31.89
due to decomposed food NOS A05.9
nervous F45.8
psychogenic F45.8
Indirect —see condition
Induration penis plastica N48.6
Induration, indurated
brain G93.89
breast (fibrous) N64.51
puerperal, postpartum O92.29
broad ligament N83.8
chancre
anus A51.1
congenital A50.07
extragenital NEC A51.2
corpora cavernosa (penis) (plastic) N48.6
liver (chronic) K76.89
lung (black) (chronic) (fibroid) (see also
Fibrosis, lung) J84.10
essential brown J84.03
penile (plastic) N48.6
phlebitic —see Phlebitis
skin R23.4
Inebriety (without dependence) —see Alcohol,
intoxication
Inefficiency, kidney N28.9
Inelasticity, skin R23.4
Inequality, leg (length) (acquired) —see also
Deformity, limb, unequal length
congenital —see Defect, reduction, lower
limb
lower leg —see Deformity, limb, unequal
length
Inertia
bladder (neurogenic) N31.2
stomach K31.89
psychogenic F45.8
uterus, uterine during labor O62.2
during latent phase of labor O62.0
primary O62.0
secondary O62.1
vesical (neurogenic) N31.2
Infancy, infantile, infantilism —see also
condition
celiac K90.0
genitalia, genitals (after puberty) E30.0
Herter's (nontropical sprue) K90.0
intestinal K90.0
Lorain E23.0
pancreatic K86.8
pelvis M95.5
with disproportion (fetopelvic) O33.1
causing obstructed labor O65.1
pituitary E23.0
renal N25.0
uterus —see Infantile, genitalia
Infant (s) —see also Infancy
excessive crying R68.11
irritable child R68.12
lack of care —see Neglect
liveborn (singleton) Z38.2
born in hospital Z38.00
by cesarean Z38.01
born outside hospital Z38.1
multiple NEC Z38.8
born in hospital Z38.68
by cesarean Z38.69
born outside hospital Z38.7
quadruplet Z38.8
born in hospital Z38.63

Infection, infected, infective (opportunistic) B99.9
- with
  - drug resistant organism —*see* Resistance (to) , drug —*see also* specific organism
  - lymphangitis —*see* Lymphangitis
  - organ dysfunction (acute) R65.20
    - with septic shock R65.21
- abscess (skin)
  - code by site under Abscess
- Absidia —*see* Mucormycosis
- Acanthamoeba —*see* Acanthamebiasis
- Acanthocheilonema (perstans) (streptocerca) B74.4
- accessory sinus (chronic) —*see* Sinusitis
- achorion —*see* Dermatophytosis
- Acremonium falciforme B47.0
- acromioclavicular M00.9
- Actinobacillus (actinomycetem-comitans) A28.8
  - mallei A24.0
  - muris A25.1
- Actinomadura B47.1
- Actinomyces (israelii) (*see also* Actinomycosis) A42.9
- Actinomycetales —*see* Actinomycosis
- actinomycotic NOS —*see* Actinomycosis
- adenoid (and tonsil) J03.90
  - chronic J35.02
- adenovirus NEC
  - as cause of disease classified elsewhere B97.0
  - unspecified nature or site B34.0
- aerogenes capsulatus A48.0
- aertrycke —*see* Infection, salmonella
- alimentary canal NOS —*see* Enteritis, infectious
- Allescheria boydii B48.2
- Alternaria B48.8
- alveolus, alveolar (process) K04.7
- Ameba, amebic (histolytica) —*see* Amebiasis
- amniotic fluid, sac or cavity O41.10
  - chorioamnionitis O41.12
  - placentitis O41.14
- amputation stump (surgical) —*see* Complication, amputation stump, infection
- Ancylostoma (duodenalis) B76.0
- Anisakiasis, Anisakis larvae B81.0
- anthrax —*see* Anthrax
- antrum (chronic) —*see* Sinusitis, maxillary
- anus, anal (papillae) (sphincter) K62.89
- arbovirus (arbor virus) A94
  - specified type NEC A93.8
- artificial insemination N98.0
- Ascaris lumbricoides —*see* Ascariasis
- Ascomycetes B47.0
- Aspergillus (flavus) (fumigatus) (terreus) — *see* Aspergillosis
- atypical
  - acid-fast (bacilli) —*see* Mycobacterium, atypical
  - mycobacteria —*see* Mycobacterium, atypical
  - virus A81.9
    - specified type NEC A81.89
- auditory meatus (external) —*see* Otitis, externa, infective
- auricle (ear) —*see* Otitis, externa, infective
- axillary gland (lymph) L04.2
- Bacillus A49.9
  - abortus A23.1
  - anthracis —*see* Anthrax

Infection, infected, infective – *continued*
- Ducrey's (any location) A57
- Flexner's A03.1
- Friedländer's NEC A49.8
- gas (gangrene) A48.0
- mallei A24.0
- melitensis A23.0
- paratyphoid, paratyphosus A01.4
  - A A01.1
  - B A01.2
  - C A01.3
- Shiga (-Kruse) A03.0
- suipestifer —*see* Infection, salmonella
- swimming pool A31.1
- typhosa A01.00
- welchii —*see* Gangrene, gas
- bacterial NOS A49.9
- as cause of disease classified elsewhere B96.89
  - Clostridium perfringens -C. perfringens] B96.7
  - Bacteroides fragilis -B. fragilis] B96.6
  - Enterobacter sakazakii B96.89
  - Enterococcus B95.2
  - Escherichia coli -E. coli] (*see also* Escherichia coli) B96.20
  - Helicobacter pylori -H. pylori] B96.81
  - Hemophilus influenzae -H. influenzae] B96.3
  - Klebsiella pneumoniae -K. pneumoniae] B96.1
  - Mycoplasma pneumoniae -M. pneumoniae] B96.0
  - Proteus (mirabilis) (morganii) B96.4
  - Pseudomonas (aeruginosa) (mallei) (pseudomallei) B96.5
  - Staphylococcus B95.8
    - aureus (methicillin susceptible) (MSSA) B95.61
      - methicillin resistant (MRSA) B95.62
    - specified NEC B95.7
  - Streptococcus B95.5
    - group A B95.0
    - group B B95.1
    - pneumoniae B95.3
    - specified NEC B95.4
  - Vibrio vulnificus B96.82
- specified NEC A48.8
- Bacterium
  - paratyphosum A01.4
    - A A01.1
    - B A01.2
    - C A01.3
  - typhosum A01.00
- Bacteroides NEC A49.8
  - fragilis, as cause of disease classified elsewhere B96.6
- Balantidium coli A07.0
- Bartholin's gland N75.8
- Basidiobolus B46.8
- bile duct (common) (hepatic) —*see* Cholangitis
- bladder —*see* Cystitis
- Blastomyces, blastomycotic —*see also* Blastomycosis
  - brasiliensis —*see* Paracoccidioidomycosis
  - dermatitidis —*see* Blastomycosis
  - European —*see* Cryptococcosis
  - Loboi B48.0
  - North American B40.9
  - South American —*see* Paracoccidioidomycosis

Infection, infected, infective – *continued*
- bleb, postprocedure —*see* Blebitis
- bone —*see* Osteomyelitis
- Bordetella —*see* Whooping cough
- Borrelia bergdorfi A69.20
- brain (*see also* Encephalitis) G04.90
  - membranes —*see* Meningitis
  - septic G06.0
    - meninges —*see* Meningitis, bacterial
- branchial cyst Q18.0
- breast —*see* Mastitis
- bronchus —*see* Bronchitis
- Brucella A23.9
  - abortus A23.1
  - canis A23.3
  - melitensis A23.0
  - mixed A23.8
  - specified NEC A23.8
  - suis A23.2
- Brugia (malayi) B74.1
  - timori B74.2
- bursa —*see* Bursitis, infective
- buttocks (skin) L08.9
- Campylobacter, intestinal A04.5
  - as cause of disease classified elsewhere B96.81
- Candida (albicans) (tropicalis) —*see* Candidiasis
- candiru B88.8
- Capillaria (intestinal) B81.1
  - hepatica B83.8
  - philippinensis B81.1
- cartilage —*see* Disorder, cartilage, specified type NEC
- catheter-related bloodstream (CRBSI) T80.211
- cat liver fluke B66.0
- cellulitis
  - code by site under Cellulitis
- central line-associated T80.219
  - bloodstream (CLABSI) T80.211
  - specified NEC T80.218
- Cephalosporium falciforme B47.0
- cerebrospinal —*see* Meningitis
- cervical gland (lymph) L04.0
- cervix —*see* Cervicitis
- cesarean delivery wound (puerperal) O86.0
- cestodes —*see* Infestation, cestodes
- chest J22
- Chilomastix (intestinal) A07.8
- Chlamydia, chlamydial A74.9
  - anus A56.3
  - genitourinary tract A56.2
    - lower A56.00
    - specified NEC A56.19
  - lymphogranuloma A55
  - pharynx A56.4
  - psittaci A70
  - rectum A56.3
  - sexually transmitted NEC A56.8
- cholera —*see* Cholera
- Cladosporium
  - bantianum (brain abscess) B43.1
  - carrionii B43.0
  - castellanii B36.1
  - trichoides (brain abscess) B43.1
  - werneckii B36.1
- Clonorchis (sinensis) (liver) B66.1
- Clostridium NEC
  - bifermentans A48.0
  - botulinum (food poisoning) A05.1
    - infant A48.51
    - wound A48.52

Infection, infected, infective – *continued*
  difficile
    as cause of disease classified elsewhere
      B96.89
    foodborne (disease) A04.7
    gas gangrene A48.0
    necrotizing enterocolitis A04.7
    sepsis A41.4
  gas-forming NEC A48.0
  histolyticum A48.0
  novyi, causing gas gangrene A48.0
  oedematiens A48.0
  perfringens
    as cause of disease classified elsewhere
      B96.7
    due to food A05.2
    foodborne (disease) A05.2
    gas gangrene A48.0
    sepsis A41.4
  septicum, causing gas gangrene A48.0
  sordellii, causing gas gangrene A48.0
  welchii
    as cause of disease classified elsewhere
      B96.7
    foodborne (disease) A05.2
    gas gangrene A48.0
    necrotizing enteritis A05.2
    sepsis A41.4
  Coccidioides (immitis) —*see*
    Coccidioidomycosis
  colon —*see* Enteritis, infectious
  colostomy K94.02
  common duct —*see* Cholangitis
  congenital P39.9
    Candida (albicans) P37.5
    cytomegalovirus P35.1
    hepatitis, viral P35.3
    herpes simplex P35.2
    infectious or parasitic disease P37.9
      specified NEC P37.8
    listeriosis (disseminated) P37.2
    malaria NEC P37.4
      falciparum P37.3
    Plasmodium falciparum P37.3
    poliomyelitis P35.8
    rubella P35.0
    skin P39.4
    toxoplasmosis (acute) (subacute) (chronic)
      P37.1
    tuberculosis P37.0
    urinary (tract) P39.3
    vaccinia P35.8
    virus P35.9
      specified type NEC P35.8
  Conidiobolus B46.8
  coronavirus NEC B34.2
    as cause of disease classified elsewhere
      B97.29
    severe acute respiratory syndrome (SARS
      associated) B97.21
  corpus luteum —*see* Salpingo-oophoritis
  Corynebacterium diphtheriae —*see*
    Diphtheria
  cotia virus B08.8
  Coxiella burnetii A78
  coxsackie —*see* Coxsackie
  Cryptococcus neoformans —*see*
    Cryptococcosis
  Cryptosporidium A07.2
  Cunninghamella —*see* Mucormycosis
  cyst —*see* Cyst
  cystic duct (*see also* Cholecystitis) K81.9

Infection, infected, infective – *continued*
  Cysticercus cellulosae —*see* Cysticercosis
  cytomegalovirus, cytomegaloviral B25.9
    congenital P35.1
    maternal, maternal care for (suspected)
    damage to fetus O35.3
    mononucleosis B27.10
      with
        complication NEC B27.19
        meningitis B27.12
        polyneuropathy B27.11
  delta-agent (acute) , in hepatitis B carrier
    B17.0
  dental (pulpal origin) K04.7
  Deuteromycetes B47.0
  Dicrocoelium dendriticum B66.2
  Dipetalonema (perstans) (streptocerca) B74.4
  diphtherial —*see* Diphtheria
  Diphyllobothrium (adult) (latum) (pacificum)
    B70.0
    larval B70.1
  Diplogonoporus (grandis) B71.8
  Dipylidium caninum B67.4
  Dirofilaria B74.8
  Dracunculus medinensis B72
  Drechslera (hawaiiensis) B43.8
  Ducrey Haemophilus (any location) A57
  due to or resulting from
    artificial insemination N98.0
    central venous catheter T80.219
      bloodstream T80.211
      exit or insertion site T80.212
      localized T80.212
      port or reservoir T80.212
      specified NEC T80.218
      tunnel T80.212
    device, implant or graft (*see also*
  Complications, by site and type, infection or
    inflammation) T85.79
      arterial graft NEC T82.7
      breast (implant) T85.79
      catheter NEC T85.79
        dialysis (renal) T82.7
          intraperitoneal T85.71
        infusion NEC T82.7
          spinal (epidural) (subdural) T85.79
        urinary (indwelling) T83.51
      electronic (electrode) (pulse generator)
    (stimulator)
        bone T84.7
        cardiac T82.7
        nervous system (brain) (peripheral nerve)
    (spinal) T85.79
        urinary T83.59
      fixation, internal (orthopedic) NEC —*see*
  Complication, fixation device, infection
      gastrointestinal (bile duct) (esophagus)
        T85.79
      genital NEC T83.6
      heart NEC T82.7
        valve (prosthesis) T82.6
          graft T82.7
      joint prosthesis —*see* Complication, joint
    prosthesis, infection
      ocular (corneal graft) (orbital implant)
        NEC T85.79
      orthopedic NEC T84.7
      specified NEC T85.79
      urinary NEC T83.59
      vascular NEC T82.7
      ventricular intracranial shunt T85.79
    Hickman catheter T80.219

Infection, infected, infective – *continued*
    bloodstream T80.211
    localized T80.212
    specified NEC T80.218
  immunization or vaccination T88.0
  infusion, injection or transfusion NEC
    T80.29
    acute T80.22
  injury NEC
  code by site under Wound, open
    peripherally inserted central catheter (PICC)
      T80.219
      bloodstream T80.211
      localized T80.212
      specified NEC T80.218
    portacath (port-a-cath) T80.219
      bloodstream T80.211
      localized T80.212
      specified NEC T80.218
    surgery T81.4
    triple lumen catheter T80.219
      bloodstream T80.211
      localized T80.212
      specified NEC T80.218
    umbilical venous catheter T80.219
      bloodstream T80.211
      localized T80.212
      specified NEC T80.218
  during labor NEC O75.3
  ear (middle) —*see also* Otitis media
    external —*see* Otitis, externa, infective
    inner —*see* subcategory H83.0
  Eberthella typhosa A01.00
  Echinococcus —*see* Echinococcus
  echovirus
    as cause of disease classified elsewhere
      B97.12
    unspecified nature or site B34.1
  endocardium I33.0
  endocervix —*see* Cervicitis
  Entamoeba —*see* Amebiasis
  enteric —*see* Enteritis, infectious
  Enterobacter sakazakii B96.89
  Enterobius vermicularis B80
  enterostomy K94.12
  enterovirus B34.1
    as cause of disease classified elsewhere
      B97.10
      coxsackievirus B97.11
      echovirus B97.12
      specified NEC B97.19
  Entomophthora B46.8
  Epidermophyton —*see* Dermatophytosis
  epididymis —*see* Epididymitis
  episiotomy (puerperal) O86.0
  Erysipelothrix (insidiosa) (rhusiopathiae) —
    see Erysipeloid
  erythema infectiosum B08.3
  Escherichia (E.) coli NEC A49.8
    as cause of disease classified elsewhere (*see
      also* Escherichia coli) B96.20
    congenital P39.8
      sepsis P36.4
    generalized A41.51
    intestinal —*see* Enteritis, infectious, due to,
      Escherichia coli
  ethmoidal (chronic) (sinus) —*see* Sinusitis,
    ethmoidal
  eustachian tube (ear) —*see* Salpingitis,
    eustachian
  external auditory canal (meatus) NEC —*see*
    Otitis, externa, infective

Infection, infected, infective – *continued*
eye (purulent) —*see* Endophthalmitis, purulent
eyelid —*see* Inflammation, eyelid
fallopian tube —*see* Salpingo-oophoritis
Fasciola (gigantica) (hepatica) (indica) B66.3
Fasciolopsis (buski) B66.5
filarial —*see* Infestation, filarial
finger (skin) L08.9
nail L03.01
fungus B35.1
fish tapeworm B70.0
larval B70.1
flagellate, intestinal A07.9
fluke —*see* Infestation, fluke
focal
teeth (pulpal origin) K04.7
tonsils J35.01
Fonsecaea (compactum) (pedrosoi) B43.0
food —*see* Intoxication, foodborne
foot (skin) L08.9
dermatophytic fungus B35.3
Francisella tularensis —*see* Tularemia
frontal (sinus) (chronic) —*see* Sinusitis, frontal
fungus NOS B49
beard B35.0
dermatophytic —*see* Dermatophytosis
foot B35.3
groin B35.6
hand B35.2
nail B35.1
pathogenic to compromised host only B48.8
perianal (area) B35.6
scalp B35.0
skin B36.9
foot B35.3
hand B35.2
toenails B35.1
Fusarium B48.8
gallbladder —*see* Cholecystitis
gas bacillus —*see* Gangrene, gas
gastrointestinal —*see* Enteritis, infectious
generalized NEC —*see* Sepsis
genital organ or tract
female —*see* Disease, pelvis, inflammatory
male N49.9
multiple sites N49.8
specified NEC N49.8
Ghon tubercle, primary A15.7
Giardia lamblia A07.1
gingiva (chronic) K05.10
acute K05.00
nonplaque induced K05.01
plaque induced K05.00
nonplaque induced K05.11
plaque induced K05.10
glanders A24.0
glenosporosis B48.0
Gnathostoma (spinigerum) B83.1
Gongylonema B83.8
gonococcal —*see* Gonococcus
gram-negative bacilli NOS A49.9
guinea worm B72
gum (chronic) K05.10
acute K05.00
nonplaque induced K05.01
plaque induced K05.00
nonplaque induced K05.11
plaque induced K05.10
Haemophilus —*see* Infection, Hemophilus
heart —*see* Carditis

Infection, infected, infective – *continued*
Helicobacter pylori A04.8
as cause of disease classified elsewhere B96.81
helminths B83.9
intestinal B82.0
mixed (types classifiable to more than one of the titles B65.0-B81.3 and B81.8) B81.4
specified type NEC B81.8
specified type NEC B83.8
Hemophilus
aegyptius, systemic A48.4
Ducrey (any location) A57
influenzae NEC A49.2
as cause of disease classified elsewhere B96.3
generalized A41.3
herpes (simplex) —*see also* Herpes
congenital P35.2
disseminated B00.7
zoster B02.9
herpesvirus, herpesviral —*see* Herpes
hip (joint) NEC M00.9
due to internal joint prosthesis
left T84.52
right T84.51
skin NEC L08.9
Heterophyes (heterophyes) B66.8
Histoplasma —*see* Histoplasmosis
American B39.4
capsulatum B39.4
hookworm B76.9
human
papilloma virus A63.0
T-cell lymphotropic virus type 1 (HTLV 1) B33.3
hydrocele N43.0
Hymenolepis B71.0
hypopharynx —*see* Pharyngitis
inguinal (lymph) glands L04.1
due to soft chancre A57
intervertebral disc, pyogenic M46.30
cervical region M46.32
cervicothoracic region M46.33
lumbar region M46.36
lumbosacral region M46.37
multiple sites M46.39
occipito-atlanto-axial region M46.31
sacrococcygeal region M46.38
thoracic region M46.34
thoracolumbar region M46.35
intestine, intestinal —*see* Enteritis, infectious
specified NEC A08.8
intra-amniotic affecting newborn NEC P39.2
Isospora belli or hominis A07.3
Japanese B encephalitis A83.0
jaw (bone) (lower) (upper) M27.2
joint NEC M00.9
due to internal joint prosthesis T84.50
kidney (cortex) (hematogenous) N15.9
with calculus N20.0
with hydronephrosis N13.6
following ectopic gestation O08.83
pelvis and ureter (cystic) N28.85
puerperal (postpartum) O86.21
specified NEC N15.8
Klebsiella (K.) pneumoniae NEC A49.8
as cause of disease classified elsewhere B96.1
knee (joint) NEC M00.9
joint M00.9

Infection, infected, infective – *continued*
due to internal joint prosthesis
left T84.54
right T84.53
skin L08.9
Koch's —*see* Tuberculosis
labia (majora) (minora) (acute) —*see* Vulvitis
lacrimal
gland —*see* Dacryoadenitis
passages (duct) (sac) —*see* Inflammation, lacrimal, passages
lancet fluke B66.2
larynx NEC J38.7
leg (skin) NOS L08.9
Legionella pneumophila A48.1
nonpneumonic A48.2
Leishmania —*see also* Leishmaniasis
aethiopica B55.1
braziliensis B55.2
chagasi B55.0
donovani B55.0
infantum B55.0
major B55.1
mexicana B55.1
tropica B55.1
lentivirus, as cause of disease classified elsewhere B97.31
Leptosphaeria senagalensis B47.0
Leptospira interrogans A27.9
autumnalis A27.89
canicola A27.89
hebdomadis A27.89
icterohaemorrhagiae A27.0
pomona A27.89
specified type NEC A27.89
leptospirochetal NEC —*see* Leptospirosis
Listeria monocytogenes —*see also* Listeriosis
congenital P37.2
Loa loa B74.3
with conjunctival infestation B74.3
eyelid B74.3
Loboa loboi B48.0
local, skin (staphylococcal) (streptococcal) L08.9
abscess
code by site under Abscess
cellulitis
code by site under Cellulitis
specified NEC L08.89
ulcer —*see* Ulcer, skin
Loefflerella mallei A24.0
lung (*see also* Pneumonia) J18.9
atypical Mycobacterium A31.0
spirochetal A69.8
tuberculous —*see* Tuberculosis, pulmonary
virus —*see* Pneumonia, viral
lymph gland —*see also* Lymphadenitis, acute
mesenteric I88.0
lymphoid tissue, base of tongue or posterior pharynx, NEC (chronic) J35.03
Madurella (grisea) (mycetomii) B47.0
major
following ectopic or molar pregnancy O08.0
puerperal, postpartum, childbirth O85
Malassezia furfur B36.0
Malleomyces
mallei A24.0
pseudomallei (whitmori) —*see* Melioidosis
mammary gland N61
Mansonella (ozzardi) (perstans) (streptocerca) B74.4
mastoid —*see* Mastoiditis
maxilla, maxillary M27.2

Infection, infected, infective – *continued*
   sinus (chronic) —*see* Sinusitis, maxillary
  mediastinum J98.5
  Medina (worm) B72
  meibomian cyst or gland —*see* Hordeolum
  meninges —*see* Meningitis, bacterial
  meningococcal (*see also* condition) A39.9
   adrenals A39.1
   brain A39.81
   cerebrospinal A39.0
   conjunctiva A39.89
   endocardium A39.51
   heart A39.50
    endocardium A39.51
    myocardium A39.52
    pericardium A39.53
   joint A39.83
   meninges A39.0
   meningococcemia A39.4
    acute A39.2
    chronic A39.3
   myocardium A39.52
   pericardium A39.53
   retrobulbar neuritis A39.82
   specified site NEC A39.89
  mesenteric lymph nodes or glands NEC I88.0
  Metagonimus B66.8
  metatarsophalangeal M00.9
  methicillin
   resistant Staphylococcus aureus (MRSA) A49.02
   susceptible Staphylococcus aureus (MSSA) A49.01
  Microsporum, microsporic —*see* Dermatophytosis
  mixed flora (bacterial) NEC A49.8
  Monilia —*see* Candidiasis
  Monosporium apiospermum B48.2
  mouth, parasitic B37.0
  Mucor —*see* Mucormycosis
  muscle NEC —*see* Myositis, infective
  mycelium NOS B49
  mycetoma B47.9
   actinomycotic NEC B47.1
   mycotic NEC B47.0
  Mycobacterium, mycobacterial —*see* Mycobacterium
  Mycoplasma NEC A49.3
   pneumoniae, as cause of disease classified elsewhere B96.0
  mycotic NOS B49
   pathogenic to compromised host only B48.8
   skin NOS B36.9
  myocardium NEC I40.0
  nail (chronic)
   with lymphangitis —*see* Lymphangitis, acute, digit
   finger L03.01
    fungus B35.1
   ingrowing L60.0
   toe L03.03
    fungus B35.1
  nasal sinus (chronic) —*see* Sinusitis
  nasopharynx —*see* Nasopharyngitis
  navel L08.82
  Necator americanus B76.1
  Neisseria —*see* Gonococcus
  Neotestudina rosatii B47.0
  newborn P39.9
   intra-amniotic NEC P39.2
   skin P39.4
   specified type NEC P39.8

Infection, infected, infective – *continued*
  nipple N61
   associated with
    lactation O91.03
    pregnancy O91.01
    puerperium O91.02
  Nocardia —*see* Nocardiosis
  obstetrical surgical wound (puerperal) O86.0
  Oesophagostomum (apiostomum) B81.8
  Oestrus ovis —*see* Myiasis
  Oidium albicans B37.9
  Onchocerca (volvulus) —*see* Onchocerciasis
  oncovirus, as cause of disease classified elsewhere B97.32
  operation wound T81.4
  Opisthorchis (felineus) (viverrini) B66.0
  orbit, orbital —*see* Inflammation, orbit
  orthopoxvirus NEC B08.09
  ovary —*see* Salpingo-oophoritis
  Oxyuris vermicularis B80
  pancreas (acute) K85.9
   abscess —*see* Pancreatitis, acute
   specified NEC K85.8
  papillomavirus, as cause of disease classified elsewhere B97.7
  papovavirus NEC B34.4
  Paracoccidioides brasiliensis —*see* Paracoccidioidomycosis
  Paragonimus (westermani) B66.4
  parainfluenza virus B34.8
  parameningococcus NOS A39.9
  parapoxvirus B08.60
   specified NEC B08.69
  parasitic B89
  Parastrongylus
   cantonensis B83.2
   costaricensis B81.3
  paratyphoid A01.4
   Type A A01.1
   Type B A01.2
   Type C A01.3
  paraurethral ducts N34.2
  parotid gland —*see* Sialoadenitis
  parvovirus NEC B34.3
   as cause of disease classified elsewhere B97.6
  Pasteurella NEC A28.0
   multocida A28.0
   pestis —*see* Plague
   pseudotuberculosis A28.0
   septica (cat bite) (dog bite) A28.0
   tularensis —*see* Tularemia
  pelvic, female —*see* Disease, pelvis, inflammatory
  Penicillium (marneffei) B48.4
  penis (glans) (retention) NEC N48.29
  periapical K04.5
  peridental, periodontal K05.20
   generalized K05.22
   localized K05.21
  perinatal period P39.9
   specified type NEC P39.8
  perineal repair (puerperal) O86.0
  periorbital —*see* Inflammation, orbit
  perirectal K62.89
  perirenal —*see* Infection, kidney
  peritoneal —*see* Peritonitis
  periureteral N28.89
  Petriellidium boydii B48.2
  pharynx —*see also* Pharyngitis
   coxsackievirus B08.5
   posterior, lymphoid (chronic) J35.03

Infection, infected, infective – *continued*
  Phialophora
   gougerotii (subcutaneous abscess or cyst) B43.2
   jeanselmei (subcutaneous abscess or cyst) B43.2
   verrucosa (skin) B43.0
  Piedraia hortae B36.3
  pinta A67.9
   intermediate A67.1
   late A67.2
   mixed A67.3
   primary A67.0
  pinworm B80
  pityrosporum furfur B36.0
  pleuro-pneumonia-like organism (PPLO) NEC A49.3
   as cause of disease classified elsewhere B96.0
  pneumococcus, pneumococcal NEC A49.1
   as cause of disease classified elsewhere B95.3
   generalized (purulent) A40.3
    with pneumonia J13
  Pneumocystis carinii (pneumonia) B59
  Pneumocystis jiroveci (pneumonia) B59
  port or reservoir T80.212
  postoperative T81.4
  postoperative wound T81.4
  postprocedural T81.4
  postvaccinal T88.0
  prepuce NEC N47.7
   with penile inflammation N47.6
  prion —*see* Disease, prion, central nervous system
  prostate (capsule) —*see* Prostatitis
  Proteus (mirabilis) (morganii) (vulgaris) NEC A49.8
   as cause of disease classified elsewhere B96.4
  protozoal NEC B64
   intestinal A07.9
    specified NEC A07.8
   specified NEC B60.8
  Pseudoallescheria boydii B48.2
  Pseudomonas NEC A49.8
   as cause of disease classified elsewhere B96.5
   mallei A24.0
   pneumonia J15.1
   pseudomallei —*see* Melioidosis
  puerperal O86.4
   genitourinary tract NEC O86.89
   major or generalized O85
   minor O86.4
   specified NEC O86.89
  pulmonary —*see* Infection, lung
  purulent —*see* Abscess
  Pyrenochaeta romeroi B47.0
  Q fever A78
  rectum (sphincter) K62.89
  renal —*see also* Infection, kidney
   pelvis and ureter (cystic) N28.85
  reovirus, as cause of disease classified elsewhere B97.5
  respiratory (tract) NEC J98.8
   acute J22
   chronic J98.8
   influenzal (upper) (acute) —*see* Influenza, with, respiratory manifestations NEC
   lower (acute) J22
    chronic —*see* Bronchitis, chronic
   rhinovirus J00

Infection, infected, infective – *continued*
syncytial virus, as cause of disease classified
elsewhere B97.4
upper (acute) NOS J06.9
chronic J39.8
streptococcal J06.9
viral NOS J06.9
resulting from
presence of internal prosthesis, implant,
graft —*see* Complications, by site and type,
infection
retortamoniasis A07.8
retroperitoneal NEC K68.9
retrovirus B33.3
as cause of disease classified elsewhere
B97.30
human
immunodeficiency, type 2 (HIV 2)
B97.35
T-cell lymphotropic
type I (HTLV-I) B97.33
type II (HTLV-II) B97.34
lentivirus B97.31
oncovirus B97.32
specified NEC B97.39
Rhinosporidium (seeberi) B48.1
rhinovirus
as cause of disease classified elsewhere
B97.89
unspecified nature or site B34.8
Rhizopus —*see* Mucormycosis
rickettsial NOS A79.9
roundworm (large) NEC B82.0
Ascariasis (*see also* Ascariasis) B77.9
rubella —*see* Rubella
Saccharomyces —*see* Candidiasis
salivary duct or gland (any) —*see*
Sialoadenitis
Salmonella (aertrycke) (arizonae)
(gallinarum) (cholerae-suis) (enteritidis)
(suipestifer) (typhimurium) A02.9
with
(gastro) enteritis A02.0
sepsis A02.1
specified manifestation NEC A02.8
due to food (poisoning) A02.9
hirschfeldii A01.3
localized A02.20
arthritis A02.23
meningitis A02.21
osteomyelitis A02.24
pneumonia A02.22
pyelonephritis A02.25
specified NEC A02.29
paratyphi A01.4
A A01.1
B A01.2
C A01.3
schottmuelleri A01.2
typhi, typhosa —*see* Typhoid
Sarcocystis A07.8
scabies B86
Schistosoma —*see* Infestation, Schistosoma
scrotum (acute) NEC N49.2
seminal vesicle —*see* Vesiculitis
septic
localized, skin —*see* Abscess
sheep liver fluke B66.3
Shigella A03.9
boydii A03.2
dysenteriae A03.0
flexneri A03.1

Infection, infected, infective – *continued*
group
A A03.0
B A03.1
C A03.2
D A03.3
Schmitz (-Stutzer) A03.0
schmitzii A03.0
shigae A03.0
sonnei A03.3
specified NEC A03.8
shoulder (joint) NEC M00.9
due to internal joint prosthesis T84.59
skin NEC L08.9
sinus (accessory) (chronic) (nasal) —*see also*
Sinusitis
pilonidal —*see* Sinus, pilonidal
skin NEC L08.89
Skene's duct or gland —*see* Urethritis
skin (local) (staphylococcal) (streptococcal)
L08.9
abscess
code by site under Abscess
cellulitis
code by site under Cellulitis
due to fungus B36.9
specified type NEC B36.8
mycotic B36.9
specified type NEC B36.8
newborn P39.4
ulcer —*see* Ulcer, skin
slow virus A81.9
specified NEC A81.89
Sparganum (mansoni) (proliferum) (baxteri)
B70.1
specific —*see also* Syphilis
to perinatal period —*see* Infection,
congenital
specified NEC B99.8
spermatic cord NEC N49.1
sphenoidal (sinus) —*see* Sinusitis, sphenoidal
spinal cord NOS (*see also* Myelitis) G04.91
abscess G06.1
meninges —*see* Meningitis
streptococcal G04.89
Spirillum A25.0
spirochetal NOS A69.9
lung A69.8
specified NEC A69.8
Spirometra larvae B70.1
spleen D73.89
Sporotrichum, Sporothrix (schenckii) —*see*
Sporotrichosis
staphylococcal, unspecified site
aureus (methicillin susceptible) (MSSA)
A49.01
methicillin resistant (MRSA) A49.02
as cause of disease classified elsewhere
B95.8
aureus (methicillin susceptible) (MSSA)
B95.61
methicillin resistant (MRSA) B95.62
specified NEC B95.7
food poisoning A05.0
generalized (purulent) A41.2
pneumonia —*see* Pneumonia,
staphylococcal
Stellantchasmus falcatus B66.8
streptobacillus moniliformis A25.1
streptococcal NEC A49.1
as cause of disease classified elsewhere
B95.5

Infection, infected, infective – *continued*
B genitourinary complicating
childbirth O98.82
pregnancy O98.81
puerperium O98.83
congenital
sepsis P36.10
group B P36.0
specified NEC P36.19
generalized (purulent) A40.9
Streptomyces B47.1
Strongyloides (stercoralis) —*see*
Strongyloidiasis
stump (amputation) (surgical) —*see*
Complication, amputation stump, infection
subcutaneous tissue, local L08.9
suipestifer —*see* Infection, salmonella
swimming pool bacillus A31.1
Taenia —*see* Infestation, Taenia
Taeniarhynchus saginatus B68.1
tapeworm —*see* Infestation, tapeworm
tendon (sheath) —*see* Tenosynovitis,
infective NEC
Ternidens diminutus B81.8
testis —*see* Orchitis
threadworm B80
throat —*see* Pharyngitis
thyroglossal duct K14.8
toe (skin) L08.9
cellulitis L03.03
fungus B35.1
nail L03.03
fungus B35.1
tongue NEC K14.0
parasitic B37.0
tonsil (and adenoid) (faucial) (lingual)
(pharyngeal) —*see* Tonsillitis
tooth, teeth K04.7
periapical K04.7
peridental, periodontal K05.20
generalized K05.22
localized K05.21
pulp K04.0
socket M27.3
TORCH —*see* Infection, congenital
without active infection P00.2
Torula histolytica —*see* Cryptococcosis
Toxocara (canis) (cati) (felis) B83.0
Toxoplasma gondii —*see* Toxoplasma
trachea, chronic J42
trematode NEC —*see* Infestation, fluke
trench fever A79.0
Treponema pallidum —*see* Syphilis
Trichinella (spiralis) B75
Trichomonas A59.9
cervix A59.09
intestine A07.8
prostate A59.02
specified site NEC A59.8
urethra A59.03
urogenitalis A59.00
vagina A59.01
vulva A59.01
Trichophyton, trichophytic —*see*
Dermatophytosis
Trichosporon (beigelii) cutaneum B36.2
Trichostrongylus B81.2
Trichuris (trichiura) B79
Trombicula (irritans) B88.0
Trypanosoma
brucei
gambiense B56.0
rhodesiense B56.1

Infection, infected, infective – *continued*
  cruzi —*see* Chagas' disease
  tubal —*see* Salpingo-oophoritis
  tuberculous NEC —*see* Tuberculosis
  tubo-ovarian —*see* Salpingo-oophoritis
  tunnel T80.212
  tunica vaginalis N49.1
  tympanic membrane NEC —*see* Myringitis
  typhoid (abortive) (ambulant) (bacillus) —*see*
  Typhoid
  typhus A75.9
    flea-borne A75.2
    mite-borne A75.3
    recrudescent A75.1
    tick-borne A77.9
      African A77.1
      North Asian A77.2
  umbilicus L08.82
  ureter N28.86
  urethra —*see* Urethritis
  urinary (tract) N39.0
    bladder —*see* Cystitis
    complicating
      pregnancy O23.4
        specified type NEC O23.3
    kidney —*see* Infection, kidney
    newborn P39.3
    puerperal (postpartum) O86.20
    tuberculous A18.13
    urethra —*see* Urethritis
  uterus, uterine —*see* Endometritis
  vaccination T88.0
  vaccinia not from vaccination B08.011
  vagina (acute) —*see* Vaginitis
  varicella B01.9
  varicose veins —*see* Varix
  vas deferens NEC N49.1
  vesical —*see* Cystitis
  Vibrio
    cholerae A00.0
      El Tor A00.1
    parahaemolyticus (food poisoning) A05.3
    vulnificus
      as cause of disease classified elsewhere
      B96.82
      foodborne intoxication A05.5
  Vincent's (gum) (mouth) (tonsil) A69.1
  virus, viral NOS B34.9
    adenovirus
      as cause of disease classified elsewhere
      B97.0
      unspecified nature or site B34.0
    arborvirus, arbovirus arthropod-borne A94
    as cause of disease classified elsewhere
    B97.89
    adenovirus B97.0
    coronavirus B97.29
      SARS-associated B97.21
    coxsackievirus B97.11
    echovirus B97.12
    enterovirus B97.10
      coxsackievirus B97.11
      echovirus B97.12
      specified NEC B97.19
    human
      immunodeficiency, type 2 (HIV 2)
      B97.35
      T-cell lymphotropic,
        type I (HTLV-I) B97.33
        type II (HTLV-II) B97.34
      metapneumovirus B97.81
      papillomavirus B97.7

Infection, infected, infective – *continued*
    parvovirus B97.6
    reovirus B97.5
    respiratory syncytial B97.4
    retrovirus B97.30
      human
        immunodeficiency, type 2 (HIV 2)
        B97.35
        T-cell lymphotropic,
          type I (HTLV-I) B97.33
          type II (HTLV-II) B97.34
      lentivirus B97.31
      oncovirus B97.32
      specified NEC B97.39
      specified NEC B97.89
    central nervous system A89
      atypical A81.9
        specified NEC A81.89
      enterovirus NEC A88.8
        meningitis A87.0
      slow virus A81.9
        specified NEC A81.89
      specified NEC A88.8
    chest J98.8
    cotia B08.8
    coxsackie (*see also* Infection, coxsackie)
    B34.1
    as cause of disease classified elsewhere
    B97.11
    ECHO
    as cause of disease classified elsewhere
    B97.12
    unspecified nature or site B34.1
    encephalitis, tick-borne A84.9
    enterovirus, as cause of disease classified
    elsewhere B97.10
      coxsackievirus B97.11
      echovirus B97.12
      specified NEC B97.19
    exanthem NOS B09
    human papilloma as cause of disease
    classified elsewhere B97.7
    human metapneumovirus as cause of disease
    classified elsewhere B97.81
    intestine —*see* Enteritis, viral
    respiratory syncytial
      as cause of disease classified elsewhere
      B97.4
      bronchopneumonia J12.1
      common cold syndrome J00
      nasopharyngitis (acute) J00
    rhinovirus
      as cause of disease classified elsewhere
      B97.89
      unspecified nature or site B34.8
    slow A81.9
      specified NEC A81.89
    specified type NEC B33.8
      as cause of disease classified elsewhere
      B97.89
      unspecified nature or site B34.8
    unspecified nature or site B34.9
    West Nile —*see* Virus, West Nile
  vulva (acute) —*see* Vulvitis
  West Nile —*see* Virus, West Nile
  pestis —*see* Plague
  pseudotuberculosis A28.2
  Zeis' gland —*see* Hordeolum
  zoonotic bacterial NOS A28.9
  Zopfia senagalensis B47.0
Infective, infectious —*see* condition

Infertility
  female N97.9
    age-related N97.8
    associated with
      anovulation N97.0
      cervical (mucus) disease or anomaly N88.3
      congenital anomaly
        cervix N88.3
        fallopian tube N97.1
        uterus N97.2
        vagina N97.8
      dysmucorrhea N88.3
      fallopian tube disease or anomaly N97.1
      pituitary-hypothalamic origin E23.0
      specified origin NEC N97.8
      Stein-Leventhal syndrome E28.2
      uterine disease or anomaly N97.2
      vaginal disease or anomaly N97.8
    due to
      cervical anomaly N88.3
      fallopian tube anomaly N97.1
      ovarian failure E28.39
      Stein-Leventhal syndrome E28.2
      uterine anomaly N97.2
      vaginal anomaly N97.8
    nonimplantation N97.2
    origin
      cervical N88.3
      tubal (block) (occlusion) (stenosis) N97.1
      uterine N97.2
      vaginal N97.8
  male N46.9
    azoospermia N46.01
      extratesticular cause N46.029
        drug therapy N46.021
        efferent duct obstruction N46.023
        infection N46.022
        radiation N46.024
        specified cause NEC N46.029
        systemic disease N46.025
    oligospermia N46.11
      extratesticular cause N46.129
        drug therapy N46.121
        efferent duct obstruction N46.123
        infection N46.122
        radiation N46.124
        specified cause NEC N46.129
        systemic disease N46.125
    specified type NEC N46.8
Infestation B88.9
  Acanthocheilonema (perstans) (streptocerca)
  B74.4
  Acariasis B88.0
    demodex folliculorum B88.0
    sarcoptes scabiei B86
    trombiculae B88.0
  Agamofilaria streptocerca B74.4
  Ancylostoma, ankylostoma (braziliense)
  (caninum) (ceylanicum) (duodenale) B76.0
    americanum B76.1
    new world B76.1
  Anisakis larvae, anisakiasis B81.0
  arthropod NEC B88.2
  Ascaris lumbricoides —*see* Ascariasis
  Balantidium coli A07.0
  beef tapeworm B68.1
  Bothriocephalus (latus) B70.0
    larval B70.1
  broad tapeworm B70.0
    larval B70.1
  Brugia (malayi) B74.1
    timori B74.2
  candiru B88.8

Infestation - *continued*
Capillaria
  hepatica B83.8
  philippinensis B81.1
cat liver fluke B66.0
cestodes B71.9
  diphyllobothrium —*see* Infestation,
diphyllobothrium
  dipylidiasis B71.1
  hymenolepiasis B71.0
  specified type NEC B71.8
chigger B88.0
chigo, chigoe B88.1
Clonorchis (sinensis) (liver) B66.1
coccidial A07.3
crab-lice B85.3
Cysticercus cellulosae —*see* Cysticercosis
Demodex (folliculorum) B88.0
Dermanyssus gallinae B88.0
Dermatobia (hominis) —*see* Myiasis
Dibothriocephalus (latus) B70.0
  larval B70.1
Dicrocoelium dendriticum B66.2
Diphyllobothrium (adult) (latum) (intestinal)
(pacificum) B70.0
  larval B70.1
Diplogonoporus (grandis) B71.8
Dipylidium caninum B67.4
Distoma hepaticum B66.3
dog tapeworm B67.4
Dracunculus medinensis B72
dragon worm B72
dwarf tapeworm B71.0
Echinococcus —*see* Echinococcus
Echinostomum ilocanum B66.8
Entamoeba (histolytica) —*see* Infection,
Ameba
Enterobius vermicularis B80
eyelid
  in (due to)
    leishmaniasis B55.1
    loiasis B74.3
    onchocerciasis B73.09
    phthiriasis B85.3
    parasitic NOS B89
eyeworm B74.3
Fasciola (gigantica) (hepatica) (indica) B66.3
Fasciolopsis (buski) (intestine) B66.5
filarial B74.9
  bancroftian B74.0
  conjunctiva B74.9
  due to
    Acanthocheilonema (perstans)
      (streptocerca) B74.4
    Brugia (malayi) B74.1
      timori B74.2
    Dracunculus medinensis B72
    guinea worm B72
    loa loa B74.3
    Mansonella (ozzardi) (perstans)
      (streptocerca) B74.4
    Onchocerca volvulus B73.00
      eye B73.00
      eyelid B73.09
    Wuchereria (bancrofti) B74.0
  Malayan B74.1
  ozzardi B74.4
  specified type NEC B74.8
fish tapeworm B70.0
  larval B70.1
fluke B66.9
  blood NOS —*see* Schistosomiasis

Infestation - *continued*
cat liver B66.0
  intestinal B66.5
liver (sheep) B66.3
  cat B66.0
  Chinese B66.1
  due to clonorchiasis B66.1
  oriental B66.1
lancet B66.2
lung (oriental) B66.4
sheep liver B66.3
specified type NEC B66.8
fly larvae —*see* Myiasis
Gasterophilus (intestinalis) —*see* Myiasis
Gastrodiscoides hominis B66.8
Giardia lamblia A07.1
Gnathostoma (spinigerum) B83.1
Gongylonema B83.8
guinea worm B72
helminth B83.9
  angiostrongyliasis B83.2
    intestinal B81.3
  gnathostomiasis B83.1
  hirudiniasis, internal B83.4
  intestinal B82.0
    angiostrongyliasis B81.3
    anisakiasis B81.0
    ascariasis —*see* Ascariasis
    capillariasis B81.1
    cysticercosis —*see* Cysticercosis
    diphyllobothriasis —*see* Infestation,
      diphyllobothriasis
    dracunculiasis B72
    echinococcus —*see* Echinococcosis
    enterobiasis B80
    filariasis
  —*see* Infestation, filarial
    fluke —*see* Infestation, fluke
    hookworm —*see* Infestation, hookworm
    mixed (types classifiable to more than one
of the titles B65.0-B81.3 and B81.8) B81.4
    onchocerciasis —*see* Onchocerciasis
    schistosomiasis —*see* Infestation,
schistosoma
    specified
      cestode NEC —*see* Infestation, cestode
      type NEC B81.8
    strongyloidiasis —*see* Strongyloidiasis
    taenia —*see* Infestation, taenia
    trichinellosis B75
    trichostrongyliasis B81.2
    trichuriasis B79
  specified type NEC B83.8
  syngamiasis B83.3
  visceral larva migrans B83.0
Heterophyes (heterophyes) B66.8
hookworm B76.9
  ancylostomiasis B76.0
  necatoriasis B76.1
  specified type NEC B76.8
Hymenolepis (diminuta) (nana) B71.0
intestinal NEC B82.9
leeches (aquatic) (land) —*see* Hirudiniasis
Leishmania —*see* Leishmaniasis
lice, louse —*see* Infestation, Pediculus
Linguatula B88.8
Liponyssoides sanguineus B88.0
Loa loa B74.3
  conjunctival B74.3
  eyelid B74.3
louse —*see* Infestation, Pediculus
maggots —*see* Myiasis

Infestation - *continued*
Mansonella (ozzardi) (perstans) (streptocerca)
B74.4
Medina (worm) B72
Metagonimus (yokogawai) B66.8
microfilaria streptocerca —*see*
Onchocerciasis
  eye B73.00
  eyelid B73.09
mites B88.9
  scabic B86
Monilia (albicans) —*see* Candidiasis
mouth B37.0
Necator americanus B76.1
nematode NEC (intestinal) B82.0
  Ancylostoma B76.0
  conjunctiva NEC B83.9
  Enterobius vermicularis B80
  Gnathostoma spinigerum B83.1
  physaloptera B80
  specified NEC B81.8
  trichostrongylus B81.2
  trichuris (trichuria) B79
Oesophagostomum (apiostomum) B81.8
Oestrus ovis (*see also* Myiasis) B87.9
Onchocerca (volvulus) —*see* Onchocerciasis
Opisthorchis (felineus) (viverrini) B66.0
orbit, parasitic NOS B89
Oxyuris vermicularis B80
Paragonimus (westermani) B66.4
parasite, parasitic B89
  eyelid B89
  intestinal NOS B82.9
  mouth B37.0
  skin B88.9
  tongue B37.0
Parastrongylus
  cantonensis B83.2
  costaricensis B81.3
Pediculus B85.2
  body B85.1
  capitis (humanus) (any site) B85.0
  corporis (humanus) (any site) B85.1
  head B85.0
  mixed (classifiable to more than one of the
titles B85.0-B85.3) B85.4
  pubis (any site) B85.3
Pentastoma B88.8
Phthirus (pubis) (any site) B85.3
  with any infestation classifiable to B85.0-
B85.2 B85.4
pinworm B80
pork tapeworm (adult) B68.0
protozoal NEC B64
  intestinal A07.9
    specified NEC A07.8
  specified NEC B60.8
pubic, louse B85.3
rat tapeworm B71.0
red bug B88.0
roundworm (large) NEC B82.0
  Ascariasis (*see also* Ascariasis) B77.9
sandflea B88.1
Sarcoptes scabiei B86
scabies B86
Schistosoma B65.9
  bovis B65.8
  cercariae B65.3
  haematobium B65.0
  intercalatum B65.8
  japonicum B65.2
  mansoni B65.1
  mattheei B65.8

Infestation - *continued*
   mekongi B65.8
   specified type NEC B65.8
   spindale B65.8
  screw worms —*see* Myiasis
  skin NOS B88.9
  Sparganum (mansoni) (proliferum) (baxteri)
    B70.1
   larval B70.1
  specified type NEC B88.8
  Spirometra larvae B70.1
  Stellantchasmus falcatus B66.8
  Strongyloides stercoralis —*see*
  Strongyloidiasis
  Taenia B68.9
   diminuta B71.0
   echinococcus —*see* Echinococcus
   mediocanellata B68.1
   nana B71.0
   saginata B68.1
   solium (intestinal form) B68.0
    larval form —*see* Cysticercosis
  Taeniarhynchus saginatus B68.1
  tapeworm B71.9
   beef B68.1
   broad B70.0
    larval B70.1
   dog B67.4
   dwarf B71.0
   fish B70.0
    larval B70.1
   pork B68.0
   rat B71.0
  Ternidens diminutus B81.8
  Tetranychus molestissimus B88.0
  threadworm B80
  tongue B37.0
  Toxocara (canis) (cati) (felis) B83.0
  trematode (s) NEC —*see* Infestation, fluke
  Trichinella (spiralis) B75
  Trichocephalus B79
  Trichomonas —*see* Trichomoniasis
  Trichostrongylus B81.2
  Trichuris (trichiura) B79
  Trombicula (irritans) B88.0
  Tunga penetrans B88.1
  Uncinaria americana B76.1
  Vandellia cirrhosa B88.8
  whipworm B79
  worms B83.9
   intestinal B82.0
  Wuchereria (bancrofti) B74.0

Infiltrate, infiltration
  amyloid (generalized) (localized) —*see*
  Amyloidosis
  calcareous NEC R89.7
   localized —*see* Degeneration, by site
  calcium salt R89.7
  cardiac
   fatty —*see* Degeneration, myocardial
   glycogenic E74.02 *[I43]*
  corneal —*see* Edema, cornea
  eyelid —*see* Inflammation, eyelid
  glycogen, glycogenic —*see* Disease, glycogen
  storage
  heart, cardiac
   fatty —*see* Degeneration, myocardial
   glycogenic E74.02 *[I43]*
  inflammatory in vitreous H43.89
  kidney N28.89
  leukemic —*see* Leukemia

Infiltrate, infiltration - *continued*
  liver K76.89
   fatty —*see* Fatty, liver NEC
   glycogen (*see also* Disease, glycogen
  storage) E74.03 *[K77]*
  lung R91.8
   eosinophilic J82
  lymphatic (*see also* Leukemia, lymphatic)
  C91.9
   gland I88.9
  muscle, fatty M62.89
  myocardium, myocardial
   fatty —*see* Degeneration, myocardial
   glycogenic E74.02 *[I43]*
  on chest x-ray R91.8
  pulmonary R91.8
   with eosinophilia J82
  skin (lymphocytic) L98.6
  thymus (gland) (fatty) E32.8
  urine R39.0
  vesicant agent
   antineoplastic chemotherapy T80.810
   other agent NEC T80.818
  vitreous body H43.89

Infirmity R68.89
  senile R54

Inflammation, inflamed, inflammatory (with exudation)
  abducent (nerve) —*see* Strabismus, paralytic, sixth nerve
  accessory sinus (chronic) —*see* Sinusitis
  adrenal (gland) E27.8
  alveoli, teeth M27.3
   scorbutic E54
  anal canal, anus K62.89
  antrum (chronic) —*see* Sinusitis, maxillary
  appendix —*see* Appendicitis
  arachnoid —*see* Meningitis
  areola N61
   puerperal, postpartum or gestational —*see*
  Infection, nipple
  areolar tissue NOS L08.9
  artery —*see* Arteritis
  auditory meatus (external) —*see* Otitis, externa
  Bartholin's gland N75.8
  bile duct (common) (hepatic) or passage —*see* Cholangitis
  bladder —*see* Cystitis
  bone —*see* Osteomyelitis
  brain —*see also* Encephalitis
   membrane —*see* Meningitis
  breast N61
   puerperal, postpartum, gestational —*see*
  Mastitis, obstetric
  broad ligament —*see* Disease, pelvis, inflammatory
  bronchi —*see* Bronchitis
  catarrhal J00
  cecum —*see* Appendicitis
  cerebral —*see also* Encephalitis
   membrane —*see* Meningitis
  cerebrospinal
   meningococcal A39.0
  cervix (uteri) —*see* Cervicitis
  chest J98.8
  chorioretinal H30.9
   cyclitis —*see* Cyclitis
   disseminated H30.10
    generalized H30.13
    peripheral H30.12
    posterior pole H30.11

Inflammation, inflamed – *continued*
  epitheliopathy —*see* Epitheliopathy
  focal H30.00
   juxtapapillary H30.01
   macular H30.04
   paramacular —*see* Inflammation, chorioretinal, focal, macular
   peripheral H30.03
   posterior pole H30.02
  specified type NEC H30.89
  choroid —*see* Inflammation, chorioretinal
  chronic, postmastoidectomy cavity —*see* Complications, postmastoidectomy, inflammation
  colon —*see* Enteritis
  connective tissue (diffuse) NEC —*see* Disorder, soft tissue, specified type NEC
  cornea —*see* Keratitis
  corpora cavernosa N48.29
  cranial nerve —*see* Disorder, nerve, cranial
  Douglas' cul-de-sac or pouch (chronic) N73.0
  due to device, implant or graft —*see also* Complications, by site and type, infection or inflammation
   arterial graft T82.7
   breast (implant) T85.79
   catheter T85.79
    dialysis (renal) T82.7
     intraperitoneal T85.71
    infusion T82.7
     spinal (epidural) (subdural) T85.79
    urinary (indwelling) T83.51
   electronic (electrode) (pulse generator) (stimulator)
    bone T84.7
    cardiac T82.7
    nervous system (brain) (peripheral nerve) (spinal) T85.79
    urinary T83.59
   fixation, internal (orthopedic) NEC —*see* Complication, fixation device, infection
   gastrointestinal (bile duct) (esophagus) T85.79
   genital NEC T83.6
   heart NEC T82.7
    valve (prosthesis) T82.6
     graft T82.7
   joint prosthesis —*see* Complication, joint prosthesis, infection
   ocular (corneal graft) (orbital implant) NEC T85.79
   orthopedic NEC T84.7
   specified NEC T85.79
   urinary NEC T83.59
   vascular NEC T82.7
   ventricular intracranial shunt T85.79
  duodenum K29.80
   with bleeding K29.81
  dura mater —*see* Meningitis
  ear (middle) —*see also* Otitis, media
   external —*see* Otitis, externa
   inner —*see* subcategory H83.0
  epididymis —*see* Epididymitis
  esophagus K20.9
  ethmoidal (sinus) (chronic) —*see* Sinusitis, ethmoidal
  eustachian tube (catarrhal) —*see* Salpingitis, eustachian
  eyelid H01.9
   abscess —*see* Abscess, eyelid
   blepharitis —*see* Blepharitis
   chalazion —*see* Chalazion

Inflammation, inflamed – *continued*
  dermatosis (noninfectious) —*see*
  Dermatosis, eyelid
    hordeolum —*see* Hordeolum
    specified NEC H01.8
  fallopian tube —*see* Salpingo-oophoritis
  fascia —*see* Myositis
  follicular, pharynx J31.2
  frontal (sinus) (chronic) —*see* Sinusitis,
  frontal
  gallbladder —*see* Cholecystitis
  gastric —*see* Gastritis
  gastrointestinal —*see* Enteritis
  genital organ (internal) (diffuse)
    female —*see* Disease, pelvis, inflammatory
    male N49.9
      multiple sites N49.8
      specified NEC N49.8
  gland (lymph) —*see* Lymphadenitis
  glottis —*see* Laryngitis
  granular, pharynx J31.2
  gum K05.10
    nonplaque induced K05.11
    plaque induced K05.10
  heart —*see* Carditis
  hepatic duct —*see* Cholangitis
  ileoanal (internal) pouch K91.850
  ileum —*see also* Enteritis
    regional or terminal —*see* Enteritis, regional
  intestine (any part) —*see* Enteritis
  intestinal pouch K91.850
  jaw (acute) (bone) (chronic) (lower)
  (suppurative) (upper) M27.2
  joint NEC —*see* Arthritis
    sacroiliac M46.1
  kidney —*see* Nephritis
  knee (joint) M13.169
    tuberculous A18.02
  labium (majus) (minus) —*see* Vulvitis
  lacrimal
    gland —*see* Dacryoadenitis
    passages (duct) (sac) —*see also*
  Dacryocystitis
    canaliculitis —*see* Canaliculitis, lacrimal
  larynx —*see* Laryngitis
  leg NOS L08.9
  lip K13.0
  liver (capsule) —*see also* Hepatitis
    chronic K73.9
    suppurative K75.0
  lung (acute) —*see also* Pneumonia
    chronic J98.4
  lymph gland or node —*see* Lymphadenitis
  lymphatic vessel —*see* Lymphangitis
  maxilla, maxillary M27.2
    sinus (chronic) —*see* Sinusitis, maxillary
  membranes of brain or spinal cord —*see*
  Meningitis
  meninges —*see* Meningitis
  mouth K12.1
  muscle —*see* Myositis
  myocardium —*see* Myocarditis
  nasal sinus (chronic) —*see* Sinusitis
  nasopharynx —*see* Nasopharyngitis
  navel L08.82
  nerve NEC —*see* Neuralgia
  nipple N61
    puerperal, postpartum or gestational —*see*
  Infection, nipple
  nose —*see* Rhinitis
  oculomotor (nerve) —*see* Strabismus,
  paralytic, third nerve

Inflammation, inflamed – *continued*
  optic nerve —*see* Neuritis, optic
  orbit (chronic) H05.10
    acute H05.00
      abscess —*see* Abscess, orbit
      cellulitis —*see* Cellulitis, orbit
      osteomyelitis —*see* Osteomyelitis, orbit
      periostitis —*see* Periostitis, orbital
      tenonitis —*see* Tenonitis, eye
    granuloma —*see* Granuloma, orbit
    myositis —*see* Myositis, orbital
  ovary —*see* Salpingo-oophoritis
  oviduct —*see* Salpingo-oophoritis
  pancreas (acute) —*see* Pancreatitis
  parametrium N73.0
  parotid region L08.9
  pelvis, female —*see* Disease, pelvis,
  inflammatory
  penis (corpora cavernosa) N48.29
  perianal K62.89
  pericardium —*see* Pericarditis
  perineum (female) (male) L08.9
  perirectal K62.89
  peritoneum —*see* Peritonitis
  periuterine —*see* Disease, pelvis,
  inflammatory
  perivesical —*see* Cystitis
  petrous bone (acute) (chronic) —*see* Petrositis
  pharynx (acute) —*see* Pharyngitis
  pia mater —*see* Meningitis
  pleura —*see* Pleurisy
  polyp, colon (*see also* Polyp, colon,
  inflammatory) K51.40
  prostate —*see also* Prostatitis
    specified type NEC N41.8
  rectosigmoid —*see* Rectosigmoiditis
  rectum (*see also* Proctitis) K62.89
  respiratory, upper (*see also* Infection,
  respiratory, upper) J06.9
    acute, due to radiation J70.0
    chronic, due to external agent —*see*
  condition, respiratory, chronic, due to
    due to
      chemicals, gases, fumes or vapors
  (inhalation) J68.2
      radiation J70.1
  retina —*see* Chorioretinitis
  retrocecal —*see* Appendicitis
  retroperitoneal —*see* Peritonitis
  salivary duct or gland (any) (suppurative) —
  see Sialoadenitis
  scorbutic, alveoli, teeth E54
  scrotum N49.2
  seminal vesicle —*see* Vesiculitis
  sigmoid —*see* Enteritis
  sinus —*see* Sinusitis
  Skene's duct or gland —*see* Urethritis
  skin L08.9
  spermatic cord N49.1
  sphenoidal (sinus) —*see* Sinusitis, sphenoidal
  spinal
    cord —*see* Encephalitis
    membrane —*see* Meningitis
    nerve —*see* Disorder, nerve
  spine —*see* Spondylopathy, inflammatory
  spleen (capsule) D73.89
  stomach —*see* Gastritis
  subcutaneous tissue L08.9
  suprarenal (gland) E27.8
  synovial —*see* Tenosynovitis
  tendon (sheath) NEC —*see* Tenosynovitis
  testis —*see* Orchitis

Inflammation, inflamed – *continued*
  throat (acute) —*see* Pharyngitis
  thymus (gland) E32.8
  thyroid (gland) —*see* Thyroiditis
  tongue K14.0
  tonsil —*see* Tonsillitis
  trachea —*see* Tracheitis
  trochlear (nerve) —*see* Strabismus, paralytic,
  fourth nerve
  tubal —*see* Salpingo-oophoritis
  tuberculous NEC —*see* Tuberculosis
  tubo-ovarian —*see* Salpingo-oophoritis
  tunica vaginalis N49.1
  tympanic membrane —*see* Tympanitis
  umbilicus, umbilical L08.82
  uterine ligament —*see* Disease, pelvis,
  inflammatory
  uterus (catarrhal) —*see* Endometritis
  uveal tract (anterior) NOS —*see also*
  Iridocyclitis
    posterior —*see* Chorioretinitis
  vagina —*see* Vaginitis
  vas deferens N49.1
  vein —*see also* Phlebitis
    intracranial or intraspinal (septic) G08
    thrombotic I80.9
      leg —*see* Phlebitis, leg
      lower extremity —*see* Phlebitis, leg
  vocal cord J38.3
  vulva —*see* Vulvitis
  Wharton's duct (suppurative) —*see*
  Sialoadenitis
Inflation, lung, imperfect (newborn) —*see*
  Atelectasis
Influenza (bronchial) (epidemic) (respiratory
  (upper)) (unidentified influenza virus) J11.1
    with
      digestive manifestations J11.2
      encephalopathy J11.81
      enteritis J11.2
      gastroenteritis J11.2
      gastrointestinal manifestations J11.2
      laryngitis J11.1
      myocarditis J11.82
      otitis media J11.83
      pharyngitis J11.1
      pneumonia J11.00
        specified type J11.08
      respiratory manifestations NEC J11.1
      specified manifestation NEC J11.89
  A/H5N1 (*see also* Influenza, due to, identified
  novel influenza A virus) J09.X2
  avian (*see also* Influenza, due to, identified
  novel influenza A virus) J09.X2
  bird (*see also* Influenza, due to, identified
  novel influenza A virus) J09.X2
  novel (2009) H1N1 influenza (*see also*
  Influenza, due to, identified influenza virus
  NEC) J10.1
  novel influenza A/H1N1 (*see also* Influenza,
  due to, identified influenza virus NEC) J10.1
    due to
      avian (*see also* Influenza, due to, identified
  novel influenza A virus) J09.X2
      identified influenza virus NEC J10.1
        with
          digestive manifestations J10.2
          encephalopathy J10.81
          enteritis J10.2
          gastroenteritis J10.2
          gastrointestinal manifestations J10.2
          laryngitis J10.1
          myocarditis J10.82

Influenza - *continued*
- otitis media J10.83
- pharyngitis J10.1
- pneumonia (unspecified type) J10.00
  - with same identified influenza virus J10.01
  - specified type NEC J10.08
- respiratory manifestations NEC J10.1
- specified manifestation NEC J10.89
- identified novel influenza A virus J09.X2
  - with
    - digestive manifestations J09.X3
    - encephalopathy J09.X9
    - enteritis J09.X3
    - gastroenteritis J09.X3
    - gastrointestinal manifestations J09.X3
    - laryngitis J09.X2
    - myocarditis J09.X9
    - otitis media J09.X9
    - pharyngitis J09.X2
    - pneumonia J09.X1
    - respiratory manifestations NEC J09.X2
    - specified manifestation NEC J09.X9
    - upper respiratory symptoms J09.X2
- of other animal origin, not bird or swine (*see also* Influenza, due to, identified novel influenza A virus) J09.X2
- swine (viruses that normally cause infections in pigs) (*see also* Influenza, due to, identified novel influenza A virus) J09.X2

Influenza-like disease —*see* Influenza

Influenzal —*see* Influenza

Infraction, Freiberg's (metatarsal head) —*see* Osteochondrosis, juvenile, metatarsus

Infraeruption of tooth (teeth) M26.34

Infusion complication, misadventure, or reaction —*see* Complications, infusion

Ingestion
- chemical —*see* Table of Drugs and Chemicals, by substance, poisoning
- drug or medicament
  - correct substance properly administered —*see* Table of Drugs and Chemicals, by drug, adverse effect
    - overdose or wrong substance given or taken —*see* Table of Drugs and Chemicals, by drug, poisoning
- foreign body —*see* Foreign body, alimentary tract
- tularemia A21.3

Ingrowing
- hair (beard) L73.1
- nail (finger) (toe) L60.0

Inguinal —*see also* condition
- testicle Q53.9
  - bilateral Q53.21
  - unilateral Q53.11

Inhalation
- anthrax A22.1
- flame T27.3
- food or foreign body —*see* Foreign body, by site
- gases, fumes, or vapors NEC T59.9
  - specified agent —*see* Table of Drugs and Chemicals, by substance
- liquid or vomitus —*see* Asphyxia
- meconium (newborn) P24.00
  - with
    - pneumonia (pneumonitis) P24.01
    - with respiratory symptoms P24.01
- mucus —*see* Asphyxia, mucus

Inhalation - *continued*
- oil or gasoline (causing suffocation) —*see* Foreign body, by site
- smoke J70.5
  - due to chemicals, gases, fumes and vapors J68.9
- steam —*see* Toxicity, vapors
- stomach contents or secretions —*see* Foreign body, by site
  - due to anesthesia (general) (local) or other sedation T88.59
    - in labor and delivery O74.0
    - in pregnancy O29.01
    - postpartum, puerperal O89.01

Inhibition, orgasm
- female F52.31
- male F52.32

Inhibitor, systemic lupus erythematosus (presence of) D68.62

Iniencephalus, iniencephaly Q00.2

Injection, traumatic jet (air) (industrial) (water) (paint or dye) T70.4

Injury (*see also* specified injury type) T14.90
- abdomen, abdominal S39.91
  - blood vessel —*see* Injury, blood vessel, abdomen
  - cavity —*see* Injury, intra-abdominal
  - contusion S30.1
  - internal —*see* Injury, intra-abdominal
  - intra-abdominal organ —*see* Injury, intra-abdominal
  - nerve —*see* Injury, nerve, abdomen
  - open —*see* Wound, open, abdomen
  - specified NEC S39.81
  - superficial —*see* Injury, superficial, abdomen
- Achilles tendon S86.00
  - laceration S86.02
  - specified type NEC S86.09
  - strain S86.01
- acoustic, resulting in deafness —*see* Injury, nerve, acoustic
- adrenal (gland) S37.819
  - contusion S37.812
  - laceration S37.813
  - specified type NEC S37.818
- alveolar (process) S09.93
- ankle S99.91
  - contusion —*see* Contusion, ankle
  - dislocation —*see* Dislocation, ankle
  - fracture —*see* Fracture, ankle
  - nerve —*see* Injury, nerve, ankle
  - open —*see* Wound, open, ankle
  - specified type NEC S99.81
  - sprain —*see* Sprain, ankle
  - superficial —*see* Injury, superficial, ankle
- anterior chamber, eye —*see* Injury, eye, specified site NEC
- anus —*see* Injury, abdomen
- aorta (thoracic) S25.00
  - abdominal S35.00
    - laceration (minor) (superficial) S35.01
      - major S35.02
    - specified type NEC S35.09
  - laceration (minor) (superficial) S25.01
    - major S25.02
  - specified type NEC S25.09
- arm (upper) S49.9
  - blood vessel —*see* Injury, blood vessel, arm
  - contusion —*see* Contusion, arm, upper
  - fracture —*see* Fracture, humerus
  - lower —*see* Injury, forearm

Injury – *continued*
- muscle —*see* Injury, muscle, shoulder
- nerve —*see* Injury, nerve, arm
- open —*see* Wound, open, arm
- specified type NEC S49.8
- superficial —*see* Injury, superficial, arm
- artery (complicating trauma) —*see also* Injury, blood vessel, by site
  - cerebral or meningeal —*see* Injury, intracranial
- auditory canal (external) (meatus) S09.91
- auricle, auris, ear S09.91
- axilla —*see* Injury, shoulder
- back —*see* Injury, back, lower
- bile duct S36.13
- birth (*see also* Birth, injury) P15.9
- bladder (sphincter) S37.20
  - at delivery O71.5
  - contusion S37.22
  - laceration S37.23
  - obstetrical trauma O71.5
  - specified type NEC S37.29
- blast (air) (hydraulic) (immersion) (underwater) NEC T14.8
  - acoustic nerve trauma —*see* Injury, nerve, acoustic
  - bladder —*see* Injury, bladder
  - brain —*see* Concussion
  - colon —*see* Injury, intestine, large, blast injury
  - ear (primary) S09.31
    - secondary S09.39
  - generalized T70.8
  - lung —*see* Injury, intrathoracic, lung, blast injury
  - multiple body organs T70.8
  - peritoneum S36.81
  - rectum S36.61
  - retroperitoneum S36.898
  - small intestine S36.419
    - duodenum S36.410
    - specified site NEC S36.418
  - specified
    - intra-abdominal organ NEC S36.898
    - pelvic organ NEC S37.899
- blood vessel NEC T14.8
  - abdomen S35.9
    - aorta —*see* Injury, aorta, abdominal
    - celiac artery —*see* Injury, blood vessel, celiac artery
    - iliac vessel —*see* Injury, blood vessel, iliac
    - laceration S35.91
    - mesenteric vessel —*see* Injury, mesenteric
    - portal vein —*see* Injury, blood vessel, portal vein
    - renal vessel —*see* Injury, blood vessel, renal
    - specified vessel NEC S35.8X
    - splenic vessel —*see* Injury, blood vessel, splenic
    - vena cava —*see* Injury, vena cava, inferior
  - ankle —*see* Injury, blood vessel, foot
  - aorta (abdominal) (thoracic) —*see* Injury, aorta
  - arm (upper) NEC S45.90
    - forearm —*see* Injury, blood vessel, forearm
    - laceration S45.91
    - specified
      - site NEC S45.80
        - laceration S45.81
        - specified type NEC S45.89
      - type NEC S45.99

Injury – *continued*
  superficial vein S45.30
    laceration S45.31
    specified type NEC S45.39
  axillary
    artery S45.00
      laceration S45.01
      specified type NEC S45.09
    vein S45.20
      laceration S45.21
      specified type NEC S45.29
  azygos vein —*see* Injury, blood vessel, thoracic, specified site NEC
  brachial
    artery S45.10
      laceration S45.11
      specified type NEC S45.19
    vein S45.20
      laceration S45.219
      specified type NEC S45.29
  carotid artery (common) (external) (internal, extracranial) S15.00
    internal, intracranial S06.8
    laceration (minor) (superficial) S15.01
      major S15.02
    specified type NEC S15.09
  celiac artery S35.219
    branch S35.299
      laceration (minor) (superficial) S35.291
        major S35.292
      specified NEC S35.298
    laceration (minor) (superficial) S35.211
      major S35.212
    specified type NEC S35.218
  cerebral —*see* Injury, intracranial
  deep plantar —*see* Injury, blood vessel, plantar artery
  digital (hand) —*see* Injury, blood vessel, finger
  dorsal
    artery (foot) S95.00
      laceration S95.01
      specified type NEC S95.09
    vein (foot) S95.20
      laceration S95.21
      specified type NEC S95.29
  due to accidental laceration during procedure —*see* Laceration, accidental complicating surgery
  extremity —*see* Injury, blood vessel, limb
  femoral
    artery (common) (superficial) S75.00
      laceration (minor) (superficial) S75.01
        major S75.02
      specified type NEC S75.09
    vein (hip level) (thigh level) S75.10
      laceration (minor) (superficial) S75.11
        major S75.12
      specified type NEC S75.19
  finger S65.50
    index S65.50
      laceration S65.51
      specified type NEC S65.59
    laceration S65.51
    little S65.50
      laceration S65.51
      specified type NEC S65.59
    middle S65.50
      laceration S65.51
      specified type NEC S65.59
    specified type NEC S65.59
    thumb —*see* Injury, blood vessel, thumb

Injury – *continued*
  foot S95.90
    dorsal
      artery —*see* Injury, blood vessel, dorsal, artery
      vein —*see* Injury, blood vessel, dorsal, vein
    laceration S95.91
    plantar artery —*see* Injury, blood vessel, plantar artery
    specified
      site NEC S95.80
        laceration S95.81
        specified type NEC S95.89
      specified type NEC S95.99
  forearm S55.90
    laceration S55.91
    radial artery —*see* Injury, blood vessel, radial artery
    specified
      site NEC S55.80
        laceration S55.81
        specified type NEC S55.89
      type NEC S55.99
    ulnar artery —*see* Injury, blood vessel, ulnar artery
      vein S55.20
        laceration S55.21
        specified type NEC S55.29
  gastric
    artery —*see* Injury, mesenteric, artery, branch
    vein —*see* Injury, blood vessel, abdomen
  gastroduodenal artery —*see* Injury, mesenteric, artery, branch
  greater saphenous vein (lower leg level) S85.30
    hip (and thigh) level S75.20
      laceration (minor) (superficial) S75.21
        major S75.22
      specified type NEC S75.29
    laceration S85.31
    specified type NEC S85.39
  hand (level) S65.90
    finger —*see* Injury, blood vessel, finger
    laceration S65.91
    palmar arch —*see* Injury, blood vessel, palmar arch
    radial artery —*see* Injury, blood vessel, radial artery, hand
    specified
      site NEC S65.80
        laceration S65.81
        specified type NEC S65.89
      type NEC S65.99
    thumb —*see* Injury, blood vessel, thumb
    ulnar artery —*see* Injury, blood vessel, ulnar artery, hand
  head S09.0
    intracranial —*see* Injury, intracranial
    multiple S09.0
  hepatic
    artery —*see* Injury, mesenteric, artery
    vein —*see* Injury, vena cava, inferior
  hip S75.90
    femoral artery —*see* Injury, blood vessel, femoral, artery
    femoral vein —*see* Injury, blood vessel, femoral, vein
    greater saphenous vein —*see* Injury, blood vessel, greater saphenous, hip level
    laceration S75.91

Injury – *continued*
  specified
    site NEC S75.80
      laceration S75.81
      specified type NEC S75.89
    type NEC S75.99
  hypogastric (artery) (vein) —*see* Injury, blood vessel, iliac
  iliac S35.5
    artery S35.51
    specified vessel NEC S35.5
    uterine vessel —*see* Injury, blood vessel, uterine
    vein S35.51
  innominate —*see* Injury, blood vessel, thoracic, innominate
  intercostal (artery) (vein) —*see* Injury, blood vessel, thoracic, intercostal
  jugular vein (external) S15.20
    internal S15.30
      laceration (minor) (superficial) S15.31
        major S15.32
      specified type NEC S15.39
    laceration (minor) (superficial) S15.21
      major S15.22
    specified type NEC S15.29
  leg (level) (lower) S85.90
    greater saphenous —*see* Injury, blood vessel, greater saphenous
    laceration S85.91
    lesser saphenous —*see* Injury, blood vessel, lesser saphenous
    peroneal artery —*see* Injury, blood vessel, peroneal artery
    popliteal
      artery —*see* Injury, blood vessel, popliteal, artery
      vein —*see* Injury, blood vessel, popliteal, vein
    specified
      site NEC S85.80
        laceration S85.81
        specified type NEC S85.89
      type NEC S85.99
    thigh —*see* Injury, blood vessel, hip
    tibial artery —*see* Injury, blood vessel, tibial artery
  lesser saphenous vein (lower leg level) S85.40
    laceration S85.41
    specified type NEC S85.49
  limb
    lower —*see* Injury, blood vessel, leg
    upper —*see* Injury, blood vessel, arm
    lower back —*see* Injury, blood vessel, abdomen
    specified NEC —*see* Injury, blood vessel, abdomen, specified, site NEC
  mammary (artery) (vein) —*see* Injury, blood vessel, thoracic, specified site NEC
  mesenteric (inferior) (superior)
    artery —*see* Injury, mesenteric, artery
    vein —*see* Injury, mesenteric, vein
  neck S15.9
    specified site NEC S15.8
  ovarian (artery) (vein) —see subcategory S35.8
  palmar arch (superficial) S65.20
    deep S65.30
      laceration S65.31
      specified type NEC S65.39
    laceration S65.21

Injury – *continued*

specified type NEC S65.29
pelvis —*see* Injury, blood vessel, abdomen
specified NEC —*see* Injury, blood vessel, abdomen, specified, site NEC
peroneal artery S85.20
  laceration S85.21
  specified type NEC S85.29
plantar artery (deep) (foot) S95.10
  laceration S95.11
  specified type NEC S95.19
popliteal
  artery S85.00
    laceration S85.01
    specified type NEC S85.09
  vein S85.50
    laceration S85.51
    specified type NEC S85.59
portal vein S35.319
  laceration S35.311
  specified type NEC S35.318
precerebral —*see* Injury, blood vessel, neck
pulmonary (artery) (vein) —*see* Injury, blood vessel, thoracic, pulmonary
radial artery (forearm level) S55.10
  hand and wrist (level) S65.10
    laceration S65.11
    specified type NEC S65.19
  laceration S55.11
  specified type NEC S55.19
renal
  artery S35.40
    laceration S35.41
    specified NEC S35.49
  vein S35.40
    laceration S35.41
    specified NEC S35.49
saphenous vein (greater) (lower leg level) —*see* Injury, blood vessel, greater saphenous
  hip and thigh level —*see* Injury, blood vessel, greater saphenous, hip level
  lesser —*see* Injury, blood vessel, lesser saphenous
shoulder
  specified NEC —*see* Injury, blood vessel, arm, specified site NEC
  superficial vein —*see* Injury, blood vessel, arm, superficial vein
specified NEC T14.8
splenic
  artery —*see* Injury, blood vessel, celiac artery, branch
  vein S35.329
    laceration S35.321
    specified NEC S35.328
subclavian —*see* Injury, blood vessel, thoracic, innominate
thigh —*see* Injury, blood vessel, hip
thoracic S25.90
  aorta S25.00
    laceration (minor) (superficial) S25.01
    major S25.02
    specified type NEC S25.09
  azygos vein —*see* Injury, blood vessel, thoracic, specified, site NEC
  innominate
    artery S25.10
      laceration (minor) (superficial) S25.11
      major S25.12
      specified type NEC S25.19
    vein S25.30
      laceration (minor) (superficial) S25.31

major S25.32
  specified type NEC S25.39
intercostal S25.50
  laceration S25.51
  specified type NEC S25.59
laceration S25.91
mammary vessel —*see* Injury, blood vessel, thoracic, specified, site NEC
pulmonary S25.40
  laceration (minor) (superficial) S25.41
  major S25.42
  specified type NEC S25.49
specified
  site NEC S25.80
    laceration S25.81
    specified type NEC S25.89
  type NEC S25.99
subclavian —*see* Injury, blood vessel, thoracic, innominate
vena cava (superior) S25.20
  laceration (minor) (superficial) S25.21
  major S25.22
  specified type NEC S25.29
thumb S65.40
  laceration S65.41
  specified type NEC S65.49
tibial artery S85.10
  anterior S85.13
    laceration S85.14
    specified injury NEC S85.15
  laceration S85.11
  posterior S85.16
    laceration S85.17
    specified injury NEC S85.18
  specified injury NEC S85.12
ulnar artery (forearm level) S55.00
  hand and wrist (level) S65.00
    laceration S65.01
    specified type NEC S65.09
  laceration S55.01
  specified type NEC S55.09
upper arm (level) —*see* Injury, blood vessel, arm
  superficial vein —*see* Injury, blood vessel, arm, superficial vein
uterine S35.5
  artery S35.53
  vein S35.53
vena cava —*see* Injury, vena cava
vertebral artery S15.10
  laceration (minor) (superficial) S15.11
  major S15.12
  specified type NEC S15.19
wrist (level) —*see* Injury, blood vessel, hand
brachial plexus S14.3
  newborn P14.3
brain (traumatic) S06.9
  diffuse (axonal) S06.2X
  focal S06.30
  traumatic —*see* category S06
brainstem S06.38
breast NOS S29.9
broad ligament —*see* Injury, pelvic organ, specified site NEC
bronchus, bronchi —*see* Injury, intrathoracic, bronchus
brow S09.90
buttock S39.92
canthus, eye S05.90
cardiac plexus —*see* Injury, nerve, thorax, sympathetic

cauda equina S34.3
cavernous sinus —*see* Injury, intracranial
cecum —*see* Injury, colon
celiac ganglion or plexus —*see* Injury, nerve, lumbosacral, sympathetic
cerebellum —*see* Injury, intracranial
cerebral —*see* Injury, intracranial
cervix (uteri) —*see* Injury, uterus
cheek (wall) S09.93
chest —*see* Injury, thorax
childbirth (newborn) —*see also* Birth, injury
  maternal NEC O71.9
chin S09.93
choroid (eye) —*see* Injury, eye, specified site NEC
clitoris S39.94
coccyx —*see also* Injury, back, lower
  complicating delivery O71.6
colon —*see* Injury, intestine, large
common bile duct —*see* Injury, liver
conjunctiva (superficial) —*see* Injury, eye, conjunctiva
conus medullaris —*see* Injury, spinal, sacral cord
  spermatic (pelvic region) S37.898
    scrotal region S39.848
  spinal —*see* Injury, spinal cord, by region
cornea —*see* Injury, eye, specified site NEC
  abrasion —*see* Injury, eye, cornea, abrasion
cortex (cerebral) —*see also* Injury, intracranial
  visual —*see* Injury, nerve, optic
costal region NEC S29.9
costochondral NEC S29.9
cranial
  cavity —*see* Injury, intracranial
  nerve —*see* Injury, nerve, cranial
crushing —*see* Crush
cutaneous sensory nerve
cystic duct —*see* Injury, liver
deep tissue —*see* Contusion, by site
  meaning pressure ulcer —*see* Ulcer, pressure, unstageable, by site
delivery (newborn) P15.9
  maternal NEC O71.9
Descemet's membrane —*see* Injury, eyeball, penetrating
diaphragm —*see* Injury, intrathoracic, diaphragm
duodenum —*see* Injury, intestine, small, duodenum
ear (auricle) (external) (canal) S09.91
  abrasion —*see* Abrasion, ear
  bite —*see* Bite, ear
  blister —*see* Blister, ear
  bruise —*see* Contusion, ear
  contusion —*see* Contusion, ear
  external constriction —*see* Constriction, external, ear
  hematoma —*see* Hematoma, ear
  inner —*see* Injury, ear, middle
  laceration —*see* Laceration, ear
  middle S09.30
    blast —*see* Injury, blast, ear
    specified NEC S09.39
  puncture —*see* Puncture, ear
  superficial —*see* Injury, superficial, ear
eighth cranial nerve (acoustic or auditory) —*see* Injury, nerve, acoustic
elbow S59.90
  contusion —*see* Contusion, elbow
  dislocation —*see* Dislocation, elbow

Injury – *continued*
  fracture —*see* Fracture, ulna, upper end
  open —*see* Wound, open, elbow
  specified NEC S59.80
  sprain —*see* Sprain, elbow
  superficial —*see* Injury, superficial, elbow
 eleventh cranial nerve (accessory) —*see*
 Injury, nerve, accessory
 epididymis S39.94
 epigastric region S39.91
 epiglottis NEC S19.89
 esophageal plexus —*see* Injury, nerve, thorax,
 sympathetic
 esophagus (thoracic part) —*see also* Injury,
 intrathoracic, esophagus
  cervical NEC S19.85
 eustachian tube S09.30
 eye S05.9
  avulsion S05.7
  ball —*see* Injury, eyeball
  conjunctiva S05.0
  cornea
   abrasion S05.0
  laceration S05.3
   with prolapse S05.2
  lacrimal apparatus S05.8X
  orbit penetration S05.4
  specified site NEC S05.8X
 eyeball S05.8X
  contusion S05.1
  penetrating S05.6
   with
    foreign body S05.5
    prolapse or loss of intraocular tissue
 S05.2
   without prolapse or loss of intraocular
 tissue S05.3
  specified type NEC S05.8
 eyebrow S09.93
 eyelid S09.93
  abrasion —*see* Abrasion, eyelid
  contusion —*see* Contusion, eyelid
  open —*see* Wound, open, eyelid
 face S09.93
 fallopian tube S37.509
  bilateral S37.502
   blast injury S37.512
   contusion S37.522
   laceration S37.532
   specified type NEC S37.592
  blast injury (primary) S37.519
   bilateral S37.512
   secondary —*see* Injury, fallopian tube,
 specified type NEC
   unilateral S37.511
  contusion S37.529
   bilateral S37.522
   unilateral S37.521
  laceration S37.539
   bilateral S37.532
   unilateral S37.531
  specified type NEC S37.599
   bilateral S37.592
   unilateral S37.591
  unilateral S37.501
   blast injury S37.511
   contusion S37.521
   laceration S37.531
   specified type NEC S37.591
 fascia —*see* Injury, muscle
 fifth cranial nerve (trigeminal) —*see* Injury,
 nerve, trigeminal

Injury – *continued*
 finger (nail) S69.9
  blood vessel —*see* Injury, blood vessel,
 finger
  contusion —*see* Contusion, finger
  dislocation —*see* Dislocation, finger
  fracture —*see* Fracture, finger
  muscle —*see* Injury, muscle, finger
  nerve —*see* Injury, nerve, digital, finger
  open —*see* Wound, open, finger
  specified NEC S69.8
  sprain —*see* Sprain, finger
  superficial —*see* Injury, superficial, finger
 first cranial nerve (olfactory) —*see* Injury,
 nerve, olfactory
 flank —*see* Injury, abdomen
 foot S99.92
  blood vessel —*see* Injury, blood vessel, foot
  contusion —*see* Contusion, foot
  dislocation —*see* Dislocation, foot
  fracture —*see* Fracture, foot
  muscle —*see* Injury, muscle, foot
  open —*see* Wound, open, foot
  specified type NEC S99.82
  sprain —*see* Sprain, foot
  superficial —*see* Injury, superficial, foot
 forceps NOS P15.9
 forearm S59.91
  blood vessel —*see* Injury, blood vessel,
 forearm
  contusion —*see* Contusion, forearm
  fracture —*see* Fracture, forearm
  muscle —*see* Injury, muscle, forearm
  nerve —*see* Injury, nerve, forearm
  open —*see* Wound, open, forearm
  specified NEC S59.81
  superficial —*see* Injury, superficial, forearm
 forehead S09.90
 fourth cranial nerve (trochlear) —*see* Injury,
 nerve, trochlear
 gallbladder S36.129
  contusion S36.122
  laceration S36.123
  specified NEC S36.128
 ganglion
  celiac, coeliac —*see* Injury, nerve,
 lumbosacral, sympathetic
   gasserian —*see* Injury, nerve, trigeminal
   stellate —*see* Injury, nerve, thorax,
 sympathetic
   thoracic sympathetic —*see* Injury, nerve,
 thorax, sympathetic
 gasserian ganglion —*see* Injury, nerve,
 trigeminal
 gastric artery —*see* Injury, blood vessel,
 celiac artery, branch
 gastroduodenal artery —*see* Injury, blood
 vessel, celiac artery, branch
 gastrointestinal tract —*see* Injury, intra-
 abdominal
  with open wound into abdominal cavity —
 see Wound, open, with penetration into
 peritoneal cavity
   colon —*see* Injury, intestine, large
   rectum —*see* Injury, intestine, large, rectum
    with open wound into abdominal cavity
 S36.61
   specified site NEC —*see* Injury, intra-
 abdominal, specified, site NEC
   stomach —*see* Injury, stomach
   small intestine —*see* Injury, intestine, small

Injury – *continued*
 genital organ (s)
  external S39.94
   specified NEC S39.848
  internal S37.90
   fallopian tube —*see* Injury, fallopian tube
   ovary —*see* Injury, ovary
   prostate —*see* Injury, prostate
   seminal vesicle —*see* Injury, pelvis, organ,
 specified site NEC
   uterus —*see* Injury, uterus
   vas deferens —*see* Injury, pelvis, organ,
 specified site NEC
  obstetrical trauma O71.9
 gland
  lacrimal laceration —*see* Injury, eye,
 specified site NEC
  salivary S09.90
  thyroid NEC S19.84
 globe (eye) S05.90
  specified NEC S05.8X
 groin —*see* Injury, abdomen
 gum S09.90
 hand S69.9
  blood vessel —*see* Injury, blood vessel,
 hand
  contusion —*see* Contusion, hand
  fracture —*see* Fracture, hand
  muscle —*see* Injury, muscle, hand
  nerve —*see* Injury, nerve, hand
  open —*see* Wound, open, hand
  specified NEC S69.8
  sprain —*see* Sprain, hand
  superficial —*see* Injury, superficial, hand
 head S09.90
  with loss of consciousness S06.9
  specified NEC S09.8
 heart S26.90
  with hemopericardium S26.00
   contusion S26.01
   laceration (mild) S26.020
    moderate S26.021
    major S26.022
   specified type NEC S26.09
  contusion S26.91
  laceration S26.92
  specified type NEC S26.99
  without hemopericardium S26.10
   contusion S26.11
   laceration S26.12
   specified type NEC S26.19
 heel —*see* Injury, foot
 hepatic
  artery —*see* Injury, blood vessel, celiac
 artery, branch
  duct —*see* Injury, liver
  vein —*see* Injury, vena cava, inferior
 hip S79.91
  blood vessel —*see* Injury, blood vessel, hip
  contusion —*see* Contusion, hip
  dislocation —*see* Dislocation, hip
  fracture —*see* Fracture, femur, neck
  muscle —*see* Injury, muscle, hip
  nerve —*see* Injury, nerve, hip
  open —*see* Wound, open, hip
  sprain —*see* Sprain, hip
  superficial —*see* Injury, superficial, hip
  specified NEC S79.81
 hymen S39.94
 hypogastric
  blood vessel —*see* Injury, blood vessel, iliac
  plexus —*see* Injury, nerve, lumbosacral,
 sympathetic

Injury – *continued*
ileum —*see* Injury, intestine, small
iliac region S39.91
instrumental (during surgery) —*see*
Laceration, accidental complicating surgery
  birth injury —*see* Birth, injury
  nonsurgical —*see* Injury, by site
  obstetrical O71.9
    bladder O71.5
    cervix O71.3
    high vaginal O71.4
    perineal NOS O70.9
    urethra O71.5
    uterus O71.5
      with rupture or perforation O71.1
internal T14.8
  aorta —*see* Injury, aorta
  bladder (sphincter) —*see* Injury, bladder
    with
      ectopic or molar pregnancy O08.6
      following ectopic or molar pregnancy
        O08.6
      obstetrical trauma O71.5
  bronchus, bronchi —*see* Injury,
intrathoracic, bronchus
  cecum —*see* Injury, intestine, large
  cervix (uteri) —*see also* Injury, uterus
    with ectopic or molar pregnancy O08.6
    following ectopic or molar pregnancy
      O08.6
    obstetrical trauma O71.3
  chest —*see* Injury, intrathoracic
  gastrointestinal tract —*see* Injury, intra-
abdominal
  heart —*see* Injury, heart
  intestine NEC —*see* Injury, intestine
  intrauterine —*see* Injury, uterus
  mesentery —*see* Injury, intra-abdominal,
specified, site NEC
  pelvis, pelvic (organ) S37.90
    following ectopic or molar pregnancy
(subsequent episode) O08.6
    obstetrical trauma NEC O71.5
      rupture or perforation O71.1
    specified NEC S39.83
  rectum —*see* Injury, intestine, large, rectum
  stomach —*see* Injury, stomach
  ureter —*see* Injury, ureter
  urethra (sphincter) following ectopic or
molar pregnancy O08.6
  uterus —*see* Injury, uterus
interscapular area —*see* Injury, thorax
intestine
  large S36.509
    ascending (right) S36.500
      blast injury (primary) S36.510
        secondary S36.590
      contusion S36.520
      laceration S36.530
      specified type NEC S36.590
    blast injury (primary) S36.519
      ascending (right) S36.510
      descending (left) S36.512
      rectum S36.61
      sigmoid S36.513
      specified site NEC S36.518
      transverse S36.511
    contusion S36.529
      ascending (right) S36.520
      descending (left) S36.522
      rectum S36.62
      sigmoid S36.523

Injury – *continued*
      specified site NEC S36.528
      transverse S36.521
    descending (left) S36.502
      blast injury (primary) S36.512
        secondary S36.592
      contusion S36.522
      laceration S36.532
      specified type NEC S36.592
    laceration S36.539
      ascending (right) S36.530
      descending (left) S36.532
      rectum S36.63
      sigmoid S36.533
      specified site NEC S36.538
      transverse S36.531
    rectum S36.60
      blast injury (primary) S36.61
        secondary S36.69
      contusion S36.62
      laceration S36.63
      specified type NEC S36.69
    sigmoid S36.503
      blast injury (primary) S36.513
        secondary S36.593
      contusion S36.523
      laceration S36.533
      specified type NEC S36.593
    specified
      site NEC S36.508
        blast injury (primary) S36.518
          secondary S36.598
        contusion S36.528
        laceration S36.538
        specified type NEC S36.598
      type NEC S36.599
        ascending (right) S36.590
        descending (left) S36.592
        rectum S36.69
        sigmoid S36.593
        specified site NEC S36.598
        transverse S36.591
    transverse S36.501
      blast injury (primary) S36.511
        secondary S36.591
      contusion S36.521
      laceration S36.531
      specified type NEC S36.591
  small S36.409
    blast injury (primary) S36.419
      duodenum S36.410
        secondary S36.499
          duodenum S36.490
          specified site NEC S36.498
      specified site NEC S36.418
    contusion S36.429
      duodenum S36.420
      specified site NEC S36.428
    duodenum S36.400
      blast injury (primary) S36.410
        secondary S36.490
      contusion S36.420
      laceration S36.430
      specified NEC S36.490
    laceration S36.439
      duodenum S36.430
      specified site NEC S36.438
    specified
      type NEC S36.499
        duodenum S36.490
        specified site NEC S36.498
      site NEC S36.408

Injury – *continued*
  intra-abdominal S36.90
    adrenal gland —*see* Injury, adrenal gland
    bladder —*see* Injury, bladder
    colon —*see* Injury, intestine, large
    contusion S36.92
    fallopian tube —*see* Injury, fallopian tube
    gallbladder —*see* Injury, gallbladder
    intestine —*see* Injury, intestine
    laceration S36.93
    liver —*see* Injury, liver
    kidney —*see* Injury, kidney
    ovary —*see* Injury, ovary
    pancreas —*see* Injury, pancreas
    pelvic NOS S37.90
    peritoneum —*see* Injury, intra-abdominal,
specified, site NEC
    prostate —*see* Injury, prostate
    rectum —*see* Injury, intestine, large, rectum
    retroperitoneum —*see* Injury, intra-
abdominal, specified, site NEC
    seminal vesicle —*see* Injury, pelvis, organ,
specified site NEC
    small intestine —*see* Injury, intestine, small
    specified
      site NEC S36.899
        contusion S36.892
        laceration S36.893
        specified type NEC S36.898
      type NEC S36.99
    pelvic S37.90
      specified
        site NEC S37.899
          specified type NEC S37.898
        type NEC S37.99
    spleen —*see* Injury, spleen
    stomach —*see* Injury, stomach
    ureter —*see* Injury, ureter
    urethra —*see* Injury, urethra
    uterus —*see* Injury, uterus
    vas deferens —*see* Injury, pelvis, organ,
specified site NEC
  intracranial (traumatic) S06.9
    cerebellar hemorrhage, traumatic —*see*
Injury, intracranial, focal
    cerebral edema, traumatic S06.1X
      diffuse S06.1X
      focal S06.1X
    diffuse (axonal) S06.2X
    epidural hemorrhage (traumatic) S06.4X
    focal brain injury S06.30
      contusion —*see* Contusion, cerebral
      laceration —*see* Laceration, cerebral
    intracerebral hemorrhage, traumatic S06.36
      left side S06.35
      right side S06.34
    subarachnoid hemorrhage, traumatic S06.6X
    subdural hemorrhage, traumatic S06.5X
  intraocular —*see* Injury, eyeball, penetrating
  intrathoracic S27.9
    bronchus S27.409
      bilateral S27.402
      blast injury (primary) S27.419
        bilateral S27.412
        secondary —*see* Injury, intrathoracic,
bronchus, specified type NEC
        unilateral S27.411
      contusion S27.429
        bilateral S27.422
        unilateral S27.421
      laceration S27.439
        bilateral S27.432
        unilateral S27.431

Injury – *continued*
  specified type NEC S27.499
    bilateral S27.492
    unilateral S27.491
    unilateral S27.401
  diaphragm S27.809
    contusion S27.802
    laceration S27.803
    specified type NEC S27.808
  esophagus (thoracic) S27.819
    contusion S27.812
    laceration S27.813
    specified type NEC S27.818
  heart —*see* Injury, heart
  hemopneumothorax S27.2
  hemothorax S27.1
  lung S27.309
    aspiration J69.0
    bilateral S27.302
    blast injury (primary) S27.319
      bilateral S27.312
      secondary —*see* Injury, intrathoracic,
lung, specified type NEC
      unilateral S27.311
    contusion S27.329
      bilateral S27.322
      unilateral S27.321
    laceration S27.339
      bilateral S27.332
      unilateral S27.331
    specified type NEC S27.399
      bilateral S27.392
      unilateral S27.391
    unilateral S27.301
  pleura S27.60
    laceration S27.63
    specified type NEC S27.69
  pneumothorax S27.0
  specified organ NEC S27.899
    contusion S27.892
    laceration S27.893
    specified type NEC S27.898
  thoracic duct —*see* Injury, intrathoracic,
specified organ NEC
  thymus gland —*see* Injury, intrathoracic,
specified organ NEC
  trachea, thoracic S27.50
    blast (primary) S27.51
    contusion S27.52
    laceration S27.53
    specified type NEC S27.59
  iris —*see* Injury, eye, specified site NEC
    penetrating —*see* Injury, eyeball,
penetrating
  jaw S09.93
  jejunum —*see* Injury, intestine, small
  joint NOS T14.8
    old or residual —*see* Disorder, joint,
specified type NEC
  kidney S37.00
    acute (nontraumatic) N17.9
    contusion —*see* Contusion, kidney
    laceration —*see* Laceration, kidney
    specified NEC S37.09
  knee S89.9
    contusion —*see* Contusion, knee
    dislocation —*see* Dislocation, knee
    meniscus (lateral) (medial) —*see* Sprain,
knee, specified site NEC
      old injury or tear —*see* Derangement,
knee, meniscus, due to old injury
    open —*see* Wound, open, knee

Injury – *continued*
    specified NEC S89.8
    sprain —*see* Sprain, knee
    superficial —*see* Injury, superficial, knee
  labium (majus) (minus) S39.94
  labyrinth, ear S09.30
  lacrimal apparatus, duct, gland, or sac —*see*
Injury, eye, specified site NEC
  larynx NEC S19.81
  leg (lower) S89.9
    blood vessel —*see* Injury, blood vessel, leg
    contusion —*see* Contusion, leg
    fracture —*see* Fracture, leg
    muscle —*see* Injury, muscle, leg
    nerve —*see* Injury, nerve, leg
    open —*see* Wound, open, leg
    specified NEC S89.8
    superficial —*see* Injury, superficial, leg
  lens, eye —*see* Injury, eye, specified site NEC
    penetrating —*see* Injury, eyeball,
penetrating
  limb NEC T14.8
  lip S09.93
  liver S36.119
    contusion S36.112
    laceration S36.113
      major (stellate) S36.116
      minor S36.114
      moderate S36.115
    specified NEC S36.118
  lower back S39.92
    specified NEC S39.82
  lumbar, lumbosacral (region) S39.92
    plexus —*see* Injury, lumbosacral plexus
  lumbosacral plexus S34.4
  lung —*see also* Injury, intrathoracic, lung
    aspiration J69.0
    transfusion-related (TRALI) J95.84
  lymphatic thoracic duct —*see* Injury,
intrathoracic, specified organ NEC
  malar region S09.93
  mastoid region S09.90
  maxilla S09.93
  mediastinum —*see* Injury, intrathoracic,
specified organ NEC
  membrane, brain —*see* Injury, intracranial
  meningeal artery —*see* Injury, intracranial,
subdural hemorrhage
  meninges (cerebral) —*see* Injury, intracranial
  mesenteric
    artery
      branch S35.299
        laceration (minor) (superficial) S35.291
          major S35.292
        specified NEC S35.298
      inferior S35.239
        laceration (minor) (superficial) S35.231
          major S35.232
        specified NEC S35.238
      superior S35.229
        laceration (minor) (superficial) S35.221
          major S35.222
        specified NEC S35.228
    plexus (inferior) (superior) —*see* Injury,
nerve, lumbosacral, sympathetic
    vein
      inferior S35.349
        laceration S35.341
        specified NEC S35.348
      superior S35.339
        laceration S35.331
        specified NEC S35.338

Injury – *continued*
  mesentery —*see* Injury, intra-abdominal,
specified site NEC
  mesosalpinx —*see* Injury, pelvic organ,
specified site NEC
  middle ear S09.30
  midthoracic region NOS S29.9
  mouth S09.93
  multiple NOS T07
  muscle (and fascia) (and tendon)
    abdomen S39.001
      laceration S39.021
      specified type NEC S39.091
      strain S39.011
    abductor
      thumb, forearm level —*see* Injury, muscle,
thumb, abductor
    adductor
      thigh S76.20
        laceration S76.22
        specified type NEC S76.29
        strain S76.21
    ankle —*see* Injury, muscle, foot
    anterior muscle group, at leg level (lower)
S86.20
      laceration S86.22
      specified type NEC S86.29
      strain S86.21
    arm (upper) —*see* Injury, muscle, shoulder
    biceps (parts NEC) S46.20
      laceration S46.22
      long head S46.10
        laceration S46.12
        strain S46.11
        specified type NEC S46.19
      specified type NEC S46.29
      strain S46.21
    extensor
      finger (s) (other than thumb) —*see* Injury,
muscle, finger by site, extensor
      forearm level, specified NEC —*see* Injury,
muscle, forearm, extensor
      thumb —*see* Injury, muscle, thumb,
extensor
      toe (large) (ankle level) (foot level) —*see*
Injury, muscle, toe, extensor
    finger
      extensor (forearm level) S56.40
        hand level S66.309
          laceration S66.329
          specified type NEC S66.399
          strain S66.319
        laceration S56.429
        specified type NEC S56.499
        strain S56.419
      flexor (forearm level) S56.10
        hand level S66.109
          laceration S66.129
          specified type NEC S66.199
          strain S66.119
        laceration S56.129
        specified type NEC S56.199
        strain S56.119
      intrinsic S66.509
        laceration S66.529
        specified type NEC S66.599
        strain S66.519
      index
        extensor (forearm level)
          hand level S66.308
            laceration S66.32
            specified type NEC S66.39
            strain S66.31

Injury – *continued*
    specified type NEC S56.492
    flexor (forearm level)
      hand level S66.108
        laceration S66.12
        specified type NEC S66.19
        strain S66.11
      specified type NEC S56.19
      strain S56.11
    intrinsic S66.50
      laceration S66.52
      specified type NEC S66.59
      strain S66.51
    little
      extensor (forearm level)
        hand level S66.30
          laceration S66.32
          specified type NEC S66.39
          strain S66.31
        laceration S56.42
        specified type NEC S56.49
        strain S56.41
      flexor (forearm level)
        hand level S66.10
          laceration S66.12
          specified type NEC S66.19
          strain S66.11
        laceration S56.12
        specified type NEC S56.19
        strain S56.11
      intrinsic S66.50
        laceration S66.52
        specified type NEC S66.59
        strain S66.51
    middle
      extensor (forearm level)
        hand level S66.30
          laceration S66.32
          specified type NEC S66.39
          strain S66.31
        laceration S56.42
        specified type NEC S56.49
        strain S56.41
      flexor (forearm level)
        hand level S66.10
          laceration S66.12
          specified type NEC S66.19
          strain S66.11
        laceration S56.12
        specified type NEC S56.19
        strain S56.11
      intrinsic S66.50
        laceration S66.52
        specified type NEC S66.59
        strain S66.51
    ring
      extensor (forearm level)
        hand level S66.30
          laceration S66.32
          specified type NEC S66.39
          strain S66.31
        laceration S56.42
        specified type NEC S56.49
        strain S56.41
      flexor (forearm level)
        hand level S66.10
          laceration S66.12
          specified type NEC S66.19
          strain S66.11
        laceration S56.12
        specified type NEC S56.19
        strain S56.11

Injury – *continued*
    intrinsic S66.50
      laceration S66.52
      specified type NEC S66.59
      strain S66.51
    flexor
      finger (s) (other than thumb) —*see* Injury, muscle, finger
      forearm level, specified NEC —*see* Injury, muscle, forearm, flexor
      thumb —*see* Injury, muscle, thumb, flexor
      toe (long) (ankle level) (foot level) —*see* Injury, muscle, toe, flexor
    foot S96.90
      intrinsic S96.20
        laceration S96.22
        specified type NEC S96.29
        strain S96.21
      laceration S96.92
      long extensor, toe —*see* Injury, muscle, toe, extensor
      long flexor, toe —*see* Injury, muscle, toe, flexor
      specified
        site NEC S96.80
          laceration S96.82
          specified type NEC S96.89
          strain S96.81
          type NEC S96.99
        strain S96.91
    forearm (level) S56.90
      extensor S56.50
        laceration S56.52
        specified type NEC S56.59
        strain S56.51
      flexor S56.20
        laceration S56.22
        specified type NEC S56.29
        strain S56.21
      laceration S56.92
      specified S56.99
        site NEC S56.80
          laceration S56.82
          strain S56.81
          type NEC S56.89
        strain S56.91
    hand (level) S66.90
      laceration S66.92
      specified
        site NEC S66.80
          laceration S66.82
          specified type NEC S66.89
          strain S66.81
          type NEC S66.99
        strain S66.91
    head S09.10
      laceration S09.12
      specified type NEC S09.19
      strain S09.11
    hip NEC S76.00
      laceration S76.02
      specified type NEC S76.09
      strain S76.01
    intrinsic
      ankle and foot level —*see* Injury, muscle, foot, intrinsic
      finger (other than thumb) —*see* Injury, muscle, finger by site, intrinsic
      foot (level) —*see* Injury, muscle, foot, intrinsic
      thumb —*see* Injury, muscle, thumb, intrinsic

Injury – *continued*
    leg (level) (lower) S86.90
      Achilles tendon —*see* Injury, Achilles tendon
      anterior muscle group —*see* Injury, muscle, anterior muscle group
      laceration S86.92
      peroneal muscle group —*see* Injury, muscle, peroneal muscle group
      posterior muscle group —*see* Injury, muscle, posterior muscle group, leg level
      specified
        site NEC S86.80
          laceration S86.82
          specified type NEC S86.89
          strain S86.81
        type NEC S86.99
      strain S86.91
    long
      extensor toe, at ankle and foot level —*see* Injury, muscle, toe, extensor
      flexor, toe, at ankle and foot level —*see* Injury, muscle, toe, flexor
      head, biceps —*see* Injury, muscle, biceps, long head
    lower back S39.002
      laceration S39.022
      specified type NEC S39.092
      strain S39.012
    neck (level) S16.9
      laceration S16.2
      specified type NEC S16.8
      strain S16.1
    pelvis S39.003
      laceration S39.023
      specified type NEC S39.093
      strain S39.013
    peroneal muscle group, at leg level (lower) S86.30
      laceration S86.32
      specified type NEC S86.39
      strain S86.31
    posterior muscle (group)
      leg level (lower) S86.10
        laceration S86.12
        specified type NEC S86.19
        strain S86.11
      thigh level S76.30
        laceration S76.32
        specified type NEC S76.39
        strain S76.31
    quadriceps (thigh) S76.10
      laceration S76.12
      specified type NEC S76.19
      strain S76.11
    shoulder S46.90
      laceration S46.92
      rotator cuff —*see* Injury, rotator cuff
      specified site NEC S46.80
        laceration S46.82
        strain S46.81
        specified type NEC S46.89
        strain S46.91
      specified type NEC S46.99
    thigh NEC (level) S76.90
      adductor —*see* Injury, muscle, adductor, thigh
      laceration S76.92
      posterior muscle (group) —*see* Injury, muscle, posterior muscle, thigh level
      quadriceps —*see* Injury, muscle, quadriceps

Injury – *continued*
  specified
    site NEC S76.80
      laceration S76.82
      specified type NEC S76.89
      strain S76.81
    type NEC S76.99
    strain S76.91
  thorax (level) S29.009
    back wall S29.002
    front wall S29.001
    laceration S29.029
      back wall S29.022
      front wall S29.021
    specified type NEC S29.099
      back wall S29.092
      front wall S29.091
    strain S29.019
      back wall S29.012
      front wall S29.011
  thumb
    abductor (forearm level) S56.30
      laceration S56.32
      specified type NEC S56.39
      strain S56.31
    extensor (forearm level) S56.30
      hand level S66.20
        laceration S66.22
        specified type NEC S66.29
        strain S66.21
      laceration S56.32
      specified type NEC S56.39
      strain S56.31
    flexor (forearm level) S56.00
      hand level S66.00
        laceration S66.02
        specified type NEC S66.09
        strain S66.01
      laceration S56.02
      specified type NEC S56.09
      strain S56.01
      wrist level —*see* Injury, muscle, thumb,
flexor, hand level
    intrinsic S66.40
      laceration S66.42
      specified type NEC S66.49
      strain S66.41
  toe —*see also* Injury, muscle, foot
    extensor, long S96.10
      laceration S96.12
      specified type NEC S96.19
      strain S96.11
    flexor, long S96.00
      laceration S96.02
      specified type NEC S96.09
      strain S96.01
  triceps S46.30
    laceration S46.32
    specified type NEC S46.39
    strain S46.31
  wrist (and hand) level —*see* Injury, muscle,
hand
  musculocutaneous nerve —*see* Injury, nerve,
musculocutaneous
  myocardium —*see* Injury, heart
  nape —*see* Injury, neck
  nasal (septum) (sinus) S09.92
  nasopharynx S09.92
  neck S19.9
    specified NEC S19.80
      specified site NEC S19.89

Injury – *continued*
  nerve NEC T14.8
    abdomen S34.9
      peripheral S34.6
      specified site NEC S34.8
    abducens S04.4
      contusion S04.4
      laceration S04.4
      specified type NEC S04.4
    abducent —*see* Injury, nerve, abducens
    accessory S04.7
      contusion S04.7
      laceration S04.7
      specified type NEC S04.7
    acoustic S04.6
      contusion S04.6
      laceration S04.6
      specified type NEC S04.6
    ankle S94.9
      cutaneous sensory S94.3
      specified site NEC —*see* subcategory
S94.8
    anterior crural, femoral —*see* Injury, nerve,
femoral
    arm (upper) S44.9
      axillary —*see* Injury, nerve, axillary
      cutaneous —*see* Injury, nerve, cutaneous,
arm
      median —*see* Injury, nerve, median, upper
arm
      musculocutaneous —*see* Injury, nerve,
musculocutaneous
      radial —*see* Injury, nerve, radial, upper
arm
      specified site NEC —*see* subcategory
S44.8
      ulnar —*see* Injury, nerve, ulnar, arm
    auditory —*see* Injury, nerve, acoustic
    axillary S44.3
    brachial plexus —*see* Injury, brachial plexus
    cervical sympathetic S14.5
    cranial S04.9
      contusion S04.9
      eighth (acoustic or auditory) —*see* Injury,
nerve, acoustic
      eleventh (accessory) —*see* Injury, nerve,
accessory
      fifth (trigeminal) —*see* Injury, nerve,
trigeminal
      first (olfactory) —*see* Injury, nerve,
olfactory
      fourth (trochlear) —*see* Injury, nerve,
trochlear
      laceration S04.9
      ninth (glossopharyngeal) —*see* Injury,
nerve, glossopharyngeal
      second (optic) —*see* Injury, nerve, optic
      seventh (facial) —*see* Injury, nerve, facial
      sixth (abducent) —*see* Injury, nerve,
abducens
      specified
        nerve NEC S04.89
          contusion S04.89
          laceration S04.89
          specified type NEC S04.89
        type NEC S04.9
      tenth (pneumogastric or vagus) —*see*
Injury, nerve, vagus
      third (oculomotor) —*see* Injury, nerve,
oculomotor
      twelfth (hypoglossal) —*see* Injury, nerve,
hypoglossal

Injury – *continued*
    cutaneous sensory
      ankle (level) S94.3
      arm (upper) (level) S44.5
      foot (level) —*see* Injury, nerve, cutaneous
sensory, ankle
      forearm (level) S54.3
      hip (level) S74.2
      leg (lower level) S84.2
      shoulder (level) —*see* Injury, nerve,
cutaneous sensory, arm
      thigh (level) —*see* Injury, nerve, cutaneous
sensory, hip
    deep peroneal —*see* Injury, nerve, peroneal,
foot
    digital
      finger S64.4
        index S64.49
        little S64.49
        middle S64.49
        ring S64.49
      thumb S64.3
      toe —*see* Injury, nerve, ankle, specified
site NEC
    eighth cranial (acoustic or auditory) —*see*
Injury, nerve, acoustic
    eleventh cranial (accessory) —*see* Injury,
nerve, accessory
    facial S04.5
      contusion S04.5
      laceration S04.5
      newborn P11.3
      specified type NEC S04.5
    femoral (hip level) (thigh level) S74.1
    fifth cranial (trigeminal) —*see* Injury, nerve,
trigeminal
    finger (digital) —*see* Injury, nerve, digital,
finger
    first cranial (olfactory) —*see* Injury, nerve,
olfactory
    foot S94.9
      cutaneous sensory S94.3
      deep peroneal S94.2
      lateral plantar S94.0
      medial plantar S94.1
      specified site NEC —*see* subcategory
S94.8
    forearm (level) S54.9
      cutaneous sensory —*see* Injury, nerve,
cutaneous sensory, forearm
      median —*see* Injury, nerve, median
      radial —*see* Injury, nerve, radial
      specified site NEC —*see* subcategory
S54.8
      ulnar —*see* Injury, nerve, ulnar
    fourth cranial (trochlear) —*see* Injury,
nerve, trochlear
    glossopharyngeal S04.89
      specified type NEC S04.89
    hand S64.9
      median —*see* Injury, nerve, median, hand
      radial —*see* Injury, nerve, radial, hand
      specified NEC —*see* subcategory S64.8
      ulnar —*see* Injury, nerve, ulnar, hand
    hip (level) S74.9
      cutaneous sensory —*see* Injury, nerve,
cutaneous sensory, hip
      femoral —*see* Injury, nerve, femoral
      sciatic —*see* Injury, nerve, sciatic
      specified site NEC —*see* subcategory
S74.8
    hypoglossal S04.89
      specified type NEC S04.89

Injury – *continued*
  lateral plantar S94.0
  leg (lower) S84.9
    cutaneous sensory —*see* Injury, nerve, cutaneous sensory, leg
    peroneal —*see* Injury, nerve, peroneal
    specified site NEC —see subcategory S84.8
    tibial —*see* Injury, nerve, tibial
    upper —*see* Injury, nerve, thigh
  lower
    back —*see* Injury, nerve, abdomen, specified site NEC
      peripheral —*see* Injury, nerve, abdomen, peripheral
    limb —*see* Injury, nerve, leg
  lumbar spinal —*see* Injury, nerve, spinal, lumbar
  lumbar plexus —*see* Injury, nerve, lumbosacral, sympathetic
  lumbosacral
    plexus —*see* Injury, nerve, lumbosacral, sympathetic
    sympathetic S34.5
  medial plantar S94.1
  median (forearm level) S54.1
    hand (level) S64.1
    upper arm (level) S44.1
    wrist (level) —*see* Injury, nerve, median, hand
  musculocutaneous S44.4
  musculospiral (upper arm level) —*see* Injury, nerve, radial, upper arm
  neck S14.9
    peripheral S14.4
    specified site NEC S14.8
    sympathetic S14.5
  ninth cranial (glossopharyngeal) —*see* Injury, nerve, glossopharyngeal
  oculomotor S04.1
    contusion S04.1
    laceration S04.1
    specified type NEC S04.1
  olfactory S04.81
    specified type NEC S04.81
  optic S04.01
    contusion S04.01
    laceration S04.01
    specified type NEC S04.01
  pelvic girdle —*see* Injury, nerve, hip
  pelvis —*see* Injury, nerve, abdomen, specified site NEC
    peripheral —*see* Injury, nerve, abdomen, peripheral
  peripheral NEC T14.8
    abdomen —*see* Injury, nerve, abdomen, peripheral
    lower back —*see* Injury, nerve, abdomen, peripheral
    neck —*see* Injury, nerve, neck, peripheral
    pelvis —*see* Injury, nerve, abdomen, peripheral
    specified NEC T14.8
  peroneal (lower leg level) S84.1
    foot S94.2
  plexus
    brachial —*see* Injury, brachial plexus
    celiac, coeliac —*see* Injury, nerve, lumbosacral, sympathetic
    mesenteric, inferior —*see* Injury, nerve, lumbosacral, sympathetic
    sacral —*see* Injury, lumbosacral plexus

Injury – *continued*
    spinal
      brachial —*see* Injury, brachial plexus
      lumbosacral —*see* Injury, lumbosacral plexus
    pneumogastric —*see* Injury, nerve, vagus
  radial (forearm level) S54.2
    hand (level) S64.2
    upper arm (level) S44.2
    wrist (level) —*see* Injury, nerve, radial, hand
  root —*see* Injury, nerve, spinal, root
  sacral plexus —*see* Injury, lumbosacral plexus
  sacral spinal —*see* Injury, nerve, spinal, sacral
  sciatic (hip level) (thigh level) S74.0
  second cranial (optic) —*see* Injury, nerve, optic
  seventh cranial (facial) —*see* Injury, nerve, facial
  shoulder —*see* Injury, nerve, arm
  sixth cranial (abducent) —*see* Injury, nerve, abducens
  spinal
    plexus —*see* Injury, nerve, plexus, spinal
    root
      cervical S14.2
      dorsal S24.2
      lumbar S34.21
      sacral S34.22
      thoracic —*see* Injury, nerve, spinal, root, dorsal
    splanchnic —*see* Injury, nerve, lumbosacral, sympathetic
    sympathetic NEC —*see* Injury, nerve, lumbosacral, sympathetic
      cervical —*see* Injury, nerve, cervical sympathetic
    tenth cranial (pneumogastric or vagus) —*see* Injury, nerve, vagus
  thigh (level) —*see* Injury, nerve, hip
    cutaneous sensory —*see* Injury, nerve, cutaneous sensory, hip
    femoral —*see* Injury, nerve, femoral
    sciatic —*see* Injury, nerve, sciatic
    specified NEC —*see* Injury, nerve, hip
  third cranial (oculomotor) —*see* Injury, nerve, oculomotor
  thorax S24.9
    peripheral S24.3
    specified site NEC S24.8
    sympathetic S24.4
  thumb, digital —*see* Injury, nerve, digital, thumb
  tibial (lower leg level) (posterior) S84.0
  toe —*see* Injury, nerve, ankle
  trigeminal S04.3
    contusion S04.3
    laceration S04.3
    specified type NEC S04.3
  trochlear S04.2
    contusion S04.2
    laceration S04.2
    specified type NEC S04.2
  twelfth cranial (hypoglossal) —*see* Injury, nerve, hypoglossal
  ulnar (forearm level) S54.0
    arm (upper) (level) S44.0
    hand (level) S64.0
    wrist (level) —*see* Injury, nerve, ulnar, hand

Injury – *continued*
  vagus S04.89
    specified type NEC S04.89
  wrist (level) —*see* Injury, nerve, hand
  ninth cranial nerve (glossopharyngeal) —*see* Injury, nerve, glossopharyngeal
  nose (septum) S09.92
  obstetrical O71.9
    specified NEC O71.89
  occipital (region) (scalp) S09.90
    lobe —*see* Injury, intracranial
  optic chiasm S04.02
  optic radiation S04.03
  optic tract and pathways S04.03
  orbit, orbital (region) —*see* Injury, eye
    penetrating (with foreign body) —*see* Injury, eye, orbit, penetrating
    specified NEC —*see* Injury, eye, specified site NEC
  ovary, ovarian S37.409
    bilateral S37.402
      contusion S37.422
      laceration S37.432
      specified type NEC S37.492
    blood vessel —*see* Injury, blood vessel, ovarian
    contusion S37.429
      bilateral S37.422
      unilateral S37.421
    laceration S37.439
      bilateral S37.432
      unilateral S37.431
    specified type NEC S37.499
      bilateral S37.492
      unilateral S37.491
    unilateral S37.401
      contusion S37.421
      laceration S37.431
      specified type NEC S37.491
  palate (hard) (soft) S09.93
  pancreas S36.209
    body S36.201
      contusion S36.221
      laceration S36.231
        major S36.261
        minor S36.241
        moderate S36.251
      specified type NEC S36.291
    contusion S36.229
    head S36.200
      contusion S36.220
      laceration S36.230
        major S36.260
        minor S36.240
        moderate S36.250
      specified type NEC S36.290
    laceration S36.239
      major S36.269
      minor S36.249
      moderate S36.259
    specified type NEC S36.299
    tail S36.202
      contusion S36.222
      laceration S36.232
        major S36.262
        minor S36.242
        moderate S36.252
      specified type NEC S36.292
  parietal (region) (scalp) S09.90
    lobe —*see* Injury, intracranial
  patellar ligament (tendon) S76.10
    laceration S76.12
    specified NEC S76.19

Injury – *continued*
  strain S76.11
  pelvis, pelvic (floor) S39.93
   complicating delivery O70.1
   joint or ligament, complicating delivery O71.6
   organ S37.90
    with ectopic or molar pregnancy O08.6
    complication of abortion —*see* Abortion
    contusion S37.92
    following ectopic or molar pregnancy O08.6
    laceration S37.93
    obstetrical trauma NEC O71.5
    specified
     site NEC S37.899
      contusion S37.892
      laceration S37.893
      specified type NEC S37.898
     type NEC S37.99
    specified NEC S39.83
  penis S39.94
  perineum S39.94
  peritoneum S36.81
   laceration S36.893
  periurethral tissue —*see* Injury, urethra
   complicating delivery O71.82
  phalanges
   foot —*see* Injury, foot
   hand —*see* Injury, hand
  pharynx NEC S19.85
  pleura —*see* Injury, intrathoracic, pleura
  plexus
   brachial —*see* Injury, brachial plexus
   cardiac —*see* Injury, nerve, thorax, sympathetic
   celiac, coeliac —*see* Injury, nerve, lumbosacral, sympathetic
   esophageal —*see* Injury, nerve, thorax, sympathetic
   hypogastric —*see* Injury, nerve, lumbosacral, sympathetic
   lumbar, lumbosacral —*see* Injury, lumbosacral plexus
   mesenteric —*see* Injury, nerve, lumbosacral, sympathetic
   pulmonary —*see* Injury, nerve, thorax, sympathetic
  postcardiac surgery (syndrome) I97.0
  prepuce S39.94
  prostate S37.829
   contusion S37.822
   laceration S37.823
   specified type NEC S37.828
  pubic region S39.94
  pudendum S39.94
  pulmonary plexus —*see* Injury, nerve, thorax, sympathetic
  rectovaginal septum NEC S39.83
  rectum —*see* Injury, intestine, large, rectum
  retina —*see* Injury, eye, specified site NEC
   penetrating —*see* Injury, eyeball, penetrating
  retroperitoneal —*see* Injury, intra-abdominal, specified site NEC
  rotator cuff (muscle(s)) (tendon(s)) S46.00
   laceration S46.02
   specified type NEC S46.09
   strain S46.01
  round ligament —*see* Injury, pelvic organ, specified site NEC

Injury – *continued*
  sacral plexus —*see* Injury, lumbosacral plexus
  salivary duct or gland S09.93
  scalp S09.90
   newborn (birth injury) P12.9
    due to monitoring (electrode) (sampling incision) P12.4
     specified NEC P12.89
      caput succedaneum P12.81
  scapular region —*see* Injury, shoulder
  sclera —*see* Injury, eye, specified site NEC
   penetrating —*see* Injury, eyeball, penetrating
  scrotum S39.94
  second cranial nerve (optic) —*see* Injury, nerve, optic
  seminal vesicle —*see* Injury, pelvic organ, specified site NEC
  seventh cranial nerve (facial) —*see* Injury, nerve, facial
  shoulder S49.9
   blood vessel —*see* Injury, blood vessel, arm
   contusion —*see* Contusion, shoulder
   dislocation —*see* Dislocation, shoulder
   fracture —*see* Fracture, shoulder
   muscle —*see* Injury, muscle, shoulder
   nerve —*see* Injury, nerve, shoulder
   open —*see* Wound, open, shoulder
   specified type NEC S49.8
   sprain —*see* Sprain, shoulder girdle
   superficial —*see* Injury, superficial, shoulder
  sinus
   cavernous —*see* Injury, intracranial
   nasal S09.92
  sixth cranial nerve (abducent) —*see* Injury, nerve, abducens
  skeleton, birth injury P13.9
   specified part NEC P13.8
  skin NEC T14.8
   surface intact —*see* Injury, superficial
  skull NEC S09.90
  specified NEC T14.8
  spermatic cord (pelvic region) S37.898
   scrotal region S39.848
  spinal (cord)
   cervical (neck) S14.109
    anterior cord syndrome S14.139
     C1 level S14.131
     C2 level S14.132
     C3 level S14.133
     C4 level S14.134
     C5 level S14.135
     C6 level S14.136
     C7 level S14.137
     C8 level S14.138
    Brown-Séquard syndrome S14.149
     C1 level S14.141
     C2 level S14.142
     C3 level S14.143
     C4 level S14.144
     C5 level S14.145
     C6 level S14.146
     C7 level S14.147
     C8 level S14.148
     C1 level S14.101
     C2 level S14.102
     C3 level S14.103
     C4 level S14.104
     C5 level S14.105
     C6 level S14.106

Injury – *continued*
     C7 level S14.107
     C8 level S14.108
    central cord syndrome S14.129
     C1 level S14.121
     C2 level S14.122
     C3 level S14.123
     C4 level S14.124
     C5 level S14.125
     C6 level S14.126
     C7 level S14.127
     C8 level S14.128
    complete lesion S14.119
     C1 level S14.111
     C2 level S14.112
     C3 level S14.113
     C4 level S14.114
     C5 level S14.115
     C6 level S14.116
     C7 level S14.117
     C8 level S14.118
    concussion S14.0
    edema S14.0
    incomplete lesion specified NEC S14.159
     C1 level S14.151
     C2 level S14.152
     C3 level S14.153
     C4 level S14.154
     C5 level S14.155
     C6 level S14.156
     C7 level S14.157
     C8 level S14.158
    posterior cord syndrome S14.159
     C1 level S14.151
     C2 level S14.152
     C3 level S14.153
     C4 level S14.154
     C5 level S14.155
     C6 level S14.156
     C7 level S14.157
     C8 level S14.158
   dorsal —*see* Injury, spinal, thoracic
   lumbar S34.109
    complete lesion S34.119
     L1 level S34.111
     L2 level S34.112
     L3 level S34.113
     L4 level S34.114
     L5 level S34.115
    concussion S34.01
    edema S34.01
    incomplete lesion S34.129
     L1 level S34.121
     L2 level S34.122
     L3 level S34.123
     L4 level S34.124
     L5 level S34.125
     L1 level S34.101
     L2 level S34.102
     L3 level S34.103
     L4 level S34.104
     L5 level S34.105
   nerve root NEC
    cervical —*see* Injury, nerve, spinal, root, cervical
    dorsal —*see* Injury, nerve, spinal, root, dorsal
    lumbar S34.21
    sacral S34.22
    thoracic —*see* Injury, nerve, spinal, root, dorsal

Injury – *continued*
  plexus
    brachial —*see* Injury, brachial plexus
    lumbosacral —*see* Injury, lumbosacral
  plexus
    sacral S34.139
      complete lesion S34.131
      incomplete lesion S34.132
    thoracic S24.109
      anterior cord syndrome S24.139
        T1 level S24.131
        T2-T6 level S24.132
        T7-T10 level S24.133
        T11-T12 level S24.134
      Brown-Séquard syndrome S24.149
        T1 level S24.141
        T2-T6 level S24.142
        T7-T10 level S24.143
        T11-T12 level S24.144
      complete lesion S24.119
        T1 level S24.111
        T2-T6 level S24.112
        T7-T10 level S24.113
        T11-T12 level S24.114
      concussion S24.0
      edema S24.0
      incomplete lesion specified NEC S24.159
        T1 level S24.151
        T2-T6 level S24.152
        T7-T10 level S24.153
        T11-T12 level S24.154
      posterior cord syndrome S24.159
        T1 level S24.151
        T2-T6 level S24.152
        T7-T10 level S24.153
        T11-T12 level S24.154
      T1 level S24.101
      T2-T6 level S24.102
      T7-T10 level S24.103
      T11-T12 level S24.104
  splanchnic nerve —*see* Injury, nerve, lumbosacral, sympathetic
  spleen S36.00
    contusion S36.029
      major S36.021
      minor S36.020
    laceration S36.039
      major (massive) (stellate) S36.032
      moderate S36.031
      superficial (capsular) (minor) S36.030
    specified type NEC S36.09
  splenic artery —*see* Injury, blood vessel, celiac artery, branch
  stellate ganglion —*see* Injury, nerve, thorax, sympathetic
  sternal region S29.9
  stomach S36.30
    contusion S36.32
    laceration S36.33
    specified type NEC S36.39
  subconjunctival —*see* Injury, eye, conjunctiva
  subcutaneous NEC T14.8
  submaxillary region S09.93
  submental region S09.93
  subungual
    fingers —*see* Injury, hand
    toes —*see* Injury, foot
  superficial NEC T14.8
    abdomen, abdominal (wall) S30.92
      abrasion S30.811
      bite S30.871
        insect S30.861

Injury – *continued*
      contusion S30.1
      external constriction S30.841
      foreign body S30.851
    abrasion —*see* Abrasion, by site
    adnexa, eye NEC —*see* Injury, eye, specified site NEC
    alveolar process —*see* Injury, superficial, oral cavity
    ankle S90.91
      abrasion —*see* Abrasion, ankle
      blister —*see* Blister, ankle
      bite —*see* Bite, ankle
      contusion —*see* Contusion, ankle
      external constriction —*see* Constriction, external, ankle
      foreign body —*see* Foreign body, superficial, ankle
    anus S30.98
    arm (upper) S40.92
      abrasion —*see* Abrasion, arm
      bite —*see* Bite, superficial, arm
      blister —*see* Blister, arm (upper)
      contusion —*see* Contusion, arm
      external constriction —*see* Constriction, external, arm
      foreign body —*see* Foreign body, superficial, arm
    auditory canal (external) (meatus) —*see* Injury, superficial, ear
    auricle —*see* Injury, superficial, ear
    axilla —*see* Injury, superficial, arm
    back —*see also* Injury, superficial, thorax, back
      lower S30.91
        abrasion S30.810
        contusion S30.0
        external constriction S30.840
        superficial
          bite NEC S30.870
          insect S30.860
          foreign body S30.830
    bite NEC —*see* Bite, superficial NEC, by site
    blister —*see* Blister, by site
    breast S20.10
      abrasion —*see* Abrasion, breast
      bite —*see* Bite, superficial, breast
      contusion —*see* Contusion, breast
      external constriction —*see* Constriction, external, breast
      foreign body —*see* Foreign body, superficial, breast
    brow —*see* Injury, superficial, head, specified NEC
    buttock S30.91
    calf —*see* Injury, superficial, leg
    canthus, eye —*see* Injury, superficial, periocular area
    cheek (external) —*see* Injury, superficial, head, specified NEC
      internal —*see* Injury, superficial, oral cavity
    chest wall —*see* Injury, superficial, thorax
    chin —*see* Injury, superficial, head NEC
    clitoris S30.95
    conjunctiva —*see* Injury, eye, conjunctiva
      with foreign body (in conjunctival sac) —*see* Foreign body, conjunctival sac
    contusion —*see* Contusion, by site
    costal region —*see* Injury, superficial, thorax

Injury – *continued*
    digit (s)
      hand —*see* Injury, superficial, finger
    ear (auricle) (canal) (external) S00.40
      abrasion —*see* Abrasion, ear
      bite —*see* Bite, superficial, ear
      contusion —*see* Contusion, ear
      external constriction —*see* Constriction, external, ear
      foreign body —*see* Foreign body, superficial, ear
    elbow S50.90
      abrasion —*see* Abrasion, elbow
      bite —*see* Bite, superficial, elbow
      blister —*see* Blister, elbow
      contusion —*see* Contusion, elbow
      external constriction —*see* Constriction, external, elbow
      foreign body —*see* Foreign body, superficial, elbow
    epididymis S30.94
    epigastric region S30.92
    epiglottis —*see* Injury, superficial, throat
    esophagus
      cervical —*see* Injury, superficial, throat
    external constriction —*see* Constriction, external, by site
    extremity NEC T14.8
    eyeball NEC —*see* Injury, eye, specified site NEC
    eyebrow —*see* Injury, superficial, periocular area
    eyelid S00.20
      abrasion —*see* Abrasion, eyelid
      bite —*see* Bite, superficial, eyelid
      contusion —*see* Contusion, eyelid
      external constriction —*see* Constriction, external, eyelid
      foreign body —*see* Foreign body, superficial, eyelid
    face NEC —*see* Injury, superficial, head, specified NEC
    finger (s) S60.949
      abrasion —*see* Abrasion, finger
      bite —*see* Bite, superficial, finger
      blister —*see* Blister, finger
      contusion —*see* Contusion, finger
      external constriction —*see* Constriction, external, finger
      foreign body —*see* Foreign body, superficial, finger
      insect bite —*see* Bite, by site, superficial, insect
      index S60.94
      little S60.94
      middle S60.94
      ring S60.94
    flank S30.92
    foot S90.92
      abrasion —*see* Abrasion, foot
      bite —*see* Bite, foot
      blister —*see* Blister, foot
      contusion —*see* Contusion, foot
      external constriction —*see* Constriction, external, foot
      foreign body —*see* Foreign body, superficial, foot
    forearm S50.91
      abrasion —*see* Abrasion, forearm
      bite —*see* Bite, forearm, superficial
      blister —*see* Blister, forearm
      contusion —*see* Contusion, forearm

Injury – *continued*

elbow only —*see* Injury, superficial, elbow
external constriction —*see* Constriction, external, forearm
foreign body —*see* Foreign body, superficial, forearm
forehead —*see* Injury, superficial, head NEC
foreign body —*see* Foreign body, superficial
genital organs, external
  female S30.97
  male S30.96
globe (eye) —*see* Injury, eye, specified site NEC
groin S30.92
gum —*see* Injury, superficial, oral cavity
hand S60.92
  abrasion —*see* Abrasion, hand
  bite —*see* Bite, superficial, hand
  contusion —*see* Contusion, hand
  external constriction —*see* Constriction, external, hand
  foreign body —*see* Foreign body, superficial, hand
head S00.90
  ear —*see* Injury, superficial, ear
  eyelid —*see* Injury, superficial, eyelid
  nose S00.30
  oral cavity S00.502
  scalp S00.00
  specified site NEC S00.80
heel —*see* Injury, superficial, foot
hip S70.91
  abrasion —*see* Abrasion, hip
  bite —*see* Bite, superficial, hip
  blister —*see* Blister, hip
  contusion —*see* Contusion, hip
  external constriction —*see* Constriction, external, hip
  foreign body —*see* Foreign body, superficial, hip
  iliac region —*see* Injury, superficial, abdomen
  inguinal region —*see* Injury, superficial, abdomen
  insect bite —*see* Bite, by site, superficial, insect
  interscapular region —*see* Injury, superficial, thorax, back
  jaw —*see* Injury, superficial, head, specified NEC
knee S80.91
  abrasion —*see* Abrasion, knee
  bite —*see* Bite, superficial, knee
  blister —*see* Blister, knee
  contusion —*see* Contusion, knee
  external constriction —*see* Constriction, external, knee
  foreign body —*see* Foreign body, superficial, knee
labium (majus) (minus) S30.95
lacrimal (apparatus) (gland) (sac) —*see* Injury, eye, specified site NEC
larynx —*see* Injury, superficial, throat
leg (lower) S80.92
  abrasion —*see* Abrasion, leg
  bite —*see* Bite, superficial, leg
  contusion —*see* Contusion, leg
  external constriction —*see* Constriction, external, leg
  foreign body —*see* Foreign body, superficial, leg

Injury – *continued*

knee —*see* Injury, superficial, knee
limb NEC T14.8
lip S00.501
lower back S30.91
lumbar region S30.91
malar region —*see* Injury, superficial, head, specified NEC
mammary —*see* Injury, superficial, breast
mastoid region —*see* Injury, superficial, head, specified NEC
mouth —*see* Injury, superficial, oral cavity
muscle NEC T14.8
nail NEC T14.8
  finger —*see* Injury, superficial, finger
  toe —*see* Injury, superficial, toe
nasal (septum) —*see* Injury, superficial, nose
neck S10.90
  specified site NEC S10.80
nose (septum) S00.30
occipital region —*see* Injury, superficial, scalp
oral cavity S00.502
orbital region —*see* Injury, superficial, periocular area
palate —*see* Injury, superficial, oral cavity
palm —*see* Injury, superficial, hand
parietal region —*see* Injury, superficial, scalp
pelvis S30.91
  girdle —*see* Injury, superficial, hip
penis S30.93
perineum
  female S30.95
  male S30.91
periocular area S00.20
  abrasion —*see* Abrasion, eyelid
  bite —*see* Bite, superficial, eyelid
  contusion —*see* Contusion, eyelid
  external constriction —*see* Constriction, external, eyelid
  foreign body —*see* Foreign body, superficial, eyelid
phalanges
  finger —*see* Injury, superficial, finger
  toe —*see* Injury, superficial, toe
pharynx —*see* Injury, superficial, throat
pinna —*see* Injury, superficial, ear
popliteal space —*see* Injury, superficial, knee
prepuce S30.93
pubic region S30.91
pudendum
  female S30.97
  male S30.96
sacral region S30.91
scalp S00.00
scapular region —*see* Injury, superficial, shoulder
sclera —*see* Injury, eye, specified site NEC
scrotum S30.94
shin —*see* Injury, superficial, leg
shoulder S40.91
  abrasion —*see* Abrasion, shoulder
  bite —*see* Bite, superficial, shoulder
  blister —*see* Blister, shoulder
  contusion —*see* Contusion, shoulder
  external constriction —*see* Constriction, external, shoulder
  foreign body —*see* Foreign body, superficial, shoulder

Injury – *continued*

skin NEC T14.8
sternal region —*see* Injury, superficial, thorax, front
subconjunctival —*see* Injury, eye, specified site NEC
subcutaneous NEC T14.8
submaxillary region —*see* Injury, superficial, head, specified NEC
submental region —*see* Injury, superficial, head, specified NEC
subungual
  finger (s) —*see* Injury, superficial, finger
  toe (s) —*see* Injury, superficial, toe
supraclavicular fossa —*see* Injury, superficial, neck
supraorbital —*see* Injury, superficial, head, specified NEC
temple —*see* Injury, superficial, head, specified NEC
temporal region —*see* Injury, superficial, head, specified NEC
testis S30.94
thigh S70.92
  abrasion —*see* Abrasion, thigh
  bite —*see* Bite, superficial, thigh
  blister —*see* Blister, thigh
  contusion —*see* Contusion, thigh
  external constriction —*see* Constriction, external, thigh
  foreign body —*see* Foreign body, superficial, thigh
thorax, thoracic (wall) S20.90
  abrasion —*see* Abrasion, thorax
  back S20.40
  bite —*see* Bite, thorax, superficial
  blister —*see* Blister, thorax
  contusion —*see* Contusion, thorax
  external constriction —*see* Constriction, external, thorax
  foreign body —*see* Foreign body, superficial, thorax
  front S20.30
throat S10.10
  abrasion S10.11
  bite S10.17
    insect S10.16
  blister S10.12
  contusion S10.0
  external constriction S10.14
  foreign body S10.15
thumb S60.93
  abrasion —*see* Abrasion, thumb
  bite —*see* Bite, superficial, thumb
  blister —*see* Blister, thumb
  contusion —*see* Contusion, thumb
  external constriction —*see* Constriction, external, thumb
  foreign body —*see* Foreign body, superficial, thumb
  insect bite —*see* Bite, by site, superficial, insect
  specified type NEC S60.39
toe (s) S90.93
  abrasion —*see* Abrasion, toe
  bite —*see* Bite, toe
  blister —*see* Blister, toe
  contusion —*see* Contusion, toe
  external constriction —*see* Constriction, external, toe
  foreign body —*see* Foreign body, superficial, toe
  great S90.93

Injury – *continued*

tongue —*see* Injury, superficial, oral cavity
tooth, teeth —*see* Injury, superficial, oral cavity
 trachea S10.10
 tunica vaginalis S30.94
 tympanum, tympanic membrane —*see* Injury, superficial, ear
 uvula —*see* Injury, superficial, oral cavity
 vagina S30.95
 vocal cords —*see* Injury, superficial, throat
 vulva S30.95
 wrist S60.91
supraclavicular region —*see* Injury, neck
supraorbital S09.93
suprarenal gland (multiple) —*see* Injury, adrenal
surgical complication (external or internal site) —*see* Laceration, accidental complicating surgery
temple S09.90
temporal region S09.90
tendon —*see also* Injury, muscle, by site
 abdomen —*see* Injury, muscle, abdomen
 Achilles —*see* Injury, Achilles tendon
 lower back —*see* Injury, muscle, lower back
 pelvic organs —*see* Injury, muscle, pelvis
tenth cranial nerve (pneumogastric or vagus) —*see* Injury, nerve, vagus
testis S39.94
thigh S79.92
 blood vessel —*see* Injury, blood vessel, hip
 contusion —*see* Contusion, thigh
 fracture —*see* Fracture, femur
 muscle —*see* Injury, muscle, thigh
 nerve —*see* Injury, nerve, thigh
 open —*see* Wound, open, thigh
 specified NEC S79.82
 superficial —*see* Injury, superficial, thigh
third cranial nerve (oculomotor) —*see* Injury, nerve, oculomotor
thorax, thoracic S29.9
 blood vessel —*see* Injury, blood vessel, thorax
 cavity —*see* Injury, intrathoracic
 dislocation —*see* Dislocation, thorax
 external (wall) S29.9
 contusion —*see* Contusion, thorax
 nerve —*see* Injury, nerve, thorax
 open —*see* Wound, open, thorax
 specified NEC S29.8
 sprain —*see* Sprain, thorax
 superficial —*see* Injury, superficial, thorax
 fracture —*see* Fracture, thorax
 internal —*see* Injury, intrathoracic
 intrathoracic organ —*see* Injury, intrathoracic
 sympathetic ganglion —*see* Injury, nerve, thorax, sympathetic
throat (*see also* Injury, neck) S19.9
thumb S69.9
 blood vessel —*see* Injury, blood vessel, thumb
 contusion —*see* Contusion, thumb
 dislocation —*see* Dislocation, thumb
 fracture —*see* Fracture, thumb
 muscle —*see* Injury, muscle, thumb
 nerve —*see* Injury, nerve, digital, thumb
 open —*see* Wound, open, thumb
 specified NEC S69.8
 sprain —*see* Sprain, thumb
 superficial —*see* Injury, superficial, thumb

Injury – *continued*

thymus (gland) —*see* Injury, intrathoracic, specified organ NEC
thyroid (gland) NEC S19.84
toe S99.92
 contusion —*see* Contusion, toe
 dislocation —*see* Dislocation, toe
 fracture —*see* Fracture, toe
 muscle —*see* Injury, muscle, toe
 open —*see* Wound, open, toe
 specified type NEC S99.82
 sprain —*see* Sprain, toe
 superficial —*see* Injury, superficial, toe
tongue S09.93
tonsil S09.93
tooth S09.93
trachea (cervical) NEC S19.82
 thoracic —*see* Injury, intrathoracic, trachea, thoracic
transfusion-related acute lung (TRALI) J95.84
tunica vaginalis S39.94
twelfth cranial nerve (hypoglossal) —*see* Injury, nerve, hypoglossal
ureter S37.10
 contusion S37.12
 laceration S37.13
 specified type NEC S37.19
urethra (sphincter) S37.30
 at delivery O71.5
 contusion S37.32
 laceration S37.33
 specified type NEC S37.39
urinary organ S37.90
 contusion S37.92
 laceration S37.93
 specified
  site NEC S37.899
   contusion S37.892
   laceration S37.893
   specified type NEC S37.898
  type NEC S37.99
uterus, uterine S37.60
 with ectopic or molar pregnancy O08.6
 blood vessel —*see* Injury, blood vessel, iliac
 contusion S37.62
 laceration S37.63
  cervix at delivery O71.3
 rupture associated with obstetrics —*see* Rupture, uterus
 specified type NEC S37.69
uvula S09.93
vagina S39.93
 abrasion S30.814
 bite S31.45
  insect S30.864
  superficial NEC S30.874
 contusion S30.23
 crush S38.03
 during delivery —*see* Laceration, vagina, during delivery
 external constriction S30.844
 insect bite S30.864
 laceration S31.41
  with foreign body S31.42
 open wound S31.40
 puncture S31.43
  with foreign body S31.44
 superficial S30.95
  foreign body S30.854
vas deferens —*see* Injury, pelvic organ, specified site NEC

Injury – *continued*

vascular NEC T14.8
vein —*see* Injury, blood vessel
vena cava (superior) S25.20
 inferior S35.10
  laceration (minor) (superficial) S35.11
   major S35.12
  specified type NEC S35.19
 laceration (minor) (superficial) S25.21
  major S25.22
 specified type NEC S25.29
vesical (sphincter) —*see* Injury, bladder
visual cortex S04.04
vitreous (humor) S05.90
 specified NEC S05.8X
vocal cord NEC S19.83
vulva S39.94
 abrasion S30.814
 bite S31.45
  insect S30.864
  superficial NEC S30.874
 contusion S30.23
 crush S38.03
 during delivery —*see* Laceration, perineum, female, during delivery
 external constriction S30.844
 insect bite S30.864
 laceration S31.41
  with foreign body S31.42
 open wound S31.40
 puncture S31.43
  with foreign body S31.44
 superficial S30.95
  foreign body S30.854
whiplash (cervical spine) S13.4
wrist S69.9
 blood vessel —*see* Injury, blood vessel, hand
 contusion —*see* Contusion, wrist
 dislocation —*see* Dislocation, wrist
 fracture —*see* Fracture, wrist
 muscle —*see* Injury, muscle, hand
 nerve —*see* Injury, nerve, hand
 open —*see* Wound, open, wrist
 specified NEC S69.8
 sprain —*see* Sprain, wrist
 superficial —*see* Injury, superficial, wrist
Inoculation —*see also* Vaccination
 complication or reaction —*see* Complications, vaccination
Insanity, insane —*see also* Psychosis
 adolescent —*see* Schizophrenia
 confusional F28
  acute or subacute F05
 delusional F22
 senile F03
Insect
 bite —*see* Bite, by site, superficial, insect
 venomous, poisoning NEC (by) —*see* Venom, arthropod
Insensitivity
 adrenocorticotropin hormone (ACTH) E27.49
 androgen E34.50
  complete E34.51
  partial E34.52
Insertion
 cord (umbilical) lateral or velamentous O43.12
 intrauterine contraceptive device (encounter for) —*see* Intrauterine contraceptive device
Insolation (sunstroke) T67.0

Insomnia (organic) G47.00
  adjustment F51.02
  adjustment disorder F51.02
  behavioral, of childhood Z73.819
    combined type Z73.812
    limit setting type Z73.811
    sleep-onset association type Z73.810
  childhood Z73.819
  chronic F51.04
    somatized tension F51.04
  conditioned F51.04
  due to
    alcohol
      abuse F10.182
      dependence F10.282
      use F10.982
    amphetamines
      abuse F15.182
      dependence F15.282
      use F15.982
    anxiety disorder F51.05
    caffeine
      abuse F15.182
      dependence F15.282
      use F15.982
    cocaine
      abuse F14.182
      dependence F14.282
      use F14.982
    depression F51.05
    drug NEC
      abuse F19.182
      dependence F19.282
      use F19.982
    medical condition G47.01
    mental disorder NEC F51.05
    opioid
      abuse F11.182
      dependence F11.282
      use F11.982
    psychoactive substance NEC
      abuse F19.182
      dependence F19.282
      use F19.982
    sedative, hypnotic, or anxiolytic
      abuse F13.182
      dependence F13.282
      use F13.982
    stimulant NEC
      abuse F15.182
      dependence F15.282
      use F15.982
  fatal familial (FFI) A81.83
  idiopathic F51.01
  learned F51.3
  nonorganic origin F51.01
  not due to a substance or known physiological
  condition F51.01
    specified NEC F51.09
  paradoxical F51.03
  primary F51.01
  psychiatric F51.05
  psychophysiologic F51.04
  related to psychopathology F51.05
  short-term F51.02
  specified NEC G47.09
  stress-related F51.02
  transient F51.02
  without objective findings F51.02
Inspiration
  food or foreign body —*see* Foreign body, by
  site
  mucus —*see* Asphyxia, mucus

Inspissated bile syndrome (newborn) P59.1
Instability
  emotional (excessive) F60.3
  joint (post-traumatic) M25.30
    ankle M25.37
    due to old ligament injury —*see* Disorder,
  ligament
    elbow M25.32
    flail —*see* Flail, joint
    foot M25.37
    hand M25.34
    hip M25.35
    knee M25.36
    lumbosacral —see subcategory M53.2
    prosthesis —*see* Complications, joint
    prosthesis, mechanical, displacement, by site
    sacroiliac —see subcategory M53.2
    secondary to
      old ligament injury —*see* Disorder,
  ligament
      removal of joint prosthesis M96.89
    shoulder (region) M25.31
    spine —see subcategory M53.2
    wrist M25.33
  knee (chronic) M23.5
  lumbosacral —see subcategory M53.2
  nervous F48.8
  personality (emotional) F60.3
  spine —*see* Instability, joint, spine
  vasomotor R55
Institutional syndrome (childhood) F94.2
Institutionalization, affecting child Z62.22
  disinhibited attachment F94.2
Insufficiency, insufficient
  accommodation, old age H52.4
  adrenal (gland) E27.40
    primary E27.1
  adrenocortical E27.40
    drug-induced E27.3
    iatrogenic E27.3
    primary E27.1
  anterior (occlusal) guidance M26.54
  anus K62.89
  aortic (valve) I35.1
    with
      mitral (valve) disease I08.0
        with tricuspid (valve) disease I08.3
      stenosis I35.2
      tricuspid (valve) disease I08.2
        with mitral (valve) disease I08.3
    congenital Q23.1
    rheumatic I06.1
      with
        mitral (valve) disease I08.0
          with tricuspid (valve) disease I08.3
        stenosis I06.2
          with mitral (valve) disease I08.0
            with tricuspid (valve) disease I08.3
        tricuspid (valve) disease I08.2
          with mitral (valve) disease I08.3
    specified cause NEC I35.1
    syphilitic A52.03
  arterial I77.1
    basilar G45.0
    carotid (hemispheric) G45.1
    cerebral I67.81
    coronary (acute or subacute) I24.8
    mesenteric K55.1
    peripheral I73.9
    precerebral (multiple) (bilateral) G45.2
    vertebral G45.0
  arteriovenous I99.8

Insufficiency, insufficient   - *continued*
  biliary K83.8
  cardiac —*see also* Insufficiency, myocardial
    due to presence of (cardiac) prosthesis
    I97.11
      postprocedural I97.11
  cardiorenal, hypertensive I13.2
  cardiovascular —*see* Disease, cardiovascular
  cerebrovascular (acute) I67.81
    with transient focal neurological signs and
  symptoms G45.8
  circulatory NEC I99.8
    newborn P29.89
  convergence H51.11
  coronary (acute or subacute) I24.8
    chronic or with a stated duration of over 4
  weeks I25.89
  corticoadrenal E27.40
    primary E27.1
  dietary E63.9
  divergence H51.8
  food T73.0
  gastroesophageal K22.8
  gonadal
    ovary E28.39
    testis E29.1
  heart —*see also* Insufficiency, myocardial
    newborn P29.0
    valve —*see* Endocarditis
  hepatic —*see* Failure, hepatic
  idiopathic autonomic G90.09
  interocclusal distance of fully erupted teeth
  (ridge) M26.36
  kidney N28.9
    acute N28.9
    chronic N18.9
  lacrimal (secretion) H04.12
    passages —*see* Stenosis, lacrimal
  liver —*see* Failure, hepatic
  lung —*see* Insufficiency, pulmonary
  mental (congenital) —*see* Disability,
  intellectual
  mesenteric K55.1
  mitral (valve) I34.0
    with
      aortic valve disease I08.0
        with tricuspid (valve) disease I08.3
      obstruction or stenosis I05.2
        with aortic valve disease I08.0
      tricuspid (valve) disease I08.1
        with aortic (valve) disease I08.3
    congenital Q23.3
    rheumatic I05.1
      with
        aortic valve disease I08.0
          with tricuspid (valve) disease I08.3
        obstruction or stenosis I05.2
          with aortic valve disease I08.0
            with tricuspid (valve) disease I08.3
        tricuspid (valve) disease I08.1
          with aortic (valve) disease I08.3
      active or acute I01.1
        with chorea, rheumatic (Sydenham's)
  I02.0
    specified cause, except rheumatic I34.0
  muscle —*see also* Disease, muscle
    heart —*see* Insufficiency, myocardial
    ocular NEC H50.9
  myocardial, myocardium (with
  arteriosclerosis) I50.9
    with
      rheumatic fever (conditions in I00) I09.0
        active, acute or subacute I01.2

Insufficiency, insufficient - *continued*
    with chorea I02.0
      inactive or quiescent (with chorea) I09.0
    congenital Q24.8
    hypertensive —*see* Hypertension, heart
    newborn P29.0
    rheumatic I09.0
      active, acute, or subacute I01.2
    syphilitic A52.06
  nourishment T73.0
  pancreatic K86.8
  parathyroid (gland) E20.9
  peripheral vascular (arterial) I73.9
  pituitary E23.0
  placental (mother) O36.51
  platelets D69.6
  prenatal care affecting management of
  pregnancy O09.3
  progressive pluriglandular E31.0
  pulmonary J98.4
    acute, following surgery (nonthoracic) J95.2
      thoracic J95.1
    chronic, following surgery J95.3
    following
      shock J98.4
      trauma J98.4
    newborn P28.5
    valve I37.1
      with stenosis I37.2
      congenital Q22.2
      rheumatic I09.89
        with aortic, mitral or tricuspid (valve)
  disease I08.8
  pyloric K31.89
  renal (acute) N28.9
    chronic N18.9
  respiratory R06.89
    newborn P28.5
  rotation —*see* Malrotation
  sleep syndrome F51.12
  social insurance Z59.7
  suprarenal E27.40
    primary E27.1
  tarso-orbital fascia, congenital Q10.3
  testis E29.1
  thyroid (gland) (acquired) E03.9
    congenital E03.1
  tricuspid (valve) (rheumatic) I07.1
    with
      aortic (valve) disease I08.2
        with mitral (valve) disease I08.3
      mitral (valve) disease I08.1
        with aortic (valve) disease I08.3
      obstruction or stenosis I07.2
        with aortic (valve) disease I08.2
          with mitral (valve) disease I08.3
    congenital Q22.8
    nonrheumatic I36.1
      with stenosis I36.2
  urethral sphincter R32
  valve, valvular (heart) —*see* Endocarditis
    congenital Q24.8
  vascular I99.8
    intestine K55.9
      acute K55.0
    mesenteric K55.1
    peripheral I73.9
    renal —*see* Hypertension, kidney
  velopharyngeal
    acquired K13.79
    congenital Q38.8

Insufficiency, insufficient - *continued*
  venous (chronic) (peripheral) I87.2
  ventricular —*see* Insufficiency, myocardial
  welfare support Z59.7
Insufflation, fallopian Z31.41
Insular —*see* condition
Insulinoma
  pancreas
    benign D13.7
    malignant C25.4
    uncertain behavior D37.8
  specified site
    benign —*see* Neoplasm, by site, benign
    malignant —*see* Neoplasm, by site,
  malignant
    uncertain behavior —*see* Neoplasm, by site,
  uncertain behavior
  unspecified site
    benign D13.7
    malignant C25.4
    uncertain behavior D37.8
Insuloma —*see* Insulinoma
Interference
  balancing side M26.56
  non-working side M26.56
Intermenstrual —*see* condition
Intermittent —*see* condition
Internal —*see* condition
Interrogation
  cardiac defibrillator (automatic) (implantable)
  Z45.02
  cardiac pacemaker Z45.018
  cardiac (event) (loop) recorder Z45.09
  infusion pump (implanted) (intrathecal) Z45.1
  neurostimulator Z46.2
Interruption
  bundle of His I44.30
  phase-shift, sleep cycle —*see* Disorder, sleep,
  circadian rhythm
  sleep phase-shift, or 24 hour sleep-wake cycle
  —*see* Disorder, sleep, circadian rhythm
Interstitial —*see* condition
Intertrigo L30.4
  labialis K13.0
Intervertebral disc —*see* condition
Intestine, intestinal —*see* condition
Intolerance
  carbohydrate K90.4
  disaccharide, hereditary E73.0
  fat NEC K90.4
    pancreatic K90.3
  food K90.4
    dietary counseling and surveillance Z71.3
  fructose E74.10
    hereditary E74.12
  glucose (-galactose) E74.39
  gluten K90.0
  lactose E73.9
    specified NEC E73.8
  lysine E72.3
  milk NEC K90.4
    lactose E73.9
  protein K90.4
  starch NEC K90.4
  sucrose (-isomaltose) E74.31
Intoxicated NEC (without dependence) —*see*
  Alcohol, intoxication
Intoxication
  acid E87.2
  alcoholic (acute) (without dependence) —*see*
  Alcohol, intoxication
  alimentary canal K52.1

Intoxication – *continued*
  amphetamine (without dependence) —*see*
  Abuse, drug, stimulant, with intoxication
    with dependence —*see* Dependence, drug,
  stimulant, with intoxication
  anxiolytic (acute) (without dependence) —*see*
  Abuse, drug, sedative, with intoxication
    with dependence —*see* Dependence, drug,
  sedative, with intoxication
  caffeine (acute) (without dependence) —*see*
  Abuse, drug, stimulant, with intoxication
    with dependence —*see* Dependence, drug,
  stimulant, with intoxication
  cannabinoids (acute) (without dependence) —
  see Abuse, drug, cannabis, with intoxication
    with dependence —*see* Dependence, drug,
  cannabis, with intoxication
  chemical —*see* Table of Drugs and Chemicals
    via placenta or breast milk —*see*
  Absorption, chemical, through placenta
  cocaine (acute) (without dependence) —*see*
  Abuse, drug, cocaine, with intoxication
    with dependence —*see* Dependence, drug,
  cocaine, with intoxication
  drug
    acute (without dependence) —*see* Abuse,
  drug, by type with intoxication
    with dependence —*see* Dependence, drug,
  by type with intoxication
    addictive
      via placenta or breast milk —*see*
  Absorption, drug, addictive, through placenta
      newborn P93.8
        gray baby syndrome P93.0
    overdose or wrong substance given or taken
  —*see* Table of Drugs and Chemicals, by drug,
  poisoning
  enteric K52.1
  foodborne A05.9
    bacterial A05.9
    classical (Clostridium botulinum) A05.1
    due to
      Bacillus cereus A05.4
      bacterium A05.9
        specified NEC A05.8
      Clostridium
        botulinum A05.1
        perfringens A05.2
        welchii A05.2
      Salmonella A02.9
        with
          (gastro) enteritis A02.0
          localized infection (s) A02.20
            arthritis A02.23
            meningitis A02.21
            osteomyelitis A02.24
            pneumonia A02.22
            pyelonephritis A02.25
            specified NEC A02.29
          sepsis A02.1
          specified manifestation NEC A02.8
      Staphylococcus A05.0
      Vibrio
        parahaemolyticus A05.3
        vulnificus A05.5
    enterotoxin, staphylococcal A05.0
    noxious —*see* Poisoning, food, noxious
  gastrointestinal K52.1
  hallucinogenic (without dependence) —*see*
  Abuse, drug, hallucinogen, with intoxication
    with dependence —*see* Dependence, drug,
  hallucinogen, with intoxication

Intoxication – *continued*
hypnotic (acute) (without dependence) —*see*
Abuse, drug, sedative, with intoxication
with dependence —*see* Dependence, drug,
sedative, with intoxication
inhalant (acute) (without dependence) —*see*
Abuse, drug, inhalant, with intoxication
with dependence —*see* Dependence, drug,
inhalant, with intoxication
meaning
inebriation —see category F10
poisoning —*see* Table of Drugs and
Chemicals
methyl alcohol (acute) (without dependence)
—*see* Alcohol, intoxication
opioid (acute) (without dependence) —*see*
Abuse, drug, opioid, with intoxication
with dependence —*see* Dependence, drug,
opioid, with intoxication
pathologic NEC (without dependence) —*see*
Alcohol, intoxication
phencyclidine (without dependence) —*see*
Abuse, drug, psychoactive NEC, with
intoxication
with dependence —*see* Dependence, drug,
psychoactive NEC, with intoxication
potassium (K) E87.5
psychoactive substance NEC (without
dependence) —*see* Abuse, drug, psychoactive
NEC, with intoxication
with dependence —*see* Dependence, drug,
psychoactive NEC, with intoxication
sedative (acute) (without dependence) —*see*
Abuse, drug, sedative, with intoxication
with dependence —*see* Dependence, drug,
sedative, with intoxication
serum (*see also* Reaction, serum) T80.69
uremic —*see* Uremia
volatile solvents (acute) (without dependence)
—*see* Abuse, drug, inhalant, with intoxication
with dependence —*see* Dependence, drug,
inhalant, with intoxication
water E87.79
Intracranial —*see* condition
Intrahepatic gallbladder Q44.1
Intraligamentous —*see* condition
Intrathoracic —*see also* condition
kidney Q63.2
Intrauterine contraceptive device
checking Z30.431
insertion Z30.430
immediately following removal Z30.433
in situ Z97.5
management Z30.431
reinsertion Z30.433
removal Z30.432
replacement Z30.433
retention in pregnancy O26.3-
Intraventricular —*see* condition
Intrinsic deformity —*see* Deformity
Intubation, difficult or failed T88.4
Intumescence, lens (eye) (cataract) —*see*
Cataract
Intussusception (bowel) (colon) (enteric)
(ileocecal) (ileocolic) (intestine) (rectum)
K56.1
appendix K38.8
congenital Q43.8
ureter (with obstruction) N13.5
Invagination (bowel, colon, intestine or
rectum) K56.1

Inversion
albumin-globulin (A-G) ratio E88.09
bladder N32.89
cecum —*see* Intussusception
cervix N88.8
chromosome in normal individual Q95.1
circadian rhythm —*see* Disorder, sleep,
circadian rhythm
nipple N64.59
congenital Q83.8
gestational —*see* Retraction, nipple
puerperal, postpartum —*see* Retraction,
nipple
nyctohemeral rhythm —*see* Disorder, sleep,
circadian rhythm
optic papilla Q14.2
organ or site, congenital NEC —*see*
Anomaly, by site
sleep rhythm —*see* Disorder, sleep, circadian
rhythm
testis (congenital) Q55.29
uterus (chronic) (postinfectional) (postpartal,
old) N85.5
postpartum O71.2
vagina (posthysterectomy) N99.3
ventricular Q20.5
Investigation (*see also* Examination) Z04.9
clinical research subject (control) (normal
comparison) (participant) Z00.6
Involuntary movement, abnormal R25.9
Involution, involutional —*see also* condition
breast, cystic —*see* Dysplasia, mammary,
specified type NEC
depression (single episode) F32.8
recurrent episode F33.9
melancholia (recurrent episode) (single
episode) F32.8
ovary, senile —*see* Atrophy, ovary
thymus failure E32.8
I.Q.
under 20 F73
20 34 F72
35 49 F71
50 69 F70
IRDS (type I) P22.0
type II P22.1
Irideremia Q13.1
Iridis rubeosis —*see* Disorder, iris, vascular
Iridochoroiditis (panuveitis) —*see* Panuveitis
Iridocyclitis H20.9
acute H20.0
hypopyon H20.05
primary H20.01
recurrent H20.02
secondary (noninfectious) H20.04
infectious H20.03
chronic H20.1
due to allergy —*see* Iridocyclitis, acute,
secondary
endogenous —*see* Iridocyclitis, acute,
primary
Fuchs' —*see* Cyclitis, Fuchs' heterochromic
gonococcal A54.32
granulomatous —*see* Iridocyclitis, chronic
herpes, herpetic (simplex) B00.51
zoster B02.32
hypopyon —*see* Iridocyclitis, acute,
hypopyon
in (due to)
ankylosing spondylitis M45.9
gonococcal infection A54.32

Iridocyclitis – *continued*
herpes (simplex) virus B00.51
zoster B02.32
infectious disease NOS B99
parasitic disease NOS B89 *[H22]*
sarcoidosis D86.83
syphilis A51.43
tuberculosis A18.54
zoster B02.32
lens-induced H20.2
nongranulomatous —*see* Iridocyclitis, acute
recurrent —*see* Iridocyclitis, acute, recurrent
rheumatic —*see* Iridocyclitis, chronic
subacute —*see* Iridocyclitis, acute
sympathetic —*see* Uveitis, sympathetic
syphilitic (secondary) A51.43
tuberculous (chronic) A18.54
Vogt-Koyanagi H20.82
Iridocyclochoroiditis (panuveitis) —*see*
Panuveitis
Iridodialysis H21.53
Iridodonesis H21.89
Iridoplegia (complete) (partial) (reflex)
H57.09
Iridoschisis H21.25
Iris —*see also* condition
bombé —*see* Membrane, pupillary
Iritis —*see also* Iridocyclitis
chronic —*see* Iridocyclitis, chronic
diabetic —*see* E08-E13 with .39
due to
herpes simplex B00.51
leprosy A30.9 *[H22]*
gonococcal A54.32
gouty M10.9
granulomatous —*see* Iridocyclitis, chronic
lens induced —*see* Iridocyclitis, lens-induced
papulosa (syphilitic) A52.71
rheumatic —*see* Iridocyclitis, chronic
syphilitic (secondary) A51.43
congenital (early) A50.01
late A52.71
tuberculous A18.54
Iron —*see* condition
Iron-miner's lung J63.4
Irradiated enamel (tooth, teeth) K03.89
Irradiation effects, adverse T66
Irreducible, irreducibility —*see* condition
Irregular, irregularity
action, heart I49.9
alveolar process K08.8
bleeding N92.6
breathing R06.89
contour of cornea (acquired) —*see* Deformity,
cornea
congenital Q13.4
contour, reconstructed breast N65.0
dentin (in pulp) K04.3
eye movements H55.89
nystagmus —*see* Nystagmus
saccadic H55.81
labor O62.2
menstruation (cause unknown) N92.6
periods N92.6
prostate N42.9
pupil —*see* Abnormality, pupillary
reconstructed breast N65.0
respiratory R06.89
septum (nasal) J34.2
shape, organ or site, congenital NEC —*see*
Distortion
sleep-wake pattern (rhythm) G47.23

Irritable, irritability R45.4
bladder N32.89
bowel (syndrome) K58.9
with diarrhea K58.0
psychogenic F45.8
bronchial —see Bronchitis
cerebral, in newborn P91.3
colon K58.9
with diarrhea K58.0
psychogenic F45.8
duodenum K59.8
heart (psychogenic) F45.8
hip —see Derangement, joint, specified type
NEC, hip
ileum K59.8
infant R68.12
jejunum K59.8
rectum K59.8
stomach K31.89
psychogenic F45.8
sympathetic G90.8
urethra N36.8
Irritation
anus K62.89
axillary nerve G54.0
bladder N32.89
brachial plexus G54.0
bronchial —see Bronchitis
cervical plexus G54.2
cervix —see Cervicitis
choroid, sympathetic —see Endophthalmitis
cranial nerve —see Disorder, nerve, cranial
gastric K31.89
psychogenic F45.8
globe, sympathetic —see Uveitis, sympathetic
labyrinth —see subcategory H83.2
lumbosacral plexus G54.1
meninges (traumatic) —see Injury,
intracranial
nontraumatic —see Meningismus
nerve —see Disorder, nerve
nervous R45.0
penis N48.89
perineum NEC L29.3
peripheral autonomic nervous system G90.8
peritoneum —see Peritonitis
pharynx J39.2
plantar nerve —see Lesion, nerve, plantar
spinal (cord) (traumatic) — see also Injury,
spinal cord, by region
nerve G58.9
root NEC —see Radiculopathy
nontraumatic —see Myelopathy
stomach K31.89
psychogenic F45.8
sympathetic nerve NEC G90.8
ulnar nerve —see Lesion, nerve, ulnar
vagina N89.8
Ischemia, ischemic I99.8
brain —see Ischemia, cerebral
bowel (transient)
acute K55.0
chronic K55.1
due to mesenteric artery insufficiency K55.1
cardiac (see Disease, heart, ischemic)
cardiomyopathy I25.5
cerebral (chronic) (generalized) I67.82
arteriosclerotic I67.2
intermittent G45.9
newborn P91.0
recurrent focal G45.8
transient G45.9

Ischemia, ischemic – *continued*
colon chronic (due to mesenteric artery
insufficiency) K55.1
coronary —see Disease, heart, ischemic
demand (coronary) (*see also* Angina) I24.8
heart (chronic or with a stated duration of
over 4 weeks) I25.9
acute or with a stated duration of 4 weeks or
less I24.9
subacute I24.9
infarction, muscle —see Infarct, muscle
intestine (large) (small) (transient) K55.9
acute K55.0
chronic K55.1
due to mesenteric artery insufficiency K55.1
kidney N28.0
mesenteric, acute K55.0
muscle, traumatic T79.6
myocardium, myocardial (chronic or with a
stated duration of over 4 weeks) I25.9
acute, without myocardial infarction I24.0
silent (asymptomatic) I25.6
transient of newborn P29.4
renal N28.0
retina, retinal —see Occlusion, artery, retina
small bowel
acute K55.0
chronic K55.1
due to mesenteric artery insufficiency K55.1
spinal cord G95.11
subendocardial —see Insufficiency, coronary
supply (coronary) (*see also* Angina) I25.9
due to vasospasm I20.1
Ischial spine —see condition
Ischialgia —see Sciatica
Ischiopagus Q89.4
Ischium, ischial —see condition
Ischuria R34
Iselin's disease or osteochondrosis —see
Osteochondrosis, juvenile, metatarsus
Islands of
parotid tissue in
lymph nodes Q38.6
neck structures Q38.6
submaxillary glands in
fascia Q38.6
lymph nodes Q38.6
neck muscles Q38.6
Islet cell tumor, pancreas D13.7
Isoimmunization NEC —see also
Incompatibility
affecting management of pregnancy (ABO)
(with hydrops fetalis) O36.11
anti-A sensitization O36.11
anti-B sensitization O36.19
anti-c sensitization O36.09
anti-C sensitization O36.09
anti-e sensitization O36.09
anti-E sensitization O36.09
Rh NEC O36.09
anti-D antibody O36.01
specified NEC O36.19
newborn P55.9
with
hydrops fetalis P56.0
kernicterus P57.0
ABO (blood groups) P55.1
Rhesus (Rh) factor P55.0
specified type NEC P55.8
Isolation, isolated
dwelling Z59.8
family Z63.79
social Z60.4

Isoleucinosis E71.19
Isomerism atrial appendages (with asplenia
or polysplenia) Q20.6
Isosporiasis, isosporosis A07.3
Isovaleric acidemia E71.110
Issue of
medical certificate Z02.79
for disability determination Z02.71
repeat prescription (appliance) (glasses)
(medicinal substance, medicament, medicine)
Z76.0
contraception —see Contraception
Itch, itching —see also Pruritus
baker's L23.6
barber's B35.0
bricklayer's L24.5
cheese B88.0
clam digger's B65.3
coolie B76.9
copra B88.0
dew B76.9
dhobi B35.6
filarial —see Infestation, filarial
grain B88.0
grocer's B88.0
ground B76.9
harvest B88.0
jock B35.6
Malabar B35.5
beard B35.0
foot B35.3
scalp B35.0
meaning scabies B86
Norwegian B86
perianal L29.0
poultry men's B88.0
sarcoptic B86
scabies B86
scrub B88.0
straw B88.0
swimmer's B65.3
water B76.9
winter L29.8
Ivemark's syndrome (asplenia with congenital
heart disease) Q89.01
Ivory bones Q78.2
Ixodiasis NEC B88.8

J

Jaccoud's syndrome —see Arthropathy,
postrheumatic, chronic
Jackson's
membrane Q43.3
paralysis or syndrome G83.89
veil Q43.3
Jacquet's dermatitis (diaper dermatitis) L22
Jadassohn-Pellizari's disease or anetoderma
L90.2
Jadassohn's
blue nevus —see Nevus
intraepidermal epithelioma —see Neoplasm,
skin, benign
Jaffe-Lichtenstein (-Uehlinger) **syndrome** —
see Dysplasia, fibrous, bone NEC
Jakob-Creutzfeldt disease or syndrome —
see Creutzfeldt-Jakob disease or syndrome
Jaksch-Luzet disease D64.89
Jamaican
neuropathy G92
paraplegic tropical ataxic-spastic syndrome
G92
Janet's disease F48.8
Janiceps Q89.4

Jansky-Bielschowsky amaurotic idiocy E75.4
Japanese
  B-type encephalitis A83.0
  river fever A75.3
Jaundice (yellow) R17
  acholuric (familial) (splenomegalic) —*see
  also* Spherocytosis
    acquired D59.8
  breast-milk (inhibitor) P59.3
  catarrhal (acute) B15.9
    with hepatic coma B15.0
  cholestatic (benign) R17
  due to or associated with
    delayed conjugation P59.8
      associated with (due to) preterm delivery
P59.0
    preterm delivery P59.0
  epidemic (catarrhal) B15.9
    with hepatic coma B15.0
    leptospiral A27.0
    spirochetal A27.0
  familial nonhemolytic (congenital) (Gilbert)
E80.4
    Crigler-Najjar E80.5
  febrile (acute) B15.9
    with hepatic coma B15.0
    leptospiral A27.0
    spirochetal A27.0
  hematogenous D59.9
  hemolytic (acquired) D59.9
    congenital —*see* Spherocytosis
  hemorrhagic (acute) (leptospiral) (spirochetal)
A27.0
  infectious (acute) (subacute) B15.9
    with hepatic coma B15.0
    leptospiral A27.0
    spirochetal A27.0
  leptospiral (hemorrhagic) A27.0
  malignant (without coma) K72.90
    with coma K72.91
  newborn P59.9
    due to or associated with
      ABO
        antibodies P55.1
        incompatibility, maternal/fetal P55.1
        isoimmunization P55.1
      absence or deficiency of enzyme system
for bilirubin conjugation (congenital) P59.8
      bleeding P58.1
      breast milk inhibitors to conjugation P59.3
        associated with preterm delivery P59.0
      bruising P58.0
      Crigler-Najjar syndrome E80.5
      delayed conjugation P59.8
        associated with preterm delivery P59.0
      drugs or toxins
        given to newborn P58.42
        transmitted from mother P58.41
      excessive hemolysis P58.9
        due to
          bleeding P58.1
          bruising P58.0
          drugs or toxins
            given to newborn P58.42
            transmitted from mother P58.41
          infection P58.2
          polycythemia P58.3
          swallowed maternal blood P58.5
        specified type NEC P58.8
      galactosemia E74.21
      Gilbert syndrome E80.4
      hemolytic disease P55.9

Jaundice – *continued*
    ABO isoimmunization P55.1
    Rh isoimmunization P55.0
      specified NEC P55.8
    hepatocellular damage P59.20
      specified NEC P59.29
    hereditary hemolytic anemia P58.8
    hypothyroidism, congenital E03.1
    incompatibility, maternal/fetal NOS P55.9
    infection P58.2
    inspissated bile syndrome P59.1
    isoimmunization NOS P55.9
    mucoviscidosis E84.9
    polycythemia P58.3
    preterm delivery P59.0
    Rh
      antibodies P55.0
      incompatibility, maternal/fetal P55.0
      isoimmunization P55.0
      specified cause NEC P59.8
      swallowed maternal blood P58.5
    spherocytosis (congenital) D58.0
  neonatal —*see* Jaundice, newborn
  nonhemolytic congenital familial (Gilbert)
E80.4
  nuclear, newborn (*see also* Kernicterus of
newborn) P57.9
  obstructive (*see also* Obstruction, bile duct)
K83.1
  post-immunization —*see* Hepatitis, viral,
type, B   post-transfusion —*see* Hepatitis,
viral, type, B
  regurgitation (*see also* Obstruction, bile duct)
K83.1
  serum (homologous) (prophylactic)
(therapeutic) —*see* Hepatitis, viral, type, B
  spirochetal (hemorrhagic) A27.0
  symptomatic R17
    newborn P59.9
Jaw —*see* condition
Jaw-winking phenomenon or syndrome
Q07.8
Jealousy
  alcoholic F10.988
  childhood F93.8
  sibling F93.8
Jejunitis —*see* Enteritis
Jejunostomy status Z93.4
Jejunum, jejunal —*see* condition
Jensen's disease —*see* Inflammation,
chorioretinal, focal, juxtapapillary
Jerks, myoclonic G25.3
Jervell-Lange-Nielsen syndrome I45.81
Jeune's disease Q77.2
Jigger disease B88.1
Job's syndrome (chronic granulomatous
disease) D71
Joint —*see also* condition
  mice —*see* Loose, body, joint
    knee M23.4
Jordan's anomaly or syndrome D72.0
Joseph-Diamond-Blackfan anemia
(congenital hypoplastic) D61.01
Jungle yellow fever A95.0
Jüngling's disease —*see* Sarcoidosis
Juvenile —*see* condition

K

Kahler's disease C90.0
Kakke E51.11
Kala-azar B55.0
Kallmann's syndrome E23.0

Kanner's syndrome (autism) —*see* Psychosis,
childhood
Kaposi's
  dermatosis (xeroderma pigmentosum) Q82.1
  lichen ruber L44.0
    acuminatus L44.0
  sarcoma
    colon C46.4
    connective tissue C46.1
    gastrointestinal organ C46.4
    lung C46.5
    lymph node (multiple) C46.3
    palate (hard) (soft) C46.2
    rectum C46.4
    skin (multiple sites) C46.0
    specified site NEC C46.7
    stomach C46.4
    unspecified site C46.9
  varicelliform eruption B00.0
  vaccinia T88.1
Kartagener's syndrome or triad (sinusitis,
bronchiectasis, situs inversus) Q89.3
Karyotype
  with abnormality except iso (Xq) Q96.2
  45,X Q96.0
  46,X
    iso (Xq) Q96.1
  46,XX Q98.3
    with streak gonads Q50.32
    hermaphrodite (true) Q99.1
    male Q98.3
  46,XY
    with streak gonads Q56.1
    female Q97.3
    hermaphrodite (true) Q99.1
  47,XXX Q97.0
  47,XXY Q98.0
  47,XYY Q98.5
Kaschin-Beck disease —*see* Disease, Kaschin-
Beck
Katayama's disease or fever B65.2
Kawasaki's syndrome M30.3
Kayser-Fleischer ring (cornea)
(pseudosclerosis) H18.04
Kaznelson's syndrome (congenital hypoplastic
anemia) D61.01
Kearns-Sayre syndrome H49.81
Kedani fever A75.3
Kelis L91.0
Kelly (-Patterson) syndrome (sideropenic
dysphagia) D50.1
Keloid, cheloid L91.0
  acne L73.0
  Addison's L94.0
  cornea —*see* Opacity, cornea
  Hawkin's L91.0
  scar L91.0
Keloma L91.0
Kenya fever A77.1
Keratectasia —*see also* Ectasia, cornea
  congenital Q13.4
Keratinization of alveolar ridge mucosa
  excessive K13.23
  minimal K13.22
Keratinized residual ridge mucosa
  excessive K13.23
  minimal K13.22
Keratitis (nodular) (nonulcerative) (simple)
(zonular) H16.9
  with ulceration (central) (marginal)
(perforated) (ring) —*see* Ulcer, cornea
  actinic —*see* Photokeratitis
  arborescens (herpes simplex) B00.52

Keratitis *- continued*
  areolar H16.11
  bullosa H16.8
  deep H16.309
    specified type NEC H16.399
  dendritic (a) (herpes simplex) B00.52
  disciform (is) (herpes simplex) B00.52
    varicella B01.81
  filamentary H16.12
  gonococcal (congenital or prenatal) A54.33
  herpes, herpetic (simplex) B00.52
    zoster B02.33
  in (due to)
    acanthamebiasis B60.13
    adenovirus B30.0
    exanthema (*see also* Exanthem) B09
    herpes (simplex) virus B00.52
    measles B05.81
    syphilis A50.31
    tuberculosis A18.52
    zoster B02.33
  interstitial (nonsyphilitic) H16.30
    diffuse H16.32
    herpes, herpetic (simplex) B00.52
      zoster B02.33
    sclerosing H16.33
    specified type NEC H16.39
    syphilitic (congenital) (late) A50.31
    tuberculous A18.52
  macular H16.11
  nummular H16.11
  oyster shuckers' H16.8
  parenchymatous —*see* Keratitis, interstitial
  petrificans H16.8
  postmeasles B05.81
  punctata
    leprosa A30.9 *[H16.14]*
    syphilitic (profunda) A50.31
  punctate H16.14
  purulent H16.8
  rosacea L71.8
  sclerosing H16.33
  specified type NEC H16.8
  stellate H16.11
  striate H16.11
  superficial H16.10
    with conjunctivitis —*see*
  Keratoconjunctivitis
    due to light   *see* Photokeratitis
  suppurative H16.8
  syphilitic (congenital) (prenatal) A50.31
  trachomatous A71.1
    sequelae B94.0
  tuberculous A18.52
  vesicular H16.8
  xerotic (*see also* Keratomalacia) H16.8
    vitamin A deficiency E50.4
Keratoacanthoma L85.8
Keratocele —*see* Descemetocele
Keratoconjunctivitis H16.20
  Acanthamoeba B60.13
  adenoviral B30.0
  epidemic B30.0
  exposure H16.21
  herpes, herpetic (simplex) B00.52
    zoster B02.33
  in exanthema (*see also* Exanthem) B09
  infectious B30.0
  lagophthalmic —*see* Keratoconjunctivitis,
  specified type NEC
  neurotrophic H16.23
  phlyctenular H16.25

Keratoconjunctivitis – *continued*
  postmeasles B05.81
  shipyard B30.0
  sicca (Sjogren's) M35.0
    not Sjogren's H16.22
  specified type NEC H16.29
  tuberculous (phlyctenular) A18.52
  vernal H16.26
Keratoconus H18.60
  congenital Q13.4
  stable H18.61
  unstable H18.62
Keratocyst (dental) (odontogenic) —*see* Cyst,
  calcifying odontogenic
Keratoderma, keratodermia (congenital)
  (palmaris et plantaris) (symmetrical) Q82.8
  acquired L85.1
    in diseases classified elsewhere L86
  climactericum L85.1
  gonococcal A54.89
  gonorrheal A54.89
  punctata L85.2
  Reiter's —*see* Reiter's disease
Keratodermatocele —*see* Descemetocele
Keratoglobus H18.79
  congenital Q15.8
    with glaucoma Q15.0
Keratohemia —*see* Pigmentation, cornea,
  stromal
Keratoiritis —*see also* Iridocyclitis
  syphilitic A50.39
  tuberculous A18.54
Keratoma L57.0
  palmaris and plantaris hereditarium Q82.8
  senile L57.0
Keratomalacia H18.44
  vitamin A deficiency E50.4
Keratomegaly Q13.4
Keratomycosis B49
  nigrans, nigricans (palmaris) B36.1
Keratopathy H18.9
  band H18.42
  bullous H18.1
  bullous (aphakic) , following cataract surgery
  H59.01
Keratoscleritis, tuberculous A18.52
Keratosis L57.0
  actinic L57.0
  arsenical L85.8
  congenital, specified NEC Q80.8
  female genital NEC N94.89
  follicularis Q82.8
    acquired L11.0
    congenita Q82.8
    et parafollicularis in cutem penetrans L87.0
    spinulosa (decalvans) Q82.8
    vitamin A deficiency E50.8
  gonococcal A54.89
  male genital (external) N50.8
  nigricans L83
  obturans, external ear (canal) —*see*
  Cholesteatoma, external ear
  palmaris et plantaris (inherited) (symmetrical)
  Q82.8
    acquired L85.1
  penile N48.89
  pharynx J39.2
  pilaris, acquired L85.8
  punctata (palmaris et plantaris) L85.2
  scrotal N50.8
  seborrheic L82.1
    inflamed L82.0

Keratosis – *continued*
  senile L57.0
  solar L57.0
  tonsillaris J35.8
  vagina N89.4
  vegetans Q82.8
  vitamin A deficiency E50.8
  vocal cord J38.3
Kerato-uveitis —*see* Iridocyclitis
Keraunoparalysis T75.09
Kerion (celsi) B35.0
Kernicterus of newborn (not due to
  isoimmunization) P57.9
  due to isoimmunization (conditions in P55.0-
  P55.9) P57.0
  specified type NEC P57.8
Keshan disease E59
Ketoacidosis E87.2
  diabetic —*see* Diabetes, by type, with
  ketoacidosis
Ketonuria R82.4
Ketosis NEC E88.89
  diabetic —*see* Diabetes, by type, with
  ketoacidosis
Kew Garden fever A79.1
Kidney —*see* condition
Kienböck's disease —*see also*
  Osteochondrosis, juvenile, hand, carpal lunate
  adult M93.1
Kimmelstiel (-Wilson) **disease** —*see* Diabetes,
  Kimmelstiel (-Wilson) disease
Kimura disease D21.9
  specified site (see Neoplasm, connective
  tissue benign)
Kink, kinking
  artery I77.1
  hair (acquired) L67.8
  ileum or intestine —*see* Obstruction, intestine
  Lane's —*see* Obstruction, intestine
  organ or site, congenital NEC —*see*
  Anomaly, by site
  ureter (pelvic junction) N13.5
    with
      hydronephrosis N13.1
        with infection N13.6
      pyelonephritis (chronic) N11.1
    congenital Q62.39
  vein (s) I87.8
    caval I87.1
    peripheral I87.1
Kinnier Wilson's disease (hepatolenticular
  degeneration) E83.01
Kissing spine M48.20
  cervical region M48.22
  cervicothoracic region M48.23
  lumbar region M48.26
  lumbosacral region M48.27
  occipito-atlanto-axial region M48.21
  thoracic region M48.24
  thoracolumbar region M48.25
Klatskin's tumor C24.0
Klauder's disease A26.8
Klebs' disease (*see also* Glomerulonephritis)
  N05.
Klebsiella (K.) **pneumoniae, as cause of
  disease classified elsewhere** B96.1
Klein (e) **-Levin syndrome** G47.13
Kleptomania F63.2
Klinefelter's syndrome Q98.4
  karyotype 47,XXY Q98.0
  male with more than two X chromosomes
  Q98.1

Klippel-Feil deficiency, disease, or syndrome (brevicollis) Q76.1
Klippel's disease I67.2
Klippel-Trenaunay (-Weber) **syndrome** Q87.2
Klumpke (-Déjerine) palsy, paralysis (birth) (newborn) P14.1
Knee —*see* condition
Knock knee (acquired) M21.06
  congenital Q74.1
Knot (s)
  intestinal, syndrome (volvulus) K56.2
  surfer S89.8
  umbilical cord (true) O69.2
Knotting (of)
  hair L67.8
  intestine K56.2
Knuckle pad (Garrod's) M72.1
Koch's
  infection —*see* Tuberculosis
  relapsing fever A68.9
Koch-Weeks' conjunctivitis —*see* Conjunctivitis, acute, mucopurulent
Köebner's syndrome Q81.8
Köenig's disease (osteochondritis dissecans) —*see* Osteochondritis, dissecans
Köhler-Pellegrini-Steida disease or syndrome (calcification, knee joint) —*see* Bursitis, tibial collateral
Köhler's disease
  patellar —*see* Osteochondrosis, juvenile, patella
  tarsal navicular —*see* Osteochondrosis, juvenile, tarsus
Koilonychia L60.3
  congenital Q84.6
Kojevnikov's, epilepsy —*see* Kozhevnikov's epilepsy
Koplik's spots B05.9
Kopp's asthma E32.8
Korsakoff's (Wernicke) disease, psychosis or syndrome (alcoholic) F10.96
  with dependence F10.26
  drug-induced
    due to drug abuse —*see* Abuse, drug, by type, with amnestic disorder
    due to drug dependence —*see* Dependence, drug, by type, with amnestic disorder
  nonalcoholic F04
Korsakov's disease, psychosis or syndrome —*see* Korsakoff's disease
Korsakow's disease, psychosis or syndrome —*see* Korsakoff's disease
Kostmann's disease or syndrome (infantile genetic agranulocytosis) —*see* Agranulocytosis
Kozhevnikov's epilepsy G40.109
  intractable G40.119
    with status epilepticus G40.111
    without status epilepticus G40.119
  not intractable G40.109
    with status epilepticus G40.101
    without status epilepticus G40.109
Krabbe's
  disease E75.23
  syndrome, congenital muscle hypoplasia Q79.8
Kraepelin-Morel disease —*see* Schizophrenia
Kraft-Weber-Dimitri disease Q85.8
Kraurosis
  ani K62.89
  penis N48.0

Kraurosis - *continued*
  vagina N89.8
  vulva N90.4
Kreotoxism A05.9
Krukenberg's
  spindle —*see* Pigmentation, cornea, posterior
  tumor C79.6
Kufs' disease E75.4
Kugelberg-Welander disease G12.1
Kuhnt-Junius degeneration (*see also* Degeneration, macula) H35.32
Kümmell's disease or spondylitis —*see* Spondylopathy, traumatic
Kupffer cell sarcoma C22.3
Kuru A81.81
Kussmaul's
  disease M30.0
  respiration E87.2
    in diabetic acidosis —*see* Diabetes, by type, with ketoacidosis
Kwashiorkor E40
  marasmic, marasmus type E42
Kyasanur Forest disease A98.2
Kyphoscoliosis, kyphoscoliotic (acquired) (*see also* Scoliosis) M41.9
  congenital Q67.5
  heart (disease) I27.1
  sequelae of rickets E64.3
  tuberculous A18.01
Kyphosis, kyphotic (acquired) M40.209
  cervical region M40.202
  cervicothoracic region M40.203
  congenital Q76.419
    cervical region Q76.412
    cervicothoracic region Q76.413
    occipito-atlanto-axial region Q76.411
    thoracic region Q76.414
    thoracolumbar region Q76.415
  Morquio-Brailsford type (spinal) (*see also* subcategory M49.8) E76.219
  postlaminectomy M96.3
  postradiation therapy M96.2
  postural (adolescent) M40.00
    cervicothoracic region M40.03
    thoracic region M40.04
    thoracolumbar region M40.05
  secondary NEC M40.10
    cervical region M40.12
    cervicothoracic region M40.13
    thoracic region M40.14
    thoracolumbar region M40.15
  sequelae of rickets E64.3
  specified type NEC M40.299
    cervical region M40.292
    cervicothoracic region M40.293
    thoracic region M40.294
    thoracolumbar region M40.295
  syphilitic, congenital A50.56
  thoracic region M40.204
  thoracolumbar region M40.205
  tuberculous A18.01
Kyrle disease L87.0

L

Labia, labium —*see* condition
Labile
  blood pressure R09.89
  vasomotor system I73.9
Labioglossal paralysis G12.29
Labium leporinum —*see* Cleft, lip
Labor —*see* Delivery
Labored breathing —*see* Hyperventilation

Labyrinthitis (circumscribed) (destructive) (diffuse) (inner ear) (latent) (purulent) (suppurative) (*see also* subcategory) H83.0
  syphilitic A52.79
Laceration
  with abortion —*see* Abortion, by type, complicated by laceration of pelvic organs
  abdomen, abdominal
    wall S31.119
      with
        foreign body S31.129
        penetration into peritoneal cavity S31.619
          with foreign body S31.629
    epigastric region S31.112
      with
        foreign body S31.122
        penetration into peritoneal cavity S31.612
          with foreign body S31.622
    left
      lower quadrant S31.114
        with
          foreign body S31.124
          penetration into peritoneal cavity S31.614
            with foreign body S31.624
      upper quadrant S31.111
        with
          foreign body S31.121
          penetration into peritoneal cavity S31.611
            with foreign body S31.621
    periumbilic region S31.115
      with
        foreign body S31.125
        penetration into peritoneal cavity S31.615
          with foreign body S31.625
    right
      lower quadrant S31.113
        with
          foreign body S31.123
          penetration into peritoneal cavity S31.613
            with foreign body S31.623
      upper quadrant S31.110
        with
          foreign body S31.120
          penetration into peritoneal cavity S31.610
            with foreign body S31.620
  accidental, complicating surgery —*see* Complications, surgical, accidental puncture or laceration
  Achilles tendon S86.02
  adrenal gland S37.813
  alveolar (process) —*see* Laceration, oral cavity
  ankle S91.01
    with
      foreign body S91.02
  antecubital space —*see* Laceration, elbow
  anus (sphincter) S31.831
    with
      ectopic or molar pregnancy O08.6
      foreign body S31.832
    complicating delivery —*see* Delivery, complicated, by, laceration, anus (sphincter)
    following ectopic or molar pregnancy O08.6
    nontraumatic, nonpuerperal —*see* Fissure, anus

Laceration - *continued*
  right S51.811
    with
      foreign body S51.821
  forehead S01.81
    with foreign body S01.82
  fourchette O70.0
    with ectopic or molar pregnancy O08.6
    complicating delivery O70.0
    following ectopic or molar pregnancy O08.6
  gallbladder S36.123
  genital organs, external
    female S31.512
      with foreign body S31.522
      vagina —*see* Laceration, vagina
      vulva —*see* Laceration, vulva
    male S31.511
      with foreign body S31.521
      penis —*see* Laceration, penis
      scrotum —*see* Laceration, scrotum
      testis —*see* Laceration, testis
  groin —*see* Laceration, abdomen, wall
  gum —*see* Laceration, oral cavity
  hand S61.419
    with
      foreign body S61.429
    finger —*see* Laceration, finger
    left S61.412
      with
        foreign body S61.422
    right S61.411
      with
        foreign body S61.421
    thumb —*see* Laceration, thumb
  head S01.91
    with foreign body S01.92
    cheek —*see* Laceration, cheek
    ear —*see* Laceration, ear
    eyelid —*see* Laceration, eyelid
    lip —*see* Laceration, lip
    nose —*see* Laceration, nose
    oral cavity —*see* Laceration, oral cavity
    scalp S01.01
      with foreign body S01.02
    specified site NEC S01.81
      with foreign body S01.82
    temporomandibular area —*see* Laceration, cheek
  heart —*see* Injury, heart, laceration
  heel —*see* Laceration, foot
  hepatic duct S36.13
  hip S71.019
    with foreign body S71.029
    left S71.012
      with foreign body S71.022
    right S71.011
      with foreign body S71.021
  hymen —*see* Laceration, vagina
  hypochondrium —*see* Laceration, abdomen, wall
  hypogastric region —*see* Laceration, abdomen, wall
  ileum S36.438
  inguinal region —*see* Laceration, abdomen, wall
  instep —*see* Laceration, foot
  internal organ —*see* Injury, by site
  interscapular region —*see* Laceration, thorax, back
  intestine
    large
      colon S36.539

Laceration - *continued*
      ascending S36.530
      descending S36.532
      sigmoid S36.533
      specified site NEC S36.538
    rectum S36.63
      transverse S36.531
    small S36.439
      duodenum S36.430
      specified site NEC S36.438
  intra-abdominal organ S36.93
    intestine —*see* Laceration, intestine
    liver —*see* Laceration, liver
    pancreas —*see* Laceration, pancreas
    peritoneum S36.81
    specified site NEC S36.893
    spleen —*see* Laceration, spleen
    stomach —*see* Laceration, stomach
  intracranial NEC —*see also* Injury, intracranial, diffuse
    birth injury P10.9
  jaw —*see* Laceration, head, specified site NEC
  jejunum S36.438
  joint capsule —*see* Sprain, by site
  kidney S37.03
    major (greater than 3 cm) (massive) (stellate) S37.06
    minor (less than 1 cm) S37.04
    moderate (1 to 3 cm) S37.05
      multiple S37.06
  knee S81.01
    with foreign body S81.02
  labium (majus) (minus) —*see* Laceration, vulva
  lacrimal duct —*see* Laceration, eyelid
  large intestine —*see* Laceration, intestine, large
  larynx S11.011
    with foreign body S11.012
  leg (lower) S81.819
    with foreign body S81.829
    foot —*see* Laceration, foot
    knee —*see* Laceration, knee
    left S81.812
      with foreign body S81.822
    right S81.811
      with foreign body S81.821
    upper —*see* Laceration, thigh
  ligament —*see* Sprain
  lip S01.511
    with foreign body S01.521
  liver S36.113
    major (stellate) S36.116
    minor S36.114
    moderate S36.115
  loin —*see* Laceration, abdomen, wall
  lower back —*see* Laceration, back, lower
  lumbar region —*see* Laceration, back, lower
  lung S27.339
    bilateral S27.332
    unilateral S27.331
  malar region —*see* Laceration, head, specified site NEC
  mammary —*see* Laceration, breast
  mastoid region —*see* Laceration, head, specified site NEC
  meninges —*see* Injury, intracranial, diffuse
  meniscus —*see* Tear, meniscus
  mesentery S36.893
  mesosalpinx S37.893
  mouth —*see* Laceration, oral cavity

Laceration - *continued*
  muscle —*see* Injury, muscle, by site, laceration
  nail
    finger —*see* Laceration, finger, with damage to nail
    toe —*see* Laceration, toe, with damage to nail
  nasal (septum) (sinus) —*see* Laceration, nose
  nasopharynx —*see* Laceration, head, specified site NEC
  neck S11.91
    with foreign body S11.92
    involving
      cervical esophagus S11.21
        with foreign body S11.22
      larynx —*see* Laceration, larynx
      pharynx —*see* Laceration, pharynx
      thyroid gland —*see* Laceration, thyroid gland
      trachea —*see* Laceration, trachea
    specified site NEC S11.81
      with foreign body S11.82
  nerve —*see* Injury, nerve
  nose (septum) (sinus) S01.21
    with foreign body S01.22
  ocular NOS S05.3
    adnexa NOS S01.11
  oral cavity S01.512
    with foreign body S01.522
  orbit (eye) —*see* Wound, open, ocular, orbit
  ovary S37.439
    bilateral S37.432
    unilateral S37.431
  palate —*see* Laceration, oral cavity
  palm —*see* Laceration, hand
  pancreas S36.239
    body S36.231
      major S36.261
      minor S36.241
      moderate S36.251
    head S36.230
      major S36.260
      minor S36.240
      moderate S36.250
      major S36.269
    minor S36.249
    moderate S36.259
    tail S36.232
      major S36.262
      minor S36.242
      moderate S36.252
  pelvic S31.010
    with
      foreign body S31.020
        penetration into retroperitoneal cavity S31.021
      penetration into retroperitoneal cavity S31.011
    floor —*see also* Laceration, back, lower
      with ectopic or molar pregnancy O08.6
      complicating delivery O70.1
      following ectopic or molar pregnancy O08.6
      old (postpartal) N81.89
    organ S37.93
      with ectopic or molar pregnancy O08.6
      adrenal gland S37.813
      bladder S37.23
      fallopian tube —*see* Laceration, fallopian tube
      following ectopic or molar pregnancy O08.6

Laceration - *continued*
- kidney —*see* Laceration, kidney
- obstetrical trauma O71.5
- ovary —*see* Laceration, ovary
- prostate S37.823
- specified site NEC S37.893
- ureter S37.13
- urethra S37.33
- uterus S37.63
- penis S31.21
  - with foreign body S31.22
- perineum
  - female S31.41
    - with
      - ectopic or molar pregnancy O08.6
      - foreign body S31.42
    - during delivery O70.9
      - first degree O70.0
      - fourth degree O70.3
      - second degree O70.1
      - third degree O70.2
    - old (postpartal) N81.89
    - postpartal N81.89
    - secondary (postpartal) O90.1
  - male S31.119
    - with foreign body S31.129
- periocular area (with or without lacrimal passages) —*see* Laceration, eyelid
- peritoneum S36.893
- periumbilic region —*see* Laceration, abdomen, wall, periumbilic
- periurethral tissue —*see* Laceration, urethra
- phalanges
  - finger —*see* Laceration, finger
  - toe —*see* Laceration, toe
- pharynx S11.21
  - with foreign body S11.22
- pinna —*see* Laceration, ear
- popliteal space —*see* Laceration, knee
- prepuce —*see* Laceration, penis
- prostate S37.823
- pubic region S31.119
  - with foreign body S31.129
- pudendum —*see* Laceration, genital organs, external
- rectovaginal septum —*see* Laceration, vagina
- rectum S36.63
- retroperitoneum S36.893
- round ligament S37.893
- sacral region —*see* Laceration, back, lower
- sacroiliac region —*see* Laceration, back, lower
- salivary gland —*see* Laceration, oral cavity
- scalp S01.01
  - with foreign body S01.02
- scapular region —*see* Laceration, shoulder
- scrotum S31.31
  - with foreign body S31.32
- seminal vesicle S37.893
- shin —*see* Laceration, leg
- shoulder S41.019
  - with foreign body S41.029
  - left S41.012
    - with foreign body S41.022
  - right S41.011
    - with foreign body S41.021
- small intestine —*see* Laceration, intestine, small
- spermatic cord —*see* Laceration, testis
- spinal cord (meninges) —*see also* Injury, spinal cord, by region
  - due to injury at birth P11.5

Laceration - *continued*
- newborn (birth injury) P11.5
- spleen S36.039
  - major (massive) (stellate) S36.032
  - moderate S36.031
  - superficial (minor) S36.030
- sternal region —*see* Laceration, thorax, front
- stomach S36.33
- submaxillary region —*see* Laceration, head, specified site NEC
- submental region —*see* Laceration, head, specified site NEC
- subungual
  - finger (s) —*see* Laceration, finger, with damage to nail
  - toe (s) —*see* Laceration, toe, with damage to nail
- suprarenal gland —*see* Laceration, adrenal gland
- temple, temporal region —*see* Laceration, head, specified site NEC
- temporomandibular area —*see* Laceration, cheek
- tendon —*see* Injury, muscle, by site, laceration
  - Achilles S86.02
- tentorium cerebelli —*see* Injury, intracranial, diffuse
- testis S31.31
  - with foreign body S31.32
- thigh S71.11
  - with foreign body S71.12
- thorax, thoracic (wall) S21.91
  - with foreign body S21.92
    - back S21.22
      - with penetration into thoracic cavity S21.42
    - front S21.12
      - with penetration into thoracic cavity S21.32
  - back S21.21
    - with
      - foreign body S21.22
        - with penetration into thoracic cavity S21.42
      - penetration into thoracic cavity S21.41
  - breast —*see* Laceration, breast
  - front S21.11
    - with
      - foreign body S21.12
        - with penetration into thoracic cavity S21.32
      - penetration into thoracic cavity S21.31
- thumb S61.019
  - with
    - damage to nail S61.119
      - with
        - foreign body S61.129
    - foreign body S61.029
  - left S61.012
    - with
      - damage to nail S61.112
        - with
          - foreign body S61.122
      - foreign body S61.022
  - right S61.011
    - with
      - damage to nail S61.111
        - with
          - foreign body S61.121
      - foreign body S61.021

Laceration - *continued*
- thyroid gland S11.11
  - with foreign body S11.12
- toe (s) S91.119
  - with
    - damage to nail S91.219
      - with
        - foreign body S91.229
    - foreign body S91.129
  - great S91.113
    - with
      - damage to nail S91.213
        - with
          - foreign body S91.223
      - foreign body S91.123
  - left S91.112
    - with
      - damage to nail S91.212
        - with
          - foreign body S91.222
      - foreign body S91.122
  - right S91.111
    - with
      - damage to nail S91.211
        - with
          - foreign body S91.221
      - foreign body S91.121
  - lesser S91.116
    - with
      - damage to nail S91.216
        - with
          - foreign body S91.226
      - foreign body S91.126
  - left S91.115
    - with
      - damage to nail S91.215
        - with
          - foreign body S91.225
      - foreign body S91.125
  - right S91.114
    - with
      - damage to nail S91.214
        - with
          - foreign body S91.224
      - foreign body S91.124
- tongue —*see* Laceration, oral cavity
- trachea S11.021
  - with foreign body S11.022
- tunica vaginalis —*see* Laceration, testis
- tympanum, tympanic membrane —*see* Laceration, ear, drum
- umbilical region S31.115
  - with foreign body S31.125
- ureter S37.13
- urethra S37.33
  - with or following ectopic or molar pregnancy O08.6
  - obstetrical trauma O71.5
- urinary organ NEC S37.893
- uterus S37.63
  - with ectopic or molar pregnancy O08.6
  - following ectopic or molar pregnancy O08.6
  - nonpuerperal, nontraumatic N85.8
  - obstetrical trauma NEC O71.81
  - old (postpartal) N85.8
- uvula —*see* Laceration, oral cavity
- vagina S31.41
  - with
    - ectopic or molar pregnancy O08.6
    - foreign body S31.42
  - during delivery O71.4
    - with perineal laceration —*see* Laceration, perineum, female, during delivery

Laceration - *continued*

following ectopic or molar pregnancy O08.6
nonpuerperal, nontraumatic N89.8
old (postpartal) N89.8
vas deferens S37.893
vesical —*see* Laceration, bladder
vocal cords S11.031
with foreign body S11.032
vulva S31.41
with
ectopic or molar pregnancy O08.6
foreign body S31.42
complicating delivery O70.0
following ectopic or molar pregnancy O08.6
nonpuerperal, nontraumatic N90.89
old (postpartal) N90.89
wrist S61.519
with
foreign body S61.529
left S61.512
with
foreign body S61.522
right S61.511
with
foreign body S61.521
Lack of
achievement in school Z55.3
adequate
food Z59.4
intermaxillary vertical dimension of fully
erupted teeth M26.36
sleep Z72.820
appetite (see Anorexia) R63.0
awareness R41.9
care
in home Z74.2
of infant (at or after birth) T76.02
confirmed T74.02
cognitive functions R41.9
coordination R27.9
ataxia R27.0
specified type NEC R27.8
development (physiological) R62.50
failure to thrive (child over 28 days old)
R62.51
adult R62.7
newborn P92.6
short stature R62.52
specified type NEC R62.59
energy R53.83
financial resources Z59.6
food T73.0
growth R62.52
heating Z59.1
housing (permanent) (temporary) Z59.0
adequate Z59.1
learning experiences in childhood Z62.898
leisure time (affecting life-style) Z73.2
material resources Z59.9
memory —*see also* Amnesia
mild, following organic brain damage F06.8
ovulation N97.0
parental supervision or control of child Z62.0
person able to render necessary care Z74.2
physical exercise Z72.3
play experience in childhood Z62.898
posterior occlusal support M26.57
relaxation (affecting life-style) Z73.2
sexual
desire F52.0
enjoyment F52.1
shelter Z59.0

Lack of - *continued*

sleep (adequate) Z72.820
supervision of child by parent Z62.0
support, posterior occlusal M26.57
water T73.1
Lacrimal —*see* condition
Lacrimation, abnormal —*see* Epiphora
Lacrimonasal duct —*see* condition
Lactation, lactating (breast) (puerperal,
postpartum)
associated
cracked nipple O92.13
retracted nipple O92.03
defective O92.4
disorder NEC O92.79
excessive O92.6
failed (complete) O92.3
partial O92.4
mastitis NEC —*see* Mastitis, obstetric
mother (care and/or examination) Z39.1
nonpuerperal N64.3
Lacticemia, excessive E87.2
Lacunar skull Q75.8
Laennec's cirrhosis K74.69
alcoholic K70.30
with ascites K70.31
Lafora's disease —*see* Epilepsy, generalized,
idiopathic
Lag, lid (nervous) —*see* Retraction, lid
Lagophthalmos (eyelid) (nervous) H02.209
cicatricial H02.219
left H02.216
lower H02.215
upper H02.214
right H02.213
lower H02.212
upper H02.211
keratoconjunctivitis —*see*
Keratoconjunctivitis
left H02.206
lower H02.205
upper H02.204
mechanical H02.229
left H02.226
lower H02.225
upper H02.224
right H02.223
lower H02.222
upper H02.221
paralytic H02.239
left H02.236
lower H02.235
upper H02.234
right H02.233
lower H02.232
upper H02.231
right H02.203
lower H02.202
upper H02.201
Laki-Lorand factor deficiency —*see* Defect,
coagulation, specified type NEC
Lalling F80.0
Lambert-Eaton syndrome —*see* Syndrome,
Lambert-Eaton
Lambliasis, lambliosis A07.1
Landau-Kleffner syndrome —*see* Epilepsy,
specified NEC
Landouzy-Déjérine dystrophy or
facioscapulohumeral atrophy G71.0
Landouzy's disease (icterohemorrhagic
leptospirosis) A27.0
Landry-Guillain-Barré, syndrome or
paralysis G61.0

Landry's disease or paralysis G61.0
Lane's
band Q43.3
kink —*see* Obstruction, intestine
syndrome K90.2
Langdon Down syndrome —*see* Trisomy, 21
Lapsed immunization schedule status Z28.3
Large
baby (regardless of gestational age) (4000g to
4499g) P08.1
ear, congenital Q17.1
physiological cup Q14.2
stature R68.89
Large-for-dates NEC (infant) (4000g to
4499g) P08.1
affecting management of pregnancy O36.6
exceptionally (4500g or more) P08.0
Larsen-Johansson disease or
osteochondrosis —*see* Osteochondrosis,
juvenile, patella
Larsen's syndrome (flattened facies and
multiple congenital dislocations) Q74.8
Larva migrans
cutaneous B76.9
Ancylostoma B76.0
visceral B83.0
Laryngeal —*see* condition
Laryngismus (stridulus) J38.5
congenital P28.89
diphtheritic A36.2
Laryngitis (acute) (edematous) (fibrinous)
(infective) (infiltrative) (malignant)
(membranous) (phlegmonous)
(pneumococcal) (pseudomembranous) (septic)
(subglottic) (suppurative) (ulcerative) J04.0
with
influenza, flu, or grippe —*see* Influenza,
with, laryngitis
tracheitis (acute) —*see* Laryngotracheitis
atrophic J37.0
catarrhal J37.0
chronic J37.0
with tracheitis (chronic) J37.1
diphtheritic A36.2
due to external agent —*see* Inflammation,
respiratory, upper, due to
Hemophilus influenzae J04.0
H. influenzae J04.0
hypertrophic J37.0
influenzal —*see* Influenza, with, respiratory
manifestations NEC
obstructive J05.0
sicca J37.0
spasmodic J05.0
acute J04.0
streptococcal J04.0
stridulous J05.0
syphilitic (late) A52.73
congenital A50.59 *[J99]*
early A50.03 *[J99]*
tuberculous A15.5
Vincent's A69.1
Laryngocele (congenital) (ventricular) Q31.3
Laryngofissure J38.7
congenital Q31.8
Laryngomalacia (congenital) Q31.5
Laryngopharyngitis (acute) J06.0
chronic J37.0
due to external agent —*see* Inflammation,
respiratory, upper, due to
Laryngoplegia J38.00
bilateral J38.02
unilateral J38.01

Laryngoptosis J38.7
Laryngospasm J38.5
Laryngostenosis J38.6
Laryngotracheitis (acute) (Infectional)
  (infective) (viral) J04.2
  atrophic J37.1
  catarrhal J37.1
  chronic J37.1
  diphtheritic A36.2
  due to external agent —*see* Inflammation,
  respiratory, upper, due to
  Hemophilus influenzae J04.2
  hypertrophic J37.1
  influenzal —*see* Influenza, with, respiratory
  manifestations NEC
  pachydermic J38.7
  sicca J37.1
  spasmodic J38.5
    acute J05.0
  streptococcal J04.2
  stridulous J38.5
  syphilitic (late) A52.73
    congenital A50.59 *[J99]*
      early A50.03 *[J99]*
  tuberculous A15.5
  Vincent's A69.1
Laryngotracheobronchitis —*see* Bronchitis
Larynx, laryngeal —*see* condition
Lassa fever A96.2
Lassitude —*see* Weakness
Late
  talker R62.0
  walker R62.0
Late effect (s) —*see* Sequelae
Latent —*see* condition
Laterocession —*see* Lateroversion
Lateroflexion —*see* Lateroversion
Lateroversion
  cervix —*see* Lateroversion, uterus
  uterus, uterine (cervix) (postinfectional)
  (postpartal, old) N85.4
    congenital Q51.818
    in pregnancy or childbirth O34.59
Lathyrism —*see* Poisoning, food, noxious,
  plant
Launois' syndrome (pituitary gigantism)
  E22.0
Launois-Bensaude adenolipomatosis E88.89
Laurence-Moon (-Bardet) -**Biedl syndrome**
  Q87.89
Lax, laxity —*see also* Relaxation
  ligament (ous) —*see also* Disorder, ligament
    familial M35.7
    knee —*see* Derangement, knee
  skin (acquired) L57.4
    congenital Q82.8
Laxative habit F55.2
Lazy leukocyte syndrome D70.8
Lead miner's lung J63.6
Leak, leakage
  air NEC J93.82
    postprocedural J95.812
  amniotic fluid —*see* Rupture, membranes,
  premature
  blood (microscopic) , fetal, into maternal
  circulation affecting management of
  pregnancy —*see* Pregnancy, complicated by
  cerebrospinal fluid G96.0
    from spinal (lumbar) puncture G97.0
  device, implant or graft —*see also*
  Complications, by site and type, mechanical

Leak, leakage – *continued*
  arterial graft NEC —*see* Complication,
  cardiovascular device, mechanical, vascular
  breast (implant) T85.43
  catheter NEC T85.638
    urinary, indwelling T83.038
      cystostomy T83.030
    dialysis (renal) T82.43
      intraperitoneal T85.631
    infusion NEC T82.534
      spinal (epidural) (subdural) T85.630
  gastrointestinal —*see* Complications,
  prosthetic device, mechanical, gastrointestinal
  device
    genital NEC T83.498
      penile prosthesis T83.490
    heart NEC —*see* Complication,
  cardiovascular device, mechanical
    joint prosthesis —*see* Complications, joint
  prosthesis, mechanical, specified NEC, by site
    ocular NEC —*see* Complications, prosthetic
  device, mechanical, ocular device
    orthopedic NEC —*see* Complication,
  orthopedic, device, mechanical
    persistent air J93.82
    specified NEC T85.638
    urinary NEC —*see also* Complication,
  genitourinary, device, urinary, mechanical
    graft T83.23
    vascular NEC —*see* Complication,
  cardiovascular device, mechanical
    ventricular intracranial shunt T85.03
  urine —*see* Incontinence
Leaky heart —*see* Endocarditis
Learning defect (specific) F81.9
Leather bottle stomach C16.9
Leber's
  congenital amaurosis H35.50
  optic atrophy (hereditary) H47.22
Lederer's anemia D59.1
Leeches (external) —*see* Hirudiniasis
Leg —*see* condition
Legg (-Calvé) -**Perthes disease, syndrome or**
  osteochondrosis M91.1
Legionellosis A48.1
  nonpneumonic A48.2
Legionnaires'
  disease A48.1
    nonpneumonic A48.2
  pneumonia A48.1
Leigh's disease G31.82
Leiner's disease L21.1
Leiofibromyoma —*see* Leiomyoma
Leiomyoblastoma —*see* Neoplasm,
  connective tissue, benign
Leiomyofibroma —*see also* Neoplasm,
  connective tissue, benign
  uterus (cervix) (corpus) D25.9
Leiomyoma —*see also* Neoplasm, connective
  tissue, benign
  bizarre —*see* Neoplasm, connective tissue,
  benign
  cellular —*see* Neoplasm, connective tissue,
  benign
  epithelioid —*see* Neoplasm, connective
  tissue, benign
  uterus (cervix) (corpus) D25.9
    intramural D25.1
    submucous D25.0
    subserosal D25.2
  vascular —*see* Neoplasm, connective tissue,
  benign

Leiomyoma, leiomyomatosis (intravascular)
  —*see* Neoplasm, connective tissue, uncertain
  behavior
Leiomyosarcoma —*see also* Neoplasm,
  connective tissue, malignant
  epithelioid —*see* Neoplasm, connective
  tissue, malignant
  myxoid —*see* Neoplasm, connective tissue,
  malignant
Leishmaniasis B55.9
  American (mucocutaneous) B55.2
    cutaneous B55.1
  Asian Desert B55.1
  Brazilian B55.2
  cutaneous (any type) B55.1
  dermal —*see also* Leishmaniasis, cutaneous
    post-kala-azar B55.0
  eyelid B55.1
  infantile B55.0
  Mediterranean B55.0
  mucocutaneous (American) (New World)
  B55.2
  naso-oral B55.2
  nasopharyngeal B55.2
  old world B55.1
  tegumentaria diffusa B55.1
  visceral B55.0
Leishmanoid, dermal —*see also*
  Leishmaniasis, cutaneous
  post-kala-azar B55.0
Lenègre's disease I44.2
Lengthening, leg —*see* Deformity, limb,
  unequal length
Lennert's lymphoma —*see* Lymphoma,
  Lennert's
Lennox-Gastaut syndrome G40.812
  intractable G40.814
    with status epilepticus G40.813
    without status epilepticus G40.814
  not intractable G40.812
    with status epilepticus G40.811
    without status epilepticus G40.812
Lens —*see* condition
Lenticonus (anterior) (posterior) (congenital)
  Q12.8
Lenticular degeneration, progressive E83.01
Lentiglobus (posterior) (congenital) Q12.8
Lentigo (congenital) L81.4
  maligna —*see also* Melanoma, in situ
  melanoma —*see* Melanoma
Lentivirus, as cause of disease classified
  elsewhere B97.31
Leontiasis
  ossium M85.2
  syphilitic (late) A52.78
    congenital A50.59
Lepothrix A48.8
Lepra —*see* Leprosy
Leprechaunism E34.8
Leprosy A30.
  with muscle disorder A30.9 *[M63.80]*
  ankle A30.9 *[M63.87]*
  foot A30.9 *[M63.87]*
  forearm A30.9 *[M63.83]*
  hand A30.9 *[M63.84]*
  lower leg A30.9 *[M63.86]*
  multiple sites A30.9 *[M63.89]*
  pelvic region A30.9 *[M63.85]*
  shoulder region A30.9 *[M63.81]*
  specified site NEC A30.9 *[M63.88]*
  thigh A30.9 *[M63.85]*
  upper arm A30.9 *[M63.82]*

Leprosy – *continued*
  anesthetic A30.9
  BB A30.3
  BL A30.4
  borderline (infiltrated) (neuritic) A30.3
    lepromatous A30.4
    tuberculoid A30.2
  BT A30.2
  dimorphous (infiltrated) (neuritic) A30.3
  I A30.0
  indeterminate (macular) (neuritic) A30.0
  lepromatous (diffuse) (infiltrated) (macular)
    (neuritic) (nodular) A30.5
  LL A30.5
  macular (early) (neuritic) (simple) A30.9
  maculoanesthetic A30.9
  mixed A30.3
  neural A30.9
  nodular A30.5
  primary neuritic A30.3
  specified type NEC A30.8
  TT A30.1
  tuberculoid (major) (minor) A30.1
Leptocytosis, hereditary D56.9
Leptomeningitis (chronic) (circumscribed)
  (hemorrhagic) (nonsuppurative) —*see*
  Meningitis
Leptomeningopathy G96.19
Leptospiral —*see* condition
Leptospirochetal —*see* condition
Leptospirosis A27.9
  canicola A27.89
  due to Leptospira interrogans serovar
  icterohaemorrhagiae A27.0
  icterohemorrhagica A27.0
  pomona A27.89
  Weil's disease A27.0
Leptus dermatitis B88.0
Leriche's syndrome (aortic bifurcation
  occlusion) I74.09
Leri's pleonosteosis Q78.8
Leri-Weill syndrome Q77.8
Lermoyez' syndrome —*see* Vertigo,
  peripheral NEC
Lesch-Nyhan syndrome E79.1
Leser-Trélat disease L82.1
  inflamed L82.0
Lesion (s) (nontraumatic)
  abducens nerve —*see* Strabismus, paralytic,
  sixth nerve
  alveolar process K08.9
  angiocentric immunoproliferative D47.Z9
  anorectal K62.9
  aortic (valve) I35.9
  auditory nerve —*see* subcategory H93.3
  basal ganglion G25.9
  bile duct —*see* Disease, bile duct
  biomechanical M99.9
    specified type NEC M99.89
      abdomen M99.89
      acromioclavicular M99.87
      cervical region M99.81
      cervicothoracic M99.81
      costochondral M99.88
      costovertebral M99.88
      head region M99.80
      hip M99.85
      lower extremity M99.86
      lumbar region M99.83
      lumbosacral M99.83
      occipitocervical M99.80
      pelvic region M99.85

Lesion – *continued*
      pubic M99.85
      rib cage M99.88
      sacral region M99.84
      sacrococcygeal M99.84
      sacroiliac M99.84
      specified NEC M99.89
      sternochondral M99.88
      sternoclavicular M99.87
      thoracic region M99.82
      thoracolumbar M99.82
      upper extremity M99.87
  bladder N32.9
  bone —*see* Disorder, bone
  brachial plexus G54.0
  brain G93.9
    congenital Q04.9
    vascular I67.9
      degenerative I67.9
      hypertensive I67.4
  buccal cavity K13.79
  calcified —*see* Calcification
  canthus —*see* Disorder, eyelid
  carate —*see* Pinta, lesions
  cardia K22.9
  cardiac (*see also* Disease, heart) I51.9
    congenital Q24.9
    valvular —*see* Endocarditis
  cauda equina G83.4
  cecum K63.9
  cerebral —*see* Lesion, brain
  cerebrovascular I67.9
    degenerative I67.9
    hypertensive I67.4
  cervical (nerve) root NEC G54.2
  chiasmal —*see* Disorder, optic, chiasm
  chorda tympani G51.8
  coin, lung R91.1
  colon K63.9
  congenital —*see* Anomaly, by site
  conjunctiva H11.9
  conus medullaris —*see* Injury, conus
  medullaris
  coronary artery —*see* Ischemia, heart
  cranial nerve G52.9
    eighth —*see* Disorder, ear
    eleventh G52.9
    fifth G50.9
    first G52.0
    fourth —*see* Strabismus, paralytic, fourth
  nerve
    seventh G51.9
    sixth —*see* Strabismus, paralytic, sixth
  nerve
    tenth G52.2
    twelfth G52.3
  cystic —*see* Cyst
  degenerative —*see* Degeneration
  duodenum K31.9
  edentulous (alveolar) ridge, associated with
  trauma, due to traumatic occlusion K06.2
  en coup de sabre L94.1
  eyelid —*see* Disorder, eyelid
  gasserian ganglion G50.8
  gastric K31.9
  gastroduodenal K31.9
  gastrointestinal K63.9
  gingiva, associated with trauma K06.2
  glomerular
    focal and segmental (*see also* N00-N07 with
  fourth character .1) N05.1
      minimal change (*see also* N00-N07 with
  fourth character .0) N05.0

Lesion – *continued*
  heart (organic) —*see* Disease, heart
  hyperchromic, due to pinta (carate) A67.1
  hyperkeratotic —*see* Hyperkeratosis
  hypothalamic E23.7
  ileocecal K63.9
  ileum K63.9
  iliohypogastric nerve G57.8
  inflammatory —*see* Inflammation
  intestine K63.9
  intracerebral —*see* Lesion, brain
  intrachiasmal (optic) —*see* Disorder, optic,
  chiasm
  intracranial, space-occupying R90.0
  joint —*see* Disorder, joint
    sacroiliac (old) M53.3
  keratotic —*see* Keratosis
  kidney —*see* Disease, renal
  laryngeal nerve (recurrent) G52.2
  lip K13.0
  liver K76.9
  lumbosacral
    plexus G54.1
    root (nerve) NEC G54.4
  lung (coin) R91.1
  maxillary sinus J32.0
  mitral I05.9
  Morel-Lavallée —*see* Hematoma, by site
  motor cortex NEC G93.89
  mouth K13.79
  nerve G58.9
    femoral G57.2
    median G56.1
      carpal tunnel syndrome —*see* Syndrome,
  carpal tunnel
    plantar G57.6
    popliteal (lateral) G57.3
      medial G57.4
    radial G56.3
    sciatic G57.0
    spinal —*see* Injury, nerve, spinal
    ulnar G56.2
  nervous system, congenital Q07.9
  nonallopathic —*see* Lesion, biomechanical
  nose (internal) J34.89
  obstructive —*see* Obstruction
  obturator nerve G57.8
  oral mucosa K13.70
  organ or site NEC —*see* Disease, by site
  osteolytic —*see* Osteolysis
  peptic K27.9
  periodontal, due to traumatic occlusion K05.5
  pharynx J39.2
  pigment, pigmented (skin) L81.9
  pinta —*see* Pinta, lesions
  polypoid —*see* Polyp
  prechiasmal (optic) —*see* Disorder, optic,
  chiasm
  primary (*see also* Syphilis, primary) A51.0
    carate A67.0
    pinta A67.0
    yaws A66.0
  pulmonary J98.4
    valve I37.9
  pylorus K31.9
  rectosigmoid K63.9
  retina, retinal H35.9
  sacroiliac (joint) (old) M53.3
  salivary gland K11.9
    benign lymphoepithelial K11.8
  saphenous nerve G57.8
  sciatic nerve G57.0

Lesion – *continued*
secondary —*see* Syphilis, secondary
shoulder (region) M75.9
  specified NEC M75.8
sigmoid K63.9
sinus (accessory) (nasal) J34.89
skin L98.9
  suppurative L08.0
SLAP S43.43
spinal cord G95.9
  congenital Q06.9
spleen D73.89
stomach K31.9
superior glenoid labrum S43.43
syphilitic —*see* Syphilis
tertiary —*see* Syphilis, tertiary
thoracic root (nerve) NEC G54.3
tonsillar fossa J35.9
tooth, teeth K08.9
  white spot
    chewing surface K02.51
    pit and fissure surface K02.51
    smooth surface K02.61
traumatic —*see* specific type of injury by site
tricuspid (valve) I07.9
  nonrheumatic I36.9
trigeminal nerve G50.9
ulcerated or ulcerative —*see* Ulcer, skin
uterus N85.9
vagus nerve G52.2
valvular —*see* Endocarditis
vascular I99.9
  affecting central nervous system I67.9
  following trauma NEC T14.8
  umbilical cord, complicating delivery O69.5
warty —*see* Verruca
white spot (tooth)
  chewing surface K02.51
  pit and fissure surface K02.51
  smooth surface K02.61
Lethargic —*see* condition
Lethargy R53.83
Letterer-Siwe's disease C96.0
Leukemia, leukemic C95.9
acute basophilic C94.8
acute bilineal C95.0
acute erythroid C94.0
acute lymphoblastic C91.0
acute megakaryoblastic C94.2
acute megakaryocytic C94.2
acute mixed lineage C95.0
acute monoblastic (monoblastic/monocytic)
  C93.0
acute monocytic (monoblastic/monocytic)
  C93.0
acute myeloblastic (minimal differentiation)
  (with maturation) C92.0
acute myeloid
  with
    11q23-abnormality C92.6
    dysplasia of remaining hematopoesis
  and/or myelodysplastic disease in its history
  C92.A
    multilineage dysplasia C92.A
    variation of MLL-gene C92.6
  M6 (a) (b) C94.0
  M7 C94.2
acute myelomonocytic C92.5
acute promyelocytic C92.4
adult T-cell (HTLV 1-associated) (acute
  variant) (chronic variant) (lymphomatoid
  variant) (smouldering variant) C91.5

Leukemia, leukemic – *continued*
aggressive NK-cell C94.8
AML (1/ETO) (M0) (M1) (M2) (without a
  FAB classification) C92.0
AML M3 C92.4
AML M4 (Eo with inv(16) or t(16;16)) C92.5
AML M5 C93.0
AML M5a C93.0
AML M5b C93.0
AML Me with t (15;17) and variants C92.4
atypical chronic myeloid, BCR/ABL-negative
  C92.2
biphenotypic acute C95.0
blast cell C95.0
Burkitt-type, mature B-cell C91.A
chronic lymphocytic, of B-cell type C91.1
chronic monocytic C93.1
chronic myelogenous (Philadelphia
  chromosome (Ph1) positive) (t(9;22))
  (q34;q11) (with crisis of blast cells) C92.1
chronic myeloid, BCR/ABL-positive C92.1
  atypical, BCR/ABL-negative C92.2
chronic myelomonocytic C93.1
chronic neutrophilic D47.1
CMML (1) (2) (with eosinophilia) C93.1
granulocytic (*see also* Category C92) C92.9
hairy cell C91.4
juvenile myelomonocytic C93.3
lymphoid C91.9
  specified NEC C91.Z
mast cell C94.3
mature B-cell, Burkitt-type C91.A
monocytic (subacute) C93.9
  specified NEC C93.Z
myelogenous (*see also* Category C92) C92.9
myeloid C92.9
  specified NEC C92.Z
plasma cell C90.1
plasmacytic C90.1
prolymphocytic
  of B-cell type C91.3
  of T-cell type C91.6
specified NEC C94.8
stem cell, of unclear lineage C95.0
subacute lymphocytic C91.9
T-cell large granular lymphocytic C91.Z
unspecified cell type C95.9
  acute C95.0
  chronic C95.1
Leukemoid reaction (*see also* Reaction,
  leukemoid) D72.823
Leukoaraiosis (hypertensive) I67.81
Leukoariosis —*see* Leukoaraiosis
Leukocoria —*see* Disorder, globe,
  degenerated condition, leucocoria
Leukocytopenia D72.819
Leukocytosis D72.829
  eosinophilic D72.1
Leukoderma, leukodermia NEC L81.5
  syphilitic A51.39
    late A52.79
Leukodystrophy E75.29
Leukoedema, oral epithelium K13.29
Leukoencephalitis G04.81
  acute (subacute) hemorrhagic G36.1
    postimmunization or postvaccinal G04.02
  postinfectious G04.01
  subacute sclerosing A81.1
  van Bogaert's (sclerosing) A81.1
Leukoencephalopathy (*see also*
  Encephalopathy) G93.49
  Binswanger's I67.3
  heroin vapor G92

Leukoencephalopathy – continued
metachromatic E75.25
multifocal (progressive) A81.2
postimmunization and postvaccinal G04.02
progressive multifocal A81.2
reversible, posterior G93.6
van Bogaert's (sclerosing) A81.1
vascular, progressive I67.3
Leukoerythroblastosis D75.9
Leukokeratosis —*see also* Leukoplakia
mouth K13.21
nicotina palati K13.24
oral mucosa K13.21
tongue K13.21
vocal cord J38.3
Leukokraurosis vulva (e) N90.4
Leukoma (cornea) —*see also* Opacity, cornea
adherent H17.0
interfering with central vision —*see* Opacity,
  cornea, central
Leukomalacia, cerebral, newborn P91.2
periventricular P91.2
Leukomelanopathy, hereditary D72.0
Leukonychia (punctata) (striata) L60.8
congenital Q84.4
Leukopathia unguium L60.8
congenital Q84.4
Leukopenia D72.819
basophilic D72.818
chemotherapy (cancer) induced D70.1
congenital D70.0
cyclic D70.0
drug induced NEC D70.2
  due to cytoreductive cancer chemotherapy
  D70.1
eosinophilic D72.818
familial D70.0
infantile genetic D70.0
malignant D70.9
periodic D70.0
transitory neonatal P61.5
Leukopenic —*see* condition
Leukoplakia
anus K62.89
bladder (postinfectional) N32.89
buccal K13.21
cervix (uteri) N88.0
esophagus K22.8
gingiva K13.21
hairy (oral mucosa) (tongue) K13.3
kidney (pelvis) N28.89
larynx J38.7
lip K13.21
mouth K13.21
oral epithelium, including tongue (mucosa)
  K13.21
palate K13.21
pelvis (kidney) N28.89
penis (infectional) N48.0
rectum K62.89
syphilitic (late) A52.79
tongue K13.21
ureter (postinfectional) N28.89
urethra (postinfectional) N36.8
uterus N85.8
vagina N89.4
vocal cord J38.3
vulva N90.4
Leukorrhea N89.8
due to Trichomonas (vaginalis) A59.00
trichomonal A59.00

Leukosarcoma C85.9
Levocardia (isolated) Q24.1
  with situs inversus Q89.3
Levotransposition Q20.5
Lev's disease or syndrome (acquired complete
  heart block) I44.2
Levulosuria —*see* Fructosuria
Levurid L30.2
Lewy body (ies) (dementia) (disease) G31.83
Leyden-Moebius dystrophy G71.0
Leydig cell
  carcinoma
    specified site —*see* Neoplasm, malignant,
    by site
      unspecified site
        female C56.9
        male C62.9
  tumor
    benign
      specified site —*see* Neoplasm, benign, by
  site
        unspecified site
          female D27.
          male D29.2
    malignant
      specified site —*see* Neoplasm, malignant,
      by site
        unspecified site
          female C56.
          male C62.9
    specified site —*see* Neoplasm, uncertain
    behavior, by site
      unspecified site
        female D39.1
        male D40.1
Leydig-Sertoli cell tumor
  specified site —*see* Neoplasm, benign, by site
  unspecified site
    female D27.
    male D29.2
LGSIL (Low grade squamous intraepithelial
  lesion on cytologic smear of)
  anus R85.612
  cervix R87.612
  vagina R87.622
Liar, pathologic F60.2
Libido
  decreased R68.82
Libman-Sacks disease M32.11
Lice (infestation) B85.2
  body (Pediculus corporis) B85.1
  crab B85.3
  head (Pediculus capitis) B85.0
  mixed (classifiable to more than one of the
    titles B85.0-B85.3) B85.4
  pubic (Phthirus pubis) B85.3
Lichen L28.0
  albus L90.0
    penis N48.0
    vulva N90.4
  amyloidosis E85.4 *[L99]*
  atrophicus L90.0
    penis N48.0
    vulva N90.4
  congenital Q82.8
  myxedematosus L98.5
  nitidus L44.1
  pilaris Q82.8
    acquired L85.8
  planopilaris L66.1
  planus (chronicus) L43.9
    annularis L43.8

Lichen – *continued*
  bullous L43.1
  follicular L66.1
  hypertrophic L43.0
  moniliformis L44.3
  of Wilson L43.9
  specified NEC L43.8
  subacute (active) L43.3
  tropicus L43.3
  ruber
    acuminatus L44.0
    moniliformis L44.3
    planus L43.9
  sclerosus (et atrophicus) L90.0
    penis N48.0
    vulva N90.4
  scrofulosus (primary) (tuberculous) A18.4
  simplex (chronicus) (circumscriptus) L28.0
  striatus L44.2
  urticatus L28.2
Lichenification L28.0
Lichenoides tuberculosis (primary) A18.4
Lichtheim's disease or syndrome —*see*
  Degeneration, combined
Lien migrans D73.89
Ligament —*see* condition
Light
  for gestational age —*see* Light for dates
  headedness R42
Light-for-dates (infant) P05.00
  with weight of
    499 grams or less P05.01
    500 749 grams P05.02
    750 999 grams P05.03
    1000 1249 grams P05.04
    1250 1499 grams P05.05
    1500 1749 grams P05.06
    1750 1999 grams P05.07
    2000 2499 grams P05.08
  and small-for-dates —*see* Small for dates
  affecting management of pregnancy O36.59
Lightning (effects) (stroke) (struck by) T75.00
  burn —*see* Burn
  foot E53.8
  shock T75.01
  specified effect NEC T75.09
Lightwood-Albright syndrome N25.89
Lightwood's disease or syndrome (renal
  tubular acidosis) N25.89
Lignac (-de Toni) (-Fanconi) (-Debré) **disease
  or syndrome** E72.09
  with cystinosis E72.04
Ligneous thyroiditis E06.5
Likoff's syndrome I20.8
Limb —*see* condition
Limbic epilepsy personality syndrome F07.0
Limitation, limited
  activities due to disability Z73.6
  cardiac reserve —*see* Disease, heart
  eye muscle duction, traumatic —*see*
    Strabismus, mechanical
  mandibular range of motion M26.52
Lindau (-von Hippel) **disease** Q85.8
Line (s)
  Beau's L60.4
  Harris' —*see* Arrest, epiphyseal
  Hudson's (cornea) —*see* Pigmentation,
    cornea, anterior
  Stähli's (cornea) —*see* Pigmentation, cornea,
    anterior
Linea corneae senilis —*see* Change, cornea,
  senile

Lingua
  geographica K14.1
  nigra (villosa) K14.3
  plicata K14.5
  tylosis K13.29
Lingual —*see* condition
Linguatulosis B88.8
Linitis (gastric) **plasticaC16.9**
Lip —*see* condition
Lipedema —*see* Edema
Lipemia —*see also* Hyperlipidemia
  retina, retinalis E78.3
Lipidosis E75.6
  cerebral (infantile) (juvenile) (late) E75.4
  cerebroretinal E75.4
  cerebroside E75.22
  cholesterol (cerebral) E75.5
  glycolipid E75.21
  hepatosplenomegalic E78.3
  sphingomyelin —*see* Niemann-Pick disease
    or syndrome
  sulfatide E75.29
Lipoadenoma —*see* Neoplasm, benign, by site
Lipoblastoma —*see* Lipoma
Lipoblastomatosis —*see* Lipoma
Lipochondrodystrophy E76.01
Lipodermatosclerosis —*see* Varix, leg, with,
  inflammation
  ulcerated —*see* Varix, leg, with, ulcer, with
    inflammation by site
Lipochrome histiocytosis (familial) D71
Lipodystrophia progressiva E88.1
Lipodystrophy (progressive) E88.1
  insulin E88.1
  intestinal K90.81
  mesenteric K65.4
Lipofibroma —*see* Lipoma
Lipofuscinosis, neuronal (with ceroidosis)
  E75.4
Lipogranuloma, sclerosing L92.8
Lipogranulomatosis E78.89
Lipoid —*see also* condition
  histiocytosis D76.3
    essential E75.29
  nephrosis N04.9
  proteinosis of Urbach E78.89
Lipoidemia —*see* Hyperlipidemia
Lipoidosis —*see* Lipidosis
Lipoma D17.9
  fetal D17.9
  fat cell D17.9
  infiltrating D17.9
  intramuscular D17.9
  pleomorphic D17.9
  site classification
    arms (skin) (subcutaneous) D17.2
    connective tissue D17.30
      intra-abdominal D17.5
      intrathoracic D17.4
      peritoneum D17.79
      retroperitoneum D17.79
      specified site NEC D17.39
      spermatic cord D17.6
    face (skin) (subcutaneous) D17.0
    genitourinary organ NEC D17.72
    head (skin) (subcutaneous) D17.0
    intra-abdominal D17.5
    intrathoracic D17.4
    kidney D17.71
    legs (skin) (subcutaneous) D17.2
    neck (skin) (subcutaneous) D17.0
    peritoneum D17.79
    retroperitoneum D17.79

Lipoma - *continued*
  skin D17.30
    specified site NEC D17.39
  specified site NEC D17.79
  spermatic cord D17.6
  subcutaneous D17.30
    specified site NEC D17.39
  trunk (skin) (subcutaneous) D17.1
  unspecified D17.9
  spindle cell D17.9
Lipomatosis E88.2
  dolorosa (Dercum) E88.2
  fetal —*see* Lipoma
  Launois-Bensaude E88.89
Lipomyoma —*see* Lipoma
Lipomyxoma —*see* Lipoma
Lipomyxosarcoma —*see* Neoplasm,
  connective tissue, malignant
Lipoprotein metabolism disorder E78.9
Lipoproteinemia E78.5
  broad-beta E78.2
  floating-beta E78.2
  hyper-pre-beta E78.1
Liposarcoma —*see also* Neoplasm, connective
  tissue, malignant
  dedifferentiated —*see* Neoplasm, connective
    tissue, malignant
  differentiated type —*see* Neoplasm,
    connective tissue, malignant
  embryonal —*see* Neoplasm, connective
    tissue, malignant
  mixed type —*see* Neoplasm, connective
    tissue, malignant
  myxoid —*see* Neoplasm, connective tissue,
    malignant
  pleomorphic —*see* Neoplasm, connective
    tissue, malignant
  round cell —*see* Neoplasm, connective tissue,
    malignant
  well differentiated type —*see* Neoplasm,
    connective tissue, malignant
Liposynovitis prepatellaris E88.89
Lipping, cervix N86
Lipschütz disease or ulcer N76.6
Lipuria R82.0
  schistosomiasis (bilharziasis) B65.0
Lisping F80.0
Lissauer's paralysis A52.17
Lissencephalia, lissencephaly Q04.3
Listeriosis, listerellosis A32.9
  congenital (disseminated) P37.2
  cutaneous A32.0
  neonatal, newborn (disseminated) P37.2
  oculoglandular A32.81
  specified NEC A32.89
Lithemia E79.0
Lithiasis —*see* Calculus
Lithosis J62.8
Lithuria R82.99
Litigation, anxiety concerning Z65.3
Little leaguer's elbow —*see* Epicondylitis,
  medial
Little's disease G80.9
Littre's
  gland —*see* condition
  hernia —*see* Hernia, abdomen
Littritis —*see* Urethritis
Livedo (annularis) (racemosa) (reticularis)
  R23.1
Liver —*see* condition
Living alone (problems with) Z60.2
  with handicapped person Z74.2

Lloyd's syndrome —*see* Adenomatosis,
  endocrine
Loa loa, loaiasis, loasis B74.3
Lobar —*see* condition
Lobomycosis B48.0
Lobo's disease B48.0
Lobotomy syndrome F07.0
Lobstein (-Ekman) **disease or syndrome**
  Q78.0
Lobster-claw hand Q71.6
Lobulation (congenital) —*see also* Anomaly,
  by site
  kidney, Q63.1
  liver, abnormal Q44.7
  spleen Q89.09
Lobule, lobular —*see* condition
Local, localized —*see* condition
Locked-in state G83.5
Locked twins causing obstructed labor
  O66.1
Locking
  joint —*see* Derangement, joint, specified type
  NEC
    knee —*see* Derangement, knee
Lockjaw —*see* Tetanus
Löffler's
  endocarditis I42.3
  eosinophilia J82
  pneumonia J82
  syndrome (eosinophilic pneumonitis) J82
Loiasis (with conjunctival infestation) (eyelid)
  B74.3
Lone Star fever A77.0
Long
  labor O63.9
    first stage O63.0
    second stage O63.1
  QT syndrome I45.81
Long-term (current) (prophylactic) drug
  therapy (use of)
  agents affecting estrogen receptors and
    estrogen levels NEC Z79.818
  anastrozole (Arimidex) Z79.811
  antibiotics Z79.2
    short-term use
  omit code
  anticoagulants Z79.01
  anti-inflammatory, non-steroidal (NSAID)
    Z79.1
  antiplatelet Z79.02
  antithrombotics Z79.02
  aromatase inhibitors Z79.811
  aspirin Z79.82
  birth control pill or patch Z79.3
  bisphosphonates Z79.83
  contraceptive, oral Z79.3
  drug, specified NEC Z79.899
  estrogen receptor downregulators Z79.818
  Evista Z79.810
  exemestane (Aromasin) Z79.811
  Fareston Z79.810
  fulvestrant (Faslodex) Z79.818
  gonadotropin-releasing hormone (GnRH)
    agonist Z79.818
  goserelin acetate (Zoladex) Z79.818
  hormone replacement (postmenopausal)
    Z79.890
  insulin Z79.4
  letrozole (Femara) Z79.811
  leuprolide acetate (leuprorelin) (Lupron)
    Z79.818
  megestrol acetate (Megace) Z79.818

Long-term – *continued*
  methadone for pain management Z79.891
  Nolvadex Z79.810
  non-steroidal anti-inflammatories (NSAID)
    Z79.1
  opiate analgesic Z79.891
  oral contraceptive Z79.3
  raloxifene (Evista) Z79.810
  selective estrogen receptor modulators
    (SERMs) Z79.810
  steroids
    inhaled Z79.51
    systemic Z79.52
  tamoxifen (Nolvadex) Z79.810
  toremifene (Fareston) Z79.810
Longitudinal stripes or grooves, nails L60.8
  congenital Q84.6
Loop
  intestine —*see* Volvulus
  vascular on papilla (optic) Q14.2
Loose —*see also* condition
  body
    joint M24.00
      ankle M24.07
      elbow M24.02
      hand M24.04
      hip M24.05
      knee M23.4
      shoulder (region) M24.01
      specified site NEC M24.08
      vertebra M24.08
      toe M24.07
      wrist M24.03
    knee M23.4
    sheath, tendon —*see* Disorder, tendon,
      specified type NEC
  cartilage —*see* Loose, body, joint
  tooth, teeth K08.8
Loosening
  aseptic
    joint prosthesis —*see* Complications, joint
    prosthesis, mechanical, loosening, by site
    epiphysis —*see* Osteochondropathy
  mechanical
    joint prosthesis —*see* Complications, joint
    prosthesis, mechanical, loosening, by site
Looser-Milkman (-Debray) **syndrome** M83.8
Lop ear (deformity) Q17.3
Lorain (-Levi) **short stature syndrome** E23.0
Lordosis M40.50
  acquired —*see* Lordosis, specified type NEC
  congenital Q76.429
    lumbar region Q76.426
    lumbosacral region Q76.427
    sacral region Q76.428
    sacrococcygeal region Q76.428
    thoracolumbar region Q76.425
  lumbar region M40.56
  lumbosacral region M40.57
  postsurgical M96.4
  postural —*see* Lordosis, specified type NEC
  rachitic (late effect) (sequelae) E64.3
  sequelae of rickets E64.3
  specified type NEC M40.40
    lumbar region M40.46
    lumbosacral region M40.47
    thoracolumbar region M40.45
  thoracolumbar region M40.55
  tuberculous A18.01 **Loss** (of)
  appetite (see Anorexia) R63.0
    hysterical F50.8
    nonorganic origin F50.8
    psychogenic F50.8

Lordosis - *continued*
blood —*see* Hemorrhage
control, sphincter, rectum R15.9
  nonorganic origin F98.1
consciousness, transient R55
  traumatic —*see* Injury, intracranial
elasticity, skin R23.4
family (member) in childhood Z62.898
fluid (acute) E86.9
  with
    hypernatremia E87.0
    hyponatremia E87.1
function of labyrinth —see subcategory H83.2
hair, nonscarring —*see* Alopecia
hearing —*see also* Deafness
  central NOS H90.5
  neural NOS H90.5
  perceptive NOS H90.5
  sensorineural NOS H90.5
  sensory NOS H90.5
height R29.890
limb or member, traumatic, current —*see*
Amputation, traumatic
love relationship in childhood Z62.898
memory —*see also* Amnesia
  mild, following organic brain damage F06.8
mind —*see* Psychosis
occlusal vertical dimension of fully erupted
teeth M26.37
organ or part —*see* Absence, by site, acquired
ossicles, ear (partial) H74.32
parent in childhood Z63.4
pregnancy, recurrent N96
  care in current pregnancy O26.2
  without current pregnancy N96
recurrent pregnancy —*see* Loss, pregnancy,
recurrent
self-esteem, in childhood Z62.898
sense of
  smell —*see* Disturbance, sensation, smell
  taste —*see* Disturbance, sensation, taste
  touch R20.8
sensory R44.9
  dissociative F44.6
sexual desire F52.0
sight (acquired) (complete) (congenital) —*see*
Blindness
substance of
  bone —*see* Disorder, bone, density and
structure, specified NEC
  cartilage —*see* Disorder, cartilage, specified
type NEC
    auricle (ear) —*see* Disorder, pinna,
specified type NEC
    vitreous (humor) H15.89
tooth, teeth —*see* Absence, teeth, acquired
vision, visual H54.7
  both eyes H54.3
  one eye H54.60
    left (normal vision on right) H54.62
    right (normal vision on left) H54.61
  specified as blindness —*see* Blindness
  subjective
    sudden H53.13
    transient H53.12
vitreous —*see* Prolapse, vitreous
voice —*see* Aphonia
weight (abnormal) (cause unknown) R63.4
Louis-Bar syndrome (ataxia-telangiectasia)
G11.3
Louping ill (encephalitis) A84.8
Louse, lousiness —*see* Lice

Low
achiever, school Z55.3
back syndrome M54.5
basal metabolic rate R94.8
birthweight (2499 grams or less) P07.10
  with weight of
    1000 1249 grams P07.14
    1250 1499 grams P07.15
    1500 1749 grams P07.16
    1750 1999 grams P07.17
    2000 2499 grams P07.18
  extreme (999 grams or less) P07.00
    with weight of
      499 grams or less P07.01
      500 749 grams P07.02
      750 999 grams P07.03
  for gestational age —*see* Light for dates
blood pressure —*see also* Hypotension
  reading (incidental) (isolated) (nonspecific)
R03.1
cardiac reserve —*see* Disease, heart
function —*see also* Hypofunction
  kidney N28.9
hematocrit D64.9
hemoglobin D64.9
income Z59.6
level of literacy Z55.0
lying
  kidney N28.89
  organ or site, congenital —*see* Malposition,
congenital
output syndrome (cardiac) —*see* Failure,
heart
platelets (blood) —*see* Thrombocytopenia
reserve, kidney N28.89
salt syndrome E87.1
self esteem R45.81
set ears Q17.4
vision H54.2
  one eye (other eye normal) H54.50
    left (normal vision on right) H54.52
    other eye blind —*see* Blindness
    right (normal vision on left) H54.51
Low-density-lipoprotein-type (LDL)
  hyperlipoproteinemia E78.0
Lowe's syndrome E72.03
Lown-Ganong-Levine syndrome I45.6
LSD reaction (acute) (without dependence)
F16.90
  with dependence F16.20
L-shaped kidney Q63.8
Ludwig's angina or disease K12.2
Lues (venerea) **, luetic** —*see* Syphilis
Luetscher's syndrome (dehydration) E86.0
Lumbago, lumbalgia M54.5
  with sciatica M54.4
    due to intervertebral disc disorder M51.17
  due to displacement, intervertebral disc
M51.27
    with sciatica M51.17
Lumbar —*see* condition
Lumbarization, vertebra, congenital Q76.49
Lumbermen's itch B88.0
Lump —*see* Mass
Lunacy —*see* Psychosis
Lung —*see* condition
Lupoid (miliary) **of Boeck** D86.3
Lupus
anticoagulant D68.62
  with
    hemorrhagic disorder D68.312
    hypercoagulable state D68.62

Lupus – *continued*
finding without diagnosis R76.0
discoid (local) L93.0
erythematosus (discoid) (local) L93.0
  disseminated —*see* Lupus, erythematosus,
systemic
  eyelid H01.129
    left H01.126
      lower H01.125
      upper H01.124
    right H01.123
      lower H01.122
      upper H01.121
  profundus L93.2
  specified NEC L93.2
  subacute cutaneous L93.1
  systemic M32.9
    with organ or system involvement M32.10
      endocarditis M32.11
      lung M32.13
      pericarditis M32.12
      renal (glomerular) M32.14
        tubulo-interstitial M32.15
      specified organ or system NEC M32.19
    drug-induced M32.0
    inhibitor (presence of) D68.62
      with
        hemorrhagic disorder D68.312
        hypercoagulable state D68.62
    finding without diagnosis R76.0
    specified NEC M32.8
exedens A18.4
hydralazine M32.0
  correct substance properly administered —
see Table of Drugs and Chemicals, by drug,
adverse effect
  overdose or wrong substance given or taken
—*see* Table of Drugs and Chemicals, by drug,
poisoning
nephritis (chronic) M32.14
nontuberculous, not disseminated L93.0
panniculitis L93.2
pernio (Besnier) D86.3
systemic —*see* Lupus, erythematosus,
systemic
tuberculous A18.4
  eyelid A18.4
vulgaris A18.4
  eyelid A18.4
Luteinoma D27.
Lutembacher's disease or syndrome (atrial
septal defect with mitral stenosis) Q21.1
Luteoma D27.
Lutz (-Splendore-de Almeida) **disease** —*see*
Paracoccidioidomycosis
Luxation —*see also* Dislocation
eyeball (nontraumatic) —*see* Luxation, globe
  birth injury P15.3
globe, nontraumatic H44.82
lacrimal gland —*see* Dislocation, lacrimal
gland
lens (old) (partial) (spontaneous)
  congenital Q12.1
  syphilitic A50.39
Lycanthropy F22
Lyell's syndrome L51.2
due to drug L51.2
  correct substance properly administered —
see Table of Drugs and Chemicals, by drug,
adverse effect
  overdose or wrong substance given or taken
—*see* Table of Drugs and Chemicals, by drug,
poisoning

Lyme disease A69.20
Lymph
  gland or node —*see* condition
  scrotum —*see* Infestation, filarial
Lymphadenitis I88.9
  with ectopic or molar pregnancy O08.0
  acute L04.9
    axilla L04.2
    face L04.0
    head L04.0
    hip L04.3
    limb
      lower L04.3
      upper L04.2
    neck L04.0
    shoulder L04.2
    specified site NEC L04.8
    trunk L04.1
  anthracosis (occupational) J60
  any site, except mesenteric I88.9
    chronic I88.1
    subacute I88.1
  breast
    gestational —*see* Mastitis, obstetric
    puerperal, postpartum (nonpurulent) O91.22
  chancroidal (congenital) A57
  chronic I88.1
    mesenteric I88.0
  due to
    Brugia (malayi) B74.1
      timori B74.2
    chlamydial lymphogranuloma A55
    diphtheria (toxin) A36.89
    lymphogranuloma venereum A55
    Wuchereria bancrofti B74.0
  following ectopic or molar pregnancy O08.0
  gonorrheal A54.89
  infective —*see* Lymphadenitis, acute
  mesenteric (acute) (chronic) (nonspecific) (subacute) I88.0
    due to Salmonella typhi A01.09
    tuberculous A18.39
  mycobacterial A31.8
  purulent —*see* Lymphadenitis, acute
  pyogenic —*see* Lymphadenitis, acute
  regional, nonbacterial I88.8
  septic —*see* Lymphadenitis, acute
  subacute, unspecified site I88.1
  suppurative —*see* Lymphadenitis, acute
  syphilitic (early) (secondary) A51.49
    late A52.79
  tuberculous —*see* Tuberculosis, lymph gland
  venereal (chlamydial) A55
Lymphadenoid goiter E06.3
Lymphadenopathy (generalized) R59.1
  angioimmunoblastic, with dysproteinemia (AILD) C86.5
  due to toxoplasmosis (acquired) B58.89
    congenital (acute) (subacute) (chronic) P37.1
  localized R59.0
  syphilitic (early) (secondary) A51.49
Lymphadenosis R59.1
Lymphangiectasis I89.0
  conjunctiva H11.89
  postinfectional I89.0
  scrotum I89.0
Lymphangiectatic elephantiasis, nonfilarial I89.0
Lymphangioendothelioma D18.1
  malignant —*see* Neoplasm, connective tissue, malignant
Lymphangioleiomyomatosis J84.81

Lymphangioma D18.1
  capillary D18.1
  cavernous D18.1
  cystic D18.1
  malignant —*see* Neoplasm, connective tissue, malignant
Lymphangiomyoma D18.1
Lymphangiomyomatosis J84.81
Lymphangiosarcoma —*see* Neoplasm, connective tissue, malignant
Lymphangitis I89.1
  with
    abscess
    code by site under Abscess
    cellulitis
    code by site under Cellulitis
    ectopic or molar pregnancy O08.0
  acute L03.91
    abdominal wall L03.321
    ankle —*see* Lymphangitis, acute, lower limb
    arm — *see* Lymphangitis, acute, upper limb
    auricle (ear) —*see* Lymphangitis, acute, ear
    axilla L03.12
    back (any part) L03.322
    buttock L03.327
    cervical (meaning neck) L03.222
    cheek (external) L03.212
    chest wall L03.323
    digit
      finger —*see* Lymphangitis, acute, finger
      toe —*see* Lymphangitis, acute, toe
    ear (external) H60.1
    external auditory canal —*see* Lymphangitis, acute, ear
    eyelid —*see* Abscess, eyelid
    face NEC L03.212
    finger (intrathecal) (periosteal) (subcutaneous) (subcuticular) L03.02
    foot —*see* Lymphangitis, acute, lower limb
    gluteal (region) L03.327
    groin L03.324
    hand —*see* Lymphangitis, acute, upper limb
    head NEC L03.891
      face (any part, except ear, eye and nose) L03.212
    heel —*see* Lymphangitis, acute, lower limb
    hip —*see* Lymphangitis, acute, lower limb
    jaw (region) L03.212
    knee —*see* Lymphangitis, acute, lower limb
    leg —*see* Lymphangitis, acute, lower limb
    lower limb L03.12
      toe —*see* Lymphangitis, acute, toe
    navel L03.326
    neck (region) L03.222
    orbit, orbital —*see* Cellulitis, orbit
    pectoral (region) L03.323
    perineal, perineum L03.325
    scalp (any part) L03.891
    shoulder —*see* Lymphangitis, acute, upper limb
    specified site NEC L03.898
    thigh —*see* Lymphangitis, acute, lower limb
    thumb (intrathecal) (periosteal) (subcutaneous) (subcuticular) —*see* Lymphangitis, acute, finger
    toe (intrathecal) (periosteal) (subcutaneous) (subcuticular) L03.04
    trunk L03.329
      abdominal wall L03.321
      back (any part) L03.322
      buttock L03.327
      chest wall L03.323

Lymphangitis – *continued*
    groin L03.324
    perineal, perineum L03.325
    umbilicus L03.326
    umbilicus L03.326
    upper limb L03.12
      axilla —*see* Lymphangitis, acute, axilla
      finger —*see* Lymphangitis, acute, finger
      thumb —*see* Lymphangitis, acute, finger
      wrist —*see* Lymphangitis, acute, upper limb
  breast
    gestational —*see* Mastitis, obstetric
  chancroidal A57
  chronic (any site) I89.1
  due to
    Brugia (malayi) B74.1
    timori B74.2
    Wuchereria bancrofti B74.0
  following ectopic or molar pregnancy O08.89
  penis
    acute N48.29
    gonococcal (acute) (chronic) A54.09
  puerperal, postpartum, childbirth O86.89
  strumous, tuberculous A18.2
  subacute (any site) I89.1
  tuberculous —*see* Tuberculosis, lymph gland
Lymphatic (vessel) —*see* condition
Lymphatism E32.8
Lymphectasia I89.0
Lymphedema (acquired) —*see also* Elephantiasis
  congenital Q82.0
  hereditary (chronic) (idiopathic) Q82.0
  postmastectomy I97.2
  praecox I89.0
  secondary I89.0
  surgical NEC I97.89
    postmastectomy (syndrome) I97.2
Lymphoblastic —*see* condition
Lymphoblastoma (diffuse) —*see* Lymphoma, lymphoblastic (diffuse)
  giant follicular —*see* Lymphoma, lymphoblastic (diffuse)
  macrofollicular —*see* Lymphoma, lymphoblastic (diffuse)
Lymphocele I89.8
Lymphocytic
  chorioencephalitis (acute) (serous) A87.2
  choriomeningitis (acute) (serous) A87.2
  meningoencephalitis A87.2
Lymphocytoma, benign cutis L98.8
Lymphocytopenia D72.810
Lymphocytosis (symptomatic) D72.820
  infectious (acute) B33.8
Lymphoepithelioma —*see* Neoplasm, malignant, by site
Lymphogranuloma (malignant) —*see also* Lymphoma, Hodgkin
  chlamydial A55
  inguinale A55
  venereum (any site) (chlamydial) (with stricture of rectum) A55
Lymphogranulomatosis (malignant) —*see also* Lymphoma, Hodgkin
  benign (Boeck's sarcoid) (Schaumann's) D86.1
Lymphohistiocytosis, hemophagocytic (familial) D76.1
Lymphoid —*see* condition

Lymphoma (of) (malignant) C85.90
  adult T-cell (HTLV 1-associated) (acute
    variant) (chronic variant) (lymphomatoid
    variant) (smouldering variant) C91.5
  anaplastic large cell
    ALK-negative C84.7
    ALK-positive C84.6
    CD30-positive C84.6
    primary cutaneous C86.6
  angioimmunoblastic T-cell C86.5
  BALT C88.4
  B-cell C85.1
  B-precursor C83.5
  blastic NK-cell C86.4
  bronchial-associated lymphoid tissue -BALT-
    lymphoma] C88.4
  Burkitt (atypical) C83.7
  Burkitt-like C83.7
  centrocytic C83.1
  cutaneous follicle center C82.6
  cutaneous T-cell C84.A
  diffuse follicle center C82.5
  diffuse large cell C83.3
    anaplastic C83.3
    B-cell C83.3
    CD30-positive C83.3
    centroblastic C83.3
    immunoblastic C83.3
    plasmablastic C83.3
    subtype not specified C83.3
    T-cell rich C83.3
  enteropathy-type (associated) (intestinal) T-
    cell C86.2
  extranodal NK/T-cell, nasal type C86.0
  extranodal marginal zone B-cell lymphoma of
    mucosa-associated lymphoid tissue -MALT-
    lymphoma] C88.4
  follicular C82.9
    grade
      I C82.0
      II C82.1
      III C82.2
      IIIa C82.3
      IIIb C82.4
    specified NEC C82.8
  hepatosplenic T-cell (alpha-beta) (gamma-
    delta) C86.1
  histiocytic C85.9
    true C96.A
  Hodgkin C81.9
    classical C81.7
      lymphocyte-rich C81.4
      lymphocyte depleted C81.3
      mixed cellularity C81.2
      nodular sclerosis C81.1
      specified NEC C81.7
    lymphocyte-rich classical C81.4
    lymphocyte depleted classical C81.3
    mixed cellularity classical C81.2
    nodular
      lymphocyte predominant C81.0
      sclerosis classical C81.1
  intravascular large B-cell C83.8
  Lennert's C84.4
  lymphoblastic B-cell C83.5
  lymphoblastic (diffuse) C83.5
  lymphoblastic T-cell C83.5
  lymphoepithelioid C84.4
  lymphoplasmacytic C83.0
    with IgM-production C88.0
  MALT C88.4
  mantle cell C83.1

Lymphoma – *continued*
  mature T-cell NEC C84.4
  mature T/NK-cell C84.9
    specified NEC C84.Z
  mediastinal (thymic) large B-cell C85.2
  Mediterranean C88.3
  mucosa-associated lymphoid tissue -MALT-
    lymphoma] C88.4
  NK/T cell C84.9
  nodal marginal zone C83.0
  non-follicular (diffuse) C83.9
    specified NEC C83.8
  non-Hodgkin (*see also* Lymphoma, by type)
    C85.9
    specified NEC C85.8
  non-leukemic variant of B-CLL C83.0
  peripheral T-cell, not classified C84.4
  primary cutaneous
    anaplastic large cell C86.6
    CD30-positive large T-cell C86.6
  primary effusion B-cell C83.8
  SALT C88.4
  skin-associated lymphoid tissue -SALT-
    lymphoma] C88.4
  small cell B-cell C83.0
  splenic marginal zone C83.0
  subcutaneous panniculitis-like T-cell C86.3
  T-precursor C83.5
  true histiocytic C96.A
Lymphomatosis —*see* Lymphoma
Lymphopathia venereum, veneris A55
Lymphopenia D72.810
Lymphoplasmacytic leukemia —*see*
  Leukemia, chronic lymphocytic, B-cell type
Lymphoproliferation, X-linked disease
  D82.3
Lymphoreticulosis, benign (of inoculation)
  A28.1
Lymphorrhea I89.8
Lymphosarcoma (diffuse) (*see also*
  Lymphoma) C85.9
Lymphostasis I89.8
Lypemania —*see* Melancholia
**Lysine and hydroxylysine metabolism
  disorder** E72.3
Lyssa —*see* Rabies

M

Macacus ear Q17.3
Maceration, wet feet, tropical (syndrome)
  T69.02
MacLeod's syndrome J43.0
Macrocephalia, macrocephaly Q75.3
Macrocheilia, macrochilia (congenital) Q18.6
Macrocolon (*see also* Megacolon) Q43.1
Macrocornea Q15.8
  with glaucoma Q15.0
Macrocytic —*see* condition
Macrocytosis D75.89
Macrodactylia, macrodactylism (fingers)
  (thumbs) Q74.0
  toes Q74.2
Macrodontia K00.2
Macrogenia M26.05
Macrogenitosomia (adrenal) (male) (praecox)
  E25.9
  congenital E25.0
Macroglobulinemia (idiopathic) (primary)
  C88.0
  monoclonal (essential) D47.2
  Waldenström C88.0
Macroglossia (congenital) Q38.2
  acquired K14.8

Macrognathia, macrognathism (congenital)
  (mandibular) (maxillary) M26.09
Macrogyria (congenital) Q04.8
Macrohydrocephalus —*see* Hydrocephalus
Macromastia —*see* Hypertrophy, breast
Macrophthalmos Q11.3
  in congenital glaucoma Q15.0
Macropsia H53.15
Macrosigmoid K59.3
  congenital Q43.2
Macrospondylitis , acromegalic E22.0
Macrostomia (congenital) Q18.4
Macrotia (external ear) (congenital) Q17.1
Macula
  cornea, corneal —*see* Opacity, cornea
  degeneration (atrophic) (exudative) (senile)
    —*see also* Degeneration, macula
  hereditary —*see* Dystrophy, retina
Maculae ceruleae
  B85.1
Maculopathy, toxic —*see* Degeneration,
  macula, toxic
Madarosis (eyelid) H02.729
  left H02.726
    lower H02.725
    upper H02.724
  right H02.723
    lower H02.722
    upper H02.721
Madelung's
  deformity (radius) Q74.0
  disease
    radial deformity Q74.0
    symmetrical lipomas, neck E88.89
Madness —*see* Psychosis
Madura
  foot B47.9
    actinomycotic B47.1
    mycotic B47.0
Maduromycosis B47.0
Maffucci's syndrome Q78.4
Magnesium metabolism disorder —*see*
  Disorder, metabolism, magnesium
Main en griffe (acquired) —*see also*
  Deformity, limb, clawhand
  congenital Q74.0
Maintenance (encounter for)
  antineoplastic chemotherapy Z51.11
  antineoplastic radiation therapy Z51.0
  methadone F11.20
Majocchi's
  disease L81.7
  granuloma B35.8
Major —*see* condition
Malabar itch (any site) B35.5
Malabsorption K90.9
  calcium K90.89
  carbohydrate K90.4
  disaccharide E73.9
  fat K90.4
  galactose E74.20
  glucose (-galactose) E74.39
  intestinal K90.9
    specified NEC K90.89
  isomaltose E74.31
  lactose E73.9
  methionine E72.19
  monosaccharide E74.39
  postgastrectomy K91.2
  postsurgical K91.2
  protein K90.4
  starch K90.4
  sucrose E74.39

Malabsorption - *continued*
  syndrome K90.9
    postsurgical K91.2
Malacia, bone (adult) M83.9
  juvenile —*see* Rickets
Malacoplakia
  bladder N32.89
  pelvis (kidney) N28.89
  ureter N28.89
  urethra N36.8
Malacosteon, juvenile —*see* Rickets
Maladaptation —*see* Maladjustment
Maladie de Roger Q21.0
Maladjustment
  conjugal Z63.0
    involving divorce or estrangement Z63.5
  educational Z55.4
  family Z63.9
  marital Z63.0
    involving divorce or estrangement Z63.5
  occupational NEC Z56.89
  simple, adult —*see* Disorder, adjustment
  situational —*see* Disorder, adjustment
  social Z60.9
    due to
      acculturation difficulty Z60.3
      discrimination and persecution (perceived)
        Z60.5
      exclusion and isolation Z60.4
      life-cycle (phase of life) transition Z60.0
      rejection Z60.4
      specified reason NEC Z60.8
Malaise R53.81
Malakoplakia —*see* Malacoplakia
Malaria, malarial (fever) B54
  with
    blackwater fever B50.8
      hemoglobinuric (bilious) B50.8
    hemoglobinuria B50.8
  accidentally induced (therapeutically)
    code by type under Malaria
  algid B50.9
  cerebral B50.0 *[G94]*
  clinically diagnosed (without parasitological
    confirmation) B54
  congenital NEC P37.4
    falciparum P37.3
  congestion, congestive B54
  continued (fever) B50.9
  estivo-autumnal B50.9
  falciparum B50.9
    with complications NEC B50.8
      cerebral B50.0 *[G94]*
      severe B50.8
  hemorrhagic B54
  malariae B52.9
    with
      complications NEC B52.8
      glomerular disorder B52.0
  malignant (tertian) —*see* Malaria, falciparum
  mixed infections
    code to first listed type in B50-B53
  ovale B53.0
  parasitologically confirmed NEC B53.8
  pernicious, acute —*see* Malaria, falciparum
  Plasmodium (P.)
    falciparum NEC —*see* Malaria, falciparum
    malariae NEC B52.9
      with Plasmodium
        falciparum (and or vivax) —*see* Malaria,
          falciparum
        vivax —*see also* Malaria, vivax

Malaria, malarial - *continued*
    and falciparum —*see* Malaria,
      falciparum
    ovale B53.0
      with Plasmodium malariae —*see also*
        Malaria, malariae
        and vivax —*see also* Malaria, vivax
        and falciparum —*see* Malaria,
          falciparum
    simian B53.1
      with Plasmodium malariae —*see also*
        Malaria, malariae
        and vivax —*see also* Malaria, vivax
        and falciparum —*see* Malaria,
          falciparum
    vivax NEC B51.9
      with Plasmodium falciparum —*see*
        Malaria, falciparum
    quartan —*see* Malaria, malariae
    quotidian —*see* Malaria, falciparum
    recurrent B54
    remittent B54
    specified type NEC (parasitologically
      confirmed) B53.8
    spleen B54
    subtertian (fever) —*see* Malaria, falciparum
    tertian (benign) —*see also* Malaria, vivax
      malignant B50.9
    tropical B50.9
    typhoid B54
    vivax B51.9
      with
        complications NEC B51.8
        ruptured spleen B51.0
Malassimilation K90.9
Malassez's disease (cystic) N50.8
Mal de los pintos —*see* Pinta
Mal de mer T75.3
Maldescent, testis Q53.9
  bilateral Q53.20
    abdominal Q53.21
    perineal Q53.22
  unilateral Q53.10
    abdominal Q53.11
    perineal Q53.12
Maldevelopment —*see also* Anomaly
  brain Q07.9
  colon Q43.9
  hip Q74.2
    congenital dislocation Q65.2
      bilateral Q65.1
      unilateral Q65.0
  mastoid process Q75.8
  middle ear Q16.4
    except ossicles Q16.4
    ossicles Q16.3
  ossicles Q16.3
  spine Q76.49
  toe Q74.2
Male type pelvis Q74.2
  with disproportion (fetopelvic) O33.3
    causing obstructed labor O65.3
Malformation (congenital) —*see also*
  Anomaly
  adrenal gland Q89.1
  affecting multiple systems with skeletal
    changes NEC Q87.5
  alimentary tract Q45.9
    specified type NEC Q45.8
    upper Q40.9
      specified type NEC Q40.8

Malformation – *continued*
  aorta Q25.9
    atresia Q25.2
    coarctation (preductal) (postductal) Q25.1
    patent ductus arteriosus Q25.0
    specified type NEC Q25.4
    stenosis (supravalvular) Q25.3
  aortic valve Q23.9
    specified NEC Q23.8
  arteriovenous, aneurysmatic (congenital)
    Q27.30
    brain Q28.2
    cerebral Q28.2
    peripheral Q27.30
      digestive system Q27.33
      lower limb Q27.32
      other specified site Q27.39
      renal vessel Q27.34
      upper limb Q27.31
    precerebral vessels (nonruptured) Q28.0
  auricle
    ear (congenital) Q17.3
      acquired H61.119
        left H61.112
          with right H61.113
        right H61.111
          with left H61.113
  bile duct Q44.5
  bladder Q64.79
    aplasia Q64.5
    diverticulum Q64.6
    exstrophy —*see* Exstrophy, bladder
    neck obstruction Q64.31
  bone Q79.9
    face Q75.9
      specified type NEC Q75.8
    skull Q75.9
      specified type NEC Q75.8
  brain (multiple) Q04.9
    arteriovenous Q28.2
    specified type NEC Q04.8
  branchial cleft Q18.2
  breast Q83.9
    specified type NEC Q83.8
  broad ligament Q50.6
  bronchus Q32.4
  bursa Q79.9
  cardiac
    chambers Q20.9
      specified type NEC Q20.8
    septum Q21.9
      specified type NEC Q21.8
  cerebral Q04.9
    vessels Q28.3
  cervix uteri Q51.9
    specified type NEC Q51.828
  Chiari
    Type I G93.5
    Type II Q07.01
  choroid (congenital) Q14.3
    plexus Q07.8
  circulatory system Q28.9
  cochlea Q16.5
  cornea Q13.4
  coronary vessels Q24.5
  corpus callosum (congenital) Q04.0
  diaphragm Q79.1
  digestive system NEC, specified type NEC
    Q45.8
  dura Q07.9
    brain Q04.9
    spinal Q06.9

Malformation – *continued*
ear Q17.9
  causing impairment of hearing Q16.9
  external Q17.9
    accessory auricle Q17.0
    causing impairment of hearing Q16.9
      absence of
        auditory canal Q16.1
        auricle Q16.0
    macrotia Q17.1
    microtia Q17.2
    misplacement Q17.4
    misshapen NEC Q17.3
    prominence Q17.5
    specified type NEC Q17.8
  inner Q16.5
  middle Q16.4
    absence of eustachian tube Q16.2
    ossicles (fusion) Q16.3
  ossicles Q16.3
  specified type NEC Q17.8
epididymis Q55.4
esophagus Q39.9
  specified type NEC Q39.8
eye Q15.9
  lid Q10.3
  specified NEC Q15.8
fallopian tube Q50.6
genital organ —*see* Anomaly, genitalia
great
  artery Q25.9
    aorta —*see* Malformation, aorta
    pulmonary artery —*see* Malformation,
pulmonary, artery
    specified type NEC Q25.8
  vein Q26.9
    anomalous
      portal venous connection Q26.5
      pulmonary venous connection Q26.4
        partial Q26.3
        total Q26.2
    persistent left superior vena cava Q26.1
    portal vein-hepatic artery fistula Q26.6
    specified type NEC Q26.8
    vena cava stenosis, congenital Q26.0
gum Q38.6
hair Q84.2
heart Q24.9
  specified type NEC Q24.8
integument Q84.9
  specified type NEC Q84.8
internal ear Q16.5
intestine Q43.9
  specified type NEC Q43.8
iris Q13.2
joint Q74.9
  ankle Q74.2
  lumbosacral Q76.49
  sacroiliac Q74.2
  specified type NEC Q74.8
kidney Q63.9
  accessory Q63.0
  giant Q63.3
  horseshoe Q63.1
  hydronephrosis Q62.0
  malposition Q63.2
  specified type NEC Q63.8
lacrimal apparatus Q10.6
lip Q38.0
lingual Q38.3
liver Q44.7
lung Q33.9

Malformation – *continued*
meninges or membrane (congenital) Q07.9
  cerebral Q04.8
  spinal (cord) Q06.9
middle ear Q16.4
  ossicles Q16.3
mitral valve Q23.9
  specified NEC Q23.8
Mondini's (congenital) (malformation,
cochlea) Q16.5
mouth (congenital) Q38.6
multiple types NEC Q89.7
musculoskeletal system Q79.9
myocardium Q24.8
nail Q84.6
nervous system (central) Q07.9
nose Q30.9
  specified type NEC Q30.8
optic disc Q14.2
orbit Q10.7
ovary Q50.39
palate Q38.5
parathyroid gland Q89.2
pelvic organs or tissues NEC
  in pregnancy or childbirth O34.8
    causing obstructed labor O65.5
penis Q55.69
  aplasia Q55.5
  curvature (lateral) Q55.61
  hypoplasia Q55.62
pericardium Q24.8
peripheral vascular system Q27.9
  specified type NEC Q27.8
pharynx Q38.8
precerebral vessels Q28.1
prostate Q55.4
pulmonary
  arteriovenous Q25.72
  artery Q25.9
    atresia Q25.5
    specified type NEC Q25.79
    stenosis Q25.6
  valve Q22.3
renal artery Q27.2
respiratory system Q34.9
retina Q14.1
scrotum —*see* Malformation, testis and
scrotum
seminal vesicles Q55.4
sense organs NEC Q07.9
skin Q82.9
specified NEC Q89.8
spinal
  cord Q06.9
  nerve root Q07.8
spine Q76.49
  kyphosis —*see* Kyphosis, congenital
  lordosis —*see* Lordosis, congenital
spleen Q89.09
stomach Q40.3
  specified type NEC Q40.2
teeth, tooth K00.9
tendon Q79.9
testis and scrotum Q55.20
  aplasia Q55.0
  hypoplasia Q55.1
  polyorchism Q55.21
  retractile testis Q55.22
  scrotal transposition Q55.23
  specified NEC Q55.29
throat Q38.8
thorax, bony Q76.9

Malformation – *continued*
thyroid gland Q89.2
tongue (congenital) Q38.3
  hypertrophy Q38.2
  tie Q38.1
trachea Q32.1
tricuspid valve Q22.9
  specified type NEC Q22.8
umbilical cord NEC (complicating delivery)
O69.89
umbilicus Q89.9
ureter Q62.8
  agenesis Q62.4
  duplication Q62.5
  malposition —*see* Malposition, congenital,
ureter
  obstructive defect —*see* Defect, obstructive,
ureter
  vesico-uretero-renal reflux Q62.7
urethra Q64.79
  aplasia Q64.5
  duplication Q64.74
  posterior valves Q64.2
  prolapse Q64.71
  stricture Q64.32
urinary system Q64.9
uterus Q51.9
  specified type NEC Q51.818
vagina Q52.4
vascular system, peripheral Q27.9
vas deferens Q55.4
  atresia Q55.3
venous —*see* Anomaly, vein(s)
vulva Q52.70

Malfunction —*see also* Dysfunction
cardiac electronic device T82.119
  electrode T82.110
  pulse generator T82.111
  specified type NEC T82.118
catheter device NEC T85.618
  cystostomy T83.010
  dialysis (renal) (vascular) T82.41
    intraperitoneal T85.611
  infusion NEC T82.514
    spinal (epidural) (subdural) T85.610
  urinary, indwelling T83.018
colostomy K94.03
  valve K94.03
cystostomy (stoma) N99.512
  catheter T83.010
enteric stoma K94.13
enterostomy K94.13
esophagostomy K94.33
gastroenteric K31.89
gastrostomy K94.23
ileostomy K94.13
  valve K94.13
jejunostomy K94.13
pacemaker —*see* Malfunction, cardiac
electronic device
prosthetic device, internal —*see*
Complications, prosthetic device, by site,
mechanical
tracheostomy J95.03
urinary device NEC —*see* Complication,
genitourinary, device, urinary, mechanical
valve
  colostomy K94.03
  heart T82.09
  ileostomy K94.13
vascular graft or shunt NEC —*see*
Complication, cardiovascular device,
mechanical, vascular

Malfunction - *continued*
ventricular (communicating shunt) T85.01
Malherbe's tumor —*see* Neoplasm, skin, benign
Malibu disease L98.8
Malignancy —*see also* Neoplasm, malignant, by site
unspecified site (primary) C80.1
Malignant —*see* condition
Malingerer, malingering Z76.5
Mallet finger (acquired) —*see* Deformity, finger, mallet finger
congenital Q74.0
sequelae of rickets E64.3
Malleus A24.0
Mallory's bodies R89.7
Mallory-Weiss syndrome K22.6
Malnutrition E46
degree
first E44.1
mild (protein) E44.1
moderate (protein) E44.0
second E44.0
severe (protein-energy) E43
intermediate form E42
with
kwashiorkor (and marasmus) E42
marasmus E41
third E43
following gastrointestinal surgery K91.2
intrauterine
light-for-dates —*see* Light for dates
small-for-dates —*see* Small for dates
lack of care, or neglect (child) (infant) T76.02
confirmed T74.02
malignant E40
protein E46
calorie E46
mild E44.1
moderate E44.0
severe E43
intermediate form E42
with
kwashiorkor (and marasmus) E42
marasmus E41
energy E46
mild E44.1
moderate E44.0
severe E43
intermediate form E42
with
kwashiorkor (and marasmus) E42
marasmus E41
severe (protein-energy) E43
with
kwashiorkor (and marasmus) E42
marasmus E41
Malocclusion (teeth) M26.4
Angle's M26.219
class I M26.211
class II M26.212
class III M26.213
due to
abnormal swallowing M26.59
mouth breathing M26.59
tongue, lip or finger habits M26.59
temporomandibular (joint) M26.69
Malposition
cervix —*see* Malposition, uterus
congenital
adrenal (gland) Q89.1
alimentary tract Q45.8

Malposition - *continued*
lower Q43.8
upper Q40.8
aorta Q25.4
appendix Q43.8
arterial trunk Q20.0
artery (peripheral) Q27.8
coronary Q24.5
digestive system Q27.8
lower limb Q27.8
pulmonary Q25.79
specified site NEC Q27.8
upper limb Q27.8
auditory canal Q17.8
causing impairment of hearing Q16.9
auricle (ear) Q17.4
causing impairment of hearing Q16.9
cervical Q18.2
biliary duct or passage Q44.5
bladder (mucosa) —*see* Exstrophy, bladder
brachial plexus Q07.8
brain tissue Q04.8
breast Q83.8
bronchus Q32.4
cecum Q43.8
clavicle Q74.0
colon Q43.8
digestive organ or tract NEC Q45.8
lower Q43.8
upper Q40.8
ear (auricle) (external) Q17.4
ossicles Q16.3
endocrine (gland) NEC Q89.2
epiglottis Q31.8
eustachian tube Q17.8
eye Q15.8
facial features Q18.8
fallopian tube Q50.6
finger (s) Q68.1
supernumerary Q69.0
foot Q66.9
gallbladder Q44.1
gastrointestinal tract Q45.8
genitalia, genital organ (s) or tract
female Q52.8
external Q52.79
internal NEC Q52.8
male Q55.8
glottis Q31.8
hand Q68.1
heart Q24.8
dextrocardia Q24.0
with complete transposition of viscera Q89.3
hepatic duct Q44.5
hip (joint) Q65.89
intestine (large) (small) Q43.8
with anomalous adhesions, fixation or malrotation Q43.3
joint NEC Q68.8
kidney Q63.2
larynx Q31.8
limb Q68.8
lower Q68.8
upper Q68.8
liver Q44.7
lung (lobe) Q33.8
nail (s) Q84.6
nerve Q07.8
nervous system NEC Q07.8
nose, nasal (septum) Q30.8

Malposition - *continued*
organ or site not listed —*see* Anomaly, by site
ovary Q50.39
pancreas Q45.3
parathyroid (gland) Q89.2
patella Q74.1
peripheral vascular system Q27.8
pituitary (gland) Q89.2
respiratory organ or system NEC Q34.8
rib (cage) Q76.6
supernumerary in cervical region Q76.5
scapula Q74.0
shoulder Q74.0
spinal cord Q06.8
spleen Q89.09
sternum NEC Q76.7
stomach Q40.2
symphysis pubis Q74.2
thymus (gland) Q89.2
thyroid (gland) (tissue) Q89.2
cartilage Q31.8
toe (s) Q66.9
supernumerary Q69.2
tongue Q38.3
trachea Q32.1
ureter Q62.60
deviation Q62.61
displacement Q62.62
ectopia Q62.63
specified type NEC Q62.69
uterus Q51.818
vein (s) (peripheral) Q27.8
great Q26.8
vena cava (inferior) (superior) Q26.8
device, implant or graft (*see also* Complications, by site and type, mechanical) T85.628
arterial graft NEC —*see* Complication, cardiovascular device, mechanical, vascular
breast (implant) T85.42
catheter NEC T85.628
cystostomy T83.020
dialysis (renal) T82.42
intraperitoneal T85.621
infusion NEC T82.524
spinal (epidural) (subdural) T85.620
urinary, indwelling T83.028
electronic (electrode) (pulse generator) (stimulator)
bone T84.320
cardiac T82.129
electrode T82.120
pulse generator T82.121
specified type NEC T82.128
nervous system —*see* Complication, prosthetic device, mechanical, electronic nervous system stimulator
urinary —*see* Complication, genitourinary, device, urinary, mechanical
fixation, internal (orthopedic) NEC —*see* Complication, fixation device, mechanical
gastrointestinal —*see* Complications, prosthetic device, mechanical, gastrointestinal device
genital NEC T83.428
intrauterine contraceptive device T83.32
penile prosthesis T83.420
heart NEC —*see* Complication, cardiovascular device, mechanical
joint prosthesis —*see* Complication, joint prosthesis, mechanical

Malposition - *continued*
  ocular NEC —*see* Complications, prosthetic device, mechanical, ocular device
  orthopedic NEC —*see* Complication, orthopedic, device, mechanical
   specified NEC T85.628
  urinary NEC —*see also* Complication, genitourinary, device, urinary, mechanical
   graft T83.22
  vascular NEC —*see* Complication, cardiovascular device, mechanical
   ventricular intracranial shunt T85.02
  fetus —*see* Pregnancy, complicated by (management affected by) , presentation, fetal
  gallbladder K82.8
  gastrointestinal tract, congenital Q45.8
  heart, congenital NEC Q24.8
  joint prosthesis —*see* Complications, joint prosthesis, mechanical, displacement, by site
  stomach K31.89
   congenital Q40.2
  tooth, teeth, fully erupted M26.30
  uterus (acute) (acquired) (adherent) (asymptomatic) (postinfectional) (postpartal, old) N85.4
   anteflexion or anteversion N85.4
    congenital Q51.818
   flexion N85.4
    lateral —*see* Lateroversion, uterus
   inversion N85.5
   lateral (flexion) (version) —*see* Lateroversion, uterus
   in pregnancy or childbirth —*see* subcategory O34.5
   retroflexion or retroversion —*see* Retroversion, uterus
Malposture R29.3
Malrotation
  cecum Q43.3
  colon Q43.3
  intestine Q43.3
  kidney Q63.2
Maltreatment
  adult
   abandonment
    confirmed T74.01
    suspected T76.01
   confirmed T74.91
   history of Z91.419
   neglect
    confirmed T74.01
    suspected T76.01
   physical abuse
    confirmed T74.11
    suspected T76.11
   psychological abuse
    confirmed T74.31
    suspected T76.31
    history of Z91.411
   sexual abuse
    confirmed T74.21
    suspected T76.21
   suspected T76.91
  child
   abandonment
    confirmed T74.02
    suspected T76.02
   confirmed T74.92
   history of —*see* History, personal (of) , abuse
   neglect
    confirmed T74.02

Maltreatment – *continued*
   history of —*see* History, personal (of) , abuse
    suspected T76.02
   physical abuse
    confirmed T74.12
    history of —*see* History, personal (of) , abuse
    suspected T76.12
   psychological abuse
    confirmed T74.32
    history of —*see* History, personal (of) , abuse
    suspected T76.32
   sexual abuse
    confirmed T74.22
    history of —*see* History, personal (of) , abuse
    suspected T76.22
   suspected T76.92
   personal history of Z91.89
Malta fever —*see* Brucellosis
Maltworker's lung J67.4
Malunion, fracture —*see* Fracture, by site
Mammillitis N61
  puerperal, postpartum O91.02
Mammitis —*see* Mastitis **Mammogram** (examination) Z12.39
  routine Z12.31
Mammoplasia N62 **Management** (of)
  bone conduction hearing device (implanted) Z45.320
  cardiac pacemaker NEC Z45.018
  cerebrospinal fluid drainage device Z45.41
  cochlear device (implanted) Z45.321
  contraceptive Z30.9
   specified NEC Z30.8
  implanted device Z45.9
   specified NEC Z45.89
  infusion pump Z45.1
  procreative Z31.9
   male factor infertility in female Z31.81
   specified NEC Z31.89
  prosthesis (external) (*see also* Fitting) Z44.9
   implanted Z45.9
    specified NEC Z45.89
  renal dialysis catheter Z49.01
  vascular access device Z45.2
Mangled —*see* specified injury by site
Mania (monopolar) —*see also* Disorder, mood, manic episode
  with psychotic symptoms F30.2
  without psychotic symptoms F30.10
   mild F30.11
   moderate F30.12
   severe F30.13
  Bell's F30.8
  chronic (recurrent) F31.89
  hysterical F44.89
  puerperal F30.8
  recurrent F31.89
Manic-depressive insanity, psychosis, or syndrome —*see* Disorder, bipolar
Mannosidosis E77.1
Mansonelliasis, mansonellosis B74.4
Manson's
  disease B65.1
  schistosomiasis B65.1
Manual —*see* condition
Maple-bark-stripper's lung (disease) J67.6
Maple-syrup-urine disease E71.0
Marable's syndrome (celiac artery compression) I77.4

Marasmus E41
  due to malnutrition E41
  intestinal E41
  nutritional E41
  senile R54
  tuberculous NEC —*see* Tuberculosis
Marble
  bones Q78.2
  skin R23.8
Marburg virus disease A98.3
March
  fracture —*see* Fracture, traumatic, stress, by site
  hemoglobinuria D59.6
Marchesani (-Weill) **syndrome** Q87.0
Marchiafava (-Bignami) **syndrome or disease** G37.1
Marchiafava-Micheli syndrome D59.5
Marcus Gunn's syndrome Q07.8
Marfan's syndrome —*see* Syndrome, Marfan's
Marie-Bamberger disease —*see* Osteoarthropathy, hypertrophic, specified NEC
Marie-Charcot-Tooth neuropathic muscular atrophy G60.0
Marie's
  cerebellar ataxia (late-onset) G11.2
  disease or syndrome (acromegaly) E22.0
Marie-Strümpell arthritis, disease or spondylitis —*see* Spondylitis, ankylosing
Marion's disease (bladder neck obstruction) N32.0
Marital conflict Z63.0
Mark
  port wine Q82.5
  raspberry Q82.5
  strawberry Q82.5
  stretch L90.6
  tattoo L81.8
Marker heterochromatin —*see* Extra, marker chromosomes
Maroteaux-Lamy syndrome (mild) (severe) E76.29
Marrow (bone)
  arrest D61.9
  poor function D75.89
Marseilles fever A77.1
Marsh fever —*see* Malaria
Marshall's (hidrotic) **ectodermal dysplasia** Q82.4
Marsh's disease (exophthalmic goiter) E05.00
  with storm E05.01
Masculinization (female) **with adrenal hyperplasia** E25.9
  congenital E25.0
Masculinovoblastoma D27.-**Masochism** (sexual) F65.51
Mason's lung J62.8
Mass
  abdominal R19.00
   epigastric R19.06
   generalized R19.07
   left lower quadrant R19.04
   left upper quadrant R19.02
   periumbilic R19.05
   right lower quadrant R19.03
   right upper quadrant R19.01
   specified site NEC R19.09
  breast N63
  chest R22.2
  cystic —*see* Cyst
  ear H93.8

Mass - *continued*
head R22.0
intra-abdominal (diffuse) (generalized) —*see* Mass, abdominal
kidney N28.89
liver R16.0
localized (skin) R22.9
chest R22.2
head R22.0
limb
lower R22.4
upper R22.3
neck R22.1
trunk R22.2
lung R91.8
malignant —*see* Neoplasm, malignant, by site
neck R22.1
pelvic (diffuse) (generalized) —*see* Mass, abdominal
specified organ NEC —*see* Disease, by site
splenic R16.1
substernal thyroid —*see* Goiter
superficial (localized) R22.9
umbilical (diffuse) (generalized) R19.09
Massive —*see* condition
Mast cell
disease, systemic tissue D47.0
leukemia C94.3
sarcoma C96.2
tumor D47.0
malignant C96.2
Mastalgia N64.4
Masters-Allen syndrome N83.8
Mastitis (acute) (diffuse) (nonpuerperal) (subacute) N61
chronic (cystic) —*see* Mastopathy, cystic
cystic (Schimmelbusch's type) —*see* Mastopathy, cystic
fibrocystic —*see* Mastopathy, cystic
infective N61
newborn P39.0
interstitial, gestational or puerperal —*see* Mastitis, obstetric
neonatal (noninfective) P83.4
infective P39.0
obstetric (interstitial) (nonpurulent)
associated with
lactation O91.23
pregnancy O91.21
puerperium O91.22
purulent
associated with
lactation O91.13
pregnancy O91.11
puerperium O91.12
periductal —*see* Ectasia, mammary duct
phlegmonous —*see* Mastopathy, cystic
plasma cell —*see* Ectasia, mammary duct
Mastocytoma D47.0
malignant C96.2
Mastocytosis Q82.2
aggressive systemic C96.2
indolent systemic D47.0
malignant C96.2
systemic, associated with clonal hematopoietic non-mast-cell disease (SM-AHNMD) D47.0
Mastodynia N64.4
Mastoid —*see* condition
Mastoidalgia —*see* subcategory H92.0

Mastoiditis (coalescent) (hemorrhagic) (suppurative) H70.9
acute, subacute H70.00
complicated NEC H70.09
subperiosteal H70.01
chronic (necrotic) (recurrent) H70.1
in (due to)
infectious disease NEC B99 *[H75.0]*
parasitic disease NEC B89 *[H75.0]*
tuberculosis A18.03
petrositis —*see* Petrositis
postauricular fistula —*see* Fistula, postauricular
specified NEC H70.89
tuberculous A18.03
Mastopathy, mastopathia N64.9
chronica cystica —*see* Mastopathy, cystic
cystic (chronic) (diffuse) N60.1
with epithelial proliferation N60.3
diffuse cystic —*see* Mastopathy, cystic
estrogenic, oestrogenica N64.89
ovarian origin N64.89
Mastoplasia, mastoplastia N62
Masturbation (excessive) F98.8
Maternal care (for) —*see* Pregnancy (complicated by) (management affected by)
Matheiu's disease (leptospiral jaundice) A27.0
Mauclaire's disease or osteochondrosis —*see* Osteochondrosis, juvenile, hand, metacarpal
Maxcy's disease A75.2
Maxilla, maxillary —*see* condition
May (-Hegglin) anomaly or syndrome D72.0
McArdle (-Schmid) (-Pearson) disease (glycogen storage) E74.04
McCune-Albright syndrome Q78.1
McQuarrie's syndrome (idiopathic familial hypoglycemia) E16.2
Meadow's syndrome Q86.1
Measles (black) (hemorrhagic) (suppressed) B05.9
with
complications NEC B05.89
encephalitis B05.0
intestinal complications B05.4
keratitis (keratoconjunctivitis) B05.81
meningitis B05.1
otitis media B05.3
pneumonia B05.2
French —*see* Rubella
German —*see* Rubella
Liberty —*see* Rubella
Meatitis, urethral —*see* Urethritis
Meatus, meatal —*see* condition
Meat-wrappers' asthma J68.9
Meckel-Gruber syndrome Q61.9
Meckel's diverticulitis, diverticulum (displaced) (hypertrophic) Q43.0
malignant —*see* Table of Neoplasms, small intestine, malignant
Meconium
ileus, newborn P76.0
in cystic fibrosis E84.11
meaning meconium plug (without cystic fibrosis) P76.0
obstruction, newborn P76.0
due to fecaliths P76.0
in mucoviscidosis E84.11
peritonitis P78.0
plug syndrome (newborn) NEC P76.0

Median —*see also* condition
arcuate ligament syndrome I77.4
bar (prostate) (vesical orifice) —*see* Hyperplasia, prostate
rhomboid glossitis K14.2
Mediastinal shift R93.8
Mediastinitis (acute) (chronic) J98.5
syphilitic A52.73
tuberculous A15.8
Mediastinopericarditis —*see also* Pericarditis
acute I30.9
adhesive I31.0
chronic I31.8
rheumatic I09.2
Mediastinum, mediastinal —*see* condition
Medicine poisoning —*see* Table of Drugs and Chemicals, by drug, poisoning
Mediterranean
fever —*see* Brucellosis
familial E85.0
tick A77.1
kala-azar B55.0
leishmaniasis B55.0
tick fever A77.1
Medulla —*see* condition
Medullary cystic kidney Q61.5
Medullated fibers
optic (nerve) Q14.8
retina Q14.1
Medulloblastoma
desmoplastic C71.6
specified site —*see* Neoplasm, malignant, by site
unspecified site C71.6
Medulloepithelioma —*see also* Neoplasm, malignant, by site
teratoid —*see* Neoplasm, malignant, by site
Medullomyoblastoma
specified site —*see* Neoplasm, malignant, by site
unspecified site C71.6
Meekeren-Ehlers-Danlos syndrome Q79.6
Megacolon (acquired) (functional) (not Hirschsprung's disease) (in) K59.3
Chagas' disease B57.32
congenital, congenitum (aganglionic) Q43.1
Hirschsprung's (disease) Q43.1
toxic NEC K59.3
due to Clostridium difficile A04.7
Megaesophagus (functional) K22.0
congenital Q39.5
in (due to) Chagas' disease B57.31
Megalencephaly Q04.5
Megalerythema (epidemic) B08.3
Megaloappendix Q43.8
Megalocephalous, megalocephaly NEC Q75.3
Megalocornea Q15.8
with glaucoma Q15.0
Megalocytic anemia D53.1
Megalodactylia (fingers) (thumbs) (congenital) Q74.0
toes Q74.2
Megaloduodenum Q43.8
Megaloesophagus (functional) K22.0
congenital Q39.5
Megalogastria (acquired) K31.89
congenital Q40.2
Megalophthalmos Q11.3
Megalopsia H53.15
Megalosplenia —*see* Splenomegaly
Megaloureter N28.82
congenital Q62.2

Megarectum K62.89
Megasigmoid K59.3
  congenital Q43.2
Megaureter N28.82
  congenital Q62.2
Megavitamin-B6 syndrome E67.2
Megrim —*see* Migraine
Meibomian
  cyst, infected —*see* Hordeolum
  gland —*see* condition
  sty, stye —*see* Hordeolum
Meibomitis —*see* Hordeolum
Meige-Milroy disease (chronic hereditary
  edema) Q82.0
Meige's syndrome Q82.0
Melalgia, nutritional E53.8
Melancholia F32.9
  climacteric (single episode) F32.8
    recurrent episode F33.9
  hypochondriac F45.29
  intermittent (single episode) F32.8
    recurrent episode F33.9
  involutional (single episode) F32.8
    recurrent episode F33.9
  menopausal (single episode) F32.8
    recurrent episode F33.9
  puerperal F32.8
  reactive (emotional stress or trauma) F32.3
  recurrent F33.9
  senile F03
  stuporous (single episode) F32.8
    recurrent episode F33.9
Melanemia R79.89
Melanoameloblastoma —*see* Neoplasm, bone,
  benign
Melanoblastoma —*see* Melanoma
Melanocarcinoma —*see* Melanoma
Melanocytoma, eyeball D31.4-**Melanocytosis,
  neurocutaneous** Q82.8
Melanoderma, melanodermia L81.4
Melanodontia, infantile K03.89
Melanodontoclasia K03.89
Melanoepithelioma —*see* Melanoma
Melanoma (malignant) C43.9
  acral lentiginous, malignant —*see* Melanoma,
  skin, by site
  amelanotic —*see* Melanoma, skin, by site
  balloon cell —*see* Melanoma, skin, by site
  benign —*see* Nevus
  desmoplastic, malignant —*see* Melanoma,
  skin, by site
  epithelioid cell —*see* Melanoma, skin, by site
    with spindle cell, mixed —*see* Melanoma,
    skin, by site
  in
    giant pigmented nevus —*see* Melanoma,
    skin, by site
    Hutchinson's melanotic freckle —*see*
    Melanoma, skin, by site
    junctional nevus —*see* Melanoma, skin, by
    site
    precancerous melanosis —*see* Melanoma,
    skin, by site
  in situ D03.9
    abdominal wall D03.59
    ala nasi D03.39
    ankle D03.7
    anus, anal (margin) (skin) D03.51
    arm D03.6
    auditory canal D03.2
    auricle (ear) D03.2
    auricular canal (external) D03.2

Melanoma – *continued*
  axilla, axillary fold D03.59
  back D03.59
  breast D03.52
  brow D03.39
  buttock D03.59
  canthus (eye) D03.1
  cheek (external) D03.39
  chest wall D03.59
  chin D03.39
  choroid D03.8
  conjunctiva D03.8
  ear (external) D03.2
  external meatus (ear) D03.2
  eye D03.8
  eyebrow D03.39
  eyelid (lower) (upper) D03.1
  face D03.30
    specified NEC D03.39
  female genital organ (external) NEC D03.8
  finger D03.6
  flank D03.59
  foot D03.7
  forearm D03.6
  forehead D03.39
  foreskin D03.8
  gluteal region D03.59
  groin D03.59
  hand D03.6
  heel D03.7
  helix D03.2
  hip D03.7
  interscapular region D03.59
  iris D03.8
  jaw D03.39
  knee D03.7
  labium (majus) (minus) D03.8
  lacrimal gland D03.8
  leg D03.7
  lip (lower) (upper) D03.0
  lower limb NEC D03.7
  male genital organ (external) NEC D03.8
  nail D03.9
    finger D03.6
    toe D03.7
  neck D03.4
  nose (external) D03.39
  orbit D03.8
  penis D03.8
  perianal skin D03.51
  perineum D03.51
  pinna D03.2
  popliteal fossa or space D03.7
  prepuce D03.8
  pudendum D03.8
  retina D03.8
  retrobulbar D03.8
  scalp D03.4
  scrotum D03.8
  shoulder D03.6
  specified site NEC D03.8
  submammary fold D03.52
  temple D03.39
  thigh D03.7
  toe D03.7
  trunk NEC D03.59
  umbilicus D03.59
  upper limb NEC D03.6
  vulva D03.8
  juvenile —*see* Nevus
  malignant, of soft parts except skin —*see*
  Neoplasm, connective tissue, malignant

Melanoma – *continued*
  metastatic
    breast C79.81
    genital organ C79.82
    specified site NEC C79.89
  neurotropic, malignant —*see* Melanoma, skin,
  by site
  nodular —*see* Melanoma, skin, by site
  regressing, malignant —*see* Melanoma, skin,
  by site
  skin C43.9
    abdominal wall C43.59
    ala nasi C43.31
    ankle C43.7
    anus, anal (skin) C43.51
    arm C43.6
    auditory canal (external) C43.2
    auricle (ear) C43.2
    auricular canal (external) C43.2
    axilla, axillary fold C43.59
    back C43.59
    breast (female) (male) C43.52
    brow C43.39
    buttock C43.59
    canthus (eye) C43.1
    cheek (external) C43.39
    chest wall C43.59
    chin C43.39
    ear (external) C43.2
    elbow C43.6
    external meatus (ear) C43.2
    eyebrow C43.39
    eyelid (lower) (upper) C43.1
    face C43.30
      specified NEC C43.39
    female genital organ (external) NEC C51.9
    finger C43.6
    flank C43.59
    foot C43.7
    forearm C43.6
    forehead C43.39
    foreskin C60.0
    glabella C43.39
    gluteal region C43.59
    groin C43.59
    hand C43.6
    heel C43.7
    helix C43.2
    hip C43.7
    interscapular region C43.59
    jaw (external) C43.39
    knee C43.7
    labium C51.9
      majus C51.0
      minus C51.1
    leg C43.7
    lip (lower) (upper) C43.0
    lower limb NEC C43.7
    male genital organ (external) NEC C63.9
    nail
      finger C43.6
      toe C43.7
    nasolabial groove C43.39
    nates C43.59
    neck C43.4
    nose (external) C43.31
    overlapping site C43.8
    palpebra C43.1
    penis C60.9
    perianal skin C43.51
    perineum C43.51
    pinna C43.2
    popliteal fossa or space C43.7

Melanoma – *continued*
  prepuce C60.0
  pudendum C51.9
  scalp C43.4
  scrotum C63.2
  shoulder C43.6
  skin NEC C43.9
  submammary fold C43.52
  temple C43.39
  thigh C43.7
  toe C43.7
  trunk NEC C43.59
  umbilicus C43.59
  upper limb NEC C43.6
  vulva C51.9
    overlapping sites C51.8
  spindle cell
    with epithelioid, mixed —*see* Melanoma, skin, by site
    type A C69.4
    type B C69.4
  superficial spreading —*see* Melanoma, skin, by site
Melanosarcoma —*see also* Melanoma
  epithelioid cell —*see* Melanoma
Melanosis L81.4
  addisonian E27.1
    tuberculous A18.7
  adrenal E27.1
  colon K63.89
  conjunctiva —*see* Pigmentation, conjunctiva
    congenital Q13.89
  cornea (presenile) (senile) —*see also* Pigmentation, cornea
    congenital Q13.4
  eye NEC H57.8
    congenital Q15.8
  lenticularis progressiva Q82.1
  liver K76.89
  precancerous —*see also* Melanoma, in situ
    malignant melanoma in —*see* Melanoma
  Riehl's L81.4
  sclera H15.89
    congenital Q13.89
  suprarenal E27.1
  tar L81.4
  toxic L81.4
Melanuria R82.99
MELAS syndrome E88.41
Melasma L81.1
  adrenal (gland) E27.1
  suprarenal (gland) E27.1
Melena K92.1
  with ulcer
  code by site under Ulcer, with hemorrhage K27.4
  due to swallowed maternal blood P78.2
  newborn, neonatal P54.1
    due to swallowed maternal blood P78.2
Meleney's
  gangrene (cutaneous) —*see* Ulcer, skin
  ulcer (chronic undermining) —*see* Ulcer, skin
Melioidosis A24.9
  acute A24.1
  chronic A24.2
  fulminating A24.1
  pneumonia A24.1
  pulmonary (chronic) A24.2
    acute A24.1
    subacute A24.2
  sepsis A24.1
  specified NEC A24.3
  subacute A24.2

Melitensis, febris A23.0
Melkersson (-Rosenthal) **syndrome** G51.2
Mellitus, diabetes —*see* Diabetes
Melorheostosis (bone) —*see* Disorder, bone, density and structure, specified NEC
Meloschisis Q18.4
Melotia Q17.4
Membrana
  capsularis lentis posterior Q13.89
  epipapillaris Q14.2
Membranacea placenta O43.19
Membranaceous uterus N85.8
Membrane (s) , **membranous** —*see also* condition
  cyclitic —*see* Membrane, pupillary
  folds, congenital —*see* Web
  Jackson's Q43.3
  over face of newborn P28.9
  premature rupture —*see* Rupture, membranes, premature
  pupillary H21.4
    persistent Q13.89
  retained (with hemorrhage) (complicating delivery) O72.2
    without hemorrhage O73.1
  secondary cataract —*see* Cataract, secondary
  unruptured (causing asphyxia) —*see* Asphyxia, newborn
  vitreous —*see* Opacity, vitreous, membranes and strands
Membranitis —*see* Chorioamnionitis
Memory disturbance, lack or loss —*see also* Amnesia
  mild, following organic brain damage F06.8
Menadione deficiency E56.1
Menarche
  delayed E30.0
  precocious E30.1
Mendacity, pathologic F60.2
Mendelson's syndrome (due to anesthesia) J95.4
  in labor and delivery O74.0
  in pregnancy O29.01
  obstetric O74.0
  postpartum, puerperal O89.01
Ménétrier's disease or syndrome K29.60
  with bleeding K29.61
Ménière's disease, syndrome or vertigo H81.0
Meninges, meningeal —*see* condition
Meningioma —*see also* Neoplasm, meninges, benign
  angioblastic —*see* Neoplasm, meninges, benign
  angiomatous —*see* Neoplasm, meninges, benign
  endotheliomatous —*see* Neoplasm, meninges, benign
  fibroblastic —*see* Neoplasm, meninges, benign
  fibrous —*see* Neoplasm, meninges, benign
  hemangioblastic —*see* Neoplasm, meninges, benign
  hemangiopericytic —*see* Neoplasm, meninges, benign
  malignant —*see* Neoplasm, meninges, malignant
  meningothelial —*see* Neoplasm, meninges, benign
  meningotheliomatous —*see* Neoplasm, meninges, benign
  mixed —*see* Neoplasm, meninges, benign

Meningioma – *continued*
  multiple —*see* Neoplasm, meninges, uncertain behavior
  papillary —*see* Neoplasm, meninges, uncertain behavior
  psammomatous —*see* Neoplasm, meninges, benign
  syncytial —*see* Neoplasm, meninges, benign
  transitional —*see* Neoplasm, meninges, benign
Meningiomatosis (diffuse) —*see* Neoplasm, meninges, uncertain behavior
Meningism —*see* Meningismus
Meningismus (infectional) (pneumococcal) R29.1
  due to serum or vaccine R29.1
  influenzal —*see* Influenza, with, manifestations NEC
Meningitis (basal) (basic) (brain) (cerebral) (cervical) (congestive) (diffuse) (hemorrhagic) (infantile) (membranous) (metastatic) (nonspecific) (pontine) (progressive) (simple) (spinal) (subacute) (sympathetic) (toxic) G03.9
  abacterial G03.0
  actinomycotic A42.81
  adenoviral A87.1
  arbovirus A87.8
  aseptic (acute) G03.0
  bacterial G00.9
    Escherichia coli (E. coli) G00.8
    Friedländer (bacillus) G00.8
    gram-negative G00.9
    H. influenzae G00.0
    Klebsiella G00.8
    pneumococcal G00.1
    specified organism NEC G00.8
    staphylococcal G00.3
    streptococcal (acute) G00.2
  benign recurrent (Mollaret) G03.2
  candidal B37.5
  caseous (tuberculous) A17.0
  cerebrospinal A39.0
  chronic NEC G03.1
  clear cerebrospinal fluid NEC G03.0
  coxsackievirus A87.0
  cryptococcal B45.1
  diplococcal (gram positive) A39.0
  echovirus A87.0
  enteroviral A87.0
  eosinophilic B83.2
  epidemic NEC A39.0
  Escherichia coli (E. coli) G00.8
  fibrinopurulent G00.9
    specified organism NEC G00.8
  Friedländer (bacillus) G00.8
  gonococcal A54.81
  gram-negative cocci G00.9
  gram-positive cocci G00.9
  Haemophilus (influenzae) G00.0
  H. influenzae G00.0
  in (due to)
    adenovirus A87.1
    African trypanosomiasis B56.9 *[G02]*
    anthrax A22.8
    bacterial disease NEC A48.8 *[G01]*
    Chagas' disease (chronic) B57.41
    chickenpox B01.0
    coccidioidomycosis B38.4
    Diplococcus pneumoniae G00.1
    enterovirus A87.0

Meningitis – *continued*
  herpes (simplex) virus B00.3
    zoster B02.1
  infectious mononucleosis B27.92
  leptospirosis A27.81
  Listeria monocytogenes A32.11
  Lyme disease A69.21
  measles B05.1
  mumps (virus) B26.1
  neurosyphilis (late) A52.13
  parasitic disease NEC B89 *[G02]*
  poliovirus A80.9 *[G02]*
  preventive immunization, inoculation or
  vaccination G03.8
  rubella B06.02
  Salmonella infection A02.21
  specified cause NEC G03.8
  typhoid fever A01.01
  varicella B01.0
  viral disease NEC A87.8
  whooping cough A37.90
  zoster B02.1
  infectious G00.9
  influenzal (H. influenzae) G00.0
  Klebsiella G00.8
  leptospiral (aseptic) A27.81
  lymphocytic (acute) (benign) (serous) A87.2
  meningococcal A39.0
  Mima polymorpha G00.8
  Mollaret (benign recurrent) G03.2
  monilial B37.5
  mycotic NEC B49 *[G02]*
  Neisseria A39.0
  nonbacterial G03.0
  nonpyogenic NEC G03.0
  ossificans G96.19
  pneumococcal G00.1
  poliovirus A80.9 *[G02]*
  postmeasles B05.1
  purulent G00.9
    specified organism NEC G00.8
  pyogenic G00.9
    specified organism NEC G00.8
  Salmonella (arizonae) (Cholerae-Suis)
  (enteritidis) (typhimurium) A02.21
  septic G00.9
    specified organism NEC G00.8
  serosa circumscripta NEC G03.0
  serous NEC G93.2
  specified organism NEC G00.8
  sporotrichosis B42.81
  staphylococcal G00.3
  sterile G03.0
  streptococcal (acute) G00.2
  suppurative G00.9
    specified organism NEC G00.8
  syphilitic (late) (tertiary) A52.13
    acute A51.41
    congenital A50.41
    secondary A51.41
  Torula histolytica (cryptococcal) B45.1
  traumatic (complication of injury) T79.8
  tuberculous A17.0
  typhoid A01.01
  viral NEC A87.9
  Yersinia pestis A20.3
Meningocele (spinal) —*see also* Spina bifida
  with hydrocephalus —*see* Spina bifida, by
  site, with hydrocephalus
  acquired (traumatic) G96.19
  cerebral —*see* Encephalocele
Meningocerebritis —*see* Meningoencephalitis

Meningococcemia A39.4
  acute A39.2
  chronic A39.3
Meningococcus, meningococcal (*see also*
  condition) A39.9
  adrenalitis, hemorrhagic A39.1
  carrier (suspected) of Z22.31
  meningitis (cerebrospinal) A39.0
Meningoencephalitis (*see also* Encephalitis)
  G04.90
  acute NEC (*see also* Encephalitis, viral) A86
  bacterial NEC G04.2
  California A83.5
  diphasic A84.1
  eosinophilic B83.2
  epidemic A39.81
  herpesviral, herpetic B00.4
    due to herpesvirus 6 B10.01
    due to herpesvirus 7 B10.09
    specified NEC B10.09
  in (due to)
    blastomycosis NEC B40.81
    diseases classified elsewhere G05.3
    free-living amebae B60.2
    Hemophilus influenzae (H .influenzae)
    G04.2
  herpes B00.4
    due to herpesvirus 6 B10.01
    due to herpesvirus 7 B10.09
    specified NEC B10.09
  H. influenzae G00.0
  Lyme disease A69.22
  mercury —*see* subcategory T56.1
  mumps B26.2
  Naegleria (amebae) (organisms) (fowleri)
    B60.2
  Parastrongylus cantonensis B83.2
  toxoplasmosis (acquired) B58.2
    congenital P37.1
  infectious (acute) (viral) A86
  influenzal (H. influenzae) G04.2
  Listeria monocytogenes A32.12
  lymphocytic (serous) A87.2
  mumps B26.2
  parasitic NEC B89 *[G05.3]*
  pneumococcal G00.1
  primary amebic B60.2
  specific (syphilitic) A52.14
  specified organism NEC G04.81
  staphylococcal G04.2
  streptococcal G04.2
  syphilitic A52.14
  toxic NEC G92
    due to mercury —*see* subcategory T56.1
  tuberculous A17.82
  virus NEC A86
Meningoencephalocele —*see also*
  Encephalocele
  syphilitic A52.19
    congenital A50.49
Meningoencephalomyelitis —*see also*
  Meningoencephalitis
  acute NEC (viral) A86
    disseminated G04.00
      postimmunization or postvaccination
    G04.02
      postinfectious G04.01
  due to
    actinomycosis A42.82
    Torula B45.1
    Toxoplasma or toxoplasmosis (acquired)
    B58.2

Meningoencephalomyelitis - *continued*
    congenital P37.1
  postimmunization or postvaccination G04.02
Meningoencephalomyelopathy G96.9
Meningoencephalopathy G96.9
Meningomyelitis —*see also*
  Meningoencephalitis
  bacterial NEC G04.2
  blastomycotic NEC B40.81
  cryptococcal B45.1
  in diseases classified elsewhere G05.4
  meningococcal A39.81
  syphilitic A52.14
  tuberculous A17.82
Meningomyelocele —*see also* Spina bifida
  syphilitic A52.19
Meningomyeloneuritis —*see*
  Meningoencephalitis
Meningoradiculitis —*see* Meningitis
Meningovascular —*see* condition
Menkes' disease or syndrome E83.09
  meaning maple-syrup-urine disease E71.0
Menometrorrhagia N92.1
Menopause, menopausal (asymptomatic)
  (state) Z78.0
  arthritis (any site) NEC —*see* Arthritis,
  specified form NEC
  bleeding N92.4
  depression (single episode) F32.8
    agitated (single episode) F32.2
      recurrent episode F33.9
    psychotic (single episode) F32.8
      recurrent episode F33.9
    recurrent episode F33.9
  melancholia (single episode) F32.8
    recurrent episode F33.9
  paranoid state F22
  premature E28.319
    asymptomatic E28.319
      postirradiation E89.40
      postsurgical E89.40
    symptomatic E28.310
      postirradiation E89.41
      postsurgical E89.41
  psychosis NEC F28
  symptomatic N95.1
  toxic polyarthritis NEC —*see* Arthritis,
  specified form NEC
Menorrhagia (primary) N92.0
  climacteric N92.4
    menopausal N92.4
  menopausal N92.4
  postclimacteric N95.0
  postmenopausal N95.0
  preclimacteric or premenopausal N92.4
  pubertal (menses retained) N92.2
Menostaxis N92.0
Menses, retention N94.89 **Menstrual** —*see*
  Menstruation
Menstruation
  absent —*see* Amenorrhea
  anovulatory N97.0
  cycle, irregular N92.6
  delayed N91.0
  disorder N93.9
    psychogenic F45.8
  during pregnancy O20.8
  excessive (with regular cycle) N92.0
    with irregular cycle N92.1
    at puberty N92.2
  frequent N92.0
  infrequent —*see* Oligomenorrhea
  irregular N92.6

Menstruation - *continued*
  specified NEC N92.5
  latent N92.5
  membranous N92.5
  painful (*see also* Dysmenorrhea) N94.6
    primary N94.4
    psychogenic F45.8
    secondary N94.5
  passage of clots N92.0
  precocious E30.1
  protracted N92.5
  rare —*see* Oligomenorrhea
  retained N94.89
  retrograde N92.5
  scanty —*see* Oligomenorrhea
  suppression N94.89
  vicarious (nasal) N94.89
Mental —*see also* condition
  deficiency —*see* Disability, intellectual
  deterioration —*see* Psychosis
  disorder —*see* Disorder, mental
  exhaustion F48.8
  insufficiency (congenital) —*see* Disability,
  intellectual
  observation without need for further medical
  care Z03.89
  retardation —*see* Disability, intellectual
  subnormality —*see* Disability, intellectual
  upset —*see* Disorder, mental
Meralgia paresthetica G57.1
Mercurial —*see* condition
Mercurialism   see subcategory T56.1
MERRF syndrome (myoclonic epilepsy
  associated with ragged-red fiber) E88.42
Merkel cell tumor —*see* Carcinoma, Merkel
cell
Merocele —*see* Hernia, femoral
Meromelia
  lower limb —*see* Defect, reduction, lower
  limb
    intercalary
      femur —*see* Defect, reduction, lower limb,
  specified type NEC
        tibiofibular (complete) (incomplete) —
  see Defect, reduction, lower limb
  upper limb —*see* Defect, reduction, upper
  limb
    intercalary, humeral, radioulnar —*see*
  Agenesis, arm, with hand present
Merzbacher-Pelizaeus disease E75.29
Mesaortitis —*see* Aortitis
Mesarteritis —*see* Arteritis
Mesencephalitis —*see* Encephalitis
Mesenchymoma —*see also* Neoplasm,
connective tissue, uncertain behavior
  benign —*see* Neoplasm, connective tissue,
  benign
  malignant —*see* Neoplasm, connective tissue,
  malignant
Mesenteritis
  retractile K65.4
  sclerosing K65.4
Mesentery, mesenteric —*see* condition
Mesiodens, mesiodentes K00.1
Mesio-occlusion M26.213
Mesocolon —*see* condition
Mesonephroma (malignant) —*see* Neoplasm,
malignant, by site
  benign —*see* Neoplasm, benign, by site
Mesophlebitis —*see* Phlebitis
Mesostromal dysgenesia Q13.89

Mesothelioma (malignant) C45.9
  benign
    mesentery D19.1
    mesocolon D19.1
    omentum D19.1
    peritoneum D19.1
    pleura D19.0
    specified site NEC D19.7
    unspecified site D19.9
  biphasic C45.9
    benign
      mesentery D19.1
      mesocolon D19.1
      omentum D19.1
      peritoneum D19.1
      pleura D19.0
      specified site NEC D19.7
      unspecified site D19.9
  cystic D48.4
  epithelioid C45.9
    benign
      mesentery D19.1
      mesocolon D19.1
      omentum D19.1
      peritoneum D19.1
      pleura D19.0
      specified site NEC D19.7
      unspecified site D19.9
  fibrous C45.9
    benign
      mesentery D19.1
      mesocolon D19.1
      omentum D19.1
      peritoneum D19.1
      pleura D19.0
      specified site NEC D19.7
      unspecified site D19.9
  site classification
    liver C45.7
    lung C45.7
    mediastinum C45.7
    mesentery C45.1
    mesocolon C45.1
    omentum C45.1
    pericardium C45.2
    peritoneum C45.1
    pleura C45.0
      parietal C45.0
    retroperitoneum C45.7
    specified site NEC C45.7
    unspecified C45.9
Metabolic syndrome E88.81
Metagonimiasis B66.8
Metagonimus infestation (intestine) B66.8
Metal
  pigmentation L81.8
  polisher's disease J62.8
Metamorphopsia H53.15
Metaplasia
  apocrine (breast) —*see* Dysplasia, mammary,
  specified type NEC
  cervix (squamous) —*see* Dysplasia, cervix
  endometrium (squamous) (uterus) N85.8
  esophagus
  kidney (pelvis) (squamous) N28.89
  myelogenous D73.1
  myeloid (agnogenic) (megakaryocytic) D73.1
  spleen D73.1
  squamous cell, bladder N32.89
Metastasis, metastatic
  abscess —*see* Abscess
  calcification E83.59

Metastasis, metastatic - *continued*
  cancer
    from specified site —*see* Neoplasm,
  malignant, by site
    to specified site —*see* Neoplasm, secondary,
    by site
  deposits (in) —*see* Neoplasm, secondary, by
  site
  disease (*see also* Neoplasm, secondary, by
  site) C79.9
  spread (to) —*see* Neoplasm, secondary, by
  site
Metastrongyliasis B83.8
Metatarsalgia M77.4
  anterior G57.6
  Morton's G57.6
Metatarsus, metatarsal —*see also* condition
  valgus (abductus) , congenital Q66.6
  varus (adductus) (congenital) Q66.2
Methadone use F11.20
Methemoglobinemia D74.9
  acquired (with sulfhemoglobinemia) D74.8
  congenital D74.0
  enzymatic (congenital) D74.0
  Hb M disease D74.0
  hereditary D74.0
  toxic D74.8
Methemoglobinuria —*see* Hemoglobinuria
Methioninemia E72.19
Methylmalonic acidemia E71.120
Metritis (catarrhal) (hemorrhagic) (septic)
  (suppurative) —*see also* Endometritis
  cervical —*see* Cervicitis
Metropathia hemorrhagica N93.8
Metroperitonitis —*see* Peritonitis, pelvic,
female
Metrorrhagia N92.1
  climacteric N92.4
  menopausal N92.4
  postpartum NEC (atonic) (following delivery
  of placenta) O72.1
    delayed or secondary O72.2
  preclimacteric or premenopausal N92.4
  psychogenic F45.8
Metrorrhexis —*see* Rupture, uterus
Metrosalpingitis N70.91
Metrostaxis N93.8
Metrovaginitis —*see* Endometritis
Meyer-Schwickerath and Weyers syndrome
Q87.0
Meynert's amentia (nonalcoholic) F04
  alcoholic F10.96
    with dependence F10.26
Mibelli's disease (porokeratosis) Q82.8
Mice, joint —*see* Loose, body, joint
  knee M23.4
Micrencephalon, micrencephaly Q02
Microalbuminuria R80.9
Microaneurysm, retinal —*see also* Disorder,
  retina, microaneurysms
  diabetic —*see* E08-E13 with .31
Microangiopathy (peripheral) I73.9
  thrombotic M31.1
Microcalcifications, breast R92.0
Microcephalus, microcephalic, microcephaly
Q02
  due to toxoplasmosis (congenital) P37.1
Microcheilia Q18.7
Microcolon (congenital) Q43.8
Microcornea (congenital) Q13.4
Microcytic —*see* condition
Microdeletions NEC Q93.88
Microdontia K00.2

Microdrepanocytosis D57.40
  with crisis (vasoocclusive pain) D57.419
    with
      acute chest syndrome D57.411
      splenic sequestration D57.412
Microembolism
  atherothrombotic —*see* Atheroembolism
  retinal —*see* Occlusion, artery, retina
Microencephalon Q02
Microfilaria streptocerca infestation —*see*
  Onchocerciasis
Microgastria (congenital) Q40.2
Microgenia M26.06
Microgenitalia, congenital
  female Q52.8
  male Q55.8
Microglioma —*see* Lymphoma, non-Hodgkin,
  specified NEC
Microglossia (congenital) Q38.3
Micrognathia, micrognathism (congenital)
  (mandibular) (maxillary) M26.09
Microgyria (congenital) Q04.3
Microinfarct of heart —*see* Insufficiency,
  coronary
Microlentia (congenital) Q12.8
Microlithiasis, alveolar, pulmonary J84.02
Micromastia N64.82
Micromyelia (congenital) Q06.8
Micropenis Q55.62
Microphakia (congenital) Q12.8
Microphthalmos, microphthalmia
  (congenital) Q11.2
  due to toxoplasmosis P37.1
Micropsia H53.15
Microscopic polyangiitis (polyarteritis) M31.7
Microsporidiosis B60.8
  intestinal A07.8
Microsporon furfur infestation B36.0
Microsporosis —*see also* Dermatophytosis
  nigra B36.1
Microstomia (congenital) Q18.5
Microtia (congenital) (external ear) Q17.2
Microtropia H50.40
Microvillus inclusion disease (MVD) (MVID)
  Q43.8
Micturition
  disorder NEC R39.19
    psychogenic F45.8
  frequency R35.0
    psychogenic F45.8
  hesitancy R39.11
  incomplete emptying R39.14
  nocturnal R35.1
  painful R30.9
    dysuria R30.0
    psychogenic F45.8
    tenesmus R30.1
  poor stream R39.12
  split stream R39.13
  straining R39.16
  urgency R39.15
Mid plane —*see* condition
Middle
  ear —*see* condition
  lobe (right) syndrome J98.19
Miescher's elastoma L87.2
Mietens' syndrome Q87.2
Migraine (idiopathic) G43.909
  with refractory migraine G43.919
    with status migrainosus G43.911
    without status migrainosus G43.919

Migraine – *continued*
  with aura (acute-onset) (prolonged) (typical)
  (without headache) G43.109
    with refractory migraine G43.119
      with status migrainosus G43.111
      without status migrainosus G43.119
    intractable G43.119
      with status migrainosus G43.111
      without status migrainosus G43.119
    not intractable G43.109
      with status migrainosus G43.101
      without status migrainosus G43.109
    persistent G43.509
      with cerebral infarction G43.609
        with refractory migraine G43.619
          with status migrainosus G43.611
          without status migrainosus G43.619
        intractable G43.619
          with status migrainosus G43.611
          without status migrainosus G43.619
        not intractable G43.609
          with status migrainosus G43.601
          without status migrainosus G43.609
        without refractory migraine G43.609
          with status migrainosus G43.601
          without status migrainosus G43.609
      without cerebral infarction G43.509
        with refractory migraine G43.519
          with status migrainosus G43.511
          without status migrainosus G43.519
        intractable G43.519
          with status migrainosus G43.511
          without status migrainosus G43.519
        not intractable G43.509
          with status migrainosus G43.501
          without status migrainosus G43.509
        without refractory migraine G43.509
          with status migrainosus G43.501
          without status migrainosus G43.509
    without mention of refractory migraine
    G43.109
      with status migrainosus G43.101
      without status migrainosus G43.109
  abdominal G43.D0
    with refractory migraine G43.D1
    intractable G43.D1
    not intractable G43.D0
    without refractory migraine G43.D0
  basilar —*see* Migraine, with aura
  classical —*see* Migraine, with aura
  common —*see* Migraine, without aura
  complicated G43.109
  equivalents —*see* Migraine, with aura
  familiar —*see* Migraine, hemiplegic
  hemiplegic G43.409
    with refractory migraine G43.419
      with status migrainosus G43.411
      without status migrainosus G43.419
    intractable G43.419
      with status migrainosus G43.411
      without status migrainosus G43.419
    not intractable G43.409
      with status migrainosus G43.401
      without status migrainosus G43.409
    without refractory migraine G43.409
      with status migrainosus G43.401
      without status migrainosus G43.409
  intractable G43.919
    with status migrainosus G43.911
    without status migrainosus G43.919
  menstrual G43.829
    with refractory migraine G43.839
      with status migrainosus G43.831

Migraine – *continued*
      without status migrainosus G43.839
    intractable G43.839
      with status migrainosus G43.831
      without status migrainosus G43.839
    not intractable 4G43.829
      with status migrainosus G43.821
      without status migrainosus G43.829
    without refractory migraine G43.829
      with status migrainosus G43.821
      without status migrainosus G43.829
  menstrually related —*see* Migraine, menstrual
  not intractable G43.909
    with status migrainosus G43.901
    without status migrainosus G43.919
  ophthalmoplegic G43.B0
    with refractory migraine G43.B1
    intractable G43.B1
    not intractable G43.B0
    without refractory migraine G43.B0
  persistent aura (with, without) cerebral
  infarction —*see* Migraine, with aura,
  persistent
  preceded or accompanied by transient focal
  neurological phenomena —*see* Migraine, with
  aura
  pre-menstrual —*see* Migraine, menstrual
  pure menstrual —*see* Migraine, menstrual
  retinal —*see* Migraine, with aura
  specified NEC G43.809
    intractable G43.819
      with status migrainosus G43.811
      without status migrainosus G43.819
    not intractable G43.809
      with status migrainosus G43.801
      without status migrainosus G43.809
  sporadic —*see* Migraine, hemiplegic
  transformed —*see* Migraine, without aura,
  chronic
  triggered seizures —*see* Migraine, with aura
  without aura G43.009
    with refractory migraine G43.019
      with status migrainosus G43.011
      without status migrainosus G43.019
    chronic G43.709
      with refractory migraine G43.719
        with status migrainosus G43.711
        without status migrainosus G43.719
      intractable
        with status migrainosus G43.711
        without status migrainosus G43.719
      not intractable
        with status migrainosus G43.701
        without status migrainosus G43.709
      without refractory migraine G43.709
        with status migrainosus G43.701
        without status migrainosus G43.709
    intractable
      with status migrainosus G43.011
      without status migrainosus G43.019
    not intractable
      with status migrainosus G43.001
      without status migrainosus G43.009
    without mention of refractory migraine
    G43.009
      with status migrainosus G43.001
      without status migrainosus G43.009
  without refractory migraine G43.909
    with status migrainosus G43.901
    without status migrainosus G43.919
Migrant, social Z59.0
Migration, anxiety concerning Z60.3

Migratory, migrating —*see also* condition
  person Z59.0
  testis Q55.29
Mikity-Wilson disease or syndrome P27.0
Mikulicz' disease or syndrome K11.8
Miliaria L74.3
  alba L74.1
  apocrine L75.2
  crystallina L74.1
  profunda L74.2
  rubra L74.0
  tropicalis L74.2
Miliary —*see* condition
Milium L72.0
  colloid L57.8
Milk
  crust L21.0
  excessive secretion O92.6
  poisoning —*see* Poisoning, food, noxious
  retention O92.79
  sickness —*see* Poisoning, food, noxious
  spots I31.0
Milk-alkali disease or syndrome E83.52
Milk-leg (deep vessels) (nonpuerperal) —*see*
  Embolism, vein, lower extremity
  complicating pregnancy O22.3
  puerperal, postpartum, childbirth O87.1
Milkman's disease or syndrome M83.8
Milky urine —*see* Chyluria
Millard-Gubler (-Foville) **paralysis or**
  syndrome G46.3
Millar's asthma J38.5
Miller Fisher syndrome G61.0
Mills' disease —*see* Hemiplegia
Millstone maker's pneumoconiosis J62.8
Milroy's disease (chronic hereditary edema)
  Q82.0
Minamata disease T26.1
Miners' asthma or lung J60
Minkowski-Chauffard syndrome —*see*
  Spherocytosis
Minor —*see* condition
Minor's disease (hematomyelia) G95.19
Minot's disease (hemorrhagic disease) ,
  newborn P53
Minot-von Willebrand-Jurgens disease or
  syndrome (angiohemophilia) D68.0
Minus (and plus) hand (intrinsic) —*see*
  Deformity, limb, specified type NEC, forearm
Miosis (pupil) H57.03
Mirizzi's syndrome (hepatic duct stenosis)
  K83.1
Mirror writing F81.0
Misadventure (of) (prophylactic) (therapeutic)
  (*see also* Complications) T88.9
  administration of insulin (by accident) —*see*
  subcategory T38.3
  infusion —*see* Complications, infusion
  local applications (of fomentations, plasters,
  etc.) T88.9
    burn or scald —*see* Burn
    specified NEC T88.8
  medical care (early) (late) T88.9
    adverse effect of drugs or chemicals —*see*
  Table of Drugs and Chemicals
  medical care (early) (late)
    burn or scald —*see* Burn
    specified NEC T88.8
  specified NEC T88.8
  surgical procedure (early) (late) —*see*
  Complications, surgical procedure
  transfusion —*see* Complications, transfusion

Misadventure – *continued*
  vaccination or other immunological procedure
  —*see* Complications, vaccination
Miscarriage O03.9
Misdirection, aqueous H40.83
Misperception, sleep state F51.02
Misplaced, misplacement
  ear Q17.4
  kidney (acquired) N28.89
    congenital Q63.2
  organ or site, congenital NEC —*see*
  Malposition, congenital
Missed
  abortion O02.1
  delivery O36.4
Missing —*see* Absence
Misuse of drugs F19.99
Mitchell's disease (erythromelalgia) I73.81
Mite (s) (infestation) B88.9
  diarrhea B88.0
  grain (itch) B88.0
  hair follicle (itch) B88.0
  in sputum B88.0
Mitral —*see* condition
Mittelschmerz N94.0
Mixed —*see* condition
MNGIE (Mitochondrial Neurogastrointestinal
  Encephalopathy) **syndrome** E88.49
Mobile, mobility
  cecum Q43.3
  excessive —*see* Hypermobility
  gallbladder, congenital Q44.1
  kidney N28.89
  organ or site, congenital NEC —*see*
  Malposition, congenital
Mobitz heart block (atrioventricular) I44.1
Moebius, Möbius
  disease (ophthalmoplegic migraine) —*see*
  Migraine, ophthalmoplegic
  syndrome Q87.0
    congenital oculofacial paralysis (with other
  anomalies) Q87.0
    ophthalmoplegic migraine —*see* Migraine,
  ophthalmoplegic
Moeller's glossitis K14.0
Mohr's syndrome (Types I and II) Q87.0
Mola destruens D39.2
Molar pregnancy O02.0
Molarization of premolars K00.2
Molding, head (during birth)   **omit code**
Mole (pigmented) —*see also* Nevus
  blood O02.0
  Breus' O02.0
  cancerous —*see* Melanoma
  carneous O02.0
  destructive D39.2
  fleshy O02.0
  hydatid, hydatidiform (benign) (complicating
  pregnancy) (delivered) (undelivered) O01.9
    classical O01.0
    complete O01.0
    incomplete O01.1
    invasive D39.2
    malignant D39.2
    partial O01.1
  intrauterine O02.0
  invasive (hydatidiform) D39.2
  malignant
    meaning
      malignant hydatidiform mole D39.2
      melanoma —*see* Melanoma
  nonhydatidiform O02.0

Mole – *continued*
  nonpigmented —*see* Nevus
  pregnancy NEC O02.0
  skin —*see* Nevus
  tubal O00.1
  vesicular —*see* Mole, hydatidiform
Molimen, molimina (menstrual) N94.3
Molluscum contagiosum (epitheliale) B08.1
Mönckeberg's arteriosclerosis, disease, or
  sclerosis —*see* Arteriosclerosis, extremities
Mondini's malformation (cochlea) Q16.5
Mondor's disease I80.8
Monge's disease T70.29
Monilethrix (congenital) Q84.1
Moniliasis (*see also* Candidiasis) B37.9
  neonatal P37.5
Monitoring (encounter for)
  therapeutic drug level Z51.81
Monkey malaria B53.1
Monkeypox B04
Monoarthritis M13.10
  ankle M13.17
  elbow M13.12
  foot joint M13.17
  hand joint M13.14
  hip M13.15
  knee M13.16
  shoulder M13.11
  wrist M13.13
Monoblastic —*see* condition
Monochromat (ism) , monochromatopsia
  (acquired) (congenital) H53.51
Monocytic —*see* condition
Monocytopenia D72.818
Monocytosis (symptomatic) D72.821
Monomania —*see* Psychosis
Mononeuritis G58.9
  cranial nerve —*see* Disorder, nerve, cranial
  femoral nerve G57.2
  lateral
    cutaneous nerve of thigh G57.1
    popliteal nerve G57.3
  lower limb G57.9
    specified nerve NEC G57.8
  medial popliteal nerve G57.4
  median nerve G56.1
  multiplex G58.7
  plantar nerve G57.6
  posterior tibial nerve G57.5
  radial nerve G56.3
  sciatic nerve G57.0
  specified NEC G58.8
  tibial nerve G57.4
  ulnar nerve G56.2
  upper limb G56.9
    specified nerve NEC G56.8
  vestibular —*see* subcategory H93.3
Mononeuropathy G58.9
  carpal tunnel syndrome —*see* Syndrome,
  carpal tunnel
  diabetic NEC —*see* E08-E13 with .41
  femoral nerve —*see* Lesion, nerve, femoral
  ilioinguinal nerve G57.8
  in diseases classified elsewhere —*see*
  category G59
  intercostal G58.0
  lower limb G57.9
    causalgia —*see* Causalgia, lower limb
    femoral nerve —*see* Lesion, nerve, femoral
    meralgia paresthetica G57.1
    plantar nerve —*see* Lesion, nerve, plantar
    popliteal nerve —*see* Lesion, nerve,
  popliteal

Mononeuropathy - *continued*
  sciatic nerve —*see* Lesion, nerve, sciatic
  specified NEC G57.8
  tarsal tunnel syndrome —*see* Syndrome,
  tarsal tunnel
  median nerve —*see* Lesion, nerve, median
  multiplex G58.7
  obturator nerve G57.8
  popliteal nerve —*see* Lesion, nerve, popliteal
  radial nerve —*see* Lesion, nerve, radial
  saphenous nerve G57.8
  specified NEC G58.8
  tarsal tunnel syndrome —*see* Syndrome,
  tarsal tunnel
  tuberculous A17.83
  ulnar nerve —*see* Lesion, nerve, ulnar
  upper limb G56.9
    carpal tunnel syndrome —*see* Syndrome,
    carpal tunnel
    causalgia —*see* Causalgia
    median nerve —*see* Lesion, nerve, median
    radial nerve —*see* Lesion, nerve, radial
    specified site NEC G56.8
    ulnar nerve —*see* Lesion, nerve, ulnar
Mononucleosis, infectious B27.90
  with
    complication NEC B27.99
    meningitis B27.92
    polyneuropathy B27.91
  cytomegaloviral B27.10
    with
      complication NEC B27.19
      meningitis B27.12
      polyneuropathy B27.11
  Epstein-Barr (virus) B27.00
    with
      complication NEC B27.09
      meningitis B27.02
      polyneuropathy B27.01
  gammaherpesviral B27.00
    with
      complication NEC B27.09
      meningitis B27.02
      polyneuropathy B27.01
  specified NEC B27.80
    with
      complication NEC B27.89
      meningitis B27.82
      polyneuropathy B27.81
Monoplegia G83.3
  congenital (cerebral) G80.8
    spastic G80.1
  embolic (current episode) I63.4
  following
    cerebrovascular disease
      cerebral infarction
        lower limb I69.34
        upper limb I69.33
      intracerebral hemorrhage
        lower limb I69.14
        upper limb I69.13
      lower limb I69.94
      nontraumatic intracranial hemorrhage NEC
        lower limb I69.24
        upper limb I69.23
      specified disease NEC
        lower limb I69.84
        upper limb I69.83
      stroke NOS
        lower limb I69.34
        upper limb I69.33
      subarachnoid hemorrhage
        lower limb I69.04

Monoplegia – *continued*
  upper limb I69.03
  upper limb I69.93
  hysterical (transient) F44.4
  lower limb G83.1
  psychogenic (conversion reaction) F44.4
  thrombotic (current episode) I63.3
  transient R29.818
  upper limb G83.2
Monorchism, monorchidism Q55.0
Monosomy (*see also* Deletion, chromosome)
  Q93.9
  specified NEC Q93.89
  whole chromosome
    meiotic nondisjunction Q93.0
    mitotic nondisjunction Q93.1
    mosaicism Q93.1
  X Q96.9
Monster, monstrosity (single) Q89.7
  acephalic Q00.0
  twin Q89.4
Monteggia's fracture (-dislocation) S52.27
Mooren's ulcer (cornea) —*see* Ulcer, cornea,
  Mooren's
Moore's syndrome —*see* Epilepsy, specified
  NEC
Mooser-Neill reaction A75.2
Mooser's bodies A75.2
Morbidity not stated or unknown R69
Morbilli —*see* Measles
Morbus —*see also* Disease
  angelicus, anglorum E55.0
  Beigel B36.2
  caducus —*see* Epilepsy
  celiacus K90.0
  comitialis —*see* Epilepsy
  cordis (*see also* Disease, heart) I51.9
    valvulorum —*see* Endocarditis
  coxae senilis M16.9
    tuberculous A18.02
  hemorrhagicus neonatorum P53
  maculosus neonatorum P54.5
Morel (-Stewart) (-Morgagni) **syndrome**
  M85.2
Morel-Kraepelin disease —*see* Schizophrenia
Morel-Moore syndrome M85.2
Morgagni's
  cyst, organ, hydatid, or appendage
    female Q50.5
    male (epididymal) Q55.4
      testicular Q55.29
  syndrome M85.2
Morgagni-Stokes-Adams syndrome I45.9
Morgagni-Stewart-Morel syndrome M85.2
Morgagni-Turner (-Albright) **syndrome**
  Q96.9
Moria F07.0
Moron (I.Q.50 69) F70
Morphea L94.0
Morphinism (without remission) F11.20
  with remission F11.21
Morphinomania (without remission) F11.20
  with remission F11.21
Morquio (-Ullrich) (-Brailsford) **disease or**
  syndrome —*see* Mucopolysaccharidosis
Mortification (dry) (moist) —*see* Gangrene
Morton's metatarsalgia (neuralgia) (neuroma)
  (syndrome) G57.6
Morvan's disease or syndrome G60.8

Mosaicism, mosaic (autosomal)
  (chromosomal)
  45,X/other cell lines NEC with abnormal sex
    chromosome Q96.4
  45,X/46,XX Q96.3
  sex chromosome
    female Q97.8
    lines with various numbers of X
      chromosomes Q97.2
    male Q98.7
  XY Q96.3
Moschowitz' disease M31.1
Mother yaw A66.0
Motion sickness (from travel, any vehicle)
  (from roundabouts or swings) T75.3
Mottled, mottling, teeth (enamel) (endemic)
  (nonendemic) K00.3
Mounier-Kuhn syndrome Q32.4
  with bronchiectasis J47.9
    exacerbation (acute) J47.1
    lower respiratory infection J47.0
  acquired J98.09
    with bronchiectasis J47.9
    with
      exacerbation (acute) J47.1
      lower respiratory infection J47.0
Mountain
  sickness T70.29
    with polycythemia , acquired (acute) D75.1
  tick fever A93.2
Mouse, joint —*see* Loose, body, joint
  knee M23.4
Mouth —*see* condition
Movable
  coccyx —see subcategory M53.2
  kidney N28.89
    congenital Q63.8
  spleen D73.89
Movements, dystonic R25.8
Moyamoya disease I67.5
MRSA (Methicillin resistant Staphylococcus
  aureus)
  infection A49.02
    as the cause of diseases classified elsewhere
      B95.62
  sepsis A41.02
MSSA (Methicillin susceptible Staphylococcus
  aureus)
  infection A49.01
    as the cause of diseases classified elsewhere
      B95.61
  sepsis A41.01
Mucha-Habermann disease L41.0
Mucinosis (cutaneous) (focal) (papular)
  (reticular erythematous) (skin) L98.5
  oral K13.79
Mucocele
  appendix K38.8
  buccal cavity K13.79
  gallbladder K82.1
  lacrimal sac, chronic H04.43
  nasal sinus J34.1
  nose J34.1
  salivary gland (any) K11.6
  sinus (accessory) (nasal) J34.1
  turbinate (bone) (middle) (nasal) J34.1
  uterus N85.8
Mucolipidosis
  I E77.1
  II, III E77.0
  IV E75.11

Mucopolysaccharidosis E76.3
  beta-gluduronidase deficiency E76.29
  cardiopathy E76.3 *[I52]*
  Hunter's syndrome E76.1
  Hurler's syndrome E76.01
  Hurler-Scheie syndrome E76.02
  Maroteaux-Lamy syndrome E76.29
  Morquio syndrome E76.219
    A E76.210
    B E76.211
    classic E76.210
  Sanfilippo syndrome E76.22
  Scheie's syndrome E76.03
  specified NEC E76.29
  type
    I
      Hurler's syndrome E76.01
      Hurler-Scheie syndrome E76.02
      Scheie's syndrome E76.03
    II E76.1
    III E76.22
    IV E76.219
    IVA E76.210
    IVB E76.211
    VI E76.29
    VII E76.29
Mucormycosis B46.5
  cutaneous B46.3
  disseminated B46.4
  gastrointestinal B46.2
  generalized B46.4
  pulmonary B46.0
  rhinocerebral B46.1
  skin B46.3
  subcutaneous B46.3
Mucositis (ulcerative) K12.30
  due to drugs NEC K12.32
  gastrointestinal K92.81
  mouth (oral) (oropharyngeal) K12.30
    due to antineoplastic therapy K12.31
    due to drugs NEC K12.32
    due to radiation K12.33
    specified NEC K12.39
    viral K12.39
  nasal J34.81
  oral cavity —*see* Mucositis, mouth
  oral soft tissues —*see* Mucositis, mouth
  vagina and vulva N76.81
Mucositis necroticans agranulocytica —*see*
  Agranulocytosis
Mucous —*see also* condition
  patches (syphilitic) A51.39
    congenital A50.07
Mucoviscidosis E84.9
  with meconium obstruction E84.11
Mucus
  asphyxia or suffocation —*see* Asphyxia,
  mucus
  in stool R19.5
  plug —*see* Asphyxia, mucus
Muguet B37.0
Mulberry molars (congenital syphilis) A50.52
Müllerian mixed tumor
  specified site —*see* Neoplasm, malignant, by
  site
  unspecified site C54.9
Multicystic kidney (development) Q61.4
Multiparity (grand) Z64.1
  affecting management of pregnancy, labor
  and delivery (supervision only) O09.4
  requiring contraceptive management —*see*
  Contraception
Multipartita placenta O43.19

Multiple, multiplex —*see also* condition
  digits (congenital) Q69.9
  endocrine neoplasia —*see* Neoplasia,
  endocrine, multiple (MEN)
  personality F44.81
Mumps B26.9
  arthritis B26.85
  complication NEC B26.89
  encephalitis B26.2
  hepatitis B26.81
  meningitis (aseptic) B26.1
  meningoencephalitis B26.2
  myocarditis B26.82
  oophoritis B26.89
  orchitis B26.0
  pancreatitis B26.3
  polyneuropathy B26.84
Mumu (*see also* Infestation, filarial) B74.9
  [N51]
Münchhausen's syndrome —*see* Disorder,
  factitious
Münchmeyer's syndrome —*see* Myositis,
  ossificans, progressiva
Mural —*see* condition
Murmur (cardiac) (heart) (organic) R01.1
  abdominal R19.15
  aortic (valve) —*see* Endocarditis, aortic
  benign R01.0
  diastolic —*see* Endocarditis
  Flint I35.1
  functional R01.0
  Graham Steell I37.1
  innocent R01.0
  mitral (valve) —*see* Insufficiency, mitral
  nonorganic R01.0
  presystolic, mitral —*see* Insufficiency, mitral
  pulmonic (valve) I37.8
  systolic (valvular) —*see* Endocarditis
  tricuspid (valve) I07.9
  valvular —*see* Endocarditis
Murri's disease (intermittent hemoglobinuria)
  D59.6
Muscle, muscular —*see also* condition
  carnitine (palmitoyltransferase) deficiency
  E71.314
Musculoneuralgia —*see* Neuralgia
Mushroom-workers' (pickers') **disease or
lung** J67.5
Mushrooming hip —*see* Derangement, joint,
  specified NEC, hip
Mutation (s)
  factor V Leiden D68.51
  surfactant, of lung J84.83
  prothrombin gene D68.52
Mutism —*see also* Aphasia
  deaf (acquired) (congenital) NEC H91.3
  elective (adjustment reaction) (childhood)
  F94.0
  hysterical F44.4
  selective (childhood) F94.0
MVD (microvillus inclusion disease) Q43.8
MVID (microvillus inclusion disease) Q43.8
Myalgia M79.1
  epidemic (cervical) B33.0
  traumatic NEC T14.8
Myasthenia G70.9
  congenital G70.2
  cordis —*see* Failure, heart
  developmental G70.2
  gravis G70.00
    with exacerbation (acute) G70.01
    in crisis G70.01

Myasthenia – *continued*
  neonatal, transient P94.0
  pseudoparalytica G70.00
    with exacerbation (acute) G70.01
    in crisis G70.01
  stomach, psychogenic F45.8
  syndrome
    in
      diabetes mellitus —*see* E08-E13 with .44
      neoplastic disease (*see also* Neoplasm)
      D49.9 *[G73.3]*
      pernicious anemia D51.0 *[G73.3]*
      thyrotoxicosis E05.90 *[G73.3]*
        with thyroid storm E05.91 *[G73.3]*
Myasthenic M62.81
Mycelium infection B49
Mycetismus —*see* Poisoning, food, noxious,
  mushroom
Mycetoma B47.9
  actinomycotic B47.1
  bone (mycotic) B47.9 *[M90.80]*
  eumycotic B47.0
  foot B47.9
    actinomycotic B47.1
    mycotic B47.0
  madurae NEC B47.9
    mycotic B47.0
  maduromycotic B47.0
  mycotic B47.0
  nocardial B47.1
Mycobacteriosis —*see* Mycobacterium
Mycobacterium, mycobacterial (infection)
  A31.9
  anonymous A31.9
  atypical A31.9
    cutaneous A31.1
    pulmonary A31.0
      tuberculous —*see* Tuberculosis, pulmonary
    specified site NEC A31.8
  avium (intracellulare complex) A31.0
  balnei A31.1
  Battey A31.0
  chelonei A31.8
  cutaneous A31.1
  extrapulmonary systemic A31.8
  fortuitum A31.8
  intracellulare (Battey bacillus) A31.0
  kansasii (yellow bacillus) A31.0
  kakaferifu A31.8
  kasongo A31.8
  leprae (*see also* Leprosy) A30.9
  luciflavum A31.1
  marinum (M. balnei) A31.1
  nonspecific —*see* Mycobacterium, atypical
  pulmonary (atypical) A31.0
    tuberculous —*see* Tuberculosis, pulmonary
  scrofulaceum A31.8
  simiae A31.8
  systemic, extrapulmonary A31.8
  szulgai A31.8
  terrae A31.8
  triviale A31.8
  tuberculosis (human, bovine)
  seeTuberculosis
  ulcerans A31.1
  xenopi A31.8
Mycoplasma (M.) **pneumoniae**, as cause of
  disease classified elsewhere B96.0
Mycosis, mycotic B49
  cutaneous NEC B36.9
  ear B36.8
  fungoides (extranodal) (solid organ) C84.0

Mycosis, mycotic – *continued*
mouth B37.0
nails B35.1
opportunistic B48.8
skin NEC B36.9
specified NEC B48.8
stomatitis B37.0
vagina, vaginitis (candidal) B37.3
Mydriasis (pupil) H57.04
Myelatelia Q06.1
Myelinolysis, pontine, central G37.2
Myelitis (acute) (ascending) (childhood)
(chronic) (descending) (diffuse)
(disseminated) (idiopathic) (pressure)
(progressive) (spinal cord) (subacute) (*see*
also Encephalitis) G04.91
herpes simplex B00.82
herpes zoster B02.24
in diseases classified elsewhere G05.4
necrotizing, subacute G37.4
optic neuritis in G36.0
post chickenpox B01.12
postherpetic B02.24
postimmunization G04.02
postinfectious NEC G04.89
postvaccinal G04.02
specified NEC G04.89
syphilitic (transverse) A52.14
toxic G92
transverse (in demyelinating diseases of
central nervous system) G37.3
tuberculous A17.82
varicella B01.12
Myeloblastic —*see* condition
Myeloblastoma
granular cell —*see also* Neoplasm, connective
tissue
malignant —*see* Neoplasm, connective
tissue, malignant
tongue D10.1
Myelocele —*see* Spina bifida
Myelocystocele —*see* Spina bifida
Myelocytic —*see* condition
Myelodysplasia D46.9
specified NEC D46.Z
spinal cord (congenital) Q06.1
Myelodysplastic syndrome D46.9
with
5q deletion D46.C
isolated del (5q) chromosomal abnormality
D46.C specified NEC D46.Z
Myeloencephalitis —*see* Encephalitis
Myelofibrosis D75.81
with myeloid metaplasia D47.4
acute C94.4
idiopathic (chronic) D47.4
primary D47.1
secondary D75.81
in myeloproliferative disease D47.4
Myelogenous —*see* condition
Myeloid —*see* condition
Myelokathexis D70.9
Myeloleukodystrophy E75.29
Myelolipoma —*see* Lipoma
Myeloma (multiple) C90.0
monostotic C90.3
plasma cell C90.0
plasma cell C90.0
solitary (*see also* Plasmacytoma, solitary)
C90.3
Myelomalacia G95.89
Myelomatosis C90.0
Myelomeningitis —*see* Meningoencephalitis

Myelomeningocele (spinal cord) —*see* Spina
bifida
Myelo-osteo-musculodysplasia hereditaria
Q79.8
Myelopathic
anemia D64.89
muscle atrophy —*see* Atrophy, muscle, spinal
pain syndrome G89.0
Myelopathy (spinal cord) G95.9
drug-induced G95.89
in (due to)
degeneration or displacement, intervertebral
disc NEC —*see* Disorder, disc, with,
myelopathy
infection —*see* Encephalitis
intervertebral disc disorder —*see also*
Disorder, disc, with, myelopathy
mercury —*see* subcategory T56.1
neoplastic disease (*see also* Neoplasm)
D49.9 *[G99.2]*
pernicious anemia D51.0 *[G99.2]*
spondylosis —*see* Spondylosis, with
myelopathy NEC
necrotic (subacute) (vascular) G95.19
radiation-induced G95.89
spondylogenic NEC —*see* Spondylosis, with
myelopathy NEC
toxic G95.89
transverse, acute G37.3
vascular G95.19
vitamin B12 E53.8 *[G32.0]*
Myelophthisis D61.82
Myeloradiculitis G04.91
Myeloradiculodysplasia (spinal) Q06.1
Myelosarcoma C92.3
Myelosclerosis D75.89
with myeloid metaplasia D47.4
disseminated, of nervous system G35
megakaryocytic D47.4
with myeloid metaplasia D47.4
Myelosis
acute C92.0
aleukemic C92.9
chronic D47.1
erythremic (acute) C94.0
megakaryocytic C94.2
nonleukemic D72.828
subacute C92.9
Myiasis (cavernous) B87.9
aural B87.4
creeping B87.0
cutaneous B87.0
dermal B87.0
ear (external) (middle) B87.4
eye B87.2
genitourinary B87.81
intestinal B87.82
laryngeal B87.3
nasopharyngeal B87.3
ocular B87.2
orbit B87.2
skin B87.0
specified site NEC B87.89
traumatic B87.1
wound B87.1
Myoadenoma, prostate —*see* Hyperplasia,
prostate
Myoblastoma
granular cell —*see also* Neoplasm, connective
tissue, benign
malignant —*see* Neoplasm, connective
tissue, malignant
tongue D10.1

Myocardial —*see* condition
Myocardiopathy (congestive) (constrictive)
(familial) (hypertrophic nonobstructive)
(idiopathic) (infiltrative) (obstructive)
(primary) (restrictive) (sporadic) (*see also*
Cardiomyopathy) I42.9
alcoholic I42.6
cobalt-beer I42.6
glycogen storage E74.02 *[I43]*
hypertrophic obstructive I42.1
in (due to)
beriberi E51.12
cardiac glycogenosis E74.02 *[I43]*
Friedreich's ataxia G11.1 *[I43]*
myotonia atrophica G71.11 *[I43]*
progressive muscular dystrophy G71.0 *[I43]*
obscure (African) I42.8
secondary I42.9
thyrotoxic E05.90 *[I43]*
with storm E05.91 *[I43]*
toxic NEC I42.7
Myocarditis (with arteriosclerosis) (chronic)
(fibroid) (interstitial) (old) (progressive)
(senile) I51.4
with
rheumatic fever (conditions in I00) I09.0
active —*see* Myocarditis, acute, rheumatic
inactive or quiescent (with chorea) I09.0
active I40.9
rheumatic I01.2
with chorea (acute) (rheumatic)
(Sydenham's) I02.0
acute or subacute (interstitial) I40.9
due to
streptococcus (beta-hemolytic) I01.2
idiopathic I40.1
rheumatic I01.2
with chorea (acute) (rheumatic)
(Sydenham's) I02.0
specified NEC I40.8
aseptic of newborn B33.22
bacterial (acute) I40.0
Coxsackie (virus) B33.22
diphtheritic A36.81
eosinophilic I40.1
epidemic of newborn (Coxsackie) B33.22
Fiedler's (acute) (isolated) I40.1
giant cell (acute) (subacute) I40.1
gonococcal A54.83
granulomatous (idiopathic) (isolated)
(nonspecific) I40.1
hypertensive —*see* Hypertension, heart
idiopathic (granulomatous) I40.1
in (due to)
diphtheria A36.81
epidemic louse-borne typhus A75.0 *[I41]*
Lyme disease A69.29
sarcoidosis D86.85
scarlet fever A38.1
toxoplasmosis (acquired) B58.81
typhoid A01.02
typhus NEC A75.9 *[I41]*
infective I40.0
influenzal —*see* Influenza, with, myocarditis
isolated (acute) I40.1
meningococcal A39.52
mumps B26.82
nonrheumatic, active I40.9
parenchymatous I40.9
pneumococcal I40.0
rheumatic (chronic) (inactive) (with chorea)
I09.0
active or acute I01.2

Myocarditis - *continued*
  with chorea (acute) (rheumatic) (Sydenham's) I02.0
  rheumatoid —*see* Rheumatoid, carditis
  septic I40.0
  staphylococcal I40.0
  suppurative I40.0
  syphilitic (chronic) A52.06
  toxic I40.8
    rheumatic —*see* Myocarditis, acute, rheumatic
  tuberculous A18.84
  typhoid A01.02
  valvular —*see* Endocarditis
  virus, viral I40.0
    of newborn (Coxsackie) B33.22
Myocardium, myocardial —*see* condition
Myocardosis —*see* Cardiomyopathy
Myoclonus, myoclonic, myoclonia (familial) (essential) (multifocal) (simplex) G25.3
  drug-induced G25.3
  epilepsy (*see also* Epilepsy, generalized, specified NEC) G40.4
    familial (progressive) G25.3
  epileptica G40.409
    with status epilepticus G40.401
  facial G51.3
  familial progressive G25.3
  Friedreich's G25.3
  jerks G25.3
  massive G25.3
  palatal G25.3
  pharyngeal G25.3
Myocytolysis I51.5
Myodiastasis —*see* Diastasis, muscle
Myoendocarditis —*see* Endocarditis
Myoepithelioma —*see* Neoplasm, benign, by site
Myofasciitis (acute) —*see* Myositis
Myofibroma —*see also* Neoplasm, connective tissue, benign
  uterus (cervix) (corpus) —*see* Leiomyoma
Myofibromatosis D48.1
  infantile Q89.8
Myofibrosis M62.89
  heart —*see* Myocarditis
  scapulohumeral —*see* Lesion, shoulder, specified NEC
Myofibrositis M79.7
  scapulohumeral —*see* Lesion, shoulder, specified NEC
Myoglobulinuria, myoglobinuria (primary) R82.1
Myokymia, facial G51.4
Myolipoma —*see* Lipoma
Myoma —*see also* Neoplasm, connective tissue, benign
  malignant —*see* Neoplasm, connective tissue, malignant
  prostate D29.1
  uterus (cervix) (corpus) —*see* Leiomyoma
Myomalacia M62.89
Myometritis —*see* Endometritis
Myometrium —*see* condition
Myonecrosis, clostridial A48.0
Myopathy G72.9
  acute
    necrotizing G72.81
    quadriplegic G72.81
  alcoholic G72.1
  benign congenital G71.2
  central core G71.2

Myopathy – *continued*
  centronuclear G71.2
  congenital (benign) G71.2
  critical illness G72.81
  distal G71.0
  drug-induced G72.0
  endocrine NEC E34.9 *[G73.7]*
  extraocular muscles H05.82
  facioscapulohumeral G71.0
  hereditary G71.9
    specified NEC G71.8
  immune NEC G72.49
  in (due to)
    Addison's disease E27.1 *[G73.7]*
    alcohol G72.1
    amyloidosis E85.0 *[G73.7]*
    cretinism E00.9 *[G73.7]*
    Cushing's syndrome E24.9 *[G73.7]*
    drugs G72.0
    endocrine disease NEC E34.9 *[G73.7]*
    giant cell arteritis M31.6 *[G73.7]*
    glycogen storage disease E74.00 *[G73.7]*
    hyperadrenocorticism E24.9 *[G73.7]*
    hyperparathyroidism NEC E21.3 *[G73.7]*
    hypoparathyroidism E20.9 *[G73.7]*
    hypopituitarism E23.0 *[G73.7]*
    hypothyroidism E03.9 *[G73.7]*
    infectious disease NEC B99 *[G73.7]*
    lipid storage disease E75.6 *[G73.7]*
    metabolic disease NEC E88.9 *[G73.7]*
    myxedema E03.9 *[G73.7]*
    parasitic disease NEC B89 *[G73.7]*
    polyarteritis nodosa M30.0 *[G73.7]*
    rheumatoid arthritis —*see* Rheumatoid, myopathy
    sarcoidosis D86.87
    scleroderma M34.82
    sicca syndrome M35.03
    Sjögren's syndrome M35.03
    systemic lupus erythematosus M32.19
    thyrotoxicosis (hyperthyroidism) E05.90 *[G73.7]*
      with thyroid storm E05.91 *[G73.7]*
    toxic agent NEC G72.2
  inflammatory NEC G72.49
  intensive care (ICU) G72.81
  limb-girdle G71.0
  mitochondrial NEC G71.3
  myotonic, proximal (PROMM) G71.11
  myotubular G71.2
  nemaline G71.2
  ocular G71.0
  oculopharyngeal G71.0
  of critical illness G72.81
  primary G71.9
    specified NEC G71.8
  progressive NEC G72.89
  proximal myotonic (PROMM) G71.11
  rod G71.2
  scapulohumeral G71.0
  specified NEC G72.89
  toxic G72.2
Myopericarditis —*see also* Pericarditis
  chronic rheumatic I09.2
Myopia (axial) (congenital) H52.1
  degenerative (malignant) H44.2
  malignant H44.2
  pernicious H44.2
  progressive high (degenerative) H44.2
Myosarcoma —*see* Neoplasm, connective tissue, malignant
Myosis (pupil) H57.03
  stromal (endolymphatic) D39.0

Myositis M60.9
  clostridial A48.0
  due to posture —*see* Myositis, specified type NEC
  epidemic B33.0
  fibrosa or fibrous (chronic) , Volkmann's T79.6
  foreign body granuloma —*see* Granuloma, foreign body
  in (due to)
    bilharziasis B65.9 *[M63.8]*
    cysticercosis B69.81
    leprosy A30.9 *[M63.8]*
    mycosis B49 *[M63.8]*
    sarcoidosis D86.87
    schistosomiasis B65.9 *[M63.8]*
    syphilis
      late A52.78
      secondary A51.49
    toxoplasmosis (acquired) B58.82
    trichinellosis B75 *[M63.8]*
    tuberculosis A18.09
  inclusion body -IBM] G72.41
  infective M60.009
    arm M60.002
      left M60.001
      right M60.000
    leg M60.005
      left M60.004
      right M60.003
    lower limb M60.005
      ankle M60.07
      foot M60.07
      lower leg M60.06
      thigh M60.05
      toe M60.07
    multiple sites M60.09
    specified site NEC M60.08
    upper limb M60.002
      finger M60.04
      forearm M60.03
      hand M60.04
      shoulder region M60.01
      upper arm M60.02
  interstitial M60.10
    ankle M60.17
    foot M60.17
    forearm M60.13
    hand M60.14
    lower leg M60.16
    multiple sites M60.19
    shoulder region M60.11
    specified site NEC M60.18
    thigh M60.15
    upper arm M60.12
  mycotic B49 *[M63.8]*
  orbital, chronic H05.12
  ossificans or ossifying (circumscripta) —*see also* Ossification, muscle, specified NEC
    in (due to)
      burns M61.30
        ankle M61.37
        foot M61.37
        forearm M61.33
        hand M61.34
        lower leg M61.36
        multiple sites M61.39
        pelvic region M61.35
        shoulder region M61.31
        specified site NEC M61.38
        thigh M61.35
        upper arm M61.32

Myositis – *continued*
  quadriplegia or paraplegia M61.20
    ankle M61.27
    foot M61.27
    forearm M61.23
    hand M61.24
    lower leg M61.26
    multiple sites M61.29
    pelvic region M61.25
    shoulder region M61.21
    specified site NEC M61.28
    thigh M61.25
    upper arm M61.22
  progressiva M61.10
    ankle M61.17
    finger M61.14
    foot M61.17
    forearm M61.13
    hand M61.14
    lower leg M61.16
    multiple sites M61.19
    pelvic region M61.15
    shoulder region M61.11
    specified site NEC M61.18
    thigh M61.15
    toe M61.17
    upper arm M61.12
  traumatica M61.00
    ankle M61.07
    foot M61.07
    forearm M61.03
    hand M61.04
    lower leg M61.06
    multiple sites M61.09
    pelvic region M61.05
    shoulder region M61.01
    specified site NEC M61.08
    thigh M61.05
    upper arm M61.02
  purulent —*see* Myositis, infective
  specified type NEC M60.80
    ankle M60.87
    foot M60.87
    forearm M60.83
    hand M60.84
    lower leg M60.86
    multiple sites M60.89
    pelvic region M60.85
    shoulder region M60.81
    specified site NEC M60.88
    thigh M60.85
    upper arm M60.82
  suppurative —*see* Myositis, infective
  traumatic (old) —*see* Myositis, specified type
  NEC
Myospasia impulsiva F95.2
Myotonia (acquisita) (intermittens) M62.89
  atrophica G71.11
  chondrodystrophic G71.13
  congenita (acetazolamide responsive)
  (dominant) (recessive) G71.12
  drug-induced G71.14
  dystrophica G71.11
  fluctuans G71.19
  levior G71.12
  permanens G71.19
  symptomatic G71.19
Myotonic pupil —*see* Anomaly, pupil,
  function, tonic pupil
Myriapodiasis B88.2

Myringitis H73.2
  with otitis media —*see* Otitis, media
  acute H73.00
    bullous H73.01
    specified NEC H73.09
  bullous —*see* Myringitis, acute, bullous
  chronic H73.1
Mysophobia F40.228
Mytilotoxism —*see* Poisoning, fish
Myxadenitis labialis K13.0
Myxedema (adult) (idiocy) (infantile)
  (juvenile) (*see also* Hypothyroidism) E03.9
  circumscribed E05.90
    with storm E05.91
  coma E03.5
  congenital E00.1
  cutis L98.5
  localized (pretibial) E05.90
    with storm E05.91
  papular L98.5
Myxochondrosarcoma —*see* Neoplasm,
  cartilage, malignant
Myxofibroma —*see* Neoplasm, connective
  tissue, benign
  odontogenic —*see* Cyst, calcifying
  odontogenic
Myxofibrosarcoma —*see* Neoplasm,
  connective tissue, malignant
Myxolipoma D17.9
Myxoliposarcoma —*see* Neoplasm,
  connective tissue, malignant
Myxoma —*see also* Neoplasm, connective
  tissue, benign
  nerve sheath —*see* Neoplasm, nerve, benign
  odontogenic —*see* Cyst, calcifying
  odontogenic
Myxosarcoma —*see* Neoplasm, connective
  tissue, malignant

N

Naegeli's
  disease Q82.8
  leukemia, monocytic C93.1
Naegleriasis (with meningoencephalitis) B60.2
Naffziger's syndrome G54.0
Naga sore —*see* Ulcer, skin
Nägele's pelvis M95.5
  with disproportion (fetopelvic) O33.0
    causing obstructed labor O65.0
Nail —*see also* condition
  biting F98.8
  patella syndrome Q87.2
Nanism, nanosomia —*see* Dwarfism
Nanophyetiasis B66.8
Nanukayami A27.89
Napkin rash L22
Narcolepsy G47.419
  with cataplexy G47.411
  in conditions classified elsewhere G47.429
    with cataplexy G47.421
Narcosis R06.89
Narcotism —*see* Dependence
NARP (Neuropathy, Ataxia and Retinitis
  pigmentosa) **syndrome** E88.49
Narrow
  anterior chamber angle H40.03
  pelvis —*see* Contraction, pelvis
Narrowing —*see also* Stenosis
  artery I77.1
    auditory, internal I65.8
    basilar —*see* Occlusion, artery, basilar
    carotid —*see* Occlusion, artery, carotid

Narrowing – *continued*
    cerebellar —*see* Occlusion, artery,
    cerebellar
    cerebral —*see* Occlusion artery, cerebral
    choroidal —*see* Occlusion, artery, cerebral,
    specified NEC
    communicating posterior —*see* Occlusion,
    artery, cerebral, specified NEC
    coronary —*see also* Disease, heart,
    ischemic, atherosclerotic
      congenital Q24.5
      syphilitic A50.54 *[I52]*
      due to syphilis NEC A52.06
    hypophyseal —*see* Occlusion, artery,
    cerebral, specified NEC
    pontine —*see* Occlusion, artery, cerebral,
    specified NEC
    precerebral —*see* Occlusion, artery,
    precerebral
    vertebral —*see* Occlusion, artery, vertebral
  auditory canal (external) —*see* Stenosis,
  external ear canal
  eustachian tube —*see* Obstruction, eustachian
  tube
  eyelid —*see* Disorder, eyelid function
  larynx J38.6
  mesenteric artery K55.0
  palate M26.89
  palpebral fissure —*see* Disorder, eyelid
  function
  ureter N13.5
    with infection N13.6
  urethra —*see* Stricture, urethra
Narrowness, abnormal, eyelid Q10.3
Nasal —*see* condition
Nasolachrymal, nasolacrimal —*see* condition
Nasopharyngeal —*see also* condition
  pituitary gland Q89.2
  torticollis M43.6
Nasopharyngitis (acute) (infective)
  (streptococcal) (subacute) J00
  chronic (suppurative) (ulcerative) J31.1
Nasopharynx, nasopharyngeal —*see*
  condition
Natal tooth, teeth K00.6
Nausea (without vomiting) R11.0
  with vomiting R11.2
  gravidarum —*see* Hyperemesis, gravidarum
  marina T75.3
  navalis T75.3
Navel —*see* condition
Neapolitan fever —*see* Brucellosis
Near drowning T75.1
Nearsightedness —*see* Myopia
Near-syncope R55
Nebula, cornea —*see* Opacity, cornea
Necator americanus infestation B76.1
Necatoriasis B76.1
Neck —*see* condition
Necrobiosis R68.89
  lipoidica NEC L92.1
    with diabetes —*see* E08-E13 with .620
Necrolysis, toxic epidermal L51.2
  due to drug
    correct substance properly administered —
    see Table of Drugs and Chemicals, by drug,
    adverse effect
    overdose or wrong substance given or taken
    —*see* Table of Drugs and Chemicals, by drug,
    poisoning
Necrophilia F65.89

Necrosis, necrotic (ischemic) —*see also*
Gangrene
   adrenal (capsule) (gland) E27.49
   amputation stump (surgical) (late) T87.50
      arm T87.5
      leg T87.5
   antrum J32.0
   aorta (hyaline) —*see also* Aneurysm, aorta
      cystic medial —*see* Dissection, aorta
   artery I77.5
   bladder (aseptic) (sphincter) N32.89
   bone (*see also* Osteonecrosis) M87.9
      aseptic or avascular —*see* Osteonecrosis
         idiopathic M87.00
      ethmoid J32.2
      jaw M27.2
      tuberculous —*see* Tuberculosis, bone
   brain I67.89
   breast (aseptic) (fat) (segmental) N64.1
   bronchus J98.09
   central nervous system NEC I67.89
   cerebellar I67.89
   cerebral I67.89
   colon K55.0
   cornea H18.40
   cortical (acute) (renal) N17.1
   cystic medial (aorta) —*see* Dissection, aorta
   dental pulp K04.1
   esophagus K22.8
   ethmoid (bone) J32.2
   eyelid —*see* Disorder, eyelid, degenerative
   fat, fatty (generalized) —*see also* Disorder,
   soft tissue, specified type NEC
      abdominal wall K65.4
      breast (aseptic) (segmental) N64.1
      localized —*see* Degeneration, by site, fatty
      mesentery K65.4
      omentum K65.4
      pancreas K86.8
      peritoneum K65.4
      skin (subcutaneous) , newborn P83.0
      subcutaneous, due to birth injury P15.6
   gallbladder —*see* Cholecystitis, acute
   heart —*see* Infarct, myocardium
   hip, aseptic or avascular —*see* Osteonecrosis,
   by type, femur
   intestine (acute) (hemorrhagic) (massive)
   K55.0
   jaw M27.2
   kidney (bilateral) N28.0
      acute N17.9
      cortical (acute) (bilateral) N17.1
         with ectopic or molar pregnancy O08.4
      medullary (bilateral) (in acute renal failure)
      (papillary) N17.2
      papillary (bilateral) (in acute renal failure)
      N17.2
      tubular N17.0
         with ectopic or molar pregnancy O08.4
         complicating
            abortion —*see* Abortion, by type,
         complicated by, tubular necrosis
            ectopic or molar pregnancy O08.4
            pregnancy —*see* Pregnancy, complicated
         by, diseases of, specified type or system NEC
            following ectopic or molar pregnancy
            O08.4
            traumatic T79.5
   larynx J38.7
   liver (with hepatic failure) (cell) —*see*
   Failure, hepatic
      hemorrhagic, central K76.2

Necrosis, necrotic – *continued*
   lung J85.0
   lymphatic gland —*see* Lymphadenitis, acute
   mammary gland (fat) (segmental) N64.1
   mastoid (chronic) —*see* Mastoiditis, chronic
   medullary (acute) (renal) N17.2
   mesentery K55.0
      fat K65.4
   mitral valve —*see* Insufficiency, mitral
   myocardium, myocardial —*see* Infarct,
   myocardium
   nose J34.0
   omentum (with mesenteric infarction) K55.0
      fat K65.4
   orbit, orbital —*see* Osteomyelitis, orbit
   ossicles, ear —*see* Abnormal, ear ossicles
   ovary N70.92
   pancreas (aseptic) (duct) (fat) K86.8
      acute (infective) —*see* Pancreatitis, acute
      infective —*see* Pancreatitis, acute
   papillary (acute) (renal) N17.2
   perineum N90.89
   peritoneum (with mesenteric infarction)
   K55.0
      fat K65.4
   pharynx J02.9
      in granulocytopenia —*see* Neutropenia
      Vincent's A69.1
   phosphorus —*see* subcategory T54.2
   pituitary (gland) (postpartum) (Sheehan)
   E23.0
   pressure —*see* Ulcer, pressure, by site
   pulmonary J85.0
   pulp (dental) K04.1
   radiation —*see* Necrosis, by site
   radium —*see* Necrosis, by site
   renal —*see* Necrosis, kidney
   sclera H15.89
   scrotum N50.8
   skin or subcutaneous tissue NEC I96
   spine, spinal (column) —*see also*
   Osteonecrosis, by type, vertebra
      cord G95.19
   spleen D73.5
   stomach K31.89
   stomatitis (ulcerative) A69.0
   subcutaneous fat, newborn P83.8
   subendocardial (acute) I21.4
      chronic I25.89
   suprarenal (capsule) (gland) E27.49
   testis N50.8
   thymus (gland) E32.8
   tonsil J35.8
   trachea J39.8
   tuberculous NEC —*see* Tuberculosis
   tubular (acute) (anoxic) (renal) (toxic) N17.0
      postprocedural N99.0
   vagina N89.8
   vertebra —*see also* Osteonecrosis, by type,
   vertebra
      tuberculous A18.01
   vulva N90.89
   X-ray —*see* Necrosis, by site
Necrospermia —*see* Infertility, male
Need (for)
   care provider because (of)
      assistance with personal care Z74.1
      continuous supervision required Z74.3
      impaired mobility Z74.09
      no other household member able to render
   care Z74.2
      specified reason NEC Z74.8

Need (for) – *continued*
   immunization —*see* Vaccination
   vaccination —*see* Vaccination
Neglect
   adult
      confirmed T74.01
      history of Z91.412
      suspected T76.01
   child (childhood)
      confirmed T74.02
      history of Z62.812
      suspected T76.02
   emotional, in childhood Z62.898
   hemispatial R41.4
   left-sided R41.4
   sensory R41.4
   visuospatial R41.4
Neisserian infection NEC —*see* Gonococcus
Nélaton's syndrome G60.8
Nelson's syndrome E24.1
Nematodiasis (intestinal) B82.0
   Ancylostoma B76.0
Neonatal —*see also* Newborn
   acne L70.4
   bradycardia P29.12
   tachycardia P29.11
   screening, abnormal findings on P09
   tooth, teeth K00.6
Neonatorum —*see* condition
Neoplasia
   endocrine, multiple (MEN) E31.20
      type I E31.21
      type IIA E31.22
      type IIB E31.23
   intraepithelial (histologically confirmed)
      anal (AIN) (histologically confirmed)
      K62.82
         grade I K62.82
         grade II K62.82
         severe D01.3
      cervical glandular (histologically confirmed)
      D06.9
      cervix (uteri) (CIN) (histologically
      confirmed) N87.9
         glandular D06.9
         grade I N87.0
         grade II N87.1
         grade III (severe dysplasia) (*see also*
      Carcinoma, cervix uteri, in situ) D06.9
      prostate (histologically confirmed) (PIN I)
      (PIN II) N42.3
         grade I N42.3
         grade II N42.3
         severe D07.5
      vagina (histologically confirmed) (VAIN)
      N89.3
         grade I N89.0
         grade II N89.1
         grade III (severe dysplasia) D07.2
      vulva (histologically confirmed) (VIN)
      N90.3
         grade I N90.0
         grade II N90.1
         grade III (severe dysplasia) D07.1
Neoplasm, neoplastic —*see also* Table of
Neoplasms
   lipomatous, benign —*see* Lipoma
Neovascularization
   ciliary body —*see* Disorder, iris, vascular
   cornea H16.40
      deep H16.44
      ghost vessels —*see* Ghost, vessels

	Malignant Primary	Malignant Secondary	Ca in Situ	Benign	Uncertain Behavior	Unspecified Behavior
Neoplasm, neoplastic	C80.1	C79.9	D09.9	D36.9	D48.9	D49.9
abdomen, abdominal	C76.2	C79.8-	D09.8	D36.7	D48.7	D49.89
cavity	C76.2	C79.8-	D09.8	D36.7	D48.7	D49.89
organ	C76.2	C79.8-	D09.8	D36.7	D48.7	D49.89
viscera	C76.2	C79.8-	D09.8	D36.7	D48.7	D49.89
wall—*see also Neoplasm, abdomen, wall, skin*	C44.509	C79.2-	D04.5	D23.5	D48.5	D49.2
connective tissue	C49.4	C79.8-	-	D21.4	D48.1	D49.2
skin	C44.509					
basal cell carcinoma	C44.519	-	-	-	-	-
specified type NEC	C44.599	-	-	-	-	-
squamous cell carcinoma	C44.529	-	-	-	-	-
abdominopelvic	C76.8	C79.8-	-	D36.7	D48.7	D49.89
accessory sinus—*see Neoplasm, sinus*						
acoustic nerve	C72.4-	C79.49	-	D33.3	D43.3	D49.7
adenoid (pharynx) (tissue)	C11.1	C79.89	D00.08	D10.6	D37.05	D49.0
adipose tissue—*see also Neoplasm, connective tissue*	C49.4	C79.89	-	D21.9	D48.1	D49.2
adnexa (uterine)	C57.4	C79.89	D07.39	D28.7	D39.8	D49.5
adrenal	C74.9-	C79.7-	D09.3	D35.0-	D44.1-	D49.7
capsule	C74.9-	C79.7-	D09.3	D35.0-	D44.1-	D49.7
cortex	C74.0-	C79.7-	D09.3	D35.0-	D44.1-	D49.7
gland	C74.9-	C79.7-	D09.3	D35.0-	D44.1-	D49.7
medulla	C74.1-	C79.7-	D09.3	D35.0-	D44.1-	D49.7
ala nasi (external)—*see also Neoplasm, skin, nose*	C44.301	C79.2	D04.39	D23.39	D48.5	D49.2
alimentary canal or tract NEC	C26.9	C78.80	D01.9	D13.9	D37.9	D49.0
alveolar	C03.9	C79.89	D00.03	D10.39	D37.09	D49.0
mucosa	C03.9	C79.89	D00.03	D10.39	D37.09	D49.0
lower	C03.1	C79.89	D00.03	D10.39	D37.09	D49.0
upper	C03.0	C79.89	D00.03	D10.39	D37.09	D49.0
ridge or process	C41.1	C79.51	-	D16.5-	D48.0	D49.2
carcinoma	C03.9	C79.8-	-	-	-	-
lower	C03.1	C79.8-	-	-	-	-
upper	C03.0	C79.8-	-	-	-	-
lower	C41.1	C79.51	-	D16.5-	D48.0	D49.2
mucosa	C03.9	C79.89	D00.03	D10.39	D37.09	D49.0
lower	C03.1	C79.89	D00.03	D10.39	D37.09	D49.0
upper	C03.0	C79.89	D00.03	D10.39	D37.09	D49.0
upper	C41.0	C79.51	-	D16.4-	D48.0	D49.2
sulcus	C06.1	C79.89	D00.02	D10.39	D37.09	D49.0
alveolus	C03.9	C79.89	D00.03	D10.39	D37.09	D49.0
lower	C03.1	C79.89	D00.03	D10.39	D37.09	D49.0
upper	C03.0	C79.89	D00.03	D10.39	D37.09	D49.0
ampulla of Vater	C24.1	C78.89	D01.5	D13.5	D37.6	D49.0
ankle NEC	C76.5-	C79.89	D04.7-	D36.7	D48.7	D49.89
anorectum, anorectal (junction)	C21.8	C78.5	D01.3	D12.9	D37.8	D49.0
antecubital fossa or space	C76.4-	C79.89	D04.6-	D36.7	D48.7	D49.89
antrum (Highmore) (maxillary)	C31.0	C78.39	D02.3	D14.0	D38.5	D49.1
pyloric	C16.3	C78.89	D00.2	D13.1	D37.1	D49.0
tympanicum	C30.1	C78.39	D02.3	D14.0	D38.5	D49.1
anus, anal	C21.0	C78.5	D01.3	D12.9	D37.8	D49.0
canal	C21.1	C78.5	D01.3	D12.9	D37.8	D49.0
cloacogenic zone	C21.2	C78.5	D01.3	D12.9	D37.8	D49.0
margin—*see also Neoplasm, anus, skin*	C44.500	C79.2	D04.5	D23.5	D48.5	D49.2
overlapping lesion with rectosigmoid junction or rectum	C21.8	-	-	-	-	-
skin	C44.500	C79.2	D04.5	D23.5	D48.5	D49.2
basal cell carcinoma	C44.510	-	-	-	-	-
specified type NEC	C44.590	-	-	-	-	-
squamous cell carcinoma	C44.520	-	-	-	-	-
sphincter	C21.1	C78.5	D01.3	D12.9	D37.8	D49.0
aorta (thoracic)	C49.3	C79.89	-	D21.3	D48.1	D49.2
abdominal	C49.4	C79.89	-	D21.4	D48.1	D49.2
aortic body	C75.5	C79.89	-	D35.6	D44.7	D49.7
aponeurosis	C49.9	C79.89	-	D21.9	D48.1	D49.2
palmar	C49.1-	C79.89	-	D21.1-	D48.1	D49.2
plantar	C49.2-	C79.89	-	D21.2-	D48.1	D49.2
appendix	C18.1	C78.5	D01.0	D12.1	D37.3	D49.0
arachnoid	C70.9	C79.49	-	D32.9	D42.9	D49.7
cerebral	C70.0	C79.32	-	D32.0	D42.0	D49.7

	Malignant Primary	Malignant Secondary	Ca in Situ	Benign	Uncertain Behavior	Unspecified Behavior
spinal	C70.1	C79.49	-	D32.1	D42.1	D49.7
areola	C50.0-	C79.81	D05.-	D24.-	D48.6-	D49.3
arm NEC	C76.4-	C79.89	D04.6-	D36.7	D48.7	D49.89
artery—see Neoplasm, connective tissue						
aryepiglottic fold	C13.1	C79.89	D00.08	D10.7	D37.05	D49.0
hypopharyngeal aspect	C13.1	C79.89	D00.08	D10.7	D37.05	D49.0
laryngeal aspect	C32.1	C78.39	D02.0	D14.1	D38.0	D49.1
marginal zone	C13.1	C79.89	D00.08	D10.7	D37.05	D49.0
arytenoid (cartilage)	C32.3	C78.39	D02.0	D14.1	D38.0	D49.1
fold—see Neoplasm, aryepiglottic						
associated with transplanted organ	C80.2	-	-	-	-	-
atlas	C41.2	C79.51	-	D16.6	D48.0	D49.2
atrium, cardiac	C38.0	C79.89	-	D15.1	D48.7	D49.89
auditory						
canal (external) (skin)A81	C44.20-	C79.2	D04.2-	D23.2-	D48.5	D49.2
internal	C30.1	C78.39	D02.3	D14.0	D38.5	D49.1
nerve	C72.4-	C79.49	-	D33.3	D43.3	D49.7
tube	C30.1	C78.39	D02.3	D14.0	D38.5	D49.1
opening	C11.2	C79.89	D00.08	D10.6	D37.05	D49.0
auricle, ear—see also Neoplasm, skin, ear	C44.20-	C79.2	D04.2-	D23.2-	D48.5	D49.2
auricular canal (external)—see also Neoplasm, skin, ear	C44.20-	C79.2	D04.2-	D23.2-	D48.5	D49.2
internal	C30.1	C78.39	D02.3	D14.0	D38.5	D49.2
autonomic nerve or nervous system NEC (see Neoplasm, nerve, peripheral)						
axilla, axillary	C76.1	C79.89	D09.8	D36.7	D48.7	D49.89
fold—see also Neoplasm, skin, trunk	C44.509	C79.2	D04.5	D23.5	D48.5	D49.2
back NEC	C76.8	C79.89	D04.5	D36.7	D48.7	D49.89
Bartholin's gland	C51.0	C79.82	D07.1	D28.0	D39.8	D49.5
basal ganglia	C71.0	C79.31	-	D33.0	D43.0	D49.6
basis pedunculi	C71.7	C79.31	-	D33.1	D43.1	D49.6
bile or biliary (tract)	C24.9	C78.89	D01.5	D13.5	D37.6	D49.0
canaliculi (biliferi) (intrahepatic)	C22.1	C78.7	D01.5	D13.4	D37.6	D49.0
canals, interlobular	C22.1	C78.89	D01.5	D13.4	D37.6	D49.0
duct or passage (common) (cystic) (extrahepatic)	C24.0	C78.89	D01.5	D13.5	D37.6	D49.0
interlobular	C22.1	C78.89	D01.5	D13.4	D37.6	D49.0
intrahepatic	C22.1	C78.7	D01.5	D13.4	D37.6	D49.0
and extrahepatic	C24.8	C78.89	D01.5	D13.5	D37.6	D49.0
bladder (urinary)	C67.9	C79.11	D09.0	D30.3	D41.4	D49.4
dome	C67.1	C79.11	D09.0	D30.3	D41.4	D49.4
neck	C67.5	C79.11	D09.0	D30.3	D41.4	D49.4
orifice	C67.9	C79.11	D09.0	D30.3	D41.4	D49.4
ureteric	C67.6	C79.11	D09.0	D30.3	D41.4	D49.4
urethral	C67.5	C79.11	D09.0	D30.3	D41.4	D49.4
overlapping lesion	C67.8	-	-	-	-	-
sphincter	C67.8	C79.11	D09.0	D30.3	D41.4	D49.4
trigone	C67.0	C79.11	D09.0	D30.3	D41.4	D49.4
urachus	C67.7	C79.11	D09.0	D30.3	D41.4	D49.4
wall	C67.9	C79.11	D09.0	D30.3	D41.4	D49.4
anterior	C67.3	C79.11	D09.0	D30.3	D41.4	D49.4
lateral	C67.2	C79.11	D09.0	D30.3	D41.4	D49.4
posterior	C67.4	C79.11	D09.0	D30.3	D41.4	D49.4
blood vessel—see Neoplasm, connective tissue						
bone (periosteum)	C41.9	C79.51	-	D16.9-	D48.0	D49.2
acetabulum	C41.4	C79.51	-	D16.8-	D48.0	D49.2
ankle	C40.3-	C79.51	-	D16.3-	-	-
arm NEC	C40.0-	C79.51	-	D16.0-	-	-
astragalus	C40.3-	C79.51	-	D16.3-	-	-
atlas	C41.2	C79.51	-	D16.6-	D48.0	D49.2
axis	C41.2	C79.51	-	D16.6-	D48.0	D49.2
back NEC	C41.2	C79.51	-	D16.6-	D48.0	D49.2
calcaneus	C40.3-	C79.51	-	D16.3-	-	-
calvarium	C41.0	C79.51	-	D16.4-	D48.0	D49.2
carpus (any)	C40.1-	C79.51	-	D16.1-	-	-
cartilage NEC	C41.9	C79.51	-	D16.9-	D48.0	D49.2
clavicle	C41.3	C79.51	-	D16.7-	D48.0	D49.2
clivus	C41.0	C79.51	-	D16.4-	D48.0	D49.2
coccygeal vertebra	C41.4	C79.51	-	D16.8-	D48.0	D49.2
coccyx	C41.4	C79.51	-	D16.8-	D48.0	D49.2

	Malignant Primary	Malignant Secondary	Ca in Situ	Benign	Uncertain Behavior	Unspecified Behavior
costal cartilage	C41.3	C79.51	-	D16.7-	D48.0	D49.2
costovertebral joint	C41.3	C79.51	-	D16.7-	D48.0	D49.2
cranial	C41.0	C79.51	-	D16.4-	D48.0	D49.2
cuboid	C40.3-	C79.51	-	D16.3-	-	-
cuneiform	C41.9	C79.51	-	D16.9-	D48.0	D49.2
elbow	C40.0-	C79.51	-	D16.0-	-	-
ethmoid (labyrinth)	C41.0	C79.51	-	D16.4-	D48.0	D49.2
face	C41.0	C79.51	-	D16.4-	D48.0	D49.2
femur (any part)	C40.2-	C79.51	-	D16.2-	-	-
fibula (any part)	C40.2-	C79.51	-	D16.2-	-	-
finger (any)	C40.1-	C79.51	-	D16.1-	-	-
foot	C40.3-	C79.51	-	D16.3-	-	-
forearm	C40.0-	C79.51	-	D16.0-	-	-
frontal	C41.0	C79.51	-	D16.4-	D48.0	D49.2
hand	C40.1-	C79.51	-	D16.1-	-	-
heel	C40.3-	C79.51	-	D16.3-	-	-
hip	C41.4	C79.51	-	D16.8-	D48.0	D49.2
humerus (any part)	C40.0-	C79.51	-	D16.0-	-	-
hyoid	C41.0	C79.51	-	D16.4-	D48.0	D49.2
ilium	C41.4	C79.51	-	D16.8-	D48.0	D49.2
innominate	C41.4	C79.51	-	D16.8-	D48.0	D49.2
intervertebral cartilage or disc	C41.2	C79.51	-	D16.6-	D48.0	D49.2
ischium	C41.4	C79.51	-	D16.8-	D48.0	D49.2
jaw (lower)	C41.1	C79.51	-	D16.5-	D48.0	D49.2
knee	C40.2-	C79.51	-	D16.2-	-	-
leg NEC	C40.2-	C79.51	-	D16.2-	-	-
limb NEC	C40.9-	C79.51	-	D16.9-	-	-
lower (long bones)	C40.2-	C79.51	-	D16.2-	-	-
short bones	C40.3-	C79.51	-	D16.3-	-	-
upper (long bones)	C40.0-	C79.51	-	D16.0-	-	-
short bones	C40.1-	C79.51	-	D16.1-	-	-
malar	C41.0	C79.51	-	D16.4-	D48.0	D49.2
mandible	C41.1	C79.51	-	D16.5-	D48.0	D49.2
marrow NEC (any bone)	C96.9	C79.52	-	-	D47.9	D49.89
mastoid	C41.0	C79.51	-	D16.4-	D48.0	D49.2
maxilla, maxillary (superior)	C41.0	C79.51	-	D16.4-	D48.0	D49.2
inferior	C41.1	C79.51	-	D16.5-	D48.0	D49.2
metacarpus (any)	C40.1-	C79.51	-	D16.1-	-	-
metatarsus (any)	C40.3-	C79.51	-	D16.3-	-	-
overlapping sites	C40.8-	-	-	-	-	-
navicular						
ankle	C40.3-	C79.51	-	-	-	-
hand	C40.1-	C79.51	-	-	-	-
nose, nasal	C41.0	C79.51	-	D16.4-	D48.0	D49.2
occipital	C41.0	C79.51	-	D16.4-	D48.0	D49.2
orbit	C41.0	C79.51	-	D16.4-	D48.0	D49.2
parietal	C41.0	C79.51	-	D16.4-	D48.0	D49.2
patella	C40.2-	C79.51	-	-	-	-
pelvic	C41.4	C79.51	-	D16.8	D48.0	D49.2
phalanges						
foot	C40.3-	C79.51	-	-	-	-
hand	C40.1-	C79.51	-	-	-	-
pubic	C41.4	C79.51	-	D16.8	D48.0	D49.2
radius (any part)	C40.0-	C79.51	-	D16.0-	-	-
rib	C41.3	C79.51	-	D16.7	D48.0	D49.2
sacral vertebra	C41.4	C79.51	-	D16.8	D48.0	D49.2
sacrum	C41.4	C79.51	-	D16.8	D48.0	D49.2
scaphoid					-	-
of ankle	C40.3-	C79.51	-	-	-	-
of hand	C40.1-	C79.51	-	-	-	-
scapula (any part)	C40.0-	C79.51	-	D16.0-	-	-
sella turcica	C41.0	C79.51	-	D16.4-	D48.0	D49.2
shoulder	C40.0-	C79.51	-	D16.0-	-	-
skull	C41.0	C79.51	-	D16.4-	D48.0	D49.2
sphenoid	C41.0	C79.51	-	D16.4-	D48.0	D49.2
spine, spinal (column)	C41.2	C79.51	-	D16.6	D48.0	D49.2
coccyx	C41.4	C79.51	-	D16.8	D48.0	D49.2
sacrum	C41.4	C79.51	-	D16.8	D48.0	D49.2

	Malignant Primary	Malignant Secondary	Ca in Situ	Benign	Uncertain Behavior	Unspecified Behavior
sternum	C41.3	C79.51	-	D16.7	D48.0	D49.2
tarsus (any)	C40.3-	C79.51	-	-	-	-
temporal	C41.0	C79.51	-	D16.4-	D48.0	D49.2
thumb	C40.1-	C79.51	-	-	-	-
tibia (any part)	C40.2-	C79.51	-	-	-	-
toe (any)	C40.3-	C79.51	-	-	-	-
trapezium	C40.1-	C79.51	-	-	-	-
trapezoid	C40.1-	C79.51	-	-	-	-
turbinate	C41.0	C79.51	-	D16.4-	D48.0	D49.2
ulna (any part)	C40.0-	C79.51	-	D16.0-	-	-
unciform	C40.1-	C79.51	-	-	-	-
vertebra (column)	C41.2	C79.51	-	D16.6	D48.0	D49.2
coccyx	C41.4	C79.51	-	D16.8	D48.0	D49.2
sacrum	C41.4	C79.51	-	D16.8	D48.0	D49.2
vomer	C41.0	C79.51	-	D16.4-	D48.0	D49.2
wrist	C40.1-	C79.51	-	-	-	-
xiphoid process	C41.3	C79.51	-	D16.7	D48.0	D49.2
zygomatic	C41.0	C79.51	-	D16.4-	D48.0	D49.2
book leaf (mouth)	C06.89	C79.89	D00.00	D10.39	D37.09	D49.0
bowel—*see Neoplasm, intestine*						
brachial plexus	C47.1-	C79.89	-	D36.12	D48.2	D49.2
brain NEC	C71.9	C79.31	-	D33.2	D43.2	D49.6
basal ganglia	C71.0	C79.31	-	D33.0	D43.0	D49.6
cerebellopontine angle	C71.6	C79.31	-	D33.1	D43.1	D49.6
cerebellum NOS	C71.6	C79.31	-	D33.1	D43.1	D49.6
cerebrum	C71.0	C79.31	-	D33.0	D43.0	D49.6
choroid plexus	C71.7	C79.31	-	D33.1	D43.1	D49.6
corpus callosum	C71.8	C79.31	-	D33.2	D43.2	D49.6
corpus striatum	C71.0	C79.31	-	D33.0	D43.0	D49.6
cortex (cerebral)	C71.0	C79.31	-	D33.0	D43.0	D49.6
frontal lobe	C71.1	C79.31	-	D33.0	D43.0	D49.6
globus pallidus	C71.0	C79.31	-	D33.0	D43.0	D49.6
hippocampus	C71.2	C79.31	-	D33.0	D43.0	D49.6
hypothalamus	C71.0	C79.31	-	D33.0	D43.0	D49.6
internal capsule	C71.0	C79.31	-	D33.0	D43.0	D49.6
medulla oblongata	C71.7	C79.31	-	D33.1	D43.1	D49.6
meninges	C70.0	C79.32	-	D32.0	D42.0	D49.7
midbrain	C71.7	C79.31	-	D33.1	D43.1	D49.6
occipital lobe	C71.4	C79.31	-	D33.0	D43.0	D49.6
overlapping lesion	C71.8	C79.31	-	-	-	-
parietal lobe	C71.3	C79.31	-	D33.0	D43.0	D49.6
peduncle	C71.7	C79.31	-	D33.1	D43.1	D49.6
pons	C71.7	C79.31	-	D33.1	D43.1	D49.6
stem	C71.7	C79.31	-	D33.1	D43.1	D49.6
tapetum	C71.8	C79.31	-	D33.2	D43.2	D49.6
temporal lobe	C71.2	C79.31	-	D33.0	D43.0	D49.6
thalamus	C71.0	C79.31	-	D33.0	D43.0	D49.6
uncus	C71.2	C79.31	-	D33.0	D43.0	D49.6
ventricle (floor)	C71.5	C79.31	-	D33.0	D43.0	D49.6
fourth	C71.7	C79.31	-	D33.1	D43.1	D49.6
branchial (cleft) (cyst) (vestiges)	C10.4	C79.89	D00.08	D10.5	D37.05	D49.0
breast (connective tissue) (glandular tissue) (soft parts)	C50.9-	C79.81	D05.-	D24.-	D48.6-	D49.3
areola	C50.0-	C79.81	D05.-	D24.-	D48.6-	D49.3
axillary tail	C50.6-	C79.81	D05.-	D24.-	D48.6-	D49.3
central portion	C50.1-	C79.81	D05.-	D24.-	D48.6-	D49.3
inner	C50.8	C79.81	D05.-	D24.-	D48.6-	D49.3
lower	C50.8-	C79.81	D05.-	D24.-	D48.6-	D49.3
lower inner quadrant	C50.3-	C79.81	D05.-	D24.-	D48.6-	D49.3
lower outer quadrant	C50.5-	C79.81	D05.-	D24.-	D48.6-	D49.3
mastectomy site (skin)—*see also Neoplasm, breast, skin*	C44.501	C79.2	-	-	-	-
specified as breast tissue	C50.8-	C79.81	-	-	-	-
midline	C50.8-	C79.81	D05.-	D24.-	D48.6-	D49.3
nipple	C50.0-	C79.81	D05.-	D24.-	D48.6-	D49.3
outer	C50.8-	C79.81	D05.-	D24.-	D48.6-	D49.3
overlapping lesion	C50.8-	-	-	-	-	-
skin	C44.501	C79.2	D04.5	D23.5	D48.5	D49.2
basal cell carcinoma	C44.511	-	-	-	-	-

	Malignant Primary	Malignant Secondary	Ca in Situ	Benign	Uncertain Behavior	Unspecified Behavior
specified type NEC	C44.591	-	-	-	-	-
squamous cell carcinoma	C44.521	-	-	-	-	-
tail (axillary)	C50.6-	C79.81	D05.-	D24.-	D48.6-	D49.3
upper	C50.8-	C79.81	D05.-	D24.-	D48.6-	D49.3
upper inner quadrant	C50.2-	C79.81	D05.-	D24.-	D48.6-	D49.3
upper outer quadrant	C50.4-	C79.81	D05.-	D24.-	D48.6-	D49.3
broad ligament	C57.1	C79.82	D07.39	D28.2	D39.8	D49.5
bronchogenic, bronchogenic (lung)	C34.9-	C78.0-	D02.2-	D14.3-	D38.1	D49.1
bronchiole	C34.9-	C78.0-	D02.2-	D14.3-	D38.1	D49.1
bronchus	C34.9-	C78.0-	D02.2-	D14.3-	D38.1	D49.1
carina	C34.0-	C78.0-	D02.2-	D14.3-	D38.1	D49.1
lower lobe of lung	C34.3-	C78.0-	D02.2-	D14.3-	D38.1	D49.1
main	C34.0-	C78.0-	D02.2-	D14.3-	D38.1	D49.1
middle lobe of lung	C34.2	C78.0-	D02.21	D14.31	D38.1	D49.1
overlapping lesion	C34.8-	-	-	-	-	-
upper lobe of lung	C34.1-	C78.0-	D02.2-	D14.3-	D38.1	D49.1
brow	C44.309	C79.2	D04.39	D23.39	D48.5	D49.2
basal cell carcinoma	C44.319	-	-	-	-	-
specified type NEC	C44.399	-	-	-	-	-
squamous cell carcinoma	C44.329	-	-	-	-	-
buccal (cavity)	C06.9	C79.89	D00.00	D10.39	D37.09	D49.0
commissure	C06.0	C79.89	D00.02	D10.39	D37.09	D49.0
groove (lower) (upper)	C06.1	C79.89	D00.02	D10.39	D37.09	D49.0
mucosa	C06.0	C79.89	D00.02	D10.39	D37.09	D49.0
sulcus (lower) (upper)	C06.1	C79.89	D00.02	D10.39	D37.09	D49.0
bulbourethral gland	C68.0	C79.19	D09.19	D30.4	D41.3	D49.5
bursa—see Neoplasm, connective tissue						
buttock NEC	C76.3	C79.89	D04.5	D36.7	D48.7	D49.89
calf	C76.5-	C79.89	D04.7-	D36.7	D48.7	D49.89
calvarium	C41.0	C79.51	-	D16.4-	D48.0	D49.2
calyx, renal	C65.-	C79.0-	D09.19	D30.1-	D41.1-	D49.5
canal						
anal	C21.1	C78.5	D01.3	D12.9	D37.8	D49.0
auditory (external)—see also Neoplasm, skin, ear	C44.20-	C79.2	D04.2-	D23.2-	D48.5	D49.2
auricular (external)—see also Neoplasm, skin, ear	C44.20-	C79.2	D04.2-	D23.2-	D48.5	D49.2
canaliculi, biliary (biliferi) (intrahepatic)	C22.1	C78.7	D01.5	D13.4	D37.6	D49.0
canthus (eye) (inner) (outer)	C44.10-	C79.2	D04.1-	D23.1-	D48.5	D49.2
basal cell carcinoma	C44.11-	-	-	-	-	-
specified type NEC	C44.19-	-	-	-	-	-
squamous cell carcinoma	C44.12-	-	-	-	-	-
capillary—see Neoplasm, connective tissue						
caput coli	C18.0	C78.5	D01.0	D12.0	D37.4	D49.0
carcinoid—see Tumor, carcinoid						
cardia (gastric)	C16.0	C78.89	D00.2	D13.1	D37.1	D49.0
cardiac orifice (stomach)	C16.0	C78.89	D00.2	D13.1	D37.1	D49.0
cardio esophageal junction	C16.0	C78.89	D00.2	D13.1	D37.1	D49.0
cardio esophagus	C16.0	C78.89	D00.2	D13.1	D37.1	D49.0
carina (bronchus)	C34.0-	C78.0-	D02.2-	D14.3-	D38.1	D49.1
carotid (artery)	C49.0	C79.89	-	D21.0	D48.1	D49.2
body	C75.4	C79.89	-	D35.5	D44.6	D49.7
carpus (any bone)	C40.1-	C79.51	-	D16.1-	-	-
cartilage (articular) (joint)NEC—see also Neoplasm, bone	C41.9	C79.51	-	D16.9-	D48.0	D49.2
arytenoid	C32.3	C78.39	D02.0	D14.1	D38.0	D49.1
auricular	C49.0	C79.89	-	D21.0	D48.1	D49.2
bronchi	C34.0-	C78.39	-	D14.3-	D38.1	D49.1
costal	C41.3	C79.51	-	D16.7	D48.0	D49.2
cricoid	C32.3	C78.39	D02.0	D14.1	D38.0	D49.1
cuneiform	C32.3	C78.39	D02.0	D14.1	D38.0	D49.1
ear (external)	C49.0	C79.89	-	D21.0	D48.1	D49.2
ensiform	C41.3	C79.51	-	D16.7	D48.0	D49.2
epiglottis	C32.1	C78.39	D02.0	D14.1	D38.0	D49.1
anterior surface	C10.1	C79.89	D00.08	D10.5	D37.05	D49.0
eyelid	C49.0	C79.89	-	D21.0	D48.1	D49.2
intervertebral	C41.2	C79.51	-	D16.6	D48.0	D49.2
larynx, laryngeal	C32.3	C78.39	D02.0	D14.1	D38.0	D49.1
nose, nasal	C30.0	C78.39	D02.3	D14.0	D38.5	D49.1
pinna	C49.0	C79.89	-	D21.0	D48.1	D49.2

	Malignant Primary	Malignant Secondary	Ca in Situ	Benign	Uncertain Behavior	Unspecified Behavior
rib	C41.3	C79.51	-	D16.7	D48.0	D49.2
semilunar (knee)	C40.2-	C79.51	-	D16.2-	D48.0	D49.2
thyroid	C32.3	C78.39	D02.0	D14.1	D38.0	D49.1
trachea	C33	C78.39	D02.1	D14.2	D38.1	D49.1
cauda equina	C72.1	C79.49	-	D33.4	D43.4	D49.7
cavity						
buccal	C06.9	C79.89	D00.00	D10.30	D37.09	D49.0
nasal	C30.0	C78.39	D02.3	D14.0	D38.5	D49.1
oral	C06.9	C79.89	D00.00	D10.30	D37.09	D49.0
peritoneal	C48.2	C78.6	-	D20.1	D48.4	D49.0
tympanic	C30.1	C78.39	D02.3	D14.0	D38.5	D49.1
cecum	C18.0	C78.5	D01.0	D12.0	D37.4	D49.0
central nervous system	C72.9	C79.40	-	-	-	-
cerebellopontine (angle)	C71.6	C79.31	-	D33.1	D43.1	D49.6
cerebellum, cerebellar	C71.6	C79.31	-	D33.1	D43.1	D49.6
cerebrum, cerebral (cortex) (hemisphere) (white matter)	C71.0	C79.31	-	D33.0	D43.0	D49.6
meninges	C70.0	C79.32	-	D32.0	D42.0	D49.7
peduncle	C71.7	C79.31	-	D33.1	D43.1	D49.6
ventricle	C71.5	C79.31	-	D33.0	D43.0	D49.6
fourth	C71.7	C79.31	-	D33.1	D43.1	D49.6
cervical region	C76.0	C79.89	D09.8	D36.7	D48.7	D49.89
cervix (cervical) (uteri) (uterus)	C53.9	C79.82	D06.9	D26.0	D39.0	D49.5
canal	C53.0	C79.82	D06.0	D26.0	D39.0	D49.5
endocervix (canal) (gland)	C53.0	C79.82	D06.0	D26.0	D39.0	D49.5
exocervix	C53.1	C79.82	D06.1	D26.0	D39.0	D49.5
external os	C53.1	C79.82	D06.1	D26.0	D39.0	D49.5
internal os	C53.0	C79.82	D06.0	D26.0	D39.0	D49.5
nabothian gland	C53.0	C79.82	D06.0	D26.0	D39.0	D49.5
overlapping lesion	C53.8	-	-	-	-	-
squamocolumnar junction	C53.8	C79.82	D06.7	D26.0	D39.0	D49.5
stump	C53.8	C79.82	D06.7	D26.0	D39.0	D49.5
cheek	C76.0	C79.89	D09.8	D36.7	D48.7	D49.89
external	C44.309	C79.2	D04.39	D23.39	D48.5	D49.2
basal cell carcinoma	C44.319	-	-	-	-	-
specified type NEC	C44.399	-	-	-	-	-
squamous cell carcinoma	C44.329	-	-	-	-	-
inner aspect	C06.0	C79.89	D00.02	D10.39	D37.09	D49.0
internal	C06.0	C79.89	D00.02	D10.39	D37.09	D49.0
mucosa	C06.0	C79.89	D00.02	D10.39	D37.09	D49.0
chest (wall)NEC	C76.1	C79.89	D09.8	D36.7	D48.7	D49.89
chiasma opticum	C72.3-	C79.49	-	D33.3	D43.3	D49.7
chin	C44.309	C79.2	D04.39	D23.39	D48.5	D49.2
basal cell carcinoma	C44.319	-	-	-	-	-
specified type NEC	C44.399	-	-	-	-	-
squamous cell carcinoma	C44.329	-	-	-	-	-
choana	C11.3	C79.89	D00.08	D10.6	D37.05	D49.0
cholangiole	C22.1	C78.89	D01.5	D13.4	D37.6	D49.0
choledochal duct	C24.0	C78.89	D01.5	D13.5	D37.6	D49.0
choroid	C69.3-	C79.49	D09.2-	D31.3-	D48.7	D49.81
plexus	C71.5	C79.31	-	D33.0	D43.0	D49.6
ciliary body	C69.4-	C79.49	D09.2-	D31.4-	D48.7	D49.89
clavicle	C41.3	C79.51	-	D16.7	D48.0	D49.2
clitoris	C51.2	C79.82	D07.1	D28.0	D39.8	D49.5
clivus	C41.0	C79.51	-	D16.4-	D48.0	D49.2
cloacogenic zone	C21.2	C78.5	D01.3	D12.9	D37.8	D49.0
coccygeal						
body or glomus	C49.5	C79.89	-	D21.5	D48.1	D49.2
vertebra	C41.4	C79.51	-	D16.8	D48.0	D49.2
coccyx	C41.4	C79.51	-	D16.8	D48.0	D49.2
colon—*see also* Neoplasm, intestine, large	C18.9	C78.5	-	-	-	-
with rectum	C19	C78.5	D01.1	D12.7	D37.5	D49.0
column, spinal—*see* Neoplasm, spine						
columnella—*see also* Neoplasm, skin, face	C44.390	C79.2	D04.39	D23.39	D48.5	D49.2
commissure						
labial, lip	C00.6	C79.89	D00.01	D10.39	D37.01	D49.0
laryngeal	C32.0	C78.39	D02.0	D14.1	D38.0	D49.1
common (bile)duct	C24.0	C78.89	D01.5	D13.5	D37.6	D49.0

	Malignant Primary	Malignant Secondary	Ca in Situ	Benign	Uncertain Behavior	Unspecified Behavior
concha—*see also Neoplasm, skin, ear*	C44.20-	C79.2	D04.2-	D23.2-	D48.5	D49.2
nose	C30.0	C78.39	D02.3	D14.0	D38.5	D49.1
conjunctiva	C69.0-	C79.49	D09.2-	D31.0-	D48.7	D49.89
connective tissue NEC	C49.9	C79.89	-	D21.9	D48.1	D49.2
Note: For neoplasms of connective tissue (blood vessel, bursa, fascia, ligament, muscle, peripheral nerves, sympathetic and parasympathetic nerves and ganglia, synovia, tendon, etc.) or of morphological types that indicate connective tissue, code according to the list under "Neoplasm, connective tissue". For sites that do not appear in this list, code to neoplasm of that site; e.g., fibrosarcoma, pancreas (C25.9)						
Note: Morphological types that indicate connective tissue appear in their proper place in the alphabetic index with the instruction "see Neoplasm, connective tissue ...."						
abdomen	C49.4	C79.89	-	D21.4	D48.1	D49.2
abdominal wall	C49.4	C79.89	-	D21.4	D48.1	D49.2
ankle	C49.2-	C79.89	-	D21.2-	D48.1	D49.2
antecubital fossa or space	C49.1-	C79.89	-	D21.1-	D48.1	D49.2
arm	C49.1-	C79.89	-	D21.1-	D48.1	D49.2
auricle (ear)	C49.0	C79.89	-	D21.0	D48.1	D49.2
axilla	C49.3	C79.89	-	D21.3	D48.1	D49.2
back	C49.6	C79.89	-	D21.6	D48.1	D49.2
breast—*see Neoplasm, breast*						
buttock	C49.5	C79.89	-	D21.5	D48.1	D49.2
calf	C49.2-	C79.89	-	D21.2-	D48.1	D49.2
cervical region	C49.0	C79.89	-	D21.0	D48.1	D49.2
cheek	C49.0	C79.89	-	D21.0	D48.1	D49.2
chest (wall)	C49.3	C79.89	-	D21.3	D48.1	D49.2
chin	C49.0	C79.89	-	D21.0	D48.1	D49.2
diaphragm	C49.3	C79.89	-	D21.3	D48.1	D49.2
ear (external)	C49.0	C79.89	-	D21.0	D48.1	D49.2
elbow	C49.1-	C79.89	-	D21.1-	D48.1	D49.2
extra rectal	C49.5	C79.89	-	D21.5	D48.1	D49.2
extremity	C49.9	C79.89	-	D21.9	D48.1	D49.2
lower	C49.2-	C79.89	-	D21.2-	D48.1	D49.2
upper	C49.1-	C79.89	-	D21.1-	D48.1	D49.2
eyelid	C49.0	C79.89	-	D21.0	D48.1	D49.2
face	C49.0	C79.89	-	D21.0	D48.1	D49.2
finger	C49.1-	C79.89	-	D21.1-	D48.1	D49.2
flank	C49.6	C79.89	-	D21.6	D48.1	D49.2
foot	C49.2-	C79.89	-	D21.2-	D48.1	D49.2
forearm	C49.1-	C79.89	-	D21.1-	D48.1	D49.2
forehead	C49.0	C79.89	-	D21.0	D48.1	D49.2
gastric	C49.4	C79.89	-	D21.4	D48.1	D49.2
gastrointestinal	C49.4	C79.89	-	D21.4	D48.1	D49.2
gluteal region	C49.5	C79.89	-	D21.5	D48.1	D49.2
great vessels NEC	C49.3	C79.89	-	D21.3	D48.1	D49.2
groin	C49.5	C79.89	-	D21.5	D48.1	D49.2
hand	C49.1-	C79.89	-	D21.1-	D48.1	D49.2
head	C49.0	C79.89	-	D21.0	D48.1	D49.2
heel	C49.2-	C79.89	-	D21.2-	D48.1	D49.2
hip	C49.2-	C79.89	-	D21.2-	D48.1	D49.2
hypochondrium	C49.4	C79.89	-	D21.4	D48.1	D49.2
iliopsoas muscle	C49.5	C79.89	-	D21.5	D48.1	D49.2
infraclavicular region	C49.3	C79.89	-	D21.3	D48.1	D49.2
inguinal (canal) (region)	C49.5	C79.89	-	D21.5	D48.1	D49.2
intestinal	C49.4	C79.89	-	D21.4	D48.1	D49.2
intrathoracic	C49.3	C79.89	-	D21.3	D48.1	D49.2
ischiorectal fossa	C49.5	C79.89	-	D21.5	D48.1	D49.2
jaw	C03.9	C79.89	D00.03	D10.39	D48.1	D49.0
knee	C49.2-	C79.89	-	D21.2-	D48.1	D49.2
leg	C49.2-	C79.89	-	D21.2-	D48.1	D49.2
limb NEC	C49.9	C79.89	-	D21.9	D48.1	D49.2
lower	C49.2-	C79.89	-	D21.2-	D48.1	D49.2
upper	C49.1-	C79.89	-	D21.1-	D48.1	D49.2
nates	C49.5	C79.89	-	D21.5	D48.1	D49.2
neck	C49.0	C79.89	-	D21.0	D48.1	D49.2

	Malignant Primary	Malignant Secondary	Ca in Situ	Benign	Uncertain Behavior	Unspecified Behavior
orbit	C69.6-	C79.49	D09.2-	D31.6-	D48.1	D49.89
overlapping lesion	C49.8	-	-	-	-	-
pararectal	C49.5	C79.89	-	D21.5	D48.1	D49.2
para urethral	C49.5	C79.89	-	D21.5	D48.1	D49.2
paravaginal	C49.5	C79.89	-	D21.5	D48.1	D49.2
pelvis (floor)	C49.5	C79.89	-	D21.5	D48.1	D49.2
pelvo abdominal	C49.8	C79.89	-	D21.6	D48.1	D49.2
perineum	C49.5	C79.89	-	D21.5	D48.1	D49.2
perirectal (tissue)	C49.5	C79.89	-	D21.5	D48.1	D49.2
periurethral (tissue)	C49.5	C79.89	-	D21.5	D48.1	D49.2
popliteal fossa or space	C49.2-	C79.89	-	D21.2-	D48.1	D49.2
presacral	C49.5	C79.89	-	D21.5	D48.1	D49.2
psoas muscle	C49.4	C79.89	-	D21.4	D48.1	D49.2
pterygoid fossa	C49.0	C79.89	-	D21.0	D48.1	D49.2
rectovaginal septum or wall	C49.5	C79.89	-	D21.5	D48.1	D49.2
rectovesical	C49.5	C79.89	-	D21.5	D48.1	D49.2
retroperitoneum	C48.0	C78.6	-	D20.0	D48.3	D49.0
sacrococcygeal region	C49.5	C79.89	-	D21.5	D48.1	D49.2
scalp	C49.0	C79.89	-	D21.0	D48.1	D49.2
scapular region	C49.3	C79.89	-	D21.3	D48.1	D49.2
shoulder	C49.1-	C79.89	-	D21.1-	D48.1	D49.2
skin (dermis)NEC—*see also Neoplasm, skin, by site*	C44.90	C79.2	D04.9	D23.9	D48.5	D49.2
stomach	C49.4	C79.89	-	D21.4	D48.1	D49.2
submental	C49.0	C79.89	-	D21.0	D48.1	D49.2
supraclavicular region	C49.0	C79.89	-	D21.0	D48.1	D49.2
temple	C49.0	C79.89	-	D21.0	D48.1	D49.2
temporal region	C49.0	C79.89	-	D21.0	D48.1	D49.2
thigh	C49.2-	C79.89	-	D21.2-	D48.1	D49.2
thoracic (duct) (wall)	C49.3	C79.89	-	D21.3	D48.1	D49.2
thorax	C49.3	C79.89	-	D21.3	D48.1	D49.2
thumb	C49.1-	C79.89	-	D21.1-	D48.1	D49.2
toe	C49.2-	C79.89	-	D21.2-	D48.1	D49.2
trunk	C49.6	C79.89	-	D21.6	D48.1	D49.2
umbilicus	C49.4	C79.89	-	D21.4	D48.1	D49.2
vesicorectal	C49.5	C79.89	-	D21.5	D48.1	D49.2
wrist	C49.1-	C79.89	-	D21.1-	D48.1	D49.2
conus medullaris	C72.0	C79.49		D33.4	D43.4	D49.7
cord (true) (vocal)	C32.0	C78.39	D02.0	D14.1	D38.0	D49.1
false	C32.1	C78.39	D02.0	D14.1	D38.0	D49.1
spermatic	C63.1-	C79.82	D07.69	D29.8	D40.8	D49.5
spinal (cervical) (lumbar) (thoracic)	C72.0	C79.49	-	D33.4	D43.4	D49.7
cornea (limbus)	C69.1-	C79.49	D09.2-	D31.1-	D48.7	D49.89
corpus						
albicans	C56.-	C79.6-	D07.39	D27.-	D39.1-	D49.5
callosum, brain	C71.0	C79.31	-	D33.2	D43.2	D49.6
cavernosum	C60.2	C79.82	D07.4	D29.0	D40.8	D49.5
gastric	C16.2	C78.89	D00.2	D13.1	D37.1	D49.0
overlapping sites	C54.8	-	-	-	-	-
penis	C60.2	C79.82	D07.4	D29.0	D40.8	D49.5
striatum, cerebrum	C71.0	C79.31	-	D33.0	D43.0	D49.6
uteri	C54.9	C79.82	D07.0	D26.1	D39.0	D49.5
isthmus	C54.0	C79.82	D07.0	D26.1	D39.0	D49.5
cortex						
adrenal	C74.0-	C79.7-	D09.3	D35.0-	D44.1-	D49.7
cerebral	C71.0	C79.31	-	D33.0	D43.0	D49.6
costal cartilage	C41.3	C79.51	-	D16.7	D48.0	D49.2
costovertebral joint	C41.3	C79.51		D16.7	D48.0	D49.2
Cowper's gland	C68.0	C79.19	D09.19	D30.4	D41.3	D49.5
cranial (fossa, any)	C71.9	C79.31	-	D33.2	D43.2	D49.6
meninges	C70.0	C79.32	-	D32.0	D42.0	D49.7
nerve	C72.50	C79.49	-	D33.3	D43.3	D49.7
specified NEC	C72.59	C79.49	-	D33.3	D43.3	D49.7
craniobuccal pouch	C75.2	C79.89	D09.3	D35.2	D44.3	D49.7
craniopharyngeal (duct) (pouch)	C75.2	C79.89	D09.3	D35.3	D44.4	D49.7
cricoid	C13.0	C79.89	D00.08	D10.7	D37.05	D49.0
cartilage	C32.3	C79.89	D02.0	D14.1	D38.0	D49.1
cricopharynx	C13.0	C79.89	D00.08	D10.7	D37.05	D49.0
crypt of Morgagni	C21.8	C78.5	D01.3	D12.9	D37.8	D49.0

	Malignant Primary	Malignant Secondary	Ca in Situ	Benign	Uncertain Behavior	Unspecified Behavior
crystalline lens	C69.4-	C79.49	D09.2-	D31.4-	D48.7	D49.89
cul de sac (Douglas')	C48.1	C78.6	-	D20.1	D48.4	D49.0
cuneiform cartilage	C32.3	C78.39	D02.0	D14.1	D38.0	D49.1
cutaneous—*see Neoplasm, skin*						
cutis—*see Neoplasm, skin*						
cystic (bile) duct (common)	C24.0	C78.89	D01.5	D13.5	D37.6	D49.0
dermis—*see Neoplasm, skin*						
diaphragm	C49.3	C79.89	-	D21.3	D48.1	D49.2
digestive organs, system, tube, or tract NEC	C26.9	C78.89	D01.9	D13.9	D37.9	D49.0
disc, intervertebral	C41.2	C79.51	-	D16.6	D48.0	D49.2
disease, generalized	C80.0	-	-	-	-	-
disseminated	C80.0	-	-	-	-	-
Douglas' cul de sac or pouch	C48.1	C78.6	-	D20.1	D48.4	D49.0
duodenojejunal junction	C17.8	C78.4	D01.49	D13.39	D37.2	D49.0
duodenum	C17.0	C78.4	D01.49	D13.2	D37.2	D49.0
dura (cranial) (mater)	C70.9	C79.49	-	D32.9	D42.9	D49.7
cerebral	C70.0	C79.32	-	D32.0	D42.0	D49.7
spinal	C70.1	C79.49	-	D32.1	D42.1	D49.7
ear (external)—*see also Neoplasm, skin, ear*	C44.20-	C79.2	D04.2-	D23.2-	D48.5	D49.2
auricle or auris—*see also Neoplasm, skin, ear*	C44.20-	C79.2	D04.2-	D23.2-	D48.5	D49.2
canal, external—*see also Neoplasm, skin, ear*	C44.20-	C79.2	D04.2-	D23.2-	D48.5	D49.2
cartilage	C49.0	C79.89	-	D21.0	D48.1	D49.2
external meatus—*see also Neoplasm, skin, ear*	C44.20-	C79.2	D04.2-	D23.2-	D48.5	D49.2
inner	C30.1	C78.39	D02.3	D14.0	D38.5	D49.1
lobule—*see also Neoplasm, skin, ear*	C44.20-	C79.2	D04.2-	D23.2-	D48.5	D49.2
middle	C30.1	C78.39	D02.3	D14.0	D38.5	D49.1
overlapping lesion with accessory sinuses	C31.8	-	-	-	-	-
skin	C44.20-	C79.2	D04.2-	D23.2-	D48.5	D49.2
basal cell carcinoma	C44.21-	-	-	-	-	-
specified type NEC	C44.29-	-	-	-	-	-
squamous cell carcinoma	C44.22-	-	-	-	-	-
earlobe	C44.20-	C79.2	D04.2-	D23.2-	D48.5	D49.2
basal cell carcinoma	C44.21-	-	-	-	-	-
specified type NEC	C44.29-	-	-	-	-	-
squamous cell carcinoma	C44.22-	-	-	-	-	-
ejaculatory duct	C63.7	C79.82	D07.69	D29.8	D40.8	D49.5
elbow NEC	C76.4-	C79.89	D04.6-	D36.7	D48.7	D49.89
endocardium	C38.0	C79.89	-	D15.1	D48.7	D49.89
endocervix (canal) (gland)	C53.0	C79.82	D06.0	D26.0	D39.0	D49.5
endocrine gland NEC	C75.9	C79.89	D09.3	D35.9	D44.9	D49.7
pluriglandular	C75.8	C79.89	D09.3	D35.7	D44.9	D49.7
endometrium (gland) (stroma)	C54.1	C79.82	D07.0	D26.1	D39.0	D49.5
ensiform cartilage	C41.3	C79.51	-	D16.7	D48.0	D49.2
enteric—*see Neoplasm, intestine*						
ependyma (brain)	C71.5	C79.31	-	D33.0	D43.0	D49.6
fourth ventricle	C71.7	C79.31	-	D33.1	D43.1	D49.6
epicardium	C38.0	C79.89	-	D15.1	D48.7	D49.89
epididymis	C63.0-	C79.82	D07.69	D29.3-	D40.8	D49.5
epidural	C72.9	C79.49	-	D33.9	D43.9	D49.7
epiglottis	C32.1	C78.39	D02.0	D14.1	D38.0	D49.1
anterior aspect or surface	C10.1	C79.89	D00.08	D10.5	D37.05	D49.0
cartilage	C32.3	C78.39	D02.0	D14.1	D38.0	D49.1
free border (margin)	C10.1	C79.89	D00.08	D10.5	D37.05	D49.0
junctional region	C10.8	C79.89	D00.08	D10.5	D37.05	D49.0
posterior (laryngeal)surface	C32.1	C78.39	D02.0	D14.1	D38.0	D49.1
suprahyoid portion	C32.1	C78.39	D02.0	D14.1	D38.0	D49.1
esophagogastric junction	C16.0	C78.89	D00.2	D13.1	D37.1	D49.0
esophagus	C15.9	C78.89	D00.1	D13.0	D37.8	D49.0
abdominal	C15.5	C78.89	D00.1	D13.0	D37.8	D49.0
cervical	C15.3	C78.89	D00.1	D13.0	D37.8	D49.0
distal (third)	C15.5	C78.89	D00.1	D13.0	D37.8	D49.0
lower (third)	C15.5	C78.89	D00.1	D13.0	D37.8	D49.0
middle (third)	C15.4	C78.89	D00.1	D13.0	D37.8	D49.0
overlapping lesion	C15.8	-	-	-	-	-
proximal (third)	C15.3	C78.89	D00.1	D13.0	D37.8	D49.0
thoracic	C15.4	C78.89	D00.1	D13.0	D37.8	D49.0
upper (third)	C15.3	C78.89	D00.1	D13.0	D37.8	D49.0
ethmoid (sinus)	C31.1	C78.39	D02.3	D14.0	D38.5	D49.1

	Malignant Primary	Malignant Secondary	Ca in Situ	Benign	Uncertain Behavior	Unspecified Behavior
bone or labyrinth	C41.0	C79.51	-	D16.4-	D48.0	D49.2
eustachian tube	C30.1	C78.39	D02.3	D14.0	D38.5	D49.1
exocervix	C53.1	C79.82	D06.1	D26.0	D39.0	D49.5
external						
meatus (ear)—*see also Neoplasm, skin, ear*	C44.20-	C79.2	D04.2-	D23.2-	D48.5	D49.2
os, cervix uteri	C53.1	C79.82	D06.1	D26.0	D39.0	D49.5
extradural	C72.9	C79.49	-	D33.9	D43.9	D49.7
extrahepatic (bile)duct	C24.0	C78.89	D01.5	D13.5	D37.6	D49.0
overlapping lesion with gallbladder	C24.8	-	-	-	-	-
extraocular muscle	C69.6-	C79.49	D09.2-	D31.6-	D48.7	D49.89
extra rectal	C76.3	C79.89	D09.8	D36.7	D48.7	D49.89
extremity	C76.8	C79.89	D04.8	D36.7	D48.7	D49.89
lower	C76.5-	C79.89	D04.7-	D36.7	D48.7	D49.89
upper	C76.4-	C79.89	D04.6-	D36.7	D48.7	D49.89
eye NEC	C69.9-	C79.49	D09.2	D31.9	D48.7	D49.89
overlapping sites	C69.8	-	-	-	-	-
eyeball	C69.9-	C79.49	D09.2-	D31.9-	D48.7	D49.89
eyebrow	C44.309	C79.2	D04.39	D23.39	D48.5	D49.2
basal cell carcinoma	C44.319	-	-	-	-	-
specified type NEC	C44.399	-	-	-	-	-
squamous cell carcinoma	C44.329	-	-	-	-	-
eyelid (lower) (skin) (upper)	C44.10-	-	-	-	-	-
basal cell carcinoma	C44.11-	-	-	-	-	-
specified type NEC	C44.19-	-	-	-	-	-
squamous cell carcinoma	C44.12-	-	-	-	-	-
cartilage	C49.0	C79.89	-	D21.0	D48.1	D49.2
face NEC	C76.0	C79.89	D04.39	D36.7	D48.7	D49.89
fallopian tube (accessory)	C57.0-	C79.82	D07.39	D28.2	D39.8	D49.5
falx (cerebella) (cerebri)	C70.0	C79.32	-	D32.0	D42.0	D49.7
fascia—*see also Neoplasm, connective tissue*						
palmar	C49.1-	C79.89	-	D21.1-	D48.1	D49.2
plantar	C49.2-	C79.89	-	D21.2-	D48.1	D49.2
fatty tissue—*see Neoplasm, connective tissue*						
fauces, faucial NEC	C10.9	C79.89	D00.08	D10.5	D37.05	D49.0
pillars	C09.1	C79.89	D00.08	D10.5	D37.05	D49.0
tonsil	C09.9	C79.89	D00.08	D10.4	D37.05	D49.0
femur (any part)	C40.2-	-	-	D16.2-	-	-
fetal membrane	C58	C79.82	D07.0	D26.7	D39.2	D49.5
fibrous tissue—*see Neoplasm, connective tissue*						
fibula (any part)	C40.2-	C79.51	-	D16.2-	-	-
filum terminale	C72.0	C79.49	-	D33.4	D43.4	D49.7
finger NEC	C76.4-	C79.89	D04.6-	D36.7	D48.7	D49.89
flank NEC	C76.8	C79.89	D04.5	D36.7	D48.7	D49.89
follicle, nabothian	C53.0	C79.82	D06.0	D26.0	D39.0	D49.5
foot NEC	C76.5-	C79.89	D04.7-	D36.7	D48.7	D49.89
forearm NEC	C76.4-	C79.89	D04.6-	D36.7	D48.7	D49.89
forehead (skin)	C44.309	C79.2	D04.39	D23.39	D48.5	D49.2
basal cell carcinoma	C44.319	-	-	-	-	-
specified type NEC	C44.399	-	-	-	-	-
squamous cell carcinoma	C44.329	-	-	-	-	-
foreskin	C60.0	C79.82	D07.4	D29.0	D40.8	D49.5
fornix						
pharyngeal	C11.3	C79.89	D00.08	D10.6	D37.05	D49.0
vagina	C52	C79.82	D07.2	D28.1	D39.8	D49.5
fossa (of)						
anterior (cranial)	C71.9	C79.31	-	D33.2	D43.2	D49.6
cranial	C71.9	C79.31	-	D33.2	D43.2	D49.6
ischiorectal	C76.3	C79.89	D09.8	D36.7	D48.7	D49.89
middle (cranial)	C71.9	C79.31	-	D33.2	D43.2	D49.6
piriform	C12	C79.89	D00.08	D10.7	D37.05	D49.0
pituitary	C75.1	C79.89	D09.3	D35.2	D44.3	D49.7
posterior (cranial)	C71.9	C79.31	-	D33.2	D43.2	D49.6
pterygoid	C49.0	C79.89	-	D21.0	D48.1	D49.2
pyriform	C12	C79.89	D00.08	D10.7	D37.05	D49.0
Rosenmüller	C11.2	C79.89	D00.08	D10.6	D37.05	D49.0
tonsillar	C09.0	C79.89	D00.08	D10.5	D37.05	D49.0
fourchette	C51.9	C79.82	D07.1	D28.0	D39.8	D49.5
frenulum						

	Malignant Primary	Malignant Secondary	Ca in Situ	Benign	Uncertain Behavior	Unspecified Behavior
labii—*see Neoplasm, lip, internal*						
linguae	C02.2	C79.89	D00.07	D10.1	D37.02	D49.0
frontal						
bone	C41.0	C79.51	-	D16.4-	D48.0	D49.2
lobe, brain	C71.1	C79.31	-	D33.0	D43.0	D49.6
pole	C71.1	C79.31	-	D33.0	D43.0	D49.6
sinus	C31.2	C78.39	D02.3	D14.0	D38.5	D49.1
fundus						
stomach	C16.1	C78.89	D00.2	D13.1	D37.1	D49.0
uterus	C54.3	C79.82	D07.0	D26.1	D39.0	D49.5
gall duct (extrahepatic)	C24.0	C78.89	D01.5	D13.5	D37.6	D49.0
intrahepatic	C22.1	C78.7	D01.5	D13.4	D37.6	D49.0
gallbladder	C23	C78.89	D01.5	D13.5	D37.6	D49.0
overlapping lesion with extrahepatic bile ducts	C24.8	-	-	-	-	-
ganglia—*see also Neoplasm, nerve, peripheral*	C47.9	C79.89	-	D36.10	D48.2	D49.2
basal	C71.0	C79.31	-	D33.0	D43.0	D49.6
cranial nerve	C72.50	C79.49	-	D33.3	D43.3	D49.7
Gartner's duct	C52	C79.82	D07.2	D28.1	D39.8	D49.5
gastric—*see Neoplasm, stomach*						
gastrocolic	C26.9	C78.89	D01.9	D13.9	D37.9	D49.0
gastroesophageal junction	C16.0	C78.89	D00.2	D13.1	D37.1	D49.0
gastrointestinal (tract)NEC	C26.9	C78.89	D01.9	D13.9	D37.9	D49.0
generalized	C80.0	-	-	-	-	-
genital organ or tract						
female NEC	C57.9	C79.82	D07.30	D28.9	D39.9	D49.5
overlapping lesion	C57.8	-	-	-	-	-
specified site NEC	C57.7	C79.82	D07.39	D28.7	D39.8	D49.5
male NEC	C63.9	C79.82	D07.60	D29.9	D40.9	D49.5
overlapping lesion	C63.8	-	-	-	-	-
specified site NEC	C63.7	C79.82	D07.69	D29.8	D40.8	D49.5
genitourinary tract						
female	C57.9	C79.82	D07.30	D28.9	D39.9	D49.5
male	C63.9	C79.82	D07.60	D29.9	D40.9	D49.5
gingiva (alveolar) (marginal)	C03.9	C79.89	D00.03	D10.39	D37.09	D49.0
lower	C03.1	C79.89	D00.03	D10.39	D37.09	D49.0
mandibular	C03.1	C79.89	D00.03	D10.39	D37.09	D49.0
maxillary	C03.0	C79.89	D00.03	D10.39	D37.09	D49.0
upper	C03.0	C79.89	D00.03	D10.39	D37.09	D49.0
gland, glandular (lymphatic) (system)—*see also Neoplasm, lymph gland*						
endocrine NEC	C75.9	C79.89	D09.3	D35.9	D44.9	D49.7
salivary—*see Neoplasm, salivary gland*						
glans penis	C60.1	C79.82	D07.4	D29.0	D40.8	D49.5
globus pallidus	C71.0	C79.31	-	D33.0	D43.0	D49.6
glomus						
coccygeal	C49.5	C79.89	-	D21.5	D48.1	D49.2
jugularis	C75.5	C79.89	-	D35.6	D44.7	D49.7
glosso epiglottic fold (s)	C10.1	C79.89	D00.08	D10.5	D37.05	D49.0
glossopalatine fold	C09.1	C79.89	D00.08	D10.5	D37.05	D49.0
glossopharyngeal sulcus	C09.0	C79.89	D00.08	D10.5	D37.05	D49.0
glottis	C32.0	C78.39	D02.0	D14.1	D38.0	D49.1
gluteal region	C76.3	C79.89	D04.5	D36.7	D48.7	D49.89
great vessels NEC	C49.3	C79.89	-	D21.3	D48.1	D49.2
groin NEC	C76.3	C79.89	D04.5	D36.7	D48.7	D49.89
gum	C03.9	C79.89	D00.03	D10.39	D37.09	D49.0
lower	C03.1	C79.89	D00.03	D10.39	D37.09	D49.0
upper	C03.0	C79.89	D00.03	D10.39	D37.09	D49.0
hand NEC	C76.4-	C79.89	D04.6-	D36.7	D48.7	D49.89
head NEC	C76.0	C79.89	D04.4	D36.7	D48.7	D49.89
heart	C38.0	C79.89	-	D15.1	D48.7	D49.89
heel NEC	C76.5-	C79.89	D04.7-	D36.7	D48.7	D49.89
helix—*see also Neoplasm, skin, ear*	C44.20-	C79.2	D04.2-	D23.2-	D48.5	D49.2
hematopoietic, hemopoietic tissue NEC	C96.9	-	-	-	-	-
specified NEC	C96.Z	-	-	-	-	-
hemisphere, cerebral	C71.0	C79.31	-	D33.0	D43.0	D49.6
hemorrhoidal zone	C21.1	C78.5	D01.3	D12.9	D37.8	D49.0
hepatic—*see also Index to disease, by histology*	C22.9	C78.7	D01.5	D13.4	D37.6	D49.0
duct (bile)	C24.0	C78.89	D01.5	D13.5	D37.6	D49.0

	Malignant Primary	Malignant Secondary	Ca in Situ	Benign	Uncertain Behavior	Unspecified Behavior
flexure (colon)	C18.3	C78.5	D01.0	D12.3	D37.4	D49.0
primary	C22.8	C78.7	D01.5	D13.4	D37.6	D49.0
hepatobiliary	C24.9	C78.89	D01.5	D13.5	D37.6	D49.0
hepatoblastoma	C22.2	C78.7	D01.5	D13.4	D37.6	D49.0
hepatoma	C22.0	C78.7	D01.5	D13.4	D37.6	D49.0
hilus of lung	C34.0-	C78.0-	D02.2-	D14.3-	D38.1	D49.1
hip NEC	C76.5-	C79.89	D04.7-	D36.7	D48.7	D49.89
hippocampus, brain	C71.2	C79.31	-	D33.0	D43.0	D49.6
humerus (any part)	C40.0-	C79.51	-	D16.0-	-	-
hymen	C52	C79.82	D07.2	D28.1	D39.8	D49.5
hypopharynx, hypopharyngeal NEC	C13.9	C79.89	D00.08	D10.7	D37.05	D49.0
overlapping lesion	C13.8	-	-	-	-	-
postcricoid region	C13.0	C79.89	D00.08	D10.7	D37.05	D49.0
posterior wall	C13.2	C79.89	D00.08	D10.7	D37.05	D49.0
pyriform fossa (sinus)	C12	C79.89	D00.08	D10.7	D37.05	D49.0
hypophysis	C75.1	C79.89	D09.3	D35.2	D44.3	D49.7
hypothalamus	C71.0	C79.31	-	D33.0	D43.0	D49.6
ileocecum, ileocecal (coil) (junction) (valve)	C18.0	C78.5	D01.0	D12.0	D37.4	D49.0
ileum	C17.2	C78.4	D01.49	D13.39	D37.2	D49.0
ilium	C41.4	C79.51	-	D16.8	D48.0	D49.2
immunoproliferative NEC	C88.9	-	-	-	-	-
infraclavicular (region)	C76.1	C79.89	D04.5	D36.7	D48.7	D49.89
inguinal (region)	C76.3	C79.89	D04.5	D36.7	D48.7	D49.89
insula	C71.0	C79.31	-	D33.0	D43.0	D49.6
insular tissue (pancreas)	C25.4	C78.89	D01.7	D13.7	D37.8	D49.0
brain	C71.0	C79.31	-	D33.0	D43.0	D49.6
interarytenoid fold	C13.1	C79.89	D00.08	D10.7	D37.05	D49.0
hypopharyngeal aspect	C13.1	C79.89	D00.08	D10.7	D37.05	D49.0
laryngeal aspect	C32.1	C79.89	D02.0	D14.1	D38.0	D49.1
marginal zone	C13.1	C79.89	D00.08	D10.7	D37.05	D49.0
interdental papillae	C03.9	C79.89	D00.03	D10.39	D37.09	D49.0
lower	C03.1	C79.89	D00.03	D10.39	D37.09	D49.0
upper	C03.0	C79.89	D00.03	D10.39	D37.09	D49.0
internal						
capsule	C71.0	C79.31	-	D33.0	D43.0	D49.6
os (cervix)	C53.0	C79.82	D06.0	D26.0	D39.0	D49.5
intervertebral cartilage or disc	C41.2	C79.51	-	D16.6	D48.0	D49.2
intestine, intestinal	C26.0	C78.80	D01.40	D13.9	D37.8	D49.0
large	C18.9	C78.5	D01.0	D12.6	D37.4	D49.0
appendix	C18.1	C78.5	D01.0	D12.1	D37.3	D49.0
caput coli	C18.0	C78.5	D01.0	D12.0	D37.4	D49.0
cecum	C18.0	C78.5	D01.0	D12.0	D37.4	D49.0
colon	C18.9	C78.5	D01.0	D12.6	D37.4	D49.0
and rectum	C19	C78.5	D01.1	D12.7	D37.5	D49.0
ascending	C18.2	C78.5	D01.0	D12.2	D37.4	D49.0
caput	C18.0	C78.5	D01.0	D12.0	D37.4	D49.0
descending	C18.6	C78.5	D01.0	D12.4	D37.4	D49.0
distal	C18.6	C78.5	D01.0	D12.4	D37.4	D49.0
left	C18.6	C78.5	D01.0	D12.4	D37.4	D49.0
overlapping lesion	C18.8	-	-	-	-	-
pelvic	C18.7	C78.5	D01.0	D12.5	D37.4	D49.0
right	C18.2	C78.5	D01.0	D12.2	D37.4	D49.0
sigmoid (flexure)	C18.7	C78.5	D01.0	D12.5	D37.4	D49.0
transverse	C18.4	C78.5	D01.0	D12.3	D37.4	D49.0
hepatic flexure	C18.3	C78.5	D01.0	D12.3	D37.4	D49.0
ileocecum, ileocecal (coil) (valve)	C18.0	C78.5	D01.0	D12.0	D37.4	D49.0
overlapping lesion	C18.8	-	-	-	-	-
sigmoid flexure (lower) (upper)	C18.7	C78.5	D01.0	D12.5	D37.4	D49.0
splenic flexure	C18.5	C78.5	D01.0	D12.3	D37.4	D49.0
small	C17.9	C78.4	D01.40	D13.30	D37.2	D49.0
duodenum	C17.0	C78.4	D01.49	D13.2	D37.2	D49.0
ileum	C17.2	C78.4	D01.49	D13.39	D37.2	D49.0
jejunum	C17.1	C78.4	D01.49	D13.39	D37.2	D49.0
overlapping lesion	C17.8	-	-	-	-	-
tract NEC	C26.0	C78.89	D01.40	D13.9	D37.8	D49.0
intra abdominal	C76.2	C79.89	D09.8	D36.7	D48.7	D49.89
intracranial NEC	C71.9	C79.31	-	D33.2	D43.2	D49.6
intrahepatic (bile)duct	C22.1	C78.7	D01.5	D13.4	D37.6	D49.0

	Malignant Primary	Malignant Secondary	Ca in Situ	Benign	Uncertain Behavior	Unspecified Behavior
intraocular	C69.9-	C79.49	D09.2-	D31.9-	D48.7	D49.89
intraorbital	C69.6-	C79.49	D09.2-	D31.6-	D48.7	D49.89
intrasellar	C75.1	C79.89	D09.3	D35.2	D44.3	D49.7
intrathoracic (cavity) (organs)	C76.1	C79.89	D09.8	D15.9	D48.7	D49.89
specified NEC	C76.1	C79.89	D09.8	D15.7	-	-
iris	C69.4-	C79.49	D09.2-	D31.4-	D48.7	D49.89
ischiorectal (fossa)	C76.3	C79.89	D09.8	D36.7	D48.7	D49.89
ischium	C41.4	C79.51	-	D16.8	D48.0	D49.2
island of Reil	C71.0	C79.31	-	D33.0	D43.0	D49.6
islands or islets of Langerhans	C25.4	C78.89	D01.7	D13.7	D37.8	D49.0
isthmus uteri	C54.0	C79.82	D07.0	D26.1	D39.0	D49.5
jaw	C76.0	C79.89	D09.8	D36.7	D48.7	D49.89
bone	C41.1	C79.51	-	D16.5-	D48.0	D49.2
lower	C41.1	C79.51	-	D16.5-	-	-
upper	C41.0	C79.51	-	D16.4-	-	-
carcinoma (any type) (lower) (upper)	C76.0	C79.89	-	-	-	-
skin—*see also Neoplasm, skin, face*	C44.309	C79.2	D04.39	D23.39	D48.5	D49.2
soft tissues	C03.9	C79.89	D00.03	D10.39	D37.09	D49.0
lower	C03.1	C79.89	D00.03	D10.39	D37.09	D49.0
upper	C03.0	C79.89	D00.03	D10.39	D37.09	D49.0
jejunum	C17.1	C78.4	D01.49	D13.39	D37.2	D49.0
joint NEC—*see also Neoplasm, bone*	C41.9	C79.51	-	D16.9-	D48.0	D49.2
acromioclavicular	C40.0-	C79.51	-	D16.0-	-	-
bursa or synovial membrane—*see Neoplasm, connective tissue*						
costovertebral	C41.3	C79.51	-	D16.7	D48.0	D49.2
sternocostal	C41.3	C79.51	-	D16.7	D48.0	D49.2
temporomandibular	C41.1	C79.51	-	D16.5-	D48.0	D49.2
junction						
anorectal	C21.8	C78.5	D01.3	D12.9	D37.8	D49.0
cardioesophageal	C16.0	C78.89	D00.2	D13.1	D37.1	D49.0
esophagogastric	C16.0	C78.89	D00.2	D13.1	D37.1	D49.0
gastroesophageal	C16.0	C78.89	D00.2	D13.1	D37.1	D49.0
hard and soft palate	C05.9	C79.89	D00.00	D10.39	D37.09	D49.0
ileocecal	C18.0	C78.5	D01.0	D12.0	D37.4	D49.0
pelvirectal	C19	C78.5	D01.1	D12.7	D37.5	D49.0
pelviureteric	C65.-	C79.0-	D09.19	D30.1-	D41.1-	D49.5
rectosigmoid	C19	C78.5	D01.1	D12.7	D37.5	D49.0
squamocolumnar, of cervix	C53.8	C79.82	D06.7	D26.0	D39.0	D49.5
Kaposi's sarcoma—*see Kaposi's, sarcoma*						
kidney (parenchymal)	C64.-	C79.0-	D09.19	D30.0-	D41.0-	D49.5
calyx	C65.-	C79.0-	D09.19	D30.1-	D41.1-	D49.5
hilus	C65.-	C79.0-	D09.19	D30.1-	D41.1-	D49.5
pelvis	C65.-	C79.0-	D09.19	D30.1-	D41.1-	D49.5
knee NEC	C76.5-	C79.89	D04.7-	D36.7	D48.7	D49.89
labia (skin)	C51.9	C79.82	D07.1	D28.0	D39.8	D49.5
majora	C51.0	C79.82	D07.1	D28.0	D39.8	D49.5
minora	C51.1	C79.82	D07.1	D28.0	D39.8	D49.5
labial—*see also Neoplasm, lip*	C00.9	C79.89	D00.01	D10.0	D37.01	D49.0
sulcus (lower) (upper)	C06.1	C79.89	D00.02	D10.39	D37.09	D49.0
labium (skin)	C51.9	C79.82	D07.1	D28.0	D39.8	D49.5
majus	C51.0	C79.82	D07.1	D28.0	D39.8	D49.5
minus	C51.1	C79.82	D07.1	D28.0	D39.8	D49.5
lacrimal						
canaliculi	C69.5-	C79.49	D09.2-	D31.5-	D48.7	D49.89
duct (nasal)	C69.5-	C79.49	D09.2-	D31.5-	D48.7	D49.89
gland	C69.5-	C79.49	D09.2-	D31.5-	D48.7	D49.89
punctum	C69.5-	C79.49	D09.2-	D31.5-	D48.7	D49.89
sac	C69.5-	C79.49	D09.2-	D31.5-	D48.7	D49.89
Langerhans, islands or islets	C25.4	C78.89	D01.7	D13.7	D37.8	D49.0
laryngopharynx	C13.9	C79.89	D00.08	D10.7	D37.05	D49.0
larynx, laryngeal NEC	C32.9	C78.39	D02.0	D14.1	D38.0	D49.1
aryepiglottic fold	C32.1	C78.39	D02.0	D14.1	D38.0	D49.1
cartilage (arytenoid) (cricoid) (cuneiform) (thyroid)	C32.3	C78.39	D02.0	D14.1	D38.0	D49.1
commissure (anterior) (posterior)	C32.0	C78.39	D02.0	D14.1	D38.0	D49.1
extrinsic NEC	C32.1	C78.39	D02.0	D14.1	D38.0	D49.1
meaning hypopharynx	C13.9	C79.89	D00.08	D10.7	D37.05	D49.0
interarytenoid fold	C32.1	C78.39	D02.0	D14.1	D38.0	D49.1

	Malignant Primary	Malignant Secondary	Ca in Situ	Benign	Uncertain Behavior	Unspecified Behavior
intrinsic	C32.0	C78.39	D02.0	D14.1	D38.0	D49.1
overlapping lesion	C32.8	-	-	-	-	-
ventricular band	C32.1	C78.39	D02.0	D14.1	D38.0	D49.1
leg NEC	C76.5-	C79.89	D04.7-	D36.7	D48.7	D49.89
lens, crystalline	C69.4-	C79.49	D09.2-	D31.4-	D48.7	D49.89
lid (lower) (upper)	C44.10-	C79.2	D04.1-	D23.1-	D48.5	D49.2
basal cell carcinoma	C44.11-	-	-	-	-	-
specified type NEC	C44.19-	-	-	-	-	-
squamous cell carcinoma	C44.12-	-	-	-	-	-
ligament—*see also Neoplasm, connective tissue*						
broad	C57.1	C79.82	D07.39	D28.2	D39.8	D49.5
Mackenrodt's	C57.7	C79.82	D07.39	D28.7	D39.8	D49.5
non uterine—*see Neoplasm, connective tissue*						
round	C57.2	C79.82	-	D28.2	D39.8	D49.5
sacro uterine	C57.3	C79.82	-	D28.2	D39.8	D49.5
uterine	C57.3	C79.82	-	D28.2	D39.8	D49.5
utero ovarian	C57.7	C79.82	D07.39	D28.2	D39.8	D49.5
uterosacral	C57.3	C79.82	-	D28.2	D39.8	D49.5
limb	C76.8	C79.89	D04.8	D36.7	D48.7	D49.89
lower	C76.5-	C79.89	D04.7-	D36.7	D48.7	D49.89
upper	C76.4-	C79.89	D04.6-	D36.7	D48.7	D49.89
limbus of cornea	C69.1-	C79.49	D09.2-	D31.1-	D48.7	D49.89
lingual NEC—*see also Neoplasm, tongue*	C02.9	C79.89	D00.07	D10.1	D37.02	D49.0
lingula, lung	C34.1-	C78.0-	D02.2-	D14.3-	D38.1	D49.1
lip	C00.9	C79.89	D00.01	D10.0	D37.01	D49.0
buccal aspect—*see Neoplasm, lip, internal*						
commissure	C00.6	C79.89	D00.01	D10.0	D37.01	D49.0
external	C00.2	C79.89	D00.01	D10.0	D37.01	D49.0
lower	C00.1	C79.89	D00.01	D10.0	D37.01	D49.0
upper	C00.0	C79.89	D00.01	D10.0	D37.01	D49.0
frenulum—*see Neoplasm, lip, internal*						
inner aspect—*see Neoplasm, lip, internal*						
internal	C00.5	C79.89	D00.01	D10.0	D37.01	D49.0
lower	C00.4	C79.89	D00.01	D10.0	D37.01	D49.0
upper	C00.3	C79.89	D00.01	D10.0	D37.01	D49.0
lipstick area	C00.2	C79.89	D00.01	D10.0	D37.01	D49.0
lower	C00.1	C79.89	D00.01	D10.0	D37.01	D49.0
upper	C00.0	C79.89	D00.01	D10.0	D37.01	D49.0
lower	C00.1	C79.89	D00.01	D10.0	D37.01	D49.0
internal	C00.4	C79.89	D00.01	D10.0	D37.01	D49.0
mucosa—*see Neoplasm, lip, internal*						
oral aspect—*see Neoplasm, lip, internal*						
overlapping lesion	C00.8	-	-	-	-	-
with oral cavity or pharynx	C14.8	-	-	-	-	-
skin (commissure) (lower) (upper)	C44.00	C79.2	D04.0	D23.0	D48.5	D49.2
basal cell carcinoma	C44.01	-	-	-	-	-
specified type NEC	C44.09	-	-	-	-	-
squamous cell carcinoma	C44.02	-	-	-	-	-
upper	C00.0	C79.89	D00.01	D10.0	D37.01	D49.0
internal	C00.3	C79.89	D00.01	D10.0	D37.01	D49.0
vermilion border	C00.2	C79.89	D00.01	D10.0	D37.01	D49.0
lower	C00.1	C79.89	D00.01	D10.0	D37.01	D49.0
upper	C00.0	C79.89	D00.01	D10.0	D37.01	D49.0
lipomatous—*see Lipoma, by site*						
liver—*see also Index to disease, by histology*	C22.9	C78.7	D01.5	D13.4	D37.6	D49.0
primary	C22.8	C78.7	D01.5	D13.4	D37.6	D49.0
lumbosacral plexus	C47.5	C79.89	-	D36.16	D48.2	D49.2
lung	C34.9-	C78.0-	D02.2-	D14.3-	D38.1	D49.1
azygos lobe	C34.1-	C78.0-	D02.2-	D14.3-	D38.1	D49.1
carina	C34.0-	C78.0-	D02.2-	D14.3-	D38.1	D49.1
hilus	C34.0-	C78.0-	D02.2-	D14.3-	D38.1	D49.1
lingula	C34.1-	C78.0-	D02.2-	D14.3-	D38.1	D49.1
lobe NEC	C34.9-	C78.0-	D02.2-	D14.3-	D38.1	D49.1
lower lobe	C34.3-	C78.0-	D02.2-	D14.3-	D38.1	D49.1
main bronchus	C34.0-	C78.0-	D02.2-	D14.3-	D38.1	D49.1
mesothelioma—*see Mesothelioma*						
middle lobe	C34.2	C78.0-	D02.21	D14.31	D38.1	D49.1
overlapping lesion	C34.8-	-	-	-	-	-

	Malignant Primary	Malignant Secondary	Ca in Situ	Benign	Uncertain Behavior	Unspecified Behavior
upper lobe	C34.1-	C78.0-	D02.2-	D14.3-	D38.1	D49.1
lymph, lymphatic channel NEC	C49.9	C79.89	-	D21.9	D48.1	D49.2
gland (secondary)	-	C77.9	-	D36.0	D48.7	D49.89
abdominal	-	C77.2	-	D36.0	D48.7	D49.89
aortic	-	C77.2	-	D36.0	D48.7	D49.89
arm	-	C77.3	-	D36.0	D48.7	D49.89
auricular (anterior) (posterior)	-	C77.0	-	D36.0	D48.7	D49.89
axilla, axillary	-	C77.3	-	D36.0	D48.7	D49.89
brachial	-	C77.3	-	D36.0	D48.7	D49.89
bronchial	-	C77.1	-	D36.0	D48.7	D49.89
bronchopulmonary	-	C77.1	-	D36.0	D48.7	D49.89
celiac	-	C77.2	-	D36.0	D48.7	D49.89
cervical	-	C77.0	-	D36.0	D48.7	D49.89
cervicofacial	-	C77.0	-	D36.0	D48.7	D49.89
Cloquet	-	C77.4	-	D36.0	D48.7	D49.89
colic	-	C77.2	-	D36.0	D48.7	D49.89
common duct	-	C77.2	-	D36.0	D48.7	D49.89
cubital	-	C77.3	-	D36.0	D48.7	D49.89
diaphragmatic	-	C77.1	-	D36.0	D48.7	D49.89
epigastric, inferior	-	C77.1	-	D36.0	D48.7	D49.89
epitrochlear	-	C77.3	-	D36.0	D48.7	D49.89
esophageal	-	C77.1	-	D36.0	D48.7	D49.89
face	-	C77.0	-	D36.0	D48.7	D49.89
femoral	-	C77.4	-	D36.0	D48.7	D49.89
gastric	-	C77.2	-	D36.0	D48.7	D49.89
groin	-	C77.4	-	D36.0	D48.7	D49.89
head	-	C77.0	-	D36.0	D48.7	D49.89
hepatic	-	C77.2	-	D36.0	D48.7	D49.89
hilar (pulmonary)	-	C77.1	-	D36.0	D48.7	D49.89
splenic	-	C77.2	-	D36.0	D48.7	D49.89
hypogastric	-	C77.5	-	D36.0	D48.7	D49.89
ileocolic	-	C77.2	-	D36.0	D48.7	D49.89
iliac	-	C77.5	-	D36.0	D48.7	D49.89
infraclavicular	-	C77.3	-	D36.0	D48.7	D49.89
inguina, inguinal	-	C77.4	-	D36.0	D48.7	D49.89
innominate	-	C77.1	-	D36.0	D48.7	D49.89
intercostal	-	C77.1	-	D36.0	D48.7	D49.89
intestinal	-	C77.2	-	D36.0	D48.7	D49.89
intraabdominal	-	C77.2	-	D36.0	D48.7	D49.89
intrapelvic	-	C77.5	-	D36.0	D48.7	D49.89
intrathoracic	-	C77.1	-	D36.0	D48.7	D49.89
jugular	-	C77.0	-	D36.0	D48.7	D49.89
leg	-	C77.4	-	D36.0	D48.7	D49.89
limb						
lower	-	C77.4	-	D36.0	D48.7	D49.89
upper	-	C77.3	-	D36.0	D48.7	D49.89
lower limb	-	C77.4	-	D36.0	D48.7	D49.89
lumbar	-	C77.2	-	D36.0	D48.7	D49.89
mandibular	-	C77.0	-	D36.0	D48.7	D49.89
mediastinal	-	C77.1	-	D36.0	D48.7	D49.89
mesenteric (inferior) (superior)	-	C77.2	-	D36.0	D48.7	D49.89
midcolic	-	C77.2	-	D36.0	D48.7	D49.89
multiple sites in categories C77.0 C77.5	-	C77.8	-	D36.0	D48.7	D49.89
neck	-	C77.0	-	D36.0	D48.7	D49.89
obturator	-	C77.5	-	D36.0	D48.7	D49.89
occipital	-	C77.0	-	D36.0	D48.7	D49.89
pancreatic	-	C77.2	-	D36.0	D48.7	D49.89
para aortic	-	C77.2	-	D36.0	D48.7	D49.89
paracervical	-	C77.5	-	D36.0	D48.7	D49.89
parametrial	-	C77.5	-	D36.0	D48.7	D49.89
parasternal	-	C77.1	-	D36.0	D48.7	D49.89
parotid	-	C77.0	-	D36.0	D48.7	D49.89
pectoral	-	C77.3	-	D36.0	D48.7	D49.89
pelvic	-	C77.5	-	D36.0	D48.7	D49.89
peri aortic	-	C77.2	-	D36.0	D48.7	D49.89
peripancreatic	-	C77.2	-	D36.0	D48.7	D49.89
popliteal	-	C77.4	-	D36.0	D48.7	D49.89
porta hepatis	-	C77.2	-	D36.0	D48.7	D49.89

	Malignant Primary	Malignant Secondary	Ca in Situ	Benign	Uncertain Behavior	Unspecified Behavior
portal	-	C77.2	-	D36.0	D48.7	D49.89
preauricular	-	C77.0	-	D36.0	D48.7	D49.89
prelaryngeal	-	C77.0	-	D36.0	D48.7	D49.89
presymphyseal	-	C77.5	-	D36.0	D48.7	D49.89
pretracheal	-	C77.0	-	D36.0	D48.7	D49.89
primary (any site)NEC	C96.9	-	-	-	-	-
pulmonary (hiler)	-	C77.1	-	D36.0	D48.7	D49.89
pyloric	-	C77.2	-	D36.0	D48.7	D49.89
retroperitoneal	-	C77.2	-	D36.0	D48.7	D49.89
retropharyngeal	-	C77.0	-	D36.0	D48.7	D49.89
Rosenmüller's	-	C77.4	-	D36.0	D48.7	D49.89
sacral	-	C77.5	-	D36.0	D48.7	D49.89
scalene	-	C77.0	-	D36.0	D48.7	D49.89
site NEC	-	C77.9	-	D36.0	D48.7	D49.89
splenic (hilar)	-	C77.2	-	D36.0	D48.7	D49.89
subclavicular	-	C77.3	-	D36.0	D48.7	D49.89
subinguinal	-	C77.4	-	D36.0	D48.7	D49.89
sublingual	-	C77.0	-	D36.0	D48.7	D49.89
submandibular	-	C77.0	-	D36.0	D48.7	D49.89
submaxillary	-	C77.0	-	D36.0	D48.7	D49.89
submental	-	C77.0	-	D36.0	D48.7	D49.89
subscapular	-	C77.3	-	D36.0	D48.7	D49.89
supraclavicular	-	C77.0	-	D36.0	D48.7	D49.89
thoracic	-	C77.1	-	D36.0	D48.7	D49.89
tibial	-	C77.4	-	D36.0	D48.7	D49.89
tracheal	-	C77.1	-	D36.0	D48.7	D49.89
tracheobronchial	-	C77.1	-	D36.0	D48.7	D49.89
upper limb	-	C77.3	-	D36.0	D48.7	D49.89
Virchow's	-	C77.0	-	D36.0	D48.7	D49.89
node—*see also Neoplasm, lymph gland*						
primary NEC	C96.9	-	-	-	-	-
vessel—*see also Neoplasm, connective tissue*	C49.9	C79.89	-	D21.9	D48.1	D49.2
Mackenrodt's ligament	C57.7	C79.82	D07.39	D28.7	D39.8	D49.5
malar	C41.0	C79.51	-	D16.4-	D48.0	D49.2
region—*see Neoplasm, cheek*						
mammary gland—*see Neoplasm, breast*						
mandible	C41.1	C79.51	-	D16.5-	D48.0	D49.2
alveolar						
mucosa (carcinoma)	C03.1	C79.89	D00.03	D10.39	D37.09	D49.0
ridge or process	C41.1	C79.51	-	D16.5-	D48.0	D49.2
marrow (bone)NEC	C96.9	C79.52	-	-	D47.9	D49.89
mastectomy site (skin)—*see also Neoplasm, breast, skin*	C44.501	C79.2	-	-	-	-
specified as breast tissue	C50.8-	C79.81	-	-	-	-
mastoid (air cells) (antrum) (cavity)	C30.1	C78.39	D02.3	D14.0	D38.5	D49.1
bone or process	C41.0	C79.51	-	D16.4-	D48.0	D49.2
maxilla, maxillary (superior)	C41.0	C79.51	-	D16.4-	D48.0	D49.2
alveolar						
mucosa	C03.0	C79.89	D00.03	D10.39	D37.09	D49.0
ridge or process (carcinoma)	C41.0	C79.51	-	D16.4-	D48.0	D49.2
antrum	C31.0	C78.39	D02.3	D14.0	D38.5	D49.1
carcinoma	C03.0	C79.51	-	-	-	-
inferior—*see Neoplasm, mandible*						
sinus	C31.0	C78.39	D02.3	D14.0	D38.5	D49.1
meatus external (ear)—*see also Neoplasm, skin, ear*	C44.20-	C79.2	D04.2-	D23.2-	D48.5	D49.2
Meckel diverticulum, malignant	C17.3	C78.4	D01.49	D13.39	D37.2	D49.0
mediastinum, mediastinal	C38.3	C78.1	-	D15.2	D38.3	D49.89
anterior	C38.1	C78.1	-	D15.2	D38.3	D49.89
posterior	C38.2	C78.1	-	D15.2	D38.3	D49.89
medulla						
adrenal	C74.1-	C79.7-	D09.3	D35.0-	D44.1-	D49.7
oblongata	C71.7	C79.31	-	D33.1	D43.1	D49.6
meibomian gland	C44.10-	C79.2	D04.1-	D23.1-	D48.5	D49.2
basal cell carcinoma	C44.11-	-	-	-	-	-
specified type NEC	C44.19-	-	-	-	-	-
squamous cell carcinoma	C44.12-	-	-	-	-	-
melanoma—*see Melanoma*						
meninges	C70.9	C79.49	-	D32.9	D42.9	D49.7

	Malignant Primary	Malignant Secondary	Ca in Situ	Benign	Uncertain Behavior	Unspecified Behavior
brain	C70.0	C79.32	-	D32.0	D42.0	D49.7
cerebral	C70.0	C79.32	-	D32.0	D42.0	D49.7
cranial	C70.0	C79.32	-	D32.0	D42.0	D49.7
intracranial	C70.0	C79.32	-	D32.0	D42.0	D49.7
spinal (cord)	C70.1	C79.49	-	D32.1	D42.1	D49.7
meniscus, knee joint (lateral) (medial)	C40.2-	C79.51	-	D16.2-	D48.0	D49.2
Merkel cell—*see Carcinoma, Merkel cell*						
mesentery, mesenteric	C48.1	C78.6	-	D20.1	D48.4	D49.0
mesoappendix	C48.1	C78.6	-	D20.1	D48.4	D49.0
mesocolon	C48.1	C78.6	-	D20.1	D48.4	D49.0
mesopharynx—*see Neoplasm, oropharynx*						
mesosalpinx	C57.1	C79.82	D07.39	D28.2	D39.8	D49.5
mesothelial tissue—*see Mesothelioma*						
mesothelioma—*see Mesothelioma*						
mesovarium	C57.1	C79.82	D07.39	D28.2	D39.8	D49.5
metacarpus (any bone)	C40.1-	C79.51	-	D16.1-	-	-
metastatic NEC—*see also Neoplasm, by site, secondary*	-	C79.9	-	-	-	-
metatarsus (any bone)	C40.3-	C79.51	-	D16.3-	-	-
midbrain	C71.7	C79.31	-	D33.1	D43.1	D49.6
milk duct—*see Neoplasm, breast*						
mons						
pubis	C51.9	C79.82	D07.1	D28.0	D39.8	D49.5
veneris	C51.9	C79.82	D07.1	D28.0	D39.8	D49.5
motor tract	C72.9	C79.49	-	D33.9	D43.9	D49.7
brain	C71.9	C79.31	-	D33.2	D43.2	D49.6
cauda equina	C72.1	C79.49	-	D33.4	D43.4	D49.7
spinal	C72.0	C79.49	-	D33.4	D43.4	D49.7
mouth	C06.9	C79.89	D00.00	D10.30	D37.09	D49.0
book leaf	C06.89	C79.89	-	-	-	-
floor	C04.9	C79.89	D00.06	D10.2	D37.09	D49.0
anterior portion	C04.0	C79.89	D00.06	D10.2	D37.09	D49.0
lateral portion	C04.1	C79.89	D00.06	D10.2	D37.09	D49.0
overlapping lesion	C04.8	-	-	-	-	-
overlapping NEC	C06.80	-	-	-	-	-
roof	C05.9	C79.89	D00.00	D10.39	D37.09	D49.0
specified part NEC	C06.89	C79.89	D00.00	D10.39	D37.09	D49.0
vestibule	C06.1	C79.89	D00.00	D10.39	D37.09	D49.0
mucosa						
alveolar (ridge or process)	C03.9	C79.89	D00.03	D10.39	D37.09	D49.0
lower	C03.1	C79.89	D00.03	D10.39	D37.09	D49.0
upper	C03.0	C79.89	D00.03	D10.39	D37.09	D49.0
buccal	C06.0	C79.89	D00.02	D10.39	D37.09	D49.0
cheek	C06.0	C79.89	D00.02	D10.39	D37.09	D49.0
lip—*see Neoplasm, lip, internal*						
nasal	C30.0	C78.39	D02.3	D14.0	D38.5	D49.1
oral	C06.0	C79.89	D00.02	D10.39	D37.09	D49.0
Mullerian duct						
female	C57.7	C79.82	D07.39	D28.7	D39.8	D49.5
male	C63.7	C79.82	D07.69	D29.8	D40.8	D49.5
muscle—*see also Neoplasm, connective tissue*						
extraocular	C69.6-	C79.49	D09.2-	D31.6-	D48.7	D49.89
myocardium	C38.0	C79.89	-	D15.1	D48.7	D49.89
myometrium	C54.2	C79.82	D07.0	D26.1	D39.0	D49.5
myopericardium	C38.0	C79.89	-	D15.1	D48.7	D49.89
nabothian gland (follicle)	C53.0	C79.82	D06.0	D26.0	D39.0	D49.5
nail—*see also Neoplasm, skin, limb*	C44.90	C79.2	D04.9	D23.9	D48.5	D49.2
finger—*see also Neoplasm, skin, limb, upper*	C44.60-	C79.2	D04.6-	D23.6-	D48.5	D49.2
toe—*see also Neoplasm, skin, limb, lower*	C44.70-	C79.2	D04.7-	D23.7-	D48.5	D49.2
nares, naris (anterior) (posterior)	C30.0	C78.39	D02.3	D14.0	D38.5	D49.1
nasal—*see Neoplasm, nose*						
nasolabial groove—*see also Neoplasm, skin, face*	C44.309	C79.2	D04.39	D23.39	D48.5	D49.2
nasolacrimal duct	C69.5-	C79.49	D09.2-	D31.5-	D48.7	D49.89
nasopharynx, nasopharyngeal	C11.9	C79.89	D00.08	D10.6	D37.05	D49.0
floor	C11.3	C79.89	D00.08	D10.6	D37.05	D49.0
overlapping lesion	C11.8	-	-	-	-	-
roof	C11.0	C79.89	D00.08	D10.6	D37.05	D49.0
wall	C11.9	C79.89	D00.08	D10.6	D37.05	D49.0

	Malignant Primary	Malignant Secondary	Ca in Situ	Benign	Uncertain Behavior	Unspecified Behavior
anterior	C11.3	C79.89	D00.08	D10.6	D37.05	D49.0
lateral	C11.2	C79.89	D00.08	D10.6	D37.05	D49.0
posterior	C11.1	C79.89	D00.08	D10.6	D37.05	D49.0
superior	C11.0	C79.89	D00.08	D10.6	D37.05	D49.0
nates—*see also Neoplasm, skin, trunk*	C44.509	C79.2	D04.5	D23.5	D48.5	D49.2
neck NEC	C76.0	C79.89	D09.8	D36.7	D48.7	D49.89
skin	C44.40	-	-	-	-	-
basal cell carcinoma	C44.41	-	-	-	-	-
specified type NEC	C44.49	-	-	-	-	-
squamous cell carcinoma	C44.42	-	-	-	-	-
nerve (ganglion)	C47.9	C79.89	-	D36.10	D48.2	D49.2
abducens	C72.59	C79.49	-	D33.3	D43.3	D49.7
accessory (spinal)	C72.59	C79.49	-	D33.3	D43.3	D49.7
acoustic	C72.4-	C79.49	-	D33.3	D43.3	D49.7
auditory	C72.4-	C79.49	-	D33.3	D43.3	D49.7
autonomic NEC—*see also Neoplasm, nerve, peripheral*	C47.9	C79.89	-	D36.10	D48.2	D49.2
brachial	C47.1-	C79.89	-	D36.12	D48.2	D49.2
cranial	C72.50	C79.49	-	D33.3	D43.3	D49.7
specified NEC	C72.59	C79.49	-	D33.3	D43.3	D49.7
facial	C72.59	C79.49	-	D33.3	D43.3	D49.7
femoral	C47.2-	C79.89	-	D36.13	D48.2	D49.2
ganglion NEC—*see also Neoplasm, nerve, peripheral*	C47.9	C79.89	-	D36.10	D48.2	D49.2
glossopharyngeal	C72.59	C79.49	-	D33.3	D43.3	D49.7
hypoglossal	C72.59	C79.49	-	D33.3	D43.3	D49.7
intercostal	C47.3	C79.89	-	D36.14	D48.2	D49.2
lumbar	C47.6	C79.89	-	D36.17	D48.2	D49.2
median	C47.1-	C79.89	-	D36.12	D48.2	D49.2
obturator	C47.2-	C79.89	-	D36.13	D48.2	D49.2
oculomotor	C72.59	C79.49	-	D33.3	D43.3	D49.7
olfactory	C47.2-	C79.49	-	D33.3	D43.3	D49.7
optic	C72.3-	C79.49	-	D33.3	D43.3	D49.7
parasympathetic NEC	C47.9	C79.89	-	D36.10	D48.2	D49.2
peripheral NEC	C47.9	C79.89	-	D36.10	D48.2	D49.2
abdomen	C47.4	C79.89	-	D36.15	D48.2	D49.2
abdominal wall	C47.4	C79.89	-	D36.15	D48.2	D49.2
ankle	C47.2-	C79.89	-	D36.13	D48.2	D49.2
antecubital fossa or space	C47.1-	C79.89	-	D36.12	D48.2	D49.2
arm	C47.1-	C79.89	-	D36.12	D48.2	D49.2
auricle (ear)	C47.0	C79.89	-	D36.11	D48.2	D49.2
axilla	C47.3	C79.89	-	D36.12	D48.2	D49.2
back	C47.6	C79.89	-	D36.17	D48.2	D49.2
buttock	C47.5	C79.89	-	D36.16	D48.2	D49.2
calf	C47.2-	C79.89	-	D36.13	D48.2	D49.2
cervical region	C47.0	C79.89	-	D36.11	D48.2	D49.2
cheek	C47.0	C79.89	-	D36.11	D48.2	D49.2
chest (wall)	C47.3	C79.89	-	D36.14	D48.2	D49.2
chin	C47.0	C79.89	-	D36.11	D48.2	D49.2
ear (external)	C47.0	C79.89	-	D36.11	D48.2	D49.2
elbow	C47.1-	C79.89	-	D36.12	D48.2	D49.2
extra rectal	C47.5	C79.89	-	D36.16	D48.2	D49.2
extremity	C47.9	C79.89	-	D36.10	D48.2	D49.2
lower	C47.2-	C79.89	-	D36.13	D48.2	D49.2
upper	C47.1-	C79.89	-	D36.12	D48.2	D49.2
eyelid	C47.0	C79.89	-	D36.11	D48.2	D49.2
face	C47.0	C79.89	-	D36.11	D48.2	D49.2
finger	C47.1-	C79.89	-	D36.12	D48.2	D49.2
flank	C47.6	C79.89	-	D36.17	D48.2	D49.2
foot	C47.2-	C79.89	-	D36.13	D48.2	D49.2
forearm	C47.1-	C79.89	-	D36.12	D48.2	D49.2
forehead	C47.0	C79.89	-	D36.11	D48.2	D49.2
gluteal region	C47.5	C79.89	-	D36.16	D48.2	D49.2
groin	C47.5	C79.89	-	D36.16	D48.2	D49.2
hand	C47.1-	C79.89	-	D36.12	D48.2	D49.2
head	C47.0	C79.89	-	D36.11	D48.2	D49.2
heel	C47.2-	C79.89	-	D36.13	D48.2	D49.2
hip	C47.2-	C79.89	-	D36.13	D48.2	D49.2
infraclavicular region	C47.3	C79.89	-	D36.14	D48.2	D49.2

	Malignant Primary	Malignant Secondary	Ca in Situ	Benign	Uncertain Behavior	Unspecified Behavior
inguinal (canal) (region)	C47.5	C79.89	-	D36.16	D48.2	D49.2
intrathoracic	C47.3	C79.89	-	D36.14	D48.2	D49.2
ischiorectal fossa	C47.5	C79.89	-	D36.16	D48.2	D49.2
knee	C47.2-	C79.89	-	D36.13	D48.2	D49.2
leg	C47.2-	C79.89	-	D36.13	D48.2	D49.2
limb NEC	C47.9	C79.89	-	D36.10	D48.2	D49.2
lower	C47.2-	C79.89	-	D36.13	D48.2	D49.2
upper	C47.1-	C79.89	-	D36.12	D48.2	D49.2
nates	C47.5	C79.89	-	D36.16	D48.2	D49.2
neck	C47.0	C79.89	-	D36.11	D48.2	D49.2
orbit	C69.6-	C79.49	-	D31.6-	D48.7	D49.2
pararectal	C47.5	C79.89	-	D36.16	D48.2	D49.2
paraurethral	C47.5	C79.89	-	D36.16	D48.2	D49.2
paravaginal	C47.5	C79.89	-	D36.16	D48.2	D49.2
pelvis (floor)	C47.5	C79.89	-	D36.16	D48.2	D49.2
pelviabdominal	C47.8	C79.89	-	D36.17	D48.2	D49.2
perineum	C47.5	C79.89	-	D36.16	D48.2	D49.2
perirectal (tissue)	C47.5	C79.89	-	D36.16	D48.2	D49.2
periurethral (tissue)	C47.5	C79.89	-	D36.16	D48.2	D49.2
popliteal fossa or space	C47.2-	C79.89	-	D36.13	D48.2	D49.2
presacral	C47.5	C79.89	-	D36.16	D48.2	D49.2
pterygoid fossa	C47.0	C79.89	-	D36.11	D48.2	D49.2
rectovaginal septum or wall	C47.5	C79.89	-	D36.16	D48.2	D49.2
rectovesical	C47.5	C79.89	-	D36.16	D48.2	D49.2
sacrococcygeal region	C47.5	C79.89	-	D36.16	D48.2	D49.2
scalp	C47.0	C79.89	-	D36.11	D48.2	D49.2
scapular region	C47.3	C79.89	-	D36.14	D48.2	D49.2
shoulder	C47.1-	C79.89	-	D36.12	D48.2	D49.2
submental	C47.0	C79.89	-	D36.11	D48.2	D49.2
supraclavicular region	C47.0	C79.89	-	D36.11	D48.2	D49.2
temple	C47.0	C79.89	-	D36.11	D48.2	D49.2
temporal region	C47.0	C79.89	-	D36.11	D48.2	D49.2
thigh	C47.2-	C79.89	-	D36.13	D48.2	D49.2
thoracic (duct) (wall)	C47.3	C79.89	-	D36.14	D48.2	D49.2
thorax	C47.3	C79.89	-	D36.14	D48.2	D49.2
thumb	C47.1-	C79.89	-	D36.12	D48.2	D49.2
toe	C47.2-	C79.89	-	D36.13	D48.2	D49.2
trunk	C47.6	C79.89	-	D36.17	D48.2	D49.2
umbilicus	C47.4	C79.89	-	D36.15	D48.2	D49.2
vesicorectal	C47.5	C79.89	-	D36.16	D48.2	D49.2
wrist	C47.1-	C79.89	-	D36.12	D48.2	D49.2
radial	C47.1-	C79.89	-	D36.12	D48.2	D49.2
sacral	C47.5	C79.89	-	D36.16	D48.2	D49.2
sciatic	C47.2-	C79.89	-	D36.13	D48.2	D49.2
spinal NEC	C47.9	C79.89	-	D36.10	D48.2	D49.2
accessory	C72.59	C79.49	-	D33.3	D43.3	D49.7
sympathetic NEC—*see also Neoplasm, nerve, peripheral*	C47.9	C79.89	-	D36.10	D48.2	D49.2
trigeminal	C72.59	C79.49	-	D33.3	D43.3	D49.7
trochlear	C72.59	C79.49	-	D33.3	D43.3	D49.7
ulnar	C47.1-	C79.89	-	D36.12	D48.2	D49.2
vagus	C72.59	C79.49	-	D33.3	D43.3	D49.7
nervous system (central)	C72.9	C79.40	-	D33.9	D43.9	D49.7
autonomic—*see Neoplasm, nerve, peripheral*						
parasympathetic—*see Neoplasm, nerve, peripheral*						
specified site NEC	-	C79.49	-	D33.7	D43.8	-
sympathetic—*see Neoplasm, nerve, peripheral*						
nevus—*see Nevus*						
nipple	C50.0-	C79.81	D05.-	D24.-	-	-
nose, nasal	C76.0	C79.89	D09.8	D36.7	D48.7	D49.89
ala (external) (nasi)—*see also Neoplasm, nose, skin*	C44.301	C79.2	D04.39	D23.39	D48.5	D49.2
bone	C41.0	C79.51	-	D16.4-	D48.0	D49.2
cartilage	C30.0	C78.39	D02.3	D14.0	D38.5	D49.1
cavity	C30.0	C78.39	D02.3	D14.0	D38.5	D49.1
choana	C11.3	C79.89	D00.08	D10.6	D37.05	D49.0
external (skin)—*see also Neoplasm, nose, skin*	C44.301	C79.2	D04.39	D23.39	D48.5	D49.2
fossa	C30.0	C78.39	D02.3	D14.0	D38.5	D49.1
internal	C30.0	C78.39	D02.3	D14.0	D38.5	D49.1

	Malignant Primary	Malignant Secondary	Ca in Situ	Benign	Uncertain Behavior	Unspecified Behavior
mucosa	C30.0	C78.39	D02.3	D14.0	D38.5	D49.1
septum	C30.0	C78.39	D02.3	D14.0	D38.5	D49.1
posterior margin	C11.3	C79.89	D00.08	D10.6	D37.05	D49.0
sinus—*see Neoplasm, sinus*						
skin	C44.301	C79.2	D04.39	D23.39	D48.5	D49.2
basal cell carcinoma	C44.311	-	-	-	-	-
specified type NEC	C44.391	-	-	-	-	-
squamous cell carcinoma	C44.321	-	-	-	-	-
turbinate (mucosa)	C30.0	C78.39	D02.3	D14.0	D38.5	D49.1
bone	C41.0	C79.51	-	D16.4-	D48.0	D49.2
vestibule	C30.0	C78.39	D02.3	D14.0	D38.5	D49.1
nostril	C30.0	C78.39	D02.3	D14.0	D38.5	D49.1
nucleus pulposus	C41.2	C79.51	-	D16.6	D48.0	D49.2
occipital						
bone	C41.0	C79.51	-	D16.4-	D48.0	D49.2
lobe or pole, brain	C71.4	C79.31	-	D33.0	D43.0	D49.6
odontogenic—*see Neoplasm, jaw bone*						
olfactory nerve or bulb	C72.2-	C79.49	-	D33.3	D43.3	D49.7
olive (brain)	C71.7	C79.31	-	D33.1	D43.1	D49.6
omentum	C48.1	C78.6	-	D20.1	D48.4	D49.0
operculum (brain)	C71.0	C79.31	-	D33.0	D43.0	D49.6
optic nerve, chiasm, or tract	C72.3-	C79.49	-	D33.3	D43.3	D49.7
oral (cavity)	C06.9	C79.89	D00.00	D10.30	D37.09	D49.0
ill defined	C14.8	C79.89	D00.00	D10.30	D37.09	D49.0
mucosa	C06.0	C79.89	D00.02	D10.39	D37.09	D49.0
orbit	C69.6-	C79.49	D09.2-	D31.6-	D48.7	D49.89
autonomic nerve	C69.6-	C79.49	-	D31.6-	D48.7	D49.2
bone	C41.0	C79.51	-	D16.4-	D48.0	D49.2
eye	C69.6-	C79.49	D09.2-	D31.6-	D48.7	D49.89
peripheral nerves	C69.6-	C79.49	-	D31.6-	D48.7	D49.2
soft parts	C69.6-	C79.49	D09.2-	D31.6-	D48.7	D49.89
organ of Zuckerkandl	C75.5	C79.89	-	D35.6	D44.7	D49.7
oropharynx	C10.9	C79.89	D00.08	D10.5	D37.05	D49.0
branchial cleft (vestige)	C10.4	C79.89	D00.08	D10.5	D37.05	D49.0
junctional region	C10.8	C79.89	D00.08	D10.5	D37.05	D49.0
lateral wall	C10.2	C79.89	D00.08	D10.5	D37.05	D49.0
overlapping lesion	C10.8	-	-	-	-	-
pillars or fauces	C09.1	C79.89	D00.08	D10.5	D37.05	D49.0
posterior wall	C10.3	C79.89	D00.08	D10.5	D37.05	D49.0
vallecula	C10.0	C79.89	D00.08	D10.5	D37.05	D49.0
os						
external	C53.1	C79.82	D06.1	D26.0	D39.0	D49.5
internal	C53.0	C79.82	D06.0	D26.0	D39.0	D49.5
ovary	C56.-	C79.6-	D07.39	D27.-	D39.1-	D49.5
oviduct	C57.0-	C79.82	D07.39	D28.2	D39.8	D49.5
palate	C05.9	C79.89	D00.00	D10.39	D37.09	D49.0
hard	C05.0	C79.89	D00.05	D10.39	D37.09	D49.0
junction of hard and soft palate	C05.9	C79.89	D00.00	D10.39	D37.09	D49.0
overlapping lesions	C05.8	-	-	-	-	-
soft	C05.1	C79.89	D00.04	D10.39	D37.09	D49.0
nasopharyngeal surface	C11.3	C79.89	D00.08	D10.6	D37.05	D49.0
posterior surface	C11.3	C79.89	D00.08	D10.6	D37.05	D49.0
superior surface	C11.3	C79.89	D00.08	D10.6	D37.05	D49.0
palatoglossal arch	C09.1	C79.89	D00.00	D10.5	D37.09	D49.0
palatopharyngeal arch	C09.1	C79.89	D00.00	D10.5	D37.09	D49.0
pallium	C71.0	C79.31	-	D33.0	D43.0	D49.6
palpebra	C44.10-	C79.2	D04.1-	D23.1-	D48.5	D49.2
basal cell carcinoma	C44.11-	-	-	-	-	-
specified type NEC	C44.19-	-	-	-	-	-
squamous cell carcinoma	C44.12-	-	-	-	-	-
pancreas	C25.9	C78.89	D01.7	D13.6	D37.8	D49.0
body	C25.1	C78.89	D01.7	D13.6	D37.8	D49.0
duct (of Santorini) (of Wirsung)	C25.3	C78.89	D01.7	D13.6	D37.8	D49.0
ectopic tissue	C25.7	C78.89	-	D13.6	D37.8	D49.0
head	C25.0	C78.89	D01.7	D13.6	D37.8	D49.0
islet cells	C25.4	C78.89	D01.7	D13.7	D37.8	D49.0
neck	C25.7	C78.89	D01.7	D13.6	D37.8	D49.0
overlapping lesion	C25.8	-	-	-	-	-

	Malignant Primary	Malignant Secondary	Ca in Situ	Benign	Uncertain Behavior	Unspecified Behavior
tail	C25.2	C78.89	D01.7	D13.6	D37.8	D49.0
para aortic body	C75.5	C79.89	-	D35.6	D44.7	D49.7
paraganglion NEC	C75.5	C79.89	-	D35.6	D44.7	D49.7
parametrium	C57.3	C79.82	-	D28.2	D39.8	D49.5
paranephric	C48.0	C78.6	-	D20.0	D48.3	D49.0
pararectal	C76.3	C79.89	-	D36.7	D48.7	D49.89
parasagittal (region)	C76.0	C79.89	D09.8	D36.7	D48.7	D49.89
parasellar	C72.9	C79.49	-	D33.9	D43.8	D49.7
parathyroid (gland)	C75.0	C79.89	D09.3	D35.1	D44.2	D49.7
paraurethral	C76.3	C79.89	-	D36.7	D48.7	D49.89
gland	C68.1	C79.19	D09.19	D30.8	D41.8	D49.5
paravaginal	C76.3	C79.89	-	D36.7	D48.7	D49.89
parenchyma, kidney	C64.-	C79.0-	D09.19	D30.0-	D41.0-	D49.5
parietal						
bone	C41.0	C79.51	-	D16.4-	D48.0	D49.2
lobe, brain	C71.3	C79.31	-	D33.0	D43.0	D49.6
paroophoron	C57.1	C79.82	D07.39	D28.2	D39.8	D49.5
parotid (duct) (gland)	C07	C79.89	D00.00	D11.0	D37.030	D49.0
parovarium	C57.1	C79.82	D07.39	D28.2	D39.8	D49.5
patella	C40.20	C79.51	-	-	-	-
peduncle, cerebral	C71.7	C79.31	-	D33.1	D43.1	D49.6
pelvirectal junction	C19	C78.5	D01.1	D12.7	D37.5	D49.0
pelvis, pelvic	C76.3	C79.89	D09.8	D36.7	D48.7	D49.89
bone	C41.4	C79.51	-	D16.8	D48.0	D49.2
floor	C76.3	C79.89	D09.8	D36.7	D48.7	D49.89
renal	C65.-	C79.0-	D09.19	D30.1-	D41.1-	D49.5
viscera	C76.3	C79.89	D09.8	D36.7	D48.7	D49.89
wall	C76.3	C79.89	D09.8	D36.7	D48.7	D49.89
pelvo abdominal	C76.8	C79.89	D09.8	D36.7	D48.7	D49.89
penis	C60.9	C79.82	D07.4	D29.0	D40.8	D49.5
body	C60.2	C79.82	D07.4	D29.0	D40.8	D49.5
corpus (cavernosum)	C60.2	C79.82	D07.4	D29.0	D40.8	D49.5
glans	C60.1	C79.82	D07.4	D29.0	D40.8	D49.5
overlapping sites	C60.8	-	-	-	-	-
skin NEC	C60.9	C79.82	D07.4	D29.0	D40.8	D49.5
periadrenal (tissue)	C48.0	C78.6	-	D20.0	D48.3	D49.0
perianal (skin)—*see also Neoplasm, anus, skin*	C44.500	C79.2	D04.5	D23.5	D48.5	D49.2
pericardium	C38.0	C79.89	-	D15.1	D48.7	D49.89
perinephric	C48.0	C78.6	-	D20.0	D48.3	D49.0
perineum	C76.3	C79.89	D09.8	D36.7	D48.7	D49.89
periodontal tissue NEC	C03.9	C79.89	D00.03	D10.39	D37.09	D49.0
periosteum—*see Neoplasm, bone*						
peripancreatic	C48.0	C78.6	-	D20.0	D48.3	D49.0
peripheral nerve NEC	C47.9	C79.89	-	D36.10	D48.2	D49.2
perirectal (tissue)	C76.3	C79.89	-	D36.7	D48.7	D49.89
perirenal (tissue)	C48.0	C78.6	-	D20.0	D48.3	D49.0
peritoneum, peritoneal (cavity)	C48.2	C78.6	-	D20.1	D48.4	D49.0
benign mesothelial tissue—*see Mesothelioma, benign*						
overlapping lesion	C48.8	-	-	-	-	-
with digestive organs	C26.9	-	-	-	-	-
parietal	C48.1	C78.6	-	D20.1	D48.4	D49.0
pelvic	C48.1	C78.6	-	D20.1	D48.4	D49.0
specified part NEC	C48.1	C78.6	-	D20.1	D48.4	D49.0
peritonsillar (tissue)	C76.0	C79.89	D09.8	D36.7	D48.7	D49.89
periurethral tissue	C76.3	C79.89	-	D36.7	D48.7	D49.89
phalanges						
foot	C40.3-	C79.51	-	D16.3-	-	-
hand	C40.1-	C79.51	-	D16.1-	-	-
pharynx, pharyngeal	C14.0	C79.89	D00.08	D10.9	D37.05	D49.0
bursa	C11.1	C79.89	D00.08	D10.6	D37.05	D49.0
fornix	C11.3	C79.89	D00.08	D10.6	D37.05	D49.0
recess	C11.2	C79.89	D00.08	D10.6	D37.05	D49.0
region	C14.0	C79.89	D00.08	D10.9	D37.05	D49.0
tonsil	C11.1	C79.89	D00.08	D10.6	D37.05	D49.0
wall (lateral) (posterior)	C14.0	C79.89	D00.08	D10.9	D37.05	D49.0
pia mater	C70.9	C79.40	-	D32.9	D42.9	D49.7
cerebral	C70.0	C79.32	-	D32.0	D42.0	D49.7

	Malignant Primary	Malignant Secondary	Ca in Situ	Benign	Uncertain Behavior	Unspecified Behavior
cranial	C70.0	C79.32	-	D32.0	D42.0	D49.7
spinal	C70.1	C79.49	-	D32.1	D42.1	D49.7
pillars of fauces	C09.1	C79.89	D00.08	D10.5	D37.05	D49.0
pineal (body) (gland)	C75.3	C79.89	D09.3	D35.4	D44.5	D49.7
pinna (ear)NEC—see also Neoplasm, skin, ear	C44.20-	C79.2	D04.2-	D23.2-	D48.5	D49.2
piriform fossa or sinus	C12	C79.89	D00.08	D10.7	D37.05	D49.0
pituitary (body) (fossa) (gland) (lobe)	C75.1	C79.89	D09.3	D35.2	D44.3	D49.7
placenta	C58	C79.82	D07.0	D26.7	D39.2	D49.5
pleura, pleural (cavity)	C38.4	C78.2	-	D19.0	D38.2	D49.1
overlapping lesion with heart or mediastinum	C38.8	-	-	-	-	-
parietal	C38.4	C78.2	-	D19.0	D38.2	D49.1
visceral	C38.4	C78.2	-	D19.0	D38.2	D49.1
plexus						
brachial	C47.1-	C79.89	-	D36.12	D48.2	D49.2
cervical	C47.0	C79.89	-	D36.11	D48.2	D49.2
choroid	C71.5	C79.31	-	D33.0	D43.0	D49.6
lumbosacral	C47.5	C79.89	-	D36.16	D48.2	D49.2
sacral	C47.5	C79.89	-	D36.16	D48.2	D49.2
pluriendocrine	C75.8	C79.89	D09.3	D35.7	D44.9	D49.7
pole						
frontal	C71.1	C79.31	-	D33.0	D43.0	D49.6
occipital	C71.4	C79.31	-	D33.0	D43.0	D49.6
pons (varolii)	C71.7	C79.31	-	D33.1	D43.1	D49.6
popliteal fossa or space	C76.5-	C79.89	D04.7-	D36.7	D48.7	D49.89
postcricoid (region)	C13.0	C79.89	D00.08	D10.7	D37.05	D49.0
posterior fossa (cranial)	C71.9	C79.31	-	D33.2	D43.2	D49.6
postnasal space	C11.9	C79.89	D00.08	D10.6	D37.05	D49.0
prepuce	C60.0	C79.82	D07.4	D29.0	D40.8	D49.5
prepylorus	C16.4	C78.89	D00.2	D13.1	D37.1	D49.0
presacral (region)	C76.3	C79.89	-	D36.7	D48.7	D49.89
prostate (gland)	C61	C79.82	D07.5	D29.1	D40.0	D49.5
utricle	C68.0	C79.19	D09.19	D30.4	D41.3	D49.5
pterygoid fossa	C49.0	C79.89	-	D21.0	D48.1	D49.2
pubic bone	C41.4	C79.51	-	D16.8	D48.0	D49.2
pudenda, pudendum (female)	C51.9	C79.82	D07.1	D28.0	D39.8	D49.5
pulmonary—see also Neoplasm, lung	C34.9-	C78.0-	D02.2-	D14.3-	D38.1	D49.1
putamen	C71.0	C79.31	-	D33.0	D43.0	D49.6
pyloric						
antrum	C16.3	C78.89	D00.2	D13.1	D37.1	D49.0
canal	C16.4	C78.89	D00.2	D13.1	D37.1	D49.0
pylorus	C16.4	C78.89	D00.2	D13.1	D37.1	D49.0
pyramid (brain)	C71.7	C79.31	-	D33.1	D43.1	D49.6
pyriform fossa or sinus	C12	C79.89	D00.08	D10.7	D37.05	D49.0
radius (any part)	C40.0-	C79.51	-	D16.0-	-	-
Rathke's pouch	C75.1	C79.89	D09.3	D35.2	D44.3	D49.7
rectosigmoid (junction)	C19	C78.5	D01.1	D12.7	D37.5	D49.0
overlapping lesion with anus or rectum	C21.8	-	-	-	-	-
rectouterine pouch	C48.1	C78.6	-	D20.1	D48.4	D49.0
rectovaginal septum or wall	C76.3	C79.89	D09.8	D36.7	D48.7	D49.89
rectovesical septum	C76.3	C79.89	D09.8	D36.7	D48.7	D49.89
rectum (ampulla)	C20	C78.5	D01.2	D12.8	D37.5	D49.0
and colon	C19	C78.5	D01.1	D12.7	D37.5	D49.0
overlapping lesion with anus or rectosigmoid junction	C21.8	-	-	-	-	-
renal	C64.-	C79.0-	D09.19	D30.0-	D41.0-	D49.5
calyx	C65.-	C79.0-	D09.19	D30.1-	D41.1-	D49.5
hilus	C65.-	C79.0-	D09.19	D30.1	D41.1	D49.5
parenchyma	C64.-	C79.0-	D09.19	D30.0-	D41.0-	D49.5
pelvis	C65.-	C79.0-	D09.19	D30.1-	D41.1-	D49.5
respiratory						
organs or system NEC	C39.9	C78.30	D02.4	D14.4	D38.6	D49.1
tract NEC	C39.9	C78.30	D02.4	D14.4	D38.5	D49.1
upper	C39.0	C78.30	D02.4	D14.4	D38.5	D49.1
retina	C69.2-	C79.49	D09.2-	D31.2-	D48.7	D49.81
retrobulbar	C69.6-	C79.49	-	D31.6-	D48.7	D49.89
retrocecal	C48.0	C78.6	-	D20.0	D48.3	D49.0
retromolar (area) (triangle) (trigone)	C06.2	C79.89	D00.00	D10.39	D37.09	D49.0
retro orbital	C76.0	C79.89	D09.8	D36.7	D48.7	D49.89

	Malignant Primary	Malignant Secondary	Ca in Situ	Benign	Uncertain Behavior	Unspecified Behavior
retroperitoneal (space) (tissue)	C48.0	C78.6	-	D20.0	D48.3	D49.0
retroperitoneum	C48.0	C78.6	-	D20.0	D48.3	D49.0
retropharyngeal	C14.0	C79.89	D00.08	D10.9	D37.05	D49.0
retrovesical (septum)	C76.3	C79.89	D09.8	D36.7	D48.7	D49.89
rhinencephalon	C71.0	C79.31	-	D33.0	D43.0	D49.6
rib	C41.3	C79.51	-	D16.7	D48.0	D49.2
Rosenmüller's fossa	C11.2	C79.89	D00.08	D10.6	D37.05	D49.0
round ligament	C57.2	C79.82	-	D28.2	D39.8	D49.5
sacrococcyx, sacrococcygeal	C41.4	C79.51	-	D16.8	D48.0	D49.2
region	C76.3	C79.89	D09.8	D36.7	D48.7	D49.89
sacrouterine ligament	C57.3	C79.82	-	D28.2	D39.8	D49.5
sacrum, sacral (vertebra)	C41.4	C79.51	-	D16.8	D48.0	D49.2
salivary gland or duct (major)	C08.9	C79.89	D00.00	D11.9	D37.039	D49.0
minor NEC	C06.9	C79.89	D00.00	D10.39	D37.04	D49.0
overlapping lesion	C08.9	-	-	-	-	-
parotid	C07	C79.89	D00.00	D11.0	D37.030	D49.0
pluriglandular	C08.9	C79.89	D00.00	D11.9	D37.039	D49.0
sublingual	C08.1	C79.89	D00.00	D11.7	D37.031	D49.0
submandibular	C08.0	C79.89	D00.00	D11.7	D37.032	D49.0
submaxillary	C08.0	C79.89	D00.00	D11.7	D37.032	D49.0
salpinx (uterine)	C57.0-	C79.82	D07.39	D28.2	D39.8	D49.5
Santorini's duct	C25.3	C78.89	D01.7	D13.6	D37.8	D49.0
scalp	C44.40	C79.2	D04.4	D23.4	D48.5	D49.2
basal cell carcinoma	C44.41	-	-	-	-	-
specified type NEC	C44.49	-	-	-	-	-
squamous cell carcinoma	C44.42	-	-	-	-	-
scapula (any part)	C40.0-	C79.51	-	D16.0-	-	-
scapular region	C76.1	C79.89	D09.8	D36.7	D48.7	D49.89
scar NEC—see also Neoplasm, skin, by site	C44.90	C79.2	D04.9	D23.9	D48.5	D49.2
sciatic nerve	C47.2-	C79.89	-	D36.13	D48.2	D49.2
sclera	C69.4-	C79.49	D09.2-	D31.4-	D48.7	D49.89
scrotum (skin)	C63.2	C79.82	D07.61	D29.4	D40.8	D49.5
sebaceous gland—see Neoplasm, skin						
sella turcica	C75.1	C79.89	D09.3	D35.2	D44.3	D49.7
bone	C41.0	C79.51	-	D16.4-	D48.0	D49.2
semilunar cartilage (knee)	C40.2-	C79.51	-	D16.2-	D48.0	D49.2
seminal vesicle	C63.7	C79.82	D07.69	D29.8	D40.8	D49.5
septum						
nasal	C30.0	C78.39	D02.3	D14.0	D38.5	D49.1
posterior margin	C11.3	C79.89	D00.08	D10.6	D37.05	D49.0
rectovaginal	C76.3	C79.89	D09.8	D36.7	D48.7	D49.89
rectovesical	C76.3	C79.89	D09.8	D36.7	D48.7	D49.89
urethrovaginal	C57.9	C79.82	D07.30	D28.9	D39.9	D49.5
vesicovaginal	C57.9	C79.82	D07.30	D28.9	D39.9	D49.5
shoulder NEC	C76.4-	C79.89	D04.6-	D36.7	D48.7	D49.89
sigmoid flexure (lower) (upper)	C18.7	C78.5	D01.0	D12.5	D37.4	D49.0
sinus (accessory)	C31.9	C78.39	D02.3	D14.0	D38.5	D49.1
bone (any)	C41.0	C79.51	-	D16.4-	D48.0	D49.2
ethmoidal	C31.1	C78.39	D02.3	D14.0	D38.5	D49.1
frontal	C31.2	C78.39	D02.3	D14.0	D38.5	D49.1
maxillary	C31.0	C78.39	D02.3	D14.0	D38.5	D49.1
nasal, paranasal NEC	C31.9	C78.39	D02.3	D14.0	D38.5	D49.1
overlapping lesion	C31.8	-	-	-	-	-
pyriform	C12	C79.89	D00.08	D10.7	D37.05	D49.0
sphenoid	C31.3	C78.39	D02.3	D14.0	D38.5	D49.1
skeleton, skeletal NEC	C41.9	C79.51	-	D16.9-	D48.0	D49.2
Skene's gland	C68.1	C79.19	D09.19	D30.8	D41.8	D49.5
skin NOS	C44.90	C79.2	D04.9	D23.9	D48.5	D49.2
abdominal wall	C44.509	C79.2	D04.5	D23.5	D48.5	D49.2
basal cell carcinoma	C44.519	-	-	-	-	-
specified type NEC	C44.599	-	-	-	-	-
squamous cell carcinoma	C44.529	-	-	-	-	-
ala nasi—see also Neoplasm, nose, skin	C44.301	C79.2	D04.39	D23.39	D48.5	D49.2
ankle—see also Neoplasm, skin, limb, lower	C44.70-	C79.2	D04.7-	D23.7-	D48.5	D49.2
antecubital space—see also Neoplasm, skin, limb, upper	C44.60-	C79.2	D04.6-	D23.6-	D48.5	D49.2
anus	C44.500	C79.2	D04.5	D23.5	D48.5	D49.2
basal cell carcinoma	C44.510	-	-	-	-	-

	Malignant Primary	Malignant Secondary	Ca in Situ	Benign	Uncertain Behavior	Unspecified Behavior
specified type NEC	C44.590	-	-	-	-	-
squamous cell carcinoma	C44.520	-	-	-	-	-
arm—*see also Neoplasm, skin, limb, upper*	C44.60-	C79.2	D04.6-	D23.6-	D48.5	D49.2
auditory canal (external)—*see also Neoplasm, skin, ear*	C44.20-	C79.2	D04.2-	D23.2-	D48.5	D49.2
auricle (ear)—*see also Neoplasm, skin, ear*	C44.20-	C79.2	D04.2-	D23.2-	D48.5	D49.2
auricular canal (external)—*see also Neoplasm, skin, ear*	C44.20-	C79.2	D04.2-	D23.2-	D48.5	D49.2
axilla, axillary fold—*see also Neoplasm, skin, trunk*	C44.509	C79.2	D04.5	D23.5	D48.5	D49.2
back—*see also Neoplasm, skin, trunk*	C44.509	C79.2	D04.5	D23.5	D48.5	D49.2
basal cell carcinoma	C44.91					
breast	C44.501	C79.2	D04.5	D23.5	D48.5	D49.2
basal cell carcinoma	C44.511	-	-	-	-	-
specified type NEC	C44.591	-	-	-	-	-
squamous cell carcinoma	C44.521	-	-	-	-	-
brow—*see also Neoplasm, skin, face*	C44.309	C79.2	D04.39	D23.39	D48.5	D49.2
buttock—*see also Neoplasm, skin, trunk*	C44.509	C79.2	D04.5	D23.5	D48.5	D49.2
calf—*see also Neoplasm, skin, limb, lower*	C44.70-	C79.2	D04.7-	D23.7-	D48.5	D49.2
canthus (eye) (inner) (outer)	C44.10-	C79.2	D04.1	D23.1	D48.5	D49.2
basal cell carcinoma	C44.11-	-	-	-	-	-
specified type NEC	C44.19-	-	-	-	-	-
squamous cell carcinoma	C44.12-	-	-	-	-	-
cervical region—*see also Neoplasm, skin, neck*	C44.40	C79.2	D04.4	D23.4	D48.5	D49.2
cheek (external)—*see also Neoplasm, skin, face*	C44.309	C79.2	D04.39	D23.39	D48.5	D49.2
chest (wall)—*see also Neoplasm, skin, trunk*	C44.509	C79.2	D04.5	D23.5	D48.5	D49.2
chin—*see also Neoplasm, skin, face*	C44.309	C79.2	D04.39	D23.39	D48.5	D49.2
clavicular area—*see also Neoplasm, skin, trunk*	C44.509	C79.2	D04.5	D23.5	D48.5	D49.2
clitoris	C51.2	C79.82	D07.1	D28.0	D39.8	D49.5
columnella—*see also Neoplasm, skin, face*	C44.309	C79.2	D04.39	D23.39	D48.5	D49.2
concha—*see also Neoplasm, skin, ear*	C44.20-	C79.2	D04.2-	D23.2-	D48.5	D49.2
ear (external)	C44.20-	C79.2	D04.2-	D23.2-	D48.5	D49.2
basal cell carcinoma	C44.21-	-	-	-	-	-
specified type NEC	C44.29-	-	-	-	-	
squamous cell carcinoma	C44.22-	-	-	-	-	-
elbow—*see also Neoplasm, skin, limb, upper*	C44.60-	C79.2	D04.6-	D23.6-	D48.5	D49.2
eyebrow—*see also Neoplasm, skin, face*	C44.309	C79.2	D04.39	D23.39	D48.5	D49.2
eyelid	C44.10-	C79.2	D04.1-	D23.1-	D48.5	D49.2
basal cell carcinoma	C44.11-	-	-	-	-	-
specified type NEC	C44.19-	-	-	-	-	
squamous cell carcinoma	C44.12-	-	-	-	-	-
face NOS	C44.300	C79.2	D04.30	D23.30	D48.5	D49.2
basal cell carcinoma	C44.310	-	-	-	-	-
specified type NEC	C44.390	-	-	-	-	-
squamous cell carcinoma	C44.320	-	-	-	-	-
female genital organs (external)	C51.9	C79.82	D07.1	D28.0	D39.8	D49.5
clitoris	C51.2	C79.82	D07.1	D28.0	D39.8	D49.5
labium NEC	C51.9	C79.82	D07.1	D28.0	D39.8	D49.5
majus	C51.0	C79.82	D07.1	D28.0	D39.8	D49.5
minus	C51.1	C79.82	D07.1	D28.0	D39.8	D49.5
pudendum	C51.9	C79.82	D07.1	D28.0	D39.8	D49.5
vulva	C51.9	C79.82	D07.1	D28.0	D39.8	D49.5
finger—*see also Neoplasm, skin, limb, upper*	C44.60-	C79.2	D04.6-	D23.6-	D48.5	D49.2
flank—*see also Neoplasm, skin, trunk*	C44.509	C79.2	D04.5	D23.5	D48.5	D49.2
foot—*see also Neoplasm, skin, limb, lower*	C44.70-	C79.2	D04.7-	D23.7-	D48.5	D49.2
forearm—*see also Neoplasm, skin, limb, upper*	C44.60-	C79.2	D04.6-	D23.6-	D48.5	D49.2
forehead—*see also Neoplasm, skin, face*	C44.309	C79.2	D04.39	D23.39	D48.5	D49.2
glabella—*see also Neoplasm, skin, face*	C44.309	C79.2	D04.39	D23.39	D48.5	D49.2
gluteal region—*see also Neoplasm, skin, trunk*	C44.509	C79.2	D04.5	D23.5	D48.5	D49.2
groin—*see also Neoplasm, skin, trunk*	C44.509	C79.2	D04.5	D23.5	D48.5	D49.2
hand—*see also Neoplasm, skin, limb, upper*	C44.60-	C79.2	D04.6-	D23.6-	D48.5	D49.2
head NEC—*see also Neoplasm, skin, scalp*	C44.40	C79.2	D04.4	D23.4	D48.5	D49.2
heel—*see also Neoplasm, skin, limb, lower*	C44.70-	C79.2	D04.7-	D23.7-	D48.5	D49.2
helix—*see also Neoplasm, skin, ear*	C44.20-	C79.2	D04.2-	D23.2-	D48.5	D49.2
hip—*see also Neoplasm, skin, limb, lower*	C44.70-	C79.2	D04.7-	D23.7-	D48.5	D49.2
infraclavicular region—*see also Neoplasm, skin, trunk*	C44.509	C79.2	D04.5	D23.5	D48.5	D49.2
inguinal region—*see also Neoplasm, skin, trunk*	C44.509	C79.2	D04.5	D23.5	D48.5	D49.2
jaw—*see also Neoplasm, skin, face*	C44.309	C79.2	D04.39	D23.39	D48.5	D49.2
Kaposi's sarcoma—*see Kaposi's, sarcoma, skin*						

	Malignant Primary	Malignant Secondary	Ca in Situ	Benign	Uncertain Behavior	Unspecified Behavior
knee—*see also Neoplasm, skin, limb, lower*	C44.70-	C79.2	D04.7-	D23.7-	D48.5	D49.2
labia						
majora	C51.0	C79.82	D07.1	D28.0	D39.8	D49.5
minora	C51.1	C79.82	D07.1	D28.0	D39.8	D49.5
leg—*see also Neoplasm, skin, limb, lower*	C44.70-	C79.2	D04.7-	D23.7-	D48.5	D49.2
lid (lower) (upper)	C44.10-	C79.2	D04.1-	D23.1-	D48.5	D49.2
basal cell carcinoma	C44.11-	-	-	-	-	-
specified type NEC	C44.19-	-	-	-	-	-
squamous cell carcinoma	C44.12-	-	-	-	-	-
limb NEC	C44.90	C79.2	D04.9	D23.9	D48.5	D49.2
basal cell carcinoma	C44.91					
lower	C44.70-	C79.2	D04.7-	D23.7-	D48.5	D49.2
basal cell carcinoma	C44.71-	-	-	-	-	-
specified type NEC	C44.79-	-	-	-	-	-
squamous cell carcinoma	C44.72-	-	-	-	-	-
upper	C44.60-	C79.2	D04.6-	D23.6-	D48.5	D49.2
basal cell carcinoma	C44.61-	-	-	-	-	-
specified type NEC	C44.69-	-	-	-	-	-
squamous cell carcinoma	C44.62-	-	-	-	-	-
lip (lower) (upper)	C44.00	C79.2	D04.0	D23.0	D48.5	D49.2
basal cell carcinoma	C44.01	-	-	-	-	-
specified type NEC	C44.09	-	-	-	-	-
squamous cell carcinoma	C44.02	-	-	-	-	-
male genital organs	C63.9	C79.82	D07.60	D29.9	D40.8	D49.5
penis	C60.9	C79.82	D07.4	D29.0	D40.8	D49.5
prepuce	C60.0	C79.82	D07.4	D29.0	D40.8	D49.5
scrotum	C63.2	C79.82	D07.61	D29.4	D40.8	D49.5
mastectomy site (skin)—*see also Neoplasm, skin, breast*	C44.501	C79.2	-	-	-	-
specified as breast tissue	C50.8-	C79.81	-	-	-	-
meatus, acoustic (external)—*see also Neoplasm, skin, ear*	C44.20-	C79.2	D04.2-	D23.2-	D48.5	D49.2
melanotic—*see Melanoma*						
Merkel cell—*see Carcinoma, Merkel cell*						
nates—*see also Neoplasm, skin, trunk*	C44.509	C79.2	D04.5	D23.5	D48.5	D49.2
neck	C44.40	C79.2	D04.4	D23.4	D48.5	D49.2
basal cell carcinoma	C44.41	-	-	-	-	-
specified type NEC	C44.49	-	-	-	-	-
squamous cell carcinoma	C44.42	-	-	-	-	-
nevus—*see Nevus, skin*						
nose (external)—*see also Neoplasm, nose, skin*	C44.301	C79.2	D04.39	D23.39	D48.5	D49.2
overlapping lesion	C44.80	-	-	-	-	-
basal cell carcinoma	C44.81	-	-	-	-	-
specified type NEC	C44.89	-	-	-	-	-
squamous cell carcinoma	C44.82	-	-	-	-	-
palm—*see also Neoplasm, skin, limb, upper*	C44.60-	C79.2	D04.6-	D23.6-	D48.5	D49.2
palpebra	C44.10-	C79.2	D04.1-	D23.1-	D48.5	D49.2
basal cell carcinoma	C44.11-	-	-	-	-	-
specified type NEC	C44.19-	-	-	-	-	-
squamous cell carcinoma	C44.12-	-	-	-	-	-
penis NEC	C60.9	C79.82	D07.4	D29.0	D40.8	D49.5
perianal—*see also Neoplasm, skin, anus*	C44.500	C79.2	D04.5	D23.5	D48.5	D49.2
perineum—*see also Neoplasm, skin, anus*	C44.500	C79.2	D04.5	D23.5	D48.5	D49.2
pinna—*see also Neoplasm, skin, ear*	C44.20-	C79.2	D04.2-	D23.2-	D48.5	D49.2
plantar—*see also Neoplasm, skin, limb, lower*	C44.70-	C79.2	D04.7-	D23.7-	D48.5	D49.2
popliteal fossa or space—*see also Neoplasm, skin, limb, lower*	C44.70-	C79.2	D04.7-	D23.7-	D48.5	D49.2
prepuce	C60.0	C79.82	D07.4	D29.0	D40.8	D49.5
pubes—*see also Neoplasm, skin, trunk*	C44.509	C79.2	D04.5	D23.5	D48.5	D49.2
sacrococcygeal region—*see also Neoplasm, skin, trunk*	C44.509	C79.2	D04.5	D23.5	D48.5	D49.2
scalp	C44.40	C79.2	D04.4	D23.4	D48.5	D49.2
basal cell carcinoma	C44.41	-	-	-	-	-
specified type NEC	C44.49	-	-	-	-	-
squamous cell carcinoma	C44.42	-	-	-	-	-
scapular region—*see also Neoplasm, skin, trunk*	C44.509	C79.2	D04.5	D23.5	D48.5	D49.2
scrotum	C63.2	C79.82	D07.61	D29.4	D40.8	D49.5
shoulder—*see also Neoplasm, skin, limb, upper*	C44.60-	C79.2	D04.6-	D23.6-	D48.5	D49.2
sole (foot)—*see also Neoplasm, skin, limb, lower*	C44.70-	C79.2	D04.7-	D23.7-	D48.5	D49.2

	Malignant Primary	Malignant Secondary	Ca in Situ	Benign	Uncertain Behavior	Unspecified Behavior
specified sites NEC	C44.80	C79.2	D04.8	D23.9	D48.5	D49.2
basal cell carcinoma	C44.81	-	-	-	-	-
specified type NEC	C44.89	-	-	-	-	-
squamous cell carcinoma	C44.82	-	-	-	-	-
specified type NEC	C44.99	-	-	-	-	-
squamous cell carcinoma	C44.92	-	-	-	-	-
submammary fold—*see also Neoplasm, skin, trunk*	C44.509	C79.2	D04.5	D23.5	D48.5	D49.2
supraclavicular region—*see also Neoplasm, skin, neck*	C44.40	C79.2	D04.4	D23.4	D48.5	D49.2
temple—*see also Neoplasm, skin, face*	C44.309	C79.2	D04.39	D23.39	D48.5	D49.2
thigh—*see also Neoplasm, skin, limb, lower*	C44.70-	C79.2	D04.7-	D23.7-	D48.5	D49.2
thoracic wall—*see also Neoplasm, skin, trunk*	C44.509	C79.2	D04.5	D23.5	D48.5	D49.2
thumb—*see also Neoplasm, skin, limb, upper*	C44.60-	C79.2	D04.6-	D23.6-	D48.5	D49.2
toe—*see also Neoplasm, skin, limb, lower*	C44.70-	C79.2	D04.7-	D23.7-	D48.5	D49.2
tragus—*see also Neoplasm, skin, ear*	C44.20-	C79.2	D04.2-	D23.2-	D48.5	D49.2
trunk	C44.509	C79.2	D04.5	D23.5	D48.5	D49.2
basal cell carcinoma	C44.519	-	-	-	-	-
specified type NEC	C44.599	-	-	-	-	-
squamous cell carcinoma	C44.529	-	-	-	-	-
umbilicus—*see also Neoplasm, skin, trunk*	C44.509	C79.2	D04.5	D23.5	D48.5	D49.2
vulva	C51.9	C79.82	D07.1	D28.0	D39.8	D49.5
overlapping lesion	C51.8	-	-	-	-	-
wrist—*see also Neoplasm, skin, limb, upper*	C44.60-	C79.2	D04.6-	D23.6-	D48.5	D49.2
skull	C41.0	C79.51	-	D16.4-	D48.0	D49.2
soft parts or tissues—*see Neoplasm, connective tissue*						
specified site NEC	C76.8	C79.89	D09.8	D36.7	D48.7	D49.89
spermatic cord	C63.1-	C79.82	D07.69	D29.8	D40.8	D49.5
sphenoid	C31.3	C78.39	D02.3	D14.0	D38.5	D49.1
bone	C41.0	C79.51	-	D16.4-	D48.0	D49.2
sinus	C31.3	C78.39	D02.3	D14.0	D38.5	D49.1
sphincter						
anal	C21.1	C78.5	D01.3	D12.9	D37.8	D49.0
of Oddi	C24.0	C78.89	D01.5	D13.5	D37.6	D49.0
spine, spinal (column)	C41.2	C79.51	-	D16.6	D48.0	D49.2
bulb	C71.7	C79.31	-	D33.1	D43.1	D49.6
coccyx	C41.4	C79.51	-	D16.8	D48.0	D49.2
cord (cervical) (lumbar) (sacral) (thoracic)	C72.0	C79.49	-	D33.4	D43.4	D49.7
dura mater	C70.1	C79.49	-	D32.1	D42.1	D49.7
lumbosacral	C41.2	C79.51	-	D16.6	D48.0	D49.2
marrow NEC	C96.9	C79.52	-	-	D47.9	D49.89
membrane	C70.1	C79.49	-	D32.1	D42.1	D49.7
meninges	C70.1	C79.49	-	D32.1	D42.1	D49.7
nerve (root)	C47.9	C79.89	-	D36.10	D48.2	D49.2
pia mater	C70.1	C79.49	-	D32.1	D42.1	D49.7
root	C47.9	C79.89	-	D36.10	D48.2	D49.2
sacrum	C41.4	C79.51	-	D16.8	D48.0	D49.2
spleen, splenic NEC	C26.1	C78.89	D01.7	D13.9	D37.8	D49.0
flexure (colon)	C18.5	C78.5	D01.0	D12.3	D37.4	D49.0
stem, brain	C71.7	C79.31	-	D33.1	D43.1	D49.6
Stensen's duct	C07	C79.89	D00.00	D11.0	D37.030	D49.0
sternum	C41.3	C79.51	-	D16.7	D48.0	D49.2
stomach	C16.9	C78.89	D00.2	D13.1	D37.1	D49.0
antrum (pyloric)	C16.3	C78.89	D00.2	D13.1	D37.1	D49.0
body	C16.2	C78.89	D00.2	D13.1	D37.1	D49.0
cardia	C16.0	C78.89	D00.2	D13.1	D37.1	D49.0
cardiac orifice	C16.0	C78.89	D00.2	D13.1	D37.1	D49.0
corpus	C16.2	C78.89	D00.2	D13.1	D37.1	D49.0
fundus	C16.1	C78.89	D00.2	D13.1	D37.1	D49.0
greater curvature NEC	C16.6	C78.89	D00.2	D13.1	D37.1	D49.0
lesser curvature NEC	C16.5	C78.89	D00.2	D13.1	D37.1	D49.0
overlapping lesion	C16.8	-	-	-	-	-
prepylorus	C16.4	C78.89	D00.2	D13.1	D37.1	D49.0
pylorus	C16.4	C78.89	D00.2	D13.1	D37.1	D49.0
wall NEC	C16.9	C78.89	D00.2	D13.1	D37.1	D49.0
anterior NEC	C16.8	C78.89	D00.2	D13.1	D37.1	D49.0
posterior NEC	C16.8	C78.89	D00.2	D13.1	D37.1	D49.0
stroma, endometrial	C54.1	C79.82	D07.0	D26.1	D39.0	D49.5
stump, cervical	C53.8	C79.82	D06.7	D26.0	D39.0	D49.5

	Malignant Primary	Malignant Secondary	Ca in Situ	Benign	Uncertain Behavior	Unspecified Behavior
subcutaneous (nodule) (tissue)NEC—*see Neoplasm, connective tissue*						
subdural	C70.9	C79.32	-	D32.9	D42.9	D49.7
subglottis, subglottic	C32.2	C78.39	D02.0	D14.1	D38.0	D49.1
sublingual	C04.9	C79.89	D00.06	D10.2	D37.09	D49.0
gland or duct	C08.1	C79.89	D00.00	D11.7	D37.031	D49.0
submandibular gland	C08.0	C79.89	D00.00	D11.7	D37.032	D49.0
submaxillary gland or duct	C08.0	C79.89	D00.00	D11.7	D37.032	D49.0
submental	C76.0	C79.89	D09.8	D36.7	D48.7	D49.89
subpleural	C34.9-	C78.0-	D02.2-	D14.3-	D38.1	D49.1
substernal	C38.1	C78.1	-	D15.2	D38.3	D49.89
sudoriferous, sudoriparous gland, site unspecified	C44.90	C79.2	D04.9	D23.9	D48.5	D49.2
specified site—*see Neoplasm, skin*						
supraclavicular region	C76.0	C79.89	D09.8	D36.7	D48.7	D49.89
supraglottis	C32.1	C78.39	D02.0	D14.1	D38.0	D49.1
suprarenal	C74.9-	C79.7-	D09.3	D35.0-	D44.1-	D49.7
capsule	C74.9-	C79.7-	D09.3	D35.0-	D44.1-	D49.7
cortex	C74.0-	C79.7-	D09.3	D35.0-	D44.1-	D49.7
gland	C74.9-	C79.7-	D09.3	D35.0-	D44.1-	D49.7
medulla	C74.1-	C79.7-	D09.3	D35.0-	D44.1-	D49.7
suprasellar (region)	C71.9	C79.31	-	D33.2	D43.2	D49.6
supratentorial (brain)NEC	C71.0	C79.31	-	D33.0	D43.0	D49.6
sweat gland (apocrine) (eccrine), site unspecified	C44.90	C79.2	D04.9	D23.9	D48.5	D49.2
specified site—*see Neoplasm, skin*						
sympathetic nerve or nervous system NEC	C47.9	C79.89	-	D36.10	D48.2	D49.2
symphysis pubis	C41.4	C79.51	-	D16.8	D48.0	D49.2
synovial membrane—*see Neoplasm, connective tissue*						
tapetum, brain	C71.8	C79.31	-	D33.2	D43.2	D49.6
tarsus (any bone)	C40.3-	C79.51	-	D16.3-	-	-
temple (skin)—*see also Neoplasm, skin, face*	C44.309	C79.2	D04.39	D23.39	D48.5	D49.2
temporal						
bone	C41.0	C79.51	-	D16.4-	D48.0	D49.2
lobe or pole	C71.2	C79.31	-	D33.0	D43.0	D49.6
region	C76.0	C79.89	D09.8	D36.7	D48.7	D49.89
skin—*see also Neoplasm, skin, face*	C44.309	C79.2	D04.39	D23.39	D48.5	D49.2
tendon (sheath)—*see Neoplasm, connective tissue*						
tentorium (cerebelli)	C70.0	C79.32	-	D32.0	D42.0	D49.7
testis, testes	C62.9-	C79.82	D07.69	D29.2-	D40.1-	D49.5
descended	C62.1-	C79.82	D07.69	D29.2-	D40.1-	D49.5
ectopic	C62.0-	C79.82	D07.69	D29.2-	D40.1-	D49.5
retained	C62.0-	C79.82	D07.69	D29.2-	D40.1-	D49.5
scrotal	C62.1-	C79.82	D07.69	D29.2-	D40.1-	D49.5
undescended	C62.0-	C79.82	D07.69	D29.2-	D40.1-	D49.5
unspecified whether descended or undescended	C62.9-	C79.82	D07.69	D29.2-	D40.1-	D49.5
thalamus	C71.0	C79.31	-	D33.0	D43.0	D49.6
thigh NEC	C76.5-	C79.89	D04.7-	D36.7	D48.7	D49.89
thorax, thoracic (cavity) (organs NEC)	C76.1	C79.89	D09.8	D36.7	D48.7	D49.89
duct	C49.3	C79.89	-	D21.3	D48.1	D49.2
wall NEC	C76.1	C79.89	D09.8	D36.7	D48.7	D49.89
throat	C14.0	C79.89	D00.08	D10.9	D37.05	D49.0
thumb NEC	C76.4-	C79.89	D04.6-	D36.7	D48.7	D49.89
thymus (gland)	C37	C79.89	D09.3	D15.0	D38.4	D49.89
thyroglossal duct	C73	C79.89	D09.3	D34	D44.0	D49.7
thyroid (gland)	C73	C79.89	D09.3	D34	D44.0	D49.7
cartilage	C32.3	C78.39	D02.0	D14.1	D38.0	D49.1
tibia (any part)	C40.2-	C79.51	-	D16.2-	-	-
toe NEC	C76.5-	C79.89	D04.7-	D36.7	D48.7	D49.89
tongue	C02.9	C79.89	D00.07	D10.1	D37.02	D49.0
anterior (two thirds)NEC	C02.3	C79.89	D00.07	D10.1	D37.02	D49.0
dorsal surface	C02.0	C79.89	D00.07	D10.1	D37.02	D49.0
ventral surface	C02.2	C79.89	D00.07	D10.1	D37.02	D49.0
base (dorsal surface)	C01	C79.89	D00.07	D10.1	D37.02	D49.0
border (lateral)	C02.1	C79.89	D00.07	D10.1	D37.02	D49.0
dorsal surface NEC	C02.0	C79.89	D00.07	D10.1	D37.02	D49.0
fixed part NEC	C01	C79.89	D00.07	D10.1	D37.02	D49.0
foramen cecum	C02.0	C79.89	D00.07	D10.1	D37.02	D49.0
frenulum linguae	C02.2	C79.89	D00.07	D10.1	D37.02	D49.0
junctional zone	C02.8	C79.89	D00.07	D10.1	D37.02	D49.0

	Malignant Primary	Malignant Secondary	Ca in Situ	Benign	Uncertain Behavior	Unspecified Behavior
margin (lateral)	C02.1	C79.89	D00.07	D10.1	D37.02	D49.0
midline NEC	C02.0	C79.89	D00.07	D10.1	D37.02	D49.0
mobile part NEC	C02.3	C79.89	D00.07	D10.1	D37.02	D49.0
overlapping lesion	C02.8	-	-	-	-	-
posterior (third)	C01	C79.89	D00.07	D10.1	D37.02	D49.0
root	C01	C79.89	D00.07	D10.1	D37.02	D49.0
surface (dorsal)	C02.0	C79.89	D00.07	D10.1	D37.02	D49.0
base	C01	C79.89	D00.07	D10.1	D37.02	D49.0
ventral	C02.2	C79.89	D00.07	D10.1	D37.02	D49.0
tip	C02.1	C79.89	D00.07	D10.1	D37.02	D49.0
tonsil	C02.4	C79.89	D00.07	D10.1	D37.02	D49.0
tonsil	C09.9	C79.89	D00.08	D10.4	D37.05	D49.0
fauces, faucial	C09.9	C79.89	D00.08	D10.4	D37.05	D49.0
lingual	C02.4	C79.89	D00.07	D10.1	D37.02	D49.0
overlapping sites	C09.8	-	-	-	-	-
palatine	C09.9	C79.89	D00.08	D10.4	D37.05	D49.0
pharyngeal	C11.1	C79.89	D00.08	D10.6	D37.05	D49.0
pillar (anterior) (posterior)	C09.1	C79.89	D00.08	D10.5	D37.05	D49.0
tonsillar fossa	C09.0	C79.89	D00.08	D10.5	D37.05	D49.0
tooth socket NEC	C03.9	C79.89	D00.03	D10.39	D37.09	D49.0
trachea (cartilage) (mucosa)	C33	C78.39	D02.1	D14.2	D38.1	D49.1
overlapping lesion with bronchus or lung	C34.8-	-	-	-	-	-
tracheobronchial	C34.8-	C78.39	D02.1	D14.2	D38.1	D49.1
overlapping lesion with lung	C34.8-	-	-	-	-	-
tragus—*see also Neoplasm, skin, ear*	C44.20-	C79.2	D04.2-	D23.2-	D48.5	D49.2
trunk NEC	C76.8	C79.89	D04.5	D36.7	D48.7	D49.89
tubo ovarian	C57.8	C79.82	D07.39	D28.7	D39.8	D49.5
tunica vaginalis	C63.7	C79.82	D07.69	D29.8	D40.8	D49.5
turbinate (bone)	C41.0	C79.51	-	D16.4-	D48.0	D49.2
nasal	C30.0	C78.39	D02.3	D14.0	D38.5	D49.1
tympanic cavity	C30.1	C78.39	D02.3	D14.0	D38.5	D49.1
ulna (any part)	C40.0-	C79.51	-	D16.0-	-	-
umbilicus, umbilical—*see also Neoplasm, skin, trunk*	C44.509	C79.2	D04.5	D23.5	D48.5	D49.2
uncus, brain	C71.2	C79.31	-	D33.0	D43.0	D49.6
unknown site or unspecified	C80.1	C79.9	D09.9	D36.9	D48.9	D49.9
urachus	C67.7	C79.11	D09.0	D30.3	D41.4	D49.4
ureter, ureteral	C66.-	C79.19	D09.19	D30.2-	D41.2-	D49.5
orifice (bladder)	C67.6	C79.11	D09.0	D30.3	D41.4	D49.4
ureter bladder (junction)	C67.6	C79.11	D09.0	D30.3	D41.4	D49.4
urethra, urethral (gland)	C68.0	C79.19	D09.19	D30.4	D41.3	D49.5
orifice, internal	C67.5	C79.11	D09.0	D30.3	D41.4	D49.4
urethrovaginal (septum)	C57.9	C79.82	D07.30	D28.9	D39.8	D49.5
urinary organ or system	C68.9	C79.10	D09.10	D30.9	D41.9	D49.5
bladder—*see Neoplasm, bladder*						
overlapping lesion	C68.8	-	-	-	-	-
specified sites NEC	C68.8	C79.19	D09.19	D30.8	D41.8	D49.5
utero ovarian	C57.8	C79.82	D07.39	D28.7	D39.8	D49.5
ligament	C57.1	C79.82	D07.39	D28.2	D39.8	D49.5
uterosacral ligament	C57.3	C79.82	-	D28.2	D39.8	D49.5
uterus, uteri, uterine	C55	C79.82	D07.0	D26.9	D39.0	D49.5
adnexa NEC	C57.4	C79.82	D07.39	D28.7	D39.8	D49.5
body	C54.9	C79.82	D07.0	D26.1	D39.0	D49.5
cervix	C53.9	C79.82	D06.9	D26.0	D39.0	D49.5
cornu	C54.9	C79.82	D07.0	D26.1	D39.0	D49.5
corpus	C54.9	C79.82	D07.0	D26.1	D39.0	D49.5
endocervix (canal) (gland)	C53.0	C79.82	D06.0	D26.0	D39.0	D49.5
endometrium	C54.1	C79.82	D07.0	D26.1	D39.0	D49.5
exocervix	C53.1	C79.82	D06.1	D26.0	D39.0	D49.5
external os	C53.1	C79.82	D06.1	D26.0	D39.0	D49.5
fundus	C54.3	C79.82	D07.0	D26.1	D39.0	D49.5
internal os	C53.0	C79.82	D06.0	D26.0	D39.0	D49.5
isthmus	C54.0	C79.82	D07.0	D26.1	D39.0	D49.5
ligament	C57.3	C79.82	-	D28.2	D39.8	D49.5
broad	C57.1	C79.82	D07.39	D28.2	D39.8	D49.5
round	C57.2	C79.82	-	D28.2	D39.8	D49.5
lower segment	C54.0	C79.82	D07.0	D26.1	D39.0	D49.5
myometrium	C54.2	C79.82	D07.0	D26.1	D39.0	D49.5
overlapping sites	C54.8	-	-	-	-	-

	Malignant Primary	Malignant Secondary	Ca in Situ	Benign	Uncertain Behavior	Unspecified Behavior
squamocolumnar junction	C53.8	C79.82	D06.7	D26.0	D39.0	D49.5
tube	C57.0-	C79.82	D07.39	D28.2	D39.8	D49.5
utricle, prostatic	C68.0	C79.19	D09.19	D30.4	D41.3	D49.5
uveal tract	C69.4-	C79.49	D09.2-	D31.4-	D48.7	D49.89
uvula	C05.2	C79.89	D00.04	D10.39	D37.09	D49.0
vagina, vaginal (fornix) (vault) (wall)	C52	C79.82	D07.2	D28.1	D39.8	D49.5
vaginovesical	C57.9	C79.82	D07.30	D28.9	D39.9	D49.5
septum	C57.9	C79.82	D07.30	D28.9	D39.9	D49.5
vallecula (epiglottis)	C10.0	C79.89	D00.08	D10.5	D37.05	D49.0
vas deferens	C63.1-	C79.82	D07.69	D29.8	D40.8	D49.5
vascular—*see Neoplasm, connective tissue*						
Vater's ampulla	C24.1	C78.89	D01.5	D13.5	D37.6	D49.0
vein, venous—*see Neoplasm, connective tissue*						
vena cava (abdominal) (inferior)	C49.4	C79.89	-	D21.4	D48.1	D49.2
superior	C49.3	C79.89	-	D21.3	D48.1	D49.2
ventricle (cerebral) (floor) (lateral) (third)	C71.5	C79.31	-	D33.0	D43.0	D49.6
cardiac (left) (right)	C38.0	C79.89	-	D15.1	D48.7	D49.89
fourth	C71.7	C79.31	-	D33.1	D43.1	D49.6
ventricular band of larynx	C32.1	C78.39	D02.0	D14.1	D38.0	D49.1
ventriculus—*see Neoplasm, stomach*						
vermillion border—*see Neoplasm, lip*						
vermis, cerebellum	C71.6	C79.31	-	D33.1	D43.1	D49.6
vertebra (column)	C41.2	C79.51	-	D16.6	D48.0	D49.2
coccyx	C41.4	C79.51	-	D16.8-	D48.0	D49.2
marrow NEC	C96.9	C79.52	-	-	D47.9	D49.89
sacrum	C41.4	C79.51	-	D16.8-	D48.0	D49.2
vesical—*see Neoplasm, bladder*						
vesicle, seminal	C63.7	C79.82	D07.69	D29.8	D40.8	D49.5
vesicocervical tissue	C57.9	C79.82	D07.30	D28.9	D39.9	D49.5
vesicorectal	C76.3	C79.82	D09.8	D36.7	D48.7	D49.89
vesicovaginal	C57.9	C79.82	D07.30	D28.9	D39.9	D49.5
septum	C57.9	C79.82	D07.30	D28.9	D39.8	D49.5
vessel (blood)—*see Neoplasm, connective tissue*						
vestibular gland, greater	C51.0	C79.82	D07.1	D28.0	D39.8	D49.5
vestibule						
mouth	C06.1	C79.89	D00.00	D10.39	D37.09	D49.0
nose	C30.0	C78.39	D02.3	D14.0	D38.5	D49.1
Virchow's gland	C77.0-	C77.0	-	D36.0	D48.7	D49.89
viscera NEC	C76.8	C79.89	D09.8	D36.7	D48.7	D49.89
vocal cords (true)	C32.0	C78.39	D02.0	D14.1	D38.0	D49.1
false	C32.1	C78.39	D02.0	D14.1	D38.0	D49.1
vomer	C41.0	C79.51	-	D16.4-	D48.0	D49.2
vulva	C51.9	C79.82	D07.1	D28.0	D39.8	D49.5
vulvovaginal gland	C51.0	C79.82	D07.1	D28.0	D39.8	D49.5
Waldeyer's ring	C14.2	C79.89	D00.08	D10.9	D37.05	D49.0
Wharton's duct	C08.0	C79.89	D00.00	D11.7	D37.032	D49.0
white matter (central) (cerebral)	C71.0	C79.31	-	D33.0	D43.0	D49.6
windpipe	C33	C78.39	D02.1	D14.2	D38.1	D49.1
Wirsung's duct	C25.3	C78.89	D01.7	D13.6	D37.8	D49.0
wolffian (body) (duct)						
female	C57.7	C79.82	D07.39	D28.7	D39.8	D49.5
male	C63.7	C79.82	D07.69	D29.8	D40.8	D49.5
womb—*see Neoplasm, uterus*						
wrist NEC	C76.4-	C79.89	D04.6-	D36.7	D48.7	D49.89
xiphoid process	C41.3	C79.51	-	D16.7	D48.0	D49.2
Zuckerkandl organ	C75.5	C79.89	-	D35.6	D44.7	D49.7

Neovascularization - *continued*
  localized H16.43
  pannus —*see* Pannus
  iris —*see* Disorder, iris, vascular
  retina H35.05
Nephralgia N23
Nephritis, nephritic (albuminuric) (azotemic)
(congenital) (disseminated) (epithelial)
(familial) (focal) (granulomatous)
(hemorrhagic) (infantile) (nonsuppurative,
excretory) (uremic) N05.9
  with
    dense deposit disease N05.6
    diffuse
      crescentic glomerulonephritis N05.7
      endocapillary proliferative
  glomerulonephritis N05.4
      membranous glomerulonephritis N05.2
      mesangial proliferative glomerulonephritis
  N05.3
      mesangiocapillary glomerulonephritis
  N05.5
    edema —*see* Nephrosis
    focal and segmental glomerular lesions
  N05.1
    foot process disease N04.9
    glomerular lesion
      diffuse sclerosing N05.8
      hypocomplementemic —*see* Nephritis,
  membranoproliferative
      IgA —*see* Nephropathy, IgA
      lobular, lobulonodular —*see* Nephritis,
  membranoproliferative
      nodular —*see* Nephritis,
  membranoproliferative
    lesion of
      glomerulonephritis, proliferative N05.8
      renal necrosis N05.9
    minor glomerular abnormality N05.0
    specified morphological changes NEC
  N05.8
  acute N00.9
    with
      dense deposit disease N00.6
      diffuse
        crescentic glomerulonephritis N00.7
        endocapillary proliferative
    glomerulonephritis N00.4
        membranous glomerulonephritis N00.2
        mesangial proliferative
    glomerulonephritis N00.3
        mesangiocapillary glomerulonephritis
    N00.5
      focal and segmental glomerular lesions
    N00.1
      minor glomerular abnormality N00.0
      specified morphological changes NEC
    N00.8
  amyloid E85.4 *[N08]*
  antiglomerular basement membrane (anti-
  GBM) antibody NEC
    in Goodpasture's syndrome M31.0
  antitubular basement membrane (tubulo-
  interstitial) NEC N12
    toxic —*see* Nephropathy, toxic
  arteriolar —*see* Hypertension, kidney
  arteriosclerotic —*see* Hypertension, kidney
  ascending —*see* Nephritis, tubulo-interstitial
  atrophic N03.9
  Balkan (endemic) N15.0
  calculous, calculus —*see* Calculus, kidney
  cardiac —*see* Hypertension, kidney

Nephritis, nephritic – *continued*
  cardiovascular —*see* Hypertension, kidney
  chronic N03.9
    with
      dense deposit disease N03.6
      diffuse
        crescentic glomerulonephritis N03.7
        endocapillary proliferative
    glomerulonephritis N03.4
        membranous glomerulonephritis N03.2
        mesangial proliferative
    glomerulonephritis N03.3
        mesangiocapillary glomerulonephritis
    N03.5
      focal and segmental glomerular lesions
    N03.1
      minor glomerular abnormality N03.0
      specified morphological changes NEC
    N03.8
  arteriosclerotic —*see* Hypertension, kidney
  cirrhotic N26.9
  complicating pregnancy O26.83
  croupous N00.9
  degenerative —*see* Nephrosis
  diffuse sclerosing N05.8
  due to
    diabetes mellitus —*see* E08-E13 with .21
    subacute bacterial endocarditis I33.0
    systemic lupus erythematosus (chronic)
  M32.14
    typhoid fever A01.09
  gonococcal (acute) (chronic) A54.21
  hypocomplementemic —*see* Nephritis,
  membranoproliferative
  IgA —*see* Nephropathy, IgA
  immune complex (circulating) NEC N05.8
  infective —*see* Nephritis, tubulo-interstitial
  interstitial —*see* Nephritis, tubulo-interstitial
  lead N14.3
  membranoproliferative (diffuse) (type 1 or 3)
  (*see also* N00-N07 with fourth character .5)
  N05.5
    type 2 (*see also* N00-N07 with fourth
  character .6) N05.6
  minimal change N05.0
  necrotic, necrotizing NEC (*see also* N00-N07
  with fourth character .8) N05.8
  nephrotic —*see* Nephrosis
  nodular —*see* Nephritis,
  membranoproliferative
  polycystic Q61.3
    adult type Q61.2
    autosomal
      dominant Q61.2
      recessive NEC Q61.19
    childhood type NEC Q61.19
    infantile type NEC Q61.19
  poststreptococcal N05.9
    acute N00.9
    chronic N03.9
    rapidly progressive N01.9
  proliferative NEC (*see also* N00-N07 with
  fourth character .8) N05.8
  purulent —*see* Nephritis, tubulo-interstitial
  rapidly progressive N01.9
    with
      dense deposit disease N01.6
      diffuse
        crescentic glomerulonephritis N01.7
        endocapillary proliferative
    glomerulonephritis N01.4
        membranous glomerulonephritis N01.2

Nephritis, nephritic – *continued*
    mesangial proliferative
  glomerulonephritis N01.3
        mesangiocapillary glomerulonephritis
  N01.5
      focal and segmental glomerular lesions
  N01.1
      minor glomerular abnormality N01.0
      specified morphological changes NEC
  N01.8
  salt losing or wasting NEC N28.89
  saturnine N14.3
  sclerosing, diffuse N05.8
  septic —*see* Nephritis, tubulo-interstitial
  specified pathology NEC (*see also* N00-N07
  with fourth character .8) N05.8
  subacute N01.9
  suppurative —*see* Nephritis, tubulo-interstitial
  syphilitic (late) A52.75
    congenital A50.59 *[N08]*
    early (secondary) A51.44
  toxic —*see* Nephropathy, toxic
  tubal, tubular —*see* Nephritis, tubulo-
  interstitial
  tuberculous A18.11
  tubulo-interstitial (in) N12
    acute (infectious) N10
    chronic (infectious) N11.9
      nonobstructive N11.8
        reflux-associated N11.0
      obstructive N11.1
      specified NEC N11.8
    due to
      brucellosis A23.9 *[N16]*
      cryoglobulinemia D89.1 *[N16]*
      glycogen storage disease E74.00 *[N16]*
      Sjögren's syndrome M35.04
    vascular —*see* Hypertension, kidney
  war N00.9
Nephroblastoma (epithelial) (mesenchymal)
C64
Nephrocalcinosis E83.59 *[N29]*
Nephrocystitis, pustular —*see* Nephritis,
tubulo-interstitial
Nephrolithiasis (congenital) (pelvis)
(recurrent) —*see also* Calculus, kidney
Nephroma C64
  mesoblastic D41.0
Nephronephritis —*see* Nephrosis
Nephronophthisis Q61.5
Nephropathia epidemica A98.5
Nephropathy (*see also* Nephritis) N28.9
  with
    edema —*see* Nephrosis
    glomerular lesion —*see* Glomerulonephritis
  amyloid, hereditary E85.0
  analgesic N14.0
    with medullary necrosis, acute N17.2
  Balkan (endemic) N15.0
  chemical —*see* Nephropathy, toxic
  diabetic —*see* E08-E13 with .21
  drug-induced N14.2
    specified NEC N14.1
  focal and segmental hyalinosis or sclerosis
  N02.1
  heavy metal-induced N14.3
  hereditary NEC N07.9
    with
      dense deposit disease N07.6
      diffuse
        crescentic glomerulonephritis N07.7
        endocapillary proliferative
  glomerulonephritis N07.4

Nephropathy - *continued*
  membranous glomerulonephritis N07.2
  mesangial proliferative
glomerulonephritis N07.3
    mesangiocapillary glomerulonephritis
N07.5
    focal and segmental glomerular lesions
N07.1
      minor glomerular abnormality N07.0
      specified morphological changes NEC
N07.8
  hypercalcemic N25.89
  hypertensive —*see* Hypertension, kidney
  hypokalemic (vacuolar) N25.89
  IgA N02.8
   with glomerular lesion N02.9
    focal and segmental hyalinosis or sclerosis
N02.1
      membranoproliferative (diffuse) N02.5
      membranous (diffuse) N02.2
      mesangial proliferative (diffuse) N02.3
      mesangiocapillary (diffuse) N02.5
      proliferative NEC N02.8
      specified pathology NEC N02.8
  lead N14.3
  membranoproliferative (diffuse) N02.5
  membranous (diffuse) N02.2
  mesangial (IgA/IgG) —*see* Nephropathy, IgA
   proliferative (diffuse) N02.3
  mesangiocapillary (diffuse) N02.5
  obstructive N13.8
  phenacetin N17.2
  phosphate-losing N25.0
  potassium depletion N25.89
  pregnancy-related O26.83
  proliferative NEC (*see also* N00-N07 with
fourth character .8) N05.8
  protein-losing N25.89
  saturnine N14.3
  sickle-cell D57. *[N08]*
  toxic NEC N14.4
   due to
    drugs N14.2
     analgesic N14.0
     specified NEC N14.1
    heavy metals N14.3
  vasomotor N17.0
  water-losing N25.89
Nephroptosis N28.83
Nephropyosis —*see* Abscess, kidney
Nephrorrhagia N28.89
Nephrosclerosis (arteriolar) (arteriosclerotic)
(chronic) (hyaline) —*see also* Hypertension,
kidney
  hyperplastic —*see* Hypertension, kidney
  senile N26.9
Nephrosis, nephrotic (Epstein's) (syndrome)
(congenital) N04.9
  with
   foot process disease N04.9
   glomerular lesion N04.1
   hypocomplementemic N04.5
  acute N04.9
  anoxic —*see* Nephrosis, tubular
  chemical —*see* Nephrosis, tubular
  cholemic K76.7
  diabetic —*see* E08-E13 with .21
  Finnish type (congenital) Q89.8
  hemoglobin N10
  hemoglobinuric —*see* Nephrosis, tubular
  in
   amyloidosis E85.4 *[N08]*

Nephrosis, nephrotic - *continued*
  diabetes mellitus —*see* E08-E13 with .21
  epidemic hemorrhagic fever A98.5
  malaria (malariae) B52.0
  ischemic —*see* Nephrosis, tubular
  lipoid N04.9
  lower nephron —*see* Nephrosis, tubular
  malarial (malariae) B52.0
  minimal change N04.0
  myoglobin N10
  necrotizing —*see* Nephrosis, tubular
  osmotic (sucrose) N25.89
  radiation N04.9
  syphilitic (late) A52.75
  toxic —*see* Nephrosis, tubular
  tubular (acute) N17.0
   postprocedural N99.0
   radiation N04.9
Nephrosonephritis, hemorrhagic (endemic)
A98.5
Nephrostomy
  attention to Z43.6
  status Z93.6
Nerve —*see also* condition
  injury —*see* Injury, nerve, by body site
Nerves R45.0
Nervous (*see also* condition) R45.0
  heart F45.8
  stomach F45.8
  tension R45.0
Nervousness R45.0
Nesidioblastoma
  pancreas D13.7
  specified site NEC —*see* Neoplasm, benign,
by site
  unspecified site D13.7
Nettleship's syndrome Q82.2
Neumann's disease or syndrome L10.1
Neuralgia, neuralgic (acute) M79.2
  accessory (nerve) G52.8
  acoustic (nerve) —*see* subcategory H93.3
  auditory (nerve) —*see* subcategory H93.3
  ciliary G44.009
   intractable G44.001
   not intractable G44.009
  cranial
   nerve —*see also* Disorder, nerve, cranial
   fifth or trigeminal —*see* Neuralgia,
trigeminal
   postherpetic, postzoster B02.29
  ear —*see* subcategory H92.0
  facialis vera G51.1
  Fothergill's —*see* Neuralgia, trigeminal
  glossopharyngeal (nerve) G52.1
  Horton's G44.099
   intractable G44.091
   not intractable G44.099
  Hunt's B02.21
  hypoglossal (nerve) G52.3
  infraorbital —*see* Neuralgia, trigeminal
  malarial —*see* Malaria
  migrainous G44.009
   intractable G44.001
   not intractable G44.009
  Morton's G57.6
  nerve, cranial —*see* Disorder, nerve, cranial
  nose G52.0
  occipital M54.81
  olfactory G52.0
  penis N48.9
  perineum R10.2

Neuralgia, neuralgic – *continued*
  postherpetic NEC B02.29
   trigeminal B02.22
  pubic region R10.2
  scrotum R10.2
  Sluder's G44.89
  specified nerve NEC G58.8
  spermatic cord R10.2
  sphenopalatine (ganglion) G90.09
  trifacial —*see* Neuralgia, trigeminal
  trigeminal G50.0
   postherpetic, postzoster B02.22
  vagus (nerve) G52.2
  writer's F48.8
   organic G25.89
Neurapraxia —*see* Injury, nerve
Neurasthenia F48.8
  cardiac F45.8
  gastric F45.8
  heart F45.8
Neurilemmoma —*see also* Neoplasm, nerve,
benign
  acoustic (nerve) D33.3
  malignant —*see also* Neoplasm, nerve,
malignant
   acoustic (nerve) C72.4
Neurilemmosarcoma —*see* Neoplasm, nerve,
malignant
Neurinoma —*see* Neoplasm, nerve, benign
Neurinomatosis —*see* Neoplasm, nerve,
uncertain behavior
Neuritis (rheumatoid) M79.2
  abducens (nerve) —*see* Strabismus, paralytic,
sixth nerve
  accessory (nerve) G52.8
  acoustic (nerve) (*see also* subcategory) H93.3
  in (due to)
   infectious disease NEC B99 *[H94.0]*
   parasitic disease NEC B89 *[H94.0]*
   syphilitic A52.15
  alcoholic G62.1
   with psychosis —*see* Psychosis, alcoholic
  amyloid, any site E85.4 *[G63]*
  auditory (nerve) —*see* subcategory H93.3
  brachial —*see* Radiculopathy
  due to displacement, intervertebral disc —
see Disorder, disc, cervical, with neuritis
  cranial nerve
   due to Lyme disease A69.22
   eighth or acoustic or auditory —*see*
subcategory H93.3
   eleventh or accessory G52.8
   fifth or trigeminal G51.0
   first or olfactory G52.0
   fourth or trochlear —*see* Strabismus,
paralytic, fourth nerve
   second or optic —*see* Neuritis, optic
   seventh or facial G51.8
    newborn (birth injury) P11.3
   sixth or abducent —*see* Strabismus,
paralytic, sixth nerve
   tenth or vagus G52.2
   third or oculomotor —*see* Strabismus,
paralytic, third nerve
   twelfth or hypoglossal G52.3
  Déjérine-Sottas G60.0
  diabetic (mononeuropathy) —*see* E08-E13
with .41
   polyneuropathy —*see* E08-E13 with .42
  due to
   beriberi E51.11

Neuritis – *continued*
  displacement, prolapse or rupture, intervertebral disc —*see* Disorder, disc, with, radiculopathy
    herniation, nucleus pulposus M51.9 *[G55]*
  endemic E51.11
  facial G51.8
    newborn (birth injury) P11.3
  general —*see* Polyneuropathy
  geniculate ganglion G51.1
    due to herpes (zoster) B02.21
  gouty M10.00 *[G63]*
  hypoglossal (nerve) G52.3
  ilioinguinal (nerve) G57.9
  infectious (multiple) NEC G61.0
  interstitial hypertrophic progressive G60.0
  lumbar M54.16
  lumbosacral M54.17
  multiple —*see also* Polyneuropathy
    endemic E51.11
    infective, acute G61.0
  multiplex endemica E51.11
  nerve root —*see* Radiculopathy
  oculomotor (nerve) —*see* Strabismus, paralytic, third nerve
  olfactory nerve G52.0
  optic (nerve) (hereditary) (sympathetic) H46.9
    with demyelination G36.0
    in myelitis G36.0
    nutritional H46.2
    papillitis —*see* Papillitis, optic
    retrobulbar H46.1
    specified type NEC H46.8
    toxic H46.3
  peripheral (nerve) G62.9
    multiple —*see* Polyneuropathy
    single —*see* Mononeuritis
  pneumogastric (nerve) G52.2
  postherpetic, postzoster B02.29
  progressive hypertrophic interstitial G60.0
  retrobulbar —*see also* Neuritis, optic, retrobulbar
    in (due to)
      late syphilis A52.15
      meningococcal infection A39.82
    meningococcal A39.82
    syphilitic A52.15
  sciatic (nerve) —*see also* Sciatica
    due to displacement of intervertebral disc —*see* Disorder, disc, with, radiculopathy
  serum (*see also* Reaction, serum) T80.69
  shoulder-girdle G54.5
  specified nerve NEC G58.8
  spinal (nerve) root —*see* Radiculopathy
  syphilitic A52.15
  thenar (median) G56.1
  thoracic M54.14
  toxic NEC G62.2
  trochlear (nerve) —*see* Strabismus, paralytic, fourth nerve
  vagus (nerve) G52.2
Neuroastrocytoma —*see* Neoplasm, uncertain behavior, by site
Neuroavitaminosis E56.9 *[G99.8]*
Neuroblastoma
  olfactory C30.0
  specified site —*see* Neoplasm, malignant, by site
  unspecified site C74.90
Neurochorioretinitis —*see* Chorioretinitis
Neurocirculatory asthenia F45.8
Neurocysticercosis B69.0
Neurocytoma —*see* Neoplasm, benign, by site

Neurodermatitis (circumscribed) (circumscripta) (local) L28.0
  atopic L20.81
  diffuse (Brocq) L20.81
  disseminated L20.81
Neuroencephalomyelopathy, optic G36.0
Neuroepithelioma —*see also* Neoplasm, malignant, by site
  olfactory C30.0
Neurofibroma —*see also* Neoplasm, nerve, benign
  melanotic —*see* Neoplasm, nerve, benign
  multiple —*see* Neurofibromatosis
  plexiform —*see* Neoplasm, nerve, benign
Neurofibromatosis (multiple) (nonmalignant) Q85.00
  acoustic Q85.02
  malignant —*see* Neoplasm, nerve, malignant
  specified NEC Q85.09
  type 1 (von Recklinghausen) Q85.01
  type 2 Q85.02
Neurofibrosarcoma —*see* Neoplasm, nerve, malignant
Neurogenic —*see also* condition
  bladder (*see also* Dysfunction, bladder, neuromuscular) N31.9
    cauda equina syndrome G83.4
  bowel NEC K59.2
  heart F45.8
Neuroglioma —*see* Neoplasm, uncertain behavior, by site
Neurolabyrinthitis (of Dix and Hallpike) —*see* Neuronitis, vestibular
Neurolathyrism —*see* Poisoning, food, noxious, plant
Neuroleprosy A30.9
Neuroma —*see also* Neoplasm, nerve, benign
  acoustic (nerve) D33.3
  amputation (stump) (traumatic) (surgical complication) (late) T87.3
    arm T87.3
    leg T87.3
  digital (toe) G57.6
  interdigital (toe) G58.8
    lower limb G57.8
    upper limb G56.8
  intermetatarsal G57.8
  Morton's G57.6
  nonneoplastic
    arm G56.9
    leg G57.9
    lower extremity G57.9
    upper extremity G56.9
  optic (nerve) D33.3
  plantar G57.6
  plexiform —*see* Neoplasm, nerve, benign
  surgical (nonneoplastic)
    arm G56.9
    leg G57.9
    lower extremity G57.9
    upper extremity G56.9
Neuromyalgia —*see* Neuralgia
Neuromyasthenia (epidemic) (postinfectious) G93.3
Neuromyelitis G36.9
  ascending G61.0
  optica G36.0
Neuromyopathy G70.9
  paraneoplastic D49.9 *[G13.0]*
Neuromyotonia (Isaacs) G71.19
Neuronevus —*see* Nevus

Neuronitis G58.9
  ascending (acute) G57.2
  vestibular H81.2
Neuroparalytic —*see* condition
Neuropathy, neuropathic G62.9
  acute motor G62.81
  alcoholic G62.1
    with psychosis —*see* Psychosis, alcoholic
  arm G56.9
  autonomic, peripheral —*see* Neuropathy, peripheral, autonomic
  axillary G56.9
  bladder N31.9
    atonic (motor) (sensory) N31.2
    autonomous N31.2
    flaccid N31.2
    nonreflex N31.2
    reflex N31.1
    uninhibited N31.0
  brachial plexus G54.0
  cervical plexus G54.2
  chronic
    progressive segmentally demyelinating G62.89
    relapsing demyelinating G62.89
  Déjérine-Sottas G60.0
  diabetic —*see* E08-E13 with .40
    mononeuropathy —*see* E08-E13 with .41
    polyneuropathy —*see* E08-E13 with .42
  entrapment G58.9
    iliohypogastric nerve G57.8
    ilioinguinal nerve G57.8
    lateral cutaneous nerve of thigh G57.1
    median nerve G56.0
    obturator nerve G57.8
    peroneal nerve G57.3
    posterior tibial nerve G57.5
    saphenous nerve G57.8
    ulnar nerve G56.2
  facial nerve G51.9
  hereditary G60.9
    motor and sensory (types I-IV) G60.0
    sensory G60.8
    specified NEC G60.8
  hypertrophic G60.0
    Charcot-Marie-Tooth G60.0
    Déjérine-Sottas G60.0
    interstitial progressive G60.0
    of infancy G60.0
    Refsum G60.1
  idiopathic G60.9
    progressive G60.3
    specified NEC G60.8
  in association with hereditary ataxia G60.2
  intercostal G58.0
  ischemic —*see* Disorder, nerve
  Jamaica (ginger) G62.2
  leg NEC G57.9
  lower extremity G57.9
  lumbar plexus G54.1
  median nerve G56.1
  motor and sensory —*see also* Polyneuropathy
    hereditary (types I-IV) G60.0
  multiple (acute) (chronic) —*see* Polyneuropathy
  optic (nerve) —*see also* Neuritis, optic
    ischemic H47.01
  paraneoplastic (sensorial) (Denny Brown) D49.9 *[G13.0]*
  peripheral (nerve) (*see also* Polyneuropathy) G62.9
    autonomic G90.9

Neuropathy, neuropathic – *continued*
  idiopathic G90.09
  in (due to)
    amyloidosis E85.4 *[G99.0]*
    diabetes mellitus —*see* E08-E13 with .43
    endocrine disease NEC E34.9 *[G99.0]*
    gout M10.00 *[G99.0]*
    hyperthyroidism E05.90 *[G99.0]*
      with thyroid storm E05.91 *[G99.0]*
    metabolic disease NEC E88.9 *[G99.0]*
  idiopathic G60.9
    progressive G60.3
  in (due to)
    antitetanus serum G62.0
    arsenic G62.2
    drugs NEC G62.0
    lead G62.2
    organophosphate compounds G62.2
    toxic agent NEC G62.2
  plantar nerves G57.6
  progressive
    hypertrophic interstitial G60.0
    inflammatory G62.81
  radicular NEC —*see* Radiculopathy
  sacral plexus G54.1
  sciatic G57.0
  serum G61.1
  toxic NEC G62.2
  trigeminal sensory G50.8
  ulnar nerve G56.2
  uremic N18.9 *[G63]*
  vitamin B12 E53.8 *[G63]*
    with anemia (pernicious) D51.0 *[G63]*
    due to dietary deficiency D51.3 *[G63]*
Neurophthisis —*see also* Disorder, nerve
  peripheral, diabetic —*see* E08-E13 with .42
Neuroretinitis —*see* Chorioretinitis
Neuroretinopathy, hereditary optic H47.22
Neurosarcoma —*see* Neoplasm, nerve,
  malignant
Neurosclerosis —*see* Disorder, nerve
Neurosis, neurotic F48.9
  anankastic F42
  anxiety (state) F41.1
    panic type F41.0
  asthenic F48.8
  bladder F45.8
  cardiac (reflex) F45.8
  cardiovascular F45.8
  character F60.9
  colon F45.8
  compensation F68.1
  compulsive, compulsion F42
  conversion F44.9
  craft F48.8
  cutaneous F45.8
  depersonalization F48.1
  depressive (reaction) (type) F34.1
  environmental F48.8
  excoriation L98.1
  fatigue F48.8
  functional —*see* Disorder, somatoform
  gastric F45.8
  gastrointestinal F45.8
  heart F45.8
  hypochondriacal F45.21
  hysterical F44.9
  incoordination F45.8
    larynx F45.8
    vocal cord F45.8
  intestine F45.8
  larynx (sensory) F45.8

Neurosis, neurotic – *continued*
  hysterical F44.4
  mixed NEC F48.8
  musculoskeletal F45.8
  obsessional F42
  obsessive-compulsive F42
  occupational F48.8
  ocular NEC F45.8
  organ —*see* Disorder, somatoform
  pharynx F45.8
  phobic F40.9
  posttraumatic (situational) F43.10
    acute F43.11
    chronic F43.12
  psychasthenic (type) F48.8
  railroad F48.8
  rectum F45.8
  respiratory F45.8
  rumination F45.8
  sexual F65.9
  situational F48.8
  social F40.10
    generalized F40.11
  specified type NEC F48.8
  state F48.9
    with depersonalization episode F48.1
  stomach F45.8
  traumatic F43.10
    acute F43.11
    chronic F43.12
  vasomotor F45.8
  visceral F45.8
  war F48.8
Neurospongioblastosis diffusa Q85.1
Neurosyphilis (arrested) (early) (gumma) (late)
  (latent) (recurrent) (relapse) A52.3
  with ataxia (cerebellar) (locomotor) (spastic)
    (spinal) A52.19
  aneurysm (cerebral) A52.05
  arachnoid (adhesive) A52.13
  arteritis (any artery) (cerebral) A52.04
  asymptomatic A52.2
  congenital A50.40
  dura (mater) A52.13
  general paresis A52.17
  hemorrhagic A52.05
  juvenile (asymptomatic) (meningeal) A50.40
  leptomeninges (aseptic) A52.13
  meningeal, meninges (adhesive) A52.13
  meningitis A52.13
  meningovascular (diffuse) A52.13
  optic atrophy A52.15
  parenchymatous (degenerative) A52.19
  paresis, paretic A52.17
    juvenile A50.45
  remission in (sustained) A52.3
  serological (without symptoms) A52.2
  specified nature or site NEC A52.19
  tabes, tabetic (dorsalis) A52.11
    juvenile A50.45
  taboparesis A52.17
    juvenile A50.45
  thrombosis (cerebral) A52.05
  vascular (cerebral) NEC A52.05
Neurothekeoma —*see* Neoplasm, nerve,
  benign
Neurotic —*see* Neurosis
Neurotoxemia —*see* Toxemia
Neutroclusion M26.211

Neutropenia, neutropenic (chronic) (genetic)
  (idiopathic) (immune) (infantile) (malignant)
  (pernicious) (splenic) D70.9
  congenital (primary) D70.0
  cyclic D70.4
  cytoreductive cancer chemotherapy sequela
    D70.1
  drug-induced D70.2
    due to cytoreductive cancer chemotherapy
      D70.1
  due to infection D70.3
  fever D70.9
  neonatal, transitory (isoimmune) (maternal
    transfer) P61.5
  periodic D70.4
  secondary (cyclic) (periodic) (splenic) D70.4
    drug-induced D70.2
      due to cytoreductive cancer chemotherapy
        D70.1
  toxic D70.8
Neutrophilia, hereditary giant D72.0
Nevocarcinoma —*see* Melanoma
Nevus D22.9
  achromic —*see* Neoplasm, skin, benign
  amelanotic —*see* Neoplasm, skin, benign
  angiomatousD18.00
    intra-abdominal D18.03
    intracranial D18.02
    skin D18.01
    specified site NEC D18.09
  araneus I78.1
  balloon cell —*see* Neoplasm, skin, benign
  bathing trunk D48.5
  blue —*see* Neoplasm, skin, benign
    cellular —*see* Neoplasm, skin, benign
    giant —*see* Neoplasm, skin, benign
    Jadassohn's —*see* Neoplasm, skin, benign
    malignant —*see* Melanoma
  capillary D18.00
    intra-abdominal D18.03
    intracranial D18.02
    skin D18.01
    specified site NEC D18.09
  cavernous D18.00
    intra-abdominal D18.03
    intracranial D18.02
    skin D18.01
    specified site NEC D18.09
  cellular —*see* Neoplasm, skin, benign
    blue —*see* Neoplasm, skin, benign
  choroid D31.3
  comedonicus Q82.5
  conjunctiva D31.0
  dermal —*see* Neoplasm, skin, benign
    with epidermal nevus —*see* Neoplasm, skin,
    benign
  dysplastic —*see* Neoplasm, skin, benign
  eye D31.9
  flammeus Q82.5
  hemangiomatous D18.00
    intra-abdominal D18.03
    intracranial D18.02
    skin D18.01
    specified site NEC D18.09
  iris D31.4
  lacrimal gland D31.5
  lymphatic D18.1
  magnocellular
    specified site —*see* Neoplasm, benign, by
    site
      unspecified site D31.40
  malignant —*see* Melanoma
  meaning hemangioma D18.00

Nevus - *continued*
  intra-abdominal D18.03
  intracranial D18.02
    skin D18.01
    specified site NEC D18.09
  mouth (mucosa) D10.30
    specified site NEC D10.39
    white sponge Q38.6
  multiplex Q85.1
  non-neoplastic I78.1
  oral mucosa D10.30
    specified site NEC D10.39
    white sponge Q38.6
  orbit D31.6
  pigmented
    giant (*see also* Neoplasm, skin, uncertain
  behavior) D48.5
      malignant melanoma in —*see* Melanoma
  port-wine Q82.5
  retina D31.2
  retrobulbar D31.6
  sanguineous Q82.5
  senile I78.1
  skin D22.9
    abdominal wall D22.5
    ala nasi D22.39
    ankle D22.7
    anus, anal D22.5
    arm D22.6
    auditory canal (external) D22.2
    auricle (ear) D22.2
    auricular canal (external) D22.2
    axilla, axillary fold D22.5
    back D22.5
    breast D22.5
    brow D22.39
    buttock D22.5
    canthus (eye) D22.1
    cheek (external) D22.39
    chest wall D22.5
    chin D22.39
    ear (external) D22.2
    external meatus (ear) D22.2
    eyebrow D22.39
    eyelid (lower) (upper) D22.1
    face D22.30
      specified NEC D22.39
    female genital organ (external) NEC D28.0
    finger D22.6
    flank D22.5
    foot D22.7
    forearm D22.6
    forehead D22.39
    foreskin D29.0
    genital organ (external) NEC
      female D28.0
      male D29.9
    gluteal region D22.5
    groin D22.5
    hand D22.6
    heel D22.7
    helix D22.2
    hip D22.7
    interscapular region D22.5
    jaw D22.39
    knee D22.7
    labium (majus) (minus) D28.0
    leg D22.7
    lip (lower) (upper) D22.0
    lower limb D22.7
    male genital organ (external) D29.9
    nail D22.9

Nevus – *continued*
  finger D22.6
  toe D22.7
  nasolabial groove D22.39
  nates D22.5
  neck D22.4
  nose (external) D22.39
  palpebra D22.1
  penis D29.0
  perianal skin D22.5
  perineum D22.5
  pinna D22.2
  popliteal fossa or space D22.7
  prepuce D29.0
  pudendum D28.0
  scalp D22.4
  scrotum D29.4
  shoulder D22.6
  submammary fold D22.5
  temple D22.39
  thigh D22.7
  toe D22.7
  trunk NEC D22.5
  umbilicus D22.5
  upper limb D22.6
  vulva D28.0
  specified site NEC —*see* Neoplasm, by site,
  benign
  spider I78.1
  stellar I78.1
  strawberry Q82.5
  Sutton's —*see* Neoplasm, skin, benign
  unius lateris Q82.5
  Unna's Q82.5
  vascular Q82.5
  verrucous Q82.5
Newborn (infant) (liveborn) (singleton) Z38.2
  acne L70.4
  abstinence syndrome P96.1
  affected by (suspected to be)
    abnormalities of membranes P02.9
      specified NEC P02.8
    abruptio placenta P02.1
    amino-acid metabolic disorder, transitory
    P74.8
    amniocentesis (while in utero) P00.6
    amnionitis P02.7
    apparent life threatening event (ALTE)
    R68.13
    bleeding (into)
      cerebral cortex P52.22
      germinal matrix P52.0
      ventricles P52.1
    breech delivery P03.0
    cardiac arrest P29.81
    cardiomyopathy I42.8
      congenital I42.4
    cerebral ischemia P91.0
    Cesarean delivery P03.4
    chemotherapy agents P04.1
    chorioamnionitis P02.7
    cocaine (crack) P04.41
    complications of labor and delivery P03.9
      specified NEC P03.89
    compression of umbilical cord NEC P02.5
    contracted pelvis P03.1
    delivery P03.9
      Cesarean P03.4
      forceps P03.2
      vacuum extractor P03.3
    environmental chemicals P04.6
    entanglement (knot) in umbilical cord P02.5

Newborn - *continued*
  fetal (intrauterine)
    growth retardation P05.9
    malnutrition not light or small for
  gestational age P05.2
  forceps delivery P03.2
  heart rate abnormalities
    bradycardia P29.12
    intrauterine P03.819
      before onset of labor P03.810
      during labor P03.811
    tachycardia P29.11
  hemorrhage (antepartum) P02.1
    cerebellar (nontraumatic) P52.6
    intracerebral (nontraumatic) P52.4
    intracranial (nontraumatic) P52.9
      specified NEC P52.8
    intraventricular (nontraumatic) P52.3
      grade 1 P52.0
      grade 2 P52.1
      grade 3 P52.21
      grade 4 P52.22
    posterior fossa (nontraumatic) P52.6
    subarachnoid (nontraumatic) P52.5
    subependymal P52.0
      with intracerebral extension P52.22
      with intraventricular extension P52.1
        with enlargement of ventricles P52.21
      without intraventricular extension P52.0
  hypoxic ischemic encephalopathy -HIE]
  P91.60
    mild P91.61
    moderate P91.62
    severe P91.63
  induction of labor P03.89
  intestinal perforation P78.0
  intrauterine (fetal) blood loss P50.9
    due to (from)
      cut end of co-twin cord P50.5
      hemorrhage into
        co-twin P50.3
        maternal circulation P50.4
      placenta P50.2
      ruptured cord blood P50.1
      vasa previa P50.0
    specified NEC P50.8
  intrauterine (fetal) hemorrhage P50.9
  intrauterine (in utero) procedure P96.5
  malpresentation (malposition) NEC P03.1
  maternal (complication of) (use of)
    alcohol P04.3
    analgesia (maternal) P04.0
    anesthesia (maternal) P04.0
    blood loss P02.1
    circulatory disease P00.3
    condition P00.9
      specified NEC P00.89
    delivery P03.9
      Cesarean P03.4
      forceps P03.2
      vacuum extractor P03.3
    diabetes mellitus (pre-existing) P70.1
    disorder P00.9
      specified NEC P00.89
    drugs (addictive) (illegal) NEC P04.49
    ectopic pregnancy P01.4
    gestational diabetes P70.0
    hemorrhage P02.1
    hypertensive disorder P00.0
    incompetent cervix P01.0
    infectious disease P00.2
    injury P00.5

Nodule (s) , nodular   *- continued*
   hip M06.35
   knee M06.36
   multiple site M06.39
   shoulder M06.31
   vertebra M06.38
   wrist M06.33
   scrotum (inflammatory) N49.2
   singer's J38.2
   solitary, lung (subsegmental branch of the
   bronchial tree) R91.1
     multiple R91.8
   subcutaneous —*see* Swelling, localized
   teacher's J38.2
   thyroid (cold) (gland) (nontoxic) E04.1
     with thyrotoxicosis E05.20
       with thyroid storm E05.21
     toxic or with hyperthyroidism E05.20
       with thyroid storm E05.21
   vocal cord J38.2
Noma (gangrenous) (hospital) (infective)
   A69.0
   auricle 196
   mouth A69.0
   pudendi N76.89
   vulvae N76.89
Nomad, nomadism Z59.0
Nonautoimmune hemolytic anemia D59.4
   drug-induced D59.2
Nonclosure —*see also* Imperfect, closure
   ductus arteriosus (Botallo's) Q25.0
   foramen
     botalli Q21.1
     ovale Q21.1
Noncompliance Z91.19
   with
     dietary regimen Z91.11
     dialysis Z91.15
     medical treatment Z91.19
     medication regimen NEC Z91.14
       underdosing (*see also* Table of Drugs and
   Chemicals, categories T36-T50, with final
   character 6) Z91.14
       intentional NEC Z91.128
         due to financial hardship of patient
   Z91.120
       unintentional NEC Z91.138
         due to patient's age related debility
   Z91.130
     renal dialysis Z91.15
Nondescent (congenital) —*see also*
   Malposition, congenital
   cecum Q43.3
   colon Q43.3
   testicle Q53.9
     bilateral Q53.20
       abdominal Q53.21
       perineal Q53.22
     unilateral Q53.10
       abdominal Q53.11
       perineal Q53.12
Nondevelopment
   brain Q02
     part of Q04.3
   heart Q24.8
   organ or site, congenital NEC —*see*
   Hypoplasia
Nonengagement
   head NEC O32.4
     in labor, causing obstructed labor O64.8
Nonexanthematous tick fever A93.2
Nonexpansion, lung (newborn) P28.0

Nonfunctioning
   cystic duct (*see also* Disease, gallbladder)
   K82.8
   gallbladder (*see also* Disease, gallbladder)
   K82.8
   kidney N28.9
   labyrinth —*see* subcategory H83.2
Non-Hodgkin lymphoma NEC —*see*
   Lymphoma, non-Hodgkin
Non-working side interference M26.56
Nonimplantation, ovum N97.2
Noninsufflation, fallopian tube N97.1
Non-ketotic hyperglycinemia E72.51
Nonne-Milroy syndrome Q82.0
Nonovulation N97.0
Nonpatent fallopian tube N97.1
Nonpneumatization, lung NEC P28.0
Nonrotation —*see* Malrotation
Nonsecretion, urine —*see* Anuria
Nonunion
   fracture —*see* Fracture, by site
   organ or site, congenital NEC —*see*
   Imperfect, closure
   symphysis pubis, congenital Q74.2
Nonvisualization, gallbladder R93.2
Nonvital, nonvitalized tooth K04.99
Noonan's syndrome Q87.1
Normocytic anemia (infectional) due to blood
   loss (chronic) D50.0
   acute D62
Norrie's disease (congenital) Q15.8
North American blastomycosis B40.9
Norwegian itch B86
Nose, nasal —*see* condition
Nosebleed R04.0
Nose-picking F98.8
Nosomania F45.21
Nosophobia F45.22
Nostalgia F43.20
Notch of iris Q13.2
Notching nose, congenital (tip) Q30.2
Nothnagel's
   syndrome —*see* Strabismus, paralytic, third
   nerve
   vasomotor acroparesthesia I73.89
Novy's relapsing fever A68.9
   louse-borne A68.0
   tick-borne A68.1
Noxious
   foodstuffs, poisoning by —*see* Poisoning,
   food, noxious, plant
   substances transmitted through placenta or
   breast milk P04.9
Nucleus pulposus —*see* condition
Numbness R20.0
Nuns' knee —*see* Bursitis, prepatellar
Nursemaid's elbow S53.03
Nutcracker esophagus K22.4
Nutmeg liver K76.1
Nutrient element deficiency E61.9
   specified NEC E61.8
Nutrition deficient or insufficient (*see also*
   Malnutrition) E46
   due to
     insufficient food T73.0
     lack of
       care (child) T76.02
         adult T76.01
       food T73.0
Nutritional stunting E45
Nyctalopia (night blindness) —*see* Blindness,
   night

Nycturia R35.1
   psychogenic F45.8
Nymphomania F52.8
Nystagmus H55.00
   benign paroxysmal —*see* Vertigo, benign
   paroxysmal
   central positional H81.4
   congenital H55.01
   dissociated H55.04
   latent H55.02
   miners' H55.09
   positional
     benign paroxysmal H81.4
     central H81.4
   specified form NEC H55.09
   visual deprivation H55.03

O

Obermeyer's relapsing fever (European)
   A68.0
Obesity E66.9
   with alveolar hyperventilation E66.2
   adrenal E27.8
   complicating
     childbirth O99.214
     pregnancy O99.21
     puerperium O99.215
   constitutional E66.8
   dietary counseling and surveillance Z71.3
   drug-induced E66.1
   due to
     drug E66.1
     excess calories E66.09
       morbid E66.01
       severe E66.01
   endocrine E66.8
   endogenous E66.8
   familial E66.8
   glandular E66.8
   hypothyroid   *see* Hypothyroidism
   morbid E66.01
     with alveolar hypoventilation E66.2
     due to excess calories E66.01
   nutritional E66.09
   pituitary E23.6
   severe E66.01
   specified type NEC E66.8
Oblique —*see* condition
Obliteration
   appendix (lumen) K38.8
   artery I77.1
   bile duct (noncalculous) K83.1
   common duct (noncalculous) K83.1
   cystic duct —*see* Obstruction, gallbladder
   disease, arteriolar I77.1
   endometrium N85.8
   eye, anterior chamber —*see* Disorder, globe,
   hypotony
   fallopian tube N97.1
   lymphatic vessel I89.0
     due to mastectomy I97.2
   organ or site, congenital NEC —*see* Atresia,
   by site
   ureter N13.5
     with infection N13.6
   urethra —*see* Stricture, urethra
   vein I87.8
   vestibule (oral) K08.8
Observation (following) (for) (without need
   for further medical care) Z04.9
   accident NEC Z04.3
     at work Z04.2
     transport Z04.1

Observation - *continued*
adverse effect of drug Z03.6
alleged rape or sexual assault (victim) , ruled out
  adult Z04.41
  child Z04.42
criminal assault Z04.8
development state
  adolescent Z00.3
  period of rapid growth in childhood Z00.2
  puberty Z00.3
disease, specified NEC Z03.89
following work accident Z04.2
growth and development state —*see* Observation, development state
injuries (accidental) NEC —*see also* Observation, accident
newborn (for suspected condition, ruled out) —*see* Newborn, affected by (suspected to be) , maternal (complication of) (use of)
postpartum
  immediately after delivery Z39.0
  routine follow-up Z39.2
pregnancy (normal) (without complication) Z34.9
  high risk O09.9
suicide attempt, alleged NEC Z03.89
  self-poisoning Z03.6
suspected, ruled out —*see also* Suspected condition, ruled out
  abuse, physical
    adult Z04.71
    child Z04.72
  accident at work Z04.2
  adult battering victim Z04.71
  child battering victim Z04.72
  condition NEC Z03.89
  newborn —*see* Newborn, affected by (suspected to be) , maternal (complication of) (use of)
  drug poisoning or adverse effect Z03.6
  exposure (to)
    anthrax Z03.810
    biological agent NEC Z03.818
  inflicted injury NEC Z04.8
  suicide attempt, alleged Z03.89
    self-poisoning Z03.6
  toxic effects from ingested substance (drug) (poison) Z03.6
  toxic effects from ingested substance (drug) (poison) Z03.6
Obsession, obsessional state F42
Obsessive-compulsive neurosis or reaction F42
Obstetric embolism, septic —*see* Embolism, obstetric, septic
Obstetrical trauma (complicating delivery) O71.9
with or following ectopic or molar pregnancy O08.6
specified type NEC O71.89
Obstipation —*see* Constipation
Obstruction, obstructed, obstructive
airway J98.8
with
  allergic alveolitis J67.9
  asthma J45.909
  with
    exacerbation (acute) J45.901
    status asthmaticus J45.902
  bronchiectasis J47.9

Obstruction, obstructed - *continued*
with
  exacerbation (acute) J47.1
  lower respiratory infection J47.0
  bronchitis (chronic) J44.9
  emphysema J43.9
chronic J44.9
with
  allergic alveolitis —*see* Pneumonitis, hypersensitivity
  bronchiectasis J47.9
  with
    exacerbation (acute) J47.1
    lower respiratory infection J47.0
due to
  foreign body —*see* Foreign body, by site, causing asphyxia
  inhalation of fumes or vapors J68.9
  laryngospasm J38.5
ampulla of Vater K83.1
aortic (heart) (valve) —*see* Stenosis, aortic
aortoiliac I74.09
aqueduct of Sylvius G91.1
  congenital Q03.0
  with spina bifida —*see* Spina bifida, by site, with hydrocephalus
Arnold-Chiari —*see* Arnold-Chiari disease
artery (see also Embolism, artery) I74.9
  basilar (complete) (partial) —*see* Occlusion, artery, basilar
  carotid (complete) (partial) —*see* Occlusion, artery, carotid
  cerebellar —*see* Occlusion, artery, cerebellar
  cerebral (anterior) (middle) (posterior) —*see* Occlusion, artery, cerebral
  precerebral —*see* Occlusion, artery, precerebral
  renal N28.0
  retinal NEC —*see* Occlusion, artery, retina
  vertebral (complete) (partial) —*see* Occlusion, artery, vertebral
band (intestinal) K56.69
bile duct or passage (common) (hepatic) (noncalculous) K83.1
  with calculus K80.51
  congenital (causing jaundice) Q44.3
biliary (duct) (tract) K83.1
  gallbladder K82.0
bladder-neck (acquired) N32.0
  congenital Q64.31
  due to hyperplasia (hypertrophy) of prostate —*see* Hyperplasia, prostate
bowel —*see* Obstruction, intestine
bronchus J98.09
canal, ear —*see* Stenosis, external ear canal
cardia K22.2
caval veins (inferior) (superior) I87.1
cecum —*see* Obstruction, intestine
circulatory I99.8
colon —*see* Obstruction, intestine
common duct (noncalculous) K83.1
coronary (artery) —*see* Occlusion, coronary
cystic duct —*see also* Obstruction, gallbladder
  with calculus K80.21
device, implant or graft (see also Complications, by site and type, mechanical) T85.698
  arterial graft NEC —*see* Complication, cardiovascular device, mechanical, vascular catheter NEC T85.628

Obstruction, obstructed - *continued*
cystostomy T83.090
dialysis (renal) T82.49
  intraperitoneal T85.691
infusion NEC T82.594
  spinal (epidural) (subdural) T85.690
urinary, indwelling T83.098
due to infection T85.79
gastrointestinal —*see* Complications, prosthetic device, mechanical, gastrointestinal device
  genital NEC T83.498
    intrauterine contraceptive device T83.39
    penile prosthesis T83.490
  heart NEC —*see* Complication, cardiovascular device, mechanical
  joint prosthesis —*see* Complications, joint prosthesis, mechanical, specified NEC, by site
  orthopedic NEC —*see* Complication, orthopedic, device, mechanical
  specified NEC T85.628
  urinary NEC —*see also* Complication, genitourinary, device, urinary, mechanical
    graft T83.29
  vascular NEC —*see* Complication, cardiovascular device, mechanical
  ventricular intracranial shunt T85.09
due to foreign body accidentally left in operative wound T81.529
duodenum K31.5
ejaculatory duct N50.8
esophagus K22.2
eustachian tube (complete) (partial) H68.10
  cartilaginous (extrinsic) H68.13
    intrinsic H68.12
  osseous H68.11
fallopian tube (bilateral) N97.1
fecal K56.41
  with hernia —*see* Hernia, by site, with obstruction
foramen of Monro (congenital) Q03.8
  with spina bifida —*see* Spina bifida, by site, with hydrocephalus
foreign body —*see* Foreign body
gallbladder K82.0
  with calculus, stones K80.21
  congenital Q44.1
gastric outlet K31.1
gastrointestinal —*see* Obstruction, intestine
hepatic K76.89
  duct (noncalculous) K83.1
hepatobiliary K83.1
ileum —*see* Obstruction, intestine
iliofemoral (artery) I74.5
intestine K56.60
with
  adhesions (intestinal) (peritoneal) K56.5
  adynamic K56.0
  by gallstone K56.3
  congenital (small) Q41.9
    large Q42.9
    specified part NEC Q42.8
  neurogenic K56.0
  Hirschsprung's disease or megacolon Q43.1
  newborn P76.9
    due to
      fecaliths P76.8
      inspissated milk P76.2
      meconium (plug) P76.0
        in mucoviscidosis E84.11
      specified NEC P76.8
  postoperative K91.3

Obstruction, obstructed   *- continued*
   reflex K56.0
     specified NEC K56.69
     volvulus K56.2
   intracardiac ball valve prosthesis T82.09
   jejunum —*see* Obstruction, intestine
   joint prosthesis —*see* Complications, joint
   prosthesis, mechanical, specified NEC, by site
   kidney (calices) N28.89
   labor —*see* Delivery
   lacrimal (passages) (duct)
     by
       dacryolith —*see* Dacryolith
       stenosis —*see* Stenosis, lacrimal
     congenital Q10.5
     neonatal H04.53
   lacrimonasal duct —*see* Obstruction, lacrimal
   lacteal, with steatorrhea K90.2
   laryngitis —*see* Laryngitis
   larynx NEC J38.6
     congenital Q31.8
   lung J98.4
     disease, chronic J44.9
   lymphatic I89.0
   meconium (plug)
     newborn P76.0
       due to fecaliths P76.0
       in mucoviscidosis E84.11
   mitral —*see* Stenosis, mitral
   nasal J34.89
   nasolacrimal duct —*see also* Obstruction,
   lacrimal
     congenital Q10.5
   nasopharynx J39.2
   nose J34.89
   organ or site, congenital NEC —*see* Atresia,
   by site
   pancreatic duct K86.8
   parotid duct or gland K11.8
   pelviureteral junction N13.5
     congenital Q62.39
   pharynx J39.2
   portal (circulation) (vein) I81
   prostate —*see also* Hyperplasia, prostate
     valve (urinary) N32.0
   pulmonary valve (heart) I37.0
   pyelonephritis (chronic) N11.1
   pylorus
     adult K31.1
     congenital or infantile Q40.0
   rectosigmoid —*see* Obstruction, intestine
   rectum K62.4
   renal N28.89
     outflow N13.8
     pelvis, congenital Q62.39
   respiratory J98.8
     chronic J44.9
   retinal (vessels) H34.9
   salivary duct (any) K11.8
     with calculus K11.5
   sigmoid —*see* Obstruction, intestine
   sinus (accessory) (nasal) J34.89
   Stensen's duct K11.8
   stomach NEC K31.89
     acute K31.0
     congenital Q40.2
     due to pylorospasm K31.3
   submandibular duct K11.8
   submaxillary gland K11.8
     with calculus K11.5
   thoracic duct I89.0
   thrombotic —*see* Thrombosis

Obstruction, obstructed   *- continued*
   trachea J39.8
   tracheostomy airway J95.03
   tricuspid (valve) —*see* Stenosis, tricuspid
   upper respiratory, congenital Q34.8
   ureter (functional) (pelvic junction) NEC
   N13.5
     with
       hydronephrosis N13.1
         with infection N13.6
       pyelonephritis (chronic) N11.1
     congenital Q62.39
     due to calculus —*see* Calculus, ureter
   urethra NEC N36.8
     congenital Q64.39
   urinary (moderate) N13.9
     due to hyperplasia (hypertrophy) of prostate
     —*see* Hyperplasia, prostate
     organ or tract (lower) N13.9
     prostatic valve N32.0
     specified NEC N13.8
   uropathy N13.9
   uterus N85.8
   vagina N89.5
   valvular —*see* Endocarditis
   vein, venous I87.1
     caval (inferior) (superior) I87.1
     thrombotic —*see* Thrombosis
   vena cava (inferior) (superior) I87.1
   vesical NEC N32.0
   vesicourethral orifice N32.0
     congenital Q64.31
   vessel NEC I99.8
Obturator —*see* condition
Occlusal wear, teeth K03.0
Occlusio pupillae —*see* Membrane, pupillary
Occlusion, occluded
   anus K62.4
     congenital Q42.3
       with fistula Q42.2
   aortoiliac (chronic) I74.09
   aqueduct of Sylvius G91.1
     congenital Q03.0
       with spina bifida —*see* Spina bifida, by
   site, with hydrocephalus
   artery (*see also* Embolism, artery) I74.9
     auditory, internal I65.8
     basilar I65.1
       with
         infarction I63.22
           due to
             embolism I63.12
             thrombosis I63.02
     brain or cerebral I66.9
       with infarction (due to) I63.5
         embolism I63.4
         thrombosis I63.3
     carotid I65.2
       with
         infarction I63.23
           due to
             embolism I63.13
             thrombosis I63.03
     cerebellar (anterior inferior) (posterior
   inferior) (superior) I66.3
       with infarction I63.54
         due to
           embolism I63.44
           thrombosis I63.34
     cerebral I66.9
       with infarction I63.50

Occlusion, occluded   *- continued*
     due to
       embolism I63.40
         specified NEC I63.49
       thrombosis I63.30
         specified NEC I63.39
     anterior I66.1
       with infarction I63.52
       due to
         embolism I63.42
         thrombosis I63.32
     middle I66.0
       with infarction I63.51
       due to
         embolism I63.41
         thrombosis I63.31
     posterior I66.2
       with infarction I63.53
       due to
         embolism I63.43
         thrombosis I63.33
     specified NEC I66.8
       with infarction I63.59
       due to
         embolism I63.4
         thrombosis I63.3
     choroidal (anterior) —*see* Occlusion, artery,
   precerebral, specified NEC
     communicating posterior —*see* Occlusion,
   artery, cerebral, specified NEC
     complete
       coronary I25.82
       extremities I70.92
     coronary (acute) (thrombotic) (without
   myocardial infarction) I24.0
       with myocardial infarction —*see*
   Infarction, myocardium
       chronic total I25.82
       complete I25.82
       healed or old I25.2
       total (chronic) I25.82
     hypophyseal —*see* Occlusion, artery,
   precerebral, specified NEC
     iliac I74.5
     lower extremities due to stenosis or stricture
   I77.1
     mesenteric (embolic) (thrombotic) K55.0
     perforating —*see* Occlusion, artery,
   cerebral, specified NEC
     peripheral I77.9
       thrombotic or embolic I74.4
     pontine —*see* Occlusion, artery, cerebral,
   specified NEC
     precerebral I65.9
       with infarction I63.20
         specified NEC I63.29
         due to
           embolism I63.10
             specified NEC I63.19
           thrombosis I63.00
             specified NEC I63.09
       basilar —*see* Occlusion, artery, basilar
       carotid —*see* Occlusion, artery, carotid
       puerperal O88.23
       specified NEC I65.8
         with infarction I63.29
           due to
             embolism I63.19
             thrombosis I63.00
       vertebral —*see* Occlusion, artery, vertebral
     renal N28.0
     retinal
       central H34.1

Occlusion, occluded *- continued*
  partial H34.21
    branch H34.23
    transient H34.0
  spinal —*see* Occlusion, artery, precerebral, vertebral
  total (chronic)
    coronary I25.82
    extremities I70.92
  vertebral I65.0
    with
      infarction I63.21
        due to
          embolism I63.11
          thrombosis I63.01
  basilar artery —*see* Occlusion, artery, basilar
  bile duct (common) (hepatic) (noncalculous) K83.1
  bowel —*see* Obstruction, intestine
  carotid (artery) (common) (internal) —*see* Occlusion, artery, carotid
  centric (of teeth) M26.59
    maximum intercuspation discrepancy M26.55
  cerebellar (artery) —*see* Occlusion, artery, cerebellar
  cerebral (artery) —*see* Occlusion, artery, cerebral
  cerebrovascular —*see also* Occlusion, artery, cerebral
    with infarction I63.5
  cervical canal —*see* Stricture, cervix
  cervix (uteri) —*see* Stricture, cervix
  choanal Q30.0
  choroidal (artery) —*see* Occlusion, artery, precerebral, specified NEC
  colon —*see* Obstruction, intestine
  communicating posterior artery —*see* Occlusion, artery, precerebral, specified NEC
  coronary (artery) (vein) (thrombotic) —*see also* Infarct, myocardium
    chronic total I25.82
    healed or old I25.2
    not resulting in infarction I24.0
    total (chronic) I25.82
  cystic duct —*see* Obstruction, gallbladder
  embolic —*see* Embolism
  fallopian tube N97.1
    congenital Q50.6
  gallbladder —*see also* Obstruction, gallbladder
    congenital (causing jaundice) Q44.1
  gingiva, traumatic K06.2
  hymen N89.6
    congenital Q52.3
  hypophyseal (artery) —*see* Occlusion, artery, precerebral, specified NEC
  iliac artery I74.5
  intestine —*see* Obstruction, intestine
  lacrimal passages —*see* Obstruction, lacrimal
  lung J98.4
  lymph or lymphatic channel I89.0
  mammary duct N64.89
  mesenteric artery (embolic) (thrombotic) K55.0
  nose J34.89
    congenital Q30.0
  organ or site, congenital NEC —*see* Atresia, by site
  oviduct N97.1
    congenital Q50.6

Occlusion, occluded *- continued*
  peripheral arteries
    due to stricture or stenosis I77.1
    upper extremity I74.2
  pontine (artery) —*see* Occlusion, artery, precerebral, specified NEC
  posterior lingual, of mandibular teeth M26.29
  precerebral artery —*see* Occlusion, artery, precerebral
  punctum lacrimale —*see* Obstruction, lacrimal
  pupil —*see* Membrane, pupillary
  pylorus, adult (*see also* Stricture, pylorus) K31.1
  renal artery N28.0
  retina, retinal
    artery —*see* Occlusion, artery, retinal
    vein (central) H34.81
      engorgement H34.82
      tributary H34.83
    vessels H34.9
  spinal artery —*see* Occlusion, artery, precerebral, vertebral
  teeth (mandibular) (posterior lingual) M26.29
  thoracic duct I89.0
  thrombotic —*see* Thrombosis, artery
  traumatic
    edentulous (alveolar) ridge K06.2
    gingiva K06.2
    periodontal K05.5
  tubal N97.1
  ureter (complete) (partial) N13.5
    congenital Q62.10
  ureteropelvic junction N13.5
    congenital Q62.11
  ureterovesical orifice N13.5
    congenital Q62.12
  urethra —*see* Stricture, urethra
  uterus N85.8
  vagina N89.5
  vascular NEC I99.8
  vein —*see* Thrombosis
    retinal —*see* Occlusion, retinal, vein
  vena cava (inferior) (superior) —*see* Embolism, vena cava
  ventricle (brain) NEC G91.1
  vertebral (artery) —*see* Occlusion, artery, vertebral
  vessel (blood) I99.8
  vulva N90.5
Occult
  blood in feces (stools) R19.5
Occupational
  problems NEC Z56.89
Ochlophobia —*see* Agoraphobia
Ochronosis (endogenous) E70.29
Ocular muscle —*see* condition
Oculogyric crisis or disturbance H51.8
  psychogenic F45.8
Oculomotor syndrome H51.9
Oculopathy
  syphilitic NEC A52.71
    congenital
      early A50.01
      late A50.30
    early (secondary) A51.43
    late A52.71
Oddi's sphincter spasm K83.4
Odontalgia K08.8
Odontoameloblastoma —*see* Cyst, calcifying odontogenic
Odontoclasia K03.89
Odontodysplasia, regional K00.4

Odontogenesis imperfecta K00.5
Odontoma (ameloblastic) (complex) (compound) (fibroameloblastic) —*see* Cyst, calcifying odontogenic
Odontomyelitis (closed) (open) K04.0
Odontorrhagia K08.8
Odontosarcoma, ameloblastic C41.1
  upper jaw (bone) C41.0
Oestriasis —*see* Myiasis
Oguchi's disease H53.63
Ohara's disease —*see* Tularemia
Oidiomycosis —*see* Candidiasis
Oidium albicans infection —*see* Candidiasis
Old age (without mention of debility) R54
  dementia F03
Old (previous) myocardial infarction I25.2
Olfactory —*see* condition
Oligemia —*see* Anemia
Oligoastrocytoma
  specified site —*see* Neoplasm, malignant, by site
  unspecified site C71.9
Oligocythemia D64.9
Oligodendroblastoma
  specified site —*see* Neoplasm, malignant
  unspecified site C71.9
Oligodendroglioma
  anaplastic type
    specified site —*see* Neoplasm, malignant, by site
    unspecified site C71.9
  specified site —*see* Neoplasm, malignant, by site
  unspecified site C71.9
Oligodontia —*see* Anodontia
Oligoencephalon Q02
Oligohidrosis L74.4
Oligohydramnios O41.0
Oligohidrosis L74.4
Oligomenorrhea N91.5
  primary N91.3
  secondary N91.4
Oligophrenia —*see also* Disability, intellectual
  phenylpyruvic E70.0
Oligospermia N46.11
  due to
    drug therapy N46.121
    efferent duct obstruction N46.123
    infection N46.122
    radiation N46.124
    specified cause NEC N46.129
    systemic disease N46.125
Oligotrichia —*see* Alopecia
Oliguria R34
  with, complicating or following ectopic or molar pregnancy O08.4
  postprocedural N99.0
Ollier's disease Q78.4
Omentitis —*see* Peritonitis
Omenotocele —*see* Hernia, abdomen, specified site NEC
Omentum, omental —*see* condition
Omphalitis (congenital) (newborn) P38.9
  with mild hemorrhage P38.1
  without hemorrhage P38.9
  not of newborn L08.82
  tetanus A33
Omphalocele Q79.2
Omphalomesenteric duct, persistent Q43.0
Omphalorrhagia, newborn P51.9
Omsk hemorrhagic fever A98.1

Onanism (excessive) F98.8
Onchocerciasis, onchocercosis B73.1
  with
    eye disease B73.00
      endophthalmitis B73.01
      eyelid B73.09
      glaucoma B73.02
      specified NEC B73.09
    eye NEC B73.00
    eyelid B73.09
Oncocytoma —*see* Neoplasm, benign, by site
Oncovirus, as cause of disease classified elsewhere B97.32
Ondine's curse —*see* Apnea, sleep
Oneirophrenia F23
Onychauxis L60.2
  congenital Q84.5
Onychia —*see also* Cellulitis, digit
  with lymphangitis —*see* Lymphangitis, acute, digit
  candidal B37.2
  dermatophytic B35.1
Onychitis —*see also* Cellulitis, digit
  with lymphangitis —*see* Lymphangitis, acute, digit
Onychocryptosis L60.0
Onychodystrophy L60.3
  congenital Q84.6
Onychogryphosis, onychogryposis L60.2
Onycholysis L60.1
Onychomadesis L60.8
Onychomalacia L60.3
Onychomycosis (finger) (toe) B35.1
Onycho-osteodysplasia Q79.8
Onychophagia F98.8
Onychophosis L60.8
Onychoptosis L60.8
Onychorrhexis L60.3
  congenital Q84.6
Onychoschizia L60.3
Onyxis (finger) (toe) L60.0
Onyxitis —*see also* Cellulitis, digit
  with lymphangitis —*see* Lymphangitis, acute, digit
Oophoritis (cystic) (infectional) (interstitial) N70.92
  with salpingitis N70.93
  acute N70.02
    with salpingitis N70.03
  chronic N70.12
    with salpingitis N70.13
  complicating abortion —*see* Abortion, by type, complicated by, oophoritis
Oophorocele N83.4
Opacity, opacities
  cornea H17.
    central H17.1
    congenital Q13.3
    degenerative —*see* Degeneration, cornea
    hereditary —*see* Dystrophy, cornea
    inflammatory —*see* Keratitis
    minor H17.81
    peripheral H17.82
    sequelae of trachoma (healed) B94.0
    specified NEC H17.89
  enamel (teeth) (fluoride) (nonfluoride) K00.3
  lens —*see* Cataract
  snowball —*see* Deposit, crystalline
  vitreous (humor) NEC H43.39
    congenital Q14.0
    membranes and strands H43.31
Opalescent dentin (hereditary) K00.5

Open, opening
  abnormal, organ or site, congenital —*see* Imperfect, closure
  angle with
    borderline
      findings
        high risk H40.02
        low risk H40.01
      intraocular pressure H40.00
    cupping of discs H40.01
    glaucoma (primary) —*see* Glaucoma, open angle
  bite
    anterior M26.220
    posterior M26.221
  false —*see* Imperfect, closure
  margin on tooth restoration K08.51
  restoration margins of tooth K08.51
  wound —*see* Wound, open
Operational fatigue F48.8
Operative —*see* condition
Operculitis —*see* Periodontitis
Operculum —*see* Break, retina
Ophiasis L63.2
Ophthalmia (*see also* Conjunctivitis) H10.9
  actinic rays —*see* Photokeratitis
  allergic (acute) —*see* Conjunctivitis, acute, atopic
  blennorrhagic (gonococcal) (neonatorum) A54.31
  diphtheritic A36.86
  Egyptian A71.1
  electrica —*see* Photokeratitis
  gonococcal (neonatorum) A54.31
  metastatic —*see* Endophthalmitis, purulent
  migraine —*see* Migraine, ophthalmoplegic
  neonatorum, newborn P39.1
    gonococcal A54.31
  nodosa H16.24
  purulent —*see* Conjunctivitis, acute, mucopurulent
  spring —*see* Conjunctivitis, acute, atopic
  sympathetic —*see* Uveitis, sympathetic
Ophthalmitis —*see* Ophthalmia
Ophthalmocele (congenital) Q15.8
Ophthalmoneuromyelitis G36.0
Ophthalmoplegia —*see also* Strabismus, paralytic
  anterior internuclear —*see* Ophthalmoplegia, internuclear
  ataxia-areflexia G61.0
  diabetic —*see* E08-E13 with .39
  exophthalmic E05.00
    with thyroid storm E05.01
  external H49.88
    progressive H49.4
      with pigmentary retinopathy —*see* Kearns-Sayre syndrome
    total H49.3
  internal (complete) (total) H52.51
  internuclear H51.2
  migraine —*see* Migraine, ophthalmoplegic
  Parinaud's H49.88
  progressive external —*see* Ophthalmoplegia, external, progressive
  supranuclear, progressive G23.1
  total (external) —*see* Ophthalmoplegia, external, total
Opioid (s)
  abuse —*see* Abuse, drug, opioids
  dependence —*see* Dependence, drug, opioids
Opisthognathism M26.09
Opisthorchiasis (felineus) (viverrini) B66.0

Opitz' disease D73.2
Opiumism —*see* Dependence, drug, opioid
Oppenheim's disease G70.2
Oppenheim-Urbach disease (necrobiosis lipoidica diabeticorum) —*see* E08-E13 with .620
Optic nerve —*see* condition
Orbit —*see* condition
Orchioblastoma C62.9
Orchitis (gangrenous) (nonspecific) (septic) (suppurative) N45.2
  blennorrhagic (gonococcal) (acute) (chronic) A54.23
  chlamydial A56.19
  filarial (*see also* Infestation, filarial) B74.9 *[N51]*
  gonococcal (acute) (chronic) A54.23
  mumps B26.0
  syphilitic A52.76
  tuberculous A18.15
Orf (virus disease) B08.02
Organic —*see also* condition
  brain syndrome F09
  heart —*see* Disease, heart
  mental disorder F09
  psychosis F09
Orgasm
  anejaculatory N53.13
Oriental
  bilharziasis B65.2
  schistosomiasis B65.2
Orifice —*see* condition
Origin of both great vessels from right ventricle Q20.1
Ormond's disease (with ureteral obstruction) N13.5
  with infection N13.6
Ornithine metabolism disorder E72.4
Ornithinemia (Type I) (Type II) E72.4
Ornithosis A70
Orotaciduria, oroticaciduria (congenital) (hereditary) (pyrimidine deficiency) E79.8
  anemia D53.0
Orthodontics
  adjustment Z46.4
  fitting Z46.4
Orthopnea R06.01
Orthopoxvirus B08.09
  specified NEC B08.09
Os, uterus —*see* condition
Osgood-Schlatter disease or osteochondrosis —*see* Osteochondrosis, juvenile, tibia
Osler (-Weber) **-Rendu disease** I78.0
Osler's nodes I33.1
Osmidrosis L75.0
Osseous —*see* condition
Ossification
  artery —*see* Arteriosclerosis
  auricle (ear) —*see* Disorder, pinna, specified type NEC
  bronchial J98.09
  cardiac —*see* Degeneration, myocardial
  cartilage (senile) —*see* Disorder, cartilage, specified type NEC
  coronary (artery) —*see* Disease, heart, ischemic, atherosclerotic
  diaphragm J98.6
  ear, middle —*see* Otosclerosis
  falx cerebri G96.19
  fontanel, premature Q75.0
  heart —*see also* Degeneration, myocardial
    valve —*see* Endocarditis

Ossification - *continued*
larynx J38.7
ligament —*see* Disorder, tendon, specified
type NEC
  posterior longitudinal —*see* Spondylopathy,
specified NEC
meninges (cerebral) (spinal) G96.19
multiple, eccentric centers —*see* Disorder,
bone, development or growth
muscle —*see also* Calcification, muscle
  due to burns —*see* Myositis, ossificans, in,
burns
  paralytic —*see* Myositis, ossificans, in,
quadriplegia
  progressive —*see* Myositis, ossificans,
progressiva
  specified NEC M61.50
    ankle M61.57
    foot M61.57
    forearm M61.53
    hand M61.54
    lower leg M61.56
    multiple sites M61.59
    pelvic region M61.55
    shoulder region M61.51
    specified site NEC M61.58
    thigh M61.55
    upper arm M61.52
  traumatic —*see* Myositis, ossificans,
traumatica
myocardium, myocardial —*see* Degeneration,
myocardial
penis N48.89
periarticular —*see* Disorder, joint, specified
type NEC
pinna —*see* Disorder, pinna, specified type
NEC
rider's bone —*see* Ossification, muscle,
specified NEC
sclera H15.89
subperiosteal, post-traumatic M89.8X
tendon —*see* Disorder, tendon, specified type
NEC
trachea J39.8
tympanic membrane —*see* Disorder,
tympanic membrane, specified NEC
vitreous (humor) —*see* Deposit, crystalline
Osteitis —*see also* Osteomyelitis
alveolar M27.3
condensans M85.30
  ankle M85.37
  foot M85.37
  forearm M85.33
  hand M85.34
  lower leg M85.36
  multiple site M85.39
  neck M85.38
  rib M85.38
  shoulder M85.31
  skull M85.38
  specified site NEC M85.38
  thigh M85.35
  toe M85.37
  upper arm M85.32
  vertebra M85.38
deformans M88.9
  in (due to)
    malignant neoplasm of bone C41.9
[M90.60]
    neoplastic disease (*see also* Neoplasm)
D49.9 *[M90.60]*
      carpus D49.9 *[M90.64]*

Osteitis - *continued*
  clavicle D49.9 *[M90.61]*
  femur D49.9 *[M90.65]*
  fibula D49.9 *[M90.66]*
  finger D49.9 *[M90.64]*
  humerus D49.9 *[M90.62]*
  ilium D49.9 *[M90.65]*
  ischium D49.9 *[M90.65]*
  metacarpus D49.9 *[M90.64]*
  metatarsus D49.9 *[M90.67]*
  multiple sites D49.9 *[M90.69]*
  neck D49.9 *[M90.68]*
  radius D49.9 *[M90.63]*
  rib D49.9 *[M90.68]*
  scapula D49.9 *[M90.61]*
  skull D49.9 *[M90.68]*
  tarsus D49.9 *[M90.67]*
  tibia D49.9 *[M90.66]*
  toe D49.9 *[M90.67]*
  ulna D49.9 *[M90.63]*
  vertebra D49.9 *[M90.68]*
skull M88.0
specified NEC —*see* Paget's disease, bone,
by site
  vertebra M88.1
due to yaws A66.6
fibrosa NEC —*see* Cyst, bone, by site
  circumscripta —*see* Dysplasia, fibrous, bone
NEC
  cystica (generalisata) E21.0
  disseminata Q78.1
  osteoplastica E21.0
fragilitans Q78.0
Garr's (sclerosing) —*see* Osteomyelitis,
specified type NEC
jaw (acute) (chronic) (lower) (suppurative)
(upper) M27.2
parathyroid E21.0
petrous bone (acute) (chronic) —*see* Petrositis
sclerotic, nonsuppurative —*see*
Osteomyelitis, specified type NEC
tuberculosa A18.09
  cystica D86.89
  multiplex cystoides D86.89
Osteoarthritis M19.90
ankle M19.07
elbow M19.02
foot joint M19.07
generalized M15.9
  erosive M15.4
  primary M15.0
  specified NEC M15.8
hand joint M19.04
  first carpometacarpal joint M18.9
hip M16.1
  bilateral M16.0
  due to hip dysplasia (unilateral) M16.3
    bilateral M16.2
interphalangeal
  distal (Heberden) M15.1
  proximal (Bouchard) M15.2
knee M17.9
  bilateral M17.0
shoulder M19.01
spine —*see* Spondylosis
wrist M19.03
post-traumatic NEC M19.92
  ankle M19.17
  elbow M19.12
  foot joint M19.17
  hand joint M19.14
    first carpometacarpal joint M18.3

Osteoarthritis - *continued*
  bilateral M18.2
  hip M16.5
    bilateral M16.4
  knee M17.3
    bilateral M17.2
  shoulder M19.11
  wrist M19.13
primary M19.91
  ankle M19.07
  elbow M19.02
  foot joint M19.07
  hand joint M19.04
    first carpometacarpal joint M18.1
      bilateral M18.0
  hip M16.1
    bilateral M16.0
  knee M17.1
    bilateral M17.0
  shoulder M19.01
  spine —*see* Spondylosis
  wrist M19.03
secondary M19.93
  ankle M19.27
  elbow M19.22
  foot joint M19.27
  hand joint M19.24
    first carpometacarpal joint M18.5
      bilateral M18.4
  hip M16.7
    bilateral M16.6
  knee M17.5
    bilateral M17.4
  multiple M15.3
  shoulder M19.21
  spine —*see* Spondylosis
  wrist M19.23
Osteoarthropathy (hypertrophic) M19.90
ankle —*see* Osteoarthritis, primary, ankle
elbow —*see* Osteoarthritis, primary, elbow
foot joint —*see* Osteoarthritis, primary, foot
hand joint —*see* Osteoarthritis, primary, hand
joint
knee joint —*see* Osteoarthritis, primary, knee
multiple site —*see* Osteoarthritis, primary,
multiple joint
pulmonary —*see also* Osteoarthropathy,
specified type NEC
  hypertrophic —*see* Osteoarthropathy,
hypertrophic, specified type NEC
secondary hypertrophic —*see*
Osteoarthropathy, specified type NEC
shoulder —*see* Osteoarthritis, primary,
shoulder
specified joint NEC —*see* Osteoarthritis,
primary, specified joint NEC
specified type NEC M89.40
  carpus M89.44
  clavicle M89.41
  femur M89.45
  fibula M89.46
  finger M89.44
  humerus M89.42
  ilium M89.459
  ischium M89.459
  metacarpus M89.44
  metatarsus M89.47
  multiple sites M89.49
  neck M89.48
  radius M89.43
  rib M89.48
  scapula M89.41
  skull M89.48

Osteoarthropathy *- continued*
  tarsus M89.47
  tibia M89.46
  toe M89.47
  ulna M89.43
  vertebra M89.48
  secondary —*see* Osteoarthropathy, specified type NEC
  spine —*see* Spondylosis
  wrist —*see* Osteoarthritis, primary, wrist
Osteoarthrosis (degenerative) (hypertrophic) (joint) —*see also* Osteoarthritis
  deformans alkaptonurica E70.29 *[M36.8]*
  erosive M15.4
  generalized M15.9
    primary M15.0
  polyarticular M15.9
  spine —*see* Spondylosis
Osteoblastoma —*see* Neoplasm, bone, benign
  aggressive —*see* Neoplasm, bone, uncertain behavior
Osteochondroarthrosis deformans endemica
  —*see* Disease, Kaschin-Beck
Osteochondritis —*see also*
  Osteochondropathy, by site
  Brailsford's —*see* Osteochondrosis, juvenile, radius
  dissecans M93.20
    ankle M93.27
    elbow M93.22
    foot M93.27
    hand M93.24
    hip M93.25
    knee M93.26
    multiple sites M93.29
    shoulder joint M93.21
    specified site NEC M93.28
    wrist M93.23
  juvenile M92.9
    patellar —*see* Osteochondrosis, juvenile, patella
  syphilitic (congenital) (early) A50.02 *[M90.80]*
    ankle A50.02 *[M90.87]*
    elbow A50.02 *[M90.82]*
    foot A50.02 *[M90.87]*
    forearm A50.02 *[M90.83]*
    hand A50.02 *[M90.84]*
    hip A50.02 *[M90.85]*
    knee A50.02 *[M90.86]*
    multiple sites A50.02 *[M90.89]*
    shoulder joint A50.02 *[M90.81]*
    specified site NEC A50.02 *[M90.88]*
Osteochondrodysplasia Q78.9
  with defects of growth of tubular bones and spine Q77.9
    specified NEC Q77.8
  specified NEC Q78.8
Osteochondrodystrophy E78.9
Osteochondrolysis —*see* Osteochondritis, dissecans
Osteochondroma —*see* Neoplasm, bone, benign
Osteochondromatosis D48.0
  syndrome Q78.4
Osteochondromyxosarcoma —*see* Neoplasm, bone, malignant
Osteochondropathy M93.90
  ankle M93.97
  elbow M93.92
  foot M93.97
  hand M93.94

Osteochondropathy *- continued*
  hip M93.95
  Kienböck's disease of adults M93.1
  knee M93.96
  multiple joints M93.99
  osteochondritis dissecans —*see* Osteochondritis, dissecans
  osteochondrosis —*see* Osteochondrosis
  shoulder region M93.91
  slipped upper femoral epiphysis —*see* Slipped, epiphysis, upper femoral
  specified joint NEC M93.98
  specified type NEC M93.80
    ankle M93.87
    elbow M93.82
    foot M93.87
    hand M93.84
    hip M93.85
    knee M93.86
    multiple joints M93.89
    shoulder region M93.81
    specified joint NEC M93.88
    wrist M93.83
  syphilitic, congenital
    early A50.02 *[M90.80]*
    late A50.56 *[M90.80]*
  wrist M93.93
Osteochondrosarcoma —*see* Neoplasm, bone, malignant
Osteochondrosis —*see also*
  Osteochondropathy, by site
  acetabulum (juvenile) M91.0
  adult —*see* Osteochondropathy, specified type NEC, by site
  astragalus (juvenile) —*see* Osteochondrosis, juvenile, tarsus
  Blount's —*see* Osteochondrosis, juvenile, tibia
  Buchanan's M91.0
  Burns' —*see* Osteochondrosis, juvenile, ulna
  calcaneus (juvenile) —*see* Osteochondrosis, juvenile, tarsus
  capitular epiphysis (femur) (juvenile) —*see* Legg-Calvé-Perthes disease
  carpal (juvenile) (lunate) (scaphoid) —*see* Osteochondrosis, juvenile, hand, carpal lunate
    adult M93.1
  coxae juvenilis —*see* Legg-Calvé-Perthes disease
  deformans juvenilis, coxae —*see* Legg-Calvé-Perthes disease
  Diaz's —*see* Osteochondrosis, juvenile, tarsus
  dissecans (knee) (shoulder) —*see* Osteochondritis, dissecans
  femoral capital epiphysis (juvenile) —*see* Legg-Calvé-Perthes disease
  femur (head) , juvenile —*see* Legg-Calvé-Perthes disease
  fibula (juvenile) —*see* Osteochondrosis, juvenile, fibula
  foot NEC (juvenile) M92.8 Freiberg's —*see* Osteochondrosis, juvenile, metatarsus
  Haas' (juvenile) —*see* Osteochondrosis, juvenile, humerus
  Haglund's —*see* Osteochondrosis, juvenile, tarsus
  hip (juvenile) —*see* Legg-Calvé-Perthes disease
  humerus (capitulum) (head) (juvenile) —*see* Osteochondrosis, juvenile, humerus
  ilium, iliac crest (juvenile) M91.0

Osteochondrosis *- continued*
  ischiopubic synchondrosis M91.0
  Iselin's —*see* Osteochondrosis, juvenile, metatarsus
  juvenile, juvenilis M92.9
    after congenital dislocation of hip reduction —*see* Osteochondrosis, juvenile, hip, specified NEC
    arm —*see* Osteochondrosis, juvenile, upper limb NEC
    capitular epiphysis (femur) —*see* Legg-Calvé-Perthes disease
    clavicle, sternal epiphysis —*see* Osteochondrosis, juvenile, upper limb NEC
    coxae —*see* Legg-Calvé-Perthes disease
    deformans M92.9
    fibula M92.5
    foot NEC M92.8
    hand M92.20
      carpal lunate M92.21
      metacarpal head M92.22
      specified site NEC M92.29
    head of femur —*see* Legg-Calvé-Perthes disease
    hip and pelvis M91.9
      coxa plana —*see* Coxa, plana
      femoral head —*see* Legg-Calvé-Perthes disease
      pelvis M91.0
      pseudocoxalgia —*see* Pseudocoxalgia
      specified NEC M91.8
    humerus M92.0
    limb
      lower NEC M92.8
      upper NEC —*see* Osteochondrosis, juvenile, upper limb NEC
    medial cuneiform bone —*see* Osteochondrosis, juvenile, tarsus
    metatarsus M92.7
    patella M92.4
    radius M92.1
    specified site NEC M92.8
    spine M42.00
      cervical region M42.02
      cervicothoracic region M42.03
      lumbar region M42.06
      lumbosacral region M42.07
      multiple sites M42.09
      occipito-atlanto-axial region M42.01
      sacrococcygeal region M42.08
      thoracic region M42.04
      thoracolumbar region M42.05
    tarsus M92.6
    tibia M92.5
    ulna M92.1
    upper limb NEC M92.3
    vertebra (body) (epiphyseal plates) (Calvé's) (Scheuermann's) —*see* Osteochondrosis, juvenile, spine
  Kienböck's —*see* Osteochondrosis, juvenile, hand, carpal lunate
    adult M93.1
  Kohler's
    patellar —*see* Osteochondrosis, juvenile, patella
    tarsal navicular —*see* Osteochondrosis, juvenile, tarsus
  Legg-Perthes (-Calvé) (-Waldenström) —*see* Legg-Calvé-Perthes disease
  limb
    lower NEC (juvenile) M92.8

Osteochondrosis - *continued*
   upper NEC (juvenile) —*see*
Osteochondrosis, juvenile, upper limb NEC
  lunate bone (carpal) (juvenile) —*see also*
Osteochondrosis, juvenile, hand, carpal lunate
   adult M93.1
  Mauclaire's —*see* Osteochondrosis, juvenile,
hand, metacarpal
  metacarpal (head) (juvenile) —*see*
Osteochondrosis, juvenile, hand, metacarpal
  metatarsus (fifth) (head) (juvenile) (second)
—*see* Osteochondrosis, juvenile, metatarsus
  navicular (juvenile) —*see* Osteochondrosis,
juvenile, tarsus
  os
   calcis (juvenile) —*see* Osteochondrosis,
juvenile, tarsus
   tibiale externum (juvenile) —*see*
Osteochondrosis, juvenile, tarsus
  Osgood-Schlatter —*see* Osteochondrosis,
juvenile, tibia
  Panner's —*see* Osteochondrosis, juvenile,
humerus
  patellar center (juvenile) (primary)
(secondary) —*see* Osteochondrosis, juvenile,
patella
  pelvis (juvenile) M91.0
  Pierson's M91.0
  radius (head) (juvenile) —*see*
Osteochondrosis, juvenile, radius
  Scheuermann's —*see* Osteochondrosis,
juvenile, spine
  Sever's —*see* Osteochondrosis, juvenile,
tarsus
  Sinding-Larsen —*see* Osteochondrosis,
juvenile, patella
  spine M42.9
   adult M42.10
    cervical region M42.12
    cervicothoracic region M42.13
    lumbar region M42.16
    lumbosacral region M42.17
    multiple sites M42.19
    occipito-atlanto-axial region M42.11
    sacrococcygeal region M42.18
    thoracic region M42.14
    thoracolumbar region M42.15
   juvenile —*see* Osteochondrosis, juvenile,
spine
  symphysis pubis (juvenile) M91.0
  syphilitic (congenital) A50.02
  talus (juvenile) —*see* Osteochondrosis,
juvenile, tarsus
  tarsus (navicular) (juvenile) —*see*
Osteochondrosis, juvenile, tarsus
  tibia (proximal) (tubercle) (juvenile) —*see*
Osteochondrosis, juvenile, tibia
  tuberculous —*see* Tuberculosis, bone
  ulna (lower) (juvenile) —*see*
Osteochondrosis, juvenile, ulna
  van Neck's M91.0
  vertebral —*see* Osteochondrosis, spine
Osteoclastoma D48.0
  malignant —*see* Neoplasm, bone, malignant
Osteodynia —*see* Disorder, bone, specified
type NEC
Osteodystrophy Q78.9
  azotemic N25.0
  congenital Q78.9
  parathyroid, secondary E21.1
  renal N25.0
Osteofibroma —*see* Neoplasm, bone, benign

Osteofibrosarcoma —*see* Neoplasm, bone,
malignant
Osteogenesis imperfecta Q78.0
Osteogenic —*see* condition
Osteolysis M89.50
  carpus M89.54
  clavicle M89.51
  femur M89.55
  fibula M89.56
  finger M89.54
  humerus M89.52
  ilium M89.559
  ischium M89.559
  joint prosthesis (periprosthetic) —*see*
Complications, joint prosthesis, mechanical,
periprosthetic, osteolysis, by site
  metacarpus M89.54
  metatarsus M89.57
  multiple sites M89.59
  neck M89.58
  periprosthetic —*see* Complications, joint
prosthesis, mechanical, periprosthetic,
osteolysis, by site
  radius M89.53
  rib M89.58
  scapula M89.51
  skull M89.58
  tarsus M89.57
  tibia M89.56
  toe M89.57
  ulna M89.53
  vertebra M89.58
Osteoma —*see also* Neoplasm, bone, benign
  osteoid —*see also* Neoplasm, bone, benign
   giant —*see* Neoplasm, bone, benign
Osteomalacia M83.9
  adult M83.9
   drug-induced NEC M83.5
   due to
    malabsorption (postsurgical) M83.2
    malnutrition M83.3
   specified NEC M83.8
  aluminium-induced M83.4
  infantile —*see* Rickets
  juvenile —*see* Rickets
  oncogenic E83.89
  pelvis M83.8
  puerperal M83.0
  senile M83.1
  vitamin-D-resistant in adults E83.31 *[M90.8]*
   carpus E83.31 *[M90.84]*
   clavicle E83.31 *[M90.81]*
   femur E83.31 *[M90.85]*
   fibula E83.31 *[M90.86]*
   finger E83.31 *[M90.84]*
   humerus E83.31 *[M90.82]*
   ilium E83.31 *[M90.859]*
   ischium E83.31 *[M90.859]*
   metacarpus E83.31 *[M90.84]*
   metatarsus E83.31 *[M90.87]*
   multiple sites E83.31 *[M90.89]*
   neck E83.31 *[M90.88]*
   radius E83.31 *[M90.83]*
   rib E83.31 *[M90.88]*
   scapula E83.31 *[M90.819]*
   skull E83.31 *[M90.88]*
   tarsus E83.31 *[M90.879]*
   tibia E83.31 *[M90.869]*
   toe E83.31 *[M90.879]*
   ulna E83.31 *[M90.839]*
   vertebra E83.31 *[M90.88]*

Osteomyelitis (general) (infective) (localized)
(neonatal) (purulent) (septic) (staphylococcal)
(streptococcal) (suppurative) (with periostitis)
M86.9
  acute M86.10
   carpus M86.14
   clavicle M86.11
   femur M86.15
   fibula M86.16
   finger M86.14
   hematogenous M86.00
    carpus M86.04
    clavicle M86.01
    femur M86.05
    fibula M86.06
    finger M86.04
    humerus M86.02
    ilium M86.059
    ischium M86.059
    mandible M27.2
    metacarpus M86.04
    metatarsus M86.07
    multiple sites M86.09
    neck M86.08
    orbit H05.02
    petrous bone —*see* Petrositis
    radius M86.03
    rib M86.08
    scapula M86.01
    skull M86.08
    tarsus M86.07
    tibia M86.06
    toe M86.07
    ulna M86.03
    vertebra —*see* Osteomyelitis, vertebra
   humerus M86.12
   ilium M86.159
   ischium M86.159
   mandible M27.2
   metacarpus M86.14
   metatarsus M86.17
   multiple sites M86.19
   neck M86.18
   orbit H05.02
   petrous bone —*see* Petrositis
   radius M86.13
   rib M86.18
   scapula M86.11
   skull M86.18
   tarsus M86.17
   tibia M86.16
   toe M86.17
   ulna M86.13
   vertebra —*see* Osteomyelitis, vertebra
  chronic (or old) M86.60
   with draining sinus M86.40
    carpus M86.44
    clavicle M86.41
    femur M86.45
    fibula M86.46
    finger M86.44
    humerus M86.42
    ilium M86.459
    ischium M86.459
    mandible M27.2
    metacarpus M86.44
    metatarsus M86.47
    multiple sites M86.49
    neck M86.48
    orbit H05.02
    petrous bone —*see* Petrositis
    radius M86.43
    rib M86.48

Osteomyelitis - *continued*
 scapula M86.41
 skull M86.48
 tarsus M86.47
 tibia M86.46
 toe M86.47
 ulna M86.43
 vertebra —*see* Osteomyelitis, vertebra
 carpus M86.64
 clavicle M86.61
 femur M86.65
 fibula M86.66
 finger M86.64
 hematogenous NEC M86.50
  carpus M86.54
  clavicle M86.51
  femur M86.55
  fibula M86.56
  finger M86.54
  humerus M86.52
  ilium M86.559
  ischium M86.559
  mandible M27.2
  metacarpus M86.54
  metatarsus M86.57
  multifocal M86.30
   carpus M86.34
   clavicle M86.31
   femur M86.35
   fibula M86.36
   finger M86.34
   humerus M86.32
   ilium M86.359
   ischium M86.359
   metacarpus M86.34
   metatarsus M86.37
   multiple sites M86.39
   neck M86.38
   radius M86.33
   rib M86.38
   scapula M86.31
   skull M86.38
   tarsus M86.37
   tibia M86.36
   toe M86.37
   ulna M86.33
   vertebra —*see* Osteomyelitis, vertebra
  multiple sites M86.59
  neck M86.58
  orbit H05.02
  petrous bone —*see* Petrositis
  radius M86.53
  rib M86.58
  scapula M86.51
  skull M86.58
  tarsus M86.57
  tibia M86.56
  toe M86.57
  ulna M86.53
  vertebra —*see* Osteomyelitis, vertebra
  humerus M86.62
  ilium M86.659
  ischium M86.659
  mandible M27.2
  metacarpus M86.64
  metatarsus M86.67
  multifocal —*see* Osteomyelitis, chronic, hematogenous, multifocal
  multiple sites M86.69
  neck M86.68
  orbit H05.02
  petrous bone —*see* Petrositis

Osteomyelitis - *continued*
 radius M86.63
 rib M86.63
 scapula M86.61
 skull M86.68
 tarsus M86.67
 tibia M86.66
 toe M86.67
 ulna M86.63
 vertebra —*see* Osteomyelitis, vertebra
 echinococcal B67.2
 Garr's —*see* Osteomyelitis, specified type NEC
 jaw (acute) (chronic) (lower) (neonatal) (suppurative) (upper) M27.2
 nonsuppurating —*see* Osteomyelitis, specified type NEC
 orbit H05.02
 petrous bone —*see* Petrositis
 Salmonella (arizonae) (cholerae-suis) (enteritidis) (typhimurium) A02.24
 sclerosing, nonsuppurative —*see* Osteomyelitis, specified type NEC
 specified type NEC (*see also* subcategory) M86.8X
  mandible M27.2
  orbit H05.02
  petrous bone —*see* Petrositis
  vertebra —*see* Osteomyelitis, vertebra
 subacute M86.20
  carpus M86.24
  clavicle M86.21
  femur M86.25
  fibula M86.26
  finger M86.24
  humerus M86.22
  mandible M27.2
  metacarpus M86.24
  metatarsus M86.27
  multiple sites M86.29
  neck M86.28
  orbit H05.02
  petrous bone —*see* Petrositis
  radius M86.23
  rib M86.28
  scapula M86.21
  skull M86.28
  tarsus M86.27
  tibia M86.26
  toe M86.27
  ulna M86.23
  vertebra —*see* Osteomyelitis, vertebra
 syphilitic A52.77
  congenital (early) A50.02 *[M90.80]*
 tuberculous —*see* Tuberculosis, bone
 typhoid A01.05
 vertebra M46.20
  cervical region M46.22
  cervicothoracic region M46.23
  lumbar region M46.26
  lumbosacral region M46.27
  occipito-atlanto-axial region M46.21
  sacrococcygeal region M46.28
  thoracic region M46.24
  thoracolumbar region M46.25
Osteomyelofibrosis D75.89
Osteomyelosclerosis D75.89
Osteonecrosis M87.9
 due to
  drugs —*see* Osteonecrosis, secondary, due to, drugs

Osteonecrosis - *continued*
 trauma —*see* Osteonecrosis, secondary, due to, trauma
 idiopathic aseptic M87.00
  ankle M87.07
  carpus M87.03
  clavicle M87.01
  femur M87.05
  fibula M87.06
  finger M87.04
  humerus M87.02
  ilium M87.050
  ischium M87.050
  metacarpus M87.04
  metatarsus M87.07
  multiple sites M87.09
  neck M87.08
  pelvis M87.050
  radius M87.03
  rib M87.08
  scapula M87.01
  skull M87.08
  tarsus M87.07
  tibia M87.06
  toe M87.07
  ulna M87.03
  vertebra M87.08
 secondary NEC M87.30
  carpus M87.33
  clavicle M87.31
  due to
   drugs M87.10
    carpus M87.13
    clavicle M87.11
    femur M87.15
    fibula M87.16
    finger M87.14
    humerus M87.12
    ilium M87.159
    ischium M87.159
    jaw M87.180
    metacarpus M87.14
    metatarsus M87.17
    multiple sites M87.19
    neck M87.18
    radius M87.13
    rib M87.18
    scapula M87.11
    skull M87.18
    tarsus M87.17
    tibia M87.16
    toe M87.17
    ulna M87.13
    vertebra M87.18
   hemoglobinopathy NEC D58.2 *[M90.50]*
    carpus D58.2 *[M90.54]*
    clavicle D58.2 *[M90.51]*
    femur D58.2 *[M90.55]*
    fibula D58.2 *[M90.56]*
    finger D58.2 *[M90.54]*
    humerus D58.2 *[M90.52]*
    ilium D58.2 *[M90.55]*
    ischium D58.2 *[M90.55]*
    metacarpus D58.2 *[M90.54]*
    metatarsus D58.2 *[M90.57]*
    multiple sites D58.2 *[M90.58]*
    neck D58.2 *[M90.58]*
    radius D58.2 *[M90.53]*
    rib D58.2 *[M90.58]*
    scapula D58.2 *[M90.51]*
    skull D58.2 *[M90.58]*
    tarsus D58.2 *[M90.57]*
    tibia D58.2 *[M90.56]*

Osteonecrosis - *continued*
  toe D58.2 *[M90.57]*
  ulna D58.2 *[M90.53]*
  vertebra D58.2 *[M90.58]*
  trauma (previous) M87.20
   carpus M87.23
   clavicle M87.21
   femur M87.25
   fibula M87.26
   finger M87.24
   humerus M87.22
   ilium M87.25
   ischium M87.25
   metacarpus M87.24
   metatarsus M87.27
   multiple sites M87.29
   neck M87.28
   radius M87.23
   rib M87.28
   scapula M87.21
   skull M87.28
   tarsus M87.27
   tibia M87.26
   toe M87.27
   ulna M87.23
   vertebra M87.28
  femur M87.35
  fibula M87.36
  finger M87.34
  humerus M87.32
  ilium M87.350
  in
   caisson disease T70.3 *[M90.50]*
    carpus T70.3 *[M90.54]*
    clavicle T70.3 *[M90.51]*
    femur T70.3 *[M90.55]*
    fibula T70.3 *[M90.56]*
    finger T70.3 *[M90.54]*
    humerus T70.3 *[M90.52]*
    ilium T70.3 *[M90.55]*
    ischium T70.3 *[M90.55]*
    metacarpus T70.3 *[M90.54]*
    metatarsus T70.3 *[M90.57]*
    multiple sites T70.3 *[M90.59]*
    neck T70.3 *[M90.58]*
    radius T70.3 *[M90.53]*
    rib T70.3 *[M90.58]*
    scapula T70.3 *[M90.51]*
    skull T70.3 *[M90.58]*
    tarsus T70.3 *[M90.57]*
    tibia T70.3 *[M90.56]*
    toe T70.3 *[M90.57]*
    ulna T70.3 *[M90.53]*
    vertebra T70.3 *[M90.58]*
  ischium M87.350
  metacarpus M87.34
  metatarsus M87.37
  multiple site M87.39
  neck M87.38
  radius M87.33
  rib M87.38
  scapula M87.319
  skull M87.38
  tarsus M87.379
  tibia M87.366
  toe M87.379
  ulna M87.33
  vertebra M87.38
 specified type NEC M87.80
  carpus M87.83
  clavicle M87.81
  femur M87.85

Osteonecrosis - *continued*
  fibula M87.86
  finger M87.84
  humerus M87.82
  ilium M87.85
  ischium M87.85
  metacarpus M87.84
  metatarsus M87.87
  multiple sites M87.89
  neck M87.88
  radius M87.83
  rib M87.88
  scapula M87.81
  skull M87.88
  tarsus M87.87
  tibia M87.86
  toe M87.87
  ulna M87.83
  vertebra M87.88
Osteo-onycho-arthro-dysplasia Q79.8
Osteo-onychodysplasia, hereditary Q79.8
Osteopathia condensans disseminata Q78.8
Osteopathy —*see also* Osteomyelitis,
  Osteonecrosis, Osteoporosis
  after poliomyelitis M89.60
   carpus M89.64
   clavicle M89.61
   femur M89.65
   fibula M89.66
   finger M89.64
   humerus M89.62
   ilium M89.659
   ischium M89.659
   metacarpus M89.64
   metatarsus M89.67
   multiple sites M89.69
   neck M89.68
   radius M89.63
   rib M89.68
   scapula M89.61
   skull M89.68
   tarsus M89.67
   tibia M89.66
   toe M89.67
   ulna M89.63
   vertebra M89.68
  in (due to)
   renal osteodystrophy N25.0
   specified diseases classified elsewhere —see
  subcategory M90.8
Osteopenia M85.8
  borderline M85.8
Osteoperiostitis —*see* Osteomyelitis, specified
  type NEC
Osteopetrosis (familial) Q78.2
Osteophyte M25.70
  ankle M25.77
  elbow M25.72
  foot joint M25.77
  hand joint M25.74
  hip M25.75
  knee M25.76
  shoulder M25.71
  spine M25.78
  vertebrae M25.78
  wrist M25.73
Osteopoikilosis Q78.8
Osteoporosis (female) (male) M81.0
  with current pathological fracture M80.00
  age-related M81.0
   with current pathologic fracture M80.00
    carpus M80.04

Osteoporosis - *continued*
  clavicle M80.01
  fibula M80.06
  finger M80.04
  humerus M80.02
  ilium M80.05
  ischium M80.05
  metacarpus M80.04
  metatarsus M80.07
  pelvis M80.05
  radius M80.03
  scapula M80.01
  tarsus M80.07
  tibia M80.06
  toe M80.07
  ulna M80.03
  vertebra M80.08
  disuse M81.8
   with current pathological fracture M80.80
    carpus M80.84
    clavicle M80.81
    fibula M80.86
    finger M80.84
    humerus M80.82
    ilium M80.85
    ischium M80.85
    metacarpus M80.84
    metatarsus M80.87
    pelvis M80.85
    radius M80.83
    scapula M80.81
    tarsus M80.87
    tibia M80.86
    toe M80.87
    ulna M80.83
    vertebra M80.88
  drug-induced —*see* Osteoporosis, specified
   type NEC
  idiopathic —*see* Osteoporosis, specified type
   NEC
  involutional —*see* Osteoporosis, age-related
  Lequesne M81.6
  localized M81.6
  postmenopausal M81.0
   with pathological fracture M80.00
    carpus M80.04
    clavicle M80.01
    fibula M80.06
    finger M80.04
    humerus M80.02
    ilium M80.05
    ischium M80.05
    metacarpus M80.04
    metatarsus M80.07
    pelvis M80.05
    radius M80.03
    scapula M80.01
    tarsus M80.07
    tibia M80.06
    toe M80.07
    ulna M80.03
    vertebra M80.08
  postoophorectomy —*see* Osteoporosis,
   specified type NEC
  postsurgical malabsorption —*see*
   Osteoporosis, specified type NEC
  post-traumatic —*see* Osteoporosis, specified
   type NEC
  senile —*see* Osteoporosis, age-related
  specified type NEC M81.8
   with pathological fracture M80.80
    carpus M80.84
    clavicle M80.81

Osteoporosis – *continued*
  fibula M80.86
  finger M80.84
  humerus M80.82
  ilium M80.85
  ischium M80.85
  metacarpus M80.84
  metatarsus M80.87
  pelvis M80.85
  radius M80.83
  scapula M80.81
  tarsus M80.87
  tibia M80.86
  toe M80.87
  ulna M80.83
  vertebra M80.88
Osteopsathyrosis (idiopathica) Q78.0
Osteoradionecrosis, jaw (acute) (chronic)
  (lower) (suppurative) (upper) M27.2
Osteosarcoma (any form) —*see* Neoplasm,
  bone, malignant
Osteosclerosis Q78.2
  acquired M85.8
  congenita Q77.4
  fragilitas (generalisata) Q78.2
  myelofibrosis D75.81
Osteosclerotic anemia D64.89
Osteosis
  cutis L94.2
  renal fibrocystic N25.0
Österreicher-Turner syndrome Q87.2
Ostium
  atrioventriculare commune Q21.2
  primum (arteriosum) (defect) (persistent)
  Q21.2
  secundum (arteriosum) (defect) (patent)
  (persistent) Q21.1
Ostrum-Furst syndrome Q75.8
Otalgia —see subcategory H92.0
Otitis (acute) H66.90
  with effusion —*see also* Otitis, media,
  nonsuppurative
    purulent —*see* Otitis, media, suppurative
  adhesive —see subcategory H74.1
  chronic —*see also* Otitis, media, chronic
    with effusion —*see also* Otitis, media,
    nonsuppurative, chronic
  externa H60.9
    abscess —*see* Abscess, ear, external
    acute (noninfective) H60.50
      actinic H60.51
      chemical H60.52
      contact H60.53
      eczematoid H60.54
      infective —*see* Otitis, externa, infective
      reactive H60.55
      specified NEC H60.59
    cellulitis —*see* Cellulitis, ear
    chronic H60.6
    diffuse —*see* Otitis, externa, infective,
    diffuse
    hemorrhagic —*see* Otitis, externa, infective,
    hemorrhagic
    in (due to)
      aspergillosis B44.89
      candidiasis B37.84
      erysipelas A46 *[H62.40]*
      herpes (simplex) virus infection B00.1
        zoster B02.8
      impetigo L01.00 *[H62.40]*
      infectious disease NEC B99 *[H62.4]*
      mycosis NEC B36.9 *[H62.40]*

Otitis – *continued*
    parasitic disease NEC B89 *[H62.40]*
    viral disease NEC B34.9 *[H62.40]*
      zoster B02.8
  infective NEC H60.39
    abscess —*see* Abscess, ear, external
    cellulitis —*see* Cellulitis, ear
    diffuse H60.31
    hemorrhagic H60.32
    swimmer's ear —*see* Swimmer's, ear
    malignant H60.2
  mycotic B36.9 *[H62.40]*
  necrotizing —*see* Otitis, externa, malignant
  Pseudomonas aeruginosa —*see* Otitis,
  externa, malignant
  reactive —*see* Otitis, externa, acute, reactive
  specified NEC —see subcategory H60.8
  tropical B36.8
  insidiosa —*see* Otosclerosis
  interna —see subcategory H83.0
  media (hemorrhagic) (staphylococcal)
  (streptococcal) H66.9
    with effusion (nonpurulent) —*see* Otitis,
    media, nonsuppurative
    acute, subacute H66.90
      allergic —*see* Otitis, media,
    nonsuppurative, acute, allergic
      exudative —*see* Otitis, media,
    nonsuppurative, acute
      mucoid —*see* Otitis, media,
    nonsuppurative, acute
      necrotizing —see also Otitis, media,
    suppurative, acute
        in
          measles B05.3
          scarlet fever A38.0
      nonsuppurative NEC —*see* Otitis, media,
    nonsuppurative, acute
      purulent —*see* Otitis, media, suppurative,
    acute
      sanguinous —*see* Otitis, media,
    nonsuppurative, acute
      secretory —*see* Otitis, media,
    nonsuppurative, acute, serous
      seromucinous —*see* Otitis, media,
    nonsuppurative, acute
      serous —*see* Otitis, media, nonsuppurative,
    acute, serous
      suppurative —*see* Otitis, media,
    suppurative, acute
      allergic —*see* Otitis, media, nonsuppurative
      catarrhal —*see* Otitis, media,
    nonsuppurative
      chronic H66.90
        with effusion (nonpurulent) —*see* Otitis,
      media, nonsuppurative, chronic
        allergic —*see* Otitis, media,
      nonsuppurative, chronic, allergic
        benign suppurative —*see* Otitis, media,
      suppurative, chronic, tubotympanic
        catarrhal —see Otitis, media,
      nonsuppurative, chronic, serous
        exudative —*see* Otitis, media,
      nonsuppurative, chronic
        mucinous —*see* Otitis, media,
      nonsuppurative, chronic, mucoid
        mucoid —*see* Otitis, media,
      nonsuppurative, chronic, mucoid
        nonsuppurative NEC —*see* Otitis, media,
      nonsuppurative, chronic
        purulent —*see* Otitis, media, suppurative,
      chronic

Otitis – *continued*
      secretory —*see* Otitis, media,
    nonsuppurative, chronic, mucoid
      seromucinous —*see* Otitis, media,
    nonsuppurative, chronic
      serous —*see* Otitis, media, nonsuppurative,
    chronic, serous
      suppurative —*see* Otitis, media,
    suppurative, chronic
      transudative —*see* Otitis, media,
    nonsuppurative, chronic, mucoid
    exudative —*see* Otitis, media,
    nonsuppurative
    in (due to) (with)
      influenza —*see* Influenza, with, otitis
    media
      measles B05.3
      scarlet fever A38.0
      tuberculosis A18.6
      viral disease NEC B34. *[H67.]*
    mucoid —*see* Otitis, media, nonsuppurative
    nonsuppurative H65.9
      acute or subacute NEC H65.19
        allergic H65.11
          recurrent H65.11
        recurrent H65.19
        secretory —*see* Otitis, media,
      nonsuppurative, serous
        serous H65.0
          recurrent H65.0
      chronic H65.49
        allergic H65.41
        mucoid H65.3
        serous H65.2
      postmeasles B05.3
      purulent —*see* Otitis, media, suppurative
      secretory —*see* Otitis, media,
    nonsuppurative
      seromucinous —*see* Otitis, media,
    nonsuppurative
      serous —*see* Otitis, media, nonsuppurative
    suppurative H66.4
      acute H66.00
        with rupture of ear drum H66.01
        recurrent H66.00
          with rupture of ear drum H66.01
      chronic (see also subcategory) H66.3
        atticoantral H66.2
        benign —*see* Otitis, media, suppurative,
      chronic, tubotympanic
        tubotympanic H66.1
      transudative —*see* Otitis, media,
    nonsuppurative
      tuberculous A18.6
Otocephaly Q18.2
Otolith syndrome —see subcategory H81.8
Otomycosis (diffuse) **NEC** B36.9 *[H62.40]*
  in
    aspergillosis B44.89
    candidiasis B37.84
    moniliasis B37.84
Otoporosis —*see* Otosclerosis
Otorrhagia (nontraumatic) H92.2
  traumatic
  code by Type of injury
Otorrhea H92.1
  cerebrospinal G96.0
Otosclerosis (general) H80.9
  cochlear (endosteal) H80.2
  involving
    otic capsule —*see* Otosclerosis, cochlear
    oval window
      nonobliterative H80.0

Otosclerosis - *continued*
  obliterative H80.1
    round window —*see* Otosclerosis, cochlear
  nonobliterative —*see* Otosclerosis, involving,
  oval window, nonobliterative
  obliterative —*see* Otosclerosis, involving,
  oval window, obliterative
  specified NEC H80.8
Otospongiosis —*see* Otosclerosis
Otto's disease or pelvis M24.7
Outcome of delivery Z37.9
  multiple births Z37.9
    all liveborn Z37.50
      quadruplets Z37.52
      quintuplets Z37.53
      sextuplets Z37.54
      specified number NEC Z37.59
      triplets Z37.51
    all stillborn Z37.7
    some liveborn Z37.60
      quadruplets Z37.62
      quintuplets Z37.63
      sextuplets Z37.64
      specified number NEC Z37.69
      triplets Z37.61
  single NEC Z37.9
    liveborn Z37.0
    stillborn Z37.1
  twins NEC Z37.9
    both liveborn Z37.2
    both stillborn Z37.4
    one liveborn, one stillborn Z37.3
Outlet —*see* condition
Ovalocytosis (congenital) (hereditary) —*see*
  Elliptocytosis
Ovarian —*see* Condition
Ovariocele N83.4
Ovaritis (cystic) —*see* Oophoritis
Ovary, ovarian —*see also* condition
  resistant syndrome E28.39
  vein syndrome N13.8
Overactive —*see also* Hyperfunction
  adrenal cortex NEC E27.0
  bladder N32.81
  hypothalamus E23.3
  thyroid —*see* Hyperthyroidism
Overactivity R46.3
  child —*see* Disorder, attention-deficit
  hyperactivity
Overbite (deep) (excessive) (horizontal)
  (vertical) M26.29
Overbreathing —*see* Hyperventilation
Overconscientious personality F60.5
Overdevelopment —*see* Hypertrophy
Overdistension —*see* Distension
Overdose, overdosage (drug) —*see* Table of
  Drugs and Chemicals, by drug, poisoning
Overeating R63.2
  nonorganic origin F50.8
  psychogenic F50.8
Overexertion (effects) (exhaustion) T73.3
Overexposure (effects) T73.9
  exhaustion T73.2
Overfeeding —*see* Overeating
  newborn P92.4
Overfill, endodontic M27.52
Overgrowth, bone —*see* Hypertrophy, bone
Overhanging of dental restorative material
  (unrepairable) K08.52
Overheated (places) (effects) —*see* Heat
Overjet (excessive horizontal) M26.23
Overlaid, overlying (suffocation) —*see*
  Asphyxia, traumatic, due to mechanical threat

Overlap, excessive horizontal (teeth) M26.23
Overlapping toe (acquired) —*see also*
  Deformity, toe, specified NEC
  congenital (fifth toe) Q66.89
Overload
  circulatory, due to transfusion (blood) (blood
  components) (TACO) E87.71
  fluid E87.70
    due to transfusion (blood) (blood
    components) E87.71
    specified NEC E87.79
  iron, due to repeated red blood cell
  transfusions E83.111
  potassium (K) E87.5
  sodium (Na) E87.0
Overnutrition —*see* Hyperalimentation
Overproduction —*see also* Hypersecretion
  ACTH E27.0
  catecholamine E27.5
  growth hormone E22.0
Overprotection, child by parent Z62.1
Overriding
  aorta Q25.4
  finger (acquired) —*see* Deformity, finger
    congenital Q68.1
  toe (acquired) —*see also* Deformity, toe,
  specified NEC
    congenital Q66.89
Overstrained R53.83
  heart —*see* Hypertrophy, cardiac
Overuse, muscle NEC M70.8
Overweight E66.3
Overworked R53.83
Oviduct —*see* condition
Ovotestis Q56.0
Ovulation (cycle)
  failure or lack of N97.0
  pain N94.0
Ovum —*see* condition
Owren's disease or syndrome
  (parahemophilia) D68.2
Ox heart —*see* Hypertrophy, cardiac
Oxalosis E72.53
Oxaluria E72.53
Oxycephaly, oxycephalic Q75.0
  syphilitic, congenital A50.02
Oxyuriasis B80
Oxyuris vermicularis (infestation) B80
Ozena J31.0

P

Pachyderma, pachydermia L85.9
  larynx (verrucosa) J38.7
Pachydermatocele (congenital) Q82.8
Pachydermoperiostosis —*see also*
  Osteoarthropathy, hypertrophic, specified type
  NEC
  clubbed nail M89.40 *[L62]*
Pachygyria Q04.3
Pachymeningitis (adhesive) (basal) (brain)
  (cervical) (chronic) (circumscribed) (external)
  (fibrous) (hemorrhagic) (hypertrophic)
  (internal) (purulent) (spinal) (suppurative) —
  see Meningitis
Pachyonychia (congenital) Q84.5
Pacinian tumor —*see* Neoplasm, skin, benign
Pad, knuckle or Garrod's M72.1
Paget-Schroetter syndrome I82.890
Paget's disease
  with infiltrating duct carcinoma —*see*
  Neoplasm, breast, malignant

Paget's disease – *continued*
  bone M88.9
    carpus M88.84
    clavicle M88.81
    femur M88.85
    fibula M88.86
    finger M88.84
    humerus M88.82
    ilium M88.85
    in neoplastic disease —*see* Osteitis,
    deformans, in neoplastic disease
    ischium M88.85
    metacarpus M88.84
    metatarsus M88.87
    multiple sites M88.89
    neck M88.88
    radius M88.83
    rib M88.88
    scapula M88.81
    skull M88.0
    tarsus M88.87
    tibia M88.86
    toe M88.87
    ulna M88.83
    vertebra M88.88
  breast (female) C50.01
    male C50.02
  extramammary —*see also* Neoplasm, skin,
  malignant
    anus C21.0
      margin C44.590
      skin C44.590
  intraductal carcinoma —*see* Neoplasm,
  breast, malignant
  malignant —*see* Neoplasm, skin, malignant
    breast (female) C50.01
      male C50.02
    unspecified site (female) C50.01
      male C50.02
  mammary —*see* Paget's disease, breast
  nipple —*see* Paget's disease, breast
  osteitis deformans —*see* Paget's disease, bone
Pain (s) (*see also* Painful) R52
  abdominal R10.9
    colic R10.83
    generalized R10.84
      with acute abdomen R10.0
    lower R10.30
      left quadrant R10.32
      pelvic or perineal R10.2
      periumbilical R10.33
      right quadrant R10.31
    rebound —*see* Tenderness, abdominal,
    rebound
    severe with abdominal rigidity R10.0
    tenderness —*see* Tenderness, abdominal
    upper R10.10
      epigastric R10.13
      left quadrant R10.12
      right quadrant R10.11
  acute R52
    due to trauma G89.11
    neoplasm related G89.3
    postprocedural NEC G89.18
    post-thoracotomy G89.12
    specified by site
  code to Pain, by site
  adnexa (uteri) R10.2
  anginoid —*see* Pain, precordial
  anus K62.89
  arm —*see* Pain, limb, upper
  axillary (axilla) M79.62
  back (postural) M54.9

Pain - *continued*
  bladder R39.89
    associated with micturition —*see*
  Micturition, painful
  bone —*see* Disorder, bone, specified type
  NEC
  breast N64.4
  broad ligament R10.2
  cancer associated (acute) (chronic) G89.3
  cecum —*see* Pain, abdominal
  cervicobrachial M53.1
  chest (central) R07.9
    anterior wall R07.89
    atypical R07.89
    ischemic I20.9
    musculoskeletal R07.89
    non-cardiac R07.89
    on breathing R07.1
    pleurodynia R07.81
    precordial R07.2
    wall (anterior) R07.89
  chronic G89.29
    associated with significant psychosocial
  dysfunction G89.4
    due to trauma G89.21
    neoplasm related G89.3
    postoperative NEC G89.28
    postprocedural NEC G89.28
    post-thoracotomy G89.22
    specified NEC G89.29
  coccyx M53.3
  colon —*see* Pain, abdominal
  coronary —*see* Angina
  costochondral R07.1
  diaphragm R07.1
  due to cancer G89.3
  due to device, implant or graft (*see also*
  Complications, by site and type, specified
  NEC) T85.84
    arterial graft NEC T82.848
    breast (implant) T85.84
    catheter NEC T85.84
      dialysis (renal) T82.848
        intraperitoneal T85.84
      infusion NEC T82.848
        spinal (epidural) (subdural) T85.84
      urinary (indwelling) T83.84
    electronic (electrode) (pulse generator)
    (stimulator)
      bone T84.84
      cardiac T82.847
      nervous system (brain) (peripheral nerve)
    (spinal) T85.84
      urinary T83.84
    fixation, internal (orthopedic) NEC T84.84
    gastrointestinal (bile duct) (esophagus)
    T85.84
      genital NEC T83.84
      heart NEC T82.847
      infusion NEC T85.84
      joint prosthesis T84.84
      ocular (corneal graft) (orbital implant) NEC
    T85.84
      orthopedic NEC T84.84
      specified NEC T85.84
      urinary NEC T83.84
      vascular NEC T82.848
      ventricular intracranial shunt T85.84
  due to malignancy (primary) (secondary)
  G89.3
  ear —see subcategory H92.0
  epigastric, epigastrium R10.13

Pain - *continued*
  eye —*see* Pain, ocular
  face, facial R51
    atypical G50.1
  female genital organs NEC N94.89
  finger —*see* Pain, limb, upper
  flank —*see* Pain, abdominal
  foot —*see* Pain, limb, lower
  gallbladder K82.9
  gas (intestinal) R14.1
  gastric —*see* Pain, abdominal
  generalized NOS R52
  genital organ
    female N94.89
    male N50.8
  groin —*see* Pain, abdominal, lower
  hand —*see* Pain, limb, upper
  head —*see* Headache
  heart —*see* Pain, precordial
  infra-orbital —*see* Neuralgia, trigeminal
  intercostal R07.82
  intermenstrual N94.0
  jaw R68.84
  joint M25.50
    ankle M25.57
    elbow M25.52
    finger M79.64
    foot M25.57
    hand M79.64
    hip M25.55
    knee M25.56
    shoulder M25.51
    toe M25.57
    wrist M25.53
  kidney N23
  laryngeal R07.0
  leg —*see* Pain, limb, lower
  limb M79.609
    lower M79.60
      foot M79.67
      lower leg M79.66
      thigh M79.65
      toe M79.67
    upper M79.60
      axilla M79.62
      finger M79.64
      forearm M79.63
      hand M79.64
      upper arm M79.62
  loin M54.5
  low back M54.5
  lumbar region M54.5
  mandibular R68.84
  mastoid —see subcategory H92.0
  maxilla R68.84
  menstrual (*see also* Dysmenorrhea) N94.6
  metacarpophalangeal (joint) —*see* Pain, joint,
  hand
  metatarsophalangeal (joint) —*see* Pain, joint,
  foot
  mouth K13.79
  muscle —*see* Myalgia
  musculoskeletal (*see also* Pain, by site) M79.1
  myofascial M79.1
  nasal J34.89
  nasopharynx J39.2
  neck NEC M54.2
  nerve NEC —*see* Neuralgia
  neuromuscular —*see* Neuralgia
  nose J34.89
  ocular H57.1
  ophthalmic —*see* Pain, ocular

Pain - *continued*
  orbital region —*see* Pain, ocular
  ovary N94.89
  over heart —*see* Pain, precordial
  ovulation N94.0
  pelvic (female) R10.2
  penis N48.89
  pericardial —*see* Pain, precordial
  perineal, perineum R10.2
  pharynx J39.2
  pleura, pleural, pleuritic R07.81
  postoperative NOS G89.18
  postprocedural NOS G89.18
  post-thoracotomy G89.12
  precordial (region) R07.2
  premenstrual N94.3
  psychogenic (persistent) (any site) F45.41
  radicular (spinal) —*see* Radiculopathy
  rectum K62.89
  respiration R07.1
  retrosternal R07.2
  rheumatoid, muscular —*see* Myalgia
  rib R07.81
  root (spinal) —*see* Radiculopathy
  round ligament (stretch) R10.2
  sacroiliac M53.3
  sciatic —*see* Sciatica
  scrotum N50.8
  seminal vesicle N50.8
  shoulder M25.51
  spermatic cord N50.8
  spinal root —*see* Radiculopathy
  spine M54.9
    cervical M54.2
    low back M54.5
      with sciatica M54.4
    thoracic M54.6
  stomach —*see* Pain, abdominal
  substernal R07.2
  temporomandibular (joint) M26.62
  testis N50.8
  thoracic spine M54.6
    with radicular and visceral pain M54.14
  throat R07.0
  tibia —*see* Pain, limb, lower
  toe —*see* Pain, limb, lower
  tongue K14.6
  tooth K08.8
  trigeminal —*see* Neuralgia, trigeminal
  tumor associated G89.3
  ureter N23
  urinary (organ) (system) N23
  uterus NEC N94.89
  vagina R10.2
  vertebrogenic (syndrome) M54.89
  vesical R39.89
    associated with micturition —*see*
  Micturition, painful
  vulva R10.2
Painful —*see also* Pain
  coitus
    female N94.1
    male N53.12
    psychogenic F52.6
  ejaculation (semen) N53.12
    psychogenic F52.6
  erection —*see* Priapism
  feet syndrome E53.8
  joint replacement (hip) (knee) T84.84
  menstruation —*see* Dysmenorrhea
    psychogenic F45.8
  micturition —*see* Micturition, painful
  respiration R07.1

Painful - *continued*
  scar NEC L90.5
  wire sutures T81.89
Painter's colic —*see* subcategory T56.0
Palate —*see* condition
Palatoplegia K13.79
Palatoschisis —*see* Cleft, palate
Palilalia R48.8
Palliative care Z51.5
Pallor R23.1
  optic disc, temporal —*see* Atrophy, optic
Palmar —*see also* condition
  fascia —*see* condition
Palpable
  cecum K63.89
  kidney N28.89
  ovary N83.8
  prostate N42.9
  spleen —*see* Splenomegaly
Palpitations (heart) R00.2
  psychogenic F45.8
Palsy (*see also* Paralysis) G83.9
  atrophic diffuse (progressive) G12.22
  Bell's —*see also* Palsy, facial
    newborn P11.3
  brachial plexus NEC G54.0
    newborn (birth injury) P14.3
  brain —*see* Palsy, cerebral
  bulbar (progressive) (chronic) G12.22
    of childhood (Fazio-Londe) G12.1
    pseudo NEC G12.29
    supranuclear (progressive) G23.1
  cerebral (congenital) G80.9
    ataxic G80.4
    athetoid G80.3
    choreathetoid G80.3
    diplegic G80.8
      spastic G80.1
    dyskinetic G80.3
      athetoid G80.3
      choreathetoid G80.3
      dystonic G80.3
    dystonic G80.3
    hemiplegic G80.8
      spastic G80.2
    mixed G80.8
    monoplegic G80.8
      spastic G80.1
    paraplegic G80.8
      spastic G80.1
    quadriplegic G80.8
      spastic G80.0
    spastic G80.1
      diplegic G80.1
      hemiplegic G80.2
      monoplegic G80.1
      quadriplegic G80.0
      specified NEC G80.1
      tetraplegic G80.0
    specified NEC G80.8
    syphilitic A52.12
      congenital A50.49
    tetraplegic G80.8
      spastic G80.0
  cranial nerve —*see also* Disorder, nerve, cranial
    multiple G52.7
      in
        infectious disease B99 *[G53]*
        neoplastic disease (*see also* Neoplasm) D49.9 *[G53]*
        parasitic disease B89 *[G53]*

Palsy - *continued*
    sarcoidosis D86.82
  creeping G12.22
  diver's T70.3
  Erb's P14.0
  facial G51.0
    newborn (birth injury) P11.3
  glossopharyngeal G52.1
  Klumpke (-Déjérine) P14.1
  lead —*see* subcategory T56.0
  median nerve (tardy) G56.1
  nerve G58.9
    specified NEC G58.8
  peroneal nerve (acute) (tardy) G57.3
  progressive supranuclear G23.1
  pseudobulbar NEC G12.29
  radial nerve (acute) G56.3
  seventh nerve —*see also* Palsy, facial
    newborn P11.3
  shaking —*see* Parkinsonism
  spastic (cerebral) (spinal) G80.1
  ulnar nerve (tardy) G56.2
  wasting G12.29
Paludism —*see* Malaria
Panangiitis M30.0
Panaris, panaritium —*see also* Cellulitis, digit
  with lymphangitis —*see* Lymphangitis, acute, digit
Panarteritis nodosa M30.0
  brain or cerebral I67.7
Pancake heart R93.1
  with cor pulmonale (chronic) I27.81
Pancarditis (acute) (chronic) I51.89
  rheumatic I09.89
    active or acute I01.8
Pancoast's syndrome or tumor C34.1
Pancolitis, ulcerative (chronic) K51.00
  with
    complication K51.019
    abscess K51.014
    fistula K51.013
    obstruction K51.012
    rectal bleeding K51.011
    specified complication NEC K51.018
Pancreas, pancreatic —*see* condition
Pancreatitis (annular) (apoplectic) (calcareous) (edematous) (hemorrhagic) (malignant) (recurrent) (subacute) (suppurative) K85.9
  acute K85.9
    alcohol induced K85.2
    biliary K85.1
    drug induced K85.3
    gallstone K85.1
    idiopathic K85.0
    specified NEC K85.8
  chronic (infectious) K86.1
    alcohol-induced K86.0
    recurrent K86.1
    relapsing K86.1
  cystic (chronic) K86.1
  cytomegaloviral B25.2
  fibrous (chronic) K86.1
  gangrenous K85.8
  gallstone K85.1
  interstitial (chronic) K86.1
    acute K85.8
  mumps B26.3
  recurrent (chronic) K86.1
  relapsing, chronic K86.1
  syphilitic A52.74
Pancreatoblastoma —*see* Neoplasm, pancreas, malignant

Pancreolithiasis K86.8
Pancytolysis D75.89
Pancytopenia (acquired) D61.818
  with
    malformations D61.09
    myelodysplastic syndrome —*see* Syndrome, myelodysplastic
  antineoplastic chemotherapy induced D61.810
  congenital D61.09
  drug-induced NEC D61.811
Panencephalitis, subacute, sclerosing A81.1
Panhematopenia D61.9
  congenital D61.09
  constitutional D61.09
  splenic, primary D73.1
Panhemocytopenia D61.9
  congenital D61.09
  constitutional D61.09
Panhypogonadism E29.1
Panhypopituitarism E23.0
  prepubertal E23.0
Panic (attack) (state) F41.0
  reaction to exceptional stress (transient) F43.0
Panmyelopathy, familial, constitutional D61.09
Panmyelophthisis D61.82
  congenital D61.09
Panmyelosis (acute) (with myelofibrosis) C94.4
Panner's disease —*see* Osteochondrosis, juvenile, humerus
Panneuritis endemica E51.11
Panniculitis (nodular) (nonsuppurative) M79.3
  back M54.00
    cervical region M54.02
    cervicothoracic region M54.03
    lumbar region M54.06
    lumbosacral region M54.07
    multiple sites M54.09
    occipito-atlanto-axial region M54.01
    sacrococcygeal region M54.08
    thoracic region M54.04
    thoracolumbar region M54.05
  lupus L93.2
  mesenteric K65.4
  neck M54.02
    cervicothoracic region M54.03
    occipito-atlanto-axial region M54.01
  relapsing M35.6
Panniculus adiposus (abdominal) E65
Pannus (allergic) (cornea) (degenerativus) (keratic) H16.42
  abdominal (symptomatic) E65
  trachomatosus, trachomatous (active) A71.1
Panophthalmitis H44.01
Pansinusitis (chronic) (hyperplastic) (nonpurulent) (purulent) J32.4
  acute J01.40
    recurrent J01.41
  tuberculous A15.8
Panuveitis (sympathetic) H44.11
Panvalvular disease I08.9
  specified NEC I08.8
Papanicolaou smear, cervix Z12.4
  as part of routine gynecological examination Z01.419
    with abnormal findings Z01.411
  for suspected neoplasm Z12.4
  nonspecific abnormal finding R87.619
  routine Z01.419
    with abnormal findings Z01.411

Papilledema (choked disc) H47.10
  associated with
    decreased ocular pressure H47.12
    increased intracranial pressure H47.11
    retinal disorder H47.13
    Foster-Kennedy syndrome H47.14
Papillitis H46.00
  anus K62.89
  chronic lingual K14.4
  necrotizing, kidney N17.2
  optic H46.0
  rectum K62.89
  renal, necrotizing N17.2
  tongue K14.0
Papilloma —*see also* Neoplasm, benign, by site
  acuminatum (female) (male) (anogenital) A63.0
  benign pinta (primary) A67.0
  bladder (urinary) (transitional cell) D41.4
  choroid plexus (lateral ventricle) (third ventricle) D33.0
    anaplastic C71.5
    fourth ventricle D33.1
    malignant C71.5
  renal pelvis (transitional cell) D41.1
    benign D30.1
  Schneiderian
    specified site —*see* Neoplasm, benign, by site
    unspecified site D14.0
  serous surface
    borderline malignancy
      specified site —*see* Neoplasm, uncertain behavior, by site
      unspecified site D39.10
    specified site —*see* Neoplasm, benign, by site
    unspecified site D27.9
  transitional (cell)
    bladder (urinary) D41.4
    inverted type —*see* Neoplasm, uncertain behavior, by site
    renal pelvis D41.1
    ureter D41.2
  ureter (transitional cell) D41.2
    benign D30.2
  urothelial —*see* Neoplasm, uncertain behavior, by site
  villous —*see* Neoplasm, uncertain behavior, by site
    adenocarcinoma in —*see* Neoplasm, malignant, by site
    in situ —*see* Neoplasm, in situ
  yaws, plantar or palmar A66.1
Papillomata, multiple, of yaws A66.1
Papillomatosis —*see also* Neoplasm, benign, by site
  confluent and reticulated L83
  cystic, breast —*see* Mastopathy, cystic
  ductal, breast —*see* Mastopathy, cystic
  intraductal (diffuse) —*see* Neoplasm, benign, by site
  subareolar duct D24
Papillomavirus, as cause of disease classified elsewhere B97.7
Papillon-Léage and Psaume syndrome Q87.0
Papule (s) R23.8
  carate (primary) A67.0
  fibrous, of nose D22.39
  Gottron's L94.4
  pinta (primary) A67.0

Papulosis
  lymphomatoid C86.6
  malignant I77.89
Papyraceous fetus O31.0
Para-albuminemia E88.09
Paracephalus Q89.7
Parachute mitral valve Q23.2
Paracoccidioidomycosis B41.9
  disseminated B41.7
  generalized B41.7
  mucocutaneous-lymphangitic B41.8
  pulmonary B41.0
  specified NEC B41.8
  visceral B41.8
Paradentosis K05.4
Paraffinoma T88.8
Paraganglioma D44.7
  adrenal D35.0
    malignant C74.1
  aortic body D44.7
    malignant C75.5
  carotid body D44.6
    malignant C75.4
  chromaffin —*see also* Neoplasm, benign, by site
    malignant —*see* Neoplasm, malignant, by site
  extra-adrenal D44.7
    malignant C75.5
      specified site —*see* Neoplasm, malignant, by site
      unspecified site C75.5
    specified site —*see* Neoplasm, uncertain behavior, by site
    unspecified site D44.7
  gangliocytic D13.2
    specified site —*see* Neoplasm, benign, by site
    unspecified site D13.2
  glomus jugulare D44.7
    malignant C75.5
  jugular D44.7
  malignant C75.5
    specified site —*see* Neoplasm, malignant, by site
    unspecified site C75.5
  nonchromaffin D44.7
    malignant C75.5
      specified site — *see* Neoplasm, malignant, by site
      unspecified site C75.5
    specified site —*see* Neoplasm, uncertain behavior, by site
    unspecified site D44.7
  parasympathetic D44.7
    specified site —*see* Neoplasm, uncertain behavior, by site
    unspecified site D44.7
  specified site —*see* Neoplasm, uncertain behavior, by site
  sympathetic D44.7
    specified site —*see* Neoplasm, uncertain behavior, by site
    unspecified site D44.7
  unspecified site D44.7
Parageusia R43.2
  psychogenic F45.8
Paragonimiasis B66.4
Paragranuloma, Hodgkin —*see* Lymphoma, Hodgkin, classical, specified NEC
Parahemophilia (*see also* Defect, coagulation) D68.2

Parakeratosis R23.4
  variegata L41.0
Paralysis, paralytic (complete) (incomplete) G83.9
  with
    syphilis A52.17
  abducens, abducent (nerve) —*see* Strabismus, paralytic, sixth nerve
  abductor, lower extremity G57.9
  accessory nerve G52.8
  accommodation —*see also* Paresis, of accommodation
    hysterical F44.89
  acoustic nerve (except Deafness) —*see* subcategory H93.3
  agitans (*see also* Parkinsonism) G20
    arteriosclerotic G21.4
  alternating (oculomotor) G83.89
  amyotrophic G12.21
  ankle G57.9
  anus (sphincter) K62.89
  arm —*see* Monoplegia, upper limb
  ascending (spinal) , acute G61.0
  association G12.29
  asthenic bulbar G70.00
    with exacerbation (acute) G70.01
    in crisis G70.01
  ataxic (hereditary) G11.9
    general (syphilitic) A52.17
  atrophic G58.9
    infantile, acute —*see* Poliomyelitis, paralytic
    progressive G12.22
    spinal (acute) —*see* Poliomyelitis, paralytic
  axillary G54.0
  Babinski-Nageotte's G83.89
  Bell's G51.0
    newborn P11.3
  Benedikt's G46.3
  birth injury P14.9
    spinal cord P11.5
  bladder (neurogenic) (sphincter) N31.2
  bowel, colon or intestine K56.0
  brachial plexus G54.0
    birth injury P14.3
    newborn (birth injury) P14.3
  brain G83.9
    diplegia G83.0
    triplegia G83.89
  bronchial J98.09
  Brown-Séquard G83.81
  bulbar (chronic) (progressive) G12.22
    infantile —*see* Poliomyelitis, paralytic
    poliomyelitic —*see* Poliomyelitis, paralytic
    pseudo G12.29
  bulbospinal G70.00
    with exacerbation (acute) G70.01
    in crisis G70.01
  cardiac (*see also* Failure, heart) I50.9
  cerebrocerebellar, diplegic G80.1
  cervical
    plexus G54.2
    sympathetic G90.09
  Céstan-Chenais G46.3
  Charcot-Marie-Tooth type G60.0
  Clark's G80.9
  colon K56.0
  compressed air T70.3
  compression
    arm G56.9
    leg G57.9
    lower extremity G57.9
    upper extremity G56.9

Paralysis, paralytic - *continued*
congenital (cerebral) —*see* Palsy, cerebral
conjugate movement (gaze) (of eye) H51.0
  cortical (nuclear) (supranuclear) H51.0
cordis —*see* Failure, heart
cranial or cerebral nerve G52.9
creeping G12.22
crossed leg G83.89
crutch —*see* Injury, brachial plexus
deglutition R13.0
  hysterical F44.4
dementia A52.17
descending (spinal) NEC G12.29
diaphragm (flaccid) J98.6
  due to accidental dissection of phrenic nerve
during procedure —*see* Puncture, accidental
complicating surgery
digestive organs NEC K59.8
diplegic —*see* Diplegia
divergence (nuclear) H51.8
diver's T70.3
Duchenne's
  birth injury P14.0
  due to or associated with
    motor neuron disease G12.22
    muscular dystrophy G71.0
due to intracranial or spinal birth injury —*see*
Palsy, cerebral
embolic (current episode) I63.4
Erb (-Duchenne) (birth) (newborn) P14.0
Erb's syphilitic spastic spinal A52.17
esophagus K22.8
eye muscle (extrinsic) H49.9
  intrinsic —*see also* Paresis, of
accommodation
facial (nerve) G51.0
  birth injury P11.3
  congenital P11.3
  following operation NEC —*see* Puncture,
accidental complicating surgery
  newborn (birth injury) P11.3
familial (recurrent) (periodic) G72.3
  spastic G11.4
fauces J39.2
finger G56.9
gait R26.1
gastric nerve (nondiabetic) G52.2
gaze, conjugate H51.0
general (progressive) (syphilitic) A52.17
  juvenile A50.45
glottis J38.00
  bilateral J38.02
  unilateral J38.01
gluteal G54.1
Gubler (-Millard) G46.3
hand —*see* Monoplegia, upper limb
heart —*see* Arrest, cardiac
hemiplegic —*see* Hemiplegia
hyperkalemic periodic (familial) G72.3
hypoglossal (nerve) G52.3
hypokalemic periodic G72.3
hysterical F44.4
ileus K56.0
infantile (*see also* Poliomyelitis, paralytic)
A80.30
  bulbar —*see* Poliomyelitis, paralytic
  cerebral —*see* Palsy, cerebral
  spastic —*see* Palsy, cerebral, spastic
infective —*see* Poliomyelitis, paralytic
inferior nuclear G83.9
internuclear —*see* Ophthalmoplegia,
internuclear

Paralysis, paralytic - *continued*
intestine K56.0
iris H57.09
  due to diphtheria (toxin) A36.89
ischemic, Volkmann's (complicating trauma)
T79.6
Jackson's G83.89
jake —*see* Poisoning, food, noxious, plant
Jamaica ginger (jake) G62.2
juvenile general A50.45
Klumpke (-Déjérine) (birth) (newborn) P14.1
labioglossal (laryngeal) (pharyngeal) G12.29
Landry's G61.0
laryngeal nerve (recurrent) (superior)
(unilateral) J38.00
  bilateral J38.02
  unilateral J38.01
larynx J38.00
  bilateral J38.02
  due to diphtheria (toxin) A36.2
  unilateral J38.01
lateral G12.21
lead —*see* subcategory T56.0
left side —*see* Hemiplegia
leg G83.1
  both —*see* Paraplegia
  crossed G83.89
  hysterical F44.4
  psychogenic F44.4
  transient or transitory R29.818
    traumatic NEC —*see* Injury, nerve, leg
levator palpebrae superioris —*see*
Blepharoptosis, paralytic
limb —*see* Monoplegia
lip K13.0
Lissauer's A52.17
lower limb —*see* Monoplegia, lower limb
  both —*see* Paraplegia
lung J98.4
median nerve G56.1
medullary (tegmental) G83.89
mesencephalic NEC G83.89
  tegmental G83.89
middle alternating G83.89
Millard-Gubler-Foville G46.3
monoplegic —*see* Monoplegia
motor G83.9
muscle, muscular NEC G72.89
  due to nerve lesion G58.9
  eye (extrinsic) H49.9
    intrinsic —*see* Paresis, of accommodation
    oblique —*see* Strabismus, paralytic, fourth
nerve
  iris sphincter H21.9
  ischemic (Volkmann's) (complicating
trauma) T79.6
  progressive G12.21
  pseudohypertrophic G71.0
musculocutaneous nerve G56.9
musculospiral G56.9
nerve —*see also* Disorder, nerve
  abducent —*see* Strabismus, paralytic, sixth
nerve
  accessory G52.8
  auditory (except Deafness) —*see*
subcategory H93.3
  birth injury P14.9
  cranial or cerebral G52.9
  facial G51.0
    birth injury P11.3
    congenital P11.3
    newborn (birth injury) P11.3

Paralysis, paralytic - *continued*
  fourth or trochlear —*see* Strabismus,
paralytic, fourth nerve
  newborn (birth injury) P14.9
  oculomotor —*see* Strabismus, paralytic,
third nerve
  phrenic (birth injury) P14.2
  radial G56.3
  seventh or facial G51.0
    newborn (birth injury) P11.3
  sixth or abducent —*see* Strabismus,
paralytic, sixth nerve
    syphilitic A52.15
  third or oculomotor —*see* Strabismus,
paralytic, third nerve
  trigeminal G50.9
  trochlear —*see* Strabismus, paralytic, fourth
nerve
  ulnar G56.2
normokalemic periodic G72.3
ocular H49.9
  alternating G83.89
oculofacial, congenital (Moebius) Q87.0
oculomotor (external bilateral) (nerve) —*see*
Strabismus, paralytic, third nerve
palate (soft) K13.79
paratrigeminal G50.9
periodic (familial) (hyperkalemic)
(hypokalemic) (myotonic) (normokalemic)
(potassium sensitive) (secondary) G72.3
peripheral autonomic nervous system —*see*
Neuropathy, peripheral, autonomic
peroneal (nerve) G57.3
pharynx J39.2
phrenic nerve G56.8
plantar nerve (s) G57.6
pneumogastric nerve G52.2
poliomyelitis (current) —*see* Poliomyelitis,
paralytic
popliteal nerve G57.3
postepileptic transitory G83.84
progressive (atrophic) (bulbar) (spinal)
G12.22
  general A52.17
  infantile acute —*see* Poliomyelitis, paralytic
  supranuclear G23.1
pseudobulbar G12.29
pseudohypertrophic (muscle) G71.0
psychogenic F44.4
quadriceps G57.9
quadriplegic —*see* Tetraplegia
radial nerve G56.3
rectus muscle (eye) H49.9
recurrent isolated sleep G47.53
respiratory (muscle) (system) (tract) R06.81
  center NEC G93.89
  congenital P28.89
  newborn P28.89
right side —*see* Hemiplegia
saturnine —*see* subcategory T56.0
sciatic nerve G57.0
senile G83.9
shaking —*see* Parkinsonism
shoulder G56.9
sleep, recurrent isolated G47.53
spastic G83.9
  cerebral —*see* Palsy, cerebral, spastic
  congenital (cerebral) —*see* Palsy, cerebral,
spastic
  familial G11.4
  hereditary G11.4
  quadriplegic G80.0
  syphilitic (spinal) A52.17

Paralysis, paralytic *- continued*
sphincter, bladder —*see* Paralysis, bladder
spinal (cord) G83.9
  accessory nerve G52.8
  acute —*see* Poliomyelitis, paralytic
  ascending acute G61.0
  atrophic (acute) —*see also* Poliomyelitis, paralytic
    spastic, syphilitic A52.17
  congenital NEC —*see* Palsy, cerebral
  infantile —*see* Poliomyelitis, paralytic
  hereditary G95.89
  progressive G12.21
  sequelae NEC G83.89
sternomastoid G52.8
stomach K31.84
  diabetic —*see* Diabetes, by type, with gastroparesis
  nerve G52.2
    diabetic —*see* Diabetes, by type, with gastroparesis
stroke —*see* Infarct, brain
subcapsularis G56.8
supranuclear (progressive) G23.1
sympathetic G90.8
  cervical G90.09
  nervous system —*see* Neuropathy, peripheral, autonomic
syndrome G83.9
  specified NEC G83.89
syphilitic spastic spinal (Erb's) A52.17
thigh G57.9
throat J39.2
  diphtheritic A36.0
  muscle J39.2
thrombotic (current episode) I63.3
thumb G56.9
tick —*see* Toxicity, venom, arthropod, specified NEC
Todd's (postepileptic transitory paralysis) G83.84
toe G57.6
tongue K14.8
transient R29.5
  arm or leg NEC R29.818
  traumatic NEC —*see* Injury, nerve
trapezius G52.8
traumatic, transient NEC —*see* Injury, nerve
trembling —*see* Parkinsonism
triceps brachii G56.9
trigeminal nerve G50.9
trochlear (nerve) —*see* Strabismus, paralytic, fourth nerve
ulnar nerve G56.2
upper limb   *see* Monoplegia, upper limb
uremic N18.9 *[G99.8]*
uveoparotitic D86.89
uvula K13.79
  postdiphtheritic A36.0
vagus nerve G52.2
vasomotor NEC G90.8
velum palati K13.79
vesical —*see* Paralysis, bladder
vestibular nerve (except Vertigo) —*see* subcategory H93.3
vocal cords J38.00
  bilateral J38.02
  unilateral J38.01
Volkmann's (complicating trauma) T79.6
wasting G12.29
Weber's G46.3
wrist G56.9
Paramedial urethrovesical orifice Q64.79

Paramenia N92.6
Parametritis (*see also* Disease, pelvis, inflammatory) N73.2
acute N73.0
complicating abortion —*see* Abortion, by type, complicated by, parametritis
Parametrium, parametric —*see* condition
Paramnesia —*see* Amnesia
Paramolar K00.1
Paramyloidosis E85.8
Paramyoclonus multiplex G25.3
Paramyotonia (congenita) G71.19
Parangi —*see* Yaws
Paranoia (querulans) F22
senile F03
Paranoid
dementia (senile) F03
  praecox —*see* Schizophrenia
personality F60.0
psychosis (climacteric) (involutional) (menopausal) F22
  psychogenic (acute) F23
  senile F03
reaction (acute) F23
  chronic F22
schizophrenia F20.0
state (climacteric) (involutional) (menopausal) (simple) F22
  senile F03
tendencies F60.0
traits F60.0
trends F60.0
type, psychopathic personality F60.0
Paraparesis —*see* Paraplegia
Paraphasia R47.02
Paraphilia F65.9
Paraphimosis (congenital) N47.2
chancroidal A57
Paraphrenia, paraphrenic (late) F22
schizophrenia F20.0
Paraplegia (lower) G82.20
ataxic —*see* Degeneration, combined, spinal cord
complete G82.21
congenital (cerebral) G80.8
  spastic G80.1
familial spastic G11.4
functional (hysterical) F44.4
hereditary, spastic G11.4
hysterical F44.4
incomplete G82.22
Pott's A18.01
psychogenic F44.4
spastic
  Erb's spinal, syphilitic A52.17
  hereditary G11.4
  tropical G04.1
syphilitic (spastic) A52.17
tropical spastic G04.1
Parapoxvirus B08.60
specified NEC B08.69
Paraproteinemia D89.2
benign (familial) D89.2
monoclonal D47.2
secondary to malignant disease D47.2
Parapsoriasis L41.9
en plaques L41.4
guttata L41.1
large plaque L41.4
retiform, retiformis L41.5
small plaque L41.3

Parapsoriasis – *continued*
specified NEC L41.8
varioliformis (acuta) L41.0
Parasitic —*see also* condition
disease NEC B89
stomatitis B37.0
sycosis (beard) (scalp) B35.0
twin Q89.4
Parasitism B89
intestinal B82.9
skin B88.9
specified —*see* Infestation
Parasitophobia F40.218
Parasomnia G47.50
due to
  alcohol
    abuse F10.182
    dependence F10.282
    use F10.982
  amphetamines
    abuse F15.182
    dependence F15.282
    use F15.982
  caffeine
    abuse F15.182
    dependence F15.282
    use F15.982
  cocaine
    abuse F14.182
    dependence F14.282
    use F14.982
  drug NEC
    abuse F19.182
    dependence F19.282
    use F19.982
  opioid
    abuse F11.182
    dependence F11.282
    use F11.982
  psychoactive substance NEC
    abuse F19.182
    dependence F19.282
    use F19.982
  sedative, hypnotic, or anxiolytic
    abuse F13.182
    dependence F13.282
    use F13.982
  stimulant NEC
    abuse F15.182
    dependence F15.282
    use F15.982
in conditions classified elsewhere G47.54
nonorganic origin F51.8
organic G47.50
specified NEC G47.59
Paraspadias Q54.9
Paraspasmus facialis G51.8
Parasuicide (attempt)
history of (personal) Z91.5
in family Z81.8
Parathyroid gland —*see* condition
Parathyroid tetany E20.9
Paratrachoma A74.0
Paratyphlitis —*see* Appendicitis
Paratyphoid (fever) —*see* Fever, paratyphoid
Paratyphus —*see* Fever, paratyphoid
Paraurethral duct Q64.79
nonorganic origin F51.5
Paraurethritis —*see also* Urethritis
gonococcal (acute) (chronic) (with abscess) A54.1
Paravaccinia NEC B08.04
Paravaginitis —*see* Vaginitis

Parencephalitis —*see also* Encephalitis
sequelae G09
Parent-child conflict —*see* Conflict, parent-
child
estrangement NEC Z62.890
Paresis —*see also* Paralysis
accommodation —*see* Paresis, of
accommodation
Bernhardt's G57.1
bladder (sphincter) —*see also* Paralysis,
bladder
tabetic A52.17
bowel, colon or intestine K56.0
extrinsic muscle, eye H49.9
general (progressive) (syphilitic) A52.17
juvenile A50.45
heart —*see* Failure, heart
insane (syphilitic) A52.17
juvenile (general) A50.45
of accommodation H52.52
peripheral progressive (idiopathic) G60.3
pseudohypertrophic G71.0
senile G83.9
syphilitic (general) A52.17
congenital A50.45
vesical NEC N31.2
Paresthesia —*see also* Disturbance, sensation
Bernhardt G57.1
Paretic —*see* condition
Parinaud's
conjunctivitis H10.89
oculoglandular syndrome H10.89
ophthalmoplegia H49.88
Parkinsonism (idiopathic) (primary) G20
with neurogenic orthostatic hypotension
(symptomatic) G90.3
arteriosclerotic G21.4
dementia G31.83 *[F02.80]*
with behavioral disturbance G31.83
[F02.81]
due to
drugs NEC G21.19
neuroleptic G21.11
neuroleptic induced G21.11
postencephalitic G21.3
secondary G21.9
due to
arteriosclerosis G21.4
drugs NEC G21.19
neuroleptic G21.11
encephalitis G21.3
external agents NEC G21.2
syphilis A52.19
specified NEC G21.8
syphilitic A52.19
treatment-induced NEC G21.19
vascular G21.4
Parkinson's disease, syndrome or tremor —
see Parkinsonism
Parodontitis —*see* Periodontitis
Parodontosis K05.4
Paronychia —*see also* Cellulitis, digit
with lymphangitis —*see* Lymphangitis, acute,
digit
candidal (chronic) B37.2
tuberculous (primary) A18.4
Parorexia (psychogenic) F50.8
Parosmia R43.1
psychogenic F45.8
Parotid gland —*see* condition

Parotitis, parotiditis (allergic) (nonspecific
toxic) (purulent) (septic) (suppurative) —*see
also* Sialoadenitis
epidemic —*see* Mumps
infectious —*see* Mumps
postoperative K91.89
surgical K91.89
Parrot fever A70
Parrot's disease (early congenital syphilitic
pseudoparalysis) A50.02
Parry-Romberg syndrome G51.8
Parry's disease or syndrome E05.00
with thyroid storm E05.01
Pars planitis —*see* Cyclitis
Parsonage (-Aldren) **-Turner syndrome**
G54.5
Parson's disease (exophthalmic goiter) E05.00
with thyroid storm E05.01
Particolored infant Q82.8
Parturition —*see* Delivery
Parulis K04.7
with sinus K04.6
Parvovirus, as cause of disease classified
elsewhere B97.6
Pasini and Pierini's atrophoderma L90.3
Passage
false, urethra N36.5
meconium (newborn) during delivery P03.82
of sounds or bougies —*see* Attention to,
artificial, opening
Passive —*see* condition
smoking Z77.22
Pasteurella septica A28.0
Pasteurellosis —*see* Infection, Pasteurella
PAT (paroxysmal atrial tachycardia) I47.1
Patau's syndrome —*see* Trisomy, 13
Patches
mucous (syphilitic) A51.39
congenital A50.07
smokers' (mouth) K13.24
Patellar —*see* condition
Patent —*see also* Imperfect, closure
canal of Nuck Q52.4
cervix N88.3
ductus arteriosus or Botallo's Q25.0
foramen
botalli Q21.1
ovale Q21.1
interauricular septum Q21.1
interventricular septum Q21.0
omphalomesenteric duct Q43.0
os (uteri) —*see* Patent, cervix
ostium secundum Q21.1
urachus Q64.4
vitelline duct Q43.0
Paterson (-Brown) (-Kelly) **syndrome or web**
D50.1
Pathologic, pathological —*see also* condition
asphyxia R09.01
fire-setting F63.1
gambling F63.0
ovum O02.0
resorption, tooth K03.3
stealing F63.2
Pathology (of) —*see* Disease
periradicular, associated with previous
endodontic treatment NEC M27.59
Pattern, sleep-wake, irregular G47.23

Patulous —*see also* Imperfect, closure
(congenital)
alimentary tract Q45.8
lower Q43.8
upper Q40.8
eustachian tube H69.0
Pause, sinoatrial I49.5
Paxton's disease B36.2
Pearl (s)
enamel K00.2
Epstein's K09.8
Pearl-worker's disease —*see* Osteomyelitis,
specified type NEC
Pectenosis K62.4
Pectoral —*see* condition
Pectus
carinatum (congenital) Q67.7
acquired M95.4
rachitic sequelae (late effect) E64.3
excavatum (congenital) Q67.6
acquired M95.4
rachitic sequelae (late effect) E64.3
recurvatum (congenital) Q67.6
Pedatrophia E41
Pederosis F65.4
Pediculosis (infestation) B85.2
capitis (head-louse) (any site) B85.0
corporis (body-louse) (any site) B85.1
eyelid B85.0
mixed (classifiable to more than one of the
titles B85.0-B85.3) B85.4
pubis (pubic louse) (any site) B85.3
vestimenti B85.1
vulvae B85.3
Pediculus (infestation) —*see* Pediculosis
Pedophilia F65.4
Peg-shaped teeth K00.2
Pelade —*see* Alopecia, areata
Pelger-Huët anomaly or syndrome D72.0
Peliosis (rheumatica) D69.0
hepatis K76.4
with toxic liver disease K71.8
Pelizaeus-Merzbacher disease E75.29
Pellagra (alcoholic) (with polyneuropathy)
E52
**Pellagra-cerebellar-ataxia-renal
aminoaciduria syndrome** E72.02
Pellegrini (-Stieda) **disease or syndrome** —
see Bursitis, tibial collateral
Pellizzi's syndrome E34.8
Pel's crisis A52.11
Pelvic —*see also* condition
examination (periodic) (routine) Z01.419
with abnormal findings Z01.411
kidney, congenital Q63.2
Pelviolithiasis —*see* Calculus, kidney
Pelviperitonitis —*see also* Peritonitis, pelvic
gonococcal A54.24
puerperal O85
Pelvis —*see* condition or type
Pemphigoid L12.9
benign, mucous membrane L12.1
bullous L12.0
cicatricial L12.1
juvenile L12.2
ocular L12.1
specified NEC L12.8
Pemphigus L10.9
benign familial (chronic) Q82.8
Brazilian L10.3
circinatus L13.0
conjunctiva L12.1
drug-induced L10.5

Pemphigus - *continued*
erythematosus L10.4
foliaceous L10.2
gangrenous —*see* Gangrene
neonatorum L01.03
ocular L12.1
paraneoplastic L10.81
specified NEC L10.89
syphilitic (congenital) A50.06
vegetans L10.1
vulgaris L10.0
wildfire L10.3
Pendred's syndrome E07.1
Pendulous
abdomen, in pregnancy —*see* Pregnancy,
complicated by, abnormal, pelvic organs or
tissues NEC
breast N64.89
Penetrating wound —*see also* Puncture
with internal injury —*see* Injury, by site
eyeball —*see* Puncture, eyeball
orbit (with or without foreign body) —*see*
Puncture, orbit
uterus by instrument with or following ectopic
or molar pregnancy O08.6
Penicillosis B48.4
Penis —*see* condition
Penitis N48.29
Pentalogy of Fallot Q21.8
Pentasomy X syndrome Q97.1
Pentosuria (essential) E74.8
Percreta placenta O43.23
Peregrinating patient —*see* Disorder,
factitious
Perforation, perforated (nontraumatic) (of)
accidental during procedure (blood vessel)
(nerve) (organ) —*see* Complication,
accidental puncture or laceration
antrum —*see* Sinusitis, maxillary
appendix K35.2
atrial septum, multiple Q21.1
attic, ear —*see* Perforation, tympanum, attic
bile duct (common) (hepatic) K83.2
cystic K82.2
bladder (urinary)
with or following ectopic or molar
pregnancy O08.6
obstetrical trauma O71.5
traumatic S37.29
at delivery O71.5
bowel K63.1
with or following ectopic or molar
pregnancy O08.6
newborn P78.0
obstetrical trauma O71.5
traumatic —*see* Laceration, intestine
broad ligament N83.8
with or following ectopic or molar
pregnancy O08.6
obstetrical trauma O71.6
by
device, implant or graft (*see also*
Complications, by site and type, mechanical)
T85.628
arterial graft NEC —*see* Complication,
cardiovascular device, mechanical, vascular
breast (implant) T85.49
catheter NEC T85.698
cystostomy T83.090
dialysis (renal) T82.49
intraperitoneal T85.691
infusion NEC T82.594

Perforation, perforated - *continued*
spinal (epidural) (subdural) T85.690
urinary, indwelling T83.098
electronic (electrode) (pulse generator)
(stimulator)
bone T84.390
cardiac T82.199
electrode T82.190
pulse generator T82.191
specified type NEC T82.198
nervous system —*see* Complication,
prosthetic device, mechanical, electronic
nervous system stimulator
urinary —*see* Complication,
genitourinary, device, urinary, mechanical
fixation, internal (orthopedic) NEC —*see*
Complication, fixation device, mechanical
gastrointestinal —*see* Complications,
prosthetic device, mechanical, gastrointestinal
device
genital NEC T83.498
intrauterine contraceptive device T83.39
penile prosthesis T83.490
heart NEC —*see* Complication,
cardiovascular device, mechanical
joint prosthesis —*see* Complications, joint
prosthesis, mechanical, specified NEC, by site
ocular NEC —*see* Complications,
prosthetic device, mechanical, ocular device
orthopedic NEC —*see* Complication,
orthopedic, device, mechanical
specified NEC T85.628
urinary NEC —*see also* Complication,
genitourinary, device, urinary, mechanical
graft T83.29
vascular NEC —*see* Complication,
cardiovascular device, mechanical
ventricular intracranial shunt T85.09
foreign body left accidentally in operative
wound T81.539
instrument (any) during a procedure,
accidental —*see* Puncture, accidental
complicating surgery
cecum K35.2
cervix (uteri) N88.8
with or following ectopic or molar
pregnancy O08.6
obstetrical trauma O71.3
colon K63.1
newborn P78.0
obstetrical trauma O71.5
traumatic —*see* Laceration, intestine, large
common duct (bile) K83.2
cornea (due to ulceration) —*see* Ulcer,
cornea, perforated
cystic duct K82.2
diverticulum (intestine) K57.80
with bleeding K57.81
large intestine K57.20
with
bleeding K57.21
small intestine K57.40
with bleeding K57.41
small intestine K57.00
with
bleeding K57.01
large intestine K57.40
with bleeding K57.41
ear drum —*see* Perforation, tympanum
esophagus K22.3
ethmoidal sinus —*see* Sinusitis, ethmoidal
frontal sinus —*see* Sinusitis, frontal

Perforation, perforated - *continued*
gallbladder K82.2
heart valve —*see* Endocarditis
ileum K63.1
newborn P78.0
obstetrical trauma O71.5
traumatic —*see* Laceration, intestine, small
instrumental, surgical (accidental) (blood
vessel) (nerve) (organ) —*see* Puncture,
accidental complicating surgery
intestine NEC K63.1
with ectopic or molar pregnancy O08.6
newborn P78.0
obstetrical trauma O71.5
traumatic —*see* Laceration, intestine
ulcerative NEC K63.1
newborn P78.0
jejunum, jejunal K63.1
obstetrical trauma O71.5
traumatic —*see* Laceration, intestine, small
ulcer —*see* Ulcer, gastrojejunal, with
perforation
joint prosthesis —*see* Complications, joint
prosthesis, mechanical, specified NEC, by site
mastoid (antrum) (cell) —*see* Disorder,
mastoid, specified NEC
maxillary sinus —*see* Sinusitis, maxillary
membrana tympani —*see* Perforation,
tympanum
nasal
septum J34.89
congenital Q30.3
syphilitic A52.73
sinus J34.89
congenital Q30.8
due to sinusitis —*see* Sinusitis
palate (*see also* Cleft, palate) Q35.9
syphilitic A52.79
palatine vault (*see also* Cleft, palate, hard)
Q35.1
syphilitic A52.79
congenital A50.59
pars flaccida (ear drum) —*see* Perforation,
tympanum, attic
pelvic
floor S31.030
with
ectopic or molar pregnancy O08.6
penetration into retroperitoneal space
S31.031
retained foreign body S31.040
with penetration into retroperitoneal
space S31.041
following ectopic or molar pregnancy
O08.6
obstetrical trauma O70.1
organ S37.99
adrenal gland S37.818
bladder —*see* Perforation, bladder
fallopian tube S37.599
bilateral S37.592
unilateral S37.591
kidney S37.09
obstetrical trauma O71.5
ovary S37.499
bilateral S37.492
unilateral S37.491
prostate S37.828
specified organ NEC S37.898
ureter —*see* Perforation, ureter
urethra —*see* Perforation, urethra
uterus —*see* Perforation, uterus

Perforation, perforated - *continued*
perineum —*see* Laceration, perineum
pharynx J39.2
rectum K63.1
  newborn P78.0
  obstetrical trauma O71.5
  traumatic S36.63
root canal space due to endodontic treatment
M27.51
sigmoid K63.1
  newborn P78.0
  obstetrical trauma O71.5
  traumatic S36.533
sinus (accessory) (chronic) (nasal) J34.89
sphenoidal sinus —*see* Sinusitis, sphenoidal
surgical (accidental) (by instrument) (blood
vessel) (nerve) (organ) —*see* Puncture,
accidental complicating surgery
traumatic
  external —*see* Puncture
  eye —*see* Puncture, eyeball
  internal organ —*see* Injury, by site
tympanum, tympanic (membrane) (persistent
post traumatic) (postinflammatory) H72.9
  attic H72.1
    multiple —*see* Perforation, tympanum,
multiple
    total —*see* Perforation, tympanum, total
  central H72.0
    multiple —*see* Perforation, tympanum,
multiple
    total —*see* Perforation, tympanum, total
  marginal NEC —see subcategory H72.2
  multiple H72.81
  pars flaccida —*see* Perforation, tympanum,
attic
  total H72.82
  traumatic, current episode S09.2
typhoid, gastrointestinal —*see* Typhoid
ulcer —*see* Ulcer, by site, with perforation
ureter N28.89
  traumatic S37.19
urethra N36.8
  with ectopic or molar pregnancy O08.6
  following ectopic or molar pregnancy O08.6
  obstetrical trauma O71.5
  traumatic S37.39
    at delivery O71.5
uterus
  with ectopic or molar pregnancy O08.6
  by intrauterine contraceptive device T83.39
  following ectopic or molar pregnancy O08.6
  obstetrical trauma O71.1
  traumatic S37.69
    obstetric O71.1
uvula K13.79
  syphilitic A52.79
vagina
  obstetrical trauma O71.4
  other trauma —*see* Puncture, vagina
Periadenitis mucosa necrotica recurrens
K12.0
Periappendicitis (acute) —*see* Appendicitis
Periarteritis nodosa (disseminated)
(infectious) (necrotizing) M30.0
Periarthritis (joint) —*see also* Enthesopathy
Duplay's M75.0
gonococcal A54.42
humeroscapularis —*see* Capsulitis, adhesive
scapulohumeral —*see* Capsulitis, adhesive
shoulder —*see* Capsulitis, adhesive
wrist M77.2

Periarthrosis (angioneural) —*see*
Enthesopathy
Pericapsulitis, adhesive (shoulder) —*see*
Capsulitis, adhesive
Pericarditis (with decompensation) (with
effusion) I31.9
with rheumatic fever (conditions in I00)
  active —*see* Pericarditis, rheumatic
  inactive or quiescent I09.2
acute (hemorrhagic) (nonrheumatic) (Sicca)
I30.9
  with chorea (acute) (rheumatic)
(Sydenham's) I02.0
  benign I30.8
  nonspecific I30.0
  rheumatic I01.0
    with chorea (acute) (Sydenham's) I02.0
adhesive or adherent (chronic) (external)
(internal) I31.0
  acute —*see* Pericarditis, acute
  rheumatic I09.2
bacterial (acute) (subacute) (with serous or
seropurulent effusion) I30.1
calcareous I31.1
cholesterol (chronic) I31.8
  acute I30.9
chronic (nonrheumatic) I31.9
  rheumatic I09.2
constrictive (chronic) I31.1
coxsackie B33.23
fibrinocaseous (tuberculous) A18.84
fibrinopurulent I30.1
fibrinous I30.8
fibrous I31.0
gonococcal A54.83
idiopathic I30.0
in systemic lupus erythematosus M32.12
infective I30.1
meningococcal A39.53
neoplastic (chronic) I31.8
  acute I30.9
obliterans, obliterating I31.0
plastic I31.0
pneumococcal I30.1
postinfarction I24.1
purulent I30.1
rheumatic (active) (acute) (with effusion)
(with pneumonia) I01.0
  with chorea (acute) (rheumatic)
(Sydenham's) I02.0
  chronic or inactive (with chorea) I09.2
rheumatoid —*see* Rheumatoid, carditis
septic I30.1
serofibrinous I30.8
staphylococcal I30.1
streptococcal I30.1
suppurative I30.1
syphilitic A52.06
tuberculous A18.84
uremic N18.9 *[I32]*
viral I30.1
Pericardium, pericardial —*see* condition
Pericellulitis —*see* Cellulitis
Pericementitis (chronic) (suppurative) —*see
also* Periodontitis
acute K05.20
  generalized K05.22
  localized K05.21
Perichondritis
auricle —*see* Perichondritis, ear
bronchus J98.09

Perichondritis - *continued*
ear (external) H61.00
  acute H61.01
  chronic H61.02
external auditory canal —*see* Perichondritis,
ear
larynx J38.7
  syphilitic A52.73
  typhoid A01.09
nose J34.89
pinna —*see* Perichondritis, ear
trachea J39.8
Periclasia K05.4
Pericoronitis —*see* Periodontitis
Pericystitis N30.90
with hematuria N30.91
Peridiverticulitis (intestine) K57.92
cecum —*see* Diverticulitis, intestine, large
colon —*see* Diverticulitis, intestine, large
duodenum —*see* Diverticulitis, intestine,
small
intestine —*see* Diverticulitis, intestine
jejunum —*see* Diverticulitis, intestine, small
rectosigmoid —*see* Diverticulitis, intestine,
large
rectum —*see* Diverticulitis, intestine, large
sigmoid —*see* Diverticulitis, intestine, large
Periendocarditis —*see* Endocarditis
Periepididymitis N45.1
Perifolliculitis L01.02
abscedens, caput, scalp L66.3
capitis, abscedens (et suffodiens) L66.3
superficial pustular L01.02
Perihepatitis K65.8
Perilabyrinthitis (acute) —*see* subcategory
H83.0
Perimeningitis —*see* Meningitis
Perimetritis —*see* Endometritis
Perimetrosalpingitis —*see* Salpingo-
oophoritis
Perineocele N81.81
Perinephric, perinephritic —*see* condition
Perinephritis —*see also* Infection, kidney
purulent —*see* Abscess, kidney
Perineum, perineal —*see* condition
Perineuritis NEC —*see* Neuralgia
Periodic —*see* condition
Periodontitis (chronic) (complex) (compound)
(local) (simplex) K05.30
acute K05.20
  generalized K05.22
  localized K05.21
apical K04.5
  acute (pulpal origin) K04.4
generalized K05.32
localized K05.31
Periodontoclasia K05.4
Periodontosis (juvenile) K05.4
Periods —*see also* Menstruation
heavy N92.0
irregular N92.6
shortened intervals (irregular) N92.1
Perionychia —*see also* Cellulitis, digit
with lymphangitis —*see* Lymphangitis, acute,
digit
Perioophoritis —*see* Salpingo-oophoritis
Periorchitis N45.2
Periosteum, periosteal —*see* condition
Periostitis (albuminosa) (circumscribed)
(diffuse) (infective) (monomelic) —*see also*
Osteomyelitis
alveolar M27.3
alveolodental M27.3

Periostitis - *continued*
  dental M27.3
  gonorrheal A54.43
  jaw (lower) (upper) M27.2
  orbit H05.03
  syphilitic A52.77
    congenital (early) A50.02 *[M90.80]*
    secondary A51.46
  tuberculous —*see* Tuberculosis, bone
  yaws (hypertrophic) (early) (late) A66.6
  [M90.80]
Periostosis (hyperplastic) —*see also* Disorder,
  bone, specified type NEC
  with osteomyelitis —*see* Osteomyelitis,
  specified type NEC
Peripartum
  cardiomyopathy O90.3
Periphlebitis —*see* Phlebitis
Periproctitis K62.89
Periprostatitis —*see* Prostatitis
Perirectal —*see* condition
Perirenal —*see* condition
Perisalpingitis —*see* Salpingo-oophoritis
Perisplenitis (infectional) D73.89
Peristalsis, visible or reversed R19.2
Peritendinitis —*see* Enthesopathy
Peritoneum, peritoneal —*see* condition
Peritonitis (adhesive) (bacterial) (fibrinous)
  (hemorrhagic) (idiopathic) (localized)
  (perforative) (primary) (with adhesions) (with
  effusion) K65.9
  with or following
    abscess K65.1
    appendicitis K35.2
      with perforation or rupture K35.2
      generalized K35.2
      localized K35.3
    diverticular disease (intestine) K57.80
      with bleeding K57.81
      large intestine K57.20
        with
          bleeding K57.21
          small intestine K57.40
            with bleeding K57.41
        small intestine K57.00
          with
            bleeding K57.01
            large intestine K57.40
              with bleeding K57.41
    ectopic or molar pregnancy O08.0
  acute (generalized) K65.0
  aseptic T81.61
  bile, biliary K65.3
  chemical T81.61
  chlamydial A74.81
  complicating abortion —*see* Abortion, by
  type, complicated by, pelvic peritonitis
  congenital P78.1
  chronic proliferative K65.8
  diaphragmatic K65.0
  diffuse K65.0
  diphtheritic A36.89
  disseminated K65.0
  due to
    bile K65.3
    foreign
      body or object accidentally left during a
      procedure (instrument) (sponge) (swab)
      T81.599
      substance accidentally left during a
      procedure (chemical) (powder) (talc) T81.61
    talc T81.61

Peritonitis - *continued*
  urine K65.8
  eosinophilic K65.8
    acute K65.0
  fibrocaseous (tuberculous) A18.31
  fibropurulent K65.0
  following ectopic or molar pregnancy O08.0
  general (ized) K65.0
  gonococcal A54.85
  meconium (newborn) P78.0
  neonatal P78.1
    meconium P78.0
  pancreatic K65.0
  paroxysmal, familial E85.0
    benign E85.0
  pelvic
    female N73.5
      acute N73.3
      chronic N73.4
        with adhesions N73.6
    male K65.0
  periodic, familial E85.0
  proliferative, chronic K65.8
  puerperal, postpartum, childbirth O85
  purulent K65.0
  septic K65.0
  specified NEC K65.8
  spontaneous bacterial K65.2
  subdiaphragmatic K65.0
  subphrenic K65.0
  suppurative K65.0
  syphilitic A52.74
    congenital (early) A50.08 *[K67]*
  talc T81.61
  tuberculous A18.31
  urine K65.8
Peritonsillar —*see* condition
Peritonsillitis J36
Perityphlitis K37
Periureteritis N28.89
Periurethral —*see* condition
Periurethritis (gangrenous) —*see* Urethritis
Periuterine —*see* condition
Perivaginitis —*see* Vaginitis
Perivasculitis, retinal H35.06
Perivasitis (chronic) N49.1
Perivesiculitis (seminal) —*see* Vesiculitis
Perlèche NEC K13.0
  due to
    candidiasis B37.83
    moniliasis B37.83
    riboflavin deficiency E53.0
    vitamin B2 (riboflavin) deficiency E53.0
Pernicious —*see* condition
Pernio, perniosis T69.1
Perpetrator (of abuse) —*see* Index to External
  Causes of Injury, Perpetrator
Persecution
  delusion F22
  social Z60.5
Perseveration (tonic) R48.8
Persistence, persistent (congenital)
  anal membrane Q42.3
    with fistula Q42.2
  arteria stapedia Q16.3
  atrioventricular canal Q21.2
  branchial cleft Q18.0
  bulbus cordis in left ventricle Q21.8
  canal of Cloquet Q14.0
  capsule (opaque) Q12.8
  cilioretinal artery or vein Q14.8
  cloaca Q43.7

Persistence, persistent - *continued*
  communication —*see* Fistula, congenital
  convolutions
    aortic arch Q25.4
    fallopian tube Q50.6
    oviduct Q50.6
    uterine tube Q50.6
  double aortic arch Q25.4
  ductus arteriosus (Botalli) Q25.0
  fetal
    circulation P29.3
    form of cervix (uteri) Q51.828
    hemoglobin, hereditary (HPFH) D56.4
  foramen
    Botalli Q21.1
    ovale Q21.1
  Gartner's duct Q52.4
  hemoglobin, fetal (hereditary) (HPFH) D56.4
  hyaloid
    artery (generally incomplete) Q14.0
    system Q14.8
  hymen, in pregnancy or childbirth —*see*
  Pregnancy, complicated by, abnormal, vulva
  lanugo Q84.2
  left
    posterior cardinal vein Q26.8
    root with right arch of aorta Q25.4
    superior vena cava Q26.1
  Meckel's diverticulum Q43.0
    malignant —*see* Table of Neoplasms, small
    intestine, malignant
  mucosal disease (middle ear) —*see* Otitis,
  media, suppurative, chronic, tubotympanic
  nail (s) , anomalous Q84.6
  omphalomesenteric duct Q43.0
  organ or site not listed —*see* Anomaly, by site
  ostium
    atrioventriculare commune Q21.2
    primum Q21.2
    secundum Q21.1
  ovarian rests in fallopian tube Q50.6
  pancreatic tissue in intestinal tract Q43.8
  primary (deciduous)
    teeth K00.6
    vitreous hyperplasia Q14.0
  pupillary membrane Q13.89
  right aortic arch Q25.4
  rhesus (Rh) titer —*see* Complication(s) ,
  transfusion, incompatibility reaction, Rh
  (factor)
  sinus
    urogenitalis
      female Q52.8
      male Q55.8
  venosus with imperfect incorporation in
  right auricle Q26.8
  thymus (gland) (hyperplasia) E32.0
  thyroglossal duct Q89.2
  thyrolingual duct Q89.2
  truncus arteriosus or communis Q20.0
  tunica vasculosa lentis Q12.2
  umbilical sinus Q64.4
  urachus Q64.4
  vitelline duct Q43.0
Person (with)
  admitted for clinical research, as a control
  subject (normal comparison) (participant)
  Z00.6
  awaiting admission to adequate facility
  elsewhere Z75.1
  concern (normal) about sick person in family
  Z63.6
  consulting on behalf of another Z71.0

Person - *continued*
feigning illness Z76.5
living (in)
  alone Z60.2
  boarding school Z59.3
  residential institution Z59.3
  without
    adequate housing (heating) (space) Z59.1
    housing (permanent) (temporary) Z59.0
    person able to render necessary care Z74.2
    shelter Z59.0
on waiting list Z75.1
sick or handicapped in family Z63.6
Personality (disorder) F60.9
accentuation of traits (type A pattern) Z73.1
affective F34.0
aggressive F60.3
amoral F60.2
anacastic, anankastic F60.5
antisocial F60.2
anxious F60.6
asocial F60.2
asthenic F60.7
avoidant F60.6
borderline F60.3
change due to organic condition (enduring)
F07.0
compulsive F60.5
cycloid F34.0
cyclothymic F34.0
dependent F60.7
depressive F34.1
dissocial F60.2
dual F44.81
eccentric F60.89
emotionally unstable F60.3
expansive paranoid F60.0
explosive F60.3
fanatic F60.0
haltose type F60.89
histrionic F60.4
hyperthymic F34.0
hypothymic F34.1
hysterical F60.4
immature F60.89
inadequate F60.7
labile (emotional) F60.3
mixed (nonspecific) F60.81
morally defective F60.2
multiple F44.81
narcissistic F60.81
obsessional F60.5
obsessive (-compulsive) F60.5
organic F07.0
overconscientious F60.5
paranoid F60.0
passive (-dependent) F60.7
passive-aggressive F60.89
pathologic F60.9
pattern defect or disturbance F60.9
pseudopsychopathic (organic) F07.0
pseudoretarded (organic) F07.0
psychoinfantile F60.4
psychoneurotic NEC F60.89
psychopathic F60.2
querulant F60.0
sadistic F60.89
schizoid F60.1
self-defeating F60.7
sensitive paranoid F60.0
sociopathic (amoral) (antisocial) (asocial)
(dissocial) F60.2

Personality - *continued*
specified NEC F60.89
type A Z73.1
unstable (emotional) F60.3
Perthes' disease —*see* Legg-Calvé-Perthes
disease
Pertussis (*see also* Whooping cough) A37.90
Perversion, perverted
appetite F50.8
  psychogenic F50.8
function
  pituitary gland E23.2
    posterior lobe E22.2
sense of smell and taste R43.8
  psychogenic F45.8
sexual —*see* Deviation, sexual
Pervious, congenital —*see also* Imperfect,
closure
ductus arteriosus Q25.0
Pes (congenital) —*see also* Talipes
acquired —*see also* Deformity, limb, foot,
specified NEC
  planus —*see* Deformity, limb, flat foot
adductus Q66.89
cavus Q66.7
deformity NEC, acquired —*see* Deformity,
limb, foot, specified NEC
planus (acquired) (any degree) —*see also*
Deformity, limb, flat foot
  rachitic sequelae (late effect) E64.3
valgus Q66.6
Pest, pestis —*see* Plague
Petechia, petechiae R23.3
newborn P54.5
Petechial typhus A75.9
Peter's anomaly Q13.4
Petit mal seizure —*see* Epilepsy, generalized,
specified NEC
Petit's hernia —*see* Hernia, abdomen,
specified site NEC
Petriellidiosis B48.2
Petrositis H70.20
acute H70.21
chronic H70.22
Peutz-Jeghers disease or syndrome Q85.8
Peyronie's disease N48.6
Pfeiffer's disease —*see* Mononucleosis,
infectious
Phagedena (dry) (moist) (sloughing) —*see*
also Gangrene
geometric L88
penis N48.29
tropical —*see* Ulcer, skin
vulva N76.6
Phagedenic —*see* condition
Phakoma H35.89
Phakomatosis (*see also* specific eponymous
syndromes) Q85.9
Bourneville's Q85.1
specified NEC Q85.8
Phantom limb syndrome (without pain)
G54.7
with pain G54.6
Pharyngeal pouch syndrome D82.1
Pharyngitis (acute) (catarrhal) (gangrenous)
(infective) (malignant) (membranous)
(phlegmonous) (pseudomembranous) (simple)
(subacute) (suppurative) (ulcerative) (viral)
J02.9
with influenza, flu, or grippe —*see* Influenza,
with, pharyngitis
aphthous B08.5

Pharyngitis - *continued*
atrophic J31.2
chlamydial A56.4
chronic (atrophic) (granular) (hypertrophic)
J31.2
coxsackievirus B08.5
diphtheritic A36.0
enteroviral vesicular B08.5
follicular (chronic) J31.2
fusospirochetal A69.1
gonococcal A54.5
granular (chronic) J31.2
herpesviral B00.2
hypertrophic J31.2
infectional, chronic J31.2
influenzal —*see* Influenza, with, respiratory
manifestations NEC
lymphonodular, acute (enteroviral) B08.8
pneumococcal J02.8
purulent J02.9
putrid J02.9
septic J02.0
sicca J31.2
specified organism NEC J02.8
staphylococcal J02.8
streptococcal J02.0
syphilitic, congenital (early) A50.03
tuberculous A15.8
vesicular, enteroviral B08.5
viral NEC J02.8
Pharyngoconjunctivitis, viral B30.2
Pharyngolaryngitis (acute) J06.0
chronic J37.0
Pharyngoplegia J39.2
Pharyngotonsillitis, herpesviral B00.2
Pharyngotracheitis, chronic J42
Pharynx, pharyngeal —*see* condition
Phenomenon
Arthus' —*see* Arthus' phenomenon
jaw-winking Q07.8
lupus erythematosus (LE) cell M32.9
Raynaud's (secondary) I73.00
  with gangrene I73.01
vasomotor R55
vasospastic I73.9
vasovagal R55
Wenckebach's I44.1
Phenylketonuria E70.1
classical E70.0
maternal E70.1
Pheochromoblastoma
specified site —*see* Neoplasm, malignant, by
site
unspecified site C74.10
Pheochromocytoma
malignant
  specified site —*see* Neoplasm, malignant,
by site
  unspecified site C74.10
specified site —*see* Neoplasm, benign, by site
unspecified site D35.00
Phaeohyphomycosis —*see* Chromomycosis
Pheomycosis —*see* Chromomycosis
Phimosis (congenital) (due to infection) N47.1
chancroidal A57
Phlebectasia —*see also* Varix
congenital Q27.4
Phlebitis (infective) (pyemic) (septic)
(suppurative) I80.9
antepartum —*see* Thrombophlebitis,
antepartum
blue —*see* Phlebitis, leg, deep
breast, superficial I80.8

Phlebitis - *continued*
cavernous (venous) sinus —*see* Phlebitis, intracranial (venous) sinus
cerebral (venous) sinus —*see* Phlebitis, intracranial (venous) sinus
chest wall, superficial I80.8
cranial (venous) sinus —*see* Phlebitis, intracranial (venous) sinus
deep (vessels) —*see* Phlebitis, leg, deep
due to implanted device —*see* Complications, by site and type, specified NEC
during or resulting from a procedure T81.72
femoral vein (superficial) I80.1
femoropopliteal vein I80.0
gestational —*see* Phlebopathy, gestational
hepatic veins I80.8
iliofemoral —*see* Phlebitis, femoral vein
intracranial (venous) sinus (any) G08
  nonpyogenic I67.6
intraspinal venous sinuses and veins G08
  nonpyogenic G95.19
lateral (venous) sinus —*see* Phlebitis, intracranial (venous) sinus
leg I80.3
  antepartum —*see* Thrombophlebitis, antepartum
  deep (vessels) NEC I80.20
    iliac I80.21
    popliteal vein I80.22
    specified vessel NEC I80.29
    tibial vein I80.23
  femoral vein (superficial) I80.1
  superficial (vessels) I80.0
longitudinal sinus —*see* Phlebitis, intracranial (venous) sinus
lower limb —*see* Phlebitis, leg
migrans, migrating (superficial) I82.1
pelvic
  with ectopic or molar pregnancy O08.0
  following ectopic or molar pregnancy O08.0
  puerperal, postpartum O87.1
popliteal vein —*see* Phlebitis, leg, deep, popliteal
portal (vein) K75.1
postoperative T81.72
pregnancy —*see* Thrombophlebitis, antepartum
puerperal, postpartum, childbirth O87.0
  deep O87.1
  pelvic O87.1
  superficial O87.0
retina —*see* Vasculitis, retina
saphenous (accessory) (great) (long) (small) —*see* Phlebitis, leg, superficial
sinus (meninges) —*see* Phlebitis, intracranial (venous) sinus
specified site NEC I80.8
syphilitic A52.09
tibial vein —*see* Phlebitis, leg, deep, tibial
ulcerative I80.9
  leg *see* Phlebitis, leg
umbilicus I80.8
uterus (septic) —*see* Endometritis
varicose (leg) (lower limb) —*see* Varix, leg, with, inflammation
Phlebofibrosis I87.8
Phleboliths I87.8
Phlebopathy,
gestational O22.9
puerperal O87.9
Phlebosclerosis I87.8

Phlebothrombosis —*see also* Thrombosis
antepartum —*see* Thrombophlebitis, antepartum
pregnancy —*see* Thrombophlebitis, antepartum
puerperal —*see* Thrombophlebitis, puerperal
Phlebotomus fever A93.1
Phlegmasia
alba dolens O87.1
  nonpuerperal —*see* Phlebitis, femoral vein
cerulea dolens —*see* Phlebitis, leg, deep
Phlegmon —*see* Abscess
Phlegmonous —*see* condition
Phlyctenulosis (allergic) (keratoconjunctivitis) (nontuberculous) —*see also* Keratoconjunctivitis
cornea —*see* Keratoconjunctivitis
tuberculous A18.52
Phobia, phobic F40.9
animal F40.218
  spiders F40.210
examination F40.298
reaction F40.9
simple F40.298
social F40.10
  generalized F40.11
specific (isolated) F40.298
  animal F40.218
    spiders F40.210
  blood F40.230
    injection F40.231
    injury F40.233
    men F40.290
  natural environment F40.228
    thunderstorms F40.220
  situational F40.248
    bridges F40.242
    closed in spaces F40.240
    flying F40.243
    heights F40.241
  specified focus NEC F40.298
  transfusion F40.231
  women F40.291
specified NEC F40.8
  medical care NEC F40.232
state F40.9
Phocas' disease —*see* Mastopathy, cystic
Phocomelia Q73.1
lower limb —*see* Agenesis, leg, with foot present
upper limb —*see* Agenesis, arm, with hand present
Phoria H50.50
Phosphate-losing tubular disorder N25.0
Phosphatemia E83.39
Phosphaturia E83.39
Photodermatitis (sun) L56.8
chronic L57.8
due to drug L56.8
light other than sun L59.8
Photokeratitis H16.13-**Photophobia** H53.14
Photophthalmia —*see* Photokeratitis
Photopsia H53.19
Photoretinitis —*see* Retinopathy, solar
Photosensitivity, photosensitization (sun)
skin L56.8
light other than sun L59.8
Phrenitis —*see* Encephalitis
Phrynoderma (vitamin A deficiency) E50.8
Phthiriasis (pubis) B85.3
with any infestation classifiable to B85.0-B85.2 B85.4
Phthirus infestation —*see* Phthiriasis

Phthisis —*see also* Tuberculosis
bulbi (infectional) —*see* Disorder, globe, degenerated condition, atrophy
eyeball (due to infection) —*see* Disorder, globe, degenerated condition, atrophy
Phycomycosis —*see* Zygomycosis
Physalopteriasis B81.8
Physical restraint status Z78.1
Phytobezoar T18.9
intestine T18.3
stomach T18.2
Pian —*see* Yaws
Pianoma A66.1
Pica F50.8
in adults F50.8
infant or child F98.3
Picking, nose F98.8
Pick-Niemann disease —*see* Niemann-Pick disease or syndrome
Pick's
cerebral atrophy G31.01 *[F02.80]*
  with behavioral disturbance G31.01 *[F02.81]*
disease or syndrome (brain) G31.01 *[F02.80]*
  with behavioral disturbance G31.01 *[F02.81]*
Pickwickian syndrome E66.2
Piebaldism E70.39
Piedra (beard) (scalp) B36.8
black B36.3
white B36.2
Pierre Robin deformity or syndrome Q87.0
Pierson's disease or osteochondrosis M91.0
Pig-bel A05.2
Pigeon
breast or chest (acquired) M95.4
  congenital Q67.7
  rachitic sequelae (late effect) E64.3
breeder's disease or lung J67.2
fancier's disease or lung J67.2
toe —*see* Deformity, toe, specified NEC
Pigmentation (abnormal) (anomaly) L81.9
conjunctiva H11.13
cornea (anterior) H18.01
  posterior H18.05
  stromal H18.06
diminished melanin formation NEC L81.6
iron L81.8
lids, congenital Q82.8
limbus corneae —*see* Pigmentation, cornea
metals L81.8
optic papilla, congenital Q14.2
retina, congenital (grouped) (nevoid) Q14.1
scrotum, congenital Q82.8
tattoo L81.8
Piles (*see also* Hemorrhoids) K64.9
Pili
annulati or torti (congenital) Q84.1
incarnati L73.1
Pill roller hand (intrinsic) —*see* Parkinsonism
Pilomatrixoma —*see* Neoplasm, skin, benign
malignant —*see* Neoplasm, skin, malignant
Pilonidal —*see* condition
Pimple R23.8
Pinched nerve —*see* Neuropathy, entrapment
Pindborg tumor —*see* Cyst, calcifying odontogenic
Pineal body or gland —*see* condition
Pinealoblastoma C75.3
Pinealoma D44.5
malignant C75.3
Pineoblastoma C75.3
Pineocytoma D44.5

Pinguecula H11.15
Pingueculitis H10.81
Pinhole meatus (*see also* Stricture, urethra) N35.9
Pink
  disease —*see* subcategory T56.1
  eye —*see* Conjunctivitis, acute, mucopurulent
Pinkus' disease (lichen nitidus) L44.1
Pinpoint
  meatus —*see* Stricture, urethra
  os (uteri) —*see* Stricture, cervix
Pins and needles R20.2
Pinta A67.9
  cardiovascular lesions A67.2
  chancre (primary) A67.0
  erythematous plaques A67.1
  hyperchromic lesions A67.1
  hyperkeratosis A67.1
  lesions A67.9
    cardiovascular A67.2
    hyperchromic A67.1
    intermediate A67.1
    late A67.2
    mixed A67.3
    primary A67.0
    skin (achromic) (cicatricial) (dyschromic) A67.2
      hyperchromic A67.1
      mixed (achromic and hyperchromic) A67.3
  papule (primary) A67.0
  skin lesions (achromic) (cicatricial) (dyschromic) A67.2
    hyperchromic A67.1
    mixed (achromic and hyperchromic) A67.3
  vitiligo A67.2
Pintids A67.1
Pinworm (disease) (infection) (infestation) B80
Piroplasmosis B60.0
Pistol wound —*see* Gunshot wound
Pitchers' elbow —*see* Derangement, joint, specified type NEC, elbow
Pithecoid pelvis Q74.2
  with disproportion (fetopelvic) O33.0
    causing obstructed labor O65.0
Pithiatism F48.8
Pitted —*see* Pitting
Pitting (*see also* Edema) R60.9
  lip R60.0
  nail L60.8
  teeth K00.4
Pituitary gland —*see* condition
Pituitary-snuff-taker's disease J67.8
Pityriasis (capitis) L21.0
  alba L30.5
  circinata (et maculata) L42
  furfuracea L21.0
  Hebra's L26
  lichenoides L41.0
    chronica L41.1
    et varioliformis (acuta) L41.0
  maculata (et circinata) L30.5
  nigra B36.1
  pilaris, Hebra's L44.0
  rosea L42
  rotunda L44.8
  rubra (Hebra) pilaris L44.0
  simplex L30.5
  specified type NEC L30.5
  streptogenes L30.5
  versicolor (scrotal) B36.0

Placenta, placental —*see* Pregnancy, complicated by (care of) (management affected by) , specified condition
Placentitis O41.14
Plagiocephaly Q67.3
Plague A20.9
  abortive A20.8
  ambulatory A20.8
  asymptomatic A20.8
  bubonic A20.0
  cellulocutaneous A20.1
  cutaneobubonic A20.1
  lymphatic gland A20.0
  meningitis A20.3
  pharyngeal A20.8
  pneumonic (primary) (secondary) A20.2
  pulmonary, pulmonic A20.2
  septicemic A20.7
  tonsillar A20.8
    septicemic A20.7
Planning, family
  contraception Z30.9
  procreation Z31.69
Plaque (s)
  artery, arterial —*see* Arteriosclerosis
  calcareous —*see* Calcification
  coronary, lipid rich I25.83
  epicardial I31.8
  erythematous, of pinta A67.1
  Hollenhorst's —*see* Occlusion, artery, retina
  lipid rich, coronary I25.83
  pleural (without asbestos) J92.9
    with asbestos J92.0
  tongue K13.29
Plasmacytoma C90.3
  extramedullary C90.2
  medullary C90.0
  solitary C90.3-**Plasmacytopenia** D72.818
Plasmacytosis D72.822
Plaster ulcer —*see* Ulcer, pressure, by site
Plateau iris syndrome (post-iridectomy) (postprocedural) (without glaucoma) H21.82
  with glaucoma H40.22
Platybasia Q75.8
Platyonychia (congenital) Q84.6
  acquired L60.8
Platypelloid pelvis M95.5
  with disproportion (fetopelvic) O33.0
    causing obstructed labor O65.0
  congenital Q74.2
Platyspondylisis Q76.49
Plaut (-Vincent) **disease** (*see also* Vincent's) A69.1
Plethora R23.2
  newborn P61.1
Pleura, pleural —*see* condition
Pleuralgia R07.81
Pleurisy (acute) (adhesive) (chronic) (costal) (diaphragmatic) (double) (dry) (fibrinous) (fibrous) (interlobar) (latent) (plastic) (primary) (residual) (sicca) (sterile) (subacute) (unresolved) R09.1
  with
    adherent pleura J86.0
    effusion J90
      chylous, chyliform J94.0
      tuberculous (non primary) A15.6
        primary (progressive) A15.7
    tuberculosis —*see* Pleurisy, tuberculous (non primary)
  encysted —*see* Pleurisy, with effusion
  exudative —*see* Pleurisy, with effusion

Pleurisy - *continued*
  fibrinopurulent, fibropurulent —*see* Pyothorax
  hemorrhagic —*see* Hemothorax
  pneumococcal J90
  purulent —*see* Pyothorax
  septic —*see* Pyothorax
  serofibrinous —*see* Pleurisy, with effusion
  seropurulent —*see* Pyothorax
  serous —*see* Pleurisy, with effusion
  staphylococcal J86.9
  streptococcal J90
  suppurative —*see* Pyothorax
  traumatic (post) (current) —*see* Injury, intrathoracic, pleura
  tuberculous (with effusion) (non primary) A15.6
    primary (progressive) A15.7
Pleuritis sicca —*see* Pleurisy
Pleurobronchopneumonia —*see* Pneumonia, broncho
Pleurodynia R07.81
  epidemic B33.0
  viral B33.0
Pleuropericarditis —*see also* Pericarditis
  acute I30.9
Pleuropneumonia (acute) (bilateral) (double) (septic) (*see also* Pneumonia) J18.8
  chronic —*see* Fibrosis, lung
Pleuro-pneumonia-like-organism (PPLO) , **as cause of disease classified elsewhere** B96.0
Pleurorrhea —*see* Pleurisy, with effusion
Plexitis, brachial G54.0
Plica
  polonica B85.0
  syndrome, knee M67.5
  tonsil J35.8
Plicated tongue K14.5
Plug
  bronchus NEC J98.09
  meconium (newborn) NEC syndrome P76.0
  mucus —*see* Asphyxia, mucus
Plumbism —see subcategory T56.0
Plummer's disease E05.20
  with thyroid storm E05.21
Plummer-Vinson syndrome D50.1
Pluricarential syndrome of infancy E40
Plus (and minus) hand (intrinsic) —*see* Deformity, limb, specified type NEC, forearm
Pneumathemia —*see* Air, embolism
Pneumatic hammer (drill) **syndrome** T75.21
Pneumatocele (lung) J98.4
  intracranial G93.89
  tension J44.9
Pneumatosis
  cystoides intestinalis K63.89
  intestinalis K63.89
  peritonei K66.8
Pneumaturia R39.89
Pneumoblastoma —*see* Neoplasm, lung, malignant
Pneumocephalus G93.89
Pneumococcemia A40.3
Pneumococcus, pneumococcal —*see* condition
Pneumoconiosis (due to) (inhalation of) J64
  with tuberculosis (any type in A15) J65
  aluminum J63.0
  asbestos J61
  bagasse, bagassosis J67.1
  bauxite J63.1
  beryllium J63.2
  coal miners' (simple) J60

Pneumoconiosis *- continued*
coal workers' (simple) J60
collier's J60
cotton dust J66.0
diatomite (diatomaceous earth) J62.8
dust
  inorganic NEC J63.6
  lime J62.8
  marble J62.8
  organic NEC J66.8
fumes or vapors (from silo) J68.9
graphite J63.3
grinder's J62.8
kaolin J62.8
mica J62.8
millstone maker's J62.8
mineral fibers NEC J61
miner's J60
moldy hay J67.0
potter's J62.8
rheumatoid —*see* Rheumatoid, lung
sandblaster's J62.8
silica, silicate NEC J62.8
  with carbon J60
stonemason's J62.8
talc (dust) J62.0
Pneumocystis carinii pneumonia B59
Pneumocystis jiroveci (pneumonia) B59
Pneumocystosis (with pneumonia) B59
Pneumohemopericardium I31.2
Pneumohemothorax J94.2
traumatic S27.2
Pneumohydropericardium —*see* Pericarditis
Pneumohydrothorax —*see* Hydrothorax
Pneumomediastinum J98.2
congenital or perinatal P25.2
Pneumomycosis B49 *[J99]*
Pneumonia (acute) (double) (migratory)
(purulent) (septic) (unresolved) J18.9
with
  lung abscess J85.1
    due to specified organism —*see*
Pneumonia, in (due to)
    influenza —*see* Influenza, with, pneumonia
adenoviral J12.0
adynamic J18.2
alba A50.04
allergic (eosinophilic) J82
alveolar —*see* Pneumonia, lobar
anaerobes J15.8
anthrax A22.1
apex, apical —*see* Pneumonia, lobar
Ascaris B77.81
aspiration J69.0
  due to
    aspiration of microorganisms
      bacterial J15.9
      viral J12.9
    food (regurgitated) J69.0
    gastric secretions J69.0
    milk (regurgitated) J69.0
    oils, essences J69.1
    solids, liquids NEC J69.8
    vomitus J69.0
  newborn P24.81
    amniotic fluid (clear) P24.11
    blood P24.21
    liquor (amnii) P24.11
    meconium P24.01
    milk P24.31
    mucus P24.11
    food (regurgitated) P24.31

Pneumonia *- continued*
specified NEC P24.81
  stomach contents P24.31
postprocedural J95.4
atypical NEC J18.9
bacillus J15.9
  specified NEC J15.8
bacterial J15.9
  specified NEC J15.8
Bacteroides (fragilis) (oralis)
(melaninogenicus) J15.8
basal, basic, basilar —*see* Pneumonia, by type
bronchiolitis obliterans organized (BOOP)
J84.89
broncho , bronchial (confluent) (croupous)
(diffuse) (disseminated) (hemorrhagic)
(involving lobes) (lobar) (terminal) J18.0
  allergic (eosinophilic) J82
  aspiration —*see* Pneumonia, aspiration
  bacterial J15.9
    specified NEC J15.8
  chronic —*see* Fibrosis, lung
  diplococcal J13
  Eaton's agent J15.7
  Escherichia coli (E. coli) J15.5
  Friedländer's bacillus J15.0
  Hemophilus influenzae J14
  hypostatic J18.2
  inhalation —*see also* Pneumonia, aspiration
    due to fumes or vapors (chemical) J68.0
    of oils or essences J69.1
  Klebsiella (pneumoniae) J15.0
  lipid, lipoid J69.1
    endogenous J84.89
  Mycoplasma (pneumoniae) J15.7
  pleuro-pneumonia-like-organisms (PPLO)
J15.7
  pneumococcal J13
  Proteus J15.6
  Pseudomonas J15.1
  Serratia marcescens J15.6
  specified organism NEC J16.8
  staphylococcal —*see* Pneumonia,
staphylococcal
  streptococcal NEC J15.4
    group B J15.3
    pneumoniae J13
  viral, virus —*see* Pneumonia, viral
Butyrivibrio (fibriosolvens) J15.8
Candida B37.1
caseous —*see* Tuberculosis, pulmonary
catarrhal —*see* Pneumonia, broncho
chlamydial J16.0
  congenital P23.1
cholesterol J84.89
cirrhotic (chronic) —*see* Fibrosis, lung
Clostridium (haemolyticum) (novyi) J15.8
confluent —*see* Pneumonia, broncho
congenital (infective) P23.9
  due to
    bacterium NEC P23.6
    Chlamydia P23.1
    Escherichia coli P23.4
    Haemophilus influenzae P23.6
    infective organism NEC P23.8
    Klebsiella pneumoniae P23.6
    Mycoplasma P23.6
    Pseudomonas P23.5
    Staphylococcus P23.2
    Streptococcus (except group B) P23.6
      group B P23.3
    viral agent P23.0

Pneumonia *- continued*
specified NEC P23.8
croupous —*see* Pneumonia, lobar
cryptogenic organizing J84.116
cytomegalic inclusion B25.0
cytomegaloviral B25.0
deglutition —*see* Pneumonia, aspiration
desquamative interstitial J84.117
diffuse —*see* Pneumonia, broncho
diplococcal, diplococcus (broncho) (lobar)
J13
disseminated (focal) —*see* Pneumonia,
broncho
Eaton's agent J15.7
embolic, embolism —*see* Embolism,
pulmonary
Enterobacter J15.6
eosinophilic J82
Escherichia coli (E. coli) J15.5
Eubacterium J15.8
fibrinous —*see* Pneumonia, lobar
fibroid, fibrous (chronic) —*see* Fibrosis, lung
Friedländer's bacillus J15.0
Fusobacterium (nucleatum) J15.8
gangrenous J85.0
giant cell (measles) B05.2
gonococcal A54.84
gram-negative bacteria NEC J15.6
  anaerobic J15.8
Hemophilus influenzae (broncho) (lobar) J14
human metapneumovirus J12.3
hypostatic (broncho) (lobar) J18.2
in (due to)
  actinomycosis A42.0
  adenovirus J12.0
  anthrax A22.1
  ascariasis B77.81
  aspergillosis B44.9
  Bacillus anthracis A22.1
  Bacterium anitratum J15.6
  candidiasis B37.1
  chickenpox B01.2
  Chlamydia J16.0
    neonatal P23.1
  coccidioidomycosis B38.2
    acute B38.0
    chronic B38.1
  cytomegalovirus disease B25.0
  Diplococcus (pneumoniae) J13
  Eaton's agent J15.7
  Enterobacter J15.6
  Escherichia coli (E. coli) J15.5
  Friedländer's bacillus J15.0
  fumes and vapors (chemical) (inhalation)
J68.0
  gonorrhea A54.84
  Hemophilus influenzae (H. influenzae) J14
  Herellea J15.6
  histoplasmosis B39.2
    acute B39.0
    chronic B39.1
  human metapneumovirus J12.3
  Klebsiella (pneumoniae) J15.0
  measles B05.2
  Mycoplasma (pneumoniae) J15.7
  nocardiosis, nocardiasis A43.0
  ornithosis A70
  parainfluenza virus J12.2
  pleuro-pneumonia-like-organism (PPLO)
J15.7
  pneumococcus J13
  pneumocystosis (Pneumocystis carinii)
(Pneumocystis jiroveci) B59

Pneumonia *- continued*
  Proteus J15.6
  Pseudomonas NEC J15.1
    pseudomallei A24.1
  psittacosis A70
  Q fever A78
  respiratory syncytial virus J12.1
  rheumatic fever I00 *[J17]*
  rubella B06.81
  Salmonella (infection) A02.22
    typhi A01.03
  schistosomiasis B65.9 *[J17]*
  Serratia marcescens J15.6
  specified
    bacterium NEC J15.8
    organism NEC J16.8
    spirochetal NEC A69.8
  Staphylococcus J15.20
    aureus (methicillin susceptible) (MSSA) J15.211
      methicillin resistant (MRSA) J15.212
    specified NEC J15.29
  Streptococcus J15.4
    group B J15.3
    pneumoniae J13
    specified NEC J15.4
  toxoplasmosis B58.3
  tularemia A21.2
  typhoid (fever) A01.03
  varicella B01.2
  virus —*see* Pneumonia, viral
  whooping cough A37.91
    due to
      Bordetella parapertussis A37.11
      Bordetella pertussis A37.01
      specified NEC A37.81
  Yersinia pestis A20.2
inhalation of food or vomit —*see* Pneumonia, aspiration
interstitial J84.9
  chronic J84.111
  desquamative J84.117
  due to
    collagen vascular disease J84.17
    known underlying cause J84.17
  idiopathic NOS J84.111
  in disease classified elsewhere J84.17
  lymphocytic (due to collagen vascular disease) (in diseases classified elsewhere) J84.17
  lymphoid J84.2
  non-specific J84.89
    due to
      collagen vascular disease J84.17
      known underlying cause J84.17
    idiopathic J84.113
    in diseases classified elsewhere J84.17
  plasma cell B59
  pseudomonas J15.1
  usual J84.112
    due to collagen vascular disease J84.17
    idiopathic J84.112
    in diseases classified elsewhere J84.17
Klebsiella (pneumoniae) J15.0
lipid, lipoid (exogenous) J69.1
  endogenous J84.89
lobar (disseminated) (double) (interstitial) J18.1
  bacterial J15.9
    specified NEC J15.8
  chronic —*see* Fibrosis, lung
  Escherichia coli (E. coli) J15.5

Pneumonia *- continued*
  Friedländer's bacillus J15.0
  Hemophilus influenzae J14
  hypostatic J18.2
  Klebsiella (pneumoniae) J15.0
  pneumococcal J13
  Proteus J15.6
  Pseudomonas J15.1
  specified organism NEC J16.8
  staphylococcal —*see* Pneumonia, staphylococcal
  streptococcal NEC J15.4
  Streptococcus pneumoniae J13
  viral, virus —*see* Pneumonia, viral
lobular —*see* Pneumonia, broncho
Löffler's J82
lymphoid interstitial J84.2
massive —*see* Pneumonia, lobar
meconium P24.01
MSSA (methicillin susceptible Staphylococcus aureus) J15.211
multilobar —*see* Pneumonia, by type
Mycoplasma (pneumoniae) J15.7
necrotic J85.0
neonatal P23.9
  aspiration —*see* Aspiration, by substance, with pneumonia
nitrogen dioxide J68.9
organizing J84.89
  due to
    collagen vascular disease J84.17
    known underlying cause J84.17
  in diseases classified elsewhere J84.17
orthostatic J18.2
parainfluenza virus J12.2
parenchymatous —*see* Fibrosis, lung
passive J18.2
patchy —*see* Pneumonia, broncho
Peptococcus J15.8
Peptostreptococcus J15.8
plasma cell (of infants) B59
pleurolobar —*see* Pneumonia, lobar
pleuro-pneumonia-like organism (PPLO) J15.7
pneumococcal (broncho) (lobar) J13
Pneumocystis (carinii) (jiroveci) B59
postinfectional NEC B99 *[J17]*
postmeasles B05.2
Proteus J15.6
Pseudomonas J15.1
psittacosis A70
radiation J70.0
respiratory syncytial virus J12.1
resulting from a procedure J95.89
rheumatic I00 *[J17]*
Salmonella (arizonae) (cholerae-suis) (enteritidis) (typhimurium) A02.22
  typhi A01.03
  typhoid fever A01.03
SARS-associated coronavirus J12.81
segmented, segmental —*see* Pneumonia, broncho
Serratia marcescens J15.6
specified NEC J18.8
  bacterium NEC J15.8
  organism NEC J16.8
  virus NEC J12.89
spirochetal NEC A69.8
staphylococcal (broncho) (lobar) J15.20
  aureus (methicillin susceptible) (MSSA) J15.211
    methicillin resistant (MRSA) J15.212

Pneumonia *- continued*
  specified NEC J15.29
static, stasis J18.2
streptococcal NEC (broncho) (lobar) J15.4
  group
    A J15.4
    B J15.3
    specified NEC J15.4
Streptococcus pneumoniae J13
syphilitic, congenital (early) A50.04
traumatic (complication) (early) (secondary) T79.8
tuberculous (any) —*see* Tuberculosis, pulmonary
tularemic A21.2
varicella B01.2
Veillonella J15.8
ventilator associated J95.851
viral, virus (broncho) (interstitial) (lobar) J12.9
  adenoviral J12.0
  congenital P23.0
  human metapneumovirus J12.3
  parainfluenza J12.2
  respiratory syncytial J12.1
  SARS-associated coronavirus J12.81
  specified NEC J12.89
white (congenital) A50.04
Pneumonic —*see* condition
Pneumonitis (acute) (primary) —*see also* Pneumonia
air-conditioner J67.7
allergic (due to) J67.9
  organic dust NEC J67.8
  red cedar dust J67.8
  sequoiosis J67.8
  wood dust J67.8
aspiration J69.0
  due to
    anesthesia J95.4
      during
        labor and delivery O74.0
        pregnancy O29.01
        puerperium O89.01
    fumes or gases J68.0
    obstetric O74.0
chemical (due to gases, fumes or vapors) (inhalation) J68.0
  due to anesthesia J95.4
cholesterol J84.89
crack (cocaine) J68.0
chronic —*see* Fibrosis, lung
congenital rubella P35.0
due to
  beryllium J68.0
  cadmium J68.0
  crack (cocaine) J68.0
  detergent J69.8
  fluorocarbon-polymer J68.0
  food, vomit (aspiration) J69.0
  fumes or vapors J68.0
  gases, fumes or vapors (inhalation) J68.0
  inhalation
    blood J69.8
    essences J69.1
    food (regurgitated) , milk, vomit J69.0
    oils, essences J69.1
    saliva J69.0
    solids, liquids NEC J69.8
  manganese J68.0
  nitrogen dioxide J68.0
  oils, essences J69.1
  solids, liquids NEC J69.8

Pneumonitis - *continued*
  toxoplasmosis (acquired) B58.3
    congenital P37.1
  vanadium J68.0
  ventilator J95.851
  eosinophilic J82
  hypersensitivity J67.9
    air conditioner lung J67.7
    bagassosis J67.1
    bird fancier's lung J67.2
    farmer's lung J67.0
    malt worker's lung J67.4
    maple bark-stripper's lung J67.6
    mushroom worker's lung J67.5
    specified organic dust NEC J67.8
    suberosis J67.3
  interstitial (chronic) J84.89
    acute J84.114
    lymphoid J84.2
    non-specific J84.89
      idiopathic J84.113
  lymphoid, interstitial J84.2
  meconium P24.01
  postanesthetic J95.4
    correct substance properly administered —
  see Table of Drugs and Chemicals, by drug,
  adverse effect
    in labor and delivery O74.0
    in pregnancy O29.01
    obstetric O74.0
    overdose or wrong substance given or taken
  (by accident) —*see* Table of Drugs and
  Chemicals, by drug, poisoning
    postpartum, puerperal O89.01
  postoperative J95.4
    obstetric O74.0
  radiation J70.0
  rubella, congenital P35.0
  ventilation (air-conditioning) J67.7
  ventilator associated J95.851
  wood-dust J67.8
Pneumonoconiosis —*see* Pneumoconiosis
Pneumoparotid K11.8
Pneumopathy NEC J98.4
  alveolar J84.09
  due to organic dust NEC J66.8
  parietoalveolar J84.09
Pneumopericarditis —*see also* Pericarditis
  acute I30.9
Pneumopericardium —*see also* Pericarditis
  congenital P25.3
  newborn P25.3
  traumatic (post) —*see* Injury, heart
Pneumophagia (psychogenic) F45.8
Pneumopleurisy, pneumopleuritis (*see also*
  Pneumonia) J18.8
Pneumopyopericardium I30.1
Pneumopyothorax —*see* Pyopneumothorax
  with fistula J86.0
Pneumorrhagia —*see also* Hemorrhage, lung
  tuberculous —*see* Tuberculosis, pulmonary
Pneumothorax NOS J93.9
  acute J93.83
  chronic J93.81
  congenital P25.1
  perinatal period P25.1
  postprocedural J95.811
  specified NEC J93.83
  spontaneous NOS J93.83
    newborn P25.1
    primary J93.11
    secondary J93.12

Pneumothorax - *continued*
  tension J93.0
  tense valvular, infectional J93.0
  tension (spontaneous) J93.0
  traumatic S27.0
    with hemothorax S27.2
  tuberculous —*see* Tuberculosis, pulmonary
Podagra (*see also* Gout) M10.9
Podencephalus Q01.9
Poikilocytosis R71.8
Poikiloderma L81.6
  Civatte's L57.3
  congenital Q82.8
  vasculare atrophicans L94.5
Poikilodermatomyositis M33.10
  with
    myopathy M33.12
    respiratory involvement M33.11
    specified organ involvement NEC M33.19
Pointed ear (congenital) Q17.3
**Poison ivy, oak, sumac or other plant
dermatitis** (allergic) (contact) L23.7
Poisoning (acute) —*see also* Table of Drugs
  and Chemicals
  algae and toxins T65.82
  Bacillus B (aertrycke) (cholerae (suis))
  (paratyphosus) (suipestifer) A02.9
    botulinus A05.1
  bacterial toxins A05.9
  berries, noxious —*see* Poisoning, food,
  noxious, berries
  botulism A05.1
  ciguatera fish T61.0
  Clostridium botulinum A05.1
  death-cap (Amanita phalloides) (Amanita
  verna) —*see* Poisoning, food, noxious,
  mushrooms
  drug —*see* Table of Drugs and Chemicals, by
  drug, poisoning
  epidemic, fish (noxious) —*see* Poisoning,
  seafood
    bacterial A05.9
  fava bean D55.0
  fish (noxious) T61.9
    bacterial —*see* Intoxication, foodborne, by
  agent
    ciguatera fish —*see* Poisoning, ciguatera
  fish
    scombroid fish —*see* Poisoning, scombroid
  fish
    specified type NEC T61.77
  food (acute) (diseased) (infected) (noxious)
  NEC T62.9
    bacterial —*see* Intoxication, foodborne, by
  agent
    due to
      Bacillus (aertrycke) (choleraesuis)
      (paratyphosus) (suipestifer) A02.9
        botulinus A05.1
      Clostridium (perfringens) (Welchii) A05.2
      salmonella (aertrycke) (gallinarum)
      (choleraesuis) (enteritidis) (paratyphi)
      (suipestifer) A02.9
        with
          gastroenteritis A02.0
          sepsis A02.1
      staphylococcus A05.0
      Vibrio
        parahaemolyticus A05.3
        vulnificus A05.5
    noxious or naturally toxic T62.9
      berries —see subcategory T62.1

Poisoning – *continued*
  fish —*see* Poisoning, seafood
  mushrooms —see subcategory T62.0X
  plants NEC —see subcategory T62.2X
  seafood —*see* Poisoning, seafood
  specified NEC —see subcategory T62.8X
  ichthyotoxism —*see* Poisoning, seafood
  kreotoxism, food A05.9
  latex T65.81
  lead T56.0
  mushroom —*see* Poisoning, food, noxious,
  mushroom
  mussels —*see also* Poisoning, shellfish
    bacterial —*see* Intoxication, foodborne, by
  agent
  nicotine (tobacco) T65.2
  noxious foodstuffs —*see* Poisoning, food,
  noxious
  plants, noxious —*see* Poisoning, food,
  noxious, plants NEC
  ptomaine —*see* Poisoning, food
  radiation J70.0
  Salmonella (arizonae) (cholerae-suis)
  (enteritidis) (typhimurium) A02.9
  scombroid fish T61.1
  seafood (noxious) T61.9
    bacterial —*see* Intoxication, foodborne, by
  agent
    fish —*see* Poisoning, fish
    shellfish —*see* Poisoning, shellfish
    specified NEC —see subcategory T61.8X
  shellfish (amnesic) (azaspiracid) (diarrheic)
  (neurotoxic) (noxious) (paralytic) T61.78
    bacterial —*see* Intoxication, foodborne, by
  agent
    ciguatera mollusk —*see* Poisoning,
  ciguatera fish
  specified substance NEC T65.891
  Staphylococcus, food A05.0
  tobacco (nicotine) T65.2
  water E87.79
Poker spine —*see* Spondylitis, ankylosing
Poland syndrome Q79.8
Polioencephalitis (acute) (bulbar) A80.9
  inferior G12.22
  influenzal —*see* Influenza, with,
  encephalopathy
  superior hemorrhagic (acute) (Wernicke's)
  E51.2
  Wernicke's E51.2
Polioencephalomyelitis (acute) (anterior)
  A80.9
  with beriberi E51.2
Polioencephalopathy, superior hemorrhagic
  E51.2
  with
    beriberi E51.11
    pellagra E52
Poliomeningoencephalitis —*see*
  Meningoencephalitis
Poliomyelitis (acute) (anterior) (epidemic)
  A80.9
  with paralysis (bulbar) —*see* Poliomyelitis,
  paralytic
  abortive A80.4
  ascending (progressive) —*see* Poliomyelitis,
  paralytic
  bulbar (paralytic) —*see* Poliomyelitis,
  paralytic
  congenital P35.8
  nonepidemic A80.9
  nonparalytic A80.4
  paralytic A80.30

Poliomyelitis *- continued*
  specified NEC A80.39
  vaccine-associated A80.0
  wild virus
    imported A80.1
    indigenous A80.2
  spinal, acute A80.9
Poliosis (eyebrow) (eyelashes) L67.1
  circumscripta, acquired L67.1
Pollakiuria R35.0
  psychogenic F45.8
Pollinosis J30.1
Pollitzer's disease L73.2
Polyadenitis *—see also* Lymphadenitis
  malignant A20.0
Polyalgia M79.89
Polyangiitis M30.0
  microscopic M31.7
  overlap syndrome M30.8
Polyarteritis
  microscopic M31.7
  nodosa M30.0
    with lung involvement M30.1
    juvenile M30.2
    related condition NEC M30.8
Polyarthralgia *—see* Pain, joint
Polyarthritis, polyarthropathy (*see also*
  Arthritis) M13.0
  due to or associated with other specified
    conditions *—see* Arthritis
  epidemic (Australian) (with exanthema)
    B33.1
  infective *—see* Arthritis, pyogenic or pyemic
  inflammatory M06.4
  juvenile (chronic) (seronegative) M08.3
  migratory *—see* Fever, rheumatic
  rheumatic, acute *—see* Fever, rheumatic
Polyarthrosis M15.9
  post-traumatic M15.3
  primary M15.0
  specified NEC M15.8
Polycarential syndrome of infancy E40
Polychondritis (atrophic) (chronic) *—see also*
  Disorder, cartilage, specified type NEC
  relapsing M94.1
Polycoria Q13.2
Polycystic (disease)
  degeneration, kidney Q61.3
    autosomal dominant (adult type) Q61.2
    autosomal recessive (infantile type) NEC
      Q61.19
  kidney Q61.3
    autosomal
      dominant Q61.2
      recessive NEC Q61.19
    autosomal dominant (adult type) Q61.2
    autosomal recessive (childhood type) NEC
      Q61.19
    infantile type NEC Q61.19
  liver Q44.6
  lung J98.4
    congenital Q33.0
  ovary, ovaries E28.2
  spleen Q89.09
Polycythemia (secondary) D75.1
  acquired D75.1
  benign (familial) D75.0
  due to
    donor twin P61.1
    erythropoietin D75.1
    fall in plasma volume D75.1
    high altitude D75.1

Polycythemia *– continued*
  maternal-fetal transfusion P61.1
    stress D75.1
  emotional D75.1
  erythropoietin D75.1
  familial (benign) D75.0
  Gaisböck's (hypertonica) D75.1
  high altitude D75.1
  hypertonica D75.1
  hypoxemic D75.1
  neonatorum P61.1
  nephrogenous D75.1
  relative D75.1
  secondary D75.1
  spurious D75.1
  stress D75.1
  vera D45
Polycytosis cryptogenica D75.1
Polydactylism, polydactyly Q69.9
  toes Q69.2
Polydipsia R63.1
Polydystrophy, pseudo-Hurler E77.0
Polyembryoma *—see* Neoplasm, malignant,
  by site
Polyglandular
  deficiency E31.0
  dyscrasia E31.9
  dysfunction E31.9
  syndrome E31.8
Polyhydramnios O40.-**Polymastia** Q83.1
Polymenorrhea N92.0
Polymyalgia M35.3
  arteritica, giant cell M31.5
  rheumatica M35.3
    with giant cell arteritis M31.5
Polymyositis (acute) (chronic) (hemorrhagic)
  M33.20
  with
    myopathy M33.22
    respiratory involvement M33.21
    skin involvement *—see*
  Dermatopolymyositis
    specified organ involvement NEC M33.29
  ossificans (generalisata) (progressiva) *—see*
  Myositis, ossificans, progressiva
Polyneuritis, polyneuritic *—see also*
  Polyneuropathy
  acute (post) infective G61.0
  alcoholic G62.1
  cranialis G52.7
  demyelinating, chronic inflammatory (CIDP)
    G61.81
  diabetic *—see* Diabetes, polyneuropathy
  diphtheritic A36.83
  due to lack of vitamin NEC E56.9 *[G63]*
  endemic E51.11
  erythredema *—see* subcategory T56.1
  febrile, acute G61.0
  hereditary ataxic G60.1
  idiopathic, acute G61.0
  infective (acute) G61.0
  inflammatory, chronic demyelinating (CIDP)
    G61.81
  nutritional E63.9 *[G63]*
  postinfective (acute) G61.0
  specified NEC G62.89
Polyneuropathy (peripheral) G62.9
  alcoholic G62.1
  amyloid (Portuguese) E85.1 *[G63]*
  arsenical G62.2
  critical illness G62.81

Polyneuropathy *– continued*
  demyelinating, chronic inflammatory (CIDP)
    G61.81
  diabetic *—see* Diabetes, polyneuropathy
  drug-induced G62.0
  hereditary G60.9
    specified NEC G60.8
  idiopathic G60.9
    progressive G60.3
  in (due to)
    alcohol G62.1
      sequelae G65.2
    amyloidosis, familial (Portuguese) E85.1
      [G63]
    antitetanus serum G61.1
    arsenic G62.2
      sequelae G65.2
    avitaminosis NEC E56.9 *[G63]*
    beriberi E51.11
    collagen vascular disease NEC M35.9 *[G63]*
    deficiency (of)
      B (-complex) vitamins E53.9 *[G63]*
      vitamin B6 E53.1 *[G63]*
    diabetes *—see* Diabetes, polyneuropathy
    diphtheria A36.83
    drug or medicament G62.0
      correct substance properly administered —
    see Table of Drugs and Chemicals, by drug,
    adverse effect
      overdose or wrong substance given or
    taken *—see* Table of Drugs and Chemicals,
    by drug, poisoning
    endocrine disease NEC E34.9 *[G63]*
    herpes zoster B02.23
    hypoglycemia E16.2 *[G63]*
    infectious
      disease NEC B99 *[G63]*
      mononucleosis B27.91
    lack of vitamin NEC E56.9 *[G63]*
    lead G62.2
      sequelae G65.2
    leprosy A30.9 *[G63]*
    Lyme disease A69.22
    metabolic disease NEC E88.9 *[G63]*
    microscopic polyangiitis M31.7 *[G63]*
    mumps B26.84
    neoplastic disease (*see also* Neoplasm)
      D49.9 *[G63]*
    nutritional deficiency NEC E63.9 *[G63]*
    organophosphate compounds G62.2
      sequelae G65.2
    parasitic disease NEC B89 *[G63]*
    pellagra E52 *[G63]*
    polyarteritis nodosa M30.0
    porphyria E80.20 *[G63]*
    radiation G62.82
    rheumatoid arthritis *—see* Rheumatoid,
      polyneuropathy
    sarcoidosis D86.89
    serum G61.1
    syphilis (late) A52.15
      congenital A50.43
    systemic
      connective tissue disorder M35.9 *[G63]*
      lupus erythematosus M32.19
    toxic agent NEC G62.2
      sequelae G65.2
    triorthocresyl phosphate G62.2
      sequelae G65.2
    tuberculosis A17.89
    uremia N18.9 *[G63]*
    vitamin B12 deficiency E53.8 *[G63]*
      with anemia (pernicious) D51.0 *[G63]*

Polyneuropathy – *continued*
    due to dietary deficiency D51.3 *[G63]*
  zoster B02.23
  inflammatory G61.9
    chronic demyelinating (CIDP) G61.81
    sequelae G65.1
    specified NEC G61.89
  lead G62.2
    sequelae G65.2
  nutritional NEC E63.9 *[G63]*
  postherpetic (zoster) B02.23
  progressive G60.3
  radiation-induced G62.82
  sensory (hereditary) (idiopathic) G60.8
  specified NEC G62.89
  syphilitic (late) A52.15
    congenital A50.43
Polyopia H53.8
Polyorchism, polyorchidism Q55.21
Polyosteoarthritis (*see also* Osteoarthritis, generalized) M15.9
  post-traumatic M15.3
  specified NEC M15.8
Polyostotic fibrous dysplasia Q78.1
Polyotia Q17.0
Polyp, polypus
  accessory sinus J33.8
  adenocarcinoma in —*see* Neoplasm, malignant, by site
  adenocarcinoma in situ in —*see* Neoplasm, in situ, by site
  adenoid tissue J33.0
  adenomatous —*see also* Neoplasm, benign, by site
    adenocarcinoma in —*see* Neoplasm, malignant, by site
    adenocarcinoma in situ in —*see* Neoplasm, in situ, by site
    carcinoma in —*see* Neoplasm, malignant, by site
    carcinoma in situ in —*see* Neoplasm, in situ, by site
    multiple —*see* Neoplasm, benign
      adenocarcinoma in —*see* Neoplasm, malignant, by site
      adenocarcinoma in situ in —*see* Neoplasm, in situ, by site
  antrum J33.8
  anus, anal (canal) K62.0
  Bartholin's gland N84.3
  bladder D41.4
  carcinoma in —*see* Neoplasm, malignant, by site
  carcinoma in situ in —*see* Neoplasm, in situ, by site
  cecum D12.0
  cervix (uteri) N84.1
    in pregnancy or childbirth —*see* Pregnancy, complicated by, abnormal, cervix
    mucous N84.1
    nonneoplastic N84.1
  choanal J33.0
  cholesterol K82.4
  clitoris N84.3
  colon K63.5
    adenomatous D12.6
    ascending D12.2
    cecum D12.0
    descending D12.4
    inflammatory K51.40
      with
        abscess K51.414

Polyp, polypus – *continued*
      complication K51.419
        specified NEC K51.418
      fistula K51.413
      intestinal obstruction K51.412
      rectal bleeding K51.411
    sigmoid D12.5
    transverse D12.3
  corpus uteri N84.0
  dental K04.0
  duodenum K31.7
  ear (middle) H74.4
  endometrium N84.0
  ethmoidal (sinus) J33.8
  fallopian tube N84.8
  female genital tract N84.9
    specified NEC N84.8
  frontal (sinus) J33.8
  gallbladder K82.4
  gingiva, gum K06.8
  labia, labium (majus) (minus) N84.3
  larynx (mucous) J38.1
    adenomatous D14.1
  malignant —*see* Neoplasm, malignant, by site
  maxillary (sinus) J33.8
  middle ear —*see* Polyp, ear (middle)
  myometrium N84.0
  nares
    anterior J33.9
    posterior J33.0
  nasal (mucous) J33.9
    cavity J33.0
    septum J33.0
  nasopharyngeal J33.0
  nose (mucous) J33.9
  oviduct N84.8
  pharynx J39.2
  placenta O90.89
  prostate —*see* Enlargement, enlarged, prostate
  pudenda, pudendum N84.3
  pulpal (dental) K04.0
  rectum (nonadenomatous) K62.1
    adenomatous —*see* Polyp, adenomatous
  septum (nasal) J33.0
  sinus (accessory) (ethmoidal) (frontal) (maxillary) (sphenoidal) J33.8
  sphenoidal (sinus) J33.8
  stomach K31.7
    adenomatous D13.1
  tube, fallopian N84.8
  turbinate, mucous membrane J33.8
  umbilical, newborn P83.6
  ureter N28.89
  urethra N36.2
  uterus (body) (corpus) (mucous) N84.0
    cervix N84.1
    in pregnancy or childbirth —*see* Pregnancy, complicated by, tumor, uterus
  vagina N84.2
  vocal cord (mucous) J38.1
  vulva N84.3
Polyphagia R63.2
Polyploidy Q92.7
Polypoid —*see* condition
Polyposis —*see also* Polyp
  coli (adenomatous) D12.6
    adenocarcinoma in C18.9
    adenocarcinoma in situ in —*see* Neoplasm, in situ, by site
    carcinoma in C18.9
  colon (adenomatous) D12.6

Polyposis – *continued*
  familial D12.6
    adenocarcinoma in situ in —*see* Neoplasm, in situ, by site
  intestinal (adenomatous) D12.6
  malignant lymphomatous C83.1
  multiple, adenomatous (*see also* Neoplasm, benign) D36.9
Polyradiculitis —*see* Polyneuropathy
Polyradiculoneuropathy (acute) (postinfective) (segmentally demyelinating) G61.0
Polyserositis
  due to pericarditis I31.1
  pericardial I31.1
  periodic, familial E85.0
  tuberculous A19.9
    acute A19.1
    chronic A19.8
Polysplenia syndrome Q89.09
Polysyndactyly (*see also* Syndactylism, syndactyly) Q70.4
Polytrichia L68.3
Polyunguia Q84.6
Polyuria R35.8
  nocturnal R35.1
  psychogenic F45.8
Pompe's disease (glycogen storage) E74.02
Pompholyx L30.1
Poncet's disease (tuberculous rheumatism) A18.09
Pond fracture —*see* Fracture, skull
Ponos B55.0
Pons, pontine —*see* condition
Poor
  aesthetic of existing restoration of tooth K08.56
  contractions, labor O62.2
  gingival margin to tooth restoration K08.51
  personal hygiene R46.0
  prenatal care, affecting management of pregnancy —*see* Pregnancy, complicated by, insufficient, prenatal care
  sucking reflex (newborn) R29.2
  urinary stream R39.12
  vision NEC H54.7
Poradenitis, nostras inguinalis or venerea A55
Porencephaly (congenital) (developmental) (true) Q04.6
  acquired G93.0
  nondevelopmental G93.0
  traumatic (post) F07.89
Porocephaliasis B88.8
Porokeratosis Q82.8
Poroma, eccrine —*see* Neoplasm, skin, benign
Porphyria (South African) E80.20
  acquired E80.20
  acute intermittent (hepatic) (Swedish) E80.21
  cutanea tarda (hereditary) (symptomatic) E80.1
  due to drugs E80.20
    correct substance properly administered — *see* Table of Drugs and Chemicals, by drug, adverse effect
    overdose or wrong substance given or taken —*see* Table of Drugs and Chemicals, by drug, poisoning
  erythropoietic (congenital) (hereditary) E80.0
  hepatocutaneous type E80.1
  secondary E80.20
  toxic NEC E80.20
  variegata E80.20

Porphyrinuria —*see* Porphyria
Porphyruria —*see* Porphyria
Portal —*see* condition
Port wine nevus, mark, or stain Q82.5
Posadas-Wernicke disease B38.9
Positive
  culture (nonspecific)
    blood R78.81
    bronchial washings R84.5
    cerebrospinal fluid R83.5
    cervix uteri R87.5
    nasal secretions R84.5
    nipple discharge R89.5
    nose R84.5
      staphylococcus (Methicillin susceptible)
      Z22.321
        Methicillin resistant Z22.322
    peritoneal fluid R85.5
    pleural fluid R84.5
    prostatic secretions R86.5
    saliva R85.5
    seminal fluid R86.5
    sputum R84.5
    synovial fluid R89.5
    throat scrapings R84.5
    urine R82.7
    vagina R87.5
    vulva R87.5
    wound secretions R89.5
  PPD (skin test) R76.11
  serology for syphilis A53.0
    false R76.8
    with signs or symptoms
  code as Syphilis, by site and stage
  skin test, tuberculin (without active
  tuberculosis) R76.11
  test, human immunodeficiency virus (HIV)
  R75
  VDRL A53.0
    with signs or symptoms
  code by site and stage under Syphilis A53.9
  Wassermann reaction A53.0
Postcardiotomy syndrome I97.0
Postcaval ureter Q62.62
Postcholecystectomy syndrome K91.5
Postclimacteric bleeding N95.0
Postcommissurotomy syndrome I97.0
Postconcussional syndrome F07.81
Postcontusional syndrome F07.81
Postcricoid region —*see* condition
Post-dates (40 42 weeks) (pregnancy)
  (mother) O48.0
  more than 42 weeks gestation O48.1
Postencephalitic syndrome F07.89
Posterior —*see* condition
Posterolateral sclerosis (spinal cord) —*see*
  Degeneration, combined
Postexanthematous —*see* condition
Postfebrile —*see* condition
Postgastrectomy dumping syndrome K91.1
Posthemiplegic chorea —*see* Monoplegia
Posthemorrhagic anemia (chronic) D50.0
  acute D62
  newborn P61.3
Postherpetic neuralgia (zoster) B02.29
  trigeminal B02.22
Posthitis N47.7
Postimmunization complication or reaction
  —*see* Complications, vaccination
Postinfectious —*see* condition
Postlaminectomy syndrome NEC M96.1
Postleukotomy syndrome F07.0

Postmastectomy lymphedema (syndrome)
  I97.2
Postmaturity, postmature (over 42 weeks)
  maternal (over 42 weeks gestation) O48.1
  newborn P08.22
Postmeasles complication NEC (*see also*
  condition) B05.89
Postmenopausal
  endometrium (atrophic) N95.8
    suppurative (*see also* Endometritis) N71.9
  osteoporosis —*see* Osteoporosis,
  postmenopausal
Postnasal drip R09.82
  due to
    allergic rhinitis —*see* Rhinitis, allergic
    common cold J00
    gastroesophageal reflux —*see* Reflux,
    gastroesophageal
    nasopharyngitis —*see* Nasopharyngitis
    other know condition
  code to condition
    sinusitis —*see* Sinusitis
Postnatal —*see* condition
Postoperative (postprocedural) —*see*
  Complication, postoperative
  pneumothorax, therapeutic Z98.3
  state NEC Z98.89
Postpancreatectomy hyperglycemia E89.1
Postpartum —*see* Puerperal
Postphlebitic syndrome —*see* Syndrome,
  postthrombotic
Postpoliomyelitic —*see also* condition
  osteopathy —*see* Osteopathy, after
  poliomyelitis
Postpolio (myelitic) syndrome G14
Postprocedural —*see also* Postoperative
  hypoinsulinemia E89.1
Postschizophrenic depression F32.8
Postsurgery status —*see also* Status (post)
  pneumothorax, therapeutic Z98.3
Post-term (40 42 weeks) (pregnancy) (mother)
  O48.0
  infant P08.21
  more than 42 weeks gestation (mother) O48.1
Post-traumatic brain syndrome,
  nonpsychotic F07.81
Post-typhoid abscess A01.09
Postures, hysterical F44.2
Postvaccinal reaction or complication —*see*
  Complications, vaccination
Postvalvulotomy syndrome I97.0
Potain's
  disease (pulmonary edema)—*see* Edema, lung
  syndrome (gastrectasis with dyspepsia) K31.0
Potter's
  asthma J62.8
  facies Q60.6
  lung J62.8
  syndrome (with renal agenesis) Q60.6
Pott's
  curvature (spinal) A18.01
  disease or paraplegia A18.01
  spinal curvature A18.01
  tumor, puffy —*see* Osteomyelitis, specified
  type NEC
Pouch
  bronchus Q32.4
  Douglas' —*see* condition
  esophagus, esophageal, congenital Q39.6
    acquired K22.5
  gastric K31.4
  Hartmann's K82.8
  pharynx, pharyngeal (congenital) Q38.7

Pouchitis K91.850
Poultry men's itch B88.0
Poverty NEC Z59.6
  extreme Z59.5
Poxvirus NEC B08.8
Prader-Willi syndrome Q87.1
Preauricular appendage or tag Q17.0
Prebetalipoproteinemia (acquired) (essential)
  (familial) (hereditary) (primary) (secondary)
  E78.1
  with chylomicronemia E78.3
Precipitate labor or delivery O62.3
Preclimacteric bleeding (menorrhagia) N92.4
Precocious
  adrenarche E30.1
  menarche E30.1
  menstruation E30.1
  pubarche E30.1
  puberty E30.1
    central E22.8
  sexual development NEC E30.1
  thelarche E30.8
Precocity, sexual (constitutional) (cryptogenic)
  (female) (idiopathic) (male) E30.1
  with adrenal hyperplasia E25.9
    congenital E25.0
Precordial pain R07.2
Predeciduous teeth K00.2
Prediabetes, prediabetic R73.09
  complicating
    pregnancy —*see* Pregnancy, complicated
    by, diseases of, specified type or system NEC
    puerperium O99.89
Predislocation status of hip at birth Q65.6
Pre-eclampsia O14.9
  with pre-existing hypertension —*see*
  Hypertension, complicating pregnancy, pre-
  existing, with, pre-eclampsia
  mild O14.0
  moderate O14.0
  severe O14.1
    with hemolysis, elevated liver enzymes and
    low platelet count (HELLP) O14.2
Pre-eruptive color change, teeth, tooth K00.8
Pre-excitation atrioventricular conduction
  I45.6
Preglaucoma H40.00
Pregnancy (single) (uterine) —*see also*
  Delivery and Puerperal
  Note: The Tabular must be reviewed for
  assignment of the appropriate character
  indicating the trimester of the pregnancy
  Note: The Tabular must be reviewed for
  assignment of appropriate seventh character
  for multiple gestation codes in Chapter 15
  abdominal (ectopic) O00.0
    with viable fetus O36.7
  ampullar O00.1
  biochemical O02.81
  broad ligament O00.8
  cervical O00.8
  chemical O02.81
  complicated NOS O26.9
  complicated by (care of) (management
  affected by)
    abnormal, abnormality
      cervix O34.4
        causing obstructed labor O65.5
      cord (umbilical) O69.9
      findings on antenatal screening of mother
      O28.9
        biochemical O28.1
        cytological O28.2

Pregnancy – *continued*

    chromosomal O28.5

    genetic O28.5

    hematological O28.0

    radiological O28.4

    specified NEC O28.8

    ultrasonic O28.3

    glucose (tolerance) NEC O99.810

    pelvic organs O34.9

      specified NEC O34.8

        causing obstructed labor O65.5

    pelvis (bony) (major) NEC O33.0

    perineum O34.7

    position

      placenta O44.1

        without hemorrhage O44.0

      uterus O34.59

    uterus O34.59

      causing obstructed labor O65.5

      congenital O34.0

    vagina O34.6

      causing obstructed labor O65.5

    vulva O34.7

      causing obstructed labor O65.5

  abruptio placentae —*see* Abruptio placentae

  abscess or cellulitis

    bladder O23.1

    breast O91.11

    genital organ or tract O23.9

  abuse

    physical O9A.31

    psychological O9A.51

    sexual O9A.41

  adverse effect anesthesia O29.9

    aspiration pneumonitis O29.01

    cardiac arrest O29.11

    cardiac complication NEC O29.19

    cardiac failure O29.12

    central nervous system complication NEC O29.29

    cerebral anoxia O29.21

    failed or difficult intubation O29.6

    inhalation of stomach contents or secretions NOS O29.01

    local, toxic reaction O29.3X

    Mendelson's syndrome O29.01

    pressure collapse of lung O29.02

    pulmonary complications NEC O29.09

    specified NEC O29.8X

    spinal and epidural type NEC O29.5X

      induced headache O29.4

  albuminuria O12.1

  alcohol use O99.31

  amnionitis O41.12

  anaphylactoid syndrome of pregnancy O88.01

  anemia (conditions in D50-D64) (pre-existing) O99.01

    complicating the puerperium O99.03

  antepartum hemorrhage O46.9

    with coagulation defect —*see* Hemorrhage, antepartum, with coagulation defect

    specified NEC O46.8X

  appendicitis O99.61

  atrophy (yellow) (acute) liver (subacute) O26.61

  bariatric surgery status O99.84

  bicornis or bicornuate uterus O34.59

  biliary tract problems O26.61

  breech presentation O32.1

  cardiovascular diseases (conditions in I00-I09, I20-I52, I70-I99) O99.41

Pregnancy – *continued*

  cerebrovascular disorders (conditions in I60-I69) O99.41

  cervical shortening O26.87

  cervicitis O23.51

  chloasma (gravidarum) O26.89

  cholestasis (intrahepatic) O26.61

  cholecystitis O99.61

  chorioamnionitis O41.12

  circulatory system disorder (conditions in I00-I09, I20-I99, O99.41)

  compound presentation O32.6

  conjoined twins O30.02

  connective system disorders (conditions in M00-M99) O99.89

  contracted pelvis (general) O33.1

    inlet O33.2

    outlet O33.3

  convulsions (eclamptic) (uremic) (*see also* Eclampsia) O15.9

  cracked nipple O92.11

  cystitis O23.1

  cystocele O34.8

  death of fetus (near term) O36.4

    early pregnancy O02.1

    of one fetus or more in multiple gestation O31.2

  deciduitis O41.14

  decreased fetal movement O36.81

  dental problems O99.61

  diabetes (mellitus) O24.91

    gestational (pregnancy induced) —*see* Diabetes, gestational

    pre-existing O24.31

      specified NEC O24.81

      type 1 O24.01

      type 2 O24.11

  digestive system disorders (conditions in K00-K93) O99.61

  diseases of —*see* Pregnancy, complicated by, specified body system disease

    biliary tract O26.61

    blood NEC (conditions in D65-D77) O99.11

    liver O26.61

    specified NEC O99.89

  disorders of —*see* Pregnancy, complicated by, specified body system disorder

    amniotic fluid and membranes O41.9

      specified NEC O41.8X

    biliary tract O26.61

    ear and mastoid process (conditions in H60-H95) O99.89

    eye and adnexa (conditions in H00-H59) O99.89

    liver O26.61

    skin (conditions in L00-L99) O99.71

    specified NEC O99.89

  displacement, uterus NEC O34.59

    causing obstructed labor O65.5

  disproportion (due to) O33.9

    fetal deformities NEC O33.7

    generally contracted pelvis O33.1

    hydrocephalic fetus O33.6

    inlet contraction of pelvis O33.2

    mixed maternal and fetal origin O33.4

    specified NEC O33.8

  double uterus O34.59

    causing obstructed labor O65.5

  drug use (conditions in F11-F19) O99.32

Pregnancy – *continued*

  eclampsia, eclamptic (coma) (convulsions) (delirium) (nephritis) (uremia) (*see also* Eclampsia) O15.

  ectopic pregnancy —*see* Pregnancy, ectopic

  edema O12.0

    with

      gestational hypertension, mild (*see also* Pre-eclampsia) O14.0

      proteinuria O12.2

  effusion, amniotic fluid —*see* Pregnancy, complicated by, premature rupture of membranes

  elderly

    multigravida O09.52

    primigravida O09.51

  embolism (*see also* Embolism, obstetric, pregnancy) O88.

  endocrine diseases NEC O99.28

  endometritis O86.12

  excessive weight gain O26.0

  exhaustion O26.81

    during labor and delivery O75.81

  face presentation O32.3

  failed induction of labor O61.9

    instrumental O61.1

    mechanical O61.1

    medical O61.0

    specified NEC O61.8

    surgical O61.1

  failed or difficult intubation for anesthesia O29.6

  false labor (pains) O47.9

    at or after 37 completed weeks of pregnancy O47.1

    before 37 completed weeks of pregnancy O47.0

  fatigue O26.81

    during labor and delivery O75.81

  fatty metamorphosis of liver O26.61

  female genital mutilation O34.8 *[N90.81]*

  fetal (maternal care for)

    abnormality or damage O35.9

      acid-base balance O68

      specified type NEC O35.8

    acidemia O68

    acidosis O68

    alkalosis O68

    anemia and thrombocytopenia O36.82

    anencephaly O35.0

    chromosomal abnormality (conditions in Q90-Q99) O35.1

    conjoined twins O30.02

    damage from

      amniocentesis O35.7

      biopsy procedures O35.7

      drug addiction O35.5

      hematological investigation O35.7

      intrauterine contraceptive device O35.7

      maternal

        alcohol addiction O35.4

        cytomegalovirus infection O35.3

        disease NEC O35.8

        drug addiction O35.5

        listeriosis O35.8

        rubella O35.3

        toxoplasmosis O35.8

        viral infection O35.3

      medical procedure NEC O35.7

      radiation O35.6

    death (near term) O36.4

      early pregnancy O02.1

Pregnancy – *continued*

decreased movement O36.81

disproportion due to deformity (fetal) O33.7

excessive growth (large for dates) O36.6

growth retardation O36.59
  light for dates O36.59
  small for dates O36.59

heart rate irregularity (bradycardia) (decelerations) (tachycardia) O76

hereditary disease O35.2

hydrocephalus O35.0

intrauterine death O36.4

poor growth O36.59
  light for dates O36.59
  small for dates O36.59

problem O36.9
  specified NEC O36.89

reduction (elective) O31.3

selective termination O31.3

spina bifida O35.0

thrombocytopenia O36.82

fibroid (tumor) (uterus) O34.1

fissure of nipple O92.11

gallstones O99.61

gastric banding status O99.84

gastric bypass status O99.84

genital herpes (asymptomatic) (history of) (inactive) O98.51

genital tract infection O23.9

glomerular diseases (conditions in N00-N07) O26.83
  with hypertension, pre-existing —*see* Hypertension, complicating, pregnancy, pre-existing, with, renal disease

gonorrhea O98.21

grand multiparity O09.4

habitual aborter —*see* Pregnancy, complicated by, recurrent pregnancy loss

HELLP syndrome (hemolysis, elevated liver enzymes and low platelet count) O14.2

hemorrhage
  antepartum —*see* Hemorrhage, antepartum
  before 20 completed weeks gestation O20.9
    specified NEC O20.8
  due to premature separation, placenta (*see also* Abruptio placentae) O45.9
    early O20.9
      specified NEC O20.8
    threatened abortion O20.0

hemorrhoids O22.4

hepatitis (viral) O98.41

herniation of uterus O34.59

high
  head at term O32.4
  risk —*see* Supervision (of) (for) , high-risk

history of in utero procedure during previous pregnancy O09.82

HIV O98.71

human immunodeficiency virus (HIV) disease O98.71

hydatidiform mole (*see also* Mole, hydatidiform) O01.9

hydramnios O40.

hydrocephalic fetus (disproportion) O33.6

hydrops
  amnii O40.
  fetalis O36.2
    associated with isoimmunization (*see also* Pregnancy, complicated by, isoimmunization) O36.11

Pregnancy – *continued*

hydrorrhea O42.90

hyperemesis (gravidarum) (mild) (*see also* Hyperemesis, gravidarum) O21.0

hypertension —*see* Hypertension, complicating pregnancy

hypertensive
  heart and renal disease, pre-existing —*see* Hypertension, complicating, pregnancy, pre-existing, with, heart disease, with renal disease
  heart disease, pre-existing —*see* Hypertension, complicating, pregnancy, pre-existing, with, heart disease
  renal disease, pre-existing —*see* Hypertension, complicating, pregnancy, pre-existing, with, renal disease

hypotension O26.5

immune disorders NEC (conditions in D80-D89) O99.11

incarceration, uterus O34.51

incompetent cervix O34.3

inconclusive fetal viability O36.80

infection (s) O98.91
  amniotic fluid or sac O41.10
  bladder O23.1
  carrier state NEC O99.830
    streptococcus B O99.820
  genital organ or tract O23.9
    specified NEC O23.59
  genitourinary tract O23.9
  gonorrhea O98.21
  hepatitis (viral) O98.41
  HIV O98.71
  human immunodeficiency virus (HIV) O98.71
  kidney O23.0
  nipple O91.01
  parasitic disease O98.91
    specified NEC O98.81
  protozoal disease O98.61
  sexually transmitted NEC O98.31
  specified type NEC O98.81
  syphilis O98.11
  tuberculosis O98.01
  urethra O23.2
  urinary (tract) O23.4
    specified NEC O23.3
  viral disease O98.51

injury or poisoning (conditions in S00-T88) O9A.21
  due to abuse
    physical O9A.31
    psychological O9A.51
    sexual O9A.41

insufficient
  prenatal care O09.3
  weight gain O26.1

insulin resistance O26.89

intrauterine fetal death (near term) O36.4
  early pregnancy O02.1
  multiple gestation (one fetus or more) O31.2

isoimmunization O36.11
  anti-A sensitization O36.11
  anti-B sensitization O36.19
  Rh O36.09
    anti-D antibody O36.01
  specified NEC O36.19

laceration of uterus NEC O71.81

Pregnancy – *continued*

malformation
  placenta, placental (vessel) O43.10
    specified NEC O43.19
  uterus (congenital) O34.0

malnutrition (conditions in E40-E46) O25.1

maternal hypotension syndrome O26.5

mental disorders (conditions in F01-F09, F20-F99) O99.34
  alcohol use O99.31
  drug use O99.32
  smoking O99.33

mentum presentation O32.3

metabolic disorders O99.28

missed
  abortion O02.1
  delivery O36.4

multiple gestations O30.9
  conjoined twins O30.02
  specified number of multiples NEC —*see* Pregnancy, multiple (gestation) , specified NEC
  quadruplet —*see* Pregnancy, quadruplet
  specified complication NEC O31.8X
  triplet —*see* Pregnancy, triplet
  twin —*see* Pregnancy, twin

musculoskeletal condition (conditions is M00-M99) O99.89

necrosis, liver (conditions in K72) O26.61

neoplasm
  benign
    cervix O34.4
    corpus uteri O34.1
    uterus O34.1
  malignant O9A.11

nephropathy NEC O26.83

nervous system condition (conditions in G00-G99) O99.35

nutritional diseases NEC O99.28

obesity (pre-existing) O99.21

obesity surgery status O99.84

oblique lie or presentation O32.2

older mother —*see* Pregnancy, complicated by, elderly

oligohydramnios O41.0
  with premature rupture of membranes (*see also* Pregnancy, complicated by, premature rupture of membranes) O42.

onset (spontaneous) of labor after 37 completed weeks of gestation but before 39 completed weeks gestation, with delivery by (planned) cesarean section O75.82

oophoritis O23.52

overdose, drug (*see also* Table of Drugs and Chemicals, by drug, poisoning) O9A.21

oversize fetus O33.5

papyraceous fetus O31.0

pelvic inflammatory disease O99.89

periodontal disease O99.61

peripheral neuritis O26.82

peritoneal (pelvic) adhesions O99.89

phlebitis O22.9

phlebopathy O22.9

phlebothrombosis (superficial) O22.2
  deep O22.3

placenta accreta O43.21

placenta increta O43.22

placenta percreta O43.23

placenta previa O44.1
  without hemorrhage O44.0

placental disorder O43.9
  specified NEC O43.89

placental dysfunction O43.89

Pregnancy – *continued*
  placental infarction O43.81
  placental insufficiency O36.51
  placental transfusion syndromes
    fetomaternal O43.01
    fetus to fetus O43.02
    maternofetal O43.01
  placentitis O41.14
  pneumonia O99.51
  poisoning (*see also* Table of Drugs and
Chemicals) O9A.21
  polyhydramnios O40
  polymorphic eruption of pregnancy O26.86
  poor obstetric history NEC O09.29
  postmaturity (post-term) (40 to 42 weeks)
    O48.0
    more than 42 completed weeks gestation
      (prolonged) O48.1
  pre-eclampsia O14.9
    mild O14.0
    moderate O14.0
    severe O14.1
    with hemolysis, elevated liver enzymes
and low platelet count (HELLP) O14.2
  premature labor —*see* Pregnancy,
complicated by, preterm labor
  premature rupture of membranes O42.90
    full-term O42.92
    with onset of labor
      within 24 hours O42.00
        after 37 weeks gestation O42.02
        pre-term (before 37 completed weeks of
gestation) O42.01
      after 24 hours O42.10
        after 37 weeks gestation O42.12
        pre-term (before 37 completed weeks of
gestation) O42.11
      after 37 weeks gestation O42.92
      pre-term (before 37 completed weeks of
gestation) O42.91
  premature separation of placenta (*see also*
Abruptio placentae) O45.9
  presentation, fetal
—*see* Delivery, complicated by, malposition
  preterm delivery O60.10
  preterm labor
    with delivery O60.10
      preterm O60.10
      term O60.20
    second trimester
      with term delivery O60.22
      without delivery O60.02
      with preterm delivery
        second trimester O60.12
        third trimester O60.13
    third trimester
      with term delivery O60.23
      without delivery O60.03
      with third trimester preterm delivery
O60.14
    without delivery O60.00
      second trimester O60.02
      third trimester O60.03
  previous history of —*see* Pregnancy,
supervision of, high-risk
  prolapse, uterus O34.52
  proteinuria (gestational) O12.1
    with edema O12.2
  pruritic urticarial papules and plaques of
pregnancy (PUPPP) O26.86
  pruritus (neurogenic) O26.89
  psychosis or psychoneurosis (puerperal) F53

Pregnancy – *continued*
  ptyalism O26.89
  PUPPP (pruritic urticarial papules and
plaques of pregnancy) O26.86
  pyelitis O23.0
  recurrent pregnancy loss O26.2
  renal disease or failure NEC O26.83
    with secondary hypertension, pre-existing
—*see* Hypertension, complicating, pregnancy,
pre-existing, secondary
      hypertensive, pre-existing —*see*
Hypertension, complicating, pregnancy, pre-
existing, with, renal disease
  respiratory condition (conditions in J00-J99)
    O99.51
  retained, retention
    dead ovum O02.0
    intrauterine contraceptive device O26.3
  retroversion, uterus O34.53
  Rh immunization, incompatibility or
sensitization NEC O36.09
    anti-D antibody O36.01
  rupture
    amnion (premature) (*see also* Pregnancy,
complicated by, premature rupture of
membranes) O42
      membranes (premature) (*see also*
Pregnancy, complicated by, premature rupture
of membranes) O42
    uterus (during labor) O71.1
      before onset of labor O71.0
  salivation (excessive) O26.89
  salpingitis O23.52
  salpingo-oophoritis O23.52
  sepsis (conditions in A40, A41) O98.81
  size date discrepancy (uterine) O26.84
  skin condition (conditions in L00-L99)
    O99.71
  smoking (tobacco) O99.33
  social problem O09.7
  specified condition NEC O26.89
  spotting O26.85
  streptococcus B carrier state O99.820
  subluxation of symphysis (pubis) O26.71
  syphilis (conditions in A50-A53) O98.11
  threatened
    abortion O20.0
    labor O47.9
      at or after 37 completed weeks of
gestation O47.1
      before 37 completed weeks of gestation
O47.0
  thrombophlebitis (superficial) O22.2
  thrombosis O22.9
    cerebral venous O22.5
    cerebrovenous sinus O22.5
    deep O22.3
  torsion of uterus O34.59
  toxemia O14.9
  transverse lie or presentation O32.2
  tuberculosis (conditions in A15-A19)
    O98.01
  tumor (benign)
    cervix O34.4
    malignant O9A.11
    uterus O34.1
  unstable lie O32.0
  upper respiratory infection O99.51
  urethritis O23.2
  uterine size date discrepancy O26.84
  vaginitis or vulvitis O23.59
  varicose veins (lower extremities) O22.0

Pregnancy – *continued*
  genitals O22.1
  legs O22.0
  perineal O22.1
  vaginal or vulval O22.1
  venereal disease NEC (conditions in A63.8)
    O98.31
  venous disorders O22.9
  specified NEC O22.8X
  viral diseases (conditions in A80-B09, B25-
B34) O98.51
  very young mother —*see* Pregnancy,
complicated by, young mother
  vomiting O21.9
    due to diseases classified elsewhere O21.8
    hyperemesis gravidarum (mild) (*see also*
Hyperemesis, gravidarum) O21.0
    late (occurring after 20 weeks of gestation)
O21.2
  young mother
    multigravida O09.62
    primigravida O09.61
concealed O09.3
continuing following
  elective fetal reduction of one or more fetus
    O31.3
  intrauterine death of one or more fetus
    O31.2
  spontaneous abortion of one or more fetus
    O31.1
cornual O00.8
ectopic (ruptured) O00.9
  abdominal O00.0
    with viable fetus O36.7
  cervical O00.8
  complicated (by) O08.9
    afibrinogenemia O08.1
    cardiac arrest O08.81
    chemical damage of pelvic organ (s) O08.6
    circulatory collapse O08.3
    defibrination syndrome O08.1
    electrolyte imbalance O08.5
    embolism (amniotic fluid) (blood clot)
      (pulmonary) (septic) O08.2
    endometritis O08.0
    genital tract and pelvic infection O08.0
    hemorrhage (delayed) (excessive) O08.1
    infection
      genital tract or pelvic O08.0
      kidney O08.83
      urinary tract O08.83
    intravascular coagulation O08.1
    laceration of pelvic organ (s) O08.6
    metabolic disorder O08.5
    oliguria O08.4
    oophoritis O08.0
    parametritis O08.0
    pelvic peritonitis O08.0
    perforation of pelvic organ (s) O08.6
    renal failure or shutdown O08.4
    salpingitis or salpingo-oophoritis O08.0
    sepsis O08.82
    shock O08.83
      septic O08.82
    specified condition NEC O08.89
    tubular necrosis (renal) O08.4
    uremia O08.4
    urinary infection O08.83
    venous complication NEC O08.7
      embolism O08.2
  cornual O00.8
  intraligamentous O00.8
  mural O00.8

Pregnancy – *continued*
  ovarian O00.2
  specified site NEC O00.8
  tubal (ruptured) O00.1
  examination (normal) Z34.9
  high-risk —*see* Pregnancy, supervision of, high-risk
    first Z34.0
    specified Z34.8
  extrauterine —*see* Pregnancy, ectopic
  fallopian O00.1
  false F45.8
  hidden O09.3
  high-risk —*see* Pregnancy, supervision of, high-risk
  incidental finding Z33.1
  interstitial O00.8
  intraligamentous O00.8
  intramural O00.8
  intraperitoneal O00.0
  isthmian O00.1
  mesometric (mural) O00.8
  molar NEC O02.0
    complicated (by) O08.9
      afibrinogenemia O08.1
      cardiac arrest O08.81
      chemical damage of pelvic organ (s) O08.6
      circulatory collapse O08.3
      defibrination syndrome O08.1
      electrolyte imbalance O08.5
      embolism (amniotic fluid) (blood clot) (pulmonary) (septic) O08.2
      endometritis O08.0
      genital tract and pelvic infection O08.0
      hemorrhage (delayed) (excessive) O08.1
      infection
        genital tract or pelvic O08.0
        kidney O08.83
        urinary tract O08.83
      intravascular coagulation O08.1
      laceration of pelvic organ (s) O08.6
      metabolic disorder O08.5
      oliguria O08.4
      oophoritis O08.0
      parametritis O08.0
      pelvic peritonitis O08.0
      perforation of pelvic organ (s) O08.6
      renal failure or shutdown O08.4
      salpingitis or salpingo-oophoritis O08.0
      sepsis O08.82
      shock O08.3
        septic O08.82
      specified condition NEC O08.89
      tubular necrosis (renal) O08.4
      uremia O08.4
      urinary infection O08.83
      venous complication NEC O08.7
        embolism O08.2
  hydatidiform (*see also* Mole, hydatidiform) O01.9
  multiple (gestation) O30.9
    greater than quadruplets —*see* Pregnancy, multiple (gestation) , specified NEC
    specified NEC O30.80
      with
        two or more monoamniotic fetuses O30.82
        two or more monochorionic fetuses O30.81
      two or more monoamniotic fetuses O30.82
      two or more monochorionic fetuses O30.81

Pregnancy – *continued*
    unable to determine number of placenta and number of amniotic sacs O30.89
    unspecified number of placenta and unspecified number of amniotic sacs O30.80
  mural O00.8
  normal (supervision of) Z34.9
  high-risk —*see* Pregnancy, supervision of, high-risk
    first Z34.0
    specified Z34.8
  ovarian O00.2
  postmature (40 to 42 weeks) O48.0
    more than 42 weeks gestation O48.1
  post-term (40 to 42 weeks) O48.0
  prenatal care only Z34.9
  high-risk —*see* Pregnancy, supervision of, high-risk
    first Z34.0
    specified Z34.8
  prolonged (more than 42 weeks gestation) O48.1
  quadruplet O30.20
    with
      two or more monoamniotic fetuses O30.22
      two or more monochorionic fetuses O30.21
    two or more monoamniotic fetuses O30.22
    two or more monochorionic fetuses O30.21
    unable to determine number of placenta and number of amniotic sacs O30.29
    unspecified number of placenta and unspecified number of amniotic sacs O30.20
  quintuplet —*see* Pregnancy, multiple (gestation) , specified NEC
  sextuplet —*see* Pregnancy, multiple (gestation) , specified NEC
  supervision of
    concealed pregnancy O09.3
    elderly mother
      multigravida O09.52
      primigravida O09.51
    hidden pregnancy O09.3
    high-risk O09.9
      due to (history of)
        ectopic pregnancy O09.1
        elderly —*see* Pregnancy, supervision, elderly mother
        grand multiparity O09.4
        infertility O09.0
        insufficient prenatal care O09.3
        in utero procedure during previous pregnancy O09.82
        in vitro fertilization O09.81
        molar pregnancy O09.1
        multiple previous pregnancies O09.4
        older mother —*see* Pregnancy, supervision of, elderly mother
        poor reproductive or obstetric history NEC O09.29
        pre-term labor O09.21
        previous
          neonatal death O09.29
        social problems O09.7
        specified NEC O09.89
        very young mother —*see* Pregnancy, supervision, young mother
      resulting from in vitro fertilization O09.81
    normal Z34.9
      first Z34.0
      specified NEC Z34.8
    young mother
      multigravida O09.62

Pregnancy – *continued*
      primigravida O09.61
  triplet O30.10
    with
      two or more monoamniotic fetuses O30.12
      two or more monochorionic fetuses O30.11
    two or more monoamniotic fetuses O30.12
    two or more monochorionic fetuses O30.11
    unable to determine number of placenta and number of amniotic sacs O30.19
    unspecified number of placenta and unspecified number of amniotic sacs O30.10
  tubal (with abortion) (with rupture) O00.1
  twin O30.00
    conjoined O30.02
    dichorionic/diamniotic (two placenta, two amniotic sacs) O30.04
    monochorionic/diamniotic (one placenta, two amniotic sacs) O30.03
    monochorionic/monoamniotic (one placenta, one amniotic sac) O30.01
    unable to determine number of placenta and number of amniotic sacs O30.09
    unspecified number of placenta and unspecified number of amniotic sacs O30.00
  unwanted Z64.0
  weeks of gestation
    8 weeks Z3A.08
    9 weeks Z3A.09
    10 weeks Z3A.10
    11 weeks Z3A.11
    12 weeks Z3A.12
    13 weeks Z3A.13
    14 weeks Z3A.14
    15 weeks Z3A.15
    16 weeks Z3A.16
    17 weeks Z3A.17
    18 weeks Z3A.18
    19 weeks Z3A.19
    20 weeks Z3A.20
    21 weeks Z3A.21
    22 weeks Z3A.22
    23 weeks Z3A.23
    24 weeks Z3A.24
    25 weeks Z3A.25
    26 weeks Z3A.26
    27 weeks Z3A.27
    28 weeks Z3A.28
    29 weeks Z3A.29
    30 weeks Z3A.30
    31 weeks Z3A.31
    32 weeks Z3A.32
    33 weeks Z3A.33
    34 weeks Z3A.34
    35 weeks Z3A.35
    36 weeks Z3A.36
    37 weeks Z3A.37
    38 weeks Z3A.38
    39 weeks Z3A.39
    40 weeks Z3A.40
    41 weeks Z3A.41
    42 weeks Z3A.42
    greater than 42 weeks Z3A.49
    less than 8 weeks Z3A.01
    not specified Z3A.00
Preiser's disease —*see* Osteonecrosis, secondary, due to, trauma, metacarpus
Pre-kwashiorkor —*see* Malnutrition, severe
Preleukemia (syndrome) D46.9
Preluxation, hip, congenital Q65.6

Premature —*see also* condition
  adrenarche E27.0
  aging E34.8
  beats I49.40
    atrial I49.1
    auricular I49.1
    supraventricular I49.1
  birth NEC —*see* Preterm, newborn
  closure, foramen ovale Q21.8
  contraction
    atrial I49.1
    atrioventricular I49.2
    auricular I49.1
    auriculoventricular I49.49
    heart (extrasystole) I49.49
    junctional I49.2
    ventricular I49.3
  delivery (*see also* Pregnancy, complicated by, preterm labor) O60.10
  ejaculation F52.4
  infant NEC —*see* Preterm, newborn
    light-for-dates —*see* Light for dates
  labor —*see* Pregnancy, complicated by, preterm labor
  lungs P28.0
  menopause E28.319
    asymptomatic E28.319
    symptomatic E28.310
  newborn
    extreme (less than 28 completed weeks) — *see* Immaturity, extreme
    less than 37 completed weeks —*see* Preterm, newborn
  puberty E30.1
  rupture membranes or amnion —*see* Pregnancy, complicated by, premature rupture of membranes
  senility E34.8
  thelarche E30.8
  ventricular systole I49.3
Prematurity NEC (less than 37 completed weeks) —*see* Preterm, newborn
  extreme (less than 28 completed weeks) —*see* Immaturity, extreme
Premenstrual
  dysphoric disorder (PMDD) N94.3
  tension (syndrome) N94.3
Premolarization, cuspids K00.2
Prenatal
  care, normal pregnancy —*see* Pregnancy, normal
  screening of mother Z36
  teeth K00.6
Preparatory care for subsequent treatment NEC
  for dialysis Z49.01
    peritoneal Z49.02
Prepartum —*see* condition
Preponderance, left or right ventricular I51.7
Prepuce —*see* condition
PRES (posterior reversible encephalopathy syndrome) I67.83
Presbycardia R54
Presbycusis, presbyacusia H91.1
Presbyesophagus K22.8
Presbyophrenia F03
Presbyopia H52.4
Prescription of contraceptives (initial) Z30.019
  emergency (postcoital) Z30.012
  implantable subdermal Z30.019

Prescription of contraceptives - *continued*
  injectable Z30.013
  intrauterine contraceptive device Z30.014
  pills Z30.011
  postcoital (emergency) Z30.012
  repeat Z30.40
    implantable subdermal Z30.49
    injectable Z30.42
    pills Z30.41
    specified type NEC Z30.49
  specified type NEC Z30.018
Presence (of)
  ankle-joint implant (functional) (prosthesis) Z96.66
  aortocoronary (bypass) graft Z95.1
  arterial-venous shunt (dialysis) Z99.2
  artificial
    eye (globe) Z97.0
    heart (fully implantable) (mechanical) Z95.812
      valve Z95.2
    larynx Z96.3
    lens (intraocular) Z96.1
    limb (complete) (partial) Z97.1
      arm Z97.1
        bilateral Z97.15
      leg Z97.1
        bilateral Z97.16
  audiological implant (functional) Z96.29
  bladder implant (functional) Z96.0
  bone
    conduction hearing device Z96.29
    implant (functional) NEC Z96.7
    joint (prosthesis) —*see* Presence, joint implant
  cardiac
    defibrillator (functional) (with synchronous cardiac pacemaker) Z95.810
    implant or graft Z95.9
      specified type NEC Z95.818
    pacemaker Z95.0
  cerebrospinal fluid drainage device Z98.2
  cochlear implant (functional) Z96.21
  contact lens (es) Z97.3
  coronary artery graft or prosthesis Z95.5
  CSF shunt Z98.2
  dental prosthesis device Z97.2
  dentures Z97.2
  device (external) NEC Z97.8
    cardiac NEC Z95.818
    heart assist Z95.811
    implanted (functional) Z96.9
      specified NEC Z96.89
    prosthetic Z97.8
  ear implant Z96.20
    cochlear implant Z96.21
    myringotomy tube Z96.22
    specified type NEC Z96.29
  elbow-joint implant (functional) (prosthesis) Z96.62
  endocrine implant (functional) NEC Z96.49
  eustachian tube stent or device (functional) Z96.29
  external hearing-aid or device Z97.4
  finger-joint implant (functional) (prosthetic) Z96.69
  functional implant Z96.9
    specified NEC Z96.89
  graft
    cardiac NEC Z95.818
    vascular NEC Z95.828

Presence (of) – *continued*
  hearing-aid or device (external) Z97.4
    implant (bone) (cochlear) (functional) Z96.21
  heart assist device Z95.811
  heart valve implant (functional) Z95.2
    prosthetic Z95.2
    specified type NEC Z95.4
    xenogenic Z95.3
  hip-joint implant (functional) (prosthesis) Z96.64
  implanted device (artificial) (functional) (prosthetic) Z96.9
    automatic cardiac defibrillator (with synchronous cardiac pacemaker) Z95.810
    cardiac pacemaker Z95.0
    cochlear Z96.21
    dental Z96.5
    heart Z95.812
    heart valve Z95.2
      prosthetic Z95.2
      specified NEC Z95.4
      xenogenic Z95.3
    insulin pump Z96.41
    intraocular lens Z96.1
    joint Z96.60
      ankle Z96.66
      elbow Z96.62
      finger Z96.69
      hip Z96.64
      knee Z96.65
      shoulder Z96.61
      specified NEC Z96.698
      wrist Z96.63
    larynx Z96.3
    myringotomy tube Z96.22
    otological Z96.20
      cochlear Z96.21
      eustachian stent Z96.29
      myringotomy Z96.22
      specified NEC Z96.29
      stapes Z96.29
    skin Z96.81
    skull plate Z96.7
    specified NEC Z96.89
    urogenital Z96.0
  insulin pump (functional) Z96.41
  intestinal bypass or anastomosis Z98.0
  intraocular lens (functional) Z96.1
  intrauterine contraceptive device (IUD) Z97.5
  intravascular implant (functional) (prosthetic) NEC Z95.9
    coronary artery Z95.5
    defibrillator (with synchronous cardiac pacemaker) Z95.810
    peripheral vessel (with angioplasty) Z95.820
  joint implant (prosthetic) (any) Z96.60
    ankle —*see* Presence, ankle joint implant
    elbow —*see* Presence, elbow joint implant
    finger —*see* Presence, finger joint implant
    hip —*see* Presence, hip joint implant
    knee —*see* Presence, knee joint implant
    shoulder —*see* Presence, shoulder joint implant
    specified joint NEC Z96.698
    wrist —*see* Presence, wrist joint implant
  knee-joint implant (functional) (prosthesis) Z96.65
  laryngeal implant (functional) Z96.3
  mandibular implant (dental) Z96.5
  myringotomy tube (s) Z96.22

Presence (of) – *continued*
orthopedic-joint implant (prosthetic) (any) — *see* Presence, joint implant
otological implant (functional) Z96.29
shoulder-joint implant (functional) (prosthesis) Z96.61
skull-plate implant Z96.7
spectacles Z97.3
stapes implant (functional) Z96.29
systemic lupus erythematosus -SLE] inhibitor D68.62
tendon implant (functional) (graft) Z96.7
tooth root (s) implant Z96.5
ureteral stent Z96.0
urethral stent Z96.0
urogenital implant (functional) Z96.0
vascular implant or device Z95.9
  access port device Z95.828
  specified type NEC Z95.828
wrist-joint implant (functional) (prosthesis) Z96.63
Presenile —*see also* condition
dementia F03
premature aging E34.8
Presentation, fetal —*see* Delivery , complicated by, malposition
Prespondylolisthesis (congenital) Q76.2
Pressure
area, skin —*see* Ulcer, pressure, by site
brachial plexus G54.0
brain G93.5
  injury at birth NEC P11.1
cerebral —*see* Pressure, brain
chest R07.89
cone, tentorial G93.5
hyposystolic —*see also* Hypotension
  incidental reading, without diagnosis of hypotension R03.1
increased
  intracranial (benign) G93.2
    injury at birth P11.0
  intraocular H40.05
lumbosacral plexus G54.1
mediastinum J98.5
necrosis (chronic) —*see* Ulcer, pressure, by site
parental, inappropriate (excessive) Z62.6
sore (chronic) —*see* Ulcer, pressure, by site
spinal cord G95.20
ulcer (chronic) —*see* Ulcer, pressure, by site
venous, increased I87.8
Pre-syncope R55
Preterm
delivery (*see also* Pregnancy, complicated by, preterm labor) O60.10
labor —*see* Pregnancy, complicated by, preterm labor
newborn (infant) P07.30
  gestational age
    28 completed weeks (28 weeks, 0 days through 28 weeks, 6 days) P07.31
    29 completed weeks (29 weeks, 0 days through 29 weeks, 6 days) P07.32
    30 completed weeks (30 weeks, 0 days through 30 weeks, 6 days) P07.33
    31 completed weeks (31 weeks, 0 days through 31 weeks, 6 days) P07.34
    32 completed weeks (32 weeks, 0 days through 32 weeks, 6 days) P07.35
    33 completed weeks (33 weeks, 0 days through 33 weeks, 6 days) P07.36

Preterm - *continued*
    34 completed weeks (34 weeks, 0 days through 34 weeks, 6 days) P07.37
    35 completed weeks (35 weeks, 0 days through 35 weeks, 6 days) P07.38
    36 completed weeks (36 weeks, 0 days through 36 weeks, 6 days) P07.39
Previa
placenta (low) (marginal) (partial) (total) (with hemorrhage) O44.1
  without hemorrhage O44.0
vasa O69.4
Priapism N48.30
due to
  disease classified elsewhere N48.32
  drug N48.33
  specified cause NEC N48.39
  trauma N48.31
Prickling sensation (skin) R20.2
Prickly heat L74.0
Primary —*see* condition
Primigravida
elderly, affecting management of pregnancy, labor and delivery (supervision only) —*see* Pregnancy, complicated by, elderly, primigravida
older, affecting management of pregnancy, labor and delivery (supervision only) —*see* Pregnancy, complicated by, elderly, primigravida
very young, affecting management of pregnancy, labor and delivery (supervision only) —*see* Pregnancy, complicated by, young mother, primigravida
Primipara
elderly, affecting management of pregnancy, labor and delivery (supervision only) —*see* Pregnancy, complicated by, elderly, primigravida
older, affecting management of pregnancy, labor and delivery (supervision only) —*see* Pregnancy, complicated by, elderly, primigravida
very young, affecting management of pregnancy, labor and delivery (supervision only) —*see* Pregnancy, complicated by, young mother, primigravida
Primus varus (bilateral) Q66.2
PRIND (Prolonged reversible ischemic neurologic deficit) I63.9
Pringle's disease (tuberous sclerosis) Q85.1
Prinzmetal angina I20.1
Prizefighter ear —*see* Cauliflower ear
Problem (with) (related to)
academic Z55.8
acculturation Z60.3
adjustment (to)
  change of job Z56.1
  life-cycle transition Z60.0
  pension Z60.0
  retirement Z60.0
adopted child Z62.821
alcoholism in family Z63.72
atypical parenting situation Z62.9
bankruptcy Z59.8
behavioral (adult) F69
  drug seeking Z72.89
birth of sibling affecting child Z62.898
care (of)
  provider dependency Z74.9
    specified NEC Z74.8
  sick or handicapped person in family or household Z63.6

Problem - *continued*
child
  abuse (affecting the child) —*see* Maltreatment, child
  custody or support proceedings Z65.3
  in welfare custody Z62.21
  in care of non-parental family member Z62.21
  in foster care Z62.21
  living in orphanage or group home Z62.22
child-rearing Z62.9
  specified NEC Z62.898
communication (developmental) F80.9
conflict or discord (with)
  boss Z56.4
  classmates Z55.4
  counselor Z64.4
  employer Z56.4
  family Z63.9
    specified NEC Z63.8
  probation officer Z64.4
  social worker Z64.4
  teachers Z55.4
  workmates Z56.4
conviction in legal proceedings Z65.0
  with imprisonment Z65.1
counselor Z64.4
creditors Z59.8
digestive K92.9
drug addict in family Z63.72
ear —*see* Disorder, ear
economic Z59.9
  affecting care Z59.9
  specified NEC Z59.8
education Z55.9
  specified NEC Z55.8
employment Z56.9
  change of job Z56.1
  discord Z56.4
  environment Z56.5
  sexual harassment Z56.81
  specified NEC Z56.89
  stress NEC Z56.6
  stressful schedule Z56.3
  threat of job loss Z56.2
  unemployment Z56.0
enuresis, child F98.0
eye H57.9
failed examinations (school) Z55.2
falling Z91.81
family (*see also* Disruption, family) Z63.9
  specified NEC Z63.8
feeding (elderly) (infant) R63.3
  newborn P92.9
    breast P92.5
    overfeeding P92.4
    slow P92.2
    specified NEC P92.8
    underfeeding P92.3
  nonorganic F50.8
finance Z59.9
  specified NEC Z59.8
foreclosure on loan Z59.8
foster child Z62.822
frightening experience (s) in childhood Z62.898
genital NEC
  female N94.9
  male N50.9
health care Z75.9
  specified NEC Z75.8
hearing —*see* Deafness
homelessness Z59.0

Problem - *continued*
  housing Z59.9
    inadequate Z59.1
    isolated Z59.8
    specified NEC Z59.8
  identity (of childhood) F93.8
  illegitimate pregnancy (unwanted) Z64.0
  illiteracy Z55.0
  impaired mobility Z74.09
  imprisonment or incarceration Z65.1
  inadequate teaching affecting education Z55.8
  inappropriate (excessive) parental pressure
    Z62.6
  influencing health status NEC Z78.9
  in-law Z63.1
  institutionalization, affecting child Z62.22
  intrafamilial communication Z63.8
  jealousy, child F93.8
  landlord Z59.2
  language (developmental) F80.9
  learning (developmental) F81.9
  legal Z65.3
    conviction without imprisonment Z65.0
    imprisonment Z65.1
    release from prison Z65.2
  life-management Z73.9
    specified NEC Z73.89
  life-style Z72.9
    gambling Z72.6
    high-risk sexual behavior (heterosexual)
      Z72.51
      bisexual Z72.53
      homosexual Z72.52
    inappropriate eating habits Z72.4
    self-damaging behavior NEC Z72.89
    specified NEC Z72.89
    tobacco use Z72.0
  literacy Z55.9
    low level Z55.0
    specified NEC Z55.8
  living alone Z60.2
  lodgers Z59.2
  loss of love relationship in childhood Z62.898
  marital Z63.0
    involving
      divorce Z63.5
      estrangement Z63.5
      gender identity F66
  mastication K08.8
  medical
    care, within family Z63.6
    facilities Z75.9
      specified NEC Z75.8
  mental F48.9
  multiparity Z64.1
  negative life events in childhood Z62.9
    altered pattern of family relationships
      Z62.898
    frightening experience Z62.898
    loss of
      love relationship Z62.898
      self-esteem Z62.898
    physical abuse (alleged) —*see*
    Maltreatment, child
    removal from home Z62.29
    specified event NEC Z62.898
  neighbor Z59.2
  neurological NEC R29.818
  new step-parent affecting child Z62.898
  none (feared complaint unfounded) Z71.1
  occupational NEC Z56.89
  parent-child —*see* Conflict, parent-child

Problem - *continued*
  personal hygiene Z91.89
  personality F69
  phase-of-life transition, adjustment Z60.0
  presence of sick or disabled person in family
  or household Z63.79
    needing care Z63.6
  primary support group (family) Z63.9
    specified NEC Z63.8
  probation officer Z64.4
  psychiatric F99
  psychosexual (development) F66
  psychosocial Z65.9
    specified NEC Z65.8
  relationship Z63.9
    childhood F93.8
  release from prison Z65.2
  removal from home affecting child Z62.29
  seeking and accepting known hazardous and
  harmful
    behavioral or psychological interventions
      Z65.8
    chemical, nutritional or physical
  interventions Z65.8
  sexual function (nonorganic) F52.9
  sight H54.7
  sleep disorder, child F51.9
  smell —*see* Disturbance, sensation, smell
  social
    environment Z60.9
      specified NEC Z60.8
    exclusion and rejection Z60.4
    worker Z64.4
  speech R47.9
    developmental F80.9
    specified NEC R47.89
  swallowing —*see* Dysphagia
  taste —*see* Disturbance, sensation, taste
  tic, child F95.0
  underachievement in school Z55.3
  unemployment Z56.0
    threatened Z56.2
  unwanted pregnancy Z64.0
  upbringing Z62.9
    specified NEC Z62.898
  urinary N39.9
  voice production R47.89
  work schedule (stressful) Z56.3
Procedure (surgical)
  for purpose other than remedying health state
    Z41.9
    specified NEC Z41.8
  not done Z53.9
    because of
      administrative reasons Z53.8
      contraindication Z53.09
        smoking Z53.01
      patient's decision Z53.20
        for reasons of belief or group pressure
          Z53.1
        left against medical advice (AMA)
          Z53.21
        specified reason NEC Z53.29
      specified reason NEC Z53.8
Procidentia (uteri) N81.3
Proctalgia K62.89
  fugax K59.4
  spasmodic K59.4
Proctitis K62.89
  amebic (acute) A06.0
  chlamydial A56.3
  gonococcal A54.6

Proctitis - *continued*
  granulomatous —*see* Enteritis, regional, large
  intestine
  herpetic A60.1
  radiation K62.7
  tuberculous A18.32
  ulcerative (chronic) K51.20
    with
      complication K51.219
        abscess K51.214
        fistula K51.213
        obstruction K51.212
        rectal bleeding K51.211
        specified NEC K51.218
Proctocele
  female (without uterine prolapse) N81.6
    with uterine prolapse N81.2
      complete N81.3
  male K62.3
Proctocolitis, mucosal —*see* Rectosigmoiditis,
  ulcerative
Proctoptosis K62.3
Proctorrhagia K62.5
Proctosigmoiditis K63.89
  ulcerative (chronic) —*see* Rectosigmoiditis,
  ulcerative
Proctospasm K59.4
  psychogenic F45.8
Profichet's disease —*see* Disorder, soft tissue,
  specified type NEC
Progeria E34.8
Prognathism (mandibular) (maxillary) M26.19
Progonoma (melanotic) —*see* Neoplasm,
  benign, by site
Progressive —*see* condition
Prolactinoma
  specified site —*see* Neoplasm, benign, by site
  unspecified site D35.2
Prolapse, prolapsed
  anus, anal (canal) (sphincter) K62.2
  arm or hand O32.2
    causing obstructed labor O64.4
  bladder (mucosa) (sphincter) (acquired)
    congenital Q79.4
    female —*see* Cystocele
    male N32.89
  breast implant (prosthetic) T85.49
  cecostomy K94.09
  cecum K63.4
  cervix, cervical (hypertrophied) N81.2
    anterior lip, obstructing labor O65.5
    congenital Q51.828
    postpartal, old N81.2
    stump N81.85
  ciliary body (traumatic) —*see* Laceration,
  eye(ball) , with prolapse or loss of interocular
  tissue
  colon (pedunculated) K63.4
  colostomy K94.09
  disc (intervertebral) —*see* Displacement,
  intervertebral disc
  eye implant (orbital) T85.398
    lens (ocular) —*see* Complications,
  intraocular lens
  fallopian tube N83.4
  gastric (mucosa) K31.89
  genital, female N81.9
    specified NEC N81.89
  globe, nontraumatic —*see* Luxation, globe
  ileostomy bud K94.19
  intervertebral disc —*see* Displacement,
  intervertebral disc
  intestine (small) K63.4

Prolapse, prolapsed - *continued*
 iris (traumatic) —*see* Laceration, eye(ball) ,
  with prolapse or loss of interocular tissue
   nontraumatic H21.89
 kidney N28.83
  congenital Q63.2
 laryngeal muscles or ventricle J38.7
 liver K76.89
 meatus urinarius N36.8
 mitral (valve) I34.1
 ocular lens implant —*see* Complications,
 intraocular lens
 organ or site, congenital NEC —*see*
 Malposition, congenital
 ovary N83.4
 pelvic floor, female N81.89
 perineum, female N81.89
 rectum (mucosa) (sphincter) K62.3
  due to trichuris trichuria B79
 spleen D73.89
 stomach K31.89
 umbilical cord
  complicating delivery O69.0
 urachus, congenital Q64.4
 ureter N28.89
  with obstruction N13.5
   with infection N13.6
 ureterovesical orifice N28.89
 urethra (acquired) (infected) (mucosa) N36.8
  congenital Q64.71
 urinary meatus N36.8
  congenital Q64.72
 uterovaginal N81.4
  complete N81.3
  incomplete N81.2
 uterus (with prolapse of vagina) N81.4
  complete N81.3
  congenital Q51.818
  first degree N81.2
  in pregnancy or childbirth —*see* Pregnancy,
 complicated by, abnormal, uterus
  incomplete N81.2
  postpartal (old) N81.4
  second degree N81.2
  third degree N81.3
 uveal (traumatic) —*see* Laceration, eye(ball) ,
 with prolapse or loss of interocular tissue
 vagina (anterior) (wall) —*see* Cystocele
  with prolapse of uterus N81.4
   complete N81.3
   incomplete N81.2
  posterior wall N81.6
  posthysterectomy N99.3
 vitreous (humor) H43.0
  in wound —*see* Laceration, eye(ball) , with
 prolapse or loss of interocular tissue
 womb —*see* Prolapse, uterus
Prolapsus, female N81.9
 specified NEC N81.89
Proliferation (s)
 primary cutaneous CD30-positive large T-cell
 C86.6
Proliferative —*see* condition
Prolonged, prolongation (of)
 bleeding (time) (idiopathic) R79.1
 coagulation (time) R79.1
 gestation (over 42 completed weeks)
  mother O48.1
  newborn P08.22
 interval I44.0
 labor O63.9
  first stage O63.0
  second stage O63.1

Prolonged continued
 partial thromboplastin time (PTT) R79.1
 pregnancy (more than 42 weeks gestation)
 O48.1
 prothrombin time R79.1
 QT interval I45.81
 uterine contractions in labor O62.4
Prominence, prominent
 auricle (congenital) (ear) Q17.5
 ischial spine or sacral promontory
  with disproportion (fetopelvic) O33.0
   causing obstructed labor O65.0
 nose (congenital) acquired M95.0
Promiscuity —*see* High, risk, sexual behavior
Pronation
 ankle —*see* Deformity, limb, foot, specified
 NEC
 foot —*see also* Deformity, limb, foot,
 specified NEC
  congenital Q74.2
Prophylactic
 administration of
  antibiotics, long-term Z79.2
   short-term use
 omit code
  drug (*see also* Long-term (current) drug
 therapy (use of)) Z79.899
 medication Z79.899
 organ removal (for neoplasia management)
  Z40.00
  breast Z40.01
  ovary Z40.02
  specified site NEC Z40.09
 surgery Z40.9
  for risk factors related to malignant
 neoplasm —*see* Prophylactic, organ removal
  specified NEC Z40.8
 vaccination Z23
Propionic acidemia E71.121
Proptosis (ocular) —*see also* Exophthalmos
 thyroid —*see* Hyperthyroidism, with goiter
Prosecution, anxiety concerning Z65.3
Prosopagnosia R48.3
Prostadynia N42.81
Prostate, prostatic —*see* condition
Prostatism —*see* Hyperplasia, prostate
Prostatitis (congestive) (suppurative) (with
 cystitis) N41.9
 acute N41.0
 cavitary N41.8
 chronic N41.1
 diverticular N41.8
 due to Trichomonas (vaginalis) A59.02
 fibrous N41.1
 gonococcal (acute) (chronic) A54.22
 granulomatous N41.4
 hypertrophic N41.1
 subacute N41.1
 trichomonal A59.02
 tuberculous A18.14
Prostatocystitis N41.3
Prostatorrhea N42.89
Prostatosis N42.82
Prostration R53.83
 heat —*see also* Heat, exhaustion
  anhydrotic T67.3
  due to
   salt (and water) depletion T67.4
   water depletion T67.3
 nervous F48.8
 senile R54
Protanomaly (anomalous trichromat) H53.54
Protanopia (complete) (incomplete) H53.54

Protection (against) (from) —*see* Prophylactic
Protein
 deficiency NEC —*see* Malnutrition
 malnutrition —*see* Malnutrition
 sickness (*see also* Reaction, serum) T80.69
Proteinemia R77.9
Proteinosis
 alveolar (pulmonary) J84.01
 lipid or lipoid (of Urbach) E78.89
Proteinuria R80.9
 Bence Jones R80.3
 complicating pregnancy —*see* Proteinuria,
 gestational
 gestational O12.1
  with edema O12.2
 idiopathic R80.0
 isolated R80.0
  with glomerular lesion N06.9
   dense deposit disease N06.6
   diffuse
    crescentic glomerulonephritis N06.7
    endocapillary proliferative
 glomerulonephritis N06.4
    mesangiocapillary glomerulonephritis
 N06.5
   focal and segmental hyalinosis or sclerosis
 N06.1
    membranous (diffuse) N06.2
    mesangial proliferative (diffuse) N06.3
    minimal change N06.0
    specified pathology NEC N06.8
 orthostatic R80.2
  with glomerular lesion —*see* Proteinuria,
 isolated, with glomerular lesion
 persistent R80.1
  with glomerular lesion —*see* Proteinuria,
 isolated, with glomerular lesion
 postural R80.2
  with glomerular lesion —*see* Proteinuria,
 isolated, with glomerular lesion
 pre-eclamptic —*see* Pre-eclampsia
 specified type NEC R80.8
Proteolysis, pathologic D65
Proteus (mirabilis) (morganii) **, as cause of**
 disease classified elsewhere B96.4
Prothrombin gene mutation D68.52
Protoporphyria, erythropoietic E80.0
Protozoal —*see also* condition
 disease B64
 specified NEC B60.8
Protrusion, protrusio
 acetabuli M24.7
 acetabulum (into pelvis) M24.7
 device, implant or graft (*see also*
 Complications, by site and type, mechanical)
 T85.698
  arterial graft NEC —*see* Complication,
 cardiovascular device, mechanical, vascular
  breast (implant) T85.49
  catheter NEC T85.698
   cystostomy T83.090
   dialysis (renal) T82.49
    intraperitoneal T85.691
   infusion NEC T82.594
    spinal (epidural) (subdural) T85.690
   urinary, indwelling T83.098
  electronic (electrode) (pulse generator)
 (stimulator)
   bone T84.390
   nervous system —*see* Complication,
 prosthetic device, mechanical, electronic
 nervous system stimulator

Protrusion, protrusion - *continued*
  fixation, internal (orthopedic) NEC —*see*
  Complication, fixation device, mechanical
  gastrointestinal —*see* Complications,
  prosthetic device, mechanical, gastrointestinal
  device
    genital NEC T83.498
      intrauterine contraceptive device T83.39
      penile prosthesis T83.490
    heart NEC —*see* Complication,
    cardiovascular device, mechanical
    joint prosthesis —*see* Complications, joint
    prosthesis, mechanical, specified NEC, by site
    ocular NEC —*see* Complications, prosthetic
    device, mechanical, ocular device
    orthopedic NEC —*see* Complication,
    orthopedic, device, mechanical
      specified NEC T85.628
    urinary NEC —*see also* Complication,
    genitourinary, device, urinary, mechanical
      graft T83.29
    vascular NEC —*see* Complication,
    cardiovascular device, mechanical
    ventricular intracranial shunt T85.09
  intervertebral disc —*see* Displacement,
  intervertebral disc
  joint prosthesis —*see* Complications, joint
  prosthesis, mechanical, specified NEC, by site
  nucleus pulposus —*see* Displacement,
  intervertebral disc
Prune belly (syndrome) Q79.4
Prurigo (ferox) (gravis) (Hebrae) (Hebra's)
  (mitis) (simplex) L28.2
  Besnier's L20.0
  estivalis L56.4
  nodularis L28.1
  psychogenic F45.8
Pruritus, pruritic (essential) L29.9
  ani, anus L29.0
    psychogenic F45.8
  anogenital L29.3
    psychogenic F45.8
  due to onchocerca volvulus B73.1
  gravidarum —*see* Pregnancy, complicated by,
  specified pregnancy-related condition NEC
  hiemalis L29.8
  neurogenic (any site) F45.8
  perianal L29.0
  psychogenic (any site) F45.8
  scroti, scrotum L29.1
    psychogenic F45.8
  senile, senilis L29.8
  specified NEC L29.8
    psychogenic F45.8
  Trichomonas A59.9
  vulva, vulvae L29.2
    psychogenic F45.8
Pseudarthrosis, pseudoarthrosis (bone) —*see*
  Nonunion, fracture
  clavicle, congenital Q74.0
  joint, following fusion or arthrodesis M96.0
Pseudoaneurysm —*see* Aneurysm
Pseudoangioma I81
Pseudoangina (pectoris) —*see* Angina
Pseudoarteriosus Q28.8
Pseudoarthrosis —*see* Pseudarthrosis
Pseudobulbar affect (PBA) F48.2
Pseudochromhidrosis L67.8
Pseudocirrhosis, liver, pericardial I31.1
Pseudocowpox B08.03
Pseudocoxalgia M91.3
Pseudocroup J38.5

Pseudo-Cushing's syndrome, alcohol-induced
  E24.4
Pseudocyesis F45.8
Pseudocyst
  lung J98.4
  pancreas K86.3
  retina —*see* Cyst, retina
Pseudoelephantiasis neuroarthritica Q82.0
Pseudoexfoliation, capsule (lens) —*see*
  Cataract, specified NEC
Pseudofolliculitis barbae L73.1
Pseudoglioma H44.89
Pseudohemophilia (Bernuth's) (hereditary)
  (type B) D68.0
  Type A D69.8
  vascular D69.8
Pseudohermaphroditism Q56.3
  adrenal E25.8
  female Q56.2
    with adrenocortical disorder E25.8
    without adrenocortical disorder Q56.2
    adrenal, congenital E25.0
  male Q56.1
    with
      adrenocortical disorder E25.8
      androgen resistance E34.51
      cleft scrotum Q56.1
      feminizing testis E34.51
      5-alpha-reductase deficiency E29.1
    without gonadal disorder Q56.1
    adrenal E25.8
Pseudo-Hurler's polydystrophy E77.0
Pseudohydrocephalus G93.2
Pseudohypertrophic muscular dystrophy
  (Erb's) G71.0
Pseudohypertrophy, muscle G71.0
Pseudohypoparathyroidism E20.1
Pseudoinsomnia F51.03
Pseudoleukemia, infantile D64.89
Pseudomembranous —*see* condition
Pseudomenses (newborn) P54.6
Pseudomenstruation (newborn) P54.6
Pseudomeningocele (cerebral) (infective)
  (post-traumatic) G96.19
  postprocedural (spinal) G97.82
Pseudomonas
  aeruginosa, as cause of disease classified
  elsewhere B96.5
  mallei infection A24.0
    as cause of disease classified elsewhere
    B96.5
  pseudomallei, as cause of disease classified
  elsewhere B96.5
Pseudomyotonia G71.19
Pseudomyxoma peritonei C78.6
Pseudoneuritis, optic (nerve) (disc) (papilla) ,
  congenital Q14.2
Pseudo-obstruction intestine (acute) (chronic)
  (idiopathic) (intermittent secondary) (primary)
  K59.8
Pseudopapilledema H47.33
  congenital Q14.2
Pseudoparalysis
  arm or leg R29.818
  atonic, congenital P94.2
Pseudopelade L66.0
Pseudophakia Z96.1
Pseudopolyarthritis, rhizomelic M35.3
Pseudopolycythemia D75.1
Pseudopseudohypoparathyroidism E20.1
Pseudopterygium H11.81
Pseudoptosis (eyelid) —*see* Blepharochalasis

Pseudopuberty, precocious
  female heterosexual E25.8
  male isosexual E25.8
Pseudorickets (renal) N25.0
Pseudorubella B08.20
Pseudosclerema, newborn P83.8
Pseudosclerosis (brain)
  of Westphal (Strümpell) E83.01
  Jakob's —*see* Creutzfeldt-Jakob disease or
  syndrome
  spastic —*see* Creutzfeldt-Jakob disease or
  syndrome
Pseudotetanus —*see* Convulsions
Pseudotetany R29.0
  hysterical F44.5
Pseudotruncus arteriosus Q25.4
Pseudotuberculosis A28.2
  enterocolitis A04.8
  pasteurella (infection) A28.0
Pseudotumor
  cerebri G93.2
  orbital H05.11
Pseudoxanthoma elasticum Q82.8
Psilosis (sprue) (tropical) K90.1
  nontropical K90.0
Psittacosis A70
Psoitis M60.88
Psoriasis L40.9
  arthropathic L40.50
    arthritis mutilans L40.52
    distal interphalangeal L40.51
    juvenile L40.54
    other specified L40.59
    spondylitis L40.53
  buccal K13.29
  flexural L40.8
  guttate L40.4
  mouth K13.29
  nummular L40.0
  plaque L40.0
  psychogenic F54
  pustular (generalized) L40.1
    palmaris et plantaris L40.3
  specified NEC L40.8
  vulgaris L40.0
Psychasthenia F48.8
Psychiatric disorder or problem F99
Psychogenic —*see also* condition
  factors associated with physical conditions
  F54
Psychological and behavioral factors
  affecting medical condition F59
Psychoneurosis, psychoneurotic —*see also*
  Neurosis
  anxiety (state) F41.1
  depersonalization F48.1
  hypochondriacal F45.21
  hysteria F44.9
  neurasthenic F48.8
  personality NEC F60.89
Psychopathy, psychopathic
  affectionless F94.2
  autistic F84.5
  constitution, post-traumatic F07.81
  personality —*see* Disorder, personality
  sexual —*see* Deviation, sexual
  state F60.2
Psychosexual identity disorder of childhood
  F64.2

Psychosis, psychotic F29
  acute (transient) F23
    hysterical F44.9
  affective —*see* Disorder, mood
  alcoholic F10.959
    with
      abuse F10.159
      anxiety disorder F10.980
        with
          abuse F10.180
          dependence F10.280
      delirium tremens F10.231
      delusions F10.950
        with
          abuse F10.150
          dependence F10.250
      dementia F10.97
        with dependence F10.27
      dependence F10.259
      hallucinosis F10.951
        with
          abuse F10.151
          dependence F10.251
      mood disorder F10.94
        with
          abuse F10.14
          dependence F10.24
      paranoia F10.950
        with
          abuse F10.150
          dependence F10.250
      persisting amnesia F10.96
        with dependence F10.26
    amnestic confabulatory F10.96
      with dependence F10.26
    delirium tremens F10.231
    Korsakoff's, Korsakov's, Korsakow's F10.26
    paranoid type F10.950
      with
        abuse F10.150
        dependence F10.250
  anergastic —*see* Psychosis, organic
  arteriosclerotic (simple type) (uncomplicated) F01.50
    with behavioral disturbance F01.51
  childhood F84.0
    atypical F84.8
  climacteric —*see* Psychosis, involutional
  confusional F29
    acute or subacute F05
    reactive F23
  cycloid F23
  depressive —*see* Disorder, depressive
  disintegrative (childhood) F84.3
  drug-induced —*see* F11-F19 with .x59
    paranoid and hallucinatory states —*see* F11-F19 with .x50 or .x51
  due to or associated with
    addiction, drug —*see* F11-F19 with .x59
    dependence
      alcohol F10.259
      drug —*see* F11-F19 with .x59
    epilepsy F06.8
    Huntington's chorea F06.8
    ischemia, cerebrovascular (generalized) F06.8
    multiple sclerosis F06.8
    physical disease F06.8
    presenile dementia F03
    senile dementia F03
    vascular disease (arteriosclerotic) (cerebral) F01.50

Psychosis, psychotic   - *continued*
  with behavioral disturbance F01.51
  epileptic F06.8
  episode F23
    due to or associated with physical condition F06.8
  exhaustive F43.0
  hallucinatory, chronic F28
  hypomanic F30.8
  hysterical (acute) F44.9
  induced F24
  infantile F84.0
    atypical F84.8
  infective (acute) (subacute) F05
  involutional F28
    depressive —*see* Disorder, depressive
    melancholic —*see* Disorder, depressive
    paranoid (state) F22
  Korsakoff's, Korsakov's, Korsakow's (nonalcoholic) F04
    alcoholic F10.96
      in dependence F10.26
    induced by other psychoactive substance —
  see categories F11-F19 with .x5x
  mania, manic (single episode) F30.2
    recurrent type F31.89
  manic-depressive —*see* Disorder, mood
  menopausal —*see* Psychosis, involutional
  mixed schizophrenic and affective F25.8
  multi-infarct (cerebrovascular) F01.50
    with behavioral disturbance F01.51
  nonorganic F29
    specified NEC F28
  organic F09
    due to or associated with
      arteriosclerosis (cerebral) —*see* Psychosis, arteriosclerotic
      cerebrovascular disease, arteriosclerotic —
  see Psychosis, arteriosclerotic
      childbirth —*see* Psychosis, puerperal
      Creutzfeldt-Jakob disease or syndrome —
  see Creutzfeldt-Jakob disease or syndrome
      dependence, alcohol F10.259
      disease
        alcoholic liver F10.259
        brain, arteriosclerotic —*see* Psychosis, arteriosclerotic
        cerebrovascular F01.50
          with behavioral disturbance F01.51
        Creutzfeldt-Jakob —*see* Creutzfeldt-Jakob disease or syndrome
      endocrine or metabolic F06.8
        acute or subacute F05
      liver, alcoholic F10.259
    epilepsy transient (acute) F05
    infection
      brain (intracranial) F06.8
      acute or subacute F05
    intoxication
      alcoholic (acute) F10.259
      drug F19 with .x59 F11
    ischemia, cerebrovascular (generalized) —
  see Psychosis, arteriosclerotic
    puerperium —*see* Psychosis, puerperal
    trauma, brain (birth) (from electric current) (surgical) F06.8
      acute or subacute F05
    infective F06.8
      acute or subacute F05
    post-traumatic F06.8
      acute or subacute F05
  paranoiac F22

Psychosis, psychotic   - *continued*
  paranoid (climacteric) (involutional) (menopausal) F22
    psychogenic (acute) F23
    schizophrenic F20.0
    senile F03
  postpartum F53
  presbyophrenic (type) F03
  presenile F03
  psychogenic (paranoid) F23
    depressive F32.3
  puerperal F53
    specified type —*see* Psychosis, by type
  reactive (brief) (transient) (emotional stress) (psychological trauma) F23
    depressive F32.3
      recurrent F33.3
    excitative type F30.8
  schizoaffective F25.9
    depressive type F25.1
    manic type F25.0
  schizophrenia, schizophrenic —*see* Schizophrenia
  schizophrenia-like, in epilepsy F06.2
  schizophreniform F20.81
    affective type F25.9
    brief F23
    confusional type F23
    depressive type F25.1
    manic type F25.0
    mixed type F25.0
  senile NEC F03
    depressed or paranoid type F03
    simple deterioration F03
    specified type
      code to condition
  shared F24
  situational (reactive) F23
  symbiotic (childhood) F84.3
  symptomatic F09
Psychosomatic —*see* Disorder, psychosomatic
Psychosyndrome, organic F07.9
Psychotic episode due to or associated with physical condition F06.8
Pterygium (eye) H11.00
  amyloid H11.01
  central H11.02
  colli Q18.3
  double H11.03
  peripheral
    progressive H11.05
    stationary H11.04
  recurrent H11.06
Ptilosis (eyelid) —*see* Madarosis
Ptomaine (poisoning) —*see* Poisoning, food
Ptosis —*see also* Blepharoptosis
  adiposa (false) —*see* Blepharoptosis
  breast N64.81
  cecum K63.4
  colon K63.4
  congenital (eyelid) Q10.0
    specified site NEC —*see* Anomaly, by site
  eyelid —*see* Blepharoptosis
    congenital Q10.0
  gastric K31.89
  intestine K63.4
  kidney N28.83
  liver K76.89
  renal N28.83
  splanchnic K63.4
  spleen D73.89
  stomach K31.89
  viscera K63.4

PTP D69.51
Ptyalism (periodic) K11.7
  hysterical F45.8
  pregnancy —see Pregnancy, complicated by,
    specified pregnancy-related condition NEC
  psychogenic F45.8
Ptyalolithiasis K11.5
Pubarche, precocious E30.1
Pubertas praecox E30.1
Puberty (development state) Z00.3
  bleeding (excessive) N92.2
  delayed E30.0
  precocious (constitutional) (cryptogenic)
  (idiopathic) E30.1
    central E22.8
    due to
      ovarian hyperfunction E28.1
        estrogen E28.0
      testicular hyperfunction E29.0
    premature E30.1
    due to
      adrenal cortical hyperfunction E25.8
      pineal tumor E34.8
      pituitary (anterior) hyperfunction E22.8
Puckering, macula —see Degeneration,
  macula, puckering
Pudenda, pudendum —see condition
Puente's disease (simple glandular cheilitis)
  K13.0
Puerperal, puerperium (complicated by,
  complications)
  abnormal glucose (tolerance test) O99.815
  abscess
    areola O91.02
      associated with lactation O91.03
    Bartholin's gland O86.19
    breast O91.12
      associated with lactation O91.13
    cervix (uteri) O86.11
    genital organ NEC O86.19
    kidney O86.21
    mammary O91.12
      associated with lactation O91.13
    nipple O91.02
      associated with lactation O91.03
    peritoneum O85
    subareolar O91.12
      associated with lactation O91.13
    urinary tract —see Puerperal, infection,
  urinary
    uterus O86.12
    vagina (wall) O86.13
    vaginorectal O86.13
    vulvovaginal gland O86.13
  adnexitis O86.19
  afibrinogenemia, or other coagulation defect
    O72.3
  albuminuria (acute) (subacute) —see
  Proteinuria, gestational
  alcohol use O99.315
  anemia O90.81
    pre-existing (pre-pregnancy) O99.03
  anesthetic death O89.8
  apoplexy O99.43
  bariatric surgery status O99.845
  blood disorder NEC O99.13
  blood dyscrasia O72.3
  cardiomyopathy O90.3
  cerebrovascular disorder (conditions in I60-
  I69) O99.43
  cervicitis O86.11
  circulatory system disorder O99.43

Puerperal, puerperium   - continued
  coagulopathy (any) O72.3
  complications O90.9
    specified NEC O90.89
  convulsions —see Eclampsia
  cystitis O86.22
  cystopyelitis O86.29
  delirium NEC F05
  diabetes O24.93
    gestational —see Puerperal, gestational
  diabetes
    pre-existing O24.33
      specified NEC O24.83
      type 1 O24.03
      type 2 O24.13
  digestive system disorder O99.63
  disease O90.9
    breast NEC O92.29
    cerebrovascular (acute) O99.43
    nonobstetric NEC O99.89
    tubo-ovarian O86.19
    Valsuani's O99.03
  disorder O90.9
    biliary tract O26.63
    lactation O92.70
    liver O26.63
    nonobstetric NEC O99.89
  disruption
    cesarean wound O90.0
    episiotomy wound O90.1
    perineal laceration wound O90.1
  drug use O99.325
  eclampsia (with pre-existing hypertension)
  O15.2
  embolism (pulmonary) (blood clot) —see
  Embolism, obstetric, puerperal
  endocrine, nutritional or metabolic disease
  NEC O99.285
  endophlebitis —see Puerperal, phlebitis
  endotrachelitis O86.11
  failure
    lactation (complete) O92.3
      partial O92.4
    renal, acute O90.4
  fever (of unknown origin) O86.4
    septic O85
  fissure, nipple O92.12
    associated with lactation O92.13
  fistula
    breast (due to mastitis) O91.12
      associated with lactation O91.13
    nipple O91.02
      associated with lactation O91.03
  galactophoritis O91.22
    associated with lactation O91.23
  galactorrhea O92.6
  gastric banding status O99.845
  gastric bypass status O99.845
  gastrointestinal disease NEC O99.63
  gestational diabetes O24.439
    diet controlled O24.430
    insulin (and diet) controlled O24.434
  gonorrhea O98.23
  hematoma, subdural O99.43
  hemiplegia, cerebral O99.355
    due to cerebrovascular disorder O99.43
  hemorrhage O72.1
    brain O99.43
    bulbar O99.43
    cerebellar O99.43
    cerebral O99.43
    cortical O99.43

Puerperal, puerperium   - continued
  delayed or secondary O72.2
    extradural O99.43
    internal capsule O99.43
    intracranial O99.43
    intrapontine O99.43
    meningeal O99.43
    pontine O99.43
    retained placenta O72.0
    subarachnoid O99.43
    subcortical O99.43
    subdural O99.43
    third stage O72.0
    uterine, delayed O72.2
    ventricular O99.43
  hemorrhoids O87.2
  hepatorenal syndrome O90.4
  hypertension —see Hypertension,
  complicating, puerperium
  hypertrophy, breast O92.29
  induration breast (fibrous) O92.29
  infection O86.4
    cervix O86.11
    generalized O85
    genital tract NEC O86.19
      obstetric surgical wound O86.0
    kidney (bacillus coli) O86.21
    maternal O98.93
      carrier state NEC O99.835
      gonorrhea O98.23
      human immunodeficiency virus (HIV)
        O98.73
      protozoal O98.63
      sexually transmitted NEC O98.33
      specified NEC O98.83
      streptococcus B carrier state O99.825
      syphilis O98.13
      tuberculosis O98.03
      viral hepatitis O98.43
      viral NEC O98.53
    nipple O91.02
      associated with lactation O91.03
    peritoneum O85
    renal O86.21
    specified NEC O86.89
    urinary (asymptomatic) (tract) NEC O86.20
      bladder O86.22
      kidney O86.21
      specified site NEC O86.29
      urethra O86.22
    vagina O86.13
    vein —see Puerperal, phlebitis
  ischemia, cerebral O99.43
  lymphangitis O86.89
    breast O91.22
      associated with lactation O91.23
  malignancy O9A.13
  malnutrition O25.3
  mammillitis O91.02
    associated with lactation O91.03
  mammitis O91.22
    associated with lactation O91.23
  mania F30.8
  mastitis O91.22
    associated with lactation O91.23
    purulent O91.12
      associated with lactation O91.13
  melancholia —see Disorder, depressive
  mental disorder NEC O99.345
  metroperitonitis O85
  metrorrhagia —see Hemorrhage, postpartum
  metrosalpingitis O86.19
  metrovaginitis O86.13

Puerperal, puerperium - *continued*
  milk leg O87.1
  monoplegia, cerebral O99.43
  mood disturbance O90.6
  necrosis, liver (acute) (subacute) (conditions in subcategory K72.0) O26.63
    with renal failure O90.4
  nervous system disorder O99.355
  neuritis O90.89
  obesity (pre-existing prior to pregnancy) O99.215
  obesity surgery status O99.845
  occlusion, precerebral artery O99.43
  paralysis
    bladder (sphincter) O90.89
    cerebral O99.43
  paralytic stroke O99.43
  parametritis O85
  paravaginitis O86.13
  pelviperitonitis O85
  perimetritis O86.12
  perimetrosalpingitis O86.19
  perinephritis O86.21
  periphlebitis —*see* Puerperal phlebitis
  peritoneal infection O85
  peritonitis (pelvic) O85
  perivaginitis O86.13
  phlebitis O87.0
    deep O87.1
    pelvic O87.1
    superficial O87.0
  phlebothrombosis, deep O87.1
  phlegmasia alba dolens O87.1
  placental polyp O90.89
  pneumonia, embolic —*see* Embolism, obstetric, puerperal
  pre-eclampsia —*see* Pre-eclampsia
  psychosis F53
  pyelitis O86.21
  pyelocystitis O86.29
  pyelonephritis O86.21
  pyelonephrosis O86.21
  pyemia O85
  pyocystitis O86.29
  pyohemia O85
  pyometra O86.12
  pyonephritis O86.21
  pyosalpingitis O86.19
  pyrexia (of unknown origin) O86.4
  renal
    disease NEC O90.89
    failure O90.4
  respiratory disease NEC O99.53
  retention
    decidua —*see* Retention, decidua
    placenta O72.0
    secundines —*see* Retention, secundines
  retracted nipple O92.02
  salpingo-ovaritis O86.19
  salpingoperitonitis O85
  secondary perineal tear O90.1
  sepsis (pelvic) O85
  sepsis O85
  septic thrombophlebitis O86.81
  skin disorder NEC O99.73
  specified condition NEC O99.89
  stroke O99.43
  subinvolution (uterus) O90.89
  subluxation of symphysis (pubis) O26.73
  suppuration —*see* Puerperal, abscess
  tetanus A34

Puerperal, puerperium - *continued*
  thelitis O91.02
    associated with lactation O91.03
  thrombocytopenia O72.3
  thrombophlebitis (superficial) O87.0
    deep O87.1
    pelvic O87.1
    septic O86.81
  thrombosis (venous) —*see* Thrombosis, puerperal
  thyroiditis O90.5
  toxemia (eclamptic) (pre-eclamptic) (with convulsions) O15.2
  trauma, non-obstetric O9A.23
    caused by abuse (physical) (suspected) O9A.33
      confirmed O9A.33
      psychological (suspected) O9A.53
        confirmed O9A.53
      sexual (suspected) O9A.43
        confirmed O9A.43
  uremia (due to renal failure) O90.4
  urethritis O86.22
  vaginitis O86.13
  varicose veins (legs) O87.4
    vulva or perineum O87.8
  venous O87.9
  vulvitis O86.19
  vulvovaginitis O86.13
  white leg O87.1
Puerperium —*see* Puerperal
Pulmolithiasis J98.4
Pulmonary —*see* condition
Pulpitis (acute) (anachoretic) (chronic) (hyperplastic) (irreversible) (putrescent) (reversible) (suppurative) (ulcerative) K04.0
Pulpless tooth K04.99
Pulse
  alternating R00.8
  bigeminal R00.8
  fast R00.0
  feeble, rapid due to shock following injury T79.4
  rapid R00.0
  weak R09.89
Pulsus alternans or trigeminus R00.8
Punch drunk F07.81
Punctum lacrimale occlusion —*see* Obstruction, lacrimal
Puncture
  abdomen, abdominal
    wall S31.139
      with
        foreign body S31.149
        penetration into peritoneal cavity S31.639
          with foreign body S31.649
      epigastric region S31.132
        with
          foreign body S31.142
          penetration into peritoneal cavity S31.632
            with foreign body S31.642
      left
        lower quadrant S31.134
          with
            foreign body S31.144
            penetration into peritoneal cavity S31.634
              with foreign body S31.644
        upper quadrant S31.131
          with
            foreign body S31.141

Puncture - *continued*
        penetration into peritoneal cavity S31.631
          with foreign body S31.641
      periumbilic region S31.135
        with
          foreign body S31.145
          penetration into peritoneal cavity S31.635
            with foreign body S31.645
      right
        lower quadrant S31.133
          with
            foreign body S31.143
            penetration into peritoneal cavity S31.633
              with foreign body S31.643
        upper quadrant S31.130
          with
            foreign body S31.140
            penetration into peritoneal cavity S31.630
              with foreign body S31.640
  accidental, complicating surgery —*see* Complication, accidental puncture or laceration
  alveolar (process) —*see* Puncture, oral cavity
  ankle S91.039
    with
      foreign body S91.049
    left S91.032
      with
        foreign body S91.042
    right S91.031
      with
        foreign body S91.041
  anus S31.833
    with foreign body S31.834
  arm (upper) S41.139
    with foreign body S41.149
    left S41.132
      with foreign body S41.142
    lower —*see* Puncture, forearm
    right S41.131
      with foreign body S41.141
  auditory canal (external) (meatus) —*see* Puncture, ear
  auricle, ear —*see* Puncture, ear
  axilla —*see* Puncture, arm
  back —*see also* Puncture, thorax, back
    lower S31.030
      with
        foreign body S31.040
          with penetration into retroperitoneal space S31.041
        penetration into retroperitoneal space S31.031
  bladder (traumatic) S37.29
    nontraumatic N32.89
  breast S21.039
    with foreign body S21.049
    left S21.032
      with foreign body S21.042
    right S21.031
      with foreign body S21.041
  buttock S31.803
    with foreign body S31.804
    left S31.823
      with foreign body S31.824
    right S31.813
      with foreign body S31.814

Puncture - *continued*

by

  device, implant or graft —*see*
Complications, by site and type, mechanical

  foreign body left accidentally in operative
wound T81.539

  instrument (any) during a procedure,
accidental —*see* Puncture, accidental

complicating surgery

calf —*see* Puncture, leg

canaliculus lacrimalis —*see* Puncture, eyelid

canthus, eye —*see* Puncture, eyelid

cervical esophagus S11.23

  with foreign body S11.24

cheek (external) S01.439

  with foreign body S01.449

  left S01.432

    with foreign body S01.442

  right S01.431

    with foreign body S01.441

  internal —*see* Puncture, oral cavity

chest wall —*see* Puncture, thorax

chin —*see* Puncture, head, specified site NEC

clitoris —*see* Puncture, vulva

costal region —*see* Puncture, thorax

digit (s)

  hand —*see* Puncture, finger

  foot —*see* Puncture, toe

ear (canal) (external) S01.339

  with foreign body S01.349

  left S01.332

    with foreign body S01.342

  right S01.331

    with foreign body S01.341

  drum S09.2

elbow S51.039

  with

    foreign body S51.049

  left S51.032

    with

      foreign body S51.042

  right S51.031

    with

      foreign body S51.041

epididymis —*see* Puncture, testis

epigastric region —*see* Puncture, abdomen, wall, epigastric

epiglottis S11.83

  with foreign body S11.84

esophagus

  cervical S11.23

    with foreign body S11.24

  thoracic S27.818

eyeball S05.6

  with foreign body S05.5

eyebrow —*see* Puncture, eyelid

eyelid S01.13

  with foreign body S01.14

  left S01.132

    with foreign body S01.142

  right S01.131

    with foreign body S01.141

face NEC —*see* Puncture, head, specified site NEC

finger (s) S61.239

  with

    damage to nail S61.339

      with

        foreign body S61.349

    foreign body S61.249

  index S61.238

with

  damage to nail S61.338

    with

      foreign body S61.348

    foreign body S61.248

  left S61.231

    with

      damage to nail S61.331

        with

          foreign body S61.341

      foreign body S61.241

  right S61.230

    with

      damage to nail S61.330

        with

          foreign body S61.340

      foreign body S61.240

little S61.238

  with

    damage to nail S61.338

      with

        foreign body S61.348

    foreign body S61.248

  left S61.237

    with

      damage to nail S61.337

        with

          foreign body S61.347

      foreign body S61.247

  right S61.236

    with

      damage to nail S61.336

        with

          foreign body S61.346

      foreign body S61.246

middle S61.238

  with

    damage to nail S61.338

      with

        foreign body S61.348

    foreign body S61.248

  left S61.233

    with

      damage to nail S61.333

        with

          foreign body S61.343

      foreign body S61.243

  right S61.232

    with

      damage to nail S61.332

        with

          foreign body S61.342

      foreign body S61.242

ring S61.238

  with

    damage to nail S61.338

      with

        foreign body S61.348

    foreign body S61.248

  left S61.235

    with

      damage to nail S61.335

        with

          foreign body S61.345

      foreign body S61.245

  right S61.234

    with

      damage to nail S61.334

        with

          foreign body S61.344

      foreign body S61.244

flank S31.139

  with foreign body S31.149

foot (except toe(s) alone) S91.339

  with foreign body S91.349

  left S91.332

    with foreign body S91.342

  right S91.331

    with foreign body S91.341

  toe —*see* Puncture, toe

forearm S51.839

  with

    foreign body S51.849

  elbow only —*see* Puncture, elbow

  left S51.832

    with

      foreign body S51.842

  right S51.831

    with

      foreign body S51.841

forehead —*see* Puncture, head, specified site NEC

genital organs, external

  female S31.532

    with foreign body S31.542

    vagina —*see* Puncture, vagina

    vulva —*see* Puncture, vulva

  male S31.531

    with foreign body S31.541

    penis —*see* Puncture, penis

    scrotum —*see* Puncture, scrotum

    testis —*see* Puncture, testis

groin —*see* Puncture, abdomen, wall

gum —*see* Puncture, oral cavity

hand S61.439

  with

    foreign body S61.449

  finger —*see* Puncture, finger

  left S61.432

    with

      foreign body S61.442

  right S61.431

    with

      foreign body S61.441

  thumb —*see* Puncture, thumb

head S01.93

  with foreign body S01.94

  cheek —*see* Puncture, cheek

  ear —*see* Puncture, ear

  eyelid —*see* Puncture, eyelid

  lip —*see* Puncture, oral cavity

  nose —*see* Puncture, nose

  oral cavity —*see* Puncture, oral cavity

  scalp S01.03

    with foreign body S01.04

  specified site NEC S01.83

    with foreign body S01.84

  temporomandibular area —*see* Puncture, cheek

heart S26.99

  with hemopericardium S26.09

  without hemopericardium S26.19

heel —*see* Puncture, foot

hip S71.039

  with foreign body S71.049

  left S71.032

    with foreign body S71.042

  right S71.031

    with foreign body S71.041

hymen —*see* Puncture, vagina

hypochondrium —*see* Puncture, abdomen, wall

Puncture - *continued*

hypogastric region —*see* Puncture, abdomen, wall
inguinal region —*see* Puncture, abdomen, wall
instep —*see* Puncture, foot
internal organs —*see* Injury, by site
interscapular region —*see* Puncture, thorax, back
intestine
  large
    colon S36.599
      ascending S36.590
      descending S36.592
      sigmoid S36.593
      specified site NEC S36.598
      transverse S36.591
    rectum S36.69
  small S36.499
    duodenum S36.490
    specified site NEC S36.498
intra-abdominal organ S36.99
  gallbladder S36.128
  intestine —*see* Puncture, intestine
  liver S36.118
  pancreas —*see* Puncture, pancreas
  peritoneum S36.81
  specified site NEC S36.898
  spleen S36.09
  stomach S36.39
jaw —*see* Puncture, head, specified site NEC
knee S81.039
  with foreign body S81.049
  left S81.032
    with foreign body S81.042
  right S81.031
    with foreign body S81.041
labium (majus) (minus) —*see* Puncture, vulva
lacrimal duct —*see* Puncture, eyelid
larynx S11.013
  with foreign body S11.014
leg (lower) S81.839
  with foreign body S81.849
  foot —*see* Puncture, foot
  knee —*see* Puncture, knee
  left S81.832
    with foreign body S81.842
  right S81.831
    with foreign body S81.841
  upper —*see* Puncture, thigh
lip S01.531
  with foreign body S01.541
loin —*see* Puncture, abdomen, wall
lower back —*see* Puncture, back, lower
lumbar region —*see* Puncture, back, lower
malar region —*see* Puncture, head, specified site NEC
mammary —*see* Puncture, breast
mastoid region —*see* Puncture, head, specified site NEC
mouth —*see* Puncture, oral cavity
nail
  finger —*see* Puncture, finger, with damage to nail
  toe —*see* Puncture, toe, with damage to nail
nasal (septum) (sinus) —*see* Puncture, nose
nasopharynx —*see* Puncture, head, specified site NEC

Puncture - *continued*

neck S11.93
  with foreign body S11.94
  involving
    cervical esophagus —*see* Puncture, cervical esophagus
    larynx —*see* Puncture, larynx
    pharynx —*see* Puncture, pharynx
    thyroid gland —*see* Puncture, thyroid gland
    trachea —*see* Puncture, trachea
  specified site NEC S11.83
    with foreign body S11.84
nose (septum) (sinus) S01.23
  with foreign body S01.24
ocular —*see* Puncture, eyeball
oral cavity S01.532
  with foreign body S01.542
orbit S05.4
palate —*see* Puncture, oral cavity
palm —*see* Puncture, hand
pancreas S36.299
  body S36.291
  head S36.290
  tail S36.292
pelvis —*see* Puncture, back, lower
penis S31.23
  with foreign body S31.24
perineum
  female S31.43
    with foreign body S31.44
  male S31.139
    with foreign body S31.149
periocular area (with or without lacrimal passages) —*see* Puncture, eyelid
phalanges
  finger —*see* Puncture, finger
  toe —*see* Puncture, toe
pharynx S11.23
  with foreign body S11.24
pinna —*see* Puncture, ear
popliteal space —*see* Puncture, knee
prepuce —*see* Puncture, penis
pubic region S31.139
  with foreign body S31.149
pudendum —*see* Puncture, genital organs, external
rectovaginal septum —*see* Puncture, vagina
sacral region —*see* Puncture, back, lower
sacroiliac region —*see* Puncture, back, lower
salivary gland —*see* Puncture, oral cavity
scalp S01.03
  with foreign body S01.04
scapular region —*see* Puncture, shoulder
scrotum S31.33
  with foreign body S31.34
shin —*see* Puncture, leg
shoulder S41.039
  with foreign body S41.049
  left S41.032
    with foreign body S41.042
  right S41.031
    with foreign body S41.041
spermatic cord —*see* Puncture, testis
sternal region —*see* Puncture, thorax, front
submaxillary region —*see* Puncture, head, specified site NEC
submental region —*see* Puncture, head, specified site NEC
subungual
  finger (s) —*see* Puncture, finger, with damage to nail
  toe —*see* Puncture, toe, with damage to nail

Puncture - *continued*

supraclavicular fossa —*see* Puncture, neck, specified site NEC
temple, temporal region —*see* Puncture, head, specified site NEC
temporomandibular area —*see* Puncture, cheek
testis S31.33
  with foreign body S31.34
thigh S71.139
  with foreign body S71.149
  left S71.132
    with foreign body S71.142
  right S71.131
    with foreign body S71.141
thorax, thoracic (wall) S21.93
  with foreign body S21.94
  back S21.23
    with
      foreign body S21.24
        with penetration S21.44
      penetration S21.43
  breast —*see* Puncture, breast
  front S21.13
    with
      foreign body S21.14
        with penetration S21.34
      penetration S21.33
throat —*see* Puncture, neck
thumb S61.039
  with
    damage to nail S61.139
      with
        foreign body S61.149
    foreign body S61.049
  left S61.032
    with
      damage to nail S61.132
        with
          foreign body S61.142
      foreign body S61.042
  right S61.031
    with
      damage to nail S61.131
        with
          foreign body S61.141
      foreign body S61.041
thyroid gland S11.13
  with foreign body S11.14
toe (s) S91.139
  with
    damage to nail S91.239
      with
        foreign body S91.249
    foreign body S91.149
  great S91.133
    with
      damage to nail S91.233
        with
          foreign body S91.243
      foreign body S91.143
  left S91.132
    with
      damage to nail S91.232
        with
          foreign body S91.242
      foreign body S91.142
  right S91.131
    with
      damage to nail S91.231
        with
          foreign body S91.241
      foreign body S91.141

Puncture - *continued*
  lesser S91.136
    with
      damage to nail S91.236
        with
          foreign body S91.246
      foreign body S91.146
  left S91.135
    with
      damage to nail S91.235
        with
          foreign body S91.245
      foreign body S91.145
  right S91.134
    with
      damage to nail S91.234
        with
          foreign body S91.244
      foreign body S91.144
  tongue —*see* Puncture, oral cavity
  trachea S11.023
    with foreign body S11.024
  tunica vaginalis —*see* Puncture, testis
  tympanum, tympanic membrane S09.2
  umbilical region S31.135
    with foreign body S31.145
  uvula —*see* Puncture, oral cavity
  vagina S31.43
    with foreign body S31.44
  vocal cords S11.033
    with foreign body S11.034
  vulva S31.43
    with foreign body S31.44
  wrist S61.539
    with
      foreign body S61.549
    left S61.532
      with
        foreign body S61.542
    right S61.531
      with
        foreign body S61.541
PUO (pyrexia of unknown origin) R50.9
Pupillary membrane (persistent) Q13.89
Pupillotonia —*see* Anomaly, pupil, function, tonic pupil
Purpura D69.2
  abdominal D69.0
  allergic D69.0
  anaphylactoid D69.0
  annularis telangiectodes L81.7
  arthritic D69.0
  autoerythrocyte sensitization D69.2
  autoimmune D69.0
  bacterial D69.0
  Bateman's (senile) D69.2
  capillary fragility (hereditary) (idiopathic) D69.8
  cryoglobulinemic D89.1
  Devil's pinches D69.2
  fibrinolytic —*see* Fibrinolysis
  fulminans, fulminous D65
  gangrenous D65
  hemorrhagic, hemorrhagica D69.3
    not due to thrombocytopenia D69.0
  Henoch (-Schönlein) (allergic) D69.0
  hypergammaglobulinemic (benign) (Waldenström) D89.0
  idiopathic (thrombocytopenic) D69.3
    nonthrombocytopenic D69.0
  immune thrombocytopenic D69.3
  infectious D69.0

Purpura – *continued*
  malignant D69.0
  neonatorum P54.5
  nervosa D69.0
  newborn P54.5
  nonthrombocytopenic D69.2
    hemorrhagic D69.0
    idiopathic D69.0
  nonthrombopenic D69.2
  peliosis rheumatica D69.0
  posttransfusion (post-transfusion) (from (fresh) whole blood or blood products) D69.51
  primary D69.49
  red cell membrane sensitivity D69.2
  rheumatica D69.0
  Schönlein (-Henoch) (allergic) D69.0
  scorbutic E54 *[D77]*
  senile D69.2
  simplex D69.2
  symptomatica D69.0
  telangiectasia annularis L81.7
  thrombocytopenic D69.49
    congenital D69.42
    hemorrhagic D69.3
    hereditary D69.42
    idiopathic D69.3
    immune D69.3
    neonatal, transitory P61.0
    thrombotic M31.1
  thrombohemolytic —*see* Fibrinolysis
  thrombolytic —*see* Fibrinolysis
  thrombopenic D69.49
  thrombotic, thrombocytopenic M31.1
  toxic D69.0
  vascular D69.0
  visceral symptoms D69.0
Purpuric spots R23.3
Purulent —*see* condition
Pus
  in
    stool R19.5
    urine N39.0
  tube (rupture) —*see* Salpingo-oophoritis
Pustular rash L08.0
Pustule (nonmalignant) L08.9
  malignant A22.0
Pustulosis palmaris et plantaris L40.3
Putnam (-Dana) disease or syndrome — *see* Degeneration, combined
Putrescent pulp (dental) K04.1
Pyarthritis, pyarthrosis —*see* Arthritis, pyogenic or pyemic
  tuberculous —*see* Tuberculosis, joint
Pyelectasis —*see* Hydronephrosis
Pyelitis (congenital) (uremic) —*see also* Pyelonephritis
  with
    calculus —*see* category N20
      with hydronephrosis N13.2
    contracted kidney N11.9
  acute N10
  chronic N11.9
    with calculus —*see* category N20
      with hydronephrosis N13.2
  cystica N28.84
  puerperal (postpartum) O86.21
  tuberculous A18.11
Pyelocystitis —*see* Pyelonephritis

Pyelonephritis —*see also* Nephritis, tubulo-interstitial
  with
    calculus —*see* category N20
      with hydronephrosis N13.2
    contracted kidney N11.9
  acute N10
  calculous —*see* category N20
    with hydronephrosis N13.2
  chronic N11.9
    with calculus —*see* category N20
      with hydronephrosis N13.2
  associated with ureteral obstruction or stricture N11.1
    nonobstructive N11.8
      with reflux (vesicoureteral) N11.0
    obstructive N11.1
    specified NEC N11.8
  in (due to)
    brucellosis A23.9 *[N16]*
    cryoglobulinemia (mixed) D89.1 *[N16]*
    cystinosis E72.04
    diphtheria A36.84
    glycogen storage disease E74.09 *[N16]*
    leukemia NEC C95.9 *[N16]*
    lymphoma NEC C85.90 *[N16]*
    multiple myeloma C90.0 *[N16]*
    obstruction N11.1
    Salmonella infection A02.25
    sarcoidosis D86.84
    sepsis A41.9 *[N16]*
    Sjögren's disease M35.04
    toxoplasmosis B58.83
    transplant rejection T86.91 *[N16]*
    Wilson's disease E83.01 *[N16]*
  nonobstructive N12
    with reflux (vesicoureteral) N11.0
    chronic N11.8
  syphilitic A52.75
Pyelonephrosis (obstructive) N11.1
  chronic N11.9
Pyelophlebitis I80.8
Pyeloureteritis cystica N28.85
Pyemia, pyemic (fever) (infection) (purulent) —*see also* Sepsis
  joint —*see* Arthritis, pyogenic or pyemic
  liver K75.1
  pneumococcal A40.3
  portal K75.1
  postvaccinal T88.0
  puerperal, postpartum, childbirth O85
  specified organism NEC A41.89
  tuberculous —*see* Tuberculosis, miliary
Pygopagus Q89.4
Pyknoepilepsy (idiopathic) —*see* Pyknolepsy
Pyknolepsy G40.A09
  intractable G40.A19
    with status epilepticus G40.A11
    without status epilepticus G40.A19
  not intractable G40.A09
    with status epilepticus G40.A01
    without status epilepticus G40.A09
Pylephlebitis K75.1
Pyle's syndrome Q78.5
Pylethrombophlebitis K75.1
Pylethrombosis K75.1
Pyloritis K29.90
  with bleeding K29.91
Pylorospasm (reflex) **NEC** K31.3
  congenital or infantile Q40.0
  newborn Q40.0
  neurotic F45.8
  psychogenic F45.8

Pylorus, pyloric —see condition
Pyoarthrosis —see Arthritis, pyogenic or pyemic
Pyocele
mastoid —see Mastoiditis, acute
sinus (accessory) —see Sinusitis
turbinate (bone) J32.9
urethra (see also Urethritis) N34.0
Pyocolpos —see Vaginitis
Pyocystitis N30.80
with hematuria N30.81
Pyoderma, pyodermia L08.0
gangrenosum L88
newborn P39.4
phagedenic L88
vegetans L08.81
Pyodermatitis L08.0
vegetans L08.81
Pyogenic —see condition
Pyohydronephrosis N13.6
Pyometra, pyometrium, pyometritis —see Endometritis
Pyomyositis (tropical) —see Myositis, infective
Pyonephritis N12
Pyonephrosis N13.6
tuberculous A18.11
Pyo-oophoritis —see Salpingo-oophoritis
Pyo-ovarium —see Salpingo-oophoritis
Pyopericarditis, pyopericardium I30.1
Pyophlebitis —see Phlebitis
Pyopneumopericardium I30.1
Pyopneumothorax (infective) J86.9
with fistula J86.0
tuberculous NEC A15.6
Pyosalpinx, pyosalpingitis —see also Salpingo-oophoritis
Pyothorax J86.9
with fistula J86.0
tuberculous NEC A15.6
Pyoureter N28.89
tuberculous A18.11
Pyramidopallidonigral syndrome G20
Pyrexia (of unknown origin) R50.9
atmospheric T67.0
during labor NEC O75.2
heat T67.0
newborn P81.9
environmentally-induced P81.0
persistent R50.9
puerperal O86.4
Pyroglobulinemia NEC E88.09
Pyromania F63.1
Pyrosis R12
Pyuria (bacterial) N39.0

Q

Q fever A78
with pneumonia A78
Quadricuspid aortic valve Q23.8
Quadrilateral fever A78
Quadriparesis —see Quadriplegia
meaning muscle weakness M62.81
Quadriplegia G82.50
complete
C1-C4 level G82.51
C5-C7 level G82.53
congenital (cerebral) (spinal) G80.8
spastic G80.0
embolic (current episode) I63.4
functional R53.2

Quadriplegia – continued
incomplete
C1-C4 level G82.52
C5-C7 level G82.54
thrombotic (current episode) I63.3
traumatic
code to injury with seventh character S
current episode —see Injury, spinal (cord) , cervical
Quadruplet, pregnancy —see Pregnancy, quadruplet
Quarrelsomeness F60.3
Queensland fever A77.3
Quervain's disease M65.4
thyroid E06.1
Queyrat's erythroplasia D07.4
penis D07.4
specified site —see Neoplasm, skin, in situ
unspecified site D07.4
Quincke's disease or edema T78.3
hereditary D84.1
Quinsy (gangrenous) J36
Quintan fever A79.0
Quintuplet, pregnancy —see Pregnancy, quintuplet

R

Rabbit fever —see Tularemia
Rabies A82.9
contact Z20.3
exposure to Z20.3
inoculation reaction —see Complications, vaccination
sylvatic A82.0
urban A82.1
Rachischisis —see Spina bifida
Rachitic —see also condition
deformities of spine (late effect) (sequelae) E64.3
pelvis (late effect) (sequelae) E64.3
with disproportion (fetopelvic) O33.0
causing obstructed labor O65.0
Rachitis, rachitism (acute) (tarda) —see also Rickets
renalis N25.0
sequelae E64.3
Radial nerve —see condition
Radiation
burn —see Burn
effects NOS T66
sickness NOS T66
therapy, encounter for Z51.0
Radiculitis (pressure) (vertebrogenic) —see Radiculopathy
Radiculomyelitis —see also Encephalitis
toxic, due to
Clostridium tetani A35
Corynebacterium diphtheriae A36.82
Radiculopathy M54.10
cervical region M54.12
cervicothoracic region M54.13
due to
disc disorder
C3 M50.11
C4 M50.11
C5 M50.12
C6 M50.12
C7 M50.12
C8 M50.13
displacement of intervertebral disc —see Disorder, disc, with, radiculopathy
leg M54.1

Radiculopathy - continued
lumbar region M54.16
lumbosacral region M54.17
occipito-atlanto-axial region M54.11
postherpetic B02.29
sacrococcygeal region M54.18
syphilitic A52.11
thoracic region (with visceral pain) M54.14
thoracolumbar region M54.15
Radiodermal burns (acute, chronic, or occupational) —see Burn
Radiodermatitis L58.9
acute L58.0
chronic L58.1
Radiotherapy session Z51.0
Rage, meaning rabies —see Rabies
Ragpicker's disease A22.1
Ragsorter's disease A22.1
Raillietiniasis B71.8
Railroad neurosis F48.8
Railway spine F48.8
Raised —see also Elevated
antibody titer R76.0
Rake teeth, tooth M26.39
Rales R09.89
Ramifying renal pelvis Q63.8
Ramsay-Hunt disease or syndrome (see also Hunt's disease) B02.21
meaning dyssynergia cerebellaris myoclonica G11.1
Ranula K11.6
congenital Q38.4
Rape
adult
confirmed T74.21
suspected T76.21
alleged, observation or examination, ruled out
adult Z04.41
child Z04.42
child
confirmed T74.22
suspected T76.22
Rapid
feeble pulse, due to shock, following injury T79.4
heart (beat) R00.0
psychogenic F45.8
second stage (delivery) O62.3
time-zone change syndrome —see Disorder, sleep, circadian rhythm, psychogenic
Rarefaction, bone —see Disorder, bone, density and structure, specified NEC
Rash (toxic) R21
canker A38.9
diaper L22
drug (internal use) L27.0
contact (see also Dermatitis, due to, drugs, external) L25.1
following immunization T88.1
food —see Dermatitis, due to, food
heat L74.0
napkin (psoriasiform) L22
nettle —see Urticaria
pustular L08.0
rose R21
epidemic B06.9
scarlet A38.9
serum (see also Reaction, serum) T80.69
wandering tongue K14.1
Rasmussen aneurysm —see Tuberculosis, pulmonary
Rasmussen encephalitis G04.81

Rat-bite fever A25.9
  due to Streptobacillus moniliformis A25.1
  spirochetal (morsus muris) A25.0
Rathke's pouch tumor D44.3
Raymond (-Céstan) **syndrome** I65.8
Raynaud's disease, phenomenon or
syndrome (secondary) I73.00
  with gangrene (symmetric) I73.01
RDS (newborn) (type I) P22.0
  type II P22.1
Reaction —see also Disorder
  adaptation —see Disorder, adjustment
  adjustment (anxiety) (conduct disorder)
  (depressiveness) (distress) —see Disorder,
  adjustment
    with
      mutism, elective (child) (adolescent) F94.0
  adverse
    food (any) (ingested) NEC T78.1
      anaphylactic —see Shock, anaphylactic,
  due to food
  affective —see Disorder, mood
  allergic —see Allergy
  anaphylactic —see Shock, anaphylactic
  anaphylactoid —see Shock, anaphylactic
  anesthesia —see Anesthesia, complication
  antitoxin (prophylactic) (therapeutic) —see
  Complications, vaccination
  anxiety F41.1
  Arthus —see Arthus' phenomenon
  asthenic F48.8
  combat and operational stress F43.0
  compulsive F42
  conversion F44.9
  crisis, acute F43.0
  deoxyribonuclease (DNA) (DNase)
  hypersensitivity D69.2
  depressive (single episode) F32.9
    affective (single episode) F31.4
      recurrent episode F33.9
    neurotic F34.1
    psychoneurotic F34.1
    psychotic F32.3
    recurrent —see Disorder, depressive,
    recurrent
  dissociative F44.9
  drug NEC T88.7
    addictive —see Dependence, drug
      transmitted via placenta or breast milk —
    see Absorption, drug, addictive, through
    placenta
    allergic —see Allergy, drug
    lichenoid L43.2
    newborn P93.8
      gray baby syndrome P93.0
    overdose or poisoning (by accident) —see
    Table of Drugs and Chemicals, by drug,
    poisoning
      photoallergic L56.1
      phototoxic L56.0
    withdrawal —see Dependence, by drug,
    with, withdrawal
      infant of dependent mother P96.1
      newborn P96.1
    wrong substance given or taken (by
    accident) —see Table of Drugs and
    Chemicals, by drug, poisoning
  fear F40.9
    child (abnormal) F93.8
  febrile nonhemolytic transfusion (FNHTR)
  R50.84
  fluid loss, cerebrospinal G97.1

Reaction - continued
  foreign
    body NEC —see Granuloma, foreign body
      in operative wound (inadvertently left) —
    see Foreign body, accidentally left during a
    procedure
      substance accidentally left during a
    procedure (chemical) (powder) (talc) T81.60
      aseptic peritonitis T81.61
      body or object (instrument) (sponge)
      (swab) —see Foreign body, accidentally
      left during a procedure
      specified reaction NEC T81.69
  grief —see Disorder, adjustment
  Herxheimer's R68.89
  hyperkinetic —see Hyperkinesia
  hypochondriacal F45.20
  hypoglycemic, due to insulin E16.0
    with coma (diabetic) —see Diabetes, coma
    nondiabetic E15
    therapeutic misadventure —see subcategory
    T38.3
  hypomanic F30.8
  hysterical F44.9
  immunization —see Complications,
  vaccination
  incompatibility
    ABO blood group (infusion) (transfusion) —
    see Complication(s), transfusion,
    incompatibility reaction, ABO
      delayed serologic T80.39
      minor blood group (Duffy) (E) (K(ell))
    (Kidd) (Lewis) (M) (N) (P) (S) T80.89
      Rh (factor) (infusion) (transfusion) —see
    Complication(s), transfusion, incompatibility
    reaction, Rh (factor)
  inflammatory —see Infection
  infusion —see Complications, infusion
  inoculation (immune serum) —see
  Complications, vaccination
  insulin T38.3
  involutional psychotic —see Disorder,
  depressive
  leukemoid D72.823
    basophilic D72.823
    lymphocytic D72.823
    monocytic D72.823
    myelocytic D72.823
    neutrophilic D72.823
  LSD (acute)
    due to drug abuse —see Abuse, drug,
    hallucinogen
    due to drug dependence —see Dependence,
    drug, hallucinogen
  lumbar puncture G97.1
  manic-depressive —see Disorder, bipolar
  neurasthenic F48.8
  neurogenic —see Neurosis
  neurotic F48.9
  neurotic-depressive F34.1
  nitritoid —see Crisis, nitritoid
  nonspecific
    to
      cell mediated immunity measurement of
    gamma interferon antigen response without
    active tuberculosis R76.12
      QuantiFERON-TB test (QFT) without
    active tuberculosis R76.12
      tuberculin test (see also Reaction,
    tuberculin skin test) R76.11
  obsessive-compulsive F42
  organic, acute or subacute —see Delirium

Reaction - continued
  paranoid (acute) F23
    chronic F22
    senile F03
  passive dependency F60.7
  phobic F40.9
  post-traumatic stress, uncomplicated Z73.3
  psychogenic F99
  psychoneurotic —see also Neurosis
    compulsive F42
    depersonalization F48.1
    depressive F34.1
    hypochondriacal F45.20
    neurasthenic F48.8
    obsessive F42
  psychophysiologic —see Disorder,
  somatoform
  psychosomatic —see Disorder, somatoform
  psychotic —see Psychosis
  scarlet fever toxin —see Complications,
  vaccination
  schizophrenic F23
    acute (brief) (undifferentiated) F23
    latent F21
    undifferentiated (acute) (brief) F23
  serological for syphilis —see Serology for
  syphilis
  serum T80.69
    anaphylactic (immediate) (see also Shock,
  anaphylactic) T80.59
    specified reaction NEC
      due to
        administration of blood and blood
  products T80.61
        immunization T80.62
        serum specified NEC T80.69
        vaccination T80.62
  situational —see Disorder, adjustment
  somatization —see Disorder, somatoform
  spinal puncture G97.1
  stress (severe) F43.9
    acute (agitation) ("daze") (disorientation)
  (disturbance of consciousness) (flight
  reaction) (fugue) F43.0
    specified NEC F43.8
  surgical procedure —see Complications,
  surgical procedure
  tetanus antitoxin —see Complications,
  vaccination
  toxic, to local anesthesia T81.89
    in labor and delivery O74.4
    in pregnancy O29.3X
    postpartum, puerperal O89.3
  toxin-antitoxin —see Complications,
  vaccination
  transfusion (blood) (bone marrow)
  (lymphocytes) (allergic) —see Complications,
  transfusion
  tuberculin skin test, abnormal R76.11
  vaccination (any) —see Complications,
  vaccination
  withdrawing, child or adolescent F93.8
Reactive airway disease —see Asthma
Reactive depression —see Reaction,
  depressive
Rearrangement
  chromosomal
    balanced (in) Q95.9
      abnormal individual (autosomal) Q95.2
      non-sex (autosomal) chromosomes Q95.2
      sex/non-sex chromosomes Q95.3
    specified NEC Q95.8

Recalcitrant patient —*see* Noncompliance
Recanalization, thrombus —*see* Thrombosis
Recession, receding
  chamber angle (eye) H21.55
  chin M26.09
  gingival (generalized) (localized)
    (postinfective) (postoperative) K06.0
Recklinghausen disease Q85.01
  bones E21.0
Reclus' disease (cystic) —*see* Mastopathy,
  cystic
Recrudescent typhus (fever) A75.1
Recruitment, auditory H93.21
Rectalgia K62.89
Rectitis K62.89
Rectocele
  female (without uterine prolapse) N81.6
    with uterine prolapse N81.4
      incomplete N81.2
  in pregnancy —*see* Pregnancy, complicated
  by, abnormal, pelvic organs or tissues NEC
  male K62.3
Rectosigmoid junction —*see* condition
Rectosigmoiditis K63.89
  ulcerative (chronic) K51.30
    with
      complication K51.319
        abscess K51.314
        fistula K51.313
        obstruction K51.312
        rectal bleeding K51.311
        specified NEC K51.318
Rectourethral —*see* condition
Rectovaginal —*see* condition
Rectovesical —*see* condition
Rectum, rectal —*see* condition
Recurrent —*see* condition
  pregnancy loss —*see* Loss (of) , pregnancy,
  recurrent
Red bugs B88.0
Red-cedar lung or pneumonitis J67.8
Red tide (*see also* Table of Drugs and
  Chemicals) T65.82
Reduced
  mobility Z74.09
  ventilatory or vital capacity R94.2
Redundant, redundancy
  anus (congenital) Q43.8
  clitoris N90.89
  colon (congenital) Q43.8
  foreskin (congenital) N47.8
  intestine (congenital) Q43.8
  labia N90.6
  organ or site, congenital NEC —*see*
  Accessory
  panniculus (abdominal) E65
  prepuce (congenital) N47.8
  pylorus K31.89
  rectum (congenital) Q43.8
  scrotum N50.8
  sigmoid (congenital) Q43.8
  skin (of face) L57.4
    eyelids —*see* Blepharochalasis
  stomach K31.89
Reduplication —*see* Duplication
Reflex R29.2
  hyperactive gag J39.2
  pupillary, abnormal —*see* Anomaly, pupil,
  function
  vasoconstriction I73.9
  vasovagal R55

Reflux K21.9
  acid K21.9
  esophageal K21.9
    with esophagitis K21.0
    newborn P78.83
  gastroesophageal K21.9
    with esophagitis K21.0
  mitral —*see* Insufficiency, mitral
  ureteral —*see* Reflux, vesicoureteral
  vesicoureteral (with scarring) N13.70
    with
      nephropathy N13.729
        with hydroureter N13.739
          bilateral N13.732
          unilateral N13.731
        bilateral N13.722
        unilateral N13.721
        without hydroureter N13.729
          bilateral N13.722
          unilateral N13.721
      pyelonephritis (chronic) N11.0
    congenital Q62.7
    without nephropathy N13.71
Reforming, artificial openings —*see*
  Attention to, artificial, opening
Refractive error —*see* Disorder, refraction
Refsum's disease or syndrome G60.1
Refusal of
  food, psychogenic F50.8
  treatment (because of) Z53.20
    left against medical advice (AMA) Z53.21
    patient's decision NEC Z53.29
    reasons of belief or group pressure Z53.1
Regional —*see* condition
Regurgitation R11.10
  aortic (valve) —*see* Insufficiency, aortic
  food —*see also* Vomiting
    with reswallowing —*see* Rumination
    newborn P92.1
  gastric contents —*see* Vomiting
  heart —*see* Endocarditis
  mitral (valve) —*see* Insufficiency, mitral
    congenital Q23.3
  myocardial —*see* Endocarditis
  pulmonary (valve) (heart) I37.1
    congenital Q22.2
    syphilitic A52.03
  tricuspid —*see* Insufficiency, tricuspid
  valve, valvular —*see* Endocarditis
    congenital Q24.8
  vesicoureteral —*see* Reflux, vesicoureteral
Reifenstein syndrome E34.52
Reinsertion, contraceptive device Z30.433
Reiter's disease, syndrome, or urethritis
  M02.30
  ankle M02.37
  elbow M02.32
  foot joint M02.37
  hand joint M02.34
  hip M02.35
  knee M02.36
  multiple site M02.39
  shoulder M02.31
  vertebra M02.38
  wrist M02.33
Reichmann's disease or syndrome K31.89
Rejection
  food, psychogenic F50.8
  transplant T86.91
    bone T86.830
      marrow T86.01
    cornea T86.840

Rejection - *continued*
  heart T86.21
    with lung (s) T86.31
  intestine T86.850
  kidney T86.11
  liver T86.41
  lung (s) T86.810
    with heart T86.31
  organ (immune or nonimmune cause)
  T86.91
  pancreas T86.890
  skin (allograft) (autograft) T86.820
  specified NEC T86.890
  stem cell (peripheral blood) (umbilical cord)
  T86.5
Relapsing fever A68.9
  Carter's (Asiatic) A68.1
  Dutton's (West African) A68.1
  Koch's A68.9
  louse-borne (epidemic) A68.0
  Novy's (American) A68.1
  Obermeyers's (European) A68.0
  Spirillum A68.9
  tick-borne (endemic) A68.1
Relationship
  occlusal
    open anterior M26.220
    open posterior M26.221
Relaxation
  anus (sphincter) K62.89
    psychogenic F45.8
  arch (foot) —*see also* Deformity, limb, flat
  foot
  back ligaments —*see* Instability, joint, spine
  bladder (sphincter) N31.2
  cardioesophageal K21.9
  cervix —*see* Incompetency, cervix
  diaphragm J98.6
  joint (capsule) (ligament) (paralytic) —*see*
  Flail, joint
    congenital NEC Q74.8
  lumbosacral (joint) —*see* subcategory M53.2
  pelvic floor N81.89
  perineum N81.89
  posture R29.3
  rectum (sphincter) K62.89
  sacroiliac (joint) —*see* subcategory M53.2
  scrotum N50.8
  urethra (sphincter) N36.44
  vesical N31.2
Release from prison, anxiety concerning
  Z65.2
Remains
  canal of Cloquet Q14.0
  capsule (opaque) Q14.8
Remittent fever (malarial) B54
Remnant
  canal of Cloquet Q14.0
  capsule (opaque) Q14.8
  cervix, cervical stump (acquired)
  (postoperative) N88.8
  cystic duct, postcholecystectomy K91.5
  fingernail L60.8
    congenital Q84.6
  meniscus, knee —*see* Derangement, knee,
  meniscus, specified NEC
  thyroglossal duct Q89.2
  tonsil J35.8
    infected (chronic) J35.01
  urachus Q64.4

Removal (from) (of)
artificial
  arm Z44.00
    complete Z44.01
    partial Z44.02
  eye Z44.2
  leg Z44.10
    complete Z44.11
    partial Z44.12
breast implant Z45.81
cardiac pulse generator (battery) (end-of-life) Z45.010
catheter (urinary) (indwelling) Z46.6
  from artificial opening —*see* Attention to, artificial, opening
  non-vascular Z46.82
  vascular NEC Z45.2
drains Z48.03
device Z46.9
  contraceptive Z30.432
  implanted NEC Z45.89
  specified NEC Z46.89
dressing (nonsurgical) Z48.00
  surgical Z48.01
external
  fixation device
code to fracture with seventh character D
prosthesis, prosthetic device Z44.9
  breast Z44.3
  specified NEC Z44.8
home in childhood (to foster home or institution) Z62.29
ileostomy Z43.2
insulin pump Z46.81
myringotomy device (stent) (tube) Z45.82
nervous system device NEC Z46.2
  brain neuropacemaker Z46.2
  visual substitution device Z46.2
    implanted Z45.31
non-vascular catheter Z46.82
orthodontic device Z46.4
organ, prophylactic (for neoplasia management) —*see* Prophylactic, organ removal
staples Z48.02
stent
  ureteral Z46.6
suture Z48.02
urinary device Z46.6
vascular access device or catheter Z45.2

Ren
arcuatus Q63.1
mobile, mobilis N28.89
  congenital Q63.8
unguliformis Q63.1

Renal —*see* condition

Rendu-Osler-Weber disease or syndrome I78.0

Reninoma D41.0

Renon-Delille syndrome E23.3

Reovirus, as cause of disease classified elsewhere B97.5

Repeated falls NEC R29.6

Replaced chromosome by dicentric ring Q93.2

Replacement by artificial or mechanical device or prosthesis of
bladder Z96.0
blood vessel NEC Z95.828
bone NEC Z96.7
cochlea Z96.21
coronary artery Z95.5

Replacement – *continued*
eustachian tube Z96.29
eye globe Z97.0
heart Z95.812
  valve Z95.2
    prosthetic Z95.2
    specified NEC Z95.4
    xenogenic Z95.3
intestine Z96.89
joint Z96.60
  hip —*see* Presence, hip joint implant
  knee —*see* Presence, knee joint implant
  specified site NEC Z96.698
larynx Z96.3
lens Z96.1
limb (s) —*see* Presence, artificial, limb
mandible NEC (for tooth root implant(s)) Z96.5
organ NEC Z96.89
peripheral vessel NEC Z95.828
stapes Z96.29
teeth Z97.2
tendon Z96.7
tissue NEC Z96.89
tooth root (s) Z96.5
vessel NEC Z95.828
  coronary (artery) Z95.5

Request for expert evidence Z04.8

Reserve, decreased or low
cardiac —*see* Disease, heart
kidney N28.89

Residual —*see also* condition
ovary syndrome N99.83
state, schizophrenic F20.5
urine R39.19

Resistance, resistant (to)
activated protein C D68.51
complicating pregnancy O26.89
insulin E88.81
organism (s)
  to
    drug
      aminoglycosides Z16.29
      amoxicillin Z16.11
      ampicillin Z16.11
      antibiotic (s) Z16.20
        multiple Z16.24
        specified NEC Z16.29
      antifungal Z16.32
      antimicrobial (single) Z16.30
        multiple Z16.35
        specified NEC Z16.39
      antimycbacterial (single) Z16.341
        multiple Z16.342
      antiparasitic Z16.31
      antiviral Z16.33
      beta lactam antibiotics Z16.10
        specified NEC Z16.19
      cephalosporins Z16.19
      extended beta lactamase (ESBL) Z16.12
      fluoroquinolones Z16.23
      macrolides Z16.29
      methicillin —*see* MRSA
      multiple drugs (MDRO)
        antibiotics Z16.24
      penicillins Z16.11
      quinine (and related compounds) Z16.31
      quinolones Z16.23
      sulfonamides Z16.29
      tetracyclines Z16.29
      tuberculostatics (single) Z16.341
        multiple Z16.342

Resistance, resistant - *continued*
      vancomycin Z16.21
        related antibiotics Z16.22
thyroid hormone E07.89

Resorption
dental (roots) K03.3
  alveoli M26.79
teeth (external) (internal) (pathological) (roots) K03.3

Respiration
Cheyne-Stokes R06.3
decreased due to shock, following injury T79.4
disorder of, psychogenic F45.8
insufficient, or poor R06.89
  newborn P28.5
painful R07.1
sighing, psychogenic F45.8

Respiratory —*see also* condition
distress syndrome (newborn) (type I) P22.0
  type II P22.1
syncytial virus, as cause of disease classified elsewhere B97.4

Respite care Z75.5

Response (drug)
photoallergic L56.1
phototoxic L56.0

Restless legs (syndrome) G25.81

Restlessness R45.1

Restriction of housing space Z59.1

Restoration (of)
dental
  aesthetically inadequate or displeasing K08.56
  defective K08.50
    specified NEC K08.59
  failure of marginal integrity K08.51
  failure of periodontal anatomical integrity K08.54
organ continuity from previous sterilization (tuboplasty) (vasoplasty) Z31.0
  aftercare Z31.42
tooth (existing)
  contours biologically incompatible with oral health K08.54
  open margins K08.51
  overhanging K08.52
  poor aesthetic K08.56
  poor gingival margins K08.51
unsatisfactory, of tooth K08.50
  specified NEC K08.59

Restorative material (dental)
allergy to K08.55
fractured K08.539
  with loss of material K08.531
  without loss of material K08.530
unrepairable overhanging of K08.52

Rests, ovarian, in fallopian tube Q50.6

Restzustand (schizophrenic) F20.5

Retained —*see also* Retention
cholelithiasis following cholecystectomy K91.86
foreign body fragments (type of) Z18.9
  acrylics Z18.2
  animal quill (s) or spines Z18.31
  cement Z18.83
  concrete Z18.83
  crystalline Z18.83
  depleted isotope Z18.09
  depleted uranium Z18.01
  diethylhexylphthalates Z18.2
  glass Z18.81
  isocyanate Z18.2

Retained - *continued*
  magnetic metal Z18.11
  metal Z18.10
  nonmagnetic metal Z18.12
  nontherapeutic radioactive Z18.09
  organic NEC Z18.39
  plastic Z18.2
  quill (s) (animal) Z18.31
  radioactive (nontherapeutic) NEC Z18.09
  specified NEC Z18.89
  spine (s) (animal) Z18.31
  stone Z18.83
  tooth (teeth) Z18.32
  wood Z18.33
 fragments (type of) Z18.9
  acrylics Z18.2
  animal quill (s) or spines Z18.31
  cement Z18.83
  concrete Z18.83
  crystalline Z18.83
  depleted isotope Z18.09
  depleted uranium Z18.01
  diethylhexylphthalates Z18.2
  glass Z18.81
  isocyanate Z18.2
  magnetic metal Z18.11
  metal Z18.10
  nonmagnetic metal Z18.12
  nontherapeutic radioactive Z18.09
  organic NEC Z18.39
  plastic Z18.2
  quill (s) (animal) Z18.31
  radioactive (nontherapeutic) NEC Z18.09
  specified NEC Z18.89
  spine (s) (animal) Z18.31
  stone Z18.83
  tooth (teeth) Z18.32
  wood Z18.33
 gallstones, following cholecystectomy K91.86
Retardation
  development, developmental, specific —*see* Disorder, developmental
  endochondral bone growth —*see* Disorder, bone, development or growth
  growth R62.50
    due to malnutrition E45
  mental —*see* Disability, intellectual
  motor function, specific F82
  physical (child) R62.52
    due to malnutrition E45
  reading (specific) F81.0
  spelling (specific) (without reading disorder) F81.81
Retching —*see* Vomiting
Retention —*see also* Retained
  bladder —*see* Retention, urine
  carbon dioxide E87.2
  cholelithiasis following cholecystectomy K91.86
  cyst —*see* Cyst
  dead
    fetus (at or near term) (mother) O36.4
      early fetal death O02.1
    ovum O02.0
  decidua (fragments) (following delivery) (with hemorrhage) O72.2
    without hemorrhage O73.1
  deciduous tooth K00.6
  dental root K08.3
  fecal —*see* Constipation
  fetus
    dead O36.4
      early O02.1

Retention - *continued*
  fluid R60.9
  foreign body —*see also* Foreign body, retained
    current trauma
  code as Foreign body, by site or type
  gallstones, following cholecystectomy K91.86
  gastric K31.89
  intrauterine contraceptive device, in pregnancy —*see* Pregnancy, complicated by, retention, intrauterine device
  membranes (complicating delivery) (with hemorrhage) O72.2
    with abortion —*see* Abortion, by type
    without hemorrhage O73.1
  meniscus —*see* Derangement, meniscus
  menses N94.89
  milk (puerperal, postpartum) O92.79
  nitrogen, extrarenal R39.2
  ovary syndrome N99.83
  placenta (total) (with hemorrhage) O72.0
    without hemorrhage O73.0
    portions or fragments (with hemorrhage) O72.2
      without hemorrhage O73.1
  products of conception
    early pregnancy (dead fetus) O02.1
    following
      delivery (with hemorrhage) O72.2
        without hemorrhage O73.1
  secundines (following delivery) (with hemorrhage) O72.0
    without hemorrhage O73.0
    complicating puerperium (delayed hemorrhage) O72.2
    partial O72.2
      without hemorrhage O73.1
  smegma, clitoris N90.89
  urine R33.9
    due to hyperplasia (hypertrophy) of prostate —*see* Hyperplasia, prostate
    drug-induced R33.0
    organic R33.8
      drug-induced R33.0
    psychogenic F45.8
    specified NEC R33.8
  water (in tissues) —*see* Edema
Reticular erythematous mucinosis L98.5
Reticulation, dust —*see* Pneumoconiosis
Reticulocytosis R70.1
Reticuloendotheliosis
  acute infantile C96.0
  leukemic C91.4
  malignant C96.9
  nonlipid C96.0
Reticulohistiocytoma (giant-cell) D76.3
Reticuloid, actinic L57.1
Reticulosis (skin)
  acute of infancy C96.0
  hemophagocytic, familial D76.1
  histiocytic medullary C96.9
  lipomelanotic I89.8
  malignant (midline) C86.0
  nonlipid C96.0
  polymorphic C86.0
  Sézary —*see* Sézary disease
Retina, retinal —*see also* condition
  dark area D49.81
Retinitis —*see also* Inflammation, chorioretinal
  albuminurica N18.9 *[H32]*
  diabetic —*see* Diabetes, retinitis

Retinitis - *continued*
  disciformis —*see* Degeneration, macula
  focal —*see* Inflammation, chorioretinal, focal
  gravidarum —*see* Pregnancy, complicated by, specified pregnancy-related condition NEC
  juxtapapillaris —*see* Inflammation, chorioretinal, focal, juxtapapillary
  luetic —*see* Retinitis, syphilitic
  pigmentosa H35.52
  proliferans —*see* Disorder, globe, degenerative, specified type NEC
  proliferating —*see* Disorder, globe, degenerative, specified type NEC
  renal N18.9 *[H32]*
  syphilitic (early) (secondary) A51.43
    central, recurrent A52.71
    congenital (early) A50.01 *[H32]*
    late A52.71
  tuberculous A18.53
Retinoblastoma C69.2
  differentiated C69.2
  undifferentiated C69.2
Retinochoroiditis —*see also* Inflammation, chorioretinal
  disseminated —*see* Inflammation, chorioretinal, disseminated
    syphilitic A52.71
  focal —*see* Inflammation, chorioretinal
  juxtapapillaris —*see* Inflammation, chorioretinal, focal, juxtapapillary
Retinopathy (background) H35.00
  arteriosclerotic I70.8 *[H35.0]*
  atherosclerotic I70.8 *[H35.0]*
  central serous —*see* Chorioretinopathy, central serous
  Coats H35.02
  diabetic —*see* Diabetes, retinopathy
  exudative H35.02
  hypertensive H35.03
  in (due to)
    diabetes —*see* Diabetes, retinopathy
    sickle-cell disorders D57. *[H36]*
  of prematurity H35.10
    stage 0 H35.11
    stage 1 H35.12
    stage 2 H35.13
    stage 3 H35.14
    stage 4 H35.15
    stage 5 H35.16
  pigmentary, congenital —*see* Dystrophy, retina
  proliferative NEC H35.2
    diabetic —*see* Diabetes, retinopathy, proliferative
    sickle-cell D57. *[H36]*
  solar H31.02
Retinoschisis H33.10
  congenital Q14.1
  specified type NEC H33.19
Retortamoniasis A07.8
Retractile testis Q55.22
Retraction
  cervix —*see* Retroversion, uterus
  drum (membrane) —*see* Disorder, tympanic membrane, specified NEC
  finger —*see* Deformity, finger
  lid H02.539
    left H02.536
      lower H02.535
      upper H02.534
    right H02.533
      lower H02.532
      upper H02.531

Retraction - continued
lung J98.4
mediastinum J98.5
nipple N64.53
associated with
lactation O92.03
pregnancy O92.01
puerperium O92.02
congenital Q83.8
palmar fascia M72.0
pleura —see Pleurisy
ring, uterus (Bandl's) (pathological) O62.4
sternum (congenital) Q76.7
acquired M95.4
uterus —see Retroversion, uterus
valve (heart) —see Endocarditis
Retrobulbar —see condition
Retrocecal —see condition
Retrocession —see Retroversion
Retrodisplacement —see Retroversion
Retroflection, retroflexion —see Retroversion
Retrognathia, retrognathism (mandibular)
(maxillary) M26.19
Retrograde menstruation N92.5
Retroperineal —see condition
Retroperitoneal —see condition
Retroperitonitis K68.9
Retropharyngeal —see condition
Retroplacental —see condition
Retroposition —see Retroversion
Retroprosthetic membrane T85.398
Retrosternal thyroid (congenital) Q89.2
Retroversion, retroverted
cervix —see Retroversion, uterus
female NEC —see Retroversion, uterus
iris H21.89
testis (congenital) Q55.29
uterus (acquired) (acute) (any degree)
(asymptomatic) (cervix) (postinfectional)
(postpartal, old) N85.4
congenital Q51.818
in pregnancy O34.53
Retrovirus, as cause of disease classified
elsewhere B97.30
human
immunodeficiency, type 2 (HIV 2) B97.35
T-cell lymphotropic
type I (HTLV-I) B97.33
type II (HTLV-II) B97.34
lentivirus B97.31
oncovirus B97.32
specified NEC B97.39
Retrusion, premaxilla (developmental)
M26.09
Rett's disease or syndrome F84.2
Reverse peristalsis R19.2
Reye's syndrome G93.7
Rh (factor)
hemolytic disease (newborn) P55.0
incompatibility, immunization or sensitization
affecting management of pregnancy NEC
O36.09
anti-D antibody O36.01
newborn P55.0
transfusion reaction —see Complication(s) ,
transfusion, incompatibility reaction, Rh
(factor)
negative mother affecting newborn P55.0
titer elevated —see Complication(s) ,
transfusion, incompatibility reaction, Rh
(factor)

Rh (factor) - continued
transfusion reaction —see Complication(s) ,
transfusion, incompatibility reaction, Rh
(factor)
Rhabdomyolysis (idiopathic) NEC M62.82
traumatic T79.6
Rhabdomyoma —see also Neoplasm,
connective tissue, benign
adult —see Neoplasm, connective tissue,
benign
fetal —see Neoplasm, connective tissue,
benign
glycogenic —see Neoplasm, connective
tissue, benign
Rhabdomyosarcoma (any type) —see
Neoplasm, connective tissue, malignant
Rhabdosarcoma —see Rhabdomyosarcoma
Rhesus (factor) **incompatibility** —see Rh,
incompatibility
Rheumatic (acute) (subacute) (chronic)
adherent pericardium I09.2
coronary arteritis I01.9
degeneration, myocardium I09.0
fever (acute) —see Fever, rheumatic
heart —see Disease, heart, rheumatic
myocardial degeneration —see Degeneration,
myocardium
myocarditis (chronic) (inactive) (with chorea)
I09.0
active or acute I01.2
with chorea (acute) (rheumatic)
(Sydenham's) I02.0
pancarditis, acute I01.8
with chorea (acute (rheumatic) Sydenham's)
I02.0
pericarditis (active) (acute) (with effusion)
(with pneumonia) I01.0
with chorea (acute) (rheumatic)
(Sydenham's) I02.0
chronic or inactive I09.2
pneumonia I00 *[J17]*
torticollis M43.6
typhoid fever A01.09
Rheumatism (articular) (neuralgic)
(nonarticular) M79.0
gout —see Arthritis, rheumatoid
intercostal, meaning Tietze's disease M94.0
palindromic (any site) M12.30
ankle M12.37
elbow M12.32
foot joint M12.37
hand joint M12.34
hip M12.35
knee M12.36
multiple site M12.39
shoulder M12.31
specified joint NEC M12.38
vertebrae M12.38
wrist M12.33
sciatic M54.4
Rheumatoid —see also condition
arthritis —see also Arthritis, rheumatoid
with involvement of organs NEC M05.60
ankle M05.67
elbow M05.62
foot joint M05.67
hand joint M05.64
hip M05.65
knee M05.66
multiple site M05.69
shoulder M05.61
vertebra —see Spondylitis, ankylosing

Rheumatoid – continued
wrist M05.63
seronegative —see Arthritis, rheumatoid,
seronegative
seropositive —see Arthritis, rheumatoid,
seropositive
carditis M05.30
ankle M05.37
elbow M05.32
foot joint M05.37
hand joint M05.34
hip M05.35
knee M05.36
multiple site M05.39
shoulder M05.31
vertebra —see Spondylitis, ankylosing
wrist M05.33
endocarditis —see Rheumatoid, carditis
lung (disease) M05.10
ankle M05.17
elbow M05.12
foot joint M05.17
hand joint M05.14
hip M05.15
knee M05.16
multiple site M05.19
shoulder M05.11
vertebra —see Spondylitis, ankylosing
wrist M05.13
myocarditis —see Rheumatoid, carditis
myopathy M05.40
ankle M05.47
elbow M05.42
foot joint M05.47
hand joint M05.44
hip M05.45
knee M05.46
multiple site M05.49
shoulder M05.41
vertebra —see Spondylitis, ankylosing
wrist M05.43
pericarditis —see Rheumatoid, carditis
polyarthritis —see Arthritis, rheumatoid
polyneuropathy M05.50
ankle M05.57
elbow M05.52
foot joint M05.57
hand joint M05.54
hip M05.55
knee M05.56
multiple site M05.59
shoulder M05.51
vertebra —see Spondylitis, ankylosing
wrist M05.53
vasculitis M05.20
ankle M05.27
elbow M05.22
foot joint M05.27
hand joint M05.24
hip M05.25
knee M05.26
multiple site M05.29
shoulder M05.21
vertebra —see Spondylitis, ankylosing
wrist M05.23
Rhinitis (atrophic) (catarrhal) (chronic)
(croupous) (fibrinous) (granulomatous)
(hyperplastic) (hypertrophic) (membranous)
(obstructive) (purulent) (suppurative)
(ulcerative) J31.0
with
sore throat —see Nasopharyngitis

Rhinitis – *continued*
acute J00
allergic J30.9
with asthma J45.909
with
exacerbation (acute) J45.901
status asthmaticus J45.902
due to
food J30.5
pollen J30.1
nonseasonal J30.89
perennial J30.89
seasonal NEC J30.2
specified NEC J30.89
infective J00
pneumococcal J00
syphilitic A52.73
congenital A50.05 [J99]
tuberculous A15.8
vasomotor J30.0
Rhinoantritis (chronic) —*see* Sinusitis,
maxillary
Rhinodacryolith —*see* Dacryolith
Rhinolith (nasal sinus) J34.89
Rhinomegaly J34.89
Rhinopharyngitis (acute) (subacute) —*see
also* Nasopharyngitis
chronic J31.1
destructive ulcerating A66.5
mutilans A66.5
Rhinophyma L71.1
Rhinorrhea J34.89
cerebrospinal (fluid) G96.0
paroxysmal —*see* Rhinitis, allergic
spasmodic —*see* Rhinitis, allergic
Rhinosalpingitis —*see* Salpingitis, eustachian
Rhinoscleroma A48.8
Rhinosporidiosis B48.1
Rhinovirus infection NEC B34.8
Rhizomelic chondrodysplasia punctata
E71.540
Rhythm
atrioventricular nodal I49.8
disorder I49.9
coronary sinus I49.8
ectopic I49.8
nodal I49.8
escape I49.9
heart, abnormal I49.9
idioventricular I44.2
nodal I49.8
sleep, inversion G47.2
nonorganic origin —*see* Disorder, sleep,
circadian rhythm, psychogenic
Rhytidosis facialis L98.8
Rib —*see also* condition
cervical Q76.5
Riboflavin deficiency E53.0
Rice bodies —*see also* Loose, body, joint
knee M23.4
Richter syndrome —*see* Leukemia, chronic
lymphocytic, B-cell type
Richter's hernia —*see* Hernia, abdomen, with
obstruction
Ricinism —*see* Poisoning, food, noxious, plant
Rickets (active) (acute) (adolescent) (chest
wall) (congenital) (current) (infantile)
(intestinal) E55.0
adult —*see* Osteomalacia
celiac K90.0
hypophosphatemic with nephrotic-glycosuric
dwarfism E72.09

Rickets – *continued*
inactive E64.3
kidney N25.0
renal N25.0
sequelae, any E64.3
vitamin-D-resistant E83.31 [M90.80]
Rickettsial disease A79.9
specified type NEC A79.89
Rickettsialpox (Rickettsia akari) A79.1
Rickettsiosis A79.9
due to
Ehrlichia sennetsu A79.81
Rickettsia akari (rickettsialpox) A79.1
specified type NEC A79.89
tick-borne A77.9
vesicular A79.1
Rider's bone —*see* Ossification, muscle,
specified NEC
Ridge, alveolus —*see also* condition
flabby K06.8
Ridged ear, congenital Q17.3
Riedel's
lobe, liver Q44.7
struma, thyroiditis or disease E06.5
Rieger's anomaly or syndrome Q13.81
Riehl's melanosis L81.4
Rietti-Greppi-Micheli anemia D56.9
Rieux's hernia —*see* Hernia, abdomen,
specified site NEC
Riga (-Fede) **disease** K14.0
Riggs' disease —*see* Periodontitis
Right middle lobe syndrome J98.11
Rigid, rigidity —*see also* condition
abdominal R19.30
with severe abdominal pain R10.0
epigastric R19.36
generalized R19.37
left lower quadrant R19.34
left upper quadrant R19.32
periumbilic R19.35
right lower quadrant R19.33
right upper quadrant R19.31
articular, multiple, congenital Q68.8
cervix (uteri) in pregnancy —*see* Pregnancy,
complicated by, abnormal, cervix
hymen (acquired) (congenital) N89.6
nuchal R29.1
pelvic floor in pregnancy —*see* Pregnancy,
complicated by, abnormal, pelvic organs or
tissues NEC
perineum or vulva in pregnancy —*see*
Pregnancy, complicated by, abnormal, vulva
spine —*see* Dorsopathy, specified NEC
vagina in pregnancy —*see* Pregnancy,
complicated by, abnormal, vagina
Rigors R68.89
with fever R50.9
Riley-Day syndrome G90.1
RIND (reversible ischemic neurologic deficit)
I63.9
Ring (s)
aorta (vascular) Q25.4
Bandl's O62.4
contraction, complicating delivery O62.4
esophageal, lower (muscular) K22.2
Fleischer's (cornea) H18.04
hymenal, tight (acquired) (congenital) N89.6
Kayser-Fleischer (cornea) H18.04
retraction, uterus, pathological O62.4
Schatzki's (esophagus) (lower) K22.2
congenital Q39.3

Ring (s) - *continued*
Soemmerring's —*see* Cataract, secondary
vascular (congenital) Q25.8
aorta Q25.4
Ringed hair (congenital) Q84.1
Ringworm B35.9
beard B35.0
black dot B35.0
body B35.4
Burmese B35.5
corporeal B35.4
foot B35.3
groin B35.6
hand B35.2
honeycomb B35.0
nails B35.1
perianal (area) B35.6
scalp B35.0
specified NEC B35.8
Tokelau B35.5
Rise, venous pressure I87.8
Risk, suicidal
meaning personal history of attempted suicide
Z91.5
meaning suicidal ideation —*see* Ideation,
suicidal
Ritter's disease L00
Rivalry, sibling Z62.891
Rivalta's disease A42.2
River blindness B73.01
Robert's pelvis Q74.2
with disproportion (fetopelvic) O33.0
causing obstructed labor O65.0
Robin (-Pierre) **syndrome** Q87.0
Robinow-Silvermann-Smith syndrome Q87.1
Robinson's (hidrotic) ectodermal dysplasia or
syndrome Q82.4
Robles' disease B73.01
Rocky Mountain (spotted) **fever** A77.0
Roetheln —*see* Rubella
Roger's disease Q21.0
Rokitansky-Aschoff sinuses (gallbladder)
K82.8
Rolando's fracture (displaced) S62.22
nondisplaced S62.22
Romano-Ward (prolonged QT interval)
syndrome I45.81
Romberg's disease or syndrome G51.8
Roof, mouth —*see* condition
Rosacea L71.9
acne L71.9
keratitis L71.8
specified NEC L71.8
Rosary, rachitic E55.0
Rose
cold J30.1
fever J30.1
rash R21
epidemic B06.9
Rosenbach's erysipeloid A26.0
Rosenthal's disease or syndrome D68.1
Roseola B09
infantum B08.20
due to human herpesvirus 6 B08.21
due to human herpesvirus 7 B08.22
Rossbach's disease K31.89
psychogenic F45.8
Ross River disease or fever B33.1
Rostan's asthma (cardiac) —*see* Failure,
ventricular, left

Rotation
anomalous, incomplete or insufficient, intestine Q43.3
cecum (congenital) Q43.3
colon (congenital) Q43.3
spine, incomplete or insufficient —see Dorsopathy, deforming, specified NEC
tooth, teeth, fully erupted M26.35
vertebra, incomplete or insufficient —see Dorsopathy, deforming, specified NEC
Rotes Quérol disease or syndrome —see Hyperostosis, ankylosing
Roth (-Bernhardt) disease or syndrome —see Meralgia paraesthetica
Rothmund (-Thomson) syndrome Q82.8
Rotor's disease or syndrome E80.6
Round
back (with wedging of vertebrae) —see Kyphosis
sequelae (late effect) of rickets E64.3
worms (large) (infestation) NEC B82.0
Ascariasis (see also Ascariasis) B77.9
Roussy-Lévy syndrome G60.0
Rubella (German measles) B06.9
complication NEC B06.09
neurological B06.00
congenital P35.0
contact Z20.4
exposure to Z20.4
maternal
manifest rubella in infant P35.0
care for (suspected) damage to fetus O35.3
suspected damage to fetus affecting management of pregnancy O35.3
specified complications NEC B06.89
Rubeola (meaning measles) —see Measles
meaning rubella —see Rubella
Rubeosis, iris —see Disorder, iris, vascular
Rubinstein-Taybi syndrome Q87.2
Rudimentary (congenital) —see also Agenesis
arm —see Defect, reduction, upper limb
bone Q79.9
cervix uteri Q51.828
eye Q11.2
lobule of ear Q17.3
patella Q74.1
respiratory organs in thoracopagus Q89.4
tracheal bronchus Q32.4
uterus Q51.818
in male Q56.1
vagina Q52.0
Ruled out condition —see Observation, suspected
Rumination R11.10
with nausea R11.2
disorder of infancy F98.21
neurotic F42
newborn P92.1
obsessional F42
psychogenic F42
Runeberg's disease D51.0
Runny nose R09.89
Rupia (syphilitic) A51.39
congenital A50.06
tertiary A52.79
Rupture, ruptured
abscess (spontaneous)
code by site under Abscess
aneurysm —see Aneurysm
anus (sphincter) —see Laceration, anus
aorta, aortic I71.8
abdominal I71.3

Rupture, ruptured - continued
arch I71.1
ascending I71.1
descending I71.8
abdominal I71.3
thoracic I71.1
syphilitic A52.01
thoracoabdominal I71.5
thorax, thoracic I71.1
transverse I71.1
traumatic —see Injury, aorta, laceration, major
valve or cusp (see also Endocarditis, aortic) I35.8
appendix (with peritonitis) K35.2
arteriovenous fistula, brain I60.8
artery I77.2
brain —see Hemorrhage, intracranial, intracerebral
coronary —see Infarct, myocardium
heart —see Infarct, myocardium
pulmonary I28.8
traumatic (complication) —see Injury, blood vessel
bile duct (common) (hepatic) K83.2
cystic K82.2
bladder (sphincter) (nontraumatic) (spontaneous) N32.89
following ectopic or molar pregnancy O08.6
obstetrical trauma O71.5
traumatic S37.29
blood vessel —see also Hemorrhage
brain —see Hemorrhage, intracranial, intracerebral
heart —see Infarct, myocardium
traumatic (complication) —see Injury, blood vessel, laceration, major, by site
bone —see Fracture
bowel (nontraumatic) K63.1
brain
aneurysm (congenital) —see also Hemorrhage, intracranial, subarachnoid
syphilitic A52.05
hemorrhagic —see Hemorrhage, intracranial, intracerebral
capillaries I78.8
cardiac (auricle) (ventricle) (wall) I23.3
with hemopericardium I23.0
infectional I40.9
traumatic —see Injury, heart
cartilage (articular) (current) —see also Sprain
knee S83.3
semilunar —see Tear, meniscus
cecum (with peritonitis) K65.0
with peritoneal abscess K35.3
traumatic S36.598
celiac artery, traumatic —see Injury, blood vessel, celiac artery, laceration, major
cerebral aneurysm (congenital) (see Hemorrhage, intracranial, subarachnoid)
cervix (uteri)
with ectopic or molar pregnancy O08.6
following ectopic or molar pregnancy O08.6
obstetrical trauma O71.3
traumatic S37.69
chordae tendineae NEC I51.1
concurrent with acute myocardial infarction —see Infarct, myocardium
following acute myocardial infarction (current complication) I23.4
choroid (direct) (indirect) (traumatic) H31.32

Rupture, ruptured - continued
circle of Willis I60.6
colon (nontraumatic) K63.1
traumatic —see Injury, intestine, large
cornea (traumatic) —see Injury, eye, laceration
coronary (artery) (thrombotic) —see Infarct, myocardium
corpus luteum (infected) (ovary) N83.1
cyst —see Cyst
cystic duct K82.2
Descemet's membrane —see Change, corneal membrane, Descemet's, rupture
traumatic —see Injury, eye, laceration
diaphragm, traumatic —see Injury, intrathoracic, diaphragm
disc —see Rupture, intervertebral disc
diverticulum (intestine) K57.80
with bleeding K57.81
bladder N32.3
large intestine K57.20
with
bleeding K57.21
small intestine K57.40
with bleeding K57.41
small intestine K57.00
with
bleeding K57.01
large intestine K57.40
with bleeding K57.41
duodenal stump K31.89
ear drum (nontraumatic) —see also Perforation, tympanum
traumatic S09.2
due to blast injury —see Injury, blast, ear
esophagus K22.3
eye (without prolapse or loss of intraocular tissue) —see Injury, eye, laceration
fallopian tube NEC (nonobstetric) (nontraumatic) N83.8
due to pregnancy O00.1
fontanel P13.1
gallbladder K82.2
traumatic S36.128
gastric —see also Rupture, stomach
vessel K92.2
globe (eye) (traumatic) —see Injury, eye, laceration
graafian follicle (hematoma) N83.0
heart —see Rupture, cardiac
hymen (nontraumatic) (nonintentional) N89.8
internal organ, traumatic —see Injury, by site
intervertebral disc —see Displacement, intervertebral disc
traumatic —see Rupture, traumatic, intervertebral disc
intestine NEC (nontraumatic) K63.1
traumatic —see Injury, intestine
iris —see also Abnormality, pupillary
traumatic —see Injury, eye, laceration
joint capsule, traumatic —see Sprain
kidney (traumatic) S37.06
birth injury P15.8
nontraumatic N28.89
lacrimal duct (traumatic) —see Injury, eye, specified site NEC
lens (cataract) (traumatic) —see Cataract, traumatic
ligament, traumatic —see Rupture, traumatic, ligament, by site
liver S36.116
birth injury P15.0

Rupture, ruptured - *continued*
  lymphatic vessel I89.8
  marginal sinus (placental) (with hemorrhage)
  —*see* Hemorrhage, antepartum, specified
  cause NEC
  membrana tympani (nontraumatic) —*see*
  Perforation, tympanum
  membranes (spontaneous)
    artificial
      delayed delivery following O75.5
    delayed delivery following —*see* Pregnancy,
  complicated by, premature rupture of
  membranes
  meningeal artery I60.8
  meniscus (knee) —*see also* Tear, meniscus
    old —*see* Derangement, meniscus
    site other than knee
  code as Sprain
  mesenteric artery, traumatic —*see* Injury,
  mesenteric, artery, laceration, major
  mesentery (nontraumatic) K66.8
    traumatic —*see* Injury, intra-abdominal,
  specified, site NEC
  mitral (valve) I34.8
  muscle (traumatic) —*see also* Strain
    diastasis —*see* Diastasis, muscle
    nontraumatic M62.10
      ankle M62.17
      foot M62.17
      forearm M62.13
      hand M62.14
      lower leg M62.16
      pelvic region M62.15
      shoulder region M62.11
      specified site NEC M62.18
      thigh M62.15
      upper arm M62.12
    traumatic —*see* Strain, by site
  musculotendinous junction NEC,
  nontraumatic —*see* Rupture, tendon,
  spontaneous
  mycotic aneurysm causing cerebral
  hemorrhage —*see* Hemorrhage, intracranial,
  subarachnoid
  myocardium, myocardial —*see* Rupture,
  cardiac
    traumatic —*see* Injury, heart
  nontraumatic, meaning hernia —*see* Hernia
  obstructed —*see* Hernia, by site, obstructed
  operation wound —*see* Disruption, wound,
  operation
  ovary, ovarian N83.8
    corpus luteum cyst N83.1
    follicle (graafian) N83.0
  oviduct (nonobstetric) (nontraumatic) N83.8
    due to pregnancy O00.1
  pancreas (nontraumatic) K86.8
    traumatic S36.299
  papillary muscle NEC I51.2
    following acute myocardial infarction
  (current complication) I23.5
  pelvic
    floor, complicating delivery O70.1
    organ NEC, obstetrical trauma O71.5
  perineum (nonobstetric) (nontraumatic)
    N90.89
    complicating delivery —*see* Delivery,
  complicated, by, laceration, anus (sphincter)
  postoperative wound —*see* Disruption,
  wound, operation
  prostate (traumatic) S37.828

Rupture, ruptured - *continued*
  pulmonary
    artery I28.8
    valve (heart) I37.8
    vein I28.8
    vessel I28.8
  pus tube —*see* Salpingitis
  pyosalpinx —*see* Salpingitis
  rectum (nontraumatic) K63.1
    traumatic S36.69
  retina, retinal (traumatic) (without
  detachment) —*see also* Break, retina
    with detachment —*see* Detachment, retina,
  with retinal, break
  rotator cuff (nontraumatic) M75.10
    complete M75.12
    incomplete M75.11
  sclera —*see* Injury, eye, laceration
  sigmoid (nontraumatic) K63.1
    traumatic S36.593
  spinal cord —*see also* Injury, spinal cord, by
  region
    due to injury at birth P11.5
    newborn (birth injury) P11.5
  spleen (traumatic) S36.09
    birth injury P15.1
    congenital (birth injury) P15.1
    due to P. vivax malaria B51.0
    nontraumatic D73.5
    spontaneous D73.5
  splenic vein R58
    traumatic —*see* Injury, blood vessel, splenic
  vein
  stomach (nontraumatic) (spontaneous) K31.89
    traumatic S36.39
  supraspinatus (complete) (incomplete)
  (nontraumatic) —*see* Tear, rotator cuff
  symphysis pubis
    obstetric O71.6
    traumatic S33.4
  synovium (cyst) M66.10
    ankle M66.17
    elbow M66.12
    finger M66.14
    foot M66.17
    forearm M66.13
    hand M66.14
    pelvic region M66.15
    shoulder region M66.11
    specified site NEC M66.18
    thigh M66.15
    toe M66.17
    upper arm M66.12
    wrist M66.13
  tendon (traumatic) —*see* Strain
    nontraumatic (spontaneous) M66.9
      ankle M66.87
      extensor M66.20
        ankle M66.27
        foot M66.27
        forearm M66.23
        hand M66.24
        lower leg M66.26
        multiple sites M66.29
        pelvic region M66.25
        shoulder region M66.21
        specified site NEC M66.28
        thigh M66.25
        upper arm M66.22
      flexor M66.30
        ankle M66.37
        foot M66.37

Rupture, ruptured - *continued*
        forearm M66.33
        hand M66.34
        lower leg M66.36
        multiple sites M66.39
        pelvic region M66.35
        shoulder region M66.31
        specified site NEC M66.38
        thigh M66.35
        upper arm M66.32
      foot M66.87
      forearm M66.83
      hand M66.84
      lower leg M66.86
      multiple sites M66.89
      pelvic region M66.85
      shoulder region M66.81
      specified
        site NEC M66.88
        tendon M66.80
      thigh M66.85
      upper arm M66.82
  thoracic duct I89.8
  tonsil J35.8
  traumatic
    aorta —*see* Injury, aorta, laceration, major
    diaphragm —*see* Injury, intrathoracic,
  diaphragm
    external site —*see* Wound, open, by site
    eye —*see* Injury, eye, laceration
    internal organ —*see* Injury, by site
    intervertebral disc
      cervical S13.0
      lumbar S33.0
      thoracic S23.0
    kidney S37.06
    ligament —*see also* Sprain
      ankle —*see* Sprain, ankle
      carpus —*see* Rupture, traumatic, ligament,
  wrist
      collateral (hand) —*see* Rupture, traumatic,
  ligament, finger, collateral
      finger (metacarpophalangeal)
  (interphalangeal) S63.40
        collateral S63.41
          index S63.41
          little S63.41
          middle S63.41
          ring S63.41
        index S63.40
        little S63.40
        middle S63.40
        palmar S63.42
          index S63.42
          little S63.42
          middle S63.42
          ring S63.42
        ring S63.40
        specified site NEC S63.499
          index S63.49
          little S63.49
          middle S63.49
          ring S63.49
        volar plate S63.43
          index S63.43
          little S63.43
          middle S63.43
          ring S63.43
      foot —*see* Sprain, foot
      radial collateral S53.2
      radiocarpal —*see* Rupture, traumatic,
  ligament, wrist, radiocarpal

Rupture, ruptured - *continued*
  ulnar collateral S53.3
  ulnocarpal —*see* Rupture, traumatic,
  ligament, wrist, ulnocarpal
    wrist S63.30
      collateral S63.31
      radiocarpal S63.32
      specified site NEC S63.39
      ulnocarpal (palmar) S63.33
  liver S36.116
  membrana tympani —*see* Rupture, ear
  drum, traumatic
  muscle or tendon —*see* Strain
  myocardium —*see* Injury, heart
  pancreas S36.299
  rectum S36.69
  sigmoid S36.593
  spleen S36.09
  stomach S36.39
  symphysis pubis S33.4
  tympanum, tympanic (membrane) —*see*
  Rupture, ear drum, traumatic
  ureter S37.19
  uterus S37.69
  vagina —*see* Injury, vagina
  vena cava —*see* Injury, vena cava,
  laceration, major
  tricuspid (heart) (valve) I07.8
  tube, tubal (nonobstetric) (nontraumatic)
  N83.8
    abscess —*see* Salpingitis
    due to pregnancy O00.1
  tympanum, tympanic (membrane)
  (nontraumatic) (*see also* Perforation,
  tympanic membrane) H72.9
    traumatic —*see* Rupture, ear drum,
  traumatic
  umbilical cord, complicating delivery O69.89
  ureter (traumatic) S37.19
    nontraumatic N28.89
  urethra (nontraumatic) N36.8
    with ectopic or molar pregnancy O08.6
    following ectopic or molar pregnancy O08.6
    obstetrical trauma O71.5
    traumatic S37.39
  uterosacral ligament (nonobstetric)
  (nontraumatic) N83.8
  uterus (traumatic) S37.69
    before labor O71.0
    during or after labor O71.1
    nonpuerperal, nontraumatic N85.8
    pregnant (during labor) O71.1
      before labor O71.0
  vagina —*see* Injury, vagina
  valve, valvular (heart) —*see* Endocarditis
  varicose vein —*see* Varix
  varix —*see* Varix
  vena cava R58
    traumatic —*see* Injury, vena cava,
  laceration, major
  vesical (urinary) N32.89
  vessel (blood) R58
    pulmonary I28.8
    traumatic —*see* Injury, blood vessel
  viscus R19.8
  vulva complicating delivery O70.0
Russell-Silver syndrome Q87.1
Russian spring-summer encephalitis A84.0
Rust's disease (tuberculous cervical
  spondylitis) A18.01
Ruvalcaba-Myhre-Smith syndrome E71.440
Rytand-Lipsitch syndrome I44.2

S

Saber, sabre shin or tibia (syphilitic) A50.56
  [M90.8]
Sac lacrimal —*see* condition
Saccharomyces infection B37.9
Saccharopinuria E72.3
Saccular —*see* condition
Sacculation
  aorta (nonsyphilitic) —*see* Aneurysm, aorta
  bladder N32.3
  intralaryngeal (congenital) (ventricular) Q31.3
  larynx (congenital) (ventricular) Q31.3
  organ or site, congenital —*see* Distortion
  pregnant uterus —*see* Pregnancy, complicated
  by, abnormal, uterus
  ureter N28.89
  urethra N36.1
  vesical N32.3
Sachs' amaurotic familial idiocy or disease
  E75.02
Sachs-Tay disease E75.02
Sacks-Libman disease M32.11
Sacralgia M53.3
Sacralization Q76.49
Sacrodynia M53.3
Sacroiliac joint —*see* condition
Sacroiliitis NEC M46.1
Sacrum —*see* condition
Saddle
  back —*see* Lordosis
  embolus
    abdominal aorta I74.01
    pulmonary artery I26.92
      with acute cor pulmonale I26.02
  injury
  code to condition
  nose M95.0
    due to syphilis A50.57
Sadism (sexual) F65.52
Sadness, postpartal O90.6
Sadomasochism F65.50
Saemisch's ulcer (cornea) —*see* Ulcer, cornea,
  central
Sahib disease B55.0
Sailors' skin L57.8
Saint
  Anthony's fire —*see* Erysipelas
  triad —*see* Hernia, diaphragm
  Vitus' dance —*see* Chorea, Sydenham's
Salaam
  attack (s) —*see* Epilepsy, spasms
  tic R25.8
Salicylism
  abuse F55.8
  overdose or wrong substance given —*see*
  Table of Drugs and Chemicals, by drug,
  poisoning
Salivary duct or gland —*see* condition
Salivation, excessive K11.7
Salmonella —*see* Infection, Salmonella
Salmonellosis A02.0
Salpingitis (catarrhal) (fallopian tube)
  (nodular) (pseudofollicular) (purulent) (septic)
  N70.91
  with oophoritis N70.93
  acute N70.01
    with oophoritis N70.03
  chlamydial A56.11
  chronic N70.11
    with oophoritis N70.13
  complicating abortion —*see* Abortion, by
  type, complicated by, salpingitis

Salpingitis - *continued*
  ear —*see* Salpingitis, eustachian
  eustachian (tube) H68.00
    acute H68.01
    chronic H68.02
  follicularis N70.11
    with oophoritis N70.13
  gonococcal (acute) (chronic) A54.24
  interstitial, chronic N70.11
    with oophoritis N70.13
  isthmica nodosa N70.11
    with oophoritis N70.13
  specific (gonococcal) (acute) (chronic)
    A54.24
  tuberculous (acute) (chronic) A18.17
  venereal (gonococcal) (acute) (chronic)
    A54.24
Salpingocele N83.4
Salpingo-oophoritis (catarrhal) (purulent)
  (ruptured) (septic) (suppurative) N70.93
  acute N70.03
    with ectopic or molar pregnancy O08.0
    following ectopic or molar pregnancy O08.0
    gonococcal A54.24
  chronic N70.13
  following ectopic or molar pregnancy O08.0
  gonococcal (acute) (chronic) A54.24
  puerperal O86.19
  specific (gonococcal) (acute) (chronic)
    A54.24
  subacute N70.03
  tuberculous (acute) (chronic) A18.17
  venereal (gonococcal) (acute) (chronic)
    A54.24
Salpingo-ovaritis —*see* Salpingo-oophoritis
Salpingoperitonitis —*see* Salpingo-oophoritis
Salzmann's nodular dystrophy —*see*
  Degeneration, cornea, nodular
Sampson's cyst or tumor N80.1
San Joaquin (Valley) fever B38.0
Sandblaster's asthma, lung or
  pneumoconiosis J62.8
Sander's disease (paranoia) F22
Sandfly fever A93.1
Sandhoff's disease E75.01
Sanfilippo (Type B) (Type C) (Type D)
  syndrome E76.22
Sanger-Brown ataxia G11.2
Sao Paulo fever or typhus A77.0
Saponification, mesenteric K65.8
Sarcocele (benign)
  syphilitic A52.76
    congenital A50.59
Sarcocystosis A07.8
Sarcoepiplocele —*see* Hernia
Sarcoepiplomphalocele Q79.2
Sarcoid —*see also* Sarcoidosis
  arthropathy D86.86
  Boeck's D86.9
  Darier-Roussy D86.3
  iridocyclitis D86.83
  meningitis D86.81
  myocarditis D86.85
  myositis D86.87
  pyelonephritis D86.84
  Spiegler-Fendt L08.89
Sarcoidosis D86.9
  with
    cranial nerve palsies D86.82
    hepatic granuloma D86.89
    polyarthritis D86.86
    tubulo-interstitial nephropathy D86.84

Sarcoidosis – *continued*
  combined sites NEC D86.89
  lung D86.0
    and lymph nodes D86.2
  lymph nodes D86.1
    and lung D86.2
  meninges D86.81
  skin D86.3
  specified type NEC D86.89
Sarcoma (of) —*see also* Neoplasm, connective
  tissue, malignant
  alveolar soft part —*see* Neoplasm, connective
  tissue, malignant
  ameloblastic C41.1
    upper jaw (bone) C41.0
  botryoid —*see* Neoplasm, connective tissue,
  malignant
  botryoides —*see* Neoplasm, connective
  tissue, malignant
  cerebellar C71.6
    circumscribed (arachnoidal) C71.6
  circumscribed (arachnoidal) cerebellar C71.6
  clear cell —*see also* Neoplasm, connective
  tissue, malignant
    kidney C64.
  dendritic cells (accessory cells) C96.4
  embryonal —*see* Neoplasm, connective
  tissue, malignant
  endometrial (stromal) C54.1
    isthmus C54.0
  epithelioid (cell) —*see* Neoplasm, connective
  tissue, malignant
  Ewing's —*see* Neoplasm, bone, malignant
  follicular dendritic cell C96.4
  germinoblastic (diffuse) —*see* Lymphoma,
  diffuse large cell
    follicular —*see* Lymphoma, follicular,
  specified NEC
  giant cell (except of bone) —*see also*
  Neoplasm, connective tissue, malignant
    bone —*see* Neoplasm, bone, malignant
  glomoid —*see* Neoplasm, connective tissue,
  malignant
  granulocytic C92.3
  hemangioendothelial —*see* Neoplasm,
  connective tissue, malignant
  hemorrhagic, multiple —*see* Sarcoma,
  Kaposi's
  histiocytic C96.A
  Hodgkin —*see* Lymphoma, Hodgkin
  immunoblastic (diffuse) —*see* Lymphoma,
  diffuse large cell
  interdigitating dendritic cell C96.4
  Kaposi's
    colon C46.4
    connective tissue C46.1
    gastrointestinal organ C46.4
    lung C46.5
    lymph node (s) C46.3
    palate (hard) (soft) C46.2
    rectum C46.4
    skin C46.0
    specified site NEC C46.7
    stomach C46.4
    unspecified site C46.9
  Kupffer cell C22.3
  Langerhans cell C96.4
  leptomeningeal —*see* Neoplasm, meninges,
  malignant
  liver NEC C22.4
  lymphangioendothelial —*see* Neoplasm,
  connective tissue, malignant

Sarcoma - *continued*
  lymphoblastic —*see* Lymphoma,
  lymphoblastic (diffuse)
  lymphocytic —*see* Lymphoma, small cell B-
  cell
  mast cell C96.2
  melanotic —*see* Melanoma
  meningeal —*see* Neoplasm, meninges,
  malignant
  meningothelial —*see* Neoplasm, meninges,
  malignant
  mesenchymal —*see also* Neoplasm,
  connective tissue, malignant
    mixed —*see* Neoplasm, connective tissue,
  malignant
  mesothelial —*see* Mesothelioma
  monstrocellular
    specified site —*see* Neoplasm, malignant,
    by site
    unspecified site C71.9
  myeloid C92.3
  neurogenic —*see* Neoplasm, nerve, malignant
  odontogenic C41.1
    upper jaw (bone) C41.0
  osteoblastic —*see* Neoplasm, bone, malignant
  osteogenic —*see also* Neoplasm, bone,
  malignant
    juxtacortical —*see* Neoplasm, bone,
  malignant
    periosteal —*see* Neoplasm, bone, malignant
  periosteal —*see also* Neoplasm, bone,
  malignant
    osteogenic —*see* Neoplasm, bone,
  malignant
  pleomorphic cell —*see* Neoplasm, connective
  tissue, malignant
  reticulum cell (diffuse) —*see* Lymphoma,
  diffuse large cell
    nodular —*see* Lymphoma, follicular
    pleomorphic cell type —*see* Lymphoma,
  diffuse large cell
  rhabdoid —*see* Neoplasm, malignant, by site
  round cell —*see* Neoplasm, connective tissue,
  malignant
  small cell —*see* Neoplasm, connective tissue,
  malignant
  soft tissue —*see* Neoplasm, connective tissue,
  malignant
  spindle cell —*see* Neoplasm, connective
  tissue, malignant
  stromal (endometrial) C54.1
    isthmus C54.0
  synovial —*see also* Neoplasm, connective
  tissue, malignant
    biphasic —*see* Neoplasm, connective tissue,
  malignant
    epithelioid cell —*see* Neoplasm, connective
  tissue, malignant
    spindle cell —*see* Neoplasm, connective
  tissue, malignant
Sarcomatosis
  meningeal —*see* Neoplasm, meninges,
  malignant
  specified site NEC —*see* Neoplasm,
  connective tissue, malignant
  unspecified site C80.1
Sarcosinemia E72.59
Sarcosporidiosis (intestinal) A07.8
Satiety, early R68.81
Saturnine —*see* condition

Saturnism
  overdose or wrong substance given or taken
    —*see* Table of Drugs and Chemicals, by drug,
  poisoning
Satyriasis F52.8
Sauriasis —*see* Ichthyosis
SBE (subacute bacterial endocarditis) I33.0
Scabs R23.4
Scabies (any site) B86
Scaglietti-Dagnini syndrome E22.0
Scald —*see* Burn
Scalenus anticus (anterior) **syndrome** G54.0
Scales R23.4
Scaling, skin R23.4
Scalp —*see* condition
Scapegoating affecting child Z62.3
Scaphocephaly Q75.0
Scapulalgia M89.8X1
Scapulohumeral myopathy G71.0
Scar, scarring (*see also* Cicatrix) L90.5
  adherent L90.5
  atrophic L90.5
  cervix
    in pregnancy or childbirth —*see* Pregnancy,
  complicated by, abnormal cervix
  cheloid L91.0
  chorioretinal H31.00
    posterior pole macula H31.01
    postsurgical H59.81
    solar retinopathy H31.02
    specified type NEC H31.09
  choroid —*see* Scar, chorioretinal
  conjunctiva H11.24
  cornea H17.9
    xerophthalmic —*see also* Opacity, cornea
    vitamin A deficiency E50.6
  duodenum, obstructive K31.5
  hypertrophic L91.0
  keloid L91.0
  labia N90.89
  lung (base) J98.4
  macula —*see* Scar, chorioretinal, posterior
  pole
  muscle M62.89
  myocardium, myocardial I25.2
  painful L90.5
  posterior pole (eye) —*see* Scar, chorioretinal,
  posterior pole
  retina —*see* Scar, chorioretinal
  trachea J39.8
  uterus N85.8
    in pregnancy O34.29
  vagina N89.8
    postoperative N99.2
  vulva N90.89
Scarabiasis B88.2
Scarlatina (anginosa) (maligna) (ulcerosa)
  A38.9
  myocarditis (acute) A38.1
    old —*see* Myocarditis
  otitis media A38.0
Scarlet fever (albuminuria) (angina) A38.9
Schamberg's disease (progressive pigmentary
  dermatosis) L81.7
Schatzki's ring (acquired) (esophagus) (lower)
  K22.2
  congenital Q39.3
Schaufenster krankheit I20.8
Schaumann's
  benign lymphogranulomatosis D86.1
  disease or syndrome —*see* Sarcoidosis
Scheie's syndrome E76.03
Schenck's disease B42.1

Scheuermann's disease or osteochondrosis
—*see* Osteochondrosis, juvenile, spine
Schilder (-Flatau) **disease** G37.0
Schilling-type monocytic leukemia C93.0
Schimmelbusch's disease, cystic mastitis, or hyperplasia —*see* Mastopathy, cystic
Schistosoma infestation —*see* Infestation, Schistosoma
Schistosomiasis B65.9
  with muscle disorder B65.9 *[M63.80]*
    ankle B65.9 *[M63.87]*
    foot B65.9 *[M63.87]*
    forearm B65.9 *[M63.83]*
    hand B65.9 *[M63.84]*
    lower leg B65.9 *[M63.86]*
    multiple sites B65.9 *[M63.89]*
    pelvic region B65.9 *[M63.85]*
    shoulder region B65.9 *[M63.81]*
    specified site NEC B65.9 *[M63.88]*
    thigh B65.9 *[M63.85]*
    upper arm B65.9 *[M63.82]*
  Asiatic B65.2
  bladder B65.0
  chestermani B65.8
  colon B65.1
  cutaneous B65.3
  due to
    S. haematobium B65.0
    S. japonicum B65.2
    S. mansoni B65.1
    S. mattheii B65.8
  Eastern B65.2
  genitourinary tract B65.0
  intestinal B65.1
  lung NEC B65.9 *[J99]*
    pneumonia B65.9 *[J17]*
  Manson's (intestinal) B65.1
  oriental B65.2
  pulmonary NEC B65.9 *[J99]*
    pneumonia B65.9
  Schistosoma
    haematobium B65.0
    japonicum B65.2
    mansoni B65.1
  specified type NEC B65.8
  urinary B65.0
  vesical B65.0
Schizencephaly Q04.6
Schizoaffective psychosis F25.9
Schizodontia K00.2
Schizoid personality F60.1
Schizophrenia, schizophrenic F20.9
  acute (brief) (undifferentiated) F23
  atypical (form) F20.3
  borderline F21
  catalepsy F20.2
  catatonic (type) (excited) (withdrawn) F20.2
  cenesthopathic, cenesthesiopathic F20.89
  childhood type F84.5
  chronic undifferentiated F20.5
  cyclic F25.0
  disorganized (type) F20.1
  flexibilitas cerea F20.2
  hebephrenic (type) F20.1
  incipient F21
  latent F21
  negative type F20.5
  paranoid (type) F20.0
  paraphrenic F20.0
  post-psychotic depression F32.8
  prepsychotic F21
  prodromal F21

Schizophrenia, schizophrenic - *continued*
  pseudoneurotic F21
  pseudopsychopathic F21
  reaction F23
  residual (state) (type) F20.5
  restzustand F20.5
  schizoaffective (type) —*see* Psychosis, schizoaffective
  simple (type) F20.89
  simplex F20.89
  specified type NEC F20.89
  stupor F20.2
  syndrome of childhood F84.5
  undifferentiated (type) F20.3
    chronic F20.5
Schizothymia (persistent) F60.1
Schlatter-Osgood disease or osteochondrosis
  —*see* Osteochondrosis, juvenile, tibia
Schlatter's tibia —*see* Osteochondrosis, juvenile, tibia
Schmidt's syndrome (polyglandular, autoimmune) E31.0
Schmincke's carcinoma or tumor —*see* Neoplasm, nasopharynx, malignant
Schmitz (-Stutzer) **dysentery** A03.0
Schmorl's disease or nodes
  lumbar region M51.46
  lumbosacral region M51.47
  sacrococcygeal region M53.3
  thoracic region M51.44
  thoracolumbar region M51.45
Schneiderian
  papilloma —*see* Neoplasm, nasopharynx, benign
    specified site —*see* Neoplasm, benign, by site
    unspecified site D14.0
  specified site —*see* Neoplasm, malignant, by site
    unspecified site C30.0
Scholte's syndrome (malignant carcinoid) E34.0
Scholz (-Bielchowsky-Henneberg) **disease or syndrome** E75.25
Schönlein (-Henoch) disease or purpura (primary) (rheumatic) D69.0
Schottmuller's disease A01.4
Schroeder's syndrome (endocrine hypertensive) E27.0
Schüller-Christian disease or syndrome C96.5
Schultze's type acroparesthesia, simple I73.89
Schultz's disease or syndrome —*see* Agranulocytosis
Schwalbe-Ziehen-Oppenheim disease G24.1
Schwannoma —*see also* Neoplasm, nerve, benign
  malignant —*see also* Neoplasm, nerve, malignant
    with rhabdomyoblastic differentiation —*see* Neoplasm, nerve, malignant
  melanocytic —*see* Neoplasm, nerve, benign
  pigmented —*see* Neoplasm, nerve, benign
Schwannomatosis Q85.03
Schwartz (-Jampel) **syndrome** G71.13
Schwartz-Bartter syndrome E22.2
Schweniger-Buzzi anetoderma L90.1
Sciatic —*see* condition
Sciatica (infective)
  with lumbago M54.4
    due to intervertebral disc disorder —*see* Disorder, disc, with, radiculopathy

Sciatica - *continued*
  due to displacement of intervertebral disc (with lumbago) —*see* Disorder, disc, with, radiculopathy
  wallet M54.3
Scimitar syndrome Q26.8
Sclera —*see* condition
Sclerectasia H15.84
Scleredema
  adultorum —*see* Sclerosis, systemic
  Buschke's —*see* Sclerosis, systemic
  newborn P83.0
Sclerema (adiposum) (edematosum) (neonatorum) (newborn) P83.0
  adultorum —*see* Sclerosis, systemic
Scleriasis —*see* Scleroderma
Scleritis H15.00
  with corneal involvement H15.04
  anterior H15.01
  brawny H15.02
  in (due to) zoster B02.34
  posterior H15.03
  specified type NEC H15.09
  syphilitic A52.71
  tuberculous (nodular) A18.51
Sclerochoroiditis H31.8
Scleroconjunctivitis —*see* Scleritis
Sclerocystic ovary syndrome E28.2
Sclerodactyly, sclerodactylia L94.3
Scleroderma, sclerodermia (acrosclerotic) (diffuse) (generalized) (progressive) (pulmonary) (*see also* Sclerosis, systemic) M34.9
  circumscribed L94.0
  linear L94.1
  localized L94.0
  newborn P83.8
  systemic M34.9
Sclerokeratitis H16.8
  tuberculous A18.52
Scleroma nasi A48.8
Scleromalacia (perforans) H15.05
Scleromyxedema L98.5
Sclérose en plaques G35
Sclerosis, sclerotic
  adrenal (gland) E27.8
  Alzheimer's —*see* Disease, Alzheimer's
  amyotrophic (lateral) G12.21
  aorta, aortic I70.0
    valve —*see* Endocarditis, aortic
  artery, arterial, arteriolar, arteriovascular —*see* Arteriosclerosis
  ascending multiple G35
  brain (generalized) (lobular) G37.9
    artery, arterial I67.2
    diffuse G37.0
    disseminated G35
    insular G35
    Krabbe's E75.23
    miliary G35
    multiple G35
    presenile (Alzheimer's) —*see* Disease, Alzheimer's, early onset
    senile (arteriosclerotic) I67.2
    stem, multiple G35
    tuberous Q85.1
  bulbar, multiple G35
  bundle of His I44.39
  cardiac —*see* Disease, heart, ischemic, atherosclerotic
  cardiorenal —*see* Hypertension, cardiorenal
  cardiovascular —*see also* Disease, cardiovascular

Sclerosis, sclerotic - *continued*
  renal —*see* Hypertension, cardiorenal
  cerebellar —*see* Sclerosis, brain
  cerebral —*see* Sclerosis, brain
  cerebrospinal (disseminated) (multiple) G35
  cerebrovascular I67.2
  choroid —*see* Degeneration, choroid
  combined (spinal cord) —*see also*
  Degeneration, combined
    multiple G35
  concentric (Balo) G37.5
  cornea —*see* Opacity, cornea
  coronary (artery) I25.10
    with angina pectoris —*see* Arteriosclerosis,
  coronary (artery)
  corpus cavernosum
    female N90.89
    male N48.6
  diffuse (brain) (spinal cord) G37.0
  disseminated G35
  dorsal G35
  dorsolateral (spinal cord) —*see* Degeneration,
  combined
  endometrium N85.5
  extrapyramidal G25.9
  eye, nuclear (senile) —*see* Cataract, senile,
  nuclear
  focal and segmental (glomerular) (*see also*
  N00-N07 with fourth character .1) N05.1
  Friedreich's (spinal cord) G11.1
  funicular (spermatic cord) N50.8
  general (vascular) —*see* Arteriosclerosis
  gland (lymphatic) I89.8
  hepatic K74.1
    alcoholic K70.2
  hereditary
    cerebellar G11.9
    spinal (Friedreich's ataxia) G11.1
  hippocampal G93.81
  insular G35
  kidney —*see* Sclerosis, renal
  larynx J38.7
  lateral (amyotrophic) (descending) (primary)
  (spinal) G12.21
  lens, senile nuclear —*see* Cataract, senile,
  nuclear
  liver K74.1
    with fibrosis K74.2
      alcoholic K70.2
    alcoholic K70.2
    cardiac K76.1
  lung —*see* Fibrosis, lung
  mastoid —*see* Mastoiditis, chronic
  mesial temporal G93.81
  mitral I05.8
  Mönckeberg's (medial) —*see*
  Arteriosclerosis, extremities
  multiple (brain stem) (cerebral) (generalized)
  (spinal cord) G35
  myocardium, myocardial —*see* Disease,
  heart, ischemic, atherosclerotic
  nuclear (senile) , eye —*see* Cataract, senile,
  nuclear
  ovary N83.8
  pancreas K86.8
  penis N48.6
  peripheral arteries —*see* Arteriosclerosis,
  extremities
  plaques G35
  pluriglandular E31.8
  polyglandular E31.8

Sclerosis, sclerotic – *continued*
  posterolateral (spinal cord) —*see*
  Degeneration, combined
  presenile (Alzheimer's) —*see* Disease,
  Alzheimer's, early onset
  primary, lateral G12.29
  progressive, systemic M34.0
  pulmonary —*see* Fibrosis, lung
    artery I27.0
    valve (heart) —*see* Endocarditis, pulmonary
  renal N26.9
    with
      cystine storage disease E72.09
      hypertensive heart disease (conditions in
      I11) —*see* Hypertension, cardiorenal
      arteriolar (hyaline) (hyperplastic) —*see*
  Hypertension, kidney
  retina (senile) (vascular) H35.00
  senile (vascular) —*see* Arteriosclerosis
  spinal (cord) (progressive) G95.89
    ascending G61.0
    combined —*see also* Degeneration,
    combined
      multiple G35
      syphilitic A52.11
    disseminated G35
    dorsolateral —*see* Degeneration, combined
    hereditary (Friedreich's) (mixed form) G11.1
    lateral (amyotrophic) G12.21
    multiple G35
    posterior (syphilitic) A52.11
  stomach K31.89
  subendocardial, congenital I42.4
  systemic M34.9
    with
      lung involvement M34.81
      myopathy M34.82
      polyneuropathy M34.83
    drug-induced M34.2
    due to chemicals NEC M34.2
    progressive M34.0
    specified NEC M34.89
  temporal (mesial) G93.81
  tricuspid (heart) (valve) I07.8
  tuberous (brain) Q85.1
  tympanic membrane —*see* Disorder,
  tympanic membrane, specified NEC
  valve, valvular (heart) —*see* Endocarditis
  vascular —*see* Arteriosclerosis
  vein I87.8
Scoliosis (acquired) (postural) M41.9
  adolescent (idiopathic) —*see* Scoliosis,
  idiopathic, juvenile
  congenital Q67.5
    due to bony malformation Q76.3
    failure of segmentation (hemivertebra)
    Q76.3
    hemivertebra fusion Q76.3
    postural Q67.5
  idiopathic M41.20
    adolescent M41.129
      cervical region M41.122
      cervicothoracic region M41.123
      lumbar region M41.126
      lumbosacral region M41.127
      thoracic region M41.124
      thoracolumbar region M41.125
    cervical region M41.22
    cervicothoracic region M41.23
    infantile M41.00
      cervical region M41.02
      cervicothoracic region M41.03

Sclerosis, sclerotic – *continued*
    lumbar region M41.06
    lumbosacral region M41.07
    sacrococcygeal region M41.08
    thoracic region M41.04
    thoracolumbar region M41.05
  juvenile M41.119
    cervical region M41.112
    cervicothoracic region M41.113
    lumbar region M41.116
    lumbosacral region M41.117
    thoracic region M41.114
    thoracolumbar region M41.115
    lumbar region M41.26
    lumbosacral region M41.27
    thoracic region M41.24
    thoracolumbar region M41.25
  neuromuscular M41.40
    cervical region M41.42
    cervicothoracic region M41.43
    lumbar region M41.46
    lumbosacral region M41.47
    occipito-atlanto-axial region M41.41
    thoracic region M41.44
    thoracolumbar region M41.45
  paralytic —*see* Scoliosis, neuromuscular
  postradiation therapy M96.5
  rachitic (late effect or sequelae) E64.3
  [M49.80]
    cervical region E64.3 *[M49.82]*
    cervicothoracic region E64.3 *[M49.83]*
    lumbar region E64.3 *[M49.86]*
    lumbosacral region E64.3 *[M49.87]*
    multiple sites E64.3 *[M49.89]*
    occipito-atlanto-axial region E64.3
  [M49.81]
    sacrococcygeal region E64.3 *[M49.88]*
    thoracic region E64.3 *[M49.84]*
    thoracolumbar region E64.3 *[M49.85]*
  sciatic M54.4
  secondary (to) NEC M41.50
    cerebral palsy, Friedreich's ataxia,
  poliomyelitis, neuromuscular disorders —*see*
  Scoliosis, neuromuscular
    cervical region M41.52
    cervicothoracic region M41.53
    lumbar region M41.56
    lumbosacral region M41.57
    thoracic region M41.54
    thoracolumbar region M41.55
  specified form NEC M41.80
    cervical region M41.82
    cervicothoracic region M41.83
    lumbar region M41.86
    lumbosacral region M41.87
    thoracic region M41.84
    thoracolumbar region M41.85
  thoracogenic M41.30
    thoracic region M41.34
    thoracolumbar region M41.35
  tuberculous A18.01
Scoliotic pelvis
  with disproportion (fetopelvic) O33.0
    causing obstructed labor O65.0
Scorbutus, scorbutic —*see also* Scurvy
  anemia D53.2
Scotoma (arcuate) (Bjerrum) (central) (ring) —
  see also Defect, visual field, localized,
  scotoma
  scintillating H53.19
Scratch —*see* Abrasion
Scratchy throat R09.89

Screening (for) Z13.9
  alcoholism Z13.89
  anemia Z13.0
  anomaly, congenital Z13.89
  antenatal, of mother Z36
  arterial hypertension Z13.6
  arthropod-borne viral disease NEC Z11.59
  bacteriuria, asymptomatic Z13.89
  behavioral disorder Z13.89
  brain injury, traumatic Z13.850
  bronchitis, chronic Z13.83
  brucellosis Z11.2
  cardiovascular disorder Z13.6
  cataract Z13.5
  chlamydial diseases Z11.8
  cholera Z11.0
  chromosomal abnormalities (nonprocreative)
      NEC Z13.79
  colonoscopy Z12.11
  congenital
    dislocation of hip Z13.89
    eye disorder Z13.5
    malformation or deformation Z13.89
  contamination NEC Z13.88
  cystic fibrosis Z13.228
  dengue fever Z11.59
  dental disorder Z13.84
  depression Z13.89
  developmental handicap Z13.4
    in early childhood Z13.4
  diabetes mellitus Z13.1
  diphtheria Z11.2
  disability, intellectual Z13.4
  disease or disorder Z13.9
    bacterial NEC Z11.2
      intestinal infectious Z11.0
      respiratory tuberculosis Z11.1
    blood or blood-forming organ Z13.0
    cardiovascular Z13.6
    Chagas' Z11.6
    chlamydial Z11.8
    dental Z13.89
    developmental Z13.4
    digestive tract NEC Z13.818
      lower GI Z13.811
      upper GI Z13.810
    ear Z13.5
    endocrine Z13.29
    eye Z13.5
    genitourinary Z13.89
    heart Z13.6
    human immunodeficiency virus (HIV)
        infection Z11.4
      immunity Z13.0
    infection
        intestinal Z11.0
        specified NEC Z11.6
      infectious Z11.9
    mental Z13.89
    metabolic Z13.228
    neurological Z13.89
    nutritional Z13.21
      metabolic Z13.228
        lipoid disorders Z13.220
    protozoal Z11.6
      intestinal Z11.0
    respiratory Z13.83
    rheumatic Z13.828
    rickettsial Z11.8
    sexually-transmitted NEC Z11.3
      human immunodeficiency virus (HIV)
          Z11.4

Screening – *continued*
  sickle-cell (trait) Z13.0
  skin Z13.89
  specified NEC Z13.89
  spirochetal Z11.8
  thyroid Z13.29
  vascular Z13.6
  venereal Z11.3
  viral NEC Z11.59
    human immunodeficiency virus (HIV)
        Z11.4
    intestinal Z11.0
  elevated titer Z13.89
  emphysema Z13.83
  encephalitis, viral (mosquito or tick-borne)
      Z11.59
  exposure to contaminants (toxic) Z13.88
  fever
    dengue Z11.59
    hemorrhagic Z11.59
    yellow Z11.59
  filariasis Z11.6
  galactosemia Z13.228
  gastrointestinal condition Z13.818
  genetic (nonprocreative)
  for procreative management —*see* Testing,
  genetic, for procreative management
    disease carrier status (nonprocreative)
        Z13.71
    specified NEC (nonprocreative) Z13.79
  genitourinary condition Z13.89
  glaucoma Z13.5
  gonorrhea Z11.3
  gout Z13.89
  helminthiasis (intestinal) Z11.6
  hematopoietic malignancy Z12.89
  hemoglobinopathies NEC Z13.0
  hemorrhagic fever Z11.59
  Hodgkin disease Z12.89
  human immunodeficiency virus (HIV) Z11.4
  human papillomavirus Z11.51
  hypertension Z13.6
  immunity disorders Z13.0
  infection
    mycotic Z11.8
    parasitic Z11.8
  ingestion of radioactive substance Z13.88
  intellectual disability Z13.4
  intestinal
    helminthiasis Z11.6
    infectious disease Z11.0
  leishmaniasis Z11.6
  leprosy Z11.2
  leptospirosis Z11.8
  leukemia Z12.89
  lymphoma Z12.89
  malaria Z11.6
  malnutrition Z13.29
    metabolic Z13.228
    nutritional Z13.21
  measles Z11.59
  mental disorder Z13.89
  metabolic errors, inborn Z13.228
  multiphasic Z13.89
  musculoskeletal disorder Z13.828
    osteoporosis Z13.820
  mycoses Z11.8
  myocardial infarction (acute) Z13.6
  neoplasm (malignant) (of) Z12.9
    bladder Z12.6
    blood Z12.89

Screening – *continued*
  breast Z12.39
    routine mammogram Z12.31
  cervix Z12.4
  colon Z12.11
  genitourinary organs NEC Z12.79
    bladder Z12.6
    cervix Z12.4
    ovary Z12.73
    prostate Z12.5
    testis Z12.71
    vagina Z12.72
  hematopoietic system Z12.89
  intestinal tract Z12.10
    colon Z12.11
    rectum Z12.12
    small intestine Z12.13
  lung Z12.2
  lymph (glands) Z12.89
  nervous system Z12.82
  oral cavity Z12.81
  prostate Z12.5
  rectum Z12.12
  respiratory organs Z12.2
  skin Z12.83
  small intestine Z12.13
  specified site NEC Z12.89
  stomach Z12.0
  nephropathy Z13.89
  nervous system disorders NEC Z13.858
  neurological condition Z13.89
  osteoporosis Z13.820
  parasitic infestation Z11.9
    specified NEC Z11.8
  phenylketonuria Z13.228
  plague Z11.2
  poisoning (chemical) (heavy metal) Z13.88
  poliomyelitis Z11.59
  postnatal, chromosomal abnormalities Z13.89
  prenatal, of mother Z36
  protozoal disease Z11.6
    intestinal Z11.0
  pulmonary tuberculosis Z11.1
  radiation exposure Z13.88
  respiratory condition Z13.83
  respiratory tuberculosis Z11.1
  rheumatoid arthritis Z13.828
  rubella Z11.59
  schistosomiasis Z11.6
  sexually-transmitted disease NEC Z11.3
    human immunodeficiency virus (HIV) Z11.4
  sickle-cell disease or trait Z13.0
  skin condition Z13.89
  sleeping sickness Z11.6
  special Z13.9
    specified NEC Z13.89
  syphilis Z11.3
  tetanus Z11.2
  trachoma Z11.8
  traumatic brain injury Z13.850
  trypanosomiasis Z11.6
  tuberculosis, respiratory Z11.1
  venereal disease Z11.3
  viral encephalitis (mosquito or tick-borne)
      Z11.59
  whooping cough Z11.2
  worms, intestinal Z11.6
  yaws Z11.8
  yellow fever Z11.59
Scrofula, scrofulosis (tuberculosis of cervical
  lymph glands) A18.2
Scrofulide (primary) (tuberculous) A18.4

Scrofuloderma, scrofulodermia (any site) (primary) A18.4
Scrofulosus lichen (primary) (tuberculous) A18.4
Scrofulous —*see* condition
Scrotal tongue K14.5
Scrotum —*see* condition
Scurvy, scorbutic E54
  anemia D53.2
  gum E54
  infantile E54
  rickets E55.0 *[M90.80]*
Sealpox B08.62
Seasickness T75.3
Seatworm (infection) (infestation) B80
Sebaceous —*see also* condition
  cyst —*see* Cyst, sebaceous
Seborrhea, seborrheic L21.9
  capillitii R23.8
  capitis L21.0
  dermatitis L21.9
    infantile L21.1
  eczema L21.9
    infantile L21.1
  sicca L21.0
Seckel's syndrome Q87.1
Seclusion, pupil —*see* Membrane, pupillary
Second hand tobacco smoke exposure (acute) (chronic) Z77.22
  in the perinatal period P96.81
Secondary
  dentin (in pulp) K04.3
  neoplasm, secondaries —*see* Table of Neoplasms, secondary
Secretion
  antidiuretic hormone, inappropriate E22.2
  catecholamine, by pheochromocytoma E27.5
  hormone
    antidiuretic, inappropriate (syndrome) E22.2
    by
      carcinoid tumor E34.0
      pheochromocytoma E27.5
    ectopic NEC E34.2
  urinary
    excessive R35.8
    suppression R34
Section
  nerve, traumatic —*see* Injury, nerve
Segmentation, incomplete (congenital) —*see also* Fusion
  bone NEC Q78.8
  lumbosacral (joint) (vertebra) Q76.49
Seitelberger's syndrome (infantile neuraxonal dystrophy) G31.89
Seizure (s) (*see also* Convulsions) R56.9
  akinetic —*see* Epilepsy, generalized, specified NEC
  atonic —*see* Epilepsy, generalized, specified NEC
  autonomic (hysterical) F44.5
  convulsive —*see* Convulsions
  cortical (focal) (motor) —*see* Epilepsy, localization-related, symptomatic, with simple partial seizures
  disorder (*see also* Epilepsy) G40.909
  due to stroke —*see* Sequelae (of) , disease, cerebrovascular, by type, specified NEC
  epileptic —*see* Epilepsy
  febrile (simple) R56.00
    with status epilepticus G40.901
    complex (atypical) (complicated) R56.01
      with status epilepticus G40.901

Seizure – *continued*
  grand mal G40.409
    intractable G40.419
      with status epilepticus G40.411
      without status epilepicus G40.419
    not intractable G40.409
      with status epilepticus G40.401
      without status epilepticus G40.409
  heart —*see* Disease, heart
  hysterical F44.5
  intractable G40.919
    with status epilepticus G40.911
  Jacksonian (focal) (motor type) (sensory type) —*see* Epilepsy, localization-related, symptomatic, with simple partial seizures
  newborn P90
  nonspecific epileptic
    atonic —*see* Epilepsy, generalized, specified NEC
    clonic —*see* Epilepsy, generalized, specified NEC
    myoclonic —*see* Epilepsy, generalized, specified NEC
    tonic —*see* Epilepsy, generalized, specified NEC
    tonic-clonic —*see* Epilepsy, generalized, specified NEC
  partial, developing into secondarily generalized seizures
    complex —*see* Epilepsy, localization-related, symptomatic, with complex partial seizures
    simple —*see* Epilepsy, localization-related, symptomatic, with simple partial seizures
  petit mal G40.409
    intractable G40.419
      with status epilepticus G40.411
      without status epilepticus G40.419
    not intractable G40.409
      with status epilepticus G40.401
      without status epilepticus G40.409
  post traumatic R56.1
  recurrent G40.909
  specified NEC G40.89
  uncinate —*see* Epilepsy, localization-related, symptomatic, with complex partial seizures
Selenium deficiency, dietary E59
Self-damaging behavior (life-style) Z72.89
Self-harm (attempted)
  history (personal) Z91.5
    in family Z81.8
Self-mutilation (attempted)
  history (personal) Z91.5
    in family Z81.8
Self-poisoning
  history (personal) Z91.5
    in family Z81.8
  observation following (alleged) attempt Z03.6
Semicoma R40.1
Seminal vesiculitis N49.0
Seminoma C62.9
  specified site —*see* Neoplasm, malignant, by site
Senear-Usher disease or syndrome L10.4
Senectus R54
Senescence (without mention of psychosis) R54
Senile, senility (*see also* condition) R41.81
  with
    acute confusional state F05
    mental changes NOS F03
    psychosis NEC —*see* Psychosis, senile

Senile, senility – *continued*
  asthenia R54
  cervix (atrophic) N88.8
  debility R54
  endometrium (atrophic) N85.8
  fallopian tube (atrophic) —*see* Atrophy, fallopian tube
  heart (failure) R54
  ovary (atrophic) —*see* Atrophy, ovary
  premature E34.8
  vagina, vaginitis (atrophic) N95.2
  wart L82.1
Sensation
  burning (skin) R20.8
    tongue K14.6
  loss of R20.8
  prickling (skin) R20.2
  tingling (skin) R20.2
Sense loss
  smell —*see* Disturbance, sensation, smell
  taste —*see* Disturbance, sensation, taste
  touch R20.8
Sensibility disturbance (cortical) (deep) (vibratory) R20.9
Sensitive, sensitivity —*see also* Allergy
  carotid sinus G90.01
  child (excessive) F93.8
  cold, autoimmune D59.1
  dentin K03.89
  latex Z91.040
  methemoglobin D74.8
  tuberculin, without clinical or radiological symptoms R76.11
  visual
    glare H53.71
    impaired contrast H53.72
Sensitiver Beziehungswahn F22
Sensitization, auto-erythrocytic D69.2
Separation
  anxiety, abnormal (of childhood) F93.0
  apophysis, traumatic
    code as Fracture, by site
  choroid —*see* Detachment, choroid
  epiphysis, epiphyseal
    nontraumatic —*see also* Osteochondropathy, specified type NEC
      upper femoral —*see* Slipped, epiphysis, upper femoral
    traumatic
      code as Fracture, by site
  fracture —*see* Fracture
  infundibulum cardiac from right ventricle by a partition Q24.3
  joint (traumatic) (current)
    code by site under Dislocation
  pubic bone, obstetrical trauma O71.6
  retina, retinal —*see* Detachment, retina
  symphysis pubis, obstetrical trauma O71.6
  tracheal ring, incomplete, congenital Q32.1
Sepsis (generalized) (unspecified organism) A41.9
  with
    organ dysfunction (acute) (multiple) R65.20
      with septic shock R65.21
  actinomycotic A42.7
  adrenal hemorrhage syndrome (meningococcal) A39.1
  anaerobic A41.4
  Bacillus anthracis A22.7
  Brucella (*see also* Brucellosis) A23.9
  candidal B37.7
  cryptogenic A41.9

Sepsis – *continued*
  due to device, implant or graft T85.79
    arterial graft NEC T82.7
    breast (implant) T85.79
    catheter NEC T85.79
      dialysis (renal) T82.7
        intraperitoneal T85.71
      infusion NEC T82.7
        spinal (epidural) (subdural) T85.79
      urinary (indwelling) T83.51
    ectopic or molar pregnancy O08.82
    electronic (electrode) (pulse generator)
        (stimulator)
      bone T84.7
      cardiac T82.7
      nervous system (brain) (peripheral nerve)
          (spinal) T85.79
      urinary T83.59
    fixation, internal (orthopedic) —*see*
Complication, fixation device, infection
    gastrointestinal (bile duct) (esophagus)
        T85.79
    genital T83.6
    heart NEC T82.7
      valve (prosthesis) T82.6
        graft T82.7
    joint prosthesis —*see* Complication, joint
prosthesis, infection
    ocular (corneal graft) (orbital implant)
        T85.79
    orthopedic NEC T84.7
      fixation device, internal —*see*
Complication, fixation device, infection
    specified NEC T85.79
    vascular T82.7
    ventricular intracranial shunt T85.79
  during labor O75.3
  Enterococcus A41.81
  Erysipelothrix (rhusiopathiae) (erysipeloid)
      A26.7
  Escherichia coli (E. coli) A41.5
  extraintestinal yersiniosis A28.2
  following
    abortion (subsequent episode) O08.0
      current episode —*see* Abortion
    ectopic or molar pregnancy O08.82
    immunization T88.0
    infusion, therapeutic injection or transfusion
NEC T80.29
  gangrenous A41.9
  gonococcal A54.86
  Gram-negative (organism) A41.5
    anaerobic A41.4
  Haemophilus influenzae A41.3
  herpesviral B00.7
  intra-abdominal K65.1
  intraocular —*see* Endophthalmitis, purulent
  Listeria monocytogenes A32.7
  localized
  code to specific localized infection
    in operation wound T81.4
    skin —*see* Abscess
  malleus A24.0
  melioidosis A24.1
  meningeal —*see* Meningitis
  meningococcal A39.4
    acute A39.2
    chronic A39.3
  MSSA (Methicillin susceptible
    Staphylococcus aureus) A41.01

Sepsis – *continued*
  newborn P36.9
    due to
      anaerobes NEC P36.5
      Escherichia coli P36.4
      Staphylococcus P36.30
        aureus P36.2
        specified NEC P36.39
      Streptococcus P36.10
        group B P36.0
        specified NEC P36.19
      specified NEC P36.8
  Pasteurella multocida A28.0
  pelvic, puerperal, postpartum, childbirth O85
  postprocedural T81.4
  pneumococcal A40.3
  puerperal, postpartum, childbirth (pelvic) O85
  Salmonella (arizonae) (cholerae-suis)
  (enteritidis) (typhimurium) A02.1
  severe R65.20
    with septic shock R65.21
  skin, localized —*see* Abscess
  Shigella (*see also* Dysentery, bacillary) A03.9
  specified organism NEC A41.89
  Staphylococcus, staphylococcal A41.2
    aureus (methicillin susceptible) (MSSA)
      A41.01
      methicillin resistant (MRSA) A41.02
    coagulase-negative A41.1
    specified NEC A41.1
  Streptococcus, streptococcal A40.9
    agalactiae A40.1
    group
      A A40.0
      B A40.1
      D A41.81
    neonatal P36.10
      group B P36.0
      specified NEC P36.19
    pneumoniae A40.3
    pyogenes A40.0
    specified NEC A40.8
  tracheostomy stoma J95.02
  tularemic A21.7
  umbilical, umbilical cord (newborn) —*see*
Sepsis, newborn
  Yersinia pestis A20.7
Septate —*see* Septum
Septic —*see* condition
  arm —*see* Cellulitis, upper limb
    with lymphangitis —*see* Lymphangitis,
acute, upper limb
  embolus —*see* Embolism
  finger —*see* Cellulitis, digit
    with lymphangitis —*see* Lymphangitis,
acute, digit
  foot —*see* Cellulitis, lower limb
    with lymphangitis —*see* Lymphangitis,
acute, lower limb
  gallbladder (acute) K81.0
  hand —*see* Cellulitis, upper limb
    with lymphangitis —*see* Lymphangitis,
acute, upper limb
  joint —*see* Arthritis, pyogenic or pyemic
  leg —*see* Cellulitis, lower limb
    with lymphangitis —*see* Lymphangitis,
acute, lower limb
  nail —*see also* Cellulitis, digit
    with lymphangitis —*see* Lymphangitis,
acute, digit

Septic – *continued*
  sore —*see also* Abscess
    throat J02.0
      streptococcal J02.0
  spleen (acute) D73.89
  teeth, tooth (pulpal origin) K04.4
  throat —*see* Pharyngitis
  thrombus —*see* Thrombosis
  toe —*see* Cellulitis, digit
    with lymphangitis —*see* Lymphangitis,
acute, digit
  tonsils, chronic J35.01
    with adenoiditis J35.03
  uterus —*see* Endometritis
Septicemia A41.9
  meaning sepsis —*see* Sepsis
Septum, septate (congenital) —*see also*
Anomaly, by site
  with fistula Q42.2
  aqueduct of Sylvius Q03.0
    with spina bifida —*see* Spina bifida, by site,
with hydrocephalus
  uterus (complete) (partial) Q51.2
  vagina Q52.10
    in pregnancy —*see* Pregnancy, complicated
by, abnormal vagina
      causing obstructed labor O65.5
    longitudinal (with or without obstruction)
        Q52.12
    transverse Q52.11
Sequelae (of) —*see also* condition
  abscess, intracranial or intraspinal (conditions
in G06) G09
  amputation
  code to injury with seventh character S
  burn and corrosion
  code to injury with seventh character S
  calcium deficiency E64.8
  cerebrovascular disease —*see* Sequelae,
disease, cerebrovascular
  childbirth O94
  contusion
  code to injury with seventh character S
  corrosion —*see* Sequelae, burn and corrosion
  crushing injury
  code to injury with seventh character S
  disease
    cerebrovascular I69.90
      alteration of sensation I69.998
      aphasia I69.920
      apraxia I69.990
      ataxia I69.993
      cognitive deficits I69.91
      disturbance of vision I69.998
      dysarthria I69.922
      dysphagia I69.991
      dysphasia I69.921
      facial droop I69.992
      facial weakness I69.992
      fluency disorder I69.923
      hemiplegia I69.95
      hemorrhage
        intracerebral —*see* Sequelae,
hemorrhage, intracerebral
        intracranial, nontraumatic NEC —*see*
Sequelae, hemorrhage, intracranial,
nontraumatic
        subarachnoid —*see* Sequelae,
hemorrhage, subarachnoid
      language deficit I69.928
      monoplegia
        lower limb I69.84
        upper limb I69.93

Sequelae - *continued*
   paralytic syndrome I69.96
   specified effect NEC I69.998
   specified type NEC I69.80
     alteration of sensation I69.898
     aphasia I69.820
     apraxia I69.890
     ataxia I69.893
     cognitive deficits I69.81
     disturbance of vision I69.898
     dysarthria I69.822
     dysphagia I69.891
     dysphasia I69.821
     facial droop I69.892
     facial weakness I69.892
     fluency disorder I69.823
     hemiplegia I69.85
     language deficit I69.828
     monoplegia
       lower limb I69.84
       upper limb I69.83
     paralytic syndrome I69.86
     specified effect NEC I69.898
     speech deficit I69.928
     speech deficit I69.828
    stroke NOS —*see* Sequelae, stroke NOS
  dislocation
  code to injury with seventh character S
  encephalitis or encephalomyelitis (conditions
  in G04) G09
   in infectious disease NEC B94.8
   viral B94.1
  external cause
  code to injury with seventh character S
  foreign body entering natural orifice
  code to injury with seventh character S
  fracture
  code to injury with seventh character S
  frostbite
  code to injury with seventh character S
  Hansen's disease B92
  hemorrhage
   intracerebral I69.10
    alteration of sensation I69.198
    aphasia I69.120
    apraxia I69.190
    ataxia I69.193
    cognitive deficits I69.11
    disturbance of vision I69.198
    dysarthria I69.122
    dysphagia I69.191
    dysphasia I69.121
    facial droop I69.192
    facial weakness I69.192
    fluency disorder I69.123
    hemiplegia I69.15
    language deficit NEC I69.128
    monoplegia
      lower limb I69.14
      upper limb I69.13
    paralytic syndrome I69.16
    specified effect NEC I69.198
    speech deficit NEC I69.128
   intracranial, nontraumatic NEC I69.20
    alteration of sensation I69.298
    aphasia I69.220
    apraxia I69.290
    ataxia I69.293
    cognitive deficits I69.21
    disturbance of vision I69.298
    dysarthria I69.222
    dysphagia I69.291

Sequelae - *continued*
    dysphasia I69.221
    facial droop I69.292
    facial weakness I69.292
    fluency disorder I69.223
    hemiplegia I69.25
    language deficit NEC I69.228
    monoplegia
      lower limb I69.24
      upper limb I69.23
    paralytic syndrome I69.26
    specified effect NEC I69.298
    speech deficit NEC I69.228
   subarachnoid I69.00
    alteration of sensation I69.098
    aphasia I69.020
    apraxia I69.090
    ataxia I69.093
    cognitive deficits I69.01
    disturbance of vision I69.098
    dysarthria I69.022
    dysphagia I69.091
    dysphasia I69.021
    facial droop I69.092
    facial weakness I69.092
    fluency disorder I69.023
    hemiplegia I69.05
    language deficit NEC I69.028
    monoplegia
      lower limb I69.04
      upper limb I69.03
    paralytic syndrome I69.06
    specified effect NEC I69.098
    speech deficit NEC I69.028
  hepatitis, viral B94.2
  hyperalimentation E68
  infarction
   cerebral I69.30
    alteration of sensation I69.398
    aphasia I69.320
    apraxia I69.390
    ataxia I69.393
    cognitive deficits I69.31
    disturbance of vision I69.398
    dysarthria I69.322
    dysphagia I69.391
    dysphasia I69.321
    facial droop I69.392
    facial weakness I69.392
    fluency disorder I69.323
    hemiplegia I69.35
    language deficit NEC I69.328
    monoplegia
      lower limb I69.34
      upper limb I69.33
    paralytic syndrome I69.36
    specified effect NEC I69.398
    speech deficit NEC I69.328
  infection, pyogenic, intracranial or intraspinal
  G09
  infectious disease B94.9
   specified NEC B94.8
  injury
  code to injury with seventh character S
  leprosy B92
  meningitis
   bacterial (conditions in G00) G09
   other or unspecified cause (conditions in
  G03) G09
  muscle (and tendon) injury
  code to injury with seventh character S
  myelitis —*see* Sequelae, encephalitis

Sequelae - *continued*
  niacin deficiency E64.8
  nutritional deficiency E64.9
   specified NEC E64.8
  obstetrical condition O94
  parasitic disease B94.9
  phlebitis or thrombophlebitis of intracranial or
  intraspinal venous sinuses and veins
  (conditions in G08) G09
  poisoning
  code to poisoning with seventh character S
   nonmedicinal substance —*see* Sequelae,
  toxic effect, nonmedicinal substance
  poliomyelitis (acute) B91
  pregnancy O94
  protein-energy malnutrition E64.0
  puerperium O94
  rickets E64.3
  selenium deficiency E64.8
  sprain and strain
  code to injury with seventh character S
  stroke NOS I69.30
   alteration in sensation I69.398
   aphasia I69.320
   apraxia I69.390
   ataxia I69.393
   cognitive deficits I69.31
   disturbance of vision I69.398
   dysarthria I69.322
   dysphagia I69.391
   dysphasia I69.321
   facial droop I69.392
   facial weakness I69.392
   hemiplegia I69.35
   language deficit NEC I69.328
   monoplegia
    lower limb I69.34
    upper limb I69.33
   paralytic syndrome I69.36
   specified effect NEC I69.398
   speech deficit NEC I69.328
  tendon and muscle injury
  code to injury with seventh character S
  thiamine deficiency E64.8
  trachoma B94.0
  tuberculosis B90.9
   bones and joints B90.2
   central nervous system B90.0
   genitourinary B90.1
   pulmonary (respiratory) B90.9
   specified organs NEC B90.8
  viral
   encephalitis B94.1
   hepatitis B94.2
  vitamin deficiency NEC E64.8
   A E64.1
   B E64.8
   C E64.2
  wound, open
  code to injury with seventh character S
Sequestration —*see also* Sequestrum
  lung, congenital Q33.2
Sequestrum
  bone —*see* Osteomyelitis, chronic
  dental M27.2
  jaw bone M27.2
  orbit —*see* Osteomyelitis, orbit
  sinus (accessory) (nasal) —*see* Sinusitis
Sequoiosis lung or pneumonitis J67.8
Serology for syphilis
  doubtful
   with signs or symptoms

Serology for syphilis - *continued*
code by site and stage under Syphilis
follow-up of latent syphilis —*see* Syphilis, latent
negative, with signs or symptoms
code by site and stage under Syphilis
positive A53.0
with signs or symptoms
code by site and stage under Syphilis
reactivated A53.0
Seroma —*see also* Hematoma
traumatic, secondary and recurrent T79.2
Seropurulent —*see* condition
Serositis, multiple K65.8
pericardial I31.1
peritoneal K65.8
Serous —*see* condition
Sertoli cell
adenoma
specified site —*see* Neoplasm, benign, by site
unspecified site
female D27.9
male D29.20
carcinoma
specified site —*see* Neoplasm, malignant, by site
unspecified site (male) C62.9
female C56.9
tumor
with lipid storage
specified site —*see* Neoplasm, benign, by site
unspecified site
female D27.9
male D29.20
specified site —*see* Neoplasm, benign, by site
unspecified site
female D27.9
male D29.20
Sertoli-Leydig cell tumor —*see* Neoplasm, benign, by site
specified site —*see* Neoplasm, benign, by site
unspecified site
female D27.9
male D29.20
Serum
allergy, allergic reaction (*see also* Reaction, serum) T80.69
shock (*see also* Shock, anaphylactic) T80.59
arthritis (*see also* Reaction, serum) T80.69
complication or reaction NEC (*see also* Reaction, serum) T80.69
disease NEC (*see also* Reaction, serum) T80.69
hepatitis —*see also* Hepatitis, viral, type B
carrier (suspected) of Z22.51
intoxication (*see also* Reaction, serum) T80.69
neuritis (*see also* Reaction, serum) T80.69
neuropathy G61.1
poisoning NEC (*see also* Reaction, serum) T80.69
rash NEC (*see also* Reaction, serum) T80.69
reaction NEC (*see also* Reaction, serum) T80.69
sickness NEC (*see also* Reaction, serum) T80.69
urticaria (*see also* Reaction, serum) T80.69
Sesamoiditis M25.8
Sever's disease or osteochondrosis —*see* Osteochondrosis, juvenile, tarsus

Severe sepsis R65.20
with septic shock R65.21
Sex
chromosome mosaics Q97.8
lines with various numbers of X chromosomes Q97.2
education Z70.8
reassignment surgery status Z87.890
Sextuplet pregnancy —*see* Pregnancy, sextuplet
Sexual
function, disorder of (psychogenic) F52.9
immaturity (female) (male) E30.0
impotence (psychogenic) organic origin NEC —*see* Dysfunction, sexual, male
precocity (constitutional) (cryptogenic) (female) (idiopathic) (male) E30.1
Sexuality, pathologic —*see* Deviation, sexual
Sézary disease C84.1
Shadow, lung R91.8
Shaking palsy or paralysis —*see* Parkinsonism
Shallowness, acetabulum —*see* Derangement, joint, specified type NEC, hip
Shaver's disease J63.1
Sheath (tendon) —*see* condition
Sheathing, retinal vessels H35.01
Shedding
nail L60.8
premature, primary (deciduous) teeth K00.6
Sheehan's disease or syndrome E23.0
Shelf, rectal K62.89
Shell teeth K00.5
Shellshock (current) F43.0
lasting state —*see* Disorder, post-traumatic stress
Shield kidney Q63.1
Shift
auditory threshold (temporary) H93.24
mediastinal R93.8
Shifting sleep-work schedule (affecting sleep) G47.26
Shiga (-Kruse) **dysentery** A03.0
Shiga's bacillus A03.0
Shigella (dysentery) —*see* Dysentery, bacillary
Shigellosis A03.9
Group A A03.0
Group B A03.1
Group C A03.2
Group D A03.3
Shin splints S86.89
Shingles —*see* Herpes, zoster
Shipyard disease or eye B30.0
Shirodkar suture, in pregnancy —*see* Pregnancy, complicated by, incompetent cervix
Shock R57.9
with ectopic or molar pregnancy O08.3
adrenal (cortical) (Addisonian) E27.2
adverse food reaction (anaphylactic) —*see* Shock, anaphylactic, due to food
allergic —*see* Shock, anaphylactic
anaphylactic T78.2
chemical —*see* Table of Drugs and Chemicals
due to drug or medicinal substance
correct substance properly administered T88.6
overdose or wrong substance given or taken (by accident) —*see* Table of Drugs and Chemicals, by drug, poisoning

Shock – *continued*
due to food (nonpoisonous) T78.00
additives T78.06
dairy products T78.07
eggs T78.08
fish T78.03
shellfish T78.02
fruit T78.04
milk T78.07
nuts T78.05
peanuts T78.01
peanuts T78.01
seeds T78.05
specified type NEC T78.09
vegetable T78.04
following sting (s) —*see* Venom
immunization T80.52
serum T80.59
blood and blood products T80.51
immunization T80.52
specified NEC T80.59
vaccination T80.52
anaphylactoid —*see* Shock, anaphylactic
anesthetic
correct substance properly administered T88.2
overdose or wrong substance given or taken —*see* Table of Drugs and Chemicals, by drug, poisoning
specified anesthetic —*see* Table of Drugs and Chemicals, by drug, poisoning
cardiogenic R57.0
chemical substance —*see* Table of Drugs and Chemicals
complicating ectopic or molar pregnancy O08.3
culture —*see* Disorder, adjustment
drug
due to correct substance properly administered T88.6
overdose or wrong substance given or taken (by accident) —*see* Table of Drugs and Chemicals, by drug, poisoning
during or after labor and delivery O75.1
electric T75.4
(taser) T75.4
endotoxic R65.21
postprocedural (during or resulting from a procedure, not elsewhere classified) T81.12
following
ectopic or molar pregnancy O08.3
injury (immediate) (delayed) T79.4
labor and delivery O75.1
food (anaphylactic) —*see* Shock, anaphylactic, due to food
from electroshock gun (taser) T75.4
gram-negative R65.21
postprocedural (during or resulting from a procedure, not elsewhere classified) T81.12
hematologic R57.8
hemorrhagic
surgery (intraoperative) (postoperative) T81.19
trauma T79.4
hypovolemic R57.1
surgical T81.19
traumatic T79.4
insulin E15
therapeutic misadventure —*see* subcategory T38.3
kidney N17.0
traumatic (following crushing) T79.5

Shock – *continued*
  lightning T75.01
  lung J80
  obstetric O75.1
    with ectopic or molar pregnancy O08.3
    following ectopic or molar pregnancy O08.3
  pleural (surgical) T81.19
    due to trauma T79.4
  postprocedural (postoperative) T81.10
    with ectopic or molar pregnancy O08.3
    cardiogenic T81.11
    endotoxic T81.12
    following ectopic or molar pregnancy O08.3
    gram-negative T81.12
    hypovolemic T81.19
    septic T81.12
    specified type NEC T81.19
  psychic F43.0
  septic (due to severe sepsis) R65.21
  specified NEC R57.8
  surgical T81.10
  taser gun (taser) T75.4
  therapeutic misadventure NEC T81.10
  thyroxin
    overdose or wrong substance given or taken
    —*see* Table of Drugs and Chemicals, by drug,
    poisoning
  toxic, syndrome A48.3
  transfusion —*see* Complications, transfusion
  traumatic (immediate) (delayed) T79.4
Shoemaker's chest M95.4
Short, shortening, shortness
  arm (acquired) —*see also* Deformity, limb,
  unequal length
    congenital Q71.81
    forearm —*see* Deformity, limb, unequal
    length
  bowel syndrome K91.2
  breath R06.02
  cervical (complicating pregnancy) O26.87
    non-gravid uterus N88.3
  common bile duct, congenital Q44.5
  cord (umbilical) , complicating delivery
  O69.3
  cystic duct, congenital Q44.5
  esophagus (congenital) Q39.8
  femur (acquired) —*see* Deformity, limb,
  unequal length, femur
    congenital —*see* Defect, reduction, lower
    limb, longitudinal, femur
  frenum, frenulum, linguae (congenital) Q38.1
  hip (acquired) —*see also* Deformity, limb,
  unequal length
    congenital Q65.89
  leg (acquired) —*see also* Deformity, limb,
  unequal length
    congenital Q72.81
    lower leg —*see also* Deformity, limb,
  unequal length
  limbed stature, with immunodeficiency D82.2
  lower limb (acquired) —*see also* Deformity,
  limb, unequal length
    congenital Q72.81
  organ or site, congenital NEC —*see*
  Distortion
  palate, congenital Q38.5
  radius (acquired) —*see also* Deformity, limb,
  unequal length
    congenital —*see* Defect, reduction, upper
    limb, longitudinal, radius
  rib syndrome Q77.2

Short, shortening, shortness - *continued*
  stature (child) (hereditary) (idiopathic) NEC
  R62.52
    constitutional E34.3
    due to endocrine disorder E34.3
    Laron-type E34.3
  tendon —*see also* Contraction, tendon
    with contracture of joint —*see* Contraction,
  joint
    Achilles (acquired) M67.0
      congenital Q66.89
    congenital Q79.8
  thigh (acquired) —*see also* Deformity, limb,
  unequal length, femur
    congenital —*see* Defect, reduction, lower
  limb, longitudinal, femur
  tibialis anterior (tendon) —*see* Contraction,
  tendon
  umbilical cord
    complicating delivery O69.3
  upper limb, congenital —*see* Defect,
  reduction, upper limb, specified type NEC
  urethra N36.8
  uvula, congenital Q38.5
  vagina (congenital) Q52.4
Shortsightedness —*see* Myopia
Shoshin (acute fulminating beriberi) E51.11
Shoulder —*see* condition
Shovel-shaped incisors K00.2
Shower, thromboembolic —*see* Embolism
Shunt
  arterial-venous (dialysis) Z99.2
  arteriovenous, pulmonary (acquired) I28.0
    congenital Q25.72
  cerebral ventricle (communicating) in situ
  Z98.2
  surgical, prosthetic, with complications —*see*
  Complications, cardiovascular, device or
  implant
Shutdown, renal N28.9
Shy-Drager syndrome G90.3
Sialadenitis, sialadenosis (any gland)
  (chronic) (periodic) (suppurative) —*see*
  Sialoadenitis
Sialectasia K11.8
Sialidosis E77.1
Sialitis, silitis (any gland) (chronic)
  (suppurative) —*see* Sialoadenitis
Sialoadenitis (any gland) (periodic)
  (suppurative) K11.20
  acute K11.21
    recurrent K11.22
  chronic K11.23
Sialadenopathy K11.9
Sialoangitis —*see* Sialoadenitis
Sialodochitis (fibrinosa) —*see* Sialoadenitis
Sialodocholithiasis K11.5
Sialolithiasis K11.5
Sialometaplasia, necrotizing K11.8
Sialorrhea —*see also* Ptyalism
  periodic —*see* Sialoadenitis
Sialosis K11.7
Siamese twin Q89.4
Sibling rivalry Z62.891
Sicard's syndrome G52.7
Sicca syndrome M35.00
  with
    keratoconjunctivitis M35.01
    lung involvement M35.02
    myopathy M35.03
    renal tubulo-interstitial disorders M35.04
  specified organ involvement NEC M35.09

Sick R69
  or handicapped person in family Z63.79
    needing care at home Z63.6
  sinus (syndrome) I49.5
Sick-euthyroid syndrome E07.81
Sickle-cell
  anemia —*see* Disease, sickle-cell
  trait D57.3
Sicklemia —*see also* Disease, sickle-cell
  trait D57.3
Sickness
  air (travel) T75.3
  airplane T75.3
  alpine T70.29
  altitude T70.20
  Andes T70.29
  aviator's T70.29
  balloon T70.29
  car T75.3
  compressed air T70.3
  decompression T70.3
  green D50.8
  milk —*see* Poisoning, food, noxious
  motion T75.3
  mountain T70.29
    acute D75.1
  protein (*see also* Reaction, serum) T80.69
  radiation T66
  roundabout (motion) T75.3
  sea T75.3
  serum NEC (*see also* Reaction, serum)
  T80.69
  sleeping (African) B56.9
    by Trypanosoma B56.9
      brucei
        gambiense B56.0
        rhodesiense B56.1
    East African B56.1
    Gambian B56.0
    Rhodesian B56.1
    West African B56.0
  swing (motion) T75.3
  train (railway) (travel) T75.3
  travel (any vehicle) T75.3
Sideropenia —*see* Anemia, iron deficiency
Siderosilicosis J62.8
Siderosis (lung) J63.4
  eye (globe) —*see* Disorder, globe,
  degenerative, siderosis
Siemens' syndrome (ectodermal dysplasia)
  Q82.8
Sighing R06.89
  psychogenic F45.8
Sigmoid —*see also* condition
  flexure —*see* condition
  kidney Q63.1
Sigmoiditis (*see also* Enteritis) K52.9
  infectious A09
  noninfectious K52.9
Silfversköld's syndrome Q78.9
Silicosiderosis J62.8
Silicosis, silicotic (simple) (complicated) J62.8
  with tuberculosis J65
Silicotuberculosis J65
Silo-fillers' disease J68.8
  bronchitis J68.0
  pneumonitis J68.0
  pulmonary edema J68.1
Silver's syndrome Q87.1
Simian malaria B53.1
Simmonds' cachexia or disease E23.0
Simons' disease or syndrome (progressive
  lipodystrophy) E88.1

Simple, simplex —*see* condition
Simulation, conscious (of illness) Z76.5
Simultanagnosia (asimultagnosia) R48.3
Sin Nombre virus disease (Hantavirus)
(cardio) -pulmonary syndrome) B33.4
Sinding-Larsen disease or osteochondrosis
—*see* Osteochondrosis, juvenile, patella
Singapore hemorrhagic fever A91
Singer's node or nodule J38.2
Single
  atrium Q21.2
  coronary artery Q24.5
  umbilical artery Q27.0
  ventricle Q20.4
Singultus R06.6
  epidemicus B33.0
Sinus —*see also* Fistula
  abdominal K63.89
  arrest I45.5
  arrhythmia I49.8
  bradycardia R00.1
  branchial cleft (internal) (external) Q18.0
  coccygeal —*see* Sinus, pilonidal
  dental K04.6
  dermal (congenital) Q06.8
    with abscess Q06.8
    coccygeal, pilonidal —*see* Sinus, coccygeal
  infected, skin NEC L08.89
  marginal, ruptured or bleeding —*see*
  Hemorrhage, antepartum, specified cause
  NEC
  medial, face and neck Q18.8
  pause I45.5
  pericranii Q01.9
  pilonidal (infected) (rectum) L05.92
    with abscess L05.02
  preauricular Q18.1
  rectovaginal N82.3
  Rokitansky-Aschoff (gallbladder) K82.8
  sacrococcygeal (dermoid) (infected) —*see*
  Sinus, pilonidal
  tachycardia R00.0
    paroxysmal I47.1
  tarsi syndrome
  M25.57
  testis N50.8
  tract (postinfective) —*see* Fistula
  urachus Q64.4
Sinusitis (accessory) (chronic) (hyperplastic)
(nasal) (nonpurulent) (purulent) J32.9
  acute J01.90
    ethmoidal J01.20
      recurrent J01.21
    frontal J01.10
      recurrent J01.11
    involving more than one sinus, other than
    pansinusitis J01.80
      recurrent J01.81
    maxillary J01.00
      recurrent J01.01
    pansinusitis J01.40
      recurrent J01.41
    recurrent J01.91
    specified NEC J01.80
      recurrent J01.81
    sphenoidal J01.30
      recurrent J01.31
  allergic —*see* Rhinitis, allergic
  due to high altitude T70.1
  ethmoidal J32.2
    acute J01.20
      recurrent J01.21

Sinusitis – *continued*
  frontal J32.1
    acute J01.10
      recurrent J01.11
  influenzal —*see* Influenza, with, respiratory
  manifestations NEC
  involving more than one sinus but not
  pansinusitis J32.8
    acute J01.80
      recurrent J01.81
  maxillary J32.0
    acute J01.00
      recurrent J01.01
  sphenoidal J32.3
    acute J01.30
      recurrent J01.31
  tuberculous, any sinus A15.8
Sinusitis-bronchiectasis-situs inversus
(syndrome) (triad) Q89.3
Sipple's syndrome E31.22
Sirenomelia (syndrome) Q87.2
Siriasis T67.0
Sirkari's disease B55.0
Siti A65
Situation, psychiatric F99
Situational
  disturbance (transient) —*see* Disorder,
  adjustment
    acute F43.0
  maladjustment —*see* Disorder, adjustment
  reaction —*see* Disorder, adjustment
    acute F43.0
Situs inversus or transversus (abdominalis)
(thoracis) Q89.3
Sixth disease B08.20
  due to human herpesvirus 6 B08.21
  due to human herpesvirus 7 B08.22
Sjögren-Larsson syndrome Q87.1
Sjögren's syndrome or disease —*see* Sicca
syndrome
Skeletal —*see* condition
Skene's gland —*see* condition
Skenitis —*see* Urethritis
Skerljevo A65
Skevas-Zerfus disease —*see* Toxicity, venom,
marine animal, sea anemone
Skin —*see also* condition
  clammy R23.1
  donor —*see* Donor, skin
  hidebound M35.9
Slate-dressers' or slate-miners' lung J62.8
Sleep
  apnea —*see* Apnea, sleep
  deprivation Z72.820
  disorder or disturbance G47.9
    child F51.9
    nonorganic origin F51.9
    specified NEC G47.8
  disturbance G47.9
    nonorganic origin F51.9
  drunkenness F51.9
  rhythm inversion G47.2
  terrors F51.4
  walking F51.3
    hysterical F44.89
Sleep hygiene
  abuse Z72.821
  inadequate Z72.821
  poor Z72.821
Sleeping sickness —*see* Sickness, sleeping
Sleeplessness —*see* Insomnia
  menopausal N95.1
Sleep-wake schedule disorder G47.20

Slim disease (in HIV infection) B20
Slipped, slipping
  epiphysis (traumatic) —*see also*
  Osteochondropathy, specified type NEC
    capital femoral (traumatic)
      acute (on chronic) S79.01
    current traumatic
    code as Fracture, by site
    upper femoral (nontraumatic) M93.00
      acute M93.01
        on chronic M93.03
      chronic M93.02
  intervertebral disc —*see* Displacement,
  intervertebral disc
  ligature, umbilical P51.8
  patella —*see* Disorder, patella, derangement
  NEC
  rib M89.8X8
  sacroiliac joint —*see* subcategory M53.2
  tendon —*see* Disorder, tendon
  ulnar nerve, nontraumatic —*see* Lesion,
  nerve, ulnar
  vertebra NEC —*see* Spondylolisthesis
Slocumb's syndrome E27.0
Sloughing (multiple) (phagedena) (skin) —*see*
also Gangrene
  abscess —*see* Abscess
  appendix K38.8
  fascia —*see* Disorder, soft tissue, specified
  type NEC
  scrotum N50.8
  tendon —*see* Disorder, tendon
  transplanted organ —*see* Rejection, transplant
  ulcer —*see* Ulcer, skin
Slow
  feeding, newborn P92.2
  flow syndrome, coronary I20.8
  heart (beat) R00.1
Slowing, urinary stream R39.19
Sluder's neuralgia (syndrome) G44.89
Slurred, slurring speech R47.81
Small (ness)
  for gestational age —*see* Small for dates
  introitus, vagina N89.6
  kidney (unknown cause) N27.9
    bilateral N27.1
    unilateral N27.0
  ovary (congenital) Q50.39
  pelvis
    with disproportion (fetopelvic) O33.1
      causing obstructed labor O65.1
  uterus N85.8
  white kidney N03.9
Small-and-light-for-dates —*see* Small for
dates
Small-for-dates (infant) P05.10
  with weight of
    499 grams or less P05.11
    500 749 grams P05.12
    750 999 grams P05.13
    1000 1249 grams P05.14
    1250 1499 grams P05.15
    1500 1749 grams P05.16
    1750 1999 grams P05.17
    2000 2499 grams P05.18
Smallpox B03
Smearing, fecal R15.1
Smith-Lemli-Opitz syndrome E78.72
Smith's fracture S52.54
Smoker —*see* Dependence, drug, nicotine

Smoker's
bronchitis J41.0
cough J41.0
palate K13.24
throat J31.2
tongue K13.24
Smoking
passive Z77.22
Smothering spells R06.81
Snaggle teeth, tooth M26.39
Snapping
finger —see Trigger finger
hip —see Derangement, joint, specified type NEC, hip
involving the iliotibial band M76.3
knee —see Derangement, knee
involving the iliotibial band M76.3
Sneddon-Wilkinson disease or syndrome
(sub-corneal pustular dermatosis) L13.1
Sneezing (intractable) R06.7
Sniffing
cocaine
abuse —see Abuse, drug, cocaine
dependence —see Dependence, drug, cocaine
gasoline
abuse —see Abuse, drug, inhalant
dependence —see Dependence, drug, inhalant
glue (airplane)
abuse —see Abuse, drug, inhalant
drug dependence —see Dependence, drug, inhalant
Sniffles
newborn P28.89
Snoring R06.83
Snow blindness —see Photokeratitis
Snuffles (non-syphilitic) R06.5
newborn P28.89
syphilitic (infant) A50.05 [J99]
Social
exclusion Z60.4
due to discrimination or persecution (perceived) Z60.5
migrant Z59.0
acculturation difficulty Z60.3
rejection Z60.4
due to discrimination or persecution Z60.5
role conflict NEC Z73.5
skills inadequacy NEC Z73.4
transplantation Z60.3
Sodoku A25.0
Soemmerring's ring —see Cataract, secondary
Soft —see also condition
nails L60.3
Softening
bone —see Osteomalacia
brain (necrotic) (progressive) G93.89
congenital Q04.8
embolic I63.4
hemorrhagic —see Hemorrhage, intracranial, intracerebral
occlusive I63.5
thrombotic I63.3
cartilage M94.2
patella M22.4
cerebellar —see Softening, brain
cerebral —see Softening, brain
cerebrospinal —see Softening, brain
myocardial, heart —see Degeneration, myocardial
spinal cord G95.89
stomach K31.89

Soldier's
heart F45.8
patches I31.0
Solitary
cyst, kidney N28.1
kidney, congenital Q60.0
Solvent abuse —see Abuse, drug, inhalant
dependence —see Dependence, drug, inhalant
Somatization reaction, somatic reaction —
see Disorder, somatoform
Somnambulism F51.3
hysterical F44.89
Somnolence R40.0
nonorganic origin F51.11
Sonne dysentery A03.3
Soor B37.0
Sore
bed —see Ulcer, pressure, by site
chiclero B55.1
Delhi B55.1
desert —see Ulcer, skin
eye H57.1
Lahore B55.1
mouth K13.79
canker K12.0
muscle M79.1
Naga —see Ulcer, skin
of skin —see Ulcer, skin
oriental B55.1
pressure —see Ulcer, pressure, by site
skin L98.9
soft A57
throat (acute) —see also Pharyngitis
with influenza, flu, or grippe —see Influenza, with, respiratory manifestations NEC
chronic J31.2
coxsackie (virus) B08.5
diphtheritic A36.0
herpesviral B00.2
influenzal —see Influenza, with, respiratory manifestations NEC
septic J02.0
streptococcal (ulcerative) J02.0
viral NEC J02.8
coxsackie B08.5
tropical —see Ulcer, skin
veldt —see Ulcer, skin
Soto's syndrome (cerebral gigantism) Q87.3
South African cardiomyopathy syndrome I42.8
Southeast Asian hemorrhagic fever A91
Spacing
abnormal, tooth, teeth, fully erupted M26.30
excessive, tooth, fully erupted M26.32
Spade-like hand (congenital) Q68.1
Spading nail L60.8
congenital Q84.6
Spanish collar N47.1
Sparganosis B70.1
Spasm (s), spastic, spasticity (see also condition) R25.2
accommodation —see Spasm, of accommodation
ampulla of Vater K83.4
anus, ani (sphincter) (reflex) K59.4
psychogenic F45.8
artery I73.9
cerebral G45.9
Bell's G51.3

Spasm (s), spastic, spasticity – continued
bladder (sphincter, external or internal) N32.89
psychogenic F45.8
bronchus, bronchiole J98.01
cardia K22.0
cardiac I20.1
carpopedal —see Tetany
cerebral (arteries) (vascular) G45.9
cervix, complicating delivery O62.4
ciliary body (of accommodation) —see Spasm, of accommodation
colon K58.9
with diarrhea K58.0
psychogenic F45.8
common duct K83.8
compulsive —see Tic
conjugate H51.8
coronary (artery) I20.1
diaphragm (reflex) R06.6
epidemic B33.0
psychogenic F45.8
duodenum K59.8
epidemic diaphragmatic (transient) B33.0
esophagus (diffuse) K22.4
psychogenic F45.8
facial G51.3
fallopian tube N83.8
gastrointestinal (tract) K31.89
psychogenic F45.8
glottis J38.5
hysterical F44.4
psychogenic F45.8
conversion reaction F44.4
reflex through recurrent laryngeal nerve J38.5
habit —see Tic
heart I20.1
hemifacial (clonic) G51.3
hourglass —see Contraction, hourglass
hysterical F44.4
infantile —see Epilepsy, spasms
inferior oblique, eye H51.8
intestinal (see also Syndrome, irritable bowel) K58.9
psychogenic F45.8
larynx, laryngeal J38.5
hysterical F44.4
psychogenic F45.8
conversion reaction F44.4
levator palpebrae superioris —see Disorder, eyelid function
muscle NEC M62.838
back M62.830
nerve, trigeminal G51.0
nervous F45.8
nodding F98.4
occupational F48.8
oculogyric H51.8
psychogenic F45.8
of accommodation H52.53
ophthalmic artery —see Occlusion, artery, retina
perineal, female N94.89
peroneo-extensor —see also Deformity, limb, flat foot
pharynx (reflex) J39.2
hysterical F45.8
psychogenic F45.8
psychogenic F45.8
pylorus NEC K31.3
adult hypertrophic K31.89
congenital or infantile Q40.0

Spasm (s), spastic, spasticity – *continued*
  psychogenic F45.8
  rectum (sphincter) K59.4
    psychogenic F45.8
  retinal (artery) —*see* Occlusion, artery, retina
  sigmoid (*see also* Syndrome, irritable bowel) K58.9
    psychogenic F45.8
  sphincter of Oddi K83.4
  stomach K31.89
    neurotic F45.8
  throat J39.2
    hysterical F45.8
    psychogenic F45.8
  tic F95.9
    chronic F95.1
    transient of childhood F95.0
  tongue K14.8
  torsion (progressive) G24.1
  trigeminal nerve —*see* Neuralgia, trigeminal
  ureter N13.5
  urethra (sphincter) N35.9
  uterus N85.8
    complicating labor O62.4
  vagina N94.2
    psychogenic F52.5
  vascular I73.9
  vasomotor I73.9
  vein NEC I87.8
  viscera —*see* Pain, abdominal
Spasmodic *see* condition
Spasmophilia —*see* Tetany
Spasmus nutans F98.4
Spastic, spasticity —*see also* Spasm
  child (cerebral) (congenital) (paralysis) G80.1
Speaker's throat R49.8
Specific, specified —*see* condition
Speech
  defect, disorder, disturbance, impediment R47.9
    psychogenic, in childhood and adolescence F98.8
      slurring R47.81
      specified NEC R47.89
Spencer's disease A08.19
Spens' syndrome (syncope with heart block) I45.9
Sperm counts (fertility testing) Z31.41
  postvasectomy Z30.8
    reversal Z31.42
Spermatic cord —*see* condition
Spermatocele N43.40
  congenital Q55.4
  multiple N43.42
  single N43.41
Spermatocystitis N49.0
Spermatocytoma C62.9
  specified site —*see* Neoplasm, malignant, site
Spermatorrhea N50.8
Sphacelus —*see* Gangrene
Sphenoidal —*see* condition
Sphenoiditis (chronic) —*see* Sinusitis, sphenoidal
Sphenopalatine ganglion neuralgia G90.09
Sphericity, increased, lens (congenital) Q12.4
Spherocytosis (congenital) (familial) (hereditary) D58.0
  hemoglobin disease D58.0
  sickle-cell (disease) D57.8
Spherophakia Q12.4
Sphincter —*see* condition
Sphincteritis, sphincter of Oddi —*see* Cholangitis

Sphingolipidosis E75.3
  specified NEC E75.29
Sphingomyelinosis E75.3
Spicule tooth K00.2
Spider
  bite —*see* Toxicity, venom, spider
  fingers —*see* Syndrome, Marfan's
  nevus I78.1
  toes —*see* Syndrome, Marfan's
  vascular I78.1
Spiegler-Fendt
  benign lymphocytoma L98.8
  sarcoid L08.89
Spielmeyer-Vogt disease E75.4
Spina bifida (aperta) Q05.9
  with hydrocephalus NEC Q05.4
  cervical Q05.5
    with hydrocephalus Q05.0
  dorsal Q05.6
    with hydrocephalus Q05.1
  lumbar Q05.7
    with hydrocephalus Q05.2
  lumbosacral Q05.7
    with hydrocephalus Q05.2
  occulta Q76.0
  sacral Q05.8
    with hydrocephalus Q05.3
  thoracic Q05.6
    with hydrocephalus Q05.1
  thoracolumbar Q05.6
    with hydrocephalus Q05.1
Spindle, Krukenberg's —*see* Pigmentation, cornea, posterior
Spine, spinal —*see* condition
Spiradenoma (eccrine) —*see* Neoplasm, skin, benign
Spirillosis A25.0
Spirillum
  minus A25.0
  obermeieri infection A68.0
Spirochetal —*see* condition
Spirochetosis A69.9
  arthritic, arthritica A69.9
  bronchopulmonary A69.8
  icterohemorrhagic A27.0
  lung A69.8
Spirometrosis B70.1
Spitting blood —*see* Hemoptysis
Splanchnoptosis K63.4
Spleen, splenic —*see* condition
Splenectasis —*see* Splenomegaly
Splenitis (interstitial) (malignant) (nonspecific) D73.89
  malarial (*see also* Malaria) B54 *[D77]*
  tuberculous A18.85
Splenocele D73.89
Splenomegaly, splenomegalia (Bengal) (cryptogenic) (idiopathic) (tropical) R16.1
  with hepatomegaly R16.2
  cirrhotic D73.2
  congenital Q89.09
  congestive, chronic D73.2
  Egyptian B65.1
  Gaucher's E75.22
  malarial (*see also* Malaria) B54 *[D77]*
  neutropenic D73.81
  Niemann-Pick —*see* Niemann-Pick disease or syndrome
  siderotic D73.2
  syphilitic A52.79
    congenital (early) A50.08 *[D77]*
Splenopathy D73.9
Splenoptosis D73.89

Splenosis D73.89
Splinter —*see* Foreign body, superficial, by site
Split, splitting
  foot Q72.7
  heart sounds R01.2
  lip, congenital —*see* Cleft, lip
  nails L60.3
  urinary stream R39.13
Spondylarthrosis —*see* Spondylosis
Spondylitis (chronic) —*see also* Spondylopathy, inflammatory
  ankylopoietica —*see* Spondylitis, ankylosing
  ankylosing (chronic) M45.9
    with lung involvement M45.9 *[J99]*
    cervical region M45.2
    cervicothoracic region M45.3
    juvenile M08.1
    lumbar region M45.6
    lumbosacral region M45.7
    multiple sites M45.0
    occipito-atlanto-axial region M45.1
    sacrococcygeal region M45.8
    thoracic region M45.4
    thoracolumbar region M45.5
  atrophic (ligamentous) —*see* Spondylitis, ankylosing
  deformans (chronic) —*see* Spondylosis
  gonococcal A54.41
  gouty M10.08
  in (due to)
    brucellosis A23.9 *[M49.80]*
      cervical region A23.9 *[M49.82]*
      cervicothoracic region A23.9 *[M49.83]*
      lumbar region A23.9 *[M49.86]*
      lumbosacral region A23.9 *[M49.87]*
      multiple sites A23.9 *[M49.89]*
      occipito-atlanto-axial region A23.9 *[M49.81]*
      sacrococcygeal region A23.9 *[M49.88]*
      thoracic region A23.9 *[M49.84]*
      thoracolumbar region A23.9 *[M49.85]*
    enterobacteria (*see also* subcategory M49.8) A04.9
    tuberculosis A18.01
  infectious NEC —*see* Spondylopathy, infective
  juvenile ankylosing (chronic) M08.1
  Kümmell's —*see* Spondylopathy, traumatic
  Marie-Strümpell —*see* Spondylitis, ankylosing
  muscularis —*see* Spondylopathy, specified NEC
  psoriatic L40.53
  rheumatoid —*see* Spondylitis, ankylosing
  rhizomelica —*see* Spondylitis, ankylosing
  sacroiliac NEC M46.1
  senescent, senile —*see* Spondylosis
  traumatic (chronic) or post-traumatic —*see* Spondylopathy, traumatic
  tuberculous A18.01
  typhosa A01.05
Spondylolisthesis (acquired) (degenerative) M43.10
  with disproportion (fetopelvic) O33.0
    causing obstructed labor O65.0
  cervical region M43.12
  cervicothoracic region M43.13
  congenital Q76.2
  lumbar region M43.16
  lumbosacral region M43.17

Spondylolisthesis – *continued*
multiple sites M43.19
occipito-atlanto-axial region M43.11
sacrococcygeal region M43.18
thoracic region M43.14
thoracolumbar region M43.15
traumatic (old) M43.10
 acute
  fifth cervical (displaced) S12.430
   nondisplaced S12.431
   specified type NEC (displaced) S12.450
    nondisplaced S12.451
   type III S12.44
  fourth cervical (displaced) S12.330
   nondisplaced S12.331
   specified type NEC (displaced) S12.350
    nondisplaced S12.351
   type III S12.34
  second cervical (displaced) S12.130
   nondisplaced S12.131
   specified type NEC (displaced) S12.150
    nondisplaced S12.151
   type III S12.14
  seventh cervical (displaced) S12.630
   nondisplaced S12.631
   specified type NEC (displaced) S12.650
    nondisplaced S12.651
   type III S12.64
  sixth cervical (displaced) S12.530
   nondisplaced S12.531
   specified type NEC (displaced) S12.550
    nondisplaced S12.551
   type III S12.54
  third cervical (displaced) S12.230
   nondisplaced S12.231
   specified type NEC (displaced) S12.250
    nondisplaced S12.251
   type III S12.24
Spondylolysis (acquired) M43.00
 cervical region M43.02
 cervicothoracic region M43.03
 congenital Q76.2
 lumbar region M43.06
 lumbosacral region M43.07
  with disproportion (fetopelvic) O33.0
   causing obstructed labor O65.8
 multiple sites M43.09
 occipito-atlanto-axial region M43.01
 sacrococcygeal region M43.08
 thoracic region M43.04
 thoracolumbar region M43.05
Spondylopathy M48.9
 infective NEC M46.50
  cervical region M46.52
  cervicothoracic region M46.53
  lumbar region M46.56
  lumbosacral region M46.57
  multiple sites M46.59
  occipito-atlanto-axial region M46.51
  sacrococcygeal region M46.58
  thoracic region M46.54
  thoracolumbar region M46.55
 inflammatory M46.90
  cervical region M46.92
  cervicothoracic region M46.93
  lumbar region M46.96
  lumbosacral region M46.97
  multiple sites M46.99
  occipito-atlanto-axial region M46.91
  sacrococcygeal region M46.98
  specified type NEC M46.80
   cervical region M46.82

Spondylopathy – *continued*
  cervicothoracic region M46.83
  lumbar region M46.86
  lumbosacral region M46.87
  multiple sites M46.89
  occipito-atlanto-axial region M46.81
  sacrococcygeal region M46.88
  thoracic region M46.84
  thoracolumbar region M46.85
 thoracic region M46.94
 thoracolumbar region M46.95
 neuropathic, in
  syringomyelia and syringobulbia G95.0
  tabes dorsalis A52.11
 specified NEC —see subcategory M48.8
 traumatic M48.30
  cervical region M48.32
  cervicothoracic region M48.33
  lumbar region M48.36
  lumbosacral region M48.37
  occipito-atlanto-axial region M48.31
  sacrococcygeal region M48.38
  thoracic region M48.34
  thoracolumbar region M48.35
Spondylosis M47.9
 with
  disproportion (fetopelvic) O33.0
   causing obstructed labor O65.0
  myelopathy NEC M47.10
   cervical region M47.12
   cervicothoracic region M47.13
   lumbar region M47.16
   occipito-atlanto-axial region M47.11
   thoracic region M47.14
   thoracolumbar region M47.15
  radiculopathy M47.20
   cervical region M47.22
   cervicothoracic region M47.23
   lumbar region M47.26
   lumbosacral region M47.27
   occipito-atlanto-axial region M47.21
   sacrococcygeal region M47.28
   thoracic region M47.24
   thoracolumbar region M47.25
 specified NEC M47.899
  cervical region M47.892
  cervicothoracic region M47.893
  lumbar region M47.896
  lumbosacral region M47.897
  occipito-atlanto-axial region M47.891
  sacrococcygeal region M47.898
  thoracic region M47.894
  thoracolumbar region M47.895
 traumatic —see Spondylopathy, traumatic
 without myelopathy or radiculopathy
 M47.819
  cervical region M47.812
  cervicothoracic region M47.813
  lumbar region M47.816
  lumbosacral region M47.817
  occipito-atlanto-axial region M47.811
  sacrococcygeal region M47.818
  thoracic region M47.814
  thoracolumbar region M47.815
Sponge
 inadvertently left in operation wound —see
 Foreign body, accidentally left during a
 procedure
 kidney (medullary) Q61.5
Sponge-diver's disease —see Toxicity,
 venom, marine animal, sea anemone

Spongioblastoma (any type) —see Neoplasm,
 malignant, by site
 specified site —see Neoplasm, malignant, by
 site
 unspecified site C71.9
Spongioneuroblastoma —see Neoplasm,
 malignant, by site
Spontaneous —see also condition
 fracture (cause unknown) —see Fracture,
 pathological
Spoon nail L60.3
 congenital Q84.6
Sporadic —see condition
Sporothrix schenckii infection —see
 Sporotrichosis
Sporotrichosis B42.9
 arthritis B42.82
 disseminated B42.7
 generalized B42.7
 lymphocutaneous (fixed) (progressive) B42.1
 pulmonary B42.0
 specified NEC B42.89
Spots, spotting (in) (of)
 Bitot's —see also Pigmentation, conjunctiva
  in the young child E50.1
  vitamin A deficiency E50.1
 café, au lait L81.3
 Cayenne pepper I78.1
 cotton wool, retina —see Occlusion, artery,
 retina
 de Morgan's (senile angiomas) I78.1
 Fuchs' black (myopic) H44.2
 intermenstrual (regular) N92.0
  irregular N92.1
 Koplik's B05.9
 liver L81.4
 pregnancy O26.85
 purpuric R23.3
 ruby I78.1
Spotted fever (see Fever, spotted) N92.3
Sprain (joint) (ligament)
 acromioclavicular joint or ligament S43.5
 ankle S93.40
  calcaneofibular ligament S93.41
  deltoid ligament S93.42
  internal collateral ligament —see Sprain,
 ankle, specified ligament NEC
  specified ligament NEC S93.49
  talofibular ligament —see Sprain, ankle,
 specified ligament NEC
  tibiofibular ligament S93.43
 anterior longitudinal, cervical S13.4
 atlas, atlanto-axial, atlanto-occipital S13.4
 breast bone —see Sprain, sternum
 calcaneofibular —see Sprain, ankle
 carpal —see Sprain, wrist
 carpometacarpal —see Sprain, hand, specified
 site NEC
 cartilage
  costal S23.41
  semilunar (knee) —see Sprain, knee,
 specified site NEC
   with current tear —see Tear, meniscus
  thyroid region S13.5
  xiphoid —see Sprain, sternum
 cervical, cervicodorsal, cervicothoracic S13.4
 chondrosternal S23.421
 coracoclavicular S43.8
 coracohumeral S43.41
 coronary, knee —see Sprain, knee, specified
 site NEC
 costal cartilage S23.41

Sprue (tropical) K90.1
  celiac K90.0
  idiopathic K90.0
  meaning thrush B37.0
  nontropical K90.0
Spur, bone —*see also* Enthesopathy
  calcaneal M77.3
  iliac crest M76.2
  nose (septum) J34.89
Spurway's syndrome Q78.0
Sputum
  abnormal (amount) (color) (odor) (purulent) R09.3
  blood-stained R04.2
  excessive (cause unknown) R09.3
Squamous —*see also* condition
  epithelium in
    cervical canal (congenital) Q51.828
    uterine mucosa (congenital) Q51.818
Squashed nose M95.0
  congenital Q67.4
Squeeze, diver's T70.3
Squint —*see also* Strabismus
  accommodative —*see* Strabismus, convergent
  concomitant
St. Hubert's disease A82.9
Stab —*see also* Laceration
  internal organs —*see* Injury, by site
Stafne's cyst or cavity M27.0
Staggering gait R26.0
  hysterical F44.4
Staghorn calculus —*see* Calculus, kidney
Stähli's line (cornea) (pigment) —*see* Pigmentation, cornea, anterior
Stain, staining
  meconium (newborn) P96.83
  port wine Q82.5
  tooth, teeth (hard tissues) (extrinsic) K03.6
    due to
      accretions K03.6
      deposits (betel) (black) (green) (materia alba) (orange) (soft) (tobacco) K03.6
      metals (copper) (silver) K03.7
      nicotine K03.6
      pulpal bleeding K03.7
      tobacco K03.6
    intrinsic K00.8
Stammering (*see also* Disorder, fluency) F80.81
Standstill
  auricular I45.5
  cardiac —*see* Arrest, cardiac
  sinoatrial I45.5
  ventricular —*see* Arrest, cardiac
Stannosis J63.5
Stanton's disease —*see* Melioidosis
Staphylitis (acute) (catarrhal) (chronic) (gangrenous) (membranous) (suppurative) (ulcerative) K12.2
Staphylococcal scalded skin syndrome L00
Staphylococcemia A41.2
Staphylococcus, staphylococcal —*see also* condition
  as cause of disease classified elsewhere B95.8
    aureus (methicillin susceptible) (MSSA) B95.61
      methicillin resistant (MRSA) B95.62
    specified NEC, as cause of disease classified elsewhere B95.7
Staphyloma (sclera)
  cornea H18.72
  equatorial H15.81

Staphyloma – *continued*
  localized (anterior) H15.82
  posticum H15.83
  ring H15.85
Stargardt's disease —*see* Dystrophy, retina
Starvation (inanition) (due to lack of food) T73.0
  edema —*see* Malnutrition, severe
Stasis
  bile (noncalculous) K83.1
  bronchus J98.09
    with infection —*see* Bronchitis
  cardiac —*see* Failure, heart, congestive
  cecum K59.8
  colon K59.8
  dermatitis —*see* Varix, leg, with, inflammation
  duodenal K31.5
  eczema —*see* Varix, leg, with, inflammation
  edema —*see* Hypertension, venous (chronic) ,
  idiopathic
  foot T69.0
  ileocecal coil K59.8
  ileum K59.8
  intestinal K59.8
  jejunum K59.8
  kidney N19
  liver (cirrhotic) K76.1
  lymphatic I89.8
  pneumonia J18.2
  pulmonary —*see* Edema, lung
  rectal K59.8
  renal N19
    tubular N17.0
  ulcer —*see* Varix, leg, with, ulcer
    without varicose veins I87.2
  urine —*see* Retention, urine
  venous I87.8
State (of)
  affective and paranoid, mixed, organic psychotic F06.8
  agitated R45.1
    acute reaction to stress F43.0
  anxiety (neurotic) F41.1
  apprehension F41.1
  burn-out Z73.0
  climacteric, female Z78.0
    symptomatic N95.1
  compulsive F42
    mixed with obsessional thoughts F42
  confusional (psychogenic) F44.89
    acute —*see also* Delirium
      with
        arteriosclerotic dementia F01.50
          with behavioral disturbance F01.51
        senility or dementia F05
      alcoholic F10.231
      epileptic F05
    reactive (from emotional stress, psychological trauma) F44.89
    subacute —*see* Delirium
  convulsive —*see* Convulsions
  crisis F43.0
  depressive F32.9
    neurotic F34.1
  dissociative F44.9
  emotional shock (stress) R45.7
  hypercoagulation —*see* Hypercoagulable
  locked-in G83.5
  menopausal Z78.0
    symptomatic N95.1

State (of) - *continued*
  neurotic F48.9
    with depersonalization F48.1
  obsessional F42
  oneiroid (schizophrenia-like) F23
  organic
    hallucinatory (nonalcoholic) F06.0
    paranoid (-hallucinatory) F06.2
  panic F41.0
  paranoid F22
    climacteric F22
    involutional F22
    menopausal F22
    organic F06.2
    senile F03
    simple F22
  persistent vegetative R40.3
  phobic F40.9
  postleukotomy F07.0
  pregnant, incidental Z33.1
  psychogenic, twilight F44.89
  psychopathic (constitutional) F60.2
  psychotic, organic —*see also* Psychosis, organic
    mixed paranoid and affective F06.8
    senile or presenile F03
    transient NEC F06.8
      with
        hallucinations F06.0
        depression F06.31
  residual schizophrenic F20.5
  restlessness R45.1
  stress (emotional) R45.7
  tension (mental) F48.9
    specified NEC F48.8
  transient organic psychotic NEC F06.8
    depressive type F06.31
    hallucinatory type F06.30
  twilight
    epileptic F05
    psychogenic F44.89
  vegetative, persistent R40.3
  vital exhaustion Z73.0
  withdrawal, —*see* Withdrawal, state
Status (post) —*see also* Presence (of)
  absence, epileptic —*see* Epilepsy, by type, with status epilepticus
  administration of tPA (rtPA) in a different facility within the last 24 hours prior to admission to current facility Z92.82
  adrenalectomy (unilateral) (bilateral) E89.6
  anastomosis Z98.0
  angioplasty (peripheral) Z98.62
    with implant Z95.820
    coronary artery Z98.61
      with implant Z95.5
  anginosus I20.9
  aortocoronary bypass Z95.1
  arthrodesis Z98.1
  artificial opening (of) Z93.9
    gastrointestinal tract Z93.4
    specified NEC Z93.8
    urinary tract Z93.6
    vagina Z93.8
  asthmaticus —*see* Asthma, by type, with status asthmaticus
  awaiting organ transplant Z76.82
  bariatric surgery Z98.84
  bed confinement Z74.01
  bleb, filtering (vitreous) , after glaucoma surgery Z98.83

Status (post) – *continued*
  breast implant Z98.82
    removal Z98.86
  cataract extraction Z98.4
  cholecystectomy Z90.49
  clitorectomy N90.811
    with excision of labia minora N90.812
  colectomy (complete) (partial) Z90.49
  colonization —*see* Carrier (suspected) of
  colostomy Z93.3
  convulsivus idiopathicus —*see* Epilepsy, by
  type, with status epilepticus
  coronary artery angioplasty —*see* Status,
  angioplasty, coronary artery
  cystectomy (urinary bladder) Z90.6
  cystostomy Z93.50
    appendico-vesicostomy Z93.52
    cutaneous Z93.51
    specified NEC Z93.59
  delinquent immunization Z28.3
  dental Z98.818
    crown Z98.811
    fillings Z98.811
    restoration Z98.811
    sealant Z98.810
    specified NEC Z98.818
  deployment (current) (military) Z56.82
  dialysis (hemodialysis) (peritoneal) Z99.2
  do not resuscitate (DNR) Z66
  donor —*see* Donor
  embedded fragments —*see* Retained, foreign
  body fragments (type of)
  embedded splinter —*see* Retained, foreign
  body fragments (type of)
  enterostomy Z93.4
  epileptic, epilepticus (*see also* Epilepsy, by
  type, with status epilepticus) G40.901
  estrogen receptor
    negative Z17.1
    positive Z17.0
  female genital cutting —*see* Female genital
  mutilation status
  female genital mutilation —*see* Female
  genital mutilation status
  filtering (vitreous) bleb after glaucoma
  surgery Z98.83
  gastrectomy (complete) (partial) Z90.3
  gastric banding Z98.84
  gastric bypass for obesity Z98.84
  gastrostomy Z93.1
  human immunodeficiency virus (HIV)
  infection, asymptomatic Z21
  hysterectomy (complete) (total) Z90.710
    partial (with remaining cervical stump)
    Z90.711
  ileostomy Z93.2
  implant
    breast Z98.82
  infibulation N90.813
  intestinal bypass Z98.0
  jejunostomy Z93.4
  laryngectomy Z90.02
  lapsed immunization schedule Z28.3
  lymphaticus E32.8
  marmoratus G80.3
  mastectomy (unilateral) (bilateral) Z90.1
  military deployment status (current) Z56.82
    in theater or in support of military war,
    peacekeeping and humanitarian operations
    Z56.82
  nephrectomy (unilateral) (bilateral) Z90.5
  nephrostomy Z93.6

Status (post) – *continued*
  obesity surgery Z98.84
  oophorectomy
    bilateral Z90.722
    unilateral Z90.721
  organ replacement
    by artificial or mechanical device or
  prosthesis of
    artery Z95.828
    bladder Z96.0
    blood vessel Z95.828
    breast Z97.8
    eye globe Z97.0
    heart Z95.812
      valve Z95.2
    intestine Z97.8
    joint Z96.60
      hip —*see* Presence, hip joint implant
      knee —*see* Presence, knee joint implant
      specified site NEC Z96.698
    kidney Z97.8
    larynx Z96.3
    lens Z96.1
    limbs —*see* Presence, artificial, limb
    liver Z97.8
    lung Z97.8
    pancreas Z97.8
    by organ transplant (heterologous)
    (homologous) —*see* Transplant
  pacemaker
    brain Z96.89
    cardiac Z95.0
    specified NEC Z96.89
  pancreatectomy Z90.410
    complete Z90.410
    partial Z90.411
    total Z90.410
  physical restraint Z78.1
  pneumonectomy (complete) (partial) Z90.2
  pneumothorax, therapeutic Z98.3
  postcommotio cerebri F07.81
  postoperative (postprocedural) NEC Z98.89
    breast implant Z98.82
    dental Z98.818
      crown Z98.811
      fillings Z98.811
      restoration Z98.811
      sealant Z98.810
      specified NEC Z98.818
    pneumothorax, therapeutic Z98.3
  postpartum (routine follow-up) Z39.2
    care immediately after delivery Z39.0
  postsurgical (postprocedural) NEC Z98.89
    pneumothorax, therapeutic Z98.3
  pregnancy, incidental Z33.1
  prosthesis coronary angioplasty Z95.5
  pseudophakia Z96.1
  renal dialysis (hemodialysis) (peritoneal)
  Z99.2
  retained foreign body —*see* Retained, foreign
  body fragments (type of)
  reversed jejunal transposition (for bypass)
  Z98.0
  salpingo-oophorectomy
    bilateral Z90.722
    unilateral Z90.721
  sex reassignment surgery status Z87.890
  shunt
    arteriovenous (for dialysis) Z99.2
    cerebrospinal fluid Z98.2
    ventricular (communicating) (for drainage)
    Z98.2

Status (post) – *continued*
  splenectomy Z90.81
  thymicolymphaticus E32.8
  thymicus E32.8
  thymolymphaticus E32.8
  thyroidectomy (hypothyroidism) E89.0
  tooth (teeth) extraction (*see also* Absence,
  teeth, acquired) K08.409
  tPA (rtPA) administration in a different
  facility within the last 24 hours prior to
  admission to current facility Z92.82
  tracheostomy Z93.0
  transplant —*see* Transplant
    organ removed Z98.85
  tubal ligation Z98.51
  underimmunization Z28.3
  ureterostomy Z93.6
  urethrostomy Z93.6
  vagina, artificial Z93.8
  vasectomy Z98.52
  wheelchair confinement Z99.3
Stealing
  child problem F91.8
    in company with others Z72.810
  pathological (compulsive) F63.2
Steam burn —*see* Burn
Steatocystoma multiplex L72.2
Steatohepatitis (nonalcoholic) (NASH)
  K75.81
Steatoma L72.3
  eyelid (cystic) —*see* Dermatosis, eyelid
  infected —*see* Hordeolum
Steatorrhea (chronic) K90.4
  with lacteal obstruction K90.2
  idiopathic (adult) (infantile) K90.0
  pancreatic K90.3
  primary K90.0
  tropical K90.1
Steatosis E88.89
  heart —*see* Degeneration, myocardial
  kidney N28.89
  liver NEC K76.0
Steele-Richardson-Olszewski disease or
  syndrome G23.1
Steinbrocker's syndrome G90.8
Steinert's disease G71.11
Stein-Leventhal syndrome E28.2
Stein's syndrome E28.2
STEMI (*see also*
  Infarct, myocardium, ST elevation) I21.3
Stenocardia I20.8
Stenocephaly Q75.8
Stenosis, stenotic (cicatricial) —*see also*
  Stricture
  ampulla of Vater K83.1
  anus, anal (canal) (sphincter) K62.4
    and rectum K62.4
    congenital Q42.3
      with fistula Q42.2
  aorta (ascending) (supraventricular)
    (congenital) Q25.3
    arteriosclerotic I70.0
    calcified I70.0
  aortic (valve) I35.0
    with insufficiency I35.2
    congenital Q23.0
    rheumatic I06.0
      with
        incompetency, insufficiency or
      regurgitation I06.2
        with mitral (valve) disease I08.0
          with tricuspid (valve) disease I08.3
        mitral (valve) disease I08.0

Stenosis, stenotic - *continued*
intervertebral disc M99.59
abdomen M99.59
cervical region M99.51
cervicothoracic M99.51
head region M99.50
lower extremity M99.56
lumbar region M99.53
lumbosacral M99.53
occipitocervical M99.50
pelvic M99.55
rib cage M99.58
sacral region M99.54
sacrococcygeal M99.54
sacroiliac M99.54
specified NEC M99.59
thoracic region M99.52
thoracolumbar M99.52
upper extremity M99.57
osseous M99.39
abdomen M99.39
cervical region M99.31
cervicothoracic M99.31
head region M99.30
lower extremity M99.36
lumbar region M99.33
lumbosacral M99.33
pelvic M99.35
rib cage M99.38
occipitocervical M99.30
sacral region M99.34
sacrococcygeal M99.34
sacroiliac M99.34
specified NEC M99.39
thoracic region M99.32
thoracolumbar M99.32
upper extremity M99.37
subluxation M99.29
cervical region M99.21
cervicothoracic M99.21
head region M99.20
lower extremity M99.26
lumbar region M99.23
lumbosacral M99.23
occipitocervical M99.20
pelvic M99.25
rib cage M99.28
sacral region M99.24
sacrococcygeal M99.24
sacroiliac M99.24
specified NEC M99.29
thoracic region M99.22
thoracolumbar M99.22
upper extremity M99.27
organ or site, congenital NEC —*see* Atresia,
by site
papilla of Vater K83.1
pulmonary (artery) (congenital) Q25.6
with ventricular septal defect, transposition
of aorta, and hypertrophy of right ventricle
Q21.3
acquired I28.8
in tetralogy of Fallot Q21.3
infundibular Q24.3
subvalvular Q24.3
supravalvular Q25.6
valve I37.0
with insufficiency I37.2
congenital Q22.1
rheumatic I09.89
with aortic, mitral or tricuspid (valve)
disease I08.8

Stenosis, stenotic - *continued*
vein, acquired I28.8
vessel NEC I28.8
pulmonic (congenital) Q22.1
infundibular Q24.3
subvalvular Q24.3
pylorus (hypertrophic) (acquired) K31.1
adult K31.1
congenital Q40.0
infantile Q40.0
rectum (sphincter) —*see* Stricture, rectum
renal artery I70.1
congenital Q27.1
salivary duct (any) K11.8
sphincter of Oddi K83.1
spinal M48.00
cervical region M48.02
cervicothoracic region M48.03
lumbar region M48.06
lumbosacral region M48.07
occipito-atlanto-axial region M48.01
sacrococcygeal region M48.08
thoracic region M48.04
thoracolumbar region M48.05
stomach, hourglass K31.2
subaortic (congenital) Q24.4
hypertrophic (idiopathic) I42.1
subglottic J38.6
congenital Q31.1
postprocedural J95.5
trachea J39.8
congenital Q32.1
syphilitic A52.73
tuberculous NEC A15.5
tracheostomy J95.03
tricuspid (valve) I07.0
with
aortic (valve) disease I08.2
incompetency, insufficiency or
regurgitation I07.2
with aortic (valve) disease I08.2
with mitral (valve) disease I08.3
mitral (valve) disease I08.1
with aortic (valve) disease I08.3
congenital Q22.4
nonrheumatic I36.0
with insufficiency I36.2
tubal N97.1
ureter —*see* Atresia, ureter
ureteropelvic junction, congenital Q62.11
ureterovesical orifice, congenital Q62.12
urethra (valve) —*see also* Stricture, urethra
congenital Q64.32
urinary meatus, congenital Q64.33
vagina N89.5
congenital Q52.4
in pregnancy —*see* Pregnancy, complicated
by, abnormal vagina
causing obstructed labor O65.5
valve (cardiac) (heart) (*see also* Endocarditis)
I38
congenital Q24.8
aortic Q23.0
mitral Q23.2
pulmonary Q22.1
tricuspid Q22.4
vena cava (inferior) (superior) I87.1
congenital Q26.0
vesicourethral orifice Q64.31
vulva N90.5
Stent jail T82.897

Stercolith (impaction) K56.41
appendix K38.1
Stercoraceous, stercoral ulcer K63.3
anus or rectum K62.6
Stereotypies NEC F98.4
Sterility —*see* Infertility
Sterilization —*see* Encounter (for) ,
sterilization
Sternalgia —*see* Angina
Sternopagus Q89.4
Sternum bifidum Q76.7
Steroid
effects (adverse) (adrenocortical) (iatrogenic)
cushingoid E24.2
correct substance properly administered —
see Table of Drugs and Chemicals, by
drug, adverse effect
overdose or wrong substance given or
taken —*see* Table of Drugs and Chemicals,
by drug, poisoning
diabetes —see category E09
correct substance properly administered —
see Table of Drugs and Chemicals, by
drug, adverse effect
overdose or wrong substance given or
taken —*see* Table of Drugs and Chemicals,
by drug, poisoning
fever R50.2
insufficiency E27.3
correct substance properly administered —
see Table of Drugs and Chemicals, by
drug, adverse effect
overdose or wrong substance given or
taken —*see* Table of Drugs and Chemicals,
by drug, poisoning
responder H40.04
Stevens-Johnson disease or syndrome L51.1
toxic epidermal necrolysis overlap L51.3
Stewart-Morel syndrome M85.2
Sticker's disease B08.3
Sticky eye —*see* Conjunctivitis, acute,
mucopurulent
Stieda's disease —*see* Bursitis, tibial collateral
Stiff neck —*see* Torticollis
Stiff-man syndrome G25.82
Stiffness, joint NEC M25.60
ankle M25.67
ankylosis —*see* Ankylosis, joint
contracture —*see* Contraction, joint
elbow M25.62
foot M25.67
hand M25.64
hip M25.65
knee M25.66
shoulder M25.61
wrist M25.63
Stigmata congenital syphilis A50.59
Stillbirth P95
Still-Felty syndrome —*see* Felty's syndrome
Still's disease or syndrome (juvenile) M08.20
adult onset M06.1
ankle M08.27
elbow M08.22
foot joint M08.27
hand joint M08.24
hip M08.25
knee M08.26
multiple site M08.29
shoulder M08.21
vertebra M08.28
wrist M08.23
Stimulation, ovary E28.1

Sting (venomous) (with allergic or anaphylactic shock) —*see* Table of Drugs and Chemicals, by animal or substance, poisoning
Stippled epiphyses Q78.8
Stitch
abscess T81.4
burst (in operation wound) —*see* Disruption, wound, operation
Stokes-Adams disease or syndrome I45.9
Stokes' disease E05.00
with thyroid storm E05.01
Stokvis (-Talma) **disease** D74.8
Stoma malfunction
colostomy K94.03
enterostomy K94.13
gastrostomy K94.23
ileostomy K94.13
tracheostomy J95.03
Stomach —*see* condition
Stomatitis (denture) (ulcerative) K12.1
angular K13.0
due to dietary or vitamin deficiency E53.0
aphthous K12.0
bovine B08.61
candidal B37.0
catarrhal K12.1
diphtheritic A36.89
due to
dietary deficiency E53.0
thrush B37.0
vitamin deficiency
B group NEC E53.9
B2 (riboflavin) E53.0
epidemic B08.8
epizootic B08.8
follicular K12.1
gangrenous A69.0
Geotrichum B48.3
herpesviral, herpetic B00.2
herpetiformis K12.0
malignant K12.1
membranous acute K12.1
monilial B37.0
mycotic B37.0
necrotizing ulcerative A69.0
parasitic B37.0
septic K12.1
spirochetal A69.1
suppurative (acute) K12.2
ulceromembranous A69.1
vesicular K12.1
with exanthem (enteroviral) B08.4
virus disease A93.8
Vincent's A69.1
Stomatocytosis D58.8
Stomatomycosis B37.0
Stomatorrhagia K13.79
Stone (s) —*see also* Calculus
bladder (diverticulum) N21.0
cystine E72.09
heart syndrome I50.1
kidney N20.0
prostate N42.0
pulpal (dental) K04.2
renal N20.0
salivary gland or duct (any) K11.5
urethra (impacted) N21.1
urinary (duct) (impacted) (passage) N20.9
bladder (diverticulum) N21.0
lower tract N21.9
specified NEC N21.8
xanthine E79.8 *[N22]*
Stonecutter's lung J62.8

Stonemason's asthma, disease, lung or pneumoconiosis J62.8
Stoppage
heart —*see* Arrest, cardiac
urine —*see* Retention, urine
Storm, thyroid —*see* Thyrotoxicosis
Strabismus (congenital) (nonparalytic) H50.9
concomitant H50.40
convergent —*see* Strabismus, convergent concomitant
divergent —*see* Strabismus, divergent concomitant
convergent concomitant H50.00
accommodative component H50.43
alternating H50.05
with
A pattern H50.06
specified nonconcomitances NEC H50.08
V pattern H50.07
monocular H50.01
with
A pattern H50.02
specified nonconcomitances NEC H50.04
V pattern H50.03
intermittent H50.31
alternating H50.32
cyclotropia H50.1
divergent concomitant H50.10
alternating H50.15
with
A pattern H50.16
specified noncomitances NEC H50.18
V pattern H50.17
monocular H50.11
with
A pattern H50.12
specified noncomitances NEC H50.14
V pattern H50.13
intermittent H50.33
alternating H50.34
Duane's syndrome H50.81
due to adhesions, scars H50.69
heterophoria H50.50
alternating H50.55
cyclophoria H50.54
esophoria H50.51
exophoria H50.52
vertical H50.53
heterotropia H50.40
intermittent H50.30
hypertropia H50.2
hypotropia —*see* Hypertropia
latent H50.50
mechanical H50.60
Brown's sheath syndrome H50.61
specified type NEC H50.69
monofixation syndrome H50.42
paralytic H49.9
abducens nerve H49.2
fourth nerve H49.1
Kearns-Sayre syndrome H49.81
ophthalmoplegia (external)
progressive H49.4
with pigmentary retinopathy H49.81
total H49.3
sixth nerve H49.2
specified type NEC H49.88
third nerve H49.0
trochlear nerve H49.1
specified type NEC H50.89
vertical H50.2

Strain
back S39.012
cervical S16.1
eye NEC —*see* Disturbance, vision, subjective
heart —*see* Disease, heart
low back S39.012
mental NOS Z73.3
work-related Z56.6
muscle (tendon) —*see* Injury, muscle, by site, strain
neck S16.1
postural —*see also* Disorder, soft tissue, due to use
physical NOS Z73.3
work-related Z56.6
psychological NEC Z73.3
tendon —*see* Injury, muscle, by site, strain
Straining, on urination R39.16
Strand, vitreous —*see* Opacity, vitreous, membranes and strands
Strangulation, strangulated —*see also* Asphyxia, traumatic
appendix K38.8
bladder-neck N32.0
bowel or colon K56.2
food or foreign body —*see* Foreign body, by site
hemorrhoids —*see* Hemorrhoids, with complication
hernia —*see also* Hernia, by site, with obstruction
with gangrene —*see* Hernia, by site, with gangrene
intestine (large) (small) K56.2
with hernia —*see also* Hernia, by site, with obstruction
with gangrene —*see* Hernia, by site, with gangrene
mesentery K56.2
mucus —*see* Asphyxia, mucus
omentum K56.2
organ or site, congenital NEC —*see* Atresia, by site
ovary —*see* Torsion, ovary
penis N48.89
foreign body T19.4
rupture —*see* Hernia, by site, with obstruction
stomach due to hernia —*see also* Hernia, by site, with obstruction
with gangrene —*see* Hernia, by site, with gangrene
vesicourethral orifice N32.0
Strangury R30.0
Straw itch B88.0 **Strawberry**
gallbladder K82.4
mark Q82.5
tongue (red) (white) K14.3
Streak (s)
macula, angioid H35.33
ovarian Q50.32
Strephosymbolia F81.0
secondary to organic lesion R48.8
Streptobacillary fever A25.1
Streptobacillosis A25.1
Streptobacillus moniliformis A25.1
Streptococcus, streptococcal —*see also* condition
as cause of disease classified elsewhere B95.5
group
A, as cause of disease classified elsewhere B95.0

Streptococcus, streptococcal *- continued*
  B, as cause of disease classified elsewhere B95.1
  D, as cause of disease classified elsewhere B95.2
  pneumoniae, as cause of disease classified elsewhere B95.3
  specified NEC, as cause of disease classified elsewhere B95.4
Streptomycosis B47.1
Streptotrichosis A48.8
Stress F43.9
  family —*see* Disruption, family
  fetal P84
    complicating pregnancy O77.9
      due to drug administration O77.1
  mental NEC Z73.3
    work-related Z56.6
  physical NEC Z73.3
    work-related Z56.6
  polycythemia D75.1
  reaction (*see also* Reaction, stress) F43.9
  work schedule Z56.3
Stretching, nerve —*see* Injury, nerve
Striae albicantes, atrophicae or distensae (cutis) L90.6
Stricture —*see also* Stenosis
  ampulla of Vater K83.1
  anus (sphincter) K62.4
    congenital Q42.3
      with fistula Q42.2
    infantile Q42.3
      with fistula Q42.2
  aorta (ascending) (congenital) Q25.3
    arteriosclerotic I70.0
    calcified I70.0
    supravalvular, congenital Q25.3
  aortic (valve) —*see* Stenosis, aortic
  aqueduct of Sylvius (congenital) Q03.0
    with spina bifida —*see* Spina bifida, by site, with hydrocephalus
    acquired G91.1
  artery I77.1
    basilar —*see* Occlusion, artery, basilar
    carotid —*see* Occlusion, artery, carotid
    celiac I77.4
    congenital (peripheral) Q27.8
      cerebral Q28.3
      coronary Q24.5
      digestive system Q27.8
      lower limb Q27.8
      retinal Q14.1
      specified site NEC Q27.8
      umbilical Q27.0
      upper limb Q27.8
    coronary —*see* Disease, heart, ischemic, atherosclerotic
      congenital Q24.5
    precerebral —*see* Occlusion, artery, precerebral
    pulmonary (congenital) Q25.6
      acquired I28.8
    renal I70.1
    vertebral —*see* Occlusion, artery, vertebral
  auditory canal (external) (congenital)
    acquired —*see* Stenosis, external ear canal
  bile duct (common) (hepatic) K83.1
    congenital Q44.3
    postoperative K91.89
  bladder N32.89
    neck N32.0
  bowel —*see* Obstruction, intestine

Stricture – *continued*
  brain G93.89
  bronchus J98.09
    congenital Q32.3
    syphilitic A52.72
  cardia (stomach) K22.2
    congenital Q39.3
  cardiac —*see also* Disease, heart
    orifice (stomach) K22.2
  cecum —*see* Obstruction, intestine
  cervix, cervical (canal) N88.2
    congenital Q51.828
    in pregnancy —*see* Pregnancy, complicated by, abnormal cervix
      causing obstructed labor O65.5
  colon —*see also* Obstruction, intestine
    congenital Q42.9
      specified NEC Q42.8
  colostomy K94.03
  common (bile) duct K83.1
  coronary (artery) —*see* Disease, heart, ischemic, atherosclerotic
  cystic duct —*see* Obstruction, gallbladder
  digestive organs NEC, congenital Q45.8
  duodenum K31.5
    congenital Q41.0
  ear canal (external) (congenital) Q16.1
    acquired —*see* Stricture, auditory canal, acquired
  ejaculatory duct N50.8
  enterostomy K94.13
  esophagus K22.2
    congenital Q39.3
    syphilitic A52.79
      congenital A50.59 [K23]
  eustachian tube —*see also* Obstruction, eustachian tube
    congenital Q17.8
  fallopian tube N97.1
    gonococcal A54.24
    tuberculous A18.17
  gallbladder —*see* Obstruction, gallbladder
  glottis J38.6
  heart —*see also* Disease, heart
    valve (*see also* Endocarditis) I38
      aortic Q23.0
      mitral Q23.4
      pulmonary Q22.1
      tricuspid Q22.4
  hepatic duct K83.1
  hourglass, of stomach K31.2
  hymen N89.6
  hypopharynx J39.2
  ileum K56.69
    congenital Q41.2
  intestine —*see also* Obstruction, intestine
    congenital (small) Q41.9
      large Q42.9
        specified NEC Q42.8
      specified NEC Q41.8
    ischemic K55.1
  jejunum K56.69
    congenital Q41.1
  lacrimal passages —*see also* Stenosis, lacrimal
    congenital Q10.5
  larynx J38.6
    congenital NEC Q31.8
      subglottic Q31.1
    syphilitic A52.73
      congenital A50.59 [J99]

Stricture – *continued*
  meatus
    ear (congenital) Q16.1
      acquired —*see* Stricture, auditory canal, acquired
    osseous (ear) (congenital) Q16.1
      acquired —*see* Stricture, auditory canal, acquired
    urinarius —*see also* Stricture, urethra
      congenital Q64.33
  mitral (valve) —*see* Stenosis, mitral
  myocardium, myocardial I51.5
    hypertrophic subaortic (idiopathic) I42.1
  nares (anterior) (posterior) J34.89
    congenital Q30.0
  nasal duct —*see also* Stenosis, lacrimal, duct
    congenital Q10.5
  nasolacrimal duct —*see also* Stenosis, lacrimal, duct
    congenital Q10.5
  nasopharynx J39.2
    syphilitic A52.73
  nose J34.89
    congenital Q30.0
  nostril (anterior) (posterior) J34.89
    congenital Q30.0
    syphilitic A52.73
      congenital A50.59 [J99]
  organ or site, congenital NEC —*see* Atresia, by site
  os uteri —*see* Stricture, cervix
  osseous meatus (ear) (congenital) Q16.1
    acquired —*see* Stricture, auditory canal, acquired
  oviduct —*see* Stricture, fallopian tube
  pelviureteric junction (congenital) Q62.11
  penis, by foreign body T19.4
  pharynx J39.2
  prostate N42.89
  pulmonary, pulmonic
    artery (congenital) Q25.6
      acquired I28.8
      noncongenital I28.8
    infundibulum (congenital) Q24.3
    valve I37.0
      congenital Q22.1
    vein, acquired I28.8
  vessel NEC I28.8
  punctum lacrimale —*see also* Stenosis, lacrimal, punctum
    congenital Q10.5
  pylorus (hypertrophic) K31.1
    adult K31.1
    congenital Q40.0
    infantile Q40.0
  rectosigmoid K56.69
  rectum (sphincter) K62.4
    congenital Q42.1
      with fistula Q42.0
    due to
      chlamydial lymphogranuloma A55
      irradiation K91.89
      lymphogranuloma venereum A55
    gonococcal A54.6
    inflammatory (chlamydial) A55
    syphilitic A52.74
    tuberculous A18.32
  renal artery I70.1
    congenital Q27.1
  salivary duct or gland (any) K11.8
  sigmoid (flexure) —*see* Obstruction, intestine
  spermatic cord N50.8

Stricture – *continued*
  stoma (following) (of)
    colostomy K94.03
    enterostomy K94.13
    gastrostomy K94.23
    ileostomy K94.13
    tracheostomy J95.03
  stomach K31.89
    congenital Q40.2
    hourglass K31.2
  subaortic Q24.4
    hypertrophic (acquired) (idiopathic) I42.1
  subglottic J38.6
  syphilitic NEC A52.79
  trachea J39.8
    congenital Q32.1
    syphilitic A52.73
    tuberculous NEC A15.5
  tracheostomy J95.03
  tricuspid (valve) —*see* Stenosis, tricuspid
  tunica vaginalis N50.8
  ureter (postoperative) N13.5
    with
      hydronephrosis N13.1
        with infection N13.6
      pyelonephritis (chronic) N11.1
    congenital —*see* Atresia, ureter
    tuberculous A18.11
  ureteropelvic junction (congenital) Q62.11
  ureterovesical orifice N13.5
    with infection N13.6
  urethra (organic) (spasmodic) N35.9
    associated with schistosomiasis B65.0 *[N37]*
    congenital Q64.39
      valvular (posterior) Q64.2
    due to
      infection —*see* Stricture, urethra,
    postinfective
      trauma —*see* Stricture, urethra, post-
    traumatic
    gonococcal, gonorrheal A54.01
    infective NEC —*see* Stricture, urethra,
    postinfective
    late effect (sequelae) of injury —*see*
    Stricture, urethra, post-traumatic
    postcatheterization —*see* Stricture, urethra,
    postprocedural
    postinfective NEC
      female N35.12
      male N35.119
        anterior urethra N35.114
        bulbous urethra N35.112
        meatal N35.111
        membranous urethra N35.113
    postobstetric N35.021
    postoperative —*see* Stricture, urethra,
    postprocedural
    postprocedural
      female N99.12
      male N99.114
        anterior urethra N99.113
        bulbous urethra N99.111
        meatal N99.110
        membranous urethra N99.112
    post-traumatic
      female N35.028
        due to childbirth N35.021
      male N35.014
        anterior urethra N35.013
        bulbous urethra N35.011
        meatal N35.010
        membranous urethra N35.012

Stricture – *continued*
  sequela (late effect) of
    childbirth N35.021
    injury —*see* Stricture, urethra, post-
    traumatic
    specified cause NEC N35.8
    syphilitic A52.76
    traumatic —*see* Stricture, urethra, post-
    traumatic
  valvular (posterior) , congenital Q64.2
  urinary meatus —*see* Stricture, urethra
  uterus, uterine (synechiae) N85.6
    os (external) (internal) —*see* Stricture,
  cervix
  vagina (outlet) —*see* Stenosis, vagina
  valve (cardiac) (heart) —*see also*
  Endocarditis
    congenital
      aortic Q23.0
      mitral Q23.2
      pulmonary Q22.1
      tricuspid Q22.4
  vas deferens N50.8
    congenital Q55.4
  vein I87.1
  vena cava (inferior) (superior) NEC I87.1
    congenital Q26.0
  vesicourethral orifice N32.0
    congenital Q64.31
  vulva (acquired) N90.5
Stridor R06.1
  congenital (larynx) P28.89
Stridulous —*see* condition
Stroke (apoplectic) (brain) (embolic)
  (ischemic) (paralytic) (thrombotic) I63.9
  epileptic —*see* Epilepsy
  heat T67.0
  in evolution I63.9
  intraoperative
    during cardiac surgery I97.810
    during other surgery I97.811
  lightning —*see* Lightning
  meaning
    cerebral hemorrhage
    code to Hemorrhage, intracranial
    cerebral infarction
    code to Infarction, cerebral
  postprocedural
    following cardiac surgery I97.820
    following other surgery I97.821
  unspecified (NOS) I63.9
Stromatosis, endometrial D39.0
Strongyloidiasis, strongyloidosis B78.9
  cutaneous B78.1
  disseminated B78.7
  intestinal B78.0
Strophulus pruriginosus L28.2
Struck by lightning —*see* Lightning
Struma —*see also* Goiter
  Hashimoto E06.3
  lymphomatosa E06.3
  nodosa (simplex) E04.9
    endemic E01.2
      multinodular E01.1
    multinodular E04.2
      iodine-deficiency related E01.1
    toxic or with hyperthyroidism E05.20
      with thyroid storm E05.21
    multinodular E05.20
      with thyroid storm E05.21
    uninodular E05.10
      with thyroid storm E05.11

Struma - *continued*
  toxicosa E05.20
    with thyroid storm E05.21
    multinodular E05.20
      with thyroid storm E05.21
    uninodular E05.10
      with thyroid storm E05.11
  uninodular E04.1
  ovarii D27.
  Riedel's E06.5
Strumipriva cachexia E03.4
Strümpell-Marie spine —*see* Spondylitis,
  ankylosing
Strümpell-Westphal pseudosclerosis E83.01
Stuart deficiency disease (factor X) D68.2
Stuart-Prower factor deficiency (factor X)
  D68.2
Student's elbow —*see* Bursitis, elbow,
  olecranon
Stump —*see* Amputation
Stunting, nutritional E45
Stupor (catatonic) R40.1
  depressive F32.8
  dissociative F44.2
  manic F30.2
  manic-depressive F31.89
  psychogenic (anergic) F44.2
  reaction to exceptional stress (transient) F43.0
Sturge (-Weber) (-Dimitri) (-Kalischer)
  disease or syndrome Q85.8
Stuttering F80.81
  adult onset F98.5
  childhood onset F80.81
  following cerebrovascular disease —*see*
  Disorder, fluency. following cerebrovascular
  disease
  in conditions classified elsewhere R47.82
Sty, stye (external) (internal) (meibomian)
  (zeisian) —*see* Hordeolum
Subacidity, gastric K31.89
  psychogenic F45.8
Subacute —*see* condition
Subarachnoid —*see* condition
Subcortical —*see* condition
Subcostal syndrome, nerve compression —
  see Mononeuropathy, upper limb, specified
  site NEC
Subcutaneous, subcuticular —*see* condition
Subdural —*see* condition
Subendocardium —*see* condition
Subependymoma
  specified site —*see* Neoplasm, uncertain
  behavior, by site
  unspecified site D43.2
Suberosis J67.3
Subglossitis —*see* Glossitis
Subhemophilia D66
Subinvolution
  breast (postlactational) (postpuerperal)
  N64.89
    puerperal O90.89
  uterus (chronic) (nonpuerperal) N85.3
    puerperal O90.89
Sublingual —*see* condition
Sublinguitis —*see* Sialoadenitis
Subluxatable hip Q65.6
Subluxation —*see also* Dislocation
  acromioclavicular S43.11
  ankle S93.0
  atlantoaxial, recurrent M43.4
    with myelopathy M43.3

Subluxation – *continued*
carpometacarpal (joint) NEC S63.05
  thumb S63.04
complex, vertebral —*see* Complex,
subluxation
congenital —*see also* Malposition, congenital
hip —*see* Dislocation, hip, congenital,
partial
  joint (excluding hip)
    lower limb Q68.8
    shoulder Q68.8
    upper limb Q68.8
elbow (traumatic) S53.10
  anterior S53.11
  lateral S53.14
  medial S53.13
  posterior S53.12
  specified type NEC S53.19
finger S63.20
  index S63.20
  interphalangeal S63.22
    distal S63.24
      index S63.24
      little S63.24
      middle S63.24
      ring S63.24
    index S63.22
    little S63.22
    middle S63.22
    proximal S63.23
      index S63.23
      little S63.23
      middle S63.23
      ring S63.23
    ring S63.22
  little S63.20
  metacarpophalangeal S63.21
    index S63.21
    little S63.21
    middle S63.21
    ring S63.21
  middle S63.20
  ring S63.20
foot S93.30
  specified site NEC S93.33
  tarsal joint S93.31
  tarsometatarsal joint S93.32
  toe —*see* Subluxation, toe
hip S73.00
  anterior S73.03
    obturator S73.02
  central S73.04
  posterior S73.01
interphalangeal (joint)
  finger S63.22
    distal joint S63.24
      index S63.24
      little S63.24
      middle S63.24
      ring S63.24
    index S63.22
    little S63.22
    middle S63.22
    proximal joint S63.23
      index S63.23
      little S63.23
      middle S63.23
      ring S63.23
    ring S63.22
  thumb S63.12
    distal joint S63.14
    proximal joint S63.13

Subluxation – *continued*
toe S93.13
  great S93.13
  lesser S93.13
joint prosthesis —*see* Complications, joint
prosthesis, mechanical, displacement, by site
knee S83.10
  cap —*see* Subluxation, patella
  patella —*see* Subluxation, patella
  proximal tibia
    anteriorly S83.11
    laterally S83.14
    medially S83.13
    posteriorly S83.12
  specified type NEC S83.19
lens —*see* Dislocation, lens, partial
ligament, traumatic —*see* Sprain, by site
metacarpal (bone)
  proximal end S63.06
metacarpophalangeal (joint)
  finger S63.21
    index S63.21
    little S63.21
    middle S63.21
    ring S63.21
  thumb S63.11
metatarsophalangeal joint S93.14
  great toe S93.14
  lesser toe S93.14
midcarpal (joint) S63.03
patella S83.00
  lateral S83.01
  recurrent (nontraumatic) —*see* Dislocation,
patella, recurrent, incomplete
  specified type NEC S83.09
pathological —*see* Dislocation, pathological
radial head S53.00
  anterior S53.01
  nursemaid's elbow S53.03
  posterior S53.02
  specified type NEC S53.09
radiocarpal (joint) S63.02
radioulnar (joint)
  distal S63.01
  proximal —*see* Subluxation, elbow
shoulder
  congenital Q68.8
  girdle S43.30
    scapula S43.31
    specified site NEC S43.39
  traumatic S43.00
    anterior S43.01
    inferior S43.03
    posterior S43.02
    specified type NEC S43.08
sternoclavicular (joint) S43.20
  anterior S43.21
  posterior S43.22
symphysis (pubis)
thumb S63.103
  interphalangeal joint —*see* Subluxation,
interphalangeal (joint) , thumb
    metacarpophalangeal joint —*see*
Subluxation, metacarpophalangeal (joint) ,
thumb
toe (s) S93.10
  great S93.10
    interphalangeal joint S93.13
    metatarsophalangeal joint S93.14
    interphalangeal joint S93.13
  lesser S93.10
    interphalangeal joint S93.13

Subluxation – *continued*
  metatarsophalangeal joint S93.14
  metatarsophalangeal joint S93.149
ulnohumeral joint —*see* Subluxation, elbow
vertebral
  recurrent NEC —*see* subcategory M43.5
  traumatic
    cervical S13.100
      atlantoaxial joint S13.120
      atlantooccipital joint S13.110
      atloido-occipital joint S13.110
      joint between
        C0 and C1 S13.110
        C1 and C2 S13.120
        C2 and C3 S13.130
        C3 and C4 S13.140
        C4 and C5 S13.150
        C5 and C6 S13.160
        C6 and C7 S13.170
        C7 and T1 S13.180
      occipitoatloid joint S13.110
    lumbar S33.100
      joint between
        L1 and L2 S33.110
        L2 and L3 S33.120
        L3 and L4 S33.130
        L4 and L5 S33.140
    thoracic S23.100
      joint between
        T1 and T2 S23.110
        T2 and T3 S23.120
        T3 and T4 S23.122
        T4 and T5 S23.130
        T5 and T6 S23.132
        T6 and T7 S23.140
        T7 and T8 S23.142
        T8 and T9 S23.150
        T9 and T10 S23.152
        T10 and T11 S23.160
        T11 and T12 S23.162
        T12 and L1 S23.170
ulna
  distal end S63.07
  proximal end —*see* Subluxation, elbow
wrist (carpal bone) S63.00
  carpometacarpal joint —*see* Subluxation,
carpometacarpal (joint)
  distal radioulnar joint —*see* Subluxation,
radioulnar (joint) , distal
  metacarpal bone, proximal —*see*
Subluxation, metacarpal (bone) , proximal end
  midcarpal —*see* Subluxation, midcarpal
(joint)
  radiocarpal joint —*see* Subluxation,
radiocarpal (joint)
  recurrent —*see* Dislocation, recurrent, wrist
  specified site NEC S63.09
  ulna —*see* Subluxation, ulna, distal end
Submaxillary —*see* condition
Submersion (fatal) (nonfatal) T75.1
Submucous   *see* condition
Subnormal, subnormality
accommodation (old age) H52.4
mental —*see* Disability, intellectual
temperature (accidental) T68
Subphrenic —*see* condition
Subscapular nerve —*see* condition
Subseptus uterus Q51.2
Subsiding appendicitis K36
Substernal thyroid E04.9
congenital Q89.2
Substitution disorder F44.9
Subtentorial —*see* condition

Subthyroidism (acquired) —*see also*
Hypothyroidism
congenital E03.1
Succenturiate placenta O43.19-**Sucking
thumb, child** (excessive) F98.8
Sudamen, sudamina L74.1
Sudanese kala-azar B55.0
Sudden
heart failure —*see* Failure, heart
hearing loss —*see* Deafness, sudden
Sudeck's atrophy, disease, or syndrome —
see Algoneurodystrophy
Suffocation —*see* Asphyxia, traumatic
Sugar
blood
high (transient) R73.9
low (transient) E16.2
in urine R81
Suicide, suicidal (attempted) T14.91
by poisoning —*see* Table of Drugs and
Chemicals
history of (personal) Z91.5
in family Z81.8
ideation —*see* Ideation, suicidal
risk
meaning personal history of attempted
suicide Z91.5
meaning suicidal ideation —*see* Ideation,
suicidal
tendencies
meaning personal history of attempted
suicide Z91.5
meaning suicidal ideation —*see* Ideation,
suicidal
trauma —*see* nature of injury by site
Suipestifer infection —*see* Infection,
salmonella
Sulfhemoglobinemia, sulphemoglobinemia
(acquired) (with methemoglobinemia) D74.8
Sumatran mite fever A75.3
Summer —*see* condition
Sunburn L55.9
first degree L55.0
second degree L55.1
third degree L55.2
SUNCT (short lasting unilateral neuralgiform
headache with conjunctival injection and
tearing) G44.059
intractable G44.051
not intractable G44.059
Sunken acetabulum —*see* Derangement,
joint, specified type NEC, hip
Sunstroke T67.0
Superfecundation —*see* Pregnancy, multiple
Superfetation —*see* Pregnancy, multiple
Superinvolution (uterus) N85.8
Supernumerary (congenital)
aortic cusps Q23.8
auditory ossicles Q16.3
bone Q79.8
breast Q83.1
carpal bones Q74.0
cusps, heart valve NEC Q24.8
aortic Q23.8
mitral Q23.2
pulmonary Q22.3
digit (s) Q69.9
ear (lobule) Q17.0
fallopian tube Q50.6
finger Q69.0
hymen Q52.4
kidney Q63.0

Supernumerary – *continued*
lacrimonasal duct Q10.6
lobule (ear) Q17.0
mitral cusps Q23.2
muscle Q79.8
nipple (s) Q83.3
organ or site not listed —*see* Accessory
ossicles, auditory Q16.3
ovary Q50.31
oviduct Q50.6
pulmonary, pulmonic cusps Q22.3
rib Q76.6
cervical or first (syndrome) Q76.5
roots (of teeth) K00.2
spleen Q89.09
tarsal bones Q74.2
teeth K00.1
testis Q55.29
thumb Q69.1
toe Q69.2
uterus Q51.2
vagina Q52.1
vertebra Q76.49
Supervision (of)
contraceptive —*see* Prescription,
contraceptives
dietary (for) Z71.3
allergy (food) Z71.3
colitis Z71.3
diabetes mellitus Z71.3
food allergy or intolerance Z71.3
gastritis Z71.3
hypercholesterolemia Z71.3
hypoglycemia Z71.3
intolerance (food) Z71.3
obesity Z71.3
specified NEC Z71.3
healthy infant or child Z76.2
foundling Z76.1
high-risk pregnancy —*see* Pregnancy,
complicated by, high, risk
lactation Z39.1
pregnancy —*see* Pregnancy, supervision of
Supplemental teeth K00.1
Suppression
binocular vision H53.34
lactation O92.5
menstruation N94.89
ovarian secretion E28.39
renal N28.9
urine, urinary secretion R34
Suppuration, suppurative —*see also*
condition
accessory sinus (chronic) —*see* Sinusitis
adrenal gland
antrum (chronic) —*see* Sinusitis, maxillary
bladder —*see* Cystitis
brain G06.0
sequelae G09
breast N61
puerperal, postpartum or gestational —*see*
Mastitis, obstetric, purulent
dental periosteum M27.3
ear (middle) —*see also* Otitis, media
external NEC —*see* Otitis, externa, infective
internal —*see* subcategory H83.0
ethmoidal (chronic) (sinus) —*see* Sinusitis,
ethmoidal
fallopian tube —*see* Salpingo-oophoritis
frontal (chronic) (sinus) —*see* Sinusitis,
frontal
gallbladder (acute) K81.0

Suppuration, suppurative – *continued*
gum K05.20
generalized K05.22
localized K05.21
intracranial G06.0
joint —*see* Arthritis, pyogenic or pyemic
labyrinthine —*see* subcategory H83.0
lung —*see* Abscess, lung
mammary gland N61
puerperal, postpartum O91.12
associated with lactation O91.13
maxilla, maxillary M27.2
sinus (chronic) —*see* Sinusitis, maxillary
muscle —*see* Myositis, infective
nasal sinus (chronic) —*see* Sinusitis
pancreas, acute K85.8
parotid gland —*see* Sialoadenitis
pelvis, pelvic
female —*see* Disease, pelvis, inflammatory
male K65.0
pericranial —*see* Osteomyelitis
salivary duct or gland (any) —*see*
Sialoadenitis
sinus (accessory) (chronic) (nasal) —*see*
Sinusitis
sphenoidal sinus (chronic) —*see* Sinusitis,
sphenoidal
thymus (gland) E32.1
thyroid (gland) E06.0
tonsil —*see* Tonsillitis
uterus —*see* Endometritis
Supraeruption of tooth (teeth) M26.34
Supraglottitis J04.30
with obstruction J04.31
Suprarenal (gland) —*see* condition
Suprascapular nerve —*see* condition
Suprasellar —*see* condition
Surfer's knots or nodules S89.8-**Surgical**
emphysema T81.82
procedures, complication or misadventure —
see Complications, surgical procedures
shock T81.10
Surveillance (of) (for) —*see also* Observation
alcohol abuse Z71.41
contraceptive —*see* Prescription,
contraceptives
dietary Z71.3
drug abuse Z71.51
Susceptibility to disease, genetic Z15.89
malignant neoplasm Z15.09
breast Z15.01
endometrium Z15.04
ovary Z15.02
prostate Z15.03
specified NEC Z15.09
multiple endocrine neoplasia Z15.81
Suspected condition, ruled out —*see also*
Observation, suspected
amniotic cavity and membrane Z03.71
cervical shortening Z03.75
fetal anomaly Z03.73
fetal growth Z03.74
maternal and fetal conditions NEC Z03.79
oligohydramnios Z03.71
placental problem Z03.72
polyhydramnios Z03.71
Suspended uterus
in pregnancy or childbirth —*see* Pregnancy,
complicated by, abnormal uterus
Sutton's nevus D22.9

Suture
　burst (in operation wound) T81.31
　　external operation wound T81.31
　　internal operation wound T81.32
　inadvertently left in operation wound —*see*
　Foreign body, accidentally left during a
　procedure
　removal Z48.02
Swab inadvertently left in operation wound
　—*see* Foreign body, accidentally left during a
　procedure
Swallowed, swallowing
　difficulty —*see* Dysphagia
　foreign body —*see* Foreign body, alimentary
　tract
Swan-neck deformity (finger) —*see*
　Deformity, finger, swan-neck
Swearing, compulsive F42
　in Gilles de la Tourette's syndrome F95.2
Sweat, sweats
　fetid L75.0
　night R61
Sweating, excessive R61
Sweeley-Klionsky disease E75.21
Sweet's disease or dermatosis L98.2
Swelling (of) R60.9
　abdomen, abdominal (not referable to any
　particular organ) —*see* Mass, abdominal
　ankle —*see* Effusion, joint, ankle
　arm M79.89
　　forearm M79.89
　breast N63
　Calabar B74.3
　cervical gland R59.0
　chest, localized R22.2
　ear H93.8
　extremity (lower) (upper) —*see* Disorder, soft
　tissue, specified type NEC
　finger M79.89
　foot M79.89
　glands R59.9
　　generalized R59.1
　　localized R59.0
　hand M79.89
　head (localized) R22.0
　inflammatory —*see* Inflammation
　intra-abdominal —*see* Mass, abdominal
　joint —*see* Effusion, joint
　leg M79.89
　　lower M79.89
　limb —*see* Disorder, soft tissue, specified
　type NEC
　localized (skin) R22.9
　　chest R22.2
　　head R22.0
　　limb
　　　lower —*see* Mass, localized, limb, lower
　　　upper —*see* Mass, localized, limb, upper
　　neck R22.1
　　trunk R22.2
　neck (localized) R22.1
　pelvic —*see* Mass, abdominal
　scrotum N50.8
　splenic —*see* Splenomegaly
　testis N50.8
　toe M79.89
　umbilical R19.09
　wandering, due to Gnathostoma (spinigerum)
　B83.1
　white —*see* Tuberculosis, arthritis

Swift (-Feer) disease
　overdose or wrong substance given or taken
　—*see* Table of Drugs and Chemicals, by drug,
　poisoning
Swimmer's
　cramp T75.1
　ear H60.33
　itch B65.3
Swimming in the head R42
Swollen —*see* Swelling
Swyer syndrome Q99.1 **Sycosis** L73.8
　barbae (not parasitic) L73.8
　contagiosa (mycotic) B35.0
　lupoides L73.8
　mycotic B35.0
　parasitic B35.0
　vulgaris L73.8
Sydenham's chorea —*see* Chorea,
　Sydenham's
Sylvatic yellow fever A95.0
Sylvest's disease B33.0
Symblepharon H11.23
　congenital Q10.3
Symond's syndrome G93.2
Sympathetic —*see* condition
Sympatheticotonia G90.8
Sympathicoblastoma
　specified site —*see* Neoplasm, malignant, by
　site
　unspecified site C74.90
Sympathogonioma —*see* Sympathicoblastoma
Symphalangy (fingers) (toes) Q70.9
Symptoms NEC R68.89
　breast NEC N64.59
　development NEC R63.8
　factitious, self-induced —*see* Disorder,
　factitious
　genital organs, female R10.2
　involving
　　abdomen NEC R19.8
　　appearance NEC R46.89
　　awareness R41.9
　　　altered mental status R41.82
　　　amnesia —*see* Amnesia
　　　borderline intellectual functioning R41.83
　　　coma —*see* Coma
　　　disorientation R41.0
　　　neurologic neglect syndrome R41.4
　　　senile cognitive decline R41.81
　　　specified symptom NEC R41.89
　　behavior NEC R46.89
　　cardiovascular system NEC R09.89
　　chest NEC R09.89
　　circulatory system NEC R09.89
　　cognitive functions R41.9
　　　altered mental status R41.82
　　　amnesia —*see* Amnesia
　　　borderline intellectual functioning R41.83
　　　coma —*see* Coma
　　　disorientation R41.0
　　　neurologic neglect syndrome R41.4
　　　senile cognitive decline R41.81
　　　specified symptom NEC R41.89
　　development NEC R62.50
　　digestive system NEC R19.8
　　emotional state NEC R45.89
　　　emotional lability R45.86
　　food and fluid intake R63.8
　　general perceptions and sensations R44.9
　　　specified NEC R44.8
　　musculoskeletal system R29.91
　　　specified NEC R29.898

Symptoms – *continued*
　nervous system R29.90
　　specified NEC R29.818
　pelvis NEC R19.8
　respiratory system NEC R09.89
　skin and integument R23.9
　urinary system R39.9
　menopausal N95.1
　metabolism NEC R63.8
　neurotic F48.8
　of infancy R68.19
　pelvis NEC, female R10.2
　skin and integument NEC R23.9
　subcutaneous tissue NEC R23.9
Sympus Q74.2
Syncephalus Q89.4
Synchondrosis
　abnormal (congenital) Q78.8
　ischiopubic M91.0
Synchysis (scintillans) (senile) (vitreous body)
　H43.89
Syncope (near) (pre) R55
　anginosa I20.8
　bradycardia R00.1
　cardiac R55
　carotid sinus G90.01
　due to spinal (lumbar) puncture G97.1
　heart R55
　heat T67.1
　laryngeal R05
　psychogenic F48.8
　tussive R05
　vasoconstriction R55
　vasodepressor R55
　vasomotor R55
　vasovagal R55
Syndactylism, syndactyly Q70.9
　complex (with synostosis)
　　fingers Q70.0
　　toes Q70.2
　simple (without synostosis)
　　fingers Q70.1
　　toes Q70.3
Syndrome —*see also* Disease
　5q minus NOS D46.C
　48,XXXX Q97.1
　49,XXXXX Q97.1
　abdominal
　　acute R10.0
　　muscle deficiency Q79.4
　abnormal innervation H02.519
　　left H02.516
　　　lower H02.515
　　　upper H02.514
　　right H02.513
　　　lower H02.512
　　　upper H02.511
　abstinence, neonatal P96.1
　acid pulmonary aspiration, obstetric O74.0
　acquired immunodeficiency —*see* Human,
　immunodeficiency virus (HIV) disease
　acute abdominal R10.0
　acute respiratory distress (adult) (child) J80
　Adair-Dighton Q78.0
　Adams-Stokes (-Morgagni) I45.9
　adiposogenital E23.6
　adrenal
　　hemorrhage (meningococcal) A39.1
　　meningococcic A39.1
　adrenocortical —*see* Cushing's, syndrome
　adrenogenital E25.9
　　congenital, associated with enzyme
　deficiency E25.0

Syndrome - *continued*
afferent loop NEC K91.89
Alagille's Q44.7
alcohol withdrawal (without convulsions) —
see Dependence, alcohol, with, withdrawal
Alder's D72.0
Aldrich (-Wiskott) D82.0
alien hand R41.4
Alport Q87.81
alveolar hypoventilation E66.2
alveolocapillary block J84.10
amnesic, amnestic (confabulatory) (due to) —
see Disorder, amnesic
amyostatic (Wilson's disease) E83.01
androgen insensitivity E34.50
  complete E34.51
  partial E34.52
androgen resistance (*see also* Syndrome,
androgen insensitivity) E34.50
Angelman Q93.5
anginal —*see* Angina
ankyloglossia superior Q38.1
anterior
  chest wall R07.89
  cord G83.82
  spinal artery G95.19
    compression M47.019
      cervical region M47.012
      cervicothoracic region M47.013
      lumbar region M47.016
      occipito-atlanto-axial region M47.011
      thoracic region M47.014
      thoracolumbar region M47.015
    tibial M76.81
antibody deficiency D80.9
  agammaglobulinemic D80.1
    hereditary D80.0
  congenital D80.0
  hypogammaglobulinemic D80.1
    hereditary D80.0
anticardiolipin (-antibody) D68.61
antiphospholipid (-antibody) D68.61
aortic
  arch M31.4
  bifurcation I74.09
aortomesenteric duodenum occlusion K31.5
apical ballooning (transient left ventricular)
I51.81
arcuate ligament I77.4
argentaffin, argintaffinoma E34.0
Arnold-Chiari —*see* Arnold-Chiari disease
Arrillaga-Ayerza I27.0
Asherman's N85.6
aspiration, of newborn —*see* Aspiration, by
substance, with pneumonia
  meconium P24.01
ataxia-telangiectasia G11.3
auriculotemporal G50.8
autoerythrocyte sensitization (Gardner-
Diamond) D69.2
autoimmune polyglandular E31.0
autoimmune lymphoproliferative -ALPS]
D89.82
autosomal —*see* Abnormal, autosomes
Avellis' G46.8
Ayerza (-Arrillaga) I27.0
Babinski-Nageotte G83.89
Bakwin-Krida Q79.8
bare lymphocyte D81.6
Barré-Guillain G61.0
Barré-Liéou M53.0
Barrett's —*see* Barrett's, esophagus

Syndrome - *continued*
Barsony-Polgar K22.4
Barsony-Teschendorf K22.4
Barth E78.71
Bartter's E26.81
basal cell nevus Q87.89
Basedow's E05.00
  with thyroid storm E05.01
basilar artery G45.0
Batten-Steinert G71.11
battered
  baby or child —*see* Maltreatment, child,
physical abuse
    spouse —*see* Maltreatment, adult, physical
abuse
Beals Q87.40
Beau's I51.5
Beck's I65.8
Benedikt's G46.3
Béquez César (-Steinbrinck-Chédiak-Higashi)
E70.330
Bernhardt-Roth —*see* Meralgia paresthetica
Bernheim's I50.9
big spleen D73.1
bilateral polycystic ovarian E28.2
Bing-Horton's —*see* Horton's headache
Birt-Hogg-Dube syndrome Q87.89
Björck (-Thorsen) E34.0
black
  lung J60
  widow spider bite —*see* Toxicity, venom,
spider, black widow
Blackfan-Diamond D61.01
blind loop K90.2
  congenital Q43.8
  postsurgical K91.2
blue sclera Q78.0
blue toe I75.02
Boder-Sedgewick G11.3
Boerhaave's K22.3
Borjeson Forssman Lehmann Q89.8
Bouillaud's I01.9
Bourneville (-Pringle) Q85.1
Bouveret (-Hoffman) I47.9
brachial plexus G54.0
bradycardia-tachycardia I49.5
brain (nonpsychotic) F09
  with psychosis, psychotic reaction F09
  acute or subacute —*see* Delirium
  congenital —*see* Disability, intellectual
  organic F09
    post-traumatic (nonpsychotic) F07.81
      psychotic F09
  personality change F07.0
  postcontusional F07.81
  post-traumatic, nonpsychotic F07.81
  psycho-organic F09
  psychotic F06.8
brain stem stroke G46.3
Brandt's (acrodermatitis enteropathica) E83.2
broad ligament laceration N83.8
Brock's J98.11
bronze baby P83.8
Brown-Sequard G83.81
bubbly lung P27.0
Buchem's M85.2
Budd-Chiari I82.0
bulbar (progressive) G12.22
Bürger-Grütz E78.3
Burke's K86.8
Burnett's (milk-alkali) E83.52
burning feet E53.9

Syndrome - *continued*
Bywaters' T79.5
Call-Fleming I67.841
carbohydrate-deficient glycoprotein (CDGS)
E77.8
carcinogenic thrombophlebitis I82.1
carcinoid E34.0
cardiac asthma I50.1
cardiacos negros I27.0
cardiofaciocutaneous Q87.89
cardiopulmonary-obesity E66.2
cardiorenal —*see* Hypertension, cardiorenal
cardiorespiratory distress (idiopathic) ,
newborn P22.0
cardiovascular renal —*see* Hypertension,
cardiorenal
carotid
  artery (hemispheric) (internal) G45.1
  body G90.01
  sinus G90.01
carpal tunnel G56.0
Cassidy (-Scholte) E34.0
cat cry Q93.4
cat eye Q92.8
cauda equina G83.4
causalgia —*see* Causalgia
celiac K90.0
  artery compression I77.4
  axis I77.4
central pain G89.0
cerebellar
  hereditary G11.9
  stroke G46.4
cerebellomedullary malformation —*see* Spina
bifida
cerebral
  artery
    anterior G46.1
    middle G46.0
    posterior G46.2
  gigantism E22.0
cervical (root) M53.1
  disc —*see* Disorder, disc, cervical, with
neuritis
  fusion Q76.1
  posterior, sympathicus M53.0
  rib Q76.5
  sympathetic paralysis G90.2
cervicobrachial (diffuse) M53.1
cervicocranial M53.0
cervicodorsal outlet G54.2
cervicothoracic outlet G54.0
Céstan (-Raymond) I65.8
Charcot's (angina cruris) (intermittent
claudication) I73.9
Charcot-Weiss-Baker G90.09
CHARGE Q89.8
Chédiak-Higashi (-Steinbrinck) E70.330
chest wall R07.1
Chiari's (hepatic vein thrombosis) I82.0
Chilaiditi's Q43.3
child maltreatment —*see* Maltreatment, child
chondrocostal junction M94.0
chondroectodermal dysplasia Q77.6
chromosome 4 short arm deletion Q93.3
chromosome 5 short arm deletion Q93.4
chronic
  pain G89.4
    personality F68.8
Clarke-Hadfield K86.8
Clerambault's automatism G93.89

Syndrome - *continued*

Clouston's (hidrotic ectodermal dysplasia) Q82.4
clumsiness, clumsy child F82
cluster headache G44.009
 intractable G44.001
 not intractable G44.009
Coffin-Lowry Q89.8
cold injury (newborn) P80.0
combined immunity deficiency D81.9
compartment (deep) (posterior) (traumatic) T79.A0
 abdomen T79.A3
 lower extremity (hip, buttock, thigh, leg, foot, toes) T79.A2
 nontraumatic
  abdomen M79.A3
  lower extremity (hip, buttock, thigh, leg, foot, toes) M79.A2
  specified site NEC M79.A9
  upper extremity (shoulder, arm, forearm, wrist, hand, fingers) M79.A1
 postprocedural —*see* Syndrome, compartment, nontraumatic
 specified site NEC T79.A9
 upper extremity (shoulder, arm, forearm, wrist, hand, fingers) T79.A1
complex regional pain —*see* Syndrome, pain, complex regional
compression T79.5
 anterior spinal —*see* Syndrome, anterior, spinal artery, compression
 cauda equina G83.4
 celiac artery I77.4
 vertebral artery M47.029
  occipito-atlanto-axial region M47.021
  cervical region M47.022
concussion F07.81
congenital
 affecting multiple systems NEC Q87.89
 central alveolar hypoventilation G47.35
 facial diplegia Q87.0
 muscular hypertrophy-cerebral Q87.89
 oculo-auriculovertebral Q87.0
 oculofacial diplegia (Moebius) Q87.0
 rubella (manifest) P35.0
congestion-fibrosis (pelvic) , female N94.89
congestive dysmenorrhea N94.6
Conn's E26.01
connective tissue M35.9
 overlap NEC M35.1
conus medullaris G95.81
cord
 anterior G83.82
 posterior G83.83
coronary
 acute NEC I24.9
 insufficiency or intermediate I20.0
 slow flow I20.8
Costen's (complex) M26.69
costochondral junction M94.0
costoclavicular G54.0
costovertebral E22.0
Cowden Q85.8
craniovertebral M53.0
Creutzfeldt-Jakob —*see* Creutzfeldt-Jakob disease or syndrome
cri-du-chat Q93.4
crib death R99
cricopharyngeal —*see* Dysphagia
croup J05.0

Syndrome - *continued*

CRPS I —*see* Syndrome, pain, complex regional I
crush T79.5
cubital tunnel —*see* Lesion, nerve, ulnar
Curschmann (-Batten) (-Steinert) G71.11
Cushing's E24.9
 alcohol-induced E24.4
 due to
  alcohol
   drugs E24.2
   ectopic ACTH E24.3
   overproduction of pituitary ACTH E24.0
 drug-induced E24.2
 overdose or wrong substance given or taken —*see* Table of Drugs and Chemicals, by drug, poisoning
 pituitary-dependent E24.0
 specified type NEC E24.8
cryptophthalmos Q87.0
cystic duct stump K91.5
Dana-Putnam D51.0
Danbolt (-Cross) (acrodermatitis enteropathica) E83.2
Dandy-Walker Q03.1
 with spina bifida Q07.01
Danlos' Q79.8
defibrination —*see also* Fibrinolysis
 with
  antepartum hemorrhage —*see* Hemorrhage, antepartum, with coagulation defect
  intrapartum hemorrhage —*see* Hemorrhage, complicating, delivery
 newborn P60
 postpartum O72.3
Degos' I77.89
Déjérine-Roussy G89.0
delayed sleep phase G47.21
demyelinating G37.9
dependence —*see* F10-F19 with fourth character .2
depersonalization (-derealization) F48.1
De Quervain E34.51
de Toni-Fanconi (-Debré) E72.09
 with cystinosis E72.04
diabetes mellitus-hypertension-nephrosis —*see* Diabetes, nephrosis
diabetes mellitus in newborn infant P70.2
diabetes-nephrosis —*see* Diabetes, nephrosis
diabetic amyotrophy —*see* Diabetes, amyotrophy
Diamond-Blackfan D61.01
Diamond-Gardener D69.2
DIC (diffuse or disseminated intravascular coagulopathy) D65
di George's D82.1
Dighton's Q78.0
disequilibrium E87.8
Döhle body-panmyelopathic D72.0
dorsolateral medullary G46.4
double athetosis G80.3
Down (*see also* Down syndrome) Q90.9
Dresbach's (elliptocytosis) D58.1
Dressler's (postmyocardial infarction) I24.1
 postcardiotomy I97.0
drug withdrawal, infant of dependent mother P96.1
dry eye H04.12
due to abnormality
 chromosomal Q99.9

Syndrome - *continued*

sex
 female phenotype Q97.9
 male phenotype Q98.9
 specified NEC Q99.8
dumping (postgastrectomy) K91.1
 nonsurgical K31.89
Dupré's (meningism) R29.1
dysmetabolic X E88.81
dyspraxia, developmental F82
Eagle-Barrett Q79.4
Eaton-Lambert —*see* Syndrome, Lambert-Eaton
Ebstein's Q22.5
ectopic ACTH E24.3
eczema-thrombocytopenia D82.0
Eddowes' Q78.0
effort (psychogenic) F45.8
Eisenmenger's I27.89
Ehlers-Danlos Q79.6
Ekman's Q78.0
electric feet E53.8
Ellis-van Creveld Q77.6
empty nest Z60.0
endocrine-hypertensive E27.0
entrapment —*see* Neuropathy, entrapment
eosinophilia-myalgia M35.8
epileptic —*see also* Epilepsy, by type
 absence G40.A09
  intractable G40.A19
   with status epilepticus G40.A11
   without status epilepticus G40.A19
  not intractable G40.A09
   with status epilepticus G40.A01
   without status epilepticus G40.A09
Erdheim-Chester (ECD) E88.89
Erdheim's E22.0
erythrocyte fragmentation D59.4
Evans D69.41
exhaustion F48.8
extrapyramidal G25.9
 specified NEC G25.89
eye retraction —*see* Strabismus
eyelid-malar-mandible Q87.0
Faber's D50.9
facial pain, paroxysmal G50.0
Fallot's Q21.3
familial eczema-thrombocytopenia (Wiskott-Aldrich) D82.0
Fanconi (-de Toni) (-Debré) E72.09
 with cystinosis E72.04
Fanconi's (anemia) (congenital pancytopenia) D61.09
fatigue
 chronic R53.82
 psychogenic F48.8
faulty bowel habit K59.3
Feil-Klippel (brevicollis) Q76.1
Felty's —*see* Felty's syndrome
fertile eunuch E23.0
fetal
 alcohol (dysmorphic) Q86.0
 hydantoin Q86.1
Fiedler's I40.1
first arch Q87.0
fish odor E72.8
Fisher's G61.0
Fitzhugh-Curtis
 due to
  Chlamydia trachomatis A74.81
  Neisseria gonorrhorea (gonococcal peritonitis) A54.85

Syndrome - *continued*
Fitz's K85.8
Flajani (-Basedow) E05.00
 with thyroid storm E05.01
flatback —*see* Flatback syndrome
floppy
 baby P94.2
 iris (intraoperative) (IFIS) H21.81
 mitral valve I34.1
flush E34.0
Foix-Alajouanine G95.19
Fong's Q79.8
foramen magnum G93.5
Foster-Kennedy H47.14
Foville's (peduncular) G46.3
fragile X Q99.2
Franceschetti Q75.4
Frey's
 auriculotemporal G50.8
 hyperhidrosis L74.52
Friderichsen-Waterhouse A39.1
Froin's G95.89
frontal lobe F07.0
Fukuhara E88.49
functional
 bowel K59.9
 prepubertal castrate E29.1
Gaisböck's D75.1
ganglion (basal ganglia brain) G25.9
 geniculi G51.1
Gardner-Diamond D69.2
gastroesophageal
 junction K22.0
 laceration-hemorrhage K22.6
gastrojejunal loop obstruction K91.89
Gee-Herter-Heubner K90.0
Gelineau's G47.419
 with cataplexy G47.411
genito-anorectal A55
Gerstmann-Sträussler-Scheinker (GSS)
A81.82
Gianotti-Crosti L44.4
giant platelet (Bernard-Soulier) D69.1
Gilles de la Tourette's F95.2
goiter-deafness E07.1
Goldberg Q89.8
Goldberg-Maxwell E34.51
Good's D83.8
Gopalan' (burning feet) E53.8
Gorlin's Q87.89
Gougerot-Blum L81.7
Gouley's I31.1
Gower's R55
gray or grey (newborn) P93.0
 platelet D69.1
Gubler-Millard G46.3
Guillain-Barré (-Strohl) G61.0
gustatory sweating G50.8
Hadfield-Clarke K86.8
hair tourniquet —*see* Constriction, external,
by site
Hamman's J98.19
hand-foot L27.1
hand-shoulder G90.8
hantavirus (cardio)
 pulmonary (HPS) (HCPS) B33.4
happy puppet Q93.5
Harada's H30.81
Hayem-Faber D50.9
headache NEC G44.89
 complicated NEC G44.59
Heberden's I20.8

Syndrome - *continued*
Hedinger's E34.0
Hegglin's D72.0
HELLP (hemolysis, elevated liver enzymes
and low platelet count) O14.2
hemolytic-uremic D59.3
hemophagocytic, infection-associated D76.2
Henoch-Schönlein D69.0
hepatic flexure K59.8
hepatopulmonary K76.81
hepatorenal K76.7
 following delivery O90.4
 postoperative or postprocedural K91.83
 postpartum, puerperal O90.4
hepatourologic K76.7
Herter (-Gee) (nontropical sprue) K90.0
Heubner-Herter K90.0
Heyd's K76.7
Hilger's G90.09
histamine-like (fish poisoning) —*see*
Poisoning, fish
histiocytic D76.3
histiocytosis NEC D76.3
HIV infection, acute B20
Hoffmann-Werdnig G12.0
Hollander-Simons E88.1
Hoppe-Goldflam G70.00
 with exacerbation (acute) G70.01
 in crisis G70.01
Horner's G90.2
hungry bone E83.81
hunterian glossitis D51.0
Hutchinson's triad A50.53
hyperabduction G54.0
hyperammonemia-hyperornithinemia-
homocitrullinemia E72.4
hypereosinophilic (idiopathic) D72.1
hyperimmunoglobulin E (IgE) D82.4
hyperkalemic E87.5
hyperkinetic —*see* Hyperkinesia
hypermobility M35.7
hypernatremia E87.0
hyperosmolarity E87.0
hyperperfusion G97.82
hypersplenic D73.1
hypertransfusion, newborn P61.1
hyperventilation F45.8
hyperviscosity (of serum)
 polycythemic D75.1
 sclerothymic D58.8
hypoglycemic (familial) (neonatal) E16.2
hypokalemic E87.6
hyponatremic E87.1
hypopituitarism E23.0
hypoplastic left-heart Q23.4
hypopotassemia E87.6
hyposmolality E87.1
hypotension, maternal O26.5
hypothenar hammer I73.89
ICF (intravascular coagulation-fibrinolysis)
D65
idiopathic
 cardiorespiratory distress, newborn P22.0
 nephrotic (infantile) N04.9
iliotibial band M76.3
immobility, immobilization (paraplegic)
M62.3
immune reconstitution D89.3
immune reconstitution inflammatory -IRIS]
D89.3
immunity deficiency, combined D81.9

Syndrome - *continued*
immunodeficiency
 acquired —*see* Human, immunodeficiency
virus (HIV) disease
 combined D81.9
impending coronary I20.0
impingement, shoulder M75.4
inappropriate secretion of antidiuretic
hormone E22.2
infant
 of diabetic mother P70.1
 gestational diabetes P70.0
infantilism (pituitary) E23.0
inferior vena cava I87.1
inspissated bile (newborn) P59.1
institutional (childhood) F94.2
insufficient sleep F51.12
intermediate coronary (artery) I20.0
interspinous ligament —*see* Spondylopathy,
specified NEC
intestinal
 carcinoid E34.0
 knot K56.2
intravascular coagulation-fibrinolysis (ICF)
D65
iodine-deficiency, congenital E00.9
 type
 mixed E00.2
 myxedematous E00.1
 neurological E00.0
IRDS (idiopathic respiratory distress,
newborn) P22.0
irritable
 bowel K58.9
 with diarrhea K58.0
 psychogenic F45.8
 heart (psychogenic) F45.8
 weakness F48.8
ischemic bowel (transient) K55.9
 chronic K55.1
 due to mesenteric artery insufficiency K55.1
IVC (intravascular coagulopathy) D65
Ivemark's Q89.01
Jaccoud's —*see* Arthropathy, postrheumatic,
chronic
Jackson's G83.89
Jakob-Creutzfeldt —*see* Creutzfeldt-Jakob
disease or syndrome
jaw-winking Q07.8
Jervell-Lange-Nielsen I45.81
jet lag G47.25
Job's D71
Joseph-Diamond-Blackfan D61.01
jugular foramen G52.7
Kabuki Q89.8
Kanner's (autism) F84.0
Kartagener's Q89.3
Kelly's D50.1
Kimmelstiel-Wilson —*see* Diabetes, specified
type, with Kimmelstiel-Wilson disease
Klein (e) -Levine G47.13
Klippel-Feil (brevicollis) Q76.1
Köhler-Pellegrini-Steida —*see* Bursitis, tibial
collateral
König's K59.8
Korsakoff (-Wernicke) (nonalcoholic) F04
 alcoholic F10.26
Kostmann's D70.0
Krabbe's congenital muscle hypoplasia Q79.8
labyrinthine —*see* subcategory H83.2
lacunar NEC G46.7

Syndrome - *continued*
- Lambert-Eaton G70.80
  - in
    - neoplastic disease G73.1
    - specified disease NEC G70.81
- Landau-Kleffner —*see* Epilepsy, specified NEC
- Larsen's Q74.8
- lateral
  - cutaneous nerve of thigh G57.1
  - medullary G46.4
- Launois' E22.0
- lazy
  - leukocyte D70.8
  - posture M62.3
- Lemiere I80.8
- Lennox-Gastaut G40.812
  - intractable G40.814
    - with status epilepticus G40.813
    - without status epilepticus G40.814
  - not intractable G40.812
    - with status epilepticus G40.811
    - without status epilepticus G40.812
- lenticular, progressive E83.01
- Leopold-Levi's E05.90
- Lev's I44.2
- Li-Fraumeni Z15.01
- Lichtheim's D51.0
- Lightwood's N25.89
- Lignac (de Toni) (-Fanconi) (-Debré) E72.09
  - with cystinosis E72.04
- Likoff's I20.8
- limbic epilepsy personality F07.0
- liver-kidney K76.7
- lobotomy F07.0
- Loffler's J82
- long arm 18 or 21 deletion Q93.89
- long QT I45.81
- Louis-Barré G11.3
- low
  - atmospheric pressure T70.29
  - back M54.5
  - output (cardiac) I50.9
- lower radicular, newborn (birth injury) P14.8
- Luetscher's (dehydration) E86.0
- Lupus anticoagulant D68.62
- Lutembacher's Q21.1
- macrophage activation D76.1
  - due to infection D76.2
- magnesium-deficiency R29.0
- Mal de Debarquement R42
- malabsorption K90.9
  - postsurgical K91.2
- malformation, congenital, due to
  - alcohol Q86.0
  - exogenous cause NEC Q86.8
  - hydantoin Q86.1
  - warfarin Q86.2
- malignant
  - carcinoid E34.0
  - neuroleptic G21.0
- Mallory-Weiss K22.6
- mandibulofacial dysostosis Q75.4
- manic-depressive —*see* Disorder, bipolar, affective
- maple-syrup-urine E71.0
- Marable's I77.4
- Marfan's Q87.40
  - with
    - cardiovascular manifestations Q87.418
      - aortic dilation Q87.410
    - ocular manifestations Q87.42

Syndrome - *continued*
- skeletal manifestations Q87.43
- Marie's (acromegaly) E22.0
- maternal hypotension —*see* Syndrome, hypotension, maternal
- May (-Hegglin) D72.0
- McArdle (-Schmidt) (-Pearson) E74.04
- McQuarrie's E16.2
- meconium plug (newborn) P76.0
- median arcuate ligament I77.4
- Meekeren-Ehlers-Danlos Q79.6
- megavitamin-B6 E67.2
- Meige G24.4
- MELAS E88.41
- Mendelson's O74.0
- MERRF (myoclonic epilepsy associated with ragged-red fibers) E88.42
- mesenteric
  - artery (superior) K55.1
  - vascular insufficiency K55.1
- metabolic E88.81
- metastatic carcinoid E34.0
- micrognathia-glossoptosis Q87.0
- midbrain NEC G93.89
- middle lobe (lung) J98.19
- middle radicular G54.0
- migraine (*see also* Migraine) G43.909
- Mikulicz' K11.8
- milk-alkali E83.52
- Millard-Gubler G46.3
- Miller-Dieker Q93.88
- Miller-Fisher G61.0
- Minkowski-Chauffard D58.0
- Mirizzi's K83.1
- MNGIE (Mitochondrial Neurogastrointestinal Encephalopathy) E88.49
- Möbius, ophthalmoplegic migraine —*see* Migraine, ophthalmoplegic
- monofixation H50.42
- Morel-Moore M85.2
- Morel-Morgagni M85.2
- Morgagni (-Morel) (-Stewart) M85.2
- Morgagni-Adams-Stokes I45.9
- mucocutaneous lymph node (acute febrile) (MCLS) M30.3
- multiple endocrine neoplasia (MEN) —*see* Neoplasia, endocrine, multiple (MEN)
- multiple operations —*see* Disorder, factitious
- Mounier-Kuhn Q32.4
  - with bronchiectasis J47.9
    - with
      - exacerbation (acute) J47.1
      - lower respiratory infection J47.0
  - acquired J98.09
    - with bronchiectasis J47.9
      - with
        - exacerbation (acute) J47.1
        - lower respiratory infection J47.0
- myasthenic G70.9
  - in
    - diabetes mellitus —*see* Diabetes, amyotrophy
    - endocrine disease NEC E34.9 *[G73.3]*
    - neoplastic disease (*see also* Neoplasm) D49.9 *[G73.3]*
    - thyrotoxicosis (hyperthyroidism) E05.90 *[G73.3]*
      - with thyroid storm E05.91 *[G73.3]*
- myelodysplastic D46.9
  - with
    - 5q deletion D46.C

Syndrome - *continued*
- isolated del (5q) chromosomal abnormality D46.C
- lesions, low grade D46.20
  - specified NEC D46.Z
- myelopathic pain G89.0
- myeloproliferative (chronic) D47.1
- myofascial pain M79.1
- Naffziger's G54.0
- nail patella Q87.2
- NARP (Neuropathy, Ataxia and Retinitis pigmentosa) E88.49
- neonatal abstinence P96.1
- nephritic —*see also* Nephritis
  - with edema —*see* Nephrosis
  - acute N00.9
  - chronic N03.9
  - rapidly progressive N01.9
- nephrotic (congenital) (*see also* Nephrosis) N04.9
  - with
    - dense deposit disease N04.6
    - diffuse
      - crescentic glomerulonephritis N04.7
      - endocapillary proliferative glomerulonephritis N04.4
      - membranous glomerulonephritis N04.2
      - mesangial proliferative glomerulonephritis N04.3
      - mesangiocapillary glomerulonephritis N04.5
    - focal and segmental glomerular lesions N04.1
    - minor glomerular abnormality N04.0
    - specified morphological changes NEC N04.8
  - diabetic —*see* Diabetes, nephrosis
- neurologic neglect R41.4
- Nezelof's D81.4
- Nonne-Milroy-Meige Q82.0
- Nothnagel's vasomotor acroparesthesia I73.89
- oculomotor H51.9
- ophthalmoplegia-cerebellar ataxia —*see* Strabismus, paralytic, third nerve
- oral-facial-digital Q87.0
- organic
  - affective F06.30
  - amnesic (not alcohol or drug-induced) F04
  - brain F09
  - depressive F06.31
  - hallucinosis F06.0
  - personality F07.0
- Ormond's N13.5
- oro-facial-digital Q87.0
- os trigonum Q68.8
- Osler-Weber-Rendu I78.0
- osteoporosis-osteomalacia M83.8
- Osterreicher-Turner Q79.8
- otolith —*see* subcategory H81.8
- oto-palatal-digital Q87.0
- outlet (thoracic) G54.0
- ovary
  - polycystic E28.2
  - resistant E28.39
  - sclerocystic E28.2
- Owren's D68.2
- Paget-Schroetter I82.890
- pain —*see also* Pain
  - complex regional I G90.50
    - lower limb G90.52
    - specified site NEC G90.59
    - upper limb G90.51
  - complex regional II —*see* Causalgia

Syndrome *- continued*
painful
  bruising D69.2
  feet E53.8
  prostate N42.81
paralysis agitans —*see* Parkinsonism
paralytic G83.9
  specified NEC G83.89
Parinaud's H51.0
parkinsonian —*see* Parkinsonism
Parkinson's —*see* Parkinsonism
paroxysmal facial pain G50.0
Parry's E05.00
  with thyroid storm E05.01
Parsonage (-Aldren) -Turner G54.5
patella clunk M25.86
Paterson (-Brown) (-Kelly) D50.1
pectoral girdle I77.89
pectoralis minor I77.89
Pelger-Huet D72.0
pellagra-cerebellar ataxia-renal aminoaciduria
E72.02
pellagroid E52
Pellegrini-Stieda —*see* Bursitis, tibial
collateral
pelvic congestion-fibrosis, female N94.89
penta X Q97.1
peptic ulcer —*see* Ulcer, peptic
perabduction I77.89
periodic headache, in adults and children —
see Headache, periodic syndromes in adults
and children
periurethral fibrosis N13.5
phantom limb (without pain) G54.7
  with pain G54.6
pharyngeal pouch D82.1
Pick's (heart) (liver) I31.1
Pickwickian E66.2
PIE (pulmonary infiltration with eosinophilia)
J82
pigmentary pallidal degeneration
(progressive) G23.0
pineal E34.8
pituitary E22.0
plantar fascia M72.2
placental transfusion —*see* Pregnancy,
complicated by, placental transfusion
syndromes
plateau iris (post-iridectomy) (postprocedural)
H21.82
Plummer-Vinson D50.1
pluricarential of infancy E40
plurideficiency E40
pluriglandular (compensatory) E31.8
  autoimmune E31.0
pneumatic hammer T75.21
polyangiitis overlap M30.8
polycarential of infancy E40
polyglandular E31.8
  autoimmune E31.0
polysplenia Q89.09
pontine NEC G93.89
popliteal
  artery entrapment I77.89
  web Q87.89
postcardiac injury
  postcardiotomy I97.0
  postmyocardial infarction I24.1
postcardiotomy I97.0
post chemoembolization
code to associated conditions
postcholecystectomy K91.5

Syndrome *- continued*
postcommissurotomy I97.0
postconcussional F07.81
postcontusional F07.81
postencephalitic F07.89
posterior
  cervical sympathetic M53.0
  cord G83.83
  fossa compression G93.5
  reversible encephalopathy (PRES) I67.83
postgastrectomy (dumping) K91.1
postgastric surgery K91.1
postinfarction I24.1
postlaminectomy NEC M96.1
postleukotomy F07.0
postmastectomy lymphedema I97.2
postmyocardial infarction I24.1
postoperative NEC T81.9
  blind loop K90.2
postpartum panhypopituitary (Sheehan) E23.0
postpolio (myelitic) G14
postthrombotic I87.009
  with
    inflammation I87.02
      with ulcer I87.03
    specified complication NEC I87.09
    ulcer I87.01
      with inflammation I87.03
  asymptomatic I87.00
postvagotomy K91.1
postvalvulotomy I97.0
postviral NEC G93.3
  fatigue G93.3
Potain's K31.0
potassium intoxication E87.5
precerebral artery (multiple) (bilateral) G45.2
preinfarction I20.0
preleukemic D46.9
premature senility E34.8
premenstrual dysphoric N94.3
premenstrual tension N94.3
Prinzmetal-Massumi R07.1
prune belly Q79.4
pseudocarpal tunnel (sublimis) —*see*
Syndrome, carpal tunnel
pseudoparalytica G70.00
  with exacerbation (acute) G70.01
  in crisis G70.01
pseudo -Turner's Q87.1
psycho-organic (nonpsychotic severity) F07.9
  acute or subacute F05
  depressive type F06.31
  hallucinatory type F06.0
  nonpsychotic severity F07.0
  specified NEC F07.89
pulmonary
  arteriosclerosis I27.0
  dysmaturity (Wilson-Mikity) P27.0
  hypoperfusion (idiopathic) P22.0
  renal (hemorrhagic) (Goodpasture's) M31.0
pure
  motor lacunar G46.5
  sensory lacunar G46.6
Putnam-Dana D51.0
pyramidopallidonigral G20
pyriformis —*see* Lesion, nerve, sciatic
QT interval prolongation I45.81
radicular NEC —*see* Radiculopathy
  upper limbs, newborn (birth injury) P14.3
rapid time-zone change G47.25
Rasmussen G04.81
Raymond (-Céstan) I65.8

Syndrome *- continued*
Raynaud's I73.00
  with gangrene I73.01
RDS (respiratory distress syndrome,
newborn) P22.0
reactive airways dysfunction J68.3
Refsum's G60.1
Reifenstein E34.52
renal glomerulohyalinosis-diabetic —*see*
Diabetes, nephrosis
Rendu-Osler-Weber I78.0
residual ovary N99.83
resistant ovary E28.39
respiratory
  distress
    acute J80
      adult J80
      child J80
    newborn (idiopathic) (type I) P22.0
      type II P22.1
restless legs G25.81
retinoblastoma (familial) C69.2
retroperitoneal fibrosis N13.5
retroviral seroconversion (acute) Z21
Reye's G93.7
Richter —*see* Leukemia, chronic
lymphocytic, B-cell type
Ridley's I50.1
right
  heart, hypoplastic Q22.6
  ventricular obstruction —*see* Failure, heart,
  congestive
Romano-Ward (prolonged QT interval)
I45.81
rotator cuff, shoulder (*see also* Tear, rotator
cuff) M75.10
Rotes Quérol —*see* Hyperostosis, ankylosing
Roth —*see* Meralgia paresthetica
rubella (congenital) P35.0
Ruvalcaba-Myhre-Smith E71.440
Rytand-Lipsitch I44.2
salt
  depletion E87.1
    due to heat NEC T67.8
      causing heat exhaustion or prostration
T67.4
  low E87.1
salt-losing N28.89
Scaglietti-Dagnini E22.0
scalenus anticus (anterior) G54.0
scapulocostal —*see* Mononeuropathy, upper
limb, specified site NEC
scapuloperoneal G71.0
schizophrenic, of childhood NEC F84.5
Schnitzler D47.2
Scholte's E34.0
Schroeder's E27.0
Schüller-Christian C96.5
Schwachman's —*see* Syndrome,
Shwachman's
Schwartz (-Jampel) G71.13
Schwartz-Bartter E22.2
scimitar Q26.8
sclerocystic ovary E28.2
Seitelberger's G31.89
septicemic adrenal hemorrhage A39.1
seroconversion, retroviral (acute) Z21
serous meningitis G93.2
severe acute respiratory (SARS) J12.81
shaken infant T74.4

Syndrome - *continued*
 shock (traumatic) T79.4
  kidney N17.0
   following crush injury T79.5
  toxic A48.3
 shock-lung J80
 Shone's
 code to specific anomalies
 short
  bowel K91.2
  rib Q77.2
 shoulder-hand —*see* Algoneurodystrophy
 Shwachman's D70.4
 sicca —*see* Sicca syndrome
 sick
  cell E87.1
  sinus I49.5
 sick-euthyroid E07.81
 sideropenic D50.1
 Siemens' ectodermal dysplasia Q82.4
 Silfversköld's Q78.9
 Simons' E88.1
 sinus tarsi
 M25.57
 sinusitis-bronchiectasis-situs inversus Q89.3
 Sipple's E31.22
 sirenomelia Q87.2
 Slocumb's E27.0
 slow flow, coronary I20.8
 Sluder's G44.89
 Smith-Magenis Q93.88
 Sneddon-Wilkinson L13.1
 Sotos' E22.0
 South African cardiomyopathy I42.8
 spasmodic
  upward movement, eyes H51.8
  winking F95.8
 Spen's I45.9
 splenic
  agenesis Q89.01
  flexure K59.8
  neutropenia D73.81
 Spurway's Q78.0
 staphylococcal scalded skin L00
 Stein-Leventhal E28.2
 Stein's E28.2
 Stevens-Johnson syndrome L51.1
  toxic epidermal necrolysis overlap L51.3
 Stewart-Morel M85.2
 Stickler Q89.8
 stiff baby Q89.8
 stiff man G25.82
 Still-Felty —*see* Felty's syndrome
 Stokes (-Adams) I45.9
 stone heart I50.1
 straight back, congenital Q76.49
 subclavian steal G45.8
 subcoracoid-pectoralis minor G54.0
 subcostal nerve compression I77.89
 subphrenic interposition Q43.3
 superior
  cerebellar artery I63.8
  mesenteric artery K55.1
  semi-circular canal dehiscence H83.8X
  vena cava I87.1
 supine hypotensive (maternal) —*see*
 Syndrome, hypotension, maternal
 suprarenal cortical E27.0
 supraspinatus (*see also* Tear, rotator cuff)
 M75.10
 Susac G93.49
 swallowed blood P78.2

Syndrome - *continued*
 sweat retention L74.0
 Swyer Q99.1
 Symond's G93.2
 sympathetic
  cervical paralysis G90.2
  pelvic, female N94.89
 systemic inflammatory response (SIRS) , of
 non-infectious origin (without organ
 dysfunction) R65.10
  with acute organ dysfunction R65.11
 tachycardia-bradycardia I49.5
 takotsubo I51.81
 TAR (thrombocytopenia with absent radius)
 Q87.2
 tarsal tunnel G57.5
 teething K00.7
 tegmental G93.89
 telangiectasic-pigmentation-cataract Q82.8
 temporal pyramidal apex —*see* Otitis, media,
 suppurative, acute
 temporomandibular joint-pain-dysfunction
 M26.62
 Terry's H44.2
 testicular feminization (*see also* Syndrome,
 androgen insensitivity) E34.51
 thalamic pain (hyperesthetic) G89.0
 thoracic outlet (compression) G54.0
 Thorson-Björck E34.0
 thrombocytopenia with absent radius (TAR)
 Q87.2
 thyroid-adrenocortical insufficiency E31.0
 tibial
  anterior M76.81
  posterior M76.82
 Tietze's M94.0
 time-zone (rapid) G47.25
 Toni-Fanconi E72.09
  with cystinosis E72.04
 Touraine's Q79.8
 tourniquet —*see* Constriction, external, by
 site
 toxic shock A48.3
 transient left ventricular apical ballooning
 I51.81
 traumatic vasospastic T75.22
 Treacher Collins Q75.4
 triple X, female Q97.0
 trisomy Q92.9
  13 Q91.7
   meiotic nondisjunction Q91.4
   mitotic nondisjunction Q91.5
   mosaicism Q91.5
   translocation Q91.6
  18 Q91.3
   meiotic nondisjunction Q91.0
   mitotic nondisjunction Q91.1
   mosaicism Q91.1
   translocation Q91.2
  20 (q) (p) Q92.8
  21 Q90.9
   meiotic nondisjunction Q90.0
   mitotic nondisjunction Q90.1
   mosaicism Q90.1
   translocation Q90.2
  22 Q92.8
 tropical wet feet T69.0
 Trousseau's I82.1
 tumor lysis (following antineoplastic
 chemotherapy) (spontaneous) NEC E88.3

Syndrome - *continued*
 Twiddler's (due to)
  automatic implantable defibrillator T82.198
  cardiac pacemaker T82.198
 Unverricht (-Lundborg) —*see* Epilepsy,
 generalized, idiopathic
 upward gaze H51.8
 uremia, chronic (*see also* Disease, kidney,
 chronic) N18.9
 urethral N34.3
 urethro-oculo-articular —*see* Reiter's disease
 urohepatic K76.7
 vago-hypoglossal G52.7
 vascular NEC in cerebrovascular disease
 G46.8
 vasoconstriction, reversible cerebrovascular
 I67.841
 vasomotor I73.9
 vasospastic (traumatic) T75.22
 vasovagal R55
 van Buchem's M85.2
 van der Hoeve's Q78.0
 VATER Q87.2
 velo-cardio-facial Q93.81
 vena cava (inferior) (superior) (obstruction)
 I87.1
 vertebral
  artery G45.0
   compression —*see* Syndrome, anterior,
 spinal artery, compression
  steal G45.0
 vertebro-basilar artery G45.0
 vertebrogenic (pain) M54.89
 vertiginous —*see* Disorder, vestibular
 function
 Vinson-Plummer D50.1
 virus B34.9
 visceral larva migrans B83.0
 visual disorientation H53.8
 vitamin B6 deficiency E53.1
 vitreal corneal H59.01
 vitreous (touch) H59.01
 Vogt-Koyanagi H20.82
 Volkmann's T79.6
 von Schroetter's I82.890
 von Willebrand (-Jürgen) D68.0
 Waldenström-Kjellberg D50.1
 Wallenberg's G46.3
 water retention E87.79
 Waterhouse (-Friderichsen) A39.1
 Weber-Gubler G46.3
 Weber-Leyden G46.3
 Weber's G46.3
 Wegener's M31.30
  with
   kidney involvement M31.31
   lung involvement M31.30
    with kidney involvement M31.31
 Weingarten's (tropical eosinophilia) J82
 Weiss-Baker G90.09
 Werdnig-Hoffman G12.0
 Wermer's E31.21
 Werner's E34.8
 Wernicke-Korsakoff (nonalcoholic) F04
  alcoholic F10.26
 West's —*see* Epilepsy, spasms
 Westphal-Strümpell E83.01
 wet
  feet (maceration) (tropical) T69.0
  lung, newborn P22.1
 whiplash S13.4
 whistling face Q87.0
 Wilkie's K55.1

Syndrome - *continued*
Wilkinson-Sneddon L13.1
Willebrand (-Jürgens) D68.0
Wilson's (hepatolenticular degeneration)
E83.01
Wiskott-Aldrich D82.0
withdrawal —*see* Withdrawal, state
  drug
    infant of dependent mother P96.1
    therapeutic use, newborn P96.2
Woakes' (ethmoiditis) J33.1
Wright's (hyperabduction) I77.89
X I20.9
XXXX Q97.1
XXXXX Q97.1
XXXXY Q98.1
XXY Q98.0
yellow nail L60.5
Zahorsky's B08.5
Zellweger syndrome E71.510
Zellweger-like syndrome E71.541
Synechia (anterior) (iris) (posterior) (pupil) —
see also Adhesions, iris
  intra-uterine (traumatic) N85.6
Synesthesia R20.8
Syngamiasis, syngamosis B83.3
Synodontia K00.2
Synorchidism, synorchism Q55.1
Synostosis (congenital) Q78.8
  astragalo-scaphoid Q74.2
  radioulnar Q74.0
Synovial sarcoma —*see* Neoplasm, connective
tissue, malignant
Synovioma (malignant) —*see also* Neoplasm,
connective tissue, malignant
  benign —*see* Neoplasm, connective tissue,
  benign
Synoviosarcoma —*see* Neoplasm, connective
tissue, malignant
Synovitis —*see also* Tenosynovitis
  crepitant
    hand M70.0
    wrist M70.03
  gonococcal A54.49
  gouty —*see* Gout, idiopathic
  in (due to)
    crystals M65.8
    gonorrhea A54.49
    syphilis (late) A52.78
  use, overuse, pressure —*see* Disorder, soft
tissue, due to use
  infective NEC —*see* Tenosynovitis, infective
NEC
  specified NEC —*see* Tenosynovitis, specified
type NEC
  syphilitic A52.78
    congenital (early) A50.02
  toxic —*see* Synovitis, transient
  transient M67.3
    ankle M67.37
    elbow M67.32
    foot joint M67.37
    hand joint M67.34
    hip M67.35
    knee M67.36
    multiple site M67.39
    pelvic region M67.35
    shoulder M67.31
    specified joint NEC M67.38
    wrist M67.33
  traumatic, current —*see* Sprain
  tuberculous —*see* Tuberculosis, synovitis

Synovitis - *continued*
  villonodular (pigmented) M12.2
    ankle M12.27
    elbow M12.22
    foot joint M12.27
    hand joint M12.24
    hip M12.25
    knee M12.26
    multiple site M12.29
    pelvic region M12.25
    shoulder M12.21
    specified joint NEC M12.28
    vertebrae M12.28
    wrist M12.23
Syphilid A51.39
  congenital A50.06
  newborn A50.06
  tubercular (late) A52.79
Syphilis, syphilitic (acquired) A53.9
  abdomen (late) A52.79
  acoustic nerve A52.15
  adenopathy (secondary) A51.49
  adrenal (gland) (with cortical hypofunction)
A52.79
  age under 2 years NOS —*see also* Syphilis,
congenital, early
    acquired A51.9
  alopecia (secondary) A51.32
  anemia (late) A52.79 *[D63.8]*
  aneurysm (aorta) (ruptured) A52.01
    central nervous system A52.05
    congenital A50.54 *[I79.0]*
  anus (late) A52.74
    primary A51.1
    secondary A51.39
  aorta (arch) (abdominal) (thoracic) A52.02
    aneurysm A52.01
  aortic (insufficiency) (regurgitation) (stenosis)
A52.03
    aneurysm A52.01
  arachnoid (adhesive) (cerebral) (spinal)
A52.13
  asymptomatic —*see* Syphilis, latent
  ataxia (locomotor) A52.11
  atrophoderma maculatum A51.39
  auricular fibrillation A52.06
  bladder (late) A52.76
  bone A52.77
    secondary A51.46
  brain A52.17
  breast (late) A52.79
  bronchus (late) A52.72
  bubo (primary) A51.0
  bulbar palsy A52.19
  bursa (late) A52.78
  cardiac decompensation A52.06
  cardiovascular A52.00
  central nervous system (late) (recurrent)
(relapse) (tertiary) A52.3
    with
      ataxia A52.11
      general paralysis A52.17
        juvenile A50.45
      paresis (general) A52.17
        juvenile A50.45
      tabes (dorsalis) A52.11
        juvenile A50.45
      taboparesis A52.17
        juvenile A50.45
    aneurysm A52.05
    congenital A50.40
    juvenile A50.40

Syphilis, syphilitic - *continued*
  remission in (sustained) A52.3
  serology doubtful, negative, or positive
A52.3
  specified nature or site NEC A52.19
  vascular A52.05
  cerebral A52.17
    meningovascular A52.13
    nerves (multiple palsies) A52.15
    sclerosis A52.17
    thrombosis A52.05
  cerebrospinal (tabetic type) A52.12
  cerebrovascular A52.05
  cervix (late) A52.76
  chancre (multiple) A51.0
    extragenital A51.2
    Rollet's A51.0
  Charcot's joint A52.16
  chorioretinitis A51.43
    congenital A50.01
    late A52.71
    prenatal A50.01
  choroiditis —*see* Syphilitic chorioretinitis
  choroidoretinitis —*see* Syphilitic
chorioretinitis
  ciliary body (secondary) A51.43
    late A52.71
  colon (late) A52.74
  combined spinal sclerosis A52.11
  condyloma (latum) A51.31
  congenital A50.9
    with
      paresis (general) A50.45
      tabes (dorsalis) A50.45
      taboparesis A50.45
    chorioretinitis, choroiditis A50.01 *[H32]*
    early, or less than 2 years after birth NEC
A50.2
      with manifestations —*see* Syphilis,
congenital, early, symptomatic
      latent (without manifestations) A50.1
        negative spinal fluid test A50.1
        serology positive A50.1
      symptomatic A50.09
        cutaneous A50.06
        mucocutaneous A50.07
        oculopathy A50.01
        osteochondropathy A50.02
        pharyngitis A50.03
        pneumonia A50.04
        rhinitis A50.05
        visceral A50.08
    interstitial keratitis A50.31
    juvenile neurosyphilis A50.45
    late, or 2 years or more after birth NEC
A50.7
      chorioretinitis, choroiditis A50.32
      interstitial keratitis A50.31
      juvenile neurosyphilis A50.45
      latent (without manifestations) A50.6
        negative spinal fluid test A50.6
        serology positive A50.6
      symptomatic or with manifestations NEC
A50.59
        arthropathy A50.55
        cardiovascular A50.54
        Clutton's joints A50.51
        Hutchinson's teeth A50.52
        Hutchinson's triad A50.53
        osteochondropathy A50.56
        saddle nose A50.57

Syphilis, syphilitic *- continued*
conjugal A53.9
  tabes A52.11
conjunctiva (late) A52.71
contact Z20.2
cord bladder A52.19
cornea, late A52.71
coronary (artery) (sclerosis) A52.06
coryza, congenital A50.05
cranial nerve A52.15
  multiple palsies A52.15
cutaneous —*see* Syphilis, skin
dacryocystitis (late) A52.71
degeneration, spinal cord A52.12
dementia paralytica A52.17
  juvenilis A50.45
destruction of bone A52.77
dilatation, aorta A52.01
due to blood transfusion A53.9
dura mater A52.13
ear A52.79
  inner A52.79
    nerve (eighth) A52.15
    neurorecurrence A52.15
early A51.9
  cardiovascular A52.00
  central nervous system A52.3
  latent (without manifestations) (less than 2
years after infection) A51.5
    negative spinal fluid test A51.5
    serological relapse after treatment A51.5
    serology positive A51.5
  relapse (treated, untreated) A51.9
  skin A51.39
  symptomatic A51.9
    extragenital chancre A51.2
    primary, except extragenital chancre A51.0
    secondary (*see also* Syphilis, secondary)
A51.39
      relapse (treated, untreated) A51.49
    ulcer A51.39
eighth nerve (neuritis) A52.15
endemic A65
endocarditis A52.03
  aortic A52.03
  pulmonary A52.03
epididymis (late) A52.76
epiglottis (late) A52.73
epiphysitis (congenital) (early) A50.02
episcleritis (late) A52.71
esophagus A52.79
eustachian tube A52.73
exposure to Z20.2
eye A52.71
eyelid (late) (with gumma) A52.71
fallopian tube (late) A52.76
fracture A52.77
gallbladder (late) A52.74
gastric (polyposis) (late) A52.74
general A53.9
  paralysis A52.17
    juvenile A50.45
genital (primary) A51.0
glaucoma A52.71
gumma NEC A52.79
  cardiovascular system A52.00
  central nervous system A52.3
  congenital A50.59
heart (block) (decompensation) (disease)
(failure) A52.06 *[I52]*
  valve NEC A52.03
hemianesthesia A52.19

Syphilis, syphilitic *- continued*
hemianopsia A52.71
hemiparesis A52.17
hemiplegia A52.17
hepatic artery A52.09
hepatis A52.74
hepatomegaly, congenital A50.08
hereditaria tarda —*see* Syphilis, congenital,
late
hereditary —*see* Syphilis, congenital
Hutchinson's teeth A50.52
hyalitis A52.71
inactive —*see* Syphilis, latent
infantum —*see* Syphilis, congenital
inherited —*see* Syphilis, congenital
internal ear A52.79
intestine (late) A52.74
iris, iritis (secondary) A51.43
  late A52.71
joint (late) A52.77
keratitis (congenital) (interstitial) (late)
A50.31
kidney (late) A52.75
lacrimal passages (late) A52.71
larynx (late) A52.73
late A52.9
  cardiovascular A52.00
  central nervous system A52.3
  kidney A52.75
  latent or 2 years or more after infection
(without manifestations) A52.8
    negative spinal fluid test A52.8
    serology positive A52.8
  paresis A52.17
  specified site NEC A52.79
  symptomatic or with manifestations A52.79
  tabes A52.11
latent A53.0
  with signs or symptoms
code by site and stage under Syphilis
  central nervous system A52.2
  date of infection unspecified A53.0
  early, or less than 2 years after infection
A51.5
  follow-up of latent syphilis A53.0
    date of infection unspecified A53.0
    late, or 2 years or more after infection
A52.8
  late, or 2 years or more after infection A52.8
  positive serology (only finding) A53.0
    date of infection unspecified A53.0
    early, or less than 2 years after infection
A51.5
    late, or 2 years or more after infection
A52.8
lens (late) A52.71
leukoderma A51.39
  late A52.79
lienitis A52.79
lip A51.39
  chancre (primary) A51.2
  late A52.79
Lissauer's paralysis A52.17
liver A52.74
locomotor ataxia A52.11
lung A52.72
lymph gland (early) (secondary) A51.49
  late A52.79
lymphadenitis (secondary) A51.49
macular atrophy of skin A51.39
  striated A52.79
mediastinum (late) A52.73

Syphilis, syphilitic *- continued*
meninges (adhesive) (brain) (spinal cord)
A52.13
meningitis A52.13
  acute (secondary) A51.41
  congenital A50.41
meningoencephalitis A52.14
meningovascular A52.13
  congenital A50.41
mesarteritis A52.09
  brain A52.04
middle ear A52.77
mitral stenosis A52.03
monoplegia A52.17
mouth (secondary) A51.39
  late A52.79
mucocutaneous (secondary) A51.39
  late A52.79
mucous
  membrane (secondary) A51.39
    late A52.79
  patches A51.39
    congenital A50.07
mulberry molars A50.52
muscle A52.78
myocardium A52.06
nasal sinus (late) A52.73
neonatorum —*see* Syphilis, congenital
nephrotic syndrome (secondary) A51.44
nerve palsy (any cranial nerve) A52.15
  multiple A52.15
nervous system, central A52.3
neuritis A52.15
  acoustic A52.15
neurorecidive of retina A52.19
neuroretinitis A52.19
newborn —*see* Syphilis, congenital
nodular superficial (late) A52.79
nonvenereal A65
nose (late) A52.73
  saddle back deformity A50.57
occlusive arterial disease A52.09
oculopathy A52.71
ophthalmic (late) A52.71
optic nerve (atrophy) (neuritis) (papilla)
A52.15
orbit (late) A52.71
organic A53.9
osseous (late) A52.77
osteochondritis (congenital) (early) A50.02
[M90.80]
osteoporosis A52.77
ovary (late) A52.76
oviduct (late) A52.76
palate (late) A52.79
pancreas (late) A52.74
paralysis A52.17
  general A52.17
    juvenile A50.45
paresis (general) A52.17
  juvenile A50.45
paresthesia A52.19
Parkinson's disease or syndrome A52.19
paroxysmal tachycardia A52.06
pemphigus (congenital) A50.06
penis (chancre) A51.0
  late A52.76
pericardium A52.06
perichondritis, larynx (late) A52.73
periosteum (late) A52.77
  congenital (early) A50.02 *[M90.80]*
  early (secondary) A51.46
peripheral nerve A52.79

Syphilis, syphilitic - *continued*
  petrous bone (late) A52.77
  pharynx (late) A52.73
    secondary A51.39
  pituitary (gland) A52.79
  pleura (late) A52.73
  pneumonia, white A50.04
  pontine lesion A52.17
  portal vein A52.09
  primary A51.0
    anal A51.1
    and secondary —*see* Syphilis, secondary
    central nervous system A52.3
    extragenital chancre NEC A51.2
    fingers A51.2
    genital A51.0
    lip A51.2
    specified site NEC A51.2
    tonsils A51.2
  prostate (late) A52.76
  ptosis (eyelid) A52.71
  pulmonary (late) A52.72
    artery A52.09
  pyelonephritis (late) A52.75
  recently acquired, symptomatic A51.9
  rectum (late) A52.74
  respiratory tract (late) A52.73
  retina, late A52.71
  retrobulbar neuritis A52.15
  salpingitis A52.76
  sclera (late) A52.71
  sclerosis
    cerebral A52.17
    coronary A52.06
    multiple A52.11
  scotoma (central) A52.71
  scrotum (late) A52.76
  secondary (and primary) A51.49
    adenopathy A51.49
    anus A51.39
    bone A51.46
    chorioretinitis, choroiditis A51.43
    hepatitis A51.45
    liver A51.45
    lymphadenitis A51.49
    meningitis (acute) A51.41
    mouth A51.39
    mucous membranes A51.39
    periosteum, periostitis A51.46
    pharynx A51.39
    relapse (treated, untreated) A51.49
    skin A51.39
    specified form NEC A51.49
    tonsil A51.39
    ulcer A51.39
    viscera NEC A51.49
    vulva A51.39
  seminal vesicle (late) A52.76
  seronegative with signs or symptoms
  code by site and stage under Syphilis
  seropositive
    with signs or symptoms
  code by site and stage under Syphilis
    follow-up of latent syphilis —*see* Syphilis,
  latent
    only finding —*see* Syphilis, latent
  seventh nerve (paralysis) A52.15
  sinus, sinusitis (late) A52.73
  skeletal system A52.77
  skin (with ulceration) (early) (secondary)
  A51.39
    late or tertiary A52.79

Syphilis, syphilitic - *continued*
  small intestine A52.74
  spastic spinal paralysis A52.17
  spermatic cord (late) A52.76
  spinal (cord) A52.12
  spleen A52.79
  splenomegaly A52.79
  spondylitis A52.77
  staphyloma A52.71
  stigmata (congenital) A50.59
  stomach A52.74
  synovium A52.78
  tabes dorsalis (late) A52.11
    juvenile A50.45
  tabetic type A52.11
    juvenile A50.45
  taboparesis A52.17
    juvenile A50.45
  tachycardia A52.06
  tendon (late) A52.78
  tertiary A52.9
    with symptoms NEC A52.79
    cardiovascular A52.00
    central nervous system A52.3
    multiple NEC A52.79
    specified site NEC A52.79
  testis A52.76
  thorax A52.73
  throat A52.73
  thymus (gland) (late) A52.79
  thyroid (late) A52.79
  tongue (late) A52.79
  tonsil (lingual) (late) A52.73
    primary A51.2
    secondary A51.39
  trachea (late) A52.73
  tunica vaginalis (late) A52.76
  ulcer (any site) (early) (secondary) A51.39
    late A52.79
    perforating A52.79
      foot A52.11
  urethra (late) A52.76
  urogenital (late) A52.76
  uterus (late) A52.76
  uveal tract (secondary) A51.43
    late A52.71
  uveitis (secondary) A51.43
    late A52.71
  uvula (late) (perforated) A52.79
  vagina A51.0
    late A52.76
  valvulitis NEC A52.03
  vascular A52.00
    brain (cerebral) A52.05
  ventriculi A52.74
  vesicae urinariae (late) A52.76
  viscera (abdominal) (late) A52.74
    secondary A51.49
  vitreous (opacities) (late) A52.71
    hemorrhage A52.71
  vulva A51.0
    late A52.76
    secondary A51.39
Syphiloma A52.79
  cardiovascular system A52.00
  central nervous system A52.3
  circulatory system A52.00
  congenital A50.59
Syphilophobia F45.29
Syringadenoma —*see also* Neoplasm, skin,
benign
  papillary —*see* Neoplasm, skin, benign

Syringobulbia G95.0
Syringocystadenoma —*see* Neoplasm, skin,
benign
  papillary —*see* Neoplasm, skin, benign
Syringoma —*see also* Neoplasm, skin, benign
  chondroid —*see* Neoplasm, skin, benign
Syringomyelia G95.0
Syringomyelitis —*see* Encephalitis
Syringomyelocele —*see* Spina bifida
Syringopontia G95.0
System, systemic —*see also* condition
  disease, combined —*see* Degeneration,
  combined
  inflammatory response syndrome (SIRS) of
  non-infectious origin (without organ
  dysfunction) R65.10
    with acute organ dysfunction R65.11
  lupus erythematosus M32.9
    inhibitor present D68.62

T

Tabacism, tabacosis, tabagism —*see also*
Poisoning, tobacco
  meaning dependence (without remission)
  F17.200
    with
      disorder F17.299
        remission F17.211
        specified disorder NEC F17.298
        withdrawal F17.203
Tabardillo A75.9
  flea-borne A75.2
  louse-borne A75.0
Tabes, tabetic A52.10
  with
    central nervous system syphilis A52.10
    Charcot's joint A52.16
    cord bladder A52.19
    crisis, viscera (any) A52.19
    paralysis, general A52.17
    paresis (general) A52.17
    perforating ulcer (foot) A52.19
  arthropathy (Charcot) A52.16
  bladder A52.19
  bone A52.11
  cerebrospinal A52.12
  congenital A50.45
  conjugal A52.10
  dorsalis A52.11
    juvenile A50.49
  juvenile A50.49
  latent A52.19
  mesenterica A18.39
  paralysis, insane, general A52.17
  spasmodic A52.17
  syphilis (cerebrospinal) A52.12
Taboparalysis A52.17
Taboparesis (remission) A52.17
  juvenile A50.45
TAC (trigeminal autonomic cephalgia) **NEC**
G44.099
  intractable G44.091
  not intractable G44.099
Tache noir S60.22
Tachyalimentation K91.2
Tachyarrhythmia, tachyrhythmia —*see*
Tachycardia
Tachycardia R00.0
  atrial (paroxysmal) I47.1
  auricular I47.1
  AV nodal re-entry (re-entrant) I47.1
  junctional (paroxysmal) I47.1
  newborn P29.11
  nodal (paroxysmal) I47.1

Tachycardia - *continued*
non-paroxysmal AV nodal I45.89
paroxysmal (sustained) (nonsustained) I47.9
  with sinus bradycardia I49.5
  atrial (PAT) I47.1
  atrioventricular (AV) (re-entrant) I47.1
    psychogenic F54
  junctional I47.1
    ectopic I47.1
  nodal I47.1
  psychogenic (atrial) (supraventricular)
  (ventricular) F54
    supraventricular (sustained) I47.1
      psychogenic F54
    ventricular I47.2
      psychogenic F54
psychogenic F45.8
sick sinus I49.5
sinoauricular NOS R00.0
  paroxysmal I47.1
sinus -sinusal] NOS R00.0
  paroxysmal I47.1
supraventricular I47.1
ventricular (paroxysmal) (sustained) I47.2
  psychogenic F54
Tachygastria K31.89
Tachypnea R06.82
hysterical F45.8
newborn (idiopathic) (transitory) P22.1
psychogenic F45.8
transitory, of newborn P22.1
Taenia (infection) (infestation) B68.9
diminuta B71.0
echinococcal infestation B67.90
mediocanellata B68.1
nana B71.0
saginata B68.1
solium (intestinal form) B68.0
  larval form —*see* Cysticercosis
Taeniasis (intestine) —*see* Taenia
TACO (transfusion associated circulatory
overload) E87.71
Tag (hypertrophied skin) (infected) L91.8
adenoid J35.8
anus K64.4
hemorrhoidal K64.4
hymen N89.8
perineal N90.89
preauricular Q17.0
sentinel K64.4
skin L91.8
  accessory (congenital) Q82.8
  anus K64.4
  congenital Q82.8
  preauricular Q17.0
tonsil J35.8
urethra, urethral N36.8
vulva N90.89
Tahyna fever B33.8
Takahara's disease E80.3
Takayasu's disease or syndrome M31.4
Talcosis (pulmonary) J62.0
Talipes (congenital) Q66.89
acquired, planus —*see* Deformity, limb, flat
foot
asymmetric Q66.89
calcaneovalgus Q66.4
calcaneovarus Q66.1
calcaneus Q66.89
cavus Q66.7
equinovalgus Q66.6
equinovarus Q66.0

Talipes - *continued*
equinus Q66.89
percavus Q66.7
planovalgus Q66.6
planus (acquired) (any degree) —*see also*
Deformity, limb, flat foot
  congenital Q66.5
  due to rickets (sequelae) E64.3
valgus Q66.6
varus Q66.3
Tall stature, constitutional E34.4
Talma's disease M62.89
Talon noir S90.3
hand S60.22
heel S90.3
toe S90.1
Tamponade, heart I31.4
Tanapox (virus disease) B08.71
Tangier disease E78.6
Tantrum, child problem F91.8
Tapeworm (infection) (infestation) —*see*
Infestation, tapeworm
Tapia's syndrome G52.7
TAR (thrombocytopenia with absent radius)
syndrome Q87.2
Tarral-Besnier disease L44.0
Tarsal tunnel syndrome —*see* Syndrome,
tarsal tunnel
Tarsalgia —*see* Pain, limb, lower
Tarsitis (eyelid) H01.8
syphilitic A52.71
tuberculous A18.4
Tartar (teeth) (dental calculus) K03.6
Tattoo (mark) L81.8
Tauri's disease E74.09
Taurodontism K00.2
Taussig-Bing syndrome Q20.1
Taybi's syndrome Q87.2
**Tay-Sachs amaurotic familial idiocy or
disease** E75.02
TBI (traumatic brain injury) —*see* category
S06
Teacher's node or nodule J38.2
Tear, torn (traumatic) —*see also* Laceration
with abortion —*see* Abortion
annular fibrosis M51.35
anus, anal (sphincter) S31.831
  complicating delivery
    with third degree perineal laceration O70.2
      with mucosa O70.3
    without third degree perineal laceration
    O70.4
  nontraumatic (healed) (old) K62.81
articular cartilage, old —*see* Derangement,
joint, articular cartilage, by site
bladder
  with ectopic or molar pregnancy O08.6
  following ectopic or molar pregnancy O08.6
  obstetrical O71.5
  traumatic —*see* Injury, bladder
bowel
  with ectopic or molar pregnancy O08.6
  following ectopic or molar pregnancy O08.6
  obstetrical trauma O71.5
broad ligament
  with ectopic or molar pregnancy O08.6
  following ectopic or molar pregnancy O08.6
  obstetrical trauma O71.6
bucket handle (knee) (meniscus) —*see* Tear,
meniscus
capsule, joint —*see* Sprain

Tear, torn – *continued*
cartilage —*see also* Sprain
  articular, old —*see* Derangement, joint,
articular cartilage, by site
cervix
  with ectopic or molar pregnancy O08.6
  following ectopic or molar pregnancy O08.6
  obstetrical trauma (current) O71.3
  old N88.1
  traumatic —*see* Injury, uterus
dural G97.41
  nontraumatic G96.11
internal organ —*see* Injury, by site
knee cartilage
  articular (current) S83.3
  old —*see* Derangement, knee, meniscus, due
to old tear
ligament —*see* Sprain
meniscus (knee) (current injury) S83.209
  bucket-handle S83.20
  lateral
    bucket-handle S83.25
    complex S83.27
    peripheral S83.26
    specified type NEC S83.28
  medial
    bucket-handle S83.21
    complex S83.23
    peripheral S83.22
    specified type NEC S83.24
  old —*see* Derangement, knee, meniscus, due
to old tear
  site other than knee
code as Sprain
  specified type NEC S83.20
muscle —*see* Strain
pelvic
  floor, complicating delivery O70.1
  organ NEC, obstetrical trauma O71.5
    with ectopic or molar pregnancy O08.6
    following ectopic or molar pregnancy
O08.6
  perineal, secondary O90.1
periurethral tissue, obstetrical trauma O71.82
  with ectopic or molar pregnancy O08.6
  following ectopic or molar pregnancy O08.6
rectovaginal septum —*see* Laceration, vagina
retina, retinal (without detachment)
(horseshoe) —*see also* Break, retina,
horseshoe
  with detachment —*see* Detachment, retina,
with retinal, break
rotator cuff (nontraumatic) M75.10
  complete M75.12
  incomplete M75.11
  traumatic S46.01
    capsule S43.42
semilunar cartilage, knee —*see* Tear,
meniscus
supraspinatus (complete) (incomplete)
(nontraumatic) (*see also* Tear, rotator cuff)
M75.10
tendon —*see* Strain
tentorial, at birth P10.4
umbilical cord
  complicating delivery O69.89
urethra
  with ectopic or molar pregnancy O08.6
  following ectopic or molar pregnancy O08.6
  obstetrical trauma O71.5
uterus —*see* Injury, uterus
vagina —*see* Laceration, vagina

Tear, torn - *continued*
  vessel, from catheter —*see* Puncture,
  accidental complicating surgery
  vulva, complicating delivery O70.0
Tear-stone —*see* Dacryolith
Teeth —*see also* condition
  grinding
    psychogenic F45.8
    sleep related G47.63
Teething (syndrome) K00.7
Telangiectasia, telangiectasis (verrucous)
  I78.1
  ataxic (cerebellar) (Louis-Bar) G11.3
  familial I78.0
  hemorrhagic, hereditary (congenital) (senile)
    I78.0
  hereditary, hemorrhagic (congenital) (senile)
    I78.0
  juxtafoveal H35.07
  macular H35.07
  parafoveal H35.07
  retinal (idiopathic) (juxtafoveal) (macular)
    (parafoveal) H35.07
  spider I78.1
Telephone scatologia F65.89
Telescoped bowel or intestine K56.1
  congenital Q43.8
Temperature
  body, high (of unknown origin) R50.9
  cold, trauma from T69.9
    newborn P80.0
    specified effect NEC T69.8
Temple —*see* condition
Temporal —*see* condition
**Temporomandibular joint pain-dysfunction
  syndrome** M26.62
Temporosphenoidal —*see* condition
Tendency
  bleeding —*see* Defect, coagulation
  suicide
    meaning personal history of attempted
    suicide Z91.5
    meaning suicidal ideation —*see* Ideation,
    suicidal
  to fall R29.6
Tenderness, abdominal R10.819
  epigastric R10.816
  generalized R10.817
  left lower quadrant R10.814
  left upper quadrant R10.812
  periumbilic R10.815
  right lower quadrant R10.813
  right upper quadrant R10.811
  rebound R10.829
    epigastric R10.826
    generalized R10.827
    left lower quadrant R10.824
    left upper quadrant R10.822
    periumbilic R10.825
    right lower quadrant R10.823
    right upper quadrant R10.821
Tendinitis, tendonitis —*see also* Enthesopathy
  Achilles M76.6
  adhesive —*see* Tenosynovitis, specified type
  NEC
    shoulder —*see* Capsulitis, adhesive
  bicipital M75.2
  calcific M65.2
    ankle M65.27
    foot M65.27
    forearm M65.23
    hand M65.24

Tendinitis, tendonitis - *continued*
  lower leg M65.26
  multiple sites M65.29
  pelvic region M65.25
  shoulder M75.3
  specified site NEC M65.28
  thigh M65.25
  upper arm M65.22
  due to use, overuse, pressure —*see also*
  Disorder, soft tissue, due to use
    specified NEC —*see* Disorder, soft tissue,
    due to use, specified NEC
  gluteal M76.0
  patellar M76.5
  peroneal M76.7
  psoas M76.1
  tibial (posterior) M76.82
    anterior M76.81
  trochanteric —*see* Bursitis, hip, trochanteric
Tendon —*see* condition
Tendosynovitis —*see* Tenosynovitis
Tenesmus (rectal) R19.8
  vesical R30.1
Tennis elbow —*see* Epicondylitis, lateral
Tenonitis —*see also* Tenosynovitis
  eye (capsule) H05.04
Tenontosynovitis —*see* Tenosynovitis
Tenontothecitis —*see* Tenosynovitis
Tenophyte —*see* Disorder, synovium,
  specified type NEC
Tenosynovitis (see also Synovitis) M65.9
  adhesive —*see* Tenosynovitis, specified type
  NEC
    shoulder —*see* Capsulitis, adhesive
  bicipital (calcifying) —*see* Tendinitis,
  bicipital
  gonococcal A54.49
  in (due to)
    crystals M65.8
    gonorrhea A54.49
    syphilis (late) A52.78
    use, overuse, pressure —*see also* Disorder,
  soft tissue, due to use
    specified NEC —*see* Disorder, soft tissue,
  due to use, specified NEC
  infective NEC M65.1
    ankle M65.17
    foot M65.17
    forearm M65.13
    hand M65.14
    lower leg M65.16
    multiple sites M65.19
    pelvic region M65.15
    shoulder region M65.11
    specified site NEC M65.18
    thigh M65.15
    upper arm M65.12
  radial styloid M65.4
  shoulder region M65.81
    adhesive —*see* Capsulitis, adhesive
  specified type NEC M65.88
    ankle M65.87
    foot M65.87
    forearm M65.83
    hand M65.84
    lower leg M65.86
    multiple sites M65.89
    pelvic region M65.85
    shoulder region M65.81
    specified site NEC M65.88
    thigh M65.85
    upper arm M65.82
  tuberculous —*see* Tuberculosis, tenosynovitis

Tenovaginitis —*see* Tenosynovitis
Tension
  arterial, high —*see also* Hypertension
    without diagnosis of hypertension R03.0
  headache G44.209
    intractable G44.201
    not intractable G44.209
  nervous R45.0
  pneumothorax J93.0
  premenstrual N94.3
  state (mental) F48.9
Tentorium —*see* condition
Teratencephalus Q89.8
Teratism Q89.7
Teratoblastoma (malignant) —*see* Neoplasm,
  malignant, by site
Teratocarcinoma —*see also* Neoplasm,
  malignant, by site
  liver C22.7
Teratoma (solid) —*see also* Neoplasm,
  uncertain behavior, by site
  with embryonal carcinoma, mixed —*see*
    Neoplasm, malignant, by site
  with malignant transformation —*see*
    Neoplasm, malignant, by site
  adult (cystic) —*see* Neoplasm, benign, by site
  benign —*see* Neoplasm, benign, by site
  combined with choriocarcinoma —*see*
    Neoplasm, malignant, by site
  cystic (adult) —*see* Neoplasm, benign, by site
  differentiated —*see* Neoplasm, benign, by site
  embryonal —*see also* Neoplasm, malignant,
    by site
    liver C22.7
  immature —*see* Neoplasm, malignant, by site
    liver C22.7
    adult, benign, cystic, differentiated type or
    mature D13.4
  malignant —*see also* Neoplasm, malignant,
    by site
    anaplastic —*see* Neoplasm, malignant, by
    site
    intermediate —*see* Neoplasm, malignant, by
    site
    specified site —*see* Neoplasm, malignant,
    by site
    unspecified site C62.90
  undifferentiated —*see* Neoplasm, malignant,
  by site
  mature —*see* Neoplasm, uncertain behavior,
  by site
    malignant —*see* Neoplasm, by site,
  malignant, by site
  ovary D27.
    embryonal, immature or malignant C56
  solid —*see* Neoplasm, uncertain behavior, by
    site
  testis C62.9
    adult, benign, cystic, differentiated type or
  mature D29.2
    scrotal C62.1
    undescended C62.0
Termination
  anomalous —*see also* Malposition, congenital
    right pulmonary vein Q26.3
  pregnancy, elective Z33.2
Ternidens diminutus infestation B81.8
Ternidensiasis B81.8
Terror (s) night (child) F51.4
Terrorism, victim of Z65.4
Terry's syndrome H44.2
Tertiary —*see* condition

Test, tests, testing (for)
  adequacy (for dialysis)
    hemodialysis Z49.31
    peritoneal Z49.32
  blood pressure Z01.30
    abnormal reading —see Blood, pressure
  blood-alcohol Z04.8
    positive —see Findings, abnormal, in blood
  blood-drug Z04.8
    positive —see Findings, abnormal, in blood
  blood typing Z01.83
    Rh typing Z01.83
  cardiac pulse generator (battery) Z45.010
  fertility Z31.41
  genetic
    disease carrier status for procreative
    management
      female Z31.430
      male Z31.440
    male partner of patient with recurrent
    pregnancy loss Z31.441
    procreative management NEC
      female Z31.438
      male Z31.448
  hearing Z01.10
    with abnormal findings NEC Z01.118
  HIV (human immunodeficiency virus)
    nonconclusive (in infants) R75
    positive Z21
    seropositive Z21
  immunity status Z01.84
  intelligence NEC Z01.89
  laboratory (as part of a general medical
  examination) Z00.00
    with abnormal finding Z00.01
    for medicolegal reason NEC Z04.8
  male partner of patient with recurrent
  pregnancy loss Z31.441
  Mantoux (for tuberculosis) Z11.1
    abnormal result R76.11
  pregnancy, positive first pregnancy —see
  Pregnancy, normal, first
  procreative Z31.49
    fertility Z31.41
  skin, diagnostic
    allergy Z01.82
      special screening examination —see
  Screening, by name of disease
    Mantoux Z11.1
    tuberculin Z11.1
  specified NEC Z01.89
  tuberculin Z11.1
    abnormal result R76.11
  vision Z01.00
    with abnormal findings Z01.01
  Wassermann Z11.3
    positive —see Serology for syphilis, positive
Testicle, testicular, testis —see also condition
  feminization syndrome (see also Syndrome,
  androgen insensitivity) E34.51
  migrans Q55.29
Tetanus, tetanic (cephalic) (convulsions) A35
  with
    abortion A34
    ectopic or molar pregnancy O08.0
    following ectopic or molar pregnancy O08.0
    inoculation reaction (due to serum) —see
  Complications, vaccination
  neonatorum A33
  obstetrical A34
  puerperal, postpartum, childbirth A34

Tetany (due to) R29.0
  alkalosis E87.3
    associated with rickets E55.0
  convulsions R29.0
    hysterical F44.5
  functional (hysterical) F44.5
  hyperkinetic R29.0
    hysterical F44.5
  hyperpnea R06.4
    hysterical F44.5
    psychogenic F45.8
  hyperventilation (see also Hyperventilation)
  R06.4
    hysterical F44.5
  neonatal (without calcium or magnesium
  deficiency) P71.3
  parathyroid (gland) E20.9
  parathyroprival E89.2
  post (para) thyroidectomy E89.2
  postoperative E89.2
  pseudotetany R29.0
  psychogenic (conversion reaction) F44.5
Tetralogy of Fallot Q21.3
Tetraplegia (chronic) (see also Quadriplegia)
  G82.50
Thailand hemorrhagic fever A91
Thalassanemia —see Thalassemia
Thalassemia (anemia) (disease) D56.9
  with other hemoglobinopathy D56.8
  alpha (major) (severe) (triple gene defect)
  D56.0
    minor D56.3
    silent carrier D56.3
    trait D56.3
  beta (severe) D56.1
    homozygous D56.1
    major D56.1
    minor D56.3
    trait D56.3
  delta-beta (homozygous) D56.2
    minor D56.3
    trait D56.3
  dominant D56.8
  hemoglobin
    C D56.8
    E-beta D56.5
  intermedia D56.1
  major D56.1
  minor D56.3
  mixed D56.8
  sickle-cell —see Disease, sickle-cell,
  thalassemia
  specified type NEC D56.8
  trait D56.3
  variants D56.8
Thanatophoric dwarfism or short stature
  Q77.1
Thaysen-Gee disease (nontropical sprue)
  K90.0
Thaysen's disease K90.0
Thecoma D27
  luteinized D27
  malignant C56
Thelarche, premature E30.8
Thelaziasis B83.8
Thelitis N61
  puerperal, postpartum or gestational —see
  Infection, nipple
Therapeutic —see condition

Therapy
  drug, long-term (current) (prophylactic)
    agents affecting estrogen receptors and
  estrogen levels NEC Z79.818
    anastrozole (Arimidex) Z79.811
    antibiotics Z79.2
      short-term use
  omit code
    anticoagulants Z79.01
    anti-inflammatory Z79.1
    antiplatelet Z79.02
    antithrombotics Z79.02
    aromatase inhibitors Z79.811
    aspirin Z79.82
    birth control pill or patch Z79.3
    bisphosphonates Z79.83
    contraceptive, oral Z79.3
    drug, specified NEC Z79.899
    estrogen receptor downregulators Z79.818
    Evista Z79.810
    exemestane (Aromasin) Z79.811
    Fareston Z79.810
    fulvestrant (Faslodex) Z79.818
    gonadotropin-releasing hormone (GnRH)
    agonist Z79.818
    goserelin acetate (Zoladex) Z79.818
    hormone replacement (postmenopausal)
    Z79.890
    insulin Z79.4
    letrozole (Femara) Z79.811
    leuprolide acetate (leuprorelin) (Lupron)
    Z79.818
    megestrol acetate (Megace) Z79.818
    methadone
      for pain management Z79.891
      maintenance therapy F11.20
    Nolvadex Z79.810
    opiate analgesic Z79.891
    oral contraceptive Z79.3
    raloxifene (Evista) Z79.810
    selective estrogen receptor modulators
    (SERMs) Z79.810
    short term
  omit code
    steroids
      inhaled Z79.51
      systemic Z79.52
    tamoxifen (Nolvadex) Z79.810
    toremifene (Fareston) Z79.810
Thermic —see condition
Thermography (abnormal) (see also
  Abnormal, diagnostic imaging) R93.8
  breast R92.8
Thermoplegia T67.0
Thesaurismosis, glycogen —see Disease,
  glycogen storage
Thiamin deficiency E51.9
  specified NEC E51.8
Thiaminic deficiency with beriberi E51.11
Thibierge-Weissenbach syndrome —see
  Sclerosis, systemic
Thickening
  bone —see Hypertrophy, bone
  breast N64.59
  endometrium R93.8
  epidermal L85.9
    specified NEC L85.8
  hymen N89.6
  larynx J38.7
  nail L60.2
    congenital Q84.5
  periosteal —see Hypertrophy, bone

Thickening – *continued*
pleura J92.9
  with asbestos J92.0
skin R23.4
subepiglottic J38.7
tongue K14.8
valve, heart —*see* Endocarditis
Thigh —*see* condition
Thinning vertebra —*see* Spondylopathy,
specified NEC
Thirst, excessive R63.1
due to deprivation of water T73.1
Thomsen disease G71.12
Thoracic —*see also* condition
kidney Q63.2
outlet syndrome G54.0
Thoracogastroschisis (congenital) Q79.8
Thoracopagus Q89.4
Thorax —*see* condition
Thorn's syndrome N28.89
Thorson-Björck syndrome E34.0
Threadworm (infection) (infestation) B80
Threatened
abortion O20.0
  with subsequent abortion O03.9
job loss, anxiety concerning Z56.2
labor (without delivery) O47.9
  after 37 completed weeks of gestation O47.1
  before 37 completed weeks of gestation
  O47.0
loss of job, anxiety concerning Z56.2
miscarriage O20.0
unemployment, anxiety concerning Z56.2
Three-day fever A93.1
Threshers' lung J67.0
Thrix annulata (congenital) Q84.1
Throat —*see* condition
Thrombasthenia (Glanzmann) (hemorrhagic)
(hereditary) D69.1
Thromboangiitis I73.1
obliterans (general) I73.1
  cerebral I67.89
  vessels
    brain I67.89
    spinal cord I67.89
Thromboarteritis —*see* Arteritis
Thromboasthenia (Glanzmann) (hemorrhagic)
(hereditary) D69.1
Thrombocytasthenia (Glanzmann) D69.1
Thrombocythemia (essential) (hemorrhagic)
(idiopathic) (primary) D47.3
Thrombocytopathy (dystrophic)
(granulopenic) D69.1
Thrombocytopenia, thrombocytopenic D69.6
with absent radius (TAR) Q87.2
congenital D69.42
dilutional D69.59
due to
  drugs D69.59
  extracorporeal circulation of blood D69.59
  (massive) blood transfusion D69.59
  platelet alloimmunization D69.59
essential D69.3
heparin induced (HIT) D75.82
hereditary D69.42
idiopathic D69.3
neonatal, transitory P61.0
  due to
    exchange transfusion P61.0
    idiopathic maternal thrombocytopenia
  P61.0
    isoimmunization P61.0

Thrombocytopenia – *continued*
primary NEC D69.49
  idiopathic D69.3
puerperal, postpartum O72.3
secondary D69.59
transient neonatal P61.0
Thrombocytosis, essential D47.3
primary D47.3
Thromboembolism —*see* Embolism
Thrombopathy (Bernard-Soulier) D69.1
constitutional D68.0
  Willebrand-Jurgens D68.0
Thrombopenia —*see* Thrombocytopenia
Thrombophilia D68.59
primary NEC D68.59
secondary NEC D68.69
specified NEC D68.69
Thrombophlebitis I80.9
antepartum O22.2
  deep O22.3
  superficial O22.2
cavernous (venous) sinus G08
  complicating pregnancy O22.5
  nonpyogenic I67.6
cerebral (sinus) (vein) G08
  nonpyogenic I67.6
  sequelae G09
due to implanted device —*see* Complications,
by site and type, specified NEC
during or resulting from a procedure NEC
T81.72
femoral vein (superficial) I80.1
femoropopliteal vein I80.0
hepatic (vein) I80.8
idiopathic, recurrent I82.1
iliofemoral I80.1
intracranial venous sinus (any) G08
  nonpyogenic I67.6
  sequelae G09
intraspinal venous sinuses and veins G08
  nonpyogenic G95.19
lateral (venous) sinus G08
  nonpyogenic I67.6
leg I80.299
  superficial I80.0
longitudinal (venous) sinus G08
  nonpyogenic I67.6
lower extremity I80.299
migrans, migrating I82.1
pelvic
  with ectopic or molar pregnancy O08.0
  following ectopic or molar pregnancy O08.0
  puerperal O87.1
popliteal vein —*see* Phlebitis, leg, deep,
popliteal
portal (vein) K75.1
postoperative T81.72
pregnancy —*see* Thrombophlebitis,
antepartum
puerperal, postpartum, childbirth O87.0
  deep O87.1
  pelvic O87.1
  septic O86.81
  superficial O87.0
saphenous (greater) (lesser) I80.0
sinus (intracranial) G08
  nonpyogenic I67.6
specified site NEC I80.8
tibial vein I80.23

Thrombosis, thrombotic (bland) (multiple)
(progressive) (silent) (vessel) I82.90
anal K64.5
antepartum —*see* Thrombophlebitis,
antepartum
aorta, aortic I74.10
  abdominal I74.09
    saddle I74.01
  bifurcation I74.09
  saddle I74.01
  specified site NEC I74.19
  terminal I74.09
  thoracic I74.11
  valve —*see* Endocarditis, aortic
apoplexy I63.3
artery, arteries (postinfectional) I74.9
  auditory, internal —*see* Occlusion, artery,
precerebral, specified NEC
  basilar —*see* Occlusion, artery, basilar
  carotid (common) (internal) —*see*
Occlusion, artery, carotid
  cerebellar (anterior inferior) (posterior
inferior) (superior) —*see* Occlusion, artery,
cerebellar
  cerebral —*see* Occlusion, artery, cerebral
  choroidal (anterior) —*see* Occlusion, artery,
cerebral, specified NEC
  communicating, posterior —*see* Occlusion,
artery, cerebral, specified NEC
  coronary —*see also* Infarct, myocardium
    not resulting in infarction I24.0
  hepatic I74.8
  hypophyseal —*see* Occlusion, artery,
cerebral, specified NEC
  iliac I74.5
  limb I74.4
    lower I74.3
    upper I74.2
  meningeal, anterior or posterior —*see*
Occlusion, artery, cerebral, specified NEC
  mesenteric (with gangrene) K55.0
  ophthalmic —*see* Occlusion, artery, retina
  pontine —*see* Occlusion, artery, cerebral,
specified NEC
  precerebral —*see* Occlusion, artery,
precerebral
  pulmonary (iatrogenic) —*see* Embolism,
pulmonary
  renal N28.0
  retinal —*see* Occlusion, artery, retina
  spinal, anterior or posterior G95.11
  traumatic NEC T14.8
  vertebral —*see* Occlusion, artery, vertebral
atrium, auricular —*see also* Infarct,
myocardium
  following acute myocardial infarction
(current complication) I23.6
  not resulting in infarction I24.0
basilar (artery) —*see* Occlusion, artery,
basilar
brain (artery) (stem) —*see also* Occlusion,
artery, cerebral
  due to syphilis A52.05
  puerperal O99.43
  sinus —*see* Thrombosis, intracranial venous
sinus
capillary I78.8
cardiac —*see also* Infarct, myocardium
  not resulting in infarction I24.0
  valve —*see* Endocarditis
carotid (artery) (common) (internal) —*see*
Occlusion, artery, carotid

Thrombosis, thrombotic - *continued*
cavernous (venous) sinus —*see* Thrombosis, intracranial venous sinus
cerebellar artery (anterior inferior) (posterior inferior) (superior) I66.3
cerebral (artery) —*see* Occlusion, artery, cerebral
cerebrovenous sinus —*see also* Thrombosis, intracranial venous sinus
  puerperium O87.3
chronic I82.91
coronary (artery) (vein) —*see also* Infarct, myocardium
  not resulting in infarction I24.0
corpus cavernosum N48.89
cortical I66.9
deep —*see* Embolism, vein, lower extremity
due to device, implant or graft (*see also* Complications, by site and type, specified NEC) T85.86
  arterial graft NEC T82.868
  breast (implant) T85.86
  catheter NEC T85.86
    dialysis (renal) T82.868
      intraperitoneal T85.86
    infusion NEC T82.868
      spinal (epidural) (subdural) T85.86
    urinary (indwelling) T83.86
  electronic (electrode) (pulse generator) (stimulator)
    bone T84.86
    cardiac T82.867
    nervous system (brain) (peripheral nerve) (spinal) T85.86
      urinary T83.86
  fixation, internal (orthopedic) NEC T84.86
  gastrointestinal (bile duct) (esophagus) T85.86
  genital NEC T83.86
  heart T82.867
  joint prosthesis T84.86
  ocular (corneal graft) (orbital implant) NEC T85.86
  orthopedic NEC T84.86
  specified NEC T85.86
  urinary NEC T83.86
  vascular NEC T82.868
  ventricular intracranial shunt T85.86
during the puerperium —*see* Thrombosis, puerperal
endocardial —*see also* Infarct, myocardium
  not resulting in infarction I24.0
eye —*see* Occlusion, retina
genital organ
  female NEC N94.89
    pregnancy —*see* Thrombophlebitis, antepartum
  male N50.1
gestational —*see* Phlebopathy, gestational
heart (chamber) —*see also* Infarct, myocardium
  not resulting in infarction I24.0
hepatic (vein) I82.0
  artery I74.8
history (of) Z86.718
intestine (with gangrene) K55.0
intracardiac NEC (apical) (atrial) (auricular) (ventricular) (old) I51.3
intracranial (arterial) I66.9
  venous sinus (any) G08
    nonpyogenic origin I67.6
    puerperium O87.3

Thrombosis, thrombotic - *continued*
intramural —*see also* Infarct, myocardium
  not resulting in infarction I24.0
intraspinal venous sinuses and veins G08
  nonpyogenic G95.19
kidney (artery) N28.0
lateral (venous) sinus —*see* Thrombosis, intracranial venous sinus
leg —*see* Thrombosis, vein, lower extremity
  arterial I74.3
liver (venous) I82.0
  artery I74.8
  portal vein I81
longitudinal (venous) sinus —*see* Thrombosis, intracranial venous sinus
lower limb —*see* Thrombosis, vein, lower extremity
lung (iatrogenic) (postoperative) —*see* Embolism, pulmonary
meninges (brain) (arterial) I66.8
mesenteric (artery) (with gangrene) K55.0
  vein (inferior) (superior) I81
mitral I34.8
mural —*see also* Infarct, myocardium
  due to syphilis A52.06
  not resulting in infarction I24.0
omentum (with gangrene) K55.0
ophthalmic —*see* Occlusion, retina
pampiniform plexus (male) N50.1
parietal —*see also* Infarct, myocardium
  not resulting in infarction I24.0
penis, superficial vein N48.81
perianal venous K64.5
peripheral arteries I74.4
  upper I74.2
personal history (of) Z86.718
portal I81
  due to syphilis A52.09
precerebral artery —*see* Occlusion, artery, precerebral
puerperal, postpartum O87.0
  brain (artery) O99.43
    venous (sinus) O87.3
  cardiac O99.43
  cerebral (artery) O99.43
    venous (sinus) O87.3
  superficial O87.0
pulmonary (artery) (iatrogenic) (postoperative) (vein) —*see* Embolism, pulmonary
renal (artery) N28.0
  vein I82.3
resulting from presence of device, implant or graft —*see* Complications, by site and type, specified NEC
retina, retinal —*see* Occlusion, retina
scrotum N50.1
seminal vesicle N50.1
sigmoid (venous) sinus —*see* Thrombosis, intracranial venous sinus
sinus, intracranial (any) —*see* Thrombosis, intracranial venous sinus
specified site NEC I82.890
  chronic I82.891
spermatic cord N50.1
spinal cord (arterial) G95.11
  due to syphilis A52.09
  pyogenic origin G06.1
spleen, splenic D73.5
  artery I74.8
testis N50.1

Thrombosis, thrombotic - *continued*
tumor —*see* Neoplasm, unspecified behavior, by site
traumatic NEC T14.8
tricuspid I07.8
tunica vaginalis N50.1
umbilical cord (vessels) , complicating delivery O69.5
vas deferens N50.1
vein (acute) I82.90
  antecubital I82.61
    chronic I82.71
  axillary I82.A1
    chronic I82.A2
  basilic I82.61
    chronic I82.71
  brachial I82.62
    chronic I82.72
  brachiocephalic (innominate) I82.290
    chronic I82.291
  cerebral, nonpyogenic I67.6
  cephalic I82.61
    chronic I82.71
  chronic I82.91
  deep (DVT) I82.40
    calf I82.4Z
      chronic I82.5Z
    lower leg I82.4Z
      chronic I82.5Z
    thigh I82.4Y
      chronic I82.5Y
    upper leg I82.4Y
      chronic I82.5y
  femoral I82.41
    chronic I82.51
  iliac (iliofemoral) I82.42
    chronic I82.52
  innominate I82.290
    chronic I82.291
  internal jugular I82.C1
    chronic I82.C2
  lower extremity
    deep I82.40
      chronic I82.50
      specified NEC I82.49
        chronic NEC I82.59
    distal
      deep I82.4Z
    proximal
      deep I82.4Y
        chronic I82.5Y
    superficial I82.81
  perianal K64.5
  popliteal I82.43
    chronic I82.53
  radial I82.62
    chronic I82.72
  renal I82.3
  saphenous (greater) (lesser) I82.81
  specified NEC I82.890
    chronic NEC I82.891
  subclavian I82.B1
    chronic I82.B2
  thoracic NEC I82.290
    chronic I82.291
  tibial I82.44
    chronic I82.54
  ulnar I82.62
    chronic I82.72
  upper extremity I82.60
    chronic I82.70
    deep I82.62
      chronic I82.72

Thrombosis, thrombotic   *- continued*
- superficial I82.61
  - chronic I82.71
- vena cava
  - inferior I82.220
    - chronic I82.221
  - superior I82.210
    - chronic I82.211
- venous, perianal K64.5
- ventricle —*see also* Infarct, myocardium
  - following acute myocardial infarction (current complication) I23.6
  - not resulting in infarction I24.0

Thrombus —*see* Thrombosis

Thrush —*see also* Candidiasis
- oral B37.0
- newborn P37.5
- vaginal B37.3

Thumb —*see also* condition
- sucking (child problem) F98.8

Thymitis E32.8

Thymoma (benign) D15.0
- malignant C37

Thymus, thymic (gland) —*see* condition

Thyrocele —*see* Goiter

Thyroglossal —*see also* condition
- cyst Q89.2
- duct, persistent Q89.2

Thyroid (gland) (body) —*see also* condition
- hormone resistance E07.89
- lingual Q89.2
- nodule (cystic) (nontoxic) (single) E04.1

Thyroiditis E06.9
- acute (nonsuppurative) (pyogenic) (suppurative) E06.0
- autoimmune E06.3
- chronic (nonspecific) (sclerosing) E06.5
  - with thyrotoxicosis, transient E06.2
  - fibrous E06.5
  - lymphadenoid E06.3
  - lymphocytic E06.3
  - lymphoid E06.3
- de Quervain's E06.1
- drug-induced E06.4
- fibrous (chronic) E06.5
- giant-cell (follicular) E06.1
- granulomatous (de Quervain) (subacute) E06.1
- Hashimoto's (struma lymphomatosa) E06.3
- iatrogenic E06.4
- ligneous E06.5
- lymphocytic (chronic) E06.3
- lymphoid E06.3
- lymphomatous E06.3
- nonsuppurative E06.1
- postpartum, puerperal O90.5
- pseudotuberculous E06.1
- pyogenic E06.0
- radiation E06.4
- Riedel's E06.5
- subacute (granulomatous) E06.1
- suppurative E06.0
- tuberculous A18.81
- viral E06.1
- woody E06.5

Thyrolingual duct, persistent Q89.2

Thyromegaly E01.0

Thyrotoxic
- crisis —*see* Thyrotoxicosis
- heart disease or failure (*see also* Thyrotoxicosis) E05.90 *[143]*
  - with thyroid storm E05.91 *[143]*

Thyrotoxic – *continued*
- storm —*see* Thyrotoxicosis

Thyrotoxicosis (recurrent) E05.90
- with
  - goiter (diffuse) E05.00
    - with thyroid storm E05.01
    - adenomatous uninodular E05.10
      - with thyroid storm E05.11
    - multinodular E05.20
      - with thyroid storm E05.21
    - nodular E05.20
      - with thyroid storm E05.21
    - uninodular E05.10
      - with thyroid storm E05.11
  - infiltrative
    - dermopathy E05.00
      - with thyroid storm E05.01
    - ophthalmopathy E05.00
      - with thyroid storm E05.01
  - single thyroid nodule E05.10
    - with thyroid storm E05.11
  - thyroid storm E05.91
- due to
  - ectopic thyroid nodule or tissue E05.30
    - with thyroid storm E05.31
  - ingestion of (excessive) thyroid material E05.40
    - with thyroid storm E05.41
  - overproduction of thyroid-stimulating hormone E05.80
    - with thyroid storm E05.81
  - specified cause NEC E05.80
    - with thyroid storm E05.81
- factitia E05.40
  - with thyroid storm E05.41
- heart E05.90 *[143]*
  - with thyroid storm E05.91 *[143]*
  - failure E05.90 *[143]*
- neonatal (transient) P72.1
- transient with chronic thyroiditis E06.2

Tibia vara —*see* Osteochondrosis, juvenile, tibia

Tic (disorder) F95.9
- breathing F95.8
- child problem F95.0
- compulsive F95.1
- de la Tourette F95.2
- degenerative (generalized) (localized) G25.69
  - facial G25.69
- disorder
  - chronic
    - motor F95.1
    - vocal F95.1
    - combined vocal and multiple motor F95.2
  - transient F95.0
- douloureux G50.0
  - atypical G50.1
  - postherpetic, postzoster B02.22
- drug-induced G25.61
- eyelid F95.8
- habit F95.9
  - chronic F95.1
  - transient of childhood F95.0
- lid, transient of childhood F95.0
- motor-verbal F95.2
- occupational F48.8
- orbicularis F95.8
  - transient of childhood F95.0
- organic origin G25.69
- postchoreic G25.69
- psychogenic, compulsive F95.1
- salaam R25.8

Tic – *continued*
- spasm (motor or vocal) F95.9
  - chronic F95.1
  - transient of childhood F95.0
- specified NEC F95.8

Tick-borne —*see* condition

Tietze's disease or syndrome M94.0

Tight, tightness
- anus K62.89
- chest R07.89
- fascia (lata) M62.89
- foreskin (congenital) N47.1
- hymen, hymenal ring N89.6
- introitus (acquired) (congenital) N89.6
- rectal sphincter K62.89
- tendon —*see* Short, tendon
- urethral sphincter N35.9

Tilting vertebra —*see* Dorsopathy, deforming, specified NEC

Timidity, child F93.8

Tin-miner's lung J63.5

Tinea (intersecta) (tarsi) B35.9
- amiantacea L44.8
- asbestina B35.0
- barbae B35.0
- beard B35.0
- black dot B35.0
- blanca B36.2
- capitis B35.0
- corporis B35.4
- cruris B35.6
- flava B36.0
- foot B35.3
- furfuracea B36.0
- imbricata (Tokelau) B35.5
- kerion B35.0
- manuum B35.2
- microsporic —*see* Dermatophytosis
- nigra B36.1
- nodosa —*see* Piedra
- pedis B35.3
- scalp B35.0
- specified site NEC B35.8
- sycosis B35.0
- tonsurans B35.0
- trichophytic —*see* Dermatophytosis
- unguium B35.1
- versicolor B36.0

Tingling sensation (skin) R20.2

Tinnitus (audible) (aurium) (subjective) —*see* subcategory H93.1

Tipped tooth (teeth) M26.33

Tipping
- pelvis M95.5
  - with disproportion (fetopelvic) O33.0
    - causing obstructed labor O65.0
- tooth (teeth) , fully erupted M26.33

Tiredness R53.83

Tissue —*see* condition

Tobacco (nicotine)
- dependence —*see* Dependence, drug, nicotine
- harmful use Z72.0
- heart —*see* Tobacco, toxic effect
- maternal use, affecting newborn P04.2
- toxic effect —*see* Table of Drugs and Chemicals, by substance, poisoning
  - chewing tobacco —*see* Table of Drugs and Chemicals, by substance, poisoning
  - cigarettes —*see* Table of Drugs and Chemicals, by substance, poisoning

Tobacco - *continued*
  use Z72.0
    complicating
      childbirth O99.334
      pregnancy O99.33
      puerperium O99.335
    counseling and surveillance Z71.6
    withdrawal state —*see* Dependence, drug,
    nicotine
Tocopherol deficiency E56.0
Todd's
  cirrhosis K74.3
  paralysis (postepileptic) (transitory) G83.84
Toe —*see* condition
Toilet, artificial opening —*see* Attention to,
  artificial, opening
Tokelau (ringworm) B35.5
Tollwut —*see* Rabies
Tommaselli's disease R31.9
  correct substance properly administered —*see*
  Table of Drugs and Chemicals, by drug,
  adverse effect
  overdose or wrong substance given or taken
  —*see* Table of Drugs and Chemicals, by drug,
  poisoning
Tongue —*see also* condition
  tie Q38.1
Tonic pupil —*see* Anomaly, pupil, function,
  tonic pupil
Toni-Fanconi syndrome (cystinosis) E72.09
  with cystinosis E72.04
Tonsil —*see* condition
Tonsillitis (acute) (catarrhal) (croupous)
  (follicular) (gangrenous) (infective) (lacunar)
  (lingual) (malignant) (membranous)
  (parenchymatous) (phlegmonous)
  (pseudomembranous) (purulent) (septic)
  (subacute) (suppurative) (toxic) (ulcerative)
  (vesicular) (viral) J03.90
  chronic J35.01
    with adenoiditis J35.03
  diphtheritic A36.0
  hypertrophic J35.01
    with adenoiditis J35.03
  recurrent J03.91
  specified organism NEC J03.80
    recurrent J03.81
  staphylococcal J03.80
    recurrent J03.81
  streptococcal J03.00
    recurrent J03.01
  tuberculous A15.8
  Vincent's A69.1
Tooth, teeth —*see* condition
Toothache K08.8
Topagnosis R20.8
Tophi —*see* Gout, chronic
TORCH infection —*see* Infection, congenital
  without active infection P00.2
Torn —*see* Tear
Tornwaldt's cyst or disease J39.2
Torsion
  accessory tube —*see* Torsion, fallopian tube
  adnexa (female) —*see* Torsion, fallopian tube
  aorta, acquired I77.1
  appendix epididymis N44.04
  appendix testis N44.03
  bile duct (common) (hepatic) K83.8
    congenital Q44.5
  bowel, colon or intestine K56.2
  cervix —*see* Malposition, uterus
  cystic duct K82.8

Torsion - *continued*
  dystonia —*see* Dystonia, torsion
  epididymis (appendix) N44.04
  fallopian tube N83.52
    with ovary N83.53
  gallbladder K82.8
    congenital Q44.1
  hydatid of Morgagni
    female N83.52
    male N44.03
  kidney (pedicle) (leading to infarction) N28.0
  Meckel's diverticulum (congenital) Q43.0
    malignant —*see* Table of Neoplasms, small
  intestine, malignant
  mesentery K56.2
  omentum K56.2
  organ or site, congenital NEC —*see*
  Anomaly, by site
  ovary (pedicle) N83.51
    with fallopian tube N83.53
    congenital Q50.2
  oviduct —*see* Torsion, fallopian tube
  penis (acquired) N48.82
    congenital Q55.63
  spasm —*see* Dystonia, torsion
  spermatic cord N44.02
    extravaginal N44.01
    intravaginal N44.02
  spleen D73.5
  testis, testicle N44.00
    appendix N44.03
  tibia —*see* Deformity, limb, specified type
  NEC, lower leg
  uterus —*see* Malposition, uterus
Torticollis (intermittent) (spastic) M43.6
  congenital (sternomastoid) Q68.0
  due to birth injury P15.8
  hysterical F44.4
  ocular R29.891
  psychogenic F45.8
    conversion reaction F44.4
  rheumatic M43.6
  rheumatoid M06.88
  spasmodic G24.3
  traumatic, current S13.4
Tortipelvis G24.1
Tortuous
  artery I77.1
  organ or site, congenital NEC —*see*
  Distortion
  retinal vessel, congenital Q14.1
  ureter N13.8
  urethra N36.8
  vein —*see* Varix
Torture, victim of Z65.4
Torula, torular (histolytica) (infection) —*see*
  Cryptococcosis
Torulosis —*see* Cryptococcosis
Torus (mandibularis) (palatinus) M27.0
  fracture —*see* Fracture, by site, torus
Touraine's syndrome Q79.8
Tourette's syndrome F95.2
Tourniquet syndrome —*see* Constriction,
  external, by site
Tower skull Q75.0
  with exophthalmos Q87.0
Toxemia R68.89
  bacterial —*see* Sepsis
  burn —*see* Burn
  eclamptic (with pre-existing hypertension) —
  see Eclampsia
  erysipelatous —*see* Erysipelas

Toxemia - *continued*
  fatigue R68.89
  food —*see* Poisoning, food
  gastrointestinal K52.1
  intestinal K52.1
  kidney —*see* Uremia
  malarial —*see* Malaria
  myocardial —*see* Myocarditis, toxic
  of pregnancy —*see* Pre-eclampsia
  pre-eclamptic —*see* Pre-eclampsia
  small intestine K52.1
  staphylococcal, due to food A05.0
  stasis R68.89
  uremic —*see* Uremia
  urinary —*see* Uremia
Toxemica cerebropathia psychica
  (nonalcoholic) F04
  alcoholic —*see* Alcohol, amnestic disorder
Toxic (poisoning) (*see also* condition) T65.91
  effect —*see* Table of Drugs and Chemicals,
  by substance, poisoning
  shock syndrome A48.3
  thyroid (gland) —*see* Thyrotoxicosis
Toxicemia —*see* Toxemia
Toxicity —*see* Table of Drugs and Chemicals,
  by substance, poisoning
  fava bean D55.0
  food, noxious —*see* Poisoning, food
  from drug or nonmedicinal substance —*see*
  Table of Drugs and Chemicals, by drug
Toxicosis —*see also* Toxemia
  capillary, hemorrhagic D69.0
Toxinfection, gastrointestinal K52.1
Toxocariasis B83.0
Toxoplasma, toxoplasmosis (acquired) B58.9
  with
    hepatitis B58.1
    meningoencephalitis B58.2
    ocular involvement B58.00
    other organ involvement B58.89
    pneumonia, pneumonitis B58.3
  congenital (acute) (subacute) (chronic) P37.1
  maternal, manifest toxoplasmosis in infant
  (acute) (subacute) (chronic) P37.1
tPA (rtPA) administration in a different
  facility within the last 24 hours prior to
  admission to current facility Z92.82
Trabeculation, bladder N32.89
Trachea —*see* condition
Tracheitis (catarrhal) (infantile) (membranous)
  (plastic) (septal) (suppurative) (viral) J04.10
  with
    bronchitis (15 years of age and above) J40
      acute or subacute —*see* Bronchitis, acute
      chronic J42
      tuberculous NEC A15.5
      under 15 years of age J20.9
    laryngitis (acute) J04.2
      chronic J37.1
      tuberculous NEC A15.5
  acute J04.10
    with obstruction J04.11
  chronic J42
    with
      bronchitis (chronic) J42
      laryngitis (chronic) J37.1
  diphtheritic (membranous) A36.89
  due to external agent —*see* Inflammation,
  respiratory, upper, due to
  syphilitic A52.73
  tuberculous A15.5
Trachelitis (nonvenereal) —*see* Cervicitis
Tracheobronchial —*see* condition

Tracheobronchitis (15 years of age and above) —*see also* Bronchitis
due to
Bordetella bronchiseptica A37.80
with pneumonia A37.81
Francisella tularensis A21.8
Tracheobronchomegaly Q32.4
with bronchiectasis J47.9
with
exacerbation (acute) J47.1
lower respiratory infection J47.0
acquired J98.09
with bronchiectasis J47.9
with
exacerbation (acute) J47.1
lower respiratory infection J47.0
Tracheobronchopneumonitis —*see*
Pneumonia, broncho
Tracheocele (external) (internal) J39.8
congenital Q32.1
Tracheomalacia J39.8
congenital Q32.0
Tracheopharyngitis (acute) J06.9
chronic J42
due to external agent —*see* Inflammation, respiratory, upper, due to
Tracheostenosis J39.8
Tracheostomy
complication —*see* Complication, tracheostomy
status Z93.0
attention to Z43.0
malfunctioning J95.03
Trachoma, trachomatous A71.9
active (stage) A71.1
contraction of conjunctiva A71.1
dubium A71.0
initial (stage) A71.0
healed or sequelae B94.0
pannus A71.1
Türck's J37.0
Traction, vitreomacular H43.82
Train sickness T75.3
Trait (s)
Hb-S D57.3
hemoglobin
abnormal NEC D58.2
with thalassemia D56.3
C —*see* Disease, hemoglobin C   S (Hb-S)
D57.3
Lepore D56.3
personality, accentuated Z73.1
sickle-cell D57.3
with elliptocytosis or spherocytosis D57.3
type A personality Z73.1
Tramp Z59.0
Trance R41.89
hysterical F44.89
Transection
abdomen (partial) S38.3
aorta (incomplete) —*see also* Injury, aorta
complete —*see* Injury, aorta, laceration, major
carotid artery (incomplete) —*see also* Injury, blood vessel, carotid, laceration
complete —*see* Injury, blood vessel, carotid, laceration, major
celiac artery (incomplete) S35.211
branch (incomplete) S35.291
complete S35.292
complete S35.212

Transection - *continued*
innominate
artery (incomplete) —*see also* Injury, blood vessel, thoracic, innominate, artery, laceration
complete —*see* Injury, blood vessel, thoracic, innominate, artery, laceration, major
vein (incomplete) —*see also* Injury, blood vessel, thoracic, innominate, vein, laceration
complete —*see* Injury, blood vessel, thoracic, innominate, vein, laceration, major
jugular vein (external) (incomplete) —*see also* Injury, blood vessel, jugular vein, laceration
complete —*see* Injury, blood vessel, jugular vein, laceration, major
internal (incomplete) —*see also* Injury, blood vessel, jugular vein, internal, laceration
complete —*see* Injury, blood vessel, jugular vein, internal, laceration, major
mesenteric artery (incomplete) —*see also* Injury, mesenteric, artery, laceration
complete —*see* Injury, mesenteric artery, laceration, major
pulmonary vessel (incomplete) —*see also* Injury, blood vessel, thoracic, pulmonary, laceration
complete —*see* Injury, blood vessel, thoracic, pulmonary, laceration, major
subclavian —*see* Transection, innominate
vena cava (incomplete) —*see also* Injury, vena cava
complete —*see* Injury, vena cava, laceration, major
vertebral artery (incomplete) —*see also* Injury, blood vessel, vertebral, laceration
complete —*see* Injury, blood vessel, vertebral, laceration, major
Transaminasemia R74.0
Transfusion
associated (red blood cell) hemochromatosis E83.111
blood
ABO incompatible —*see* Complication(s), transfusion, incompatibility reaction, ABO
minor blood group (Duffy) (E) (K(ell)) (Kidd) (Lewis) (M) (N) (P) (S) T80.89
reaction or complication —*see* Complications, transfusion
fetomaternal (mother) —*see* Pregnancy, complicated by, placenta, transfusion syndrome
maternofetal (mother) —*see* Pregnancy, complicated by, placenta, transfusion syndrome
placental (syndrome) (mother) —*see* Pregnancy, complicated by, placenta, transfusion syndrome
reaction (adverse) —*see* Complications, transfusion
related acute lung injury (TRALI) J95.84
twin-to-twin —*see* Pregnancy, complicated by, placenta, transfusion syndrome, fetus to fetus
Transient (meaning homeless) (*see also* condition) Z59.0
Translocation
balanced autosomal Q95.9
in normal individual Q95.0
chromosomes NEC Q99.8
balanced and insertion in normal individual Q95.0
Down syndrome Q90.2

Translocation - *continued*
trisomy
13 Q91.6
18 Q91.2
21 Q90.2
Translucency, iris —*see* Degeneration, iris
Transmission of chemical substances through the placenta —*see* Absorption, chemical, through placenta
Transparency, lung, unilateral J43.0
Transplant (ed) (status) Z94.9
awaiting organ Z76.82
bone Z94.6
marrow Z94.81
candidate Z76.82
complication —*see* Complication, transplant
cornea Z94.7
heart Z94.1
and lung (s) Z94.3
valve Z95.2
prosthetic Z95.2
specified NEC Z95.4
xenogenic Z95.3
intestine Z94.82
kidney Z94.0
liver Z94.4
lung (s) Z94.2
and heart Z94.3
organ (failure) (infection) (rejection) Z94.9
removal status Z98.85
pancreas Z94.83
skin Z94.5
social Z60.3
specified organ or tissue NEC Z94.89
stem cells Z94.84
tissue Z94.9
Transplants, ovarian, endometrial N80.1
Transposed —*see* Transposition
Transposition (congenital) —*see also* Malposition, congenital
abdominal viscera Q89.3
aorta (dextra) Q20.3
appendix Q43.8
colon Q43.8
corrected Q20.5
great vessels (complete) (partial) Q20.3
heart Q24.0
with complete transposition of viscera Q89.3
intestine (large) (small) Q43.8
reversed jejunal (for bypass) (status) Z98.0
scrotum Q55.23
stomach Q40.2
with general transposition of viscera Q89.3
tooth, teeth, fully erupted M26.30
vessels, great (complete) (partial) Q20.3
viscera (abdominal) (thoracic) Q89.3
Transsexualism F64.1
Transverse —*see also* condition
arrest (deep) , in labor O64.0
lie (mother) O32.2
causing obstructed labor O64.8
Transvestism, transvestitism (dual-role) F64.1
fetishistic F65.1
Trapped placenta (with hemorrhage) O72.0
without hemorrhage O73.0
Trauma, traumatism —*see also* Injury
acoustic —*see* subcategory H83.3
birth —*see* Birth, injury
complicating ectopic or molar pregnancy O08.6
during delivery O71.9

Trauma, traumatism – *continued*
  following ectopic or molar pregnancy O08.6
  obstetric O71.9
    specified NEC O71.89
Traumatic —*see also* condition
  brain injury —see category S06
Treacher Collins syndrome Q75.4
Treitz's hernia —*see* Hernia, abdomen,
  specified site NEC
Trematode infestation —*see* Infestation, fluke
Trematodiasis —*see* Infestation, fluke
Trembling paralysis —*see* Parkinsonism
Tremor (s) R25.1
  drug induced G25.1
  essential (benign) G25.0
  familial G25.0
  hereditary G25.0
  hysterical F44.4
  intention G25.2
  medication induced postural G25.1
  mercurial —see subcategory T56.1
  Parkinson's —*see* Parkinsonism
  psychogenic (conversion reaction) F44.4
  senilis R54
  specified type NEC G25.2
Trench
  fever A79.0
  foot —*see* Immersion, foot
  mouth A69.1
Treponema pallidum infection —*see* Syphilis
Treponematosis
  due to
    T. pallidum —*see* Syphilis
    T. pertenue —*see* Yaws
Triad
  Hutchinson's (congenital syphilis) A50.53
  Kartagener's Q89.3
  Saint's —*see* Hernia, diaphragm
Trichiasis (eyelid) H02.059
  with entropion —*see* Entropion
  left H02.056
    lower H02.055
    upper H02.054
  right H02.053
    lower H02.052
    upper H02.051
Trichinella spiralis (infection) (infestation)
  B75
**Trichinellosis, trichiniasis, trichinelliasis,
  trichinosis** B75
  with muscle disorder B75 *[M63.80]*
    ankle B75 *[M63.87]*
    foot B75 *[M63.87]*
    forearm B75 *[M63.83]*
    hand B75 *[M63.84]*
    lower leg B75 *[M63.86]*
    multiple sites B75 *[M63.89]*
    pelvic region B75 *[M63.85]*
    shoulder region B75 *[M63.81]*
    specified site NEC B75 *[M63.88]*
    thigh B75 *[M63.85]*
    upper arm B75 *[M63.82]*
Trichobezoar T18.9
  intestine T18.3
  stomach T18.2
Trichocephaliasis, trichocephalosis B79
Trichocephalus infestation B79
Trichoclasis L67.8
Trichoepithelioma —*see also* Neoplasm, skin,
  benign
  malignant —*see* Neoplasm, skin, malignant
Trichofolliculoma —*see* Neoplasm, skin,
  benign

Tricholemmoma —*see* Neoplasm, skin,
  benign
Trichomoniasis A59.9
  bladder A59.03
  cervix A59.09
  intestinal A07.8
  prostate A59.02
  seminal vesicles A59.09
  specified site NEC A59.8
  urethra A59.03
  urogenitalis A59.00
  vagina A59.01
  vulva A59.01
Trichomycosis
  axillaris A48.8
  nodosa, nodularis B36.8
Trichonodosis L67.8
Trichophytid, trichophyton infection —*see*
  Dermatophytosis
Trichophytobezoar T18.9
  intestine T18.3
  stomach T18.2
Trichophytosis —*see* Dermatophytosis
Trichoptilosis L67.8
Trichorrhexis (nodosa) (invaginata) L67.0
Trichosis axillaris A48.8
Trichosporosis nodosa B36.2
Trichostasis spinulosa (congenital) Q84.1
Trichostrongyliasis, trichostrongylosis (small
  intestine) B81.2
Trichostrongylus infection B81.2
Trichotillomania F63.3
Trichromat, trichromatopsia, anomalous
  (congenital) H53.55
Trichuriasis B79
Trichuris trichiura (infection) (infestation)
  (any site) B79
Tricuspid (valve) —*see* condition
Trifid —*see also* Accessory
  kidney (pelvis) Q63.8
  tongue Q38.3
Trigeminal neuralgia —*see* Neuralgia,
  trigeminal
Trigeminy R00.8
Trigger finger (acquired) M65.30
  congenital Q74.0
  index finger M65.32
  little finger M65.35
  middle finger M65.33
  ring finger M65.34
  thumb M65.31
Trigonitis (bladder) (chronic)
  (pseudomembranous) N30.30
  with hematuria N30.31
Trigonocephaly Q75.0
Trilocular heart —*see* Cor triloculare
Trimethylaminuria E72.52
Tripartite placenta O43.19-**Triphalangeal
  thumb** Q74.0
Triple —*see also* Accessory
  kidneys Q63.0
  uteri Q51.818
  X, female Q97.0
Triplegia G83.89
  congenital G80.8
Triplet (newborn) —*see also* Newborn, triplet
  complicating pregnancy —*see* Pregnancy,
  triplet
Triplication —*see* Accessory
Triploidy Q92.7
Trismus R25.2
  neonatorum A33
  newborn A33

Trisomy (syndrome) Q92.9
  autosomes Q92.9
  chromosome specified NEC Q92.8
    partial Q92.2
      due to unbalanced translocation Q92.5
    whole (nonsex chromosome)
      meiotic nondisjunction Q92.0
      mitotic nondisjunction Q92.1
      mosaicism Q92.1
    specified NEC Q92.8
  due to
    dicentrics —*see* Extra, marker chromosomes
    extra rings —*see* Extra, marker
  chromosomes
    isochromosomes —*see* Extra, marker
  chromosomes
  specified NEC Q92.8
  whole chromosome Q92.9
    meiotic nondisjunction Q92.0
    mitotic nondisjunction Q92.1
    mosaicism Q92.1
    partial Q92.9
    specified NEC Q92.8
  13 (partial) Q91.7
    meiotic nondisjunction Q91.4
    mitotic nondisjunction Q91.5
    mosaicism Q91.5
    translocation Q91.6
  18 (partial) Q91.3
    meiotic nondisjunction Q91.4
    mitotic nondisjunction Q91.1
    mosaicism Q91.1
    translocation Q91.2
  20 Q92.8
  21 (partial) Q90.9
    meiotic nondisjunction Q90.0
    mitotic nondisjunction Q90.1
    mosaicism Q90.1
    translocation Q90.2
  22 Q92.8
Tritanomaly, tritanopia H53.55
Trombiculosis, trombiculiasis, trombidiosis
  B88.0
Trophedema (congenital) (hereditary) Q82.0
Trophoblastic disease (*see also* Mole,
  hydatidiform) O01.9
Tropholymphedema Q82.0
Trophoneurosis NEC G96.8
  disseminated M34.9
Tropical —*see* condition
Trouble —*see also* Disease
  heart —*see* Disease, heart
  kidney —*see* Disease, renal
  nervous R45.0
  sinus —*see* Sinusitis
Trousseau's syndrome (thrombophlebitis
  migrans) I82.1
Truancy, childhood
  from school Z72.810
Truncus
  arteriosus (persistent) Q20.0
  communis Q20.0
Trunk —*see* condition
Trypanosomiasis
  African B56.9
    by Trypanosoma brucei
      gambiense B56.0
      rhodesiense B56.1
  American —*see* Chagas' disease
  Brazilian —*see* Chagas' disease
  by Trypanosoma
    brucei gambiense B56.0
    brucei rhodesiense B56.1

Trypanosomiasis *- continued*
cruzi —*see* Chagas' disease
gambiensis, Gambian B56.0
rhodesiensis, Rhodesian B56.1
South American —*see* Chagas' disease
where
   African trypanosomiasis is prevalent B56.9
   Chagas' disease is prevalent B57.2
T-shaped incisors K00.2
Tsutsugamushi (disease) (fever) A75.3
Tube, tubal, tubular —*see* condition
Tubercle —*see also* Tuberculosis
brain, solitary A17.81
Darwin's Q17.8
Ghon, primary infection A15.7
Tuberculid, tuberculide (indurating,
subcutaneous) (lichenoid) (miliary)
(papulonecrotic) (primary) (skin) A18.4
Tuberculoma —*see also* Tuberculosis
brain A17.81
meninges (cerebral) (spinal) A17.1
spinal cord A17.81
Tuberculosis, tubercular, tuberculous
(calcification) (calcified) (caseous)
(chromogenic acid-fast bacilli) (degeneration)
(fibrocaseous) (fistula) (interstitial) (isolated
circumscribed lesions) (necrosis)
(parenchymatous) (ulcerative) A15.9
with pneumoconiosis (any condition in J60-
J64) J65
abdomen (lymph gland) A18.39
abscess (respiratory) A15.9
  bone A18.03
    hip A18.02
    knee A18.02
    sacrum A18.01
    specified site NEC A18.03
    spinal A18.01
    vertebra A18.01
  brain A17.81
  breast A18.89
  Cowper's gland A18.15
  dura (mater) (cerebral) (spinal) A17.81
  epidural (cerebral) (spinal) A17.81
  female pelvis A18.17
  frontal sinus A15.8
  genital organs NEC A18.10
  genitourinary A18.10
  gland (lymphatic) —*see* Tuberculosis,
lymph gland
  hip A18.02
  intestine A18.32
  ischiorectal A18.32
  joint NEC A18.02
    hip A18.02
    knee A18.02
    specified NEC A18.02
    vertebral A18.01
  kidney A18.11
  knee A18.02
  latent R76.11
  lumbar (spine) A18.01
  lung —*see* Tuberculosis, pulmonary
  meninges (cerebral) (spinal) A17.0
  muscle A18.09
  perianal (fistula) A18.32
  perinephritic A18.11
  perirectal A18.32
  rectum A18.32
  retropharyngeal A15.8
  sacrum A18.01
  scrofulous A18.2

Tuberculosis, tubercular – *continued*
scrotum A18.15
skin (primary) A18.4
spinal cord A17.81
spine or vertebra (column) A18.01
subdiaphragmatic A18.31
testis A18.15
urinary A18.13
uterus A18.17
accessory sinus —*see* Tuberculosis, sinus
Addison's disease A18.7
adenitis —*see* Tuberculosis, lymph gland
adenoids A15.8
adenopathy —*see* Tuberculosis, lymph gland
adherent pericardium A18.84
adnexa (uteri) A18.17
adrenal (capsule) (gland) A18.7
alimentary canal A18.32
anemia A18.89
ankle (joint) (bone) A18.02
anus A18.32
apex, apical —*see* Tuberculosis, pulmonary
appendicitis, appendix A18.32
arachnoid A17.0
artery, arteritis A18.89
  cerebral A18.89
arthritis (chronic) (synovial) A18.02
  spine or vertebra (column) A18.01
articular —*see* Tuberculosis, joint
ascites A18.31
asthma —*see* Tuberculosis, pulmonary
axilla, axillary (gland) A18.2
bladder A18.12
bone A18.03
  hip A18.02
  knee A18.02
  limb NEC A18.03
  sacrum A18.01
  spine or vertebral column A18.01
bowel (miliary) A18.32
brain A17.81
breast A18.89
broad ligament A18.17
bronchi, bronchial, bronchus A15.5
  ectasia, ectasis (bronchiectasis) —*see*
Tuberculosis, pulmonary
  fistula A15.5
    primary (progressive) A15.7
  gland or node A15.4
    primary (progressive) A15.7
  lymph gland or node A15.4
    primary (progressive) A15.7
bronchiectasis —*see* Tuberculosis, pulmonary
bronchitis A15.5
bronchopleural A15.6
bronchopneumonia, bronchopneumonic —*see*
Tuberculosis, pulmonary
bronchorrhagia A15.5
bronchotracheal A15.5
bronze disease A18.7
buccal cavity A18.83
bulbourethral gland A18.15
bursa A18.09
cachexia A15.9
cardiomyopathy A18.84
caries —*see* Tuberculosis, bone
cartilage A18.02
  intervertebral A18.01
catarrhal —*see* Tuberculosis, respiratory
cecum A18.32
cellulitis (primary) A18.4
cerebellum A17.81

Tuberculosis, tubercular – *continued*
cerebral, cerebrum A17.81
cerebrospinal A17.81
  meninges A17.0
cervical (lymph gland or node) A18.2
cervicitis, cervix (uteri) A18.16
chest —*see* Tuberculosis, respiratory
chorioretinitis A18.53
choroid, choroiditis A18.53
ciliary body A18.54
colitis A18.32
collier's J65
colliquativa (primary) A18.4
colon A18.32
complex, primary A15.7
congenital P37.0
conjunctiva A18.59
connective tissue (systemic) A18.89
contact Z20.1
cornea (ulcer) A18.52
Cowper's gland A18.15
coxae A18.02
coxalgia A18.02
cul-de-sac of Douglas A18.17
curvature, spine A18.01
cutis (colliquativa) (primary) A18.4
cyst, ovary A18.18
cystitis A18.12
dactylitis A18.03
diarrhea A18.32
diffuse —*see* Tuberculosis, miliary
digestive tract A18.32
disseminated —*see* Tuberculosis, miliary
duodenum A18.32
dura (mater) (cerebral) (spinal) A17.0
  abscess (cerebral) (spinal) A17.81
dysentery A18.32
ear (inner) (middle) A18.6
  bone A18.03
  external (primary) A18.4
  skin (primary) A18.4
elbow A18.02
emphysema —*see* Tuberculosis, pulmonary
empyema A15.6
encephalitis A17.82
endarteritis A18.89
endocarditis A18.84
  aortic A18.84
  mitral A18.84
  pulmonary A18.84
  tricuspid A18.84
endocrine glands NEC A18.82
endometrium A18.17
enteric, enterica, enteritis A18.32
enterocolitis A18.32
epididymis, epididymitis A18.15
epidural abscess (cerebral) (spinal) A17.81
epiglottis A15.5
episcleritis A18.51
erythema (induratum) (nodosum) (primary)
A18.4
esophagus A18.83
eustachian tube A18.6
exposure (to) Z20.1
exudative —*see* Tuberculosis, pulmonary
eye A18.50
eyelid (primary) (lupus) A18.4
fallopian tube (acute) (chronic) A18.17
fascia A18.09
fauces A15.8
female pelvic inflammatory disease A18.17
finger A18.03

Tuberculosis, tubercular – *continued*
first infection A15.7
gallbladder A18.83
ganglion A18.09
gastritis A18.83
gastrocolic fistula A18.32
gastroenteritis A18.32
gastrointestinal tract A18.32
general, generalized —*see* Tuberculosis, miliary
genital organs A18.10
genitourinary A18.10
genu A18.02
glandula suprarenalis A18.7
glandular, general A18.2
glottis A15.5
grinder's J65
gum A18.83
hand A18.03
heart A18.84
hematogenous —*see* Tuberculosis, miliary
hemoptysis —*see* Tuberculosis, pulmonary
hemorrhage NEC —*see* Tuberculosis, pulmonary
hemothorax A15.6
hepatitis A18.83
hilar lymph nodes A15.4
  primary (progressive) A15.7
hip (joint) (disease) (bone) A18.02
hydropneumothorax A15.6
hydrothorax A15.6
hypoadrenalism A18.7
hypopharynx A15.8
ileocecal (hyperplastic) A18.32
ileocolitis A18.32
ileum A18.32
iliac spine (superior) A18.03
immunological findings only A15.7
indurativa (primary) A18.4
infantile A15.7
infection A15.9
  without clinical manifestations A15.7
infraclavicular gland A18.2
inguinal gland A18.2
inguinalis A18.2
intestine (any part) A18.32
iridocyclitis A18.54
iris, iritis A18.54
ischiorectal A18.32
jaw A18.03
jejunum A18.32
joint A18.02
  vertebral A18.01
keratitis (interstitial) A18.52
keratoconjunctivitis A18.52
kidney A18.11
knee (joint) A18.02
kyphosis, kyphoscoliosis A18.01
laryngitis A15.5
larynx A15.5
latent R76.11
leptomeninges, leptomeningitis (cerebral) (spinal) A17.0
lichenoides (primary) A18.4
linguae A18.83
lip A18.83
liver A18.83
lordosis A18.01
lung —*see* Tuberculosis, pulmonary
lupus vulgaris A18.4
lymph gland or node (peripheral) A18.2
  abdomen A18.39

Tuberculosis, tubercular – *continued*
bronchial A15.4
  primary (progressive) A15.7
cervical A18.2
hilar A15.4
  primary (progressive) A15.7
intrathoracic A15.4
  primary (progressive) A15.7
mediastinal A15.4
  primary (progressive) A15.7
mesenteric A18.39
retroperitoneal A18.39
tracheobronchial A15.4
  primary (progressive) A15.7
lymphadenitis —*see* Tuberculosis, lymph gland
lymphangitis —*see* Tuberculosis, lymph gland
lymphatic (gland) (vessel) —*see* Tuberculosis, lymph gland
mammary gland A18.89
marasmus A15.9
mastoiditis A18.03
mediastinal lymph gland or node A15.4
  primary (progressive) A15.7
mediastinitis A15.8
  primary (progressive) A15.7
mediastinum A15.8
  primary (progressive) A15.7
medulla A17.81
melanosis, Addisonian A18.7
meninges, meningitis (basilar) (cerebral) (cerebrospinal) (spinal) A17.0
meningoencephalitis A17.82
mesentery, mesenteric (gland or node) A18.39
miliary A19.9
  acute A19.2
    multiple sites A19.1
    single specified site A19.0
  chronic A19.8
  specified NEC A19.8
millstone makers' J65
miner's J65
molder's J65
mouth A18.83
multiple A19.9
  acute A19.1
  chronic A19.8
muscle A18.09
myelitis A17.82
myocardium, myocarditis A18.84
nasal (passage) (sinus) A15.8
nasopharynx A15.8
neck gland A18.2
nephritis A18.11
nerve (mononeuropathy) A17.83
nervous system A17.9
nose (septum) A15.8
ocular A18.50
omentum A18.31
oophoritis (acute) (chronic) A18.17
optic (nerve trunk) (papilla) A18.59
orbit A18.59
orchitis A18.15
organ, specified NEC A18.89
osseous —*see* Tuberculosis, bone
osteitis —*see* Tuberculosis, bone
osteomyelitis —*see* Tuberculosis, bone
otitis media A18.6
ovary, ovaritis (acute) (chronic) A18.17
oviduct (acute) (chronic) A18.17
pachymeningitis A17.0

Tuberculosis, tubercular – *continued*
palate (soft) A18.83
pancreas A18.83
papulonecrotic (a) (primary) A18.4
parathyroid glands A18.82
paronychia (primary) A18.4
parotid gland or region A18.83
pelvis (bony) A18.03
penis A18.15
peribronchitis A15.5
pericardium, pericarditis A18.84
perichondritis, larynx A15.5
periostitis —*see* Tuberculosis, bone
perirectal fistula A18.32
peritoneum NEC A18.31
peritonitis A18.31
pharynx, pharyngitis A15.8
phlyctenulosis (keratoconjunctivitis) A18.52
phthisis NEC —*see* Tuberculosis, pulmonary
pituitary gland A18.82
pleura, pleural, pleurisy, pleuritis (fibrinous) (obliterative) (purulent) (simple plastic) (with effusion) A15.6
  primary (progressive) A15.7
pneumonia, pneumonic —*see* Tuberculosis, pulmonary
pneumothorax (spontaneous) (tense valvular) —*see* Tuberculosis, pulmonary
polyneuropathy A17.89
polyserositis A19.9
  acute A19.1
  chronic A19.8
potter's J65
prepuce A18.15
primary (complex) A15.7
proctitis A18.32
prostate, prostatitis A18.14
pulmonalis —*see* Tuberculosis, pulmonary
pulmonary (cavitated) (fibrotic) (infiltrative) (nodular) A15.0
  childhood type or first infection A15.7
  primary (complex) A15.7
pyelitis A18.11
pyelonephritis A18.11
pyemia —*see* Tuberculosis, miliary
pyonephrosis A18.11
pyopneumothorax A15.6
pyothorax A15.6
rectum (fistula) (with abscess) A18.32
reinfection stage —*see* Tuberculosis, pulmonary
renal A18.11
renis A18.11
respiratory A15.9
  primary A15.7
  specified site NEC A15.8
retina, retinitis A18.53
retroperitoneal (lymph gland or node) A18.39
rheumatism NEC A18.09
rhinitis A15.8
sacroiliac (joint) A18.01
sacrum A18.01
salivary gland A18.83
salpingitis (acute) (chronic) A18.17
sandblaster's J65
sclera A18.51
scoliosis A18.01
scrofulous A18.2
scrotum A18.15
seminal tract or vesicle A18.15
senile A15.9
septic —*see* Tuberculosis, miliary

Tuberculosis, tubercular – *continued*
  shoulder (joint) A18.02
    blade A18.03
  sigmoid A18.32
  sinus (any nasal) A15.8
    bone A18.03
    epididymis A18.15
  skeletal NEC A18.03
  skin (any site) (primary) A18.4
  small intestine A18.32
  soft palate A18.83
  spermatic cord A18.15
  spine, spinal (column) A18.01
    cord A17.81
    medulla A17.81
    membrane A17.0
    meninges A17.0
  spleen, splenitis A18.85
  spondylitis A18.01
  sternoclavicular joint A18.02
  stomach A18.83
  stonemason's J65
  subcutaneous tissue (cellular) (primary)
    A18.4
  subcutis (primary) A18.4
  subdeltoid bursa A18.83
  submaxillary (region) A18.83
  supraclavicular gland A18.2
  suprarenal (capsule) (gland) A18.7
  swelling, joint (see also category M01) (*see*
    also Tuberculosis, joint) A18.02
  symphysis pubis A18.02
  synovitis A18.09
    articular A18.02
    spine or vertebra A18.01
  systemic —*see* Tuberculosis, miliary
  tarsitis A18.4
  tendon (sheath) —*see* Tuberculosis,
    tenosynovitis
  tenosynovitis A18.09
    spine or vertebra A18.01
  testis A18.15
  throat A15.8
  thymus gland A18.82
  thyroid gland A18.81
  tongue A18.83
  tonsil, tonsillitis A15.8
  trachea, tracheal A15.5
    lymph gland or node A15.4
      primary (progressive) A15.7
  tracheobronchial A15.5
    lymph gland or node A15.4
      primary (progressive) A15.7
  tubal (acute) (chronic) A18.17
  tunica vaginalis A18.15
  ulcer (skin) (primary) A18.4
    bowel or intestine A18.32
    specified NEC
  code under Tuberculosis, by site
  unspecified site A15.9
  ureter A18.11
  urethra, urethral (gland) A18.13
  urinary organ or tract A18.13
  uterus A18.17
  uveal tract A18.54
  uvula A18.83
  vagina A18.18
  vas deferens A18.15
  verruca, verrucosa (cutis) (primary) A18.4
  vertebra (column) A18.01
  vesiculitis A18.15
  vulva A18.18

Tuberculosis, tubercular – *continued*
  wrist (joint) A18.02
Tuberculum
  Carabelli (*see* Note at) K00.2
  occlusal (*see* Note at) K00.2
  paramolare K00.2
Tuberosity, entire maxillary M26.07
Tuberous sclerosis (brain) Q85.1
Tubo-ovarian —*see* condition
Tuboplasty, after previous sterilization
  Z31.0
  aftercare Z31.42
Tubotympanitis, catarrhal (chronic) —*see*
  Otitis, media, nonsuppurative, chronic, serous
Tularemia A21.9
  with
    conjunctivitis A21.1
    pneumonia A21.2
  abdominal A21.3
  bronchopneumonic A21.2
  conjunctivitis A21.1
  cryptogenic A21.3
  enteric A21.3
  gastrointestinal A21.3
  generalized A21.7
  ingestion A21.3
  intestinal A21.3
  oculoglandular A21.1
  ophthalmic A21.1
  pneumonia (any) , pneumonic A21.2
  pulmonary A21.2
  sepsis A21.7
  specified NEC A21.8
  typhoidal A21.7
  ulceroglandular A21.0
Tularensis conjunctivitis A21.1
Tumefaction —*see also* Swelling
  liver —*see* Hypertrophy, liver
Tumor —*see also* Neoplasm, unspecified
  behavior, by site
  acinar cell —*see* Neoplasm, uncertain
    behavior, by site
  acinic cell —*see* Neoplasm, uncertain
    behavior, by site
  adenocarcinoid —*see* Neoplasm, malignant,
    by site
  adenomatoid —*see also* Neoplasm, benign,
    by site
    odontogenic —*see* Cyst, calcifying
  odontogenic
  adnexal (skin) —*see* Neoplasm, skin, benign,
    by site
  adrenal
    cortical (benign) D35.0
      malignant C74.0
    rest —*see* Neoplasm, benign, by site
  alpha-cell
    malignant
      pancreas C25.4
      specified site NEC —*see* Neoplasm,
    malignant, by site
      unspecified site C25.4
    pancreas D13.7
    specified site NEC —*see* Neoplasm, benign,
      by site
    unspecified site D13.7
  aneurysmal —*see* Aneurysm
  aortic body D44.7
    malignant C75.5
  Askin's —*see* Neoplasm, connective tissue,
    malignant

Tumor – *continued*
  basal cell (*see also* Neoplasm, skin, uncertain
    behavior) D48.5
  Bednar —*see* Neoplasm, skin, malignant
  benign (unclassified) —*see* Neoplasm,
    benign, by site
  beta-cell
    malignant
      pancreas C25.4
      specified site NEC —*see* Neoplasm,
    malignant, by site
      unspecified site C25.4
    pancreas D13.7
    specified site NEC —*see* Neoplasm, benign,
      by site
    unspecified site D13.7
  Brenner D27.9
    borderline malignancy D39.1
    malignant C56
    proliferating D39.1
  bronchial alveolar, intravascular D38.1
  Brooke's —*see* Neoplasm, skin, benign
  brown fat —*see* Lipoma
  Burkitt —*see* Lymphoma, Burkitt
  calcifying epithelial odontogenic —*see* Cyst,
    calcifying odontogenic
  carcinoid
    benign D3A.00
      appendix D3A.020
      ascending colon D3A.022
      bronchus (lung) D3A.090
      cecum D3A.021
      colon D3A.029
      descending colon D3A.024
      duodenum D3A.010
      foregut NOS D3A.094
      hindgut NOS D3A.096
      ileum D3A.012
      jejunum D3A.011
      kidney D3A.093
      large intestine D3A.029
      lung (bronchus) D3A.090
      midgut NOS D3A.095
      rectum D3A.026
      sigmoid colon D3A.025
      small intestine D3A.019
      specified NEC D3A.098
      stomach D3A.092
      thymus D3A.091
      transverse colon D3A.023
    malignant C7A.00
      appendix C7A.020
      ascending colon C7A.022
      bronchus (lung) C7A.090
      cecum C7A.021
      colon C7A.029
      descending colon C7A.024
      duodenum C7A.010
      foregut NOS C7A.094
      hindgut NOS C7A.096
      ileum C7A.012
      jejunum C7A.011
      kidney C7A.093
      large intestine C7A.029
      lung (bronchus) C7A.090
      midgut NOS C7A.095
      rectum C7A.026
      sigmoid colon C7A.025
      small intestine C7A.019
      specified NEC C7A.098
      stomach C7A.092
      thymus C7A.091

Tumor – *continued*

transverse colon C7A.023
mesentery metastasis C7B.04
secondary C7B.00
bone C7B.03
distant lymph nodes C7B.01
liver C7B.02
peritoneum C7B.04
specified NEC C7B.09
carotid body D44.6
malignant C75.4
cells —*see also* Neoplasm, unspecified behavior, by site
benign —*see* Neoplasm, benign, by site
malignant —*see* Neoplasm, malignant, by site
uncertain whether benign or malignant —*see* Neoplasm, uncertain behavior, by site
cervix, in pregnancy or childbirth —*see* Pregnancy, complicated by, tumor, cervix
chondromatous giant cell —*see* Neoplasm, bone, benign
chromaffin —*see also* Neoplasm, benign, by site
malignant —*see* Neoplasm, malignant, by site
Cock's peculiar L72.3
Codman's —*see* Neoplasm, bone, benign
dentigerous, mixed —*see* Cyst, calcifying odontogenic
dermoid —*see* Neoplasm, benign, by site
with malignant transformation C56
desmoid (extra-abdominal) —*see also* Neoplasm, connective tissue, uncertain behavior
abdominal —*see* Neoplasm, connective tissue, uncertain behavior
embolus —*see* Neoplasm, secondary, by site
embryonal (mixed) —*see also* Neoplasm, uncertain behavior, by site
liver C22.7
endodermal sinus
specified site —*see* Neoplasm, malignant, by site
unspecified site
female C56.
male C62.90
epithelial
benign —*see* Neoplasm, benign, by site
malignant —*see* Neoplasm, malignant, by site
Ewing's —*see* Neoplasm, bone, malignant, by site
fatty —*see* Lipoma
fibroid —*see* Leiomyoma
G cell
malignant
pancreas C25.4
specified site NEC —*see* Neoplasm, malignant, by site
unspecified site C25.4
specified site —*see* Neoplasm, uncertain behavior, by site
unspecified site D37.8
germ cell —*see also* Neoplasm, malignant, by site
mixed —*see* Neoplasm, malignant, by site
ghost cell, odontogenic —*see* Cyst, calcifying odontogenic
giant cell —*see also* Neoplasm, uncertain behavior, by site

bone D48.0
malignant —*see* Neoplasm, bone, malignant
chondromatous —*see* Neoplasm, bone, benign
malignant —*see* Neoplasm, malignant, by site
soft parts —*see* Neoplasm, connective tissue, uncertain behavior
malignant —*see* Neoplasm, connective tissue, malignant
glomus D18.00
intra-abdominal D18.03
intracranial D18.02
jugulare D44.7
malignant C75.5
skin D18.01
specified site NEC D18.09
gonadal stromal —*see* Neoplasm, uncertain behavior, by site
granular cell —*see also* Neoplasm, connective tissue, benign
malignant —*see* Neoplasm, connective tissue, malignant
granulosa cell D39.1
juvenile D39.1
malignant C56
granulosa cell-theca cell D39.1
malignant C56
Grawitz's C64
hemorrhoidal —*see* Hemorrhoids
hilar cell D27
hilus cell D27
Hürthle cell (benign) D34
malignant C73
hydatid —*see* Echinococcus
hypernephroid —*see also* Neoplasm, uncertain behavior, by site
interstitial cell —*see also* Neoplasm, uncertain behavior, by site
benign —*see* Neoplasm, benign, by site
malignant —*see* Neoplasm, malignant, by site
intravascular bronchial alveolar D38.1
islet cell —*see* Neoplasm, benign, by site
malignant —*see* Neoplasm, malignant, by site
pancreas C25.4
specified site NEC —*see* Neoplasm, malignant, by site
unspecified site C25.4
pancreas D13.7
specified site NEC —*see* Neoplasm, benign, by site
unspecified site D13.7
juxtaglomerular D41.0
Klatskin's C24.0
Krukenberg's C79.6
Leydig cell —*see* Neoplasm, uncertain behavior, by site
benign —*see* Neoplasm, benign, by site
specified site —*see* Neoplasm, benign, by site
unspecified site
female D27.9
male D29.20
malignant —*see* Neoplasm, malignant, by site
specified site —*see* Neoplasm, malignant, by site

unspecified site
female C56.9
male C62.90
specified site —*see* Neoplasm, uncertain behavior, by site
unspecified site
female D39.10
male D40.10
lipid cell, ovary D27
lipoid cell, ovary D27
malignant (*see also* Neoplasm, malignant, by site) C80.1
fusiform cell (type) C80.1
giant cell (type) C80.1
localized, plasma cell —*see* Plasmacytoma, solitary
mixed NEC C80.1
small cell (type) C80.1
spindle cell (type) C80.1
unclassified C80.1
mast cell D47.0
malignant C96.2
melanotic, neuroectodermal —*see* Neoplasm, benign, by site
Merkel cell —*see* Carcinoma, Merkel cell
mesenchymal
malignant —*see* Neoplasm, connective tissue, malignant
mixed —*see* Neoplasm, connective tissue, uncertain behavior
mesodermal, mixed —*see also* Neoplasm, malignant, by site
liver C22.4
mesonephric —*see also* Neoplasm, uncertain behavior, by site
malignant —*see* Neoplasm, malignant, by site
metastatic
from specified site —*see* Neoplasm, malignant, by site
of specified site —*see* Neoplasm, malignant, by site
to specified site —*see* Neoplasm, secondary, by site
mixed NEC —*see also* Neoplasm, benign, by site
malignant —*see* Neoplasm, malignant, by site
mucinous of low malignant potential
specified site —*see* Neoplasm, malignant, by site
unspecified site C56.9
mucocarcinoid
specified site —*see* Neoplasm, malignant, by site
unspecified site C18.1
mucoepidermoid —*see* Neoplasm, uncertain behavior, by site
Müllerian, mixed
specified site —*see* Neoplasm, malignant, by site
unspecified site C54.9
myoepithelial —*see* Neoplasm, benign, by site
neuroectodermal (peripheral) —*see* Neoplasm, malignant, by site
primitive
specified site —*see* Neoplasm, malignant, by site
unspecified site C71.9

Tumor – *continued*
  neuroendocrine D3A.8
    malignant poorly differentiated C7A.1
    secondary NEC C7B.8
    specified NEC C7A.8
  neurogenic olfactory C30.0
  nonencapsulated sclerosing C73
  odontogenic (adenomatoid) (benign)
  (calcifying epithelial) (keratocystic)
  (squamous) —*see* Cyst, calcifying
  odontogenic
    malignant C41.1
      upper jaw (bone) C41.0
  ovarian stromal D39.1
  ovary, in pregnancy —*see* Pregnancy,
  complicated by
  pacinian —*see* Neoplasm, skin, benign
  Pancoast's —*see* Pancoast's syndrome
  papillary —*see also* Papilloma
    cystic D37.9
    mucinous of low malignant potential C56
      specified site —*see* Neoplasm, malignant,
  by site
      unspecified site C56.9
    serous of low malignant potential
      specified site —*see* Neoplasm, malignant,
  by site
      unspecified site C56.9
  pelvic, in pregnancy or childbirth —*see*
  Pregnancy, complicated by
  phantom F45.8
  phyllodes D48.6
    benign D24
    malignant —*see* Neoplasm, breast,
  malignant
  Pindborg —*see* Cyst, calcifying odontogenic
  placental site trophoblastic D39.2
  plasma cell (malignant) (localized) —*see*
  Plasmacytoma, solitary
  polyvesicular vitelline
    specified site —*see* Neoplasm, malignant,
  by site
    unspecified site
      female C56.9
      male C62.90
  Pott's puffy —*see* Osteomyelitis, specified
  NEC
  Rathke's pouch D44.3
  retinal anlage —*see* Neoplasm, benign, by site
  salivary gland type, mixed —*see* Neoplasm,
  salivary gland, benign
    malignant —*see* Neoplasm, salivary gland,
  malignant
  Sampson's N80.1
  Schmincke's —*see* Neoplasm, nasopharynx,
  malignant
  sclerosing stromal D27
  sebaceous —*see* Cyst, sebaceous
  secondary —*see* Neoplasm, secondary, by site
    carcinoid C7B.00
      bone C7B.03
      distant lymph nodes C7B.01
      liver C7B.02
      peritoneum C7B.04
      specified NEC C7B.09
    neuroendocrine NEC C7B.8
  serous of low malignant potential
    specified site —*see* Neoplasm, malignant,
  by site
    unspecified site C56.9

Tumor – *continued*
  Sertoli cell —*see* Neoplasm, benign, by site
    with lipid storage
      specified site —*see* Neoplasm, benign, by
  site
      unspecified site
        female D27.9
        male D29.20
    specified site —*see* Neoplasm, benign, by
  site
    unspecified site
      female D27.9
      male D29.20
  Sertoli-Leydig cell —*see* Neoplasm, benign,
  by site
    specified site —*see* Neoplasm, benign, by
  site
    unspecified site
      female D27.9
      male D29.20
  sex cord (-stromal) —*see* Neoplasm,
  uncertain behavior, by site
    with annular tubules D39.1
  skin appendage —*see* Neoplasm, skin, benign
  smooth muscle —*see* Neoplasm, connective
  tissue, uncertain behavior
  soft tissue
    benign —*see* Neoplasm, connective tissue,
  benign
    malignant —*see* Neoplasm, connective
  tissue, malignant
  sternomastoid (congenital) Q68.0
  stromal
    endometrial D39.0
    gastric D48.1
      benign D21.4
      malignant C16.9
      uncertain behavior D48.1
    gastrointestinal
      benign D21.4
      malignant C49.4
      uncertain behavior D48.1
    intestine
      benign D21.4
      malignant C49.4
      uncertain behavior D48.1
    ovarian D39.1
    stomach
      benign D21.4
      malignant C16.9
      uncertain behavior D48.1
  testicular D40.10
  sweat gland —*see also* Neoplasm, skin,
  uncertain behavior
    benign —*see* Neoplasm, skin, benign
    malignant —*see* Neoplasm, skin, malignant
  syphilitic, brain A52.17
  testicular stromal D40.1
  theca cell D27.
  theca cell-granulosa cell D39.1
  Triton, malignant —*see* Neoplasm, nerve,
  malignant
  trophoblastic, placental site D39.2
  turban D23.4
  uterus (body) , in pregnancy or childbirth —
  see Pregnancy, complicated by, tumor, uterus
  vagina, in pregnancy or childbirth —*see*
  Pregnancy, complicated by
  varicose —*see* Varix
  von Recklinghausen's —*see*
  Neurofibromatosis

Tumor – *continued*
  vulva or perineum, in pregnancy or childbirth
  —*see* Pregnancy, complicated by
    causing obstructed labor O65.5
  Warthin's —*see* Neoplasm, salivary gland,
  benign
  Wilms' C64
  yolk sac —*see* Neoplasm, malignant, by site
    specified site —*see* Neoplasm, malignant,
  by site
    unspecified site
      female C56.9
      male C62.90
Tumor lysis syndrome (following
  antineoplastic chemotherapy) (spontaneous)
  NEC E88.3
Tumorlet —*see* Neoplasm, uncertain behavior,
  by site
Tungiasis B88.1
Tunica vasculosa lentis Q12.2
Turban tumor D23.4
Türck's trachoma J37.0
Turner-Kieser syndrome Q79.8
Turner-like syndrome Q87.1
Turner's
  hypoplasia (tooth) K00.4
  syndrome Q96.9
    specified NEC Q96.8
  tooth K00.4
Turner-Ullrich syndrome Q96.9
Tussis convulsiva —*see* Whooping cough
Twiddler's syndrome (due to)
  automatic implantable defibrillator T82.198
  cardiac pacemaker T82.198
Twilight state
  epileptic F05
  psychogenic F44.89
Twin (newborn) —*see also* Newborn, twin
  conjoined Q89.4
  pregnancy —*see* Pregnancy, twin, conjoined
Twinning, teeth K00.2
Twist, twisted
  bowel, colon or intestine K56.2
  hair (congenital) Q84.1
  mesentery K56.2
  omentum K56.2
  organ or site, congenital NEC —*see*
  Anomaly, by site
  ovarian pedicle —*see* Torsion, ovary
Twitching R25.3
Tylosis (acquired) L84
  buccalis K13.29
  linguae K13.29
  palmaris et plantaris (congenital) (inherited)
  Q82.8
    acquired L85.1
Tympanism R14.0
Tympanites (abdominal) (intestinal) R14.0
Tympanitis —*see* Myringitis
Tympanosclerosis —*see* subcategory H74.0
Tympanum —*see* condition
Tympany
  abdomen R14.0
  chest R09.89
Type A behavior pattern Z73.1
Typhlitis —*see* Appendicitis
Typhoenteritis —*see* Typhoid
Typhoid (abortive) (ambulant) (any site)
  (clinical) (fever) (hemorrhagic) (infection)
  (intermittent) (malignant) (rheumatic) (Widal
  negative) A01.00
  with pneumonia A01.03
  abdominal A01.09

Typhoid - *continued*
arthritis A01.04
carrier (suspected) of Z22.0
cholecystitis (current) A01.09
endocarditis A01.02
heart involvement A01.02
inoculation reaction —*see* Complications, vaccination
meningitis A01.01
mesenteric lymph nodes A01.09
myocarditis A01.02
osteomyelitis A01.05
perichondritis, larynx A01.09
pneumonia A01.03
spine A01.05
specified NEC A01.09
ulcer (perforating) A01.09
Typhomalaria (fever) —*see* Malaria
Typhomania A01.00
Typhoperitonitis A01.09
Typhus (fever) A75.9
abdominal, abdominalis —*see* Typhoid
African tick A77.1
amarillic A95.9
brain A75.9 *[G94]*
cerebral A75.9 *[G94]*
classical A75.0
due to Rickettsia
prowazekii A75.0
recrudescent A75.1
tsutsugamushi A75.3
typhi A75.2
endemic (flea-borne) A75.2
epidemic (louse-borne) A75.0
exanthematic NEC A75.0
exanthematicus SAI A75.0
brillii SAI A75.1
mexicanus SAI A75.2
typhus murinus A75.2
flea-borne A75.2
India tick A77.1
Kenya (tick) A77.1
louse-borne A75.0
Mexican A75.2
mite-borne A75.3
murine A75.2
North Asian tick-borne A77.2
petechial A75.9
Queensland tick A77.3
rat A75.2
recrudescent A75.1
recurrens —*see* Fever, relapsing
Sao Paulo A77.0
scrub (China) (India) (Malaysia) (New Guinea) A75.3
shop (of Malaysia) A75.2
Siberian tick A77.2
tick-borne A77.9
tropical (mite-borne) A75.3
Tyrosinemia E70.21
newborn, transitory P74.5
Tyrosinosis E70.21
Tyrosinuria E70.29

U

Uhl's anomaly or disease Q24.8
Ulcer, ulcerated, ulcerating, ulceration, ulcerative
alveolar process M27.3
amebic (intestine) A06.1
skin A06.7
anastomotic —*see* Ulcer, gastrojejunal

Ulcer, ulcerated - *continued*
anorectal K62.6
antral —*see* Ulcer, stomach
anus (sphincter) (solitary) K62.6
aorta —*see* Aneurysm
aphthous (oral) (recurrent) K12.0
genital organ (s)
female N76.6
male N50.8
artery I77.2
atrophic —*see* Ulcer, skin
decubitus —*see* Ulcer, pressure, by site
back L98.429
with
bone necrosis L98.424
exposed fat layer L98.422
muscle necrosis L98.423
skin breakdown only L98.421
Barrett's (esophagus) K22.10
with bleeding K22.11
bile duct (common) (hepatic) K83.8
bladder (solitary) (sphincter) NEC N32.89
bilharzial B65.9 *[N33]*
in schistosomiasis (bilharzial) B65.9 *[N33]*
submucosal —*see* Cystitis, interstitial
tuberculous A18.12
bleeding K27.4
bone —*see* Osteomyelitis, specified type NEC
bowel —*see* Ulcer, intestine
breast N61
bronchus J98.09
buccal (cavity) (traumatic) K12.1
Buruli A31.1
buttock L98.419
with
bone necrosis L98.414
exposed fat layer L98.412
muscle necrosis L98.413
skin breakdown only L98.411
cancerous —*see* Neoplasm, malignant, by site
cardia K22.10
with bleeding K22.11
cardioesophageal (peptic) K22.10
with bleeding K22.11
cecum —*see* Ulcer, intestine
cervix (uteri) (decubitus) (trophic) N86
with cervicitis N72
chancroidal A57
chiclero B55.1
chronic (cause unknown) —*see* Ulcer, skin
Cochin-China B55.1
colon —*see* Ulcer, intestine
conjunctiva H10.89
cornea H16.00
with hypopyon H16.03
central H16.01
dendritic (herpes simplex) B00.52
marginal H16.04
Mooren's H16.05
mycotic H16.06
perforated H16.07
ring H16.02
tuberculous (phlyctenular) A18.52
corpus cavernosum (chronic) N48.5
crural —*see* Ulcer, lower limb
Curling's —*see* Ulcer, peptic, acute
Cushing's —*see* Ulcer, peptic, acute
cystic duct K82.8
cystitis (interstitial) —*see* Cystitis, interstitial
decubitus —*see* Ulcer, pressure, by site
dendritic, cornea (herpes simplex) B00.52
diabetes, diabetic —*see* Diabetes, ulcer

Ulcer, ulcerated - *continued*
Dieulafoy's K25.0
due to
infection NEC —*see* Ulcer, skin
radiation NEC L59.8
trophic disturbance (any region) —*see* Ulcer, skin
X-ray L58.1
duodenum, duodenal (eroded) (peptic) K26.9
with
hemorrhage K26.4
and perforation K26.6
perforation K26.5
acute K26.3
with
hemorrhage K26.0
and perforation K26.2
perforation K26.1
chronic K26.7
with
hemorrhage K26.4
and perforation K26.6
perforation K26.5
dysenteric A09
elusive —*see* Cystitis, interstitial
endocarditis (acute) (chronic) (subacute) I28.8
epiglottis J38.7
esophagus (peptic) K22.10
with bleeding K22.11
due to
aspirin K22.10
with bleeding K22.11
gastrointestinal reflux disease K21.0
ingestion of chemical or medicament K22.10
with bleeding K22.11
fungal K22.10
with bleeding K22.11
infective K22.10
with bleeding K22.11
varicose —*see* Varix, esophagus
eyelid (region) H01.8
fauces J39.2
Fenwick (-Hunner) (solitary) —*see* Cystitis, interstitial
fistulous —*see* Ulcer, skin
foot (indolent) (trophic) —*see* Ulcer, lower limb
frambesial, initial A66.0
frenum (tongue) K14.0
gallbladder or duct K82.8
gangrenous —*see* Gangrene
gastric —*see* Ulcer, stomach
gastrocolic —*see* Ulcer, gastrojejunal
gastroduodenal —*see* Ulcer, peptic
gastroesophageal —*see* Ulcer, stomach
gastrointestinal —*see* Ulcer, gastrojejunal
gastrojejunal (peptic) K28.9
with
hemorrhage K28.4
and perforation K28.6
perforation K28.5
acute K28.3
with
hemorrhage K28.0
and perforation K28.2
perforation K28.1
chronic K28.7
with
hemorrhage K28.4
and perforation K28.6
perforation K28.5

Ulcer, ulcerated *- continued*
gastrojejunocolic —*see* Ulcer, gastrojejunal
gingiva K06.8
gingivitis K05.10
  nonplaque induced K05.11
  plaque induced K05.10
glottis J38.7
granuloma of pudenda A58
gum K06.8
gumma, due to yaws A66.4
heel —*see* Ulcer, lower limb
hemorrhoid (*see also* Hemorrhoids, by degree) K64.8
Hunner's —*see* Cystitis, interstitial
hypopharynx J39.2
hypopyon (chronic) (subacute) —*see* Ulcer, cornea, with hypopyon
hypostaticum —*see* Ulcer, varicose
ileum —*see* Ulcer, intestine
intestine, intestinal K63.3
  with perforation K63.1
  amebic A06.1
  duodenal —*see* Ulcer, duodenum
  granulocytopenic (with hemorrhage) —*see* Neutropenia
  marginal —*see* Ulcer, gastrojejunal
  perforating K63.1
    newborn P78.0
  primary, small intestine K63.3
  rectum K62.6
  stercoraceous, stercoral K63.3
  tuberculous A18.32
  typhoid (fever) —*see* Typhoid
  varicose I86.8
jejunum, jejunal —*see* Ulcer, gastrojejunal
keratitis —*see* Ulcer, cornea
knee —*see* Ulcer, lower limb
labium (majus) (minus) N76.6
laryngitis —*see* Laryngitis
larynx (aphthous) (contact) J38.7
  diphtheritic A36.2
leg —*see* Ulcer, lower limb
lip K13.0
Lipschütz's N76.6
lower limb (atrophic) (chronic) (neurogenic) (perforating) (pyogenic) (trophic) (tropical) L97.909
  with
    bone necrosis L97.904
    exposed fat layer L97.902
    muscle necrosis L97.903
    skin breakdown only L97.901
  ankle L97.309
    with
      bone necrosis L97.304
      exposed fat layer L97.302
      muscle necrosis L97.303
      skin breakdown only L97.301
    left L97.329
      with
        bone necrosis L97.324
        exposed fat layer L97.322
        muscle necrosis L97.323
        skin breakdown only L97.321
    right L97.319
      with
        bone necrosis L97.314
        exposed fat layer L97.312
        muscle necrosis L97.313
        skin breakdown only L97.311

Ulcer, ulcerated *- continued*
calf L97.209
  with
    bone necrosis L97.204
    exposed fat layer L97.202
    muscle necrosis L97.203
    skin breakdown only L97.201
  left L97.229
    with
      bone necrosis L97.224
      exposed fat layer L97.222
      muscle necrosis L97.223
      skin breakdown only L97.221
  right L97.219
    with
      bone necrosis L97.214
      exposed fat layer L97.212
      muscle necrosis L97.213
      skin breakdown only L97.211
decubitus —*see* Ulcer, pressure, by site
foot specified NEC L97.509
  with
    bone necrosis L97.504
    exposed fat layer L97.502
    muscle necrosis L97.503
    skin breakdown only L97.501
  left L97.529
    with
      bone necrosis L97.524
      exposed fat layer L97.522
      muscle necrosis L97.523
      skin breakdown only L97.521
  right L97.519
    with
      bone necrosis L97.514
      exposed fat layer L97.512
      muscle necrosis L97.513
      skin breakdown only L97.511
heel L97.409
  with
    bone necrosis L97.404
    exposed fat layer L97.402
    muscle necrosis L97.403
    skin breakdown only L97.401
  left L97.429
    with
      bone necrosis L97.424
      exposed fat layer L97.422
      muscle necrosis L97.423
      skin breakdown only L97.421
  right L97.419
    with
      bone necrosis L97.414
      exposed fat layer L97.412
      muscle necrosis L97.413
      skin breakdown only L97.411
left L97.929
  with
    bone necrosis L97.924
    exposed fat layer L97.922
    muscle necrosis L97.923
    skin breakdown only L97.921
lower leg NOS L97.909
  with
    bone necrosis L97.904
    exposed fat layer L97.902
    muscle necrosis L97.903
    skin breakdown only L97.901
left L97.929
  with
    bone necrosis L97.924
    exposed fat layer L97.922

Ulcer, ulcerated *- continued*
    muscle necrosis L97.923
    skin breakdown only L97.921
  right L97.919
    with
      bone necrosis L97.914
      exposed fat layer L97.912
      muscle necrosis L97.913
      skin breakdown only L97.911
specified site NEC L97.809
  with
    bone necrosis L97.804
    exposed fat layer L97.802
    muscle necrosis L97.803
    skin breakdown only L97.801
  left L97.829
    with
      bone necrosis L97.824
      exposed fat layer L97.822
      muscle necrosis L97.823
      skin breakdown only L97.821
  right L97.819
    with
      bone necrosis L97.814
      exposed fat layer L97.812
      muscle necrosis L97.813
      skin breakdown only L97.811
midfoot L97.409
  with
    bone necrosis L97.404
    exposed fat layer L97.402
    muscle necrosis L97.403
    skin breakdown only L97.401
  left L97.429
    with
      bone necrosis L97.424
      exposed fat layer L97.422
      muscle necrosis L97.423
      skin breakdown only L97.421
  right L97.419
    with
      bone necrosis L97.414
      exposed fat layer L97.412
      muscle necrosis L97.413
      skin breakdown only L97.411
right L97.919
  with
    bone necrosis L97.914
    exposed fat layer L97.912
    muscle necrosis L97.913
    skin breakdown only L97.911
thigh L97.109
  with
    bone necrosis L97.104
    exposed fat layer L97.102
    muscle necrosis L97.103
    skin breakdown only L97.101
  left L97.129
    with
      bone necrosis L97.124
      exposed fat layer L97.122
      muscle necrosis L97.123
      skin breakdown only L97.121
  right L97.119
    with
      bone necrosis L97.114
      exposed fat layer L97.112
      muscle necrosis L97.113
      skin breakdown only L97.111

Ulcer, ulcerated   - continued
  toe L97.509
    with
      bone necrosis L97.504
      exposed fat layer L97.502
      muscle necrosis L97.503
      skin breakdown only L97.501
    left L97.529
      with
        bone necrosis L97.524
        exposed fat layer L97.522
        muscle necrosis L97.523
        skin breakdown only L97.521
    right L97.519
      with
        bone necrosis L97.514
        exposed fat layer L97.512
        muscle necrosis L97.513
        skin breakdown only L97.511
  leprous A30.1
  syphilitic A52.19
  varicose —see Varix, leg, with, ulcer
  luetic —see Ulcer, syphilitic
  lung J98.4
    tuberculous —see Tuberculosis, pulmonary
  malignant —see Neoplasm, malignant, by site
  marginal NEC —see Ulcer, gastrojejunal
  meatus (urinarius) N34.2
  Meckel's diverticulum Q43.0
    malignant —see Table of Neoplasms, small
  intestine, malignant
  Meleney's (chronic undermining) —see Ulcer,
  skin
  Mooren's (cornea) —see Ulcer, cornea,
  Mooren's
  mycobacterial (skin) A31.1
  nasopharynx J39.2
  neck, uterus N86
  neurogenic NEC —see Ulcer, skin
  nose, nasal (passage) (infective) (septum)
  J34.0
    skin —see Ulcer, skin
    spirochetal A69.8
    varicose (bleeding) I86.8
  oral mucosa (traumatic) K12.1
  palate (soft) K12.1
  penis (chronic) N48.5
  peptic (site unspecified) K27.9
    with
      hemorrhage K27.4
        and perforation K27.6
      perforation K27.5
    acute K27.3
      with
        hemorrhage K27.0
          and perforation K27.2
        perforation K27.1
    chronic K27.7
      with
        hemorrhage K27.4
          and perforation K27.6
        perforation K27.5
    esophagus K22.10
      with bleeding K22.11
    newborn P78.82
    perforating K27.5
    skin —see Ulcer, skin
  peritonsillar J35.8
  phagedenic (tropical) —see Ulcer, skin
  pharynx J39.2
  phlebitis —see Phlebitis

Ulcer, ulcerated   - continued
  plaster —see Ulcer, pressure, by site
  popliteal space —see Ulcer, lower limb
  postpyloric —see Ulcer, duodenum
  prepuce N47.7
  prepyloric —see Ulcer, stomach
  pressure (pressure area) L89.9
    ankle L89.5
    back L89.1
    buttock L89.3
    coccyx L89.15
    contiguous site of back, buttock, hip L89.4
    elbow L89.0
    face L89.81
    head L89.81
    heel L89.6
    hip L89.2
    sacral region (tailbone) L89.15
    specified site NEC L89.89
    stage 1 (healing) (pre-ulcer skin changes
  limited to persistent focal edema)
    ankle L89.5
    back L89.1
    buttock L89.3
    coccyx L89.15
    contiguous site of back, buttock, hip L89.4
    elbow L89.0
    face L89.81
    head L89.81
    heel L89.6
    hip L89.2
    sacral region (tailbone) L89.15
    specified site NEC L89.89
    stage 2 (healing) (abrasion, blister, partial
  thickness skin loss involving epidermis and/or
  dermis)
    ankle L89.5
    back L89.1
    buttock L89.3
    coccyx L89.15
    contiguous site of back, buttock, hip L89.4
    elbow L89.0
    face L89.81
    head L89.81
    heel L89.6
    hip L89.2
    sacral region (tailbone) L89.15
    specified site NEC L89.89
    stage 3 (healing) (full thickness skin loss
  involving damage or necrosis of subcutaneous
  tissue)
    ankle L89.5
    back L89.1
    buttock L89.3
    coccyx L89.15
    contiguous site of back, buttock, hip L89.4
    elbow L89.0
    face L89.81
    head L89.81
    heel L89.6
    hip L89.2
    sacral region (tailbone) L89.15
    specified site NEC L89.89
    stage 4 (healing) (necrosis of soft tissues
  through to underlying muscle, tendon, or
  bone)
    ankle L89.5
    back L89.1
    buttock L89.3
    coccyx L89.15
    contiguous site of back, buttock, hip L89.4
    elbow L89.0

Ulcer, ulcerated   - continued
    face L89.81
    head L89.81
    heel L89.6
    hip L89.2
    sacral region (tailbone) L89.15
    specified site NEC L89.89
    unspecified stage
    ankle L89.5
    back L89.1
    buttock L89.3
    coccyx L89.15
    contiguous site of back, buttock, hip L89.4
    elbow L89.0
    face L89.81
    head L89.81
    heel L89.6
    hip L89.2
    sacral region (tailbone) L89.15
    specified site NEC L89.89
    unstageable
    ankle L89.5
    back L89.1
    buttock L89.3
    coccyx L89.15
    contiguous site of back, buttock, hip L89.4
    elbow L89.0
    face L89.81
    head L89.81
    heel L89.6
    hip L89.2
    sacral region (tailbone) L89.15
    specified site NEC L89.89
  primary of intestine K63.3
    with perforation K63.1
  prostate N41.9
  pyloric —see Ulcer, stomach
  rectosigmoid K63.3
    with perforation K63.1
  rectum (sphincter) (solitary) K62.6
    stercoraceous, stercoral K62.6
  retina —see Inflammation, chorioretinal
  rodent —see also Neoplasm, skin, malignant
  sclera —see Scleritis
  scrofulous (tuberculous) A18.2
  scrotum N50.8
    tuberculous A18.15
    varicose I86.1
  seminal vesicle N50.8
  sigmoid —see Ulcer, intestine
  skin (atrophic) (chronic) (neurogenic) (non-
  healing) (perforating) (pyogenic) (trophic)
  (tropical) L98.499
    with gangrene —see Gangrene
    amebic A06.7
    back —see Ulcer, back
    buttock —see Ulcer, buttock
    decubitus —see Ulcer, pressure
    lower limb —see Ulcer, lower limb
    mycobacterial A31.1
    specified site NEC L98.499
      with
        bone necrosis L98.494
        exposed fat layer L98.492
        muscle necrosis L98.493
        skin breakdown only L98.491
    tuberculous (primary) A18.4
    varicose —see Ulcer, varicose
    sloughing —see Ulcer, skin
  solitary, anus or rectum (sphincter) K62.6
  sore throat J02.9
    streptococcal J02.0

Ulcer, ulcerated *- continued*
　spermatic cord N50.8
　spine (tuberculous) A18.01
　stasis (venous) —*see* Varix, leg, with, ulcer
　　without varicose veins I87.2
　stercoraceous, stercoral K63.3
　　with perforation K63.1
　　anus or rectum K62.6
　stoma, stomal —*see* Ulcer, gastrojejunal
　stomach (eroded) (peptic) (round) K25.9
　　with
　　　hemorrhage K25.4
　　　　and perforation K25.6
　　　perforation K25.5
　　acute K25.3
　　　with
　　　　hemorrhage K25.0
　　　　　and perforation K25.2
　　　　perforation K25.1
　　chronic K25.7
　　　with
　　　　hemorrhage K25.4
　　　　　and perforation K25.6
　　　　perforation K25.5
　stomal —*see* Ulcer, gastrojejunal
　stomatitis K12.1
　stress —*see* Ulcer, peptic
　strumous (tuberculous) A18.2
　submucosal, bladder —*see* Cystitis, interstitial
　syphilitic (any site) (early) (secondary)
　　A51.39
　　late A52.79
　　　perforating A52.79
　　　　foot A52.11
　testis N50.8
　thigh —*see* Ulcer, lower limb
　throat J39.2
　　diphtheritic A36.0
　toe —*see* Ulcer, lower limb
　tongue (traumatic) K14.0
　tonsil J35.8
　　diphtheritic A36.0
　trachea J39.8
　trophic —*see* Ulcer, skin
　tropical —*see* Ulcer, skin
　tuberculous —*see* Tuberculosis, ulcer
　tunica vaginalis N50.8
　turbinate J34.89
　typhoid (perforating) —*see* Typhoid
　unspecified site —*see* Ulcer, skin
　urethra (meatus) —*see* Urethritis
　uterus N85.8
　　cervix N86
　　　with cervicitis N72
　　neck N86
　　　with cervicitis N72
　vagina N76.5
　　in Behçet's disease M35.2 *[N77.0]*
　　pessary N89.8
　valve, heart I33.0
　varicose (lower limb, any part) —*see also*
　　Varix, leg, with, ulcer
　　broad ligament I86.2
　　esophagus —*see* Varix, esophagus
　　inflamed or infected —*see* Varix, leg, with
　ulcer, with inflammation
　　nasal septum I86.8
　　perineum I86.3
　　scrotum I86.1
　　specified site NEC I86.8
　　sublingual I86.0
　　vulva I86.3

Ulcer, ulcerated *- continued*
　vas deferens N50.8
　vulva (acute) (infectional) N76.6
　　in (due to)
　　　Behçet's disease M35.2 *[N77.0]*
　　　herpesviral (herpes simplex) infection
　　A60.04
　　　　tuberculosis A18.18
　vulvobuccal, recurring N76.6
　X-ray L58.1
　yaws A66.4
Ulcerosa scarlatina A38.8
Ulcus —*see also* Ulcer
　cutis tuberculosum A18.4
　duodeni —*see* Ulcer, duodenum
　durum (syphilitic) A51.0
　　extragenital A51.2
　gastrojejunale —*see* Ulcer, gastrojejunal
　hypostaticum —*see* Ulcer, varicose
　molle (cutis) (skin) A57
　serpens corneae —*see* Ulcer, cornea, central
　ventriculi —*see* Ulcer, stomach
Ulegyria Q04.8
Ulerythema
　ophryogenes, congenital Q84.2
　sycosiforme L73.8
Ullrich (-Bonnevie) (-Turner) syndrome
　Q87.1
Ullrich-Feichtiger syndrome Q87.0
Ulnar —*see* condition
Ulorrhagia, ulorrhea K06.8
Umbilicus, umbilical —*see* condition
Unacceptable
　contours of tooth K08.54
　morphology of tooth K08.54
Unavailability (of)
　bed at medical facility Z75.1
　health service-related agencies Z75.4
　medical facilities (at) Z75.3
　　due to
　　　investigation by social service agency
　　Z75.2
　　　lack of services at home Z75.0
　　　remoteness from facility Z75.3
　　　waiting list Z75.1
　　home Z75.0
　　outpatient clinic Z75.3
　schooling Z55.1
　social service agencies Z75.4
Uncinaria americana infestation B76.1
Uncinariasis B76.9
Uncongenial work Z56.5
Unconscious (ness) —*see* Coma
Under observation —*see* Observation
Underachievement in school Z55.3
Underdevelopment —*see also* Undeveloped
　nose Q30.1
　sexual E30.0
Underdosing (*see also* Table of Drugs and
　Chemicals, categories T36-T50, with final
　character 6) Z91.14
　intentional NEC Z91.128
　　due to financial hardship of patient Z91.120
　unintentional NEC Z91.138
　　due to patient's age related debility Z91.130
Underfeeding, newborn P92.3
Underfill, endodontic M27.53
Underimmunization status Z28.3
Undernourishment —*see* Malnutrition
Undernutrition —*see* Malnutrition
Underweight R63.6
　for gestational age —*see* Light for dates
Underwood's disease P83.0

Undescended —*see also* Malposition,
　congenital
　cecum Q43.3
　colon Q43.3
　testicle —*see* Cryptorchid
Undeveloped, undevelopment —*see also*
　Hypoplasia
　brain (congenital) Q02
　cerebral (congenital) Q02
　heart Q24.8
　lung Q33.6
　testis E29.1
　uterus E30.0
Undiagnosed (disease) R69
Undulant fever —*see* Brucellosis
Unemployment, anxiety concerning Z56.0
　threatened Z56.2
Unequal length (acquired) (limb) —*see also*
　Deformity, limb, unequal length
　leg —*see also* Deformity, limb, unequal
　length
　　congenital Q72.9
Unextracted dental root K08.3
Unguis incarnatus L60.0
Unhappiness R45.2
Unicornate uterus Q51.4
Unilateral —*see also* condition
　development, breast N64.89
　organ or site, congenital NEC —*see* Agenesis,
　by site
Unilocular heart Q20.8
Union, abnormal —*see also* Fusion
　larynx and trachea Q34.8
Universal mesentery Q43.3
Unrepairable overhanging of dental
　restorative materials K08.52
Unsatisfactory
　restoration of tooth K08.50
　　specified NEC K08.59
　sample of cytologic smear
　　anus R85.615
　　cervix R87.615
　　vagina R87.625
　surroundings Z59.1
　work Z56.5
Unsoundness of mind —*see* Psychosis
Unstable
　back NEC —*see* Instability, joint, spine
　hip (congenital) Q65.6
　　acquired —*see* Derangement, joint,
　specified type NEC, hip
　joint —*see* Instability, joint
　　secondary to removal of joint prosthesis
　M96.89
　lie (mother) O32.0
　lumbosacral joint (congenital)
　　acquired —*see* subcategory M53.2
　sacroiliac —*see* subcategory M53.2
　spine NEC —*see* Instability, joint, spine
Unsteadiness on feet R26.81
Untruthfulness, child problem F91.8
Unverricht (-Lundborg) disease or epilepsy
　—*see* Epilepsy, generalized, idiopathic
Unwanted pregnancy Z64.0
Upbringing, institutional Z62.22
　away from parents NEC Z62.29
　in care of non-parental family member Z62.21
　in foster care Z62.21
　in orphanage or group home Z62.22
　in welfare custody Z62.21
Upper respiratory —*see* condition

Upset
  gastric K30
  gastrointestinal K30
    psychogenic F45.8
  intestinal (large) (small) K59.9
    psychogenic F45.8
  menstruation N93.9
  mental F48.9
  stomach K30
    psychogenic F45.8
Urachus —*see also* condition
  patent or persistent Q64.4
Urbach-Oppenheim disease (necrobiosis
  lipoidica diabeticorum) —*see* E08-E13 with
  .620
Urbach's lipoid proteinosis E78.89
Urbach-Wiethe disease E78.89
Urban yellow fever A95.1
Urea
  blood, high —*see* Uremia
  cycle metabolism disorder —*see* Disorder,
  urea cycle metabolism
Uremia, uremic N19
  with
    ectopic or molar pregnancy O08.4
    polyneuropathy N18.9 *[G63]*
  chronic (*see also* Disease, kidney, chronic)
  N18.9
    due to hypertension —*see* Hypertensive,
    kidney
  complicating
    ectopic or molar pregnancy O08.4
  congenital P96.0
  extrarenal R39.2
  following ectopic or molar pregnancy O08.4
  newborn P96.0
  prerenal R39.2
Ureter, ureteral —*see* condition
Ureteralgia N23
Ureterectasis —*see* Hydroureter
Ureteritis N28.89
  cystica N28.86
  due to calculus N20.1
    with calculus, kidney N20.2
      with hydronephrosis N13.2
  gonococcal (acute) (chronic) A54.21
  nonspecific N28.89
Ureterocele N28.89
  congenital (orthotopic) Q62.31
  ectopic Q62.32
Ureterolith, ureterolithiasis —*see* Calculus,
  ureter
Ureterostomy
  attention to Z43.6
  status Z93.6
Urethra, urethral —*see* condition
Urethralgia R39.89
Urethritis (anterior) (posterior) N34.2
  calculous N21.1
  candidal B37.41
  chlamydial A56.01
  diplococcal (gonococcal) A54.01
    with abscess (accessory gland) (periurethral)
    A54.1
  gonococcal A54.01
    with abscess (accessory gland) (periurethral)
    A54.1
  nongonococcal N34.1
    Reiter's —*see* Reiter's disease
  nonspecific N34.1
  nonvenereal N34.1
  postmenopausal N34.2

Urethritis – *continued*
  puerperal O86.22
  Reiter's —*see* Reiter's disease
  specified NEC N34.2
  trichomonal or due to Trichomonas
    (vaginalis) A59.03
Urethrocele N81.0
  with
    cystocele —*see* Cystocele
    prolapse of uterus —*see* Prolapse, uterus
Urethrolithiasis (with colic or infection)
  N21.1
Urethrorectal —*see* condition
Urethrorrhagia N36.8
Urethrorrhea R36.9
Urethrostomy
  attention to Z43.6
  status Z93.6
Urethrotrigonitis —*see* Trigonitis
Urethrovaginal —*see* condition
Urgency
  fecal R15.2
  hypertensive —*see* Hypertension
  urinary N39.41
Urhidrosis, uridrosis L74.8
Uric acid in blood (increased) E79.0
Uricacidemia (asymptomatic) E79.0
Uricemia (asymptomatic) E79.0
Uricosuria R82.99
Urinary —*see* condition
Urination
  frequent R35.0
  painful R30.9
Urine
  blood in —*see* Hematuria
  discharge, excessive R35.8
  enuresis, nonorganic origin F98.0
  extravasation R39.0
  frequency R35.0
  incontinence R32
    nonorganic origin F98.0
  intermittent stream R39.19
  pus in N39.0
  retention or stasis R33.9
    organic R33.8
      drug-induced R33.0
    psychogenic F45.8
  secretion
    deficient R34
    excessive R35.8
    frequency R35.0
  stream
    intermittent R39.19
    slowing R39.19
    splitting R39.13
    weak R39.12
Urinemia —*see* Uremia
Urinoma, urethra N36.8
Uroarthritis, infectious (Reiter's) —*see*
  Reiter's disease
Urodialysis R34
Urolithiasis —*see* Calculus, urinary
Uronephrosis —*see* Hydronephrosis
Uropathy N39.9
  obstructive N13.9
    specified NEC N13.8
  reflux N13.9
    specified NEC N13.8
  vesicoureteral reflux-associated —*see* Reflux,
  vesicoureteral
Urosepsis   code to condition

Urticaria L50.9
  with angioneurotic edema T78.3
    hereditary D84.1
  allergic L50.0
  cholinergic L50.5
  chronic L50.8
  cold, familial L50.2
  contact L50.6
  dermatographic L50.3
  due to
    cold or heat L50.2
    drugs L50.0
    food L50.0
    inhalants L50.0
    plants L50.6
    serum (*see also* Reaction, serum) T80.69
  factitial L50.3
  giant T78.3
    hereditary D84.1
  gigantea T78.3
  idiopathic L50.1
  larynx T78.3
    hereditary D84.1
  neonatorum P83.8
  nonallergic L50.1
  papulosa (Hebra) L28.2
  pigmentosa Q82.2
  recurrent periodic L50.8
  serum (*see also* Reaction, serum) T80.69
  solar L56.3
  specified type NEC L50.8
  thermal (cold) (heat) L50.2
  vibratory L50.4
  xanthelasmoidea Q82.2
Use (of)
  alcohol F10.99
    with sleep disorder F10.982
    harmful —*see* Abuse, alcohol
  amphetamines —*see* Use, stimulant NEC
  caffeine —*see* Use, stimulant NEC
  cannabis F12.90
    with
      anxiety disorder F12.980
      intoxication F12.929
        with
          delirium F12.921
          perceptual disturbance F12.922
        uncomplicated F12.920
      other specified disorder F12.988
      psychosis F12.959
        delusions F12.950
        hallucinations F12.951
      unspecified disorder F12.99
  cocaine F14.90
    with
      anxiety disorder F14.980
      intoxication F14.929
        with
          delirium F14.921
          perceptual disturbance F14.922
        uncomplicated F14.920
      other specified disorder F14.988
      psychosis F14.959
        delusions F14.950
        hallucinations F14.951
      sexual dysfunction F14.981
      sleep disorder F14.982
      unspecified disorder F14.99
    harmful —*see* Abuse, drug, cocaine
  drug (s) NEC F19.90
    with sleep disorder F19.982
    harmful —*see* Abuse, drug, by type

Use (of) *- continued*
  hallucinogen NEC F16.90
    with
      anxiety disorder F16.980
      intoxication F16.929
        with
          delirium F16.921
        uncomplicated F16.920
      mood disorder F16.94
      other specified disorder F16.988
      perception disorder (flashbacks) F16.983
      psychosis F16.959
        delusions F16.950
        hallucinations F16.951
      unspecified disorder F16.99
    harmful —*see* Abuse, drug, hallucinogen
NEC
  inhalants F18.90
    with
      anxiety disorder F18.980
      intoxication F18.929
        with delirium F18.921
        uncomplicated F18.920
      mood disorder F18.94
      other specified disorder F18.988
      persisting dementia F18.97
      psychosis F18.959
        delusions F18.950
        hallucinations F18.951
      unspecified disorder F18.99
    harmful —*see* Abuse, drug, inhalant
  methadone F11.20
  nonprescribed drugs F19.90
    harmful —*see* Abuse, non-psychoactive
substance
  opioid F11.90
    with
      disorder F11.99
        mood F11.94
        sleep F11.982
        specified type NEC F11.988
      intoxication F11.929
        with
          delirium F11.921
          perceptual disturbance F11.922
        uncomplicated F11.920
      withdrawal F11.93
    harmful —*see* Abuse, drug, opioid
  patent medicines F19.90
    harmful —*see* Abuse, non-psychoactive
substance
  psychoactive drug NEC F19.90
    with
      anxiety disorder F19.980
      intoxication F19.929
        with
          delirium F19.921
          perceptual disturbance F19.922
        uncomplicated F19.920
      mood disorder F19.94
      other specified disorder F19.988
      persisting
        amnestic disorder F19.96
        dementia F19.97
      psychosis F19.959
        delusions F19.950
        hallucinations F19.951
      sexual dysfunction F19.981
      sleep disorder F19.982
      unspecified disorder F19.99
      withdrawal F19.939
        with

Use (of) *- continued*
        delirium F19.931
          perceptual disturbance F19.932
        uncomplicated F19.930
    harmful —*see* Abuse, drug NEC,
psychoactive NEC
  sedative, hypnotic, or anxiolytic F13.90
    with
      anxiety disorder F13.980
      intoxication F13.929
        with
          delirium F13.921
        uncomplicated F13.920
      other specified disorder F13.988
      persisting
        amnestic disorder F13.96
        dementia F13.97
      psychosis F13.959
        delusions F13.950
        hallucinations F13.951
      sexual dysfunction F13.981
      sleep disorder F13.982
      unspecified disorder F13.99
    harmful —*see* Abuse, drug, sedative,
hypnotic, or anxiolytic
  stimulant NEC F15.90
    with
      anxiety disorder F15.980
      intoxication F15.929
        with
          delirium F15.921
          perceptual disturbance F15.922
        uncomplicated F15.920
      mood disorder F15.94
      other specified disorder F15.988
      psychosis F15.959
        delusions F15.950
        hallucinations F15.951
      sexual dysfunction F15.981
      sleep disorder F15.982
      unspecified disorder F15.99
      withdrawal F15.93
    harmful —*see* Abuse, drug, stimulant NEC
  volatile solvents (*see also* Use, inhalant)
F18.90
    harmful —*see* Abuse, drug, inhalant
  tobacco Z72.0
    with dependence —*see* Dependence, drug,
nicotine
Usher-Senear disease or syndrome L10.4
Uta B55.1
Uteromegaly N85.2
Uterovaginal —*see* condition
Uterovesical —*see* condition
Uveal —*see* condition
Uveitis (anterior) —*see also* Iridocyclitis
  acute —*see* Iridocyclitis, acute
  chronic —*see* Iridocyclitis, chronic
  due to toxoplasmosis (acquired) B58.09
    congenital P37.1
  granulomatous —*see* Iridocyclitis, chronic
  heterochromic —*see* Cyclitis, Fuchs'
heterochromic
  lens-induced —*see* Iridocyclitis, lens-induced
  posterior —*see* Chorioretinitis
  sympathetic H44.13
  syphilitic (secondary) A51.43
    congenital (early) A50.01
    late A52.71
  tuberculous A18.54
Uveoencephalitis —*see* Inflammation,
  chorioretinal
Uveokeratitis —*see* Iridocyclitis

Uveoparotitis D86.89
Uvula —*see* condition
Uvulitis (acute) (catarrhal) (chronic)
  (membranous) (suppurative) (ulcerative)
  K12.2

V

Vaccination (prophylactic)
  complication or reaction —*see*
  Complications, vaccination
  delayed Z28.9
  encounter for Z23
  not done —*see* Immunization, not done,
  because (of)
Vaccinia (generalized) (localized) T88.1
  congenital P35.8
  without vaccination B08.011
Vacuum, in sinus (accessory) (nasal) J34.89
Vagabond, vagabondage Z59.0
Vagabond's disease B85.1
Vagina, vaginal — *see* condition
Vaginalitis (tunica) (testis) N49.1
Vaginismus (reflex) N94.2
  functional F52.5
  nonorganic F52.5
  psychogenic F52.5
  secondary N94.2
Vaginitis (acute) (circumscribed) (diffuse)
  (emphysematous) (nonvenereal) (ulcerative)
  N76.0
  with ectopic or molar pregnancy O08.0
  amebic A06.82
  atrophic, postmenopausal N95.2
  bacterial N76.0
  blennorrhagic (gonococcal) A54.02
  candidal B37.3
  chlamydial A56.02
  chronic N76.1
  due to Trichomonas (vaginalis) A59.01
  following ectopic or molar pregnancy O08.0
  gonococcal A54.02
    with abscess (accessory gland) (periurethral)
  A54.1
  granuloma A58
  in (due to)
    candidiasis B37.3
    herpesviral (herpes simplex) infection
  A60.04
    pinworm infection B80 *[N77.1]*
  monilial B37.3
  mycotic (candidal) B37.3
  postmenopausal atrophic N95.2
  puerperal (postpartum) O86.13
  senile (atrophic) N95.2
  subacute or chronic N76.1
  syphilitic (early) A51.0
    late A52.76
  trichomonal A59.01
  tuberculous A18.18
Vaginosis —*see* Vaginitis
Vagotonia G52.2
Vagrancy Z59.0
VAIN —*see* Neoplasia, intraepithelial, vagina
Vallecula —*see* condition
Valley fever B38.0
Valsuani's disease —*see* Anemia, obstetric
Valve, valvular (formation) —*see also*
  condition
  cerebral ventricle (communicating) in situ
  Z98.2
  cervix, internal os Q51.828

Valve, valvular - *continued*
  congenital NEC —*see* Atresia, by site
  ureter (pelvic junction) (vesical orifice)
    Q62.39
  urethra (congenital) (posterior) Q64.2
Valvulitis (chronic) —*see* Endocarditis
Valvulopathy —*see* Endocarditis
Van Bogaert's leukoencephalopathy
  (sclerosing) (subacute) A81.1
Van Bogaert-Scherer-Epstein disease or
  syndrome E75.5
Van Buchem's syndrome M85.2
Van Creveld-von Gierke disease E74.01
Van der Hoeve (-de Kleyn) **syndrome** Q78.0
Van der Woude's syndrome Q38.0
Van Neck's disease or osteochondrosis
  M91.0
Vanishing lung J44.9
Vapor asphyxia or suffocation T59.9
  specified agent —*see* Table of Drugs and
    Chemicals
Variance, lethal ball, prosthetic heart valve
  T82.09
Variants, thalassemic D56.8
Variations in hair color L67.1
Varicella B01.9
  with
    complications NEC B01.89
    encephalitis B01.11
    encephalomyelitis B01.11
    meningitis B01.0
    myelitis B01.12
    pneumonia B01.2
  congenital P35.8
Varices —*see* Varix
Varicocele (scrotum) (thrombosed) I86.1
  ovary I86.2
  perineum I86.3
  spermatic cord (ulcerated) I86.1
Varicose
  aneurysm (ruptured) I77.0
  dermatitis —*see* Varix, leg, with,
  inflammation
  eczema —*see* Varix, leg, with, inflammation
  phlebitis —*see* Varix, with, inflammation
  tumor —*see* Varix
  ulcer (lower limb, any part) —*see also* Varix,
  leg, with, ulcer
    anus (*see also* Hemorrhoids) K64.8
    esophagus —*see* Varix, esophagus
    inflamed or infected —*see* Varix, leg, with
    ulcer, with inflammation
    nasal septum I86.8
    perineum I86.3
    scrotum I86.1
    specified site NEC I86.8
    vein —*see* Varix
    vessel —*see* Varix, leg
Varicosis, varicosities, varicosity —*see* Varix
Variola (major) (minor) B03
Varioloid B03
Varix (lower limb) (ruptured) I83.90
  with
    edema I83.899
    inflammation I83.10
      with ulcer (venous) I83.209
    pain I83.819
    specified complication NEC I83.899
    stasis dermatitis I83.10
      with ulcer (venous) I83.209
    swelling I83.899

Varix - *continued*
  ulcer I83.009
    with inflammation I83.209
  aneurysmal I77.0
  asymptomatic I83.9
  bladder I86.2
  broad ligament I86.2
  complicating
    childbirth (lower extremity) O87.4
      anus or rectum O87.2
      genital (vagina, vulva or perineum) O87.8
    pregnancy (lower extremity) O22.0
      anus or rectum O22.4
      genital (vagina, vulva or perineum) O22.1
    puerperium (lower extremity) O87.4
      anus or rectum O87.2
      genital (vagina, vulva, perineum) O87.8
  congenital (any site) Q27.8
  esophagus (idiopathic) (primary) (ulcerated)
    I85.00
    bleeding I85.01
    congenital Q27.8
    in (due to)
      alcoholic liver disease I85.10
        bleeding I85.11
      cirrhosis of liver I85.10
        bleeding I85.11
      portal hypertension I85.10
        bleeding I85.11
      schistosomiasis I85.10
        bleeding I85.11
      toxic liver disease I85.10
        bleeding I85.11
    secondary I85.10
      bleeding I85.11
  gastric I86.4
  inflamed or infected I83.10
    ulcerated I83.209
  labia (majora) I86.3
  leg (asymptomatic) I83.90
    with
      edema I83.899
      inflammation I83.10
        with ulcer —*see* Varix, leg, with, ulcer,
    with inflammation by site
      pain I83.819
      specified complication NEC I83.899
      swelling I83.899
      ulcer I83.009
        with inflammation I83.209
        ankle I83.003
          with inflammation I83.203
        calf I83.002
          with inflammation I83.202
        foot NEC I83.005
          with inflammation I83.205
        heel I83.004
          with inflammation I83.204
        lower leg NEC I83.008
          with inflammation I83.208
        midfoot I83.004
          with inflammation I83.204
        thigh I83.001
          with inflammation I83.201
  bilateral (asymptomatic) I83.93
    with
      edema I83.893
      pain I83.813
      specified complication NEC I83.893
      swelling I83.893
      ulcer I83.009
        with inflammation I83.209

Varix - *continued*
  left (asymptomatic) I83.92
    with
      edema I83.892
      pain I83.812
      specified complication NEC I83.892
      swelling I83.892
      inflammation I83.12
        with ulcer —*see* Varix, leg, with, ulcer,
    with inflammation by site
      ulcer I83.029
        with inflammation I83.229
        ankle I83.023
          with inflammation I83.223
        calf I83.022
          with inflammation I83.222
        foot NEC I83.025
          with inflammation I83.225
        heel I83.024
          with inflammation I83.224
        lower leg NEC I83.028
          with inflammation I83.228
        midfoot I83.024
          with inflammation I83.224
        thigh I83.021
          with inflammation I83.221
  right (asymptomatic) I83.91
    with
      edema I83.891
      pain I83.811
      specified complication NEC I83.891
      swelling I83.891
      inflammation I83.11
        with ulcer —*see* Varix, leg, with, ulcer,
    with inflammation by site
      ulcer I83.019
        with inflammation I83.219
        ankle I83.013
          with inflammation I83.213
        calf I83.012
          with inflammation I83.212
        foot NEC I83.015
          with inflammation I83.215
        heel I83.014
          with inflammation I83.214
        lower leg NEC I83.018
          with inflammation I83.218
        midfoot I83.014
          with inflammation I83.214
        thigh I83.011
          with inflammation I83.211
  nasal septum I86.8
  orbit I86.8
    congenital Q27.8
  ovary I86.2
  papillary I78.1
  pelvis I86.2
  perineum I86.3
  pharynx I86.8
  placenta O43.89
  renal papilla I86.8
  retina H35.09
  scrotum (ulcerated) I86.1
  sigmoid colon I86.8
  specified site NEC I86.8
  spinal (cord) (vessels) I86.8
  spleen, splenic (vein) (with phlebolith) I86.8
  stomach I86.4
  sublingual I86.0
  ulcerated I83.009
    inflamed or infected I83.209
  uterine ligament I86.2

Varix *- continued*
  vagina I86.8
  vocal cord I86.8
  vulva I86.3
Vas deferens —*see* condition
Vas deferentitis N49.1
Vasa previa O69.4
  hemorrhage from, affecting newborn P50.0
Vascular —*see also* condition
  loop on optic papilla Q14.2
  spasm I73.9
  spider I78.1
Vascularization, cornea —*see*
  Neovascularization, cornea
Vasculitis I77.6
  allergic D69.0
  cryoglobulinemic D89.1
  disseminated I77.6
  hypocomplementemic M31.8
  kidney I77.89
  livedoid L95.0
  nodular L95.8
  retina H35.06
  rheumatic —*see* Fever, rheumatic
  rheumatoid —*see* Rheumatoid, vasculitis
  skin (limited to) L95.9
    specified NEC L95.8
Vasculopathy, necrotizing M31.9
  cardiac allograft T86.290
  specified NEC M31.8
Vasitis (nodosa) N49.1
  tuberculous A18.15
Vasodilation I73.9
Vasomotor —*see* condition
Vasoplasty, after previous sterilization Z31.0
  aftercare Z31.42
Vasospasm (vasoconstriction) I73.9
  cerebral (cerebrovascular) (artery) I67.848
    reversible I67.841
  coronary I20.1
  nerve
    arm —*see* Mononeuropathy, upper limb
    brachial plexus G54.0
    cervical plexus G54.2
    leg —*see* Mononeuropathy, lower limb
    peripheral NOS I73.9
  retina (artery) —*see* Occlusion, artery, retina
Vasospastic —*see* condition
Vasovagal attack (paroxysmal) R55
  psychogenic F45.8
VATER syndrome Q87.2
Vater's ampulla —*see* condition
Vegetation, vegetative
  adenoid (nasal fossa) J35.8
  endocarditis (acute) (any valve) (subacute)
    I33.0
  heart (mycotic) (valve) I33.0
Veil
  Jackson's Q43.3
Vein, venous —*see* condition
Veldt sore —*see* Ulcer, skin
Velpeau's hernia —*see* Hernia, femoral
Venereal
  bubo A55
  disease A64
  granuloma inguinale A58
  lymphogranuloma (Durand-Nicolas-Favre)
    A55
Venofibrosis I87.8
Venom, venomous —*see* Table of Drugs and
  Chemicals, by animal or substance, poisoning
Venous —*see* condition
Ventilator lung, newborn P27.8

Ventral —*see* condition
Ventricle, ventricular —*see also* condition
  escape I49.3
  inversion Q20.5
Ventriculitis (cerebral) (*see also* Encephalitis)
  G04.90
Ventriculostomy status Z98.2
Vernet's syndrome G52.7
Verneuil's disease (syphilitic bursitis) A52.78
Verruca (due to HPV) (filiformis) (simplex)
  (viral) (vulgaris) B07.9
  acuminata A63.0
  necrogenica (primary) (tuberculosa) A18.4
  plana B07.8
  plantaris B07.0
  seborrheica L82.1
    inflamed L82.0
  senile (seborrheic) L82.1
    inflamed L82.0
  tuberculosa (primary) A18.4
  venereal A63.0
Verrucosities —*see* Verruca
Verruga peruana, peruviana A44.1
Version
  with extraction
  cervix —*see* Malposition, uterus
  uterus (postinfectional) (postpartal, old) —*see*
    Malposition, uterus
Vertebra, vertebral —*see* condition
Vertical talus (congenital) Q66.80
  left foot Q66.82
  right foot Q66.81
Vertigo R42
  auditory —*see* Vertigo, aural
  aural H81.31
  benign paroxysmal (positional) H81.1
  central (origin) H81.4
  cerebral H81.4
  Dix and Hallpike (epidemic) —*see*
    Neuronitis, vestibular
  due to infrasound T75.23
  epidemic A88.1
    Dix and Hallpike —*see* Neuronitis,
    vestibular
    Pedersen's —*see* Neuronitis, vestibular
    vestibular neuronitis —*see* Neuronitis,
    vestibular
  hysterical F44.89
  infrasound T75.23
  labyrinthine —*see* subcategory H81.0
  laryngeal R05
  malignant positional H81.4
  Ménière's —*see* subcategory H81.0
  menopausal N95.1
  otogenic —*see* Vertigo, aural
  paroxysmal positional, benign —*see* Vertigo,
    benign paroxysmal
  Pedersen's (epidemic) —*see* Neuronitis,
    vestibular
  peripheral NEC H81.39
  positional
    benign paroxysmal —*see* Vertigo, benign
    paroxysmal
    malignant H81.4
Very-low-density-lipoprotein-type (VLDL)
  hyperlipoproteinemia E78.1
Vesania —*see* Psychosis
Vesical —*see* condition
Vesicle
  cutaneous R23.8
  seminal —*see* condition
  skin R23.8
Vesicocolic —*see* condition

Vesicoperineal —*see* condition
Vesicorectal —*see* condition
Vesicourethrorectal —*see* condition
Vesicovaginal —*see* condition
Vesicular —*see* condition
Vesiculitis (seminal) N49.0
  amebic A06.82
  gonorrheal (acute) (chronic) A54.23
  trichomonal A59.09
  tuberculous A18.15
Vestibulitis (ear) (*see also* subcategory) H83.0
  nose (external) J34.89
  vulvar N94.810
Vestibulopathy, acute peripheral (recurrent)
  —*see* Neuronitis, vestibular
Vestige, vestigial —*see also* Persistence
  branchial Q18.0
  structures in vitreous Q14.0
Vibration
  adverse effects T75.20
    pneumatic hammer syndrome T75.21
    specified effect NEC T75.29
    vasospastic syndrome T75.22
    vertigo from infrasound T75.23
  exposure (occupational) Z57.7
  vertigo T75.23
Vibriosis A28.9
Victim (of)
  crime Z65.4
  disaster Z65.5
  terrorism Z65.4
  torture Z65.4
  war Z65.5
Vidal's disease L28.0
Villaret's syndrome G52.7
Villous —*see* condition
VIN —*see* Neoplasia, intraepithelial, vulva
Vincent's infection (angina) (gingivitis) A69.1
  stomatitis NEC A69.1
Vinson-Plummer syndrome D50.1
Violence, physical R45.6
Viosterol deficiency —*see* Deficiency,
  calciferol
Vipoma —*see* Neoplasm, malignant, by site
Viremia B34.9
Virilism (adrenal) E25.9
  congenital E25.0
Virilization (female) (suprarenal) E25.9
  congenital E25.0
  isosexual E28.2
Virulent bubo A57
Virus, viral —*see also* condition
  as cause of disease classified elsewhere
    B97.89
  cytomegalovirus B25.9
  human immunodeficiency (HIV) —*see*
    Human, immunodeficiency virus (HIV)
    disease
  infection —*see* Infection, virus
  specified NEC B34.8
  swine influenza (viruses that normally cause
    infections in pigs) (*see also* Influenza, due to,
    identified novel influenza A virus) J09.X2
  West Nile (fever) A92.30
    with
      complications NEC A92.39
      cranial nerve disorders A92.32
      encephalitis A92.31
      encephalomyelitis A92.31
      neurologic manifestation NEC A92.32
      optic neuritis A92.32
      polyradiculitis A92.32

Viscera, visceral —*see* condition
Visceroptosis K63.4
Visible peristalsis R19.2
Vision, visual
  binocular, suppression H53.34
  blurred, blurring H53.8
    hysterical F44.6
  defect, defective NEC H54.7
  disorientation (syndrome) H53.8
  disturbance H53.9
    hysterical F44.6
  double H53.2
  examination Z01.00
    with abnormal findings Z01.01
  field, limitation (defect) —*see* Defect, visual
  field
  hallucinations R44.1
  halos H53.19
  loss —*see* Loss, vision
    sudden —*see* Disturbance, vision,
  subjective, loss, sudden
  low (both eyes) —*see* Low, vision
  perception, simultaneous without fusion
  H53.33
Vitality, lack or want of R53.83
  newborn P96.89
Vitamin deficiency —*see* Deficiency, vitamin
Vitelline duct, persistent Q43.0
Vitiligo L80
  eyelid H02.739
    left H02.736
      lower H02.735
      upper H02.734
    right H02.733
      lower H02.732
      upper H02.731
  pinta A67.2
  vulva N90.89
Vitreal corneal syndrome H59.01
Vitreoretinopathy, proliferative —*see also*
  Retinopathy, proliferative
  with retinal detachment —*see* Detachment,
  retina, traction
Vitreous —*see also* condition
  touch syndrome —*see* Complication,
  postprocedural, following cataract surgery
Vocal cord —*see* condition
Vogt-Koyanagi syndrome H20.82
Vogt's disease or syndrome G80.3
Vogt-Spielmeyer amaurotic idiocy or disease
  E75.4
Voice
  change R49.9
    specified NEC R49.8
  loss —*see* Aphonia
Volhynian fever A79.0
Volkmann's ischemic contracture or
  paralysis (complicating trauma) T79.6
Volvulus (bowel) (colon) (duodenum)
  (intestine) K56.2
  with perforation K56.2
  congenital Q43.8
  fallopian tube —*see* Torsion, fallopian tube
  oviduct —*see* Torsion, fallopian tube
  stomach (due to absence of gastrocolic
  ligament) K31.89
Vomiting R11.10
  with nausea R11.2
  asphyxia —*see* Foreign body, by site, causing
  asphyxia, gastric contents
  bilious (cause unknown) R11.14
    in newborn P92.01

Vomiting   *- continued*
  following gastro-intestinal surgery K91.0
  blood —*see* Hematemesis
  causing asphyxia, choking, or suffocation —
  see Foreign body, by site
  cyclical G43.A0
    with refractory migraine G43.A1
    intractable G43.A1
    not intractable G43.A0
    psychogenic F50.8
    without refractory migraine G43.A0
  fecal mater R11.13
  following gastrointestinal surgery K91.0
    psychogenic F50.8
  functional K31.89
  hysterical F50.8
  nervous F50.8
  neurotic F50.8
  newborn NEC P92.09
    bilious P92.01
  periodic R11.10
    psychogenic F50.8
  projectile R11.12
  psychogenic F50.8
  uremic —*see* Uremia
  without nausea R11.11
Vomito negro —*see* Fever, yellow
Von Bezold's abscess —*see* Mastoiditis, acute
Von Economo-Cruchet disease A85.8
Von Eulenburg's disease G71.19
Von Gierke's disease E74.01
Von Hippel (-Lindau) **disease or syndrome**
  Q85.8
Von Jaksch's anemia or disease D64.89
Von Recklinghausen
  disease (neurofibromatosis) Q85.01
    bones E21.0
Von Schroetter's syndrome I82.890
Von Willebrand (-Jurgens) (-Minot) **disease**
  or syndrome D68.0
Von Zumbusch's disease L40.1
Voyeurism F65.3
Vrolik's disease Q78.0
Vulva —*see* condition
Vulvismus N94.2
Vulvitis (acute) (allergic) (atrophic)
  (hypertrophic) (intertriginous) (senile) N76.2
  with ectopic or molar pregnancy O08.0
  adhesive, congenital Q52.79
  blennorrhagic (gonococcal) A54.02
  candidal B37.3
  chlamydial A56.02
  due to Haemophilus ducreyi A57
  following ectopic or molar pregnancy O08.0
  gonococcal A54.02
    with abscess (accessory gland) (periurethral)
  A54.1
  herpesviral A60.04
  leukoplakic N90.4
  monilial B37.3
  puerperal (postpartum) O86.19
  subacute or chronic N76.3
  syphilitic (early) A51.0
    late A52.76
  trichomonal A59.01
  tuberculous A18.18
Vulvodynia N94.819
  specified NEC N94.818
Vulvorectal —*see* condition
Vulvovaginitis (acute) —*see* Vaginitis

W

Waiting list, person on Z75.1
  for organ transplant Z76.82
  undergoing social agency investigation Z75.2
Waldenström-Kjellberg syndrome D50.1
Waldenström
  hypergammaglobulinemia D89.0
  syndrome or macroglobulinemia C88.0
Walking
  difficulty R26.2
    psychogenic F44.4
  sleep F51.3
    hysterical F44.89
Wall, abdominal —*see* condition
Wallenberg's disease or syndrome G46.3
Wallgren's disease I87.8
Wandering
  gallbladder, congenital Q44.1
  in diseases classified elsewhere Z91.83
  kidney, congenital Q63.8
  organ or site, congenital NEC —*see*
  Malposition, congenital, by site
  pacemaker (heart) I49.8
  spleen D73.89
War neurosis F48.8
Wart (due to HPV) (filiform) (infectious)
  (viral) B07.9
  anogenital region (venereal) A63.0
  common B07.8
  external genital organs (venereal) A63.0
  flat B07.8
  Hassal-Henle's (of cornea) H18.49
  Peruvian A44.1
  plantar B07.0
  prosector (tuberculous) A18.4
  seborrheic L82.1
    inflamed L82.0
  senile (seborrheic) L82.1
    inflamed L82.0
  tuberculous A18.4
  venereal A63.0
Warthin's tumor —*see* Neoplasm, salivary
  gland, benign
Wassilieff's disease A27.0
Wasting
  disease R64
    due to malnutrition E41
  extreme (due to malnutrition) E41
  muscle NEC —*see* Atrophy, muscle
Water
  clefts (senile cataract) —*see* Cataract, senile,
  incipient
  deprivation of T73.1
  intoxication E87.79
  itch B76.9
  lack of T73.1
  loading E87.70
  on
    brain —*see* Hydrocephalus
    chest J94.8
  poisoning E87.79
Waterbrash R12
Waterhouse (-Friderichsen) syndrome or
  disease (meningococcal) A39.1
Water-losing nephritis N25.89
Watermelon stomach K31.819
  with hemorrhage K31.811
  without hemorrhage K31.819
Watsoniasis B66.8
Wax in ear —*see* Impaction, cerumen

Weak, weakening, weakness (generalized) R53.1
  arches (acquired) —*see also* Deformity, limb, flat foot
  bladder (sphincter) R32
  facial R29.810
    following
      cerebrovascular disease I69.992
        cerebral infarction I69.392
        intracerebral hemorrhage I69.192
        nontraumatic intracranial hemorrhage NEC I69.292
        specified disease NEC I69.892
        stroke I69.392
        subarachnoid hemorrhage I69.092
  foot (double) —*see* Weak, arches
  heart, cardiac —*see* Failure, heart
  mind F70
  muscle M62.81
  myocardium —*see* Failure, heart
  newborn P96.89
  pelvic fundus N81.89
  pubocervical tissue N81.82
  senile R54
  rectovaginal tissue N81.83
  urinary stream R39.12
  valvular —*see* Endocarditis
Wear, worn (with normal or routine use)
  articular bearing surface of internal joint prosthesis —*see* Complications, joint prosthesis, mechanical, wear of articular bearing surfaces, by site
  device, implant or graft —*see* Complications, by site, mechanical complication
  tooth, teeth (approximal) (hard tissues) (interproximal) (occlusal) K03.0
Weather, weathered
  effects of
    cold T69.9
      specified effect NEC T69.8
    hot —*see* Heat
  skin L57.8
Weaver's syndrome Q87.3
Web, webbed (congenital)
  duodenal Q43.8
  esophagus Q39.4
  fingers Q70.1
  larynx (glottic) (subglottic) Q31.0
  neck (pterygium colli) Q18.3
  Paterson-Kelly D50.1
  popliteal syndrome Q87.89
  toes Q70.3
Weber-Christian disease M35.6
Weber-Cockayne syndrome (epidermolysis bullosa) Q81.8
Weber-Gubler syndrome G46.3
Weber-Leyden syndrome G46.3
Weber-Osler syndrome I78.0
Weber's paralysis or syndrome G46.3
Wedge-shaped or wedging vertebra —*see* Collapse, vertebra NEC
Wegener's granulomatosis or syndrome M31.30
  with
    kidney involvement M31.31
    lung involvement M31.30
      with kidney involvement M31.31
Wegner's disease A50.02
Weight
  1000 2499 grams at birth (low) —*see* Low, birthweight

Weight – *continued*
  999 grams or less at birth (extremely low) —*see* Low, birthweight, extreme
  gain (abnormal) (excessive) R63.5
    in pregnancy —*see* Pregnancy, complicated by, excessive weight gain
      low —*see* Pregnancy, complicated by, insufficient, weight gain
  loss (abnormal) (cause unknown) R63.4
Weightlessness (effect of) T75.82
Weil (l) -Marchesani syndrome Q87.1
Weil's disease A27.0
Weingarten's syndrome J82
Weir Mitchell's disease I73.81
Weiss-Baker syndrome G90.09
Wells' disease L98.3
Wen —*see* Cyst, sebaceous
Wenckebach's block or phenomenon I44.1
Werdnig-Hoffmann syndrome (muscular atrophy) G12.0
Werlhof's disease D69.3
Wermer's disease or syndrome E31.21
Werner-His disease A79.0
Werner's disease or syndrome E34.8
Wernicke-Korsakoff's syndrome or psychosis (alcoholic) F10.96
  with dependence F10.26
  drug-induced
    due to drug abuse —*see* Abuse, drug, by type, with amnestic disorder
    due to drug dependence —*see* Dependence, drug, by type, with amnestic disorder
  nonalcoholic F04
Wernicke-Posadas disease B38.9
Wernicke's
  developmental aphasia F80.2
  disease or syndrome E51.2
  encephalopathy E51.2
  polioencephalitis, superior E51.2
West African fever B50.8
Westphal-Strümpell syndrome E83.01
West's syndrome —*see* Epilepsy, spasms
Wet
  feet, tropical (maceration) (syndrome) —*see* Immersion, foot
  lung (syndrome) , newborn P22.1
Wharton's duct —*see* condition
Wheal —*see* Urticaria
Wheezing R06.2
Whiplash injury S13.4
Whipple's disease (*see also* subcategory M14.8) K90.81
Whipworm (disease) (infection) (infestation) B79
Whistling face Q87.0
White —*see also* condition
  kidney, small N03.9
  leg, puerperal, postpartum, childbirth O87.1
  mouth B37.0
  patches of mouth K13.29
  spot lesions, teeth
    chewing surface K02.51
    pit and fissure surface K02.51
    smooth surface K02.61
Whitehead L70.0
Whitlow —*see also* Cellulitis, digit
  with lymphangitis —*see* Lymphangitis, acute, digit
  herpesviral B00.89
Whitmore's disease or fever —*see* Melioidosis

Whooping cough A37.90
  with pneumonia A37.91
  due to Bordetella
    bronchiseptica A37.81
    parapertussis A37.11
    pertussis A37.01
    specified organism NEC A37.81
  due to
    Bordetella
      bronchiseptica A37.80
        with pneumonia A37.81
      parapertussis A37.10
        with pneumonia A37.11
      pertussis A37.00
        with pneumonia A37.01
      specified NEC A37.80
        with pneumonia A37.81
Wichman's asthma J38.5
Wide cranial sutures, newborn P96.3
Widening aorta —*see* Ectasia, aorta
  with aneurysm —*see* Aneurysm, aorta
Wilkie's disease or syndrome K55.1
Wilkinson-Sneddon disease or syndrome L13.1
Willebrand (-Jürgens) thrombopathy D68.0
Willige-Hunt disease or syndrome G23.1
Wilms' tumor C64
Wilson-Mikity syndrome P27.0
Wilson's
  disease or syndrome E83.01
  hepatolenticular degeneration E83.01
  lichen ruber L43.9
Window —*see also* Imperfect, closure
  aorticopulmonary Q21.4
Winter —*see* condition
Wiskott-Aldrich syndrome D82.0
Withdrawal state —*see also* Dependence, drug by type, with withdrawal
  newborn
    correct therapeutic substance properly administered P96.2
    infant of dependent mother P96.1
  therapeutic substance, neonatal P96.2
Witts' anemia D50.8
Witzelsucht F07.0
Woakes' ethmoiditis or syndrome J33.1
Wolff-Hirschorn syndrome Q93.3
Wolff-Parkinson-White syndrome I45.6
Wolhynian fever A79.0
Wolman's disease E75.5
Wood lung or pneumonitis J67.8
Woolly, wooly hair (congenital) (nevus) Q84.1
Woolsorter's disease A22.1
Word
  blindness (congenital) (developmental) F81.0
  deafness (congenital) (developmental) H93.25
Worm (s) (infection) (infestation) —*see also* Infestation, helminth
  guinea B72
  in intestine NEC B82.0
Worm-eaten soles A66.3
Worn out —*see* Exhaustion
  cardiac
    defibrillator (with synchronous cardiac pacemaker) Z45.02
    pacemaker
      battery Z45.010
      lead Z45.018
  device, implant or graft —*see* Complications, by site, mechanical
Worried well Z71.1
Worries R45.82

Wound, open
abdomen, abdominal
wall S31.109
with penetration into peritoneal cavity
S31.609
bite —*see* Bite, abdomen, wall
epigastric region S31.102
with penetration into peritoneal cavity
S31.602
bite —*see* Bite, abdomen, wall, epigastric
region
laceration —*see* Laceration, abdomen,
wall, epigastric region
puncture —*see* Puncture, abdomen, wall,
epigastric region
laceration —*see* Laceration, abdomen, wall
left
lower quadrant S31.104
with penetration into peritoneal cavity
S31.604
bite —*see* Bite, abdomen, wall, left,
lower quadrant
laceration —*see* Laceration, abdomen,
wall, left, lower quadrant
puncture —*see* Puncture, abdomen,
wall, left, lower quadrant
upper quadrant S31.101
with penetration into peritoneal cavity
S31.601
bite —*see* Bite, abdomen, wall, left,
upper quadrant
laceration —*see* Laceration, abdomen,
wall, left, upper quadrant
puncture —*see* Puncture, abdomen,
wall, left, upper quadrant
periumbilic region S31.105
with penetration into peritoneal cavity
S31.605
bite —*see* Bite, abdomen, wall,
periumbilic region
laceration —*see* Laceration, abdomen,
wall, periumbilic region
puncture —*see* Puncture, abdomen, wall,
periumbilic region
puncture —*see* Puncture, abdomen, wall
right
lower quadrant S31.103
with penetration into peritoneal cavity
S31.603
bite —*see* Bite, abdomen, wall, right,
lower quadrant
laceration —*see* Laceration, abdomen,
wall, right, lower quadrant
puncture —*see* Puncture, abdomen,
wall, right, lower quadrant
upper quadrant S31.100
with penetration into peritoneal cavity
S31.600
bite —*see* Bite, abdomen, wall, right,
upper quadrant
laceration —*see* Laceration, abdomen,
wall, right, upper quadrant
puncture —*see* Puncture, abdomen,
wall, right, upper quadrant
alveolar (process) —*see* Wound, open, oral
cavity
ankle S91.00
bite —*see* Bite, ankle
laceration —*see* Laceration, ankle
puncture —*see* Puncture, ankle
antecubital space —*see* Wound, open, elbow

Wound, open - *continued*
anterior chamber, eye —*see* Wound, open,
ocular
anus S31.839
bite S31.835
laceration —*see* Laceration, anus
puncture —*see* Puncture, anus
arm (upper) S41.10
with amputation —*see* Amputation,
traumatic, arm
bite —*see* Bite, arm
forearm —*see* Wound, open, forearm
laceration —*see* Laceration, arm
puncture —*see* Puncture, arm
auditory canal (external) (meatus) —*see*
Wound, open, ear
auricle, ear —*see* Wound, open, ear
axilla —*see* Wound, open, arm
back —*see also* Wound, open, thorax, back
lower S31.000
with penetration into retroperitoneal space
S31.001
bite —*see* Bite, back, lower
laceration —*see* Laceration, back, lower
puncture —*see* Puncture, back, lower
bite —*see* Bite
blood vessel —*see* Injury, blood vessel
breast S21.00
with amputation —*see* Amputation,
traumatic, breast
bite —*see* Bite, breast
laceration —*see* Laceration, breast
puncture —*see* Puncture, breast
buttock S31.809
bite —*see* Bite, buttock
laceration —*see* Laceration, buttock
left S31.829
puncture —*see* Puncture, buttock
right S31.819
calf —*see* Wound, open, leg
canaliculus lacrimalis —*see* Wound, open,
eyelid
canthus, eye —*see* Wound, open, eyelid
cervical esophagus S11.20
bite S11.25
laceration —*see* Laceration, esophagus,
traumatic, cervical
puncture —*see* Puncture, cervical esophagus
cheek (external) S01.40
bite —*see* Bite, cheek
laceration —*see* Laceration, cheek
puncture —*see* Puncture, cheek
internal —*see* Wound, open, oral cavity
chest wall —*see* Wound, open, thorax
chin —*see* Wound, open, head, specified site
NEC
choroid —*see* Wound, open, ocular
ciliary body (eye) —*see* Wound, open, ocular
clitoris S31.40
with amputation —*see* Amputation,
traumatic, clitoris
bite S31.45
laceration —*see* Laceration, vulva
puncture —*see* Puncture, vulva
conjunctiva —*see* Wound, open, ocular
cornea —*see* Wound, open, ocular
costal region —*see* Wound, open, thorax
Descemet's membrane —*see* Wound, open,
ocular
digit (s)
foot —*see* Wound, open, toe
hand —*see* Wound, open, finger

Wound, open - *continued*
ear (canal) (external) S01.30
with amputation —*see* Amputation,
traumatic, ear
bite —*see* Bite, ear
laceration —*see* Laceration, ear
puncture —*see* Puncture, ear
drum S09.2
elbow S51.00
bite —*see* Bite, elbow
laceration —*see* Laceration, elbow
puncture —*see* Puncture, elbow
epididymis —*see* Wound, open, testis
epigastric region S31.102
with penetration into peritoneal cavity
S31.602
bite —*see* Bite, abdomen, wall, epigastric
region
laceration —*see* Laceration, abdomen, wall,
epigastric region
puncture —*see* Puncture, abdomen, wall,
epigastric region
epiglottis —*see* Wound, open, neck, specified
site NEC
esophagus (thoracic) S27.819
cervical —*see* Wound, open, cervical
esophagus
laceration S27.813
specified type NEC S27.818
eye —*see* Wound, open, ocular
eyeball —*see* Wound, open, ocular
eyebrow —*see* Wound, open, eyelid
eyelid S01.10
bite —*see* Bite, eyelid
laceration —*see* Laceration, eyelid
puncture —*see* Puncture, eyelid
face NEC —*see* Wound, open, head, specified
site NEC
finger (s) S61.209
with
amputation —*see* Amputation, traumatic,
finger
damage to nail S61.309
bite —*see* Bite, finger
index S61.208
with
damage to nail S61.308
left S61.201
with
damage to nail S61.301
right S61.200
with
damage to nail S61.300
laceration —*see* Laceration, finger
little S61.208
with
damage to nail S61.308
left S61.207
with damage to nail S61.307
right S61.206
with damage to nail S61.306
middle S61.208
with
damage to nail S61.308
left S61.203
with damage to nail S61.303
right S61.202
with damage to nail S61.302
puncture —*see* Puncture, finger
ring S61.208
with
damage to nail S61.308

Wound, open - *continued*
   left S61.205
     with damage to nail S61.305
   right S61.204
     with damage to nail S61.304
  flank —*see* Wound, open, abdomen, wall
  foot (except toe(s) alone) S91.30
   with amputation —*see* Amputation, traumatic, foot
   bite —*see* Bite, foot
   laceration —*see* Laceration, foot
   puncture —*see* Puncture, foot
   toe —*see* Wound, open, toe
  forearm S51.80
   with
    amputation —*see* Amputation, traumatic, forearm
   bite —*see* Bite, forearm
   elbow only —*see* Wound, open, elbow
   laceration —*see* Laceration, forearm
   puncture —*see* Puncture, forearm
  forehead —*see* Wound, open, head, specified site NEC
  genital organs, external
   with amputation —*see* Amputation, traumatic, genital organs
   bite —*see* Bite, genital organ
   female S31.502
    vagina S31.40
    vulva S31.40
   laceration —*see* Laceration, genital organ
   male S31.501
    penis S31.20
    scrotum S31.30
    testes S31.30
   puncture —*see* Puncture, genital organ
  globe (eye) —*see* Wound, open, ocular
  groin —*see* Wound, open, abdomen, wall
  gum —*see* Wound, open, oral cavity
  hand S61.40
   with
    amputation —*see* Amputation, traumatic, hand
   bite —*see* Bite, hand
   finger (s) —*see* Wound, open, finger
   laceration —*see* Laceration, hand
   puncture —*see* Puncture, hand
   thumb —*see* Wound, open, thumb
  head S01.90
   bite —*see* Bite, head
   cheek —*see* Wound, open, cheek
   ear —*see* Wound, open, ear
   eyelid —*see* Wound, open, eyelid
   laceration —*see* Laceration, head
   lip —*see* Wound, open, lip
   nose S01.20
   oral cavity —*see* Wound, open, oral cavity
   puncture —*see* Puncture, head
   scalp —*see* Wound, open, scalp
   specified site NEC S01.80
   temporomandibular area —*see* Wound, open, cheek
  heel —*see* Wound, open, foot
  hip S71.00
   with amputation —*see* Amputation, traumatic, hip
   bite —*see* Bite, hip
   laceration —*see* Laceration, hip
   puncture —*see* Puncture, hip
  hymen S31.40
   bite —*see* Bite, vulva
   laceration —*see* Laceration, vagina

   puncture —*see* Puncture, vagina
  hypochondrium S31.109
   bite —*see* Bite, hypochondrium
   laceration —*see* Laceration, hypochondrium
   puncture —*see* Puncture, hypochondrium
  hypogastric region S31.109
   bite —*see* Bite, hypogastric region
   laceration —*see* Laceration, hypogastric region
   puncture —*see* Puncture, hypogastric region
  iliac (region) —*see* Wound, open, inguinal region
  inguinal region S31.109
   bite —*see* Bite, abdomen, wall, lower quadrant
   laceration —*see* Laceration, inguinal region
   puncture —*see* Puncture, inguinal region
  instep —*see* Wound, open, foot
  interscapular region —*see* Wound, open, thorax, back
  intraocular —*see* Wound, open, ocular
  iris —*see* Wound, open, ocular
  jaw —*see* Wound, open, head, specified site NEC
  knee S81.00
   bite —*see* Bite, knee
   laceration —*see* Laceration, knee
   puncture —*see* Puncture, knee
  labium (majus) (minus) —*see* Wound, open, vulva
  laceration —*see* Laceration, by site
  lacrimal duct —*see* Wound, open, eyelid
  larynx S11.019
   bite —*see* Bite, larynx
   laceration —*see* Laceration, larynx
   puncture —*see* Puncture, larynx
  left
   lower quadrant S31.104
    with penetration into peritoneal cavity S31.604
   bite —*see* Bite, abdomen, wall, left, lower quadrant
   laceration —*see* Laceration, abdomen, wall, left, lower quadrant
   puncture —*see* Puncture, abdomen, wall, left, lower quadrant
   upper quadrant S31.101
    with penetration into peritoneal cavity S31.601
   bite —*see* Bite, abdomen, wall, left, upper quadrant
   laceration —*see* Laceration, abdomen, wall, left, upper quadrant
   puncture —*see* Puncture, abdomen, wall, left, upper quadrant
  leg (lower) S81.80
   with amputation —*see* Amputation, traumatic, leg
   ankle —*see* Wound, open, ankle
   bite —*see* Bite, leg
   foot —*see* Wound, open, foot
   knee —*see* Wound, open, knee
   laceration —*see* Laceration, leg
   puncture —*see* Puncture, leg
   toe —*see* Wound, open, toe
   upper —*see* Wound, open, thigh
  lip S01.501
   bite —*see* Bite, lip
   laceration —*see* Laceration, lip
   puncture —*see* Puncture, lip

  loin S31.109
   bite —*see* Bite, abdomen, wall
   laceration —*see* Laceration, loin
   puncture —*see* Puncture, loin
  lower back —*see* Wound, open, back, lower
  lumbar region —*see* Wound, open, back, lower
  malar region —*see* Wound, open, head, specified site NEC
  mammary —*see* Wound, open, breast
  mastoid region —*see* Wound, open, head, specified site NEC
  mouth —*see* Wound, open, oral cavity
  nail
   finger —*see* Wound, open, finger, with damage to nail
   toe —*see* Wound, open, toe, with damage to nail
  nape (neck) —*see* Wound, open, neck
  nasal (septum) (sinus) —*see* Wound, open, nose
  nasopharynx —*see* Wound, open, head, specified site NEC
  neck S11.90
   bite —*see* Bite, neck
   involving
    cervical esophagus S11.20
    larynx —*see* Wound, open, larynx
    pharynx S11.20
    thyroid S11.10
    trachea (cervical) S11.029
     bite —*see* Bite, trachea
     laceration S11.021
      with foreign body S11.022
     puncture S11.023
      with foreign body S11.024
   laceration —*see* Laceration, neck
   puncture —*see* Puncture, neck
   specified site NEC S11.80
   specified type NEC S11.89
  nose (septum) (sinus) S01.20
   with amputation —*see* Amputation, traumatic, nose
   bite —*see* Bite, nose
   laceration —*see* Laceration, nose
   puncture —*see* Puncture, nose
  ocular S05.90
   avulsion (traumatic enucleation) S05.7
   eyeball S05.6
    with foreign body S05.5
   eyelid —*see* Wound, open, eyelid
   laceration and rupture S05.3
    with prolapse or loss of intraocular tissue S05.2
   orbit (penetrating) (with or without foreign body) S05.4
   periocular area —*see* Wound, open, eyelid
   specified NEC S05.8X
  oral cavity S01.502
   bite S01.552
   laceration —*see* Laceration, oral cavity
   puncture —*see* Puncture, oral cavity
  orbit —*see* Wound, open, ocular, orbit
  palate —*see* Wound, open, oral cavity
  palm —*see* Wound, open, hand
  pelvis, pelvic —*see also* Wound, open, back, lower
   girdle —*see* Wound, open, hip
  penetrating —*see* Puncture, by site

Wound, open - *continued*
  penis S31.20
    with amputation —*see* Amputation, traumatic, penis
    bite S31.25
    laceration —*see* Laceration, penis
    puncture —*see* Puncture, penis
  perineum
    bite —*see* Bite, perineum
    female S31.502
    laceration —*see* Laceration, perineum
    male S31.501
    puncture —*see* Puncture, perineum
  periocular area (with or without lacrimal passages) —*see* Wound, open, eyelid
  periumbilic region S31.105
    with penetration into peritoneal cavity S31.605
    bite —*see* Bite, abdomen, wall, periumbilic region
    laceration —*see* Laceration, abdomen, wall, periumbilic region
    puncture —*see* Puncture, abdomen, wall, periumbilic region
  phalanges
    finger —*see* Wound, open, finger
    toe —*see* Wound, open, toe
  pharynx S11.20
  pinna —*see* Wound, open, ear
  popliteal space —*see* Wound, open, knee
  prepuce —*see* Wound, open, penis
  pubic region —*see* Wound, open, back, lower
  pudendum —*see* Wound, open, genital organs, external
  puncture wound —*see* Puncture
  rectovaginal septum —*see* Wound, open, vagina
  right
    lower quadrant S31.103
      with penetration into peritoneal cavity S31.603
      bite —*see* Bite, abdomen, wall, right, lower quadrant
      laceration —*see* Laceration, abdomen, wall, right, lower quadrant
      puncture —*see* Puncture, abdomen, wall, right, lower quadrant
    upper quadrant S31.100
      with penetration into peritoneal cavity S31.600
      bite —*see* Bite, abdomen, wall, right, upper quadrant
      laceration —*see* Laceration, abdomen, wall, right, upper quadrant
      puncture —*see* Puncture, abdomen, wall, right, upper quadrant
  sacral region —*see* Wound, open, back, lower
  sacroiliac region —*see* Wound, open, back, lower
  salivary gland —*see* Wound, open, oral cavity
  scalp S01.00
    bite S01.05
    laceration —*see* Laceration, scalp
    puncture —*see* Puncture, scalp
  scalpel, newborn (birth injury) P15.8
  scapular region —*see* Wound, open, shoulder
  sclera —*see* Wound, open, ocular
  scrotum S31.30
    with amputation —*see* Amputation, traumatic, scrotum
    bite S31.35
    laceration —*see* Laceration, scrotum

Wound, open - *continued*
    puncture —*see* Puncture, scrotum
  shin —*see* Wound, open, leg
  shoulder S41.00
    with amputation —*see* Amputation, traumatic, arm
    bite —*see* Bite, shoulder
    laceration —*see* Laceration, shoulder
    puncture —*see* Puncture, shoulder
  skin NOS T14.8
  spermatic cord —*see* Wound, open, testis
  sternal region —*see* Wound, open, thorax, front wall
  submaxillary region —*see* Wound, open, head, specified site NEC
  submental region —*see* Wound, open, head, specified site NEC
  subungual
    finger (s) —*see* Wound, open, finger
    toe (s) —*see* Wound, open, toe
  supraclavicular region —*see* Wound, open, neck, specified site NEC
  temple, temporal region —*see* Wound, open, head, specified site NEC
  temporomandibular area —*see* Wound, open, cheek
  testis S31.30
    with amputation —*see* Amputation, traumatic, testes
    bite S31.35
    laceration —*see* Laceration, testis
    puncture —*see* Puncture, testis
  thigh S71.10
    with amputation —*see* Amputation, traumatic, hip
    bite —*see* Bite, thigh
    laceration —*see* Laceration, thigh
    puncture —*see* Puncture, thigh
  thorax, thoracic (wall) S21.90
    back S21.20
      with penetration S21.40
    bite —*see* Bite, thorax
    breast —*see* Wound, open, breast
    front S21.10
      with penetration S21.30
    laceration —*see* Laceration, thorax
    puncture —*see* Puncture, thorax
  throat —*see* Wound, open, neck
  thumb S61.009
    with
      amputation —*see* Amputation, traumatic, thumb
      damage to nail S61.109
    bite —*see* Bite, thumb
    laceration —*see* Laceration, thumb
    left S61.002
      with
        damage to nail S61.102
    puncture —*see* Puncture, thumb
    right S61.001
      with
        damage to nail S61.101
  thyroid (gland) —*see* Wound, open, neck, thyroid
  toe (s) S91.109
    with
      amputation —*see* Amputation, traumatic, toe
      damage to nail S91.209
    bite —*see* Bite, toe
    great S91.103
      with

Wound, open - *continued*
    damage to nail S91.203
    left S91.102
      with
        damage to nail S91.202
    right S91.101
      with
        damage to nail S91.201
    laceration —*see* Laceration, toe
    lesser S91.106
      with
        damage to nail S91.206
    left S91.105
      with
        damage to nail S91.205
    right S91.104
      with
        damage to nail S91.204
    puncture —*see* Puncture, toe
  tongue —*see* Wound, open, oral cavity
  trachea (cervical region) —*see* Wound, open, neck, trachea
  tunica vaginalis —*see* Wound, open, testis
  tympanum, tympanic membrane S09.2
    laceration —*see* Laceration, ear, drum
    puncture —*see* Puncture, tympanum
  umbilical region —*see* Wound, open, abdomen, wall, periumbilic region
  uvula —*see* Wound, open, oral cavity
  vagina S31.40
    bite S31.45
    laceration —*see* Laceration, vagina
    puncture —*see* Puncture, vagina
  vocal cord S11.039
    bite —*see* Bite, vocal cord
    laceration S11.031
      with foreign body S11.032
    puncture S11.033
      with foreign body S11.034
  vitreous (humor) —*see* Wound, open, ocular
  vulva S31.40
    with amputation —*see* Amputation, traumatic, vulva
    bite S31.45
    laceration —*see* Laceration, vulva
    puncture —*see* Puncture, vulva
  wrist S61.50
    bite —*see* Bite, wrist
    laceration —*see* Laceration, wrist
    puncture —*see* Puncture, wrist
Wound, superficial —*see* Injury —*see also* specified injury type
Wright's syndrome G54.0
Wrist —*see* condition
Wrong drug (by accident) (given in error) — *see* Table of Drugs and Chemicals, by drug, poisoning
Wry neck —*see* Torticollis
Wuchereria (bancrofti) **infestation** B74.0
Wuchereriasis B74.0
Wuchernde Struma Langhans C73

X

Xanthelasma (eyelid) (palpebrarum) H02.60
  left H02.66
    lower H02.65
    upper H02.64
  right H02.63
    lower H02.62
    upper H02.61
Xanthelasmatosis (essential) E78.2
Xanthinuria, hereditary E79.8

Xanthoastrocytoma
  specified site —*see* Neoplasm, malignant, by site
  unspecified site C71.9
Xanthofibroma —*see* Neoplasm, connective tissue, benign
Xanthogranuloma D76.3
Xanthoma (s) , xanthomatosis (primary) (familial) (hereditary) E75.5
  with
    hyperlipoproteinemia
      Type I E78.3
      Type III E78.2
      Type IV E78.1
      Type V E78.3
  bone (generalisata) C96.5
  cerebrotendinous E75.5
  cutaneotendinous E75.5
  disseminatum (skin) E78.2
  eruptive E78.2
  hypercholesterinemic E78.0
  hypercholesterolemic E78.0
  hyperlipidemic E78.5
  joint E75.5
  multiple (skin) E78.2
  tendon (sheath) E75.5
  tubo-eruptive E78.2
  tuberosum E78.2
  tuberous E78.2
  verrucous, oral mucosa K13.4
Xanthosis R23.8
Xenophobia F40.10
Xeroderma —*see also* Ichthyosis
  acquired L85.0
    eyelid H01.149
      left H01.146
        lower H01.145
        upper H01.144
      right H01.143
        lower H01.142
        upper H01.141
  pigmentosum Q82.1
  vitamin A deficiency E50.8
Xerophthalmia (vitamin A deficiency) E50.7
  unrelated to vitamin A deficiency —*see* Keratoconjunctivitis
Xerosis
  conjunctiva H11.14
    with Bitot's spots —*see also* Pigmentation, conjunctiva
      vitamin A deficiency E50.1
      vitamin A deficiency E50.0
  cornea H18.89
    with ulceration —*see* Ulcer, cornea
      vitamin A deficiency E50.3
      vitamin A deficiency E50.2
  cutis L85.3
  skin L85.3
Xerostomia K11.7
Xiphopagus Q89.4
XO syndrome Q96.9
X-ray (of)
  abnormal findings —*see* Abnormal, diagnostic imaging
  breast (mammogram) (routine) Z12.31
  chest
    routine (as part of a general medical examination) Z00.00
      with abnormal findings Z00.01
    routine (as part of a general medical examination) Z00.00
      with abnormal findings Z00.01
XXXXY syndrome Q98.1

XXY syndrome Q98.0

Y

Yaba pox (virus disease) B08.72
Yatapoxvirus B08.70
  specified NEC B08.79
Yawning R06.89
  psychogenic F45.8
Yaws A66.9
  bone lesions A66.6
  butter A66.1
  chancre A66.0
  cutaneous, less than five years after infection A66.2
  early (cutaneous) (macular) (maculopapular) (micropapular) (papular) A66.2
    frambeside A66.2
    skin lesions NEC A66.2
  eyelid A66.2
  ganglion A66.6
  gangosis, gangosa A66.5
  gumma, gummata A66.4
    bone A66.6
  gummatous
    frambeside A66.4
    osteitis A66.6
    periostitis A66.6
  hydrarthrosis (*see also* subcategory M14.8) A66.6
  hyperkeratosis (early) (late) A66.3
  initial lesions A66.0
  joint lesions (*see also* subcategory M14.8) A66.6
  juxta-articular nodules A66.7
  late nodular (ulcerated) A66.4
  latent (without clinical manifestations) (with positive serology) A66.8
  mother A66.0
  mucosal A66.7
  multiple papillomata A66.1
  nodular, late (ulcerated) A66.4
  osteitis A66.6
  papilloma, plantar or palmar A66.1
  periostitis (hypertrophic) A66.6
  specified NEC A66.7
  ulcers A66.4
  wet crab A66.1
Yeast infection (*see also* Candidiasis) B37.9
Yellow
  atrophy (liver) —*see* Failure, hepatic
  fever —*see* Fever, yellow
  jack —*see* Fever, yellow
  jaundice —*see* Jaundice
  nail syndrome L60.5
Yersiniosis —*see also* Infection, Yersinia
  extraintestinal A28.2
  intestinal A04.6

Z

Zahorsky's syndrome (herpangina) B08.5
Zellweger's syndrome Q87.89
Zenker's diverticulum (esophagus) K22.5
Ziehen-Oppenheim disease G24.1
Zieve's syndrome K70.0
Zinc
  deficiency, dietary E60
  metabolism disorder E83.2
Zollinger-Ellison syndrome E16.4
Zona —*see* Herpes, zoster
Zoophobia F40.218
Zoster (herpes) —*see* Herpes, zoster
Zygomycosis B46.9
  specified NEC B46.8
Zymotic —*see* condition

ALPHABETIC INDEX TO POISONING AND EXTERNAL CAUSES OF
ADVERSE EFFECTS OF DRUGS AND OTHER CHEMICAL SUBSTANCES

Substance	Poisoning, Accidental (unintentional)	Poisoning, Intentional Self-harm	Poisoning, Assault	Poisoning, Undetermined	Adverse effect	Underdosing
1-propanol	T51.3X1	T51.3X2	T51.3X3	T51.3X4	--	--
2-propanol	T51.2X1	T51.2X2	T51.2X3	T51.2X4	--	--
2,4-D (dichlorophen-oxyacetic acid)	T60.3X1	T60.3X2	T60.3X3	T60.3X4	--	--
2,4-toluene diisocyanate	T65.0X1	T65.0X2	T65.0X3	T65.0X4	--	--
2,4,5-T (trichloro-phenoxyacetic acid)	T60.1X1	T60.1X2	T60.1X3	T60.1X4	--	--
14-hydroxydihydro-morphinone	T40.2X1	T40.2X2	T40.2X3	T40.2X4	T40.2X5	T40.2X6
ABOB	T37.5X1	T37.5X2	T37.5X3	T37.5X4	T37.5X5	T37.5X6
Abrine	T62.2X1	T62.2X2	T62.2X3	T62.2X4	--	--
Abrus (seed)	T62.2X1	T62.2X2	T62.2X3	T62.2X4	--	--
Absinthe	T51.0X1	T51.0X2	T51.0X3	T51.0X4	--	--
- beverage	T51.0X1	T51.0X2	T51.0X3	T51.0X4	--	--
Acaricide	T60.8X1	T60.8X2	T60.8X3	T60.8X4	--	--
Acebutolol	T44.7X1	T44.7X2	T44.7X3	T44.7X4	T44.7X5	T44.7X6
Acecarbromal	T42.6X1	T42.6X2	T42.6X3	T42.6X4	T42.6X5	T42.6X6
Aceclidine	T44.1X1	T44.1X2	T44.1X3	T44.1X4	T44.1X5	T44.1X6
Acedapsone	T37.0X1	T37.0X2	T37.0X3	T37.0X4	T37.0X5	T37.0X6
Acefylline piperazine	T48.6X1	T48.6X2	T48.6X3	T48.6X4	T48.6X5	T48.6X6
Acemorphan	T40.2X1	T40.2X2	T40.2X3	T40.2X4	T40.2X5	T40.2X6
Acenocoumarin	T45.511	T45.512	T45.513	T45.514	T45.515	T45.516
Acenocoumarol	T45.511	T45.512	T45.513	T45.514	T45.515	T45.516
Acepifylline	T48.6X1	T48.6X2	T48.6X3	T48.6X4	T48.6X5	T48.6X6
Acepromazine	T43.3X1	T43.3X2	T43.3X3	T43.3X4	T43.3X5	T43.3X6
Acesulfamethoxypyridazine	T37.0X1	T37.0X2	T37.0X3	T37.0X4	T37.0X5	T37.0X6
Acetal	T52.8X1	T52.8X2	T52.8X3	T52.8X4	--	--
Acetaldehyde (vapor)	T52.8X1	T52.8X2	T52.8X3	T52.8X4	--	--
- liquid	T65.891	T65.892	T65.893	T65.894	--	--
P-Acetamidophenol	T39.1X1	T39.1X2	T39.1X3	T39.1X4	T39.1X5	T39.1X6
Acetaminophen	T39.1X1	T39.1X2	T39.1X3	T39.1X4	T39.1X5	T39.1X6
Acetaminosalol	T39.1X1	T39.1X2	T39.1X3	T39.1X4	T39.1X5	T39.1X6
Acetanilide	T39.1X1	T39.1X2	T39.1X3	T39.1X4	T39.1X5	T39.1X6
Acetarsol	T37.3X1	T37.3X2	T37.3X3	T37.3X4	T37.3X5	T37.3X6
Acetazolamide	T50.2X1	T50.2X2	T50.2X3	T50.2X4	T50.2X5	T50.2X6
Acetiamine	T45.2X1	T45.2X2	T45.2X3	T45.2X4	T45.2X5	T45.2X6
Acetic						
- acid	T54.2X1	T54.2X2	T54.2X3	T54.2X4	--	--
- - with sodium acetate (ointment)	T49.3X1	T49.3X2	T49.3X3	T49.3X4	T49.3X5	T49.3X6
- - ester (solvent) (vapor)	T52.8X1	T52.8X2	T52.8X3	T52.8X4	--	--
- - irrigating solution	T50.3X1	T50.3X2	T50.3X3	T50.3X4	T50.3X5	T50.3X6
- - medicinal (lotion)	T49.2X1	T49.2X2	T49.2X3	T49.2X4	T49.2X5	T49.2X6
- anhydride	T65.891	T65.892	T65.893	T65.894	--	--
- ether (vapor)	T52.8X1	T52.8X2	T52.8X3	T52.8X4	--	--
Acetohexamide	T38.3X1	T38.3X2	T38.3X3	T38.3X4	T38.3X5	T38.3X6
Acetohydroxamic acid	T50.991	T50.992	T50.993	T50.994	T50.995	T50.996
Acetomenaphthone	T45.7X1	T45.7X2	T45.7X3	T45.7X4	T45.7X5	T45.7X6
Acetomorphine	T40.1X1	T40.1X2	T40.1X3	T40.1X4	T40.1X5	--
Acetone (oils)	T52.4X1	T52.4X2	T52.4X3	T52.4X4	--	--
- chlorinated	T52.4X1	T52.4X2	T52.4X3	T52.4X4	--	--
- vapor	T52.4X1	T52.4X2	T52.4X3	T52.4X4	--	--
Acetonitrile	T52.8X1	T52.8X2	T52.8X3	T52.8X4	--	--
Acetophenazine	T43.3X1	T43.3X2	T43.3X3	T43.3X4	T43.3X5	T43.3X6
Acetophenetedin	T39.1X1	T39.1X2	T39.1X3	T39.1X4	T39.1X5	T39.1X6
Acetophenone	T52.4X1	T52.4X2	T52.4X3	T52.4X4	--	--
Acetorphine	T40.2X1	T40.2X2	T40.2X3	T40.2X4	--	--
Acetosulfone (sodium)	T37.1X1	T37.1X2	T37.1X3	T37.1X4	T37.1X5	T37.1X6
Acetrizoate (sodium)	T50.8X1	T50.8X2	T50.8X3	T50.8X4	T50.8X5	T50.8X6
Acetrizoic acid	T50.8X1	T50.8X2	T50.8X3	T50.8X4	T50.8X5	T50.8X6
Acetyl						
- bromide	T53.6X1	T53.6X2	T53.6X3	T53.6X4	--	--
- chloride	T53.6X1	T53.6X2	T53.6X3	T53.6X4	--	--
Acetylcarbromal	T42.6X1	T42.6X2	T42.6X3	T42.6X4	T42.6X5	T42.6X6
Acetylcholine						
- chloride	T44.1X1	T44.1X2	T44.1X3	T44.1X4	T44.1X5	T44.1X6
- derivative	T44.1X1	T44.1X2	T44.1X3	T44.1X4	T44.1X5	T44.1X6
Acetylcysteine	T48.4X1	T48.4X2	T48.4X3	T48.4X4	T48.4X5	T48.4X6
Acetyldigitoxin	T46.0X1	T46.0X2	T46.0X3	T46.0X4	T46.0X5	T46.0X6

Substance	Poisoning, Accidental (unintentional)	Poisoning, Intentional Self-harm	Poisoning, Assault	Poisoning, Undetermined	Adverse effect	Underdosing
Acetyldigoxin	T46.0X1	T46.0X2	T46.0X3	T46.0X4	T46.0X5	T46.0X6
Acetyldihydrocodeine	T40.2X1	T40.2X2	T40.2X3	T40.2X4	--	--
Acetyldihydrocodeinone	T40.2X1	T40.2X2	T40.2X3	T40.2X4	--	--
Acetylene (gas)	T59.891	T59.892	T59.893	T59.894	--	--
- dichloride	T53.6X1	T53.6X2	T53.6X3	T53.6X4	--	--
- incomplete combustion of	T58.11	T58.12	T58.13	T58.14	--	--
- industrial	T59.891	T59.892	T59.893	T59.894	--	--
- tetrachloride	T53.6X1	T53.6X2	T53.6X3	T53.6X4	--	--
- - vapor	T53.6X1	T53.6X2	T53.6X3	T53.6X4	--	--
Acetylpheneturide	T42.6X1	T42.6X2	T42.6X3	T42.6X4	T42.6X5	T42.6X6
Acetylphenylhydrazine	T39.8X1	T39.8X2	T39.8X3	T39.8X4	T39.8X5	T39.8X6
Acetylsalicylic acid (salts)	T39.011	T39.012	T39.013	T39.014	T39.015	T39.016
- enteric coated	T39.011	T39.012	T39.013	T39.014	T39.015	T39.016
Acetylsulfamethoxypyridazine	T37.0X1	T37.0X2	T37.0X3	T37.0X4	T37.0X5	T37.0X6
Achromycin	T36.4X1	T36.4X2	T36.4X3	T36.4X4	T36.4X5	T36.4X6
- ophthalmic preparation	T49.5X1	T49.5X2	T49.5X3	T49.5X4	T49.5X5	T49.5X6
- topical NEC	T49.0X1	T49.0X2	T49.0X3	T49.0X4	T49.0X5	T49.0X6
Aciclovir	T37.5X1	T37.5X2	T37.5X3	T37.5X4	T37.5X5	T37.5X6
Acid (corrosive) NEC	T54.2X1	T54.2X2	T54.2X3	T54.2X4	--	--
Acidifying agent NEC	T50.901	T50.902	T50.903	T50.904	T50.905	T50.906
Acipimox	T46.6X1	T46.6X2	T46.6X3	T46.6X4	T46.6X5	T46.6X6
Acitretin	T50.991	T50.992	T50.993	T50.994	T50.995	T50.996
Aclarubicin	T45.1X1	T45.1X2	T45.1X3	T45.1X4	T45.1X5	T45.1X6
Aclatonium napadisilate	T48.1X1	T48.1X2	T48.1X3	T48.1X4	T48.1X5	T48.1X6
Aconite (wild)	T46.991	T46.992	T46.993	T46.994	T46.995	T46.996
Aconitine	T46.991	T46.992	T46.993	T46.994	T46.995	T46.996
Aconitum ferox	T46.991	T46.992	T46.993	T46.994	T46.995	T46.996
Acridine	T65.6X1	T65.6X2	T65.6X3	T65.6X4	--	--
- vapor	T59.891	T59.892	T59.893	T59.894	--	--
Acriflavine	T37.91	T37.92	T37.93	T37.94	T37.95	T37.96
Acriflavinium chloride	T49.0X1	T49.0X2	T49.0X3	T49.0X4	T49.0X5	T49.0X6
Acrinol	T49.0X1	T49.0X2	T49.0X3	T49.0X4	T49.0X5	T49.0X6
Acrisorcin	T49.0X1	T49.0X2	T49.0X3	T49.0X4	T49.0X5	T49.0X6
Acrivastine	T45.0X1	T45.0X2	T45.0X3	T45.0X4	T45.0X5	T45.0X6
Acrolein (gas)	T59.891	T59.892	T59.893	T59.894	--	--
- liquid	T54.1X1	T54.1X2	T54.1X3	T54.1X4	--	--
Acrylamide	T65.891	T65.892	T65.893	T65.894	--	--
Acrylic resin	T49.3X1	T49.3X2	T49.3X3	T49.3X4	T49.3X5	T49.3X6
Acrylonitrile	T65.891	T65.892	T65.893	T65.894	--	--
Actaea spicata	T62.2X1	T62.2X2	T62.2X3	T62.2X4	--	--
- berry	T62.1X1	T62.1X2	T62.1X3	T62.1X4	--	--
Acterol	T37.3X1	T37.3X2	T37.3X3	T37.3X4	T37.3X5	T37.3X6
ACTH	T38.811	T38.812	T38.813	T38.814	T38.815	T38.816
Actinomycin C	T45.1X1	T45.1X2	T45.1X3	T45.1X4	T45.1X5	T45.1X6
Actinomycin D	T45.1X1	T45.1X2	T45.1X3	T45.1X4	T45.1X5	T45.1X6
Activated charcoal—see also Charcoal, medicinal	T47.6X1	T47.6X2	T47.6X3	T47.6X4	T47.6X5	T47.6X6
Acyclovir	T37.5X1	T37.5X2	T37.5X3	T37.5X4	T37.5X5	T37.5X6
Adenine	T45.2X1	T45.2X2	T45.2X3	T45.2X4	T45.2X5	T45.2X6
- arabinoside	T37.5X1	T37.5X2	T37.5X3	T37.5X4	T37.5X5	T37.5X6
Adenosine (phosphate)	T46.2X1	T46.2X2	T46.2X3	T46.2X4	T46.2X5	T46.2X6
ADH	T38.891	T38.892	T38.893	T38.894	T38.895	T38.896
Adhesive NEC	T65.891	T65.892	T65.893	T65.894	--	--
Adicillin	T36.0X1	T36.0X2	T36.0X3	T36.0X4	T36.0X5	T36.0X6
Adiphenine	T44.3X1	T44.3X2	T44.3X3	T44.3X4	T44.3X5	T44.3X6
Adipiodone	T50.8X1	T50.8X2	T50.8X3	T50.8X4	T50.8X5	T50.8X6
Adjunct, pharmaceutical	T50.901	T50.902	T50.903	T50.904	T50.905	T50.906
Adrenal (extract, cortex or medulla) (glucocorticoids)(hormones)(mineralocorticoids)	T38.0X1	T38.0X2	T38.0X3	T38.0X4	T38.0X5	T38.0X6
- ENT agent	T49.6X1	T49.6X2	T49.6X3	T49.6X4	T49.6X5	T49.6X6
- ophthalmic preparation	T49.5X1	T49.5X2	T49.5X3	T49.5X4	T49.5X5	T49.5X6
- topical NEC	T49.0X1	T49.0X2	T49.0X3	T49.0X4	T49.0X5	T49.0X6
Adrenaline	T44.5X1	T44.5X2	T44.5X3	T44.5X4	T44.5X5	T44.5X6
Adrenalin—see Adrenaline						
Adrenergic NEC	T44.901	T44.902	T44.903	T44.904	T44.905	T44.906
- blocking agent NEC	T44.8X1	T44.8X2	T44.8X3	T44.8X4	T44.8X5	T44.8X6

Substance	Poisoning, Accidental (unintentional)	Poisoning, Intentional Self-harm	Poisoning, Assault	Poisoning, Undetermined	Adverse effect	Underdosing
- - beta, heart	T44.7X1	T44.7X2	T44.7X3	T44.7X4	T44.7X5	T44.7X6
- specified NEC	T44.991	T44.992	T44.993	T44.994	T44.995	T44.996
Adrenochrome						
- (mono) semicarbazone	T46.991	T46.992	T46.993	T46.994	T46.995	T46.996
- derivative	T46.991	T46.992	T46.993	T46.994	T46.995	T46.996
Adrenocorticotrophic hormone	T38.811	T38.812	T38.813	T38.814	T38.815	T38.816
Adrenocorticotrophin	T38.811	T38.812	T38.813	T38.814	T38.815	T38.816
Adriamycin	T45.1X1	T45.1X2	T45.1X3	T45.1X4	T45.1X5	T45.1X6
Aerosol spray NEC	T65.91	T65.92	T65.93	T65.94	--	--
Aerosporin	T36.8X1	T36.8X2	T36.8X3	T36.8X4	T36.8X5	T36.8X6
- ENT agent	T49.6X1	T49.6X2	T49.6X3	T49.6X4	T49.6X5	T49.6X6
- ophthalmic preparation	T49.5X1	T49.5X2	T49.5X3	T49.5X4	T49.5X5	T49.5X6
- topical NEC	T49.0X1	T49.0X2	T49.0X3	T49.0X4	T49.0X5	T49.0X6
Aethusa cynapium	T62.2X1	T62.2X2	T62.2X3	T62.2X4	--	--
Afghanistan black	T40.7X1	T40.7X2	T40.7X3	T40.7X4	T40.7X5	T40.7X6
Aflatoxin	T64.01	T64.02	T64.03	T64.04	--	--
Afloqualone	T42.8X1	T42.8X2	T42.8X3	T42.8X4	T42.8X5	T42.8X6
African boxwood	T62.2X1	T62.2X2	T62.2X3	T62.2X4	--	--
Agar	T47.4X1	T47.4X2	T47.4X3	T47.4X4	T47.4X5	T47.4X6
Agonist						
- predominantly						
- - alpha-adrenoreceptor	T44.4X1	T44.4X2	T44.4X3	T44.4X4	T44.4X5	T44.4X6
- - beta-adrenoreceptor	T44.5X1	T44.5X2	T44.5X3	T44.5X4	T44.5X5	T44.5X6
Agricultural agent NEC	T65.91	T65.92	T65.93	T65.94	--	--
Agrypnal	T42.3X1	T42.3X2	T42.3X3	T42.3X4	T42.3X5	T42.3X6
AHLG	T50.Z11	T50.Z12	T50.Z13	T50.Z14	T50.Z15	T50.Z16
Air contaminant (s) , source/type NOS	T65.91	T65.92	T65.93	T65.94	--	--
Ajmaline	T46.2X1	T46.2X2	T46.2X3	T46.2X4	T46.2X5	T46.2X6
Akee	T62.1X1	T62.1X2	T62.1X3	T62.1X4	--	--
Akrinol	T49.0X1	T49.0X2	T49.0X3	T49.0X4	T49.0X5	T49.0X6
Akritoin	T37.8X1	T37.8X2	T37.8X3	T37.8X4	T37.8X5	T37.8X6
Alacepril	T46.4X1	T46.4X2	T46.4X3	T46.4X4	T46.4X5	T46.4X6
Alantolactone	T37.4X1	T37.4X2	T37.4X3	T37.4X4	T37.4X5	T37.4X6
Albamycin	T36.8X1	T36.8X2	T36.8X3	T36.8X4	T36.8X5	T36.8X6
Albendazole	T37.4X1	T37.4X2	T37.4X3	T37.4X4	T37.4X5	T37.4X6
Albumin						
- bovine	T45.8X1	T45.8X2	T45.8X3	T45.8X4	T45.8X5	T45.8X6
- human serum	T45.8X1	T45.8X2	T45.8X3	T45.8X4	T45.8X5	T45.8X6
- - salt-poor	T45.8X1	T45.8X2	T45.8X3	T45.8X4	T45.8X5	T45.8X6
- normal human serum	T45.8X1	T45.8X2	T45.8X3	T45.8X4	T45.8X5	T45.8X6
Albuterol	T48.6X1	T48.6X2	T48.6X3	T48.6X4	T48.6X5	T48.6X6
Albutoin	T42.0X1	T42.0X2	T42.0X3	T42.0X4	T42.0X5	T42.0X6
Alclometasone	T49.0X1	T49.0X2	T49.0X3	T49.0X4	T49.0X5	T49.0X6
Alcohol	T51.91	T51.92	T51.93	T51.94	--	--
- absolute	T51.0X1	T51.0X2	T51.0X3	T51.0X4	--	--
- - beverage	T51.0X1	T51.0X2	T51.0X3	T51.0X4	--	--
- allyl	T51.8X1	T51.8X2	T51.8X3	T51.8X4	--	--
- amyl	T51.3X1	T51.3X2	T51.3X3	T51.3X4	--	--
- antifreeze	T51.1X1	T51.1X2	T51.1X3	T51.1X4	--	--
- beverage	T51.0X1	T51.0X2	T51.0X3	T51.0X4	--	--
- butyl	T51.3X1	T51.3X2	T51.3X3	T51.3X4	--	--
- dehydrated	T51.0X1	T51.0X2	T51.0X3	T51.0X4	--	--
- - beverage	T51.0X1	T51.0X2	T51.0X3	T51.0X4		--
- denatured	T51.0X1	T51.0X2	T51.0X3	T51.0X4	--	--
- deterrent NEC	T50.6X1	T50.6X2	T50.6X3	T50.6X4	T50.6X5	T50.6X6
- diagnostic (gastric function)	T50.8X1	T50.8X2	T50.8X3	T50.8X4	T50.8X5	T50.8X6
- ethyl	T51.0X1	T51.0X2	T51.0X3	T51.0X4	--	--
- - beverage	T51.0X1	T51.0X2	T51.0X3	T51.0X4	--	--
- grain	T51.0X1	T51.0X2	T51.0X3	T51.0X4	--	--
- - beverage	T51.0X1	T51.0X2	T51.0X3	T51.0X4	--	--
- industrial	T51.0X1	T51.0X2	T51.0X3	T51.0X4	--	--
- isopropyl	T51.2X1	T51.2X2	T51.2X3	T51.2X4	--	--
- methyl	T51.1X1	T51.1X2	T51.1X3	T51.1X4	--	--
- preparation for consumption	T51.0X1	T51.0X2	T51.0X3	T51.0X4	--	--
- propyl	T51.3X1	T51.3X2	T51.3X3	T51.3X4	--	--

TABLE OF DRUGS AND CHEMICALS

Substance	Poisoning, Accidental (unintentional)	Poisoning, Intentional Self-harm	Poisoning, Assault	Poisoning, Undetermined	Adverse effect	Underdosing
- - secondary	T51.2X1	T51.2X2	T51.2X3	T51.2X4	--	--
- radiator	T51.1X1	T51.1X2	T51.1X3	T51.1X4	--	--
- rubbing	T51.2X1	T51.2X2	T51.2X3	T51.2X4	--	--
- specified type NEC	T51.8X1	T51.8X2	T51.8X3	T51.8X4	--	--
- surgical	T51.0X1	T51.0X2	T51.0X3	T51.0X4	--	--
- vapor (from any type of Alcohol)	T59.891	T59.892	T59.893	T59.894	--	--
- wood	T51.1X1	T51.1X2	T51.1X3	T51.1X4	--	--
Alcuronium (chloride)	T48.1X1	T48.1X2	T48.1X3	T48.1X4	T48.1X5	T48.1X6
Aldactone	T50.0X1	T50.0X2	T50.0X3	T50.0X4	T50.0X5	T50.0X6
Aldesulfone sodium	T37.1X1	T37.1X2	T37.1X3	T37.1X4	T37.1X5	T37.1X6
Aldicarb	T60.0X1	T60.0X2	T60.0X3	T60.0X4	--	--
Aldomet	T46.5X1	T46.5X2	T46.5X3	T46.5X4	T46.5X5	T46.5X6
Aldosterone	T50.0X1	T50.0X2	T50.0X3	T50.0X4	T50.0X5	T50.0X6
Aldrin (dust)	T60.1X1	T60.1X2	T60.1X3	T60.1X4	--	--
Aleve—see Naproxen						
Alexitol sodium	T47.1X1	T47.1X2	T47.1X3	T47.1X4	T47.1X5	T47.1X6
Alfacalcidol	T45.2X1	T45.2X2	T45.2X3	T45.2X4	T45.2X5	T45.2X6
Alfadolone	T41.1X1	T41.1X2	T41.1X3	T41.1X4	T41.1X5	T41.1X6
Alfaxalone	T41.1X1	T41.1X2	T41.1X3	T41.1X4	T41.1X5	T41.1X6
Alfentanil	T40.4X1	T40.4X2	T40.4X3	T40.4X4	T40.4X5	T40.4X6
Alfuzosin (hydrochloride)	T44.8X1	T44.8X2	T44.8X3	T44.8X4	T44.8X5	T44.8X6
Algae (harmful) (toxin)	T65.821	T65.822	T65.823	T65.824	--	--
Algeldrate	T47.1X1	T47.1X2	T47.1X3	T47.1X4	T47.1X5	T47.1X6
Algin	T47.8X1	T47.8X2	T47.8X3	T47.8X4	T47.8X5	T47.8X6
Alglucerase	T45.3X1	T45.3X2	T45.3X3	T45.3X4	T45.3X5	T45.3X6
Alidase	T45.3X1	T45.3X2	T45.3X3	T45.3X4	T45.3X5	T45.3X6
Alimemazine	T43.3X1	T43.3X2	T43.3X3	T43.3X4	T43.3X5	T43.3X6
Aliphatic thiocyanates	T65.0X1	T65.0X2	T65.0X3	T65.0X4	--	--
Alizapride	T45.0X1	T45.0X2	T45.0X3	T45.0X4	T45.0X5	T45.0X6
Alkali (caustic)	T54.3X1	T54.3X2	T54.3X3	T54.3X4	--	--
Alkaline antiseptic solution (aromatic)	T49.6X1	T49.6X2	T49.6X3	T49.6X4	T49.6X5	T49.6X6
Alkalinizing agents (medicinal)	T50.901	T50.902	T50.903	T50.904	T50.905	T50.906
Alkalizing agent NEC	T50.901	T50.902	T50.903	T50.904	T50.905	T50.906
Alka-seltzer	T39.011	T39.012	T39.013	T39.014	T39.015	T39.016
Alkavervir	T46.5X1	T46.5X2	T46.5X3	T46.5X4	T46.5X5	T46.5X6
Alkonium (bromide)	T49.0X1	T49.0X2	T49.0X3	T49.0X4	T49.0X5	T49.0X6
Alkylating drug NEC	T45.1X1	T45.1X2	T45.1X3	T45.1X4	T45.1X5	T45.1X6
- antimyeloproliferative	T45.1X1	T45.1X2	T45.1X3	T45.1X4	T45.1X5	T45.1X6
- lymphatic	T45.1X1	T45.1X2	T45.1X3	T45.1X4	T45.1X5	T45.1X6
Alkylisocyanate	T65.0X1	T65.0X2	T65.0X3	T65.0X4	--	--
Allantoin	T49.4X1	T49.4X2	T49.4X3	T49.4X4	T49.4X5	T49.4X6
Allegron	T43.011	T43.012	T43.013	T43.014	T43.015	T43.016
Allethrin	T49.0X1	T49.0X2	T49.0X3	T49.0X4	T49.0X5	T49.0X6
Allobarbital	T42.3X1	T42.3X2	T42.3X3	T42.3X4	T42.3X5	T42.3X6
Allopurinol	T50.4X1	T50.4X2	T50.4X3	T50.4X4	T50.4X5	T50.4X6
Allyl						
- Alcohol	T51.8X1	T51.8X2	T51.8X3	T51.8X4	--	--
- disulfide	T46.6X1	T46.6X2	T46.6X3	T46.6X4	T46.6X5	T46.6X6
Allylestrenol	T38.5X1	T38.5X2	T38.5X3	T38.5X4	T38.5X5	T38.5X6
Allylisopropylacetylurea	T42.6X1	T42.6X2	T42.6X3	T42.6X4	T42.6X5	T42.6X6
Allylisopropylmalonylurea	T42.3X1	T42.3X2	T42.3X3	T42.3X4	T42.3X5	T42.3X6
Allylthiourea	T49.3X1	T49.3X2	T49.3X3	T49.3X4	T49.3X5	T49.3X6
Allyltribromide	T42.6X1	T42.6X2	T42.6X3	T42.6X4	T42.6X5	T42.6X6
Allypropymal	T42.3X1	T42.3X2	T42.3X3	T42.3X4	T42.3X5	T42.3X6
Almagate	T47.1X1	T47.1X2	T47.1X3	T47.1X4	T47.1X5	T47.1X6
Almasilate	T47.1X1	T47.1X2	T47.1X3	T47.1X4	T47.1X5	T47.1X6
Almitrine	T50.7X1	T50.7X2	T50.7X3	T50.7X4	T50.7X5	T50.7X6
Aloes	T47.2X1	T47.2X2	T47.2X3	T47.2X4	T47.2X5	T47.2X6
Aloglutamol	T47.1X1	T47.1X2	T47.1X3	T47.1X4	T47.1X5	T47.1X6
Aloin	T47.2X1	T47.2X2	T47.2X3	T47.2X4	T47.2X5	T47.2X6
Aloxidone	T42.2X1	T42.2X2	T42.2X3	T42.2X4	T42.2X5	T42.2X6
Alpha						
- acetyldigoxin	T46.0X1	T46.0X2	T46.0X3	T46.0X4	T46.0X5	T46.0X6
- adrenergic blocking drug	T44.6X1	T44.6X2	T44.6X3	T44.6X4	T44.6X5	T44.6X6
- amylase	T45.3X1	T45.3X2	T45.3X3	T45.3X4	T45.3X5	T45.3X6

TABLE OF DRUGS AND CHEMICALS

Substance	Poisoning, Accidental (unintentional)	Poisoning, Intentional Self-harm	Poisoning, Assault	Poisoning, Undetermined	Adverse effect	Underdosing
- tocoferol (acetate)	T45.2X1	T45.2X2	T45.2X3	T45.2X4	T45.2X5	T45.2X6
- tocopherol	T45.2X1	T45.2X2	T45.2X3	T45.2X4	T45.2X5	T45.2X6
Alphadolone	T41.1X1	T41.1X2	T41.1X3	T41.1X4	T41.1X5	T41.1X6
Alphaprodine	T40.4X1	T40.4X2	T40.4X3	T40.4X4	T40.4X5	T40.4X6
Alphaxalone	T41.1X1	T41.1X2	T41.1X3	T41.1X4	T41.1X5	T41.1X6
Alprazolam	T42.4X1	T42.4X2	T42.4X3	T42.4X4	T42.4X5	T42.4X6
Alprenolol	T44.7X1	T44.7X2	T44.7X3	T44.7X4	T44.7X5	T44.7X6
Alprostadil	T46.7X1	T46.7X2	T46.7X3	T46.7X4	T46.7X5	T46.7X6
Alsactide	T38.811	T38.812	T38.813	T38.814	T38.815	T38.816
Alseroxylon	T46.5X1	T46.5X2	T46.5X3	T46.5X4	T46.5X5	T46.5X6
Alteplase	T45.611	T45.612	T45.613	T45.614	T45.615	T45.616
Altizide	T50.2X1	T50.2X2	T50.2X3	T50.2X4	T50.2X5	T50.2X6
Altretamine	T45.1X1	T45.1X2	T45.1X3	T45.1X4	T45.1X5	T45.1X6
Alum (medicinal)	T49.4X1	T49.4X2	T49.4X3	T49.4X4	T49.4X5	T49.4X6
- nonmedicinal (ammonium) (potassium)	T56.891	T56.892	T56.893	T56.894	--	--
Aluminium, aluminum						
- acetate	T49.2X1	T49.2X2	T49.2X3	T49.2X4	T49.2X5	T49.2X6
- - solution	T49.0X1	T49.0X2	T49.0X3	T49.0X4	T49.0X5	T49.0X6
- aspirin	T39.011	T39.012	T39.013	T39.014	T39.015	T39.016
- bis (acetylsalicylate)	T39.011	T39.012	T39.013	T39.014	T39.015	T39.016
- carbonate (gel, basic)	T47.1X1	T47.1X2	T47.1X3	T47.1X4	T47.1X5	T47.1X6
- chlorhydroxide-complex	T47.1X1	T47.1X2	T47.1X3	T47.1X4	T47.1X5	T47.1X6
- chloride	T49.2X1	T49.2X2	T49.2X3	T49.2X4	T49.2X5	T49.2X6
- clofibrate	T46.6X1	T46.6X2	T46.6X3	T46.6X4	T46.6X5	T46.6X6
- diacetate	T49.2X1	T49.2X2	T49.2X3	T49.2X4	T49.2X5	T49.2X6
- glycinate	T47.1X1	T47.1X2	T47.1X3	T47.1X4	T47.1X5	T47.1X6
- hydroxide (gel)	T47.1X1	T47.1X2	T47.1X3	T47.1X4	T47.1X5	T47.1X6
- hydroxide-magnesium carb. gel	T47.1X1	T47.1X2	T47.1X3	T47.1X4	T47.1X5	T47.1X6
- magnesium silicate	T47.1X1	T47.1X2	T47.1X3	T47.1X4	T47.1X5	T47.1X6
- nicotinate	T46.7X1	T46.7X2	T46.7X3	T46.7X4	T46.7X5	T46.7X6
- ointment (surgical) (topical)	T49.3X1	T49.3X2	T49.3X3	T49.3X4	T49.3X5	T49.3X6
- phosphate	T47.1X1	T47.1X2	T47.1X3	T47.1X4	T47.1X5	T47.1X6
- salicylate	T39.091	T39.092	T39.093	T39.094	T39.095	T39.096
- silicate	T47.1X1	T47.1X2	T47.1X3	T47.1X4	T47.1X5	T47.1X6
- sodium silicate	T47.1X1	T47.1X2	T47.1X3	T47.1X4	T47.1X5	T47.1X6
- subacetate	T49.2X1	T49.2X2	T49.2X3	T49.2X4	T49.2X5	T49.2X6
- sulfate	T49.0X1	T49.0X2	T49.0X3	T49.0X4	T49.0X5	T49.0X6
- tannate	T47.6X1	T47.6X2	T47.6X3	T47.6X4	T47.6X5	T47.6X6
- topical NEC	T49.3X1	T49.3X2	T49.3X3	T49.3X4	T49.3X5	T49.3X6
Alurate	T42.3X1	T42.3X2	T42.3X3	T42.3X4	T42.3X5	T42.3X6
Alverine	T44.3X1	T44.3X2	T44.3X3	T44.3X4	T44.3X5	T44.3X6
Alvodine	T40.2X1	T40.2X2	T40.2X3	T40.2X4	T40.2X5	T40.2X6
Amanita phalloides	T62.0X1	T62.0X2	T62.0X3	T62.0X4	--	--
Amanitine	T62.0X1	T62.0X2	T62.0X3	T62.0X4	--	--
Amantadine	T42.8X1	T42.8X2	T42.8X3	T42.8X4	T42.8X5	T42.8X6
Ambazone	T49.6X1	T49.6X2	T49.6X3	T49.6X4	T49.6X5	T49.6X6
Ambenonium (chloride)	T44.0X1	T44.0X2	T44.0X3	T44.0X4	T44.0X5	T44.0X6
Ambroxol	T48.4X1	T48.4X2	T48.4X3	T48.4X4	T48.4X5	T48.4X6
Ambuphylline	T48.6X1	T48.6X2	T48.6X3	T48.6X4	T48.6X5	T48.6X6
Ambutonium bromide	T44.3X1	T44.3X2	T44.3X3	T44.3X4	T44.3X5	T44.3X6
Amcinonide	T49.0X1	T49.0X2	T49.0X3	T49.0X4	T49.0X5	T49.0X6
Amdinocilline	T36.0X1	T36.0X2	T36.0X3	T36.0X4	T36.0X5	T36.0X6
Ametazole	T50.8X1	T50.8X2	T50.8X3	T50.8X4	T50.8X5	T50.8X6
Amethocaine	T41.3X1	T41.3X2	T41.3X3	T41.3X4	T41.3X5	T41.3X6
- regional	T41.3X1	T41.3X2	T41.3X3	T41.3X4	T41.3X5	T41.3X6
- spinal	T41.3X1	T41.3X2	T41.3X3	T41.3X4	T41.3X5	T41.3X6
Amethopterin	T45.1X1	T45.1X2	T45.1X3	T45.1X4	T45.1X5	T45.1X6
Amezinium metilsulfate	T44.991	T44.992	T44.993	T44.994	T44.995	T44.996
Amfebutamone	T43.291	T43.292	T43.293	T43.294	T43.295	T43.296
Amfepramone	T50.5X1	T50.5X2	T50.5X3	T50.5X4	T50.5X5	T50.5X6
Amfetamine	T43.621	T43.622	T43.623	T43.624	T43.625	T43.626
Amfetaminil	T43.621	T43.622	T43.623	T43.624	T43.625	T43.626
Amfomycin	T36.8X1	T36.8X2	T36.8X3	T36.8X4	T36.8X5	T36.8X6
Amidefrine mesilate	T48.5X1	T48.5X2	T48.5X3	T48.5X4	T48.5X5	T48.5X6
Amidone	T40.3X1	T40.3X2	T40.3X3	T40.3X4	T40.3X5	T40.3X6

Substance	Poisoning, Accidental (unintentional)	Poisoning, Intentional Self-harm	Poisoning, Assault	Poisoning, Undetermined	Adverse effect	Underdosing
Amidopyrine	T39.2X1	T39.2X2	T39.2X3	T39.2X4	T39.2X5	T39.2X6
Amidotrizoate	T50.8X1	T50.8X2	T50.8X3	T50.8X4	T50.8X5	T50.8X6
Amiflamine	T43.1X1	T43.1X2	T43.1X3	T43.1X4	T43.1X5	T43.1X6
Amikacin	T36.5X1	T36.5X2	T36.5X3	T36.5X4	T36.5X5	T36.5X6
Amikhelline	T46.3X1	T46.3X2	T46.3X3	T46.3X4	T46.3X5	T46.3X6
Amiloride	T50.2X1	T50.2X2	T50.2X3	T50.2X4	T50.2X5	T50.2X6
Aminacrine	T49.0X1	T49.0X2	T49.0X3	T49.0X4	T49.0X5	T49.0X6
Amineptine	T43.011	T43.012	T43.013	T43.014	T43.015	T43.016
Aminitrozole	T37.3X1	T37.3X2	T37.3X3	T37.3X4	T37.3X5	T37.3X6
Amino acids	T50.3X1	T50.3X2	T50.3X3	T50.3X4	T50.3X5	T50.3X6
Aminoacetic acid (derivatives)	T50.3X1	T50.3X2	T50.3X3	T50.3X4	T50.3X5	T50.3X6
Aminoacridine	T49.0X1	T49.0X2	T49.0X3	T49.0X4	T49.0X5	T49.0X6
Aminobenzoic acid (-p)	T49.3X1	T49.3X2	T49.3X3	T49.3X4	T49.3X5	T49.3X6
4-Aminobutyric acid	T43.8X1	T43.8X2	T43.8X3	T43.8X4	T43.8X5	T43.8X6
Aminocaproic acid	T45.621	T45.622	T45.623	T45.624	T45.625	T45.626
Aminoethylisothiourium	T45.8X1	T45.8X2	T45.8X3	T45.8X4	T45.8X5	T45.8X6
Aminofenazone	T39.2X1	T39.2X2	T39.2X3	T39.2X4	T39.2X5	T39.2X6
Aminoglutethimide	T45.1X1	T45.1X2	T45.1X3	T45.1X4	T45.1X5	T45.1X6
Aminohippuric acid	T50.8X1	T50.8X2	T50.8X3	T50.8X4	T50.8X5	T50.8X6
Aminomethylbenzoic acid	T45.691	T45.692	T45.693	T45.694	T45.695	T45.696
Aminometradine	T50.2X1	T50.2X2	T50.2X3	T50.2X4	T50.2X5	T50.2X6
Aminopentamide	T44.3X1	T44.3X2	T44.3X3	T44.3X4	T44.3X5	T44.3X6
Aminophenazone	T39.2X1	T39.2X2	T39.2X3	T39.2X4	T39.2X5	T39.2X6
Aminophenol	T54.0X1	T54.0X2	T54.0X3	T54.0X4	--	--
4-Aminophenol derivatives	T39.1X1	T39.1X2	T39.1X3	T39.1X4	T39.1X5	T39.1X6
Aminophenylpyridone	T43.591	T43.592	T43.593	T43.594	T43.595	T43.596
Aminophylline	T48.6X1	T48.6X2	T48.6X3	T48.6X4	T48.6X5	T48.6X6
Aminopterin sodium	T45.1X1	T45.1X2	T45.1X3	T45.1X4	T45.1X5	T45.1X6
Aminopyrine	T39.2X1	T39.2X2	T39.2X3	T39.2X4	T39.2X5	T39.2X6
8-Aminoquinoline drugs	T37.2X1	T37.2X2	T37.2X3	T37.2X4	T37.2X5	T37.2X6
Aminorex	T50.5X1	T50.5X2	T50.5X3	T50.5X4	T50.5X5	T50.5X6
Aminosalicylic acid	T37.1X1	T37.1X2	T37.1X3	T37.1X4	T37.1X5	T37.1X6
Aminosalylum	T37.1X1	T37.1X2	T37.1X3	T37.1X4	T37.1X5	T37.1X6
Amiodarone	T46.2X1	T46.2X2	T46.2X3	T46.2X4	T46.2X5	T46.2X6
Amiphenazole	T50.7X1	T50.7X2	T50.7X3	T50.7X4	T50.7X5	T50.7X6
Amiquinsin	T46.5X1	T46.5X2	T46.5X3	T46.5X4	T46.5X5	T46.5X6
Amisometradine	T50.2X1	T50.2X2	T50.2X3	T50.2X4	T50.2X5	T50.2X6
Amisulpride	T43.591	T43.592	T43.593	T43.594	T43.595	T43.596
Amitriptyline	T43.011	T43.012	T43.013	T43.014	T43.015	T43.016
Amitriptylinoxide	T43.011	T43.012	T43.013	T43.014	T43.015	T43.016
Amlexanox	T48.6X1	T48.6X2	T48.6X3	T48.6X4	T48.6X5	T48.6X6
Ammonia (fumes) (gas) (vapor)	T59.891	T59.892	T59.893	T59.894	--	--
- aromatic spirit	T48.991	T48.992	T48.993	T48.994	T48.995	T48.996
- liquid (household)	T54.3X1	T54.3X2	T54.3X3	T54.3X4	--	--
Ammoniated mercury	T49.0X1	T49.0X2	T49.0X3	T49.0X4	T49.0X5	T49.0X6
Ammonium						
- acid tartrate	T49.5X1	T49.5X2	T49.5X3	T49.5X4	T49.5X5	T49.5X6
- bromide	T42.6X1	T42.6X2	T42.6X3	T42.6X4	T42.6X5	T42.6X6
- carbonate	T54.3X1	T54.3X2	T54.3X3	T54.3X4	--	--
- chloride	T50.991	T50.992	T50.993	T50.994	T50.995	T50.996
- - expectorant	T48.4X1	T48.4X2	T48.4X3	T48.4X4	T48.4X5	T48.4X6
- compounds (household) NEC	T54.3X1	T54.3X2	T54.3X3	T54.3X4	--	--
- - fumes (any usage)	T59.891	T59.892	T59.893	T59.894	--	--
- - industrial	T54.3X1	T54.3X2	T54.3X3	T54.3X4	--	--
- ichthyosulronate	T49.4X1	T49.4X2	T49.4X3	T49.4X4	T49.4X5	T49.4X6
- mandelate	T37.91	T37.92	T37.93	T37.94	T37.95	T37.96
- sulfamate	T60.3X1	T60.3X2	T60.3X3	T60.3X4	--	--
- sulfonate resin	T47.8X1	T47.8X2	T47.8X3	T47.8X4	T47.8X5	T47.8X6
Amobarbital (sodium)	T42.3X1	T42.3X2	T42.3X3	T42.3X4	T42.3X5	T42.3X6
Amodiaquine	T37.2X1	T37.2X2	T37.2X3	T37.2X4	T37.2X5	T37.2X6
Amopyroquin (e)	T37.2X1	T37.2X2	T37.2X3	T37.2X4	T37.2X5	T37.2X6
Amoxapine	T43.011	T43.012	T43.013	T43.014	T43.015	T43.016
Amoxicillin	T36.0X1	T36.0X2	T36.0X3	T36.0X4	T36.0X5	T36.0X6
Amperozide	T43.591	T43.592	T43.593	T43.594	T43.595	T43.596
Amphenidone	T43.591	T43.592	T43.593	T43.594	T43.595	T43.596

Substance	Poisoning, Accidental (unintentional)	Poisoning, Intentional Self-harm	Poisoning, Assault	Poisoning, Undetermined	Adverse effect	Underdosing
Amphetamine NEC	T43.621	T43.622	T43.623	T43.624	T43.625	T43.626
Amphomycin	T36.8X1	T36.8X2	T36.8X3	T36.8X4	T36.8X5	T36.8X6
Amphotalide	T37.4X1	T37.4X2	T37.4X3	T37.4X4	T37.4X5	T37.4X6
Amphotericin B	T36.7X1	T36.7X2	T36.7X3	T36.7X4	T36.7X5	T36.7X6
- topical	T49.0X1	T49.0X2	T49.0X3	T49.0X4	T49.0X5	T49.0X6
Ampicillin	T36.0X1	T36.0X2	T36.0X3	T36.0X4	T36.0X5	T36.0X6
Amprotropine	T44.3X1	T44.3X2	T44.3X3	T44.3X4	T44.3X5	T44.3X6
Amsacrine	T45.1X1	T45.1X2	T45.1X3	T45.1X4	T45.1X5	T45.1X6
Amygdaline	T62.2X1	T62.2X2	T62.2X3	T62.2X4	--	--
Amyl						
- acetate	T52.8X1	T52.8X2	T52.8X3	T52.8X4	--	--
- - vapor	T59.891	T59.892	T59.893	T59.894	--	--
- alcohol	T51.3X1	T51.3X2	T51.3X3	T51.3X4	--	--
- chloride	T53.6X1	T53.6X2	T53.6X3	T53.6X4	--	--
- formate	T52.8X1	T52.8X2	T52.8X3	T52.8X4	--	--
- nitrite	T46.3X1	T46.3X2	T46.3X3	T46.3X4	T46.3X5	T46.3X6
- propionate	T65.891	T65.892	T65.893	T65.894	--	--
Amylase	T47.5X1	T47.5X2	T47.5X3	T47.5X4	T47.5X5	T47.5X6
Amyleine, regional	T41.3X1	T41.3X2	T41.3X3	T41.3X4	T41.3X5	T41.3X6
Amylene						
- dichloride	T53.6X1	T53.6X2	T53.6X3	T53.6X4	--	--
- hydrate	T51.3X1	T51.3X2	T51.3X3	T51.3X4	--	--
Amylmetacresol	T49.6X1	T49.6X2	T49.6X3	T49.6X4	T49.6X5	T49.6X6
Amylobarbitone	T42.3X1	T42.3X2	T42.3X3	T42.3X4	T42.3X5	T42.3X6
Amylocaine, regional	T41.3X1	T41.3X2	T41.3X3	T41.3X4	T41.3X5	T41.3X6
- infiltration (subcutaneous)	T41.3X1	T41.3X2	T41.3X3	T41.3X4	T41.3X5	T41.3X6
- nerve block (peripheral) (plexus)	T41.3X1	T41.3X2	T41.3X3	T41.3X4	T41.3X5	T41.3X6
- spinal	T41.3X1	T41.3X2	T41.3X3	T41.3X4	T41.3X5	T41.3X6
- topical (surface)	T41.3X1	T41.3X2	T41.3X3	T41.3X4	T41.3X5	T41.3X6
Amylopectin	T47.6X1	T47.6X2	T47.6X3	T47.6X4	T47.6X5	T47.6X6
Amytal (sodium)	T42.3X1	T42.3X2	T42.3X3	T42.3X4	T42.3X5	T42.3X6
Anabolic steroid	T38.7X1	T38.7X2	T38.7X3	T38.7X4	T38.7X5	T38.7X6
Analeptic NEC	T50.7X1	T50.7X2	T50.7X3	T50.7X4	T50.7X5	T50.7X6
Analgesic	T39.91	T39.92	T39.93	T39.94	T39.95	T39.96
- anti-inflammatory NEC	T39.91	T39.92	T39.93	T39.94	T39.95	T39.96
- - propionic acid derivative	T39.311	T39.312	T39.313	T39.314	T39.315	T39.316
- antirheumatic NEC	T39.4X1	T39.4X2	T39.4X3	T39.4X4	T39.4X5	T39.4X6
- aromatic NEC	T39.1X1	T39.1X2	T39.1X3	T39.1X4	T39.1X5	T39.1X6
- narcotic NEC	T40.601	T40.602	T40.603	T40.604	T40.605	T40.606
- - combination	T40.601	T40.602	T40.603	T40.604	T40.605	T40.606
- - obstetric	T40.601	T40.602	T40.603	T40.604	T40.605	T40.606
- non-narcotic NEC	T39.91	T39.92	T39.93	T39.94	T39.95	T39.96
- - combination	T39.91	T39.92	T39.93	T39.94	T39.95	T39.96
- pyrazole	T39.2X1	T39.2X2	T39.2X3	T39.2X4	T39.2X5	T39.2X6
- specified NEC	T39.8X1	T39.8X2	T39.8X3	T39.8X4	T39.8X5	T39.8X6
Analgin	T39.2X1	T39.2X2	T39.2X3	T39.2X4	T39.2X5	T39.2X6
Anamirta cocculus	T62.1X1	T62.1X2	T62.1X3	T62.1X4	--	--
Ancillin	T36.0X1	T36.0X2	T36.0X3	T36.0X4	T36.0X5	T36.0X6
Ancrod	T45.691	T45.692	T45.693	T45.694	T45.695	T45.696
Androgen	T38.7X1	T38.7X2	T38.7X3	T38.7X4	T38.7X5	T38.7X6
Androgen-estrogen mixture	T38.7X1	T38.7X2	T38.7X3	T38.7X4	T38.7X5	T38.7X6
Androstalone	T38.7X1	T38.7X2	T38.7X3	T38.7X4	T38.7X5	T38.7X6
Androstanolone	T38.7X1	T38.7X2	T38.7X3	T38.7X4	T38.7X5	T38.7X6
Androsterone	T38.7X1	T38.7X2	T38.7X3	T38.7X4	T38.7X5	T38.7X6
Anemone pulsatilla	T62.2X1	T62.2X2	T62.2X3	T62.2X4	--	--
Anesthesia						
- caudal	T41.3X1	T41.3X2	T41.3X3	T41.3X4	T41.3X5	T41.3X6
- endotracheal	T41.0X1	T41.0X2	T41.0X3	T41.0X4	T41.0X5	T41.0X6
- epidural	T41.3X1	T41.3X2	T41.3X3	T41.3X4	T41.3X5	T41.3X6
- inhalation	T41.0X1	T41.0X2	T41.0X3	T41.0X4	T41.0X5	T41.0X6
- local	T41.3X1	T41.3X2	T41.3X3	T41.3X4	T41.3X5	T41.3X6
- mucosal	T41.3X1	T41.3X2	T41.3X3	T41.3X4	T41.3X5	T41.3X6
- muscle relaxation	T48.1X1	T48.1X2	T48.1X3	T48.1X4	T48.1X5	T48.1X6
- nerve blocking	T41.3X1	T41.3X2	T41.3X3	T41.3X4	T41.3X5	T41.3X6
- plexus blocking	T41.3X1	T41.3X2	T41.3X3	T41.3X4	T41.3X5	T41.3X6

Substance	Poisoning, Accidental (unintentional)	Poisoning, Intentional Self-harm	Poisoning, Assault	Poisoning, Undetermined	Adverse effect	Underdosing
- potentiated	T41.201	T41.202	T41.203	T41.204	T41.205	T41.206
- rectal	T41.201	T41.202	T41.203	T41.204	T41.205	T41.206
- - general	T41.201	T41.202	T41.203	T41.204	T41.205	T41.206
- - local	T41.3X1	T41.3X2	T41.3X3	T41.3X4	T41.3X5	T41.3X6
- regional	T41.3X1	T41.3X2	T41.3X3	T41.3X4	T41.3X5	T41.3X6
- surface	T41.3X1	T41.3X2	T41.3X3	T41.3X4	T41.3X5	T41.3X6
Anesthetic NEC—see also Anesthesia	T41.41	T41.42	T41.43	T41.44	T41.45	T41.46
- with muscle relaxant	T41.201	T41.202	T41.203	T41.204	T41.205	T41.206
- - general	T41.201	T41.202	T41.203	T41.204	T41.205	T41.206
- - local	T41.3X1	T41.3X2	T41.3X3	T41.3X4	T41.3X5	T41.3X6
- gaseous NEC	T41.0X1	T41.0X2	T41.0X3	T41.0X4	T41.0X5	T41.0X6
- general NEC	T41.201	T41.202	T41.203	T41.204	T41.205	T41.206
- halogenated hydrocarbon derivatives NEC	T41.0X1	T41.0X2	T41.0X3	T41.0X4	T41.0X5	T41.0X6
- infiltration NEC	T41.3X1	T41.3X2	T41.3X3	T41.3X4	T41.3X5	T41.3X6
- intravenous NEC	T41.1X1	T41.1X2	T41.1X3	T41.1X4	T41.1X5	T41.1X6
- local NEC	T41.3X1	T41.3X2	T41.3X3	T41.3X4	T41.3X5	T41.3X6
- rectal	T41.201	T41.202	T41.203	T41.204	T41.205	T41.206
- - general	T41.201	T41.202	T41.203	T41.204	T41.205	T41.206
- - local	T41.3X1	T41.3X2	T41.3X3	T41.3X4	T41.3X5	T41.3X6
- regional NEC	T41.3X1	T41.3X2	T41.3X3	T41.3X4	T41.3X5	T41.3X6
- spinal NEC	T41.3X1	T41.3X2	T41.3X3	T41.3X4	T41.3X5	T41.3X6
- thiobarbiturate	T41.1X1	T41.1X2	T41.1X3	T41.1X4	T41.1X5	T41.1X6
- topical	T41.3X1	T41.3X2	T41.3X3	T41.3X4	T41.3X5	T41.3X6
Aneurine	T45.2X1	T45.2X2	T45.2X3	T45.2X4	T45.2X5	T45.2X6
Angio-Conray	T50.8X1	T50.8X2	T50.8X3	T50.8X4	T50.8X5	T50.8X6
Angiotensin	T44.5X1	T44.5X2	T44.5X3	T44.5X4	T44.5X5	T44.5X6
Angiotensinamide	T44.991	T44.992	T44.993	T44.994	T44.995	T44.996
Anhydrohydroxy-progesterone	T38.5X1	T38.5X2	T38.5X3	T38.5X4	T38.5X5	T38.5X6
Anhydron	T50.2X1	T50.2X2	T50.2X3	T50.2X4	T50.2X5	T50.2X6
Anileridine	T40.4X1	T40.4X2	T40.4X3	T40.4X4	T40.4X5	T40.4X6
Aniline (dye) (liquid)	T65.3X1	T65.3X2	T65.3X3	T65.3X4	--	--
- analgesic	T39.1X1	T39.1X2	T39.1X3	T39.1X4	T39.1X5	T39.1X6
- derivatives, therapeutic NEC	T39.1X1	T39.1X2	T39.1X3	T39.1X4	T39.1X5	T39.1X6
- vapor	T65.3X1	T65.3X2	T65.3X3	T65.3X4	--	--
Aniscoropine	T44.3X1	T44.3X2	T44.3X3	T44.3X4	T44.3X5	T44.3X6
Anise oil	T47.5X1	T47.5X2	T47.5X3	T47.5X4	T47.5X5	T47.5X6
Anisidine	T65.3X1	T65.3X2	T65.3X3	T65.3X4	--	--
Anisindione	T45.511	T45.512	T45.513	T45.514	T45.515	T45.516
Anisotropine methyl-bromide	T44.3X1	T44.3X2	T44.3X3	T44.3X4	T44.3X5	T44.3X6
Anistreplase	T45.611	T45.612	T45.613	T45.614	T45.615	T45.616
Anorexiant (central)	T50.5X1	T50.5X2	T50.5X3	T50.5X4	T50.5X5	T50.5X6
Anorexic agents	T50.5X1	T50.5X2	T50.5X3	T50.5X4	T50.5X5	T50.5X6
Ansamycin	T36.6X1	T36.6X2	T36.6X3	T36.6X4	T36.6X5	T36.6X6
Ant (bite) (sting)	T63.421	T63.422	T63.423	T63.424	--	--
Ant poison—see Insecticide						
Antabuse	T50.6X1	T50.6X2	T50.6X3	T50.6X4	T50.6X5	T50.6X6
Antacid NEC	T47.1X1	T47.1X2	T47.1X3	T47.1X4	T47.1X5	T47.1X6
Antagonist						
- Aldosterone	T50.0X1	T50.0X2	T50.0X3	T50.0X4	T50.0X5	T50.0X6
- alpha-adrenoreceptor	T44.6X1	T44.6X2	T44.6X3	T44.6X4	T44.6X5	T44.6X6
- anticoagulant	T45.7X1	T45.7X2	T45.7X3	T45.7X4	T45.7X5	T45.7X6
- beta-adrenoreceptor	T44.7X1	T44.7X2	T44.7X3	T44.7X4	T44.7X5	T44.7X6
- extrapyramidal NEC	T44.3X1	T44.3X2	T44.3X3	T44.3X4	T44.3X5	T44.3X6
- folic acid	T45.1X1	T45.1X2	T45.1X3	T45.1X4	T45.1X5	T45.1X6
- H2 receptor	T47.0X1	T47.0X2	T47.0X3	T47.0X4	T47.0X5	T47.0X6
- heavy metal	T45.8X1	T45.8X2	T45.8X3	T45.8X4	T45.8X5	T45.8X6
- narcotic analgesic	T50.7X1	T50.7X2	T50.7X3	T50.7X4	T50.7X5	T50.7X6
- opiate	T50.7X1	T50.7X2	T50.7X3	T50.7X4	T50.7X5	T50.7X6
- pyrimidine	T45.1X1	T45.1X2	T45.1X3	T45.1X4	T45.1X5	T45.1X6
- serotonin	T46.5X1	T46.5X2	T46.5X3	T46.5X4	T46.5X5	T46.5X6
Antazolin (e)	T45.0X1	T45.0X2	T45.0X3	T45.0X4	T45.0X5	T45.0X6
Anterior pituitary hormone NEC	T38.811	T38.812	T38.813	T38.814	T38.815	T38.816
Anthelmintic NEC	T37.4X1	T37.4X2	T37.4X3	T37.4X4	T37.4X5	T37.4X6
Anthiolimine	T37.4X1	T37.4X2	T37.4X3	T37.4X4	T37.4X5	T37.4X6
Anthralin	T49.4X1	T49.4X2	T49.4X3	T49.4X4	T49.4X5	T49.4X6

Substance	Poisoning, Accidental (unintentional)	Poisoning, Intentional Self-harm	Poisoning, Assault	Poisoning, Undetermined	Adverse effect	Underdosing
Anthramycin	T45.1X1	T45.1X2	T45.1X3	T45.1X4	T45.1X5	T45.1X6
Antiadrenergic NEC	T44.8X1	T44.8X2	T44.8X3	T44.8X4	T44.8X5	T44.8X6
Antiallergic NEC	T45.0X1	T45.0X2	T45.0X3	T45.0X4	T45.0X5	T45.0X6
Anti-anemic (drug) (preparation)	T45.8X1	T45.8X2	T45.8X3	T45.8X4	T45.8X5	T45.8X6
Antiandrogen NEC	T38.6X1	T38.6X2	T38.6X3	T38.6X4	T38.6X5	T38.6X6
Antianxiety drug NEC	T43.501	T43.502	T43.503	T43.504	T43.505	T43.506
Antiaris toxicaria	T65.891	T65.892	T65.893	T65.894	--	--
Antiarteriosclerotic drug	T46.6X1	T46.6X2	T46.6X3	T46.6X4	T46.6X5	T46.6X6
Antiasthmatic drug NEC	T48.6X1	T48.6X2	T48.6X3	T48.6X4	T48.6X5	T48.6X6
Antibiotic NEC	T36.91	T36.92	T36.93	T36.94	T36.95	T36.96
- aminoglycoside	T36.5X1	T36.5X2	T36.5X3	T36.5X4	T36.5X5	T36.5X6
- anticancer	T45.1X1	T45.1X2	T45.1X3	T45.1X4	T45.1X5	T45.1X6
- antifungal	T36.7X1	T36.7X2	T36.7X3	T36.7X4	T36.7X5	T36.7X6
- antimycobacterial	T36.5X1	T36.5X2	T36.5X3	T36.5X4	T36.5X5	T36.5X6
- antineoplastic	T45.1X1	T45.1X2	T45.1X3	T45.1X4	T45.1X5	T45.1X6
- cephalosporin (group)	T36.1X1	T36.1X2	T36.1X3	T36.1X4	T36.1X5	T36.1X6
- chloramphenicol (group)	T36.2X1	T36.2X2	T36.2X3	T36.2X4	T36.2X5	T36.2X6
- ENT	T49.6X1	T49.6X2	T49.6X3	T49.6X4	T49.6X5	T49.6X6
- eye	T49.5X1	T49.5X2	T49.5X3	T49.5X4	T49.5X5	T49.5X6
- fungicidal (local)	T49.0X1	T49.0X2	T49.0X3	T49.0X4	T49.0X5	T49.0X6
- intestinal	T36.8X1	T36.8X2	T36.8X3	T36.8X4	T36.8X5	T36.8X6
- b-lactam NEC	T36.1X1	T36.1X2	T36.1X3	T36.1X4	T36.1X5	T36.1X6
- local	T49.0X1	T49.0X2	T49.0X3	T49.0X4	T49.0X5	T49.0X6
- macrolides	T36.3X1	T36.3X2	T36.3X3	T36.3X4	T36.3X5	T36.3X6
- polypeptide	T36.8X1	T36.8X2	T36.8X3	T36.8X4	T36.8X5	T36.8X6
- specified NEC	T36.8X1	T36.8X2	T36.8X3	T36.8X4	T36.8X5	T36.8X6
- tetracycline (group)	T36.4X1	T36.4X2	T36.4X3	T36.4X4	T36.4X5	T36.4X6
- throat	T49.6X1	T49.6X2	T49.6X3	T49.6X4	T49.6X5	T49.6X6
Anticancer agents NEC	T45.1X1	T45.1X2	T45.1X3	T45.1X4	T45.1X5	T45.1X6
Anticholesterolemic drug NEC	T46.6X1	T46.6X2	T46.6X3	T46.6X4	T46.6X5	T46.6X6
Anticholinergic NEC	T44.3X1	T44.3X2	T44.3X3	T44.3X4	T44.3X5	T44.3X6
Anticholinesterase	T44.0X1	T44.0X2	T44.0X3	T44.0X4	T44.0X5	T44.0X6
- organophosphorus	T44.0X1	T44.0X2	T44.0X3	T44.0X4	T44.0X5	T44.0X6
- - insecticide	T60.0X1	T60.0X2	T60.0X3	T60.0X4	--	--
- - nerve gas	T59.891	T59.892	T59.893	T59.894		
- reversible	T44.0X1	T44.0X2	T44.0X3	T44.0X4	T44.0X5	T44.0X6
- - ophthalmological	T49.5X1	T49.5X2	T49.5X3	T49.5X4	T49.5X5	T49.5X6
Anticoagulant NEC	T45.511	T45.512	T45.513	T45.514	T45.515	T45.516
- Antagonist	T45.7X1	T45.7X2	T45.7X3	T45.7X4	T45.7X5	T45.7X6
Anti-common-cold drug NEC	T48.5X1	T48.5X2	T48.5X3	T48.5X4	T48.5X5	T48.5X6
Anticonvulsant	T42.71	T42.72	T42.73	T42.74	T42.75	T42.76
- barbiturate	T42.3X1	T42.3X2	T42.3X3	T42.3X4	T42.3X5	T42.3X6
- combination (with barbiturate)	T42.3X1	T42.3X2	T42.3X3	T42.3X4	T42.3X5	T42.3X6
- hydantoin	T42.0X1	T42.0X2	T42.0X3	T42.0X4	T42.0X5	T42.0X6
- hypnotic NEC	T42.6X1	T42.6X2	T42.6X3	T42.6X4	T42.6X5	T42.6X6
- oxazolidinedione	T42.2X1	T42.2X2	T42.2X3	T42.2X4	T42.2X5	T42.2X6
- pyrimidinedione	T42.6X1	T42.6X2	T42.6X3	T42.6X4	T42.6X5	T42.6X6
- specified NEC	T42.6X1	T42.6X2	T42.6X3	T42.6X4	T42.6X5	T42.6X6
- succinimide	T42.2X1	T42.2X2	T42.2X3	T42.2X4	T42.2X5	T42.2X6
Anti-D immunoglobulin (human)	T50.Z11	T50.Z12	T50.Z13	T50.Z14	T50.Z15	T50.Z16
Antidepressant	T43.201	T43.202	T43.203	T43.204	T43.205	T43.206
- monoamine oxidase inhibitor	T43.1X1	T43.1X2	T43.1X3	T43.1X4	T43.1X5	T43.1X6
- selective serotonin norepinephrine reuptake inhibitor	T43.211	T43.212	T43.213	T43.214	T43.215	T43.216
- selective serotonin reuptake inhibitor	T43.221	T43.222	T43.223	T43.224	T43.225	T43.226
- specified NEC	T43.291	T43.292	T43.293	T43.294	T43.295	T43.296
- tetracyclic	T43.021	T43.022	T43.023	T43.024	T43.025	T43.026
- triazolopyridine	T43.211	T43.212	T43.213	T43.214	T43.215	T43.216
- tricyclic	T43.011	T43.012	T43.013	T43.014	T43.015	T43.016
Antidiabetic NEC	T38.3X1	T38.3X2	T38.3X3	T38.3X4	T38.3X5	T38.3X6
- biguanide	T38.3X1	T38.3X2	T38.3X3	T38.3X4	T38.3X5	T38.3X6
- - and sulfonyl combined	T38.3X1	T38.3X2	T38.3X3	T38.3X4	T38.3X5	T38.3X6
- combined	T38.3X1	T38.3X2	T38.3X3	T38.3X4	T38.3X5	T38.3X6
- sulfonylurea	T38.3X1	T38.3X2	T38.3X3	T38.3X4	T38.3X5	T38.3X6
Antidiarrheal drug NEC	T47.6X1	T47.6X2	T47.6X3	T47.6X4	T47.6X5	T47.6X6

Substance	Poisoning, Accidental (unintentional)	Poisoning, Intentional Self-harm	Poisoning, Assault	Poisoning, Undetermined	Adverse effect	Underdosing
- absorbent	T47.6X1	T47.6X2	T47.6X3	T47.6X4	T47.6X5	T47.6X6
Antidiphtheria serum	T50.Z11	T50.Z12	T50.Z13	T50.Z14	T50.Z15	T50.Z16
Antidiuretic hormone	T38.891	T38.892	T38.893	T38.894	T38.895	T38.896
Antidote NEC	T50.6X1	T50.6X2	T50.6X3	T50.6X4	T50.6X5	T50.6X6
- heavy metal	T45.8X1	T45.8X2	T45.8X3	T45.8X4	T45.8X5	T45.8X6
Antidysrhythmic NEC	T46.2X1	T46.2X2	T46.2X3	T46.2X4	T46.2X5	T46.2X6
Antiemetic drug	T45.0X1	T45.0X2	T45.0X3	T45.0X4	T45.0X5	T45.0X6
Antiepilepsy agent	T42.71	T42.72	T42.73	T42.74	T42.75	T42.76
- combination	T42.5X1	T42.5X2	T42.5X3	T42.5X4	T42.5X5	T42.5X6
- mixed	T42.5X1	T42.5X2	T42.5X3	T42.5X4	T42.5X5	T42.5X6
- specified, NEC	T42.6X1	T42.6X2	T42.6X3	T42.6X4	T42.6X5	T42.6X6
Antiestrogen NEC	T38.6X1	T38.6X2	T38.6X3	T38.6X4	T38.6X5	T38.6X6
Antifertility pill	T38.4X1	T38.4X2	T38.4X3	T38.4X4	T38.4X5	T38.4X6
Antifibrinolytic drug	T45.621	T45.622	T45.623	T45.624	T45.625	T45.626
Antifilarial drug	T37.4X1	T37.4X2	T37.4X3	T37.4X4	T37.4X5	T37.4X6
Antiflatulent	T47.5X1	T47.5X2	T47.5X3	T47.5X4	T47.5X5	T47.5X6
Antifreeze	T65.91	T65.92	T65.93	T65.94	--	--
- alcohol	T51.1X1	T51.1X2	T51.1X3	T51.1X4	--	--
- ethylene glycol	T51.8X1	T51.8X2	T51.8X3	T51.8X4	--	--
Antifungal						
- antibiotic (systemic)	T36.7X1	T36.7X2	T36.7X3	T36.7X4	T36.7X5	T36.7X6
- anti-infective NEC	T37.91	T37.92	T37.93	T37.94	T37.95	T37.96
- disinfectant, local	T49.0X1	T49.0X2	T49.0X3	T49.0X4	T49.0X5	T49.0X6
- nonmedicinal (spray)	T60.3X1	T60.3X2	T60.3X3	T60.3X4	--	--
- topical	T49.0X1	T49.0X2	T49.0X3	T49.0X4	T49.0X5	T49.0X6
Anti-gastric-secretion drug NEC	T47.1X1	T47.1X2	T47.1X3	T47.1X4	T47.1X5	T47.1X6
Antigonadotrophin NEC	T38.6X1	T38.6X2	T38.6X3	T38.6X4	T38.6X5	T38.6X6
Antihallucinogen	T43.501	T43.502	T43.503	T43.504	T43.505	T43.506
Antihelmintics	T37.4X1	T37.4X2	T37.4X3	T37.4X4	T37.4X5	T37.4X6
Antihemophilic						
- factor	T45.8X1	T45.8X2	T45.8X3	T45.8X4	T45.8X5	T45.8X6
- fraction	T45.8X1	T45.8X2	T45.8X3	T45.8X4	T45.8X5	T45.8X6
- globulin concentrate	T45.7X1	T45.7X2	T45.7X3	T45.7X4	T45.7X5	T45.7X6
- human plasma	T45.8X1	T45.8X2	T45.8X3	T45.8X4	T45.8X5	T45.8X6
- plasma, dried	T45.7X1	T45.7X2	T45.7X3	T45.7X4	T45.7X5	T45.7X6
Antihemorrhoidal preparation	T49.2X1	T49.2X2	T49.2X3	T49.2X4	T49.2X5	T49.2X6
Antiheparin drug	T45.7X1	T45.7X2	T45.7X3	T45.7X4	T45.7X5	T45.7X6
Antihistamine	T45.0X1	T45.0X2	T45.0X3	T45.0X4	T45.0X5	T45.0X6
Antihookworm drug	T37.4X1	T37.4X2	T37.4X3	T37.4X4	T37.4X5	T37.4X6
Anti-human lymphocytic globulin	T50.Z11	T50.Z12	T50.Z13	T50.Z14	T50.Z15	T50.Z16
Antihyperlipidemic drug	T46.6X1	T46.6X2	T46.6X3	T46.6X4	T46.6X5	T46.6X6
Antihypertensive drug NEC	T46.5X1	T46.5X2	T46.5X3	T46.5X4	T46.5X5	T46.5X6
Anti-infective NEC	T37.91	T37.92	T37.93	T37.94	T37.95	T37.96
- anthelmintic	T37.4X1	T37.4X2	T37.4X3	T37.4X4	T37.4X5	T37.4X6
- antibiotics	T36.91	T36.92	T36.93	T36.94	T36.95	T36.96
- - specified NEC	T36.8X1	T36.8X2	T36.8X3	T36.8X4	T36.8X5	T36.8X6
- antimalarial	T37.2X1	T37.2X2	T37.2X3	T37.2X4	T37.2X5	T37.2X6
- antimycobacterial NEC	T37.1X1	T37.1X2	T37.1X3	T37.1X4	T37.1X5	T37.1X6
- - antibiotics	T36.5X1	T36.5X2	T36.5X3	T36.5X4	T36.5X5	T36.5X6
- antiprotozoal NEC	T37.3X1	T37.3X2	T37.3X3	T37.3X4	T37.3X5	T37.3X6
- - blood	T37.2X1	T37.2X2	T37.2X3	T37.2X4	T37.2X5	T37.2X6
- antiviral	T37.5X1	T37.5X2	T37.5X3	T37.5X4	T37.5X5	T37.5X6
- arsenical	T37.8X1	T37.8X2	T37.8X3	T37.8X4	T37.8X5	T37.8X6
- bismuth, local	T49.0X1	T49.0X2	T49.0X3	T49.0X4	T49.0X5	T49.0X6
- ENT	T49.6X1	T49.6X2	T49.6X3	T49.6X4	T49.6X5	T49.6X6
- eye NEC	T49.5X1	T49.5X2	T49.5X3	T49.5X4	T49.5X5	T49.5X6
- heavy metals NEC	T37.8X1	T37.8X2	T37.8X3	T37.8X4	T37.8X5	T37.8X6
- local NEC	T49.0X1	T49.0X2	T49.0X3	T49.0X4	T49.0X5	T49.0X6
- - specified NEC	T49.0X1	T49.0X2	T49.0X3	T49.0X4	T49.0X5	T49.0X6
- mixed	T37.91	T37.92	T37.93	T37.94	T37.95	T37.96
- ophthalmic preparation	T49.5X1	T49.5X2	T49.5X3	T49.5X4	T49.5X5	T49.5X6
- topical NEC	T49.0X1	T49.0X2	T49.0X3	T49.0X4	T49.0X5	T49.0X6
Anti-inflammatory drug NEC	T39.391	T39.392	T39.393	T39.394	T39.395	T39.396
- local	T49.0X1	T49.0X2	T49.0X3	T49.0X4	T49.0X5	T49.0X6
- nonsteroidal NEC	T39.391	T39.392	T39.393	T39.394	T39.395	T39.396

Substance	Poisoning, Accidental (unintentional)	Poisoning, Intentional Self-harm	Poisoning, Assault	Poisoning, Undetermined	Adverse effect	Underdosing
- - propionic acid derivative	T39.311	T39.312	T39.313	T39.314	T39.315	T39.316
- specified NEC	T39.391	T39.392	T39.393	T39.394	T39.395	T39.396
Antikaluretic	T50.3X1	T50.3X2	T50.3X3	T50.3X4	T50.3X5	T50.3X6
Antiknock (tetraethyl lead)	T56.0X1	T56.0X2	T56.0X3	T56.0X4	--	--
Antilipemic drug NEC	T46.6X1	T46.6X2	T46.6X3	T46.6X4	T46.6X5	T46.6X6
Antimalarial	T37.2X1	T37.2X2	T37.2X3	T37.2X4	T37.2X5	T37.2X6
- prophylactic NEC	T37.2X1	T37.2X2	T37.2X3	T37.2X4	T37.2X5	T37.2X6
- pyrimidine derivative	T37.2X1	T37.2X2	T37.2X3	T37.2X4	T37.2X5	T37.2X6
Antimetabolite	T45.1X1	T45.1X2	T45.1X3	T45.1X4	T45.1X5	T45.1X6
Antimitotic agent	T45.1X1	T45.1X2	T45.1X3	T45.1X4	T45.1X5	T45.1X6
Antimony (compounds) (vapor) NEC	T56.891	T56.892	T56.893	T56.894	--	--
- anti-infectives	T37.8X1	T37.8X2	T37.8X3	T37.8X4	T37.8X5	T37.8X6
- dimercaptosuccinate	T37.3X1	T37.3X2	T37.3X3	T37.3X4	T37.3X5	T37.3X6
- hydride	T56.891	T56.892	T56.893	T56.894	--	--
- pesticide (vapor)	T60.8X1	T60.8X2	T60.8X3	T60.8X4	--	--
- potassium (sodium) tartrate	T37.8X1	T37.8X2	T37.8X3	T37.8X4	T37.8X5	T37.8X6
- sodium dimercaptosuccinate	T37.3X1	T37.3X2	T37.3X3	T37.3X4	T37.3X5	T37.3X6
- tartrated	T37.8X1	T37.8X2	T37.8X3	T37.8X4	T37.8X5	T37.8X6
Antimuscarinic NEC	T44.3X1	T44.3X2	T44.3X3	T44.3X4	T44.3X5	T44.3X6
Antimycobacterial drug NEC	T37.1X1	T37.1X2	T37.1X3	T37.1X4	T37.1X5	T37.1X6
- antibiotics	T36.5X1	T36.5X2	T36.5X3	T36.5X4	T36.5X5	T36.5X6
- combination	T37.1X1	T37.1X2	T37.1X3	T37.1X4	T37.1X5	T37.1X6
Antinausea drug	T45.0X1	T45.0X2	T45.0X3	T45.0X4	T45.0X5	T45.0X6
Antinematode drug	T37.4X1	T37.4X2	T37.4X3	T37.4X4	T37.4X5	T37.4X6
Antineoplastic NEC	T45.1X1	T45.1X2	T45.1X3	T45.1X4	T45.1X5	T45.1X6
- alkaloidal	T45.1X1	T45.1X2	T45.1X3	T45.1X4	T45.1X5	T45.1X6
- antibiotics	T45.1X1	T45.1X2	T45.1X3	T45.1X4	T45.1X5	T45.1X6
- combination	T45.1X1	T45.1X2	T45.1X3	T45.1X4	T45.1X5	T45.1X6
- - estrogen	T38.5X1	T38.5X2	T38.5X3	T38.5X4	T38.5X5	T38.5X6
- steroid	T38.7X1	T38.7X2	T38.7X3	T38.7X4	T38.7X5	T38.7X6
Antiparasitic drug (systemic)	T37.91	T37.92	T37.93	T37.94	T37.95	T37.96
- local	T49.0X1	T49.0X2	T49.0X3	T49.0X4	T49.0X5	T49.0X6
- specified NEC	T37.8X1	T37.8X2	T37.8X3	T37.8X4	T37.8X5	T37.8X6
Antiparkinsonism drug NEC	T42.8X1	T42.8X2	T42.8X3	T42.8X4	T42.8X5	T42.8X6
Antiperspirant NEC	T49.2X1	T49.2X2	T49.2X3	T49.2X4	T49.2X5	T49.2X6
Antiphlogistic NEC	T39.4X1	T39.4X2	T39.4X3	T39.4X4	T39.4X5	T39.4X6
Antiplatyhelmintic drug	T37.4X1	T37.4X2	T37.4X3	T37.4X4	T37.4X5	T37.4X6
Antiprotozoal drug NEC	T37.3X1	T37.3X2	T37.3X3	T37.3X4	T37.3X5	T37.3X6
- blood	T37.2X1	T37.2X2	T37.2X3	T37.2X4	T37.2X5	T37.2X6
- local	T49.0X1	T49.0X2	T49.0X3	T49.0X4	T49.0X5	T49.0X6
Antipruritic drug NEC	T49.1X1	T49.1X2	T49.1X3	T49.1X4	T49.1X5	T49.1X6
Antipsychotic drug	T43.501	T43.502	T43.503	T43.504	T43.505	T43.506
- specified NEC	T43.591	T43.592	T43.593	T43.594	T43.595	T43.596
Antipyretic	T39.91	T39.92	T39.93	T39.94	T39.95	T39.96
- specified NEC	T39.8X1	T39.8X2	T39.8X3	T39.8X4	T39.8X5	T39.8X6
Antipyrine	T39.2X1	T39.2X2	T39.2X3	T39.2X4	T39.2X5	T39.2X6
Antirabies hyperimmune serum	T50.Z11	T50.Z12	T50.Z13	T50.Z14	T50.Z15	T50.Z16
Antirheumatic NEC	T39.4X1	T39.4X2	T39.4X3	T39.4X4	T39.4X5	T39.4X6
Antirigidity drug NEC	T42.8X1	T42.8X2	T42.8X3	T42.8X4	T42.8X5	T42.8X6
Antischistosomal drug	T37.4X1	T37.4X2	T37.4X3	T37.4X4	T37.4X5	T37.4X6
Antiscorpion sera	T50.Z11	T50.Z12	T50.Z13	T50.Z14	T50.Z15	T50.Z16
Antiseborrheics	T49.4X1	T49.4X2	T49.4X3	T49.4X4	T49.4X5	T49.4X6
Antiseptics (external) (medicinal)	T49.0X1	T49.0X2	T49.0X3	T49.0X4	T49.0X5	T49.0X6
Antistine	T45.0X1	T45.0X2	T45.0X3	T45.0X4	T45.0X5	T45.0X6
Antitapeworm drug	T37.4X1	T37.4X2	T37.4X3	T37.4X4	T37.4X5	T37.4X6
Antitetanus immunoglobulin	T50.Z11	T50.Z12	T50.Z13	T50.Z14	T50.Z15	T50.Z16
Antithyroid drug NEC	T38.2X1	T38.2X2	T38.2X3	T38.2X4	T38.2X5	T38.2X6
Antitoxin	T50.Z11	T50.Z12	T50.Z13	T50.Z14	T50.Z15	T50.Z16
- diphtheria	T50.Z11	T50.Z12	T50.Z13	T50.Z14	T50.Z15	T50.Z16
- gas gangrene	T50.Z11	T50.Z12	T50.Z13	T50.Z14	T50.Z15	T50.Z16
- tetanus	T50.Z11	T50.Z12	T50.Z13	T50.Z14	T50.Z15	T50.Z16
Antitrichomonal drug	T37.3X1	T37.3X2	T37.3X3	T37.3X4	T37.3X5	T37.3X6
Antituberculars	T37.1X1	T37.1X2	T37.1X3	T37.1X4	T37.1X5	T37.1X6
- antibiotics	T36.5X1	T36.5X2	T36.5X3	T36.5X4	T36.5X5	T36.5X6
Antitussive NEC	T48.3X1	T48.3X2	T48.3X3	T48.3X4	T48.3X5	T48.3X6

Substance	Poisoning, Accidental (unintentional)	Poisoning, Intentional Self-harm	Poisoning, Assault	Poisoning, Undetermined	Adverse effect	Underdosing
- codeine mixture	T40.2X1	T40.2X2	T40.2X3	T40.2X4	T40.2X5	T40.2X6
- opiate	T40.2X1	T40.2X2	T40.2X3	T40.2X4	T40.2X5	T40.2X6
Antivaricose drug	T46.8X1	T46.8X2	T46.8X3	T46.8X4	T46.8X5	T46.8X6
Antivenin, antivenom (sera)	T50.Z11	T50.Z12	T50.Z13	T50.Z14	T50.Z15	T50.Z16
- crotaline	T50.Z11	T50.Z12	T50.Z13	T50.Z14	T50.Z15	T50.Z16
- spider bite	T50.Z11	T50.Z12	T50.Z13	T50.Z14	T50.Z15	T50.Z16
Antivertigo drug	T45.0X1	T45.0X2	T45.0X3	T45.0X4	T45.0X5	T45.0X6
Antiviral drug NEC	T37.5X1	T37.5X2	T37.5X3	T37.5X4	T37.5X5	T37.5X6
- eye	T49.5X1	T49.5X2	T49.5X3	T49.5X4	T49.5X5	T49.5X6
Antiwhipworm drug	T37.4X1	T37.4X2	T37.4X3	T37.4X4	T37.4X5	T37.4X6
Antrol—see also by specific chemical	T60.91	T60.92	T60.93	T60.94	--	--substance
- fungicide	T60.91	T60.92	T60.93	T60.94	--	--
ANTU (alpha naphthylthiourea)	T60.4X1	T60.4X2	T60.4X3	T60.4X4	--	--
Apalcillin	T36.0X1	T36.0X2	T36.0X3	T36.0X4	T36.0X5	T36.0X6
APC	T48.5X1	T48.5X2	T48.5X3	T48.5X4	T48.5X5	T48.5X6
Aplonidine	T44.4X1	T44.4X2	T44.4X3	T44.4X4	T44.4X5	T44.4X6
Apomorphine	T47.7X1	T47.7X2	T47.7X3	T47.7X4	T47.7X5	T47.7X6
Appetite depressants, central	T50.5X1	T50.5X2	T50.5X3	T50.5X4	T50.5X5	T50.5X6
Apraclonidine (hydrochloride)	T44.4X1	T44.4X2	T44.4X3	T44.4X4	T44.4X5	T44.4X6
Apresoline	T46.5X1	T46.5X2	T46.5X3	T46.5X4	T46.5X5	T46.5X6
Aprindine	T46.2X1	T46.2X2	T46.2X3	T46.2X4	T46.2X5	T46.2X6
Aprobarbital	T42.3X1	T42.3X2	T42.3X3	T42.3X4	T42.3X5	T42.3X6
Apronalide	T42.6X1	T42.6X2	T42.6X3	T42.6X4	T42.6X5	T42.6X6
Aprotinin	T45.621	T45.622	T45.623	T45.624	T45.625	T45.626
Aptocaine	T41.3X1	T41.3X2	T41.3X3	T41.3X4	T41.3X5	T41.3X6
Aqua fortis	T54.2X1	T54.2X2	T54.2X3	T54.2X4	--	--
Ara-A	T37.5X1	T37.5X2	T37.5X3	T37.5X4	T37.5X5	T37.5X6
Ara-C	T45.1X1	T45.1X2	T45.1X3	T45.1X4	T45.1X5	T45.1X6
Arachis oil	T49.3X1	T49.3X2	T49.3X3	T49.3X4	T49.3X5	T49.3X6
- cathartic	T47.4X1	T47.4X2	T47.4X3	T47.4X4	T47.4X5	T47.4X6
Aralen	T37.2X1	T37.2X2	T37.2X3	T37.2X4	T37.2X5	T37.2X6
Arecoline	T44.1X1	T44.1X2	T44.1X3	T44.1X4	T44.1X5	T44.1X6
Arginine	T50.991	T50.992	T50.993	T50.994	T50.995	T50.996
- glutamate	T50.991	T50.992	T50.993	T50.994	T50.995	T50.996
Argyrol	T49.0X1	T49.0X2	T49.0X3	T49.0X4	T49.0X5	T49.0X6
- EN	T agent	T49.6X1	T49.6X2	T49.6X3	T49.6X4	T49.6X5
T49.6X6						
- ophthalmic preparation	T49.5X1	T49.5X2	T49.5X3	T49.5X4	T49.5X5	T49.5X6
Aristocort	T38.0X1	T38.0X2	T38.0X3	T38.0X4	T38.0X5	T38.0X6
- ENT agent	T49.6X1	T49.6X2	T49.6X3	T49.6X4	T49.6X5	T49.6X6
- ophthalmic preparation	T49.5X1	T49.5X2	T49.5X3	T49.5X4	T49.5X5	T49.5X6
- topical NEC	T49.0X1	T49.0X2	T49.0X3	T49.0X4	T49.0X5	T49.0X6
Aromatics, corrosive	T54.1X1	T54.1X2	T54.1X3	T54.1X4	--	--
- disinfectants	T54.1X1	T54.1X2	T54.1X3	T54.1X4	--	--
Arsenate of lead	T57.0X1	T57.0X2	T57.0X3	T57.0X4	--	--
- herbicide	T57.0X1	T57.0X2	T57.0X3	T57.0X4	--	--
Arsenic, arsenicals (compounds) (dust) (vapor) NEC	T57.0X1	T57.0X2	T57.0X3	T57.0X4	--	--
- anti-infectives	T37.8X1	T37.8X2	T37.8X3	T37.8X4	T37.8X5	T37.8X6
- pesticide (dust) (fumes)	T57.0X1	T57.0X2	T57.0X3	T57.0X4	--	--
Arsine (gas)	T57.0X1	T57.0X2	T57.0X3	T57.0X4	--	--
Arsphenamine (silver)	T37.8X1	T37.8X2	T37.8X3	T37.8X4	T37.8X5	T37.8X6
Arsthinol	T37.3X1	T37.3X2	T37.3X3	T37.3X4	T37.3X5	T37.3X6
Artane	T44.3X1	T44.3X2	T44.3X3	T44.3X4	T44.3X5	T44.3X6
Arthropod (venomous) NEC	T63.481	T63.482	T63.483	T63.484	--	--
Articaine	T41.3X1	T41.3X2	T41.3X3	T41.3X4	T41.3X5	T41.3X6
Asbestos	T57.8X1	T57.8X2	T57.8X3	T57.8X4	--	--
Ascaridole	T37.4X1	T37.4X2	T37.4X3	T37.4X4	T37.4X5	T37.4X6
Ascorbic acid	T45.2X1	T45.2X2	T45.2X3	T45.2X4	T45.2X5	T45.2X6
Asiaticoside	T49.0X1	T49.0X2	T49.0X3	T49.0X4	T49.0X5	T49.0X6
Asparaginase	T45.1X1	T45.1X2	T45.1X3	T45.1X4	T45.1X5	T45.1X6
Aspidium (oleoresin)	T37.4X1	T37.4X2	T37.4X3	T37.4X4	T37.4X5	T37.4X6
Aspirin (aluminum) (soluble)	T39.011	T39.012	T39.013	T39.014	T39.015	T39.016
Aspoxicillin	T36.0X1	T36.0X2	T36.0X3	T36.0X4	T36.0X5	T36.0X6
Astemizole	T45.0X1	T45.0X2	T45.0X3	T45.0X4	T45.0X5	T45.0X6

Substance	Poisoning, Accidental (unintentional)	Poisoning, Intentional Self-harm	Poisoning, Assault	Poisoning, Undetermined	Adverse effect	Underdosing
Astringent (local)	T49.2X1	T49.2X2	T49.2X3	T49.2X4	T49.2X5	T49.2X6
- specified NEC	T49.2X1	T49.2X2	T49.2X3	T49.2X4	T49.2X5	T49.2X6
Astromicin	T36.5X1	T36.5X2	T36.5X3	T36.5X4	T36.5X5	T36.5X6
Ataractic drug NEC	T43.501	T43.502	T43.503	T43.504	T43.505	T43.506
Atenolol	T44.7X1	T44.7X2	T44.7X3	T44.7X4	T44.7X5	T44.7X6
Atonia drug, intestinal	T47.4X1	T47.4X2	T47.4X3	T47.4X4	T47.4X5	T47.4X6
Atophan	T50.4X1	T50.4X2	T50.4X3	T50.4X4	T50.4X5	T50.4X6
Atracurium besilate	T48.1X1	T48.1X2	T48.1X3	T48.1X4	T48.1X5	T48.1X6
Atropine	T44.3X1	T44.3X2	T44.3X3	T44.3X4	T44.3X5	T44.3X6
- derivative	T44.3X1	T44.3X2	T44.3X3	T44.3X4	T44.3X5	T44.3X6
- methonitrate	T44.3X1	T44.3X2	T44.3X3	T44.3X4	T44.3X5	T44.3X6
Attapulgite	T47.6X1	T47.6X2	T47.6X3	T47.6X4	T47.6X5	T47.6X6
Auramine	T65.891	T65.892	T65.893	T65.894	--	--
- dye	T65.6X1	T65.6X2	T65.6X3	T65.6X4	--	--
- fungicide	T60.3X1	T60.3X2	T60.3X3	T60.3X4	--	--
Auranofin	T39.4X1	T39.4X2	T39.4X3	T39.4X4	T39.4X5	T39.4X6
Aurantiin	T46.991	T46.992	T46.993	T46.994	T46.995	T46.996
Aureomycin	T36.4X1	T36.4X2	T36.4X3	T36.4X4	T36.4X5	T36.4X6
- ophthalmic preparation	T49.5X1	T49.5X2	T49.5X3	T49.5X4	T49.5X5	T49.5X6
- topical NEC	T49.0X1	T49.0X2	T49.0X3	T49.0X4	T49.0X5	T49.0X6
Aurothioglucose	T39.4X1	T39.4X2	T39.4X3	T39.4X4	T39.4X5	T39.4X6
Aurothioglycanide	T39.4X1	T39.4X2	T39.4X3	T39.4X4	T39.4X5	T39.4X6
Aurothiomalate sodium	T39.4X1	T39.4X2	T39.4X3	T39.4X4	T39.4X5	T39.4X6
Aurotioprol	T39.4X1	T39.4X2	T39.4X3	T39.4X4	T39.4X5	T39.4X6
Automobile fuel	T52.0X1	T52.0X2	T52.0X3	T52.0X4	--	--
Autonomic nervous system agent NEC	T44.901	T44.902	T44.903	T44.904	T44.905	T44.906
Avlosulfon	T37.1X1	T37.1X2	T37.1X3	T37.1X4	T37.1X5	T37.1X6
Avomine	T42.6X1	T42.6X2	T42.6X3	T42.6X4	T42.6X5	T42.6X6
Axerophthol	T45.2X1	T45.2X2	T45.2X3	T45.2X4	T45.2X5	T45.2X6
Azacitidine	T45.1X1	T45.1X2	T45.1X3	T45.1X4	T45.1X5	T45.1X6
Azacyclonol	T43.591	T43.592	T43.593	T43.594	T43.595	T43.596
Azadirachta	T60.2X1	T60.2X2	T60.2X3	T60.2X4	--	--
Azanidazole	T37.3X1	T37.3X2	T37.3X3	T37.3X4	T37.3X5	T37.3X6
Azapetine	T46.7X1	T46.7X2	T46.7X3	T46.7X4	T46.7X5	T46.7X6
Azapropazone	T39.2X1	T39.2X2	T39.2X3	T39.2X4	T39.2X5	T39.2X6
Azaribine	T45.1X1	T45.1X2	T45.1X3	T45.1X4	T45.1X5	T45.1X6
Azaserine	T45.1X1	T45.1X2	T45.1X3	T45.1X4	T45.1X5	T45.1X6
Azatadine	T45.0X1	T45.0X2	T45.0X3	T45.0X4	T45.0X5	T45.0X6
Azatepa	T45.1X1	T45.1X2	T45.1X3	T45.1X4	T45.1X5	T45.1X6
Azathioprine	T45.1X1	T45.1X2	T45.1X3	T45.1X4	T45.1X5	T45.1X6
Azelaic acid	T49.0X1	T49.0X2	T49.0X3	T49.0X4	T49.0X5	T49.0X6
Azelastine	T45.0X1	T45.0X2	T45.0X3	T45.0X4	T45.0X5	T45.0X6
Azidocillin	T36.0X1	T36.0X2	T36.0X3	T36.0X4	T36.0X5	T36.0X6
Azidothymidine	T37.5X1	T37.5X2	T37.5X3	T37.5X4	T37.5X5	T37.5X6
Azinphos (ethyl) (methyl)	T60.0X1	T60.0X2	T60.0X3	T60.0X4	--	--
Aziridine (chelating)	T54.1X1	T54.1X2	T54.1X3	T54.1X4	--	--
Azithromycin	T36.3X1	T36.3X2	T36.3X3	T36.3X4	T36.3X5	T36.3X6
Azlocillin	T36.0X1	T36.0X2	T36.0X3	T36.0X4	T36.0X5	T36.0X6
Azobenzene smoke	T65.3X1	T65.3X2	T65.3X3	T65.3X4	--	--
- acaricide	T60.8X1	T60.8X2	T60.8X3	T60.8X4	--	--
Azosulfamide	T37.0X1	T37.0X2	T37.0X3	T37.0X4	T37.0X5	T37.0X6
AZT	T37.5X1	T37.5X2	T37.5X3	T37.5X4	T37.5X5	T37.5X6
Aztreonam	T36.1X1	T36.1X2	T36.1X3	T36.1X4	T36.1X5	T36.1X6
Azulfidine	T37.0X1	T37.0X2	T37.0X3	T37.0X4	T37.0X5	T37.0X6
Azurcsin	T50.8X1	T50.8X2	T50.8X3	T50.8X4	T50.8X5	T50.8X6
Bacampicillin	T36.0X1	T36.0X2	T36.0X3	T36.0X4	T36.0X5	T36.0X6
Bacillus						
- lactobacillus	T47.8X1	T47.8X2	T47.8X3	T47.8X4	T47.8X5	T47.8X6
- subtilis	T47.6X1	T47.6X2	T47.6X3	T47.6X4	T47.6X5	T47.6X6
Bacimycin	T49.0X1	T49.0X2	T49.0X3	T49.0X4	T49.0X5	T49.0X6
- ophthalmic preparation	T49.5X1	T49.5X2	T49.5X3	T49.5X4	T49.5X5	T49.5X6
Bacitracin zinc	T49.0X1	T49.0X2	T49.0X3	T49.0X4	T49.0X5	T49.0X6
- with neomycin	T49.0X1	T49.0X2	T49.0X3	T49.0X4	T49.0X5	T49.0X6
- ENT agent	T49.6X1	T49.6X2	T49.6X3	T49.6X4	T49.6X5	T49.6X6
- ophthalmic preparation	T49.5X1	T49.5X2	T49.5X3	T49.5X4	T49.5X5	T49.5X6

Substance	Poisoning, Accidental (unintentional)	Poisoning, Intentional Self-harm	Poisoning, Assault	Poisoning, Undetermined	Adverse effect	Underdosing
- topical NEC	T49.0X1	T49.0X2	T49.0X3	T49.0X4	T49.0X5	T49.0X6
Baclofen	T42.8X1	T42.8X2	T42.8X3	T42.8X4	T42.8X5	T42.8X6
Baking soda	T50.991	T50.992	T50.993	T50.994	T50.995	T50.996
BAL	T45.8X1	T45.8X2	T45.8X3	T45.8X4	T45.8X5	T45.8X6
Bambuterol	T48.6X1	T48.6X2	T48.6X3	T48.6X4	T48.6X5	T48.6X6
Bamethan (sulfate)	T46.7X1	T46.7X2	T46.7X3	T46.7X4	T46.7X5	T46.7X6
Bamifylline	T48.6X1	T48.6X2	T48.6X3	T48.6X4	T48.6X5	T48.6X6
Bamipine	T45.0X1	T45.0X2	T45.0X3	T45.0X4	T45.0X5	T45.0X6
Baneberry—see Actaea spicata						
Banewort—see Belladonna						
Barbenyl	T42.3X1	T42.3X2	T42.3X3	T42.3X4	T42.3X5	T42.3X6
Barbexaclone	T42.6X1	T42.6X2	T42.6X3	T42.6X4	T42.6X5	T42.6X6
Barbital	T42.3X1	T42.3X2	T42.3X3	T42.3X4	T42.3X5	T42.3X6
- sodium	T42.3X1	T42.3X2	T42.3X3	T42.3X4	T42.3X5	T42.3X6
Barbitone	T42.3X1	T42.3X2	T42.3X3	T42.3X4	T42.3X5	T42.3X6
Barbiturate NEC	T42.3X1	T42.3X2	T42.3X3	T42.3X4	T42.3X5	T42.3X6
- with tranquilizer	T42.3X1	T42.3X2	T42.3X3	T42.3X4	T42.3X5	T42.3X6
- anesthetic (intravenous)	T41.1X1	T41.1X2	T41.1X3	T41.1X4	T41.1X5	T41.1X6
Barium (carbonate) (chloride) (sulfite)	T57.8X1	T57.8X2	T57.8X3	T57.8X4	--	--
- diagnostic agent	T50.8X1	T50.8X2	T50.8X3	T50.8X4	T50.8X5	T50.8X6
- pesticide	T60.4X1	T60.4X2	T60.4X3	T60.4X4	--	--
- rodenticide	T60.4X1	T60.4X2	T60.4X3	T60.4X4	--	--
- sulfate (medicinal)	T50.8X1	T50.8X2	T50.8X3	T50.8X4	T50.8X5	T50.8X6
Barrier cream	T49.3X1	T49.3X2	T49.3X3	T49.3X4	T49.3X5	T49.3X6
Basic fuchsin	T49.0X1	T49.0X2	T49.0X3	T49.0X4	T49.0X5	T49.0X6
Battery acid or fluid	T54.2X1	T54.2X2	T54.2X3	T54.2X4	--	--
Bay rum	T51.8X1	T51.8X2	T51.8X3	T51.8X4	--	--
BCG (vaccine)	T50.A91	T50.A92	T50.A93	T50.A94	T50.A95	T50.A96
BCNU	T45.1X1	T45.1X2	T45.1X3	T45.1X4	T45.1X5	T45.1X6
Bearsfoot	T62.2X1	T62.2X2	T62.2X3	T62.2X4	--	--
Beclamide	T42.6X1	T42.6X2	T42.6X3	T42.6X4	T42.6X5	T42.6X6
Beclomethasone	T44.5X1	T44.5X2	T44.5X3	T44.5X4	T44.5X5	T44.5X6
Bee (sting) (venom)	T63.441	T63.442	T63.443	T63.444	--	--
Befunolol	T49.5X1	T49.5X2	T49.5X3	T49.5X4	T49.5X5	T49.5X6
Bekanamycin	T36.5X1	T36.5X2	T36.5X3	T36.5X4	T36.5X5	T36.5X6
Belladonna—see also Nightshade						
- alkaloids	T44.3X1	T44.3X2	T44.3X3	T44.3X4	T44.3X5	T44.3X6
- extract	T44.3X1	T44.3X2	T44.3X3	T44.3X4	T44.3X5	T44.3X6
- herb	T44.3X1	T44.3X2	T44.3X3	T44.3X4	T44.3X5	T44.3X6
Bemegride	T50.7X1	T50.7X2	T50.7X3	T50.7X4	T50.7X5	T50.7X6
Benactyzine	T44.3X1	T44.3X2	T44.3X3	T44.3X4	T44.3X5	T44.3X6
Benadryl	T45.0X1	T45.0X2	T45.0X3	T45.0X4	T45.0X5	T45.0X6
Benaprizine	T44.3X1	T44.3X2	T44.3X3	T44.3X4	T44.3X5	T44.3X6
Benazepril	T46.4X1	T46.4X2	T46.4X3	T46.4X4	T46.4X5	T46.4X6
Bencyclane	T46.7X1	T46.7X2	T46.7X3	T46.7X4	T46.7X5	T46.7X6
Bendazol	T46.3X1	T46.3X2	T46.3X3	T46.3X4	T46.3X5	T46.3X6
Bendrofluazide	T50.2X1	T50.2X2	T50.2X3	T50.2X4	T50.2X5	T50.2X6
Bendroflumethiazide	T50.2X1	T50.2X2	T50.2X3	T50.2X4	T50.2X5	T50.2X6
Benemid	T50.4X1	T50.4X2	T50.4X3	T50.4X4	T50.4X5	T50.4X6
Benethamine penicillin	T36.0X1	T36.0X2	T36.0X3	T36.0X4	T36.0X5	T36.0X6
Benexate	T47.1X1	T47.1X2	T47.1X3	T47.1X4	T47.1X5	T47.1X6
Benfluorex	T46.6X1	T46.6X2	T46.6X3	T46.6X4	T46.6X5	T46.6X6
Benfotiamine	T45.2X1	T45.2X2	T45.2X3	T45.2X4	T45.2X5	T45.2X6
Benisone	T49.0X1	T49.0X2	T49.0X3	T49.0X4	T49.0X5	T49.0X6
Benomyl	T60.0X1	T60.0X2	T60.0X3	T60.0X4	--	--
Benoquin	T49.8X1	T49.8X2	T49.8X3	T49.8X4	T49.8X5	T49.8X6
Benoxinate	T41.3X1	T41.3X2	T41.3X3	T41.3X4	T41.3X5	T41.3X6
Benperidol	T43.4X1	T43.4X2	T43.4X3	T43.4X4	T43.4X5	T43.4X6
Benproperine	T48.3X1	T48.3X2	T48.3X3	T48.3X4	T48.3X5	T48.3X6
Benserazide	T42.8X1	T42.8X2	T42.8X3	T42.8X4	T42.8X5	T42.8X6
Bentazepam	T42.4X1	T42.4X2	T42.4X3	T42.4X4	T42.4X5	T42.4X6
Bentiromide	T50.8X1	T50.8X2	T50.8X3	T50.8X4	T50.8X5	T50.8X6
Bentonite	T49.3X1	T49.3X2	T49.3X3	T49.3X4	T49.3X5	T49.3X6
Benzalbutyramide	T46.6X1	T46.6X2	T46.6X3	T46.6X4	T46.6X5	T46.6X6
Benzalkonium (chloride)	T49.0X1	T49.0X2	T49.0X3	T49.0X4	T49.0X5	T49.0X6

Substance	Poisoning, Accidental (unintentional)	Poisoning, Intentional Self-harm	Poisoning, Assault	Poisoning, Undetermined	Adverse effect	Underdosing
- ophthalmic preparation	T49.5X1	T49.5X2	T49.5X3	T49.5X4	T49.5X5	T49.5X6
Benzamidosalicylate (calcium)	T37.1X1	T37.1X2	T37.1X3	T37.1X4	T37.1X5	T37.1X6
Benzamine	T41.3X1	T41.3X2	T41.3X3	T41.3X4	T41.3X5	T41.3X6
- lactate	T49.1X1	T49.1X2	T49.1X3	T49.1X4	T49.1X5	T49.1X6
Benzamphetamine	T50.5X1	T50.5X2	T50.5X3	T50.5X4	T50.5X5	T50.5X6
Benzapril hydrochloride	T46.5X1	T46.5X2	T46.5X3	T46.5X4	T46.5X5	T46.5X6
Benzathine benzylpenicillin	T36.0X1	T36.0X2	T36.0X3	T36.0X4	T36.0X5	T36.0X6
Benzathine penicillin	T36.0X1	T36.0X2	T36.0X3	T36.0X4	T36.0X5	T36.0X6
Benzatropine	T42.8X1	T42.8X2	T42.8X3	T42.8X4	T42.8X5	T42.8X6
Benzbromarone	T50.4X1	T50.4X2	T50.4X3	T50.4X4	T50.4X5	T50.4X6
Benzcarbimine	T45.1X1	T45.1X2	T45.1X3	T45.1X4	T45.1X5	T45.1X6
Benzedrex	T44.991	T44.992	T44.993	T44.994	T44.995	T44.996
Benzedrine (amphetamine)	T43.621	T43.622	T43.623	T43.624	T43.625	T43.626
Benzenamine	T65.3X1	T65.3X2	T65.3X3	T65.3X4	--	--
Benzene	T52.1X1	T52.1X2	T52.1X3	T52.1X4	--	--
- homologues (acetyl) (dimethyl) (methyl) (solvent)	T52.2X1	T52.2X2	T52.2X3	T52.2X4	--	--
Benzethonium (chloride)	T49.0X1	T49.0X2	T49.0X3	T49.0X4	T49.0X5	T49.0X6
Benzfetamine	T50.5X1	T50.5X2	T50.5X3	T50.5X4	T50.5X5	T50.5X6
Benzhexol	T44.3X1	T44.3X2	T44.3X3	T44.3X4	T44.3X5	T44.3X6
Benzhydramine (chloride)	T45.0X1	T45.0X2	T45.0X3	T45.0X4	T45.0X5	T45.0X6
Benzidine	T65.891	T65.892	T65.893	T65.894	--	--
Benzilonium bromide	T44.3X1	T44.3X2	T44.3X3	T44.3X4	T44.3X5	T44.3X6
Benzimidazole	T60.3X1	T60.3X2	T60.3X3	T60.3X4	--	--
Benzin (e) —see Ligroin						
Benziodarone	T46.3X1	T46.3X2	T46.3X3	T46.3X4	T46.3X5	T46.3X6
Benznidazole	T37.3X1	T37.3X2	T37.3X3	T37.3X4	T37.3X5	T37.3X6
Benzocaine	T41.3X1	T41.3X2	T41.3X3	T41.3X4	T41.3X5	T41.3X6
Benzodiapin	T42.4X1	T42.4X2	T42.4X3	T42.4X4	T42.4X5	T42.4X6
Benzodiazepine NEC	T42.4X1	T42.4X2	T42.4X3	T42.4X4	T42.4X5	T42.4X6
Benzoic acid	T49.0X1	T49.0X2	T49.0X3	T49.0X4	T49.0X5	T49.0X6
- with salicylic acid	T49.0X1	T49.0X2	T49.0X3	T49.0X4	T49.0X5	T49.0X6
Benzoin (tincture)	T48.5X1	T48.5X2	T48.5X3	T48.5X4	T48.5X5	T48.5X6
Benzol (benzene)	T52.1X1	T52.1X2	T52.1X3	T52.1X4	--	--
- vapor	T52.0X1	T52.0X2	T52.0X3	T52.0X4	--	--
Benzomorphan	T40.2X1	T40.2X2	T40.2X3	T40.2X4	T40.2X5	T40.2X6
Benzonatate	T48.3X1	T48.3X2	T48.3X3	T48.3X4	T48.3X5	T48.3X6
Benzophenones	T49.3X1	T49.3X2	T49.3X3	T49.3X4	T49.3X5	T49.3X6
Benzopyrone	T46.991	T46.992	T46.993	T46.994	T46.995	T46.996
Benzothiadiazides	T50.2X1	T50.2X2	T50.2X3	T50.2X4	T50.2X5	T50.2X6
Benzoxonium chloride	T49.0X1	T49.0X2	T49.0X3	T49.0X4	T49.0X5	T49.0X6
Benzoyl peroxide	T49.0X1	T49.0X2	T49.0X3	T49.0X4	T49.0X5	T49.0X6
Benzoylpas calcium	T37.1X1	T37.1X2	T37.1X3	T37.1X4	T37.1X5	T37.1X6
Benzperidin	T43.591	T43.592	T43.593	T43.594	T43.595	T43.596
Benzperidol	T43.591	T43.592	T43.593	T43.594	T43.595	T43.596
Benzphetamine	T50.5X1	T50.5X2	T50.5X3	T50.5X4	T50.5X5	T50.5X6
Benzpyrinium bromide	T44.1X1	T44.1X2	T44.1X3	T44.1X4	T44.1X5	T44.1X6
Benzquinamide	T45.0X1	T45.0X2	T45.0X3	T45.0X4	T45.0X5	T45.0X6
Benzthiazide	T50.2X1	T50.2X2	T50.2X3	T50.2X4	T50.2X5	T50.2X6
Benztropine						
- anticholinergic	T44.3X1	T44.3X2	T44.3X3	T44.3X4	T44.3X5	T44.3X6
- antiparkinson	T42.8X1	T42.8X2	T42.8X3	T42.8X4	T42.8X5	T42.8X6
Benzydamine	T49.0X1	T49.0X2	T49.0X3	T49.0X4	T49.0X5	T49.0X6
Benzyl						
- acetate	T52.8X1	T52.8X2	T52.8X3	T52.8X4	--	--
alcohol	T49.0X1	T49.0X2	T49.0X3	T49.0X4	T49.0X5	T49.0X6
- benzoate	T49.0X1	T49.0X2	T49.0X3	T49.0X4	T49.0X5	T49.0X6
- Benzoic acid	T49.0X1	T49.0X2	T49.0X3	T49.0X4	T49.0X5	T49.0X6
- morphine	T40.2X1	T40.2X2	T40.2X3	T40.2X4	--	--
- nicotinate	T46.6X1	T46.6X2	T46.6X3	T46.6X4	T46.6X5	T46.6X6
- penicillin	T36.0X1	T36.0X2	T36.0X3	T36.0X4	T36.0X5	T36.0X6
Benzylhydrochlorthia-zide	T50.2X1	T50.2X2	T50.2X3	T50.2X4	T50.2X5	T50.2X6
Benzylpenicillin	T36.0X1	T36.0X2	T36.0X3	T36.0X4	T36.0X5	T36.0X6
Benzylthiouracil	T38.2X1	T38.2X2	T38.2X3	T38.2X4	T38.2X5	T38.2X6
Bephenium hydroxy-naphthoate	T37.4X1	T37.4X2	T37.4X3	T37.4X4	T37.4X5	T37.4X6
Bepridil	T46.1X1	T46.1X2	T46.1X3	T46.1X4	T46.1X5	T46.1X6

Substance	Poisoning, Accidental (unintentional)	Poisoning, Intentional Self-harm	Poisoning, Assault	Poisoning, Undetermined	Adverse effect	Underdosing
Bergamot oil	T65.891	T65.892	T65.893	T65.894	--	--
Bergapten	T50.991	T50.992	T50.993	T50.994	T50.995	T50.996
Berries, poisonous	T62.1X1	T62.1X2	T62.1X3	T62.1X4	--	--
Beryllium (compounds)	T56.7X1	T56.7X2	T56.7X3	T56.7X4	--	--
b-acetyldigoxin	T46.0X1	T46.0X2	T46.0X3	T46.0X4	T46.0X5	T46.0X6
beta adrenergic blocking agent, heart	T44.7X1	T44.7X2	T44.7X3	T44.7X4	T44.7X5	T44.7X6
b-benzalbutyramide	T46.6X1	T46.6X2	T46.6X3	T46.6X4	T46.6X5	T46.6X6
Betacarotene	T45.2X1	T45.2X2	T45.2X3	T45.2X4	T45.2X5	T45.2X6
b-eucaine	T49.1X1	T49.1X2	T49.1X3	T49.1X4	T49.1X5	T49.1X6
Beta-Chlor	T42.6X1	T42.6X2	T42.6X3	T42.6X4	T42.6X5	T42.6X6
b-galactosidase	T47.5X1	T47.5X2	T47.5X3	T47.5X4	T47.5X5	T47.5X6
Betahistine	T46.7X1	T46.7X2	T46.7X3	T46.7X4	T46.7X5	T46.7X6
Betaine	T47.5X1	T47.5X2	T47.5X3	T47.5X4	T47.5X5	T47.5X6
Betamethasone	T49.0X1	T49.0X2	T49.0X3	T49.0X4	T49.0X5	T49.0X6
- topical	T49.0X1	T49.0X2	T49.0X3	T49.0X4	T49.0X5	T49.0X6
Betamicin	T36.8X1	T36.8X2	T36.8X3	T36.8X4	T36.8X5	T36.8X6
Betanidine	T46.5X1	T46.5X2	T46.5X3	T46.5X4	T46.5X5	T46.5X6
b-sitosterol (s)	T46.6X1	T46.6X2	T46.6X3	T46.6X4	T46.6X5	T46.6X6
Betaxolol	T44.7X1	T44.7X2	T44.7X3	T44.7X4	T44.7X5	T44.7X6
Betazole	T50.8X1	T50.8X2	T50.8X3	T50.8X4	T50.8X5	T50.8X6
Bethanechol	T44.1X1	T44.1X2	T44.1X3	T44.1X4	T44.1X5	T44.1X6
- chloride	T44.1X1	T44.1X2	T44.1X3	T44.1X4	T44.1X5	T44.1X6
Bethanidine	T46.5X1	T46.5X2	T46.5X3	T46.5X4	T46.5X5	T46.5X6
Betoxycaine	T41.3X1	T41.3X2	T41.3X3	T41.3X4	T41.3X5	T41.3X6
Betula oil	T49.3X1	T49.3X2	T49.3X3	T49.3X4	T49.3X5	T49.3X6
Bevantolol	T44.7X1	T44.7X2	T44.7X3	T44.7X4	T44.7X5	T44.7X6
Bevonium metilsulfate	T44.3X1	T44.3X2	T44.3X3	T44.3X4	T44.3X5	T44.3X6
Bezafibrate	T46.6X1	T46.6X2	T46.6X3	T46.6X4	T46.6X5	T46.6X6
Bezitramide	T40.4X1	T40.4X2	T40.4X3	T40.4X4	T40.4X5	T40.4X6
BHA	T50.991	T50.992	T50.993	T50.994	T50.995	T50.996
Bhang	T40.7X1	T40.7X2	T40.7X3	T40.7X4	T40.7X5	T40.7X6
BHC (medicinal)	T49.0X1	T49.0X2	T49.0X3	T49.0X4	T49.0X5	T49.0X6
- nonmedicinal (vapor)	T53.6X1	T53.6X2	T53.6X3	T53.6X4	--	--
Bialamicol	T37.3X1	T37.3X2	T37.3X3	T37.3X4	T37.3X5	T37.3X6
Bibenzonium bromide	T48.3X1	T48.3X2	T48.3X3	T48.3X4	T48.3X5	T48.3X6
Bibrocathol	T49.5X1	T49.5X2	T49.5X3	T49.5X4	T49.5X5	T49.5X6
Bichloride of mercury—see Mercury, chloride						
Bichromates (calcium) (potassium) (sodium)	T57.8X1	T57.8X2	T57.8X3	T57.8X4	--	-- (crystals)
- fumes	T56.2X1	T56.2X2	T56.2X3	T56.2X4	--	--
Biclotymol	T49.6X1	T49.6X2	T49.6X3	T49.6X4	T49.6X5	T49.6X6
Bicuculline	T50.7X1	T50.7X2	T50.7X3	T50.7X4	T50.7X5	T50.7X6
Bifemelane	T43.291	T43.292	T43.293	T43.294	T43.295	T43.296
Biguanide derivatives, oral	T38.3X1	T38.3X2	T38.3X3	T38.3X4	T38.3X5	T38.3X6
Bile salts	T47.5X1	T47.5X2	T47.5X3	T47.5X4	T47.5X5	T47.5X6
Biligrafin	T50.8X1	T50.8X2	T50.8X3	T50.8X4	T50.8X5	T50.8X6
Bilopaque	T50.8X1	T50.8X2	T50.8X3	T50.8X4	T50.8X5	T50.8X6
Binifibrate	T46.6X1	T46.6X2	T46.6X3	T46.6X4	T46.6X5	T46.6X6
Binitrobenzol	T65.3X1	T65.3X2	T65.3X3	T65.3X4	--	--
Bioflavonoid (s)	T46.991	T46.992	T46.993	T46.994	T46.995	T46.996
Biological substance NEC	T50.901	T50.902	T50.903	T50.904	T50.905	T50.906
Biotin	T45.2X1	T45.2X2	T45.2X3	T45.2X4	T45.2X5	T45.2X6
Biperiden	T44.3X1	T44.3X2	T44.3X3	T44.3X4	T44.3X5	T44.3X6
Bisacodyl	T47.2X1	T47.2X2	T47.2X3	T47.2X4	T47.2X5	T47.2X6
Bisbentiamine	T45.2X1	T45.2X2	T45.2X3	T45.2X4	T45.2X5	T45.2X6
Bisbutiamine	T45.2X1	T45.2X2	T45.2X3	T45.2X4	T45.2X5	T45.2X6
Bisdequalinium (salts) (diacetate)	T49.6X1	T49.6X2	T49.6X3	T49.6X4	T49.6X5	T49.6X6
Bishydroxycoumarin	T45.511	T45.512	T45.513	T45.514	T45.515	T45.516
Bismarsen	T37.8X1	T37.8X2	T37.8X3	T37.8X4	T37.8X5	T37.8X6
Bismuth salts	T47.6X1	T47.6X2	T47.6X3	T47.6X4	T47.6X5	T47.6X6
- aluminate	T47.1X1	T47.1X2	T47.1X3	T47.1X4	T47.1X5	T47.1X6
- anti-infectives	T37.8X1	T37.8X2	T37.8X3	T37.8X4	T37.8X5	T37.8X6
- formic iodide	T49.0X1	T49.0X2	T49.0X3	T49.0X4	T49.0X5	T49.0X6
- glycolylarsenate	T49.0X1	T49.0X2	T49.0X3	T49.0X4	T49.0X5	T49.0X6
- nonmedicinal (compounds) NEC	T65.91	T65.92	T65.93	T65.94	--	--
- subcarbonate	T47.6X1	T47.6X2	T47.6X3	T47.6X4	T47.6X5	T47.6X6

Substance	Poisoning, Accidental (unintentional)	Poisoning, Intentional Self-harm	Poisoning, Assault	Poisoning, Undetermined	Adverse effect	Underdosing
- subsalicylate	T37.8X1	T37.8X2	T37.8X3	T37.8X4	T37.8X5	T37.8X6
- sulfarsphenamine	T37.8X1	T37.8X2	T37.8X3	T37.8X4	T37.8X5	T37.8X6
Bisoprolol	T44.7X1	T44.7X2	T44.7X3	T44.7X4	T44.7X5	T44.7X6
Bisoxatin	T47.2X1	T47.2X2	T47.2X3	T47.2X4	T47.2X5	T47.2X6
Bisulepin (hydrochloride)	T45.0X1	T45.0X2	T45.0X3	T45.0X4	T45.0X5	T45.0X6
Bithionol	T37.8X1	T37.8X2	T37.8X3	T37.8X4	T37.8X5	T37.8X6
- anthelminthic	T37.4X1	T37.4X2	T37.4X3	T37.4X4	T37.4X5	T37.4X6
Bitolterol	T48.6X1	T48.6X2	T48.6X3	T48.6X4	T48.6X5	T48.6X6
Bitoscanate	T37.4X1	T37.4X2	T37.4X3	T37.4X4	T37.4X5	T37.4X6
Bitter almond oil	T62.8X1	T62.8X2	T62.8X3	T62.8X4	--	--
Bittersweet	T62.2X1	T62.2X2	T62.2X3	T62.2X4	--	--
Black						
- flag	T60.91	T60.92	T60.93	T60.94	--	--
- henbane	T62.2X1	T62.2X2	T62.2X3	T62.2X4	--	--
- leaf (40)	T60.91	T60.92	T60.93	T60.94	--	--
- widow spider (bite)	T63.311	T63.312	T63.313	T63.314	--	--
antivenin	T50.Z11	T50.Z12	T50.Z13	T50.Z14	T50.Z15	T50.Z16
Blast furnace gas (carbon monoxide from)	T58.8X1	T58.8X2	T58.8X3	T58.8X4	--	--
Bleach	T54.91	T54.92	T54.93	T54.94		
Bleaching agent (medicinal)	T49.4X1	T49.4X2	T49.4X3	T49.4X4	T49.4X5	T49.4X6
Bleomycin	T45.1X1	T45.1X2	T45.1X3	T45.1X4	T45.1X5	T45.1X6
Blockain	T41.3X1	T41.3X2	T41.3X3	T41.3X4	T41.3X5	T41.3X6
- infiltration (subcutaneous)	T41.3X1	T41.3X2	T41.3X3	T41.3X4	T41.3X5	T41.3X6
- nerve block (peripheral) (plexus)	T41.3X1	T41.3X2	T41.3X3	T41.3X4	T41.3X5	T41.3X6
- topical (surface)	T41.3X1	T41.3X2	T41.3X3	T41.3X4	T41.3X5	T41.3X6
Blockers, calcium channel	T46.1X1	T46.1X2	T46.1X3	T46.1X4	T46.1X5	T46.1X6
Blood (derivatives) (natural) (plasma) (whole)	T45.8X1	T45.8X2	T45.8X3	T45.8X4	T45.8X5	T45.8X6
- dried	T45.8X1	T45.8X2	T45.8X3	T45.8X4	T45.8X5	T45.8X6
- drug affecting NEC	T45.91	T45.92	T45.93	T45.94	T45.95	T45.96
- expander NEC	T45.8X1	T45.8X2	T45.8X3	T45.8X4	T45.8X5	T45.8X6
- fraction NEC	T45.8X1	T45.8X2	T45.8X3	T45.8X4	T45.8X5	T45.8X6
- substitute (macromolecular)	T45.8X1	T45.8X2	T45.8X3	T45.8X4	T45.8X5	T45.8X6
Blue velvet	T40.2X1	T40.2X2	T40.2X3	T40.2X4	--	--
Bone meal	T62.8X1	T62.8X2	T62.8X3	T62.8X4	--	--
Bonine	T45.0X1	T45.0X2	T45.0X3	T45.0X4	T45.0X5	T45.0X6
Bopindolol	T44.7X1	T44.7X2	T44.7X3	T44.7X4	T44.7X5	T44.7X6
Boracic acid	T49.0X1	T49.0X2	T49.0X3	T49.0X4	T49.0X5	T49.0X6
- ENT agent	T49.6X1	T49.6X2	T49.6X3	T49.6X4	T49.6X5	T49.6X6
- ophthalmic preparation	T49.5X1	T49.5X2	T49.5X3	T49.5X4	T49.5X5	T49.5X6
Borane complex	T57.8X1	T57.8X2	T57.8X3	T57.8X4	--	--
Borate (s)	T57.8X1	T57.8X2	T57.8X3	T57.8X4	--	--
- buffer	T50.991	T50.992	T50.993	T50.994	T50.995	T50.996
- cleanser	T54.91	T54.92	T54.93	T54.94	--	--
- sodium	T57.8X1	T57.8X2	T57.8X3	T57.8X4	--	--
Borax (cleanser)	T54.91	T54.92	T54.93	T54.94	--	--
Bordeaux mixture	T60.3X1	T60.3X2	T60.3X3	T60.3X4	--	--
Boric acid	T49.0X1	T49.0X2	T49.0X3	T49.0X4	T49.0X5	T49.0X6
- ENT agent	T49.6X1	T49.6X2	T49.6X3	T49.6X4	T49.6X5	T49.6X6
- ophthalmic preparation	T49.5X1	T49.5X2	T49.5X3	T49.5X4	T49.5X5	T49.5X6
Bornaprine	T44.3X1	T44.3X2	T44.3X3	T44.3X4	T44.3X5	T44.3X6
Boron	T57.8X1	T57.8X2	T57.8X3	T57.8X4	--	--
- hydride NEC	T57.8X1	T57.8X2	T57.8X3	T57.8X4	--	--
- - fumes or gas	T57.8X1	T57.8X2	T57.8X3	T57.8X4	--	--
- trifluoride	T59.891	T59.892	T59.893	T59.894	--	--
Botox	T48.291	T48.292	T48.293	T48.294	T48.295	T48.296
Botulinus anti-toxin (type A, B)	T50.Z11	T50.Z12	T50.Z13	T50.Z14	T50.Z15	T50.Z16
Brake fluid vapor	T59.891	T59.892	T59.893	T59.894	--	--
Brallobarbital	T42.3X1	T42.3X2	T42.3X3	T42.3X4	T42.3X5	T42.3X6
Bran (wheat)	T47.4X1	T47.4X2	T47.4X3	T47.4X4	T47.4X5	T47.4X6
Brass (fumes)	T56.891	T56.892	T56.893	T56.894	--	--
Brasso	T52.0X1	T52.0X2	T52.0X3	T52.0X4	--	--
Bretylium tosilate	T46.2X1	T46.2X2	T46.2X3	T46.2X4	T46.2X5	T46.2X6
Brevital (sodium)	T41.1X1	T41.1X2	T41.1X3	T41.1X4	T41.1X5	T41.1X6
Brinase	T45.3X1	T45.3X2	T45.3X3	T45.3X4	T45.3X5	T45.3X6
British antilewisite	T45.8X1	T45.8X2	T45.8X3	T45.8X4	T45.8X5	T45.8X6

Substance	Poisoning, Accidental (unintentional)	Poisoning, Intentional Self-harm	Poisoning, Assault	Poisoning, Undetermined	Adverse effect	Underdosing
Brodifacoum	T60.4X1	T60.4X2	T60.4X3	T60.4X4	--	--
Bromal (hydrate)	T42.6X1	T42.6X2	T42.6X3	T42.6X4	T42.6X5	T42.6X6
Bromazepam	T42.4X1	T42.4X2	T42.4X3	T42.4X4	T42.4X5	T42.4X6
Bromazine	T45.0X1	T45.0X2	T45.0X3	T45.0X4	T45.0X5	T45.0X6
Brombenzylcyanide	T59.3X1	T59.3X2	T59.3X3	T59.3X4	--	--
Bromelains	T45.3X1	T45.3X2	T45.3X3	T45.3X4	T45.3X5	T45.3X6
Bromethalin	T60.4X1	T60.4X2	T60.4X3	T60.4X4	--	--
Bromhexine	T48.4X1	T48.4X2	T48.4X3	T48.4X4	T48.4X5	T48.4X6
Bromide salts	T42.6X1	T42.6X2	T42.6X3	T42.6X4	T42.6X5	T42.6X6
Bromindione	T45.511	T45.512	T45.513	T45.514	T45.515	T45.516
Bromine						
- compounds (medicinal)	T42.6X1	T42.6X2	T42.6X3	T42.6X4	T42.6X5	T42.6X6
- sedative	T42.6X1	T42.6X2	T42.6X3	T42.6X4	T42.6X5	T42.6X6
- vapor	T59.891	T59.892	T59.893	T59.894	--	--
Bromisoval	T42.6X1	T42.6X2	T42.6X3	T42.6X4	T42.6X5	T42.6X6
Bromisovalum	T42.6X1	T42.6X2	T42.6X3	T42.6X4	T42.6X5	T42.6X6
Bromobenzylcyanide	T59.3X1	T59.3X2	T59.3X3	T59.3X4	--	--
Bromochlorosalicylani-lide	T49.0X1	T49.0X2	T49.0X3	T49.0X4	T49.0X5	T49.0X6
Bromocriptine	T42.8X1	T42.8X2	T42.8X3	T42.8X4	T42.8X5	T42.8X6
Bromodiphenhydramine	T45.0X1	T45.0X2	T45.0X3	T45.0X4	T45.0X5	T45.0X6
Bromoform	T42.6X1	T42.6X2	T42.6X3	T42.6X4	T42.6X5	T42.6X6
Bromophenol blue reagent	T50.991	T50.992	T50.993	T50.994	T50.995	T50.996
Bromopride	T47.8X1	T47.8X2	T47.8X3	T47.8X4	T47.8X5	T47.8X6
Bromosalicylchloranitide	T49.0X1	T49.0X2	T49.0X3	T49.0X4	T49.0X5	T49.0X6
Bromosalicylhydroxamic acid	T37.1X1	T37.1X2	T37.1X3	T37.1X4	T37.1X5	T37.1X6
Bromo-seltzer	T39.1X1	T39.1X2	T39.1X3	T39.1X4	T39.1X5	T39.1X6
Bromoxynil	T60.3X1	T60.3X2	T60.3X3	T60.3X4	--	--
Bromperidol	T43.4X1	T43.4X2	T43.4X3	T43.4X4	T43.4X5	T43.4X6
Brompheniramine	T45.0X1	T45.0X2	T45.0X3	T45.0X4	T45.0X5	T45.0X6
Bromsulfophthalein	T50.8X1	T50.8X2	T50.8X3	T50.8X4	T50.8X5	T50.8X6
Bromural	T42.6X1	T42.6X2	T42.6X3	T42.6X4	T42.6X5	T42.6X6
Bromvaletone	T42.6X1	T42.6X2	T42.6X3	T42.6X4	T42.6X5	T42.6X6
Bronchodilator NEC	T48.6X1	T48.6X2	T48.6X3	T48.6X4	T48.6X5	T48.6X6
Brotizolam	T42.4X1	T42.4X2	T42.4X3	T42.4X4	T42.4X5	T42.4X6
Brovincamine	T46.7X1	T46.7X2	T46.7X3	T46.7X4	T46.7X5	T46.7X6
Brown recluse spider (bite) (venom)	T63.331	T63.332	T63.333	T63.334	--	--
Brown spider (bite) (venom)	T63.391	T63.392	T63.393	T63.394	--	--
Broxaterol	T48.6X1	T48.6X2	T48.6X3	T48.6X4	T48.6X5	T48.6X6
Broxuridine	T45.1X1	T45.1X2	T45.1X3	T45.1X4	T45.1X5	T45.1X6
Broxyquinoline	T37.8X1	T37.8X2	T37.8X3	T37.8X4	T37.8X5	T37.8X6
Bruceine	T48.291	T48.292	T48.293	T48.294	T48.295	T48.296
Brucia	T62.2X1	T62.2X2	T62.2X3	T62.2X4	--	--
Brucine	T65.1X1	T65.1X2	T65.1X3	T65.1X4	--	--
Brunswick green—see Copper						
Bruten—see Ibuprofen						
Bryonia	T47.2X1	T47.2X2	T47.2X3	T47.2X4	T47.2X5	T47.2X6
Buclizine	T45.0X1	T45.0X2	T45.0X3	T45.0X4	T45.0X5	T45.0X6
Buclosamide	T49.0X1	T49.0X2	T49.0X3	T49.0X4	T49.0X5	T49.0X6
Budesonide	T44.5X1	T44.5X2	T44.5X3	T44.5X4	T44.5X5	T44.5X6
Budralazine	T46.5X1	T46.5X2	T46.5X3	T46.5X4	T46.5X5	T46.5X6
Bufferin	T39.011	T39.012	T39.013	T39.014	T39.015	T39.016
Buflomedil	T46.7X1	T46.7X2	T46.7X3	T46.7X4	T46.7X5	T46.7X6
Buformin	T38.3X1	T38.3X2	T38.3X3	T38.3X4	T38.3X5	T38.3X6
Bufotenine	T40.991	T40.992	T40.993	T40.994	--	--
Bufrolin	T48.6X1	T48.6X2	T48.6X3	T48.6X4	T48.6X5	T48.6X6
Bufylline	T48.6X1	T48.6X2	T48.6X3	T48.6X4	T48.6X5	T48.6X6
Bulk filler	T50.5X1	T50.5X2	T50.5X3	T50.5X4	T50.5X5	T50.5X6
- cathartic	T47.4X1	T47.4X2	T47.4X3	T47.4X4	T47.4X5	T47.4X6
Bumetanide	T50.1X1	T50.1X2	T50.1X3	T50.1X4	T50.1X5	T50.1X6
Bunaftine	T46.2X1	T46.2X2	T46.2X3	T46.2X4	T46.2X5	T46.2X6
Bunamiodyl	T50.8X1	T50.8X2	T50.8X3	T50.8X4	T50.8X5	T50.8X6
Bunazosin	T44.6X1	T44.6X2	T44.6X3	T44.6X4	T44.6X5	T44.6X6
Bunitrolol	T44.7X1	T44.7X2	T44.7X3	T44.7X4	T44.7X5	T44.7X6
Buphenine	T46.7X1	T46.7X2	T46.7X3	T46.7X4	T46.7X5	T46.7X6
Bupivacaine	T41.3X1	T41.3X2	T41.3X3	T41.3X4	T41.3X5	T41.3X6

Substance	Poisoning, Accidental (unintentional)	Poisoning, Intentional Self-harm	Poisoning, Assault	Poisoning, Undetermined	Adverse effect	Underdosing
- infiltration (subcutaneous)	T41.3X1	T41.3X2	T41.3X3	T41.3X4	T41.3X5	T41.3X6
- nerve block (peripheral) (plexus)	T41.3X1	T41.3X2	T41.3X3	T41.3X4	T41.3X5	T41.3X6
- spinal	T41.3X1	T41.3X2	T41.3X3	T41.3X4	T41.3X5	T41.3X6
Bupranolol	T44.7X1	T44.7X2	T44.7X3	T44.7X4	T44.7X5	T44.7X6
Buprenorphine	T40.4X1	T40.4X2	T40.4X3	T40.4X4	T40.4X5	T40.4X6
Bupropion	T43.291	T43.292	T43.293	T43.294	T43.295	T43.296
Burimamide	T47.1X1	T47.1X2	T47.1X3	T47.1X4	T47.1X5	T47.1X6
Buserelin	T38.891	T38.892	T38.893	T38.894	T38.895	T38.896
Buspirone	T43.591	T43.592	T43.593	T43.594	T43.595	T43.596
Busulfan, busulphan	T45.1X1	T45.1X2	T45.1X3	T45.1X4	T45.1X5	T45.1X6
Butabarbital (sodium)	T42.3X1	T42.3X2	T42.3X3	T42.3X4	T42.3X5	T42.3X6
Butabarbitone	T42.3X1	T42.3X2	T42.3X3	T42.3X4	T42.3X5	T42.3X6
Butabarpal	T42.3X1	T42.3X2	T42.3X3	T42.3X4	T42.3X5	T42.3X6
Butacaine	T41.3X1	T41.3X2	T41.3X3	T41.3X4	T41.3X5	T41.3X6
Butalamine	T46.7X1	T46.7X2	T46.7X3	T46.7X4	T46.7X5	T46.7X6
Butalbital	T42.3X1	T42.3X2	T42.3X3	T42.3X4	T42.3X5	T42.3X6
Butallylonal	T42.3X1	T42.3X2	T42.3X3	T42.3X4	T42.3X5	T42.3X6
Butamben	T41.3X1	T41.3X2	T41.3X3	T41.3X4	T41.3X5	T41.3X6
Butamirate	T48.3X1	T48.3X2	T48.3X3	T48.3X4	T48.3X5	T48.3X6
Butane (distributed in mobile container)	T59.891	T59.892	T59.893	T59.894	--	--
- distributed through pipes	T59.891	T59.892	T59.893	T59.894	--	--
- incomplete combustion	T58.11	T58.12	T58.13	T58.14	--	--
Butanilicaine	T41.3X1	T41.3X2	T41.3X3	T41.3X4	T41.3X5	T41.3X6
Butanol	T51.3X1	T51.3X2	T51.3X3	T51.3X4	--	--
Butanone, 2-butanone	T52.4X1	T52.4X2	T52.4X3	T52.4X4	--	--
Butantrone	T49.4X1	T49.4X2	T49.4X3	T49.4X4	T49.4X5	T49.4X6
Butaperazine	T43.3X1	T43.3X2	T43.3X3	T43.3X4	T43.3X5	T43.3X6
Butazolidin	T39.2X1	T39.2X2	T39.2X3	T39.2X4	T39.2X5	T39.2X6
Butetamate	T48.6X1	T48.6X2	T48.6X3	T48.6X4	T48.6X5	T48.6X6
Butethal	T42.3X1	T42.3X2	T42.3X3	T42.3X4	T42.3X5	T42.3X6
Butethamate	T44.3X1	T44.3X2	T44.3X3	T44.3X4	T44.3X5	T44.3X6
Buthalitone (sodium)	T41.1X1	T41.1X2	T41.1X3	T41.1X4	T41.1X5	T41.1X6
Butisol (sodium)	T42.3X1	T42.3X2	T42.3X3	T42.3X4	T42.3X5	T42.3X6
Butizide	T50.2X1	T50.2X2	T50.2X3	T50.2X4	T50.2X5	T50.2X6
Butobarbital	T42.3X1	T42.3X2	T42.3X3	T42.3X4	T42.3X5	T42.3X6
- sodium	T42.3X1	T42.3X2	T42.3X3	T42.3X4	T42.3X5	T42.3X6
Butobarbitone	T42.3X1	T42.3X2	T42.3X3	T42.3X4	T42.3X5	T42.3X6
Butoconazole (nitrate)	T49.0X1	T49.0X2	T49.0X3	T49.0X4	T49.0X5	T49.0X6
Butorphanol	T40.4X1	T40.4X2	T40.4X3	T40.4X4	T40.4X5	T40.4X6
Butriptyline	T43.011	T43.012	T43.013	T43.014	T43.015	T43.016
Butropium bromide	T44.3X1	T44.3X2	T44.3X3	T44.3X4	T44.3X5	T44.3X6
Butter of antimony—see Antimony						
Buttercups	T62.2X1	T62.2X2	T62.2X3	T62.2X4	--	--
Butyl						
- acetate (secondary)	T52.8X1	T52.8X2	T52.8X3	T52.8X4	--	--
- alcohol	T51.3X1	T51.3X2	T51.3X3	T51.3X4	--	--
- aminobenzoate	T41.3X1	T41.3X2	T41.3X3	T41.3X4	T41.3X5	T41.3X6
- butyrate	T52.8X1	T52.8X2	T52.8X3	T52.8X4	--	--
- carbinol	T51.3X1	T51.3X2	T51.3X3	T51.3X4	--	--
- carbitol	T52.3X1	T52.3X2	T52.3X3	T52.3X4	--	--
- cellosolve	T52.3X1	T52.3X2	T52.3X3	T52.3X4	--	--
- chloral (hydrate)	T42.6X1	T42.6X2	T42.6X3	T42.6X4	T42.6X5	T42.6X6
- formate	T52.8X1	T52.8X2	T52.8X3	T52.8X4	--	--
- lactate	T52.8X1	T52.8X2	T52.8X3	T52.8X4	--	--
- propionate	T52.8X1	T52.8X2	T52.8X3	T52.8X4	--	--
- scopolamine bromide	T44.3X1	T44.3X2	T44.3X3	T44.3X4	T44.3X5	T44.3X6
- thiobarbital sodium	T41.1X1	T41.1X2	T41.1X3	T41.1X4	T41.1X5	T41.1X6
Butylated hydroxy-anisole	T50.991	T50.992	T50.993	T50.994	T50.995	T50.996
Butylchloral hydrate	T42.6X1	T42.6X2	T42.6X3	T42.6X4	T42.6X5	T42.6X6
Butyltoluene	T52.2X1	T52.2X2	T52.2X3	T52.2X4	--	--
Butyn	T41.3X1	T41.3X2	T41.3X3	T41.3X4	T41.3X5	T41.3X6
Butyrophenone (-based tranquilizers)	T43.4X1	T43.4X2	T43.4X3	T43.4X4	T43.4X5	T43.4X6
Cabergoline	T42.8X1	T42.8X2	T42.8X3	T42.8X4	T42.8X5	T42.8X6
Cacodyl, cacodylic acid	T57.0X1	T57.0X2	T57.0X3	T57.0X4	--	--
Cactinomycin	T45.1X1	T45.1X2	T45.1X3	T45.1X4	T45.1X5	T45.1X6

Substance	Poisoning, Accidental (unintentional)	Poisoning, Intentional Self-harm	Poisoning, Assault	Poisoning, Undetermined	Adverse effect	Underdosing
Cade oil	T49.4X1	T49.4X2	T49.4X3	T49.4X4	T49.4X5	T49.4X6
Cadexomer iodine	T49.0X1	T49.0X2	T49.0X3	T49.0X4	T49.0X5	T49.0X6
Cadmium (chloride) (fumes) (oxide)	T56.3X1	T56.3X2	T56.3X3	T56.3X4	--	--
- sulfide (medicinal) NEC	T49.4X1	T49.4X2	T49.4X3	T49.4X4	T49.4X5	T49.4X6
Cadralazine	T46.5X1	T46.5X2	T46.5X3	T46.5X4	T46.5X5	T46.5X6
Caffeine	T43.611	T43.612	T43.613	T43.614	T43.615	T43.616
Calabar bean	T62.2X1	T62.2X2	T62.2X3	T62.2X4	--	--
Caladium seguinum	T62.2X1	T62.2X2	T62.2X3	T62.2X4	--	--
Calamine (lotion)	T49.3X1	T49.3X2	T49.3X3	T49.3X4	T49.3X5	T49.3X6
Calcifediol	T45.2X1	T45.2X2	T45.2X3	T45.2X4	T45.2X5	T45.2X6
Calciferol	T45.2X1	T45.2X2	T45.2X3	T45.2X4	T45.2X5	T45.2X6
Calcitonin	T50.991	T50.992	T50.993	T50.994	T50.995	T50.996
Calcitriol	T45.2X1	T45.2X2	T45.2X3	T45.2X4	T45.2X5	T45.2X6
Calcium	T50.3X1	T50.3X2	T50.3X3	T50.3X4	T50.3X5	T50.3X6
- actylsalicylate	T39.011	T39.012	T39.013	T39.014	T39.015	T39.016
- benzamidosalicylate	T37.1X1	T37.1X2	T37.1X3	T37.1X4	T37.1X5	T37.1X6
- bromide	T42.6X1	T42.6X2	T42.6X3	T42.6X4	T42.6X5	T42.6X6
- bromolactobionate	T42.6X1	T42.6X2	T42.6X3	T42.6X4	T42.6X5	T42.6X6
- carbaspirin	T39.011	T39.012	T39.013	T39.014	T39.015	T39.016
- carbimide	T50.6X1	T50.6X2	T50.6X3	T50.6X4	T50.6X5	T50.6X6
- carbonate	T47.1X1	T47.1X2	T47.1X3	T47.1X4	T47.1X5	T47.1X6
- chloride	T50.991	T50.992	T50.993	T50.994	T50.995	T50.996
- - anhydrous	T50.991	T50.992	T50.993	T50.994	T50.995	T50.996
- cyanide	T57.8X1	T57.8X2	T57.8X3	T57.8X4	--	--
- dioctyl sulfosuccinate	T47.4X1	T47.4X2	T47.4X3	T47.4X4	T47.4X5	T47.4X6
- disodium edathamil	T45.8X1	T45.8X2	T45.8X3	T45.8X4	T45.8X5	T45.8X6
- disodium edetate	T45.8X1	T45.8X2	T45.8X3	T45.8X4	T45.8X5	T45.8X6
- dobesilate	T46.991	T46.992	T46.993	T46.994	T46.995	T46.996
- EDTA	T45.8X1	T45.8X2	T45.8X3	T45.8X4	T45.8X5	T45.8X6
- ferrous citrate	T45.4X1	T45.4X2	T45.4X3	T45.4X4	T45.4X5	T45.4X6
- folinate	T45.8X1	T45.8X2	T45.8X3	T45.8X4	T45.8X5	T45.8X6
- glubionate	T50.3X1	T50.3X2	T50.3X3	T50.3X4	T50.3X5	T50.3X6
- gluconate	T50.3X1	T50.3X2	T50.3X3	T50.3X4	T50.3X5	T50.3X6
- gluconogalactogluc-onate	T50.3X1	T50.3X2	T50.3X3	T50.3X4	T50.3X5	T50.3X6
- hydrate, hydroxide	T54.3X1	T54.3X2	T54.3X3	T54.3X4	--	--
- hypochlorite	T54.3X1	T54.3X2	T54.3X3	T54.3X4	--	--
- iodide	T48.4X1	T48.4X2	T48.4X3	T48.4X4	T48.4X5	T48.4X6
- ipodate	T50.8X1	T50.8X2	T50.8X3	T50.8X4	T50.8X5	T50.8X6
- lactate	T50.3X1	T50.3X2	T50.3X3	T50.3X4	T50.3X5	T50.3X6
- leucovorin	T45.8X1	T45.8X2	T45.8X3	T45.8X4	T45.8X5	T45.8X6
- mandelate	T37.91	T37.92	T37.93	T37.94	T37.95	T37.96
- oxide	T54.3X1	T54.3X2	T54.3X3	T54.3X4	--	--
- pantothenate	T45.2X1	T45.2X2	T45.2X3	T45.2X4	T45.2X5	T45.2X6
- phosphate	T50.3X1	T50.3X2	T50.3X3	T50.3X4	T50.3X5	T50.3X6
- salicylate	T39.091	T39.092	T39.093	T39.094	T39.095	T39.096
- salts	T50.3X1	T50.3X2	T50.3X3	T50.3X4	T50.3X5	T50.3X6
Calculus-dissolving drug	T50.991	T50.992	T50.993	T50.994	T50.995	T50.996
Calomel	T49.0X1	T49.0X2	T49.0X3	T49.0X4	T49.0X5	T49.0X6
Caloric agent	T50.3X1	T50.3X2	T50.3X3	T50.3X4	T50.3X5	T50.3X6
Calusterone	T38.7X1	T38.7X2	T38.7X3	T38.7X4	T38.7X5	T38.7X6
Camazepam	T42.4X1	T42.4X2	T42.4X3	T42.4X4	T42.4X5	T42.4X6
Camomile	T49.0X1	T49.0X2	T49.0X3	T49.0X4	T49.0X5	T49.0X6
Camoquin	T37.2X1	T37.2X2	T37.2X3	T37.2X4	T37.2X5	T37.2X6
Camphor						
- insecticide	T60.2X1	T60.2X2	T60.2X3	T60.2X4	--	--
- medicinal	T49.8X1	T49.8X2	T49.8X3	T49.8X4	T49.8X5	T49.8X6
Camylofin	T44.3X1	T44.3X2	T44.3X3	T44.3X4	T44.3X5	T44.3X6
Cancer chemotherapy drug regimen	T45.1X1	T45.1X2	T45.1X3	T45.1X4	T45.1X5	T45.1X6
Candeptin	T49.0X1	T49.0X2	T49.0X3	T49.0X4	T49.0X5	T49.0X6
Candicidin	T49.0X1	T49.0X2	T49.0X3	T49.0X4	T49.0X5	T49.0X6
Cannabinol	T40.7X1	T40.7X2	T40.7X3	T40.7X4	T40.7X5	T40.7X6
Cannabis (derivatives)	T40.7X1	T40.7X2	T40.7X3	T40.7X4	T40.7X5	T40.7X6
Canned heat	T51.1X1	T51.1X2	T51.1X3	T51.1X4	--	--
Canrenoic acid	T50.0X1	T50.0X2	T50.0X3	T50.0X4	T50.0X5	T50.0X6
Canrenone	T50.0X1	T50.0X2	T50.0X3	T50.0X4	T50.0X5	T50.0X6

Substance	Poisoning, Accidental (unintentional)	Poisoning, Intentional Self-harm	Poisoning, Assault	Poisoning, Undetermined	Adverse effect	Underdosing
Cantharides, cantharidin, cantharis	T49.8X1	T49.8X2	T49.8X3	T49.8X4	T49.8X5	T49.8X6
Canthaxanthin	T50.991	T50.992	T50.993	T50.994	T50.995	T50.996
Capillary-active drug NEC	T46.901	T46.902	T46.903	T46.904	T46.905	T46.906
Capreomycin	T36.8X1	T36.8X2	T36.8X3	T36.8X4	T36.8X5	T36.8X6
Capsicum	T49.4X1	T49.4X2	T49.4X3	T49.4X4	T49.4X5	T49.4X6
Captafol	T60.3X1	T60.3X2	T60.3X3	T60.3X4	--	--
Captan	T60.3X1	T60.3X2	T60.3X3	T60.3X4	--	--
Captodiame, captodiamine	T43.591	T43.592	T43.593	T43.594	T43.595	T43.596
Captopril	T46.4X1	T46.4X2	T46.4X3	T46.4X4	T46.4X5	T46.4X6
Caramiphen	T44.3X1	T44.3X2	T44.3X3	T44.3X4	T44.3X5	T44.3X6
Carazolol	T44.7X1	T44.7X2	T44.7X3	T44.7X4	T44.7X5	T44.7X6
Carbachol	T44.1X1	T44.1X2	T44.1X3	T44.1X4	T44.1X5	T44.1X6
Carbacrylamine (resin)	T50.3X1	T50.3X2	T50.3X3	T50.3X4	T50.3X5	T50.3X6
Carbamate (insecticide)	T60.0X1	T60.0X2	T60.0X3	T60.0X4	--	--
Carbamate (sedative)	T42.6X1	T42.6X2	T42.6X3	T42.6X4	T42.6X5	T42.6X6
- herbicide	T60.0X1	T60.0X2	T60.0X3	T60.0X4	--	--
- insecticide	T60.0X1	T60.0X2	T60.0X3	T60.0X4	--	--
Carbamazepine	T42.1X1	T42.1X2	T42.1X3	T42.1X4	T42.1X5	T42.1X6
Carbamide	T47.3X1	T47.3X2	T47.3X3	T47.3X4	T47.3X5	T47.3X6
- peroxide	T49.0X1	T49.0X2	T49.0X3	T49.0X4	T49.0X5	T49.0X6
- topical	T49.8X1	T49.8X2	T49.8X3	T49.8X4	T49.8X5	T49.8X6
Carbamylcholine chloride	T44.1X1	T44.1X2	T44.1X3	T44.1X4	T44.1X5	T44.1X6
Carbaril	T60.0X1	T60.0X2	T60.0X3	T60.0X4	--	--
Carbarsone	T37.3X1	T37.3X2	T37.3X3	T37.3X4	T37.3X5	T37.3X6
Carbaryl	T60.0X1	T60.0X2	T60.0X3	T60.0X4	--	--
Carbaspirin	T39.011	T39.012	T39.013	T39.014	T39.015	T39.016
Carbazochrome (salicylate) (sodium sulfonate)	T49.4X1	T49.4X2	T49.4X3	T49.4X4	T49.4X5	T49.4X6
Carbenicillin	T36.0X1	T36.0X2	T36.0X3	T36.0X4	T36.0X5	T36.0X6
Carbenoxolone	T47.1X1	T47.1X2	T47.1X3	T47.1X4	T47.1X5	T47.1X6
Carbetapentane	T48.3X1	T48.3X2	T48.3X3	T48.3X4	T48.3X5	T48.3X6
Carbethyl salicylate	T39.091	T39.092	T39.093	T39.094	T39.095	T39.096
Carbidopa (with levodopa)	T42.8X1	T42.8X2	T42.8X3	T42.8X4	T42.8X5	T42.8X6
Carbimazole	T38.2X1	T38.2X2	T38.2X3	T38.2X4	T38.2X5	T38.2X6
Carbinol	T51.1X1	T51.1X2	T51.1X3	T51.1X4	--	--
Carbinoxamine	T45.0X1	T45.0X2	T45.0X3	T45.0X4	T45.0X5	T45.0X6
Carbiphene	T39.8X1	T39.8X2	T39.8X3	T39.8X4	T39.8X5	T39.8X6
Carbitol	T52.3X1	T52.3X2	T52.3X3	T52.3X4	--	--
Carbo medicinalis	T47.6X1	T47.6X2	T47.6X3	T47.6X4	T47.6X5	T47.6X6
Carbocaine	T41.3X1	T41.3X2	T41.3X3	T41.3X4	T41.3X5	T41.3X6
- infiltration (subcutaneous)	T41.3X1	T41.3X2	T41.3X3	T41.3X4	T41.3X5	T41.3X6
- nerve block (peripheral) (plexus)	T41.3X1	T41.3X2	T41.3X3	T41.3X4	T41.3X5	T41.3X6
- topical (surface)	T41.3X1	T41.3X2	T41.3X3	T41.3X4	T41.3X5	T41.3X6
Carbocisteine	T48.4X1	T48.4X2	T48.4X3	T48.4X4	T48.4X5	T48.4X6
Carbocromen	T46.3X1	T46.3X2	T46.3X3	T46.3X4	T46.3X5	T46.3X6
Carbol fuchsin	T49.0X1	T49.0X2	T49.0X3	T49.0X4	T49.0X5	T49.0X6
Carbolic acid—see also Phenol	T54.0X1	T54.0X2	T54.0X3	T54.0X4	--	--
Carbolonium (bromide)	T48.1X1	T48.1X2	T48.1X3	T48.1X4	T48.1X5	T48.1X6
Carbomycin	T36.8X1	T36.8X2	T36.8X3	T36.8X4	T36.8X5	T36.8X6
- bisulfide (liquid)	T65.4X1	T65.4X2	T65.4X3	T65.4X4	--	--
- - vapor	T65.4X1	T65.4X2	T65.4X3	T65.4X4	--	--
- dioxide (gas)	T59.7X1	T59.7X2	T59.7X3	T59.7X4	--	--
- - medicinal	T41.5X1	T41.5X2	T41.5X3	T41.5X4	T41.5X5	T41.5X6
- - nonmedicinal	T59.7X1	T59.7X2	T59.7X3	T59.7X4	--	--
snow	T49.4X1	T49.4X2	T49.4X3	T49.4X4	T49.4X5	T49.4X6
- disulfide (liquid)	T65.4X1	T65.4X2	T65.4X3	T65.4X4	--	--
- - vapor	T65.4X1	T65.4X2	T65.4X3	T65.4X4	--	--
- monoxide (from incomplete combustion)	T58.91	T58.92	T58.93	T58.94	--	--
- - blast furnace gas	T58.8X1	T58.8X2	T58.8X3	T58.8X4	--	--
- - butane (distributed in mobile container)	T58.11	T58.12	T58.13	T58.14	--	--
- - - distributed through pipes	T58.11	T58.12	T58.13	T58.14	--	--
- - charcoal fumes	T58.2X1	T58.2X2	T58.2X3	T58.2X4	--	--
- - coal	T58.2X1	T58.2X2	T58.2X3	T58.2X4	--	--
- - coke (in domestic stoves, fireplaces)	T58.2X1	T58.2X2	T58.2X3	T58.2X4	--	--
- - gas (piped)	T58.11	T58.12	T58.13	T58.14	--	--
- - solid (in domestic stoves, fireplaces)	T58.2X1	T58.2X2	T58.2X3	T58.2X4	--	--

Substance	Poisoning, Accidental (unintentional)	Poisoning, Intentional Self-harm	Poisoning, Assault	Poisoning, Undetermined	Adverse effect	Underdosing
- - exhaust gas (motor) not in transit	T58.01	T58.02	T58.03	T58.04	--	--
- - - combustion engine, any not in watercraft	T58.01	T58.02	T58.03	T58.04	--	--
- - - farm tractor, not in transit	T58.01	T58.02	T58.03	T58.04	--	--
- - - gas engine	T58.01	T58.02	T58.03	T58.04	--	--
- - - motor pump	T58.01	T58.02	T58.03	T58.04	--	--
- - - motor vehicle, not in transit	T58.01	T58.02	T58.03	T58.04	--	--
- - fuel (in domestic use)	T58.2X1	T58.2X2	T58.2X3	T58.2X4	--	--
- - - gas (piped)	T58.11	T58.12	T58.13	T58.14	--	--
- - - - in mobile container	T58.11	T58.12	T58.13	T58.14	--	--
- - - piped (natural)	T58.11	T58.12	T58.13	T58.14	--	--
- - - utility	T58.11	T58.12	T58.13	T58.14	--	--
- - - - in mobile container	T58.11	T58.12	T58.13	T58.14	--	--
- - illuminating gas	T58.11	T58.12	T58.13	T58.14	--	--
- - industrial fuels or gases, any	T58.8X1	T58.8X2	T58.8X3	T58.8X4	--	--
- - kerosene (in domestic stoves, fireplaces)	T58.2X1	T58.2X2	T58.2X3	T58.2X4	--	--
- - kiln gas or vapor	T58.8X1	T58.8X2	T58.8X3	T58.8X4	--	--
- - motor exhaust gas, not in transit	T58.01	T58.02	T58.03	T58.04	--	--
- - piped gas (manufactured) (natural)	T58.11	T58.12	T58.13	T58.14	--	--
- - producer gas	T58.8X1	T58.8X2	T58.8X3	T58.8X4	--	--
- - propane (distributed in mobile container)	T58.11	T58.12	T58.13	T58.14	--	--
- - - distributed through pipes	T58.11	T58.12	T58.13	T58.14	--	--
- - specified source NEC	T58.8X1	T58.8X2	T58.8X3	T58.8X4	--	--
- - stove gas	T58.11	T58.12	T58.13	T58.14	--	--
- - - piped	T58.11	T58.12	T58.13	T58.14	--	--
- - utility gas	T58.11	T58.12	T58.13	T58.14	--	--
- - - piped	T58.11	T58.12	T58.13	T58.14	--	--
- - water gas	T58.11	T58.12	T58.13	T58.14	--	--
- - wood (in domestic stoves, fireplaces)	T58.2X1	T58.2X2	T58.2X3	T58.2X4	--	--
- tetrachloride (vapor) NEC	T53.0X1	T53.0X2	T53.0X3	T53.0X4	--	--
- - liquid (cleansing agent) NEC	T53.0X1	T53.0X2	T53.0X3	T53.0X4	--	--
- - solvent	T53.0X1	T53.0X2	T53.0X3	T53.0X4	--	--
Carbonic acid gas	T59.7X1	T59.7X2	T59.7X3	T59.7X4	--	--
- anhydrase inhibitor NEC	T50.2X1	T50.2X2	T50.2X3	T50.2X4	T50.2X5	T50.2X6
Carbophenothion	T60.0X1	T60.0X2	T60.0X3	T60.0X4	--	--
Carboplatin	T45.1X1	T45.1X2	T45.1X3	T45.1X4	T45.1X5	T45.1X6
Carboprost	T48.0X1	T48.0X2	T48.0X3	T48.0X4	T48.0X5	T48.0X6
Carboquone	T45.1X1	T45.1X2	T45.1X3	T45.1X4	T45.1X5	T45.1X6
Carbowax	T49.3X1	T49.3X2	T49.3X3	T49.3X4	T49.3X5	T49.3X6
Carboxymethyl-cellulose	T47.4X1	T47.4X2	T47.4X3	T47.4X4	T47.4X5	T47.4X6
S-Carboxymethyl-cysteine	T48.4X1	T48.4X2	T48.4X3	T48.4X4	T48.4X5	T48.4X6
Carbrital	T42.3X1	T42.3X2	T42.3X3	T42.3X4	T42.3X5	T42.3X6
Carbromal	T42.6X1	T42.6X2	T42.6X3	T42.6X4	T42.6X5	T42.6X6
Carbutamide	T38.3X1	T38.3X2	T38.3X3	T38.3X4	T38.3X5	T38.3X6
Carbuterol	T48.6X1	T48.6X2	T48.6X3	T48.6X4	T48.6X5	T48.6X6
Cardiac						
- depressants	T46.2X1	T46.2X2	T46.2X3	T46.2X4	T46.2X5	T46.2X6
- rhythm regulator	T46.2X1	T46.2X2	T46.2X3	T46.2X4	T46.2X5	T46.2X6
- - specified NEC	T46.2X1	T46.2X2	T46.2X3	T46.2X4	T46.2X5	T46.2X6
Cardiografin	T50.8X1	T50.8X2	T50.8X3	T50.8X4	T50.8X5	T50.8X6
Cardio-green	T50.8X1	T50.8X2	T50.8X3	T50.8X4	T50.8X5	T50.8X6
Cardiotonic (glycoside) NEC	T46.0X1	T46.0X2	T46.0X3	T46.0X4	T46.0X5	T46.0X6
Cardiovascular drug NEC	T46.901	T46.902	T46.903	T46.904	T46.905	T46.906
Cardrase	T50.2X1	T50.2X2	T50.2X3	T50.2X4	T50.2X5	T50.2X6
Carfecillin	T36.0X1	T36.0X2	T36.0X3	T36.0X4	T36.0X5	T36.0X6
Carfenazine	T43.3X1	T43.3X2	T43.3X3	T43.3X4	T43.3X5	T43.3X6
Carfusin	T49.0X1	T49.0X2	T49.0X3	T49.0X4	T49.0X5	T49.0X6
Carindacillin	T36.0X1	T36.0X2	T36.0X3	T36.0X4	T36.0X5	T36.0X6
Carisoprodol	T42.8X1	T42.8X2	T42.8X3	T42.8X4	T42.8X5	T42.8X6
Carmellose	T47.4X1	T47.4X2	T47.4X3	T47.4X4	T47.4X5	T47.4X6
Carminative	T47.5X1	T47.5X2	T47.5X3	T47.5X4	T47.5X5	T47.5X6
Carmofur	T45.1X1	T45.1X2	T45.1X3	T45.1X4	T45.1X5	T45.1X6
Carmustine	T45.1X1	T45.1X2	T45.1X3	T45.1X4	T45.1X5	T45.1X6
Carotene	T45.2X1	T45.2X2	T45.2X3	T45.2X4	T45.2X5	T45.2X6
Carphenazine	T43.3X1	T43.3X2	T43.3X3	T43.3X4	T43.3X5	T43.3X6
Carpipramine	T42.4X1	T42.4X2	T42.4X3	T42.4X4	T42.4X5	T42.4X6

Substance	Poisoning, Accidental (unintentional)	Poisoning, Intentional Self-harm	Poisoning, Assault	Poisoning, Undetermined	Adverse effect	Underdosing
Carprofen	T39.311	T39.312	T39.313	T39.314	T39.315	T39.316
Carpronium chloride	T44.3X1	T44.3X2	T44.3X3	T44.3X4	T44.3X5	T44.3X6
Carrageenan	T47.8X1	T47.8X2	T47.8X3	T47.8X4	T47.8X5	T47.8X6
Carteolol	T44.7X1	T44.7X2	T44.7X3	T44.7X4	T44.7X5	T44.7X6
Carter's Little Pills	T47.2X1	T47.2X2	T47.2X3	T47.2X4	T47.2X5	T47.2X6
Cascara (sagrada)	T47.2X1	T47.2X2	T47.2X3	T47.2X4	T47.2X5	T47.2X6
Cassava	T62.2X1	T62.2X2	T62.2X3	T62.2X4	--	--
Castellani's paint	T49.0X1	T49.0X2	T49.0X3	T49.0X4	T49.0X5	T49.0X6
Castor						
- bean	T62.2X1	T62.2X2	T62.2X3	T62.2X4	--	--
- oil	T47.2X1	T47.2X2	T47.2X3	T47.2X4	T47.2X5	T47.2X6
Catalase	T45.3X1	T45.3X2	T45.3X3	T45.3X4	T45.3X5	T45.3X6
Caterpillar (sting)	T63.431	T63.432	T63.433	T63.434	--	--
Catha (edulis) (tea)	T43.691	T43.692	T43.693	T43.694	--	--
Cathartic NEC	T47.4X1	T47.4X2	T47.4X3	T47.4X4	T47.4X5	T47.4X6
- anthacene derivative	T47.2X1	T47.2X2	T47.2X3	T47.2X4	T47.2X5	T47.2X6
- bulk	T47.4X1	T47.4X2	T47.4X3	T47.4X4	T47.4X5	T47.4X6
- contact	T47.2X1	T47.2X2	T47.2X3	T47.2X4	T47.2X5	T47.2X6
- emollient NEC	T47.4X1	T47.4X2	T47.4X3	T47.4X4	T47.4X5	T47.4X6
- irritant NEC	T47.2X1	T47.2X2	T47.2X3	T47.2X4	T47.2X5	T47.2X6
- mucilage	T47.4X1	T47.4X2	T47.4X3	T47.4X4	T47.4X5	T47.4X6
- saline	T47.3X1	T47.3X2	T47.3X3	T47.3X4	T47.3X5	T47.3X6
- vegetable	T47.2X1	T47.2X2	T47.2X3	T47.2X4	T47.2X5	T47.2X6
Cathine	T50.5X1	T50.5X2	T50.5X3	T50.5X4	T50.5X5	T50.5X6
Cathomycin	T36.8X1	T36.8X2	T36.8X3	T36.8X4	T36.8X5	T36.8X6
Cation exchange resin	T50.3X1	T50.3X2	T50.3X3	T50.3X4	T50.3X5	T50.3X6
Caustic (s) NEC	T54.91	T54.92	T54.93	T54.94	--	--
- alkali	T54.3X1	T54.3X2	T54.3X3	T54.3X4	--	--
- hydroxide	T54.3X1	T54.3X2	T54.3X3	T54.3X4	--	--
- potash	T54.3X1	T54.3X2	T54.3X3	T54.3X4	--	--
- soda	T54.3X1	T54.3X2	T54.3X3	T54.3X4	--	--
specified NEC	T54.91	T54.92	T54.93	T54.94	--	--
Ceepryn	T49.0X1	T49.0X2	T49.0X3	T49.0X4	T49.0X5	T49.0X6
- ENT agent	T49.6X1	T49.6X2	T49.6X3	T49.6X4	T49.6X5	T49.6X6
- lozenges	T49.6X1	T49.6X2	T49.6X3	T49.6X4	T49.6X5	T49.6X6
Cefacetrile	T36.1X1	T36.1X2	T36.1X3	T36.1X4	T36.1X5	T36.1X6
Cefaclor	T36.1X1	T36.1X2	T36.1X3	T36.1X4	T36.1X5	T36.1X6
Cefadroxil	T36.1X1	T36.1X2	T36.1X3	T36.1X4	T36.1X5	T36.1X6
Cefalexin	T36.1X1	T36.1X2	T36.1X3	T36.1X4	T36.1X5	T36.1X6
Cefaloglycin	T36.1X1	T36.1X2	T36.1X3	T36.1X4	T36.1X5	T36.1X6
Cefaloridine	T36.1X1	T36.1X2	T36.1X3	T36.1X4	T36.1X5	T36.1X6
Cefalosporins	T36.1X1	T36.1X2	T36.1X3	T36.1X4	T36.1X5	T36.1X6
Cefalotin	T36.1X1	T36.1X2	T36.1X3	T36.1X4	T36.1X5	T36.1X6
Cefamandole	T36.1X1	T36.1X2	T36.1X3	T36.1X4	T36.1X5	T36.1X6
Cefamycin antibiotic	T36.1X1	T36.1X2	T36.1X3	T36.1X4	T36.1X5	T36.1X6
Cefapirin	T36.1X1	T36.1X2	T36.1X3	T36.1X4	T36.1X5	T36.1X6
Cefatrizine	T36.1X1	T36.1X2	T36.1X3	T36.1X4	T36.1X5	T36.1X6
Cefazedone	T36.1X1	T36.1X2	T36.1X3	T36.1X4	T36.1X5	T36.1X6
Cefazolin	T36.1X1	T36.1X2	T36.1X3	T36.1X4	T36.1X5	T36.1X6
Cefbuperazone	T36.1X1	T36.1X2	T36.1X3	T36.1X4	T36.1X5	T36.1X6
Cefetamet	T36.1X1	T36.1X2	T36.1X3	T36.1X4	T36.1X5	T36.1X6
Cefixime	T36.1X1	T36.1X2	T36.1X3	T36.1X4	T36.1X5	T36.1X6
Cefmenoxime	T36.1X1	T36.1X2	T36.1X3	T36.1X4	T36.1X5	T36.1X6
Cefmetazole	T36.1X1	T36.1X2	T36.1X3	T36.1X4	T36.1X5	T36.1X6
Cefminox	T36.1X1	T36.1X2	T36.1X3	T36.1X4	T36.1X5	T36.1X6
Cefonicid	T36.1X1	T36.1X2	T36.1X3	T36.1X4	T36.1X5	T36.1X6
Cefoperazone	T36.1X1	T36.1X2	T36.1X3	T36.1X4	T36.1X5	T36.1X6
Ceforanide	T36.1X1	T36.1X2	T36.1X3	T36.1X4	T36.1X5	T36.1X6
Cefotaxime	T36.1X1	T36.1X2	T36.1X3	T36.1X4	T36.1X5	T36.1X6
Cefotetan	T36.1X1	T36.1X2	T36.1X3	T36.1X4	T36.1X5	T36.1X6
Cefotiam	T36.1X1	T36.1X2	T36.1X3	T36.1X4	T36.1X5	T36.1X6
Cefoxitin	T36.1X1	T36.1X2	T36.1X3	T36.1X4	T36.1X5	T36.1X6
Cefpimizole	T36.1X1	T36.1X2	T36.1X3	T36.1X4	T36.1X5	T36.1X6
Cefpiramide	T36.1X1	T36.1X2	T36.1X3	T36.1X4	T36.1X5	T36.1X6
Cefradine	T36.1X1	T36.1X2	T36.1X3	T36.1X4	T36.1X5	T36.1X6

Substance	Poisoning, Accidental (unintentional)	Poisoning, Intentional Self-harm	Poisoning, Assault	Poisoning, Undetermined	Adverse effect	Underdosing
Cefroxadine	T36.1X1	T36.1X2	T36.1X3	T36.1X4	T36.1X5	T36.1X6
Cefsulodin	T36.1X1	T36.1X2	T36.1X3	T36.1X4	T36.1X5	T36.1X6
Ceftazidime	T36.1X1	T36.1X2	T36.1X3	T36.1X4	T36.1X5	T36.1X6
Cefteram	T36.1X1	T36.1X2	T36.1X3	T36.1X4	T36.1X5	T36.1X6
Ceftezole	T36.1X1	T36.1X2	T36.1X3	T36.1X4	T36.1X5	T36.1X6
Ceftizoxime	T36.1X1	T36.1X2	T36.1X3	T36.1X4	T36.1X5	T36.1X6
Ceftriaxone	T36.1X1	T36.1X2	T36.1X3	T36.1X4	T36.1X5	T36.1X6
Cefuroxime	T36.1X1	T36.1X2	T36.1X3	T36.1X4	T36.1X5	T36.1X6
Cefuzonam	T36.1X1	T36.1X2	T36.1X3	T36.1X4	T36.1X5	T36.1X6
Celestone	T38.0X1	T38.0X2	T38.0X3	T38.0X4	T38.0X5	T38.0X6
- topical	T49.0X1	T49.0X2	T49.0X3	T49.0X4	T49.0X5	T49.0X6
Celiprolol	T44.7X1	T44.7X2	T44.7X3	T44.7X4	T44.7X5	T44.7X6
Cell stimulants and proliferants	T49.8X1	T49.8X2	T49.8X3	T49.8X4	T49.8X5	T49.8X6
Cellosolve	T52.91	T52.92	T52.93	T52.94	--	--
Cellulose						
- cathartic	T47.4X1	T47.4X2	T47.4X3	T47.4X4	T47.4X5	T47.4X6
- hydroxyethyl	T47.4X1	T47.4X2	T47.4X3	T47.4X4	T47.4X5	T47.4X6
- nitrates (topical)	T49.3X1	T49.3X2	T49.3X3	T49.3X4	T49.3X5	T49.3X6
- oxidized	T49.4X1	T49.4X2	T49.4X3	T49.4X4	T49.4X5	T49.4X6
Centipede (bite)	T63.411	T63.412	T63.413	T63.414	--	--
Central nervous system						
- depressants	T42.71	T42.72	T42.73	T42.74	T42.75	T42.76
- - anesthetic (general) NEC	T41.201	T41.202	T41.203	T41.204	T41.205	T41.206
- - - gases NEC	T41.0X1	T41.0X2	T41.0X3	T41.0X4	T41.0X5	T41.0X6
- - - intravenous	T41.1X1	T41.1X2	T41.1X3	T41.1X4	T41.1X5	T41.1X6
- - barbiturates	T42.3X1	T42.3X2	T42.3X3	T42.3X4	T42.3X5	T42.3X6
- - benzodiazepines	T42.4X1	T42.4X2	T42.4X3	T42.4X4	T42.4X5	T42.4X6
- - bromides	T42.6X1	T42.6X2	T42.6X3	T42.6X4	T42.6X5	T42.6X6
- - cannabis sativa	T40.7X1	T40.7X2	T40.7X3	T40.7X4	T40.7X5	T40.7X6
- - chloral hydrate	T42.6X1	T42.6X2	T42.6X3	T42.6X4	T42.6X5	T42.6X6
- - ethanol	T51.0X1	T51.0X2	T51.0X3	T51.0X4	--	--
- - hallucinogenics	T40.901	T40.902	T40.903	T40.904	T40.905	T40.906
- - hypnotics	T42.71	T42.72	T42.73	T42.74	T42.75	T42.76
- - - specified NEC	T42.6X1	T42.6X2	T42.6X3	T42.6X4	T42.6X5	T42.6X6
- - muscle relaxants	T42.8X1	T42.8X2	T42.8X3	T42.8X4	T42.8X5	T42.8X6
- - paraldehyde	T42.6X1	T42.6X2	T42.6X3	T42.6X4	T42.6X5	T42.6X6
- - sedatives; sedative-hypnotics	T42.71	T42.72	T42.73	T42.74	T42.75	T42.76
- - - mixed NEC	T42.6X1	T42.6X2	T42.6X3	T42.6X4	T42.6X5	T42.6X6
- - - specified NEC	T42.6X1	T42.6X2	T42.6X3	T42.6X4	T42.6X5	T42.6X6
- muscle-tone depressants	T42.8X1	T42.8X2	T42.8X3	T42.8X4	T42.8X5	T42.8X6
- stimulants	T43.601	T43.602	T43.603	T43.604	T43.605	T43.606
- - amphetamines	T43.621	T43.622	T43.623	T43.624	T43.625	T43.626
- - analeptics	T50.7X1	T50.7X2	T50.7X3	T50.7X4	T50.7X5	T50.7X6
- - antidepressants	T43.201	T43.202	T43.203	T43.204	T43.205	T43.206
- - opiate antagonists	T50.7X1	T50.7X2	T50.7X3	T50.7X4	T50.7X5	T50.7X6
- - specified NEC	T43.691	T43.692	T43.693	T43.694	T43.695	T43.696
Cephalexin	T36.1X1	T36.1X2	T36.1X3	T36.1X4	T36.1X5	T36.1X6
Cephaloglycin	T36.1X1	T36.1X2	T36.1X3	T36.1X4	T36.1X5	T36.1X6
Cephaloridine	T36.1X1	T36.1X2	T36.1X3	T36.1X4	T36.1X5	T36.1X6
Cephalosporins	T36.1X1	T36.1X2	T36.1X3	T36.1X4	T36.1X5	T36.1X6
- N (adicillin)	T36.0X1	T36.0X2	T36.0X3	T36.0X4	T36.0X5	T36.0X6
Cephalothin	T36.1X1	T36.1X2	T36.1X3	T36.1X4	T36.1X5	T36.1X6
Cephalotin	T36.1X1	T36.1X2	T36.1X3	T36.1X4	T36.1X5	T36.1X6
Cephradine	T36.1X1	T36.1X2	T36.1X3	T36.1X4	T36.1X5	T36.1X6
Cerbera (odallam)	T62.2X1	T62.2X2	T62.2X3	T62.2X4	--	--
Cerberin	T46.0X1	T46.0X2	T46.0X3	T46.0X4	T46.0X5	T46.0X6
Cerebral stimulants	T43.601	T43.602	T43.603	T43.604	T43.605	T43.606
- psychotherapeutic	T43.601	T43.602	T43.603	T43.604	T43.605	T43.606
- specified NEC	T43.691	T43.692	T43.693	T43.694	T43.695	T43.696
Cerium oxalate	T45.0X1	T45.0X2	T45.0X3	T45.0X4	T45.0X5	T45.0X6
Cerous oxalate	T45.0X1	T45.0X2	T45.0X3	T45.0X4	T45.0X5	T45.0X6
Ceruletide	T50.8X1	T50.8X2	T50.8X3	T50.8X4	T50.8X5	T50.8X6
Cetalkonium (chloride)	T49.0X1	T49.0X2	T49.0X3	T49.0X4	T49.0X5	T49.0X6
Cethexonium chloride	T49.0X1	T49.0X2	T49.0X3	T49.0X4	T49.0X5	T49.0X6
Cetiedil	T46.7X1	T46.7X2	T46.7X3	T46.7X4	T46.7X5	T46.7X6

Substance	Poisoning, Accidental (unintentional)	Poisoning, Intentional Self-harm	Poisoning, Assault	Poisoning, Undetermined	Adverse effect	Underdosing
Cetirizine	T45.0X1	T45.0X2	T45.0X3	T45.0X4	T45.0X5	T45.0X6
Cetomacrogol	T50.991	T50.992	T50.993	T50.994	T50.995	T50.996
Cetotiamine	T45.2X1	T45.2X2	T45.2X3	T45.2X4	T45.2X5	T45.2X6
Cetoxime	T45.0X1	T45.0X2	T45.0X3	T45.0X4	T45.0X5	T45.0X6
Cetraxate	T47.1X1	T47.1X2	T47.1X3	T47.1X4	T47.1X5	T47.1X6
Cetrimide	T49.0X1	T49.0X2	T49.0X3	T49.0X4	T49.0X5	T49.0X6
Cetrimonium (bromide)	T49.0X1	T49.0X2	T49.0X3	T49.0X4	T49.0X5	T49.0X6
Cetylpyridinium chloride	T49.0X1	T49.0X2	T49.0X3	T49.0X4	T49.0X5	T49.0X6
- ENT agent	T49.6X1	T49.6X2	T49.6X3	T49.6X4	T49.6X5	T49.6X6
- lozenges	T49.6X1	T49.6X2	T49.6X3	T49.6X4	T49.6X5	T49.6X6
Cevadilla—see Sabadilla						
Cevitamic acid	T45.2X1	T45.2X2	T45.2X3	T45.2X4	T45.2X5	T45.2X6
Chalk, precipitated	T47.1X1	T47.1X2	T47.1X3	T47.1X4	T47.1X5	T47.1X6
Chamomile	T49.0X1	T49.0X2	T49.0X3	T49.0X4	T49.0X5	T49.0X6
Ch'an su	T46.0X1	T46.0X2	T46.0X3	T46.0X4	T46.0X5	T46.0X6
Charcoal	T47.6X1	T47.6X2	T47.6X3	T47.6X4	T47.6X5	T47.6X6
- activated—see also Charcoal, medicinal	T47.6X1	T47.6X2	T47.6X3	T47.6X4	T47.6X5	T47.6X6
- fumes (Carbon monoxide)	T58.2X1	T58.2X2	T58.2X3	T58.2X4	--	--
- - industrial	T58.8X1	T58.8X2	T58.8X3	T58.8X4	--	--
- medicinal (activated)	T47.6X1	T47.6X2	T47.6X3	T47.6X4	T47.6X5	T47.6X6
- - antidiarrheal	T47.6X1	T47.6X2	T47.6X3	T47.6X4	T47.6X5	T47.6X6
- - poison control	T47.8X1	T47.8X2	T47.8X3	T47.8X4	T47.8X5	T47.8X6
- - specified use other than for diarrhea	T47.8X1	T47.8X2	T47.8X3	T47.8X4	T47.8X5	T47.8X6
- - topical	T49.8X1	T49.8X2	T49.8X3	T49.8X4	T49.8X5	T49.8X6
Chaulmosulfone	T37.1X1	T37.1X2	T37.1X3	T37.1X4	T37.1X5	T37.1X6
Chelating agent NEC	T50.6X1	T50.6X2	T50.6X3	T50.6X4	T50.6X5	T50.6X6
Chelidonium majus	T62.2X1	T62.2X2	T62.2X3	T62.2X4	--	--
Chemical substance NEC	T65.91	T65.92	T65.93	T65.94	--	--
Chenodeoxycholic acid	T47.5X1	T47.5X2	T47.5X3	T47.5X4	T47.5X5	T47.5X6
Chenodiol	T47.5X1	T47.5X2	T47.5X3	T47.5X4	T47.5X5	T47.5X6
Chenopodium	T37.4X1	T37.4X2	T37.4X3	T37.4X4	T37.4X5	T37.4X6
Cherry laurel	T62.2X1	T62.2X2	T62.2X3	T62.2X4	--	--
Chinidin (e)	T46.2X1	T46.2X2	T46.2X3	T46.2X4	T46.2X5	T46.2X6
Chiniofon	T37.8X1	T37.8X2	T37.8X3	T37.8X4	T37.8X5	T37.8X6
Chlophedianol	T48.3X1	T48.3X2	T48.3X3	T48.3X4	T48.3X5	T48.3X6
Chloral	T42.6X1	T42.6X2	T42.6X3	T42.6X4	T42.6X5	T42.6X6
- derivative	T42.6X1	T42.6X2	T42.6X3	T42.6X4	T42.6X5	T42.6X6
- hydrate	T42.6X1	T42.6X2	T42.6X3	T42.6X4	T42.6X5	T42.6X6
Chloralamide	T42.6X1	T42.6X2	T42.6X3	T42.6X4	T42.6X5	T42.6X6
Chloralodol	T42.6X1	T42.6X2	T42.6X3	T42.6X4	T42.6X5	T42.6X6
Chloralose	T60.4X1	T60.4X2	T60.4X3	T60.4X4	--	--
Chlorambucil	T45.1X1	T45.1X2	T45.1X3	T45.1X4	T45.1X5	T45.1X6
Chloramine	T57.8X1	T57.8X2	T57.8X3	T57.8X4	--	--
- T	T49.0X1	T49.0X2	T49.0X3	T49.0X4	T49.0X5	T49.0X6
- topical	T49.0X1	T49.0X2	T49.0X3	T49.0X4	T49.0X5	T49.0X6
Chloramphenicol	T36.2X1	T36.2X2	T36.2X3	T36.2X4	T36.2X5	T36.2X6
- ENT agent	T49.6X1	T49.6X2	T49.6X3	T49.6X4	T49.6X5	T49.6X6
- ophthalmic preparation	T49.5X1	T49.5X2	T49.5X3	T49.5X4	T49.5X5	T49.5X6
- topical NEC	T49.0X1	T49.0X2	T49.0X3	T49.0X4	T49.0X5	T49.0X6
Chlorate (potassium) (sodium) NEC	T60.3X1	T60.3X2	T60.3X3	T60.3X4	--	--
- herbicide	T60.3X1	T60.3X2	T60.3X3	T60.3X4	--	--
Chlorazanil	T50.2X1	T50.2X2	T50.2X3	T50.2X4	T50.2X5	T50.2X6
Chlorbenzene, chlorbenzol	T53.7X1	T53.7X2	T53.7X3	T53.7X4	--	--
Chlorbenzoxamine	T44.3X1	T44.3X2	T44.3X3	T44.3X4	T44.3X5	T44.3X6
Chlorbutol	T42.6X1	T42.6X2	T42.6X3	T42.6X4	T42.6X5	T42.6X6
Chlorcyclizine	T45.0X1	T45.0X2	T45.0X3	T45.0X4	T45.0X5	T45.0X6
Chlordan (e) (dust)	T60.1X1	T60.1X2	T60.1X3	T60.1X4	--	--
Chlordantoin	T49.0X1	T49.0X2	T49.0X3	T49.0X4	T49.0X5	T49.0X6
Chlordiazepoxide	T42.4X1	T42.4X2	T42.4X3	T42.4X4	T42.4X5	T42.4X6
Chlordiethyl benzamide	T49.3X1	T49.3X2	T49.3X3	T49.3X4	T49.3X5	T49.3X6
Chloresium	T49.8X1	T49.8X2	T49.8X3	T49.8X4	T49.8X5	T49.8X6
Chlorethiazol	T42.6X1	T42.6X2	T42.6X3	T42.6X4	T42.6X5	T42.6X6
Chlorethyl—see Ethyl chloride						
Chloretone	T42.6X1	T42.6X2	T42.6X3	T42.6X4	T42.6X5	T42.6X6
Chlorex	T53.6X1	T53.6X2	T53.6X3	T53.6X4	--	--

Substance	Poisoning, Accidental (unintentional)	Poisoning, Intentional Self-harm	Poisoning, Assault	Poisoning, Undetermined	Adverse effect	Underdosing
- insecticide	T60.1X1	T60.1X2	T60.1X3	T60.1X4	--	--
Chlorfenvinphos	T60.0X1	T60.0X2	T60.0X3	T60.0X4	--	--
Chlorhexadol	T42.6X1	T42.6X2	T42.6X3	T42.6X4	T42.6X5	T42.6X6
Chlorhexamide	T45.1X1	T45.1X2	T45.1X3	T45.1X4	T45.1X5	T45.1X6
Chlorhexidine	T49.0X1	T49.0X2	T49.0X3	T49.0X4	T49.0X5	T49.0X6
Chlorhydroxyquinolin	T49.0X1	T49.0X2	T49.0X3	T49.0X4	T49.0X5	T49.0X6
Chloride of lime (bleach)	T54.3X1	T54.3X2	T54.3X3	T54.3X4	--	--
Chlorimipramine	T43.011	T43.012	T43.013	T43.014	T43.015	T43.016
Chlorinated						
- camphene	T53.6X1	T53.6X2	T53.6X3	T53.6X4	--	--
- diphenyl	T53.7X1	T53.7X2	T53.7X3	T53.7X4	--	--
- hydrocarbons NEC	T53.91	T53.92	T53.93	T53.94	--	--
- - solvents	T53.91	T53.92	T53.93	T53.94	--	--
- lime (bleach)	T54.3X1	T54.3X2	T54.3X3	T54.3X4	--	--
- - and boric acid solution	T49.0X1	T49.0X2	T49.0X3	T49.0X4	T49.0X5	T49.0X6
- naphthalene (insecticide)	T60.1X1	T60.1X2	T60.1X3	T60.1X4	--	--
- - industrial (non-pesticide)	T53.7X1	T53.7X2	T53.7X3	T53.7X4	--	--
- pesticide NEC	T60.8X1	T60.8X2	T60.8X3	T60.8X4	--	--
- soda—see also sodium hypochlorite						
- - solution	T49.0X1	T49.0X2	T49.0X3	T49.0X4	T49.0X5	T49.0X6
Chlorine (fumes) (gas)	T59.4X1	T59.4X2	T59.4X3	T59.4X4	--	--
- bleach	T54.3X1	T54.3X2	T54.3X3	T54.3X4	--	--
- compound gas NEC	T59.4X1	T59.4X2	T59.4X3	T59.4X4	--	--
- disinfectant	T59.4X1	T59.4X2	T59.4X3	T59.4X4	--	--
- releasing agents NEC	T59.4X1	T59.4X2	T59.4X3	T59.4X4	--	--
Chlorisondamine chloride	T46.991	T46.992	T46.993	T46.994	T46.995	T46.996
Chlormadinone	T38.5X1	T38.5X2	T38.5X3	T38.5X4	T38.5X5	T38.5X6
Chlormephos	T60.0X1	T60.0X2	T60.0X3	T60.0X4	--	--
Chlormerodrin	T50.2X1	T50.2X2	T50.2X3	T50.2X4	T50.2X5	T50.2X6
Chlormethiazole	T42.6X1	T42.6X2	T42.6X3	T42.6X4	T42.6X5	T42.6X6
Chlormethine	T45.1X1	T45.1X2	T45.1X3	T45.1X4	T45.1X5	T45.1X6
Chlormethylenecycline	T36.4X1	T36.4X2	T36.4X3	T36.4X4	T36.4X5	T36.4X6
Chlormezanone	T42.6X1	T42.6X2	T42.6X3	T42.6X4	T42.6X5	T42.6X6
Chloroacetic acid	T60.3X1	T60.3X2	T60.3X3	T60.3X4	--	--
Chloroacetone	T59.3X1	T59.3X2	T59.3X3	T59.3X4	--	--
Chloroacetophenone	T59.3X1	T59.3X2	T59.3X3	T59.3X4	--	--
Chloroaniline	T53.7X1	T53.7X2	T53.7X3	T53.7X4	--	--
Chlorobenzene, chlorobenzol	T53.7X1	T53.7X2	T53.7X3	T53.7X4	--	--
Chlorobromomethane (fire extinguisher)	T53.6X1	T53.6X2	T53.6X3	T53.6X4	--	--
Chlorobutanol	T49.0X1	T49.0X2	T49.0X3	T49.0X4	T49.0X5	T49.0X6
Chlorocresol	T49.0X1	T49.0X2	T49.0X3	T49.0X4	T49.0X5	T49.0X6
Chlorodehydro-methyltestosterone	T38.7X1	T38.7X2	T38.7X3	T38.7X4	T38.7X5	T38.7X6
Chlorodinitrobenzene	T53.7X1	T53.7X2	T53.7X3	T53.7X4	--	--
- dust or vapor	T53.7X1	T53.7X2	T53.7X3	T53.7X4	--	--
Chlorodiphenyl	T53.7X1	T53.7X2	T53.7X3	T53.7X4	--	--
Chloroethane—see Ethyl chloride						
Chloroethylene	T53.6X1	T53.6X2	T53.6X3	T53.6X4	--	--
Chlorofluorocarbons	T53.5X1	T53.5X2	T53.5X3	T53.5X4	--	--
Chloroform (fumes) (vapor)	T53.1X1	T53.1X2	T53.1X3	T53.1X4	--	--
- anesthetic	T41.0X1	T41.0X2	T41.0X3	T41.0X4	T41.0X5	T41.0X6
- solvent	T53.1X1	T53.1X2	T53.1X3	T53.1X4	--	--
- water, concentrated	T41.0X1	T41.0X2	T41.0X3	T41.0X4	T41.0X5	T41.0X6
Chloroguanide	T37.2X1	T37.2X2	T37.2X3	T37.2X4	T37.2X5	T37.2X6
Chloromycetin	T36.2X1	T36.2X2	T36.2X3	T36.2X4	T36.2X5	T36.2X6
- ENT agent	T49.6X1	T49.6X2	T49.6X3	T49.6X4	T49.6X5	T49.6X6
- ophthalmic preparation	T49.5X1	T49.5X2	T49.5X3	T49.5X4	T49.5X5	T49.5X6
- otic solution	T49.6X1	T49.6X2	T49.6X3	T49.6X4	T49.6X5	T49.6X6
- topical NEC	T49.0X1	T49.0X2	T49.0X3	T49.0X4	T49.0X5	T49.0X6
Chloronitrobenzene	T53.7X1	T53.7X2	T53.7X3	T53.7X4	--	--
- dust or vapor	T53.7X1	T53.7X2	T53.7X3	T53.7X4	--	--
Chlorophacinone	T60.4X1	T60.4X2	T60.4X3	T60.4X4	--	--
Chlorophenol	T53.7X1	T53.7X2	T53.7X3	T53.7X4	--	--
Chlorophenothane	T60.1X1	T60.1X2	T60.1X3	T60.1X4	--	--
Chlorophyll	T50.991	T50.992	T50.993	T50.994	T50.995	T50.996
Chloropicrin (fumes)	T53.6X1	T53.6X2	T53.6X3	T53.6X4	--	--

Substance	Poisoning, Accidental (unintentional)	Poisoning, Intentional Self-harm	Poisoning, Assault	Poisoning, Undetermined	Adverse effect	Underdosing
- fumigant	T60.8X1	T60.8X2	T60.8X3	T60.8X4	--	--
- fungicide	T60.3X1	T60.3X2	T60.3X3	T60.3X4	--	--
- pesticide	T60.8X1	T60.8X2	T60.8X3	T60.8X4	--	--
Chloroprocaine	T41.3X1	T41.3X2	T41.3X3	T41.3X4	T41.3X5	T41.3X6
- infiltration (subcutaneous)	T41.3X1	T41.3X2	T41.3X3	T41.3X4	T41.3X5	T41.3X6
- nerve block (peripheral) (plexus)	T41.3X1	T41.3X2	T41.3X3	T41.3X4	T41.3X5	T41.3X6
- spinal	T41.3X1	T41.3X2	T41.3X3	T41.3X4	T41.3X5	T41.3X6
Chloroptic	T49.5X1	T49.5X2	T49.5X3	T49.5X4	T49.5X5	T49.5X6
Chloropurine	T45.1X1	T45.1X2	T45.1X3	T45.1X4	T45.1X5	T45.1X6
Chloropyramine	T45.0X1	T45.0X2	T45.0X3	T45.0X4	T45.0X5	T45.0X6
Chloropyrifos	T60.0X1	T60.0X2	T60.0X3	T60.0X4	--	--
Chloropyrilene	T45.0X1	T45.0X2	T45.0X3	T45.0X4	T45.0X5	T45.0X6
Chloroquine	T37.2X1	T37.2X2	T37.2X3	T37.2X4	T37.2X5	T37.2X6
Chlorothalonil	T60.3X1	T60.3X2	T60.3X3	T60.3X4	--	--
Chlorothen	T45.0X1	T45.0X2	T45.0X3	T45.0X4	T45.0X5	T45.0X6
Chlorothiazide	T50.2X1	T50.2X2	T50.2X3	T50.2X4	T50.2X5	T50.2X6
Chlorothymol	T49.4X1	T49.4X2	T49.4X3	T49.4X4	T49.4X5	T49.4X6
Chlorotrianisene	T38.5X1	T38.5X2	T38.5X3	T38.5X4	T38.5X5	T38.5X6
Chlorovinyldichloro-arsinc, not in war	T57.0X1	T57.0X2	T57.0X3	T57.0X4	--	--
Chloroxine	T49.4X1	T49.4X2	T49.4X3	T49.4X4	T49.4X5	T49.4X6
Chloroxylenol	T49.0X1	T49.0X2	T49.0X3	T49.0X4	T49.0X5	T49.0X6
Chlorphenamine	T45.0X1	T45.0X2	T45.0X3	T45.0X4	T45.0X5	T45.0X6
Chlorphenesin	T42.8X1	T42.8X2	T42.8X3	T42.8X4	T42.8X5	T42.8X6
- topical (antifungal)	T49.0X1	T49.0X2	T49.0X3	T49.0X4	T49.0X5	T49.0X6
Chlorpheniramine	T45.0X1	T45.0X2	T45.0X3	T45.0X4	T45.0X5	T45.0X6
Chlorphenoxamine	T45.0X1	T45.0X2	T45.0X3	T45.0X4	T45.0X5	T45.0X6
Chlorphentermine	T50.5X1	T50.5X2	T50.5X3	T50.5X4	T50.5X5	T50.5X6
Chlorprocaine—see Chloroprocaine						
Chlorproguanil	T37.2X1	T37.2X2	T37.2X3	T37.2X4	T37.2X5	T37.2X6
Chlorpromazine	T43.3X1	T43.3X2	T43.3X3	T43.3X4	T43.3X5	T43.3X6
Chlorpropamide	T38.3X1	T38.3X2	T38.3X3	T38.3X4	T38.3X5	T38.3X6
Chlorprothixene	T43.4X1	T43.4X2	T43.4X3	T43.4X4	T43.4X5	T43.4X6
Chlorquinaldol	T49.0X1	T49.0X2	T49.0X3	T49.0X4	T49.0X5	T49.0X6
Chlorquinol	T49.0X1	T49.0X2	T49.0X3	T49.0X4	T49.0X5	T49.0X6
Chlortalidone	T50.2X1	T50.2X2	T50.2X3	T50.2X4	T50.2X5	T50.2X6
Chlortetracycline	T36.4X1	T36.4X2	T36.4X3	T36.4X4	T36.4X5	T36.4X6
Chlorthalidone	T50.2X1	T50.2X2	T50.2X3	T50.2X4	T50.2X5	T50.2X6
Chlorthiophos	T60.0X1	T60.0X2	T60.0X3	T60.0X4	--	--
Chlortrianisene	T38.5X1	T38.5X2	T38.5X3	T38.5X4	T38.5X5	T38.5X6
Chlor-Trlmeton	T45.0X1	T45.0X2	T45.0X3	T45.0X4	T45.0X5	T45.0X6
Chlorthion	T60.0X1	T60.0X2	T60.0X3	T60.0X4	--	--
Chlorzoxazone	T42.8X1	T42.8X2	T42.8X3	T42.8X4	T42.8X5	T42.8X6
Choke damp	T59.7X1	T59.7X2	T59.7X3	T59.7X4	--	--
Cholagogues	T47.5X1	T47.5X2	T47.5X3	T47.5X4	T47.5X5	T47.5X6
Cholebrine	T50.8X1	T50.8X2	T50.8X3	T50.8X4	T50.8X5	T50.8X6
Cholecalciferol	T45.2X1	T45.2X2	T45.2X3	T45.2X4	T45.2X5	T45.2X6
Cholecystokinin	T50.8X1	T50.8X2	T50.8X3	T50.8X4	T50.8X5	T50.8X6
Cholera vaccine	T50.A91	T50.A92	T50.A93	T50.A94	T50.A95	T50.A96
Choleretic	T47.5X1	T47.5X2	T47.5X3	T47.5X4	T47.5X5	T47.5X6
Cholesterol-lowering agents	T46.6X1	T46.6X2	T46.6X3	T46.6X4	T46.6X5	T46.6X6
Cholestyramine (resin)	T46.6X1	T46.6X2	T46.6X3	T46.6X4	T46.6X5	T46.6X6
Cholic acid	T47.5X1	T47.5X2	T47.5X3	T47.5X4	T47.5X5	T47.5X6
Choline	T48.6X1	T48.6X2	T48.6X3	T48.6X4	T48.6X5	T48.6X6
- chloride	T50.991	T50.992	T50.993	T50.994	T50.995	T50.996
- dihydrogen citrate	T50.991	T50.992	T50.993	T50.994	T50.995	T50.996
- salicylate	T39.091	T39.092	T39.093	T39.094	T39.095	T39.096
- theophyllinate	T48.6X1	T48.6X2	T48.6X3	T48.6X4	T48.6X5	T48.6X6
Cholinergic (drug) NEC	T44.1X1	T44.1X2	T44.1X3	T44.1X4	T44.1X5	T44.1X6
- muscle tone enhancer	T44.1X1	T44.1X2	T44.1X3	T44.1X4	T44.1X5	T44.1X6
- organophosphorus	T44.0X1	T44.0X2	T44.0X3	T44.0X4	T44.0X5	T44.0X6
- - insecticide	T60.0X1	T60.0X2	T60.0X3	T60.0X4	--	--
- - nerve gas	T59.891	T59.892	T59.893	T59.894	--	--
- trimethyl ammonium propanediol	T44.1X1	T44.1X2	T44.1X3	T44.1X4	T44.1X5	T44.1X6
Cholinesterase reactivator	T50.6X1	T50.6X2	T50.6X3	T50.6X4	T50.6X5	T50.6X6
Cholografin	T50.8X1	T50.8X2	T50.8X3	T50.8X4	T50.8X5	T50.8X6

Substance	Poisoning, Accidental (unintentional)	Poisoning, Intentional Self-harm	Poisoning, Assault	Poisoning, Undetermined	Adverse effect	Underdosing
Chorionic gonadotropin	T38.891	T38.892	T38.893	T38.894	T38.895	T38.896
Chromate	T56.2X1	T56.2X2	T56.2X3	T56.2X4	--	--
- dust or mist	T56.2X1	T56.2X2	T56.2X3	T56.2X4	--	--
- lead—see also lead	T56.0X1	T56.0X2	T56.0X3	T56.0X4	--	--
- - paint	T56.0X1	T56.0X2	T56.0X3	T56.0X4	--	--
Chromic						
- acid	T56.2X1	T56.2X2	T56.2X3	T56.2X4	--	--
- - dust or mist	T56.2X1	T56.2X2	T56.2X3	T56.2X4	--	--
- phosphate 32P	T45.1X1	T45.1X2	T45.1X3	T45.1X4	T45.1X5	T45.1X6
Chromium	T56.2X1	T56.2X2	T56.2X3	T56.2X4	--	
- compounds—see Chromate						
- sesquioxide	T50.8X1	T50.8X2	T50.8X3	T50.8X4	T50.8X5	T50.8X6
Chromomycin A3	T45.1X1	T45.1X2	T45.1X3	T45.1X4	T45.1X5	T45.1X6
Chromonar	T46.3X1	T46.3X2	T46.3X3	T46.3X4	T46.3X5	T46.3X6
Chromyl chloride	T56.2X1	T56.2X2	T56.2X3	T56.2X4	--	--
Chrysarobin	T49.4X1	T49.4X2	T49.4X3	T49.4X4	T49.4X5	T49.4X6
Chrysazin	T47.2X1	T47.2X2	T47.2X3	T47.2X4	T47.2X5	T47.2X6
Chymar	T45.3X1	T45.3X2	T45.3X3	T45.3X4	T45.3X5	T45.3X6
- ophthalmic preparation	T49.5X1	T49.5X2	T49.5X3	T49.5X4	T49.5X5	T49.5X6
Chymopapain	T45.3X1	T45.3X2	T45.3X3	T45.3X4	T45.3X5	T45.3X6
Chymotrypsin	T45.3X1	T45.3X2	T45.3X3	T45.3X4	T45.3X5	T45.3X6
- ophthalmic preparation	T49.5X1	T49.5X2	T49.5X3	T49.5X4	T49.5X5	T49.5X6
Cianidanol	T50.991	T50.992	T50.993	T50.994	T50.995	T50.996
Cianopramine	T43.011	T43.012	T43.013	T43.014	T43.015	T43.016
Cibenzoline	T46.2X1	T46.2X2	T46.2X3	T46.2X4	T46.2X5	T46.2X6
Ciclacillin	T36.0X1	T36.0X2	T36.0X3	T36.0X4	T36.0X5	T36.0X6
Ciclobarbital—see Hexobarbital						
Ciclonicate	T46.7X1	T46.7X2	T46.7X3	T46.7X4	T46.7X5	T46.7X6
Ciclopirox (olamine)	T49.0X1	T49.0X2	T49.0X3	T49.0X4	T49.0X5	T49.0X6
Ciclosporin	T45.1X1	T45.1X2	T45.1X3	T45.1X4	T45.1X5	T45.1X6
Cicuta maculata or virosa	T62.2X1	T62.2X2	T62.2X3	T62.2X4	--	--
Cicutoxin	T62.2X1	T62.2X2	T62.2X3	T62.2X4	--	--
Cigarette lighter fluid	T52.0X1	T52.0X2	T52.0X3	T52.0X4	--	--
Cigarettes (tobacco)	T65.221	T65.222	T65.223	T65.224	--	--
Ciguatoxin	T61.01	T61.02	T61.03	T61.04	--	--
Cilazapril	T46.4X1	T46.4X2	T46.4X3	T46.4X4	T46.4X5	T46.4X6
Cimetidine	T47.0X1	T47.0X2	T47.0X3	T47.0X4	T47.0X5	T47.0X6
Cimetropium bromide	T44.3X1	T44.3X2	T44.3X3	T44.3X4	T44.3X5	T44.3X6
Cinchocaine	T41.3X1	T41.3X2	T41.3X3	T41.3X4	T41.3X5	T41.3X6
- topical (surface)	T41.3X1	T41.3X2	T41.3X3	T41.3X4	T41.3X5	T41.3X6
Cinchona	T37.2X1	T37.2X2	T37.2X3	T37.2X4	T37.2X5	T37.2X6
Cinchonine alkaloids	T37.2X1	T37.2X2	T37.2X3	T37.2X4	T37.2X5	T37.2X6
Cinchophen	T50.4X1	T50.4X2	T50.4X3	T50.4X4	T50.4X5	T50.4X6
Cinepazide	T46.7X1	T46.7X2	T46.7X3	T46.7X4	T46.7X5	T46.7X6
Cinnamedrine	T48.5X1	T48.5X2	T48.5X3	T48.5X4	T48.5X5	T48.5X6
Cinnarizine	T45.0X1	T45.0X2	T45.0X3	T45.0X4	T45.0X5	T45.0X6
Cinoxacin	T37.8X1	T37.8X2	T37.8X3	T37.8X4	T37.8X5	T37.8X6
Ciprofibrate	T46.6X1	T46.6X2	T46.6X3	T46.6X4	T46.6X5	T46.6X6
Ciprofloxacin	T36.8X1	T36.8X2	T36.8X3	T36.8X4	T36.8X5	T36.8X6
Cisapride	T47.8X1	T47.8X2	T47.8X3	T47.8X4	T47.8X5	T47.8X6
Cisplatin	T45.1X1	T45.1X2	T45.1X3	T45.1X4	T45.1X5	T45.1X6
Citalopram	T43.221	T43.222	T43.223	T43.224	T43.225	T43.226
Citanest	T41.3X1	T41.3X2	T41.3X3	T41.3X4	T41.3X5	T41.3X6
- infiltration (subcutaneous)	T41.3X1	T41.3X2	T41.3X3	T41.3X4	T41.3X5	T41.3X6
- nerve block (peripheral) (plexus)	T41.3X1	T41.3X2	T41.3X3	T41.3X4	T41.3X5	T41.3X6
Citric acid	T47.5X1	T47.5X2	T47.5X3	T47.5X4	T47.5X5	T47.5X6
Citrovorum (factor)	T45.8X1	T45.8X2	T45.8X3	T45.8X4	T45.8X5	T45.8X6
Claviceps purpurea	T62.2X1	T62.2X2	T62.2X3	T62.2X4	--	--
Clavulanic acid	T36.1X1	T36.1X2	T36.1X3	T36.1X4	T36.1X5	T36.1X6
Cleaner, cleansing agent, type not specified	T65.891	T65.892	T65.893	T65.894	--	--
- of paint or varnish	T52.91	T52.92	T52.93	T52.94	--	--
- specified type NEC	T65.891	T65.892	T65.893	T65.894	--	--
Clebopride	T47.8X1	T47.8X2	T47.8X3	T47.8X4	T47.8X5	T47.8X6
Clefamide	T37.3X1	T37.3X2	T37.3X3	T37.3X4	T37.3X5	T37.3X6
Clemastine	T45.0X1	T45.0X2	T45.0X3	T45.0X4	T45.0X5	T45.0X6

Substance	Poisoning, Accidental (unintentional)	Poisoning, Intentional Self-harm	Poisoning, Assault	Poisoning, Undetermined	Adverse effect	Underdosing
Clematis vitalba	T62.2X1	T62.2X2	T62.2X3	T62.2X4	--	--
Clemizole	T45.0X1	T45.0X2	T45.0X3	T45.0X4	T45.0X5	T45.0X6
- penicillin	T36.0X1	T36.0X2	T36.0X3	T36.0X4	T36.0X5	T36.0X6
Clenbuterol	T48.6X1	T48.6X2	T48.6X3	T48.6X4	T48.6X5	T48.6X6
Clidinium bromide	T44.3X1	T44.3X2	T44.3X3	T44.3X4	T44.3X5	T44.3X6
Clindamycin	T36.8X1	T36.8X2	T36.8X3	T36.8X4	T36.8X5	T36.8X6
Clinofibrate	T46.6X1	T46.6X2	T46.6X3	T46.6X4	T46.6X5	T46.6X6
Clioquinol	T37.8X1	T37.8X2	T37.8X3	T37.8X4	T37.8X5	T37.8X6
Cliradon	T40.2X1	T40.2X2	T40.2X3	T40.2X4	--	--
Clobazam	T42.4X1	T42.4X2	T42.4X3	T42.4X4	T42.4X5	T42.4X6
Clobenzorex	T50.5X1	T50.5X2	T50.5X3	T50.5X4	T50.5X5	T50.5X6
Clobetasol	T49.0X1	T49.0X2	T49.0X3	T49.0X4	T49.0X5	T49.0X6
Clobetasone	T49.0X1	T49.0X2	T49.0X3	T49.0X4	T49.0X5	T49.0X6
Clobutinol	T48.3X1	T48.3X2	T48.3X3	T48.3X4	T48.3X5	T48.3X6
Clocortolone	T38.0X1	T38.0X2	T38.0X3	T38.0X4	T38.0X5	T38.0X6
Clodantoin	T49.0X1	T49.0X2	T49.0X3	T49.0X4	T49.0X5	T49.0X6
Clodronic acid	T50.991	T50.992	T50.993	T50.994	T50.995	T50.996
Clofazimine	T37.1X1	T37.1X2	T37.1X3	T37.1X4	T37.1X5	T37.1X6
Clofedanol	T48.3X1	T48.3X2	T48.3X3	T48.3X4	T48.3X5	T48.3X6
Clofenamide	T50.2X1	T50.2X2	T50.2X3	T50.2X4	T50.2X5	T50.2X6
Clofenotane	T49.0X1	T49.0X2	T49.0X3	T49.0X4	T49.0X5	T49.0X6
Clofezone	T39.2X1	T39.2X2	T39.2X3	T39.2X4	T39.2X5	T39.2X6
Clofibrate	T46.6X1	T46.6X2	T46.6X3	T46.6X4	T46.6X5	T46.6X6
Clofibride	T46.6X1	T46.6X2	T46.6X3	T46.6X4	T46.6X5	T46.6X6
Cloforex	T50.5X1	T50.5X2	T50.5X3	T50.5X4	T50.5X5	T50.5X6
Clomethiazole	T42.6X1	T42.6X2	T42.6X3	T42.6X4	T42.6X5	T42.6X6
Clometocillin	T36.0X1	T36.0X2	T36.0X3	T36.0X4	T36.0X5	T36.0X6
Clomifene	T38.5X1	T38.5X2	T38.5X3	T38.5X4	T38.5X5	T38.5X6
Clomiphene	T38.5X1	T38.5X2	T38.5X3	T38.5X4	T38.5X5	T38.5X6
Clomipramine	T43.011	T43.012	T43.013	T43.014	T43.015	T43.016
Clomocycline	T36.4X1	T36.4X2	T36.4X3	T36.4X4	T36.4X5	T36.4X6
Clonazepam	T42.4X1	T42.4X2	T42.4X3	T42.4X4	T42.4X5	T42.4X6
Clonidine	T46.5X1	T46.5X2	T46.5X3	T46.5X4	T46.5X5	T46.5X6
Clonixin	T39.8X1	T39.8X2	T39.8X3	T39.8X4	T39.8X5	T39.8X6
Clopamide	T50.2X1	T50.2X2	T50.2X3	T50.2X4	T50.2X5	T50.2X6
Clopenthixol	T43.4X1	T43.4X2	T43.4X3	T43.4X4	T43.4X5	T43.4X6
Cloperastine	T48.3X1	T48.3X2	T48.3X3	T48.3X4	T48.3X5	T48.3X6
Clophedianol	T48.3X1	T48.3X2	T48.3X3	T48.3X4	T48.3X5	T48.3X6
Cloponone	T36.2X1	T36.2X2	T36.2X3	T36.2X4	T36.2X5	T36.2X6
Cloprednol	T38.0X1	T38.0X2	T38.0X3	T38.0X4	T38.0X5	T38.0X6
Cloral betaine	T42.6X1	T42.6X2	T42.6X3	T42.6X4	T42.6X5	T42.6X6
Cloramfenicol	T36.2X1	T36.2X2	T36.2X3	T36.2X4	T36.2X5	T36.2X6
Clorazepate (dipotassium)	T42.4X1	T42.4X2	T42.4X3	T42.4X4	T42.4X5	T42.4X6
Clorexolone	T50.2X1	T50.2X2	T50.2X3	T50.2X4	T50.2X5	T50.2X6
Clorfenamine	T45.0X1	T45.0X2	T45.0X3	T45.0X4	T45.0X5	T45.0X6
Clorgiline	T43.1X1	T43.1X2	T43.1X3	T43.1X4	T43.1X5	T43.1X6
Clorotepine	T44.3X1	T44.3X2	T44.3X3	T44.3X4	T44.3X5	T44.3X6
Clorox (bleach)	T54.91	T54.92	T54.93	T54.94	--	--
Clorprenaline	T48.6X1	T48.6X2	T48.6X3	T48.6X4	T48.6X5	T48.6X6
Clortermine	T50.5X1	T50.5X2	T50.5X3	T50.5X4	T50.5X5	T50.5X6
Clotiapine	T43.591	T43.592	T43.593	T43.594	T43.595	T43.596
Clotiazepam	T42.4X1	T42.4X2	T42.4X3	T42.4X4	T42.4X5	T42.4X6
Clotibric acid	T46.6X1	T46.6X2	T46.6X3	T46.6X4	T46.6X5	T46.6X6
Clotrimazole	T49.0X1	T49.0X2	T49.0X3	T49.0X4	T49.0X5	T49.0X6
Cloxacillin	T36.0X1	T36.0X2	T36.0X3	T36.0X4	T36.0X5	T36.0X6
Cloxazolam	T42.4X1	T42.4X2	T42.4X3	T42.4X4	T42.4X5	T42.4X6
Cloxiquine	T49.0X1	T49.0X2	T49.0X3	T49.0X4	T49.0X5	T49.0X6
Clozapine	T42.4X1	T42.4X2	T42.4X3	T42.4X4	T42.4X5	T42.4X6
Coagulant NEC	T45.7X1	T45.7X2	T45.7X3	T45.7X4	T45.7X5	T45.7X6
Coal (carbon monoxide from) —see also Carbon, monoxide, coal	T58.2X1	T58.2X2	T58.2X3	T58.2X4	--	--
- oil—see Kerosene						
- tar	T49.1X1	T49.1X2	T49.1X3	T49.1X4	T49.1X5	T49.1X6
- - fumes	T59.891	T59.892	T59.893	T59.894	--	--
- - medicinal (ointment)	T49.4X1	T49.4X2	T49.4X3	T49.4X4	T49.4X5	T49.4X6

Substance	Poisoning, Accidental (unintentional)	Poisoning, Intentional Self-harm	Poisoning, Assault	Poisoning, Undetermined	Adverse effect	Underdosing
- - - analgesics NEC	T39.2X1	T39.2X2	T39.2X3	T39.2X4	T39.2X5	T39.2X6
- - naphtha (solvent)	T52.0X1	T52.0X2	T52.0X3	T52.0X4	--	--
Cobalamine	T45.2X1	T45.2X2	T45.2X3	T45.2X4	T45.2X5	T45.2X6
Cobalt (nonmedicinal) (fumes) (industrial)	T56.891	T56.892	T56.893	T56.894	--	--
- medicinal (trace) (chloride)	T45.8X1	T45.8X2	T45.8X3	T45.8X4	T45.8X5	T45.8X6
Cobra (venom)	T63.041	T63.042	T63.043	T63.044	--	--
Coca (leaf)	T40.5X1	T40.5X2	T40.5X3	T40.5X4	T40.5X5	T40.5X6
Cocaine	T40.5X1	T40.5X2	T40.5X3	T40.5X4	T40.5X5	T40.5X6
- topical anesthetic	T41.3X1	T41.3X2	T41.3X3	T41.3X4	T41.3X5	T41.3X6
Cocarboxylase	T45.3X1	T45.3X2	T45.3X3	T45.3X4	T45.3X5	T45.3X6
Coccidioidin	T50.8X1	T50.8X2	T50.8X3	T50.8X4	T50.8X5	T50.8X6
Cocculus indicus	T62.1X1	T62.1X2	T62.1X3	T62.1X4	--	--
Cochineal	T65.6X1	T65.6X2	T65.6X3	T65.6X4	--	--
- medicinal products	T50.991	T50.992	T50.993	T50.994	T50.995	T50.996
Codcine	T40.2X1	T40.2X2	T40.2X3	T40.2X4	T40.2X5	T40.2X6
Cod-liver oil	T45.2X1	T45.2X2	T45.2X3	T45.2X4	T45.2X5	T45.2X6
Coenzyme A	T50.991	T50.992	T50.993	T50.994	T50.995	T50.996
Coffee	T62.8X1	T62.8X2	T62.8X3	T62.8X4	--	--
Cogalactoiso-merase	T50.991	T50.992	T50.993	T50.994	T50.995	T50.996
Cogentin	T44.3X1	T44.3X2	T44.3X3	T44.3X4	T44.3X5	T44.3X6
Coke fumes or gas (carbon monoxide)	T58.2X1	T58.2X2	T58.2X3	T58.2X4		--
- industrial use	T58.8X1	T58.8X2	T58.8X3	T58.8X4	--	--
Colace	T47.4X1	T47.4X2	T47.4X3	T47.4X4	T47.4X5	T47.4X6
Colaspase	T45.1X1	T45.1X2	T45.1X3	T45.1X4	T45.1X5	T45.1X6
Colchicine	T50.4X1	T50.4X2	T50.4X3	T50.4X4	T50.4X5	T50.4X6
Colchicum	T62.2X1	T62.2X2	T62.2X3	T62.2X4	--	--
Cold cream	T49.3X1	T49.3X2	T49.3X3	T49.3X4	T49.3X5	T49.3X6
Colecalciferol	T45.2X1	T45.2X2	T45.2X3	T45.2X4	T45.2X5	T45.2X6
Colestipol	T46.6X1	T46.6X2	T46.6X3	T46.6X4	T46.6X5	T46.6X6
Colestyramine	T46.6X1	T46.6X2	T46.6X3	T46.6X4	T46.6X5	T46.6X6
Colimycin	T36.8X1	T36.8X2	T36.8X3	T36.8X4	T36.8X5	T36.8X6
Colistimethate	T36.8X1	T36.8X2	T36.8X3	T36.8X4	T36.8X5	T36.8X6
Colistin	T36.8X1	T36.8X2	T36.8X3	T36.8X4	T36.8X5	T36.8X6
- sulfate (eye preparation)	T49.5X1	T49.5X2	T49.5X3	T49.5X4	T49.5X5	T49.5X6
Collagen	T50.991	T50.992	T50.993	T50.994	T50.995	T50.996
Collagenase	T49.4X1	T49.4X2	T49.4X3	T49.4X4	T49.4X5	T49.4X6
Collodion	T49.3X1	T49.3X2	T49.3X3	T49.3X4	T49.3X5	T49.3X6
Colocynth	T47.2X1	T47.2X2	T47.2X3	T47.2X4	T47.2X5	T47.2X6
Colophony adhesive	T49.3X1	T49.3X2	T49.3X3	T49.3X4	T49.3X5	T49.3X6
Colorant—see also Dye	T50.991	T50.992	T50.993	T50.994	T50.995	T50.996
Coloring matter—see Dye (s)						
Combustion gas (after combustion) —see Carbon, monoxide						
- prior to combustion	T59.891	T59.892	T59.893	T59.894	--	--
Compazine	T43.3X1	T43.3X2	T43.3X3	T43.3X4	T43.3X5	T43.3X6
Compound						
- 42 (warfarin)	T60.4X1	T60.4X2	T60.4X3	T60.4X4	--	--
- 269 (endrin)	T60.1X1	T60.1X2	T60.1X3	T60.1X4	--	--
- 497 (dieldrin)	T60.1X1	T60.1X2	T60.1X3	T60.1X4	--	--
- 1080 (sodium fluoroacetate)	T60.4X1	T60.4X2	T60.4X3	T60.4X4	--	--
- 3422 (parathion)	T60.0X1	T60.0X2	T60.0X3	T60.0X4	--	--
- 3911 (phorate)	T60.0X1	T60.0X2	T60.0X3	T60.0X4	--	--
- 3956 (toxaphene)	T60.1X1	T60.1X2	T60.1X3	T60.1X4	--	--
- 4049 (malathion)	T60.0X1	T60.0X2	T60.0X3	T60.0X4	--	--
- 4069 (malathion)	T60.0X1	T60.0X2	T60.0X3	T60.0X4	--	--
- 4124 (dicapthon)	T60.0X1	T60.0X2	T60.0X3	T60.0X4	--	--
- E (cortisone)	T38.0X1	T38.0X2	T38.0X3	T38.0X4	T38.0X5	T38.0X6
- F (hydrocortisone)	T38.0X1	T38.0X2	T38.0X3	T38.0X4	T38.0X5	T38.0X6
Congener, anabolic	T38.7X1	T38.7X2	T38.7X3	T38.7X4	T38.7X5	T38.7X6
Congo red	T50.8X1	T50.8X2	T50.8X3	T50.8X4	T50.8X5	T50.8X6
Coniine, conine	T62.2X1	T62.2X2	T62.2X3	T62.2X4	--	--
Conium (maculatum)	T62.2X1	T62.2X2	T62.2X3	T62.2X4	--	--
Conjugated estrogenic substances	T38.5X1	T38.5X2	T38.5X3	T38.5X4	T38.5X5	T38.5X6
Contac	T48.5X1	T48.5X2	T48.5X3	T48.5X4	T48.5X5	T48.5X6
Contact lens solution	T49.5X1	T49.5X2	T49.5X3	T49.5X4	T49.5X5	T49.5X6

Substance	Poisoning, Accidental (unintentional)	Poisoning, Intentional Self-harm	Poisoning, Assault	Poisoning, Undetermined	Adverse effect	Underdosing
Contraceptive (oral)	T38.4X1	T38.4X2	T38.4X3	T38.4X4	T38.4X5	T38.4X6
- vaginal	T49.8X1	T49.8X2	T49.8X3	T49.8X4	T49.8X5	T49.8X6
Contrast medium, radiography	T50.8X1	T50.8X2	T50.8X3	T50.8X4	T50.8X5	T50.8X6
Convallaria glycosides	T46.0X1	T46.0X2	T46.0X3	T46.0X4	T46.0X5	T46.0X6
Convallaria majalis	T62.2X1	T62.2X2	T62.2X3	T62.2X4	--	--
- berry	T62.1X1	T62.1X2	T62.1X3	T62.1X4	--	--
Copper (dust) (fumes) (nonmedicinal) NEC	T56.4X1	T56.4X2	T56.4X3	T56.4X4	--	--
- arsenate, arsenite	T57.0X1	T57.0X2	T57.0X3	T57.0X4	--	--
- - insecticide	T60.2X1	T60.2X2	T60.2X3	T60.2X4	--	--
- emetic	T47.7X1	T47.7X2	T47.7X3	T47.7X4	T47.7X5	T47.7X6
- fungicide	T60.3X1	T60.3X2	T60.3X3	T60.3X4	--	--
- gluconate	T49.0X1	T49.0X2	T49.0X3	T49.0X4	T49.0X5	T49.0X6
- insecticide	T60.2X1	T60.2X2	T60.2X3	T60.2X4	--	--
- medicinal (trace)	T45.8X1	T45.8X2	T45.8X3	T45.8X4	T45.8X5	T45.8X6
- oleate	T49.0X1	T49.0X2	T49.0X3	T49.0X4	T49.0X5	T49.0X6
- sulfate	T56.4X1	T56.4X2	T56.4X3	T56.4X4	--	--
- - cupric	T56.4X1	T56.4X2	T56.4X3	T56.4X4	--	--
- - - fungicide	T60.3X1	T60.3X2	T60.3X3	T60.3X4	--	--
- - - medicinal						
- - - - ear	T49.6X1	T49.6X2	T49.6X3	T49.6X4	T49.6X5	T49.6X6
- - - - emetic	T47.7X1	T47.7X2	T47.7X3	T47.7X4	T47.7X5	T47.7X6
- - - - eye	T49.5X1	T49.5X2	T49.5X3	T49.5X4	T49.5X5	T49.5X6
- - cuprous	T56.4X1	T56.4X2	T56.4X3	T56.4X4	--	--
- - fungicide	T60.3X1	T60.3X2	T60.3X3	T60.3X4	--	--
- - medicinal						
- - - ear	T49.6X1	T49.6X2	T49.6X3	T49.6X4	T49.6X5	T49.6X6
- - - emetic	T47.7X1	T47.7X2	T47.7X3	T47.7X4	T47.7X5	T47.7X6
- - - eye	T49.5X1	T49.5X2	T49.5X3	T49.5X4	T49.5X5	T49.5X6
Copperhead snake (bite) (venom)	T63.061	T63.062	T63.063	T63.064	--	--
Coral (sting)	T63.691	T63.692	T63.693	T63.694	--	--
- snake (bite) (venom)	T63.021	T63.022	T63.023	T63.024	--	--
Corbadrine	T49.6X1	T49.6X2	T49.6X3	T49.6X4	T49.6X5	T49.6X6
Cordite	T65.891	T65.892	T65.893	T65.894	--	--
- vapor	T59.891	T59.892	T59.893	T59.894	--	--
Cordran	T49.0X1	T49.0X2	T49.0X3	T49.0X4	T49.0X5	T49.0X6
Corn cures	T49.4X1	T49.4X2	T49.4X3	T49.4X4	T49.4X5	T49.4X6
Corn starch	T49.3X1	T49.3X2	T49.3X3	T49.3X4	T49.3X5	T49.3X6
Cornhusker's lotion	T49.3X1	T49.3X2	T49.3X3	T49.3X4	T49.3X5	T49.3X6
Coronary vasodilator NEC	T46.3X1	T46.3X2	T46.3X3	T46.3X4	T46.3X5	T46.3X6
Corrosive NEC	T54.91	T54.92	T54.93	T54.94	--	--
- acid NEC	T54.2X1	T54.2X2	T54.2X3	T54.2X4	--	--
- aromatics	T54.1X1	T54.1X2	T54.1X3	T54.1X4	--	--
- - disinfectant	T54.1X1	T54.1X2	T54.1X3	T54.1X4	--	--
- fumes NEC	T54.91	T54.92	T54.93	T54.94	--	--
- specified NEC	T54.91	T54.92	T54.93	T54.94	--	--
- sublimate	T56.1X1	T56.1X2	T56.1X3	T56.1X4	--	--
Cortate	T38.0X1	T38.0X2	T38.0X3	T38.0X4	T38.0X5	T38.0X6
Cort-Dome	T38.0X1	T38.0X2	T38.0X3	T38.0X4	T38.0X5	T38.0X6
- ENT agent	T49.6X1	T49.6X2	T49.6X3	T49.6X4	T49.6X5	T49.6X6
- ophthalmic preparation	T49.5X1	T49.5X2	T49.5X3	T49.5X4	T49.5X5	T49.5X6
- topical NEC	T49.0X1	T49.0X2	T49.0X3	T49.0X4	T49.0X5	T49.0X6
Cortef	T38.0X1	T38.0X2	T38.0X3	T38.0X4	T38.0X5	T38.0X6
- ENT agent	T49.6X1	T49.6X2	T49.6X3	T49.6X4	T49.6X5	T49.6X6
- ophthalmic preparation	T49.5X1	T49.5X2	T49.5X3	T49.5X4	T49.5X5	T49.5X6
- topical NEC	T49.0X1	T49.0X2	T49.0X3	T49.0X4	T49.0X5	T49.0X6
Corticosteroid	T38.0X1	T38.0X2	T38.0X3	T38.0X4	T38.0X5	T38.0X6
- ENT agent	T49.6X1	T49.6X2	T49.6X3	T49.6X4	T49.6X5	T49.6X6
- mineral	T50.0X1	T50.0X2	T50.0X3	T50.0X4	T50.0X5	T50.0X6
- ophthalmic	T49.5X1	T49.5X2	T49.5X3	T49.5X4	T49.5X5	T49.5X6
- topical NEC	T49.0X1	T49.0X2	T49.0X3	T49.0X4	T49.0X5	T49.0X6
Corticotropin	T38.811	T38.812	T38.813	T38.814	T38.815	T38.816
Cortisol	T49.0X1	T49.0X2	T49.0X3	T49.0X4	T49.0X5	T49.0X6
- ENT agent	T49.6X1	T49.6X2	T49.6X3	T49.6X4	T49.6X5	T49.6X6
- ophthalmic preparation	T49.5X1	T49.5X2	T49.5X3	T49.5X4	T49.5X5	T49.5X6
- topical NEC	T49.0X1	T49.0X2	T49.0X3	T49.0X4	T49.0X5	T49.0X6

Substance	Poisoning, Accidental (unintentional)	Poisoning, Intentional Self-harm	Poisoning, Assault	Poisoning, Undetermined	Adverse effect	Underdosing
Cortisone (acetate)	T38.0X1	T38.0X2	T38.0X3	T38.0X4	T38.0X5	T38.0X6
- ENT agent	T49.6X1	T49.6X2	T49.6X3	T49.6X4	T49.6X5	T49.6X6
- ophthalmic preparation	T49.5X1	T49.5X2	T49.5X3	T49.5X4	T49.5X5	T49.5X6
- topical NEC	T49.0X1	T49.0X2	T49.0X3	T49.0X4	T49.0X5	T49.0X6
Cortivazol	T38.0X1	T38.0X2	T38.0X3	T38.0X4	T38.0X5	T38.0X6
Cortogen	T38.0X1	T38.0X2	T38.0X3	T38.0X4	T38.0X5	T38.0X6
- ENT agent	T49.6X1	T49.6X2	T49.6X3	T49.6X4	T49.6X5	T49.6X6
- ophthalmic preparation	T49.5X1	T49.5X2	T49.5X3	T49.5X4	T49.5X5	T49.5X6
Cortone	T38.0X1	T38.0X2	T38.0X3	T38.0X4	T38.0X5	T38.0X6
- ENT agent	T49.6X1	T49.6X2	T49.6X3	T49.6X4	T49.6X5	T49.6X6
- ophthalmic preparation	T49.5X1	T49.5X2	T49.5X3	T49.5X4	T49.5X5	T49.5X6
Cortril	T38.0X1	T38.0X2	T38.0X3	T38.0X4	T38.0X5	T38.0X6
- ENT agent	T49.6X1	T49.6X2	T49.6X3	T49.6X4	T49.6X5	T49.6X6
- ophthalmic preparation	T49.5X1	T49.5X2	T49.5X3	T49.5X4	T49.5X5	T49.5X6
- topical NEC	T49.0X1	T49.0X2	T49.0X3	T49.0X4	T49.0X5	T49.0X6
Corynebacterium parvum	T45.1X1	T45.1X2	T45.1X3	T45.1X4	T45.1X5	T45.1X6
Cosmetic preparation	T49.8X1	T49.8X2	T49.8X3	T49.8X4	T49.8X5	T49.8X6
Cosmetics	T49.8X1	T49.8X2	T49.8X3	T49.8X4	T49.8X5	T49.8X6
Cosyntropin	T38.811	T38.812	T38.813	T38.814	T38.815	T38.816
Cotarnine	T45.7X1	T45.7X2	T45.7X3	T45.7X4	T45.7X5	T45.7X6
Co-trimoxazole	T36.8X1	T36.8X2	T36.8X3	T36.8X4	T36.8X5	T36.8X6
Cottonseed oil	T49.3X1	T49.3X2	T49.3X3	T49.3X4	T49.3X5	T49.3X6
Cough mixture (syrup)	T48.4X1	T48.4X2	T48.4X3	T48.4X4	T48.4X5	T48.4X6
- containing opiates	T40.2X1	T40.2X2	T40.2X3	T40.2X4	T40.2X5	T40.2X6
- expectorants	T48.4X1	T48.4X2	T48.4X3	T48.4X4	T48.4X5	T48.4X6
Coumadin	T45.511	T45.512	T45.513	T45.514	T45.515	T45.516
- rodenticide	T60.4X1	T60.4X2	T60.4X3	T60.4X4	--	--
Coumaphos	T60.0X1	T60.0X2	T60.0X3	T60.0X4	--	--
Coumarin	T45.511	T45.512	T45.513	T45.514	T45.515	T45.516
Coumetarol	T45.511	T45.512	T45.513	T45.514	T45.515	T45.516
Cowbane	T62.2X1	T62.2X2	T62.2X3	T62.2X4	--	--
Cozyme	T45.2X1	T45.2X2	T45.2X3	T45.2X4	T45.2X5	T45.2X6
Crack	T40.5X1	T40.5X2	T40.5X3	T40.5X4	--	--
Crataegus extract	T46.0X1	T46.0X2	T46.0X3	T46.0X4	T46.0X5	T46.0X6
Creolin	T54.1X1	T54.1X2	T54.1X3	T54.1X4	--	--
- disinfectant	T54.1X1	T54.1X2	T54.1X3	T54.1X4	--	--
Creosol (compound)	T49.0X1	T49.0X2	T49.0X3	T49.0X4	T49.0X5	T49.0X6
Creosote (coal tar) (beechwood)	T49.0X1	T49.0X2	T49.0X3	T49.0X4	T49.0X5	T49.0X6
- medicinal (expectorant)	T48.4X1	T48.4X2	T48.4X3	T48.4X4	T48.4X5	T48.4X6
- syrup	T48.4X1	T48.4X2	T48.4X3	T48.4X4	T48.4X5	T48.4X6
Cresol (s)	T49.0X1	T49.0X2	T49.0X3	T49.0X4	T49.0X5	T49.0X6
- and soap solution	T49.0X1	T49.0X2	T49.0X3	T49.0X4	T49.0X5	T49.0X6
Cresyl acetate	T49.0X1	T49.0X2	T49.0X3	T49.0X4	T49.0X5	T49.0X6
Cresylic acid	T49.0X1	T49.0X2	T49.0X3	T49.0X4	T49.0X5	T49.0X6
Crimidine	T60.4X1	T60.4X2	T60.4X3	T60.4X4	--	--
Croconazole	T37.8X1	T37.8X2	T37.8X3	T37.8X4	T37.8X5	T37.8X6
Cromoglicic acid	T48.6X1	T48.6X2	T48.6X3	T48.6X4	T48.6X5	T48.6X6
Cromolyn	T48.6X1	T48.6X2	T48.6X3	T48.6X4	T48.6X5	T48.6X6
Cromonar	T46.3X1	T46.3X2	T46.3X3	T46.3X4	T46.3X5	T46.3X6
Cropropamide	T39.8X1	T39.8X2	T39.8X3	T39.8X4	T39.8X5	T39.8X6
- with crotethamide	T50.7X1	T50.7X2	T50.7X3	T50.7X4	T50.7X5	T50.7X6
Crotamiton	T49.0X1	T49.0X2	T49.0X3	T49.0X4	T49.0X5	T49.0X6
Crotethamide	T39.8X1	T39.8X2	T39.8X3	T39.8X4	T39.8X5	T39.8X6
- with cropropamide	T50.7X1	T50.7X2	T50.7X3	T50.7X4	T50.7X5	T50.7X6
Croton (oil)	T47.2X1	T47.2X2	T47.2X3	T47.2X4	T47.2X5	T47.2X6
- chloral	T42.6X1	T42.6X2	T42.6X3	T42.6X4	T42.6X5	T42.6X6
Crude oil	T52.0X1	T52.0X2	T52.0X3	T52.0X4	--	--
Cryogenine	T39.8X1	T39.8X2	T39.8X3	T39.8X4	T39.8X5	T39.8X6
Cryolite (vapor)	T60.1X1	T60.1X2	T60.1X3	T60.1X4	--	--
- insecticide	T60.1X1	T60.1X2	T60.1X3	T60.1X4	--	--
Cryptenamine (tannates)	T46.5X1	T46.5X2	T46.5X3	T46.5X4	T46.5X5	T46.5X6
Crystal violet	T49.0X1	T49.0X2	T49.0X3	T49.0X4	T49.0X5	T49.0X6
Cuckoopint	T62.2X1	T62.2X2	T62.2X3	T62.2X4	--	--
Cumetharol	T45.511	T45.512	T45.513	T45.514	T45.515	T45.516
Cupric						

Substance	Poisoning, Accidental (unintentional)	Poisoning, Intentional Self-harm	Poisoning, Assault	Poisoning, Undetermined	Adverse effect	Underdosing
- acetate	T60.3X1	T60.3X2	T60.3X3	T60.3X4	--	--
- acetoarsenite	T57.0X1	T57.0X2	T57.0X3	T57.0X4	--	--
- arsenate	T57.0X1	T57.0X2	T57.0X3	T57.0X4	--	--
- gluconate	T49.0X1	T49.0X2	T49.0X3	T49.0X4	T49.0X5	T49.0X6
- oleate	T49.0X1	T49.0X2	T49.0X3	T49.0X4	T49.0X5	T49.0X6
- sulfate	T56.4X1	T56.4X2	T56.4X3	T56.4X4	--	--
Cuprous sulfate—see also Copper sulfate	T56.4X1	T56.4X2	T56.4X3	T56.4X4	--	--
Curare, curarine	T48.1X1	T48.1X2	T48.1X3	T48.1X4	T48.1X5	T48.1X6
Cyamemazine	T43.3X1	T43.3X2	T43.3X3	T43.3X4	T43.3X5	T43.3X6
Cyamopsis tetragono-loba	T46.6X1	T46.6X2	T46.6X3	T46.6X4	T46.6X5	T46.6X6
Cyanacetyl hydrazide	T37.1X1	T37.1X2	T37.1X3	T37.1X4	T37.1X5	T37.1X6
Cyanic acid (gas)	T59.891	T59.892	T59.893	T59.894	--	--
Cyanide (s) (compounds) (potassium) (sodium) NEC	T65.0X1	T65.0X2	T65.0X3	T65.0X4	--	--
- dust or gas (inhalation) NEC	T57.3X1	T57.3X2	T57.3X3	T57.3X4	--	--
- fumigant	T65.0X1	T65.0X2	T65.0X3	T65.0X4	--	--
- hydrogen	T57.3X1	T57.3X2	T57.3X3	T57.3X4	--	--
- mercuric—see Mercury						
- pesticide (dust) (fumes)	T65.0X1	T65.0X2	T65.0X3	T65.0X4	--	--
Cyanoacrylate adhesive	T49.3X1	T49.3X2	T49.3X3	T49.3X4	T49.3X5	T49.3X6
Cyanocobalamin	T45.8X1	T45.8X2	T45.8X3	T45.8X4	T45.8X5	T45.8X6
Cyanogen (chloride) (gas) NEC	T59.891	T59.892	T59.893	T59.894	--	--
Cyclacillin	T36.0X1	T36.0X2	T36.0X3	T36.0X4	T36.0X5	T36.0X6
Cyclaine	T41.3X1	T41.3X2	T41.3X3	T41.3X4	T41.3X5	T41.3X6
Cyclamate	T50.991	T50.992	T50.993	T50.994	T50.995	T50.996
Cyclamen europaeum	T62.2X1	T62.2X2	T62.2X3	T62.2X4	--	--
Cyclandelate	T46.7X1	T46.7X2	T46.7X3	T46.7X4	T46.7X5	T46.7X6
Cyclazocine	T50.7X1	T50.7X2	T50.7X3	T50.7X4	T50.7X5	T50.7X6
Cyclizine	T45.0X1	T45.0X2	T45.0X3	T45.0X4	T45.0X5	T45.0X6
Cyclobarbital	T42.3X1	T42.3X2	T42.3X3	T42.3X4	T42.3X5	T42.3X6
Cyclobarbitone	T42.3X1	T42.3X2	T42.3X3	T42.3X4	T42.3X5	T42.3X6
Cyclobenzaprine	T48.1X1	T48.1X2	T48.1X3	T48.1X4	T48.1X5	T48.1X6
Cyclodrine	T44.3X1	T44.3X2	T44.3X3	T44.3X4	T44.3X5	T44.3X6
Cycloguanil embonate	T37.2X1	T37.2X2	T37.2X3	T37.2X4	T37.2X5	T37.2X6
Cyclohexane	T52.8X1	T52.8X2	T52.8X3	T52.8X4	--	--
Cyclohexanol	T51.8X1	T51.8X2	T51.8X3	T51.8X4	--	--
Cyclohexanone	T52.4X1	T52.4X2	T52.4X3	T52.4X4	--	--
Cycloheximide	T60.3X1	T60.3X2	T60.3X3	T60.3X4	--	--
Cyclohexyl acetate	T52.8X1	T52.8X2	T52.8X3	T52.8X4	--	--
Cycloleucin	T45.1X1	T45.1X2	T45.1X3	T45.1X4	T45.1X5	T45.1X6
Cyclomethycaine	T41.3X1	T41.3X2	T41.3X3	T41.3X4	T41.3X5	T41.3X6
Cyclopentamine	T44.4X1	T44.4X2	T44.4X3	T44.4X4	T44.4X5	T44.4X6
Cyclopenthiazide	T50.2X1	T50.2X2	T50.2X3	T50.2X4	T50.2X5	T50.2X6
Cyclopentolate	T44.3X1	T44.3X2	T44.3X3	T44.3X4	T44.3X5	T44.3X6
Cyclophosphamide	T45.1X1	T45.1X2	T45.1X3	T45.1X4	T45.1X5	T45.1X6
Cycloplegic drug	T49.5X1	T49.5X2	T49.5X3	T49.5X4	T49.5X5	T49.5X6
Cyclopropane	T41.291	T41.292	T41.293	T41.294	T41.295	T41.296
Cyclopyrabital	T39.8X1	T39.8X2	T39.8X3	T39.8X4	T39.8X5	T39.8X6
Cycloserine	T37.1X1	T37.1X2	T37.1X3	T37.1X4	T37.1X5	T37.1X6
Cyclosporin	T45.1X1	T45.1X2	T45.1X3	T45.1X4	T45.1X5	T45.1X6
Cyclothiazide	T50.2X1	T50.2X2	T50.2X3	T50.2X4	T50.2X5	T50.2X6
Cycrimine	T44.3X1	T44.3X2	T44.3X3	T44.3X4	T44.3X5	T44.3X6
Cyhalothrin	T60.1X1	T60.1X2	T60.1X3	T60.1X4	--	--
Cymarin	T46.0X1	T46.0X2	T46.0X3	T46.0X4	T46.0X5	T46.0X6
Cypermethrin	T60.1X1	T60.1X2	T60.1X3	T60.1X4	--	--
Cyphenothrin	T60.2X1	T60.2X2	T60.2X3	T60.2X4	--	--
Cyproheptadine	T45.0X1	T45.0X2	T45.0X3	T45.0X4	T45.0X5	T45.0X6
Cyproterone	T38.6X1	T38.6X2	T38.6X3	T38.6X4	T38.6X5	T38.6X6
Cysteamine	T50.6X1	T50.6X2	T50.6X3	T50.6X4	T50.6X5	T50.6X6
Cytarabine	T45.1X1	T45.1X2	T45.1X3	T45.1X4	T45.1X5	T45.1X6
Cytisus						
- laburnum	T62.2X1	T62.2X2	T62.2X3	T62.2X4	--	--
- scoparius	T62.2X1	T62.2X2	T62.2X3	T62.2X4	--	--
Cytochrome C	T47.5X1	T47.5X2	T47.5X3	T47.5X4	T47.5X5	T47.5X6
Cytomel	T38.1X1	T38.1X2	T38.1X3	T38.1X4	T38.1X5	T38.1X6

Substance	Poisoning, Accidental (unintentional)	Poisoning, Intentional Self-harm	Poisoning, Assault	Poisoning, Undetermined	Adverse effect	Underdosing
Cytosine arabinoside	T45.1X1	T45.1X2	T45.1X3	T45.1X4	T45.1X5	T45.1X6
Cytoxan	T45.1X1	T45.1X2	T45.1X3	T45.1X4	T45.1X5	T45.1X6
Cytozyme	T45.7X1	T45.7X2	T45.7X3	T45.7X4	T45.7X5	T45.7X6
2,4-D	T60.3X1	T60.3X2	T60.3X3	T60.3X4	--	--
Dacarbazine	T45.1X1	T45.1X2	T45.1X3	T45.1X4	T45.1X5	T45.1X6
Dactinomycin	T45.1X1	T45.1X2	T45.1X3	T45.1X4	T45.1X5	T45.1X6
DADPS	T37.1X1	T37.1X2	T37.1X3	T37.1X4	T37.1X5	T37.1X6
Dakin's solution	T49.0X1	T49.0X2	T49.0X3	T49.0X4	T49.0X5	T49.0X6
Dalapon (sodium)	T60.3X1	T60.3X2	T60.3X3	T60.3X4	--	--
Dalmane	T42.4X1	T42.4X2	T42.4X3	T42.4X4	T42.4X5	T42.4X6
Danazol	T38.6X1	T38.6X2	T38.6X3	T38.6X4	T38.6X5	T38.6X6
Danilone	T45.511	T45.512	T45.513	T45.514	T45.515	T45.516
Danthron	T47.2X1	T47.2X2	T47.2X3	T47.2X4	T47.2X5	T47.2X6
Dantrolene	T42.8X1	T42.8X2	T42.8X3	T42.8X4	T42.8X5	T42.8X6
Dantron	T47.2X1	T47.2X2	T47.2X3	T47.2X4	T47.2X5	T47.2X6
Daphne (gnidium) (mezereum)	T62.2X1	T62.2X2	T62.2X3	T62.2X4	--	--
- berry	T62.1X1	T62.1X2	T62.1X3	T62.1X4	--	--
Dapsone	T37.1X1	T37.1X2	T37.1X3	T37.1X4	T37.1X5	T37.1X6
Daraprim	T37.2X1	T37.2X2	T37.2X3	T37.2X4	T37.2X5	T37.2X6
Darnel	T62.2X1	T62.2X2	T62.2X3	T62.2X4	--	--
Darvon	T39.8X1	T39.8X2	T39.8X3	T39.8X4	T39.8X5	T39.8X6
Daunomycin	T45.1X1	T45.1X2	T45.1X3	T45.1X4	T45.1X5	T45.1X6
Daunorubicin	T45.1X1	T45.1X2	T45.1X3	T45.1X4	T45.1X5	T45.1X6
DBI	T38.3X1	T38.3X2	T38.3X3	T38.3X4	T38.3X5	T38.3X6
D-Con	T60.91	T60.92	T60.93	T60.94	--	--
- insecticide	T60.2X1	T60.2X2	T60.2X3	T60.2X4	--	--
- rodenticide	T60.4X1	T60.4X2	T60.4X3	T60.4X4	--	--
DDAVP	T38.891	T38.892	T38.893	T38.894	T38.895	T38.896
DDE (bis (chlorophenyl) -dichloroethylene)	T60.2X1	T60.2X2	T60.2X3	T60.2X4	--	--
DDS	T37.1X1	T37.1X2	T37.1X3	T37.1X4	T37.1X5	T37.1X6
DDT (dust)	T60.1X1	T60.1X2	T60.1X3	T60.1X4	--	--
Deadly nightshade—see also Belladonna	T62.2X1	T62.2X2	T62.2X3	T62.2X4	--	--
- berry	T62.1X1	T62.1X2	T62.1X3	T62.1X4	--	--
Deamino-D-arginine vasopressin	T38.891	T38.892	T38.893	T38.894	T38.895	T38.896
Deanol (aceglumate)	T50.991	T50.992	T50.993	T50.994	T50.995	T50.996
Debrisoquine	T46.5X1	T46.5X2	T46.5X3	T46.5X4	T46.5X5	T46.5X6
Decaborane	T57.8X1	T57.8X2	T57.8X3	T57.8X4	--	--
- fumes	T59.891	T59.892	T59.893	T59.894	--	--
Decadron	T38.0X1	T38.0X2	T38.0X3	T38.0X4	T38.0X5	T38.0X6
- ENT agent	T49.6X1	T49.6X2	T49.6X3	T49.6X4	T49.6X5	T49.6X6
- ophthalmic preparation	T49.5X1	T49.5X2	T49.5X3	T49.5X4	T49.5X5	T49.5X6
- topical NEC	T49.0X1	T49.0X2	T49.0X3	T49.0X4	T49.0X5	T49.0X6
Decahydronaphthalene	T52.8X1	T52.8X2	T52.8X3	T52.8X4	--	--
Decalin	T52.8X1	T52.8X2	T52.8X3	T52.8X4	--	--
Decamethonium (bromide)	T48.1X1	T48.1X2	T48.1X3	T48.1X4	T48.1X5	T48.1X6
Decholin	T47.5X1	T47.5X2	T47.5X3	T47.5X4	T47.5X5	T47.5X6
Declomycin	T36.4X1	T36.4X2	T36.4X3	T36.4X4	T36.4X5	T36.4X6
Decongestant, nasal (mucosa)	T48.5X1	T48.5X2	T48.5X3	T48.5X4	T48.5X5	T48.5X6
- combination	T48.5X1	T48.5X2	T48.5X3	T48.5X4	T48.5X5	T48.5X6
Deet	T60.8X1	T60.8X2	T60.8X3	T60.8X4	--	--
Deferoxamine	T45.8X1	T45.8X2	T45.8X3	T45.8X4	T45.8X5	T45.8X6
Deflazacort	T38.0X1	T38.0X2	T38.0X3	T38.0X4	T38.0X5	T38.0X6
Deglycyrrhizinized extract of licorice	T48.4X1	T48.4X2	T48.4X3	T48.4X4	T48.4X5	T48.4X6
Dehydrocholic acid	T47.5X1	T47.5X2	T47.5X3	T47.5X4	T47.5X5	T47.5X6
Dehydroemetine	T37.3X1	T37.3X2	T37.3X3	T37.3X4	T37.3X5	T37.3X6
Dekalin	T52.8X1	T52.8X2	T52.8X3	T52.8X4	--	--
Delalutin	T38.5X1	T38.5X2	T38.5X3	T38.5X4	T38.5X5	T38.5X6
Delorazepam	T42.4X1	T42.4X2	T42.4X3	T42.4X4	T42.4X5	T42.4X6
Delphinium	T62.2X1	T62.2X2	T62.2X3	T62.2X4	--	--
Deltamethrin	T60.1X1	T60.1X2	T60.1X3	T60.1X4	--	--
Deltasone	T38.0X1	T38.0X2	T38.0X3	T38.0X4	T38.0X5	T38.0X6
Deltra	T38.0X1	T38.0X2	T38.0X3	T38.0X4	T38.0X5	T38.0X6
Delvinal	T42.3X1	T42.3X2	T42.3X3	T42.3X4	T42.3X5	T42.3X6
Demecarium (bromide)	T49.5X1	T49.5X2	T49.5X3	T49.5X4	T49.5X5	T49.5X6
Demeclocycline	T36.4X1	T36.4X2	T36.4X3	T36.4X4	T36.4X5	T36.4X6

Substance	Poisoning, Accidental (unintentional)	Poisoning, Intentional Self-harm	Poisoning, Assault	Poisoning, Undetermined	Adverse effect	Underdosing
Demecolcine	T45.1X1	T45.1X2	T45.1X3	T45.1X4	T45.1X5	T45.1X6
Demegestone	T38.5X1	T38.5X2	T38.5X3	T38.5X4	T38.5X5	T38.5X6
Demelanizing agents	T49.8X1	T49.8X2	T49.8X3	T49.8X4	T49.8X5	T49.8X6
Demephion -O and -S	T60.0X1	T60.0X2	T60.0X3	T60.0X4	--	--
Demerol	T40.2X1	T40.2X2	T40.2X3	T40.2X4	T40.2X5	T40.2X6
Demethylchlortetracycline	T36.4X1	T36.4X2	T36.4X3	T36.4X4	T36.4X5	T36.4X6
Demethyltetracycline	T36.4X1	T36.4X2	T36.4X3	T36.4X4	T36.4X5	T36.4X6
Demeton -O and -S	T60.0X1	T60.0X2	T60.0X3	T60.0X4	--	--
Demulcent (external)	T49.3X1	T49.3X2	T49.3X3	T49.3X4	T49.3X5	T49.3X6
- specified NEC	T49.3X1	T49.3X2	T49.3X3	T49.3X4	T49.3X5	T49.3X6
Demulen	T38.4X1	T38.4X2	T38.4X3	T38.4X4	T38.4X5	T38.4X6
Denatured alcohol	T51.0X1	T51.0X2	T51.0X3	T51.0X4	--	--
Dendrid	T49.5X1	T49.5X2	T49.5X3	T49.5X4	T49.5X5	T49.5X6
Dental drug, topical application NEC	T49.7X1	T49.7X2	T49.7X3	T49.7X4	T49.7X5	T49.7X6
Dentifrice	T49.7X1	T49.7X2	T49.7X3	T49.7X4	T49.7X5	T49.7X6
Deodorant spray (feminine hygiene)	T49.8X1	T49.8X2	T49.8X3	T49.8X4	T49.8X5	T49.8X6
Deoxycortone	T50.0X1	T50.0X2	T50.0X3	T50.0X4	T50.0X5	T50.0X6
2-Deoxy-5-fluorouridine	T45.1X1	T45.1X2	T45.1X3	T45.1X4	T45.1X5	T45.1X6
5-Deoxy-5-fluorouridine	T45.1X1	T45.1X2	T45.1X3	T45.1X4	T45.1X5	T45.1X6
Deoxyribonuclease (pancreatic)	T45.3X1	T45.3X2	T45.3X3	T45.3X4	T45.3X5	T45.3X6
Depilatory	T49.4X1	T49.4X2	T49.4X3	T49.4X4	T49.4X5	T49.4X6
Deprenalin	T42.8X1	T42.8X2	T42.8X3	T42.8X4	T42.8X5	T42.8X6
Deprenyl	T42.8X1	T42.8X2	T42.8X3	T42.8X4	T42.8X5	T42.8X6
Depressant, appetite	T50.5X1	T50.5X2	T50.5X3	T50.5X4	T50.5X5	T50.5X6
Depressant						
- appetite (central)	T50.5X1	T50.5X2	T50.5X3	T50.5X4	T50.5X5	T50.5X6
- cardiac	T46.2X1	T46.2X2	T46.2X3	T46.2X4	T46.2X5	T46.2X6
-central nervous system (anesthetic) —see also Central nervous system, depressants	T42.71	T42.72	T42.73	T42.74	T42.75	T42.76
- - general anesthetic	T41.201	T41.202	T41.203	T41.204	T41.205	T41.206
- - muscle tone	T42.8X1	T42.8X2	T42.8X3	T42.8X4	T42.8X5	T42.8X6
- muscle tone, central	T42.8X1	T42.8X2	T42.8X3	T42.8X4	T42.8X5	T42.8X6
- psychotherapeutic	T43.501	T43.502	T43.503	T43.504	T43.505	T43.506
Deptropine	T45.0X1	T45.0X2	T45.0X3	T45.0X4	T45.0X5	T45.0X6
Dequalinium (chloride)	T49.0X1	T49.0X2	T49.0X3	T49.0X4	T49.0X5	T49.0X6
Derris root	T60.2X1	T60.2X2	T60.2X3	T60.2X4	--	--
Deserpidine	T46.5X1	T46.5X2	T46.5X3	T46.5X4	T46.5X5	T46.5X6
Desferrioxamine	T45.8X1	T45.8X2	T45.8X3	T45.8X4	T45.8X5	T45.8X6
Desipramine	T43.011	T43.012	T43.013	T43.014	T43.015	T43.016
Deslanoside	T46.0X1	T46.0X2	T46.0X3	T46.0X4	T46.0X5	T46.0X6
Desloughing agent	T49.4X1	T49.4X2	T49.4X3	T49.4X4	T49.4X5	T49.4X6
Desmethylimipramine	T43.011	T43.012	T43.013	T43.014	T43.015	T43.016
Desmopressin	T38.891	T38.892	T38.893	T38.894	T38.895	T38.896
Desocodeine	T40.2X1	T40.2X2	T40.2X3	T40.2X4	T40.2X5	T40.2X6
Desogestrel	T38.5X1	T38.5X2	T38.5X3	T38.5X4	T38.5X5	T38.5X6
Desomorphine	T40.2X1	T40.2X2	T40.2X3	T40.2X4	--	--
Desonide	T49.0X1	T49.0X2	T49.0X3	T49.0X4	T49.0X5	T49.0X6
Desoximetasone	T49.0X1	T49.0X2	T49.0X3	T49.0X4	T49.0X5	T49.0X6
Desoxycorticosteroid	T50.0X1	T50.0X2	T50.0X3	T50.0X4	T50.0X5	T50.0X6
Desoxycortone	T50.0X1	T50.0X2	T50.0X3	T50.0X4	T50.0X5	T50.0X6
Desoxyephedrine	T43.621	T43.622	T43.623	T43.624	T43.625	T43.626
Detaxtran	T46.6X1	T46.6X2	T46.6X3	T46.6X4	T46.6X5	T46.6X6
Detergent	T49.2X1	T49.2X2	T49.2X3	T49.2X4	T49.2X5	T49.2X6
- external medication	T49.2X1	T49.2X2	T49.2X3	T49.2X4	T49.2X5	T49.2X6
- local	T49.2X1	T49.2X2	T49.2X3	T49.2X4	T49.2X5	T49.2X6
- medicinal	T49.2X1	T49.2X2	T49.2X3	T49.2X4	T49.2X5	T49.2X6
- nonmedicinal	T55.1X1	T55.1X2	T55.1X3	T55.1X4	--	--
- specified NEC	T55.1X1	T55.1X2	T55.1X3	T55.1X4	--	--
Deterrent, alcohol	T50.6X1	T50.6X2	T50.6X3	T50.6X4	T50.6X5	T50.6X6
Detoxifying agent	T50.6X1	T50.6X2	T50.6X3	T50.6X4	T50.6X5	T50.6X6
Detrothyronine	T38.1X1	T38.1X2	T38.1X3	T38.1X4	T38.1X5	T38.1X6
Dettol (external medication)	T49.0X1	T49.0X2	T49.0X3	T49.0X4	T49.0X5	T49.0X6
Dexamethasone	T38.0X1	T38.0X2	T38.0X3	T38.0X4	T38.0X5	T38.0X6

Substance	Poisoning, Accidental (unintentional)	Poisoning, Intentional Self-harm	Poisoning, Assault	Poisoning, Undetermined	Adverse effect	Underdosing
- ENT agent	T49.6X1	T49.6X2	T49.6X3	T49.6X4	T49.6X5	T49.6X6
- ophthalmic preparation	T49.5X1	T49.5X2	T49.5X3	T49.5X4	T49.5X5	T49.5X6
- topical NEC	T49.0X1	T49.0X2	T49.0X3	T49.0X4	T49.0X5	T49.0X6
Dexamfetamine	T43.621	T43.622	T43.623	T43.624	T43.625	T43.626
Dexamphetamine	T43.621	T43.622	T43.623	T43.624	T43.625	T43.626
Dexbrompheniramine	T45.0X1	T45.0X2	T45.0X3	T45.0X4	T45.0X5	T45.0X6
Dexchlorpheniramine	T45.0X1	T45.0X2	T45.0X3	T45.0X4	T45.0X5	T45.0X6
Dexedrine	T43.621	T43.622	T43.623	T43.624	T43.625	T43.626
Dexetimide	T44.3X1	T44.3X2	T44.3X3	T44.3X4	T44.3X5	T44.3X6
Dexfenfluramine	T50.5X1	T50.5X2	T50.5X3	T50.5X4	T50.5X5	T50.5X6
Dexpanthenol	T45.2X1	T45.2X2	T45.2X3	T45.2X4	T45.2X5	T45.2X6
Dextran (40) (70) (150)	T45.8X1	T45.8X2	T45.8X3	T45.8X4	T45.8X5	T45.8X6
Dextriferron	T45.4X1	T45.4X2	T45.4X3	T45.4X4	T45.4X5	T45.4X6
Dextro calcium pantothenate	T45.2X1	T45.2X2	T45.2X3	T45.2X4	T45.2X5	T45.2X6
Dextro pantothenyl alcohol	T45.2X1	T45.2X2	T45.2X3	T45.2X4	T45.2X5	T45.2X6
Dextroamphetamine	T43.621	T43.622	T43.623	T43.624	T43.625	T43.626
Dextromethorphan	T48.3X1	T48.3X2	T48.3X3	T48.3X4	T48.3X5	T48.3X6
Dextromoramide	T40.4X1	T40.4X2	T40.4X3	T40.4X4	--	--
- topical	T49.8X1	T49.8X2	T49.8X3	T49.8X4	T49.8X5	T49.8X6
Dextropropoxyphene	T40.4X1	T40.4X2	T40.4X3	T40.4X4	T40.4X5	T40.4X6
Dextrorphan	T40.2X1	T40.2X2	T40.2X3	T40.2X4	T40.2X5	T40.2X6
Dextrose	T50.3X1	T50.3X2	T50.3X3	T50.3X4	T50.3X5	T50.3X6
- concentrated solution, intravenous	T46.8X1	T46.8X2	T46.8X3	T46.8X4	T46.8X5	T46.8X6
Dextrothyroxin	T38.1X1	T38.1X2	T38.1X3	T38.1X4	T38.1X5	T38.1X6
Dextrothyroxine sodium	T38.1X1	T38.1X2	T38.1X3	T38.1X4	T38.1X5	T38.1X6
DFP	T44.0X1	T44.0X2	T44.0X3	T44.0X4	T44.0X5	T44.0X6
DHE	T37.3X1	T37.3X2	T37.3X3	T37.3X4	T37.3X5	T37.3X6
- 45	T46.5X1	T46.5X2	T46.5X3	T46.5X4	T46.5X5	T46.5X6
Diabinese	T38.3X1	T38.3X2	T38.3X3	T38.3X4	T38.3X5	T38.3X6
Diacetone alcohol	T52.4X1	T52.4X2	T52.4X3	T52.4X4	--	--
Diacetyl monoxime	T50.991	T50.992	T50.993	T50.994	--	--
Diacetylmorphine	T40.1X1	T40.1X2	T40.1X3	T40.1X4	T40.1X5	--
Diachylon plaster	T49.4X1	T49.4X2	T49.4X3	T49.4X4	T49.4X5	T49.4X6
Diaethylstilboestrolum	T38.5X1	T38.5X2	T38.5X3	T38.5X4	T38.5X5	T38.5X6
Diagnostic agent NEC	T50.8X1	T50.8X2	T50.8X3	T50.8X4	T50.8X5	T50.8X6
Dial (soap)	T49.2X1	T49.2X2	T49.2X3	T49.2X4	T49.2X5	T49.2X6
- sedative	T42.3X1	T42.3X2	T42.3X3	T42.3X4	T42.3X5	T42.3X6
Dialkyl carbonate	T52.91	T52.92	T52.93	T52.94	--	--
Diallylbarbituric acid	T42.3X1	T42.3X2	T42.3X3	T42.3X4	T42.3X5	T42.3X6
Diallymal	T42.3X1	T42.3X2	T42.3X3	T42.3X4	T42.3X5	T42.3X6
Dialysis solution (intraperitoneal)	T50.3X1	T50.3X2	T50.3X3	T50.3X4	T50.3X5	T50.3X6
Diaminodiphenylsulfone	T37.1X1	T37.1X2	T37.1X3	T37.1X4	T37.1X5	T37.1X6
Diamorphine	T40.1X1	T40.1X2	T40.1X3	T40.1X4	T40.1X5	--
Diamox	T50.2X1	T50.2X2	T50.2X3	T50.2X4	T50.2X5	T50.2X6
Diamthazole	T49.0X1	T49.0X2	T49.0X3	T49.0X4	T49.0X5	T49.0X6
Dianthone	T47.2X1	T47.2X2	T47.2X3	T47.2X4	T47.2X5	T47.2X6
Diaphenylsulfone	T37.0X1	T37.0X2	T37.0X3	T37.0X4	T37.0X5	T37.0X6
Diasone (sodium)	T37.1X1	T37.1X2	T37.1X3	T37.1X4	T37.1X5	T37.1X6
Diastase	T47.5X1	T47.5X2	T47.5X3	T47.5X4	T47.5X5	T47.5X6
Diatrizoate	T50.8X1	T50.8X2	T50.8X3	T50.8X4	T50.8X5	T50.8X6
Diazepam	T42.4X1	T42.4X2	T42.4X3	T42.4X4	T42.4X5	T42.4X6
Diazinon	T60.0X1	T60.0X2	T60.0X3	T60.0X4	--	--
Diazomethane (gas)	T59.891	T59.892	T59.893	T59.894	--	--
Diazoxide	T46.5X1	T46.5X2	T46.5X3	T46.5X4	T46.5X5	T46.5X6
Dibekacin	T36.5X1	T36.5X2	T36.5X3	T36.5X4	T36.5X5	T36.5X6
Dibenamine	T44.6X1	T44.6X2	T44.6X3	T44.6X4	T44.6X5	T44.6X6
Dibenzepin	T43.011	T43.012	T43.013	T43.014	T43.015	T43.016
Dibenzheptropine	T45.0X1	T45.0X2	T45.0X3	T45.0X4	T45.0X5	T45.0X6
Dibenzyline	T44.6X1	T44.6X2	T44.6X3	T44.6X4	T44.6X5	T44.6X6
Diborane (gas)	T59.891	T59.892	T59.893	T59.894	--	--
Dibromochloropropane	T60.8X1	T60.8X2	T60.8X3	T60.8X4	--	--
Dibromodulcitol	T45.1X1	T45.1X2	T45.1X3	T45.1X4	T45.1X5	T45.1X6
Dibromoethane	T53.6X1	T53.6X2	T53.6X3	T53.6X4	--	--
Dibromomannitol	T45.1X1	T45.1X2	T45.1X3	T45.1X4	T45.1X5	T45.1X6
Dibromopropamidine isethionate	T49.0X1	T49.0X2	T49.0X3	T49.0X4	T49.0X5	T49.0X6

Substance	Poisoning, Accidental (unintentional)	Poisoning, Intentional Self-harm	Poisoning, Assault	Poisoning, Undetermined	Adverse effect	Underdosing
Dibrompropamidine	T49.0X1	T49.0X2	T49.0X3	T49.0X4	T49.0X5	T49.0X6
Dibucaine	T41.3X1	T41.3X2	T41.3X3	T41.3X4	T41.3X5	T41.3X6
- topical (surface)	T41.3X1	T41.3X2	T41.3X3	T41.3X4	T41.3X5	T41.3X6
Dibunate sodium	T48.3X1	T48.3X2	T48.3X3	T48.3X4	T48.3X5	T48.3X6
Dibutoline sulfate	T44.3X1	T44.3X2	T44.3X3	T44.3X4	T44.3X5	T44.3X6
Dicamba	T60.3X1	T60.3X2	T60.3X3	T60.3X4	--	--
Dicapthon	T60.0X1	T60.0X2	T60.0X3	T60.0X4	--	--
Dichlobenil	T60.3X1	T60.3X2	T60.3X3	T60.3X4	--	--
Dichlone	T60.3X1	T60.3X2	T60.3X3	T60.3X4	--	--
Dichloralphenozone	T42.6X1	T42.6X2	T42.6X3	T42.6X4	T42.6X5	T42.6X6
Dichlorbenzidine	T65.3X1	T65.3X2	T65.3X3	T65.3X4	--	--
Dichlorhydrin	T52.8X1	T52.8X2	T52.8X3	T52.8X4	--	--
Dichlorhydroxyquinoline	T37.8X1	T37.8X2	T37.8X3	T37.8X4	T37.8X5	T37.8X6
Dichlorobenzene	T53.7X1	T53.7X2	T53.7X3	T53.7X4	--	--
Dichlorobenzyl alcohol	T49.6X1	T49.6X2	T49.6X3	T49.6X4	T49.6X5	T49.6X6
Dichlorodifluoromethane	T53.5X1	T53.5X2	T53.5X3	T53.5X4	--	--
Dichloroethane	T52.8X1	T52.8X2	T52.8X3	T52.8X4	--	--
Sym-Dichloroethyl ether	T53.6X1	T53.6X2	T53.6X3	T53.6X4	--	--
Dichloroethyl sulfide, not in war	T59.891	T59.892	T59.893	T59.894	--	--
Dichloroethylene	T53.6X1	T53.6X2	T53.6X3	T53.6X4	--	--
Dichloroformoxine, not in war	T59.891	T59.892	T59.893	T59.894	--	--
Dichlorohydrin, alpha-dichlorohydrin	T52.8X1	T52.8X2	T52.8X3	T52.8X4	--	--
Dichloromethane (solvent)	T53.4X1	T53.4X2	T53.4X3	T53.4X4	--	--
- vapor	T53.4X1	T53.4X2	T53.4X3	T53.4X4	--	--
Dichloronaphthoquinone	T60.3X1	T60.3X2	T60.3X3	T60.3X4	--	--
Dichlorophen	T37.4X1	T37.4X2	T37.4X3	T37.4X4	T37.4X5	T37.4X6
2,4-Dichlorophenoxyacetic acid	T60.3X1	T60.3X2	T60.3X3	T60.3X4	--	--
Dichloropropene	T60.3X1	T60.3X2	T60.3X3	T60.3X4	--	--
Dichloropropionic acid	T60.3X1	T60.3X2	T60.3X3	T60.3X4	--	--
Dichlorphenamide	T50.2X1	T50.2X2	T50.2X3	T50.2X4	T50.2X5	T50.2X6
Dichlorvos	T60.0X1	T60.0X2	T60.0X3	T60.0X4	--	--
Diclofenac	T39.391	T39.392	T39.393	T39.394	T39.395	T39.396
Diclofenamide	T50.2X1	T50.2X2	T50.2X3	T50.2X4	T50.2X5	T50.2X6
Diclofensine	T43.291	T43.292	T43.293	T43.294	T43.295	T43.296
Diclonixine	T39.8X1	T39.8X2	T39.8X3	T39.8X4	T39.8X5	T39.8X6
Dicloxacillin	T36.0X1	T36.0X2	T36.0X3	T36.0X4	T36.0X5	T36.0X6
Dicophane	T49.0X1	T49.0X2	T49.0X3	T49.0X4	T49.0X5	T49.0X6
Dicoumarol, dicoumarin, dicumarol	T45.511	T45.512	T45.513	T45.514	T45.515	T45.516
Dicrotophos	T60.0X1	T60.0X2	T60.0X3	T60.0X4	--	--
Dicyanogen (gas)	T65.0X1	T65.0X2	T65.0X3	T65.0X4	--	--
Dicyclomine	T44.3X1	T44.3X2	T44.3X3	T44.3X4	T44.3X5	T44.3X6
Dicycloverine	T44.3X1	T44.3X2	T44.3X3	T44.3X4	T44.3X5	T44.3X6
Dideoxycytidine	T37.5X1	T37.5X2	T37.5X3	T37.5X4	T37.5X5	T37.5X6
Dideoxyinosine	T37.5X1	T37.5X2	T37.5X3	T37.5X4	T37.5X5	T37.5X6
Dieldrin (vapor)	T60.1X1	T60.1X2	T60.1X3	T60.1X4	--	--
Diemal	T42.3X1	T42.3X2	T42.3X3	T42.3X4	T42.3X5	T42.3X6
Dienestrol	T38.5X1	T38.5X2	T38.5X3	T38.5X4	T38.5X5	T38.5X6
Dienoestrol	T38.5X1	T38.5X2	T38.5X3	T38.5X4	T38.5X5	T38.5X6
Dietetic drug NEC	T50.901	T50.902	T50.903	T50.904	T50.905	T50.906
Diethazine	T42.8X1	T42.8X2	T42.8X3	T42.8X4	T42.8X5	T42.8X6
Diethyl						
- barbituric acid	T42.3X1	T42.3X2	T42.3X3	T42.3X4	T42.3X5	T42.3X6
- carbamazine	T37.4X1	T37.4X2	T37.4X3	T37.4X4	T37.4X5	T37.4X6
carbinol	T51.3X1	T51.3X2	T51.3X3	T51.3X4	--	--
- carbonate	T52.8X1	T52.8X2	T52.8X3	T52.8X4	--	--
- ether (vapor) —see also ether	T41.0X1	T41.0X2	T41.0X3	T41.0X4	T41.0X5	T41.0X6
- oxide	T52.8X1	T52.8X2	T52.8X3	T52.8X4	--	--
- propion	T50.5X1	T50.5X2	T50.5X3	T50.5X4	T50.5X5	T50.5X6
- stilbestrol	T38.5X1	T38.5X2	T38.5X3	T38.5X4	T38.5X5	T38.5X6
- toluamide (nonmedicinal)	T60.8X1	T60.8X2	T60.8X3	T60.8X4	--	--
- - medicinal	T49.3X1	T49.3X2	T49.3X3	T49.3X4	T49.3X5	T49.3X6
Diethylcarbamazine	T37.4X1	T37.4X2	T37.4X3	T37.4X4	T37.4X5	T37.4X6
Diethylene						
- dioxide	T52.8X1	T52.8X2	T52.8X3	T52.8X4	--	--

Substance	Poisoning, Accidental (unintentional)	Poisoning, Intentional Self-harm	Poisoning, Assault	Poisoning, Undetermined	Adverse effect	Underdosing
- glycol (monoacetate) (monobutyl ether) (monoethyl ether)	T52.3X1	T52.3X2	T52.3X3	T52.3X4	--	--
Diethylhexylphthalate	T65.891	T65.892	T65.893	T65.894	--	--
Diethylpropion	T50.5X1	T50.5X2	T50.5X3	T50.5X4	T50.5X5	T50.5X6
Diethylstilbestrol	T38.5X1	T38.5X2	T38.5X3	T38.5X4	T38.5X5	T38.5X6
Diethylstilboestrol	T38.5X1	T38.5X2	T38.5X3	T38.5X4	T38.5X5	T38.5X6
Diethylsulfone-diethylmethane	T42.6X1	T42.6X2	T42.6X3	T42.6X4	T42.6X5	T42.6X6
Diethyltoluamide	T49.0X1	T49.0X2	T49.0X3	T49.0X4	T49.0X5	T49.0X6
Diethyltryptamine (DET)	T40.991	T40.992	T40.993	T40.994	--	--
Difebarbamate	T42.3X1	T42.3X2	T42.3X3	T42.3X4	T42.3X5	T42.3X6
Difencloxazine	T40.2X1	T40.2X2	T40.2X3	T40.2X4	T40.2X5	T40.2X6
Difenidol	T45.0X1	T45.0X2	T45.0X3	T45.0X4	T45.0X5	T45.0X6
Difenoxin	T47.6X1	T47.6X2	T47.6X3	T47.6X4	T47.6X5	T47.6X6
Difetarsone	T37.3X1	T37.3X2	T37.3X3	T37.3X4	T37.3X5	T37.3X6
Diffusin	T45.3X1	T45.3X2	T45.3X3	T45.3X4	T45.3X5	T45.3X6
Diflorasone	T49.0X1	T49.0X2	T49.0X3	T49.0X4	T49.0X5	T49.0X6
Diflos	T44.0X1	T44.0X2	T44.0X3	T44.0X4	T44.0X5	T44.0X6
Diflubenzuron	T60.1X1	T60.1X2	T60.1X3	T60.1X4	--	--
Diflucortolone	T49.0X1	T49.0X2	T49.0X3	T49.0X4	T49.0X5	T49.0X6
Diflunisal	T39.091	T39.092	T39.093	T39.094	T39.095	T39.096
Difluoromethyldopa	T42.8X1	T42.8X2	T42.8X3	T42.8X4	T42.8X5	T42.8X6
Difluorophate	T44.0X1	T44.0X2	T44.0X3	T44.0X4	T44.0X5	T44.0X6
Digestant NEC	T47.5X1	T47.5X2	T47.5X3	T47.5X4	T47.5X5	T47.5X6
Digitalin (e)	T46.0X1	T46.0X2	T46.0X3	T46.0X4	T46.0X5	T46.0X6
Digitalis (leaf) (glycoside)	T46.0X1	T46.0X2	T46.0X3	T46.0X4	T46.0X5	T46.0X6
- lanata	T46.0X1	T46.0X2	T46.0X3	T46.0X4	T46.0X5	T46.0X6
- purpurea	T46.0X1	T46.0X2	T46.0X3	T46.0X4	T46.0X5	T46.0X6
Digitoxin	T46.0X1	T46.0X2	T46.0X3	T46.0X4	T46.0X5	T46.0X6
Digitoxose	T46.0X1	T46.0X2	T46.0X3	T46.0X4	T46.0X5	T46.0X6
Digoxin	T46.0X1	T46.0X2	T46.0X3	T46.0X4	T46.0X5	T46.0X6
Digoxine	T46.0X1	T46.0X2	T46.0X3	T46.0X4	T46.0X5	T46.0X6
Dihydralazine	T46.5X1	T46.5X2	T46.5X3	T46.5X4	T46.5X5	T46.5X6
Dihydrazine	T46.5X1	T46.5X2	T46.5X3	T46.5X4	T46.5X5	T46.5X6
Dihydrocodeine	T40.2X1	T40.2X2	T40.2X3	T40.2X4	T40.2X5	T40.2X6
Dihydrocodeinone	T40.2X1	T40.2X2	T40.2X3	T40.2X4	T40.2X5	T40.2X6
Dihydroergocornine	T46.7X1	T46.7X2	T46.7X3	T46.7X4	T46.7X5	T46.7X6
Dihydroergocristine (mesilate)	T46.7X1	T46.7X2	T46.7X3	T46.7X4	T46.7X5	T46.7X6
Dihydroergokryptine	T46.7X1	T46.7X2	T46.7X3	T46.7X4	T46.7X5	T46.7X6
Dihydroergotamine	T46.5X1	T46.5X2	T46.5X3	T46.5X4	T46.5X5	T46.5X6
Dihydroergotoxine	T46.7X1	T46.7X2	T46.7X3	T46.7X4	T46.7X5	T46.7X6
- mesilate	T46.7X1	T46.7X2	T46.7X3	T46.7X4	T46.7X5	T46.7X6
Dihydrohydroxycodeinone	T40.2X1	T40.2X2	T40.2X3	T40.2X4	T40.2X5	T40.2X6
Dihydrohydroxymorphinone	T40.2X1	T40.2X2	T40.2X3	T40.2X4	T40.2X5	T40.2X6
Dihydroisocodeine	T40.2X1	T40.2X2	T40.2X3	T40.2X4	T40.2X5	T40.2X6
Dihydromorphine	T40.2X1	T40.2X2	T40.2X3	T40.2X4	--	--
Dihydromorphinone	T40.2X1	T40.2X2	T40.2X3	T40.2X4	T40.2X5	T40.2X6
Dihydrostreptomycin	T36.5X1	T36.5X2	T36.5X3	T36.5X4	T36.5X5	T36.5X6
Dihydrotachysterol	T45.2X1	T45.2X2	T45.2X3	T45.2X4	T45.2X5	T45.2X6
Dihydroxyaluminum aminoacetate	T47.1X1	T47.1X2	T47.1X3	T47.1X4	T47.1X5	T47.1X6
Dihydroxyaluminum sodium carbonate	T47.1X1	T47.1X2	T47.1X3	T47.1X4	T47.1X5	T47.1X6
Dihydroxyanthraquinone	T47.2X1	T47.2X2	T47.2X3	T47.2X4	T47.2X5	T47.2X6
Dihydroxycodeinone	T40.2X1	T40.2X2	T40.2X3	T40.2X4	T40.2X5	T40.2X6
Dihydroxypropyl theophylline	T50.2X1	T50.2X2	T50.2X3	T50.2X4	T50.2X5	T50.2X6
Diiodohydroxyquin	T37.8X1	T37.8X2	T37.8X3	T37.8X4	T37.8X5	T37.8X6
- topical	T49.0X1	T49.0X2	T49.0X3	T49.0X4	T49.0X5	T49.0X6
Diiodohydroxyquinoline	T37.8X1	T37.8X2	T37.8X3	T37.8X4	T37.8X5	T37.8X6
Diiodotyrosine	T38.2X1	T38.2X2	T38.2X3	T38.2X4	T38.2X5	T38.2X6
Diisopromine	T44.3X1	T44.3X2	T44.3X3	T44.3X4	T44.3X5	T44.3X6
Diisopropylamine	T46.3X1	T46.3X2	T46.3X3	T46.3X4	T46.3X5	T46.3X6
Diisopropylfluorophos-phonate	T44.0X1	T44.0X2	T44.0X3	T44.0X4	T44.0X5	T44.0X6
Dilantin	T42.0X1	T42.0X2	T42.0X3	T42.0X4	T42.0X5	T42.0X6
Dilaudid	T40.2X1	T40.2X2	T40.2X3	T40.2X4	T40.2X5	T40.2X6
Dilazep	T46.3X1	T46.3X2	T46.3X3	T46.3X4	T46.3X5	T46.3X6
Dill	T47.5X1	T47.5X2	T47.5X3	T47.5X4	T47.5X5	T47.5X6
Diloxanide	T37.3X1	T37.3X2	T37.3X3	T37.3X4	T37.3X5	T37.3X6

Substance	Poisoning, Accidental (unintentional)	Poisoning, Intentional Self-harm	Poisoning, Assault	Poisoning, Undetermined	Adverse effect	Underdosing
Diltiazem	T46.1X1	T46.1X2	T46.1X3	T46.1X4	T46.1X5	T46.1X6
Dimazole	T49.0X1	T49.0X2	T49.0X3	T49.0X4	T49.0X5	T49.0X6
Dimefline	T50.7X1	T50.7X2	T50.7X3	T50.7X4	T50.7X5	T50.7X6
Dimefox	T60.0X1	T60.0X2	T60.0X3	T60.0X4	--	--
Dimemorfan	T48.3X1	T48.3X2	T48.3X3	T48.3X4	T48.3X5	T48.3X6
Dimenhydrinate	T45.0X1	T45.0X2	T45.0X3	T45.0X4	T45.0X5	T45.0X6
Dimercaprol (British anti-lewisite)	T45.8X1	T45.8X2	T45.8X3	T45.8X4	T45.8X5	T45.8X6
Dimercaptopropanol	T45.8X1	T45.8X2	T45.8X3	T45.8X4	T45.8X5	T45.8X6
Dimestrol	T38.5X1	T38.5X2	T38.5X3	T38.5X4	T38.5X5	T38.5X6
Dimetane	T45.0X1	T45.0X2	T45.0X3	T45.0X4	T45.0X5	T45.0X6
Dimethicone	T47.1X1	T47.1X2	T47.1X3	T47.1X4	T47.1X5	T47.1X6
Dimethindene	T45.0X1	T45.0X2	T45.0X3	T45.0X4	T45.0X5	T45.0X6
Dimethisoquin	T49.1X1	T49.1X2	T49.1X3	T49.1X4	T49.1X5	T49.1X6
Dimethisterone	T38.5X1	T38.5X2	T38.5X3	T38.5X4	T38.5X5	T38.5X6
Dimethoate	T60.0X1	T60.0X2	T60.0X3	T60.0X4	--	--
Dimethocaine	T41.3X1	T41.3X2	T41.3X3	T41.3X4	T41.3X5	T41.3X6
Dimethoxanate	T48.3X1	T48.3X2	T48.3X3	T48.3X4	T48.3X5	T48.3X6
Dimethyl						
- arsine, arsinic acid	T57.0X1	T57.0X2	T57.0X3	T57.0X4	--	--
- carbinol	T51.2X1	T51.2X2	T51.2X3	T51.2X4	--	--
- carbonate	T52.8X1	T52.8X2	T52.8X3	T52.8X4	--	--
- diguanide	T38.3X1	T38.3X2	T38.3X3	T38.3X4	T38.3X5	T38.3X6
- ketone	T52.4X1	T52.4X2	T52.4X3	T52.4X4	--	--
- - vapor	T52.4X1	T52.4X2	T52.4X3	T52.4X4	--	--
- meperidine	T40.2X1	T40.2X2	T40.2X3	T40.2X4	T40.2X5	T40.2X6
- parathion	T60.0X1	T60.0X2	T60.0X3	T60.0X4	--	--
- phthlate	T49.3X1	T49.3X2	T49.3X3	T49.3X4	T49.3X5	T49.3X6
- polysiloxane	T47.8X1	T47.8X2	T47.8X3	T47.8X4	T47.8X5	T47.8X6
- sulfate (fumes)	T59.891	T59.892	T59.893	T59.894	--	--
- - liquid	T65.891	T65.892	T65.893	T65.894	--	--
- sulfoxide (nonmedicinal)	T52.8X1	T52.8X2	T52.8X3	T52.8X4	--	--
- - medicinal	T49.4X1	T49.4X2	T49.4X3	T49.4X4	T49.4X5	T49.4X6
- tryptamine	T40.991	T40.992	T40.993	T40.994	--	--
- tubocurarine	T48.1X1	T48.1X2	T48.1X3	T48.1X4	T48.1X5	T48.1X6
Dimethylamine sulfate	T49.4X1	T49.4X2	T49.4X3	T49.4X4	T49.4X5	T49.4X6
Dimethylformamide	T52.8X1	T52.8X2	T52.8X3	T52.8X4	--	--
Dimethyltubocurarinium chloride	T48.1X1	T48.1X2	T48.1X3	T48.1X4	T48.1X5	T48.1X6
Dimeticone	T47.1X1	T47.1X2	T47.1X3	T47.1X4	T47.1X5	T47.1X6
Dimetilan	T60.0X1	T60.0X2	T60.0X3	T60.0X4	--	--
Dimetindene	T45.0X1	T45.0X2	T45.0X3	T45.0X4	T45.0X5	T45.0X6
Dimetotiazine	T43.3X1	T43.3X2	T43.3X3	T43.3X4	T43.3X5	T43.3X6
Dimorpholamine	T50.7X1	T50.7X2	T50.7X3	T50.7X4	T50.7X5	T50.7X6
Dimoxyline	T46.3X1	T46.3X2	T46.3X3	T46.3X4	T46.3X5	T46.3X6
Dinitrobenzene	T65.3X1	T65.3X2	T65.3X3	T65.3X4	--	--
- vapor	T59.891	T59.892	T59.893	T59.894	--	--
Dinitrobenzol	T65.3X1	T65.3X2	T65.3X3	T65.3X4	--	--
- vapor	T59.891	T59.892	T59.893	T59.894	--	--
Dinitrobutylphenol	T65.3X1	T65.3X2	T65.3X3	T65.3X4	--	--
Dinitro (-ortho-) cresol (pesticide) (spray)	T65.3X1	T65.3X2	T65.3X3	T65.3X4	--	--
Dinitrocyclohexylphenol	T65.3X1	T65.3X2	T65.3X3	T65.3X4	--	--
Dinitrophenol	T65.3X1	T65.3X2	T65.3X3	T65.3X4	--	--
Dinoprost	T48.0X1	T48.0X2	T48.0X3	T48.0X4	T48.0X5	T48.0X6
Dinoprostone	T48.0X1	T48.0X2	T48.0X3	T48.0X4	T48.0X5	T48.0X6
Dinoseb	T60.3X1	T60.3X2	T60.3X3	T60.3X4	--	--
Dioctyl sulfosuccinate (calcium) (sodium)	T47.4X1	T47.4X2	T47.4X3	T47.4X4	T47.4X5	T47.4X6
Diodone	T50.8X1	T50.8X2	T50.8X3	T50.8X4	T50.8X5	T50.8X6
Diodoquin	T37.8X1	T37.8X2	T37.8X3	T37.8X4	T37.8X5	T37.8X6
Dionin	T40.2X1	T40.2X2	T40.2X3	T40.2X4	T40.2X5	T40.2X6
Diosmin	T46.991	T46.992	T46.993	T46.994	T46.995	T46.996
Dioxane	T52.8X1	T52.8X2	T52.8X3	T52.8X4	--	--
Dioxathion	T60.0X1	T60.0X2	T60.0X3	T60.0X4	--	--
Dioxin	T53.7X1	T53.7X2	T53.7X3	T53.7X4	--	--
Dioxopromethazine	T43.3X1	T43.3X2	T43.3X3	T43.3X4	T43.3X5	T43.3X6
Dioxyline	T46.3X1	T46.3X2	T46.3X3	T46.3X4	T46.3X5	T46.3X6
Dipentene	T52.8X1	T52.8X2	T52.8X3	T52.8X4	--	--

Substance	Poisoning, Accidental (unintentional)	Poisoning, Intentional Self-harm	Poisoning, Assault	Poisoning, Undetermined	Adverse effect	Underdosing
Diperodon	T41.3X1	T41.3X2	T41.3X3	T41.3X4	T41.3X5	T41.3X6
Diphacinone	T60.4X1	T60.4X2	T60.4X3	T60.4X4	--	--
Diphemanil	T44.3X1	T44.3X2	T44.3X3	T44.3X4	T44.3X5	T44.3X6
- metilsulfate	T44.3X1	T44.3X2	T44.3X3	T44.3X4	T44.3X5	T44.3X6
Diphenadione	T45.511	T45.512	T45.513	T45.514	T45.515	T45.516
- rodenticide	T60.4X1	T60.4X2	T60.4X3	T60.4X4	--	--
Diphenhydramine	T45.0X1	T45.0X2	T45.0X3	T45.0X4	T45.0X5	T45.0X6
Diphenidol	T45.0X1	T45.0X2	T45.0X3	T45.0X4	T45.0X5	T45.0X6
Diphenoxylate	T47.6X1	T47.6X2	T47.6X3	T47.6X4	T47.6X5	T47.6X6
Diphenylamine	T65.3X1	T65.3X2	T65.3X3	T65.3X4	--	--
Diphenylbutazone	T39.2X1	T39.2X2	T39.2X3	T39.2X4	T39.2X5	T39.2X6
Diphenylchloroarsine, not in war	T57.0X1	T57.0X2	T57.0X3	T57.0X4	--	--
Diphenylhydantoin	T42.0X1	T42.0X2	T42.0X3	T42.0X4	T42.0X5	T42.0X6
Diphenylmethane dye	T52.1X1	T52.1X2	T52.1X3	T52.1X4	--	--
Diphenylpyraline	T45.0X1	T45.0X2	T45.0X3	T45.0X4	T45.0X5	T45.0X6
Diphtheria						
- antitoxin	T50.Z11	T50.Z12	T50.Z13	T50.Z14	T50.Z15	T50.Z16
- toxoid	T50.A91	T50.A92	T50.A93	T50.A94	T50.A95	T50.A96
- - with tetanus toxoid	T50.A21	T50.A22	T50.A23	T50.A24	T50.A25	T50.A26
- - - with pertussis component	T50.A11	T50.A12	T50.A13	T50.A14	T50.A15	T50.A16
- vaccine	T50.A91	T50.A92	T50.A93	T50.A94	T50.A95	T50.A96
- - combination						
- - - including pertussis	T50.A11	T50.A12	T50.A13	T50.A14	T50.A15	T50.A16
- - - without pertussis	T50.A21	T50.A22	T50.A23	T50.A24	T50.A25	T50.A26
Diphylline	T50.2X1	T50.2X2	T50.2X3	T50.2X4	T50.2X5	T50.2X6
Dipipanone	T40.4X1	T40.4X2	T40.4X3	T40.4X4	--	--
Dipivefrine	T49.5X1	T49.5X2	T49.5X3	T49.5X4	T49.5X5	T49.5X6
Diplovax	T50.B91	T50.B92	T50.B93	T50.B94	T50.B95	T50.B96
Diprophylline	T50.2X1	T50.2X2	T50.2X3	T50.2X4	T50.2X5	T50.2X6
Dipropyline	T48.291	T48.292	T48.293	T48.294	T48.295	T48.296
Dipyridamole	T46.3X1	T46.3X2	T46.3X3	T46.3X4	T46.3X5	T46.3X6
Dipyrone	T39.2X1	T39.2X2	T39.2X3	T39.2X4	T39.2X5	T39.2X6
Diquat (dibromide)	T60.3X1	T60.3X2	T60.3X3	T60.3X4	--	--
Disinfectant	T65.891	T65.892	T65.893	T65.894	--	--
- alkaline	T54.3X1	T54.3X2	T54.3X3	T54.3X4	--	--
- aromatic	T54.1X1	T54.1X2	T54.1X3	T54.1X4	--	--
- intestinal	T37.8X1	T37.8X2	T37.8X3	T37.8X4	T37.8X5	T37.8X6
Disipal	T42.8X1	T42.8X2	T42.8X3	T42.8X4	T42.8X5	T42.8X6
Disodium edetate	T50.6X1	T50.6X2	T50.6X3	T50.6X4	T50.6X5	T50.6X6
Disoprofol	T41.291	T41.292	T41.293	T41.294	T41.295	T41.296
Disopyramide	T46.2X1	T46.2X2	T46.2X3	T46.2X4	T46.2X5	T46.2X6
Distigmine (bromide)	T44.0X1	T44.0X2	T44.0X3	T44.0X4	T44.0X5	T44.0X6
Disulfamide	T50.2X1	T50.2X2	T50.2X3	T50.2X4	T50.2X5	T50.2X6
Disulfanilamide	T37.0X1	T37.0X2	T37.0X3	T37.0X4	T37.0X5	T37.0X6
Disulfiram	T50.6X1	T50.6X2	T50.6X3	T50.6X4	T50.6X5	T50.6X6
Disulfoton	T60.0X1	T60.0X2	T60.0X3	T60.0X4	--	--
Dithiazanine iodide	T37.4X1	T37.4X2	T37.4X3	T37.4X4	T37.4X5	T37.4X6
Dithiocarbamate	T60.0X1	T60.0X2	T60.0X3	T60.0X4	--	--
Dithranol	T49.4X1	T49.4X2	T49.4X3	T49.4X4	T49.4X5	T49.4X6
Diucardin	T50.2X1	T50.2X2	T50.2X3	T50.2X4	T50.2X5	T50.2X6
Diupres	T50.2X1	T50.2X2	T50.2X3	T50.2X4	T50.2X5	T50.2X6
Diuretic NEC	T50.2X1	T50.2X2	T50.2X3	T50.2X4	T50.2X5	T50.2X6
- benzothiadiazine	T50.2X1	T50.2X2	T50.2X3	T50.2X4	T50.2X5	T50.2X6
- carbonic acid anhydrase inhibitors	T50.2X1	T50.2X2	T50.2X3	T50.2X4	T50.2X5	T50.2X6
- furfuryl NEC	T50.2X1	T50.2X2	T50.2X3	T50.2X4	T50.2X5	T50.2X6
- loop (high-ceiling)	T50.1X1	T50.1X2	T50.1X3	T50.1X4	T50.1X5	T50.1X6
- mercurial NEC	T50.2X1	T50.2X2	T50.2X3	T50.2X4	T50.2X5	T50.2X6
- osmotic	T50.2X1	T50.2X2	T50.2X3	T50.2X4	T50.2X5	T50.2X6
- purine NEC	T50.2X1	T50.2X2	T50.2X3	T50.2X4	T50.2X5	T50.2X6
- saluretic NEC	T50.2X1	T50.2X2	T50.2X3	T50.2X4	T50.2X5	T50.2X6
- sulfonamide	T50.2X1	T50.2X2	T50.2X3	T50.2X4	T50.2X5	T50.2X6
- thiazide NEC	T50.2X1	T50.2X2	T50.2X3	T50.2X4	T50.2X5	T50.2X6
- xanthine	T50.2X1	T50.2X2	T50.2X3	T50.2X4	T50.2X5	T50.2X6
Diurgin	T50.2X1	T50.2X2	T50.2X3	T50.2X4	T50.2X5	T50.2X6
Diuril	T50.2X1	T50.2X2	T50.2X3	T50.2X4	T50.2X5	T50.2X6

Substance	Poisoning, Accidental (unintentional)	Poisoning, Intentional Self-harm	Poisoning, Assault	Poisoning, Undetermined	Adverse effect	Underdosing
Diuron	T60.3X1	T60.3X2	T60.3X3	T60.3X4	--	--
Divalproex	T42.6X1	T42.6X2	T42.6X3	T42.6X4	T42.6X5	T42.6X6
Divinyl ether	T41.0X1	T41.0X2	T41.0X3	T41.0X4	T41.0X5	T41.0X6
Dixanthogen	T49.0X1	T49.0X2	T49.0X3	T49.0X4	T49.0X5	T49.0X6
Dixyrazine	T43.3X1	T43.3X2	T43.3X3	T43.3X4	T43.3X5	T43.3X6
D-lysergic acid diethylamide	T40.8X1	T40.8X2	T40.8X3	T40.8X4	T40.8X5	--
DMCT	T36.4X1	T36.4X2	T36.4X3	T36.4X4	T36.4X5	T36.4X6
DMSO—see Dimethyl sulfoxide						
DNBP	T60.3X1	T60.3X2	T60.3X3	T60.3X4	--	--
DNOC	T65.3X1	T65.3X2	T65.3X3	T65.3X4	--	--
Dobutamine	T44.5X1	T44.5X2	T44.5X3	T44.5X4	T44.5X5	T44.5X6
DOCA	T38.0X1	T38.0X2	T38.0X3	T38.0X4	T38.0X5	T38.0X6
Docusate sodium	T47.4X1	T47.4X2	T47.4X3	T47.4X4	T47.4X5	T47.4X6
Dodicin	T49.0X1	T49.0X2	T49.0X3	T49.0X4	T49.0X5	T49.0X6
Dofamium chloride	T49.0X1	T49.0X2	T49.0X3	T49.0X4	T49.0X5	T49.0X6
Dolophine	T40.3X1	T40.3X2	T40.3X3	T40.3X4	T40.3X5	T40.3X6
Doloxene	T39.8X1	T39.8X2	T39.8X3	T39.8X4	T39.8X5	T39.8X6
Domestic gas (after combustion) —see Gas, utility						
- prior to combustion	T59.891	T59.892	T59.893	T59.894	--	--
Domiodol	T48.4X1	T48.4X2	T48.4X3	T48.4X4	T48.4X5	T48.4X6
Domiphen (bromide)	T49.0X1	T49.0X2	T49.0X3	T49.0X4	T49.0X5	T49.0X6
Domperidone	T45.0X1	T45.0X2	T45.0X3	T45.0X4	T45.0X5	T45.0X6
Dopa	T42.8X1	T42.8X2	T42.8X3	T42.8X4	T42.8X5	T42.8X6
Dopamine	T44.991	T44.992	T44.993	T44.994	T44.995	T44.996
Doriden	T42.6X1	T42.6X2	T42.6X3	T42.6X4	T42.6X5	T42.6X6
Dormiral	T42.3X1	T42.3X2	T42.3X3	T42.3X4	T42.3X5	T42.3X6
Dormison	T42.6X1	T42.6X2	T42.6X3	T42.6X4	T42.6X5	T42.6X6
Dornase	T48.4X1	T48.4X2	T48.4X3	T48.4X4	T48.4X5	T48.4X6
Dorsacaine	T41.3X1	T41.3X2	T41.3X3	T41.3X4	T41.3X5	T41.3X6
Dosulepin	T43.011	T43.012	T43.013	T43.014	T43.015	T43.016
Dothiepin	T43.011	T43.012	T43.013	T43.014	T43.015	T43.016
Doxantrazole	T48.6X1	T48.6X2	T48.6X3	T48.6X4	T48.6X5	T48.6X6
Doxapram	T50.7X1	T50.7X2	T50.7X3	T50.7X4	T50.7X5	T50.7X6
Doxazosin	T44.6X1	T44.6X2	T44.6X3	T44.6X4	T44.6X5	T44.6X6
Doxepin	T43.011	T43.012	T43.013	T43.014	T43.015	T43.016
Doxifluridine	T45.1X1	T45.1X2	T45.1X3	T45.1X4	T45.1X5	T45.1X6
Doxorubicin	T45.1X1	T45.1X2	T45.1X3	T45.1X4	T45.1X5	T45.1X6
Doxycycline	T36.4X1	T36.4X2	T36.4X3	T36.4X4	T36.4X5	T36.4X6
Doxylamine	T45.0X1	T45.0X2	T45.0X3	T45.0X4	T45.0X5	T45.0X6
Dramamine	T45.0X1	T45.0X2	T45.0X3	T45.0X4	T45.0X5	T45.0X6
Drano (drain cleaner)	T54.3X1	T54.3X2	T54.3X3	T54.3X4	--	--
Dressing, live pulp	T49.7X1	T49.7X2	T49.7X3	T49.7X4	T49.7X5	T49.7X6
Drocode	T40.2X1	T40.2X2	T40.2X3	T40.2X4	T40.2X5	T40.2X6
Dromoran	T40.2X1	T40.2X2	T40.2X3	T40.2X4	T40.2X5	T40.2X6
Dromostanolone	T38.7X1	T38.7X2	T38.7X3	T38.7X4	T38.7X5	T38.7X6
Dronabinol	T40.7X1	T40.7X2	T40.7X3	T40.7X4	T40.7X5	T40.7X6
Droperidol	T43.591	T43.592	T43.593	T43.594	T43.595	T43.596
Dropropizine	T48.3X1	T48.3X2	T48.3X3	T48.3X4	T48.3X5	T48.3X6
Drostanolone	T38.7X1	T38.7X2	T38.7X3	T38.7X4	T38.7X5	T38.7X6
Drotaverine	T44.3X1	T44.3X2	T44.3X3	T44.3X4	T44.3X5	T44.3X6
Drotrecogin alfa	T45.511	T45.512	T45.513	T45.514	T45.515	T45.516
Drug NEC	T50.901	T50.902	T50.903	T50.904	T50.905	T50.906
- specified NEC	T50.991	T50.992	T50.993	T50.994	T50.995	T50.996
DTIC	T45.1X1	T45.1X2	T45.1X3	T45.1X4	T45.1X5	T45.1X6
Duboisine	T44.3X1	T44.3X2	T44.3X3	T44.3X4	T44.3X5	T44.3X6
Dulcolax	T47.2X1	T47.2X2	T47.2X3	T47.2X4	T47.2X5	T47.2X6
Duponol (C) (EP)	T49.2X1	T49.2X2	T49.2X3	T49.2X4	T49.2X5	T49.2X6
Durabolin	T38.7X1	T38.7X2	T38.7X3	T38.7X4	T38.7X5	T38.7X6
Dyclone	T41.3X1	T41.3X2	T41.3X3	T41.3X4	T41.3X5	T41.3X6
Dyclonine	T41.3X1	T41.3X2	T41.3X3	T41.3X4	T41.3X5	T41.3X6
Dydrogesterone	T38.5X1	T38.5X2	T38.5X3	T38.5X4	T38.5X5	T38.5X6
Dye NEC	T65.6X1	T65.6X2	T65.6X3	T65.6X4	--	--
- antiseptic	T49.0X1	T49.0X2	T49.0X3	T49.0X4	T49.0X5	T49.0X6
- diagnostic agents	T50.8X1	T50.8X2	T50.8X3	T50.8X4	T50.8X5	T50.8X6
- pharmaceutical NEC	T50.901	T50.902	T50.903	T50.904	T50.905	T50.906

Substance	Poisoning, Accidental (unintentional)	Poisoning, Intentional Self-harm	Poisoning, Assault	Poisoning, Undetermined	Adverse effect	Underdosing
Dyflos	T44.0X1	T44.0X2	T44.0X3	T44.0X4	T44.0X5	T44.0X6
Dymelor	T38.3X1	T38.3X2	T38.3X3	T38.3X4	T38.3X5	T38.3X6
Dynamite	T65.3X1	T65.3X2	T65.3X3	T65.3X4	--	--
- fumes	T59.891	T59.892	T59.893	T59.894	--	--
Dyphylline	T44.3X1	T44.3X2	T44.3X3	T44.3X4	T44.3X5	T44.3X6
Ear drug NEC	T49.6X1	T49.6X2	T49.6X3	T49.6X4	T49.6X5	T49.6X6
Ear preparations	T49.6X1	T49.6X2	T49.6X3	T49.6X4	T49.6X5	T49.6X6
Echothiophate, echothiopate, ecothiopate	T49.5X1	T49.5X2	T49.5X3	T49.5X4	T49.5X5	T49.5X6
Econazole	T49.0X1	T49.0X2	T49.0X3	T49.0X4	T49.0X5	T49.0X6
Ecothiopate iodide	T49.5X1	T49.5X2	T49.5X3	T49.5X4	T49.5X5	T49.5X6
Ecstasy	T43.621	T43.622	T43.623	T43.624	T43.625	T43.626
Ectylurea	T42.6X1	T42.6X2	T42.6X3	T42.6X4	T42.6X5	T42.6X6
Edathamil disodium	T45.8X1	T45.8X2	T45.8X3	T45.8X4	T45.8X5	T45.8X6
Edecrin	T50.1X1	T50.1X2	T50.1X3	T50.1X4	T50.1X5	T50.1X6
Edetate, disodium (calcium)	T45.8X1	T45.8X2	T45.8X3	T45.8X4	T45.8X5	T45.8X6
Edoxudine	T49.5X1	T49.5X2	T49.5X3	T49.5X4	T49.5X5	T49.5X6
Edrophonium	T44.0X1	T44.0X2	T44.0X3	T44.0X4	T44.0X5	T44.0X6
- chloride	T44.0X1	T44.0X2	T44.0X3	T44.0X4	T44.0X5	T44.0X6
EDTA	T50.6X1	T50.6X2	T50.6X3	T50.6X4	T50.6X5	T50.6X6
Eflornithine	T37.2X1	T37.2X2	T37.2X3	T37.2X4	T37.2X5	T37.2X6
Efloxate	T46.3X1	T46.3X2	T46.3X3	T46.3X4	T46.3X5	T46.3X6
Elase	T49.8X1	T49.8X2	T49.8X3	T49.8X4	T49.8X5	T49.8X6
Elastase	T47.5X1	T47.5X2	T47.5X3	T47.5X4	T47.5X5	T47.5X6
Elaterium	T47.2X1	T47.2X2	T47.2X3	T47.2X4	T47.2X5	T47.2X6
Elcatonin	T50.991	T50.992	T50.993	T50.994	T50.995	T50.996
Elder	T62.2X1	T62.2X2	T62.2X3	T62.2X4	--	--
- berry, (unripe)	T62.1X1	T62.1X2	T62.1X3	T62.1X4	--	--
Electrolyte balance drug	T50.3X1	T50.3X2	T50.3X3	T50.3X4	T50.3X5	T50.3X6
Electrolytes NEC	T50.3X1	T50.3X2	T50.3X3	T50.3X4	T50.3X5	T50.3X6
Electrolytic agent NEC	T50.3X1	T50.3X2	T50.3X3	T50.3X4	T50.3X5	T50.3X6
Elemental diet	T50.902	T50.902	T50.903	T50.904	T50.905	T50.906
Elliptinium acetate	T45.1X1	T45.1X2	T45.1X3	T45.1X4	T45.1X5	T45.1X6
Embramine	T45.0X1	T45.0X2	T45.0X3	T45.0X4	T45.0X5	T45.0X6
Emepronium (salts)	T44.3X1	T44.3X2	T44.3X3	T44.3X4	T44.3X5	T44.3X6
- bromide	T44.3X1	T44.3X2	T44.3X3	T44.3X4	T44.3X5	T44.3X6
Emetic NEC	T47.7X1	T47.7X2	T47.7X3	T47.7X4	T47.7X5	T47.7X6
Emetine	T37.3X1	T37.3X2	T37.3X3	T37.3X4	T37.3X5	T37.3X6
Emollient NEC	T49.3X1	T49.3X2	T49.3X3	T49.3X4	T49.3X5	T49.3X6
Emorfazone	T39.8X1	T39.8X2	T39.8X3	T39.8X4	T39.8X5	T39.8X6
Emylcamate	T43.591	T43.592	T43.593	T43.594	T43.595	T43.596
Enalapril	T46.4X1	T46.4X2	T46.4X3	T46.4X4	T46.4X5	T46.4X6
Enalaprilat	T46.4X1	T46.4X2	T46.4X3	T46.4X4	T46.4X5	T46.4X6
Encainide	T46.2X1	T46.2X2	T46.2X3	T46.2X4	T46.2X5	T46.2X6
Endocaine	T41.3X1	T41.3X2	T41.3X3	T41.3X4	T41.3X5	T41.3X6
Endosulfan	T60.2X1	T60.2X2	T60.2X3	T60.2X4	--	--
Endothall	T60.3X1	T60.3X2	T60.3X3	T60.3X4	--	--
Endralazine	T46.5X1	T46.5X2	T46.5X3	T46.5X4	T46.5X5	T46.5X6
Endrin	T60.1X1	T60.1X2	T60.1X3	T60.1X4	--	--
Enflurane	T41.0X1	T41.0X2	T41.0X3	T41.0X4	T41.0X5	T41.0X6
Enhexymal	T42.3X1	T42.3X2	T42.3X3	T42.3X4	T42.3X5	T42.3X6
Enocitabine	T45.1X1	T45.1X2	T45.1X3	T45.1X4	T45.1X5	T45.1X6
Enovid	T38.4X1	T38.4X2	T38.4X3	T38.4X4	T38.4X5	T38.4X6
Enoxacin	T36.8X1	T36.8X2	T36.8X3	T36.8X4	T36.8X5	T36.8X6
Enoxaparin (sodium)	T45.511	T45.512	T45.513	T45.514	T45.515	T45.516
Enpiprazole	T43.591	T43.592	T43.593	T43.594	T43.595	T43.596
Enprofylline	T48.6X1	T48.6X2	T48.6X3	T48.6X4	T48.6X5	T48.6X6
Enprostil	T47.1X1	T47.1X2	T47.1X3	T47.1X4	T47.1X5	T47.1X6
ENT preparations (anti-infectives)	T49.6X1	T49.6X2	T49.6X3	T49.6X4	T49.6X5	T49.6X6
Enterogastrone	T38.891	T38.892	T38.893	T38.894	T38.895	T38.896
Enviomycin	T36.8X1	T36.8X2	T36.8X3	T36.8X4	T36.8X5	T36.8X6
Enzodase	T45.3X1	T45.3X2	T45.3X3	T45.3X4	T45.3X5	T45.3X6
Enzyme NEC	T45.3X1	T45.3X2	T45.3X3	T45.3X4	T45.3X5	T45.3X6
- depolymerizing	T49.8X1	T49.8X2	T49.8X3	T49.8X4	T49.8X5	T49.8X6
- fibrolytic	T45.3X1	T45.3X2	T45.3X3	T45.3X4	T45.3X5	T45.3X6
- gastric	T47.5X1	T47.5X2	T47.5X3	T47.5X4	T47.5X5	T47.5X6

Substance	Poisoning, Accidental (unintentional)	Poisoning, Intentional Self-harm	Poisoning, Assault	Poisoning, Undetermined	Adverse effect	Underdosing
- intestinal	T47.5X1	T47.5X2	T47.5X3	T47.5X4	T47.5X5	T47.5X6
- local action	T49.4X1	T49.4X2	T49.4X3	T49.4X4	T49.4X5	T49.4X6
- proteolytic	T49.4X1	T49.4X2	T49.4X3	T49.4X4	T49.4X5	T49.4X6
- thrombolytic	T45.3X1	T45.3X2	T45.3X3	T45.3X4	T45.3X5	T45.3X6
EPAB	T41.3X1	T41.3X2	T41.3X3	T41.3X4	T41.3X5	T41.3X6
Epanutin	T42.0X1	T42.0X2	T42.0X3	T42.0X4	T42.0X5	T42.0X6
Ephedra	T44.991	T44.992	T44.993	T44.994	T44.995	T44.996
Ephedrine	T44.991	T44.992	T44.993	T44.994	T44.995	T44.996
Epichlorhydrin, epichlorohydrin	T52.8X1	T52.8X2	T52.8X3	T52.8X4	--	--
Epicillin	T36.0X1	T36.0X2	T36.0X3	T36.0X4	T36.0X5	T36.0X6
Epiestriol	T38.5X1	T38.5X2	T38.5X3	T38.5X4	T38.5X5	T38.5X6
Epilim—see Sodium valproate						
Epimestrol	T38.5X1	T38.5X2	T38.5X3	T38.5X4	T38.5X5	T38.5X6
Epinephrine	T44.5X1	T44.5X2	T44.5X3	T44.5X4	T44.5X5	T44.5X6
Epirubicin	T45.1X1	T45.1X2	T45.1X3	T45.1X4	T45.1X5	T45.1X6
Epitiostanol	T38.7X1	T38.7X2	T38.7X3	T38.7X4	T38.7X5	T38.7X6
Epitizide	T50.2X1	T50.2X2	T50.2X3	T50.2X4	T50.2X5	T50.2X6
EPN	T60.0X1	T60.0X2	T60.0X3	T60.0X4	--	--
EPO	T45.8X1	T45.8X2	T45.8X3	T45.8X4	T45.8X5	T45.8X6
Epoetin alpha	T45.8X1	T45.8X2	T45.8X3	T45.8X4	T45.8X5	T45.8X6
Epomediol	T50.991	T50.992	T50.993	T50.994	T50.995	T50.996
Epoprostenol	T45.521	T45.522	T45.523	T45.524	T45.525	T45.526
Epoxy resin	T65.891	T65.892	T65.893	T65.894	--	--
Eprazinone	T48.4X1	T48.4X2	T48.4X3	T48.4X4	T48.4X5	T48.4X6
Epsilon amino-caproic acid	T45.621	T45.622	T45.623	T45.624	T45.625	T45.626
Epsom salt	T47.3X1	T47.3X2	T47.3X3	T47.3X4	T47.3X5	T47.3X6
Eptazocine	T40.4X1	T40.4X2	T40.4X3	T40.4X4	T40.4X5	T40.4X6
Equanil	T43.591	T43.592	T43.593	T43.594	T43.595	T43.596
Equisetum	T62.2X1	T62.2X2	T62.2X3	T62.2X4	--	--
- diuretic	T50.2X1	T50.2X2	T50.2X3	T50.2X4	T50.2X5	T50.2X6
Ergobasine	T48.0X1	T48.0X2	T48.0X3	T48.0X4	T48.0X5	T48.0X6
Ergocalciferol	T45.2X1	T45.2X2	T45.2X3	T45.2X4	T45.2X5	T45.2X6
Ergoloid mesylates	T46.7X1	T46.7X2	T46.7X3	T46.7X4	T46.7X5	T46.7X6
Ergometrine	T48.0X1	T48.0X2	T48.0X3	T48.0X4	T48.0X5	T48.0X6
Ergonovine	T48.0X1	T48.0X2	T48.0X3	T48.0X4	T48.0X5	T48.0X6
Ergot NEC	T64.81	T64.82	T64.83	T64.84	--	--
- derivative	T48.0X1	T48.0X2	T48.0X3	T48.0X4	T48.0X5	T48.0X6
- medicinal (alkaloids)	T48.0X1	T48.0X2	T48.0X3	T48.0X4	T48.0X5	T48.0X6
- prepared	T48.0X1	T48.0X2	T48.0X3	T48.0X4	T48.0X5	T48.0X6
Ergotamine	T46.5X1	T46.5X2	T46.5X3	T46.5X4	T46.5X5	T46.5X6
Ergotocine	T48.0X1	T48.0X2	T48.0X3	T48.0X4	T48.0X5	T48.0X6
Ergotrate	T48.0X1	T48.0X2	T48.0X3	T48.0X4	T48.0X5	T48.0X6
Eritrityl tetranitrate	T46.3X1	T46.3X2	T46.3X3	T46.3X4	T46.3X5	T46.3X6
Erythrityl tetranitrate	T46.3X1	T46.3X2	T46.3X3	T46.3X4	T46.3X5	T46.3X6
Erythrol tetranitrate	T46.3X1	T46.3X2	T46.3X3	T46.3X4	T46.3X5	T46.3X6
Erythromycin (salts)	T36.3X1	T36.3X2	T36.3X3	T36.3X4	T36.3X5	T36.3X6
- ophthalmic preparation	T49.5X1	T49.5X2	T49.5X3	T49.5X4	T49.5X5	T49.5X6
- topical NEC	T49.0X1	T49.0X2	T49.0X3	T49.0X4	T49.0X5	T49.0X6
Erythropoietin	T45.8X1	T45.8X2	T45.8X3	T45.8X4	T45.8X5	T45.8X6
- human	T45.8X1	T45.8X2	T45.8X3	T45.8X4	T45.8X5	T45.8X6
Escin	T46.991	T46.992	T46.993	T46.994	T46.995	T46.996
Esculin	T45.2X1	T45.2X2	T45.2X3	T45.2X4	T45.2X5	T45.2X6
Esculoside	T45.2X1	T45.2X2	T45.2X3	T45.2X4	T45.2X5	T45.2X6
ESDT (ether-soluble tar distillate)	T49.1X1	T49.1X2	T49.1X3	T49.1X4	T49.1X5	T49.1X6
Eserine	T49.5X1	T49.5X2	T49.5X3	T49.5X4	T49.5X5	T49.5X6
Esflurbiprofen	T39.311	T39.312	T39.313	T39.314	T39.315	T39.316
Eskabarb	T42.3X1	T42.3X2	T42.3X3	T42.3X4	T42.3X5	T42.3X6
Eskalith	T43.8X1	T43.8X2	T43.8X3	T43.8X4	T43.8X5	T43.8X6
Esmolol	T44.7X1	T44.7X2	T44.7X3	T44.7X4	T44.7X5	T44.7X6
Estanozolol	T38.7X1	T38.7X2	T38.7X3	T38.7X4	T38.7X5	T38.7X6
Estazolam	T42.4X1	T42.4X2	T42.4X3	T42.4X4	T42.4X5	T42.4X6
Estradiol	T38.5X1	T38.5X2	T38.5X3	T38.5X4	T38.5X5	T38.5X6
- with testosterone	T38.7X1	T38.7X2	T38.7X3	T38.7X4	T38.7X5	T38.7X6
- benzoate	T38.5X1	T38.5X2	T38.5X3	T38.5X4	T38.5X5	T38.5X6
Estramustine	T45.1X1	T45.1X2	T45.1X3	T45.1X4	T45.1X5	T45.1X6

Substance	Poisoning, Accidental (unintentional)	Poisoning, Intentional Self-harm	Poisoning, Assault	Poisoning, Undetermined	Adverse effect	Underdosing
Estriol	T38.5X1	T38.5X2	T38.5X3	T38.5X4	T38.5X5	T38.5X6
Estrogen	T38.5X1	T38.5X2	T38.5X3	T38.5X4	T38.5X5	T38.5X6
- with progesterone	T38.5X1	T38.5X2	T38.5X3	T38.5X4	T38.5X5	T38.5X6
- conjugated	T38.5X1	T38.5X2	T38.5X3	T38.5X4	T38.5X5	T38.5X6
Estrone	T38.5X1	T38.5X2	T38.5X3	T38.5X4	T38.5X5	T38.5X6
Estropipate	T38.5X1	T38.5X2	T38.5X3	T38.5X4	T38.5X5	T38.5X6
Etacrynate sodium	T50.1X1	T50.1X2	T50.1X3	T50.1X4	T50.1X5	T50.1X6
Etacrynic acid	T50.1X1	T50.1X2	T50.1X3	T50.1X4	T50.1X5	T50.1X6
Etafedrine	T48.6X1	T48.6X2	T48.6X3	T48.6X4	T48.6X5	T48.6X6
Etafenone	T46.3X1	T46.3X2	T46.3X3	T46.3X4	T46.3X5	T46.3X6
Etambutol	T37.1X1	T37.1X2	T37.1X3	T37.1X4	T37.1X5	T37.1X6
Etamiphyllin	T48.6X1	T48.6X2	T48.6X3	T48.6X4	T48.6X5	T48.6X6
Etamivan	T50.7X1	T50.7X2	T50.7X3	T50.7X4	T50.7X5	T50.7X6
Etamsylate	T45.7X1	T45.7X2	T45.7X3	T45.7X4	T45.7X5	T45.7X6
Etebenecid	T50.4X1	T50.4X2	T50.4X3	T50.4X4	T50.4X5	T50.4X6
Ethacridine	T49.0X1	T49.0X2	T49.0X3	T49.0X4	T49.0X5	T49.0X6
Ethacrynic acid	T50.1X1	T50.1X2	T50.1X3	T50.1X4	T50.1X5	T50.1X6
Ethadione	T42.2X1	T42.2X2	T42.2X3	T42.2X4	T42.2X5	T42.2X6
Ethambutol	T37.1X1	T37.1X2	T37.1X3	T37.1X4	T37.1X5	T37.1X6
Ethamide	T50.2X1	T50.2X2	T50.2X3	T50.2X4	T50.2X5	T50.2X6
Ethamivan	T50.7X1	T50.7X2	T50.7X3	T50.7X4	T50.7X5	T50.7X6
Ethamsylate	T45.7X1	T45.7X2	T45.7X3	T45.7X4	T45.7X5	T45.7X6
Ethanol	T51.0X1	T51.0X2	T51.0X3	T51.0X4	--	--
- beverage	T51.0X1	T51.0X2	T51.0X3	T51.0X4	--	--
Ethanolamine oleate	T46.8X1	T46.8X2	T46.8X3	T46.8X4	T46.8X5	T46.8X6
Ethaverine	T44.3X1	T44.3X2	T44.3X3	T44.3X4	T44.3X5	T44.3X6
Ethchlorvynol	T42.6X1	T42.6X2	T42.6X3	T42.6X4	T42.6X5	T42.6X6
Ethebenecid	T50.4X1	T50.4X2	T50.4X3	T50.4X4	T50.4X5	T50.4X6
Ether (vapor)	T41.0X1	T41.0X2	T41.0X3	T41.0X4	T41.0X5	T41.0X6
- anesthetic	T41.0X1	T41.0X2	T41.0X3	T41.0X4	T41.0X5	T41.0X6
- divinyl	T41.0X1	T41.0X2	T41.0X3	T41.0X4	T41.0X5	T41.0X6
- ethyl (medicinal)	T41.0X1	T41.0X2	T41.0X3	T41.0X4	T41.0X5	T41.0X6
- - nonmedicinal	T52.8X1	T52.8X2	T52.8X3	T52.8X4	--	--
- petroleum—see Ligroin						
- solvent	T52.8X1	T52.8X2	T52.8X3	T52.8X4	--	--
Ethiazide	T50.2X1	T50.2X2	T50.2X3	T50.2X4	T50.2X5	T50.2X6
Ethidium chloride (vapor)	T59.891	T59.892	T59.893	T59.894	--	--
Ethinamate	T42.6X1	T42.6X2	T42.6X3	T42.6X4	T42.6X5	T42.6X6
Ethinylestradiol, ethinyloestradiol	T38.5X1	T38.5X2	T38.5X3	T38.5X4	T38.5X5	T38.5X6
- with						
- - levonorgestrel	T38.4X1	T38.4X2	T38.4X3	T38.4X4	T38.4X5	T38.4X6
- - norethisterone	T38.4X1	T38.4X2	T38.4X3	T38.4X4	T38.4X5	T38.4X6
Ethiodized oil (131 I)	T50.8X1	T50.8X2	T50.8X3	T50.8X4	T50.8X5	T50.8X6
Ethion	T60.0X1	T60.0X2	T60.0X3	T60.0X4	--	--
Ethionamide	T37.1X1	T37.1X2	T37.1X3	T37.1X4	T37.1X5	T37.1X6
Ethioniamide	T37.1X1	T37.1X2	T37.1X3	T37.1X4	T37.1X5	T37.1X6
Ethisterone	T38.5X1	T38.5X2	T38.5X3	T38.5X4	T38.5X5	T38.5X6
Ethobral	T42.3X1	T42.3X2	T42.3X3	T42.3X4	T42.3X5	T42.3X6
Ethocaine (infiltration) (topical)	T41.3X1	T41.3X2	T41.3X3	T41.3X4	T41.3X5	T41.3X6
- nerve block (peripheral) (plexus)	T41.3X1	T41.3X2	T41.3X3	T41.3X4	T41.3X5	T41.3X6
- spinal	T41.3X1	T41.3X2	T41.3X3	T41.3X4	T41.3X5	T41.3X6
Ethoheptazine	T40.4X1	T40.4X2	T40.4X3	T40.4X4	T40.4X5	T40.4X6
Ethopropazine	T44.3X1	T44.3X2	T44.3X3	T44.3X4	T44.3X5	T44.3X6
Ethosuximide	T42.2X1	T42.2X2	T42.2X3	T42.2X4	T42.2X5	T42.2X6
Ethotoin	T42.0X1	T42.0X2	T42.0X3	T42.0X4	T42.0X5	T42.0X6
Ethoxazene	T37.91	T37.92	T37.93	T37.94	T37.95	T37.96
Ethoxazorutoside	T46.991	T46.992	T46.993	T46.994	T46.995	T46.996
2-Ethoxyethanol	T52.3X1	T52.3X2	T52.3X3	T52.3X4	--	--
Ethoxzolamide	T50.2X1	T50.2X2	T50.2X3	T50.2X4	T50.2X5	T50.2X6
Ethyl						
- acetate	T52.8X1	T52.8X2	T52.8X3	T52.8X4	--	--
- alcohol	T51.0X1	T51.0X2	T51.0X3	T51.0X4	--	--
- - beverage	T51.0X1	T51.0X2	T51.0X3	T51.0X4	--	--
- aldehyde (vapor)	T59.891	T59.892	T59.893	T59.894	--	--
- - liquid	T52.8X1	T52.8X2	T52.8X3	T52.8X4	--	--

Substance	Poisoning, Accidental (unintentional)	Poisoning, Intentional Self-harm	Poisoning, Assault	Poisoning, Undetermined	Adverse effect	Underdosing
- aminobenzoate	T41.3X1	T41.3X2	T41.3X3	T41.3X4	T41.3X5	T41.3X6
- aminophenothiazine	T43.3X1	T43.3X2	T43.3X3	T43.3X4	T43.3X5	T43.3X6
- benzoate	T52.8X1	T52.8X2	T52.8X3	T52.8X4	--	--
- biscoumacetate	T45.511	T45.512	T45.513	T45.514	T45.515	T45.516
- bromide (anesthetic)	T41.0X1	T41.0X2	T41.0X3	T41.0X4	T41.0X5	T41.0X6
- carbamate	T45.1X1	T45.1X2	T45.1X3	T45.1X4	T45.1X5	T45.1X6
- carbinol	T51.3X1	T51.3X2	T51.3X3	T51.3X4	--	--
- carbonate	T52.8X1	T52.8X2	T52.8X3	T52.8X4	--	--
- chaulmoograte	T37.1X1	T37.1X2	T37.1X3	T37.1X4	T37.1X5	T37.1X6
- chloride (anesthetic)	T41.0X1	T41.0X2	T41.0X3	T41.0X4	T41.0X5	T41.0X6
- - anesthetic (local)	T41.3X1	T41.3X2	T41.3X3	T41.3X4	T41.3X5	T41.3X6
- - - inhaled	T41.0X1	T41.0X2	T41.0X3	T41.0X4	T41.0X5	T41.0X6
- - local	T49.4X1	T49.4X2	T49.4X3	T49.4X4	T49.4X5	T49.4X6
- - solvent	T53.6X1	T53.6X2	T53.6X3	T53.6X4	--	--
- dibunate	T48.3X1	T48.3X2	T48.3X3	T48.3X4	T48.3X5	T48.3X6
- dichloroarsine (vapor)	T57.0X1	T57.0X2	T57.0X3	T57.0X4	--	--
- estranol	T38.7X1	T38.7X2	T38.7X3	T38.7X4	T38.7X5	T38.7X6
- ether—see also ether	T52.8X1	T52.8X2	T52.8X3	T52.8X4	--	--
- formate NEC (solvent)	T52.0X1	T52.0X2	T52.0X3	T52.0X4	--	--
- fumarate	T49.4X1	T49.4X2	T49.4X3	T49.4X4	T49.4X5	T49.4X6
- hydroxyisobutyrate NEC (solvent)	T52.8X1	T52.8X2	T52.8X3	T52.8X4	--	--
- iodoacetate	T59.3X1	T59.3X2	T59.3X3	T59.3X4	--	--
- lactate NEC (solvent)	T52.8X1	T52.8X2	T52.8X3	T52.8X4	--	--
- loflazepate	T42.4X1	T42.4X2	T42.4X3	T42.4X4	T42.4X5	T42.4X6
- mercuric chloride	T56.1X1	T56.1X2	T56.1X3	T56.1X4	--	--
- methylcarbinol	T51.8X1	T51.8X2	T51.8X3	T51.8X4	--	--
- morphine	T40.2X1	T40.2X2	T40.2X3	T40.2X4	T40.2X5	T40.2X6
- noradrenaline	T48.6X1	T48.6X2	T48.6X3	T48.6X4	T48.6X5	T48.6X6
- oxybutyrate NEC (solvent)	T52.8X1	T52.8X2	T52.8X3	T52.8X4	--	--
Ethylene (gas)	T59.891	T59.892	T59.893	T59.894	--	--
- anesthetic (general)	T41.0X1	T41.0X2	T41.0X3	T41.0X4	T41.0X5	T41.0X6
- chlorohydrin	T52.8X1	T52.8X2	T52.8X3	T52.8X4	--	--
- - vapor	T53.6X1	T53.6X2	T53.6X3	T53.6X4	--	--
- dichloride	T52.8X1	T52.8X2	T52.8X3	T52.8X4	--	--
- - vapor	T53.6X1	T53.6X2	T53.6X3	T53.6X4	--	--
- dinitrate	T52.3X1	T52.3X2	T52.3X3	T52.3X4	--	--
- glycol (s)	T52.8X1	T52.8X2	T52.8X3	T52.8X4	--	--
- - dinitrate	T52.3X1	T52.3X2	T52.3X3	T52.3X4	--	--
- - monobutyl ether	T52.3X1	T52.3X2	T52.3X3	T52.3X4	--	--
- imine	T54.1X1	T54.1X2	T54.1X3	T54.1X4	--	--
- oxide (fumigant) (nonmedicinal)	T59.891	T59.892	T59.893	T59.894	--	--
- - medicinal	T49.0X1	T49.0X2	T49.0X3	T49.0X4	T49.0X5	T49.0X6
Ethylenediamine theophylline	T48.6X1	T48.6X2	T48.6X3	T48.6X4	T48.6X5	T48.6X6
Ethylenediaminetetra-acetic acid	T50.6X1	T50.6X2	T50.6X3	T50.6X4	T50.6X5	T50.6X6
Ethylenedinitrilotetra-acetate	T50.6X1	T50.6X2	T50.6X3	T50.6X4	T50.6X5	T50.6X6
Ethylestrenol	T38.7X1	T38.7X2	T38.7X3	T38.7X4	T38.7X5	T38.7X6
Ethylhydroxycellulose	T47.4X1	T47.4X2	T47.4X3	T47.4X4	T47.4X5	T47.4X6
Ethylidene						
- chloride NEC	T53.6X1	T53.6X2	T53.6X3	T53.6X4	--	--
- diacetate	T60.3X1	T60.3X2	T60.3X3	T60.3X4	--	--
- dicoumarin	T45.511	T45.512	T45.513	T45.514	T45.515	T45.516
- dicoumarol	T45.511	T45.512	T45.513	T45.514	T45.515	T45.516
- diethyl ether	T52.0X1	T52.0X2	T52.0X3	T52.0X4	--	--
Ethylmorphine	T40.2X1	T40.2X2	T40.2X3	T40.2X4	T40.2X5	T40.2X6
Ethylnorepinephrine	T48.6X1	T48.6X2	T48.6X3	T48.6X4	T48.6X5	T48.6X6
Ethylparachlorophen-oxyisobutyrate	T46.6X1	T46.6X2	T46.6X3	T46.6X4	T46.6X5	T46.6X6
Ethynodiol	T38.4X1	T38.4X2	T38.4X3	T38.4X4	T38.4X5	T38.4X6
- with mestranol diacetate	T38.4X1	T38.4X2	T38.4X3	T38.4X4	T38.4X5	T38.4X6
Etidocaine	T41.3X1	T41.3X2	T41.3X3	T41.3X4	T41.3X5	T41.3X6
- infiltration (subcutaneous)	T41.3X1	T41.3X2	T41.3X3	T41.3X4	T41.3X5	T41.3X6
- nerve (peripheral) (plexus)	T41.3X1	T41.3X2	T41.3X3	T41.3X4	T41.3X5	T41.3X6
Etidronate	T50.991	T50.992	T50.993	T50.994	T50.995	T50.996
Etidronic acid (disodium salt)	T50.991	T50.992	T50.993	T50.994	T50.995	T50.996
Etifoxine	T42.6X1	T42.6X2	T42.6X3	T42.6X4	T42.6X5	T42.6X6
Etilefrine	T44.4X1	T44.4X2	T44.4X3	T44.4X4	T44.4X5	T44.4X6

Substance	Poisoning, Accidental (unintentional)	Poisoning, Intentional Self-harm	Poisoning, Assault	Poisoning, Undetermined	Adverse effect	Underdosing
Etilfen	T42.3X1	T42.3X2	T42.3X3	T42.3X4	T42.3X5	T42.3X6
Etinodiol	T38.4X1	T38.4X2	T38.4X3	T38.4X4	T38.4X5	T38.4X6
Etiroxate	T46.6X1	T46.6X2	T46.6X3	T46.6X4	T46.6X5	T46.6X6
Etizolam	T42.4X1	T42.4X2	T42.4X3	T42.4X4	T42.4X5	T42.4X6
Etodolac	T39.391	T39.392	T39.393	T39.394	T39.395	T39.396
Etofamide	T37.3X1	T37.3X2	T37.3X3	T37.3X4	T37.3X5	T37.3X6
Etofibrate	T46.6X1	T46.6X2	T46.6X3	T46.6X4	T46.6X5	T46.6X6
Etofylline	T46.7X1	T46.7X2	T46.7X3	T46.7X4	T46.7X5	T46.7X6
- clofibrate	T46.6X1	T46.6X2	T46.6X3	T46.6X4	T46.6X5	T46.6X6
Etoglucid	T45.1X1	T45.1X2	T45.1X3	T45.1X4	T45.1X5	T45.1X6
Etomidate	T41.1X1	T41.1X2	T41.1X3	T41.1X4	T41.1X5	T41.1X6
Etomide	T39.8X1	T39.8X2	T39.8X3	T39.8X4	T39.8X5	T39.8X6
Etomidoline	T44.3X1	T44.3X2	T44.3X3	T44.3X4	T44.3X5	T44.3X6
Etoposide	T45.1X1	T45.1X2	T45.1X3	T45.1X4	T45.1X5	T45.1X6
Etorphine	T40.2X1	T40.2X2	T40.2X3	T40.2X4	T40.2X5	T40.2X6
Etoval	T42.3X1	T42.3X2	T42.3X3	T42.3X4	T42.3X5	T42.3X6
Etozolin	T50.1X1	T50.1X2	T50.1X3	T50.1X4	T50.1X5	T50.1X6
Etretinate	T50.991	T50.992	T50.993	T50.994	T50.995	T50.996
Etryptamine	T43.691	T43.692	T43.693	T43.694	T43.695	T43.696
Etybenzatropine	T44.3X1	T44.3X2	T44.3X3	T44.3X4	T44.3X5	T44.3X6
Etynodiol	T38.4X1	T38.4X2	T38.4X3	T38.4X4	T38.4X5	T38.4X6
Eucaine	T41.3X1	T41.3X2	T41.3X3	T41.3X4	T41.3X5	T41.3X6
Eucalyptus oil	T49.7X1	T49.7X2	T49.7X3	T49.7X4	T49.7X5	T49.7X6
Eucatropine	T49.5X1	T49.5X2	T49.5X3	T49.5X4	T49.5X5	T49.5X6
Eucodal	T40.2X1	T40.2X2	T40.2X3	T40.2X4	T40.2X5	T40.2X6
Euneryl	T42.3X1	T42.3X2	T42.3X3	T42.3X4	T42.3X5	T42.3X6
Euphthalmine	T44.3X1	T44.3X2	T44.3X3	T44.3X4	T44.3X5	T44.3X6
Eurax	T49.0X1	T49.0X2	T49.0X3	T49.0X4	T49.0X5	T49.0X6
Euresol	T49.4X1	T49.4X2	T49.4X3	T49.4X4	T49.4X5	T49.4X6
Euthroid	T38.1X1	T38.1X2	T38.1X3	T38.1X4	T38.1X5	T38.1X6
Evans blue	T50.8X1	T50.8X2	T50.8X3	T50.8X4	T50.8X5	T50.8X6
Evipal	T42.3X1	T42.3X2	T42.3X3	T42.3X4	T42.3X5	T42.3X6
- sodium	T41.1X1	T41.1X2	T41.1X3	T41.1X4	T41.1X5	T41.1X6
Evipan	T42.3X1	T42.3X2	T42.3X3	T42.3X4	T42.3X5	T42.3X6
- sodium	T41.1X1	T41.1X2	T41.1X3	T41.1X4	T41.1X5	T41.1X6
Exalamide	T49.0X1	T49.0X2	T49.0X3	T49.0X4	T49.0X5	T49.0X6
Exalgin	T39.1X1	T39.1X2	T39.1X3	T39.1X4	T39.1X5	T39.1X6
Excipients, pharmaceutical	T50.901	T50.902	T50.903	T50.904	T50.905	T50.906
Exhaust gas (engine) (motor vehicle)	T58.01	T58.02	T58.03	T58.04	--	--
Ex-Lax (phenolphthalein)	T47.2X1	T47.2X2	T47.2X3	T47.2X4	T47.2X5	T47.2X6
Expectorant NEC	T48.4X1	T48.4X2	T48.4X3	T48.4X4	T48.4X5	T48.4X6
Extended insulin zinc suspension	T38.3X1	T38.3X2	T38.3X3	T38.3X4	T38.3X5	T38.3X6
External medications (skin) (mucous membrane)	T49.91	T49.92	T49.93	T49.94	T49.95	T49.96
- dental agent	T49.7X1	T49.7X2	T49.7X3	T49.7X4	T49.7X5	T49.7X6
- ENT agent	T49.6X1	T49.6X2	T49.6X3	T49.6X4	T49.6X5	T49.6X6
- ophthalmic preparation	T49.5X1	T49.5X2	T49.5X3	T49.5X4	T49.5X5	T49.5X6
- specified NEC	T49.8X1	T49.8X2	T49.8X3	T49.8X4	T49.8X5	T49.8X6
Extrapyramidal antagonist NEC	T44.3X1	T44.3X2	T44.3X3	T44.3X4	T44.3X5	T44.3X6
Eye agents (anti-infective)	T49.5X1	T49.5X2	T49.5X3	T49.5X4	T49.5X5	T49.5X6
Eye drug NEC	T49.5X1	T49.5X2	T49.5X3	T49.5X4	T49.5X5	T49.5X6
FAC (fluorouracil + doxorubicin + cyclophosphamide)	T45.1X1	T45.1X2	T45.1X3	T45.1X4	T45.1X5	T45.1X6
Factor						
- I (fibrinogen)	T45.8X1	T45.8X2	T45.8X3	T45.8X4	T45.8X5	T45.8X6
- III (thromboplastin)	T45.8X1	T45.8X2	T45.8X3	T45.8X4	T45.8X5	T45.8X6
- VIII (antihemophilic Factor) (concentrate)	T45.8X1	T45.8X2	T45.8X3	T45.8X4	T45.8X5	T45.8X6
- IX complex	T45.7X1	T45.7X2	T45.7X3	T45.7X4	T45.7X5	T45.7X6
- - human	T45.8X1	T45.8X2	T45.8X3	T45.8X4	T45.8X5	T45.8X6
Famotidine	T47.0X1	T47.0X2	T47.0X3	T47.0X4	T47.0X5	T47.0X6
Fat suspension, intravenous	T50.991	T50.992	T50.993	T50.994	T50.995	T50.996
Fazadinium bromide	T48.1X1	T48.1X2	T48.1X3	T48.1X4	T48.1X5	T48.1X6
Febarbamate	T42.3X1	T42.3X2	T42.3X3	T42.3X4	T42.3X5	T42.3X6
Fecal softener	T47.4X1	T47.4X2	T47.4X3	T47.4X4	T47.4X5	T47.4X6
Fedrilate	T48.3X1	T48.3X2	T48.3X3	T48.3X4	T48.3X5	T48.3X6
Felodipine	T46.1X1	T46.1X2	T46.1X3	T46.1X4	T46.1X5	T46.1X6

Substance	Poisoning, Accidental (unintentional)	Poisoning, Intentional Self-harm	Poisoning, Assault	Poisoning, Undetermined	Adverse effect	Underdosing
Felypressin	T38.891	T38.892	T38.893	T38.894	T38.895	T38.896
Femoxetine	T43.221	T43.222	T43.223	T43.224	T43.225	T43.226
Fenalcomine	T46.3X1	T46.3X2	T46.3X3	T46.3X4	T46.3X5	T46.3X6
Fenamisal	T37.1X1	T37.1X2	T37.1X3	T37.1X4	T37.1X5	T37.1X6
Fenazone	T39.2X1	T39.2X2	T39.2X3	T39.2X4	T39.2X5	T39.2X6
Fenbendazole	T37.4X1	T37.4X2	T37.4X3	T37.4X4	T37.4X5	T37.4X6
Fenbutrazate	T50.5X1	T50.5X2	T50.5X3	T50.5X4	T50.5X5	T50.5X6
Fencamfamine	T43.691	T43.692	T43.693	T43.694	T43.695	T43.696
Fendiline	T46.1X1	T46.1X2	T46.1X3	T46.1X4	T46.1X5	T46.1X6
Fenetylline	T43.691	T43.692	T43.693	T43.694	T43.695	T43.696
Fenflumizole	T39.391	T39.392	T39.393	T39.394	T39.395	T39.396
Fenfluramine	T50.5X1	T50.5X2	T50.5X3	T50.5X4	T50.5X5	T50.5X6
Fenobarbital	T42.3X1	T42.3X2	T42.3X3	T42.3X4	T42.3X5	T42.3X6
Fenofibrate	T46.6X1	T46.6X2	T46.6X3	T46.6X4	T46.6X5	T46.6X6
Fenoprofen	T39.311	T39.312	T39.313	T39.314	T39.315	T39.316
Fenoterol	T48.6X1	T48.6X2	T48.6X3	T48.6X4	T48.6X5	T48.6X6
Fenoverine	T44.3X1	T44.3X2	T44.3X3	T44.3X4	T44.3X5	T44.3X6
Fenoxazoline	T48.5X1	T48.5X2	T48.5X3	T48.5X4	T48.5X5	T48.5X6
Fenproporex	T50.5X1	T50.5X2	T50.5X3	T50.5X4	T50.5X5	T50.5X6
Fenquizone	T50.2X1	T50.2X2	T50.2X3	T50.2X4	T50.2X5	T50.2X6
Fentanyl	T40.4X1	T40.4X2	T40.4X3	T40.4X4	T40.4X5	T40.4X6
Fentazin	T43.3X1	T43.3X2	T43.3X3	T43.3X4	T43.3X5	T43.3X6
Fenthion	T60.0X1	T60.0X2	T60.0X3	T60.0X4	--	--
Fenticlor	T49.0X1	T49.0X2	T49.0X3	T49.0X4	T49.0X5	T49.0X6
Fenylbutazone	T39.2X1	T39.2X2	T39.2X3	T39.2X4	T39.2X5	T39.2X6
Feprazone	T39.2X1	T39.2X2	T39.2X3	T39.2X4	T39.2X5	T39.2X6
Fer de lance (bite) (venom)	T63.061	T63.062	T63.063	T63.064	--	--
Ferric—see also Iron						
- chloride	T45.4X1	T45.4X2	T45.4X3	T45.4X4	T45.4X5	T45.4X6
- citrate	T45.4X1	T45.4X2	T45.4X3	T45.4X4	T45.4X5	T45.4X6
- hydroxide						
- - colloidal	T45.4X1	T45.4X2	T45.4X3	T45.4X4	T45.4X5	T45.4X6
- - polymaltose	T45.4X1	T45.4X2	T45.4X3	T45.4X4	T45.4X5	T45.4X6
- pyrophosphate	T45.4X1	T45.4X2	T45.4X3	T45.4X4	T45.4X5	T45.4X6
Ferritin	T45.4X1	T45.4X2	T45.4X3	T45.4X4	T45.4X5	T45.4X6
Ferrocholinate	T45.4X1	T45.4X2	T45.4X3	T45.4X4	T45.4X5	T45.4X6
Ferrodextrane	T45.4X1	T45.4X2	T45.4X3	T45.4X4	T45.4X5	T45.4X6
Ferropolimaler	T45.4X1	T45.4X2	T45.4X3	T45.4X4	T45.4X5	T45.4X6
Ferrous—see also Iron						
- phosphate	T45.4X1	T45.4X2	T45.4X3	T45.4X4	T45.4X5	T45.4X6
- salt	T45.4X1	T45.4X2	T45.4X3	T45.4X4	T45.4X5	T45.4X6
- - with folic acid	T45.4X1	T45.4X2	T45.4X3	T45.4X4	T45.4X5	T45.4X6
Ferrous fumarate, gluconate, lactate, salt NEC, sulfate (medicinal)	T45.4X1	T45.4X2	T45.4X3	T45.4X4	T45.4X5	T45.4X6
Ferrovanadium (fumes)	T59.891	T59.892	T59.893	T59.894	--	--
Ferrum—see Iron						
Fertilizers NEC	T65.891	T65.892	T65.893	T65.894	--	--
- with herbicide mixture	T60.3X1	T60.3X2	T60.3X3	T60.3X4	--	--
Fetoxilate	T47.6X1	T47.6X2	T47.6X3	T47.6X4	T47.6X5	T47.6X6
Fiber, dietary	T47.4X1	T47.4X2	T47.4X3	T47.4X4	T47.4X5	T47.4X6
Fiberglass	T65.831	T65.832	T65.833	T65.834	--	--
Fibrinogen (human)	T45.8X1	T45.8X2	T45.8X3	T45.8X4	T45.8X5	T45.8X6
Fibrinolysin (human)	T45.691	T45.692	T45.693	T45.694	T45.695	T45.696
Fibrinolysis						
- affecting drug	T45.601	T45.602	T45.603	T45.604	T45.605	T45.606
- inhibitor NEC	T45.621	T45.622	T45.623	T45.624	T45.625	T45.626
Fibrinolytic drug	T45.611	T45.612	T45.613	T45.614	T45.615	T45.616
Filix mas	T37.4X1	T37.4X2	T37.4X3	T37.4X4	T37.4X5	T37.4X6
Filtering cream	T49.3X1	T49.3X2	T49.3X3	T49.3X4	T49.3X5	T49.3X6
Fiorinal	T39.011	T39.012	T39.013	T39.014	T39.015	T39.016
Firedamp	T59.891	T59.892	T59.893	T59.894	--	--
Fish, noxious, nonbacterial	T61.91	T61.92	T61.93	T61.94	--	--
- ciguatera	T61.01	T61.02	T61.03	T61.04	--	--
- scombroid	T61.11	T61.12	T61.13	T61.14	--	--
- shell	T61.781	T61.782	T61.783	T61.784	--	--

Substance	Poisoning, Accidental (unintentional)	Poisoning, Intentional Self-harm	Poisoning, Assault	Poisoning, Undetermined	Adverse effect	Underdosing
- specified NEC	T61.771	T61.772	T61.773	T61.774	--	--
Flagyl	T37.3X1	T37.3X2	T37.3X3	T37.3X4	T37.3X5	T37.3X6
Flavine adenine dinucleotide	T45.2X1	T45.2X2	T45.2X3	T45.2X4	T45.2X5	T45.2X6
Flavodic acid	T46.991	T46.992	T46.993	T46.994	T46.995	T46.996
Flavoxate	T44.3X1	T44.3X2	T44.3X3	T44.3X4	T44.3X5	T44.3X6
Flaxedil	T48.1X1	T48.1X2	T48.1X3	T48.1X4	T48.1X5	T48.1X6
Flaxseed (medicinal)	T49.3X1	T49.3X2	T49.3X3	T49.3X4	T49.3X5	T49.3X6
Flecainide	T46.2X1	T46.2X2	T46.2X3	T46.2X4	T46.2X5	T46.2X6
Fleroxacin	T36.8X1	T36.8X2	T36.8X3	T36.8X4	T36.8X5	T36.8X6
Floctafenine	T39.8X1	T39.8X2	T39.8X3	T39.8X4	T39.8X5	T39.8X6
Flomax	T44.6X1	T44.6X2	T44.6X3	T44.6X4	T44.6X5	T44.6X6
Flomoxef	T36.1X1	T36.1X2	T36.1X3	T36.1X4	T36.1X5	T36.1X6
Flopropione	T44.3X1	T44.3X2	T44.3X3	T44.3X4	T44.3X5	T44.3X6
Florantyrone	T47.5X1	T47.5X2	T47.5X3	T47.5X4	T47.5X5	T47.5X6
Floraquin	T37.8X1	T37.8X2	T37.8X3	T37.8X4	T37.8X5	T37.8X6
Florinef	T38.0X1	T38.0X2	T38.0X3	T38.0X4	T38.0X5	T38.0X6
- ENT agent	T49.6X1	T49.6X2	T49.6X3	T49.6X4	T49.6X5	T49.6X6
- ophthalmic preparation	T49.5X1	T49.5X2	T49.5X3	T49.5X4	T49.5X5	T49.5X6
- topical NEC	T49.0X1	T49.0X2	T49.0X3	T49.0X4	T49.0X5	T49.0X6
Flowers of sulfur	T49.4X1	T49.4X2	T49.4X3	T49.4X4	T49.4X5	T49.4X6
Floxuridine	T45.1X1	T45.1X2	T45.1X3	T45.1X4	T45.1X5	T45.1X6
Fluanisone	T43.4X1	T43.4X2	T43.4X3	T43.4X4	T43.4X5	T43.4X6
Flubendazole	T37.4X1	T37.4X2	T37.4X3	T37.4X4	T37.4X5	T37.4X6
Fluclorolone acetonide	T49.0X1	T49.0X2	T49.0X3	T49.0X4	T49.0X5	T49.0X6
Flucloxacillin	T36.0X1	T36.0X2	T36.0X3	T36.0X4	T36.0X5	T36.0X6
Fluconazole	T37.8X1	T37.8X2	T37.8X3	T37.8X4	T37.8X5	T37.8X6
Flucytosine	T37.8X1	T37.8X2	T37.8X3	T37.8X4	T37.8X5	T37.8X6
Fludeoxyglucose (18F)	T50.8X1	T50.8X2	T50.8X3	T50.8X4	T50.8X5	T50.8X6
Fludiazepam	T42.4X1	T42.4X2	T42.4X3	T42.4X4	T42.4X5	T42.4X6
Fludrocortisone	T50.0X1	T50.0X2	T50.0X3	T50.0X4	T50.0X5	T50.0X6
- ENT agent	T49.6X1	T49.6X2	T49.6X3	T49.6X4	T49.6X5	T49.6X6
- ophthalmic preparation	T49.5X1	T49.5X2	T49.5X3	T49.5X4	T49.5X5	T49.5X6
- topical NEC	T49.0X1	T49.0X2	T49.0X3	T49.0X4	T49.0X5	T49.0X6
Fludroxycortide	T49.0X1	T49.0X2	T49.0X3	T49.0X4	T49.0X5	T49.0X6
Flufenamic acid	T39.391	T39.392	T39.393	T39.394	T39.395	T39.396
Fluindione	T45.511	T45.512	T45.513	T45.514	T45.515	T45.516
Flumequine	T37.8X1	T37.8X2	T37.8X3	T37.8X4	T37.8X5	T37.8X6
Flumethasone	T49.0X1	T49.0X2	T49.0X3	T49.0X4	T49.0X5	T49.0X6
Flumethiazide	T50.2X1	T50.2X2	T50.2X3	T50.2X4	T50.2X5	T50.2X6
Flumidin	T37.5X1	T37.5X2	T37.5X3	T37.5X4	T37.5X5	T37.5X6
Flunarizine	T46.7X1	T46.7X2	T46.7X3	T46.7X4	T46.7X5	T46.7X6
Flunidazole	T37.8X1	T37.8X2	T37.8X3	T37.8X4	T37.8X5	T37.8X6
Flunisolide	T48.6X1	T48.6X2	T48.6X3	T48.6X4	T48.6X5	T48.6X6
Flunitrazepam	T42.4X1	T42.4X2	T42.4X3	T42.4X4	T42.4X5	T42.4X6
Fluocinolone (acetonide)	T49.0X1	T49.0X2	T49.0X3	T49.0X4	T49.0X5	T49.0X6
Fluocinonide	T49.0X1	T49.0X2	T49.0X3	T49.0X4	T49.0X5	T49.0X6
Fluocortin (butyl)	T49.0X1	T49.0X2	T49.0X3	T49.0X4	T49.0X5	T49.0X6
Fluocortolone	T49.0X1	T49.0X2	T49.0X3	T49.0X4	T49.0X5	T49.0X6
Fluohydrocortisone	T38.0X1	T38.0X2	T38.0X3	T38.0X4	T38.0X5	T38.0X6
- ENT agent	T49.6X1	T49.6X2	T49.6X3	T49.6X4	T49.6X5	T49.6X6
- ophthalmic preparation	T49.5X1	T49.5X2	T49.5X3	T49.5X4	T49.5X5	T49.5X6
- topical NEC	T49.0X1	T49.0X2	T49.0X3	T49.0X4	T49.0X5	T49.0X6
Fluonid	T49.0X1	T49.0X2	T49.0X3	T49.0X4	T49.0X5	T49.0X6
Fluopromazine	T43.3X1	T43.3X2	T43.3X3	T43.3X4	T43.3X5	T43.3X6
Fluoracetate	T60.8X1	T60.8X2	T60.8X3	T60.8X4	--	--
Fluorescein	T50.8X1	T50.8X2	T50.8X3	T50.8X4	T50.8X5	T50.8X6
Fluorhydrocortisone	T50.0X1	T50.0X2	T50.0X3	T50.0X4	T50.0X5	T50.0X6
Fluoride (nonmedicinal) (pesticide) (sodium) NEC	T60.8X1	T60.8X2	T60.8X3	T60.8X4	--	--
- hydrogen—see Hydrofluoric acid						
- medicinal NEC	T50.991	T50.992	T50.993	T50.994	T50.995	T50.996
- - dental use	T49.7X1	T49.7X2	T49.7X3	T49.7X4	T49.7X5	T49.7X6
- not pesticide NEC	T54.91	T54.92	T54.93	T54.94	--	--
- stannous	T49.7X1	T49.7X2	T49.7X3	T49.7X4	T49.7X5	T49.7X6
Fluorinated corticosteroids	T38.0X1	T38.0X2	T38.0X3	T38.0X4	T38.0X5	T38.0X6
Fluorine (gas)	T59.5X1	T59.5X2	T59.5X3	T59.5X4	--	--

Substance	Poisoning, Accidental (unintentional)	Poisoning, Intentional Self-harm	Poisoning, Assault	Poisoning, Undetermined	Adverse effect	Underdosing
- salt—see Fluoride (s)						
Fluoristan	T49.7X1	T49.7X2	T49.7X3	T49.7X4	T49.7X5	T49.7X6
Fluormetholone	T49.0X1	T49.0X2	T49.0X3	T49.0X4	T49.0X5	T49.0X6
Fluoroacetate	T60.8X1	T60.8X2	T60.8X3	T60.8X4	--	--
Fluorocarbon monomer	T53.6X1	T53.6X2	T53.6X3	T53.6X4	--	--
Fluorocytosine	T37.8X1	T37.8X2	T37.8X3	T37.8X4	T37.8X5	T37.8X6
Fluorodeoxyuridine	T45.1X1	T45.1X2	T45.1X3	T45.1X4	T45.1X5	T45.1X6
Fluorometholone	T49.0X1	T49.0X2	T49.0X3	T49.0X4	T49.0X5	T49.0X6
Fluorophosphate insecticide	T60.0X1	T60.0X2	T60.0X3	T60.0X4	--	--
Fluorosol	T46.3X1	T46.3X2	T46.3X3	T46.3X4	T46.3X5	T46.3X6
Fluorouracil	T45.1X1	T45.1X2	T45.1X3	T45.1X4	T45.1X5	T45.1X6
Fluorphenylalanine	T49.5X1	T49.5X2	T49.5X3	T49.5X4	T49.5X5	T49.5X6
Fluothane	T41.0X1	T41.0X2	T41.0X3	T41.0X4	T41.0X5	T41.0X6
Fluoxetine	T43.221	T43.222	T43.223	T43.224	T43.225	T43.226
Fluoxymesterone	T38.7X1	T38.7X2	T38.7X3	T38.7X4	T38.7X5	T38.7X6
Flupenthixol	T43.4X1	T43.4X2	T43.4X3	T43.4X4	T43.4X5	T43.4X6
Flupentixol	T43.4X1	T43.4X2	T43.4X3	T43.4X4	T43.4X5	T43.4X6
Fluphenazine	T43.3X1	T43.3X2	T43.3X3	T43.3X4	T43.3X5	T43.3X6
Fluprednidene	T49.0X1	T49.0X2	T49.0X3	T49.0X4	T49.0X5	T49.0X6
Fluprednisolone	T38.0X1	T38.0X2	T38.0X3	T38.0X4	T38.0X5	T38.0X6
Fluradoline	T39.8X1	T39.8X2	T39.8X3	T39.8X4	T39.8X5	T39.8X6
Flurandrenolide	T49.0X1	T49.0X2	T49.0X3	T49.0X4	T49.0X5	T49.0X6
Flurandrenolone	T49.0X1	T49.0X2	T49.0X3	T49.0X4	T49.0X5	T49.0X6
Flurazepam	T42.4X1	T42.4X2	T42.4X3	T42.4X4	T42.4X5	T42.4X6
Flurbiprofen	T39.311	T39.312	T39.313	T39.314	T39.315	T39.316
Flurobate	T49.0X1	T49.0X2	T49.0X3	T49.0X4	T49.0X5	T49.0X6
Fluroxene	T41.0X1	T41.0X2	T41.0X3	T41.0X4	T41.0X5	T41.0X6
Fluspirilene	T43.591	T43.592	T43.593	T43.594	T43.595	T43.596
Flutamide	T38.6X1	T38.6X2	T38.6X3	T38.6X4	T38.6X5	T38.6X6
Flutazolam	T42.4X1	T42.4X2	T42.4X3	T42.4X4	T42.4X5	T42.4X6
Fluticasone propionate	T49.1X1	T49.1X2	T49.1X3	T49.1X4	T49.1X5	T49.1X6
Flutoprazepam	T42.4X1	T42.4X2	T42.4X3	T42.4X4	T42.4X5	T42.4X6
Flutropium bromide	T48.6X1	T48.6X2	T48.6X3	T48.6X4	T48.6X5	T48.6X6
Fluvoxamine	T43.221	T43.222	T43.223	T43.224	T43.225	T43.226
Folacin	T45.8X1	T45.8X2	T45.8X3	T45.8X4	T45.8X5	T45.8X6
Folic acid	T45.8X1	T45.8X2	T45.8X3	T45.8X4	T45.8X5	T45.8X6
- with ferrous salt	T45.2X1	T45.2X2	T45.2X3	T45.2X4	T45.2X5	T45.2X6
- antagonist	T45.1X1	T45.1X2	T45.1X3	T45.1X4	T45.1X5	T45.1X6
Folinic acid	T45.8X1	T45.8X2	T45.8X3	T45.8X4	T45.8X5	T45.8X6
Folium stramoniae	T48.6X1	T48.6X2	T48.6X3	T48.6X4	T48.6X5	T48.6X6
Follicle-stimulating hormone, human	T38.811	T38.812	T38.813	T38.814	T38.815	T38.816
Folpet	T60.3X1	T60.3X2	T60.3X3	T60.3X4	--	--
Fominoben	T48.3X1	T48.3X2	T48.3X3	T48.3X4	T48.3X5	T48.3X6
Food, foodstuffs, noxious, nonbacterial, NEC	T62.91	T62.92	T62.93	T62.94	--	--
- berries	T62.1X1	T62.1X2	T62.1X3	T62.1X4	--	--
- fish—see also Fish	T61.91	T61.92	T61.93	T61.94	--	--
- mushrooms	T62.0X1	T62.0X2	T62.0X3	T62.0X4	--	--
- plants	T62.2X1	T62.2X2	T62.2X3	T62.2X4	--	--
- seafood	T61.91	T61.92	T61.93	T61.94	--	--
- - specified NEC	T61.8X1	T61.8X2	T61.8X3	T61.8X4	--	--
- seeds	T62.2X1	T62.2X2	T62.2X3	T62.2X4	--	--
- shellfish	T61.781	T61.782	T61.783	T61.784	--	--
- specified NEC	T62.8X1	T62.8X2	T62.8X3	T62.8X4	--	--
Fool's parsley	T62.2X1	T62.2X2	T62.2X3	T62.2X4	--	--
Formaldehyde (solution), gas or vapor	T59.2X1	T59.2X2	T59.2X3	T59.2X4	--	--
- fungicide	T60.3X1	T60.3X2	T60.3X3	T60.3X4	--	--
Formalin	T59.2X1	T59.2X2	T59.2X3	T59.2X4	--	--
- fungicide	T60.3X1	T60.3X2	T60.3X3	T60.3X4	--	--
- vapor	T59.2X1	T59.2X2	T59.2X3	T59.2X4	--	--
Formic acid	T54.2X1	T54.2X2	T54.2X3	T54.2X4	--	--
- vapor	T59.891	T59.892	T59.893	T59.894	--	--
Foscarnet sodium	T37.5X1	T37.5X2	T37.5X3	T37.5X4	T37.5X5	T37.5X6
Fosfestrol	T38.5X1	T38.5X2	T38.5X3	T38.5X4	T38.5X5	T38.5X6
Fosfomycin	T36.8X1	T36.8X2	T36.8X3	T36.8X4	T36.8X5	T36.8X6
Fosfonet sodium	T37.5X1	T37.5X2	T37.5X3	T37.5X4	T37.5X5	T37.5X6

Substance	Poisoning, Accidental (unintentional)	Poisoning, Intentional Self-harm	Poisoning, Assault	Poisoning, Undetermined	Adverse effect	Underdosing
Fosinopril	T46.4X1	T46.4X2	T46.4X3	T46.4X4	T46.4X5	T46.4X6
- sodium	T46.4X1	T46.4X2	T46.4X3	T46.4X4	T46.4X5	T46.4X6
Fowler's solution	T57.0X1	T57.0X2	T57.0X3	T57.0X4	--	--
Foxglove	T62.2X1	T62.2X2	T62.2X3	T62.2X4		
Framycetin	T36.5X1	T36.5X2	T36.5X3	T36.5X4	T36.5X5	T36.5X6
Frangula	T47.2X1	T47.2X2	T47.2X3	T47.2X4	T47.2X5	T47.2X6
- extract	T47.2X1	T47.2X2	T47.2X3	T47.2X4	T47.2X5	T47.2X6
Frei antigen	T50.8X1	T50.8X2	T50.8X3	T50.8X4	T50.8X5	T50.8X6
Freon	T53.5X1	T53.5X2	T53.5X3	T53.5X4	--	--
Fructose	T50.3X1	T50.3X2	T50.3X3	T50.3X4	T50.3X5	T50.3X6
Frusemide	T50.1X1	T50.1X2	T50.1X3	T50.1X4	T50.1X5	T50.1X6
FSH	T38.811	T38.812	T38.813	T38.814	T38.815	T38.816
Ftorafur	T45.1X1	T45.1X2	T45.1X3	T45.1X4	T45.1X5	T45.1X6
Fuel						
- automobile	T52.0X1	T52.0X2	T52.0X3	T52.0X4	--	--
- - exhaust gas, not in transit	T58.01	T58.02	T58.03	T58.04	--	--
- - vapor NEC	T52.0X1	T52.0X2	T52.0X3	T52.0X4	--	--
- gas (domestic use) —see also Carbon, monoxide, fuel, utility	T59.891	T59.892	T59.893	T59.894	--	--
- - utility	T59.891	T59.892	T59.893	T59.894	--	--
- - - in mobile container	T59.891	T59.892	T59.893	T59.894	--	--
- - - incomplete combustion of—see Carbon, monoxide, fuel, utility						
- - - piped (natural)	T59.891	T59.892	T59.893	T59.894	--	--
- industrial, incomplete combustion	T58.8X1	T58.8X2	T58.8X3	T58.8X4	--	--
Fugillin	T36.8X1	T36.8X2	T36.8X3	T36.8X4	T36.8X5	T36.8X6
Fulminate of mercury	T56.1X1	T56.1X2	T56.1X3	T56.1X4	--	--
Fulvicin	T36.7X1	T36.7X2	T36.7X3	T36.7X4	T36.7X5	T36.7X6
Fumadil	T36.8X1	T36.8X2	T36.8X3	T36.8X4	T36.8X5	T36.8X6
Fumagillin	T36.8X1	T36.8X2	T36.8X3	T36.8X4	T36.8X5	T36.8X6
Fumaric acid	T49.4X1	T49.4X2	T49.4X3	T49.4X4	T49.4X5	T49.4X6
Fumes (from)	T59.91	T59.92	T59.93	T59.94	--	--
- carbon monoxide—see Carbon, monoxide						
- charcoal (domestic use) —see Charcoal, fumes						
- chloroform—see Chloroform						
- coke (in domestic stoves, fireplaces) —see Coke fumes						
- corrosive NEC	T54.91	T54.92	T54.93	T54.94	--	--
- ether—see ether						
- freons	T53.5X1	T53.5X2	T53.5X3	T53.5X4	--	--
- hydrocarbons	T59.891	T59.892	T59.893	T59.894	--	--
- - petroleum (liquefied)	T59.891	T59.892	T59.893	T59.894	--	--
- - - distributed through pipes (pure or mixed with air)	T59.891	T59.892	T59.893	T59.894	--	--
- lead—see lead						
- metal—see Metals, or the specified metal						
- nitrogen dioxide	T59.0X1	T59.0X2	T59.0X3	T59.0X4	--	--
- pesticides—see Pesticides						
- petroleum (liquefied)	T59.891	T59.892	T59.893	T59.894	--	--
- - distributed through pipes (pure or mixed with air)	T59.891	T59.892	T59.893	T59.894	--	--
- polyester	T59.891	T59.892	T59.893	T59.894	--	--
- specified source NEC—see also substance specified	T59.891	T59.892	T59.893	T59.894	--	--
- sulfur dioxide	T59.1X1	T59.1X2	T59.1X3	T59.1X4	--	--
Fumigant NEC	T60.91	T60.92	T60.93	T60.94	--	--
Fungi, noxious, used as food	T62.0X1	T62.0X2	T62.0X3	T62.0X4	--	--
Fungicide NEC (nonmedicinal)	T60.3X1	T60.3X2	T60.3X3	T60.3X4	--	--
Fungizone	T36.7X1	T36.7X2	T36.7X3	T36.7X4	T36.7X5	T36.7X6
- topical	T49.0X1	T49.0X2	T49.0X3	T49.0X4	T49.0X5	T49.0X6
Furacin	T49.0X1	T49.0X2	T49.0X3	T49.0X4	T49.0X5	T49.0X6
Furadantin	T37.91	T37.92	T37.93	T37.94	T37.95	T37.96
Furazolidone	T37.8X1	T37.8X2	T37.8X3	T37.8X4	T37.8X5	T37.8X6
Furazolium chloride	T49.0X1	T49.0X2	T49.0X3	T49.0X4	T49.0X5	T49.0X6
Furfural	T52.8X1	T52.8X2	T52.8X3	T52.8X4	--	--
Furnace (coal burning) (domestic) , gas from	T58.2X1	T58.2X2	T58.2X3	T58.2X4	--	--
- industrial	T58.8X1	T58.8X2	T58.8X3	T58.8X4	--	--

Substance	Poisoning, Accidental (unintentional)	Poisoning, Intentional Self-harm	Poisoning, Assault	Poisoning, Undetermined	Adverse effect	Underdosing
Furniture polish	T65.891	T65.892	T65.893	T65.894	--	--
Furosemide	T50.1X1	T50.1X2	T50.1X3	T50.1X4	T50.1X5	T50.1X6
Furoxone	T37.91	T37.92	T37.93	T37.94	T37.95	T37.96
Fursultiamine	T45.2X1	T45.2X2	T45.2X3	T45.2X4	T45.2X5	T45.2X6
Fusafungine	T36.8X1	T36.8X2	T36.8X3	T36.8X4	T36.8X5	T36.8X6
Fusel oil (any) (amyl) (butyl) (propyl) , vapor	T51.3X1	T51.3X2	T51.3X3	T51.3X4	--	--
Fusidate (ethanolamine) (sodium)	T36.8X1	T36.8X2	T36.8X3	T36.8X4	T36.8X5	T36.8X6
Fusidic acid	T36.8X1	T36.8X2	T36.8X3	T36.8X4	T36.8X5	T36.8X6
Fytic acid, nonasodium	T50.6X1	T50.6X2	T50.6X3	T50.6X4	T50.6X5	T50.6X6
GABA	T43.8X1	T43.8X2	T43.8X3	T43.8X4	T43.8X5	T43.8X6
Gadopentetic acid	T50.8X1	T50.8X2	T50.8X3	T50.8X4	T50.8X5	T50.8X6
Galactose	T50.3X1	T50.3X2	T50.3X3	T50.3X4	T50.3X5	T50.3X6
b-Galactosidase	T47.5X1	T47.5X2	T47.5X3	T47.5X4	T47.5X5	T47.5X6
Galantamine	T44.0X1	T44.0X2	T44.0X3	T44.0X4	T44.0X5	T44.0X6
Gallamine (triethiodide)	T48.1X1	T48.1X2	T48.1X3	T48.1X4	T48.1X5	T48.1X6
Gallium citrate	T50.991	T50.992	T50.993	T50.994	T50.995	T50.996
Gallopamil	T46.1X1	T46.1X2	T46.1X3	T46.1X4	T46.1X5	T46.1X6
Gamboge	T47.2X1	T47.2X2	T47.2X3	T47.2X4	T47.2X5	T47.2X6
Gamimune	T50.Z11	T50.Z12	T50.Z13	T50.Z14	T50.Z15	T50.Z16
Gamma globulin	T50.Z11	T50.Z12	T50.Z13	T50.Z14	T50.Z15	T50.Z16
Gamma-aminobutyric acid	T43.8X1	T43.8X2	T43.8X3	T43.8X4	T43.8X5	T43.8X6
Gamma-benzene hexachloride (medicinal)	T49.0X1	T49.0X2	T49.0X3	T49.0X4	T49.0X5	T49.0X6
- nonmedicinal, vapor	T53.6X1	T53.6X2	T53.6X3	T53.6X4	--	--
Gamma-BHC (medicinal) —see also Gamma-benzene hexachloride	T49.0X1	T49.0X2	T49.0X3	T49.0X4	T49.0X5	T49.0X6
Gamulin	T50.Z11	T50.Z12	T50.Z13	T50.Z14	T50.Z15	T50.Z16
Ganciclovir (sodium)	T37.5X1	T37.5X2	T37.5X3	T37.5X4	T37.5X5	T37.5X6
Ganglionic blocking drug NEC	T44.2X1	T44.2X2	T44.2X3	T44.2X4	T44.2X5	T44.2X6
- specified NEC	T44.2X1	T44.2X2	T44.2X3	T44.2X4	T44.2X5	T44.2X6
Ganja	T40.7X1	T40.7X2	T40.7X3	T40.7X4	T40.7X5	T40.7X6
Garamycin	T36.5X1	T36.5X2	T36.5X3	T36.5X4	T36.5X5	T36.5X6
- ophthalmic preparation	T49.5X1	T49.5X2	T49.5X3	T49.5X4	T49.5X5	T49.5X6
- topical NEC	T49.0X1	T49.0X2	T49.0X3	T49.0X4	T49.0X5	T49.0X6
Gardenal	T42.3X1	T42.3X2	T42.3X3	T42.3X4	T42.3X5	T42.3X6
Gardepanyl	T42.3X1	T42.3X2	T42.3X3	T42.3X4	T42.3X5	T42.3X6
Gas	T59.91	T59.92	T59.93	T59.94	--	--
- acetylene	T59.891	T59.892	T59.893	T59.894	--	--
- - incomplete combustion of	T58.11	T58.12	T58.13	T58.14	--	--
- air contaminants, source or type not specified	T59.91	T59.92	T59.93	T59.94	--	--
- anesthetic	T41.0X1	T41.0X2	T41.0X3	T41.0X4	T41.0X5	T41.0X6
- blast furnace	T58.8X1	T58.8X2	T58.8X3	T58.8X4	--	--
- butane—see butane						
- carbon monoxide—see Carbon, monoxide						
- chlorine	T59.4X1	T59.4X2	T59.4X3	T59.4X4	--	--
- coal	T58.2X1	T58.2X2	T58.2X3	T58.2X4	--	--
- cyanide	T57.3X1	T57.3X2	T57.3X3	T57.3X4	--	--
dicyanogen	T65.0X1	T65.0X2	T65.0X3	T65.0X4	--	--
- domestic—see Domestic gas						
- exhaust	T58.01	T58.02	T58.03	T58.04	--	--
- from utility (for cooking, heating, or lighting) (after combustion) —see Carbon, monoxide, fuel, utility						
- - prior to combustion	T59.891	T59.892	T59.893	T59.894	--	--
- from wood- or coal-burning stove or fireplace	T58.2X1	T58.2X2	T58.2X3	T58.2X4	--	--
- fuel (domestic use) (after combustion) —see also Carbon, monoxide, fuel						
- - industrial use	T58.8X1	T58.8X2	T58.8X3	T58.8X4	--	--
- - prior to combustion	T59.891	T59.892	T59.893	T59.894	--	--
- - utility	T59.891	T59.892	T59.893	T59.894	--	--
- - - in mobile container	T59.891	T59.892	T59.893	T59.894	--	--
- - - incomplete combustion of—see Carbon, monoxide, fuel, utility						
- - - piped (natural)	T59.891	T59.892	T59.893	T59.894	--	--
- garage	T58.01	T58.02	T58.03	T58.04	--	--
- hydrocarbon NEC	T59.891	T59.892	T59.893	T59.894	--	--

Substance	Poisoning, Accidental (unintentional)	Poisoning, Intentional Self-harm	Poisoning, Assault	Poisoning, Undetermined	Adverse effect	Underdosing
- - incomplete combustion of—see Carbon, monoxide, fuel, utility						
- - liquefied—see butane						
- - - piped	T59.891	T59.892	T59.893	T59.894	--	--
- hydrocyanic acid	T65.0X1	T65.0X2	T65.0X3	T65.0X4	--	--
- illuminating (after combustion)	T58.11	T58.12	T58.13	T58.14	--	--
- - prior to combustion	T59.891	T59.892	T59.893	T59.894	--	--
- incomplete combustion, any—see Carbon, monoxide						
- kiln	T58.8X1	T58.8X2	T58.8X3	T58.8X4	--	--
- lacrimogenic	T59.3X1	T59.3X2	T59.3X3	T59.3X4	--	--
- liquefied petroleum—see butane						
- marsh	T59.891	T59.892	T59.893	T59.894	--	--
- motor exhaust, not in transit	T58.01	T58.02	T58.03	T58.04	--	--
- mustard, not in war	T59.891	T59.892	T59.893	T59.894	--	--
- natural	T59.891	T59.892	T59.893	T59.894	--	--
- nerve, not in war	T59.91	T59.92	T59.93	T59.94	--	--
- oil	T52.0X1	T52.0X2	T52.0X3	T52.0X4	--	--
- petroleum (liquefied) (distributed in mobile containers)	T59.891	T59.892	T59.893	T59.894	--	--
- - piped (pure or mixed with air)	T59.891	T59.892	T59.893	T59.894	--	--
- piped (manufactured) (natural) NEC	T59.891	T59.892	T59.893	T59.894	--	--
- producer	T58.8X1	T58.8X2	T58.8X3	T58.8X4	--	--
- propane—see propane						
- refrigerant (chlorofluoro-carbon)	T53.5X1	T53.5X2	T53.5X3	T53.5X4	--	--
- - - not chlorofluoro-carbon	T59.891	T59.892	T59.893	T59.894	--	--
- sewer	T59.91	T59.92	T59.93	T59.94	--	--
- specified source NEC	T59.91	T59.92	T59.93	T59.94	--	--
- stove (after combustion)	T58.11	T58.12	T58.13	T58.14	--	--
- - prior to combustion	T59.891	T59.892	T59.893	T59.894	--	--
- tear	T59.3X1	T59.3X2	T59.3X3	T59.3X4	--	--
- therapeutic	T41.5X1	T41.5X2	T41.5X3	T41.5X4	T41.5X5	T41.5X6
- utility (for cooking, heating, or lighting) (piped) NEC	T59.891	T59.892	T59.893	T59.894	--	--
- - in mobile container	T59.891	T59.892	T59.893	T59.894	--	--
- - incomplete combustion of—see Carbon, monoxide, fuel, utilty						
- - piped (natural)	T59.891	T59.892	T59.893	T59.894	--	--
- water	T58.11	T58.12	T58.13	T58.14	--	--
- - incomplete combustion of—see Carbon, monoxide, fuel, utility						
Gaseous substance—see Gas						
Gasoline	T52.0X1	T52.0X2	T52.0X3	T52.0X4		
- vapor	T52.0X1	T52.0X2	T52.0X3	T52.0X4	--	--
Gastric enzymes	T47.5X1	T47.5X2	T47.5X3	T47.5X4	T47.5X5	T47.5X6
Gastrografin	T50.8X1	T50.8X2	T50.8X3	T50.8X4	T50.8X5	T50.8X6
Gastrointestinal drug	T47.91	T47.92	T47.93	T47.94	T47.95	T47.96
- biological	T47.8X1	T47.8X2	T47.8X3	T47.8X4	T47.8X5	T47.8X6
- specified NEC	T47.8X1	T47.8X2	T47.8X3	T47.8X4	T47.8X5	T47.8X6
Gaultheria procumbens	T62.2X1	T62.2X2	T62.2X3	T62.2X4	--	--
Gefarnate	T44.3X1	T44.3X2	T44.3X3	T44.3X4	T44.3X5	T44.3X6
Gelatin (intravenous)	T45.8X1	T45.8X2	T45.8X3	T45.8X4	T45.8X5	T45.8X6
- absorbable (sponge)	T45.7X1	T45.7X2	T45.7X3	T45.7X4	T45.7X5	T45.7X6
Gelfilm	T49.8X1	T49.8X2	T49.8X3	T49.8X4	T49.8X5	T49.8X6
Gelfoam	T45.7X1	T45.7X2	T45.7X3	T45.7X4	T45.7X5	T45.7X6
Gelsemine	T50.991	T50.992	T50.993	T50.994	T50.995	T50.996
Gelsemium (sempervirens)	T62.2X1	T62.2X2	T62.2X3	T62.2X4	--	--
Gemeprost	T48.0X1	T48.0X2	T48.0X3	T48.0X4	T48.0X5	T48.0X6
Gemfibrozil	T46.6X1	T46.6X2	T46.6X3	T46.6X4	T46.6X5	T46.6X6
Gemonil	T42.3X1	T42.3X2	T42.3X3	T42.3X4	T42.3X5	T42.3X6
Gentamicin	T36.5X1	T36.5X2	T36.5X3	T36.5X4	T36.5X5	T36.5X6
- ophthalmic preparation	T49.5X1	T49.5X2	T49.5X3	T49.5X4	T49.5X5	T49.5X6
- topical NEC	T49.0X1	T49.0X2	T49.0X3	T49.0X4	T49.0X5	T49.0X6
Gentian	T47.5X1	T47.5X2	T47.5X3	T47.5X4	T47.5X5	T47.5X6
- violet	T49.0X1	T49.0X2	T49.0X3	T49.0X4	T49.0X5	T49.0X6

Substance	Poisoning, Accidental (unintentional)	Poisoning, Intentional Self-harm	Poisoning, Assault	Poisoning, Undetermined	Adverse effect	Underdosing
Gepefrine	T44.4X1	T44.4X2	T44.4X3	T44.4X4	T44.4X5	T44.4X6
Gestonorone caproate	T38.5X1	T38.5X2	T38.5X3	T38.5X4	T38.5X5	T38.5X6
Gexane	T49.0X1	T49.0X2	T49.0X3	T49.0X4	T49.0X5	T49.0X6
Gila monster (venom)	T63.111	T63.112	T63.113	T63.114	--	--
Ginger	T47.5X1	T47.5X2	T47.5X3	T47.5X4	T47.5X5	T47.5X6
- Jamaica—see Jamaica, ginger						
Gitalin	T46.0X1	T46.0X2	T46.0X3	T46.0X4	T46.0X5	T46.0X6
- amorphous	T46.0X1	T46.0X2	T46.0X3	T46.0X4	T46.0X5	T46.0X6
Gitaloxin	T46.0X1	T46.0X2	T46.0X3	T46.0X4	T46.0X5	T46.0X6
Gitoxin	T46.0X1	T46.0X2	T46.0X3	T46.0X4	T46.0X5	T46.0X6
Glafenine	T39.8X1	T39.8X2	T39.8X3	T39.8X4	T39.8X5	T39.8X6
Glandular extract (medicinal) NEC	T50.Z91	T50.Z92	T50.Z93	T50.Z94	T50.Z95	T50.Z96
Glaucarubin	T37.3X1	T37.3X2	T37.3X3	T37.3X4	T37.3X5	T37.3X6
Glibenclamide	T38.3X1	T38.3X2	T38.3X3	T38.3X4	T38.3X5	T38.3X6
Glibornuride	T38.3X1	T38.3X2	T38.3X3	T38.3X4	T38.3X5	T38.3X6
Gliclazide	T38.3X1	T38.3X2	T38.3X3	T38.3X4	T38.3X5	T38.3X6
Glimidine	T38.3X1	T38.3X2	T38.3X3	T38.3X4	T38.3X5	T38.3X6
Glipizide	T38.3X1	T38.3X2	T38.3X3	T38.3X4	T38.3X5	T38.3X6
Gliquidone	T38.3X1	T38.3X2	T38.3X3	T38.3X4	T38.3X5	T38.3X6
Glisolamide	T38.3X1	T38.3X2	T38.3X3	T38.3X4	T38.3X5	T38.3X6
Glisoxepide	T38.3X1	T38.3X2	T38.3X3	T38.3X4	T38.3X5	T38.3X6
Globin zinc insulin	T38.3X1	T38.3X2	T38.3X3	T38.3X4	T38.3X5	T38.3X6
Globulin						
- antilymphocytic	T50.Z11	T50.Z12	T50.Z13	T50.Z14	T50.Z15	T50.Z16
- antirhesus	T50.Z11	T50.Z12	T50.Z13	T50.Z14	T50.Z15	T50.Z16
- antivenin	T50.Z11	T50.Z12	T50.Z13	T50.Z14	T50.Z15	T50.Z16
- antiviral	T50.Z11	T50.Z12	T50.Z13	T50.Z14	T50.Z15	T50.Z16
Glucagon	T38.3X1	T38.3X2	T38.3X3	T38.3X4	T38.3X5	T38.3X6
Glucocorticoids	T38.0X1	T38.0X2	T38.0X3	T38.0X4	T38.0X5	T38.0X6
Glucocorticosteroid	T38.0X1	T38.0X2	T38.0X3	T38.0X4	T38.0X5	T38.0X6
Gluconic acid	T50.991	T50.992	T50.993	T50.994	T50.995	T50.996
Glucosamine sulfate	T39.4X1	T39.4X2	T39.4X3	T39.4X4	T39.4X5	T39.4X6
Glucose	T50.3X1	T50.3X2	T50.3X3	T50.3X4	T50.3X5	T50.3X6
- with sodium chloride	T50.3X1	T50.3X2	T50.3X3	T50.3X4	T50.3X5	T50.3X6
Glucosulfone sodium	T37.1X1	T37.1X2	T37.1X3	T37.1X4	T37.1X5	T37.1X6
Glucurolactone	T47.8X1	T47.8X2	T47.8X3	T47.8X4	T47.8X5	T47.8X6
Glue NEC	T52.8X1	T52.8X2	T52.8X3	T52.8X4	--	--
Glutamic acid	T47.5X1	T47.5X2	T47.5X3	T47.5X4	T47.5X5	T47.5X6
Glutaral (medicinal)	T49.0X1	T49.0X2	T49.0X3	T49.0X4	T49.0X5	T49.0X6
- nonmedicinal	T65.891	T65.892	T65.893	T65.894	--	--
Glutaraldehyde (nonmedicinal)	T65.891	T65.892	T65.893	T65.894	--	--
- medicinal	T49.0X1	T49.0X2	T49.0X3	T49.0X4	T49.0X5	T49.0X6
Glutathione	T50.6X1	T50.6X2	T50.6X3	T50.6X4	T50.6X5	T50.6X6
Glutethimide	T42.6X1	T42.6X2	T42.6X3	T42.6X4	T42.6X5	T42.6X6
Glyburide	T38.3X1	T38.3X2	T38.3X3	T38.3X4	T38.3X5	T38.3X6
Glycerin	T47.4X1	T47.4X2	T47.4X3	T47.4X4	T47.4X5	T47.4X6
Glycerol	T47.4X1	T47.4X2	T47.4X3	T47.4X4	T47.4X5	T47.4X6
- borax	T49.6X1	T49.6X2	T49.6X3	T49.6X4	T49.6X5	T49.6X6
- intravenous	T50.3X1	T50.3X2	T50.3X3	T50.3X4	T50.3X5	T50.3X6
- iodinated	T48.4X1	T48.4X2	T48.4X3	T48.4X4	T48.4X5	T48.4X6
Glycerophosphate	T50.991	T50.992	T50.993	T50.994	T50.995	T50.996
Glyceryl						
- gualacolate	T48.4X1	T48.4X2	T48.4X3	T48.4X4	T48.4X5	T48.4X6
- nitrate	T46.3X1	T46.3X2	T46.3X3	T46.3X4	T46.3X5	T46.3X6
- triacetate (topical)	T49.0X1	T49.0X2	T49.0X3	T49.0X4	T49.0X5	T49.0X6
- trinitrate	T46.3X1	T46.3X2	T46.3X3	T46.3X4	T46.3X5	T46.3X6
Glycine	T50.3X1	T50.3X2	T50.3X3	T50.3X4	T50.3X5	T50.3X6
Glyclopyramide	T38.3X1	T38.3X2	T38.3X3	T38.3X4	T38.3X5	T38.3X6
Glycobiarsol	T37.3X1	T37.3X2	T37.3X3	T37.3X4	T37.3X5	T37.3X6
Glycols (ether)	T52.3X1	T52.3X2	T52.3X3	T52.3X4	--	--
Glyconiazide	T37.1X1	T37.1X2	T37.1X3	T37.1X4	T37.1X5	T37.1X6
Glycopyrrolate	T44.3X1	T44.3X2	T44.3X3	T44.3X4	T44.3X5	T44.3X6
Glycopyrronium	T44.3X1	T44.3X2	T44.3X3	T44.3X4	T44.3X5	T44.3X6
- bromide	T44.3X1	T44.3X2	T44.3X3	T44.3X4	T44.3X5	T44.3X6
Glycoside, cardiac (stimulant)	T46.0X1	T46.0X2	T46.0X3	T46.0X4	T46.0X5	T46.0X6

Substance	Poisoning, Accidental (unintentional)	Poisoning, Intentional Self-harm	Poisoning, Assault	Poisoning, Undetermined	Adverse effect	Underdosing
Glycyclamide	T38.3X1	T38.3X2	T38.3X3	T38.3X4	T38.3X5	T38.3X6
Glycyrrhiza extract	T48.4X1	T48.4X2	T48.4X3	T48.4X4	T48.4X5	T48.4X6
Glycyrrhizic acid	T48.4X1	T48.4X2	T48.4X3	T48.4X4	T48.4X5	T48.4X6
Glycyrrhizinate potassium	T48.4X1	T48.4X2	T48.4X3	T48.4X4	T48.4X5	T48.4X6
Glymidine sodium	T38.3X1	T38.3X2	T38.3X3	T38.3X4	T38.3X5	T38.3X6
Glyphosate	T60.3X1	T60.3X2	T60.3X3	T60.3X4	--	--
Glyphylline	T48.6X1	T48.6X2	T48.6X3	T48.6X4	T48.6X5	T48.6X6
Gold						
- colloidal (l98Au)	T45.1X1	T45.1X2	T45.1X3	T45.1X4	T45.1X5	T45.1X6
- salts	T39.4X1	T39.4X2	T39.4X3	T39.4X4	T39.4X5	T39.4X6
Golden sulfide of antimony	T56.891	T56.892	T56.893	T56.894	--	--
Goldylocks	T62.2X1	T62.2X2	T62.2X3	T62.2X4	--	--
Gonadal tissue extract	T38.901	T38.902	T38.903	T38.904	T38.905	T38.906
- female	T38.5X1	T38.5X2	T38.5X3	T38.5X4	T38.5X5	T38.5X6
- male	T38.7X1	T38.7X2	T38.7X3	T38.7X4	T38.7X5	T38.7X6
Gonadorelin	T38.891	T38.892	T38.893	T38.894	T38.895	T38.896
Gonadotropin	T38.891	T38.892	T38.893	T38.894	T38.895	T38.896
- chorionic	T38.891	T38.892	T38.893	T38.894	T38.895	T38.896
- pituitary	T38.811	T38.812	T38.813	T38.814	T38.815	T38.816
Goserelin	T45.1X1	T45.1X2	T45.1X3	T45.1X4	T45.1X5	T45.1X6
Grain alcohol	T51.0X1	T51.0X2	T51.0X3	T51.0X4	--	--
Gramicidin	T49.0X1	T49.0X2	T49.0X3	T49.0X4	T49.0X5	T49.0X6
Granisetron	T45.0X1	T45.0X2	T45.0X3	T45.0X4	T45.0X5	T45.0X6
Gratiola officinalis	T62.2X1	T62.2X2	T62.2X3	T62.2X4	--	--
Grease	T65.891	T65.892	T65.893	T65.894	--	--
Green hellebore	T62.2X1	T62.2X2	T62.2X3	T62.2X4	--	--
Green soap	T49.2X1	T49.2X2	T49.2X3	T49.2X4	T49.2X5	T49.2X6
Grifulvin	T36.7X1	T36.7X2	T36.7X3	T36.7X4	T36.7X5	T36.7X6
Griseofulvin	T36.7X1	T36.7X2	T36.7X3	T36.7X4	T36.7X5	T36.7X6
Growth hormone	T38.811	T38.812	T38.813	T38.814	T38.815	T38.816
Guaiac reagent	T50.991	T50.992	T50.993	T50.994	T50.995	T50.996
Guaiacol derivatives	T48.4X1	T48.4X2	T48.4X3	T48.4X4	T48.4X5	T48.4X6
Guaifenesin	T48.4X1	T48.4X2	T48.4X3	T48.4X4	T48.4X5	T48.4X6
Guaimesal	T48.4X1	T48.4X2	T48.4X3	T48.4X4	T48.4X5	T48.4X6
Guaiphenesin	T48.4X1	T48.4X2	T48.4X3	T48.4X4	T48.4X5	T48.4X6
Guamecycline	T36.4X1	T36.4X2	T36.4X3	T36.4X4	T36.4X5	T36.4X6
Guanabenz	T46.5X1	T46.5X2	T46.5X3	T46.5X4	T46.5X5	T46.5X6
Guanacline	T46.5X1	T46.5X2	T46.5X3	T46.5X4	T46.5X5	T46.5X6
Guanadrel	T46.5X1	T46.5X2	T46.5X3	T46.5X4	T46.5X5	T46.5X6
Guanatol	T37.2X1	T37.2X2	T37.2X3	T37.2X4	T37.2X5	T37.2X6
Guanethidine	T46.5X1	T46.5X2	T46.5X3	T46.5X4	T46.5X5	T46.5X6
Guanfacine	T46.5X1	T46.5X2	T46.5X3	T46.5X4	T46.5X5	T46.5X6
Guano	T65.891	T65.892	T65.893	T65.894	--	--
Guanochlor	T46.5X1	T46.5X2	T46.5X3	T46.5X4	T46.5X5	T46.5X6
Guanoclor	T46.5X1	T46.5X2	T46.5X3	T46.5X4	T46.5X5	T46.5X6
Guanoctine	T46.5X1	T46.5X2	T46.5X3	T46.5X4	T46.5X5	T46.5X6
Guanoxabenz	T46.5X1	T46.5X2	T46.5X3	T46.5X4	T46.5X5	T46.5X6
Guanoxan	T46.5X1	T46.5X2	T46.5X3	T46.5X4	T46.5X5	T46.5X6
Guar gum (medicinal)	T46.6X1	T46.6X2	T46.6X3	T46.6X4	T46.6X5	T46.6X6
Hachimycin	T36.7X1	T36.7X2	T36.7X3	T36.7X4	T36.7X5	T36.7X6
Hair						
- dye	T49.4X1	T49.4X2	T49.4X3	T49.4X4	T49.4X5	T49.4X6
- preparation NEC	T49.4X1	T49.4X2	T49.4X3	T49.4X4	T49.4X5	T49.4X6
Halazepam	T42.4X1	T42.4X2	T42.4X3	T42.4X4	T42.4X5	T42.4X6
Halcinolone	T49.0X1	T49.0X2	T49.0X3	T49.0X4	T49.0X5	T49.0X6
Halcinonide	T49.0X1	T49.0X2	T49.0X3	T49.0X4	T49.0X5	T49.0X6
Halethazole	T49.0X1	T49.0X2	T49.0X3	T49.0X4	T49.0X5	T49.0X6
Hallucinogen NEC	T40.901	T40.902	T40.903	T40.904	T40.905	T40.906
Halofantrine	T37.2X1	T37.2X2	T37.2X3	T37.2X4	T37.2X5	T37.2X6
Halofenate	T46.6X1	T46.6X2	T46.6X3	T46.6X4	T46.6X5	T46.6X6
Halometasone	T49.0X1	T49.0X2	T49.0X3	T49.0X4	T49.0X5	T49.0X6
Haloperidol	T43.4X1	T43.4X2	T43.4X3	T43.4X4	T43.4X5	T43.4X6
Haloprogin	T49.0X1	T49.0X2	T49.0X3	T49.0X4	T49.0X5	T49.0X6
Halotex	T49.0X1	T49.0X2	T49.0X3	T49.0X4	T49.0X5	T49.0X6
Halothane	T41.0X1	T41.0X2	T41.0X3	T41.0X4	T41.0X5	T41.0X6

Substance	Poisoning, Accidental (unintentional)	Poisoning, Intentional Self-harm	Poisoning, Assault	Poisoning, Undetermined	Adverse effect	Underdosing
Haloxazolam	T42.4X1	T42.4X2	T42.4X3	T42.4X4	T42.4X5	T42.4X6
Halquinols	T49.0X1	T49.0X2	T49.0X3	T49.0X4	T49.0X5	T49.0X6
Hamamelis	T49.2X1	T49.2X2	T49.2X3	T49.2X4	T49.2X5	T49.2X6
Haptendextran	T45.8X1	T45.8X2	T45.8X3	T45.8X4	T45.8X5	T45.8X6
Harmonyl	T46.5X1	T46.5X2	T46.5X3	T46.5X4	T46.5X5	T46.5X6
Hartmann's solution	T50.3X1	T50.3X2	T50.3X3	T50.3X4	T50.3X5	T50.3X6
Hashish	T40.7X1	T40.7X2	T40.7X3	T40.7X4	T40.7X5	T40.7X6
Hawaiian Woodrose seeds	T40.991	T40.992	T40.993	T40.994	--	--
HCB	T60.3X1	T60.3X2	T60.3X3	T60.3X4	--	--
HCH	T53.6X1	T53.6X2	T53.6X3	T53.6X4	--	--
- medicinal	T49.0X1	T49.0X2	T49.0X3	T49.0X4	T49.0X5	T49.0X6
HCN	T57.3X1	T57.3X2	T57.3X3	T57.3X4	--	--
Headache cures, drugs, powders NEC	T50.901	T50.902	T50.903	T50.904	T50.905	T50.906
Heavenly Blue (morning glory)	T40.991	T40.992	T40.993	T40.994	--	--
Heavy metal antidote	T45.8X1	T45.8X2	T45.8X3	T45.8X4	T45.8X5	T45.8X6
Hedaquinium	T49.0X1	T49.0X2	T49.0X3	T49.0X4	T49.0X5	T49.0X6
Hedge hyssop	T62.2X1	T62.2X2	T62.2X3	T62.2X4		
Heet	T49.8X1	T49.8X2	T49.8X3	T49.8X4	T49.8X5	T49.8X6
Helenin	T37.4X1	T37.4X2	T37.4X3	T37.4X4	T37.4X5	T37.4X6
Helium (nonmedicinal) NEC	T59.891	T59.892	T59.893	T59.894	--	--
- medicinal	T48.991	T48.992	T48.993	T48.994	T48.995	T48.996
Hellebore (black) (green) (white)	T62.2X1	T62.2X2	T62.2X3	T62.2X4	--	--
Hematin	T45.8X1	T45.8X2	T45.8X3	T45.8X4	T45.8X5	T45.8X6
Hematinic preparation	T45.8X1	T45.8X2	T45.8X3	T45.8X4	T45.8X5	T45.8X6
Hematological agent	T45.91	T45.92	T45.93	T45.94	T45.95	T45.96
- specified NEC	T45.8X1	T45.8X2	T45.8X3	T45.8X4	T45.8X5	T45.8X6
Hemlock	T62.2X1	T62.2X2	T62.2X3	T62.2X4	--	--
Hemostatic	T45.621	T45.622	T45.623	T45.624	T45.625	T45.626
- drug, systemic	T45.621	T45.622	T45.623	T45.624	T45.625	T45.626
Hemostyptic	T49.4X1	T49.4X2	T49.4X3	T49.4X4	T49.4X5	T49.4X6
Henbane	T62.2X1	T62.2X2	T62.2X3	T62.2X4	--	--
Heparin (sodium)	T45.511	T45.512	T45.513	T45.514	T45.515	T45.516
- action reverser	T45.7X1	T45.7X2	T45.7X3	T45.7X4	T45.7X5	T45.7X6
Heparin-fraction	T45.511	T45.512	T45.513	T45.514	T45.515	T45.516
Heparinoid (systemic)	T45.511	T45.512	T45.513	T45.514	T45.515	T45.516
Hepatic secretion stimulant	T47.8X1	T47.8X2	T47.8X3	T47.8X4	T47.8X5	T47.8X6
Hepatitis B						
- immune globulin	T50.Z11	T50.Z12	T50.Z13	T50.Z14	T50.Z15	T50.Z16
- vaccine	T50.B91	T50.B92	T50.B93	T50.B94	T50.B95	T50.B96
Hepronicate	T46.7X1	T46.7X2	T46.7X3	T46.7X4	T46.7X5	T46.7X6
Heptabarb	T42.3X1	T42.3X2	T42.3X3	T42.3X4	T42.3X5	T42.3X6
Heptabarbital	T42.3X1	T42.3X2	T42.3X3	T42.3X4	T42.3X5	T42.3X6
Heptabarbitone	T42.3X1	T42.3X2	T42.3X3	T42.3X4	T42.3X5	T42.3X6
Heptachlor	T60.1X1	T60.1X2	T60.1X3	T60.1X4	--	--
Heptalgin	T40.2X1	T40.2X2	T40.2X3	T40.2X4	T40.2X5	T40.2X6
Heptaminol	T46.3X1	T46.3X2	T46.3X3	T46.3X4	T46.3X5	T46.3X6
Herbicide NEC	T60.3X1	T60.3X2	T60.3X3	T60.3X4	--	--
Heroin	T40.1X1	T40.1X2	T40.1X3	T40.1X4	T40.1X5	--
Herplex	T49.5X1	T49.5X2	T49.5X3	T49.5X4	T49.5X5	T49.5X6
HES	T45.8X1	T45.8X2	T45.8X3	T45.8X4	T45.8X5	T45.8X6
Hesperidin	T46.991	T46.992	T46.993	T46.994	T46.995	T46.996
Hetacillin	T36.0X1	T36.0X2	T36.0X3	T36.0X4	T36.0X5	T36.0X6
Hetastarch	T45.8X1	T45.8X2	T45.8X3	T45.8X4	T45.8X5	T45.8X6
HETP	T60.0X1	T60.0X2	T60.0X3	T60.0X4	--	--
Hexachlorobenzene (vapor)	T60.3X1	T60.3X2	T60.3X3	T60.3X4	--	--
Hexachlorocyclohexane	T53.6X1	T53.6X2	T53.6X3	T53.6X4	--	--
Hexachlorophene	T49.0X1	T49.0X2	T49.0X3	T49.0X4	T49.0X5	T49.0X6
Hexadiline	T46.3X1	T46.3X2	T46.3X3	T46.3X4	T46.3X5	T46.3X6
Hexadimethrine (bromide)	T45.7X1	T45.7X2	T45.7X3	T45.7X4	T45.7X5	T45.7X6
Hexadylamine	T46.3X1	T46.3X2	T46.3X3	T46.3X4	T46.3X5	T46.3X6
Hexaethyl tetraphos-phate	T60.0X1	T60.0X2	T60.0X3	T60.0X4	--	--
Hexafluorenium bromide	T48.1X1	T48.1X2	T48.1X3	T48.1X4	T48.1X5	T48.1X6
Hexafluronium (bromide)	T48.1X1	T48.1X2	T48.1X3	T48.1X4	T48.1X5	T48.1X6
Hexa-germ	T49.2X1	T49.2X2	T49.2X3	T49.2X4	T49.2X5	T49.2X6
Hexahydrobenzol	T52.8X1	T52.8X2	T52.8X3	T52.8X4	--	--

Substance	Poisoning, Accidental (unintentional)	Poisoning, Intentional Self-harm	Poisoning, Assault	Poisoning, Undetermined	Adverse effect	Underdosing
Hexahydrocresol (s)	T51.8X1	T51.8X2	T51.8X3	T51.8X4	--	--
- arsenide	T57.0X1	T57.0X3	T57.0X3	T57.0X4	--	--
- arseniurated	T57.0X1	T57.0X2	T57.0X3	T57.0X4	--	--
- cyanide	T57.3X1	T57.3X2	T57.3X3	T57.3X4	--	--
- - gas	T59.891	T59.892	T59.893	T59.894	--	--
- Fluoride (liquid)	T57.8X1	T57.8X2	T57.8X3	T57.8X4	--	--
- - vapor	T59.891	T59.892	T59.893	T59.894	--	--
- phophorated	T60.0X1	T60.0X2	T60.0X3	T60.0X4	--	--
- sulfate	T57.8X1	T57.8X2	T57.8X3	T57.8X4	--	--
- sulfide (gas)	T59.6X1	T59.6X2	T59.6X3	T59.6X4	--	--
- - arseniurated	T57.0X1	T57.0X2	T57.0X3	T57.0X4	--	--
- sulfurated	T57.8X1	T57.8X2	T57.8X3	T57.8X4	--	--
Hexahydrophenol	T51.8X1	T51.8X2	T51.8X3	T51.8X4	--	--
Hexalen	T51.8X1	T51.8X2	T51.8X3	T51.8X4	--	--
Hexamethonium bromide	T44.2X1	T44.2X2	T44.2X3	T44.2X4	T44.2X5	T44.2X6
Hexamethylene	T52.8X1	T52.8X2	T52.8X3	T52.8X4	--	--
Hexamethylmelamine	T45.1X1	T45.1X2	T45.1X3	T45.1X4	T45.1X5	T45.1X6
Hexamidine	T49.0X1	T49.0X2	T49.0X3	T49.0X4	T49.0X5	T49.0X6
Hexamine (mandelate)	T37.8X1	T37.8X2	T37.8X3	T37.8X4	T37.8X5	T37.8X6
Hexanone, 2-hexanone	T52.4X1	T52.4X2	T52.4X3	T52.4X4	--	--
Hexanuorenium	T48.1X1	T48.1X2	T48.1X3	T48.1X4	T48.1X5	T48.1X6
Hexapropymate	T42.6X1	T42.6X2	T42.6X3	T42.6X4	T42.6X5	T42.6X6
Hexasonium iodide	T44.3X1	T44.3X2	T44.3X3	T44.3X4	T44.3X5	T44.3X6
Hexcarbacholine bromide	T48.1X1	T48.1X2	T48.1X3	T48.1X4	T48.1X5	T48.1X6
Hexemal	T42.3X1	T42.3X2	T42.3X3	T42.3X4	T42.3X5	T42.3X6
Hexestrol	T38.5X1	T38.5X2	T38.5X3	T38.5X4	T38.5X5	T38.5X6
Hexethal (sodium)	T42.3X1	T42.3X2	T42.3X3	T42.3X4	T42.3X5	T42.3X6
Hexetidine	T37.8X1	T37.8X2	T37.8X3	T37.8X4	T37.8X5	T37.8X6
Hexobarbital	T42.3X1	T42.3X2	T42.3X3	T42.3X4	T42.3X5	T42.3X6
- rectal	T41.291	T41.292	T41.293	T41.294	T41.295	T41.296
- sodium	T41.1X1	T41.1X2	T41.1X3	T41.1X4	T41.1X5	T41.1X6
Hexobendine	T46.3X1	T46.3X2	T46.3X3	T46.3X4	T46.3X5	T46.3X6
Hexocyclium	T44.3X1	T44.3X2	T44.3X3	T44.3X4	T44.3X5	T44.3X6
- metilsulfate	T44.3X1	T44.3X2	T44.3X3	T44.3X4	T44.3X5	T44.3X6
Hexoestrol	T38.5X1	T38.5X2	T38.5X3	T38.5X4	T38.5X5	T38.5X6
Hexone	T52.4X1	T52.4X2	T52.4X3	T52.4X4	--	--
Hexoprenaline	T48.6X1	T48.6X2	T48.6X3	T48.6X4	T48.6X5	T48.6X6
Hexylcaine	T41.3X1	T41.3X2	T41.3X3	T41.3X4	T41.3X5	T41.3X6
Hexylresorcinol	T52.2X1	T52.2X2	T52.2X3	T52.2X4	--	--
HGH (human growth hormone)	T38.811	T38.812	T38.813	T38.814	T38.815	T38.816
Hinkle's pills	T47.2X1	T47.2X2	T47.2X3	T47.2X4	T47.2X5	T47.2X6
Histalog	T50.8X1	T50.8X2	T50.8X3	T50.8X4	T50.8X5	T50.8X6
Histamine (phosphate)	T50.8X1	T50.8X2	T50.8X3	T50.8X4	T50.8X5	T50.8X6
Histoplasmin	T50.8X1	T50.8X2	T50.8X3	T50.8X4	T50.8X5	T50.8X6
Holly berries	T62.2X1	T62.2X2	T62.2X3	T62.2X4	--	--
Homatropine	T44.3X1	T44.3X2	T44.3X3	T44.3X4	T44.3X5	T44.3X6
- methylbromide	T44.3X1	T44.3X2	T44.3X3	T44.3X4	T44.3X5	T44.3X6
Homochlorcyclizine	T45.0X1	T45.0X2	T45.0X3	T45.0X4	T45.0X5	T45.0X6
Homosalate	T49.3X1	T49.3X2	T49.3X3	T49.3X4	T49.3X5	T49.3X6
Homo-tet	T50.Z11	T50.Z12	T50.Z13	T50.Z14	T50.Z15	T50.Z16
Hormone	T38.801	T38.802	T38.803	T38.804	T38.805	T38.806
- adrenal cortical steroids	T38.0X1	T38.0X2	T38.0X3	T38.0X4	T38.0X5	T38.0X6
- androgenic	T38.7X1	T38.7X2	T38.7X3	T38.7X4	T38.7X5	T38.7X6
- anterior pituitary NEC	T38.811	T38.812	T38.813	T38.814	T38.815	T38.816
- antidiabetic agents	T38.3X1	T38.3X2	T38.3X3	T38.3X4	T38.3X5	T38.3X6
- antidiuretic	T38.891	T38.892	T38.893	T38.894	T38.895	T38.896
- cancer therapy	T45.1X1	T45.1X2	T45.1X3	T45.1X4	T45.1X5	T45.1X6
- follicle stimulating	T38.811	T38.812	T38.813	T38.814	T38.815	T38.816
- gonadotropic	T38.891	T38.892	T38.893	T38.894	T38.895	T38.896
- - pituitary	T38.811	T38.812	T38.813	T38.814	T38.815	T38.816
- growth	T38.811	T38.812	T38.813	T38.814	T38.815	T38.816
- luteinizing	T38.811	T38.812	T38.813	T38.814	T38.815	T38.816
- ovarian	T38.5X1	T38.5X2	T38.5X3	T38.5X4	T38.5X5	T38.5X6
- oxytocic	T48.0X1	T48.0X2	T48.0X3	T48.0X4	T48.0X5	T48.0X6
- parathyroid (derivatives)	T50.991	T50.992	T50.993	T50.994	T50.995	T50.996

Substance	Poisoning, Accidental (unintentional)	Poisoning, Intentional Self-harm	Poisoning, Assault	Poisoning, Undetermined	Adverse effect	Underdosing
- pituitary (posterior) NEC	T38.891	T38.892	T38.893	T38.894	T38.895	T38.896
- - anterior	T38.811	T38.812	T38.813	T38.814	T38.815	T38.816
- specified, NEC	T38.891	T38.892	T38.893	T38.894	T38.895	T38.896
- thyroid	T38.1X1	T38.1X2	T38.1X3	T38.1X4	T38.1X5	T38.1X6
Hornet (sting)	T63.451	T63.452	T63.453	T63.454	--	--
Horse anti-human lymphocytic serum	T50.Z11	T50.Z12	T50.Z13	T50.Z14	T50.Z15	T50.Z16
Horticulture agent NEC	T65.91	T65.92	T65.93	T65.94	--	--
- with pesticide	T60.91	T60.92	T60.93	T60.94	--	--
Human						
- albumin	T45.8X1	T45.8X2	T45.8X3	T45.8X4	T45.8X5	T45.8X6
- growth hormone (HGH)	T38.811	T38.812	T38.813	T38.814	T38.815	T38.816
- immune serum	T50.Z11	T50.Z12	T50.Z13	T50.Z14	T50.Z15	T50.Z16
Hyaluronidase	T45.3X1	T45.3X2	T45.3X3	T45.3X4	T45.3X5	T45.3X6
Hyazyme	T45.3X1	T45.3X2	T45.3X3	T45.3X4	T45.3X5	T45.3X6
Hycodan	T40.2X1	T40.2X2	T40.2X3	T40.2X4	T40.2X5	T40.2X6
Hydantoin derivative NEC	T42.0X1	T42.0X2	T42.0X3	T42.0X4	T42.0X5	T42.0X6
Hydeltra	T38.0X1	T38.0X2	T38.0X3	T38.0X4	T38.0X5	T38.0X6
Hydergine	T44.6X1	T44.6X2	T44.6X3	T44.6X4	T44.6X5	T44.6X6
Hydrabamine penicillin	T36.0X1	T36.0X2	T36.0X3	T36.0X4	T36.0X5	T36.0X6
Hydralazine	T46.5X1	T46.5X2	T46.5X3	T46.5X4	T46.5X5	T46.5X6
Hydrargaphen	T49.0X1	T49.0X2	T49.0X3	T49.0X4	T49.0X5	T49.0X6
Hydrargyri amino-chloridum	T49.0X1	T49.0X2	T49.0X3	T49.0X4	T49.0X5	T49.0X6
Hydrastine	T48.291	T48.292	T48.293	T48.294	T48.295	T48.296
Hydrazine	T54.1X1	T54.1X2	T54.1X3	T54.1X4	--	--
- monoamine oxidase inhibitors	T43.1X1	T43.1X2	T43.1X3	T43.1X4	T43.1X5	T43.1X6
Hydrazoic acid, azides	T54.2X1	T54.2X2	T54.2X3	T54.2X4	--	--
Hydriodic acid	T48.4X1	T48.4X2	T48.4X3	T48.4X4	T48.4X5	T48.4X6
Hydrocarbon gas	T59.891	T59.892	T59.893	T59.894	--	--
- incomplete combustion of—see Carbon, monoxide, fuel, utility						
- liquefied (mobile container)	T59.891	T59.892	T59.893	T59.894	--	--
- - piped (natural)	T59.891	T59.892	T59.893	T59.894	--	--
Hydrochloric acid (liquid)	T54.2X1	T54.2X2	T54.2X3	T54.2X4	--	--
- medicinal (digestant)	T47.5X1	T47.5X2	T47.5X3	T47.5X4	T47.5X5	T47.5X6
- vapor	T59.891	T59.892	T59.893	T59.894	--	--
Hydrochlorothiazide	T50.2X1	T50.2X2	T50.2X3	T50.2X4	T50.2X5	T50.2X6
Hydrocodone	T40.2X1	T40.2X2	T40.2X3	T40.2X4	T40.2X5	T40.2X6
Hydrocortisone (derivatives)	T49.0X1	T49.0X2	T49.0X3	T49.0X4	T49.0X5	T49.0X6
- aceponate	T49.0X1	T49.0X2	T49.0X3	T49.0X4	T49.0X5	T49.0X6
- ENT agent	T49.6X1	T49.6X2	T49.6X3	T49.6X4	T49.6X5	T49.6X6
- ophthalmic preparation	T49.5X1	T49.5X2	T49.5X3	T49.5X4	T49.5X5	T49.5X6
- topical NEC	T49.0X1	T49.0X2	T49.0X3	T49.0X4	T49.0X5	T49.0X6
Hydrocortone	T38.0X1	T38.0X2	T38.0X3	T38.0X4	T38.0X5	T38.0X6
- ENT agent	T49.6X1	T49.6X2	T49.6X3	T49.6X4	T49.6X5	T49.6X6
- ophthalmic preparation	T49.5X1	T49.5X2	T49.5X3	T49.5X4	T49.5X5	T49.5X6
- topical NEC	T49.0X1	T49.0X2	T49.0X3	T49.0X4	T49.0X5	T49.0X6
Hydrocyanic acid (liquid)	T57.3X1	T57.3X2	T57.3X3	T57.3X4	--	--
- gas	T65.0X1	T65.0X2	T65.0X3	T65.0X4	--	--
Hydroflumethiazide	T50.2X1	T50.2X2	T50.2X3	T50.2X4	T50.2X5	T50.2X6
Hydrofluoric acid (liquid)	T54.2X1	T54.2X2	T54.2X3	T54.2X4	--	--
- vapor	T59.891	T59.892	T59.893	T59.894	--	--
Hydrogen	T59.891	T59.892	T59.893	T59.894	--	--
- arsenide	T57.0X1	T57.0X2	T57.0X3	T57.0X4	--	--
arseniureted	T57.0X1	T57.0X2	T57.0X3	T57.0X4	--	--
- chloride	T57.8X1	T57.8X2	T57.8X3	T57.8X4		--
- cyanide (salts)	T57.3X1	T57.3X2	T57.3X3	T57.3X4	--	--
- - gas	T57.3X1	T57.3X2	T57.3X3	T57.3X4	--	--
- Fluoride	T59.5X1	T59.5X2	T59.5X3	T59.5X4	--	--
- - vapor	T59.5X1	T59.5X2	T59.5X3	T59.5X4	--	--
- peroxide	T49.0X1	T49.0X2	T49.0X3	T49.0X4	T49.0X5	T49.0X6
- phosphureted	T57.1X1	T57.1X2	T57.1X3	T57.1X4	--	--
- sulfide	T59.6X1	T59.6X2	T59.6X3	T59.6X4	--	--
- - arseniureted	T57.0X1	T57.0X2	T57.0X3	T57.0X4	--	--
- sulfureted	T59.6X1	T59.6X2	T59.6X3	T59.6X4	--	--
Hydromethylpyridine	T46.7X1	T46.7X2	T46.7X3	T46.7X4	T46.7X5	T46.7X6

Substance	Poisoning, Accidental (unintentional)	Poisoning, Intentional Self-harm	Poisoning, Assault	Poisoning, Undetermined	Adverse effect	Underdosing
Hydromorphinol	T40.2X1	T40.2X2	T40.2X3	T40.2X4	--	--
Hydromorphinone	T40.2X1	T40.2X2	T40.2X3	T40.2X4	T40.2X5	T40.2X6
Hydromorphone	T40.2X1	T40.2X2	T40.2X3	T40.2X4	T40.2X5	T40.2X6
Hydromox	T50.2X1	T50.2X2	T50.2X3	T50.2X4	T50.2X5	T50.2X6
Hydrophilic lotion	T49.3X1	T49.3X2	T49.3X3	T49.3X4	T49.3X5	T49.3X6
Hydroquinidine	T46.2X1	T46.2X2	T46.2X3	T46.2X4	T46.2X5	T46.2X6
Hydroquinone	T52.2X1	T52.2X2	T52.2X3	T52.2X4	--	--
- vapor	T59.891	T59.892	T59.893	T59.894	--	--
Hydrosulfuric acid (gas)	T59.6X1	T59.6X2	T59.6X3	T59.6X4	--	--
Hydrotalcite	T47.1X1	T47.1X2	T47.1X3	T47.1X4	T47.1X5	T47.1X6
Hydrous wool fat	T49.3X1	T49.3X2	T49.3X3	T49.3X4	T49.3X5	T49.3X6
Hydroxide, caustic	T54.3X1	T54.3X2	T54.3X3	T54.3X4	--	--
Hydroxocobalamin	T45.8X1	T45.8X2	T45.8X3	T45.8X4	T45.8X5	T45.8X6
Hydroxyamphetamine	T49.5X1	T49.5X2	T49.5X3	T49.5X4	T49.5X5	T49.5X6
Hydroxycarbamide	T45.1X1	T45.1X2	T45.1X3	T45.1X4	T45.1X5	T45.1X6
Hydroxychloroquine	T37.8X1	T37.8X2	T37.8X3	T37.8X4	T37.8X5	T37.8X6
Hydroxydihydrocodeinone	T40.2X1	T40.2X2	T40.2X3	T40.2X4	T40.2X5	T40.2X6
Hydroxyestrone	T38.5X1	T38.5X2	T38.5X3	T38.5X4	T38.5X5	T38.5X6
Hydroxyethyl starch	T45.8X1	T45.8X2	T45.8X3	T45.8X4	T45.8X5	T45.8X6
Hydroxymethylpenta-none	T52.4X1	T52.4X2	T52.4X3	T52.4X4	--	--
Hydroxyphenamate	T43.591	T43.592	T43.593	T43.594	T43.595	T43.596
Hydroxyphenylbutazone	T39.2X1	T39.2X2	T39.2X3	T39.2X4	T39.2X5	T39.2X6
Hydroxyprogesterone	T38.5X1	T38.5X2	T38.5X3	T38.5X4	T38.5X5	T38.5X6
- caproate	T38.5X1	T38.5X2	T38.5X3	T38.5X4	T38.5X5	T38.5X6
Hydroxyquinoline (derivatives) NEC	T37.8X1	T37.8X2	T37.8X3	T37.8X4	T37.8X5	T37.8X6
Hydroxystilbamidine	T37.3X1	T37.3X2	T37.3X3	T37.3X4	T37.3X5	T37.3X6
Hydroxytoluene (nonmedicinal)	T54.0X1	T54.0X2	T54.0X3	T54.0X4	--	--
- medicinal	T49.0X1	T49.0X2	T49.0X3	T49.0X4	T49.0X5	T49.0X6
Hydroxyurea	T45.1X1	T45.1X2	T45.1X3	T45.1X4	T45.1X5	T45.1X6
Hydroxyzine	T43.591	T43.592	T43.593	T43.594	T43.595	T43.596
Hyoscine	T44.3X1	T44.3X2	T44.3X3	T44.3X4	T44.3X5	T44.3X6
Hyoscyamine	T44.3X1	T44.3X2	T44.3X3	T44.3X4	T44.3X5	T44.3X6
Hyoscyamus	T44.3X1	T44.3X2	T44.3X3	T44.3X4	T44.3X5	T44.3X6
- dry extract	T44.3X1	T44.3X2	T44.3X3	T44.3X4	T44.3X5	T44.3X6
Hypaque	T50.8X1	T50.8X2	T50.8X3	T50.8X4	T50.8X5	T50.8X6
Hypertussis	T50.Z11	T50.Z12	T50.Z13	T50.Z14	T50.Z15	T50.Z16
Hypnotic	T42.71	T42.72	T42.73	T42.74	T42.75	T42.76
- anticonvulsant	T42.71	T42.72	T42.73	T42.74	T42.75	T42.76
- specified NEC	T42.6X1	T42.6X2	T42.6X3	T42.6X4	T42.6X5	T42.6X6
Hypochlorite	T49.0X1	T49.0X2	T49.0X3	T49.0X4	T49.0X5	T49.0X6
Hypophysis, posterior	T38.891	T38.892	T38.893	T38.894	T38.895	T38.896
Hypotensive NEC	T46.5X1	T46.5X2	T46.5X3	T46.5X4	T46.5X5	T46.5X6
Hypromellose	T49.5X1	T49.5X2	T49.5X3	T49.5X4	T49.5X5	T49.5X6
Ibacitabine	T37.5X1	T37.5X2	T37.5X3	T37.5X4	T37.5X5	T37.5X6
Ibopamine	T44.991	T44.992	T44.993	T44.994	T44.995	T44.996
Ibufenac	T39.311	T39.312	T39.313	T39.314	T39.315	T39.316
Ibuprofen	T39.311	T39.312	T39.313	T39.314	T39.315	T39.316
Ibuproxam	T39.311	T39.312	T39.313	T39.314	T39.315	T39.316
Ibuterol	T48.6X1	T48.6X2	T48.6X3	T48.6X4	T48.6X5	T48.6X6
Ichthammol	T49.0X1	T49.0X2	T49.0X3	T49.0X4	T49.0X5	T49.0X6
Ichthyol	T49.4X1	T49.4X2	T49.4X3	T49.4X4	T49.4X5	T49.4X6
Idarubicin	T45.1X1	T45.1X2	T45.1X3	T45.1X4	T45.1X5	T45.1X6
Idrocilamide	T42.8X1	T42.8X2	T42.8X3	T42.8X4	T42.8X5	T42.8X6
Ifenprodil	T46.7X1	T46.7X2	T46.7X3	T46.7X4	T46.7X5	T46.7X6
Ifosfamide	T45.1X1	T45.1X2	T45.1X3	T45.1X4	T45.1X5	T45.1X6
Iletin	T38.3X1	T38.3X2	T38.3X3	T38.3X4	T38.3X5	T38.3X6
Ilex	T62.2X1	T62.2X2	T62.2X3	T62.2X4	--	--
Illuminating gas (after combustion)	T58.11	T58.12	T58.13	T58.14	--	--
- prior to combustion	T59.891	T59.892	T59.893	T59.894	--	--
Ilopan	T45.2X1	T45.2X2	T45.2X3	T45.2X4	T45.2X5	T45.2X6
Iloprost	T46.7X1	T46.7X2	T46.7X3	T46.7X4	T46.7X5	T46.7X6
Ilotycin	T36.3X1	T36.3X2	T36.3X3	T36.3X4	T36.3X5	T36.3X6
- ophthalmic preparation	T49.5X1	T49.5X2	T49.5X3	T49.5X4	T49.5X5	T49.5X6
- topical NEC	T49.0X1	T49.0X2	T49.0X3	T49.0X4	T49.0X5	T49.0X6
Imidazole-4-carboxamide	T45.1X1	T45.1X2	T45.1X3	T45.1X4	T45.1X5	T45.1X6

TABLE OF DRUGS AND CHEMICALS

Substance	Poisoning, Accidental (unintentional)	Poisoning, Intentional Self-harm	Poisoning, Assault	Poisoning, Undetermined	Adverse effect	Underdosing
Imipenem	T36.0X1	T36.0X2	T36.0X3	T36.0X4	T36.0X5	T36.0X6
Imipramine	T43.011	T43.012	T43.013	T43.014	T43.015	T43.016
Iminostilbene	T42.1X1	T42.1X2	T42.1X3	T42.1X4	T42.1X5	T42.1X6
Immu-G	T50.Z11	T50.Z12	T50.Z13	T50.Z14	T50.Z15	T50.Z16
Immuglobin	T50.Z11	T50.Z12	T50.Z13	T50.Z14	T50.Z15	T50.Z16
Immune						
- globulin	T50.Z11	T50.Z12	T50.Z13	T50.Z14	T50.Z15	T50.Z16
- serum globulin	T50.Z11	T50.Z12	T50.Z13	T50.Z14	T50.Z15	T50.Z16
Immunoglobin human (intravenous) (normal)	T50.Z11	T50.Z12	T50.Z13	T50.Z14	T50.Z15	T50.Z16
- unmodified	T50.Z11	T50.Z12	T50.Z13	T50.Z14	T50.Z15	T50.Z16
Immunosuppressive drug	T45.1X1	T45.1X2	T45.1X3	T45.1X4	T45.1X5	T45.1X6
Immu-tetanus	T50.Z11	T50.Z12	T50.Z13	T50.Z14	T50.Z15	T50.Z16
Indalpine	T43.221	T43.222	T43.223	T43.224	T43.225	T43.226
Indanazoline	T48.5X1	T48.5X2	T48.5X3	T48.5X4	T48.5X5	T48.5X6
Indandione (derivatives)	T45.511	T45.512	T45.513	T45.514	T45.515	T45.516
Indapamide	T46.5X1	T46.5X2	T46.5X3	T46.5X4	T46.5X5	T46.5X6
Indendione (derivatives)	T45.511	T45.512	T45.513	T45.514	T45.515	T45.516
Indenolol	T44.7X1	T44.7X2	T44.7X3	T44.7X4	T44.7X5	T44.7X6
Inderal	T44.7X1	T44.7X2	T44.7X3	T44.7X4	T44.7X5	T44.7X6
Indian						
- hemp	T40.7X1	T40.7X2	T40.7X3	T40.7X4	T40.7X5	T40.7X6
- tobacco	T62.2X1	T62.2X2	T62.2X3	T62.2X4	--	--
Indigo carmine	T50.8X1	T50.8X2	T50.8X3	T50.8X4	T50.8X5	T50.8X6
Indobufen	T45.521	T45.522	T45.523	T45.524	T45.525	T45.526
Indocln	T39.2X1	T39.2X2	T39.2X3	T39.2X4	T39.2X5	T39.2X6
Indocyanine green	T50.8X1	T50.8X2	T50.8X3	T50.8X4	T50.8X5	T50.8X6
Indometacin	T39.391	T39.392	T39.393	T39.394	T39.395	T39.396
Indomethacin	T39.391	T39.392	T39.393	T39.394	T39.395	T39.396
- farnesil	T39.4X1	T39.4X2	T39.4X3	T39.4X4	T39.4X5	T39.4X6
Indoramin	T44.6X1	T44.6X2	T44.6X3	T44.6X4	T44.6X5	T44.6X6
Industrial						
- alcohol	T51.0X1	T51.0X2	T51.0X3	T51.0X4	--	--
- fumes	T59.891	T59.892	T59.893	T59.894	--	--
- solvents (fumes) (vapors)	T52.91	T52.92	T52.93	T52.94	--	--
Influenza vaccine	T50.B91	T50.B92	T50.B93	T50.B94	T50.B95	T50.B96
Ingested substance NEC	T65.91	T65.92	T65.93	T65.94	--	--
INH	T37.1X1	T37.1X2	T37.1X3	T37.1X4	T37.1X5	T37.1X6
Inhalation, gas (noxious) —see Gas Inhibitor						
- angiotensin-converting enzyme	T46.4X1	T46.4X2	T46.4X3	T46.4X4	T46.4X5	T46.4X6
- carbonic anhydrase	T50.2X1	T50.2X2	T50.2X3	T50.2X4	T50.2X5	T50.2X6
- fibrinolysis	T45.621	T45.622	T45.623	T45.624	T45.625	T45.626
- monoamine oxidase NEC	T43.1X1	T43.1X2	T43.1X3	T43.1X4	T43.1X5	T43.1X6
- - hydrazine	T43.1X1	T43.1X2	T43.1X3	T43.1X4	T43.1X5	T43.1X6
- postsynaptic	T43.8X1	T43.8X2	T43.8X3	T43.8X4	T43.8X5	T43.8X6
- prothrombin synthesis	T45.511	T45.512	T45.513	T45.514	T45.515	T45.516
Ink	T65.891	T65.892	T65.893	T65.894	--	--
Inorganic substance NEC	T57.91	T57.92	T57.93	T57.94	--	--
Inosine pranobex	T37.5X1	T37.5X2	T37.5X3	T37.5X4	T37.5X5	T37.5X6
Inositol	T50.991	T50.992	T50.993	T50.994	T50.995	T50.996
- nicotinate	T46.7X1	T46.7X2	T46.7X3	T46.7X4	T46.7X5	T46.7X6
Inproquone	T45.1X1	T45.1X2	T45.1X3	T45.1X4	T45.1X5	T45.1X6
Insect (sting) , venomous	T63.481	T63.482	T63.483	T63.484	--	--
- ant	T63.421	T63.422	T63.423	T63.424	--	--
- bee	T63.441	T63.442	T63.443	T63.444	--	--
- caterpillar	T63.431	T63.432	T63.433	T63.434	--	--
- hornet	T63.451	T63.452	T63.453	T63.454	--	--
- wasp	T63.461	T63.462	T63.463	T63.464	--	--
Insecticide NEC	T60.91	T60.92	T60.93	T60.94	--	--
- carbamate	T60.0X1	T60.0X2	T60.0X3	T60.0X4	--	--
- chlorinated	T60.1X1	T60.1X2	T60.1X3	T60.1X4	--	--
- mixed	T60.91	T60.92	T60.93	T60.94	--	--
- organochlorine	T60.1X1	T60.1X2	T60.1X3	T60.1X4	--	--
- organophosphorus	T60.0X1	T60.0X2	T60.0X3	T60.0X4	--	--
Insular tissue extract	T38.3X1	T38.3X2	T38.3X3	T38.3X4	T38.3X5	T38.3X6
Insulin (amorphous) (globin) (isophane) (Lente)	T38.3X1	T38.3X2	T38.3X3	T38.3X4	T38.3X5	T38.3X6

Substance	Poisoning, Accidental (unintentional)	Poisoning, Intentional Self-harm	Poisoning, Assault	Poisoning, Undetermined	Adverse effect	Underdosing
(NPH) (Semilente) (Ultralente)						
- defalan	T38.3X1	T38.3X2	T38.3X3	T38.3X4	T38.3X5	T38.3X6
- human	T38.3X1	T38.3X2	T38.3X3	T38.3X4	T38.3X5	T38.3X6
- injection, soluble	T38.3X1	T38.3X2	T38.3X3	T38.3X4	T38.3X5	T38.3X6
- - biphasic	T38.3X1	T38.3X2	T38.3X3	T38.3X4	T38.3X5	T38.3X6
- intermediate acting	T38.3X1	T38.3X2	T38.3X3	T38.3X4	T38.3X5	T38.3X6
- protamine zinc	T38.3X1	T38.3X2	T38.3X3	T38.3X4	T38.3X5	T38.3X6
- slow acting	T38.3X1	T38.3X2	T38.3X3	T38.3X4	T38.3X5	T38.3X6
- zinc						
- - protamine injection	T38.3X1	T38.3X2	T38.3X3	T38.3X4	T38.3X5	T38.3X6
- - suspension (amorphous) (crystalline)	T38.3X1	T38.3X2	T38.3X3	T38.3X4	T38.3X5	T38.3X6
Interferon (alpha) (beta) (gamma)	T37.5X1	T37.5X2	T37.5X3	T37.5X4	T37.5X5	T37.5X6
Intestinal motility control drug	T47.6X1	T47.6X2	T47.6X3	T47.6X4	T47.6X5	T47.6X6
- biological	T47.8X1	T47.8X2	T47.8X3	T47.8X4	T47.8X5	T47.8X6
Intranarcon	T41.1X1	T41.1X2	T41.1X3	T41.1X4	T41.1X5	T41.1X6
Intravenous						
- amino acids	T50.991	T50.992	T50.993	T50.994	T50.995	T50.996
- fat suspension	T50.991	T50.992	T50.993	T50.994	T50.995	T50.996
Inulin	T50.8X1	T50.8X2	T50.8X3	T50.8X4	T50.8X5	T50.8X6
Invert sugar	T50.3X1	T50.3X2	T50.3X3	T50.3X4	T50.3X5	T50.3X6
Inza—see Naproxen						
Iobenzamic acid	T50.8X1	T50.8X2	T50.8X3	T50.8X4	T50.8X5	T50.8X6
Iocarmic acid	T50.8X1	T50.8X2	T50.8X3	T50.8X4	T50.8X5	T50.8X6
Iocetamic acid	T50.8X1	T50.8X2	T50.8X3	T50.8X4	T50.8X5	T50.8X6
Iodamide	T50.8X1	T50.8X2	T50.8X3	T50.8X4	T50.8X5	T50.8X6
Iodide NEC—see also Iodine	T49.0X1	T49.0X2	T49.0X3	T49.0X4	T49.0X5	T49.0X6
- mercury (ointment)	T49.0X1	T49.0X2	T49.0X3	T49.0X4	T49.0X5	T49.0X6
- methylate	T49.0X1	T49.0X2	T49.0X3	T49.0X4	T49.0X5	T49.0X6
- potassium (expectorant) NEC	T48.4X1	T48.4X2	T48.4X3	T48.4X4	T48.4X5	T48.4X6
Iodinated						
- contrast medium	T50.8X1	T50.8X2	T50.8X3	T50.8X4	T50.8X5	T50.8X6
- glycerol	T48.4X1	T48.4X2	T48.4X3	T48.4X4	T48.4X5	T48.4X6
- human serum albumin (131I)	T50.8X1	T50.8X2	T50.8X3	T50.8X4	T50.8X5	T50.8X6
Iodine (antiseptic, external) (tincture) NEC	T49.0X1	T49.0X2	T49.0X3	T49.0X4	T49.0X5	T49.0X6
- 125—see also Radiation sickness, and Exposure to radioactivce isotopes	T50.8X1	T50.8X2	T50.8X3	T50.8X4	T50.8X5	T50.8X6
- - therapeutic	T50.991	T50.992	T50.993	T50.994	T50.995	T50.996
- 131—see also Radiation sickness, and Exposure to radioactivce isotopes	T50.8X1	T50.8X2	T50.8X3	T50.8X4	T50.8X5	T50.8X6
- - therapeutic	T38.2X1	T38.2X2	T38.2X3	T38.2X4	T38.2X5	T38.2X6
- diagnostic	T50.8X1	T50.8X2	T50.8X3	T50.8X4	T50.8X5	T50.8X6
- for thyroid conditions (antithyroid)	T38.2X1	T38.2X2	T38.2X3	T38.2X4	T38.2X5	T38.2X6
- solution	T49.0X1	T49.0X2	T49.0X3	T49.0X4	T49.0X5	T49.0X6
- vapor	T59.891	T59.892	T59.893	T59.894	--	--
Iodipamide	T50.8X1	T50.8X2	T50.8X3	T50.8X4	T50.8X5	T50.8X6
Iodized (poppy seed) oil	T50.8X1	T50.8X2	T50.8X3	T50.8X4	T50.8X5	T50.8X6
Iodobismitol	T37.8X1	T37.8X2	T37.8X3	T37.8X4	T37.8X5	T37.8X6
Iodochlorhydroxyquin	T37.8X1	T37.8X2	T37.8X3	T37.8X4	T37.8X5	T37.8X6
- topical	T49.0X1	T49.0X2	T49.0X3	T49.0X4	T49.0X5	T49.0X6
Iodochlorhydroxyquinoline	T37.8X1	T37.8X2	T37.8X3	T37.8X4	T37.8X5	T37.8X6
Iodocholesterol (131I)	T50.8X1	T50.8X2	T50.8X3	T50.8X4	T50.8X5	T50.8X6
Iodoform	T49.0X1	T49.0X2	T49.0X3	T49.0X4	T49.0X5	T49.0X6
Iodohippuric acid	T50.8X1	T50.8X2	T50.8X3	T50.8X4	T50.8X5	T50.8X6
Iodopanoic acid	T50.8X1	T50.8X2	T50.8X3	T50.8X4	T50.8X5	T50.8X6
Iodophthalein (sodium)	T50.8X1	T50.8X2	T50.8X3	T50.8X4	T50.8X5	T50.8X6
Iodopyracet	T50.8X1	T50.8X2	T50.8X3	T50.8X4	T50.8X5	T50.8X6
Iodoquinol	T37.8X1	T37.8X2	T37.8X3	T37.8X4	T37.8X5	T37.8X6
Iodoxamic acid	T50.8X1	T50.8X2	T50.8X3	T50.8X4	T50.8X5	T50.8X6
Iofendylate	T50.8X1	T50.8X2	T50.8X3	T50.8X4	T50.8X5	T50.8X6
Ioglycamic acid	T50.8X1	T50.8X2	T50.8X3	T50.8X4	T50.8X5	T50.8X6
Iohexol	T50.8X1	T50.8X2	T50.8X3	T50.8X4	T50.8X5	T50.8X6
Ion exchange resin						
- anion	T47.8X1	T47.8X2	T47.8X3	T47.8X4	T47.8X5	T47.8X6
- cation	T50.3X1	T50.3X2	T50.3X3	T50.3X4	T50.3X5	T50.3X6
- cholestyramine	T46.6X1	T46.6X2	T46.6X3	T46.6X4	T46.6X5	T46.6X6

Substance	Poisoning, Accidental (unintentional)	Poisoning, Intentional Self-harm	Poisoning, Assault	Poisoning, Undetermined	Adverse effect	Underdosing
- intestinal	T47.8X1	T47.8X2	T47.8X3	T47.8X4	T47.8X5	T47.8X6
Iopamidol	T50.8X1	T50.8X2	T50.8X3	T50.8X4	T50.8X5	T50.8X6
Iopanoic acid	T50.8X1	T50.8X2	T50.8X3	T50.8X4	T50.8X5	T50.8X6
Iophenoic acid	T50.8X1	T50.8X2	T50.8X3	T50.8X4	T50.8X5	T50.8X6
Iopodate, sodium	T50.8X1	T50.8X2	T50.8X3	T50.8X4	T50.8X5	T50.8X6
Iopodic acid	T50.8X1	T50.8X2	T50.8X3	T50.8X4	T50.8X5	T50.8X6
Iopromide	T50.8X1	T50.8X2	T50.8X3	T50.8X4	T50.8X5	T50.8X6
Iopydol	T50.8X1	T50.8X2	T50.8X3	T50.8X4	T50.8X5	T50.8X6
Iotalamic acid	T50.8X1	T50.8X2	T50.8X3	T50.8X4	T50.8X5	T50.8X6
Iothalamate	T50.8X1	T50.8X2	T50.8X3	T50.8X4	T50.8X5	T50.8X6
Iothiouracil	T38.2X1	T38.2X2	T38.2X3	T38.2X4	T38.2X5	T38.2X6
Iotrol	T50.8X1	T50.8X2	T50.8X3	T50.8X4	T50.8X5	T50.8X6
Iotrolan	T50.8X1	T50.8X2	T50.8X3	T50.8X4	T50.8X5	T50.8X6
Iotroxate	T50.8X1	T50.8X2	T50.8X3	T50.8X4	T50.8X5	T50.8X6
Iotroxic acid	T50.8X1	T50.8X2	T50.8X3	T50.8X4	T50.8X5	T50.8X6
Ioversol	T50.8X1	T50.8X2	T50.8X3	T50.8X4	T50.8X5	T50.8X6
Ioxaglate	T50.8X1	T50.8X2	T50.8X3	T50.8X4	T50.8X5	T50.8X6
Ioxaglic acid	T50.8X1	T50.8X2	T50.8X3	T50.8X4	T50.8X5	T50.8X6
Ioxitalamic acid	T50.8X1	T50.8X2	T50.8X3	T50.8X4	T50.8X5	T50.8X6
Ipecac	T47.7X1	T47.7X2	T47.7X3	T47.7X4	T47.7X5	T47.7X6
Ipecacuanha	T48.4X1	T48.4X2	T48.4X3	T48.4X4	T48.4X5	T48.4X6
Ipodate, calcium	T50.8X1	T50.8X2	T50.8X3	T50.8X4	T50.8X5	T50.8X6
Ipral	T42.3X1	T42.3X2	T42.3X3	T42.3X4	T42.3X5	T42.3X6
Ipratropium (bromide)	T48.6X1	T48.6X2	T48.6X3	T48.6X4	T48.6X5	T48.6X6
Ipriflavone	T46.3X1	T46.3X2	T46.3X3	T46.3X4	T46.3X5	T46.3X6
Iprindole	T43.011	T43.012	T43.013	T43.014	T43.015	T43.016
Iproclozide	T43.1X1	T43.1X2	T43.1X3	T43.1X4	T43.1X5	T43.1X6
Iprofenin	T50.8X1	T50.8X2	T50.8X3	T50.8X4	T50.8X5	T50.8X6
Iproheptine	T49.2X1	T49.2X2	T49.2X3	T49.2X4	T49.2X5	T49.2X6
Iproniazid	T43.1X1	T43.1X2	T43.1X3	T43.1X4	T43.1X5	T43.1X6
Iproplatin	T45.1X1	T45.1X2	T45.1X3	T45.1X4	T45.1X5	T45.1X6
Iproveratril	T46.1X1	T46.1X2	T46.1X3	T46.1X4	T46.1X5	T46.1X6
Iron (compounds) (medicinal) NEC	T45.4X1	T45.4X2	T45.4X3	T45.4X4	T45.4X5	T45.4X6
- ammonium	T45.4X1	T45.4X2	T45.4X3	T45.4X4	T45.4X5	T45.4X6
- dextran injection	T45.4X1	T45.4X2	T45.4X3	T45.4X4	T45.4X5	T45.4X6
- nonmedicinal	T56.891	T56.892	T56.893	T56.894	--	--
- salts	T45.4X1	T45.4X2	T45.4X3	T45.4X4	T45.4X5	T45.4X6
- sorbitex	T45.4X1	T45.4X2	T45.4X3	T45.4X4	T45.4X5	T45.4X6
- sorbitol citric acid complex	T45.4X1	T45.4X2	T45.4X3	T45.4X4	T45.4X5	T45.4X6
Irrigating fluid (vaginal)	T49.8X1	T49.8X2	T49.8X3	T49.8X4	T49.8X5	T49.8X6
- eye	T49.5X1	T49.5X2	T49.5X3	T49.5X4	T49.5X5	T49.5X6
Isepamicin	T36.5X1	T36.5X2	T36.5X3	T36.5X4	T36.5X5	T36.5X6
Isoaminile (citrate)	T48.3X1	T48.3X2	T48.3X3	T48.3X4	T48.3X5	T48.3X6
Isoamyl nitrite	T46.3X1	T46.3X2	T46.3X3	T46.3X4	T46.3X5	T46.3X6
Isobenzan	T60.1X1	T60.1X2	T60.1X3	T60.1X4	--	--
Isobutyl acetate	T52.8X1	T52.8X2	T52.8X3	T52.8X4	--	--
Isocarboxazid	T43.1X1	T43.1X2	T43.1X3	T43.1X4	T43.1X5	T43.1X6
Isoconazole	T49.0X1	T49.0X2	T49.0X3	T49.0X4	T49.0X5	T49.0X6
Isocyanate	T65.0X1	T65.0X2	T65.0X3	T65.0X4	--	--
Isoephedrine	T44.991	T44.992	T44.993	T44.994	T44.995	T44.996
Isoetarine	T48.6X1	T48.6X2	T48.6X3	T48.6X4	T48.6X5	T48.6X6
Isoethadione	T42.2X1	T42.2X2	T42.2X3	T42.2X4	T42.2X5	T42.2X6
Isoetharine	T44.5X1	T44.5X2	T44.5X3	T44.5X4	T44.5X5	T44.5X6
Isoflurane	T41.0X1	T41.0X2	T41.0X3	T41.0X4	T41.0X5	T41.0X6
Isoflurophate	T44.0X1	T44.0X2	T44.0X3	T44.0X4	T44.0X5	T44.0X6
Isomaltose, ferric complex	T45.4X1	T45.4X2	T45.4X3	T45.4X4	T45.4X5	T45.4X6
Isometheptene	T44.3X1	T44.3X2	T44.3X3	T44.3X4	T44.3X5	T44.3X6
Isoniazid	T37.1X1	T37.1X2	T37.1X3	T37.1X4	T37.1X5	T37.1X6
- with						
- - rifampicin	T36.6X1	T36.6X2	T36.6X3	T36.6X4	T36.6X5	T36.6X6
- - thioacetazone	T37.1X1	T37.1X2	T37.1X3	T37.1X4	T37.1X5	T37.1X6
Isonicotinic acid hydrazide	T37.1X1	T37.1X2	T37.1X3	T37.1X4	T37.1X5	T37.1X6
Isonipecaine	T40.4X1	T40.4X2	T40.4X3	T40.4X4	T40.4X5	T40.4X6
Isopentaquine	T37.2X1	T37.2X2	T37.2X3	T37.2X4	T37.2X5	T37.2X6
Isophane insulin	T38.3X1	T38.3X2	T38.3X3	T38.3X4	T38.3X5	T38.3X6

Substance	Poisoning, Accidental (unintentional)	Poisoning, Intentional Self-harm	Poisoning, Assault	Poisoning, Undetermined	Adverse effect	Underdosing
Isophorone	T65.891	T65.892	T65.893	T65.894	--	--
Isophosphamide	T45.1X1	T45.1X2	T45.1X3	T45.1X4	T45.1X5	T45.1X6
Isopregnenone	T38.5X1	T38.5X2	T38.5X3	T38.5X4	T38.5X5	T38.5X6
Isoprenaline	T48.6X1	T48.6X2	T48.6X3	T48.6X4	T48.6X5	T48.6X6
Isopromethazine	T43.3X1	T43.3X2	T43.3X3	T43.3X4	T43.3X5	T43.3X6
Isopropamide	T44.3X1	T44.3X2	T44.3X3	T44.3X4	T44.3X5	T44.3X6
- iodide	T44.3X1	T44.3X2	T44.3X3	T44.3X4	T44.3X5	T44.3X6
Isopropanol	T51.2X1	T51.2X2	T51.2X3	T51.2X4	--	--
Isopropyl						
- acetate	T52.8X1	T52.8X2	T52.8X3	T52.8X4	--	--
- alcohol	T51.2X1	T51.2X2	T51.2X3	T51.2X4	--	--
- - medicinal	T49.4X1	T49.4X2	T49.4X3	T49.4X4	T49.4X5	T49.4X6
- ether	T52.8X1	T52.8X2	T52.8X3	T52.8X4	--	--
Isopropylaminophenazone	T39.2X1	T39.2X2	T39.2X3	T39.2X4	T39.2X5	T39.2X6
Isoproterenol	T48.6X1	T48.6X2	T48.6X3	T48.6X4	T48.6X5	T48.6X6
Isosorbide dinitrate	T46.3X1	T46.3X2	T46.3X3	T46.3X4	T46.3X5	T46.3X6
Isothipendyl	T45.0X1	T45.0X2	T45.0X3	T45.0X4	T45.0X5	T45.0X6
Isotretinoin	T50.991	T50.992	T50.993	T50.994	T50.995	T50.996
Isoxazolyl penicillin	T36.0X1	T36.0X2	T36.0X3	T36.0X4	T36.0X5	T36.0X6
Isoxicam	T39.391	T39.392	T39.393	T39.394	T39.395	T39.396
Isoxsuprine	T46.7X1	T46.7X2	T46.7X3	T46.7X4	T46.7X5	T46.7X6
Ispagula	T47.4X1	T47.4X2	T47.4X3	T47.4X4	T47.4X5	T47.4X6
- husk	T47.4X1	T47.4X2	T47.4X3	T47.4X4	T47.4X5	T47.4X6
Isradipine	T46.1X1	T46.1X2	T46.1X3	T46.1X4	T46.1X5	T46.1X6
I-thyroxine sodium	T38.1X1	T38.1X2	T38.1X3	T38.1X4	T38.1X5	T38.1X6
Itraconazole	T37.8X1	T37.8X2	T37.8X3	T37.8X4	T37.8X5	T37.8X6
Itramin tosilate	T46.3X1	T46.3X2	T46.3X3	T46.3X4	T46.3X5	T46.3X6
Ivermectin	T37.4X1	T37.4X2	T37.4X3	T37.4X4	T37.4X5	T37.4X6
Izoniazid	T37.1X1	T37.1X2	T37.1X3	T37.1X4	T37.1X5	T37.1X6
- with thioacetazone	T37.1X1	T37.1X2	T37.1X3	T37.1X4	T37.1X5	T37.1X6
Jalap	T47.2X1	T47.2X2	T47.2X3	T47.2X4	T47.2X5	T47.2X6
Jamaica						
- dogwood (bark)	T39.8X1	T39.8X2	T39.8X3	T39.8X4	T39.8X5	T39.8X6
- ginger	T65.891	T65.892	T65.893	T65.894	--	--
- - root	T62.2X1	T62.2X2	T62.2X3	T62.2X4	--	--
Jatropha	T62.2X1	T62.2X2	T62.2X3	T62.2X4	--	--
- curcas	T62.2X1	T62.2X2	T62.2X3	T62.2X4	--	--
Jectofer	T45.4X1	T45.4X2	T45.4X3	T45.4X4	T45.4X5	T45.4X6
Jellyfish (sting)	T63.621	T63.622	T63.623	T63.624	--	--
Jequirity (bean)	T62.2X1	T62.2X2	T62.2X3	T62.2X4	--	--
Jimson weed (stramonium)	T62.2X1	T62.2X2	T62.2X3	T62.2X4	--	--
- seeds	T62.2X1	T62.2X2	T62.2X3	T62.2X4	--	--
Josamycin	T36.3X1	T36.3X2	T36.3X3	T36.3X4	T36.3X5	T36.3X6
Juniper tar	T49.1X1	T49.1X2	T49.1X3	T49.1X4	T49.1X5	T49.1X6
Kallidinogenase	T46.7X1	T46.7X2	T46.7X3	T46.7X4	T46.7X5	T46.7X6
Kallikrein	T46.7X1	T46.7X2	T46.7X3	T46.7X4	T46.7X5	T46.7X6
Kanamycin	T36.5X1	T36.5X2	T36.5X3	T36.5X4	T36.5X5	T36.5X6
Kantrex	T36.5X1	T36.5X2	T36.5X3	T36.5X4	T36.5X5	T36.5X6
Kaolin	T47.6X1	T47.6X2	T47.6X3	T47.6X4	T47.6X5	T47.6X6
- light	T47.6X1	T47.6X2	T47.6X3	T47.6X4	T47.6X5	T47.6X6
Karaya (gum)	T47.4X1	T47.4X2	T47.4X3	T47.4X4	T47.4X5	T47.4X6
Kebuzone	T39.2X1	T39.2X2	T39.2X3	T39.2X4	T39.2X5	T39.2X6
Kelevan	T60.1X1	T60.1X2	T60.1X3	T60.1X4	--	--
Kemithal	T41.1X1	T41.1X2	T41.1X3	T41.1X4	T41.1X5	T41.1X6
Kenacort	T38.0X1	T38.0X2	T38.0X3	T38.0X4	T38.0X5	T38.0X6
Keratolytic drug NEC	T49.4X1	T49.4X2	T49.4X3	T49.4X4	T49.4X5	T49.4X6
- anthracene	T49.4X1	T49.4X2	T49.4X3	T49.4X4	T49.4X5	T49.4X6
Keratoplastic NEC	T49.4X1	T49.4X2	T49.4X3	T49.4X4	T49.4X5	T49.4X6
Kerosene, kerosine (fuel) (solvent) NEC	T52.0X1	T52.0X2	T52.0X3	T52.0X4	--	--
- insecticide	T52.0X1	T52.0X2	T52.0X3	T52.0X4	--	--
- vapor	T52.0X1	T52.0X2	T52.0X3	T52.0X4	--	--
Ketamine	T41.291	T41.292	T41.293	T41.294	T41.295	T41.296
Ketazolam	T42.4X1	T42.4X2	T42.4X3	T42.4X4	T42.4X5	T42.4X6
Ketazon	T39.2X1	T39.2X2	T39.2X3	T39.2X4	T39.2X5	T39.2X6
Ketobemidone	T40.4X1	T40.4X2	T40.4X3	T40.4X4	--	--

TABLE OF DRUGS AND CHEMICALS

Substance	Poisoning, Accidental (unintentional)	Poisoning, Intentional Self-harm	Poisoning, Assault	Poisoning, Undetermined	Adverse effect	Underdosing
Ketoconazole	T49.0X1	T49.0X2	T49.0X3	T49.0X4	T49.0X5	T49.0X6
Ketols	T52.4X1	T52.4X2	T52.4X3	T52.4X4	--	--
Ketone oils	T52.4X1	T52.4X2	T52.4X3	T52.4X4	--	--
Ketoprofen	T39.311	T39.312	T39.313	T39.314	T39.315	T39.316
Ketorolac	T39.8X1	T39.8X2	T39.8X3	T39.8X4	T39.8X5	T39.8X6
Ketotifen	T45.0X1	T45.0X2	T45.0X3	T45.0X4	T45.0X5	T45.0X6
Khat	T43.691	T43.692	T43.693	T43.694	--	--
Khellin	T46.3X1	T46.3X2	T46.3X3	T46.3X4	T46.3X5	T46.3X6
Khelloside	T46.3X1	T46.3X2	T46.3X3	T46.3X4	T46.3X5	T46.3X6
Kiln gas or vapor (carbon monoxide)	T58.8X1	T58.8X2	T58.8X3	T58.8X4	--	--
Kitasamycin	T36.3X1	T36.3X2	T36.3X3	T36.3X4	T36.3X5	T36.3X6
Konsyl	T47.4X1	T47.4X2	T47.4X3	T47.4X4	T47.4X5	T47.4X6
Kosam seed	T62.2X1	T62.2X2	T62.2X3	T62.2X4	--	--
Krait (venom)	T63.091	T63.092	T63.093	T63.094	--	--
Kwell (insecticide)	T60.1X1	T60.1X2	T60.1X3	T60.1X4	--	--
- anti-infective (topical)	T49.0X1	T49.0X2	T49.0X3	T49.0X4	T49.0X5	T49.0X6
Labetalol	T44.8X1	T44.8X2	T44.8X3	T44.8X4	T44.8X5	T44.8X6
Laburnum (seeds)	T62.2X1	T62.2X2	T62.2X3	T62.2X4	--	--
- leaves	T62.2X1	T62.2X2	T62.2X3	T62.2X4	--	--
Lachesine	T49.5X1	T49.5X2	T49.5X3	T49.5X4	T49.5X5	T49.5X6
Lacidipine	T46.5X1	T46.5X2	T46.5X3	T46.5X4	T46.5X5	T46.5X6
Lacquer	T65.6X1	T65.6X2	T65.6X3	T65.6X4	--	--
Lacrimogenic gas	T59.3X1	T59.3X2	T59.3X3	T59.3X4	--	--
Lactated potassic saline	T50.3X1	T50.3X2	T50.3X3	T50.3X4	T50.3X5	T50.3X6
Lactic acid	T49.8X1	T49.8X2	T49.8X3	T49.8X4	T49.8X5	T49.8X6
Lactobacillus						
- acidophilus	T47.6X1	T47.6X2	T47.6X3	T47.6X4	T47.6X5	T47.6X6
- - compound	T47.6X1	T47.6X2	T47.6X3	T47.6X4	T47.6X5	T47.6X6
- bifidus, lyophilized	T47.6X1	T47.6X2	T47.6X3	T47.6X4	T47.6X5	T47.6X6
- bulgaricus	T47.6X1	T47.6X2	T47.6X3	T47.6X4	T47.6X5	T47.6X6
- sporogenes	T47.6X1	T47.6X2	T47.6X3	T47.6X4	T47.6X5	T47.6X6
Lactoflavin	T45.2X1	T45.2X2	T45.2X3	T45.2X4	T45.2X5	T45.2X6
Lactose (as excipient)	T50.901	T50.902	T50.903	T50.904	T50.905	T50.906
Lactuca (virosa) (extract)	T42.6X1	T42.6X2	T42.6X3	T42.6X4	T42.6X5	T42.6X6
Lactucarium	T42.6X1	T42.6X2	T42.6X3	T42.6X4	T42.6X5	T42.6X6
Lactulose	T47.3X1	T47.3X2	T47.3X3	T47.3X4	T47.3X5	T47.3X6
Laevo—see Levo-						
Lanatosides	T46.0X1	T46.0X2	T46.0X3	T46.0X4	T46.0X5	T46.0X6
Lanolin	T49.3X1	T49.3X2	T49.3X3	T49.3X4	T49.3X5	T49.3X6
Largactil	T43.3X1	T43.3X2	T43.3X3	T43.3X4	T43.3X5	T43.3X6
Larkspur	T62.2X1	T62.2X2	T62.2X3	T62.2X4	--	--
Laroxyl	T43.011	T43.012	T43.013	T43.014	T43.015	T43.016
Lasix	T50.1X1	T50.1X2	T50.1X3	T50.1X4	T50.1X5	T50.1X6
Lassar's paste	T49.4X1	T49.4X2	T49.4X3	T49.4X4	T49.4X5	T49.4X6
Latamoxef	T36.1X1	T36.1X2	T36.1X3	T36.1X4	T36.1X5	T36.1X6
Latex	T65.811	T65.812	T65.813	T65.814	--	--
Lathyrus (seed)	T62.2X1	T62.2X2	T62.2X3	T62.2X4	--	--
Laudanum	T40.0X1	T40.0X2	T40.0X3	T40.0X4	T40.0X5	T40.0X6
Laudexium	T48.1X1	T48.1X2	T48.1X3	T48.1X4	T48.1X5	T48.1X6
Laughing gas	T41.0X1	T41.0X2	T41.0X3	T41.0X4	T41.0X5	T41.0X6
Laurel, black or cherry	T62.2X1	T62.2X2	T62.2X3	T62.2X4	--	--
Laurolinium	T49.0X1	T49.0X2	T49.0X3	T49.0X4	T49.0X5	T49.0X6
Lauryl sulfoacetate	T49.2X1	T49.2X2	T49.2X3	T49.2X4	T49.2X5	T49.2X6
Laxative NEC	T47.4X1	T47.4X2	T47.4X3	T47.4X4	T47.4X5	T47.4X6
- osmotic	T47.3X1	T47.3X2	T47.3X3	T47.3X4	T47.3X5	T47.3X6
- saline	T47.3X1	T47.3X2	T47.3X3	T47.3X4	T47.3X5	T47.3X6
- stimulant	T47.2X1	T47.2X2	T47.2X3	T47.2X4	T47.2X5	T47.2X6
L-dopa	T42.8X1	T42.8X2	T42.8X3	T42.8X4	T42.8X5	T42.8X6
Lead (dust) (fumes) (vapor) NEC	T56.0X1	T56.0X2	T56.0X3	T56.0X4	--	--
- acetate	T49.2X1	T49.2X2	T49.2X3	T49.2X4	T49.2X5	T49.2X6
- alkyl (fuel additive)	T56.0X1	T56.0X2	T56.0X3	T56.0X4	--	--
- anti-infectives	T37.8X1	T37.8X2	T37.8X3	T37.8X4	T37.8X5	T37.8X6
- antiknock compound (tetraethyl)	T56.0X1	T56.0X2	T56.0X3	T56.0X4	--	--
- arsenate, arsenite (dust) (herbicide) (insecticide) (vapor)	T57.0X1	T57.0X2	T57.0X3	T57.0X4	--	--

Substance	Poisoning, Accidental (unintentional)	Poisoning, Intentional Self-harm	Poisoning, Assault	Poisoning, Undetermined	Adverse effect	Underdosing
- carbonate	T56.0X1	T56.0X2	T56.0X3	T56.0X4	--	--
- - paint	T56.0X1	T56.0X2	T56.0X3	T56.0X4	--	--
- chromate	T56.0X1	T56.0X2	T56.0X3	T56.0X4	--	--
- - paint	T56.0X1	T56.0X2	T56.0X3	T56.0X4	--	--
- dioxide	T56.0X1	T56.0X2	T56.0X3	T56.0X4	--	--
- inorganic	T56.0X1	T56.0X2	T56.0X3	T56.0X4	--	--
- iodide	T56.0X1	T56.0X2	T56.0X3	T56.0X4	--	--
- - pigment (paint)	T56.0X1	T56.0X2	T56.0X3	T56.0X4	--	--
- monoxide (dust)	T56.0X1	T56.0X2	T56.0X3	T56.0X4	--	--
- - paint	T56.0X1	T56.0X2	T56.0X3	T56.0X4	--	--
- organic	T56.0X1	T56.0X2	T56.0X3	T56.0X4	--	--
- oxide	T56.0X1	T56.0X2	T56.0X3	T56.0X4	--	--
- - paint	T56.0X1	T56.0X2	T56.0X3	T56.0X4	--	--
- paint	T56.0X1	T56.0X2	T56.0X3	T56.0X4	--	--
- salts	T56.0X1	T56.0X2	T56.0X3	T56.0X4	--	--
- specified compound NEC	T56.0X1	T56.0X2	T56.0X3	T56.0X4	--	--
- tetra-ethyl	T56.0X1	T56.0X2	T56.0X3	T56.0X4	--	--
Lebanese red	T40.7X1	T40.7X2	T40.7X3	T40.7X4	T40.7X5	T40.7X6
Lefetamine	T39.8X1	T39.8X2	T39.8X3	T39.8X4	T39.8X5	T39.8X6
Lenperone	T43.4X1	T43.4X2	T43.4X3	T43.4X4	T43.4X5	T43.4X6
Lente lietin (insulin)	T38.3X1	T38.3X2	T38.3X3	T38.3X4	T38.3X5	T38.3X6
Leptazol	T50.7X1	T50.7X2	T50.7X3	T50.7X4	T50.7X5	T50.7X6
Leptophos	T60.0X1	T60.0X2	T60.0X3	T60.0X4	--	--
Leritine	T40.2X1	T40.2X2	T40.2X3	T40.2X4	T40.2X5	T40.2X6
Letosteine	T48.4X1	T48.4X2	T48.4X3	T48.4X4	T48.4X5	T48.4X6
Letter	T38.1X1	T38.1X2	T38.1X3	T38.1X4	T38.1X5	T38.1X6
Lettuce opium	T42.6X1	T42.6X2	T42.6X3	T42.6X4	T42.6X5	T42.6X6
Leucinocaine	T41.3X1	T41.3X2	T41.3X3	T41.3X4	T41.3X5	T41.3X6
Leucocianidol	T46.991	T46.992	T46.993	T46.994	T46.995	T46.996
Leucovorin (factor)	T45.8X1	T45.8X2	T45.8X3	T45.8X4	T45.8X5	T45.8X6
Leukeran	T45.1X1	T45.1X2	T45.1X3	T45.1X4	T45.1X5	T45.1X6
Leuprolide	T38.891	T38.892	T38.893	T38.894	T38.895	T38.896
Levalbuterol	T48.6X1	T48.6X2	T48.6X3	T48.6X4	T48.6X5	T48.6X6
Levallorphan	T50.7X1	T50.7X2	T50.7X3	T50.7X4	T50.7X5	T50.7X6
Levamisole	T37.4X1	T37.4X2	T37.4X3	T37.4X4	T37.4X5	T37.4X6
Levanil	T42.6X1	T42.6X2	T42.6X3	T42.6X4	T42.6X5	T42.6X6
Levarterenol	T44.4X1	T44.4X2	T44.4X3	T44.4X4	T44.4X5	T44.4X6
Levdropropizine	T48.3X1	T48.3X2	T48.3X3	T48.3X4	T48.3X5	T48.3X6
Levobunolol	T49.5X1	T49.5X2	T49.5X3	T49.5X4	T49.5X5	T49.5X6
Levocabastine (hydrochloride)	T45.0X1	T45.0X2	T45.0X3	T45.0X4	T45.0X5	T45.0X6
Levocarnitine	T50.991	T50.992	T50.993	T50.994	T50.995	T50.996
Levodopa	T42.8X1	T42.8X2	T42.8X3	T42.8X4	T42.8X5	T42.8X6
- with carbidopa	T42.8X1	T42.8X2	T42.8X3	T42.8X4	T42.8X5	T42.8X6
Levo-dromoran	T40.2X1	T40.2X2	T40.2X3	T40.2X4	T40.2X5	T40.2X6
Levoglutamide	T50.991	T50.992	T50.993	T50.994	T50.995	T50.996
Levoid	T38.1X1	T38.1X2	T38.1X3	T38.1X4	T38.1X5	T38.1X6
Levo-iso-methadone	T40.3X1	T40.3X2	T40.3X3	T40.3X4	T40.3X5	T40.3X6
Levomepromazine	T43.3X1	T43.3X2	T43.3X3	T43.3X4	T43.3X5	T43.3X6
Levonordefrin	T49.6X1	T49.6X2	T49.6X3	T49.6X4	T49.6X5	T49.6X6
Levonorgestrel	T38.4X1	T38.4X2	T38.4X3	T38.4X4	T38.4X5	T38.4X6
- with ethinylestradiol	T38.5X1	T38.5X2	T38.5X3	T38.5X4	T38.5X5	T38.5X6
Levopromazine	T43.3X1	T43.3X2	T43.3X3	T43.3X4	T43.3X5	T43.3X6
Levoprome	T42.6X1	T42.6X2	T42.6X3	T42.6X4	T42.6X5	T42.6X6
Levopropoxyphene	T40.4X1	T40.4X2	T40.4X3	T40.4X4	T40.4X5	T40.4X6
Levopropylhexedrine	T50.5X1	T50.5X2	T50.5X3	T50.5X4	T50.5X5	T50.5X6
Levoproxyphylline	T48.6X1	T48.6X2	T48.6X3	T48.6X4	T48.6X5	T48.6X6
Levorphanol	T40.4X1	T40.4X2	T40.4X3	T40.4X4	T40.4X5	T40.4X6
Levothyroxine	T38.1X1	T38.1X2	T38.1X3	T38.1X4	T38.1X5	T38.1X6
- sodium	T38.1X1	T38.1X2	T38.1X3	T38.1X4	T38.1X5	T38.1X6
Levsin	T44.3X1	T44.3X2	T44.3X3	T44.3X4	T44.3X5	T44.3X6
Levulose	T50.3X1	T50.3X2	T50.3X3	T50.3X4	T50.3X5	T50.3X6
Lewisite (gas) , not in war	T57.0X1	T57.0X2	T57.0X3	T57.0X4	--	--
Librium	T42.4X1	T42.4X2	T42.4X3	T42.4X4	T42.4X5	T42.4X6
Lidex	T49.0X1	T49.0X2	T49.0X3	T49.0X4	T49.0X5	T49.0X6
Lidocaine	T41.3X1	T41.3X2	T41.3X3	T41.3X4	T41.3X5	T41.3X6

Substance	Poisoning, Accidental (unintentional)	Poisoning, Intentional Self-harm	Poisoning, Assault	Poisoning, Undetermined	Adverse effect	Underdosing
- regional	T41.3X1	T41.3X2	T41.3X3	T41.3X4	T41.3X5	T41.3X6
- spinal	T41.3X1	T41.3X2	T41.3X3	T41.3X4	T41.3X5	T41.3X6
Lidofenin	T50.8X1	T50.8X2	T50.8X3	T50.8X4	T50.8X5	T50.8X6
Lidoflazine	T46.1X1	T46.1X2	T46.1X3	T46.1X4	T46.1X5	T46.1X6
Lighter fluid	T52.0X1	T52.0X2	T52.0X3	T52.0X4	--	--
Lignin hemicellulose	T47.6X1	T47.6X2	T47.6X3	T47.6X4	T47.6X5	T47.6X6
Lignocaine	T41.3X1	T41.3X2	T41.3X3	T41.3X4	T41.3X5	T41.3X6
- regional	T41.3X1	T41.3X2	T41.3X3	T41.3X4	T41.3X5	T41.3X6
- spinal	T41.3X1	T41.3X2	T41.3X3	T41.3X4	T41.3X5	T41.3X6
Ligroin (e) (solvent)	T52.0X1	T52.0X2	T52.0X3	T52.0X4	--	--
- vapor	T59.891	T59.892	T59.893	T59.894	--	--
Ligustrum vulgare	T62.2X1	T62.2X2	T62.2X3	T62.2X4	--	--
Lily of the valley	T62.2X1	T62.2X2	T62.2X3	T62.2X4	--	--
Lime (chloride)	T54.3X1	T54.3X2	T54.3X3	T54.3X4	--	--
Limonene	T52.8X1	T52.8X2	T52.8X3	T52.8X4	--	--
Lincomycin	T36.8X1	T36.8X2	T36.8X3	T36.8X4	T36.8X5	T36.8X6
Lindane (insecticide) (nonmedicinal) (vapor)	T53.6X1	T53.6X2	T53.6X3	T53.6X4	--	--
- medicinal	T49.0X1	T49.0X2	T49.0X3	T49.0X4	T49.0X5	T49.0X6
Liniments NEC	T49.91	T49.92	T49.93	T49.94	T49.95	T49.96
Linoleic acid	T46.6X1	T46.6X2	T46.6X3	T46.6X4	T46.6X5	T46.6X6
Linolenic acid	T46.6X1	T46.6X2	T46.6X3	T46.6X4	T46.6X5	T46.6X6
Linseed	T47.4X1	T47.4X2	T47.4X3	T47.4X4	T47.4X5	T47.4X6
Liothyronine	T38.1X1	T38.1X2	T38.1X3	T38.1X4	T38.1X5	T38.1X6
Liotrix	T38.1X1	T38.1X2	T38.1X3	T38.1X4	T38.1X5	T38.1X6
Lipancreatin	T47.5X1	T47.5X2	T47.5X3	T47.5X4	T47.5X5	T47.5X6
Lipo-alprostadil	T46.7X1	T46.7X2	T46.7X3	T46.7X4	T46.7X5	T46.7X6
Lipo-Lutin	T38.5X1	T38.5X2	T38.5X3	T38.5X4	T38.5X5	T38.5X6
Lipotropic drug NEC	T50.901	T50.902	T50.903	T50.904	T50.905	T50.906
Liquefied petroleum gases	T59.891	T59.892	T59.893	T59.894	--	--
- piped (pure or mixed with air)	T59.891	T59.892	T59.893	T59.894	--	--
Liquid						
- paraffin	T47.4X1	T47.4X2	T47.4X3	T47.4X4	T47.4X5	T47.4X6
- petrolatum	T47.4X1	T47.4X2	T47.4X3	T47.4X4	T47.4X5	T47.4X6
- - topical	T49.3X1	T49.3X2	T49.3X3	T49.3X4	T49.3X5	T49.3X6
- specified NEC	T65.891	T65.892	T65.893	T65.894	--	--
- substance	T65.91	T65.92	T65.93	T65.94	--	--
Liquor creosolis compositus	T65.891	T65.892	T65.893	T65.894	--	--
Liquorice	T48.4X1	T48.4X2	T48.4X3	T48.4X4	T48.4X5	T48.4X6
- extract	T47.8X1	T47.8X2	T47.8X3	T47.8X4	T47.8X5	T47.8X6
Lisinopril	T46.4X1	T46.4X2	T46.4X3	T46.4X4	T46.4X5	T46.4X6
Lisuride	T42.8X1	T42.8X2	T42.8X3	T42.8X4	T42.8X5	T42.8X6
Lithane	T43.8X1	T43.8X2	T43.8X3	T43.8X4	T43.8X5	T43.8X6
Lithium	T56.891	T56.892	T56.893	T56.894	--	--
- gluconate	T43.591	T43.592	T43.593	T43.594	T43.595	T43.596
- salts (carbonate)	T43.591	T43.592	T43.593	T43.594	T43.595	T43.596
Lithonate	T43.8X1	T43.8X2	T43.8X3	T43.8X4	T43.8X5	T43.8X6
Liver						
- extract	T45.8X1	T45.8X2	T45.8X3	T45.8X4	T45.8X5	T45.8X6
- - for parenteral use	T45.8X1	T45.8X2	T45.8X3	T45.8X4	T45.8X5	T45.8X6
- fraction 1	T45.8X1	T45.8X2	T45.8X3	T45.8X4	T45.8X5	T45.8X6
- hydrolysate	T45.8X1	T45.8X2	T45.8X3	T45.8X4	T45.8X5	T45.8X6
Lizard (bite) (venom)	T63.121	T63.122	T63.123	T63.124	--	--
LMD	T45.8X1	T45.8X2	T45.8X3	T45.8X4	T45.8X5	T45.8X6
Lobelia	T62.2X1	T62.2X2	T62.2X3	T62.2X4	--	--
Lobeline	T50.7X1	T50.7X2	T50.7X3	T50.7X4	T50.7X5	T50.7X6
Local action drug NEC	T49.8X1	T49.8X2	T49.8X3	T49.8X4	T49.8X5	T49.8X6
Locorten	T49.0X1	T49.0X2	T49.0X3	T49.0X4	T49.0X5	T49.0X6
Lofepramine	T43.011	T43.012	T43.013	T43.014	T43.015	T43.016
Lolium temulentum	T62.2X1	T62.2X2	T62.2X3	T62.2X4	--	--
Lomotil	T47.6X1	T47.6X2	T47.6X3	T47.6X4	T47.6X5	T47.6X6
Lomustine	T45.1X1	T45.1X2	T45.1X3	T45.1X4	T45.1X5	T45.1X6
Lonidamine	T45.1X1	T45.1X2	T45.1X3	T45.1X4	T45.1X5	T45.1X6
Loperamide	T47.6X1	T47.6X2	T47.6X3	T47.6X4	T47.6X5	T47.6X6
Loprazolam	T42.4X1	T42.4X2	T42.4X3	T42.4X4	T42.4X5	T42.4X6
Lorajmine	T46.2X1	T46.2X2	T46.2X3	T46.2X4	T46.2X5	T46.2X6

Substance	Poisoning, Accidental (unintentional)	Poisoning, Intentional Self-harm	Poisoning, Assault	Poisoning, Undetermined	Adverse effect	Underdosing
Loratidine	T45.0X1	T45.0X2	T45.0X3	T45.0X4	T45.0X5	T45.0X6
Lorazepam	T42.4X1	T42.4X2	T42.4X3	T42.4X4	T42.4X5	T42.4X6
Lorcainide	T46.2X1	T46.2X2	T46.2X3	T46.2X4	T46.2X5	T46.2X6
Lormetazepam	T42.4X1	T42.4X2	T42.4X3	T42.4X4	T42.4X5	T42.4X6
Lotions NEC	T49.91	T49.92	T49.93	T49.94	T49.95	T49.96
Lotusate	T42.3X1	T42.3X2	T42.3X3	T42.3X4	T42.3X5	T42.3X6
Lovastatin	T46.6X1	T46.6X2	T46.6X3	T46.6X4	T46.6X5	T46.6X6
Lowila	T49.2X1	T49.2X2	T49.2X3	T49.2X4	T49.2X5	T49.2X6
Loxapine	T43.591	T43.592	T43.593	T43.594	T43.595	T43.596
Lozenges (throat)	T49.6X1	T49.6X2	T49.6X3	T49.6X4	T49.6X5	T49.6X6
LSD	T40.8X1	T40.8X2	T40.8X3	T40.8X4	T40.8X5	--
L-Tryptophan—see amino acid						
Lubricant, eye	T49.5X1	T49.5X2	T49.5X3	T49.5X4	T49.5X5	T49.5X6
Lubricating oil NEC	T52.0X1	T52.0X2	T52.0X3	T52.0X4	--	--
Lucanthone	T37.4X1	T37.4X2	T37.4X3	T37.4X4	T37.4X5	T37.4X6
Luminal	T42.3X1	T42.3X2	T42.3X3	T42.3X4	T42.3X5	T42.3X6
Lung irritant (gas) NEC	T59.91	T59.92	T59.93	T59.94	--	--
Luteinizing hormone	T38.811	T38.812	T38.813	T38.814	T38.815	T38.816
Lutocylol	T38.5X1	T38.5X2	T38.5X3	T38.5X4	T38.5X5	T38.5X6
Lutromone	T38.5X1	T38.5X2	T38.5X3	T38.5X4	T38.5X5	T38.5X6
Lututrin	T48.291	T48.292	T48.293	T48.294	T48.295	T48.296
Lye (concentrated)	T54.3X1	T54.3X2	T54.3X3	T54.3X4	--	--
Lygranum (skin test)	T50.8X1	T50.8X2	T50.8X3	T50.8X4	T50.8X5	T50.8X6
Lymecycline	T36.4X1	T36.4X2	T36.4X3	T36.4X4	T36.4X5	T36.4X6
Lymphogranuloma venereum antigen	T50.8X1	T50.8X2	T50.8X3	T50.8X4	T50.8X5	T50.8X6
Lynestrenol	T38.4X1	T38.4X2	T38.4X3	T38.4X4	T38.4X5	T38.4X6
Lyovac Sodium Edecrin	T50.1X1	T50.1X2	T50.1X3	T50.1X4	T50.1X5	T50.1X6
Lypressin	T38.891	T38.892	T38.893	T38.894	T38.895	T38.896
Lysergic acid diethylamide	T40.8X1	T40.8X2	T40.8X3	T40.8X4	T40.8X5	--
Lysergide	T40.8X1	T40.8X2	T40.8X3	T40.8X4	T40.8X5	--
Lysine vasopressin	T38.891	T38.892	T38.893	T38.894	T38.895	T38.896
Lysol	T54.1X1	T54.1X2	T54.1X3	T54.1X4	--	--
Lysozyme	T49.0X1	T49.0X2	T49.0X3	T49.0X4	T49.0X5	T49.0X6
Lytta (vitatta)	T49.8X1	T49.8X2	T49.8X3	T49.8X4	T49.8X5	T49.8X6
Mace	T59.3X1	T59.3X2	T59.3X3	T59.3X4	--	--
Macrogol	T50.991	T50.992	T50.993	T50.994	T50.995	T50.996
Macrolide						
- anabolic drug	T38.7X1	T38.7X2	T38.7X3	T38.7X4	T38.7X5	T38.7X6
- antibiotic	T36.3X1	T36.3X2	T36.3X3	T36.3X4	T36.3X5	T36.3X6
Mafenide	T49.0X1	T49.0X2	T49.0X3	T49.0X4	T49.0X5	T49.0X6
Magaldrate	T47.1X1	T47.1X2	T47.1X3	T47.1X4	T47.1X5	T47.1X6
Magic mushroom	T40.991	T40.992	T40.993	T40.994	--	--
Magnamycin	T36.8X1	T36.8X2	T36.8X3	T36.8X4	T36.8X5	T36.8X6
Magnesia magma	T47.1X1	T47.1X2	T47.1X3	T47.1X4	T47.1X5	T47.1X6
Magnesium NEC	T56.891	T56.892	T56.893	T56.894	--	--
- carbonate	T47.1X1	T47.1X2	T47.1X3	T47.1X4	T47.1X5	T47.1X6
- citrate	T47.4X1	T47.4X2	T47.4X3	T47.4X4	T47.4X5	T47.4X6
- hydroxide	T47.1X1	T47.1X2	T47.1X3	T47.1X4	T47.1X5	T47.1X6
- oxide	T47.1X1	T47.1X2	T47.1X3	T47.1X4	T47.1X5	T47.1X6
- peroxide	T49.0X1	T49.0X2	T49.0X3	T49.0X4	T49.0X5	T49.0X6
- salicylate	T39.091	T39.092	T39.093	T39.094	T39.095	T39.096
- silicofluoride	T50.3X1	T50.3X2	T50.3X3	T50.3X4	T50.3X5	T50.3X6
- sulfate	T47.4X1	T47.4X2	T47.4X3	T47.4X4	T47.4X5	T47.4X6
- thiosulfate	T45.0X1	T45.0X2	T45.0X3	T45.0X4	T45.0X5	T45.0X6
- trisilicate	T47.1X1	T47.1X2	T47.1X3	T47.1X4	T47.1X5	T47.1X6
Malathion (medicinal)	T49.0X1	T49.0X2	T49.0X3	T49.0X4	T49.0X5	T49.0X6
- insecticide	T60.0X1	T60.0X2	T60.0X3	T60.0X4	--	--
Male fern extract	T37.4X1	T37.4X2	T37.4X3	T37.4X4	T37.4X5	T37.4X6
M-AMSA	T45.1X1	T45.1X2	T45.1X3	T45.1X4	T45.1X5	T45.1X6
Mandelic acid	T37.8X1	T37.8X2	T37.8X3	T37.8X4	T37.8X5	T37.8X6
Manganese (dioxide) (salts)	T57.2X1	T57.2X2	T57.2X3	T57.2X4	--	--
- medicinal	T50.991	T50.992	T50.993	T50.994	T50.995	T50.996
Mannitol	T47.3X1	T47.3X2	T47.3X3	T47.3X4	T47.3X5	T47.3X6
- hexanitrate	T46.3X1	T46.3X2	T46.3X3	T46.3X4	T46.3X5	T46.3X6
Mannomustine	T45.1X1	T45.1X2	T45.1X3	T45.1X4	T45.1X5	T45.1X6

Substance	Poisoning, Accidental (unintentional)	Poisoning, Intentional Self-harm	Poisoning, Assault	Poisoning, Undetermined	Adverse effect	Underdosing
MAO inhibitors	T43.1X1	T43.1X2	T43.1X3	T43.1X4	T43.1X5	T43.1X6
Mapharsen	T37.8X1	T37.8X2	T37.8X3	T37.8X4	T37.8X5	T37.8X6
Maphenide	T49.0X1	T49.0X2	T49.0X3	T49.0X4	T49.0X5	T49.0X6
Maprotiline	T43.021	T43.022	T43.023	T43.024	T43.025	T43.026
Marcaine	T41.3X1	T41.3X2	T41.3X3	T41.3X4	T41.3X5	T41.3X6
- infiltration (subcutaneous)	T41.3X1	T41.3X2	T41.3X3	T41.3X4	T41.3X5	T41.3X6
- nerve block (peripheral) (plexus)	T41.3X1	T41.3X2	T41.3X3	T41.3X4	T41.3X5	T41.3X6
Marezine	T45.0X1	T45.0X2	T45.0X3	T45.0X4	T45.0X5	T45.0X6
Marihuana	T40.7X1	T40.7X2	T40.7X3	T40.7X4	T40.7X5	T40.7X6
Marijuana	T40.7X1	T40.7X2	T40.7X3	T40.7X4	T40.7X5	T40.7X6
Marine (sting)	T63.691	T63.692	T63.693	T63.694	--	--
- animals (sting)	T63.691	T63.692	T63.693	T63.694	--	--
- plants (sting)	T63.711	T63.712	T63.713	T63.714	--	--
Marplan	T43.1X1	T43.1X2	T43.1X3	T43.1X4	T43.1X5	T43.1X6
Marsh gas	T59.891	T59.892	T59.893	T59.894	--	--
Marsilid	T43.1X1	T43.1X2	T43.1X3	T43.1X4	T43.1X5	T43.1X6
Matulane	T45.1X1	T45.1X2	T45.1X3	T45.1X4	T45.1X5	T45.1X6
Mazindol	T50.5X1	T50.5X2	T50.5X3	T50.5X4	T50.5X5	T50.5X6
MCPA	T60.3X1	T60.3X2	T60.3X3	T60.3X4	--	--
MDMA	T43.621	T43.622	T43.623	T43.624	T43.625	T43.626
Meadow saffron	T62.2X1	T62.2X2	T62.2X3	T62.2X4	--	--
Measles virus vaccine (attenuated)	T50.B91	T50.B92	T50.B93	T50.B94	T50.B95	T50.B96
Meat, noxious	T62.8X1	T62.8X2	T62.8X3	T62.8X4	--	--
Meballymal	T42.3X1	T42.3X2	T42.3X3	T42.3X4	T42.3X5	T42.3X6
Mebanazine	T43.1X1	T43.1X2	T43.1X3	T43.1X4	T43.1X5	T43.1X6
Mebaral	T42.3X1	T42.3X2	T42.3X3	T42.3X4	T42.3X5	T42.3X6
Mebendazole	T37.4X1	T37.4X2	T37.4X3	T37.4X4	T37.4X5	T37.4X6
Mebeverine	T44.3X1	T44.3X2	T44.3X3	T44.3X4	T44.3X5	T44.3X6
Mebhydrolin	T45.0X1	T45.0X2	T45.0X3	T45.0X4	T45.0X5	T45.0X6
Mebumal	T42.3X1	T42.3X2	T42.3X3	T42.3X4	T42.3X5	T42.3X6
Mebutamate	T43.591	T43.592	T43.593	T43.594	T43.595	T43.596
Mecamylamine	T44.2X1	T44.2X2	T44.2X3	T44.2X4	T44.2X5	T44.2X6
Mechlorethamine	T45.1X1	T45.1X2	T45.1X3	T45.1X4	T45.1X5	T45.1X6
Mecillinam	T36.0X1	T36.0X2	T36.0X3	T36.0X4	T36.0X5	T36.0X6
Meclizine (hydrochloride)	T45.0X1	T45.0X2	T45.0X3	T45.0X4	T45.0X5	T45.0X6
Meclocycline	T36.4X1	T36.4X2	T36.4X3	T36.4X4	T36.4X5	T36.4X6
Meclofenamate	T39.391	T39.392	T39.393	T39.394	T39.395	T39.396
Meclofenamic acid	T39.391	T39.392	T39.393	T39.394	T39.395	T39.396
Meclofenoxate	T43.691	T43.692	T43.693	T43.694	T43.695	T43.696
Meclozine	T45.0X1	T45.0X2	T45.0X3	T45.0X4	T45.0X5	T45.0X6
Mecobalamin	T45.8X1	T45.8X2	T45.8X3	T45.8X4	T45.8X5	T45.8X6
Mecoprop	T60.3X1	T60.3X2	T60.3X3	T60.3X4	--	--
Mecrilate	T49.3X1	T49.3X2	T49.3X3	T49.3X4	T49.3X5	T49.3X6
Mecysteine	T48.4X1	T48.4X2	T48.4X3	T48.4X4	T48.4X5	T48.4X6
Medazepam	T42.4X1	T42.4X2	T42.4X3	T42.4X4	T42.4X5	T42.4X6
Medicament NEC	T50.901	T50.902	T50.903	T50.904	T50.905	T50.906
Medinal	T42.3X1	T42.3X2	T42.3X3	T42.3X4	T42.3X5	T42.3X6
Medomin	T42.3X1	T42.3X2	T42.3X3	T42.3X4	T42.3X5	T42.3X6
Medrogestone	T38.5X1	T38.5X2	T38.5X3	T38.5X4	T38.5X5	T38.5X6
Medroxalol	T44.8X1	T44.8X2	T44.8X3	T44.8X4	T44.8X5	T44.8X6
Medroxyprogesterone acetate (depot)	T38.5X1	T38.5X2	T38.5X3	T38.5X4	T38.5X5	T38.5X6
Medrysone	T49.0X1	T49.0X2	T49.0X3	T49.0X4	T49.0X5	T49.0X6
Mefenamic acid	T39.391	T39.392	T39.393	T39.394	T39.395	T39.396
Mefenorex	T50.5X1	T50.5X2	T50.5X3	T50.5X4	T50.5X5	T50.5X6
Mefloquine	T37.2X1	T37.2X2	T37.2X3	T37.2X4	T37.2X5	T37.2X6
Mefruside	T50.2X1	T50.2X2	T50.2X3	T50.2X4	T50.2X5	T50.2X6
Megahallucinogen	T40.901	T40.902	T40.903	T40.904	T40.905	T40.906
Megestrol	T38.5X1	T38.5X2	T38.5X3	T38.5X4	T38.5X5	T38.5X6
Meglumine						
- antimoniate	T37.8X1	T37.8X2	T37.8X3	T37.8X4	T37.8X5	T37.8X6
- diatrizoate	T50.8X1	T50.8X2	T50.8X3	T50.8X4	T50.8X5	T50.8X6
- iodipamide	T50.8X1	T50.8X2	T50.8X3	T50.8X4	T50.8X5	T50.8X6
- iotroxate	T50.8X1	T50.8X2	T50.8X3	T50.8X4	T50.8X5	T50.8X6
MEK (methyl ethyl ketone)	T52.4X1	T52.4X2	T52.4X3	T52.4X4	--	--
Meladinin	T49.3X1	T49.3X2	T49.3X3	T49.3X4	T49.3X5	T49.3X6

Substance	Poisoning, Accidental (unintentional)	Poisoning, Intentional Self-harm	Poisoning, Assault	Poisoning, Undetermined	Adverse effect	Underdosing
Meladrazine	T44.3X1	T44.3X2	T44.3X3	T44.3X4	T44.3X5	T44.3X6
Melaleuca alternifolia oil	T49.0X1	T49.0X2	T49.0X3	T49.0X4	T49.0X5	T49.0X6
Melanizing agents	T49.3X1	T49.3X2	T49.3X3	T49.3X4	T49.3X5	T49.3X6
Melanocyte-stimulating hormone	T38.891	T38.892	T38.893	T38.894	T38.895	T38.896
Melarsonyl potassium	T37.3X1	T37.3X2	T37.3X3	T37.3X4	T37.3X5	T37.3X6
Melarsoprol	T37.3X1	T37.3X2	T37.3X3	T37.3X4	T37.3X5	T37.3X6
Melia azedarach	T62.2X1	T62.2X2	T62.2X3	T62.2X4	--	--
Melitracen	T43.011	T43.012	T43.013	T43.014	T43.015	T43.016
Mellaril	T43.3X1	T43.3X2	T43.3X3	T43.3X4	T43.3X5	T43.3X6
Meloxine	T49.3X1	T49.3X2	T49.3X3	T49.3X4	T49.3X5	T49.3X6
Melperone	T43.4X1	T43.4X2	T43.4X3	T43.4X4	T43.4X5	T43.4X6
Melphalan	T45.1X1	T45.1X2	T45.1X3	T45.1X4	T45.1X5	T45.1X6
Memantine	T43.8X1	T43.8X2	T43.8X3	T43.8X4	T43.8X5	T43.8X6
Menadiol	T45.7X1	T45.7X2	T45.7X3	T45.7X4	T45.7X5	T45.7X6
- sodium sulfate	T45.7X1	T45.7X2	T45.7X3	T45.7X4	T45.7X5	T45.7X6
Menadione	T45.7X1	T45.7X2	T45.7X3	T45.7X4	T45.7X5	T45.7X6
- sodium bisulfite	T45.7X1	T45.7X2	T45.7X3	T45.7X4	T45.7X5	T45.7X6
Menaphthone	T45.7X1	T45.7X2	T45.7X3	T45.7X4	T45.7X5	T45.7X6
Menaquinone	T45.7X1	T45.7X2	T45.7X3	T45.7X4	T45.7X5	T45.7X6
Menatetrenone	T45.7X1	T45.7X2	T45.7X3	T45.7X4	T45.7X5	T45.7X6
Meningococcal vaccine	T50.A91	T50.A92	T50.A93	T50.A94	T50.A95	T50.A96
Menningovax (-AC) (-C)	T50.A91	T50.A92	T50.A93	T50.A94	T50.A95	T50.A96
Menotropins	T38.811	T38.812	T38.813	T38.814	T38.815	T38.816
Menthol	T48.5X1	T48.5X2	T48.5X3	T48.5X4	T48.5X5	T48.5X6
Mepacrine	T37.2X1	T37.2X2	T37.2X3	T37.2X4	T37.2X5	T37.2X6
Meparfynol	T42.6X1	T42.6X2	T42.6X3	T42.6X4	T42.6X5	T42.6X6
Mepartricin	T36.7X1	T36.7X2	T36.7X3	T36.7X4	T36.7X5	T36.7X6
Mepazine	T43.3X1	T43.3X2	T43.3X3	T43.3X4	T43.3X5	T43.3X6
Mepenzolate	T44.3X1	T44.3X2	T44.3X3	T44.3X4	T44.3X5	T44.3X6
- bromide	T44.3X1	T44.3X2	T44.3X3	T44.3X4	T44.3X5	T44.3X6
Meperidine	T40.4X1	T40.4X2	T40.4X3	T40.4X4	T40.4X5	T40.4X6
Mephebarbital	T42.3X1	T42.3X2	T42.3X3	T42.3X4	T42.3X5	T42.3X6
Mephenamin (e)	T42.8X1	T42.8X2	T42.8X3	T42.8X4	T42.8X5	T42.8X6
Mephenesin	T42.8X1	T42.8X2	T42.8X3	T42.8X4	T42.8X5	T42.8X6
Mephenhydramine	T45.0X1	T45.0X2	T45.0X3	T45.0X4	T45.0X5	T45.0X6
Mephenoxalone	T42.8X1	T42.8X2	T42.8X3	T42.8X4	T42.8X5	T42.8X6
Mephentermine	T44.991	T44.992	T44.993	T44.994	T44.995	T44.996
Mephenytoin	T42.0X1	T42.0X2	T42.0X3	T42.0X4	T42.0X5	T42.0X6
- with phenobarbital	T42.3X1	T42.3X2	T42.3X3	T42.3X4	T42.3X5	T42.3X6
Mephobarbital	T42.3X1	T42.3X2	T42.3X3	T42.3X4	T42.3X5	T42.3X6
Mephosfolan	T60.0X1	T60.0X2	T60.0X3	T60.0X4	--	--
Mepindolol	T44.7X1	T44.7X2	T44.7X3	T44.7X4	T44.7X5	T44.7X6
Mepiperphenidol	T44.3X1	T44.3X2	T44.3X3	T44.3X4	T44.3X5	T44.3X6
Mepitiostane	T38.7X1	T38.7X2	T38.7X3	T38.7X4	T38.7X5	T38.7X6
Mepivacaine	T41.3X1	T41.3X2	T41.3X3	T41.3X4	T41.3X5	T41.3X6
- epidural	T41.3X1	T41.3X2	T41.3X3	T41.3X4	T41.3X5	T41.3X6
Meprednisone	T38.0X1	T38.0X2	T38.0X3	T38.0X4	T38.0X5	T38.0X6
Meprobam	T43.591	T43.592	T43.593	T43.594	T43.595	T43.596
Meprobamate	T43.591	T43.592	T43.593	T43.594	T43.595	T43.596
Meproscillarin	T46.0X1	T46.0X2	T46.0X3	T46.0X4	T46.0X5	T46.0X6
Meprylcaine	T41.3X1	T41.3X2	T41.3X3	T41.3X4	T41.3X5	T41.3X6
Meptazinol	T39.8X1	T39.8X2	T39.8X3	T39.8X4	T39.8X5	T39.8X6
Mepyramine	T45.0X1	T45.0X2	T45.0X3	T45.0X4	T45.0X5	T45.0X6
Mequitazine	T43.3X1	T43.3X2	T43.3X3	T43.3X4	T43.3X5	T43.3X6
Meralluride	T50.2X1	T50.2X2	T50.2X3	T50.2X4	T50.2X5	T50.2X6
Merbaphen	T50.2X1	T50.2X2	T50.2X3	T50.2X4	T50.2X5	T50.2X6
Merbromin	T49.0X1	T49.0X2	T49.0X3	T49.0X4	T49.0X5	T49.0X6
Mercaptobenzothiazole salts	T49.0X1	T49.0X2	T49.0X3	T49.0X4	T49.0X5	T49.0X6
Mercaptomerin	T50.2X1	T50.2X2	T50.2X3	T50.2X4	T50.2X5	T50.2X6
Mercaptopurine	T45.1X1	T45.1X2	T45.1X3	T45.1X4	T45.1X5	T45.1X6
Mercumatilin	T50.2X1	T50.2X2	T50.2X3	T50.2X4	T50.2X5	T50.2X6
Mercuramide	T50.2X1	T50.2X2	T50.2X3	T50.2X4	T50.2X5	T50.2X6
Mercurochrome	T49.0X1	T49.0X2	T49.0X3	T49.0X4	T49.0X5	T49.0X6
Mercurophylline	T50.2X1	T50.2X2	T50.2X3	T50.2X4	T50.2X5	T50.2X6
Mercury, mercurial, mercuric, mercurous	T56.1X1	T56.1X2	T56.1X3	T56.1X4	--	--

Substance	Poisoning, Accidental (unintentional)	Poisoning, Intentional Self-harm	Poisoning, Assault	Poisoning, Undetermined	Adverse effect	Underdosing
(compounds) (cyanide) (fumes) (nonmedicinal) (vapor) NEC						
- ammoniated	T49.0X1	T49.0X2	T49.0X3	T49.0X4	T49.0X5	T49.0X6
- anti-infective						
- - local	T49.0X1	T49.0X2	T49.0X3	T49.0X4	T49.0X5	T49.0X6
- - systemic	T37.8X1	T37.8X2	T37.8X3	T37.8X4	T37.8X5	T37.8X6
- - topical	T49.0X1	T49.0X2	T49.0X3	T49.0X4	T49.0X5	T49.0X6
- chloride (ammoniated)	T49.0X1	T49.0X2	T49.0X3	T49.0X4	T49.0X5	T49.0X6
- - fungicide	T56.1X1	T56.1X2	T56.1X3	T56.1X4	--	--
- diuretic NEC	T50.2X1	T50.2X2	T50.2X3	T50.2X4	T50.2X5	T50.2X6
- fungicide	T56.1X1	T56.1X2	T56.1X3	T56.1X4	--	--
- organic (fungicide)	T56.1X1	T56.1X2	T56.1X3	T56.1X4	--	--
- oxide, yellow	T49.0X1	T49.0X2	T49.0X3	T49.0X4	T49.0X5	T49.0X6
Mersalyl	T50.2X1	T50.2X2	T50.2X3	T50.2X4	T50.2X5	T50.2X6
Merthiolate	T49.0X1	T49.0X2	T49.0X3	T49.0X4	T49.0X5	T49.0X6
- ophthalmic preparation	T49.5X1	T49.5X2	T49.5X3	T49.5X4	T49.5X5	T49.5X6
Meruvax	T50.B91	T50.B92	T50.B93	T50.B94	T50.B95	T50.B96
Mesalazine	T47.8X1	T47.8X2	T47.8X3	T47.8X4	T47.8X5	T47.8X6
Mescal buttons	T40.991	T40.992	T40.993	T40.994	--	--
Mescaline	T40.991	T40.992	T40.993	T40.994	--	--
Mesna	T48.4X1	T48.4X2	T48.4X3	T48.4X4	T48.4X5	T48.4X6
Mesoglycan	T46.6X1	T46.6X2	T46.6X3	T46.6X4	T46.6X5	T46.6X6
Mesoridazine	T43.3X1	T43.3X2	T43.3X3	T43.3X4	T43.3X5	T43.3X6
Mestanolone	T38.7X1	T38.7X2	T38.7X3	T38.7X4	T38.7X5	T38.7X6
Mesterolone	T38.7X1	T38.7X2	T38.7X3	T38.7X4	T38.7X5	T38.7X6
Mestranol	T38.5X1	T38.5X2	T38.5X3	T38.5X4	T38.5X5	T38.5X6
Mesulergine	T42.8X1	T42.8X2	T42.8X3	T42.8X4	T42.8X5	T42.8X6
Mesulfen	T49.0X1	T49.0X2	T49.0X3	T49.0X4	T49.0X5	T49.0X6
Mesuximide	T42.2X1	T42.2X2	T42.2X3	T42.2X4	T42.2X5	T42.2X6
Metabutethamine	T41.3X1	T41.3X2	T41.3X3	T41.3X4	T41.3X5	T41.3X6
Metactesylacetate	T49.0X1	T49.0X2	T49.0X3	T49.0X4	T49.0X5	T49.0X6
Metacycline	T36.4X1	T36.4X2	T36.4X3	T36.4X4	T36.4X5	T36.4X6
Metaldehyde (snail killer) NEC	T60.8X1	T60.8X2	T60.8X3	T60.8X4	--	--
Metals (heavy) (nonmedicinal)	T56.91	T56.92	T56.93	T56.94	--	--
- dust, fumes, or vapor NEC	T56.91	T56.92	T56.93	T56.94	--	--
- light NEC	T56.91	T56.92	T56.93	T56.94	--	--
- - dust, fumes, or vapor NEC	T56.91	T56.92	T56.93	T56.94	--	--
- specified NEC	T56.891	T56.892	T56.893	T56.894	--	--
- thallium	T56.811	T56.812	T56.813	T56.814	--	--
Metamfetamine	T43.621	T43.622	T43.623	T43.624	T43.625	T43.626
Metamizole sodium	T39.2X1	T39.2X2	T39.2X3	T39.2X4	T39.2X5	T39.2X6
Metampicillin	T36.0X1	T36.0X2	T36.0X3	T36.0X4	T36.0X5	T36.0X6
Metamucil	T47.4X1	T47.4X2	T47.4X3	T47.4X4	T47.4X5	T47.4X6
Metandienone	T38.7X1	T38.7X2	T38.7X3	T38.7X4	T38.7X5	T38.7X6
Metandrostenolone	T38.7X1	T38.7X2	T38.7X3	T38.7X4	T38.7X5	T38.7X6
Metaphen	T49.0X1	T49.0X2	T49.0X3	T49.0X4	T49.0X5	T49.0X6
Metaphos	T60.0X1	T60.0X2	T60.0X3	T60.0X4	--	--
Metapramine	T43.011	T43.012	T43.013	T43.014	T43.015	T43.016
Metaproterenol	T48.291	T48.292	T48.293	T48.294	T48.295	T48.296
Metaraminol	T44.4X1	T44.4X2	T44.4X3	T44.4X4	T44.4X5	T44.4X6
Metaxalone	T42.8X1	T42.8X2	T42.8X3	T42.8X4	T42.8X5	T42.8X6
Metenolone	T38.7X1	T38.7X2	T38.7X3	T38.7X4	T38.7X5	T38.7X6
Metergoline	T42.8X1	T42.8X2	T42.8X3	T42.8X4	T42.8X5	T42.8X6
Metescufylline	T46.991	T46.992	T46.993	T46.994	T46.995	T46.996
Metetoin	T42.0X1	T42.0X2	T42.0X3	T42.0X4	T42.0X5	T42.0X6
Metformin	T38.3X1	T38.3X2	T38.3X3	T38.3X4	T38.3X5	T38.3X6
Methacholine	T44.1X1	T44.1X2	T44.1X3	T44.1X4	T44.1X5	T44.1X6
Methacycline	T36.4X1	T36.4X2	T36.4X3	T36.4X4	T36.4X5	T36.4X6
Methadone	T40.3X1	T40.3X2	T40.3X3	T40.3X4	T40.3X5	T40.3X6
Methallenestril	T38.5X1	T38.5X2	T38.5X3	T38.5X4	T38.5X5	T38.5X6
Methallenoestril	T38.5X1	T38.5X2	T38.5X3	T38.5X4	T38.5X5	T38.5X6
Methamphetamine	T43.621	T43.622	T43.623	T43.624	T43.625	T43.626
Methampyrone	T39.2X1	T39.2X2	T39.2X3	T39.2X4	T39.2X5	T39.2X6
Methandienone	T38.7X1	T38.7X2	T38.7X3	T38.7X4	T38.7X5	T38.7X6
Methandriol	T38.7X1	T38.7X2	T38.7X3	T38.7X4	T38.7X5	T38.7X6

Substance	Poisoning, Accidental (unintentional)	Poisoning, Intentional Self-harm	Poisoning, Assault	Poisoning, Undetermined	Adverse effect	Underdosing
Methandrostenolone	T38.7X1	T38.7X2	T38.7X3	T38.7X4	T38.7X5	T38.7X6
Methane	T59.891	T59.892	T59.893	T59.894	--	--
Methanethiol	T59.891	T59.892	T59.893	T59.894	--	--
Methaniazide	T37.1X1	T37.1X2	T37.1X3	T37.1X4	T37.1X5	T37.1X6
Methanol (vapor)	T51.1X1	T51.1X2	T51.1X3	T51.1X4	--	--
Methantheline	T44.3X1	T44.3X2	T44.3X3	T44.3X4	T44.3X5	T44.3X6
Methanthelinium bromide	T44.3X1	T44.3X2	T44.3X3	T44.3X4	T44.3X5	T44.3X6
Methaphenilene	T45.0X1	T45.0X2	T45.0X3	T45.0X4	T45.0X5	T45.0X6
Methapyrilene	T45.0X1	T45.0X2	T45.0X3	T45.0X4	T45.0X5	T45.0X6
Methaqualone (compound)	T42.6X1	T42.6X2	T42.6X3	T42.6X4	T42.6X5	T42.6X6
Metharbital	T42.3X1	T42.3X2	T42.3X3	T42.3X4	T42.3X5	T42.3X6
Methazolamide	T50.2X1	T50.2X2	T50.2X3	T50.2X4	T50.2X5	T50.2X6
Methdilazine	T43.3X1	T43.3X2	T43.3X3	T43.3X4	T43.3X5	T43.3X6
Methedrine	T43.621	T43.622	T43.623	T43.624	T43.625	T43.626
Methenamine (mandelate)	T37.8X1	T37.8X2	T37.8X3	T37.8X4	T37.8X5	T37.8X6
Methenolone	T38.7X1	T38.7X2	T38.7X3	T38.7X4	T38.7X5	T38.7X6
Methergine	T48.0X1	T48.0X2	T48.0X3	T48.0X4	T48.0X5	T48.0X6
Methetoin	T42.0X1	T42.0X2	T42.0X3	T42.0X4	T42.0X5	T42.0X6
Methiacil	T38.2X1	T38.2X2	T38.2X3	T38.2X4	T38.2X5	T38.2X6
Methicillin	T36.0X1	T36.0X2	T36.0X3	T36.0X4	T36.0X5	T36.0X6
Methimazole	T38.2X1	T38.2X2	T38.2X3	T38.2X4	T38.2X5	T38.2X6
Methiodal sodium	T50.8X1	T50.8X2	T50.8X3	T50.8X4	T50.8X5	T50.8X6
Methionine	T50.991	T50.992	T50.993	T50.994	T50.995	T50.996
Methisazone	T37.5X1	T37.5X2	T37.5X3	T37.5X4	T37.5X5	T37.5X6
Methisoprinol	T37.5X1	T37.5X2	T37.5X3	T37.5X4	T37.5X5	T37.5X6
Methitural	T42.3X1	T42.3X2	T42.3X3	T42.3X4	T42.3X5	T42.3X6
Methixene	T44.3X1	T44.3X2	T44.3X3	T44.3X4	T44.3X5	T44.3X6
Methobarbital, methobarbitone	T42.3X1	T42.3X2	T42.3X3	T42.3X4	T42.3X5	T42.3X6
Methocarbamol	T42.8X1	T42.8X2	T42.8X3	T42.8X4	T42.8X5	T42.8X6
- skeletal muscle relaxant	T48.1X1	T48.1X2	T48.1X3	T48.1X4	T48.1X5	T48.1X6
Methohexital	T41.1X1	T41.1X2	T41.1X3	T41.1X4	T41.1X5	T41.1X6
Methohexitone	T41.1X1	T41.1X2	T41.1X3	T41.1X4	T41.1X5	T41.1X6
Methoin	T42.0X1	T42.0X2	T42.0X3	T42.0X4	T42.0X5	T42.0X6
Methopholine	T39.8X1	T39.8X2	T39.8X3	T39.8X4	T39.8X5	T39.8X6
Methopromazine	T43.3X1	T43.3X2	T43.3X3	T43.3X4	T43.3X5	T43.3X6
Methorate	T48.3X1	T48.3X2	T48.3X3	T48.3X4	T48.3X5	T48.3X6
Methoserpidine	T46.5X1	T46.5X2	T46.5X3	T46.5X4	T46.5X5	T46.5X6
Methotrexate	T45.1X1	T45.1X2	T45.1X3	T45.1X4	T45.1X5	T45.1X6
Methotrimeprazine	T43.3X1	T43.3X2	T43.3X3	T43.3X4	T43.3X5	T43.3X6
Methoxa-Dome	T49.3X1	T49.3X2	T49.3X3	T49.3X4	T49.3X5	T49.3X6
Methoxamine	T44.4X1	T44.4X2	T44.4X3	T44.4X4	T44.4X5	T44.4X6
Methoxsalen	T50.991	T50.992	T50.993	T50.994	T50.995	T50.996
Methoxyaniline	T65.3X1	T65.3X2	T65.3X3	T65.3X4	--	--
Methoxybenzyl penicillin	T36.0X1	T36.0X2	T36.0X3	T36.0X4	T36.0X5	T36.0X6
Methoxychlor	T53.7X1	T53.7X2	T53.7X3	T53.7X4	--	--
Methoxy-DDT	T53.7X1	T53.7X2	T53.7X3	T53.7X4	--	--
2-Methoxyethanol	T52.3X1	T52.3X2	T52.3X3	T52.3X4	--	--
Methoxyflurane	T41.0X1	T41.0X2	T41.0X3	T41.0X4	T41.0X5	T41.0X6
Methoxyphenamine	T48.6X1	T48.6X2	T48.6X3	T48.6X4	T48.6X5	T48.6X6
Methoxypromazine	T43.3X1	T43.3X2	T43.3X3	T43.3X4	T43.3X5	T43.3X6
5-Methoxypsoralen (5-MOP)	T50.991	T50.992	T50.993	T50.994	T50.995	T50.996
8-Methoxypsoralen (8-MOP)	T50.991	T50.992	T50.993	T50.994	T50.995	T50.996
Methscopolamine bromide	T44.3X1	T44.3X2	T44.3X3	T44.3X4	T44.3X5	T44.3X6
Methsuximide	T42.2X1	T42.2X2	T42.2X3	T42.2X4	T42.2X5	T42.2X6
Methyclothiazide	T50.2X1	T50.2X2	T50.2X3	T50.2X4	T50.2X5	T50.2X6
Methyl						
- acetate	T52.4X1	T52.4X2	T52.4X3	T52.4X4	--	--
- acetone	T52.4X1	T52.4X2	T52.4X3	T52.4X4	--	--
- acrylate	T65.891	T65.892	T65.893	T65.894	--	--
- alcohol	T51.1X1	T51.1X2	T51.1X3	T51.1X4	--	--
- aminophenol	T65.3X1	T65.3X2	T65.3X3	T65.3X4	--	--
- amphetamine	T43.621	T43.622	T43.623	T43.624	T43.625	T43.626
- androstanolone	T38.7X1	T38.7X2	T38.7X3	T38.7X4	T38.7X5	T38.7X6
- atropine	T44.3X1	T44.3X2	T44.3X3	T44.3X4	T44.3X5	T44.3X6
- benzene	T52.2X1	T52.2X2	T52.2X3	T52.2X4	--	--

Substance	Poisoning, Accidental (unintentional)	Poisoning, Intentional Self-harm	Poisoning, Assault	Poisoning, Undetermined	Adverse effect	Underdosing
- benzoate	T52.8X1	T52.8X2	T52.8X3	T52.8X4	--	--
- benzol	T52.2X1	T52.2X2	T52.2X3	T52.2X4	--	--
- bromide (gas)	T59.891	T59.892	T59.893	T59.894	--	--
- - fumigant	T60.8X1	T60.8X2	T60.8X3	T60.8X4	--	--
- butanol	T51.3X1	T51.3X2	T51.3X3	T51.3X4	--	--
- carbinol	T51.1X1	T51.1X2	T51.1X3	T51.1X4	--	--
- carbonate	T52.8X1	T52.8X2	T52.8X3	T52.8X4	--	--
- CCNU	T45.1X1	T45.1X2	T45.1X3	T45.1X4	T45.1X5	T45.1X6
- cellosolve	T52.91	T52.92	T52.93	T52.94	--	--
- cellulose	T47.4X1	T47.4X2	T47.4X3	T47.4X4	T47.4X5	T47.4X6
- chloride (gas)	T59.891	T59.892	T59.893	T59.894	--	--
- chloroformate	T59.3X1	T59.3X2	T59.3X3	T59.3X4	--	--
- cyclohexane	T52.8X1	T52.8X2	T52.8X3	T52.8X4	--	--
- cyclohexanol	T51.8X1	T51.8X2	T51.8X3	T51.8X4	--	--
- cyclohexanone	T52.8X1	T52.8X2	T52.8X3	T52.8X4	--	--
- cyclohexyl acetate	T52.8X1	T52.8X2	T52.8X3	T52.8X4	--	--
- demeton	T60.0X1	T60.0X2	T60.0X3	T60.0X4	--	--
- dihydromorphinone	T40.2X1	T40.2X2	T40.2X3	T40.2X4	T40.2X5	T40.2X6
- ergometrine	T48.0X1	T48.0X2	T48.0X3	T48.0X4	T48.0X5	T48.0X6
- ergonovine	T48.0X1	T48.0X2	T48.0X3	T48.0X4	T48.0X5	T48.0X6
- ethyl ketone	T52.4X1	T52.4X2	T52.4X3	T52.4X4	--	--
- glucamine antimonate	T37.8X1	T37.8X2	T37.8X3	T37.8X4	T37.8X5	T37.8X6
- hydrazine	T65.891	T65.892	T65.893	T65.894	--	--
- iodide	T65.891	T65.892	T65.893	T65.894	--	--
- isobutyl ketone	T52.4X1	T52.4X2	T52.4X3	T52.4X4	--	--
- isothiocyanate	T60.3X1	T60.3X2	T60.3X3	T60.3X4	--	--
- mercaptan	T59.891	T59.892	T59.893	T59.894	--	--
- morphine NEC	T40.2X1	T40.2X2	T40.2X3	T40.2X4	T40.2X5	T40.2X6
- nicotinate	T49.4X1	T49.4X2	T49.4X3	T49.4X4	T49.4X5	T49.4X6
- paraben	T49.0X1	T49.0X2	T49.0X3	T49.0X4	T49.0X5	T49.0X6
- parafynol	T42.6X1	T42.6X2	T42.6X3	T42.6X4	T42.6X5	T42.6X6
- parathion	T60.0X1	T60.0X2	T60.0X3	T60.0X4	--	--
- peridol	T43.4X1	T43.4X2	T43.4X3	T43.4X4	T43.4X5	T43.4X6
- phenidate	T43.631	T43.632	T43.633	T43.634	T43.635	T43.636
- prednisolone	T38.0X1	T38.0X2	T38.0X3	T38.0X4	T38.0X5	T38.0X6
- - ENT agent	T49.6X1	T49.6X2	T49.6X3	T49.6X4	T49.6X5	T49.6X6
- - ophthalmic preparation	T49.5X1	T49.5X2	T49.5X3	T49.5X4	T49.5X5	T49.5X6
- - topical NEC	T49.0X1	T49.0X2	T49.0X3	T49.0X4	T49.0X5	T49.0X6
- propylcarbinol	T51.3X1	T51.3X2	T51.3X3	T51.3X4	--	--
- rosaniline NEC	T49.0X1	T49.0X2	T49.0X3	T49.0X4	T49.0X5	T49.0X6
- salicylate	T49.2X1	T49.2X2	T49.2X3	T49.2X4	T49.2X5	T49.2X6
- sulfate (fumes)	T59.891	T59.892	T59.893	T59.894	--	--
- - liquid	T52.8X1	T52.8X2	T52.8X3	T52.8X4	--	--
- sulfonal	T42.6X1	T42.6X2	T42.6X3	T42.6X4	T42.6X5	T42.6X6
- testosterone	T38.7X1	T38.7X2	T38.7X3	T38.7X4	T38.7X5	T38.7X6
- thiouracil	T38.2X1	T38.2X2	T38.2X3	T38.2X4	T38.2X5	T38.2X6
Methylamphetamine	T43.621	T43.622	T43.623	T43.624	T43.625	T43.626
Methylated spirit	T51.1X1	T51.1X2	T51.1X3	T51.1X4	--	--
Methylatropine nitrate	T44.3X1	T44.3X2	T44.3X3	T44.3X4	T44.3X5	T44.3X6
Methylbenactyzium bromide	T44.3X1	T44.3X2	T44.3X3	T44.3X4	T44.3X5	T44.3X6
Methylbenzethonium chloride	T49.0X1	T49.0X2	T49.0X3	T49.0X4	T49.0X5	T49.0X6
Methylcellulose	T47.4X1	T47.4X2	T47.4X3	T47.4X4	T47.4X5	T47.4X6
- laxative	T47.4X1	T47.4X2	T47.4X3	T47.4X4	T47.4X5	T47.4X6
Methylchlorophenoxy-acetic acid	T60.3X1	T60.3X2	T60.3X3	T60.3X4	--	--
Methyldopa	T46.5X1	T46.5X2	T46.5X3	T46.5X4	T46.5X5	T46.5X6
Methyldopate	T46.5X1	T46.5X2	T46.5X3	T46.5X4	T46.5X5	T46.5X6
Methylene						
- blue	T50.6X1	T50.6X2	T50.6X3	T50.6X4	T50.6X5	T50.6X6
- chloride or dichloride (solvent) NEC	T53.4X1	T53.4X2	T53.4X3	T53.4X4	--	--
Methylenedioxyamphetamine	T43.621	T43.622	T43.623	T43.624	T43.625	T43.626
Methylenedioxymethamphetamine	T43.621	T43.622	T43.623	T43.624	T43.625	T43.626
Methylergometrine	T48.0X1	T48.0X2	T48.0X3	T48.0X4	T48.0X5	T48.0X6
Methylergonovine	T48.0X1	T48.0X2	T48.0X3	T48.0X4	T48.0X5	T48.0X6
Methylestrenolone	T38.5X1	T38.5X2	T38.5X3	T38.5X4	T38.5X5	T38.5X6
Methylethyl cellulose	T50.991	T50.992	T50.993	T50.994	T50.995	T50.996

Substance	Poisoning, Accidental (unintentional)	Poisoning, Intentional Self-harm	Poisoning, Assault	Poisoning, Undetermined	Adverse effect	Underdosing
Methylhexabital	T42.3X1	T42.3X2	T42.3X3	T42.3X4	T42.3X5	T42.3X6
Methylmorphine	T40.2X1	T40.2X2	T40.2X3	T40.2X4	T40.2X5	T40.2X6
Methylparaben (ophthalmic)	T49.5X1	T49.5X2	T49.5X3	T49.5X4	T49.5X5	T49.5X6
Methylparafynol	T42.6X1	T42.6X2	T42.6X3	T42.6X4	T42.6X5	T42.6X6
Methylpentynol, methylpenthynol	T42.6X1	T42.6X2	T42.6X3	T42.6X4	T42.6X5	T42.6X6
Methylphenidate	T43.631	T43.632	T43.633	T43.634	T43.635	T43.636
Methylphenobarbital	T42.3X1	T42.3X2	T42.3X3	T42.3X4	T42.3X5	T42.3X6
Methylpolysiloxane	T47.1X1	T47.1X2	T47.1X3	T47.1X4	T47.1X5	T47.1X6
Methylprednisolone—see Methyl, prednisolone						
Methylrosaniline	T49.0X1	T49.0X2	T49.0X3	T49.0X4	T49.0X5	T49.0X6
Methylrosanilinium chloride	T49.0X1	T49.0X2	T49.0X3	T49.0X4	T49.0X5	T49.0X6
Methyltestosterone	T38.7X1	T38.7X2	T38.7X3	T38.7X4	T38.7X5	T38.7X6
Methylthionine chloride	T50.6X1	T50.6X2	T50.6X3	T50.6X4	T50.6X5	T50.6X6
Methylthioninium chloride	T50.6X1	T50.6X2	T50.6X3	T50.6X4	T50.6X5	T50.6X6
Methylthiouracil	T38.2X1	T38.2X2	T38.2X3	T38.2X4	T38.2X5	T38.2X6
Methyprylon	T42.6X1	T42.6X2	T42.6X3	T42.6X4	T42.6X5	T42.6X6
Methysergide	T46.5X1	T46.5X2	T46.5X3	T46.5X4	T46.5X5	T46.5X6
Metiamide	T47.1X1	T47.1X2	T47.1X3	T47.1X4	T47.1X5	T47.1X6
Meticillin	T36.0X1	T36.0X2	T36.0X3	T36.0X4	T36.0X5	T36.0X6
Meticrane	T50.2X1	T50.2X2	T50.2X3	T50.2X4	T50.2X5	T50.2X6
Metildigoxin	T46.0X1	T46.0X2	T46.0X3	T46.0X4	T46.0X5	T46.0X6
Metipranolol	T49.5X1	T49.5X2	T49.5X3	T49.5X4	T49.5X5	T49.5X6
Metirosine	T46.5X1	T46.5X2	T46.5X3	T46.5X4	T46.5X5	T46.5X6
Metisazone	T37.5X1	T37.5X2	T37.5X3	T37.5X4	T37.5X5	T37.5X6
Metixene	T44.3X1	T44.3X2	T44.3X3	T44.3X4	T44.3X5	T44.3X6
Metizoline	T48.5X1	T48.5X2	T48.5X3	T48.5X4	T48.5X5	T48.5X6
Metoclopramide	T45.0X1	T45.0X2	T45.0X3	T45.0X4	T45.0X5	T45.0X6
Metofenazate	T43.3X1	T43.3X2	T43.3X3	T43.3X4	T43.3X5	T43.3X6
Metofoline	T39.8X1	T39.8X2	T39.8X3	T39.8X4	T39.8X5	T39.8X6
Metolazone	T50.2X1	T50.2X2	T50.2X3	T50.2X4	T50.2X5	T50.2X6
Metopon	T40.2X1	T40.2X2	T40.2X3	T40.2X4	T40.2X5	T40.2X6
Metoprine	T45.1X1	T45.1X2	T45.1X3	T45.1X4	T45.1X5	T45.1X6
Metoprolol	T44.7X1	T44.7X2	T44.7X3	T44.7X4	T44.7X5	T44.7X6
Metrifonate	T60.0X1	T60.0X2	T60.0X3	T60.0X4	--	--
Metrizamide	T50.8X1	T50.8X2	T50.8X3	T50.8X4	T50.8X5	T50.8X6
Metrizoic acid	T50.8X1	T50.8X2	T50.8X3	T50.8X4	T50.8X5	T50.8X6
Metronidazole	T37.8X1	T37.8X2	T37.8X3	T37.8X4	T37.8X5	T37.8X6
Metycaine	T41.3X1	T41.3X2	T41.3X3	T41.3X4	T41.3X5	T41.3X6
- infiltration (subcutaneous)	T41.3X1	T41.3X2	T41.3X3	T41.3X4	T41.3X5	T41.3X6
- nerve block (peripheral) (plexus)	T41.3X1	T41.3X2	T41.3X3	T41.3X4	T41.3X5	T41.3X6
- topical (surface)	T41.3X1	T41.3X2	T41.3X3	T41.3X4	T41.3X5	T41.3X6
Metyrapone	T50.8X1	T50.8X2	T50.8X3	T50.8X4	T50.8X5	T50.8X6
Mevinphos	T60.0X1	T60.0X2	T60.0X3	T60.0X4	--	--
Mexazolam	T42.4X1	T42.4X2	T42.4X3	T42.4X4	T42.4X5	T42.4X6
Mexenone	T49.3X1	T49.3X2	T49.3X3	T49.3X4	T49.3X5	T49.3X6
Mexiletine	T46.2X1	T46.2X2	T46.2X3	T46.2X4	T46.2X5	T46.2X6
Mezereon	T62.2X1	T62.2X2	T62.2X3	T62.2X4	--	--
- berries	T62.1X1	T62.1X2	T62.1X3	T62.1X4	--	--
Mezlocillin	T36.0X1	T36.0X2	T36.0X3	T36.0X4	T36.0X5	T36.0X6
Mianserin	T43.021	T43.022	T43.023	T43.024	T43.025	T43.026
Micatin	T49.0X1	T49.0X2	T49.0X3	T49.0X4	T49.0X5	T49.0X6
Miconazole	T49.0X1	T49.0X2	T49.0X3	T49.0X4	T49.0X5	T49.0X6
Micronomicin	T36.5X1	T36.5X2	T36.5X3	T36.5X4	T36.5X5	T36.5X6
Midazolam	T42.4X1	T42.4X2	T42.4X3	T42.4X4	T42.4X5	T42.4X6
Midecamycin	T36.3X1	T36.3X2	T36.3X3	T36.3X4	T36.3X5	T36.3X6
Mifepristone	T38.6X1	T38.6X2	T38.6X3	T38.6X4	T38.6X5	T38.6X6
Milk of magnesia	T47.1X1	T47.1X2	T47.1X3	T47.1X4	T47.1X5	T47.1X6
Millipede (tropical) (venomous)	T63.411	T63.412	T63.413	T63.414	--	--
Miltown	T43.591	T43.592	T43.593	T43.594	T43.595	T43.596
Milverine	T44.3X1	T44.3X2	T44.3X3	T44.3X4	T44.3X5	T44.3X6
Minaprine	T43.291	T43.292	T43.293	T43.294	T43.295	T43.296
Minaxolone	T41.291	T41.292	T41.293	T41.294	T41.295	T41.296
Mineral						
- acids	T54.2X1	T54.2X2	T54.2X3	T54.2X4	--	--
- oil (laxative) (medicinal)	T47.4X1	T47.4X2	T47.4X3	T47.4X4	T47.4X5	T47.4X6

Substance	Poisoning, Accidental (unintentional)	Poisoning, Intentional Self-harm	Poisoning, Assault	Poisoning, Undetermined	Adverse effect	Underdosing
- - emulsion	T47.2X1	T47.2X2	T47.2X3	T47.2X4	T47.2X5	T47.2X6
- - nonmedicinal	T52.0X1	T52.0X2	T52.0X3	T52.0X4	--	--
- - topical	T49.3X1	T49.3X2	T49.3X3	T49.3X4	T49.3X5	T49.3X6
- salt NEC	T50.3X1	T50.3X2	T50.3X3	T50.3X4	T50.3X5	T50.3X6
- spirits	T52.0X1	T52.0X2	T52.0X3	T52.0X4	--	--
Mineralocorticosteroid	T50.0X1	T50.0X2	T50.0X3	T50.0X4	T50.0X5	T50.0X6
Minocycline	T36.4X1	T36.4X2	T36.4X3	T36.4X4	T36.4X5	T36.4X6
Minoxidil	T46.7X1	T46.7X2	T46.7X3	T46.7X4	T46.7X5	T46.7X6
Miokamycin	T36.3X1	T36.3X2	T36.3X3	T36.3X4	T36.3X5	T36.3X6
Miotic drug	T49.5X1	T49.5X2	T49.5X3	T49.5X4	T49.5X5	T49.5X6
Mipafox	T60.0X1	T60.0X2	T60.0X3	T60.0X4	--	--
Mirex	T60.1X1	T60.1X2	T60.1X3	T60.1X4	--	--
Mirtazapine	T43.021	T43.022	T43.023	T43.024	T43.025	T43.026
Misonidazole	T37.3X1	T37.3X2	T37.3X3	T37.3X4	T37.3X5	T37.3X6
Misoprostol	T47.1X1	T47.1X2	T47.1X3	T47.1X4	T47.1X5	T47.1X6
Mithramycin	T45.1X1	T45.1X2	T45.1X3	T45.1X4	T45.1X5	T45.1X6
Mitobronitol	T45.1X1	T45.1X2	T45.1X3	T45.1X4	T45.1X5	T45.1X6
Mitoguazone	T45.1X1	T45.1X2	T45.1X3	T45.1X4	T45.1X5	T45.1X6
Mitolactol	T45.1X1	T45.1X2	T45.1X3	T45.1X4	T45.1X5	T45.1X6
Mitomycin	T45.1X1	T45.1X2	T45.1X3	T45.1X4	T45.1X5	T45.1X6
Mitopodozide	T45.1X1	T45.1X2	T45.1X3	T45.1X4	T45.1X5	T45.1X6
Mitotane	T45.1X1	T45.1X2	T45.1X3	T45.1X4	T45.1X5	T45.1X6
Mitoxantrone	T45.1X1	T45.1X2	T45.1X3	T45.1X4	T45.1X5	T45.1X6
Mivacurium chloride	T48.1X1	T48.1X2	T48.1X3	T48.1X4	T48.1X5	T48.1X6
Miyari bacteria	T47.6X1	T47.6X2	T47.6X3	T47.6X4	T47.6X5	T47.6X6
Moclobemide	T43.1X1	T43.1X2	T43.1X3	T43.1X4	T43.1X5	T43.1X6
Moderil	T46.5X1	T46.5X2	T46.5X3	T46.5X4	T46.5X5	T46.5X6
Mofebutazone	T39.2X1	T39.2X2	T39.2X3	T39.2X4	T39.2X5	T39.2X6
Mogadon—see Nitrazepam						
Molindone	T43.591	T43.592	T43.593	T43.594	T43.595	T43.596
Molsidomine	T46.3X1	T46.3X2	T46.3X3	T46.3X4	T46.3X5	T46.3X6
Mometasone	T49.0X1	T49.0X2	T49.0X3	T49.0X4	T49.0X5	T49.0X6
Monistat	T49.0X1	T49.0X2	T49.0X3	T49.0X4	T49.0X5	T49.0X6
Monkshood	T62.2X1	T62.2X2	T62.2X3	T62.2X4	--	--
Monoamine oxidase inhibitor NEC	T43.1X1	T43.1X2	T43.1X3	T43.1X4	T43.1X5	T43.1X6
- hydrazine	T43.1X1	T43.1X2	T43.1X3	T43.1X4	T43.1X5	T43.1X6
Monobenzone	T49.4X1	T49.4X2	T49.4X3	T49.4X4	T49.4X5	T49.4X6
Monochloroacetic acid	T60.3X1	T60.3X2	T60.3X3	T60.3X4	--	--
Monochlorobenzene	T53.7X1	T53.7X2	T53.7X3	T53.7X4	--	--
Monoethanolamine	T46.8X1	T46.8X2	T46.8X3	T46.8X4	T46.8X5	T46.8X6
- oleate	T46.8X1	T46.8X2	T46.8X3	T46.8X4	T46.8X5	T46.8X6
Monooctanoin	T50.991	T50.992	T50.993	T50.994	T50.995	T50.996
Monophenylbutazone	T39.2X1	T39.2X2	T39.2X3	T39.2X4	T39.2X5	T39.2X6
Monosodium glutamate	T65.891	T65.892	T65.893	T65.894	--	--
Monosulfiram	T49.0X1	T49.0X2	T49.0X3	T49.0X4	T49.0X5	T49.0X6
Monoxide, carbon—see Carbon, monoxide						
Monoxidine hydrochloride	T46.1X1	T46.1X2	T46.1X3	T46.1X4	T46.1X5	T46.1X6
Monuron	T60.3X1	T60.3X2	T60.3X3	T60.3X4	--	--
Moperone	T43.4X1	T43.4X2	T43.4X3	T43.4X4	T43.4X5	T43.4X6
Mopidamol	T45.1X1	T45.1X2	T45.1X3	T45.1X4	T45.1X5	T45.1X6
MOPP (mechloreth-amine + vincristine + prednisone + procarba-zine)	T45.1X1	T45.1X2	T45.1X3	T45.1X4	T45.1X5	T45.1X6
Morfin	T40.2X1	T40.2X2	T40.2X3	T40.2X4	T40.2X5	T40.2X6
Morinamide	T37.1X1	T37.1X2	T37.1X3	T37.1X4	T37.1X5	T37.1X6
Morning glory seeds	T40.991	T40.992	T40.993	T40.994	--	--
Moroxydine	T37.5X1	T37.5X2	T37.5X3	T37.5X4	T37.5X5	T37.5X6
Morphazinamide	T37.1X1	T37.1X2	T37.1X3	T37.1X4	T37.1X5	T37.1X6
Morphine	T40.2X1	T40.2X2	T40.2X3	T40.2X4	T40.2X5	T40.2X6
- antagonist	T50.7X1	T50.7X2	T50.7X3	T50.7X4	T50.7X5	T50.7X6
Morpholinylethylmorphine	T40.2X1	T40.2X2	T40.2X3	T40.2X4	--	--
Morsuximide	T42.2X1	T42.2X2	T42.2X3	T42.2X4	T42.2X5	T42.2X6
Mosapramine	T43.591	T43.592	T43.593	T43.594	T43.595	T43.596
Moth balls—see also Pesticides	T60.2X1	T60.2X2	T60.2X3	T60.2X4	--	--
- naphthalene	T60.2X1	T60.2X2	T60.2X3	T60.2X4	--	--
- paradichlorobenzene	T60.1X1	T60.1X2	T60.1X3	T60.1X4	--	--

Substance	Poisoning, Accidental (unintentional)	Poisoning, Intentional Self-harm	Poisoning, Assault	Poisoning, Undetermined	Adverse effect	Underdosing
Motor exhaust gas	T58.01	T58.02	T58.03	T58.04	--	--
Mouthwash (antiseptic) (zinc chloride)	T49.6X1	T49.6X2	T49.6X3	T49.6X4	T49.6X5	T49.6X6
Moxastine	T45.0X1	T45.0X2	T45.0X3	T45.0X4	T45.0X5	T45.0X6
Moxaverine	T44.3X1	T44.3X2	T44.3X3	T44.3X4	T44.3X5	T44.3X6
Moxisylyte	T46.7X1	T46.7X2	T46.7X3	T46.7X4	T46.7X5	T46.7X6
Mucilage, plant	T47.4X1	T47.4X2	T47.4X3	T47.4X4	T47.4X5	T47.4X6
Mucolytic drug	T48.4X1	T48.4X2	T48.4X3	T48.4X4	T48.4X5	T48.4X6
Mucomyst	T48.4X1	T48.4X2	T48.4X3	T48.4X4	T48.4X5	T48.4X6
Mucous membrane agents (external)	T49.91	T49.92	T49.93	T49.94	T49.95	T49.96
- specified NEC	T49.8X1	T49.8X2	T49.8X3	T49.8X4	T49.8X5	T49.8X6
Mumps						
- immune globulin (human)	T50.Z11	T50.Z12	T50.Z13	T50.Z14	T50.Z15	T50.Z16
- skin test antigen	T50.8X1	T50.8X2	T50.8X3	T50.8X4	T50.8X5	T50.8X6
- vaccine	T50.B91	T50.B92	T50.B93	T50.B94	T50.B95	T50.B96
Mumpsvax	T50.B91	T50.B92	T50.B93	T50.B94	T50.B95	T50.B96
Mupirocin	T49.0X1	T49.0X2	T49.0X3	T49.0X4	T49.0X5	T49.0X6
Muriatic acid—see Hydrochloric acid						
Muromonab-CD3	T45.1X1	T45.1X2	T45.1X3	T45.1X4	T45.1X5	T45.1X6
Muscle-action drug NEC	T48.201	T48.202	T48.203	T48.204	T48.205	T48.206
Muscle affecting agents NEC	T48.201	T48.202	T48.203	T48.204	T48.205	T48.206
- oxytocic	T48.0X1	T48.0X2	T48.0X3	T48.0X4	T48.0X5	T48.0X6
- relaxants	T48.201	T48.202	T48.203	T48.204	T48.205	T48.206
- - central nervous system	T42.8X1	T42.8X2	T42.8X3	T42.8X4	T42.8X5	T42.8X6
- - skeletal	T48.1X1	T48.1X2	T48.1X3	T48.1X4	T48.1X5	T48.1X6
- - smooth	T44.3X1	T44.3X2	T44.3X3	T44.3X4	T44.3X5	T44.3X6
Muscle relaxant—see Relaxant, muscle						
Muscle-tone depressant, central NEC	T42.8X1	T42.8X2	T42.8X3	T42.8X4	T42.8X5	T42.8X6
- specified NEC	T42.8X1	T42.8X2	T42.8X3	T42.8X4	T42.8X5	T42.8X6
Mushroom, noxious	T62.0X1	T62.0X2	T62.0X3	T62.0X4	--	--
Mussel, noxious	T61.781	T61.782	T61.783	T61.784	--	--
Mustard (emetic)	T47.7X1	T47.7X2	T47.7X3	T47.7X4	T47.7X5	T47.7X6
- black	T47.7X1	T47.7X2	T47.7X3	T47.7X4	T47.7X5	T47.7X6
- gas, not in war	T59.91	T59.92	T59.93	T59.94	--	--
- nitrogen	T45.1X1	T45.1X2	T45.1X3	T45.1X4	T45.1X5	T45.1X6
Mustine	T45.1X1	T45.1X2	T45.1X3	T45.1X4	T45.1X5	T45.1X6
M-vac	T45.1X1	T45.1X2	T45.1X3	T45.1X4	T45.1X5	T45.1X6
Mycifradin	T36.5X1	T36.5X2	T36.5X3	T36.5X4	T36.5X5	T36.5X6
- topical	T49.0X1	T49.0X2	T49.0X3	T49.0X4	T49.0X5	T49.0X6
Mycitracin	T36.8X1	T36.8X2	T36.8X3	T36.8X4	T36.8X5	T36.8X6
- ophthalmic preparation	T49.5X1	T49.5X2	T49.5X3	T49.5X4	T49.5X5	T49.5X6
Mycostatin	T36.7X1	T36.7X2	T36.7X3	T36.7X4	T36.7X5	T36.7X6
- topical	T49.0X1	T49.0X2	T49.0X3	T49.0X4	T49.0X5	T49.0X6
Mycotoxins	T64.81	T64.82	T64.83	T64.84	--	--
- aflatoxin	T64.01	T64.02	T64.03	T64.04	--	--
- specified NEC	T64.81	T64.82	T64.83	T64.84	--	--
Mydriacyl	T44.3X1	T44.3X2	T44.3X3	T44.3X4	T44.3X5	T44.3X6
Mydriatic drug	T49.5X1	T49.5X2	T49.5X3	T49.5X4	T49.5X5	T49.5X6
Myelobromal	T45.1X1	T45.1X2	T45.1X3	T45.1X4	T45.1X5	T45.1X6
Myleran	T45.1X1	T45.1X2	T45.1X3	T45.1X4	T45.1X5	T45.1X6
Myochrysin (e)	T39.2X1	T39.2X2	T39.2X3	T39.2X4	T39.2X5	T39.2X6
Myoneural blocking agents	T48.1X1	T48.1X2	T48.1X3	T48.1X4	T48.1X5	T48.1X6
Myralact	T49.0X1	T49.0X2	T49.0X3	T49.0X4	T49.0X5	T49.0X6
Myristica fragrans	T62.2X1	T62.2X2	T62.2X3	T62.2X4	--	--
Myristicin	T65.891	T65.892	T65.893	T65.894	--	--
Mysoline	T42.3X1	T42.3X2	T42.3X3	T42.3X4	T42.3X5	T42.3X6
Nabilone	T40.7X1	T40.7X2	T40.7X3	T40.7X4	T40.7X5	T40.7X6
Nabumetone	T39.391	T39.392	T39.393	T39.394	T39.395	T39.396
Nadolol	T44.7X1	T44.7X2	T44.7X3	T44.7X4	T44.7X5	T44.7X6
Nafcillin	T36.0X1	T36.0X2	T36.0X3	T36.0X4	T36.0X5	T36.0X6
Nafoxidine	T38.6X1	T38.6X2	T38.6X3	T38.6X4	T38.6X5	T38.6X6
Naftazone	T46.991	T46.992	T46.993	T46.994	T46.995	T46.996
Naftidrofuryl (oxalate)	T46.7X1	T46.7X2	T46.7X3	T46.7X4	T46.7X5	T46.7X6
Naftifine	T49.0X1	T49.0X2	T49.0X3	T49.0X4	T49.0X5	T49.0X6
Nail polish remover	T52.91	T52.92	T52.93	T52.94	--	--
Nalbuphine	T40.4X1	T40.4X2	T40.4X3	T40.4X4	T40.4X5	T40.4X6

TABLE OF DRUGS AND CHEMICALS

Substance	Poisoning, Accidental (unintentional)	Poisoning, Intentional Self-harm	Poisoning, Assault	Poisoning, Undetermined	Adverse effect	Underdosing
Naled	T60.0X1	T60.0X2	T60.0X3	T60.0X4	--	--
Nalidixic acid	T37.8X1	T37.8X2	T37.8X3	T37.8X4	T37.8X5	T37.8X6
Nalorphine	T50.7X1	T50.7X2	T50.7X3	T50.7X4	T50.7X5	T50.7X6
Naloxone	T50.7X1	T50.7X2	T50.7X3	T50.7X4	T50.7X5	T50.7X6
Naltrexone	T50.7X1	T50.7X2	T50.7X3	T50.7X4	T50.7X5	T50.7X6
Namenda	T43.8X1	T43.8X2	T43.8X3	T43.8X4	T43.8X5	T43.8X6
Nandrolone	T38.7X1	T38.7X2	T38.7X3	T38.7X4	T38.7X5	T38.7X6
Naphazoline	T48.5X1	T48.5X2	T48.5X3	T48.5X4	T48.5X5	T48.5X6
Naphtha (painters') (petroleum)	T52.0X1	T52.0X2	T52.0X3	T52.0X4	--	--
- solvent	T52.0X1	T52.0X2	T52.0X3	T52.0X4	--	--
- vapor	T52.0X1	T52.0X2	T52.0X3	T52.0X4	--	--
Naphthalene (non-chlorinated)	T60.2X1	T60.2X2	T60.2X3	T60.2X4	--	--
- chlorinated	T60.1X1	T60.1X2	T60.1X3	T60.1X4	--	--
- - vapor	T60.1X1	T60.1X2	T60.1X3	T60.1X4	--	--
- insecticide or moth repellent	T60.2X1	T60.2X2	T60.2X3	T60.2X4	--	--
- - chlorinated	T60.1X1	T60.1X2	T60.1X3	T60.1X4	--	--
- vapor	T60.2X1	T60.2X2	T60.2X3	T60.2X4	--	--
- - chlorinated	T60.1X1	T60.1X2	T60.1X3	T60.1X4	--	--
Naphthol	T65.891	T65.892	T65.893	T65.894	--	--
Naphthylamine	T65.891	T65.892	T65.893	T65.894	--	--
Naphthylthiourea (ANTU)	T60.4X1	T60.4X2	T60.4X3	T60.4X4	--	--
Naprosyn—see Naproxen						
Naproxen	T39.311	T39.312	T39.313	T39.314	T39.315	T39.316
Narcotic (drug)	T40.601	T40.602	T40.603	T40.604	T40.605	T40.606
- analgesic NEC	T40.601	T40.602	T40.603	T40.604	T40.605	T40.606
- antagonist	T50.7X1	T50.7X2	T50.7X3	T50.7X4	T50.7X5	T50.7X6
- specified NEC	T40.691	T40.692	T40.693	T40.694	T40.695	T40.696
- synthetic	T40.4X1	T40.4X2	T40.4X3	T40.4X4	T40.4X5	T40.4X6
Narcotine	T48.3X1	T48.3X2	T48.3X3	T48.3X4	T48.3X5	T48.3X6
Nardil	T43.1X1	T43.1X2	T43.1X3	T43.1X4	T43.1X5	T43.1X6
Nasal drug NEC	T49.6X1	T49.6X2	T49.6X3	T49.6X4	T49.6X5	T49.6X6
Natamycin	T49.0X1	T49.0X2	T49.0X3	T49.0X4	T49.0X5	T49.0X6
Natrium cyanide—see Cyanide (s)						
Natural						
- blood (product)	T45.8X1	T45.8X2	T45.8X3	T45.8X4	T45.8X5	T45.8X6
- gas (piped)	T59.891	T59.892	T59.893	T59.894	--	--
- - incomplete combustion	T58.11	T58.12	T58.13	T58.14	--	--
Nealbarbital	T42.3X1	T42.3X2	T42.3X3	T42.3X4	T42.3X5	T42.3X6
Nectadon	T48.3X1	T48.3X2	T48.3X3	T48.3X4	T48.3X5	T48.3X6
Nedocromil	T48.6X1	T48.6X2	T48.6X3	T48.6X4	T48.6X5	T48.6X6
Nefopam	T39.8X1	T39.8X2	T39.8X3	T39.8X4	T39.8X5	T39.8X6
Nematocyst (sting)	T63.691	T63.692	T63.693	T63.694	--	--
Nembutal	T42.3X1	T42.3X2	T42.3X3	T42.3X4	T42.3X5	T42.3X6
Nemonapride	T43.591	T43.592	T43.593	T43.594	T43.595	T43.596
Neoarsphenamine	T37.8X1	T37.8X2	T37.8X3	T37.8X4	T37.8X5	T37.8X6
Neocinchophen	T50.4X1	T50.4X2	T50.4X3	T50.4X4	T50.4X5	T50.4X6
Neomycin (derivatives)	T36.5X1	T36.5X2	T36.5X3	T36.5X4	T36.5X5	T36.5X6
- with						
- - bacitracin	T49.0X1	T49.0X2	T49.0X3	T49.0X4	T49.0X5	T49.0X6
- - neostigmine	T44.0X1	T44.0X2	T44.0X3	T44.0X4	T44.0X5	T44.0X6
- ENT agent	T49.6X1	T49.6X2	T49.6X3	T49.6X4	T49.6X5	T49.6X6
- ophthalmic preparation	T49.5X1	T49.5X2	T49.5X3	T49.5X4	T49.5X5	T49.5X6
- topical NEC	T49.0X1	T49.0X2	T49.0X3	T49.0X4	T49.0X5	T49.0X6
Neonal	T42.3X1	T42.3X2	T42.3X3	T42.3X4	T42.3X5	T42.3X6
Neoprontosil	T37.0X1	T37.0X2	T37.0X3	T37.0X4	T37.0X5	T37.0X6
Neosalvarsan	T37.8X1	T37.8X2	T37.8X3	T37.8X4	T37.8X5	T37.8X6
Neosilversalvarsan	T37.8X1	T37.8X2	T37.8X3	T37.8X4	T37.8X5	T37.8X6
Neosporin	T36.8X1	T36.8X2	T36.8X3	T36.8X4	T36.8X5	T36.8X6
- ENT agent	T49.6X1	T49.6X2	T49.6X3	T49.6X4	T49.6X5	T49.6X6
- opthalmic preparation	T49.5X1	T49.5X2	T49.5X3	T49.5X4	T49.5X5	T49.5X6
- topical NEC	T49.0X1	T49.0X2	T49.0X3	T49.0X4	T49.0X5	T49.0X6
Neostigmine bromide	T44.0X1	T44.0X2	T44.0X3	T44.0X4	T44.0X5	T44.0X6
Neraval	T42.3X1	T42.3X2	T42.3X3	T42.3X4	T42.3X5	T42.3X6
Neravan	T42.3X1	T42.3X2	T42.3X3	T42.3X4	T42.3X5	T42.3X6
Nerium oleander	T62.2X1	T62.2X2	T62.2X3	T62.2X4	--	--

Substance	Poisoning, Accidental (unintentional)	Poisoning, Intentional Self-harm	Poisoning, Assault	Poisoning, Undetermined	Adverse effect	Underdosing
Nerve gas, not in war	T59.91	T59.92	T59.93	T59.94	--	--
Nesacaine	T41.3X1	T41.3X2	T41.3X3	T41.3X4	T41.3X5	T41.3X6
- infiltration (subcutaneous)	T41.3X1	T41.3X2	T41.3X3	T41.3X4	T41.3X5	T41.3X6
- nerve block (peripheral) (plexus)	T41.3X1	T41.3X2	T41.3X3	T41.3X4	T41.3X5	T41.3X6
Netilmicin	T36.5X1	T36.5X2	T36.5X3	T36.5X4	T36.5X5	T36.5X6
Neurobarb	T42.3X1	T42.3X2	T42.3X3	T42.3X4	T42.3X5	T42.3X6
Neuroleptic drug NEC	T43.501	T43.502	T43.503	T43.504	T43.505	T43.506
Neuromuscular blocking drug	T48.1X1	T48.1X2	T48.1X3	T48.1X4	T48.1X5	T48.1X6
Neutral insulin injection	T38.3X1	T38.3X2	T38.3X3	T38.3X4	T38.3X5	T38.3X6
Neutral spirits	T51.0X1	T51.0X2	T51.0X3	T51.0X4	--	--
- beverage	T51.0X1	T51.0X2	T51.0X3	T51.0X4	--	--
Niacin	T46.7X1	T46.7X2	T46.7X3	T46.7X4	T46.7X5	T46.7X6
Niacinamide	T45.2X1	T45.2X2	T45.2X3	T45.2X4	T45.2X5	T45.2X6
Nialamide	T43.1X1	T43.1X2	T43.1X3	T43.1X4	T43.1X5	T43.1X6
Niaprazine	T42.6X1	T42.6X2	T42.6X3	T42.6X4	T42.6X5	T42.6X6
Nicametate	T46.7X1	T46.7X2	T46.7X3	T46.7X4	T46.7X5	T46.7X6
Nicardipine	T46.1X1	T46.1X2	T46.1X3	T46.1X4	T46.1X5	T46.1X6
Nicergoline	T46.7X1	T46.7X2	T46.7X3	T46.7X4	T46.7X5	T46.7X6
Nickel (carbonyl) (tetra-carbonyl) (fumes) (vapor)	T56.891	T56.892	T56.893	T56.894	--	--
Nickelocene	T56.891	T56.892	T56.893	T56.894	--	--
Niclosamide	T37.4X1	T37.4X2	T37.4X3	T37.4X4	T37.4X5	T37.4X6
Nicofuranose	T46.7X1	T46.7X2	T46.7X3	T46.7X4	T46.7X5	T46.7X6
Nicomorphine	T40.2X1	T40.2X2	T40.2X3	T40.2X4	--	--
Nicorandil	T46.3X1	T46.3X2	T46.3X3	T46.3X4	T46.3X5	T46.3X6
Nicotiana (plant)	T62.2X1	T62.2X2	T62.2X3	T62.2X4	--	--
Nicotinamide	T45.2X1	T45.2X2	T45.2X3	T45.2X4	T45.2X5	T45.2X6
Nicotine (insecticide) (spray) (sulfate) NEC	T60.2X1	T60.2X2	T60.2X3	T60.2X4	--	--
- from tobacco	T65.291	T65.292	T65.293	T65.294	--	--
- - cigarettes	T65.221	T65.222	T65.223	T65.224	--	--
- not insecticide	T65.291	T65.292	T65.293	T65.294	--	--
Nicotinic acid	T46.7X1	T46.7X2	T46.7X3	T46.7X4	T46.7X5	T46.7X6
Nicotinyl alcohol	T46.7X1	T46.7X2	T46.7X3	T46.7X4	T46.7X5	T46.7X6
Nicoumalone	T45.511	T45.512	T45.513	T45.514	T45.515	T45.516
Nifedipine	T46.1X1	T46.1X2	T46.1X3	T46.1X4	T46.1X5	T46.1X6
Nifenazone	T39.2X1	T39.2X2	T39.2X3	T39.2X4	T39.2X5	T39.2X6
Nifuraldezone	T37.91	T37.92	T37.93	T37.94	T37.95	T37.96
Nifuratel	T37.8X1	T37.8X2	T37.8X3	T37.8X4	T37.8X5	T37.8X6
Nifurtimox	T37.3X1	T37.3X2	T37.3X3	T37.3X4	T37.3X5	T37.3X6
Nifurtoinol	T37.8X1	T37.8X2	T37.8X3	T37.8X4	T37.8X5	T37.8X6
Nightshade, deadly (solanum) —see also Belladonna	T62.2X1	T62.2X2	T62.2X3	T62.2X4	--	--
- berry	T62.1X1	T62.1X2	T62.1X3	T62.1X4	--	--
Nikethamide	T50.7X1	T50.7X2	T50.7X3	T50.7X4	T50.7X5	T50.7X6
Nilstat	T36.7X1	T36.7X2	T36.7X3	T36.7X4	T36.7X5	T36.7X6
- topical	T49.0X1	T49.0X2	T49.0X3	T49.0X4	T49.0X5	T49.0X6
Nilutamide	T38.6X1	T38.6X2	T38.6X3	T38.6X4	T38.6X5	T38.6X6
Nimesulide	T39.391	T39.392	T39.393	T39.394	T39.395	T39.396
Nimetazepam	T42.4X1	T42.4X2	T42.4X3	T42.4X4	T42.4X5	T42.4X6
Nimodipine	T46.1X1	T46.1X2	T46.1X3	T46.1X4	T46.1X5	T46.1X6
Nimorazole	T37.3X1	T37.3X2	T37.3X3	T37.3X4	T37.3X5	T37.3X6
Nimustine	T45.1X1	T45.1X2	T45.1X3	T45.1X4	T45.1X5	T45.1X6
Niridazole	T37.4X1	T37.4X2	T37.4X3	T37.4X4	T37.4X5	T37.4X6
Nisentil	T40.2X1	T40.2X2	T40.2X3	T40.2X4	T40.2X5	T40.2X6
Nisoldipine	T46.1X1	T46.1X2	T46.1X3	T46.1X4	T46.1X5	T46.1X6
Nitramine	T65.3X1	T65.3X2	T65.3X3	T65.3X4	--	--
Nitrate, organic	T46.3X1	T46.3X2	T46.3X3	T46.3X4	T46.3X5	T46.3X6
Nitrazepam	T42.4X1	T42.4X2	T42.4X3	T42.4X4	T42.4X5	T42.4X6
Nitrefazole	T50.6X1	T50.6X2	T50.6X3	T50.6X4	T50.6X5	T50.6X6
Nitrendipine	T46.1X1	T46.1X2	T46.1X3	T46.1X4	T46.1X5	T46.1X6
Nitric						
- acid (liquid)	T54.2X1	T54.2X2	T54.2X3	T54.2X4	--	--
- - vapor	T59.891	T59.892	T59.893	T59.894	--	--
- oxide (gas)	T59.0X1	T59.0X2	T59.0X3	T59.0X4	--	--
Nitrimidazine	T37.3X1	T37.3X2	T37.3X3	T37.3X4	T37.3X5	T37.3X6
Nitrite, amyl (medicinal) (vapor)	T46.3X1	T46.3X2	T46.3X3	T46.3X4	T46.3X5	T46.3X6

Substance	Poisoning, Accidental (unintentional)	Poisoning, Intentional Self-harm	Poisoning, Assault	Poisoning, Undetermined	Adverse effect	Underdosing
Nitroaniline	T65.3X1	T65.3X2	T65.3X3	T65.3X4	--	--
- vapor	T59.891	T59.892	T59.893	T59.894	--	--
Nitrobenzene, nitrobenzol	T65.3X1	T65.3X2	T65.3X3	T65.3X4	--	--
- vapor	T65.3X1	T65.3X2	T65.3X3	T65.3X4	--	--
Nitrocellulose	T65.891	T65.892	T65.893	T65.894	--	--
- lacquer	T65.891	T65.892	T65.893	T65.894	--	--
Nitrodiphenyl	T65.3X1	T65.3X2	T65.3X3	T65.3X4	--	--
Nitrofural	T49.0X1	T49.0X2	T49.0X3	T49.0X4	T49.0X5	T49.0X6
Nitrofurantoin	T37.8X1	T37.8X2	T37.8X3	T37.8X4	T37.8X5	T37.8X6
Nitrofurazone	T49.0X1	T49.0X2	T49.0X3	T49.0X4	T49.0X5	T49.0X6
Nitrogen	T59.0X1	T59.0X2	T59.0X3	T59.0X4	--	--
- mustard	T45.1X1	T45.1X2	T45.1X3	T45.1X4	T45.1X5	T45.1X6
Nitroglycerin, nitro-glycerol (medicinal)	T46.3X1	T46.3X2	T46.3X3	T46.3X4	T46.3X5	T46.3X6
- nonmedicinal	T65.5X1	T65.5X2	T65.5X3	T65.5X4	--	--
- - fumes	T65.5X1	T65.5X2	T65.5X3	T65.5X4	--	--
Nitroglycol	T52.3X1	T52.3X2	T52.3X3	T52.3X4	--	--
Nitrohydrochloric acid	T54.2X1	T54.2X2	T54.2X3	T54.2X4	--	--
Nitromersol	T49.0X1	T49.0X2	T49.0X3	T49.0X4	T49.0X5	T49.0X6
Nitronaphthalene	T65.891	T65.892	T65.893	T65.894	--	--
Nitrophenol	T54.0X1	T54.0X2	T54.0X3	T54.0X4	--	--
Nitropropane	T52.8X1	T52.8X2	T52.8X3	T52.8X4	--	--
Nitroprusside	T46.5X1	T46.5X2	T46.5X3	T46.5X4	T46.5X5	T46.5X6
Nitrosodimethylamine	T65.3X1	T65.3X2	T65.3X3	T65.3X4	--	--
Nitrothiazol	T37.4X1	T37.4X2	T37.4X3	T37.4X4	T37.4X5	T37.4X6
Nitrotoluene, nitrotoluol	T65.3X1	T65.3X2	T65.3X3	T65.3X4	--	--
- vapor	T65.3X1	T65.3X2	T65.3X3	T65.3X4	--	--
Nitrous						
- acid (liquid)	T54.2X1	T54.2X2	T54.2X3	T54.2X4	--	--
- - fumes	T59.891	T59.892	T59.893	T59.894	--	--
- ether spirit	T46.3X1	T46.3X2	T46.3X3	T46.3X4	T46.3X5	T46.3X6
- oxide	T41.0X1	T41.0X2	T41.0X3	T41.0X4	T41.0X5	T41.0X6
Nitroxoline	T37.8X1	T37.8X2	T37.8X3	T37.8X4	T37.8X5	T37.8X6
Nitrozone	T49.0X1	T49.0X2	T49.0X3	T49.0X4	T49.0X5	T49.0X6
Nizatidine	T47.0X1	T47.0X2	T47.0X3	T47.0X4	T47.0X5	T47.0X6
Nizofenone	T43.8X1	T43.8X2	T43.8X3	T43.8X4	T43.8X5	T43.8X6
Noctec	T42.6X1	T42.6X2	T42.6X3	T42.6X4	T42.6X5	T42.6X6
Noludar	T42.6X1	T42.6X2	T42.6X3	T42.6X4	T42.6X5	T42.6X6
Nomegestrol	T38.5X1	T38.5X2	T38.5X3	T38.5X4	T38.5X5	T38.5X6
Nomifensine	T43.291	T43.292	T43.293	T43.294	T43.295	T43.296
Nonoxinol	T49.8X1	T49.8X2	T49.8X3	T49.8X4	T49.8X5	T49.8X6
Nonylphenoxy (polyethoxy-ethanol)	T49.8X1	T49.8X2	T49.8X3	T49.8X4	T49.8X5	T49.8X6
Noptil	T42.3X1	T42.3X2	T42.3X3	T42.3X4	T42.3X5	T42.3X6
Noradrenaline	T44.4X1	T44.4X2	T44.4X3	T44.4X4	T44.4X5	T44.4X6
Noramidopyrine	T39.2X1	T39.2X2	T39.2X3	T39.2X4	T39.2X5	T39.2X6
- methanesulfonate sodium	T39.2X1	T39.2X2	T39.2X3	T39.2X4	T39.2X5	T39.2X6
Norbormide	T60.4X1	T60.4X2	T60.4X3	T60.4X4	--	--
Nordazepam	T42.4X1	T42.4X2	T42.4X3	T42.4X4	T42.4X5	T42.4X6
Norepinephrine	T44.4X1	T44.4X2	T44.4X3	T44.4X4	T44.4X5	T44.4X6
Norethandrolone	T38.7X1	T38.7X2	T38.7X3	T38.7X4	T38.7X5	T38.7X6
Norethindrone	T38.4X1	T38.4X2	T38.4X3	T38.4X4	T38.4X5	T38.4X6
Norethisterone (acetate) (enantate)	T38.4X1	T38.4X2	T38.4X3	T38.4X4	T38.4X5	T38.4X6
- with ethinylestradiol	T38.5X1	T38.5X2	T38.5X3	T38.5X4	T38.5X5	T38.5X6
Noretynodrel	T38.5X1	T38.5X2	T38.5X3	T38.5X4	T38.5X5	T38.5X6
Norfenefrine	T44.4X1	T44.4X2	T44.4X3	T44.4X4	T44.4X5	T44.4X6
Norfloxacin	T36.8X1	T36.8X2	T36.8X3	T36.8X4	T36.8X5	T36.8X6
Norgestrel	T38.4X1	T38.4X2	T38.4X3	T38.4X4	T38.4X5	T38.4X6
Norgestrienone	T38.4X1	T38.4X2	T38.4X3	T38.4X4	T38.4X5	T38.4X6
Norlestrin	T38.4X1	T38.4X2	T38.4X3	T38.4X4	T38.4X5	T38.4X6
Norlutin	T38.4X1	T38.4X2	T38.4X3	T38.4X4	T38.4X5	T38.4X6
Normal serum albumin (human) , salt-poor	T45.8X1	T45.8X2	T45.8X3	T45.8X4	T45.8X5	T45.8X6
Normethandrone	T38.5X1	T38.5X2	T38.5X3	T38.5X4	T38.5X5	T38.5X6
Normison—see Benzodiazepines						
Normorphine	T40.2X1	T40.2X2	T40.2X3	T40.2X4	--	--
Norpseudoephedrine	T50.5X1	T50.5X2	T50.5X3	T50.5X4	T50.5X5	T50.5X6
Nortestosterone (furanpropionate)	T38.7X1	T38.7X2	T38.7X3	T38.7X4	T38.7X5	T38.7X6

Substance	Poisoning, Accidental (unintentional)	Poisoning, Intentional Self-harm	Poisoning, Assault	Poisoning, Undetermined	Adverse effect	Underdosing
Nortriptyline	T43.011	T43.012	T43.013	T43.014	T43.015	T43.016
Noscapine	T48.3X1	T48.3X2	T48.3X3	T48.3X4	T48.3X5	T48.3X6
Nose preparations	T49.6X1	T49.6X2	T49.6X3	T49.6X4	T49.6X5	T49.6X6
Novobiocin	T36.5X1	T36.5X2	T36.5X3	T36.5X4	T36.5X5	T36.5X6
Novocain (infiltration) (topical)	T41.3X1	T41.3X2	T41.3X3	T41.3X4	T41.3X5	T41.3X6
- nerve block (peripheral) (plexus)	T41.3X1	T41.3X2	T41.3X3	T41.3X4	T41.3X5	T41.3X6
- spinal	T41.3X1	T41.3X2	T41.3X3	T41.3X4	T41.3X5	T41.3X6
Noxious foodstuff	T62.91	T62.92	T62.93	T62.94	--	--
- specified NEC	T62.8X1	T62.8X2	T62.8X3	T62.8X4	--	--
Noxiptiline	T43.011	T43.012	T43.013	T43.014	T43.015	T43.016
Noxytiolin	T49.0X1	T49.0X2	T49.0X3	T49.0X4	T49.0X5	T49.0X6
NPH lletin (insulin)	T38.3X1	T38.3X2	T38.3X3	T38.3X4	T38.3X5	T38.3X6
Numorphan	T40.2X1	T40.2X2	T40.2X3	T40.2X4	T40.2X5	T40.2X6
Nunol	T42.3X1	T42.3X2	T42.3X3	T42.3X4	T42.3X5	T42.3X6
Nupercaine (spinal anesthetic)	T41.3X1	T41.3X2	T41.3X3	T41.3X4	T41.3X5	T41.3X6
- topical (surface)	T41.3X1	T41.3X2	T41.3X3	T41.3X4	T41.3X5	T41.3X6
Nutmeg oil (liniment)	T49.3X1	T49.3X2	T49.3X3	T49.3X4	T49.3X5	T49.3X6
Nutritional supplement	T50.901	T50.902	T50.903	T50.904	T50.905	T50.906
Nux vomica	T65.1X1	T65.1X2	T65.1X3	T65.1X4	--	--
Nydrazid	T37.1X1	T37.1X2	T37.1X3	T37.1X4	T37.1X5	T37.1X6
Nylidrin	T46.7X1	T46.7X2	T46.7X3	T46.7X4	T46.7X5	T46.7X6
Nystatin	T36.7X1	T36.7X2	T36.7X3	T36.7X4	T36.7X5	T36.7X6
- topical	T49.0X1	T49.0X2	T49.0X3	T49.0X4	T49.0X5	T49.0X6
Nytol	T45.0X1	T45.0X2	T45.0X3	T45.0X4	T45.0X5	T45.0X6
Obidoxime chloride	T50.6X1	T50.6X2	T50.6X3	T50.6X4	T50.6X5	T50.6X6
Octafonium (chloride)	T49.3X1	T49.3X2	T49.3X3	T49.3X4	T49.3X5	T49.3X6
Octamethyl pyrophos-phoramide	T60.0X1	T60.0X2	T60.0X3	T60.0X4	--	--
Octanoin	T50.991	T50.992	T50.993	T50.994	T50.995	T50.996
Octatropine methyl-bromide	T44.3X1	T44.3X2	T44.3X3	T44.3X4	T44.3X5	T44.3X6
Octotiamine	T45.2X1	T45.2X2	T45.2X3	T45.2X4	T45.2X5	T45.2X6
Octoxinol (9)	T49.8X1	T49.8X2	T49.8X3	T49.8X4	T49.8X5	T49.8X6
Octreotide	T38.991	T38.992	T38.993	T38.994	T38.995	T38.996
Octyl nitrite	T46.3X1	T46.3X2	T46.3X3	T46.3X4	T46.3X5	T46.3X6
Oestradiol	T38.5X1	T38.5X2	T38.5X3	T38.5X4	T38.5X5	T38.5X6
Oestriol	T38.5X1	T38.5X2	T38.5X3	T38.5X4	T38.5X5	T38.5X6
Oestrogen	T38.5X1	T38.5X2	T38.5X3	T38.5X4	T38.5X5	T38.5X6
Oestrone	T38.5X1	T38.5X2	T38.5X3	T38.5X4	T38.5X5	T38.5X6
Ofloxacin	T36.8X1	T36.8X2	T36.8X3	T36.8X4	T36.8X5	T36.8X6
Oil (of)	T65.891	T65.892	T65.893	T65.894	--	--
- bitter almond	T62.8X1	T62.8X2	T62.8X3	T62.8X4	--	--
- cloves	T49.7X1	T49.7X2	T49.7X3	T49.7X4	T49.7X5	T49.7X6
- colors	T65.6X1	T65.6X2	T65.6X3	T65.6X4	--	--
- fumes	T59.891	T59.892	T59.893	T59.894	--	--
- lubricating	T52.0X1	T52.0X2	T52.0X3	T52.0X4	--	--
- Niobe	T52.8X1	T52.8X2	T52.8X3	T52.8X4	--	--
- vitriol (liquid)	T54.2X1	T54.2X2	T54.2X3	T54.2X4	--	--
- - fumes	T54.2X1	T54.2X2	T54.2X3	T54.2X4	--	--
- wintergreen (bitter) NEC	T49.3X1	T49.3X2	T49.3X3	T49.3X4	T49.3X5	T49.3X6
Oily preparation (for skin)	T49.3X1	T49.3X2	T49.3X3	T49.3X4	T49.3X5	T49.3X6
Ointment NEC	T49.3X1	T49.3X2	T49.3X3	T49.3X4	T49.3X5	T49.3X6
Olanzapine	T43.591	T43.592	T43.593	T43.594	T43.595	T43.596
Oleander	T62.2X1	T62.2X2	T62.2X3	T62.2X4	--	--
Oleandomycin	T36.3X1	T36.3X2	T36.3X3	T36.3X4	T36.3X5	T36.3X6
Oleandrin	T46.0X1	T46.0X2	T46.0X3	T46.0X4	T46.0X5	T46.0X6
Oleic acid	T46.6X1	T46.6X2	T46.6X3	T46.6X4	T46.6X5	T46.6X6
Oleovitamin A	T45.2X1	T45.2X2	T45.2X3	T45.2X4	T45.2X5	T45.2X6
Oleum ricini	T47.2X1	T47.2X2	T47.2X3	T47.2X4	T47.2X5	T47.2X6
Olive oil (medicinal) NEC	T47.4X1	T47.4X2	T47.4X3	T47.4X4	T47.4X5	T47.4X6
Olivomycin	T45.1X1	T45.1X2	T45.1X3	T45.1X4	T45.1X5	T45.1X6
Olsalazine	T47.8X1	T47.8X2	T47.8X3	T47.8X4	T47.8X5	T47.8X6
Omeprazole	T47.1X1	T47.1X2	T47.1X3	T47.1X4	T47.1X5	T47.1X6
OMPA	T60.0X1	T60.0X2	T60.0X3	T60.0X4	--	--
Oncovin	T45.1X1	T45.1X2	T45.1X3	T45.1X4	T45.1X5	T45.1X6
Ondansetron	T45.0X1	T45.0X2	T45.0X3	T45.0X4	T45.0X5	T45.0X6
Ophthaine	T41.3X1	T41.3X2	T41.3X3	T41.3X4	T41.3X5	T41.3X6

Substance	Poisoning, Accidental (unintentional)	Poisoning, Intentional Self-harm	Poisoning, Assault	Poisoning, Undetermined	Adverse effect	Underdosing
Ophthetic	T41.3X1	T41.3X2	T41.3X3	T41.3X4	T41.3X5	T41.3X6
Opiate NEC	T40.601	T40.602	T40.603	T40.604	T40.605	T40.606
- antagonists	T50.7X1	T50.7X2	T50.7X3	T50.7X4	T50.7X5	T50.7X6
Opioid NEC	T40.2X1	T40.2X2	T40.2X3	T40.2X4	T40.2X5	T40.2X6
Opipramol	T43.011	T43.012	T43.013	T43.014	T43.015	T43.016
Opium alkaloids (total)	T40.0X1	T40.0X2	T40.0X3	T40.0X4	T40.0X5	T40.0X6
- standardized powdered	T40.0X1	T40.0X2	T40.0X3	T40.0X4	T40.0X5	T40.0X6
- tincture (camphorated)	T40.0X1	T40.0X2	T40.0X3	T40.0X4	T40.0X5	T40.0X6
Oracon	T38.4X1	T38.4X2	T38.4X3	T38.4X4	T38.4X5	T38.4X6
Oragrafin	T50.8X1	T50.8X2	T50.8X3	T50.8X4	T50.8X5	T50.8X6
Oral contraceptives	T38.4X1	T38.4X2	T38.4X3	T38.4X4	T38.4X5	T38.4X6
Oral rehydration salts	T50.3X1	T50.3X2	T50.3X3	T50.3X4	T50.3X5	T50.3X6
Orazamide	T50.991	T50.992	T50.993	T50.994	T50.995	T50.996
Orciprenaline	T48.291	T48.292	T48.293	T48.294	T48.295	T48.296
Organidin	T48.4X1	T48.4X2	T48.4X3	T48.4X4	T48.4X5	T48.4X6
Organonitrate NEC	T46.3X1	T46.3X2	T46.3X3	T46.3X4	T46.3X5	T46.3X6
Organophosphates	T60.0X1	T60.0X2	T60.0X3	T60.0X4	--	--
Orimune	T50.B91	T50.B92	T50.B93	T50.B94	T50.B95	T50.B96
Orinase	T38.3X1	T38.3X2	T38.3X3	T38.3X4	T38.3X5	T38.3X6
Ormeloxifene	T38.6X1	T38.6X2	T38.6X3	T38.6X4	T38.6X5	T38.6X6
Ornidazole	T37.3X1	T37.3X2	T37.3X3	T37.3X4	T37.3X5	T37.3X6
Ornithine aspartate	T50.991	T50.992	T50.993	T50.994	T50.995	T50.996
Ornoprostil	T47.1X1	T47.1X2	T47.1X3	T47.1X4	T47.1X5	T47.1X6
Orphenadrine (hydrochloride)	T42.8X1	T42.8X2	T42.8X3	T42.8X4	T42.8X5	T42.8X6
Ortal (sodium)	T42.3X1	T42.3X2	T42.3X3	T42.3X4	T42.3X5	T42.3X6
Orthoboric acid	T49.0X1	T49.0X2	T49.0X3	T49.0X4	T49.0X5	T49.0X6
- ENT agent	T49.6X1	T49.6X2	T49.6X3	T49.6X4	T49.6X5	T49.6X6
- ophthalmic preparation	T49.5X1	T49.5X2	T49.5X3	T49.5X4	T49.5X5	T49.5X6
Orthocaine	T41.3X1	T41.3X2	T41.3X3	T41.3X4	T41.3X5	T41.3X6
Orthodichlorobenzene	T53.7X1	T53.7X2	T53.7X3	T53.7X4	--	--
Ortho-Novum	T38.4X1	T38.4X2	T38.4X3	T38.4X4	T38.4X5	T38.4X6
Orthotolidine (reagent)	T54.2X1	T54.2X2	T54.2X3	T54.2X4	--	--
Osmic acid (liquid)	T54.2X1	T54.2X2	T54.2X3	T54.2X4	--	--
- fumes	T54.2X1	T54.2X2	T54.2X3	T54.2X4	--	--
Osmotic diuretics	T50.2X1	T50.2X2	T50.2X3	T50.2X4	T50.2X5	T50.2X6
Otilonium bromide	T44.3X1	T44.3X2	T44.3X3	T44.3X4	T44.3X5	T44.3X6
Otorhinolaryngological drug NEC	T49.6X1	T49.6X2	T49.6X3	T49.6X4	T49.6X5	T49.6X6
Ouabain (e)	T46.0X1	T46.0X2	T46.0X3	T46.0X4	T46.0X5	T46.0X6
Ovarian						
- hormone	T38.5X1	T38.5X2	T38.5X3	T38.5X4	T38.5X5	T38.5X6
- stimulant	T38.5X1	T38.5X2	T38.5X3	T38.5X4	T38.5X5	T38.5X6
Ovral	T38.4X1	T38.4X2	T38.4X3	T38.4X4	T38.4X5	T38.4X6
Ovulen	T38.4X1	T38.4X2	T38.4X3	T38.4X4	T38.4X5	T38.4X6
Oxacillin	T36.0X1	T36.0X2	T36.0X3	T36.0X4	T36.0X5	T36.0X6
Oxalic acid	T54.2X1	T54.2X2	T54.2X3	T54.2X4	--	--
- ammonium salt	T50.991	T50.992	T50.993	T50.994	T50.995	T50.996
Oxamniquine	T37.4X1	T37.4X2	T37.4X3	T37.4X4	T37.4X5	T37.4X6
Oxanamide	T43.591	T43.592	T43.593	T43.594	T43.595	T43.596
Oxandrolone	T38.7X1	T38.7X2	T38.7X3	T38.7X4	T38.7X5	T38.7X6
Oxantel	T37.4X1	T37.4X2	T37.4X3	T37.4X4	T37.4X5	T37.4X6
Oxapium iodide	T44.3X1	T44.3X2	T44.3X3	T44.3X4	T44.3X5	T44.3X6
Oxaprotiline	T43.021	T43.022	T43.023	T43.024	T43.025	T43.026
Oxaprozin	T39.311	T39.312	T39.313	T39.314	T39.315	T39.316
Oxatomide	T45.0X1	T45.0X2	T45.0X3	T45.0X4	T45.0X5	T45.0X6
Oxazepam	T42.4X1	T42.4X2	T42.4X3	T42.4X4	T42.4X5	T42.4X6
Oxazimedrine	T50.5X1	T50.5X2	T50.5X3	T50.5X4	T50.5X5	T50.5X6
Oxazolam	T42.4X1	T42.4X2	T42.4X3	T42.4X4	T42.4X5	T42.4X6
Oxazolidine derivatives	T42.2X1	T42.2X2	T42.2X3	T42.2X4	T42.2X5	T42.2X6
Oxazolidinedione (derivative)	T42.2X1	T42.2X2	T42.2X3	T42.2X4	T42.2X5	T42.2X6
Ox bile extract	T47.5X1	T47.5X2	T47.5X3	T47.5X4	T47.5X5	T47.5X6
Oxcarbazepine	T42.1X1	T42.1X2	T42.1X3	T42.1X4	T42.1X5	T42.1X6
Oxedrine	T44.4X1	T44.4X2	T44.4X3	T44.4X4	T44.4X5	T44.4X6
Oxeladin (citrate)	T48.3X1	T48.3X2	T48.3X3	T48.3X4	T48.3X5	T48.3X6
Oxendolone	T38.5X1	T38.5X2	T38.5X3	T38.5X4	T38.5X5	T38.5X6
Oxetacaine	T41.3X1	T41.3X2	T41.3X3	T41.3X4	T41.3X5	T41.3X6

Substance	Poisoning, Accidental (unintentional)	Poisoning, Intentional Self-harm	Poisoning, Assault	Poisoning, Undetermined	Adverse effect	Underdosing
Oxethazine	T41.3X1	T41.3X2	T41.3X3	T41.3X4	T41.3X5	T41.3X6
Oxetorone	T39.8X1	T39.8X2	T39.8X3	T39.8X4	T39.8X5	T39.8X6
Oxiconazole	T49.0X1	T49.0X2	T49.0X3	T49.0X4	T49.0X5	T49.0X6
Oxidizing agent NEC	T54.91	T54.92	T54.93	T54.94	--	--
Oxipurinol	T50.4X1	T50.4X2	T50.4X3	T50.4X4	T50.4X5	T50.4X6
Oxitriptan	T43.291	T43.292	T43.293	T43.294	T43.295	T43.296
Oxitropium bromide	T48.6X1	T48.6X2	T48.6X3	T48.6X4	T48.6X5	T48.6X6
Oxodipine	T46.1X1	T46.1X2	T46.1X3	T46.1X4	T46.1X5	T46.1X6
Oxolamine	T48.3X1	T48.3X2	T48.3X3	T48.3X4	T48.3X5	T48.3X6
Oxolinic acid	T37.8X1	T37.8X2	T37.8X3	T37.8X4	T37.8X5	T37.8X6
Oxomemazine	T43.3X1	T43.3X2	T43.3X3	T43.3X4	T43.3X5	T43.3X6
Oxophenarsine	T37.3X1	T37.3X2	T37.3X3	T37.3X4	T37.3X5	T37.3X6
Oxprenolol	T44.7X1	T44.7X2	T44.7X3	T44.7X4	T44.7X5	T44.7X6
Oxsoralen	T49.3X1	T49.3X2	T49.3X3	T49.3X4	T49.3X5	T49.3X6
Oxtriphyllinc	T48.6X1	T48.6X2	T48.6X3	T48.6X4	T48.6X5	T48.6X6
Oxybate sodium	T41.291	T41.292	T41.293	T41.294	T41.295	T41.296
Oxybuprocaine	T41.3X1	T41.3X2	T41.3X3	T41.3X4	T41.3X5	T41.3X6
Oxybutynin	T44.3X1	T44.3X2	T44.3X3	T44.3X4	T44.3X5	T44.3X6
Oxychlorosene	T49.0X1	T49.0X2	T49.0X3	T49.0X4	T49.0X5	T49.0X6
Oxycodone	T40.2X1	T40.2X2	T40.2X3	T40.2X4	T40.2X5	T40.2X6
Oxyfedrine	T46.3X1	T46.3X2	T46.3X3	T46.3X4	T46.3X5	T46.3X6
Oxygen	T41.5X1	T41.5X2	T41.5X3	T41.5X4	T41.5X5	T41.5X6
Oxylone	T49.0X1	T49.0X2	T49.0X3	T49.0X4	T49.0X5	T49.0X6
- ophthalmic preparation	T49.5X1	T49.5X2	T49.5X3	T49.5X4	T49.5X5	T49.5X6
Oxymesterone	T38.7X1	T38.7X2	T38.7X3	T38.7X4	T38.7X5	T38.7X6
Oxymetazoline	T48.5X1	T48.5X2	T48.5X3	T48.5X4	T48.5X5	T48.5X6
Oxymetholone	T38.7X1	T38.7X2	T38.7X3	T38.7X4	T38.7X5	T38.7X6
Oxymorphone	T40.2X1	T40.2X2	T40.2X3	T40.2X4	T40.2X5	T40.2X6
Oxypertine	T43.591	T43.592	T43.593	T43.594	T43.595	T43.596
Oxyphenbutazone	T39.2X1	T39.2X2	T39.2X3	T39.2X4	T39.2X5	T39.2X6
Oxyphencyclimine	T44.3X1	T44.3X2	T44.3X3	T44.3X4	T44.3X5	T44.3X6
Oxyphenisatine	T47.2X1	T47.2X2	T47.2X3	T47.2X4	T47.2X5	T47.2X6
Oxyphenonium bromide	T44.3X1	T44.3X2	T44.3X3	T44.3X4	T44.3X5	T44.3X6
Oxypolygelatin	T45.8X1	T45.8X2	T45.8X3	T45.8X4	T45.8X5	T45.8X6
Oxyquinoline (derivatives)	T37.8X1	T37.8X2	T37.8X3	T37.8X4	T37.8X5	T37.8X6
Oxytetracycline	T36.4X1	T36.4X2	T36.4X3	T36.4X4	T36.4X5	T36.4X6
Oxytocic drug NEC	T48.0X1	T48.0X2	T48.0X3	T48.0X4	T48.0X5	T48.0X6
Oxytocin (synthetic)	T48.0X1	T48.0X2	T48.0X3	T48.0X4	T48.0X5	T48.0X6
Ozone	T59.891	T59.892	T59.893	T59.894	--	--
PABA	T49.3X1	T49.3X2	T49.3X3	T49.3X4	T49.3X5	T49.3X6
Packed red cells	T45.8X1	T45.8X2	T45.8X3	T45.8X4	T45.8X5	T45.8X6
Padimate	T49.3X1	T49.3X2	T49.3X3	T49.3X4	T49.3X5	T49.3X6
Paint NEC	T65.6X1	T65.6X2	T65.6X3	T65.6X4	--	--
- cleaner	T52.91	T52.92	T52.93	T52.94	--	--
- fumes NEC	T59.891	T59.892	T59.893	T59.894	--	--
- lead (fumes)	T56.0X1	T56.0X2	T56.0X3	T56.0X4	--	--
- solvent NEC	T52.8X1	T52.8X2	T52.8X3	T52.8X4	--	--
- stripper	T52.8X1	T52.8X2	T52.8X3	T52.8X4	--	--
Palfium	T40.2X1	T40.2X2	T40.2X3	T40.2X4	--	--
Palm kernel oil	T50.991	T50.992	T50.993	T50.994	T50.995	T50.996
Paludrine	T37.2X1	T37.2X2	T37.2X3	T37.2X4	T37.2X5	T37.2X6
PAM (pralidoxime)	T50.6X1	T50.6X2	T50.6X3	T50.6X4	T50.6X5	T50.6X6
Pamaquine (naphthoute)	T37.2X1	T37.2X2	T37.2X3	T37.2X4	T37.2X5	T37.2X6
Panadol	T39.1X1	T39.1X2	T39.1X3	T39.1X4	T39.1X5	T39.1X6
Pancreatic						
- digestive secretion stimulant	T47.8X1	T47.8X2	T47.8X3	T47.8X4	T47.8X5	T47.8X6
- dornase	T45.3X1	T45.3X2	T45.3X3	T45.3X4	T45.3X5	T45.3X6
Pancreatin	T47.5X1	T47.5X2	T47.5X3	T47.5X4	T47.5X5	T47.5X6
Pancrelipase	T47.5X1	T47.5X2	T47.5X3	T47.5X4	T47.5X5	T47.5X6
Pancuronium (bromide)	T48.1X1	T48.1X2	T48.1X3	T48.1X4	T48.1X5	T48.1X6
Pangamic acid	T45.2X1	T45.2X2	T45.2X3	T45.2X4	T45.2X5	T45.2X6
Panthenol	T45.2X1	T45.2X2	T45.2X3	T45.2X4	T45.2X5	T45.2X6
- topical	T49.8X1	T49.8X2	T49.8X3	T49.8X4	T49.8X5	T49.8X6
Pantopon	T40.0X1	T40.0X2	T40.0X3	T40.0X4	T40.0X5	T40.0X6
Pantothenic acid	T45.2X1	T45.2X2	T45.2X3	T45.2X4	T45.2X5	T45.2X6

Substance	Poisoning, Accidental (unintentional)	Poisoning, Intentional Self-harm	Poisoning, Assault	Poisoning, Undetermined	Adverse effect	Underdosing
Panwarfin	T45.511	T45.512	T45.513	T45.514	T45.515	T45.516
Papain	T47.5X1	T47.5X2	T47.5X3	T47.5X4	T47.5X5	T47.5X6
- digestant	T47.5X1	T47.5X2	T47.5X3	T47.5X4	T47.5X5	T47.5X6
Papaveretum	T40.0X1	T40.0X2	T40.0X3	T40.0X4	T40.0X5	T40.0X6
Papaverine	T44.3X1	T44.3X2	T44.3X3	T44.3X4	T44.3X5	T44.3X6
Para-acetamidophenol	T39.1X1	T39.1X2	T39.1X3	T39.1X4	T39.1X5	T39.1X6
Para-aminobenzoic acid	T49.3X1	T49.3X2	T49.3X3	T49.3X4	T49.3X5	T49.3X6
Para-aminophenol derivatives	T39.1X1	T39.1X2	T39.1X3	T39.1X4	T39.1X5	T39.1X6
Para-aminosalicylic acid	T37.1X1	T37.1X2	T37.1X3	T37.1X4	T37.1X5	T37.1X6
Paracetaldehyde	T42.6X1	T42.6X2	T42.6X3	T42.6X4	T42.6X5	T42.6X6
Paracetamol	T39.1X1	T39.1X2	T39.1X3	T39.1X4	T39.1X5	T39.1X6
Parachlorophenol (camphorated)	T49.0X1	T49.0X2	T49.0X3	T49.0X4	T49.0X5	T49.0X6
Paracodin	T40.2X1	T40.2X2	T40.2X3	T40.2X4	T40.2X5	T40.2X6
Paradione	T42.2X1	T42.2X2	T42.2X3	T42.2X4	T42.2X5	T42.2X6
Paraffin (s) (wax)	T52.0X1	T52.0X2	T52.0X3	T52.0X4	--	--
- liquid (medicinal)	T47.4X1	T47.4X2	T47.4X3	T47.4X4	T47.4X5	T47.4X6
- - nonmedicinal	T52.0X1	T52.0X2	T52.0X3	T52.0X4	--	--
Paraformaldehyde	T60.3X1	T60.3X2	T60.3X3	T60.3X4	--	--
Paraldehyde	T42.6X1	T42.6X2	T42.6X3	T42.6X4	T42.6X5	T42.6X6
Paramethadione	T42.2X1	T42.2X2	T42.2X3	T42.2X4	T42.2X5	T42.2X6
Paramethasone	T38.0X1	T38.0X2	T38.0X3	T38.0X4	T38.0X5	T38.0X6
- acetate	T49.0X1	T49.0X2	T49.0X3	T49.0X4	T49.0X5	T49.0X6
Paraoxon	T60.0X1	T60.0X2	T60.0X3	T60.0X4	--	--
Paraquat	T60.3X1	T60.3X2	T60.3X3	T60.3X4	--	--
Parasympatholytic NEC	T44.3X1	T44.3X2	T44.3X3	T44.3X4	T44.3X5	T44.3X6
Parasympathomimetic drug NEC	T44.1X1	T44.1X2	T44.1X3	T44.1X4	T44.1X5	T44.1X6
Parathion	T60.0X1	T60.0X2	T60.0X3	T60.0X4	--	--
Parathormone	T50.991	T50.992	T50.993	T50.994	T50.995	T50.996
Parathyroid extract	T50.991	T50.992	T50.993	T50.994	T50.995	T50.996
Paratyphoid vaccine	T50.A91	T50.A92	T50.A93	T50.A94	T50.A95	T50.A96
Paredrine	T44.4X1	T44.4X2	T44.4X3	T44.4X4	T44.4X5	T44.4X6
Paregoric	T40.0X1	T40.0X2	T40.0X3	T40.0X4	T40.0X5	T40.0X6
Pargyline	T46.5X1	T46.5X2	T46.5X3	T46.5X4	T46.5X5	T46.5X6
Paris green	T57.0X1	T57.0X2	T57.0X3	T57.0X4	--	--
- insecticide	T57.0X1	T57.0X2	T57.0X3	T57.0X4	--	--
Parnate	T43.1X1	T43.1X2	T43.1X3	T43.1X4	T43.1X5	T43.1X6
Paromomycin	T36.5X1	T36.5X2	T36.5X3	T36.5X4	T36.5X5	T36.5X6
Paroxypropione	T45.1X1	T45.1X2	T45.1X3	T45.1X4	T45.1X5	T45.1X6
Parzone	T40.2X1	T40.2X2	T40.2X3	T40.2X4	T40.2X5	T40.2X6
PAS	T37.1X1	T37.1X2	T37.1X3	T37.1X4	T37.1X5	T37.1X6
Pasiniazid	T37.1X1	T37.1X2	T37.1X3	T37.1X4	T37.1X5	T37.1X6
PBB (polybrominated biphenyls)	T65.891	T65.892	T65.893	T65.894	--	--
PCB	T65.891	T65.892	T65.893	T65.894	--	--
PCP						
- meaning pentachlorophenol	T60.1X1	T60.1X2	T60.1X3	T60.1X4	--	--
- - fungicide	T60.3X1	T60.3X2	T60.3X3	T60.3X4	--	--
- - herbicide	T60.3X1	T60.3X2	T60.3X3	T60.3X4	--	--
- - insecticide	T60.1X1	T60.1X2	T60.1X3	T60.1X4	--	--
- meaning phencyclidine	T40.991	T40.992	T40.993	T40.994	--	--
Peach kernel oil (emulsion)	T47.4X1	T47.4X2	T47.4X3	T47.4X4	T47.4X5	T47.4X6
Peanut oil (emulsion) NEC	T47.4X1	T47.4X2	T47.4X3	T47.4X4	T47.4X5	T47.4X6
- topical	T49.3X1	T49.3X2	T49.3X3	T49.3X4	T49.3X5	T49.3X6
Pearly Gates (morning glory seeds)	T40.991	T40.992	T40.993	T40.994	--	--
Pecazine	T43.3X1	T43.3X2	T43.3X3	T43.3X4	T43.3X5	T43.3X6
Pectin	T47.6X1	T47.6X2	T47.6X3	T47.6X4	T47.6X5	T47.6X6
Pefloxacin	T37.8X1	T37.8X2	T37.8X3	T37.8X4	T37.8X5	T37.8X6
Pegademase, bovine	T50.Z91	T50.Z92	T50.Z93	T50.Z94	T50.Z95	T50.Z96
Pelletierine tannate	T37.4X1	T37.4X2	T37.4X3	T37.4X4	T37.4X5	T37.4X6
Pemirolast (potassium)	T48.6X1	T48.6X2	T48.6X3	T48.6X4	T48.6X5	T48.6X6
Pemoline	T50.7X1	T50.7X2	T50.7X3	T50.7X4	T50.7X5	T50.7X6
Pempidine	T44.2X1	T44.2X2	T44.2X3	T44.2X4	T44.2X5	T44.2X6
Penamecillin	T36.0X1	T36.0X2	T36.0X3	T36.0X4	T36.0X5	T36.0X6
Penbutolol	T44.7X1	T44.7X2	T44.7X3	T44.7X4	T44.7X5	T44.7X6
Penethamate	T36.0X1	T36.0X2	T36.0X3	T36.0X4	T36.0X5	T36.0X6
Penfluridol	T43.591	T43.592	T43.593	T43.594	T43.595	T43.596

Substance	Poisoning, Accidental (unintentional)	Poisoning, Intentional Self-harm	Poisoning, Assault	Poisoning, Undetermined	Adverse effect	Underdosing
Penflutizide	T50.2X1	T50.2X2	T50.2X3	T50.2X4	T50.2X5	T50.2X6
Pengitoxin	T46.0X1	T46.0X2	T46.0X3	T46.0X4	T46.0X5	T46.0X6
Penicillamine	T50.6X1	T50.6X2	T50.6X3	T50.6X4	T50.6X5	T50.6X6
Penicillin (any)	T36.0X1	T36.0X2	T36.0X3	T36.0X4	T36.0X5	T36.0X6
Penicillinase	T45.3X1	T45.3X2	T45.3X3	T45.3X4	T45.3X5	T45.3X6
Penicilloyl polylysine	T50.8X1	T50.8X2	T50.8X3	T50.8X4	T50.8X5	T50.8X6
Penimepicycline	T36.4X1	T36.4X2	T36.4X3	T36.4X4	T36.4X5	T36.4X6
Pentachloroethane	T53.6X1	T53.6X2	T53.6X3	T53.6X4	--	--
Pentachloronaphthalene	T53.7X1	T53.7X2	T53.7X3	T53.7X4	--	--
Pentachlorophenol (pesticide)	T60.1X1	T60.1X2	T60.1X3	T60.1X4	--	--
- fungicide	T60.3X1	T60.3X2	T60.3X3	T60.3X4	--	--
- herbicide	T60.3X1	T60.3X2	T60.3X3	T60.3X4	--	--
- insecticide	T60.1X1	T60.1X2	T60.1X3	T60.1X4	--	--
Pentaerythritol	T46.3X1	T46.3X2	T46.3X3	T46.3X4	T46.3X5	T46.3X6
- chloral	T42.6X1	T42.6X2	T42.6X3	T42.6X4	T42.6X5	T42.6X6
- tetranitrate NEC	T46.3X1	T46.3X2	T46.3X3	T46.3X4	T46.3X5	T46.3X6
Pentaerythrityl tetranitrate	T46.3X1	T46.3X2	T46.3X3	T46.3X4	T46.3X5	T46.3X6
Pentagastrin	T50.8X1	T50.8X2	T50.8X3	T50.8X4	T50.8X5	T50.8X6
Pentalin	T53.6X1	T53.6X2	T53.6X3	T53.6X4	--	--
Pentamethonium bromide	T44.2X1	T44.2X2	T44.2X3	T44.2X4	T44.2X5	T44.2X6
Pentamidine	T37.3X1	T37.3X2	T37.3X3	T37.3X4	T37.3X5	T37.3X6
Pentanol	T51.3X1	T51.3X2	T51.3X3	T51.3X4	--	--
Pentapyrrolinium (bitartrate)	T44.2X1	T44.2X2	T44.2X3	T44.2X4	T44.2X5	T44.2X6
Pentaquine	T37.2X1	T37.2X2	T37.2X3	T37.2X4	T37.2X5	T37.2X6
Pentazocine	T40.4X1	T40.4X2	T40.4X3	T40.4X4	T40.4X5	T40.4X6
Pentetrazole	T50.7X1	T50.7X2	T50.7X3	T50.7X4	T50.7X5	T50.7X6
Penthienate bromide	T44.3X1	T44.3X2	T44.3X3	T44.3X4	T44.3X5	T44.3X6
Pentifylline	T46.7X1	T46.7X2	T46.7X3	T46.7X4	T46.7X5	T46.7X6
Pentobarbital	T42.3X1	T42.3X2	T42.3X3	T42.3X4	T42.3X5	T42.3X6
- sodium	T42.3X1	T42.3X2	T42.3X3	T42.3X4	T42.3X5	T42.3X6
Pentobarbitone	T42.3X1	T42.3X2	T42.3X3	T42.3X4	T42.3X5	T42.3X6
Pentolonium tartrate	T44.2X1	T44.2X2	T44.2X3	T44.2X4	T44.2X5	T44.2X6
Pentosan polysulfate (sodium)	T39.8X1	T39.8X2	T39.8X3	T39.8X4	T39.8X5	T39.8X6
Pentostatin	T45.1X1	T45.1X2	T45.1X3	T45.1X4	T45.1X5	T45.1X6
Pentothal	T41.1X1	T41.1X2	T41.1X3	T41.1X4	T41.1X5	T41.1X6
Pentoxifylline	T46.7X1	T46.7X2	T46.7X3	T46.7X4	T46.7X5	T46.7X6
Pentoxyverine	T48.3X1	T48.3X2	T48.3X3	T48.3X4	T48.3X5	T48.3X6
Pentrinat	T46.3X1	T46.3X2	T46.3X3	T46.3X4	T46.3X5	T46.3X6
Pentylenetetrazole	T50.7X1	T50.7X2	T50.7X3	T50.7X4	T50.7X5	T50.7X6
Pentylsalicylamide	T37.1X1	T37.1X2	T37.1X3	T37.1X4	T37.1X5	T37.1X6
Pentymal	T42.3X1	T42.3X2	T42.3X3	T42.3X4	T42.3X5	T42.3X6
Peplomycin	T45.1X1	T45.1X2	T45.1X3	T45.1X4	T45.1X5	T45.1X6
Peppermint (oil)	T47.5X1	T47.5X2	T47.5X3	T47.5X4	T47.5X5	T47.5X6
Pepsin	T47.5X1	T47.5X2	T47.5X3	T47.5X4	T47.5X5	T47.5X6
- digestant	T47.5X1	T47.5X2	T47.5X3	T47.5X4	T47.5X5	T47.5X6
Pepstatin	T47.1X1	T47.1X2	T47.1X3	T47.1X4	T47.1X5	T47.1X6
Peptavlon	T50.8X1	T50.8X2	T50.8X3	T50.8X4	T50.8X5	T50.8X6
Perazine	T43.3X1	T43.3X2	T43.3X3	T43.3X4	T43.3X5	T43.3X6
Percaine (spinal)	T41.3X1	T41.3X2	T41.3X3	T41.3X4	T41.3X5	T41.3X6
- topical (surface)	T41.3X1	T41.3X2	T41.3X3	T41.3X4	T41.3X5	T41.3X6
Perchloroethylene	T53.3X1	T53.3X2	T53.3X3	T53.3X4	--	--
- medicinal	T37.4X1	T37.4X2	T37.4X3	T37.4X4	T37.4X5	T37.4X6
- vapor	T53.3X1	T53.3X2	T53.3X3	T53.3X4	--	--
Percodan	T40.2X1	T40.2X2	T40.2X3	T40.2X4	T40.2X5	T40.2X6
Percogesic—see also acetaminophen	T45.0X1	T45.0X2	T45.0X3	T45.0X4	T45.0X5	T45.0X6
Percorten	T38.0X1	T38.0X2	T38.0X3	T38.0X4	T38.0X5	T38.0X6
Pergolide	T42.8X1	T42.8X2	T42.8X3	T42.8X4	T42.8X5	T42.8X6
Pergonal	T38.811	T38.812	T38.813	T38.814	T38.815	T38.816
Perhexilene	T46.3X1	T46.3X2	T46.3X3	T46.3X4	T46.3X5	T46.3X6
Perhexiline (maleate)	T46.3X1	T46.3X2	T46.3X3	T46.3X4	T46.3X5	T46.3X6
Periactin	T45.0X1	T45.0X2	T45.0X3	T45.0X4	T45.0X5	T45.0X6
Periciazine	T43.3X1	T43.3X2	T43.3X3	T43.3X4	T43.3X5	T43.3X6
Periclor	T42.6X1	T42.6X2	T42.6X3	T42.6X4	T42.6X5	T42.6X6
Perindopril	T46.4X1	T46.4X2	T46.4X3	T46.4X4	T46.4X5	T46.4X6
Perisoxal	T39.8X1	T39.8X2	T39.8X3	T39.8X4	T39.8X5	T39.8X6

Substance	Poisoning, Accidental (unintentional)	Poisoning, Intentional Self-harm	Poisoning, Assault	Poisoning, Undetermined	Adverse effect	Underdosing
Peritoneal dialysis solution	T50.3X1	T50.3X2	T50.3X3	T50.3X4	T50.3X5	T50.3X6
Peritrate	T46.3X1	T46.3X2	T46.3X3	T46.3X4	T46.3X5	T46.3X6
Perlapine	T42.4X1	T42.4X2	T42.4X3	T42.4X4	T42.4X5	T42.4X6
Permanganate	T65.891	T65.892	T65.893	T65.894	--	--
Permethrin	T60.1X1	T60.1X2	T60.1X3	T60.1X4	--	--
Pernocton	T42.3X1	T42.3X2	T42.3X3	T42.3X4	T42.3X5	T42.3X6
Pernoston	T42.3X1	T42.3X2	T42.3X3	T42.3X4	T42.3X5	T42.3X6
Peronine	T40.2X1	T40.2X2	T40.2X3	T40.2X4	--	--
Perphenazine	T43.3X1	T43.3X2	T43.3X3	T43.3X4	T43.3X5	T43.3X6
Pertofrane	T43.011	T43.012	T43.013	T43.014	T43.015	T43.016
Pertussis						
- immune serum (human)	T50.Z11	T50.Z12	T50.Z13	T50.Z14	T50.Z15	T50.Z16
- vaccine (with diphtheria toxoid) (with tetanus toxoid)	T50.A11	T50.A12	T50.A13	T50.A14	T50.A15	T50.A16
Peruvian balsam	T49.0X1	T49.0X2	T49.0X3	T49.0X4	T49.0X5	T49.0X6
Peruvoside	T46.0X1	T46.0X2	T46.0X3	T46.0X4	T46.0X5	T46.0X6
Pesticide (dust) (fumes) (vapor) NEC	T60.91	T60.92	T60.93	T60.94	--	
- arsenic	T57.0X1	T57.0X2	T57.0X3	T57.0X4	--	--
- chlorinated	T60.1X1	T60.1X2	T60.1X3	T60.1X4	--	--
- cyanide	T65.0X1	T65.0X2	T65.0X3	T65.0X4	--	--
- kerosene	T52.0X1	T52.0X2	T52.0X3	T52.0X4	--	--
- mixture (of compounds)	T60.91	T60.92	T60.93	T60.94	--	--
- naphthalene	T60.2X1	T60.2X2	T60.2X3	T60.2X4	--	--
- organochlorine (compounds)	T60.1X1	T60.1X2	T60.1X3	T60.1X4	--	--
- petroleum (distillate) (products) NEC	T60.8X1	T60.8X2	T60.8X3	T60.8X4	--	--
- specified ingredient NEC	T60.8X1	T60.8X2	T60.8X3	T60.8X4	--	--
- strychnine	T65.1X1	T65.1X2	T65.1X3	T65.1X4	--	--
- thallium	T60.4X1	T60.4X2	T60.4X3	T60.4X4	--	--
Pethidine	T40.4X1	T40.4X2	T40.4X3	T40.4X4	T40.4X5	T40.4X6
Petrichloral	T42.6X1	T42.6X2	T42.6X3	T42.6X4	T42.6X5	T42.6X6
Petrol	T52.0X1	T52.0X2	T52.0X3	T52.0X4	--	--
- vapor	T52.0X1	T52.0X2	T52.0X3	T52.0X4	--	--
Petrolatum	T49.3X1	T49.3X2	T49.3X3	T49.3X4	T49.3X5	T49.3X6
- hydrophilic	T49.3X1	T49.3X2	T49.3X3	T49.3X4	T49.3X5	T49.3X6
- liquid	T47.4X1	T47.4X2	T47.4X3	T47.4X4	T47.4X5	T47.4X6
- - topical	T49.3X1	T49.3X2	T49.3X3	T49.3X4	T49.3X5	T49.3X6
- nonmedicinal	T52.0X1	T52.0X2	T52.0X3	T52.0X4	--	--
- red veterinary	T49.3X1	T49.3X2	T49.3X3	T49.3X4	T49.3X5	T49.3X6
- white	T49.3X1	T49.3X2	T49.3X3	T49.3X4	T49.3X5	T49.3X6
Petroleum (products) NEC	T52.0X1	T52.0X2	T52.0X3	T52.0X4	--	--
- benzine (s) —see Ligroin						
- ether—see Ligroin						
- jelly—see Petrolatum						
- naphtha—see Ligroin						
- pesticide	T60.8X1	T60.8X2	T60.8X3	T60.8X4	--	--
- solids	T52.0X1	T52.0X2	T52.0X3	T52.0X4	--	--
- solvents	T52.0X1	T52.0X2	T52.0X3	T52.0X4	--	--
- vapor	T52.0X1	T52.0X2	T52.0X3	T52.0X4	--	--
Peyote	T40.991	T40.992	T40.993	T40.994	--	--
Phanodorm, phanodorn	T42.3X1	T42.3X2	T42.3X3	T42.3X4	T42.3X5	T42.3X6
Phanquinone	T37.3X1	T37.3X2	T37.3X3	T37.3X4	T37.3X5	T37.3X6
Phanquone	T37.3X1	T37.3X2	T37.3X3	T37.3X4	T37.3X5	T37.3X6
Pharmaceutical						
- adjunct NEC	T50.901	T50.902	T50.903	T50.904	T50.905	T50.906
- excipient NEC	T50.901	T50.902	T50.903	T50.904	T50.905	T50.906
- sweetener	T50.901	T50.902	T50.903	T50.904	T50.905	T50.906
- viscous agent	T50.901	T50.902	T50.903	T50.904	T50.905	T50.906
Phemitone	T42.3X1	T42.3X2	T42.3X3	T42.3X4	T42.3X5	T42.3X6
Phenacaine	T41.3X1	T41.3X2	T41.3X3	T41.3X4	T41.3X5	T41.3X6
Phenacemide	T42.6X1	T42.6X2	T42.6X3	T42.6X4	T42.6X5	T42.6X6
Phenacetin	T39.1X1	T39.1X2	T39.1X3	T39.1X4	T39.1X5	T39.1X6
Phenadoxone	T40.2X1	T40.2X2	T40.2X3	T40.2X4	--	--
Phenaglycodol	T43.591	T43.592	T43.593	T43.594	T43.595	T43.596
Phenantoin	T42.0X1	T42.0X2	T42.0X3	T42.0X4	T42.0X5	T42.0X6
Phenaphthazine reagent	T50.991	T50.992	T50.993	T50.994	T50.995	T50.996

Substance	Poisoning, Accidental (unintentional)	Poisoning, Intentional Self-harm	Poisoning, Assault	Poisoning, Undetermined	Adverse effect	Underdosing
Phenazocine	T40.4X1	T40.4X2	T40.4X3	T40.4X4	T40.4X5	T40.4X6
Phenazone	T39.2X1	T39.2X2	T39.2X3	T39.2X4	T39.2X5	T39.2X6
Phenazopyridine	T39.8X1	T39.8X2	T39.8X3	T39.8X4	T39.8X5	T39.8X6
Phenbenicillin	T36.0X1	T36.0X2	T36.0X3	T36.0X4	T36.0X5	T36.0X6
Phenbutrazate	T50.5X1	T50.5X2	T50.5X3	T50.5X4	T50.5X5	T50.5X6
Phencyclidine	T40.991	T40.992	T40.993	T40.994	T40.995	T40.996
Phendimetrazine	T50.5X1	T50.5X2	T50.5X3	T50.5X4	T50.5X5	T50.5X6
Phenelzine	T43.1X1	T43.1X2	T43.1X3	T43.1X4	T43.1X5	T43.1X6
Phenemal	T42.3X1	T42.3X2	T42.3X3	T42.3X4	T42.3X5	T42.3X6
Phenergan	T42.6X1	T42.6X2	T42.6X3	T42.6X4	T42.6X5	T42.6X6
Pheneticillin	T36.0X1	T36.0X2	T36.0X3	T36.0X4	T36.0X5	T36.0X6
Pheneturide	T42.6X1	T42.6X2	T42.6X3	T42.6X4	T42.6X5	T42.6X6
Phenformin	T38.3X1	T38.3X2	T38.3X3	T38.3X4	T38.3X5	T38.3X6
Phenglutarimide	T44.3X1	T44.3X2	T44.3X3	T44.3X4	T44.3X5	T44.3X6
Phenicarbazide	T39.8X1	T39.8X2	T39.8X3	T39.8X4	T39.8X5	T39.8X6
Phenindamine	T45.0X1	T45.0X2	T45.0X3	T45.0X4	T45.0X5	T45.0X6
Phenindione	T45.511	T45.512	T45.513	T45.514	T45.515	T45.516
Pheniprazine	T43.1X1	T43.1X2	T43.1X3	T43.1X4	T43.1X5	T43.1X6
Pheniramine	T45.0X1	T45.0X2	T45.0X3	T45.0X4	T45.0X5	T45.0X6
Phenisatin	T47.2X1	T47.2X2	T47.2X3	T47.2X4	T47.2X5	T47.2X6
Phenmetrazine	T50.5X1	T50.5X2	T50.5X3	T50.5X4	T50.5X5	T50.5X6
Phenobal	T42.3X1	T42.3X2	T42.3X3	T42.3X4	T42.3X5	T42.3X6
Phenobarbital	T42.3X1	T42.3X2	T42.3X3	T42.3X4	T42.3X5	T42.3X6
- with						
- - mephenytoin	T42.3X1	T42.3X2	T42.3X3	T42.3X4	T42.3X5	T42.3X6
- - phenytoin	T42.3X1	T42.3X2	T42.3X3	T42.3X4	T42.3X5	T42.3X6
- sodium	T42.3X1	T42.3X2	T42.3X3	T42.3X4	T42.3X5	T42.3X6
Phenobarbitone	T42.3X1	T42.3X2	T42.3X3	T42.3X4	T42.3X5	T42.3X6
Phenobutiodil	T50.8X1	T50.8X2	T50.8X3	T50.8X4	T50.8X5	T50.8X6
Phenoctide	T49.0X1	T49.0X2	T49.0X3	T49.0X4	T49.0X5	T49.0X6
Phenol	T49.0X1	T49.0X2	T49.0X3	T49.0X4	T49.0X5	T49.0X6
- disinfectant	T54.0X1	T54.0X2	T54.0X3	T54.0X4	--	--
- in oil injection	T46.8X1	T46.8X2	T46.8X3	T46.8X4	T46.8X5	T46.8X6
- medicinal	T49.1X1	T49.1X2	T49.1X3	T49.1X4	T49.1X5	T49.1X6
- nonmedicinal NEC	T54.0X1	T54.0X2	T54.0X3	T54.0X4	--	--
- pesticide	T60.8X1	T60.8X2	T60.8X3	T60.8X4	--	--
- red	T50.8X1	T50.8X2	T50.8X3	T50.8X4	T50.8X5	T50.8X6
Phenolic preparation	T49.1X1	T49.1X2	T49.1X3	T49.1X4	T49.1X5	T49.1X6
Phenolphthalein	T47.2X1	T47.2X2	T47.2X3	T47.2X4	T47.2X5	T47.2X6
Phenolsulfonphthalein	T50.8X1	T50.8X2	T50.8X3	T50.8X4	T50.8X5	T50.8X6
Phenomorphan	T40.2X1	T40.2X2	T40.2X3	T40.2X4	--	--
Phenonyl	T42.3X1	T42.3X2	T42.3X3	T42.3X4	T42.3X5	T42.3X6
Phenoperidine	T40.4X1	T40.4X2	T40.4X3	T40.4X4	--	--
Phenopyrazone	T46.991	T46.992	T46.993	T46.994	T46.995	T46.996
Phenoquin	T50.4X1	T50.4X2	T50.4X3	T50.4X4	T50.4X5	T50.4X6
Phenothiazine (psychotropic) NEC	T43.3X1	T43.3X2	T43.3X3	T43.3X4	T43.3X5	T43.3X6
- insecticide	T60.2X1	T60.2X2	T60.2X3	T60.2X4	--	--
Phenothrin	T49.0X1	T49.0X2	T49.0X3	T49.0X4	T49.0X5	T49.0X6
Phenoxybenzamine	T46.7X1	T46.7X2	T46.7X3	T46.7X4	T46.7X5	T46.7X6
Phenoxyethanol	T49.0X1	T49.0X2	T49.0X3	T49.0X4	T49.0X5	T49.0X6
Phenoxymethyl penicillin	T36.0X1	T36.0X2	T36.0X3	T36.0X4	T36.0X5	T36.0X6
Phenprobamate	T42.8X1	T42.8X2	T42.8X3	T42.8X4	T42.8X5	T42.8X6
Phenprocoumon	T45.511	T45.512	T45.513	T45.514	T45.515	T45.516
Phensuximide	T42.2X1	T42.2X2	T42.2X3	T42.2X4	T42.2X5	T42.2X6
Phentermine	T50.5X1	T50.5X2	T50.5X3	T50.5X4	T50.5X5	T50.5X6
Phenthicillin	T36.0X1	T36.0X2	T36.0X3	T36.0X4	T36.0X5	T36.0X6
Phentolamine	T46.7X1	T46.7X2	T46.7X3	T46.7X4	T46.7X5	T46.7X6
Phenyl						
- butazone	T39.2X1	T39.2X2	T39.2X3	T39.2X4	T39.2X5	T39.2X6
- enediamine	T65.3X1	T65.3X2	T65.3X3	T65.3X4	--	--
- hydrazine	T65.3X1	T65.3X2	T65.3X3	T65.3X4	--	--
- - antineoplastic	T45.1X1	T45.1X2	T45.1X3	T45.1X4	T45.1X5	T45.1X6
- mercuric compounds—see Mercury						
- salicylate	T49.3X1	T49.3X2	T49.3X3	T49.3X4	T49.3X5	T49.3X6
Phenylalanine mustard	T45.1X1	T45.1X2	T45.1X3	T45.1X4	T45.1X5	T45.1X6

TABLE OF DRUGS AND CHEMICALS

Substance	Poisoning, Accidental (unintentional)	Poisoning, Intentional Self-harm	Poisoning, Assault	Poisoning, Undetermined	Adverse effect	Underdosing
Phenylbutazone	T39.2X1	T39.2X2	T39.2X3	T39.2X4	T39.2X5	T39.2X6
Phenylenediamine	T65.3X1	T65.3X2	T65.3X3	T65.3X4	--	--
Phenylephrine	T44.4X1	T44.4X2	T44.4X3	T44.4X4	T44.4X5	T44.4X6
Phenylethylbiguanide	T38.3X1	T38.3X2	T38.3X3	T38.3X4	T38.3X5	T38.3X6
Phenylmercuric						
- acetate	T49.0X1	T49.0X2	T49.0X3	T49.0X4	T49.0X5	T49.0X6
- borate	T49.0X1	T49.0X2	T49.0X3	T49.0X4	T49.0X5	T49.0X6
- nitrate	T49.0X1	T49.0X2	T49.0X3	T49.0X4	T49.0X5	T49.0X6
Phenylmethylbarbitone	T42.3X1	T42.3X2	T42.3X3	T42.3X4	T42.3X5	T42.3X6
Phenylpropanol	T47.5X1	T47.5X2	T47.5X3	T47.5X4	T47.5X5	T47.5X6
Phenylpropanolamine	T44.991	T44.992	T44.993	T44.994	T44.995	T44.996
Phenylsulfthion	T60.0X1	T60.0X2	T60.0X3	T60.0X4	--	--
Phenyltoloxamine	T45.0X1	T45.0X2	T45.0X3	T45.0X4	T45.0X5	T45.0X6
Phenyramidol, phenyramidon	T39.8X1	T39.8X2	T39.8X3	T39.8X4	T39.8X5	T39.8X6
Phenytoin	T42.0X1	T42.0X2	T42.0X3	T42.0X4	T42.0X5	T42.0X6
- with Phenobarbital	T42.3X1	T42.3X2	T42.3X3	T42.3X4	T42.3X5	T42.3X6
pHisoHex	T49.2X1	T49.2X2	T49.2X3	T49.2X4	T49.2X5	T49.2X6
Pholcodine	T48.3X1	T48.3X2	T48.3X3	T48.3X4	T48.3X5	T48.3X6
Pholedrine	T46.991	T46.992	T46.993	T46.994	T46.995	T46.996
Phorate	T60.0X1	T60.0X2	T60.0X3	T60.0X4	--	--
Phosdrin	T60.0X1	T60.0X2	T60.0X3	T60.0X4	--	--
Phosfolan	T60.0X1	T60.0X2	T60.0X3	T60.0X4	--	--
Phosgene (gas)	T59.891	T59.892	T59.893	T59.894	--	--
Phosphamidon	T60.0X1	T60.0X2	T60.0X3	T60.0X4	--	--
Phosphate	T65.891	T65.892	T65.893	T65.894	--	--
- laxative	T47.4X1	T47.4X2	T47.4X3	T47.4X4	T47.4X5	T47.4X6
- organic	T60.0X1	T60.0X2	T60.0X3	T60.0X4	--	--
- solvent	T52.91	T52.92	T52.93	T52.94	--	--
- tricresyl	T65.891	T65.892	T65.893	T65.894	--	--
Phosphine	T57.1X1	T57.1X2	T57.1X3	T57.1X4	--	--
- fumigant	T57.1X1	T57.1X2	T57.1X3	T57.1X4	--	--
Phospholine	T49.5X1	T49.5X2	T49.5X3	T49.5X4	T49.5X5	T49.5X6
Phosphoric acid	T54.2X1	T54.2X2	T54.2X3	T54.2X4	--	--
Phosphorus (compound) NEC	T57.1X1	T57.1X2	T57.1X3	T57.1X4	--	--
- pesticide	T60.0X1	T60.0X2	T60.0X3	T60.0X4	--	--
Phthalates	T65.891	T65.892	T65.893	T65.894	--	--
Phthalic anhydride	T65.891	T65.892	T65.893	T65.894	--	--
Phthalimidoglutarimide	T42.6X1	T42.6X2	T42.6X3	T42.6X4	T42.6X5	T42.6X6
Phthalylsulfathiazole	T37.0X1	T37.0X2	T37.0X3	T37.0X4	T37.0X5	T37.0X6
Phylloquinone	T45.7X1	T45.7X2	T45.7X3	T45.7X4	T45.7X5	T45.7X6
Physeptone	T40.3X1	T40.3X2	T40.3X3	T40.3X4	T40.3X5	T40.3X6
Physostigma venenosum	T62.2X1	T62.2X2	T62.2X3	T62.2X4	--	--
Physostigmine	T49.5X1	T49.5X2	T49.5X3	T49.5X4	T49.5X5	T49.5X6
Phytolacca decandra	T62.2X1	T62.2X2	T62.2X3	T62.2X4	--	--
- berries	T62.1X1	T62.1X2	T62.1X3	T62.1X4	--	--
Phytomenadione	T45.7X1	T45.7X2	T45.7X3	T45.7X4	T45.7X5	T45.7X6
Phytonadione	T45.7X1	T45.7X2	T45.7X3	T45.7X4	T45.7X5	T45.7X6
Picoperine	T48.3X1	T48.3X2	T48.3X3	T48.3X4	T48.3X5	T48.3X6
Picosulfate (sodium)	T47.2X1	T47.2X2	T47.2X3	T47.2X4	T47.2X5	T47.2X6
Picric (acid)	T54.2X1	T54.2X2	T54.2X3	T54.2X4	--	--
Picrotoxin	T50.7X1	T50.7X2	T50.7X3	T50.7X4	T50.7X5	T50.7X6
Piketoprofen	T49.0X1	T49.0X2	T49.0X3	T49.0X4	T49.0X5	T49.0X6
Pilocarpine	T44.1X1	T44.1X2	T44.1X3	T44.1X4	T44.1X5	T44.1X6
Pilocarpus (jaborandi) extract	T44.1X1	T44.1X2	T44.1X3	T44.1X4	T44.1X5	T44.1X6
Pilsicainide (hydrochloride)	T46.2X1	T46.2X2	T46.2X3	T46.2X4	T46.2X5	T46.2X6
Pimaricin	T36.7X1	T36.7X2	T36.7X3	T36.7X4	T36.7X5	T36.7X6
Pimeclone	T50.7X1	T50.7X2	T50.7X3	T50.7X4	T50.7X5	T50.7X6
Pimelic ketone	T52.8X1	T52.8X2	T52.8X3	T52.8X4	--	--
Pimethixene	T45.0X1	T45.0X2	T45.0X3	T45.0X4	T45.0X5	T45.0X6
Piminodine	T40.2X1	T40.2X2	T40.2X3	T40.2X4	T40.2X5	T40.2X6
Pimozide	T43.591	T43.592	T43.593	T43.594	T43.595	T43.596
Pinacidil	T46.5X1	T46.5X2	T46.5X3	T46.5X4	T46.5X5	T46.5X6
Pinaverium bromide	T44.3X1	T44.3X2	T44.3X3	T44.3X4	T44.3X5	T44.3X6
Pinazepam	T42.4X1	T42.4X2	T42.4X3	T42.4X4	T42.4X5	T42.4X6
Pindolol	T44.7X1	T44.7X2	T44.7X3	T44.7X4	T44.7X5	T44.7X6

Substance	Poisoning, Accidental (unintentional)	Poisoning, Intentional Self-harm	Poisoning, Assault	Poisoning, Undetermined	Adverse effect	Underdosing
Pindone	T60.4X1	T60.4X2	T60.4X3	T60.4X4	--	--
Pine oil (disinfectant)	T65.891	T65.892	T65.893	T65.894	--	--
Pinkroot	T37.4X1	T37.4X2	T37.4X3	T37.4X4	T37.4X5	T37.4X6
Pipadone	T40.2X1	T40.2X2	T40.2X3	T40.2X4	--	
Pipamazine	T45.0X1	T45.0X2	T45.0X3	T45.0X4	T45.0X5	T45.0X6
Pipamperone	T43.4X1	T43.4X2	T43.4X3	T43.4X4	T43.4X5	T43.4X6
Pipazetate	T48.3X1	T48.3X2	T48.3X3	T48.3X4	T48.3X5	T48.3X6
Pipemidic acid	T37.8X1	T37.8X2	T37.8X3	T37.8X4	T37.8X5	T37.8X6
Pipenzolate bromide	T44.3X1	T44.3X2	T44.3X3	T44.3X4	T44.3X5	T44.3X6
Piperacetazine	T43.3X1	T43.3X2	T43.3X3	T43.3X4	T43.3X5	T43.3X6
Piperacillin	T36.0X1	T36.0X2	T36.0X3	T36.0X4	T36.0X5	T36.0X6
Piperazine	T37.4X1	T37.4X2	T37.4X3	T37.4X4	T37.4X5	T37.4X6
- estrone sulfate	T38.5X1	T38.5X2	T38.5X3	T38.5X4	T38.5X5	T38.5X6
Piper cubeba	T62.2X1	T62.2X2	T62.2X3	T62.2X4	--	--
Piperidione	T48.3X1	T48.3X2	T48.3X3	T48.3X4	T48.3X5	T48.3X6
Piperidolate	T44.3X1	T44.3X2	T44.3X3	T44.3X4	T44.3X5	T44.3X6
Piperocaine	T41.3X1	T41.3X2	T41.3X3	T41.3X4	T41.3X5	T41.3X6
- infiltration (subcutaneous)	T41.3X1	T41.3X2	T41.3X3	T41.3X4	T41.3X5	T41.3X6
- nerve block (peripheral) (plexus)	T41.3X1	T41.3X2	T41.3X3	T41.3X4	T41.3X5	T41.3X6
- topical (surface)	T41.3X1	T41.3X2	T41.3X3	T41.3X4	T41.3X5	T41.3X6
Piperonyl butoxide	T60.8X1	T60.8X2	T60.8X3	T60.8X4	--	--
Pipethanate	T44.3X1	T44.3X2	T44.3X3	T44.3X4	T44.3X5	T44.3X6
Pipobroman	T45.1X1	T45.1X2	T45.1X3	T45.1X4	T45.1X5	T45.1X6
Pipotiazine	T43.3X1	T43.3X2	T43.3X3	T43.3X4	T43.3X5	T43.3X6
Pipoxizine	T45.0X1	T45.0X2	T45.0X3	T45.0X4	T45.0X5	T45.0X6
Pipradrol	T43.691	T43.692	T43.693	T43.694	T43.695	T43.696
Piprinhydrinate	T45.0X1	T45.0X2	T45.0X3	T45.0X4	T45.0X5	T45.0X6
Pirarubicin	T45.1X1	T45.1X2	T45.1X3	T45.1X4	T45.1X5	T45.1X6
Pirazinamide	T37.1X1	T37.1X2	T37.1X3	T37.1X4	T37.1X5	T37.1X6
Pirbuterol	T48.6X1	T48.6X2	T48.6X3	T48.6X4	T48.6X5	T48.6X6
Pirenzepine	T47.1X1	T47.1X2	T47.1X3	T47.1X4	T47.1X5	T47.1X6
Piretanide	T50.1X1	T50.1X2	T50.1X3	T50.1X4	T50.1X5	T50.1X6
Piribedil	T42.8X1	T42.8X2	T42.8X3	T42.8X4	T42.8X5	T42.8X6
Piridoxilate	T46.3X1	T46.3X2	T46.3X3	T46.3X4	T46.3X5	T46.3X6
Piritramide	T40.4X1	T40.4X2	T40.4X3	T40.4X4	--	--
Piromidic acid	T37.8X1	T37.8X2	T37.8X3	T37.8X4	T37.8X5	T37.8X6
Piroxicam	T39.391	T39.392	T39.393	T39.394	T39.395	T39.396
- beta-cyclodextrin complex	T39.8X1	T39.8X2	T39.8X3	T39.8X4	T39.8X5	T39.8X6
Pirozadil	T46.6X1	T46.6X2	T46.6X3	T46.6X4	T46.6X5	T46.6X6
Piscidia (bark) (erythrina)	T39.8X1	T39.8X2	T39.8X3	T39.8X4	T39.8X5	T39.8X6
Pitch	T65.891	T65.892	T65.893	T65.894	--	--
Pitkin's solution	T41.3X1	T41.3X2	T41.3X3	T41.3X4	T41.3X5	T41.3X6
Pitocin	T48.0X1	T48.0X2	T48.0X3	T48.0X4	T48.0X5	T48.0X6
Pitressin (tannate)	T38.891	T38.892	T38.893	T38.894	T38.895	T38.896
Pituitary extracts (posterior)	T38.891	T38.892	T38.893	T38.894	T38.895	T38.896
- anterior	T38.811	T38.812	T38.813	T38.814	T38.815	T38.816
Pituitrin	T38.891	T38.892	T38.893	T38.894	T38.895	T38.896
Pivampicillin	T36.0X1	T36.0X2	T36.0X3	T36.0X4	T36.0X5	T36.0X6
Pivmecillinam	T36.0X1	T36.0X2	T36.0X3	T36.0X4	T36.0X5	T36.0X6
Placental hormone	T38.891	T38.892	T38.893	T38.894	T38.895	T38.896
Placidyl	T42.6X1	T42.6X2	T42.6X3	T42.6X4	T42.6X5	T42.6X6
Plague vaccine	T50.A91	T50.A92	T50.A93	T50.A94	T50.A95	T50.A96
Plant						
- food or fertilizer NEC	T65.891	T65.892	T65.893	T65.894	--	--
- - containing herbicide	T60.3X1	T60.3X2	T60.3X3	T60.3X4	--	--
- noxious, used as food	T62.2X1	T62.2X2	T62.2X3	T62.2X4	--	--
- - berries	T62.1X1	T62.1X2	T62.1X3	T62.1X4	--	--
- - seeds	T62.2X1	T62.2X2	T62.2X3	T62.2X4	--	--
- - specified type NEC	T62.2X1	T62.2X2	T62.2X3	T62.2X4	--	--
Plasma	T45.8X1	T45.8X2	T45.8X3	T45.8X4	T45.8X5	T45.8X6
- expander NEC	T45.8X1	T45.8X2	T45.8X3	T45.8X4	T45.8X5	T45.8X6
- protein fraction (human)	T45.8X1	T45.8X2	T45.8X3	T45.8X4	T45.8X5	T45.8X6
Plasmanate	T45.8X1	T45.8X2	T45.8X3	T45.8X4	T45.8X5	T45.8X6
Plasminogen (tissue) activator	T45.611	T45.612	T45.613	T45.614	T45.615	T45.616
Plaster dressing	T49.3X1	T49.3X2	T49.3X3	T49.3X4	T49.3X5	T49.3X6

Substance	Poisoning, Accidental (unintentional)	Poisoning, Intentional Self-harm	Poisoning, Assault	Poisoning, Undetermined	Adverse effect	Underdosing
Plastic dressing	T49.3X1	T49.3X2	T49.3X3	T49.3X4	T49.3X5	T49.3X6
Plegicil	T43.3X1	T43.3X2	T43.3X3	T43.3X4	T43.3X5	T43.3X6
Plicamycin	T45.1X1	T45.1X2	T45.1X3	T45.1X4	T45.1X5	T45.1X6
Podophyllotoxin	T49.8X1	T49.8X2	T49.8X3	T49.8X4	T49.8X5	T49.8X6
Podophyllum (resin)	T49.4X1	T49.4X2	T49.4X3	T49.4X4	T49.4X5	T49.4X6
Poison NEC	T65.91	T65.92	T65.93	T65.94	--	--
Poisonous berries	T62.1X1	T62.1X2	T62.1X3	T62.1X4	--	--
Pokeweed (any part)	T62.2X1	T62.2X2	T62.2X3	T62.2X4	--	--
Poldine metilsulfate	T44.3X1	T44.3X2	T44.3X3	T44.3X4	T44.3X5	T44.3X6
Polidexide (sulfate)	T46.6X1	T46.6X2	T46.6X3	T46.6X4	T46.6X5	T46.6X6
Polidocanol	T46.8X1	T46.8X2	T46.8X3	T46.8X4	T46.8X5	T46.8X6
Poliomyelitis vaccine	T50.B91	T50.B92	T50.B93	T50.B94	T50.B95	T50.B96
Polish (car) (floor) (furni-ture) (metal) (porcelain) (silver)	T65.891	T65.892	T65.893	T65.894	--	--
- abrasive	T65.891	T65.892	T65.893	T65.894	--	--
- porcelain	T65.891	T65.892	T65.893	T65.894	--	--
Poloxalkol	T47.4X1	T47.4X2	T47.4X3	T47.4X4	T47.4X5	T47.4X6
Poloxamer	T47.4X1	T47.4X2	T47.4X3	T47.4X4	T47.4X5	T47.4X6
Polyaminostyrene resins	T50.3X1	T50.3X2	T50.3X3	T50.3X4	T50.3X5	T50.3X6
Polycarbophil	T47.4X1	T47.4X2	T47.4X3	T47.4X4	T47.4X5	T47.4X6
Polychlorinated biphenyl	T65.891	T65.892	T65.893	T65.894	--	--
Polycycline	T36.4X1	T36.4X2	T36.4X3	T36.4X4	T36.4X5	T36.4X6
Polyester fumes	T59.891	T59.892	T59.893	T59.894	--	--
Polyester resin hardener	T52.91	T52.92	T52.93	T52.94	--	--
- fumes	T59.891	T59.892	T59.893	T59.894	--	--
Polyestradiol phosphate	T38.5X1	T38.5X2	T38.5X3	T38.5X4	T38.5X5	T38.5X6
Polyethanolamine alkyl sulfate	T49.2X1	T49.2X2	T49.2X3	T49.2X4	T49.2X5	T49.2X6
Polyethylene adhesive	T49.3X1	T49.3X2	T49.3X3	T49.3X4	T49.3X5	T49.3X6
Polyferose	T45.4X1	T45.4X2	T45.4X3	T45.4X4	T45.4X5	T45.4X6
Polygeline	T45.8X1	T45.8X2	T45.8X3	T45.8X4	T45.8X4	T45.8X6
Polymyxin	T36.8X1	T36.8X2	T36.8X3	T36.8X4	T36.8X5	T36.8X6
- B	T36.8X1	T36.8X2	T36.8X3	T36.8X4	T36.8X5	T36.8X6
- - ENT agent	T49.6X1	T49.6X2	T49.6X3	T49.6X4	T49.6X5	T49.6X6
- - topical NEC	T49.0X1	T49.0X2	T49.0X3	T49.0X4	T49.0X5	T49.0X6
- E sulfate (eye preparation)	T49.5X1	T49.5X2	T49.5X3	T49.5X4	T49.5X5	T49.5X6
Polynoxylin	T49.0X1	T49.0X2	T49.0X3	T49.0X4	T49.0X5	T49.0X6
Polyoestradiol phosphate	T38.5X1	T38.5X2	T38.5X3	T38.5X4	T38.5X5	T38.5X6
Polyoxymethyleneurea	T49.0X1	T49.0X2	T49.0X3	T49.0X4	T49.0X5	T49.0X6
Polysilane	T47.8X1	T47.8X2	T47.8X3	T47.8X4	T47.8X5	T47.8X6
Polytetrafluoroethylene (inhaled)	T59.891	T59.892	T59.893	T59.894	--	--
Polythiazide	T50.2X1	T50.2X2	T50.2X3	T50.2X4	T50.2X5	T50.2X6
Polyvidone	T45.8X1	T45.8X2	T45.8X3	T45.8X4	T45.8X5	T45.8X6
Polyvinylpyrrolidone	T45.8X1	T45.8X2	T45.8X3	T45.8X4	T45.8X5	T45.8X6
Pontocaine (hydrochloride) (infiltration) (topical)	T41.3X1	T41.3X2	T41.3X3	T41.3X4	T41.3X5	T41.3X6
- nerve block (peripheral) (plexus)	T41.3X1	T41.3X2	T41.3X3	T41.3X4	T41.3X5	T41.3X6
- spinal	T41.3X1	T41.3X2	T41.3X3	T41.3X4	T41.3X5	T41.3X6
Porfiromycin	T45.1X1	T45.1X2	T45.1X3	T45.1X4	T45.1X5	T45.1X6
Posterior pituitary hormone NEC	T38.891	T38.892	T38.893	T38.894	T38.895	T38.896
Pot	T40.7X1	T40.7X2	T40.7X3	T40.7X4	T40.7X5	T40.7X6
Potash (caustic)	T54.3X1	T54.3X2	T54.3X3	T54.3X4	--	--
Potassic saline injection (lactated)	T50.3X1	T50.3X2	T50.3X3	T50.3X4	T50.3X5	T50.3X6
Potassium (salts) NEC	T50.3X1	T50.3X2	T50.3X3	T50.3X4	T50.3X5	T50.3X6
- aminobenzoate	T45.8X1	T45.8X2	T45.8X3	T45.8X4	T45.8X5	T45.8X6
- aminosalicylate	T37.1X1	T37.1X2	T37.1X3	T37.1X4	T37.1X5	T37.1X6
- antimony ' tartrate'	T37.8X1	T37.8X2	T37.8X3	T37.8X4	T37.8X5	T37.8X6
- arsenite (solution)	T57.0X1	T57.0X2	T57.0X3	T57.0X4	--	--
- bichromate	T56.2X1	T56.2X2	T56.2X3	T56.2X4	--	--
- bisulfate	T47.3X1	T47.3X2	T47.3X3	T47.3X4	T47.3X5	T47.3X6
- bromide	T42.6X1	T42.6X2	T42.6X3	T42.6X4	T42.6X5	T42.6X6
- canrenoate	T50.0X1	T50.0X2	T50.0X3	T50.0X4	T50.0X5	T50.0X6
- carbonate	T54.3X1	T54.3X2	T54.3X3	T54.3X4	--	--
- chlorate NEC	T65.891	T65.892	T65.893	T65.894	--	--
- chloride	T50.3X1	T50.3X2	T50.3X3	T50.3X4	T50.3X5	T50.3X6
- citrate	T50.991	T50.992	T50.993	T50.994	T50.995	T50.996
- cyanide	T65.0X1	T65.0X2	T65.0X3	T65.0X4	--	--

Substance	Poisoning, Accidental (unintentional)	Poisoning, Intentional Self-harm	Poisoning, Assault	Poisoning, Undetermined	Adverse effect	Underdosing
- ferric hexacyanoferrate (medicinal)	T50.6X1	T50.6X2	T50.6X3	T50.6X4	T50.6X5	T50.6X6
- - nonmedicinal	T65.891	T65.892	T65.893	T65.894	--	--
- Fluoride	T57.8X1	T57.8X2	T57.8X3	T57.8X4	--	--
- glucaldrate	T47.1X1	T47.1X2	T47.1X3	T47.1X4	T47.1X5	T47.1X6
- hydroxide	T54.3X1	T54.3X2	T54.3X3	T54.3X4	--	--
- iodate	T49.0X1	T49.0X2	T49.0X3	T49.0X4	T49.0X5	T49.0X6
- iodide	T48.4X1	T48.4X2	T48.4X3	T48.4X4	T48.4X5	T48.4X6
- nitrate	T57.8X1	T57.8X2	T57.8X3	T57.8X4	--	--
- oxalate	T65.891	T65.892	T65.893	T65.894	--	--
- perchlorate (nonmedicinal) NEC	T65.891	T65.892	T65.893	T65.894	--	--
- - antithyroid	T38.2X1	T38.2X2	T38.2X3	T38.2X4	T38.2X5	T38.2X6
- - medicinal	T38.2X1	T38.2X2	T38.2X3	T38.2X4	T38.2X5	T38.2X6
- Permanganate (nonmedicinal)	T65.891	T65.892	T65.893	T65.894	--	--
- - medicinal	T49.0X1	T49.0X2	T49.0X3	T49.0X4	T49.0X5	T49.0X6
- sulfate	T47.2X1	T47.2X2	T47.2X3	T47.2X4	T47.2X5	T47.2X6
Potassium-removing resin	T50.3X1	T50.3X2	T50.3X3	T50.3X4	T50.3X5	T50.3X6
Potassium-retaining drug	T50.3X1	T50.3X2	T50.3X3	T50.3X4	T50.3X5	T50.3X6
Povidone	T45.8X1	T45.8X2	T45.8X3	T45.8X4	T45.8X5	T45.8X6
- iodine	T49.0X1	T49.0X2	T49.0X3	T49.0X4	T49.0X5	T49.0X6
Practolol	T44.7X1	T44.7X2	T44.7X3	T44.7X4	T44.7X5	T44.7X6
Prajmalium bitartrate	T46.2X1	T46.2X2	T46.2X3	T46.2X4	T46.2X5	T46.2X6
Pralidoxime (iodide)	T50.6X1	T50.6X2	T50.6X3	T50.6X4	T50.6X5	T50.6X6
- chloride	T50.6X1	T50.6X2	T50.6X3	T50.6X4	T50.6X5	T50.6X6
Pramiverine	T44.3X1	T44.3X2	T44.3X3	T44.3X4	T44.3X5	T44.3X6
Pramocaine	T49.1X1	T49.1X2	T49.1X3	T49.1X4	T49.1X5	T49.1X6
Pramoxine	T49.1X1	T49.1X2	T49.1X3	T49.1X4	T49.1X5	T49.1X6
Prasterone	T38.7X1	T38.7X2	T38.7X3	T38.7X4	T38.7X5	T38.7X6
Pravastatin	T46.6X1	T46.6X2	T46.6X3	T46.6X4	T46.6X5	T46.6X6
Prazepam	T42.4X1	T42.4X2	T42.4X3	T42.4X4	T42.4X5	T42.4X6
Praziquantel	T37.4X1	T37.4X2	T37.4X3	T37.4X4	T37.4X5	T37.4X6
Prazitone	T43.291	T43.292	T43.293	T43.294	T43.295	T43.296
Prazosin	T44.6X1	T44.6X2	T44.6X3	T44.6X4	T44.6X5	T44.6X6
Prednicarbate	T49.0X1	T49.0X2	T49.0X3	T49.0X4	T49.0X5	T49.0X6
Prednimustine	T45.1X1	T45.1X2	T45.1X3	T45.1X4	T45.1X5	T45.1X6
Prednisolone	T38.0X1	T38.0X2	T38.0X3	T38.0X4	T38.0X5	T38.0X6
- ENT agent	T49.6X1	T49.6X2	T49.6X3	T49.6X4	T49.6X5	T49.6X6
- ophthalmic preparation	T49.5X1	T49.5X2	T49.5X3	T49.5X4	T49.5X5	T49.5X6
- steaglate	T49.0X1	T49.0X2	T49.0X3	T49.0X4	T49.0X5	T49.0X6
- topical NEC	T49.0X1	T49.0X2	T49.0X3	T49.0X4	T49.0X5	T49.0X6
Prednisone	T38.0X1	T38.0X2	T38.0X3	T38.0X4	T38.0X5	T38.0X6
Prednylidene	T38.0X1	T38.0X2	T38.0X3	T38.0X4	T38.0X5	T38.0X6
Pregnandiol	T38.5X1	T38.5X2	T38.5X3	T38.5X4	T38.5X5	T38.5X6
Pregneninolone	T38.5X1	T38.5X2	T38.5X3	T38.5X4	T38.5X5	T38.5X6
Preludin	T43.691	T43.692	T43.693	T43.694	T43.695	T43.696
Premarin	T38.5X1	T38.5X2	T38.5X3	T38.5X4	T38.5X5	T38.5X6
Premedication anesthetic	T41.201	T41.202	T41.203	T41.204	T41.205	T41.206
Prenalterol	T44.5X1	T44.5X2	T44.5X3	T44.5X4	T44.5X5	T44.5X6
Prenoxdiazine	T48.3X1	T48.3X2	T48.3X3	T48.3X4	T48.3X5	T48.3X6
Prenylamine	T46.3X1	T46.3X2	T46.3X3	T46.3X4	T46.3X5	T46.3X6
Preparation H	T49.8X1	T49.8X2	T49.8X3	T49.8X4	T49.8X5	T49.8X6
Preparation, local	T49.4X1	T49.4X2	T49.4X3	T49.4X4	T49.4X5	T49.4X6
Preservative (nonmedicinal)	T65.891	T65.892	T65.893	T65.894	--	--
- medicinal	T50.901	T50.902	T50.903	T50.904	T50.905	T50.906
- wood	T60.91	T60.92	T60.93	T60.94	--	--
Prethcamide	T50.7X1	T50.7X2	T50.7X3	T50.7X4	T50.7X5	T50.7X6
Pride of China	T62.2X1	T62.2X2	T62.2X3	T62.2X4	--	--
Pridinol	T44.3X1	T44.3X2	T44.3X3	T44.3X4	T44.3X5	T44.3X6
Prifinium bromide	T44.3X1	T44.3X2	T44.3X3	T44.3X4	T44.3X5	T44.3X6
Prilocaine	T41.3X1	T41.3X2	T41.3X3	T41.3X4	T41.3X5	T41.3X6
- infiltration (subcutaneous)	T41.3X1	T41.3X2	T41.3X3	T41.3X4	T41.3X5	T41.3X6
- nerve block (peripheral) (plexus)	T41.3X1	T41.3X2	T41.3X3	T41.3X4	T41.3X5	T41.3X6
- regional	T41.3X1	T41.3X2	T41.3X3	T41.3X4	T41.3X5	T41.3X6
Primaquine	T37.2X1	T37.2X2	T37.2X3	T37.2X4	T37.2X5	T37.2X6
Primidone	T42.6X1	T42.6X2	T42.6X3	T42.6X4	T42.6X5	T42.6X6
Primula (veris)	T62.2X1	T62.2X2	T62.2X3	T62.2X4	--	--

Substance	Poisoning, Accidental (unintentional)	Poisoning, Intentional Self-harm	Poisoning, Assault	Poisoning, Undetermined	Adverse effect	Underdosing
Prinadol	T40.2X1	T40.2X2	T40.2X3	T40.2X4	T40.2X5	T40.2X6
Priscol, Priscoline	T44.6X1	T44.6X2	T44.6X3	T44.6X4	T44.6X5	T44.6X6
Pristinamycin	T36.3X1	T36.3X2	T36.3X3	T36.3X4	T36.3X5	T36.3X6
Privet	T62.2X1	T62.2X2	T62.2X3	T62.2X4	--	--
- berries	T62.1X1	T62.1X2	T62.1X3	T62.1X4	--	--
Privine	T44.4X1	T44.4X2	T44.4X3	T44.4X4	T44.4X5	T44.4X6
Pro-Banthine	T44.3X1	T44.3X2	T44.3X3	T44.3X4	T44.3X5	T44.3X6
Probarbital	T42.3X1	T42.3X2	T42.3X3	T42.3X4	T42.3X5	T42.3X6
Probenecid	T50.4X1	T50.4X2	T50.4X3	T50.4X4	T50.4X5	T50.4X6
Probucol	T46.6X1	T46.6X2	T46.6X3	T46.6X4	T46.6X5	T46.6X6
Procainamide	T46.2X1	T46.2X2	T46.2X3	T46.2X4	T46.2X5	T46.2X6
Procaine	T41.3X1	T41.3X2	T41.3X3	T41.3X4	T41.3X5	T41.3X6
- benzylpenicillin	T36.0X1	T36.0X2	T36.0X3	T36.0X4	T36.0X5	T36.0X6
- nerve block (periphreal) (plexus)	T41.3X1	T41.3X2	T41.3X3	T41.3X4	T41.3X5	T41.3X6
- penicillin G	T36.0X1	T36.0X2	T36.0X3	T36.0X4	T36.0X5	T36.0X6
- regional	T41.3X1	T41.3X2	T41.3X3	T41.3X4	T41.3X5	T41.3X6
- spinal	T41.3X1	T41.3X2	T41.3X3	T41.3X4	T41.3X5	T41.3X6
Procalmidol	T43.591	T43.592	T43.593	T43.594	T43.595	T43.596
Procarbazine	T45.1X1	T45.1X2	T45.1X3	T45.1X4	T45.1X5	T45.1X6
Procaterol	T44.5X1	T44.5X2	T44.5X3	T44.5X4	T44.5X5	T44.5X6
Prochlorperazine	T43.3X1	T43.3X2	T43.3X3	T43.3X4	T43.3X5	T43.3X6
Procyclidine	T44.3X1	T44.3X2	T44.3X3	T44.3X4	T44.3X5	T44.3X6
Producer gas	T58.8X1	T58.8X2	T58.8X3	T58.8X4	--	--
Profadol	T40.4X1	T40.4X2	T40.4X3	T40.4X4	T40.4X5	T40.4X6
Profenamine	T44.3X1	T44.3X2	T44.3X3	T44.3X4	T44.3X5	T44.3X6
Profenil	T44.3X1	T44.3X2	T44.3X3	T44.3X4	T44.3X5	T44.3X6
Proflavine	T49.0X1	T49.0X2	T49.0X3	T49.0X4	T49.0X5	T49.0X6
Progabide	T42.6X1	T42.6X2	T42.6X3	T42.6X4	T42.6X5	T42.6X6
Progesterone	T38.5X1	T38.5X2	T38.5X3	T38.5X4	T38.5X5	T38.5X6
Progestin	T38.5X1	T38.5X2	T38.5X3	T38.5X4	T38.5X5	T38.5X6
- oral contraceptive	T38.4X1	T38.4X2	T38.4X3	T38.4X4	T38.4X5	T38.4X6
Progestogen NEC	T38.5X1	T38.5X2	T38.5X3	T38.5X4	T38.5X5	T38.5X6
Progestone	T38.5X1	T38.5X2	T38.5X3	T38.5X4	T38.5X5	T38.5X6
Proglumide	T47.1X1	T47.1X2	T47.1X3	T47.1X4	T47.1X5	T47.1X6
Proguanil	T37.2X1	T37.2X2	T37.2X3	T37.2X4	T37.2X5	T37.2X6
Prolactin	T38.811	T38.812	T38.813	T38.814	T38.815	T38.816
Prolintane	T43.691	T43.692	T43.693	T43.694	T43.695	T43.696
Proloid	T38.1X1	T38.1X2	T38.1X3	T38.1X4	T38.1X5	T38.1X6
Proluton	T38.5X1	T38.5X2	T38.5X3	T38.5X4	T38.5X5	T38.5X6
Promacetin	T37.1X1	T37.1X2	T37.1X3	T37.1X4	T37.1X5	T37.1X6
Promazine	T43.3X1	T43.3X2	T43.3X3	T43.3X4	T43.3X5	T43.3X6
Promedol	T40.2X1	T40.2X2	T40.2X3	T40.2X4	--	--
Promegestone	T38.5X1	T38.5X2	T38.5X3	T38.5X4	T38.5X5	T38.5X6
Promethazine (teoclate)	T43.3X1	T43.3X2	T43.3X3	T43.3X4	T43.3X5	T43.3X6
Promin	T37.1X1	T37.1X2	T37.1X3	T37.1X4	T37.1X5	T37.1X6
Pronase	T45.3X1	T45.3X2	T45.3X3	T45.3X4	T45.3X5	T45.3X6
Pronestyl (hydrochloride)	T46.2X1	T46.2X2	T46.2X3	T46.2X4	T46.2X5	T46.2X6
Pronetalol	T44.7X1	T44.7X2	T44.7X3	T44.7X4	T44.7X5	T44.7X6
Prontosil	T37.0X1	T37.0X2	T37.0X3	T37.0X4	T37.0X5	T37.0X6
Propachlor	T60.3X1	T60.3X2	T60.3X3	T60.3X4	--	--
Propafenone	T46.2X1	T46.2X2	T46.2X3	T46.2X4	T46.2X5	T46.2X6
Propallylonal	T42.3X1	T42.3X2	T42.3X3	T42.3X4	T42.3X5	T42.3X6
Propamidine	T49.0X1	T49.0X2	T49.0X3	T49.0X4	T49.0X5	T49.0X6
Propane (distributed in mobile container)	T59.891	T59.892	T59.893	T59.894	--	--
- distributed through pipes	T59.891	T59.892	T59.893	T59.894		
- incomplete combustion	T58.11	T58.12	T58.13	T58.14	--	--
Propanidid	T41.291	T41.292	T41.293	T41.294	T41.295	T41.296
Propanil	T60.3X1	T60.3X2	T60.3X3	T60.3X4	--	--
1-Propanol	T51.3X1	T51.3X2	T51.3X3	T51.3X4	--	--
2-Propanol	T51.2X1	T51.2X2	T51.2X3	T51.2X4	--	--
Propantheline	T44.3X1	T44.3X2	T44.3X3	T44.3X4	T44.3X5	T44.3X6
- bromide	T44.3X1	T44.3X2	T44.3X3	T44.3X4	T44.3X5	T44.3X6
Proparacaine	T41.3X1	T41.3X2	T41.3X3	T41.3X4	T41.3X5	T41.3X6
Propatylnitrate	T46.3X1	T46.3X2	T46.3X3	T46.3X4	T46.3X5	T46.3X6
Propicillin	T36.0X1	T36.0X2	T36.0X3	T36.0X4	T36.0X5	T36.0X6

Substance	Poisoning, Accidental (unintentional)	Poisoning, Intentional Self-harm	Poisoning, Assault	Poisoning, Undetermined	Adverse effect	Underdosing
Propiolactone	T49.0X1	T49.0X2	T49.0X3	T49.0X4	T49.0X5	T49.0X6
Propiomazine	T45.0X1	T45.0X2	T45.0X3	T45.0X4	T45.0X5	T45.0X6
Propionaidehyde (medicinal)	T42.6X1	T42.6X2	T42.6X3	T42.6X4	T42.6X5	T42.6X6
Propionate (calcium) (sodium)	T49.0X1	T49.0X2	T49.0X3	T49.0X4	T49.0X5	T49.0X6
Propion gel	T49.0X1	T49.0X2	T49.0X3	T49.0X4	T49.0X5	T49.0X6
Propitocaine	T41.3X1	T41.3X2	T41.3X3	T41.3X4	T41.3X5	T41.3X6
- infiltration (subcutaneous)	T41.3X1	T41.3X2	T41.3X3	T41.3X4	T41.3X5	T41.3X6
- nerve block (peripheral) (plexus)	T41.3X1	T41.3X2	T41.3X3	T41.3X4	T41.3X5	T41.3X6
Propofol	T41.291	T41.292	T41.293	T41.294	T41.295	T41.296
Propoxur	T60.0X1	T60.0X2	T60.0X3	T60.0X4	--	--
Propoxycaine	T41.3X1	T41.3X2	T41.3X3	T41.3X4	T41.3X5	T41.3X6
- infiltration (subcutaneous)	T41.3X1	T41.3X2	T41.3X3	T41.3X4	T41.3X5	T41.3X6
- nerve block (peripheral) (plexus)	T41.3X1	T41.3X2	T41.3X3	T41.3X4	T41.3X5	T41.3X6
- topical (surface)	T41.3X1	T41.3X2	T41.3X3	T41.3X4	T41.3X5	T41.3X6
Propoxyphene	T40.4X1	T40.4X2	T40.4X3	T40.4X4	T40.4X5	T40.4X6
Propranolol	T44.7X1	T44.7X2	T44.7X3	T44.7X4	T44.7X5	T44.7X6
Propyl						
- alcohol	T51.3X1	T51.3X2	T51.3X3	T51.3X4	--	--
- carbinol	T51.3X1	T51.3X2	T51.3X3	T51.3X4	--	--
- hexadrine	T44.4X1	T44.4X2	T44.4X3	T44.4X4	T44.4X5	T44.4X6
- iodone	T50.8X1	T50.8X2	T50.8X3	T50.8X4	T50.8X5	T50.8X6
- thiouracil	T38.2X1	T38.2X2	T38.2X3	T38.2X4	T38.2X5	T38.2X6
Propylaminopheno-thiazine	T43.3X1	T43.3X2	T43.3X3	T43.3X4	T43.3X5	T43.3X6
Propylene	T59.891	T59.892	T59.893	T59.894	--	--
Propylhexedrine	T48.5X1	T48.5X2	T48.5X3	T48.5X4	T48.5X5	T48.5X6
Propyliodone	T50.8X1	T50.8X2	T50.8X3	T50.8X4	T50.8X5	T50.8X6
Propylparaben (ophthalmic)	T49.5X1	T49.5X2	T49.5X3	T49.5X4	T49.5X5	T49.5X6
Propylthiouracil	T38.2X1	T38.2X2	T38.2X3	T38.2X4	T38.2X5	T38.2X6
Propyphenazone	T39.2X1	T39.2X2	T39.2X3	T39.2X4	T39.2X5	T39.2X6
Proquazone	T39.391	T39.392	T39.393	T39.394	T39.395	T39.396
Proscillaridin	T46.0X1	T46.0X2	T46.0X3	T46.0X4	T46.0X5	T46.0X6
Prostacyclin	T45.521	T45.522	T45.523	T45.524	T45.525	T45.526
Prostaglandin (I2)	T45.521	T45.522	T45.523	T45.524	T45.525	T45.526
- E1	T46.7X1	T46.7X2	T46.7X3	T46.7X4	T46.7X5	T46.7X6
- E2	T48.0X1	T48.0X2	T48.0X3	T48.0X4	T48.0X5	T48.0X6
- F2 alpha	T48.0X1	T48.0X2	T48.0X3	T48.0X4	T48.0X5	T48.0X6
Prostigmin	T44.0X1	T44.0X2	T44.0X3	T44.0X4	T44.0X5	T44.0X6
Prosultiamine	T45.2X1	T45.2X2	T45.2X3	T45.2X4	T45.2X5	T45.2X6
Protamine sulfate	T45.7X1	T45.7X2	T45.7X3	T45.7X4	T45.7X5	T45.7X6
- zinc insulin	T38.3X1	T38.3X2	T38.3X3	T38.3X4	T38.3X5	T38.3X6
Protease	T47.5X1	T47.5X2	T47.5X3	T47.5X4	T47.5X5	T47.5X6
Protectant, skin NEC	T49.3X1	T49.3X2	T49.3X3	T49.3X4	T49.3X5	T49.3X6
Protein hydrolysate	T50.991	T50.992	T50.993	T50.994	T50.995	T50.996
Prothiaden—see Dothiepin hydrochloride						
Prothionamide	T37.1X1	T37.1X2	T37.1X3	T37.1X4	T37.1X5	T37.1X6
Prothipendyl	T43.591	T43.592	T43.593	T43.594	T43.595	T43.596
Prothoate	T60.0X1	T60.0X2	T60.0X3	T60.0X4	--	--
Prothrombin						
- activator	T45.7X1	T45.7X2	T45.7X3	T45.7X4	T45.7X5	T45.7X6
- synthesis inhibitor	T45.511	T45.512	T45.513	T45.514	T45.515	T45.516
Protionamide	T37.1X1	T37.1X2	T37.1X3	T37.1X4	T37.1X5	T37.1X6
Protirelin	T38.891	T38.892	T38.893	T38.894	T38.895	T38.896
Protokylol	T48.6X1	T48.6X2	T48.6X3	T48.6X4	T48.6X5	T48.6X6
Protopam	T50.6X1	T50.6X2	T50.6X3	T50.6X4	T50.6X5	T50.6X6
Protoveratrine (s) (A) (B)	T46.5X1	T46.5X2	T46.5X3	T46.5X4	T46.5X5	T46.5X6
Protriptyline	T43.011	T43.012	T43.013	T43.014	T43.015	T43.016
Provera	T38.5X1	T38.5X2	T38.5X3	T38.5X4	T38.5X5	T38.5X6
Provitamin A	T45.2X1	T45.2X2	T45.2X3	T45.2X4	T45.2X5	T45.2X6
Proxibarbal	T42.3X1	T42.3X2	T42.3X3	T42.3X4	T42.3X5	T42.3X6
Proxymetacaine	T41.3X1	T41.3X2	T41.3X3	T41.3X4	T41.3X5	T41.3X6
Proxyphylline	T48.6X1	T48.6X2	T48.6X3	T48.6X4	T48.6X5	T48.6X6
Prozac—see Fluoxetine hydrochloride						
Prunus						
- laurocerasus	T62.2X1	T62.2X2	T62.2X3	T62.2X4	--	--
- virginiana	T62.2X1	T62.2X2	T62.2X3	T62.2X4	--	--

Substance	Poisoning, Accidental (unintentional)	Poisoning, Intentional Self-harm	Poisoning, Assault	Poisoning, Undetermined	Adverse effect	Underdosing
Prussian blue						
- commercial	T65.891	T65.892	T65.893	T65.894	--	--
- therapeutic	T50.6X1	T50.6X2	T50.6X3	T50.6X4	T50.6X5	T50.6X6
Prussic acid	T65.0X1	T65.0X2	T65.0X3	T65.0X4	--	--
- vapor	T57.3X1	T57.3X2	T57.3X3	T57.3X4	--	--
Pseudoephedrine	T44.991	T44.992	T44.993	T44.994	T44.995	T44.996
Psilocin	T40.991	T40.992	T40.993	T40.994	--	--
Psilocybin	T40.991	T40.992	T40.993	T40.994	--	--
Psilocybine	T40.991	T40.992	T40.993	T40.994	--	--
Psoralene (nonmedicinal)	T65.891	T65.892	T65.893	T65.894	--	--
Psoralens (medicinal)	T50.991	T50.992	T50.993	T50.994	T50.995	T50.996
PSP (phenolsulfonphthalein)	T50.8X1	T50.8X2	T50.8X3	T50.8X4	T50.8X5	T50.8X6
Psychodysleptic drug NEC	T40.901	T40.902	T40.903	T40.904	T40.905	T40.906
Psychostimulant	T43.601	T43.602	T43.603	T43.604	T43.605	T43.606
- amphetamine	T43.621	T43.622	T43.623	T43.624	T43.625	T43.626
- caffeine	T43.611	T43.612	T43.613	T43.614	T43.615	T43.616
- methylphenidate	T43.631	T43.632	T43.633	T43.634	T43.635	T43.636
- specified NEC	T43.691	T43.692	T43.693	T43.694	T43.695	T43.696
Psychotherapeutic drug NEC	T43.91	T43.92	T43.93	T43.94	T43.95	T43.96
- antidepressants—see also Antidepressant	T43.201	T43.202	T43.203	T43.204	T43.205	T43.206
- specified NEC	T43.8X1	T43.8X2	T43.8X3	T43.8X4	T43.8X5	T43.8X6
- tranquilizers NEC	T43.501	T43.502	T43.503	T43.504	T43.505	T43.506
Psychotomimetic agents	T40.901	T40.902	T40.903	T40.904	T40.905	T40.906
Psychotropic drug NEC	T43.91	T43.92	T43.93	T43.94	T43.95	T43.96
- specified NEC	T43.8X1	T43.8X2	T43.8X3	T43.8X4	T43.8X5	T43.8X6
Psyllium hydrophilic mucilloid	T47.4X1	T47.4X2	T47.4X3	T47.4X4	T47.4X5	T47.4X6
Pteroylglutamic acid	T45.8X1	T45.8X2	T45.8X3	T45.8X4	T45.8X5	T45.8X6
Pteroyltriglutamate	T45.1X1	T45.1X2	T45.1X3	T45.1X4	T45.1X5	T45.1X6
PTFE—see Polytetrafluoroethylene						
Pulp						
- devitalizing paste	T49.7X1	T49.7X2	T49.7X3	T49.7X4	T49.7X5	T49.7X6
- dressing	T49.7X1	T49.7X2	T49.7X3	T49.7X4	T49.7X5	T49.7X6
Pulsatilla	T62.2X1	T62.2X2	T62.2X3	T62.2X4	--	--
Pumpkin seed extract	T37.4X1	T37.4X2	T37.4X3	T37.4X4	T37.4X5	T37.4X6
Purex (bleach)	T54.91	T54.92	T54.93	T54.94	--	--
Purgative NEC—see also Cathartic	T47.4X1	T47.4X2	T47.4X3	T47.4X4	T47.4X5	T47.4X6
Purine analogue (antineoplastic)	T45.1X1	T45.1X2	T45.1X3	T45.1X4	T45.1X5	T45.1X6
Purine diuretics	T50.2X1	T50.2X2	T50.2X3	T50.2X4	T50.2X5	T50.2X6
Purinethol	T45.1X1	T45.1X2	T45.1X3	T45.1X4	T45.1X5	T45.1X6
PVP	T45.8X1	T45.8X2	T45.8X3	T45.8X4	T45.8X5	T45.8X6
Pyrabital	T39.8X1	T39.8X2	T39.8X3	T39.8X4	T39.8X5	T39.8X6
Pyramidon	T39.2X1	T39.2X2	T39.2X3	T39.2X4	T39.2X5	T39.2X6
Pyrantel	T37.4X1	T37.4X2	T37.4X3	T37.4X4	T37.4X5	T37.4X6
Pyrathiazine	T45.0X1	T45.0X2	T45.0X3	T45.0X4	T45.0X5	T45.0X6
Pyrazinamide	T37.1X1	T37.1X2	T37.1X3	T37.1X4	T37.1X5	T37.1X6
Pyrazinoic acid (amide)	T37.1X1	T37.1X2	T37.1X3	T37.1X4	T37.1X5	T37.1X6
Pyrazole (derivatives)	T39.2X1	T39.2X2	T39.2X3	T39.2X4	T39.2X5	T39.2X6
Pyrazolone analgesic NEC	T39.2X1	T39.2X2	T39.2X3	T39.2X4	T39.2X5	T39.2X6
Pyrethrin, pyrethrum (nonmedicinal)	T60.2X1	T60.2X2	T60.2X3	T60.2X4	--	--
Pyrethrum extract	T49.0X1	T49.0X2	T49.0X3	T49.0X4	T49.0X5	T49.0X6
Pyribenzamine	T45.0X1	T45.0X2	T45.0X3	T45.0X4	T45.0X5	T45.0X6
Pyridine	T52.8X1	T52.8X2	T52.8X3	T52.8X4	--	--
- aldoxime methiodide	T50.6X1	T50.6X2	T50.6X3	T50.6X4	T50.6X5	T50.6X6
- aldoxime methyl chloride	T50.6X1	T50.6X2	T50.6X3	T50.6X4	T50.6X5	T50.6X6
- vapor	T59.891	T59.892	T59.893	T59.894	--	--
Pyridium	T39.8X1	T39.8X2	T39.8X3	T39.8X4	T39.8X5	T39.8X6
Pyridostigmine bromide	T44.0X1	T44.0X2	T44.0X3	T44.0X4	T44.0X5	T44.0X6
Pyridoxal phosphate	T45.2X1	T45.2X2	T45.2X3	T45.2X4	T45.2X5	T45.2X6
Pyridoxine	T45.2X1	T45.2X2	T45.2X3	T45.2X4	T45.2X5	T45.2X6
Pyrilamine	T45.0X1	T45.0X2	T45.0X3	T45.0X4	T45.0X5	T45.0X6
Pyrimethamine	T37.2X1	T37.2X2	T37.2X3	T37.2X4	T37.2X5	T37.2X6
- with sulfadoxine	T37.2X1	T37.2X2	T37.2X3	T37.2X4	T37.2X5	T37.2X6
Pyrimidine antagonist	T45.1X1	T45.1X2	T45.1X3	T45.1X4	T45.1X5	T45.1X6
Pyriminil	T60.4X1	T60.4X2	T60.4X3	T60.4X4	--	--
Pyrithione zinc	T49.4X1	T49.4X2	T49.4X3	T49.4X4	T49.4X5	T49.4X6

Substance	Poisoning, Accidental (unintentional)	Poisoning, Intentional Self-harm	Poisoning, Assault	Poisoning, Undetermined	Adverse effect	Underdosing
Pyrithyldione	T42.6X1	T42.6X2	T42.6X3	T42.6X4	T42.6X5	T42.6X6
Pyrogallic acid	T49.0X1	T49.0X2	T49.0X3	T49.0X4	T49.0X5	T49.0X6
Pyrogallol	T49.0X1	T49.0X2	T49.0X3	T49.0X4	T49.0X5	T49.0X6
Pyroxylin	T49.3X1	T49.3X2	T49.3X3	T49.3X4	T49.3X5	T49.3X6
Pyrrobutamine	T45.0X1	T45.0X2	T45.0X3	T45.0X4	T45.0X5	T45.0X6
Pyrrolizidine alkaloids	T62.8X1	T62.8X2	T62.8X3	T62.8X4	--	--
Pyrvinium chloride	T37.4X1	T37.4X2	T37.4X3	T37.4X4	T37.4X5	T37.4X6
PZI	T38.3X1	T38.3X2	T38.3X3	T38.3X4	T38.3X5	T38.3X6
Quaalude	T42.6X1	T42.6X2	T42.6X3	T42.6X4	T42.6X5	T42.6X6
Quarternary ammonium						
- anti-infective	T49.0X1	T49.0X2	T49.0X3	T49.0X4	T49.0X5	T49.0X6
- ganglion blocking	T44.2X1	T44.2X2	T44.2X3	T44.2X4	T44.2X5	T44.2X6
- parasympatholytic	T44.3X1	T44.3X2	T44.3X3	T44.3X4	T44.3X5	T44.3X6
Quazepam	T42.4X1	T42.4X2	T42.4X3	T42.4X4	T42.4X5	T42.4X6
Quicklime	T54.3X1	T54.3X2	T54.3X3	T54.3X4	--	--
Quillaja extract	T48.4X1	T48.4X2	T48.4X3	T48.4X4	T48.4X5	T48.4X6
Quinacrine	T37.2X1	T37.2X2	T37.2X3	T37.2X4	T37.2X5	T37.2X6
Quinaglute	T46.2X1	T46.2X2	T46.2X3	T46.2X4	T46.2X5	T46.2X6
Quinalbarbital	T42.3X1	T42.3X2	T42.3X3	T42.3X4	T42.3X5	T42.3X6
Quinalbarbitone sodium	T42.3X1	T42.3X2	T42.3X3	T42.3X4	T42.3X5	T42.3X6
Quinalphos	T60.0X1	T60.0X2	T60.0X3	T60.0X4	--	--
Quinapril	T46.4X1	T46.4X2	T46.4X3	T46.4X4	T46.4X5	T46.4X6
Quinestradiol	T38.5X1	T38.5X2	T38.5X3	T38.5X4	T38.5X5	T38.5X6
Quinestradol	T38.5X1	T38.5X2	T38.5X3	T38.5X4	T38.5X5	T38.5X6
Quinestrol	T38.5X1	T38.5X2	T38.5X3	T38.5X4	T38.5X5	T38.5X6
Quinethazone	T50.2X1	T50.2X2	T50.2X3	T50.2X4	T50.2X5	T50.2X6
Quingestanol	T38.4X1	T38.4X2	T38.4X3	T38.4X4	T38.4X5	T38.4X6
Quinidine	T46.2X1	T46.2X2	T46.2X3	T46.2X4	T46.2X5	T46.2X6
Quinine	T37.2X1	T37.2X2	T37.2X3	T37.2X4	T37.2X5	T37.2X6
Quiniobine	T37.8X1	T37.8X2	T37.8X3	T37.8X4	T37.8X5	T37.8X6
Quinisocaine	T49.1X1	T49.1X2	T49.1X3	T49.1X4	T49.1X5	T49.1X6
Quinocide	T37.2X1	T37.2X2	T37.2X3	T37.2X4	T37.2X5	T37.2X6
Quinoline (derivatives) NEC	T37.8X1	T37.8X2	T37.8X3	T37.8X4	T37.8X5	T37.8X6
Quinupramine	T43.011	T43.012	T43.013	T43.014	T43.015	T43.016
Quotane	T41.3X1	T41.3X2	T41.3X3	T41.3X4	T41.3X5	T41.3X6
Rabies						
- immune globulin (human)	T50.Z11	T50.Z12	T50.Z13	T50.Z14	T50.Z15	T50.Z16
- vaccine	T50.B91	T50.B92	T50.B93	T50.B94	T50.B95	T50.B96
Racemoramide	T40.2X1	T40.2X2	T40.2X3	T40.2X4	--	--
Racemorphan	T40.2X1	T40.2X2	T40.2X3	T40.2X4	T40.2X5	T40.2X6
Racepinefrin	T44.5X1	T44.5X2	T44.5X3	T44.5X4	T44.5X5	T44.5X6
Raclopride	T43.591	T43.592	T43.593	T43.594	T43.595	T43.596
Radiator alcohol	T51.1X1	T51.1X2	T51.1X3	T51.1X4	--	--
Radioactive drug NEC	T50.8X1	T50.8X2	T50.8X3	T50.8X4	T50.8X5	T50.8X6
Radio-opaque (drugs) (materials)	T50.8X1	T50.8X2	T50.8X3	T50.8X4	T50.8X5	T50.8X6
Ramifenazone	T39.2X1	T39.2X2	T39.2X3	T39.2X4	T39.2X5	T39.2X6
Ramipril	T46.4X1	T46.4X2	T46.4X3	T46.4X4	T46.4X5	T46.4X6
Ranitidine	T47.0X1	T47.0X2	T47.0X3	T47.0X4	T47.0X5	T47.0X6
Ranunculus	T62.2X1	T62.2X2	T62.2X3	T62.2X4	--	--
Rat poison NEC	T60.4X1	T60.4X2	T60.4X3	T60.4X4	--	--
Rattlesnake (venom)	T63.011	T63.012	T63.013	T63.014	--	--
Raubasine	T46.7X1	T46.7X2	T46.7X3	T46.7X4	T46.7X5	T46.7X6
Raudixin	T46.5X1	T46.5X2	T46.5X3	T46.5X4	T46.5X5	T46.5X6
Rautensin	T46.5X1	T46.5X2	T46.5X3	T46.5X4	T46.5X5	T46.5X6
Rautina	T46.5X1	T46.5X2	T46.5X3	T46.5X4	T46.5X5	T46.5X6
Rautotal	T46.5X1	T46.5X2	T46.5X3	T46.5X4	T46.5X5	T46.5X6
Rauwiloid	T46.5X1	T46.5X2	T46.5X3	T46.5X4	T46.5X5	T46.5X6
Rauwoldin	T46.5X1	T46.5X2	T46.5X3	T46.5X4	T46.5X5	T46.5X6
Rauwolfia (alkaloids)	T46.5X1	T46.5X2	T46.5X3	T46.5X4	T46.5X5	T46.5X6
Razoxane	T45.1X1	T45.1X2	T45.1X3	T45.1X4	T45.1X5	T45.1X6
Realgar	T57.0X1	T57.0X2	T57.0X3	T57.0X4	--	--
Recombinant (R) —see specific protein						
Red blood cells, packed	T45.8X1	T45.8X2	T45.8X3	T45.8X4	T45.8X5	T45.8X6
Red squill (scilliroside)	T60.4X1	T60.4X2	T60.4X3	T60.4X4	--	--
Reducing agent, industrial NEC	T65.891	T65.892	T65.893	T65.894	--	--

Substance	Poisoning, Accidental (unintentional)	Poisoning, Intentional Self-harm	Poisoning, Assault	Poisoning, Undetermined	Adverse effect	Underdosing
Refrigerant gas (chlorofluoro-carbon)	T53.5X1	T53.5X2	T53.5X3	T53.5X4	--	--
- not chlorofluoro-carbon	T59.891	T59.892	T59.893	T59.894	--	--
Regroton	T50.2X1	T50.2X2	T50.2X3	T50.2X4	T50.2X5	T50.2X6
Rehydration salts (oral)	T50.3X1	T50.3X2	T50.3X3	T50.3X4	T50.3X5	T50.3X6
Rela	T42.8X1	T42.8X2	T42.8X3	T42.8X4	T42.8X5	T42.8X6
Relaxant, muscle						
- anesthetic	T48.1X1	T48.1X2	T48.1X3	T48.1X4	T48.1X5	T48.1X6
- central nervous system	T42.8X1	T42.8X2	T42.8X3	T42.8X4	T42.8X5	T42.8X6
- skeletal NEC	T48.1X1	T48.1X2	T48.1X3	T48.1X4	T48.1X5	T48.1X6
- smooth NEC	T44.3X1	T44.3X2	T44.3X3	T44.3X4	T44.3X5	T44.3X6
Remoxipride	T43.591	T43.592	T43.593	T43.594	T43.595	T43.596
Renese	T50.2X1	T50.2X2	T50.2X3	T50.2X4	T50.2X5	T50.2X6
Renografin	T50.8X1	T50.8X2	T50.8X3	T50.8X4	T50.8X5	T50.8X6
Replacement solution	T50.3X1	T50.3X2	T50.3X3	T50.3X4	T50.3X5	T50.3X6
Reproterol	T48.6X1	T48.6X2	T48.6X3	T48.6X4	T48.6X5	T48.6X6
Rescinnamine	T46.5X1	T46.5X2	T46.5X3	T46.5X4	T46.5X5	T46.5X6
Reserpin (e)	T46.5X1	T46.5X2	T46.5X3	T46.5X4	T46.5X5	T46.5X6
Resorcin, resorcinol (nonmedicinal)	T65.891	T65.892	T65.893	T65.894	--	--
- medicinal	T49.4X1	T49.4X2	T49.4X3	T49.4X4	T49.4X5	T49.4X6
Respaire	T48.4X1	T48.4X2	T48.4X3	T48.4X4	T48.4X5	T48.4X6
Respiratory drug NEC	T48.901	T48.902	T48.903	T48.904	T48.905	T48.906
- antiasthmatic NEC	T48.6X1	T48.6X2	T48.6X3	T48.6X4	T48.6X5	T48.6X6
- anti-common-cold NEC	T48.5X1	T48.5X2	T48.5X3	T48.5X4	T48.5X5	T48.5X6
- expectorant NEC	T48.4X1	T48.4X2	T48.4X3	T48.4X4	T48.4X5	T48.4X6
- stimulant	T48.901	T48.902	T48.903	T48.904	T48.905	T48.906
Retinoic acid	T49.0X1	T49.0X2	T49.0X3	T49.0X4	T49.0X5	T49.0X6
Retinol	T45.2X1	T45.2X2	T45.2X3	T45.2X4	T45.2X5	T45.2X6
Rh (D) immune globulin (human)	T50.Z11	T50.Z12	T50.Z13	T50.Z14	T50.Z15	T50.Z16
Rhodine	T39.011	T39.012	T39.013	T39.014	T39.015	T39.016
RhoGAM	T50.Z11	T50.Z12	T50.Z13	T50.Z14	T50.Z15	T50.Z16
Rhubarb						
- dry extract	T47.2X1	T47.2X2	T47.2X3	T47.2X4	T47.2X5	T47.2X6
- tincture, compound	T47.2X1	T47.2X2	T47.2X3	T47.2X4	T47.2X5	T47.2X6
Ribavirin	T37.5X1	T37.5X2	T37.5X3	T37.5X4	T37.5X5	T37.5X6
Riboflavin	T45.2X1	T45.2X2	T45.2X3	T45.2X4	T45.2X5	T45.2X6
Ribostamycin	T36.5X1	T36.5X2	T36.5X3	T36.5X4	T36.5X5	T36.5X6
Ricin	T62.2X1	T62.2X2	T62.2X3	T62.2X4	--	--
Ricinus communis	T62.2X1	T62.2X2	T62.2X3	T62.2X4	--	--
Rickettsial vaccine NEC	T50.A91	T50.A92	T50.A93	T50.A94	T50.A95	T50.A96
Rifabutin	T36.6X1	T36.6X2	T36.6X3	T36.6X4	T36.6X5	T36.6X6
Rifamide	T36.6X1	T36.6X2	T36.6X3	T36.6X4	T36.6X5	T36.6X6
Rifampicin	T36.6X1	T36.6X2	T36.6X3	T36.6X4	T36.6X5	T36.6X6
- with isoniazid	T37.1X1	T37.1X2	T37.1X3	T37.1X4	T37.1X5	T37.1X6
Rifampin	T36.6X1	T36.6X2	T36.6X3	T36.6X4	T36.6X5	T36.6X6
Rifamycin	T36.6X1	T36.6X2	T36.6X3	T36.6X4	T36.6X5	T36.6X6
Rifaximin	T36.6X1	T36.6X2	T36.6X3	T36.6X4	T36.6X5	T36.6X6
Rimantadine	T37.5X1	T37.5X2	T37.5X3	T37.5X4	T37.5X5	T37.5X6
Rimazolium metilsulfate	T39.8X1	T39.8X2	T39.8X3	T39.8X4	T39.8X5	T39.8X6
Rimifon	T37.1X1	T37.1X2	T37.1X3	T37.1X4	T37.1X5	T37.1X6
Rimiterol	T48.6X1	T48.6X2	T48.6X3	T48.6X4	T48.6X5	T48.6X6
Ringer (lactate) solution	T50.3X1	T50.3X2	T50.3X3	T50.3X4	T50.3X5	T50.3X6
Ristocetin	T36.8X1	T36.8X2	T36.8X3	T36.8X4	T36.8X5	T36.8X6
Ritalin	T43.631	T43.632	T43.633	T43.634	T43.635	T43.636
Ritodrine	T44.5X1	T44.5X2	T44.5X3	T44.5X4	T44.5X5	T44.5X6
Roach killer—see Insecticide						
Rociverine	T44.3X1	T44.3X2	T44.3X3	T44.3X4	T44.3X5	T44.3X6
Rocky Mountain spotted fever vaccine	T50.A91	T50.A92	T50.A93	T50.A94	T50.A95	T50.A96
Rodenticide NEC	T60.4X1	T60.4X2	T60.4X3	T60.4X4	--	--
Rohypnol	T42.4X1	T42.4X2	T42.4X3	T42.4X4	T42.4X5	T42.4X6
Rokitamycin	T36.3X1	T36.3X2	T36.3X3	T36.3X4	T36.3X5	T36.3X6
Rolaids	T47.1X1	T47.1X2	T47.1X3	T47.1X4	T47.1X5	T47.1X6
Rolitetracycline	T36.4X1	T36.4X2	T36.4X3	T36.4X4	T36.4X5	T36.4X6
Romilar	T48.3X1	T48.3X2	T48.3X3	T48.3X4	T48.3X5	T48.3X6
Ronifibrate	T46.6X1	T46.6X2	T46.6X3	T46.6X4	T46.6X5	T46.6X6
Rosaprostol	T47.1X1	T47.1X2	T47.1X3	T47.1X4	T47.1X5	T47.1X6

Substance	Poisoning, Accidental (unintentional)	Poisoning, Intentional Self-harm	Poisoning, Assault	Poisoning, Undetermined	Adverse effect	Underdosing
Rose bengal sodium (131I)	T50.8X1	T50.8X2	T50.8X3	T50.8X4	T50.8X5	T50.8X6
Rose water ointment	T49.3X1	T49.3X2	T49.3X3	T49.3X4	T49.3X5	T49.3X6
Rosoxacin	T37.8X1	T37.8X2	T37.8X3	T37.8X4	T37.8X5	T37.8X6
Rotenone	T60.2X1	T60.2X2	T60.2X3	T60.2X4	--	--
Rotoxamine	T45.0X1	T45.0X2	T45.0X3	T45.0X4	T45.0X5	T45.0X6
Rough-on-rats	T60.4X1	T60.4X2	T60.4X3	T60.4X4	--	--
Roxatidine	T47.0X1	T47.0X2	T47.0X3	T47.0X4	T47.0X5	T47.0X6
Roxithromycin	T36.3X1	T36.3X2	T36.3X3	T36.3X4	T36.3X5	T36.3X6
Rt-PA	T45.611	T45.612	T45.613	T45.614	T45.615	T45.616
Rubbing alcohol	T51.2X1	T51.2X2	T51.2X3	T51.2X4	--	--
Rubefacient	T49.4X1	T49.4X2	T49.4X3	T49.4X4	T49.4X5	T49.4X6
Rubella vaccine	T50.B91	T50.B92	T50.B93	T50.B94	T50.B95	T50.B96
Rubeola vaccine	T50.B91	T50.B92	T50.B93	T50.B94	T50.B95	T50.B96
Rubidium chloride Rb82	T50.8X1	T50.8X2	T50.8X3	T50.8X4	T50.8X5	T50.8X6
Rubidomycin	T45.1X1	T45.1X2	T45.1X3	T45.1X4	T45.1X5	T45.1X6
Rue	T62.2X1	T62.2X2	T62.2X3	T62.2X4	--	--
Rufocromomycin	T45.1X1	T45.1X2	T45.1X3	T45.1X4	T45.1X5	T45.1X6
Russel's viper venin	T45.7X1	T45.7X2	T45.7X3	T45.7X4	T45.7X5	T45.7X6
Ruta (graveolens)	T62.2X1	T62.2X2	T62.2X3	T62.2X4	--	--
Rutinum	T46.991	T46.992	T46.993	T46.994	T46.995	T46.996
Rutoside	T46.991	T46.992	T46.993	T46.994	T46.995	T46.996
Sabadilla (plant)	T62.2X1	T62.2X2	T62.2X3	T62.2X4	--	--
- pesticide	T60.2X1	T60.2X2	T60.2X3	T60.2X4	--	--
Saccharated iron oxide	T45.8X1	T45.8X2	T45.8X3	T45.8X4	T45.8X5	T45.8X6
Saccharin	T50.901	T50.902	T50.903	T50.904	T50.905	T50.906
Saccharomyces boulardii	T47.6X1	T47.6X2	T47.6X3	T47.6X4	T47.6X5	T47.6X6
Safflower oil	T46.6X1	T46.6X2	T46.6X3	T46.6X4	T46.6X5	T46.6X6
Safrazine	T43.1X1	T43.1X2	T43.1X3	T43.1X4	T43.1X5	T43.1X6
Salazosulfapyridine	T37.0X1	T37.0X2	T37.0X3	T37.0X4	T37.0X5	T37.0X6
Salbutamol	T48.6X1	T48.6X2	T48.6X3	T48.6X4	T48.6X5	T48.6X6
Salicylamide	T39.091	T39.092	T39.093	T39.094	T39.095	T39.096
Salicylate NEC	T39.091	T39.092	T39.093	T39.094	T39.095	T39.096
- methyl	T49.3X1	T49.3X2	T49.3X3	T49.3X4	T49.3X5	T49.3X6
- theobromine calcium	T50.2X1	T50.2X2	T50.2X3	T50.2X4	T50.2X5	T50.2X6
Salicylazosulfapyridine	T37.0X1	T37.0X2	T37.0X3	T37.0X4	T37.0X5	T37.0X6
Salicylhydroxamic acid	T49.0X1	T49.0X2	T49.0X3	T49.0X4	T49.0X5	T49.0X6
Salicylic acid	T49.4X1	T49.4X2	T49.4X3	T49.4X4	T49.4X5	T49.4X6
- with benzoic acid	T49.4X1	T49.4X2	T49.4X3	T49.4X4	T49.4X5	T49.4X6
- congeners	T39.091	T39.092	T39.093	T39.094	T39.095	T39.096
- derivative	T39.091	T39.092	T39.093	T39.094	T39.095	T39.096
- salts	T39.091	T39.092	T39.093	T39.094	T39.095	T39.096
Salinazid	T37.1X1	T37.1X2	T37.1X3	T37.1X4	T37.1X5	T37.1X6
Salmeterol	T48.6X1	T48.6X2	T48.6X3	T48.6X4	T48.6X5	T48.6X6
Salol	T49.3X1	T49.3X2	T49.3X3	T49.3X4	T49.3X5	T49.3X6
Salsalate	T39.091	T39.092	T39.093	T39.094	T39.095	T39.096
Salt substitute	T50.901	T50.902	T50.903	T50.904	T50.905	T50.906
Salt-replacing drug	T50.901	T50.902	T50.903	T50.904	T50.905	T50.906
Salt-retaining mineralocorticoid	T50.0X1	T50.0X2	T50.0X3	T50.0X4	T50.0X5	T50.0X6
Saluretic NEC	T50.2X1	T50.2X2	T50.2X3	T50.2X4	T50.2X5	T50.2X6
Saluron	T50.2X1	T50.2X2	T50.2X3	T50.2X4	T50.2X5	T50.2X6
Salvarsan 606 (neosilver) (silver)	T37.8X1	T37.8X2	T37.8X3	T37.8X4	T37.8X5	T37.8X6
Sambucus canadensis	T62.2X1	T62.2X2	T62.2X3	T62.2X4	--	--
- berry	T62.1X1	T62.1X2	T62.1X3	T62.1X4	--	--
Sandril	T46.5X1	T46.5X2	T46.5X3	T46.5X4	T46.5X5	T46.5X6
Sanguinaria canadensis	T62.2X1	T62.2X2	T62.2X3	T62.2X4	--	--
Saniflush (cleaner)	T54.2X1	T54.2X2	T54.2X3	T54.2X4	--	--
Santonin	T37.4X1	T37.4X2	T37.4X3	T37.4X4	T37.4X5	T37.4X6
Santyl	T49.8X1	T49.8X2	T49.8X3	T49.8X4	T49.8X5	T49.8X6
Saralasin	T46.5X1	T46.5X2	T46.5X3	T46.5X4	T46.5X5	T46.5X6
Sarcolysin	T45.1X1	T45.1X2	T45.1X3	T45.1X4	T45.1X5	T45.1X6
Sarkomycin	T45.1X1	T45.1X2	T45.1X3	T45.1X4	T45.1X5	T45.1X6
Saroten	T43.011	T43.012	T43.013	T43.014	T43.015	T43.016
Saturnine—see Lead						
Savin (oil)	T49.4X1	T49.4X2	T49.4X3	T49.4X4	T49.4X5	T49.4X6
Scammony	T47.2X1	T47.2X2	T47.2X3	T47.2X4	T47.2X5	T47.2X6

TABLE OF DRUGS AND CHEMICALS

Substance	Poisoning, Accidental (unintentional)	Poisoning, Intentional Self-harm	Poisoning, Assault	Poisoning, Undetermined	Adverse effect	Underdosing
Scarlet red	T49.8X1	T49.8X2	T49.8X3	T49.8X4	T49.8X5	T49.8X6
Scheele's green	T57.0X1	T57.0X2	T57.0X3	T57.0X4	--	--
- insecticide	T57.0X1	T57.0X2	T57.0X3	T57.0X4	--	--
Schizontozide (blood) (tissue)	T37.2X1	T37.2X2	T37.2X3	T37.2X4	T37.2X5	T37.2X6
Schradan	T60.0X1	T60.0X2	T60.0X3	T60.0X4	--	--
Schweinfurth green	T57.0X1	T57.0X2	T57.0X3	T57.0X4	--	--
- insecticide	T57.0X1	T57.0X2	T57.0X3	T57.0X4	--	--
Scilla, rat poison	T60.4X1	T60.4X2	T60.4X3	T60.4X4	--	--
Scillaren	T60.4X1	T60.4X2	T60.4X3	T60.4X4	--	--
Sclerosing agent	T46.8X1	T46.8X2	T46.8X3	T46.8X4	T46.8X5	T46.8X6
Scombrotoxin	T61.11	T61.12	T61.13	T61.14	--	--
Scopolamine	T44.3X1	T44.3X2	T44.3X3	T44.3X4	T44.3X5	T44.3X6
Scopolia extract	T44.3X1	T44.3X2	T44.3X3	T44.3X4	T44.3X5	T44.3X6
Scouring powder	T65.891	T65.892	T65.893	T65.894	--	--
Sea						
- anemone (sting)	T63.631	T63.632	T63.633	T63.634	--	--
- cucumber (sting)	T63.691	T63.692	T63.693	T63.694	--	--
- snake (bite) (venom)	T63.091	T63.092	T63.093	T63.094	--	--
- urchin spine (puncture)	T63.691	T63.692	T63.693	T63.694	--	--
Seafood	T61.91	T61.92	T61.93	T61.94	--	--
- specified NEC	T61.8X1	T61.8X2	T61.8X3	T61.8X4	--	--
Secbutabarbital	T42.3X1	T42.3X2	T42.3X3	T42.3X4	T42.3X5	T42.3X6
Secbutabarbitone	T42.3X1	T42.3X2	T42.3X3	T42.3X4	T42.3X5	T42.3X6
Secnidazole	T37.3X1	T37.3X2	T37.3X3	T37.3X4	T37.3X5	T37.3X6
Secobarbital	T42.3X1	T42.3X2	T42.3X3	T42.3X4	T42.3X5	T42.3X6
Seconal	T42.3X1	T42.3X2	T42.3X3	T42.3X4	T42.3X5	T42.3X6
Secretin	T50.8X1	T50.8X2	T50.8X3	T50.8X4	T50.8X5	T50.8X6
Sedative NEC	T42.71	T42.72	T42.73	T42.74	T42.75	T42.76
- mixed NEC	T42.6X1	T42.6X2	T42.6X3	T42.6X4	T42.6X5	T42.6X6
Sedormid	T42.6X1	T42.6X2	T42.6X3	T42.6X4	T42.6X5	T42.6X6
Seed disinfectant or dressing	T60.8X1	T60.8X2	T60.8X3	T60.8X4	--	--
Seeds (poisonous)	T62.2X1	T62.2X2	T62.2X3	T62.2X4	--	--
Selegiline	T42.8X1	T42.8X2	T42.8X3	T42.8X4	T42.8X5	T42.8X6
Selenium NEC	T56.891	T56.892	T56.893	T56.894	--	--
- disulfide or sulfide	T49.4X1	T49.4X2	T49.4X3	T49.4X4	T49.4X5	T49.4X6
- fumes	T59.891	T59.892	T59.893	T59.894	--	--
- sulfide	T49.4X1	T49.4X2	T49.4X3	T49.4X4	T49.4X5	T49.4X6
Selenomethionine (75Se)	T50.8X1	T50.8X2	T50.8X3	T50.8X4	T50.8X5	T50.8X6
Selsun	T49.4X1	T49.4X2	T49.4X3	T49.4X4	T49.4X5	T49.4X6
Semustine	T45.1X1	T45.1X2	T45.1X3	T45.1X4	T45.1X5	T45.1X6
Senega syrup	T48.4X1	T48.4X2	T48.4X3	T48.4X4	T48.4X5	T48.4X6
Senna	T47.2X1	T47.2X2	T47.2X3	T47.2X4	T47.2X5	T47.2X6
Sennoside A+B	T47.2X1	T47.2X2	T47.2X3	T47.2X4	T47.2X5	T47.2X6
Septisol	T49.2X1	T49.2X2	T49.2X3	T49.2X4	T49.2X5	T49.2X6
Seractide	T38.811	T38.812	T38.813	T38.814	T38.815	T38.816
Serax	T42.4X1	T42.4X2	T42.4X3	T42.4X4	T42.4X5	T42.4X6
Serenesil	T42.6X1	T42.6X2	T42.6X3	T42.6X4	T42.6X5	T42.6X6
Serenium (hydrochloride)	T37.91	T37.92	T37.93	T37.94	T37.95	T37.96
Serepax—see Oxazepam						
Sermorelin	T38.891	T38.892	T38.893	T38.894	T38.895	T38.896
Sernyl	T41.1X1	T41.1X2	T41.1X3	T41.1X4	T41.1X5	T41.1X6
Serotonin	T50.991	T50.992	T50.993	T50.994	T50.995	T50.996
Serpasil	T46.5X1	T46.5X2	T46.5X3	T46.5X4	T46.5X5	T46.5X6
Serrapeptase	T45.3X1	T45.3X2	T45.3X3	T45.3X4	T45.3X5	T45.3X6
Serum						
- antibotulinus	T50.Z11	T50.Z12	T50.Z13	T50.Z14	T50.Z15	T50.Z16
- anticytotoxic	T50.Z11	T50.Z12	T50.Z13	T50.Z14	T50.Z15	T50.Z16
- antidiphtheria	T50.Z11	T50.Z12	T50.Z13	T50.Z14	T50.Z15	T50.Z16
- antimeningococcus	T50.Z11	T50.Z12	T50.Z13	T50.Z14	T50.Z15	T50.Z16
- anti-Rh	T50.Z11	T50.Z12	T50.Z13	T50.Z14	T50.Z15	T50.Z16
- anti-snake-bite	T50.Z11	T50.Z12	T50.Z13	T50.Z14	T50.Z15	T50.Z16
- antitetanic	T50.Z11	T50.Z12	T50.Z13	T50.Z14	T50.Z15	T50.Z16
- antitoxic	T50.Z11	T50.Z12	T50.Z13	T50.Z14	T50.Z15	T50.Z16
- complement (inhibitor)	T45.8X1	T45.8X2	T45.8X3	T45.8X4	T45.8X5	T45.8X6
- convalescent	T50.Z11	T50.Z12	T50.Z13	T50.Z14	T50.Z15	T50.Z16

Substance	Poisoning, Accidental (unintentional)	Poisoning, Intentional Self-harm	Poisoning, Assault	Poisoning, Undetermined	Adverse effect	Underdosing
- hemolytic complement	T45.8X1	T45.8X2	T45.8X3	T45.8X4	T45.8X5	T45.8X6
- immune (human)	T50.Z11	T50.Z12	T50.Z13	T50.Z14	T50.Z15	T50.Z16
- protective NEC	T50.Z11	T50.Z12	T50.Z13	T50.Z14	T50.Z15	T50.Z16
Setastine	T45.0X1	T45.0X2	T45.0X3	T45.0X4	T45.0X5	T45.0X6
Setoperone	T43.591	T43.592	T43.593	T43.594	T43.595	T43.596
Sewer gas	T59.91	T59.92	T59.93	T59.94	--	--
Shampoo	T55.0X1	T55.0X2	T55.0X3	T55.0X4	--	--
Shellfish, noxious, nonbacterial	T61.781	T61.782	T61.783	T61.784	--	--
Sildenafil	T46.7X1	T46.7X2	T46.7X3	T46.7X4	T46.7X5	T46.7X6
Silibinin	T50.991	T50.992	T50.993	T50.994	T50.995	T50.996
Silicone NEC	T65.891	T65.892	T65.893	T65.894	--	--
- medicinal	T49.3X1	T49.3X2	T49.3X3	T49.3X4	T49.3X5	T49.3X6
Silvadene	T49.0X1	T49.0X2	T49.0X3	T49.0X4	T49.0X5	T49.0X6
Silver	T49.0X1	T49.0X2	T49.0X3	T49.0X4	T49.0X5	T49.0X6
- anti-infectives	T49.0X1	T49.0X2	T49.0X3	T49.0X4	T49.0X5	T49.0X6
- arsphenamine	T37.8X1	T37.8X2	T37.8X3	T37.8X4	T37.8X5	T37.8X6
- colloidal	T49.0X1	T49.0X2	T49.0X3	T49.0X4	T49.0X5	T49.0X6
- nitrate	T49.0X1	T49.0X2	T49.0X3	T49.0X4	T49.0X5	T49.0X6
- - ophthalmic preparation	T49.5X1	T49.5X2	T49.5X3	T49.5X4	T49.5X5	T49.5X6
- - toughened (keratolytic)	T49.4X1	T49.4X2	T49.4X3	T49.4X4	T49.4X5	T49.4X6
- nonmedicinal (dust)	T56.891	T56.892	T56.893	T56.894	--	--
- protein	T49.5X1	T49.5X2	T49.5X3	T49.5X4	T49.5X5	T49.5X6
- salvarsan	T37.8X1	T37.8X2	T37.8X3	T37.8X4	T37.8X5	T37.8X6
- sulfadiazine	T49.4X1	T49.4X2	T49.4X3	T49.4X4	T49.4X5	T49.4X6
Silymarin	T50.991	T50.992	T50.993	T50.994	T50.995	T50.996
Simaldrate	T47.1X1	T47.1X2	T47.1X3	T47.1X4	T47.1X5	T47.1X6
Simazine	T60.3X1	T60.3X2	T60.3X3	T60.3X4	--	--
Simethicone	T47.1X1	T47.1X2	T47.1X3	T47.1X4	T47.1X5	T47.1X6
Simfibrate	T46.6X1	T46.6X2	T46.6X3	T46.6X4	T46.6X5	T46.6X6
Simvastatin	T46.6X1	T46.6X2	T46.6X3	T46.6X4	T46.6X5	T46.6X6
Sincalide	T50.8X1	T50.8X2	T50.8X3	T50.8X4	T50.8X5	T50.8X6
Sinequan	T43.011	T43.012	T43.013	T43.014	T43.015	T43.016
Singoserp	T46.5X1	T46.5X2	T46.5X3	T46.5X4	T46.5X5	T46.5X6
Sintrom	T45.511	T45.512	T45.513	T45.514	T45.515	T45.516
Sisomicin	T36.5X1	T36.5X2	T36.5X3	T36.5X4	T36.5X5	T36.5X6
Sitosterols	T46.6X1	T46.6X2	T46.6X3	T46.6X4	T46.6X5	T46.6X6
Skeletal muscle relaxants	T48.1X1	T48.1X2	T48.1X3	T48.1X4	T48.1X5	T48.1X6
Skin						
- agents (external)	T49.91	T49.92	T49.93	T49.94	T49.95	T49.96
- - specified NEC	T49.8X1	T49.8X2	T49.8X3	T49.8X4	T49.8X5	T49.8X6
- test antigen	T50.8X1	T50.8X2	T50.8X3	T50.8X4	T50.8X5	T50.8X6
Sleep-eze	T45.0X1	T45.0X2	T45.0X3	T45.0X4	T45.0X5	T45.0X6
Sleeping draught, pill	T42.71	T42.72	T42.73	T42.74	T42.75	T42.76
Smallpox vaccine	T50.B11	T50.B12	T50.B13	T50.B14	T50.B15	T50.B16
Smelter fumes NEC	T56.91	T56.92	T56.93	T56.94	--	--
Smog	T59.1X1	T59.1X2	T59.1X3	T59.1X4	--	--
Smoke NEC	T59.811	T59.812	T59.813	T59.814	--	--
Smooth muscle relaxant	T44.3X1	T44.3X2	T44.3X3	T44.3X4	T44.3X5	T44.3X6
Snail killer NEC	T60.8X1	T60.8X2	T60.8X3	T60.8X4	--	--
Snake venom or bite	T63.001	T63.002	T63.003	T63.004	--	--
- hemocoagulase	T45.7X1	T45.7X2	T45.7X3	T45.7X4	T45.7X5	T45.7X6
Snuff	T65.211	T65.212	T65.213	T65.214	--	--
Soap (powder) (product)	T55.0X1	T55.0X2	T55.0X3	T55.0X4	--	--
- enema	T47.4X1	T47.4X2	T47.4X3	T47.4X4	T47.4X5	T47.4X6
- medicinal, soft	T49.2X1	T49.2X2	T49.2X3	T49.2X4	T49.2X5	T49.2X6
- superfatted	T49.2X1	T49.2X2	T49.2X3	T49.2X4	T49.2X5	T49.2X6
Sobrerol	T48.4X1	T48.4X2	T48.4X3	T48.4X4	T48.4X5	T48.4X6
Soda (caustic)	T54.3X1	T54.3X2	T54.3X3	T54.3X4	--	--
- bicarb	T47.1X1	T47.1X2	T47.1X3	T47.1X4	T47.1X5	T47.1X6
- chlorinated—see Sodium, hypochlorite						
Sodium						
- acetosulfone	T37.1X1	T37.1X2	T37.1X3	T37.1X4	T37.1X5	T37.1X6
- acetrizoate	T50.8X1	T50.8X2	T50.8X3	T50.8X4	T50.8X5	T50.8X6
- acid phosphate	T50.3X1	T50.3X2	T50.3X3	T50.3X4	T50.3X5	T50.3X6
- alginate	T47.8X1	T47.8X2	T47.8X3	T47.8X4	T47.8X5	T47.8X6

Substance	Poisoning, Accidental (unintentional)	Poisoning, Intentional Self-harm	Poisoning, Assault	Poisoning, Undetermined	Adverse effect	Underdosing
- amidotrizoate	T50.8X1	T50.8X2	T50.8X3	T50.8X4	T50.8X5	T50.8X6
- aminopterin	T45.1X1	T45.1X2	T45.1X3	T45.1X4	T45.1X5	T45.1X6
- amylosulfate	T47.8X1	T47.8X2	T47.8X3	T47.8X4	T47.8X5	T47.8X6
- amytal	T42.3X1	T42.3X2	T42.3X3	T42.3X4	T42.3X5	T42.3X6
- antimony gluconate	T37.3X1	T37.3X2	T37.3X3	T37.3X4	T37.3X5	T37.3X6
- arsenate	T57.0X1	T57.0X2	T57.0X3	T57.0X4	--	--
- aurothiomalate	T39.4X1	T39.4X2	T39.4X3	T39.4X4	T39.4X5	T39.4X6
- aurothiosulfate	T39.4X1	T39.4X2	T39.4X3	T39.4X4	T39.4X5	T39.4X6
- barbiturate	T42.3X1	T42.3X2	T42.3X3	T42.3X4	T42.3X5	T42.3X6
- basic phosphate	T47.4X1	T47.4X2	T47.4X3	T47.4X4	T47.4X5	T47.4X6
- bicarbonate	T47.1X1	T47.1X2	T47.1X3	T47.1X4	T47.1X5	T47.1X6
- bichromate	T57.8X1	T57.8X2	T57.8X3	T57.8X4	--	--
- biphosphate	T50.3X1	T50.3X2	T50.3X3	T50.3X4	T50.3X5	T50.3X6
- bisulfate	T65.891	T65.892	T65.893	T65.894	--	--
- borate						
- - - cleanser	T57.8X1	T57.8X2	T57.8X3	T57.8X4	--	
- - - eye	T49.5X1	T49.5X2	T49.5X3	T49.5X4	T49.5X5	T49.5X6
- - - therapeutic	T49.8X1	T49.8X2	T49.8X3	T49.8X4	T49.8X5	T49.8X6
- bromide	T42.6X1	T42.6X2	T42.6X3	T42.6X4	T42.6X5	T42.6X6
- cacodylate (nonmedicinal) NEC	T50.8X1	T50.8X2	T50.8X3	T50.8X4	T50.8X5	T50.8X6
- - anti-infective	T37.8X1	T37.8X2	T37.8X3	T37.8X4	T37.8X5	T37.8X6
- - herbicide	T60.3X1	T60.3X2	T60.3X3	T60.3X4	--	--
- calcium edetate	T45.8X1	T45.8X2	T45.8X3	T45.8X4	T45.8X5	T45.8X6
- carbonate NEC	T54.3X1	T54.3X2	T54.3X3	T54.3X4	--	--
- chlorate NEC	T65.891	T65.892	T65.893	T65.894	--	--
- - herbicide	T54.91	T54.92	T54.93	T54.94	--	--
- chloride	T50.3X1	T50.3X2	T50.3X3	T50.3X4	T50.3X5	T50.3X6
- - with glucose	T50.3X1	T50.3X2	T50.3X3	T50.3X4	T50.3X5	T50.3X6
- chromate	T65.891	T65.892	T65.893	T65.894	--	--
- citrate	T50.991	T50.992	T50.993	T50.994	T50.995	T50.996
- cromoglicate	T48.6X1	T48.6X2	T48.6X3	T48.6X4	T48.6X5	T48.6X6
- cyanide	T65.0X1	T65.0X2	T65.0X3	T65.0X4	--	--
- cyclamate	T50.3X1	T50.3X2	T50.3X3	T50.3X4	T50.3X5	T50.3X6
- dehydrocholate	T45.8X1	T45.8X2	T45.8X3	T45.8X4	T45.8X5	T45.8X6
- diatrizoate	T50.8X1	T50.8X2	T50.8X3	T50.8X4	T50.8X5	T50.8X6
- dibunate	T48.4X1	T48.4X2	T48.4X3	T48.4X4	T48.4X5	T48.4X6
- dioctyl sulfosuccinate	T47.4X1	T47.4X2	T47.4X3	T47.4X4	T47.4X5	T47.4X6
- dipantoyl ferrate	T45.8X1	T45.8X2	T45.8X3	T45.8X4	T45.8X5	T45.8X6
- edetate	T45.8X1	T45.8X2	T45.8X3	T45.8X4	T45.8X5	T45.8X6
- ethacrynate	T50.1X1	T50.1X2	T50.1X3	T50.1X4	T50.1X5	T50.1X6
- feredetate	T45.8X1	T45.8X2	T45.8X3	T45.8X4	T45.8X5	T45.8X6
- Fluoride—see Fluoride						
- fluoroacetate (dust) (pesticide)	T60.4X1	T60.4X2	T60.4X3	T60.4X4	--	--
- free salt	T50.3X1	T50.3X2	T50.3X3	T50.3X4	T50.3X5	T50.3X6
- fusidate	T36.8X1	T36.8X2	T36.8X3	T36.8X4	T36.8X5	T36.8X6
- glucaldrate	T47.1X1	T47.1X2	T47.1X3	T47.1X4	T47.1X5	T47.1X6
- glucosulfone	T37.1X1	T37.1X2	T37.1X3	T37.1X4	T37.1X5	T37.1X6
- glutamate	T45.8X1	T45.8X2	T45.8X3	T45.8X4	T45.8X5	T45.8X6
- hydrogen carbonate	T50.3X1	T50.3X2	T50.3X3	T50.3X4	T50.3X5	T50.3X6
- hydroxide	T54.3X1	T54.3X2	T54.3X3	T54.3X4	--	--
- hypochlorite (bleach) NEC	T54.3X1	T54.3X2	T54.3X3	T54.3X4	--	--
- - disinfectant	T54.3X1	T54.3X2	T54.3X3	T54.3X4	--	--
- - medicinal (anti-infective) (external)	T49.0X1	T49.0X2	T49.0X3	T49.0X4	T49.0X5	T49.0X6
- - vapor	T54.3X1	T54.3X2	T54.3X3	T54.3X4	--	--
- hyposulfite	T49.0X1	T49.0X2	T49.0X3	T49.0X4	T49.0X5	T49.0X6
- indigotin disulfonate	T50.8X1	T50.8X2	T50.8X3	T50.8X4	T50.8X5	T50.8X6
- iodide	T50.991	T50.992	T50.993	T50.994	T50.995	T50.996
- - I-131	T50.8X1	T50.8X2	T50.8X3	T50.8X4	T50.8X5	T50.8X6
- - - therapeutic	T38.2X1	T38.2X2	T38.2X3	T38.2X4	T38.2X5	T38.2X6
- iodohippurate (131I)	T50.8X1	T50.8X2	T50.8X3	T50.8X4	T50.8X5	T50.8X6
- iopodate	T50.8X1	T50.8X2	T50.8X3	T50.8X4	T50.8X5	T50.8X6
- iothalamate	T50.8X1	T50.8X2	T50.8X3	T50.8X4	T50.8X5	T50.8X6
- iron edetate	T45.4X1	T45.4X2	T45.4X3	T45.4X4	T45.4X5	T45.4X6
- lactate (compound solution)	T45.8X1	T45.8X2	T45.8X3	T45.8X4	T45.8X5	T45.8X6
- lauryl (sulfate)	T49.2X1	T49.2X2	T49.2X3	T49.2X4	T49.2X5	T49.2X6

Substance	Poisoning, Accidental (unintentional)	Poisoning, Intentional Self-harm	Poisoning, Assault	Poisoning, Undetermined	Adverse effect	Underdosing
- L-triiodothyronine	T38.1X1	T38.1X2	T38.1X3	T38.1X4	T38.1X5	T38.1X6
- magnesium citrate	T50.991	T50.992	T50.993	T50.994	T50.995	T50.996
- mersalate	T50.2X1	T50.2X2	T50.2X3	T50.2X4	T50.2X5	T50.2X6
- metasilicate	T65.891	T65.892	T65.893	T65.894	--	--
- metrizoate	T50.8X1	T50.8X2	T50.8X3	T50.8X4	T50.8X5	T50.8X6
- monofluoroacetate (pesticide)	T60.1X1	T60.1X2	T60.1X3	T60.1X4	--	--
- morrhuate	T46.8X1	T46.8X2	T46.8X3	T46.8X4	T46.8X5	T46.8X6
- nafcillin	T36.0X1	T36.0X2	T36.0X3	T36.0X4	T36.0X5	T36.0X6
- nitrate (oxidizing agent)	T65.891	T65.892	T65.893	T65.894	--	--
- nitrite	T50.6X1	T50.6X2	T50.6X3	T50.6X4	T50.6X5	T50.6X6
- nitroferricyanide	T46.5X1	T46.5X2	T46.5X3	T46.5X4	T46.5X5	T46.5X6
- nitroprusside	T46.5X1	T46.5X2	T46.5X3	T46.5X4	T46.5X5	T46.5X6
- oxalate	T65.891	T65.892	T65.893	T65.894	--	--
- oxide/peroxide	T65.891	T65.892	T65.893	T65.894	--	--
- oxybate	T41.291	T41.292	T41.293	T41.294	T41.295	T41.296
- para-aminohippurate	T50.8X1	T50.8X2	T50.8X3	T50.8X4	T50.8X5	T50.8X6
- perborate (nonmedicinal) NEC	T65.891	T65.892	T65.893	T65.894	--	--
- - medicinal	T49.0X1	T49.0X2	T49.0X3	T49.0X4	T49.0X5	T49.0X6
- - soap	T55.0X1	T55.0X2	T55.0X3	T55.0X4	--	--
- percarbonate—see Sodium, perborate						
- pertechnetate Tc99m	T50.8X1	T50.8X2	T50.8X3	T50.8X4	T50.8X5	T50.8X6
- phosphate						
- - cellulose	T45.8X1	T45.8X2	T45.8X3	T45.8X4	T45.8X5	T45.8X6
- - dibasic	T47.2X1	T47.2X2	T47.2X3	T47.2X4	T47.2X5	T47.2X6
- - monobasic	T47.2X1	T47.2X2	T47.2X3	T47.2X4	T47.2X5	T47.2X6
- phytate	T50.6X1	T50.6X2	T50.6X3	T50.6X4	T50.6X5	T50.6X6
- picosulfate	T47.2X1	T47.2X2	T47.2X3	T47.2X4	T47.2X5	T47.2X6
- polyhydroxyaluminium monocarbonate	T47.1X1	T47.1X2	T47.1X3	T47.1X4	T47.1X5	T47.1X6
- polystyrene sulfonate	T50.3X1	T50.3X2	T50.3X3	T50.3X4	T50.3X5	T50.3X6
- propionate	T49.0X1	T49.0X2	T49.0X3	T49.0X4	T49.0X5	T49.0X6
- propyl hydroxybenzoate	T50.991	T50.992	T50.993	T50.994	T50.995	T50.996
- psylliate	T46.8X1	T46.8X2	T46.8X3	T46.8X4	T46.8X5	T46.8X6
- removing resins	T50.3X1	T50.3X2	T50.3X3	T50.3X4	T50.3X5	T50.3X6
- salicylate	T39.091	T39.092	T39.093	T39.094	T39.095	T39.096
- salt NEC	T50.3X1	T50.3X2	T50.3X3	T50.3X4	T50.3X5	T50.3X6
- selenate	T60.2X1	T60.2X2	T60.2X3	T60.2X4	--	--
- stibogluconate	T37.3X1	T37.3X2	T37.3X3	T37.3X4	T37.3X5	T37.3X6
- sulfate	T47.4X1	T47.4X2	T47.4X3	T47.4X4	T47.4X5	T47.4X6
- sulfoxone	T37.1X1	T37.1X2	T37.1X3	T37.1X4	T37.1X5	T37.1X6
- tetradecyl sulfate	T46.8X1	T46.8X2	T46.8X3	T46.8X4	T46.8X5	T46.8X6
- thiopental	T41.1X1	T41.1X2	T41.1X3	T41.1X4	T41.1X5	T41.1X6
- thiosalicylate	T39.091	T39.092	T39.093	T39.094	T39.095	T39.096
- thiosulfate	T50.6X1	T50.6X2	T50.6X3	T50.6X4	T50.6X5	T50.6X6
- tolbutamide	T38.3X1	T38.3X2	T38.3X3	T38.3X4	T38.3X5	T38.3X6
- (L) -triiodothyronine	T38.1X1	T38.1X2	T38.1X3	T38.1X4	T38.1X5	T38.1X6
- tyropanoate	T50.8X1	T50.8X2	T50.8X3	T50.8X4	T50.8X5	T50.8X6
- valproate	T42.6X1	T42.6X2	T42.6X3	T42.6X4	T42.6X5	T42.6X6
- versenate	T50.6X1	T50.6X2	T50.6X3	T50.6X4	T50.6X5	T50.6X6
Sodium-free salt	T50.901	T50.902	T50.903	T50.904	T50.905	T50.906
Sodium-removing resin	T50.3X1	T50.3X2	T50.3X3	T50.3X4	T50.3X5	T50.3X6
Soft soap	T55.0X1	T55.0X2	T55.0X3	T55.0X4	--	--
Solanine	T62.2X1	T62.2X2	T62.2X3	T62.2X4	--	--
- berries	T62.1X1	T62.1X2	T62.1X3	T62.1X4	--	--
Solanum dulcamara	T62.2X1	T62.2X2	T62.2X3	T62.2X4	--	--
- berries	T62.1X1	T62.1X2	T62.1X3	T62.1X4	--	--
Solapsone	T37.1X1	T37.1X2	T37.1X3	T37.1X4	T37.1X5	T37.1X6
Solar lotion	T49.3X1	T49.3X2	T49.3X3	T49.3X4	T49.3X5	T49.3X6
Solasulfone	T37.1X1	T37.1X2	T37.1X3	T37.1X4	T37.1X5	T37.1X6
Soldering fluid	T65.891	T65.892	T65.893	T65.894	--	--
Solid substance	T65.91	T65.92	T65.93	T65.94	--	--
- specified NEC	T65.891	T65.892	T65.893	T65.894	--	--
Solvent, industrial NEC	T52.91	T52.92	T52.93	T52.94	--	--
- naphtha	T52.0X1	T52.0X2	T52.0X3	T52.0X4	--	--
- petroleum	T52.0X1	T52.0X2	T52.0X3	T52.0X4	--	--
- specified NEC	T52.8X1	T52.8X2	T52.8X3	T52.8X4	--	--

Substance	Poisoning, Accidental (unintentional)	Poisoning, Intentional Self-harm	Poisoning, Assault	Poisoning, Undetermined	Adverse effect	Underdosing
Soma	T42.8X1	T42.8X2	T42.8X3	T42.8X4	T42.8X5	T42.8X6
Somatorelin	T38.891	T38.892	T38.893	T38.894	T38.895	T38.896
Somatostatin	T38.991	T38.992	T38.993	T38.994	T38.995	T38.996
Somatotropin	T38.811	T38.812	T38.813	T38.814	T38.815	T38.816
Somatrem	T38.811	T38.812	T38.813	T38.814	T38.815	T38.816
Somatropin	T38.811	T38.812	T38.813	T38.814	T38.815	T38.816
Sominex	T45.0X1	T45.0X2	T45.0X3	T45.0X4	T45.0X5	T45.0X6
Somnos	T42.6X1	T42.6X2	T42.6X3	T42.6X4	T42.6X5	T42.6X6
Somonal	T42.3X1	T42.3X2	T42.3X3	T42.3X4	T42.3X5	T42.3X6
Soneryl	T42.3X1	T42.3X2	T42.3X3	T42.3X4	T42.3X5	T42.3X6
Soothing syrup	T50.901	T50.902	T50.903	T50.904	T50.905	T50.906
Sopor	T42.6X1	T42.6X2	T42.6X3	T42.6X4	T42.6X5	T42.6X6
Soporific	T42.71	T42.72	T42.73	T42.74	T42.75	T42.76
Soporific drug	T42.71	T42.72	T42.73	T42.74	T42.75	T42.76
- specified type NEC	T42.6X1	T42.6X2	T42.6X3	T42.6X4	T42.6X5	T42.6X6
Sorbide nitrate	T46.3X1	T46.3X2	T46.3X3	T46.3X4	T46.3X5	T46.3X6
Sorbitol	T47.4X1	T47.4X2	T47.4X3	T47.4X4	T47.4X5	T47.4X6
Sotalol	T44.7X1	T44.7X2	T44.7X3	T44.7X4	T44.7X5	T44.7X6
Sotradecol	T46.8X1	T46.8X2	T46.8X3	T46.8X4	T46.8X5	T46.8X6
Soysterol	T46.6X1	T46.6X2	T46.6X3	T46.6X4	T46.6X5	T46.6X6
Spacoline	T44.3X1	T44.3X2	T44.3X3	T44.3X4	T44.3X5	T44.3X6
Spanish fly	T49.8X1	T49.8X2	T49.8X3	T49.8X4	T49.8X5	T49.8X6
Sparine	T43.3X1	T43.3X2	T43.3X3	T43.3X4	T43.3X5	T43.3X6
Sparteine	T48.0X1	T48.0X2	T48.0X3	T48.0X4	T48.0X5	T48.0X6
Spasmolytic						
- anticholinergics	T44.3X1	T44.3X2	T44.3X3	T44.3X4	T44.3X5	T44.3X6
- autonomic	T44.3X1	T44.3X2	T44.3X3	T44.3X4	T44.3X5	T44.3X6
- bronchial NEC	T48.6X1	T48.6X2	T48.6X3	T48.6X4	T48.6X5	T48.6X6
- quaternary ammonium	T44.3X1	T44.3X2	T44.3X3	T44.3X4	T44.3X5	T44.3X6
- skeletal muscle NEC	T48.1X1	T48.1X2	T48.1X3	T48.1X4	T48.1X5	T48.1X6
Spectinomycin	T36.5X1	T36.5X2	T36.5X3	T36.5X4	T36.5X5	T36.5X6
Speed	T43.621	T43.622	T43.623	T43.624	T43.625	T43.626
Spermicide	T49.8X1	T49.8X2	T49.8X3	T49.8X4	T49.8X5	T49.8X6
Spider (bite) (venom)	T63.391	T63.392	T63.393	T63.394	--	--
- antivenin	T50.Z11	T50.Z12	T50.Z13	T50.Z14	T50.Z15	T50.Z16
Spigelia (root)	T37.4X1	T37.4X2	T37.4X3	T37.4X4	T37.4X5	T37.4X6
Spindle inactivator	T50.4X1	T50.4X2	T50.4X3	T50.4X4	T50.4X5	T50.4X6
Spiperone	T43.4X1	T43.4X2	T43.4X3	T43.4X4	T43.4X5	T43.4X6
Spiramycin	T36.3X1	T36.3X2	T36.3X3	T36.3X4	T36.3X5	T36.3X6
Spirapril	T46.4X1	T46.4X2	T46.4X3	T46.4X4	T46.4X5	T46.4X6
Spirilene	T43.591	T43.592	T43.593	T43.594	T43.595	T43.596
Spirit (s) (neutral) NEC	T51.0X1	T51.0X2	T51.0X3	T51.0X4	--	--
- beverage	T51.0X1	T51.0X2	T51.0X3	T51.0X4	--	--
- industrial	T51.0X1	T51.0X2	T51.0X3	T51.0X4	--	--
- mineral	T52.0X1	T52.0X2	T52.0X3	T52.0X4	--	--
- of salt—see Hydrochloric acid						
- surgical	T51.0X1	T51.0X2	T51.0X3	T51.0X4	--	--
Spironolactone	T50.0X1	T50.0X2	T50.0X3	T50.0X4	T50.0X5	T50.0X6
Spiroperidol	T43.4X1	T43.4X2	T43.4X3	T43.4X4	T43.4X5	T43.4X6
Sponge, absorbable (gelatin)	T45.7X1	T45.7X2	T45.7X3	T45.7X4	T45.7X5	T45.7X6
Sporostacin	T49.0X1	T49.0X2	T49.0X3	T49.0X4	T49.0X5	T49.0X6
Spray (aerosol)	T65.91	T65.92	T65.93	T65.94	--	--
- cosmetic	T65.891	T65.892	T65.893	T65.894	--	
- medicinal NEC	T50.901	T50.902	T50.903	T50.904	T50.905	T50.906
- pesticides—see Pesticides						
- specified content—see specific substance						
Spurge flax	T62.2X1	T62.2X2	T62.2X3	T62.2X4	--	--
Spurges	T62.2X1	T62.2X2	T62.2X3	T62.2X4	--	--
Sputum viscosity-lowering drug	T48.4X1	T48.4X2	T48.4X3	T48.4X4	T48.4X5	T48.4X6
Squill	T46.0X1	T46.0X2	T46.0X3	T46.0X4	T46.0X5	T46.0X6
- rat poison	T60.4X1	T60.4X2	T60.4X3	T60.4X4	--	--
Squirting cucumber (cathartic)	T47.2X1	T47.2X2	T47.2X3	T47.2X4	T47.2X5	T47.2X6
Stains	T65.6X1	T65.6X2	T65.6X3	T65.6X4	--	--
Stannous fluoride	T49.7X1	T49.7X2	T49.7X3	T49.7X4	T49.7X5	T49.7X6
Stanolone	T38.7X1	T38.7X2	T38.7X3	T38.7X4	T38.7X5	T38.7X6

Substance	Poisoning, Accidental (unintentional)	Poisoning, Intentional Self-harm	Poisoning, Assault	Poisoning, Undetermined	Adverse effect	Underdosing
Stanozolol	T38.7X1	T38.7X2	T38.7X3	T38.7X4	T38.7X5	T38.7X6
Staphisagria or stavesacre (pediculicide)	T49.0X1	T49.0X2	T49.0X3	T49.0X4	T49.0X5	T49.0X6
Starch	T50.901	T50.902	T50.903	T50.904	T50.905	T50.906
Stelazine	T43.3X1	T43.3X2	T43.3X3	T43.3X4	T43.3X5	T43.3X6
Stemetil	T43.3X1	T43.3X2	T43.3X3	T43.3X4	T43.3X5	T43.3X6
Stepronin	T48.4X1	T48.4X2	T48.4X3	T48.4X4	T48.4X5	T48.4X6
Sterculia	T47.4X1	T47.4X2	T47.4X3	T47.4X4	T47.4X5	T47.4X6
Sternutator gas	T59.891	T59.892	T59.893	T59.894	--	--
Steroid	T38.0X1	T38.0X2	T38.0X3	T38.0X4	T38.0X5	T38.0X6
- anabolic	T38.7X1	T38.7X2	T38.7X3	T38.7X4	T38.7X5	T38.7X6
- androgenic	T38.7X1	T38.7X2	T38.7X3	T38.7X4	T38.7X5	T38.7X6
- antineoplastic, hormone	T38.7X1	T38.7X2	T38.7X3	T38.7X4	T38.7X5	T38.7X6
- - estrogen	T38.5X1	T38.5X2	T38.5X3	T38.5X4	T38.5X5	T38.5X6
- ENT agent	T49.6X1	T49.6X2	T49.6X3	T49.6X4	T49.6X5	T49.6X6
- ophthalmic preparation	T49.5X1	T49.5X2	T49.5X3	T49.5X4	T49.5X5	T49.5X6
- topical NEC	T49.0X1	T49.0X2	T49.0X3	T49.0X4	T49.0X5	T49.0X6
Stibine	T56.891	T56.892	T56.893	T56.894	--	--
Stibogluconate	T37.3X1	T37.3X2	T37.3X3	T37.3X4	T37.3X5	T37.3X6
Stibophen	T37.4X1	T37.4X2	T37.4X3	T37.4X4	T37.4X5	T37.4X6
Stilbamidine (isetionate)	T37.3X1	T37.3X2	T37.3X3	T37.3X4	T37.3X5	T37.3X6
Stilbestrol	T38.5X1	T38.5X2	T38.5X3	T38.5X4	T38.5X5	T38.5X6
Stilboestrol	T38.5X1	T38.5X2	T38.5X3	T38.5X4	T38.5X5	T38.5X6
Stimulant						
- central nervous system—see also Psychostimulant	T43.601	T43.602	T43.603	T43.604	T43.605	T43.606
- - analeptics	T50.7X1	T50.7X2	T50.7X3	T50.7X4	T50.7X5	T50.7X6
- - opiate antagonist	T50.7X1	T50.7X2	T50.7X3	T50.7X4	T50.7X5	T50.7X6
- - psychotherapeutic NEC—see also Psychotherapeutic drug	T43.601	T43.602	T43.603	T43.604	T43.605	T43.606
- - specified NEC	T43.691	T43.692	T43.693	T43.694	T43.695	T43.696
- respiratory	T48.901	T48.902	T48.903	T48.904	T48.905	T48.906
Stone-dissolving drug	T50.901	T50.902	T50.903	T50.904	T50.905	T50.906
Storage battery (cells) (acid)	T54.2X1	T54.2X2	T54.2X3	T54.2X4	--	--
Stovaine	T41.3X1	T41.3X2	T41.3X3	T41.3X4	T41.3X5	T41.3X6
- infiltration (subcutaneous)	T41.3X1	T41.3X2	T41.3X3	T41.3X4	T41.3X5	T41.3X6
- nerve block (peripheral) (plexus)	T41.3X1	T41.3X2	T41.3X3	T41.3X4	T41.3X5	T41.3X6
- spinal	T41.3X1	T41.3X2	T41.3X3	T41.3X4	T41.3X5	T41.3X6
- topical (surface)	T41.3X1	T41.3X2	T41.3X3	T41.3X4	T41.3X5	T41.3X6
Stovarsal	T37.8X1	T37.8X2	T37.8X3	T37.8X4	T37.8X5	T37.8X6
Stove gas—see Gas, stove						
Stoxil	T49.5X1	T49.5X2	T49.5X3	T49.5X4	T49.5X5	T49.5X6
Stramonium	T48.6X1	T48.6X2	T48.6X3	T48.6X4	T48.6X5	T48.6X6
- natural state	T62.2X1	T62.2X2	T62.2X3	T62.2X4	--	--
Streptodornase	T45.3X1	T45.3X2	T45.3X3	T45.3X4	T45.3X5	T45.3X6
Streptoduocin	T36.5X1	T36.5X2	T36.5X3	T36.5X4	T36.5X5	T36.5X6
Streptokinase	T45.611	T45.612	T45.613	T45.614	T45.615	T45.616
Streptomycin (derivative)	T36.5X1	T36.5X2	T36.5X3	T36.5X4	T36.5X5	T36.5X6
Streptonivicin	T36.5X1	T36.5X2	T36.5X3	T36.5X4	T36.5X5	T36.5X6
Streptovarycin	T36.5X1	T36.5X2	T36.5X3	T36.5X4	T36.5X5	T36.5X6
Streptozocin	T45.1X1	T45.1X2	T45.1X3	T45.1X4	T45.1X5	T45.1X6
Streptozotocin	T45.1X1	T45.1X2	T45.1X3	T45.1X4	T45.1X5	T45.1X6
Stripper (paint) (solvent)	T52.8X1	T52.8X2	T52.8X3	T52.8X4	--	--
Strobane	T60.1X1	T60.1X2	T60.1X3	T60.1X4	--	--
Strofantina	T46.0X1	T46.0X2	T46.0X3	T46.0X4	T46.0X5	T46.0X6
Strophanthin (g) (k)	T46.0X1	T46.0X2	T46.0X3	T46.0X4	T46.0X5	T46.0X6
Strophanthus	T46.0X1	T46.0X2	T46.0X3	T46.0X4	T46.0X5	T46.0X6
Strophantin	T46.0X1	T46.0X2	T46.0X3	T46.0X4	T46.0X5	T46.0X6
Strophantin-g	T46.0X1	T46.0X2	T46.0X3	T46.0X4	T46.0X5	T46.0X6
Strychnine (nonmedicinal) (pesticide) (salts)	T65.1X1	T65.1X2	T65.1X3	T65.1X4	--	--
- medicinal	T48.291	T48.292	T48.293	T48.294	T48.295	T48.296
Strychnos (ignatii) —see Strychnine						
Styramate	T42.8X1	T42.8X2	T42.8X3	T42.8X4	T42.8X5	T42.8X6
Styrene	T65.891	T65.892	T65.893	T65.894	--	--
Succinimide, antiepileptic or anticonvulsant	T42.2X1	T42.2X2	T42.2X3	T42.2X4	T42.2X5	T42.2X6
- mercuric—see Mercury						
Succinylcholine	T48.1X1	T48.1X2	T48.1X3	T48.1X4	T48.1X5	T48.1X6

Substance	Poisoning, Accidental (unintentional)	Poisoning, Intentional Self-harm	Poisoning, Assault	Poisoning, Undetermined	Adverse effect	Underdosing
Succinylsulfathiazole	T37.0X1	T37.0X2	T37.0X3	T37.0X4	T37.0X5	T37.0X6
Sucralfate	T47.1X1	T47.1X2	T47.1X3	T47.1X4	T47.1X5	T47.1X6
Sucrose	T50.3X1	T50.3X2	T50.3X3	T50.3X4	T50.3X5	T50.3X6
Sufentanil	T40.4X1	T40.4X2	T40.4X3	T40.4X4	T40.4X5	T40.4X6
Sulbactam	T36.0X1	T36.0X2	T36.0X3	T36.0X4	T36.0X5	T36.0X6
Sulbenicillin	T36.0X1	T36.0X2	T36.0X3	T36.0X4	T36.0X5	T36.0X6
Sulbentine	T49.0X1	T49.0X2	T49.0X3	T49.0X4	T49.0X5	T49.0X6
Sulfacetamide	T49.0X1	T49.0X2	T49.0X3	T49.0X4	T49.0X5	T49.0X6
- ophthalmic preparation	T49.5X1	T49.5X2	T49.5X3	T49.5X4	T49.5X5	T49.5X6
Sulfachlorpyridazine	T37.0X1	T37.0X2	T37.0X3	T37.0X4	T37.0X5	T37.0X6
Sulfacitine	T37.0X1	T37.0X2	T37.0X3	T37.0X4	T37.0X5	T37.0X6
Sulfadiasulfone sodium	T37.0X1	T37.0X2	T37.0X3	T37.0X4	T37.0X5	T37.0X6
Sulfadiazine	T37.0X1	T37.0X2	T37.0X3	T37.0X4	T37.0X5	T37.0X6
- silver (topical)	T49.0X1	T49.0X2	T49.0X3	T49.0X4	T49.0X5	T49.0X6
Sulfadimethoxine	T37.0X1	T37.0X2	T37.0X3	T37.0X4	T37.0X5	T37.0X6
Sulfadimidine	T37.0X1	T37.0X2	T37.0X3	T37.0X4	T37.0X5	T37.0X6
Sulfadoxlne	T37.0X1	T37.0X2	T37.0X3	T37.0X4	T37.0X5	T37.0X6
- with pyrimethamine	T37.2X1	T37.2X2	T37.2X3	T37.2X4	T37.2X5	T37.2X6
Sulfaethidole	T37.0X1	T37.0X2	T37.0X3	T37.0X4	T37.0X5	T37.0X6
Sulfafurazole	T37.0X1	T37.0X2	T37.0X3	T37.0X4	T37.0X5	T37.0X6
Sulfaguanidine	T37.0X1	T37.0X2	T37.0X3	T37.0X4	T37.0X5	T37.0X6
Sulfalene	T37.0X1	T37.0X2	T37.0X3	T37.0X4	T37.0X5	T37.0X6
Sulfaloxate	T37.0X1	T37.0X2	T37.0X3	T37.0X4	T37.0X5	T37.0X6
Sulfaloxic acid	T37.0X1	T37.0X2	T37.0X3	T37.0X4	T37.0X5	T37.0X6
Sulfamazone	T39.2X1	T39.2X2	T39.2X3	T39.2X4	T39.2X5	T39.2X6
Sulfamerazine	T37.0X1	T37.0X2	T37.0X3	T37.0X4	T37.0X5	T37.0X6
Sulfameter	T37.0X1	T37.0X2	T37.0X3	T37.0X4	T37.0X5	T37.0X6
Sulfamethazine	T37.0X1	T37.0X2	T37.0X3	T37.0X4	T37.0X5	T37.0X6
Sulfamethizole	T37.0X1	T37.0X2	T37.0X3	T37.0X4	T37.0X5	T37.0X6
Sulfamethoxazole	T37.0X1	T37.0X2	T37.0X3	T37.0X4	T37.0X5	T37.0X6
- with trimethoprim	T36.8X1	T36.8X2	T36.8X3	T36.8X4	T36.8X5	T36.8X6
Sulfamethoxydiazine	T37.0X1	T37.0X2	T37.0X3	T37.0X4	T37.0X5	T37.0X6
Sulfamethoxypyridazine	T37.0X1	T37.0X2	T37.0X3	T37.0X4	T37.0X5	T37.0X6
Sulfamethylthiazole	T37.0X1	T37.0X2	T37.0X3	T37.0X4	T37.0X5	T37.0X6
Sulfametoxydiazine	T37.0X1	T37.0X2	T37.0X3	T37.0X4	T37.0X5	T37.0X6
Sulfamidopyrine	T39.2X1	T39.2X2	T39.2X3	T39.2X4	T39.2X5	T39.2X6
Sulfamonomethoxine	T37.0X1	T37.0X2	T37.0X3	T37.0X4	T37.0X5	T37.0X6
Sulfamoxole	T37.0X1	T37.0X2	T37.0X3	T37.0X4	T37.0X5	T37.0X6
Sulfamylon	T49.0X1	T49.0X2	T49.0X3	T49.0X4	T49.0X5	T49.0X6
Sulfan blue (diagnostic dye)	T50.8X1	T50.8X2	T50.8X3	T50.8X4	T50.8X5	T50.8X6
Sulfanilamide	T37.0X1	T37.0X2	T37.0X3	T37.0X4	T37.0X5	T37.0X6
Sulfanilylguanidine	T37.0X1	T37.0X2	T37.0X3	T37.0X4	T37.0X5	T37.0X6
Sulfaperin	T37.0X1	T37.0X2	T37.0X3	T37.0X4	T37.0X5	T37.0X6
Sulfaphcnazolc	T37.0X1	T37.0X2	T37.0X3	T37.0X4	T37.0X5	T37.0X6
Sulfaphenylthiazole	T37.0X1	T37.0X2	T37.0X3	T37.0X4	T37.0X5	T37.0X6
Sulfaproxyline	T37.0X1	T37.0X2	T37.0X3	T37.0X4	T37.0X5	T37.0X6
Sulfapyridine	T37.0X1	T37.0X2	T37.0X3	T37.0X4	T37.0X5	T37.0X6
Sulfapyrimidine	T37.0X1	T37.0X2	T37.0X3	T37.0X4	T37.0X5	T37.0X6
Sulfarsphenamine	T37.8X1	T37.8X2	T37.8X3	T37.8X4	T37.8X5	T37.8X6
Sulfasalazine	T37.0X1	T37.0X2	T37.0X3	T37.0X4	T37.0X5	T37.0X6
Sulfasuxidine	T37.0X1	T37.0X2	T37.0X3	T37.0X4	T37.0X5	T37.0X6
Sulfasymazine	T37.0X1	T37.0X2	T37.0X3	T37.0X4	T37.0X5	T37.0X6
Sulfated amylopectin	T47.8X1	T47.8X2	T47.8X3	T47.8X4	T47.8X5	T47.8X6
Sulfathiazole	T37.0X1	T37.0X2	T37.0X3	T37.0X4	T37.0X5	T37.0X6
Sulfatostearate	T49.2X1	T49.2X2	T49.2X3	T49.2X4	T49.2X5	T49.2X6
Sulfinpyrazone	T50.4X1	T50.4X2	T50.4X3	T50.4X4	T50.4X5	T50.4X6
Sulfiram	T49.0X1	T49.0X2	T49.0X3	T49.0X4	T49.0X5	T49.0X6
Sulfisomidine	T37.0X1	T37.0X2	T37.0X3	T37.0X4	T37.0X5	T37.0X6
Sulfisoxazole	T37.0X1	T37.0X2	T37.0X3	T37.0X4	T37.0X5	T37.0X6
- ophthalmic preparation	T49.5X1	T49.5X2	T49.5X3	T49.5X4	T49.5X5	T49.5X6
Sulfobromophthalein (sodium)	T50.8X1	T50.8X2	T50.8X3	T50.8X4	T50.8X5	T50.8X6
Sulfobromphthalein	T50.8X1	T50.8X2	T50.8X3	T50.8X4	T50.8X5	T50.8X6
Sulfogaiacol	T48.4X1	T48.4X2	T48.4X3	T48.4X4	T48.4X5	T48.4X6
Sulfomyxin	T36.8X1	T36.8X2	T36.8X3	T36.8X4	T36.8X5	T36.8X6
Sulfonal	T42.6X1	T42.6X2	T42.6X3	T42.6X4	T42.6X5	T42.6X6

Substance	Poisoning, Accidental (unintentional)	Poisoning, Intentional Self-harm	Poisoning, Assault	Poisoning, Undetermined	Adverse effect	Underdosing
Sulfonamide NEC	T37.0X1	T37.0X2	T37.0X3	T37.0X4	T37.0X5	T37.0X6
- eye	T49.5X1	T49.5X2	T49.5X3	T49.5X4	T49.5X5	T49.5X6
Sulfonazide	T37.1X1	T37.1X2	T37.1X3	T37.1X4	T37.1X5	T37.1X6
Sulfones	T37.1X1	T37.1X2	T37.1X3	T37.1X4	T37.1X5	T37.1X6
Sulfonethylmethane	T42.6X1	T42.6X2	T42.6X3	T42.6X4	T42.6X5	T42.6X6
Sulfonmethane	T42.6X1	T42.6X2	T42.6X3	T42.6X4	T42.6X5	T42.6X6
Sulfonphthal, sulfonphthol	T50.8X1	T50.8X2	T50.8X3	T50.8X4	T50.8X5	T50.8X6
Sulfonylurea derivatives, oral	T38.3X1	T38.3X2	T38.3X3	T38.3X4	T38.3X5	T38.3X6
Sulforidazine	T43.3X1	T43.3X2	T43.3X3	T43.3X4	T43.3X5	T43.3X6
Sulfoxone	T37.1X1	T37.1X2	T37.1X3	T37.1X4	T37.1X5	T37.1X6
Sulfur, sulfurated, sulfuric, sulfurous, sulfuryl (compounds NEC) (medicinal)	T49.4X1	T49.4X2	T49.4X3	T49.4X4	T49.4X5	T49.4X6
- acid	T54.2X1	T54.2X2	T54.2X3	T54.2X4	--	--
- dioxide (gas)	T59.1X1	T59.1X2	T59.1X3	T59.1X4	--	--
- ether—see Ether (s)						
- hydrogen	T59.6X1	T59.6X2	T59.6X3	T59.6X4	--	--
- medicinal (keratolytic) (ointment) NEC	T49.4X1	T49.4X2	T49.4X3	T49.4X4	T49.4X5	T49.4X6
- ointment	T49.0X1	T49.0X2	T49.0X3	T49.0X4	T49.0X5	T49.0X6
- pesticide (vapor)	T60.91	T60.92	T60.93	T60.94	--	--
- vapor NEC	T59.891	T59.892	T59.893	T59.894	--	--
Sulfuric acid	T54.2X1	T54.2X2	T54.2X3	T54.2X4	--	--
Sulglicotide	T47.1X1	T47.1X2	T47.1X3	T47.1X4	T47.1X5	T47.1X6
Sulindac	T39.391	T39.392	T39.393	T39.394	T39.395	T39.396
Sulisatin	T47.2X1	T47.2X2	T47.2X3	T47.2X4	T47.2X5	T47.2X6
Sulisobenzone	T49.3X1	T49.3X2	T49.3X3	T49.3X4	T49.3X5	T49.3X6
Sulkowitch's reagent	T50.8X1	T50.8X2	T50.8X3	T50.8X4	T50.8X5	T50.8X6
Sulmetozine	T44.3X1	T44.3X2	T44.3X3	T44.3X4	T44.3X5	T44.3X6
Suloctidil	T46.7X1	T46.7X2	T46.7X3	T46.7X4	T46.7X5	T46.7X6
Sulph—see also Sulf-						
Sulphadiazine	T37.0X1	T37.0X2	T37.0X3	T37.0X4	T37.0X5	T37.0X6
Sulphadimethoxine	T37.0X1	T37.0X2	T37.0X3	T37.0X4	T37.0X5	T37.0X6
Sulphadimidine	T37.0X1	T37.0X2	T37.0X3	T37.0X4	T37.0X5	T37.0X6
Sulphadione	T37.1X1	T37.1X2	T37.1X3	T37.1X4	T37.1X5	T37.1X6
Sulphafurazole	T37.0X1	T37.0X2	T37.0X3	T37.0X4	T37.0X5	T37.0X6
Sulphamethizole	T37.0X1	T37.0X2	T37.0X3	T37.0X4	T37.0X5	T37.0X6
Sulphamethoxazole	T37.0X1	T37.0X2	T37.0X3	T37.0X4	T37.0X5	T37.0X6
Sulphan blue	T50.8X1	T50.8X2	T50.8X3	T50.8X4	T50.8X5	T50.8X6
Sulphaphenazole	T37.0X1	T37.0X2	T37.0X3	T37.0X4	T37.0X5	T37.0X6
Sulphapyridine	T37.0X1	T37.0X2	T37.0X3	T37.0X4	T37.0X5	T37.0X6
Sulphasalazine	T37.0X1	T37.0X2	T37.0X3	T37.0X4	T37.0X5	T37.0X6
Sulphinpyrazone	T50.4X1	T50.4X2	T50.4X3	T50.4X4	T50.4X5	T50.4X6
Sulpiride	T43.591	T43.592	T43.593	T43.594	T43.595	T43.596
Sulprostone	T48.0X1	T48.0X2	T48.0X3	T48.0X4	T48.0X5	T48.0X6
Sulpyrine	T39.2X1	T39.2X2	T39.2X3	T39.2X4	T39.2X5	T39.2X6
Sultamicillin	T36.0X1	T36.0X2	T36.0X3	T36.0X4	T36.0X5	T36.0X6
Sulthiame	T42.6X1	T42.6X2	T42.6X3	T42.6X4	T42.6X5	T42.6X6
Sultiame	T42.6X1	T42.6X2	T42.6X3	T42.6X4	T42.6X5	T42.6X6
Sultopride	T43.591	T43.592	T43.593	T43.594	T43.595	T43.596
Sumatriptan	T39.8X1	T39.8X2	T39.8X3	T39.8X4	T39.8X5	T39.8X6
Sunflower seed oil	T46.6X1	T46.6X2	T46.6X3	T46.6X4	T46.6X5	T46.6X6
Superinone	T48.4X1	T48.4X2	T48.4X3	T48.4X4	T48.4X5	T48.4X6
Suprofen	T39.311	T39.312	T39.313	T39.314	T39.315	T39.316
Suramin (sodium)	T37.4X1	T37.4X2	T37.4X3	T37.4X4	T37.4X5	T37.4X6
Surfacaine	T41.3X1	T41.3X2	T41.3X3	T41.3X4	T41.3X5	T41.3X6
Surital	T41.1X1	T41.1X2	T41.1X3	T41.1X4	T41.1X5	T41.1X6
Sutilains	T45.3X1	T45.3X2	T45.3X3	T45.3X4	T45.3X5	T45.3X6
Suxamethonium (chloride)	T48.1X1	T48.1X2	T48.1X3	T48.1X4	T48.1X5	T48.1X6
Suxethonium (chloride)	T48.1X1	T48.1X2	T48.1X3	T48.1X4	T48.1X5	T48.1X6
Suxibuzone	T39.2X1	T39.2X2	T39.2X3	T39.2X4	T39.2X5	T39.2X6
Sweet niter spirit	T46.3X1	T46.3X2	T46.3X3	T46.3X4	T46.3X5	T46.3X6
Sweet oil (birch)	T49.3X1	T49.3X2	T49.3X3	T49.3X4	T49.3X5	T49.3X6
Sweetener	T50.901	T50.902	T50.903	T50.904	T50.905	T50.906
Sym-dichloroethyl ether	T53.6X1	T53.6X2	T53.6X3	T53.6X4	--	--
Sympatholytic NEC	T44.8X1	T44.8X2	T44.8X3	T44.8X4	T44.8X5	T44.8X6
- haloalkylamine	T44.8X1	T44.8X2	T44.8X3	T44.8X4	T44.8X5	T44.8X6

Substance	Poisoning, Accidental (unintentional)	Poisoning, Intentional Self harm	Poisoning, Assault	Poisoning, Undetermined	Adverse effect	Underdosing
Sympathomimetic NEC	T44.901	T44.902	T44.903	T44.904	T44.905	T44.906
- anti-common-cold	T48.5X1	T48.5X2	T48.5X3	T48.5X4	T48.5X5	T48.5X6
- bronchodilator	T48.6X1	T48.6X2	T48.6X3	T48.6X4	T48.6X5	T48.6X6
- specified NEC	T44.991	T44.992	T44.993	T44.994	T44.995	T44.996
Synagis	T50.B91	T50.B92	T50.B93	T50.B94	T50.B95	T50.B96
Synalar	T49.0X1	T49.0X2	T49.0X3	T49.0X4	T49.0X5	T49.0X6
Synthroid	T38.1X1	T38.1X2	T38.1X3	T38.1X4	T38.1X5	T38.1X6
Syntocinon	T48.0X1	T48.0X2	T48.0X3	T48.0X4	T48.0X5	T48.0X6
Syrosingopine	T46.5X1	T46.5X2	T46.5X3	T46.5X4	T46.5X5	T46.5X6
Systemic drug	T45.91	T45.92	T45.93	T45.94	T45.95	T45.96
- specified NEC	T45.8X1	T45.8X2	T45.8X3	T45.8X4	T45.8X5	T45.8X6
2,4,5-T	T60.3X1	T60.3X2	T60.3X3	T60.3X4	--	--
Tablets—see also specified substance	T50.901	T50.902	T50.903	T50.904	T50.905	T50.906
Tace	T38.5X1	T38.5X2	T38.5X3	T38.5X4	T38.5X5	T38.5X6
Tacrine	T44.0X1	T44.0X2	T44.0X3	T44.0X4	T44.0X5	T44.0X6
Tadalafil	T46.7X1	T46.7X2	T46.7X3	T46.7X4	T46.7X5	T46.7X6
Talampicillin	T36.0X1	T36.0X2	T36.0X3	T36.0X4	T36.0X5	T36.0X6
Talbutal	T42.3X1	T42.3X2	T42.3X3	T42.3X4	T42.3X5	T42.3X6
Talc powder	T49.3X1	T49.3X2	T49.3X3	T49.3X4	T49.3X5	T49.3X6
Talcum	T49.3X1	T49.3X2	T49.3X3	T49.3X4	T49.3X5	T49.3X6
Taleranol	T38.6X1	T38.6X2	T38.6X3	T38.6X4	T38.6X5	T38.6X6
Tamoxifen	T38.6X1	T38.6X2	T38.6X3	T38.6X4	T38.6X5	T38.6X6
Tamsulosin	T44.6X1	T44.6X2	T44.6X3	T44.6X4	T44.6X5	T44.6X6
Tandearil, tanderil	T39.2X1	T39.2X2	T39.2X3	T39.2X4	T39.2X5	T39.2X6
Tannic acid	T49.2X1	T49.2X2	T49.2X3	T49.2X4	T49.2X5	T49.2X6
- medicinal (astringent)	T49.2X1	T49.2X2	T49.2X3	T49.2X4	T49.2X5	T49.2X6
Tannin—see Tannic acid						
Tansy	T62.2X1	T62.2X2	T62.2X3	T62.2X4	--	--
TAO	T36.3X1	T36.3X2	T36.3X3	T36.3X4	T36.3X5	T36.3X6
Tapazole	T38.2X1	T38.2X2	T38.2X3	T38.2X4	T38.2X5	T38.2X6
Tar NEC	T52.0X1	T52.0X2	T52.0X3	T52.0X4	--	--
- camphor	T60.1X1	T60.1X2	T60.1X3	T60.1X4	--	--
- distillate	T49.1X1	T49.1X2	T49.1X3	T49.1X4	T49.1X5	T49.1X6
- fumes	T59.891	T59.892	T59.893	T59.894	--	--
- medicinal	T49.1X1	T49.1X2	T49.1X3	T49.1X4	T49.1X5	T49.1X6
- ointment	T49.1X1	T49.1X2	T49.1X3	T49.1X4	T49.1X5	T49.1X6
Taractan	T43.591	T43.592	T43.593	T43.594	T43.595	T43.596
Tarantula (venomous)	T63.321	T63.322	T63.323	T63.324	--	--
Tartar emetic	T37.8X1	T37.8X2	T37.8X3	T37.8X4	T37.8X5	T37.8X6
Tartaric acid	T65.891	T65.892	T65.893	T65.894	--	--
Tartrate, laxative	T47.4X1	T47.4X2	T47.4X3	T47.4X4	T47.4X5	T47.4X6
Tartrated antimony (anti-infective)	T37.8X1	T37.8X2	T37.8X3	T37.8X4	T37.8X5	T37.8X6
Tauromustine	T45.1X1	T45.1X2	T45.1X3	T45.1X4	T45.1X5	T45.1X6
TCA see Trichloroacetic acid						
TCDD	T53.7X1	T53.7X2	T53.7X3	T53.7X4	--	--
TDI (vapor)	T65.0X1	T65.0X2	T65.0X3	T65.0X4	--	--
Tear						
- gas	T59.3X1	T59.3X2	T59.3X3	T59.3X4	--	--
- solution	T49.5X1	T49.5X2	T49.5X3	T49.5X4	T49.5X5	T49.5X6
Teclothiazide	T50.2X1	T50.2X2	T50.2X3	T50.2X4	T50.2X5	T50.2X6
Teclozan	T37.3X1	T37.3X2	T37.3X3	T37.3X4	T37.3X5	T37.3X6
Tegafur	T45.1X1	T45.1X2	T45.1X3	T45.1X4	T45.1X5	T45.1X6
Tegretol	T42.1X1	T42.1X2	T42.1X3	T42.1X4	T42.1X5	T42.1X6
Teicoplanin	T36.8X1	T36.8X2	T36.8X3	T36.8X4	T36.8X5	T36.8X6
Telepaque	T50.8X1	T50.8X2	T50.8X3	T50.8X4	T50.8X5	T50.8X6
Tellurium	T56.891	T56.892	T56.893	T56.894	--	--
- fumes	T56.891	T56.892	T56.893	T56.894	--	--
TEM	T45.1X1	T45.1X2	T45.1X3	T45.1X4	T45.1X5	T45.1X6
Temazepam	T42.4X1	T42.4X2	T42.4X3	T42.4X4	T42.4X5	T42.4X6
Temocillin	T36.0X1	T36.0X2	T36.0X3	T36.0X4	T36.0X5	T36.0X6
Tenamfetamine	T43.621	T43.622	T43.623	T43.624	T43.625	T43.626
Teniposide	T45.1X1	T45.1X2	T45.1X3	T45.1X4	T45.1X5	T45.1X6
Tenitramine	T46.3X1	T46.3X2	T46.3X3	T46.3X4	T46.3X5	T46.3X6
Tenoglicin	T48.4X1	T48.4X2	T48.4X3	T48.4X4	T48.4X5	T48.4X6
Tenonitrozole	T37.3X1	T37.3X2	T37.3X3	T37.3X4	T37.3X5	T37.3X6

Substance	Poisoning, Accidental (unintentional)	Poisoning, Intentional Self-harm	Poisoning, Assault	Poisoning, Undetermined	Adverse effect	Underdosing
Tenoxicam	T39.391	T39.392	T39.393	T39.394	T39.395	T39.396
TEPA	T45.1X1	T45.1X2	T45.1X3	T45.1X4	T45.1X5	T45.1X6
TEPP	T60.0X1	T60.0X2	T60.0X3	T60.0X4	--	--
Teprotide	T46.5X1	T46.5X2	T46.5X3	T46.5X4	T46.5X5	T46.5X6
Terazosin	T44.6X1	T44.6X2	T44.6X3	T44.6X4	T44.6X5	T44.6X6
Terbufos	T60.0X1	T60.0X2	T60.0X3	T60.0X4	--	--
Terbutaline	T48.6X1	T48.6X2	T48.6X3	T48.6X4	T48.6X5	T48.6X6
Terconazole	T49.0X1	T49.0X2	T49.0X3	T49.0X4	T49.0X5	T49.0X6
Terfenadine	T45.0X1	T45.0X2	T45.0X3	T45.0X4	T45.0X5	T45.0X6
Teriparatide (acetate)	T50.991	T50.992	T50.993	T50.994	T50.995	T50.996
Terizidone	T37.1X1	T37.1X2	T37.1X3	T37.1X4	T37.1X5	T37.1X6
Terlipressin	T38.891	T38.892	T38.893	T38.894	T38.895	T38.896
Terodiline	T46.3X1	T46.3X2	T46.3X3	T46.3X4	T46.3X5	T46.3X6
Teroxalene	T37.4X1	T37.4X2	T37.4X3	T37.4X4	T37.4X5	T37.4X6
Terpin (cis) hydrate	T48.4X1	T48.4X2	T48.4X3	T48.4X4	T48.4X5	T48.4X6
Terramycin	T36.4X1	T36.4X2	T36.4X3	T36.4X4	T36.4X5	T36.4X6
Tertatolol	T44.7X1	T44.7X2	T44.7X3	T44.7X4	T44.7X5	T44.7X6
Tessalon	T48.3X1	T48.3X2	T48.3X3	T48.3X4	T48.3X5	T48.3X6
Testolactone	T38.7X1	T38.7X2	T38.7X3	T38.7X4	T38.7X5	T38.7X6
Testosterone	T38.7X1	T38.7X2	T38.7X3	T38.7X4	T38.7X5	T38.7X6
Tetanus toxoid or vaccine	T50.A91	T50.A92	T50.A93	T50.A94	T50.A95	T50.A96
- antitoxin	T50.Z11	T50.Z12	T50.Z13	T50.Z14	T50.Z15	T50.Z16
- immune globulin (human)	T50.Z11	T50.Z12	T50.Z13	T50.Z14	T50.Z15	T50.Z16
- toxoid	T50.A91	T50.A92	T50.A93	T50.A94	T50.A95	T50.A96
- - with diphtheria toxoid	T50.A21	T50.A22	T50.A23	T50.A24	T50.A25	T50.A26
- - - with pertussis	T50.A11	T50.A12	T50.A13	T50.A14	T50.A15	T50.A16
Tetrabenazine	T43.591	T43.592	T43.593	T43.594	T43.595	T43.596
Tetracaine	T41.3X1	T41.3X2	T41.3X3	T41.3X4	T41.3X5	T41.3X6
- nerve block (peripheral) (plexus)	T41.3X1	T41.3X2	T41.3X3	T41.3X4	T41.3X5	T41.3X6
- regional	T41.3X1	T41.3X2	T41.3X3	T41.3X4	T41.3X5	T41.3X6
- spinal	T41.3X1	T41.3X2	T41.3X3	T41.3X4	T41.3X5	T41.3X6
Tetrachlorethylene—see Tetrachloroethylene						
Tetrachlormethiazide	T50.2X1	T50.2X2	T50.2X3	T50.2X4	T50.2X5	T50.2X6
2,3,7,8-Tetrachlorodibenzo-p-dioxin	T53.7X1	T53.7X2	T53.7X3	T53.7X4	--	--
Tetrachloroethane	T53.6X1	T53.6X2	T53.6X3	T53.6X4	--	--
- vapor	T53.6X1	T53.6X2	T53.6X3	T53.6X4	--	--
- - paint or varnish	T53.6X1	T53.6X2	T53.6X3	T53.6X4	--	--
Tetrachloroethylene (liquid)	T53.3X1	T53.3X2	T53.3X3	T53.3X4	--	--
- medicinal	T37.4X1	T37.4X2	T37.4X3	T37.4X4	T37.4X5	T37.4X6
- vapor	T53.3X1	T53.3X2	T53.3X3	T53.3X4	--	--
Tetrachloromethane—see Carbon tetrachloride						
Tetracosactide	T38.811	T38.812	T38.813	T38.814	T38.815	T38.816
Tetracosactrin	T38.811	T38.812	T38.813	T38.814	T38.815	T38.816
Tetracycline	T36.4X1	T36.4X2	T36.4X3	T36.4X4	T36.4X5	T36.4X6
- ophthalmic preparation	T49.5X1	T49.5X2	T49.5X3	T49.5X4	T49.5X5	T49.5X6
- topical NEC	T49.0X1	T49.0X2	T49.0X3	T49.0X4	T49.0X5	T49.0X6
Tetradifon	T60.8X1	T60.8X2	T60.8X3	T60.8X4	--	--
Tetradotoxin	T61.771	T61.772	T61.773	T61.774	--	--
Tetraethyl						
- lead	T56.0X1	T56.0X2	T56.0X3	T56.0X4	--	--
- pyrophosphate	T60.0X1	T60.0X2	T60.0X3	T60.0X4	--	--
Tetraethylammonium chloride	T44.2X1	T44.2X2	T44.2X3	T44.2X4	T44.2X5	T44.2X6
Tetraethylthiuram disulfide	T50.6X1	T50.6X2	T50.6X3	T50.6X4	T50.6X5	T50.6X6
Tetrahydroaminoacridine	T44.0X1	T44.0X2	T44.0X3	T44.0X4	T44.0X5	T44.0X6
Tetrahydrocannabinol	T40.7X1	T40.7X2	T40.7X3	T40.7X4	T40.7X5	T40.7X6
Tetrahydrofuran	T52.8X1	T52.8X2	T52.8X3	T52.8X4	--	--
Tetrahydronaphthalene	T52.8X1	T52.8X2	T52.8X3	T52.8X4	--	--
Tetrahydrozoline	T49.5X1	T49.5X2	T49.5X3	T49.5X4	T49.5X5	T49.5X6
Tetralin	T52.8X1	T52.8X2	T52.8X3	T52.8X4	--	--
Tetramethrin	T60.2X1	T60.2X2	T60.2X3	T60.2X4	--	--
Tetramethylthiuram (disulfide) NEC	T60.3X1	T60.3X2	T60.3X3	T60.3X4	--	--
- medicinal	T49.0X1	T49.0X2	T49.0X3	T49.0X4	T49.0X5	T49.0X6
Tetramisole	T37.4X1	T37.4X2	T37.4X3	T37.4X4	T37.4X5	T37.4X6
Tetranicotinoyl fructose	T46.7X1	T46.7X2	T46.7X3	T46.7X4	T46.7X5	T46.7X6
Tetrazepam	T42.4X1	T42.4X2	T42.4X3	T42.4X4	T42.4X5	T42.4X6

Substance	Poisoning, Accidental (unintentional)	Poisoning, Intentional Self-harm	Poisoning, Assault	Poisoning, Undetermined	Adverse effect	Underdosing
Tetronal	T42.6X1	T42.6X2	T42.6X3	T42.6X4	T42.6X5	T42.6X6
Tetryl	T65.3X1	T65.3X2	T65.3X3	T65.3X4	--	--
Tetrylammonium chloride	T44.2X1	T44.2X2	T44.2X3	T44.2X4	T44.2X5	T44.2X6
Tetryzoline	T49.5X1	T49.5X2	T49.5X3	T49.5X4	T49.5X5	T49.5X6
Thalidomide	T45.1X1	T45.1X2	T45.1X3	T45.1X4	T45.1X5	T45.1X6
Thallium (compounds) (dust) NEC	T56.811	T56.812	T56.813	T56.814	--	--
- pesticide	T60.4X1	T60.4X2	T60.4X3	T60.4X4	--	--
THC	T40.7X1	T40.7X2	T40.7X3	T40.7X4	T40.7X5	T40.7X6
Thebacon	T48.3X1	T48.3X2	T48.3X3	T48.3X4	T48.3X5	T48.3X6
Thebaine	T40.2X1	T40.2X2	T40.2X3	T40.2X4	T40.2X5	T40.2X6
Thenoic acid	T49.6X1	T49.6X2	T49.6X3	T49.6X4	T49.6X5	T49.6X6
Thenyldiamine	T45.0X1	T45.0X2	T45.0X3	T45.0X4	T45.0X5	T45.0X6
Theobromine (calcium salicylate)	T48.6X1	T48.6X2	T48.6X3	T48.6X4	T48.6X5	T48.6X6
- sodium salicylate	T48.6X1	T48.6X2	T48.6X3	T48.6X4	T48.6X5	T48.6X6
Theophyllamine	T48.6X1	T48.6X2	T48.6X3	T48.6X4	T48.6X5	T48.6X6
Theophylline	T48.6X1	T48.6X2	T48.6X3	T48.6X4	T48.6X5	T48.6X6
- aminobenzoic acid	T48.6X1	T48.6X2	T48.6X3	T48.6X4	T48.6X5	T48.6X6
- ethylenediamine	T48.6X1	T48.6X2	T48.6X3	T48.6X4	T48.6X5	T48.6X6
- piperazine p-amino-benzoate	T48.6X1	T48.6X2	T48.6X3	T48.6X4	T48.6X5	T48.6X6
Thiabendazole	T37.4X1	T37.4X2	T37.4X3	T37.4X4	T37.4X5	T37.4X6
Thialbarbital	T41.1X1	T41.1X2	T41.1X3	T41.1X4	T41.1X5	T41.1X6
Thiamazole	T38.2X1	T38.2X2	T38.2X3	T38.2X4	T38.2X5	T38.2X6
Thiambutosine	T37.1X1	T37.1X2	T37.1X3	T37.1X4	T37.1X5	T37.1X6
Thiamine	T45.2X1	T45.2X2	T45.2X3	T45.2X4	T45.2X5	T45.2X6
Thiamphenicol	T36.2X1	T36.2X2	T36.2X3	T36.2X4	T36.2X5	T36.2X6
Thiamylal	T41.1X1	T41.1X2	T41.1X3	T41.1X4	T41.1X5	T41.1X6
- sodium	T41.1X1	T41.1X2	T41.1X3	T41.1X4	T41.1X5	T41.1X6
Thiazesim	T43.291	T43.292	T43.293	T43.294	T43.295	T43.296
Thiazides (diuretics)	T50.2X1	T50.2X2	T50.2X3	T50.2X4	T50.2X5	T50.2X6
Thiazinamium metilsulfate	T43.3X1	T43.3X2	T43.3X3	T43.3X4	T43.3X5	T43.3X6
Thiethylperazine	T43.3X1	T43.3X2	T43.3X3	T43.3X4	T43.3X5	T43.3X6
Thimerosal	T49.0X1	T49.0X2	T49.0X3	T49.0X4	T49.0X5	T49.0X6
- ophthalmic preparation	T49.5X1	T49.5X2	T49.5X3	T49.5X4	T49.5X5	T49.5X6
Thioacetazone	T37.1X1	T37.1X2	T37.1X3	T37.1X4	T37.1X5	T37.1X6
- with isoniazid	T37.1X1	T37.1X2	T37.1X3	T37.1X4	T37.1X5	T37.1X6
Thiobarbital sodium	T41.1X1	T41.1X2	T41.1X3	T41.1X4	T41.1X5	T41.1X6
Thiobarbiturate anesthetic	T41.1X1	T41.1X2	T41.1X3	T41.1X4	T41.1X5	T41.1X6
Thiobismol	T37.8X1	T37.8X2	T37.8X3	T37.8X4	T37.8X5	T37.8X6
Thiobutabarbital sodium	T41.1X1	T41.1X2	T41.1X3	T41.1X4	T41.1X5	T41.1X6
Thiocarbamate (insecticide)	T60.0X1	T60.0X2	T60.0X3	T60.0X4	--	--
Thiocarbamide	T38.2X1	T38.2X2	T38.2X3	T38.2X4	T38.2X5	T38.2X6
Thiocarbarsone	T37.8X1	T37.8X2	T37.8X3	T37.8X4	T37.8X5	T37.8X6
Thiocarlide	T37.1X1	T37.1X2	T37.1X3	T37.1X4	T37.1X5	T37.1X6
Thioctamide	T50.991	T50.992	T50.993	T50.994	T50.995	T50.996
Thioctic acid	T50.991	T50.992	T50.993	T50.994	T50.995	T50.996
Thiofos	T60.0X1	T60.0X2	T60.0X3	T60.0X4	--	--
Thioglycolate	T49.4X1	T49.4X2	T49.4X3	T49.4X4	T49.4X5	T49.4X6
Thioglycolic acid	T65.891	T65.892	T65.893	T65.894	--	--
Thioguanine	T45.1X1	T45.1X2	T45.1X3	T45.1X4	T45.1X5	T45.1X6
Thiomercaptomerin	T50.2X1	T50.2X2	T50.2X3	T50.2X4	T50.2X5	T50.2X6
Thiomerin	T50.2X1	T50.2X2	T50.2X3	T50.2X4	T50.2X5	T50.2X6
Thiomersal	T49.0X1	T49.0X2	T49.0X3	T49.0X4	T49.0X5	T49.0X6
Thionazin	T60.0X1	T60.0X2	T60.0X3	T60.0X4	--	--
Thiopental (sodium)	T41.1X1	T41.1X2	T41.1X3	T41.1X4	T41.1X5	T41.1X6
Thiopentone (sodium)	T41.1X1	T41.1X2	T41.1X3	T41.1X4	T41.1X5	T41.1X6
Thiopropazate	T43.3X1	T43.3X2	T43.3X3	T43.3X4	T43.3X5	T43.3X6
Thioproperazine	T43.3X1	T43.3X2	T43.3X3	T43.3X4	T43.3X5	T43.3X6
Thioridazine	T43.3X1	T43.3X2	T43.3X3	T43.3X4	T43.3X5	T43.3X6
Thiosinamine	T49.3X1	T49.3X2	T49.3X3	T49.3X4	T49.3X5	T49.3X6
Thiotepa	T45.1X1	T45.1X2	T45.1X3	T45.1X4	T45.1X5	T45.1X6
Thiothixene	T43.4X1	T43.4X2	T43.4X3	T43.4X4	T43.4X5	T43.4X6
Thiouracil (benzyl) (methyl) (propyl)	T38.2X1	T38.2X2	T38.2X3	T38.2X4	T38.2X5	T38.2X6
Thiourea	T38.2X1	T38.2X2	T38.2X3	T38.2X4	T38.2X5	T38.2X6
Thiphenamil	T44.3X1	T44.3X2	T44.3X3	T44.3X4	T44.3X5	T44.3X6
Thiram	T60.3X1	T60.3X2	T60.3X3	T60.3X4	--	--

Substance	Poisoning, Accidental (unintentional)	Poisoning, Intentional Self-harm	Poisoning, Assault	Poisoning, Undetermined	Adverse effect	Underdosing
- medicinal	T49.2X1	T49.2X2	T49.2X3	T49.2X4	T49.2X5	T49.2X6
Thonzylamine (systemic)	T45.0X1	T45.0X2	T45.0X3	T45.0X4	T45.0X5	T45.0X6
- mucosal decongestant	T48.5X1	T48.5X2	T48.5X3	T48.5X4	T48.5X5	T48.5X6
Thorazine	T43.3X1	T43.3X2	T43.3X3	T43.3X4	T43.3X5	T43.3X6
Thorium dioxide suspension	T50.8X1	T50.8X2	T50.8X3	T50.8X4	T50.8X5	T50.8X6
Thornapple	T62.2X1	T62.2X2	T62.2X3	T62.2X4	--	--
Throat drug NEC	T49.6X1	T49.6X2	T49.6X3	T49.6X4	T49.6X5	T49.6X6
Thrombin	T45.7X1	T45.7X2	T45.7X3	T45.7X4	T45.7X5	T45.7X6
Thrombolysin	T45.611	T45.612	T45.613	T45.614	T45.615	T45.616
Thromboplastin	T45.7X1	T45.7X2	T45.7X3	T45.7X4	T45.7X5	T45.7X6
Thurfyl nicotinate	T46.7X1	T46.7X2	T46.7X3	T46.7X4	T46.7X5	T46.7X6
Thymol	T49.0X1	T49.0X2	T49.0X3	T49.0X4	T49.0X5	T49.0X6
Thymopentin	T37.5X1	T37.5X2	T37.5X3	T37.5X4	T37.5X5	T37.5X6
Thymoxamine	T46.7X1	T46.7X2	T46.7X3	T46.7X4	T46.7X5	T46.7X6
Thymus extract	T38.891	T38.892	T38.893	T38.894	T38.895	T38.896
Thyreotrophic hormone	T38.811	T38.812	T38.813	T38.814	T38.815	T38.816
Thyroglobulin	T38.1X1	T38.1X2	T38.1X3	T38.1X4	T38.1X5	T38.1X6
Thyroid (hormone)	T38.1X1	T38.1X2	T38.1X3	T38.1X4	T38.1X5	T38.1X6
Thyrolar	T38.1X1	T38.1X2	T38.1X3	T38.1X4	T38.1X5	T38.1X6
Thyrotrophin	T38.811	T38.812	T38.813	T38.814	T38.815	T38.816
Thyrotropic hormone	T38.811	T38.812	T38.813	T38.814	T38.815	T38.816
Thyroxine	T38.1X1	T38.1X2	T38.1X3	T38.1X4	T38.1X5	T38.1X6
Tiabendazole	T37.4X1	T37.4X2	T37.4X3	T37.4X4	T37.4X5	T37.4X6
Tiamizide	T50.2X1	T50.2X2	T50.2X3	T50.2X4	T50.2X5	T50.2X6
Tianeptine	T43.291	T43.292	T43.293	T43.294	T43.295	T43.296
Tiapamil	T46.1X1	T46.1X2	T46.1X3	T46.1X4	T46.1X5	T46.1X6
Tiapride	T43.591	T43.592	T43.593	T43.594	T43.595	T43.596
Tiaprofenic acid	T39.311	T39.312	T39.313	T39.314	T39.315	T39.316
Tiaramide	T39.8X1	T39.8X2	T39.8X3	T39.8X4	T39.8X5	T39.8X6
Ticarcillin	T36.0X1	T36.0X2	T36.0X3	T36.0X4	T36.0X5	T36.0X6
Ticlatone	T49.0X1	T49.0X2	T49.0X3	T49.0X4	T49.0X5	T49.0X6
Ticlopidine	T45.521	T45.522	T45.523	T45.524	T45.525	T45.526
Ticrynafen	T50.1X1	T50.1X2	T50.1X3	T50.1X4	T50.1X5	T50.1X6
Tidiacic	T50.991	T50.992	T50.993	T50.994	T50.995	T50.996
Tiemonium	T44.3X1	T44.3X2	T44.3X3	T44.3X4	T44.3X5	T44.3X6
- iodide	T44.3X1	T44.3X2	T44.3X3	T44.3X4	T44.3X5	T44.3X6
Tienilic acid	T50.1X1	T50.1X2	T50.1X3	T50.1X4	T50.1X5	T50.1X6
Tifenamil	T44.3X1	T44.3X2	T44.3X3	T44.3X4	T44.3X5	T44.3X6
Tigan	T45.0X1	T45.0X2	T45.0X3	T45.0X4	T45.0X5	T45.0X6
Tigloidine	T44.3X1	T44.3X2	T44.3X3	T44.3X4	T44.3X5	T44.3X6
Tilactase	T47.5X1	T47.5X2	T47.5X3	T47.5X4	T47.5X5	T47.5X6
Tiletamine	T41.291	T41.292	T41.293	T41.294	T41.295	T41.296
Tilidine	T40.4X1	T40.4X2	T40.4X3	T40.4X4	--	--
Timepidium bromide	T44.3X1	T44.3X2	T44.3X3	T44.3X4	T44.3X5	T44.3X6
Timiperone	T43.4X1	T43.4X2	T43.4X3	T43.4X4	T43.4X5	T43.4X6
Timolol	T44.7X1	T44.7X2	T44.7X3	T44.7X4	T44.7X5	T44.7X6
Tin (chloride) (dust) (oxide) NEC	T56.6X1	T56.6X2	T56.6X3	T56.6X4	--	--
- anti-infectives	T37.8X1	T37.8X2	T37.8X3	T37.8X4	T37.8X5	T37.8X6
Tincture, iodine—see Iodine						
Tindal	T43.3X1	T43.3X2	T43.3X3	T43.3X4	T43.3X5	T43.3X6
Tinidazole	T37.3X1	T37.3X2	T37.3X3	T37.3X4	T37.3X5	T37.3X6
Tinoridine	T39.8X1	T39.8X2	T39.8X3	T39.8X4	T39.8X5	T39.8X6
Tiocarlide	T37.1X1	T37.1X2	T37.1X3	T37.1X4	T37.1X5	T37.1X6
Tioclomarol	T45.511	T45.512	T45.513	T45.514	T45.515	T45.516
Tioconazole	T49.0X1	T49.0X2	T49.0X3	T49.0X4	T49.0X5	T49.0X6
Tioguanine	T45.1X1	T45.1X2	T45.1X3	T45.1X4	T45.1X5	T45.1X6
Tiopronin	T50.991	T50.992	T50.993	T50.994	T50.995	T50.996
Tiotixene	T43.4X1	T43.4X2	T43.4X3	T43.4X4	T43.4X5	T43.4X6
Tioxolone	T49.4X1	T49.4X2	T49.4X3	T49.4X4	T49.4X5	T49.4X6
Tipepidine	T48.3X1	T48.3X2	T48.3X3	T48.3X4	T48.3X5	T48.3X6
Tiquizium bromide	T44.3X1	T44.3X2	T44.3X3	T44.3X4	T44.3X5	T44.3X6
Tiratricol	T38.1X1	T38.1X2	T38.1X3	T38.1X4	T38.1X5	T38.1X6
Tisopurine	T50.4X1	T50.4X2	T50.4X3	T50.4X4	T50.4X5	T50.4X6
Titanium (compounds) (vapor)	T56.891	T56.892	T56.893	T56.894	--	--
- dioxide	T49.3X1	T49.3X2	T49.3X3	T49.3X4	T49.3X5	T49.3X6

Substance	Poisoning, Accidental (unintentional)	Poisoning, Intentional Self-harm	Poisoning, Assault	Poisoning, Undetermined	Adverse effect	Underdosing
- ointment	T49.3X1	T49.3X2	T49.3X3	T49.3X4	T49.3X5	T49.3X6
- oxide	T49.3X1	T49.3X2	T49.3X3	T49.3X4	T49.3X5	T49.3X6
- tetrachloride	T56.891	T56.892	T56.893	T56.894	--	--
Titanocene	T56.891	T56.892	T56.893	T56.894	--	--
Titroid	T38.1X1	T38.1X2	T38.1X3	T38.1X4	T38.1X5	T38.1X6
Tizanidine	T42.8X1	T42.8X2	T42.8X3	T42.8X4	T42.8X5	T42.8X6
TMTD	T60.3X1	T60.3X2	T60.3X3	T60.3X4	--	--
TNT (fumes)	T65.3X1	T65.3X2	T65.3X3	T65.3X4	--	--
Toadstool	T62.0X1	T62.0X2	T62.0X3	T62.0X4	--	--
Tobacco NEC	T65.291	T65.292	T65.293	T65.294	--	--
- cigarettes	T65.221	T65.222	T65.223	T65.224	--	--
- Indian	T62.2X1	T62.2X2	T62.2X3	T62.2X4	--	--
- smoke, second-hand	T65.221	T65.222	T65.223	T65.224	--	--
Tobramycin	T36.5X1	T36.5X2	T36.5X3	T36.5X4	T36.5X5	T36.5X6
Tocainide	T46.2X1	T46.2X2	T46.2X3	T46.2X4	T46.2X5	T46.2X6
Tocoferol	T45.2X1	T45.2X2	T45.2X3	T45.2X4	T45.2X5	T45.2X6
Tocopherol	T45.2X1	T45.2X2	T45.2X3	T45.2X4	T45.2X5	T45.2X6
- acetate	T45.2X1	T45.2X2	T45.2X3	T45.2X4	T45.2X5	T45.2X6
Tocosamine	T48.0X1	T48.0X2	T48.0X3	T48.0X4	T48.0X5	T48.0X6
Todralazine	T46.5X1	T46.5X2	T46.5X3	T46.5X4	T46.5X5	T46.5X6
Tofisopam	T42.4X1	T42.4X2	T42.4X3	T42.4X4	T42.4X5	T42.4X6
Tofranil	T43.011	T43.012	T43.013	T43.014	T43.015	T43.016
Toilet deodorizer	T65.891	T65.892	T65.893	T65.894	--	--
Tolamolol	T44.7X1	T44.7X2	T44.7X3	T44.7X4	T44.7X5	T44.7X6
Tolazamide	T38.3X1	T38.3X2	T38.3X3	T38.3X4	T38.3X5	T38.3X6
Tolazoline	T46.7X1	T46.7X2	T46.7X3	T46.7X4	T46.7X5	T46.7X6
Tolbutamide (sodium)	T38.3X1	T38.3X2	T38.3X3	T38.3X4	T38.3X5	T38.3X6
Tolciclate	T49.0X1	T49.0X2	T49.0X3	T49.0X4	T49.0X5	T49.0X6
Tolmetin	T39.391	T39.392	T39.393	T39.394	T39.395	T39.396
Tolnaftate	T49.0X1	T49.0X2	T49.0X3	T49.0X4	T49.0X5	T49.0X6
Tolonidine	T46.5X1	T46.5X2	T46.5X3	T46.5X4	T46.5X5	T46.5X6
Toloxatone	T42.6X1	T42.6X2	T42.6X3	T42.6X4	T42.6X5	T42.6X6
Tolperisone	T44.3X1	T44.3X2	T44.3X3	T44.3X4	T44.3X5	T44.3X6
Tolserol	T42.8X1	T42.8X2	T42.8X3	T42.8X4	T42.8X5	T42.8X6
Toluene (liquid)	T52.2X1	T52.2X2	T52.2X3	T52.2X4	--	--
- diisocyanate	T65.0X1	T65.0X2	T65.0X3	T65.0X4	--	--
Toluidine	T65.891	T65.892	T65.893	T65.894	--	--
- vapor	T59.891	T59.892	T59.893	T59.894	--	--
Toluol (liquid)	T52.2X1	T52.2X2	T52.2X3	T52.2X4	--	--
- vapor	T52.2X1	T52.2X2	T52.2X3	T52.2X4	--	--
Toluylenediamine	T65.3X1	T65.3X2	T65.3X3	T65.3X4	--	--
Tolylene-2,4-diisocyanate	T65.0X1	T65.0X2	T65.0X3	T65.0X4	--	--
Tonic NEC	T50.901	T50.902	T50.903	T50.904	T50.905	T50.906
Topical action drug NEC	T49.91	T49.92	T49.93	T49.94	T49.95	T49.96
- ear, nose or throat	T49.6X1	T49.6X2	T49.6X3	T49.6X4	T49.6X5	T49.6X6
- eye	T49.5X1	T49.5X2	T49.5X3	T49.5X4	T49.5X5	T49.5X6
- skin	T49.91	T49.92	T49.93	T49.94	T49.95	T49.96
- specified NEC	T49.8X1	T49.8X2	T49.8X3	T49.8X4	T49.8X5	T49.8X6
Toquizine	T44.3X1	T44.3X2	T44.3X3	T44.3X4	T44.3X5	T44.3X6
Toremifene	T38.6X1	T38.6X2	T38.6X3	T38.6X4	T38.6X5	T38.6X6
Tosylchloramide sodium	T49.8X1	T49.8X2	T49.8X3	T49.8X4	T49.8X5	T49.8X6
Toxaphene (dust) (spray)	T60.1X1	T60.1X2	T60.1X3	T60.1X4	--	--
Toxin, diphtheria (Schick Test)	T50.8X1	T50.8X2	T50.8X3	T50.8X4	T50.8X5	T50.8X6
Toxoid						
- combined	T50.A21	T50.A22	T50.A23	T50.A24	T50.A25	T50.A26
- diphtheria	T50.A91	T50.A92	T50.A93	T50.A94	T50.A95	T50.A96
- tetanus	T50.A91	T50.A92	T50.A93	T50.A94	T50.A95	T50.A96
Trace element NEC	T45.8X1	T45.8X2	T45.8X3	T45.8X4	T45.8X5	T45.8X6
Tractor fuel NEC	T52.0X1	T52.0X2	T52.0X3	T52.0X4	--	--
Tragacanth	T50.991	T50.992	T50.993	T50.994	T50.995	T50.996
Tramadol	T40.4X1	T40.4X2	T40.4X3	T40.4X4	T40.4X5	T40.4X6
Tramazoline	T48.5X1	T48.5X2	T48.5X3	T48.5X4	T48.5X5	T48.5X6
Tranexamic acid	T45.621	T45.622	T45.623	T45.624	T45.625	T45.626
Tranilast	T45.0X1	T45.0X2	T45.0X3	T45.0X4	T45.0X5	T45.0X6
Tranquilizer NEC	T43.501	T43.502	T43.503	T43.504	T43.505	T43.506

Substance	Poisoning, Accidental (unintentional)	Poisoning, Intentional Self-harm	Poisoning, Assault	Poisoning, Undetermined	Adverse effect	Underdosing
- with hypnotic or sedative	T42.6X1	T42.6X2	T42.6X3	T42.6X4	T42.6X5	T42.6X6
- benzodiazepine NEC	T42.4X1	T42.4X2	T42.4X3	T42.4X4	T42.4X5	T42.4X6
- butyrophenone NEC	T43.4X1	T43.4X2	T43.4X3	T43.4X4	T43.4X5	T43.4X6
- carbamate	T43.591	T43.592	T43.593	T43.594	T43.595	T43.596
- dimethylamine	T43.3X1	T43.3X2	T43.3X3	T43.3X4	T43.3X5	T43.3X6
- ethylamine	T43.3X1	T43.3X2	T43.3X3	T43.3X4	T43.3X5	T43.3X6
- hydroxyzine	T43.591	T43.592	T43.593	T43.594	T43.595	T43.596
- major NEC	T43.501	T43.502	T43.503	T43.504	T43.505	T43.506
- penothiazine NEC	T43.3X1	T43.3X2	T43.3X3	T43.3X4	T43.3X5	T43.3X6
- phenothiazine-based	T43.3X1	T43.3X2	T43.3X3	T43.3X4	T43.3X5	T43.3X6
- piperazine NEC	T43.3X1	T43.3X2	T43.3X3	T43.3X4	T43.3X5	T43.3X6
- piperidine	T43.3X1	T43.3X2	T43.3X3	T43.3X4	T43.3X5	T43.3X6
- propylamine	T43.3X1	T43.3X2	T43.3X3	T43.3X4	T43.3X5	T43.3X6
- specified NEC	T43.591	T43.592	T43.593	T43.594	T43.595	T43.596
- thioxanthene NEC	T43.591	T43.592	T43.593	T43.594	T43.595	T43.596
Tranxene	T42.4X1	T42.4X2	T42.4X3	T42.4X4	T42.4X5	T42.4X6
Tranylcypromine	T43.1X1	T43.1X2	T43.1X3	T43.1X4	T43.1X5	T43.1X6
Trapidil	T46.3X1	T46.3X2	T46.3X3	T46.3X4	T46.3X5	T46.3X6
Trasentine	T44.3X1	T44.3X2	T44.3X3	T44.3X4	T44.3X5	T44.3X6
Travert	T50.3X1	T50.3X2	T50.3X3	T50.3X4	T50.3X5	T50.3X6
Trazodone	T43.211	T43.212	T43.213	T43.214	T43.215	T43.216
Trecator	T37.1X1	T37.1X2	T37.1X3	T37.1X4	T37.1X5	T37.1X6
Treosulfan	T45.1X1	T45.1X2	T45.1X3	T45.1X4	T45.1X5	T45.1X6
Tretamine	T45.1X1	T45.1X2	T45.1X3	T45.1X4	T45.1X5	T45.1X6
Tretinoin	T49.0X1	T49.0X2	T49.0X3	T49.0X4	T49.0X5	T49.0X6
Tretoquinol	T48.6X1	T48.6X2	T48.6X3	T48.6X4	T48.6X5	T48.6X6
Triacetin	T49.0X1	T49.0X2	T49.0X3	T49.0X4	T49.0X5	T49.0X6
Triacetoxyanthracene	T49.4X1	T49.4X2	T49.4X3	T49.4X4	T49.4X5	T49.4X6
Triacetyloleandomycin	T36.3X1	T36.3X2	T36.3X3	T36.3X4	T36.3X5	T36.3X6
Triamcinolone	T49.0X1	T49.0X2	T49.0X3	T49.0X4	T49.0X5	T49.0X6
- ENT agent	T49.6X1	T49.6X2	T49.6X3	T49.6X4	T49.6X5	T49.6X6
- hexacetonide	T49.0X1	T49.0X2	T49.0X3	T49.0X4	T49.0X5	T49.0X6
- ophthalmic preparation	T49.5X1	T49.5X2	T49.5X3	T49.5X4	T49.5X5	T49.5X6
- topical NEC	T49.0X1	T49.0X2	T49.0X3	T49.0X4	T49.0X5	T49.0X6
Triampyzine	T44.3X1	T44.3X2	T44.3X3	T44.3X4	T44.3X5	T44.3X6
Triamterene	T50.2X1	T50.2X2	T50.2X3	T50.2X4	T50.2X5	T50.2X6
Triazine (herbicide)	T60.3X1	T60.3X2	T60.3X3	T60.3X4	--	--
Triaziquone	T45.1X1	T45.1X2	T45.1X3	T45.1X4	T45.1X5	T45.1X6
Triazolam	T42.4X1	T42.4X2	T42.4X3	T42.4X4	T42.4X5	T42.4X6
Triazole (herbicide)	T60.3X1	T60.3X2	T60.3X3	T60.3X4	--	--
Tribenoside	T46.991	T46.992	T46.993	T46.994	T46.995	T46.996
Tribromacetaldehyde	T42.6X1	T42.6X2	T42.6X3	T42.6X4	T42.6X5	T42.6X6
Tribromoethanol, rectal	T41.291	T41.292	T41.293	T41.294	T41.295	T41.296
Tribromomethane	T42.6X1	T42.6X2	T42.6X3	T42.6X4	T42.6X5	T42.6X6
Trichlorethane	T53.2X1	T53.2X2	T53.2X3	T53.2X4	--	--
Trichlorethylene	T53.2X1	T53.2X2	T53.2X3	T53.2X4	--	--
Trichlorfon	T60.0X1	T60.0X2	T60.0X3	T60.0X4	--	--
Trichlormethiazide	T50.2X1	T50.2X2	T50.2X3	T50.2X4	T50.2X5	T50.2X6
Trichlormethine	T45.1X1	T45.1X2	T45.1X3	T45.1X4	T45.1X5	T45.1X6
Trichloroacetic acid, Trichloracetic acid	T54.2X1	T54.2X2	T54.2X3	T54.2X4	--	--
- medicinal	T49.4X1	T49.4X2	T49.4X3	T49.4X4	T49.4X5	T49.4X6
Trichloroethane	T53.2X1	T53.2X2	T53.2X3	T53.2X4	--	--
Trichloroethanol	T42.6X1	T42.6X2	T42.6X3	T42.6X4	T42.6X5	T42.6X6
Trichloroethyl phosphate	T42.6X1	T42.6X2	T42.6X3	T42.6X4	T42.6X5	T42.6X6
Trichloroethylene (liquid) (vapor)	T53.2X1	T53.2X2	T53.2X3	T53.2X4	--	--
- anesthetic (gas)	T41.0X1	T41.0X2	T41.0X3	T41.0X4	T41.0X5	T41.0X6
- vapor NEC	T53.2X1	T53.2X2	T53.2X3	T53.2X4	--	--
Trichlorofluoromethane NEC	T53.5X1	T53.5X2	T53.5X3	T53.5X4	--	--
Trichloronate	T60.0X1	T60.0X2	T60.0X3	T60.0X4	--	--
2,4,5-Trichlorophen-oxyacetic acid	T60.3X1	T60.3X2	T60.3X3	T60.3X4	--	--
Trichloropropane	T53.6X1	T53.6X2	T53.6X3	T53.6X4	--	--
Trichlorotriethylamine	T45.1X1	T45.1X2	T45.1X3	T45.1X4	T45.1X5	T45.1X6
Trichomonacides NEC	T37.3X1	T37.3X2	T37.3X3	T37.3X4	T37.3X5	T37.3X6
Trichomycin	T36.7X1	T36.7X2	T36.7X3	T36.7X4	T36.7X5	T36.7X6
Triclobisonium chloride	T49.0X1	T49.0X2	T49.0X3	T49.0X4	T49.0X5	T49.0X6

Substance	Poisoning, Accidental (unintentional)	Poisoning, Intentional Self-harm	Poisoning, Assault	Poisoning, Undetermined	Adverse effect	Underdosing
Triclocarban	T49.0X1	T49.0X2	T49.0X3	T49.0X4	T49.0X5	T49.0X6
Triclofos	T42.6X1	T42.6X2	T42.6X3	T42.6X4	T42.6X5	T42.6X6
Triclosan	T49.0X1	T49.0X2	T49.0X3	T49.0X4	T49.0X5	T49.0X6
Tricresyl phosphate	T65.891	T65.892	T65.893	T65.894	--	--
- solvent	T52.91	T52.92	T52.93	T52.94	--	--
Tricyclamol chloride	T44.3X1	T44.3X2	T44.3X3	T44.3X4	T44.3X5	T44.3X6
Tridesilon	T49.0X1	T49.0X2	T49.0X3	T49.0X4	T49.0X5	T49.0X6
Tridihexethyl iodide	T44.3X1	T44.3X2	T44.3X3	T44.3X4	T44.3X5	T44.3X6
Tridione	T42.2X1	T42.2X2	T42.2X3	T42.2X4	T42.2X5	T42.2X6
Trientine	T45.8X1	T45.8X2	T45.8X3	T45.8X4	T45.8X5	T45.8X6
Triethanolamine NEC	T54.3X1	T54.3X2	T54.3X3	T54.3X4	--	--
- detergent	T54.3X1	T54.3X2	T54.3X3	T54.3X4	--	--
- trinitrate (biphosphate)	T46.3X1	T46.3X2	T46.3X3	T46.3X4	T46.3X5	T46.3X6
Triethanomelamine	T45.1X1	T45.1X2	T45.1X3	T45.1X4	T45.1X5	T45.1X6
Triethylenemelamine	T45.1X1	T45.1X2	T45.1X3	T45.1X4	T45.1X5	T45.1X6
Triethylenephosphoramide	T45.1X1	T45.1X2	T45.1X3	T45.1X4	T45.1X5	T45.1X6
Triethylenethiophosphoramide	T45.1X1	T45.1X2	T45.1X3	T45.1X4	T45.1X5	T45.1X6
Trifluoperazine	T43.3X1	T43.3X2	T43.3X3	T43.3X4	T43.3X5	T43.3X6
Trifluorocthyl vinyl ether	T41.0X1	T41.0X2	T41.0X3	T41.0X4	T41.0X5	T41.0X6
Trifluperidol	T43.4X1	T43.4X2	T43.4X3	T43.4X4	T43.4X5	T43.4X6
Triflupromazine	T43.3X1	T43.3X2	T43.3X3	T43.3X4	T43.3X5	T43.3X6
Trifluridine	T37.5X1	T37.5X2	T37.5X3	T37.5X4	T37.5X5	T37.5X6
Triflusal	T45.521	T45.522	T45.523	T45.524	T45.525	T45.526
Trihexyphenidyl	T44.3X1	T44.3X2	T44.3X3	T44.3X4	T44.3X5	T44.3X6
Triiodothyronine	T38.1X1	T38.1X2	T38.1X3	T38.1X4	T38.1X5	T38.1X6
Trilene	T41.0X1	T41.0X2	T41.0X3	T41.0X4	T41.0X5	T41.0X6
Trilostane	T38.991	T38.992	T38.993	T38.994	T38.995	T38.996
Trimebutine	T44.3X1	T44.3X2	T44.3X3	T44.3X4	T44.3X5	T44.3X6
Trimecaine	T41.3X1	T41.3X2	T41.3X3	T41.3X4	T41.3X5	T41.3X6
Trimeprazine (tartrate)	T44.3X1	T44.3X2	T44.3X3	T44.3X4	T44.3X5	T44.3X6
Trimetaphan camsilate	T44.2X1	T44.2X2	T44.2X3	T44.2X4	T44.2X5	T44.2X6
Trimetazidine	T46.7X1	T46.7X2	T46.7X3	T46.7X4	T46.7X5	T46.7X6
Trimethadione	T42.2X1	T42.2X2	T42.2X3	T42.2X4	T42.2X5	T42.2X6
Trimethaphan	T44.2X1	T44.2X2	T44.2X3	T44.2X4	T44.2X5	T44.2X6
Trimethidinium	T44.2X1	T44.2X2	T44.2X3	T44.2X4	T44.2X5	T44.2X6
Trimethobenzamide	T45.0X1	T45.0X2	T45.0X3	T45.0X4	T45.0X5	T45.0X6
Trimethoprim	T37.8X1	T37.8X2	T37.8X3	T37.8X4	T37.8X5	T37.8X6
- with sulfamethoxazole	T36.8X1	T36.8X2	T36.8X3	T36.8X4	T36.8X5	T36.8X6
Trimethylcarbinol	T51.3X1	T51.3X2	T51.3X3	T51.3X4	--	--
Trimethylpsoralen	T49.3X1	T49.3X2	T49.3X3	T49.3X4	T49.3X5	T49.3X6
Trimeton	T45.0X1	T45.0X2	T45.0X3	T45.0X4	T45.0X5	T45.0X6
Trimetrexate	T45.1X1	T45.1X2	T45.1X3	T45.1X4	T45.1X5	T45.1X6
Trimipramine	T43.011	T43.012	T43.013	T43.014	T43.015	T43.016
Trimustine	T45.1X1	T45.1X2	T45.1X3	T45.1X4	T45.1X5	T45.1X6
Trinitrine	T46.3X1	T46.3X2	T46.3X3	T46.3X4	T46.3X5	T46.3X6
Trinitrobenzol	T65.3X1	T65.3X2	T65.3X3	T65.3X4	--	--
Trinitrophenol	T65.3X1	T65.3X2	T65.3X3	T65.3X4	--	--
Trinitrotoluene (fumes)	T65.3X1	T65.3X2	T65.3X3	T65.3X4	--	--
Trional	T42.6X1	T42.6X2	T42.6X3	T42.6X4	T42.6X5	T42.6X6
Triorthocresyl phosphate	T65.891	T65.892	T65.893	T65.894	--	--
Trioxide of arsenic	T57.0X1	T57.0X2	T57.0X3	T57.0X4	--	--
Trioxysalen	T49.4X1	T49.4X2	T49.4X3	T49.4X4	T49.4X5	T49.4X6
Tripamide	T50.2X1	T50.2X2	T50.2X3	T50.2X4	T50.2X5	T50.2X6
Triparanol	T46.6X1	T46.6X2	T46.6X3	T46.6X4	T46.6X5	T46.6X6
Tripelennamine	T45.0X1	T45.0X2	T45.0X3	T45.0X4	T45.0X5	T45.0X6
Triperiden	T44.3X1	T44.3X2	T44.3X3	T44.3X4	T44.3X5	T44.3X6
Triperidol	T43.4X1	T43.4X2	T43.4X3	T43.4X4	T43.4X5	T43.4X6
Triphenylphosphate	T65.891	T65.892	T65.893	T65.894	--	--
Triple						
- bromides	T42.6X1	T42.6X2	T42.6X3	T42.6X4	T42.6X5	T42.6X6
- carbonate	T47.1X1	T47.1X2	T47.1X3	T47.1X4	T47.1X5	T47.1X6
- vaccine						
- - DPT	T50.A11	T50.A12	T50.A13	T50.A14	T50.A15	T50.A16
- - including pertussis	T50.A11	T50.A12	T50.A13	T50.A14	T50.A15	T50.A16
- - MMR	T50.B91	T50.B92	T50.B93	T50.B94	T50.B95	T50.B96

Substance	Poisoning, Accidental (unintentional)	Poisoning, Intentional Self-harm	Poisoning, Assault	Poisoning, Undetermined	Adverse effect	Underdosing
Triprolidine	T45.0X1	T45.0X2	T45.0X3	T45.0X4	T45.0X5	T45.0X6
Trisodium hydrogen edetate	T50.6X1	T50.6X2	T50.6X3	T50.6X4	T50.6X5	T50.6X6
Trisoralen	T49.3X1	T49.3X2	T49.3X3	T49.3X4	T49.3X5	T49.3X6
Trisulfapyrimidines	T37.0X1	T37.0X2	T37.0X3	T37.0X4	T37.0X5	T37.0X6
Trithiozine	T44.3X1	T44.3X2	T44.3X3	T44.3X4	T44.3X5	T44.3X6
Tritiozine	T44.3X1	T44.3X2	T44.3X3	T44.3X4	T44.3X5	T44.3X6
Tritoqualine	T45.0X1	T45.0X2	T45.0X3	T45.0X4	T45.0X5	T45.0X6
Trofosfamide	T45.1X1	T45.1X2	T45.1X3	T45.1X4	T45.1X5	T45.1X6
Troleandomycin	T36.3X1	T36.3X2	T36.3X3	T36.3X4	T36.3X5	T36.3X6
Trolnitrate (phosphate)	T46.3X1	T46.3X2	T46.3X3	T46.3X4	T46.3X5	T46.3X6
Tromantadine	T37.5X1	T37.5X2	T37.5X3	T37.5X4	T37.5X5	T37.5X6
Trometamol	T50.2X1	T50.2X2	T50.2X3	T50.2X4	T50.2X5	T50.2X6
Tromethamine	T50.2X1	T50.2X2	T50.2X3	T50.2X4	T50.2X5	T50.2X6
Tronothane	T41.3X1	T41.3X2	T41.3X3	T41.3X4	T41.3X5	T41.3X6
Tropacine	T44.3X1	T44.3X2	T44.3X3	T44.3X4	T44.3X5	T44.3X6
Tropatepine	T44.3X1	T44.3X2	T44.3X3	T44.3X4	T44.3X5	T44.3X6
Tropicamide	T44.3X1	T44.3X2	T44.3X3	T44.3X4	T44.3X5	T44.3X6
Trospium chloride	T44.3X1	T44.3X2	T44.3X3	T44.3X4	T44.3X5	T44.3X6
Troxerutin	T46.991	T46.992	T46.993	T46.994	T46.995	T46.996
Troxidone	T42.2X1	T42.2X2	T42.2X3	T42.2X4	T42.2X5	T42.2X6
Tryparsamide	T37.3X1	T37.3X2	T37.3X3	T37.3X4	T37.3X5	T37.3X6
Trypsin	T45.3X1	T45.3X2	T45.3X3	T45.3X4	T45.3X5	T45.3X6
Tryptizol	T43.011	T43.012	T43.013	T43.014	T43.015	T43.016
TSH	T38.811	T38.812	T38.813	T38.814	T38.815	T38.816
Tuaminoheptane	T48.5X1	T48.5X2	T48.5X3	T48.5X4	T48.5X5	T48.5X6
Tuberculin, purified protein derivative (PPD)	T50.8X1	T50.8X2	T50.8X3	T50.8X4	T50.8X5	T50.8X6
Tubocurare	T48.1X1	T48.1X2	T48.1X3	T48.1X4	T48.1X5	T48.1X6
Tubocurarine (chloride)	T48.1X1	T48.1X2	T48.1X3	T48.1X4	T48.1X5	T48.1X6
Tulobuterol	T48.6X1	T48.6X2	T48.6X3	T48.6X4	T48.6X5	T48.6X6
Turpentine (spirits of)	T52.8X1	T52.8X2	T52.8X3	T52.8X4	--	--
- vapor	T52.8X1	T52.8X2	T52.8X3	T52.8X4	--	--
Tybamate	T43.591	T43.592	T43.593	T43.594	T43.595	T43.596
Tyloxapol	T48.4X1	T48.4X2	T48.4X3	T48.4X4	T48.4X5	T48.4X6
Tymazoline	T48.5X1	T48.5X2	T48.5X3	T48.5X4	T48.5X5	T48.5X6
Typhoid-paratyphoid vaccine	T50.A91	T50.A92	T50.A93	T50.A94	T50.A95	T50.A96
Typhus vaccine	T50.A91	T50.A92	T50.A93	T50.A94	T50.A95	T50.A96
Tyropanoate	T50.8X1	T50.8X2	T50.8X3	T50.8X4	T50.8X5	T50.8X6
Tyrothricin	T49.6X1	T49.6X2	T49.6X3	T49.6X4	T49.6X5	T49.6X6
- ENT agent	T49.6X1	T49.6X2	T49.6X3	T49.6X4	T49.6X5	T49.6X6
- ophthalmic preparation	T49.5X1	T49.5X2	T49.5X3	T49.5X4	T49.5X5	T49.5X6
Ufenamate	T39.391	T39.392	T39.393	T39.394	T39.395	T39.396
Ultraviolet light protectant	T49.3X1	T49.3X2	T49.3X3	T49.3X4	T49.3X5	T49.3X6
Undecenoic acid	T49.0X1	T49.0X2	T49.0X3	T49.0X4	T49.0X5	T49.0X6
Undecoylium	T49.0X1	T49.0X2	T49.0X3	T49.0X4	T49.0X5	T49.0X6
Undecylenic acid (derivatives)	T49.0X1	T49.0X2	T49.0X3	T49.0X4	T49.0X5	T49.0X6
Unna's boot	T49.3X1	T49.3X2	T49.3X3	T49.3X4	T49.3X5	T49.3X6
Unsaturated fatty acid	T46.6X1	T46.6X2	T46.6X3	T46.6X4	T46.6X5	T46.6X6
Uracil mustard	T45.1X1	T45.1X2	T45.1X3	T45.1X4	T45.1X5	T45.1X6
Uramustine	T45.1X1	T45.1X2	T45.1X3	T45.1X4	T45.1X5	T45.1X6
Urapidil	T46.5X1	T46.5X2	T46.5X3	T46.5X4	T46.5X5	T46.5X6
Urari	T48.1X1	T48.1X2	T48.1X3	T48.1X4	T48.1X5	T48.1X6
Urate oxidase	T50.4X1	T50.4X2	T50.4X3	T50.4X4	T50.4X5	T50.4X6
Urea	T47.3X1	T47.3X2	T47.3X3	T47.3X4	T47.3X5	T47.3X6
- peroxide	T49.0X1	T49.0X2	T49.0X3	T49.0X4	T49.0X5	T49.0X6
- stibamine	T37.4X1	T37.4X2	T37.4X3	T37.4X4	T37.4X5	T37.4X6
- topical	T49.8X1	T49.8X2	T49.8X3	T49.8X4	T49.8X5	T49.8X6
Urethane	T45.1X1	T45.1X2	T45.1X3	T45.1X4	T45.1X5	T45.1X6
Urginea (maritima) (scilla) —see Squill						
Uric acid metabolism drug NEC	T50.4X1	T50.4X2	T50.4X3	T50.4X4	T50.4X5	T50.4X6
Uricosuric agent	T50.4X1	T50.4X2	T50.4X3	T50.4X4	T50.4X5	T50.4X6
Urinary anti-infective	T37.8X1	T37.8X2	T37.8X3	T37.8X4	T37.8X5	T37.8X6
Urofollitropin	T38.811	T38.812	T38.813	T38.814	T38.815	T38.816
Urokinase	T45.611	T45.612	T45.613	T45.614	T45.615	T45.616
Urokon	T50.8X1	T50.8X2	T50.8X3	T50.8X4	T50.8X5	T50.8X6
Ursodeoxycholic acid	T50.991	T50.992	T50.993	T50.994	T50.995	T50.996

Substance	Poisoning, Accidental (unintentional)	Poisoning, Intentional Self-harm	Poisoning, Assault	Poisoning, Undetermined	Adverse effect	Underdosing
Ursodiol	T50.991	T50.992	T50.993	T50.994	T50.995	T50.996
Urtica	T62.2X1	T62.2X2	T62.2X3	T62.2X4	--	--
Utility gas—see Gas, utility						
Vaccine NEC	T50.Z91	T50.Z92	T50.Z93	T50.Z94	T50.Z95	T50.Z96
- antineoplastic	T50.Z91	T50.Z92	T50.Z93	T50.Z94	T50.Z95	T50.Z96
- bacterial NEC	T50.A91	T50.A92	T50.A93	T50.A94	T50.A95	T50.A96
- - with						
- - - other bacterial component	T50.A21	T50.A22	T50.A23	T50.A24	T50.A25	T50.A26
- - - pertussis component	T50.A11	T50.A12	T50.A13	T50.A14	T50.A15	T50.A16
- - - viral-rickettsial component	T50.A21	T50.A22	T50.A23	T50.A24	T50.A25	T50.A26
- - mixed NEC	T50.A21	T50.A22	T50.A23	T50.A24	T50.A25	T50.A26
- BCG	T50.A91	T50.A92	T50.A93	T50.A94	T50.A95	T50.A96
- cholera	T50.A91	T50.A92	T50.A93	T50.A94	T50.A95	T50.A96
- diphtheria	T50.A91	T50.A92	T50.A93	T50.A94	T50.A95	T50.A96
- - with tetanus	T50.A21	T50.A22	T50.A23	T50.A24	T50.A25	T50.A26
- - - and pertussis	T50.A11	T50.A12	T50.A13	T50.A14	T50.A15	T50.A16
- influenza	T50.B91	T50.B92	T50.B93	T50.D94	T50.B95	T50.B96
- measles	T50.B91	T50.B92	T50.B93	T50.B94	T50.B95	T50.B96
- - with mumps and rubella	T50.B91	T50.B92	T50.B93	T50.B94	T50.B95	T50.B96
- meningococcal	T50.A91	T50.A92	T50.A93	T50.A94	T50.A95	T50.A96
- mumps	T50.B91	T50.B92	T50.B93	T50.B94	T50.B95	T50.B96
- paratyphoid	T50.A91	T50.A92	T50.A93	T50.A94	T50.A95	T50.A96
- pertussis	T50.A11	T50.A12	T50.A13	T50.A14	T50.A15	T50.A16
- - with diphtheria	T50.A11	T50.A12	T50.A13	T50.A14	T50.A15	T50.A16
- - - and tetanus	T50.A11	T50.A12	T50.A13	T50.A14	T50.A15	T50.A16
- - with other component	T50.A11	T50.A12	T50.A13	T50.A14	T50.A15	T50.A16
- plague	T50.A91	T50.A92	T50.A93	T50.A94	T50.A95	T50.A96
- poliomyelitis	T50.B91	T50.B92	T50.B93	T50.B94	T50.B95	T50.B96
- poliovirus	T50.B91	T50.B92	T50.B93	T50.B94	T50.B95	T50.B96
- rabies	T50.B91	T50.B92	T50.B93	T50.B94	T50.B95	T50.B96
- respiratory syncytial virus	T50.B91	T50.B92	T50.B93	T50.B94	T50.B95	T50.B96
- rickettsial NEC	T50.A91	T50.A92	T50.A93	T50.A94	T50.A95	T50.A96
- - with						
- - - bacterial component	T50.A21	T50.A22	T50.A23	T50.A24	T50.A25	T50.A26
- Rocky Mountain spotted fever	T50.A91	T50.A92	T50.A93	T50.A94	T50.A95	T50.A96
- rubella	T50.B91	T50.B92	T50.B93	T50.B94	T50.B95	T50.B96
- sabin oral	T50.B91	T50.B92	T50.B93	T50.B94	T50.B95	T50.B96
- smallpox	T50.B11	T50.B12	T50.B13	T50.B14	T50.B15	T50.B16
- TAB	T50.A91	T50.A92	T50.A93	T50.A94	T50.A95	T50.A96
- tetanus	T50.A91	T50.A92	T50.A93	T50.A94	T50.A95	T50.A96
- typhoid	T50.A91	T50.A92	T50.A93	T50.A94	T50.A95	T50.A96
- typhus	T50.A91	T50.A92	T50.A93	T50.A94	T50.A95	T50.A96
- viral NEC	T50.B91	T50.B92	T50.B93	T50.B94	T50.B95	T50.B96
- yellow fever	T50.B91	T50.B92	T50.B93	T50.B94	T50.B95	T50.B96
Vaccinia immune globulin	T50.Z11	T50.Z12	T50.Z13	T50.Z14	T50.Z15	T50.Z16
Vaginal contraceptives	T49.8X1	T49.8X2	T49.8X3	T49.8X4	T49.8X5	T49.8X6
Valerian						
- root	T42.6X1	T42.6X2	T42.6X3	T42.6X4	T42.6X5	T42.6X6
- tincture	T42.6X1	T42.6X2	T42.6X3	T42.6X4	T42.6X5	T42.6X6
Valethamate bromide	T44.3X1	T44.3X2	T44.3X3	T44.3X4	T44.3X5	T44.3X6
Valisone	T49.0X1	T49.0X2	T49.0X3	T49.0X4	T49.0X5	T49.0X6
Valium	T42.4X1	T42.4X2	T42.4X3	T42.4X4	T42.4X5	T42.4X6
Valmid	T42.6X1	T42.6X2	T42.6X3	T42.6X4	T42.6X5	T42.6X6
Valnoctamide	T42.6X1	T42.6X2	T42.6X3	T42.6X4	T42.6X5	T42.6X6
Valproate (sodium)	T42.6X1	T42.6X2	T42.6X3	T42.6X4	T42.6X5	T42.6X6
Valproic acid	T42.6X1	T42.6X2	T42.6X3	T42.6X4	T42.6X5	T42.6X6
Valpromide	T42.6X1	T42.6X2	T42.6X3	T42.6X4	T42.6X5	T42.6X6
Vanadium	T56.891	T56.892	T56.893	T56.894	--	--
Vancomycin	T36.8X1	T36.8X2	T36.8X3	T36.8X4	T36.8X5	T36.8X6
Vapor—see also Gas	T59.91	T59.92	T59.93	T59.94	--	--
- kiln (carbon monoxide)	T58.8X1	T58.8X2	T58.8X3	T58.8X4	--	--
- lead—see lead						
- specified source NEC	T59.891	T59.892	T59.893	T59.894	--	--
Vardenafil	T46.7X1	T46.7X2	T46.7X3	T46.7X4	T46.7X5	T46.7X6
Varicose reduction drug	T46.8X1	T46.8X2	T46.8X3	T46.8X4	T46.8X5	T46.8X6

Substance	Poisoning, Accidental (unintentional)	Poisoning, Intentional Self-harm	Poisoning, Assault	Poisoning, Undetermined	Adverse effect	Underdosing
Varnish	T65.4X1	T65.4X2	T65.4X3	T65.4X4	--	--
- cleaner	T52.91	T52.92	T52.93	T52.94	--	--
Vaseline	T49.3X1	T49.3X2	T49.3X3	T49.3X4	T49.3X5	T49.3X6
Vasodilan	T46.7X1	T46.7X2	T46.7X3	T46.7X4	T46.7X5	T46.7X6
Vasodilator						
- coronary NEC	T46.3X1	T46.3X2	T46.3X3	T46.3X4	T46.3X5	T46.3X6
- peripheral NEC	T46.7X1	T46.7X2	T46.7X3	T46.7X4	T46.7X5	T46.7X6
Vasopressin	T38.891	T38.892	T38.893	T38.894	T38.895	T38.896
Vasopressor drugs	T38.891	T38.892	T38.893	T38.894	T38.895	T38.896
Vecuronium bromide	T48.1X1	T48.1X2	T48.1X3	T48.1X4	T48.1X5	T48.1X6
Vegetable extract, astringent	T49.2X1	T49.2X2	T49.2X3	T49.2X4	T49.2X5	T49.2X6
Venlafaxine	T43.211	T43.212	T43.213	T43.214	T43.215	T43.216
Venom, venomous (bite) (sting)	T63.91	T63.92	T63.93	T63.94	--	--
- amphibian NEC	T63.831	T63.832	T63.833	T63.834	--	--
- animal NEC	T63.891	T63.892	T63.893	T63.894	--	--
- ant	T63.421	T63.422	T63.423	T63.424	--	--
- arthropod NEC	T63.481	T63.482	T63.483	T63.484	--	--
- bee	T63.441	T63.442	T63.443	T63.444	--	--
- centipede	T63.411	T63.412	T63.413	T63.414	--	--
- fish	T63.591	T63.592	T63.593	T63.594	--	--
- frog	T63.811	T63.812	T63.813	T63.814	--	--
- hornet	T63.451	T63.452	T63.453	T63.454	--	--
- insect NEC	T63.481	T63.482	T63.483	T63.484	--	--
- lizard	T63.121	T63.122	T63.123	T63.124	--	--
- marine						
- - animals	T63.691	T63.692	T63.693	T63.694	--	--
- - - bluebottle	T63.611	T63.612	T63.613	T63.614	--	--
- - - jellyfish NEC	T63.621	T63.622	T63.623	T63.624	--	--
- - - Portugese Man-o-war	T63.611	T63.612	T63.613	T63.614	--	--
- - - sea anemone	T63.631	T63.632	T63.633	T63.634	--	--
- - - specified NEC	T63.691	T63.692	T63.693	T63.694	--	--
- - fish	T63.591	T63.592	T63.593	T63.594	--	--
- - plants	T63.711	T63.712	T63.713	T63.714	--	--
- - sting ray	T63.511	T63.512	T63.513	T63.514	--	--
- millipede (tropical)	T63.411	T63.412	T63.413	T63.414	--	--
- plant NEC	T63.791	T63.792	T63.793	T63.794	--	--
- - marine	T63.711	T63.712	T63.713	T63.714	--	--
- reptile	T63.191	T63.192	T63.193	T63.194	--	--
- - gila monster	T63.111	T63.112	T63.113	T63.114	--	--
- - lizard NEC	T63.121	T63.122	T63.123	T63.124	--	--
- scorpion	T63.2X1	T63.2X2	T63.2X3	T63.2X4	--	--
- snake	T63.001	T63.002	T63.003	T63.004	--	--
- - African NEC	T63.081	T63.082	T63.083	T63.084	--	--
- - American (North) (South) NEC	T63.061	T63.062	T63.063	T63.064	--	--
- - Asian	T63.081	T63.082	T63.083	T63.084	--	--
- - Australian	T63.071	T63.072	T63.073	T63.074	--	--
- - cobra	T63.041	T63.042	T63.043	T63.044	--	--
- - coral snake	T63.021	T63.022	T63.023	T63.024	--	--
- - rattlesnake	T63.011	T63.012	T63.013	T63.014	--	--
- - specified NEC	T63.091	T63.092	T63.093	T63.094	--	--
- - taipan	T63.031	T63.032	T63.033	T63.034	--	--
- specified NEC	T63.891	T63.892	T63.893	T63.894	--	--
- spider	T63.301	T63.302	T63.303	T63.304	--	--
- - black widow	T63.311	T63.312	T63.313	T63.314	--	--
- - brown recluse	T63.331	T63.332	T63.333	T63.334	--	--
- - specified NEC	T63.391	T63.392	T63.393	T63.394	--	--
- - tarantula	T63.321	T63.322	T63.323	T63.324	--	--
- sting ray	T63.511	T63.512	T63.513	T63.514	--	--
- toad	T63.821	T63.822	T63.823	T63.824	--	--
- wasp	T63.461	T63.462	T63.463	T63.464	--	--
Venous sclerosing drug NEC	T46.8X1	T46.8X2	T46.8X3	T46.8X4	T46.8X5	T46.8X6
Ventolin—see Albuterol						
Veramon	T42.3X1	T42.3X2	T42.3X3	T42.3X4	T42.3X5	T42.3X6
Verapamil	T46.1X1	T46.1X2	T46.1X3	T46.1X4	T46.1X5	T46.1X6
Veratrine	T46.5X1	T46.5X2	T46.5X3	T46.5X4	T46.5X5	T46.5X6

Substance	Poisoning, Accidental (unintentional)	Poisoning, Intentional Self-harm	Poisoning, Assault	Poisoning, Undetermined	Adverse effect	Underdosing
Veratrum						
- album	T62.2X1	T62.2X2	T62.2X3	T62.2X4	--	--
- alkaloids	T46.5X1	T46.5X2	T46.5X3	T46.5X4	T46.5X5	T46.5X6
- viride	T62.2X1	T62.2X2	T62.2X3	T62.2X4	--	--
Verdigris	T60.3X1	T60.3X2	T60.3X3	T60.3X4	--	
Veronal	T42.3X1	T42.3X2	T42.3X3	T42.3X4	T42.3X5	T42.3X6
Veroxil	T37.4X1	T37.4X2	T37.4X3	T37.4X4	T37.4X5	T37.4X6
Versenate	T50.6X1	T50.6X2	T50.6X3	T50.6X4	T50.6X5	T50.6X6
Versidyne	T39.8X1	T39.8X2	T39.8X3	T39.8X4	T39.8X5	T39.8X6
Vetrabutine	T48.0X1	T48.0X2	T48.0X3	T48.0X4	T48.0X5	T48.0X6
Vidarabine	T37.5X1	T37.5X2	T37.5X3	T37.5X4	T37.5X5	T37.5X6
Vienna						
- green	T57.0X1	T57.0X2	T57.0X3	T57.0X4	--	--
- - insecticide	T60.2X1	T60.2X2	T60.2X3	T60.2X4	--	--
- red	T57.0X1	T57.0X2	T57.0X3	T57.0X4	--	
- - pharmaceutical dye	T50.991	T50.992	T50.993	T50.994	T50.995	T50.996
Vigabatrin	T42.6X1	T42.6X2	T42.6X3	T42.6X4	T42.6X5	T42.6X6
Viloxazine	T43.291	T43.292	T43.293	T43.294	T43.295	T43.296
Viminol	T39.8X1	T39.8X2	T39.8X3	T39.8X4	T39.8X5	T39.8X6
Vinbarbital, vinbarbitone	T42.3X1	T42.3X2	T42.3X3	T42.3X4	T42.3X5	T42.3X6
Vinblastine	T45.1X1	T45.1X2	T45.1X3	T45.1X4	T45.1X5	T45.1X6
Vinburnine	T46.7X1	T46.7X2	T46.7X3	T46.7X4	T46.7X5	T46.7X6
Vincamine	T45.1X1	T45.1X2	T45.1X3	T45.1X4	T45.1X5	T45.1X6
Vincristine	T45.1X1	T45.1X2	T45.1X3	T45.1X4	T45.1X5	T45.1X6
Vindesine	T45.1X1	T45.1X2	T45.1X3	T45.1X4	T45.1X5	T45.1X6
Vinesthene, vinethene	T41.0X1	T41.0X2	T41.0X3	T41.0X4	T41.0X5	T41.0X6
Vinorelbine tartrate	T45.1X1	T45.1X2	T45.1X3	T45.1X4	T45.1X5	T45.1X6
Vinpocetine	T46.7X1	T46.7X2	T46.7X3	T46.7X4	T46.7X5	T46.7X6
Vinyl						
- acetate	T65.891	T65.892	T65.893	T65.894	--	--
- bital	T42.3X1	T42.3X2	T42.3X3	T42.3X4	T42.3X5	T42.3X6
- bromide	T65.891	T65.892	T65.893	T65.894	--	--
- chloride	T59.891	T59.892	T59.893	T59.894	--	--
- ether	T41.0X1	T41.0X2	T41.0X3	T41.0X4	T41.0X5	T41.0X6
Vinylbital	T42.3X1	T42.3X2	T42.3X3	T42.3X4	T42.3X5	T42.3X6
Vinylidene chloride	T65.891	T65.892	T65.893	T65.894	--	--
Vioform	T37.8X1	T37.8X2	T37.8X3	T37.8X4	T37.8X5	T37.8X6
- topical	T49.0X1	T49.0X2	T49.0X3	T49.0X4	T49.0X5	T49.0X6
Viomycin	T36.8X1	T36.8X2	T36.8X3	T36.8X4	T36.8X5	T36.8X6
Vlosterol	T45.2X1	T45.2X2	T45.2X3	T45.2X4	T45.2X5	T45.2X6
Viper (venom)	T63.091	T63.092	T63.093	T63.094	--	--
Viprynium	T37.4X1	T37.4X2	T37.4X3	T37.4X4	T37.4X5	T37.4X6
Viquidil	T46.7X1	T46.7X2	T46.7X3	T46.7X4	T46.7X5	T46.7X6
Viral vaccine NEC	T50.B91	T50.B92	T50.B93	T50.B94	T50.B95	T50.B96
Virginiamycin	T36.8X1	T36.8X2	T36.8X3	T36.8X4	T36.8X5	T36.8X6
Virugon	T37.5X1	T37.5X2	T37.5X3	T37.5X4	T37.5X5	T37.5X6
Viscous agent	T50.901	T50.902	T50.903	T50.904	T50.905	T50.906
Visine	T49.5X1	T49.5X2	T49.5X3	T49.5X4	T49.5X5	T49.5X6
Visnadine	T46.3X1	T46.3X2	T46.3X3	T46.3X4	T46.3X5	T46.3X6
Vitamin NEC	T45.2X1	T45.2X2	T45.2X3	T45.2X4	T45.2X5	T45.2X6
- A	T45.2X1	T45.2X2	T45.2X3	T45.2X4	T45.2X5	T45.2X6
- B NEC	T45.2X1	T45.2X2	T45.2X3	T45.2X4	T45.2X5	T45.2X6
- - nicotinic acid	T46.7X1	T46.7X2	T46.7X3	T46.7X4	T46.7X5	T46.7X6
- B1	T45.2X1	T45.2X2	T45.2X3	T45.2X4	T45.2X5	T45.2X6
- B2	T45.2X1	T45.2X2	T45.2X3	T45.2X4	T45.2X5	T45.2X6
- B6	T45.2X1	T45.2X2	T45.2X3	T45.2X4	T45.2X5	T45.2X6
- B12	T45.2X1	T45.2X2	T45.2X3	T45.2X4	T45.2X5	T45.2X6
- B15	T45.2X1	T45.2X2	T45.2X3	T45.2X4	T45.2X5	T45.2X6
- C	T45.2X1	T45.2X2	T45.2X3	T45.2X4	T45.2X5	T45.2X6
- D	T45.2X1	T45.2X2	T45.2X3	T45.2X4	T45.2X5	T45.2X6
- D2	T45.2X1	T45.2X2	T45.2X3	T45.2X4	T45.2X5	T45.2X6
- D3	T45.2X1	T45.2X2	T45.2X3	T45.2X4	T45.2X5	T45.2X6
- E	T45.2X1	T45.2X2	T45.2X3	T45.2X4	T45.2X5	T45.2X6
- E acetate	T45.2X1	T45.2X2	T45.2X3	T45.2X4	T45.2X5	T45.2X6
- hematopoietic	T45.8X1	T45.8X2	T45.8X3	T45.8X4	T45.8X5	T45.8X6

Substance	Poisoning, Accidental (unintentional)	Poisoning, Intentional Self-harm	Poisoning, Assault	Poisoning, Undetermined	Adverse effect	Underdosing
- K NEC	T45.7X1	T45.7X2	T45.7X3	T45.7X4	T45.7X5	T45.7X6
- K1	T45.7X1	T45.7X2	T45.7X3	T45.7X4	T45.7X5	T45.7X6
- K2	T45.7X1	T45.7X2	T45.7X3	T45.7X4	T45.7X5	T45.7X6
- PP	T45.2X1	T45.2X2	T45.2X3	T45.2X4	T45.2X5	T45.2X6
- ulceroprotectant	T47.1X1	T47.1X2	T47.1X3	T47.1X4	T47.1X5	T47.1X6
Vleminckx's solution	T49.4X1	T49.4X2	T49.4X3	T49.4X4	T49.4X5	T49.4X6
Voltaren—see Diclofenac sodium						
Warfarin	T45.511	T45.512	T45.513	T45.514	T45.515	T45.516
- rodenticide	T60.4X1	T60.4X2	T60.4X3	T60.4X4	--	--
- sodium	T60.4X1	T60.4X2	T60.4X3	T60.4X4	--	--
Wasp (sting)	T63.461	T63.462	T63.463	T63.464	--	--
Water						
- balance drug	T50.3X1	T50.3X2	T50.3X3	T50.3X4	T50.3X5	T50.3X6
- distilled	T50.3X1	T50.3X2	T50.3X3	T50.3X4	T50.3X5	T50.3X6
- gas—see Gas, water						
- - incomplete combustion of—see Carbon, monoxide, fuel, utility						
- hemlock	T62.2X1	T62.2X2	T62.2X3	T62.2X4	--	--
- moccasin (venom)	T63.061	T63.062	T63.063	T63.064	--	--
- purified	T50.3X1	T50.3X2	T50.3X3	T50.3X4	T50.3X5	T50.3X6
Wax (paraffin) (petroleum)	T52.0X1	T52.0X2	T52.0X3	T52.0X4	--	--
- automobile	T65.891	T65.892	T65.893	T65.894	--	--
- floor	T52.0X1	T52.0X2	T52.0X3	T52.0X4	--	--
Weed killers NEC	T60.3X1	T60.3X2	T60.3X3	T60.3X4	--	--
Welldorm	T42.6X1	T42.6X2	T42.6X3	T42.6X4	T42.6X5	T42.6X6
White						
- arsenic	T57.0X1	T57.0X2	T57.0X3	T57.0X4	--	--
- hellebore	T62.2X1	T62.2X2	T62.2X3	T62.2X4	--	--
- lotion (keratolytic)	T49.4X1	T49.4X2	T49.4X3	T49.4X4	T49.4X5	T49.4X6
- spirit	T52.0X1	T52.0X2	T52.0X3	T52.0X4	--	--
Whitewash	T65.891	T65.892	T65.893	T65.894	--	--
Whole blood (human)	T45.8X1	T45.8X2	T45.8X3	T45.8X4	T45.8X5	T45.8X6
Wild						
- black cherry	T62.2X1	T62.2X2	T62.2X3	T62.2X4	--	--
- poisonous plants NEC	T62.2X1	T62.2X2	T62.2X3	T62.2X4	--	--
Window cleaning fluid	T65.891	T65.892	T65.893	T65.894	--	--
Wintergreen (oil)	T49.3X1	T49.3X2	T49.3X3	T49.3X4	T49.3X5	T49.3X6
Wisterine	T62.2X1	T62.2X2	T62.2X3	T62.2X4	--	--
Witch hazel	T49.2X1	T49.2X2	T49.2X3	T49.2X4	T49.2X5	T49.2X6
Wood alcohol or spirit	T51.1X1	T51.1X2	T51.1X3	T51.1X4	--	--
Wool fat (hydrous)	T49.3X1	T49.3X2	T49.3X3	T49.3X4	T49.3X5	T49.3X6
Woorali	T48.1X1	T48.1X2	T48.1X3	T48.1X4	T48.1X5	T48.1X6
Wormseed, American	T37.4X1	T37.4X2	T37.4X3	T37.4X4	T37.4X5	T37.4X6
Xamoterol	T44.5X1	T44.5X2	T44.5X3	T44.5X4	T44.5X5	T44.5X6
Xanthine diuretics	T50.2X1	T50.2X2	T50.2X3	T50.2X4	T50.2X5	T50.2X6
Xanthinol nicotinate	T46.7X1	T46.7X2	T46.7X3	T46.7X4	T46.7X5	T46.7X6
Xanthotoxin	T49.3X1	T49.3X2	T49.3X3	T49.3X4	T49.3X5	T49.3X6
Xantinol nicotinate	T46.7X1	T46.7X2	T46.7X3	T46.7X4	T46.7X5	T46.7X6
Xantocillin	T36.0X1	T36.0X2	T36.0X3	T36.0X4	T36.0X5	T36.0X6
Xenon (127Xe) (133Xe)	T50.8X1	T50.8X2	T50.8X3	T50.8X4	T50.8X5	T50.8X6
Xenysalate	T49.4X1	T49.4X2	T49.4X3	T49.4X4	T49.4X5	T49.4X6
Xibornol	T37.8X1	T37.8X2	T37.8X3	T37.8X4	T37.8X5	T37.8X6
Xigris	T45.511	T45.512	T45.513	T45.514	T45.515	T45.516
Xipamide	T50.2X1	T50.2X2	T50.2X3	T50.2X4	T50.2X5	T50.2X6
Xylene (vapor)	T52.2X1	T52.2X2	T52.2X3	T52.2X4	--	--
Xylocaine (infiltration) (topical)	T41.3X1	T41.3X2	T41.3X3	T41.3X4	T41.3X5	T41.3X6
- nerve block (peripheral) (plexus)	T41.3X1	T41.3X2	T41.3X3	T41.3X4	T41.3X5	T41.3X6
- spinal	T41.3X1	T41.3X2	T41.3X3	T41.3X4	T41.3X5	T41.3X6
Xylol (vapor)	T52.2X1	T52.2X2	T52.2X3	T52.2X4	--	--
Xylometazoline	T48.5X1	T48.5X2	T48.5X3	T48.5X4	T48.5X5	T48.5X6
Yeast	T45.2X1	T45.2X2	T45.2X3	T45.2X4	T45.2X5	T45.2X6
- dried	T45.2X1	T45.2X2	T45.2X3	T45.2X4	T45.2X5	T45.2X6
Yellow						
- fever vaccine	T50.B91	T50.B92	T50.B93	T50.B94	T50.B95	T50.B96
- jasmine	T62.2X1	T62.2X2	T62.2X3	T62.2X4	--	--

Substance	Poisoning, Accidental (unintentional)	Poisoning, Intentional Self-harm	Poisoning, Assault	Poisoning, Undetermined	Adverse effect	Underdosing
- phenolphthalein	T47.2X1	T47.2X2	T47.2X3	T47.2X4	T47.2X5	T47.2X6
Yew	T62.2X1	T62.2X2	T62.2X3	T62.2X4	--	--
Yohimbic acid	T40.991	T40.992	T40.993	T40.994	T40.995	T40.996
Zactane	T39.8X1	T39.8X2	T39.8X3	T39.8X4	T39.8X5	T39.8X6
Zalcitabine	T37.5X1	T37.5X2	T37.5X3	T37.5X4	T37.5X5	T37.5X6
Zaroxolyn	T50.2X1	T50.2X2	T50.2X3	T50.2X4	T50.2X5	T50.2X6
Zephiran (topical)	T49.0X1	T49.0X2	T49.0X3	T49.0X4	T49.0X5	T49.0X6
- ophthalmic preparation	T49.5X1	T49.5X2	T49.5X3	T49.5X4	T49.5X5	T49.5X6
Zeranol	T38.7X1	T38.7X2	T38.7X3	T38.7X4	T38.7X5	T38.7X6
Zerone	T51.1X1	T51.1X2	T51.1X3	T51.1X4	--	--
Zidovudine	T37.5X1	T37.5X2	T37.5X3	T37.5X4	T37.5X5	T37.5X6
Zimeldine	T43.221	T43.222	T43.223	T43.224	T43.225	T43.226
Zinc (compounds) (fumes) (vapor) NEC	T56.5X1	T56.5X2	T56.5X3	T56.5X4	--	--
- anti-infectives	T49.0X1	T49.0X2	T49.0X3	T49.0X4	T49.0X5	T49.0X6
- antivaricose	T46.8X1	T46.8X2	T46.8X3	T46.8X4	T46.8X5	T46.8X6
- bacitracin	T49.0X1	T49.0X2	T49.0X3	T49.0X4	T49.0X5	T49.0X6
- chloride (mouthwash)	T49.6X1	T49.6X2	T49.6X3	T49.6X4	T49.6X5	T49.6X6
- chromate	T56.5X1	T56.5X2	T56.5X3	T56.5X4	--	--
- gelatin	T49.3X1	T49.3X2	T49.3X3	T49.3X4	T49.3X5	T49.3X6
- oxide	T49.3X1	T49.3X2	T49.3X3	T49.3X4	T49.3X5	T49.3X6
- - plaster	T49.3X1	T49.3X2	T49.3X3	T49.3X4	T49.3X5	T49.3X6
- peroxide	T49.0X1	T49.0X2	T49.0X3	T49.0X4	T49.0X5	T49.0X6
- pesticides	T56.5X1	T56.5X2	T56.5X3	T56.5X4	--	--
- phosphide	T60.4X1	T60.4X2	T60.4X3	T60.4X4	--	--
- pyrithionate	T49.4X1	T49.4X2	T49.4X3	T49.4X4	T49.4X5	T49.4X6
- stearate	T49.3X1	T49.3X2	T49.3X3	T49.3X4	T49.3X5	T49.3X6
- sulfate	T49.5X1	T49.5X2	T49.5X3	T49.5X4	T49.5X5	T49.5X6
- - ENT agent	T49.6X1	T49.6X2	T49.6X3	T49.6X4	T49.6X5	T49.6X6
- - ophthalmic solution	T49.5X1	T49.5X2	T49.5X3	T49.5X4	T49.5X5	T49.5X6
- - topical NEC	T49.0X1	T49.0X2	T49.0X3	T49.0X4	T49.0X5	T49.0X6
- undecylenate	T49.0X1	T49.0X2	T49.0X3	T49.0X4	T49.0X5	T49.0X6
Zineb	T60.0X1	T60.0X2	T60.0X3	T60.0X4	--	--
Zinostatin	T45.1X1	T45.1X2	T45.1X3	T45.1X4	T45.1X5	T45.1X6
Zipeprol	T48.3X1	T48.3X2	T48.3X3	T48.3X4	T48.3X5	T48.3X6
Zofenopril	T46.4X1	T46.4X2	T46.4X3	T46.4X4	T46.4X5	T46.4X6
Zolpidem	T42.6X1	T42.6X2	T42.6X3	T42.6X4	T42.6X5	T42.6X6
Zomepirac	T39.391	T39.392	T39.393	T39.394	T39.395	T39.396
Zopiclone	T42.6X1	T42.6X2	T42.6X3	T42.6X4	T42.6X5	T42.6X6
Zorubicin	T45.1X1	T45.1X2	T45.1X3	T45.1X4	T45.1X5	T45.1X6
Zotepine	T43.591	T43.592	T43.593	T43.594	T43.595	T43.596
Zovant	T45.511	T45.512	T45.513	T45.514	T45.515	T45.516
Zoxazolamine	T42.8X1	T42.8X2	T42.8X3	T42.8X4	T42.8X5	T42.8X6
Zuclopenthixol	T43.4X1	T43.4X2	T43.4X3	T43.4X4	T43.4X5	T43.4X6
Zygadenus (venenosus)	T62.2X1	T62.2X2	T62.2X3	T62.2X4		--
Zyprexa	T43.591	T43.592	T43.593	T43.594	T43.595	T43.596

A

Abandonment (causing exposure to weather conditions) (with intent to injure or kill) NEC X58

Abuse (adult) (child) (mental) (physical) (sexual) X58

Accident (to) X58
  aircraft (in transit) (powered) —see also Accident, transport, aircraft
    due to, caused by cataclysm —see Forces of nature, by type
  animal-rider — see Accident, transport, animal-rider
  animal-drawn vehicle —see Accident, transport, animal-drawn vehicle occupant
  automobile —see Accident, transport, car occupant
  bare foot water skier V94.4
  boat, boating —see also Accident, watercraft
    striking swimmer
      powered V94.11
      unpowered V94.12
  bus —see Accident, transport, bus occupant
  cable car, not on rails V98.0
    on rails —see Accident, transport, streetcar occupant
  car —see Accident, transport, car occupant
  caused by, due to
    animal NEC W64
    chain hoist W24.0
    cold (excessive) —see Exposure, cold
    corrosive liquid, substance —see Table of drugs and chemicals
    cutting or piercing instrument —see Contact, with, by type of instrument
    drive belt W24.0
    electric
      current —see Exposure, electric current
      motor (see also Contact, with, by type of machine) W31.3
        current (of) W86.8
    environmental factor NEC X58
    explosive material —see Explosion
    fire, flames —see Exposure, fire
    firearm missile —see Discharge, firearm by type
    heat (excessive) —see Heat
    hot —see Contact, with, hot
    ignition —see Ignition
    lifting device W24.0
    lightning —see subcategory T75.0
      causing fire —see Exposure, fire
    machine, machinery —see Contact, with, by type of machine
    natural factor NEC X58
    pulley (block) W24.0
    radiation —see Radiation
    steam X13.1
      inhalation X13.0
      pipe X16
    thunderbolt —see subcategory T75.0
      causing fire —see Exposure, fire
    transmission device W24.1
  coach —see Accident, transport, bus occupant
  coal car —see Accident, transport, industrial vehicle occupant
  diving —see also Fall, into, water
    with
      drowning or submersion —see Drowning
  forklift —see Accident, transport, industrial vehicle occupant

Accident - continued
  heavy transport vehicle NOS —see Accident, transport, truck occupant
  ice yacht V98.2
  in
    medical, surgical procedure
      as, or due to misadventure —see Misadventure
      causing an abnormal reaction or later complication without mention of misadventure (see also Complication of or following, by type of procedure) Y84.9
  land yacht V98.1
  late effect of —see W00
  X58 with 7th character S
  logging car —see Accident, transport, industrial vehicle occupant
  machine, machinery —see also Contact, with, by type of machine
    on board watercraft V93.69
      explosion —see Explosion, in, watercraft
      fire —see Burn, on board watercraft
      powered craft V93.63
        ferry boat V93.61
        fishing boat V93.62
        jet skis V93.63
        liner V93.61
        merchant ship V93.60
        passenger ship V93.61
        sailboat V93.64
  mine tram —see Accident, transport, industrial vehicle occupant
  mobility scooter (motorized) —see Accident, transport, pedestrian, conveyance, specified type NEC
  motor scooter —see Accident, transport, motorcyclist
  motor vehicle NOS (traffic) (see also Accident, transport) V89.2
    nontraffic V89.0
    three-wheeled NOS —see Accident, transport, three-wheeled motor vehicle occupant
  motorcycle NOS —see Accident, transport, motorcyclist
  nonmotor vehicle NOS (nontraffic) (see also Accident, transport) V89.1
    traffic NOS V89.3
  nontraffic (victim's mode of transport NOS) V88.9
    collision (between) V88.7
      bus and truck V88.5
      car and:
        bus V88.3
        pickup V88.2
        three-wheeled motor vehicle V88.0
        train V88.6
        truck V88.4
        two-wheeled motor vehicle V88.0
        van V88.2
      specified vehicle NEC and:
        three-wheeled motor vehicle V88.1
        two-wheeled motor vehicle V88.1
    known mode of transport —see Accident, transport, by type of vehicle
    noncollision V88.8
  on board watercraft V93.89
    powered craft V93.83
      ferry boat V93.81
      fishing boat V93.82
      jet skis V93.83
      liner V93.81
      merchant ship V93.80

Accident - continued
      passenger ship V93.81
    unpowered craft V93.88
      canoe V93.85
      inflatable V93.86
      in tow
        recreational V94.31
        specified NEC V94.32
      kayak V93.85
      sailboat V93.84
      surf-board V93.88
      water skis V93.87
      windsurfer V93.88
  parachutist V97.29
    entangled in object V97.21
    injured on landing V97.22
  pedal cycle —see Accident, transport, pedal cyclist
  pedestrian (on foot)
    with
      another pedestrian W51
        with fall W03
          due to ice or snow W00.0
      on pedestrian conveyance NEC V00.09
      roller skater (in-line) V00.01
      skate boarder V00.02
      transport vehicle —see Accident, transport
    on pedestrian conveyance —see Accident, transport, pedestrian, conveyance
  pick-up truck or van —see Accident, transport, pickup truck occupant
  quarry truck —see Accident, transport, industrial vehicle occupant
  railway vehicle (any) (in motion) —see Accident, transport, railway vehicle occupant
    due to cataclysm —see Forces of nature, by type
  scooter (non-motorized) —see Accident, transport, pedestrian, conveyance, scooter
  sequelae of —see W00
  X58 with 7th character S
  skateboard —see Accident, transport, pedestrian, conveyance, skateboard
  ski (ing) —see Accident, transport, pedestrian, conveyance
    lift V98.3
  specified cause NEC X58
  streetcar —see Accident, transport, streetcar occupant
  traffic (victim's mode of transport NOS) V87.9
    collision (between) V87.7
      bus and truck V87.5
      car and:
        bus V87.3
        pickup V87.2
        three-wheeled motor vehicle V87.0
        train V87.6
        truck V87.4
        two-wheeled motor vehicle V87.0
        van V87.2
      specified vehicle NEC and:
        three-wheeled motor vehicle V87.1
        two-wheeled motor vehicle V87.1
    known mode of transport —see Accident, transport, by type of vehicle
    noncollision V87.8
  transport (involving injury to) V99
    18 wheeler —see Accident, transport, truck occupant
    agricultural vehicle occupant (nontraffic) V84.9
      driver V84.5

Accident - *continued*
  hanger-on V84.7
  passenger V84.6
  traffic V84.3
    driver V84.0
    hanger-on V84.2
    passenger V84.1
  while boarding or alighting V84.4
aircraft NEC V97.89
  military NEC V97.818
    with civilian aircraft V97.810
    civilian injured by V97.811
  occupant injured (in)
    nonpowered craft accident V96.9
      balloon V96.00
        collision V96.03
        crash V96.01
        explosion V96.05
        fire V96.04
        forced landing V96.02
        specified type NEC V96.09
      glider V96.20
        collision V96.23
        crash V96.21
        explosion V96.25
        fire V96.24
        forced landing V96.22
        specified type NEC V96.29
      hang glider V96.10
        collision V96.13
        crash V96.11
        explosion V96.15
        fire V96.14
        forced landing V96.12
        specified type NEC V96.19
      specified craft NEC V96.8
    powered craft accident V95.9
      fixed wing NEC
        commercial V95.30
          collision V95.33
          crash V95.31
          explosion V95.35
          fire V95.34
          forced landing V95.32
          specified type NEC V95.39
        private V95.20
          collision V95.23
          crash V95.21
          explosion V95.25
          fire V95.24
          forced landing V95.22
          specified type NEC V95.29
      glider V95.10
        collision V95.13
        crash V95.11
        explosion V95.15
        fire V95.14
        forced landing V95.12
        specified type NEC V95.19
      helicopter V95.00
        collision V95.03
        crash V95.01
        explosion V95.05
        fire V95.04
        forced landing V95.02
        specified type NEC V95.09
      spacecraft V95.40
        collision V95.43
        crash V95.41
        explosion V95.45
        fire V95.44
        forced landing V95.42
        specified type NEC V95.49

Accident - *continued*
      specified craft NEC V95.8
    ultralight V95.10
      collision V95.13
      crash V95.11
      explosion V95.15
      fire V95.14
      forced landing V95.12
      specified type NEC V95.19
  specified accident NEC V97.0
  while boarding or alighting V97.1
  person (injured by)
    falling from, in or on aircraft V97.0
    machinery on aircraft V97.89
    on ground with aircraft involvement V97.39
    rotating propeller V97.32
    struck by object falling from aircraft V97.31
    sucked into aircraft jet V97.33
    while boarding or alighting aircraft V97.1
  airport (battery-powered) passenger vehicle —
    see Accident, transport, industrial vehicle
    occupant
  all-terrain vehicle occupant (nontraffic) V86.99
    driver V86.59
    dune buggy —*see* Accident, transport, dune
    buggy occupant
    hanger-on V86.79
    passenger V86.69
    snowmobile —*see* Accident, transport,
    snowmobile occupant
    traffic V86.39
      driver V86.09
      hanger-on V86.29
      passenger V86.19
    while boarding or alighting V86.49
  ambulance occupant (traffic) V86.31
    driver V86.01
    hanger-on V86.21
    nontraffic V86.91
      driver V86.51
      hanger-on V86.71
      passenger V86.61
    passenger V86.11
    while boarding or alighting V86.41
  animal-drawn vehicle occupant (in) V80.929
    collision (with)
      animal V80.12
        being ridden V80.711
      animal-drawn vehicle V80.721
      bus V80.42
      car V80.42
      fixed or stationary object V80.82
      military vehicle V80.920
      nonmotor vehicle V80.791
      pedal cycle V80.22
      pedestrian V80.12
      pickup V80.42
      railway train or vehicle V80.62
      specified motor vehicle NEC V80.52
      streetcar V80.731
      truck V80.42
      two or three-wheeled motor vehicle V80.32
      van V80.42
    noncollision V80.02
    specified circumstance NEC V80.928
  animal-rider V80.919
    collision (with)
      animal V80.11
        being ridden V80.710
      animal-drawn vehicle V80.720

Accident - *continued*
      bus V80.41
      car V80.41
      fixed or stationary object V80.81
      military vehicle V80.910
      nonmotor vehicle V80.790
      pedal cycle V80.21
      pedestrian V80.11
      pickup V80.41
      railway train or vehicle V80.61
      specified motor vehicle NEC V80.51
      streetcar V80.730
      truck V80.41
      two or three-wheeled motor vehicle V80.31
      van V80.41
    noncollision V80.018
      specified as horse rider V80.010
      specified circumstance NEC V80.918
  armored car —*see* Accident, transport, truck
    occupant
  battery-powered truck (baggage) (mail) —*see*
    Accident, transport, industrial vehicle occupant
  bus occupant V79.9
    collision (with)
      animal (traffic) V70.9
        being ridden (traffic) V76.9
          nontraffic V76.3
            while boarding or alighting V76.4
        nontraffic V70.3
          while boarding or alighting V70.4
      animal-drawn vehicle (traffic) V76.9
        nontraffic V76.3
          while boarding or alighting V76.4
      bus (traffic) V74.9
        nontraffic V74.3
          while boarding or alighting V74.4
      car (traffic) V73.9
        nontraffic V73.3
          while boarding or alighting V73.4
      motor vehicle NOS (traffic) V79.60
        nontraffic V79.20
        specified type NEC (traffic) V79.69
          nontraffic V79.29
      pedal cycle (traffic) V71.9
        nontraffic V71.3
          while boarding or alighting V71.4
      pickup truck (traffic) V73.9
        nontraffic V73.3
          while boarding or alighting V73.4
      railway vehicle (traffic) V75.9
        nontraffic V75.3
          while boarding or alighting V75.4
      specified vehicle NEC (traffic) V76.9
        nontraffic V76.3
          while boarding or alighting V76.4
      stationary object (traffic) V77.9
        nontraffic V77.3
          while boarding or alighting V77.4
      streetcar (traffic) V76.9
        nontraffic V76.3
          while boarding or alighting V76.4
      three wheeled motor vehicle (traffic) V72.9
        nontraffic V72.3
          while boarding or alighting V72.4
      truck (traffic) V74.9
        nontraffic V74.3
          while boarding or alighting V74.4
      two wheeled motor vehicle (traffic) V72.9
        nontraffic V72.3
          while boarding or alighting V72.4
      van (traffic) V73.9
        nontraffic V73.3

Accident - *continued*
  while boarding or alighting V73.4
  driver
   collision (with)
    animal (traffic) V70.5
     being ridden (traffic) V76.5
      nontraffic V76.0
     nontraffic V70.0
    animal-drawn vehicle (traffic) V76.5
     nontraffic V76.0
    bus (traffic) V74.5
     nontraffic V74.0
    car (traffic) V73.5
     nontraffic V73.0
    motor vehicle NOS (traffic) V79.40
     nontraffic V79.00
      specified type NEC (traffic) V79.49
       nontraffic V79.09
    pedal cycle (traffic) V71.5
     nontraffic V71.0
    pickup truck (traffic) V73.5
     nontraffic V73.0
    railway vehicle (traffic) V75.5
     nontraffic V75.0
    specified vehicle NEC (traffic) V76.5
     nontraffic V76.0
    stationary object (traffic) V77.5
     nontraffic V77.0
    streetcar (traffic) V76.5
     nontraffic V76.0
    three wheeled motor vehicle (traffic)
     V72.5
     nontraffic V72.0
    truck (traffic) V74.5
     nontraffic V74.0
    two wheeled motor vehicle (traffic) V72.5
     nontraffic V72.0
    van (traffic) V73.5
     nontraffic V73.0
   noncollision accident (traffic) V78.5
    nontraffic V78.0
  noncollision accident (traffic) V78.9
   nontraffic V78.3
   while boarding or alighting V78.4
  nontraffic V79.3
  hanger-on
   collision (with)
    animal (traffic) V70.7
     being ridden (traffic) V76.7
      nontraffic V76.2
     nontraffic V70.2
    animal-drawn vehicle (traffic) V76.7
     nontraffic V76.2
    bus (traffic) V74.7
     nontraffic V74.2
    car (traffic) V73.7
     nontraffic V73.2
    pedal cycle (traffic) V71.7
     nontraffic V71.2
    pickup truck (traffic) V73.7
     nontraffic V73.2
    railway vehicle (traffic) V75.7
     nontraffic V75.2
    specified vehicle NEC (traffic) V76.7
     nontraffic V76.2
    stationary object (traffic) V77.7
     nontraffic V77.2
    streetcar (traffic) V76.7
     nontraffic V76.2
    three wheeled motor vehicle (traffic)
     V72.7
     nontraffic V72.2
    truck (traffic) V74.7

Accident - *continued*
     nontraffic V74.2
    two wheeled motor vehicle (traffic) V72.7
     nontraffic V72.2
    van (traffic) V73.7
     nontraffic V73.2
   noncollision accident (traffic) V78.7
    nontraffic V78.2
  passenger
   collision (with)
    animal (traffic) V70.6
     being ridden (traffic) V76.6
      nontraffic V76.1
     nontraffic V70.1
    animal-drawn vehicle (traffic) V76.6
     nontraffic V76.1
    bus (traffic) V74.6
     nontraffic V74.1
    car (traffic) V73.6
     nontraffic V73.1
    motor vehicle NOS (traffic) V79.50
     nontraffic V79.10
      specified type NEC (traffic) V79.59
       nontraffic V79.19
    pedal cycle (traffic) V71.6
     nontraffic V71.1
    pickup truck (traffic) V73.6
     nontraffic V73.1
    railway vehicle (traffic) V75.6
     nontraffic V75.1
    specified vehicle NEC (traffic) V76.6
     nontraffic V76.1
    stationary object (traffic) V77.6
     nontraffic V77.1
    streetcar (traffic) V76.6
     nontraffic V76.1
    three wheeled motor vehicle (traffic)
     V72.6
     nontraffic V72.1
    truck (traffic) V74.6
     nontraffic V74.1
    two wheeled motor vehicle (traffic) V72.6
     nontraffic V72.1
    van (traffic) V73.6
     nontraffic V73.1
   noncollision accident (traffic) V78.6
    nontraffic V78.1
  specified type NEC V79.88
   military vehicle V79.81
  cable car, not on rails V98.0
  on rails —*see* Accident, transport, streetcar
 occupant
  car occupant V49.9
   ambulance occupant —*see* Accident,
 transport, ambulance occupant
   collision (with)
    animal (traffic) V40.9
     being ridden (traffic) V46.9
      nontraffic V46.3
      while boarding or alighting V46.4
     nontraffic V40.3
     while boarding or alighting V40.4
    animal-drawn vehicle (traffic) V46.9
     nontraffic V46.3
     while boarding or alighting V46.4
    bus (traffic) V44.9
     nontraffic V44.3
     while boarding or alighting V44.4
    car (traffic) V43.92
     nontraffic V43.32
     while boarding or alighting V43.42
    motor vehicle NOS (traffic) V49.60
     nontraffic V49.20

Accident - *continued*
     specified type NEC (traffic) V49.69
     nontraffic V49.29
    pedal cycle (traffic) V41.9
     nontraffic V41.3
     while boarding or alighting V41.4
    pickup truck (traffic) V43.93
     nontraffic V43.33
     while boarding or alighting V43.43
    railway vehicle (traffic) V45.9
     nontraffic V45.3
     while boarding or alighting V45.4
    specified vehicle NEC (traffic) V46.9
     nontraffic V46.3
     while boarding or alighting V46.4
    sport utility vehicle (traffic) V43.91
     nontraffic V43.31
     while boarding or alighting V43.41
    stationary object (traffic) V47.92
     nontraffic V47.32
     while boarding or alighting V47.4
    streetcar (traffic) V46.9
     nontraffic V46.3
     while boarding or alighting V46.4
    three wheeled motor vehicle (traffic) V42.9
     nontraffic V42.3
     while boarding or alighting V42.4
    truck (traffic) V44.9
     nontraffic V44.3
     while boarding or alighting V44.4
    two wheeled motor vehicle (traffic) V42.9
     nontraffic V42.3
     while boarding or alighting V42.4
    van (traffic) V43.94
     nontraffic V43.34
     while boarding or alighting V43.44
   driver
    collision (with)
     animal (traffic) V40.5
      being ridden (traffic) V46.5
       nontraffic V46.0
      nontraffic V40.0
     animal-drawn vehicle (traffic) V46.5
      nontraffic V46.0
     bus (traffic) V44.5
      nontraffic V44.0
     car (traffic) V43.52
      nontraffic V43.02
     motor vehicle NOS (traffic) V49.40
      nontraffic V49.00
       specified type NEC (traffic) V49.49
        nontraffic V49.09
     pedal cycle (traffic) V41.5
      nontraffic V41.0
     pickup truck (traffic) V43.53
      nontraffic V43.03
     railway vehicle (traffic) V45.5
      nontraffic V45.0
     specified vehicle NEC (traffic) V46.5
      nontraffic V46.0
     sport utility vehicle (traffic) V43.51
      nontraffic V43.01
     stationary object (traffic) V47.52
      nontraffic V47.02
     streetcar (traffic) V46.5
      nontraffic V46.0
     three wheeled motor vehicle (traffic)
      V42.5
      nontraffic V42.0
     truck (traffic) V44.5
      nontraffic V44.0
     two wheeled motor vehicle (traffic) V42.5
      nontraffic V42.0

Accident - *continued*
  van (traffic) V43.54
    nontraffic V43.04
  noncollision accident (traffic) V48.5
    nontraffic V48.0
  noncollision accident (traffic) V48.9
    nontraffic V48.3
    while boarding or alighting V48.4
  nontraffic V49.3
  hanger-on
    collision (with)
      animal (traffic) V40.7
        being ridden (traffic) V46.7
          nontraffic V46.2
        nontraffic V40.2
      animal-drawn vehicle (traffic) V46.7
        nontraffic V46.2
      bus (traffic) V44.7
        nontraffic V44.2
      car (traffic) V43.72
        nontraffic V43.22
      pedal cycle (traffic) V41.7
        nontraffic V41.2
      pickup truck (traffic) V43.73
        nontraffic V43.23
      railway vehicle (traffic) V45.7
        nontraffic V45.2
      specified vehicle NEC (traffic) V46.7
        nontraffic V46.2
      sport utility vehicle (traffic) V43.71
        nontraffic V43.21
      stationary object (traffic) V47.7
        nontraffic V47.2
      streetcar (traffic) V46.7
        nontraffic V46.2
      three wheeled motor vehicle (traffic)
        V42.7
        nontraffic V42.2
      truck (traffic) V44.7
        nontraffic V44.2
      two wheeled motor vehicle (traffic) V42.7
        nontraffic V42.2
      van (traffic) V43.74
        nontraffic V43.24
    noncollision accident (traffic) V48.7
      nontraffic V48.2
  passenger
    collision (with)
      animal (traffic) V40.6
        being ridden (traffic) V46.6
          nontraffic V46.1
        nontraffic V40.1
      animal-drawn vehicle (traffic) V46.6
        nontraffic V46.1
      bus (traffic) V44.6
        nontraffic V44.1
      car (traffic) V43.62
        nontraffic V43.12
      motor vehicle NOS (traffic) V49.50
        nontraffic V49.10
        specified type NEC (traffic) V49.59
          nontraffic V49.19
      pedal cycle (traffic) V41.6
        nontraffic V41.1
      pickup truck (traffic) V43.63
        nontraffic V43.13
      railway vehicle (traffic) V45.6
        nontraffic V45.1
      specified vehicle NEC (traffic) V46.6
        nontraffic V46.1
      sport utility vehicle (traffic) V43.61
        nontraffic V43.11
      stationary object (traffic) V47.62

Accident - *continued*
      nontraffic V47.12
      streetcar (traffic) V46.6
        nontraffic V46.1
      three wheeled motor vehicle (traffic)
        V42.6
        nontraffic V42.1
      truck (traffic) V44.6
        nontraffic V44.1
      two wheeled motor vehicle (traffic) V42.6
        nontraffic V42.1
      van (traffic) V43.64
        nontraffic V43.14
    noncollision accident (traffic) V48.6
      nontraffic V48.1
    specified type NEC V49.88
      military vehicle V49.81
  coal car —*see* Accident, transport, industrial
  vehicle occupant
  construction vehicle occupant (nontraffic)
    V85.9
    driver V85.5
    hanger-on V85.7
    passenger V85.6
    traffic V85.3
      ·driver V85.0
      hanger-on V85.2
      passenger V85.1
    while boarding or alighting V85.4
  dirt bike rider —*see* Accident, transport, all-
  terrain vehicle occupant
  due to cataclysm —*see* Forces of nature, by
  type
    dune buggy occupant (nontraffic) V86.93
      driver V86.53
      hanger-on V86.73
      passenger V86.63
      traffic V86.33
        driver V86.03
        hanger-on V86.23
        passenger V86.13
      while boarding or alighting V86.43
  forklift —*see* Accident, transport, industrial
  vehicle occupant
  go cart —*see* Accident, transport, all-terrain
  vehicle occupant
  golf cart —*see* Accident, transport, all-terrain
  vehicle occupant
  heavy transport vehicle occupant —*see*
  Accident, transport, truck occupant
  ice yacht V98.2
  industrial vehicle occupant (nontraffic) V83.9
    driver V83.5
    hanger-on V83.7
    passenger V83.6
    traffic V83.3
      driver V83.0
      hanger-on V83.2
      passenger V83.1
    while boarding or alighting V83.4
  interurban electric car —*see* Accident,
  transport, streetcar
  land yacht V98.1
  logging car —*see* Accident, transport,
  industrial vehicle occupant
  military vehicle occupant (traffic) V86.34
    driver V86.04
    hanger-on V86.24
    nontraffic V86.94
      driver V86.54
      hanger-on V86.74
      passenger V86.64
    passenger V86.14

Accident - *continued*
    while boarding or alighting V86.44
  mine tram —*see* Accident, transport, industrial
  vehicle occupant
  motorcoach —*see* Accident, transport, bus
  occupant
  motorcyclist V29.9
    collision (with)
      animal (traffic) V20.9
        being ridden (traffic) V26.9
          nontraffic V26.2
          while boarding or alighting V26.3
        nontraffic V20.2
        while boarding or alighting V20.3
      animal-drawn vehicle (traffic) V26.9
        nontraffic V26.2
        while boarding or alighting V26.3
      bus (traffic) V24.9
        nontraffic V24.2
        while boarding or alighting V24.3
      car (traffic) V23.9
        nontraffic V23.2
        while boarding or alighting V23.3
      motor vehicle NOS (traffic) V29.60
        nontraffic V29.20
        specified type NEC (traffic) V29.69
          nontraffic V29.29
      pedal cycle (traffic) V21.9
        nontraffic V21.2
        while boarding or alighting V21.3
      pickup truck (traffic) V23.9
        nontraffic V23.2
        while boarding or alighting V23.3
      railway vehicle (traffic) V25.9
        nontraffic V25.2
        while boarding or alighting V25.3
      specified vehicle NEC (traffic) V26.9
        nontraffic V26.2
        while boarding or alighting V26.3
      stationary object (traffic) V27.9
        nontraffic V27.2
        while boarding or alighting V27.3
      streetcar (traffic) V26.9
        nontraffic V26.2
        while boarding or alighting V26.3
      three wheeled motor vehicle (traffic) V22.9
        nontraffic V22.2
        while boarding or alighting V22.3
      truck (traffic) V24.9
        nontraffic V24.2
        while boarding or alighting V24.3
      two wheeled motor vehicle (traffic) V22.9
        nontraffic V22.2
        while boarding or alighting V22.3
      van (traffic) V23.9
        nontraffic V23.2
        while boarding or alighting V23.3
    driver
      collision (with)
        animal (traffic) V20.4
          being ridden (traffic) V26.4
            nontraffic V26.0
          nontraffic V20.0
        animal-drawn vehicle (traffic) V26.4
          nontraffic V26.0
        bus (traffic) V24.4
          nontraffic V24.0
        car (traffic) V23.4
          nontraffic V23.0
        motor vehicle NOS (traffic) V29.40
          nontraffic V29.00
          specified type NEC (traffic) V29.49
            nontraffic V29.09

Accident - *continued*

heavy transport —*see* Accident, transport, truck occupant

motor (traffic) NEC V89.2

nontraffic NEC V89.0

watercraft NOS V94.9

causing drowning —*see* Drowning, resulting from accident to boat

parachutist V97.29

after accident to aircraft —*see* Accident, transport, aircraft

entangled in object V97.21

injured on landing V97.22

pedal cyclist V19.9

collision (with)

animal (traffic) V10.9

being ridden (traffic) V16.9

nontraffic V16.2

while boarding or alighting V16.3

nontraffic V10.2

while boarding or alighting V10.3

animal-drawn vehicle (traffic) V16.9

nontraffic V16.2

while boarding or alighting V16.3

bus (traffic) V14.9

nontraffic V14.2

while boarding or alighting V14.3

car (traffic) V13.9

nontraffic V13.2

while boarding or alighting V13.3

motor vehicle NOS (traffic) V19.60

nontraffic V19.20

specified type NEC (traffic) V19.69

nontraffic V19.29

pedal cycle (traffic) V11.9

nontraffic V11.2

while boarding or alighting V11.3

pickup truck (traffic) V13.9

nontraffic V13.2

while boarding or alighting V13.3

railway vehicle (traffic) V15.9

nontraffic V15.2

while boarding or alighting V15.3

specified vehicle NEC (traffic) V16.9

nontraffic V16.2

while boarding or alighting V16.3

stationary object (traffic) V17.9

nontraffic V17.2

while boarding or alighting V17.3

streetcar (traffic) V16.9

nontraffic V16.2

while boarding or alighting V16.3

three wheeled motor vehicle (traffic) V12.9

nontraffic V12.2

while boarding or alighting V12.3

truck (traffic) V14.9

nontraffic V14.2

while boarding or alighting V14.3

two wheeled motor vehicle (traffic) V12.9

nontraffic V12.2

while boarding or alighting V12.3

van (traffic) V13.9

nontraffic V13.2

while boarding or alighting V13.3

driver

collision (with)

animal (traffic) V10.4

being ridden (traffic) V16.4

nontraffic V16.0

nontraffic V10.0

animal-drawn vehicle (traffic) V16.4

nontraffic V16.0

bus (traffic) V14.4

Accident - *continued*

nontraffic V14.0

car (traffic) V13.4

nontraffic V13.0

motor vehicle NOS (traffic) V19.40

nontraffic V19.00

specified type NEC (traffic) V19.49

nontraffic V19.09

pedal cycle (traffic) V11.4

nontraffic V11.0

pickup truck (traffic) V13.4

nontraffic V13.0

railway vehicle (traffic) V15.4

nontraffic V15.0

specified vehicle NEC (traffic) V16.4

nontraffic V16.0

stationary object (traffic) V17.4

nontraffic V17.0

streetcar (traffic) V16.4

nontraffic V16.0

three wheeled motor vehicle (traffic) V12.4

nontraffic V12.0

truck (traffic) V14.4

nontraffic V14.0

two wheeled motor vehicle (traffic) V12.4

nontraffic V12.0

van (traffic) V13.4

nontraffic V13.0

noncollision accident (traffic) V18.4

nontraffic V18.0

noncollision accident (traffic) V18.9

nontraffic V18.2

while boarding or alighting V18.3

nontraffic V19.3

passenger

collision (with)

animal (traffic) V10.5

being ridden (traffic) V16.5

nontraffic V16.1

nontraffic V10.1

animal-drawn vehicle (traffic) V16.5

nontraffic V16.1

bus (traffic) V14.5

nontraffic V14.1

car (traffic) V13.5

nontraffic V13.1

motor vehicle NOS (traffic) V19.50

nontraffic V19.10

specified type NEC (traffic) V19.59

nontraffic V19.19

pedal cycle (traffic) V11.5

nontraffic V11.1

pickup truck (traffic) V13.5

nontraffic V13.1

railway vehicle (traffic) V15.5

nontraffic V15.1

specified vehicle NEC (traffic) V16.5

nontraffic V16.1

stationary object (traffic) V17.5

nontraffic V17.1

streetcar (traffic) V16.5

nontraffic V16.1

three wheeled motor vehicle (traffic) V12.5

nontraffic V12.1

truck (traffic) V14.5

nontraffic V14.1

two wheeled motor vehicle (traffic) V12.5

nontraffic V12.1

van (traffic) V13.5

nontraffic V13.1

noncollision accident (traffic) V18.5

Accident - *continued*

nontraffic V18.1

specified type NEC V19.88

military vehicle V19.81

pedestrian

conveyance (occupant) V09.9

babystroller V00.828

collision (with) V09.9

animal being ridden or animal drawn vehicle V06.99

nontraffic V06.09

traffic V06.19

bus or heavy transport V04.99

nontraffic V04.09

traffic V04.19

car V03.99

nontraffic V03.09

traffic V03.19

pedal cycle V01.99

nontraffic V01.09

traffic V01.19

pick-up truck or van V03.99

nontraffic V03.09

traffic V03.19

railway (train) (vehicle) V05.99

nontraffic V05.09

traffic V05.19

streetcar V06.99

nontraffic V06.09

traffic V06.19

stationary object V00.822

two or three-wheeled motor vehicle V02.99

nontraffic V02.09

traffic V02.19

vehicle V09.9

animal-drawn V06.99

nontraffic V06.09

traffic V06.19

motor

nontraffic V09.00

traffic V09.20

fall V00.821

nontraffic V09.1

involving motor vehicle NEC V09.00

traffic V09.3

involving motor vehicle NEC V09.20

flat-bottomed NEC V00.388

collision (with) V09.9

animal being ridden or animal drawn vehicle V06.99

nontraffic V06.09

traffic V06.19

bus or heavy transport V04.99

nontraffic V04.09

traffic V04.19

car V03.99

nontraffic V03.09

traffic V03.19

pedal cycle V01.99

nontraffic V01.09

traffic V01.19

pick-up truck or van V03.99

nontraffic V03.09

traffic V03.19

railway (train) (vehicle) V05.99

nontraffic V05.09

traffic V05.19

stationary object V00.382

streetcar V06.99

nontraffic V06.09

traffic V06.19

Accident - *continued*
   two or three-wheeled motor vehicle
     V02.99
      nontraffic V02.09
      traffic V02.19
   vehicle V09.9
     animal-drawn V06.99
      nontraffic V06.09
      traffic V06.19
     motor
      nontraffic V09.00
      traffic V09.20
  fall V00.381
  nontraffic V09.1
   involving motor vehicle NEC V09.00
  snow
   board —*see* Accident, transport,
    pedestrian, conveyance, snow board
   ski —*see* Accident, transport,
    pedestrian, conveyance, skis (snow)
  traffic V09.3
   involving motor vehicle NEC V09.20
 gliding type NEC V00.288
  collision (with) V09.9
   animal being ridden or animal drawn
    vehicle V06.99
     nontraffic V06.09
     traffic V06.19
   bus or heavy transport V04.99
    nontraffic V04.09
    traffic V04.19
   car V03.99
    nontraffic V03.09
    traffic V03.19
   pedal cycle V01.99
    nontraffic V01.09
    traffic V01.19
   pick-up truck or van V03.99
    nontraffic V03.09
    traffic V03.19
   railway (train) (vehicle) V05.99
    nontraffic V05.09
    traffic V05.19
   stationary object V00.282
   streetcar V06.99
    nontraffic V06.09
    traffic V06.19
   two or three-wheeled motor vehicle
    V02.99
     nontraffic V02.09
     traffic V02.19
   vehicle V09.9
    animal-drawn V06.99
     nontraffic V06.09
     traffic V06.19
    motor
     nontraffic V09.00
     traffic V09.20
  fall V00.281
  heelies —*see* Accident, transport,
   pedestrian, conveyance, heelies
  ice skate —*see* Accident, transport,
   pedestrian, conveyance, ice skate
  nontraffic V09.1
   involving motor vehicle NEC V09.00
  sled —*see* Accident, transport, pedestrian,
   conveyance, sled
  traffic V09.3
   involving motor vehicle NEC V09.20
  wheelies —*see* Accident, transport,
   pedestrian, conveyance, heelies
 heelies V00.158
  colliding with stationary object V00.152

Accident - *continued*
  fall V00.151
 ice skates V00.218
  collision (with) V09.9
   animal being ridden or animal drawn
    vehicle V06.99
     nontraffic V06.09
     traffic V06.19
   bus or heavy transport V04.99
    nontraffic V04.09
    traffic V04.19
   car V03.99
    nontraffic V03.09
    traffic V03.19
   pedal cycle V01.99
    nontraffic V01.09
    traffic V01.19
   pick-up truck or van V03.99
    nontraffic V03.09
    traffic V03.19
   railway (train) (vehicle) V05.99
    nontraffic V05.09
    traffic V05.19
   streetcar V06.99
    nontraffic V06.09
    traffic V06.19
   stationary object V00.212
   two or three-wheeled motor vehicle
    V02.99
     nontraffic V02.09
     traffic V02.19
   vehicle V09.9
    animal-drawn V06.99
     nontraffic V06.09
     traffic V06.19
    motor
     nontraffic V09.00
     traffic V09.20
  fall V00.211
  nontraffic V09.1
   involving motor vehicle NEC V09.00
  traffic V09.3
   involving motor vehicle NEC V09.20
 motorized mobility scooter V00.838
  collision with stationary object V00.832
  fall from V00.831
  nontraffic V09.1
   involving motor vehicle V09.00
    military V09.01
    specified type NEC V09.09
 roller skates (non in-line) V00.128
  collision (with) V09.9
   animal being ridden or animal drawn
    vehicle V06.91
     nontraffic V06.01
     traffic V06.11
   bus or heavy transport V04.91
    nontraffic V04.01
    traffic V04.11
   car V03.91
    nontraffic V03.01
    traffic V03.11
   pedal cycle V01.91
    nontraffic V01.01
    traffic V01.11
   pick-up truck or van V03.91
    nontraffic V03.01
    traffic V03.11
   railway (train) (vehicle) V05.91
    nontraffic V05.01
    traffic V05.11
   streetcar V06.91
    nontraffic V06.01

Accident - *continued*
    traffic V06.11
   stationary object V00.122
   two or three-wheeled motor vehicle
    V02.91
     nontraffic V02.01
     traffic V02.11
   vehicle V09.9
    animal-drawn V06.91
     nontraffic V06.01
     traffic V06.11
    motor
     nontraffic V09.00
     traffic V09.20
  fall V00.121
  in-line V00.118
   collision —*see also* Accident, transport,
    pedestrian, conveyance occupant, roller
    skates, collision
    with stationary object V00.112
   fall V00.111
   nontraffic V09.1
    involving motor vehicle NEC V09.00
   traffic V09.3
    involving motor vehicle NEC V09.20
 rolling shoes V00.158
  colliding with stationary object V00.152
  fall V00.151
 rolling type NEC V00.188
  collision (with) V09.9
   animal being ridden or animal drawn
    vehicle V06.99
     nontraffic V06.09
     traffic V06.19
   bus or heavy transport V04.99
    nontraffic V04.09
    traffic V04.19
   car V03.99
    nontraffic V03.09
    traffic V03.19
   pedal cycle V01.99
    nontraffic V01.09
    traffic V01.19
   pick-up truck or van V03.99
    nontraffic V03.09
    traffic V03.19
   railway (train) (vehicle) V05.99
    nontraffic V05.09
    traffic V05.19
   stationary object V00.182
   streetcar V06.99
    nontraffic V06.09
    traffic V06.19
   two or three-wheeled motor vehicle
    V02.99
     nontraffic V02.09
     traffic V02.19
   vehicle V09.9
    animal-drawn V06.99
     nontraffic V06.09
     traffic V06.19
    motor
     nontraffic V09.00
     traffic V09.20
  fall V00.181
  in-line roller skate —*see* Accident,
   transport, pedestrian, conveyance, roller
   skate, in-line
  nontraffic V09.1
   involving motor vehicle NEC V09.00
  roller skate —*see* Accident, transport,
   pedestrian, conveyance, roller skate

Accident - *continued*
  nontraffic V54.0
  car (traffic) V53.5
   nontraffic V53.0
  motor vehicle NOS (traffic) V59.40
   nontraffic V59.00
   specified type NEC (traffic) V59.49
    nontraffic V59.09
  pedal cycle (traffic) V51.5
   nontraffic V51.0
  pickup truck (traffic) V53.5
   nontraffic V53.0
  railway vehicle (traffic) V55.5
   nontraffic V55.0
  specified vehicle NEC (traffic) V56.5
   nontraffic V56.0
  stationary object (traffic) V57.5
   nontraffic V57.0
  streetcar (traffic) V56.5
   nontraffic V56.0
  three wheeled motor vehicle (traffic)
   V52.5
   nontraffic V52.0
  truck (traffic) V54.5
   nontraffic V54.0
  two wheeled motor vehicle (traffic) V52.5
   nontraffic V52.0
  van (traffic) V53.5
   nontraffic V53.0
 noncollision accident (traffic) V58.5
  nontraffic V58.0
 noncollision accident (traffic) V58.9
  nontraffic V58.3
  while boarding or alighting V58.4
 nontraffic V59.3
 hanger-on
  collision (with)
   animal (traffic) V50.7
    being ridden (traffic) V56.7
     nontraffic V56.2
    nontraffic V50.2
   animal-drawn vehicle (traffic) V56.7
    nontraffic V56.2
   bus (traffic) V54.7
    nontraffic V54.2
   car (traffic) V53.7
    nontraffic V53.2
   pedal cycle (traffic) V51.7
    nontraffic V51.2
   pickup truck (traffic) V53.7
    nontraffic V53.2
   railway vehicle (traffic) V55.7
    nontraffic V55.2
   specified vehicle NEC (traffic) V56.7
    nontraffic V56.2
   stationary object (traffic) V57.7
    nontraffic V57.2
   streetcar (traffic) V56.7
    nontraffic V56.2
   three wheeled motor vehicle (traffic)
    V52.7
    nontraffic V52.2
   truck (traffic) V54.7
    nontraffic V54.2
   two wheeled motor vehicle (traffic) V52.7
    nontraffic V52.2
   van (traffic) V53.7
    nontraffic V53.2
   noncollision accident (traffic) V58.7
    nontraffic V58.2
 passenger
  collision (with)
   animal (traffic) V50.6

Accident - *continued*
   being ridden (traffic) V56.6
    nontraffic V56.1
    nontraffic V50.1
   animal-drawn vehicle (traffic) V56.6
    nontraffic V56.1
   bus (traffic) V54.6
    nontraffic V54.1
   car (traffic) V53.6
    nontraffic V53.1
   motor vehicle NOS (traffic) V59.50
    nontraffic V59.10
    specified type NEC (traffic) V59.59
     nontraffic V59.19
   pedal cycle (traffic) V51.6
    nontraffic V51.1
   pickup truck (traffic) V53.6
    nontraffic V53.1
   railway vehicle (traffic) V55.6
    nontraffic V55.1
   specified vehicle NEC (traffic) V56.6
    nontraffic V56.1
   stationary object (traffic) V57.6
    nontraffic V57.1
   streetcar (traffic) V56.6
    nontraffic V56.1
   three wheeled motor vehicle (traffic)
    V52.6
    nontraffic V52.1
   truck (traffic) V54.6
    nontraffic V54.1
   two wheeled motor vehicle (traffic) V52.6
    nontraffic V52.1
   van (traffic) V53.6
    nontraffic V53.1
  noncollision accident (traffic) V58.6
   nontraffic V58.1
  specified type NEC V59.88
  military vehicle V59.81
 quarry truck —*see* Accident, transport,
 industrial vehicle occupant
 race car —*see* Accident, transport, motor
 vehicle NEC occupant
 railway vehicle occupant V81.9
  collision (with) V81.3
   motor vehicle (non-military) (traffic) V81.1
   military V81.83
   nontraffic V81.0
   rolling stock V81.2
   specified object NEC V81.3
   during derailment V81.7
   with antecedent collision —*see* Accident,
 transport, railway vehicle occupant, collision
   explosion V81.81
   fall (in railway vehicle) V81.5
    during derailment V81.7
    with antecedent collision —*see* Accident,
 transport, railway vehicle occupant, collision
    from railway vehicle V81.6
    during derailment V81.7
     with antecedent collision —*see*
 Accident, transport, railway vehicle occupant,
 collision
   while boarding or alighting V81.4
   fire V81.81
   object falling onto train V81.82
   specified type NEC V81.89
   while boarding or alighting V81.4
 ski lift V98.3
 snowmobile occupant (nontraffic) V86.92
  driver V86.52
  hanger-on V86.72
  passenger V86.62

Accident - *continued*
  traffic V86.32
  driver V86.02
  hanger-on V86.22
  passenger V86.12
  while boarding or alighting V86.42
  specified NEC V98.8
 sport utility vehicle occupant —*see also*
 Accident, transport, car occupant
  collision (with)
   stationary object (traffic) V47.91
    nontraffic V47.31
  driver
   collision (with)
    stationary object (traffic) V47.51
     nontraffic V47.01
  passenger
   collision (with)
    stationary object (traffic) V47.61
     nontraffic V47.11
 streetcar occupant V82.9
  collision (with) V82.3
   motor vehicle (traffic) V82.1
   nontraffic V82.0
   rolling stock V82.2
  during derailment V82.7
   with antecedent collision —*see* Accident,
   transport, streetcar occupant, collision
  fall (in streetcar) V82.5
   during derailment V82.7
   with antecedent collision —*see* Accident,
 transport, streetcar occupant, collision
   from streetcar V82.6
   during derailment V82.7
    with antecedent collision —*see*
 Accident, transport, streetcar occupant, collision
   while boarding or alighting V82.4
  while boarding or alighting V82.4
  specified type NEC V82.8
  while boarding or alighting V82.4
 three-wheeled motor vehicle occupant V39.9
  collision (with)
   animal (traffic) V30.9
    being ridden (traffic) V36.9
     nontraffic V36.3
     while boarding or alighting V36.4
    nontraffic V30.3
    while boarding or alighting V30.4
   animal-drawn vehicle (traffic) V36.9
    nontraffic V36.3
    while boarding or alighting V36.4
   bus (traffic) V34.9
    nontraffic V34.3
    while boarding or alighting V34.4
   car (traffic) V33.9
    nontraffic V33.3
    while boarding or alighting V33.4
   motor vehicle NOS (traffic) V39.60
    nontraffic V39.20
    specified type NEC (traffic) V39.69
     nontraffic V39.29
   pedal cycle (traffic) V31.9
    nontraffic V31.3
    while boarding or alighting V31.4
   pickup truck (traffic) V33.9
    nontraffic V33.3
    while boarding or alighting V33.4
   railway vehicle (traffic) V35.9
    nontraffic V35.3
    while boarding or alighting V35.4
   specified vehicle NEC (traffic) V36.9
    nontraffic V36.3
    while boarding or alighting V36.4

Accident - *continued*
  stationary object (traffic) V37.9
    nontraffic V37.3
    while boarding or alighting V37.4
  streetcar (traffic) V36.9
    nontraffic V36.3
    while boarding or alighting V36.4
  three wheeled motor vehicle (traffic) V32.9
    nontraffic V32.3
    while boarding or alighting V32.4
  truck (traffic) V34.9
    nontraffic V34.3
    while boarding or alighting V34.4
  two wheeled motor vehicle (traffic) V32.9
    nontraffic V32.3
    while boarding or alighting V32.4
  van (traffic) V33.9
    nontraffic V33.3
    while boarding or alighting V33.4
driver
  collision (with)
    animal (traffic) V30.5
      being ridden (traffic) V36.5
        nontraffic V36.0
      nontraffic V30.0
    animal-drawn vehicle (traffic) V36.5
      nontraffic V36.0
    bus (traffic) V34.5
      nontraffic V34.0
    car (traffic) V33.5
      nontraffic V33.0
    motor vehicle NOS (traffic) V39.40
      nontraffic V39.00
      specified type NEC (traffic) V39.49
        nontraffic V39.09
    pedal cycle (traffic) V31.5
      nontraffic V31.0
    pickup truck (traffic) V33.5
      nontraffic V33.0
    railway vehicle (traffic) V35.5
      nontraffic V35.0
    specified vehicle NEC (traffic) V36.5
      nontraffic V36.0
    stationary object (traffic) V37.5
      nontraffic V37.0
    streetcar (traffic) V36.5
      nontraffic V36.0
    three wheeled motor vehicle (traffic) V32.5
      nontraffic V32.0
    truck (traffic) V34.5
      nontraffic V34.0
    two wheeled motor vehicle (traffic) V32.5
      nontraffic V32.0
    van (traffic) V33.5
      nontraffic V33.0
  noncollision accident (traffic) V38.5
    nontraffic V38.0
  noncollision accident (traffic) V38.9
    nontraffic V38.3
    while boarding or alighting V38.4
  nontraffic V39.3
hanger-on
  collision (with)
    animal (traffic) V30.7
      being ridden (traffic) V36.7
        nontraffic V36.2
      nontraffic V30.2
    animal-drawn vehicle (traffic) V36.7
      nontraffic V36.2
    bus (traffic) V34.7
      nontraffic V34.2
    car (traffic) V33.7

Accident - *continued*
    nontraffic V33.2
  pedal cycle (traffic) V31.7
    nontraffic V31.2
  pickup truck (traffic) V33.7
    nontraffic V33.2
  railway vehicle (traffic) V35.7
    nontraffic V35.2
  specified vehicle NEC (traffic) V36.7
    nontraffic V36.2
  stationary object (traffic) V37.7
    nontraffic V37.2
  streetcar (traffic) V36.7
    nontraffic V36.2
  three wheeled motor vehicle (traffic)
    V32.7
    nontraffic V32.2
  truck (traffic) V34.7
    nontraffic V34.2
  two wheeled motor vehicle (traffic) V32.7
    nontraffic V32.2
  van (traffic) V33.7
    nontraffic V33.2
  noncollision accident (traffic) V38.7
    nontraffic V38.2
passenger
  collision (with)
    animal (traffic) V30.6
      being ridden (traffic) V36.6
        nontraffic V36.1
      nontraffic V30.1
    animal-drawn vehicle (traffic) V36.6
      nontraffic V36.1
    bus (traffic) V34.6
      nontraffic V34.1
    car (traffic) V33.6
      nontraffic V33.1
    motor vehicle NOS (traffic) V39.50
      nontraffic V39.10
      specified type NEC (traffic) V39.59
        nontraffic V39.19
    pedal cycle (traffic) V31.6
      nontraffic V31.1
    pickup truck (traffic) V33.6
      nontraffic V33.1
    railway vehicle (traffic) V35.6
      nontraffic V35.1
    specified vehicle NEC (traffic) V36.6
      nontraffic V36.1
    stationary object (traffic) V37.6
      nontraffic V37.1
    streetcar (traffic) V36.6
      nontraffic V36.1
    three wheeled motor vehicle (traffic)
      V32.6
      nontraffic V32.1
    truck (traffic) V34.6
      nontraffic V34.1
    two wheeled motor vehicle (traffic) V32.6
      nontraffic V32.1
    van (traffic) V33.6
      nontraffic V33.1
  noncollision accident (traffic) V38.6
    nontraffic V38.1
  specified type NEC V39.89
    military vehicle V39.81
  tractor (farm) (and trailer) —*see* Accident,
    transport, agricultural vehicle occupant
  tram —*see* Accident, transport, streetcar
    in mine or quarry —*see* Accident, transport,
  industrial vehicle occupant
    trolley —*see* Accident, transport, streetcar

Accident - *continued*
  in mine or quarry —*see* Accident, transport,
  industrial vehicle occupant
truck (heavy) occupant V69.9
  collision (with)
    animal (traffic) V60.9
      being ridden (traffic) V66.9
        nontraffic V66.3
        while boarding or alighting V66.4
      nontraffic V60.3
      while boarding or alighting V60.4
    animal-drawn vehicle (traffic) V66.9
      nontraffic V66.3
      while boarding or alighting V66.4
    bus (traffic) V64.9
      nontraffic V64.3
      while boarding or alighting V64.4
    car (traffic) V63.9
      nontraffic V63.3
      while boarding or alighting V63.4
    motor vehicle NOS (traffic) V69.60
      nontraffic V69.20
      specified type NEC (traffic) V69.69
        nontraffic V69.29
    pedal cycle (traffic) V61.9
      nontraffic V61.3
      while boarding or alighting V61.4
    pickup truck (traffic) V63.9
      nontraffic V63.3
      while boarding or alighting V63.4
    railway vehicle (traffic) V65.9
      nontraffic V65.3
      while boarding or alighting V65.4
    specified vehicle NEC (traffic) V66.9
      nontraffic V66.3
      while boarding or alighting V66.4
    stationary object (traffic) V67.9
      nontraffic V67.3
      while boarding or alighting V67.4
    streetcar (traffic) V66.9
      nontraffic V66.3
      while boarding or alighting V66.4
    three wheeled motor vehicle (traffic) V62.9
      nontraffic V62.3
      while boarding or alighting V62.4
    truck (traffic) V64.9
      nontraffic V64.3
      while boarding or alighting V64.4
    two wheeled motor vehicle (traffic) V62.9
      nontraffic V62.3
      while boarding or alighting V62.4
    van (traffic) V63.9
      nontraffic V63.3
      while boarding or alighting V63.4
  driver
    collision (with)
      animal (traffic) V60.5
        being ridden (traffic) V66.5
          nontraffic V66.0
        nontraffic V60.0
      animal-drawn vehicle (traffic) V66.5
        nontraffic V66.0
      bus (traffic) V64.5
        nontraffic V64.0
      car (traffic) V63.5
        nontraffic V63.0
      motor vehicle NOS (traffic) V69.40
        nontraffic V69.00
        specified type NEC (traffic) V69.49
          nontraffic V69.09
      pedal cycle (traffic) V61.5
        nontraffic V61.0
      pickup truck (traffic) V63.5

Activity - *continued*
vacuuming Y93.E3
volleyball (beach) (court) Y93.68
wake boarding Y93.17
walking an animal Y93.K1
walking (on level or elevated terrain) Y93.01
an animal Y93.K1
wall climbing Y93.31
warm up and cool down exercises Y93.A2
water NEC Y93.19
aerobics Y93.14
craft NEC Y93.19
exercise Y93.14
polo Y93.13
skiing Y93.17
sliding Y93.18
survival training and testing Y93.19
weeding (garden and lawn) Y93.H2
wind instrument playing Y93.J4
windsurfing Y93.18
wrestling Y93.72
yoga Y93.42
Adverse effect of drugs —*see* Table of Drugs and Chemicals
Aerosinusitis
—*see* Air, pressure
After-effect, late —*see* Sequelae
Air
blast in war operations —*see* War operations, air blast
pressure
change, rapid
during
ascent W94.29
while (in) (surfacing from)
aircraft W94.23
deep water diving W94.21
underground W94.22
descent W94.39
in
aircraft W94.31
water W94.32
high, prolonged W94.0
low, prolonged W94.12
due to residence or long visit at high altitude W94.11
Alpine sickness W94.11
Altitude sickness W94.11
Anaphylactic shock, anaphylaxis —*see* Table of drugs and chemicals
Andes disease W94.11
Arachnidism, arachnoidism X58
Arson (with intent to injure or kill) X97
Asphyxia, asphyxiation
by
food (bone) (seed) (*see* categories T17 and) T18
gas —*see also* Table of drugs and chemicals
legal
execution —*see* Legal, intervention, gas
intervention —*see* Legal, intervention, gas
from
fire —*see also* Exposure, fire
in war operations —*see* War operations, fire
ignition —*see* Ignition
vomitus T17.81
in war operations —*see* War operations, restriction of airway
Aspiration
food (any type) (into respiratory tract) (with asphyxia, obstruction respiratory tract, suffocation) (*see* categories T17 and) T18
foreign body —*see* Foreign body, aspiration

Aspiration - *continued*
vomitus (with asphyxia, obstruction respiratory tract, suffocation) T17.81
Assassination (attempt) —*see* Assault
Assault (homicidal) (by) (in) Y09
arson X97
bite (of human being) Y04.1
bodily force Y04.8
bite Y04.1
bumping into Y04.2
sexual (*see* subcategories T74.0,) T76.0
unarmed fight Y04.0
bomb X96.9
antipersonnel X96.0
fertilizer X96.3
gasoline X96.1
letter X96.2
petrol X96.1
pipe X96.3
specified NEC X96.8
brawl (hand) (fists) (foot) (unarmed) Y04.0
burning, burns (by fire) NEC X97
acid Y08.89
caustic, corrosive substance Y08.89
chemical from swallowing caustic, corrosive substance —*see* Table of drugs and chemicals
cigarette (s) X97
hot object X98.9
fluid NEC X98.2
household appliance X98.3
specified NEC X98.8
steam X98.0
tap water X98.1
vapors X98.0
scalding —*see* Assault, burning
steam X98.0
vitriol Y08.89
caustic, corrosive substance (gas) Y08.89
crashing of
aircraft Y08.81
motor vehicle Y03.8
pushed in front of Y02.0
run over Y03.0
specified NEC Y03.8
cutting or piercing instrument X99.9
dagger X99.2
glass X99.0
knife X99.1
specified NEC X99.8
sword X99.2
dagger X99.2
drowning (in) X92.9
bathtub X92.0
natural water X92.3
specified NEC X92.8
swimming pool X92.1
following fall X92.2
dynamite X96.8
explosive (s) (material) X96.9
fight (hand) (fists) (foot) (unarmed) Y04.0
with weapon —*see* Assault, by type of weapon
fire X97
firearm X95.9
airgun X95.01
handgun X93
hunting rifle X94.1
larger X94.9
specified NEC X94.8
machine gun X94.2
shotgun X94.0
specified NEC X95.8
gunshot (wound) NEC —*see* Assault, firearm, by type

Assault - *continued*
incendiary device X97
injury Y09
to child due to criminal abortion attempt NEC Y08.89
knife X99.1
late effect of —*see* X92
Y08 with 7th character S
placing before moving object NEC Y02.8
motor vehicle Y02.0
poisoning —*see* categories T36
T65 with 7th character S
puncture, any part of body —*see* Assault, cutting or piercing instrument
pushing
before moving object NEC Y02.8
motor vehicle Y02.0
subway train Y02.1
train Y02.1
from high place Y01
rape T74.2
scalding —*see* Assault, burning
sequelae of —*see* X92
Y08 with 7th character S
sexual (by bodily force) T74.2
shooting —*see* Assault, firearm
specified means NEC Y08.89
stab, any part of body —*see* Assault, cutting or piercing instrument
steam X98.0
striking against
other person Y04.2
sports equipment Y08.09
baseball bat Y08.02
hockey stick Y08.01
struck by
sports equipment Y08.09
baseball bat Y08.02
hockey stick Y08.01
submersion —*see* Assault, drowning
violence Y09
weapon Y09
blunt Y00
cutting or piercing —*see* Assault, cutting or piercing instrument
firearm —*see* Assault, firearm
wound Y09
cutting —*see* Assault, cutting or piercing instrument
gunshot —*see* Assault, firearm
knife X99.1
piercing —*see* Assault, cutting or piercing instrument
puncture —*see* Assault, cutting or piercing instrument
stab —*see* Assault, cutting or piercing instrument
Attack by mammals NEC W55.89
Avalanche —*see* Landslide
Aviator's disease —*see* Air, pressure

B

Barotitis, barodontalgia, barosinusitis, barotrauma (otitic) (sinus) —*see* Air, pressure
Battered (baby) (child) (person) (syndrome) X58
Bayonet wound W26.1
in
legal intervention —*see* Legal, intervention, sharp object, bayonet
war operations —*see* War operations, combat

Bayonet wound - *continued*
stated as undetermined whether accidental or intentional Y28.8
suicide (attempt) X78.2
Bean in nose (*see* categories T17 and) T18
Bed set on fire NEC —*see* Exposure, fire, uncontrolled, building, bed
Beheading (by guillotine)
homicide X99.9
legal execution —*see* Legal, intervention
Bending, injury in —*see* category Y93
Bends —*see* Air, pressure, change
Bite, bitten by
alligator W58.01
arthropod (nonvenomous) NEC W57
bull W55.21
cat W55.01
cow W55.21
crocodile W58.11
dog W54.0
goat W55.31
hoof stock NEC W55.31
horse W55.11
human being (accidentally) W50.3
with intent to injure or kill Y04.1
as, or caused by, a crowd or human stampede (with fall) W52
assault Y04.1
homicide (attempt) Y04.1
in
fight Y04.1
insect (nonvenomous) W57
lizard (nonvenomous) W59.01
mammal NEC W55.81
marine W56.31
marine animal (nonvenomous) W56.81
millipede W57
moray eel W56.51
mouse W53.01
person (s) (accidentally) W50.3
with intent to injure or kill Y04.1
as, or caused by, a crowd or human stampede (with fall) W52
assault Y04.1
homicide (attempt) Y04.1
in
fight Y04.1
pig W55.41
raccoon W55.51
rat W53.11
reptile W59.81
lizard W59.01
snake W59.11
turtle W59.21
terrestrial W59.81
rodent W53.81
mouse W53.01
rat W53.11
specified NEC W53.81
squirrel W53.21
shark W56.41
sheep W55.31
snake (nonvenomous) W59.11
spider (nonvenomous) W57
squirrel W53.21
Blast (air) in war operations —*see* War operations, blast
Blizzard X37.2
Blood alcohol level Y90.9
less than 20mg/100ml Y90.0
presence in blood, level not specified Y90.9
20 39mg/100ml Y90.1
40 59mg/100ml Y90.2

Bite, bitten by - *continued*
60 79mg/100ml Y90.3
80 99mg/100ml Y90.4
100 119mg/100ml Y90.5
120 199mg/100ml Y90.6
200 239mg/100ml Y90.7
Blow X58
by law-enforcing agent, police (on duty) —*see* Legal, intervention, manhandling
blunt object —*see* Legal, intervention, blunt object
Blowing up —*see* Explosion
Brawl (hand) (fists) (foot) Y04.0
Breakage (accidental) (part of) ladder (causing fall) W11
scaffolding (causing fall) W12
Broken
glass, contact with —*see* Contact, with, glass
power line (causing electric shock) W85
Bumping against, into (accidentally)
object NEC W22.8
with fall —*see* Fall, due to, bumping against, object
caused by crowd or human stampede (with fall) W52
sports equipment W21.9
person (s) W51
with fall W03
due to ice or snow W00.0
assault Y04.2
caused by, a crowd or human stampede (with fall) W52
homicide (attempt) Y04.2
sports equipment W21.9
Burn, burned, burning (accidental) (by) (from) (on)
acid NEC —*see* Table of drugs and chemicals
bed linen —*see* Exposure, fire, uncontrolled, in building, bed
blowtorch X08.8
with ignition of clothing NEC X06.2
nightwear X05
bonfire, campfire (controlled) —*see also* Exposure, fire, controlled, not in building
uncontrolled —*see* Exposure, fire, uncontrolled, not in building
candle X08.8
with ignition of clothing NEC X06.2
nightwear X05
caustic liquid, substance (external) (internal) NEC —*see* Table of drugs and chemicals
chemical (external) (internal) —*see also* Table of drugs and chemicals
in war operations —*see* War operations. fire
cigar (s) or cigarette (s) X08.8
with ignition of clothing NEC X06.2
nightwear X05
clothes, clothing NEC (from controlled fire) X06.2
with conflagration —*see* Exposure, fire, uncontrolled, building
not in building or structure —*see* Exposure, fire, uncontrolled, not in building
cooker (hot) X15.8
stated as undetermined whether accidental or intentional Y27.3
suicide (attempt) X77.3
electric blanket X16
engine (hot) X17
fire, flames —*see* Exposure, fire
flare, Very pistol —*see* Discharge, firearm NEC
heat
from appliance (electrical) (household) X15.8

Burn, burned, burning (accidental) - *continued*
cooker X15.8
hotplate X15.2
kettle X15.8
light bulb X15.8
saucepan X15.3
skillet X15.3
stove X15.0
stated as undetermined whether accidental or intentional Y27.3
suicide (attempt) X77.3
toaster X15.1
in local application or packing during medical or surgical procedure Y63.5
heating
appliance, radiator or pipe X16
homicide (attempt) —*see* Assault, burning
hot
air X14.1
cooker X15.8
drink X10.0
engine X17
fat X10.2
fluid NEC X12
food X10.1
gases X14.1
heating appliance X16
household appliance NEC X15.8
kettle X15.8
liquid NEC X12
machinery X17
metal (molten) (liquid) NEC X18
object (not producing fire or flames) NEC X19
oil (cooking) X10.2
pipe (s) X16
radiator X16
saucepan (glass) (metal) X15.3
stove (kitchen) X15.0
substance NEC X19
caustic or corrosive NEC —*see* Table of drugs and chemicals
toaster X15.1
tool X17
vapor X13.1
water (tap) —*see* Contact, with, hot, tap water
hotplate X15.2
suicide (attempt) X77.3
ignition —*see* Ignition
in war operations —*see* War operations, fire inflicted by other person X97
by hot objects, hot vapor, and steam —*see* Assault, burning, hot object
internal, from swallowed caustic, corrosive liquid, substance —*see* Table of drugs and chemicals
iron (hot) X15.8
stated as undetermined whether accidental or intentional Y27.3
suicide (attempt) X77.3
kettle (hot) X15.8
stated as undetermined whether accidental or intentional Y27.3
suicide (attempt) X77.3
lamp (flame) X08.8
with ignition of clothing NEC X06.2
nightwear X05
lighter (cigar) (cigarette) X08.8
with ignition of clothing NEC X06.2
nightwear X05
lightning —*see* subcategory T75.0
causing fire —*see* Exposure, fire
liquid (boiling) (hot) NEC X12

Burn, burned, burning (accidental) - *continued*
  stated as undetermined whether accidental or intentional Y27.2
    suicide (attempt) X77.2
  local application of externally applied substance in medical or surgical care Y63.5
  on board watercraft
    due to
      accident to watercraft V91.09
        powered craft V91.03
          ferry boat V91.01
          fishing boat V91.02
          jet skis V91.03
          liner V91.01
          merchant ship V91.00
          passenger ship V91.01
        unpowered craft V91.08
          canoe V91.05
          inflatable V91.06
          kayak V91.05
          sailboat V91.04
          surf-board V91.08
          water skis V91.07
          windsurfer V91.08
      fire on board V93.09
        ferry boat V93.01
        fishing boat V93.02
        jet skis V93.03
        liner V93.01
        merchant ship V93.00
        passenger ship V93.01
        powered craft NEC V93.03
        sailboat V93.04
      specified heat source NEC on board V93.19
        ferry boat V93.11
        fishing boat V93.12
        jet skis V93.13
        liner V93.11
        merchant ship V93.10
        passenger ship V93.11
        powered craft NEC V93.13
        sailboat V93.14
  machinery (hot) X17
  matches X08.8
    with ignition of clothing NEC X06.2
      nightwear X05
  mattress —*see* Exposure, fire, uncontrolled, building, bed
  medicament, externally applied Y63.5
  metal (hot) (liquid) (molten) NEC X18
  nightwear (nightclothes, nightdress, gown, pajamas, robe) X05
  object (hot) NEC X19
  pipe (hot) X16
    smoking X08.8
      with ignition of clothing NEC X06.2
        nightwear X05
  powder —*see* Powder burn
  radiator (hot) X16
  saucepan (hot) (glass) (metal) X15.3
    stated as undetermined whether accidental or intentional Y27.3
      suicide (attempt) X77.3
      self-inflicted X76
    stated as undetermined whether accidental or intentional Y26
  steam X13.1
    pipe X16
      stated as undetermined whether accidental or intentional Y27.8
    stated as undetermined whether accidental or intentional Y27.0
      suicide (attempt) X77.0

Burn, burned, burning (accidental) - *continued*
  stove (hot) (kitchen) X15.0
    stated as undetermined whether accidental or intentional Y27.3
      suicide (attempt) X77.3
  substance (hot) NEC X19
    boiling X12
      stated as undetermined whether accidental or intentional Y27.2
        suicide (attempt) X77.2
    molten (metal) X18
  suicide (attempt) NEC X76
  hot
    household appliance X77.3
    object X77.9
  stated as undetermined whether accidental or intentional Y27.0
  therapeutic misadventure
    heat in local application or packing during medical or surgical procedure Y63.5
    overdose of radiation Y63.2
  toaster (hot) X15.1
    stated as undetermined whether accidental or intentional Y27.3
      suicide (attempt) X77.3
  tool (hot) X17
  torch, welding X08.8
    with ignition of clothing NEC X06.2
      nightwear X05
  trash fire (controlled) —*see* Exposure, fire, controlled, not in building
    uncontrolled —*see* Exposure, fire, uncontrolled, not in building
  vapor (hot) X13.1
    stated as undetermined whether accidental or intentional Y27.0
      suicide (attempt) X77.0
  Very pistol —*see* Discharge, firearm NEC
Butted by animal W55.82
  bull W55.22
  cow W55.22
  goat W55.32
  horse W55.12
  pig W55.42
  sheep W55.32

C

Caisson disease
  —*see* Air, pressure, change
Campfire (exposure to) (controlled) —*see also* Exposure, fire, controlled, not in building
  uncontrolled —*see* Exposure, fire, uncontrolled, not in building
Capital punishment (any means) —*see* Legal, intervention
Car sickness T75.3
Casualty (not due to war) NEC X58
  war —*see* War operations
Cat
  bite W55.01
  scratch W55.03
Cataclysm, cataclysmic (any injury) NEC —*see* Forces of nature
Catching fire —*see* Exposure, fire
Caught
  between
    folding object W23.0
    objects (moving) (stationary and moving) W23.0
      and machinery —*see* Contact, with, by type of machine
        stationary W23.1
    sliding door and door frame W23.0

Caught - *continued*
  by, in
    machinery (moving parts of) —*see* Contact, with, by type of machine
      washing-machine wringer W23.0
    under packing crate (due to losing grip) W23.1
Cave-in caused by cataclysmic earth surface movement or eruption —*see* Landslide
Change (s) in air pressure —*see* Air, pressure, change
Choked, choking (on) (any object except food or vomitus)
  food (bone) (seed) (*see* categories T17 and) T18
Choked - *continued*
  vomitus T17.81
Civil insurrection —*see* War operations
Cloudburst (any injury) X37.8
Cold, exposure to (accidental) (excessive) (extreme) (natural) (place) NEC —*see* Exposure, cold
Collapse
  building W20.1
    burning (uncontrolled fire) X00.2
  dam or man-made structure (causing earth movement) X36.0
  machinery —*see* Contact, with, by type of machine
  structure W20.1
    burning (uncontrolled fire) X00.2
Collision (accidental) NEC (*see also* Accident, transport) V89.9
  pedestrian W51
    with fall W03
      due to ice or snow W00.0
      involving pedestrian conveyance —*see* Accident, transport, pedestrian, conveyance
    and
      crowd or human stampede (with fall) W52
      object W22.8
        with fall —*see* Fall, due to, bumping against, object
  person (s) —*see* Collision, pedestrian
  transport vehicle NEC V89.9
    and
      avalanche, fallen or not moving —*see* Accident, transport
        falling or moving —*see* Landslide
      landslide, fallen or not moving —*see* Accident, transport
        falling or moving —*see* Landslide
    due to cataclysm —*see* Forces of nature, by type
    intentional, purposeful suicide (attempt) —*see* Suicide, collision
Combustion, spontaneous —*see* Ignition
Complication (delayed) of or following (medical or surgical procedure) Y84.9
  with misadventure —*see* Misadventure
  amputation of limb (s) Y83.5
  anastomosis (arteriovenous) (blood vessel) (gastrojejunal) (tendon) (natural or artificial material) Y83.2
  aspiration (of fluid) Y84.4
    tissue Y84.8
  biopsy Y84.8
  blood
    sampling Y84.7
    transfusion
      procedure Y84.8
  bypass Y83.2
  catheterization (urinary) Y84.6
    cardiac Y84.0
  colostomy Y83.3

Complication - *continued*
cystostomy Y83.3
dialysis (kidney) Y84.1
drug —*see* Table of drugs and chemicals
due to misadventure —*see* Misadventure
duodenostomy Y83.3
electroshock therapy Y84.3
external stoma, creation of Y83.3
formation of external stoma Y83.3
gastrostomy Y83.3
graft Y83.2
hypothermia (medically-induced) Y84.8
implant, implantation (of)
  artificial
    internal device (cardiac pacemaker)
(electrodes in brain) (heart valve prosthesis)
(orthopedic) Y83.1
      material or tissue (for anastomosis or bypass)
        Y83.2
        with creation of external stoma Y83.3
    natural tissues (for anastomosis or bypass)
      Y83.2
      with creation of external stoma Y83.3
  infusion
    procedure Y84.8
  injection —*see* Table of drugs and chemicals
    procedure Y84.8
  insertion of gastric or duodenal sound Y84.5
  insulin-shock therapy Y84.3
  paracentesis (abdominal) (thoracic) (aspirative)
    Y84.4
  procedures other than surgical operation —*see*
Complication of or following, by type of
procedure
  radiological procedure or therapy Y84.2
  removal of organ (partial) (total) NEC Y83.6
  sampling
    blood Y84.7
    fluid NEC Y84.4
    tissue Y84.8
  shock therapy Y84.3
  surgical operation NEC (*see also* Complication
of or following, by type of operation) Y83.9
    reconstructive NEC Y83.4
      with
        anastomosis, bypass or graft Y83.2
        formation of external stoma Y83.3
      specified NEC Y83.8
  transfusion —*see also* Table of drugs and
chemicals
    procedure Y84.8
  transplant, transplantation (heart) (kidney)
(liver) (whole organ, any) Y83.0
    partial organ Y83.4
  ureterostomy Y83.3
  vaccination —*see also* Table of drugs and
chemicals
    procedure Y84.8
Compression
divers' squeeze
—*see* Air, pressure, change
trachea by
  food (lodged in esophagus) (*see* categories
T17 and) T18
  vomitus (lodged in esophagus) T17.81
Conflagration —*see* Exposure, fire, uncontrolled
Constriction (external)
hair W49.01
jewelry W49.04
ring W49.04
rubber band W49.03
specified item NEC W49.09
string W49.02

Constriction (external) - *continued*
thread W49.02
Contact (accidental) with
abrasive wheel (metalworking) W31.1
alligator W58.09
  bite W58.01
  crushing W58.03
  strike W58.02
amphibian W62.9
  frog W62.0
  toad W62.1
animal (nonvenomous) NEC W64
  marine W56.89
    bite W56.81
    dolphin —*see* Contact, with, dolphin
    fish NEC —*see* Contact, with, fish
    mammal —*see* Contact, with, mammal,
marine
      orca —*see* Contact, with, orca
      sea lion —*see* Contact, with, sea lion
      shark —*see* Contact, with, shark
      strike W56.82
animate mechanical force NEC W64
arrow W21.89
  not thrown, projected or falling W45.8
arthropods (nonvenomous) W57
axe W27.0
band-saw (industrial) W31.2
bayonet —*see* Bayonet wound
bee (s) X58
bench-saw (industrial) W31.2
bird W61.99
  bite W61.91
  chicken —*see* Contact, with, chicken
  duck —*see* Contact, with, duck
  goose —*see* Contact, with, goose
  macaw —*see* Contact, with, macaw
  parrot —*see* Contact, with, parrot
  psittacine —*see* Contact, with, psittacine
  strike W61.92
  turkey —*see* Contact, with, turkey
blender W29.0
boiling water X12
  stated as undetermined whether accidental or
intentional Y27.2
  suicide (attempt) X77.2
bore, earth-drilling or mining (land) (seabed)
  W31.0
buffalo —*see* Contact, with, hoof stock NEC
bull W55.29
  bite W55.21
  gored W55.22
  strike W55.22
bumper cars W31.81
camel —*see* Contact, with, hoof stock NEC
can
  lid W45.2
  opener W27.4
    powered W29.0
cat W55.09
  bite W55.01
  scratch W55.03
caterpillar (venomous) X58
centipede (venomous) X58
chain
  hoist W24.0
    agricultural operations W30.89
  saw W29.3
chicken W61.39
  peck W61.33
  strike W61.32
chisel W27.0
circular saw W31.2

Contact (accidental) - *continued*
cobra X58
combine (harvester) W30.0
conveyer belt W24.1
cooker (hot) X15.8
  stated as undetermined whether accidental or
intentional Y27.3
  suicide (attempt) X77.3
coral X58
cotton gin W31.82
cow W55.29
  bite W55.21
  strike W55.22
crane W24.0
  agricultural operations W30.89
crocodile W58.19
  bite W58.11
  crushing W58.13
  strike W58.12
dagger W26.1
  stated as undetermined whether accidental or
intentional Y28.2
  suicide (attempt) X78.2
dairy equipment W31.82
dart W21.89
  not thrown, projected or falling W45.8
deer —*see* Contact, with, hoof stock NEC
derrick W24.0
  agricultural operations W30.89
    hay W30.2
dog W54.8
  bite W54.0
  strike W54.1
dolphin W56.09
  bite W56.01
  strike W56.02
donkey —*see* Contact, with, hoof stock NEC
drill (powered) W29.8
  earth (land) (seabed) W31.0
    nonpowered W27.8
drive belt W24.0
  agricultural operations W30.89
dry ice —*see* Exposure, cold, man-made
dryer (clothes) (powered) (spin) W29.2
duck W61.69
  bite W61.61
  strike W61.62
earth ( )
  drilling machine (industrial) W31.0
  scraping machine in stationary use W31.83
edge of stiff paper W45.1
electric
  beater W29.0
  blanket X16
  fan W29.2
    commercial W31.82
  knife W29.1
  mixer W29.0
elevator (building) W24.0
  agricultural operations W30.89
    grain W30.3
engine (s) , hot NEC X17
excavating machine W31.0
farm machine W30.9
feces —*see* Contact, with, by type of animal
fer de lance X58
fish W56.59
  bite W56.51
  shark —*see* Contact, with, shark
  strike W56.52
flying horses W31.81
forging (metalworking) machine W31.1
fork W27.4

Contact (accidental) - *continued*
  forklift (truck) W24.0
    agricultural operations W30.89
  frog W62.0
  garden
    cultivator (powered) W29.3
      riding W30.89
    fork W27.1
  gas turbine W31.3
  Gila monster X58
  giraffe —*see* Contact, with, hoof stock NEC
  glass (sharp) (broken) W25
    with subsequent fall W18.02
    assault X99.0
    due to fall —*see* Fall, by type
    stated as undetermined whether accidental or
  intentional Y28.0
    suicide (attempt) X78.0
  goat W55.39
    bite W55.31
    strike W55.32
  goose W61.59
    bite W61.51
    strike W61.52
  hand
    saw W27.0
    tool (not powered) NEC W27.8
      powered W29.8
  harvester W30.0
  hay-derrick W30.2
  heat NEC X19
    from appliance (electrical) (household) —*see*
  Contact, with, hot, household appliance
      heating appliance X16
  heating
    appliance (hot) X16
    pad (electric) X16
  hedge-trimmer (powered) W29.3
  hoe W27.1
  hoist (chain) (shaft) NEC W24.0
    agricultural W30.89
  hoof stock NEC W55.39
    bite W55.31
    strike W55.32
  hornet (s) X58
  horse W55.19
    bite W55.11
    strike W55.12
  hot
    air X14.1
      inhalation X14.0
    cooker X15.8
    drinks X10.0
    engine X17
    fats X10.2
    fluids NEC X12
      assault X98.2
      suicide (attempt) X77.2
      undetermined whether accidental or
  intentional Y27.2
    food X10.1
    gases X14.1
      inhalation X14.0
    heating appliance X16
    household appliance X15.8
      assault X98.3
      cooker X15.8
      hotplate X15.2
      kettle X15.8
      light bulb X15.8
      object NEC X19
        assault X98.8

    stated as undetermined whether accidental
  or intentional Y27.9
      suicide (attempt) X77.8
    saucepan X15.3
    skillet X15.3
    stove X15.0
    stated as undetermined whether accidental
  or intentional Y27.3
      suicide (attempt) X77.3
    toaster X15.1
    kettle X15.8
    light bulb X15.8
    liquid NEC (*see also* Burning) X12
      drinks X10.0
      stated as undetermined whether accidental
  or intentional Y27.2
        suicide (attempt) X77.2
      tap water X11.8
        stated as undetermined whether accidental
  or intentional Y27.1
          suicide (attempt) X77.1
    machinery X17
    metal (molten) (liquid) NEC X18
    object (not producing fire or flames) NEC
  X19
    oil (cooking) X10.2
    pipe X16
    plate X15.2
    radiator X16
    saucepan (glass) (metal) X15.3
    skillet X15.3
    stove (kitchen) X15.0
    substance NEC X19
    tap-water X11.8
      assault X98.1
      heated on stove X12
        stated as undetermined whether accidental
  or intentional Y27.2
          suicide (attempt) X77.2
      in bathtub X11.0
      running X11.1
        stated as undetermined whether accidental
  or intentional Y27.1
          suicide (attempt) X77.1
    toaster X15.1
    tool X17
    vapors X13.1
      inhalation X13.0
    water (tap) X11.8
      boiling X12
        stated as undetermined whether accidental
  or intentional Y27.2
          suicide (attempt) X77.2
      heated on stove X12
        stated as undetermined whether accidental
  or intentional Y27.2
          suicide (attempt) X77.2
      in bathtub X11.0
      running X11.1
        stated as undetermined whether accidental
  or intentional Y27.1
          suicide (attempt) X77.1
    hotplate X15.2
    ice-pick W27.4
    insect (nonvenomous) NEC W57
    kettle (hot) X15.8
    knife W26.0
      assault X99.1
      electric W29.1
      stated as undetermined whether accidental or
  intentional Y28.1
        suicide (attempt) X78.1

  lathe (metalworking) W31.1
    turnings W45.8
    woodworking W31.2
  lawnmower (powered) (ridden) W28
    causing electrocution W86.8
      suicide (attempt) X83.1
    unpowered W27.1
  lift, lifting (devices) W24.0
    agricultural operations W30.89
    shaft W24.0
  liquefied gas —*see* Exposure, cold, man-made
  liquid air, hydrogen, nitrogen —*see* Exposure,
  cold, man-made
  lizard (nonvenomous) W59.09
    bite W59.01
    strike W59.02
  llama —*see* Contact, with, hoof stock NEC
  macaw W61.19
    bite W61.11
    strike W61.12
  machine, machinery W31.9
    abrasive wheel W31.1
    agricultural including animal-powered W30.9
      combine harvester W30.0
      grain storage elevator W30.3
      hay derrick W30.2
      power take-off device W30.1
      reaper W30.0
      specified NEC W30.89
      thresher W30.0
      transport vehicle, stationary W30.81
    band saw W31.2
    bench saw W31.2
    circular saw W31.2
    commercial NEC W31.82
    drilling, metal (industrial) W31.1
    earth-drilling W31.0
    earthmoving or scraping W31.89
    excavating W31.89
    forging machine W31.1
    gas turbine W31.3
    hot X17
    internal combustion engine W31.3
    land drill W31.0
    lathe W31.1
    lifting (devices) W24.0
    metal drill W31.1
    metalworking (industrial) W31.1
    milling, metal W31.1
    mining W31.0
    molding W31.2
    overhead plane W31.2
    power press, metal W31.1
    prime mover W31.3
    printing W31.89
    radial saw W31.2
    recreational W31.81
    roller-coaster W31.81
    rolling mill, metal W31.1
    sander W31.2
    seabed drill W31.0
    shaft
      hoist W31.0
      lift W31.0
    specified NEC W31.89
    spinning W31.89
    steam engine W31.3
    transmission W24.1
    undercutter W31.0
    water driven turbine W31.3
    weaving W31.89
    woodworking or forming (industrial) W31.2

Contact (accidental) - *continued*
  mammal (feces) (urine) W55.89
    bull —*see* Contact, with, bull
    cat —*see* Contact, with, cat
    cow —*see* Contact, with, cow
    goat —*see* Contact, with, goat
    hoof stock —*see* Contact, with, hoof stock
    horse —*see* Contact, with, horse
    marine W56.39
     dolphin —*see* Contact, with, dolphin
     orca —*see* Contact, with, orca
     sea lion —*see* Contact, with, sea lion
     specified NEC W56.39
      bite W56.31
      strike W56.32
    pig —*see* Contact, with, pig
    raccoon —*see* Contact, with, raccoon
    rodent —*see* Contact, with, rodent
    sheep —*see* Contact, with, sheep
    specified NEC W55.89
     bite W55.81
     strike W55.82
  marine
    animal W56.89
     bite W56.81
     dolphin —*see* Contact, with, dolphin
     fish NEC —*see* Contact, with, fish
     mammal —*see* Contact, with, mammal, marine
     orca —*see* Contact, with, orca
     sea lion —*see* Contact, with, sea lion
     shark —*see* Contact, with, shark
     strike W56.82
  meat
    grinder (domestic) W29.0
     industrial W31.82
     nonpowered W27.4
    slicer (domestic) W29.0
     industrial W31.82
  merry go round W31.81
  metal, hot (liquid) (molten) NEC X18
  millipede W57
  nail W45.0
    gun W29.4
  needle (sewing) W27.3
    hypodermic W46.0
     contaminated W46.1
  object (blunt) NEC
    hot NEC X19
    legal intervention —*see* Legal, intervention, blunt object
    sharp NEC W45.8
     inflicted by other person NEC W45.8
      stated as
       intentional homicide (attempt) —*see* Assault, cutting or piercing instrument
     legal intervention —*see* Legal, intervention, sharp object
     self-inflicted X78.9
  orca W56.29
    bite W56.21
    strike W56.22
  overhead plane W31.2
  paper (as sharp object) W45.1
  paper-cutter W27.5
  parrot W61.09
    bite W61.01
    strike W61.02
  pig W55.49
    bite W55.41
    strike W55.42
  pipe, hot X16
  pitchfork W27.1

Contact (accidental) - *continued*
  plane (metal) (wood) W27.0
    overhead W31.2
  plant thorns, spines, sharp leaves or other mechanisms W60
  powered
    garden cultivator W29.3
    household appliance, implement, or machine W29.8
    saw (industrial) W31.2
     hand W29.8
  printing machine W31.89
  psittacine bird W61.29
    bite W61.21
    macaw —*see* Contact, with, macaw
    parrot —*see* Contact, with, parrot
    strike W61.22
  pulley (block) (transmission) W24.0
    agricultural operations W30.89
  raccoon W55.59
    bite W55.51
    strike W55.52
  radial-saw (industrial) W31.2
  radiator (hot) X16
  rake W27.1
  rattlesnake X58
  reaper W30.0
  reptile W59.89
    lizard —*see* Contact, with, lizard
    snake —*see* Contact, with, snake
    specified NEC W59.89
     bite W59.81
     crushing W59.83
     strike W59.82
    turtle —*see* Contact, with, turtle
  rivet gun (powered) W29.4
  road scraper —*see* Accident, transport, construction vehicle
  rodent (feces) (urine) W53.89
    bite W53.81
    mouse W53.09
     bite W53.01
    rat W53.19
     bite W53.11
    specified NEC W53.89
     bite W53.81
    squirrel W53.29
     bite W53.21
  roller coaster W31.81
  rope NEC W24.0
    agricultural operations W30.89
  saliva —*see* Contact, with, by type of animal
  sander W29.8
    industrial W31.2
  saucepan (hot) (glass) (metal) X15.3
  saw W27.0
    band (industrial) W31.2
    bench (industrial) W31.2
    chain W29.3
    hand W27.0
  sawing machine, metal W31.1
  scissors W27.2
  scorpion X58
  screwdriver W27.0
    powered W29.8
  sea
    anemone, cucumber or urchin (spine) X58
    lion W56.19
     bite W56.11
     strike W56.12
  serpent —*see* Contact, with, snake, by type
  sewing-machine (electric) (powered) W29.2
    not powered W27.8

Contact (accidental) - *continued*
  shaft (hoist) (lift) (transmission) NEC W24.0
    agricultural W30.89
  shark W56.49
    bite W56.41
    strike W56.42
  shears (hand) W27.2
    powered (industrial) W31.1
     domestic W29.2
  sheep W55.39
    bite W55.31
    strike W55.32
  shovel W27.8
    steam —*see* Accident, transport, construction vehicle
  snake (nonvenomous) W59.19
    bite W59.11
    crushing W59.13
    strike W59.12
  spade W27.1
  spider (venomous) X58
  spin-drier W29.2
  spinning machine W31.89
  splinter W45.8
  sports equipment W21.9
  staple gun (powered) W29.8
  steam X13.1
    engine W31.3
    inhalation X13.0
    pipe X16
    shovel W31.89
  stove (hot) (kitchen) X15.0
  substance, hot NEC X19
    molten (metal) X18
  sword W26.1
    assault X99.2
    stated as undetermined whether accidental or intentional Y28.2
    suicide (attempt) X78.2
  tarantula X58
  thresher W30.0
  tin can lid W45.2
  toad W62.1
  toaster (hot) X15.1
  tool W27.8
    hand (not powered) W27.8
     auger W27.0
     axe W27.0
     can opener W27.4
     chisel W27.0
     fork W27.4
     garden W27.1
     handsaw W27.0
     hoe W27.1
     ice-pick W27.4
     kitchen utensil W27.4
     manual
      lawn mower W27.1
      sewing machine W27.8
     meat grinder W27.4
     needle (sewing) W27.3
      hypodermic W46.0
       contaminated W46.1
     paper cutter W27.5
     pitchfork W27.1
     rake W27.1
     scissors W27.2
     screwdriver W27.0
     specified NEC W27.8
     workbench W27.0
    hot X17
    powered W29.8
     blender W29.0

Contact (accidental) - *continued*
- commercial W31.82
- can opener W29.0
  - commercial W31.82
- chainsaw W29.3
- clothes dryer W29.2
  - commercial W31.82
- dishwasher W29.2
  - commercial W31.82
- edger W29.3
- electric fan W29.2
  - commercial W31.82
- electric knife W29.1
- food processor W29.0
  - commercial W31.82
- garbage disposal W29.0
  - commercial W31.82
- garden tool W29.3
- hedge trimmer W29.3
- ice maker W29.0
  - commercial W31.82
- kitchen appliance W29.0
  - commercial W31.82
- lawn mower W28
- meat grinder W29.0
  - commercial W31.82
- mixer W29.0
  - commercial W31.82
- rototiller W29.3
- sewing machine W29.2
  - commercial W31.82
- washing machine W29.2
  - commercial W31.82
- transmission device (belt, cable, chain, gear, pinion, shaft) W24.1
  - agricultural operations W30.89
- turbine (gas) (water-driven) W31.3
- turkey W61.49
  - peck W61.43
  - strike W61.42
- turtle (nonvenomous) W59.29
  - bite W59.21
  - strike W59.22
  - terrestrial W59.89
    - bite W59.81
    - crushing W59.83
    - strike W59.82
  - under-cutter W31.0
- urine —*see* Contact, with, by type of animal
- vehicle
  - agricultural use (transport) —*see* Accident, transport, agricultural vehicle
    - not on public highway W30.81
  - industrial use (transport) —*see* Accident, transport, industrial vehicle
    - not on public highway W31.83
  - off-road use (transport) —*see* Accident, transport, all-terrain or off-road vehicle
    - not on public highway W31.83
  - special construction use (transport) —*see* Accident, transport, construction vehicle
    - not on public highway W31.83
- venomous
  - animal X58
  - arthropods X58
  - lizard X58
  - marine animal NEC X58
  - marine plant NEC X58
  - millipedes (tropical) X58
  - plant (s) X58
  - snake X58
  - spider X58
  - viper X58

Contact (accidental) - *continued*
- washing-machine (powered) W29.2
- wasp X58
- weaving-machine W31.89
- winch W24.0
  - agricultural operations W30.89
- wire NEC W24.0
  - agricultural operations W30.89
- wood slivers W45.8
- yellow jacket X58
- zebra —*see* Contact, with, hoof stock NEC

Coup de soleil X32

Crash
- aircraft (in transit) (powered) V95.9
  - balloon V96.01
  - fixed wing NEC (private) V95.21
    - commercial V95.31
  - glider V96.21
    - hang V96.11
    - powered V95.11
  - helicopter V95.01
  - in war operations —*see* War operations, destruction of aircraft
  - microlight V95.11
  - nonpowered V96.9
    - specified NEC V96.8
  - powered NEC V95.8
  - stated as
    - homicide (attempt) Y08.81
    - suicide (attempt) X83.0
  - ultralight V95.11
- spacecraft V95.41
- transport vehicle NEC (*see also* Accident, transport) V89.9
  - homicide (attempt) Y03.8
  - motor NEC (traffic) V89.2
    - homicide (attempt) Y03.8
  - suicide (attempt) —*see* Suicide, collision

Cruelty (mental) (physical) (sexual) X58

Crushed (accidentally) X58
- between objects (moving) (stationary and moving) W23.0
  - stationary W23.1
- by
  - alligator W58.03
  - avalanche NEC —*see* Landslide
  - cave-in W20.0
    - caused by cataclysmic earth surface movement —*see* Landslide
  - crocodile W58.13
  - crowd or human stampede W52
  - falling
    - aircraft V97.39
      - in war operations —*see* War operations, destruction of aircraft
    - earth, material W20.0
      - caused by cataclysmic earth surface movement —*see* Landslide
    - object NEC W20.8
  - landslide NEC —*see* Landslide
  - lizard (nonvenomous) W59.09
  - machinery —*see* Contact, with, by type of machine
  - reptile NEC W59.89
  - snake (nonvenomous) W59.13
- in
  - machinery —*see* Contact, with, by type of machine

Cut, cutting (any part of body) (accidental) — *see also* Contact, with, by object or machine
- during medical or surgical treatment as misadventure —*see* Misadventure, cut, by type of procedure

Cut, cutting - *continued*
- homicide (attempt) —*see* Assault, cutting or piercing instrument
- inflicted by other person —*see* Assault, cutting or piercing instrument
- legal
  - execution —*see* Legal, intervention
  - intervention —*see* Legal, intervention, sharp object
- machine NEC (*see also* Contact, with, by type of machine) W31.9
- self-inflicted —*see* Suicide, cutting or piercing instrument
- suicide (attempt) —*see* Suicide, cutting or piercing instrument

Cyclone (any injury) X37.1

D

Decapitation (accidental circumstances) NEC X58
- homicide X99.9
- legal execution —*see* Legal, intervention

Dehydration from lack of water X58

Deprivation X58

Derailment (accidental)
- railway (rolling stock) (train) (vehicle) (without antecedent collision) V81.7
  - with antecedent collision —*see* Accident, transport, railway vehicle occupant
- streetcar (without antecedent collision) V82.7
  - with antecedent collision —*see* Accident, transport, streetcar occupant

Descent
- parachute (voluntary) (without accident to aircraft) V97.29
  - due to accident to aircraft —*see* Accident, transport, aircraft

Desertion X58

Destitution X58

Disability, late effect or sequela of injury —*see* Sequelae

Discharge (accidental)
- airgun W34.010
  - assault X95.01
    - homicide (attempt) X95.01
  - stated as undetermined whether accidental or intentional Y24.0
  - suicide (attempt) X74.01
- BB gun —*see* Discharge, airgun
- firearm (accidental) W34.00
  - assault X95.9
  - handgun (pistol) (revolver) W32.0
    - assault X93
      - homicide (attempt) X93
    - legal intervention —*see* Legal, intervention, firearm, handgun
    - stated as undetermined whether accidental or intentional Y22
    - suicide (attempt) X72
  - homicide (attempt) X95.9
  - hunting rifle W33.02
    - assault X94.1
      - homicide (attempt) X94.1
    - legal intervention
      - injuring
        - bystander Y35.032
        - law enforcement personnel Y35.031
        - suspect Y35.033
    - stated as undetermined whether accidental or intentional Y23.1
    - suicide (attempt) X73.1
  - larger W33.00
    - assault X94.9

Drowning (accidental) - *continued*

accident to watercraft —*see* Drowning, due to, accident to, watercraft
being washed overboard (from) V92.29
  powered craft V92.23
    ferry boat V92.21
    liner V92.21
    merchant ship V92.20
    passenger ship V92.21
    fishing boat V92.22
    jet skis V92.23
  unpowered craft V92.28
    canoe V92.25
    inflatable V92.26
    kayak V92.25
    sailboat V92.24
    surf-board V92.28
    water skis V92.27
    windsurfer V92.28
motion of watercraft V92.19
  powered craft V92.13
    ferry boat V92.11
    liner V92.11
    merchant ship V92.10
    passenger ship V92.11
    fishing boat V92.12
    jet skis V92.13
  unpowered craft
    canoe V92.15
    inflatable V92.16
    kayak V92.15
    sailboat V92.14
hurricane X37.0
jumping into water from watercraft (involved in accident) —*see also* Drowning, due to, accident to, watercraft
  without accident to or on watercraft W16.711
tidal wave NEC —*see* Forces of nature, tidal wave
torrential rain X37.8
following
  fall
    into
      bathtub W16.211
      bucket W16.221
      fountain —*see* Drowning, following, fall, into, water, specified NEC
      quarry —*see* Drowning, following, fall, into, water, specified NEC
      reservoir —*see* Drowning, following, fall, into, water, specified NEC
      swimming-pool W16.011
        striking
          bottom W16.021
          wall W16.031
        stated as undetermined whether accidental or intentional Y21.3
        suicide (attempt) X71.2
      water NOS W16.41
      natural (lake) (open sea) (river) (stream) (pond) W16.111
        striking
          bottom W16.121
          side W16.131
      specified NEC W16.311
        striking
          bottom W16.321
          wall W16.331
    overboard NEC —*see* Drowning, due to, fall overboard
jump or dive
  from boat W16.711
    striking bottom W16.721

Drowning (accidental) - *continued*

into
  fountain —*see* Drowning, following, jump or dive, into, water, specified NEC
  quarry —*see* Drowning, following, jump or dive, into, water, specified NEC
  reservoir —*see* Drowning, following, jump or dive, into, water, specified NEC
  swimming-pool W16.511
    striking
      bottom W16.521
      wall W16.531
    suicide (attempt) X71.2
  water NOS W16.91
  natural (lake) (open sea) (river) (stream) (pond) W16.611
    specified NEC W16.811
      striking
        bottom W16.821
        wall W16.831
      striking bottom W16.621
homicide (attempt) X92.9
in
 bathtub (accidental) W65
  assault X92.0
  following fall W16.211
  stated as undetermined whether accidental or intentional Y21.1
  stated as undetermined whether accidental or intentional Y21.0
  suicide (attempt) X71.0
 lake —*see* Drowning, in, natural water
 natural water (lake) (open sea) (river) (stream) (pond) W69
  assault X92.3
  following
    dive or jump W16.611
      striking bottom W16.621
    fall W16.111
      striking
        bottom W16.121
        side W16.131
  stated as undetermined whether accidental or intentional Y21.4
  suicide (attempt) X71.3
 quarry —*see* Drowning, in, specified place NEC
 quenching tank —*see* Drowning, in, specified place NEC
 reservoir —*see* Drowning, in, specified place NEC
 river —*see* Drowning, in, natural water
 sea —*see* Drowning, in, natural water
 specified place NEC W73
  assault X92.8
  following
    dive or jump W16.811
      striking
        bottom W16.821
        wall W16.831
    fall W16.311
      striking
        bottom W16.321
        wall W16.331
  stated as undetermined whether accidental or intentional Y21.8
  suicide (attempt) X71.8
 stream —*see* Drowning, in, natural water
 swimming-pool W67
  assault X92.1
  following fall X92.2
  following
    dive or jump W16.511

Drowning (accidental) - *continued*

striking
  bottom W16.521
  wall W16.531
fall W16.011
  striking
    bottom W16.021
    wall W16.031
stated as undetermined whether accidental or intentional Y21.2
  following fall Y21.3
  suicide (attempt) X71.1
  following fall X71.2
war operations —*see* War operations, restriction of airway
resulting from accident to watercraft see Drowning, due to, accident, watercraft
self-inflicted X71.9
stated as undetermined whether accidental or intentional Y21.9
suicide (attempt) X71.9

E

Earth (surface) movement NEC —*see* Forces of nature, earth movement
Earth falling (on) W20.0
caused by cataclysmic earth surface movement or eruption —*see* Landslide
Earthquake (any injury) X34
Effect (s) (adverse) of
air pressure (any) —*see* Air, pressure
cold, excessive (exposure to) —*see* Exposure, cold
heat (excessive) —*see* Heat
hot place (weather) —*see* Heat
insolation X30
late —*see* Sequelae
motion —*see* Motion
nuclear explosion or weapon in war operations —*see* War operations, nuclear weapon
radiation —*see* Radiation
travel —*see* Travel
Electric shock (accidental) (by) (in) —*see* Exposure, electric current
Electrocution (accidental) —*see* Exposure, electric current
Endotracheal tube wrongly placed during anesthetic procedure
Entanglement
in
 bed linen, causing suffocation —*see* category T71
 wheel of pedal cycle V19.88
Entry of foreign body or material —*see* Foreign body
Environmental pollution related condition see Z57
Execution, legal (any method) —*see* Legal, intervention
Exhaustion
cold —*see* Exposure, cold
due to excessive exertion —*see* category Y93
heat —*see* Heat
Explosion (accidental) (of) (with secondary fire) W40.9
acetylene W40.1
aerosol can W36.1
air tank (compressed) (in machinery) W36.2
aircraft (in transit) (powered) NEC V95.9
 balloon V96.05
 fixed wing NEC (private) V95.25
  commercial V95.35
 glider V96.25

Explosion (accidental) - *continued*
  hang V96.15
    powered V95.15
  helicopter V95.05
  in war operations —*see* War operations, destruction of aircraft
  microlight V95.15
  nonpowered V96.9
    specified NEC V96.8
  powered NEC V95.8
  stated as
    homicide (attempt) Y03.8
    suicide (attempt) X83.0
  ultralight V95.15
  anesthetic gas in operating room W40.1
  antipersonnel bomb W40.8
    assault X96.0
    homicide (attempt) X96.0
    suicide (attempt) X75
  assault X96.9
  bicycle tire W37.0
  blasting (cap) (materials) W40.0
  boiler (machinery) , not on transport vehicle W35
    on watercraft —*see* Explosion, in, watercraft
  butane W40.1
  caused by other person X96.9
  coal gas W40.1
  detonator W40.0
  dump (munitions) W40.8
  dynamite W40.0
  in
    assault X96.8
    homicide (attempt) X96.8
    legal intervention
      injuring
        bystander Y35.112
        law enforcement personnel Y35.111
        suspect Y35.113
    suicide (attempt) X75
  explosive (material) W40.9
    gas W40.1
    in blasting operation W40.0
    specified NEC W40.8
    in
      assault X96.8
      homicide (attempt) X96.8
      legal intervention
        injuring
          bystander Y35.192
          law enforcement personnel Y35.191
          suspect Y35.193
      suicide (attempt) X75
  factory (munitions) W40.8
  fertilizer bomb W40.8
    assault X96.3
    homicide (attempt) X96.3
    suicide (attempt) X75
  firearm (parts) NEC W34.19
    airgun W34.110
    BB gun W34.110
    gas, air or spring-operated gun NEC W34.118
    handgun W32.1
    hunting rifle W33.12
    larger firearm W33.10
      specified NEC W33.19
    machine gun W33.13
    paintball gun W34.111
    pellet gun W34.110
    shotgun W33.11
    Very pistol [flare] W34.19
  fire-damp W40.1
  fireworks W39

Explosion (accidental) - *continued*
  gas (coal) (explosive) W40.1
    cylinder W36.9
      aerosol can W36.1
      air tank W36.2
      pressurized W36.3
      specified NEC W36.8
  gasoline (fumes) (tank) not in moving motor vehicle W40.1
    bomb W40.8
    assault X96.1
    homicide (attempt) X96.1
    suicide (attempt) X75
    in motor vehicle —*see* Accident, transport, by type of vehicle
  grain store W40.8
  grenade W40.8
    in
      assault X96.8
      homicide (attempt) X96.8
      legal intervention
        injuring
          bystander Y35.192
          law enforcement personnel Y35.191
          suspect Y35.193
      suicide (attempt) X75
  handgun (parts) —*see* Explosion, firearm,
  handgun (parts)   homicide (attempt) X96.9
    antipersonnel bomb —*see* Explosion, antipersonnel bomb
    fertilizer bomb —*see* Explosion, fertilizer bomb
    gasoline bomb —*see* Explosion, gasoline bomb
    letter bomb —*see* Explosion, letter bomb
    pipe bomb —*see* Explosion, pipe bomb
    specified NEC X96.8
  hose, pressurized W37.8
  hot water heater, tank (in machinery) W35
    on watercraft —*see* Explosion, in, watercraft
  in, on
    dump W40.8
    factory W40.8
    mine (of explosive gases) NEC W40.1
    watercraft V93.59
      powered craft V93.53
      ferry boat V93.51
      fishing boat V93.52
      jet skis V93.53
      liner V93.51
      merchant ship V93.50
      passenger ship V93.51
      sailboat V93.54
  letter bomb W40.8
    assault X96.2
    homicide (attempt) X96.2
    suicide (attempt) X75
  machinery —*see also* Contact, with, by type of machine
    on board watercraft —*see* Explosion, in, watercraft
    pressure vessel —*see* Explosion, by type of vessel
  methane W40.1
  mine W40.1
  missile NEC W40.8
  mortar bomb W40.8
    in
      assault X96.8
      homicide (attempt) X96.8
      legal intervention
        injuring
          bystander Y35.192

Explosion (accidental) - *continued*
    law enforcement personnel Y35.191
    suspect Y35.193
    suicide (attempt) X75
  munitions (dump) (factory) W40.8
  pipe, pressurized W37.8
    bomb W40.8
    assault X96.4
    homicide (attempt) X96.4
    suicide (attempt) X75
  pressure, pressurized
    cooker W38
    gas tank (in machinery) W36.3
    hose W37.8
    pipe W37.8
    specified device NEC W38
    tire W37.8
      bicycle W37.0
    vessel (in machinery) W38
  propane W40.1
  self-inflicted X75
  shell (artillery) NEC W40.8
    during war operations —*see* War operations, explosion
    in
      legal intervention
        injuring
          bystander Y35.122
          law enforcement personnel Y35.121
          suspect Y35.123
    war —*see* War operations, explosion
  spacecraft V95.45
  steam or water lines (in machinery) W37.8
  stove W40.9
  stated as undetermined whether accidental or intentional Y25
  suicide (attempt) X75
  tire, pressurized W37.8
    bicycle W37.0
  undetermined whether accidental or intentional Y25
  vehicle tire NEC W37.8
    bicycle W37.0
  war operations —*see* War operations, explosion

Exposure (to) X58
  air pressure change —*see* Air, pressure
  cold (accidental) (excessive) (extreme) (natural) (place) X31
    assault Y08.89
    due to
      man-made conditions W93.8
      dry ice (contact) W93.01
        inhalation W93.02
      liquid air (contact) (hydrogen) (nitrogen) W93.11
        inhalation W93.12
      refrigeration unit (deep freeze) W93.2
    suicide (attempt) X83.2
    weather (conditions) X31
    homicide (attempt) Y08.89
    self-inflicted X83.2
  due to abandonment or neglect X58
  electric current W86.8
    appliance (faulty) W86.8
      domestic W86.0
    caused by other person Y08.89
    conductor (faulty) W86.1
    control apparatus (faulty) W86.1
    electric power generating plant, distribution station W86.1
    electroshock gun —*see* Exposure, electric current, taser
    high-voltage cable W85

Exposure (to) - *continued*
  homicide (attempt) Y08.89
  legal execution —*see* Legal, intervention,
specified means NEC
  lightning —see subcategory T75.0
  live rail W86.8
  misadventure in medical or surgical procedure
in electroshock therapy Y63.4
    motor (electric) (faulty) W86.8
      domestic W86.0
    self-inflicted X83.1
    specified NEC W86.8
      domestic W86.0
    stun gun —*see* Exposure, electric current, taser
    suicide (attempt) X83.1
    taser W86.8
      assault Y08.89
      legal intervention —see category Y35
      self-harm (intentional) X83.8
      undetermined intent Y33
    third rail W86.8
    transformer (faulty) W86.1
    transmission lines W85
  environmental tobacco smoke X58
  excessive
    cold —*see* Exposure, cold
    heat (natural) NEC X30
      man-made W92
  factor (s) NOS X58
    environmental NEC X58
    man-made NEC W99
    natural NEC —*see* Forces of nature
  specified NEC X58
  fire, flames (accidental) X08.8
    assault X97
    campfire —*see* Exposure, fire, controlled, not
in building
    controlled (in)
      with ignition (of) clothing (*see also* Ignition,
clothes) X06.2
        nightwear X05
      bonfire —*see* Exposure, fire, controlled, not
in building
      brazier (in building or structure) —*see also*
      Exposure, fire, controlled, building
      not in building or structure —*see* Exposure,
      fire, controlled, not in building
      building or structure X02.0
        with
          fall from building X02.3
          injury due to building collapse X02.2
          from building X02.5
          smoke inhalation X02.1
        hit by object from building X02.4
        specified mode of injury NEC X02.8
      fireplace, furnace or stove —*see* Exposure,
fire, controlled, building
      not in building or structure X03.0
        with
          fall X03.3
          smoke inhalation X03.1
        hit by object X03.4
        specified mode of injury NEC X03.8
      trash —*see* Exposure, fire, controlled, not in
building
      fireplace —*see* Exposure, fire, controlled,
building
      fittings or furniture (in building or structure)
(uncontrolled) —*see* Exposure, fire,
uncontrolled, building
      forest (uncontrolled) —*see* Exposure, fire,
uncontrolled, not in building

Exposure (to) - *continued*
    grass (uncontrolled) —*see* Exposure, fire,
uncontrolled, not in building
    hay (uncontrolled) —*see* Exposure, fire,
uncontrolled, not in building
    homicide (attempt) X97
    ignition of highly flammable material X04
    in, of, on, starting in
      machinery —*see* Contact, with, by type of
machine
      motor vehicle (in motion) (*see also* Accident,
transport, occupant by type of vehicle) V87.8
        with collision —*see* Collision
      railway rolling stock, train, vehicle V81.81
        with collision —*see* Accident, transport,
        railway vehicle occupant
      street car (in motion) V82.8
        with collision —*see* Accident, transport,
        streetcar occupant
      transport vehicle NEC —*see also* Accident,
transport
        with collision —*see* Collision
      war operations —*see also* War operations,
fire
        from nuclear explosion —*see* War
operations, nuclear weapons
      watercraft (in transit) (not in transit) V91.09
        localized —*see* Burn, on board watercraft,
due to, fire on board
        powered craft V91.03
          ferry boat V91.01
          fishing boat V91.02
          jet skis V91.03
          liner V91.01
          merchant ship V91.00
          passenger ship V91.01
        unpowered craft V91.08
          canoe V91.05
          inflatable V91.06
          kayak V91.05
          sailboat V91.04
          surf-board V91.08
          waterskis V91.07
          windsurfer V91.08
    lumber (uncontrolled) —*see* Exposure, fire,
uncontrolled, not in building
    mine (uncontrolled) —*see* Exposure, fire,
uncontrolled, not in building
    prairie (uncontrolled) —*see* Exposure, fire,
uncontrolled, not in building
    resulting from
      explosion —*see* Explosion
      lightning X08.8
    self-inflicted X76
    specified NEC X08.8
    started by other person X97
    stove —*see* Exposure, fire, controlled,
building
    stated as undetermined whether accidental or
intentional Y26
    suicide (attempt) X76
    tunnel (uncontrolled) —*see* Exposure, fire,
uncontrolled, not in building
    uncontrolled
      in building or structure X00.0
        with
          fall from building X00.3
          injury due to building collapse X00.2
          jump from building X00.5
          smoke inhalation X00.1
        bed X08.00
          due to
            cigarette X08.01

Exposure (to) - *continued*
          specified material NEC X08.09
        furniture NEC X08.20
          due to
            cigarette X08.21
            specified material NEC X08.29
        hit by object from building X00.4
        sofa X08.10
          due to
            cigarette X08.11
            specified material NEC X08.19
        specified mode of injury NEC X00.8
      not in building or structure (any) X01.0
        with
          fall X01.3
          smoke inhalation X01.1
        hit by object X01.4
        specified mode of injury NEC X01.8
      undetermined whether accidental or intentional
Y26
    forces of nature NEC —*see* Forces of nature
    G-forces (abnormal) W49.9
    gravitational forces (abnormal) W49.9
    heat (natural) NEC —*see* Heat
    high-pressure jet (hydraulic) (pneumatic) W49.9
    hydraulic jet W49.9
    inanimate mechanical force W49.9
    jet, high-pressure (hydraulic) (pneumatic)
W49.9
    lightning —see subcategory T75.0
      causing fire —*see* Exposure, fire
    mechanical forces NEC W49.9
      animate NEC W64
      inanimate NEC W49.9
    noise W42.9
      supersonic W42.0
    noxious substance —*see* Table of drugs and
chemical
    pneumatic jet W49.9
    prolonged in deep-freeze unit or refrigerator
W93.2
    radiation —*see* Radiation
    smoke —*see also* Exposure, fire
      tobacco, second hand Z77.22
    specified factors NEC X58
    sunlight X32
      man-made (sun lamp) W89.8
        tanning bed W89.1
    supersonic waves W42.0
    transmission line (s), electric W85
    vibration W49.9
    waves
      infrasound W49.9
      sound W42.9
      supersonic W42.0
    weather NEC —*see* Forces of nature
External cause status Y99.9
  child assisting in compensated work for family
Y99.8
  civilian activity done for financial or other
compensation Y99.0
  civilian activity done for income or pay Y99.0
  family member assisting in compensated work
for other family member Y99.8
  hobby not done for income Y99.8
  leisure activity Y99.8
  military activity Y99.1
  off-duty activity of military personnel Y99.8
  recreation or sport not for income or while a
student Y99.8
  specified NEC Y99.8
  student activity Y99.8
  volunteer activity Y99.2

F

Factors, supplemental
alcohol
 blood level
  less than 20mg/100ml Y90.0
  presence in blood, level not specified Y90.9
  20 39mg/100ml Y90.1
  40 59mg/100ml Y90.2
  60 79mg/100ml Y90.3
  80 99mg/100ml Y90.4
  100 119mg/100ml Y90.5
  120 199mg/100ml Y90.6
  200 239mg/100ml Y90.7
  240mg/100ml or more Y90.8
 presence in blood, but level not specified
 Y90.9
environmental-pollution-related condition see
Z57
nosocomial condition Y95
work-related condition Y99.0
Failure
in suture or ligature during surgical procedure
Y65.2
mechanical, of instrument or apparatus (any)
(during any medical or surgical procedure)
Y65.8
sterile precautions (during medical and surgical
care) —*see* Misadventure, failure, sterile
precautions, by type of procedure
to
 introduce tube or instrument Y65.4
  endotracheal tube during anesthesia Y65.3
 make curve (transport vehicle) NEC —*see*
Accident, transport
 remove tube or instrument Y65.4
Fall, falling (accidental) W19
building W20.1
 burning (uncontrolled fire) X00.3
down
 embankment W17.81
 escalator W10.0
 hill W17.81
 ladder W11
 ramp W10.2
 stairs, steps W10.9
due to
 bumping against
  object W18.00
   sharp glass W18.02
   specified NEC W18.09
   sports equipment W18.01
  person W03
   due to ice or snow W00.0
   on pedestrian conveyance —*see* Accident,
  transport, pedestrian, conveyance
 collision with another person W03
  due to ice or snow W00.0
  involving pedestrian conveyance —*see*
  Accident, transport, pedestrian, conveyance
 grocery cart tipping over W17.82
 ice or snow W00.9
  from one level to another W00.2
   on stairs or steps W00.1
  involving pedestrian conveyance —*see*
  Accident, transport, pedestrian, conveyance
  on same level W00.0
 slipping (on moving sidewalk) W01.0
  with subsequent striking against object
  W01.10
   furniture W01.190
   sharp object W01.119

Fall, falling (accidental) - *continued*
 glass W01.110
  power tool or machine W01.111
  specified NEC W01.118
 specified NEC W01.198
striking against
 object W18.00
  sharp glass W18.02
  specified NEC W18.09
  sports equipment W18.01
 person W03
  due to ice or snow W00.0
  on pedestrian conveyance —*see* Accident,
transport, pedestrian, conveyance
earth (with asphyxia or suffocation (by pressure)
—*see* Earth, falling
from, off, out of
aircraft NEC (with accident to aircraft NEC)
V97.0
 while boarding or alighting V97.1
balcony W13.0
bed W06
boat, ship, watercraft NEC (with drowning or
submersion) —*see* Drowning, due to, fall
overboard
 with hitting bottom or object V94.0
bridge W13.1
building W13.9
 burning (uncontrolled fire) X00.3
cavity W17.2
chair W07
cherry picker W17.89
cliff W15
dock W17.4
embankment W17.81
escalator W10.0
flagpole W13.8
furniture NEC W08
grocery cart W17.82
haystack W17.89
high place NEC W17.89
 stated as undetermined whether accidental or
intentional Y30
hole W17.2
incline W10.2
ladder W11
lifting device W17.89
machine, machinery —*see also* Contact, with,
by type of machine
 not in operation W17.89
manhole W17.1
mobile elevated work platform [MEWP]
W17.89
motorized mobility scooter W05.2
one level to another NEC W17.89
 intentional, purposeful, suicide (attempt) X80
 stated as undetermined whether accidental or
intentional Y30
pit W17.2
playground equipment W09.8
 jungle gym W09.2
 slide W09.0
 swing W09.1
quarry W17.89
railing W13.9
ramp W10.2
roof W13.2
scaffolding W12
scooter (nonmotorized) W05.1
 motorized mobility W05.2
sky lift W17.89
stairs, steps W10.9
 curb W10.1

Fall, falling (accidental) - *continued*
 due to ice or snow W00.1
 escalator W10.0
 incline W10.2
 ramp W10.2
 sidewalk curb W10.1
 specified NEC W10.8
stepladder W11
storm drain W17.1
streetcar NEC V82.6
 with antecedent collision —*see* Accident,
 transport, streetcar occupant
 while boarding or alighting V82.4
structure NEC W13.8
 burning (uncontrolled fire) X00.3
table W08
toilet W18.11
 with subsequent striking against object
 W18.12
train NEC V81.6
 during derailment (without antecedent
 collision) V81.7
 with antecedent collision —*see* Accident,
 transport, railway vehicle occupant
 while boarding or alighting V81.4
transport vehicle after collision —*see*
Accident, transport, by type of vehicle, collision
tree W14
vehicle (in motion) NEC (*see also* Accident,
transport) V89.9
 motor NEC (*see also* Accident, transport,
occupant, by type of vehicle) V87.8
 stationary W17.89
 while boarding or alighting —*see* Accident,
transport, by type of vehicle, while boarding or
alighting
viaduct W13.8
wall W13.8
watercraft —*see also* Drowning, due to, fall
overboard
 with hitting bottom or object V94.0
well W17.0
wheelchair, non-moving W05.0
 powered —*see* Accident, transport,
 pedestrian, conveyance occupant, specified
 type NEC
window W13.4
in, on
aircraft NEC V97.0
 with accident to aircraft V97.0
 while boarding or alighting V97.1
bathtub (empty) W18.2
 filled W16.212
  causing drowning W16.211
escalator W10.0
incline W10.2
ladder W11
machine, machinery —*see* Contact, with, by
type of machine
object, edged, pointed or sharp (with cut) —
 see Fall, by type
playground equipment W09.8
 jungle gym W09.2
 slide W09.0
 swing W09.1
ramp W10.2
scaffolding W12
shower W18.2
 causing drowning W16.211
staircase, stairs, steps W10.9
 curb W10.1
 due to ice or snow W00.1
 escalator W10.0

Incident, adverse - *continued*
   miscellaneous Y75.8
   monitoring Y75.0
   prosthetic Y75.2
   rehabilitative Y75.1
   surgical Y75.3
   therapeutic Y75.1
  obstetrical Y76.8
   accessory Y76.2
   diagnostic Y76.0
   miscellaneous Y76.8
   monitoring Y76.0
   prosthetic Y76.2
   rehabilitative Y76.1
   surgical Y76.3
   therapeutic Y76.1
  ophthalmic Y77.8
   accessory Y77.2
   diagnostic Y77.0
   miscellaneous Y77.8
   monitoring Y77.0
   prosthetic Y77.2
   rehabilitative Y77.1
   surgical Y77.3
   therapeutic Y77.1
  orthopedic Y79.8
   accessory Y79.2
   diagnostic Y79.0
   miscellaneous Y79.8
   monitoring Y79.0
   prosthetic Y79.2
   rehabilitative Y79.1
   surgical Y79.3
   therapeutic Y79.1
  otorhinolaryngological Y72.8
   accessory Y72.2
   diagnostic Y72.0
   miscellaneous Y72.8
   monitoring Y72.0
   prosthetic Y72.2
   rehabilitative Y72.1
   surgical Y72.3
   therapeutic Y72.1
  personal use Y74.8
   accessory Y74.2
   diagnostic Y74.0
   miscellaneous Y74.8
   monitoring Y74.0
   prosthetic Y74.2
   rehabilitative Y74.1
   surgical Y74.3
   therapeutic Y74.1
  physical medicine Y80.8
   accessory Y80.2
   diagnostic Y80.0
   miscellaneous Y80.8
   monitoring Y80.0
   prosthetic Y80.2
   rehabilitative Y80.1
   surgical Y80.3
   therapeutic Y80.1
  plastic surgical Y81.8
   accessory Y81.2
   diagnostic Y81.0
   miscellaneous Y81.8
   monitoring Y81.0
   prosthetic Y81.2
   rehabilitative Y81.1
   surgical Y81.3
   therapeutic Y81.1
  radiological Y78.8
   accessory Y78.2
   diagnostic Y78.0

Incident, adverse - *continued*
   miscellaneous Y78.8
   monitoring Y78.0
   prosthetic Y78.2
   rehabilitative Y78.1
   surgical Y78.3
   therapeutic Y78.1
  urology Y73.8
   accessory Y73.2
   diagnostic Y73.0
   miscellaneous Y73.8
   monitoring Y73.0
   prosthetic Y73.2
   rehabilitative Y73.1
   surgical Y73.3
   therapeutic Y73.1
Incineration (accidental) —*see* Exposure, fire
Infanticide —*see* Assault
Infrasound waves (causing injury) W49.9
Ingestion
  foreign body (causing injury) (with obstruction) —*see* Foreign body, alimentary canal
  poisonous
   plant (s) X58
   substance NEC —*see* Table of drugs and chemicals
Inhalation
  excessively cold substance, man-made —*see* Exposure, cold, man-made
  food (any type) (into respiratory tract) (with asphyxia, obstruction respiratory tract, suffocation) (*see* categories T17 and) T18
  foreign body —*see* Foreign body, aspiration
  gastric contents (with asphyxia, obstruction respiratory passage, suffocation) T17.81
  hot air or gases X14.0
  liquid air, hydrogen, nitrogen W93.12
   suicide (attempt) X83.2
  steam X13.0
   assault X98.0
   stated as undetermined whether accidental or intentional Y27.0
   suicide (attempt) X77.0
  toxic gas —*see* Table of drugs and chemicals
  vomitus (with asphyxia, obstruction respiratory passage, suffocation) T17.81
Injury, injured (accidental (ly)) NOS X58
  by, caused by, from
   assault —*see* Assault
   law-enforcing agent, police, in course of legal intervention —*see* Legal intervention
   suicide (attempt) X83.8
  due to, in
   civil insurrection —*see* War operations
   fight (*see also* Assault, fight) Y04.0
   war operations —*see* War operations
  homicide (*see also* Assault) Y09
  inflicted (by)
   in course of arrest (attempted) , suppression of disturbance, maintenance of order, by law-enforcing agents —*see* Legal intervention
   other person
    stated as
     accidental X58
     intentional, homicide (attempt) —*see* Assault
     undetermined whether accidental or intentional Y33
   purposely (inflicted) by other person (s) —*see* Assault
  self-inflicted X83.8
   stated as accidental X58
  specified cause NEC X58

Inhalation - *continued*
  undetermined whether accidental or intentional Y33
Insolation, effects X30
Insufficient nourishment X58
Interruption of respiration (by)
  food (lodged in esophagus) (*see* categories T17 and) T18
  vomitus (lodged in esophagus) T17.81
Intervention, legal —*see* Legal intervention
Intoxication
  drug —*see* Table of drugs and chemicals
  poison —*see* Table of drugs and chemicals

J

Jammed (accidentally)
  between objects (moving) (stationary and moving) W23.0
   stationary W23.1
Jumped, jumping
  before moving object NEC X81.8
   motor vehicle X81.0
   subway train X81.1
   train X81.1
   undetermined whether accidental or intentional Y31
  from
   boat (into water) voluntarily, without accident (to or on boat) W16.712
    with
     accident to or on boat —*see* Accident, watercraft
     drowning or submersion W16.711
      suicide (attempt) X71.3
     striking bottom W16.722
      causing drowning W16.721
   building (*see also* Jumped, from, high place) W13.9
    burning (uncontrolled fire) X00.5
   high place NEC W17.89
    suicide (attempt) X80
    undetermined whether accidental or intentional Y30
   structure (*see also* Jumped, from, high place) W13.9
    burning (uncontrolled fire) X00.5
  into water W16.92
   causing drowning W16.91
   from, off watercraft —*see* Jumped, from, boat
   in
    natural body W16.612
     causing drowning W16.611
     striking bottom W16.622
      causing drowning W16.621
    specified place NEC W16.812
     causing drowning W16.811
     striking
      bottom W16.822
       causing drowning W16.821
      wall W16.832
       causing drowning W16.831
    swimming pool W16.512
     causing drowning W16.511
     striking
      bottom W16.522
       causing drowning W16.521
      wall W16.532
       causing drowning W16.531
  suicide (attempt) X71.3

K

Kicked by
  animal NEC W55.82

Kicked by - *continued*
person (s) (accidentally) W50.1
with intent to injure or kill Y04.0
as, or caused by, a crowd or human stampede (with fall) W52
assault Y04.0
homicide (attempt) Y04.0
in
fight Y04.0
legal intervention
injuring
bystander Y35.812
law enforcement personnel Y35.811
suspect Y35.813
Kicking against
object W22.8
sports equipment W21.9
stationary wW22.09
sports equipment W21.89
person —*see* Striking against, person
sports equipment W21.9
Killed, killing (accidentally) NOS (*see also* Injury) X58
in
action —*see* War operations
brawl, fight (hand) (fists) (foot) Y04.0
by weapon —*see also* Assault
cutting, piercing —*see* Assault, cutting or piercing instrument
firearm —*see* Discharge, firearm, by type, homicide
self
stated as
accident NOS X58
suicide —*see* Suicide
undetermined whether accidental or intentional Y33
Knocked down (accidentally) (by) NOS X58
animal (not being ridden) NEC —*see also* Struck by, by type of animal
crowd or human stampede W52
person W51
in brawl, fight Y04.0
transport vehicle NEC (*see also* Accident, transport) V09.9

L

Laceration NEC —*see* Injury
Lack of
care (helpless person) (infant) (newborn) X58
food except as result of abandonment or neglect X58
due to abandonment or neglect X58
water except as result of transport accident X58
due to transport accident —*see* Accident, transport, by type
helpless person, infant, newborn X58
Landslide (falling on transport vehicle) X36.1
caused by collapse of man-made structure X36.0 **Late effect** —*see* Sequelae
Legal
execution (any method) —*see* Legal, intervention
intervention (by)
baton —*see* Legal, intervention, blunt object, baton
bayonet —*see* Legal, intervention, sharp object, bayonet
blow —*see* Legal, intervention, manhandling
nt object
on
ring
nder Y35.312

Legal - *continued*
law enforcement personnel Y35.311
suspect Y35.313
injuring
bystander Y35.302
law enforcement personnel Y35.301
suspect Y35.303
specified NEC
injuring
bystander Y35.392
law enforcement personnel Y35.391
suspect Y35.393
stave
injuring
bystander Y35.392
law enforcement personnel Y35.391
suspect Y35.393
bomb —*see* Legal, intervention, explosive
cutting or piercing instrument —*see* Legal, intervention, sharp object
dynamite —*see* Legal, intervention, explosive, dynamite
explosive (s)   dynamite
injuring
bystander Y35.112
law enforcement personnel Y35.111
suspect Y35.113
grenade
injuring
bystander Y35.192
law enforcement personnel Y35.191
suspect Y35.193
injuring
bystander Y35.102
law enforcement personnel Y35.101
suspect Y35.103
mortar bomb
injuring
bystander Y35.192
law enforcement personnel Y35.191
suspect Y35.193
shell
injuring
bystander Y35.122
law enforcement personnel Y35.121
suspect Y35.123
specified NEC
injuring
bystander Y35.192
law enforcement personnel Y35.191
suspect Y35.193
firearm (s) (discharge)   handgun
injuring
bystander Y35.022
law enforcement personnel Y35.021
suspect Y35.023
injuring
bystander Y35.002
law enforcement personnel Y35.001
suspect Y35.003
machine gun
injuring
bystander Y35.012
law enforcement personnel Y35.011
suspect Y35.013
rifle pellet
injuring
bystander Y35.032
law enforcement personnel Y35.031
suspect Y35.033
rubber bullet
injuring
bystander Y35.042

Legal - *continued*
law enforcement personnel Y35.041
suspect Y35.043
shotgun —*see* Legal, intervention, firearm, specified NEC
specified NEC
injuring
bystander Y35.092
law enforcement personnel Y35.091
suspect Y35.093
gas (asphyxiation) (poisoning)   injuring
bystander Y35.202
law enforcement personnel Y35.201
suspect Y35.203
specified NEC
injuring
bystander Y35.292
law enforcement personnel Y35.291
suspect Y35.293
tear gas
injuring
bystander Y35.212
law enforcement personnel Y35.211
suspect Y35.213
grenade —*see* Legal, intervention, explosive, grenade
injuring
bystander Y35.92
law enforcement personnel Y35.91
suspect Y35.93
late effect (of) (*see with 7th character S*) Y35
manhandling
injuring
bystander Y35.812
law enforcement personnel Y35.811
suspect Y35.813
sequelae (of) (*see with 7th character S*) Y35
sharp objects
bayonet
injuring
bystander Y35.412
law enforcement personnel Y35.411
suspect Y35.413
injuring
bystander Y35.402
law enforcement personnel Y35.401
suspect Y35.403
specified NEC
injuring
bystander Y35.492
law enforcement personnel Y35.491
suspect Y35.493
specified means NEC
injuring
bystander Y35.892
law enforcement personnel Y35.891
suspect Y35.893
stabbing —*see* Legal, intervention, sharp object
stave —*see* Legal, intervention, blunt object, stave
tear gas —*see* Legal, intervention, gas, tear gas
truncheon —*see* Legal, intervention, blunt object, stave
Lightning (shock) (stroke) (struck by) —*see* subcategory T75.0
causing fire —*see* Exposure, fire
Loss of control (transport vehicle) NEC —*see* Accident, transport
Lost at sea NOS —*see* Drowning, due to, fall overboard

Low
  pressure (effects) —*see* Air, pressure, low
  temperature (effects) —*see* Exposure, cold
Lying before train, vehicle or other moving object X81.8
  subway train X81.1
  train X81.1
  undetermined whether accidental or intentional Y31
Lynching —*see* Assault

M

Malfunction (mechanism or component) (of)
  firearm W34.10
    airgun W34.110
    BB gun W34.110
    gas, air or spring-operated gun NEC W34.118
    handgun W32.1
    hunting rifle W33.12
    larger firearm W33.10
      specified NEC W33.19
    machine gun W33.13
    paintball gun W34.111
    pellet gun W34.110
    shotgun W33.11
    specified NEC W34.19
    Very pistol [flare] W34.19
  handgun —*see* Malfunction, firearm, handgun
Maltreatment —*see* Perpetrator
Mangled (accidentally) NOS X58
Manhandling (in brawl, fight) Y04.0
  legal intervention —*see* Legal, intervention, manhandling
Manslaughter (nonaccidental) —*see* Assault
Mauled by animal NEC W55.89
Medical procedure, complication of (delayed or as an abnormal reaction without mention of misadventure) —*see* Complication of or following, by specified type of procedure
  due to or as a result of misadventure —*see* Misadventure
Melting (due to fire) —*see also* Exposure, fire
  apparel NEC X06.3
  clothes, clothing NEC X06.3
    nightwear X05
  fittings or furniture (burning building) (uncontrolled fire) X00.8
  nightwear X05
  plastic jewelry X06.1
Mental cruelty X58
Military operations (injuries to military and civilians occurring during peacetime on military property and during routine military exercises and operations) (by) (from) (involving) Y37.90
  air blast Y37.20
  aircraft
  destruction —*see* Military operations, destruction of aircraft
  airway restriction —*see* Military operations, restriction of airways
  asphyxiation —*see* Military operations, restriction of airways
  biological weapons Y37.6X
    blast Y37.20
    blast fragments Y37.20
    blast wave Y37.20
    blast wind Y37.20
    bomb Y37.20
    dirty Y37.50
    gasoline Y37.31
    incendiary Y37.31
      petrol Y37.31

Military operations - *continued*
  bullet Y37.43
    incendiary Y37.32
    rubber Y37.41
  chemical weapons Y37.7X
  combat
  hand to hand (unarmed) combat Y37.44
    using blunt or piercing object Y37.45
  conflagration —*see* Military operations, fire
  conventional warfare NEC Y37.49
  depth-charge Y37.01
    destruction of aircraft Y37.10
    due to
    air to air missile Y37.11
      collision with other aircraft Y37.12
      detonation (accidental) of onboard munitions and explosives Y37.14
      enemy fire or explosives Y37.11
      explosive placed on aircraft Y37.11
      onboard fire Y37.13
      rocket propelled grenade [RPG] Y37.11
      small arms fire Y37.11
      surface to air missile Y37.11
      specified NEC Y37.19
  detonation (accidental) of
  onboard marine weapons Y37.05
    own munitions or munitions launch device Y37.24
  dirty bomb Y37.50
  explosion (of) Y37.20
    aerial bomb Y37.21
    bomb NOS (*see also* Military operations, bomb (s)) Y37.20
    own munitions or munitions launch device (accidental) Y37.24
    fragments Y37.20
    grenade Y37.29
    guided missile Y37.22
    improvised explosive device [IED] (person-borne) (roadside) (vehicle-borne) Y37.23
    land mine Y37.29
    marine mine (at sea) (in harbor) Y37.02
    marine weapon Y37.00
      specified NEC Y37.09
    sea-based artillery shell Y37.03
    specified NEC Y37.29
    torpedo Y37.04
  fire Y37.30
    specified NEC Y37.39
  firearms
  discharge Y37.43
    pellets Y37.42
  flamethrower Y37.33
  fragments (from) (of)
  improvised explosive device [IED] (person-borne) (roadside) (vehicle-borne) Y37.26
    munitions Y37.25
    specified NEC Y37.29
    weapons Y37.27
  friendly fire Y37.92
  hand to hand (unarmed) combat Y37.44
  hot substances —*see* Military operations, fire
  incendiary bullet Y37.32
  nuclear weapon (effects of) Y37.50
    acute radiation exposure Y37.54
    blast pressure Y37.51
    direct blast Y37.51
    direct heat Y37.53
    fallout exposure Y37.54
    fireball Y37.53
    indirect blast (struck or crushed by blast debris) (being thrown by blast) Y37.52

Military operations - *continued*
    ionizing radiation (immediate exposure) Y37.54
    nuclear radiation Y37.54
    radiation
    ionizing (immediate exposure) Y37.54
      nuclear Y37.54
      thermal Y37.53
      specified NEC Y37.59
    secondary effects Y37.54
    thermal radiation Y37.53
  restriction of air (airway)
    intentional Y37.46
    unintentional Y37.47
  rubber bullets Y37.41
  shrapnel NOS Y37.29
  suffocation —*see* Military operations, restriction of airways
  unconventional warfare NEC Y37.7X
  underwater blast NOS Y37.00
  warfare
  conventional NEC Y37.49
  unconventional NEC Y37.7X
  weapons
  biological weapons Y37.6X
  chemical Y37.7X
  nuclear (effects of) Y37.50
    acute radiation exposure Y37.54
    blast pressure Y37.51
    direct blast Y37.51
    direct heat Y37.53
    fallout exposure Y37.54
    fireball Y37.53
    indirect blast (struck or crushed by blast debris) (being thrown by blast) Y37.52
    radiation
    ionizing (immediate exposure) Y37.54
      nuclear Y37.54
      thermal Y37.53
    secondary effects Y37.54
    specified NEC Y37.59
  of mass destruction [WMD] Y37.91
  weapon of mass destruction [WMD] Y37.91
Misadventure (s) to patient (s) during surgical or medical care Y69
  contaminated medical or biological substance (blood, drug, fluid) Y64.9
    administered (by) NEC Y64.9
    immunization Y64.1
    infusion Y64.0
    injection Y64.1
    specified means NEC Y64.8
    transfusion Y64.0
    vaccination Y64.1
  excessive amount of blood or other fluid during transfusion or infusion Y63.0
  failure
  in dosage Y63.9
    electroshock therapy Y63.4
    inappropriate temperature (too hot or too cold) in local application and packing Y63.5
    infusion
      excessive amount of fluid Y63.0
      incorrect dilution of fluid Y63.1
    insulin-shock therapy Y63.4
    nonadministration of necessary drug or biological substance Y63.6
    overdose —*see* Table of drugs and chemicals radiation, in therapy Y63.2
    radiation
      overdose Y63.2
    specified procedure NEC Y63.8
    transfusion

Misadventure (s) to patient (s) - *continued*
　　excessive amount of blood Y63.0
　　mechanical, of instrument or apparatus (any)
(during any procedure) Y65.8
　　　sterile precautions (during procedure) Y62.9
　　　　aspiration of fluid or tissue (by puncture or
catheterization, except heart) Y62.6
　　　　　biopsy (except needle aspiration) Y62.8
　　　　　　needle (aspirating) Y62.6
　　　　　blood sampling Y62.6
　　　　　catheterization Y62.6
　　　　　　heart Y62.5
　　　　　dialysis (kidney) Y62.2
　　　　　endoscopic examination Y62.4
　　　　　enema Y62.8
　　　　　immunization Y62.3
　　　　　infusion Y62.1
　　　　　injection Y62.3
　　　　　needle biopsy Y62.6
　　　　　paracentesis (abdominal) (thoracic) Y62.6
　　　　　perfusion Y62.2
　　　　　puncture (lumbar) Y62.6
　　　　　removal of catheter or packing Y62.8
　　　　　specified procedure NEC Y62.8
　　　　　surgical operation Y62.0
　　　　　transfusion Y62.1
　　　　　vaccination Y62.3
　　suture or ligature during surgical procedure
Y65.2
　　to introduce or to remove tube or instrument
—*see* Failure, to
　hemorrhage —*see* Misadventure, cut, by type of
procedure
　inadvertent exposure of patient to radiation
Y63.3
　inappropriate
　　operation performed —*see* Inappropriate
operation performed
　　temperature (too hot or too cold) in local
application or packing Y63.5
　infusion (*see also* Misadventure, by type,
infusion) Y69
　　excessive amount of fluid Y63.0
　　incorrect dilution of fluid Y63.1
　　wrong fluid Y65.1
　mismatched blood in transfusion Y65.0
　nonadministration of necessary drug or
biological substance Y63.6
　overdose —*see* Table of drugs and chemicals
　　radiation (in therapy) Y63.2
　perforation —*see* Misadventure, cut, by type of
procedure
　performance of inappropriate operation —*see*
Inappropriate operation performed
　puncture —*see* Misadventure, cut, by type of
procedure
　specified type NEC Y65.8
　　failure
　　　suture or ligature during surgical operation
Y65.2
　　　to introduce or to remove tube or instrument
—*see* Failure, to
　　infusion of wrong fluid Y65.1
　　performance of inappropriate operation —*see*
Inappropriate operation performed
　　transfusion of mismatched blood Y65.0
　　wrong
　　　fluid in infusion Y65.1
　　　placement of endotracheal tube during
anesthetic procedure Y65.3
　　~~sfusion~~ —*see* Misadventure, by type,
　　~~sion~~
　　~~ve~~ amount of blood Y63.0

Misadventure (s) to patient (s) - *continued*
　mismatched blood Y65.0
　wrong
　　drug given in error —*see* Table of drugs and
chemicals
　　fluid in infusion Y65.1
　　placement of endotracheal tube during
anesthetic procedure Y65.3
Mismatched blood in transfusion Y65.0
Motion sickness T75.3
Mountain sickness W94.11
Mudslide (of cataclysmic nature) —*see*
Landslide
Murder (attempt) —*see* Assault

N

Nail, contact with W45.0
　gun W29.4
Neglect (criminal) (homicidal intent) X58
Noise (causing injury) (pollution) W42.9
　supersonic W42.0
Nonadministration (of)
　drug or biological substance (necessary) Y63.6
　surgical and medical care Y66
Nosocomial condition Y95

O

Object
　falling
　　from, in, on, hitting
　　　machinery —*see* Contact, with, by type of
machine
　set in motion by
　　accidental explosion or rupture of pressure
vessel W38
　　　firearm —*see* Discharge, firearm, by type
　　　machine (ry) —*see* Contact, with, by type of
machine
Overdose (drug) —*see* Table of drugs and
chemicals
　radiation Y63.2
Overexertion —see category Y93
Overexposure (accidental) (to)
　cold (*see also* Exposure, cold) X31
　　due to man-made conditions —*see* Exposure,
cold, man-made
　heat (*see also* Heat) X30
　radiation —*see* Radiation
　radioactivity W88.0
　sun (sunburn) X32
　weather NEC —*see* Forces of nature
　wind NEC —*see* Forces of nature
Overheated —*see* Heat
Overturning (accidental)
　machinery —*see* Contact, with, by type of
machine
　transport vehicle NEC (*see also* Accident,
transport) V89.9
　watercraft (causing drowning, submersion) —
see also Drowning, due to, accident to,
watercraft, overturning
　　causing injury except drowning or submersion
—*see* Accident, watercraft, causing, injury NEC

P

**Parachute descent (voluntary) (without
accident to aircraft)** V97.29
　due to accident to aircraft —*see* Accident,
transport, aircraft
Pecked by bird W61.99
**Perforation during medical or surgical
treatment as misadventure** —*see*
Misadventure, cut, by type of procedure

**Perpetrator, perpetration, of assault,
maltreatment and neglect (by)** Y07.9
　boyfriend Y07.03
　brother Y07.410
　　stepbrother Y07.435
　coach Y07.53
　cousin
　　female Y07.491
　　male Y07.490
　daycare provider Y07.519
　　at-home
　　　adult care Y07.512
　　　childcare Y07.510
　　care center
　　　adult care Y07.513
　　　childcare Y07.511
　family member NEC Y07.499
　father Y07.11
　　adoptive Y07.13
　　foster Y07.420
　　stepfather Y07.430
　foster father Y07.420
　foster mother Y07.421
　girl friend Y07.04
　healthcare provider Y07.529
　　mental health Y07.521
　　specified NEC Y07.528
　husband Y07.01
　instructor Y07.53
　mother Y07.12
　　adoptive Y07.14
　　foster Y07.421
　　stepmother Y07.433
　nonfamily member Y07.50
　　specified NEC Y07.59
　nurse Y07.528
　occupational therapist Y07.528
　partner of parent
　　female Y07.434
　　male Y07.432
　physical therapist Y07.528
　sister Y07.411
　speech therapist Y07.528
　stepbrother Y07.435
　stepfather Y07.430
　stepmother Y07.433
　stepsister Y07.436
　teacher Y07.53
　wife Y07.02
Piercing —*see* Contact, with, by type of object or
machine
Pinched
　between objects (moving) (stationary and
moving) W23.0
　　stationary W23.1
Pinned under machine (ry) —*see* Contact, with,
by type of machine
Place of occurrence Y92.9
　abandoned house Y92.89
　airplane Y92.813
　airport Y92.520
　ambulatory health services establishment NEC
Y92.538
　ambulatory surgery center Y92.530
　amusement park Y92.831
　apartment (co-op) —*see* Place of occurrence,
residence, apartment
　assembly hall Y92.29
　bank Y92.510
　barn Y92.71
　baseball field Y92.320
　basketball court Y92.310
　beach Y92.832

Place of occurrence - *continued*
boarding house —*see* Place of occurrence, residence, boarding house
boat Y92.814
bowling alley Y92.39
bridge Y92.89
building under construction Y92.61
bus Y92.811
  station Y92.521
cafe Y92.511
campsite Y92.833
campus —*see* Place of occurrence, school
canal Y92.89
car Y92.810
casino Y92.59
children's home —*see* Place of occurrence, residence, institutional, orphanage
church Y92.22
cinema Y92.26
clubhouse Y92.29
coal pit Y92.64
college (community) Y92.214
condominium —*see* Place of occurrence, residence, apartment
construction area —*see* Place of occurrence, industrial and construction area
convalescent home —*see* Place of occurrence, residence, institutional, nursing home
court-house Y92.240
cricket ground Y92.328
cultural building Y92.258
  art gallery Y92.250
  museum Y92.251
  music hall Y92.252
  opera house Y92.253
  specified NEC Y92.258
  theater Y92.254
dancehall Y92.252
day nursery Y92.210
dentist office Y92.531
derelict house Y92.89
desert Y92.820
dock NOS Y92.89
dockyard Y92.62
doctor's office Y92.531
dormitory —*see* Place of occurrence, residence, institutional, school dormitory
dry dock Y92.62
factory (building) (premises) Y92.63
farm (land under cultivation) (outbuildings) Y92.79
  barn Y92.71
  chicken coop Y92.72
  field Y92.73
  hen house Y92.72
  house —*see* Place of occurrence, residence, house
  orchard Y92.74
  specified NEC Y92.79
football field Y92.321
forest Y92.821
freeway Y92.411
gallery Y92.250
garage (commercial) Y92.59
  boarding house Y92.044
  military base Y92.135
  mobile home Y92.025
  nursing home Y92.124
  orphanage Y92.114
  private house Y92.015
  reform school Y92.155
gas station Y92.524
gasworks Y92.69

Place of occurrence - *continued*
golf course Y92.39
gravel pit Y92.64
grocery Y92.512
gymnasium Y92.39
handball court Y92.318
harbor Y92.89
harness racing course Y92.39
healthcare provider office Y92.531
highway (interstate) Y92.411
hill Y92.828
hockey rink Y92.330
home —*see* Place of occurrence, residence
hospice —*see* Place of occurrence, residence, institutional, nursing home
hospital Y92.239
  cafeteria Y92.233
  corridor Y92.232
  operating room Y92.234
  patient
    bathroom Y92.231
    room Y92.230
  specified NEC Y92.238
hotel Y92.59
house —*see also* Place of occurrence, residence
  abandoned Y92.89
  under construction Y92.61
industrial and construction area (yard) Y92.69
  building under construction Y92.61
  dock Y92.62
  dry dock Y92.62
  factory Y92.63
  gasworks Y92.69
  mine Y92.64
  oil rig Y92.65
  pit Y92.64
  power station Y92.69
  shipyard Y92.62
  specified NEC Y92.69
  tunnel under construction Y92.69
  workshop Y92.69
kindergarten Y92.211
lacrosse field Y92.328
lake Y92.828
library Y92.241
mall Y92.59
market Y92.512
marsh Y92.828
military
  base —*see* Place of occurrence, residence, institutional, military base
  training ground Y92.84
mine Y92.64
mosque Y92.22
motel Y92.59
motorway (interstate) Y92.411
mountain Y92.828
movie-house Y92.26
museum Y92.251
music-hall Y92.252
not applicable Y92.9
nuclear power station Y92.69
nursing home —*see* Place of occurrence, residence, institutional, nursing home
office building Y92.59
offshore installation Y92.65
oil rig Y92.65
old people's home —*see* Place of occurrence, residence, institutional, specified NEC
opera-house Y92.253
orphanage —*see* Place of occurrence, residence, institutional, orphanage
outpatient surgery center Y92.530

Place of occurrence - *continued*
park (public) Y92.830
  amusement Y92.831
parking garage Y92.89
  lot Y92.481
pavement Y92.480
physician office Y92.531
polo field Y92.328
pond Y92.828
post office Y92.242
power station Y92.69
prairie Y92.828
prison —*see* Place of occurrence, residence, institutional, prison
public
  administration building Y92.248
    city hall Y92.243
    courthouse Y92.240
    library Y92.241
    post office Y92.242
    specified NEC Y92.248
  building NEC Y92.29
  hall Y92.29
  place NOS Y92.89
race course Y92.39
radio station Y92.59
railway line (bridge) Y92.85
ranch (outbuildings) —*see* Place of occurrence, farm
recreation area Y92.838
  amusement park Y92.831
  beach Y92.832
  campsite Y92.833
  park (public) Y92.830
  seashore Y92.832
  specified NEC Y92.838
religious institution Y92.22
reform school
—*see* Place of occurrence, residence, institutional, reform school
residence (non-institutional) (private) Y92.009
  apartment Y92.039
    bathroom Y92.031
    bedroom Y92.032
    kitchen Y92.030
    specified NEC Y92.038
  bathroom Y92.002
  bedroom Y92.003
  boarding house Y92.049
    bathroom Y92.041
    bedroom Y92.042
    driveway Y92.043
    garage Y92.044
    garden Y92.046
    kitchen Y92.040
    specified NEC Y92.048
    swimming pool Y92.045
    yard Y92.046
  dining room Y92.001
  garden Y92.007
  home Y92.009
  house, single family Y92.019
    bathroom Y92.012
    bedroom Y92.013
    dining room Y92.011
    driveway Y92.014
    garage Y92.015
    garden Y92.017
    kitchen Y92.010
    specified NEC Y92.018
    swimming pool Y92.016
    yard Y92.017
  institutional Y92.10

Place of occurrence - *continued*
  truck Y92.812
  warehouse Y92.59
  water reservoir Y92.89
  wilderness area Y92.828
    desert Y92.820
    forest Y92.821
    marsh Y92.828
    mountain Y92.828
    prairie Y92.828
    specified NEC Y92.828
    swamp Y92.828
  workshop Y92.69
  yard, private Y92.096
    boarding house Y92.046
    single family house Y92.017
    mobile home Y92.027
  youth center Y92.29
  zoo (zoological garden) Y92.834
Plumbism —*see* Table of drugs and chemicals,
lead
Poisoning (accidental) (by) —*see also* Table of
drugs and chemicals
  by plant, thorns, spines, sharp leaves or other
  mechanisms NEC X58
  carbon monoxide
    generated by
      motor vehicle —*see* Accident, transport
      watercraft (in transit) (not in transit) V93.89
        ferry boat V93.81
        fishing boat V93.82
        jet skis V93.83
        liner V93.81
        merchant ship V93.80
        passenger ship V93.81
        powered craft NEC V93.83
  caused by injection of poisons into skin by plant
  thorns, spines, sharp leaves X58
    marine or sea plants (venomous) X58
  exhaust gas
    generated by
      motor vehicle —*see* Accident, transport
      watercraft (in transit) (not in transit) V93.89
        ferry boat V93.81
        fishing boat V93.82
        jet skis V93.83
        liner V93.81
        merchant ship V93.80
        passenger ship V93.81
        powered craft NEC V93.83
  fumes or smoke due to
    explosion (*see also* Explosion) W40.9
    fire —*see* Exposure, fire
    ignition —*see* Ignition
  gas
    in legal intervention —*see* Legal, intervention,
    gas
      legal execution —*see* Legal, intervention, gas
    in war operations —*see* War operations
  legal
    execution —*see* Legal, intervention, gas
    intervention
      by gas —*see* Legal, intervention, gas
      other specified means —*see* Legal,
    intervention, specified means NEC
Powder burn (by) (from)
  airgun W34.110
  BB gun W34.110
  firearm NEC W34.19
  gas, air or spring-operated gun NEC W34.118
  handgun W32.1
  hunting rifle W33.12
  larger firearm W33.10

Powder burn - *continued*
    specified NEC W33.19
  machine gun W33.13
  paintball gun W34.111
  pellet gun W34.110
  shotgun W33.11
  Very pistol [flare] W34.19
Premature cessation (of) surgical and medical
care Y66
Privation (food) (water) X58
Procedure (operation)
  correct, on wrong side or body part (wrong side)
  (wrong site) Y65.53
  intended for another patient done on wrong
  patient Y65.52
  performed on patient not scheduled for surgery
  Y65.52
  performed on wrong patient Y65.52
  wrong, performed on correct patient Y65.51
Prolonged
  sitting in transport vehicle —*see* Travel, by type
  of vehicle
  stay in
    high altitude as cause of anoxia, barodontalgia,
    barotitis or hypoxia W94.11
    weightless environment X52
Pulling, excessive —see category Y93
Puncture, puncturing —*see also* Contact, with,
by type of object or machine
  by
    plant thorns, spines, sharp leaves or other
  mechanisms NEC W60
  during medical or surgical treatment as
  misadventure —*see* Misadventure, cut, by type
  of procedure
Pushed, pushing (accidental) (injury in)
(overexertion) —see category Y93
  by other person (s) (accidental) W51
    with fall W03
      due to ice or snow W00.0
    as, or caused by, a crowd or human stampede
  (with fall) W52
      before moving object NEC Y02.8
        motor vehicle Y02.0
        subway train Y02.1
        train Y02.1
      from
        high place NEC
          in accidental circumstances W17.89
          stated as
            intentional, homicide (attempt) Y01
            undetermined whether accidental or
      intentional Y30
        transport vehicle NEC (*see also* Accident,
        transport) V89.9
          stated as
            intentional, homicide (attempt) Y08.89

R
Radiation (exposure to)   arc lamps W89.0
  atomic power plant (malfunction) NEC W88.1
  complication of or abnormal reaction to medical
  radiotherapy Y84.2
  electromagnetic, ionizing W88.0
  gamma rays W88.1
  in
    war operations (from or following nuclear
      explosion) —*see* War operations
  inadvertent exposure of patient (receiving test or
  therapy) Y63.3
  infrared (heaters and lamps) W90.1
    excessive heat from W92

Radiation (exposure to) - *continued*
  ionized, ionizing (particles, artificially
  accelerated)   radioisotopes W88.1
    specified NEC W88.8
    x-rays W88.0
  isotopes, radioactive —*see* Radiation,
  radioactive isotopes
  laser (s) W90.2
    in war operations —*see* War operations
    misadventure in medical care Y63.2
  light sources (man-made visible and ultraviolet)
  W89.9
    natural X32
    specified NEC W89.8
    tanning bed W89.1
    welding light W89.0
  man-made visible light W89.9
    specified NEC W89.8
    tanning bed W89.1
    welding light W89.0
  microwave W90.8
  misadventure in medical or surgical procedure
  Y63.2
  natural NEC X39.08
    radon X39.01
  overdose (in medical or surgical procedure)
  Y63.2
  radar W90.0
  radioactive isotopes (any) W88.1
    atomic power plant malfunction W88.1
    misadventure in medical or surgical treatment
  Y63.2
  radiofrequency W90.0
  radium NEC W88.1
  sun X32
  ultraviolet (light) (man-made) W89.9
    natural X32
    specified NEC W89.8
    tanning bed W89.1
    welding light W89.0
  welding arc, torch, or light W89.0
    excessive heat from W92
  x-rays (hard) (soft) W88.0
Range disease W94.11
Rape (attempted) T74.2
Rat bite W53.11
Reaction, abnormal to medical procedure (*see*
  also Complication of or following, by type of
  procedure) Y84.9
  with misadventure —*see* Misadventure
  biologicals —*see* Table of drugs and chemicals
  drugs —*see* Table of drugs and chemicals
  vaccine —*see* Table of drugs and chemicals
Recoil
  airgun W34.110
  BB gun W34.110
  firearm NEC W34.19
  gas, air or spring-operated gun NEC W34.118
  handgun W32.1
  hunting rifle W33.12
  larger firearm W33.10
    specified NEC W33.19
  machine gun W33.13
  paintball gun W34.111
  pellet W34.110
  shotgun W33.11
  Very pistol [flare] W34.19
Reduction in
  atmospheric pressure
  —*see* Air, pressure, change
Rock falling on or hitting (accidentally)
(person) W20.8
  in cave-in W20.0

Run over (accidentally) (by)
  animal (not being ridden) NEC W55.89
  machinery —*see* Contact, with, by specified
  type of machine
  transport vehicle NEC (*see also* Accident,
  transport) V09.9
    intentional homicide (attempt) Y03.0
    motor NEC V09.20
      intentional homicide (attempt) Y03.0
Running
  before moving object X81.8
Running - continued
  motor vehicle X81.0
Running off, away
  animal (being ridden) (*see also* Accident,
  transport) V80.918
    not being ridden W55.89
  animal-drawn vehicle NEC (*see also* Accident,
  transport) V80.928
  highway, road (way) , street
    transport vehicle NEC (*see also* Accident,
    transport) V89.9
Rupture pressurized devices —*see* Explosion,
  by type of device

S

Saturnism —*see* Table of drugs and chemicals, lead
Scald, scalding (accidental) (by) (from) (in) X19
  air (hot) X14.1
  gases (hot) X14.1
  homicide (attempt) —*see* Assault, burning, hot object
  inflicted by other person
    stated as intentional, homicide (attempt) —*see* Assault, burning, hot object
  liquid (boiling) (hot) NEC X12
    stated as undetermined whether accidental or intentional Y27.2
    suicide (attempt) X77.2
  local application of externally applied substance in medical or surgical care Y63.5
  metal (molten) (liquid) (hot) NEC X18
  self-inflicted X77.9
  stated as undetermined whether accidental or intentional Y27.8
  steam X13.1
    assault X98.0
    stated as undetermined whether accidental or intentional Y27.0
    suicide (attempt) X77.0
  suicide (attempt) X77.9
  vapor (hot) X13.1
    assault X98.0
    stated as undetermined whether accidental or intentional Y27.0
    suicide (attempt) X77.0
Scratched by
  cat W55.03
  person (s) (accidentally) W50.4
    with intent to injure or kill Y04.0
    as, or caused by, a crowd or human stampede (with fall) W52
    assault Y04.0
    homicide (attempt) Y04.0
    in
      fight Y04.0
      legal intervention
        injuring
          bystander Y35.892
          law enforcement personnel Y35.891
          suspect Y35.893

Seasickness T75.3
Self-harm NEC —*see also* External cause by type, undetermined whether accidental or intentional
  intentional —*see* Suicide
  poisoning NEC —*see* Table of drugs and biologicals, accident
Self-inflicted (injury) NEC —*see also* External cause by type, undetermined whether accidental or intentional
  intentional —*see* Suicide
Self-inflicted (injury) - continued
  poisoning NEC —*see* Table of drugs and biologicals, accident
Sequelae (of)
  accident NEC —*see* W00
  X58 with 7th character S
  assault (homicidal) (any means) —*see* X92
  Y08 with 7th character S
  homicide, attempt (any means) —*see* X92
  Y08 with 7th character S
  injury undetermined whether accidentally or purposely inflicted —*see* Y21
  Y33 with 7th character S
  intentional self-harm (classifiable to X71 X83) —*see* X71
  X83 with 7th character S
  legal intervention (*see* with 7th character S) Y35
  motor vehicle accident —*see* V00
  V99 with 7th character S
  suicide, attempt (any means) —*see* X71
  X83 with 7th character S
  transport accident —*see* V00
  V99 with 7th character S
  war operations —*see* War operations
Shock
  electric —*see* Exposure, electric current
  from electric appliance (any) (faulty) W86.8
    domestic W86.0
    suicide (attempt) X83.1
Shooting, shot (accidental (ly)) —*see also* Discharge, firearm, by type
  herself or himself —*see* Discharge, firearm by type, self-inflicted
  homicide (attempt) —*see* Discharge, firearm by type, homicide
  in war operations —*see* War operations
  inflicted by other person —*see* Discharge, firearm by type, homicide
    accidental —*see* Discharge, firearm, by type of firearm
  legal
    execution —*see* Legal, intervention, firearm
    intervention —*see* Legal, intervention, firearm
  self-inflicted —*see* Discharge, firearm by type, suicide
    accidental —*see* Discharge, firearm, by type of firearm
  suicide (attempt) —*see* Discharge, firearm by type, suicide
Shoving (accidentally) by other person —*see* Pushing, by other person
Sickness
  alpine W94.11
  motion —*see* Motion
  mountain W94.11
Sinking (accidental)
  watercraft (causing drowning, submersion) —*see also* Drowning, due to, accident to, watercraft, sinking
    causing injury except drowning or submersion —*see* Accident, watercraft, causing, injury NEC
Siriasis X32

Slashed wrists —*see* Cut, self-inflicted
Slipping (accidental) (on same level) (with fall) W01.0
  on
    ice W00.0
      with skates —*see* Accident, transport, pedestrian, conveyance
    mud W01.0
    oil W01.0
    snow W00.0
      with skis —*see* Accident, transport, pedestrian, conveyance
    surface (slippery) (wet) NEC W01.0
  without fall W18.40
    due to
      specified NEC W18.49
      stepping from one level to another W18.43
      stepping into hole or opening W18.42
      stepping on object W18.41
Sliver, wood, contact with W45.8
Smoldering (due to fire) —*see* Exposure, fire
Sodomy (attempted) by force T74.2
Sound waves (causing injury) W42.9
  supersonic W42.0
Splinter, contact with W45.8
Stab, stabbing —*see* Cut
Starvation X58
Status of external cause Y99.9
  child assisting in compensated work for family Y99.8
  civilian activity done for financial or other compensation Y99.0
  civilian activity done for income or pay Y99.0
  family member assisting in compensated work for other family member Y99.8
  hobby not done for income Y99.8
  leisure activity Y99.8
  military activity Y99.1
  off-duty activity of military personnel Y99.8
  recreation or sport not for income or while a student Y99.8
  specified NEC Y99.8
  student activity Y99.8
  volunteer activity Y99.2
Stepped on
  by
    animal (not being ridden) NEC W55.89
    crowd or human stampede W52
    person W50.0
Stepping on
  object W22.8
    with fall W18.31
    sports equipment W21.9
    stationary W22.09
      sports equipment W21.89
  person W51
    by crowd or human stampede W52
  sports equipment W21.9
Sting
  arthropod, nonvenomous W57
  insect, nonvenomous W57
Storm (cataclysmic) —*see* Forces of nature, cataclysmic storm
Straining, excessive —see category Y93
Strangling —*see* Strangulation
Strangulation (accidental) —see category T71
Strenuous movements —see category Y93
Striking against
  airbag (automobile) W22.10
    driver side W22.11
    front passenger side W22.12
    specified NEC W22.19
  bottom when

Striking against - *continued*
 diving or jumping into water (in) W16.822
  causing drowning W16.821
  from boat W16.722
   causing drowning W16.721
  natural body W16.622
   causing drowning W16.821
  swimming pool W16.522
   causing drowning W16.521
 falling into water (in) W16.322
  causing drowning W16.321
  fountain —*see* Striking against, bottom
 when, falling into water, specified NEC
  natural body W16.122
   causing drowning W16.121
  reservoir —*see* Striking against, bottom
 when, falling into water, specified NEC
  specified NEC W16.322
   causing drowning W16.321
  swimming pool W16.022
   causing drowning W16.021
 diving board (swimming-pool) W21.4
 object W22.8
  with
   drowning or submersion —*see* Drowning
   fall —*see* Fall, due to, bumping against,
 object
  caused by crowd or human stampede (with
 fall) W52
   furniture W22.03
   lamppost W22.02
   sports equipment W21.9
   stationary W22.09
    sports equipment W21.89
   wall W22.01
 person (s) W51
  with fall W03
   due to ice or snow W00.0
  as, or caused by, a crowd or human stampede
 (with fall) W52
  assault Y04.2
  homicide (attempt) Y04.2
 sports equipment W21.9
 wall (when) W22.01
  diving or jumping into water (in) W16.832
   causing drowning W16.831
   swimming pool W16.532
    causing drowning W16.531
  falling into water (in) W16.332
   causing drowning W16.331
  fountain —*see* Striking against, wall when,
 falling into water, specified NEC
   natural body W16.132
    causing drowning W16.131
  reservoir —*see* Striking against, wall when,
 falling into water, specified NEC
  specified NEC W16.332
   causing drowning W16.331
  swimming pool W16.032
   causing drowning W16.031
 swimming pool (when) W22.042
  causing drowning W22.041
  diving or jumping into water W16.532
   causing drowning W16.531
  falling into water W16.032
   causing drowning W16.031

Struck (accidentally) by
 airbag (automobile) W22.10
  driver side W22.11
  front passenger side W22.12
  specified NEC W22.19
 alligator W58.02
 animal (not being ridden) NEC W55.89

Struck (accidentally) by - *continued*
 avalanche —*see* Landslide
 ball (hit) (thrown) W21.00
  assault Y08.09
  baseball W21.03
  basketball W21.05
  golf ball W21.04
  football W21.01
  soccer W21.02
  softball W21.07
  specified NEC W21.09
  volleyball W21.06
 bat or racquet
  baseball bat W21.11
   assault Y08.02
  golf club W21.13
   assault Y08.09
  specified NEC W21.19
   assault Y08.09
  tennis racquet W21.12
   assault Y08.09
 bullet —*see also* Discharge, firearm by type
  in war operations —*see* War operations
 crocodile W58.12
 dog W54.1
 flare, Very pistol —*see* Discharge, firearm NEC
 hailstones X39.8
 hockey (ice) field
   puck W21.221
   stick W21.211
  puck W21.220
  stick W21.210
   assault Y08.01
 landslide —*see* Landslide
 law-enforcement agent (on duty) —*see* Legal,
 intervention, manhandling
  with blunt object —*see* Legal, intervention,
 blunt object
 lightning —see subcategory T75.0
  causing fire —*see* Exposure, fire
 machine —*see* Contact, with, by type of
 machine
 mammal NEC W55.89
  marine W56.32
 marine animal W56.82
 missile
  firearm —*see* Discharge, firearm by type
  in war operations —*see* War operations,
 missile
 object W22.8
  blunt W22.8
   assault Y00
   suicide (attempt) X79
   undetermined whether accidental or
 intentional Y29
  falling W20.8
   from, in, on
    building W20.1
     burning (uncontrolled fire) X00.4
    cataclysmic
     earth surface movement NEC —*see*
 Landslide
     storm *see* Forces of nature, cataclysmic
 storm
    cave-in W20.0
    earthquake X34
    machine (in operation) —*see* Contact, with,
 by type of machine
    structure W20.1
     burning X00.4
    transport vehicle (in motion) —*see*
 Accident, transport, by type of vehicle
     watercraft V93.49

Struck (accidentally) by - *continued*
 due to
  accident to craft V91.39
   powered craft V91.33
    ferry boat V91.31
    fishing boat V91.32
    jet skis V91.33
    liner V91.31
    merchant ship V91.30
    passenger ship V91.31
   unpowered craft V91.38
    canoe V91.35
    inflatable V91.36
    kayak V91.35
    sailboat V91.34
    surf-board V91.38
    windsurfer V91.38
  powered craft V93.43
   ferry boat V93.41
   fishing boat V93.42
   jet skis V93.43
   liner V93.41
   merchant ship V93.40
   passenger ship V93.41
  unpowered craft V93.48
   sailboat V93.44
   surf-board V93.48
   windsurfer V93.48
 moving NEC W20.8
 projected W20.8
  assault Y00
  in sports W21.9
   assault Y08.09
  ball W21.00
   baseball W21.03
   basketball W21.05
   football W21.01
   golf ball W21.04
   soccer W21.02
   softball W21.07
   specified NEC W21.09
   volleyball W21.06
  bat or racquet
   baseball bat W21.11
    assault Y08.02
   golf club W21.13
    assault Y08.09
   specified NEC W21.19
    assault Y08.09
   tennis racquet W21.12
    assault Y08.09
  hockey (ice)
   field
    puck W21.221
    stick W21.211
   puck W21.220
   stick W21.210
    assault Y08.01
  specified NEC W21.89
 set in motion by explosion —*see* Explosion
 thrown W20.8
  assault Y00
  in sports W21.9
   assault Y08.09
  ball W21.00
   baseball W21.03
   basketball W21.05
   football W21.01
   golf ball W21.04
   soccer W21.02
   soft ball W21.07
   specified NEC W21.09
   volleyball W21.06

Struck (accidentally) by - *continued*
  bat or racquet
    baseball bat W21.11
      assault Y08.02
    golf club W21.13
      assault Y08.09
    specified NEC W21.19
      assault Y08.09
    tennis racquet W21.12
      assault Y08.09
  hockey (ice)
    field
      puck W21.221
      stick W21.211
    puck W21.220
    stick W21.210
      assault Y08.01
    specified NEC W21.89
  other person (s) W50.0
  with
    blunt object W22.8
      intentional, homicide (attempt) Y00
      sports equipment W21.9
      undetermined whether accidental or
  intentional Y29
    fall W03
      due to ice or snow W00.0
  as, or caused by, a crowd or human stampede
  (with fall) W52
    assault Y04.2
    homicide (attempt) Y04.2
  in legal intervention
    injuring
      bystander Y35.812
      law enforcement personnel Y35.811
      suspect Y35.813
  sports equipment W21.9
  police (on duty) —*see* Legal, intervention,
  manhandling
    with blunt object —*see* Legal, intervention,
  blunt object
  sports equipment W21.9
    assault Y08.09
    ball W21.00
      baseball W21.03
      basketball W21.05
      football W21.01
      golf ball W21.04
      soccer W21.02
      soft ball W21.07
      specified NEC W21.09
      volleyball W21.06
    bat or racquet
      baseball bat W21.11
        assault Y08.02
      golf club W21.13
        assault Y08.09
      specified NEC W21.19
      tennis racquet W21.12
        assault Y08.09
    cleats (shoe) W21.31
    foot wear NEC W21.39
    football helmet W21.81
    hockey (ice)
      field
        puck W21.221
        stick W21.211
      puck W21.220
      stick W21.210
        assault Y08.01
    skate blades W21.32
    ~cified NEC W21.89
    ~ult Y08.09

Struck (accidentally) by - *continued*
  thunderbolt —see subcategory T75.0
    causing fire —*see* Exposure, fire
  transport vehicle NEC (*see also* Accident,
  transport) V09.9
    intentional, homicide (attempt) Y03.0
    motor NEC (*see also* Accident, transport)
  V09.20
      homicide Y03.0
  vehicle (transport) NEC —*see* Accident,
  transport, by type of vehicle
    stationary (falling from jack, hydraulic lift,
    ramp) W20.8
Stumbling
  over
    animal NEC W01.0
      with fall W18.09
    carpet, rug or (small) object W22.8
      with fall W18.09
    person W51
      with fall W03
        due to ice or snow W00.0
  without fall W18.40
    due to
      specified NEC W18.49
      stepping from one level to another W18.43
      stepping into hole or opening W18.42
      stepping on object W18.41
Submersion (accidental) —*see* Drowning
Suffocation (accidental) (by external means)
(by pressure) (mechanical) (*see also* category)
T71
  due to, by
    avalanche —*see* Landslide
    explosion —*see* Explosion
    fire —*see* Exposure, fire
    food, any type (aspiration) (ingestion)
    (inhalation) (*see* categories T17 and) T18
    ignition —*see* Ignition
    landslide —*see* Landslide
    machine (ry) —*see* Contact, with, by type of
  machine
    vomitus (aspiration) (inhalation) T17.81
    in
      burning building X00.8
Suicide, suicidal (attempted) (by) X83.8
  blunt object X79
  burning, burns X76
    hot object X77.9
      fluid NEC X77.2
      household appliance X77.3
      specified NEC X77.8
      steam X77.0
      tap water X77.1
      vapors X77.0
  caustic substance —*see* Table of drugs and
  chemicals
  cold, extreme X83.2
  collision of motor vehicle with
    motor vehicle X82.0
    specified NEC X82.8
    train X82.1
    tree X82.2
  crashing of aircraft X83.0
  cut (any part of body) X78.9
  cutting or piercing instrument X78.9
    dagger X78.2
    glass X78.0
    knife X78.1
    specified NEC X78.8
    sword X78.2
  drowning (in) X71.9
    bathtub X71.0

Suicide, suicidal (attempted) - *continued*
  natural water X71.3
  specified NEC X71.8
  swimming pool X71.1
    following fall X71.2
  electrocution X83.1
  explosive (s) (material) X75
  fire, flames X76
  firearm X74.9
    airgun X74.01
    handgun X72
    hunting rifle X73.1
    larger X73.9
      specified NEC X73.8
    machine gun X73.2
    shotgun X73.0
    specified NEC X74.8
  hanging X83.8
  hot object —*see* Suicide, burning, hot object
  jumping
    before moving object X81.8
      motor vehicle X81.0
      subway train X81.1
      train X81.1
    from high place X80
  late effect of attempt —*see* X71
  X83 with 7th character S
  lying before moving object, train, vehicle X81.8
  poisoning —*see* Table of drugs and chemicals
  puncture (any part of body) —*see* Suicide,
  cutting or piercing instrument
  scald —*see* Suicide, burning, hot object
  sequelae of attempt —*see* X71
  X83 with 7th character S
  sharp object (any) —*see* Suicide, cutting or
  piercing instrument
  shooting —*see* Suicide, firearm
  specified means NEC X83.8
  stab (any part of body) —*see* Suicide, cutting or
  piercing instrument
  steam, hot vapors X77.0
  strangulation X83.8
  submersion —*see* Suicide, drowning
  suffocation X83.8
  wound NEC X83.8
Sunstroke X32
Supersonic waves (causing injury) W42.0
Surgical procedure, complication of (delayed
or as an abnormal reaction without mention
of misadventure) —*see also* Complication of
  or following, by type of procedure
  due to or as a result of misadventure —*see*
  Misadventure
Swallowed, swallowing
  foreign body —*see* Foreign body, alimentary
  canal
  poison —*see* Table of drugs and chemicals
  substance
    caustic or corrosive —*see* Table of drugs and
  chemicals
    poisonous —*see* Table of drugs and chemicals

T

Tackle in sport W03
Terrorism (involving) Y38.80
  biological weapons Y38.6X
    chemical weapons Y38.7X
    conflagration Y38.3X
    drowning and submersion Y38.89
    explosion Y38.2X
      destruction of aircraft Y38.1X
      marine weapons Y38.0X
    fire Y38.3X

Terrorism (involving) - *continued*
   firearms Y38.4X
   hot substances Y38.5X   lasers Y38.89
   nuclear weapons Y38.5X
   piercing or stabbing instruments Y38.89
   secondary effects Y38.9X
   specified method NEC Y38.89
   suicide bomber Y38.81
Thirst X58
Threat to breathing
   aspiration —*see* Aspiration
   due to cave-in, falling earth or substance NEC
   —see category T71
Thrown (accidentally)
   against part (any) of or object in transport
   vehicle (in motion) NEC —*see also* Accident,
   transport
   from
     high place, homicide (attempt) Y01
     machinery —*see* Contact, with, by type of
     machine
     transport vehicle NEC (*see also* Accident,
     transport) V89.9
   off —*see* Thrown, from
Thunderbolt —see subcategory T75.0
   causing fire —*see* Exposure, fire
Tidal wave (any injury) NEC —*see* Forces of
   nature, tidal wave
Took
   overdose (drug) —*see* Table of drugs and
   chemicals
   poison —*see* Table of drugs and chemicals
Tornado (any injury) X37.1
Torrential rain (any injury) X37.8
Torture X58
Trampled by animal NEC W55.89
Trapped (accidentally)
   between objects (moving) (stationary and
   moving) —*see* Caught
   by part (any) of
     motorcycle V29.88
     pedal cycle V19.88
     transport vehicle NEC (*see also* Accident,
     transport) V89.9
Travel (effects) (sickness) T75.3
Tree falling on or hitting (accidentally)
(person) W20.8
Tripping
   over
     animal W01.0
      with fall W01.0
     carpet, rug or (small) object W22.8
      with fall W18.09
     person W51
      with fall W03
       due to ice or snow W00.0
     without fall W18.40
     due to
      specified NEC W18.49
      stepping from one level to another W18.43
      stepping into hole or opening W18.42
      stepping on object W18.41
Twisted by person (s) (accidentally) W50.2
   with intent to injure or kill Y04.0
   as, or caused by, a crowd or human stampede
   (with fall) W52
   assault Y04.0
   homicide (attempt) Y04.0
   in
     fight Y04.0
     legal intervention —*see* Legal, intervention,
     manhandling
Twisting, excessive —see category Y93

U

Underdosing of necessary drugs, medicaments
or biological substances Y63.6
Undetermined intent (contact) (exposure)
   automobile collision Y32
   blunt object Y29
   drowning (submersion) (in) Y21.9
     bathtub Y21.0
      after fall Y21.1
     natural water (lake) (ocean) (pond) (river)
     (stream) Y21.4
     specified place NEC Y21.8
     swimming pool Y21.2
      after fall Y21.3
   explosive material Y25
   fall, jump or push from high place Y30
   falling, lying or running before moving object
   Y31
   fire Y26
   firearm discharge Y24.9
     airgun (BB) (pellet) Y24.0
     handgun (pistol) (revolver) Y22
     hunting rifle Y23.1
     larger Y23.9
      hunting rifle Y23.1
      machine gun Y23.3
      military Y23.2
      shotgun Y23.0
      specified type NEC Y23.8
     machine gun Y23.3
     military Y23.2
     shotgun Y23.0
     specified type NEC Y24.8
     Very pistol Y24.8
   hot object Y27.9
     fluid NEC Y27.2
     household appliance Y27.3
     specified object NEC Y27.8
     steam Y27.0
     tap water Y27.1
     vapor Y27.0
   jump, fall or push from high place Y30
   lying, falling or running before moving object
   Y31
   motor vehicle crash Y32
   push, fall or jump from high place Y30
   running, falling or lying before moving object
   Y31
   sharp object Y28.9
     dagger Y28.2
     glass Y28.0
     knife Y28.1
     specified object NEC Y28.8
     sword Y28.2
   smoke Y26
   specified event NEC Y33

V

Vibration (causing injury) W49.9
Victim (of)
   avalanche —*see* Landslide
   earth movements NEC —*see* Forces of nature,
   earth movement
   earthquake X34
   flood —*see* Flood
   landslide —*see* Landslide
   lightning —see subcategory T75.0
     causing fire —*see* Exposure, fire
   storm (cataclysmic) NEC —*see* Forces of
   nature, cataclysmic storm
   volcanic eruption X35
Volcanic eruption (any injury) X35

Vomitus, gastric contents in air passages (with
asphyxia, obstruction or suffocation) T17.81

W

Walked into stationary object (any) W22.09
   furniture W22.03
   lamppost W22.02
   wall W22.01
War operations (injuries to military personnel
and civilians during war, civil insurrection
and peacekeeping missions) (by) (from)
(involving) Y36.90
   after cessation of hostilities Y36.89
     explosion (of)
      bomb placed during war operations Y36.82
      mine placed during war operations Y36.81
      specified NEC Y36.88
   air blast Y36.20
   aircraft
     destruction —*see* War operations, destruction
   of aircraft
   airway restriction —*see* War operations,
   restriction of airways
   asphyxiation —*see* War operations, restriction
   of airways
   biological weapons Y36.6X
   blast Y36.20
   blast fragments Y36.20
   blast wave Y36.20
   blast wind Y36.20
   bomb Y36.20
     dirty Y36.50
     gasoline Y36.31
     incendiary Y36.31
     petrol Y36.31
   bullet Y36.43
     incendiary Y36.32
     rubber Y36.41
   chemical weapons Y36.7X   combat
   hand to hand (unarmed) combat Y36.44
     using blunt or piercing object Y36.45
   conflagration —*see* War operations, fire
   conventional warfare NEC Y36.49
   depth-charge Y36.01
   destruction of aircraft Y36.10
     due to
      air to air missile Y36.11
      collision with other aircraft Y36.12
      detonation (accidental) of onboard
     munitions and explosives Y36.14
      enemy fire or explosives Y36.11
      explosive placed on aircraft Y36.11
      onboard fire Y36.13
      rocket propelled grenade [RPG] Y36.11
      small arms fire Y36.11
      surface to air missile Y36.11
      specified NEC Y36.19
   detonation (accidental) of
   onboard marine weapons Y36.05
   own munitions or munitions launch device
   Y36.24
   dirty bomb Y36.50
   explosion (of) Y36.20
     after cessation of hostilities
     bomb placed during war operations Y36.82
     mine placed during war operations Y36.81
     aerial bomb Y36.21
     bomb NOS (*see also* War operations, bomb
     (s)) Y36.20
     own munitions or munitions launch device
     (accidental) Y36.24
     fragments Y36.20
     grenade Y36.29

War operations - *continued*

  guided missile Y36.22

  improvised explosive device [IED] (person-borne) (roadside) (vehicle-borne) Y36.23

  land mine Y36.29

  marine mine (at sea) (in harbor) Y36.02

  marine weapon Y36.00

   specified NEC Y36.09

  sea-based artillery shell Y36.03

  specified NEC Y36.29

  torpedo Y36.04

  fire Y36.30

   specified NEC Y36.39

  firearms

  discharge Y36.43

   pellets Y36.42

  flamethrower Y36.33

  fragments (from) (of)

  improvised explosive device [IED] (person-borne) (roadside) (vehicle-borne) Y36.26

   munitions Y36.25

   specified NEC Y36.29

   weapons Y36.27

  friendly fire Y36.92

hand to hand (unarmed) combat Y36.44

  hot substances —*see* War operations, fire

incendiary bullet Y36.32

  nuclear weapon (effects of) Y36.50

   acute radiation exposure Y36.54

   blast pressure Y36.51

   direct blast Y36.51

   direct heat Y36.53

   fallout exposure Y36.54

   fireball Y36.53

   indirect blast (struck or crushed by blast debris) (being thrown by blast) Y36.52

   ionizing radiation (immediate exposure) Y36.54

   nuclear radiation Y36.54

   radiation

   ionizing (immediate exposure) Y36.54

    nuclear Y36.54

    thermal Y36.53

   specified NEC Y36.59

   secondary effects Y36.54

   thermal radiation Y36.53

  restriction of air (airway)

  intentional Y36.46

   unintentional Y36.47

  rubber bullets Y36.41

  shrapnel NOS Y36.29

  suffocation —*see* War operations, restriction of airways

unconventional warfare NEC Y36.7X

  underwater blast NOS Y36.00

  warfare

  conventional NEC Y36.49

   unconventional NEC Y36.7X

  weapons

  biological weapons Y36.6X

   chemical Y36.7X

   nuclear (effects of) Y36.50

    acute radiation exposure Y36.54

    blast pressure Y36.51

    direct blast Y36.51

    direct heat Y36.53

    fallout exposure Y36.54

    fireball Y36.53

    indirect blast (struck or crushed by blast debris) (being thrown by blast) Y36.52

    radiation

    ionizing (immediate exposure) Y36.54

     nuclear Y36.54

War operations - *continued*

   thermal Y36.53

   secondary effects Y36.54

   specified NEC Y36.59

  of mass destruction [WMD] Y36.91

 weapon of mass destruction [WMD] Y36.91

Washed

 away by flood —*see* Flood

 off road by storm (transport vehicle) —*see* Forces of nature, cataclysmic storm

Weather exposure NEC —*see* Forces of nature

Weightlessness (causing injury) (effects of) (in spacecraft, real or simulated) X52

Work related condition Y99.0

Wound (accidental) NEC (*see also* Injury) X58

 battle (*see also* War operations) Y36.90

 gunshot —*see* Discharge, firearm by type

Wreck transport vehicle NEC (*see also* Accident, transport) V89.9

Wrong

 device implanted into correct surgical site Y65.51

 fluid in infusion Y65.1

 procedure (operation) on correct patient Y65.51

 patient, procedure performed on Y65.52

LIST OF THREE DIGIT CATEGORIES

CHAPTER 1: CERTAIN INFECTIOUS AND PARASITIC DISEASES (A00-B99)

A00	Cholera
A01	Typhoid and paratyphoid fevers
A02	Other salmonella infections
A03	Shigellosis
A04	Other bacterial intestinal infections
A05	Other bacterial foodborne intoxications, not elsewhere classified
A06	Amebiasis
A07	Other protozoal intestinal diseases
A08	Viral and other specified intestinal infections
A09	Infectious gastroenteritis and colitis unspecified
A15	Respiratory tuberculosis
A17	Tuberculosis of nervous system
A18	Tuberculosis of other organs
A19	Miliary tuberculosis
A20	Plague
A21	Tularemia
A22	Anthrax
A23	Brucellosis
A24	Glanders and melioidosis
A25	Rat-bite fever
A26	Erysipeloid
A27	Leptospirosis
A28	Other zoonotic bacterial diseases, not elsewhere classified
A30	Leprosy (Hansen's disease)
A31	Infection due to other mycobacteria
A32	Listeriosis
A33	Tetanus neonatorum
A34	Obstetrical tetanus
A35	Other tetanus
A36	Diphtheria
A37	Whooping cough
A38	Scarlet fever
A39	Meningococcal infection
A40	Streptococcal sepsis
A41	Other sepsis
A42	Actinomycosis
A43	Nocardiosis
A44	Bartonellosis
A46	Erysipelas
A48	Other bacterial diseases, not elsewhere classified
A49	Staphylococcal infection of unspecified site
A50	Congenital syphilis
A51	Early syphilis
A52	Late syphilis
A53	Other and unspecified syphilis
A54	Gonococcal infection
A55	Chlamydial lymphogranuloma (venereum)
A56	Other sexually transmitted chlamydial diseases
A57	Chancroid
A58	Granuloma inguinale
A59	Trichomoniasis
A60	Anogenital herpesviral [herpes simplex] infections
A63	Other predominantly sexually transmitted diseases, not elsewhere classified
A64	Unspecified sexually transmitted disease
A65	Nonvenereal syphilis
A66	Yaws
A67	Pinta [carate]
A68	Relapsing fevers
A69	Other spirochetal infections
A70	Chlamydia psittaci infections
A71	Trachoma
A74	Other diseases caused by chlamydiae
A75	Typhus fever
A77	Spotted fever [tick-borne rickettsioses]
A78	Q fever
A79	Other rickettsioses
A80	Acute poliomyelitis
A81	Atypical virus infections of central nervous system
A82	Rabies
A83	Mosquito-borne viral encephalitis
A84	Tick-borne viral encephalitis
A85	Other viral encephalitis, not elsewhere classified
A86	Unspecified viral encephalitis
A87	Viral meningitis
A88	Other viral infections of central nervous system, not elsewhere classified
A89	Unspecified viral infection of central nervous system
A90	Dengue fever [classical dengue]
A91	Dengue hemorrhagic fever
A92	Other mosquito-borne viral fevers
A93	Other arthropod-borne viral fevers, not elsewhere classified
A94	Unspecified arthropod-borne viral fever
A95	Yellow fever
A96	Arenaviral hemorrhagic fever
A98	Other viral hemorrhagic fevers, not elsewhere classified
A99	Unspecified viral hemorrhagic fever
B00	Herpesviral [herpes simplex] infections
B01	Varicella [chickenpox]
B02	Zoster [herpes zoster]
B03	Smallpox
B04	Monkeypox
B05	Measles
B06	Rubella [German measles]
B07	Viral warts
B08	Cowpox
B09	Other human herpesviruses
B10	Other human herpesviruses
B15	Acute hepatitis A
B16	Acute hepatitis B
B17	Other acute viral hepatitis
B18	Chronic viral hepatitis
B19	Unspecified viral hepatitis
B20	Human immunodeficiency virus [HIV] disease
B25	Cytomegaloviral disease
B26	Mumps
B27	Infectious mononucleosis
B30	Viral conjunctivitis
B33	Other viral diseases, not elsewhere classified
B34	Viral infection of unspecified site
B35	Dermatophytosis
B36	Other superficial mycoses
B37	Candidiasis
B38	Coccidioidomycosis

B39	Histoplasmosis
B40	Blastomycosis
B41	Paracoccidioidomycosis
B42	Sporotrichosis
B43	Chromomycosis and pheomycotic abscess
B44	Aspergillosis
B45	Cryptococcosis
B46	Zygomycosis
B47	Mycetoma
B48	Other mycoses, not elsewhere classified
B49	Unspecified mycosis
B50	Plasmodium falciparum malaria
B51	Plasmodium vivax malaria
B52	Plasmodium malariae malaria
B53	Other specified malaria
B54	Unspecified malaria
B55	Leishmaniasis
B56	African trypanosomiasis
B57	Chagas' disease
B58	Toxoplasmosis
B59	Pneumocystosis
B60	Other protozoal diseases, not elsewhere classified
B64	Unspecified protozoal disease
B65	Schistosomiasis [bilharziasis]
B66	Other fluke infections
B67	Echinococcosis
B68	Taeniasis
B69	Cysticercosis
B70	Diphyllobothriasis and sparganosis
B71	Other cestode infections
B72	Dracunculiasis
B73	Onchocerciasis
B74	Filariasis
B75	Trichinellosis
B76	Hookworm diseases
B77	Ascariasis
B78	Strongyloidiasis
B79	Trichuriasis
B80	Enterobiasis
B81	Other intestinal helminthiases, not elsewhere classified
B82	Unspecified intestinal parasitism
B83	Other helminthiases
B85	Pediculosis and phthiriasis
B86	Scabies
B87	Myiasis
B88	Other infestations
B89	Unspecified parasitic disease
B90	Sequelae of tuberculosis
B91	Sequelae of poliomyelitis
B92	Sequelae of leprosy
B94	Sequelae of other and unspecified infectious and parasitic diseases
B95	Streptococcus, Staphylococcus, and Enterococcus as the cause of diseases classified elsewhere
B96	Other bacterial agents as the cause of diseases classified elsewhere
B97	Viral agents as the cause of diseases classified elsewhere
B99	Other and unspecified infectious diseases

CHAPTER 2: NEOPLASMS (C00-D49)

C00	Malignant neoplasm of lip
C01	Malignant neoplasm of base of tongue
C02	Malignant neoplasm of other and unspecified parts of tongue
C03	Malignant neoplasm of gum
C04	Malignant neoplasm of floor of mouth
C05	Malignant neoplasm of palate
C06	Malignant neoplasm of other and unspecified parts of mouth
C07	Malignant neoplasm of parotid gland
C08	Malignant neoplasm of other and unspecified major salivary glands
C09	Malignant neoplasm of tonsil
C10	Malignant neoplasm of oropharynx
C11	Malignant neoplasm of nasopharynx
C12	Malignant neoplasm of pyriform sinus
C13	Malignant neoplasm of hypopharynx
C14	Malignant neoplasm of other and ill-defined sites in the lip, oral cavity and pharynx
C15	Malignant neoplasm of esophagus
C16	Malignant neoplasm of stomach
C17	Malignant neoplasm of small intestine
C18	Malignant neoplasm of colon
C19	Malignant neoplasm of rectosigmoid junction
C20	Malignant neoplasm of rectum
C21	Malignant neoplasm of anus and anal canal
C22	Malignant neoplasm of liver and intrahepatic bile ducts
C23	Malignant neoplasm of gallbladder
C24	Malignant neoplasm of other and unspecified parts of biliary tract
C25	Malignant neoplasm of pancreas
C26	Malignant neoplasm of other and ill-defined digestive organs
C30	Malignant neoplasm of nasal cavity and middle ear
C31	Malignant neoplasm of accessory sinuses
C32	Malignant neoplasm of larynx
C33	Malignant neoplasm of trachea
C34	Malignant neoplasm of bronchus and lung
C37	Malignant neoplasm of thymus
C38	Malignant neoplasm of heart, mediastinum and pleura
C39	Malignant neoplasm of other and ill-defined sites in the respiratory system and intrathoracic organs
C40	Malignant neoplasm of bone and articular cartilage of limbs
C41	Malignant neoplasm of bone and articular cartilage of other and unspecified sites
C43	Malignant melanoma of skin
C44	Other and unspecified malignant neoplasm of skin
C45	Mesothelioma
C46	Kaposi's sarcoma
C47	Malignant neoplasm of peripheral nerves and autonomic nervous system
C48	Malignant neoplasm of retroperitoneum and peritoneum
C49	Malignant neoplasm of other connective and soft tissue
C4A	Merkel cell carcinoma
C50	Malignant neoplasm of breast
C52	Malignant neoplasm of vagina
C53	Malignant neoplasm of cervix uteri

C54	Malignant neoplasm of corpus uteri
C55	Malignant neoplasm of uterus, part unspecified
C56	Malignant neoplasm of ovary
C57	Malignant neoplasm of other and unspecified female genital organs
C58	Malignant neoplasm of placenta
C60	Malignant neoplasm of penis
C61	Malignant neoplasm of prostate
C62	Malignant neoplasm of testis
C63	Malignant neoplasm of other and unspecified male genital organs
C64	Malignant neoplasm of kidney, except renal pelvis
C65	Malignant neoplasm of renal pelvis
C66	Malignant neoplasm of ureter
C67	Malignant neoplasm of bladder
C68	Malignant neoplasm of other and unspecified urinary organs
C69	Malignant neoplasm of eye and adnexa
C70	Malignant neoplasm of meninges
C71	Malignant neoplasm of brain
C72	Malignant neoplasm of spinal cord, cranial nerves and other parts of central nervous system
C73	Malignant neoplasm of thyroid gland
C74	Malignant neoplasm of adrenal gland
C75	Malignant neoplasm of other endocrine glands and related structures
C76	Malignant neoplasm of other and ill-defined sites
C77	Secondary and unspecified malignant neoplasm of lymph nodes
C78	Secondary malignant neoplasm of respiratory and digestive organs
C79	Secondary malignant neoplasm of other and unspecified sites
C7A	Malignant neuroendocrine tumors
C7B	Secondary neuroendocrine tumors
C80	Malignant neoplasm without specification of site
C81	Hodgkin lymphoma
C82	Follicular lymphoma
C83	Non-follicular lymphoma
C84	Mature T/NK-cell lymphomas
C85	Other specified and unspecified types of non-Hodgkin lymphoma
C86	Other specified types of T/NK-cell lymphoma
C88	Malignant immunoproliferative diseases and certain other B-cell lymphomas
C90	Multiple myeloma and malignant plasma cell neoplasms
C91	Lymphoid leukemia
C92	Myeloid leukemia
C93	Monocytic leukemia
C94	Other leukemias of specified cell type
C95	Leukemia of unspecified cell type
C96	Other and unspecified malignant neoplasms of lymphoid, hematopoietic and related tissue
D00	Carcinoma in situ of oral cavity, esophagus and stomach
D01	Carcinoma in situ of other and unspecified digestive organs
D02	Carcinoma in situ of middle ear and respiratory system
D03	Melanoma in situ
D04	Carcinoma in situ of skin
D05	Carcinoma in situ of breast
D06	Carcinoma in situ of cervix uteri
D07	Carcinoma in situ of other and unspecified genital organs

D09	Carcinoma in situ of other and unspecified sites
D10	Benign neoplasm of mouth and pharynx
D11	Benign neoplasm of major salivary glands
D12	Benign neoplasm of colon, rectum, anus and anal canal
D13	Benign neoplasm of other and ill-defined parts of digestive system
D14	Benign neoplasm of middle ear and respiratory system
D15	Benign neoplasm of other and unspecified intrathoracic organs
D16	Benign neoplasm of bone and articular cartilage
D17	Benign lipomatous neoplasm
D18	Hemangioma and lymphangioma, any site
D19	Benign neoplasm of mesothelial tissue
D20	Benign neoplasm of soft tissue of retroperitoneum and peritoneum
D21	Other benign neoplasms of connective and other soft tissue
D22	Melanocytic nevi
D23	Other benign neoplasms of skin
D24	Benign neoplasm of breast
D25	Leiomyoma of uterus
D26	Other benign neoplasms of uterus
D27	Benign neoplasm of ovary
D28	Benign neoplasm of other and unspecified female genital organs
D29	Benign neoplasm of male genital organs
D30	Benign neoplasm of urinary organs
D31	Benign neoplasm of eye and adnexa
D32	Benign neoplasm of meninges
D33	Benign neoplasm of brain and other parts of central nervous system
D34	Benign neoplasm of thyroid gland
D35	Benign neoplasm of other and unspecified endocrine glands
D36	Benign neoplasm of other and unspecified sites
D37	Neoplasm of uncertain behavior of oral cavity and digestive organs
D38	Neoplasm of uncertain behavior of middle ear and respiratory and intrathoracic organs
D39	Neoplasm of uncertain behavior of female genital organs
D3A	Benign carcinoid tumor of unspecified site
D40	Neoplasm of uncertain behavior of male genital organs
D41	Neoplasm of uncertain behavior of urinary organs
D42	Neoplasm of uncertain behavior of meninges
D43	Neoplasm of uncertain behavior of brain and central nervous system
D44	Neoplasm of uncertain behavior of endocrine glands
D45	Polycythemia vera
D46	Myelodysplastic syndromes
D47	Other neoplasms of uncertain behavior of lymphoid, hematopoietic and related tissue
D48	Neoplasm of uncertain behavior of other and unspecified sites
D49	Neoplasms of unspecified behavior

CHAPTER 3: DISEASES OF THE BLOOD AND BLOOD-FORMING ORGANS AND CERTAIN DISORDERS INVOLVING THE IMMUNE MECHANISM (D50-D89)

D50	Iron deficiency anemia
D51	Vitamin B12 deficiency anemia

D52	Folate deficiency anemia	**E16**	Other disorders of pancreatic internal secretion
D53	Other nutritional anemias	**E20**	Hypoparathyroidism
D55	Anemia due to enzyme disorders	**E21**	Hyperparathyroidism and other disorders of parathyroid gland
D56	Thalassemia		
D57	Sickle-cell disorders	**E22**	Hyperfunction of pituitary gland
D58	Other hereditary hemolytic anemias	**E23**	Hypofunction and other disorders of the pituitary gland
D59	Acquired hemolytic anemia	**E24**	Cushing's syndrome
D60	Acquired pure red cell aplasia [erythroblastopenia]	**E25**	Adrenogenital disorders
D61	Other aplastic anemias and other bone marrow failure syndromes	**E26**	Hyperaldosteronism
		E27	Other disorders of adrenal gland
D62	Acute posthemorrhagic anemia	**E28**	Ovarian dysfunction
D63	Anemia in chronic diseases classified elsewhere	**E29**	Testicular dysfunction
D64	Other anemias	**E30**	Disorders of puberty, not elsewhere classified
D65	Disseminated intravascular coagulation [defibrination syndrome]	**E31**	Polyglandular dysfunction
		E32	Diseases of thymus
D66	Hereditary factor VIII deficiency	**E34**	Other endocrine disorders
D67	Hereditary factor IX deficiency	**E35**	Disorders of endocrine glands in diseases classified elsewhere
D68	Other coagulation defects		
D69	Purpura and other hemorrhagic conditions	**E36**	Intraoperative complications of endocrine system
D70	Neutropenia	**E40**	Kwashiorkor
D71	Functional disorders of polymorphonuclear neutrophils	**E41**	Nutritional marasmus
		E42	Marasmic kwashiorkor
D72	Other disorders of white blood cells	**E43**	Unspecified severe protein-calorie malnutrition
D73	Diseases of spleen	**E44**	Protein-calorie malnutrition of moderate and mild degree
D74	Methemoglobinemia		
D75	Other and unspecified diseases of blood and blood-forming organs	**E45**	Retarded development following protein-calorie malnutrition
D76	Other specified diseases with participation of lymphoreticular and reticulohistiocytic tissue	**E46**	Unspecified protein-calorie malnutrition
		E50	Vitamin A deficiency
D77	Other disorders of blood and blood-forming organs in diseases classified elsewhere	**E51**	Thiamine deficiency
		E52	Niacin deficiency [pellagra]
D78	Intraoperative and postprocedural complications of the spleen	**E53**	Deficiency of other B group vitamins
		E54	Ascorbic acid deficiency
D80	Immunodeficiency with predominantly antibody defects	**E55**	Vitamin D deficiency
D81	Combined immunodeficiencies	**E56**	Other vitamin deficiencies
D82	Immunodeficiency associated with other major defects	**E58**	Dietary calcium deficiency
		E59	Dietary selenium deficiency
D83	Common variable immunodeficiency	**E60**	Dietary zinc deficiency
D84	Other immunodeficiencies	**E61**	Deficiency of other nutrient elements
D86	Sarcoidosis	**E63**	Other nutritional deficiencies
D89	Other disorders involving the immune mechanism, not elsewhere classified	**E64**	Sequelae of malnutrition and other nutritional deficiencies
		E65	Localized adiposity
		E66	Overweight and obesity
		E67	Other hyperalimentation
		E68	Sequelae of hyperalimentation

CHAPTER 4: ENDOCRINE, NUTRITIONAL AND METABOLIC DISEASES (E00-E89)

E00	Congenital iodine-deficiency syndrome	**E70**	Disorders of aromatic amino-acid metabolism
E01	Iodine-deficiency related thyroid disorders and allied conditions	**E71**	Disorders of branched-chain amino-acid metabolism and fatty-acid metabolism
E02	Subclinical iodine-deficiency hypothyroidism	**E72**	Other disorders of amino-acid metabolism
E03	Other hypothyroidism	**E73**	Lactose intolerance
E04	Other nontoxic goiter	**E74**	Other disorders of carbohydrate metabolism
E05	Thyrotoxicosis [hyperthyroidism]	**E75**	Disorders of sphingolipid metabolism and other lipid storage disorders
E06	Thyroiditis		
E07	Other disorders of thyroid	**E76**	Disorders of glycosaminoglycan metabolism
E08	Diabetes mellitus due to underlying condition	**E77**	Disorders of glycoprotein metabolism
E09	Drug or chemical induced diabetes mellitus	**E78**	Disorders of lipoprotein metabolism and other lipidemias
E10	Type 1 diabetes mellitus	**E79**	Disorders of purine and pyrimidine metabolism
E11	Type 2 diabetes mellitus	**E80**	Disorders of porphyrin and bilirubin metabolism
E13	Other specified diabetes mellitus		
E15	Nondiabetic hypoglycemic coma	**E83**	Disorders of mineral metabolism
		E84	Cystic fibrosis

E85	Amyloidosis
E86	Volume depletion
E87	Other disorders of fluid, electrolyte and acid-base balance
E88	Other and unspecified metabolic disorders
E89	Postprocedural endocrine and metabolic complications and disorders, not elsewhere classified

CHAPTER 5: MENTAL, BEHAVIORAL AND NEURODEVELOPMENTAL DISORDERS (F01-F99)

F01	Vascular dementia
F02	Dementia in other diseases classified elsewhere
F03	Unspecified dementia
F04	Amnestic disorder due to known physiological condition
F05	Delirium due to known physiological condition
F06	Unspecified dementia
F07	Other mental disorders due to known physiological condition
F09	Personality and behavioral disorders due to known physiological condition
F10	Alcohol related disorders
F11	Opioid related disorders
F12	Cannabis related disorders
F13	Sedative, hypnotic, or anxiolytic related disorders
F14	Cocaine related disorders
F15	Other stimulant related disorders
F16	Hallucinogen related disorders
F17	Nicotine dependence
F18	Inhalant related disorders
F19	Other psychoactive substance related disorders
F21	Schizotypal disorder
F22	Delusional disorders
F23	Brief psychotic disorder
F24	Shared psychotic disorder
F25	Schizoaffective disorders
F28	Other psychotic disorder not due to a substance or known physiological condition
F29	Unspecified psychosis not due to a substance or known physiological condition
F30	Manic episode
F31	Bipolar disorder
F32	Major depressive disorder, single episode
F33	Major depressive disorder, recurrent
F34	Persistent mood [affective] disorders
F39	Unspecified mood [affective] disorder
F40	Phobic anxiety disorders
F41	Other anxiety disorders
F42	Obsessive-compulsive disorder
F43	Reaction to severe stress, and adjustment disorders
F44	Dissociative and conversion disorders
F45	Somatoform disorders
F48	Other nonpsychotic mental disorders
F50	Eating disorders
F51	Sleep disorders not due to a substance or known physiological condition
F52	Sexual dysfunction not due to a substance or known physiological condition
F53	Puerperal psychosis

F54	Psychological and behavioral factors associated with disorders or diseases classified elsewhere
F55	Abuse of non-psychoactive substances
F59	Unspecified behavioral syndromes associated with physiological disturbances and physical factors
F60	Specific personality disorders
F63	Impulse disorders
F64	Gender identity disorders
F65	Paraphilias
F66	Other sexual disorders
F68	Other disorders of adult personality and behavior
F69	Unspecified disorder of adult personality and behavior
F70	Mild intellectual disabilities
F71	Moderate mental retardation
F72	Severe intellectual disabilities
F73	Profound intellectual disabilities
F78	Other intellectual disabilities
F79	Unspecified intellectual disabilities
F80	Specific developmental disorders of speech and language
F81	Specific developmental disorders of scholastic skills
F82	Specific developmental disorder of motor function
F84	Pervasive developmental disorders
F88	Other disorders of psychological development
F89	Unspecified disorder of psychological development
F90	Attention-deficit hyperactivity disorders
F91	Conduct disorders
F93	Emotional disorders with onset specific to childhood
F94	Disorders of social functioning with onset specific to childhood and adolescence
F95	Tic disorder
F98	Other behavioral and emotional disorders with onset usually occurring in childhood and adolescence
F99	Mental disorder not otherwise specified

CHAPTER 6: DISEASES OF THE NERVOUS SYSTEM (G00-G99)

G00	Bacterial meningitis, not elsewhere classified
G01	Meningitis in bacterial diseases classified elsewhere
G02	Meningitis in other infectious and parasitic diseases classified elsewhere
G03	Meningitis due to other and unspecified causes
G04	Encephalitis, myelitis and encephalomyelitis
G05	Encephalitis, myelitis and encephalomyelitis in diseases classified elsewhere
G06	Intracranial and intraspinal abscess and granuloma
G07	Intracranial and intraspinal abscess and granuloma in diseases classified elsewhere
G08	Intracranial and intraspinal phlebitis and thrombophlebitis
G09	Sequelae of inflammatory diseases of central nervous system
G10	Huntington's disease
G11	Hereditary ataxia
G12	Spinal muscular atrophy and related syndromes
G13	Systemic atrophies primarily affecting central nervous system in diseases classified elsewhere
G14	Postpolio syndrome
G20	Parkinson's disease
G21	Secondary parkinsonism
G23	Other degenerative diseases of basal ganglia

G24	Dystonia
G25	Other extrapyramidal and movement disorders
G26	Extrapyramidal and movement disorders in diseases classified elsewhere
G30	Alzheimer's disease
G31	Other degenerative diseases of nervous system, not elsewhere classified
G32	Other degenerative disorders of nervous system in diseases classified elsewhere
G35	Multiple sclerosis
G36	Other acute disseminated demyelination
G37	Other demyelinating diseases of central nervous system
G40	Epilepsy and recurrent seizures
G43	Migraine
G44	Other headache syndromes
G45	Transient cerebral ischemic attacks and related syndromes
G46	Vascular syndromes of brain in cerebrovascular diseases
G47	Sleep disorders
G50	Disorders of trigeminal nerve
G51	Facial nerve disorders
G52	Disorders of other cranial nerves
G53	Cranial nerve disorders in diseases classified elsewhere
G54	Nerve root and plexus disorders
G55	Mononeuropathies of upper limb
G56	Mononeuropathies of lower limb
G57	Mononeuropathy in diseases classified elsewhere
G58	Other mononeuropathies
G59	Hereditary and idiopathic neuropathy
G60	Disorders of trigeminal nerve
G61	Inflammatory polyneuropathy
G62	Other and unspecified polyneuropathies
G63	Polyneuropathy in diseases classified elsewhere
G64	Other disorders of peripheral nervous system
G65	Sequelae of inflammatory and toxic polyneuropathies
G70	Myasthenia gravis and other myoneural disorders
G71	Primary disorders of muscles
G72	Other and unspecified myopathies
G73	Malignant neoplasm of thyroid gland
G80	Cerebral palsy
G81	Hemiplegia and hemiparesis
G82	Paraplegia (paraparesis) and quadriplegia (quadriparesis)
G83	Other paralytic syndromes
G89	Pain, not elsewhere classified
G90	Disorders of autonomic nervous system
G91	Hydrocephalus
G92	Toxic encephalopathy
G93	Other disorders of brain
G94	Other disorders of brain in diseases classified elsewhere
G95	Other and unspecified diseases of spinal cord
G96	Other disorders of central nervous system
G97	Intraoperative and postprocedural complications and disorders of nervous system, not elsewhere classified
G98	Other disorders of nervous system not elsewhere classified
G99	Other disorders of nervous system in diseases classified elsewhere

CHAPTER 7: DISEASES OF THE EYE AND ADNEXA (H00-H59)

H00	Hordeolum and chalazion
H01	Other inflammation of eyelid
H02	Other disorders of eyelid
H04	Disorders of lacrimal system
H05	Disorders of orbit
H10	Conjunctivitis
H11	Other disorders of conjunctiva
H15	Disorders of sclera
H16	Keratitis
H17	Corneal scars and opacities
H18	Other disorders of cornea
H20	Iridocyclitis
H21	Other disorders of iris and ciliary body
H22	Disorders of iris and ciliary body in diseases classified elsewhere
H25	Age-related cataract
H26	Other cataract
H27	Other disorders of lens
H28	Cataract in diseases classified elsewhere
H30	Chorioretinal inflammation
H31	Other disorders of choroid
H32	Chorioretinal disorders in diseases classified elsewhere
H33	Retinal detachments and breaks
H34	Retinal vascular occlusions
H35	Other retinal disorders
H36	Retinal disorders in diseases classified elsewhere
H40	Glaucoma
H42	Glaucoma in diseases classified elsewhere
H43	Disorders of vitreous body
H44	Disorders of globe
H46	Optic neuritis
H47	Other disorders of optic [2nd] nerve and visual pathways
H49	Paralytic strabismus
H50	Other strabismus
H51	Other disorders of binocular movement
H52	Disorders of refraction and accommodation
H53	Visual disturbances
H54	Blindness and low vision
H55	Nystagmus and other irregular eye movements
H57	Other disorders of eye and adnexa
H59	Intraoperative and postprocedural complications and disorders of eye and adnexa, not elsewhere classified

CHAPTER 8: DISEASES OF THE EAR AND MASTOID PROCESS (H60-H95)

H60	Otitis externa
H61	Other disorders of external ear
H62	Disorders of external ear in diseases classified elsewhere
H65	Nonsuppurative otitis media
H66	Suppurative and unspecified otitis media
H67	Otitis media in diseases classified elsewhere
H68	Eustachian salpingitis and obstruction
H69	Other and unspecified disorders of Eustachian tube
H70	Mastoiditis and related conditions
H71	Cholesteatoma of middle ear

H72	Perforation of tympanic membrane
H73	Other disorders of tympanic membrane
H74	Other disorders of middle ear mastoid
H75	Other disorders of middle ear and mastoid in diseases classified elsewhere
H80	Otosclerosis
H81	Disorders of vestibular function
H82	Vertiginous syndromes in diseases classified elsewhere
H83	Other diseases of inner ear
H90	Conductive and sensorineural hearing loss
H91	Other and unspecified hearing loss
H92	Otalgia and effusion of ear
H93	Other disorders of ear, not elsewhere classified
H94	Other disorders of ear in diseases classified elsewhere
H95	Intraoperative and postprocedural complications and disorders of ear and mastoid process, not elsewhere classified

CHAPTER 9: DISEASES OF THE CIRCULATORY SYSTEM (I00-I99)

I00	Rheumatic fever without heart involvement
I01	Rheumatic fever with heart involvement
I02	Rheumatic chorea
I05	Rheumatic mitral valve diseases
I06	Rheumatic aortic valve diseases
I07	Rheumatic tricuspid valve diseases
I08	Multiple valve diseases
I09	Other rheumatic heart diseases
I10	Essential (primary) hypertension
I11	Hypertensive heart disease
I12	Hypertensive chronic kidney disease
I13	Hypertensive heart and chronic kidney disease
I15	Secondary hypertension
I20	Angina pectoris
I21	ST elevation (STEMI) and non-ST elevation (NSTEMI) myocardial infarction
I22	Subsequent ST elevation (STEMI) and non-ST elevation (NSTEMI) myocardial infarction
I23	Certain current complications following ST elevation (STEMI) and non-ST elevation (NSTEMI) myocardial infarction (within the 28 day period)
I24	Other acute ischemic heart diseases
I25	Chronic ischemic heart disease
I26	Pulmonary embolism
I27	Other pulmonary heart diseases
I28	Other diseases of pulmonary vessels
I30	Acute pericarditis
I31	Other diseases of pericardium
I32	Pericarditis in diseases classified elsewhere
I33	Acute and subacute endocarditis
I34	Nonrheumatic mitral valve disorders
I35	Nonrheumatic aortic valve disorders
I36	Nonrheumatic tricuspid valve disorders
I37	Nonrheumatic pulmonary valve disorders
I38	Endocarditis, valve unspecified
I39	Endocarditis and heart valve disorders in diseases classified elsewhere
I40	Acute myocarditis

I41	Myocarditis in diseases classified elsewhere
I42	Cardiomyopathy
I43	Cardiomyopathy in diseases classified elsewhere
I44	Atrioventricular and left bundle-branch block
I45	Other conduction disorders
I46	Cardiac arrest
I47	Paroxysmal tachycardia
I48	Atrial fibrillation and flutter
I49	Other cardiac arrhythmias
I50	Heart failure
I51	Complications and ill-defined descriptions of heart disease
I52	Other heart disorders in diseases classified elsewhere
I60	Nontraumatic subarachnoid hemorrhage
I61	Nontraumatic intracerebral hemorrhage
I62	Other and unspecified nontraumatic intracranial hemorrhage
I63	Cerebral infarction
I65	Occlusion and stenosis of precerebral arteries, not resulting in cerebral infarction
I66	Occlusion and stenosis of cerebral arteries, not resulting in cerebral infarction
I67	Other cerebrovascular diseases
I68	Cerebrovascular disorders in diseases classified elsewhere
I69	Sequelae of cerebrovascular disease
I70	Atherosclerosis
I71	Aortic aneurysm and dissection
I72	Other aneurysm
I73	Other peripheral vascular diseases
I74	Arterial embolism and thrombosis
I75	Atheroembolism
I76	Other disorders of arteries and arterioles
I77	Diseases of capillaries
I78	Disorders of arteries, arterioles and capillaries in diseases classified elsewhere
I79	Disorders of arteries, arterioles and capillaries in diseases classified elsewhere
I80	Phlebitis and thrombophlebitis
I81	Portal vein thrombosis
I82	Other venous embolism and thrombosis
I83	Varicose veins of lower extremities
I84	Unspecified thrombosed hemorrhoids
I85	Esophageal varices
I86	Varicose veins of other sites
I87	Other disorders of veins
I88	Nonspecific lymphadenitis
I89	Other noninfective disorders of lymphatic vessels and lymph nodes
I95	Hypotension
I96	Gangrene, not elsewhere classified
I97	Intraoperative and postprocedural complications and disorders of circulatory system, not elsewhere classified
I99	Other and unspecified disorders of circulatory system

CHAPTER 10: DISEASES OF THE RESPIRATORY SYSTEM (J00-J99)

J00	Acute nasopharyngitis [common cold]
J01	Acute sinusitis
J02	Acute nasopharyngitis [common cold]
J03	Acute tonsillitis

J04	Acute laryngitis and tracheitis
J05	Acute obstructive laryngitis [croup] and epiglottitis
J06	Acute upper respiratory infections of multiple and unspecified sites
J09	Influenza due to certain identified influenza viruses
J10	Influenza due to other identified influenza virus
J12	Viral pneumonia, not elsewhere classified
J13	Pneumonia due to Streptococcus pneumoniae
J14	Pneumonia due to Hemophilus influenzae
J15	Bacterial pneumonia, not elsewhere classified
J16	Pneumonia due to other infectious organisms, not elsewhere classified
J17	Pneumonia in diseases classified elsewhere
J18	Pneumonia, unspecified organism
J20	Acute bronchitis
J21	Acute bronchiolitis
J22	Unspecified acute lower respiratory infection
J30	Vasomotor and allergic rhinitis
J31	Chronic rhinitis, nasopharyngitis and pharyngitis
J32	Chronic sinusitis
J33	Nasal polyp
J34	Other and unspecified disorders of nose and nasal sinuses
J35	Chronic diseases of tonsils and adenoids
J36	Peritonsillar abscess
J37	Chronic laryngitis and laryngotracheitis
J38	Diseases of vocal cords and larynx, not elsewhere classified
J39	Other diseases of upper respiratory tract
J40	Bronchitis, not specified as acute or chronic
J41	Simple and mucopurulent chronic bronchitis
J42	Unspecified chronic bronchitis
J43	Emphysema
J44	Other chronic obstructive pulmonary disease
J45	Asthma
J47	Bronchiectasis
J60	Coalworker's pneumoconiosis
J61	Pneumoconiosis due to asbestos and other mineral fibers
J62	Pneumoconiosis due to dust containing silica
J63	Pneumoconiosis due to other inorganic dusts
J64	Unspecified pneumoconiosis
J65	Pneumoconiosis associated with tuberculosis
J66	Airway disease due to specific organic dust
J67	Hypersensitivity pneumonitis due to organic dust
J68	Respiratory conditions due to inhalation of chemicals, gases, fumes and vapors
J69	Pneumonitis due to solids and liquids
J70	Respiratory conditions due to other external agents
J80	Acute respiratory distress syndrome
J81	Pulmonary edema
J82	Pulmonary eosinophilia, not elsewhere classified
J84	Other interstitial pulmonary diseases
J85	Abscess of lung and mediastinum
J86	Pyothorax
J90	Pleural effusion, not elsewhere classified
J91	Pleural effusion in conditions classified elsewhere
J92	Pleural plaque
J93	Pneumothorax and air leak
J94	Other pleural conditions
J95	Intraoperative and postprocedural complications and disorders of respiratory system, not elsewhere classified
J96	Respiratory failure, not elsewhere classified
J98	Other respiratory disorders
J99	Respiratory disorders in diseases classified elsewhere

CHAPTER 11: DISEASES OF THE DIGESTIVE SYSTEM (K00-K95)

K00	Disorders of tooth development and eruption
K01	Embedded and impacted teeth
K02	Dental caries
K03	Other diseases of hard tissues of teeth
K04	Diseases of pulp and periapical tissues
K05	Gingivitis and periodontal diseases
K06	Other disorders of gingiva and edentulous alveolar ridge
K08	Other disorders of teeth and supporting structures
K09	Cysts of oral region, not elsewhere classified
K11	Diseases of salivary glands
K12	Stomatitis and related lesions
K13	Other diseases of lip and oral mucosa
K14	Diseases of tongue
K20	Esophagitis
K21	Gastro-esophageal reflux disease
K22	Other diseases of esophagus
K23	Disorders of esophagus in diseases classified elsewhere
K25	Gastric ulcer
K26	Duodenal ulcer
K27	Peptic ulcer, site unspecified
K28	Gastrojejunal ulcer
K29	Gastritis and duodenitis
K30	Functional dyspepsia
K31	Other diseases of stomach and duodenum
K35	Acute appendicitis
K36	Other appendicitis
K37	Unspecified appendicitis
K38	Other diseases of appendix
K40	Inguinal hernia
K41	Femoral hernia
K42	Umbilical hernia
K43	Ventral hernia
K44	Diaphragmatic hernia
K45	Other abdominal hernia
K46	Unspecified abdominal hernia
K50	Crohn's disease [regional enteritis]
K51	Ulcerative colitis
K52	Other and unspecified noninfective gastroenteritis and colitis
K55	Vascular disorders of intestine
K56	Paralytic ileus and intestinal obstruction without hernia
K57	Diverticular disease of intestine
K58	Irritable bowel syndrome
K59	Fissure and fistula of anal and rectal regions
K60	Abscess of anal and rectal regions
K61	Other diseases of anus and rectum
K62	Other diseases of intestine
K63	Hemorrhoids and perianal venous thrombosis
K65	Peritonitis
K66	Other disorders of peritoneum
K67	Disorders of peritoneum in infectious diseases classified elsewhere

K68	Disorders of retroperitoneum	L49	Exfoliation due to erythematous conditions according to extent of body surface involved
K70	Alcoholic liver disease	L50	Urticaria
K71	Toxic liver disease	L51	Erythema multiforme
K72	Hepatic failure, not elsewhere classified	L52	Erythema nodosum
K73	Chronic hepatitis, not elsewhere classified	L53	Other erythematous conditions
K74	Fibrosis and cirrhosis of liver	L54	Erythema in diseases classified elsewhere
K75	Other inflammatory liver diseases	L55	Sunburn
K76	Other diseases of liver	L56	Other acute skin changes due to ultraviolet radiation
K77	Liver disorders in diseases classified elsewhere	L57	Skin changes due to chronic exposure to nonionizing radiation
K80	Cholelithiasis	L58	Radiodermatitis
K81	Cholecystitis	L59	Other disorders of skin and subcutaneous tissue related to radiation
K82	Other diseases of gallbladder	L60	Nail disorders
K83	Other diseases of biliary tract	L62	Nail disorders in diseases classified elsewhere
K85	Acute pancreatitis	L63	Alopecia areata
K86	Other diseases of pancreas	L64	Androgenic alopecia
K87	Disorders of gallbladder biliary tract and pancreas in diseases classified elsewhere	L65	Other nonscarring hair loss
K90	Intestinal malabsorption	L66	Cicatricial alopecia [scarring hair loss]
K91	Intraoperative and postprocedural complications and disorders of digestive system, not elsewhere classified	L67	Hair color and hair shaft abnormalities
		L68	Hypertrichosis
K92	Other diseases of digestive system	L70	Acne
K94	Complications of artificial openings of the digestive system	L71	Rosacea
K95	Complications of bariatric procedures	L72	Follicular cysts of skin and subcutaneous tissue
		L73	Other follicular disorders
		L74	Eccrine sweat disorders
		L75	Apocrine sweat disorders

CHAPTER 12: DISEASES OF THE SKIN AND SUBCUTANEOUS TISSUE (L00-L99)

		L76	Intraoperative and postprocedural complications of skin and subcutaneous tissue
L00	Staphylococcal scalded skin syndrome	L80	Vitiligo
L01	Impetigo	L81	Other disorders of pigmentation
L02	Cutaneous abscess, furuncle and carbuncle	L82	Seborrheic keratosis
L03	Cellulitis and acute lymphangitis	L83	Acanthosis nigricans
L04	Acute lymphadenitis	L84	Corns and callosities
L05	Pilonidal cyst and sinus	L85	Other epidermal thickening
L08	Other local infections of skin and subcutaneous tissue	L86	Keratoderma in diseases classified elsewhere
L08	Other specified local infections of the skin and subcutaneous tissue	L87	Transepidermal elimination disorders
		L88	Pyoderma gangrenosum
L10	Pemphigus	L89	Pressure ulcer
L11	Other acantholytic disorders	L90	Atrophic disorders of skin
L12	Pemphigoid	L91	Hypertrophic disorders of skin
L13	Other bullous disorders	L92	Granulomatous disorders of skin and subcutaneous tissue
L14	Bullous disorders in diseases classified elsewhere	L93	Lupus erythematosus
L20	Atopic dermatitis	L94	Other localized connective tissue disorders
L21	Seborrheic dermatitis	L95	Vasculitis limited to skin, not elsewhere classified
L22	Diaper dermatitis	L97	Non-pressure chronic ulcer of lower limb, not elsewhere classified
L23	Allergic contact dermatitis		
L24	Irritant contact dermatitis	L98	Other disorders of skin and subcutaneous tissue, not elsewhere classified
L25	Unspecified contact dermatitis		
L26	Exfoliative dermatitis	L99	Other disorders of skin and subcutaneous tissue in diseases classified elsewhere
L27	Dermatitis due to substances taken internally		
L28	Lichen simplex chronicus and prurigo		
L29	Pruritus		
L30	Other and unspecified dermatitis		

CHAPTER 13: DISEASES OF THE MUSCULOSKELETAL SYSTEM AND CONNECTIVE TISSUE (M00-M99)

L40	Psoriasis		
L41	Parapsoriasis	M00	Pyogenic arthritis
L42	Pityriasis rosea	M01	Direct infections of joint in infectious and parasitic diseases classified elsewhere
L43	Lichen planus		
L44	Other papulosquamous disorders		
L45	Papulosquamous disorders in diseases classified elsewhere		

M02	Postinfective and reactive arthropathies
M05	Rheumatoid arthritis with rheumatoid factor
M06	Other rheumatoid arthritis
M07	Enteropathic arthropathies
M08	Juvenile arthritis
M10	Idiopathic gout unspecified site
M11	Other crystal arthropathies
M12	Other and unspecified arthropathy
M13	Other arthritis
M14	Arthropathies in other diseases classified elsewhere
M15	Polyosteoarthritis
M16	Osteoarthritis of hip
M17	Osteoarthritis of knee
M18	Osteoarthritis of first carpometacarpal joint
M19	Other and unspecified osteoarthritis
M1A	Idiopathic chronic gout unspecified site without tophus (tophi)
M20	Acquired deformities of fingers and toes
M21	Other acquired deformities of limbs
M22	Disorder of patella
M23	Internal derangement of knee
M24	Other specific joint derangements
M25	Other joint disorder, not elsewhere classified
M26	Dentofacial anomalies [including malocclusion]
M27	Other diseases of jaws
M30	Polyarteritis nodosa and related conditions
M31	Other necrotizing vasculopathies
M32	Systemic lupus erythematosus (SLE)
M33	Dermatopolymyositis
M34	Systemic sclerosis [scleroderma]
M35	Other systemic involvement of connective tissue
M36	Systemic disorders of connective tissue in diseases classified elsewhere
M40	Kyphosis and lordosis
M41	Scoliosis
M42	Spinal osteochondrosis
M43	Other deforming dorsopathies
M45	Ankylosing spondylitis
M46	Other inflammatory spondylopathies
M47	Spondylosis
M48	Other spondylopathies
M49	Spondylopathies in diseases classified elsewhere
M50	Cervical disc disorders
M51	Thoracic, thoracolumbar, and lumbosacral intervertebral disc disorders
M53	Other and unspecified dorsopathies, not elsewhere classified
M54	Dorsalgia
M60	Myositis
M61	Calcification and ossification of muscle
M62	Other disorders of muscle
M63	Disorders of muscle in diseases classified elsewhere
M65	Synovitis and tenosynovitis
M66	Spontaneous rupture of synovium and tendon
M67	Other disorders of synovium and tendon
M70	Soft tissue disorders related to use, overuse and pressure
M71	Other bursopathies
M72	Fibroblastic disorders
M75	Shoulder lesions
M76	Enthesopathies, lower limb, excluding foot
M77	Other enthesopathies
M79	Other and unspecified soft tissue disorders, not elsewhere classified
M80	Osteoporosis with current pathological fracture
M81	Osteoporosis without current pathological fracture
M83	Puerperal osteomalacia
M84	Disorder of continuity of bone
M85	Other disorders of bone density and structure
M86	Osteomyelitis
M87	Osteonecrosis
M88	Osteitis deformans [Paget's disease of bone]
M89	Other disorders of bone
M90	Osteopathies in diseases classified elsewhere
M91	Juvenile osteochondrosis of hip and pelvis
M92	Other juvenile osteochondrosis
M93	Other osteochondropathies
M94	Other disorders of cartilage
M95	Other acquired deformities of musculoskeletal system and connective tissue
M96	Intraoperative and postprocedural complications and disorders of musculoskeletal system, not elsewhere classified
M99	Biomechanical lesions, not elsewhere classified

CHAPTER 14: DISEASES OF THE GENITOURINARY SYSTEM (N00-N99)

N00	Acute nephritic syndrome
N01	Rapidly progressive nephritic syndrome
N02	Recurrent and persistent hematuria
N03	Chronic nephritic syndrome
N04	Nephrotic syndrome
N05	Unspecified nephritic syndrome
N06	Isolated proteinuria with specified morphological lesion
N07	Hereditary nephropathy, not elsewhere classified
N08	Glomerular disorders in diseases classified elsewhere
N10	Acute tubulointerstitial nephritis
N11	Chronic tubulointerstitial nephritis
N12	Tubulo-interstitial nephritis not specified as acute or chronic
N13	Obstructive and reflux uropathy
N14	Drug- and heavy-metal-induced tubulointerstitial and tubular conditions
N15	Other renal tubulointerstitial diseases
N16	Renal tubulointerstitial disorders in diseases classified elsewhere
N17	Acute kidney failure
N18	Chronic kidney disease (CKD)
N19	Unspecified kidney failure
N20	Calculus of kidney and ureter
N21	Calculus of lower urinary tract
N22	Calculus of urinary tract in diseases classified elsewhere
N23	Unspecified renal colic
N25	Disorders resulting from impaired renal tubular function
N26	Unspecified contracted kidney
N27	Small kidney of unknown cause
N28	Other disorders of kidney and ureter, not elsewhere classified
N29	Other disorders of kidney and ureter in diseases classified elsewhere

N30	Cystitis
N31	Neuromuscular dysfunction of bladder, not elsewhere classified
N32	Other disorders of bladder
N34	Urethritis and urethral syndrome
N35	Urethral stricture
N36	Other disorders of urethra
N37	Urethral disorders in diseases classified elsewhere
N39	Other disorders of urinary system
N40	Enlarged prostate
N41	Inflammatory diseases of prostate
N42	Other and unspecified disorders of prostate
N43	Hydrocele and spermatocele
N44	Noninflammatory disorders of testis
N45	Orchitis and epididymitis
N46	Male infertility
N47	Disorders of prepuce
N48	Other disorders of penis
N49	Inflammatory disorders of male genital organs, not elsewhere classified
N50	Other and unspecified disorders of male genital organs
N51	Disorders of male genital organs in diseases classified elsewhere
N52	Male erectile dysfunction
N53	Other male sexual dysfunction
N60	Benign mammary dysplasia
N61	Inflammatory disorders of breast
N62	Hypertrophy of breast
N63	Unspecified lump in breast
N64	Other disorders of breast
N65	Deformity and disproportion of reconstructed breast
N70	Salpingitis and oophoritis
N71	Acute inflammatory disease of uterus
N72	Inflammatory disease of cervix uteri
N73	Other female pelvic inflammatory diseases
N74	Female pelvic inflammatory disorders in diseases classified elsewhere
N75	Diseases of Bartholin's gland
N76	Other inflammation of vagina and vulva
N77	Vulvovaginal ulceration and inflammation in diseases classified elsewhere
N80	Endometriosis
N81	Female genital prolapse
N82	Fistulae involving female genital tract
N83	Noninflammatory disorders of ovary, fallopian tube and broad ligament
N84	Polyp of female genital tract
N85	Other noninflammatory disorders of uterus, except cervix
N86	Erosion and ectropion of cervix uteri
N87	Dysplasia of cervix uteri
N88	Other noninflammatory disorders of cervix uteri
N89	Other noninflammatory disorders of vagina
N90	Other noninflammatory disorders of vulva and perineum
N91	Absent, scanty and rare menstruation
N92	Excessive, frequent and irregular menstruation
N93	Other abnormal uterine and vaginal bleeding
N94	Pain and other conditions associated with female genital organs and menstrual cycle
N95	Menopausal and other perimenopausal disorders
N96	Recurrent pregnancy loss
N97	Female infertility
N98	Complications associated with artificial fertilization
N99	Intraoperative and postprocedural complications and disorders of genitourinary system, not elsewhere classified

CHAPTER 15: PREGNANCY, CHILDBIRTH AND THE PUERPERIUM (O00-O9A)

O00	Ectopic pregnancy
O00	Anencephaly and similar malformations
O01	Hydatidiform mole
O02	Other abnormal products of conception
O03	Spontaneous abortion
O04	Complications following (induced) termination of pregnancy
O07	Failed attempted termination of pregnancy
O07	Other congenital malformations of nervous system
O08	Complications following ectopic and molar pregnancy
O09	Supervision of high risk pregnancy
O10	Pre-existing hypertension complicating pregnancy, childbirth and the puerperium
O11	Pre-existing hypertension with pre-eclampsia
O12	Gestational [pregnancy-induced] edema and proteinuria without hypertension
O13	Gestational [pregnancy-induced] hypertension without significant proteinuria
O14	Pre-eclampsia
O15	Eclampsia
O16	Unspecified maternal hypertension
O20	Hemorrhage in early pregnancy
O21	Excessive vomiting in pregnancy
O22	Venous complications and hemorrhoids in pregnancy
O23	Infections of genitourinary tract in pregnancy
O24	Diabetes mellitus in pregnancy, childbirth, and the puerperium
O25	Malnutrition in pregnancy, childbirth and the puerperium
O26	Maternal care for other conditions predominantly related to pregnancy
O28	Abnormal findings on antenatal screening of mother
O29	Complications of anesthesia during pregnancy
O30	Multiple gestation
O31	Complications specific to multiple gestation
O32	Maternal care for malpresentation of fetus
O33	Maternal care for disproportion
O34	Maternal care for abnormality of pelvic organs
O35	Maternal care for known or suspected fetal abnormality and damage
O36	Maternal care for other fetal problems
O40	Polyhydramnios
O41	Other disorders of amniotic fluid and membranes
O42	Premature rupture of membranes
O43	Placental disorders
O44	Placenta previa
O45	Premature separation of placenta [abruptio placentae]
O46	Antepartum hemorrhage, not elsewhere classified
O47	False labor
O48	Late pregnancy
O60	Preterm labor

O61	Failed induction of labor
O62	Abnormalities of forces of labor
O63	Long labor
O64	Obstructed labor due to malposition and malpresentation of fetus
O65	Obstructed labor due to maternal pelvic abnormality
O66	Other obstructed labor
O67	Labor and delivery complicated by intrapartum hemorrhage, not elsewhere classified
O68	Labor and delivery complicated by abnormality of fetal acid-base balance
O69	Labor and delivery complicated by umbilical cord complications
O70	Perineal laceration during delivery
O71	Other obstetric trauma
O72	Postpartum hemorrhage
O73	Retained placenta and membranes, without hemorrhage
O74	Complications of anesthesia during labor and delivery
O75	Other complications of labor and delivery, not elsewhere classified
O76	Abnormality in fetal heart rate and rhythm complicating labor and delivery
O77	Other fetal stress complicating labor and delivery
O80	Encounter for full-term uncomplicated delivery
O82	Encounter for cesarean delivery without indication
O85	Puerperal sepsis
O86	Other puerperal infections
O87	Venous complications and hemorrhoids in the puerperium
O88	Obstetric embolism
O89	Complications of anesthesia during the puerperium
O90	Complications of the puerperium, not elsewhere classified
O91	Infections of breast associated with pregnancy, the puerperium and lactation
O92	Other disorders of breast and disorders of lactation associated with pregnancy and the puerperium
O94	Sequelae of complication of pregnancy, childbirth, and the puerperium
O98	Maternal infectious and parasitic diseases classifiable elsewhere but complicating pregnancy, childbirth and the puerperium
O99	Other maternal diseases classifiable elsewhere but complicating pregnancy, childbirth and the puerperium
O9A	Maternal malignant neoplasms, traumatic injuries and abuse classifiable elsewhere but complicating pregnancy, childbirth and the puerperium

CHAPTER 16: CERTAIN CONDITIONS ORIGINATING IN THE PERINATAL PERIOD (P00-P96)

P00	Newborn (suspected to be) affected by maternal conditions that may be unrelated to present pregnancy
P01	Newborn (suspected to be) affected by maternal complications of pregnancy
P02	Newborn (suspected to be) affected by complications of placenta, cord and membranes
P03	Newborn (suspected to be) affected by other complications of labor and delivery
P04	Newborn (suspected to be) affected by noxious substances transmitted via placenta or breast milk

P05	Disorders of newborn related to slow fetal growth and fetal malnutrition
P07	Disorders of newborn related to short gestation and low birth weight, not elsewhere classified
P08	Disorders of newborn related to long gestation and high birth weight
P09	Abnormal findings on neonatal screening
P10	Intracranial laceration and hemorrhage due to birth injury
P11	Other birth injuries to central nervous system
P12	Birth injury to scalp
P13	Birth injury to skeleton
P14	Birth injury to peripheral nervous system
P15	Other birth injuries
P19	Metabolic acidemia in newborn
P22	Respiratory distress of newborn
P23	Congenital pneumonia
P24	Neonatal aspiration
P25	Interstitial emphysema and related conditions originating in the perinatal period
P26	Pulmonary hemorrhage originating in the perinatal period
P27	Chronic respiratory disease originating in the perinatal period
P28	Other respiratory conditions originating in the perinatal period
P29	Cardiovascular disorders originating in the perinatal period
P35	Congenital viral diseases
P36	Bacterial sepsis of newborn
P37	Other congenital infectious and parasitic diseases
P38	Omphalitis of newborn
P39	Other infections specific to the perinatal period
P50	Newborn affected by intrauterine (fetal) blood loss
P51	Umbilical hemorrhage of newborn
P52	Intracranial nontraumatic hemorrhage of newborn
P53	Hemorrhagic disease of newborn
P54	Other neonatal hemorrhages
P55	Hemolytic disease of newborn
P56	Hydrops fetalis due to hemolytic disease
P57	Kernicterus
P58	Neonatal jaundice due to other excessive hemolysis
P59	Neonatal jaundice from other and unspecified causes
P60	Disseminated intravascular coagulation of newborn
P61	Other perinatal hematological disorders
P70	Transitory disorders of carbohydrate metabolism specific to newborn
P71	Transitory neonatal disorders of calcium and magnesium metabolism
P72	Other transitory neonatal endocrine disorders
P74	Other transitory neonatal electrolyte and metabolic disturbances
P76	Other intestinal obstruction of newborn
P77	Necrotizing enterocolitis of newborn
P78	Other perinatal digestive system disorders
P80	Hypothermia of newborn
P81	Other disturbances of temperature regulation of newborn
P83	Other conditions of integument specific to newborn
P84	Other problems with newborn
P90	Convulsions of newborn
P91	Other disturbances of cerebral status of newborn
P92	Feeding problems of newborn

P93 Reactions and intoxications due to drugs administered to newborn

P94 Disorders of muscle tone of newborn

P95 Stillbirth

P96 Other conditions originating in the perinatal period

CHAPTER 17: CONGENITAL MALFORMATIONS, DEFORMATIONS AND CHROMOSOMAL ABNORMALITIES (Q00-Q99)

Q01 Encephalocele

Q02 Microcephaly

Q03 Congenital hydrocephalus

Q04 Other congenital malformations of brain

Q05 Spina bifida

Q06 Other congenital malformations of spinal cord

Q10 Congenital malformations of eyelid, lacrimal apparatus and orbit

Q11 Anophthalmos, microphthalmos and macrophthalmos

Q12 Congenital lens malformations

Q13 Congenital malformations of anterior segment of eye

Q14 Congenital malformations of posterior segment of eye

Q15 Other congenital malformations of eye

Q16 Congenital malformations of ear causing impairment of hearing

Q17 Other congenital malformations of ear

Q18 Other congenital malformations of face and neck

Q20 Congenital malformations of cardiac chambers and connections

Q21 Congenital malformations of cardiac septa

Q22 Congenital malformations of pulmonary and tricuspid valves

Q23 Congenital malformations of aortic and mitral valves

Q24 Other congenital malformations of heart

Q25 Congenital malformations of great arteries

Q26 Congenital malformations of great veins

Q27 Other congenital malformations of peripheral vascular system

Q28 Other congenital malformations of circulatory system

Q30 Congenital malformations of nose

Q31 Congenital malformations of larynx

Q32 Congenital malformations of trachea and bronchus

Q33 Congenital malformations of lung

Q34 Other congenital malformations of respiratory system

Q35 Cleft palate

Q36 Cleft lip

Q37 Cleft palate with cleft lip

Q38 Other congenital malformations of tongue, mouth and pharynx

Q39 Congenital malformations of esophagus

Q40 Other congenital malformations of upper alimentary tract

Q41 Congenital absence, atresia and stenosis of small intestine

Q42 Congenital absence, atresia and stenosis of large intestine

Q43 Other congenital malformations of intestine

Q44 Congenital malformations of gallbladder, bile ducts and liver

Q45 Other congenital malformations of digestive system

Q50 Congenital malformations of ovaries, fallopian tubes and broad ligaments

Q51 Congenital malformations of uterus and cervix

Q52 Other congenital malformations of female genitalia

Q53 Undescended and ectopic testicle

Q54 Hypospadias

Q55 Other congenital malformations of male genital organs

Q56 Indeterminate sex and pseudohermaphroditism

Q60 Renal agenesis and other reduction defects of kidney

Q61 Cystic kidney disease

Q62 Congenital obstructive defects of renal pelvis and congenital malformations of ureter

Q63 Other congenital malformations of kidney

Q64 Other congenital malformations of urinary system

Q65 Congenital deformities of hip

Q66 Congenital deformities of feet

Q67 Congenital musculoskeletal deformities of head, face, spine and chest

Q68 Other congenital musculoskeletal deformities

Q69 Polydactyly

Q70 Syndactyly

Q71 Reduction defects of upper limb

Q72 Reduction defects of lower limb

Q73 Reduction defects of unspecified limb

Q74 Other congenital malformations of limb(s)

Q75 Other congenital malformations of skull and face bones

Q76 Congenital malformations of spine and bony thorax

Q77 Osteochondrodysplasia with defects of growth of tubular bones and spine

Q78 Other osteochondrodysplasias

Q79 Congenital malformations of musculoskeletal system, not elsewhere classified

Q80 Congenital ichthyosis

Q81 Epidermolysis bullosa

Q82 Other congenital malformations of skin

Q83 Congenital malformations of breast

Q84 Other congenital malformations of integument

Q85 Phakomatoses, not elsewhere classified

Q86 Congenital malformation syndromes due to known exogenous causes, not elsewhere classified

Q87 Other specified congenital malformation syndromes affecting multiple systems

Q89 Other congenital malformations, not elsewhere classified

Q90 Down syndrome

Q91 Trisomy 18 and Trisomy 13

Q92 Other trisomies and partial trisomies of the autosomes, not elsewhere classified

Q93 Monosomies and deletions from the autosomes, not elsewhere classified

Q95 Balanced rearrangements and structural markers, not elsewhere classified

Q96 Turner's syndrome

Q97 Other sex chromosome abnormalities, female phenotype, not elsewhere classified

Q98 Other sex chromosome abnormalities, male phenotype, not elsewhere classified

Q99 Other chromosome abnormalities, not elsewhere classified

CHAPTER 18: SYMPTOMS, SIGNS AND ABNORMAL CLINICAL AND LABORATORY FINDINGS, NOT ELSEWHERE CLASSIFIED (R00-R99)

R00 Abnormalities of heart beat

R01	Cardiac murmurs and other cardiac sounds	R57	Shock, not elsewhere classified
R03	Abnormal blood-pressure reading, without diagnosis	R58	Hemorrhage not elsewhere classified
R04	Hemorrhage from respiratory passages	R59	Enlarged lymph nodes
R05	Cough	R60	Edema, not elsewhere classified
R06	Abnormalities of breathing	R61	Generalized hyperhidrosis
R07	Pain in throat and chest	R62	Lack of expected normal physiological development in childhood and adults
R09	Other symptoms and signs involving the circulatory and respiratory system	R63	Symptoms and signs concerning food and fluid intake
R10	Abdominal and pelvic pain	R64	Cachexia
R11	Nausea and vomiting	R65	Symptoms and signs specifically associated with systemic inflammation and infection
R12	Heartburn		
R13	Aphagia and dysphagia	R68	Other general symptoms and signs
R14	Flatulence and related conditions	R70	Elevated erythrocyte sedimentation rate and abnormality of plasma viscosity
R15	Fecal incontinence		
R16	Hepatomegaly and splenomegaly, not elsewhere classified	R71	Abnormality of red blood cells
R17	Unspecified jaundice	R73	Elevated blood glucose level
R18	Ascites	R74	Abnormal serum enzyme levels
R19	Other symptoms and signs involving the digestive system and abdomen	R75	Inconclusive laboratory evidence of human immunodeficiency virus [HIV]
R20	Disturbances of skin sensation	R76	Other abnormal immunological findings in serum
R21	Rash and other nonspecific skin eruption	R77	Other abnormalities of plasma proteins
R22	Localized swelling, mass and lump of skin and subcutaneous tissue	R78	Findings of drugs and other substances, not normally found in blood
R23	Other skin changes	R79	Other abnormal findings of blood chemistry
R25	Abnormal involuntary movements	R80	Proteinuria
R26	Abnormalities of gait and mobility	R81	Glycosuria
R27	Other lack of coordination	R82	Other and unspecified abnormal findings in urine
R29	Other symptoms and signs involving the nervous and musculoskeletal systems	R83	Abnormal findings in cerebrospinal fluid
R30	Pain associated with micturition	R84	Abnormal findings in specimens from respiratory organs and thorax
R31	Hematuria	R85	Abnormal findings in specimens from digestive organs and abdominal cavity
R32	Unspecified urinary incontinence		
R33	Retention of urine	R86	Abnormal findings in specimens from male genital organs
R34	Polyuria	R87	Abnormal findings in specimens from female genital organs
R35	Polyuria	R88	Abnormal findings in other body fluids and substances
R36	Urethral discharge	R89	Abnormal findings in specimens from other organs, systems and tissues
R37	Sexual dysfunction, unspecified		
R39	Other and unspecified symptoms and signs involving the genitourinary system	R90	Abnormal findings on diagnostic imaging of central nervous system
R40	Somnolence, stupor and coma	R91	Abnormal findings on diagnostic imaging of lung
R41	Other symptoms and signs involving cognitive functions and awareness	R92	Abnormal and inconclusive findings on diagnostic imaging of breast
R42	Dizziness and giddiness	R93	Abnormal findings on diagnostic imaging of other body structures
R43	Disturbances of smell and taste		
R44	Other symptoms and signs involving general sensations and perceptions	R94	Abnormal results of function studies
		R97	Abnormal tumor markers
R45	Symptoms and signs involving emotional state	R99	Ill-defined and unknown cause of mortality
R46	Symptoms and signs involving appearance and behavior		
R47	Speech disturbances, not elsewhere classified		
R48	Dyslexia and other symbolic dysfunctions, not elsewhere classified		

CHAPTER 19: INJURY, POISONING AND CERTAIN OTHER CONSEQUENCES OF EXTERNAL CAUSES (S00-T88)

R49	Voice and resonance disorders
R50	Fever of other and unknown origin
R51	Headache
R52	Pain, unspecified
R53	Malaise and fatigue
R54	Age-related physical debility
R55	Syncope and collapse
R56	Convulsions, not elsewhere classified

S00	Superficial injury of head
S00	Insect bite (nonvenomous) of scalp, initial encounter
S01	Open wound of head
S02	Fracture of skull and facial bones
S03	Dislocation and sprain of joints and ligaments of head
S04	Injury of cranial nerve
S05	Injury of eye and orbit
S06	Intracranial injury

S07	Crushing injury of head	S53	Dislocation and sprain of joints and ligaments of elbow
S08	Avulsion and traumatic amputation of part of head	S54	Injury of nerves at forearm level
S09	Other and unspecified injuries of head	S55	Injury of blood vessels at forearm level
S10	Superficial injury of neck	S56	Injury of muscle, fascia and tendon at forearm level
S10	Abrasion of unspecified part of neck, initial encounter	S57	Crushing injury of elbow and forearm
S11	Open wound of neck	S58	Traumatic amputation of elbow and forearm
S12	Fracture of cervical vertebra and other parts of neck	S59	Other and unspecified injuries of elbow and forearm
S13	Dislocation and sprain of joints and ligaments at neck level	S60	Superficial injury of wrist, hand and fingers
S14	Injury of nerves and spinal cord at neck level	S61	Open wound of wrist, hand and fingers
S15	Injury of blood vessels at neck level	S62	Fracture at wrist and hand level
S16	Injury of muscle, fascia and tendon at neck level	S63	Dislocation and sprain of joints and ligaments at wrist and hand level
S17	Crushing injury of neck	S64	Injury of nerves at wrist and hand level
S19	Other specified and unspecified injuries of neck	S65	Injury of blood vessels at wrist and hand level
S20	Superficial injury of thorax	S66	Injury of muscle, fascia and tendon at wrist and hand level
S20	Abrasion of unspecified parts of thorax, initial encounter	S67	Crushing injury of wrist, hand and fingers
S21	Open wound of thorax	S68	Traumatic amputation of wrist, hand and fingers
S22	Fracture of rib(s), sternum and thoracic spine	S69	Other and unspecified injuries of wrist, hand and finger(s)
S23	Dislocation and sprain of joints and ligaments of thorax	S70	Superficial injury of hip and thigh
S24	Injury of nerves and spinal cord at thorax level	S71	Open wound of hip and thigh
S25	Injury of blood vessels of thorax	S72	Fracture of femur
S26	Injury of heart	S73	Dislocation and sprain of joint and ligaments of hip
S27	Injury of other and unspecified intrathoracic organs	S74	Injury of nerves at hip and thigh level
S28	Crushing injury of thorax, and traumatic amputation of part of thorax	S75	Injury of blood vessels at hip and thigh level
S29	Other and unspecified injuries of thorax	S76	Injury of muscle, fascia and tendon at hip and thigh level
S30	Superficial injury of abdomen, lower back, pelvis and external genitals	S77	Crushing injury of hip and thigh
S30	Blister (nonthermal) of lower back and pelvis, initial encounter	S78	Traumatic amputation of hip and thigh
		S79	Other and unspecified injuries of hip and thigh
S31	Open wound of abdomen, lower back, pelvis and external genitals	S80	Superficial injury of knee and lower leg
S32	Fracture of lumbar spine and pelvis	S81	Open wound of knee and lower leg
S33	Dislocation and sprain of joints and ligaments of lumbar spine and pelvis	S82	Fracture of lower leg, including ankle
		S83	Dislocation and sprain of joints and ligaments of knee
S34	Injury of lumbar and sacral spinal cord and nerves at abdomen, lower back and pelvis level	S84	Injury of nerves at lower leg level
		S85	Injury of blood vessels at lower leg level
S35	Injury of blood vessels at abdomen, lower back and pelvis level	S86	Injury of muscle, fascia and tendon at lower leg level
		S87	Crushing injury of lower leg
S36	Injury of intra-abdominal organs	S88	Traumatic amputation of lower leg
S36	Injury of intra-abdominal organs	S89	Other and unspecified injuries of lower leg
S37	Injury of urinary and pelvic organs	S90	Superficial injury of ankle, foot and toes
S38	Crushing injury and traumatic amputation of abdomen, lower back, pelvis and external genitals	S91	Open wound of ankle, foot and toes
		S92	Fracture of foot and toe, except ankle
S39	Other and unspecified injuries of abdomen, lower back, pelvis and external genitals	S93	Dislocation and sprain of joints and ligaments at ankle, foot and toe level
S40	Superficial injury of shoulder and upper arm	S93	Dislocation and sprain of joints and ligaments at ankle, foot and toe
S41	Open wound of shoulder and upper arm	S94	Injury of nerves at ankle and foot level
S42	Fracture of shoulder and upper arm	S95	Injury of blood vessels at ankle and foot level
S43	Dislocation and sprain of joints and ligaments of shoulder girdle	S96	Injury of muscle and tendon at ankle and foot level
		S97	Crushing injury of ankle and foot
S44	Injury of nerves at shoulder and upper arm level	S98	Traumatic amputation of ankle and foot
S45	Injury of blood vessels at shoulder and upper arm level	S99	Other and unspecified injuries of ankle and foot
S46	Injury of muscle, fascia and tendon at shoulder and upper arm level	T07	Unspecified multiple injuries
		T14	Injury of unspecified body region
S47	Crushing injury of shoulder and upper arm	T15	Foreign body on external eye
S48	Traumatic amputation of shoulder and upper arm	T16	Foreign body in ear
S49	Other and unspecified injuries of shoulder and upper arm	T17	Foreign body in respiratory tract
S50	Superficial injury of elbow and forearm	T18	Foreign body in alimentary tract
S51	Open wound of elbow and forearm	T19	Foreign body in genitourinary tract
S52	Fracture of forearm	T20	Burn and corrosion of head, face, and neck

T21	Burn and corrosion of trunk	T59	Toxic effect of other gases, fumes and vapors
T22	Burn and corrosion of shoulder and upper limb, except wrist and hand	T60	Toxic effect of pesticides
T23	Burn and corrosion of wrist and hand	T61	Toxic effect of noxious substances eaten as seafood
T24	Burn and corrosion of lower limb, except ankle and foot	T62	Toxic effect of other noxious substances eaten as food
T25	Burn and corrosion of ankle and foot	T63	Toxic effect of contact with venomous animals and plants
T26	Burn and corrosion confined to eye and adnexa	T64	Toxic effect of aflatoxin and other mycotoxin food contaminants
T27	Burn and corrosion of respiratory tract	T65	Toxic effect of other and unspecified substances
T28	Burn and corrosion of other internal organs	T66	Radiation sickness, unspecified
T30	Burn and corrosion, body region unspecified	T67	Effects of heat and light
T31	Burns classified according to extent of body surface involved	T68	Hypothermia
T32	Corrosions classified according to extent of body surface involved	T69	Other effects of reduced temperature
		T70	Effects of air pressure and water pressure
T33	Superficial frostbite	T71	Asphyxiation
T34	Frostbite with tissue necrosis	T73	Effects of other deprivation
T36	Poisoning by, adverse effect of and underdosing of systemic antibiotics	T74	Adult and child abuse, neglect and other maltreatment, confirmed
T37	Poisoning by, adverse effect of and underdosing of other systemic anti- infectives and antiparasitics	T75	Other and unspecified effects of other external causes
T38	Poisoning by, adverse effect of and underdosing of hormones and their synthetic substitutes and antagonists, not elsewhere classified	T76	Adult and child abuse, neglect and other maltreatment, suspected
		T78	Adverse effects, not elsewhere classified
T39	Poisoning by, adverse effect of and underdosing of nonopioid analgesics, antipyretics and antirheumatics	T79	Certain early complications of trauma, not elsewhere classified
T40	Poisoning by, adverse effect of and underdosing of narcotics and psychodysleptics [hallucinogens]	T80	Complications following infusion, transfusion and therapeutic injection
T41	Poisoning by, adverse effect of and underdosing of anesthetics and therapeutic gases	T81	Complications of procedures, not elsewhere classified
T42	Poisoning by, adverse effect of and underdosing of antiepileptic, sedative- hypnotic and antiparkinsonism drugs	T82	Complications of cardiac and vascular prosthetic devices, implants and grafts
T43	Poisoning by, adverse effect of and underdosing of psychotropic drugs, not elsewhere classified	T83	Complications of genitourinary prosthetic devices, implants and grafts
T44	Poisoning by, adverse effect of and underdosing of drugs primarily affecting the autonomic nervous system	T84	Complications of internal orthopedic prosthetic devices, implants and grafts
T45	Poisoning by, adverse effect of and underdosing of primarily systemic and hematological agents, not elsewhere classified	T85	Complications of other internal prosthetic devices, implants and grafts
		T86	Complications of transplanted organs and tissue
T46	Poisoning by, adverse effect of and underdosing of agents primarily affecting the cardiovascular system	T87	Complications peculiar to reattachment and amputation
T47	Poisoning by, adverse effect of and underdosing of agents primarily affecting the gastrointestinal system	T88	Other complications of surgical and medical care, not elsewhere classified
T48	Poisoning by, adverse effect of and underdosing of agents primarily acting on smooth and skeletal muscles and the respiratory system		

CHAPTER 20: EXTERNAL CAUSES OF MORBIDITY (V00-Y99)

T49	Poisoning by, adverse effect of and underdosing of topical agents primarily affecting skin and mucous membrane and by ophthalmological, otorhinolaryngological and dental drugs
V00	Pedestrian conveyance accident
V01	Pedestrian injured in collision with pedal cycle
V03	Pedestrian injured in collision with car, pick-up truck or van
V05	Pedestrian injured in collision with railway train or railway vehicle
T50	Poisoning by, adverse effect of and underdosing of diuretics and other and unspecified drugs, medicaments and biological substances
V06	Pedestrian injured in collision with other nonmotor vehicle
V09	Pedestrian injured in other and unspecified transport accidents
T51	Toxic effect of alcohol
V10	Pedal cycle rider injured in collision with pedestrian or animal
T52	Toxic effect of organic solvents
T53	Toxic effect of halogen derivatives of aliphatic and aromatic hydrocarbons
V13	Pedal cycle rider injured in collision with car, pick-up truck or van
T54	Toxic effect of corrosive substances
V15	Pedal cycle rider injured in collision with railway train or railway vehicle
T55	Toxic effect of soaps and detergents
T56	Toxic effect of metals
V17	Pedal cycle rider injured in collision with fixed or stationary object
T57	Toxic effect of other inorganic substances
T58	Toxic effect of carbon monoxide
V18	Pedal cycle rider injured in noncollision transport accident

V19	Pedal cycle rider injured in other and unspecified transport accidents
V20	Motorcycle rider injured in collision with pedestrian or animal
V21	Motorcycle rider injured in collision with pedal cycle
V23	Motorcycle rider injured in collision with car, pick-up truck or van
V25	Motorcycle rider injured in collision with railway train or railway vehicle
V26	Motorcycle rider injured in collision with other nonmotor vehicle
V27	Motorcycle rider injured in collision with fixed or stationary object
V28	Motorcycle rider injured in noncollision transport accident
V29	Motorcycle rider injured in other and unspecified transport accidents
V40	Car occupant injured in collision with pedestrian or animal
V43	Car occupant injured in collision with car, pick-up truck or van
V45	Car occupant injured in collision with railway train or railway vehicle
V46	Car occupant injured in collision with other nonmotor vehicle
V47	Car occupant injured in collision with fixed or stationary object
V48	Car occupant injured in noncollision transport accident
V49	Car occupant injured in other and unspecified transport accidents
V57	Occupant of pick-up truck or van injured in collision with fixed or stationary object
V58	Occupant of pick-up truck or van injured in noncollision transport accident
V59	Occupant of pick-up truck or van injured in other and unspecified transport accidents
V69	Occupant of heavy transport vehicle injured in other and unspecified transport accidents
V78	Bus occupant injured in noncollision transport accident
V80	Animal-rider or occupant of animal-drawn vehicle injured in transport accident
V81	Occupant of railway train or railway vehicle injured in transport accident
V82	Occupant of powered streetcar injured in transport accident
V83	Occupant of special vehicle mainly used on industrial premises injured in transport accident
V86	Occupant of special all-terrain or other off-road motor vehicle, injured in transport accident
V87	Traffic accident of specified type but victim's mode of transport unknown
V88	Nontraffic accident of specified type but victim's mode of transport unknown
V89	Motor- or nonmotor-vehicle accident, type of vehicle unspecified
V90	Drowning and submersion due to accident to watercraft
V91	Other injury due to accident to watercraft
V92	Drowning and submersion due to accident on board watercraft, without accident to watercraft
V93	Other injury due to accident on board watercraft, without accident to watercraft
V94	Other and unspecified water transport accidents
V95	Accident to powered aircraft causing injury to occupant
V96	Accident to nonpowered aircraft causing injury to occupant
V97	Other specified air transport accidents
V98	Other specified transport accidents
V99	Unspecified transport accident
W01	Fall on same level from slipping, tripping and stumbling
W03	Other fall on same level due to collision with another person
W05	Fall from non-moving wheelchair, nonmotorized scooter and motorized mobility scooter
W06	Fall from bed
W07	Fall from chair
W08	Fall from other furniture
W09	Fall on and from playground equipment
W10	Fall on and from stairs and steps
W11	Fall on and from ladder
W12	Fall on and from scaffolding
W13	Fall from, out of or through building or structure
W14	Fall from tree
W15	Fall from cliff
W16	Fall, jump or diving into water
W17	Other fall from one level to another
W18	Other slipping, tripping and stumbling and falls
W19	Unspecified fall
W20	Struck by thrown, projected or falling object
W21	Striking against or struck by sports equipment
W22	Striking against or struck by other objects
W23	Caught, crushed, jammed or pinched in or between objects
W24	Contact with lifting and transmission devices, not elsewhere classified
W26	Contact with knife, sword or dagger
W27	Contact with nonpowered hand tool
W28	Contact with powered lawn mower
W29	Contact with other powered hand tools and household machinery
W30	Contact with agricultural machinery
W31	Contact with other and unspecified machinery
W32	Accidental handgun discharge and malfunction
W33	Accidental rifle, shotgun and larger firearm discharge and malfunction
W34	Accidental discharge and malfunction from other and unspecified firearms and guns
W35	Explosion and rupture of boiler
W36	Explosion and rupture of gas cylinder
W38	Explosion and rupture of other specified pressurized devices
W39	Discharge of firework
W40	Explosion of other materials
W42	Exposure to noise
W45	Foreign body or object entering through skin
W46	Contact with hypodermic needle
W49	Exposure to other inanimate mechanical forces
W50	Accidental hit, strike, kick, twist, bite or scratch by another person
W51	Accidental striking against or bumped into by another person
W52	Crushed, pushed or stepped on by crowd or human stampede
W53	Contact with rodent
W54	Contact with dog
W55	Contact with other mammals
W57	Bitten or stung by nonvenomous insect and other nonvenomous arthropods

W59	Contact with other nonvenomous reptiles	**X97**	Assault by smoke, fire and flames
W64	Exposure to other animate mechanical forces	**X98**	Assault by steam, hot vapors and hot objects
W65	Accidental drowning and submersion while in bath-tub	**X99**	Assault by sharp object
W67	Accidental drowning and submersion while in swimming-pool	**Y00**	Assault by blunt object
W69	Accidental drowning and submersion while in natural water	**Y01**	Assault by pushing from high place
		Y03	Assault by crashing of motor vehicle
W74	Unspecified cause of accidental drowning and submersion	**Y04**	Assault by bodily force
W85	Exposure to electric transmission lines	**Y07**	Perpetrator of assault, maltreatment and neglect
W86	Exposure to other specified electric current	**Y08**	Assault by other specified means
W88	Exposure to ionizing radiation	**Y22**	Handgun discharge, undetermined intent
W89	Exposure to man-made visible and ultraviolet light	**Y23**	Rifle, shotgun and larger firearm discharge, undetermined intent
W90	Exposure to other nonionizing radiation	**Y24**	Other and unspecified firearm discharge, undetermined intent
W92	Exposure to excessive heat of man-made origin	**Y25**	Contact with explosive material, undetermined intent
W93	Exposure to excessive cold of man-made origin	**Y26**	Exposure to smoke, fire and flames, undetermined intent
W94	Exposure to high and low air pressure and changes in air pressure	**Y27**	Contact with steam, hot vapors and hot objects, undetermined intent
W99	Exposure to other man-made environmental factors	**Y28**	Contact with sharp object, undetermined intent
X00	Exposure to uncontrolled fire in building or structure	**Y30**	Falling, jumping or pushed from a high place, undetermined intent
X01	Exposure to uncontrolled fire, not in building or structure	**Y31**	Falling, lying or running before or into moving object, undetermined intent
X02	Exposure to controlled fire in building or structure	**Y32**	Crashing of motor vehicle, undetermined intent
X03	Exposure to controlled fire, not in building or structure	**Y33**	Other specified events, undetermined intent
X04	Exposure to ignition of highly flammable material	**Y35**	Legal intervention
X05	Exposure to ignition or melting of nightwear	**Y36**	Operations of war
X06	Exposure to ignition or melting of other clothing and apparel	**Y38**	Terrorism
		Y62	Failure of sterile precautions during surgical and medical care
X08	Exposure to other specified smoke, fire and flames	**Y63**	Failure in dosage during surgical and medical care
X11	Contact with hot tap-water	**Y64**	Contaminated medical or biological substances
X12	Contact with other hot fluids	**Y65**	Other misadventures during surgical and medical care
X19	Contact with other heat and hot substances	**Y69**	Unspecified misadventure during surgical and medical care
X30	Exposure to excessive natural heat	**Y83**	Surgical operation and other surgical procedures as the cause of abnormal reaction of the patient, or of later
X31	Exposure to excessive natural cold	
X34	Earthquake	**Y84**	Other medical procedures as the cause of abnormal reaction of the patient, or of later complication, without
X35	Volcanic eruption	
X36	Avalanche, landslide and other earth movements	**Y92**	Place of occurrence of the external cause
X37	Cataclysmic storm	**Y93**	Activity codes
X38	Flood	**Y99**	External cause status
X39	Exposure to other forces of nature		
X52	Prolonged stay in weightless environment		
X58	Exposure to other specified factors		

CHAPTER 21: FACTORS INFLUENCING HEALTH STATUS AND CONTACT WITH HEALTH SERVICES (Z00-Z99)

X71	Intentional self-harm by drowning and submersion		
X72	Intentional self-harm by handgun discharge	**Z00**	Encounter for general examination without complaint, suspected or reported diagnosis
X73	Intentional self-harm by rifle, shotgun and larger firearm discharge	**Z01**	Encounter for other special examination without complaint, suspected or reported diagnosis
X74	Intentional self-harm by other and unspecified firearm and gun discharge	**Z02**	Encounter for administrative examination
X75	Intentional self-harm by explosive material	**Z03**	Encounter for medical observation for suspected diseases and conditions ruled out
X76	Intentional self-harm by smoke, fire and flames	**Z04**	Encounter for examination and observation for other reasons
X77	Intentional self-harm by steam, hot vapors and hot objects	**Z08**	Encounter for follow-up examination after completed treatment for malignant neoplasm
X78	Intentional self-harm by sharp object	
X80	Intentional self-harm by jumping from a high place	**Z09**	Encounter for follow-up examination after completed treatment for conditions other than malignant neoplasm
X81	Intentional self-harm by jumping or lying in front of moving object	
X82	Intentional self-harm by crashing of motor vehicle	**Z11**	Encounter for screening for infectious and parasitic diseases
X83	Intentional self-harm by other specified means	
X92	Assault by drowning and submersion		
X93	Assault by handgun discharge		
X94	Assault by rifle, shotgun and larger firearm discharge		
X95	Assault by other and unspecified firearm and gun discharge		
X96	Assault by explosive material		

Z12	Encounter for screening for malignant neoplasms		Z71	Persons encountering health services for other counseling and medical advice, not elsewhere classified
Z13	Encounter for screening for other diseases and disorders		Z72	Problems related to lifestyle
Z14	Genetic carrier		Z73	Problems related to life management difficulty
Z15	Genetic susceptibility to disease		Z74	Problems related to care provider dependency
Z16	Resistance to antimicrobial drugs		Z75	Problems related to medical facilities and other health care
Z17	Estrogen receptor status		Z76	Persons encountering health services in other circumstances
Z18	Retained foreign body fragments		Z77	Other contact with and (suspected) exposures hazardous to health
Z20	Contact with and (suspected) exposure to communicable diseases		Z78	Other specified health status
Z21	Asymptomatic human immunodeficiency virus [HIV] infection status		Z79	Long term (current) drug therapy
Z22	Encounter for immunization		Z80	Family history of primary malignant neoplasm
Z23	Immunization not carried out and underimmunization status		Z81	Family history of mental and behavioral disorders
Z28	Immunization not carried out and underimmunization status		Z82	Family history of certain disabilities and chronic diseases (leading to disablement)
Z30	Encounter for contraceptive management		Z83	Family history of other specific disorders
Z31	Encounter for procreative management		Z84	Family history of other conditions
Z32	Encounter for pregnancy test and childbirth and childcare instruction		Z85	Personal history of malignant neoplasm
Z33	Pregnant state		Z86	Personal history of certain other diseases
Z34	Encounter for supervision of normal pregnancy		Z87	Personal history of other diseases and conditions
Z36	Encounter for antenatal screening of mother		Z88	Allergy status to drugs, medicaments and biological substances
Z37	Outcome of delivery		Z89	Acquired absence of limb
Z38	Liveborn infants according to place of birth and type of delivery		Z90	Acquired absence of organs, not elsewhere classified
Z39	Encounter for maternal postpartum care and examination		Z91	Personal risk factors, not elsewhere classified
Z40	Encounter for prophylactic surgery		Z92	Personal history of medical treatment
Z41	Encounter for procedures for purposes other than remedying health state		Z93	Artificial opening status
Z42	Encounter for plastic and reconstructive surgery following medical procedure		Z94	Transplanted organ and tissue status
Z43	Encounter for attention to artificial openings		Z95	Presence of cardiac and vascular implants and grafts
Z44	Encounter for fitting and adjustment of external prosthetic device		Z96	Presence of other functional implants
Z45	Encounter for adjustment and management of implanted device		Z97	Presence of other devices
Z46	Encounter for fitting and adjustment of other devices		Z98	Other postprocedural states
Z47	Orthopedic aftercare		Z99	Dependence on enabling machines and devices, not elsewhere classified
Z48	Encounter for other postprocedural aftercare			
Z49	Encounter for attention to artificial openings			
Z51	Encounter for other aftercare			
Z52	Donors of organs and tissues			
Z53	Persons encountering health services for specific procedures and treatment, not carried out			
Z55	Problems related to education and literacy			
Z56	Problems related to employment and unemployment			
Z57	Occupational exposure to risk factors			
Z59	Problems related to housing and economic circumstances			
Z60	Problems related to social environment			
Z62	Problems related to upbringing			
Z63	Other problems related to primary support group, including family circumstances			
Z64	Problems related to certain psychosocial circumstances			
Z65	Problems related to other psychosocial services			
Z65	Problems related to other psychosocial circumstances			
Z68	Body mass index [BMI]			
Z69	Encounter for mental health services for victim and perpetrator of abuse			
Z70	Counseling related to sexual attitude, behavior and orientation			

SUMMARY OF ADDITIONS, DELETIONS AND
REVISIONS TO ICD-10-CM 2014

L70.5   **Acne excoriee des jeunes filles**
Revised description

M08.88   **Other juvenile arthritis, other specified site**
Revised description

M12.08   **Chronic postrheumatic arthropathy [Jaccoud], other specified site**
Revised description

M12.28   **Villonodular synovitis (pigmented), other specified site**
Revised description

M12.38   **Palindromic rheumatism, other specified site**
Revised description

M12.58   **Traumatic arthropathy, other specified site**
Revised description

M12.88   **Other specific arthropathies, not elsewhere classified, other specified site**
Revised description

M25.08   **Hemarthrosis, other specified site**
Revised description

M25.18   **Fistula, other specified site**
Revised description

M47.17   **Other spondylosis with myelopathy, lumbosacral region**
Code deleted 2014

M47.18   **Other spondylosis with myelopathy, sacral and sacrococcygeal region**
Code deleted 2014

M50.01   **Cervical disc disorder with myelopathy, high cervical region**
Revised description

M50.11   **Cervical disc disorder with radiculopathy, high cervical region**
Revised description

M50.21   **Other cervical disc displacement, high cervical region**
Revised description

M50.31   **Other cervical disc degeneration, high cervical region**
Revised description

M50.81   **Other cervical disc disorders, high cervical region**
Revised description

M50.91   **Cervical disc disorder, unspecified, high cervical region**
Revised description

M51.07   **Intervertebral disc disorders with myelopathy, lumbosacral region**
Code deleted 2014

M84.58XA   **Pathological fracture in neoplastic disease, other specified site, initial encounter for fracture**
Revised description

M84.58XD   **Pathological fracture in neoplastic disease, other specified site, subsequent encounter for fracture with routine healing**
Revised description

M84.58XG   **Pathological fracture in neoplastic disease, other specified site, subsequent encounter for fracture with delayed healing**
Revised description

M84.58XK   **Pathological fracture in neoplastic disease, other specified site, subsequent encounter for fracture with nonunion**
Revised description

M84.58XP   **Pathological fracture in neoplastic disease, other specified site, subsequent encounter for fracture with malunion**
Revised description

M84.58XS   **Pathological fracture in neoplastic disease, other specified site, sequela**
Revised description

T20.56XA   **Corrosion of first degree of forehead and cheek, initial encounter**
Revised description

T20.56XD   **Corrosion of first degree of forehead and cheek, subsequent encounter**
Revised description

T20.56XS   **Corrosion of first degree of forehead and cheek, sequela**
Revised description

T40.1X5A   **Adverse effect of heroin, initial encounter**
Code deleted 2014

T40.1X5D **Adverse effect of heroin, subsequent encounter**
Code deleted 2014

T40.1X5S **Adverse effect of heroin, sequela**
Code deleted 2014

T40.8X5A **Adverse effect of lysergide [LSD], initial encounter**
Code deleted 2014

T40.8X5D **Adverse effect of lysergide [LSD], subsequent encounter**
Code deleted 2014

T40.8X5S **Adverse effect of lysergide [LSD], sequela**
Code deleted 2014

W94.31XA **Exposure to sudden change in air pressure in aircraft during descent, initial encounter**
Revised description

W94.31XD **Exposure to sudden change in air pressure in aircraft during descent, subsequent encounter**
Revised description

W94.31XS **Exposure to sudden change in air pressure in aircraft during descent, sequela**
Revised description

Y92.002 **Bathroom of unspecified non-institutional (private) residence single-family (private) house as the place of occurrence of the external cause**
Revised description